# Cardiovascular Emergencies

## Recognition and Management

### Volume 1

# Cardiovascular Emergencies

## Recognition and Management

## Volume 1

**K C Verma**
MBBS, DCH, MD, DM (Cardiology)
FICP (USA), FRST M&H (Lond.), FCSI (India)
Senior Consulting Heart Specialist and
Former Professor in Cardiovascular and Thoracic Unit
Government Medical College
Jammu (J&K)

CBS

**CBS Publishers & Distributors** Pvt Ltd

New Delhi • Bengaluru • Chennai • Kochi • Kolkata • Mumbai
Bhopal • Bhubaneswar • Hyderabad • Jharkhand • Nagpur • Patna • Pune • Uttarakhand • Dhaka (Bangladesh)

*Disclaimer*

Science and technology are constantly changing fields. New research and experience broaden the scope of information and knowledge. The author has tried his best in giving information available to him while preparing the material for this book. Although, all efforts have been made to ensure optimum accuracy of the material, yet it is quite possible some errors might have been left uncorrected. The publisher, the printer and the author will not be held responsible for any inadvertent errors, omissions or inaccuracies.

**Cardiovascular Emergencies**

**Recognition and Management**

Volume 1

ISBN: 978-93-88725-61-3



**First Edition:** 2019



Published by Satish Kumar Jain and produced by Varun Jain for
**CBS Publishers & Distributors** Pvt Ltd
4819/XI Prahlad Street, 24 Ansari Road, Daryaganj, New Delhi 110 002, India
Ph: 23289259, 23266861, 23266867 Website: www.cbspd.com
Fax: 011-23243014 e-mail: delhi@cbspd.com; cbspubs@airtelmail.in

*Corporate Office:* 204 FIE, Industrial Area, Patparganj, Delhi 110 092
Ph: 4934 4934 Fax: 4934 4935 e-mail: publishing@cbspd.com; publicity@cbspd.com

***Branches***

- **Bengaluru:** Seema House 2975, 17th Cross, K.R. Road, Banasankari 2nd Stage, Bengaluru 560 070, Karnataka
  Ph: +91-80-26771678/79 Fax: +91-80-26771680 e-mail: bangalore@cbspd.com
- **Chennai:** 7, Subbaraya Street, Shenoy Nagar, Chennai 600 030, Tamil Nadu
  Ph: +91-44-26680620/26681266 Fax: +91-44-42032115 e-mail: chennai@cbspd.com
- **Kochi:** 42/1325, 1326, Power House Road, Opp KSEB, Power House, Ernakulam 682 018, Kochi, Kerala
  Ph: +91-484-4059061-65 Fax: +91-484-4059065 e-mail: kochi@cbspd.com
- **Kolkata:** 6/B, Ground Floor, Rameswar Shaw Road, Kolkata 700 014, West Bengal
  Ph: +91-33-22891126, 22891127, 22891128 e-mail: kolkata@cbspd.com
- **Mumbai:** 83-C, Dr E Moses Road, Worli, Mumbai 400018, Maharashtra
  Ph: +91-22-24902340/41 Fax: +91-22-24902342 e-mail: mumbai@cbspd.com

*Representatives*

| | | | | | | | |
|---|---|---|---|---|---|---|---|
| • **Bhopal** | 0-8319310552 | • **Bhubaneswar** | 0-9911037372 | • **Hyderabad** | 0-9885175004 | • **Jharkhand** | 0-9811541605 |
| • **Nagpur** | 0-9421945513 | • **Patna** | 0-9334159340 | • **Pune** | 0-9623451994 | • **Uttarakhand** | 0-9716462459 |
| • **Dhaka (Bangladesh)** | 01912-003485 | | | | | | |

*Printed at:* Nutech Print Services, Faridabad, Haryana, India

*to*

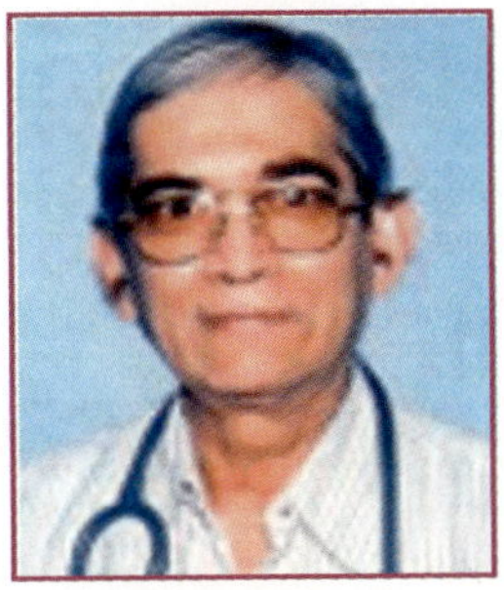

**Prof. T K Lahri**

*Eminent cardiothoracic surgeon and a great teacher*

Tapan Kumar Lahri is an Indian cardiothoracic surgeon, medical and academic writer. He is ex-Professor and Head, Department of Cardiothoracic Surgery, Institute of Medical Sciences, Banaras Hindu University, Varanasi. Born in Varanasi, Uttar Pradesh, he secured MS in general surgery in 1969 from All India Institute of Medical Sciences, New Delhi, and MCh in thoracic surgery in 1972 from the same institution before starting his career as a member of the faculty at Institute of Medical Sciences, Banaras Hindu University, where he held the posts of reader, assistant professor, professor and head of the department of cardiothoracic surgery. After his retirement in 2003, he was made professor emeritus of the institution. Government of India awarded him the fourth highest civilian honour of Padma Shri in 2016 for his contributions to medicine.

# Foreword

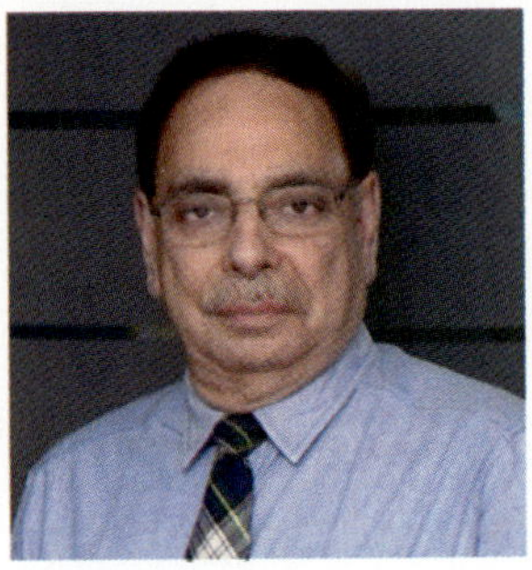

Dr KC Verma, an eminent cardiologist practising in Jammu (J&K), has done a commendable job in writing this book *Cardiovascular Emergencies: Recognition and Management*. The book is an exhaustive work covering all aspects of the management. It starts from basics like history and clinical evaluation and goes on in depth of all varieties of cardiopulmonary emergencies. I find it a very lucid and comprehensive work.

I know Dr Verma for more than 3 decades and always found him a very inquisitive person very well read and always practising ethical medicine. He has been an excellent teacher for his younger colleagues.

The book should be a great help for practising physicians as a day-to-day reference book while handling medical emergencies with cardiac issues. Many such patients would eventually need referral to higher centres for management. The initial management, however, is very important and a working knowledge of starting the correct treatment early can make all the difference in the final outcomes.

I recommend this very well written book for all the busy physicians and cardiologists who want evidence-based guidance for treating their patients.

**Prof. Upendra Kaul**
MD DM FCSI FSCAI FAPSIC FACC FAMS
Awarded Padma Shri and Dr BC Roy Award
*Chairman*
Batra Heart Centre
*Dean*
Academics and Research, Batra Hospital and
Medical Research Centre, New Delhi

# Preface

Cardiac emergencies pose a special challenge to the physician both at tehsil and district headquarters and to the cardiologist in any of the established ICUs of the country and are a leading cause for emergent visits in any emergency department. Failure to quickly recognize them with rapid and appropriate therapy and delay in referring to an appropriate emergency medical care centre can have devastating results. This subject of cardiac emergencies, is therefore, an important curriculum in training ICU nurse, ICU health workers, and both undergraduate and postgraduate medical students in the field of cardiovascular emegency situations. With these objectives in mind, I have chosen most common topics in cardiac emergencies to publish it as a ready guide for the learners.

This book on cardiac emergencies begins with a brief overview of history taking, physical examination, and investigative techniques just as in any other book in discipline of medicine. Most frequently and day-to-day encountered emergencies include acute coronary syndrome, angina pectoris, myocardial infarction, venus thrombosis and pulmonary embolism, complete heart block and accelerated hypertensive vascular emergencies. These chapters have been written with easily understandable text supported with lucid graphs, line diagrams, photographs, latest noninvasive and invasive investigative techniques supported with bibliography for individual chapter for further readings.

'Percutaneous coronary interventions' remain the cornerstone in the management of both acute and chronic coronary obstructions, congenital anomalies, optical coherence tomography, IVUS and fractional flow reserve (FFR) in any of the cardiac catheterization laboratories, but till recently coronary angioplasty has also been performed with robotic interventions. A brief description of these procedures has been recorded in this book. The heart failure which is often the terminal event of many congenital and acquired heart disorders is yet another cardiac emergency which attracts physician, cardiologist, or cardiac surgeon's attention in emergency department all over the world. This subject has been written with utmost care giving details of its recognition with international recommendations and medical and surgical interventions in its management.

Cardiac arrhythmias both in children and adults are not only difficult to diagnose but also to manage these rhythm disturbances with emergent treatment. This book, therefore, describes details of investigations and pharmacological and catheter-based technologies of their respective management.

A brief description of infections leading to varying cardiac complications such as myocarditis, endocarditis, pericarditis, cardiac tamponade, and additionally DCM, valvular and vascular emergencies, hypothermia and cardiogenic shock, have been included in this book. I felt that I could do injustice to this subject of cardiac emergencies if I do not include the description of invasive procedures and noninvasive cardiovascular imaging techniques which are most essential in any emergency department.

Cardiac resuscitation is the most essential part of management of cardiac emergencies both on road side and inside ICU, hence I have been able to describe in detail the techniques of cardiopulmonary resuscitation, non-invasive ventilation, 'ECMO therapy' in acute cardiopulmonary failure.

Radiotherapy and chemotherapy are most important modes of treatment of systemic malignancy disorders and lead to varying grades of cardiac complications. This book includes the brief account of side effects and their respective management.

In emergency department the attending physician or on-duty medical officer may find young children and adolescents admitted with either heart failure, cardiac arrhythmias, intoxicated with frequently prescribed drugs such as digitalis, calcium channel blockers, β-blockers and other antiarrhythmics for their respective treatment or other addictions such as alcohol and cocaine. This book, therefore, records their brief account under separate chapters of 'cardiac emergencies in children and adolescents' and toxicological emergencies in general. Subject of 'telemedicine in emergency cardiology' is quite newer in India, where a patient with fresh cardiac problem and those with operative interventions can contact their cardiologist and cardiac surgeon immediately for remedy. With this view, a chapter on telemedicine with possible inputs including technique of setting and operating has been introduced among the list of other chapters.

In view of the abovementioned chapters included in this book of cardiac emergencies, I am very confident that readers would find it a most valuable and perfect guide and ready-reckoner in obtaining knowledge for the day-to-day management of cardiac emergencies at any level of posting in their service. Besides, it would be very useful book for ICU nurse, ICU technical officers, undergraduate and postgraduate medical students, cardiac fellows, during DM examination, and physicians posted at tehsil and district headquarter medical services.

**KC Verma**

# Acknowledgements

I am very grateful to my wife Dr (Mrs) Urmil Kanta Verma, former professor in department of blood transfusion medicine and pathology, for providing me a perfect congenital atmosphere and all material and moral support needed for writing such a basic book on *Cardiovascular Emergencies: Recognition and Management* which I am sure would prove very helpful in the workup of a heart patient.

To my lovely grandchildren — Adwita, Sidhant, Deven, Leena and Meera. I also appreciate the support of concerned staff of CBS Publishers & Distributors Pvt. Ltd., New Delhi, for their timely guidance in its perfect designing, typesetting, preparation of lucid figures and line diagrams, which itself was a big challenging task and is, therefore, joyfully acknowledged.

**KC Verma**

# Contents

# Cardiovascular Emergencies in India (An Overview)

Cardiovascular emergencies are life-threatening disorders that must be recognized immediately to avoid delay in treatment and to minimize morbidity and mortality. The terms like 'The Golden Hour' and the 'Platinum Ten Minutes' that typify the importance of emergency medical services (EMS) all over the world. It is a well-accepted fact that a patient who receives basic care from trained professionals and is transported to the nearest healthcare facility within 15–20 minutes of an emergency has the greatest chance of survival. EMS is an essential part of the overall healthcare system, as it saves lives by providing care immediately. It's this recognition that has led to research and development in EMS. Over the years several advancements have been made and research is underway to create services that provide medical assistance to patients at the earliest. However, the state of EMS varies drastically from developed to developing countries like India. In spite of the development in the healthcare sector over the past decade, India is yet to create a single, comprehensive EMS that can be accessed throughout the country.

Patients may present with severe hypertension, chest pain, dysrhythmia or cardiopulmonary arrest. It is estimated that by 2020, cardiovascular disease (CVD) will be the largest cause of disability and death in India. The country already has more than 118 million people with hypertension, which is expected to increase to 213 million by 2025. Within CVD, coronary heart disease (CHD) and congestive heart failure are major contributors to the disease burden. CHD has led to an estimated 23% of deaths across all age ranges and 32% of adult deaths from 2010 to 2013. In 2010, it was the leading cause of disability-adjusted life years worldwide (up from fourth in 1990 and increased by 29%).

In cardiac emergencies, ambulance based emergency medical services are the important link in the chain of survival. In view of the time sensitive interventions required in cardiac emergencies and anticipated growing burden of CVDs, such EMS services should be available throughout the country including rural areas on high priority.

Close monitoring of the response time of EMS is critical. Plans should be in place to further reduce the current response times. Training of emergency response officers and involvement of emergency response center physicians in cardiac emergencies may have higher survival rates and desired prognosis.

Bystander cardiopulmonary resuscitation (CPR), public access automatic external defibrillation (AED) and telephone CPR are strongly recommended in case of sudden cardiac arrest situations. Emergency medical techniques (EMT)

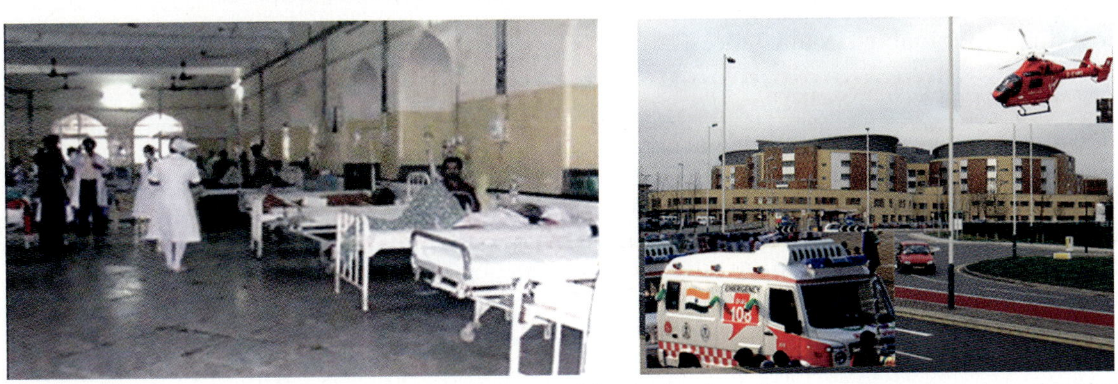

**Fig. 1:** Indoor and outdoor scenes of an emergency wing of one of the Indian hospitals including air and road ambulance services

education and re-education should remain to be a continuous endeavor. Protocol adherence by prehospital care providers and equity, reciprocity and competition (ERC) physicians in providing online medical direction, can reduce deaths and enable appropriate management of cardiac emergencies. Pre-arrival information including ECG transmission should be considered even in India at the earliest. Communities, EMS and hospital based care should have care continuum. Cardiac emergency education, training and research at basic and advanced levels of care should remain high in non-communicable diseases agenda at the national level.

Emergency medical services are an essential part of the overall healthcare system, as it saves lives by providing care immediately. These services are not limited to actual in-hospital treatment, from hospital arrival to stabilization, but include prehospital care and transportation. The World Health Organization regards EMS systems as an integral part of any effective and functional healthcare system. It is the first point of contact for the majority of people to healthcare services during emergencies and life-threatening injuries and can connect people to necessary secondary and tertiary healthcare services. India faces a growing number of emergencies amenable to EMS care and requires a stronger EMS system. GVK Emergency Management and Research Institute (GVK EMRI) has been providing comprehensive emergency services, in partnership with various state governments, by running a single toll-free number 108 in 17 states and union territories across India. The aim of this study is to describe the epidemiology of suspected cardiac emergencies presenting to GVK EMRI across 11 states in India in 2015.

The importance of a reliable EMS cannot be over emphasised, especially in India where the government has the responsibility of caring for a majority of the population. It can be argued that a nation of a over billion people has been deprived of a decent EMS for too long now and it is high time the government takes definitive action. The success of a few services is evident enough of the need for EMS and what it will take to ensure that it works as expected. In a healthcare system that is sprouting and experiencing the benefits of involving private players, a public-private partnership framework could be the right way forward for policy-makers. At a time when the emphasis on preventing damage is greater than ever, the provision of prehospital care will be the key to ensure that lives are not lost due to avoidable circumstances.*

## TYPES OF CARDIAC EMERGENCIES IN INDIA

Listed below are conditions that constitute a possible medical emergency and may require immediate first aid, emergency room care, surgery, or care by a physician or nurse. Not all medical emergencies are life-threatening; some conditions require medical attention in order to prevent significant and long-lasting effects on physical or mental health. However, comprehensive reviews of different cardiovascular emergencies has been done separately in this book (*see* chapters of this book).

### Angina Pectoris

Although, James B. Herrick identified clinical features of angina as early as 1912, but William Heberden is still considered as the first person who drew attention of the world towards this condition for the first time in the history of medical science delivering his classical lecture on angina pectoris before the August audience of Royal College of Physician in 1968 in London Angina pectoris is the result of myocardial ischemia caused by an imbalance between myocardial blood supply and oxygen demand. Angina is a common presenting symptom (typically, chest pain) among patients with coronary artery disease. A comprehensive approach to diagnosis and to medical management of angina pectoris is an integral part of the daily responsibilities of physicians.

### Acute Coronary Syndrome

Acute coronary syndrome (ACS) refers to a spectrum of clinical presentations ranging from those for ST-segment elevation myocardial infarction (STEMI) to presentations found in non-ST-segment elevation myocardial infarction (NSTEMI) or in unstable angina. In terms of pathology, ACS is almost always associated with rupture of an atherosclerotic plaque and partial or complete thrombosis of the infarct-related artery.

### Percutaneous Coronary Interventions (Balloon Angioplasty and Stentoplasty)

Grüntzig's first successful coronary angioplasty treatment on a human was performed in 1977, in Zurich, Switzerland. He expanded a short, about 3 mm, non-branching section of the left anterior descending (LAD) artery (the front branch of the left coronary artery), which supplies the front wall and tip of the heart which had a high grade stenosis, about 80%, of the lumen. Dr Grüntzig presented the results of his first four angioplasty cases at the 1977 American Heart Association (AHA) meeting, which led to widespread acknowledgement of his pioneering work.

### Acute Pulmonary Edema

Pulmonary edema is the term used when edema happens in the lungs. The immediate area outside of the small blood vessels in the lungs is occupied by very tiny air sacs called the alveoli. This is where oxygen from the air is picked up by the blood passing by, and carbon dioxide in the blood is passed into the alveoli to be exhaled out. Alveoli normally have a thin wall that allows for this air exchange, and fluids are usually kept out of the alveoli unless these walls lose their integrity. Pulmonary edema occurs when the alveoli fill up with excess fluid seeped out of the blood vessels in the lung instead of air. This can cause problems with the exchange of gas (oxygen and carbon dioxide), resulting in breathing difficulty and poor oxygenation of blood.

*Prasanthi P. "Emergency Services in India-Counting on betterment," Asian Hospital and Healthcare Management. Available from: *http://www.asianhhm.com/healthcare-management/emergency-services-india* [Last accessed on 2016 Jul 16].

Sometimes, this can be referred to as 'water in the lungs' when describing the condition to patients. Pulmonary edema can be caused by many different factors. It can be related to heart failure, called cardiogenic pulmonary edema, or related to other causes, referred to as non-cardiogenic pulmonary edema.

## Heart Failure

Heart failure is the pathophysiologic state in which the heart, via an abnormality of cardiac function (detectable or not), fails to pump blood at a rate commensurate with the requirements of the metabolizing tissues or is able to do so only with an elevated diastolic filling pressure. Heart failure is a common condition, affecting up to 3 per cent of the population aged 45 and older, and is associated with high mortality and poor quality of life. Major diagnostic and therapeutic advances have been made over the past three decades, but international and national audits suggest that many patients are incompletely investigated and treated. Heart failure may be caused by myocardial failure but may also occur in the presence of near-normal cardiac function under conditions of high demand. Heart failure always causes circulatory failure, but the converse is not necessarily the case, because various noncardiac conditions (e.g. hypovolemic shock, septic shock) can produce circulatory failure in the presence of normal, modestly impaired, or even supranormal cardiac function.

## Syncopal Attacks

Syncope is defined as a partial or complete loss of consciousness with interruption of awareness of oneself and ones surroundings. When the loss of consciousness is temporary and there is spontaneous recovery, it is referred to as syncope or, in nonmedical quarters, fainting. Syncope accounts for one in every 30 visits to an emergency room. It is pronounced sin-ko-pea.

Syncope is due to a temporary reduction in blood flow and, therefore, a shortage of oxygen to the brain. Determining that certain individuals are at 'low mortality risk' and often benign from a mortality perspective, tends to recur, is associated with risk of physical injury, diminishes quality-of-life and might lead to restriction from employment or avocation.

## Cardiac Temponade

Cardiac tamponade is a medical emergency. Early diagnosis and treatment are crucial to reduce morbidity and mortality. Untreated, it is rapidly and universally fatal. Cardiac tamponade is a clinical syndrome caused by the accumulation of fluid in the pericardial space, resulting in reduced ventricular filling and subsequent hemodynamic compromise. Cardiac tamponade is a medical emergency. The overall risk of death depends on the speed of diagnosis, the treatment provided and the underlying cause of the tamponade.

## Cardiac Arrhythmia

Arrhythmias may cause you to feel premature or extra heartbeats, or you may feel that your heart is racing or beating too slowly. Other signs and symptoms may be related to your heart not pumping effectively due to the fast or slow heartbeat. These include shortness of breath, weakness, dizziness, lightheadedness, fainting or near fainting and chest pain or discomfort.

Seek urgent medical care, if you suddenly or frequently experience any of these signs and symptoms at a time when you wouldn't expect to feel them. Ventricular fibrillation is one type of arrhythmia that can be deadly. It occurs when the heart beats with rapid, erratic electrical impulses. This causes pumping chambers in your heart (the ventricles) to quiver uselessly instead of pumping blood. Without an effective heartbeat, blood pressure plummets, cutting off blood supply to your vital organs.

## Cardiopulmonary Arrest

Cardiopulmonary arrest is a sudden and unexpected loss of perfusing pulsatile blood flow attributable to cessation of cardiac mechanical activity. It occurs as a result of a multitude of cardiovascular, metabolic, infectious, neurologic, inflammatory and traumatic diseases. These diseases can be generally classified into '5 Hs' and '4 Ts' [Hypovolemia, Hypoxemia, Hydrogen ion (acidosis), Hypokalemia or Hyperkalemia, Hypothermia, Tension pneumothorax, Tamponade, Toxins and Thrombosis–both pulmonary and cardiac]. The endpoint of these disorders is commonly pulseless ventricular tachycardia (VT) or ventricular fibrillation (VF), pulseless electrical activity or asystole.

## Hypertensive Emergency

A hypertensive emergency is an acute, severe elevation in blood pressure accompanied by end-organ compromise. It is usually associated with a systolic blood pressure (SBP) equal to or higher than 180 mmHg and/or a diastolic blood pressure (DBP) equal to or higher than 120 mmHg. End-organ compromise includes acute renal failure due to nephrosclerosis, ocular involvement with retinal exudates, hemorrhages, or papilledema, hypertensive encephalopathy, acute stroke or intracranial hemorrhage, acute myocardial infarction, aortic dissection and eclampsia. Hypertensive encephalopathy signals the presence of cerebral edema and loss of vascular integrity. If left untreated, hypertensive encephalopathy may progress to seizure and coma. Aortic dissection is associated with severe elevations in systemic blood pressure and wall stress, requiring immediate lowering of the blood pressure and emergent surgery for type-A dissection to reduce morbidity and mortality. Eclampsia, the second most common cause of maternal death, occurs from the second trimester to the peripartum period. It is characterized by the presence of seizures, coma, or both, in the setting of pre-eclampsia. Delivery remains its only cure.

## Aortic Dissection

Aortic dissection is a tear of the aortic intima that allows the shear forces of blood flow to dissect the intima from the media and, in some cases, penetrate the diseased media with resultant rupture and hemorrhage. 65% of dissections originate in the ascending aorta, 20% in the descending aorta, 10% in the aortic arch, and the remainder in the abdominal aorta. While some older classification systems of aortic dissection (such as Stanford and DeBakey) still exist and are used, they seem anachronistic in the current era of advanced imaging. The most commonly used old classification system is the Stanford system; a dissection that involves the ascending aorta is classified as type-A, and one that does not, only affecting the aorta distal to the left subclavian artery, is classified as type-B. Dissections are further classified by chronicity as acute (<2 weeks) or chronic (>2 weeks); mortality peaks at 80% after 2 weeks, and then levels off.

### Cardiogenic Shock

Cardiogenic shock is a major, and frequently fatal complication of a variety of acute and chronic disorders, that impair the ability of the heart to maintain adequate tissue perfusion. Cardiac failure with cardiogenic shock continues to be a frustrating clinical problem; the management of this condition requires a rapid and well-organized approach. Cardiogenic shock is a physiologic state in which inadequate tissue perfusion results from cardiac dysfunction, most commonly following acute myocardial infarction (MI). Although ST-elevation MI (STEM, previously termed Q-wave MI) is encountered in most patients, cardiogenic shock may also develop in patients with non-ST-elevation acute coronary syndrome (NSTEMI, NSTACS or unstable angina).

### Cardiac Valvular Emergencies

Chronic rheumatic valvular dysfunctions can lead to very high morbidity and mortality among patients unless they are helped with either reconstructive surgery or replacement of an artificial valve. Two types of artificial valves which are available today have their own limitations and till date there is no ideal valve which could closely resemble with natural valve in terms of cost and post-operative long term out come. Recently attempts have been made in constructing artificial heart valves with the help of stem cell modification and genetic engineering techniques though long term follow up is still awaited.

In developing countries, rheumatic process is so extensive that often more than one valves (multi-valvular) are affected which further complicates the final management of the patients besides the cost implications among poor patients.

### Deep Vein Thrombosis and Pulmonary Embolism

Pulmonary embolism (PE) is a blockage of the main artery of the lung or one of its branches by a substance that has travelled from elsewhere in the body through the bloodstream (embolism). PE most commonly results from deep vein thrombosis (a blood clot in the deep veins of the legs or pelvis) that breaks off and migrates to the lung, a process termed venous thromboembolism (VTE). A small proportion of cases are caused by the embolization of air, fat, or talc in drugs of intravenous drug abusers or amniotic fluid.

### Peripheral Vascular Disease and Endovascular Therapy

Peripheral vascular diseases (PVDs) are circulation disorders that affect blood vessels outside of the heart and brain. PVD typically strikes the veins and arteries that supply the arms, legs and organs located below your stomach. These are the blood vessels that are distant from the heart. They are known as peripheral vessels. In PVD, blood vessels are narrowed. Narrowing is usually caused by arteriosclerosis. Arteriosclerosis is a condition, where plaque builds up inside a vessel. It is also called 'hardening of the arteries.' Plaque decreases the amount of blood and oxygen supplied to the arms and legs. As plaque growth progresses, clots may develop. This further restricts the affected vessel. Eventually, arteries can become obstructed. PVD that develops only in the arteries is called peripheral arterial disease (PAD). This is the most common form of PVD. Approximately, 12–20% of people over age 65 have PAD. PVD that develops in the deep veins in the body is usually caused from claudication and is called deep vein thrombosis (DVT) Aggressive treatment of existing conditions that may aggravate PVD, such as diabetes, hypertension, and hyperlipidemia (elevated blood cholesterol). Medications for improving blood flow, such as antiplatelet agents (blood thinners) and medications that relax the blood vessel walls Some cases who do not responde to medical therapy, are subjected to catheter/laser based endovascular therapy.

### Extracorporeal Membrane Oxygenation Support in Critically Ill Patients

The term extracorporeal membrane oxygenation (ECMO) was initially used to describe long-term extracorporeal support that focused on the function of oxygenation. Subsequently, in some patients, the emphasis shifted to carbon dioxide removal, and the term extracorporeal carbon dioxide removal was coined. Extracorporeal support was later used for postoperative support in patients following cardiac surgery. Other variations of its capabilities have been tested and used over the last few years, making it an important tool in the armamentarium of life and organ support measures for clinicians. With all of these uses for extracorporeal circuitry, a new term, extracorporeal life support (ECLS), has come into vogue to describe this technology. In emergency medicine, ECMO is an extracorporeal technique of providing both cardiac and respiratory support oxygen to patients whose heart and lungs are so severely diseased or damaged that they can no longer serve their function. Initial cannulation of a patient receiving ECMO is performed by a surgeon and maintenance of the patient is the responsibility of the ECMO specialist and gives 24/7 monitoring care for the duration of the ECMO treatment.

### First Heart Transplant in India

AIIMS is the first Indian center to perform a successful cardiac transplant. The surgery was performed by Dr Panangipalli Venugopal, the ex-director of AIIMS in 1994. The Organ Transplant Bill 1994, was passed in the Indian Parliament in May 1994, which legalized the organ transplants in India. The Bill was on the Table of the President of India for final approval when Dr Venugopal led a team of doctors to perform the first successful heart transplant in India on 3 August 1994. This was the first of the 26 heart transplant procedures performed by Dr Venugopal. Another heart surgeon from India, i.e. Dr KM Cherian performed the first coronary artery bypass surgery in India in 1975. He also performed the country's first heart transplant, first infant cardiac surgery and the first heart and lung transplant (1999). Pioneering pediatric cardiac surgery in India, Cherian has pioneered the first coronary artery bypass surgery in India, as well as the first heart transplant after the legislation of Brain Death in India; the first bilateral lung transplant; the first pediatric heart transplant; the first auto-transplant; and the first heart and lung transplant (1999).

### Emergencies Among Patients on Anticoagulant Therapies

Thromboembolism is a common complication of heart disease. The decision to prescribe an anticoagulant to prevent thromboemboli should be based on a particular patient's risk without treatment and the likely benefit and side effects of the proposed treatment. In this article, we will discuss the use of warfarin and heparin in patients with heart disease.

- Whether anticoagulant treatment should be started depends on the balance between the risk of thromboemboli without treatment and the likely benefits of treatment in each patient.
- Factors increasing the risk of bleeding include serious concomitant disease, previous gastrointestinal bleeding, uncontrolled hypertension and immobility.
- Factors that cumulatively increase the risk of thromboembolism in non-rheumatic atrial fibrillation include age over 60, recent congestive heart failure, hypertension (treated or untreated), previous thromboembolism, and the presence of a large atrium or of global left ventricular dysfunction.
- Cardioversion of non-rheumatic atrial fibrillation (including fibrillation of new onset) is associated with an increased thromboembolic risk, which is reduced by anticoagulant treatment.
- Heparin and aspirin are both beneficial in unstable angina.
- Anticoagulants should be considered after myocardial infarction in patients with an increased risk of thromboemboli—patients in atrial fibrillation and those with persistent heart failure.

**KC Verma**

# 1 History Taking, Symptoms, Signs and Investigations in a Heart Patient (An Overview)

In order to arrive at an accurate diagnosis of heart disease among patients, it is important for the physician/cardiologist to follow the set clinical procedures of extracting accurate clinical history, thorough clinical examination supported with basic biochemical investigation. This provisional diagnosis is further confirmed with the help of specialised invasive techniques, such as cardiac catheterisation and angiocardiography and noninvasive tests like echocardiography, CMRI and MD/CT. The following are the different clinical and investigative steps which could help physician/cardiologist to arrive at a correct diagnosis.

## HISTORY TAKING

### BEDSIDE HISTORY

A painstaking and problem-oriented history taking is often helpful in the diagnosis. Family history and attention to pertinent symptomatology in the various age-groups, such as cyanosis, poor feeding, tachypnoea and orthopnea, cyanotic spells, squatting, growth retardation, easy fatigability, recurrent pneumonia and congestive failure, may offer clues for the presence of heart disease. It is necessary to establish whether the disease is congenital or acquired. This can be achieved by a good history and a well conducted physical examination (Fig. 1.1).

The presence of a murmur especially below the age of 1 year, cyanosis and parasternal murmurs are suggestive of congenital heart disease. Even apical murmurs do not exclude the presence of congenital heart disease and have to be carefully evaluated.

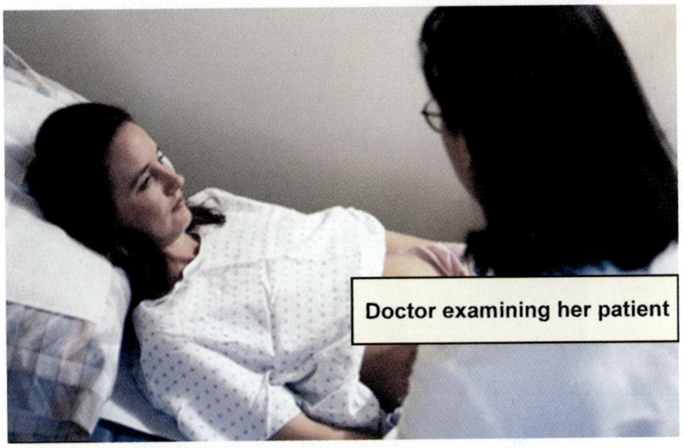


**Fig. 1.1:** Doctor examining an adolescent admitted with recurrent palpitation

#### History of Rheumatic Fever

1. Chorea twitches or clumsiness for a few months in childhood. Epistaxis. Frequent sore throats. Tonsillectomy and adenoidectomy.
2. Growing pains (i.e. nocturnal pains or aches in the legs). (Arthritis or other joint involvement in daytime suggests rheumatic fever.)
3. Was the diagnosis of rheumatic fever based merely on signs of fever and murmur or were actually red swollen, painful joints and rash?
4. What was the therapy given? (Aspirin, steroids, prophylactic penicillin and prolonged bed rest.)
5. Is there a family history of rheumatic fever? (This is almost as suggestive of a rheumatic origin of a patient's murmur as a history of rheumatic fever in the patient.)

#### History of Rheumatic Heart Disease

1. Murmurs heard on previous examination (school, operation, hospitalization, insurance or military service).
2. Carditis with Caray-Coombs murmur and rheumatic nodules (Fig. 1.2).
3. Results of cardiac catheterization. When and where was it done?

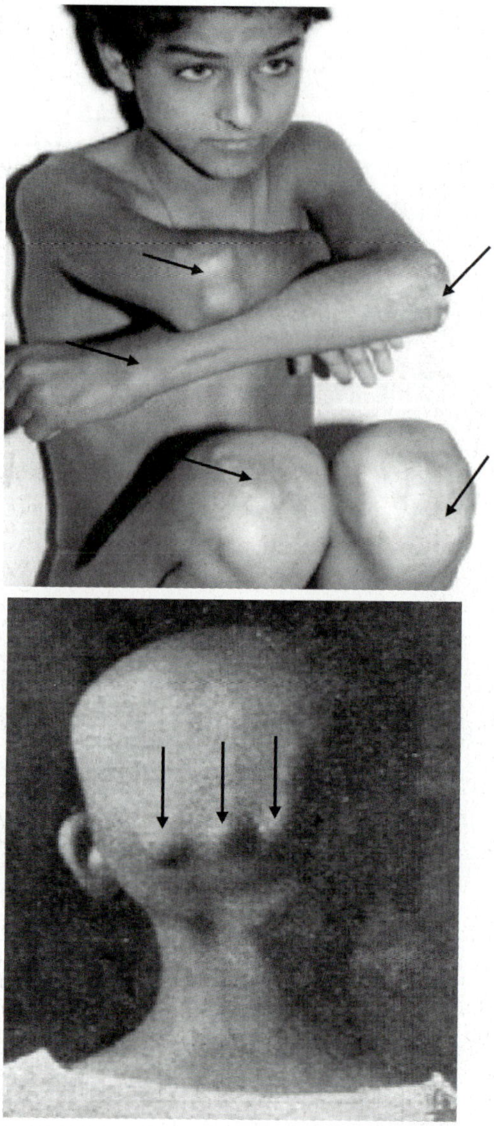

**Fig. 1.2:** Multiple rheumatic nodules over both elbows, wrist, knee joints and occiput regions in active rheumatic fever

## Complications of Rheumatic Heart Disease

1. In the presence of mitral disease
   a. Hemoptysis: Is it mixed or pure? Quantity, color and frequency. (If this occurs with dyspnea or pleuritic pain, consider pulmonary infarction. If it arises from the submucosal bronchial veins, the blood is dark, and the cause is usually raised left atrial pressure due to mitral stenosis).
   b. Hoarseness of voice: Without obvious upper respiratory infection? The cardio-vocal syndrome, due to the pressure of a large left atrium on an enlarged pulmonary artery, which in turn may press on the peribronchial lymph nodes to compress the recurrent laryngeal nerve. Dysphagia may be due to both pressure by a large left atrium and stretch of the autonomic fibers to the esophagus.
   c. Winter bronchitis or wheezing.
   d. Ruptured chordae tendinae suggested by sudden worsening of dyspnea orthopnea, or paroxysmal nocturnal dyspnea (PND).
   e. Embolic phenomena: Hematuria, pleurisy and unilateral weakness. Sudden loss of vision or loss in one visual field of one eye.
2. In the presence of aortic stenosis, angina, exertional syncope, or dyspnea (a classic triad).
3. In the presence of aortic regurgitation nocturnal angina [but is a sign of vasospastic angina if no aortic regurgiatation (AR)].
4. Awareness of large pulsations in arms, neck or cheek.
5. Epilepsy (increased incidence with mitral stenosis).
6. Possible infective endocarditis (Fig. 1.3).
   a. Fever and night sweats (enough to require change of pajamas).
   b. Tooth extraction or cleaning or other possible causes of bacteremia.
   c. Prolonged treatment with penicillin or other antibiotic.
   d. Embolic phenomena, hematuria, back pain, splinter hemorrhages, petechiae, tender finger pads, or cerebro-vascular accident (unilateral weakness, paralysis or speech difficulty).
   e. Seagull murmur usually is indicative of aortic valvulitis.

## Could it be a Congenital Heart Disease?

To be asked, if patient is an infant.

1. Growth and development: High birth weight suggests transposition of the great vessels.
2. Mother's pregnancy:
   a. Stilbestrol in pregnancy has been linked to transposition of great vessels.
   b. Viral illness

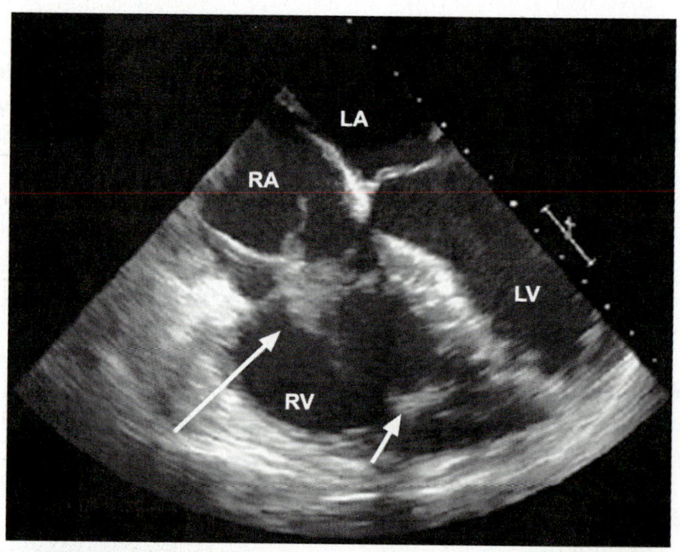


**Fig. 1.3:** Transesophageal echocardiography—4-chamber view shows multiple vegetations on the tricuspid valve (long arrow) and pacing leads (short arrow)

c. Diabetes in pregnancy suggests transposition of great vessels combined with high birth weight.
3. Frequent pneumonias.
4. Excessive sweating. Asthmatic attacks in newborn.
5. Has mother been aware of infant's heart beating against chest wall or the vibrations or a thrill?

### To be Asked if Patient is a Child or Adult

1. *Mother's pregnancy:* Rubella in first trimester.
2. *Family history:* Congenital heart disease or murmur in family.
3. *Cyanosis:* When did it begin? [Cyanosis either from birth or within a few days of birth, suggests transposition of the great vessels (TGV)]. Delayed for years and associated with palpitations suggests Ebstein's anomaly, especially if present with little dyspnoea on exertion (DOE). If delayed until adolescence of middle age, suggests atrial septal defect with Eisenmenger's reaction or syndrome. Does it occur with crying, feeding or warm bath or only with syncope? (Suggests tetralogy of Fallot.) Differential cyanosis and clubbing suggests patent ductus arteriosus with Eisenmenger's syndrome, especially if there is unexpectedly little DOE. Frequent phlebotomies.
4. *Syncope or faintness:* Do these signs occur on exposure to cold or only during effort or excitement? (Sugggests primary pulmonary hypertension.) With straining, after a long sleep and with cyanosis? (Suggests tetralogy of Fallot or complete atrioventricular block.) Only with effort (suggests severe aortic stenosis, pulmonary stenosis, or primary pulmonary hypertension).
5. Angina (suggests severe aortic or pulmonary stenosis)
6. Exact day the murmur was first heard. (Stenotic murmurs are heard in newborn nursery; left-to-right shunt murmurs are often delayed a few weeks.) Was it discovered by a physician who had seen the patient before or by a physician seeing the patient for the first time?
7. *Squatting or knee-chest position frequent* (suggests decreased pulmonary flow due to tetralogy or Fallot or more rarely, due to tricuspid atresia).
8. Headaches, epistaxis, leg fatigue or aches after exercise, cold legs, or claudication (suggests aortic coarctation. Epistaxis alone suggests rheumatic fever).
9. When and where was cardiac catheterization done?
10. *Dysphagia* (consider coarctation, with the right subclavian artery passing behind the esophagus).
11. *Awareness of pulsations in the neck* (consider coarctation, aortic regurgitation, thyrotoxicosis or the venous pulsations or gaint A waves in primary pulmonary hypertension or severe pulmonary stenosis).
12. *Strokes* (consider emboli from endoardial fibroelastosis if patient is an infant or emboli from idiopathic cardiomyopathy if patient is a child. May be due to paradoxical emboli or cerebral abscess if patient is cyanotic. Somnolence with cyanosis suggests cerebral abscess).
13. *Hoarseness of voice* (suggests primary pulmonary hypertension or large patent ductus arteriosus).
14. *Surgery:* When, where and by whom? What were the symptomatic results?
15. *Mental retardation* (consider Down's syndrome or supravalvular aortic stenosis).
16. *Swelling, pain, warmth and tenderness of lower extremities* (hypertrophic osteo-orthropathy suggests patent ductus arteriosus with Eisenmenger's syndrome).
17. Recurrent bleeding from the nose, lips or mouth with hemoptysis or melena, multiple cerebral symptoms such as dizziness and visual disturbances and a family history of epistaxis (this complex of symptoms comprises hereditary hemorrhagic telangiectasis or Rendu-Osler-Weber disease and suggests a pulmonary arteriovenous fistula, especially if the patient is cyanotic)
18. *Weakness and incoordination* (suggests the cardiomyopathy of Friedreich's ataxia or muscular dystrophy).

## SPLINTER HEMORRHAGES

Splinter hemorrhages (or haemorrhages) are tiny lines that run vertically under nails (Fig. 1.4). Splinter hemorrhage is a nonspecific finding and can be associated with subacute bacterial endocarditis, scleroderma, trichinosis, systemic lupus erythematosus (SLE), rheumatoid arthritis, psoriatic nails, antiphospholipid syndrome, and trauma. At first they are usually plum-colored, but then darken to brown or black in a couple of days. In certain conditions (in particular, infective endocarditis), clots can migrate from the affected heart valve and find their way into various parts of the body. If this happens in the finger, it can cause damage to the capillaries resulting in a splinter hemorrhage.

There are a number of other causes for splinter hemorrhages.

They could be due to hitting the nail ('trauma'), a sign of inflammation in blood vessels all around the body ('systemic vasculitis'), or they could be where a bit of

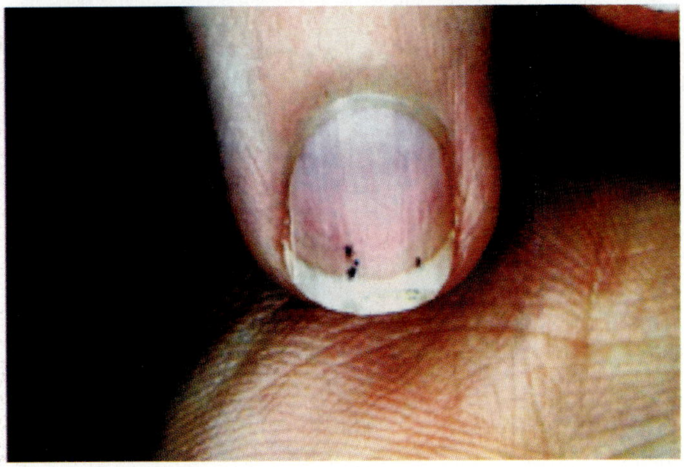

**Fig. 1.4:** Thumb showing splinter hemorrhage under nail in patient with infective endocarditis

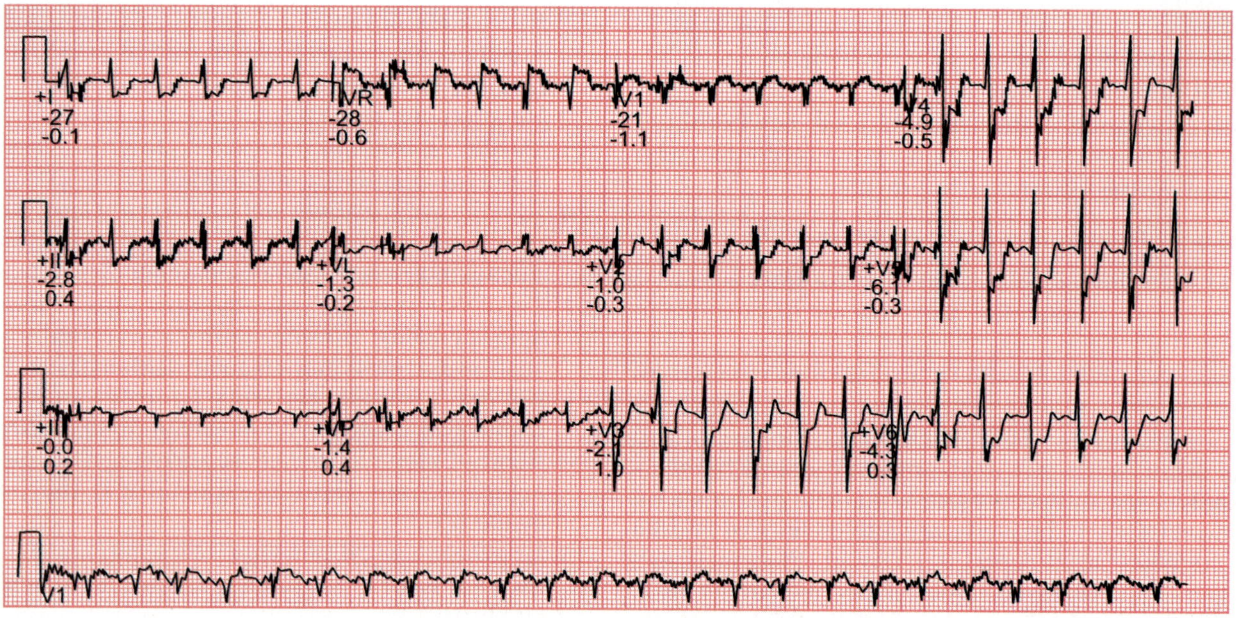


**Fig. 1.5:** ST-depression in leads 1, 11, aVF and V3–V6 strongly positive TMT in a patient with cardiac syndrome X

cholesterol has got lodged in the finger's capillaries. Even if a patient does have infective endocarditis, probably 5 in every 6 patients won't have splinter hemorrhages.

## CARDIAC SYNDROME X (ANGINA WITH NORMAL CORONARY ARTERIES)

Cardiac syndrome X (CSX) (not to be confused with metabolic syndrome X, or metabolic syndrome) is the name given to a clinical condition which produces angina-like chest pain, often with signs of cardiac ischemia (i.e. poor blood flow in the heart muscle) in the absence of coronary artery disease (Figs 1.5 and 1.6). The chief characteristics of CSX are as follows:

- Angina-line chest pain during exertion
- Characteristic ECG changes during exercise testing
- Normal coronary arteries on cardiac catheterization
- No inducible coronary artery spasm during catheterization

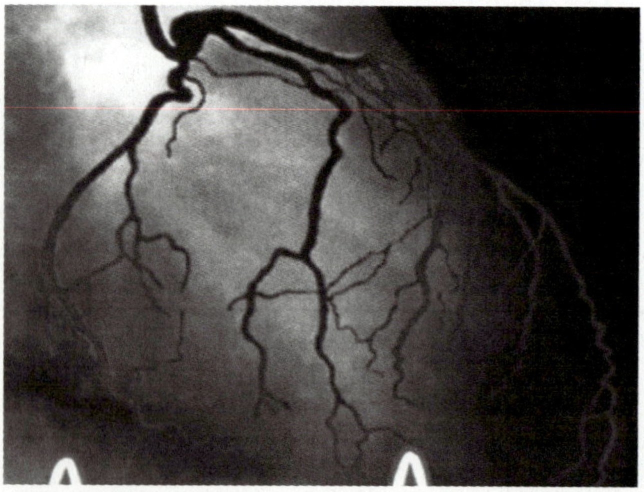

**Fig. 1.6:** Angiogram showing normal coronary vessels in a patient with chest pain in syndrome X with positive TMT results

## INTERMITTENT CLAUDICATION

Intermittent claudication (*Latin:* claudicatio intermittens) is a clinical diagnosis given for muscle pain (ache, cramp, numbness or sense of fatigue), classically in the calf muscle, which occurs during exercise and is relieved by a short period of rest (Fig. 1.7). Claudication derives from the *Latin* verb claudicare, 'to limp'.

### Signs

One of the hallmarks of arterial claudication is that, it occurs intermittently. It disappears after a brief rest and the patient can start walking again until the pain recurs. The following are the general signs of atherosclerosis of the lower extremity arteries:

- Cyanosis
- Atrophic changes like loss of hair, shiny skin
- Decreased temperature
- Decreased pulse
- Redness when limb is returned to a 'dependent' position

All the 'Ps' are

1. Increase in Pallor
2. Decrease in Pulses
3. Perishing cold
4. Pain
5. Paraesthesia
6. Paralysis

### Causes

Most commonly, intermittent (or vascular or venous) claudication is due to peripheral arterial disease which

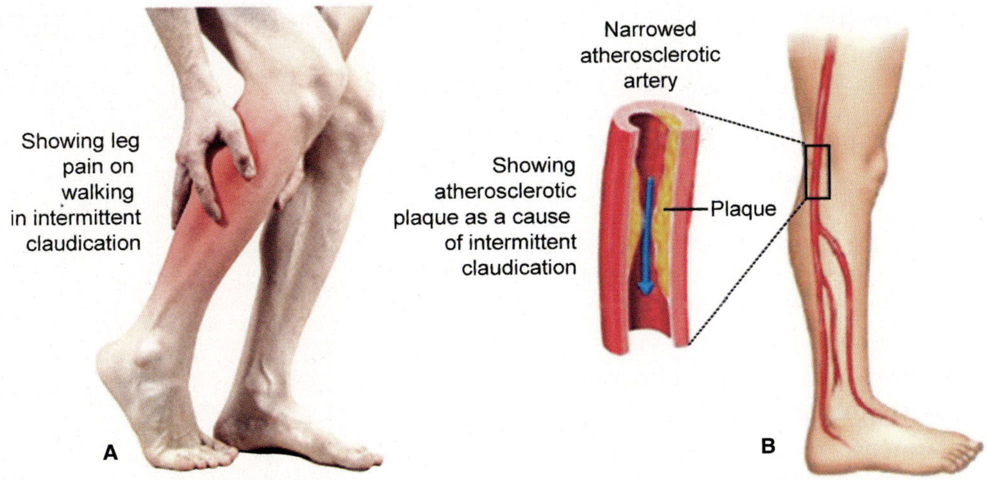


**Fig. 1.7:** (A) Patient is feeling severe leg pain during walking. (B) Atherosclerotic obstruction as a cause of intermittent claudication

implies significant atherosclerotic blockages resulting in arterial insufficiency. It is distinct from neurogenic claudication, which is associated with lumbar spinal stenosis.

### Epidemiology

Atherosclerosis affects up to 10% of the western population older than 65 years and for intermittent claudication this number is around 5%. Intermittent claudication most commonly manifests in men older than 50 years.

### Peripheral, Venous Congestion or Pseudo-right Heart Failure Possibilities

1. *Peripheral edema:* Maximum and minimum weight. Reasons for any weight gain or loss.
2. *Ascites* (if this occurs before or simultaneously with orthopnea or dyspnea, consider tamponade)
3. *Upper abdominal pain, especially on exercise* (this suggests increased stretch of liver capsule due to hepatomegaly.)
4. *Bending or stooping discomfort* (suggests hepatomegaly)
5. Positive hepato-jugular reflux.

### Low Output State Possibilities

1. *Weakness and fatigue:* Do these occur only in the morning (depression)? Is afternoon nap necessary? If these signs occur only in the afternoon, they suggest low blood sugar or hypothyroidism. Is the patient on drugs that would cause weakness (i.e. digitalis, diuretics, β-blockers, or tranquilizers)? Is there only psychoneurotic basis (relationship to family, spouse, work supervisor)? Is the patient taking a contraceptive pill, diphenylhydantion and spironolactone?
2. *Coldness of extremities:* For how long?
3. *Excessive perspiration* (a common sign of failure in infants. If recent in an adult and not due to hyperthyroidism or neurosis; it suggests severe failure. With warm hands, it suggests thyrotoxicosis; with cold hands it suggests psychoneurosis or heart failure.)
4. Insomnia due to hyperpnea on going to sleep or dozing. It should be asked to his wife or closely associated family member.
5. Nocturia with polyuria.

### Possibilities of Fixed Output State

1. Syncope, faintness or dizzines.
2. Chest pain tightness, pressure or discomfort. Could it be a high out put failure?
   a. Anemia
      i. Has the patient ever been told that he has anemia? Pins and needles? Bleeding from menorrhagia, hemorrhoids, or ulcers. Is anemia being treated?
      ii. Bone marrow or metabolic disorders; upper GIT surgery in the past (leading to B12 deficiency), sickle cell disease in self or family, contact with lead or radiation.
   b. Thyrotoxicosis
   c. Beriberi

## EXPLORING HYPERTENSIVE HEART DISEASE

1. When was the patient first told? Under what circumstances was it discovered?
2. Has treatment been taken regularly? What drugs in what dosage have been taken?
3. Has there been a previous kidney infection or nephritis, or back injury in sport or accident?
4. Frequency of urination or nocturia, polyuria, kidney X-rays, renal calculi, gout, severe diabetes.
5. Family history of hypertension. At what age the patient was told?
6. Coarctation of aorta; cold legs or intermittent claudication, nosebleeds, shoulder girdle pains. Have angiograms been done?

7. Pheochromocytoma; flushing with pounding headaches, dizziness, sweating, palpitations, nausea, chest pain and paresthesia. Weight loss. Elevated blood sugar.
8. Cushing syndrome hirsutism, corticosteroid intake, easy bruising slow wound healing, acne, muscle weakness, kidney stones, emotional unstability or depression.
9. Past blood pressure reading. Visual problems, convulsions, strokes, head aches, dyspnea on exertion, orthopnea, post-nasal drip (PND) or epistaxis.
10. Known X-ray or EKG abnormalities.
11. Amount of success of medical or surgical therapy
12. Metabolic syndrome and obesity
13. Side effects of treatment; muscle aches and pains, weakness, sleepiness, postural hypotension, nausea, nasal stuffiness, impotence or palpitation.

## ENQUIRING FOR COR PULMONALE

1. Chronic obstructive pulmonary disease; pulmonary function tests. Easier to breathe leaning forward? Smoking history. Chronic cough and sputum.
2. Asthma, wheezing or dyspnea relieved by bronchodilators.
3. Ever worked in a soft or hard coal mine.
4. Pulmonary emboli. History of phlebitis. Marked diuresis with diuretics. On contraceptive pills. Ever sudden dyspnea at rest with palpitations pleurisy, faintness, cold sweat, or hemoptysis. Recurrent stabbing groin pains. Recent trauma or surgery. Pregnancy or long automobile trip.
5. History of lung infiltrate or tuberculosis.
6. Bilateral rales over the bases of the chest.

## CARDIAC CHAMBER ENLARGEMENT POSSIBILITIES

1. Trepopnea (certain positions in bed cause discomfort).
2. Palpitations or awareness of heart beat.
3. Has patient been told of an enlarged heart? When was he first told? If yes, was it after an ECG or X-ray or echocardiogram. Where and when done?
4. Has an X-ray examination been done? When and where was first and last one done?

## HOW TO KNOW ABOUT PAST CARDIAC SURGERY?

1. Date and place of surgery. Type of operation or prosthesis. Name of surgeon.
2. Heart failure or other cardiac symptoms present before surgery. Which symptoms were present, and for how long?
3. Was patient catheterized before or after surgery? Was he told about the results of the studies?
4. Complications after surgery; embolic phenomenon, infections or other.
5. What treatment was given after surgery (anti-coagulants, digitalis, diuretics)? For how long? (Fig. 1.8)

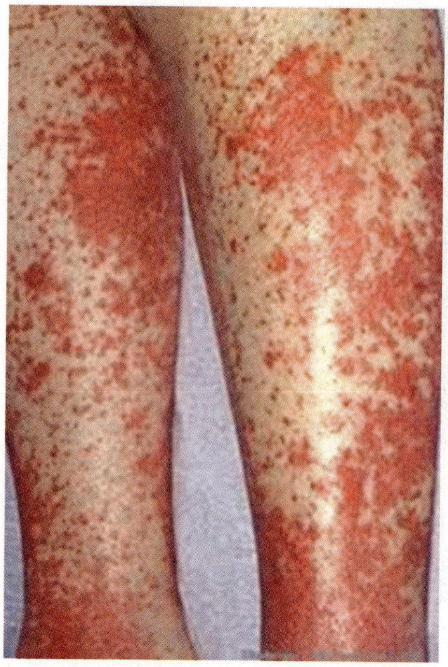

**Fig. 1.8:** Ecchymosis over the legs in an adolescent patient with consumption of anticoagulants after corrective surgery

## PERICARDITIS, EFFUSION CONSTRICTION OR TAMPONADE POSSIBILITIES

History of chest trauma, recent heart surgery. (The postcardiotomy syndrome, fever, pleurisy, pericarditis and polyserositis may occur as long as 2 months after heart surgery). Myocardial infarction (Dressler's syndrome, which is the same as postcardiotomy syndrome but follows myocardial infarction, now extremely rare), radiation to chest in past few months, uremia, metastatic cancer, lymphoma, leukemia, myxedema, scleroderma, lupus, rheumatoid arthritis, and contact with tuberculosis, or recent viral infection Is patient taking drugs that would produce lupus erythematosus syndrome procainamide, hydralazine, penicillin and isoniazid? Is he on drug, like minoxidil? (Fig. 1.9)

### Symptoms of Pericarditis

1. Chest pain on exertion, swallowing or deep breathing.
2. Joint symptoms (with facial rash suggests possible lupus erythematosus; with rash on limbs or body, rheumatic fever).
3. Past history of pericarditis (in about one-fourth of cases idiopathic pericarditis is recurrent).
4. Epigastric pain for 1–3 days before the chest pain (this is the initial manifestation in one-third of patients with acute idiopathic pericarditis. Pain may occur alone in the abdomen).

### Symptoms of Tamponade

1. Dyspnea on exertion (DOE).
2. Edema or ascites preceding dyspnea. Abdominal swelling before or simultaneous with edema (highly suggestive of tamponade).

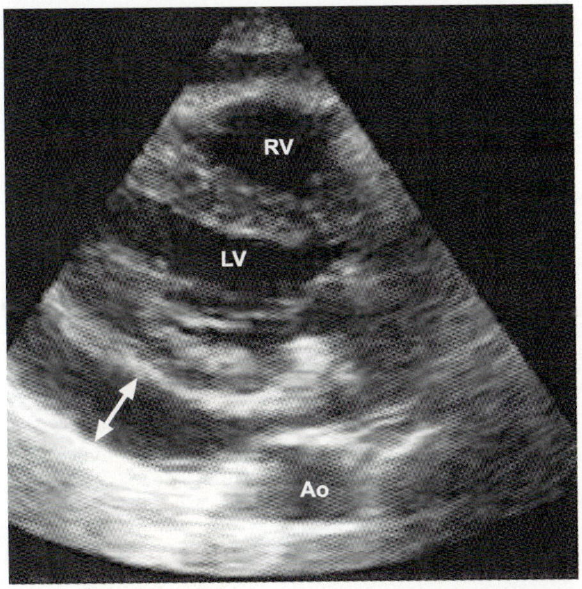


**Fig. 1.9:** LPS LAX echo scan showing large pericardial effusion (arrow)

3. Does DOE stop immediately when the patient stops moving (rare sign)?

## Myocarditis, Endocarditis and Other Heart Disease Possibilities

1. *Acute myocarditis:* Recent influenza-like illness with myalgia.
2. *Infective endocarditis:* Has patient ever been told about it or cardiac murmur? Drug addiction, fevers, surgical or dental cause of bacteremia, prolonged penicillin treatment hematuria, back pain, petechiae, strokes? (Fig. 1.10).
3. *'Collagen' disease:* Raynaud's phenomenon, dysphagia, arthritis, or arthralgias tight skin epistaxis, rash in sunlight?
4. *Ankylosing spondylitis:* Pain in the hip or sciatic region, or low back pain. Does the pain awaken patient in the early morning hours? Morning back stiffness. Pain increased on coughing.

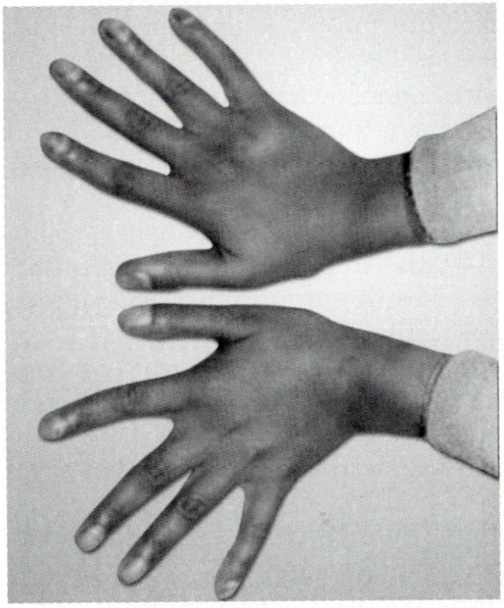

**Fig 1.10:** Bilateral clubbing of fingers in infective endocarditis in patient with chronic rheumatic valvular dysfunction

5. *Carcinoid heart disease:* Diarrhoea, bronchospasm, flushing of the upper chest and head that lasts from minutes to days.
6. *Parasitic disease (trichinosis or Chagas' disease):* Consumption of special meat preparation. Foreign travel.
7. *Hypophosphatemia:* High intake of phosphorus-binding antacids, aluminum hydroxide gel. Acute alcohol excess.
8. *Atrial myxoma:* Embolic phenomena, recurrent fevers, arthralgias, or skin lesions of a vasculitis type. Paresthesias in hands. Pulsations in neck (giant A waves, as in tricuspid stenosis) (Fig. 1.11).
9. Syncope or faintness on changing body position.
10. *Hemochromatosis:* History of diabetes especially, if patient is insulin resistant. Skin color changes. Liver failure and enlargement symptoms; upper abdominal

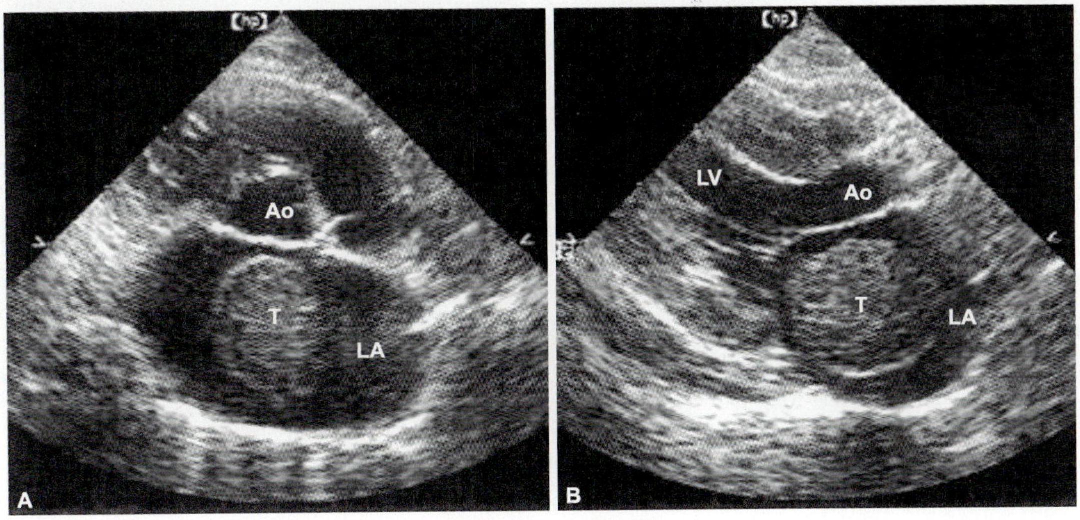


**Fig. 1.11:** Echocardiogram short axis (A) and parasternal long-axis, (B) show tumor mass in LA

pain, sexual impotence or gynecomastia? Frequent transfusions.

11. *Sarcoidosis:* Syncope (due to complete atrioventricular block). Known bundle branch block. Abnormal chest radiograph. Cough. Kidney stones or eye symptoms (uveitis).
12. Hypertrophic subaortic stenosis family history of sudden death. Angina or syncope after but not during exercise intermittent murmur. Do symptoms become worse on digitalis? (Fig. 1.12)
13. Amyloid heart disease; postural hypertension with peripheral neuropathy. Skin lesions, especially if there is bleeding on scratching.
14. Aortic regurgitation or aneurysm. History of venereal disease or positive serology.
15. Hoarseness due to recurrent laryngeal nerve compression by aneurysm.
16. Traumatic tricuspid regurgitation may not cause cardiac sympoms for up to 3 years after the accident.

## NEW YORK HEART ASSOCIATION FUNCTIONAL AND THERAPEUTIC CLASSIFICATION

### Functional Classification

This functional classification refers to fatigue, dyspnea or angina. The original classification is too long to grasp and a simplified one follows.

*Class 1:* The patient is asymptomatic, or symptoms occur on extraordinary exertion (there is no class, or classification for a patient with a normal heart).
*Class 2:* Symptoms occur on ordinary exertion.
*Class 3:* Symptoms occur on less than ordinary exertion.
*Class 4:* Symptoms occur even at rest.

***Note:*** The functional classification is easily remembered, if one simply remembers the words ordinary exertion, because class 1 simply adds extra in front of ordinary class 2 adds no words in front of ordinary, and class 3 adds less than in front of ordinary.

### Therapeutic Classification

It also refers only to patients with abnormal heart.
Class A: No restriction
Class B: Severe effort restricted
Class C: Ordinary effort moderately restricted
Class D: Ordinary effort markedly restricted
Class E: Confined to chair.

Enquiring about the symptoms of the heart disease. The nature of the underlying physiological disturbances can often be assessed from the symptoms. For example:

1. Raised pulmonary venous pressure
   a. Dyspnea
   b. Orthopnea
   c. Paroxysmal nocturnal dyspnea
   d. Cough
   e. Haemoptysis
2. Inadequate coronary blood flow; angina pectoris
3. Congestive cardiac failure; ankle swelling, hepatic pain.
4. Right to left intracardiac shunt;
   a. Cyanosis
   b. Dyspnea
   c. Squatting
   d. Syncopal attacks.

## SYMPTOMS RESULTING FROM A RAISED PULMONARY VENOUS PRESSURE

## DYSPNEA

### Definition

Dyspnea is an uncomfortable and inappropriate awareness of respiration. Dyspnea can result from several physiological disturbances, the most frequent cause in cardiac disease being a high pulmonary venous pressure.

### Mechanism

Any rise in pressure in the left atrium and pulmonary veins is transmitted to the pulmonary capillaries, increasing the

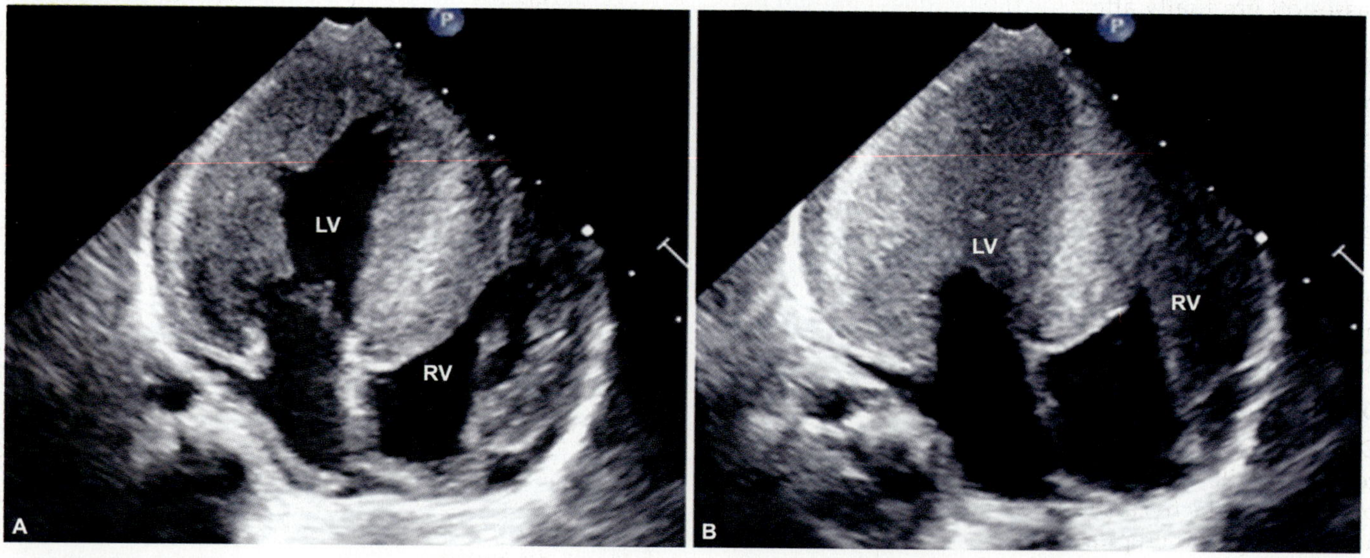


**Fig. 1.12:** Transthoracic echocardiogram. Apical 4-chamber view shows LV hypertrophy in HOCM. LV=left ventricle, RV=right ventricle

transudation of fluid from the capillaries into the interstitial tissues of the lung. The lungs then offer more resistance to inflation and deflation and the greater muscular effort required gives the patient the sensation of dyspnea. Frank pulmonary oedema represents the extreme situation when severe elevation of the pulmonary venous pressure forces large amounts of fluid into the alveoli.

### Types

Orthopnea and paroxysmal nocturnal dyspnea describe specific forms of dyspnea arising from a high pulmonary venous pressure. The presence of either or both is evidence that the patient's dyspnoea is caused by a high pulmonary venous pressure.

## ORTHOPNOEA

### Definition

It may be defined as respiratory difficulty while lying flat and relieved while sitting up.

### Mechanism

In normal subjects the volume of blood in the lungs is increased by lying flat, right atrial filling pressure is increased and the increased filling of the right atrium and ventricle is passed on into the lungs. The pulmonary blood volume is already large in patients with a high pulmonary venous pressure and the further volume change on lying flat adds to the stiffness of the lungs.

## PAROXYSMAL NOCTURNAL DYSPNEA

It is that kind of acute dyspnea in which the patient feels uncomfortable during awakening from sleep.

### Description

Acute dyspnea, awakening the patient from sleep, forcing him to sit upright or stand out of bed for relief. A dry cough and wheeze are commonly present during the attack, which passes off gradually after 10–20 minutes.

### Mechanism

During the night the circulation of blood volume increases in heart failure as interstitial fluid returns to the blood, and the pulmonary venous pressure may build up to high levels. The reduced awareness during sleep allows high levels to be reached before dyspnea awakens the patient.

## ACUTE PULMONARY EDEMA

Figure 1.13 shows chest X-ray depicting bilateral acute pulmonary edema.

### Description

Dyspnea is acute and is accompanied by cough and a copious white or pink frothy sputum. There is cyanosis, perspiration, tachycardia, raised systemic blood pressure and wide spread crepitations over the lungs.

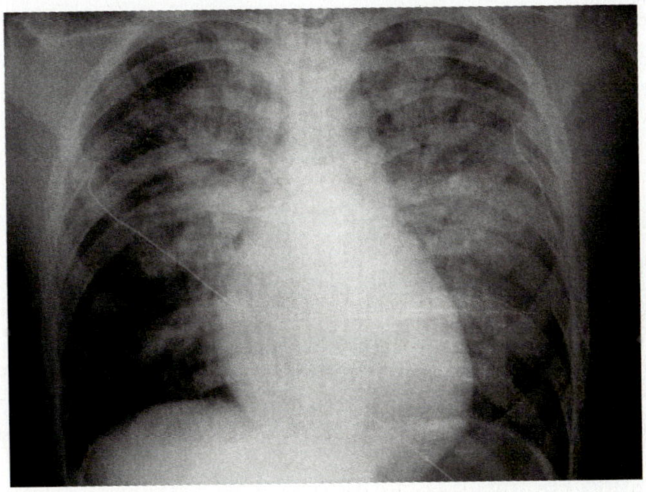

**Fig. 1.13:** Chest X-ray showing bilateral acute pulmonary edema

### Mechanism

When levels of pressure of 40 mmHg, are exceeded in the pulmonary veins, the osmotic pressure of the plasma is overcome and fluid transits from the lungs capillaries into the alveoli in large quantities. Rupture of pulmonary capillaries from the high pressures produces pink expectorated sputum.

## GRADATION OF DYSPNEA

Useful information about the severity of heart disease is obtained by grading the severity of dyspnea. The following workable categories have been found useful in clinical practice.

- *Grade 1 (Mild dyspnea):* When undertaking unusual exertion (running, walking and scrubbing).
- *Grade 2 (Moderate):* Walking on the level causes dyspnea
- *Grade 3 (Severe):* Unable to continue walking even slowly on the level.
- *Grade 4 (Gross):* The slight effort induces severe breathlessness. The patient is practically confined to bed by dyspnea. A history of nocturnal dyspnea or acute pulmonary oedema places the patient in the severe grade and irrespective of the effort tolerance.

## COUGH

Two types of cough may be caused by a high pulmonary venous pressure. Dry cough during exertion. Cough, producing expectoration along with wheezing.

### Mechanism

The bronchial venous return is mainly drained into the pulmonary veins, so that when the pulmonary venous pressure rises during exertion there is engorgement of the bronchial mucosa. This activates the cough reflex resulting in a troublesome dry cough. Chronic elevation of the bronchial venous pressure results in an edematous mucosa offering less resistance to infection and prone to repeated attacks of bronchitis.

## HAEMOPTYSIS (COUGHING OUT OF BLOOD)

As a result of the high venous pressure a bronchial vein may rupture and cause a small or large haemoptysis.

1. Diseases associated with a raised pulmonary venous pressure.
2. Left ventricular failure. The high filling pressure required for the failing left ventricle results in an increased pressure in the left atrium and the pulmonary veins which in turn leads to left ventricular failure.
3. Obstruction to blood flow from the lungs. The pressure in the pulmonary veins proximal to any obstruction is high, e.g. mitral stenosis, left atrial myxoma.

## SYMPTOMS OF AN INADEQUATE CORONARY BLOOD FLOW

### Angina Pectoris (Figs 1.14 and 1.15)

Four major characteristics are:

1. *Quality:* A crushing pain or a tight constricting sensation.
2. *Site:* Pain is maximum behind the sternum or across the front of the chest.
3. *Radiation:* Radiates into the shoulders, the neck, jaw and the fingers and through to the back of the chest.
4. *Relation to exertion:* Pain is experienced during exertion. When exertion is discontinued, the pain wears off in 2–3 minutes, pain may also be provoked by anger or excitement.

## SYMPTOMS OF RIGHT TO LEFT INTRACARDIAC SHUNTS

### Central Cyanosis

Blue discoloration of skin, nail beds and mucous membrane which is more marked on exertion or during crying. Central cyanosis in congenital heart disease implies that blood low in oxygen content reaches the systemic arteries without first passing through the lungs.

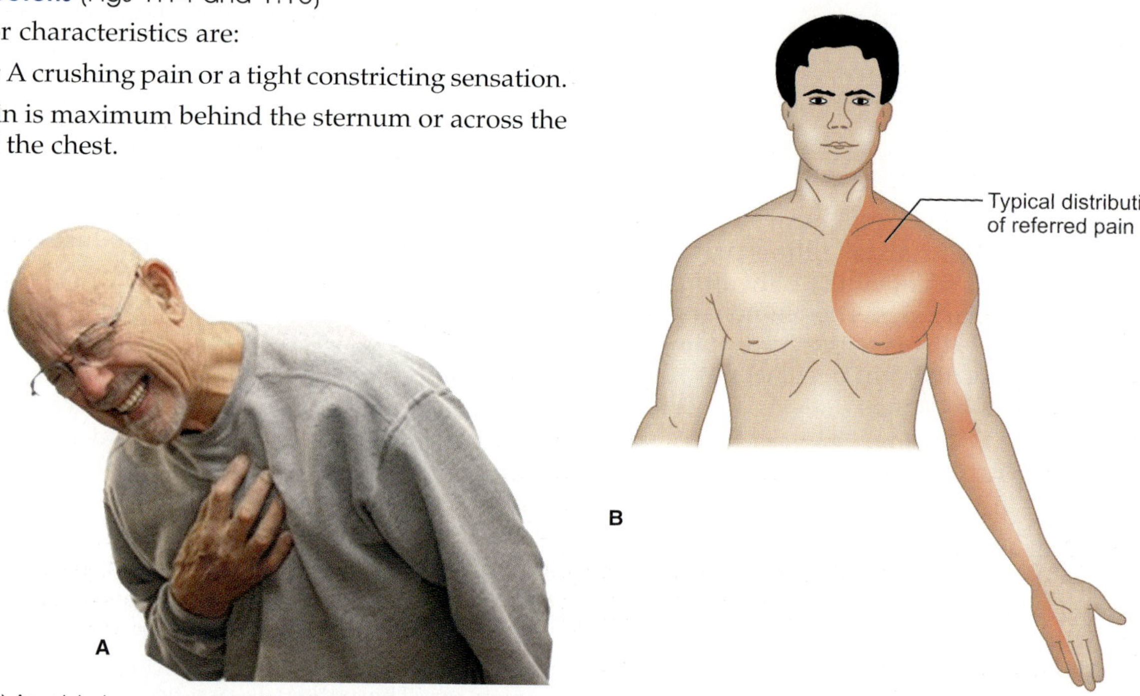


Fig. 1.14: (A) An elderly person experiencing an excruciating retrosternal chest pain with bending farward posture in angina pectoris. (B) Classical radiating pain of angina pectoris over the shoulder, neck and medial side of left arm and hand

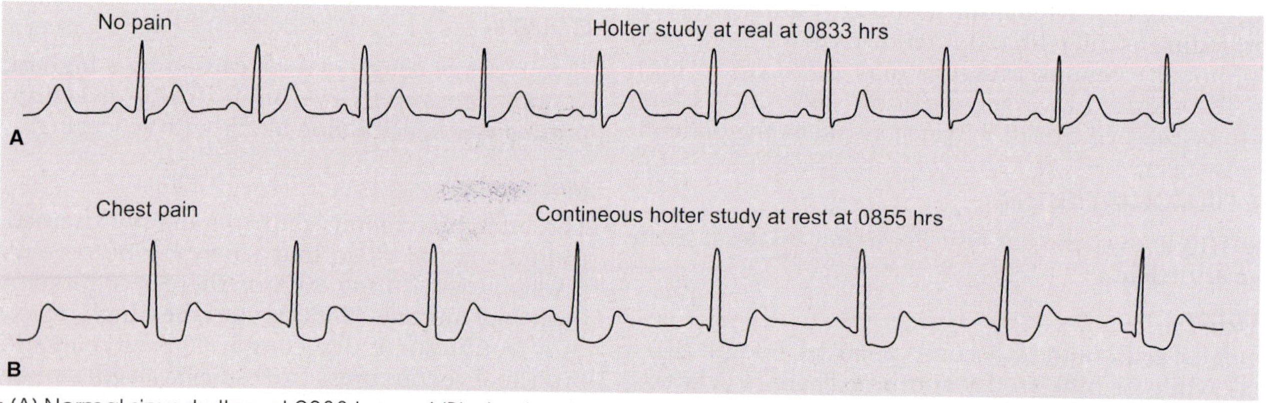


Fig. 1.15: (A) Normal sinus rhythm at 0833 hrs and (B) chest pain with significant ST-segment depression at 0855 hrs on Holter monitor recording of a patient with angina pectoris

### Dyspnea

Breathlessness on exertion is present with all right to left intracardiac shunts. The reduced oxygen content of the arterial blood causes breathlessness by stimulating the chemoreceptors of the carotid body and the respiratory centre.

*Squatting*—characteristic posture of children who crawl on their heels when breathless, particularly after exertion. Squatting is most commonly seen in Fallot's tetralogy, but is not specific to this condition, being occasionally seen in other forms of cyanotic congenital heart disease. By squatting the arterial oxygen saturation is improved during the compression of the great vessels of the lower extremities particularly over the femoral vessels thereby decreasing the input of the right ventricle and raising the systemic blood pressure, hence both leading to better oxygenation in a squatting posture. However, precise mechanism is not known.

## SYMPTOMS OF CONGESTIVE HEART FAILURE

Congestive heart failure (CHF) symptoms are illustrated in Figs 1.16–1.18.

### Ankle Swelling

An excess of tissue fluid follows abnormal retention of sodium and water by the kidneys in heart failure, and this tissue fluid tends to localise under the influence of gravity into the most dependent parts of the body (Fig. 1.16).

Thus, the ambulant patient develops swelling of the feet and legs which is most marked in the evenings, whereas the patient confined to bed has a pad of edema overlying the sacrum. Edema over the ankles due to congestive cardiac failure (CCF) should be differentiated from other causes, such as:

1. Renal disease
2. Deficient lymphatic drainage of legs

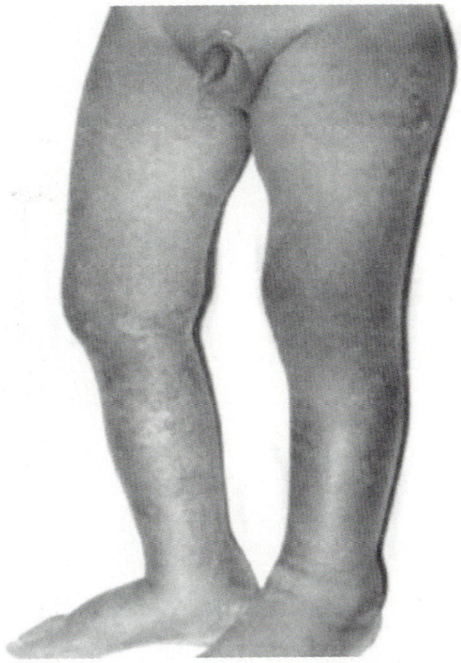

**Fig 1.16:** Edema of ankles and lower legs in patient with congestive cardiac failure

3. Deep vein thrombosis of the legs or severe varicose veins
4. Cirrhosis of the liver
5. Ankle swelling in normal individual after standing for much of the day.

### Abdominal Pain due to Hepatic Distension

The high systemic venous pressure due to right heart failure causes hepatic enlargement and distension of the hepatic capsule. This is responsible for a dull ache in the epigastrium and the right hypochondrium. It is often aggravated by exertion which, further increases the systemic venous pressure.

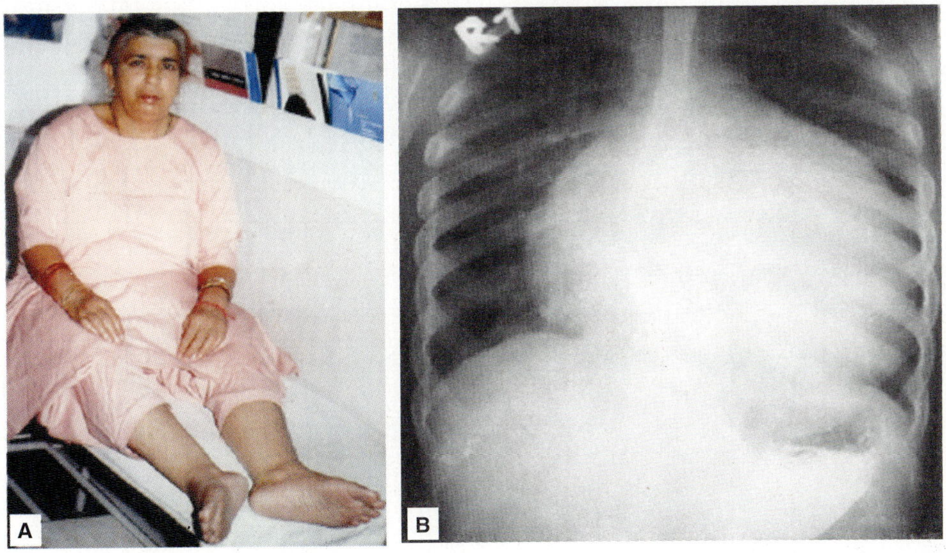


**Fig. 1.17:** (A) Rough, dry hair, skin, facial puffiness, edema of whole body and cardiomegaly in a middle-aged lady with hypothyroidism and heart failure. (B) Chest X-ray of patient with gross diffuse cardiomegaly who presented with grade-4 type of dyspnea

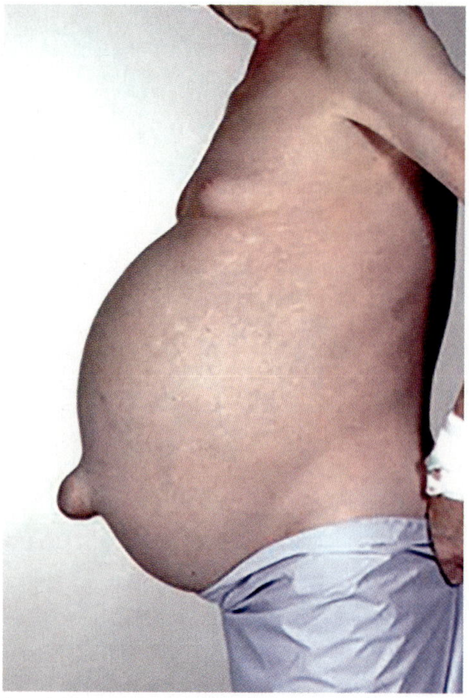

**Fig. 1.18:** A middle-aged patient showing protruded umbilicus due to ascites in congestive heart failure

### Ascites

It is also one of the features of right heart failure (Fig. 1.18).

### Symptoms of Low Cardiac Output

*Fatigue:* A low cardiac output has the effect of producing a constant feeling of fatigue, presumably related to the poor blood supply to muscles and other organs. However, the symptom of tiredness is so usual in all types of illness, including psychological illness, that it cannot be regarded as reliable evidence of a low cardiac output.

### Dyspnea

The tissue anoxia of low cardiac output may lead to mild dyspnea.

### Symptoms of Cardiac Arrhythmia (Figs 1.19–1.21)

Palpitations is a frequently used term for any increased beats of the heart. Occasional extra beats are described as the heart 'seeming to miss a beat', or as the heart 'turning over in the chest'. The sudden onset of faster heart rate may represent the onset of an attack of paroxysmal tachycardia or of atrial fibrillation.

## CARDIAC SYNCOPE

### Definition

Syncope resulting from the sudden cessation of cerebral blood flow when there is an arrest of the cardiac pumping action (Figs 1.22–1.24 and Table 1.1).

### Description

There is an abrupt loss of consciousness with extreme pallor. The pupils dilate and epileptiform convulsions may occur. When efficient cardiac pumping action returns, there is abrupt restoration of consciousness, accompanied by a red flush of the skin as blood flows into vessels widely dilated by the accumulation of metabolites during the brief period of circulatory arrest.

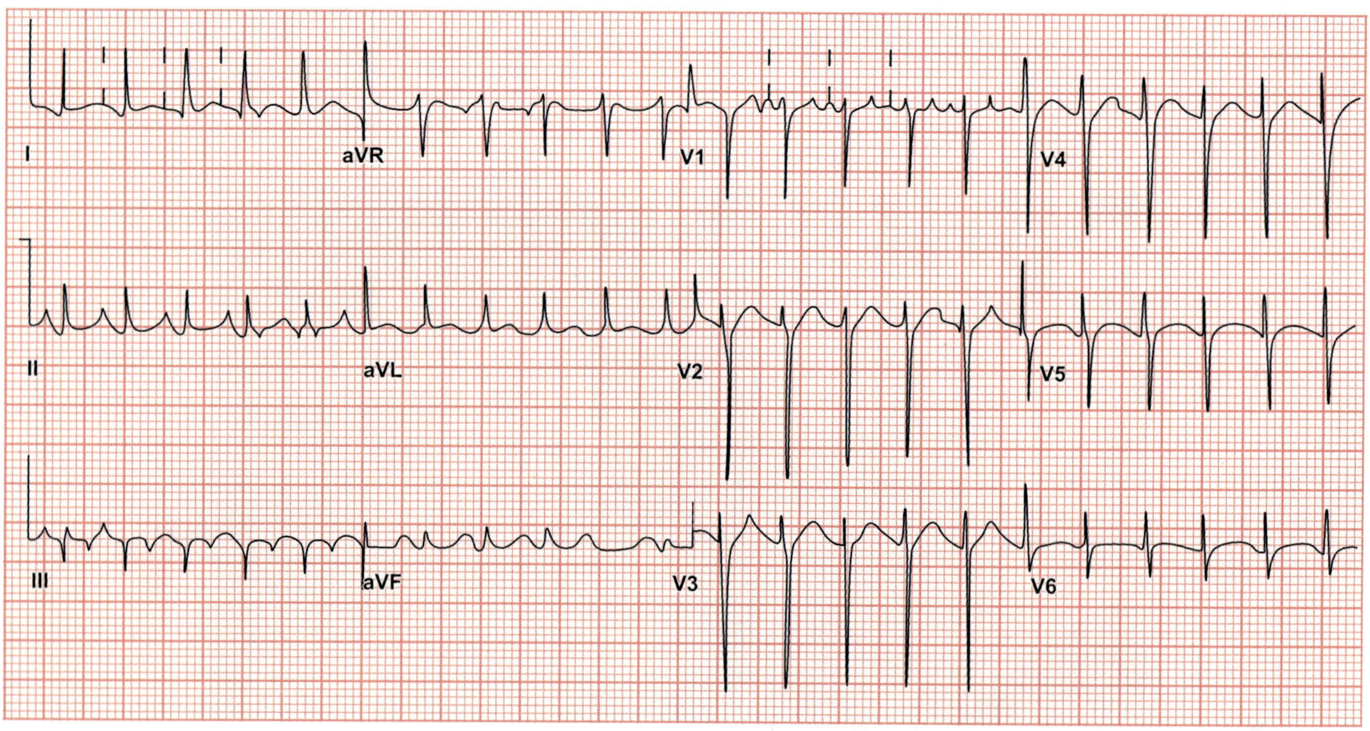


**Fig. 1.19:** ECG showing features of focal atrial tachycardia with 1:1 conduction. Note the narrow and regular tachycardia. The P-waves are marked with arrows (long-RP interval), and the P-wave morphology differs from that of sinus rhythm

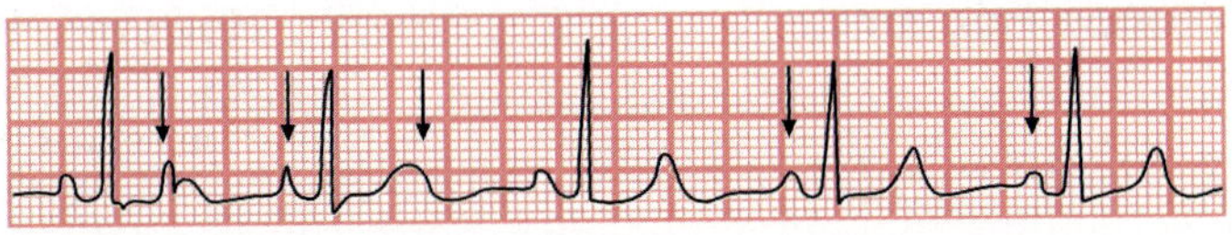

**Fig. 1.20:** ECG graph showing complete heart block respectively presenting syncopal attack

Sudden attacks of loss of consciousness are common in children suffering from Fallot's tetralogy, during the atack the child has a pallid cyanosis and profound desaturation of the arterial blood at a normal blood pressure. These attacks occur with emotion, stress, being particularly common in hospital and may be due to spasm of the infundibulum of the right ventricle. The blood flow is then greatly reduced through the lungs most of the blood passing across the ventricular septal defect into the aorta. Cerebral anoxia produces syncope and if the attack is prolonged death may also occur.

## Causes

1. Complete heart block (Stokes Adams attack): Short episodes of cardiac arrest or of ventricular fibrillation are particularly frequent at the onset of complete heart block before the ventricular pacemaker has become well established.
2. Severe aortic stenosis: The syncope of severe aortic stenosis during exertion is a result of brief attacks of ventricular arrhythmias in some patients.
3. Paroxysmal tachycardia: Occasionally, the cardiac output is so reduced at the onset of fast arrhythmia that syncope results.
4. Left atrial thrombus, and left atrial myxoma: Impaction of these structures in the mitral valve orifice is a rare cause of syncope.

**Table 1.1:** Cardiovascular causes of syncope

*Neurally-mediated (vasovagal)*
- Situational
  - Micturition
  - Defecation
  - Postprandial
  - Swallowing
  - Coughing
  - Sneezing
- Glossopharyngeal neuralgia
- Orthostatic syncope
- Carotid sinus syncope
  - Cardioinhibitory
  - Vasodepressor
  - Mixed

*Mechanical*
- Aortic stenosis
- Hypertrophic cardiomyopathy
- Left atrial myxoma
- Mitral stenosis
- Pulmonic stenosis
- Pulmonary hypertension or embolism
- Right atrial myxoma
- Myocardial infarction
- Cardiac tamponade

*Electrical*
- Second- and third-degree atrioventricular block
- Sick sinus syndrome
- Supraventricular tachycardia
- Ventricular tachycardia
- Torsade de pointes
- Pacemaker malfunction

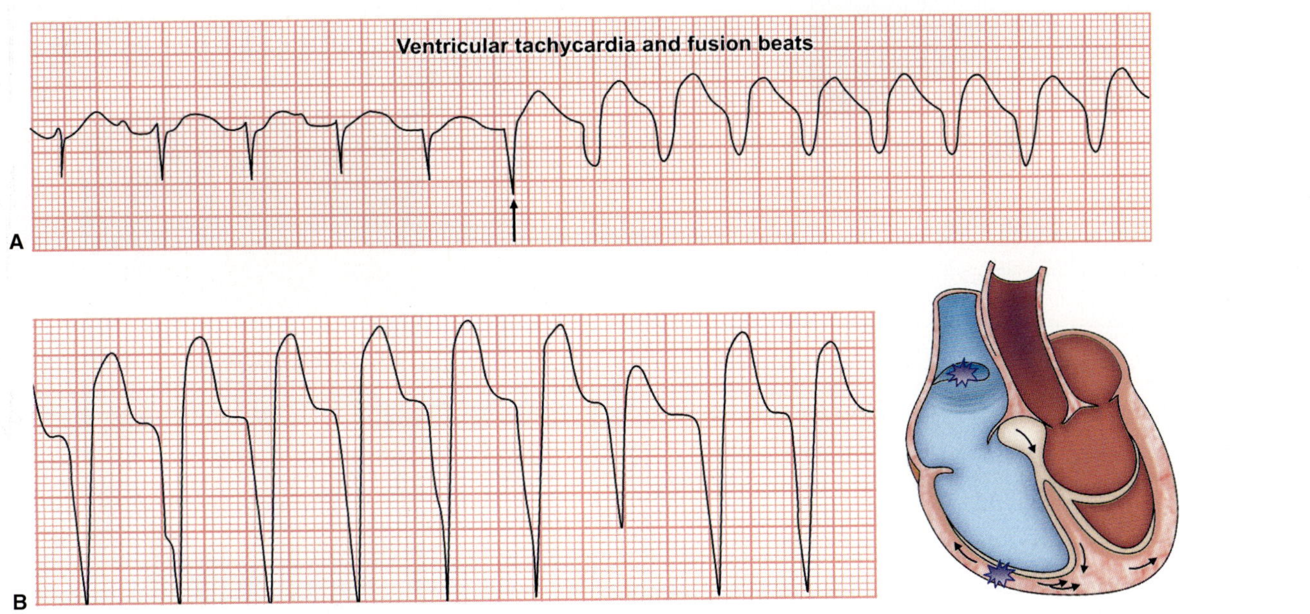


**Fig. 1.21:** ECG showing (A) ventricular tachycardia and fusion beat as indicated and (B) diagram showing the genesis of fusion beats

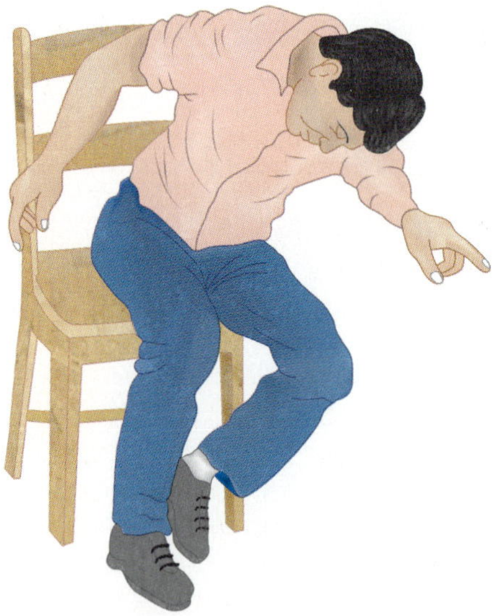

**Fig. 1.22:** Illustration showing syncopal attack, becoming temporarily unconcious, toneless and tendency to fall on the ground

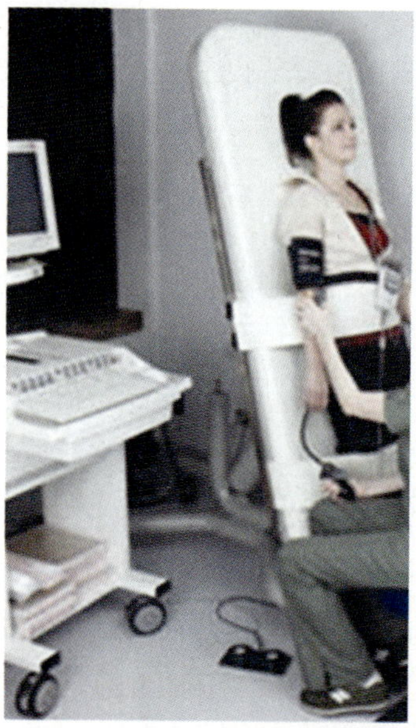

**Fig. 1.23:** Performance of HUTT test a young lady with syncopal attack

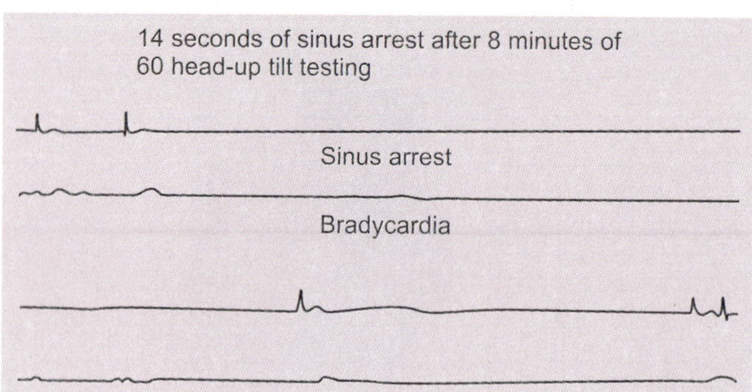


**Fig. 1.24:** EC graph depicting 14 second sinus arrest and critical bradycardia in positive head up tilt test for investigation of cardiogenic syncope

### Balance Problems

*Other names:* Dizziness, unsteadiness, lightheadedness.

*Description:* Inability to walk or stand without holding on to something to maintain balance. Some causes related to cardiovascular disease can be seen after stroke, or due to general weakness caused by low cardiac output or low blood pressure. Some causes related to other disorders can be seen with several neurological problems or with inner ear problems, as well as to numerous general medical problems.

Significance: Many significant medical problems can cause problems with balance. This symptom always needs to be carefully evaluated by a physician.

## GENERAL PHYSICAL EXAMINATION

### Physical Examination

Chronic severe heart failure may cause emaciation, and cyanotic congenital heart disease may be responsible for stunted growth and poor development (Figs 1.25–1.35).

Obesity aggravates the effect of cardiac disease.

### Anatomical Abnormalities

*Anatomical abnormalities,* i.e. anatomical defects. Absence or hypoplasia of one or both upper limbs are associated with intracardiac defects such as atrial septal defect (ASD) or ventricular septal defect (VSD) (Holt-Oram syndrome).

### Genetic Abnormalities

Many genetically determined disorders are easily recognised from their effects on the general body configuration. The cardiac malformations commonly associated with specific genetic defects are given below.

#### *Chromosome Disorders*

*Mongolism* is also known as Down syndrome is caused by a random error in cell division that results in the presence of an extra copy of chromosome 21. The type of error is

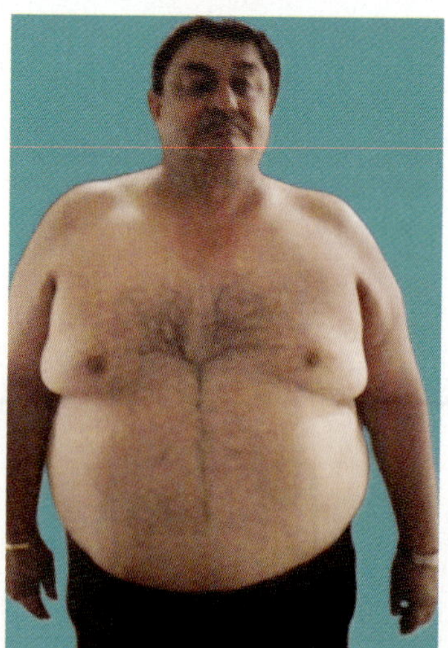

**Fig. 1.25:** An obese patient with metabolic syndrome

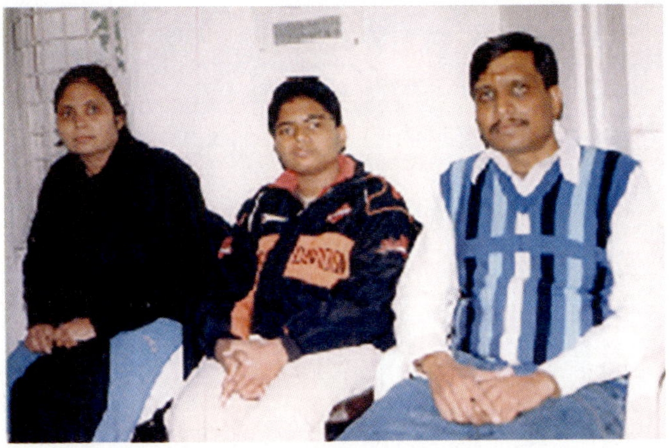

**Fig. 1.26:** Genetically transmitted hypothyroidism in husband, wife and son (middle)

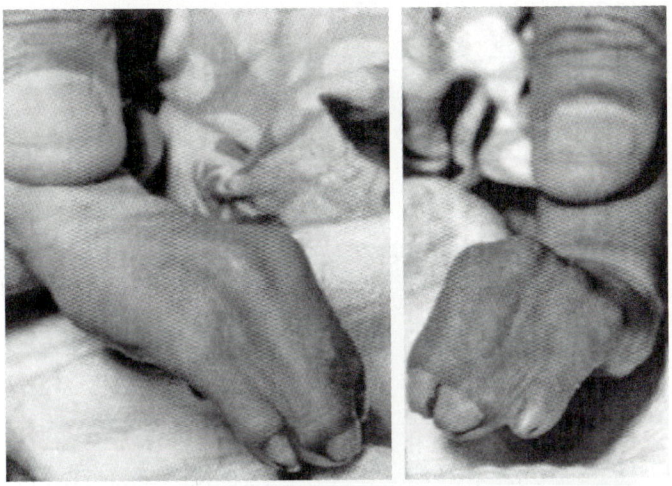

**Fig. 1.27:** A child with syndactylism in Apert syndrome

called nondisjunction (pronounced non-dis-JUHNGK-shuhn). Usually, when one cell divides in two, pairs of chromosomes are split so that one of the pair goes to one cell, and the other from the pair goes to the other cell. In nondisjunction, something goes wrong and both chromosomes from one pair go into one cell and no chromosomes for that pair go into the other cell.

*Heart defects.* Endocardial cushion defects. Turner's syndrome (XO) coarctation of the aorta pulmonary stenosis.

### DiGeorge Syndrome

DiGeorge syndrome, additionally known as 22q11.2 deletion syndrome, could be a disorder caused by a defect in chromosome 22. It ends up in the poor development of several body systems. Medical problems usually associated with DiGeorge syndrome embrace heart defects, poor immune system performance, a cleft palate, complications associated with low levels of calcium in the blood, and delayed development with behavioral and emotional problems. The quantity and severity of symptoms related to DiGeorge syndrome vary greatly.

*Heart defects.* DiGeorge syndrome typically causes heart defects that end in an meagre supply of oxygen-rich blood. These defects might include a hole between the lower chambers of the heart (ventricular septal defect); only one large vessel, instead of two vessels, leading out of the heart (truncus arteriosus); or a mixture of four abnormal structural heart defects (tetralogy of Fallot). DiGeorge syndrome will cause smaller than traditional parathyroid glands that secrete insufficient parathyroid hormone (PTH), leading to a condition called hypoparathyroidism. This condition ends up in low levels of calcium and high levels of phosphorus in your blood. In children with DiGeorge syndrome, the thymus gland could also be small

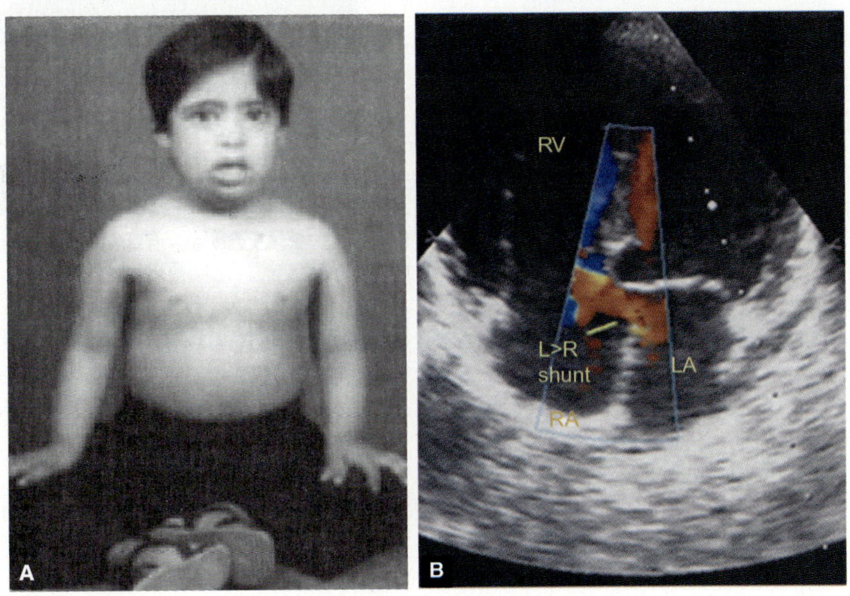


**Fig. 1.28:** (A) Stunted growth, polydactylism and chest deformity in a child with endocardial cushion defect, (B) Color flow apical 4C views in dual scan showing large septum primum defect with almost single dilated atrium, dilated LV with gross mitral regurgitation in patient with endocardial cushion defect

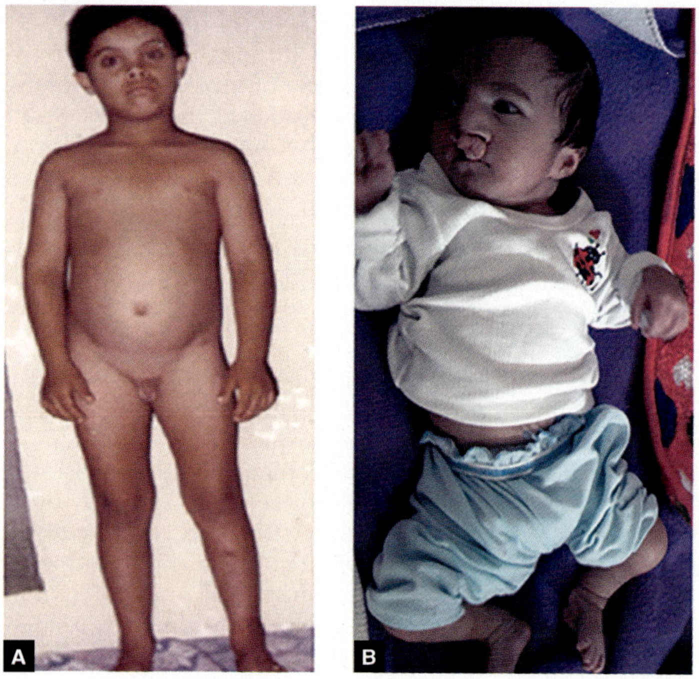


**Fig. 1.29:** (A) Physical features of mongolism associated with VSD, (B) DiGeorge syndrome with cleft lip, hypoparathyroidism, hemitruncus, VSD, pulmonary stenosis and hypoplasia of left sided upper and lower limbs with poor physical growth

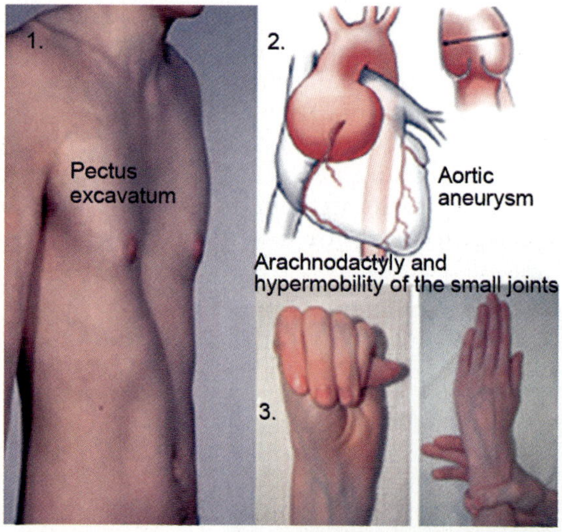


**Fig. 1.30A:** Different clinical features of Mafan syndrome

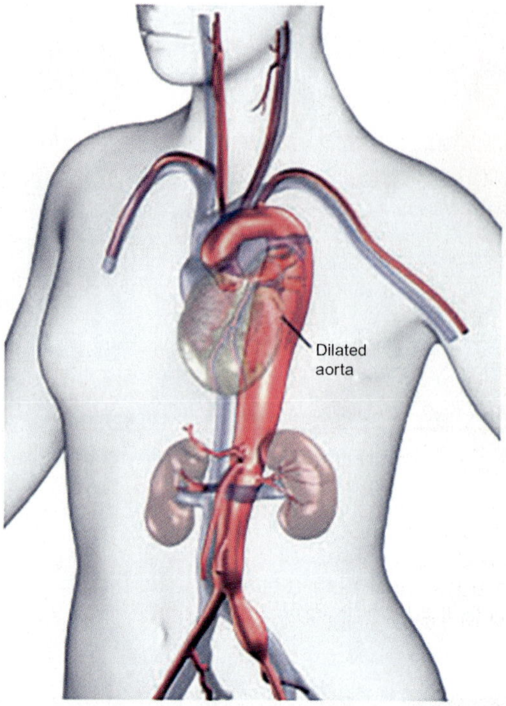


**Fig. 1.30B:** Dilation of aorta in Mafan syndrome

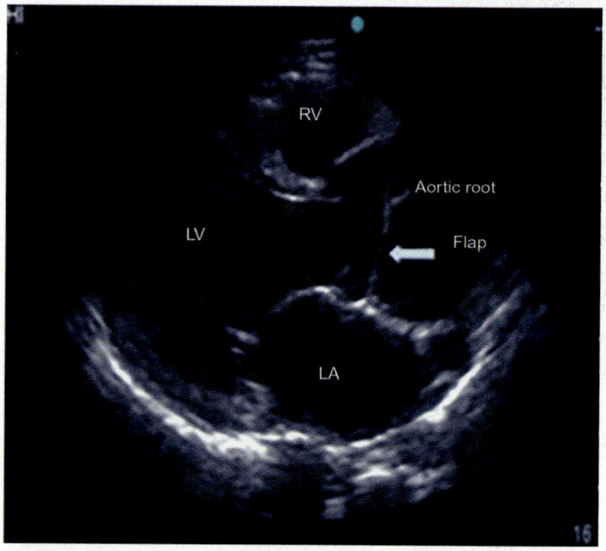


**Fig. 1.30C:** Echo scan showing dilated aortic root in Mafan syndrome

or missing, leading to poor immune functions and frequent, severe infections.

### Single Gene Disorders

*Marfan syndrome:* Aortic ectasia, dissecting aneurysm of the aorta. Hereditary haemorrhagic telangiectasia, pulmonary arteriovenous fistulae, neurofibromatosis phaeochromocytoma, polydactyly common atrium, atrial septal defect etc.

*Rubella infection* Lesions such as mental deficiency, nerve deafnes and cataract in a child suggest that the mother was infected during early pregnancy by rubella. In such cases there is a strong likelihood of congenital heart disease (Fig. 1.31).

The common cardiac lesions produced by the virus are:

- Patent ductus arteriosus
- Pulmonary Valve Stenosis
- Pulmonary artery branch stenosis

### Thoracic Deformity

Massive enlargement of the heart in infancy can produce a permanent deformity of the overlying chest wall with a forward bulge of the precordium to the left of the sternum.

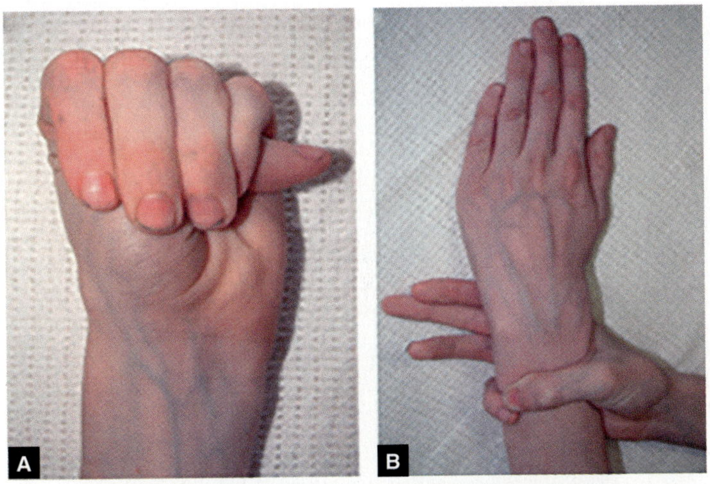

**Fig. 1.30D:** Arachnodactyly. (A) Steinberg thumb sign. Entire thumb nail protrudes beyond ulnar border of hand, (B) Walker-Murdoch wrist sign. Thumb and fifth finger can overlap around wrist. Both signs must be present to diagnose arachnodactyly according to the Ghent Marfan diagnostic criteria

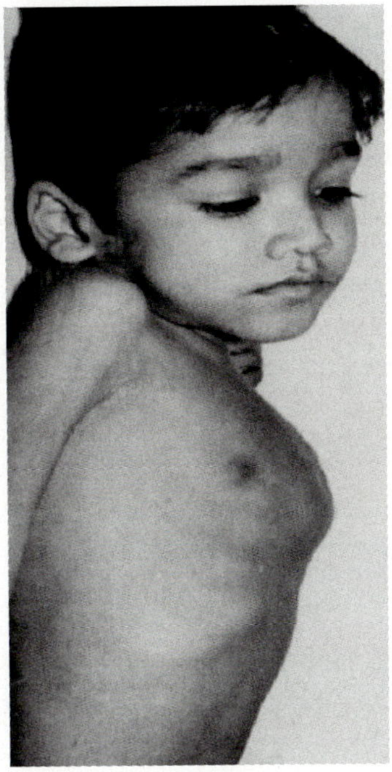

**Fig. 1.32:** Pigeon chest deformity

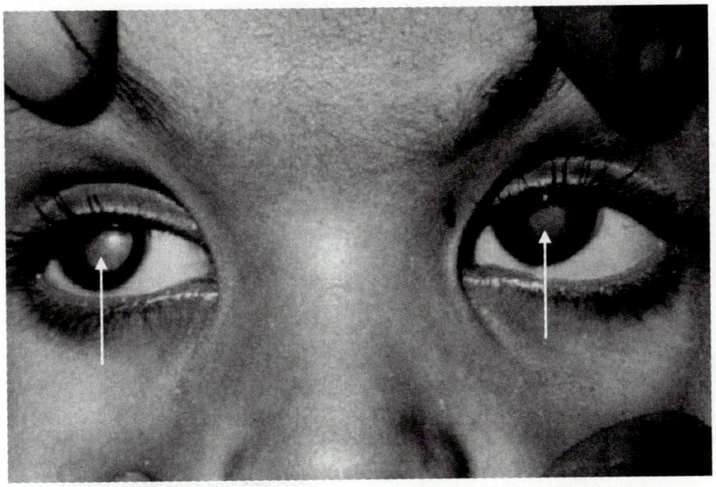

**Fig. 1.31:** Bilateral congenital cataracts in congenital Rubella syndrome with PDA (arrows)

Pulmonary hypertension complicating a left to right intracardiac to right intracardiac shunt may result in an abnormally rounded configuration of the front of the chest in children. Pectus excavatum type of chest deformity may also be associated with high incidence of mitral valve prolapse (MVP) and ASD (Fig. 1.32).

*Earlobe crease:* Taken in conjunction, most of the studies conducted clearly show an association between earlobe creases and heart disease. In fact, most studies including the larger ones-suggest that this association is true and conclude the association cannot be explained by other risk factors. Unfortunately, although research supports an association as of yet we don't have a convincing explanation as to why earlobe crease would be associated with heart disease.

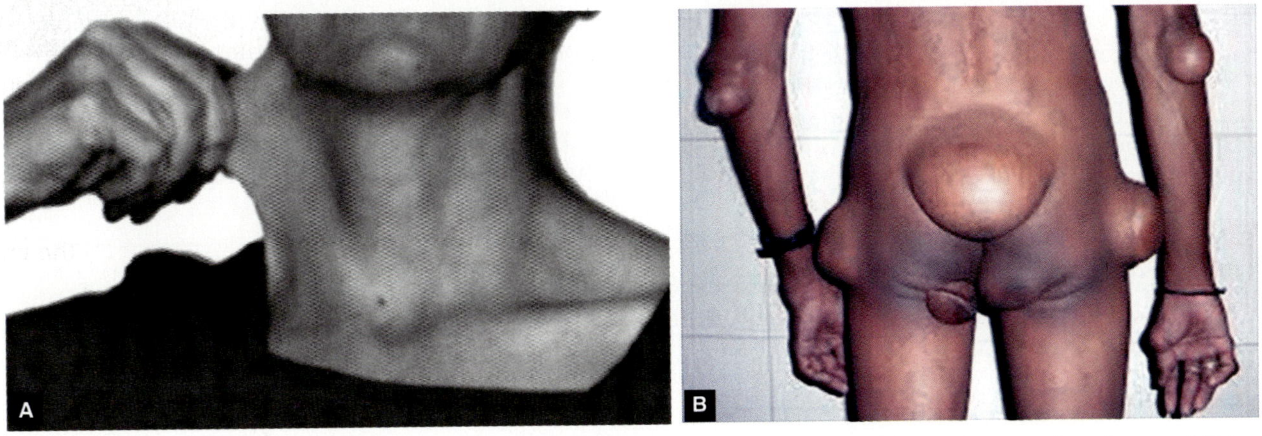

**Fig. 1.33:** (A) Feature of cutus hyperelastica. The vascular type 111 is considered one of the more serious forms of Ehlers-Danlos syndrome because blood vessels and organs are fragile and prone to tearing (rupture). (B) Multiple swellings over extensor aspects of limbs and buttocks in hereditary tuberous xanthomas

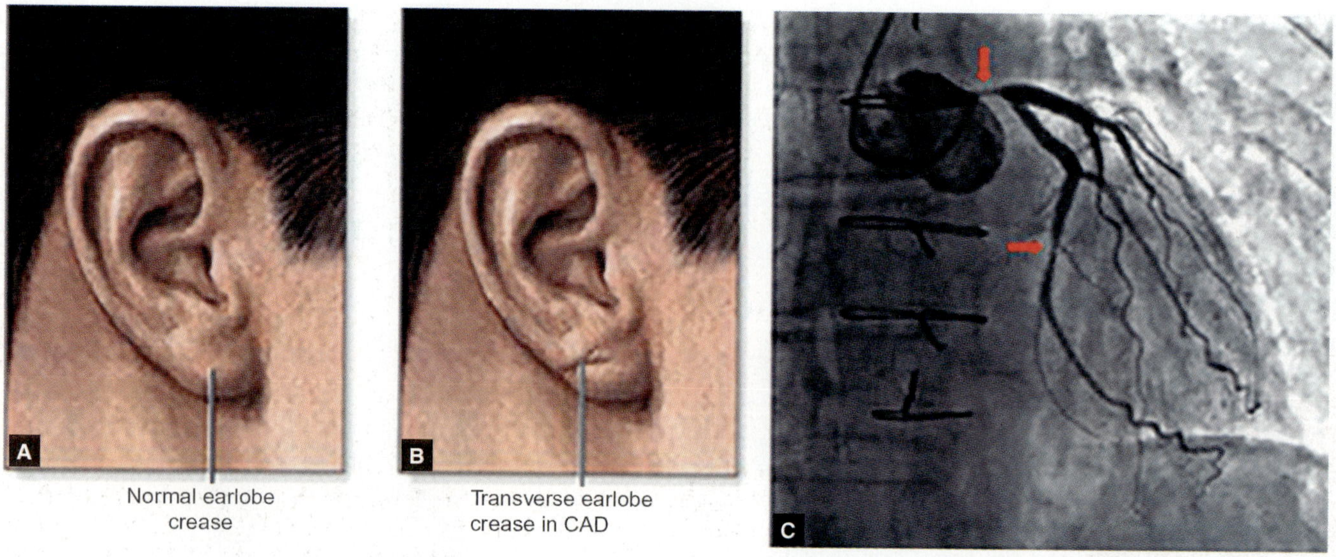


**Fig. 1.34:** (A) Normal earlobe crease, (B) transverse earlobe crease as a physical sign in coronary artery disease and (C) coronary angiography of a critical sub-occlusion of the common trunk of the left coronary artery and the circumflex artery (see arrows)

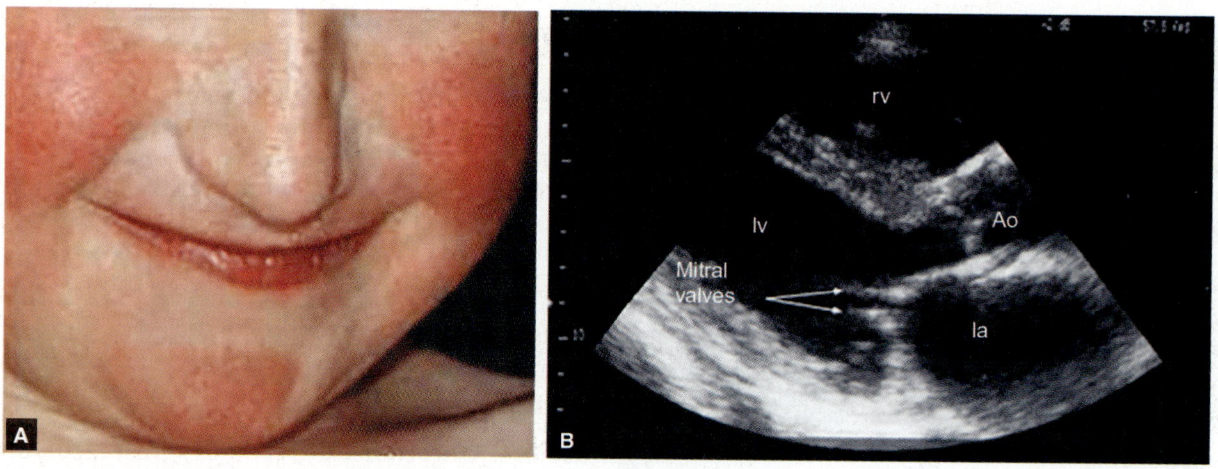


**Fig. 1.35:** (A) Photograph of a young lady suffering from chronic rheumatic mitral stenosis with facial redness as malar flush. (B) Echo scan in LAX view showing thickened and restricted opening of both AML and PML in mitral stenosis

### *Malar Flush*

Patients with a chronic low cardiac output have a dusky flush of the cheeks. This color is the result of dilated capillaries in the dermis, in which the circulation of blood is slow, and is most commonly seen in mitral stenosis complicated by pulmonary hypertension.

## CYANOSIS

A blue discoloration of the skin and mucous membranes caused by 5.0 g or more of reduced haemoglobin per 100 ml of blood in the skin capillaries (Fig. 1.36).

### Peripheral Cyanosis

There is a slow circulation of blood to the cyanosed part and, because the blood is in prolonged contact with the tissues, the extraction of oxygen is more complete than nomal. The blood in the capillaries thus has an increased proportion of reduced haemoglobin. Vasoconstriction due to cold or as compensation for a low cardiac output is the usual cause of peripheral cyanosis, which is best seen in the lobes of the ears, the nose and the fingers.

### *1. Central Cyanosis*

#### *Definition*

Central cyanosis is defined as cyanosis caused by a reduced oxygen saturation of the systemic arterial blood.

#### *Clinical Features*

The following features accompany central cyanosis and distinguish it from peripheral cyanosis.

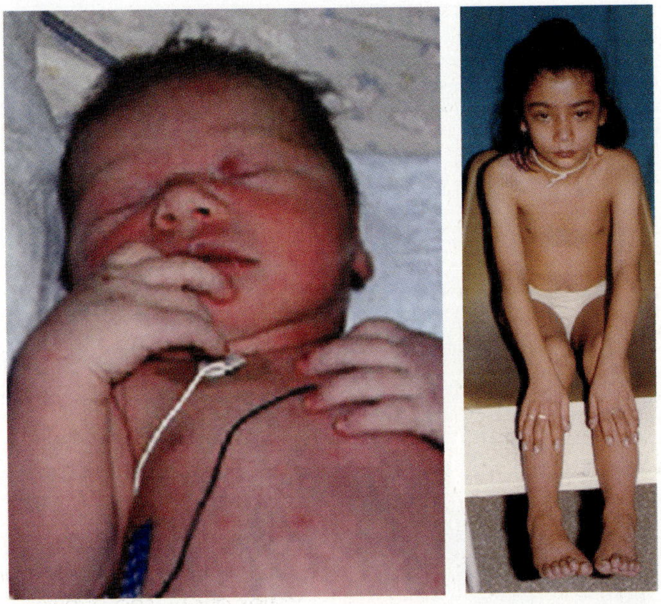

**Fig. 1.36:** Two children having central cyanosis with congenital heart diseases

*Finger clubbing:* Warm mucous membranes, blue tongue, lips and conjunctiva. Polycythaemia is present with abnormally raised haemoglobin and haematocrit. Arteries blood, obtained by needle puncture from a peripheral artery, is desaturated, this is the absolute differentiating test in doubtful cases.

### Causes

*Cardiac disease:* Venous blood entering the left heart without passing through the lungs, i.e. right to left shunting of blood through abnormal communication in the heart.

### Pulmonary Disease

Inadequate oxygenation of the blood as the blood passes through the lungs. The breathing of oxygen for a few minutes increases the oxygen tension in the alveoli of the lungs thus compensating for poor lung functions. Cyanosis due to lung disease is markedely improved with $O_2$ therapy while cyanosis caused by a right to left intracardiac shunt is little affected.

## 2. *Differential Cyanosis*

This condition is depicted in Fig. 1.37.

### Definition

Cyanosis is more intense in the feet than in the hands when both are warm.

### Cause

Differential cyanosis implies that the oxygen content of the arterial blood in the legs is lower than in the arms. Blood low in oxygen will pass from the pulmonary artery through a persistent ductus arteriosus only when there is severe pulmonary hypertension. The presence of differerential cyanosis is therefore, diagnostic of persistent ductus arteriosus with pulmonary hypertension.

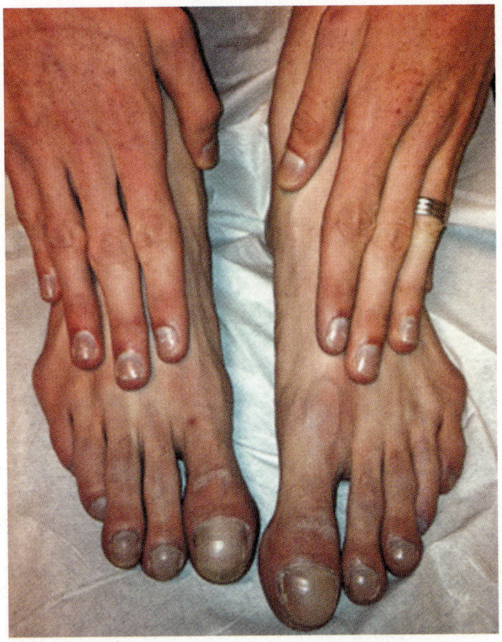

**Fig. 1.37:** Differential cyanosis in a patient with patent ductus arteriosus, severe pH, and right to left shunt (Eisenmenger syndrome). Note the severe clubbing and cyanosis of the toes as compared to the lesser degree of clubbing and cyanosis of the fingers

## CLUBBING OF THE FINGERS

Clubbing of the fingers is shown in Figs 1.38–1.41.

### Stages

1. Obliteration of the normal angle between the finger nail and skin on the dorsum of the finger by an increase in the soft tissues underneath the nail bed.
2. The nail becomes curved longitudinally.
3. Swelling of soft tissues of the terminal phalanges gives a drum stick appearance to the digits.

### Causes

The exact stimulus producing finger clubbing is not known. Heart disease finger clubbing is due to cyanotic heart disease, bacterial endocarditis or left atrial myxoma. However, rarely it may be of a heredito-familial .

## ABDOMINAL PAIN

*Description:* Pain or discomfort in or around the abdominal area (Fig. 1.42).

*Causes related to cardiovascular disease:* Vascular disease can cause abdominal pain in several ways. Blockage or partial blockage (due to atherosclerosis) of arteries supplying the vital organs can cause those organs to become ischemic, and therefore painful. This type of pain is usually greater after a meal. An aneurysm of the abdominal aorta can cause pain, especially if the aneurysm begins to tear or rupture. This pain is often very severe, and sudden in onset. It is a medical emergency.

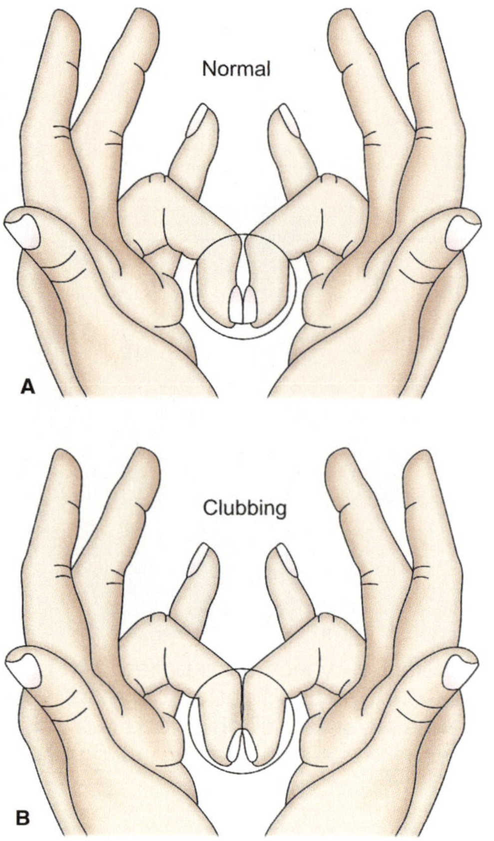


**Fig. 1.38:** (A) Normal curvatures of the ring fingers of both hands in flexion. (B) Clubbing of fingers

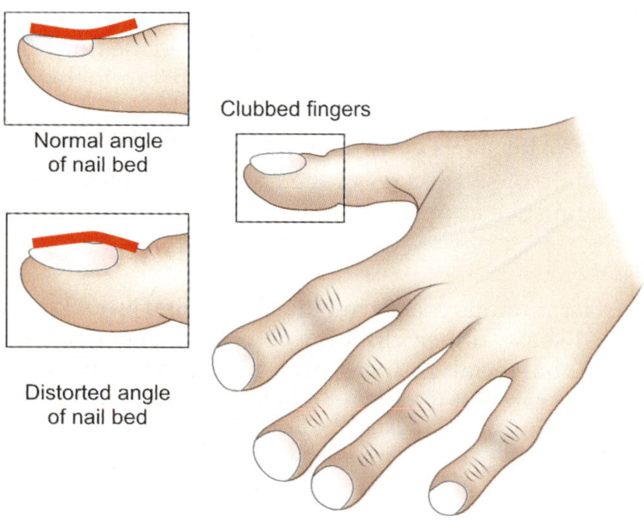


**Fig. 1.39:** Features of clubbing of fingers

*Causes related to other disorders:* Numerous disorders of abdominal organs—stomach, intestines, bowel, liver, spleen, gallbladder, reproductive organs, can cause pain.

*Significance:* Vascular disease involving the abdominal blood vessels is always significant, and potentially dangerous medical problem. A ruptured or torn abdominal aortic aneurysm is often fatal. Many non-cardiovascular diseases causing pain in abdominal organs are also medically significant. Any unexplained abdominal pain that is severe, frequent, prolonged or persistent needs to be evaluated by a physician.

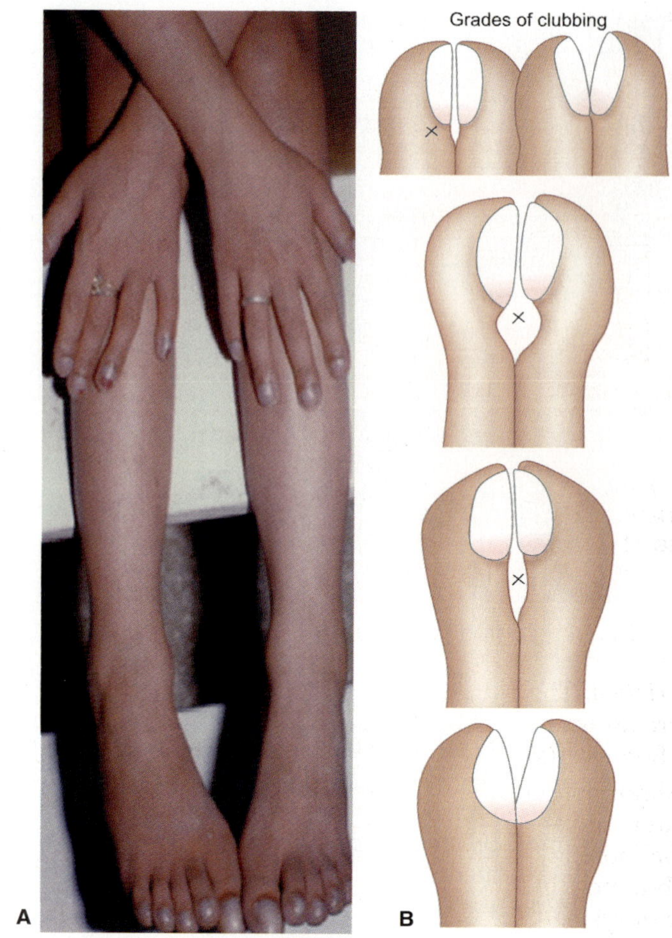


**Fig. 1.40:** Bilateral digital clubbing and central cyanosis in patient with Fallot's tetralogy (A) and graphic representation of various grades of digital clubbing (B)

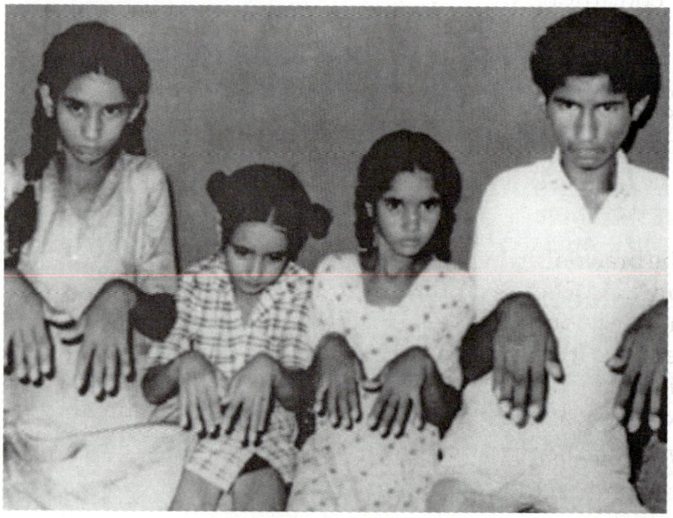

**Fig. 1.41:** Hereditary transmitted bilateral congenital clubbing among all the members of a family

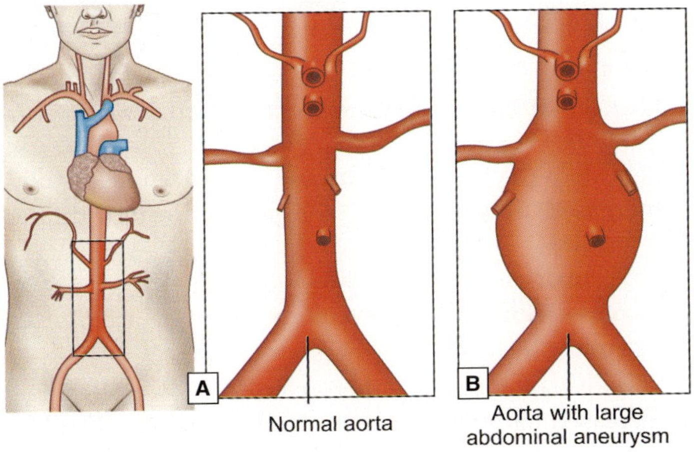


**Fig. 1.42:** (A) Normal thoracic and abdominal aorta. (B) Aneurysmal dilatation of thoracic and abdominal aorta as a cause of abdominal pain and abnormal pulsations

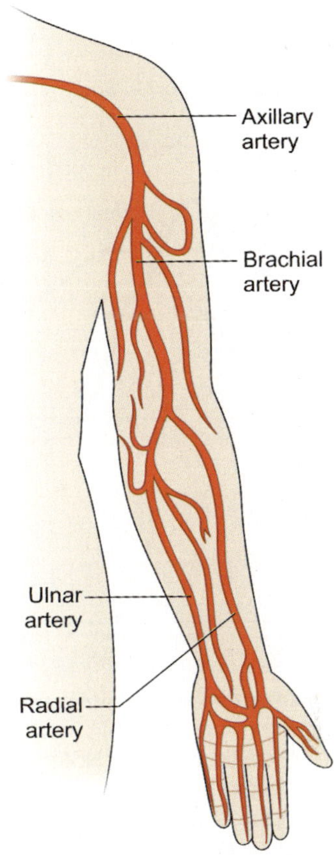


**Fig. 1.43:** Anatomy of axillary/brachial and radial arteries which are used in clinical assessment of peripheral arterial diseases

## ABNORMAL PULSE

*Description:* The patient notices an area in or on the body where an unusual or a vigorous pulsation can be seen or felt. Some causes related to cardiovascular disease are:

- Abnormal pulsations can be related to vascular disease, such as an aneurysm (an abnormal dilation or 'ballooning' of an artery). Abnormal pulsations in the abdomen, in particular, are often indicative of an aortic aneurysm. A 'bounding' pulse can also be felt in patients who have aortic insufficiency (a 'leaky' aortic valve.)
- Some causes related to other disorders: Any condition that leads to particularly vigorous pumping of the heart can create an unusual awareness of the pulse. Such conditions include anemia, thyroid disease, hypertension, anxiety, or other medical problems.

*Significance:* A persistent abnormal pulsation can indicate significant medical disease, and should be reported to a doctor.

## THE ARTERIAL PULSE

The brachial arterial pulse: It is larger and more convenient for detailed study than the radial. For maximum information, the palpating finger should compress the vessel with just sufficient force to collapse the lumen in diastole. The rise in pressure with each heart beat forcibly expands the wall against the finger (Figs 1.43–1.45).

*The carotid pulse:* It is also examined and other arterial pulses are compared with each other.

The brachial pulse is analysed under four headings:

1. Rate
2. Rhythm
3. Amplitude
4. Waveform

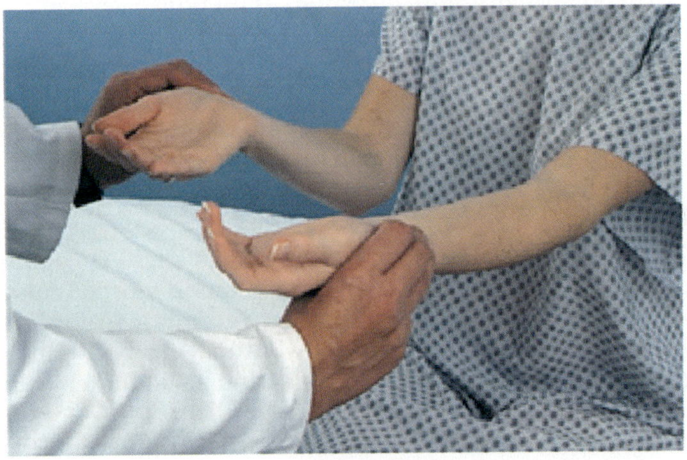

**Fig. 1.44:** The radial pulse is palpable over the lateral wrist

### Rate

1. An abnormally fast pulse may represent:
   a. Sinus tachycardia (sinoatrial node remains in control), e.g. excitement, fever, exertion, thyrotoxicosis and haemorrhage.
   b. Arrhythmia (an ectopic focus in the heart has taken over the pacemaking function from the sinoatrial node),

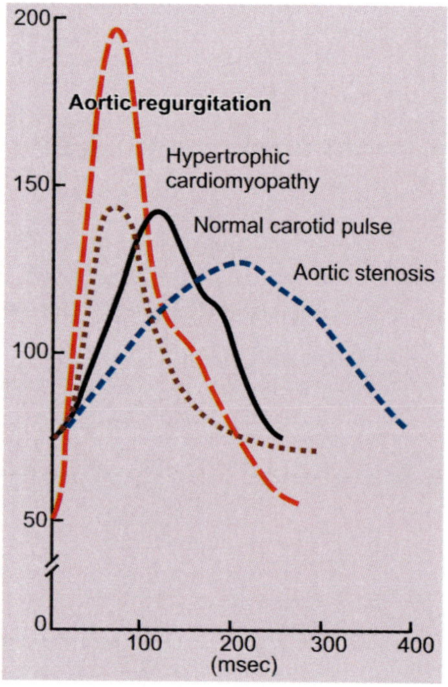


**Fig. 1.45:** The normal carotid arterial pulse recording compared with recordings in hypertrophic cardiomyopathy, aortic regurgitation and aortic stenosis. Note the very rapid upstroke of the pulse in hypertrophic cardiomyopathy and aortic regurgitation compared with the slow upstroke in aortic stenosis. The pulse pressure in aortic regurgitation is widened because of the exaggerated systolic peak and the diastolic collapse

e.g. paroxysmal atrial tachycardia and atrial flutter, atrial fibrillation, ventricular tachycardia.

2. An abnormally slow pulse may represent:
   a. Sinus bradycardia (sinoatrial node remains in control), e.g. trained athletes, increased intracranial pressure, jaundice.
   b. Arrhythmia (a pulse rate below 40 beats per minute usually means complete heart block).

### Rhythm

The normal pulse is regular apart from a slight speeding up on inspiration and slowing on expiration most obvious in younger individuals (sinus arrhythmia). Complete irregularity indicates atrial fibrillation, but both sinus rhythm with multiple extrasystoles and atrial flutter with changing block can simulate atrial fibrillation.

During exercise, a patient with atrial fibrillation, the irregularity of the pulse is accentuated, atrial extrasystoles, disappear, so that the pulse become regular. In atrial flutter, regular degree of atrioventricular (AV) block becomes established, and the pulse becomes regular.

### Amplitude

The amplitude of the pulse is judged by the movement of the palpating finger produced by the arrival of the pulse wave. A large amplitude pulse means that the pressure wave is large, i.e. there is a large difference between systolic and diastolic blood pressures.

## LARGE AMPLITUDE PULSE

### Causes

1. Leakage of blood from the aorta in aortic valve regurgitation
2. Persistent ductus arteriosus and arteriovenous fistula
3. Increased flow of blood from aorta through dilated arterioles
4. Thyrotoxicosis and other high output states
5. Increased left ventricular volume
6. Complete heart block
7. Raigidity of aorta, i.e. atherosclerosis
8. Increased left ventricular stroke volume-heart block

### Mechanism

The rapid escape of blood from the aorta in the first two groups results in a low pressure in the arterial system by the end of diastole and the large left ventricular stroke volume ejected into the aorta causes a high systolic pressure. The very large stroke volume of complete heart block gives an abnormally large pressure peak in the aorta. A normal stroke volume produces an abnormal great pressure rise when the aorta has lost its elasticity.

## SMALL AMPLITUDE PULSE

### Cause

Low left ventricular stroke volume (shock, tachycardia and mitral stenosis). Obstruction to left ventricular ejection (aortic stenosis).

### Mechanism

In the low cardiac output states, the volume of blood ejected into the aorta with each beat is small and the pressure rise also tends to be small.

Obstruction to left ventricular ejection reduces the speed of blood flow into the aorta during systole, thereby producing a smaller and slower than normal pressurise in aortic stenosis.

## PULSE VARYING IN AMPLITUDE

### A. Pulsus Alternans

#### *Description*

The amplitude of the pulse wave, in a patient in sinus rhythm is large and small alternately.

#### *Mechanism*

Usually, in a patient with heart failure, an episode of alternans is initiated by an extra systole. In the succeeding pause, there is excessive filling of the left ventricle and the next ventricular contraction is powerful and prolonged because of the large volume to be expelled. The period available for diastolic filling of the ventricle prior to the next beat is therefore short and the contraction less forceful.

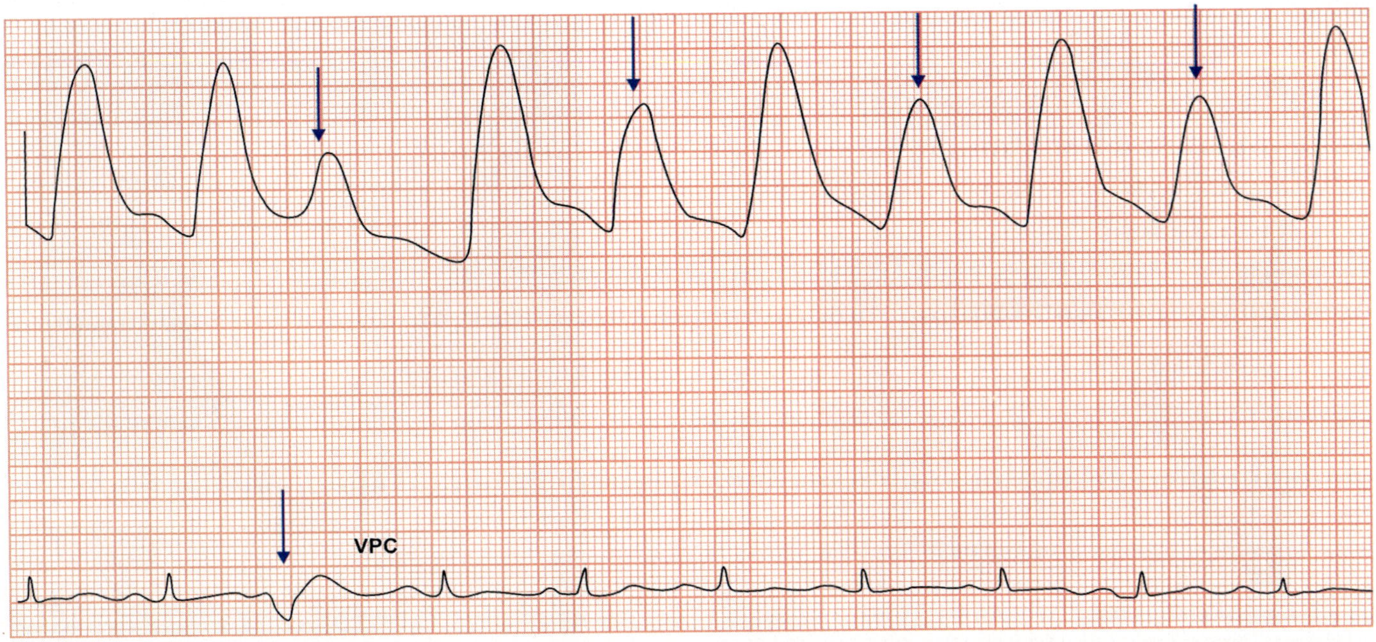


**Fig. 1.46:** Hemodynamic study shows an alternating pulse-arterial pressure recording in severe left ventricular failure. After the second beat a ventricular premature beat triggers an episode of alternating pulse

### *Significance*

Pulsus alternans is a good evidence of left ventricular failure (Fig. 1.46).

## B. Pulsus Paradoxus

### *Description*

A marked accentuation of the normal decrease in the amplitude of the arterial pulse during quiet inspiration.

### *Causes*

1. Increased inspiratory effort (laryngeal stridor, severe asthma)
2. Restriction of diastolic filling of the heart (cardiac tamponade, constrictive pericarditis)
3. Occasionally present in right ventricular failure.

### *Mechanism*

1. *Pulsus paradoxus in asthma:* The powerful inspiratory effort to overcome airway obstruction considerably increases the capacity of the lung vessels and thereby reduces the flow of blood out of the lungs to the left heart. The systemic arterial pulse pressure is then diminished during inspiration.
2. *Pulsus paradoxus in tamponade:* When the diastolic volume of the heart is limited by a pericardial effusion or a rigid pericardium, the normal increased filling of the right atrium and right ventricle during inspiration leaves less available volume for the left atrium and the left ventricle. Left ventricular stroke volume is reduced during inspiration and pulsus paradoxus is produced.
3. *Pulsus paradoxus in right ventricular failure:* If the failing right ventricle does not increase its output during inspiration, the normal increase in the capacity of the lung vessels will restrict the flow out of the lungs into the left heart and the left ventricular stroke output will decrease resulting into formation of pulsus paradoxus.

### *Pulse Varying in Waveforms*

The shape of the pressure wave is of diagnostic value as many abnormalities of the circulation produce characteristic changes in the form of the pulse wave which are readily detected by palpation. The normal brachial pulse has a smooth fairly sharp upstroke, a momentarily sustained peak and a quick downstroke. The dicrotic notch, representing aortic valve closure, cannot be detected clinically, but the other features are readily analysed.

## ANACROTIC PULSE (PLATEAU PULSE, SLOW RISING PULSE)

### Description

The upstroke is slow with often a distinct notch on it. The time taken to reach the peak is prolonged and the entire pulse wave is of small amplitude.

### Causes

Aortic valve stenosis. The rate of ejection of blood into the aorta is decreased so that the ejection is prolonged and the amplitude of the pulse is diminished.

## WATER HAMMER PULSE (COLLAPSING PULSE)

### Description

The upstroke is more abrupt and steep than normal. The peak is reached early, is not sustained and the downstroke is also rapid. The amplitude is usually abnormally large. The examiner's finger appreciates the sharper than normal upstroke rather than the downstroke and experiences a sharp tap with each pulse beat (Fig. 1.47).

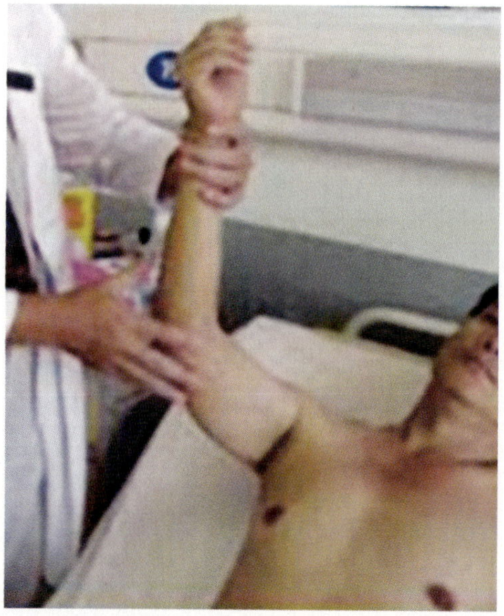

**Fig. 1.47:** The collapsing pulse. The collapsing pulse is best elicited by grabbing the patient's left wrist with your left hand (bottom, left). After you have detected the pulsation of his radial pulse in your palm, gradually relax the grip of your hand until the radial pulse just disappear. Then with the help of your right hand, lift the patient's arm in the air (bottom, right) while maintaining the same grip pressure. If the pulse returns, it has become more forceful and thus deemed collapsing

### Causes

The sharp upstroke represents the rapid ejection of blood into an empty arterial system and the rapid downstroke indicates abnormally fast escape of blood from the arteries during diastole. A water hammer or bounding pulse is found in:

1. Aortic valve regurgitation
2. Persistent ductus arteriosus
3. Systemic arteriovenous fistula
4. Pregnancy
5. Fever
6. Thyrotoxicosis (Fig. 1.48)
7. Anemia
8. Anoxic lung disease

## PULSUS BISFERIENS

### Description

The upstroke is sharp to a high peak, the pressure then falls and rises again to a second peak of about the same height as the first peak before falling off. The amplitude of the pulse wave is large and the palpating finger experiences two distinct impulses with each pulse beat.

### Cause

This waveform indicates combined stenosis and incompetence of the aortic valve, both lesions being severe. The exact mechanism producing pulsus bisferiens is unknown.

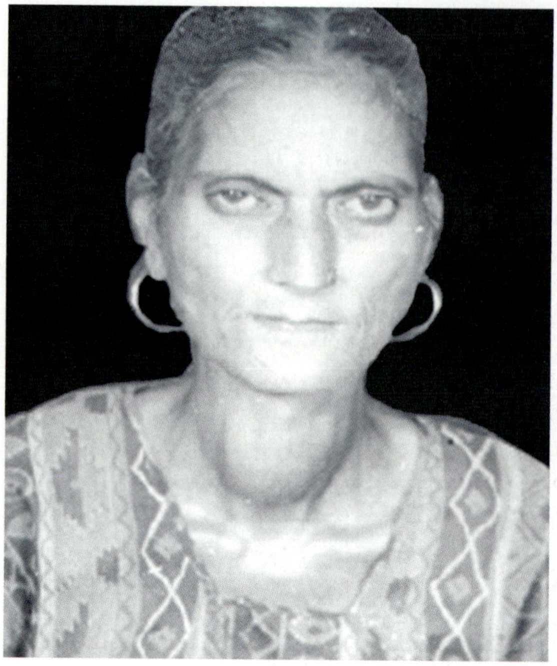

**Fig. 1.48:** Enlargement of thyroid gland, mild exophthalmos, thin physique in 40-year-old female suffering from hyperthyroidism who clinically presented with atrial fibrillation and cardiomegaly and water-hammer type of pulse

## DICROTIC PULSE

### Description

A secondary pressure wave follows the dicrotic notch (later than the second peak of the bisferiens pulse) so that two impulses are felt with each pulse beat and may give the impression that the heart rate is twice as fast as it really is.

### Cause

The normal very small secondary pressure wave produced by aortic valve closure is accentuated during its transmission

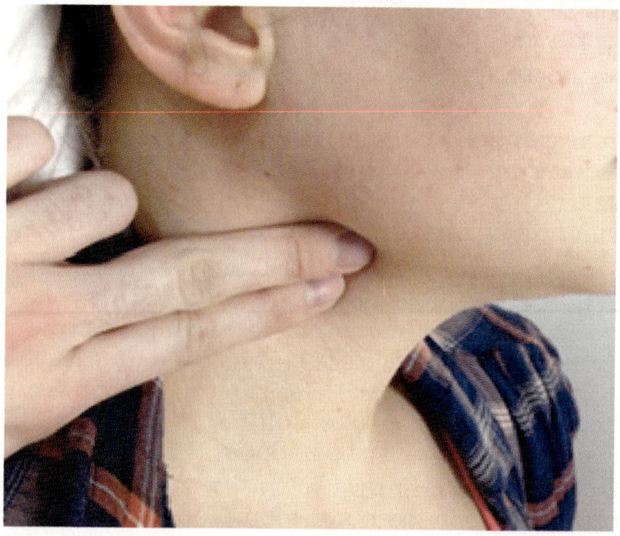

**Fig. 1.49:** Palpation of carotid arteries in a young child

to the peripheral arteries when the tone of the arterial system is low, classically in typhoid fever.

## CAROTID PULSE

Carotid arterial pulsation is normally visible in the neck (Fig. 1.49).

1. Invisible carotid pulsation—small pulse pressure, e.g. aortic stenosis.
2. Prominent carotid pulsation—large pulse pressure, e.g. aortic regurgitation, persistent ductus arteriosus, heart block, excitement, or loss of elascity of the aorta, e.g. atheroma of the aorta and coarctation of the aorta.
3. Unequal carotid pulses:
   a. Atheroma of innominate or common carotid arteries,
   b. Aortic arch syndrome
   c. Dissecting aneurysm

## COMPARISON OF THE PULSES

The radial pulses are compared one with the other and with the femoral pulses. The pulsations of both carotid arteries are also compared (Figs 1.50–1.52).

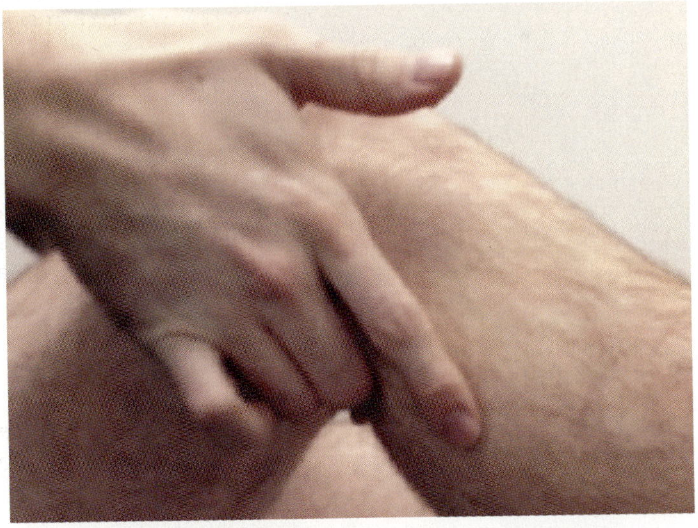

**Fig. 1.50:** The popliteal pulse is palpable in the popliteal fossa whilst holding the bent knee with both hands

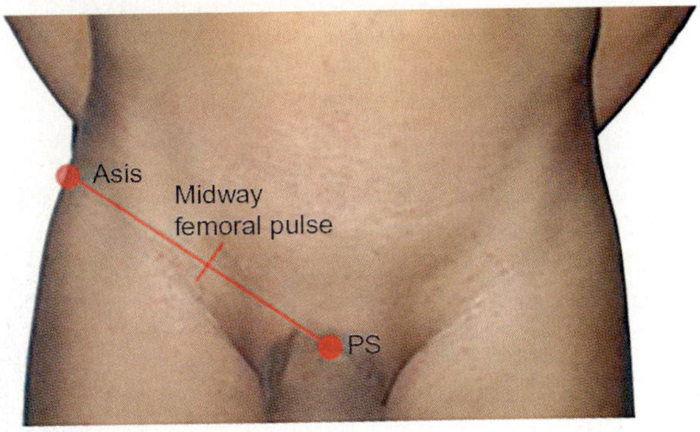


**Fig. 1.51:** The femoral pulse is palpable at the mid-inguinal point, halfway between the pubic symphysis (PS) and the anterior superior iliac spine (ASIS)

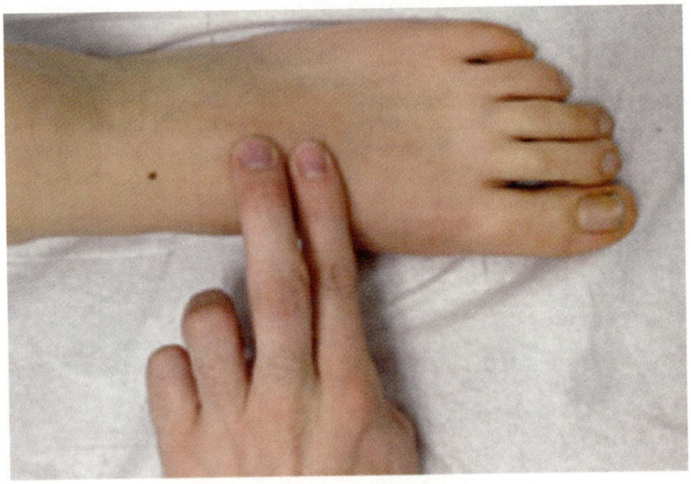

**Fig. 1.52:** The dorsalis pedis pulse is palpable over the foot, lateral to the path taken by the extensor hallicus longus (the muscle which supplies the big toe)

1. Unequal or delayed radial pulsation on one side indicates obstruction
   a. At origin of a subclavian artery, e.g. atheromatous plaque; involvement of the origin by an aortic aneurysm and origin of a subclavian artery below a coarctation of the aorta.
   b. Distal to origin of subclavian artery, e.g. subclavian or brachial embolus.
2. Femoral pulses small or delayed compared with radial pulses
   a. Coarctation of the aorta (obstruction to blood flow in the thoracic aorta)
   b. Saddle embolus

## BLOOD PRESSURE

Blood pressure is the pressure exerted by circulating blood upon the walls of blood vessels. When used without further specification, 'blood pressure' usually

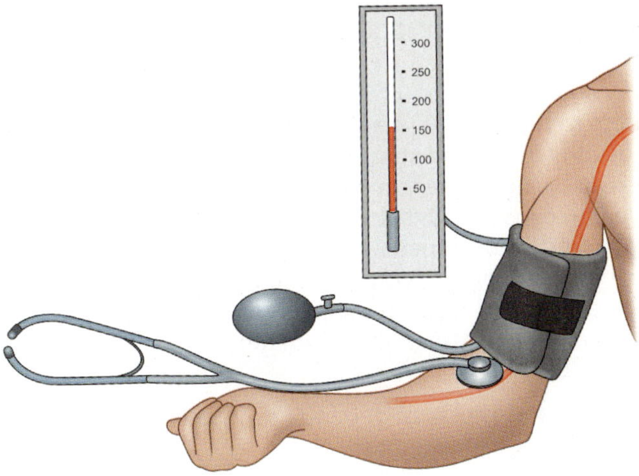


**Fig. 1.53:** Application of sphygmomanometer a common instrument for measuring systolic and diastolic blood pressure in human body

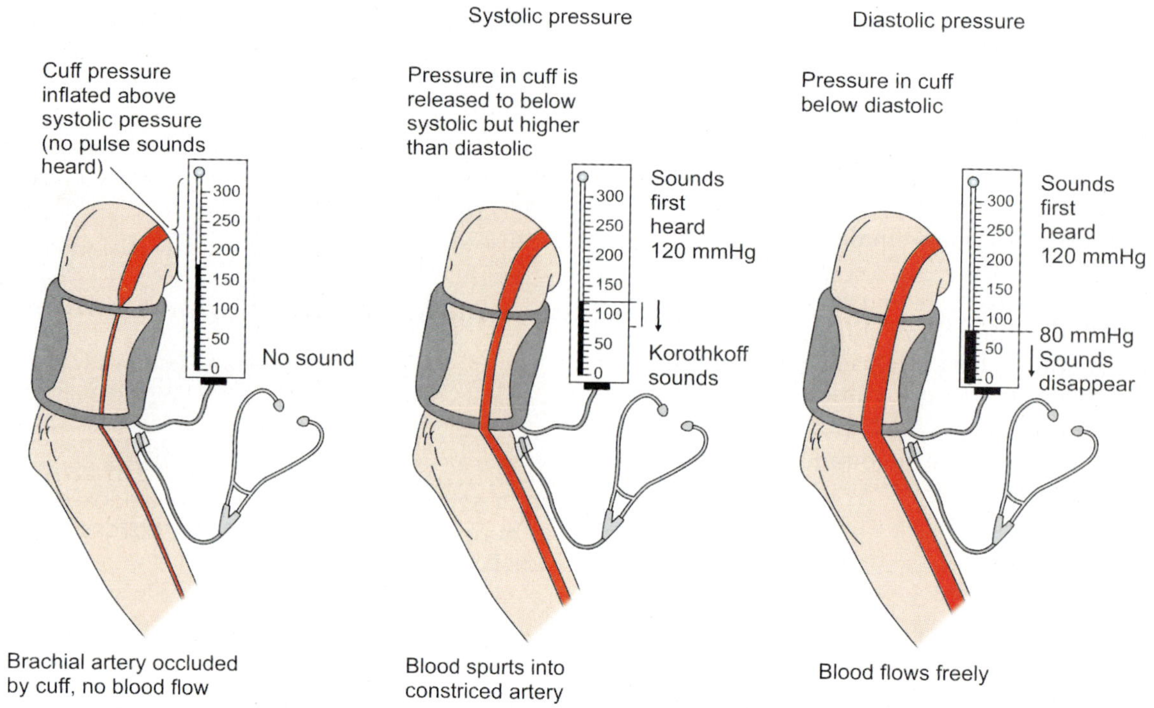


**Fig. 1.54:** Technique of measuring systolic and diastolic blood pressure

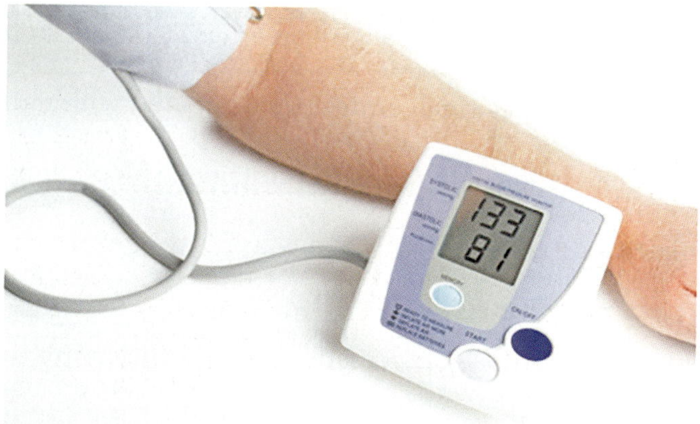


**Fig. 1.55:** Technique of measuring systolic and diastolic blood pressures with an automatic electronic instrument

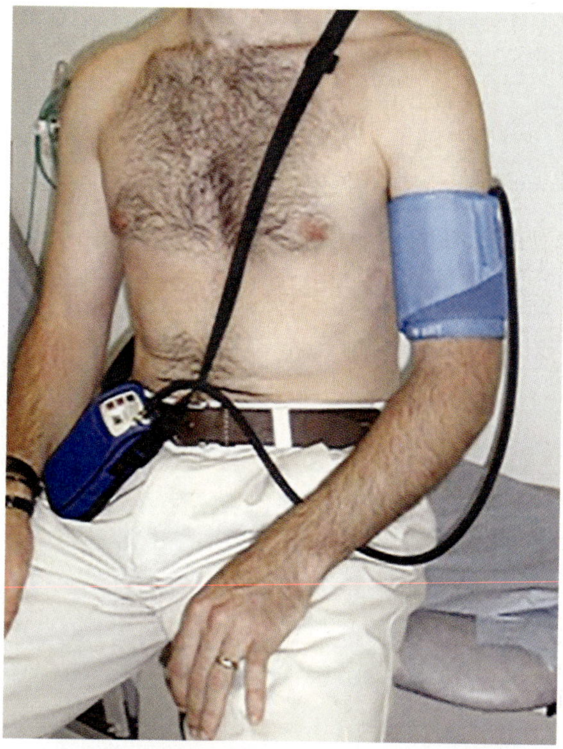

**Fig. 1.56:** Placing the BP monitoring equipment for 24 hours. The diagnostic test begins with fitting a patient with a portable monitor and BP cuff

refers to the arterial pressure in the systemic circulation. It is usually measured at a person's upper arm. Blood pressure is usually expressed in terms of the systolic (maximum) pressure overdiastolic (minimum) pressure and is measured in millimeters of mercury (mmHg). It is one of the vital signs along with respiratory rate, heart rate, oxygen saturation, and body temperature. Normal resting blood pressure in an adult is approximately under 140/90 mmHg (Figs 1.53–1.58).

The blood pressure depends primarily on the

1. Cardiac output
2. Peripheral resistance
3. Elasticity of the aorta, the blood volume
4. Blood viscosity

### Types of Blood Pressure

a. The systolic blood pressure is the peak pressure achieved during the ejection of blood from the ventricle into the aorta.

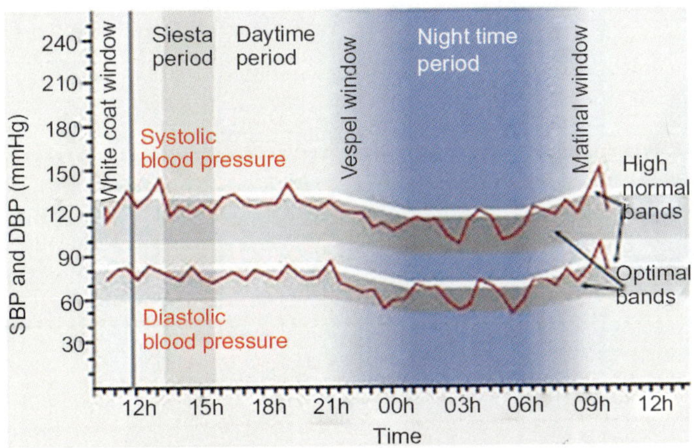


**Fig. 1.57:** ABPM suggests low daytime systolic and diastolic blood pressure (100 mmHg/59 mmHg) and moderate night time systolic and diastolic hypertension (146 mmHg/89 mmHg) with a white-coat effect (181 mmHg/102 mmHg). Reverse dipping pattern

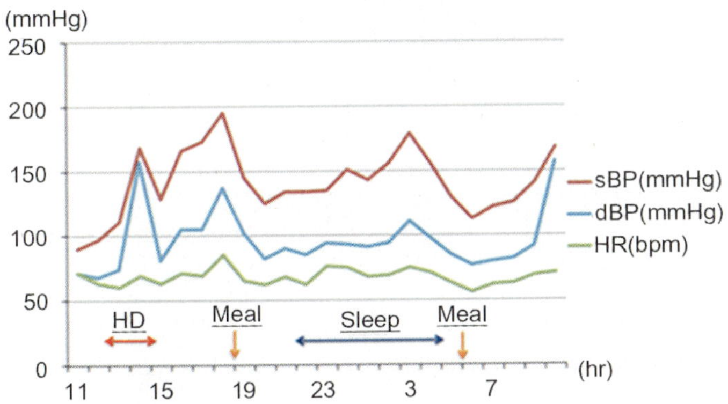


**Fig. 1.58:** The data of 24-hour ambulatory blood pressure monitoring (24-hour ABPM). This is the data of 24-hour ABPM on dialysis day. There was an extreme change in blood pressure during the day and the patient experienced hypotensive episodes several times. Most episodes were after inserting meal from PEG and after lying in bed, when vagus nerve was stimulated. These episodes also indicate that the patient was unable to have vasovagal reflex when there was vagus nerve stimulation

b. The diastolic blood pressure varies with the peripheral resistance. If there is a rapid escape of blood from the aorta, there will be a low pressure at the end of diastole. In the absence of anatomical leaks (persistent ductus arteriosus, arteriovenous fistula) the peripheral resistance is governed by the arterioles, vasodilatation lowering the diastolic pressure.

### Measurement

An inflatable cuff firmly bound to the upper arm and connected to a mercury column is used for measurement of the arterial pressure in the arm. For accurate results, the width of the sphygmomanometer cuff must be appropriate to the circumference of the arm. A cuff 5 inches in width is correct for a normal sized adult and smaller cuffs are necessary for the children since a large cuff gives a falsely low reading. The systolic pressure is the highest pressure at which successive sounds are heard when auscultating over the brachial artery, and the diastolic pressure is taken at the point when sounds abruptly become dull and muffled.

Doppler technique may be employed when pulses are weak. Such as in pulseless disease. In the adult, top normal pressure should probably be taken to be about 120/80 mmHg. Whereas in infants and children one may apply the rule that by age one year the systolic pressure is about 90 mmHg. and increases by 5 mmHg. about every 3 years, so that by the age of 13 or 14, it has reached to adult level.

### Ambulatory Blood Pressure Monitoring

It provides accurate and reliable blood pressure day and night. Ambulatory blood pressure monitoring (ABPM) is considered the gold standard for measuring blood pressure by clinicians worldwide. It provides valuable diagnostic information that in-clinic and home blood pressure monitoring systems are incapable of measuring including:

1. Blood pressure variability and a more accurate estimation of true blood pressure
2. Overnight changes in blood pressure (dipper status)
3. Morning surges in blood pressure
4. In general, ABPM is recognized in the medical community as a valuable tool for supporting the management of appropriate pharmacologic treatment as well as the assessment of 1 and 2.
5. 'White coat' hypertension, when elevated blood pressure measurements are recorded in the physican's office environment while blood pressure readings outside the physician's office are within a normal range.
6. Resistant hypertension, when multiple anti-hypertensive medications fail to adequately control high blood pressure.
7. Masked hypertension, when in-office measurements fall within an acceptable range, but the mean blood pressure is actually above the acceptable range.
8. Hypotensive symptoms with hypertensive medications.

The diagnostic test begins with fitting a patient with a portable monitor and BP cuff. The patient leaves and returns the next day. Over this period of time, the monitor takes measurements periodically as programmed by the clinician, generally each 15–30 minutes during awake hours and 30–45 minutes during sleeping hours. When the patient returns, these measurements are transferred to a computer, where they can be easily viewed and documented in a report using the enclosed AccuWin Pro™ software. The results of ambulatory blood pressure testing provide the most comprehensive representation of a patient's complete blood pressure profile.

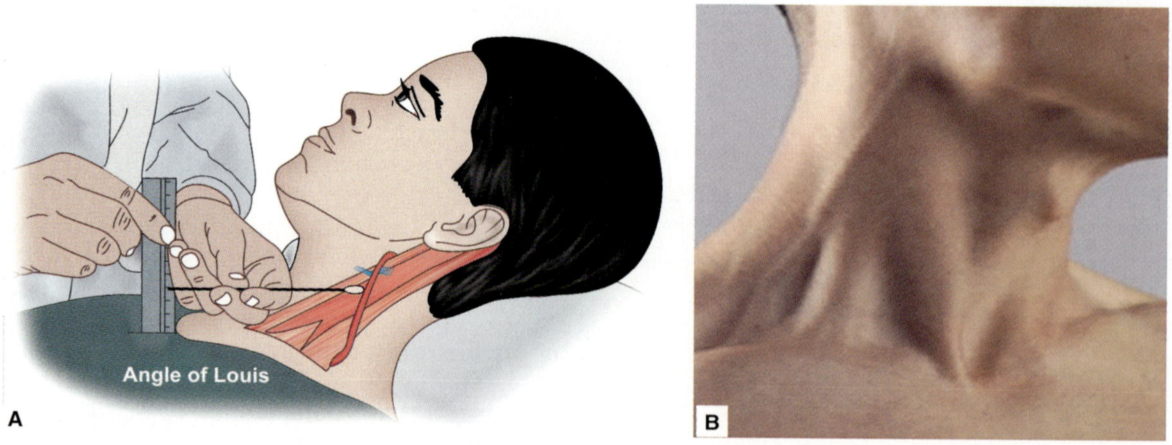


Fig. 1.59: (A) Demonstrating the RA pressure in relation to anatomical position of both RA, RV and internal jugular vein to the body positioned at 45°, (B) showing raised internal jugular venous pressure in a person with CHF

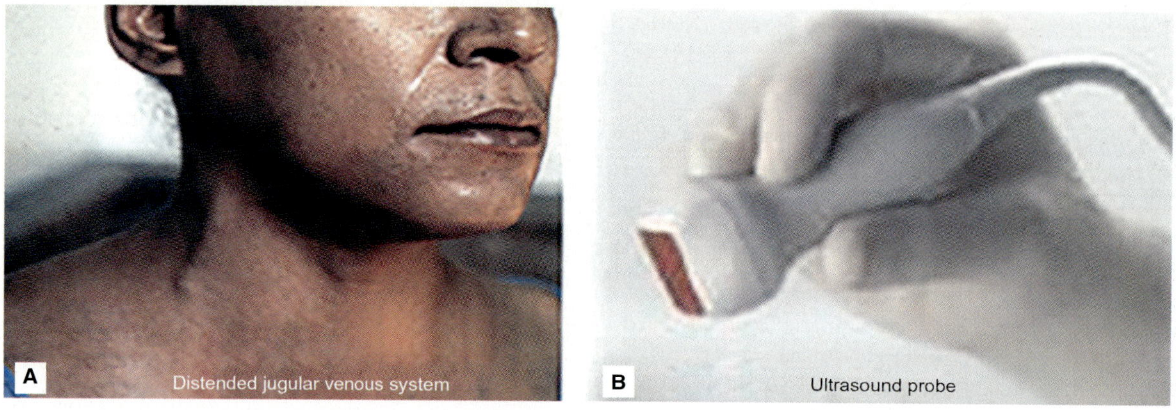


Fig. 1.60: (A) Looking at the neck veins for hours together has been a favorite pastime of our cardiology ancestors. Thanks to those sharp intellect, that has led us to this height of cardiovascular revolution. Measuring JV pressure by itself was considered a big science. Putting a patient at 45°, marking the sternal angle, identify the oscillating venous column, measuring the vertical distance, etc. Now in 2010, with bedside hand-held echo (B) one can rapidly rule out an elevated central venous pressure by imaging the jugular vein directly

## JUGULAR VENOUS PRESSURE

Jugular venous pressure is depicted in Figs 1.59–1.63.

### Measurement

The patient is placed at an angle of 45° with the head supported on a pillow and the pulsations of the internal jugular vein in the neck are usually visible. The internal jugular vein is collapsed except for its lower part, where the pressure from the right atrium keeps it distended. The right atrial pressure fluctuates throughout the cardiac cycle and the changing level of distension of the internal jugular vein imparts a gentle undulation to the skin of the neck which is readily distinguishable from the single sharp movement produced by carotid arterial pulsation. The vertical distance in centimetres between the top of this undulation and the sternal angle is called the jugular venous pressure and is a measurement of the pressure in the right atrium. The external jugular vein is often partially kinked and obstructed near the root of the neck and is a less reliable measure of the right atrial pressure. The jugular venous pulse is analysed for height above the sternal angel and for waveform. The normal mean pressure is 0–2 cm above sternal sangle and the waveform reveals 'a' and 'v' waves of approximately equal height. Many other workers refer the figure of 4.6 cm at 45° inclination.

### Causes of a Raised Mean Jugular Venous Pressure

1. *High right ventricular filling pressure:*
   a. Right ventricular failure: Failing right ventricle requires a diastolic pressure as high as 4.0 mmHg to maintain a cardiac output of 4.0 litres per minute. The whole circulation adjusts to maintain a high right atrial filling pressure under these circumstances.
   b. High output states: A slight increase in right atrial filling pressure is required even in normal hearts for the right ventricle to maintain a high cardiac output.

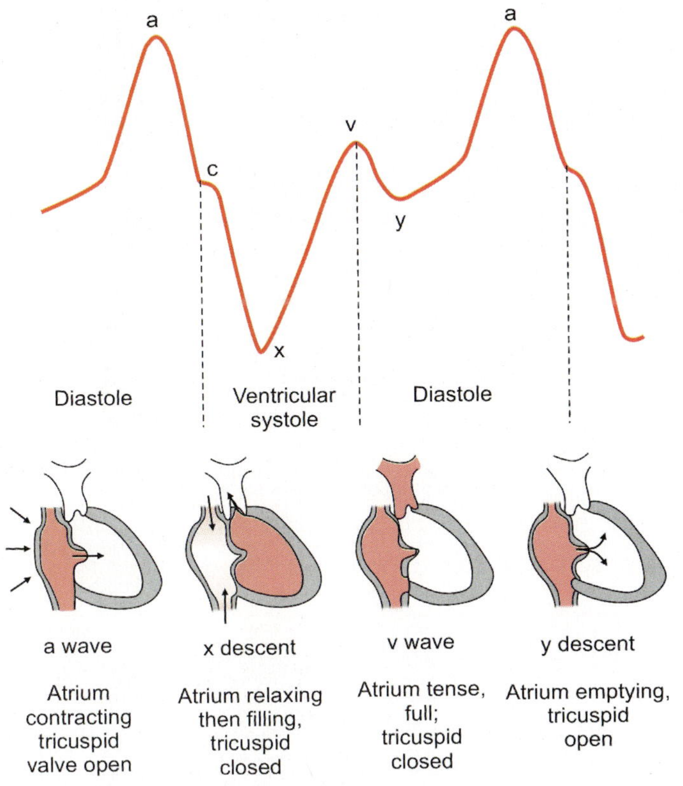


**Fig. 1.61:** Illustration showing graphic presentation of genesis of various waveforms in relation to cardiac contraction undulation and the sternal angle is called the jugular venous pressure and is a measurement of the pressure in the right atrium. The external jugular vein is often partially kinked and obstructed near the root of the neck and is a less reliable measure of the right atrial pressure. The jugular venous pulse is analysed for height above the sternal angel and for wave form. The normal mean pressure is 0–2 cm above sternal angle and the waveform reveals 'a' and 'v' waves of approximately equal height. Many other workers refer the figure of 4.6 cm at 45° inclination

c. Increased blood volume (over transfusion, acute nephritis). Until the blood vessels dilate to accommodate the increased volume, there is an increased venous return and a raised right atrial pressure.

d. Restriction of relaxation of the heart in diastole: Normal filling of the heart is impeded during diastole in tamponade and in constrictive pericarditis.

2. *Obstruction to blood flow from right atrium to right ventricle (tricuspid stenosis, right atrial myxoma):* A high right atrial pressure serves to maintain the blood flow across the obstructed region.
3. *Superior vena cava obstruction (involvement by or retrosternal thyroid gland enlargement):* The distended veins do not pulsate which distinguishes this cause of an elevated venous pressure.
4. *Loss of negative intrathoracic pressure (emphysema, pleural effusion and pneumothorax):* Any rise in pressure within the thorax is transmitted to the right atrium.

## ABNORMALITIES OF WAVEFORM IN THE JUGULAR

### Venous Pulse

#### *Normal*

Two peaks (a and v) and two troughs (x and y) are seen during each cardiac cycle. The waves are timed by relating them to the carotid pulse. The a wave precedes the carotid arterial pulse and is the pressure wave of right atrial systole. A fall in pressure follows, the x descent, during which the right atrium relaxes. The v wave is the positive pressure wave immediately after the carotid pulse and represents the rise in pressure in the right atrium, as it fills with the tricuspid valve closed during ventricular systole. At the termination of ventricular systole with the opening of the tricuspid valve, blood leaves the right atrium and its pressure falls, producing the y descent. The a and v waves are of approximately equal height and do not rise more than 2 cm above the sternal angle.

#### *Abnormalities of the a Wave*

1. *Large a wave (powerful right atrial contraction):* This implies an increase resistance to blood flow from right atrium to right ventricle. The resistance may be at valve level

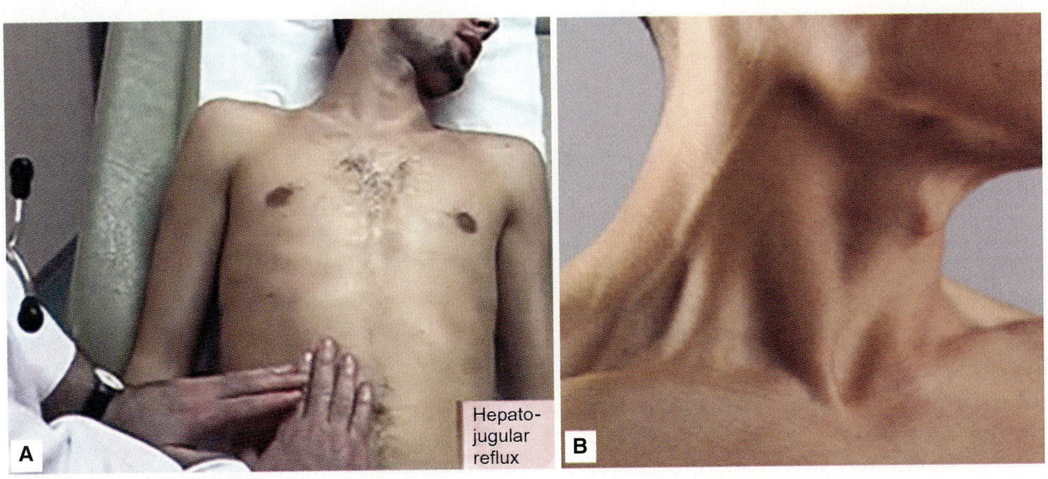


**Fig. 1.62:** (A) Doctor is pressing over the liver area and looking for distension of neck veins to demonstrate hepatojugular reflux in an adolescent with congestive heart failure and (B) engorged jugular vein in intractable heart failure

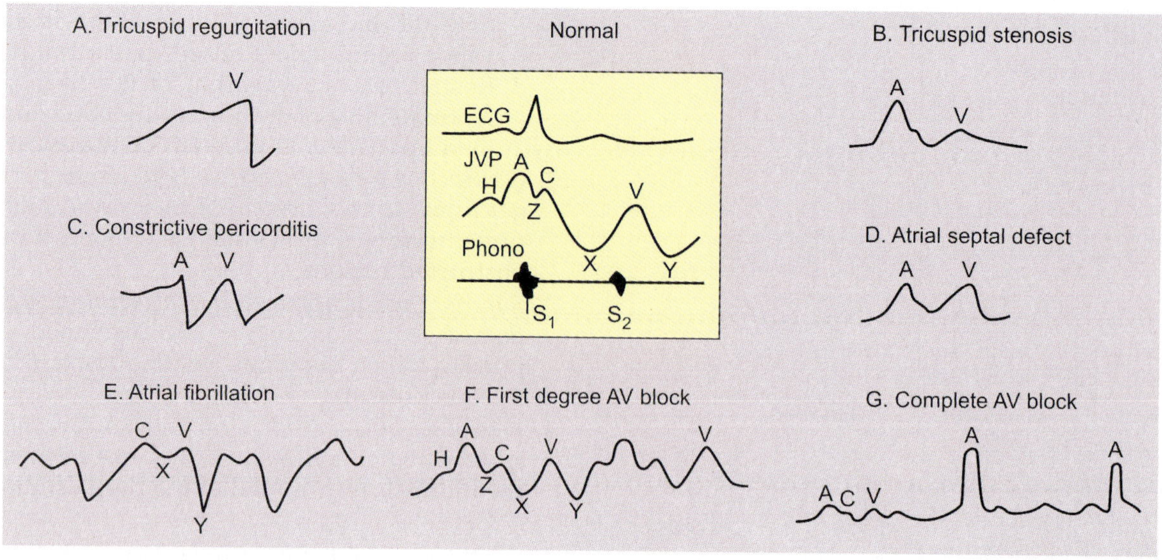


**Fig. 1.63:** Schematic representation of the normal jugular venous pulse (JVP), four types of abnormal JVPs, and the JVPs in three arrhythmias

(tricuspid stenosis, tricuspid atresia), or the right ventricle may offer more resistance to filing when its walls are hypertrophied (pulmonary stenosis, pulmonary hypertension).

2. Absent a wave non-coordinated contraction of the right atrium), i.e. atrial fibrillation.

### Abnormalities of the v Wave

Large v waves indicate considerable reflux of blood into the right atrium during ventricular systole, i.e. tricuspid valvular regurgitation (TR).

### Abnormalities of the x Descent

It is absent in atrial fibrillation. Accentuated in tamponade and in some cases of constrictive pericarditis. During ventricular systole, blood is ejected from the heart into the pulmonary artery and into the aorta. The decrease in volume of the ventricles with the rigid pericardial sac creates more volume available for filling of the right atrium from the great veins.

### Abnormalities of the y Descent

1. *Sharp y descent:* The higher the venous pressure the more abrupt is the fall in pressure when the tricuspid valve opens, provided there is no obstruction to flow from the right atrium into the right ventricle.
2. *Slow y descent:* This provides evidence of obstruction to flow from right atriam into right ventricle and is found in tricuspid stenosis or when there is tumor mass within the right atrium.

## Cannon Waves

Large venous pressure waves synchronous with the carotid pulse, produced by atrial contraction against a closed tricuspid valve. A cannon wave, therefore, implies atrial contraction coinciding with ventricular systole (Fig. 1.64).

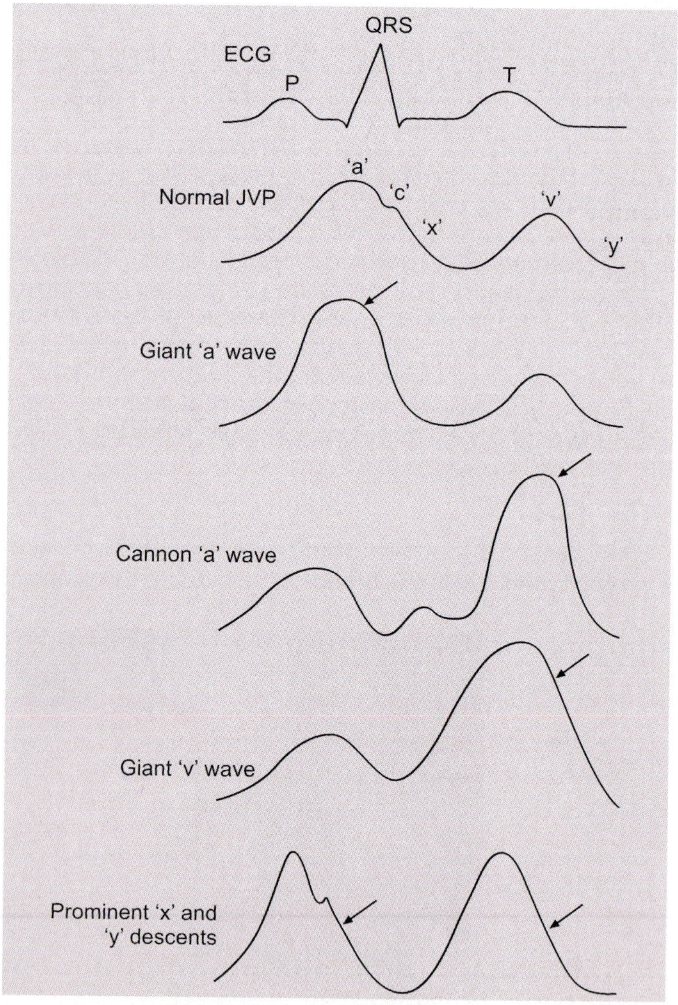


**Fig. 1.64:** The jugular venous pulse (JVP). Electrical events always precede mechanical events. Thus, the P-wave of the ECG (representing atrial depolarization) and the ORS complex (representing ventricular depolarization) precede the 'a' wave and the 'v' wave of the JVP, respectively

### *Causes of Cannon Waves*

Regular fast cannon waves are found in paroxysmal nodal tachycardia. Occasional irregular cannon waves are also encountred in complete heart block. Cannon waves are only seen when atrial and ventricular systole happen to coincide.

### *Respiratory Variation and Kussmaul's Sign*

The mean jugular venous pressure normally falls with inspiration, passively following the intrathoracic pressure. In some patients with decreased RV compliance, the relative height of the 'a' wave will increase with inspiration even though the mean venous pressure falls. This is considered to be related to an enhancement in the force of atrial contraction wth atrial distention caused by the ventilatory increase in the venous return. Subjects with a marked decrease in RV compliance, such as those with constrictive pericarditis. In the later, there is a rise in the mean height of the jugular venous pulse during inspiration. This is known as Kussmaul's sign and is observed approximately 40% of the patients with constrictive pericarditis. Kussmaul's sign is generally not seen in patients with pericardial tamponade or massive pericardial effusion (Fig. 1.65).

## NORMAL PRECORDIAL ACTIVITY

Examination of the heart begins with observation and palpation of the chest for abnormal impulses and thrills The palpable apical impulse in a normal subject is produced by an anterior movement of the left ventricle during early systole. As isovolumic intraventricular pressure rises, the left ventricle rotates in a counterclockwise direction on its long axis as the cardiac apex lifts and makes contact with the left anterior chest wall following aortic valve opening and the first half of ejection, the LV chamber moves away from the chest wall and continues to diminish in size until systole is completed. Thus, the impulse felt or recorded on the precordium is made up of an early outward thrust followed by retraction during the last part of systole; normal palpable cardiac activity occurs only during the first half of systole. The retraction wave can be seen but is not felt. Diastolic events, such as the LV rapid filling phase or left atrial contraction, are normally not palpable. In angiographic studies, the interventricular septum (composed mostly of LV muscle) and the anteroseptal aspect of the left ventricle makes contact with the inner thoracic cage to form the palpable apical impulse. The true anatomical LV apex is actually slightly lower and more lateral than the palpable apical impulse.

### How to Examine the Precordium

For optimal precordial examination, it is important for the examiner and the patient to be relaxed. The room should be confortably warm. Clothing and undergarments must be removed to allow wider inspection and palpation of the chest. Because the examiner must be prepared, e.g. to count intercostal spaces, measure the distance of the precordial impulse from the sternum or axillary line, and chest exposure should be maximal. The patient should be lying comfortably, in the supine position or with the thorax elevated not more than 30°. Perloff suggests that the 30° position is preferable because precordial examination in this position may bring out abnormalities more often than

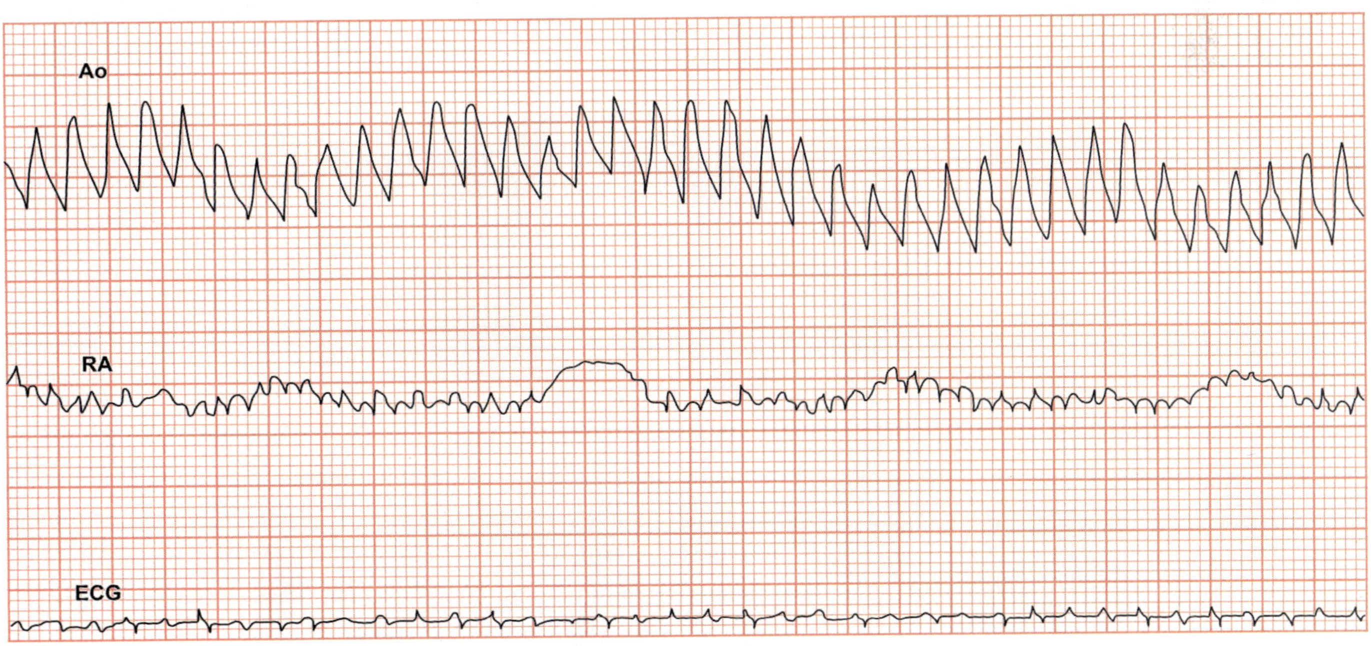


**Fig. 1.65:** Paradoxical pulse and Kussmaul's sign. Pericardial effusion (evidenced by the small voltage deflexions on the ECGI has caused tamponade. Respiratory fluctuations in the aortic (Ao) and right atrial (RA) pressure signals are seen. During inspiration aortic pressure falls markedly (paradoxical pulse) and right atrial pressure rises (Kussmaul's sign)

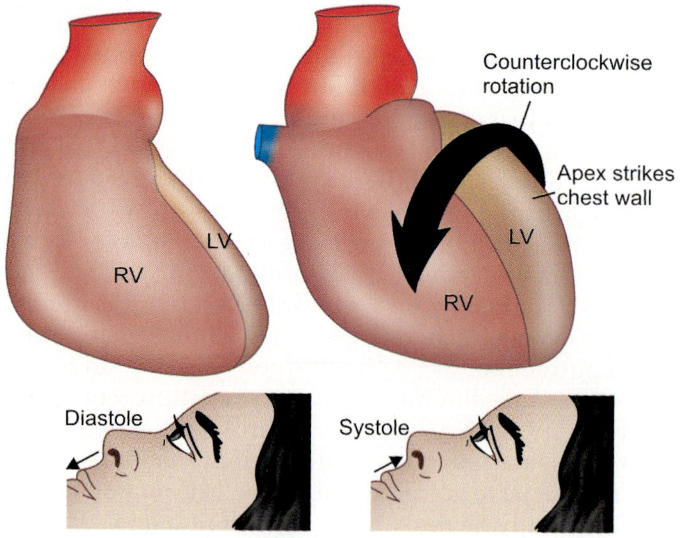


**Fig. 1.66:** Diagrammatic demonstration of apical movements in syslole and diastole during cardiac cycle

when the patient is lying supine. In a given patient, cardiovascular diseases should routinely be examined in the left lateral decubitus position; the subject should be instructed to turn on his or her left side at a 45° to 60° angle with the examining table, elevating the left arm over the head, so that the examiner may have unobstructed access to the left precordium (Fig. 1.66).

## 1. INSPECTION

Careful inspection of the chest is useful in the precordial examination, particularly after preliminary palpation has identified the site of the apical beat or any other impulses that may be present. Retraction movements, which may be more obvious than outward motion are quite prominent in severe degrees of LV enlargement. Tangential lighting with the examining lamp or a pen torch may accentuate visible movements on the chest wall (Figs 1.67, 1.68 and Table 1.2).

## 2. PALPATION

The physician should be standing comfortably at the patient's right side. Both the palm of the hand and the ventral aspect of the proximal metacarpals and fingers should be used for palpation (Figs 1.69–1.71). One must learn which aspect the hand has the best sense of touch, it is advisable to use the pads of the fingers for precise localization and assessment of LV and RV activity. The palm and proximal metacarpals are usually best used to localize palpable cardiac motion as well as to detect precordial thrills. Varying pressure with the hand should be applied once a precordial impulse has been identified.

High frequency sounds, such as an increased S1, and opening snap, or a transmitted thrill, are best localized with the hand firmly applied to the chest. However, the subtle, low frequency motion of a palpable S3 or S4 or double systolic apical impulse will be felt only with light pressure of the fingers and may be totally obscured if the examination is not performed correctly. In most normal subjects, parasternal activity is not usually detectable. However, in young or thin people, a gentle shock or tap at the lower left sternal border may be felt, and, occasionally, a pulmonary artery mpulse in the second to third left intercostal space adjacent to the sternum may be detected. Forceful, unstained, or high amplitude parasternal motion is always an abnormal finding.

### *Point of Maximum Impulse (PMI)*

Many textbooks use the term for PMI, the same as the apical beat. Although not ideal, this expression is so frequently

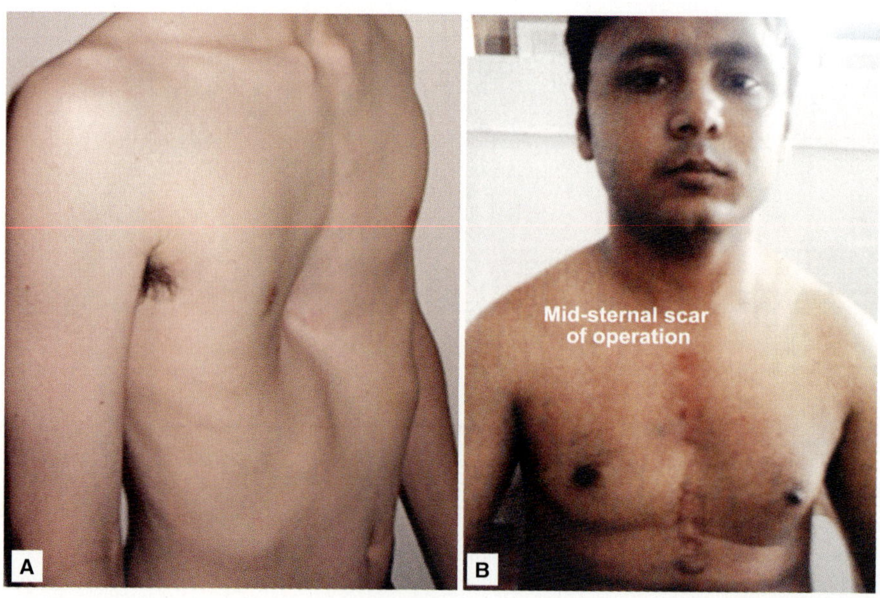


**Fig. 1.67:** (A) Pectus excavatum deformity of chest in VSD. (B) Photograph of 20 years old male had bicuspid aortic stenosis with AR with LVH. He was successfully operated with AVR and regular follow up for more than 6 years maintained good health

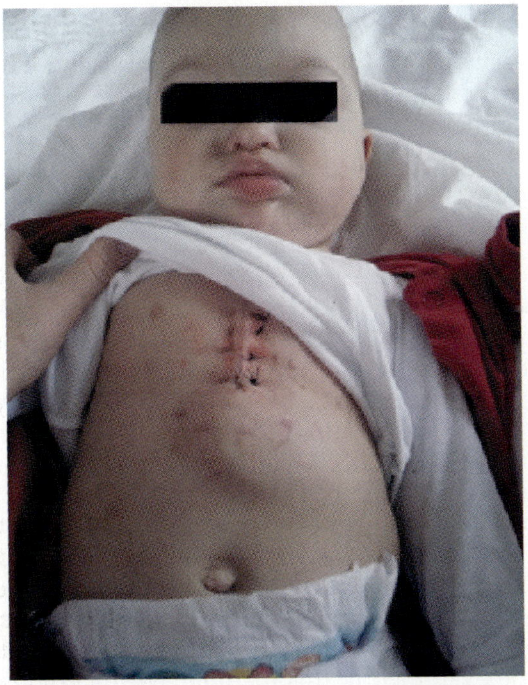

**Fig 1.68:** Dual chamber pacemaker with epicardial electrodes implanted through a median sternotomy in a newborn with complete heart block

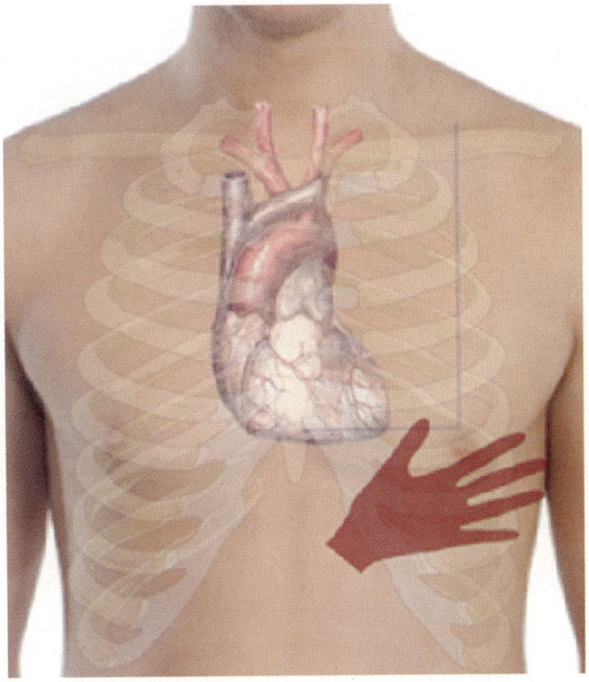

**Fig. 1.69:** The apex beat is the lowest, most lateral point where the heartbeat can be felt

used that it has become acceptable to many. Nevertheless, it should be recognized that the terms PMI and apical impulse are not necessarily synonymous. In some patients, the most prominent, 'maximal', impulse may actually reflect ectopic LV motion, RV activity, or a vascular impulse.

### Other Palpable Events

In a subject with suspected cardiac disease. the examiner should explore the entire precordium with firm pressure of the hand and proximal fingers, separating the aortic, pulmonic, lower sternal and apical regions. In this way, the unexpected vascular impulse, such as a dilated or aneurysmal ascending aorta or pulmonary artery, may be detected. Particular attention should be given to the upper sternal area, to the manubrium, and to the adjacent first to second intercostal spaces below the medial aspect of the clavicles. Aortic pulsations and systolic thrills are often found there. If a patient has coronary artery disease, particularly with a prior myocardial infraction, careful

**Table 1.2:** Clinical classification and causes of precordial impulses

| Site of impulse | Sustained | Hyperdynamic | Late systole |
|---|---|---|---|
| 1. Parasternal area | *Pressure overload:*<br>Pulmonary hypertension<br>Cor pulmonale<br>Mitral stenosis<br>Pulmonary emboli<br>Cardiomyopathy | Hyperkinetic circulatory states in young subjects<br><br>*Volume overload:*<br>Atrial septal defect<br>Tricuspid regurgitation | Severe mitral regurgitation |
| 2. LV (apical beat) | *Pressure overload:*<br>Hypertension aortic stenosis<br>Chronic or severe<br><br>*Volume overload:*<br>LV dilatation,<br>especially with decreased ejection fraction<br>LV dysfunction<br>LV aneurysm | Hyperkinetic circulatory states<br>Thin chest wall<br>Pectus excavatum<br><br>*Volume overload:*<br>Aortic regurgitation<br>Mitral regurgitation<br>Ventricular septal defect | LV dyssynergy HOCM<br><br>Mitral valve prolapse (uncommon) |

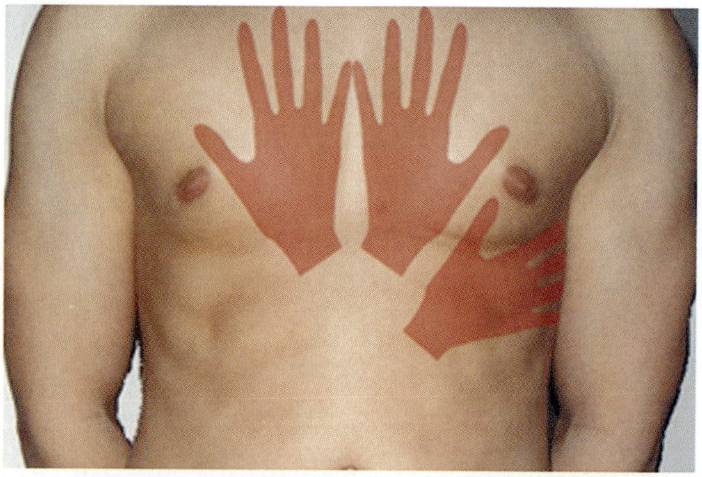

**Fig. 1.70:** Heaves and thrills can be detected by placing the hand flat against either side of the sternum and over the apex of the heart

examination for ectopic impulse should be carried out. These typically occur medial and superior to the ectopic impulse. The use of the entire palm and proximal metacarpals will help to detect the diffuse lift of a very large left or right ventricle. At times the entire anterior precordium will move in systole. This technique is also suited for detection of thrills and palpable heart sounds.

### *Assessment of the Apical Cardiac Impulse*

The assessment of the apical cardiac impulse should include analysis of the following headings:

- Location
- Size
- Force
- Duration
- Contour

In addition, there should be visual inspection of the chest for the presence of prominent retraction waves as well as for systolic and diastolic events.Timing of precordial events is best carried out by simultaneously palpating the carotid arterial pulse with the left hand. Some find that concomitant auscultation of S1 and S2 is useful for timing purposes. Application of the stethoscope chest piece directly on the apical impulse can help identify systole.

It is desirable to use held end expiration for the RV examination. Firm pressure, using the heel of the hand with the wrist turned upward, is advisable. The lower sternum and adjacent third through fifth rib and left interspaces should be examined in this manner. The examining hand and fingers should be carefully observed, as low amplitude RV activity is often found in epigastric region, with the extended fingers oriented superiorly; the patient should be instructed to hold his breath in end-inspiration and careful palpation for the descending right ventricle is

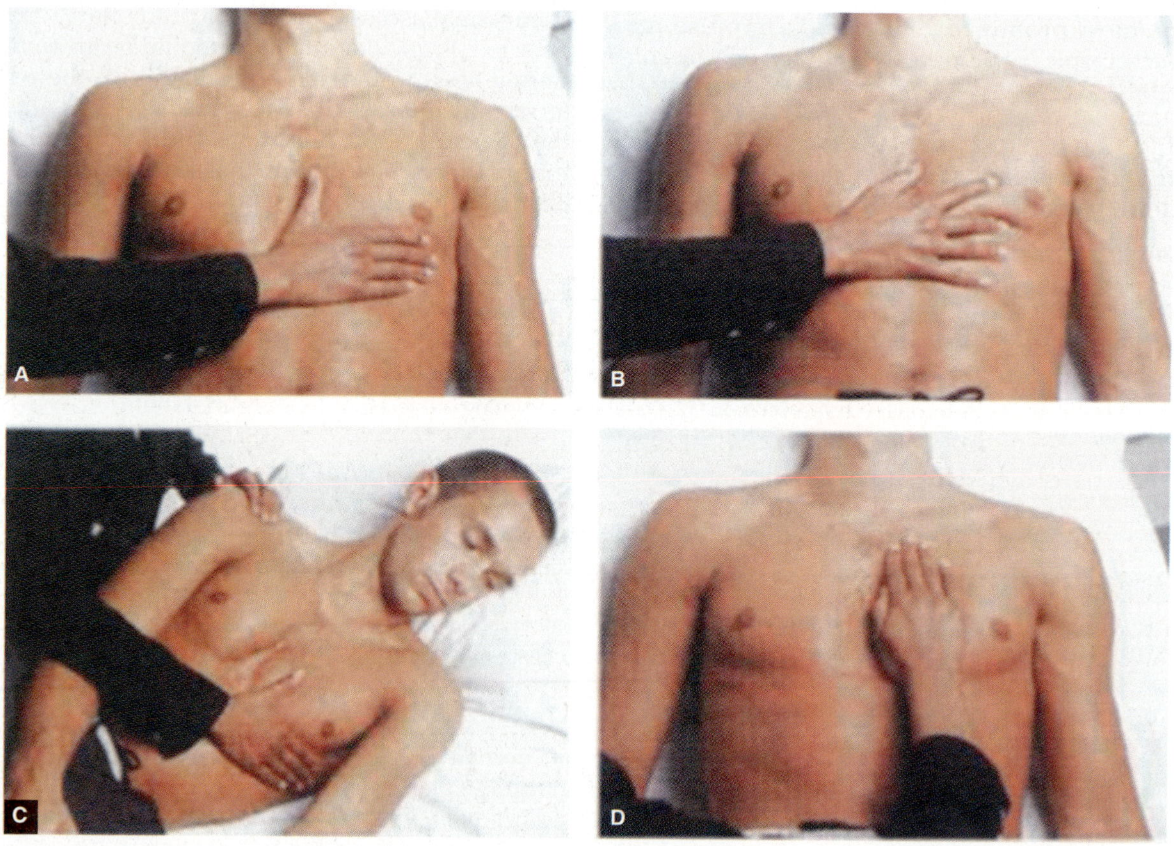


**Fig. 1.71:** Palpating the heart. (A) Use the hand to palpate the cardiac impulse. (B) Localise the apex beat with a middle finger. (C) If necessary, roll the patient into the left lateral position. (D) Palpate from apex to sternum for parasternal pulsations

performed. This technique is particularly useful in patients with an increased anteroposterior diameter, obesity or chronic obstructive lung disease.

### Characteristics of the Normal Apical Impulse

1. A gentle, nonsustained tap.
2. An early systolic anterior motion that ends before the last third of systole.
3. Location within 10 cm of the midsternal line in the fourth or fifth left intercostal space.
4. A palpable area less than 2–2.5 cm$^2$ and detectable in only 1 intercostal space.
5. RV motion that is not normally palpable.
6. Diastolic events that are normally palpable.
7. Complete absence in some older individuals.

### Location

To identify the site of the apical impulse on the thorax with respect to both the longitudinal and horizontal axes of the patient. To note in which intercostal space the, PMI or apical beat is located; occasionally a large heart will result in detectable precordial activity in 2 or even 3 intercostal spaces. Localize the apical impulse with reference to the mid-clavicular line, distance from the midsternum or relationship to the left anterior axillary line.

### Size

If the apical impulse is larger than normal, it is useful to note the area of contact with the chest. Any area greater than 2–2.5 cm$^2$ in the supine position, or greater than 3 cm$^2$ in the left decubitus position, represents cardiac enlargement.

### Force or Amplitude

Is the apical beat a soft, unimpressive impulse? Or Does it lift the examining fingers off the chest well? Is the anterior or outward excursion greater than normal or consistent with a hyperdynamic or hyperkinetic PMI? An increase in force is consistent with LV hypertrophy with preserved systolic functions. Assessment of the force of contraction is the most subjective and least quantifiable aspect of precordial examination.

### Duration

The duration of the systolic outward motion is probably the most important feature of the precordial examination, although cardiomegaly or hypertrophy can exist in the presence of a brief 'normal' outward movement, or even when the PMI is absent, truly sustained LV impulse in the supine or 30° elevation position is distinctly abnormal. Such findings suggest a pressure overstressed ventricle (e.g. aortic stenosis, hypertension or an LV chamber with a depressed ejection fraction and a substantialy dilated cavity. A Study by 'Conn' demonstrated that a sustained apex impulse in the supine position was highly correlated with an increase in angiographically determined LV mass, and this observation was actually more sensitive than the electrocardiogram (ECG) in the diagnosis of LV hypertrophy. The critical point to assess is whether or not the impulse 'stays up' into the second half of systole. Timing that uses simultaenous auscultation of S1 and S2 is essential in making this observation. With practice, one can be quite accurate in assessing the actual duration of the apical impulse. Simple observation of movement of the chest piece of the stethoscope resting on the PMI may be helpful.

### Left Lateral Decubitus Position

It is unclear whether LV impulse that becomes sustained when the patient is turned into left lateral position which is of normal duration in the supine position, has the same specificity for LV enlargement as a sustained impulse (LV heave) that is present when the patient is lying flat. Since the left decubitus position causes the heart to approximate the chest wall more closely, many experts feels that the observation of a prolonged impulse in this position has little diagnostic value. Some believe that a definite sustained impulse in the left lateral position is highly indicative of true LV dilatation. False positives may occur, however, echocardiography is recommended in equivocal cases.

### Contour

The normal apical impulse is a brief, nonsustained anterior motion in early systole. A sustained LV movement is the commonest abnormality of contour, but occasionally other different types are also recorded.

### A Double Systolic Impulse or Bifid Impulse

It may be seen in hypertrophic obstructive cardiomyopathy (IHSS) and occasionally in some patients with severe LV dyssnergy or LV aneurysm in coronary artery disease. Presystolic distention is commonly found in the left lateral position in subjects who have decreased LV compliance, complicated from coronary artery disease, hypertensive heart disease, or aortic valve disease. Palpable diastolic events, such as an S3 or a pericardial knock, also fall into the general category of contour variations.

### Palpable a Wave (Presystolic Distention)

Palpable a waves are usually detected in the left posture. The apical beat is carefully localised, and varying pressure is applied with the pads of the fingers at the site of the LV impulse. A double early systolic impulse is noted, feeling like a 'shelf or ridge' on the upstroke of the beat. Usually, this low amplitude finding will best be felt when finger pressure is light; firm pressure with the fingers may make the finding more difficult or impossible to feel. On occasion, this presystolic distention can be quite prominent. The palpable a wave reflects a high LV end-diastolic pressure and decrease LV compliance. It is important observation because it documents a definite abnormality that usually implies LV hypertrophy and increased chamber stiffness. The audibility of the S4 does not correlate with palpability; presystolic distention may be detectable when the S4 is quite soft. Occasionally, one may not be able to hear an S4 at all, even though it is palpable; this is because the frequency of the diastolic filling event is extremely low (usually, less than 60 cycles per second).

### Palpable S3

The S3 is less often palpable than an S4. It is most often observed in severe mitral regurgitation or in a markedly dilated cardiomyopathic ventricle. As with S4, palpation is greater enhanced in the left decubitus position. The S4, appears as a brief outward motion in early systole, gently tapping the examining finger pads, but not displacing the fingers, since it is usually not forceful.

### Palpable S4

A palpable S4 is related to decreased LV compliance usually as a result of hypertrophy without dilatation or ischemia with increased, diastolic stiffness. A palpable S4 is always associated with LV end-diastolic pressure that is elevated, sometimes strikingly so, although early and mid-diastolic pressure is often normal in hypertensive heart disease, coronary artery disease, and occasionally, in congestive cardiomyopathy. The implications of a palpable S4 are quite different from those of a palpable S3 in the former case, LV systolic function is usually well preserved and the ejection fraction is normal. A palpable S3 (in the absence of significant mitral regurgitation) is associated with high LV filling pressurs, as in dilated ventricle, and decreased systolic function.

### Palpable Right Ventricle (S3 and S4)

The pathophysiology of palpable S3 and S4 generated in the right ventricle is similar to that in the left heart. Compliance changes (RV hypertrophy secondary to pulmonay hypertension) may result in a palpable RV S4. Increased blood flow across the tricuspid valve may produce a prominent S3. Tricuspid regurgitation is a good example. A large left-to-right shunt and atrial septal defect may also occasionally produce a palpable RV S3. In severe RV dysfunction, an S3 may be heard and felt. Classically, RV events are marked by inspiratory augmentation and expiratory attenuation or disappearance.

### Other Causes of Palpable Cardiovascular Activity

In addition to the tactile precordial phenomena related to LV and RV systolic and diastolic events palpable precordial activity is occasionally detectable as a result of vascular pulsations or ectopic LV wall motion abnormalities.

### Palpable Cardiovascular Events at the Level

#### *Aorta*

When either the ascending aorta or the aortic arch is enlarged or dilated, palpable systolic pulsations may be detected. Thus, with aortic aneurysms, diffuse aortic dilatation, or aortic dissection, a systolic impulse may be felt in the right first or second intercostal space, in the right or left sternoclavicular junction, or in the suprasternal areas. Dilatation or enlargement of the brachiocephalic vessels may also cause prominent vascular pulsations at the supersternal notch or above the clavicles.

#### *Pulmonary Artery*

Dilatation or enlargement of the pulmonary artery is usually associated with pulmonary hypertension, which itself may resuit from hyperkinetic; high flow states or from increased pulmonary vascular resistance. Idiopathic dilatation of the pulmonary artery results in an enlarged proximal pulmonary artery segment. All these conditions may produce a palpable systolic impulse in the second to third left intercostal space just to the left of the sternal edge. This is easily detectable in thin subjects.

#### *Left Ventricular Ectopic Impulse*

Focal wall-motion abnormalities or big LV aneurysms may produce systolic impulses that are detectable at sites away from the LV apical beat, usually medial and superior to the apical area. With anteroseptal LV scarring or dyskinesis, the ectopic impulse may be found at the lower parasternal edge and thus may simulate RV activity.

#### *Palpable Heart Sounds and Murmurs*

Loud sounds, such as an increased S1, A2 or P2 are often readily palpable. An opening snap is commonly palpable in mitral stenosis, as a loud S1, on occasion the diagnosis of this valve lesion can be made prior to using the stethoscope. Ejection clicks may be easily felt; the aortic ejection sound is detected at the LV apex, while a pulmonic ejection sound is palpable at the upper left sternal border.

#### *Thrills*

Any loud murmur may be transmitted to the chest wall, where it can produce a vibratory sensation to the examining hand. These palpable murmurs or thrills correlate with a murmur intensity of grade IV/VI or greater. Such murmurs may be felt at the apex (mitral regurgitation, hypertrophic obstructive cardiomyopathy), left sternal border (ventricular septal defect) or cardiac base (pulmonic stenosis, aortic stenosis). Obviously, in thin subjects the likelihood of a thrill is greater than in muscular or bulky patients. A diastolic thrill may occasionally be felt usually a the apex with the subject in the lateral decubitus position in mitral stenosis, or at the lower left sternal border in acute aortic regurgitation secondary to a perforated or ruptured aortic cusp.

## PERCUSSION

Under ordinary circumstances, percussion is neither necessary nor useful. When a PMI cannot be identified, however, the technique may help establish the presence or absence of cardiomegaly and will identify the approximate left border of the heart. In patients with a large pericardial effusion, the apex beat may actually be detected inside the lateral border of the cardiac silhouette, as determined by percussion (Figs 1.72 and 1.73).

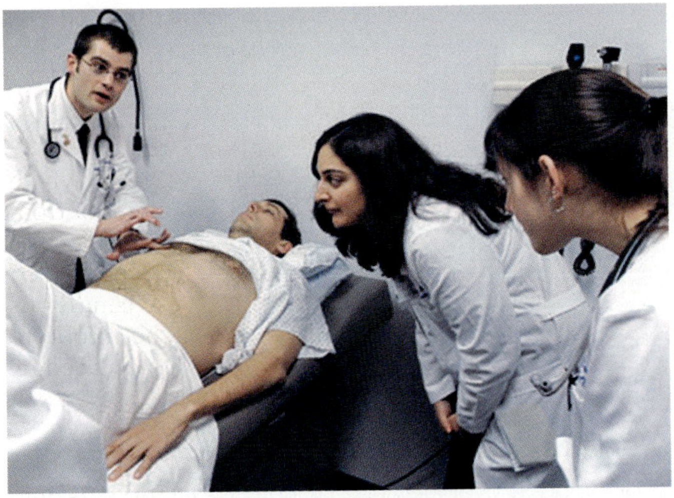

Fig. 1.72: Senior resident in cardiology is demonstrating to the medical students the clinical technique of percussion on the chest of one of the patients admitted to the medical college hospital

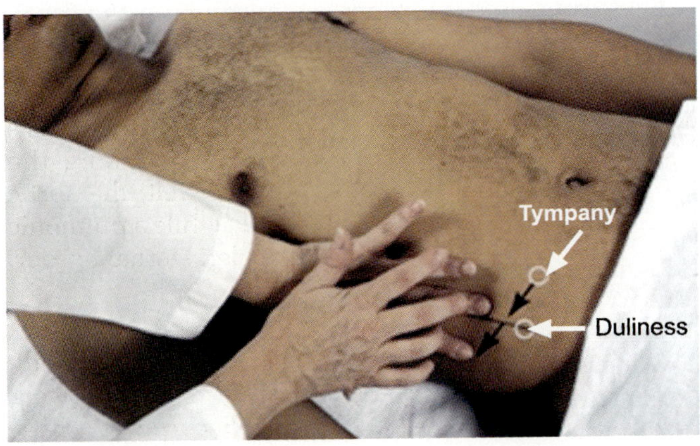


Fig. 1.73: Method of percussion over lower lung and liver areas for fluid and enlargement in patient with heart failure

## AUSCULTATION

Auscultation is depicted with Figs 1.74–1.85.

### Stethoscope

The chest piece should have a diaphragm and a bell. High frequency sounds and murmurs are heard better with the diaphragm, e.g. opening snap and aortic diastolic murmur. The bell transmits low frequency sounds better, e.g. gallop sounds, and mitral diastolic murmur. The bell should be applied very lightly to the chest when listening for these low frequency sounds.

### New Visual, Amplified Stethoscope for Hearing Impaired Clinicians

Properly diagnosing the patients using a stethoscope requires good hearing to discern the murmurs from normal heart sounds. Yet many doctors and nurses suffer from poor

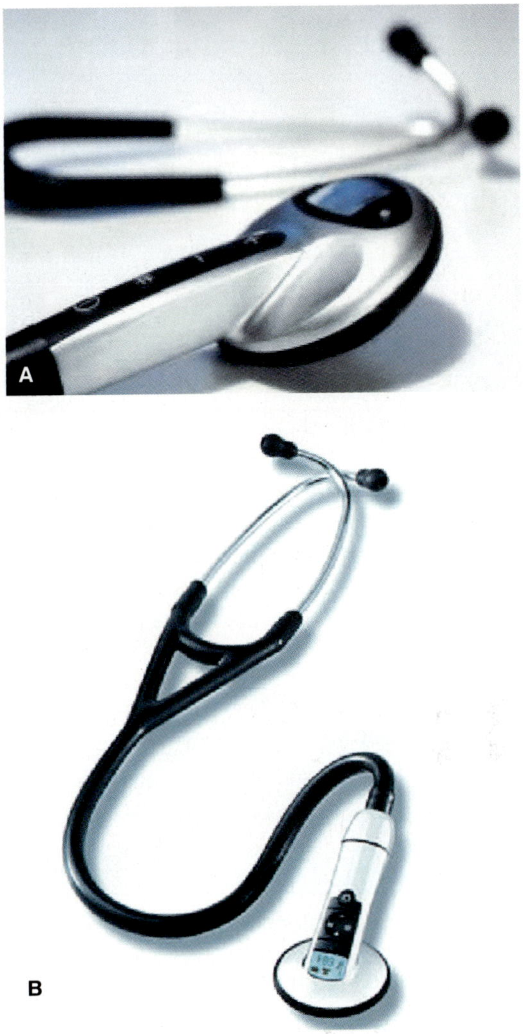


Fig. 1.74: (A) Conventional stethoscope used by the doctors for auscultation. (B) 3M Littmann Scope-to-Scope Tele-Auscultation System for remote diagnosis

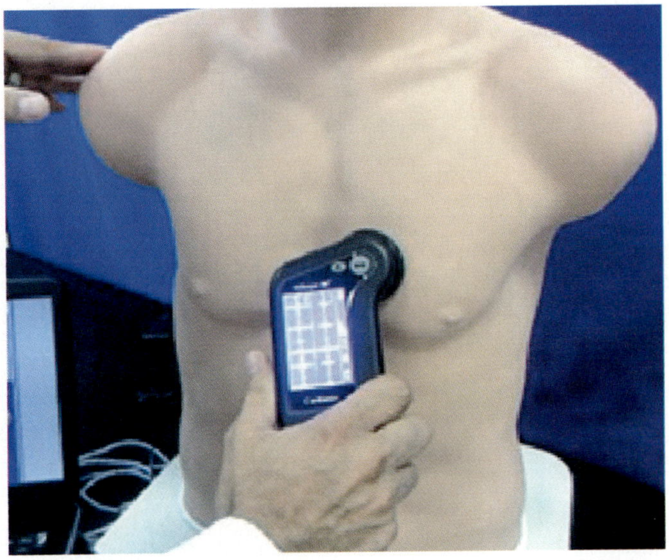

Fig. 1.75: New visual, amplified stethoscope for hearing impaired clinicians

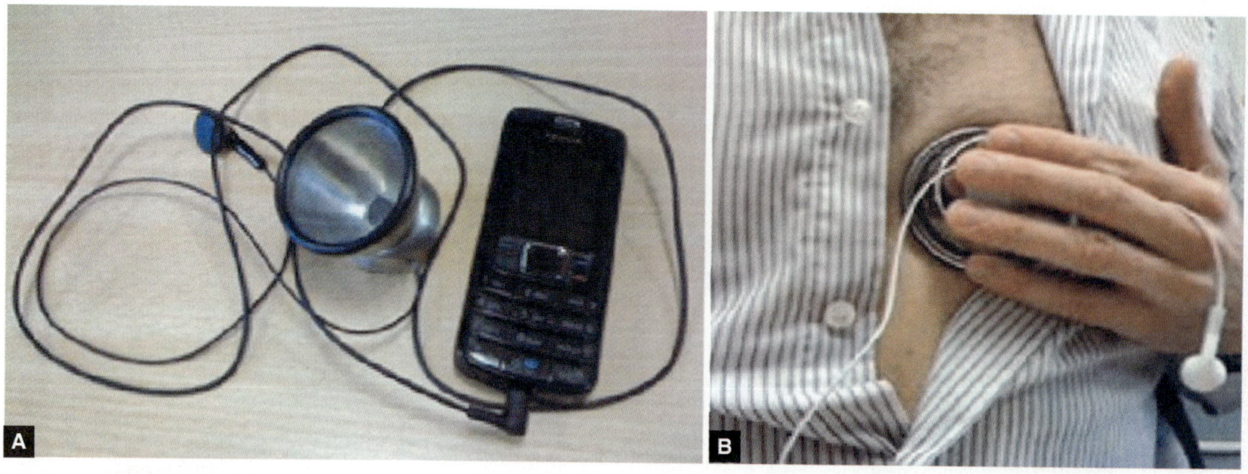


**Fig. 1.76:** (A) Mobile phone stethoscopes, and (B) its applicability over the chest of the patient

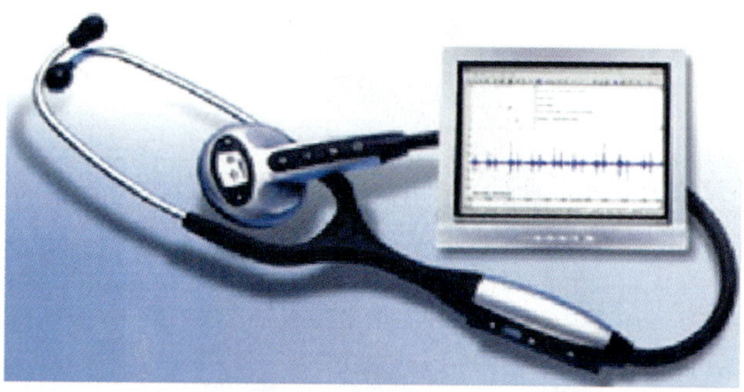

**Fig. 1.77:** Heart murmur detection software designed to support physicians in analyzing cardiac sounds for the identification and classification of suspected murmurs

hearing, making it difficult to auscultate their patients, seriously hampering their ability to perform a basic screening. The Cardionics ViScope aims to solve that problem by providing both amplification of the audio signal and a visual display of the phonocardiogram or phonopneumogram.

The device is compatible with in-the-ear or open fit behind-the-ear hearing aids, offering the ability to boost the signal 30 times over a conventional stethoscope. Visualization assists the listener in identifying the position of clicks, rubs, knocks, snaps or murmurs in the cardiac cycle. Murmurs such as aortic stenosis, aortic regurgitation or mitral regurgitation are clearly seen. Pediatric sounds including atrial septal defect, ventricular septal defect and primary pulmonary hypertension are easily identified.

*How it works:* Simply place the stethoscope on the chest and as the sounds are detected, the phonocardiogram of heart sounds will be displayed on the screen. Sounds can be downloaded to the ViScope-100 software for storage and recall. With a resolution of 1024×768 pixels, the software allows the trace to be enlarged for a better view. Calipers allow measurement of events such as the opening snap of mitral stenosis.

## Mobile Phone Stethoscopes

A team of researchers from the University of Oxford have developed a new kind of stethoscope that uses the micro-

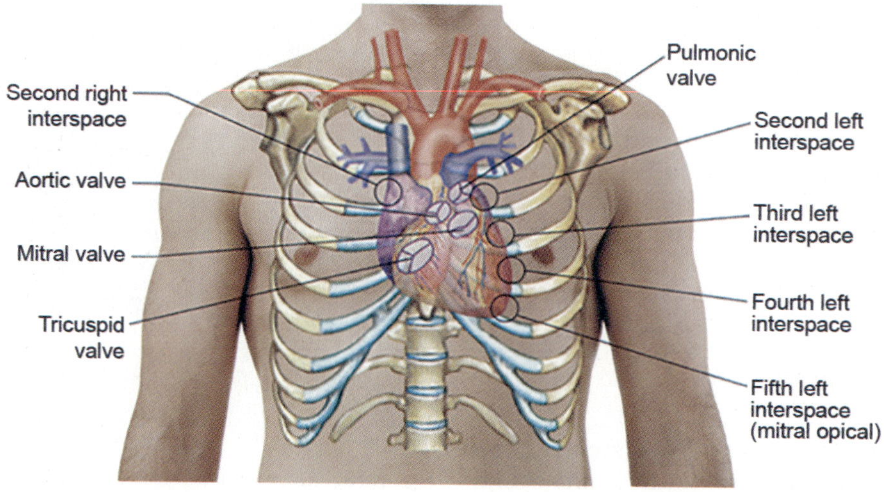


**Fig. 1.78:** Diagrammatic representation of conventional area of auscultation

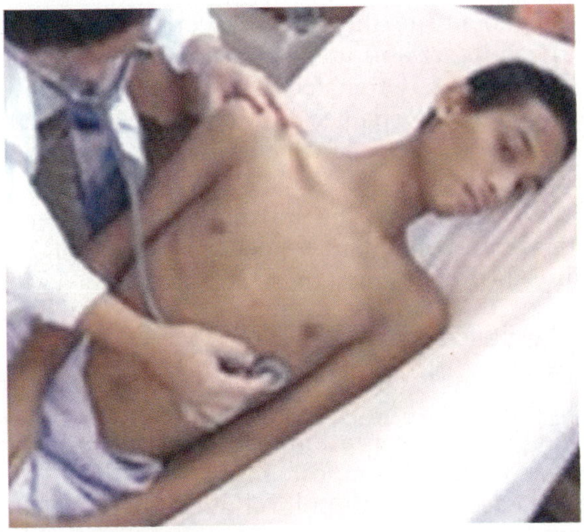

**Fig. 1.79:** Method of auscultation lying left lateral position for augmentation of apical events

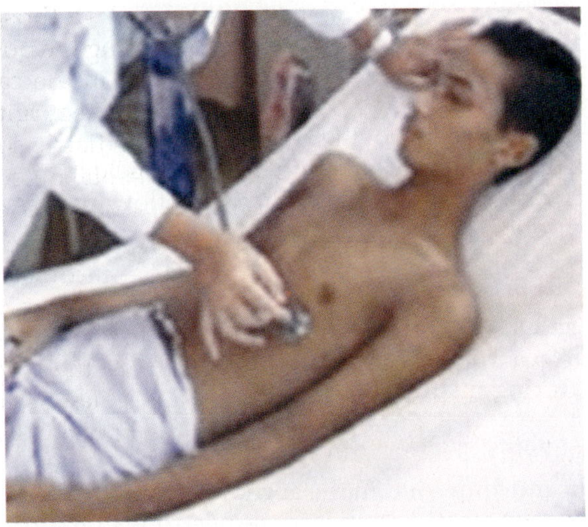

**Fig. 1.80:** Method of auscultation lying supine in the bed at 45° position for apical events

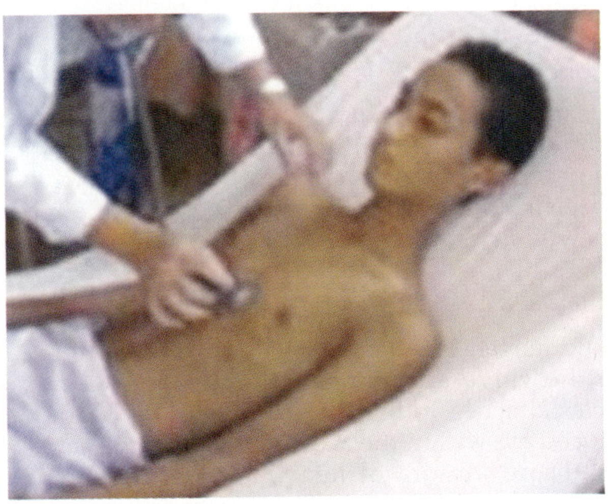

**Fig. 1.81:** Method of auscultation for mitral and tricuspid valvular defects

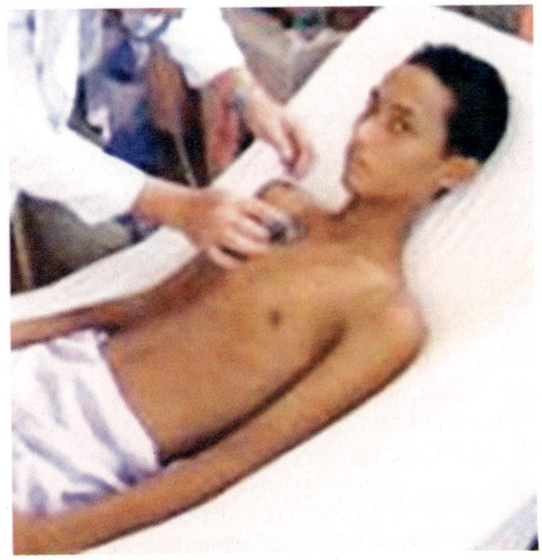

**Fig. 1.82:** Method of auscultation for aortic defects

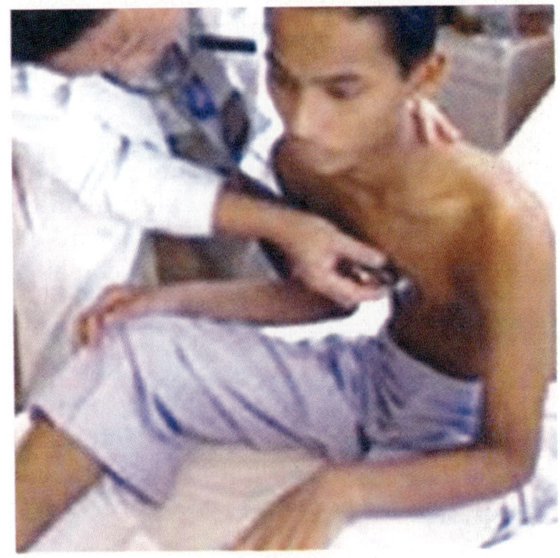

**Fig. 1.83:** Method of auscultation while sitting and leaning farward posture for augmentation of aortic and pulmonary events

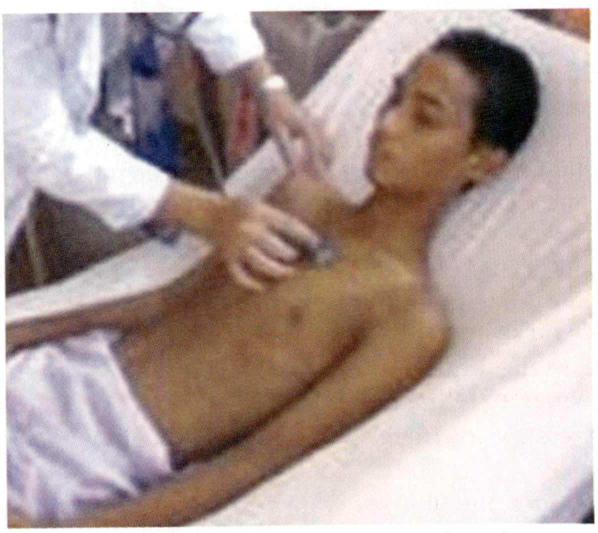

**Fig. 1.84:** Method of auscultation for pulmonary valve

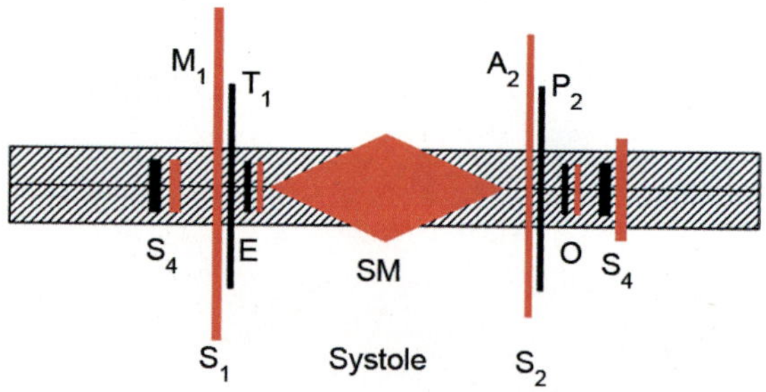


**Fig 1.85:** Heart sound events represented graphically. The red bars represent left-side events, and the black bars represent right-side events. The gray area is normally inaudible. The first heart sound (S1) contains two components—the mitral valve closure sound (M1) and the tricuspid valve closure sound (T1). The second heart sound (S2) contains two components—the aortic valve closure sound (A2) followed by the pulmonary valve closure sound (P2). The presystolic (atrial) gallop sound (S4) is normally inaudible. The prodiastolic (ventricular) gallop (S3) may be audible and is normal in children. Innocent systolic murmur (SM) is a common normal finding, especially in children. Ejection sounds (E) are normally inaudible. Opening snaps (O), if audible, indicate some level of pathology. Adapted from Leatham

phone input of a cell phone. The rudimentary stethoscope is basically a cell phone with an external microphone attached to the base of an egg-cup to focus and collect the sounds. The phonocardiograms recorded can be analyzed by a computer to filter out distortion and noise and process the signal to identify heart rate and abnormal heart sounds. So far, the stethoscope has been tested with an iPhone 3G and a Nokia 3100 Classic. Surprisingly, the Nokia 3100 Classic outperformed a 3M Littmann Electronic Stethoscope in detecting heart rate. According to Oxford, an Android version of the phonocardiogram processing software is also in the work.

### A New Littmann Scope-to-Scope Tele Auscultation System

It allows physicians to remotely listen to patients using a stethoscope as though they are on-site. Using bluetooth connectivity, the system transfers the real time audio gathered on one Littmann Model 3200 stethoscope to another, anywhere in the world. It is truly amazing how the stethoscope, from being a medical diagnostic device, has moved to also become a communication and telemedicine device.

- Allows clinicians to provide world-class patient care by hearing internal sounds of the body clearly across data networks in real-time, from anywhere in the world.
- Uses the bluetooth enabled Littmann Model 3200 electronic stethoscope.
- Offers a user-friendly design and phenomenal sound quality.
- Requires one-time software set-up that takes only a few minutes to complete.
- At the patient site, the scope-to-scope software digitally captures heart sound with a state-of-the-art sound sensor, wirelessly transfers the sound to software using the bluetooth → enabled Littmann → Model 3200 electronic stethoscope, and sends the sound across the internet securely.
- At the consultant site, the sound is delivered to the eartips of the consultant, who hears the patient's internal sounds as if the patient were in the room.

### Site of Auscultation

The site of maximum intensity of a sound of murmur is important in deciding its origin, but it cannot be taken as reliable clinical observation, e.g. the murmur of aortic stenosis is frequently loudest at the apex. The diagnosis of the basic defect accounting for a murmur is considerably more accurate when the murmur is also analysed for:

- Timing
- Quality
- Direction of selective propagation
- Influence of respiration.

#### *Mitral Events*

Loudest in the region of the apex beat heard with the patient turned on the left side and with the breath held in expiration (heart nearest chest wall with increased flow through valve on expiration).

#### Tricuspid Events

Localised to the fourth left intercostal space at the sternal edge. Accentuated by inspiration (increased flow across valve during inspiration) (Fig. 1.81).

#### Aortic Events

Systolic murmur loud in the aortic area, at the cardiac apex and over the carotid arteries in the neck (Figs 1.82 and 1.83).

Regurgitant murmur loudest in third and fourth left intercostals spaces at the sternal edge with the patient leaning forward in expiration (direction of the turbulent jet).

#### Pulmonary Events

Loudest in the pulmonary area and usually localised to it. Accentuated during inspiration. Low pressures in the right heart produce soft noises which are not conducted widely, but become louder with the increased blood flow into the lungs with inspiration (Fig. 1.84).

## THE HEART SOUNDS

The sudden tensing of a heart valve produces vibrations to both the valve and chordae tendineae and papillary muscles attached to the valve. Many of the vibrations, so produced are within the acoustic range of the ear, and the normal and abnormal heart sounds are the audible vibrations produced in this way from the four valves of the heart (Figs 1.85–1.89 and Tables 1.3 and 1.4).

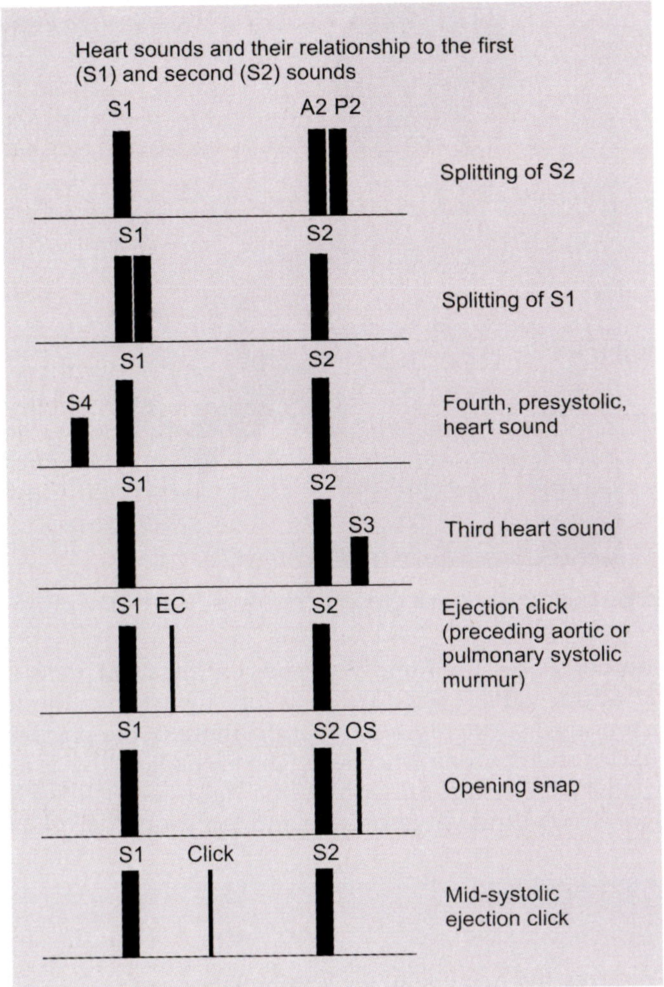


**Fig 1.86:** Diagrammatic representation of various types of ejection clicks, sounds and their splitting, along with opening snap at different timings of human cardiac cycle

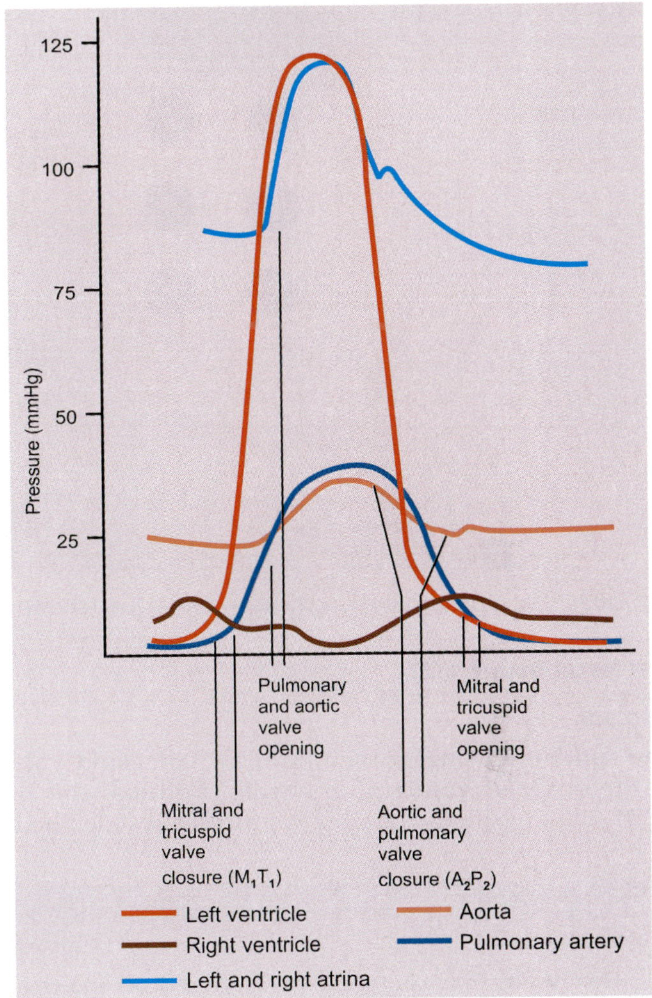


**Fig. 1.87:** Intracardiac tracings of LV, RV, RA, LA, aorta and pulmonary artery demonstrating opening and closure of mitral and tricuspid valve (M1-T1) and opening and closure of aortic and pulmonary valves (A2- P2) in cardiac cycle of normal person

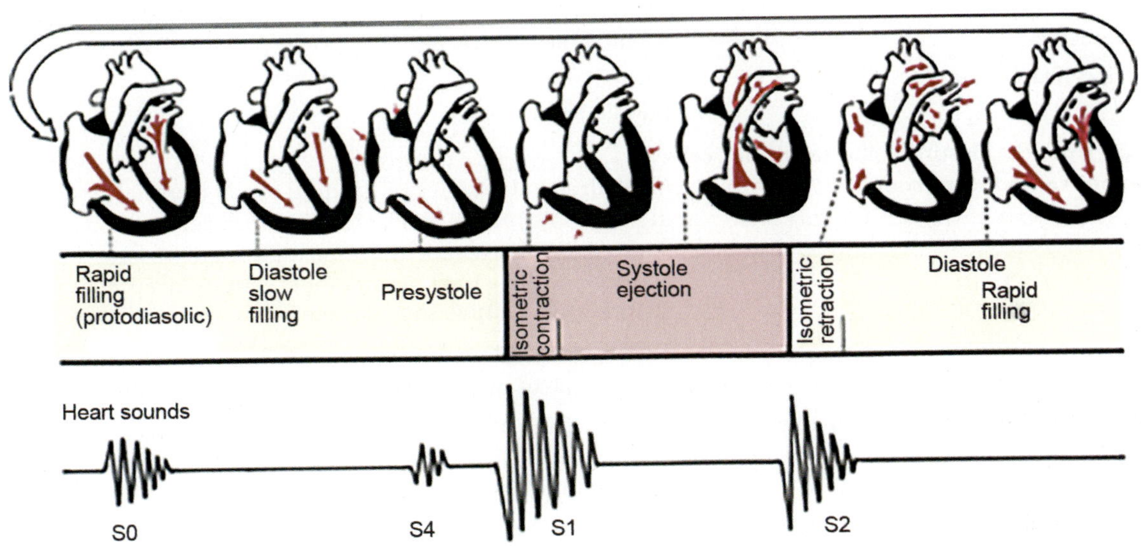


**Fig. 1.88:** Cardiac sounds and associated cardiac physiological changes are part of the cardiac cycle (From Jarvis C: Physical examination and health assessment, 5th edition, Philadelphia, Saunders, 2008)

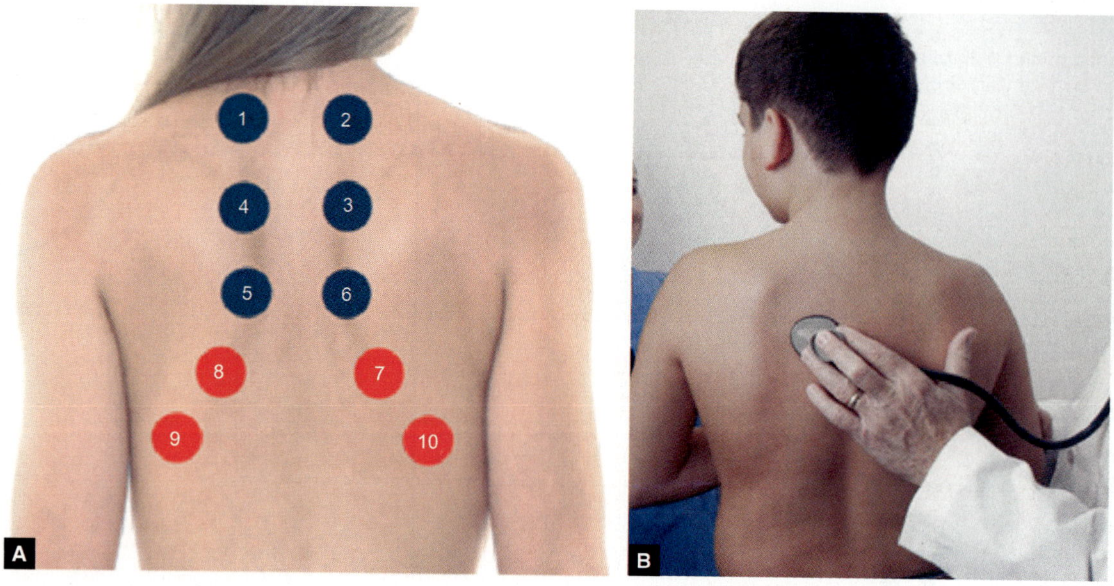


**Fig. 1.89:** Auscultation of the lung bases—zones 7–10 shown (A) should be performed in a thorough cardiovascular examination (B)

## First Heart Sound (S1)

### *Normal*

The sudden tensing of the mitral and tricuspid valves at the onset of ventricular systole produces the first heart sound. With the onset of ventricular systole, the left ventricular pressure rapidly exceeds the left atrial pressure. The mitral valve cusps are therefore thrust into the left atrium until suddenly held in apposition by the papillary muscles and chordae tendineae. The tricuspid valve is also closed by the rising pressure in the right ventricle within 20 msec of mitral valve closure and the sounds produced

**Table 1.3:** Heart sounds and their causes

| Heart sounds | Causes |
|---|---|
| **$S_1$: This results from contraction of the ventricles and closure of AV valves and opening of the semilunar valves** | |
| | 1. The heart beats force fully in exerciseor excitement, fever or anemia<br>2. Mitral stenosis when it is 'booming' |
| **Decreased in intensity** | 1. Pericardial effusion<br>2. Constrictive pericarditis<br>3. When P-R interval is prolonged in acute rheumatic fever<br>4. Myocarditis. |
| **Varying in intensity** | Congenital heart block |
| **Splitting of first heart sound** | 1. Normal in healthy children<br>2. Bundle branch block |
| **$S_2$: This results from the closure of the semilunar valves** | |
| **Wide splitting of second heart sound** | 1. In children mild degree of splitting of S2 is normal<br>2. Right bundle branch block (splitting increased with inspiration)<br>3. Any condition where there is increased flow of blood to the right ventricle (ASD, VSD, anomalous venous drainage) in ASD both the factors are operative so that there is a wide splitting of S2 |
| **Single $P_2$** | 1. Tetralogy of Fallot<br>2. Severe type of pulmonary stenosis/pulmonary atresia |
| **$S_3$: This results from the vibrations of the heart during rapid filling of the ventricles** | |
| | It is heard at the apex and latter in the cardiac cycle in about 20% of the normal children and about 30% among children with rheumatic carditis |
| **$S_4$: This results from the high atrial pressurewave which is reflected back from the ventricles** | |
| | 1. Left ventricle stress<br>2. Systemic hypertension, ischemic heart disease and aortic stenosis |

**Table 1.4:** Reversed splitting of S2

**Delayed A2**

- Delayed electric activation of the left ventricle
- Complete left bundle branch block
- RV paced beats
- RV ectopic beats

**Prolonged LV mechanical systole**

- Compete left bundle branch block
- LV outflow tract obstruction
- Hypertensive cardiovascular disease
- Arteriosclerotic heart disease
- Chronic ischemic heart disease
- Angina pectoris

**Decreased impedance of the systemic vascular bed (increasead hangout)**

- Poststenotic dilation of the aorta as a result of aortic stenosis or regurgitatation
- Patent ductus arteriosus

**Early P2**

- Early electric—activation of the right ventricle
- Wolf-Parkinson-White's syndrome type B

by these two valves are heard as a single sound, i.e. the first heart sound (S1).

## Loud S1

### *Mechanism*

At the commencement of ventricular systole the valves are already almost in apposition as blood flowing into the ventricles has practically ceased. If the cusps still wide apart at the onset of ventricular systole with slack chordae, an abnormally loud first sound is produced when they are abruptly tensed.

### *Causes*

Mitral stenosis, tricuspid stenosis; high cardiac output states (the flow of blood through the valve in late diastole remains high, keeping the cusps wide open); short PR interval (atrial contraction maintains a high flow of blood through the valve in late diastole, keeping the mitral and tricuspid valves wide apart).

## Soft S1

### *Mechanism*

If the valve cusps are rigid and incapable of much movement, or if the cusps are already close together before the onset of ventricular systole, the first heart sound is soft.

### *Causes*

- Calcification or fibrosis of the mitral valve cusps in some of the patients with mitral stenosis limit valve movement. The valve cusps are nearly closed before the onset of ventricular systole when the PR interval is long, i.e. in first degree heart block.
- The varying PR interval of complete heart block has the effect of modifying the intensity of the first heart sound from loud, when the interval is short, to soft when the PR interval is long.

## Splitting of S1

Normally the tricuspid valve closes within 0.02 sec of the mitral valve and only one sound is heard. Asynchronous contraction of the ventricles in bundle branch block particularly right bundle branch block, may produce appreciable splitting of the first heart sound.

## Ejection Clicks

An ejection click is a short, high frequency clicking occurring shortly after the first heart sound and it arises from abnormal semilunar valves or from dilated great vessels.

### *Mechanism*

- When the ventricular pressures exceed the aortic and pulmonary artery pressures in early systole, the normal aortic and pulmonary valve cusps open widely against the vessel wall so that there is no obstruction to flow. Fusion of the cusps of these valves prevents their full opening and the abrupt arrest of the valve dome in a semi-open position produces a high pitched sound soon after the first heart sound.
- Ejection clicks can also arise from the ejection of blood into a dilated aortic root or into a dilated pulmonary artery.

### *Types of Ejection Clicks*

Aortic ejection click, arising from an abnormal aortic valve or from a dilated aorta. This click is loudest at the apex and at the lower left sternal edge.

Pulmonary ejection click, arising from an abnormal pulmonary valve or from a dilated pulmonary artery. A pulmonary ejection click is loudest at the pulmonary area and often heard only during expiration.

### *Causes*

- Aortic click
- Aortic valve stenosis
- Bicuspid aortic valve (a bicuspid valve cannot open completely)
- Dilated ascending aorta, e.g. systemic hypertension
- Pulmonary click
- Pulmonary valve stenosis
- Pulmonary hypertension (dilated main pulmonary artery)

## Second Heart Sound (S2)

### *Normal*

The vibrations produced by closure of the aortic and pulmonary valves give rise to the second heart sound. The aortic valve closes at the end of left ventricular systole when the left ventricular pressure falls below the aortic pressure and the pulmonary valve closes at the end of right ventricular systole.

In expiration, both valves close almost simultaneously and the sound is single. During inspiration the systemic venous return to the right ventricle is increased, and right ventricular systole is prolonged. Accordingly pulmonary valve closure is delayed and the second heart sound becomes split during inspiration into an aortic component (A2) and a pulmonary component (P2) which A2 by 0.04 seconds or more.

Normal splitting of the second heart sound on inspiration is usual at all ages, but is most frequent in the younger subjects. It is best heard in the pulmonary area.

Loud S2, when the sound splits on inspiration. It is possible to determine which of the valve closures sounds is loud. A2 is loud in systemic hypertension (more forceful closures of the aortic valve). P2 is loud in pulmonary hypertension. P2 is soft and not heard at the cardiac apex unless there is pulmonary hypertension.

### Splitting of S2

A constant gap between A2 and P2 throughout all phases of respiration is the characteristic feature of an ASD.

When the defect is large the right and left atria act as one common chamber and the increased return of blood to the right atrium during inspiration increased blood flow equally to both right and left ventricles. It therefore, results into the prolongation of both right and left ventricular systole and the gap between A2 and P2 does not alter.

### Reversed Splitting S2

#### Description

In reversed splitting, second heart sound is single on inspiration and clearly split into two components during expiration.

#### Mechanism

Reversed splitting implies that the aortic valve closes after the pulmonary valve. This occurs when left ventricular systole is prolonged or when the left ventricle contracts after the right ventricle.

#### Causes

Myocardial ischaemia or infarction, aortic stenosis, coarctation of the aorta (increased resistance to ejection) and large persistent ductus arteriosus (increase in left ventricular volume load). Left bundle branch block (delay in a activation of the left ventricle).

### Wide Splitting of S2

This is heard when pulmonary valve closure is delayed either because of prolonged right ventricular systole (pulmonary stenosis) or delay in onset of right ventricular systole (right bundle branch block).

### Opening Snap

Opening snap (OS) is a short, high-pitched, clicking sound closely following the second heart sound (0.06–0.12 seconds), heard loudest medial to the apex or at the lower left sternal border.

#### Mechanism

The sound is heard in mitral stenosis provided the fused valve cusps retain pliability. When the left ventricular pressure falls below the left atrial pressure, the mobile valve is pushed downward into the left ventricular cavity until it suddenly tightens in its most fully open position with a high pitched snapping sound.

#### Causes

*Mitral stenosis:* The opening snap is absent if the valve pliability is reduced by calcification or fibrosis.

*Tricuspid stenosis:* A tricuspid opening snap is only occasionally present and is difficult clinically to differentiate it from a mitral snap. A low frequency, soft thud, late after the second sound and heard at the apex (left ventricular third sound) or at the tricuspid area (right ventricular third sound).

### Third Heart Sound (LVS3)

#### Mechanism

During the rapid inflow phase of early diastole, the left ventricle elongates. The apex moving downward and the mitral valve ring upward. This phase of rapid ventricular filling ends when the mitral valve cusps are suddenly drawn taut, stretched between the apex and the mitral valve ring, by the papillary muscles and chordae tendinae. The vibrations produced may be audible as third heart sound which occurs about 0.16 seconds after A2 at the end of the rapid ventricular filling phase. Similarly, rapid filling of the right ventricle may produce a third heart sound from tautening of the tricuspid valve.

#### Causes

Physiological third heart sound heard at the apex in most children and in few young adults.The early filling phase of the ventricle is more rapid due to altered myocardial tone and the raised filling pressure.

Abnormally, large flow in the filling phase (mitral incompetence, aortic incompetence, ventricular septal defect, persistent ductus arteriosus) result into left ventricular third heart sound.

#### Causes of Right Ventricular Third Sound (RVS3)

1. Right ventricular failure
2. Constrictive pericarditis

This sound has a different mechanism and is of higher pitch and earlier than the usual third sound (0.1 second after A2). Sudden restriction of filling of the ventricle by the rigid pericardium plays some part in this.

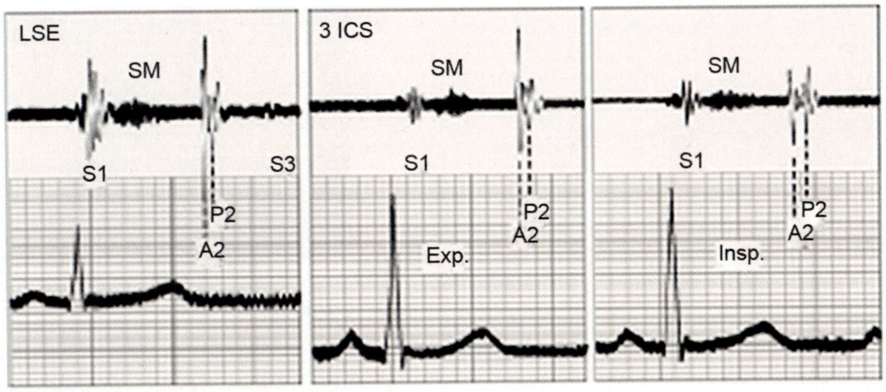


**Fig. 1.90:** A vibratory midsystolic murmur (SM) from a healthy 7-year-old boy. The murmur is maximal along the lower left sternal edge (LSE) and is accompanied by a physiologic third heart sound (S3) and normal respiratory splitting of the second heart sound. (A2/P2=aortic and pulmonary components; 3 ICS=third intercostal space)

### Fourth Heart Sound (Atrial Sound) (S4)

A low frequency, soft sound preceding the first heart sound.

#### *Mechanism*

This sound is heard when the left or right atrium contracts more forcefully than normal. A high atrial pressure wave reflected back from the ventricle tenses the mitral or tricuspid valve to produce the fourth heart sound. The sound is presystolic in timing, coincides with atrial systole and is heard when a ventricle is under stress.

#### *Causes of a Left Ventricular Fourth Sound*

Left ventricular stress, systemic hypertension, ischaemic heart disease and aortic stenosis.

#### *Causes of a Right Ventricular Fourth Sound*

1. Right ventricular stress
2. Pulmonary hypertension
3. Embolism
4. Pulmonary stenosis

## GALLOP RHYTHM

The presence of a third or fourth heart sound (or both) in addition to the usual first and second sounds is referred to as a gallop rhythm. By convention the term is used to imply a pathological condition. However, physiological third sound of the young is not called a gallop.

### Summation Gallop

At faster heart rate, an inaudible fourth sound may be superimposed on a normally inaudible third sound, the combined effect being the production of a gallop rhythm. The summation gallop disappears with slowing of the heart and does not necessarily mean ventricular stress

## CARDIAC MURMURS

Cardiac murmurs are depicted in Figs 1.90–1.98 and briefly described in Tables 1.5 and 1.6.

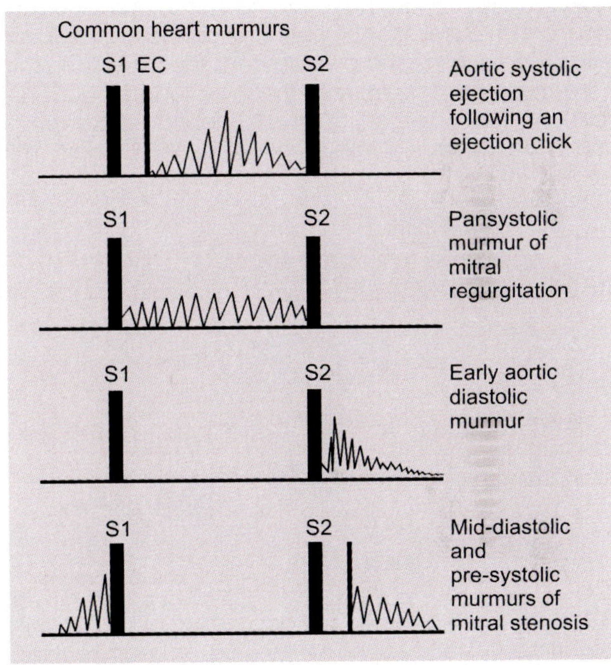


**Fig. 1.91:** Graphic representation of common heart murmurs in clinical practice

### How to diagnose innocent versus/pathological murmurs?

How should a clinician distinguish between innocent murmurs and pathological murmurs, and what factors should be evaluated? If the primary care physician is unsure whether the murmur is innocent, then referral to a pediatric cardiologist is the next step. Murmurs are common findings in infants and children. Most murmurs in infants and children originate through normal flow patterns with no structural or anatomic abnormalities of the heart or vessels and are referred to as 'innocent', 'physiological', or 'normal' murmurs. 'Innocent' is the preferred term because it strongly conveys that nothing is abnormal, as opposed to the older term 'functional', which is not always understood clearly by parents and patients as being 'normal'. Although

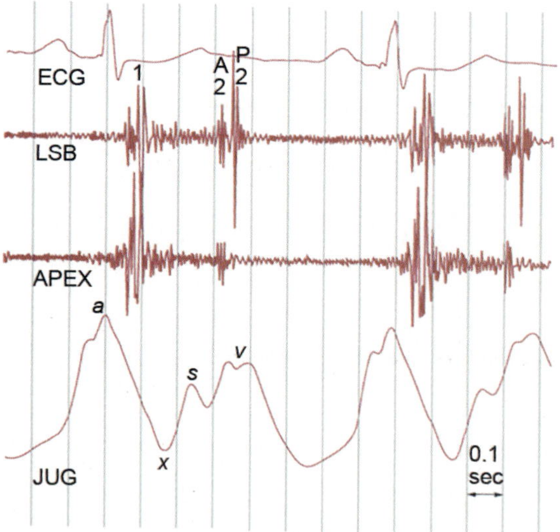


**Fig. 1.92:** Jugular venous pulse tracing from a patient with mitral stenosis and tricuspid regurgitation secondary to pulmonary hypertension. Note the shallow x descent, the midsystolic s wave, and the respiratory increase in the v wave (reproduced, with permission, from Tavel ME. Clinical Phonocardiography and External Pulse Recording. Year book Medical Publishers, 1978)

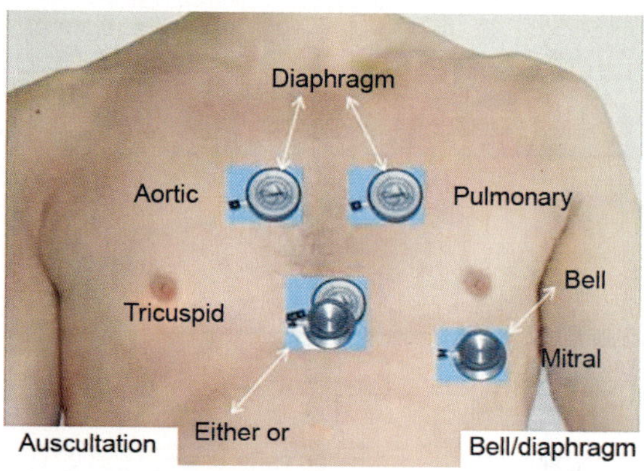


**Fig. 1.93:** Selective approach of application of bell/diaphragm of the Littmann stethoscope in listening of heart sounds and murmurs over the chest

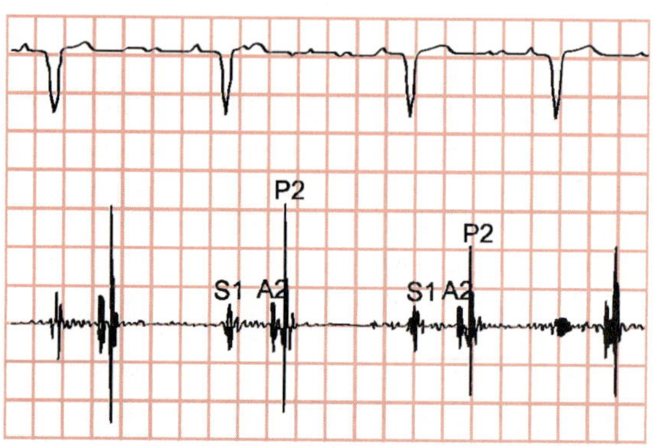


**Fig. 1.94:** Split second heart sound in a patient with severe pulmonary hypertension associated with a reversed patent ductus arteriosus. S1, first heart sound; A2, aortic component of second heart sound; P2, pulmonic component of second heart sound

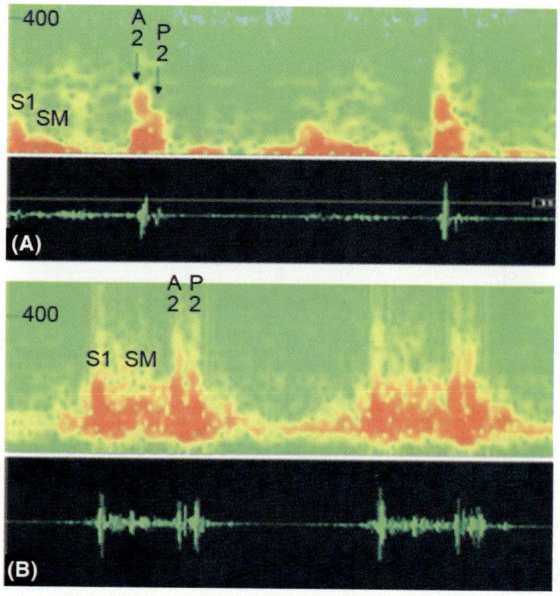


**Fig. 1.95A:** Examples of second heart sound characteristics, normal and abnormal. (A) Normal second sound, demonstrating both aortic (A2) and pulmonic (P2) components. Peak frequencies of the aortic component exceed those of the pulmonic. (B) Spectral display from a patient with an atrial septal defect. In this example, the second sound is widely split, with the peak frequency of the pulmonic component equaling or exceeding that of the aortic component. A systolic ejection murmur (SM) is also displayed in this instance, which contains relatively low peak frequencies in the range of 250 Hz. S1 indicates first heart sound

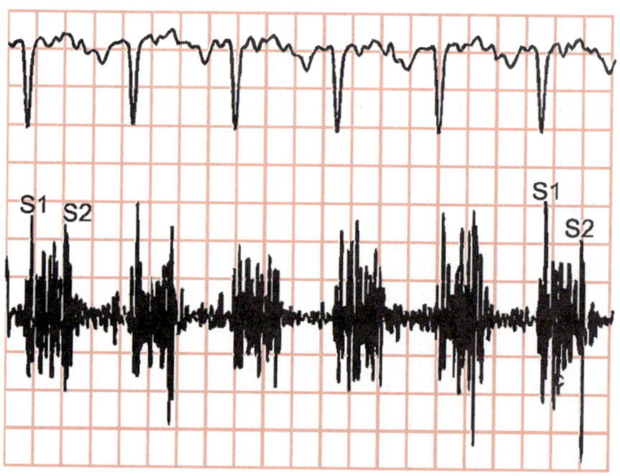


**Fig. 1.95B:** Phonocardiographic tracing of the plateau-shaped systolic murmur of mitral regurgitation. S1=first heart sound; S2= second heart sound; M=systolic murmur

murmurs may be heard in virtually anyone, they are most commonly heard in children. Virtually all children will have a murmur sometime while they are growing up. Conversely, murmurs may be created by abnormal flow patterns in the heart and vessels resulting from congenital heart abnormalities, valve disease, or other acquired conditions. In evaluating the infant or child with a murmur, the clinician must make a complete assessment of the cardiovascular system—not just listen to the murmurs because there are some serious cardiovascular abnor-

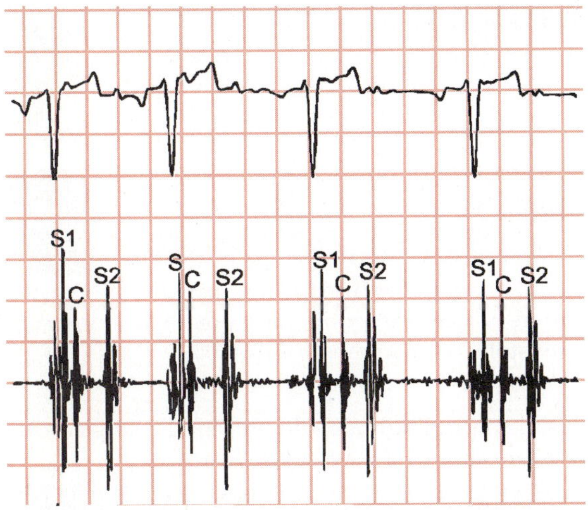


**Fig. 1.96:** Phonocardiogram showing high-frequency systolic clicks occurring at various points within systole. Midsystolic clicks are caused by valvular prolapse in patients with degenerative valve disease. S1, first heart sound; S2, second heart sound; C, systolic click

malities, that may have no murmurs. Looking for clues of heart disease, the clinician must obtain a focused history from the patient's parents. For infants, this history will include birth history, feeding patterns, breathing difficulties, color changes, growth pattern and activity levels. Changes in feeding patterns, particularly a progressively longer time to complete the feeding, may be an early sign of congestive heart failure. For children,

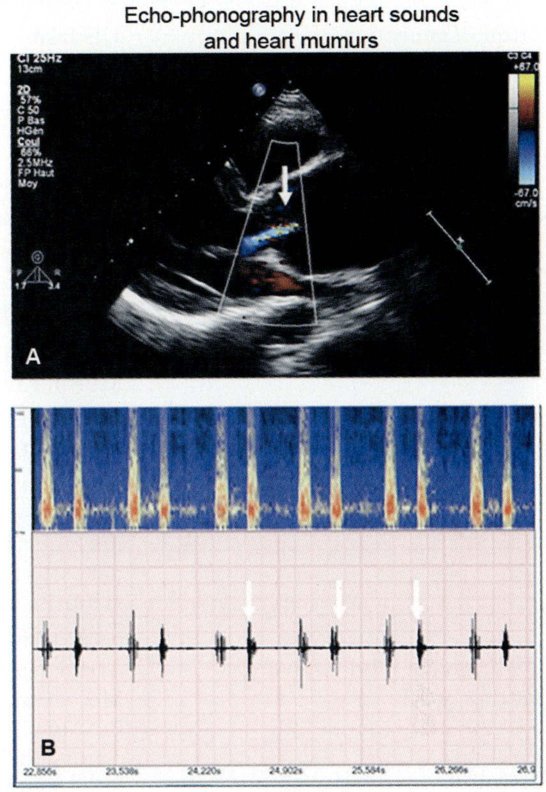


**Fig. 1.98:** Aortic insufficiency (indicated by white arrows) not heard with the acoustic stethoscope, but visualized using our intelligent stethoscope prototype and confirmed by echocardiography

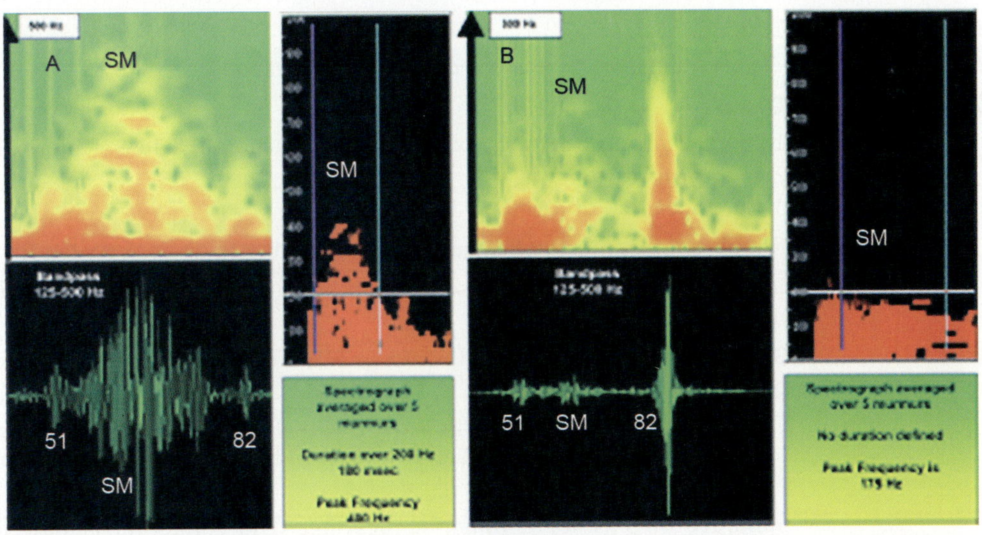


**Fig. 1.97:** (A) An example of a spectral display (upper left panel) recorded simultaneously with a waveform display (below) in a patient with severe aortic stenosis. The waveform image was obtained with a band-pass filter (125–500 Hz). A systolic murmur is noted that has a crescendo-decrescendo contour in the waveform display, whereas it also shows a crescendo-decrescendo frequency pattern in the spectral image. This latter image presents a colored plot, in which the relative signal intensities correlate with the colors, i.e. greater intensity is shown in orange and lesser intensity in yellow. Absence of sound is shown in green. The panel at the right shows a spectral average of murmurs derived from multiple cycles in this case. It is color coded to demonstrate only more intense frequencies uniformly in red, i.e. after a given 'cutoff' attenuation (–25 dB in this example), the red changes abruptly to black. Displayed in this way, this latter image shows a relatively high-peak frequency of 400 Hz (vertical scale at the left). This display also allows for measurement of the time duration for the murmur to exceed any arbitrary frequency level, in this case 200 Hz. (B) An example demonstrating a similar display for an individual with an innocent murmur, which appears primarily in early systole and does not reach a peak frequency of 200 Hz. SM indicates systolic murmur

**Table 1.5:** Heart murmurs in congenital heart diseases

| Description of murmurs | Disease |
|---|---|
| Continuous murmur with thrill | 1. PDA<br>2. Tetralogy of Fallot<br>3. Venous hum<br>4. Pulmonary arteriovenous fistula |
| Pansystolic murmur | *Ventricular septal defect*<br>Plateua throughout systole, loud, harsh in the third and fourth left intercostal space close the left lower sternal border. P2 heard in pulmonary area with normal split—if not obscured by the murmur. Systolic thrill in most cases (80%). |
| Mid or late systolic murmur with thrill | *Pulmonary stenosis*<br>Murmur in second left intercostal space. Thrill may be present. P2 single or may be split in moderate stenosis. In severe cases, P2 may not be heard. |
| Ejection systolic murmur (moderate or harsh) | *Fallot's tetralogy*<br>Systolic murmur in the third or fourth left intercostal space in 25% of cases the murmur is in the second left intercostal space due to valvular stenosis shorter than the murmur of the pulmonary stenosis. Murmur fainter or abscent when the pulmonary valve is much narrowed. The murmur is lower down in the cases of infundibular stenosis. The murmur is abscent in pulmonary atresia, P2 is single and loud in 20% of cases. Thrill is not common in infancy. |
| Systolic murmur of loud intensity, wide splitting of P2 | *Atrial septal defect*<br>Moderate or Faint systolic murmur in second left intercostal space with widely P2. Apical diastolic murmur is an indication of rapid inflow at the begining of diastole, occurs in larger defects of ASD and VSD. Associated systolic thrill indicates pulmonary stenosis. |
| Loud, harsh systolic murmur with a thrill in the first and second right interspace | *Congenital aortic stenosis*<br>Loud, harsh, systolic murmur in aortic area ending before second sound; systolic thrill present over the aortic area and transmitted to the neck over the carotids. |

**Table 1.6:** Heart murmurs (acquired heart disease)

| Description of murmur | Disease |
|---|---|
| Mitral systotic | 1. In mitral insufficiency (apex, blowing-conduction to axilla or inferior angle of scapula)<br>2. In any myocarditis<br>3. In endocardial fibrucelastosis |
| Mitral presystolic | Mitral stenosis, presystolic and crescendo leading to an accentuated first sound |
| Mitral mid-diastolic | In rheumatic heart disease of some standing but not yet full blown picture of mitral stenosis; first sound accentuated. |
| Mitral early diastolic | Short, faint, with a third sound occurs in 30% of acute rheumatic fever and disappears during convalescence. |
| Aortic diastolic | Occurs in 10% of children with acute rheumatic fever, collapsing pulse, etc. only later on. Decrescendo, often faint and best heard down the left sternal border with breath held at the end of expiration. |
| Pulmonary diastolic | Same features as aortic diastolic, best heard in congenital hearts and severe anemia. Also right ventricle hypertrophy and prominent pulmonary artery with pulsating hilar shadows. |

parents should be asked about activity capacity. Can the child keep up with peers while playing vigorously? Have there been complaints of shortness of breath, palpitations, or chest pain? Chest pain is a common complaint, but a cardiac cause is found in less than 1% of children complaining of chest pain.

Blood flow through the cardiac chambers is normally systematically streamlined. Murmurs are produced when there is turbulence of the blood flow. The origin of murmurs is determined by the application of the following parameters.

1. Timing in the cardiac cycle

2. Site of maximal intensity and conduction
3. Loudness and quality
4. Influence of respiration
5. Timing in cardiac cycle

Auscultation begins with listening for the normal sounds of the valves closing and for S1 and S2. It is important not to focus on murmurs initially. Atrial septal defect accounts for about one-third of the congenital defects first detected in adulthood. This is because the characteristic murmur, a pulmonary flow murmur, also is one of the most common childhood innocent murmurs. The key to diagnosis is appreciating the wide fixedly split-second heart sound resulting from right volume overload. This will not be easily appreciated if the clinician focuses on murmurs before defining the heart sounds. Gallop sounds also may be present, signaling difficulty in keeping up with the demands placed on the heart. Conversely, isolated S3 gallop sounds may be heard in healthy adolescents.

### Site of Maximal Intensity and Conduction of the Murmur

This is helpful in identifying the origin of murmurs but is unreliable if used in isolation from the other features, e.g. aortic systolic murmurs are often loudest at the apex and aortic diastolic murmurs are loudest at the fourth left interspace close to the sternum.

### Loudness and Quality

The loudness of a murmur correlates poorly with the severity of the lesion producing it. A very loud murmur may be produced by turbulent blood flow through a small ventricular septal defect whereas the murmur is softer with larger defects. Similarly the loudness of a mitral pansystolic murmur is a poor guide to the severity of the regurgitation.

### The Quality or Pitch of a Murmur Aids in its Identification

High pitched murmurs indicate a stream of blood under high pressure (aortic incompetence, mitral incompetence). Low-pitched murmurs are indicative of a turbulent blood flow under low pressure (mitral stenosis, diastolic flow murmurs).

### Influence of Respiration

With inspiration, the negative pressure in the thorax, sucks more blood into the right atrium from the superior and inferior venae cavae. The blood flowing across the tricuspid and pulmonary valves is, therefore, increased during inspiration and increases the intensity of pulmonary and tricuspid murmurs, making this a useful clinical sign. Inspiration also brings the lung over the heart, which tends to make all sounds less well heard on the chest wall and this at times leads to confusion.

In general, right sided events are louder or unchanged on inspiration and left-sided events are louder on expiration.

## Classic Types of Innocent or Flow Murmurs

*Presence or absence:* Innocent murmurs are murmurs produced by normal flow. Changing the flow should therefore change the intensity of the murmur. Characteristically, maneuvers that decrease the flow of blood returning to the heart through the venous system will decrease the intensity of flow murmurs, suggesting that the murmur is flow related or innocent. Changing the child's position from supine to sitting, then to standing, and finally to squatting during the examination will change the flow and is useful in helping to define innocent murmurs. The child may be asked to push out the abdomen or bear down to perform a Valsalva maneuver, which reduces venous blood flow to the heart and the intensity of innocent murmurs. An examiner can coax even a young toddler into doing this by placing a hand on the child's abdomen and asking the child to push it out.

### Still's Murmurs

These murmurs are low-pitched sounds heard at the lower left sternal area. They are musical or have a relatively pure tone in quality or may be squeaky. These most commonly occur between age of 3 and adolescence.

Because of low-pitched, they are heard best with the bell of the stethoscope. They are related to flow, and they can change with position alteration and then can decrease or disappear with the Valsalva maneuver. No clicks are present. Pulmonary flow murmurs. These are high-pitched, harsher murmurs heard at the upper left sternal border. Because they are high pitched, they are heard best with the diaphragm of the stethoscope. They are flow-dependent and also will change with position alteration and decrease or disappear with the Valsalva maneuver. These murmurs originate from the right ventricular outflow tract and radiate along the pulmonary arteries and, thus may be well heard in the back and axilla bilaterally. They are differentiated from pulmonic stenosis by their quality and from valvar pulmonic stenosis by the absence of an ejection click. Pulmonary flow murmurs can occur at any age, but they are common particularly in adolescents or in children with pectus excavatum. They are prominent in high-flow situations, such as when a child has a fever or is anemic, because flow increases in these situations. In infants, these sounds may be most prominent in the back or axilla because turbulence occurs when the blood flows from the larger main pulmonary artery to the smaller, less well-developed distal pulmonary arteries. In fetal life, the main pulmonary artery transports about 90% of the blood to the ductus arteriosus and only about 10% to the distal pulmonary arteries. The main pulmonary artery is thus large, whereas the distal pulmonary arteries are relatively smaller and come off at more acute angles than they do later as the child's chest grows. An analogy from nature would be the noise, that is created as a large stream narrows into smaller streams. This innocent murmur has been termed 'benign peripheral pulmonary stenosis of the newborn' to differentiate it from true anatomic obstructions to distal pulmonary arteries that occur in pathological conditions such as congenital rubella syndrome.

Systolic murmurs occur during ventricular systole. Diastolic murmurs occur in ventricular diastole. Continuous murmurs are heard throughout the cardiac cycle. Systolic Murmurs (Pansystolic, Ejection and Late systotic).

### Grading and Types of Murmurs

Murmurs are graded on a four point or, more commonly, a six-point scale. A common six-point scale is:

- Grade 1—audible with difficulty
- Grade 2—faint but recognizable
- Grade 3—moderate intensity
- Grade 4—loud
- Grade 5—louder, but still needing a stethoscope
- Grade 6—audible without a stethoscope

### Pansystolic Murmur

The pansystolic murmur beings with the first heart sound and remains of uniform intensity throughout systole up to the second heart sound A pansystolic murmur is caused by a 'leaking ventricle' (mitral incompetence tricuspid incompetence, ventricular septal defect). Blood escapes from the ventricle as soon as it begins to contract (first sound) and continues to escape until the pressures equalise between the ventricle and atrium (just after second sound). Left ventricular pressure exceeds left atrial pressure throughout systole from the first heart sound untill after A2 and blood escapes through the mitral valve into the left atrium giving rise to a murmur throughout systole).

A pansystolic murmur is heard in the following conditions:

*Mitral incompetence:* The murmur is maximal at the apex, loudest on expiration and conducted into the axila.

*Tricuspid incompetence:* The murmur is maximal at the lower left sternal edge and becomes louder during inspiration.

*Ventricular septal defect:* The murmur is classically loud and rasping in quality, maximal at the lower left sternal edge and loudest on expiration.

### Ejection Murmur

There is a short gap between the first heart sound and the beginning of the murmur.

The murmur begins slowly, reaches highest intensity in midsystole and ends before the second heart sound. An ejection systolic murmur arises at the aortic or pulmonary valves when the blood flow through them is turbulent. This may be caused by narrowing of the valve orifice (aortic stenosis and pulmonary stenosis) or by a greatly increased flow through an orifice of normal size (high cardiac output states and left to right shunts). The murmur begins when the aortic or pulmonary valve opens, reaches its maximum with top most flow in midsystole and becomes soft again towards the end of systole. An ejection murmur must cease when flow across the valve ceases, that is, before the end of second sound which indicates closure of that valve.

### Late Systolic Murmur

This murmur likely to start well after the first heart sound and thereafter increases in intensity up to the second sound. It is characteristic of mild mitral regurgitation, when the greatest regurgitant flow occurs in late systole as seen in mitral valve prolapse.

### Diastolic Murmurs

*Early diastolic (regurgitant):* The murmur begins immediately after the second sound and is loudest at its onset, but may extend throughout diastole. High frequency and blowing in quality, the murmur is maximal usually in the third and fourth intercostal spaces close to the sternum, and may also be heard in the aortic area and at apex.

A leaking aortic or pulmonary valve allows blood to flow back into the ventricle as soon as the valve closes (second sound), and is loudest at the beginning when the aortic or pulmonary artery pressure is highest, becoming softer as the pressure falls in diastole.

An early diastolic murmur is heard in either aortic valve regurgitation or pulmonary valve regurgitation, usually as a result of pulmonary hypertension.

The murmurs of aortic and pulmonary regurgitation are so similar that differentiation is made on other evidence, such as a water hammer pulse favouring aortic in-competence, and evidence of pulmonary hypertension suggesting pulmonary incompetence.

### Mid-diastolic Murmur

The diastolic murmur begins some time after the second heart sound (Fig. 1.98). Delayed diastolic murmur is a more accurate description than mid-diastolic since the murmur may be short or may extend throughout the remainder of diastole. It is characteristically low-pitched rumbling in character.

The murmur from a stenosed mitral or tricuspid valve begins with the resumption of flow through valve at the end of isometric relaxation of the ventricle. The opening snap indicates the end of isometric relaxation and is followed by the murmur, loudest at its onset when the atrial pressure is greatest, becoming softer as the pressure gradient between atrium and ventricle falls during diastole. The length of the murmur is determined by the time taken for the left atrial pressure to equalize with left ventricular pressure. When stenosis is severe the left atrial pressure does not fall to the left ventricular diastolic level in the time available and the diastolic murmur persists up to the first heart sound.

#### *Causes of a Mid-diastolic and Flow Murmurs*

*Mitral stenosis:* Murmur is maximal at the apex.

*Tricuspid stenosis:* Murmur maximal at the lower left sternal edge and becoming louder during inspiration. Increased blood flow across normal mitral and tricuspid valve (flow murmurs). Flow murmurs are low pitched, usually short and occur at the time when blood flow through the valve is rapid, that is, around mid-diastole. Mitral flow murmurs are present when there is an increased flow across that valve due to a left to right intracardiac shunt (ventricular septal defect and persistent ductus arteriosus) or due to a generalised high cardiac output states (thyrotoxicosis, anemia and systemic arteriovenous fistula). Tricuspid flow murmurs are usually the result of an increased flow over the tricuspid valve resulting from an atrial septal defect.

### Presystolic Murmur

This murmur begins in late diastole and is at its loudest just before the first heart sound.

The presystolic murmur is the result of atrial systole due to flow of blood through a narrowed mitral or tricuspid valve. Atrial systole causes an increase in blood flow across the valve just before the first heart sound, provided the PR interval is normal. There is no presystolic murmur if atrial contraction is absent as in atrial fibrillation.

#### Causes

*Mitral stenosis:* Murmur maximal at the apex.

*Tricuspid stenosis:* Murmur maximal at the lower left sternal edge and louder during inspiration.

### Austin Flint Murmur

A presystolic murmur or a low rumbling diastolic murmur maximal at the apex and indistinguishable from the murmur of mitral stenosis.

This murmur is heard when there is free regurgitation at the aortic valve. The regurgitant stream impinges on the anterior cusp of the mitral valve and tends to hold it closed. Under these circumstances the diastolic murmur of mitral stenosis can be produced by a normal mitral valve.

### Continuous Murmurs

A continuous murmur extends uninterrupted from systole into diastole and is often heard throughout all phases of the cardiac cycle. When a communication exists between two parts of the circulation, one of which is at a higher pressure than the other throughout the cardiac cycle, blood flows uninterruptedly which results into a continuous murmur.

#### Causes

1. *Escape of blood from aorta:* Persistent ductus arteriosus. Blood flow through the ductus is maximal towards the end of systole when aortic pressure is highest. The murmur is heard below the left clavicle and is loudest in late systole.
2. *Pulmonary atresia:* Blood flows from high pressure aortic bronchial arteries into the lungs. Again loudest in systole, often heard below the right left clavicles or in the interscapular region at the back.
3. *Ruptured aortic sinus of valsalva:* Coronary artenovenous fistula and any other large systemic arteriovenous fistula.
4. Blood flowing from a high to a low pressure region in the lungs.
   a. Pulmonary artery branch stenosis
   b. Pulmonary arteriovenous fistula.

## SYSTEMIC FLOW MURMURS (SUPRACLAVICULAR SYSTEMIC BRUITS)

The systemic flow murmurs are harsh high-pitched murmurs caused by normal blood flow into the aorta and into the head and neck vessels and are heard best high up in the chest and above the clavicles (Figs 1.99–1.101). They are also heard best with the diaphragm of the stethoscope. No ejection click is associated with these murmurs. They are transmitted to the arch vessels and are heard when listening over the carotid arteries of the neck. It has been said that because of these sounds 'all children have carotid bruits'; however, the sounds differ in quality from true carotid bruits and are not associated with aortic outflow pathology.

## VENOUS HUM

It is common in children; mimics a continuous murmur and is caused by blood flowing through the great veins in the neck and the innominate veins (Fig. 1.102).

It can be distinguished from the murmur of a persistent ductus arteriosus by the following features; variations in posture and placing the head in different positions markedly affect the venous hum. Light pressure on the neck reduces venous return from the jugular veins and may abolish the venous hum. These are low-pitched continuous murmurs made by blood returning from the great veins to the heart. They are heard best with the bell of the stethoscope. By changing the position of the patient's head or by pressing in the area of the major neck veins, the flow may be changed and these murmurs will change or

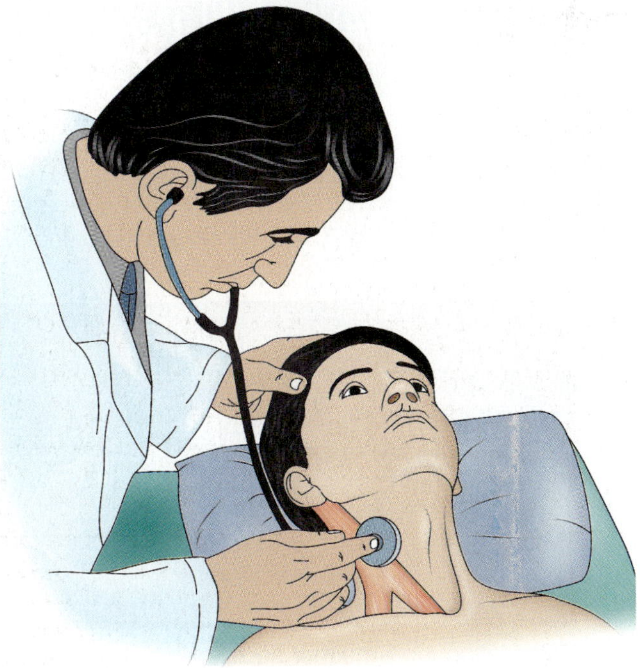

**Fig. 1.99:** Auscultation over the carotid artery

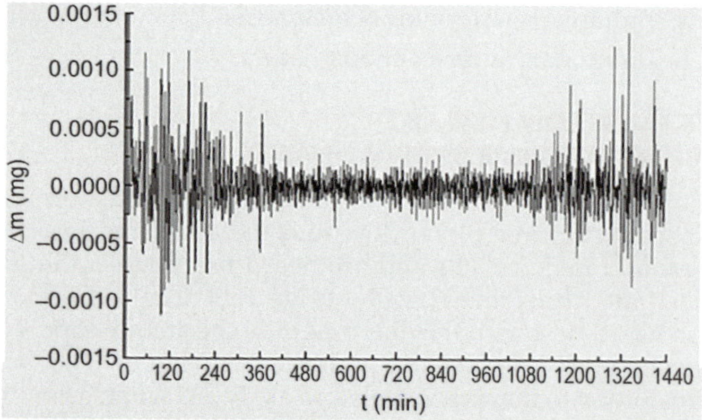


**Fig. 1.100:** A carotid bruit is an abnormal sound from the heart. The sound is in synchronization with the heartbeat. It is generally caused by turbulent blood flow, such as caused by irregularities in the wall of the blood vessel or by an abnormal connection (fistula) between an artery and vein. A bruit that is normally heard over the carotid artery is a sign that there are fats in the wall of the vessel. The bruit can be heard by using a stethoscope to listen to blood flow in the carotid artery. The carotid artery is the main artery in the neck region and is responsible for bringing blood to the head. A bruit indicates a fatty buildup (atherosclerosis) in the artery. Carotid bruit is a sign of the person's higher stroke risk

disappear. Having the child look down or to the side while listening will often make these murmurs or sounds disappear. They are differentiated from the murmurs of patent ductus arteriosus in that they are louder in diastole, when maximal flow occurs in the venous system, and are often heard bilaterally. Venous hums are sensitive to posture and head and neck position, whereas the murmur of patent ductus is not. Although an ECG is usually part of the evaluation and may be helpful, further testing is not needed in the overwhelming majority of infants and children to distinguish between normal or pathological hearts. It has been shown that a competent pediatric cardiologist can determine with a high degree of certainty, whether there is heart disease. Because of the characteristics of the sounds and the maneuvers that can be used to facilitate identifying them as flow-related phenomenon, these murmurs can be correctly identified without further testing. After concluding that the murmur or murmurs (a child may have more than one kind) are innocent, the practitioner should explain the findings to the parents and child. The practitioner should emphasize during the discussion that murmurs simply mean sounds or noises and that in and of themselves they are not synonymous with abnormalities of the heart. The clinician should stress

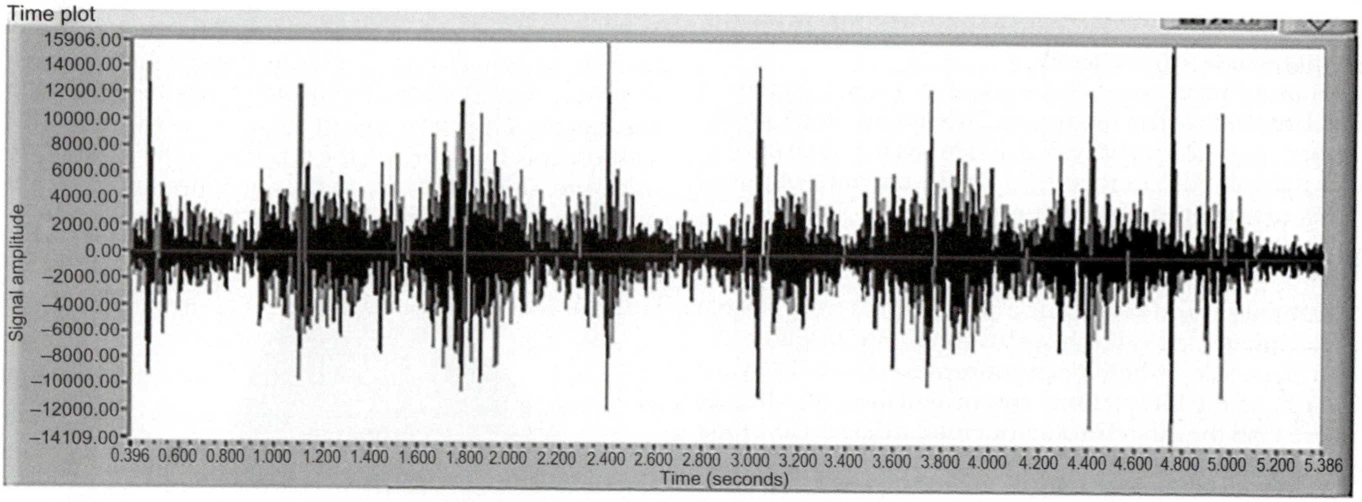


**Fig. 1.101:** Phonogram showing systo-diastolic murmur heard over the clavicle

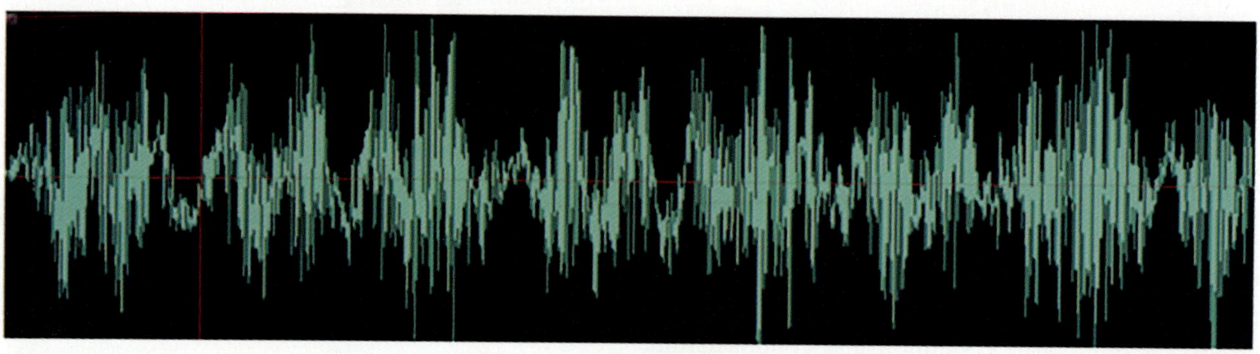

**Fig. 1.102:** Friction rub—murmur heard in a continuous fashion, regardless of cardiac cycle and may change in character in different patient positions (supine, on side, sitting, etc.)

that although a large percentage of infants and children have murmurs, less than 1% are born with the congenital heart defects that are the most common cause of heart disease in children. Parents should not be promised that their children will outgrow these murmurs because this is not necessarily true; adults can have innocent murmurs as well. Assurances should be given that because the heart is normal, whether or not the murmur disappears or changes is of no consequence. In addition, because flow changes the murmur, with growth and the changing configuration of chest and heart dynamics, murmurs may change, disappear, and reappear at various times-further evidence that the murmurs are indeed flow related and innocent.

## PERICARDIAL FRICTION RUB

The pericardial friction rub is a superficial sound produced by the rubbing together of inflammed surfaces of the pericardium (Fig. 1.102). It may be heard anywhere over the precordium and usually has two components during each cardiac cycle. It is often soft, localised to one small area, and the rub can be abolished by a pericardial effusion separating the inflammed surfaces. The superficial quality and timing of the sound, which is confined neither to systole nor diastole, distinguishes it from a murmur. It is commonly found in pericarditis of different aetiology.

## INVESTIGATIONS REQUIRED IN ESTABLISHING DIAGNOSIS

These investigations are depicted in Figs 1.103–1.114.

### Routine Laboratory Tests

Estemation of Hb%, packed cell volume (PCV), HIV screening and blood group typying are most most essential part of a preoperative work up in both acquired and congenital heart ailments.

### Chest X-ray

The interpretation of chest films requires lot of experience and proper technique. It is difficult to obtain a satisfactory film in the newborn and young in fants (Fig. 1.103).

Likewise, a film taken in expiration may produce a false picture of cardiac enlargement, or suggestive of congenital heart disease, because of the large thymic and cardiac silhouette. Dark films may create difficulties in detection of pulmonary vascularity. It is also worthwhile remembering that the cardiothoracic ratio is 55% in infants. After this age period a cardiothoracic ratio of 50% or less can be taken as normal. For a proper evaluation at least four views—posterior, anterior, lateral and oblique views may be necessary. In addition, these views of the chest may have to be supplemented with a barium swallow.

### Electrocardiogram

The electrocardiogram is an important diagnostic aid in the evaluation of the cardiovascular system and is a must for the diagnosis of arrhythmias (Fig. 1.104).

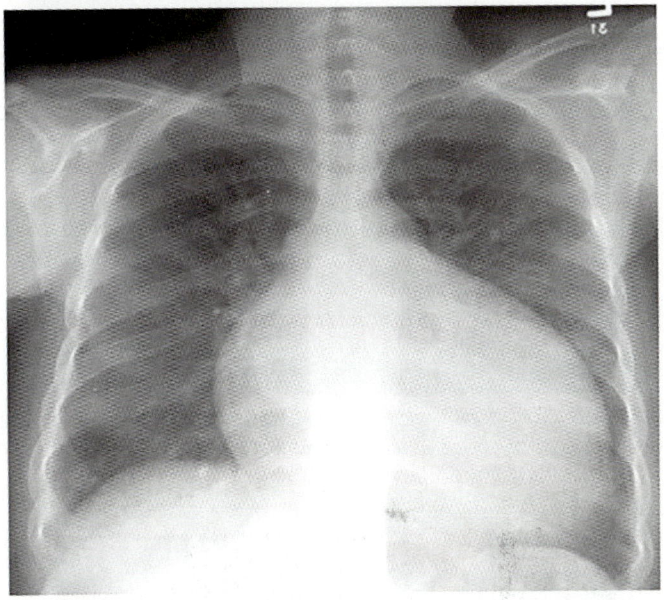

**Fig. 1.103:** X-ray chest (PA view). Showing cardiomegaly with enlargement of left ventricle with dilated main pulmonary artery along with congested lung fields in left to right shunt

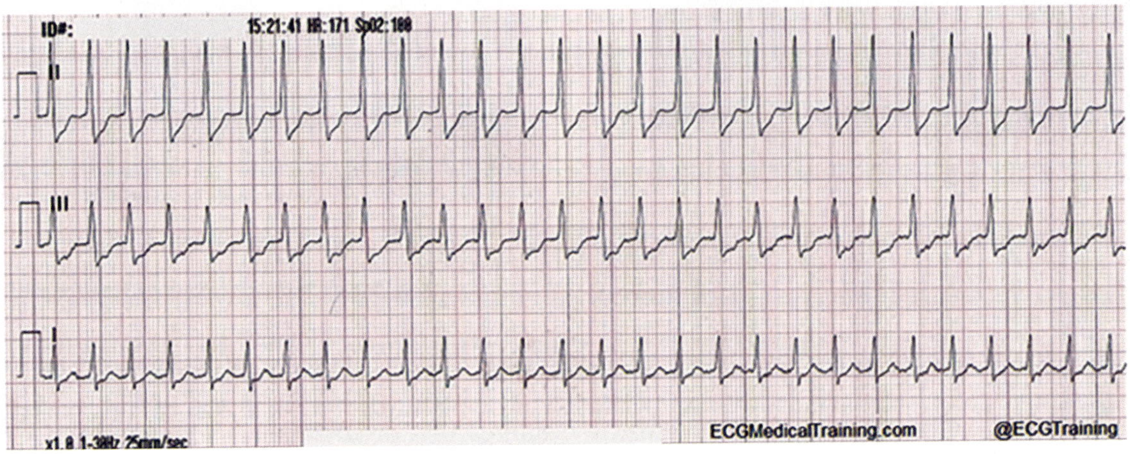


**Fig. 1.104:** ECG trace showing re-entrant SVT due to AVNRT

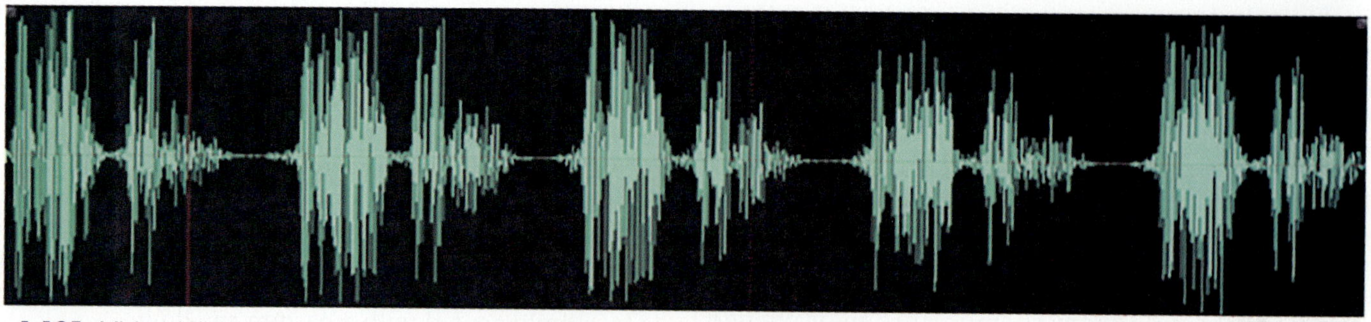

**Fig. 1.105:** Mid-systolic murmur—murmur heard in systole, in a crescendo-decrescendo fashion. The murmur is mid-systolic and NOT associated with a click. Ejection systolic murmurs indicate shunting of blood between two structures in which the pressure in one structure is higher than the other in mid-systole, e.g. Increase volume of blood flowing through normal valves ASD, this murmur is associated with a mid-diastolic murmur and fixed splitting of second heart sound. Anemia or small VSD, which is not open throughout systole due to constricting effecting of contracting myocardial fibers

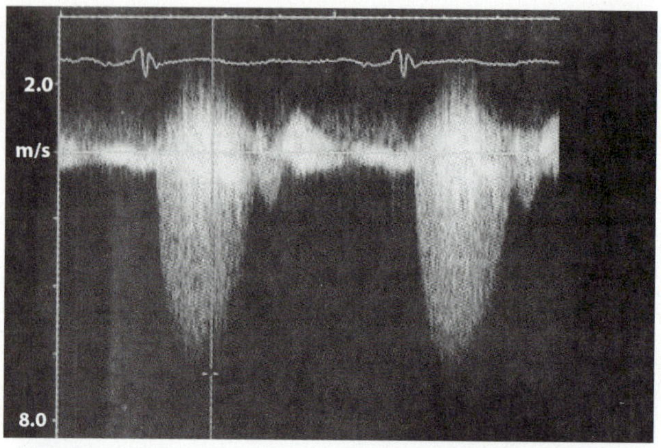


**Fig. 1.106:** Continuous-wave Doppler recording across a severely stenosed aortic valve showing an instantaneous pressure gradient by the application of Bernoulli equation

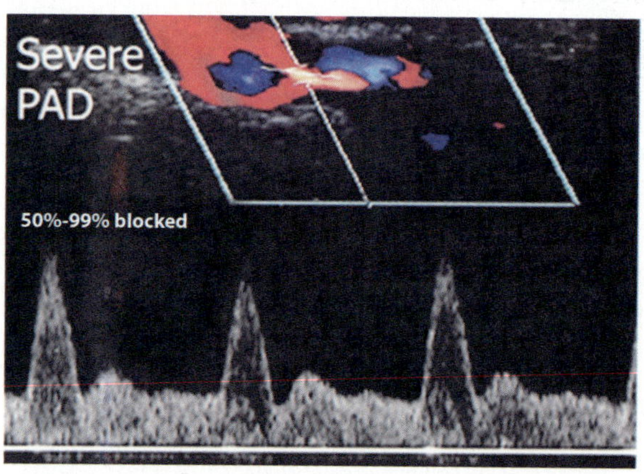


**Fig. 1.107:** A duplex ultrasound image of an artery that has been almost completely blocked by peripheral arterial disease (PAD). The blue areas indicate slow blood flow, and not much blood flow is visible beyond the blockage because PAD has nearly closed off the artery

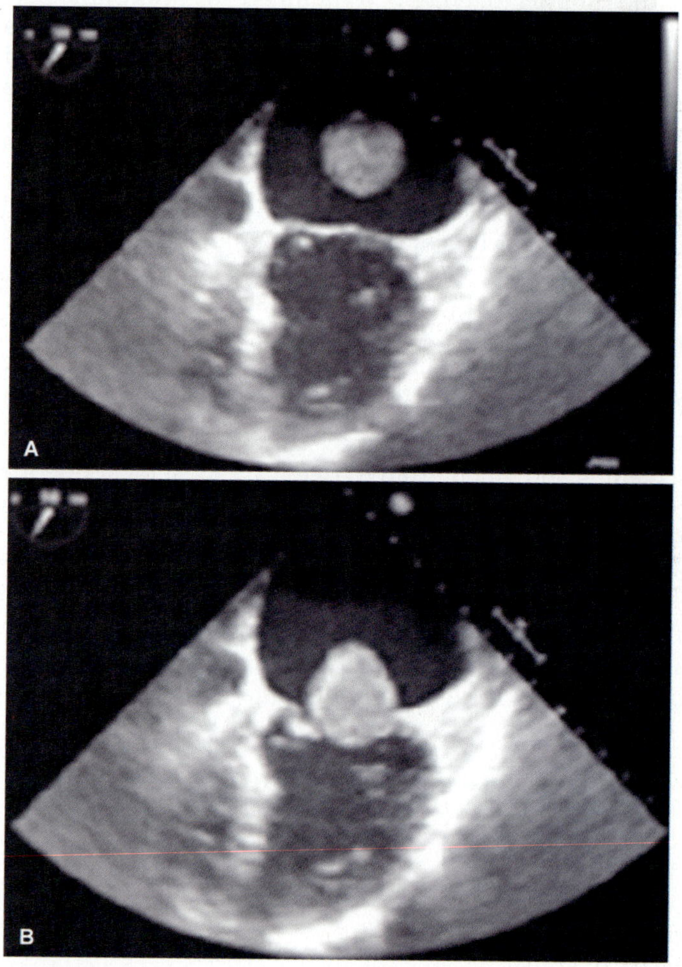


**Fig. 1.108:** Intraoperative transesophageal echocardiogram showing the free-floating myxoma in the left atrium (A) and the myxoma obstructing the mitral valve orifice at end-diastole (B)

Phonocardiogram is also a useful aid, as there is a close correlation between visual and acoustic events. The severity of lesion can also be assessed by this method besides obtaining graphic record of heart sounds and murmurs (Fig. 1.105).

Echocardiogmphy is being widely used at present and makes use of ultrasonic sounds for the detection of anatomic and physiologic abnormalities. Measurements the dimensions of the ventricles, the outflow tracts,

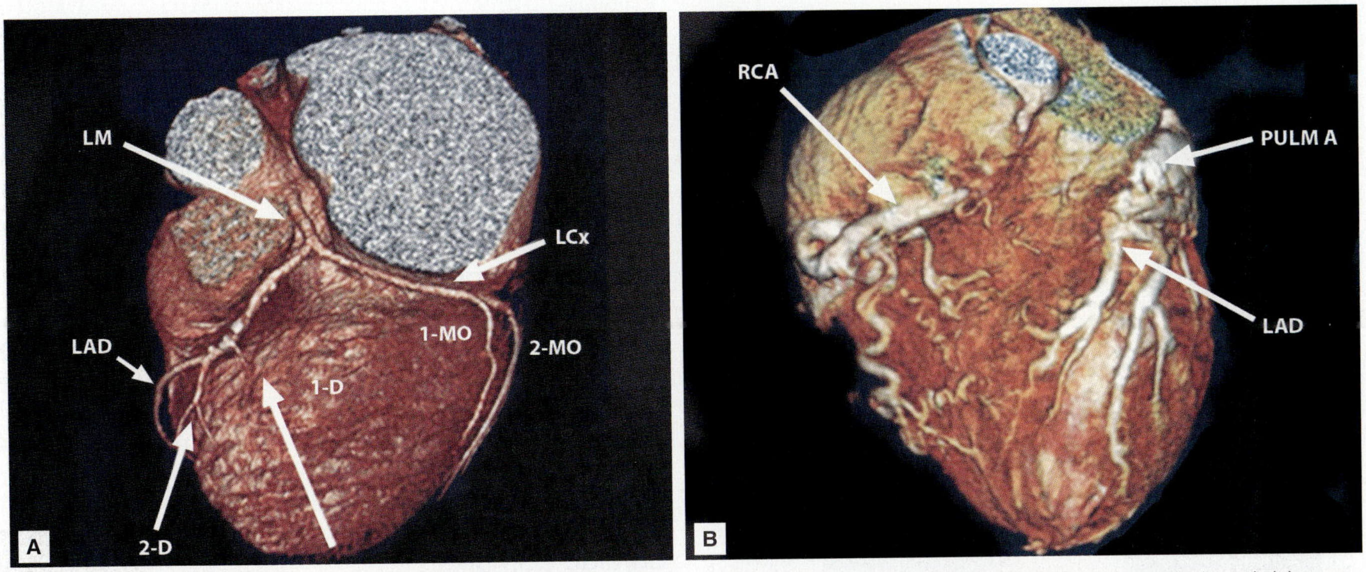


**Fig. 1.109:** (A) Volume-rendered CT image (right anterior oblique view with cranial angulation) shows the arteries: right coronary artery (RCA), marginal acute branch (MAb), left anterior descending (LAD) and second diagonal (2-D). (B) CT angiography volume rendered image. Right coronary artery is dilated and tortious with a large number of collaterals feeding the left coronary system. Left coronary artery is emerging from pulmonary artery trunk. The left anterior descending artery and their diagonal branches are also dilated and tortious

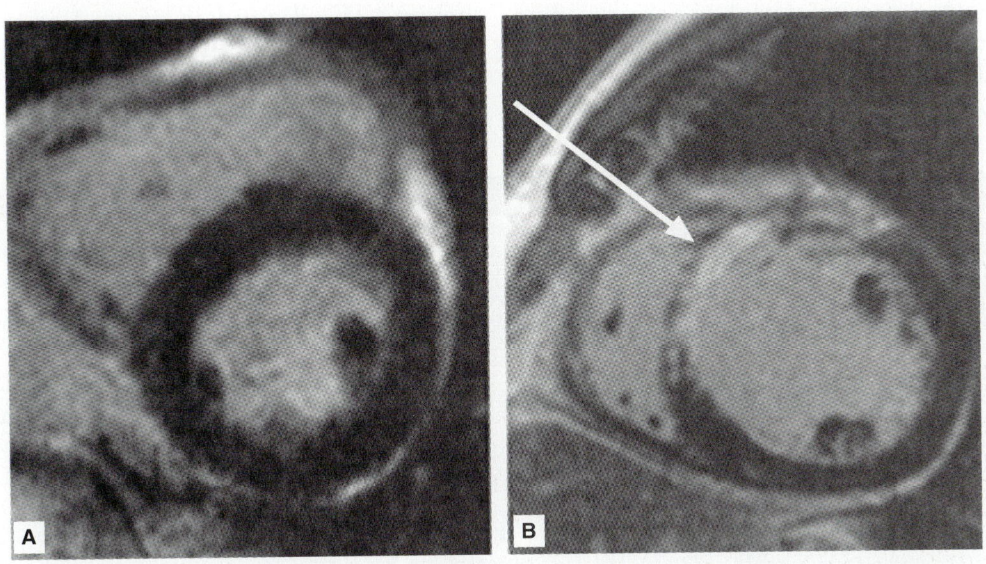


**Fig. 1.110:** Cardiac MRI—(A) normal heart muscle, (B) scarring after a heart attack

detection of pericardial effusion, congenital and acquired heart dysfunctions are now possible with this technique without risk or injury to the body tissues (Figs 1.106–1.108).

## Computed Tomography and MRI

It is one of the most useful noninvasive techniques employed in the assessment of cardiac fuctions and its great vessels. In children, it is being used in the diagnosis of congenital and acquired cardiac dysfunctions with least discomfort. It also gives most useful information before and after cardiac surgery and medical therapy (Figs 1.109–1.111).

Radioisotopic studies using technitium 99 m is useful for delineating left to right shunts as well as the vessels and location of cardiac chambers (Fig. 1.112).

## *Cath Laboratory Procedures*

Cardiac catheterisation aims at defining the anatomical and physiological variation of congenital heart disease and is undertaken only in specialised cardiac centres. It is indicated in infants and children with progressive lesions, complex malformations, severe degrees of cyanosis, severe degrees of refractory heart failure and in those in whom early surgery is contemplated (Fig. 1.113).

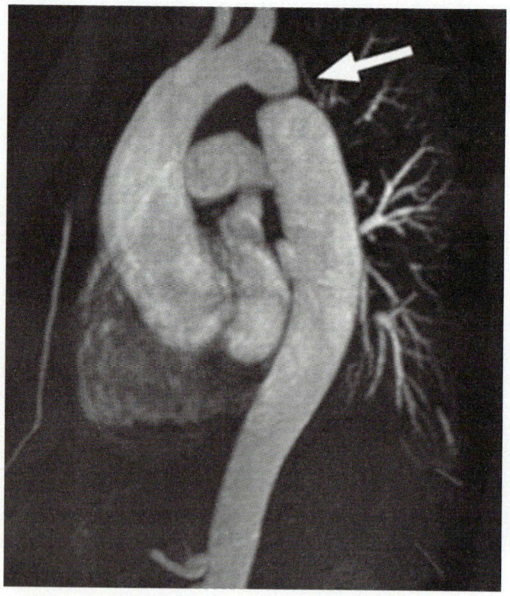

**Fig. 1.111:** MR angiography of the thoracic aorta with gadolinium-enhanced 3D gradient-echo imaging. in a 47-year-old man with recurrent aortic coarctation (arrow)

In competent hands, the technique is low risk procedure and provides data regarding $O_2$ content in the various chambers, systemic and pulmonary vascular resistance. Special techniques, such as the hydrogen electrode catheter (for very small L-R shunts) and the indicator dilution curves, detection of shunts as well as cardiac outputs, are employed when special indication exists. Cardiac catheterisation is also used for injection of contrast material for angiography and percutaneous introduction of intracardiac devices in the management of congenital and acquired heart defects.

## Angiocardiography

Injection of contrast media into the required chambers or great vessels permits identification of specific anomalies (selective angiocardiography) producing pictures without shadows from other areas of the caxdiovascular system. A number of serial X-ray films (6–14/sec and even faster) are taken. Cineangiocardiography is being employed on a large scale in well-equipped centres (Fig. 1.114).

## Cardiac Biomarkers

The use of cardiac biomarkers for the diagnosis and risk stratification of patients in the emergency department (ED) is evolving rapidly. Previously, the role of cardiac enzymes was restricted to the diagnosis of acute myocardial infarction (AMI). The identification of new biomarkers and more sensitive assays has extended the use of biomarkers beyond the diagnosis of cardiac necrosis. As novel biomarkers are identified, emergency physicians should be aware of both the potential clinical usefulness and the limitations of promising biomarkers. Testing should always

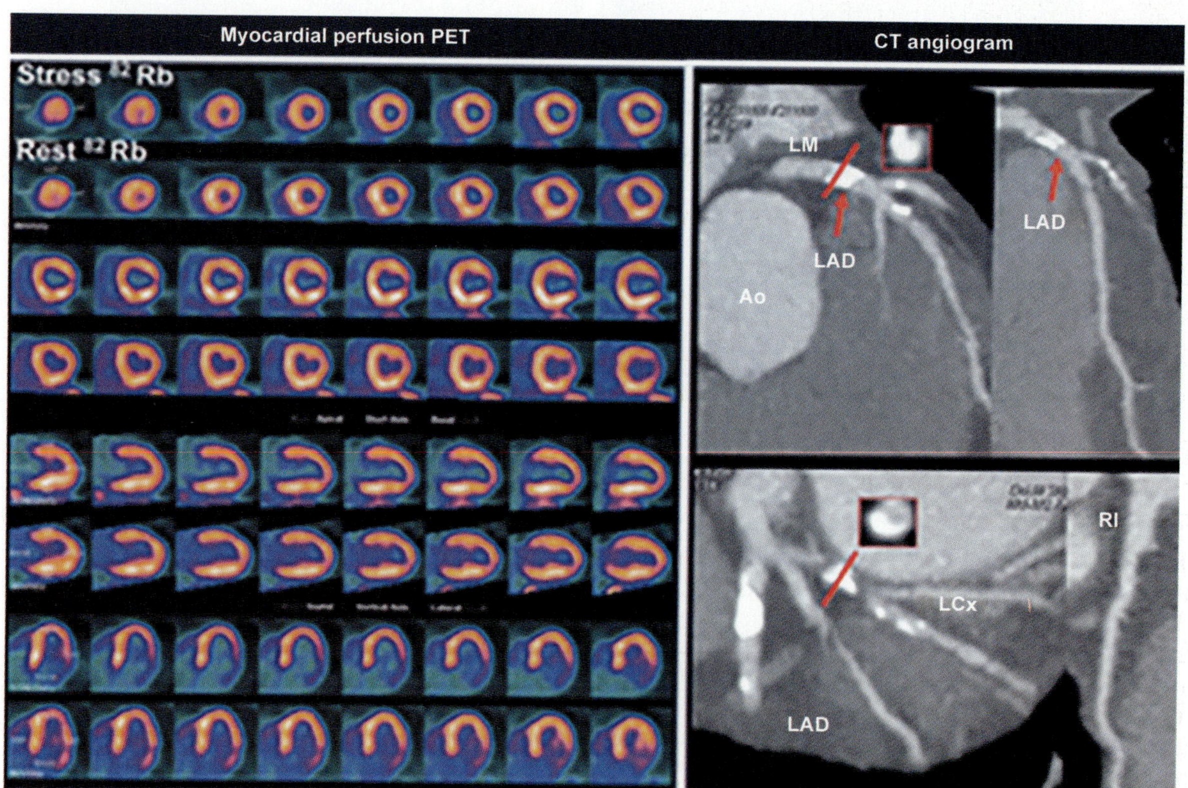


**Fig. 1.112:** Well-correlated myocardial perfusion with PET and CT coronary angiography of an obstructed and calcified left anterior descending artery

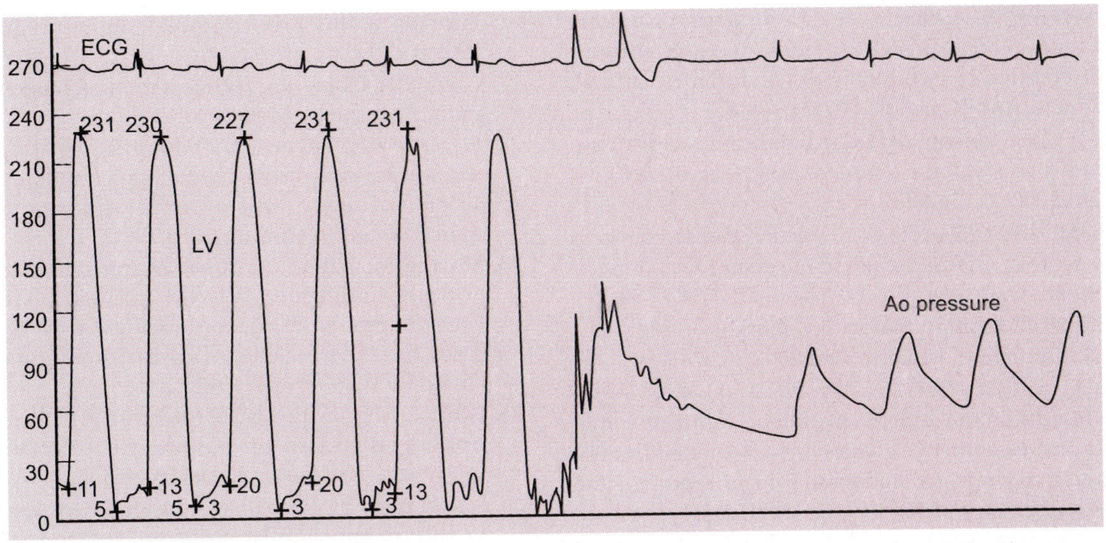


**Fig. 1.113:** Pullback catheter pressure trace across an aortic valve showing a peak-to-peak pressure gradient in excess of 110 mmHg indicating severe stenosis (LV=left ventricular pressure; Ao=aorta)

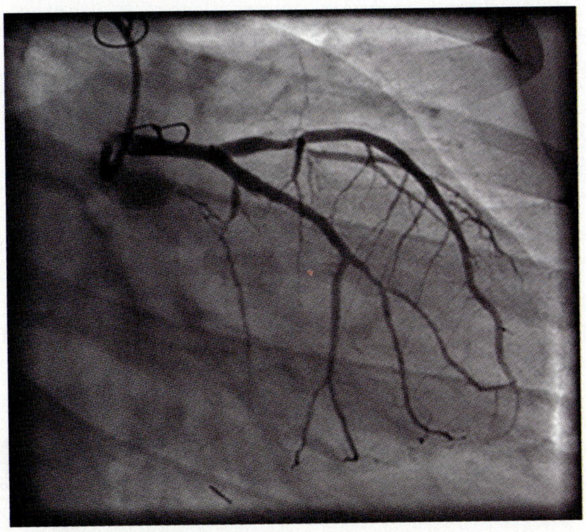

**Fig. 1.114:** Cine-angiography of coronary system showing osteal circumflex artery obstruction

be guided by a patient's history and physical examination to avoid misusing biomarkers as 'screening' tools in critically ill patients. This update focuses on the present and future value of cardiac biomarkers in the care of patients who have suspected cardiac and cardiac-related diseases in the emergency department.

**Galectin-3, a biomarker:** Galectin-3 is a protein that binds and activates myofibroblasts in damaged heart tissue, which leads to collagen synthesis and subsequently problematic fibrosis. Though, the current use case for galectin-3 is simply to get a better sense for the probability of adverse disease outcomes in patients with heart failure, ideally, treatments would be found that work best in patients with high galectin-3 levels. Believers include Abbott, Alere and bioMérieux, who have all entered agreements with BG Medicine to commercialize the assay for use in their own systems. From the press release, galectin-3 is a protein that has been shown to play an important role in the development and progression of heart failure in approximately 30% of the patients diagnosed with heart failure. (i) This galectin-3, mediated form of heart failure is associated with progressive fibrosis, or stiffening, in the heart muscle, which impairs the heart's ability to pump. (ii) The role of galectin-3 in heart failure was first established in 2004. (iii) The clearance of the company's galectin-3, blood test now for the first time allows physicians to use this product in the evaluation of patients diagnosed with heart failure. The availability of a galectin-3 test to identify high risk patients with cardiovascular disease and myocardial fibrosis represents another step toward the goal of enabling more efficient targeting of therapeutic approaches to reduce fibrosis in patients with chronic heart failure.

## BIBLIOGRAPHY


1. A viles RJ, Askari AT, Lindahl B, et al. Troponin T levels in patients with acute coronary syndromes, with or without renal dysfunction. N Engl J Med 2002;346:2047–52.
2. Alpert LS, Thygesen K, Antman E, et al. Myocardial infarction redefined: a consensus document of The 10 Int. European Society of Cardiology/American College of Cardiology Committee for the redefinition of myocardial infarction. Am Coil Cardio 2000;36:959–69.
3. Ammann P, Sabine M, Kraus M, et al. Characteristics and prognosis of myocardial infarction in patients with normal coronary arteries. Chest 2000;117:333.
4. Antman EM, Tanasijevic MJ, Thompson B, et al. Cardiac-specific troponin I levels to predict the risk of mortality in patients with acute coronary syndromes. N Engl J Med 1996; 335: 1342–9.
5. Apple FS, Murakami MM, Pearce LA, et al. Predictive value of cardiac troponin I and T for subsequent death in end-stage renal disease. Circulation 2002;106:2941–5.

6. Aviles R1, Wright RS, Aviles M, et al. Long-term prognosis of patients with clinical unstable angina pectoris without elevation of creatine kinase but with elevation of cardiac troponin I levels. Am J Cardiol 2002;90:875–8.
7. Azzazy HM, Christenson RH. Cardiac markers of acute coronary syndromes: is there a case for point-of-care testing? Clin Biochem 2002;35:13–27.
8. Balk EM, Ioannidis P, Salem D, et al. Accuracy of biomarkers to diagnose acute cardiac ischemia in the emergency department: a meta-analysis. Ann Emerg Med 2001;37:478–94.
9. Blake GJ, Ridker PM. Inflammatory bio-markers and cardiovascular risk prediction. J Intern Med 2002;252:283–94.
10. Braunwald E, Antman EM, Beasley W, et al. ACC/AHA guidelines for the management of patients with unstable angina and non-ST-segment elevation myocardial infarction: executive summary and recommendations: a report of the American College of Cardiology/American Heart Association task force on practice guidelines (committee on the management of patients with unstable angina). Circulation 2000;102:1193–209.
11. Cantwell RV, Aviles RL, Bjornsson L, et al. Cardiac amyloidsis presenting with elevations of cardiac troponin I and angina pectoris. Clin Cardiol 2002;25:33–7.
12. Cheitlin MD, Alpert JS, Armstrong WF, et al. ACC/AHA Guidelines for the clinical application of echocardiography. A report of the American College of Cardiology/American Heart Association Task Force on Practice Guidelines (Committee on Clinical Application of Echocardiography). Developed in collaboration with the American Society of Echocardiography. Circulation 1997;95:1686.
13. Chou TM, Amidon TM. Evaluating coronary artery disease noninvasively: which test for whom? West J Med 1994; 161:173.
14. Diamond GA, Forrester JS. Analysis of probability as an aid in the clinical diagnosis of coronary artery disease. N Engl J Med 1979;300:1350.
15. Donnino MW, Karriem-Norwood V, Rivers EP, et al. Prevalence of elevated troponin I in end-stage renal disease patients receiving hemodialysis. Acad Emerg Med 2004; II:979–81.
16. Garber AM, Solomon NA. Cost effectiveness of alternative test strategies for the diagnosis of coronary artery disease. Ann Intern Med 1999;130:719.
17. Geleijnse ML, Elhendy A, Fioretti PM, et al. Dobutamine stress myocardial perfusion imaging. J Am Coll Cardiol 2000;36:2017.
18. Gianrossi R, Detrano R, Mulvihil D, et al. Exercise-induced ST-depression in the diagnosis of coronary artery disease: a meta-analysis. Circulation 1989;80:87.
19. Gibbons RJ, Balady GJ, Beasley JW, et al. ACC/AHA guidelines for exercise testing: a report of the American College of Cardiology/American Heart Association Task Force on Practice Guidelines (Committee on Exercise Testing). J Am Coll Cardiol 1997;30:260.
20. Gibbons RJ, Chatterjee K, Daley J, et al. ACC/AHA/ACP-ASIM guidelines for the management of patients with chronic stable angina: a report of the American College of Cardiology/American Heart Association Task Force on Practice Guidelines (Committee on the Management of Patients with Chronic Stable Angina). J Am Coll Cardiol 1999;33:2092.
21. Goyal RK. Changing focus on unexplained esophageal chest pain. Ann Intern Med 1996;124:1008.
22. Hertzer NR, Beven EG, Young JR, et al. Coronary artery disease in peripheral vascular patients: a classification of 1,000 coronary angiograms and results of surgical management. Ann Surg 1984;199:223.
23. Hwang SJ, Ballantyne CM, Sharrett AR, et al. Circulating adhesion molecules VCAM-I, CAM-I, and E-selectin in carotid atherosclerosis and incident coronary heart disease cases: the Atherosclerosis Risk In Communities (ARIC) study. Circulation 1997;96:4219–25.
24. Kontos MC, Fritz LM, Anderson FP, et al. Impact of the troponin standard on the prevalence of acute myocardial infarction. Am Heart 2003;146:446–52.
25. Koukkunen H, Penttila K, Kemppainen A, et al. Differences in the diagnosis of myocardial infarction by troponin T compared with clinical and epidemiologic criteria. Am 1 Cardiol 2001;88:727–31.
26. Kwok Y, Kim C, Grady D, et al. Meta-analysis of exercise testing to detect coronary artery disease in women. Am J Cardiol 1999;83:660.
27. Laffe AS, Katus H. Acute coronary syndrome biomarkers: the need for more adequate reporting. Circulation 2004; 110:104–6.
28. Laffe AS, Ravkilde, Roberts R, et al. It's time for a change to a troponin standard. Circulation 2000;102:1216–20.
29. Lee TH, Goldman L. Evaluation of the patient with acute chest pain. N Engl J Med 2000;341:1187.
30. Lee-Lewandrowski E, Corboy D, Lewandrowski K, et al. Implementation of a point-of-care satellite laboratory in the emergency department of an academic medical center: impact on test turnaround time and patient emergency department length of stay. Arch Pathol Lab Med 2003; 127:456–60.
31. Libby P. Inflammation in atherosclerosis. Nature 2002;420: 868–74.
32. Newby LK. Markers of cardiac ischemia, injury, and inflammation. Prog Cardiovasc Dis 2004;46:404–16.
33. Nissen SE, Grines CL, Gurley JC, et al. Application of a new phased-array ultrasound catheter in the assessHamm CW, Giannitsis E, Katus HA. Cardiac troponin elevations in patients without acute coronary syndrome. Circulation 2002; 106:2871–2.
34. Panteghini M. Acute coronary syndrome: biochemical strategies in the troponin era. Chest 2002; 122: 1428–35.
35. Panteghini M. Role and importance of biochemical markers in clinical cardiology. Eur Heart J. 2004;25:1187–96.
36. Polanczyk CA, Lee TH, Cook EF, et al. Cardiac troponin I as a predictor of major cardiac events in emergency department patients with acute chest pain. J Am Coli Cardiol 1998; 32:8–14.
37. Pryor DB, Harrell FE, Lee KL, et al. Estimating the likelihood of significant coronary artery disease. Am J Med 1983;75:771.
38. Quiles J, Roy D, Gaze D, et al. Relation of ischemia-modified albumin (IMA) levels following elective angioplasty for stable angina pectoris duration of balloon-induced myocardial ischemia. Am J Cardiol 2003;92:322–4.

39. Ridker PM, Brown NJ, Vaughan DE, et al. Established and emerging plasma biomarkers in the prediction of first atherothrombotic events. Circulation 2004; 109:IV6–19.
40. Ridker PM, Hennekens CH, Buring JE, et al. C-reactive protein and other markers of inflammation in the prediction of cardiovascular disease in women. N Engl J Med 2000;342: 836–43.
41. Ridker PM, Hennekens CH, Roitman-Johnson B, et al. Plasma concentration of soluble intercellular adhesion molecule I and risks of future myocardial infarction in apparently healthy men. Lancet 1998;351:88–92.
42. Roongsritong C, Warraich I, Bradley C. Common causes of troponin elevations in the absence of acute myocardial infarction: incidence and clinical significance. Chest 2004; 125: 1877–84.
43. Ross R. Atherosclerosis-an inflammatory disease. N Engl J Med 1999;340:115–26.
44. Roy D, Quiles J, Aldama G, et al. Ischemia modified albumin for the assessment of patients presenting to the emergency department with acute chest pain but normal or non-diagnostic 12-lead electrocardiograms and negative cardiac troponin T. Int J Cardiol 2004;97:297–301.
45. Sinha MK, Gaze DC, Tippins JR, et al. Ischemia modified albumin is a sensitive marker of myocardial ischemia after percutaneous coronary intervention. Circulation 2003;107: 2403–5.
46. Smith SC Jr, Anderson JL, Cannon RO III, et al. CDC/AHA workshop on markers of inflammation and cardiovascular disease: application to clinical and public health practice: report from the clinical practice discussion group. Circulation 2004;110:e550–3.
47. Wu AH, Apple FS, Gibler WB, et al. National Academy of Clinical Biochemistry Standards of Laboratory Practice: recommendations for the use of cardiac markers in coronary artery diseases. Clin Chem 1999;45:1104–21.
48. Wu AH, Smith A, Christenson RH, et al. Evaluation of a point-of-care assay for cardiac markers for patients suspected of acute myocardial infarction. Clin Chem Acta 2004;346: 211–9.

# 2 Recognition and Management of Angina Pectoris

Although James B. Herrick identified clinical features of angina as early as 1912, but William Heberden is still considered as the first person who drew attention of the world towards this condition for the first time in the history of medical science delivering his classical lecture on angina pectoris before the August audience of Royal College of Physician in 1968 in London. Since then, its spectrum of manifestation and modalities of treatment have been the attraction of the various medical scientists from time to time. Angina pectoris may be called symptom complex in which sensation of 'strangling' or 'squeezing' in restro-stemal area of the chest remains the dominant symptom. It is a symptom and not a disease. Although the most common cause of the angina is coronary artery disease due to atheroma, it is important not to overlook other conditions that give rise to angina. These include valvular heart disease, congenital coronary artery anomalies syphilitic aortitis, cardiomyopathy and coronary artery vasculitis. Several 'anginal equivalents', such as dyspnea on exertion and exhaustion, that are not associated with chest discomfort, but are caused by myocardial ischemia also occur. Angina pectoris is the result of myocardial ischemia caused by an imbalance between myocardial blood supply and oxygen demand. Angina is a common presenting symptom (typically, chest pain) among patients with coronary artery disease. A comprehensive approach to diagnosis and to medical management of angina pectoris is an integral part of the daily responsibilities of physicians (Figs 2.1, 2.2 and Tables 2.1–2.5).

## MAIN CATEGORIES OF ANGINA PECTORIS

The major types of angina are stable, unstable, variant (Prinzmetal's), and microvascular. Their knowledge is important due to the fact that they have different symptoms and require different treatments (Figs 2.3 and 2.8).

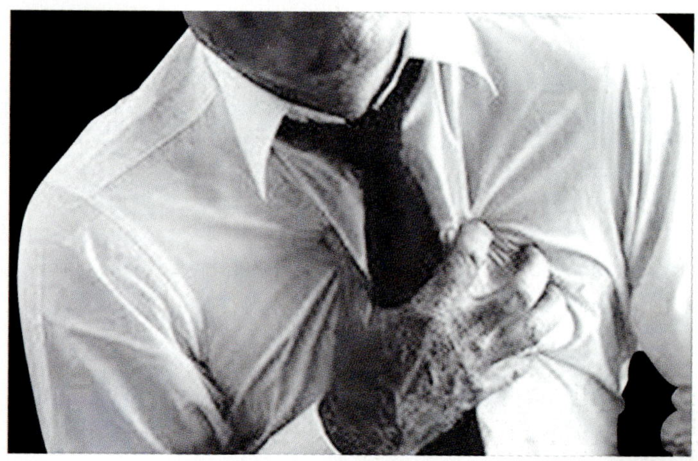

**Fig, 2.1:** A middle-aged man experiencing excruciating chest pain in angina pectoris

### 1. Stable Angina

It is the commonest type of angina, and occurs when the heart is working harder than usual. It has a regular pattern. ('Pattern' refers to how often the angina occurs, how severe it is, and what factors trigger it.)

If somebody is suffering with stable angina, one can learn its pattern and predict when the pain will happen. The pain usually goes away a few minutes after you rest or take your angina medicine.

It cannot be considered as a heart attack, but it can warn the person for heart attack, which is more likely to happen in the future.

### 2. Unstable Angina

**Unstable angina** is defined as new-onset angina (i.e. within 2 months of initial presentation) of at least class III severity, significant recent increase in frequency and severity of

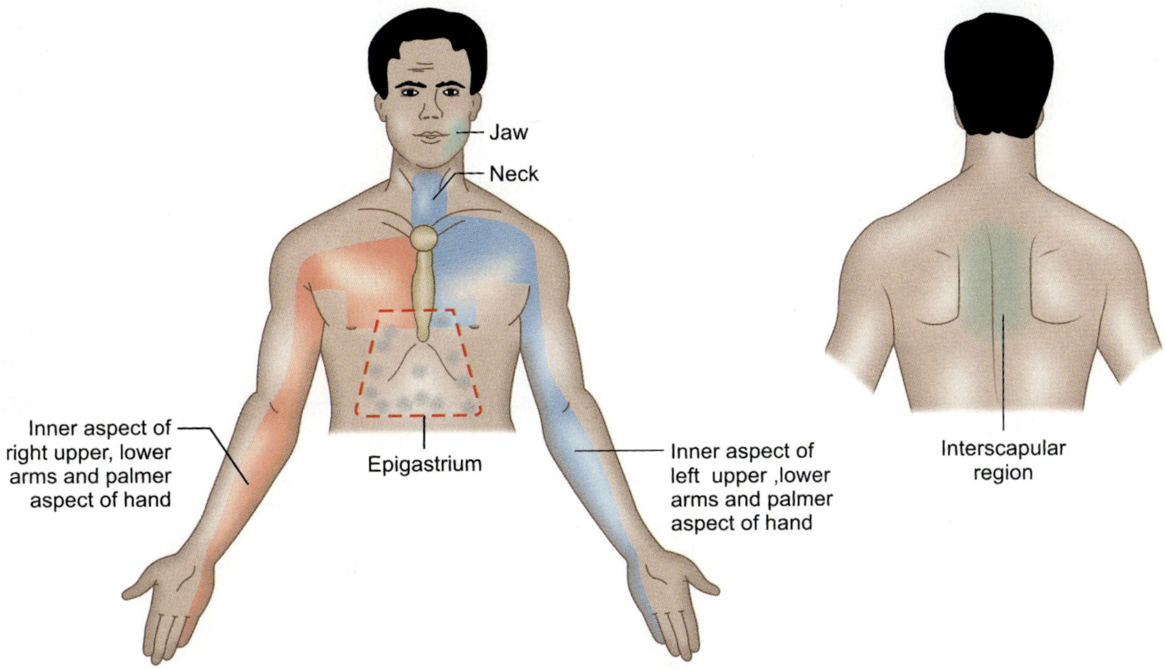


**Fig. 2.2:** Diagrammatic representation of regional distribution of anginal pain

**Table 2.1:** Classification of unstable angina

| | |
|---|---|
| **Severity** | |
| Class I | New-onset, severe or accelerated angina<br>Patients with angina of less than 2 months' duration, severe or occurring 3 or more times per day, or angina that is distinctly more frequent and precipitated by distinctly less exertion. No rest pain in the last 2 months. |
| Class II | Angina at rest, subacute<br>Patients with 1 or more episodes of antina at rest during preceding month but not within 48 hours. |
| Class III | Angina at rest, acute.<br>Patients with 1 or more episodes of angina at rest within the preceding 48 hours. |
| **Clinical circumstances** | |
| Class A | Secondary unstable angina<br>A clearly identified condition extrinsic to the coronary vascular bed that has intensified myocardial ischemia, such as anemia, infection, fever, hypotension, tacharrhythmia, thyrotoxicosis, and hypoxemia due to respiratory failure. |
| Class B | Primary unstable angina |
| Class C | Postinfarction unstable angina (within 2 weeks of documented myocardial infarction). |
| **Intensity of treatment** | |
| 1. | Absence of treatment or minimal treatment |
| 2. | Occurring in the presence of standard therapy for chronic stable angina (conventional doses of oral β-adrenergic blockers, nitrates and calcium antagonists). |
| 3. | Occurring despite maximally tolerated doses of all three categories of oral therapy, including intravenous nitroglycerin. |

angina, or angina at rest. Unstable angina does not follow a fixed pattern. It may occur more often and be more severe than stable angina. Unstable angina can also occur with or without physical exertion, and rest or medicine may not relieve the pain. It is usually fatal and needs an urgent management. Unstable angina is a sign that a heart attack may happen soon.

### 3. Variant (Prinzmetal's) Angina

This type of angina is very uncommon. A spasm in a coronary artery leads to this type of angina. Variant angina usually occurs while one is resting and the pain can be severe. It usually happens between midnight and early morning. Coronary vasodilators can relieve the pain of this type of angina. Electrocardiogram reveals ST-segment

**Table 2.2:** Differential diagnosis of chest pain

| |
|---|
| ***Life-threatening causes*** |
| Acute coronary syndrome and aortic dissection |
| Pulmonary embolus |
| Tension pneumothorax |
| ***Other cardiovascular and nonischemic causes*** |
| Pericarditis |
| Atypical angina |
| Hypertrophic cardiomyopathy |
| Vasospastic angina |
| ***Other noncardiac causes*** |
| Boerhaave's syndrome (esophageal rupture with mediastinitis) |
| Gastroesophageal reflux and spasm |
| Chest-wall pain |
| Pleurisy |
| Peptic ulcer disease |
| Panic attack |
| Biliary or pancreatic pain |
| Cervical disc or neuropathic pain |
| Somatization and psychogenic pain disorder |

**Table 2.3:** The New York Heart Association classification

| | |
|---|---|
| **Class I** | No limitation of physical activity (ordinary physical activity does not cause symptoms) |
| **Class II** | Slight limitation of physical activity (ordinary physical activity causes symptoms) |
| **Class III** | Moderate limitation of activity (patient is comfortable at rest, but less than ordinary activities cause symptoms.) |
| **Class IV** | Unable to perform any physical activity without discomfort, therefore severe limitation (patient may be symptomatic even at rest) |

**Table 2.4:** Canadian cardiovascular society angina grading scale

The Canadian Cardiovascular Society Angina Grading Scale is commonly used for the classification of severity of angina.

| | |
|---|---|
| **Class I** | Angina only during strenuous or prolonged physical activity |
| **Class II** | Slight limitation, with angina only during vigorous physical activity |
| **Class III** | Symptoms with everyday living activities, i.e. moderate limitation |
| **Class IV** | Inability to perform any activity without angina or angina at rest, i.e. severe limitation |

**Table 2.5:** Comparative features between Prinzmetal's classic effort angina and variant angina

| **Effort angina** | **Variant angina** |
|---|---|
| 1. Its occurance at time of day | |
| Ischaemic episodes cluster in early hours the day (6 am to noon) | Attacks usually cluster in very early of the day (mid-night to 6 am) |
| 2. Pain | |
| Brought on by exertion or emotion | Occur at rest |
| Less severe | Frequently more severe |
| Shorter duration | Longer duration |
| Relieved after the exertion or emotional stress is taken away | |
| Non-cyclic | May occur in cycles |
| 3. ECG | |
| ST-segments usually depressed without reciprocal changes | ST-segments is typically elevated with reciprocal depression |
| 4. Holter monitoring | |
| Approximately 70% ST-segment depression without symptoms | ST-segment equally elevated and depressed (90%) without symptoms |
| 5. Cardiac arrhythmia | |
| Hardly associated with cardiac arrhythmia | In about 50% of the cases cardiac arrhythmia occures either during or immediately after the attack |
| 6. Treadmill testing | |
| There is ST-segment depression and/or precordial pain | Usually there is no ST-segment shift and/or chest pain |

elevation caused by focal coronary artery spasm. Although, most patients had coronary lesions, some have angiographically normal coronary arteries. Different types of mechanisms have been been cited for Prinzmetal angina, such as focal deficiency of nitric oxide production, hyperinsulinemia, low intracellular magnesium levels, smoking cigarettes and using cocaine. Approximately, 30% of patients with chest pain referred for cardiac catheterization have normal or minimal atherosclerosis of coronary arteries. A subset of these patients demonstrates reduced coronary flow reserve (CFR), which is considered due to functional and structural changes of small coronary arteries and arterioles (i.e. resistance vessels). Normally, resistance vessels are responsible for as much as 95% of coronary

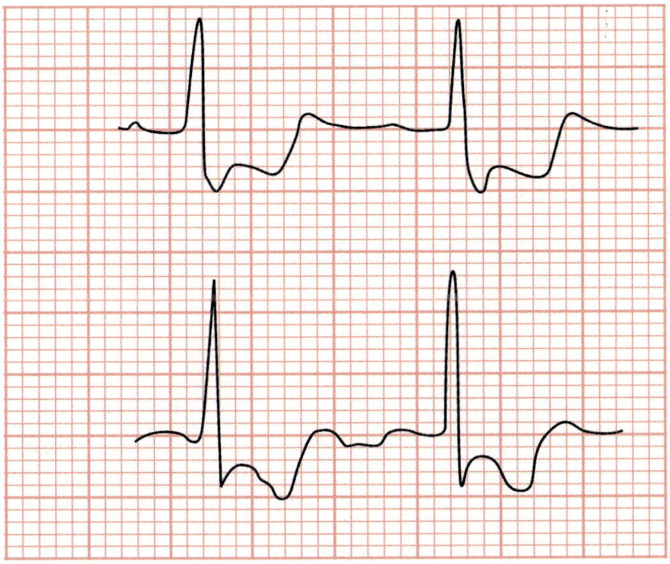

**Fig. 2.3:** Substantial ST-segment depression in patient with angina pectoris

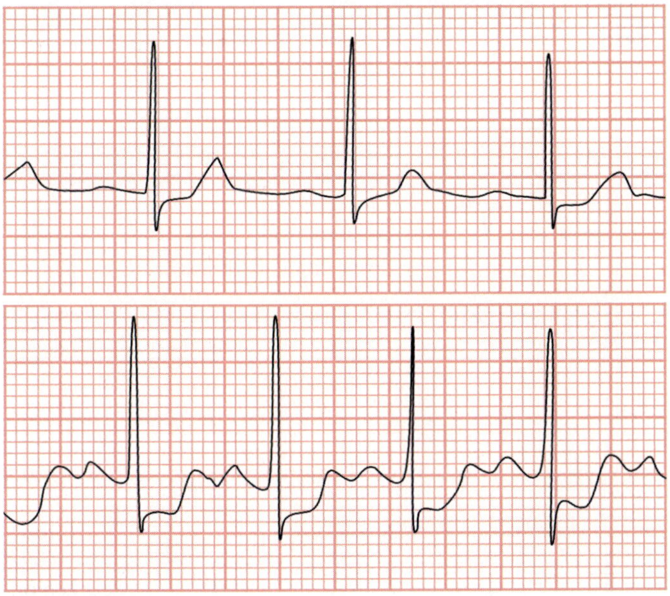

**Fig. 2.4:** Electrocardiogram showing stress induced ST-depression in patient with stable angina

artery resistance, with the remaining 5% being from epicardial coronary arteries (i.e. conductive vessels). The former is not visualized during regular coronary catheterization.

Angina which results from dysfunction of small coronary arteries and arterioles is called microvascular angina. Several diseases, such as diabetes mellitus, hypertension and systemic collagen vascular diseases (e.g. systemic lupus erythematosus, polyarteritis nodosa), are thought to produce microvascular abnormalities with subsequent reduction in CFR.

### 4. Microvascular Angina

Microvascular angina (MVA) can be considered as a result of microvascular disease (MVD) of the coronary artery. It

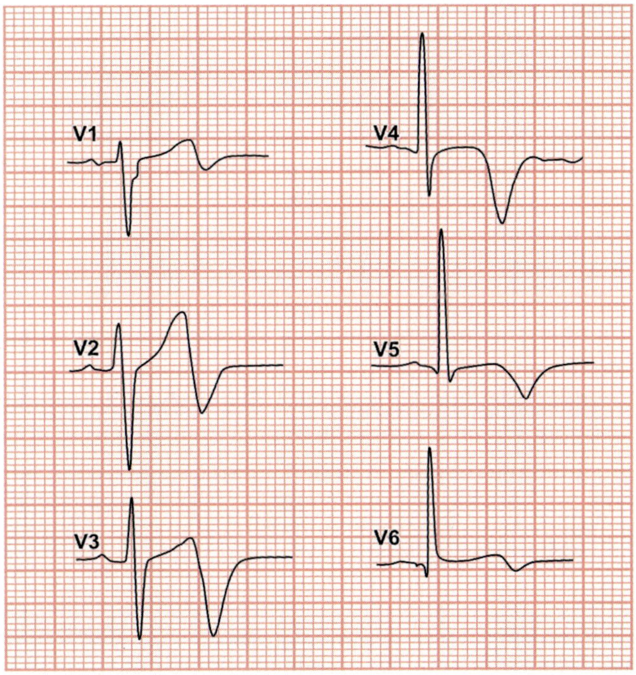


**Fig. 2.5:** Biphasic T-waves in patient with unstable angina

is a type of heart disease that affects the heart's smallest coronary arteries. Reduction in blood supply of the smaller coronary arteries may cause microvascular angina. Later can occur due to factors, such as plaque in the arteries, artery spasms, or damaged or diseased artery walls.

### 5. Angina Decubitus

Angina decubitus is a variant of angina pectoris that happens at night while the patient is in a recumbent posture. It is thought to be induced by an increase in myocardial oxygen demand due to expansion of the blood volume with increased venous return at recumbency. This type of angina is found equally among both the sexes. It can be a sign of coronary heart disease (CHD), irrespective of initial tests do not point to the disease. However, not all chest pain or discomfort is a sign of coronary artery disease.

Other conditions can also cause chest pain, such as

- Pulmonary embolism (a blockage in a lung artery)
- A lung infection
- Aortic dissection (tearing of a major artery)
- Aortic stenosis (narrowing of the heart's aortic valve)
- Hypertrophic cardiomyopathy (KAR-de-o-mi-OP-ah-thee; heart muscle disease)
- Pericarditis (inflammation in the tissues that surround the heart)
- A panic attack

## MYOCARDIAL ISCHEMIA IN ANGINA PECTORIS

It can result due to the following reasons:

1. A reduction of coronary blood flow caused by fixed and/or dynamic epicardial coronary artery (i.e. conductive vessel) stenosis

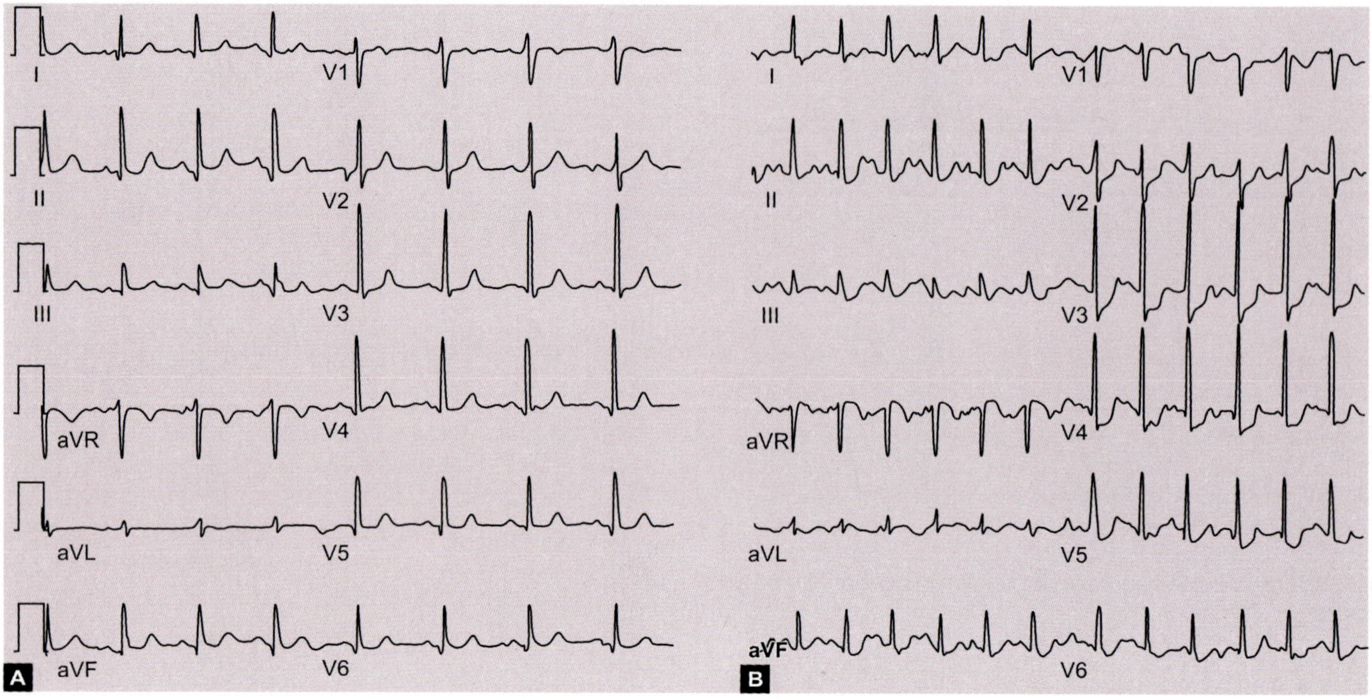


**Fig. 2.6:** ECG showing endothelial vascular angina with normal coronary arteries

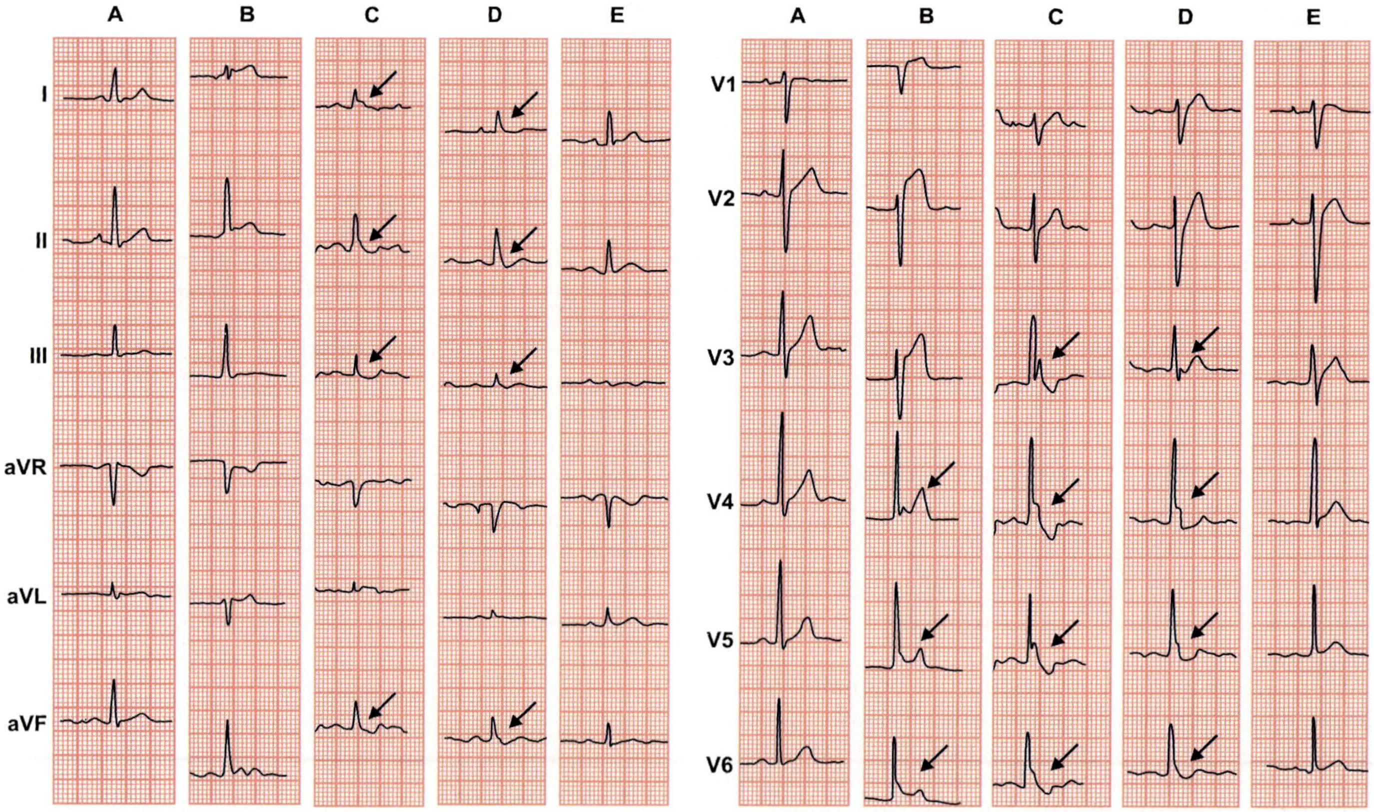


**Fig. 2.7:** The time course of twelve-lead ECG in a 52-year-old man with vasospastic angina. ECGs were obtained prior to the ischemic attack (A), at the onset of chest pressure (B), immediately before ventricular fibrillation (C), after defibrillation and administration of intravenous lidocaine and magnesium (D), and 2 days after the episode (E). Osborn waves (arrowheads) were best seen in the inferior and lateral leads around the occurrence of ventricular fibrillation. In contrast to hypothermic patients, the tracing shows sinus tachycardia and short QT

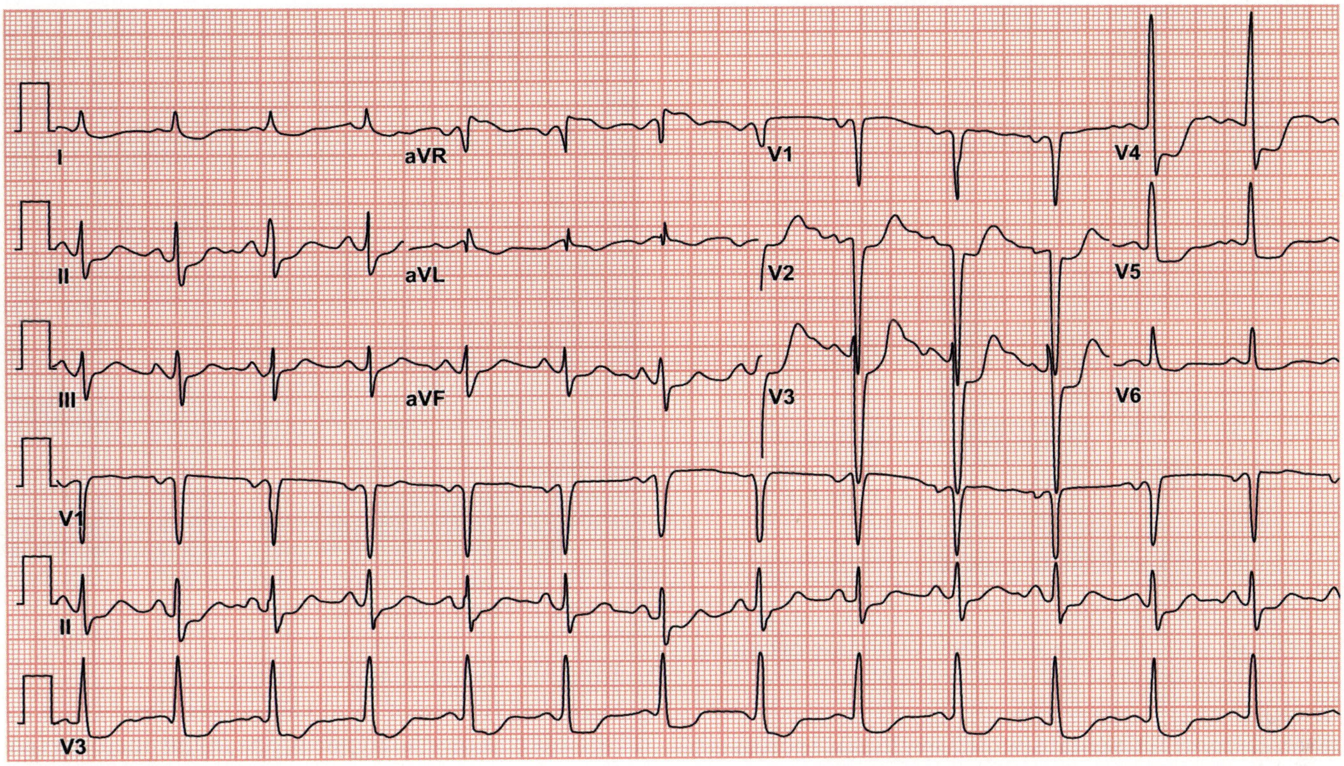


**Fig. 2.8:** A 12-lead electrocardiogram example of ischemic anterolateral ST-segment depression in a patient with known case of chronic stable angina

2. Abnormal constriction or deficient relaxation of coronary microcirculation (i.e. resistance vessels), or
3. Reduced oxygen-carrying capacity of the blood

Atherosclerosis is the most common cause of epicardial coronary artery stenosis and, hence, angina pectoris. Patients with a fixed coronary atherosclerotic lesion of at least 50% show myocardial ischemia during increased myocardial metabolic demand as the result of a significant reduction in CFR. These patients are notable to increase their coronary blood flow during stress to match the increased myocardial metabolic demand, thus they experience angina. Fixed atherosclerotic lesions of at least 90% almost completely abolish the flow reserve; patients with these lesions may experience angina at rest.

Coronary spasm can also reduce CFR significantly by causing dynamic stenosis of coronary arteries.

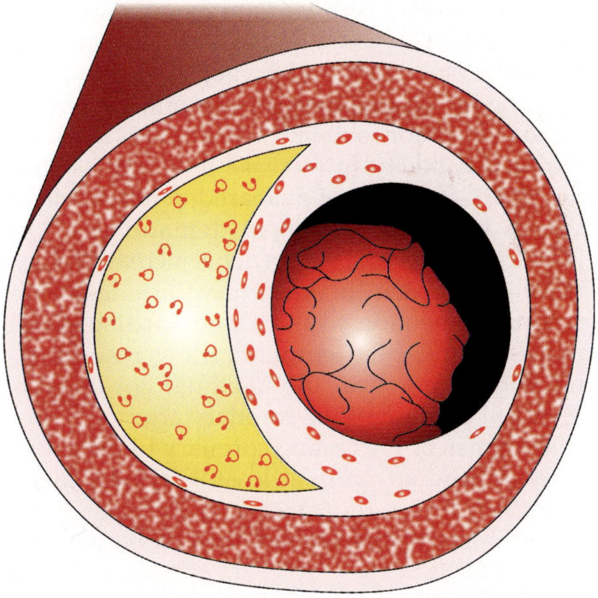

**Fig. 2.9:** Cross-section of an artery with an atherosclerotic lesion with a narrowed lumen in the genesis of angina pectoris

## PATHOGENESIS IN ANGINA PECTORIS

Reduction in blood supply to heart muscle can occur when coronary blood flow becomes insufficient to meet myocardial oxygen demand. It can lead to myocardial cells to switch from aerobic to anaerobic metabolism, with a progressive impairment of metabolic, mechanical and electrical functions. It is the most common clinical presentation of myocardial ischemia. It is caused by chemical and mechanical stimulation of sensory afferent nerve endings in the coronary vessels and myocardium. These nerve fibers extend from the first to fourth thoracic spinal nerves, ascending via the spinal cord to the thalamus, and from there to the cerebral cortex. Currently it has been demonstrated that adenosine may be the main chemical mediator of anginal pain. At the time of ischemia, ATP is degraded to adenosine, which after diffusion to the extracellular space, causes arteriolar dilation and anginal pain. Adenosine induces angina mainly due to stimulating the A1 receptors in cardiac afferent nerve endings. The major determinants of myocardial metabolic activity are myocardial oxygen demand. Increases in the heart rate and

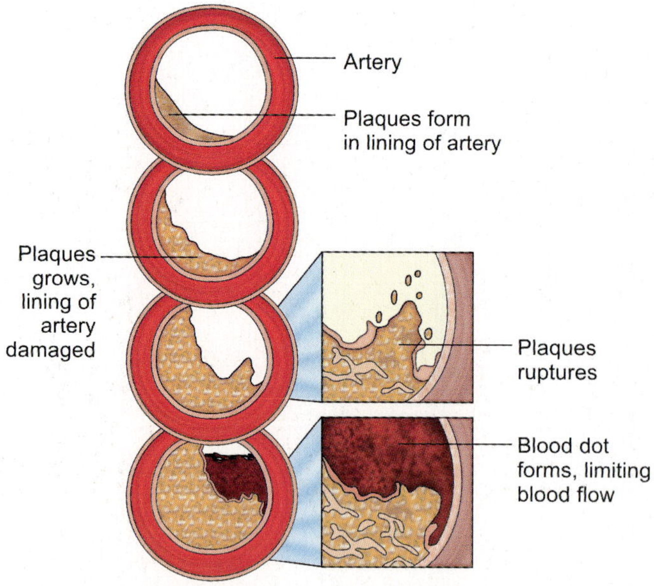


**Fig. 2.10:** Gradual onset of atherosclerosis in an artery with plaque buildup. It finally leads to blockage of artery with rupture of plaque and terminal unstable angina or myocardial infarction

myocardial contractile state which result in increased myocardial oxygen demand. Increases in both afterload (i.e. aortic pressure) and preload (i.e. ventricular end-diastolic volume) result in a proportional elevation of myocardial wall tension which in turn leads to increased myocardial oxygen demand. Oxygen supply to any organ system is determined by blood flow and oxygen extraction. Since the resting coronary venous oxygen saturation is already set at its lower level approximately (30%), the myocardium has a limited capacity to increase its oxygen extraction during certain situations of increased demand. Hence, an increase in myocardial oxygen demand (e.g. during exercise) must be met by a proportional increase in coronary blood flow. The capacity of the coronary arteries to enhance blood flow in reaction to increased cardiac metabolic demand is often called coronary flow reserve (CFR). Among normal persons, the maximal coronary blood flow after full dilation of the coronary arteries is approximately 4–6 times of the resting coronary blood flow. CFR is usually dependant upon at least 3 factors: Large and small coronary artery resistance, extravascular (i.e. myocardial and interstitial) resistance, and blood composition (Figs 2.9 and 2.10).

## Syndrome X

The signs and symptoms comprising of syndrome X include angina pectoris, ischemia like ST-segment changes and/or myocardial perfusion defects during stress testing, and angiographically normal coronary arteries (Figs 2.11 and 2.12). In majority, patients with this syndrome are postmenopausal women, and they usually carry an excellent prognosis. Syndrome X is thought to be caused by microvascular angina. The following are the different mechanisms which can result this type of syndrome:

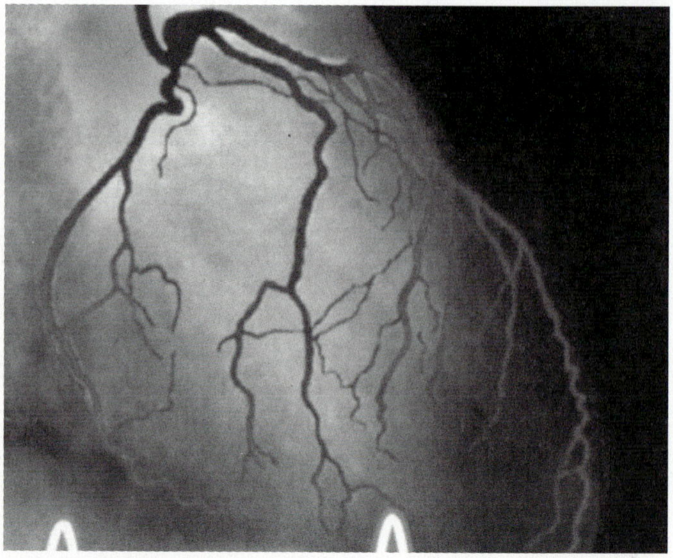

**Fig. 2.11:** Angiogram showing normal coronary vessels in patient with atypical noncardiac chest pain

1. Impaired endothelial dysfunction
2. Increased release of local vasoconstrictors
3. Fibrosis and medial hypertrophy of the microcirculation
4. Abnormal cardiac adrenergic nerve function, and/of
5. Estrogen deficiency

Many of the extravascular forces produced by contraction of adjacent myocardium and intraventricular pressures can affect coronary microcirculation resistance and thus lead to fall in CFR. Extravascular compressive forces are highest in the subendocardium and decrease toward the subepicardium. Left ventricular (LV) hypertrophy together with a higher myocardial oxygen demand (e.g. during tachycardia) can result in greater susceptibility to reduced blood supply in the region of subendocardial layers. Reduction in blood supply to the myocardium can also be due to other factors affecting blood composition, such as reduced oxygen carrying capacity of blood, as is observed with severe anemia (hemoglobin, <8 g/dl), or elevated levels of carboxyhemoglobin. The latter may be the result of inhalation of carbon monoxide in a closed area or of long-term smoking. Holter Electrocardiographic Monitoring Study has revealed that silent ischemia is a common phenomenon among patients with established coronary artery disease. In one particular study some workers had demonstrated as many as 75% of episodes of ischemia (defined as transient ST-depression of ≥1 mm persisting for at least 1 min) happening in patients with stable angina were clinically silent. Silent ischemia occurs most frequently in early morning hours and may result in transient myocardial contractile dysfunction (i.e. stunning). The exact pathophysiology for silent ischemia is not very well known. However, autonomic dysfunction (especially in diabetic patients, a higher pain threshold in some individuals, and the production of excessive quantities of endorphins are the popular hypotheses in silent myocardial ischemia.

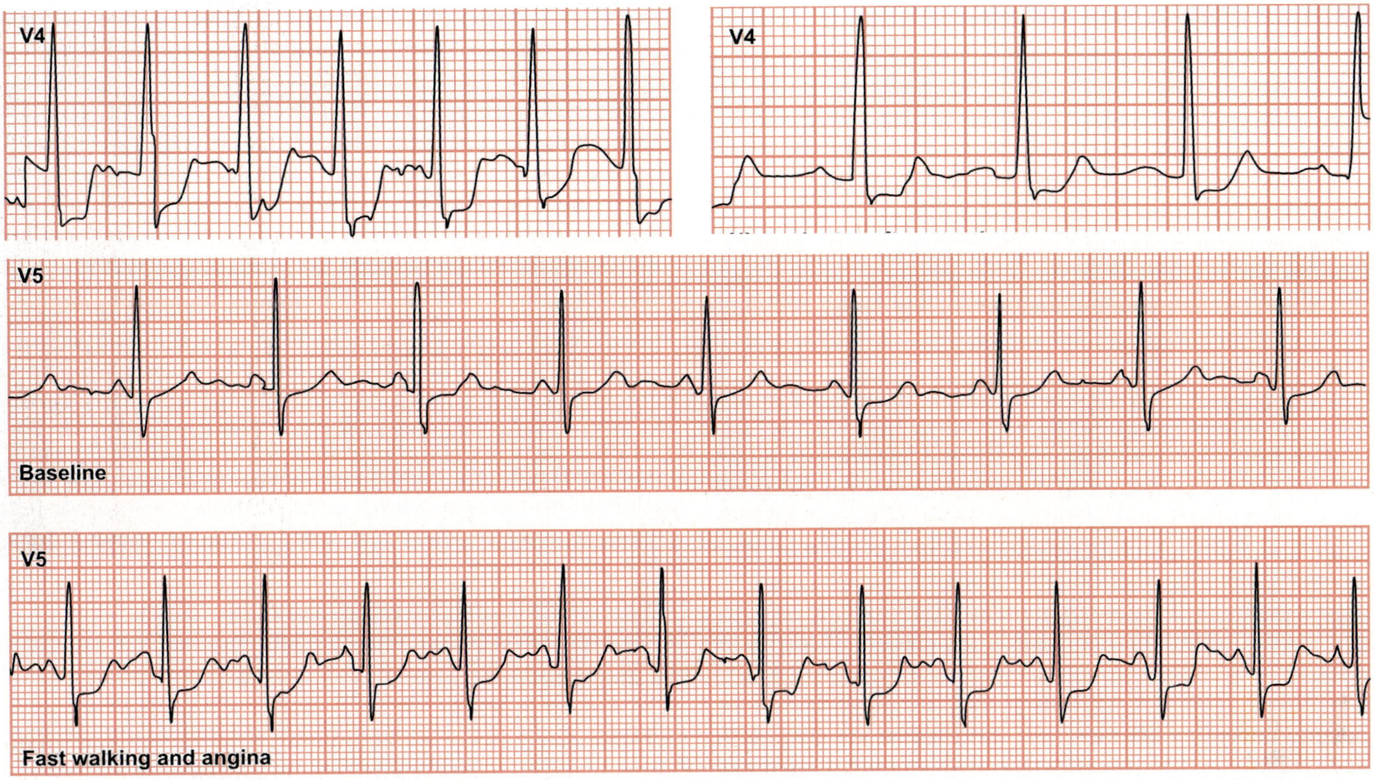


**Fig. 2.12:** (Top) Syndrome X'-exercise testing in a patient with angina and angiographically normal coronary arteries showed CAD-like ST-segment depression. Similarly, transient ischemia like ST-segment changes were recorded during 24-hours ECG monitoring in another patient with exertional chest pain and normal coronary angiograms (bottom)

## INCIDENCE OF ANGINA PECTORIS

Approximately, 6.3 million Americans are estimated to experience angina. An estimated 350,000 new cases of angina occur every year. Each year, 1.1 million new and recurrent cases of an acute coronary event occur, of which more than 40% are fatal. Roughly, more than 12 million had a history of myocardial infarction (MI) and/or angina pectoris in the year 2000.

*Mortality/Morbidity:* Coronary artery disease is the single most common cause of death in most of developed and developing countries, accounting for almost one death per minute. More than half of those who die suddenly from coronary artery disease have no previous symptoms.

*Race:* The rate of angina pectoris in women older than 2 years ranges from 3.9% in non-Hispanic white women to 6.2% in non-Hispanic black women and 5.5% in Mexican American women. The rates of angina pectoris for men in the same ethnic groups are 2.6%, 3.1% and 4.1%, respectively. Among American Indians aged 65–74 years, the rates (per 1000 persons) of new and recurrent heart attacks are 25.1% for men and 9.1% for women.

*Gender:* Angina pectoris is more often the presenting symptom of coronary artery disease in women than in men, with a female-to-male ratio of 1.7:1. It has a prevalence of 3.9 million in women and 2.3 million in men. The frequency of atypical presentations is also more common among women compared with men. Women have a slightly higher rate of mortality from coronary artery disease compared with men, in part because of an older age at presentation and a frequent lack of classic anginal symptoms. The estimated age-adjusted prevalence of angina is greater in women than in men.

*Age:* The prevalence of angina pectoris increases with age. Age is a strong independent risk factor in ischemic heart disease.

## HISTORY IN ANGINA PECTORIS

Most patients with angina pectoris report of retrosternal chest discomfort rather than frank pain. The former is usually described as a pressure, heaviness, squeezing, burning, or choking sensation. Anginal pain may be localized primarily in the epigastrium, back, neck, jaw, or shoulders. Typical locations for radiation of pain are arms, shoulders and neck.

Typically, angina is precipitated by exertion, eating, exposure to cold, or emotional stress. It lasts for approximately 1–5 minutes and is relieved by rest or nitroglycerin. Chest pain lasting only a few seconds is not usually angina pectoris. The intensity of angina does not change with respiration, cough, or change in position. Pain above the mandible and below the epigastrium is rarely anginal in nature. Ask patients about the frequency of angina, severity of pain, and number of nitroglycerin pills used during angina episodes.

## PHYSICAL EXAMINATION IN ANGINA PECTORIS

For most patients with stable angina, physical examination findings are normal. Diagnosing secondary causes of angina, such as aortic stenosis, is important.

**A positive Levine sign** (characterized by the patient's fist clenched over the sternum when describing the discomfort) is suggestive of angina pectoris. Look for physical signs of abnormal lipid metabolism (e.g. xanthelasma, xanthoma) or of diffuse atherosclerosis (e.g. absence or diminished peripheral pulses, increased light reflexes or arteriovenous nicking upon ophthalmic examination and carotid bruit).

Clinical examination of patients during the angina attack may be more contributory. Examination findings, which are most important include third and/or fourth heart sounds due to LV systolic and/or diastolic dysfunction and mitral regurgitation secondary to papillary muscle dysfunction. Pain which is produced with pressure on the chest wall is usually of chest wall diseases. Factors leading to angina pectoris decrease in myocardial blood supply due to increased coronary resistance in large and small coronary arteries.

Significant coronary atherosclerotic lesion in the large epicardial coronary arteries (i.e. conductive vessels) with at least a 50% reduction in arterial diameter. Coronary spasm (i.e. Prinzmetal angina), abnormal constriction or deficient endothelial-dependent relaxation of resistant vessels associated with diffuse vascular disease (i.e. microvascular angina) syndrome X. Systemic inflammatory or collagen vascular disease, such as scleroderma, systemic lupus Erythematous, Kawasaki disease, polyarteritis nodosa, and Takayasu arteritis. Increased extravascular forces, such as severe LV hypertrophy caused by hypertension, aortic stenosis, or hypertrophic cardiomyopathy, or increased LV diastolic pressures. Reduction in the oxygen-carrying capacity of blood, such as elevated carboxyhemoglobin or severe anemia (hemoglobin, < 8 g/dl)

The following are congenital anomalies of the origin and/or course of the major epicardial coronary arteries:

1. Structural abnormalities of the coronary arteries
2. Congenital coronary artery aneurysm or fistula
3. Coronary artery ectasia
4. Coronary artery fibrosis after chest radiation
5. Coronary intimal fibrosis following cardiac transplantation

## RISK FACTORS

Major risk factors which can lead to atherosclerosis are:

1. Family history of premature coronary artery disease,
2. Cigarette smoking
3. Diabetes mellitus
4. Hypercholesterolemia or
5. Systemic hypertension
6. Other risk factors include LV hypertrophy, obesity, and elevated serum levels of homocysteine, lipoprotein (a), plasminogen activator inhibitor, fibrinogen, serum triglycerides, or low high-density lipoprotein (HDL).

*Metabolic syndrome:* The main features of this syndrome are the presence of hyperinsulinemia (fasting glucose level ≥110 mg/dl), abdominal obesity (waist circumference >40 inches for men or >35 inches for women) decreased HDL cholesterol levels (<40 mg/dl for men or <50 mg/dl for women), hypertriglyceridemia (>150 mg/dl), and hypertension (≥130/85 mmHg). Patients with the metabolic syndrome have a 3-fold increased risk for coronary atherosclerosis and stroke compared with those without these features.

*Precipitating factors:* The factors which can precipitate angina pectoris are severe anemia, fever, tachyarrhythmias, catecholamines, emotional stress, and hyperthyroidism, due to increase in myocardial oxygen demand.

*Preventive factors:* Factors associated with reduced risk of atherosclerosis are a high serum HDL cholesterol level, physical activity, estrogen, and moderate alcohol intake (1–2 drinks/day).

*Other problems to be considered*

1. Esophageal spasm
2. Esophageal rupture
3. Costochondritis
4. Herpes zoster
5. Pneumonia with pleural involvement

## LABORATORY INVESTIGATIONS

*Chest radiography:* Findings are usually normal in patients. However, they may show cardiomegaly in patients with previous MI, ischemic cardiomyopathy, pericardial effusion or acute pulmonary edema. Calcification of coronary arteries frequently correlates with major coronary artery disease with angina pectoris.

### Imaging Studies

*Exercise stress testing*: When performed alone, exercise stress testing generally has somewhat lower sensitivity and

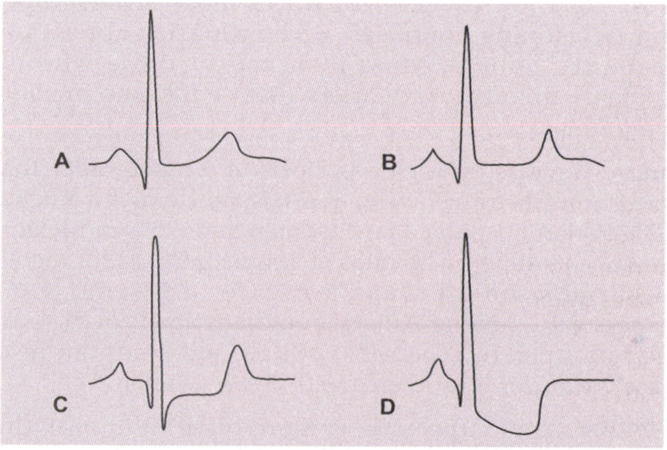


**Fig. 2.13:** (A) ST changes with ischemia depicting normal waveforms, (B) Flattening of ST-segment, (C) Making T-wave more prominent, horizontal ST-segment depression, (D) Down slopping ST-segment depression

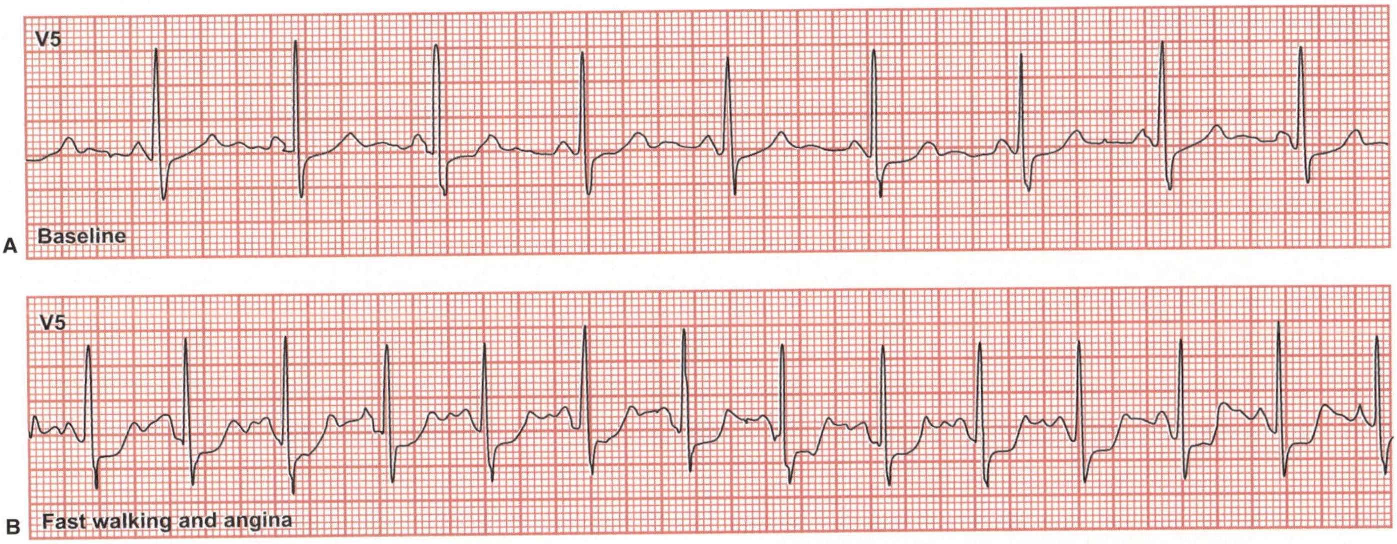


**Fig. 2.14:** (A) ECG showing normal STT changes at rest and (B) marked ST-depression in a in stable angina patient with exercise

specificity, but it is cheaper and therefore is a reasonable option in patient with a low probability of disease. It can be performed alone and in conjunction with echocardiography or myocardial perfusion scintigraphy tests. Stress echocardiography has an overall sensitivity of 78% and specificity of 86%; myocardial perfusion scintigraphy has an overall sensitivity of 83% and specificity of 77%. Test results must be interpreted with the background of patient's history and physical examination. In population with low prevalence, the predictive abilities of these tests are low; however, in patients with a high likelihood of coronary artery disease, the predictive value is much higher (Figs 2.13 and 2.14).

*Stress echocardiography:* It can be used to evaluate segmental wall motion during exercise. It detects changes in regional wall motion that occur during myocardial ischemia. Normal myocardium becomes hyperdynamic during exercise; ischemic segments become hypokinetic or akinetic (Fig. 2.15).

It has the advantage of simultaneous evaluation of LV function, cardiac dimensions,valvular disease, in patients with baseline ECG abnormalities and those with systolic murmurs suggestive of aortic stenosis or hypertrophic cardiomyopathy. It is also helpful for localizing ischemia and evaluating its severity. During exercise stress echocardiography signs of severe coronary artery disease include LV dilation, a decrease in global systolic function, and new or worsening mitral regurgitation. However, with dobutamine stress echocardiography, even in patients with severe coronary artery disease, the LV cavity may not dilate and global systolic function may improve. A major problem with stress echocardiography is the technical difficulty with obtaining adequate images in some patients.

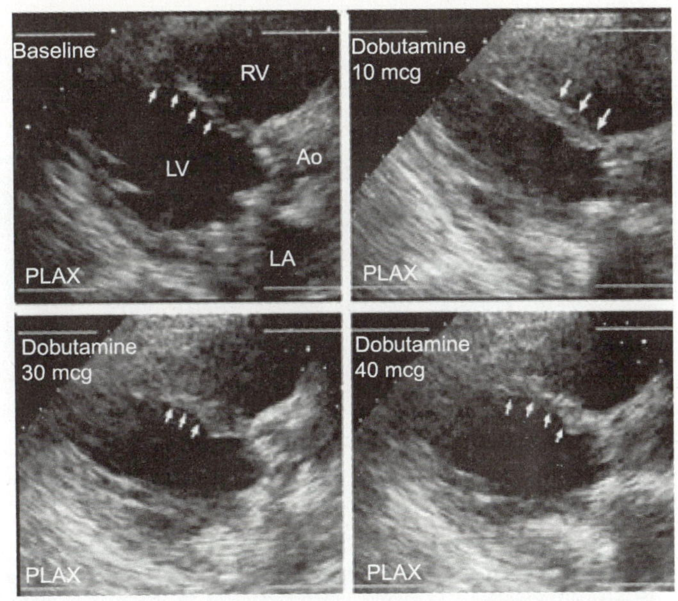


**Fig. 2.15:** Dobutamine stress echocardiogram—biphasic response. A biphasic response on dobutamine stress echoardiography in an anginal patient who is considered as a candidate for coronary artery revascularization procedures

*Nuclear evaluation in anginal patient:* These are the most frequently used myocardial perfusion scintigraphy tests. These tests are especially useful in patients with baseline ECG abnormalities, to localize the region of ischemia, and as prognostic indicators (Figs 2.16 and 2.20).

The presence of increased lung uptake upon thallium imaging is associated with a poor prognosis. Increased lung uptake, together with post-stress dilation of the LV and multiple perfusion defects, is suggestive of either left main coronary artery disease or severe three-vessel disease. The number of affected myocardial segments is predictive of long-term survival. Smaller perfusion defects are usually associated with peripheral coronary artery lesions, which are associated with a better prognosis. The absence of perfusion defects even in the presence of symptoms indicates an excellent prognosis. The frequency of infarction or death is 1 case per 10,000 stress tests. Absolute contra-

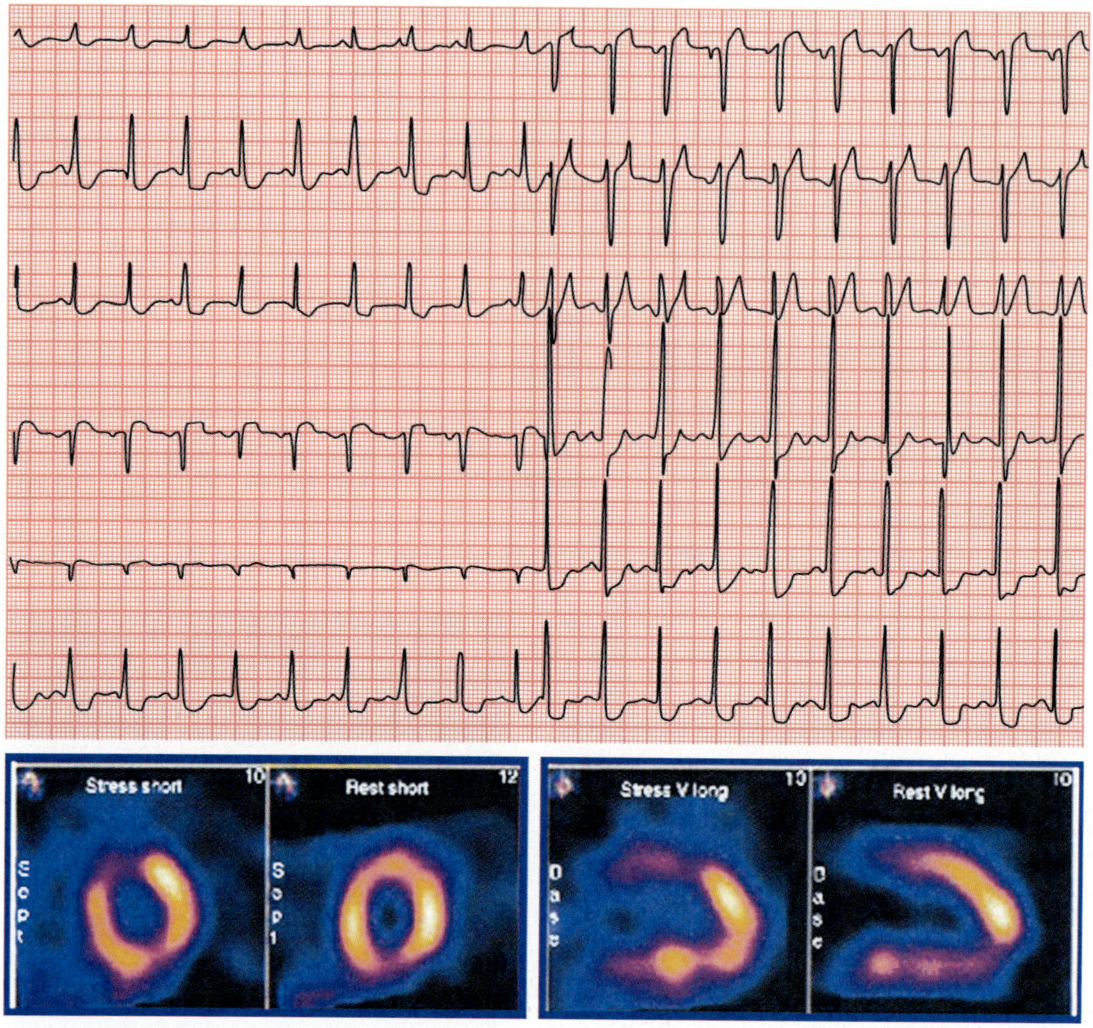


**Fig. 2.16:** Effort ECG and (upper panel) corresponding myocardial SPECT (lower panel) of the DM2 patient. At maximal exercise, ECG shows diffuse ST-segment depression. At the same time, SPECT reveals septal myocardial perfusion defect which is reversible at rest

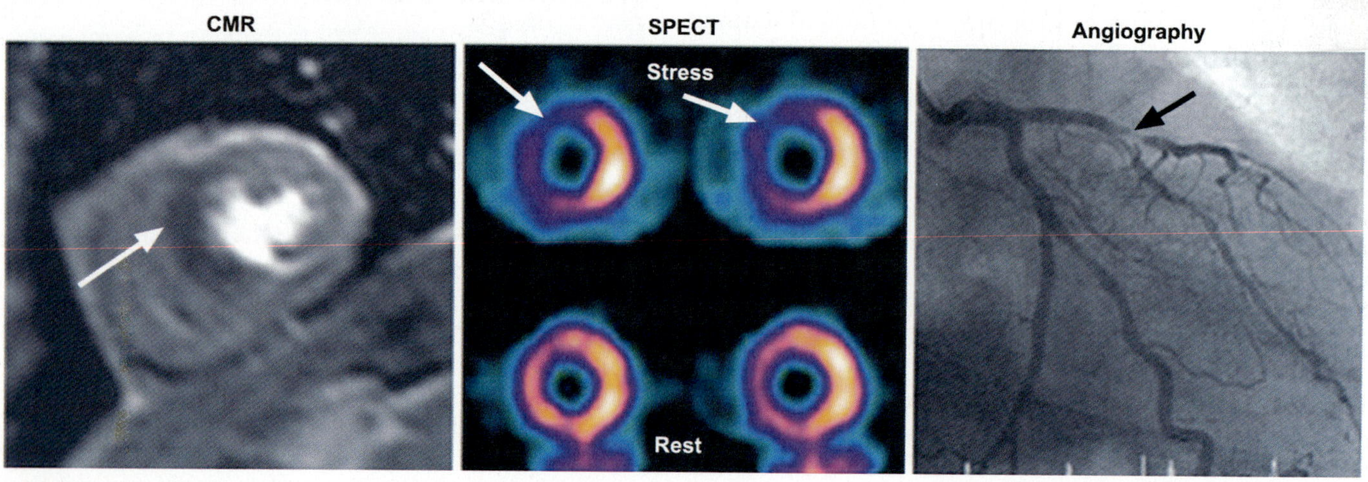


**Fig. 2.17:** Hypoperfusion of the anterior wall and septum seen on MRI (left) and SPECT (centre). Angiography demonstrates this to be due to LAD and diagonal disease

indications include symptomatic cardiac arrhythmias, severe aortic stenosis, acute MI within the previous 2 days, acute myocarditis, or pericarditis. Discontinue the exercise stress test in the presence of chest pain, a drop in systolic blood pressure of more than 10 mmHg, severe shortness of breath, fatigue, dizziness or near syncope, ST-depression

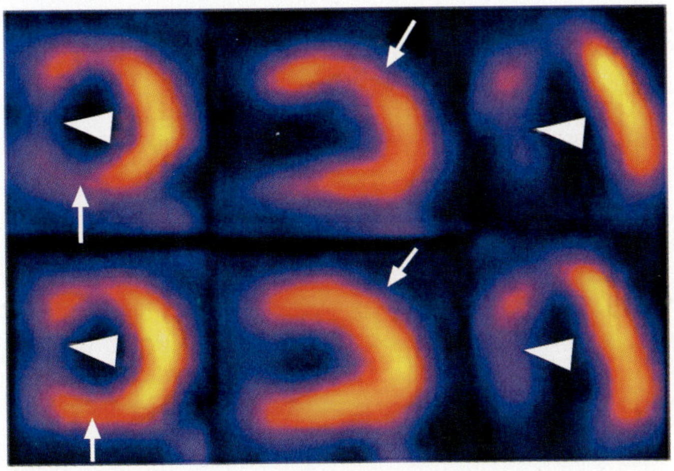

**Fig. 2.18:** Example of a patient with a reversible defect as well as an irreversible defect on perfusion SPECT. Example of a patient with reversible perfusion defect in the inferior (white arrows short-axis images) and anterior wall (white arrows vertical long-axis images), and an irreversible perfusion defect in the septum (arrow heads short-axis and horizontal long-axis images). The upper panel shows from left to right the short axis, the vertical long axis and the horizontal long axis reconstructions after stress and the lower panel shows the same reconstructions during rest

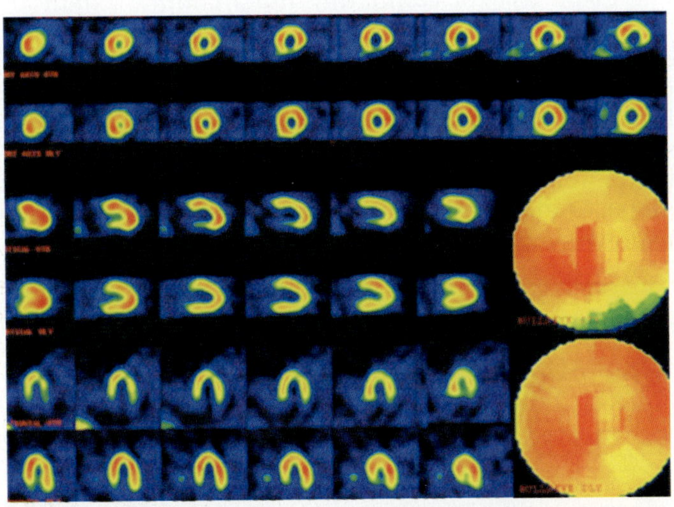

**Fig. 2.19:** A patient with multiple perfusion defects with different degrees of severity. The upper images are stress phase and lower images are rest or delayed images. There is moderate ischemia in the mid-anterolateral and mid-inferolateral walls. Also there is severe ischemia in the basal inferior wall. Mild ischemia in the apex, apical septal and basal anterolateral are also noted

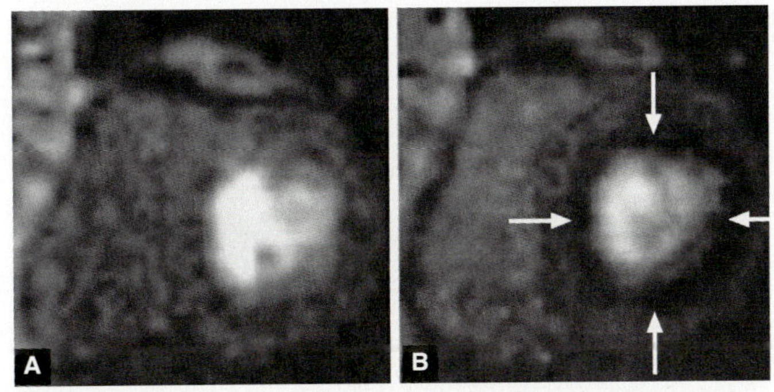


**Fig. 2.20:** Images of myocardium at peak myocardial enhancement during the first pass of gadolinium in a patient with syndrome X at rest (A) and during stress (B), showing a ring of delayed subendocardial enhancement (arrows in B)

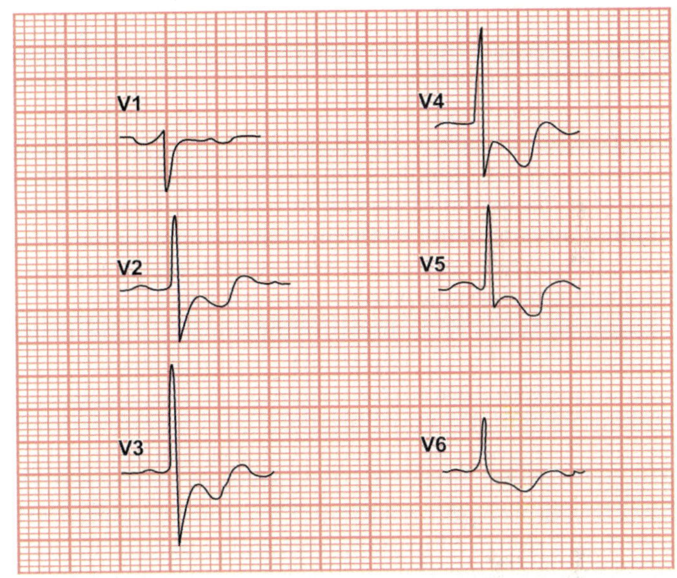


**Fig. 2.21:** Widespread ST-segment depression in patient with unstable angina

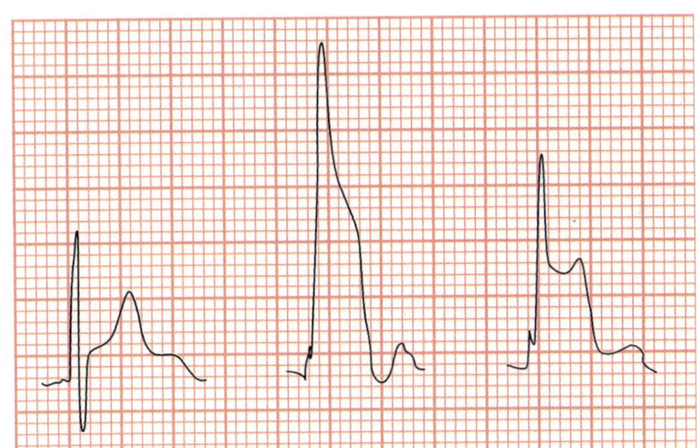

**Fig. 2.22:** Reversible ST-segment alterations in patient with chest pain; the ST-segment elevation returns to normal as the pain subsides

of more than 2 mm, ST-elevation of at least 1 mm without diagnostic Q-waves, or development of ventricular tachyarrhythmia.

### Other Tests

*Electrocardiography:* It is a useful tool for evaluating persons with angina pectoris; however, findings are variable among patients (Figs 2.21 and 2.22). Approximately 50% of patients with angina pectoris have normal findings after a resting ECG. However, abnormalities, such as evidence for prior MI, intraventricular conduction delay, various degrees of atrioventricular block, arrhythmias, or

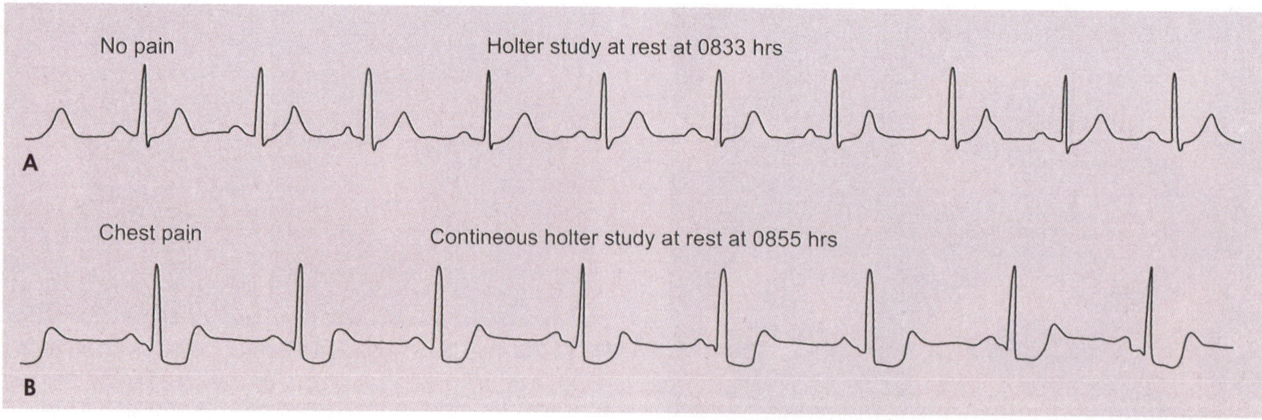


**Fig. 2.23:** (A) normal sinus rhythm at 0833 hrs and (B) chest pain with significant ST-segment depression at 0855 hours on Holter monitor recording of a patient with angina pectoris

ST-T-wave changes may be seen. During an attack of angina pectoris, 50% of patients with normal findings after resting ECG show abnormalities. A 1 mm or greater depression of the ST-segment below the baseline, measured 80 milliseconds from the J point, is the most characteristic change. Reversible ST-segment elevation occurs with Prinzmetal angina. Some patients with coronary artery disease may show pseudo-normalization of the resting ECG ST-T-wave abnormalities during episodes of chest pain.

Exercise with ECG monitoring alone is the initial procedure of choice in patients without baseline ST-segment abnormalities or in whom anatomic localization of ischemia is not a consideration. Horizontal or down-sloping ST-segment depression of at least 1 mm, measured 80 milliseconds from the J point, is considered the characteristic ischemic response. ST-segment depression of more than 2 mm at a low workload or that persists for more than 5 minutes after termination of exercise and a failure of blood pressure to rise or an actual drop in blood pressure are signs of severe ischemic heart disease and a poor prognosis. Withhold beta-blockers for approximately 48 hours before the stress test, whenever possible. Patients on digoxin and those with LV hypertrophy with repolarization abnormalities more often show positive results. Exercise stress tests have lower sensitivity and specificity in women and in patients with left bundle-branch block.

*Ambulatory ECG monitoring*: It can be used for diagnostic purposes in patients with chest pain suggestive of Prinzmetal angina but is primarily used to evaluate the frequency of silent ischemia (Fig. 2.23). Silent ischemia has been shown to be an independent predictor of mortality in patients with angina pectoris.

Several studies have shown that calcium in the coronary arteries as detected by electron-beam computed tomography is an important indicator of coronary artery stenosis. In these studies, the sensitivity of a positive electron-beam computed tomography scan ranged from 85% to 100% and the specificity varied from 41% to 76%, while the positiv predictive value varied from 55% to 84% and the negative predictive value varied from 84% to 100%. However, several studies, have shown inconsistent reproducibility in repeated measures of coronary calcium with electron-beam computed tomography. Thus, its proper role at this time remains controversial.

### Procedures

*Selective coronary angiography:* It is the definitive diagnostic test for evaluating the anatomic extent and severity of coronary artery disease. Consider coronary angiography in symptomatic patients with inconclusive noninvasive study results, in survivors of sudden cardiac death, in those who are considered to have a poor prognosis based on the results of noninvasive studies, in those with occupational requirements for a definite diagnosis (e.g. pilots), or in patients with coronary artey disease who are severely symptomatic despite maximal medical therapy.

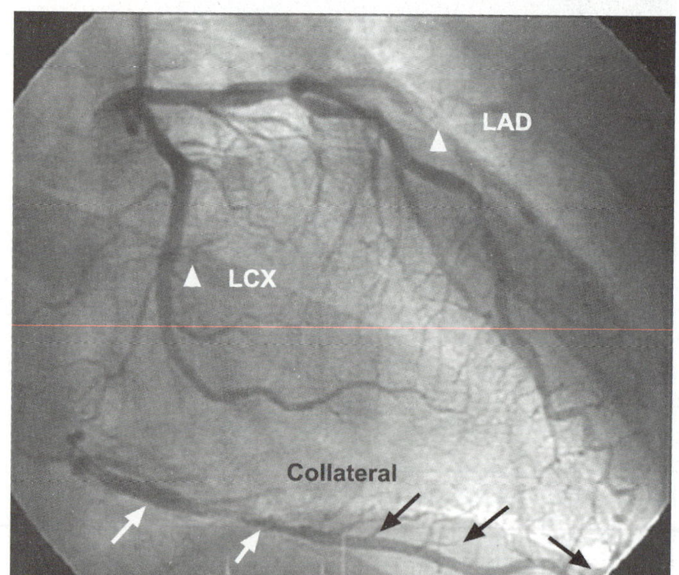


**Fig. 2.24:** Representative coronary angiography for collaterals. The patient is a 42-year-old man. His right coronary artery is totally occluded, but Rentrop grade III collateral (arrowheads) can be seen from the left coronary artery. His left ventricular ejection fraction is 60%. LAD, left anterior descending coronary artery; LCX, left circumflex coronary artery

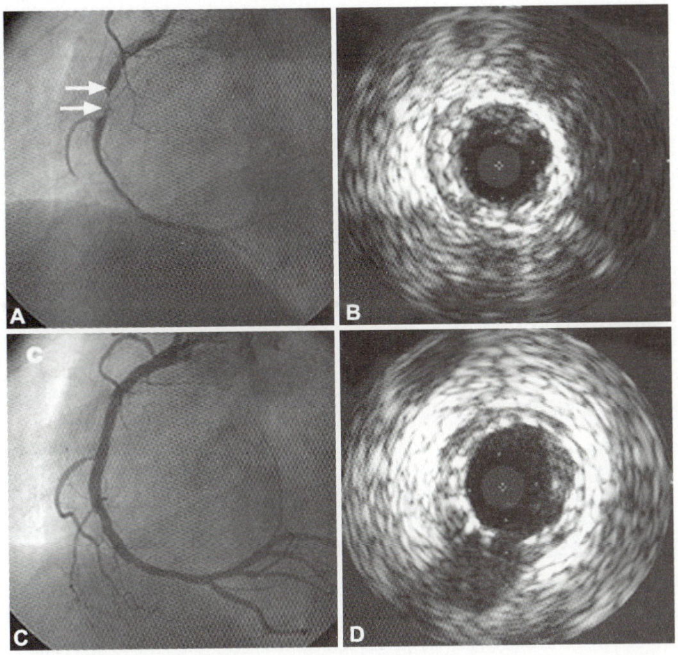

Fig. 2.25: (A) Right coronary angiogram showing very late stent thrombosis in RCA stent, (B) IVUS showing neointima breakdown and ruptured plaque within the RCA stent, (C) Coronary angiography after plain old balloon angioplasty (POBA). Final coronary angiogram showed good distal flow, (D) IVUS showed markedly decreased residual stenosis

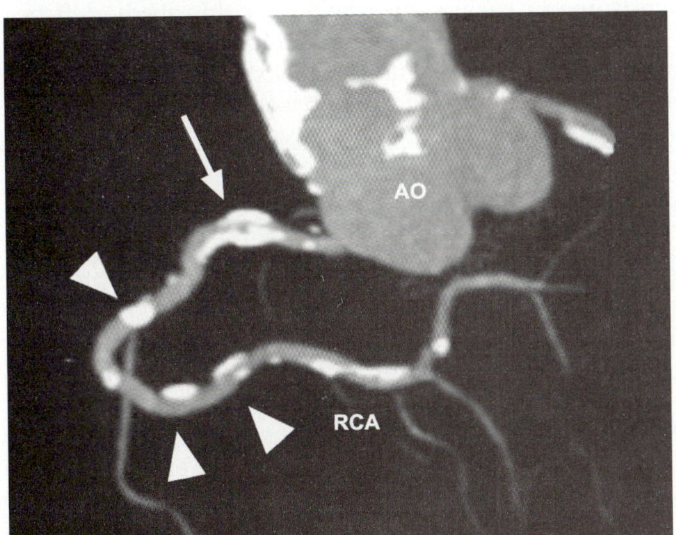


Fig. 2.26: A 58-year-old man with stable angina. Diffuse calcification (arrow and arrowheads) was detected in right coronary artery (RCA) on MDCT angiography maximum-intensity-projection (MIP) image. AO=aorta

In patients in whom Prinzmetal angina is suggested, provocative testing with ergonovine maleate during coronary angiography may be useful (Figs 2.24–2.32).

*Optical coherence tomography in angina:* It is an excellent investigation in the evaluation of ruptured plaque of stent complication in unstable angina and other complications in coronary artery disease (Figs 2.33 and 2.35).

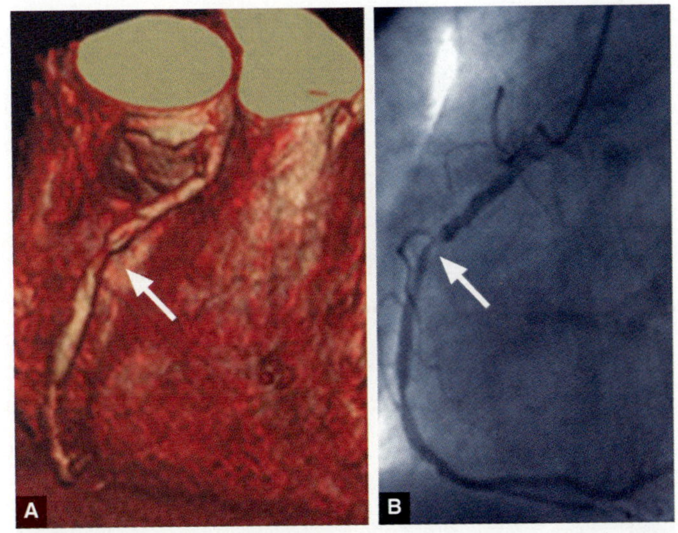

Fig. 2.27: Multislice computed tomography study. 3-D volumetric image (A) and angiographic image (B) showing occlusive stenosis in the right coronary artery (arrow)

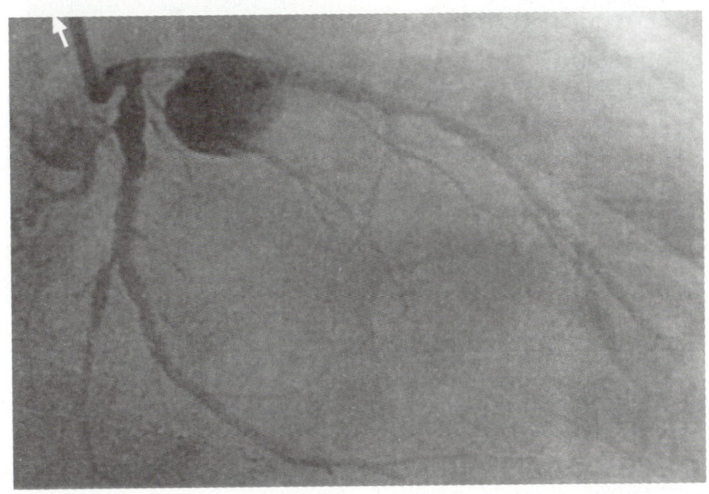

Fig. 2.28: Giant aneurysm proximal to stent and progression of lesion in LAD and LCx arteries in patient with persistent angia pectoris even after stentoplasty for the treatment of effort angia

## MANAGEMENT OF ANGINA PECTORIS

*Enhanced external counterpulsation (EECP):* It is a non-invasive technique that reduces angina and extends time to exercise-induced myocardial ischemia in patients with symptomatic coronary disease (Figs 2.36 and 2.39). EECP uses the sequential inflation of 3 sets of pneumatic cuffs wrapped around the lower extremities. The cuffs are inflated sequentially (from calf to thigh to buttock) at the onset of diastole, producing aortic counterpulsation, diastolic augmentation, and increased venous return. At the onset of systole, the external pressure in the cuffs is released rapidly, producing a decrease in systolic pressure. It has been hypothesized that the sustained benefits of EECP result from effective diastolic augmentation that may promote collateral development or improve endothelial

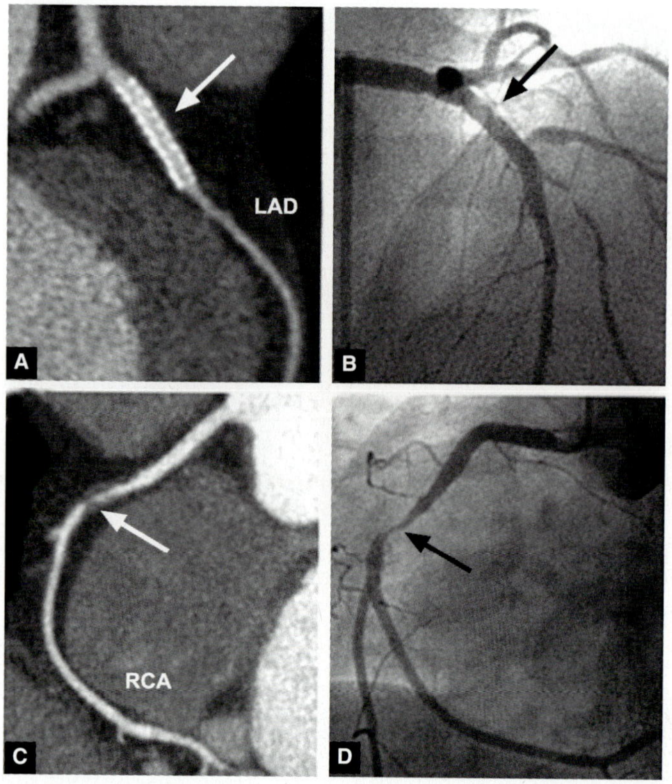


Fig. 2.29: MDCT and invasive angiographic findings in a 51-year-old woman with atypical chest pain and nondiagnostic stress test 7 months after anterior myocardial infarction and PCI to the left anterior descending (LAD) coronary artery. MDCT (A) and invasive angiography (B) showed patent LAD stent (arrow) but new soft noncalcified plaque (arrow), (C) in right coronary artery (RCA) causing severe RCA stenosis (C, D)

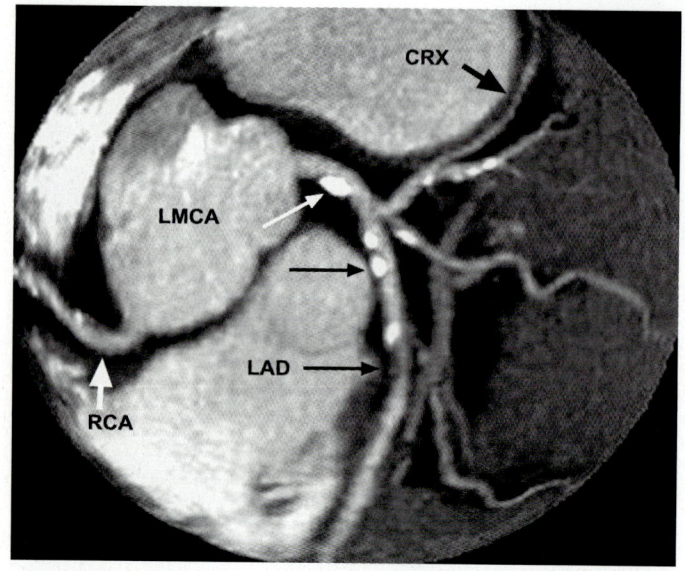


Fig. 2.30: A 72-year-old man with unstable angina pectoris shows several nonsignificant calcified plaques in left main and proximal left anterior descending (LAD) coronary arteries (dotted arrows) and significant heterogenous plaque in mid-left anterior descending coronary artery (solid arrows) that is causing 60% diameter stenosis detected on MDCT angiography maximum-intensity-projection (MIP) image

function. Most studies have shown that patients with higher levels of diastolic augmentation measured by finger plethysmography have improved early and late clinical outcomes.

In practice, EECP is limited to treating outpatients with chronic stable angina pectoris. Early external counter pulsation models involving a lower-extremity hydraulic water-compression system were shown to provide clinical benefit in a small sample of patients with either acute myocardial infarction or cardiogenic shock. Whether the acute hemodynamic effects of the sequential, pneumatic EECP device could benefit inpatients with these acute cardiac disorders is not known.

Measurements of the acute hemodynamic effects during EECP have been limited to noninvasive finger plethysmography, thoracic electrical bioimpedance methodology, echocardiography, right heart catheterization, and radial artery catheterization. Because the EECP cuffs cover the femoral site, invasive left heart catheterization or intracoronary hemodynamic studies during EECP have not been performed previously. The purpose of this study was to assess intracoronary, central aortic and cardiac hemodynamics during EECP and to determine whether these acute hemodynamic effects of EECP will have a favorable profile for patients with disorders such as acute coronary syndrome or cardiogenic shock. For this study, left heart catheterization and measurements of intracoronary pressure and Doppler flow velocity were performed from the right radial arterial site at baseline and during EECP.

*Clinical indications of enhanced external electro-counterpulsation therapy:*

1. Those who have been advised bypass surgery and choose not to have it.
2. Those who cannot afford the cost of bypass surgery.
3. Those who have other diseases which make them unfit for surgery, e.g. coexisting diabetes mellitus, bronchial asthma, kidney failure, rhyroid disorders, old age, i.e. more than 80 years.
4. Those who have already had bypass surgery done a few years earlier and don't want to suffer the experience again.
5. Those patients who cannot afford the exorbitant cost of angioplasty with two cipher stents.
6. Those patients who have chest pain or breathlessness of cardiac origin and do not wish to undergo any further investigation can go for EECP directly.
7. Patients whose stents have got blocked again.

*Intra-aortic balloon counterpulsation:* It can be used in patients who continue to have unstable angina pectoris despite maximal medical treatment (Fig. 2.40). This procedure should be followed promptly by coronary angiography with possible coronary revascularization.

In patients whose angina is refractory to medical therapy who are not suitable candidates for either percutaneous or surgical revascularization.

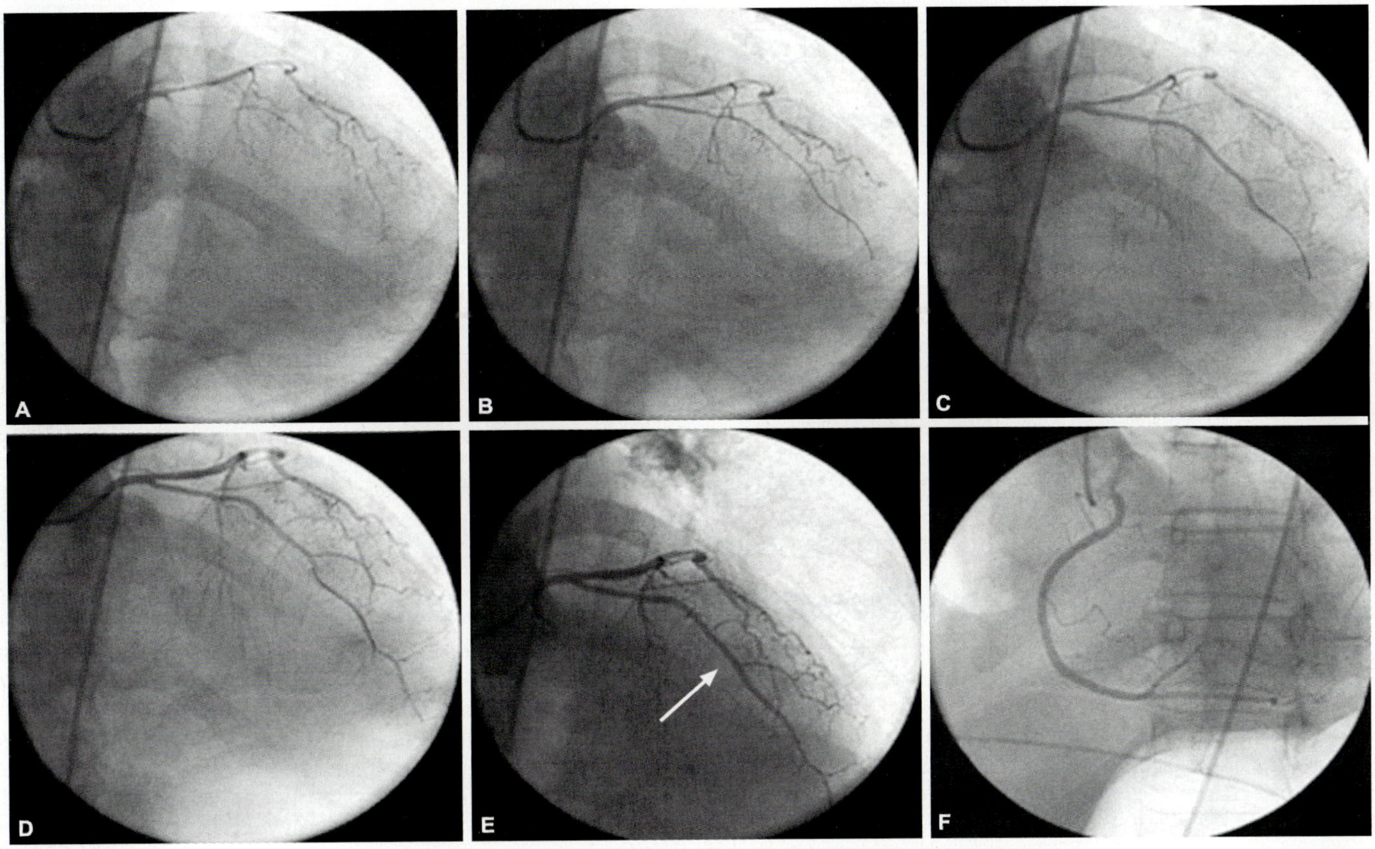


**Fig. 2.31:** Coronary vasospasm is a well-known cause of exercise-induced angina pectoris, Prinzmetal's unstable angina, and myocardial infarction. In general, the prognosis of patients with isolated coronary vasospasm is good, although in the setting of myocardial infarction, mechanical complications, such as free wall or interventricular septal rupture, malignant arrhythmias, and sudden death can occur

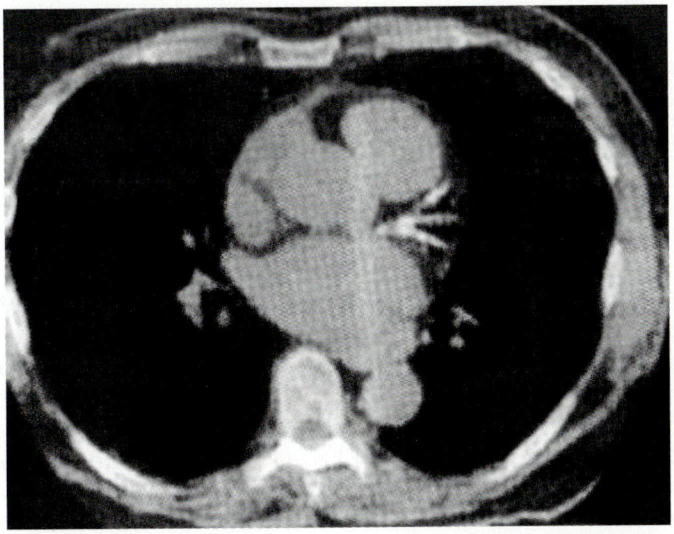

**Fig. 2.32:** MRI scan for coronary arteries showing significantly thickened and calcified major coronary vessels in patient with effort angina

## Surgical Care

*Revascularization therapy* (i.e. coronary revascularization): It can be considered in patients with left main artery stenosis greater than 50%, 2- or 3-vessel disease and LV dysfunction (ejection fraction, <45%), poor prognostic signs during noninvasive studies, or severe symptoms despite maximum medical therapy (Fig. 2.41). The two main coronary revascularization procedures are percutaneous transluminal coronary angioplasty, with or without coronary stenting, and coronary artery bypass grafting.

Patients with 1- or 2-vessel disease and normal LV function, who have anatomically suitable lesions are candidates for percutaneous transluminal coronary angioplasty and coronary stenting. Restenosis is the major complication, with symptomatic restenosis occurring in 20–25% of patients. Restenosis mostly occurs during the first 6 months after the procedure and can be managed by repeat angioplasty. Several recent trials have demonstrated that the use of drug-eluting stents (e.g. sirolimus-eluting stents and paclitaxel-coated stents) can remarkably reduce the rate of in-stent restenosis. Recently, with the introduction of these drug-coated stents, patients with multivessel coronary artery disease are more frequently treated with percutaneous revascularization as opposed to the surgical revascularization.

Patients with single-vessel disease and normal ventricular function treated with percutaneous transluminal coronary angioplasty show improved exercise tolerance and fewer episodes of angina compared with those who receive medical treatment. However, no difference in the

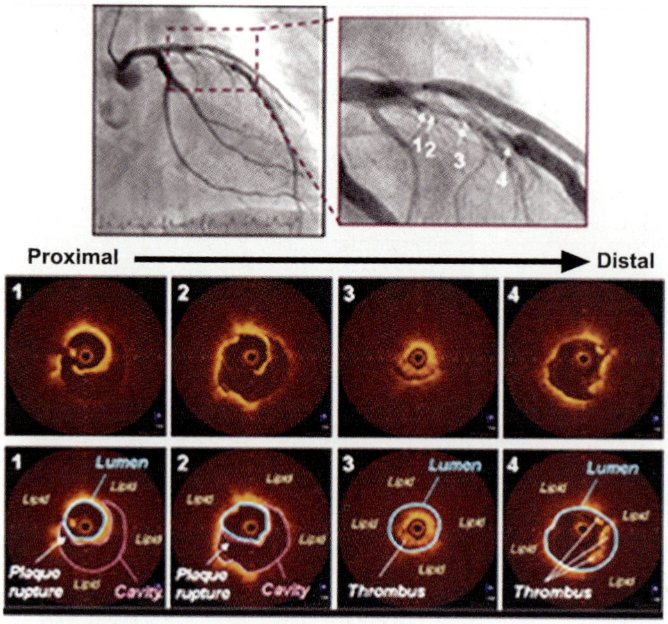


**Fig. 2.33:** Representative OCT images of plaque rupture in unstable angina pectoris. Angiography showed a complex lesion in the left anterior descending coronary artery. OCT revealed a plaque rupture with a residual fibrous-cap and plaque cavity (#1 and #2), and intracoronary thrombi (#3 and #4). Schemas demonstrate plaque rupture, lumen, ruptured cavity, lipid, and thrombi. Plaque rupture was observed at the minimal lumen area site [minimal lumen area = 1.83 mm$^2$ (#1); maximal ruptured cavity area = 3.26 mm$^2$ (#2)]. The plaque was considered to contain abundant lipid (number of lipid quadrants = 4). Thrombi occupied coronary lumen distal to the plaque rupture

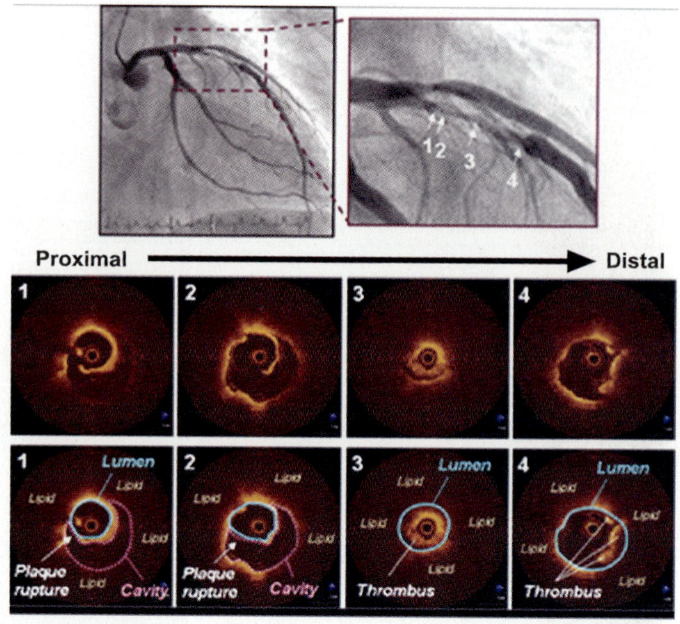


**Fig. 2.34:** Representative OCT images of plaque rupture in stable angina pectoris. Angiography showed an eccentric stenosis in the left anterior descending coronary artery. OCT revealed a plaque rupture with a residual fibrous-cap and plaque cavity (#1, #2 and #3). Schemas demonstrate plaque rupture, lumen, ruptured cavity, 3-layered coronary artery wall, lipid, and calcification. Plaque rupture was located proximally to the minimal lumen area site [maximal ruptured cavity area = 0.45 mm$^2$; (#2) minimal lumen area = 2.59 mm$^2$ (#4)]. The plaque contained lipdic tissue (number of lipid quadrants = 2) and calcium. Intracoronary thrombi were not detected in the lesion with plaque rupture

frequency of MI or death has been shown between these two groups.

Patients with significant left main coronary artery disease, 2- or 3-vessel disease and LV dysfunction, diabetes mellitus, or lesions anatomically unsuitable for percutaneous transluminal coronary angioplasty have better results with coronary artery bypass grafting. The overall operative mortality rate for coronary artery bypass grafting is approximately 1.3%. The rate of graft patency 10 years after surgery is less than 50% for vein grafting, although more than 90% of grafts using internal mammary arteries are patent at 10 years. In recent years, interest has increased regarding surgery without cardiopulmonary bypass (i.e. off-pump) in an attempt to avoid the morbidity associated with cardiopulmonary bypass. A recent randomized study demonstrated that off-pump coronary surgery was as safe as on-pump surgery and caused less myocardial damage. However, the graft-patency rate was lower at 3 months in the off-pump group than in the on-pump group.

Recently, laser transmyocardial revascularization has been used as an experimental therapy for the treatment of severe, chronic, stable angina refractory to medical or other therapies. This technique has been performed with either an epicardial surgical technique or by a percutaneous approach. In both approaches, a series of transmural endomyocardial channels are created to improve myocardial perfusion. The surgical transmyocardial revascularization technique has been associated with symptomatic relief for end-stage chronic angina in the short term. However, no published data address the long-term efficacy of surgical transmyocardial revascularization. Nonetheless, this technique appears to provide at least symptomatic relief for end-stage chronic angina in the short term (Fig. 2.42).

*General measures:* Smoking cessation results in a significant reduction of acute adverse effects on the heart and may reverse, or at least slow, atherosclerosis. Strongly encourage patients to quit smoking, and take an active role in helping them to achieve this goal. Treat risk factors, including hypertension, diabetes mellitus, obesity, and hyperlipidemia. Several clinical trials have shown that in patients with established coronary artery disease, reduction of low-density lipoprotein (LDL) level with a beta-hydroxy-beta-methylglutaryl coenzyme A reductase inhibitor (i.e. statin) is associated with significant reductions in both mortality rate and major cardiac events. These benefits are present even in patients with mild-to-moderate elevations of LDL cholesterol level.

*Diet:* A diet low in saturated fat and dietary cholesterol is the mainstay of the step I and step II diet from the American Heart Association.

*Activity:* The level of activity that aggravates anginal symptoms is different for each patient. However, most

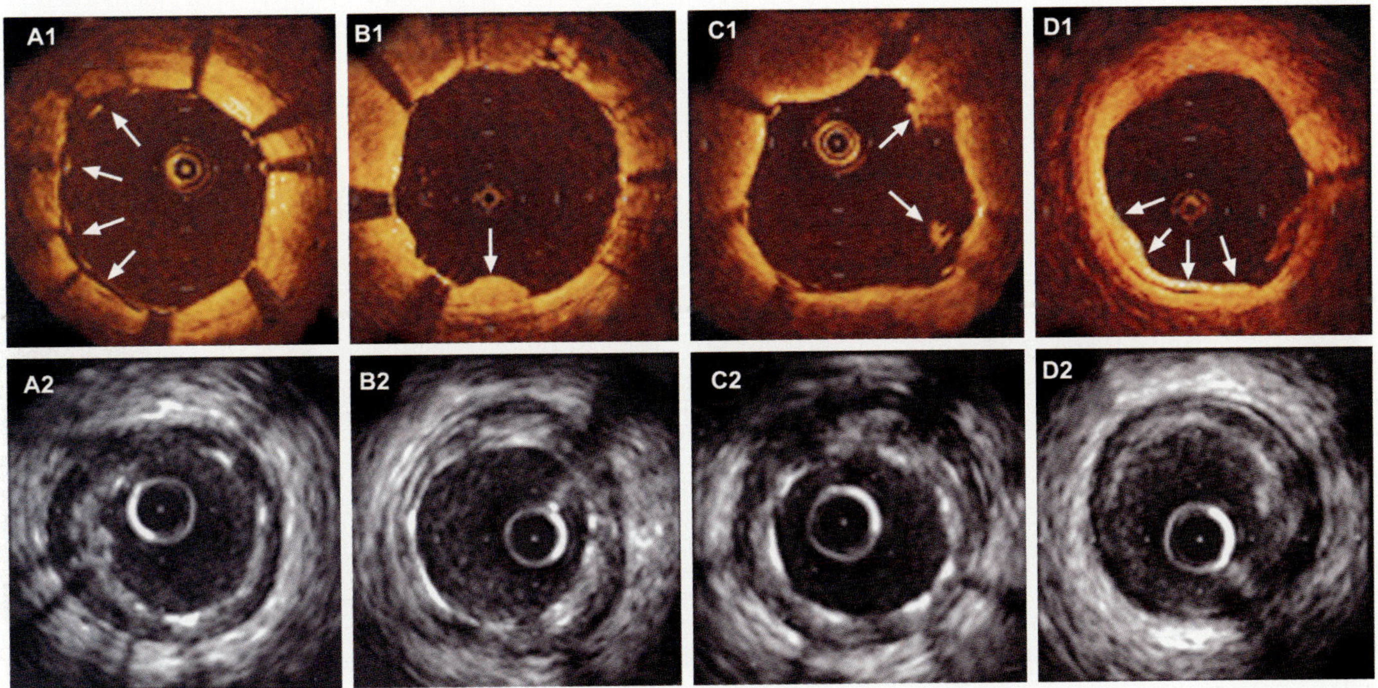


**Fig. 2.35:** Representative OCT images of stented lesions after PCI and corresponding IVUS images. (A1) OCT-visualized inadequate stent strut apposition (arrows). (A-2) It was not shown clearly on IVUS. (B1) Tissue protrusion between stent struts was observed in OCT image (arrow). (B2) It was not evident in the IVUS image. (C1) Intracoronary thrombi were identified as intraluminal mass images with signal-free shadow by OCT (arrows). (C2) They were not detected by IVUS. (D1) Coronary dissection at the site of stent edge was demonstrated by OCT (arrows). (D2) IVUS documented dissection (5 o'clock) and clot (2 o'clock). IVUS=intravascular ultrasound; OCT=optical coherence tomography; PCI=percutaneous coronary intervention

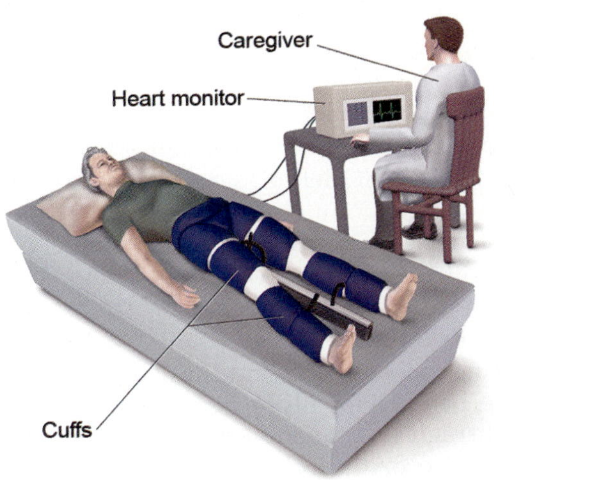


**Fig. 2.36:** Patient with chronic angina pectoris has been connected with EECP equipment ready to perform the application. Patient receives treatment of 1 hour daily for 35 days course

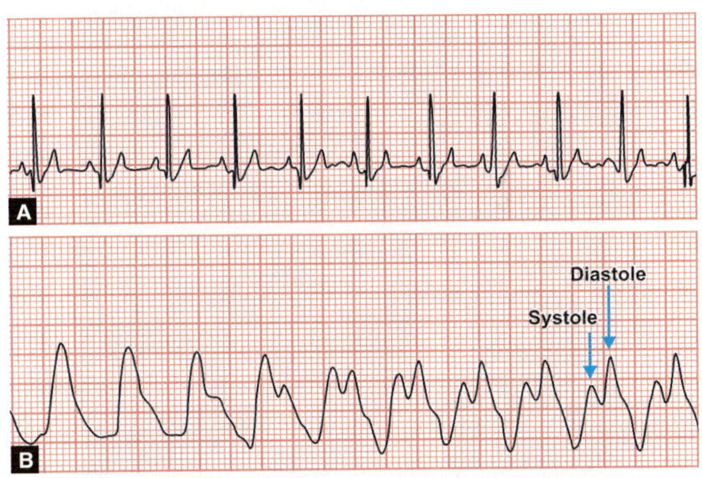


**Fig. 2.37:** Electrocardiogram (A) and finger plethysmographic recording (B) after initiation of enhanced external counterpulsation (EECP). Enhanced external counterpulsation leads to an increase in diastolic pressure (diastolic augmentation) and a decrease in systolic pressure (systolic unloading). The magnitude of EECP-induced hemodynamic changes is commonly assessed by measuring the diastolic-to-systolic effectiveness ratio, which is calculated by dividing the peak diastolic amplitude by the peak systolic amplitude of the finger plethysmographic signal

patients with stable angina can avoid symptoms during daily activities simply by reducing the speed of activity.The goals of pharmacotherapy are to reduce morbidity and to prevent complications.

## Medical Care

The main goals of treatment in angina pectoris are to relieve the symptoms, slow the progression of disease, and reduce the possibility of future events, especially MI and premature death.

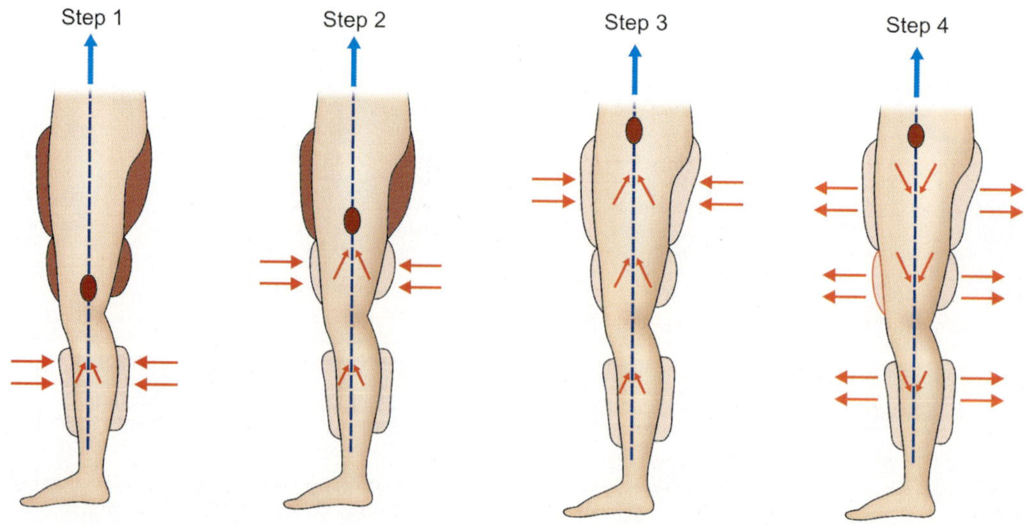


**Fig. 2.38:** Technique of EECP—three pairs of pneumatic cuffs are applied to the calves, lower thighs and upper thighs. The cuffs are inflated sequentially during diastole, distal to proximal. The compression of the lower-extremity vascular bed increases diastolic pressure and flow, and increases venous return. The pressure is then released at the onset of systole. Inflation and deflation are timed according to the R-wave on the patient's cardiac monitor. The pressures applied and the inflation–deflation timing can be altered by using the pressure waveforms and electrocardiogram on the enhanced external counterpulsation (EECP) therapy monitor

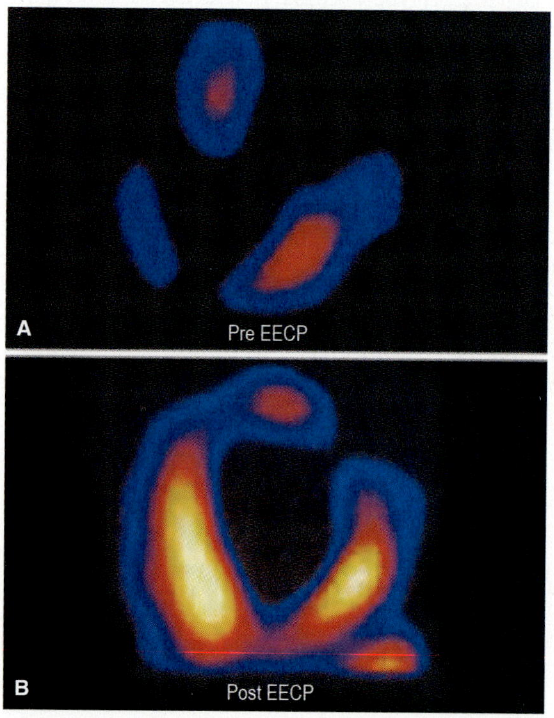


**Fig. 2.39:** (A) Nuclear scan prior to the application of EECP and (B) improvement in angina patient after the application of EECP

*Recent trials with cholesterol-lowering agents* have confirmed the benefits of the therapeutic LDL lowering in older persons.

*Angiographic studies* demonstrate that a reduction of the LDL level in patients with coronary artery disease could cause slowing of progression, stabilization, or even regression of coronary artery lesions.

A recent study demonstrates a significant reduction of symptomatic myocardial ischemia in patients with unstable angina or non-Q-wave infarction with the administration of a statin during the early acute phase.

In a more recent study of 10,001 patients with stable coronary artery disease, an aggressive cholesterol-lowering approach with atorvastatin 80 mg daily (mean cholesterol level of 77 mg/dl) compared to a less-aggressive approach with atorvastatin 10 mg daily (mean cholesterol level of 101 mg/dl) resulted in a 2.2% absolute reduction and a 22% relative reduction in the occurrence of a first major cardiovascular event (define as death from coronary heart disease; nonfatal, non-procedure-related myocardial infarction; resuscitation from cardiac arrest; or fatal or nonfatal stroke). This occurred with a greater incidence of elevated aminotransferase levels with the aggressive cholesterol-lowering approach (1.2% vs 0.2%, $p<0.001$).

On the basis of several recent studies that have demonstrated the benefits of more aggressive LDL-lowering therapies in high-risk patients with coronary artery disease, the Committee of the National Cholesterol Education Program recently made the following modifications to the Adult Treatment Panel III (ATP III) guidelines. In high-risk patients, a serum LDL cholesterol level of less than 100 mg/dl is the goal.

In very high-risk patients, an LDL cholesterol level goal of less than 70 mg/dl is a therapeutic option. Patients in the category of very high risk are those with established coronary artery disease with one of the following:

- Multiple major risk factors (especially diabetes)
- Severe and poorly controlled risk factors (especially continued cigarette smoking)
- Multiple risk factors of the metabolic syndrome (especially high triglyceride levels ≥200 mg/dl plus non-

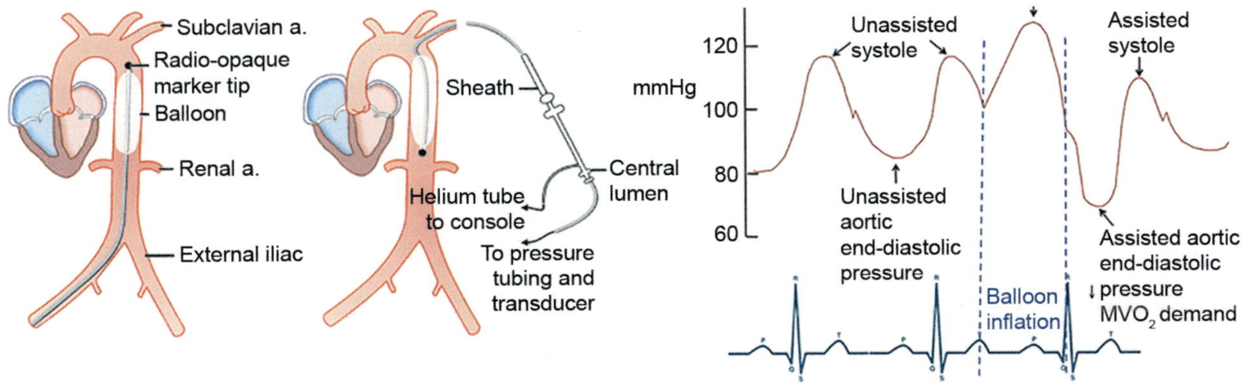


**Fig. 2.40:** Illustrations showing application of intra-aortic balloon counterpulsation in the tratment of unstable angina

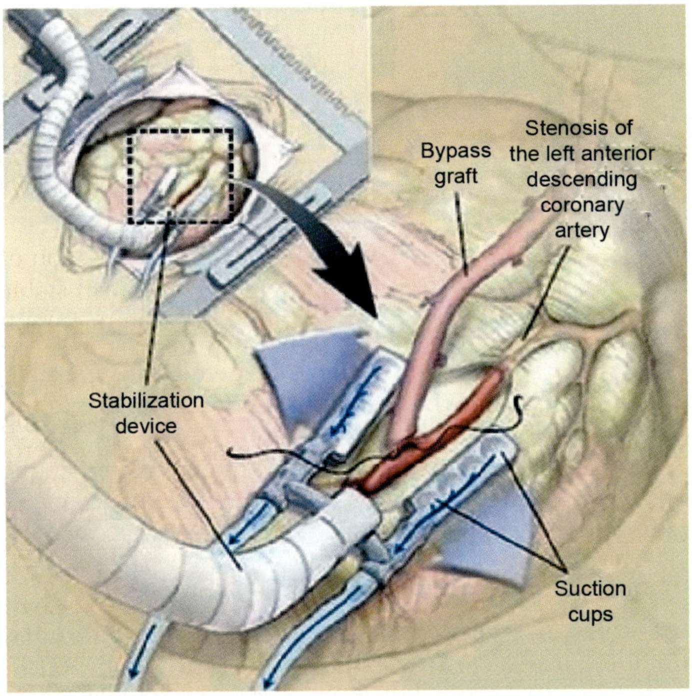


**Fig. 2.41:** Bypass graft to critically stenosed LAD in a patient with exercise stress positive test

HDL cholesterol level ≥130 mg/dl with low HDL cholesterol level <40 mg/dl)
- Patients with acute coronary syndromes.

For moderately high-risk persons (2+ risk factors), the recommended LDL cholesterol level is <130 mg/dl, but an LDL cholesterol level of 100 mg/dl is a therapeutic option. Some triglyceride-rich lipoproteins, including partially degraded very LDL levels, are believed to be independent risk factors for coronary artery disease. In daily practice, non-HDL cholesterol level (i.e. LDL + very LDL cholesterol [total cholesterol-HDL cholesterol]) is the most readily available measure of the total pool of these atherogenic lipoproteins. Thus, the ATP III has identified non-HDL cholesterol level as a secondary target of therapy in persons with high triglyceride levels (>200 mg/dl). The goal for non-HDL cholesterol level (for persons with serum triglyceride levels >200 mg/dl) is 30 mg/dl higher than the identified.

LDL cholesterol level goal. Patients with established coronary disease and low HDL/cholesterol levels are at high risk for recurrent events and should be targeted for aggressive nonpharmacological (i.e. dietary modification, weight loss, physical exercise) and pharmacological treatment.

A recent study demonstrated that in patients with established coronary artery disease who have low HDL and low-risk LDL levels, drug therapy with medications that raise HDL cholesterol levels and lower triglyceride levels but have no effect on LDL cholesterol levels (e.g. gemfibrozil) could significantly reduce the risk of major cardiac events.

Currently, the accepted approach to the management of patients with coronary artery disease and low HDL levels is as follows.

In all persons with low HDL cholesterol levels, the primary target of therapy is to achieve the ATP III guideline LDL cholesterol level goals with diet, exercise, and drug therapy as needed. After reaching the targeted LDL level goal, emphasis shifts to other issues. That is, in patients with low HDL cholesterol levels, who have associated high triglyceride levels (>200 mg/dl), the secondary priority is to achieve the non-HDL cholesterol level goal of 30 mg/dl higher than the identified LDL cholesterol level goal. In patients with isolated low HDL cholesterol levels (triglycerides <200 mg/dl), drugs to raise the HDL cholesterol level (e.g. gemfibrozil and nicotinic acid) can be considered. Exercise training results in improvement of symptoms, increase in the threshold of ischemia, and improvement of patients' sense of well-being. However, before enrolling a patient in an exercise-training program, perform an exercise tolerance test to establish the safety of such a program. Consider enteric-coated aspirin at a dose of 80–325 mg/day for all patients with stable angina, who have no contraindications to its use. In patients in whom aspirin cannot be used because of allergy or gastrointestinal complications, consider clopidogrel. Although, early observational studies suggested a cardiovascular protective effect with the use of hormone replacement therapy, recent large randomized trials failed to demonstrate any benefit with hormone replacement therapy in the primary or secondary prevention of cardiovascular disease.

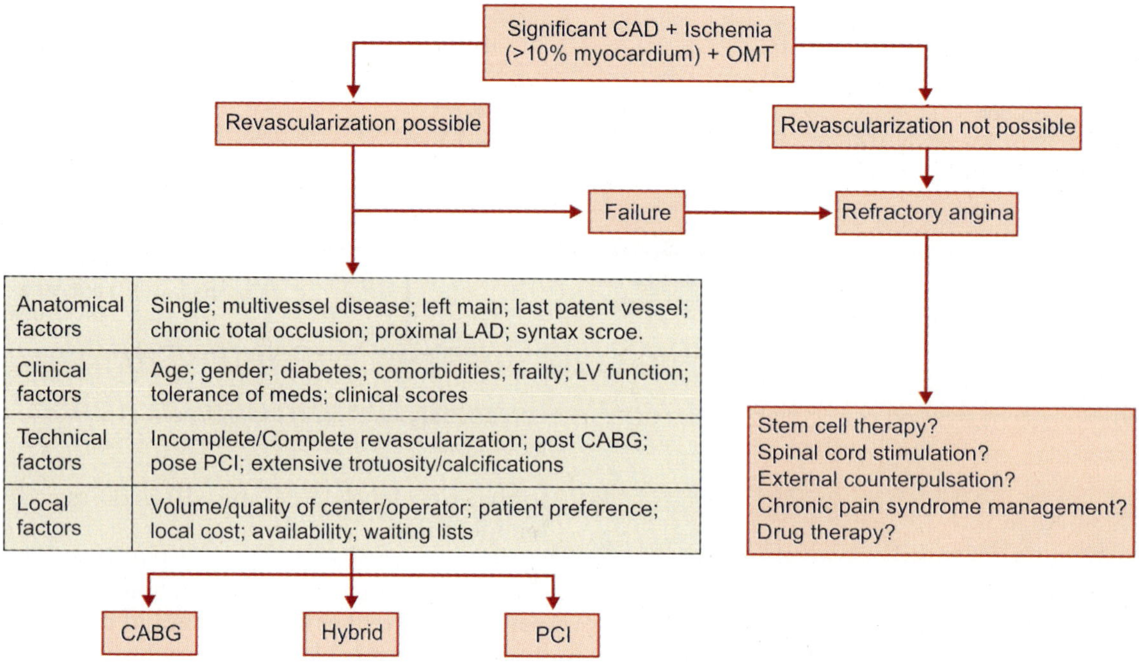


**Fig. 2.42:** Indications of revascularization therapy

In fact, these studies even demonstrated an increased risk of coronary artery disease and stroke in patients on hormone replacement therapy.

The women's health initiative study demonstrated that the use of hormone replacement therapy for 1 year in 10,000 healthy postmenopausal women is associated with 7 more instances of coronary artery disease, 8 more strokes, 8 more pulmonary emboli, 8 more invasive breast cancers, 5 fewer hip fractures, and 6 fewer colorectal cancers.

Based on these data, the risks and benefits of hormone replacement therapy must be assessed on an individual basis for each patient.

*Sublingual nitroglycerin:* It has been the mainstay of treatment for angina pectoris. Sublingual nitroglycerin can be used for acute relief of angina and prophylactically before activities that may precipitate angina. No evidence indicates that long-acting nitrates improve survival in patients with coronary artery disease.

*Beta-blockers:* These are also used for symptomatic relief of angina and prevention of ischemic events. They work by reducing myocardial oxygen demand and by decreasing the heart rate and myocardial contractility. Beta-blockers have been shown to reduce the rates of mortality and morbidity following acute MI.

Long-acting calcium channel blockers can be used to control anginal symptoms in patients with a contra-indication to beta-blockers and in those in whom symptomatic relief of angina cannot be achieved with the use of beta-blockers, nitrates, or both. Avoid short-acting dihydropyridine calcium channel blockers because they have been shown to increase the risk of adverse cardiac events.

Anginal symptoms in patients with Prinzmetal angina can be treated with calcium channel blockers with or without nitrates. In one study, supplemental vitamin E added to a calcium channel blocker significantly reduced anginal symptoms among such patients.

In patients with syndrome X and hypertension, angiotensin converting enzyme (ACE) inhibitors may normalize thallium perfusion defects and increase exercise capacity.

## Antianginal Pharmacology

*Antiplatelet agents:* Prevent thrombus formation by inhibiting platelet aggregation. Aspirin is proven beneficial in primary and secondary prevention of coronary artery disease. In patients with aspirin intolerance, use clopidogrel. Clopidogrel is also used in combination with aspirin after coronary stent placement. Recently, clopidogrel use in addition to aspirin has been shown to be significantly superior to aspirin alone in patients with acute coronary syndrome without ST-segment elevation MI.

*Aspirin (bayer, empirin and anacin):* Prevents platelet aggregation by irreversible cyclooxygenase inhibition with subsequent suppression of thromboxane A2. Antiplatelet effects can last as along as 7 days.

**Adult dose:** 81–325 mg PO qd

*Clopidogrel (plavix):* Selectively inhibits ADP binding to platelet receptor and subsequent ADP-mediated activation of GPIIb/IIIa complex, thereby inhibiting platelet aggregation. Consider in patients with contraindication to aspirin.

**Adult dose:** 75 mg PO qd

*Beta-adrenergic blocking agents:* These work by competing with endogenous catecholamines for beta-adrenergic receptors. Reduce myocardial oxygen consumption via several effects, including decrease in resting and exercise heart rates and reductions in myocardial contractility and afterload. Classified as non-selective, beta-1 selective and having intrinsic sympathomimetic effects.

*Metoprolol (lopressor, toprol XL):* Selective beta-1 adrenergic receptor blocker that decreases automaticity of contractions. It is lipophilic and penetrates CNS.

**Adult dose:** 50–200 mg PO bid

*Atenolol (tenormin):* It selectively blocks beta-1 receptors with little or no effect on beta-2 receptors. It is hydrophilic and does not penetrate CNS.

**Adult dose:** 50–200 mg PO qd

*Propranolol (inderal):* Non-selective beta-blocker that is lipophilic (penetrates CNS). Although, generally short-acting agent, long-acting preparations also available.

**Adult dose:** Immediate release: 40–160 mg PO bid
Sustained release: 60–320 mg PO qd

*Calcium channel blockers:* They reduce transmembrane flux of calcium via calcium channels. Cause smooth muscle relaxation, resulting in peripheral arterial vasodilation and afterload reduction. Indicated when symptoms persist despite treatment with beta-blockers or when beta-blockers are contraindicated. Also indicated in patients with Prinzmetal angina with or without nitrates.

*Amlodipine (Norvasc):* During depolarization, inhibits calcium ions from entering slow channels and voltage-sensitive areas of vascular smooth muscle and myocardium.

**Adult dose:** 5–10 mg PO qd

*Diltiazem (cardizem CD, dilacor):* During depolarization, inhibits calcium ions from entering slow channels and voltage-sensitive areas of vascular smooth muscle and myocardium.

**Adult dose:** Immediate release (IR): 120–360 mg PO divided tid/qid
Sustained release (SR): 120–480 mg PO qd

*Verapamil (calan, covera):* During depolarization, inhibits calcium ion from entering slow channels or voltage-sensitive areas of vascular smooth muscle and myocardium.

**Adult dose:** Immediate release: 80–120 mg PO tid/qid
Sustained release: 120–240 mg PO qd/bid

*Short-acting nitroglycerins:* Suitable for immediate relief of exertional or rest angina. Can also be used for prophylaxis several minutes before planned exercise to avoid angina. Reduce myocardial oxygen demand by reduction of LV and arterial pressure, primarily by reducing preload.

*Nitroglycerin (nitrostat, nitro-bid, nitrol):* It causes relaxation of vascular smooth muscle by stimulating intracellular cyclic GMP production. Result is decrease in BP.

**Adult dose:** 0.3–0.6 mg SL prn 0.4 mg metered-dose spray PO prn 0.1–0.8 mg/h patch TD qd 1

*Long-acting nitroglycerins:* These reduce LV preload and afterload by venous and arterial dilation, which subsequently reduces myocardial oxygen consumption and relieves angina. Also cause dilation of epicardial coronary arteries, which is beneficial in patients with coronary spasm. In addition, nitroglycerin has antithrombotic and anti-platelet effects in patients with angina pectoris. No evidence suggests that nitrates improve survival or slow progression of coronary artery disease.

*Isosorbide [isordil, isosorbide mononitrate (ISMO)]:* It relaxes vascular smooth muscle by stimulating intracellular cyclic guanosine monophosphate (GMP). Decreases LV pressure (i.e. preload) and arterial resistance (i.e. afterload). Reduces cardiac oxygen demand by decreasing LV pressure and dilating arteries.

**Adult dose:** *Isosorbide dinitrate:* 2.5–10 mg SL prn IR 10–30 mg PO bid/tid SR 80–120 mg PO qd.
*Isosorbide mononitrate:* 10–20 mg PO bid SR 30–120 mg PO qd

*Angiotensin-converting enzyme inhibitors:* Recently, shown to reduce rates of death, MI, stroke and need for revascularization procedures in patients with coronary artery disease or diabetes mellitus and at least one other cardiovascular risk factor, irrespective of the presence of hypertension or heart failure.

*Ramipril (altace):* Prevents conversion of angiotensin I to angiotensin II, a potent vasoconstrictor, resulting in lower aldosterone secretion.

**Adult dose:** 2.5–5 mg PO qd not to exceed 20 mg/d

*Anti-ischemic agents, miscellaneous:* Ranolazine elicits action unlike beta-blockers, calcium antagonists, or nitrates. It does not affect hemodynamics or contractile and conduction parameters.

*Ranolazine (Ranexa):* Cardioselective anti-ischemic agent (piperazine derivative) that partially inhibits fatty acid oxidation. Also inhibits late sodium current into myocardial cells and prolongs QTc interval. Indicated for chronic angina unresponsive to other antianginal treatments. Used in combination with amlodipine, beta-blockers, or nitrates. Unlike beta-blockers, calcium channel blockers and nitrates, does not reduce blood pressure or heart rate. Effect on angina rate or exercise tolerance appears to be smaller in women than in men. Absorption is highly variable but unaffected by food.

**Adult dose:** 500 mg PO bid initially; if necessary, may increase to 1000 mg PO bid

*Contraindications:* Documented hypersensitivity; pre-existing QT prolongation; hepatic impairment [Child-Pugh class A (mild), B (moderate), or C (severe)]; QT-prolonging drugs (see interactions); potent or moderate CYP4503A inhibitors (e.g. ketoconazole and diltiazem).

*Interactions:* CYP4503A and P-gp substrate; potent CYP3A inhibitors (e.g. ketoconazole at 200 mg bid) increase levels approximately 3.2-fold, moderate CYP3A inhibitors (e.g. diltiazem at 180–360 mg/day) increase levels approximately 1.8- to 2.3-fold, and verapamil (a CYP3A and P-gp inhibitor) increases levels approximately 2-fold; caution with other P-gp inhibitors (e.g. ritonavir, cyclosporine); toxicity may occur when coadministered with other drugs that increase QTc interval (e.g. class I and III antiarrhythmic agents, certain macrolide and quinolone antibiotics, phenothiazines, TCAs). Inhibits CYP4503A, CYP 4502D6, and P-gp; may increase plasma levels of digoxin, simvastatin, dextromethorphan, TCAs, and antipsychotics.

*Precautions:* Causes dose-related QTc-interval prolongation (obtain baseline and follow-up ECGs to monitor for torsades de pointes and potential for sudden death; mild and moderate hepatic impairment increases QTc interval compared with normal hepatic function at the same plasma level; increases blood pressure by approximately 15 mmHg in persons with severe renal impairment; common adverse effects include dizziness, headache, constipation, and nausae.

*Prevention:* Coronary atherosclerosis is the main preventable cause of mortality in the United States. A rigorous effort to address correctable risk factors is the mainstay of preventive cardiovascular medicine. Smoking cessation is the single most effective preventive intervention to reduce coronary atherosclerosis prevalence. It has been associated with a coronary artery disease reduction of 7–47% in primary prevention settings.

- Aggressive treatment of diabetes mellitus, hypertension, LV hypertrophy, hyperlipidemia, and obesity has an important role in the prevention of coronary artery disease.
- The most important recent development in coronary atherosclerosis risk modification is the introduction of inhibitors of beta-hydroxy-beta-methylglutaryl coenzyme A reductase. Reductions of total and LDL cholesterol levels by 25% and 35%, respectively, can achieve a similar reduction in rates of total and coronary mortality, MI, and need for coronary revascularization.

*Optimal medical therapy for stable coronary artery disease versus PCI or CABG (STICH Trial 2011):*

Medical, percutaneous interventional and surgical treatments for the management of coronary heart disease have progressed markedly during the past decade. There is evidence to suggest that for patients with stable coronary heart disease optimal medical therapy is equal in effectiveness for lowering the risk of major cardiovascular events, such as cardiovascular death, myocardial infarction, and stroke, as are revascularization procedures, such as coronary artery bypass grafting or percutaneous coronary intervention. The landmark surgical treatment for ischemic heart failure (STICH) trial found no significant difference between medical therapy alone and medical therapy plus coronary artery bypass grafting with respect to the primary end point of death from any cause (all-cause mortality). However, secondary outcomes showed fewer deaths from cardiovascular causes in the surgical group versus the medical group. Medical therapy has improved over time, as have surgical techniques including myocardial preservation, and both approaches have their place, especially since chest pain relief and quality of life may benefit more in some cases by revascularization. Certainly, coronary artery bypass grafting has general acceptance for three-vessel coronary heart disease, and percutaneous coronary artery intervention is the standard of care for the involved artery in acute ST-segment elevation myocardial infarction when the intervention can be accomplished rapidly. Medical management includes lifestyle changes that benefit coronary heart disease, drug therapy to improve prognosis, and drug therapy to improve symptoms. The key to clinical management is the selection of the procedure and/or medical management strategy that is in the best interest of the individual cardiovascular patient. In addition, discussing with patients their options and considering what best fits their wishes is especially critical when there is no clear-cut best strategy. Continued collaboration between cardiologists concentrating on medical approaches with interventionists and cardiac surgeons (heart team approach) is essential for optimal management for each individual patient.

The abstract of complete results of FAME II Study revealed that in patients with stable coronary artery disease and at least one stenosis with a fraction flow reserve (FFR) <0.80, optimal medical therapy (OMT) alone was associated with a more than fourfold larger hazard of major adverse cardiac events than FFR-guided percutaneous coronary intervention (PCI) with drug-eluting stents plus OMT. This difference was driven by a difference in unplanned hospitalization with urgent revascularisation. In contrast, in patients with hemodynamically non-significant stenoses (FFR >0.80), OMT alone was associated with a favorable clinical outcome (Table 2.6).

*Complications:* Complications of angina pectoris include unstable angina, MI, and death.

*Prognosis:* Important prognostic indicators in patients with angina pectoris include LV function, severity and location of atherosclerotic lesions, and response of symptoms to medical treatment.

Left ventricular function is the strongest predictor of long-term survival. Elevated LV end-diastolic pressure and volume along with reduced LV ejection fraction (<40%) are poor prognostic signs.

Critical lesions of left main and proximal left anterior descending coronary arteries are associated with a greater risk. Mortality rates are also directly associated with the number of epicardial arteries involved.

Unstable angina, recent MI, or both is a sign of atherosclerotic plaque instability, which is a strong predictor of increased risk of short-term coronary events.

A number of signs during noninvasive testing is predictive of a higher risk of coronary events, including ST-segment depression of more than 2 mm at a low workload, ST-segment depression that persists for more

**Table 2.6:** Indications for diagnostic testing in patients with suspected CAD and stable symptoms

| | *Asymptomatic*[a] | | *Smptomatic* | | | | | |
|---|---|---|---|---|---|---|---|---|
| | | | **Probability of significant disease**[b] | | | | | |
| | | | Low (<15%) | | Intermediate (15–85%) | | High (>85%) | |
| | Class[c] | Level[d] | Class[c] | Level[d] | Class[c] | Level[d] | Class[c] | Level[d] |
| **Anatomical detection of CAD** | | | | | | | | |
| **Invasive angiography** | III | A | III | A | IIb | A | I | A |
| **CT angiography**[e] | III | B | III | C | IIa | A | III | B |
| **Functional test** | | | | | | | | |
| **Stress echo** | III | A | III | A | I | A | III | A |
| **Nuclear imaging** | III | A | III | A | I | A | III | A |
| **Stress MRI** | III | B | III | C | I | A | III | B |
| **PET perfusion** | III | B | III | C | I | A | III | B |
| **Combined or hybrid imaging test** | | | | | | | | |
| | III | C | III | C | IIa | B | III | B |

a = In asymptomatic patients, the decision will be guided by the extent of ischemia on stress testing; b = with documented ischemia or FFR <0.80 for angiographic diameter stenoses 50–90%; c = as assessed by noninvasive test (SPECT, MRI and stress echocardiography); d =class of recommendation; e =level of evidence. (Adapted from 2013 ESC guidelines on the management of stable coronary artery disease)

than 5 minutes after termination of exercise, and failure of blood pressure to rise or an actual drop in blood pressure.

- Patients who continue to smoke after MI have a 22–47% increased risk of reinfarction and death.
- In general, Prinzmetal angina and syndrome X are associated with excellent long-term prognoses.

*Patient education:* Educating patients about the benefits of smoking cessation, a low-cholesterol diet, physical activity, and periodic screening for diabetes mellitus and hypertension is the prime component of a long-term management plan.

*Medical/Legal Pitfalls*

- In patients with stable angina pectoris, even the most carefully performed history and physical examination have limitations. Classification of these patients solely on the basis of history and physical examination findings may lead to serious mistakes. Some type of stress testing is usually indicated to confirm the diagnosis and quantitate the severity of ischemia.
- In women, elderly persons, and diabetic patients, coronary artery disease may manifest with atypical presentations other than angina pectoris, such as silent ischemia or infarction. Physicians should use a careful approach when evaluating these patients.

**KEY POINTS**

- Angina pectoris occurs when cardiac workload exceeds the ability of coronary arteries to supply an adequate amount of oxygenated blood.
- Symptoms of stable angina pectoris range from a vague, barely troublesome ache to a severe, intense precordial crushing sensation; they are typically precipitated by exertion, last no more than a few minutes, and subside with rest.
- Do stress testing with ECG for patients with normal resting ECG or with myocardial imaging (e.g. echocardiography, radionuclide imaging, and MRI) for patients with abnormal resting ECG.
- Do coronary angiography when revascularization (percutaneous intervention or coronary artery bypass grafting) is being considered.
- Give nitroglycerin for immediate relief of angina.
- Maintain patients on an antiplatelet drug, a β-blocker, and a statin, and add a Ca channel blocker for further symptom prevention if needed.
- Consider revascularization if significant angina persists despite drug therapy or if lesions noted during angiography indicate high risk of mortality.

## BIBLIOGRAPHY


1. Allen KB, Dowling RD, Fudge TL, et al. Comparison of transmyocardial revascularization with medical therapy in patients with refractory angina. N Engl J Med 1999;341(14):1029–36.
2. Ambrosio G, Betocchi S, Pace L, et al. Prolonged impairment of regional contractile function after resolution of exercise-induced angina. Evidence of myocardial stunning in patients with coronary artery disease. Circulation 1996;94(10):2455–64.
3. Anderson HV. Angiotensin-converting enzyme inhibitors: ischemia is not the correct measure of benefit. J Am Coll Cardiol 2003;42(12):2060–2.
4. Arora RR, Chou TM, Jain D, et al. The multicenter study of enhanced external counterpulsation (MUST-EECP): effect of EECP on exercise-induced myocardial ischemia and anginal episodes. J Am Coll Cardiol 1999;33(7):1833–40.
5. Borden WB, Redberg RF, Mushlin AI, et al. Patterns and Intensity of Medical Therapy in Patients Undergoing Percutaneous Coronary Intervention. JAMA 2011;305:1882–9.
6. Brown G, Albers JJ, Fisher LD, et al. Regression of coronary artery disease as a result of intensive lipid-lowering therapy in men with high levels of apolipoprotein B. N Engl J Med 1990;323(19):1289–98.
7. Califf RM, Armstrong PW, Carver JR, et al. 27th Bethesda Conference: matching the intensity of risk factor management with the hazard for coronary disease events. Task Force 5. Stratification of patients into high, medium and low risk subgroups for purposes of risk factor management. J Am Coll Cardiol 1996;27(5):1007–19.
8. Cannon CP, Braunwald E, McCabe CH, et al. Intensive versus moderate lipid lowering with statins after acute coronary syndromes. N Engl J Med 2004;350(15):1495–504.
9. Chauhan A, Mullins PA, Taylor G, et al. Both endothelium-dependent and endothelium-independent function is impaired in patients with angina pectoris and normal coronary angiograms. Eur Heart J 1997;18(1):60–8.
10. Connolly DC, Elveback LR, Oxman HA. Coronary heart disease in residents of Rochester, Minnesota. IV. Prognostic value of the resting electrocardiogram at the time of initial diagnosis of angina pectoris. Mayo Clin Proc 1984;59(4):247–50.
11. Crea F, Pupita G, Galassi AR, et al. Role of adenosine in pathogenesis of anginal pain. Circulation 1990;81(1):164–72.
12. de Bruyne B, Pijls NH, Kalesan B, et al. Fractional flow reserve-guided PCI versus medical therapy in stable coronary disease. N Eng J Med 2012;367:991–1001.
13. Deedwania PC, Carbajal EV. Silent ischemia during daily life is an independent predictor of mortality in stable angina. Circulation 1990;81(3):748–56.
14. Frileux S, Munoz Sastre MT, Mullet E, et al. The impact of the preventive medical message on intention to change behavior. Patient Educ Couns 2004;52(1):79–88.
15. Gibbons RJ, Abrams J, Chatterjee K, et al. ACC/AHA 2002 guideline update for the management of patients with chronic stable angina—summary article: a report of the American College of Cardiology/American Heart Association Task Force on practice guidelines (Committee on the Management of Patients. J Am Coll Cardiol 2003;41(1):159–68.
16. Gibbons RJ, Balady GJ, Bricker JT, et al. ACC/AHA 2002 guideline update for exercise testing: summary article: a report of the American College of Cardiology/American Heart Association Task Force on Practice.
17. Guidelines (Committee to Update the 1997 Exercise Testing Guidelines). Circulation 2002.;106(14):1883–92.
18. Grundy SM, Cleeman JI, Merz CN, et al. Implications of recent clinical trials for the National Cholesterol Education Program Adult Treatment Panel III Guidelines. J Am Coll Cardiol 2004;44(3):720–32.
19. Hamm CW, Bassand JP, Agewall S, et al. ESC Guidelines for the management of acute coronary syndromes in patients presenting without persistent ST-segment elevation: The Task Force for the management of acute coronary syndromes (ACS) in patients presenting without persistent ST-segment elevation of the European Society of Cardiology (ESC). Eur Heart J 2011;32:2999–3054.
20. Juul-Moller S, Edvardsson N, Jahnmatz B, et al. Double-blind trial of aspirin in primary prevention of myocardial infarction in patients with stable chronic angina pectoris. The Swedish Angina Pectoris Aspirin Trial (SAPAT) Group. Lancet 1992;340(8833):1421–5.
21. Kannel WB, Feinleib M. Natural history of angina pectoris in the Framingham study. Prognosis and survival. Am J Cardiol 1972;29(2):154–63.
22. Kaski JC, Elliott PM, Salomone O, et al. Concentration of circulating plasma endothelin in patients with angina and normal coronary angiograms. Br Heart J 1995;74(6):620–4.
23. Kaski JC, Rosano G, Gavrielides S, et al. Effects of angiotensin-converting enzyme inhibition on exercise-induced angina and ST-segment depression in patients with microvascular angina. J Am Coll Cardiol 1994;23(3):652–7.
24. Khan NE, De Souza A, Mister R, et al. A randomized comparison of off-pump and on-pump multivessel coronary-artery bypass surgery. N Engl J Med 2004;350(1):21–8.
25. Kugiyama K, Yasue H, Okumura K, et al. Nitric oxide activity is deficient in spasm arteries of patients with coronary spastic angina. Circulation 1996;94(3):266–71.
26. Kuo L, Davis MJ, Chilian WM. Longitudinal gradients for endothelium-dependent and -independent vascular responses in the coronary microcirculation. Circulation 1995;92(3):518–25.
27. Lacoste LL, Theroux P, Lidon RM, et al. Antithrombotic properties of transdermal nitroglycerin in stable angina pectoris. Am J Cardiol 1994.;73(15):1058–62.
28. Lanza GA, Giordano A, Pristipino C, et al. Abnormal cardiac adrenergic nerve function in patients with syndrome X detected by $^{123}$I metaiodobenzylguanidine myocardial scintigraphy. Circulation 1997;96(3):821–6.
29. LaRosa JC, Grundy SM, Waters DD, et al. Intensive lipid lowering with atorvastatin in patients with stable coronary disease. N Engl J Med 2005;352(14):1425–35.
30. Margolis JR, Chen JT, Kong Y, et al. The diagnostic and prognostic significance of coronary artery calcification. A report of 800 cases. Radiology 1980;137(3):609–16.
31. Mark DB, Califf RM, Morris KG, et al. Clinical characteristics and long-term survival of patients with variant angina. Circulation 1984;69(5):880–8.

32. Maseri A, Crea F, Kaski JC, et al. Mechanisms and significance of cardiac ischemic pain. Prog Cardiovasc Dis 1992; 35(1):1–18.
33. Miwa K, Miyagi Y, Igawa A, et al. Vitamin E deficiency in variant angina. Circulation 1996;94(1):14–8.
34. Morice MC, Serruys PW, Sousa JE, et al. A randomized comparison of a sirolimus-eluting stent with a standard stent for coronary revascularization. N Engl J Med 2002;346(23): 1773–80.
35. National Cholesterol Education Program. Executive Summary of The Third Report of The National Cholesterol Education Program (NCEP) Expert Panel on Detection, Evaluation, And Treatment of High Blood Cholesterol In Adults (Adult Treatment Panel III). JAMA 2001;285(19):2486–97.
36. Ndrepepa G, Braun S, Mehilli J, et al. Prognostic value of sensitive troponin T in patients with stable and unstable angina and undetectable conventional troponin. Am Heart J 2011;161:68–75.
37. Norwegian Multicenter Study Group. Timolol-induced reduction in mortality and reinfarction in patients surviving acute myocardial infarction. N Engl J Med 1981;304(14): 801–7.
38. O'Keefe JH, Barnhart CS, Bateman TM. Comparison stress echocardiography and stress myocardial perfusion scintigraphy for diagnosing coronary artery disease and assessing its severity. Am J Cardiol 1995;75(11):25D–34D.
39. Oesterle SN, Sanborn TA, Ali N, et al. Percutaneous transmyocardial laser revascularisation for severe angina: the PACIFIC randomised trial. Potential Class Improvement From Intramyocardial Channels. Lancet 2000;356(9243): 1705–10.
40. Piatti P, Fragasso G, Monti LD, et al. Endothelial and metabolic characteristics of patients with angina and angiographically normal coronary arteries: comparison with subjects with insulin resistance syndrome and normal controls. J Am Coll Cardiol 1999;34(5):1452–60.
41. Ridker PM, Manson JE, Gaziano JM, et al. Low-dose aspirin therapy for chronic stable angina. A randomized, placebo-controlled clinical trial. Ann Intern Med 1991;114(10):835–9.
42. Rocco MB, Nabel EG, Campbell S, et al. Prognostic importance of myocardial ischemia detected by ambulatory monitoring in patients with stable coronary artery disease. Circulation 1988;78(4):877–84.
43. Rosano GM, Collins P, Kaski JC, et al. Syndrome X in women is associated with oestrogen deficiency. Eur Heart J 1995; 16(5):610–4.
44. Rossouw JE, Anderson GL, Prentice RL, et al. Risks and benefits of estrogen plus progestin in healthy postmenopausal women: principal results From the Women's Health Initiative randomized controlled trial. JAMA 2002;288(3):321–33.
45. Rubins HB, Robins SJ, Collins D, et al. Gemfibrozil for the secondary prevention of coronary heart disease in men with low levels of high-density lipoprotein cholesterol. Veterans Affairs High-Density Lipoprotein Cholesterol Intervention Trial Study Group. N Engl J Med 1999;341(6):410–8.
46. Scandinavian Simvastatin Survival Study Group. Randomised trial of cholesterol lowering in 4444 patients with coronary heart disease: the Scandinavian Simvastatin Survival Study (4S). Lancet 1994;344(8934):1383–9.
47. Schwartz GG, Olsson AG, Ezekowitz MD, et al. Effects of atorvastatin on early recurrent ischemic events in acute coronary syndromes: the MIRACL study: a randomized controlled trial. JAMA 2001;285(13):1711–8.
48. Sever PS, Dahlof B, Poulter NR, et al. Prevention of coronary and stroke events with atorvastatin in hypertensive patients who have average or lower-than-average cholesterol concentrations, in the Anglo-Scandinavian Cardiac Outcomes Trial—Lipid Lowering Arm (ASCOT-LLA): a multicentre randomi. Lancet 2003;361(9364):1149–58.
49. Shepherd J, Blauw GJ, Murphy MB, et al. Pravastatin in elderly individuals at risk of vascular disease (PROSPER): a randomised controlled trial. Lancet 2002; 360(9346):1623–30.

# 3 Recognition and Management of Acute Coronary Syndrome

Acute coronary syndrome (ACS) refers to a spectrum of clinical presentations ranging from those for ST-segment elevation myocardial infarction (STEMI) to presentations found in non-ST-segment elevation myocardial infarction (NSTEMI) or in unstable angina. In terms of pathology, ACS is almost always associated with rupture of an atherosclerotic plaque and partial or complete thrombosis of the infarct-related artery. Components of acute coronary syndrome are:

1. **ST-segment elevation myocardial infarction (STEMI)**
2. **Non-ST-segment elevation myocardial infarction (NSTEMI)**
3. **Unstable angina**

In some instances, however, stable coronary artery disease (CAD) may result in ACS in the absence of plaque rupture and thrombosis, when physiologic stress (e.g. trauma, blood loss, anemia, infection, tachyarrhythmia) increases demands on the heart. The diagnosis of acute myocardial infarction in this setting requires a finding of the typical rise and fall of biochemical markers of myocardial necrosis in addition to at least one of the following (Figs 3.1–3.3):

- Ischemic symptoms
- Development of pathologic Q-waves

Ischemic ST-segment changes on electrocardiogram (ECG) or in the setting of a coronary intervention. The terms *transmural* and *nontransmural* (subendocardial) myocardial infarction are no longer used because ECG findings in patients with this condition are not closely correlated with pathologic changes in the myocardium. Therefore, a transmural infarct may occur in the absence of Q-waves on ECGs, and many Q-wave myocardial infarctions may be subendocardial, as noted on pathologic examination. Because elevation of the ST-segment during ACS is correlated with coronary occlusion and because it affects

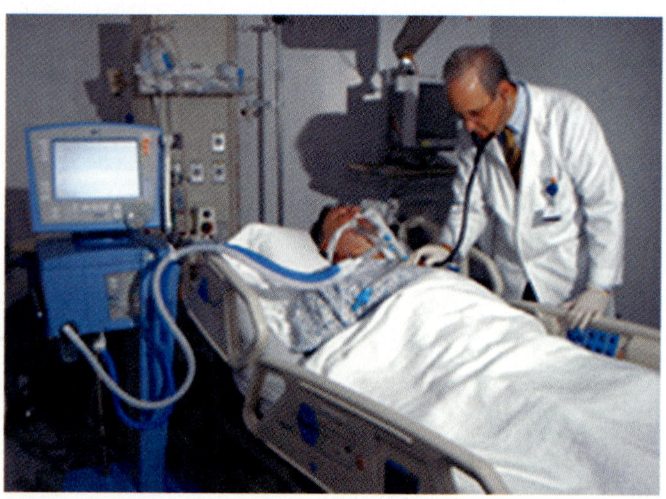

**Fig. 3.1:** Doctor examining a middle-aged patient admitted in ICCU with acute coronary syndrome in a stage of shock

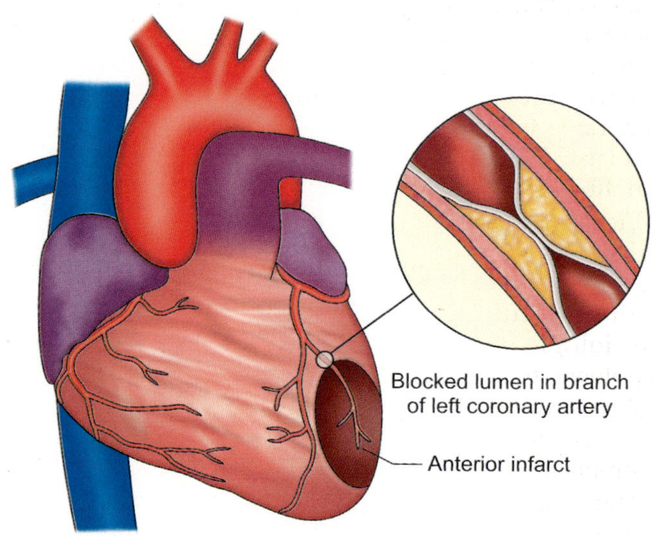


**Fig. 3.2:** Left ventricular infarct due to obstructed lumen of the left coronary artery

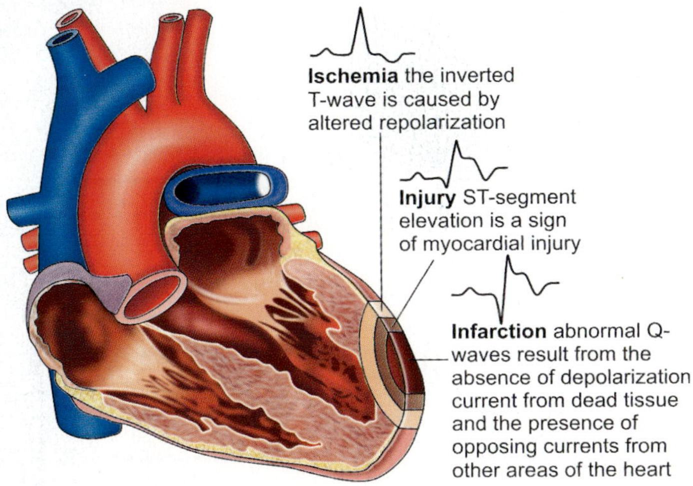


**Fig. 3.3:** Left ventricular infarct due to obstructed lumen of the left coronary artery (left) and ECG morphology showing various stages of ST- and T-waves changes in its resolution (right)

the choice of therapy (urgent reperfusion therapy), ACS-related myocardial infarction should be designated STEMI or NSTEMI.

Attention to the underlying mechanisms of ischemia is important when managing ACS. A simple predictor of demand is rate-pressure product, which can be lowered by beta blockers (e.g. metoprolol or atenolol) and pain/stress relievers (e.g. morphine), while supply may be improved by oxygen, adequate hematocrit, blood thinners (e.g. heparin, IIb/IIIa agents, such as abciximab, eptifibatide, tirofiban, or thrombolytics), and/or vasodilators (e.g. nitrates, amlodipine).

In 2010, the American Heart Association (AHA) published new guideline recommendations for the diagnosis and treatment of ACS.

### Etiological Factors

Acute coronary syndrome is caused primarily by atherosclerosis. Most cases of ACS occur from disruption of a previously nonsevere lesion (an atherosclerotic lesion that was previously hemodynamically insignificant yet vulnerable to rupture). The vulnerable plaque is typified by a large lipid pool, numerous inflammatory cells, and a thin, fibrous cap.

Elevated demand can produce ACS in the presence of a high-grade fixed coronary obstruction, due to increased myocardial oxygen and nutrition requirements, such as those resulting from exertion, emotional stress, or physiologic stress (e.g. from dehydration, blood loss, hypotension, infection, thyrotoxicosis, or surgery).

Acute coronary syndrome without elevation in demand requires a new impairment in supply, typically due to thrombosis and/or plaque hemorrhage.

The major trigger for coronary thrombosis is considered to be plaque rupture caused by the dissolution of the fibrous cap, the dissolution itself being the result of the release of metalloproteinases (collagenases) from activated inflammatory cells. This event is followed by platelet activation and aggregation, activation of the coagulation pathway, and vasoconstriction. This process culminates in coronary intraluminal thrombosis and variable degrees of vascular occlusion. Distal embolization may occur. The severity and duration of coronary arterial obstruction, the volume of myocardium affected, the level of demand on the heart, and the ability of the rest of the heart to compensate are major determinants of a patient's clinical presentation and outcome. (Anemia and hypoxemia can precipitate myocardial ischemia in the absence of severe reduction in coronary artery blood flow.)

A syndrome consisting of chest pain, ischemic ST-segment and T-wave changes, elevated levels of biomarkers of myocyte injury, and transient left ventricular apical ballooning (Takotsubo syndrome) has been shown to occur in the absence of clinical CAD, after emotional or physical stress. The etiology of this syndrome is not well understood, but is thought to relate to a surge of catechol stress hormones and/or high sensitivity to those hormones.

## PATHOGENESIS AND PATHOPHYSIOLOGY

The factors responsible for the sudden thrombotic occlusion of a coronary artery have only recently been elucidated. Atherosclerotic plaques rich in foam cells (lipid-laden macrophages) are susceptible to sudden plaque rupture and hemorrhage into the vessel wall, which may result in the sudden partial or total occlusion of the coronary artery. Although severe stenosis of a coronary artery (i.e. stenosis 70% of the diameter of the artery) is generally required to produce anginal symptoms, such stenoses tend to have dense fibrotic caps and are less prone to rupture than mild to moderate stenoses, which are generally more lipid laden. Studies of patients in whom angiography was performed before and after a myocardial infarction revealed that in most cases, acute coronary artery occlusion occurred at sites in the coronary artery circulation with stenoses of less than 70%, as demonstrated on the preinfarction angiogram. Although patients who have unstable anginal syndromes with increasingly frequent and severe angina are clearly at increased risk for myocardial infarction (MI), the ability of physicians to predict which patients with stable anginal syndromes are likely to experience infarction and which coronary artery stenoses are likely to result in acute thrombotic occlusion is poor.

Atherosclerosis is the disease primarily responsible for most ACS cases. Approximately 90% of MIs result from an acute thrombus that obstructs an atherosclerotic coronary artery. Plaque rupture is considered to be the major trigger of coronary thrombosis. Following plaque rupture, platelet activation and aggregation, coagulation pathway activation, and endothelial vasoconstriction occur and lead to coronary thrombosis and occlusion. Consider nonatherosclerotic causes of acute MIs in younger patients or if no evidence of atherosclerosis is noted. Such causes include coronary emboli from sources, such as an infected cardiac valve, coronary occlusion secondary to vasculitis, primary coronary vasospasm (variant angina), cocaine use, or other factors leading to mismatch of oxygen supply and demand, as may occur with a significant gastrointestinal (GI) bleed (Figs 3.4–3.9 and Table 3.1).

## DIAGNOSTIC APPROACH IN ACS

As many as half of all cases of ACS are clinically silent in that they do not cause the classic symptoms of this syndrome. Consequently, ACS goes unrecognized by the patient. Maintain a high index of suspicion for ACS, especially when evaluating women, patients with diabetes, older patients, patients with dementia, and those with a history of heart failure.

Although, ST-segment and T-wave changes are associated with CAD, alternative causes of these findings are left ventricular aneurysm, pericarditis, Prinzmetal angina, early repolarization, Wolff-Parkinson-White syndrome, and drug therapy (e.g. with tricyclic antidepressants, phenothiazines).

Increasing public awareness of the typical and atypical presentations of ACS is of the utmost importance for optimal and timely treatment. Many patients do not recognize that their symptoms are cardiac in origin and

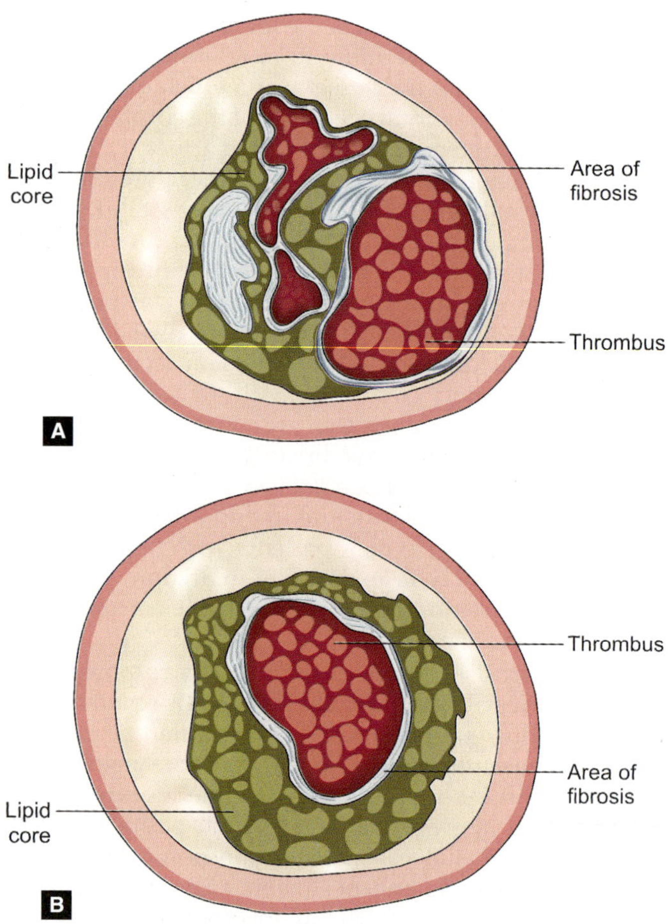


**Fig. 3.4:** Diagrams showing the two mechanisms of coronary total occlusion formation—(A) late evolution of an acute occlusion of an eccentric stenosis, (B) progressive occlusion of a long standing concentric stenosis

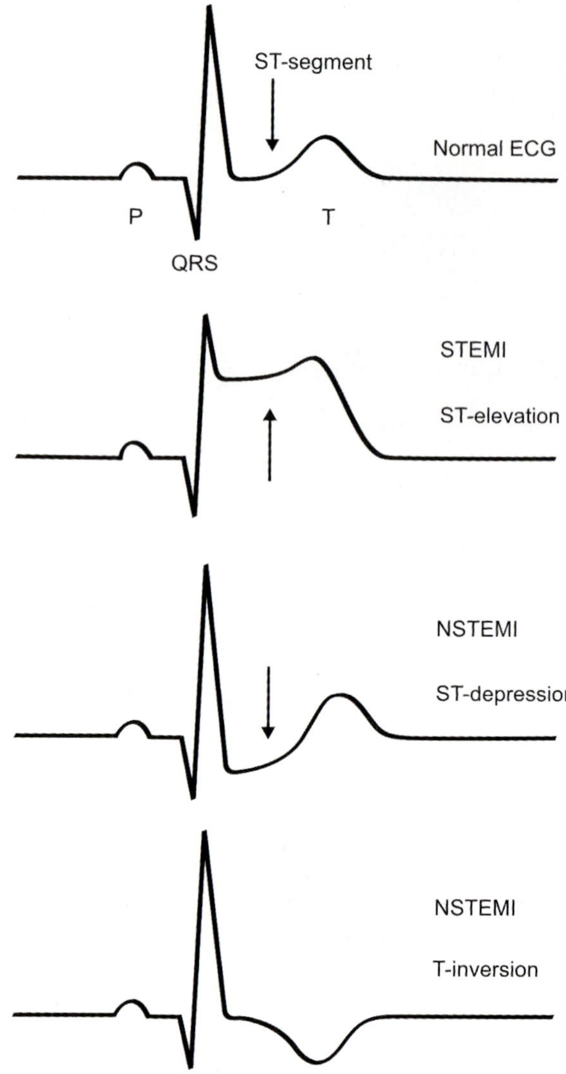


**Unstable Angina or Pre-infarction Syndrome**

- **Diagnosis:** Transient ECG changes—these are 'ST' elevation/ depression and 'T' inversion.
- Changes revert back to normal in 24 hours
- Since no necarosis

**Suspect MI when:**

- ECG changes no revert back in 24 hours
- Cardiac enzymes levels are increased

**Fig. 3.5:** ECG diagram showing diagnosis of acute coronary syndrome. When ECG shows transient ST-elevation/depression and T-wave inversion without elevation of cardiac markers, it is classified as unstale angina pectoris and when markers are elevated, it could be either Q-/non-Q-wave STEMI or non-Q-wave NSTEMI

therefore may delay seeking medical help. Guidelines from the European Society of Cardiology (ESC)/American College of Cardiology (ACC)/American Heart Association (AHA) recommend that patients with established CAD call emergency medical services if they have chest pain that does not resolve after they take a sublingual nitroglycerin tablet.

In patients presenting to the emergency department (ED) with chest pain, a structured diagnostic approach that

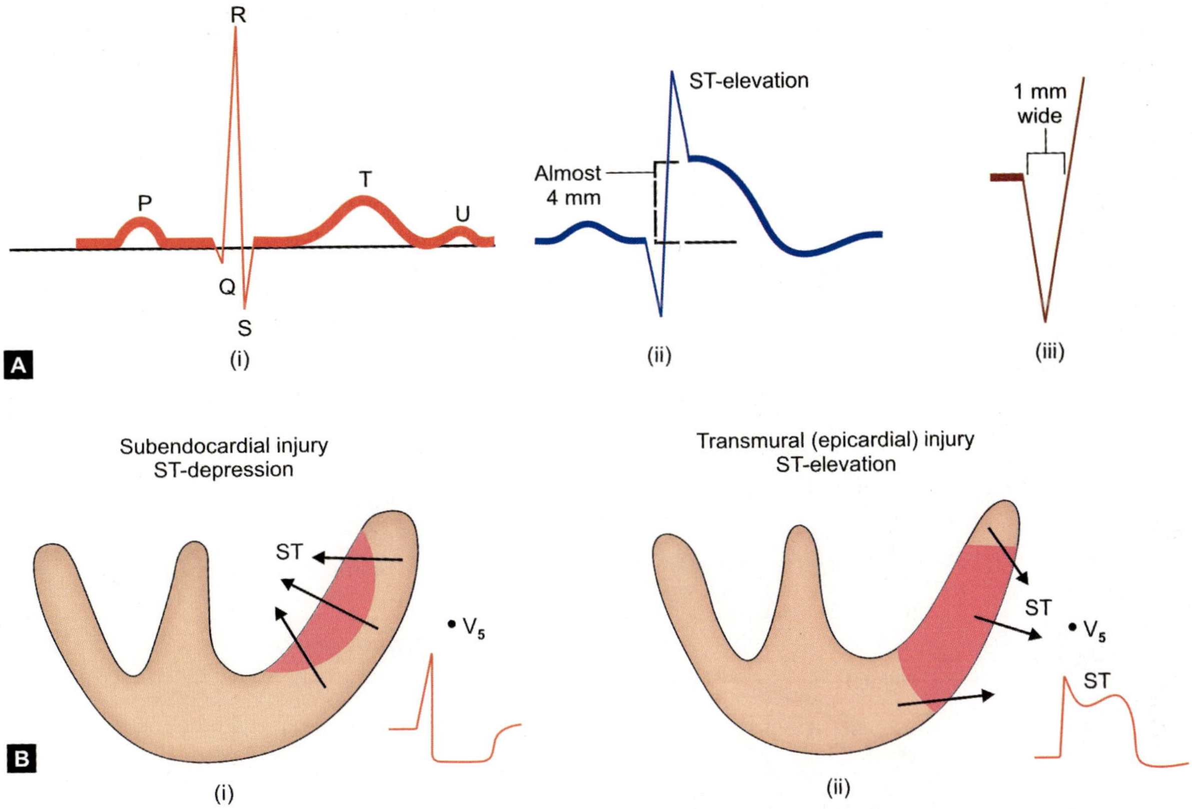


**Fig. 3.6:** (A) (i) ECG tracing showing normal P, Q, R, S, and T-waves. (ii) ST-elevation with acute ischemia. (iii) Q-wave with acute myocardial infarction. (B) Current-of-injury patterns with acute ischemia. With predominant subendocardial ischemia (i), the resultant ST-segment is directed toward the inner layer of the affected ventricle and the ventricular cavity. Overlying leads therefore record ST-segment depression. With ischemia involving the outer ventricular layer (ii) (transmural or epicardial injury), the ST vector is directed outward. Overlying leads record ST-segment elevation. *Credit: (Bottom) adapted from Braunwald E, Zipes DP, Libby P [2002]. (Heart disease: A textbook of cardiovascular medicine) [6th ed. p. 108]. Philadelphia: WB Saunders*

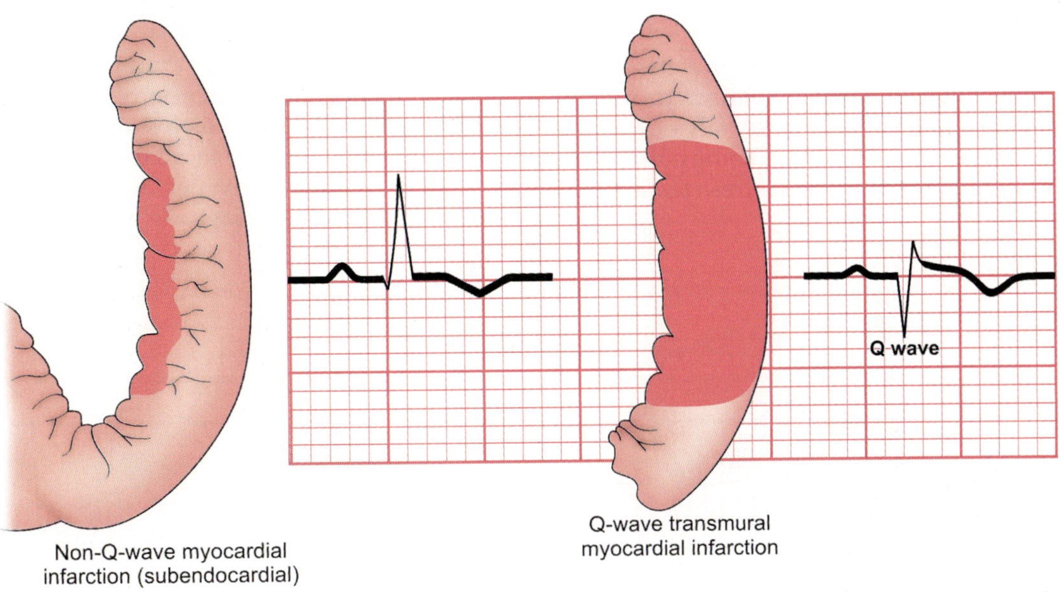


**Fig. 3.7:** ECG tracing showing subendocardial (non-Q-wave) versus a transmural (Q-wave) myocardial infarction

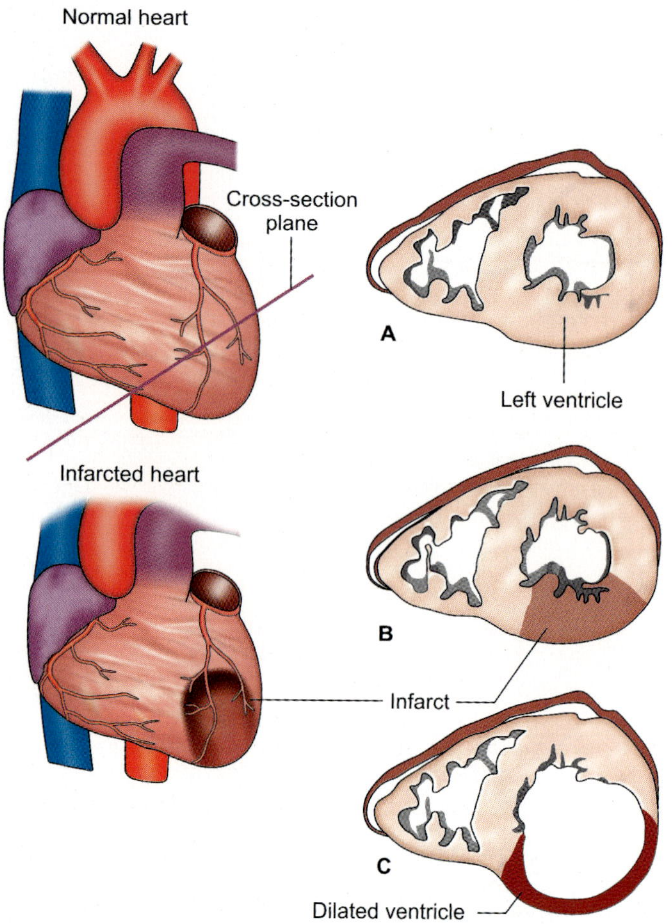


**Fig 3.8:** Normal vs infarcted heart. (A) The left ventricle has a thick muscular wall, shown in cross-section. (B) After a myocardial infarction (heart attack), heart muscle cells in the left ventricle are deprived of oxygen and die. (C) Eventually causing the ventricular wall to become thinner

**Table 3.1:** Different risk factors for atherosclerosis

| |
|---|
| ***Non-modifiable risk factors for atherosclerosis*** |
| Age |
| Sex |
| Family history of premature coronary heart disease |
| ***Modifiable risk factors for atherosclerosis*** |
| Smoking or other tobacco use |
| Diabetes mellitus |
| Hypertension |
| Dyslipidemia |
| Obesity |
| ***New and other risk factors for atherosclerosis*** |
| Elevated homocysteine levels |
| Male pattern baldness |
| Sedentary lifestyle and/or lack of exercise |
| Psychosocial stress |
| Presence of peripheral vascular disease |
| Poor oral hygiene |
| ***Non-atherosclerotic causes*** |
| Vasculitis |
| Coronary emboli |
| Congenital coronary anomalies |
| Coronary trauma |
| Coronary spasm |
| Drug use (cocaine) |

includes time-focused ED decision points, brief observation, and selective application of early outpatient provocative testing appeared both safe and diagnostically efficient in a study by Scheuermeyer et al. However, some patients with ACS may be discharged for outpatient stress testing on the index ED visit.

## Clinical History

The severity and duration of coronary artery obstruction, the volume of myocardium affected, the level of demand, and the ability of the rest of the heart to compensate are major determinants of a patient's clinical presentation and outcome. A patient may present to the ED because of a change in pattern or severity of symptoms.

Typically, angina is a symptom of myocardial ischemia that appears in circumstances of increased oxygen demand. It is usually described as a sensation of chest pressure or heaviness that is reproduced by activities or conditions that increase myocardial oxygen demand. A new case of angina is more difficult to diagnose because symptoms are often

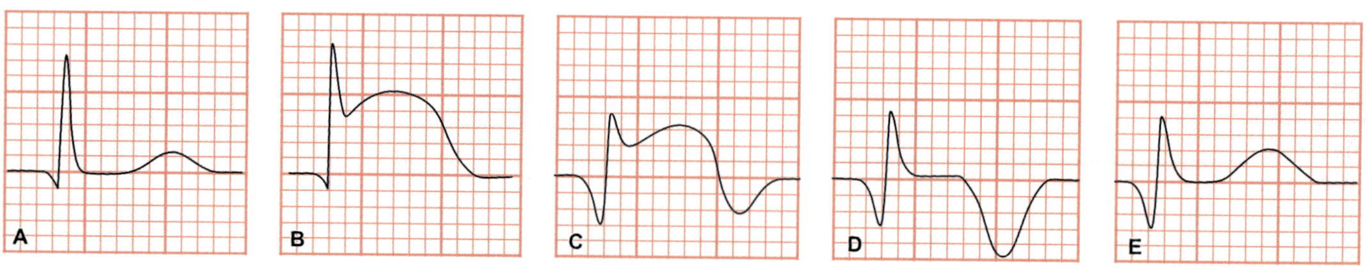


**Fig. 3.9:** ECG showing the evolution of an infarct on the ECG. ST-elevation, Q-wave formation, T-wave inversion, normalisation with a persistent Q-wave

vague and similar to those caused by other conditions (e.g. indigestion and anxiety).

However, not all patients experience chest pain. They may present with only neck, jaw, ear, arm, or epigastric discomfort. Some patients, including some who are elderly or who have diabetes, present with no pain, complaining only of episodic shortness of breath, severe weakness, lightheadedness, diaphoresis, or nausea and vomiting. Elderly persons may also present only with altered mental status. Those with preexisting altered mental status or dementia may have no recollection of recent symptoms and may have no complaints.

In addition, evidence exists that women more often have coronary events without typical symptoms, which may explain the frequent failure of clinicians to initially diagnose ACS in women.

**A summary of patient's complaints is as follows:**
- Palpitations
- Pain, which is usually described as pressure, squeezing, or a burning sensation across the precordium and may radiate to the neck, shoulder, jaw, back, upper abdomen, or either arm
- Exertional dyspnea that resolves with pain or rest
- Diaphoresis from sympathetic discharge
- Nausea from vagal stimulation
- Decreased exercise tolerance

Stable angina involves episodic pain lasting 5–15 minutes, is provoked by exertion, and is relieved by rest or nitroglycerin. In unstable angina, patients have increased risk for adverse cardiac events, such as myocardial infarction or death. New-onset exertional angina can occur at rest and is of increasing frequency or duration or is refractory to nitroglycerin. Variant angina (Prinzmetal angina) occurs primarily at rest, is triggered by smoking, and is thought to be due to coronary vasospasm.

## Physical Examination

Physical examination (Fig. 3.10) results are frequently normal. If chest pain is ongoing, the patient will usually lie quietly in bed and may appear anxious, diaphoretic, and pale. Physical findings can vary from normal to any of the following:
- Hypotension: Indicates ventricular dysfunction due to myocardial ischemia, infarction, or acute valvular dysfunction
- Hypertension: May precipitate angina or reflect elevated catecholamine levels due to anxiety or to exogenous sympathomimetic stimulation
- Diaphoresis
- Pulmonary edema and other signs of left heart failure
- Extracardiac vascular disease
- Jugular venous distention
- Cool, clammy skin and diaphoresis in patients with cardiogenic shock

In addition, a third heart sound (S3) may be present, and frequently, a fourth heart sound (S4) exists. The latter is especially prevalent in patients with inferior-wall ischemia and may be heard in patients with ischemia or systolic murmur secondary to mitral regurgitation.

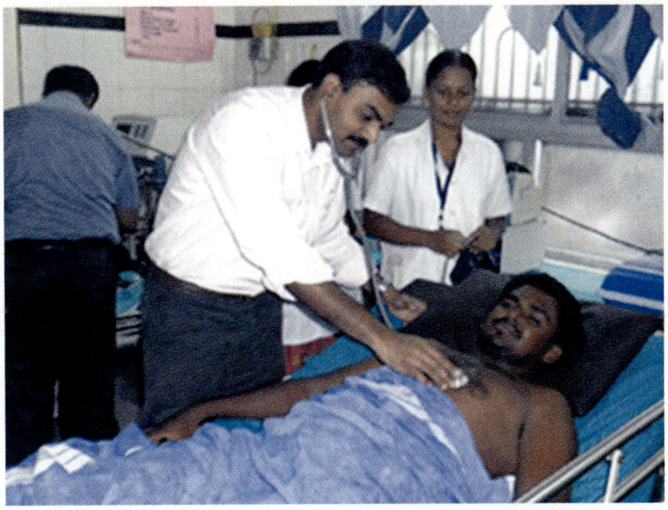

**Fig. 3.10:** A patient with acute coronary syndrome is being examined by the attending doctor after resuscitation in a recovery unit of the hospital

A systolic murmur related to dynamic obstruction of the left ventricular (LV) outflow tract may also occur. It is caused by hyperdynamic motion of the basal left ventricular myocardium and may be heard in patients with an apical infarct.

A new murmur may reflect papillary muscle dysfunction. Rales on pulmonary examination may suggest LV dysfunction or mitral regurgitation.

Patients who present to the ED with chest pain who have a low short-term risk of a major adverse cardiac event must be identified to facilitate early discharge in order to avoid lengthy and costly hospital stays. The ASPECT study tested a 2-hour, accelerated diagnostic protocol (ADP) that included the use of a structured pretest probability scoring method, electrocardiography, and a point-of-care biomarker panel that included troponin, creatine kinase MB, and myoglobin levels. The study suggests that ADP can identify patients at low risk for a short-term major adverse cardiac event who may be suitable for early discharge; such an approach could be used to decrease the overall observation periods and admissions for chest pain and has the potential to affect health-service delivery worldwide.

## Differential Diagnosis in ACS

- Anxiety
- Aortic stenosis
- Asthma
- Cardiomyopathy, dilated
- Esophagitis
- Gastroenteritis
- Hypertensive emergencies in emergency medicine
- Myocardial infarction
- Myocarditis
- Pericarditis and cardiac tamponade

## Laboratory Blood Tests

### Measurement of CK-MB Levels

CK-MB, the isoenzyme specific to the heart muscle, was the principal biomarker of cardiac injury until troponin supplemented it.

In the setting of myocardial infarction, plasma CK-MB concentrations typically rise about 4–6 hours after the onset of chest pain. They peak within 12–24 hours and return to baseline levels within 24–48 hours. Serial measurements obtained every 6–8 hours (at least 3 times) are warranted until peak values are determined.

The area under the concentration-time curve for CK-MB created with serial measurements of blood enzyme levels provides a reliable estimate of the size of the infarct.

Clinical settings other than ACS, such as trauma, heavy exertion, and skeletal muscle disease (e.g. rhabdomyolysis), may elevate CK-MB values.

Determination of subforms of CK-MB (CK-MB2 that is more specific to heart muscle) may improve the sensitivity of this test (Fig. 3.11).

### Measurement of Troponin Levels

The troponins are regulatory proteins found in skeletal and cardiac muscle. The three subunits that have been identified include troponin I (TnI), troponin T (TnT), and troponin C (TnC). The genes that code for the skeletal and cardiac isoforms of TnC are identical; thus, no structural difference exists between them. However, the skeletal and cardiac subforms for TnI and TnT are distinct, and immunoassays have been designed to differentiate between them. This explains the cardiospecificity of the cardiac troponins. Skeletal TnI and TnT are structurally different. No cross-reactivity occurs between skeletal and cardiac TnI and TnT with the current assays.

The cardiac troponins are sensitive, cardiospecific, and provide prognostic information for patients with ACS.

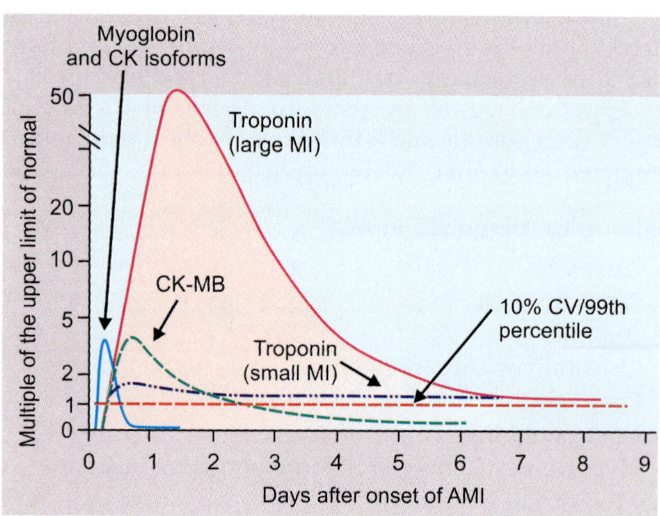


**Fig. 3.11:** Elevation of different biomarkers at different ACS

They have become the cardiac markers of choice for patients with ACS.

Early studies on the release kinetics of the cardiac troponins indicated that they were not early markers of myocardial necrosis. The early generation troponin assays yielded positive results within 4–8 hours after symptom onset, similar in timing to the release of CK-MB; however, they remained elevated for as long as 7–10 days post-myocardial infarction.

Initial studies on the cardiac troponins revealed a subset of patients with rest unstable angina in whom CK-MB levels were normal, but who had elevated troponin levels. These patients had higher adverse cardiac event rates (acute myocardial infarction, death) within the 30 days after the index admission and a natural history that closely resembled patients with NSTEMI.

As previously mentioned, an elevated troponin level also enables risk stratification of patients with ACS and identifies patients at high risk for adverse cardiac events (i.e. myocardial infarction, death) up to 6 months after the index event.

In a study by Antman et al. the initial TnI level on admission in patients with ACS correlated with mortality at 6 weeks. CK-MB levels, although sensitive and specific for the diagnosis of acute myocardial infarction (AMI), were not predictive of adverse cardiac events and had no prognostic value. The relationship between TnI levels and risk of cardiac events and mortality is demonstrated in the graphs shown in Fig. 3.11.

Use of cardiac markers in the ED. Troponin I levels and cardiac mortality in ACS. Cardiac event rates in the platelet receptor inhibition for ischemic syndrome (PRISM) study based on TnI results.

Data from a meta-analysis indicated that an elevated troponin level in patients without ST-segment elevation is associated with a nearly fourfold increase in cardiac mortality rate. For the composite end point of acute myocardial infarction or death, an elevated troponin level was associated with an odds ratio of 3.3.

The TIMI IIIB, GUSTO IIa, GUSTO IV ACS, and Fragmin during instability in coronary artery disease (FRISC) trial all demonstrated a direct correlation between the level of TnI or TnT and the adverse cardiac event rate and mortality rate in ACS. These studies confirmed the use of the cardiac troponins, i.e. TnI and TnT in risk stratification and therapeutic decision making.

Studies by Ohman et al. and Stubbs et al. revealed that an elevated troponin level at baseline was an independent predictor of mortality even in patients with chest pain and acute myocardial infarction with ST-segment elevation who were eligible for reperfusion therapy.

With the introduction of increasingly sensitive and precise troponin assays, up to 80% of patients with acute myocardial infarction will be found to have an elevated troponin within 2–3 hours of ED arrival. With this improved clinical performance in cardiac troponin assays, the so-called rapidly rising cardiac biomarkers, such as myoglobin or CK-MB isoforms, have a little clinical utility. In a prospective multicenter study, patients with ACS who presented with acute chest pain to the ED were followed for 12 months. The study found that patients with normal high-sensitivity cardiac troponin T (hs-cTnT) levels at presentation have low mortality rates but an increased rate of acute myocardial infarction during the subsequent 360 days. As a result, some authorities have called for a troponin standard alone and recommend eliminating CK-MB.

Many patients with acute myocardial infarction present with equivocal ECG patterns, making prehospital ECG diagnosis difficult. A study by Sorensen et al. suggests prehospital TnT testing may improve diagnosis in patients with chest pain transported by ambulance. When quantitative TnT was measured at hospital arrival in 958 patients after 8 and 24 hours, a diagnosis of acute myocardial infarction was established in 208 of 258 patients with increased TnT levels, showing prehospital TnT testing is feasible with a high success rate. Prehospital implementation of quantitative tests, with lower detection limits, may identify most patients with acute myocardial infarction irrespective of ECG changes.

The 2007 American College of Cardiology (ACC) guidelines for NSTEMI recommend that serial troponins be obtained for a definitive rule out at baseline and 6–9 hours later. To establish the diagnosis of acute myocardial infarction, only one elevated level above the established cutoff is required. The demonstration of a rising or falling level is needed to distinguish persistently elevated troponin levels (e.g. in some patients with renal failure) from those patients with acute myocardial infarction.

If myocardial injury is suspected despite negative cardiac-specific troponin findings, additional, sensitive laboratory assays are indicated.

### *Measurement of Myoglobin Levels*

Myoglobin is not cardiac specific, but it may be detected as early as 2 hours after myocardial necrosis starts. However, myoglobin results should be supplemented with other, more specific cardiac biomarkers, such as CK-MB or troponin.

Myoglobin values have a high negative predictive value when blood is sampled in the first 4–8 hours after onset.

## Complete Blood Count Determination

The complete blood count (CBC) helps in ruling out anemia as a secondary cause of ACS. Leukocytosis has prognostic value in the setting of acute myocardial infarction.

### *Basic Metabolic Panel*

Obtain a basic metabolic profile, including a check of blood glucose level, renal function, and electrolytes levels, for patients with new-onset angina. Close monitoring of potassium and magnesium levels is important in patients with ACS because low levels may predispose them to ventricular arrhythmias. Routine measurement of serum potassium levels and prompt correction are recommended.

Creatinine levels must be considered before using an angiotensin-converting enzyme (ACE) inhibitor and particularly if cardiac catheterization is considered. Use of N -acetylcysteine and adequate hydration can help prevent contrast material-induced nephropathy.

**Other useful metabolic profiles include amylase and lipase.**

A study by Charpentier et al. suggests that a serum glucose level of more than 140 mg/dl is associated with non-ST-elevation ACS in patients admitted to an ED for chest pain. However, when this level of blood glucose is added to the conventional diagnostic tools, the result is only a small increase in the ability to classify ACS.

### *New Biomarkers*

Levels of brain natriuretic peptide (BNP) and N-terminal pro-BNP (NT-pro-BNP) are elevated in acute MI and provide predictive information for risk stratification across the spectrum of ACS. However, a single, low BNP level obtained within 4 hours of a patient presenting to the ED does not identify the patient as low-risk for 30-day acute myocardial infarction or death.

In the future, a combination of levels of troponin (a biomarker for myocardial necrosis), NT-pro-BNP (an indicator of elevated LV end-diastolic pressure and wall stress), and C-reactive protein (CRP, an estimate of the extent of systemic inflammation) may prove useful for predicting the outcome of patients with ACS.

**Routine measurement of BNP and CRP levels in patients with ACS is not warranted.**

**Interleukin-6** is the major determinant of acute-phase reactant proteins in the liver, and serum amyloid A is another acute-phase reactant. Elevations of either of these can be predictive in determining increased risk of adverse outcomes in patients with unstable angina.

Cavusoqlu et al. suggests that elevated baseline levels of plasma interleukin-10 are associated with long-term adverse outcomes in patients with ACS.

Several other biomarkers with variable sensitivity and specificity have been investigated, including **sCD40** ligand, myeloperoxidase, pregnancy-associated plasma protein-A, choline, placental growth factor, cystatin C, fatty acid binding protein, ischemia modified albumin, chemokines ligand-5 and -18 (mediators of monocyte recruitment induced by ischemia), angiogenin, SCUBE1 (a novel platelet protein), and others. In a study that included 107 patients presenting to an emergency department with chest pain, ischemia modified albumin was not found to have superior sensitivity and specificity over traditional biomarkers, with a sensitivity of 0.86 and specificity of 0.49.

## Noninvasive and Invasive Laboratory Procedures

### *Chest Radiography*

Chest radiography (Figs 3.13 and 3.14) helps in assessing cardiomegaly and pulmonary edema, or it may reveal complications of ischemia, such as pulmonary edema. It may also provide clues to alternative causes of symptoms,

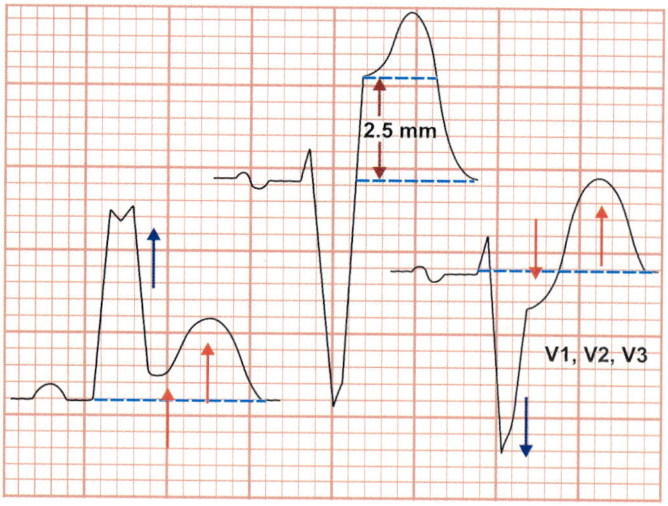


**Fig. 3.12:** Diagrammatic ECG criteria. The three criteria used to diagnose infarction in patients with LBBB are—concordant ST-elevation >1 mm in leads with a positive QRS complex (score 5) concordant ST depression >1 mm in V1–V3 (score 3), and excessively discordant ST-elevation >5 mm in leads with a negative QRS complex (score 2). This criterion is sensitive, but not specific for ischemia in LBBB. It is however associated with a worse prognosis, when present in LBBB during ischemia. A total score of >3 has a specificity of 90% for diagnosing MI

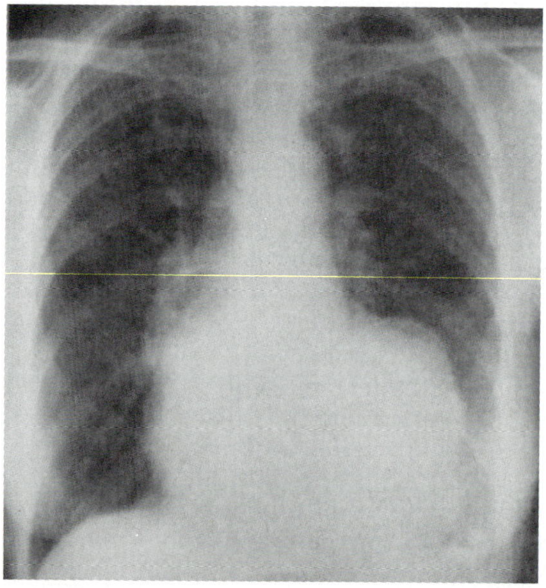

**Fig. 3.13:** Chest X-ray (PA) view showing bulge in the region of anterolateral border of LV in patient with aneurysm of LV wall following chronic MI

such as thoracic aneurysm or pneumonia (which can be a precipitating cause of ACS).

### Electrocardiography

ECGs should be reviewed promptly (Figs 3.15–3.31 and Table 3.2). Involve a cardiologist when in doubt.

Recording an ECG during an episode of the presenting symptoms is valuable. Transient ST-segment changes

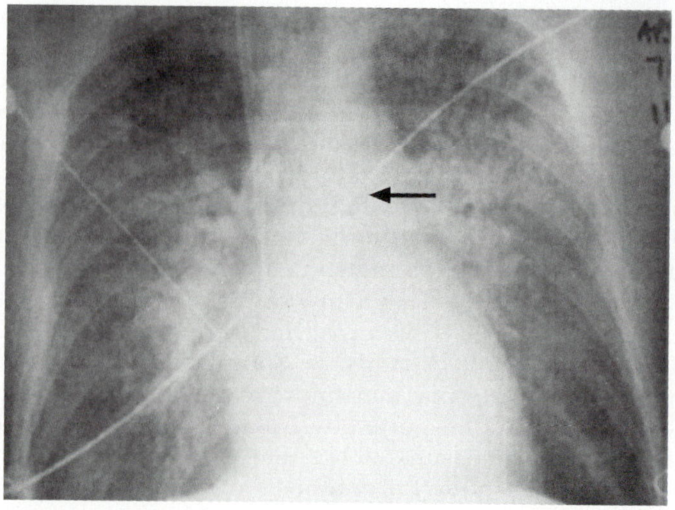

**Fig. 3.14:** Cardiogenic alveolar edema. Symmetrical airspace opacity with perihilar predominance is one characteristic pattern produced by cardiogenic edema

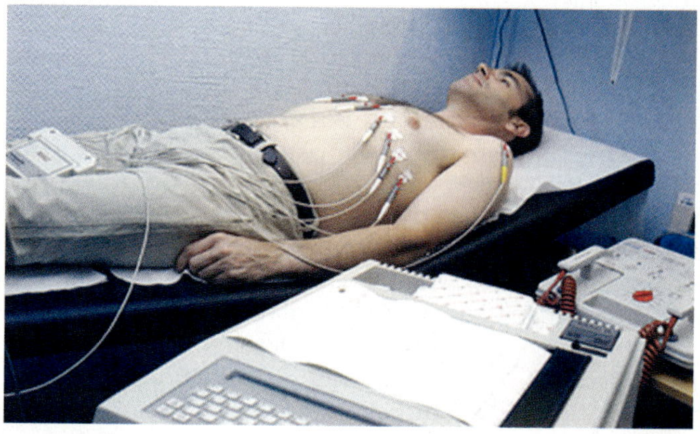

**Fig. 3.15:** An electrocardiogram (ECG) test records the electrical activity of the heart in a young patient with ACS

(>0.05 mV) that develop during a symptomatic period and that resolve when the symptoms are strongly predictive of underlying CAD and have prognostic value. Comparison with previous ECGs is often helpful.

Alternative causes of ST-segment and T-wave changes are left ventricular aneurysm, pericarditis, Prinzmetal angina, early repolarization, Wolff-Parkinson-White syndrome, and drug therapy (e.g. with tricyclic antidepressants, phenothiazines).

In the emergency setting, ECG is the most important ED diagnostic test for angina. It may show change during symptoms and in response to treatment, confirm a cardiac basis for symptoms. It may also demonstrate preexisting structural or ischemic heart disease (left ventricular hypertrophy, Q-waves). A normal ECG or one that remains unchanged from the baseline does not exclude the possibility that chest pain is ischemic in origin. Changes that may be seen during anginal episodes are given in Fig. 3.31.

- Transient ST-segment elevations

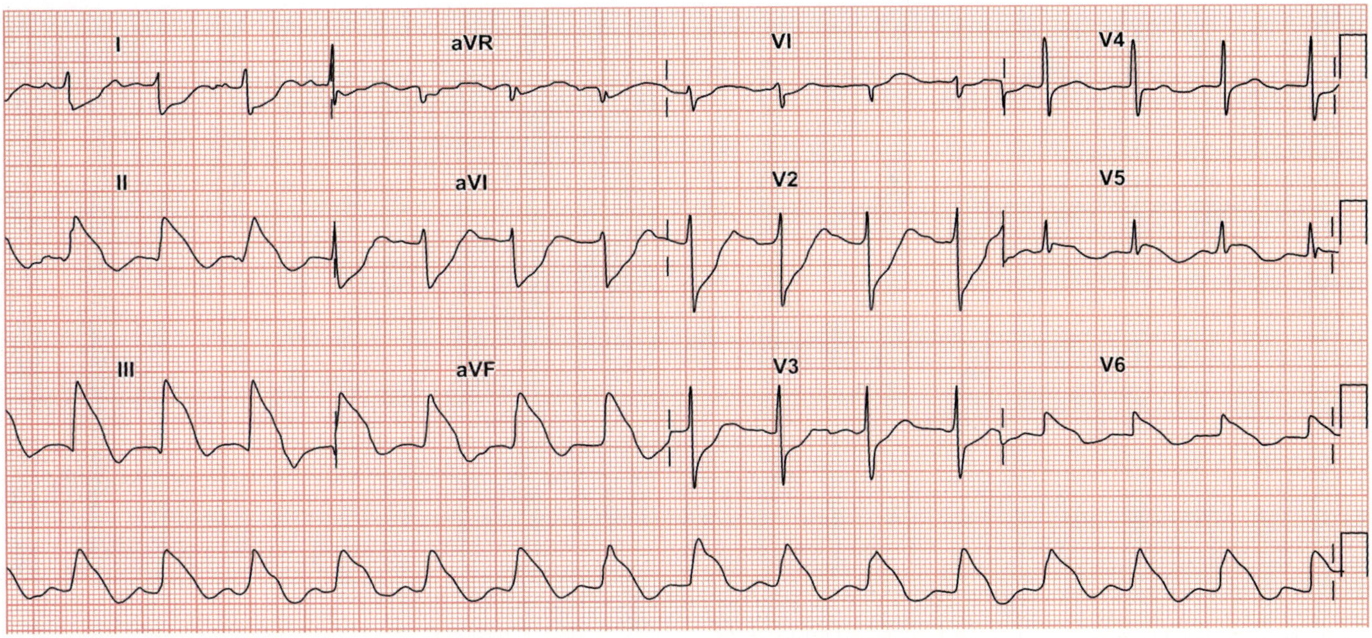


**Fig. 3.16:** Inferior wall MI—tombstone ST-elevation is an unusual morphological ECG appearance of acute myocardial infarction. The ST-segment is convexed upwards and the peak of the convexed ST-segment is often higher than the preceding R-wave, which is less than 0.04 s and small in amplitude

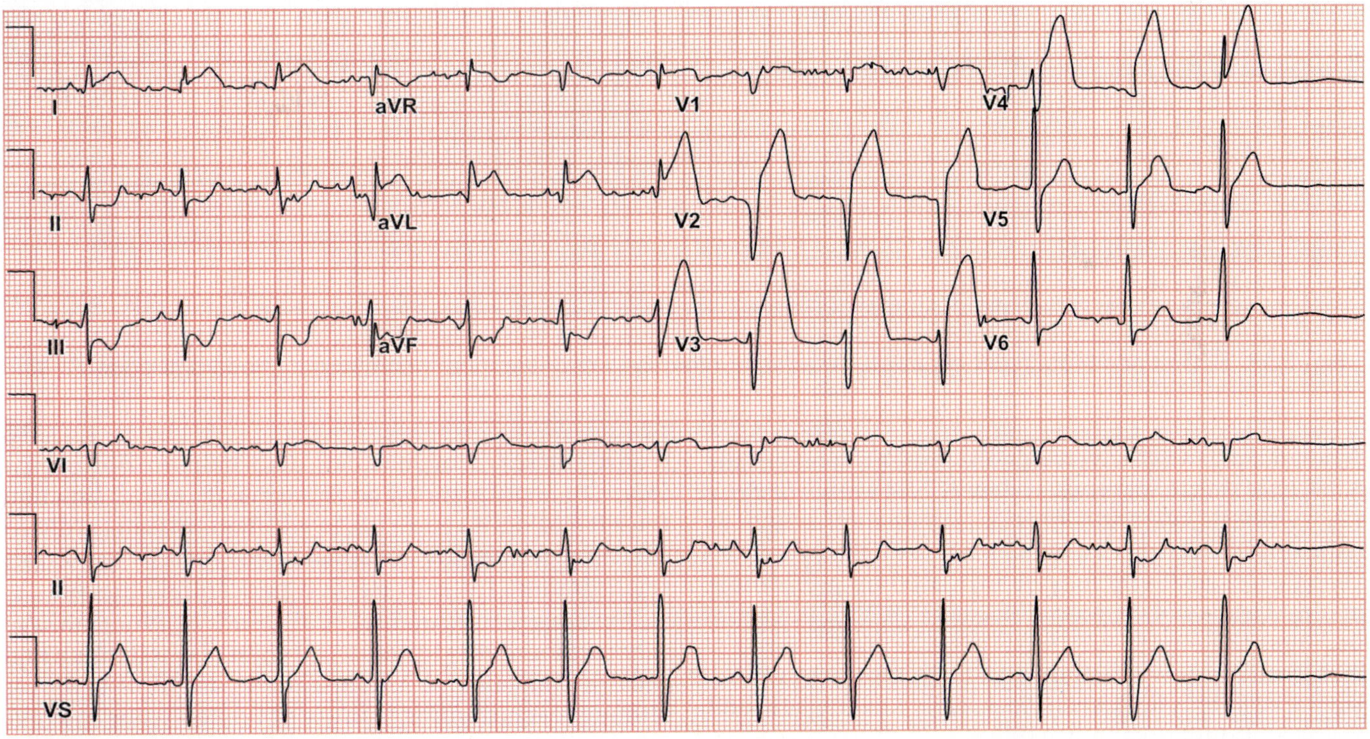


**Fig. 3.17:** Anterior wall MI—tombstone ST-elevation is an unusual morphological ECG appearance of acute myocardial infarction. The ST-segment is convexed upwards and the peak of the convexed ST-segment is often higher than the preceding R-wave, which is less than 0.04 s and small in amplitude. This type of tombstone pattern is associated with reperfusion polymorphous ventricular tachyarrhythmias and is thought to represent extensive and rapid myocardial damage after the ischemic episode. At coronary angiography, patients with tombstoning are likely to have high grade stenosis of the proximal left anterior descending artery

- Dynamic T-wave changes: Inversions, normalizations, or hyperacute changes
- ST-depressions: May be junctional, downsloping, or horizontal.

In patients with transient ST-segment elevations, consider LV aneurysm, pericarditis, Prinzmetal angina, early repolarization, and Wolff-Parkinson-White syndrome as possible diagnoses. Fixed changes suggest acute myocardial infarction.

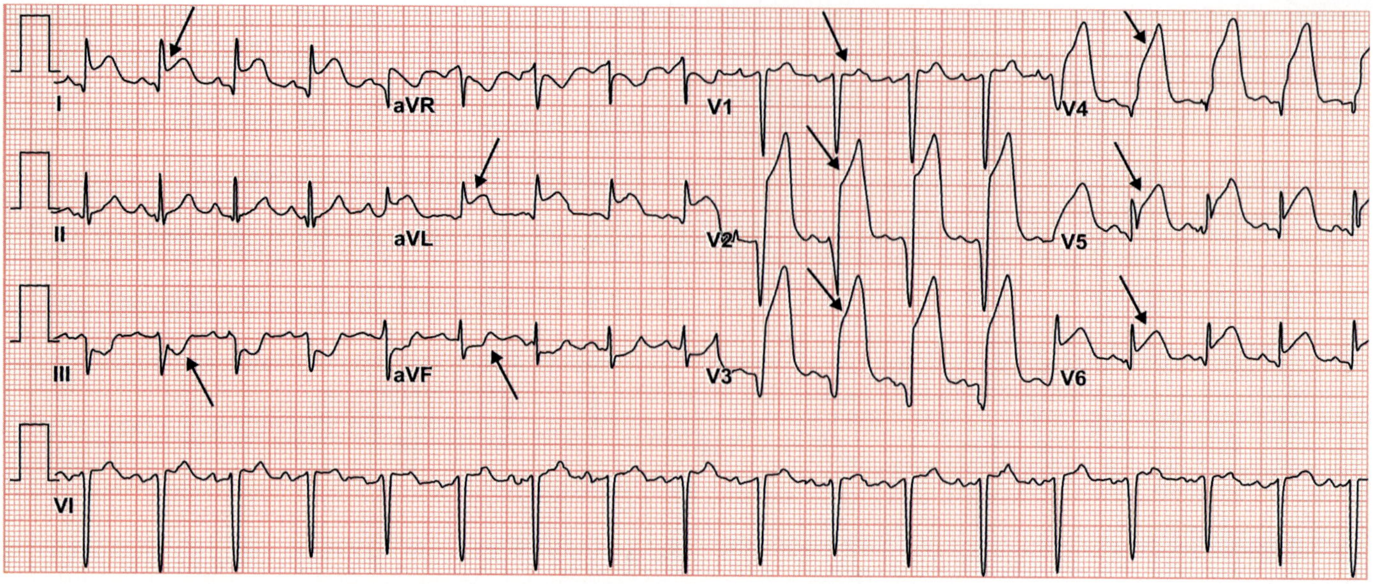


**Fig. 3.18:** ECG of ST-segment elevation myocardial infarction

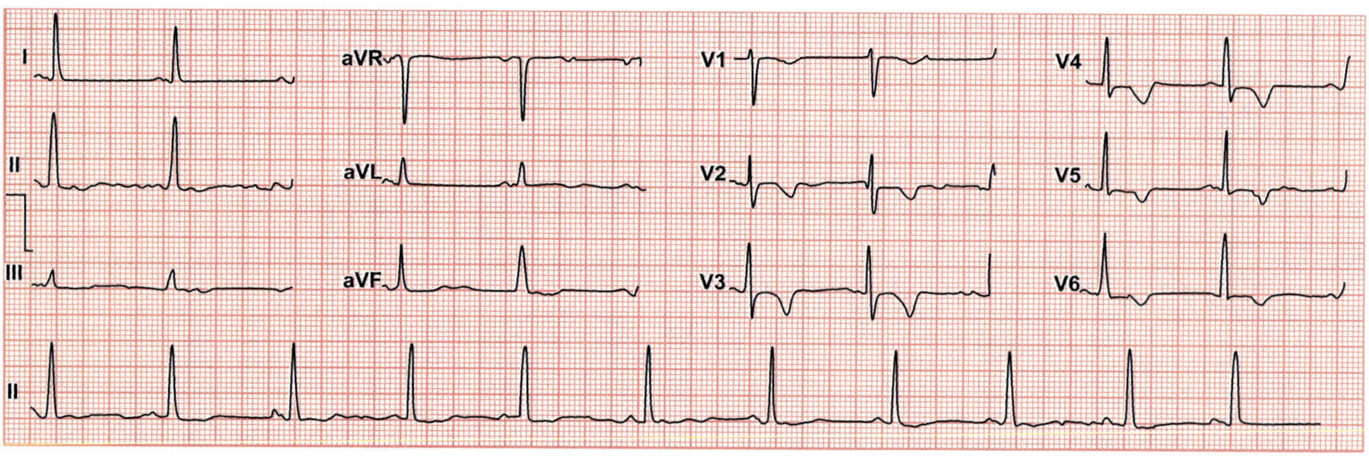


**Fig. 3.19:** ECG of non-ST-segment elevation myocardial infarction with ST-segment depression in precordial leads V2–V6

When deep T-wave inversions are present, consider the possibility of central nervous system (CNS) events or drug therapy with tricyclic antidepressants or phenothiazines as the cause.

Diagnostic sensitivity may be increased by performing right-sided leads (V4 R), posterior leads (V8, V9), and serial recordings.

In difficult cases with nondiagnostic ECGs, such as those involving a left bundle-branch block, early imaging is useful to assess wall-motion abnormalities.

An important use of noninvasive imaging is to classify a patient having NSTEMI or true STEMI.

## Echocardiography

Echocardiograms (Figs 3.32–3.35) may play an important role in the setting of ACS. Regional wall-motion abnormalities can be identified with this modality, and echocardiograms are especially helpful if the diagnosis is questionable.

An echocardiogram can also help in defining the extent of an infarction and in assessing overall function of the left and right ventricles. In addition, an echocardiogram can help to identify complications, such as acute mitral regurgitation, LV rupture, and pericardial effusion.

Absence of segmental wall-motion abnormality on echocardiography during active chest discomfort is a highly reliable indicator of a nonischemic origin of symptoms; although, echocardiography is of limited value in patients whose symptoms have resolved or who have pre-existing wall-motion abnormalities.

## Myocardial Perfusion Imaging

Radionuclide myocardial perfusion imaging has been shown to have favorable diagnostic and prognostic value in the emergent setting, with an excellent early sensitivity in the detection of acute myocardial infarction not found in other testing modalities (Figs 3.36–3.41).

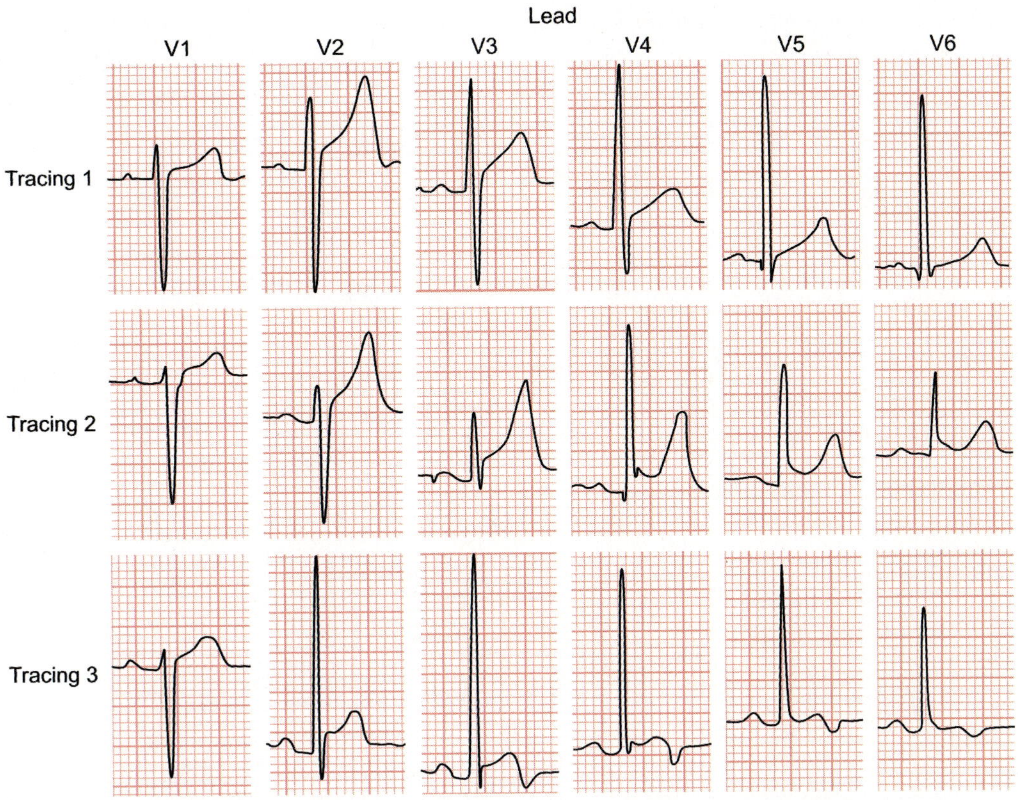


**Fig. 3.20:** Unstable angina (UA). Non-ST-elevation (non-Q-wave) myocardial infarction (NSTEMI) are part of the continuum of ACS

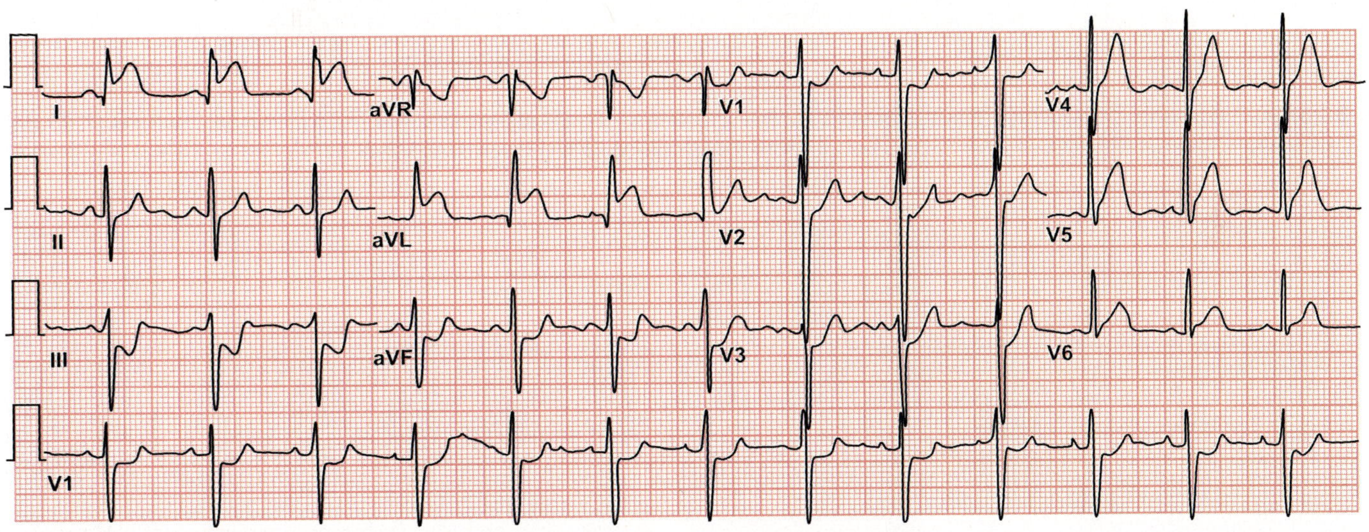


**Fig. 3.21:** ECG shows high lateral STEMI—ST-elevation is present in the high lateral leads (I and aVL). There is also subtle ST-elevation with hyperacute T-waves in V5–6. There is reciprocal ST depression in the inferior leads (III and aVF) with associated ST depression in V1–3 (which could represent anterior ischaemia or reciprocal change). This pattern is consistent with an acute infarction localised to the superior portion of the lateral wall of the left ventricle (high lateral STEMI). The culprit vessel in this case was an occluded first diagonal branch of the LAD

A normal resting perfusion imaging study has been shown to have a negative predictive value of more than 99% excluding myocardial infarction. Observational and randomized trials of rest and stress imaging in the ED evaluation of patients with chest pain have demonstrated reductions in unnecessary hospitalizations and cost savings compared with routine care.

Perfusion imaging has also been used in risk stratification after myocardial infarction and for measurement of infarct size to evaluate reperfusion therapies. Novel 'hot spot' imaging radiopharmaceuticals that visualize infarction or ischemia are currently undergoing evaluation and hold promise for future imaging of ACS.

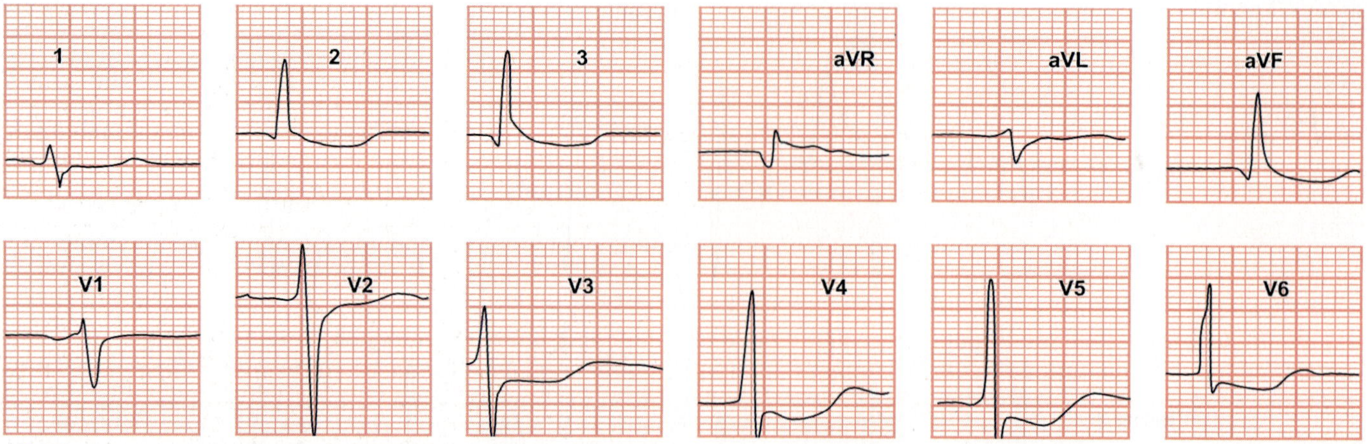


**Fig. 3.22:** ECG showing classical subendocardial (non-Q-wave) infarction manifested by abnormal ST-segment depressionin all leads except AVR, which showed ST-segment elevation

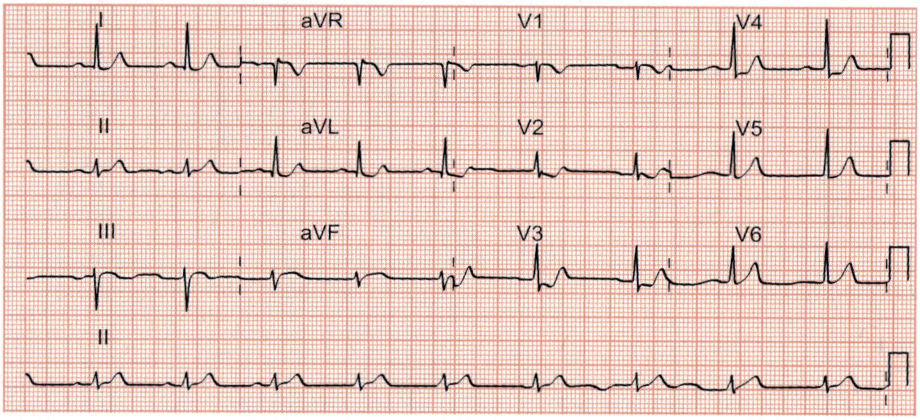


**Fig. 3.23:** ECG showing posterior MI. It is suggested by the presence of—ST-depression in V2–3 tall, broad R-waves (>30 ms) in V2–3, dominant R-wave (R/S ratio >) in V2, and upright terminal portions of the T-waves in V2–3

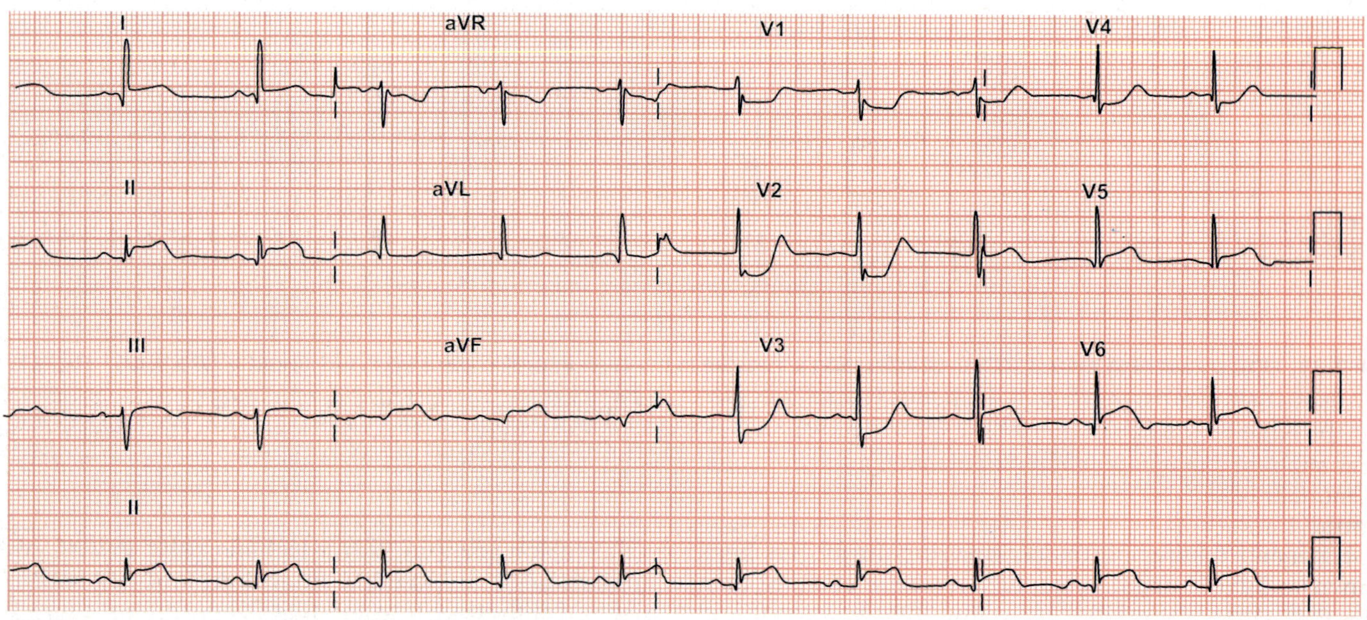


**Fig. 3.24:** ECG showing inferoposterolateral STEMI—ST-elevation is present in the inferior (II, III and aVF) and lateral leads (I, V5–6). ST-depression in V1–3 with tall, broad R-waves and upright T-waves and a R/S ratio >1 in V2 indicate concomitant posterior infarction (this patient also had ST-elevation in the posterior leads V7–9). These changes are consistent with a massive infarction involving the inferior, lateral, and posterior walls of the left ventricle.The culprit vessel is again very likely to be an occluded proximal circumflex artery

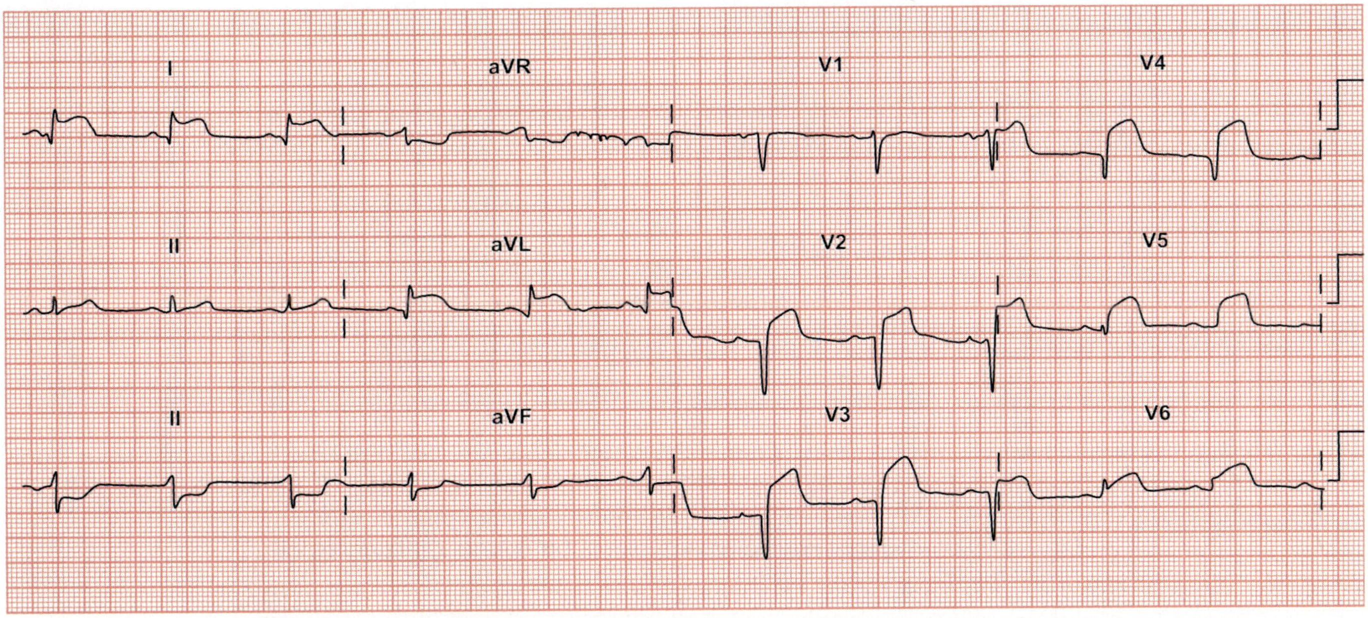


**Fig. 3.25:** ECG showing anterolateral STEMI—ST-elevation is present in the anterior (V2–4) and lateral leads (I, aVL, V5–6). Q-waves are present in both the anterior and lateral leads, most prominently in V2–4. There is reciprocal ST depression in the inferior leads (III and aVF). This pattern indicates an extensive infarction involving the anterior and lateral walls of the left ventricle. ST-elevation in the precordial leads plus the high lateral leads (I and aVL) is strongly suggestive of an acute proximal LAD occlusion (this combination predicts a proximal LAD lesion 87% of the time)

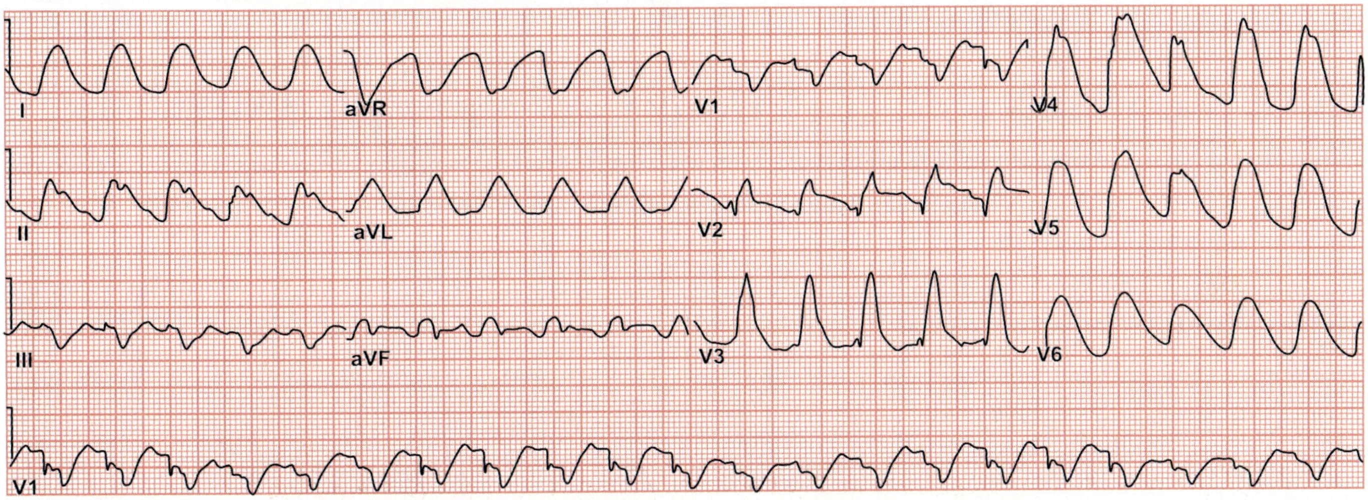


**Fig. 3.26:** Wide complex tachycardia, acute myocardial infarction

## Cardiac Catheterization and Angiography

Cardiac catheterization helps in defining coronary anatomy and the extent of a patient's disease. Patients with cardiogenic shock, intractable angina (despite medication), severe pulmonary congestion, or right ventricular (RV) infarction should immediately undergo cardiac catheterization. (Cardiogenic shock is defined as a systolic BP of less than 90 mmHg in the presence of organ hypoperfusion) (Figs 3.42–3.48).

For high-risk patients with ACS without persistent ST-elevation, angiography with glycoprotein IIb/IIIa inhibition has been recommended. Earlier that coronary angiography is performed, the lower the risk of recurrent ischemia. This also shortens the hospital stay for those patients.

Most patients benefit from angiography when they have a thrombolysis in myocardial infarction (TIMI) risk score of <3 points.

## Computed Tomographic, Coronary Artery Angiography and Calcium Scoring

Dual-source 64-slice CT scanners can do a full scan in 10 seconds and produce high-resolution images that allow fine details of the patient's coronary arteries to be seen. This technology allows for noninvasive and early diagnosis of CAD and thus earlier treatment before the coronary

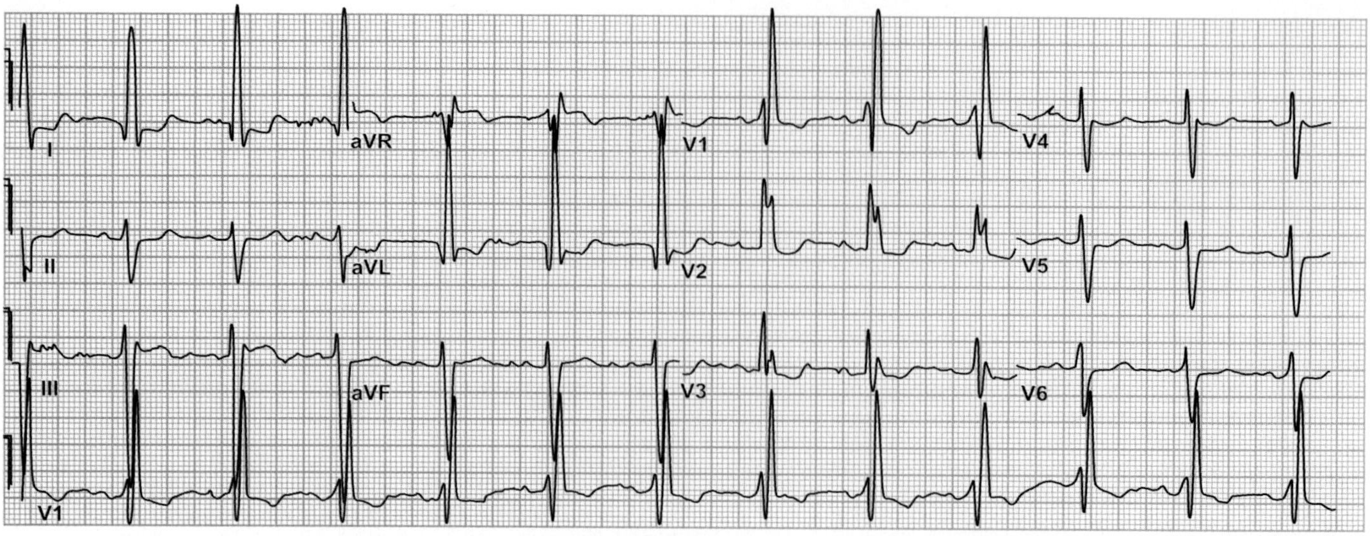


**Fig. 3.27:** Showing right bundle branch block, left anterior divisional block

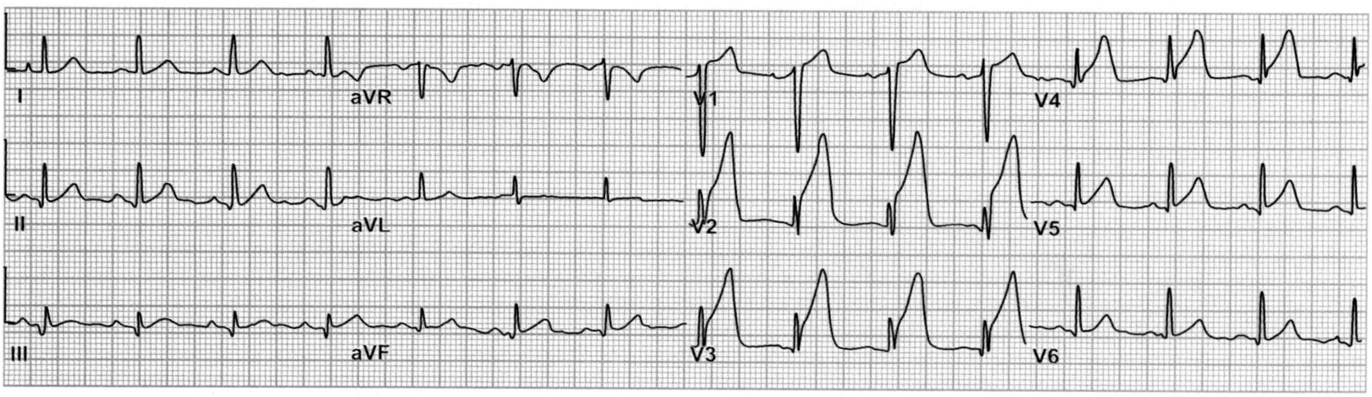


**Fig. 3.28:** Showing anteroseptal myocardial infarction

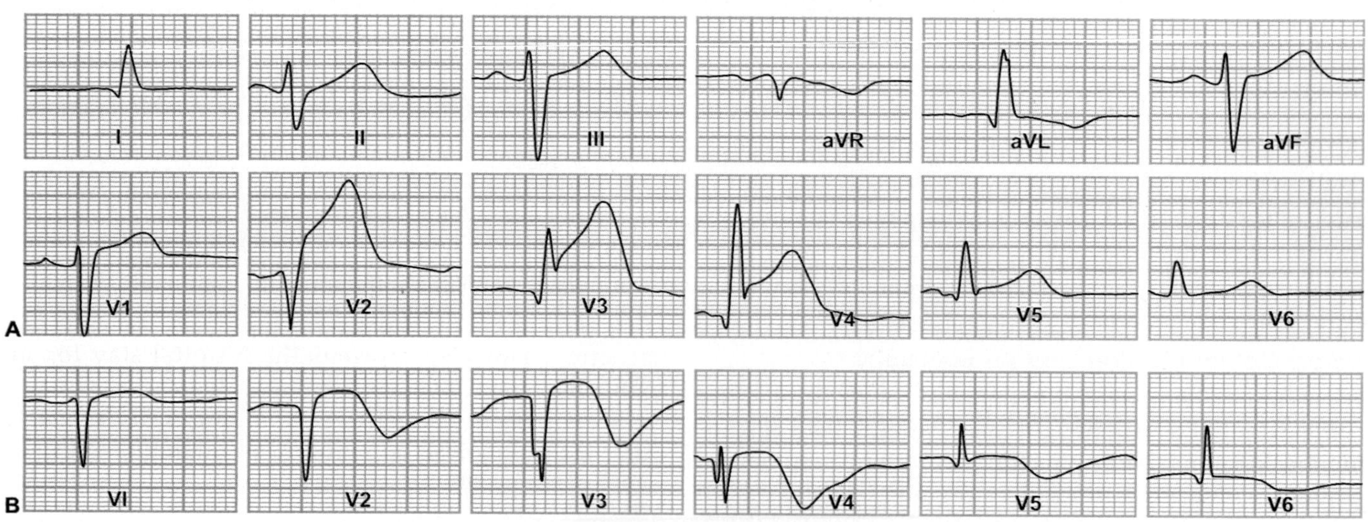


**Fig. 3.29:** Showing acute extensive anterior myocardial infarction

arteries become more or completely occluded. It permits direct visualization of not only the lumen of the coronary arteries but also plaque within the artery. Dual-source 64-slice CT scanning is being used with intravenous (IV) contrast to determine if a stent or graft is open or closed.

CT coronary artery scoring is emerging as an attractive risk stratification tool in patients who are at low risk for ACS. This imaging modality exposes the patient to very little radiation (1–2 msV). No contrast is needed, and the study does not have a requirement for heart rate (Figs 3.49–3.52).

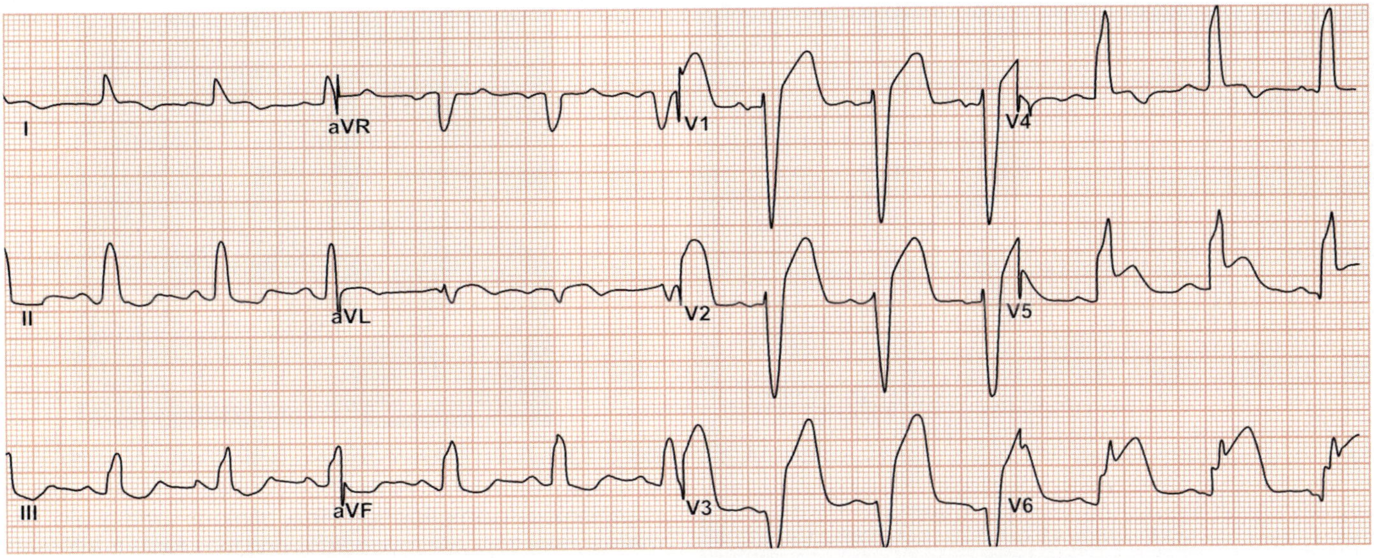


**Fig. 3.30:** Acute anteroseptal myocardial infarction—see the tall T-waves in V2–V4

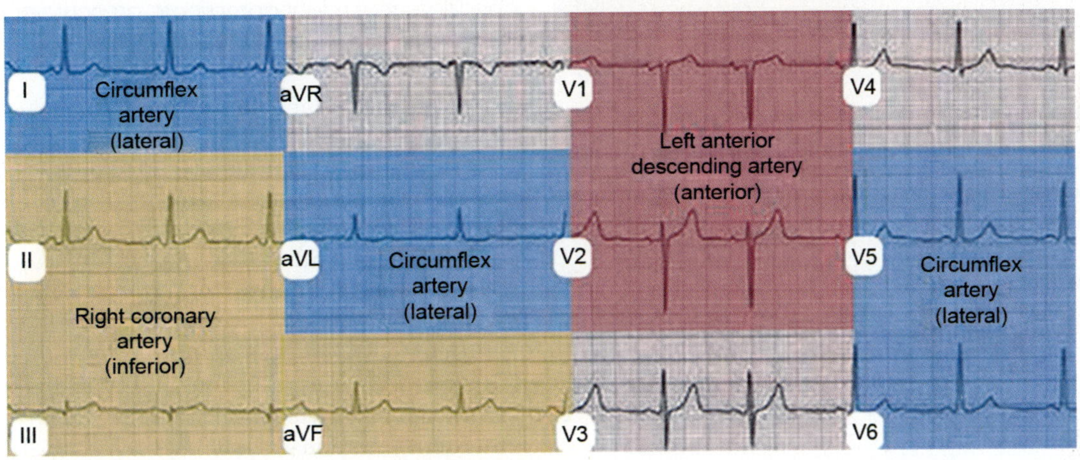


**Fig. 3.31:** Color map showing regional involvement of heart in relation to branches of coronary arteries involved

**Table 3.2:** ECG changes during myocardial infarction

| Location of MI | Leads affected | Vessel involved | ECG changes |
|---|---|---|---|
| Anterior wall | V2–V4 | • Left anterior descending artery (LAD) – Diagonal branch | • Poor R-wave progression<br>• ST-segment elevation<br>• T-wave inversion |
| Septal wall | V1 and V2 | • Left anterior descending artery (LAD) – Septal branch | • R-wave disappears<br>• ST-segment rises<br>• T-wave inverts |
| Lateral wall | I, aVL, V5, V6 | • Left coronary artery (LCA) – Circumflex branch | • ST-segment elevation |
| Inferior wall | II, III, aVF | • Right coronary artery (RCA) – Posterior descending branch | • T-wave inversion<br>• ST-segment elevation |
| Posterior wall | V1–V4 | • Left coronary artery (LCA) – Circumflex branch<br>• Right coronary artery (RCA) – Posterior descending branch | • Tall R-waves<br>• ST-segment depression<br>• Upright T-waves |

## Coronary Angioscopy and Optical Coherence Tomography

These investigations are helpful when others fail to contribute in the final diagnosis of acute coronary syndrome (Figs 3.53–3.54).

## *Cardiac MRI in Acute Coronary Syndrome*

Resting cardiac MRI exhibited diagnostic operating characteristics suitable for triage of patients with chest pain in the emergency department. Performed urgently to evaluate

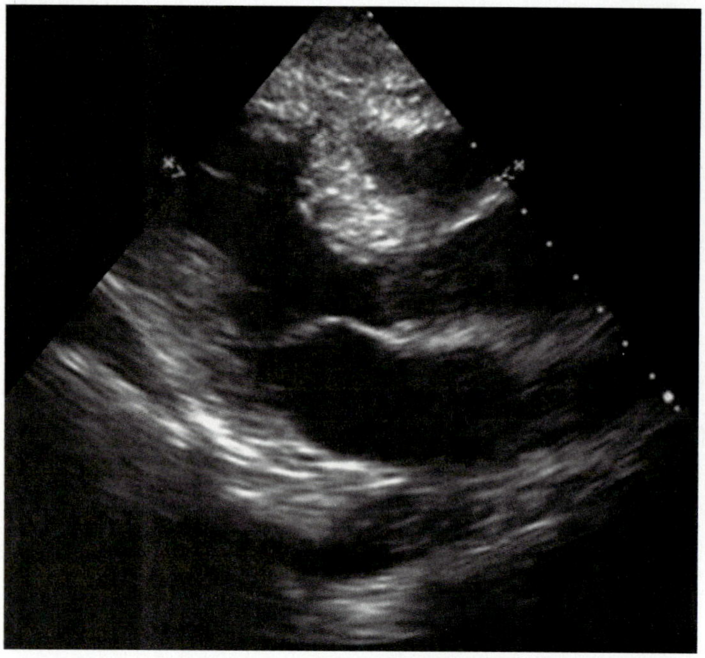

**Fig. 3.32:** Regional wall motion abnormalities in LAD territory in ACS

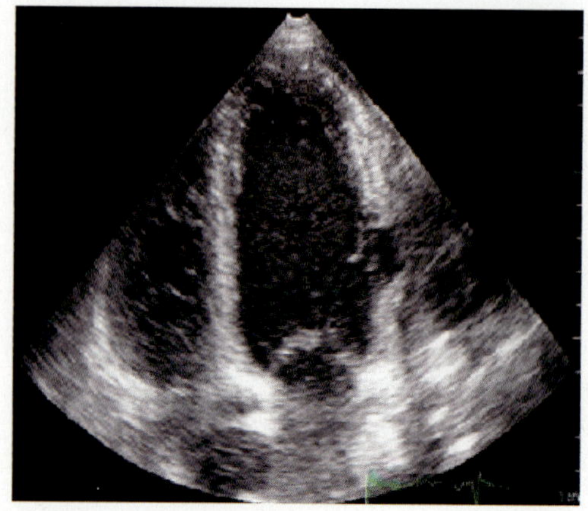

**Fig. 3.33:** This is a case of acute coronary syndrome in a patient with respiratory tract infection further complicated by a mechanical complication. The clinical setting led to the misdiagnosis of acute myocarditis and the proper treatment was delayed until a mechanical complication of the myocardial infarction appeared. This case indicates the multiplicity of clinical conditions that might complicate an acute coronary syndrome and obscure early diagnosis and treatment

chest pain, MRI accurately detected a high fraction of patients with acute coronary syndrome, including patients with enzyme-negative unstable angina (Figs 3.55–3.58).

## Complications in ACS

Complications of ischemia include pulmonary edema, while those of myocardial infarction include rupture of the papillary muscle, left ventricular free wall, and ventricular septum (Figs 3.59–3.70).

### *Arrhythmias*

**Classification of peri-infarction arrhythmias**: Peri-infarction arrhythmias can be broadly classified into the following categories (Figs 3.59–3.65 and Table 3.3):

- **Supraventricular tachyarrhythmias,** including sinus tachycardia, premature atrial contractions, paroxysmal supraventricular tachycardia, atrial flutter, and atrial fibrillation
- **Accelerated junctional rhythms**
- Bradyarrhythmias, including sinus bradycardia and junctional bradycardia
- **Atrioventricular (AV) blocks,** including first-degree AV block, second-degree AV block, and third-degree AV block
- **Intraventricular blocks,** including left anterior fascicular block, right bundle branch block (RBBB), and left bundle branch block (LBBB)
- **Ventricular arrhythmias,** including premature ventricular contractions (PVCs), accelerated idioventricular rhythm, ventricular tachycardia, and ventricular fibrillation
- **Reperfusion arrhythmias**

## Ventricular Arrhythmias

Ventricular arrhythmias are a frequent cause of death in the earliest stages of acute myocardial infarction. The development of coronary care units, continuous ECG surveillance, and defibrillators in the 1960s led to a reduction in mortality from acute myocardial infarction through the prompt identification and treatment of ventricular arrhythmia; and emergency medical technicians have reduced outpatient mortality in the earliest minutes of myocardial infarction. In cities with well-developed emergency response systems, such as Seattle, Washington, and Rochester, Minnesota, where the average response time is less than 5 minutes, survival of patients with myocardial infarction complicated by cardiac arrest has increased. In fact, long-term survival of patients who have undergone rapid defibrillation after out-of-hospital cardiac arrest is similar to that of age-, sex-, and disease-matched patients who did not have out-of-hospital cardiac arrest; the quality of life of the majority of survivors is similar to that of the general population.

## Ventricular Fibrillation

In the setting of acute myocardial infarction, ventricular fibrillation is often described as either primary, when it occurs in the absence of hypotension or heart failure, or secondary, when hypotension or heart failure is present. Primary ventricular fibrillation occurs in approximately 3–5% of patients with acute myocardial infarction; the peak incidence is in the first 4 hours of infarction. Primary ventricular fibrillation is infrequent more than 24 hours after symptom onset. Mortality is increased in patients who suffer this complication. In patients who are successfully resuscitated and survive to hospital discharge, however,

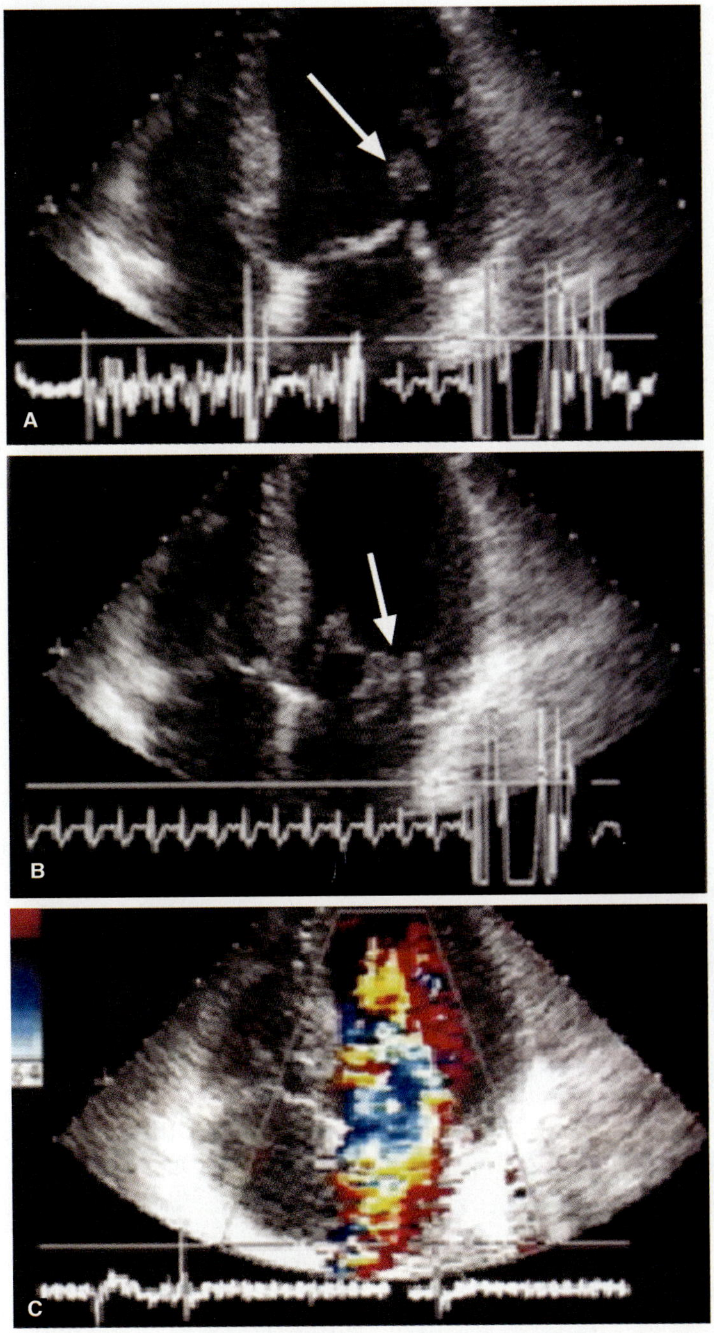


**Fig. 3.34:** Transthoracic echocardiography showed complete rupture of the anterolateral papillary muscle (arrow in A), prolapse of the muscle into the left atrium (arrow in BI), and severe mitral regurgitation (C)

the long-term prognosis does not appear to be affected. Although lidocaine was shown to reduce the occurrence of primary ventricular fibrillation, mortality in patients receiving lidocaine increased because of an increase in fatal bradycardia and asystole; therefore, prophylactic lidocaine is no longer recommended if defibrillation can rapidly be performed. Beta blockers may reduce the early occurrence of ventricular fibrillation and should be administered to patients who have no contraindications.

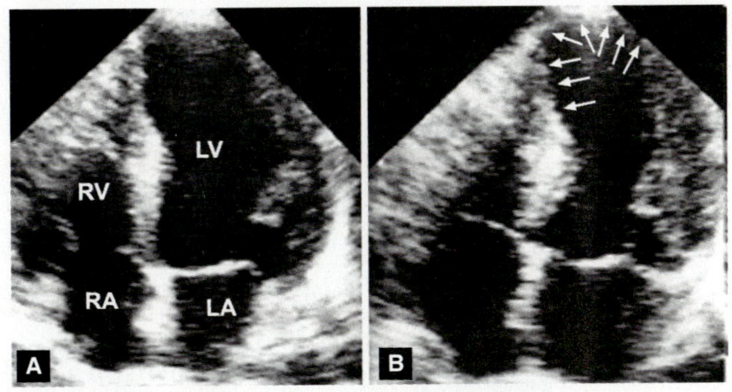


**Fig. 3.35:** Echocardiographic wall motion abnormality coronary artery disease. (A) Two-dimensional echocardiographic apical four-chamber view at end-diastole. (B) Two-dimensional echocardiographic apical four-chamber view at end-systole. The right ventricle (RV) and the septal and lateral walls at the base of the left ventricle (LV) demonstrate normal inward motion from diastole through systole; however, the distal septum and apex demonstrate akinesis (arrows in B). The wall motion. abnormality demonstrated in this frame was caused by ischemia from a lesion in the mid-left anterior descending artery. LA=left atrium; RA=right atrium

Hypokalemia is a risk factor for primary ventricular fibrillation and should be rapidly corrected if present. When ventricular fibrillation occurs, rapid defibrillation with 200–300 joules should be attempted, and repeated shocks of 360 joules should be administered. The advanced cardiac life support (ACLS) guidelines recommend medical therapy, including epinephrine, lidocaine, and bretylium; in addition, IV amiodarone should be considered in patients in whom defibrillation is initially unsuccessful. Secondary ventricular fibrillation is associated with a high mortality, in part because of the underlying hypotension and heart failure. Treatment must be aimed not only at terminating the arrhythmia but also at treating the hemodynamic abnormalities and their causes.

### Ventricular Tachycardia

Ventricular tachycardia (three or more consecutive ventricular ectopic beats) is common in patients with acute myocardial infarction; however, short runs of nonsustained ventricular tachycardia are no longer believed to predispose a patient to sustained ventricular tachycardia or ventricular fibrillation. In patients in whom sustained or hemodynamically significant ventricular tachycardia occurs, prompt electrical cardioversion should be performed. If the ventricular tachycardia is monomorphic, synchronic cardioversion with 100 joules should first be attempted. As with ventricular fibrillation, polymorphic ventricular tachycardia should be treated with unsynchronized discharge. Prolonged runs of asymptomatic ventricular tachycardia can be initially treated with IV lidocaine, procainamide, or amiodarone. These medications may also be helpful in reducing recurrent ventricular tachycardia.

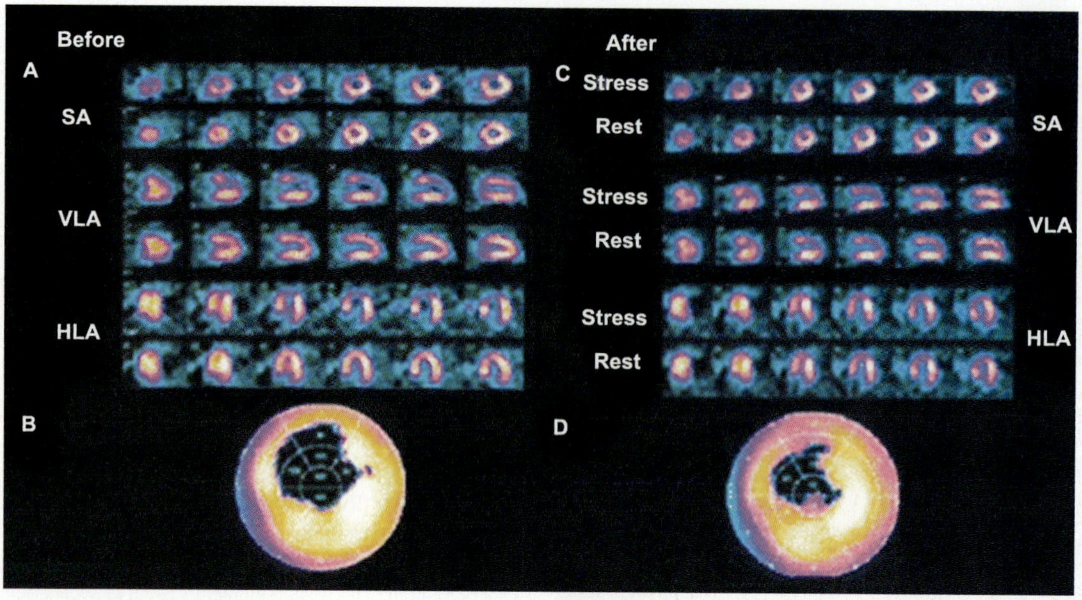


**Fig. 3.36:** Baseline and follow-up stress/rest SPECT sestamibi MPI after medical therapy. (A) A patient's baseline stress/rest SPECT sestamibi perfusion images showing large ischemia of the left anterior descending artery territory; the top rows show stress images and the bottom rows show rest images. (B) Polar maps estimated the extent of total ischemia to be 31% of left ventricular myocardium. The left ventricular ejection fraction was 62% by gated SPECT. (C) SPECT sestamibi MPI at 6-month follow-up with maximal medical therapy including statin, beta-blockers, and nitrates. The ischemia (same format as A) is less. (D) Polar maps estimated extent of total abnormality to be 21%, ischemia 16%, and scar 5%. The left ventricular ejection fraction was 67%. HLA=horizontal long axis; MPI=myocardial perfusion imaging; SAX=short axis; SPECT=single-photon emission computed tomography; VLA=vertical long axis

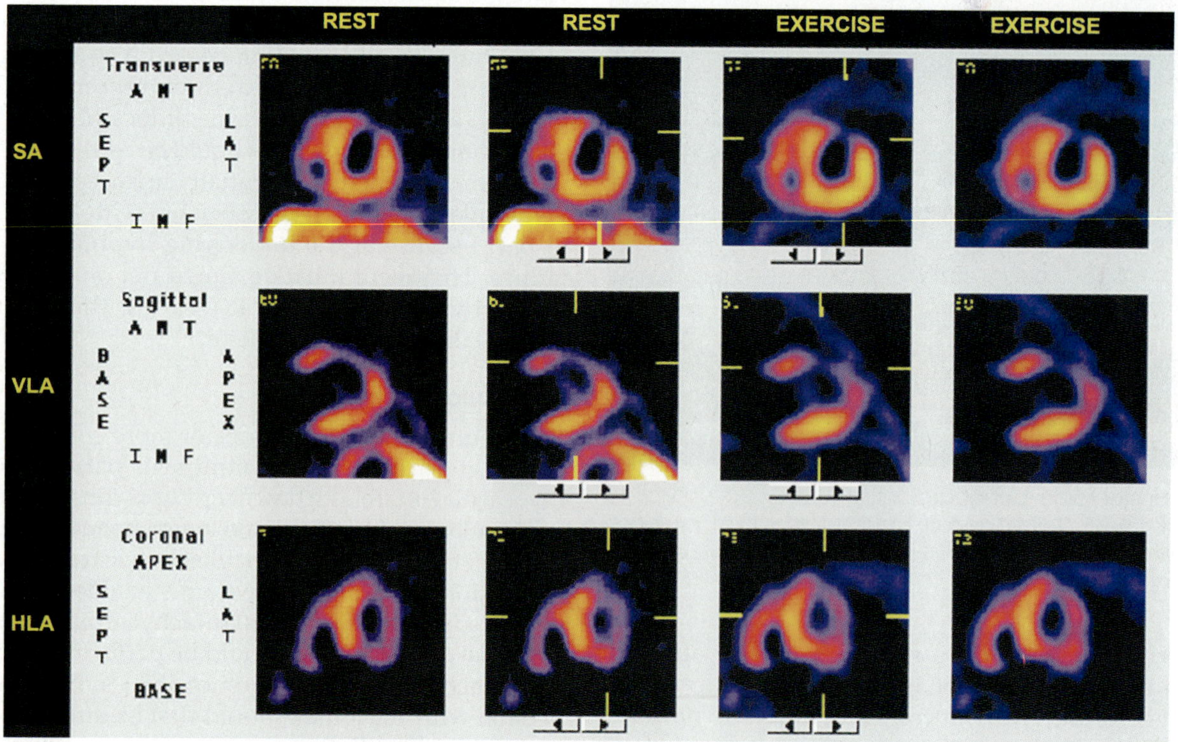


**Fig. 3.37:** Eleven days after PTCA, a second rest-exercise myocardial scintigraphy with Tc-99m sestamibi showed a fixed perfusion defect in the anterolateral segment of the left ventricle (shown by thin arrows) with no other significant abnormalities. Ischemia in the apical portion of the anterior wall is no longer seen (thick arrows). (The second study was obtained with different system than the first study.) A concomitant echocardiographic study demonstrated left ventricle hypertrophy with an ejection fraction of approximately 61%, hypokinesis of the anterolateral wall and abnormal septal motion

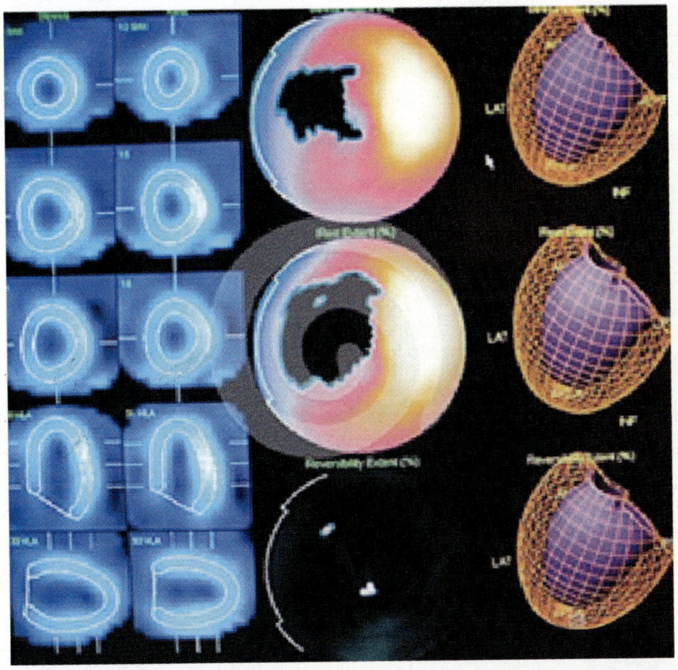

**Fig. 3.38:** Myocardial perfusion nuclear scan, rest and stress part presented myocardial scar as evidence of heart attack in past, the black spots are on both parts of test in the same areas of upper and lower circles of image

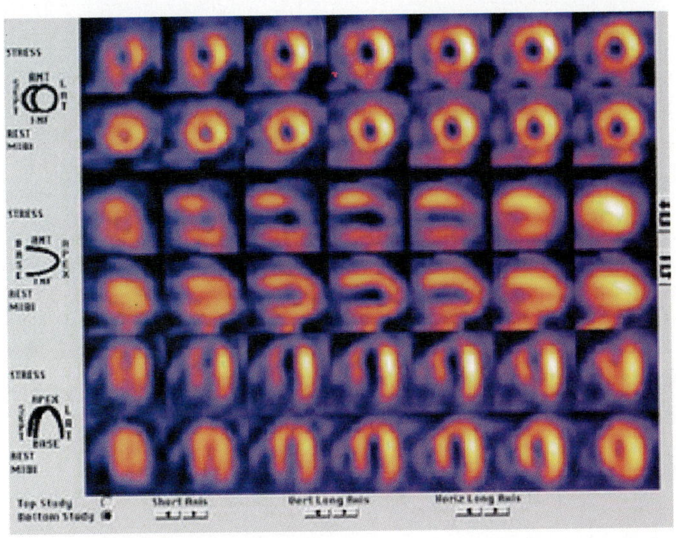


**Fig. 3.39:** A SPECT perfusion study in a patient with a large degree of tracer redistribution affecting the left anterior descending and right coronary artery territories

## ATRIAL ARRHYTHMIA

### Atrial Fibrillation

Atrial fibrillation is the most common atrial arrhythmia in acute myocardial infarction, occurring in 10–16% of patients. Atrial fibrillation may result either from an acute increase in left atrial pressure caused by left ventricular dysfunction or from atrial ischemia as a result of occlusion of a coronary artery (usually the right coronary artery) proximal to the origin of atrial branches. The incidence of

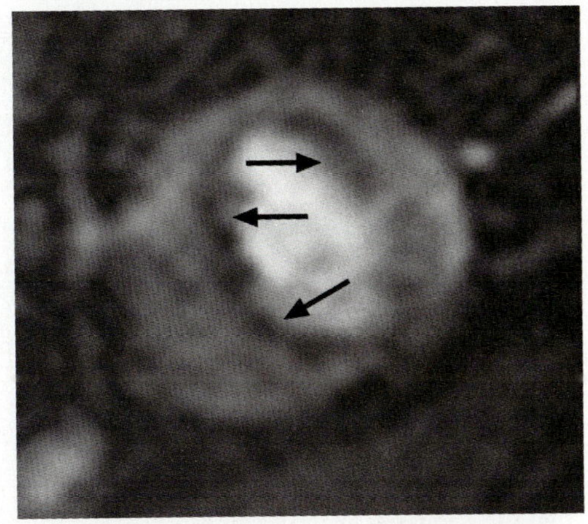

**Fig. 3.40:** Perfusion defect in myocardial infarction. Short-axis SSFP first-pass perfusion imaging at rest in a 43-year-old male with chest pain shows a perfusion defect (arrows) in the apical anterior, septal, and inferior segments (arrows), consistent with myocardial infarction in left anterior descending (LAD) artery territory

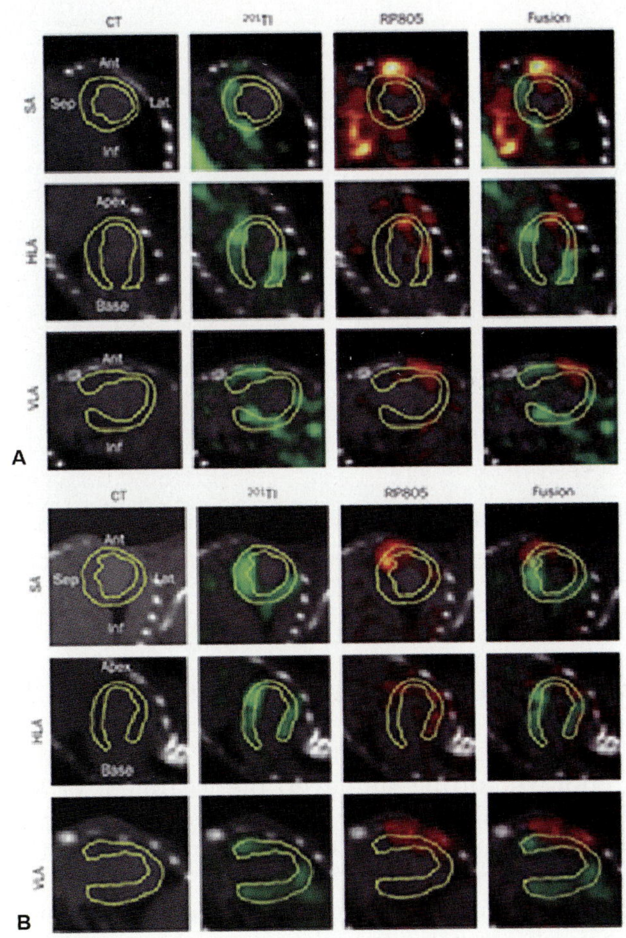


**Fig. 3.41:** The contrast agent permitted better definition of the left ventricular myocardium (highlighted by yellow line). Representative short-axis (SA), horizontal long-axis (HLA), and vertical long-axis (VLA) images are shown. Focal uptake of 99mTc-RP805 targeted at matrix metalloproteinases is seen within the central infarct and peri-infarct regions, which corresponds to 201Tl perfusion defect

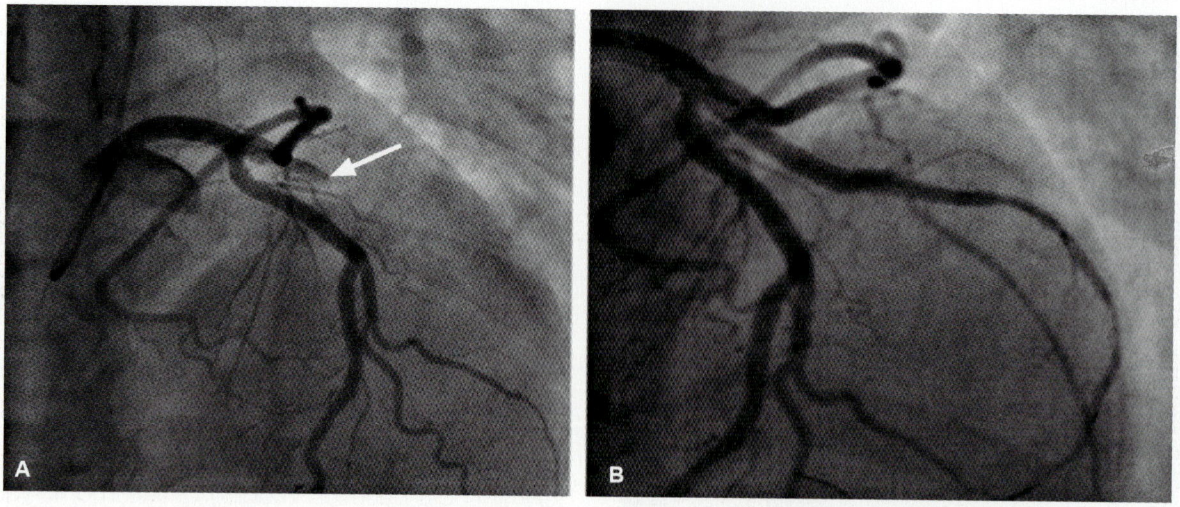


**Fig. 3.42:** Occlusive concomitant dissections of the carotid and coronary arteries treated with stent placement in a 60-year-old male with ACS

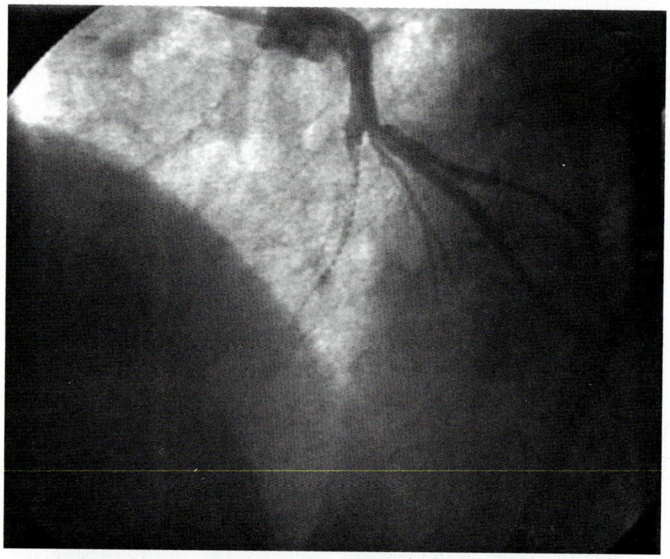

**Fig. 3.43:** Left selective coronary angiogram in left anterior oblique cranial projection (48° LAO, 33° ocranial) showing the no-reflow phenomenon in the LAD after stent deployment

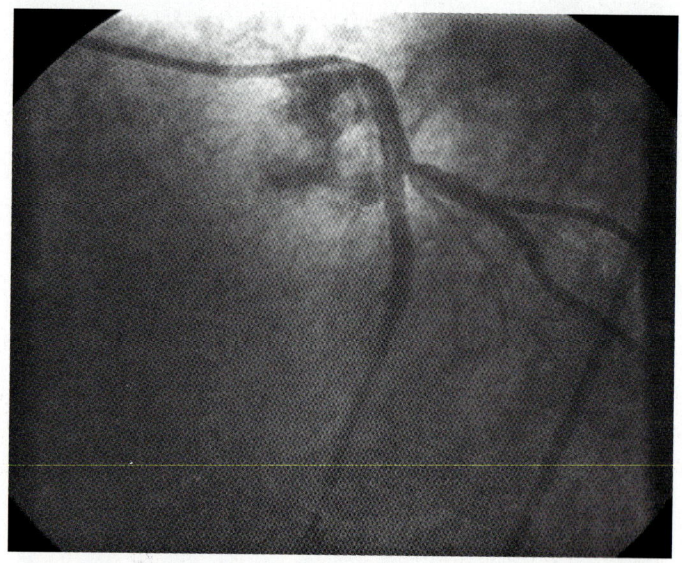

**Fig. 3.44:** Left selective coronary angiogram in left anterior oblique cranial projection (48° LAO, 33° cranial) showing TIMI 3 flow in LAD after balloon angioplasty and stenting of severe distal disease

atrial fibrillation is decreased in patients given thrombolytic therapy.

The treatment of atrial fibrillation in acute myocardial infarction should be similar to the treatment of atrial fibrillation in other settings. When there is hemodynamic compromise caused by loss of atrial systole or a rapid ventricular response with a reduction.

In cardiac output, cardioversion should be performed immediately. In patients with preserved left ventricular function in whom the atrial fibrillation is well tolerated, beta-blocker therapy is indicated. Verapamil and diltiazem may also be effective in such patients. In patients with congestive heart failure (CHF), digoxin is a reasonable alternative and may slow the ventricular response. If atrial fibrillation recurs, antiarrhythmic agents may be used, although their impact on clinical outcomes is unproved. The atrial fibrillation follow-up investigation of rhythm management (AFFIRM) investigators randomized 4,060 patients to either rhythm-control or rate-control treatment strategies. The rhythm-control strategy achieved no survival advantage over the rate-control strategy and there were both fewer hospital admissions and fewer adverse drug reactions in the rate-control group.

### Bradyarrhythmias and Heart Block

Sinus bradycardia is common in acute myocardial infarction, particularly in patients with inferior myocardial infarction. However, treatment with atropine and a temporary pacemaker is required infrequently and, generally,

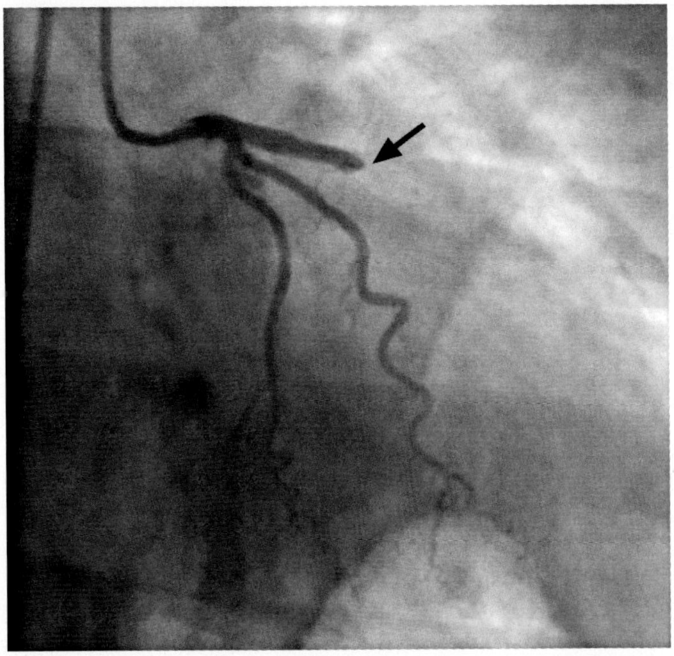

**Fig. 3.45:** Angiography revealed obstruction (arrow) in LAD artery in patient with acute myocardial infarction

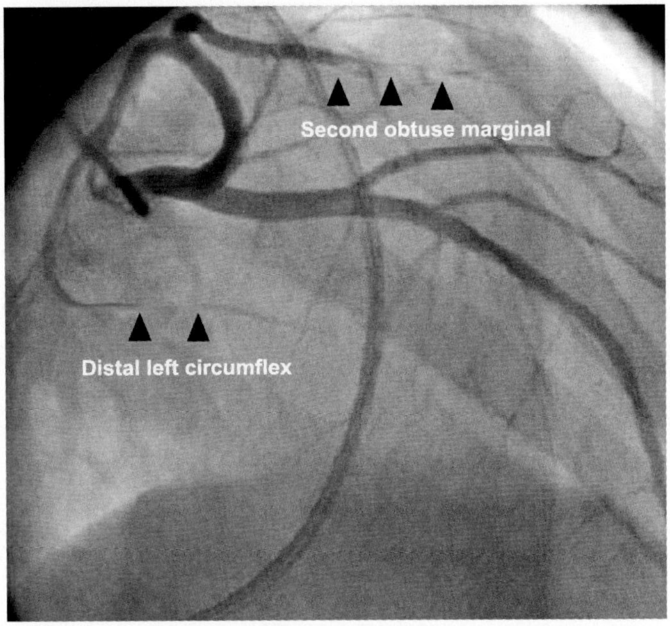


**Fig. 3.47:** Coronary angiogram showing an RAO cranial view of the left coronary artery and its branches, the left circumfled (LCX) and the left anterior descending arteries. Multiple thrombi are noted within the LCX arterial system (arrowheads)

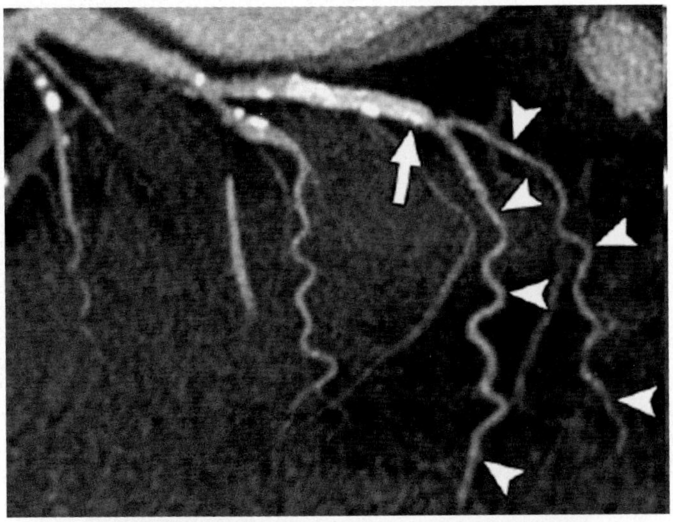

**Fig. 3.46:** Multiplanar reformation image of coronary artery shows stent implantation (arrow) and good enhancement over distal branches of circumflex artery (arrowheads)

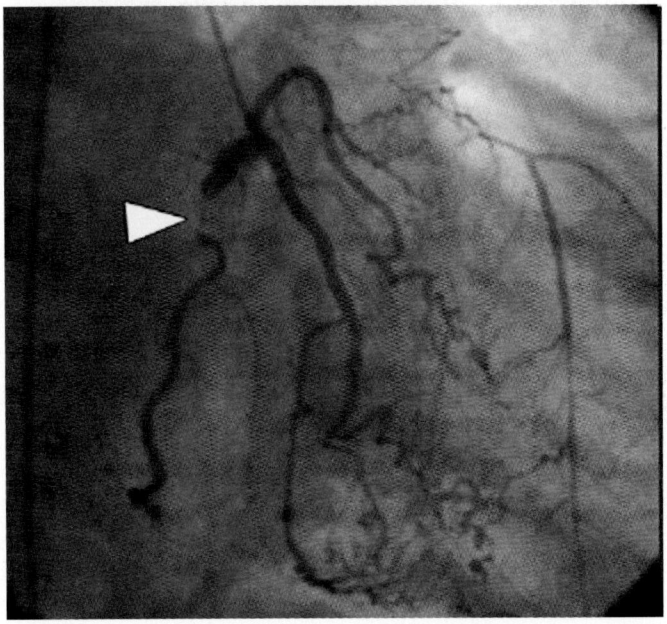

**Fig. 3.48:** A 75-year-old woman with unstable angina pectoris and three-vessel disease. Coronary angiography image shows severe stenosis at proximal portion (arrowhead) and total occlusion of distal portion and collateral vessels to distal LAD branch. Coronary angiography could not clear culprit lesion because there were critical stenoses in three vessels

only in patients with significant hemodynamic compromise manifested by increased angina, hypotension, or congestive heart failure. High-degree (second- or third-degree) heart block occurs in approximately 20% of patients with inferior infarction; it is uncommon with infarction at other sites. About half of the cases of heart block seen with inferior infarction are Wenckebach-type second-degree heart block; the remainder are cases of third-degree heart block. The heart block is often easily treated with atropine, but a temporary pacemaker is required in as many as 50% of cases. The heart block generally lasts for hours to days; placement of a permanent pacemaker is needed in fewer than 1% of cases. However, the development of heart block with inferior infarction is associated with a threefold to fourfold increase in in-hospital mortality over inferior

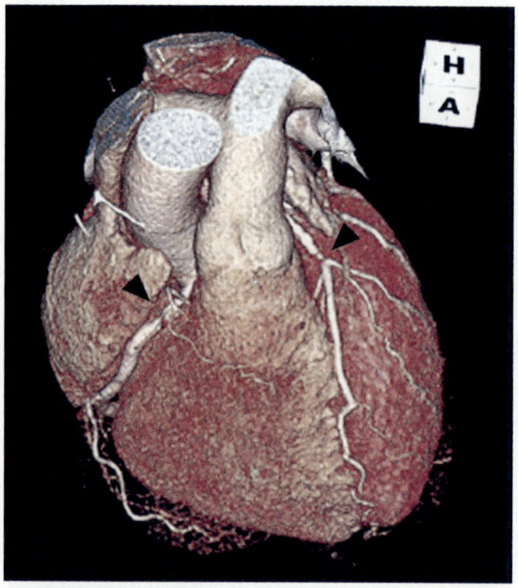


**Fig. 3.49:** 64-slice computed tomography can detect severe coronary artery stenosis (arrowheads)

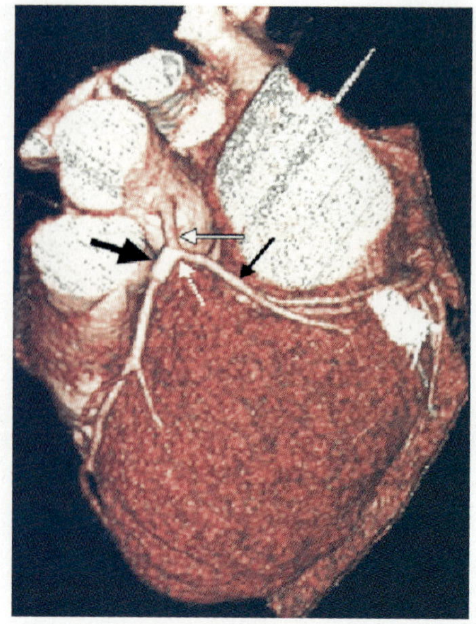

**Fig. 3.51:** A 59-year-old man 2 days after percutaneous transluminal coronary angioplasty and stent placement in proximal left anterior descending artery. Volume-rendered CT angiogram shows stent in proximal left anterior descending artery (thick black arrow). Note protrusion of proximal end of stent (dotted white arrow) into proximal left circumflex artery (thin black arrow). Also note left main coronary artery (solid white arrow)

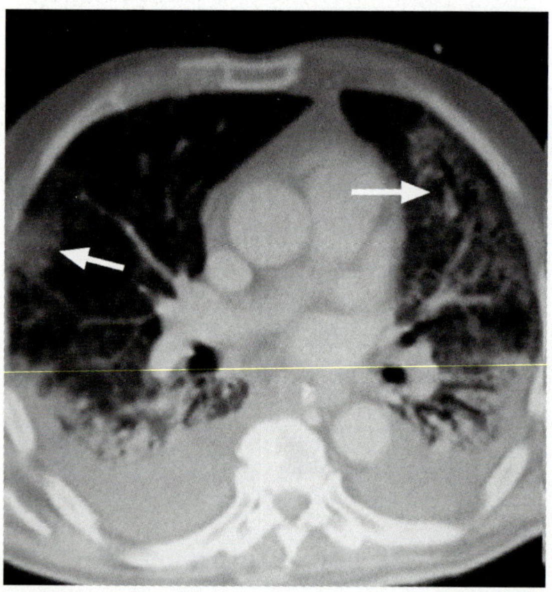

**Fig. 3.50:** An old man of 76 years with acute coronary syndrome. CT scan taken several days after showed ground-glass patch lesions (arrows) due to pulmonary hemorrhage and parenchymal opacifications interpreted as adult respiratory distress syndrome

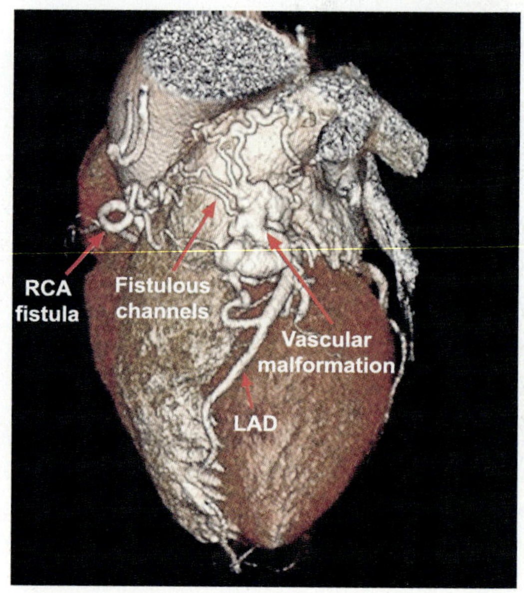


**Fig. 3.52:** Acute coronary syndrome in a patient with a large intercommunicating coronary vascular malformation: imaging with 320-slice CT

infarction without heart block. The increased mortality appears to result from the association between heart block and more severe left and right ventricular infarction rather than from the heart block itself or treatment of the heart block. Heart block during anterior infarction is uncommon, occurring in fewer than 1% of cases. It is generally associated with extensive left ventricular myocardial infarction involving the conduction system below the atrioventricular node and carries a very poor prognosis.

## Mitral Regurgitation

Mitral regurgitation may result from injury to any of the components of the mitral valve apparatus, including the papillary muscles and ventricular walls to which they attach. Mild mitral regurgitation is common in acute myocardial infarction and is present in nearly 50% of patients. Severe mitral regurgitation caused by acute

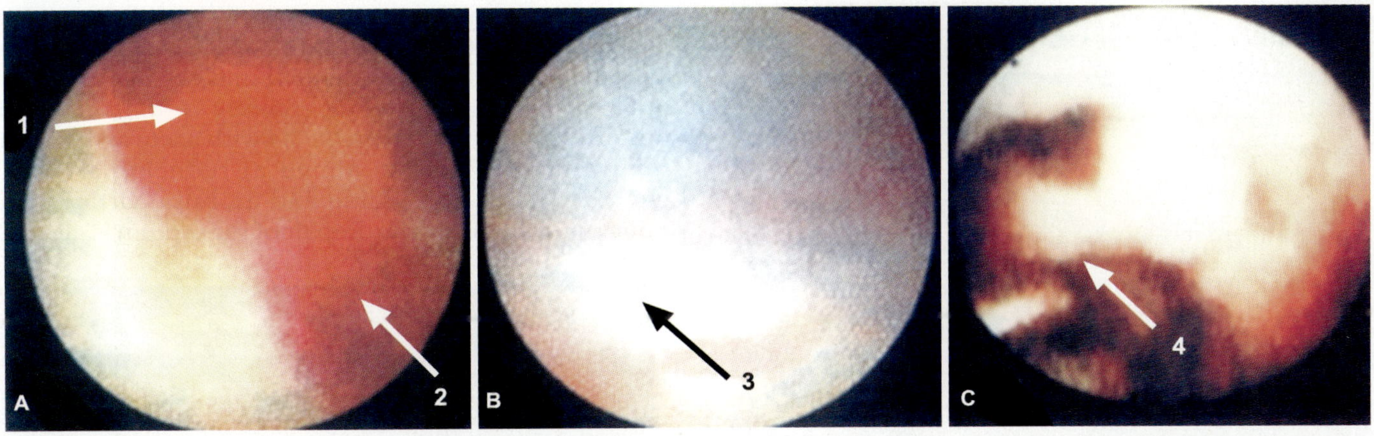


**Fig. 3.53:** Angioscopy shows (A) a red thrombus on a plaque (1) blocking a part of the lumen (2) after removal of thrombus and plaque with atherectomy, (B) a white flap is visible (3) post-angioplasty angioscopy, (C) can show a dissecting flap (4) within the lumen

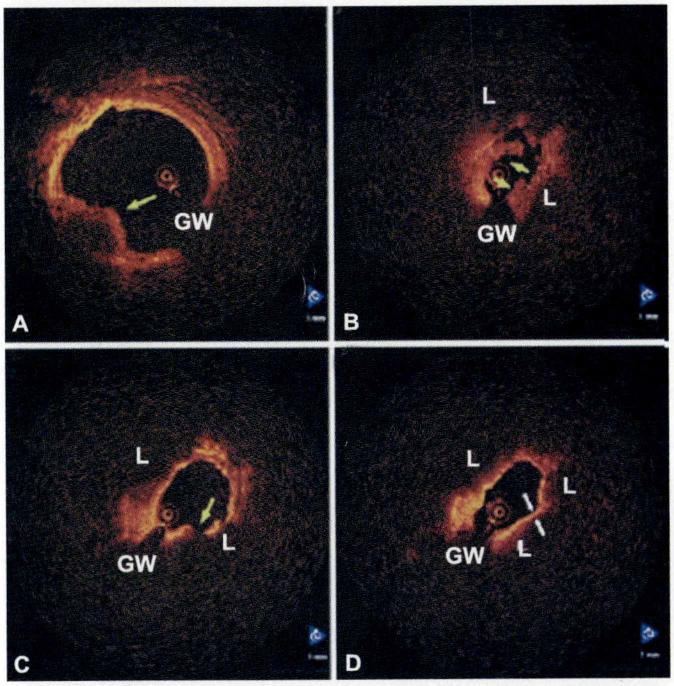


**Fig. 3.54:** Multiple plaque morphologies assessed by optical coherence tomography in a patient with acute coronary syndrome

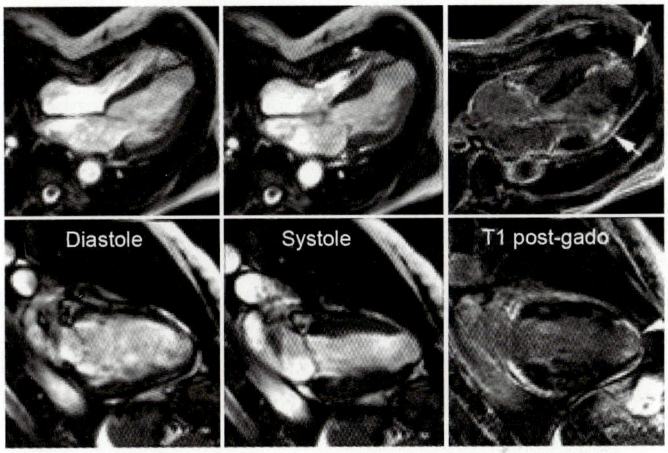


**Fig. 3.55:** Cine-MR four-chamber and vertical long-axis diastolic and systolic views, with marked left ventricular wall thinning and dyskinesia at the apex and at the mid-lateral part of the left ventricle. T1-weighted images 10 minutes after gadolinium injection (right panel) show transmural hyper-enhancement in the same apical and lateral segments, related to gadolinium retention in scarred infarcted tissue (arrows)

myocardial infarction is rare and generally results from partial or complete rupture of a papillary muscle. The characteristic murmur of severe chronic mitral regurgitation may not be present with acute rupture of a papillary muscle. Instead, a decrescendo systolic murmur is often present, extending less throughout systole as systemic arterial pressure falls and left arterial pressure rises. In many cases, the significance of the murmur is not recognized. The blood supply of the anterior papillary muscle arises from branches of both the left anterior descending and the circumflex arteries; therefore, rupture of the anterior papillary muscle is rare. However, the posterior papillary muscle receives blood only from the dominant coronary artery (the right coronary artery in nearly 90% of patients); thrombotic occlusion of this artery may cause rupture of the posterior papillary muscle, resulting in severe mitral regurgitation. Severe mitral regurgitation is 10 times more likely to occur with inferior infarction than with anterior infarction. Acute severe mitral regurgitation is poorly tolerated and generally results in pulmonary edema, often with cardiogenic shock. Prompt surgical repair is recommended. Although the mortality associated with mitral valve surgery is high in this setting, approaching 50%, survival appears to be greater than with medical therapy alone. Therapy aimed at reducing left ventricular afterload, such as use of IV nitroprusside and an intra-aortic balloon pump, reduces the regurgitant volume and increases forward blood flow and cardiac output and may be helpful as a temporizing measure.

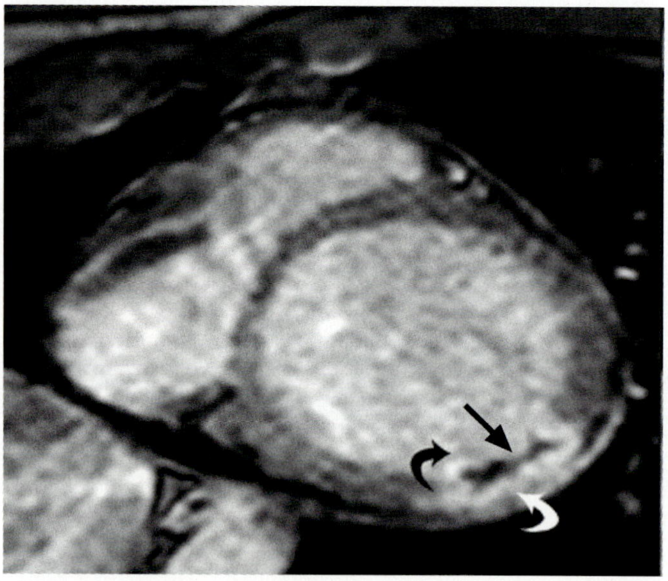

**Fig. 3.56:** Microvascular obstruction. Short-axis PSIR image in a 47-year-old male with acute chest pain and ST-segment elevation reveals dark nonenhancing tissue (straight arrow) located within bright enhancing scar (curved arrow), consistent with microvascular obstruction within an area of myocardial infarction in the left circumflex artery territory

### Ventricular Septal Defects (Figs 3.66–3.68)

Ventricular septal defects are slightly more frequent in patients with anterior infarction than in patients with inferior infarction. The characteristic holosystolic murmur of ventricular septal defects may be difficult to distinguish from that of severe mitral regurgitation; however, ventricular septal defects are generally better tolerated and less frequently result in severe congestive heart failure. Surgical repair is recommended and results in the best outcome when repaired emergently in the hemodynamically compromised patient. As with acute severe mitral regurgitation, therapy aimed at reducing afterload, including IV nitroprusside and an intra-aortic balloon pump, may be beneficial. Repair of the septum is generally

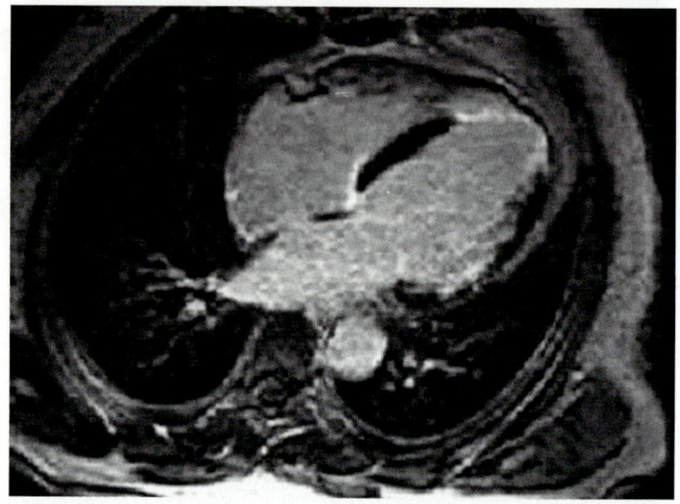

**Fig. 3.58:** Four-chamber view with the late enhancement technique in a patient with myocardial infarction. 10 minutes after contrast agent injection normal myocardium remains black, whereas fibrosis enhances due to the accumulation of contrast agent in the enlarged interstitial space. Note the transmural infarction in the apex and the subendocardial pronounciation of the infarction in the lateral wall

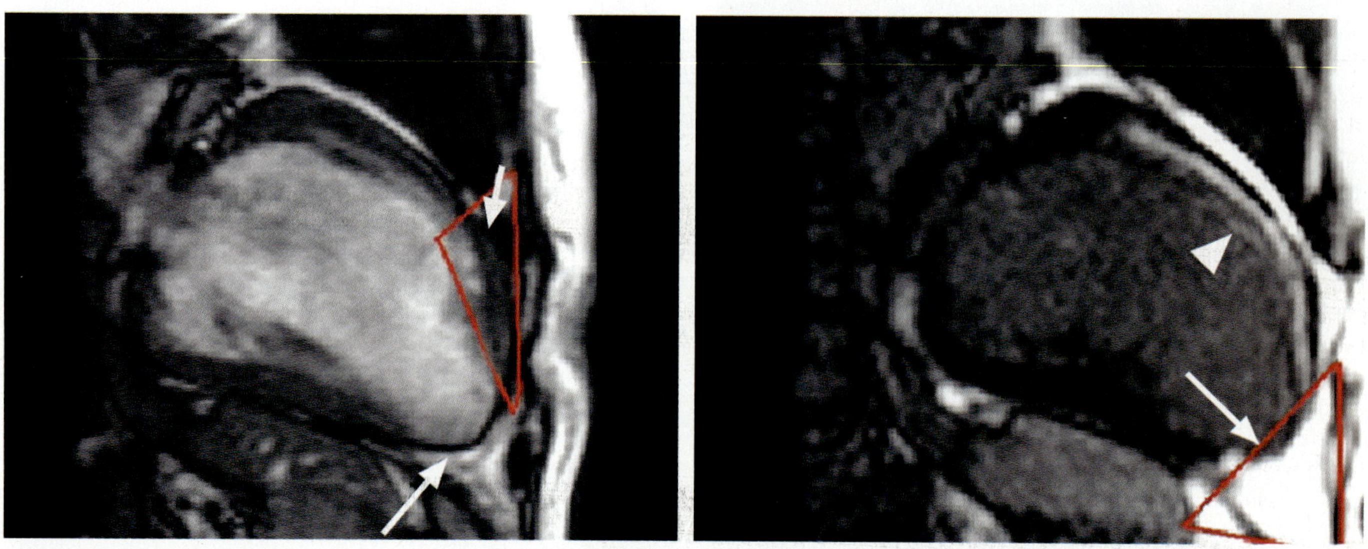

**Fig. 3.57:** Cardiac MRI to determine myocardium viability before revascularization. The whole concept of viability on cardiac MRI is based on the fact that all infarcts enhance vividly 10–15 minutes after intravenous contrast administration. Cardiac MRI shows the transmural extent of the infarct very reliably. It tells you that: *'white is dead' (all infarcts irrespective of age enhance)* in areas of hypokinesia, if there is a rim of 'black' or non-infarcted myocardium that is not contracting well, it indicates the presence of hibernating myocardium, which is likely to improve after revascularization of the artery supplying that particular territory. Viability imaging reliably allows identification of areas of hibernation and viable or nonviable myocardium. All infarcts irrespective of age enhance. The percentage involvement of the myocardial wall thickness by an infarct determines viability

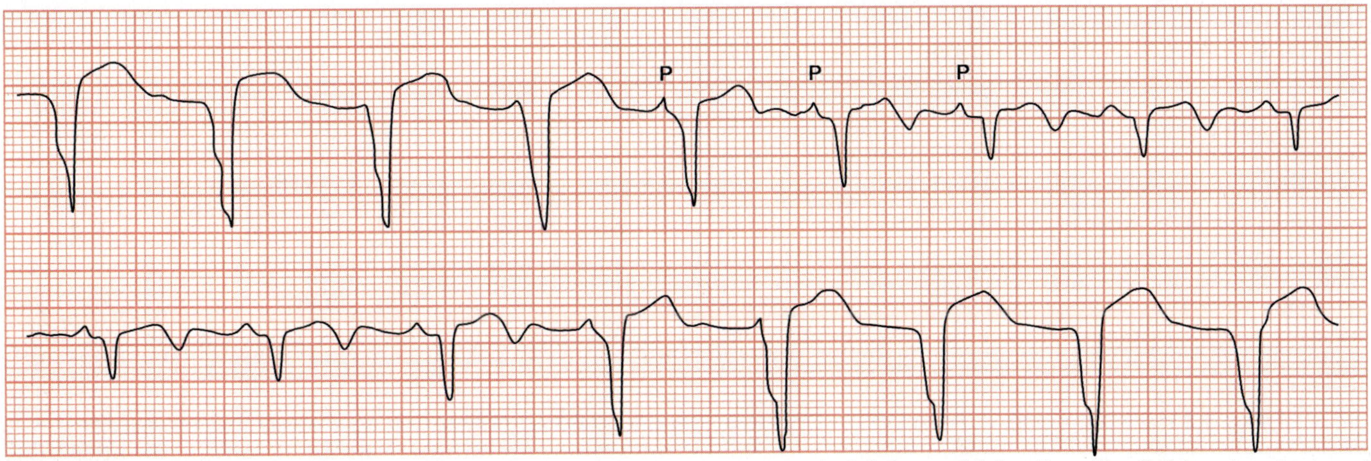


**Fig. 3.59:** Accelerated idioventricular rhythm (AIVR) in a patient with an acute inferior wall infarction. The first four beats show the typical pattern, followed by a return of sinus rhythm, then the reappearance of the AIVR. Notice that the fifth, sixth, twelfth, and thirteenth QRS complexes are 'fusion beats' because of the nearly simultaneous occurrence of a sinus beat and a ventricular beat (P/P-wave)

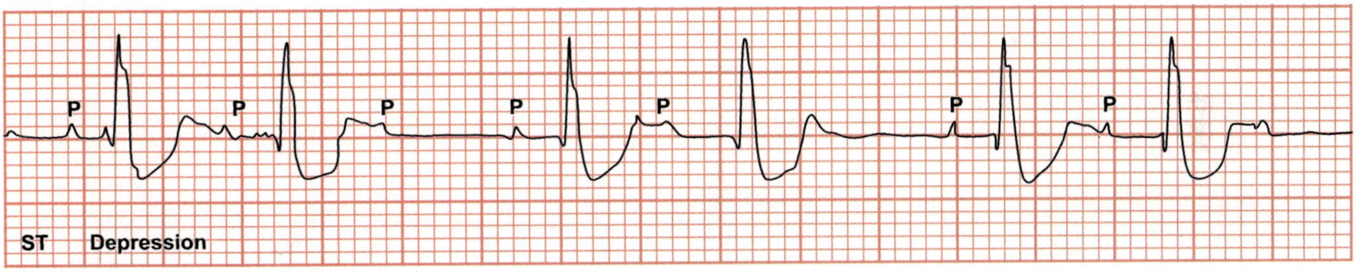


**Fig. 3.60:** Mobitz type 1 (Wenckebach) second-degree heart block in an acute myocardial infarction. The patient had a recent inferior infarct. The Wenckebach cycles are indicated in each of which progressive prolongation of the P–R interval culminates in a dropped beat

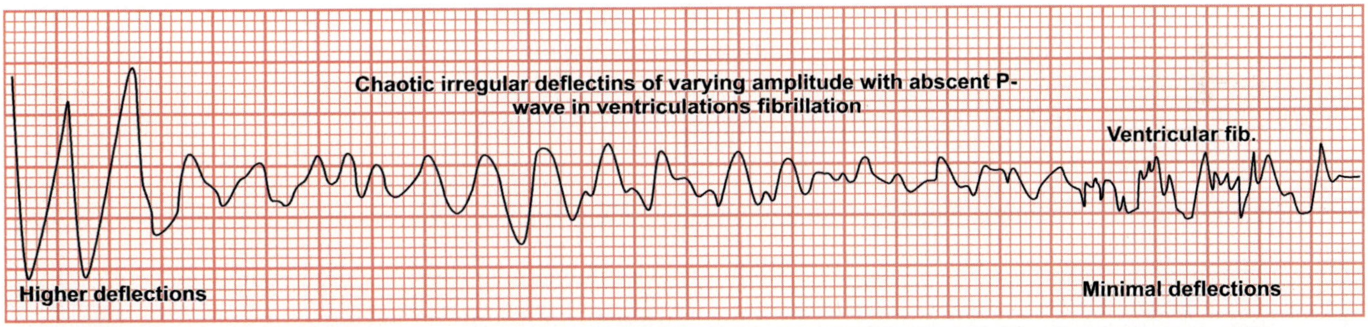


**Fig. 3.61:** Showing ventricular fibrillation. Chaotic irregular deflections of varying amplitude. No identifiable P-waves, QRS complexes or T-waves rate 150 to 500 per minute

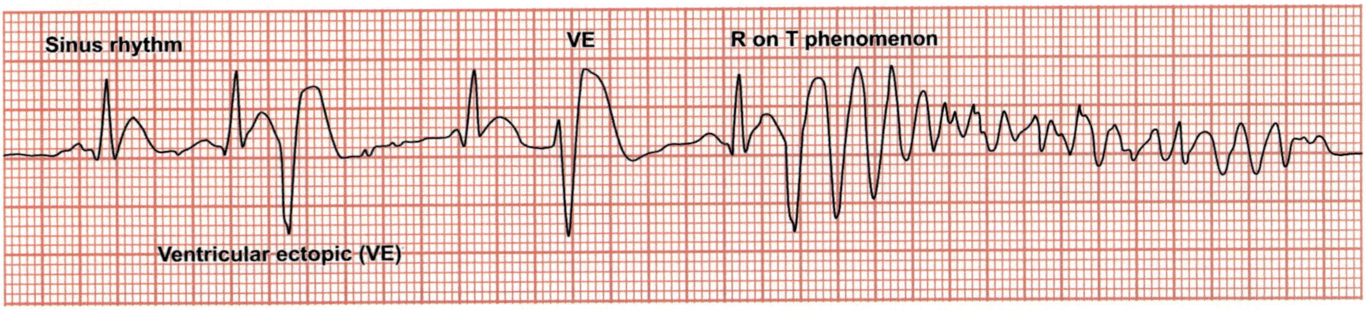


**Fig. 3.62:** ECG trace showing R on T phenomenon (arrow) giving rise to ventricular fibrillation (arrow) in AMI

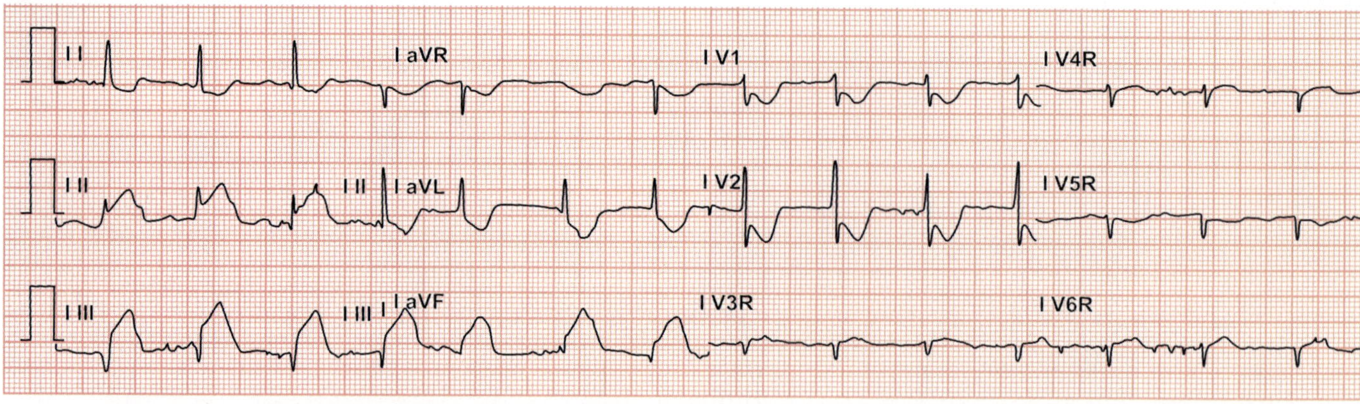


**Fig. 3.63:** ECG showing St-elevation in V3 and V4, II, III and aVF in a patient with right ventricular infarction

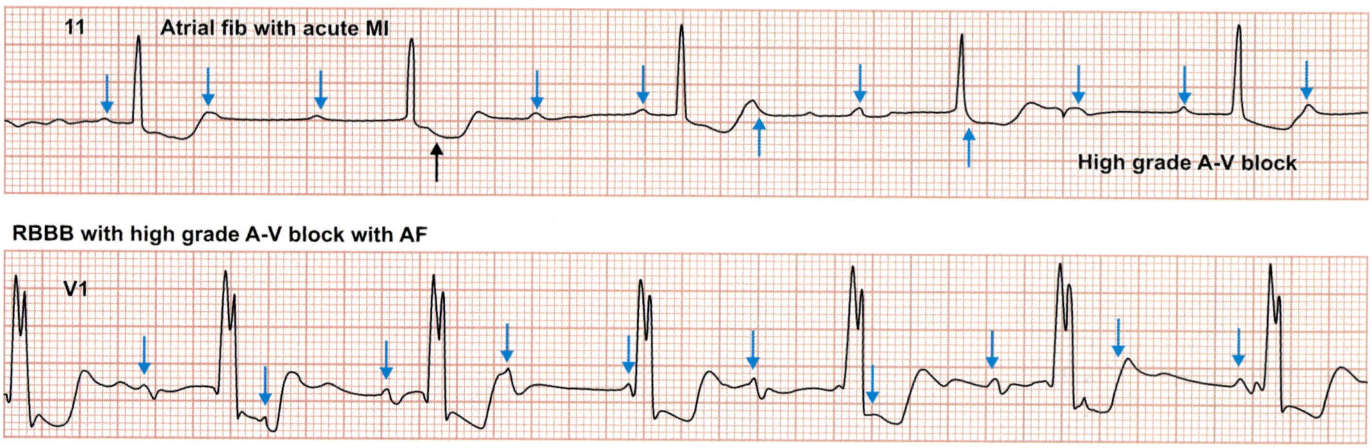


**Fig. 3.64:** ECG showing atrial fibrillation and high grade A-V block in patient with acute AMI who needed temporary pacemaker as an emergent life support

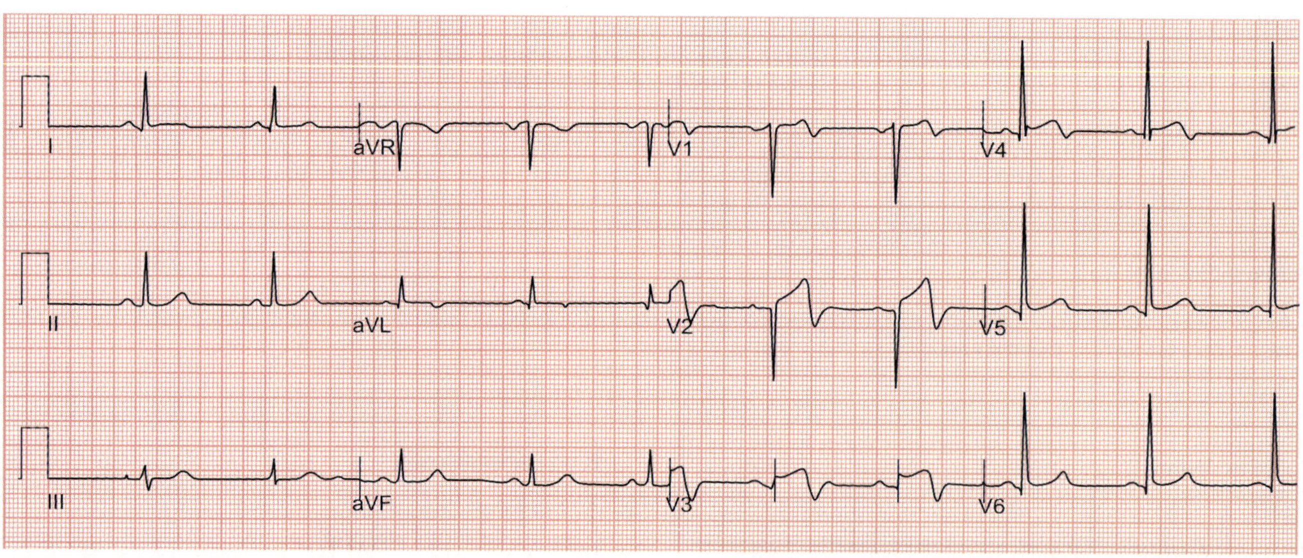


**Fig. 3.65A:** Wellens syndrome (type A pattern). Biphasic precordial T-waves with terminal negativity, most prominent in V2–3. Minor precordial ST elevation. Preserved R wave progression (R wave in V3 >3 mm)

more difficult when associated with inferior infarction, because there may not be a viable rim of myocardial tissue beneath the defect to facilitate repair. The surgical mortality associated with repair of a postinfarction ventricular septal defect is approximately 20%, but is largely related to the age of the patient, whether cardiogenic shock is present,

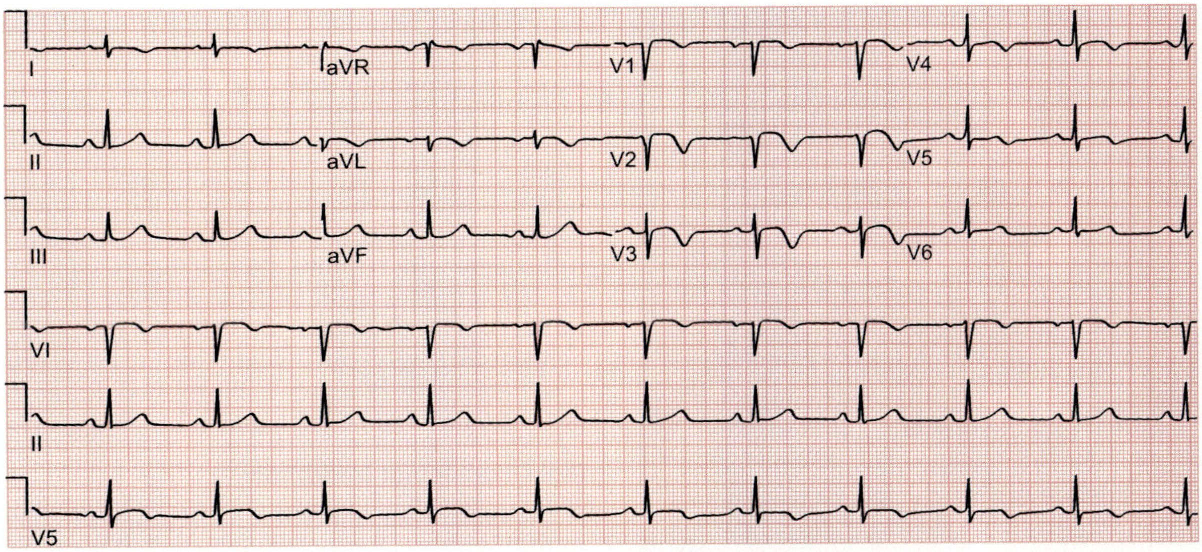


**Fig. 3.65B:** Wellens syndrome (type B pattern). There are deep, symmetrical T-wave inversions in leads V2–V3

**Table 3.3:** Indications of temporary pacing in acute MI

*Class I*

1. Asystole
2. Symptomatic bradycardia (includes sinus bradycardia with hypotension and type I second degree AV block with hypotension not responsive to atropine)
3. Bilateral bundle branch block [BBB; alternating BBB or right BBB (RBBB) with alternating left anterior fascicular block (LAFB) left posterior fascicular block (LPFB)] (any age)
4. New bundle branch block with Mobitz II second-degree AV block
5. RBBB plus fascicular block with Mobitz II second-degree AV block

*Class IIa*

1. Narrow QRS plus Mobitz II second-degree AV block
2. Old or new fascicular block with Mobitz II second degree AV block and anterior MI
3. Old bundle branch block and Mobitz II second degree AV block
4. New bundle branch block plus first-degree AV block
5. New bundle branch block plus Mobitz I second-degree AV block
6. RBBB plus LAFB or LPFB (new or indeterminate) with first-degree AV block
7. RBBB plus LAFB or LPFB (new or indeterminate) with Mobitz I second-degree AV block

*Class IIb*

1. Bifascicular block of indeteminate age and Mobitz II second-degree AV block
2. Old bundle branch block and first-degree AV block or second-degree AV block

*Class III*

1. First-degree heart block
2. Type I second-degree AV block
3. Accelerated idioventricular rhythm
4. BBB or fascicular block known to exist before acute myocardial infarction without conduction system disease

the infarction site, and the severity of the underlying coronary artery disease.

### Myocardial Rupture

As more and more patients survive the acute phase of myocardial infarction because reperfusion therapy reduces myocardial infarct size, myocardial rupture has increased in frequency as a cause of early death. Myocardial rupture has been reported to account for more than 20% of in-hospital deaths in some series in the thrombolytic era. Physicians must have a heightened awareness of the diagnosis if a patient is to survive this catastrophic

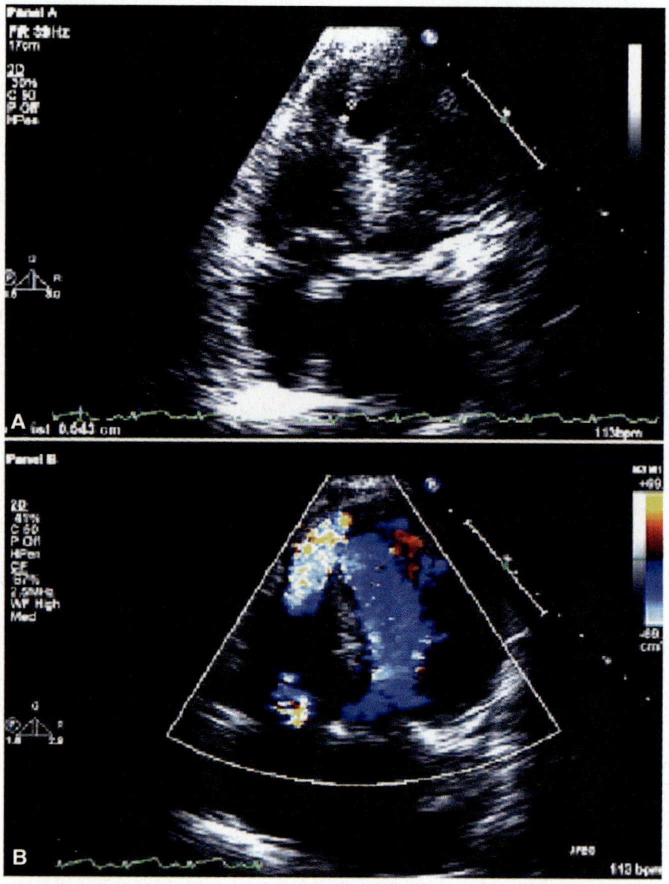


Fig. 3.66: Modified two-dimensional (A) echocardiogram and color flow Doppler image (B). Apical 4-chamber views show a breach in the interventricular septum and free communication between ventricles through a large apical septum ventricular septal defect in a patient who recently had an anterior myocardial infarction

occurrence, because emergency surgery is required. Symptoms suggestive of rupture include repetitive vomiting, pleuritic chest pain, restlessness, and agitation. ECG evidence of rupture includes a deviation from the normal pattern of ST-segment and T-wave evolution. Resolution of ST-segment elevation and T-wave inversion, with maximal T-wave negativity in the leads with maximal ST-segment elevation, should normally occur; however, in patients with rupture, there is progressive or recurrent ST-segment elevation and persistently positive T-wave deflections or reversal of initially inverted T-waves. Echocardiography can quickly confirm the diagnosis. Even when emergency surgery is performed, fewer than 50% of patients survive to discharge.

## Right Ventricular Infarction

Right ventricular infarction occurs in approximately one-third of patients with acute inferior left ventricular infarction and is hemodynamically significant in approximately 50% of affected patients. Hemodynamically significant right ventricular infarction associated with anterior infarction or isolated right ventricular infarction is rare. The classic findings associated with hemodynamically significant right ventricular infarction are hypotension with clear lung fields and an elevated jugular venous pressure, often with the Kussmaul sign. Although, nearly all patients with right ventricular infarction suffer both right and left ventricular infarction, the characteristic hemodynamic findings of right ventricular infarction generally dominate the clinical course and must be the main focus of therapy. Right ventricular involvement during inferior myocardial infarction is associated with a significant increase in mortality, and aggressive attempts at early reperfusion should be pursued. Prompt recognition of right ventricular involvement is

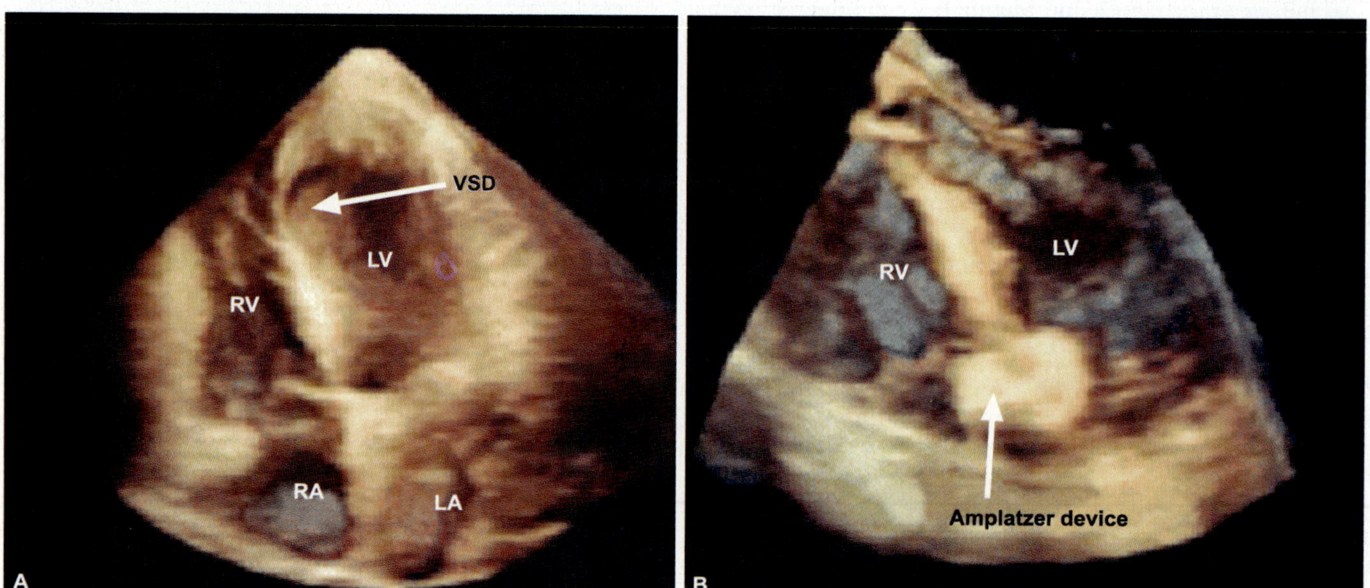


Fig. 3.67: Transcatheter closure of postmyocardial infarction muscular ventricular septal defects. Real-time 3D transthoracic echocardiography demonstrates the apical septal thinning and ventricular septal defect. (A) After the transcatheter closure, real-time 3D transoesophageal echocardiography demonstrates the final position of the deployed occluder device. (B) Adapted with permission from Halpern et al. LA, left atrium; LV=left ventricle; RA=right atrium; RV=right ventricle; VSD=ventricular septal defect

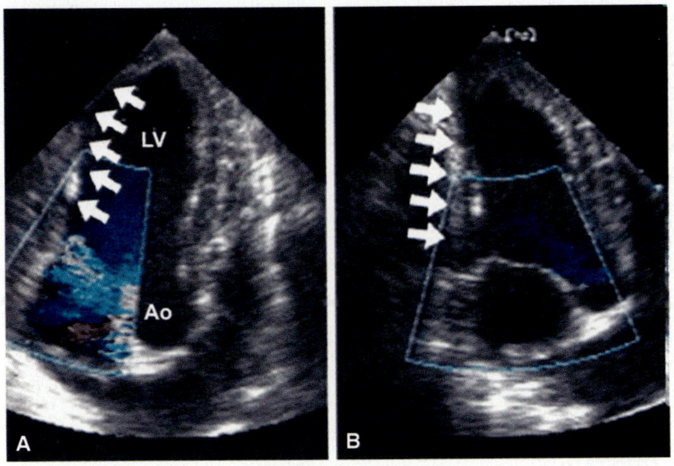


**Fig. 3.68:** Epicardial echocardiography 8 weeks after inferior infarction (A) and acutely after balloon-patch device placement (B). Before patching, the inferior wall bulges out, the posterior PM is displaced away from the annulus, and severe MR is seen. After patching, the inferior wall is straightened, the PM is realigned, and MR is absent. LV=left ventricle; Ao=aorta

clinically important because therapy that reduces right ventricular filling, such as use of nitrates or diuretics, should be avoided. Volume therapy should be administered to maintain cardiac output; in patients whose hypotension is refractory to volume therapy, dopamine may be beneficial. Heart block, which occurs in as many as 50% of patients with right ventricular infarction, should be treated rapidly, and maintenance of atrioventricular synchrony with dual atrial and ventricular pacing is often required to maintain filling of the ischemic noncompliant right ventricle and an adequate cardiac output.

Cardiogenic shock resulting from right ventricular infarction is generally reversible with these measures. Improvement in right ventricular function generally occurs over time, particularly in patients in whom reperfusion therapy was successful in achieving vessel patency. In patients who survive the initial hospitalization, left ventricular function is the most potent predictor of long-term outcome.

### Stroke

Extensive infarction of the anterior wall and apex of the left ventricle leads to thrombus formation in the apex of the left ventricle in approximately 30% of patients; systemic embolization occurs in about 15% of these patients. Left ventricular thrombus formation is much less common after inferior infarction. The thrombus generally appears within the first several days after infarction; it is more likely to embolize and cause stroke if it is pedunculated, protrudes into the left ventricular cavity, or is mobile. Left ventricular thrombus is an indication for anticoagulation with IV heparin, followed by warfarin therapy for 3–6 months.

Therapy that reduces infarct size, such as thrombolytic therapy, reduces the frequency of thrombus formation and therefore the risk of systemic embolization and stroke. However, in 0.3–1.0% of patients, thrombolytic therapy causes hemorrhagic stroke, most commonly in the 24 hours after its administration, which is fatal in more than 50% of cases. Hemorrhagic stroke is rare in acute myocardial infarction except as a consequence of thrombolytic therapy, although an ischemic stroke may become hemorrhagic because of thrombolytic, antiplatelet, and anticoagulation therapy. Hemorrhagic stroke, the most feared complication of thrombolytic therapy, is more likely in elderly patients; in patients with low body weight, with hypertension, or who have previously had a stroke; and in those on warfarin. Although thrombolytic therapy decreases the risk of ischemic stroke, there is a slight net increase in the overall risk of stroke because of the risk of hemorrhagic stroke. Primary coronary angioplasty is believed to reduce the incidence of ischemic stroke without increasing the risk of hemorrhagic stroke.

### Therapeutic Approaches in Acute Coronary Syndrome

Initial therapy for acute coronary syndrome should focus on stabilizing the patient's condition, relieving ischemic pain, and providing antithrombotic therapy to reduce myocardial damage and prevent further ischemia. Morphine (or fentanyl) for pain control, oxygen, sublingual and/or IV nitroglycerin, soluble aspirin 162–325 mg, and clopidogrel with a 300–600 mg loading dose are given as initial treatment.

In complete vessel occlusion without collateralization of the infarct-related vessel, there is a little utility in 'pushing nitrates'.

High-risk patients with non-ST-segment elevation myocardial infarction acute coronary syndrome (NSTEMI-ACS) should receive aggressive care, including aspirin, clopidogrel, unfractionated heparin or low-molecular weight heparin (LMWH), intravenous platelet glycoprotein IIb/IIIa complex blockers (e.g. tirofiban, eptifibatide), and a beta-blocker. The goal is early revascularization.

Intermediate-risk patients with NSTEMI-ACS should rapidly undergo diagnostic evaluation and further assessment to determine their appropriate risk category.

Low-risk patients with NSTEMI-ACS should undergo further follow-up with biomarkers and clinical assessment. Optimal medical therapies include use of standard medical therapies, including beta-blockers, aspirin, and unfractionated heparin or LMWH. The clopidogrel in unstable angina to prevent recurrent events (CURE) study showed that clopidogrel would be beneficial even in low-risk patients. If no further pain occurs, and follow-up studies are negative, a stress study should drive further management.

Monitor and immediately treat arrhythmias in the first 48 hours. Pay attention to exacerbating factors, such as disturbances in electrolytes (especially potassium and magnesium), hypoxemia, drugs, or acidosis. Correct these factors accordingly.

Humidified oxygen may reduce the risk of nosebleeds in patients with ACS who are receiving antiplatelet and antithrombin therapy.

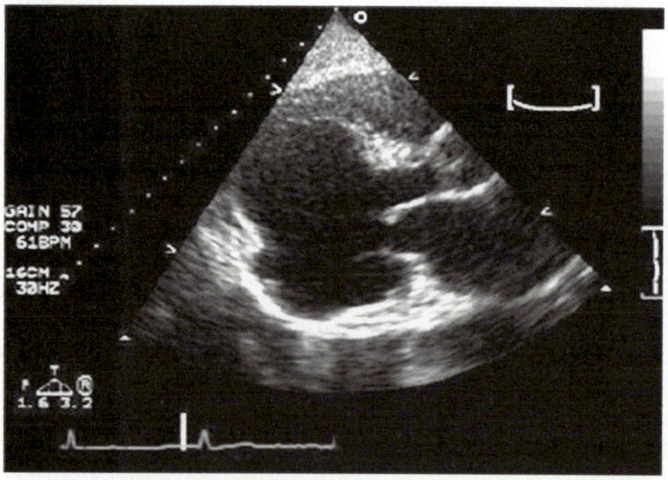

**Fig. 3.69:** Parasternal long-axis view of the left ventricle demonstrates a large inferobasal aneurysm. Note the wide neck and base of the aneurysm

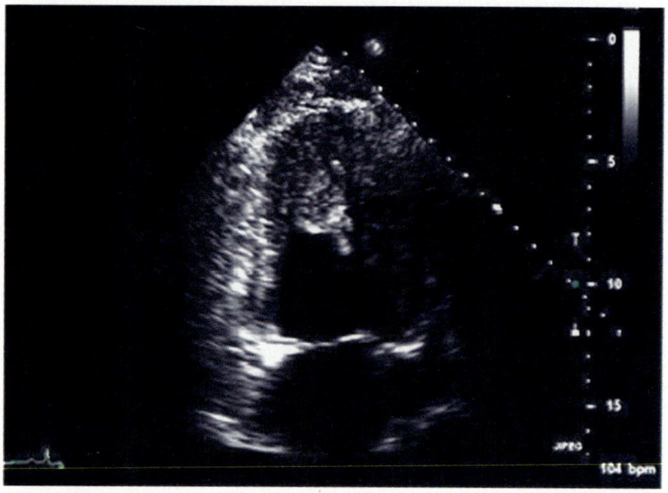

**Fig. 3.70:** Apical 2-chamber view depicts a large left ventricular apical thrombus with mobile extensions

Do not administer nitrates if the patient is hypotensive (systolic BP < 90 mmHg); if RV infarction, large pericardial effusion, or severe aortic stenosis is suspected; or if the patient recently received phosphodiesterase-5 inhibitors (e.g. sildenafil).

Patients with known hypersensitivity to antiplatelet agents, active internal bleeding, and bleeding disorders should not receive antiplatelet or antithrombotic therapy. Some patients with intractable chest pain or severe hypotension may require the insertion of an intra-aortic balloon pump. The EuroHeart survey showed a nearly 40% reduction in the risk of death in patients with ACS who received support with an intra-aortic balloon pump. This benefit was independent of the status of the ST-segment.

Congestive heart failure can be due to systolic dysfunction or diastolic dysfunction in the setting of myocardial infarction. Aggressive treatment is indicated to prevent worsening of the situation.

Patients presenting with cardiogenic shock should undergo percutaneous coronary intervention (PCI) as soon as possible. Cardiogenic shock is associated with a high mortality rate. Pressor agents, such as dopamine, and inotropic agents, such as dobutamine, may be needed. In a prospective, natural-history study of coronary atherosclerosis, patients underwent 3-vessel coronary angiography and gray-scale and radiofrequency intravascular ultrasonographic imaging after PCI.

Recurrent ischemia may be due to incomplete reperfusion. In the setting of PCI, consider stent thrombosis as a possible cause. Whether drug-eluting stents have an increased rate of thrombosis compared with bare metal stents is unclear.

Drug-eluting stents are linked with fewer periprocedural risks but tend to have high incidence of postprocedural complications including myocardial infarction, repeat procedures, and 12-month major adverse cardiac and brain complications, compared with coronary bypass surgery.

One study by Ribichini et al. suggests that prednisone treatment after bare metal stents or drug-eluting stent implantation results in a better event-free survival at 1 year.

In the final report of the HORIZONS-AMI trial, which assessed the 3 years outcomes of the effectiveness and safety of bivalirudin monotherapy and paclitaxel-eluting stenting, outcomes were sustained for patients with STEMI undergoing primary PCI.

**Table 3.4:** Differential diagnosis of ventricular septal defect and papillary muscle rupture

| | Ventricular septal defect | Papillary muscle rupture |
|---|---|---|
| Murmur | Left stenal edge | Apex |
| Heart | Dominantly right-sided often with minimal pulmonary edema | Dominantly left-sided always with severe pulomnary edema |
| Infarct location | Anterior or inferior | Inferior |
| Right heart catheter | Step-up in oxygen saturation in right ventricle | Dominant V-wave in pulmonary artery wedge pressure trace |
| Echocardiography | Permits direct visualization of defect in some cases | Demonstrates flail valve leaflet |
| Doppler study | Demonstrates high-velocity jet across defect | Demonstrates high velocity regurgitant jet |

In a study of 3031 patients, Mehta et al. found that early intervention (coronary angiography < or = 24-hour after randomization) in patients with ACS did not differ greatly from delayed intervention (coronary angiography > or = 36-hour randomization) in the prevention of primary outcomes (i.e. composite of death, myocardial infarction, or stroke at 6 months). Early intervention did reduce the rate of secondary outcomes (i.e. death, myocardial infarction, or refractory ischemia at 6 months) and improved primary outcomes in patients who were at highest risk (i.e. GRACE risk score >140).

In a Swedish registry of patients with STEMI from 1996–2007, reported an increase in the prevalence of evidence-based treatments. The use of aspirin, clopidogrel, beta- blockers, statins, and ACE inhibitors all increased. Clopidogrel increased from 0% to 82%, statins increased from 23% to 83%, and various ACE inhibitors increased by a large margin. A decrease was reported in 30-day and 1-year mortality that was sustained during long-term follow-up. By following the proper guidelines, patients who have experienced STEMI have higher survival rates.

## PHARMACOLOGIC ANTI-ISCHEMIC THERAPY

The pharmacologic anti-ischemic therapy is listed in Table 3.5.

### Nitrates

Nitrates do not improve mortality. However, they provide symptomatic relief by means of several mechanisms, including coronary vasodilation, improved collateral blood flow, decrease in preload (venodilation and reduced venous return), and decrease in afterload (arterial vasodilation). Care should be taken to avoid hypotension, because this can potentially reduce coronary perfusion pressure (diastolic BP-LV diastolic pressure).

### Beta-blockers

Beta-blockers are indicated in all patients unless they have the following contraindications:

- Systolic blood pressure less than 90 mmHg
- Cardiogenic shock
- Severe bradycardia
- Second- or third-degree heart block
- Asthma or emphysema that is sensitive to beta agonists
- Peripheral vascular disease
- Uncompensated CHF

Beta-blockers reduce oxygen demand and ventricular wall tension. They also decrease mortality and adverse cardiovascular events. These drugs may prevent mechanical complications of myocardial infarction, including rupture of the papillary muscle, left ventricular free wall, and ventricular septum. Beta-blockers meliorate dynamic obstruction of the left ventricular outflow tract in patients with apical infarct and hyperdynamic basal segments.

The most frequently used regimen is IV metoprolol 2–5 mg given every 5 minutes (up to 15 mg total) followed by 25–100 mg given orally twice a day.

Beta-blockers should not be used acutely in patients with cardiogenic shock or signs of heart failure on presentation.

## PHARMACOLOGIC ANTI-THROMBOTIC THERAPY

### Aspirin

Aspirin permanently impairs the cyclooxygenase pathway of thromboxane A2 production in platelets, in this way inhibiting platelet function. Aspirin reduces morbidity and mortality and is continued indefinitely (Table 3.5).

### Clopidogrel

Clopidogrel (thienopyridine) inhibits adenosine 5'-diphosphate (ADP) dependent activation of the glycoprotein IIb/IIIa complex, a necessary step for platelet aggregation. This process results in intense inhibition of platelet function, particularly in combination with aspirin. In the CURE trial, thienopyridine reduced the rate of myocardial infarction by 20%.

Clopidogrel is a class I recommendation for patients when an early noninterventional approach is planned in therapy for at least 1 month and ideally up to 1 year. When percutaneous coronary intervention (PCI) is planned, clopidogrel 300–600 mg should be given as early as possible before or at the time of PCI. Clopidogrel, 75 mg daily, is

**Table 3.5:** Therapeutic interventions in acute myocardial infarction

*Immediate measures to incraease safety and comfort*

- Intravenous access
- Access to advanced life support and defibrillation
- Analgsia
- Antiemetic
- Oxygen
- Nitrates

*Immediate measures to initiate and maintain reperfusion of the ischemic myocardium*

- Anti-platelet therapy
- Thrombolysis
- Primary angioplasty
- Heparin

*Immediate measurs to protect ischemic myocardium*

- β-adrenoceptor blockers
- Magnesium sulphate
- Insulin

*Early adjunctive treatment for heart failure*

- ACE inhibitors

*Later measures to prevent reinfarction (secondary prevention)*

- Aspirin
- β-adrenoceptor blockers
- ACE inhibitors
- Cholesterol-lowering drugs
- Lifestyle modifications (smoking, diet, weight, and exercise)
- Also to be considered: anticoagulants/amiodarone/oestrogens/antioxidants

continued for at least 12 months after PCI, if the patient is not at high risk for bleeding, according to 2011 ACCF/AHA guidelines (class I recommendation). Early discontinuation should be considered if the risk of bleeding-related morbidity outweighs the anticipated benefits.

The optimal loading dose for clopidogrel is still being evaluated. Reports show that a loading dose of 600 mg might be more beneficial than 300 mg. Withhold clopidogrel for at least 5 days before elective coronary artery bypass grafting (CABG). Since 12% of patients with non-ST-elevation ACS have coronary anatomy that favors CABG, the use of clopidogrel is withheld until coronary angiography at some institutions.

A meta-analysis of 34 studies analyzed the safety of CABG among patients with ACS continuing clopidogrel. The investigators found that although mortality is increased in those receiving clopidogrel, it is influenced by ACS status and case urgency in primarily nonrandomized studies. Among patients with ACS, no differences in mortality or postoperative myocardial infarction or stroke rates were found. This suggests that in patients with ACS who require urgent CABG, proceeding despite the continuation of clopidogrel is likely safe.

Clopidogrel can be considered an alternative to aspirin in patients with aspirin intolerance or who are allergic to aspirin.

Patients with chronic kidney disease who have low platelet response to clopidogrel tend to have worse outcomes after PCI. A consensus statement issued by the American College of Cardiology, American College of Gastroenterology, and American Heart Association in November 2010 addresses the issue of concomitant use of proton pump inhibitors (PPIs) and thienopyridine antiplatelet drugs.

Evidence has shown that dexlansoprazole and lansoprazole do not significantly reduce the conversion of clopidogrel to its active metabolite (reduced by 9% and 14%, respectively), and no dose adjustment of clopidogrel is required.

The group's findings and recommendations are listed as follows:

- Clopidogrel reduces major CV events compared with placebo or aspirin.
- Dual antiplatelet therapy with clopidogrel and aspirin, compared with aspirin alone, reduces major CV events in patients with established ischemic heart disease, and it reduces coronary stent thrombosis but is not routinely recommended for patients with prior ischemic stroke because of the risk of bleeding.
- Clopidogrel alone, aspirin alone, and their combination are all associated with increased risk of GI bleeding.
- Clopidogrel requires metabolic activation by cytochrome P450 2C19 (CYP2C19). PPIs that inhibit CYP2C19 are commonly coadministered with clopidogrel to reduce the risk of GI bleeding. A study by Simon et al. showed that PPI use is not associated with an increased risk of cardiovascular events or mortality in patients who have been treated with clopidogrel for a recent MI, regardless of CYP2C19 genotype.
- Patients with prior GI bleeding are at highest risk for recurrent bleeding on antiplatelet therapy; other risk factors include advanced age, concurrent use of anticoagulants, steroids, or NSAIDs including aspirin, and Helicobacter pylori infection; risk increases as the number of risk factors increases.
- Use of PPIs or histamine H2 receptor antagonists (H2RAs) reduces the risk of upper GI bleeding compared with no therapy; PPIs reduce upper GI bleeding to a greater degree than do H2Ras.
- PPIs are recommended to reduce GI bleeding among patients with a history of upper GI bleeding; PPIs are appropriate in patients with multiple risk factors for GI bleeding who require antiplatelet therapy.
- Routine use of either a PPI or an H2RA is not recommended for patients at lower risk of upper GI bleeding, who have much less potential to benefit from prophylactic therapy.
- Clinical decisions regarding concomitant use of PPIs and thienopyridines must balance overall risks and benefits, considering both CV and GI complications.
- Pharmacokinetic and pharmacodynamic studies, using platelet assays as surrogate endpoints, suggest that concomitant use of clopidogrel and a PPI reduces the antiplatelet effects of clopidogrel; the strongest evidence for an interaction is between omeprazole and clopidogrel; it is not established that changes in these surrogate endpoints translate into clinically meaningful differences.
- Observational studies and a single randomized clinical trial have shown inconsistent effects on CV outcomes of concomitant use of thienopyridines and PPIs; a clinically important interaction cannot be excluded, particularly in certain subgroups, such as poor metabolizers of clopidogrel.
- The role of either pharmacogenomic testing or platelet function testing in managing therapy with thienopyridines and PPIs has not yet been established.

### Prasugrel

Like clopidogrel, prasugrel is a thienopyridine ADP receptor inhibitor that inhibits platelet aggregation. It has been approved in the United States and has been shown to reduce new and recurrent myocardial infarctions. The loading dose is 60 mg PO once and maintenance is 10 mg PO qd (given with aspirin 75–325 mg/d). Prasugrel is indicated for the reduction of thrombotic cardiovascular events (including stent thrombosis) with ACS that is managed with PCI.

The 2011 ACF/AHA guidelines advise that a loading dose of prasugrel be given as soon as possible, once coronary anatomy is defined and a decision is made to proceed with PCI. Prasugrel should be administered no later than 1 hour after PCI. Maintenance therapy with prasugrel is continued for at least 1 year after PCI. Early discontinuation should be considered if the risk of bleeding-related morbidity outweighs the anticipated benefits.

One study, however, found that significant, sometimes fatal, bleeding occurred more frequently with prasugrel than with clopidogrel, although the overall mortality rate did not differ significantly between a treatment group receiving prasugrel and another receiving clopidogrel.

### Ticagrelor

Ticagrelor (Brilinta) was approved by the US Food and Drug Administration in July 2011 and is the first reversible oral P2Y receptor antagonist. Results from the platelet inhibition and patient outcomes (PLATO) trial showed ticagrelor provides faster, greater, and more consistent ADP-receptor inhibition than clopidogrel.

The difference between treatments on the composite resulted from effects on CV death and MI; each was statistically significant when considered as a secondary endpoint and there was no beneficial effect on strokes. For all-cause mortality, the benefit was also statistically significant of 9.8% for ticagrelor and 11.7% for clopidogrel ($p = 0.0003$) with a hazard ratio of 0.78.

Bleeding risk was assessed in the PLATO trial and ticagrelor increased the overall risk of bleeding (major + minor) to a somewhat greater extent than did clopidogrel. The increase was seen for non-CABG-related bleeding but not for CABG-related bleeding. Fatal and life-threatening bleeding rates were not increased.

### Abciximab, Eptifibatide, and Tirofiban

Glycoprotein IIb/IIIa receptor antagonists include abciximab, eptifibatide, and tirofiban. These drugs inhibit the glycoprotein IIb/IIIa receptor, which is involved in the final common pathway for platelet adhesion and aggregation.

Use of cardiac markers in the ED. Effect of time to use of cardiac markers in the ED. Effect of time to treatment in patients with acute coronary syndrome (ACS) who are treated with the GIIb/IIIa inhibitor eptifibatide.

Use eptifibatide or tirofiban in patients with high-risk features in whom invasive treatment is not planned.

The use of eptifibatide 12 hours or more before angiography was not superior to the provisional use of eptifibatide after angiography, according to results from the EARLY ACS trial. The study compared a strategy of early, routine administration of eptifibatide with delayed, provisional administration in patients who had ACS without ST-segment elevation and who were assigned to an invasive strategy. The study also found that early use of eptifibatide was associated with an increased risk of non-life-threatening bleeding and the need for transfusion.

Two trials with tirofiban and 1 trial with eptifibatide documented their efficacy in unstable angina/NSTEMI patients, only some of whom underwent interventions. These antagonists are a class I recommendation in patients in whom catheterization and PCI are planned. Intermediate- and high-risk patients appear to respond favorably to glycoprotein IIb/IIIa inhibitors. They include patients with ST-segment depression, elevated risk scores, elevated serum troponin levels, and/or diabetes mellitus.

Currently, IIb/IIIb antagonists in combination with aspirin are considered standard antiplatelet therapy for patients at high risk for unstable angina.

## PHARMACOLOGIC ANTICOAGULATION THERAPY

### Unfractionated Heparin

A study by Oler et al. found that unfractionated heparin was associated with a 33% reduction in the risk of myocardial infarction or death in patients with unstable angina who were treated with aspirin plus heparin, compared with patients who were treated with aspirin alone. The FUTURA/OASIS-8 randomized trial found that low-dose unfractionated heparin, 50 U/kg (regardless of use of glycoprotein (Gp) IIb/IIIa inhibitors), compared with standard-dose unfractionated heparin, 85 U/kg (60 U/kg with Gp IIb/IIIa inhibitors), did not reduce major peri-PCI bleeding and vascular access-site complications.

### Low Molecular Weight Heparin

Low molecular weight heparins (LMWHs) might be superior to unfractionated heparin in reducing cardiovascular outcomes, with a safety profile similar to that of heparin in patients receiving medical care.

Conflicting results emerged from 9 randomized trials directly comparing LMWH with unfractionated heparin. Two trials evaluated dalteparin, another evaluated nadroparin, and 6 evaluated enoxaparin. Trials with dalteparin and nadroparin reported similar rates of nonfatal myocardial infarction or death compared with heparin, whereas 5 of 6 trials of enoxaparin found point estimates for death or nonfatal myocardial infarction that favored enoxaparin over heparin. The benefit of enoxaparin appeared to be driven largely by a reduction in nonfatal myocardial infarction, especially in the cohort of patients who had not received any open-label anticoagulant therapy before randomization.

In addition, a systematic review comparing LMWH with unfractionated heparin found no significant difference in benefits between the two drugs.

Aside from the possible medical benefits of using LMWH in place of unfractionated heparin, advantages of LMWH include ease of administration, absence of need for anticoagulation monitoring, and potential for overall cost savings. Although LMWHs are approved for use in the United States, only enoxaparin is currently approved for use in unstable angina. Lev et al. found that the combination of eptifibatide with enoxaparin appears to have a more potent antithrombotic effect than that of eptifibatide and unfractionated heparin.

The role of LMWHs in patients for whom PCI is scheduled is relatively ill defined. However, it is likely to be at least equivalent to that of heparin. It appears reasonable to minimize the risk of excessive anticoagulation during PCI by avoiding crossover of anticoagulants (i.e. maintain consistent anticoagulant therapy from the pre-

PCI phase throughout the procedure itself). Additional experience with regard to the safety and efficacy of the concomitant administration of LMWHs with Gp IIb/IIIa antagonists and fibrinolytic agents is currently being acquired.

Adding apixaban (5 mg twice daily) to antiplatelet therapy in high-risk patients after ACS may increase the number of major bleeding events without significantly reducing recurrent ischemic events.

### Factor Xa Inhibitors

Use of the oral Xa inhibitor, rivaroxaban (Xarelto), in addition to dual antiplatelet therapy in patients with ACS was recently investigated in the ATLAS ACS2-TIMI 51 trial. Low-dose rivaroxaban (2.5 mg twice daily) resulted in a significant reduction in overall and cardiac mortality, whereas use of the higher dose (5 mg twice daily) did not result in a significant mortality reduction. However, both doses were associated with an increased risk of bleeding compared with placebo. Rivaroxaban is not currently approved by the US Food and Drug Administration (FDA) for use in ACS.

Another factor Xda inhibitor, fondaparinux (Arixtra), has been studied for use in patients with STEMI who do not undergo PCI. In the Fifth Organization to Assess Strategies in Ischemic Syndromes (OASIS-5) trial, fondaparinux reduced major bleeding and improved net clinical outcome compared with enoxaparin in patients receiving.

Glycoprotein IIb/IIIa inhibitors or thienopyridines for ACS. Fondaparinux is not currently FDA approved for use in ACS.

## THROMBOLYSIS

Prehospital thrombolysis allows eligible patients to receive thrombolysis 30–60 minutes sooner than if treatment were given in the ED; however, prehospital thrombolysis is still under investigation and has not become a trend, as a result of unproven benefit and an increase in the availability of PCI in many medical centers as an alternative to thrombolysis for STEMI (Table 3.6).

The remodeling with erythropoietin after large myocardial infarction (REVEAL) trial evaluated the safety and efficacy of a single intravenous bolus of epoetin alfa in patients with STEMI who had successful reperfusion with primary or rescue PCI. A single intravenous bolus of epoetin alfa within 4 hours of PCI did not reduce infarct size and was associated with higher rates of adverse cardiovascular events.

Although PCI is the preferred treatment for STEMI, the distance to primary PCI centers and the inherent time delay in delivering primary PCI limits widespread use of this treatment. Pre-hospital electrocardiographic (ECG) diagnosis and direct referral for primary PCI enables patients with STEMI living far from a PCI center to achieve a system delay comparable to patients who are closer to a PCI center.

**Table 3.6:** Thrombolytic therapy for acute myocardial infarction

***Standard indications***

1. Chest pain typical of myocardial ischemia. Discomfort from peptic ulcer disease or aortic dissection is a contraindication.
2. Suspicion of Q-wave infarction, i.e. ST-segment elevation in two contiguous ECG leads (benefit of thrombolysis in non-Q-wave infarction and unstable angina is under investigation.
3. Therapy can be administered within 6 hours after onset (but later treatment may confer benefit; actual time constraint is unclear)

***Contraindications***

1. History of cerebrovascular accident
2. Surgery, invasive procedure, or prolonged cardiopulmonary resuscitation in preceding 2 weeks
3. Systolic blood pressure >180
4. Diastolic blood pressure >110
5. Bleeding risk

***Dosage (intravenous)***

1. *Streptokinase:* 1.5 million units over 1 hours
2. *Tissue plasminogen activator:* 10 mg/h/bolus, followed by 50 mg over first hour and 20 mg/h for next 2 hours
3. *Anisolyated plasminogen streptokinase activator complex:* 30 units over 5 minutes

### Concomitant Therapy

Current guidelines for patients with moderate- or high-risk ACS recommend an early invasive. approach with concomitant antithrombotic therapy, including aspirin, clopidogrel, and unfractionated or LMWH. The Acute Catheterization and Urgent Intervention Triage Strategy (ACUITY) trial evaluated the role of thrombin-specific anticoagulation with bivalirudin in this patient population. In patients with moderate- or high-risk ACS who were undergoing invasive treatment with glycoprotein IIb/IIIa inhibitors, bivalirudin was associated with rates of ischemia and bleeding that were similar to those with heparin. Bivalirudin alone was associated with similar rates of ischemia and significantly lower rates of bleeding. Further, glycoprotein IIb/IIIa inhibitors can be initiated at the time of angiography; routine administration 12–24 hours before the procedure carries an increased risk of bleeding and no improvement in outcome.

Kastrati et al. compared the combination of Gp IIb/IIIa inhibitors and heparin with bivalirudin, specifically among patients with NSTEMI undergoing PCI. In a double-blind manner, 1721 patients with acute NSTEMI were randomly assigned to receive abciximab plus unfractionated heparin (861 patients) or bivalirudin (860 patients). The study concluded that abciximab and unfractionated heparin, compared with bivalirudin, failed to reduce death, large recurrent myocardial infarction, urgent target-vessel revascularization, or major bleeding within 30 days. It also increased the risk of bleeding among patients with NSTEMI who were undergoing PCI.

The goals of treatment are to preserve patency of the coronary artery, augment blood flow through stenotic lesions, and reduce myocardial oxygen demand. All patients should receive antiplatelet agents, and patients with evidence of ongoing ischemia should receive aggressive medical intervention until signs of ischemia, as determined by symptoms and ECG resolve.

## ANTIPLATELET AGENTS

Antiplatelets inhibit the cyclooxygenase system, decreasing the level of thromboxane A2, which is a potent platelet activator. Antiplatelet therapy reduces mortality by reducing the risk of fatal strokes and fatal myocardial infarctions.

### Aspirin (Anacin, Ascriptin and Bayer Aspirin)

Early administration of aspirin (e.g. anacin, ascriptin and Bayer aspirin) in patients with acute myocardial infarction may reduce cardiac mortality in the first month. The adult dose is 160–324 mg PO or chewed. It can be administered as a suppository if the patient is unable to take PO medications. Aspirin reduces morbidity and mortality and is continued indefinitely. If administered with ticagrelor (Brilinta), do not exceed 100 mg/day after a one-time loading dose of 325 mg.

Nitrates oppose coronary artery spasm and reduce myocardial oxygen demand by reducing preload and afterload.

### Nitroglycerin Topical (Nitro-Bid)

Nitroglycerin (Nitro-Bid) causes relaxation of the vascular smooth muscle via stimulation of intracellular cyclic guanosine monophosphate production, causing a decrease in blood pressure. Nitrates do not improve mortality. However, they provide symptomatic relief by means of several mechanisms, including coronary vasodilation, improved collateral blood flow, decrease in preload (venodilation and reduced venous return), and decrease in afterload (arterial vasodilation). Care should be taken to avoid hypotension, because this can potentially reduce coronary perfusion pressure (diastolic BP-LV diastolic pressure).

## ANALGESICS

These agents reduce pain which decreases sympathetic stress, in addition to providing some preload reduction.

Morphine sulfate (duramorph, astramorph and MS Contin) is the drug of choice for narcotic analgesia because of its reliable and predictable effects, safety profile, and ease of reversibility with naloxone. Morphine sulfate administered intravenously may be dosed in a number of ways and commonly titrated until the desired effect is obtained.

## BETA-ADRENERGIC BLOCKERS

Beta-blockers have antiarrhythmic and antihypertensive properties, as well as the ability to reduce ischemia. They minimize the imbalance between myocardial supply and demand by reducing afterload and wall stress. In patients with acute MI, they decrease infarct size as well as short- and long-term mortality, which is a function of their anti-ischemic and antiarrhythmic properties. These drugs may prevent mechanical complications of myocardial infarction, including rupture of the papillary muscle, left ventricular free wall, and ventricular septum. Beta blockers ameliorate dynamic obstruction of the left ventricular outflow tract in patients with apical infarct and hyperdynamic basal segments. They should not be used acutely in patients with cardiogenic shock or signs of heart failure on presentation.

### Metoprolol (Lopressor)

Metoprolol (lopressor) is a selective beta1-adrenergic receptor blocker that decreases the automaticity of contractions. During IV administration, blood pressure, heart rate, and ECG should be carefully monitored. The goal of treatment is to reduce the patient's heart rate to 60–90 beats/min.

### Esmolol (Brevibloc)

Esmolol (brevibloc) is an excellent drug for use in patients at risk for complications from beta-blockers, particularly reactive airway disease, mild to moderate LV dysfunction, and peripheral vascular disease. Its short half-life of 8 minutes allows for titration to desired effect with the ability to stop quickly.

### Glycoprotein IIB/IIIA Inhibitors

Glycoprotein IIb/IIIa receptor antagonists include abciximab eptifibatide, and tirofiban. Glycoprotein IIb/IIIa antagonists prevent the binding of fibrinogen, thereby blocking platelet aggregation. These drugs inhibit the glycoprotein IIb/IIIa receptor, which is involved in the final common pathway for platelet adhesion and aggregation. Currently, Gp IIb/IIIb receptor antagonists in combination with aspirin are considered standard antiplatelet therapy for patients at high risk for unstable angina.

### Abciximab (ReoPro)

Abciximab (ReoPro) is a chimeric human-murine monoclonal antibody. It binds to receptors with high affinity and reduces platelet aggregation by 80%. Inhibition of platelet aggregation persists for up to 48 hours after the end of infusion. Abciximab has been approved for use in elective/urgent/emergent percutaneous coronary intervention.

### Eptifibatide (Integrilin)

Eptifibatide (integrilin) is an antagonist of the platelet Gp IIb/IIIa receptor; it reversibly prevents von Willebrand factor, fibrinogen, and other adhesion ligands from binding to the Gp IIb/IIIa receptor. The end effect is the inhibition of platelet aggregation. The effects persist over the duration of maintenance infusion and are reversed when infusion ends. Use eptifibatide (or tirofiban, see below) in patients with high-risk features in whom invasive treatment is not planned.

### Tirofiban (Aggrastat)

Tirofiban (aggrastat) is a nonpeptide antagonist of the Gp IIb/IIIa receptor. It is a reversible antagonist of fibrinogen binding. When administered intravenously, more than 90% of platelet aggregation is inhibited. Tirofiban has been approved for use in combination with heparin for patients with unstable angina who are being treated medically and for patients undergoing percutaneous coronary intervention.

## ANTICOAGULANTS

Anticoagulants are used to prevent recurrence of clot after a spontaneous fibrinolysis.

### Heparin

Heparin augments the activity of antithrombin III and prevents the conversion of fibrinogen to fibrin. It does not actively lyse but is able to inhibit further thrombogenesis. This agent prevents recurrence of a clot after spontaneous fibrinolysis.

### Low Molecular Weight Heparins

LMWH is indicated for treatment of ST-segment elevation myocardial infarction (STEMI) managed medically or with subsequent PCI. It is also indicated as prophylaxis for ischemic complications caused by unstable angina and non-Q-wave myocardial infarction.

Aside from the possible medical benefits of using LMWH in place of unfractionated heparin, advantages of LMWH include ease of administration, absence of need for anticoagulation monitoring, and potential for overall cost savings. Although LMWHs are approved for use in the United States, only enoxaparin is currently approved for use in unstable angina.

### Enoxaparin (Lovenox)

Low molecular weight heparin (enoxaparin; lovenox), which is produced by partial chemical or enzymatic depolymerization of unfractionated heparin, binds to antithrombin III, enhancing its therapeutic effect. The heparin-antithrombin III complex binds to and inactivates activated factor X (Xa) and factor II (thrombin). LMWH differs from unfractionated heparin by having a higher ratio of antifactor Xa to antifactor IIa than does unfractionated heparin. Maximum antifactor Xa and antithrombin activities occur 3–5 hours after administration.

### Direct Thrombin Inhibitors

Direct thrombin inhibitors bind directly to the anion binding site and the catalytic sites of thrombin to produce potent and predictable anticoagulation.

### Hirudin (Lepirudin, Refludan)

Hirudin (lepirudin, refludan) is the prototype of direct thrombin inhibitors. Hirudin binds directly to the anion binding site and the catalytic sites of thrombin to produce potent and predictable anticoagulation. Currently, hirudin is indicated only in patients who are unable to receive heparin because of heparin-induced thrombocytopenia.

### Bivalirudin (Angiomax)

Bivalirudin (angiomax) is a synthetic analogue of recombinant hirudin. It inhibits thrombin and is used for anticoagulation in unstable angina in patients undergoing PTCA. Potential advantages over conventional heparin therapy include more predictable and precise levels of anticoagulation, activity against clot-bound thrombin, absence of natural inhibitors (e.g. platelet factor 4, heparinase), and continued efficacy following clearance from plasma (because of binding to thrombin).

## ADENOSINE DIPHOSPHATE RECEPTOR ANTAGONISTS

Thienopyridine adenosine 5′-diphosphate (ADP) antagonists approved for antiplatelet activity in the United States include clopidogrel, ticlopidine, prasugrel, and ticagrelor. All but ticagrelor have irreversible antiplatelet activity and take several days to manifest an effect, whereas ticagrelor is a reversible P2Y12 receptor inhibitor. A potential additive benefit exists when ADP antagonists are used in conjunction with aspirin. These drugs may be considered alternatives to aspirin in patients with aspirin intolerance or who are allergic to aspirin.

### Clopidogrel (Plavix)

Clopidogrel (plavix) inhibits ADP-dependent activation of the glycoprotein IIb/IIIa complex, a necessary step for platelet aggregation. This process results in intense inhibition of platelet function, particularly in combination with aspirin.

Clopidogrel can be considered an alternative to aspirin in patients with aspirin intolerance or who are allergic to aspirin. The CURRENT-OASIS 7 trial suggests that a 7-day double-dose clopidogrel regimen can be considered for patients with acute coronary syndromes, as the efficacy and safety did not differ from that of a high- and low-dose aspirin regimen. However, there is no benefit in the double-dose treatment for patients who are undergoing an early invasive strategy.

Clopidogrel is a class I recommendation for patients when an early noninterventional approach is planned in therapy. When percutaneous coronary intervention (PCI) is planned, clopidogrel is started and continued for at least 1 month and for up to 9 months, if the patient is not at high risk for bleeding.

Clopidogrel is generally preferred over ticlopidine (ticlid), because it more rapidly inhibits platelets and appears to have a more favorable safety profile.

Clopidogrel has been suggested to be less effective in reducing the rate of cardiovascular events in individuals who carry the loss-of-function CYP2C19 alleles. However, a 2010 study concluded that patients with ACS or atrial fibrillation respond well to clopidogrel, regardless of CYP2C19 loss-of-function carrier status.

### Ticlopidine (Ticlid)

Beneficial effects were noted in patients with unstable angina (UA) after 2 weeks of use in one randomized trial. When compared to controls, ticlopidine use decreased vascular deaths and nonfatal MIs.

### Prasugrel (Effient)

Thienopyridine drug that inhibits platelet activation and aggregation through the irreversible binding of its active metabolite to ADP platelet receptors (specifically the P2Y12 receptor). Platelet inhibition is the result of this action.

Indicated to reduce thrombotic cardiovascular (CV) events (including stent thrombosis) with acute coronary syndrome (ACS) that is managed with percutaneous coronary intervention (PCI). Specifically for unstable angina or non-ST-elevation myocardial infarction (NSTEMI) or with ST-elevation myocardial infarction (STEMI) when managed with primary or delayed PCI.

Reduces rate of combined endpoint of CV death, nonfatal MI, or nonfatal stroke compared with clopidogrel.

### Ticagrelor (Brilinta)

Ticagrelor and its major metabolite reversibly interact with the platelet P2Y12 ADP-receptor to prevent signal transduction and platelet activation. Indicated to reduce the rate of thrombotic cardiovascular events in patients with ACS (unstable angina, non-ST-elevation MI, or ST-elevation MI).

Clinical trial results showed a reduced rate of combined endpoint of cardiovascular death, MI, or stroke compared to clopidogrel. Difference between treatments was driven by CV death and MI with no difference in stroke. In patients treated with PCI, ticagrelor also reduces the rate of stent thrombosis.

The drug is administered with aspirin (loading dose of 325 mg PO once, then 75–100 mg/day). Note that exceeding an aspirin dose of 100 mg/day decreases ticagrelor effectiveness.

## MANAGEMENT OF NON-ST-ELEVATION ACUTE CORONARY SYNDROMES (ACSS)

In 2015, the American College of Cardiology/American Heart Association (ACC/AHA) released the guidelines recommendations on the management of non-ST-elevation acute coronary syndromes (ACSs) to assist in maximizing patient outcomes, including the following:

Standard initial medical therapies include supplemental oxygen for arterial oxygen saturation < 90% or respiratory distress; sublingual nitroglycerin; oral beta-blocker therapy within the first 24 hours in the absence of heart failure, low output state, increased risk for cardiogenic shock, or other contraindications to beta-blockade; nondihydropyridine calcium channel blocker for continuing or recurrent ischemia and contraindication to beta-blockade (in the absence of clinically significant left ventricular dysfunction).

Nonsteroidal anti-inflammatory drugs (except aspirin) should not be initiated and should be discontinued during the hospitalization for NSTE-ACS, because of the increased risk of major adverse cardiac events associated with their use.

Initial antiplatelet/anticoagulant therapy includes 325 mg chewable aspirin at presentation, followed by a daily maintenance dose of aspirin at 81–126 mg daily. A P2Y12 inhibitor (clopidogrel or ticagrelor) should be used in addition to aspirin for up to 12 months in patients treated with either an early-invasive or ischemia-guided strategy. In addition to antiplatelet therapy, parenteral anticoagulation is indicated with enoxaparin, bivalirudin, fondaparinux, or unfractionated heparin.

A high-intensity statin should be initiated or continued in all patients without contraindications. Angiotensin-converting enzyme inhibitors should be started and continued indefinitely with a left ventricular ejection fraction = 40% or hypertension, diabetes, or stable chronic kidney disease unless contraindicated.

An early invasive strategy is indicated for patients with refractory angina or hemodynamic or electrical instability and those at elevated risk for clinical events. An early invasive strategy is not recommended for patients with extensive comorbidities (e.g. hepatic, renal, or pulmonary failure; cancer) in whom the risks of revascularization and comorbid conditions are likely to outweigh the benefits of revascularization. An ischemia-guided strategy is appropriate for low-risk score patients (thrombolysis in myocardial infarction or global registry of acute coronary events), for low-risk troponin-negative women, and by patient or clinician preference in the absence of high-risk features. When an ischemia-guided strategy is chosen, noninvasive stress testing is recommended prior to hospital discharge to detect severe ischemia occurring at a low-stress threshold.

Patients undergoing percutaneous coronary intervention (PCI) should be treated with a P2Y12 inhibitor: clopidogrel, prasugrel, or ticagrelor. Discharge planning should include detailed patient education about symptoms, lifestyle interventions, standard medication with dual antiplatelet therapy, cholesterol management, referral to cardiac rehabilitation, timely follow-up with the healthcare team, and influenza and pneumococcal vaccines.

Non-ST-elevation-ACS patients with prior revascularization PCI or coronary artery bypass grafting should receive antiplatelet and anticoagulant therapy and be strongly considered for an early invasive strategy because of their increased risk. Medical treatment in the acute phase of NSTE-ACS and decisions to perform stress testing, angiography, and revascularization should be similar in patients with and without diabetes mellitus.

Patients who develop NSTE-ACS following noncardiac surgery should receive guideline-directed medical therapy, with additional management directed at the underlying cause of the pathophysiologic process.

Older patients with NSTE-ACS, because of their high-risk status, should be treated with guideline-directed medical therapy and an early invasive strategy with revascularization as appropriate; pharmacotherapy should be individualized and dose adjusted by weight and creatinine clearance to reduce adverse events. Management decisions should be patient centered, incorporating patient preferences, comorbidities, functional and cognitive status, and life expectancy.

Women with NSTE-ACS should be managed with the same pharmacologic therapy as men for acute care and secondary prevention, with attention to weight and/or renally calculated doses of antiplatelet and anticoagulant agents to reduce bleeding risk. Women with NSTE-ACS and high-risk features (e.g. troponin positive) should undergo an early invasive strategy.

Initial therapy for ACS should focus on stabilizing the patient's condition, relieving ischemic pain, and providing antithrombotic therapy to reduce myocardial damage and prevent further ischemia. Morphine (or fentanyl) for pain control, oxygen, sublingual or intravenous (IV) nitroglycerin, soluble aspirin 162–325 mg, and clopidogrel with a 300–600 mg loading dose are given as initial treatment.

In complete vessel occlusion without collateralization of the infarct-related vessel, there is a little utility in 'pushing nitrates'.

High-risk patients with non-ST-segment elevation myocardial infarction (NSTEMI ACS) should receive aggressive care, including aspirin, clopidogrel, unfractionated heparin or low molecular weight heparin (LMWH), IV platelet Gp IIb/IIIa complex blockers (e.g. tirofiban and eptifibatide), and a beta-blocker. The goal is early revascularization.

Intermediate-risk patients with NSTEMI ACS should rapidly undergo diagnostic evaluation and further assessment to determine their appropriate risk category.

Low-risk patients with NSTEMI ACS should undergo further follow-up with biomarkers and clinical assessment. Optimal medical therapies include use of standard medical therapies, including beta blockers, aspirin, and unfractionated heparin or LMWH. The clopidogrel in Unstable Angina to Prevent Recurrent Events CURE study showed that clopidogrel would be beneficial even in low-risk patients. If no further pain occurs, and follow-up studies are negative, a stress study should drive further management.

Monitor and immediately treat arrhythmias in the first 48 hours. Pay attention to exacerbating factors, such as disturbances in electrolytes (especially potassium and magnesium), hypoxemia, drugs, or acidosis. Correct these factors accordingly.

Humidified oxygen may reduce the risk of nosebleeds in patients with ACS who are receiving antiplatelet and antithrombin therapy.

Do not administer nitrates if the patient is hypotensive (systolic BP < 90 mmHg); if RV infarction, large pericardial effusion, or severe aortic stenosis is suspected; or if the patient recently received phosphodiesterase-5 inhibitors (e.g. sildenafil).

Patients with known hypersensitivity to antiplatelet agents, active internal bleeding, and bleeding disorders should not receive antiplatelet or antithrombotic therapy.

Some patients with intractable chest pain or severe hypotension may require the insertion of an intra-aortic balloon pump. The EuroHeart survey showed a nearly 40% reduction in the risk of death in patients with ACS who received support with an intra-aortic balloon pump. This benefit was independent of the status of the ST-segment.

Congestive heart failure can be due to systolic dysfunction or diastolic dysfunction in the setting of myocardial infarction. Aggressive treatment is indicated to prevent worsening of the situation.

Patients presenting with cardiogenic shock should undergo percutaneous coronary intervention (PCI) as soon as possible. Cardiogenic shock is associated with a high mortality rate. Pressor agents, such as dopamine, and inotropic agents, such as dobutamine, may be needed. In a prospective, natural-history study of coronary atherosclerosis, patients underwent 3-vessel coronary angiography and gray-scale and radiofrequency intravascular ultrasonographic imaging after PCI.

Recurrent ischemia may be due to incomplete reperfusion. In the setting of PCI, consider stent thrombosis as a possible cause. Whether drug-eluting stents have an increased rate of thrombosis compared with bare metal stents is unclear.

The clinical significance of incomplete coronary revascularization (ICR) following PCI in patients with ACS was examined in 2,954 patients from the Acute Catheterization and Urgent Intervention Triage Strategy (ACUITS) trial. At one year follow-up, ICR was strongly associated with ischemia-driven unplanned revascularization, myocardial infarction and major adverse cardiac events.

Drug-eluting stents are linked with fewer periprocedural risks but tend to have high incidence of postprocedural complications including myocardial infarction, repeat procedures, and 12-month major adverse cardiac and brain complications, compared with coronary bypass surgery.

One study by Ribichini et al. suggests that prednisone treatment after bare metal stents or drug-eluting stent implantation results in a better event-free survival at 1 year.

In the final report of the HORIZONS-AMI trial, which assessed the 3-year outcomes of the effectiveness and safety of bivalirudin monotherapy and paclitaxel-eluting stenting, outcomes were sustained for patients with STEMI undergoing primary PCI.

In a study of 3031 patients, Mehta et al. found that early intervention (coronary angiography < or = 24 hours after randomization) in patients with ACS did not differ greatly from delayed intervention (coronary angiography > or = 36-hour randomization) in the prevention of primary outcomes (i.e. composite of death, myocardial infarction, or stroke at 6 months). Early intervention did reduce the rate of secondary outcomes (i.e. death, myocardial infarction, or refractory ischemia at 6 months) and improved primary outcomes in patients who were at highest risk (i.e. GRACE risk score >140).

In a Swedish registry of patients with STEMI from 1996–2007, reported an increase in the prevalence of evidence-based treatments. The use of aspirin, clopidogrel, beta-blockers, statins, and ACE inhibitors all increased. Clopidogrel increased from 0% to 82%, statins increased from 23% to 83%, and various ACE inhibitors increased by a large margin. A decrease was reported in 30-day and 1-year mortality that was sustained during long-term follow-up. By following the proper guidelines, patients who have experienced STEMI have higher survival rates.

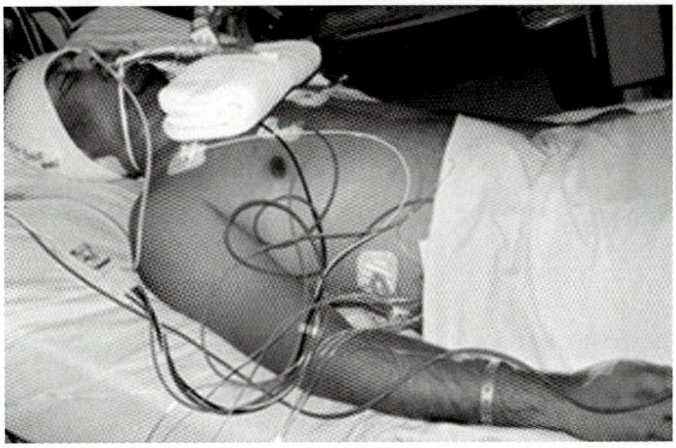

**Fig. 3.71:** A middle-aged-patient with acute myocardial infarction has been selected by doctors for primary angioplasty

## CORONARY INTERVENTIONS

An early invasive strategy (i.e. diagnostic angiography with intent to perform revascularization) is indicated in unstable angina/NSTEMI patients who have refractory angina or hemodynamic or electrical instability without serious comorbidities or contraindications to such procedures. An early invasive strategy is also indicated in initially stabilized unstable angina/NSTEMI patients who do not have serious comorbidities or contraindications to such procedures and who have an elevated risk for clinical events (Figs 3.71–3.78 and Table 3.7).

According to the 2011 American College of Cardiology Foundation (ACCF)/American Heart Association (AHA) guidelines, an early invasive strategy (i.e. within 12–24 hours of admission) is a reasonable choice for initially stabilized high-risk patients with unstable angina/NSTEMI; for patients not at high risk, a delayed invasive approach is also reasonable (class IIa recommendation).

In NSTEMI ACS, early revascularization reduces myocardial infarction and death rates compared with a more selective strategy, particularly in high-risk patients. Use of Gp IIb/IIIa blockers followed by early invasive catheterization is the most logical approach. An early invasive strategy should be considered in patients with large myocardial infarction, hypotension, shock, RV infarction, and refractory chest pain.

In the invasive versus conservative treatment in unstable coronary syndromes (ICTUS) trial, an early invasive strategy had no apparent long-term benefit in reducing death or myocardial infarction. After stratification for risk, analysis of 5-year clinical outcomes in patients presenting with non-ST-segment elevation ACS and elevated troponin T (TnT) level showed that cumulative myocardial infarction or death rates were 22.3% in the early invasive group versus 18.1% in the selective invasive group. No difference was observed in mortality or myocardial infarction.

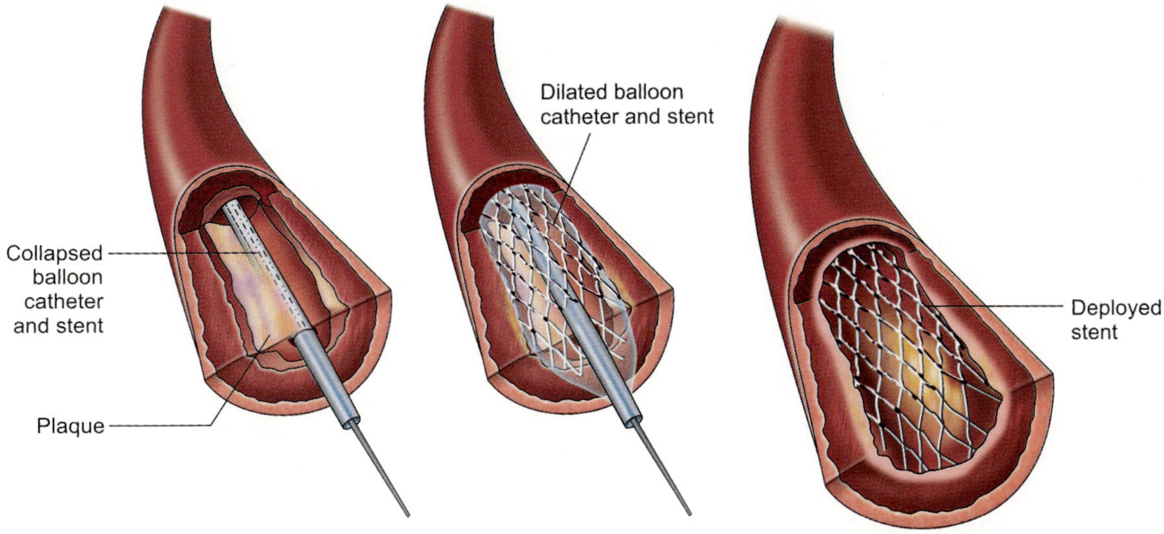


**Fig. 3.72:** The stent is a self-expanding—its shape and diameter can adapt to the anatomical changes of coronary arteries during the post-infarction phase, so as to stay permanently in contact with the vessel wall. It also avoids, thanks to a mesh made of micro-connectors, blocking the access to lateral branches

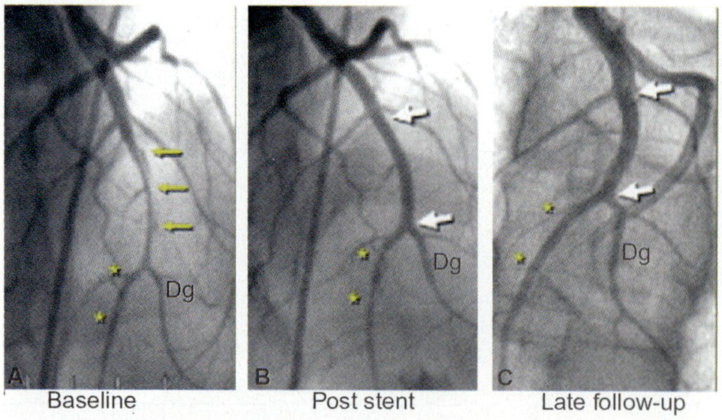


**Fig. 3.73:** SCD in the left anterior descending coronary artery requiring coronary stenting for ongoing ischemia. (A) Before intervention, a clear angiographic flap is detected (yellow arrows) together with a smooth vessel narrowing (asterisks) distal to the second diagonal branch (Dg). (B) Result after stenting (white arrows). The diagonal branch became transiently occluded and required additional stent implantation in its proximal segment. (C) Late angiographic follow-up. Notice the enlargement of lumen diameter at the distal vessel (asterisks), suggesting resolution of intramural hematoma. I-SCD=isolated spontaneous coronary artery dissection

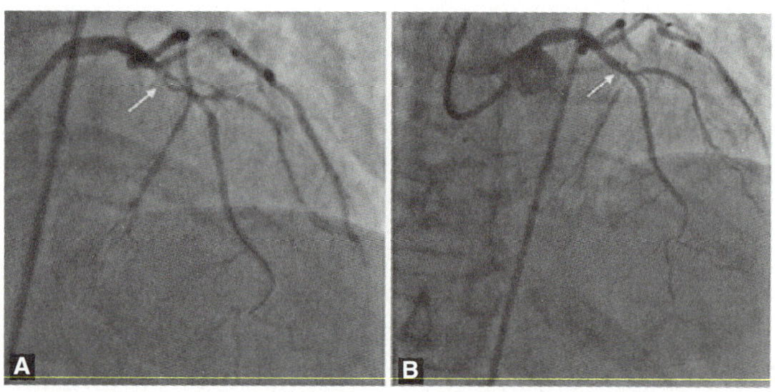


**Fig. 3.74:** (A) Left anterior descending coronary artery with type B dissection postangiosplasty. Note double lumen (arrow) without flow compromise. (B) Left anterior descending coronary artery after stenting (arrow)

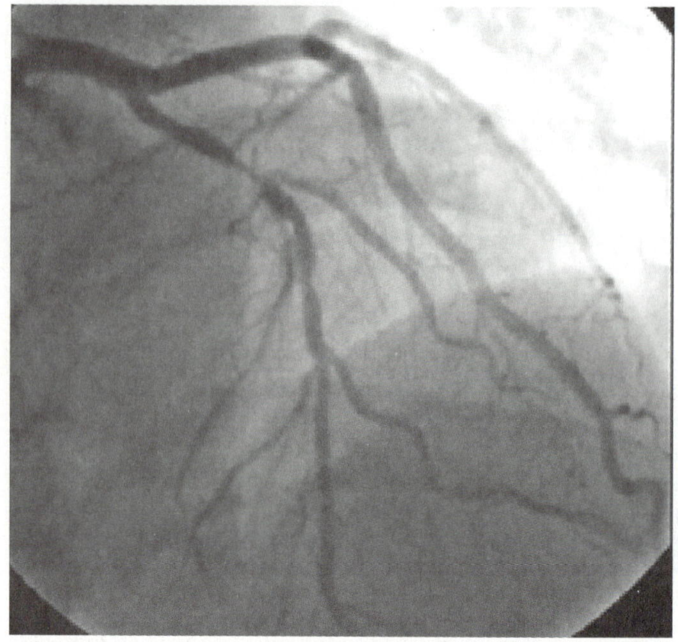

**Fig. 3.75:** UC San Diego performs first robotically assisted double vessel coronary stenting after a heart attack procedure in California by Dr Sie Hing Tanga and published on August 31, 2014

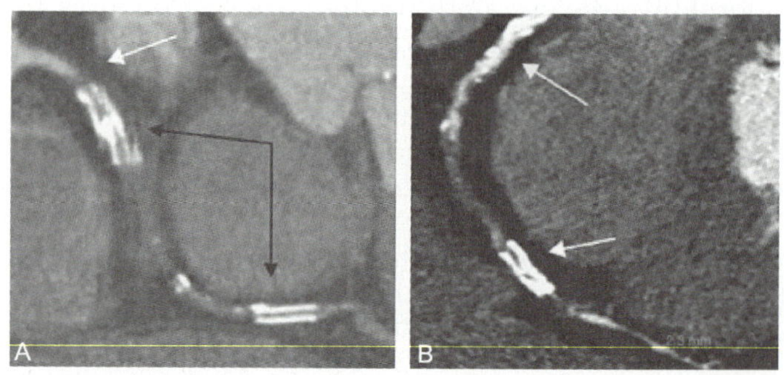


**Fig. 3.76:** Occluded coronary arteries with previously implanted stent. (A) Right coronary, middle and distal stent; high-density image (black arrows), occlusion of the artery immediately proximal to the first stent (white arrow). (B) Total chronic coronary occlusion difficult to evaluate because of an intense proximal calcification (yellow arrow) of the vessel, middle occlusion, and distal stent (white arrow)

## Primary Coronary Angioplasty

Coronary angioplasty without antecedent thrombolytic therapy, termed primary or direct coronary angioplasty, has been studied in the treatment of acute myocardial infarction. In prospective, randomized trials comparing primary coronary angioplasty with different thrombolytic agents, primary coronary angioplasty was associated with a lower morbidity and mortality than thrombolytic therapy. Although most of the individual trials were too small to detect statistically significant differences in mortality, pooled data from these trials suggest that primary coronary angioplasty is the preferred therapy for acute myocardial infarction at institutions where it can be performed without delay. However, the degree of benefit associated with primary coronary angioplasty was much smaller than that seen in the earlier randomized studies; this finding was in part related to the lower frequency with which patients assigned to undergo angioplasty in GUSTO-IIb actually underwent the procedure and in part related to the lower frequency with which normal antegrade coronary blood flow was achieved in patients who did undergo coronary angioplasty.

The consistency of the results favoring primary coronary angioplasty and the greater speed and frequency with which coronary angioplasty can restore flow to an occluded coronary artery support the conclusion that primary coronary angioplasty is preferable to thrombolytic therapy

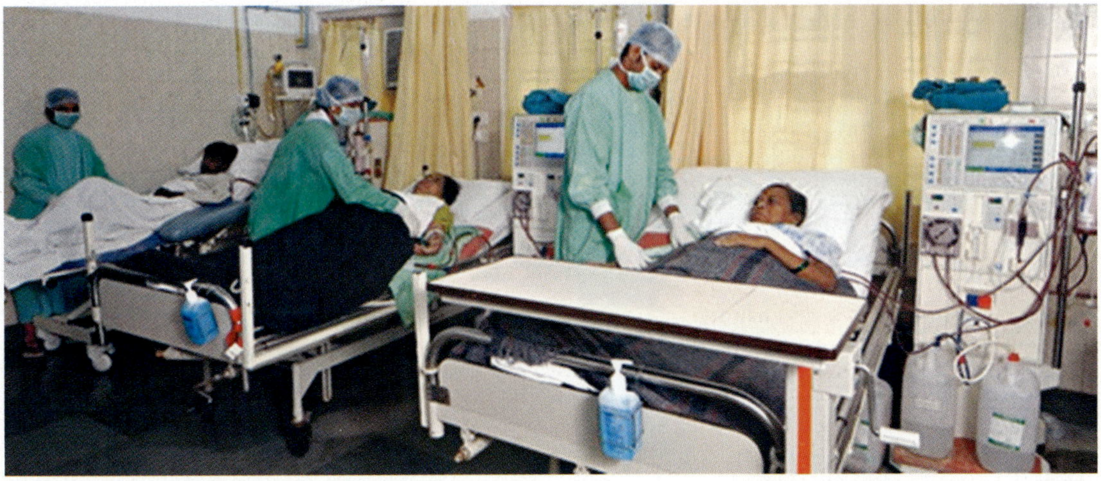

**Fig. 3.77:** All patients with acute coronary syndrome who are managed with angioplasty are being monitored in intensive coronary care unit

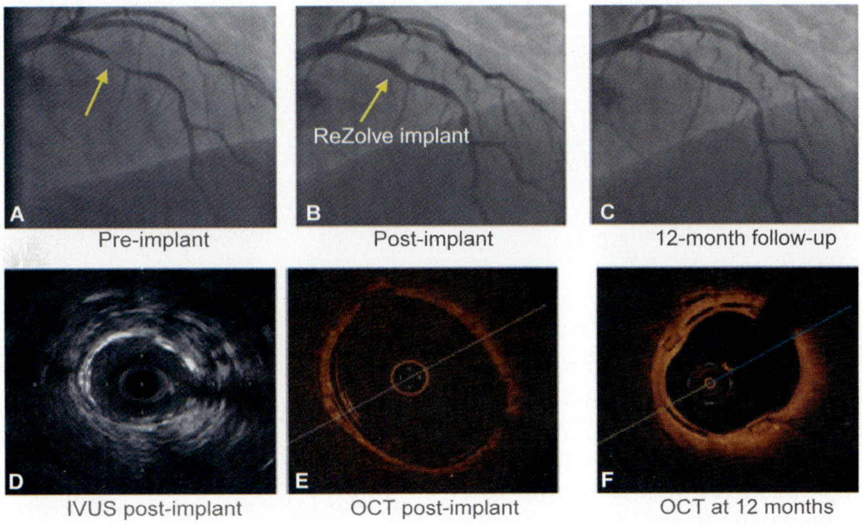


**Fig. 3.78:** Angiographic, intravascular ultrasound (IVUS), and optical coherence tomography (OCT) illustrations of a case with ReZolve® bioresorbable scaffold. Angiogram revealed a 90% stenosis (A) which was treated with implantation of ReZolve bioresorbable scaffold. (B) showed good angiographic results at 12-month follow-up. (C) Representative intravascular ultrasound. (D) Optical coherence tomography sections post-implant. (E) At 12 months, and (F) are shown (*Courtesy:* Alexandre Abizaid)

at institutions where it can be performed quickly with a high success rate. Studies have shown that excessive delay in performing primary coronary angioplasty and operator inexperience lead to a higher mortality than that seen when primary coronary angioplasty is performed rapidly by experienced operators. It has been recommended that primary angioplasty be performed only in hospitals where a high success rate and low complication rate can be demonstrated and where primary angioplasty is performed in at least 80–90% of patients in whom acute myocardial infarction is confirmed. The need for surgical backup is controversial, as excellent results have been obtained at centers without surgical backup. However, surgical backup is recommended because approximately 5% of patients with acute myocardial infarction who undergo immediate coronary angiography require emergency surgery either for angioplasty that has failed or, more commonly, because lethal coronary anatomy precludes primary angioplasty. Immediate transfer for primary angioplasty is an alternative treatment strategy for patients with STEMI initially assessed at a hospital without on-site cardiac surgery facilities.

### Glycoprotein IIb/IIIa Inhibitor Therapy and Primary Angioplasty for Acute Myocardial Infarction

The role of the platelet glycoprotein inhibitor abciximab in conjunction with primary coronary angioplasty has been examined in the randomized, placebo-controlled trial of

**Table 3.7:** Recommendations for early conservative versus invasive treatment strategies

*Class I*

- An early invasive strategy is indicated in patients who have unstable angina/NSTEMI and any of the following high-risk indicators (level of evidence: A)
- Recurrent angina/ischemia at rest or with low-level activities despite intensive anti-ischemic therapy.
- Elevated troponin T or troponin I
- New or presumably new ST-segment depression
- Recurrent angina/ischemia with symptoms of chronic heart failure, an S3 gallop, pulmonary edema, worsening rales, or new or worsening mitral regurgitation
- High-risk findings on noninvasive stress testing
- Depressed left ventricular systolic function (e.g. ejection fraction <0.40 on noninvasive study)
- Hemodynamic instability
- Sustained ventricular tachycardia
- PCI within 6 months
- Prior coronary artery bypass graft surgery
- In the absence of these findings, either an early conservative or an early invasive strategy is indicated in hospitalized patients who do not have contraindications for revascularization (level of evidence: B)

*Class IIa*

- An early invasive strategy is indicated in patiets who have repeated presentations ofr ACS despite therapy and without evidence for ongoing ischemia or high risk (level of evidence: C)

*Class III*

- Coronary angiography is indicated in patients who have extensive comobidities (e.e. liver or pulmonary failure, cancer), in whom the risks of revascularization are not likely to outweigh the benefits (level of evidence: C)
- Coronary angiography is recommended in patients who have acute chest pain and a lowlikelihood of ACS (level of evidence: C)
- Coronary angiography is indicated in patients who will not consent to revascularization regardless of athe findings (level of evidence: C).

abciximab with primary angioplasty for acute myocardial infarction (RAPPORT), the intracoronary stenting and antithrombotic regimen-2 (ISAR-2) study, the abciximab before direct angioplasty and stenting in myocardial infarction adverse events, but the benefit appeared to be limited to patients undergoing balloon angioplasty without stent placement. This would suggest that glycoprotein IIb/IIIa inhibitors should be beneficial in this setting. Taken together, the results of these studies that are currently available suggest that abciximab is beneficial in patients with acute myocardial infarction but that the benefit in patients undergoing balloon angioplasty alone may differ from that in patients who undergo balloon angioplasty with stent placement. Clearly, however, stents markedly reduce the frequency with which a repeat revascularization procedure is needed in the months after the angioplasty procedure. The combined use of stents and platelet glycoprotein inhibitors may maximize the frequency with which normal antegrade blood flow is achieved while reducing the need for repeat procedures in the following year. One study compared the outcome of thrombolytic therapy using t-PA with that of primary angioplasty utilizing both stents and abciximab. The reduction in infarct size was far greater in the group undergoing primary angioplasty; the clinical outcome was also better in the patients who underwent angioplasty.

## Rescue Coronary Angioplasty

Depending on the regimen used, only 33–60% of patients treated with thrombolytic therapy have restoration of normal antegrade flow in the infarct-related artery 90 minutes after the initiation of therapy. Accordingly, immediate coronary angiography has been studied to determine whether patients with persistent occlusion of the infarct-related artery benefit from coronary angioplasty; this procedure has been termed rescue angioplasty. A single small, randomized trial has examined the clinical outcome of patients with anterior infarction and coronary occlusion that persist despite thrombolytic therapy. Patients were randomized to either undergo rescue coronary angioplasty or receive continued medical therapy alone. The results of the trial suggested improved outcome with rescue angioplasty, although the benefits were not compelling. Three additional randomized trials evaluated the role of rescue angioplasty. Analyzed together, the four trials suggest that rescue angioplasty offers benefit, although the data are not compelling. Although use of coronary stents and platelet glycoprotein inhibitors improves the results of percutaneous revascularization procedures and would be expected to further increase the benefit of angioplasty after failed thrombolytic therapy, this has not yet been proved. There are insufficient data to recommend immediate angiography and angioplasty in all patients early after thrombolytic therapy. Immediate angiography is most likely to be beneficial in patients with large myocardial infarctions in whom persistent pain, ST-segment elevation, or hemodynamic compromise is present more than 90 minutes after the administration of a thrombolytic agent. The routine performance of angioplasty immediately after the administration of thrombolytic therapy in all patients with a significant residual stenosis (not just those patients with occluded coronary arteries) has been well studied in three prospectives, randomized trials and has been found to be either of no benefit or deleterious. Angioplasty should not be routinely performed in such patients. Stents appear to improve the ability to achieve arterial patency early after thrombolytic therapy, as compared with balloon angioplasty alone, therapy with a glycoprotein IIb/IIIa inhibitor may also do so, although an increase in bleeding has been seen when glycoprotein IIb/IIIa inhibitors are used early after full-dose thrombolytic therapy. Data from several pilot studies suggest that the combination of a fibrin-specific thrombolytic agent, either t-PA or reteplase, combined with the glycoprotein IIb/IIIa inhibitor abciximab, may actually facilitate the performance of angioplasty rather than reduce its safety and efficacy, as was seen when balloon angioplasty was performed after thrombolytic therapy. Hence, the term facilitated angioplasty has been coined for the routine performance of angioplasty after the combination of half-dose thrombolytic therapy with a glycoprotein IIb/IIIa inhibitor.

The plasminogen-activator angioplasty compatibility trial (PACT) investigators randomized 606 patients to a reduced dose of a short-acting fibrinolytic regimen (50 mg bolus of reteplase) or a placebo followed by immediate angiography with angioplasty, if needed. In the group receiving reduced-dose reteplase, there was no increase in the incidence of stroke or major bleeding, and convalescent left-ventricular ejection fraction was higher, as evidenced by a patent infarct-related artery (TIMI-3 flow) on arrival in the catheterization laboratory (62%) or a TIMI-3 flow that was achieved by angioplasty within 1 hour after administration of the drug bolus (58%). However, only 12% of successful angioplasty procedures resulted in a patent infarct-related artery within 1 hour, because of routine delay in transfer to the catheterization laboratory, and there was no difference between the two treatment groups by a traditional intention-to-treat analysis. The Southwest German Study in Acute Myocardial Infarction III (SIAM III) investigators randomized 163 patients initially treated with thrombolysis at a community hospital with no on-site PCI facilities either to hospital transfer and immediate stenting within 6-hours of thrombolysis or to delayed, elective stenting approximately 2 weeks after acute myocardial infarction. Transfer and immediate stenting were associated with a statistically significant reduction in the incidence of the composite primary end-point (i.e. death, reinfarction, ischemic events, and target-lesion revascularization at 6 months), as compared with delayed stenting (25.6% versus 50.6%; $P = 0.001$). The difference in outcome was driven by events occurring during the 2 weeks that patients waited for elective stenting in the deferred PCI group. This trial design does not address whether PCI performed 1–2 days after thrombolytic therapy, as is usual in the United States, is as effective as PCI performed immediately after thrombolytic therapy. A randomized trial that analyzed the use of combination therapy (half-dose thrombolytic therapy with full-dose abciximab) before routinely performing primary PCI was recently reported. In the Bavarian reperfusion alternatives evaluation (BRAVE) trial, patients with STEMI were randomly assigned to receive either half-dose reteplase and full-dose abciximab or abciximab alone, and all patients underwent PCI as rapidly as possible. No advantage was seen with combination therapy; in fact, more bleeding complications occurred in this group. The results argue against the use of a facilitated PCI approach using the combination regimen of reteplase and abciximab.

### Bioresorbable Scaffolds

Current generation of drug-eluting stents has significantly improved the outcomes of percutaneous coronary intervention by substantially reducing in-stent restenosis and stent thrombosis. However, a potential limitation of these stents is the permanent presence of a metallic foreign body within the artery, which may cause vascular inflammation, restenosis, thrombosis, and neoatherosclerosis. The permanent stents also indefinitely impair the physiological vasomotor function of the vessel and future potential of grafting the stented segment. Bioresorbable scaffolds (BRSs) have the potential to overcome these limitations as they provide temporary scaffolding and then disappear, liberating the treated vessel from its cage and restoring pulsatility, cyclical strain, physiological shear stress, and mechanotransduction. While a number of BRSs are under development, two devices with substantial clinical data have already received a Conformité Européenne marking. This review article presents the current status of these devices and evaluates the challenges that need to be overcome before BRSs can become the workhorse device in coronary intervention.

## ADJUNCTIVE MEDICAL THERAPY

### Intravenous Heparin

The need for IV heparin after thrombolytic therapy varies with the thrombolytic agents used. A retrospective analysis of the GUSTO-I trial suggested that IV heparin with a partial thromboplastin time of 50–70 seconds was associated with the best clinical outcome in patients treated with t-PA. Data from GUSTO-I also suggest that IV heparin is not required when IV streptokinase is used, although heparin is recommended in patients with large anterior infarctions to prevent the development of apical mural thrombus and embolization. In patients in whom IV heparin is not administered, subcutaneous heparin should be administered during the period of bedrest to reduce the risk of deep vein thrombosis.

The optimal duration of IV heparin therapy is unclear. Standard practice was to administer IV heparin for 3–5 days, although patients are now often discharged after only 3 days. It is recommended that heparin be discontinued more than 24 hours before patient discharge from the hospital because of the possibility of a rebound effect and recurrent thrombosis within 24 hours after cessation of heparin therapy.

Randomized studies from the prethrombolytic era suggested that administration of IV heparin reduces mortality and reinfarction in patients not treated with thrombolytic agents. Aspirin and beta-blockers were not routinely administered in those early trials; consequently, the true benefits of heparin when these drugs are administered are unknown. However, on the basis of the early data, IV heparin is generally recommended for patients with suspected myocardial infarction who are not treated with thrombolytic therapy.

### Low Molecular Weight Heparin

Low molecular weight heparins (depolymerized unfractionated heparin with a mean molecular weight of approximately 5,000) have a number of potential pharmacokinetic advantages over the parent molecule, including decreased binding to plasma proteins, decreased sensitivity to platelet factor 4, enhanced factor Xa activity, and improved bioavailability. These factors are associated with a predictable dose-response relationship and, combined with the ease of administration (once or twice daily SC dosing regimens) and lower rates of heparin-induced thrombocytopenia, have increased investigators' interest in low molecular weight heparins in preference to unfractionated heparin for the treatment of myocardial infarction. The results of four large randomized trials comparing three different low molecular weight heparins with unfractionated heparin have suggested that low molecular-weight heparin is at least as effective in reducing ischemic events in patients with NSTEMI acute coronary syndromes. Following patients with STEMI, the second trial of heparin and aspirin reperfusion therapy (HART II) and the Acute Myocardial Infarction-Streptokinase (AMI-SK) trial demonstrated evidence of improved rates of reperfusion when the low-molecular-weight heparin enoxaparin was combined with t-PA or streptokinase, respectively. The ASSENT-3 trial compared three regimens: full-dose tenecteplase and enoxaparin, full-dose tenecteplase and unfractionated heparin, and half-dose tenecteplase and abciximab for the treatment of thrombolytic-eligible STEMI; the study revealed that enoxaparin fared better than unfractionated heparin in terms of 30-day mortality, in-hospital reinfarction, and in-hospital refractory ischemia ($P = 0.0001$) at 30 days. However, at 1 year, the benefits had diminished, and the mortality with enoxaparin was identical to that with unfractionated heparin. In addition, when the data from ASSENT-3 and ASSENT-3-PLUS (a study examining the administration of tenecteplase with enoxaparin in the prehospital setting) were pooled, a marked and prohibitive increase in the risk of intracerebral hemorrhage was seen in the elderly. As a result, ongoing trials utilizing enoxaparin with a fibrinolytic agent have adjusted the dose of enoxaparin downward in elderly patients. At present, the adjunctive anticoagulant that should be administered with fibrinolytic therapy and its optimal dose is not known.

### Direct Thrombin Inhibitors

Direct thrombin inhibitors are an attractive alternative to indirect thrombin inhibitors, such as heparin or low molecular weight heparins, particularly because they block both circulating and clot-bound thrombin. A collaborative meta-analysis of phase-3 trials of direct thrombin inhibitors for the treatment of acute coronary artery syndromes demonstrated superiority over unfractionated heparin for the prevention of the composite end-point of death or myocardial infarction. The Hirulog and early reperfusion or occlusion (HERO)-2 trial demonstrated a similar benefit in comparison to bivalirudin with heparin in patients with STEMI bivalirudin was associated with a 30% reduction in the incidence of reinfarction, but mortality did not decrease; however, the bivalirudin arm of the study exhibited a trend toward more bleeding events.

### Beta-blockers

Numerous studies of beta-blocker therapy in patients with acute myocardial infarction have documented significant reductions in in-hospital and long-term mortality. Early administration of beta-blockers has been promoted because it may reduce infarct size by reducing heart rate, blood pressure, and myocardial contractility, all of which diminish myocardial oxygen demand. Meta-analysis of the effects of early administration of IV beta blockers in 27, 486 patients with acute myocardial infarction enrolled in 28 randomized trials revealed a 14% reduction in mortality during the first week of therapy; reinfarction was reduced by 18%.

The TIMI-II study compared immediate beta-blocker therapy with deferred beta-blocker therapy in acute myocardial infarction; all patients also received IV t-PA. Results indicated that immediate beta-blocker therapy reduced the incidence of nonfatal reinfarction and recurrent ischemia, compared with oral metoprolol therapy begun on the sixth hospital day; as in earlier studies, only about 40% of patients with acute myocardial infarction were eligible for acute beta-blocker therapy. There are also data suggesting that immediate beta-blocker therapy reduces the risk of intracranial hemorrhage after lytic therapy. It is recommended that all patients with acute myocardial infarction without contraindications receive IV beta-blockers as early as possible, whether or not they receive reperfusion therapy.

In patients in whom contraindications preclude early beta-blocker therapy, reevaluation should take place before discharge. Many patients will no longer have contraindications at the time of discharge. Patients without contraindications should be routinely started on beta-blocker therapy before discharge from the hospital. The optimal duration of benefit remains unclear, but it appears that the benefit of beta-blocker therapy is maintained for years. Patients with the largest infarctions benefit the most from the use of beta-blockers. Current recommendations are that beta-blocker therapy be continued indefinitely in the absence of contraindications or side-effects.

### Angiotensin-converting Enzyme Inhibitors

Several large randomized, controlled clinical trials evaluating the use of angiotensin-converting enzyme (ACE) inhibitors early after acute myocardial infarction have been performed; all but one trial revealed a significant reduction in mortality. Meta-analysis of these large trials and many smaller trials, which together included over 100,000 patients, suggested a 6.5% reduction in deaths, with an absolute reduction in mortality of 4.6 deaths per 1,000 patients among those treated with an ACE inhibitor. All patients with significant ventricular dysfunction (an ejection fraction < 40%) without contraindications should be treated with an ACE inhibitor; treatment should begin within the first 48 hours of infarction and be increased cautiously to avoid hypotension. If hypotension results from the early administration of ACE inhibitors, short-term mortality may be increased.

The benefit of ACE inhibitors is clear in patients with large anterior infarctions and an ejection fraction less than 40%; whether patients with an ejection fraction greater than 40% benefit from ACE inhibitor therapy is less clear. However, the results of two large trials suggest that patients with a normal ejection fraction after myocardial infarction, as well as even patients with coronary artery disease without a previous myocardial infarction, have a reduction in mortality when treated with an ACE inhibitor. Treatment with perindopril was associated with a highly statistically significant reduction in the incidence of fatal and nonfatal myocardial infarction at 4 years. Whether these favorable results are unique to tissue-specific ACE inhibitors or represent a class effect is unknown.

### Intravenous Nitroglycerin

Randomized studies examining the role of IV nitroglycerin in acute myocardial infarction revealed beneficial effects on left ventricular function and a reduction in infarct size and mortality. However, these studies were small and were performed before the reperfusion era. To determine whether nitroglycerin therapy is beneficial in patients treated with reperfusion, 58,050 patients with acute myocardial infarction in the fourth International Study of Infarct Survival (ISIS-4) were randomized to receive either oral controlled-release mononitrate therapy or placebo; thrombolytic therapy was administered to patients in both groups. The results of this study revealed no benefit to the routine administration of oral nitrate therapy in this setting. Similar results were seen among 19, 000 patients in the third Gruppo Italiano per lo Studio della Sopravvivenza nell' Infarto Miocardico (GISSI-3) Study, in whom IV nitroglycerin was administered for the first 24 hours, followed by transdermal nitrates. Whether these disappointing results in the ISIS-4 and GISSI-3 trials were caused by the routes of administration of the nitroglycerin preparation or the administration of thrombolytic therapy is unknown. However, on the basis of existing data, it does not appear that the routine administration of nitroglycerin to patients receiving early thrombolytic therapy is beneficial. IV nitroglycerin is probably most likely to be beneficial in patients with persistent or recurrent chest pain after reperfusion therapy and in patients in whom reperfusion therapy is not administered.

### Insulin Therapy

Diabetic patients have a significantly worse prognosis after myocardial infarction than those without diabetes, mainly because of greater left ventricular dysfunction and increased reinfarction rates. This applies to both patients who are newly diagnosed on the coronary care unit and those already diagnosed. Recent evidence from the DIGAMI study suggests that a more intensive approach to achieving metabolic control in patients presenting with hyperglycaemia may be beneficial. Six hundred and twenty patients presenting within 24 hours of a myocardial infarction with a blood glucose concentration greater than 11 mmol/L (whether known to have diabetes mellitus or not) were randomised to receive a glucose-insulin infusion followed by subcutaneous insulin four times daily for at least 3 months. Patients in the control group only received insulin if indicated by normal clinical practice. The mean time to randomisation was 13 hours after the onset of symptoms. The target range plasma glucose was 7–10.9 mmol/L, with 2 hours monitoring of plasma glucose for at least 24 hours. There were hypoglycaemic episodes in 15% of patients receiving intensive therapy. Mortality at 1 year was 29% lower in the intervention group than in the control group (95% CI 4%, 51%). After a mean follow-up of 3.4 years there was a 28% relative risk reduction in mortality in the glucose insulin treatment group (95% CI 8%, 45%). The benefit was particularly apparent in the low risk patients (age < 70, no previous infarct, no heart failure) who were not previously using insulin (51% reduction, 95% CI 19, 70%). In this group the benefit was already apparent at the time of hospital discharge and continued to 5 years of follow-up. The results suggest that diabetic patients are likely to benefit from an early intensive approach to metabolic control although this is likely to pose logistic problems for many units.

### Prophylactic Antiarrhythmic Therapy

Previously, routine prophylactic antiarrhythmic therapy with IV lidocaine was recommended for all patients in the early stages of acute myocardial infarction. However, studies have revealed that prophylactic therapy with lidocaine does not reduce and may actually increase mortality because of an increase in the occurrence of fatal bradyarrhythmia and asystole. Neither IV lidocaine nor other antiarrhythmic agents are recommended as prophylactic therapy for patients without malignant ventricular ectopy.

### Calcium Channel Antagonists

Calcium channel antagonists should not be routinely administered for acute myocardial infarction. Calcium channel antagonists have been studied in prospective, doubleblind, placebo-controlled trials; and neither verapamil nifedipine nor diltiazem appears to reduce postinfarction mortality. Verapamil and diltiazem may be useful in patients with preserved left ventricular function and no heart failure in whom contraindications to beta-blockers exist. However, the data are insufficient to recommend the routine administration of these agents. On the basis of existing data, treatment with calcium channel blockers should be reserved for patients with ischemia that persists despite use of aspirin, beta-blockers, nitrate therapy, and IV heparin and for patients with other indications for their administration.

### Magnesium

Magnesium has been studied in many prospective, randomized trials of acute myocardial infarction, and the results have been conflicting. Magnesium is involved in hundreds of enzymatic steps and produces systemic and coronary vasodilatation, inhibits platelet function, and reduces reperfusion injury. Meta-analysis of seven prospective, randomized trials revealed a significant reduction in mortality with the use of magnesium. It is possible that magnesium is of benefit, particularly in patients not receiving reperfusion therapy. Magnesium is clearly indicated in patients with myocardial infarction who have torsade de pointes-type ventricular tachycardia and in patients with magnesium deficiency.

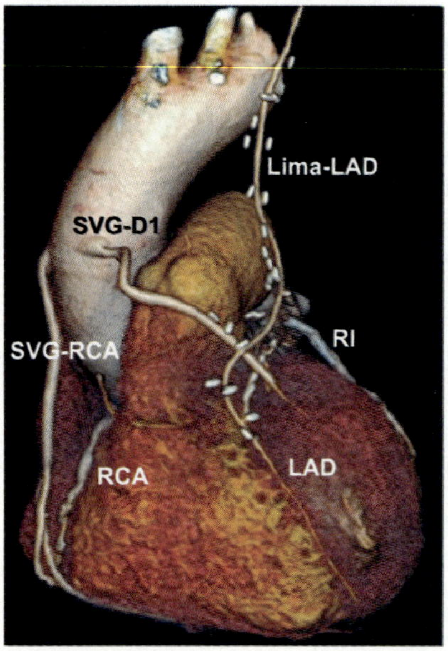


**Fig. 3.79:** CABG: MD.CT 64 slices of the LV and aorta showing CABG with intact grafts from ascending aorta to the proximal of of the obstructed right coronary artery and left anterior descending artery in the process of perfusion plan in the management of ischemic myocardiumas a result of myocardial infarction

### Coronary Artery Bypass Surgery

Coronary artery bypass surgery can restore blood flow in an occluded infarct-related artery. However, because of the time required to perform coronary angiography and to transport patients to the operating room, reperfusion is achieved more slowly with bypass surgery than with thrombolytic therapy and primary coronary angioplasty. Emergency coronary artery bypass surgery should generally be reserved for patients in whom immediate angiography reveals coronary anatomy that precludes primary coronary angioplasty; for patients in whom angioplasty has failed; and for patients with a ventricular septal defect, severe mitral regurgitation, or myocardial rupture.

### Prognosis in ACS

Six-month mortality rates in the global registry of acute coronary events (GRACE) were 13% for patients with NSTEMI ACS and 8% for those with unstable angina.

An elevated level of troponin (a type of regulatory protein found in skeletal and cardiac muscle) permits risk stratification of patients with ACS and identifies patients at high risk for adverse cardiac events (i.e. myocardial infarction, death) up to 6 months after the index event.

The PROVE IT-TIMI trial found that after ACS, a J-shaped or U-shaped curve association is observed between BP and the risk of future cardiovascular events.

LeLeiko et al. determined that serum choline and free F(2)-isoprostane are also predictors of cardiac events in ACS. The authors evaluated the prognostic value of vascular inflammation and oxidative stress biomarkers in patients with ACS to determine their role in predicting 30-day clinical outcomes. Serum F(2)-isoprostane had an optimal cutoff level of 124.5 pg/ml, and serum choline had a cutoff level of 30.5 μmol/L. Choline and F(2)-isoprostane had a positive predictive value of 44% and 57% and a negative predictive value of 89% and 90%, respectively.

Testosterone deficiency is common in patients with coronary disease and has a significant negative impact on mortality. Further study is needed to assess the effect of treatment on survival.

A study by Sanchis et al. suggests renal dysfunction, dementia, peripheral artery disease, previous heart failure, and previous myocardial infarction are the comorbid conditions that predict mortality in NSTEMI ACS. In patients with comorbid conditions, the highest risk period was in the first weeks after NSTEMI ACS. In-hospital management of patients with comorbid conditions merits further investigation.

Patients with end-stage renal disease often develop ACS, and little is known about the natural history of ACS in patients receiving dialysis.

NSTEMI ACS was the most common in patients receiving dialysis, occurring in 50% of patients (290 of 579) versus 33% of those not receiving dialysis. The in-hospital mortality rates were higher among patients receiving dialysis (12% vs 4.8%; $p < 0.0001$). Higher 6-month mortality

**Table 3.8:** Adverse prognostic features in myocardial infarction

- Advanced age
- Diabetes
- Left ventricular failure
- Systolic hypotension
- anterior full-thickness infarction
- Left bundle brench block
- History of previous myocardial infarction (complex ventricular arrhythmias, particulary those occuring late >36 hours) after myocardial infarction

rates (13% vs 4.2%; $p < 0.0001$), recurrent myocardial infarction incidence (7.6% vs 2.9%; $p < 0.0001$), and unplanned rehospitalizations (31% vs 18%; $p < 0.0001$) were found among those who survived to discharge. Outcomes in patients who received dialysis was worse than was predicted by the calculated GRACE risk score for in-hospital mortality (7.8% predicted vs 12% observed; $p < 0.05$). This suggests that the GRACE risk score underestimated the risk of major events in these patients (Table 3.8).

In a study that assessed the impact of prehospital time on STEMI outcome, Chughatai et al. suggest that 'total time to treatment' should be used as a core measure instead of 'door-to-balloon time'. This is because on-scene time was the biggest fraction of 'prehospital time'. The study compared groups with total time to treatment of more than 120 minutes compared with 120 minutes or less and found mortalities were 4 compared with 0 and transfers to a tertiary care facility were 3 compared with 1, respectively.

### Telemedicine and Newer ECG Techniques in Fighting Acute Coronary Syndromes

Transmitting 12-lead ECGs from the community directly to attending cardiologists should become routine. Time to reperfusion in STEMI has decreased, explaining much of the observed decrease in STEMI mortality. This technology allows for increasingly complex and individualized prehospital medical care and could be expanded to a broader number of cardiovascular diagnoses (Figs 3.80–3.83).

### Automated, Implantable Cardioverter-defibrillator (Fig. 3.84)

Automated implantable cardioverter-defibrillators are of proven benefit in patients with coronary artery disease, reduced left ventricular ejection fraction, nonsustained ventricular tachycardia, and inducible ventricular tachycardia. It has been proposed that patients with a prior myocardial infarction and advanced left ventricular dysfunction may benefit from prophylactic implantation of a defibrillator (in the absence of electrophysiologic testing to induce arrhythmias). Prophylactic implantation of a defibrillator is a recommended therapy in this patient population.

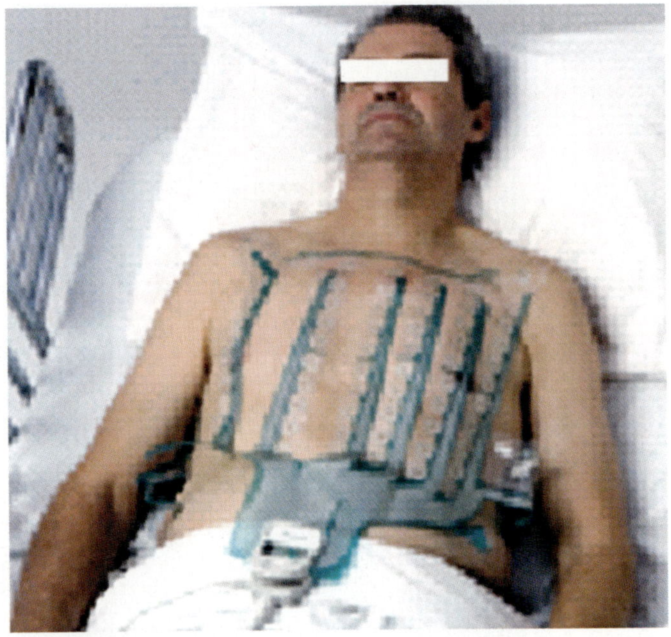

**Fig. 3.80:** Showing ECG 80 leads placement on patient with chest pain of recent onset

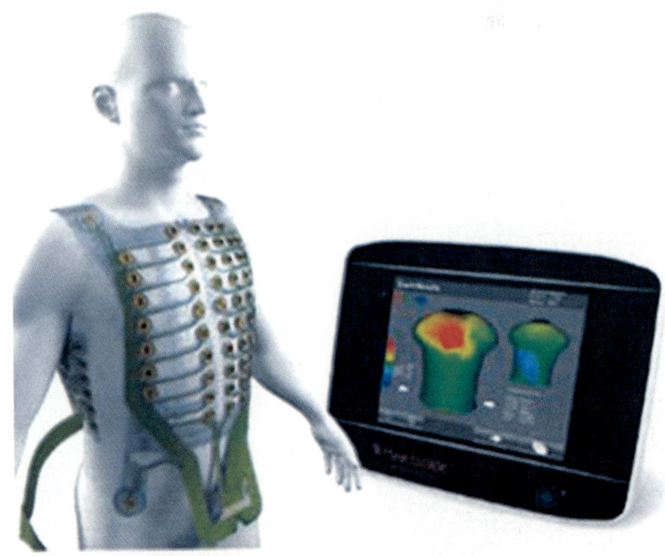

**Fig. 3.81:** Heartscape 80-lead 3D ECG system, Heartscape 80-lead 3D ECG system. The concept is not entirely new, as it is the successor to the PRIME ECG system which has the same amount of leads, and has been available since 2003. The Heartscape 3D ECG System aims to give a 360 degree electrocardiographic view of the heart, to helping in identifying myocardial infarcts without ST-segment elevation on traditional 12-lead ECGs, and in patients with left bundle branch block.Compared to traditional 12-lead ECG's, the system has shown to be more sensitive while retaining comparable specificity in detecting acute infarcts

### Patient Education

Patient education of risk factors is important, but more attention is needed regarding delays in door-to-balloon time, and one major barrier to improving this delay is patient education regarding his or her symptoms. Lack of

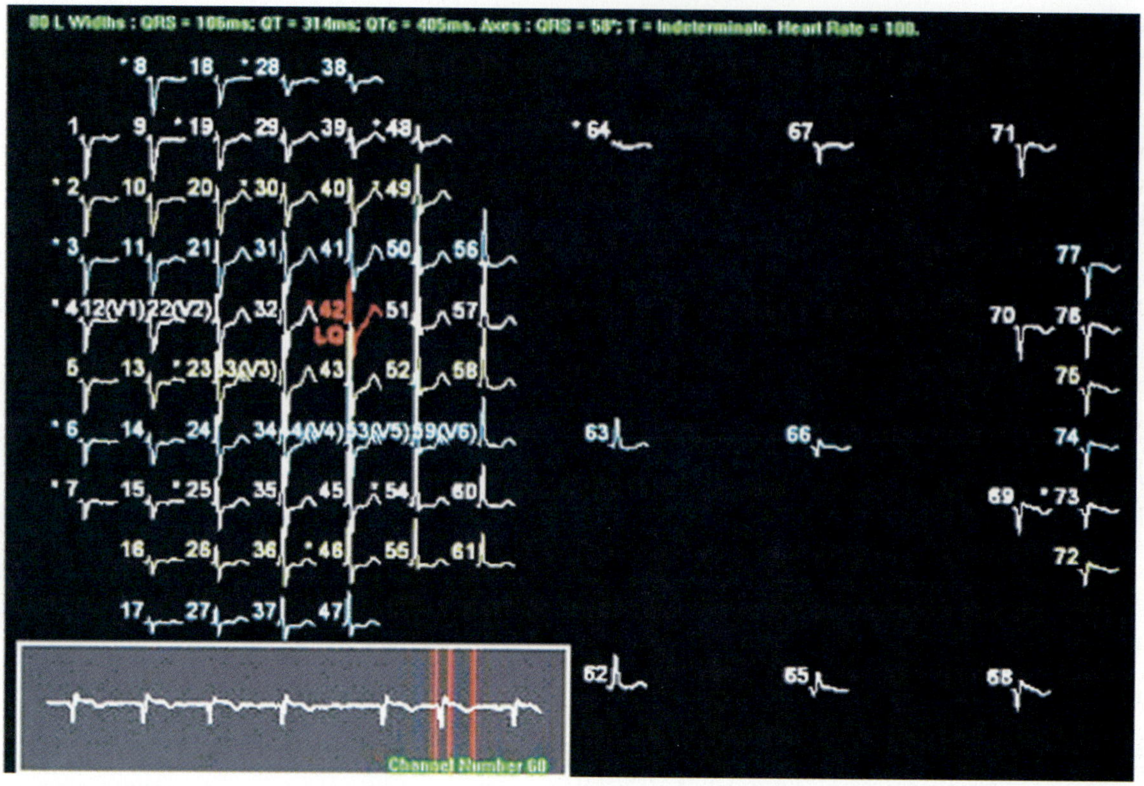


**Fig. 3.82:** Example of a STEMI missed on 12-lead EKG detected on 80-Lead EKG. An 80-lead EKG system shown to the right are the 80-EKG lead tracings displayed individually. The anterior leads is displayed on the left-hand side. The posterior or back of the heart leads are displayed on the right-hand side of the figure. For instance lead-68 shows ST-elevation. Posterior and right-sided leads reveal ST-elevation, where the 12-lead was silent

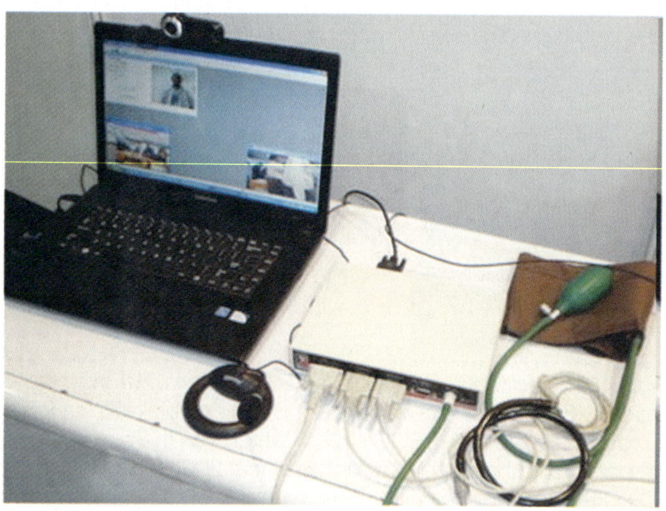

**Fig. 3.83:** Laboratory equipment in telemedicine

recognition of symptoms may cause tremendous delays in seeking medical attention.

Educate patients about the dangers of cigarette smoking, a major risk factor for coronary artery disease (CAD). The risk of recurrent coronary events decreases 50% at 1 year after smoking cessation. Provide all patients who smoke with guidance, education, and support to avoid smoking. Smoking-cessation classes should be offered to help patients avoid smoking after a myocardial infarction. Bupropion increases the likelihood of successful smoking cessation.

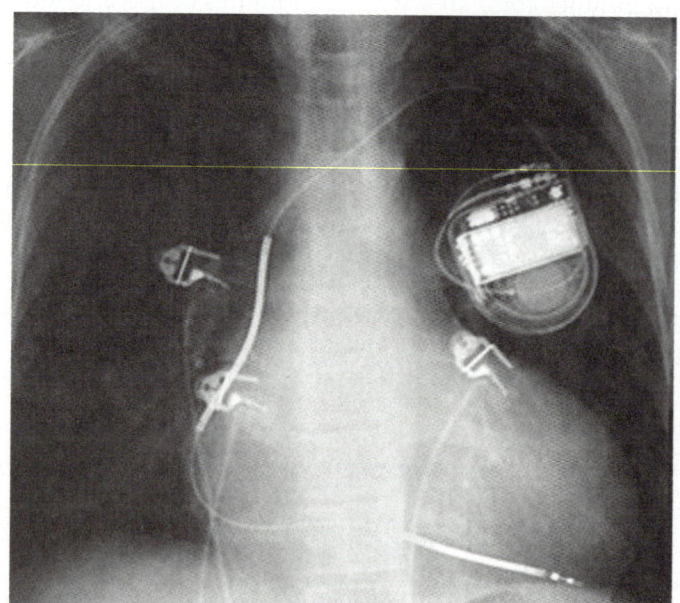

**Fig. 3.84:** Frontal view of the chest shows a typical automatic implantable cardioverter defibrillator

Diet plays an important role in the development of CAD. Therefore, prior to hospital discharge, a patient who has had a myocardial infarction should be evaluated by a dietitian. Patients should be informed about the benefits of a low-cholesterol, low-salt diet. In addition, educate patients about AHA dietary guidelines regarding a low-fat, low-cholesterol diet.

A cardiac rehabilitation program after discharge may reinforce education and enhance compliance.

The following mnemonic may useful in educating patients with CAD regarding treatments and lifestyle changes necessitated by their condition:

A = Aspirin and antianginals

B = Beta-blockers and blood pressure (BP)

C = Cholesterol and cigarettes

D = Diet and diabetes

E = Exercise and education

For patients being discharged home, emphasize the following:

- Timely follow-up with primary care provider
- Compliance with discharge medications, specifically aspirin and other medications used to control symptoms
- Need to return to the ED for any change in frequency or severity of symptoms

## Current Techniques in the Revival of Myocardial Damage after Myocardial Infarction Under Trials

### *Myogenesis in the Heart Muscle*

Myoblasts are super powerhouse cells that originate from human body's muscle stem cells. These cells have the ability to take on the properties of the other cells, such as cardiac muscle cells that make up the heart. The myoblasts can be transplanted from the skeletal muscles into heart and can stimulate myogenesis. Other trials, such as intracoronary stem cell implantation and genetic transformation into myocardfial cells are under review (Fig. 3.85).

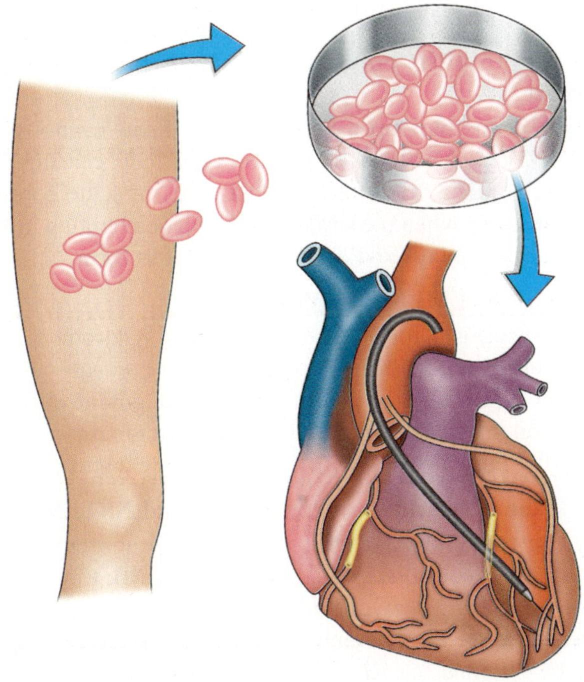

**Fig. 3.85:** Diagrammatic depiction of myogenesis in the heart muscle. Myoblasts are super powerhouse cells that originate from human body's muscle stem cells. These cells have the ability to take on the properties of the other cells, such as cardiac muscle cells that make up the heart. The myoblasts can be transplanted from the skeletal muscles into heart and can stimulate myogenesis. A biopsy of muscle cells from patient thigh is taken and isolated, and expanded in culture in a special cell laboratory for 3 weeks. These multiple cells are injected directly into the areas of heart where the muscle is damaged

## Percutaneous Coronary Intervention Versus Optimal Medical Therapy in Stable Coronary Artery Disease (Systematic Review and Meta-analysis of Randomized Clinical Trials 2012)

In summary, in patients with stable CAD there is no definitive evidence of an added benefit of PCI to reduce the risk of mortality, cardiac death, nonfatal MI, and need for revascularization, when compared with medical therapy alone. PCI appeared to show a benefit for all-cause mortality and cardiac death that was attenuated when recent studies (with more aggressive medical therapy) with a high proportion of stent use were analyzed. However, PCI provides a benefit over medical therapy in symptom relief of angina in patients with stable CAD.

A greater understanding of the pathophysiology of atherosclerosis has led to advancements in PCI with the advent of DES and improvements in medical therapies. In addition, the prior strategy trials have been criticized for enrolling participants after cardiac catheterization (creating selection bias), enrolling lower risk individuals (without significant ischemia) and with the use of DES (only first generation) in a small fraction of the cohort. Ongoing trials, such as the International Study of Comparative Health Effectiveness with Medical and Invasive Approaches (ISCHEMIA), will test treatment strategies upstream of cardiac catheterization and involve patients with at least moderate ischemia, with the use of contemporary optimal medical and optimal revascularization strategies, with a sample size (N=8000) large enough to detect small differences in outcomes.

**QUICK READINGS**

**BOX 3.1:** Frequent questions to be asked by the reader in acute coronary syndrome

**What is an acute coronary syndrome?**

ACS includes myocardial infarction (MI), also known as a heart attack, and unstable angina, or sudden, severe chest pain that typically occurs when a person is at rest. Every year, ACS affects an estimated 1.4 million people in the United States and another 1.4 million people in Europe.

*Contd...*

*Contd...*

**What is the most common cause of acute coronary syndrome?**

Eventually, this buildup means that your heart cannot pump enough oxygen-rich blood to the rest of your body, causing chest pain (angina) or a heart attack. Most cases of acute coronary syndrome occur when the surface of the plaque buildup in your heart arteries ruptures and causes blood clot to form.

**What is a NSTEMI heart attack?**

A heart attack is a form of acute coronary syndrome (ACS), where there is a significant blockage in the coronary arteries. There are three main types of ACS: ST-segment elevation myocardial infarction (STEMI), non-ST-segment elevation myocardial infarction (NSTEMI) and unstable angina.

**What is the difference between STEMI and NSTEMI?**

There are two types, STEMI, which is the abbreviation of ST-elevation myocardial infarction, and NSTEMI, which stands for non-ST-elevation myocardial infarction. The names reflect differences in the ECG tracings—specifically whether a portion of the ECG called the ST-segment is elevated above baseline, or not.

**BOX 3.2:** Key points in heart attack treatment guidelines

The American College of Cardiology and the American Heart Association, in collaboration with the Society for Cardiovascular Angiography and Intervention, and the American Association of Cardiovascular and Pulmonary Rehabilitation, have developed a series of guidelines that address the treatment of heart attack. These guidelines apply to most patients, but also give your doctor the flexibility to tailor treatment to your specific clinical needs. Below is a summary of key information and recommendations.

**Early hospital care**

When you arrive at the hospital you will have blood tests called cardiac biomarkers to check for damage to your heart muscle.

- Have an **electrocardiogram (ECG)** to evaluate your heart's rhythm and look for abnormalities in the heart's electrical system
- Be treated with several medications that protect your heart and relieve pain. These may include a beta-blocker, nitroglycerin, and morphine. You will also be given an aspirin tablet to chew, if you have not taken one already.
- If your heart stopped beating during or after your heart attack (cardiac arrest), your doctor may use a treatment called therapeutic hypothermia. This involves infusion of a liquid into your blood vessels that cools your body to about 90°F for up to 24 hours. Cooling your body will help protect against brain damage that can occur when the brain is deprived of blood during cardiac arrest.
- The next steps in your treatment will depend on what type of heart attack you are having. There are two types, STEMI, which is short-hand for ST-elevation myocardial infarction, and NSTEMI, which stands for non-ST-elevation myocardial infarction. The names reflect differences in the ECG tracings—specifically whether a portion of the ECG called the ST-segment is elevated above baseline, or not. More important, there are differences in the underlying cause of these two types of heart attack and, therefore, in the initial treatment.

**STEMI**

A STEMI heart attack is caused when a blood clot suddenly forms, completely blocking an artery in the heart. This can result in damage that covers a large area of the heart and extends deep into the heart muscle. The priority in treating a STEMI heart attack is to open the artery quickly, saving as much heart muscle as possible. Treatment options include percutaneous coronary intervention (PCI), a term that encompasses both angioplasty and stenting; clot-busting medication; and coronary artery bypass graft surgery (CABG).

***PCI***

PCI is the first choice for the treatment of STEMI, if it is available. The goal is to open the artery within 90 minutes of the patient first receiving care by emergency medical workers, including ambulance personnel.

If your hospital does not have a PCI program, the next best option may be rapid transfer to a nearby medical center that is experienced and prepared to use PCI to treat heart attack. The goal in this case is to open the artery within 2 hours of the patient first receiving care by emergency medical workers. In many areas of the country, regional STEMI networks are being set up to make transport to a PCI hospital fast and efficient.

***Clot-busting medication***

Most hospitals do not have a cardiac catheterization laboratory available 24 hours a day to treat heart attack patients. If you seek emergency treatment at a hospital that is not equipped to perform PCI, and the nearest PCI-capable hospital is too far away to meet the goal of opening the artery within 2 hours, clot-busting medications are an effective treatment option. These medications, also called fibrinolytics, open the artery by dissolving the clot. The goal is to infuse clot-busting medications within 30 minutes of a patient's arrival at the hospital.

In some cases, your doctor may decide that you should have PCI in addition to treatment with clot-busting medication. With this 'pharmacoinvasive strategy', clot-busting medication is used at the first hospital to initially restore blood flow to your heart, then after transport to a PCI-capable hospital, PCI is performed within 24 hours to make sure the artery is fully open and supported with a stent.

***Coronary Artery Bypass Graft Surgery (CABG)***

In some cases, emergency **bypass surgery** may be the best option, especially if you are medically unstable and cannot be treated with PCI or clot-busting medications, or when these treatments fail. Emergency CABG may also be needed if serious complications develop after a heart attack, such as shock, life-threatening abnormalities of the heart rhythm, or rupture of heart tissues. Your doctor may also recommend having CABG surgery within the first 2 days of a heart attack if you have several clogged arteries and start experiencing a return of chest pain while resting quietly.

*Contd...*

*Contd...*

**NSTEMI**

NSTEMI heart attacks are different from STEMI heart attacks in several ways, not just how they appear on the ECG. With NSTEMI, the heart attack damage usually does not extend through the full depth of the heart muscle. Equally important, NSTEMI heart attacks are caused by different types of blood clots than STEMI heart attacks, with differing amounts of clotting proteins and platelet blood cells. Therefore, the treatment of NSTEMI heart attacks differs from the treatment of STEMI heart attacks. Clot-busting medications, for example, are not effective, and although PCI may be part of the treatment, opening the artery within 90 minutes is not a primary goal.

Diagnosis of NSTEMI can be complex, as the diagnostic signs do not always show up right away. Your doctor may repeat the ECG and cardiac biomarker blood tests several times, and carefully analyze the pattern and severity of your chest pain, your other symptoms, and your history of heart disease to determine your level of risk. You may be transferred to a special chest pain unit for observation for several hours. After that, if your chest pain has not returned and the diagnosis is still unclear, your doctor may order an imaging test of your heart (a **nuclear scan**, a type of ultrasound known as **echocardiography,** or a **treadmill stress test**). This will help to determine a final diagnosis.

Once the diagnosis of NSTEMI has been made, you will be admitted to the hospital. Medications to protect your heart and reduce its workload (beta-blockers, nitroglycerin, and possibly an angiotensin-converting-enzyme (ACE) inhibitor or angiotensin-receptor blocker) will be continued. Your doctors will also add one or more **anti-clotting medication**s to prevent blood clots.

Within the first 12–24 hours of your hospital stay, your doctor will select one of two main treatment strategies. One option is continued treatment with medications that protect your heart, reduce its workload, and prevent blood clots. This is a reasonable strategy if your condition is stable and you are not at high risk for serious cardiac complications.

The second treatment option is an 'early invasive' strategy. This means that you will go to the cardiac catheterization laboratory for **angiography,** a procedure that enables your doctor to see inside the arteries of your heart. Usually angiography is followed by PCI and stenting to widen clogged, inflamed portions of the arteries where blood clots may have formed. The 'invasive' strategy is a reasonable option if you are continuing to have chest pain, are medically unstable, or have a high-risk history of heart disease.

**During your hospital stay**

Whether you have a STEMI or NSTEMI heart attack, you will begin to take steps toward recovery and a healthy new lifestyle while you are still in the hospital. You will learn about your medications and begin eating a heart-healthy diet that is low in sodium, cholesterol, and fat (especially 'saturated' animal fats). As soon as it is safe, you will also begin mild exercise, such as walking in the hallway. In addition, your doctor will refer you to a cardiac rehab program, so that you can continue. You may have an imaging test while in the hospital, or shortly after discharge, to evaluate how efficiently your heart is pumping blood. This information, known as the ejection fraction or systolic function, will guide your doctor in prescribing medications and other treatments.

**Discharge from the hospital**

When you are ready to go home, you will be prescribed several medications that have been proven to protect the heart, help it to function better, and prevent repeat heart attacks. Your medications will include some or all of the following:

- Aspirin, to keep platelets in the blood from clumping together and forming blood clots
- Another anticlotting medication such as clopidogrel or prasugrel, or ticagrelor. How much anticlotting medication you take, which specific drug, and how long you take it will depend on your medical condition and whether you were treated with a stenting procedure.
- Beta-blocker
- Cholesterol-lowering therapy
- Angiotensin-converting-enzyme (ACE) inhibitor or angiotensin-receptor blocker (ARB), if your heart is not pumping as strongly as it should

Certain medications used to treat heartburn—called proton pump inhibitors—may reduce the effectiveness of anti-clotting medications. Talk to your doctor about what type of heartburn medication is safe to use.

**Staying healthy after the hospital**

Participating in a cardiac rehabilitation program a high priority for anyone who has had a heart attack. Not only will cardiac rehab help you to feel healthy and strong again, it can actually help you to live longer. Your cardiac rehab program will teach you to:

- Stop smoking and/or using tobacco products
- Follow a heart-healthy diet
- Exercise safely, guided by specially trained physical therapists, nurses, and doctors
- Manage stress and anxiety
- Safely resume your sex life
- Avoid a second heart attack
- In addition to participating in a cardiac rehab program, the following steps will help prevent a second heart attack and keep your arteries from becoming clogged with atherosclerotic plaque:
  - Quit smoking, and avoid second-hand smoke
  - Keep blood pressure under 140/90 mmHg (or lower, if you have diabetes or heart failure)
  - Keep LDL ('bad') cholesterol under 100 mg/dl, or under 70 mg/dl if you are at high risk. This is generally accomplished through the use of statin medications.
  - Exercise for 30–60 minutes at least 5 days a week. The exercise should be moderate-intensity, such as brisk walking.

*Contd...*

*Contd...*

- Maintain a normal body weight
- Maintain good diabetes control
- Take low-dose aspirin daily to prevent unwanted blood clots, plus additional anticlotting medication if advised by your doctor
- Take an ACE inhibitor or ARB, if your heart's pumping ability is abnormal or you have heart failure
- Take beta-blockers to protect the heart and reduce its workload
- Get an annual flu shot
- Seek treatment for depression

## BIBLIOGRAPHY


1. Alpert JS, Thygesen K, Antman E, et al. Myocardial infarction redefined—a consensus document of The Joint European Society of Cardiology/American College of Cardiology Committee for the redefinition of myocardial infarction. J Am Coll Cardiol 2000;36(3):959–69.
2. Antman EM, Tanasijevic MJ, Thompson B, Schactman M, McCabe CH, Cannon CP, et al. Cardiac-specific troponin I levels to predict the risk of mortality in patients with acute coronary syndromes. N Engl J Med 1996;335(18):1342–9.
3. Bangalore S, Qin J, Sloan S, et al. What is the optimal blood pressure in patients after acute coronary syndromes?: Relationship of blood pressure and cardio-vascular events in the PRavastatin OR atorVastatin Evaluation and Infection Therapy—Thrombolysis In Myocardial Infarction (PROVE IT-TIMI) 22 trial. Circulation 2010;122(21):2142–51.
4. Chughtai H, Ratner D, Pozo M, et al. Prehospital delay and its impact on time to treatment in ST-elevation myocardial infarction. Am J Emerg Med 2011;29(4):396–400.
5. Damman P, Holmvang L, Tijssen JG, et al. Usefulness of the Admission Electrocardiogram to Predict Long-Term Outcomes After Non-ST-Elevation Acute Coronary Syndrome (from the FRISC II, ICTUS, and RITA-3 [FIR] Trials). Am J Cardiol 2012;109(1):6–12.
6. Gurm HS, Gore JM, Anderson FA Jr, et al. Comparison of Acute Coronary Syndrome in Patients Receiving Versus Not Receiving Chronic Dialysis (from the Global Registry of Acute Coronary Events [GRACE] Registry). Am J Cardiol 2012;109(1):19–25.
7. Hamm CW, Bassand JP, Agewall S, et al. ESC Guidelines for the management of acute coronary syndromes in patients presenting without persistent ST-segment elevation: The Task Force for the management of acute coronary syndromes (ACS) in patients presenting without persistent ST-segment elevation of the European Society of Cardiology (ESC). Eur Heart J 2011.
8. Heidenreich PA, Alloggiamento T, Melsop K, et al. The prognostic value of troponin in patients with non-ST-elevation acute coronary syndromes: a meta-analysis. J Am Coll Cardiol 2001;38(2):478–85.
9. Iliou MC, Fumeron C, Benoit MO, Tuppin P, et al. Prognostic value of cardiac markers in ESRD: Chronic Hemodialysis and New Cardiac Markers Evaluation (CHANCE) study. Am J Kidney Dis 2003;42(3):513–23.
10. Keller T, Zeller T, Ojeda F, et al. Serial changes in highly sensitive troponin I assay and early diagnosis of myocardial infarction. JAMA 2011;306(24):2684–93.
11. LeLeiko RM, Vaccari CS, Sola S, et al. Useful-ness of elevations in serum choline and free F2—isoprostane to predict 30-day cardiovascular outcomes in patients with acute coronary syndrome. Am J Cardiol 2009;104(5):638–43. [Best Evidence]
12. Lindahl B, Toss H, Siegbahn A, et al. Markers of myocardial damage and inflammation in relation to long-term mortality in unstable coronary artery disease. FRISC Study Group. Fragmin during Instability in Coronary Artery Disease. N Engl J Med 2000;343(16):1139–47.
13. Ma RC, Tong PC. Testosterone levels and cardiovascular disease. Heart 2010;96(22):1787–8 [Medline].
14. Newby LK, Christenson RH, Ohman EM, et al. Value of serial troponin T measures for early and late risk stratification in patients with acute coronary syndromes. The GUSTO-IIa Investigators. Circulation 1998;98(18):1853–9.
15. O'Connor RE, Bossaert L, Arntz HR, et al. Part 9: acute coronary syndromes: 2010 International Consensus on Cardiopulmonary Resuscitation and Emergency Cardio-vascular Care Science with Treatment Recommendations. Circulation 2010;122 (16 Suppl 2): S422–65.
16. Ohman EM, Armstrong PW, Christenson RH, et al. Cardiac troponin T levels for risk stratification in acute myocardial ischemia. GUSTO IIA Investigators. N Engl J Med 1996; 335(18):1333–41.
17. O'Neil BJ, Hoekstra J, Pride YB, et al. Incremental benefit of 80-lead electrocardio-gram body surface mapping over the 12-lead electro-cardiogram in the detection of acute coronary syndromes in patients without ST-elevation myocardial infarction: Results from the Optimal Cardiovascular Diag-nostic Evaluation Enabling Faster Treatment of Myocardial Infarction (OCCULT MI) trial. Acad Emerg Med2010;17(9): 932–9.
18. Sanchis J, Nunez J, Bodí V, et al. Influence of comorbid conditions on one-year outcomes in non-ST-segment elevation acute coronary syndrome. Mayo Clin Proc 2011;86(4):291–6.
19. Scheuermeyer FX, Innes G, Grafstein E, et al. Safety and efficiency of a chest pain diagnostic algorithm with selective outpatient stress testing for emergency department patients with potential ischemic chest pain. Ann Emerg Med 2012.
20. Than M, Cullen L, Reid CM, et al. A 2-h diagnostic protocol to assess patients with chest pain symptoms in the Asia-Pacific region (ASPECT): a pros-pective observational validation study. Lancet 2011;377(9771):1077–84.

# 4 Invasive and Noninvasive Coronary Angiography

## HISTORICAL BACKGROUND

The technique of angiography was first developed in 1927 by the Portuguese physician Egas Moniz at the University of Lisbon to provide contrasted X-ray in order to diagnose nervous diseases, such as tumors, coronary heart disease and arteriovenous malformations. He is recognized as one of the pioneers in this field. Coronary catheterization was further explored in 1929 when the German physician Werner Forssmann inserted a plastic tube in his cubital vein and guided it to the right chamber of the heart. He took an X-ray to prove his success and published it on November 5th, 1929 with the title 'Über die Sondierung des rechten Herzens' (About probing of the right heart) (Fig. 4.1).

The coronarography of the left heart was introduced in 1953 with the report by a Portuguese group, published in Cardiologia, International Archives of Cardiology vol. 22, pp 45–61, by E. Coelho et al. entitled "Arteriografia das coronárias no homem vivo/L'artériograpie des coronaires chez l'homme vivant" (arteriography of the coronaries in the living man). They were the first to nonselectively inject radiocontrast in the coronary arteries. In 1960, F. Mason Sones, a pediatric cardiologist at the Cleveland Clinic, accidentally injected radiocontrast in a coronary artery instead of the left ventricle. Although the patient had a reversible cardiac arrest, Sones and Shirey developed the procedure further, and are credited with the discovery (Connolly 2002); they published a series of 1,000 patents in 1966 (Proudfit et al.). Since the late 1970s, building on the pioneering work of Charles Dotter in 1964 and especially Andreas Gruentzig starting in 1977, coronary catheterization has been extended to therapeutic uses.

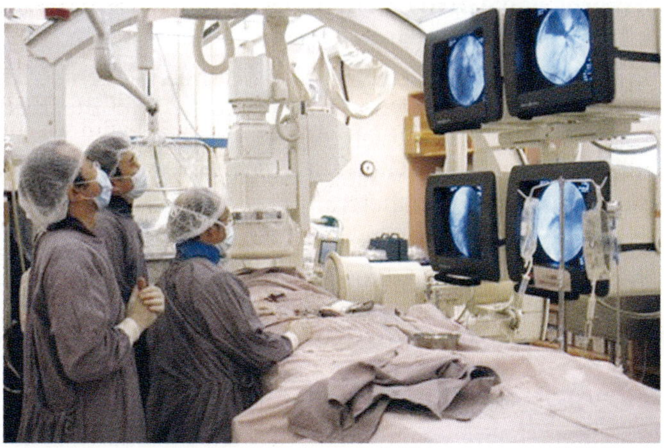

**Fig. 4.1:** Catheterization laboratory and busy medical personnel in preparing patient for heart catheterization

- The performance of less invasive physical treatment for angina and some of the complications of severe atherosclerosis
- Treating heart attacks before complete damage has occurred
- Research for better understanding of the pathology of coronary artery disease and atherosclerosis
- In the early 1960s, cardiac catheterization frequently took several hours and involved significant complications for as many as 2–3% of patients. With multiple incremental improvements over time, simple coronary catheterization examinations are now commonly done more rapidly and with significantly improved outcomes.

### Basics of Coronary Anatomy

The trileaflet aortic valve gives rise to 3 cusp or sinuses in the aortic root. The left coronary and right coronary cusp give rise to their respective coronary arteries while the noncoronary cusp which arises from the posterior root usually does not give rise to a coronary artery (Fig. 4.2).

The major epicardial vessels supplying the myocardium are the left main coronary artery that divides into the left anterior descending artery and left circumflex artery, and the right coronary artery. These arteries lie on the epicardial surface and supply smaller branch vessels that eventually give rise to the microvascular network supplying the

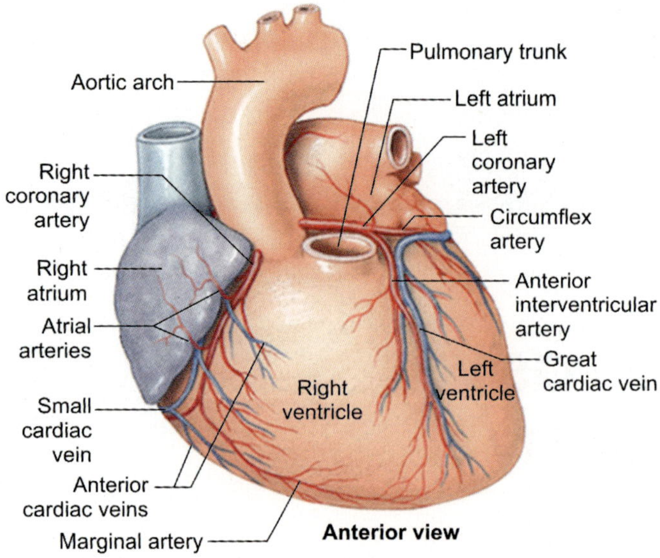


**Fig. 4.2:** Anatomy of main coronary arteries which are usually visualized by coronary angiography

myocardium. Coronary dominance is based on the vessel that gives rise to the posterior descending artery (PDA) which travels in the posterior interventricular groove and supplies the atrioventricular node (AV node). This vessel, which can be recognized by the presence of septal perforating branches, arises from the right coronary artery (RCA) in 80% of the population and the left circumflex (LCx) in 10% of the population. Co-dominance of the arterial circulation is found in 10% of the population where the posterior interventricular artery is formed by both the RCA and LCx. The left main coronary artery or left main trunk (LMT) originates from the left coronary cusp and bifurcates to give rise to the left anterior descending (LAD) and left circumflex (LCx) coronary arteries. Occasionally, a third branch vessel, the ramus intermedius (RI) arises from the LMT. The LMT varies in length in many patients and in a small number of patients, the two major branch vessels arise from separate origins.

The left anterior descending coronary artery provides blood supply to the anterior wall of the left ventricle. As it courses through the anterior intraventricular groove it provides multiple septal branches to the interventricular septum and diagonal branches to the anterior lateral wall. The LAD then courses to the ventricular apex and in some patients wraps around the apex to supply a small amount of the posterior apex.

The left circumflex coronary artery courses around the lateral or left atrioventricular groove and gives rise to multiple marginal or lateral branches. The branches are termed obtuse marginal (OM) or lateral branches depending on institutional preference. OM branches are sequentially numbered (OM1, OM2, etc.) while lateral branches are termed based on the segment of the lateral wall they supply (high lateral, lateral, and posterior lateral). As the LCx courses the AV groove it also gives rise to several atrial branches, and occasionally the sino-atrial branch (40% of the population).

The right coronary artery arises from the right coronary cusp. This vessel follows the right AV groove and provides branches to the right ventricle. The most proximal branches of the RCA are the conus-branch which supplies the right ventricular outflow tract and a branch that supplies the sinoatrial (SA) node (60% of patients). The RCA then courses through the interventricular and gives rise to marginal branches and branches to the atrium. Manipulation of the coronary arteries in 3-dimensions via spacial reconstructions of the coronary arteries is helpful in interpreting coronary angiographic images.

## MAIN OBJECTIVE OF CORONARY ANGIOGRAPHY

1. Coronary luminal obstruction:
   - Guide revascularization decisions
   - Severity of luminal narrowing
   - Distribution of stenotic lesions
   - Identification of acute thrombotic lesion
2. Coronary blood flow
3. LV systolic and diastolic function, ejection fraction, and regional wall motion
4. Anomalous vessel
5. Coronary collateral circulation

The first attempts to visualize the coronary arteries in living humans were published in 1945 by Radner S, who used trans-sternal punctures to inject contrast material into the ascending aorta. High complication rate with poor results, the technique was abandoned. The first selective coronary angiogram was performed by Mason Sones in 1959 through the brachial cut-down technique. With the prior introduction of the Seldinger wire cannulation method for vascular cannulation percutaneous transfemoral catheterization technique was developed. Judkins, Amplatz, Abrams and others invented preformed catheters that could be passed with great ease from the femoral artery to the coronary ostium. Arterial access most commonly femoral, brachial or radial arteries can also be used. Catheter size depends on several patient variables including:

1. Aortic root size and shape
2. Aortic valve plane orientation
3. Angle of coronary ostial origin

Typically, left and right Judkins catheters are used to engage the left coronary artery (LCA) and the right coronary artery respectively.

Provides excellent delineation of coronary anatomy in vessels >400 um in diameter.

*Major deficiencies include:*

- Mainly shows the anatomy of the arterial lumen opposed to the wall of the artery.
- It is a 2D shadow of a 3D object.

### Explanation of Test to the Patient

The patient being examined or treated is usually awake during coronary catheterization, ideally with only local anesthesia, such as lidocaine and minimal general sedation, throughout the procedure. Performing the procedure with the patient awake is safer as the patient can immediately report any discomfort or problems and thereby facilitate rapid correction of any undesirable events. Medical monitors fail to give a comprehensive view of the patient's immediate well-being; how the patient feels is often a most reliable indicator of procedural safety. Death, myocardial infarction, stroke, serious ventricular arrhythmia, and major vascular complications, each occur in less than 1% of patients undergoing catheterization. However, though the imaging portion of the examination is often brief, because of setup and safety issues the patient is often in the lab for 20–45 minutes. Any of multiple technical difficulties, while not endangering the patient (indeed added to protect the patient's interests) can significantly increase the examination time.

### *Equipment required for the procedure*

Coronary catheterization is performed in a cardiac catheterization lab, usually located within a hospital. With current designs, the patient must lie relatively flat on a narrow, minimally padded, radiolucent (transparent to X-ray) table. The X-ray source and imaging camera equipment are on opposite sides of the patient's chest and freely move, under motorized control, around the patient's chest so images can be taken quickly from multiple angles. More advanced equipment, termed a bi-plane cath lab, uses two sets of X-ray source and imaging cameras, each free to move independently which allows two sets of images to be taken with each injection of radiocontrast agent (Figs 4.3 and 4.4).

## Standard Angiographic Views

For the beginner angiographer the anatomic landmarks formed by the spine, catheter and diaphragm, provide information to discern which tomographic view from which the image is obtained. In the left anterior oblique (LAO) view the catheter and spine are seen on the right side of the image, while in the right anterior oblique (RAO) they are found on the right. PA imaging places these landmarks in the center of the image. Cranial angulation can usually be distinguished from caudal angulation by the presence of the diaphragm. For cranial imaging, the patient should be asked to inspire to remove the diaphragmatic shadow from the image (Figs 4.5 and 4.6) .

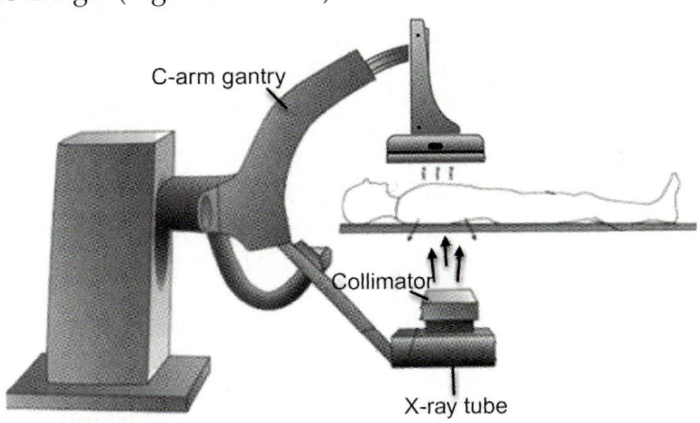


**Fig. 4.3:** Schematic of radiographic imaging system

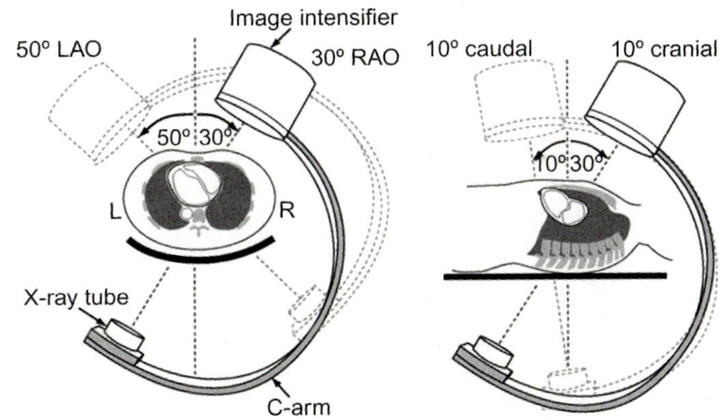


**Fig. 4.4:** Relationship among the patient, X-ray tube, and image intensifier during coronary angiography. LAO=left anterior oblique; RAO=right anterior oblique. The X-ray beam is generated by an X-ray tube. The beam passes through a collimator where lead apertures form and limit the beam. On intersection with the patient, most of the beam is reflected or absorbed. The remaining photons pass through the image intensifier. Thirty to sixty exposures are needed to give appearance of a live continuous image

## INDICATIONS

1. Acute ST-segment elevation myocardial infarction (STEMI) to identify and reperfuse the infarct-related artery
2. Acute STEMI who have received lytic or medical therapy and have-recurrent angina-heart failure-Arrhythmia or for risk stratification purposes
3. Non-ST-segment elevation myocardial infarction (NSTEMI) or unstable angina in whom an invasive management strategy is chosen
4. Evaluation of select stable angina patients with or without a prior, abnormal noninvasive test
5. Evaluation of certain 'high-risk' asymptomatic patients
6. Patients with chest pain syndromes and abnormal or nondiagnostic noninvasive tests
7. Preoperative evaluation for select patients undergoing noncardiac surgery
8. Preoperative evaluation for select patients undergoing cardiac surgery
9. Evaluation of heart failure syndromes to exclude significant coronary disease
10. Other conditions (hypertrophic obstructive cardiomyopathy, aortic dissection, and chest trauma)

## CONTRAINDICATIONS

These are listed in Table 4.1.

1. Patients who do not desire or who are not candidates for revascularization
2. Patients in whom revascularization is unlikely to improve quality/duration of life
3. As a screening test for CAD in asymptomatic patients
4. Routine angiography within 24 hours of lytic therapy in the absence of ongoing ischemia
5. Acute renal failure, marked electrolyte imbalance, or metabolic disarray

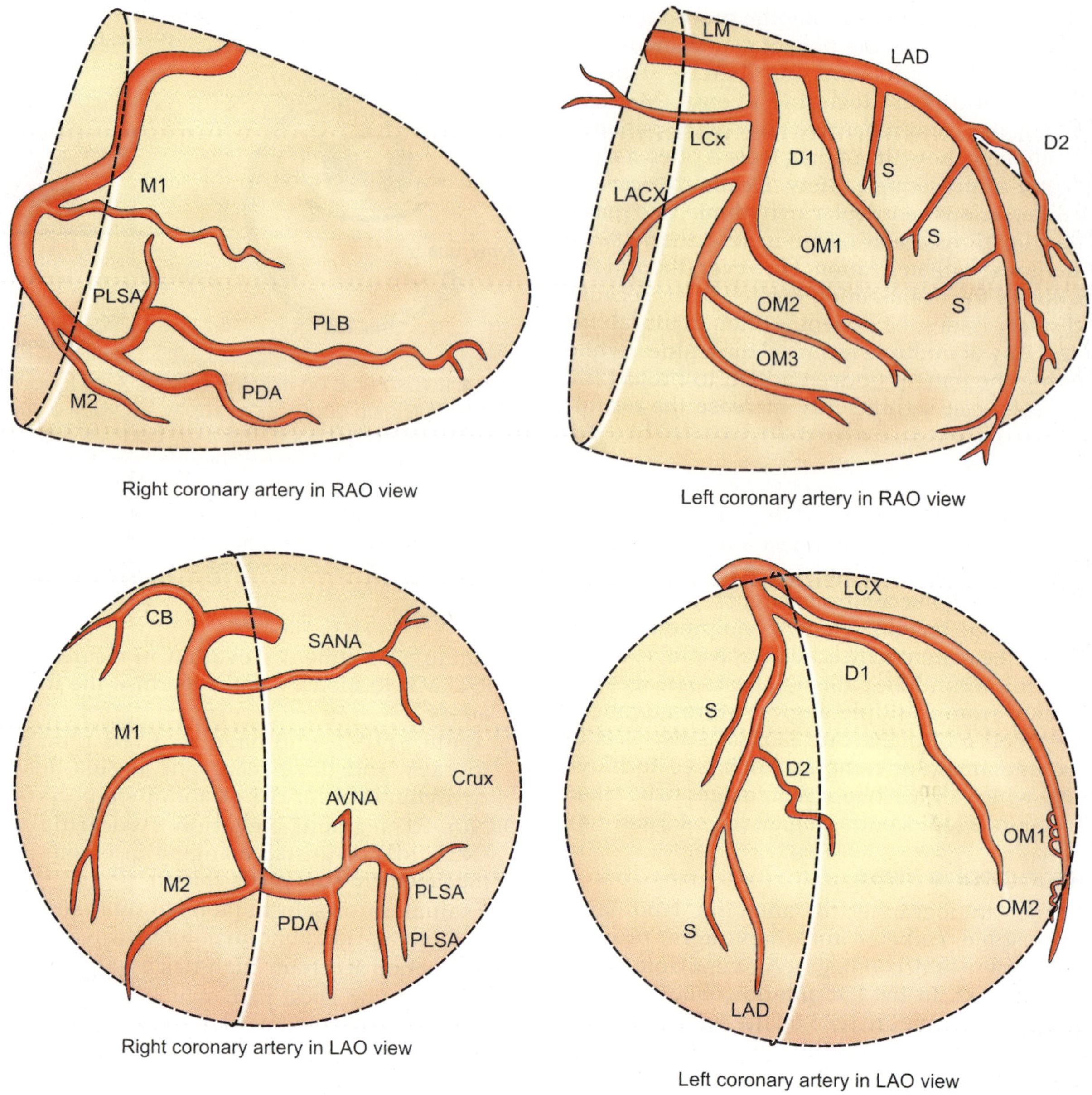


**Fig. 4.5:** Various branches of left and right major coronary arteries. LM=left main, SN=sinus node branch, D=diagnol, S=septal branches, LAD=left anterior descending, OM=obtuse marginal, RV=right-ventricular branch, AC=atrial circumflex, M=marginal, PDA=posterior descending artery, AVNA=atrioventricular nodal artery, LCX=left circumflex artery, SANA=Sinoatrial nodal artery

6. Active bleeding or severe coagulopathy
7. Prior cholesterol embolization syndrome or anaphylaxis to contrast
8. Active infection or unexplained fever
9. Decompensated respiratory status, heart failure, or uncontrolled hypertension
10. Changing mental status or inability to cooperate

### Catheters

Catheter selection for a routine left heart catheterization is generally straight forward. Most often, Judkins catheter types are most routinely used (Figs 4.7 and 4.8). For engagement of the left main coronary artery, a Judkins left size 4 (JL4) catheter will generally engaged the left coronary artery in most patients with relative ease. Increasing catheter size (JL5) for tall patients or patients with dilated aorta or decreasing size (JL3.5) in small patients is sometimes required. Engagement of the LMT is usually most straightforward in the LAO projection. For extremely dilated roots or anomalous arteries other catheters such as Amplatz catheters can be used. For the right coronary artery, a Judkins right size 4 (JR4) is most often used. The right coronary artery is engaged in the LAO projection. Usually slow clockwise rotation of the JR4 in the aortic root will engage the ostium of the RCA. Specialized catheters are available to engage anomalous origins of coronary arteries and saphenous and internal mammary artery bypass grafts. Once the artery is engaged, it is important to examine the pressure waveform. Normally, the waveform should mimic

**Table 4.1:** Relative contraindications to coronary angiography

- Acute renal failure
- Chronic renal failure secondary to diabetes
- Active gastrointestinal bleeding
- Unexplained fever, which may be due to infection
- Untreated active infection
- Acute stroke
- Severe anemia
- Severe uncontrolled hypertension
- Severe symptomatic electrolyte imbalance
- Severe lack of cooperation by patient due to psychological or severe systemic illness
- Severe concomitant illness that drastically shortens life expectancy or increases risk of therapeutic interventions
- Refusal of patient to consider definitive therapy such as PTCA, CABG, or valve replacement
- Digitalis intoxication
- Documented anaphylactoid reaction to angiographic contrast media
- Severe peripheral vascular disease limiting vascular access
- Decompensated congestive heart failure or acute pulmonary edema
- Severe coagulopathy
- Aortic valve endocarditis

PTCA=percutaneous transluminal coronary angioplasty; CABG= coronary artery bypass graft.

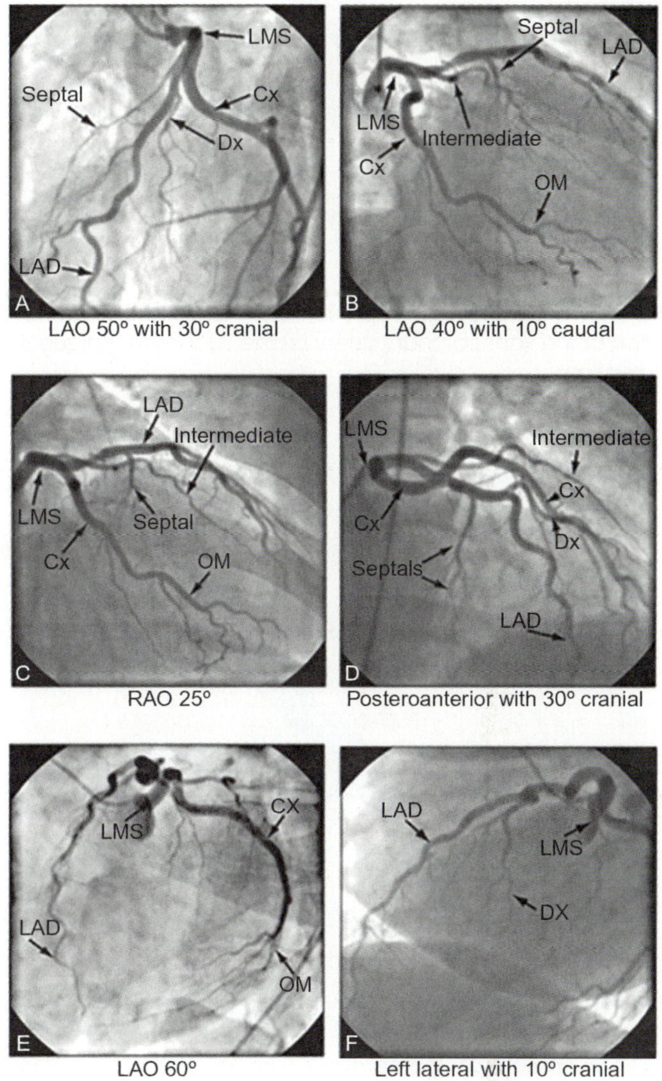


**Fig. 4.6:** (A–F) Angiography of the left coronary arterial system. Cx=circumflex coronary artery, Dx=diagonal coronary artery, LAD=left anterior descending coronary artery, LAO=left anterior oblique projection, LMS=left main stem coronary artery, OM=obtuse marginal coronary artery; RAO=right anterior oblique projection

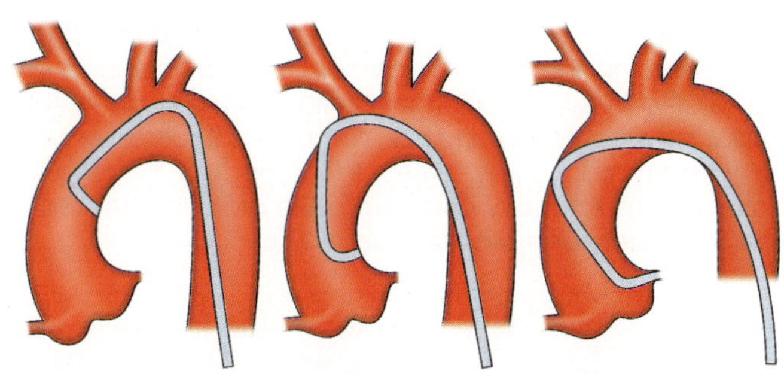

**Fig. 4.7:** Selective catheterization of the left coronary artery by the Judkins technique. In LAO position,the catheter is rotated so that it appears unfolded and enface; it is then slowly advanced until it engages the left coronary orifice. A size 4 (4 cm curve) catheter is adequate for most patients, but with moderate or severe aortic dilatation, a size 5 or 6 catheter may be required

aortic root pressure. Dampening or ventricularization of the pressure waveform may indicate over engagement of the catheter or significant vessel stenosis. Extreme care should be taken before instillation of contrast medium without normal pressure waveforms.

## Technique in Coronary Angiography

### *Vascular Access* (Figs 4.9 to 4.12)

Common femoral arterial access is the most common arterial access for performing left heart catheterization. The original catheterization procedure was performed via brachial access. This site is still commonly used in patients with lower extremity peripheral access issues. Arm access also facilitates internal mammary access, especially in patients with tortuous innominant or subclavian arteries. Radial artery access is also used commonly in some practice settings. Before radial access is performed, competence of the radial artery arch should be assessed with the Allen test. Use of pulse oximetry can facilitate interpretation of the test. Anatomic landmarks are used to identify the correct site of arterial puncture.

For the femoral artery access, the femoral head provides the best visible landmark. Arterial puncture at this site remains below the inguinal ligament, is generally above the bifurcation of the superfical femoral and deep femoral arteries, and allows for hemostasis. It is recommended that this site should be observed under floroscopy in any patient prior to access. In obese patients the inguinal skin crease is generally too low. After the administration of subcutaneous anesthetic, an 18G Cook® needle is used to puncture the

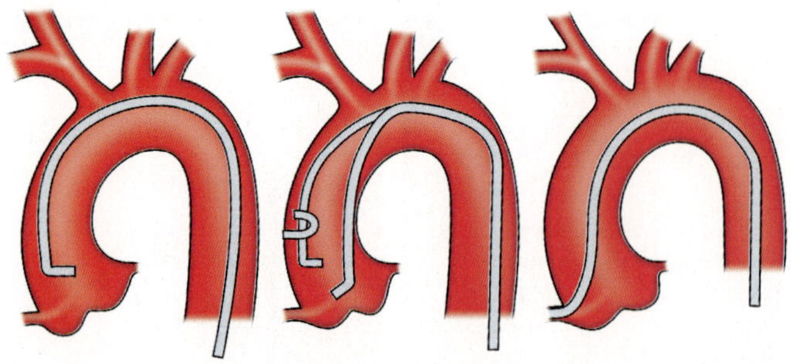

Fig. 4.8: Diagrammatic representation of selective catheterization of the right coronary artery by the Judkins technique (LAO projection)

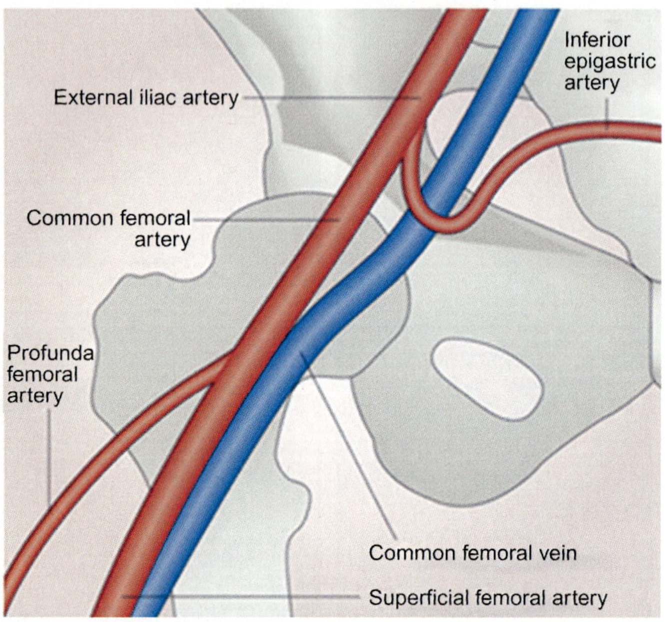


Fig. 4.9: Anatomy of the common femoral artery. The common femoral artery is the terminal branch of the external iliac artery, and provides the main arterial supply to the lower limb. The common femoral artery enters the femoral triangle deep to the midpoint of the inguinal ligament, posterior to the deep fascia, and overlying the head of the femur bone. These features facilitate arterial puncture, but necessitate deep pressure for compression hemostasis. At this point, the artery has adiameter of 7–10 mm and lies within the femoral sheath close to the common femoral vein and the femoral nerve and its branches. Just proximal to the inguinal ligament, the external iliac artery gives off the clinically important inferior epigastric artery, which courses superomedially and anastomoses with distal end of the internal mammary artery. Inferior to the neck of the femur, the common femoral artery divides into the profunda femoris and superficial artery end branches

front wall of the artery. This technique is known as the modified Seldinger technique and prevents posterior arterial bleeding or venous communication from the puncture. Complications from arterial access include arterial dissection, AV fistula formation, retroperitoneal hemmorrhage, and pseudoaneurysm formation. Once access is obtained, the Cook needle is steadied while the artery is accessed with a wire through the lumen of the Cook

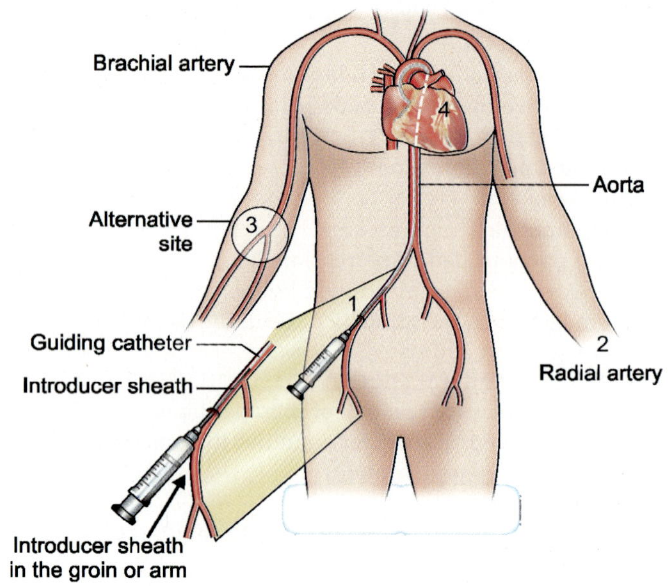


Fig. 4.10: Different catheter routes of cardiac catheterization including coronary angiography. Catheter in—(1) groin, (2) radial artery, (3) brachial artery, and (4) heart

needle. The Cook needle is then removed and a sheath is inserted into the artery. Under floroscopy, catheters are then introduced using an 0.35 J-tipped guide wire into the aortic root. The catheters are then attached to a 3-way manifold. Manifold used allows for continuous pressure monitoring, saline flush instillation, and contrast administration through the catheter tip (Figs 4.9–4.12).

## LEFT CORONARY SYSTEM

### LEFT CORONARY ARTERY

The left main coronary artery gives rise to the left anterior descending artery and the left circumflex coronary artery. Complete visualization of these arteries and their branches requires care and rigor to ensure complete anatomical documentation. Often bifurcations and vessel foreshortening and overlap cause errors in stenosis estimation. There are no steadfast rules in which tomographic views are most useful. Generally, for circumflex and proximal epicardial visualization the caudal views are most useful. For LAD and LAD/diagonal bifurcation visualization the cranial views are most useful. Overall, if there is not a significant limitation on contrast utilization, standard 'around the world' angiography using a selection of the following angiographic views will document left coronary anatomy (Figs 4.13–4.20).

- Left main stem
  - Best seen in posteroanterior (PA) view or very shallow oblique projection (either RAO or LAO)
- Left anterior descending coronary artery
  - RAO or PA view
  - Steep LAO view (40°) with severe cranial angulation (40°) for LAD and diagonal bifurcation

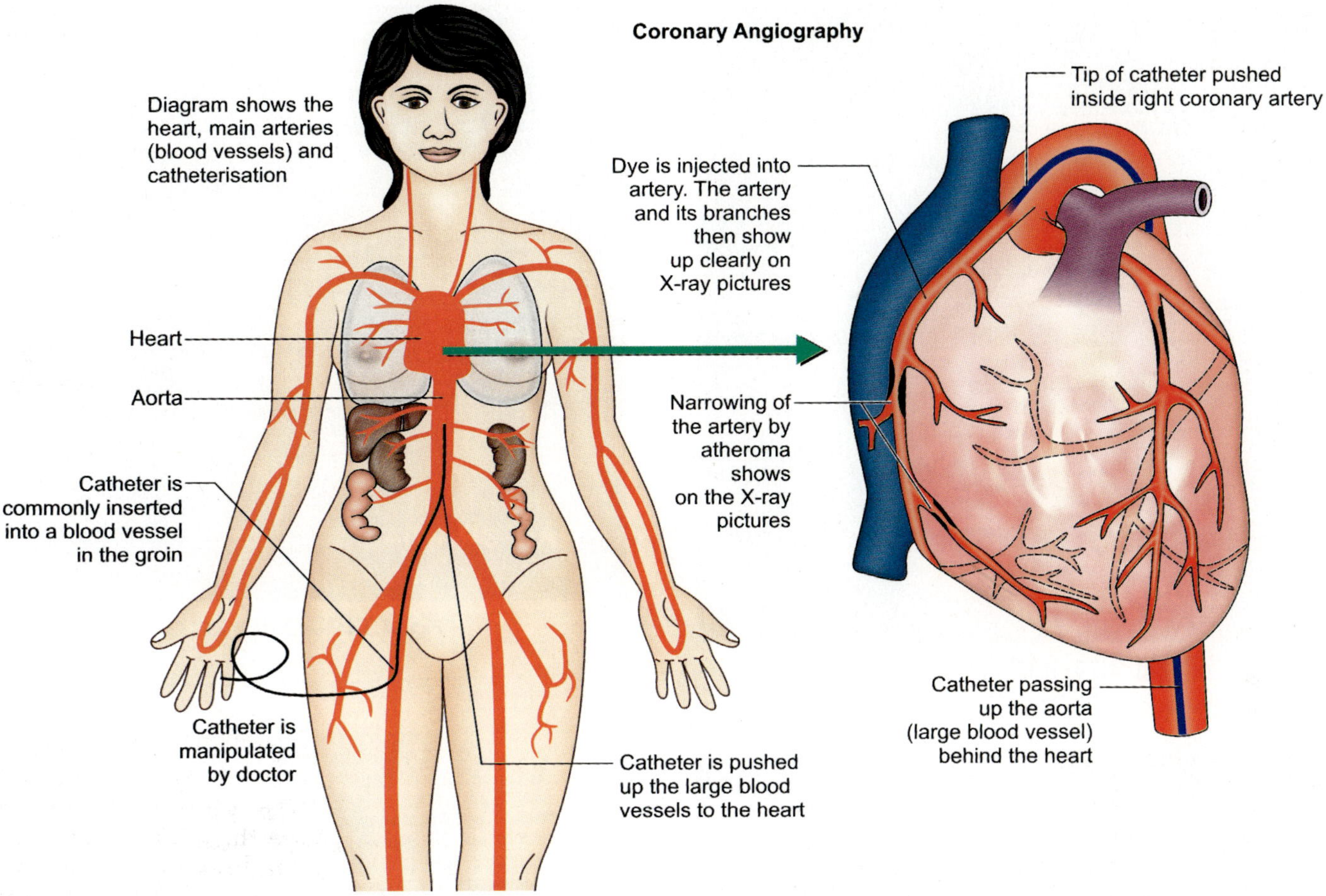


**Fig. 4.11:** Diagrammatic representation of procedure in coronary angiogram

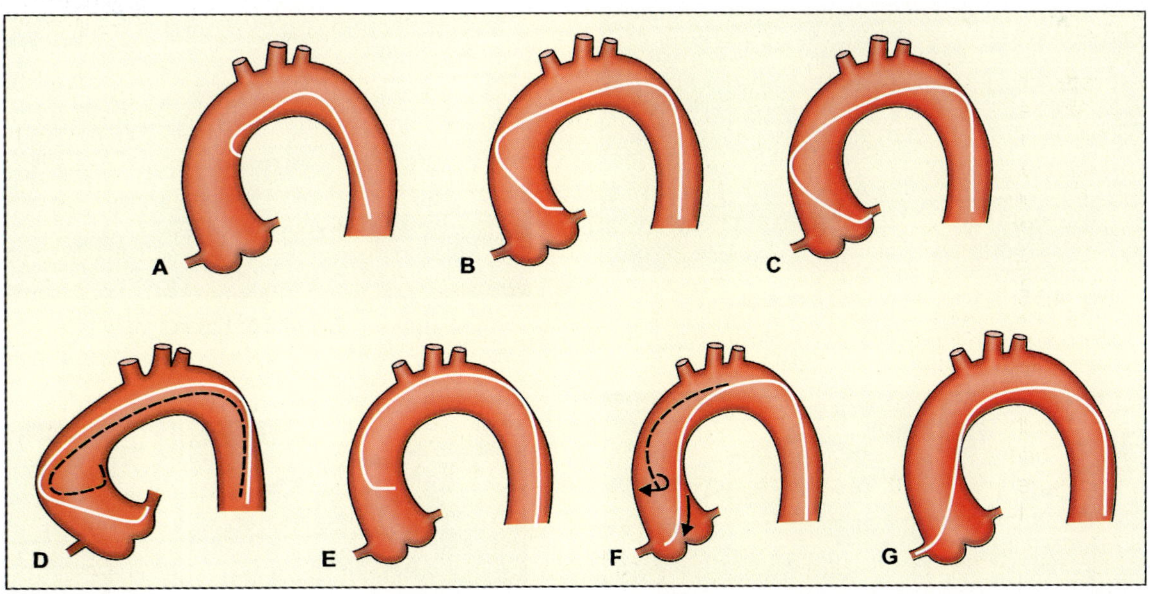


**Fig. 4.12:** (A–G) Left and right Judkins catheters engagement at the mouth of left and right coronary arteries in obtaining coronary angiogram

- LAO 40°, caudal 40° (spider view) for bifurcation of LMS, proximal circumflex and LAD and at times distal LAD

- Circumflex coronary artery
  - RAO 20° or 30° angulation with 20°–30° caudal angulation

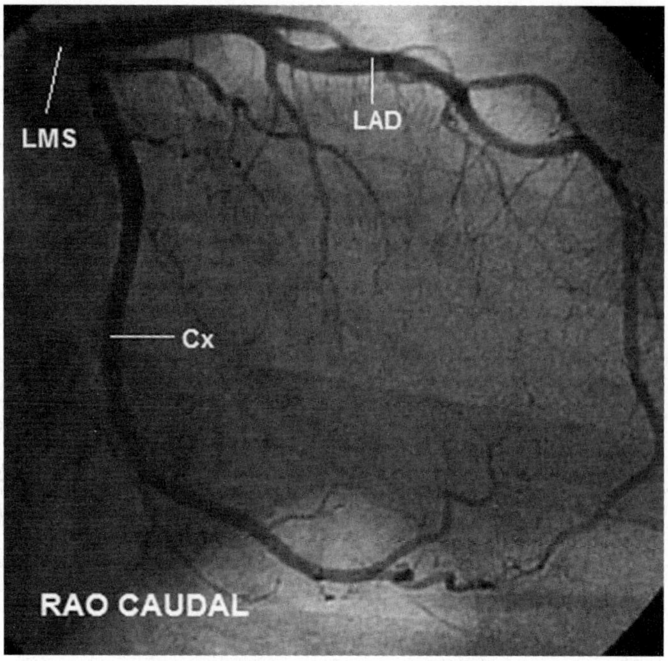


**Fig. 4.13:** RAO caudal-LCA

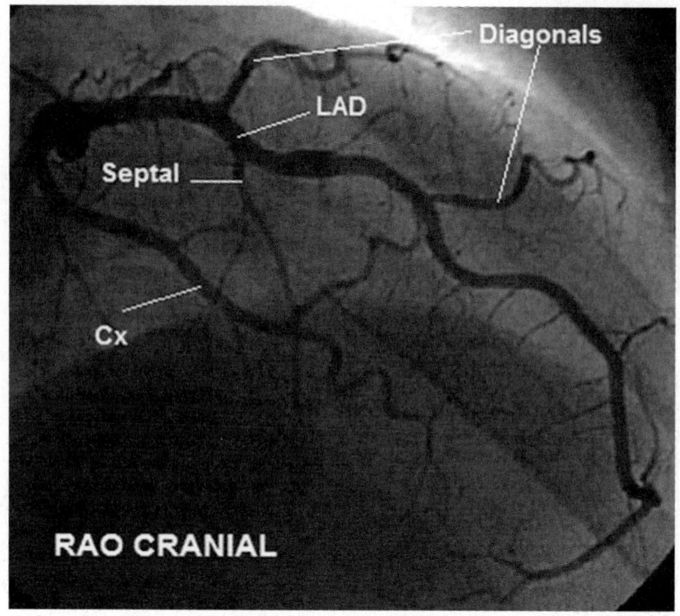


**Fig. 4.14:** RAO cranial-LCA

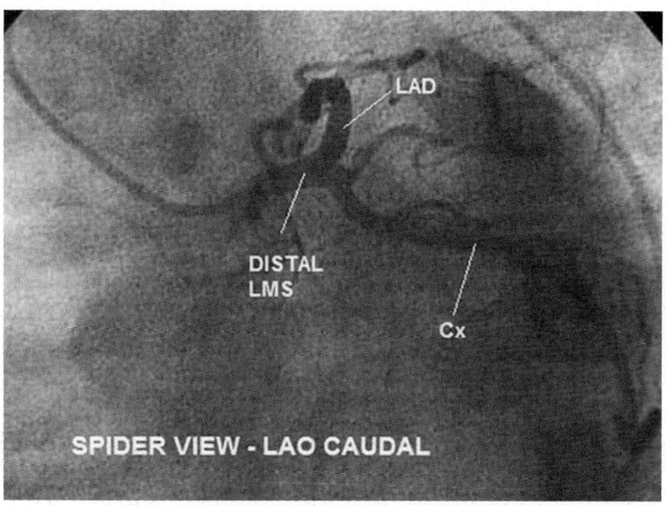


**Fig. 4.15:** Spider view-LAO caudal

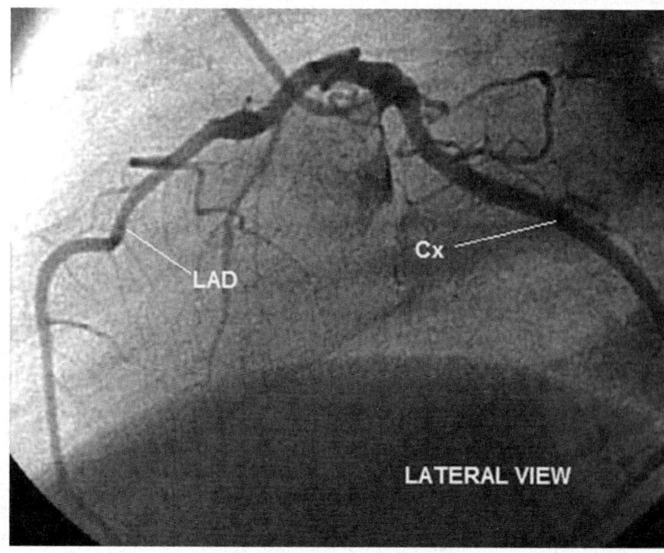


**Fig. 4.16:** Lateral view-LCA

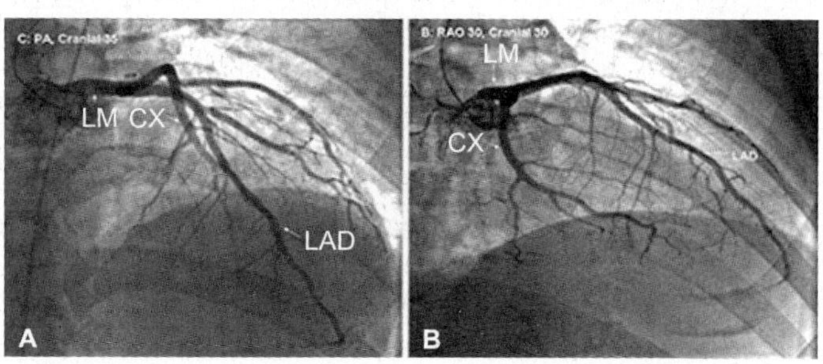


**Fig. 4.17:** (A) Normal left coronary artery viewed in the PA projection with 35° cranial angulation, (B) Left coronary angiogram viewed with 30° RAO and 30° cranial angulation delineating the course of the LAD

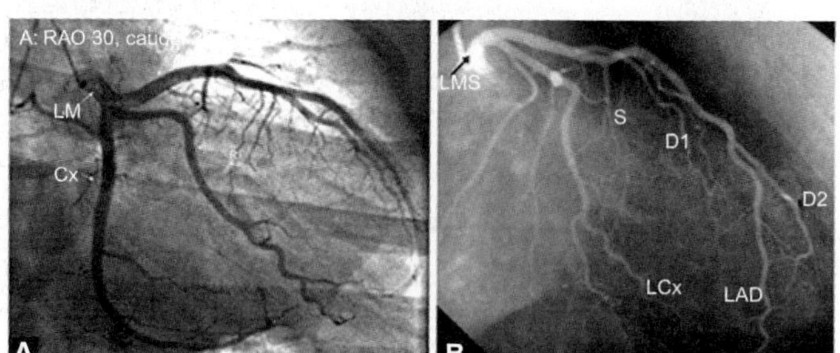


**Fig. 4.18:** (A) Selective left coronary angiogram viewed with 30° RAO and 20° caudal angulation viewing the circumflex artery, (B) LCA-RAO (30°) straight LCA-RAO (30°) straight

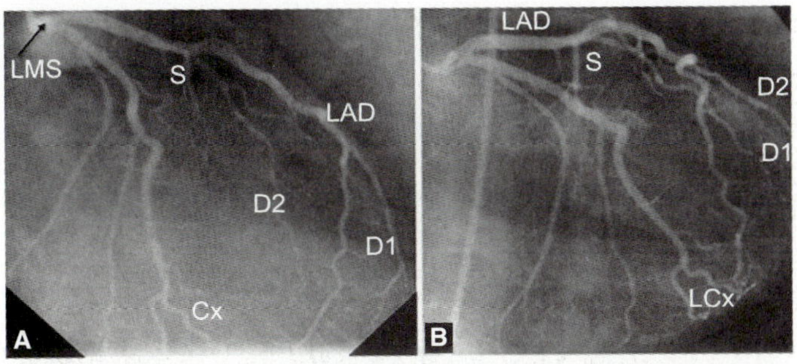


**Fig. 4.19:** (A) LCA-RAO (30°) caudal (30°),(B) LCA-AP caudal (30°)

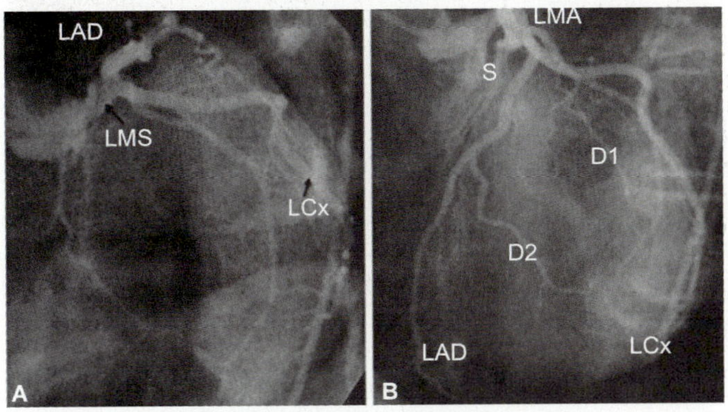


**Fig. 4.20:** (A) LCA-LAO (50°) caudal (30°), (B) LCA-LAO (60°) straight

## RIGHT CORONARY SYSTEM

### RIGHT CORONARY ARTERY

The right coronary artery is engaged in the LAO position (Figs 4.21–4.23). Initial angiographic imaging of the RCA in this view (LAO 30) gives the best view of significant ostial and proximal RCA disease. The mid-RCA is best visualized in the straight RAO 30 position.

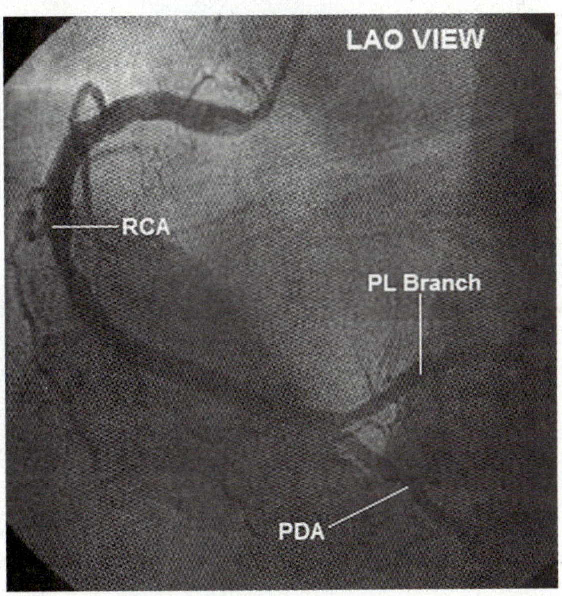


**Fig. 4.21:** LAO view—RCA

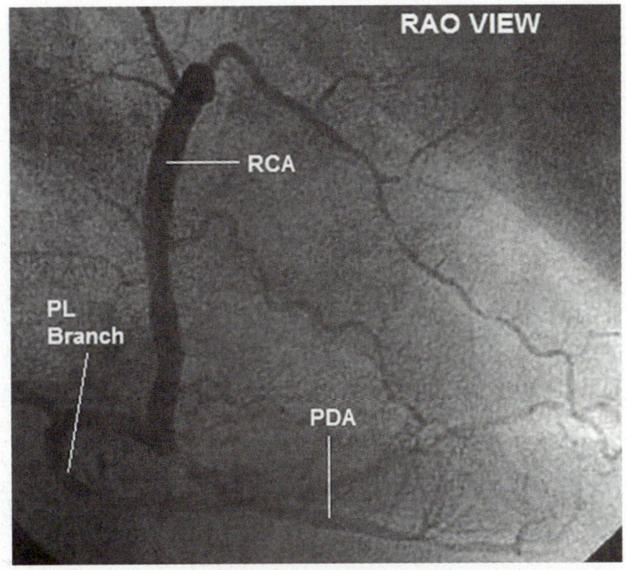


**Fig. 4.22:** RAO view—RC

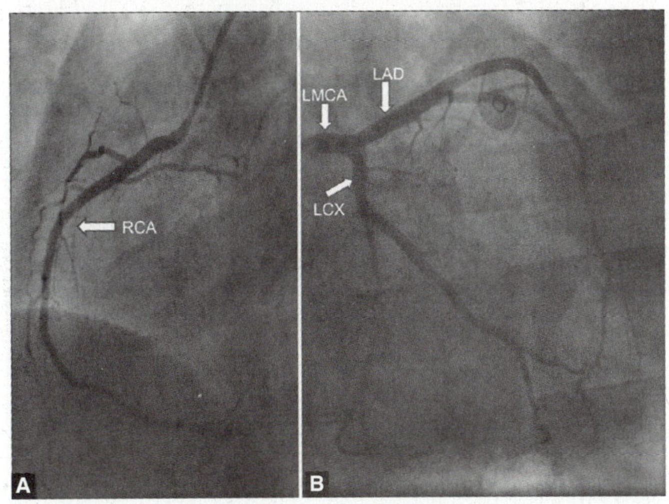


**Fig. 4.23:** Coronary angiogram showing normal filling of (A) right and (B) left coronary arteries. RCA=right coronary artery, LMCA=left main coronary artery, LAD=left anterior descending artery, LCX=left circumflex artery

### COMPLICATIONS IN CORONARY ANGIOGRAPHY

Coronary arteriography is generally a safe procedure (Figs 4.24–4.30). The overall incidence of complications and mortality increases directly with:

1. Extent of coronary artery disease, particularly left main coronary stenosis
2. Presence of coexistent significant valvular disease
3. Reduced ventricular ejection fraction
4. Reduced functional state
5. Advancing age

This include:

- Arrhythmia
- Coronary artery dissection or embolization

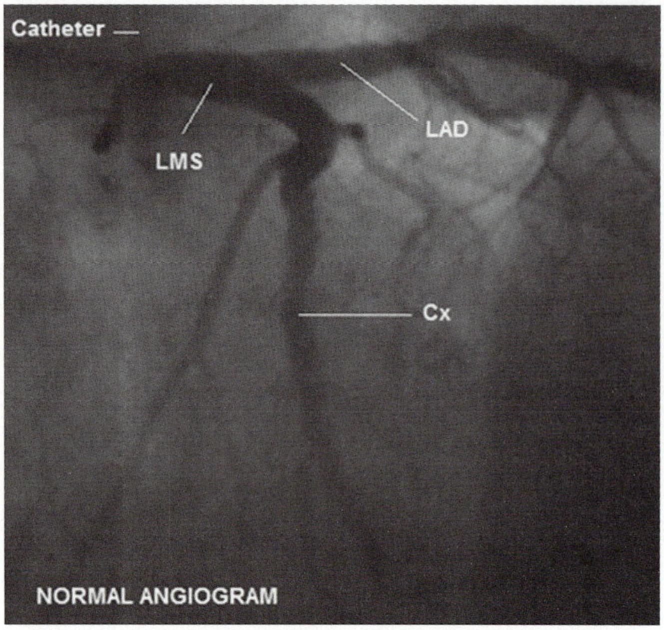


**Fig. 4.24:** Normal angiogram

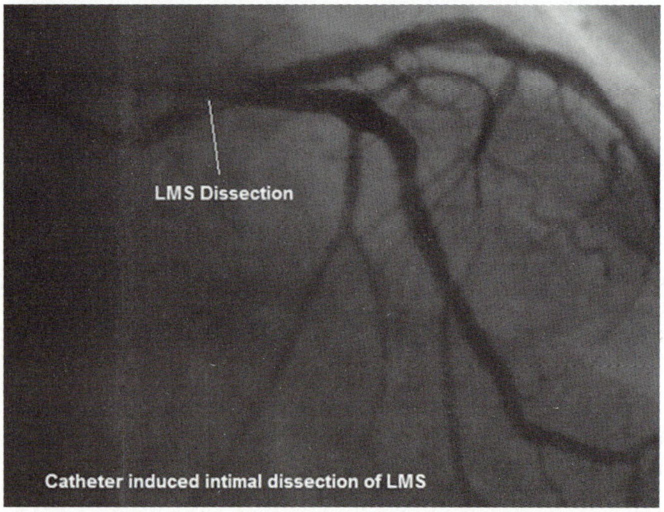


**Fig. 4.25:** Catheter-induced intimal dissection of left main artery

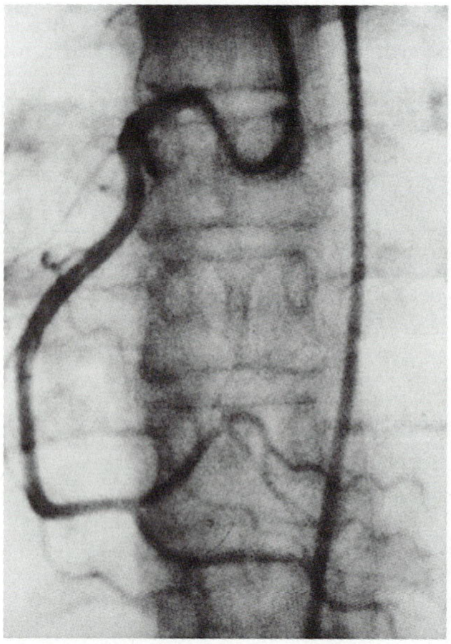

**Fig. 4.26:** RC arteriogram in frontal projection showing a fine line of radiolucency within the artery, suggesting a coronary arterial dissecting aneurysm

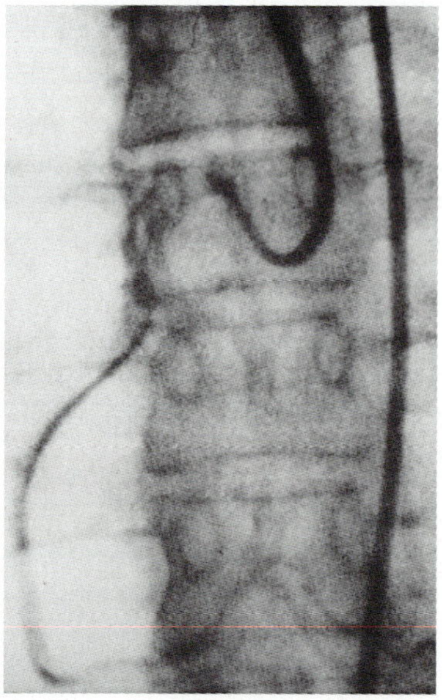

**Fig. 4.27:** RC arteriogram demonstrating slower flow in the false channel (dissection) than in the principal one

- Myocardial infarction
- Heart failure
- Death
- Stroke
- Contrast toxicity/reaction:
  i. Hypotension and myocardial depression
  ii. ST/T wave changes
  iii. Allergic reaction (urticaria, bronchospasm, angioedema, laryngospasm, and anaphylaxis)
- Renal failure
- Vascular complications:
  i. Hematoma, AV fistula, and pseudoaneurysm
  ii. Local femoral or brachial artery injury from arterial cannulation and compression for hemostasis
- Neurologic:
  i. Ulnar nerve compression from prolonged procedures
  ii. Transient ischemic attacks and strokes: mostly embolic from the aorta

## ACC and AHA Update Guidelines for Coronary Angiography

The American College of Cardiology (ACC) and the American Heart Association (AHA) have updated their guidelines for coronary angiography (Figs 4.31–4.36). The executive summary and recommendations are published

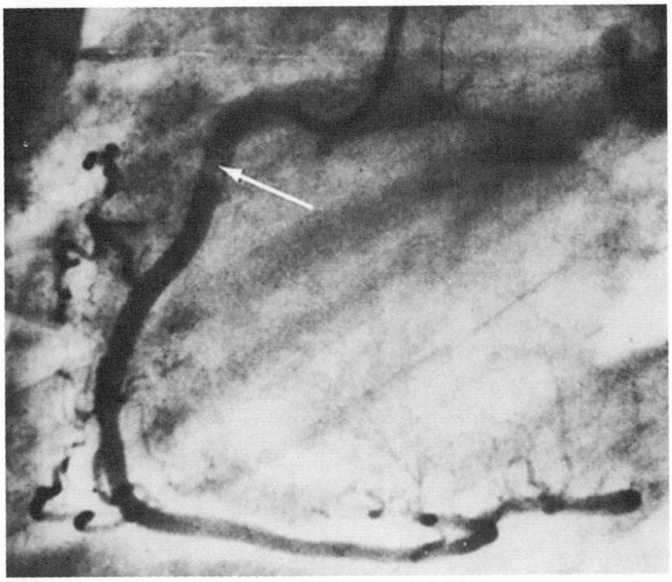

**Fig. 4.28:** LAO view of RC arteriogram. Evidence of embolic material probably from a catheter thrombus, or less likely, from an atherosclerotic plaque; large RCA

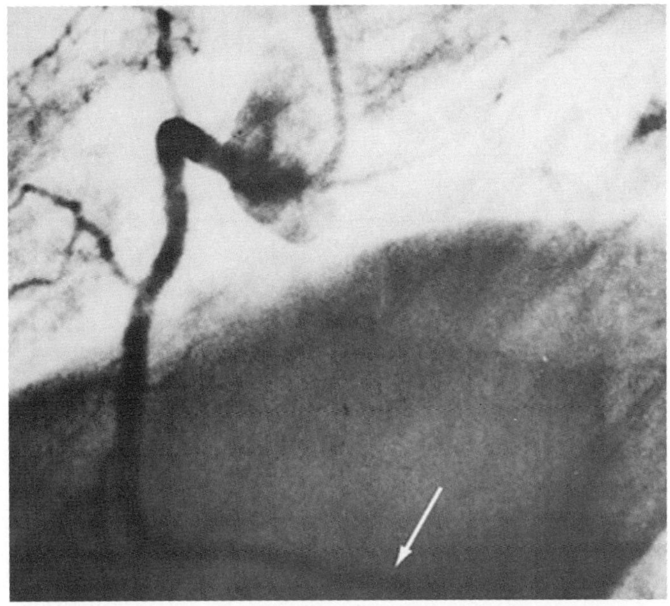

**Fig. 4.29:** LAO view of RC arteriogram. Repeat injection now shows occlusion (arrow) of the PDA filling defect (arrow) can be seen clearly and was observed to migrate toward the periphery

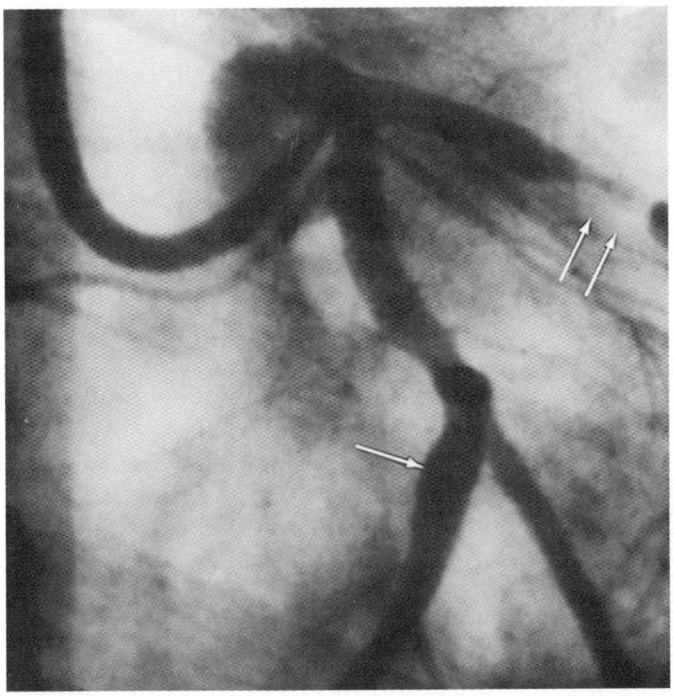

**Fig. 4.30:** Air embolism magnification coronary arteriography of a patient with localized stenosis of the LAD (double arrow). A small air bubble can be seen migrating through the Cx (arrow)

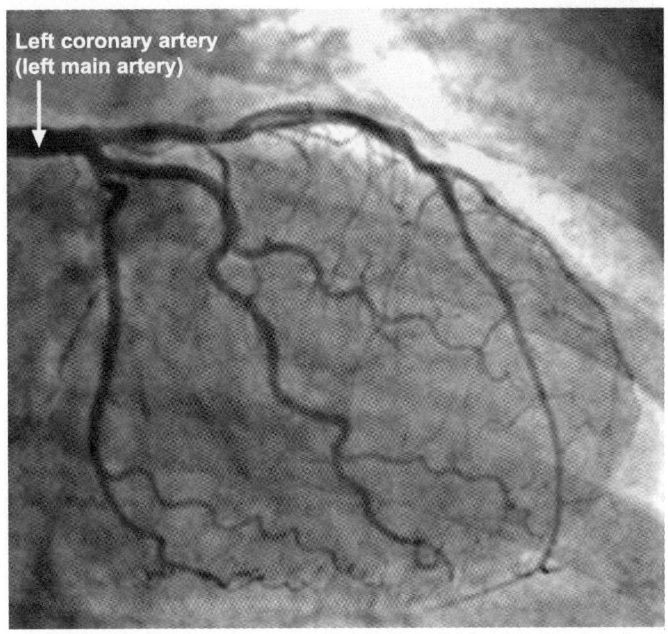


**Fig. 4.31:** Left coronary angiography showing left main coronary artery

in the May 4th, 1999, issue of Circulation. The entire guidelines are published in the May 1999 issue of the Journal of the American College of Cardiology. The ACC/AHA coronary angiography guidelines represent an update of the 1987 guidelines. In addition to reviewing the previous guidelines, the 12-member ACC/AHA Committee on coronary angiography also conducted a search of the pertinent literature for the previous 10 years. The weight of evidence in support of each recommendation was then ranked into three categories—(A) the presence of multiple randomized clinical trials; (B) the presence of a single randomized trial or nonrandomized studies; and (C) expert consensus.

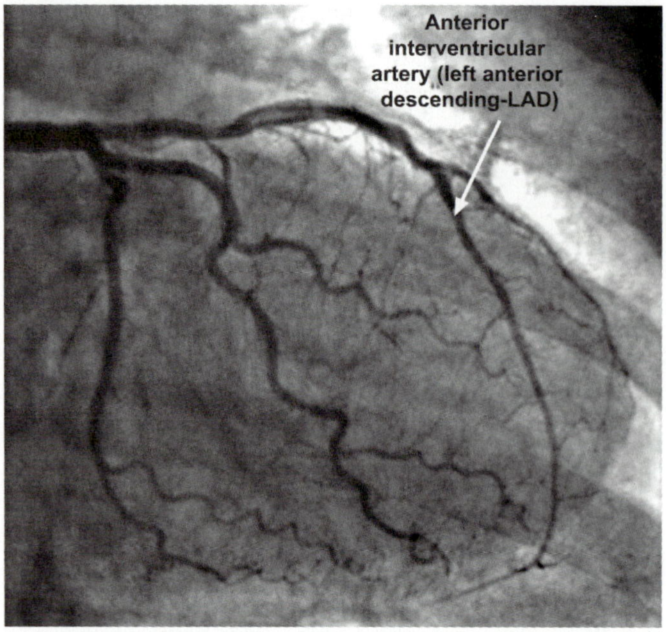


**Fig. 4.32:** Left coronary angiography showing left anterior descending artery

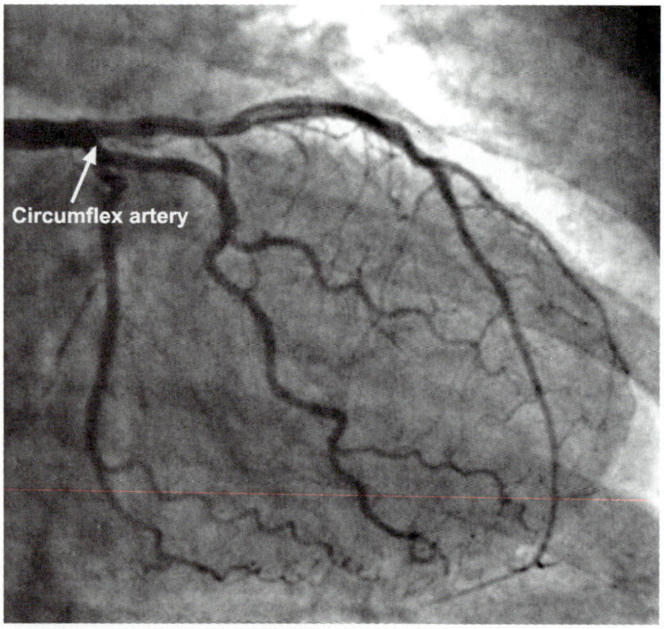


**Fig. 4.33:** Left coronary angiography showing circumflex artery

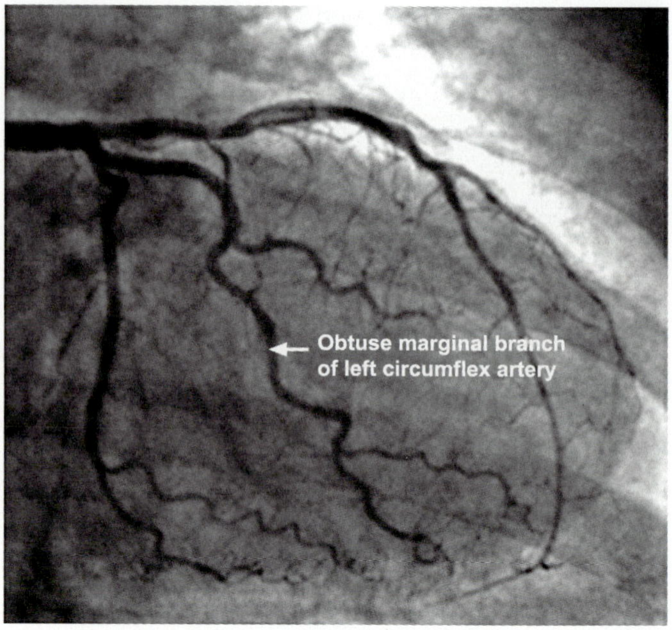


**Fig. 4.34:** Left coronary angiography showing obtuse marginal branch of left coronary artyery

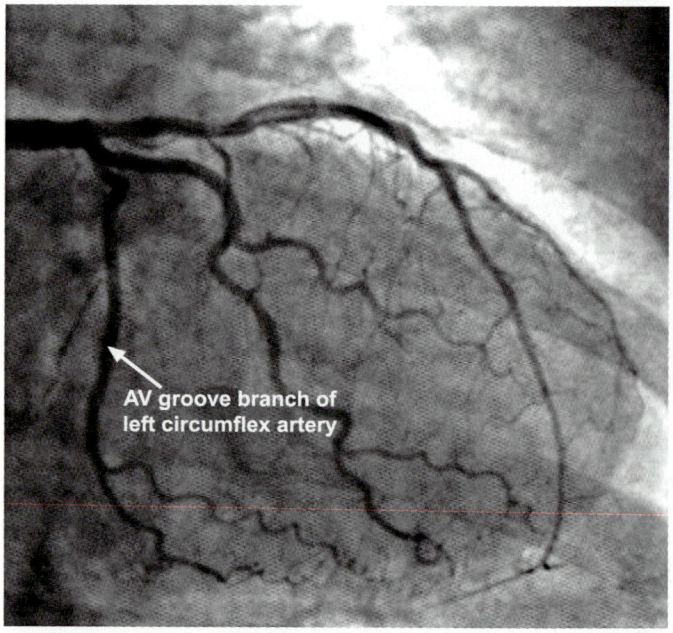


**Fig. 4.35:** Left coronary angiography showing AV groove branch of left coronary artyery

### The Recommendations are also Classified on the Basis of Conditions for which Coronary Angiography has Demonstrated Usefulness/Efficacy.

The definitions of these categories are as follows:

- **Class I:** Conditions for which there is evidence and/or general agreement that this procedure is useful and effective
- **Class II:** Conditions for which there is conflicting evidence and/or a divergence of opinion about the usefulness/efficacy of the procedure
- **Class IIa:** The weight of evidence/opinion is in favor of usefulness/efficacy
- **Class IIb:** Usefulness/efficacy is less well established by evidence/opinion

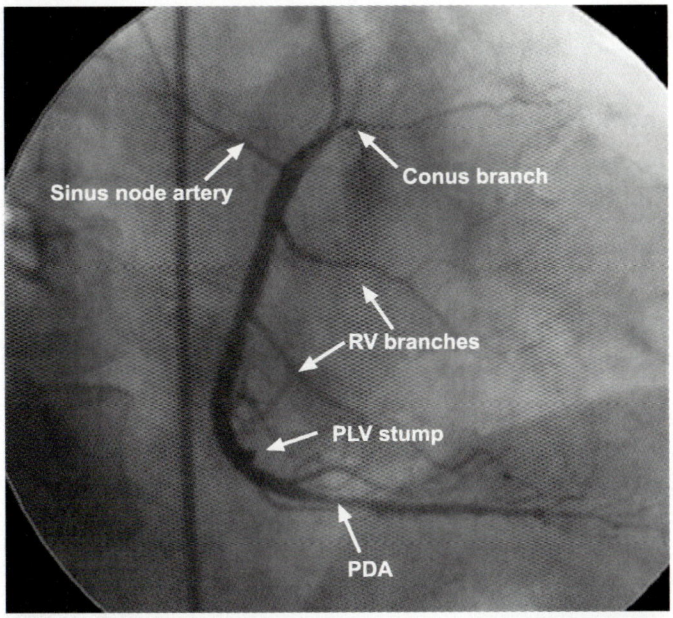


**Fig. 4.36:** Angiogram showing branches of the right coronary artery as indicated on the skiagram

- **Class III:** Conditions for which there is evidence and/or general agreement that the procedure is not useful/effective and in some cases may be harmful.

## Recommendations for Coronary Angiography When Coronary Artery Disease is Suspected

The algorithm on the following page gives a scheme for the noninvasive evaluation of a patient with suspected coronary artery disease. The following is an excerpt of the recommendations for coronary angiography in the evaluation of patients with known or suspected coronary artery disease who are asymptomatic or have stable angina.

### *Class I*

1. Canadian Cardiovascular Society (CCS) class III and class IV angina on medical treatment (level of evidence: B)
2. High-risk criteria on noninvasive testing regardless of angina severity (level of evidence: A)
3. Patients who have been successfully resuscitated from sudden cardiac death or have sustained (more than 30 seconds) monomorphic ventricular tachycardia or nonsustained (less than 30 seconds) polymorphic ventricular tachycardia (level of evidence: B).

### *Class IIa*

1. CCS class III or IV angina, which improves to class I or II with medical therapy (level of evidence: C)
2. Serial noninvasive testing with identical testing protocols, at the same level of medical therapy, showing progressively worsening abnormalities (level of evidence: C).
3. Patients with angina and suspected coronary disease who because of disability, illness or physical challenge, cannot be adequately risk-stratified by other means (level of evidence: C)
4. CCS class I or II angina with intolerance to adequate medical therapy or with failure to respond, or patients who have recurrence of symptoms during adequate medical therapy (level of evidence: C)
5. Individuals whose occupation involves the safety of others (e.g. pilots, bus drivers) who have abnormal but not high-risk stress test results or multiple clinical features that suggest high risk (level of evidence: C).

### *Class IIb*

1. CCS class I or II angina with demonstrable ischemia but no high-risk criteria on noninvasive testing (level of evidence: C)
2. An asymptomatic man or postmenopausal woman without known coronary heart disease with two or more major clinical risk factors and abnormal, but not high-risk criteria on noninvasive testing (performed for indications stated in the ACC/AHA noninvasive testing guidelines) (level of evidence: C)
3. Asymptomatic patients with prior myocardial infarction with normal resting left ventricular function and ischemia on noninvasive testing but without high-risk criteria (level of evidence: C)
4. Periodic evaluation after cardiac transplantation (level of evidence: C)
5. Candidate for liver, lung or renal transplant 40 years of age or older as part of the evaluation for transplantation (level of evidence: C).

### *Class III*

1. Angina in patients who prefer to avoid revascularization even though it might be appropriate (level of evidence: C)
2. Angina in patients who are not candidates for coronary revascularization or in whom revascularization is not likely to improve the quality or duration of life (level of evidence: C)
3. As a screening test for coronary artery disease in asymptomatic patients (level of evidence: C)
4. After coronary artery bypass grafting or angioplasty when there is no evidence of ischemia on noninvasive testing, unless there is informed consent for research purposes (level of evidence: C)
5. Coronary calcification on fluoroscopy, electron-beam computed tomography or other screening tests without criteria listed above (level of evidence: C).

## *Coronary Angiography for Specific Conditions*

### *Known or suspected CAD**

Coronary atherosclerosis is a slowly progressive process that can be clinically inapparent for long periods of time. Coronary disease often becomes clinically evident because of the occurrence of symptoms, such as angina or those associated with MI. Patients with known coronary artery disease (CAD) are those in whom the disease has been documented by either angiography or MI (i.e. using WHO criteria). 'Suspected coronary disease' means that a patient's symptoms or other clinical characteristics suggest a high likelihood for significant CAD and its related adverse outcomes but that evidence of CAD has not yet been documented as defined above (Figs 4.37–4.53).

Patients may develop symptoms at one point in time but may become asymptomatic thereafter as the result of a change in the disease or as the result of therapy. For instance, many patients are asymptomatic after an uncomplicated MI, as patients with mild angina, can be rendered asymptomatic by medications. The severity of clinical presentations and the degree of provokable ischemia on noninvasive testing are the principal factors used in determining the appropriateness of coronary angiography. Although the extent of coronary disease defined by coronary angiography does predict outcome, use of coronary angiography as a 'screening tool' in unselected populations is neither prudent nor cost-effective. The same can be stated regarding the routine use of exercise testing, radionuclide imaging and stress echocardiography in unselected patients. With only a few exceptions, coronary angiography is not clearly indicated in asymptomatic

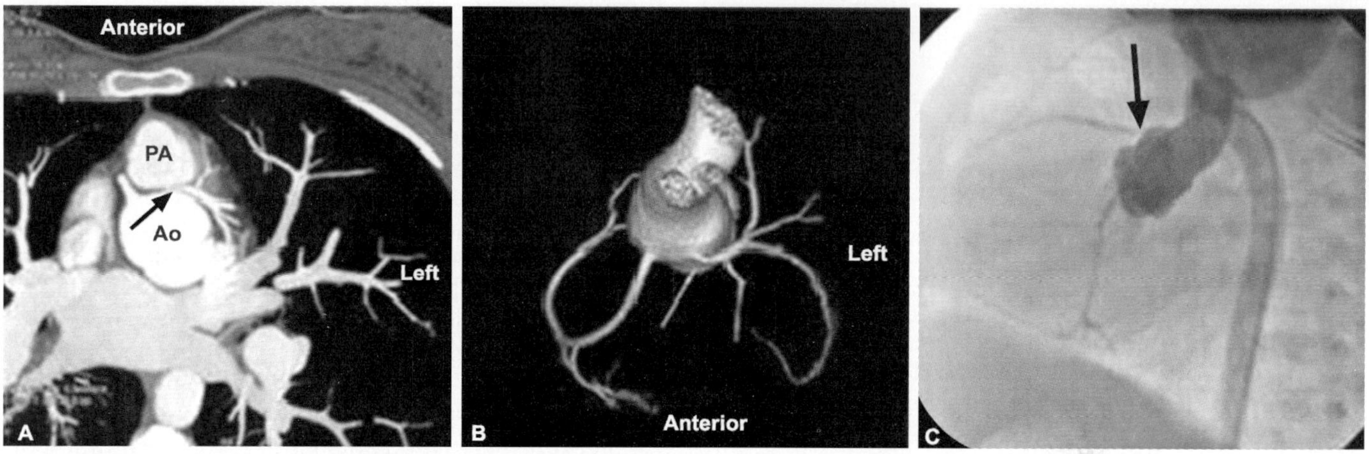


**Fig. 4.37:** Ostial stenosis of the left main coronary artery. Axial cross-section (A) and 3-dimensional reconstructed image in anterosuperior orientation, (B) showing a tight stenosis (arrow) at the ostium of the left coronary artery. Please note that the left ostium is reimplanted at an anterior 12 o'clock position so that it is localized between the great arteries. (C) corresponding invasive aortography showing the tight stenosis of the left coronary artery ostium

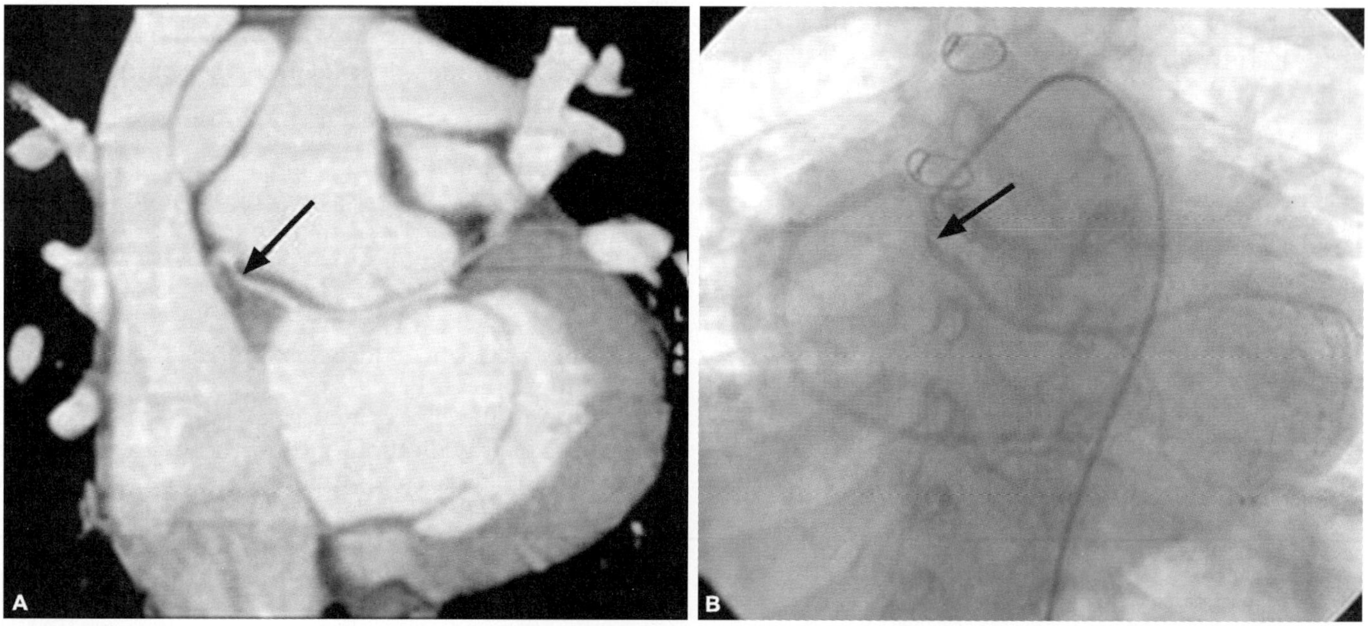


**Fig. 4.38:** Stretching of the circumflex artery. Oblique multiplanar reconstruction (A) showing the origin of the right coronary artery in a child presenting with a Yacoub type D coronary distribution. The left circumflex artery arises from the right neosinus and follows a long retroaortic course with substantial stretching of its proximal segment (arrow). A neosinus had been surgically created to treat a stenosis of the right ostium, (B) Corresponding invasive angiogram: selective catheterization of the right neosinus, showing the right coronary artery and the stenosis (arrow) of the proximal segment of the retroaortic circumflex artery

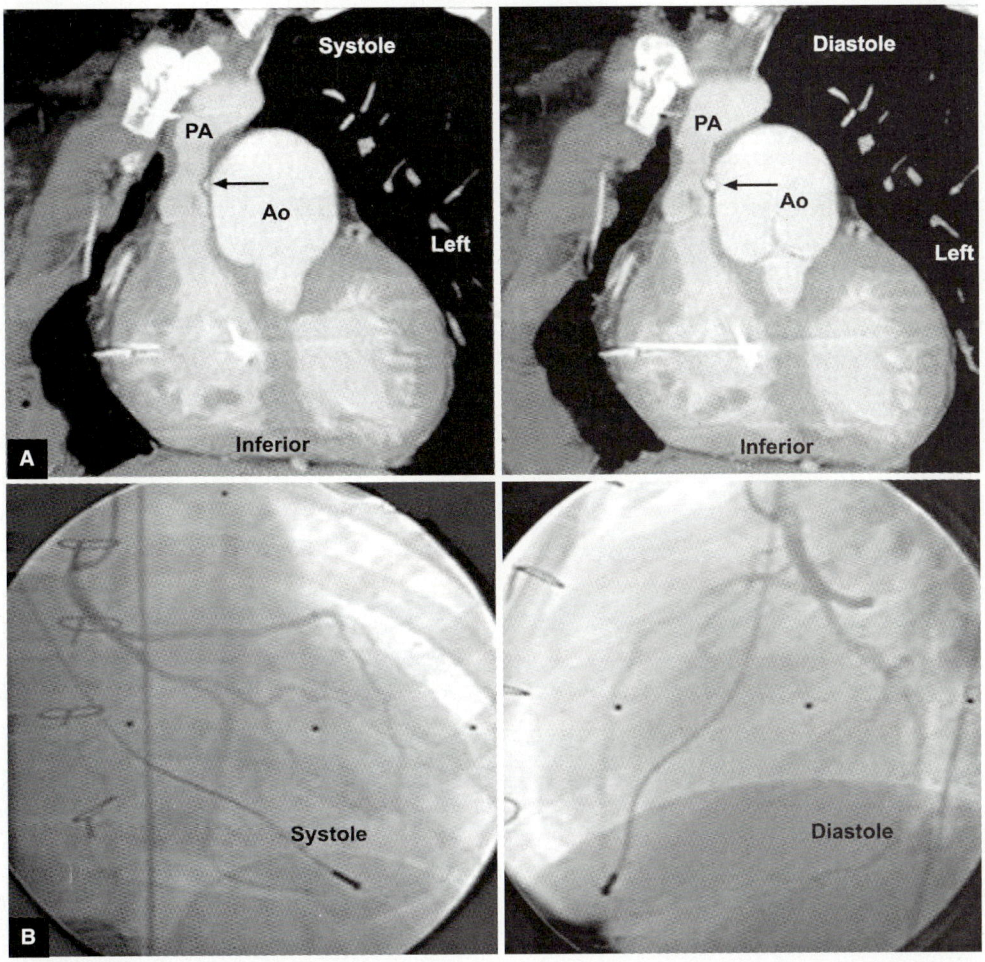


**Fig. 4.39:** Systolic compression of the left coronary artery (A) sagittal oblique cross-section on CT. Note the banana-shape of the left coronary artery (arrow) caused by systolic compression between the anterior pulmonary artery and the posterior aorta (left panel). During diastole, caliber and shape of the coronary artery are normal (right panel), (B) corresponding invasive angiogram: the systolic compression of the proximal segment of the left coronary artery appears nonsignificant

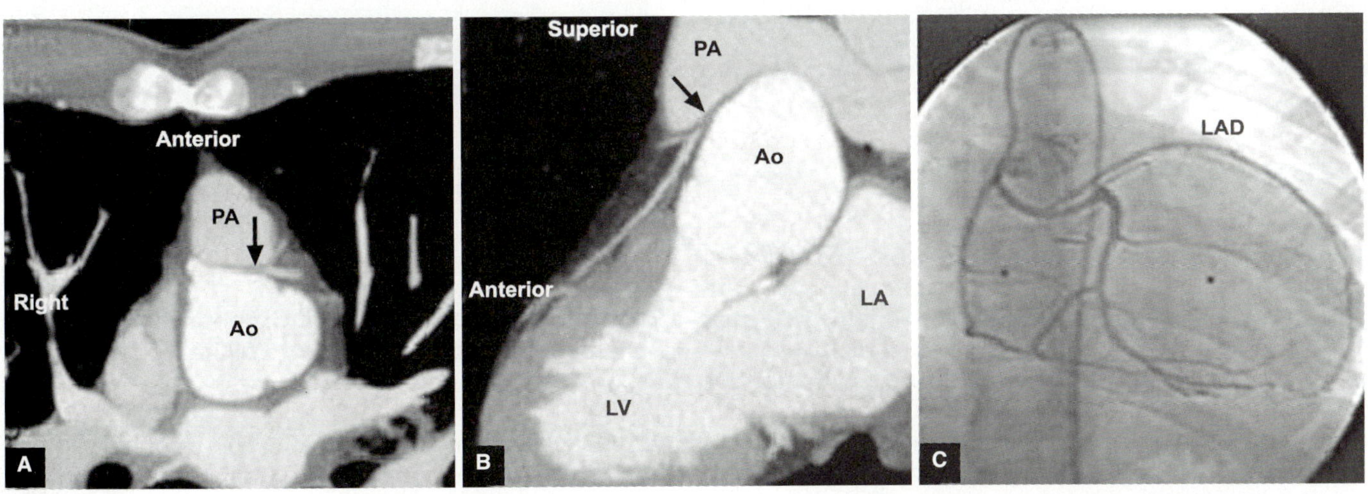


**Fig. 4.40:** Left main coronary artery with a course between aorta and pulmonary artery axial (A) and sagittal oblique (B) cross-section through the origin of the left coronary artery. The left coronary artery displays a tight stenosis (arrow) and follows a course between the aorta and pulmonary artery. (C) Corresponding invasive angiogram: selective catheterization of the left coronary ostium was not achieved. Selective right coronary angiography shows a dominant right coronary artery giving rise to a circumflex artery retrogradely filling the left anterior descending artery. Ao=aorta; LA=left atrium; LAD=left anterior descending coronary artery; LV=left ventricle, PA=pulmonary artery

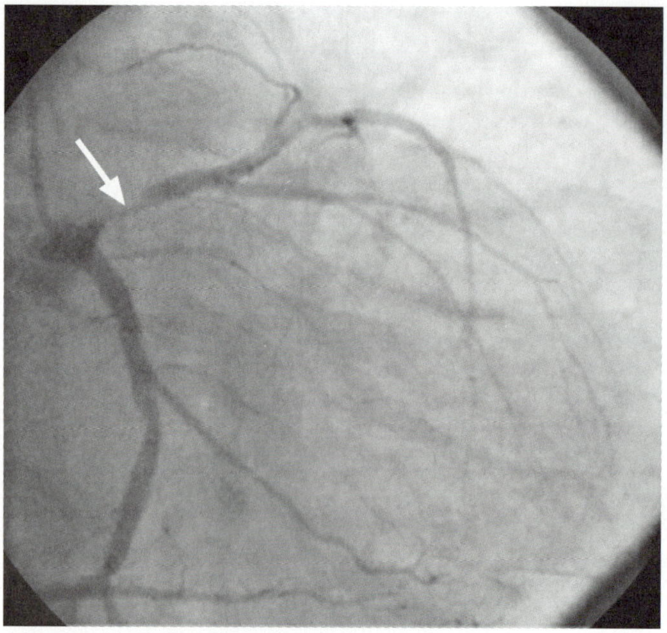

**Fig. 4.41:** Caudal view in selective coronary angiogram showing subtotal paraosteal occlusion of LAD

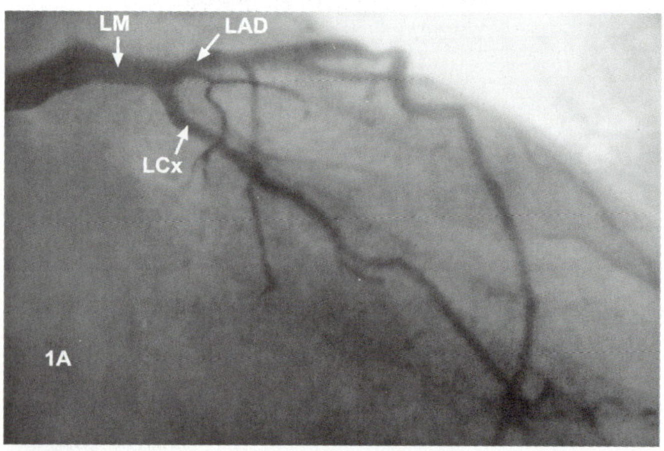


**Fig. 4.42:** 1A showing the origin of left circumflex artery from left main coronary artery LCx=left circumflex artery, LAD=left anterior descending artery, LM=left main

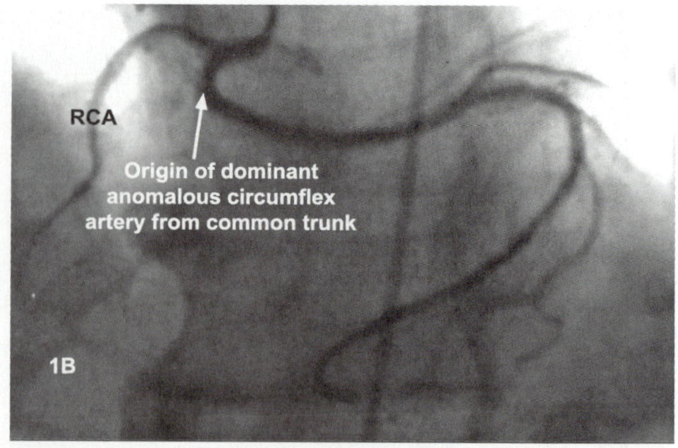


**Fig. 4.43:** 1B showing the origin of dominant anomalous circumflex artery from a common trunk originating from the right coronary cusp. RCA=right coronary artery

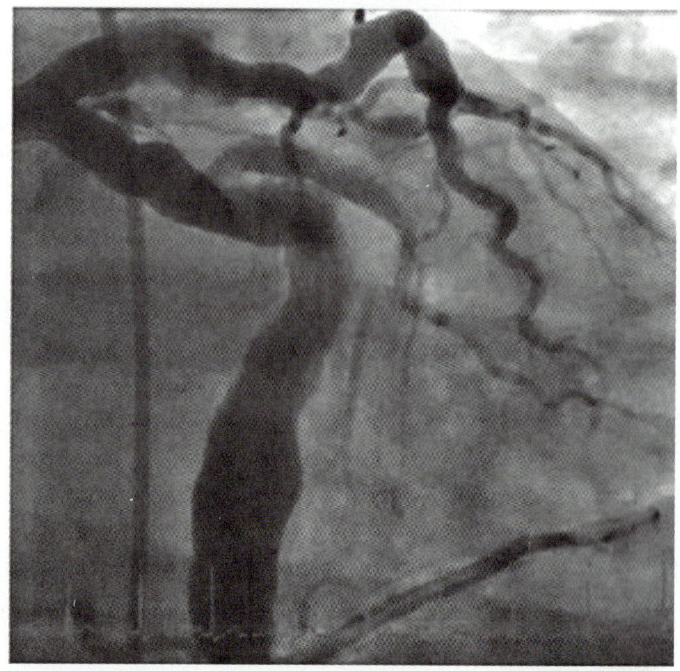

**Fig. 4.44:** Heart catheterization image showing severe diffuse coronary artery ectasia with left circumflex dominant circulation in a patient with adult Kawasaki's disease

patients with either known or suspected CAD, unless noninvasive testing (performed as recommended in the ACC/AHA noninvasive guidelines), reveals findings that suggest a high risk for adverse outcome. Coronary angiography is also frequently done during evaluation for other cardiac conditions, such as valvular heart disease, congestive heart failure, or assessment of congenital heart disease. In this setting, angiography may be performed in asymptomatic patients. The details of indications for coronary angiography in specific conditions are described ahead.

### Recommendations for Use of Coronary Angiography in Patients with Congestive Heart Failure

*Class I*

1. Congestive heart failure due to systolic dysfunction with angina or with regional wall motion abnormalities and/or scintigraphic evidence of reversible myocardial ischemia when revascularization is being considered (level of evidence: B).

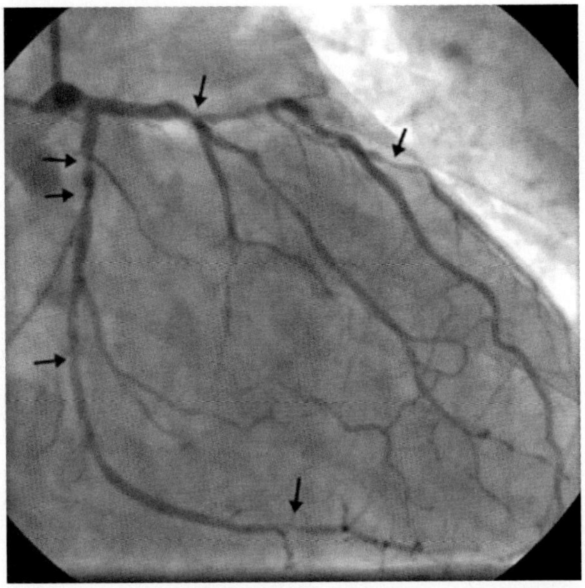

**Fig. 4.45:** Extensive coronary artery disease. Multiple stenoses are present; they involve the left anterior descending coronary artery and the circumflex coronary artery and their branches. Some of the more severe lesions are identified by arrows. Projection: RAO 2

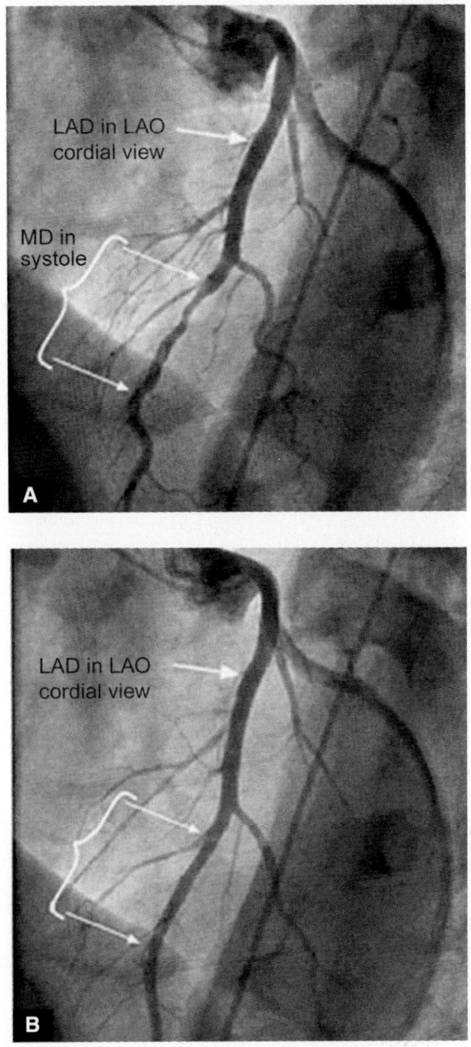


**Fig. 4.46:** (A) Selective angiography showing coronary constriction (terminal part of LAD) during systole and normal lumen during diastole, (B) in a patient who presented with angina pectoris, HT and nonspecific ECG alterations in anterolateral leads and finally found to have muscular banding of LAD

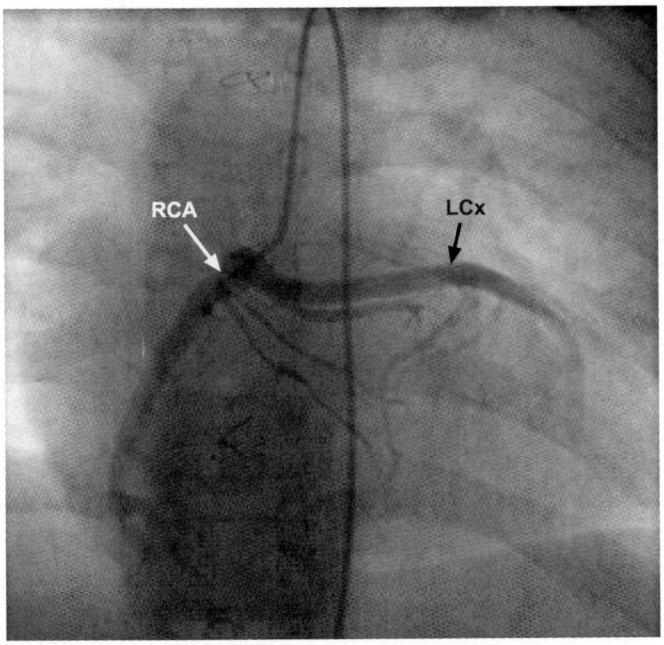


**Fig. 4.47:** Selective right coronary angiography, early phase, the left circumflex artery (LCx) originating from the right coronary artery (RC)

2. Before cardiac transplantation (level of evidence: C)
3. Congestive heart failure secondary to postinfarction ventricular aneurysm or other mechanical complications of MI (level of evidence: C).

*Class IIa*

1. Systolic dysfunction with unexplained cause despite noninvasive testing (level of evidence: C).

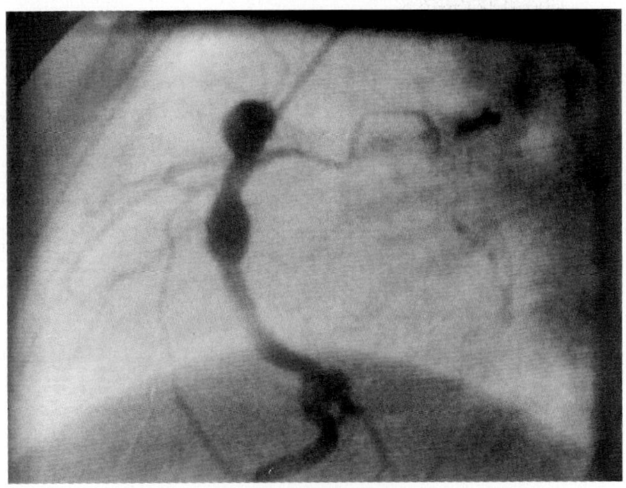

**Fig. 4.48:** Aneurysm and stenosis affecting right coronary artery and obliterated left anterior descending

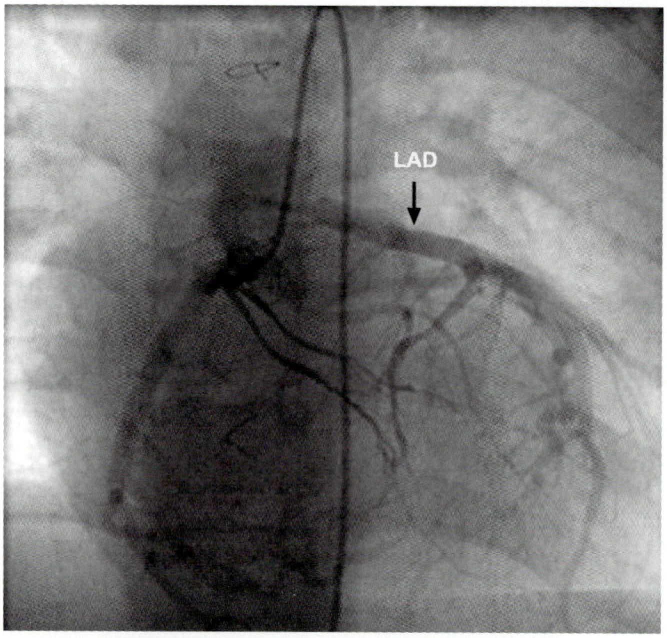


**Fig. 4.49:** Late phase of contrast injection to the right coronary artery demonstrated retrograde filling of the left anterior descending coronary artery (LAD) via intramyocardial collaterals and shunting to pulmonary artery

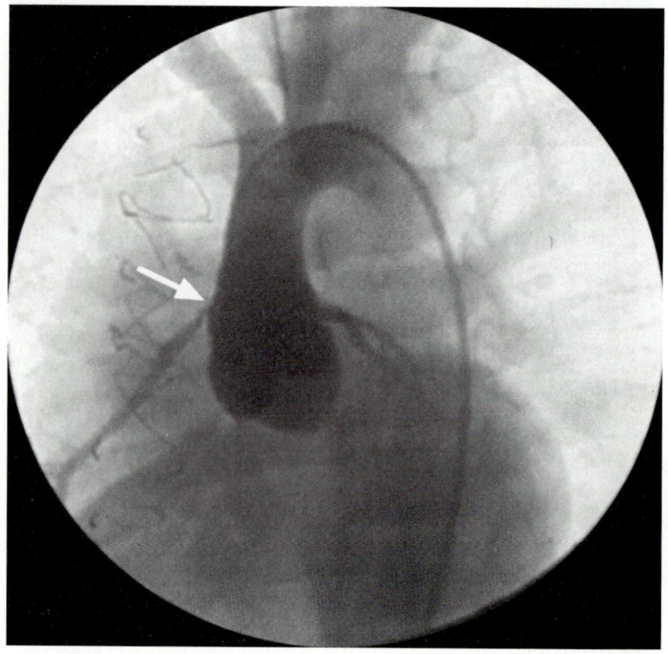

**Fig. 4.51:** Late assessment after the arterial switch operation for transposition of the great arteries, coronary angiogram shows lumen reduction at the origin of the right coronary artery

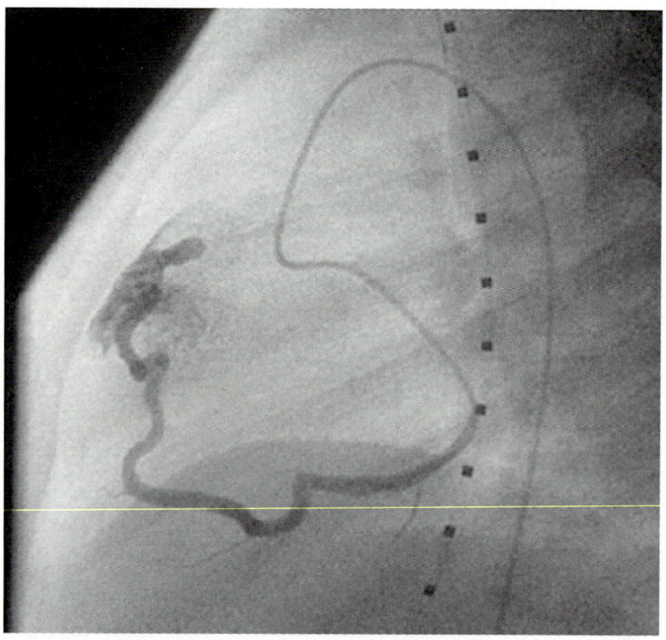

**Fig. 4.50:** Coronary angiogram during interventional catheterisation in a patient with coronary artery fistula

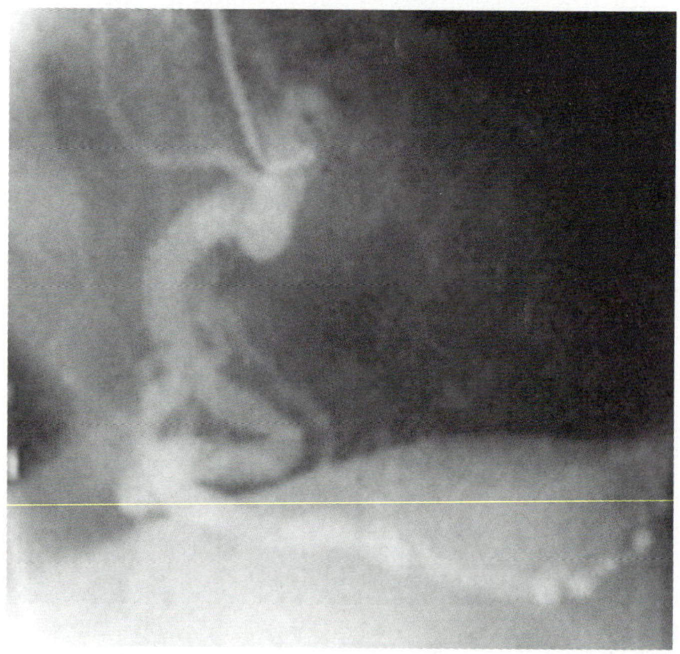

**Fig. 4.52:** Dilated right coronary artery associated with ALCAPA

2. Normal systolic function, but episodic heart failure raises suspicion of ischemically mediated left ventricular dysfunction (level of evidence: C).

*Class III*

Congestive heart failure with previous coronary angiograms showing normal coronary arteries, with no new evidence to suggest ischemic heart disease (level of evidence: C).

## Conditions Associated with Coronary Artery Involvement

### *Aortic Dissection*

The need for coronary angiography before surgical treatment for aortic dissection remains controversial

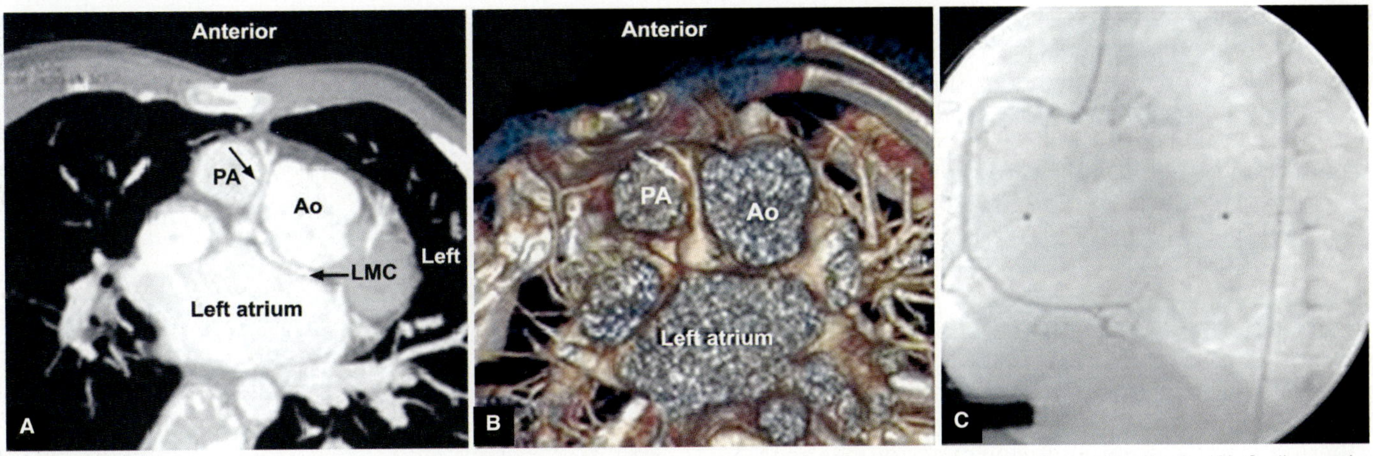


**Fig. 4.53:** Mild compression of the right coronary artery axial cross-section (maximum intensity projection). (A) 3-dimensional reconstruction, (B) showing a single coronary ostium from which both the right and left coronary arteries arise. There is mild compression of a long segment of the right coronary artery between the great arteries. The left coronary artery has a retroaortic loop with no stretching or compression, and (C) selective invasive angiogram of the right coronary artery: the proximal segment was classified as normal

because there are no large trials to support its use. In young patients with dissection due to Marfan syndrome or in dissection in peripartum females, coronary angiography is unnecessary unless there is suspicion that the dissection has affected one or both coronary ostia. In older patients, in whom dissection is usually related to hypertension, coronary angiography is often necessary, especially if patients are suspected of having coronary disease because of a history of angina or objective evidence of myocardial ischemia. In patients who have no history of coronary disease, the indications for coronary angiography are much less certain. Because of the high incidence of coronary disease in older patients with dissection, some studies have advocated routine coronary angiography, whereas others have found increased mortality when angiography is performed (Fig. 4.54).

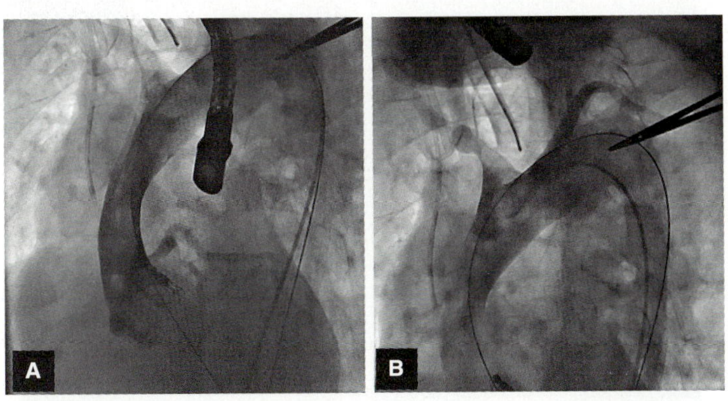


**Fig. 4.54:** Intraprocedural angiography demonstrating typical findings of ascending aortic dissection. Early phase of the injection of contrast medium into the proximal ascending aorta through a pigtail catheter showed only antegrade perfusion of the true lumen and smooth walls excluding the presence of the intimal tear ('entry') in the ascending aorta (A). The late phase revealed no malperfusion of the great vessels of the aortic arch and their perfusion from the true lumen (B)

### *Arteritis*

Some patients with inflammatory processes affecting the aorta, such as Takayasu arteritis, may have coronary artery involvement requiring coronary artery revascularization. In such patients, coronary angiography is required before the surgical procedure. Kawasaki disease can result in coronary artery aneurysm and coronary artery stenosis producing myocardial ischemia or silent occlusion and may require coronary angiographic assessment (Fig. 4.55).

### *Hypertrophic Cardiomyopathy*

Significant CAD due to atherosclerosis is found in 25% of patients aged >45 years with hypertrophic cardiomyopathy.

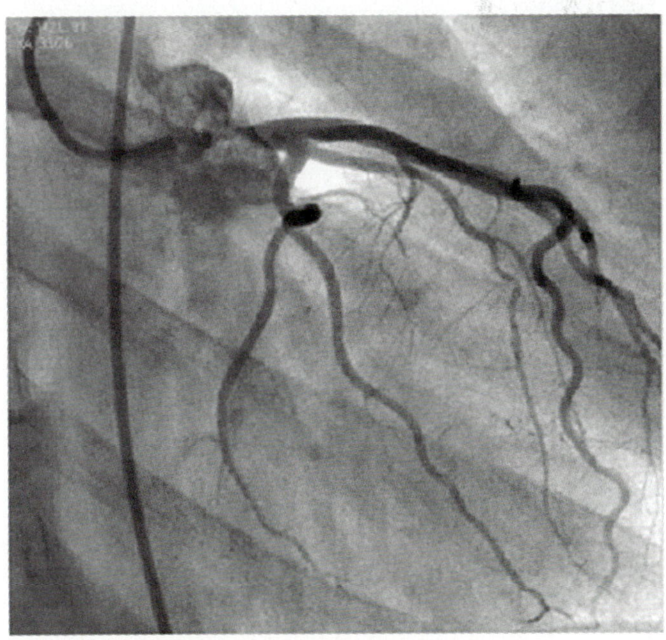

**Fig. 4.55:** A coronary angiography was performed, which showed in-stent restenosis with 90% obstruction in the left main coronary artery in a patient with Takayasu arteritis

Because symptoms due to CAD and hypertrophic cardiomyopathy are similar, patients with ischemic symptoms not well controlled with medical therapy may require coronary angiography to resolve the cause of chest pain. Coronary angiography also is indicated in patients with chest discomfort and hypertrophic cardiomyopathy in whom a surgical procedure is planned to correct outflow tract obstruction (Fig. 4.56).

### Chest Trauma

Patients who have an acute MI shortly after blunt or penetrating chest trauma may have atherosclerotic CAD, but coronary artery obstruction or damage has been reported in the absence of coronary atherosclerosis. Furthermore, myocardial contusion may simulate acute MI. Infrequently, coronary angiography is indicated in the management of such patients (Fig. 4.57).

### Miscellaneous Conditions

Preoperative coronary angiography may be indicated in patients undergoing cardiac operations such as pericardiectomy or removal of chronic pulmonary emboli if they have 1 risk factor for coronary disease, especially advanced age. Because of the concern about transplanting a donor heart affected by coronary disease, many advocate coronary angiography before transplantation, at least for those donors with a significant likelihood of CAD (Figs 4.58–4.60) .

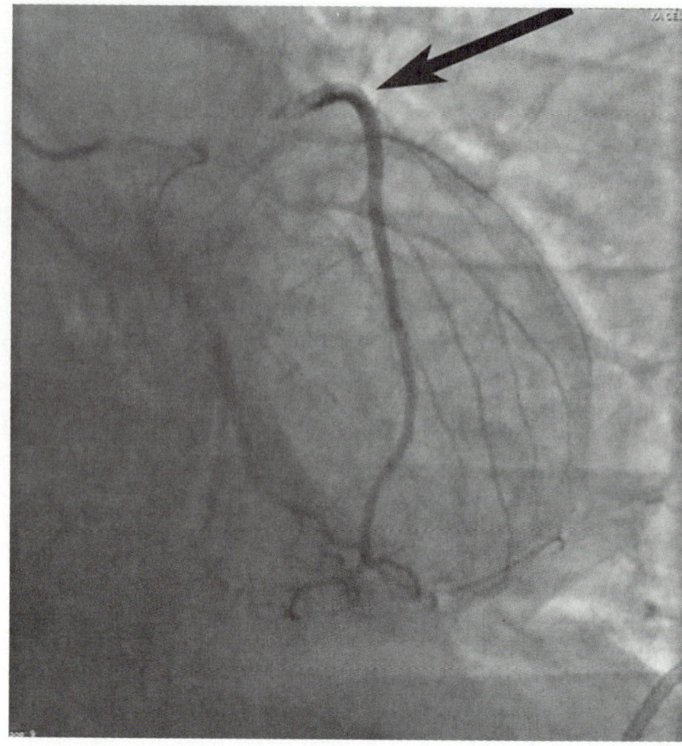

**Fig. 4.57:** Coronary artery dissection and acute myocardial infarction following blunt chest trauma. Coronary angiogram showing dissection of the middle part of the left anterior descending coronary artery (arrow)

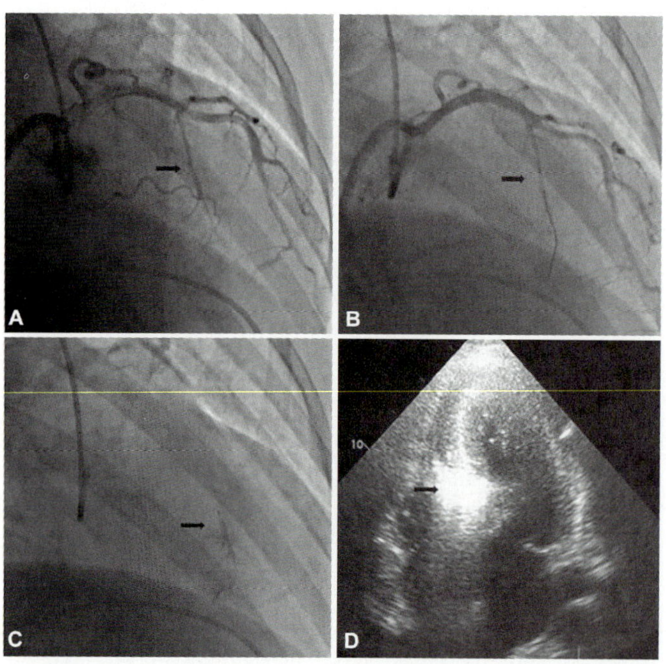


**Fig. 4.56:** Procedure: (A) angiography, right oblique cranial view of the left coronary artery, showing the target vessel; (B) selective catheterization of the target vessel and placement of balloon catheter; (C) selective angiography of the target vessel, showing injection of contrast through the lumen of the balloon catheter; (D) transthoracic echocardiography, 4-chamber view, showing hyperechogenic basal septum after injection of contrast

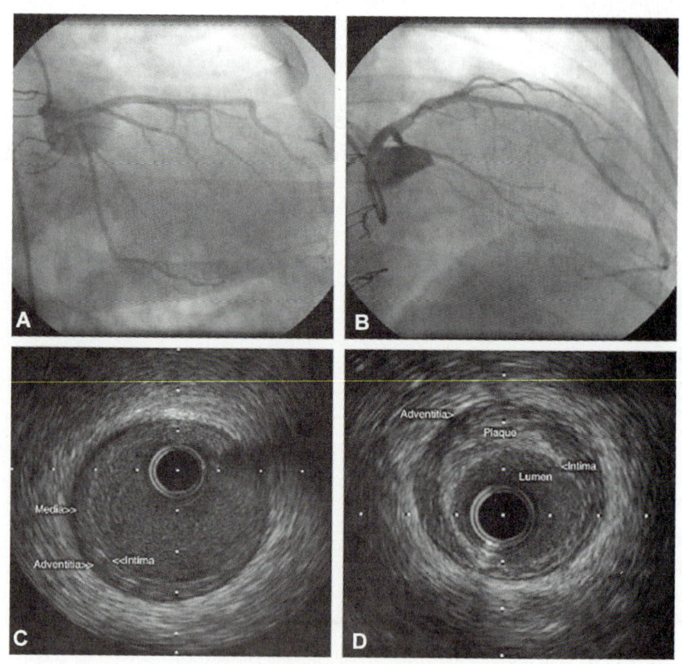


**Fig. 4.58:** Intravascular ultrasound images of the anterior descending artery in a patient transplanted 5 years previously, showing both the concentric intimal thickening typical of cardiac allograft vasculopathy (A) and an eccentric plaque typical of atherosclerotic coronary disease (B). Coronary angiography did not suggest disease in this artery (C and D)

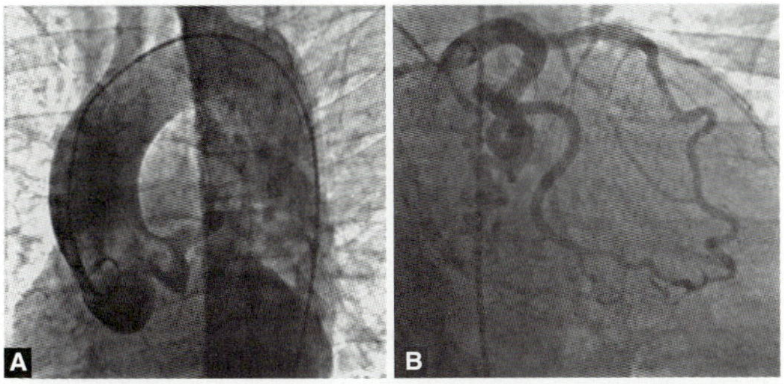

**Fig. 4.59:** Anomalous right coronary artery arising from the pulmonary artery. Aortography demonstrated the absence of a right coronary system but the presence of left coronary system. (A) Selective coronary angiography illustrated a dilated left coronary system with large collaterals to the right coronary territory. (B) A subsequent pulmonary angiogram showed constrast entering the right coronary artery from the main pulmonary trunk

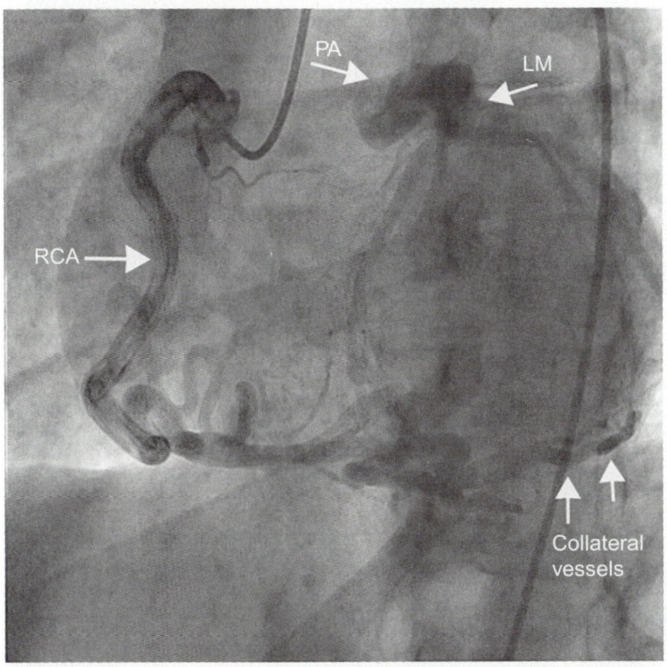


**Fig. 4.60:** Coronary angiography. Coronary angiography of the right coronary artery with collateral filling of the left coronary vascular territory, which connects directly to the pulmonary trunk

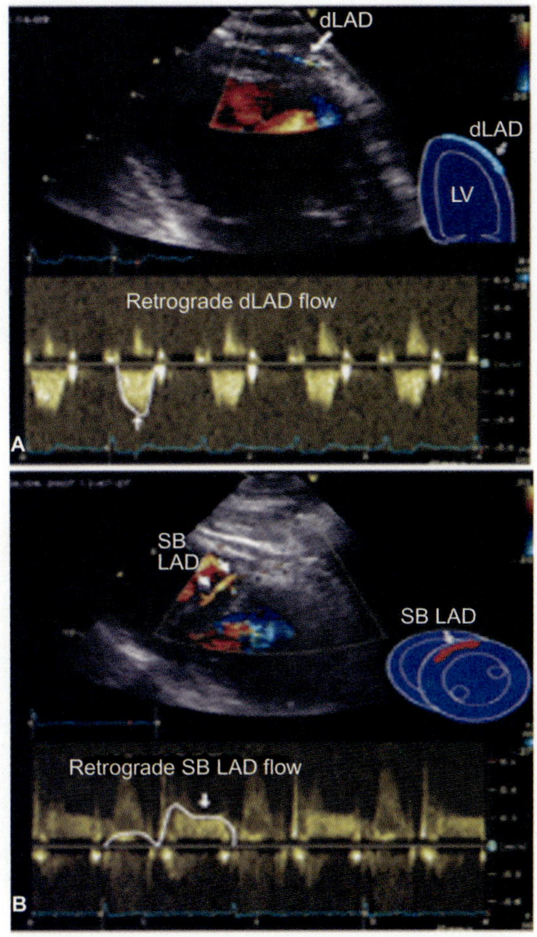


**Fig. 4.61:** Proximal occlusion of the left anterior descending coronary artery (LAD). Examples of color Doppler mapping (top) and Doppler spectrum (bottom) of the retrograde coronary blood flow. (A) Epicardial collateral vessel: distal LAD (dLAD); (B) intramyocardial collateral vessel: septal branch of the LAD (SB LAD)

## Recommendations for Intracoronary Doppler Ultrasound

Following are the recommendations for intracoronary Doppler ultrasound (Fig. 4.61):

- Class I: None.
- Class IIa: Assessment of the physiological effects of intermediate coronary stenoses (30–70% luminal narrowing) in patients with anginal symptoms. Doppler velocimetry may also be useful as an alternative to performing a noninvasive functional study to determine whether an intervention is warranted for intermediate lesions (or when the functional study is ambiguous) (level of evidence: C)
- Class IIb:
  1. Evaluation of the success of percutaneous coronary revascularization in restoring flow reserve and to predict the risk of restenosis (level of evidence: C).
  2. After cardiac transplantation, diagnosis of impaired CFR in patients with anginal symptoms but no apparent angiographic culprit lesion (level of evidence: C)
  3. Assessment of the severity of coronary flow abnormalities in patients with anginal symptoms and a positive noninvasive functional study but no apparent angiographic lesion (level of evidence: C)
- Class III: Routine assessment of the severity of angiographic disease in patients with a positive noninvasive functional study (level of evidence: C).

## Coronary Angioscopy

Coronary angioscopy uses visible light conducted through fiberoptic filaments to provide direct visual assessment of the surface characteristics and intraluminal morphology in vivo (Figs 4.62–4.63A, B and Table 4.2). The images appear

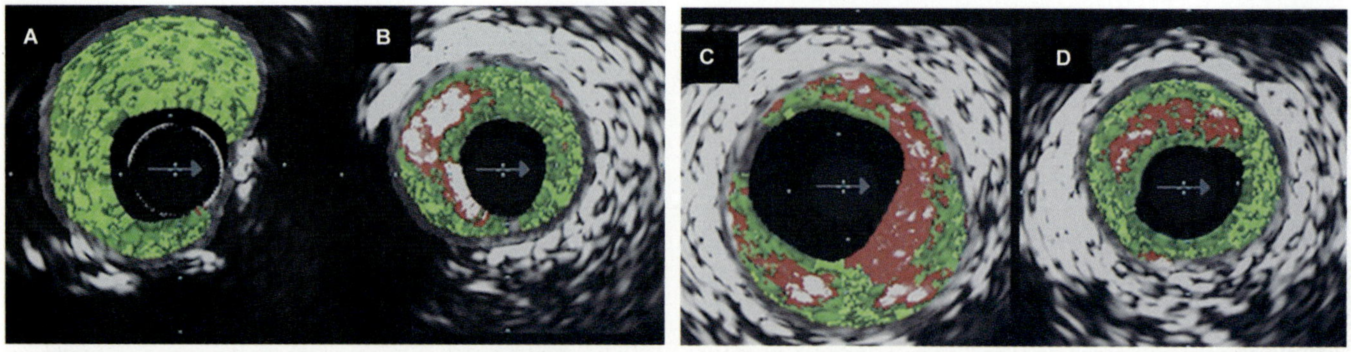


**Fig. 4.62:** Types of atherosclerotic plaque characterized by intravascular ultrasound virtual histology: (A) fibrotic plaque, (B) fibrocalcific plaque, (C) thin-cap fibroatheroma, (D) thick-cap fibroatheroma

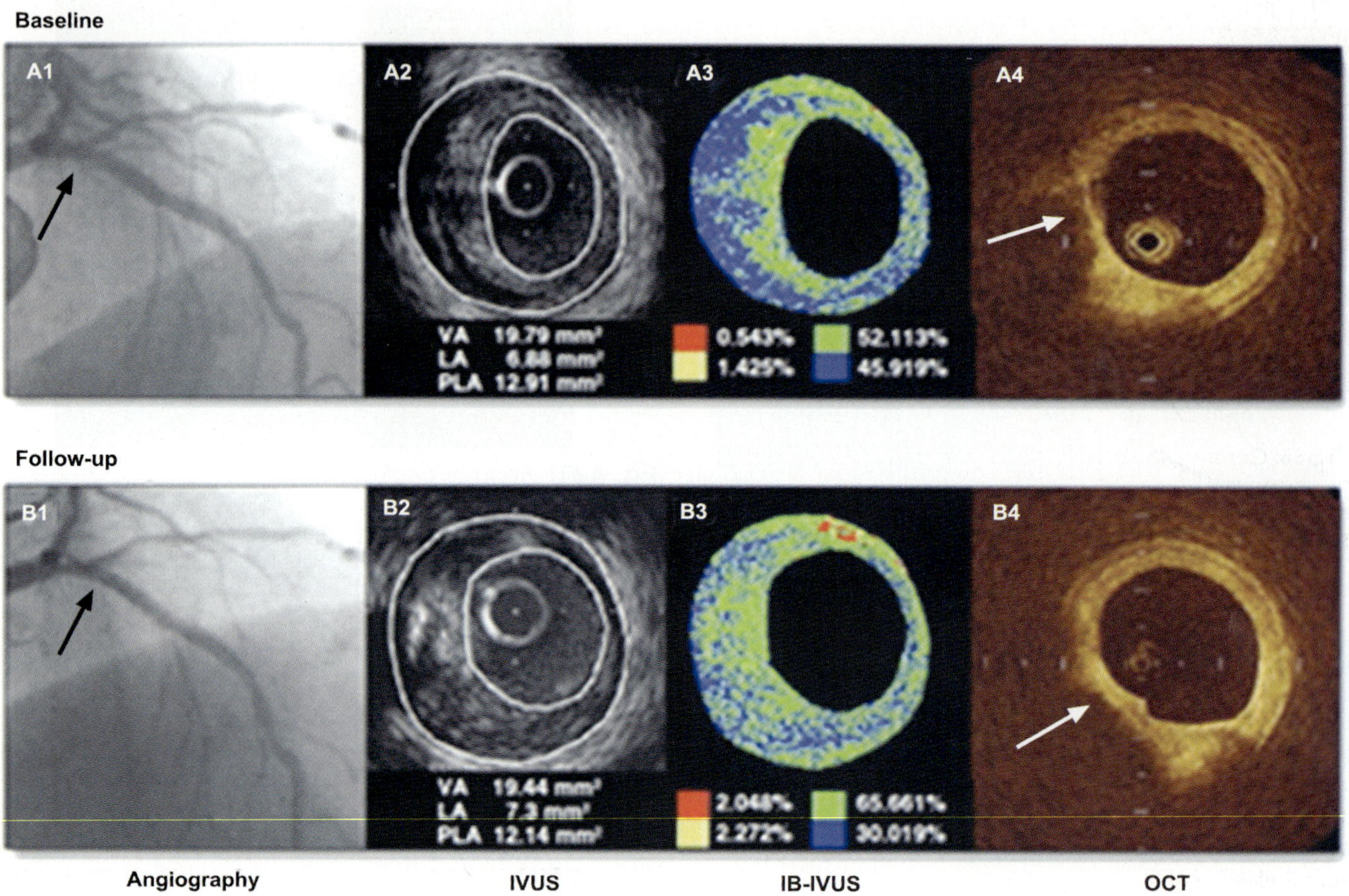


**Fig. 4.63A:** Coronary angiographic, grayscale IVUS, IB-IVUS, and OCT at baseline and follow-up for the pitavastatin group, while no significant difference was found between baseline and follow-up angiography (A1, B1), plaque volume index (i.e. plaque area in this slice) decreased from 12.9 mm$^2$ to 12.1 mm$^2$ by grayscale IVUS during follow-up (A2 and B2). Lipid (blue) volume index decreased from 45.9% to 30.0%, while fibrous (green) volume index increased from 52.1% to 65.6% by IB-IVUS (A3 and B3). OCT revealed that the fibrous cap thickness increased from 80 micm to 220 micm during follow-up (arrows in A4 and B4). IB-IVUS=integrated backscatter-intravascular ultrasound, IVUS=intravascular ultrasound, LA=lumen area, OCT=optical coherence tomography, PLA=plaque area; VA=vessel area

in color on a television monitor, which enables examination of the hue of the target lesion and associated plaques. Although difficult to use, angioscopy allows the differentiation of platelet-rich from fibrin-rich thrombus, and it may provide evidence of atheroma rupture, intraplaque hemorrhage, and coronary dissection. Accordingly, this diagnostic imaging modality yields information on the pathogenesis of acute coronary syndromes.

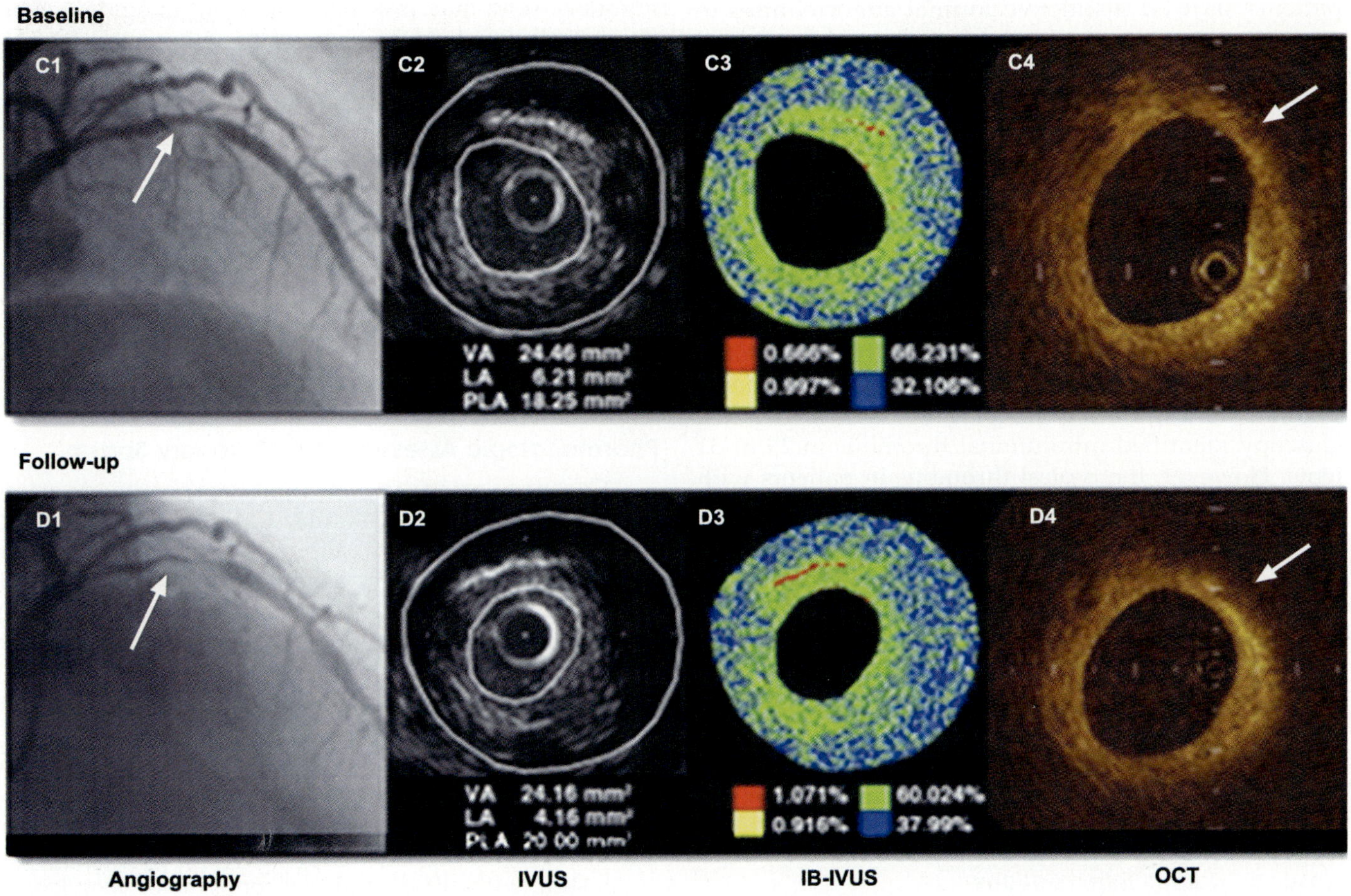


**Fig. 4.63B:** Coronary angiographic, grayscale IVUS, IB-IVUS, and OCT at baseline and follow-Up for the dietary group, whilst significant progression was observed by angiography during follow-up (C1 and C2), plaque volume index (e.g. plaque area in this slice) increased from 18.2 mm$^2$ to 20.0 mm$^2$ by grayscale IVUS during follow-up (C2 and D2). Lipid (blue) volume index increased from 32.1% to 37.9%, whereas fibrous (green) volume index decreased from 66.2% to 60.0% by IB-IVUS (C3 and D3). OCT revealed that the fibrous cap thickness of 110 micm did not change during follow-up (arrows in C4 and D4)

**Table 4.2:** Differences between cardiac allograft vasculopathy and atherosclerotic coronary disease

| | **Cardiac allograft vasculopathy** | **Atherosclerotic coronary disease** |
|---|---|---|
| Location | Distal epicardial and intramyocardial vessels | Proximal epicardial vessels |
| Plaque type | Diffuse, concentric | Focal, eccentric |
| Inflammation | Yes | Rarely |
| Vasculitis | Infrequently | Never |
| Internal elastic lamina | Intact | Disrupted |
| Calcium deposits | No | Yes |

### *Angioscopy Equipment and Technique*

All angioscopes require a blood-free field for clear visualization of the arterial wall. This is obtained by inflating a proximal balloon to temporarily occlude blood flow, followed by continuous saline irrigation, which requires a second catheter lumen. Two additional lumens are required for the optical fibers, one for visualization and another to serve as a light source. Videotape recording allows for more detailed offline analysis. A commonly used device is a 120-cm-long 4.5 monorail catheter with an imaging bundle containing 3,000 fibers that permits a viewing arc of 55° and a depth-of-field of 0.5 mm. A video camera displays the images in real time on a color monitor, while videotape recording allows for more detailed offline analysis.

### *Angioscopy of Unstable Coronary Syndromes*

Small-scale studies of fiberoptic angioscopy demonstrate differences in the intraluminal appearance of stable versus unstable coronary lesions. An intraoperative study of

32 patients showed distinctive intimal abnormalities in all 10 patient's with unstable angina: four patients had 'complex plaque' and seven had overt intraluminal thrombus. Neither complex plaques nor thrombi were observed by angioscopy in any patient with stable coronary disease. These findings were later confirmed by percutaneous angioscopy. In 16 patients with unstable angina, 50% had thrombus and 14% had overt dissection. Neither thrombus nor dissection was seen in any of the 4 patients with stable angina.

In addition to identifying the presence of thrombus, angioscopy can differentiate platelet-rich from fibrin-rich thrombi. Mizuno et al. performed angioscopy in 15 patients with unstable angina and 16 patients with acute MI. Angioscopy identified intraluminal thrombus in 29 of 31 patients. However, the typical thrombus in patients with unstable angina was grayish-white in color, suggesting the predominance of platelets, whereas in patients with acute MI, angioscopy identified a preponderance of red thrombi, suggesting an erythrocyte and fibrin-rich clot. Angioscopy can distinguish other surface features of coronary atheromata. Stable plaques are recognized by their elevated contour, smooth configuration, and yellowish-white color. In a study of 199 patients, those with predominantly yellow plaques were found to have higher low-density lipoprotein (LDL) cholesterol and apolipoprotein B levels.

### *Angioscopy during Interventions*

Assessment of lesions before or after coronary intervention represents the most commonly reported application of coronary angioscopy. Angioscopy after balloon angioplasty demonstrates that dissections and thrombus are present in almost all cases. However, no prospective data exist that demonstrate a different outcome for patients on the basis of angioscopic findings. The preprocedural identification of thrombus may also prove useful in selecting candidates for coronary stenting and for the use of any of the new antiplatelet agents. Although the value of angioscopy in identifying thrombus is well established, no data exist to suggest that angioscopy can reduce stent-related complications.

## Limitations of Coronary Angioscopy

Despite recent technical advances, angioscopy is still limited to the proximal and midportions of relatively straight, large epicardial coronary arteries. Furthermore, the rapid development of ischemia during balloon inflation limits the time of examination. For successful imaging, lesions need to be located 20 mm distal to the balloon site, which makes it impossible to visualize ostial or very proximal lesions. Angioscopy shows only the surface characteristics of plaques and cannot discern the underlying atheroma morphology. Accordingly, it remains unproved whether visualization of surface anatomy alone warrants the time, expense and risk of angioscopy. In addition, occlusion of coronary flow may produce important imaging artifacts. A recently published study of the European Working Group on Coronary Angioscopy demonstrated that the identification of red thrombus and dissection has relatively close interobserver agreement. However, other angioscopic diagnoses have wide interobserver variability.

## Recommendations for Coronary Angioscopy

- Class I: None
- Class II: None
- Class III: Coronary angioscopy should be considered a research tool for which there are no established clinical indications.

## Pharmacologic Assessment of Coronary Spasm

a. **Coronary artery spasm:** Epicardial coronary arteries exhibit vasoactivity similar to that of many systemic arteries of a similar caliber. The presence of atherosclerotic plaque is associated with endothelial dysfunction, which can increase or decrease segmental responses to endogenous and exogenous vasoactive substances. Thus, patients with coronary atherosclerosis may have spontaneous increases in coronary vasomotor tone, resulting in myocardial ischemia. These regional coronary vasospastic events can cause ischemia associated with a variety of ST and T-wave changes. Tobacco and cocaine abuse are important risk factors for the provocation of vasospasm. Provocative testing with either methylergonovine or acetylcholine often demonstrates the presence of coronary spasm. Although vasomotion can result in as much as a 20% change in lumen diameter, coronary spasm is considered to be present when a reduction in lumen caliber of >50% occurs during a provocative test and reversal is achieved with intracoronary nitroglycerin. Prinzmetal variant angina is a clinical syndrome occurring in a small percentage of patients without angiographic evidence of significant stenosis or normal angiograms in whom ischemia is caused by severe spasm of an epicardial coronary artery. Variant angina, as described by Prinzmetal in 1959 is an unusual syndrome characterized by ischemic myocardial pain that usually occurs at rest, with accompanying ECG ST-segment elevation.

Basal coronary artery vasoreactivity and tone are increased in variant angina. Studies using $^{123}$I metaiodobenzylguanidine ($^{123}$I MIBG) SPECT demonstrate regional myocardial sympathetic dysinnervation in patients with variant angina. Tobacco and cocaine may cause episodes of variant angina, the latter because it blocks presynaptic uptake of norepinephrine and dopamine, thereby facilitating alpha-adrenergically mediated vasospasm. Cardiac arrhythmias, including ventricular tachycardia and fibrillation, heart block, acute infarction and sudden death, may occur in association with variant angina. Studies using $^{123}$I BMIPP, a branched fatty acid, have demonstrated

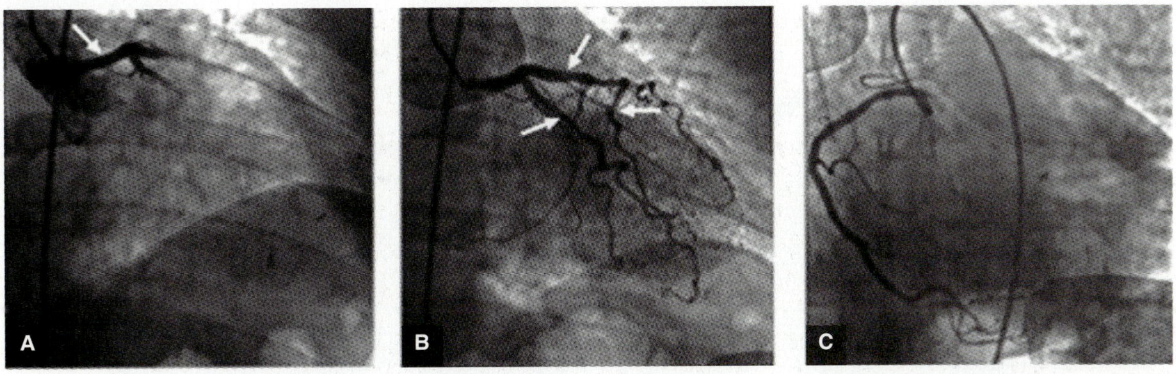

**Fig. 4.64:** (A) angiography of the left coronary arterial system showed total occlusions of the proximal left anterior descending coronary artery (LAD) and left circumflex artery (LCX). (B) An immediate left coronary artery angiography revealed complete restoration of coronary artery occlusion, suggesting resolution of the acute coronary spasm C. Her proximal LAD had mild luminal irregularities, with up to 30% luminal stenosis, near the site of the previously seen spasm. Her right coronary angiogram was widely patent at the stent site, with only a 20–30% eccentric luminal narrowing at the distal end of the stent

myocardial injury in association with some episodes of variant angina (Fig. 4.64).

b. **Provocative testing for spasm:** Of the tests available to demonstrate coronary spasm, provocation by ergonovine maleate, methylergonovine maleate, acetylcholine or hyperventilation are the most useful (Figs 4.65 and 4.66). Ergonovine maleate for injection is no longer available, and the availability of methylergonovine is limited. The intravenous administration of incremental doses of methylergonovine starting at 0.05 mg to a maximum of 0.40 mg is both sensitive and specific, and there is an inverse relationship between the dose required to provoke spasm in the laboratory and the frequency of spontaneous episodes experienced by the patient. To ensure a valid test, nitrates and calcium antagonists must be withdrawn for 48 hours before testing. Women are more sensitive than men to methylergonovine The intracoronary route of administration of methylergonovine for provocation of spasm is safe, sensitive, and specific. This route is preferable in hypertensive patients and affords the opportunity to evaluate the left and right coronary circulations separately. Small dosing increments of 5–10 µg are used, with a total dose not to exceed 50 µg.

Absolute contraindications to methylergonovine include pregnancy, severe hypertension, severe left ventricular dysfunction, moderate to severe aortic stenosis and high-grade left main coronary stenosis. Relative contra-indications include uncontrolled or unstable angina, uncontrolled ventricular arrhythmia, recent MI and advanced coronary disease. Alternatively, intracoronary acetylcholine can be used as a provocative test for spasm, and its effectiveness is comparable to methylergonovine. Acetylcholine is infused over 1 minute into a coronary

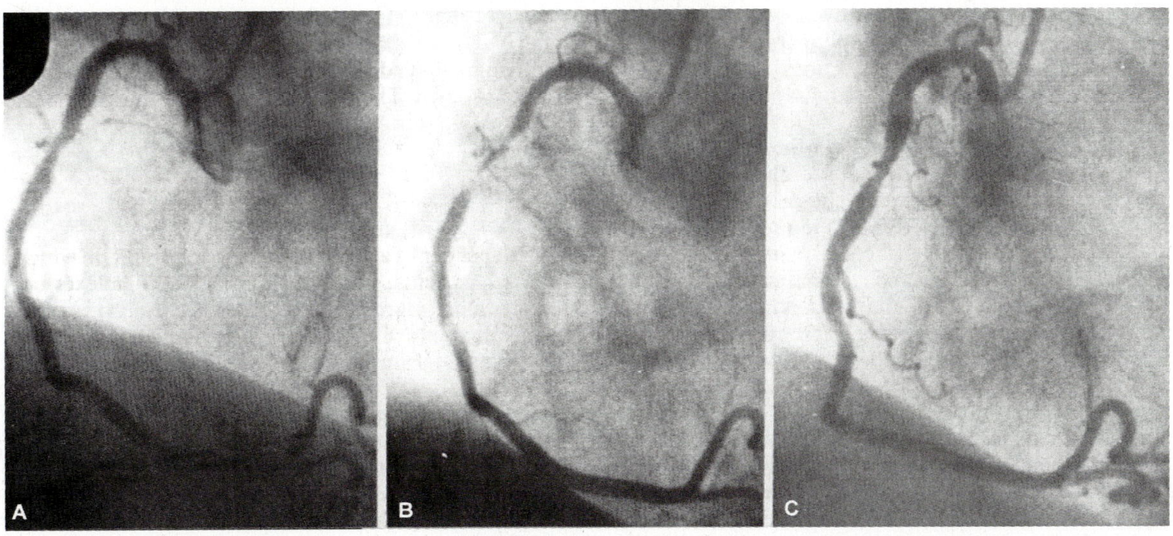

**Fig. 4.65:** A sequence of right coronary arteriograms in the 60° left anterior oblique projection which demonstrates (A) approximately 60% narrowing of the diameter of the right coronary artery before ergonovine maleate (EM), (B) greater than 95% focal narrowing following a cumulative dose of 0.40 mg EM at the site of narrowing demonstrated in (A), and (C) diffuse dilatation and dilatation at the site offocal spasm after 0.40 mg sublingual nitroglycerin

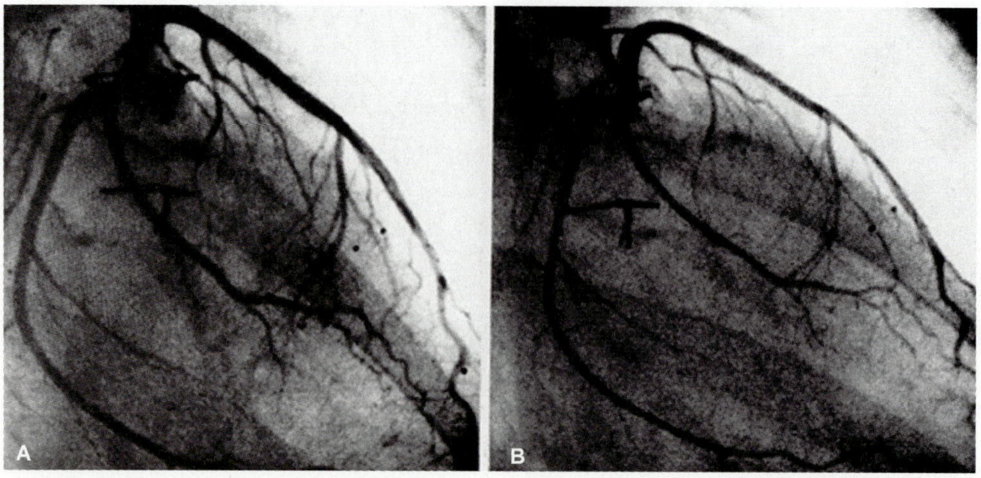


**Fig. 4.66:** Left coronary artery arteriograms of a heart transplant recipient in the 30° right anterior oblique view: (A) before administering ergonovine maleate (EM) and (B) 3 minutes after a cumulative dose of 0.40 mg EM, which demonstrates the same degree of mild, diffuse narrowing of coronary arteries observed after EM administration in patients with normally innervated hearts. The small densities which outline the left ventricle are tantallum markers within the left ventricular myocardium

artery in incremental doses of 10, 25, 50 and 100 µg. Doses should be separated by 5-minute intervals. The same procedural safeguards must be used with acetylcholine and methylergonovine. In patients with 1 episode of variant angina per day, the hyperventilation provocative test is nearly as effective as methylergonovine in causing vasospasm. In patients with less frequent attacks, hyperventilation is less sensitive. The test requires a patient to hyperventilate vigorously at 30 respirations per minute for 5 minutes. With this degree of hyperventilation, arterial pH will increase to 7.60 and $pCO_2$ will decrease to 20 mmHg. Variant angina, if provoked, will occur during hyperventilation and will subside more rapidly than after methylergonovine infusion. The cold presser test can also provoke coronary spasm but is less reliable than pharmacologic techniques.

In patients with ST-segment elevation during episodes of chest pain and a normal coronary angiogram, provocative tests are usually not necessary, because ample clinical evidence is present to confirm the diagnosis of coronary spasm.

## FRACTIONAL FLOW RESERVE

The measurement of pressure gradients across coronary stenoses was the earliest method used to assess the

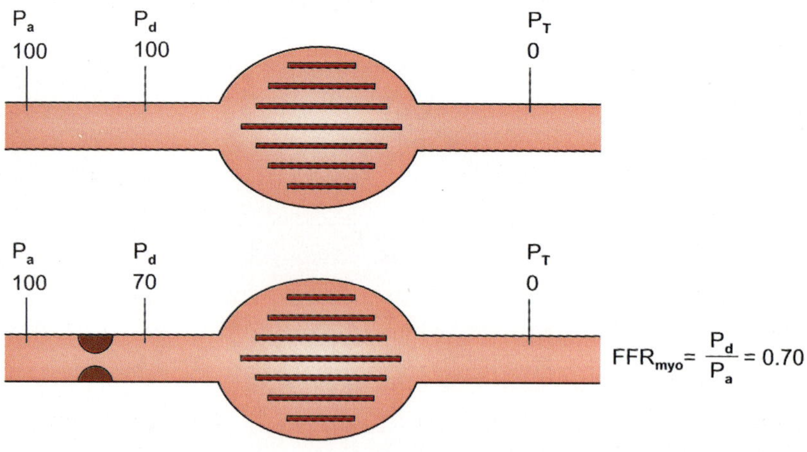


**Fig. 4.67:** Simplified illustration of a coronary artery and the dependent myocardial bed. If that system is studied under conditions of maximum arteriolar vasodilatation, myocardial resistance will be minimal and equal to Rmin. Under such circumstances the flow limiting effect of the epicardial stenosis is maximal, as is the pressure drop across the lesion, expressed as the ratio of driving pressure to resistance, maximum attainable blood flow through the myocardium equals the ratio of the perfusion pressure across the myocardium (distal coronary pressure minus central venous pressure) and the resistance Rmin. If there is no epicardial stenosis, the perfusion pressure across the myocardium equals PaPv where Pa is mean aortic pressure and Pv is central venous pressure. In the presence of a coronary stenosis, the perfusion pressure across the myocardium has decreased to PdPv, where Pd represents hyperaemic coronary pressure distal to the stenosis

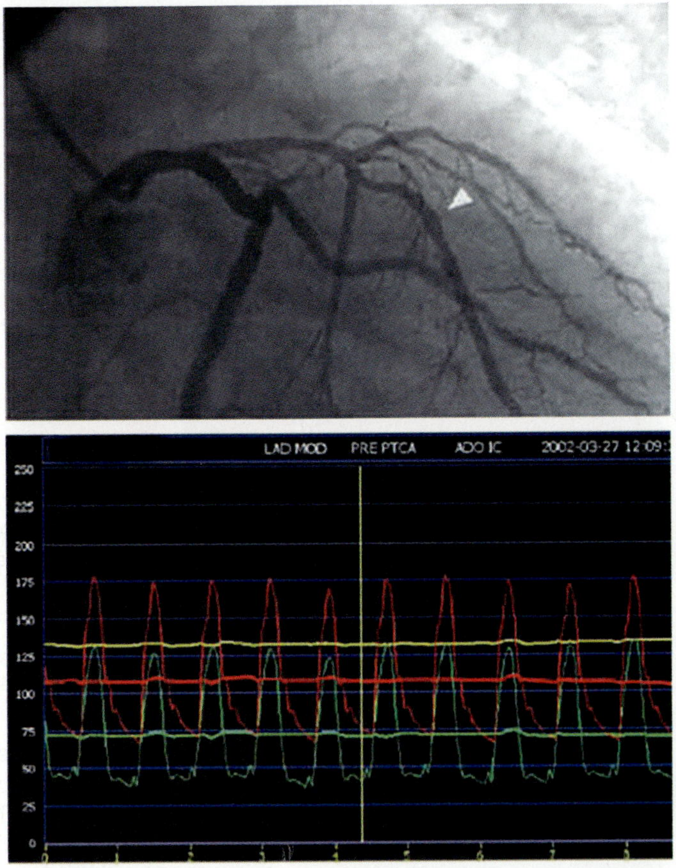


**Fig. 4.68:** Anterior right oblique projection showing an intermediate lesion in the middle third of the anterior descending coronary artery, distal to a well-developed septal branch. There is also another mild lesion close to the septal branch. After positioning the transducer of the pressure guidewire distal to the stenosis (arrowhead) and inducing maximum hyperemia with intravenous adenosine, a mean pressure of 71 mmHg was recorded by the pressure guidewire transducer and 108 mmHg by the catheter guidewire. The ratio of the two values for myocardial fractional flow reserve (MFFR) was 0.66, indicating a significant lesion

adequacy of coronary angioplasty. However, because of the size of the catheter and changes in technology, angiographic and now ultrasonic assessments are more commonly used. Recently, small catheters and guidewires have been developed to more accurately measure pressure gradients across stenoses before and after interventional procedures. Pijls and colleagues demonstrated that just as with CFR measurements by Doppler ultrasound, fractional flow reserve (FFR) is useful in assessing the severity of a coronary stenosis (Figs 4.67 and 4.74). The ratio of the mean pressure distal to a coronary stenosis to that proximal to the stenosis, usually measured through the guiding catheter after maximal vasodilation induced by adenosine or papaverine, can assess the severity of the stenosis. When this ratio falls below 75%, there is an 88% sensitivity and an 84% specificity for an abnormal exercise test. Similar correlations have been made with positron emission tomography (PET) and CFR measured by Doppler ultrasound. The technique is easier

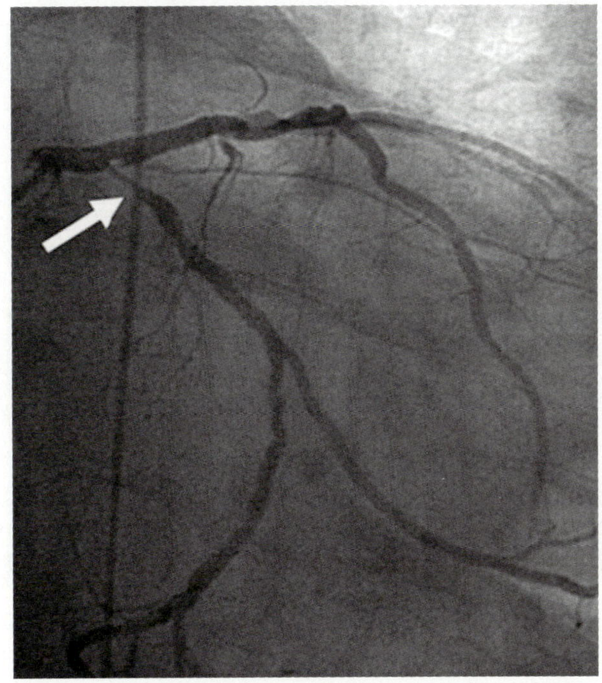

**Fig. 4.69:** Invasive coronary angiogram in a patient demonstrates moderate lesion in the proximal left circumflex coronary artery (arrow), which was hemodynamically significant (FFR, 0.67)

to use than Doppler ultrasound. Although it is still in development and validation, it appears likely to be a useful tool in the future to assess coronary stenoses.

### *What is Fractional Flow Reserve?*

Myocardial fractional flow reserve is a new index of the functional severity of a coronary stenosis that is calculated from pressure measurements made during coronary arteriography. This new approach enables an 'on the spot' diagnosis as to what extent a given stenosis (coronary blockage) contributes to reversible myocardial ischemia and the decision whether revascularization of the stenosis is warranted.

### *How does FFR work?*

- Fractional flow reserve (FFR) closely relates distal coronary pressure to myocardial blood flow during maximum arteriolar vasodilatation.
- The functional state of a patient with a coronary artery stenosis is determined by the maximum blood flow that can reach the heart muscle. As soon as maximum achievable blood flow, at a given level of exercise, is no longer sufficient to match oxygen demand, myocardial ischemia and angina will occur.

### *How are FFR measurements performed?*

- FFR can be measured during a routine cardiac catheterization
- The stenosis is crossed with an 0.014 inch pressure guidewire for recording the trans-stenotic pressure, and administering a maximum hyperemic stimulus (intracoronary adenosine 12–20 µg or intravenous adenosine 140 µg/kg/min infused into the femoral vein).

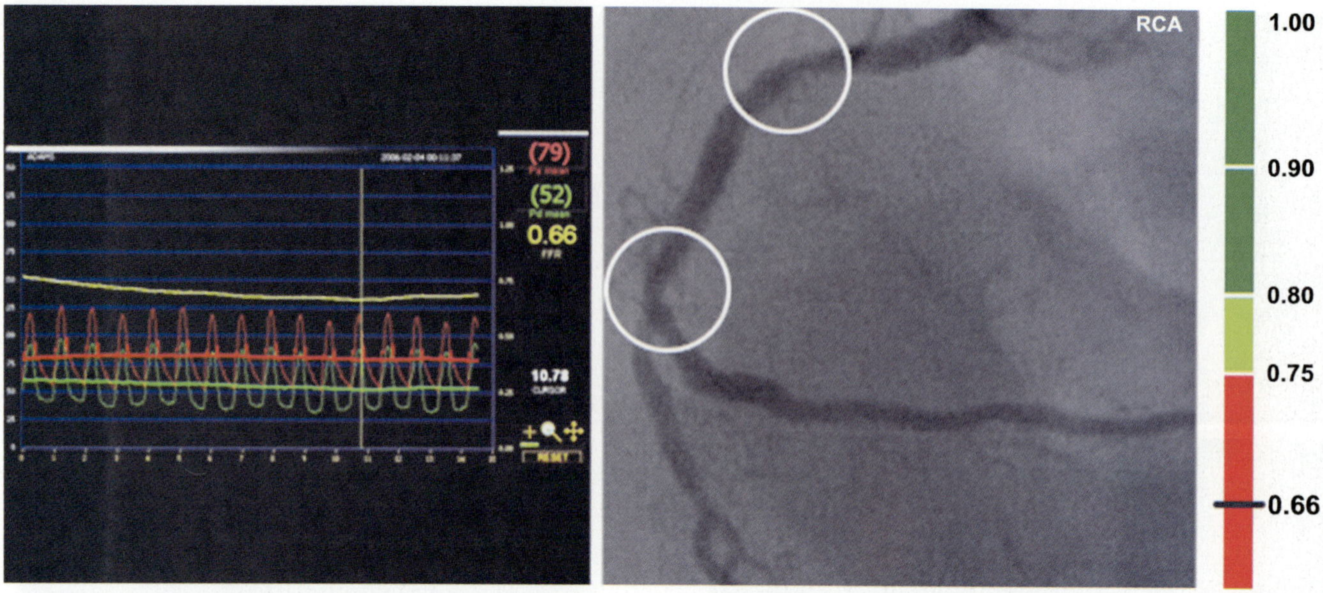


**Fig. 4.70:** The FFR in the RCA was well below 0.75. The most proximal stenosis was stented first and a new FFR measurement was performed. A continued low FFR prompted stenting of the distal lesion as well

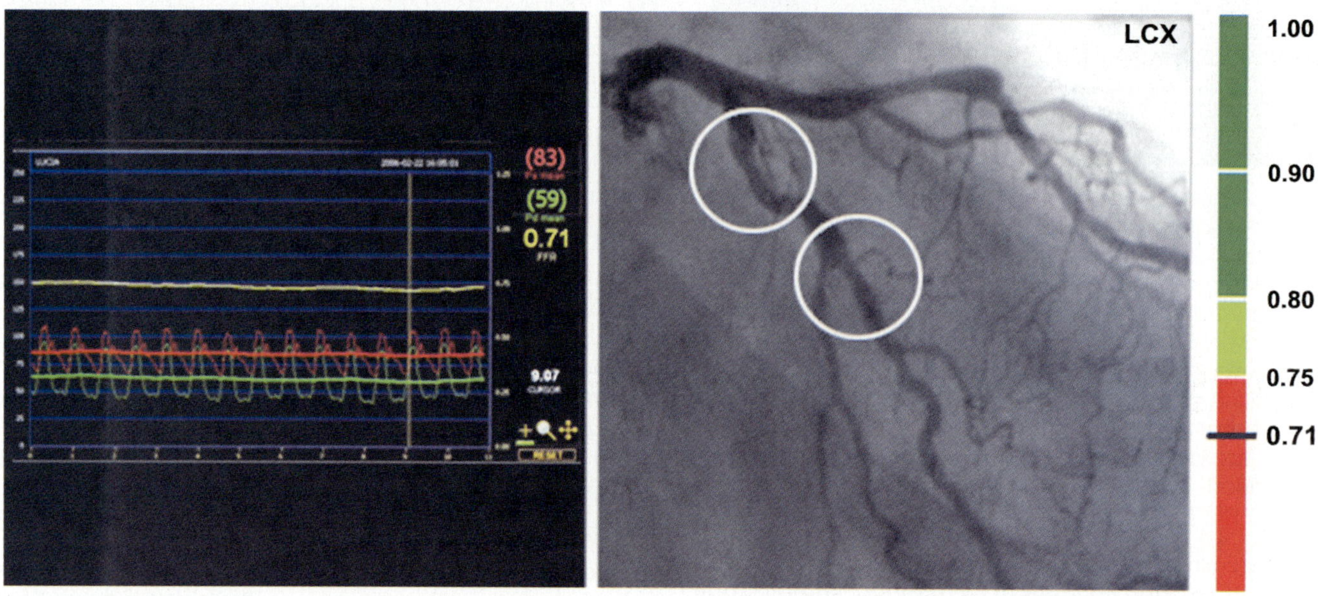


**Fig. 4.71:** The FFR in the LCX was below 0.75 and a pressure pullback recording showed both lesions to be significant. Two stents were placed satisfactorily as confirmed by FFR >0.90

*What do the FFR values mean?*

- FFR value <0.75 discriminates functionally significant lesions
- FFR >0.75 means the blockage is not severe enough to limit blood flow to the heart
- FFR <0.75 means that the blockage is severe enough to limit blood flow to the heart and should be opened if possible.

*What are the benefits of FFR?*

- FFR is a specific index for the epicardial stenosis and therefore better indicates to what degree a patient can be helped by revascularization
- FFR has a normal value of 1.0 in every patient and every coronary artery
- FFR is independent of changes in heart rate, blood pressure, and contractility
- FFR takes into account the contribution of the collateral flow
- FFR can be applied in multivessel disease and for serial lesions within one vessel.

*How are FFR measurements performed?*

- FFR can be measured during a routine cardiac catheterization

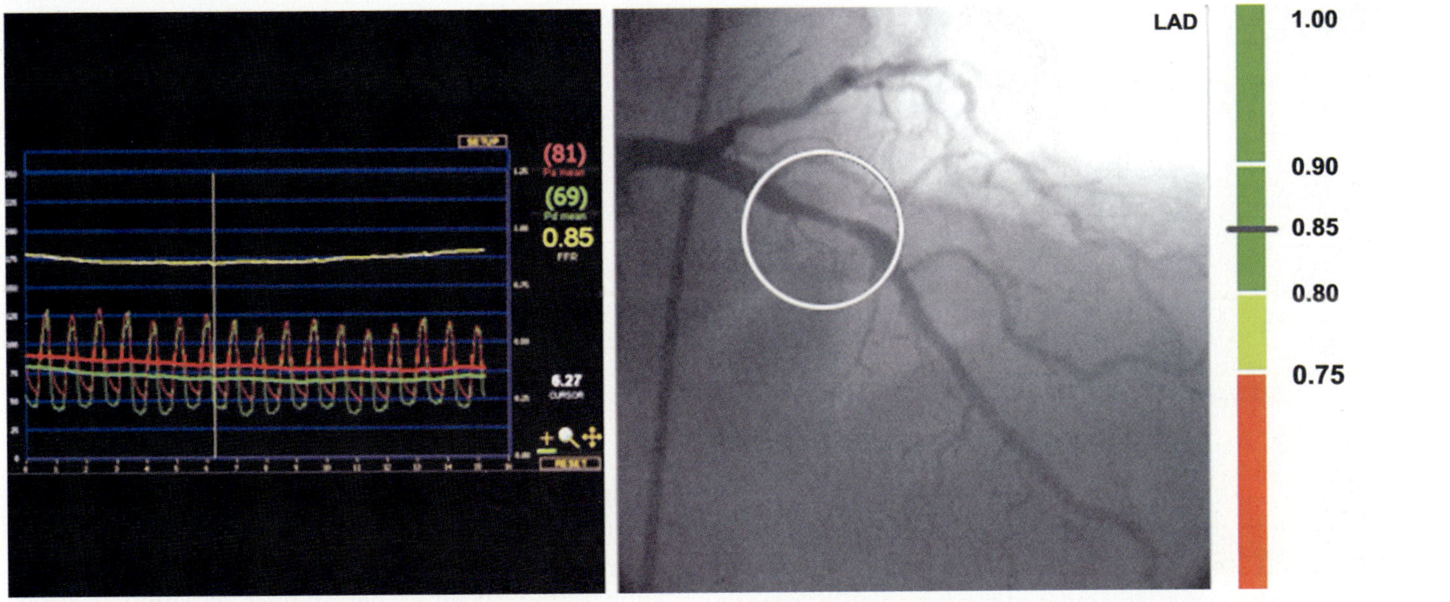


**Fig. 4.72:** Angiography showed three diseased vessels. FFR helped to identify which lesions required treatment. A pressure pullback in the long disease segment of the LAD revealed that there was no significant reduction in flow in this vessel (FFR >0.75)

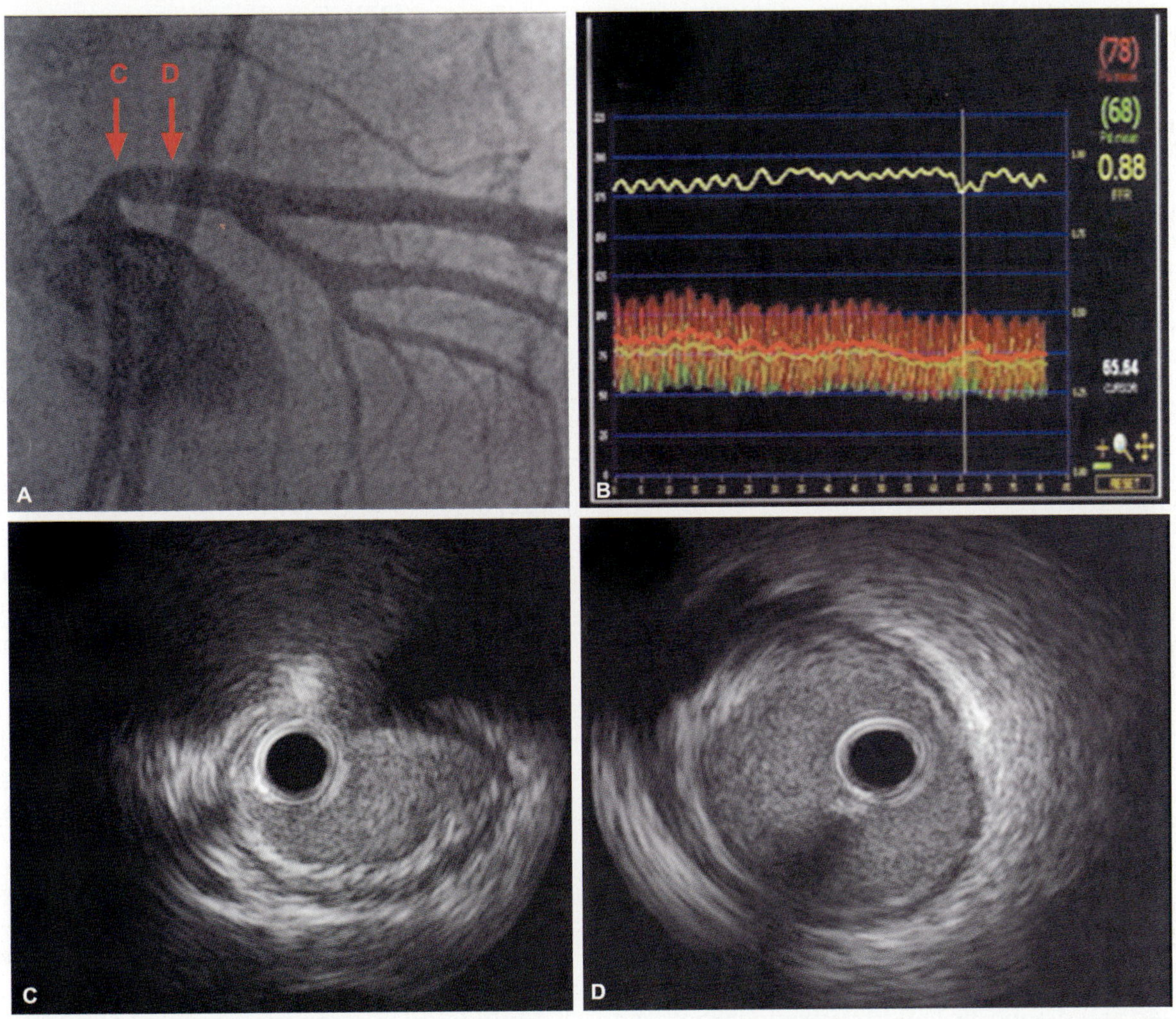


**Fig. 4.73:** Angiographic intermediate ostial left main lesion. An example of an angiographic intermediate ostial left main lesion (A) that was investigated by FFR (B), and IVUS (C, D). FFR was 0.88, and IVUS demonstrated mild plaque with significant negative remodeling resulting in an MLA of 8.9 mm$^2$. The red arrows (A) indicate the location of IVUS frames displayed in C and D. The patient was medically managed and revascularization was deferred

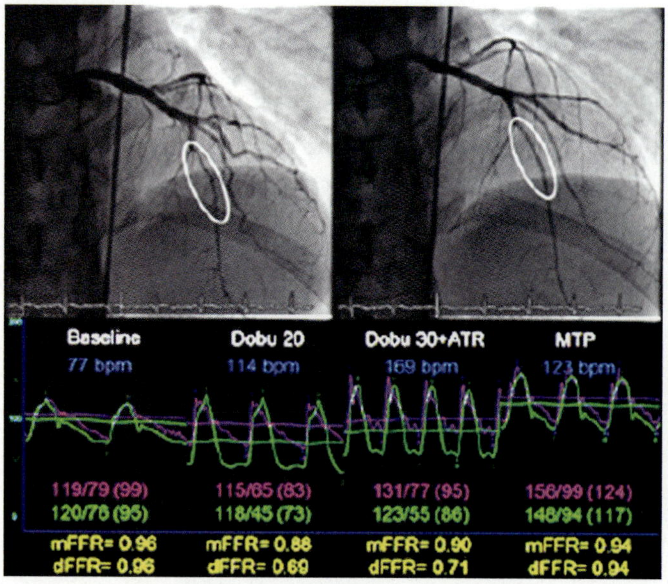


**Fig. 4.74:** Left, midsystolic image of the left coronary artery in anteroposterior view, with 20° of cranial inclination. Just distal to a septal branch, myocardial bridging and 'milking' is observed in the left anterior descending artery (encircled in white). Right, end-diastolic view in the same incidence. The segment just distal to the septal branch is smooth and free of atherosclerotic disease. The lower insert of the figure depicts the pressure tracings and their respective values in mmHg at the level of the aorta (in purple) and in the left anterior descending artery distal to the segment with systolic compression (in green). The ratio of distal pressure to aortic pressure (FFR) is depicted in yellow. Values are mentioned for mean and diastolic pressures (mFFR and dFFR, respectively). The distal measurements were obtained using a 0.014 inch pressure wire, after induction of maximum hyperemia with an intracoronary bolus of adenosine. Left to right—measurements in baseline condition, during intravenous infusion of dobutamine at 20 micg/kg/min, during intravenous infusion of dobutamine at 30 micg/kg/min and administration of 1 mg of atropine, and finally after intravenous administration of 10 mg of metoprolol. The respective heart rates (bpm) are mentioned in blue. At a dose of 20 micg/kg/min of dobutamine, systolic pressure overshoots distally to the dynamic lesion with a diastolic pressure gradient $<0.75$. At the highest dose of dobutamine and after administration of atropine, an important diastolic pressure gradient is seen (55/77=0.71), indicating impaired myocardial perfusion by the myocardial bridge. This gradient disappeared almost instantly after the intravenous administration of metoprolol, despite a higher heart rate than that during the intravenous infusion of dobutamine at a dose of 20 micg/kg/min

- The stenosis is crossed with an 0.014" pressure guidewire for recording the trans-stenotic pressure, and administering a maximum hyperemic stimulus (intracoronary adenosine 12–20 µg or intravenous adenosine 140 µg/kg/min infused into the femoral vein).

*When is FFR used?*

- FFR is used as a diagnostic tool to determine whether a particular coronary stenosis, found at angiography, is responsible for reversible ischemia (and consequently should be dilated or bypassed if medical treatment fails)
    - Specifically in respect to intermediate stenosis
    - Identification of the culprit lesion in case of multivessel disease
    - Justification to perform (or avoid) angioplasty in a patient without documented evidence of ischemia at noninvasive testing
    - To indicate the exact location of a lesion in case of overprojection and other situations where the angiographic image is unclear.
- Coronary intervention
    - A high value of FFR after regular balloon angioplasty is associated with a favorable long term outcome.
- Coronary stenting
    - Evaluation of optimum stent deployment.

### Computed Fractional Flow Reserve Derived from Coronary CT Angiography

Recent advances in image-based modeling and computational fluid dynamics permit the calculation of coronary artery pressure and flow from typically acquired coronary computed tomography (CT) scans. Computed fractional flow reserve (FFRCT) is the ratio of mean coronary artery pressure divided by mean aortic pressure under conditions of simulated maximal coronary hyperemia, thus providing a noninvasive estimate of fractional flow reserve (FFRCT) at every point in the coronary tree. Prospective multicenter clinical trials have shown that computed FFRCT improves diagnostic accuracy and discrimination compared to CT stenosis alone for the diagnosis of hemodynamically significant coronary artery disease (CAD), when compared to invasive FFR as the reference gold standard. This promising new technology provides a combined anatomic and physiologic assessment of CAD in a single noninvasive test that can help select patients for invasive angiography and revascularization or best medical therapy. Further evaluation of the clinical effectiveness and economic implications of noninvasive FFRCT are now being explored (Fig. 4.75).

### Noninvasive Coronary Artery Disease with Multidetector CT Angiography in Patients with Noncoronary Cardiovascular Surgery (Figs 4.76 and 4.94)

Preoperative evaluation of patients scheduled to undergo noncoronary cardiovascular surgery includes the use of invasive coronary angiography (ICA) to rule out the coexistence of significant coronary artery disease Despite the absence of apparent clinical symptoms of angina, prevalence of significant CAD in this population has been reported to be between 8% and 41%. The relevance of this finding lies in the observation that revascularization in these patients in addition to the procedure of noncoronary cardiovascular surgery reduces the occurrence of peri- and postoperative adverse major clinical events.

Multidetector coronary computed tomographic angiography of the coronary arteries is nowadays a reliable technique to rule out significant CAD, with a proved high negative predictive value, particularly in patients with low

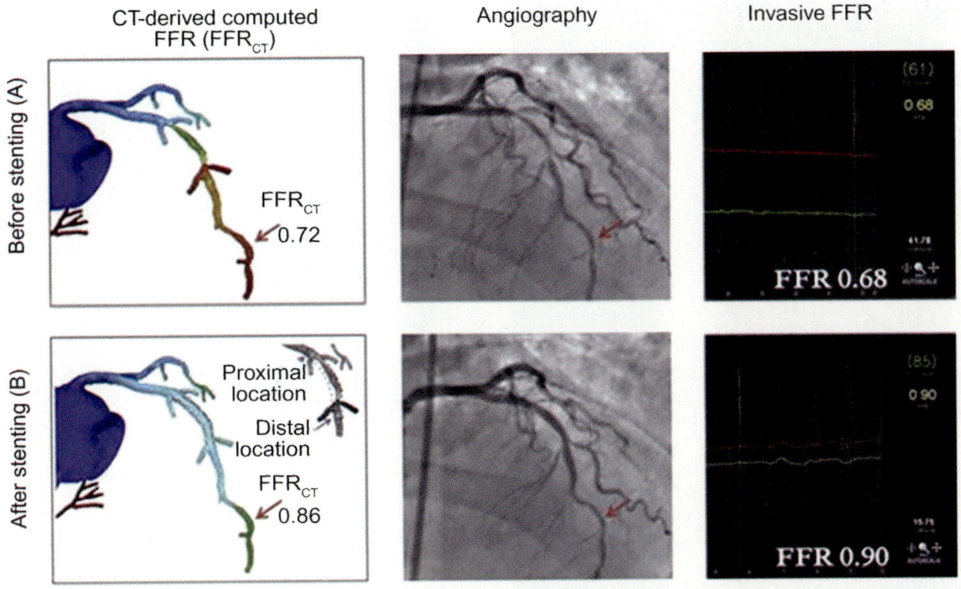


**Fig. 4.75:** Invasive and noninvasive functional assessment before and after revascularization. (A) Noninvasive fractional flow reserve (FFR) from coronary computed tomographic angiography data (FFRCT) of the left anterior descending (LAD) coronary artery was 0.72. Invasive coronary angiography and FFR confirmed the functionally significant LAD stenosis. (B) FFRCT demonstrated no ischemia in the LAD after virtual stenting, with a computed value of 0.86. Invasive FFR after stent implantation was 0.90

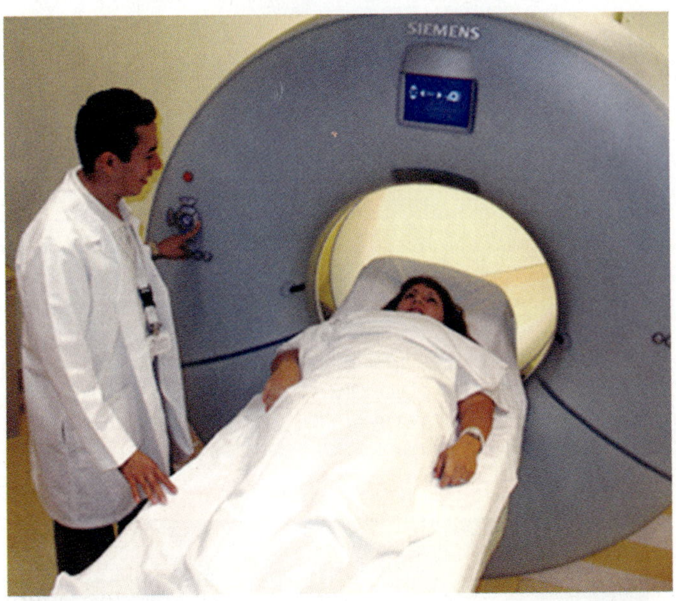


**Fig. 4.76:** Photograph of a CT scan machine. Noninvasive coronary multidetector CT angiography in patients with noncoronary cardiovascular surgery

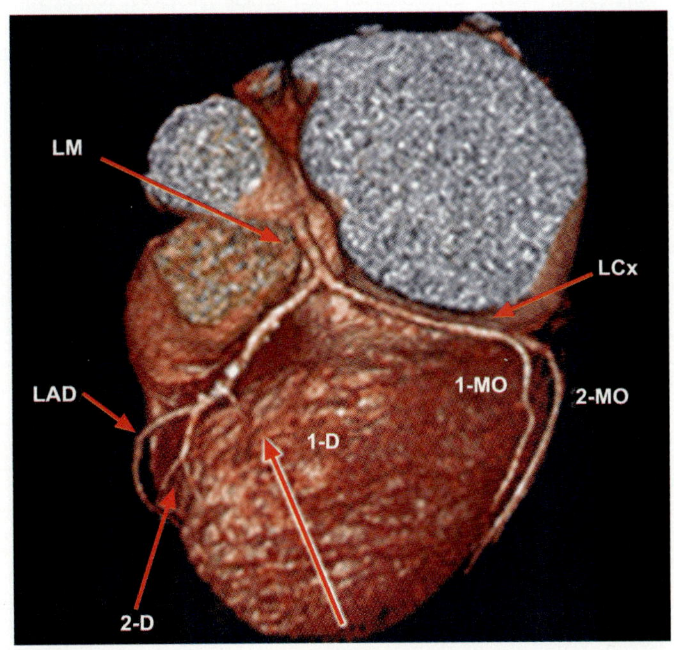


**Fig. 4.77:** Coronary CT angiographic results in patient with a dilated left atrium and atrial fibrillation with mean heart rate of 73 beats per minute at coronary CT angiographic acquisition. Volume-rendered CT image (left anterior oblique view with cranial angulation) shows the arteries—left main (LM), left anterior descending (LAD), first diagonal (1-D), second diagonal (2-D), left circumflex (LCx), and first and second marginal obtuse branches (1-MO, 2-MO)

or intermediate pretest probability of disease. Thus, the technique has been applied in the preoperative screening of noncoronary cardiovascular surgery, although initial reports are limited to patients with valvular heart disease, in regular sinus rhythm. In the largest study to date, patients with atrial fibrillation also were included. All these studies, however, consist basically of a comparison between ICA and coronary CT angiography, without testing the actual value of coronary CT angiography in terms of avoiding routine ICA in these patients.

The findings of the various studies can be summarized as—first, preoperative routine ICA can be safely avoided in a considerable number of patients scheduled to undergo noncoronary cardiovascular surgery by use of coronary CT

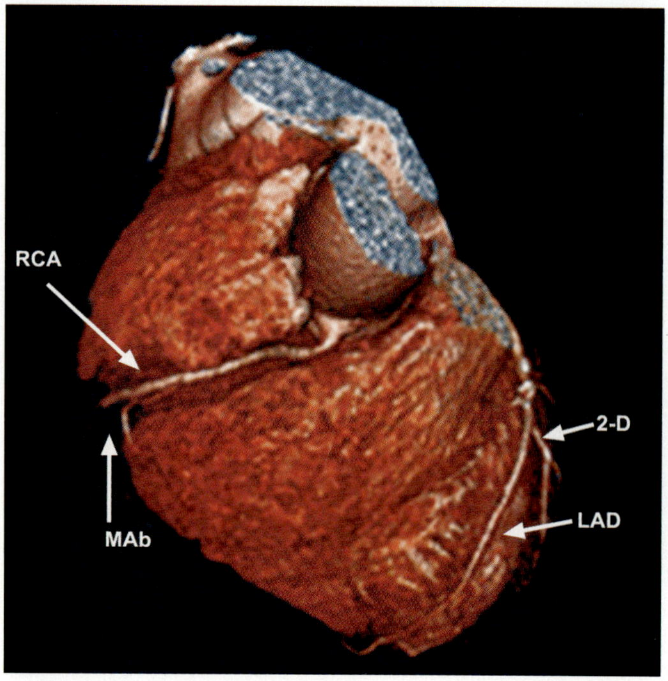


Fig. 4.78: Coronary CT angiographic results in patient with a dilated left atrium and atrial fibrillation with mean heart rate of 73 beats per minute at coronary CT angiographic acquisition. Volume-rendered CT image (right anterior oblique view with cranial angulation) shows the arteries—right coronary artery (RCA), marginal acute branch (MAb), left anterior descending (LAD), and second diagonal (2-D)

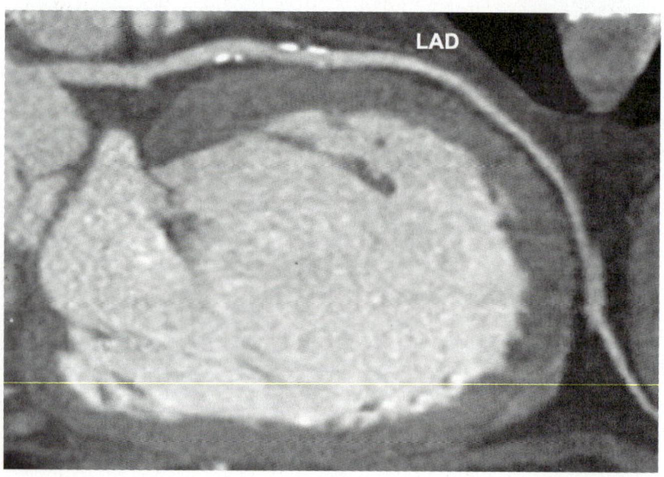


Fig. 4.79: Coronary CT angiographic results in patient with a dilated left atrium and atrial fibrillation with mean heart rate of 73 beats per minute at coronary CT angiographic acquisition. Curved multiplanar reconstruction of left anterior descending coronary

angiography; second, the presence of a controlled atrial fibrillation does not preclude performing diagnostic coronary CT angiographic examination; third, an Agatston score of coronary calcification higher than 579 significantly increases the likelihood of a subsequent nondiagnostic coronary CT angiography.

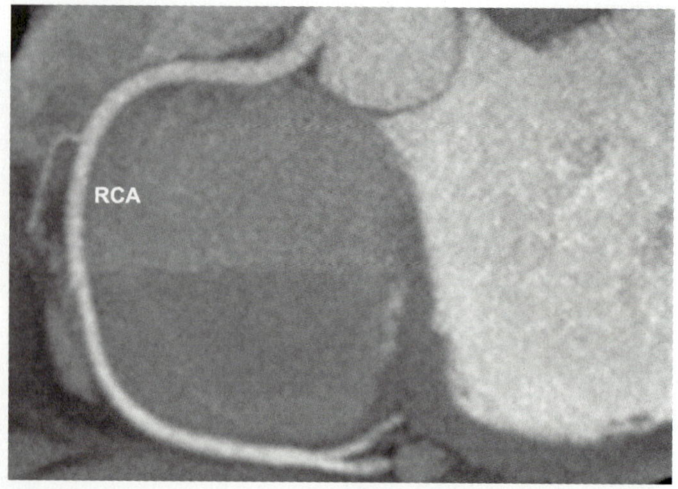


Fig. 4.80: Coronary CT angiographic results in patient with a dilated left atrium and atrial fibrillation with mean heart rate of 73 beats per minute at coronary CT angiographic acquisition. Maximum intensity projection of right coronary artery

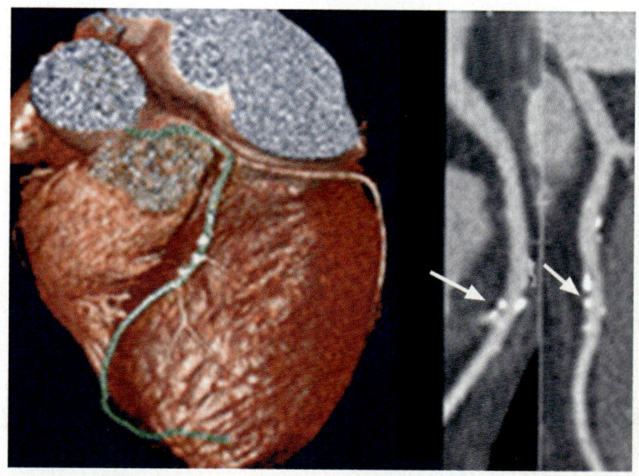

Fig. 4.81: Noninvasive coronary multidetector CT angiographic images of diagnostic categories. Left anterior descending coronary artery with nonsignificant stenosis (arrows)

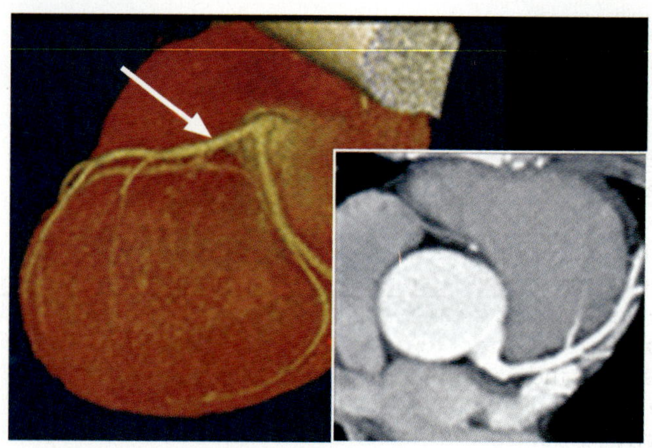

Fig. 4.82: Noninvasive coronary multidetector CT angiographic images of diagnostic categories. Normal left anterior descending coronary artery (arrow)

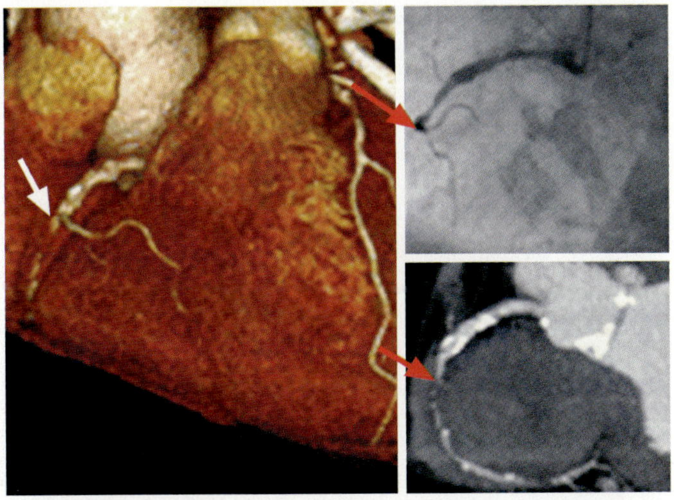

**Fig. 4.83:** Noninvasive coronary multidetector CT angiographic images of diagnostic categories. Right coronary artery with a significant stenosis; a total occlusion of the midpart of the right coronary artery (arrows). Top right—ICA image

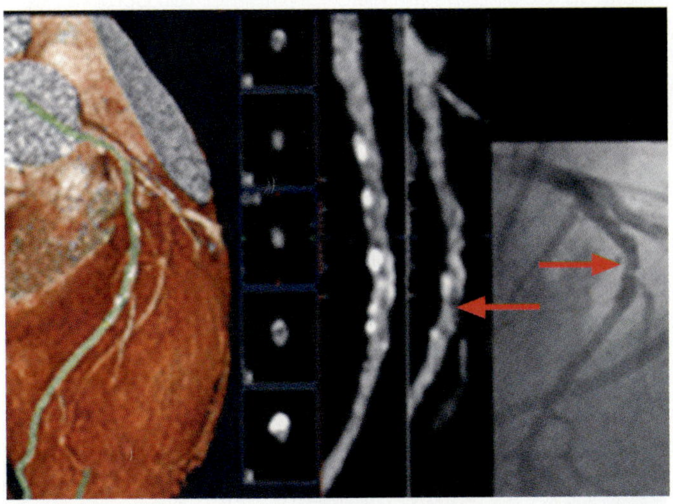

**Fig. 4.84:** Noninvasive coronary multidetector CT angiographic images of diagnostic categories. Coronary CT angiogram is nondiagnostic because of severe calcification and shows significant stenosis (arrows) on ICA image (far right)

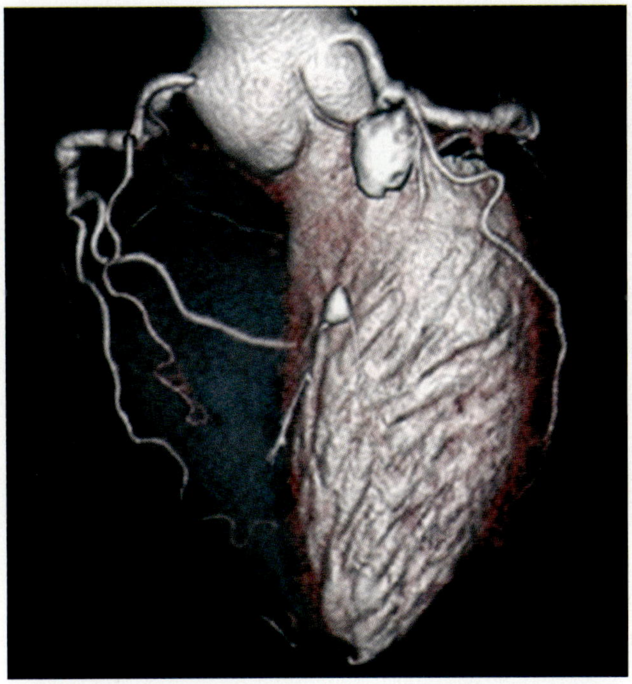

**Fig. 4.85:** 20-year-adolescent with Kawasaki disease. VR image show partly calcified thrombosed saccular aneurysm in proximal LAD. He has another fusiform aneurysm in the right coronary artery

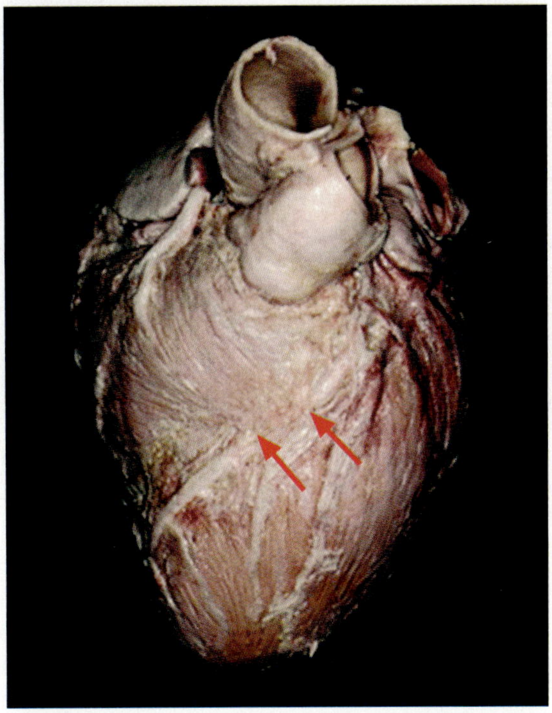

**Fig. 4.86:** MB in the LAD of an autopsied heart. The epicardial adipose tissues were manually removed after fixation with formaldehyde. The two arrows indicate the entrance and exit of the MB, respectively

The performance of ICA as a screening preoperative test before major noncoronary cardiovascular surgery in patients at risk for CAD is recommended. The rationale for this approach lies in the proved adverse prognosis after surgery in patients with undetected CAD and in the reduction in terms of mortality observed when coronary revascularization is performed simultaneously with noncoronary cardiovascular surgery Although noninvasive tests for inducible ischemia could represent an alternative to ICA, its usefulness is limited in practice because of a proved suboptimal predictive value of postoperative complications in these patients.

As an invasive procedure, ICA is costly and carries a small but definite risk of complications (1.5%) and even a certain mortality risk (0.15%), and these numbers are higher when the population involved has an increased associated comorbidity, as is the case in those patients scheduled to

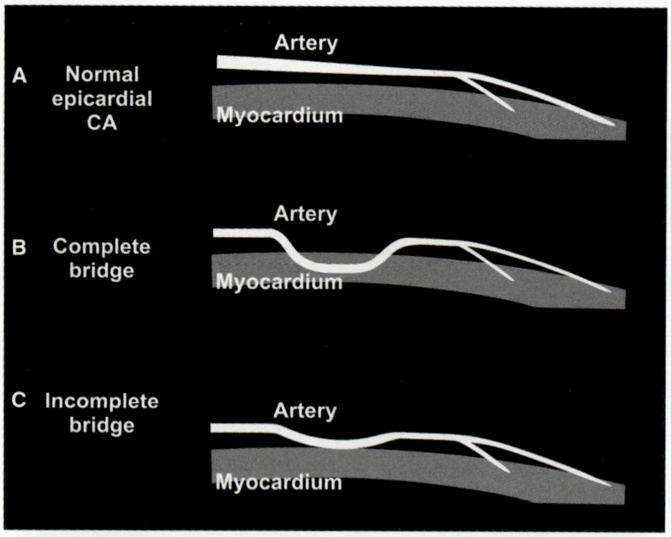


**Fig. 4.87:** (A) Normal epicardial artery. (B) Complete bridging of the artery. (C) Incomplete bridging of the epicardial artery

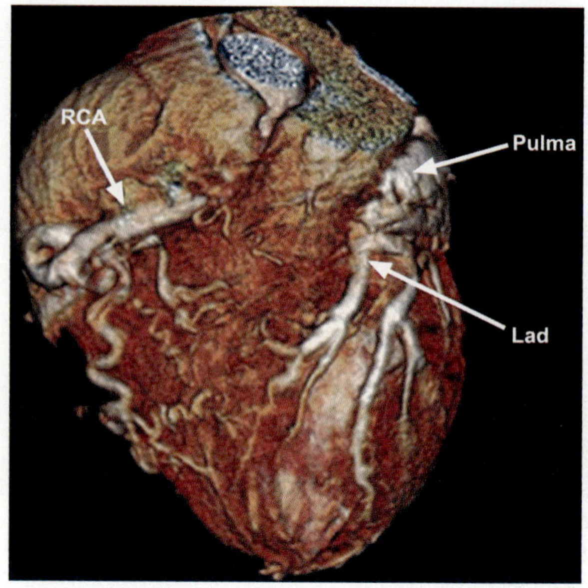


**Fig. 4.89:** CT angiography volume rendered image. Right coronary artery is dilated and tortious with a large number of collaterals feeding the left coronary system. Left coronary artery is emerging from pulmonary artery trunk. The left anterior descending artery and their diagonal branches are also dilated and tortuous

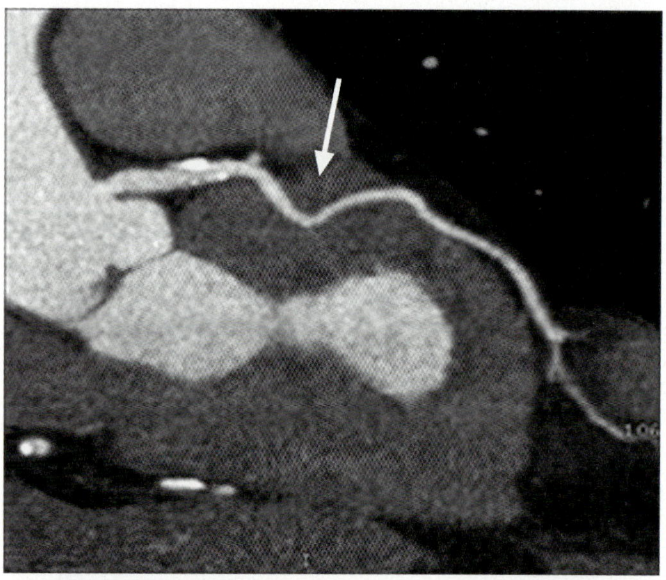

**Fig. 4.88:** An adolescent with suspected coronary artery disease. Curved MPR shows long segment of myocardial bridging of mid LAD

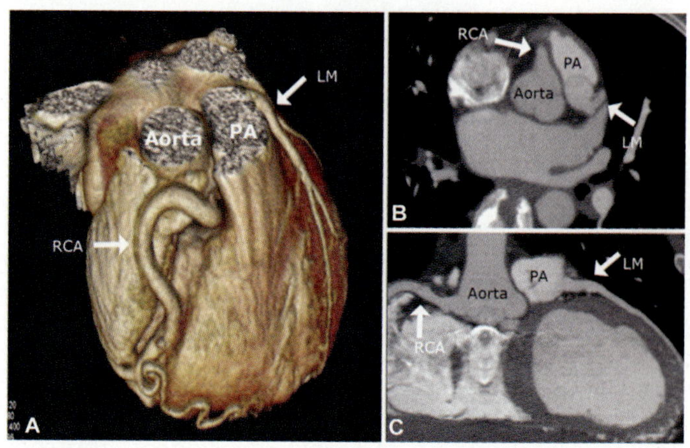


**Fig. 4.90:** CT-angiography before operation. Coronary CT-angiography showing an anomalous origin of the left main coronary artery (LM) from the pulmonary artery (PA). Normal course of a very large right coronary artery (RCA) is seen. Volume-rendered reformation (A), axial (B), and curved multiplanar reconstruction (C)

undergo noncoronary cardiovascular surgery. Furthermore, most of these patients will have normal results at ICA examination; the prevalence of significant CAD in these patients has been reported to range between 10% and 20%.

Because coronary CT angiography has recently emerged as a valuable noninvasive tool for the diagnosis of CAD in symptomatic patients with low to intermediate pretest risk, it seems appropriate to apply the technique to rule out CAD in patients scheduled to undergo noncoronary cardiovascular surgery. Some previous studies have shown a good correlation between coronary CT angiographic and ICA results in selected groups of patients submitted to undergo noncoronary cardiovascular surgery. Of note, in our study, patients did not undergo preoperative ICA if deemed to be free of significant CAD after diagnostic coronary CT angiographic examination. Most important, none of these patients had peri- or postoperative complications potentially because of CAD, thus proving the safety of this approach. ICA was performed, in addition to coronary CT angiography, in a total of 40 patients. In those with nondiagnostic coronary CT angiographic studies, ICA

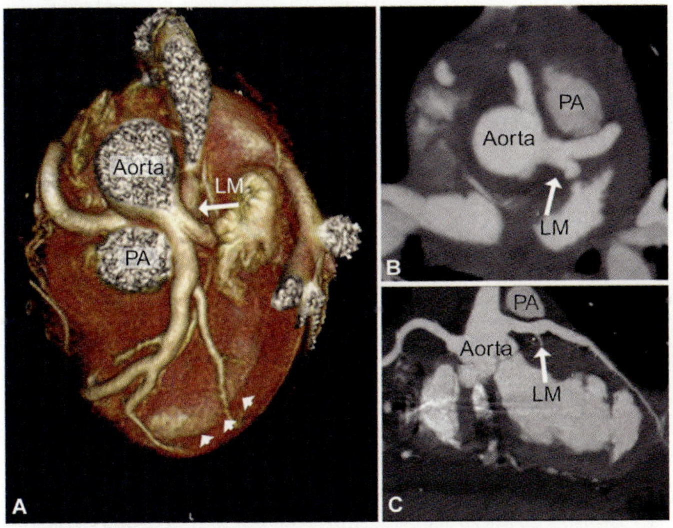


**Fig. 4.91:** CT-angiography after operation. Coronary CT-angiography after aortic reimplantation of the left coronary artery confirms patency. Note the myocardial wall thinning in the apical anterior part of the left ventricle demonstrating the old infarction (arrowheads). Volume-rendered reformation (A), axial (B) and curved multiplanar reconstruction (C)

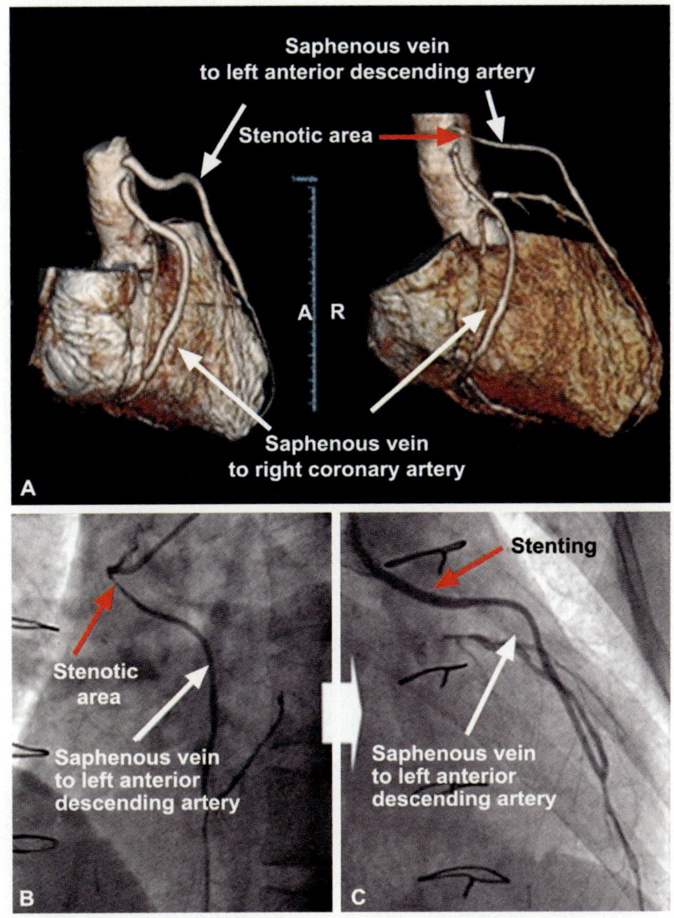


**Fig. 4.92:** Chronic occlusion of left saphenous vein graft (SVG). (A–left panel) Immediate after CABG surgery, three-dimensional volume-rendered image showed that left saphenous vein graft (SVG) was patent with its anastomosis to the mid-portion of left anterior descending (LAD) artery. There was a patent right saphenous vein graft (SVG), which was attached to the distal-portion of right coronary artery (RCA). (A–right panel) At 8 months after CABG surgery, three-dimensional volume-rendered image showed severe stenosis at proximal-portion of left saphenous vein graft (SVG), which was attached to the midportion of left anterior descending (LAD) artery. Right saphenous vein graft (SVG) was still patent despite the graft had diffuse mild narrowing from proximal anastomosis site to distal anastomosis site, (B) invasive coronary angiography showed the proximal-portion of left saphenous vein graft (SVG) was severely occluded, and (C) percutaneous coronary intervention was performed successfully. Note that the findings of invasive coronary angiography is similar to those of three-dimensional volume-rendered images of 64-MDCT

results showed a relatively low (5 of 25) prevalence of significant CAD. In most of those patients catheterized because of apparently significant CAD at coronary CT angiography (11 of 15), severity of CAD was confirmed. This is in agreement with the reported suboptimal positive predictive value of coronary CT angiography for defining significant coronary artery lesions. In practice, however, this is not a major limitation in the setting of noninvasive preoperative screening for CAD, where it is more relevant to avoid underdiagnosis of CAD rather than overdiagnosis. The consequence will be that a small proportion of patients without significant CAD will still be referred to undergo ICA.

Most important, preoperative coronary CT angiography provides additional information about the thoracic aorta and other mediastinal structures, which is relevant for the cardiac surgeon's choice of cannulation and cross-clamping sites.

The consecutive recruitment of subjects without exclusions due to atrial fibrillation, which was present in nearly half of our population, is also important. Atrial fibrillation has been traditionally considered a relative contraindication to coronary CT angiographic examination. However, when the mean heart rate is appropriately controlled by means of medical therapy, the deleterious effect of an irregular heart rhythm on the quality of the images is notably minimized. The availability of systems for editing ECG synchronization improves the retrospective reconstruction in cases of arrhythmia. This is proved by the results of our study, which showed a similar proportion of nondiagnostic studies in patients with sinus rhythm and in those with controlled atrial fibrillation.

Nondiagnostic coronary CT angiography accounted for 19% of patients studied. The amount of coronary artery calcium, quantified by means of the Agatston score, was the determinant for a diagnostic study, with a cutoff of 579 being the best predictor. In view of these data, it could be questionable to proceed with noninvasive coronary CT angiography after coronary calcium scanning yielded an Agatston score higher than this value. For example, a rise

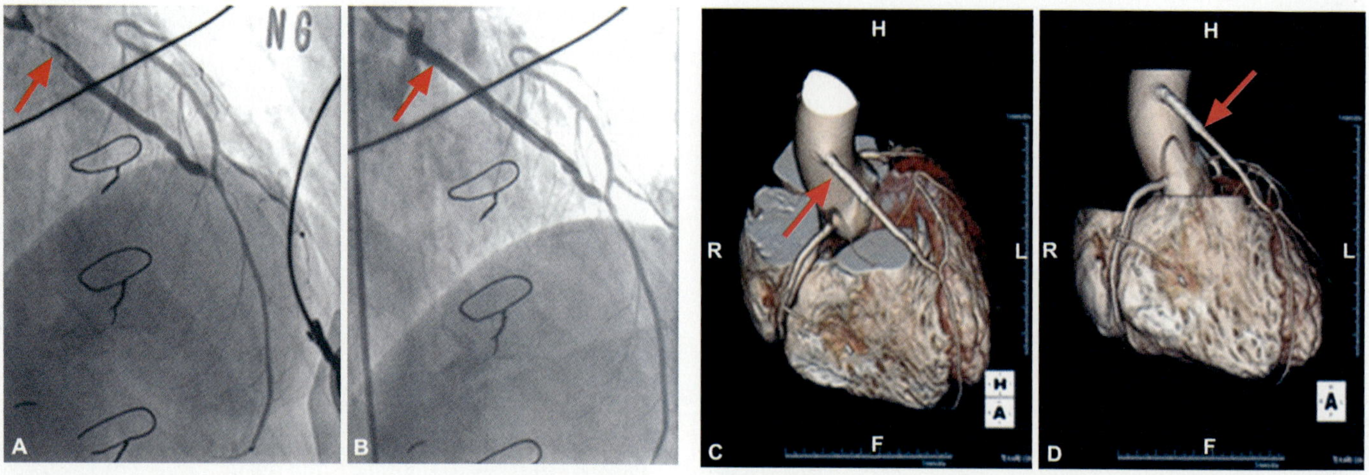


**Fig. 4.93:** Acute occlusion of saphenous vein graft (SVG). (A) Invasive coronary angiography showed the proximal-portion of saphenous vein graft (SVG) was severely occluded with thrombi. (B) After successful percutaneous coronary intervention (PCI), invasive coronary angiography showed the proximal portion of saphenous vein graft (SVG) with stenting was patent. (C, D) At 6-month follow-up, three-dimensional volume-rendered image showed the proximal portion of saphenous vein graft (SVG) with stenting was still patent. Note that the findings of invasive coronary angiography is similar to those of three-dimensional volume-rendered images of 64-MDCT. The figures also demonstrate that 64-MDCT has a useful role to follow-up of patients who have undergone percutaneous intervention for bypass graft stenosis and occlusion

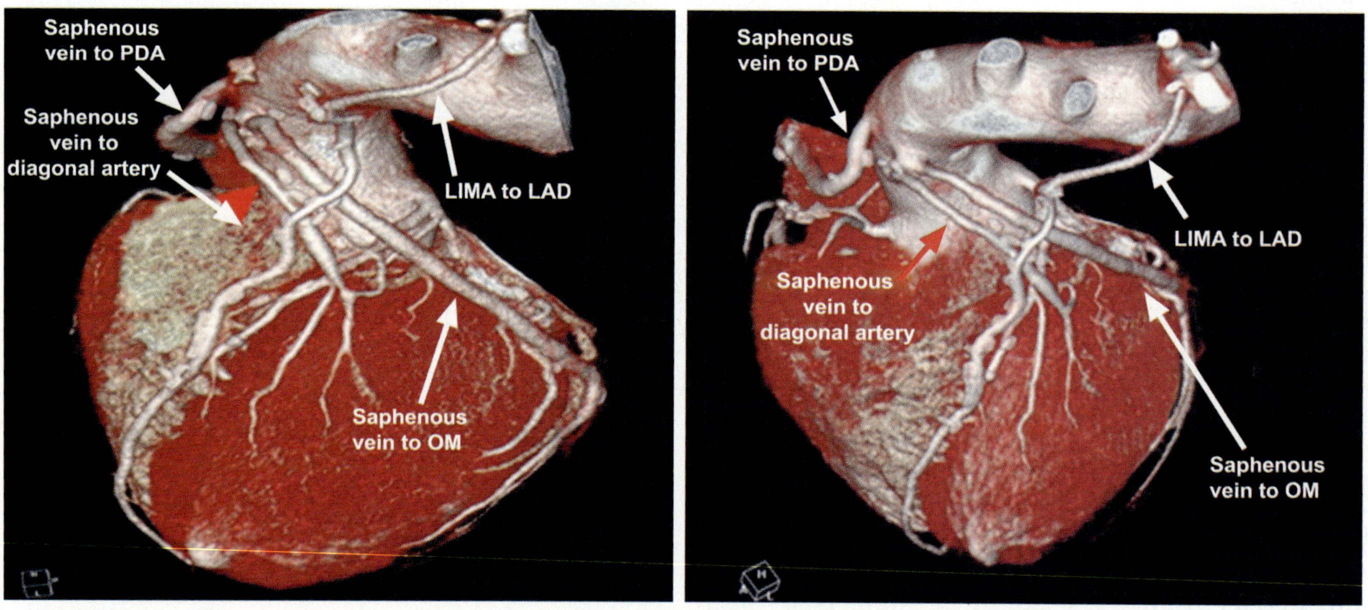


**Fig. 4.94:** Left internal mammary artery (IMA) graft. Three-dimensional volume-rendered images show the left IMA graft from its origin at the left subclavian artery to its anastomosis with the left anterior descending (LAD) artery. There is also a right saphenous vein graft (SVG) sutured to the anterior aorta with its anastomosis with the posterior descending artery (PDA). The left saphenous vein grafts (SVG) are attached to diagonal artery and the obtuse marginal (OM) artery

in the Agatston score from 579 to 1000 or 1500 increases two- and sixfold, respectively, the risk of nondiagnostic coronary CT angiography. As with any other procedure that involves CT, radiation associated with coronary CT angiography is an issue of concern. In particular, the estimated doses of radiation in our study proved to be significantly higher than those reported for diagnostic ICA. Strategies to limit radiation dose include reduction of tube current or voltage, which is not always feasible in patients with large body mass, and the use of prospective X-ray tube current modulation, which cannot be used in patients with atrial fibrillation, which is a frequent occurrence in this clinical setting. The new generation of CT systems already available, which are based on a single heart beat volume acquisition, will greatly overcome this limitation by means of an important reduction of radiation.

A potential limitation of the study was that its results cannot be extrapolated to other populations of patients usually submitted to preoperative ICA, as those scheduled to undergo major vascular surgery, in whom the presumably higher prevalence of significant CAD would probably lead to a lower number of avoided ICA studies. A further study particularly addressing this issue is warranted.

## SUMMARY

In conclusion, in patients scheduled to undergo noncoronary cardiovascular surgery, including those with controlled atrial fibrillation, the presence or absence of CAD can be reliably assessed preoperatively by using coronary CT angiography in a majority of cases. Preoperative ICA was safely avoided in those patients without significant CAD. A proportion of nondiagnostic coronary CT angiographic studies still remained, mainly because of severe coronary calcification, and a high Agatston score was the only predictor of an adequate coronary CT angiographic examination.

### Advances in Knowledge

- In patients scheduled to undergo noncoronary cardiovascular surgery, coronary CT angiograms are of diagnostic image quality in 81% of cases.
- The presence of atrial fibrillation is not a limitation for performing diagnostic coronary CT angiography, provided that the ventricular heart rate is adequately controlled to less than 70 beats per minute.
- The presence of severe coronary artery calcification is the only independent predictor of nondiagnostic coronary CT angiography; an Agatston score cutoff of about 600 shows the best predictive accuracy for performing diagnostic coronary CT angiography.
- Preoperative invasive coronary angiography can be safely omitted in patients without significant CAD (defined as >50% stenosis) by using coronary CT angiography.

### *Implications for Patient Care*

- Coronary CT angiography is a useful preoperative test for safely avoiding ICA in most of the patients scheduled to undergo noncoronary cardiovascular surgery.
- Coronary CT angiography provides additional anatomic information on extracoronary structures that may be relevant in relation to the surgical procedure.

## BIBLIOGRAPHY


1. American Heart Association. Heart and Stroke Facts: 1996 Statistical Supplement. Dallas, TX: American Heart Association. 1996;22.
2. Bates DW, Bernstein SJ. Coronary Angiography in Acute Myocardial Infarction: A Review of the Literature Regarding Efficacy and Risks. Boston, MA: Harvard Medical School, Department of Health Care Policy; 1995.
3. Bettencourt N, Rocha J, Carvalho M, et al. Multislice computed tomography in the exclusion of coronary artery disease in patients with presurgical valve disease. Circ Cardiovasc Imaging 2009;2(4):306–13.
4. Bettmann MA. Safety and efficacy of iodinated contrast agents. Invest Radiol 1994;29:S33–S36.
5. Blustein J. High-technology cardiac procedures: the impact of service availability on service use in New York State. JAMA 1993;270:344–9.
6. Bonow RO, Carabello BA, Chatterjee K, et al. ACC/AHA 2006 guidelines for the management of patients with valvular heart disease: a report of the ACC/AHA Task Force on Pactice guide-lines (Writing Committee to revise the 1998 Guidelines for the Management of Patients With Valvular Heart Disease) developed in collaboration with the Society of Cardiovascular Anesthesiologists endorsed by the Society for Cardiovascular Angiography and Interventions and the Society of Thoracic Surgeons. J Am Coll Cardiol 2006;48:e1-e148.
7. Budoff MJ, Dowe D, Jollis JG, et al. Diagnostic performance of 64-multidetector row coronary computed tomographic angiography for evaluation of coronary artery stenosis in individuals without known coronary artery disease: results from the prospective multicenter ACCURACY (Assessment by Coronary Computed Tomographic Angiography of Individuals Undergoing Invasive Coronary Angiography) trial. J Am Coll Cardiol 2008;52(21):1724–32.
8. Califf RM, Phillips HR III, Hindman MC, et al. Prognostic value of a coronary artery jeopardy score. J Am Coll Cardiol 1985;5:1055–63.
9. Czer LS, Gray RJ, Stewart ME, De Robertis M, Chaux A, Matloff JM. Reduction in sudden late death by concomitant revascularization with aortic valve replacement. J Thorac Cardiovasc Surg 1988;95(3):390–401.
10. Deray G, Jacobs C. Radiocontrast nephrotoxicity: a review. Invest Radiol 1995;30:221–5.
11. DiSalvo TT, Paul SD, Lloyd-Jones D, et al. Care of acute myocardial infarction by noninvasive and invasive cardiologists: procedure use, cost and outcome. J Am Coll Cardiol 1996;27:262–9.
12. Emond M, Mock MB, Davis KB, et al. Long-term survival of medically treated patients in the Coronary Artery Surgery Study (CASS) Registry. Circulation 1994;90:2645–57.
13. Every NR, Larson EB, Litwin PE, et al. The association between on-site cardiac catheterization facilities and the use of coronary angiography after acute myocardial infarction: Myocardial Infarction Triage and Intervention Project Investigators. N Engl J Med 1993;329:546–51.
14. Gaur S, Achenbach S, Leipsic J, et al. Rationale and design of the Heart Flow NXT (Heart Flow analysis of coronary blood flow using CT angiography: NeXt sTeps) study. J Cardiovasc Comput Tomogr 2013;7:279–88.
15. Gensini GG. Coronary Angiography. Mount Kisco, NY: Futura Publishing; 1996.
16. Graves EJ. National hospital discharge survey: annual summary, 1993. Vital Health Stat 13 1995;1–63.
17. Greenberger PA, Patterson R, Tapio CM. Prophylaxis against repeated radiocontrast media reactions in 857 cases: adverse experience with cimetidine and safety of beta-adrenergic antagonists. Arch Intern Med 1985;145:2197–200.

18. Greenberger PA, Patterson R. Adverse reactions to radiocontrast media. Prog Cardiovasc Dis 1988;31:239–48.
19. Grossman WB, Baim DS. Cardiac Catheterization, Angiography and Intervention. Philadelphia, Pa: Lea & Febiger; 1991.
20. Guadagnoli E, Hauptman PJ, Ayanian JZ, et al. Variation in the use of cardiac procedures after acute myocardial infarction. N Engl J Med 1995;333:573–8.
21. Guidelines for professional staff privileges in the cardiac catheterization laboratory: Laboratory Performance Standards Committee. Cathet Cardiovasc Diagn 1990;21: 203–4.
22. Hanley PC, Vlietstra RE, Fisher LD, Smith HC. Indications for coronary angiography: changes in laboratory practice over a decade. Mayo Clin Proc. 1986;61:248–53.
23. Hirshfeld JW Jr, Ellis SG, Faxon DP. Recommendations for the assessment and maintenance of proficiency in coronary interventional procedures: statement of the American College of Cardiology. J Am Coll Cardiol 1998;31:722–743.
24. Johnson LW, Lozner EC, Johnson S, et al. Coronary arterio-graphy 1984–1987: a report of the Registry of the Society for Cardiac Angiography and Interventions, I: results and complications. Cathet Cardiovasc Diagn 1989;17:5–10.
25. Kimmel SE, Berlin JA, Laskey WK. The relationship between coronary angioplasty procedure volume and major compli-cations. JAMA 1995;274:1137–42.
26. Koo BK, Erglis A, Doh JH, et al. Diagnosis of ischemia-causing coronary stenoses by noninvasive fractional flow reserve computed from coronary computed tomographic angiograms. Results from the prospective multicenter DISCOVER-FLOW (Diagnosis of Ischemia-Causing Stenoses Obtained Via Noninvasive Fractional Flow Reserve) study. J Am Coll Cardiol 2011;58:1989-97.
27. Laskey W, Boyle J, Johnson LW. Multivariable model for prediction of risk of significant complication during diag-nostic cardiac catheterization: the Registry Committee of the Society for Cardiac Angiography and Interventions. Cathet Cardiovasc Diagn 1993;30:185–90.
28. Lasser EC, Berry CC, Talner LB, et al. Pretreatment with corticosteroids to alleviate reactions to intravenous contrast material. N Engl J Med 1987;317:845–9.
29. Leape LL, Park RE, Solomon DH, et al. Does inappropriate use explain small-area variations in the use of health care services? JAMA 1990;263: 669–72.
30. Marcus ML, Schelbert HR, Skorton DJ, et al. Cardiac Imaging: A Companion to Braunwald's Heart Disease. Philadelphia, Pa: WB Saunders; 1991.
31. Mark DB, Naylor CD, Hlatky MA, et al. Use of medical resources and quality of life after acute myocardial infarction in Canada and the United States. N Engl J Med 1994;331: 1130–35.
32. Matthai WH Jr, Kussmaul WG III, Krol J, Goin JE, Schwartz JS, Hirshfeld JW Jr. A comparison of low-with high-osmolality contrast agents in cardiac angiography: identification of criteria for selective use. Circulation 1994;89:291–301.
33. Medicare claims data. Provided by the Physician Payment Review Commission. 1996.
34. Meijboom WB, Mollet NR, Van Mieghem CA, et al. Pre-operative computed tomography coronary angiography to detect significant coronary artery disease in patients referred for cardiac valve surgery. J Am Coll Cardiol 2006;48(8): 1658–65.
35. Meijboom WB, van Mieghem CA, Mollet NR, et al. 64-slice computed tomography coronary angiography in patients with high, intermediate, or low pretest probability of significant coronary artery disease. J Am Coll Cardiol 2007;50(15): 1469–75.
36. Mikkonen R, Kontkanen T, Kivisaari L. Acute and late adverse reactions to low-osmolal contrast media. Acta Radiol 1995;36:72–6.
37. Min JK, Leipsic J, Pencina MJ, et al. Diagnostic accuracy of fractional flow reserve from anatomic CT angiography. JAMA 2012;308:1237–45.
38. Myers GE, Bloom FL. Cimetidine (Tagamet) combined with steroids and H1 antihistamines for the prevention of serious radiographic contrast material reactions. Cathet Cardiovasc Diagn 1981;7:65–9.
39. National Heart, Lung, and Blood Institute Coronary Artery Surgery Study. A multicenter comparison of the effects of randomized medical and surgical treatment of mildly sympto-matic patients with coronary artery disease and a registry of consecutive patients undergoing coronary angiography. Circulation 1981;63:I-1–I-81 Monograph 79.
40. Norgaard BL, Leipsic J, Sengupta S, et al. Quantitative assess-ment of image quality for determination of FFR by coronary computed tomography angiography (abstr). J Cardiovasc Comput Tomogr 2013;3(Suppl):233.
41. Noto TJ Jr, Johnson LW, Krone R, et al. Cardiac catheterization 1990: a report of the Registry of the Society for Cardiac Angiography and Interventions (SCA&I). Cathet Cardiovasc Diagn 1991;24:75–83.
42. Parfrey PS, Griffiths SM, Barrett BJ, et al. Contrast material-induced renal failure in patients with diabetes mellitus, renal insufficiency, or both: a prospective controlled study. N Engl J Med 1989;320:143–9.
43. Pashos CL, Newhouse JP, McNeil BJ. Temporal changes in the care and outcomes of elderly patients with acute myocardial infarction, 1987 through 1990. JAMA 1993;270: 1832–6.
44. Pepine CJ, Allen HD, Bashore TM, et al. ACC/AHA guidelines for cardiac catheterization and cardiac catheterization laboratories: American College of Cardiology/American Heart Association Ad Hoc Task Force on Cardiac Catheterization. J Am Coll Cardiol 1991;18:1149–82.
45. Pilote L, Califf RM, Sapp S, et al. Regional variation across the United States in the management of acute myocardial infarction: GUSTO-1 Investigators. Global Utilization of Streptokinase and Tissue Plasminogen Activator for Occluded Coronary Arteries. N Engl J Med 1995;333:565–72.
46. Potter DD, Sundt TM 3rd., Zehr KJ, et al. Operative risk of reoperative aortic valve replacement. J Thorac Cardiovasc Surg 2005;129(1):94–103.
47. Ringqvist I, Fisher LD, Mock M, et al. Prognostic value of angiographic indices of coronary artery disease from the Coronary Artery Surgery Study (CASS). J Clin Invest 1983;71:1854–66.
48. Ritchie JL, Phillips KA, Luft HS. Coronary angioplasty: statewide experience in California. Circulation 1993;88:2735–43.
49. Ross J Jr, Brandenburg RO, Dinsmore RE, et al. ACC/AHA Guidelines for coronary angiography. A report of the

American College of Cardiology/American Heart Association Task Force on Assessment of Diagnostic and Therapeutic Cardiovascular Procedures (Subcommittee on Coronary Angiography). J Am Coll Cardiol 1987;10:935–9502.

50. Rouleau JL, Moye LA, Pfeffer MA, et al. A comparison of management patterns after acute myocardial infarction in Canada and the United States: the SAVE investigators. N Engl J Med 1993;328:779–84.
51. Rudnick MR, Goldfarb S, Wexler L, et al. Nephrotoxicity of ionic and nonionic contrast media in 1,196 patients: a randomized trial. The Iohexol Cooperative Study. Kidney Int 1995;47:254–61.
52. Russo V, Gostoli V, Lovato L, et al. Clinical value of multidetector CT coronary angiography as a preoperative screening test before non-coronary cardiac surgery. Heart 2007; 93(12):1591–8.
53. Salas-Lara VM, Rangel-Abundis A, Solorio-Meza S, Albarrán-López H. Assessment of a predictive index for coronary artery disease in patients with rheumatic valvular disease. Cir Cir 2005;73(2):85–9.
54. Schwab SJ, Hlatky MA, Pieper KS, et al. Contrast nephro-toxicity: a randomized controlled trial of a nonionic and an ionic radiographic contrast agent. N Engl J Med 1989;320:149–53.
55. Selby JV, Fireman BH, Lundstrom RJ, et al. Variation among hospitals in coronary-angiography practices and outcomes after myocardial infarction in a large health maintenance organization. N Engl J Med 1996;335:1888–96.
56. Selker HP, Zalenski RJ, Antman EM, et al. An evaluation of technologies for identifying acute cardiac ischemia in the emergency department: executive summary of a National Heart Attack Alert Program Working Group Report. Ann Emerg Med 1997;29:1–12.
57. Solomon R, Werner C, Mann D, et al. Effects of saline, mannitol, and furosemide to prevent acute decreases in renal function induced by radiocontrast agents. N Engl J Med 1994;331:1416–20.
58. Spertus JA, Weiss NS, Every NR, Weaver WD. The influence of clinical risk factors on the use of angiography and revascularization after acute myocardial infarction: Myocardial Infarction Triage and Intervention Project Investigators. Arch Intern Med 1995;155:2309–16.
59. Taliercio CP, Vlietstra RE, Fisher LD, et al. Risks for renal dysfunction with cardiac angiography. Ann Intern Med 1986;104:501–4.
60. Tommaso CL. Contrast-induced nephrotoxicity in patients undergoing cardiac catheterization. Cathet Cardiovasc Diagn 1994;31:316–321.
61. Tu JV, Pashos CL, Naylor CD, et al. Use of cardiac procedures and outcomes in elderly patients with myocardial infarction in the United States and Canada. N Engl J Med 1997;336: 1500–05.
62. Vahanian A, Baumgartner H, Bax J, et al. Guidelines on the management of valvular heart disease: The Task Force on the Management of Valvular Heart Disease of the European Society of Cardiology. Eur Heart J 2007;28(2):230–68.
63. Wittbrodt ET, Spinler SA. Prevention of anaphylactoid reactions in high-risk patients receiving radiographic contrast media. Ann Pharmacother 1994;28:236–41.

# 5 Right Ventricular Infarction

Right ventricular infarction was first recognized in a subgroup of patients with inferior wall myocardial infarctions who demonstrated right ventricular failure and elevated right ventricular filling pressures despite relatively normal left ventricular filling pressures. Increasing recognition of right ventricular infarction, either in association with left ventricular infarction or as an isolated event, emphasizes the clinical significance of the right ventricle to total cardiac function.

Interest in recognizing right ventricular infarction noninvasively has grown because of the therapeutic implications of distinguishing patients with right ventricular dysfunction from those with the more usual clinical presentation of left ventricular dysfunction. Patients with right ventricular infarctions associated with inferior infarctions have much higher rates of significant hypotension, bradycardia requiring pacing support, and in-hospital mortality than isolated inferior infarctions.

## PATHOPHYSIOLOGY (Figs 5.1 and 5.2)

The right ventricle is a thin-walled chamber that functions at low oxygen demands and pressure. It is perfused throughout the cardiac cycle in both systole and diastole, and its ability to extract oxygen is increased during hemodynamic stress. All of these factors make the right ventricle less susceptible to infarction than the left ventricle.

The posterior descending branch of the right coronary artery usually supplies the inferior and posterior walls of the right ventricle. The marginal branches of the right coronary artery supply the lateral wall of the right ventricle. The anterior wall of the right ventricle has a dual blood supply—the conus branch of the right coronary artery and the moderator branch artery, which courses from the left anterior descending artery.

Interestingly, right ventricular infarction noted at necropsy usually involves the posterior septum and posterior wall rather than the right free wall. The relative sparing of the right ventricular anterior wall apparently arises from a high degree of collateralization. This collateral blood flow is thought to be derived from the thebesian veins and diffusion of oxygen directly from the ventricular cavity. A direct correlation exists between the anatomic site of right coronary artery occlusion and the extent of right ventricular

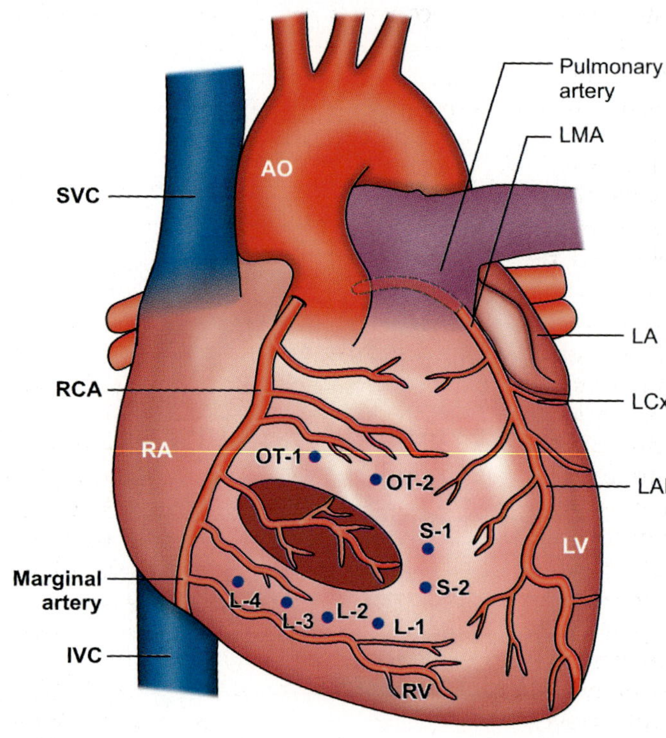


**Fig. 5.1:** Diagram showing heart viewed from the right anterolateral aspect. Sites of electrode placement; shaded area, region of infarction. Ao=aorta; SVC=superior vena cava; IVC=inferior vena cava; RA=right atrium; OT=outflow tract; S=septal; L=lateral; LMA=left main coronary artery; LCx=left circumflex coronary artery; and LA=left atrium

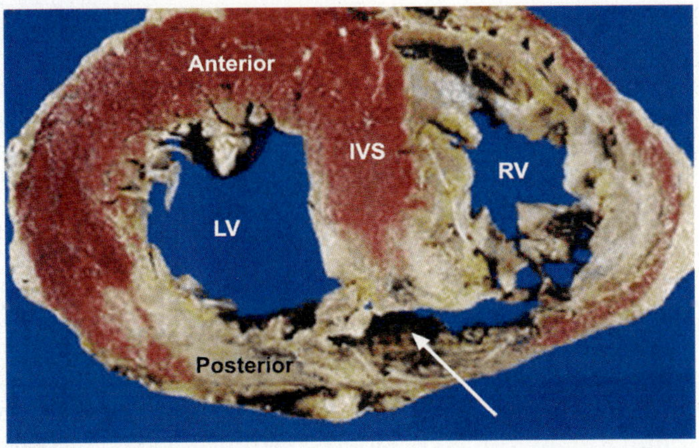


**Fig. 5.2:** Gross findings in a patient with a posterior ventricular septal rupture. There is an infarction involving the basal inferior septum, the basal posteroinferior wall, and the right ventricle (RV). The ventricular septal rupture (arrow) is complex, with an irregular, serpiginous tract at the junction of the inferior wall and the interventricular septum (IVS). LV denotes left ventricle

infarction. Studies have demonstrated that more proximal right coronary artery occlusions result in larger right ventricular infarctions. On occasion, the right ventricle can be subjected to infarction from occlusion of the left circumflex coronary artery.

Because the right ventricle is considered a low-pressure volume pump, its contractility is highly dependent on diastolic pressure. Hence, when contractility and associated diastolic dysfunction are impaired attendant to right ventricular infarction, the right ventricular diastolic pressure increases substantially and systolic pressure decreases. In such a scenario, concomitant left ventricular dysfunction, with increase in right ventricular afterload, is possible. In such a setting, right ventricular output can decrease dramatically, and the only driving force remaining is elevated right atrial pressure. In such a circumstance, the right ventricle serves as a poorly functioning conduit between the right atrium and the pulmonary artery.

Elevation of right atrial pressure secondary to right ventricular infarction has been noted to serve as a stimulus for secretion of atrial natriuretic factor. Increased levels of this polypeptide can be detrimental to normal left ventricular filling pressures. This occurs by virtue of the potent vasodilating, natriuretic, diuretic, and aldosterone-inhibiting properties of atrial natriuretic factor. Inappropriately elevated levels of atrial natriuretic factor may worsen the clinical syndrome of right ventricular infarction. The potential hemodynamic derangements associated with right ventricular infarction render the afflicted patient unusually sensitive to diminished preload (i.e. volume) and loss of atrioventricular synchrony. These two circumstances can result in a severe decrease in right and, secondarily, left, ventricular output.

Early thrombolysis or mechanical reperfusion of an occluded coronary artery resulting in right ventricular infarction is associated with prompt reduction in right atrial pressure. This is extremely important because persistently elevated right atrial pressure has been associated with increased in-hospital mortality rate when associated with myocardial infarction. The extent of right ventricular infarction varies greatly and is dependent on the site of occlusion of the right ventricular arterial supply. If occlusion occurs before the right ventricular marginal branches, and collateral blood flow from the left anterior descending coronary artery is absent, then the size of infarction generally is greater. Extent of infarction depends somewhat on flow through the thebesian veins.In general, any major reduction in blood supply to the right ventricular free wall portends an adverse prognosis in association with this disorder.

## FREQUENCY

Isolated infarction of the right ventricle is extremely rare; right ventricular infarction usually is noted in association with inferior wall myocardial infarction. The incidence of right ventricular infarction in such cases ranges from 10% to 50%, depending on the series.

The frequency of right ventricular infarction, which can be detected by right-sided precordial leads, in association with non-ST-segment elevation or non-Q-wave myocardial infarction is not known and currently is being investigated. Although right ventricular infarction is clinically evident in a sizable number of cases, the incidence is considerably less than that found at autopsy. A major reason for the discrepancy is the difficulty in establishing the presence of right ventricular infarction in living subjects. Additionally, right ventricular dysfunction and stunning frequently is of a transient nature, such that estimation of its true incidence is even more difficult.

Criteria have been set forth to diagnose right ventricular infarction; even when strictly employed, however, the criteria lead to underestimation of the true incidence of right ventricular infarction.

## HISTORY

- Although right ventricular infarction occurs in more than 30% of patients with inferior posterior left ventricular myocardial infarction, hemodynamically significant right ventricular infarction occurs in less than 10% of these patients.
- A right ventricular infarct should be considered in all patients who present with an acute inferior wall myocardial infarction, especially in the setting of a low cardiac output.
- Patients may describe symptoms consistent with hypotension.
- A subtle clue to the presence of hemodynamically significant right ventricular infarction is a marked sensitivity to preload-reducing agents such as nitrates, morphine, or diuretics.
- Other presentations include high-grade atrioventricular block, tricuspid regurgitation, cardiogenic shock, right ventricular free wall rupture, and cardiac tamponade.
- Should a patient with right ventricular infarction experience unexplained hypoxia despite administration of 100% oxygen, right-to-left shunting at the atrial

level in the presence of right ventricular failure and increased right atrial pressure must be considered. Despite its rarity, this complication of right ventricular infarction must always be considered when a patient with myocardial infarction is thought to have hypoxia secondary to clinically silent pulmonary emboli. The mechanism for right-to-left shunting in the absence of increased pulmonary arterial pressure resides in patency of the foramen ovale in association with poor right ventricular compliance and increased right atrial filling pressures.

- Patients with extensive right ventricular necrosis are at risk for right ventricular catheter-related perforation, and passage of a floating balloon catheter or pacemaker must always be performed with great care in such a setting.

## PHYSICAL EXAMINATION

The clinical triad of hypotension, clear lung fields, and elevated jugular venous pressure has been traditionally considered as a maker of RV infarction in patients with inferior wall myocardial infarction (IWMI). However, this triad has high specificity (96%) but very low sensitivity (25%). Kussmaul's venous sign (distension of the jugular vein on inspiration), a feature of constrictive pericarditis, may also occur with RV infarction. Electrocardiography and other noninvasive imaging modalities continue to be the cornerstones of the diagnosis of RV infarction because of the high specificity but low sensitivity associated with physical examination.

## IMAGING STUDIES

### Electrocardiography

In clinical practice, RV infarction is frequently diagnosed electrocardiographically. An ST-segment elevation of >1 mm in lead V4R is considered significant and correlates closely with other noninvasive evidences of RV dysfunction. This electrocardiographic finding is also a strong independent predictor of major complications and in-hospital mortality. This ST-segment elevation is thought to represent an ischemic injury of the posterobasal septum, since this area of contiguous myocardium is invariably damaged in patients who have pathological evidence of IWMI involving the RV (Figs 5.3–5.11).

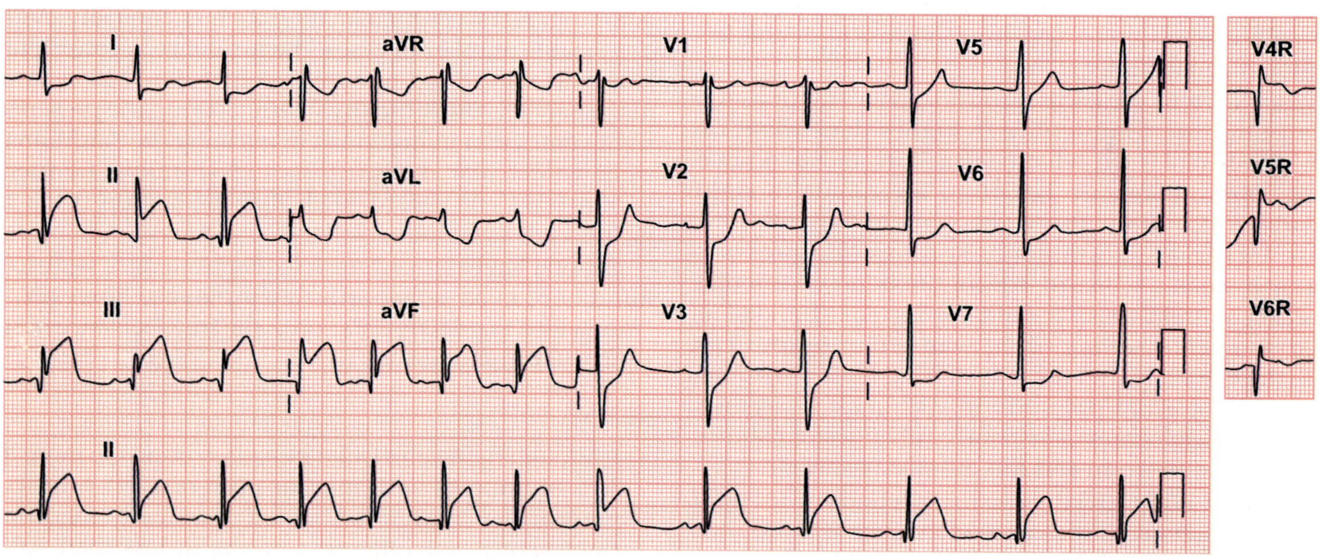


| | | | |
|---|---|---|---|
| ST-depression I + aVL>2mm | I + aVL >2mm | ST-elevation in aVF > ST depression in lead V2 | aVF > V2 |
| ST-elevation ≥ 1mm in V4R | ≥1mm V4R | ST-depression V3 < ½ ST-elevation lead III | V3 < ½ III |
| ST-elevation lead III> elevation at lead II | III > II | QRS prolongation in R precordial leads | V4R > V6 |
| Reciprocal depression at lateral leads | V6 | Epsilon waves in R precordial leads | V4R |

**Fig. 5.3:** Illustration showing various ECG criteria in the diagnosis of right ventricular myocardial infarction

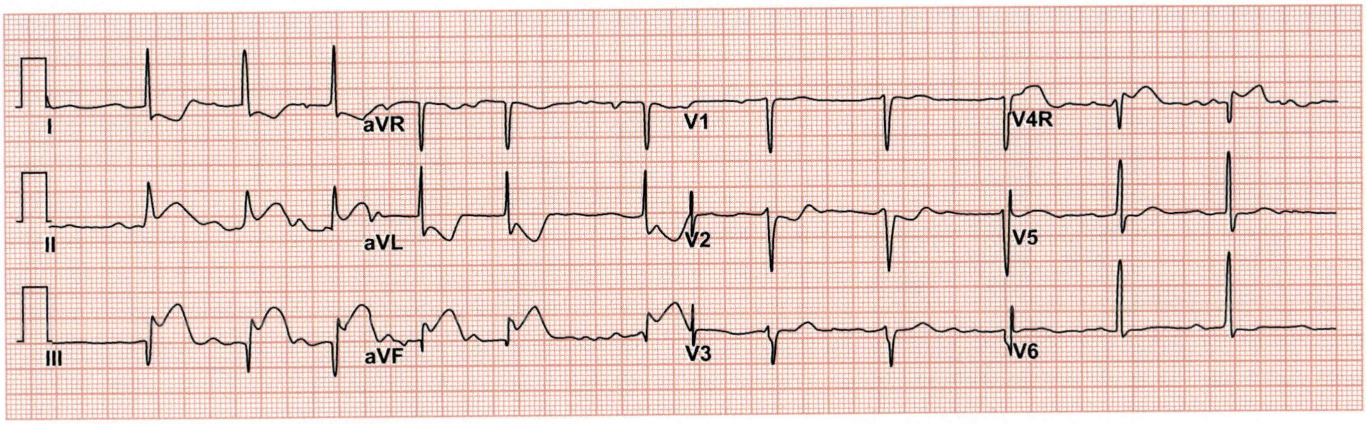


**Fig. 5.4:** ECG showing right ventricular MI—there is an inferior STEMI with ST-elevation in lead III >lead II. There is subtle ST-elevation in V1 with ST-depression in V2. There is ST-elevation in V4R

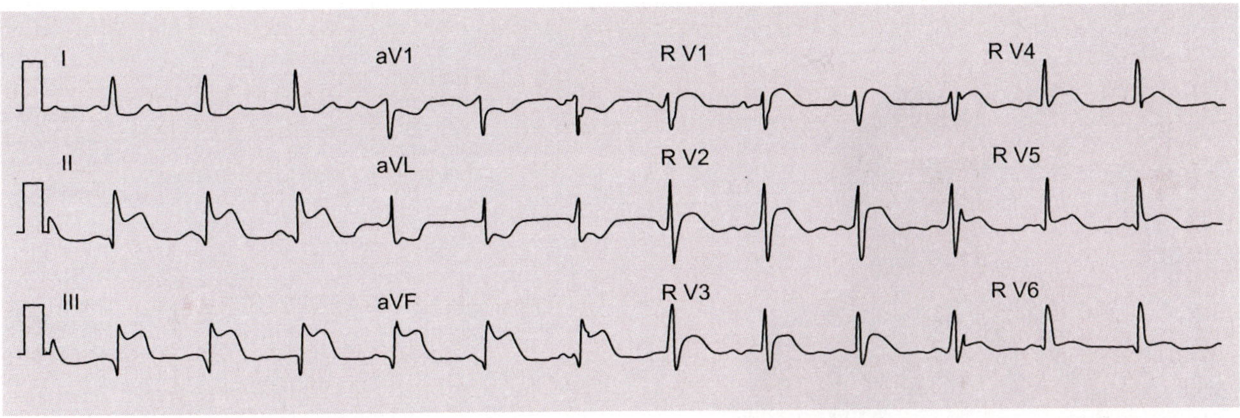


**Fig. 5.5:** ECG suggestive of RV infarction-ST-segment elevation (0.1 mV) in lead II, III and aVF (inferior leads)-coexistent ST-segment elevation in lead VR1–VR6 suggests right ventricular involvement pathological Q-waves formation in inferior leads—reciprocal ST-segment depression in lead I and aVL

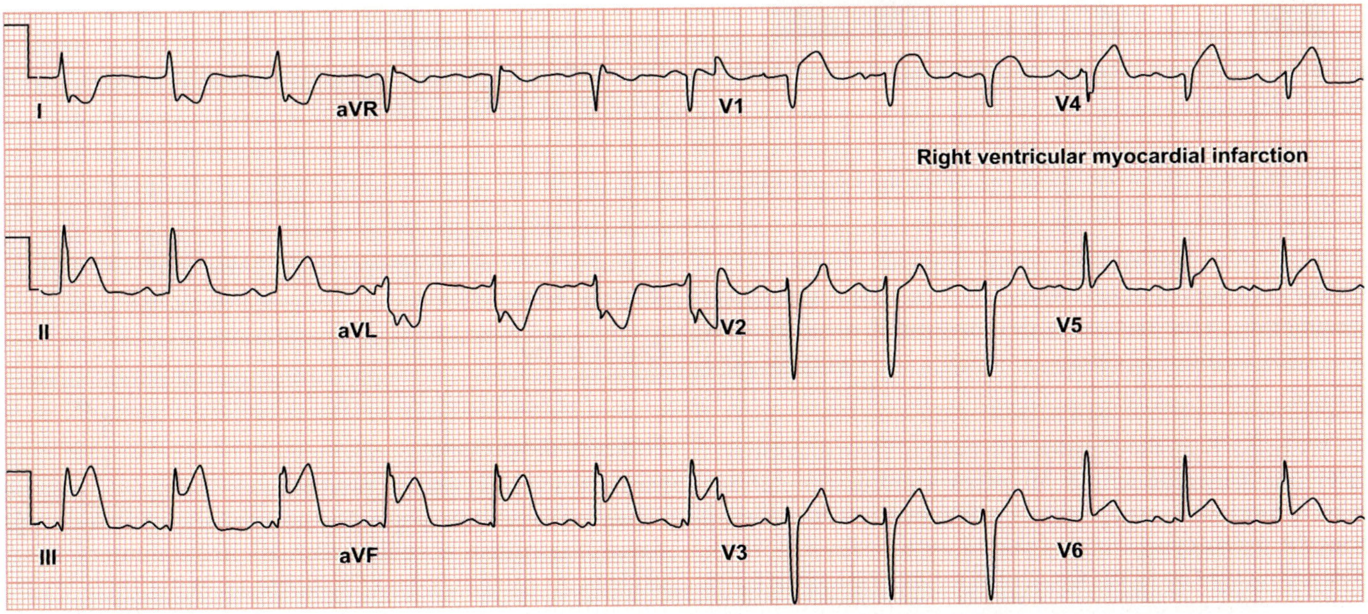


**Fig. 5.6:** ECG showing right ventricular myocardial infarction. ST-elevation in lead V1 and high R/S ratio in V1

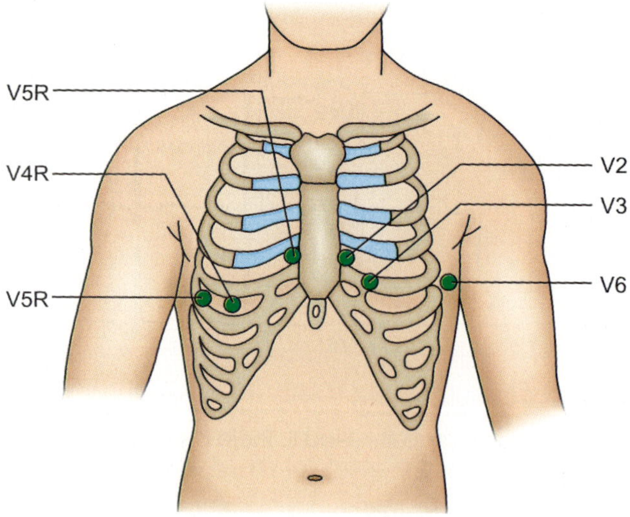


Fig. 5.7: Right-sided ECG leads placement on chest for diagnosis of RV infarct

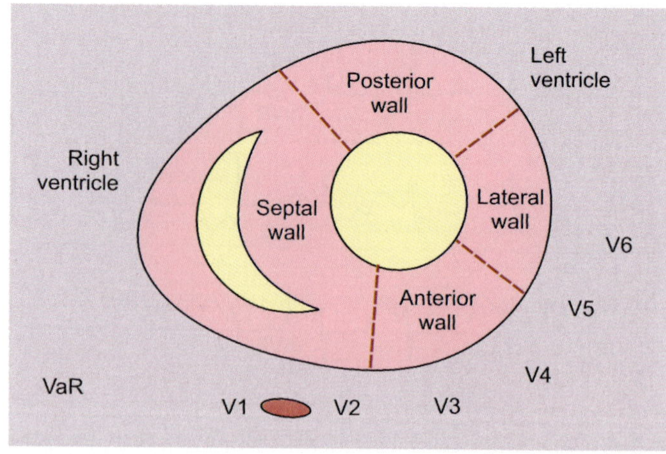


Fig. 5.9: Different regions of right and left ventricles and lead placement over the chest for diagnosis of myocardial injury

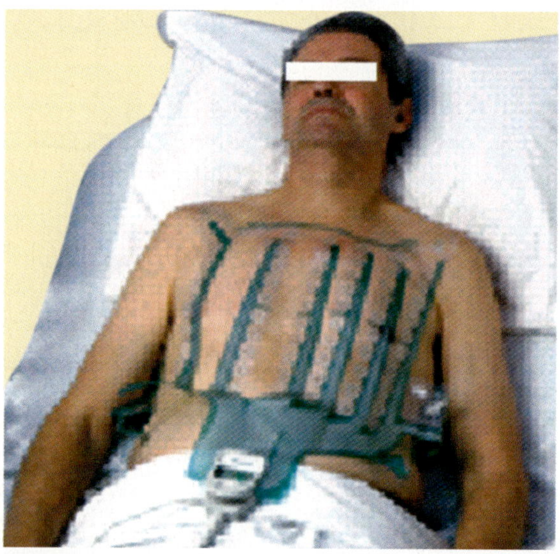

Fig. 5.8: ECG 80 leads placement on patient with chest pain of recent onset

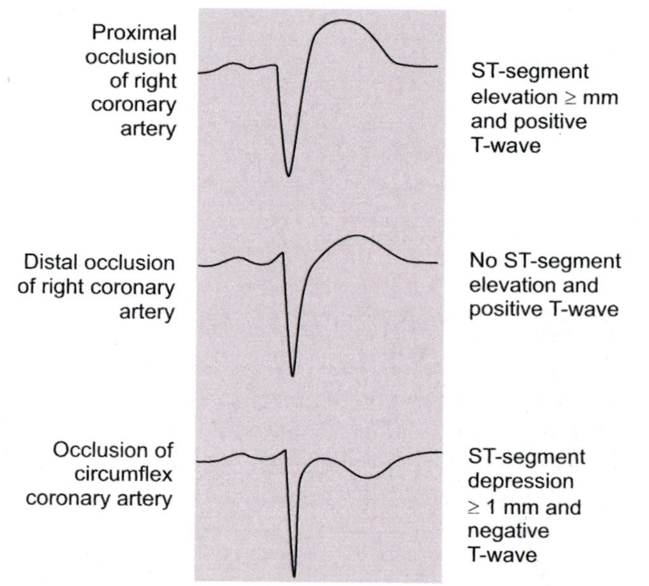


Fig. 5.10: ECG morphologies of segmental occlusion of right coronary and circumflex arteries

Notably, most of the so-called RV 'infarctions', indicated by right-sided ST-segment changes or pathological Q-waves, do not progress to an actual infarction (e.g. myocardial necrosis and scar formation); these electrocardiographic findings usually represent an early, transient phenomenon. This has been demonstrated recently in a study with sequential cardiac magnetic resonance (CMR) imaging. Several unique anatomic and physiological characteristics of the right ventricle contribute to recovery from RV infarction. First, pulmonary circulation is approximately one-tenth the length of systemic circulation, and a 5 mmHg perfusion gradient is sufficient to propel blood across the pulmonary circuit. Second, unlike diastolic flow in the left ventricle (LV), the thin RV free wall allows the biphasic perfusion of coronary blood, with approximately equal contributions during systole and diastole. Third, the right ventricle has rich collaterals from the left anterior descending artery in addition to right coronary artery (RCA) blood flow. Thus, RV infarcts may be clinically suspected in many patients with a stunned or hibernating RV free wall.

## Chest X-ray

Chest X-ray is shown in Fig. 5.12.

### *Echocardiography*

Since the late 1980s, considerable progress has been achieved in echocardiography and radionuclide techniques; these modalities revealed that RV involvement may be present in as much as 59% of the patients with IWMI at the initial presentation (Figs 5.13–5.15). In particular, echocardiography is a widely available and inexpensive

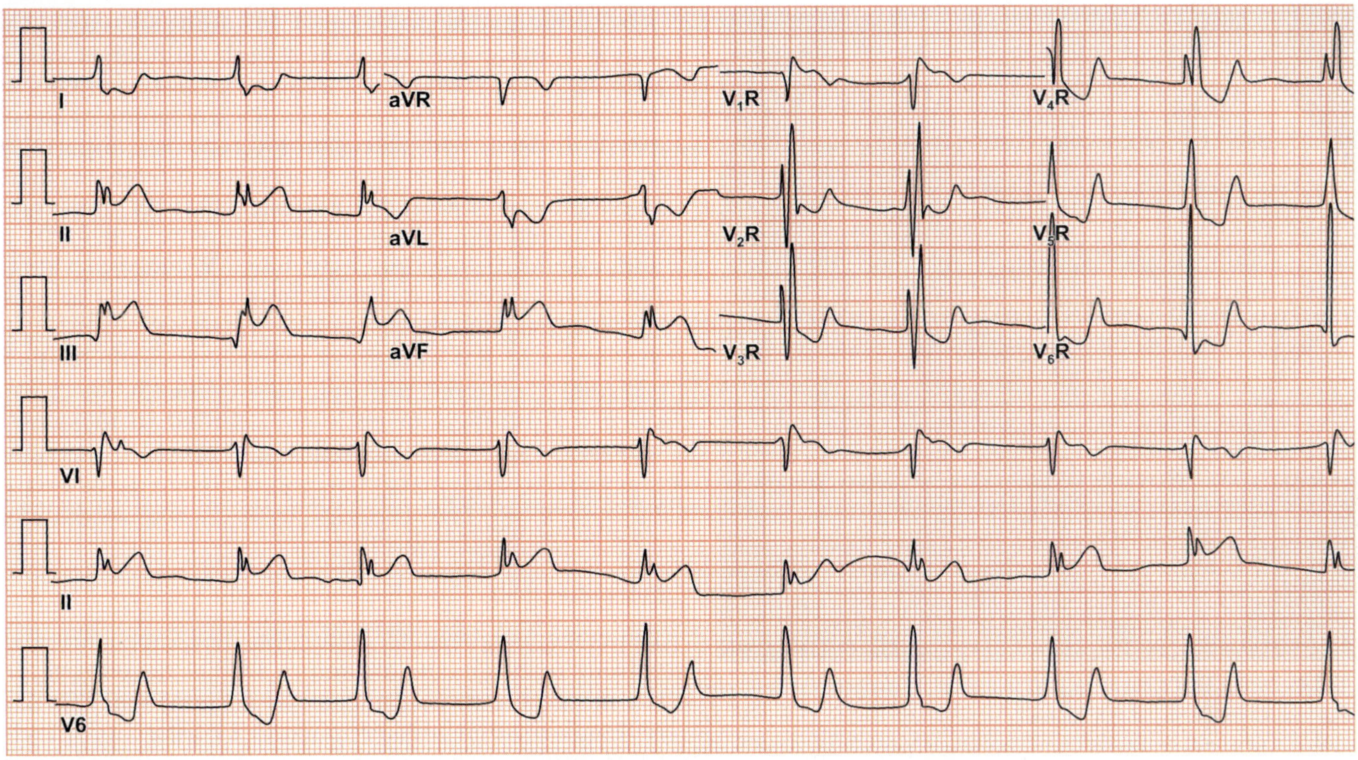


**Fig. 5.11:** ECG shows an inferior wall infarct, i.e. ST-segment elevation in leads II, III and aVF. The precordial V leads are actually right sided on this ECG. This is evident because the tracing in V6 does not resemble lead I and aVL. Also the P-waves in V4 to V6 are flat. ST-depression in I and aVL along with ST-elevation in right sided V3–V6 indicates right ventricular infarct

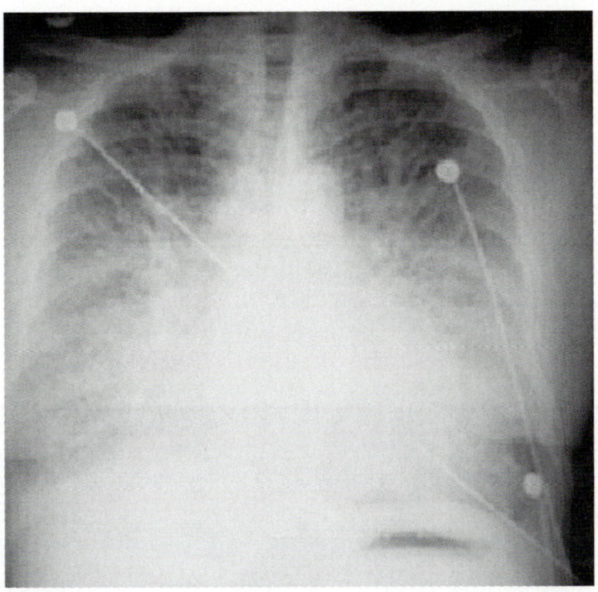

**Fig. 5.12:** Skiagram of chest PA view showing cardiomegaly with pulmonary edema in RV infarction

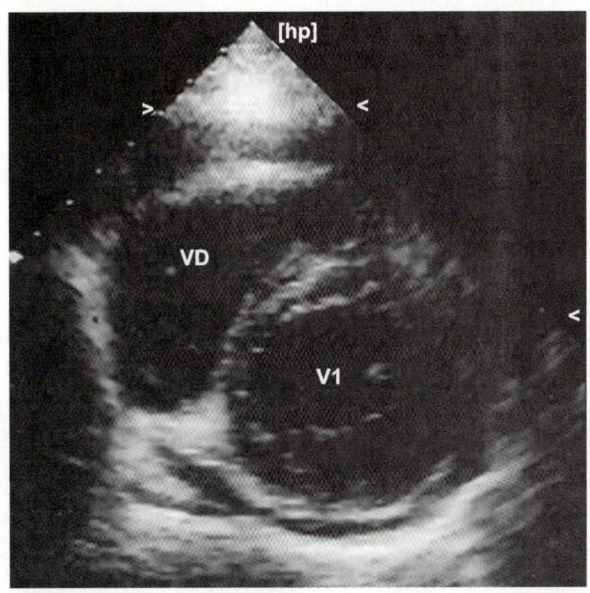


**Fig. 5.13:** Parasternal echocardiogram in the short axis. The right ventricle appears dilated, with a crescent-moon morphology. Real-time images revealed reduced motion and/or a lack of systolic thickening in the compromised walls in a patient with RV infarction

tool for the comprehensive evaluation of the size and function of the right ventricle. However, echocardiographic imaging of the RV has technical challenges due to the chamber's complex shape; the RV cannot be completely visualized in any single two-dimensional (2D) echocardiographic view. Furthermore, although RV infarction inherently complicates the initial management in cases of acute infarction, echocardiographic abnormalities can be temporary and resolve within a few hours. Therefore, information from all available acoustic windows is necessary for the complete assessment of the RV. Although not validated in acute situations, three-dimensional (3D)

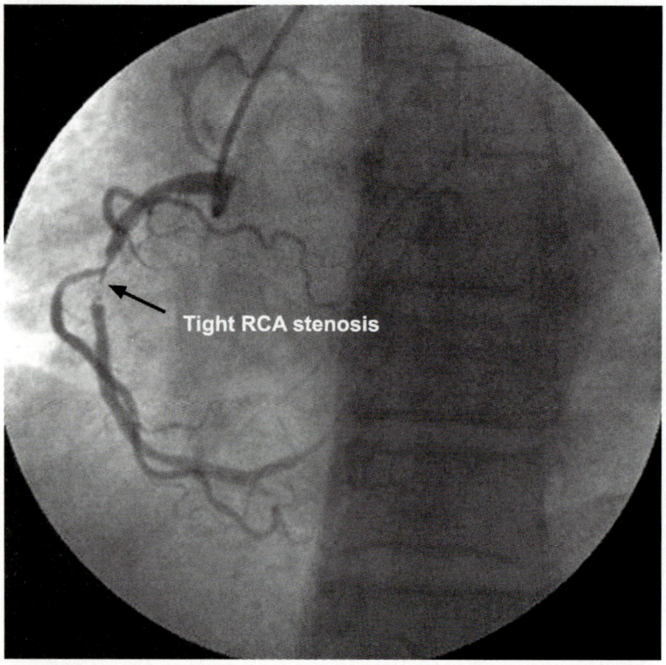


**Fig. 5.14:** Tissue Doppler imaging is useful in determining myocardial velocities and for ventricular function evaluation. In RVMI, the systolic and early diastolic velocities, myocardial velocities for the free right wall are decreased. Tissue Doppler echocardiography can also demonstrate ventricular asynchrony by using septal and left ventricular free wall measurements. In RVMI, the typical apex-base gradient is inverted and high flow velocities are found at the apex and in the outflow tract. In PE, an increase in myocardial strain-rate is noticed with the decrease of maximal systolic strain indicating a reduction in cardiac output. The profile changes from protomezosystolic to telesystolic and even protodiastolic (postsystolic shortening)

echocardiographic RV volumes are comparable to those derived by CMR and are probably more accurate than 2D echocardiographic volumes.

### Cardiac Magnetic Resonance

Cardiac magnetic resonance (CMR) using late gadolinium enhancement imaging enables the accurate characterization of ischemic myocardial injury. CMR studies have indicated that RV infarction occurs in a high number of cases in patients with IWMI (47–57%) and that some patients with anterior MI (11–65%) also have RV involvement to some extent. Indeed, two observational reports comparing the frequency of RV involvement between different modalities in patients with acute MI indicated that RV involvement was detected significantly more frequently with CMR than with electrocardiography or echocardiography. Although the recent advances in CMR may contribute to understanding the pathology as well as providing a more accurate diagnosis of RV infarction, further investigations are essential to establish the usefulness of the CMR technique, since the numbers of patients included in these observational studies were limited (Fig. 5.16).

*Cine-angiography:* It would be helpful in profiling coronary arteries (Fig. 5.17).

## MANAGEMENT

The management of RV infarction should be started with volume replacement, and recent studies have highlighted the adverse effect of excessive volume loading. Early revascularization is also applied to RV infarction, in which the complete revascularization of the affected vessels, including the major RV branch, plays an important role in the recovery of RV function. Electrical stabilization, including adequate heart rate and the maintenance of atrioventricular synchrony, is another key factor for preserving cardiac output in RV infarction. Furthermore, various extracorporeal support devices have been used to support RV failure secondary to RV infarction and contributed to the improvement of RV shock.

### Volume Replacement

When RV infarction is complicated by acute MI, it is widely recognized that adequate therapy can be achieved only by expanding the plasma volume, ideally with the aid of invasive monitoring. However, fluid replacement can be challenging in some patients with RV infarction, particularly in the presence of severe RV dysfunction. The

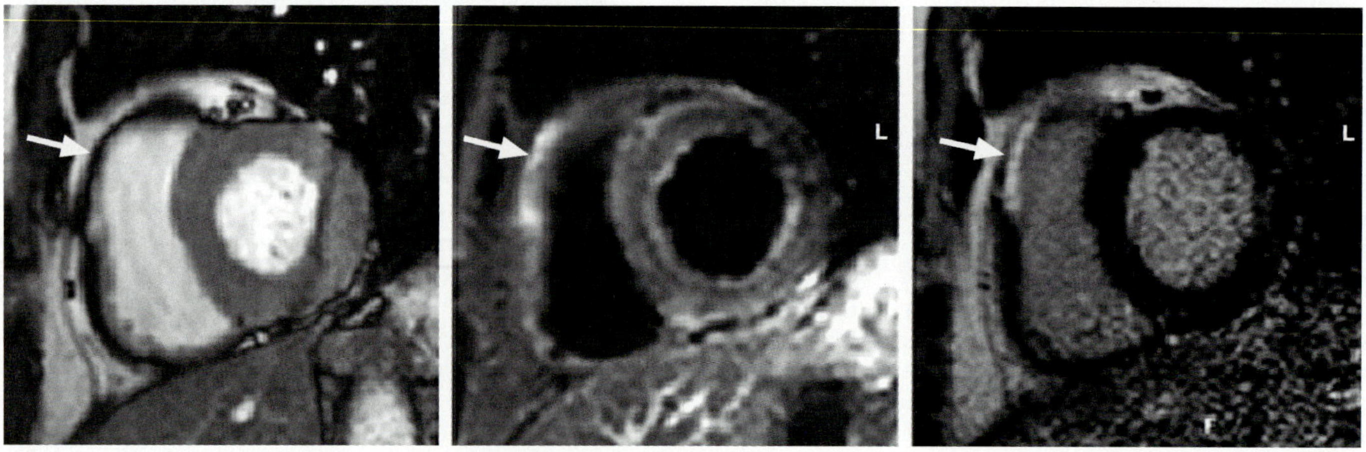


**Fig. 5.15:** RV failure. (A) Showing speckle tracking of 2D echocardiographic image of the right ventricle. (B) Strain vs time plotted for various regions of the RV. It shows delay in time to peak strain in the septum compared to the RV free wall

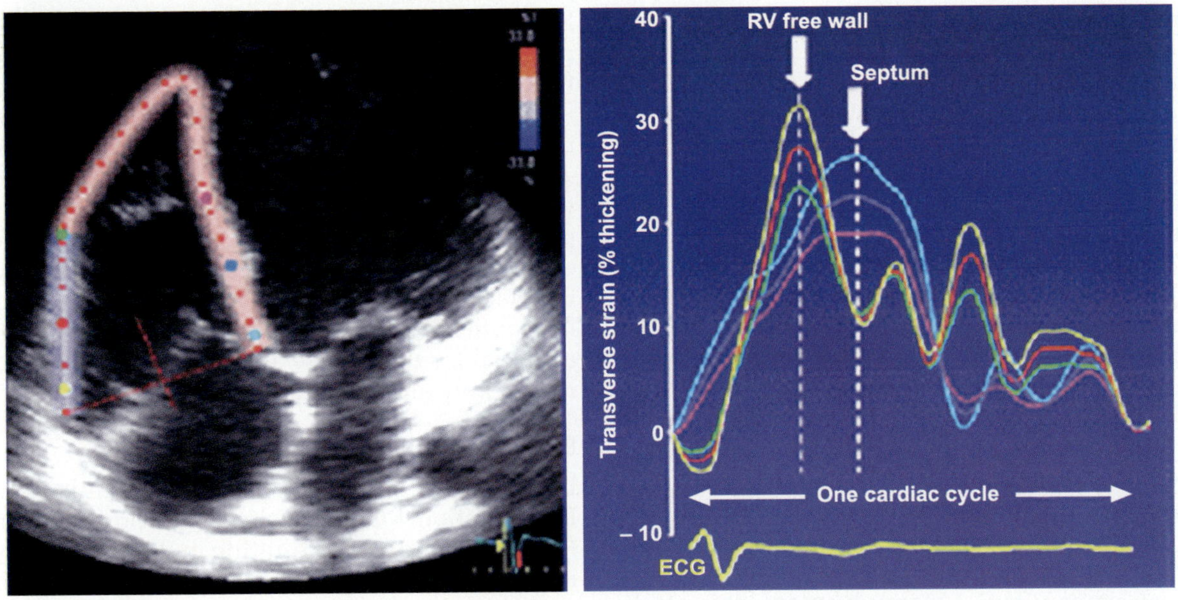


**Fig. 5.16:** CMR images from a patient with acute non-STEMI, evidenced by a rise in cardiac enzymes and nonspecific ST-segment changes on an ECG. Invasive coronary angiography revealed 3-vessel CAD with an occluded proximal RV branch of the right coronary artery. A cine CMR image (A) in systole shows a subtle wall motion abnormality in the anterior RV free wall (arrow). The T2-weighted image (B) shows high signal in this area with corresponding high signal on the late gadolinium-enhanced image. There is no evidence of scar in the left ventricle, suggesting isolated RV infarction

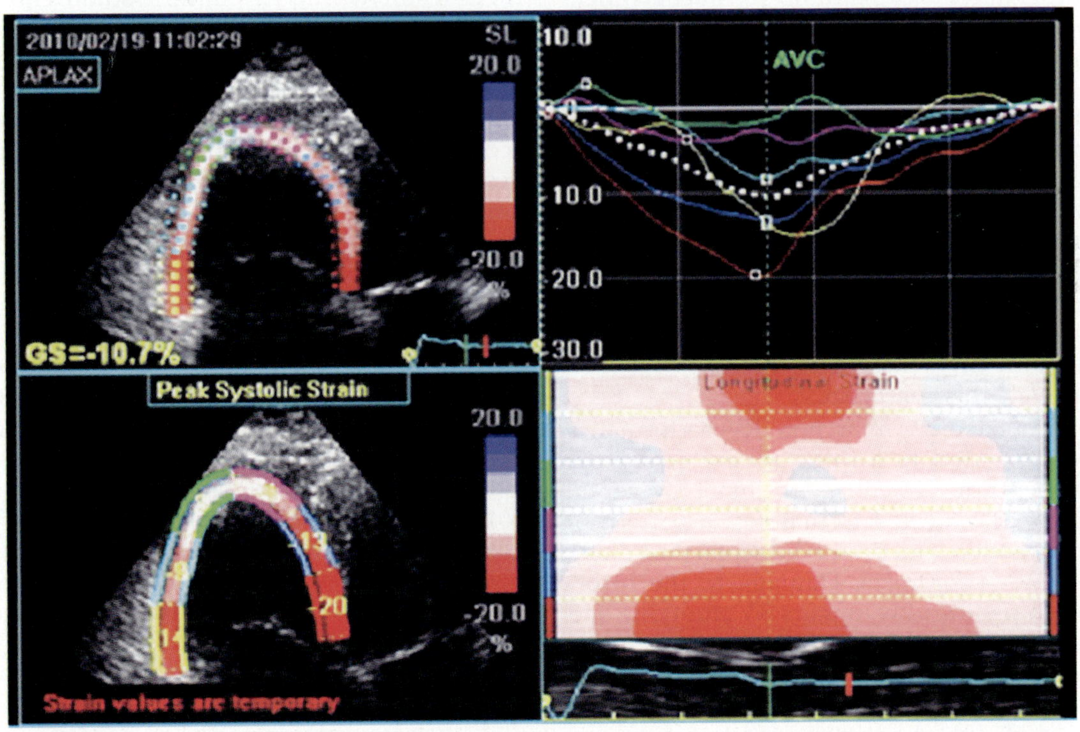


**Fig. 5.17:** Angiography showing tight stenosis of right coronary artery disease in RV infarction

concept of fluid replacement was first described as a treatment option approximately 25 years ago with the development of pulmonary artery catheterization. Since then, several studies have validated the usefulness of volume loading for ischemic RV dysfunction. Therefore, the initial therapy for hypotension in patients with RV infarction without pulmonary congestion has traditionally been volume expansion, particularly if the estimated central venous pressure was <15 mmHg. In previous studies, maintenance of the RV preload with volume loading and normal saline alone was thought to resolve the accompanying hypotension and improve the cardiac output. The typical regimen consisted of normal saline (40 ml/min, up to total of 2 l, intravenously), while maintaining the right atrial pressure (RAP) at <18 mmHg to prevent volume overload. However, later clinical studies reported variable responses to aggressive fluid therapy with a target pulmonary wedge pressure (PWP) of 18–24 mmHg. Some studies, including two prospective ones, showed that volume loading further elevates the right-sided filling pressure without improving cardiac output Berisha and associates in a study of 41 patients who fulfilled the diagnostic electrocardiographic and hemodynamic criteria for RV infarction, reported that the maximal RV stroke work index occurred when the filling pressure was 10–14 mmHg, and a mean RAP of >14 mmHg was almost always associated with a reduced RV stroke work index. Although, the hemodynamic characteristics of RV infarction may be extremely variable, depending on the patient's state of hydration and the degree of concomitant LV involvement, this study indicated that the mean optimal PWP, which corresponds to the maximum LV stroke work index in each patient, was 16 mmHg.

### Clinical Implications of Biventricular Interdependence

Two physiological concepts explain the detrimental effect of excessive volume loading in patients with RV infarction. First, data from animal studies suggest that excessive RV dilatation can further compromise LV output because of pericardial restraining effects. Biventricular interdependence is mediated by the shared interventricular septum and the surrounding pericardium. The disproportionate elevation of RV filling pressure because of surplus volume loading can lead to marked RV dilatation, elevation of intrapericardial pressure, and subsequent equalization of RV and LV diastolic pressures. By compromising LV filling, this situation will precipitate a low-output state. The resultant impairment of interventricular septal motion can further aggravate this condition.

In addition, in isolated RV infarction, RV performance can be largely attributed to a force generated by the interventricular septum. Patients with intact LV-septal contraction would be expected to manifest a pattern of paradoxical septal motion with preserved septal thickening portending a better prognosis. Damage to the interventricular septum significantly impairs RV emptying and exacerbates diastolic dysfunction, with an increase in the filling pressure. In RV infarction associated with septal dysfunction, compensation from LV-septal contraction transmitted through systolic ventricular interaction is lacking, and these patients usually present with hypotension and low cardiac output that are refractory to initial volume loading. Under these circumstances, inotropic stimulation of contractility, usually with dobutamine, has consistently improved RV performance by enhancing global LV contraction and increasing paradoxical septal displacement into the right ventricle. These important impacts of the interventricular septum on RV performance after acute MI were observed in a study using echocardiography, in which the recovery of RV function was best correlated with the improvement of the interventricular septum wall. In earlier studies, RV infarction was defined by hemodynamic criteria, such as an elevated RAP or PWP. At present, in most coronary units, physicians are able to identify RV infarction more precisely using noninvasive imaging techniques (e.g. echocardiography, radionuclide imaging, cardiac magnetic resonance), as discussed earlier. With these noninvasive modalities, the extent of interventricular involvement is essential for the precise assessment of fluid balance, early risk stratification, and prognostic evaluation.

### Early Revascularization

In the typical situation of a hemodynamically significant RV infarction, RCA occlusion compromises right atrial and RV branch perfusion, resulting in RV ischemic dysfunction related to the loss of the critical compensatory contribution of augmented right atrial contraction. Patients with proximal RCA culprit lesions have worse baseline characteristics, less spontaneous recanalization, and a greater clot burden than those without occlusion.

Although the relative prognostic impact of RV infarction has been more prominent, successful mechanical reperfusion has improved the absolute clinical outcome as a whole, in relation to RV infarction. Because of the higher reperfusion rate achieved with primary angioplasty, the mortality among patients treated with this method has been relatively low. In addition, the clinical outcomes have been acceptable in patients with proximal RCA culprit lesions, despite their worse baseline characteristics; these outcomes have been similar to those of patients with nonproximal RCA culprit lesions. Technically, a shorter time taken to reperfusion and complete revascularization of the affected vessels, including the major RV branch, play an important role in the recovery of RV function. Early revascularization leads to an immediate recovery of RV function; conversely, late revascularization is associated with higher RV dysfunction and complications. Asalli and colleagues reported that complete revascularization of the RCA, including the major RV branch, was more closely associated with a higher recovery rate of RV function by echocardiography and better 30-day mortality than incomplete revascularization in patients with RV infarction. Further, in cases of complication with ventricular arrhythmia, reperfusion results in a better prognosis. Thus, prompt, successful, complete revascularization seems to benefit all patients with RV infarction.

### Surgical Intervention

The current treatment of RVMI patients, other than the optimization of RV and LV preload with intravenous fluids, the administration of inotropic agents, and revascularization, includes the maintenance of atrioventricular synchrony, intra-aortic balloon pump counterpulsation, and more intensive mechanical support, including an emergent cardiopulmonary bypass and use of a ventricular assist device (VAD). In this section, we summarize the newly developing modalities for patients with RV shock as follows: (1) electrical stabilization device, including adequate heart rate and the maintenance of atrioventricular synchrony; (2) percutaneous implantable VAD (especially focused on Tandem-Heart); and (3) percutaneous cardiopulmonary support (PCPS).

An adequate heart rate and the maintenance of atrioventricular synchrony can play an important role in sustaining a sufficient cardiac output. Patients with RV infarction tend to have bradyarrhythmia. In addition, the ischemic right ventricle and, consequently, the preload-deprived left ventricle have a relatively fixed stroke volume, and cardiac output strongly depends on the heart rate Therefore, an adequate heart rate with pacing is essential for patients with RV infarction, regardless of the presence or absence of bradyarrhythmia. Moreover, several investigators have shown that atrioventricular sequential pacing in patients with a complete atrioventricular block associated with RV infarction leads to a significant improvement in the cardiac output and recovery from shock when ventricular pacing alone has no benefit. Unfortunately, transvenous pacing may prove problematic due to ventricular sensing failure from the ischemic right ventricle and difficulties with lead positioning after right atrial enlargement.

Surgically implanted right VADs have been used mostly for the support of surgical or pretransplant patients. They have been less commonly used in the management of shock or for the post-cardiopulmonary arrest syndrome. However, in recent years, very few papers have described the use of percutaneous VAD implantation using Tandem-Heart (Cardiac Assist, Pittsburgh, PA, USA) for RV infarction Tandem-Heart is a temporary, external, continuous-flow, centrifugal pump that is placed nonsurgically in the catheterization laboratory through the femoral vein; it was originally intended for stabilizing critically ill patients who require short-term left heart support. The cannulas can be placed in the right atrium and pulmonary artery to support the right ventricle, as indicated in case reports. Percutaneous VADs are expected to allow time for the recovery of RV function in acute conditions or to serve as a bridge to other interventions, such as surgical VAD implantation.

PCPS has also been used successfully to provide support for patients with refractory RV failure secondary to RV infarction. A PCPS is a compact, portable heart-lung machine that can be quickly installed using a thin-walled cannula inserted via the femoral vessels. Cannulas are advanced in the right atrium and femoral artery, and oxygenated blood is transmitted from the femoral artery in a retrograde fashion. Although the installation of the Tandem Heart for left ventricular support requires a trans-septal puncture to place the blood removal cannula into the left atrium, such techniques are not required to install a PCPS, which has been used to apply shock or for cardiopulmonary arrest due to accessibility issues. Suguta and colleagues reported the first case of cardiogenic shock caused by RV infarction treated with a PCPS, which is now recognized as one of the therapeutic options.

## SUMMARY

In patients with MI, especially those with IWMI, RV involvement is an important contributor to shock, which significantly increases the risk of mortality. The recent advances in noninvasive modalities, such as CMR, provide a more accurate diagnosis of RV infarction, which in turn helps elucidate the precise pathophysiology. Although volume loading has long been considered the cornerstone of management in these cases, we can apprehend the harmful aspects of this therapy by understanding its effect on the interventricular septum. Early successful reperfusion, especially using revascularization, contributes to the recovery from shock associated with RV infarctions, which thus results in an improved prognosis. On the other hand, the importance of RV infarction is highlighted in this mechanical reperfusion era. The maintenance of an adequate heart rate and atrioventricular synchrony is another key factor for sustaining a sufficient cardiac output in patients with RV infarction. In refractory cases, more intensive mechanical support, including Tandem-Heart or PCPS, has been applied and is recognized as new therapeutic options.

### Cardiovascular Agents

Dobutamine is an inotropic agent used to improve right ventricular contractility and maintain cardiac output. Sodium nitroprusside reduces afterload.

- **Dobutamine:** Produces vasodilation and increases inotropic state. At higher dosages, may cause increased heart rate, exacerbating myocardial ischemia.
- **Adult:** 0.5 mcg/kg/min IV initial; titrate until desired effect attained
- **Beta-adrenergic blockers**: They antagonize effects; general anesthetics may increase toxicity
- ***Documented hypersensitivity***: Idiopathic hypertrophic subaortic stenosis; atrial fibrillation or flutter
- **Pregnancy:** B-Fetal risk not confirmed in studies in humans but has been shown in some studies in animals

### Precautions

Caution following MI; hypovolemic state should be corrected before using:

- **Nitroprusside (nitropress):** Produces vasodilation and increases inotropic activity of heart. At higher doses, may exacerbate myocardial ischemia by increasing heart rate. Infusion rates >10 mcg/kg/min may lead to cyanide toxicity.
- **Adult:** 0.3–0.5 mcg/kg/min IV initial infusion; use 0.5 mcg/kg/min increments and titrate to desired effect; average dose is 1–6 mcg/kg/min
- Coadministration with other hypotensive agents may have additive effects

- **Documented hypersensitivity:** Subaortic stenosis; idiopathic hypertrophic subaortic stenosis; decreased cerebral perfusion; arteriovenous shunt or coarctation of aorta (e.g. compensatory hypertension); atrial fibrillation or flutter
- **Pregnancy:** C-Fetal risk revealed in studies in animals but not established or not studied in humans; may use if benefits outweigh risk to fetus.

### Precautions

Caution in increased intracranial pressure, hepatic failure, severe renal impairment, and hypothyroidism; in renal or hepatic insufficiency, nitroprusside levels may increase and can cause cyanide toxicity; sodium nitroprusside has ability to lower blood pressure and should be used only in patients with mean arterial pressures >70 mmHg.

### Tissue Plasminogen Activators

These agents bind to fibrin and convert plasminogen to plasmin, which in turn initiates local fibrinolysis with limited systemic proteolysis.

- ***Alteplase (Activase):*** Tissue plasminogen activator (t-PA) used in management of acute myocardial infarction, acute ischemic stroke, and pulmonary embolism. May administer heparin or aspirin with and after alteplase infusions to reduce risk of rethrombosis. Safety and efficacy of concomitant administration of heparin or aspirin during first 24 h after symptom onset have not been investigated.
- ***Adult:*** 0.9 mg/kg (not to exceed 90 mg) IV infusion over 60 minutes with 10% of total dose administered as initial IV bolus over 1 minute.

## BIBLIOGRAPHY


1. Andersen HR, Falk E, Nielsen D. Right ventricular infarction: frequency, size and topography in coronary heart disease: a prospective study comprising 107 consecutive autopsies from a coronary care unit. J Am Coll Cardiol 1987;10(6): 1223–32.
2. Andersen HR, Nielsen D, Falk E, et al. Right ventricular infarction: larger enzyme release with posterior than with anterior involvement. Int J Cardiol 1989;22(3):347–55.
3. Andersen HR, Nielsen D, Lund O. Prognostic significance of right ventricular infarction diagnosed by ST-elevation in right chest leads V3R to V7R. Int J Cardiol 1989;23(3): 349–56.
4. Bates ER. Revisiting reperfusion therapy in inferior myocardial infarction. J Am Coll Cardiol 1997;30(2):334–42.
5. Birnbaum Y, Wagner GS, Barbash GI. Correlation of angiographic findings and right (V1 to V3) versus left (V4 to V6) precordial ST-segment depression in inferior wall acute myocardial infarction. Am J Cardiol 1999;83(2):143–8.
6. Braat SH, Brugada P, de Zwaan C. Value of electrocardiogram in diagnosing right ventricular involvement in patients with an acute inferior wall myocardial infarction. Br Heart J 1983;49(4):368–72.
7. Braat SH, Brugada P, den Dulk K. Value of lead V4R for recognition of the infarct coronary artery in acute inferior myocardial infarction. Am J Cardiol 1984;53(11):1538–41.
8. Chockalingam A, Gnanavelu G, Alagesan R, Subramaniam T. Myocardial performance index in evaluation of acute right ventricular myocardial infarction. Echocardiography 2004; 21(6):487–94.
9. Chockalingam A, Gnanavelu G, Subramaniam T, et al. Right ventricular myocardial infarction: presentation and acute outcomes. Angiology 2005;56(4):371–6.
10. Dokainish H, Abbey H, Gin K, et al. Usefulness of tissue Doppler imaging in the diagnosis and prognosis of acute right ventricular infarction with inferior wall acute left ventri-cular infarction. Am J Cardiol 2005;95(9):1039–42.
11. Elkayam U, Halprin SL, Frishman W. Echocardiographic findings in cardiogenic shock due to right ventricular myocardial infarction. Cathet Cardiovasc Diagn 1979;5(3): 289–94.
12. Forman MB, Goodin J, Phelan B. Electrocardiographic changes associated with isolated right ventricular infarction. J Am Coll Cardiol 1984;4(3):640-3.
13. Garty I, Barzilay J, Bloch L. The diagnosis and early complications of right ventricular infarction. Eur J Nucl Med 1984;9(10):453–60.
14. Giannitsis E, Potratz J, Wiegand U. Impact of early accelerated dose tissue plasminogen activator on in-hospital patency of the infarcted vessel in patients with acute right ventricular infarction. Heart 1997;77(6):512–6.
15. Haupt HM, Hutchins GM, Moore GW. Right ventricular infarction: role of the moderator band artery in determining infarct size. Circulation 1983;67(6):1268–72.
16. Hirsowitz GS, Lakier JB, Goldstein S. Right ventricular function evaluated by radionuclide angiography in acute myocardial infarction. Am Heart J 1984;108(4 Pt 1):949–54.
17. Hurst JW. Comments about the electrocardiographic signs of right ventricular infarction. Clin Cardiol 1998;21(4): 289–91.
18. Iqbal MZ, Liebson PR. Counterpulsation and dobutamine. Their use in treatment of cardiogenic shock due to right ventricular infarct. Arch Intern Med 1981;141(2):247–9.
19. Kinn JW, Ajluni SC, Samyn JG. Rapid hemodynamic improvement after reperfusion during right ventricular infarction. J Am Coll Cardiol 1995;26(5):1230–4.
20. Lisbona R, Sniderman A, Derbekyan V. Phase and amplitude imaging in the diagnosis of acute right ventricular damage in inferior infarction. Clin Nucl Med 1983;8(11):517–20.
21. Martin W, Tweddel A, McGhie I. The evaluation of right ventricular function in acute myocardial infarction by xenon-133. Nucl Med Commun 1989;10(1):35–43.
22. Mavric Z, Zaputovic L, Matana A. Prognostic significance of complete atrioventricular block in patients with acute inferior myocardial infarction with and without right ventri-cular involvement. Am Heart J 1990;119(4):823–8.
23. Mittal SR. Isolated right ventricular infarction. Int J Cardiol 1994;46(1):53–60.
24. Nader DA, Ceretto WJ, Vieweg WV. Atrial pacing in the manage-ment of right ventricular infarction. South Med J 1981;74(3):362–3.
25. Pfisterer M, Emmenegger H, Muller-Brand J. Prevalence and extent of right ventricular dysfunction after myocardial

infarction—relation to location and extent of infarction and left ventricular function. Int J Cardiol 1990;28(3):325–32.

26. Robalino BD, Petrella RW, Jubran FY. Atrial natriuretic factor in patients with right ventricular infarction. J Am Coll Cardiol 1990;15(3):546–53.
27. Roth A, Miller HI, Kaluski E. Early thrombolytic therapy does not enhance the recovery of the right ventricle in patients with acute inferior myocardial infarction and predominant right ventricular involvement. Cardiology 1990; 77(1):40–9.
28. Singhal AM, Ilangovan S, Mehta S. Isolated right ventricular infarction followed by posterior left ventricular infarction after a few days. Acta Cardiol 1984;39(4):307–12.
29. Strauss HD, Sobel BE, Roberts R. The influence of occult right ventricular infarction on enzymatically estimated infarct size, hemodynamics and prognosis. Circulation 1980;62(3): 503–8.
30. Sugimoto T, Ogawa K, Asada T. Surgical treatment of ventricular septal perforation with right ventricular infarction. J Cardiovasc Surg (Torino) 1996;37(1):71–4.

# 6 Percutaneous Coronary Interventions (Balloon Angioplasty and Stentoplasty)

Grüntzig's first successful coronary angioplasty treatment on a human was performed in 1977, in Zurich, Switzerland. He expanded a short, about 3 mm, nonbranching section of the left anterior descending (LAD) artery (the front branch of the left coronary artery) which supplies the front wall and tip of the heart which had a high grade stenosis, about 80%, of the lumen. Dr Grüntzig presented the results of his first four angioplasty cases at the 1977 American Heart Association (AHA) meeting, which led to widespread acknowledgement of his pioneering work ( Fig. 6.1).

The immediate results of this treatment, despite using only a carefully *kitchen built* catheter (crude by current standards), was quite good. The patient became and remained angina free after this treatment. This initial patient's result was electively rechecked, by angiography at Emory University, on the 10 year anniversary of the initial treatment. The LAD narrowing, after this 10 year timespan, remained almost perfectly expanded. There was minimal residual narrowing, probably less than 10%, as seen in similar angle and multiple different views comparing with photographs of the original, 10 years earlier, before and after results. The excellent results of this initial and subsequent patients were critical to the rapid development and growing acceptance of the angioplasty treatment option. Dr Grüntzig recognized multiple important issues early—(a) the treatment would not be readily accepted by most physicians, especially bypass surgeons, (b) it could easily lead to bad outcomes without great care in selection of which patients/lesions to treat and of the treating physicians, and (c) it required careful teaching of the technique and its potential difficulties and pitfalls to other physicians, so as to proactively reduce the occurrence of poor results. Understanding these issues and tireless effort on his part are widely recognized in cardiology for being of fundamental importance to the ultimate success of the technique.

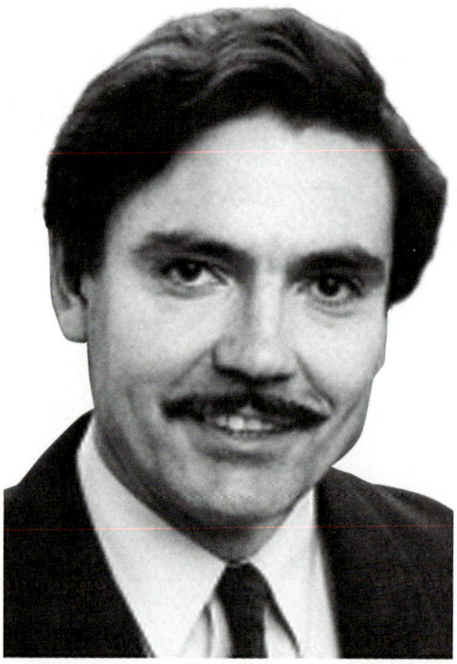

**Fig. 6.1:** Andreas Roland Grüntzig (June 25, 1939–October 27, 1985) was a German cardiologist who first developed successful balloon angioplasty for expanding lumens of narrowed arteries

By about 1990, lumen stenosis of the coronary arteries was more commonly treated by the angioplasty technique than by coronary artery bypass surgery. This treatment approach is now referred to as plain old balloon angioplasty (POBA).

In the 1990s, further major improvements, both immediate and especially long term became possible with better understanding of disease as a result of clinical research trials using intravascular ultrasonography (IVUS) and the development of stents to mechanically support POBA results. Since the later 1990s, most angioplasties also involve a stent over the angioplasty balloon; the balloon is hydraulically (typically 6 up to 25 atmospheres of internal pressure) expanded, then deflated and removed while the stent remains behind to mechanically support the lumen remaining in the new, more open shape as created by the hydraulically expanded balloon. Grüntzig's success remains a major breakthrough and great contribution to the field of medicine in demonstrating that doctors could work inside of the arteries safely, without the need for open surgery. By utilizing the arterial circulation as a 'therapeutic highway', many types of devices and drugs can now be delivered directly to the heart, kidneys, carotid arteries, brain, legs, and aorta without the need for major surgery and general anesthesia.

Since the first human percutaneous transluminal coronary angioplasty (PTCA) procedure was performed in 1977, the use of percutaneous coronary intervention (PCI) has increased dramatically, becoming one of the most common medical interventions performed. The technique, originally developed in Switzerland by Andreas Gruentzig, has transformed the practice of revascularization for coronary artery disease (CAD). Initially used in the treatment of patients with stable angina and discrete lesions in a single coronary artery, coronary angioplasty has multiple indications today, including unstable angina, acute myocardial infarction (MI), and multivessel coronary artery disease. With the combination of sophisticated equipment, experienced operators, and modern drug therapy, PCI has evolved into an effective nonsurgical modality for treating patients with coronary artery disease. Recent advances in guidewires, stents, and devices to cross chronically occluded arteries are evolving, so that more patients with chronic total occlusions (CTOs) are now being successfully treated percutaneously. Improvements in catheter technique and the development of new devices, wires, stents, drug-eluting stents, and medications have occurred parallel to advances in the understanding of cardiovascular physiology, the pathogenesis of atherosclerosis, and the body's response to vascular injury. Intracoronary stents and atherectomy devices were developed to increase the success rate of, and decrease the complications associated with, conventional balloon dilation and to expand the indications for revascularization. These devices have enabled the interventionalist to safely treat more complex coronary lesions and restenosis. Stents have evolved to a level where the problems of restenosis seen with bare metal stents are a les frequent occurrence after drug-eluting stents are implanted. At the same time, advances in intravascular ultrasonography and fractional flow reserve evaluation have improved the understanding of coronary plaque morphology, plaque vulnerability, and coronary physiology. Furthermore, many of these technologies are able to help identify patients who will benefit most from PCI, coronary bypass surgery, or medical therapy. Adjunctive pharmacologic therapies aimed at preventing acute reocclusion have also improved the safety and efficacy of coronary angioplasty. The growth of PCIs has been remarkable andwill likely be sustained, as new technologies have resulted in improved outcomes. Since 1994, the use of intracoronary stents has risen dramatically, and now with drug-eluting stents, stents are used in more than 80% of PCI cases in the United States. Innovations in PCIs over the past 2 decades have been paralleled by a dramatic reduction in 30-day death, myocardial infarction, and target-vessel revascularization rates.

## INDICATIONS FOR PCI

*Clinical indications for PCI include the following:*

1. Acute ST-elevation myocardial infarction (STEMI)
2. Non ST-elevation acute coronary syndrome
3. Stable angina
4. Anginal equivalent (e.g. dyspnea, arrhythmia, dizziness/syncope)
5. Asymptomatic or mildly symptomatic patients with objective evidence of a moderate to large area of viable myocardium or moderate to severe ischemia on noninvasive testing
6. Angiographic indications include hemodynamically significant lesions in vessels serving viable myocardium (vessel diameter >1.5 mm)

## CONTRAINDICATIONS TO PCI

Clinical contraindications include significant comorbidities (relative contraindication).

*Angiographic contraindications include the following:*

- Left main stenosis in a patient who is a surgical candidate (coronary artery bypass graft [CABG] surgery is still the preferred treatment for left main stenosis; however, this area is rapidly evolving toward safe and feasible PCI options)
- Diffusely diseased small-caliber artery or vein graft
- Other coronary anatomy not amenable to percutaneous intervention

## PREPARATION IN PERCUTANEOUS CORONARY BALLOON ANGIOPLASTY EQUIPMENT (Figs 6.2 to 6.4)

The original description of angioplasty by Dotter and Judkins described enlargement of the vessel lumen through a mechanism of atheromatous plaque compression. This mechanism is also partially responsible for luminal enlargement with balloon angioplasty. In addition, however, improvement in luminal diameter following balloon angioplasty also results from stretching of the vessel wall by the balloon. Balloon inflation actually results in overstretching of the vessel wall and partial disruption of not only the intimal plaque but also the media and adventitia, resulting in enlargement of the lumen and the outer diameter of the vessel.

Axial redistribution of plaque material also contributes to improvements in lumen diameter. Atherectomy devices and, subsequently, intracoronary stents were developed, in part, to decrease the early and late loss in luminal diameter observed with conventional balloon angioplasty. Several different balloon catheter designs have existed (over-the-wire, monorail, and fixed wire) with balloon materials that have different compliance characteristics allowing various degrees of expansion with increasing pressure. Irrespective of the balloon design, a steerable

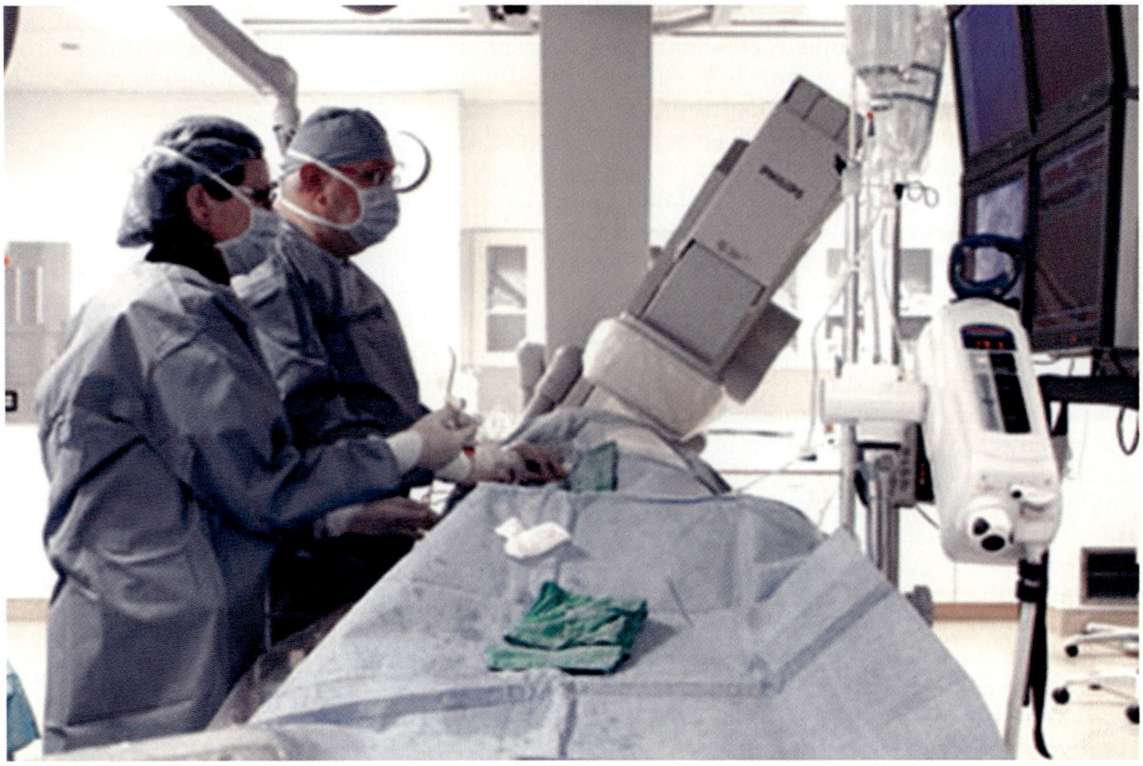

**Fig. 6.2:** Interventional laboratory for conducting percutaneous coronary interventions

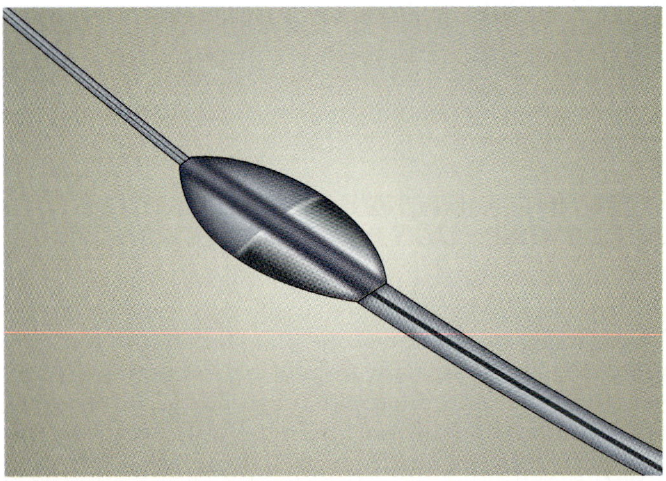

**Fig. 6.3:** Percutaneous transluminal coronary angioplasty (PTCA). The rotational atherectomy catheter (rotablator) is a device designed for the removal of plaque from coronary arteries. This tip, rotates at about 160,000 rpm and is particularly well suited for ablation of calcific or fibrotic plaque material

guidewire precedes the balloon into the artery and allows navigation through a considerable portion of the coronary tree. The development of balloon catheters that bend, allowing easy advancement through tortuous vascular segments (trackability), and that have increased shaft stiffness (pushability), allowing the catheter to be forced through stenotic lesions, has increased their versatility significantly. Another evolving feature of catheter design has been a reduction in the diameter of the deflated balloon, allowing easier passage through very stenotic lesions. Improvements in catheter design have been partially responsible for the improved success rates of PCIs.

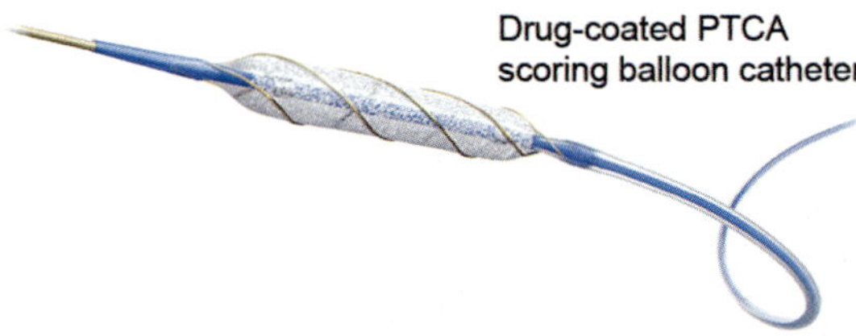


**Fig. 6.4:** Features of drug-coated PTCA scoring balloon catheter

The balloon catheter also serves as an adjunctive device for many other interventional therapies, including atherectomy and coronary stents.

*Technique of percutaneous coronary intervention:* Different technical stepts (Fig. 6.5) which are employed in cardiac catheterization laboratory are described below as:

- **Angioplasty procedure, step 1:** While the patient is awake and pain-free (local anesthesia), a catheter is inserted into an artery at the top of the leg (the femoral artery). The procedure begins with the doctor injecting some local anesthesia into the groin area and putting a needle into the femoral artery (the blood vessel that runs from the heart down the leg). Once the needle is inserted, a guide wire is placed through the needle, into the blood vessel. Following this step, the guide wire is left in the blood vessel and the needle is removed. A large needle

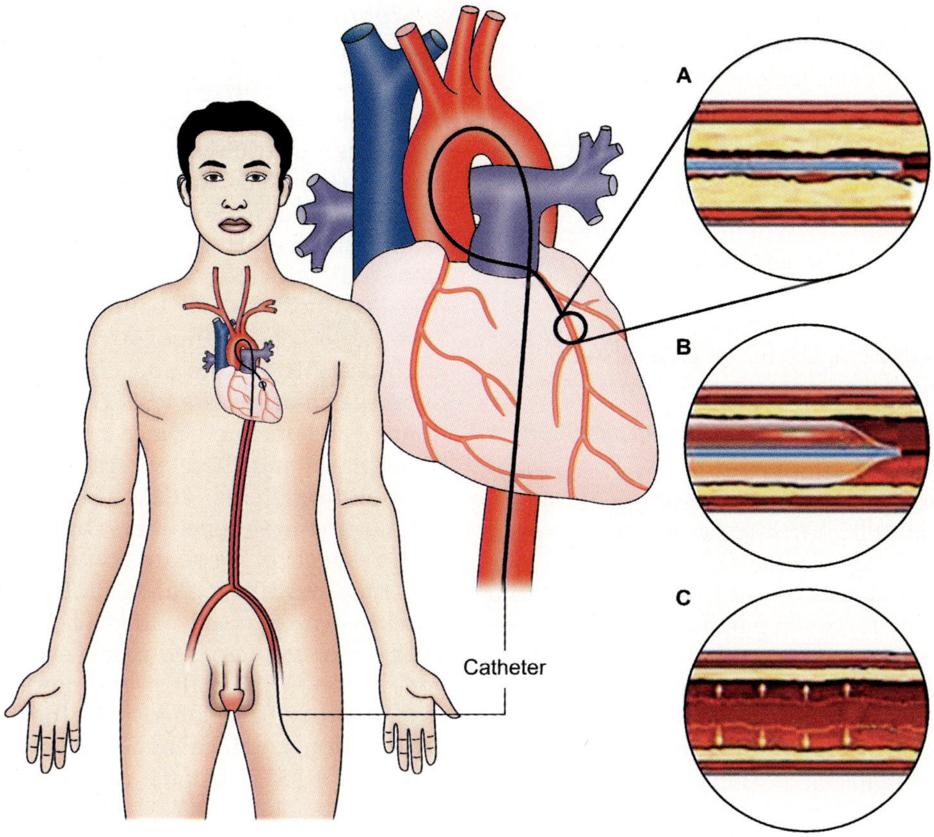


**Fig. 6.5:** Technique of percutaneous coronary angioplasty

called an introducer is then placed over the guide wire and the guide wire is removed.

- **Angioplasty procedure, step 2:** Next, a diagnostic catheter, which is a long narrow tube, is advanced through the introducer over a .035" guidewire, into the blood vessel. This catheter is then guided to the aorta and the guidewire is removed. Once the catheter is placed in the opening or ostium of one of the coronary arteries, the doctor injects dye and takes a series of X-rays films.
- **Angioplasty procedure, step 3:** After visualising the culprit vessel an appropriate sized balloon over the catheter is inserted and the vessel is then dilated with desired pressure to its fullest intraluminal size. This procedure can greatly improve the blood flow through the coronary arteries and to the heart tissue in about 90% of patients and may eliminate the need for coronary artery bypass surgery. The outcome is relief from chest pain symptoms and an improved exercise capacity. In 2 out of 3 cases, the procedure is considered successful with complete elimination of the narrowing or blockage.

### Coronary Physiologic Assessment

Intracoronary Doppler pressure wires are able to characterize coronary lesion physiology and to estimate lesion severity. Comparison of pressure distal to a lesion with aortic pressure enables determination of fractional flow reserve (FFR) (see the Fig. 6.6). A measurement below 0.75–0.80 during maximal hyperemia (induced via administration of adenosine) is consistent with a hemodynamically significant lesion. This determination is useful in deciding whether to perform PCI in an angiographic intermediate lesion. Clinical data, namely the DEFER study, support using this approach, with a low event rate seen in medically managed patients with angina and an FFR measurement greater than 0.75. Fractional flow ratio (FFR). Pressure wire is advanced across left anterior descending (LAD) stenosis and intracoronary adenosine is given. FFR ratio is recorded at baseline and then after adenosine push is given. Here, LAD lesion and FFR postadenosine is shown.

The fractional flow reserve versus angiography for guiding PCI in patients with multivessel coronary artery disease (FAME) trial showed that routine measurement of FFR during angioplasty reduced the risk of death, myocardial infarction, or repeat revascularization by 30% and death or myocardial infarction by 35%, compared with the current practice of using angiography to guide stenting decisions. In this study, a cut-off of FFR greater than 0.80 was used to define a nonischemic lesion. Two-year follow-up of the FAME trial showed continuing significant reductions in the combined endpoint of death and myocardial infarction with the use of FFR compared with standard angiography-guided PCI.

This form of physiologic lesion assessment is also useful for defining optimal stenting, assessing the angiographic severity of jailed side branch lesions, helping guide the decision for multivessel percutaneous coronary intervention or coronary artery bypass graft in multiple intermediate lesions, and assessing the severity of instant restenosis. FFR measurements have excellent correlation with IVUS analysis, especially when determining lesion severity, such as in ambiguous left main coronary artery anatomy (Fig. 6.6).

## TYPES OF INTERVENTIONS EMPLOYED IN CORONARY ARTERY DISEASE

### *1. Percutaneous Transluminal Coronary Angioplasty*

Angioplasty (or balloon angioplasty) is an *endovascular procedure* to widen narrowed or obstructed arteries or veins, typically to treat arterial *atherosclerosis*. An empty, collapsed balloon, known as a *balloon catheter*, is passed over a wire into the narrowed locations and then inflated to a fixed size. The balloon forces expansion of the *stenosis* (narrowing) within the vessel and the surrounding muscular wall, opening up the blood vessel for improved flow, and the balloon is then deflated and withdrawn. A *stent* may or may not be inserted at the time of ballooning to ensure the vessel remains open (Figs 6.7–6.12).

### *2. Stentoplasty*

Coronary stents were first developed in the mid 1980s to overcome the inherent limitations of balloon angioplasty, including elastic recoil and vessel closure in the acute phase, as well as constrictive remodeling and restenosis in the late phase. In the 1990s, this technology became widely accepted as a promising treatment strategy for patients with coronary artery disease after the landmark Belgian Netherlands Stent trial, which demonstrated the superiority of the bare metal stent (BMS) over balloon angioplasty (Figs 6.13–6.31 and Table 6.1). Although coronary stenting improved angiographic results and clinical outcomes, neointimal hyperplasia and restenosis continued to be major limitations of this technology. In order to minimize neointimal hyperplasia and thereby reduce repeat revascularization, drug-eluting stents (DES) were developed. Early pivotal trials of the first generation DES showed excellent results with respect to the reduction of in-stent restenosis, such that they rapidly replaced BMS. In the year 2006, safety concerns were raised with DES following reports linking their use to an increased risk of stent thrombosis (ST). First generation DES, with permanent polymers, have been associated with delayed endothelialization, endothelial dysfunction, and local hypersensitivity reactions, resulting in an increased risk of ST and the need for prolongation of

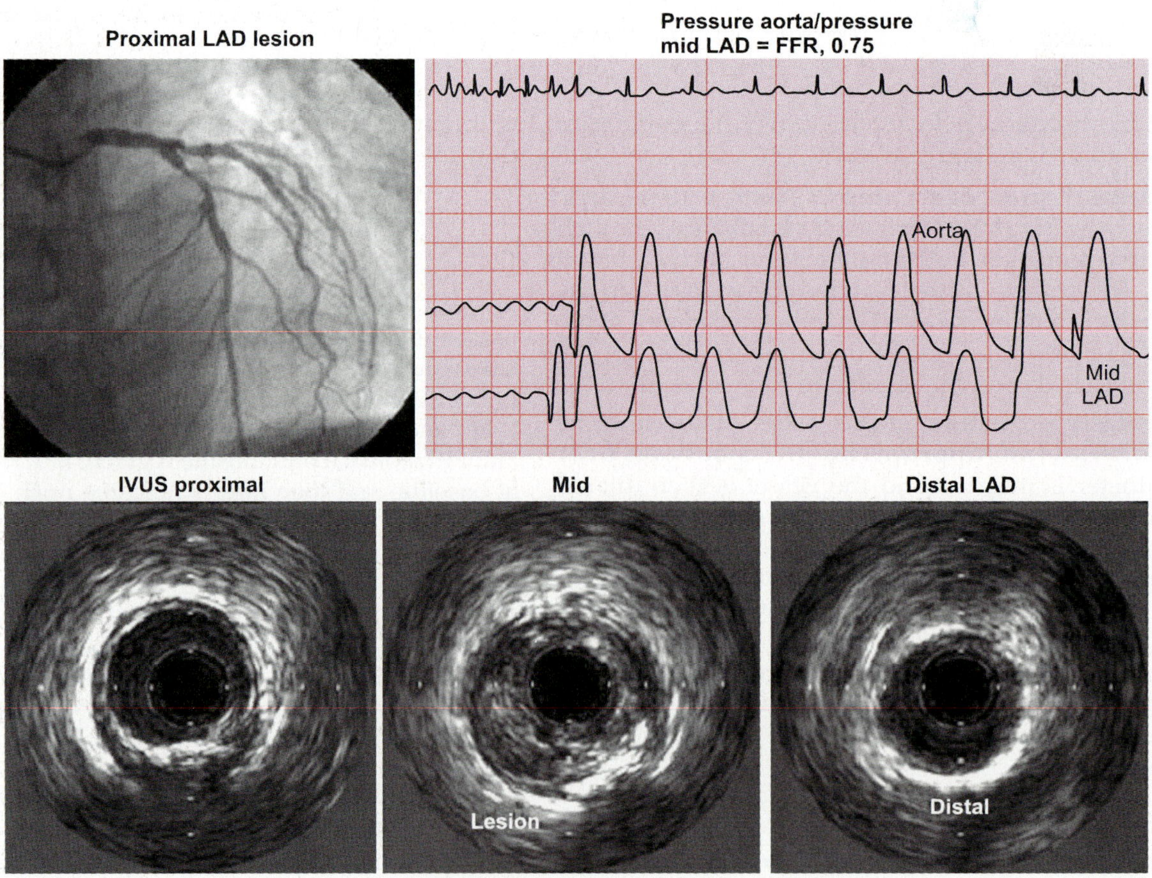


**Fig. 6.6:** Fractional flow ratio (FFR). Pressure wire is advanced across left anterior descending (LAD) stenosis and intracoronary adenosine is given. FFR ratio is recorded at baseline and then after adenosine push is given. Here, LAD lesion and FFR postadenosine is shown

**Table 6.1:** Types of coronary stents and selected antirestenosis devices

| Stent type | Description |
|---|---|
| Drug-eluting stent | A stent that slowly releases a drug to block cell proliferation and/or restenosis |
| Bare metal stent, stainless steel | A vascular thin metal wire or mesh stent without a coating, typically first-generation technology |
| Bare metal stent, CoCr | A vascular thin metal wire or mesh without a coating, typially next-generation technology |
| Absorbable stent | Completely biodegradable, bioabsorbable stent, typically polymer or magnesium, sometimes coated with anti-restenotic agent |
| Bioactive stent | A stent that reacts with the body's natural processes to achieve an antirestenotic effect |
| Radioactive stent | Stent with a radiation-emitting coating |
| Drug-eluting balloon | Angioplasty balloon that, after deflation, leaves behind an antirestenotic drug |

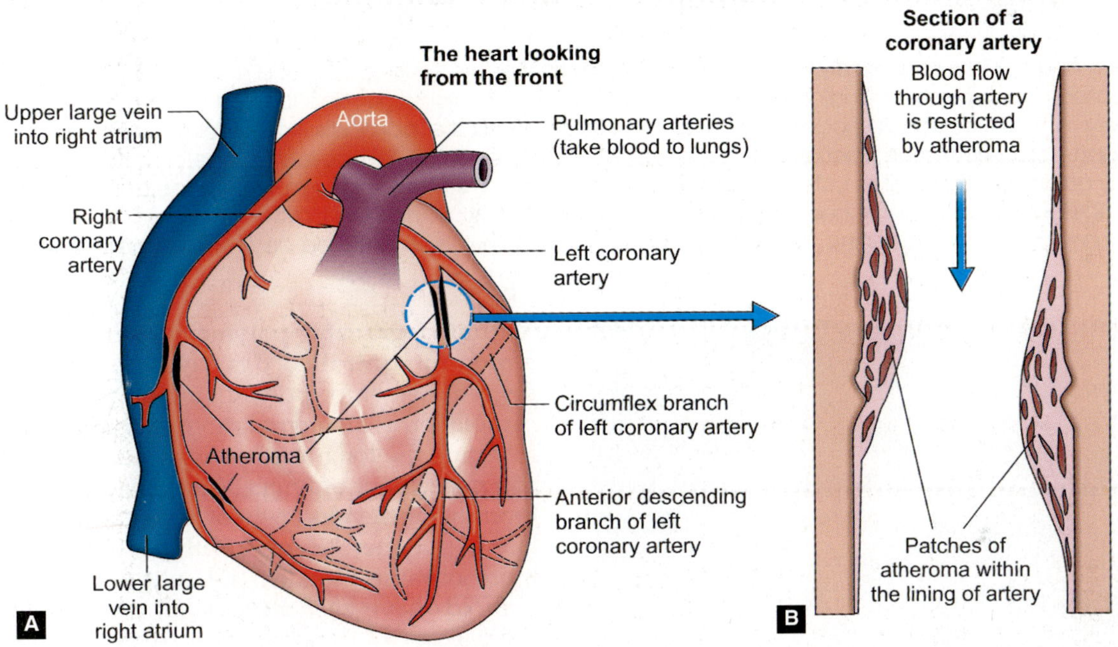


**Fig. 6.7:** (A) Anatomical localisation of atherosclerosed coronary arteries, and (B) morphology of section of atheromatous coronary artery

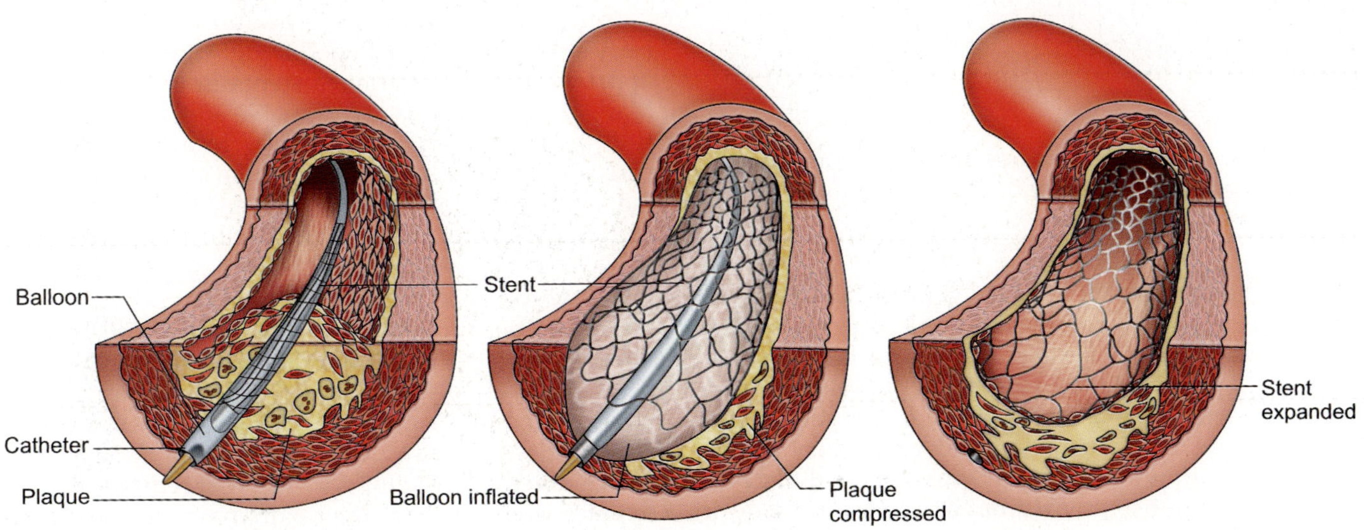


**Fig. 6.8:** Stepwise opening of obstructed coronary artery after stent has been installed in the lumen of the artery

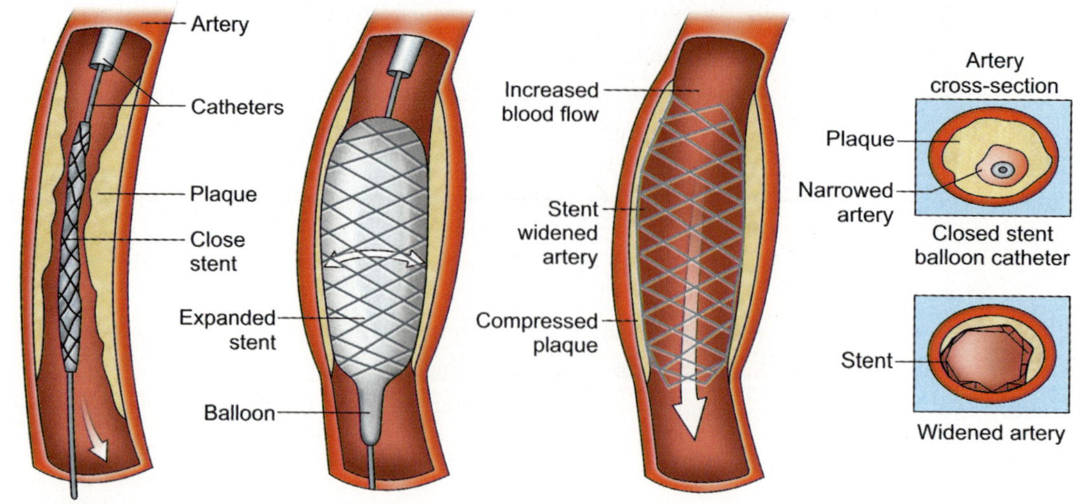


**Fig. 6.9:** Balloon angioplasty. Angioplasty is a minimally invasive procedure used to open up clogged arteries in almost any part of the body. In balloon angioplasty, a small balloon is guided to the site of blockage, and inflated to compress the plaque and thus widen the artery. A small incision is made in the groin or wrist, following the administration of local anesthesia. A balloon-tipped catheter (balloon catheter) is then inserted into an artery of the leg or arms. The balloon catheter is threaded to the blockage site under X-ray guidance. Once at the site of blockage, a dye may be inserted at the site so as to determine the exact location of the blockage. The balloon catheter is then positioned at the precise location, and the balloon is inflated. As a result the surrounding plaque gets compressed, thus widening the arterial lumen. The balloon is then deflated and removed along with the catheter

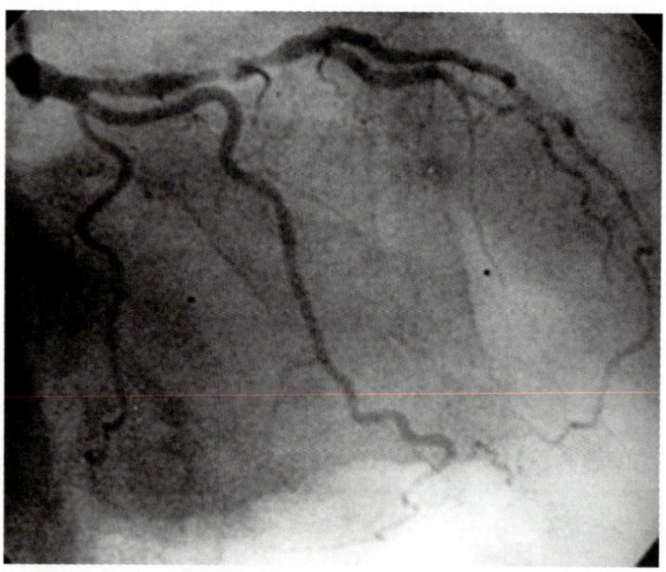

**Fig. 6.10:** Coronary angiography revealed diffuse irregular 73% luminal narrowing of the proximal left anterior descending coronary artery

dual antiplatelet therapy. Newer generation DES, with thinner struts and more biocompatible polymers, have considerably improved their safety profile. However, concerns still persist over the presence of durable polymers, as evidence from animal and human studies still suggest that these durable polymers may cause persistent arterial wall inflammation and delayed vascular healing, both of which may subsequently have a potential role in precipitating ST and delayed in-stent restenosis (i.e. late catch-up phenomenon). Newer generation DES, coated with biodegradable polymers, offer the attractive combination of controlled drug elution in parallel with biodegradation of the polymer into inert monomers. After the completion of biodegradation, only a BMS remains, thereby reducing the long-term risks associated with the presence of a permanent polymer. An extension of this concept has brought the development of newer DES that are completely free of polymer, or come with novel coatings. In addition, bioresorbable metallic (i.e. magnesium) and polymeric scaffolds have been developed, which initially safeguard the patency of the treated vessel and then disappear. The aim of this article is to review new stent technologies that are currently undergoing clinical investigation and discuss their future perspectives in interventional cardiology.

Intracoronary stents have been used widely since the early 1990s [the original Food Drug Administration (FDA) approval for intracoronary stents in the US was 1994]. Many different stents are available and differ in composition (e.g. stainless steel, cobalt chromium, and nickel chromium), architectural design, and stent delivery system (i.e. the balloon catheter that delivers it). The development of drug-eluting stents has revolutionized coronary intervention to the extent that balloon angioplasty and bare metal stents did in the 1980s and 1990s.

Today, four types of drug-eluting stents are available in the United States, the sirolimus-eluting stent (Cypher), the paclitaxel-eluting stent (Taxus), and the newer-generation zotarolimus-eluting stent (Endeavor) and everolimus-eluting stent (Xience V). These stents comprise a metal stent with a polymer that elutes a drug that reduces neointimal hyperplasia. Drug-eluting stents have been extensively tested in a wide spectrum of coronary lesions, all of which have demonstrated significant reductions in restenosis and

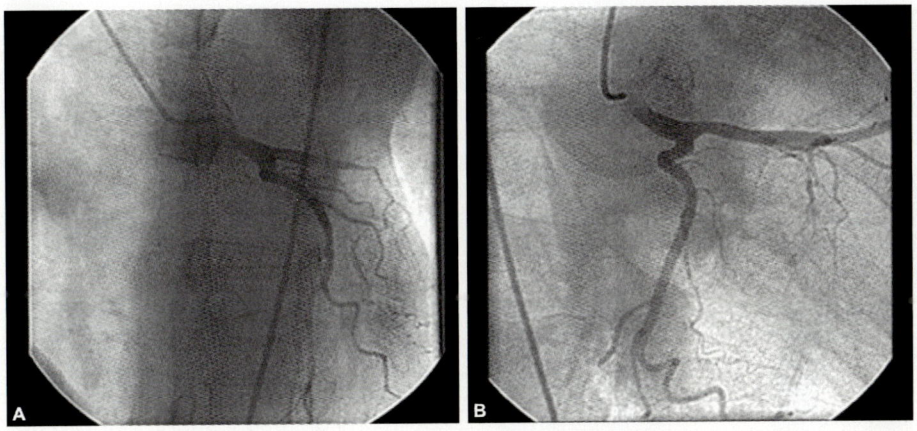


**Fig. 6.11:** (A) Coronary angiogram confirming a severe ostial stenosis of the LMCA, with extensive right-to-left collaterals to the left anterior descending (LAD) and left anterior circumflex (LCX) vessels. (B) Coronary angiogram showing the final result of the percutaneous coronary intervention

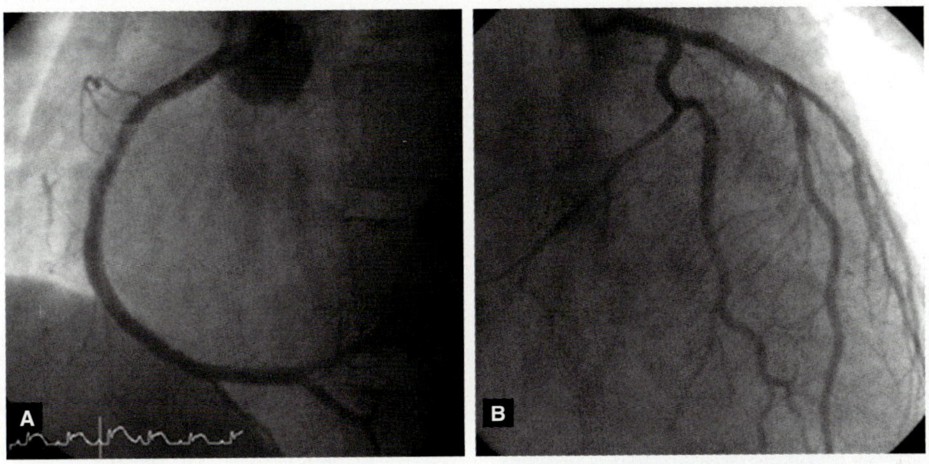


**Fig. 6.12:** After balloon angioplasty, the distal flow was restored to TIMI III in both coronary artery, but some residual thrombi were remained. (A) LAO view of RCA, (B) RAO caudal view of LAD

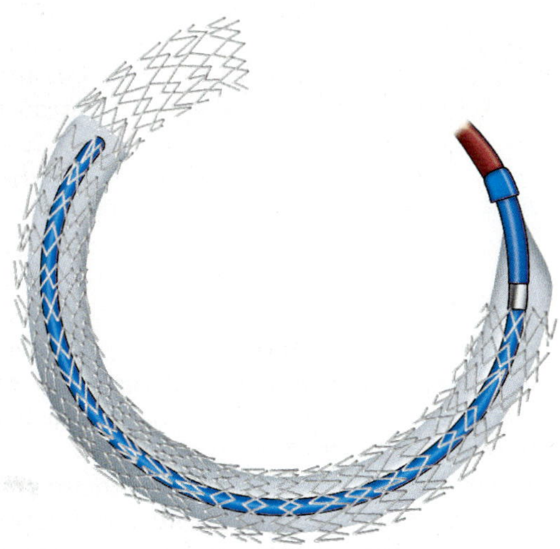

**Fig. 6.13:** Promus premier stent system is designed to provide physicians improved drug-eluting stent performance in treating patients with coronary artery disease. It is the only platform to feature a customised platinum chromium stent architecture, the market-leading everolimus drug coating and fluorinated co-polymer, and an enhanced stent delivery system

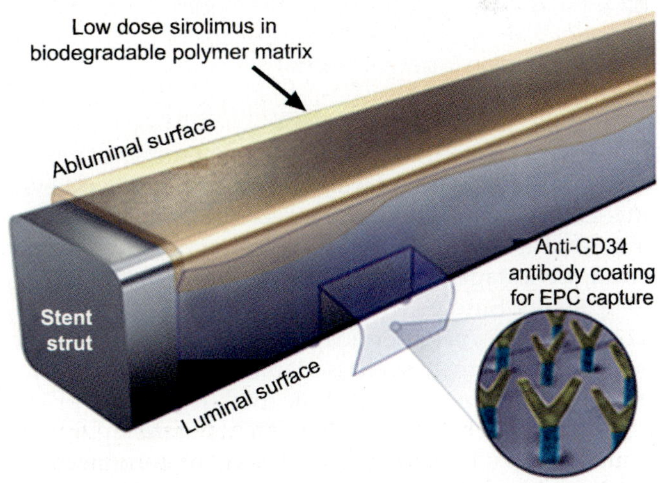


**Fig. 6.14:** The combo dual therapy device is hailed by OrbusNeich (Hoevelaken, Netherlands) as the first example of a dual therapy stent. The product combines abluminal sirolimus drug elution for the control of neointimal proliferation with the company's proprietary Genous prohealing technology to promote endothelial coverage. On the luminal side of the stent are immobilized antibodies that capture circulating endothelial progenitor cells

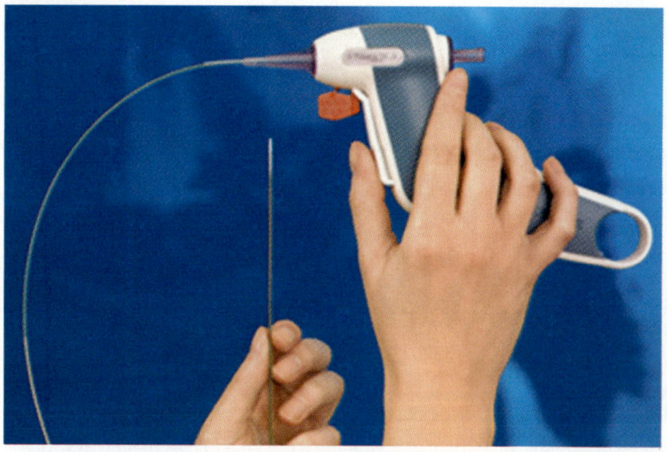

**Fig. 6.15:** Self-expanding Nitinol stent Pulsar-18 Fracture Resistant by Design Asymmetrical s-shape articulations and peak-to-valley design prevent fish-scaling. Small design modifications allow for better fatigue resistance through improved axial and bending flexibility

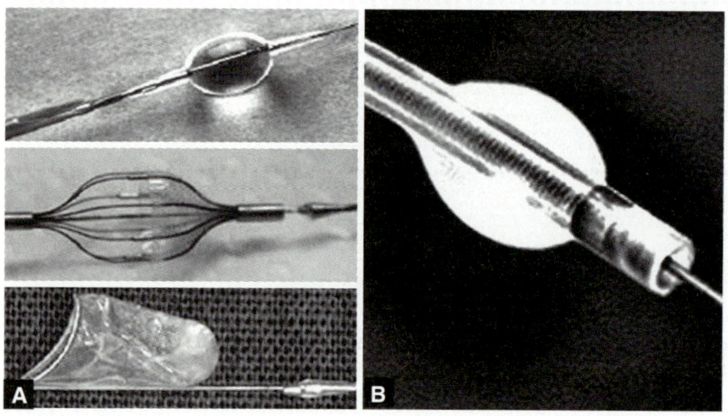


**Fig. 6.16:** The commonly used protection devices during vein graft interventions—(A) Percu-Surge (Guardwire Medtronic), Angioguard XP (Cordis), Filterwire EX (Boston). (B) The Proxis Embolic Protection System (St. Jude)

target-lesion revascularization rates when compared with bare metal stents. The zotarolimus-eluting stent and everolimus-eluting stent have improved deliverability, thinner struts, and a thinner polymer layer, and they may have clinical advantages over sirolimus-eluting and paclitaxel-eluting stents. Studies with drug-eluting stents are ongoing and include efforts to define safety and outcomes in every range of PCI setting, such as stable and unstable lesions, small vessels, vein grafts, chronic total occlusions, primary PCI, and comparing drug-eluting stent technologies with a coronary artery bypass graft in left main coronary artery disease and in diabetes patients with multivessel coronary artery disease. Although stents are conventionally placed after balloon predilation, a meta-analysis by Piscione et al. suggests that, in selected coronary lesions, direct stenting may lead to better outcomes. Myocardial infarction rates were lower with direct stenting (3.16% *vs* 4.04% with conventional stenting), while rates of target vessel revascularization were similar.

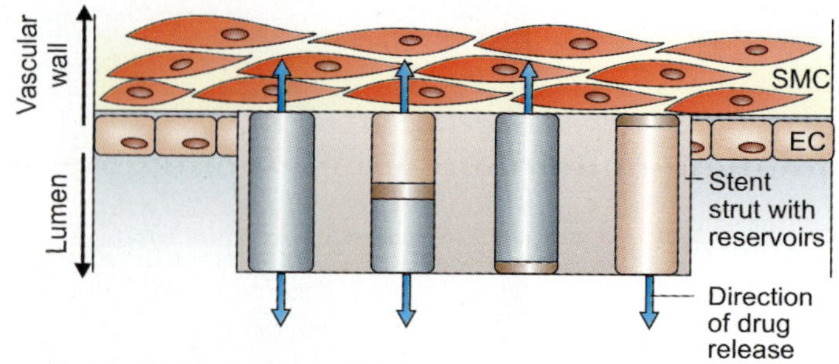


**Fig. 6.17:** This technology allows a targeted therapeutic approach, for example, by delivery of an agent that inhibits SMC proliferation via the ablumenal route of the stent surface. Concomitantly, an agent that promotes endothelial recovery can be released via the lumenal route. Furthermore, downstream drug delivery to tissue seems to be feasible (preferably at the lumenal side). The lateral view of a stent strut in the blood vessel exemplifies the diversity of drug delivery options (from left to right)— bidirectional delivery of one drug to both the ablumenal and lumenal side (blue), ablumenal delivery of one drug (orange) and lumenal delivery of a different drug (blue) where the drugs are separated in the reservoir to avoid mixing, or ablumenal delivery of one drug only (blue) and lumenal delivery of one drug only (orange). Reservoirs are sealed and drugs are separated by a layer of biodegradable polymer (brown disk). (EC=endothelial cell; SMC=smooth muscle cell)

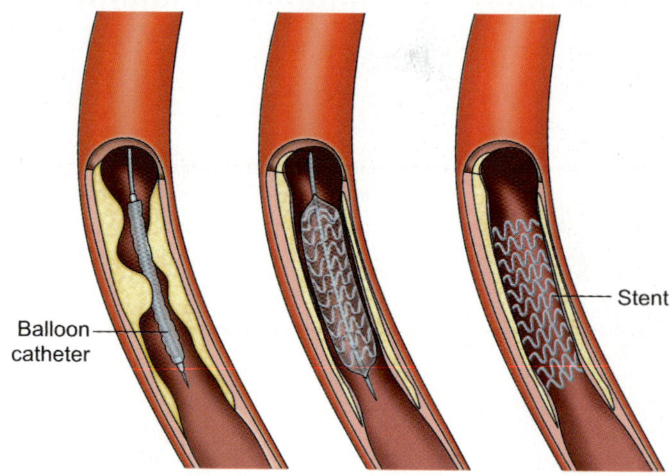


**Fig. 6.18:** Atheromated blocked coronary artery opened with stentoplasty

## The Stent of the Future

First generation drug-eluting stents have considerably reduced in-stent restenosis and broadened the applications of percutaneous coronary interventions for the treatment of coronary artery disease. The polymer is an integral part of drug-eluting stents in that, it controls the release of an antiproliferative drug. The main safety concern of first generation drug-eluting stents with permanent polymers (stent thrombosis) has been caused by local hypersensitivity, delayed vessel healing, and endothelial dysfunction. This has prompted the development of newer generation drug-eluting stents with biodegradable polymers or even polymer-free drug-eluting stents. Recent clinical trials have shown the safety and efficacy of drug-eluting stents with

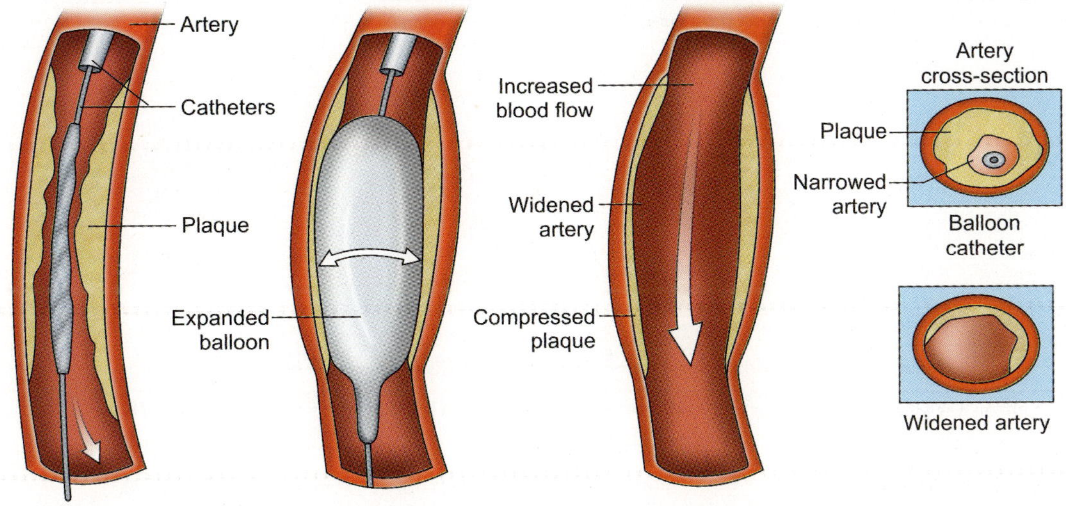


**Fig 6.19:** Stent angioplasty. This procedure is similar to balloon angioplasty, but involves the use of a small, expandable metallic mesh called 'stent', along with the balloon. The stent is placed around the balloon in a compressed form, and this assembly is placed at the tip of a catheter. It is then guided to the site of blockage as done during a balloon angioplasty. When the balloon is inflated, the stent expands and compresses the plaque. The balloon is then deflated and removed, leaving behind the stent which acts as a support and helps to keep the artery open

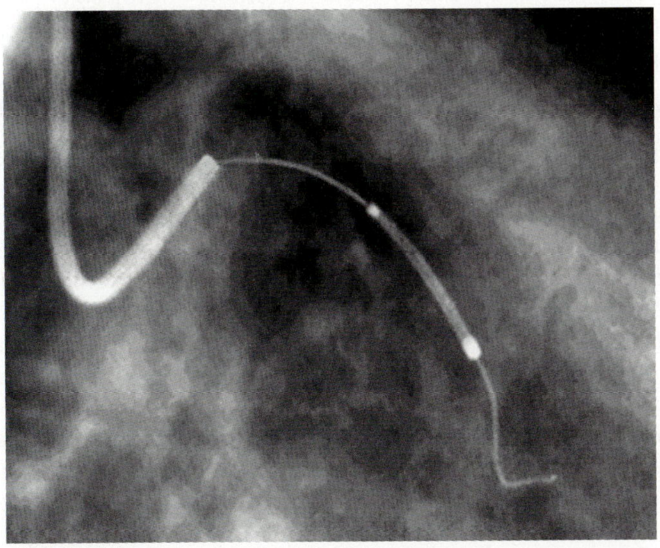

**Fig. 6.20:** Coronary angioplasty. X-ray angiogram of a balloon catheter and stent (white tipped tube, centre right) being placed within a coronary artery of a heart. They will be used to treat stenosis (narrowing) of the artery. The flexible catheter used to place them there is seen snaking down from top left. The inflation of the balloon catheter will expand the artery and restore normal blood flow. The stent is a hollow tube mesh, expanded by the balloon catheter, that stays in the artery and supports it after the balloon catheter has been withdrawn. Arterial stenosis may arise from arterial disease. X-ray angiography injects a radio-opaque contrast medium to highlight blood vessels on X-rays

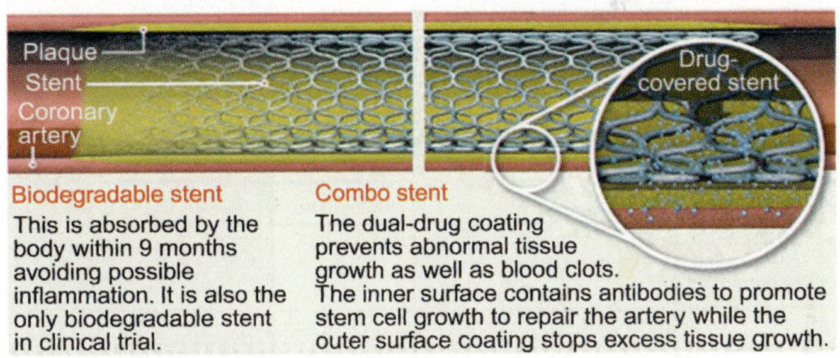


**Fig. 6.21:** Biodegradable coronary stents

biodegradable polymer, with proven reductions in very late stent thrombosis as compared to first generation drug-eluting stents. However, the concept of using a permanent metallic prosthesis implies major drawbacks, such as the presence of a foreign material within the native coronary artery that causes vascular inflammation and neoatherosclerosis, and also impedes the restoration of the vasomotor function of the stented segment. Bioresorbable scaffolds have been introduced to overcome these limitations, since they provide temporary scaffolding and then disappear, liberating the treated vessel from its cage.

## Future Perspectives in Stents

Newer generation DES, with biodegradable polymers, have shown an impressive reduction in very late stent thrombosis (VLST), contributing to improved long-term outcomes, as compared to first generation DES. The polymer-free DES or BRS are relatively new technologies, with many trials still in progress. The currently available angiographic, intravascular imaging, and clinical data, suggest acceptable safety and efficacy of these new technologies. However, it remains unclear as to whether biodegradable-polymer DES or polymer-free DES can minimize late ST events, particularly as these late events have also been observed in patients receiving BMS. Furthermore, considering the fatal consequences of ST, focus should be maintained on the eradication, rather than the minimization of this serious complication. There is a fundamental difference in concept between the DES and

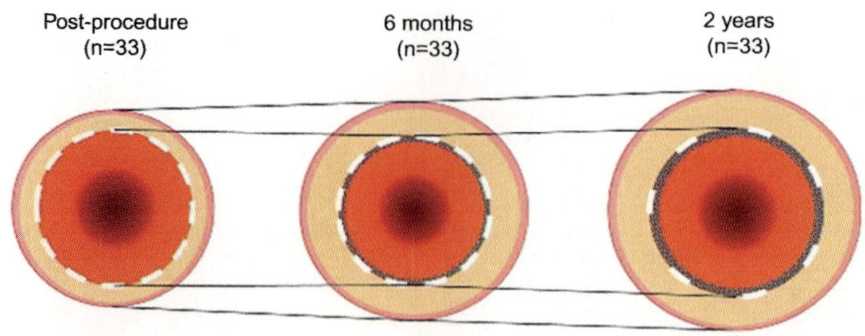


**IVUS measurements**

| | Post-procedure | | 6 months | | 2 years |
|---|---|---|---|---|---|
| Mean vessel area (mm$^2$) | 14.04 (3.80) | *P*=.008 → | 14.44 (3.82) | *P*<.001 → | 15.35 (4.05) |
| Mean scaffold area (mm$^2$) | 6.53 (1.23) | *P*=.06 → | 6.42 (1.17) | *P*<.001 → | 7.08 (1.73) |
| Mean plaque area (mm$^2$) | 7.51 (2.85) | *P*<.001 → | 8.02 (2.89) | *P*=.03 → | 8.27 (2.87) |
| Mean lumen area (mm$^2$) | 6.53 (1.24) | *P*=.02 → | 6.36 (1.18) | *P*=.01 → | 6.85 (1.78) |
| Mean NIH area (mm$^2$) | | | 0.08 (0.13) | *P*<.001 → | 0.25 (0.27) |

**Fig. 6.22:** Serial changes in intravascular ultrasound measurements over postprocedure, 6 months, and 2 years after absorb BVS implantation (NIH=neointimal hyperplasia, IVUS=intravascular ultrasound)

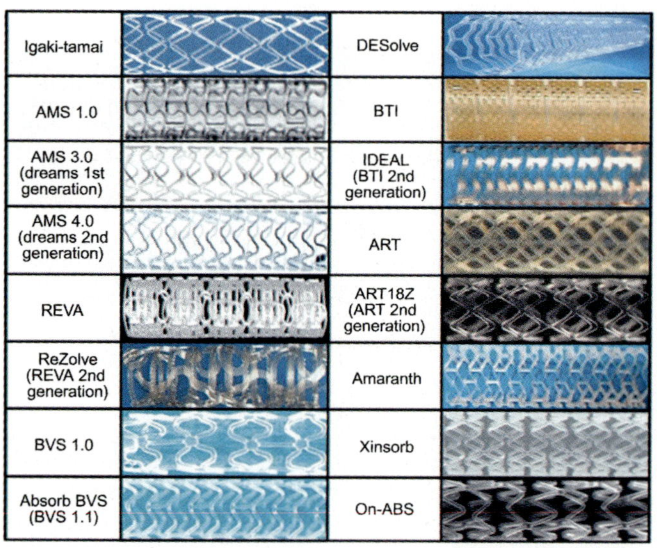


**Fig. 6.23:** Bioresorbable scaffolds under clinical or preclinical investigation

the BRS technologies, with the latter having a capability of liberating the vessel from a permanent metallic cage. Therefore, BRS technology has a theoretical advantage in reducing ST by means of endoluminal prosthesis elimination. BRS also facilitates the restoration of vasomotor function, which indirectly results in the completeness of vessel healing. The entire process of this treatment has been hence named as vascular reparative therapy.

Stents, particularly stents coated with materials to reduce inflammatory and cell growth responses, have resulted in greatly improved outcomes.

## Technique of Atherectomy

As a result of technical challenges, suboptimal clinical outcomes, and the significant rates of restenosis following percutaneous coronary artery balloon angioplasty, two innovative types of devices were developed: those used for atherectomy and coronary stents.

The idea behind atherectomy devices was to physically remove atheroma, calcium, and excess cellular material from the site of a coronary occlusion or stenosis (Figs 6.32–6.34). Both mechanical and laser-based approaches are used. An alternative approach developed at about the same time was intracoronary stent placement, based on the notion that permanent implantation of a scaffold to hold open the coronary artery at the site of an intervention would improve outcomes. Long-term outcomes from atherectomy alone have been disappointing and, in most cases, little better than balloon angioplasty. The rotational atherectomy catheter (Rotablator) is designed for the removal of plaque from coronary arteries. This device, which has a diamond-studded burr at its tip, rotates at about 160,000 rpm and is particularly well-suited for ablation of calcific or fibrotic plaque material. Unlike other atherectomy devices that rely on tissue cutting, the rotational atherectomy device relies on plaque abrasion and pulverization. Rotational atherectomy is successful in 92–97% of these cases, with a low incidence of major complications. It causes dislodgement of particles into the microcirculation, which occasionally may lead to infarction and no reflow (impaired distal coronary flow). Currently, the use of rotational atherectomy is largely confined to fibrotic or heavily calcified lesions that can be wired but not crossed or dilated by a balloon catheter.

Long-term outcomes from atherectomy alone have been disappointing and little better than balloon angioplasty in most cases. Stents, particularly stents coated with materials to reduce inflammatory and cell growth responses, have resulted in greatly improved outcomes. Atherectomy is still used for specific, niche indications, but the most common intracoronary device used today is a stent.

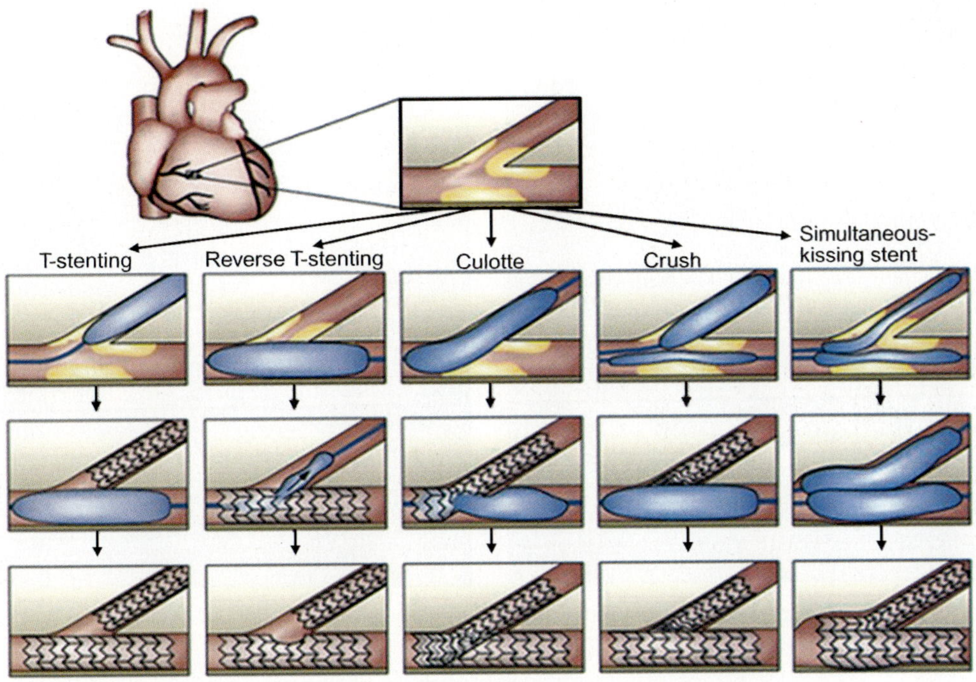


**Fig. 6.24:** Features of a bifurcated self-expanding coronary stent

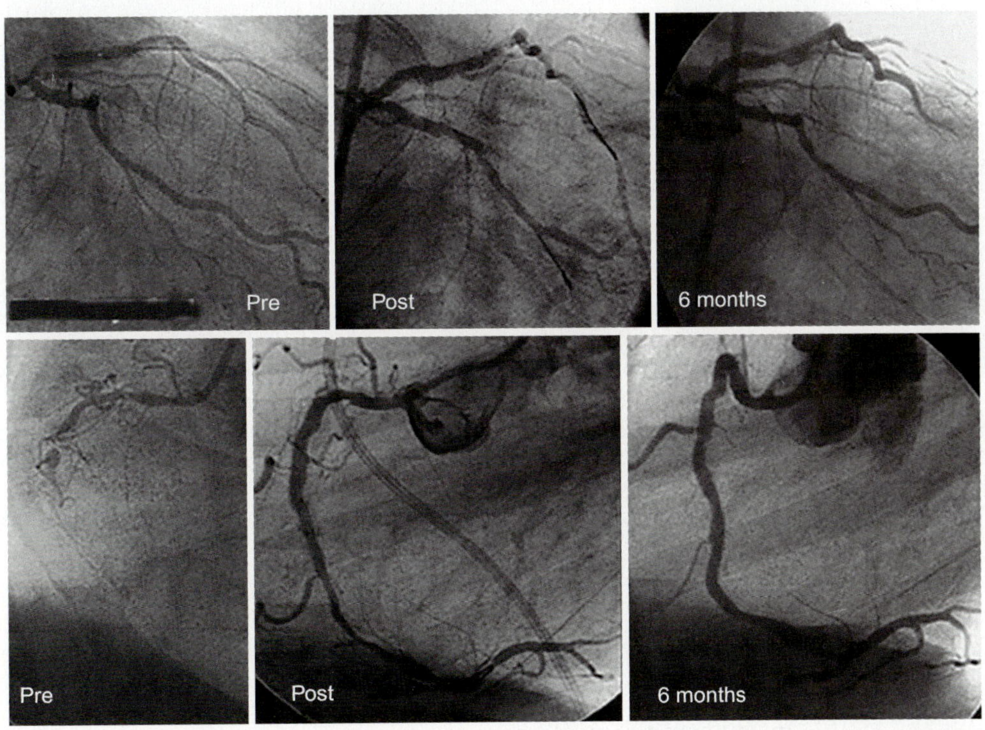


**Fig. 6.25:** A patient recently revascularized 20 years after the first angioplasty. The patient presents a severe bifurcation lesion in the left main coronary artery that is severely calcified. The right coronary artery also contains an occlusion that is more than 3 months old. The bifurcation of the artery is resolved by implantation of a rapamycin-coated stent close to the anterior descending artery and balloon angioplasty at the origin of the circumflex artery. The occlusion of the right coronary artery was crossed using a Safe-Cross radio frequency guidewire and the procedure was completed through implantation of rapamycin-coated stents. Excellent results were seen in both treated lesions by angiography at 6 months. The results obtained during follow-up would have been unthinkable 20 years earlier using percutaneous revascularization techniques

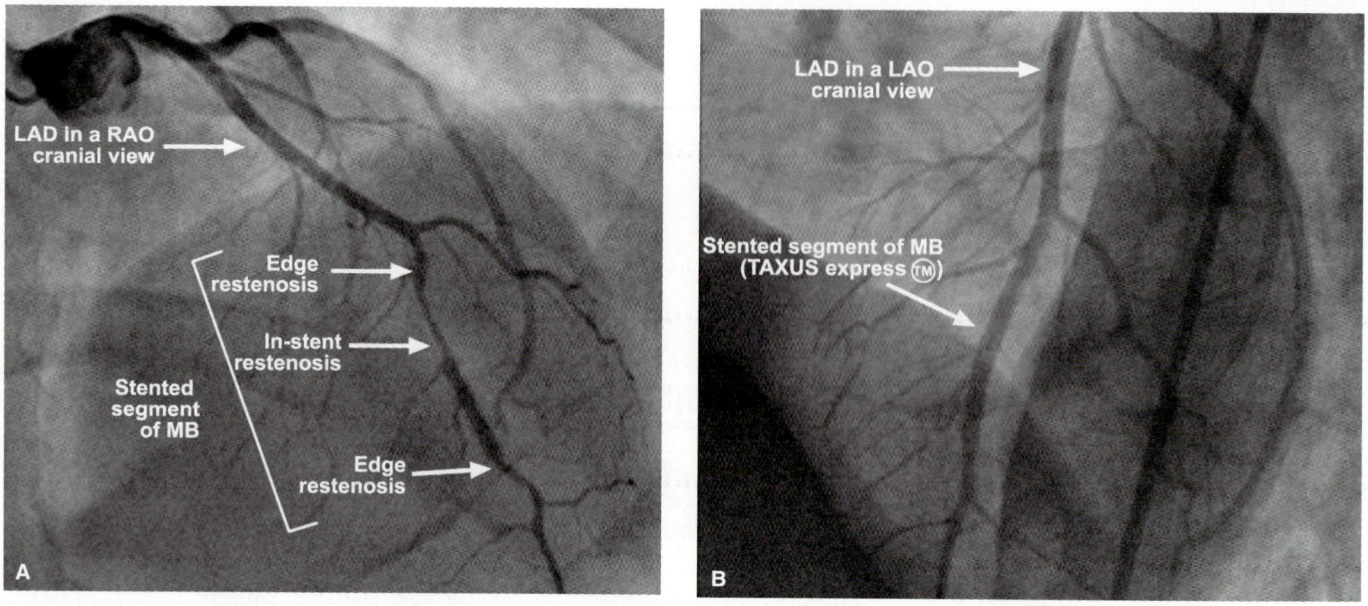


**Fig. 6.26:** (A) Stent restenosis of LAD artery in myocardial bridging, (B) successful stenting of segment in myocardial bridging (MB)

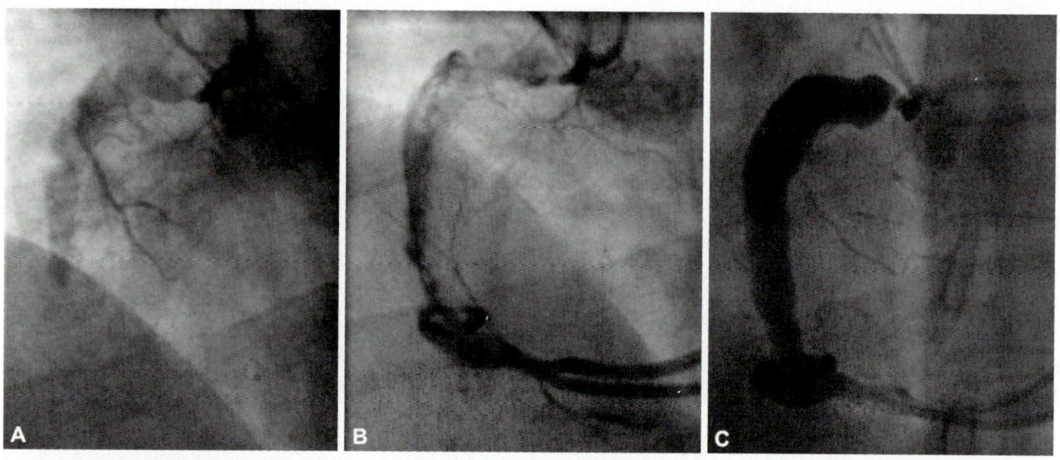


**Fig. 6.27:** Occlusion of the RCA. Angiogram of occluded right coronary artery (RCA) aneurysm in a 33-year-old man who experienced a Kawasaki disease—compatible illness at age 6 years (diagnosed as nonspecific viral illness) and was asymptomatic until his myocardial infarction. (A) Injection of the occluded RCA, (B) RCA after percutaneous transluminal coronary angioplasty with reestablished distal flow. Note smooth appearance of distal branches of the RCA, (C) Patent RCA aneurysm 1 month after percutaneous transluminal coronary angioplasty, aspirin, and warfarin therapy maintaining an international normalized ratio of 2–2.5

## Intravascular Ultrasonography

Coronary angiography provides a display of luminal narrowing in multiple planes and is useful in guiding coronary interventions. However, angiography cannot provide information about the vessel wall, which is where the atherosclerotic process resides. Intravascular ultrasonography (IVUS) was developed to provide information about the plaque, the vessel wall, and the degree of luminal narrowing. It provides a tomographic cross-section of the vessel, allowing operators to gather significant qualitative and quantitative information that is potentially valuable in assessing stenosis severity and the true extent of atherosclerotic involvement of main vessel (Figs 6.35–6.38).

Identification of the lumen border and the media-adventitia interface form the key landmarks during interpretation. Plaque can be distinguished from the lumen by differences in echogenicity. In addition to providing information about the amount and distribution of plaque, IVUS can identify features of plaque composition, such as calcification and lipid collections, which may not be appreciated by angiography alone. Frequent uses of IVUS include the assessment of indeterminate lesions and the evaluation of adequate stent deployment. The latter has become increasingly important, since proper deployment of drug-eluting stents is critical to reduction in rates of thrombosis. Recent developments in ultrasonography (e.g.

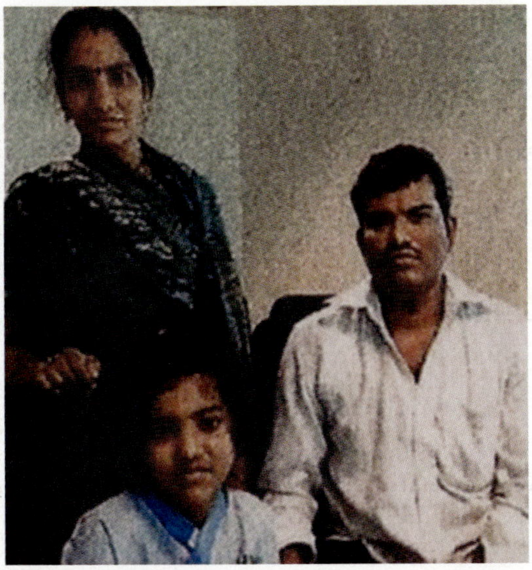

**Fig. 6.28:** Youngest child to receive coronary stent Deepa alongwith her parents (street bender) in whom bioabsorable stent was fitted to open her coronary artery blocked due to familial hypercholesterolemia

virtual histology) and other technologies (e.g. optical coherence tomography, plaque thermography) have led to ways of characterizing and identifying vulnerable segments of plaque that may pose a risk for future cardiac events.

### Comparison of (ERBAC), Excimer Laser, Rotational Atherectomy, and Balloon Angioplasty Study (Fig. 6.39)

This showed that rotational atherectomy was associated with a higher short-term success rate than balloon angioplasty (90% *vs* 80%), but major ischemic complications and repeat revascularization were higher 6 months after

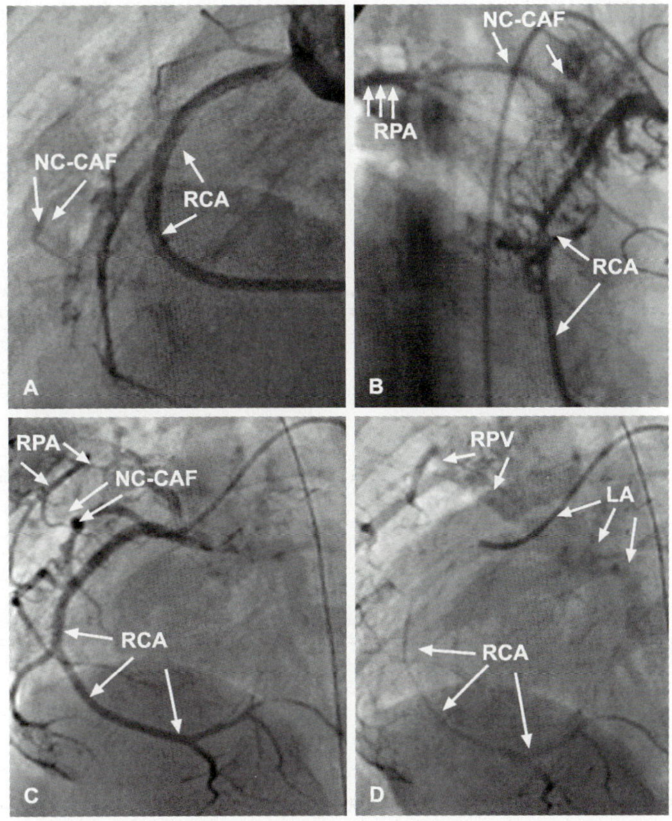



**Fig. 6.29:** Examples of noncameral coronary artery fistulae (NC-CAFs) are shown in 3 patients—(A) a small NC-CAF from the right coronary artery (RCA) with flow into the right lung field, but no clear identification of a pulmonary vessel; (B) a moderate NC-CAF with a diffuse connection originating from the RCA and filling an identifiable right pulmonary artery (RPA) branch; and (C–D) a large NC-CAF from the RCA (C) filling a RPA branch, (D) and then on levophase of the same angiogram

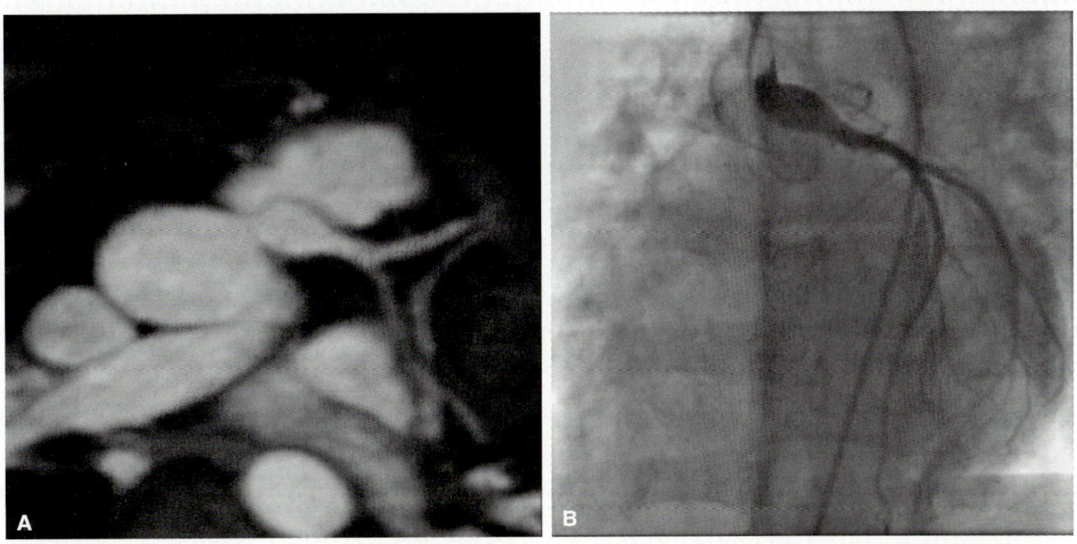



**Fig. 6.30:** 3D b-SSFP whole heart images, magnetic resonance coronary angiography (MRCA)—(A) shows large patent, reconstructed, reimplanted left coronary artery into the left coronary sinus. (B) Findings confirmed on X-ray coronary angiography

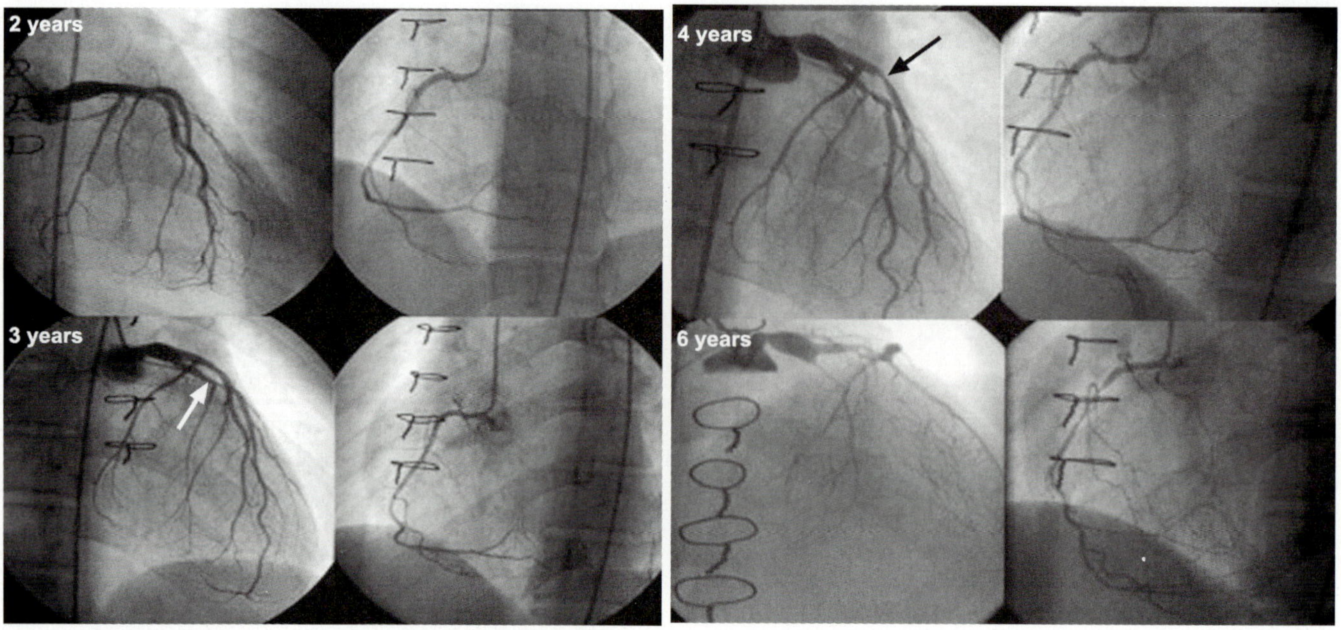


**Fig. 6.31:** The progressive nature of allograft vasculopathy. At 2 years after heart transplantation, there is ectasia of the left main coronary artery but no evidence of allograft vasculopathy. At 3 years, the left anterior descending coronary artery developed mild disease at the bifurcation of the septal artery (white arrow). At 4 years, the first obtuse marginal branch of the circumflex has an additional lesion (black arrow). At 6 years, the left anterior descending coronary artery is occluded totally and the circumflex is diseased severely. The right coronary artery is also diseased diffusely, including the smaller secondary branches, with abrupt cut-off in some of them. Unfortunately, this patient had a fatal myocardial infarction a few weeks after

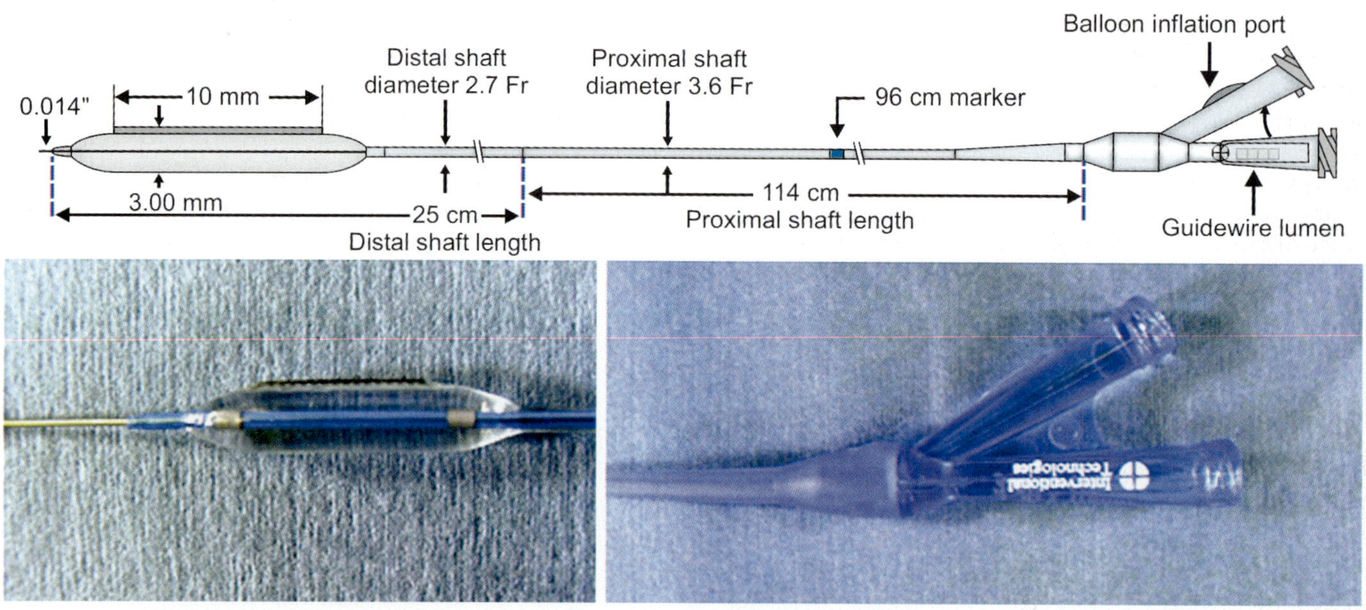


**Fig. 6.32:** Athertomy device. The SBC is an over-the-wire type catheter with a single blade attached to the surface of a noncompliant balloon. The blade is 10 mm in length and runs along the same side and axis as the balloon inflation port. The polysulfone balloon shaft is 3.6 Fr proximal and 2.7 Fr distal and is compatible with a 6 Fr guiding catheter. The working height and width of the blade are identical to those used for the current cutting balloon, namely 0.005-0.006 inches in height and 0.003 inches thick

treatment (46% vs 37%). A meta-analysis failed to show any significant difference in mortality, major adverse cardiovascular events (MACE), or revascularization rates in patients treated with rotational atherectomy, laser, or cutting balloon angioplasty when compared with balloon angioplasty alone. In some cases, rotational atherectomy was actually associated with an increase in periprocedural myocardial infarction. However, none of these trials compared stent-related outcomes. In fact, many of these devices may be used to facilitate stent delivery in complex lesions, especially when balloon angioplasty alone has failed. Since 1987, directional coronary atherectomy (DCA) has been used to debulk coronary plaques. A steel fenestrated cage housing a cup-shaped blade is positioned

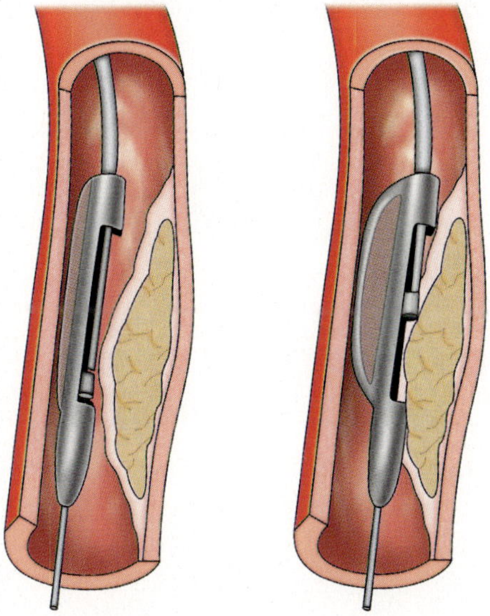

Fig. 6.33: Working of directional atherotomy device in removing the plaque from the occluded artery

against the coronary lesion by a low-pressure positioning balloon, allowing any protruding plaque to be removed.

Atherectomy is typically followed by balloon dilation and stenting. The acute gain, therefore, is a combination of the removal of atheromatous plaque and radial displacement of plaque from dilation. Major complication rates associated with directional atherectomy are low and similar to those associated with conventional balloon angioplasty. Other complications (e.g. distal embolization of plaque, transient side-branch occlusion, coronary vasospasm, the no-reflow phenomenon, non-Q-wave myocardial infarction) are greater with DCA than with balloon angioplasty. Because of the increased complication rates and the greater technical demands of DCA compared with balloon angioplasty or stenting, the use of DCAs has greatly decreased in recent years. A 2006 meta-analysis demonstrated that DCA is superior to stenting alone with regard to acute angiographic results and target-lesion revascularization with a similar prevalence of late MACEs. There was, however, a higher prevalence of early MACEs with DCA before stenting, which probably related to distal embolization Although initial excitement about the development of laser atherectomy was considerable, it is not used widely because of the technical demands of this device and no clear improvements in outcome over therapy with other devices.

## POST-PROCEDURE OUTCOME OF PCI

A major 2009 task force report viewed favorably, in general, the use of coronary revascularization for patients with acute coronary syndromes and combinations of significant symptoms and/or ischemia. However, revascularization of asymptomatic patients or patients with low-risk findings on noninvasive testing and minimal medical therapy were viewed less favorably (Figs 6.40–6.44).

## FIRST-IN-HUMAN EVALUATION OF A NOVEL ROBOT-ASSISTED CORONARY ANGIOPLASTY SYSTEM

The main aim of a novel robotic-assisted coronary angioplasty is to evaluate the safety and feasibility of a robotic angioplasty system in delivery and manipulation of coronary guidewires, balloons, and stents in patients undergoing elective percutaneous coronary intervention (PCI) (Fig 6.45).

### Background

A remote-control, robotic-assisted angioplasty system is under development to address some of the procedural challenges and occupational hazards associated with traditional PCI.

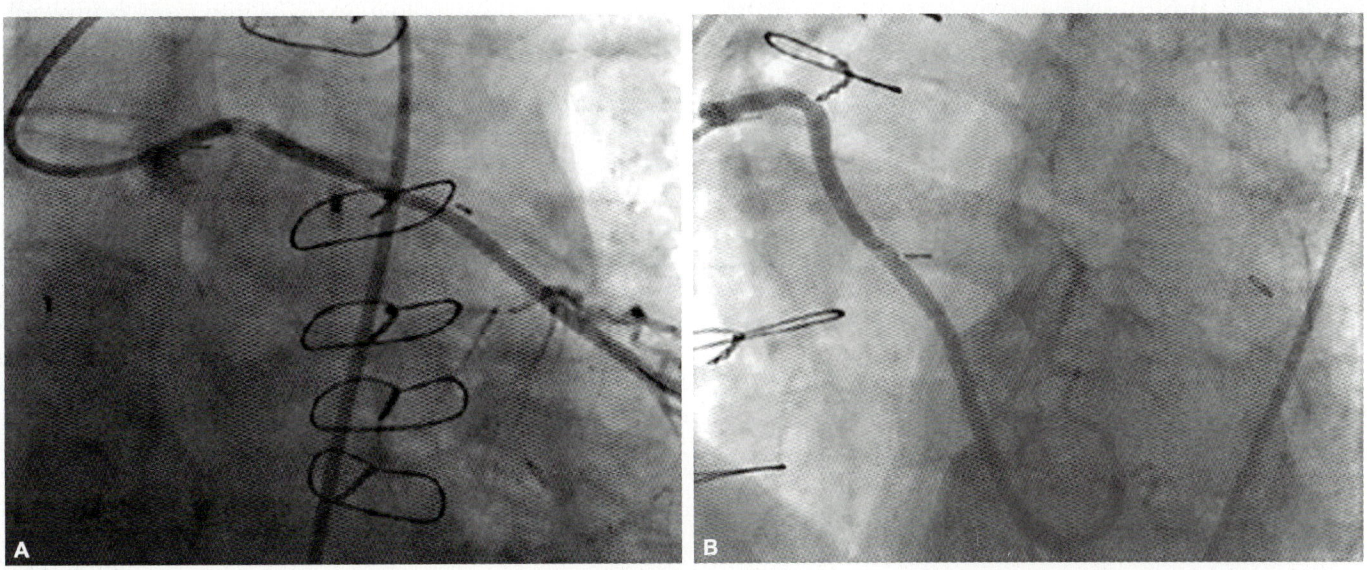


Fig. 6.34: (A) Vein graft deply intubated to allow the Rotablator burr to be advanced, (B) final result after rotational atherectomy and stent placement

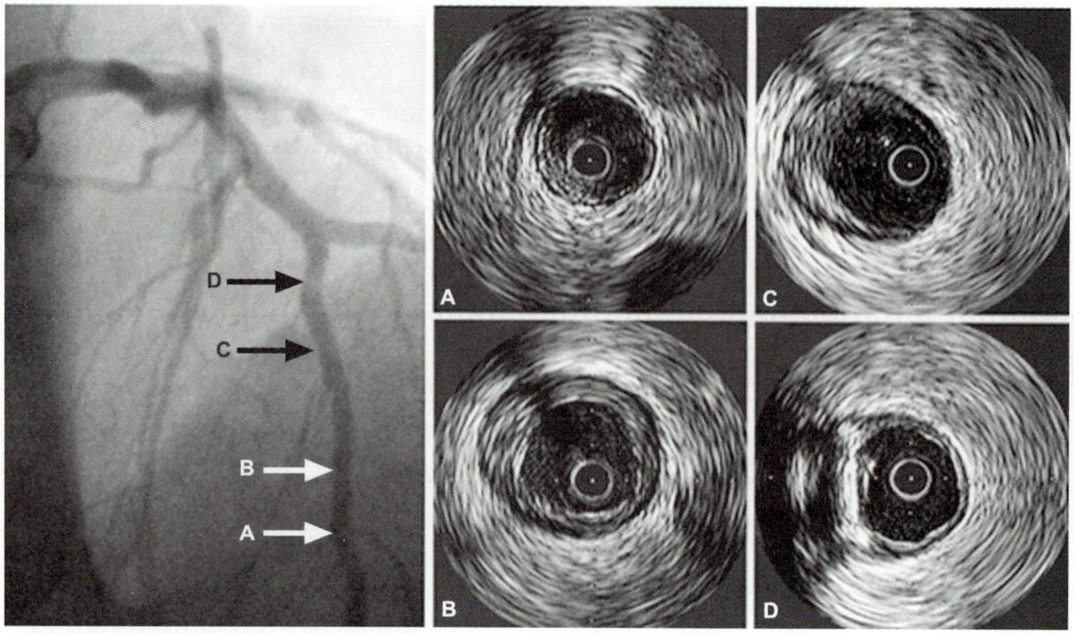


**Fig. 6.35:** Intravascular ultrasound (IVUS) at multiple sites in an angiographically normal artery. The 4 images obtained from sites A through D exhibit various degrees of atherosclerotic involvement, despite a normal-appearing angiogram. The IVUS images were obtained via a motorized pullback

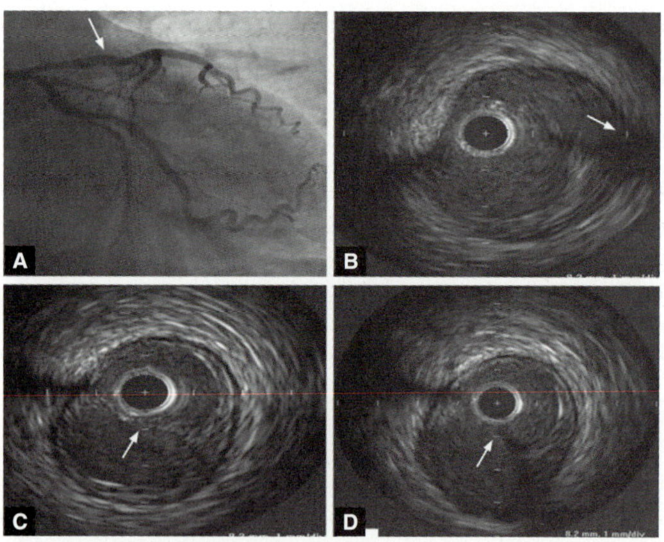


**Fig. 6.36:** (A) Intimal dissection (arrow) in proximal left anterior descending artery (LAD) by coronary angiography, (B) entry (arrow) of intimal tear of the proximal to dissection site in the LAD by intravascular ultrasonography (IVUS), (C) intimal flap (arrow) dividing between true lumen and false lumen in the dissection site by IVUS, (D) reentry (arrow) of intimal tear of the distal to dissection site by IVUS

### *Clinical Utility of Robotic Systems*

Robotic systems have been suggested to enhance the precision of cardiovascular procedures with increased accuracy. One of the technical features of the robotic system is the capability to control and accurately position (1 mm steps) the stent delivery system. The recent stent deployment techniques on clinical outcomes of patients treated with the cypher stent (STLLR) trial highlighted the impact on clinical outcomes of geographic miss and stent misplacement. Although endovascular imaging guidance is likely necessary to improve the precision of stent placement, the robotically assisted system facilitates the positioning of the stent delivery system with a high degree of accuracy. In addition, robotic systems have been suggested to reduce radiation exposure.

Despite the significant evolution in interventional device technologies, the actual procedural methodology and workflow in the catheterization laboratory has remained unchanged in the last 25 years. As the current practice of interventional cardiology evolves into more complex PCI procedures, interventional cardiologists, the professional societies US Food and Drug Administration, and International Atomic Energy Agency called for enhanced catheterization laboratory safety by reducing radiation exposure to both patients and operators and making the overall catheterization laboratory environment more ergonomically friendly through technological innovations. Incorporating a remote-control, robotic-assisted PCI system into the catheterization laboratory might address some of the procedural deficiencies and occupational hazards associated with traditional PCI in addition to contributing to a higher degree of precision and control for the interventional procedure.

### Technique of Robot-assisted Coronary Angioplasty

Patients with coronary artery disease and clinical indication for elective PCI were enrolled. The coronary angioplasty procedure was performed with the CorPath 200 robotic system (Corindus, Inc., Natick, Massachusetts).

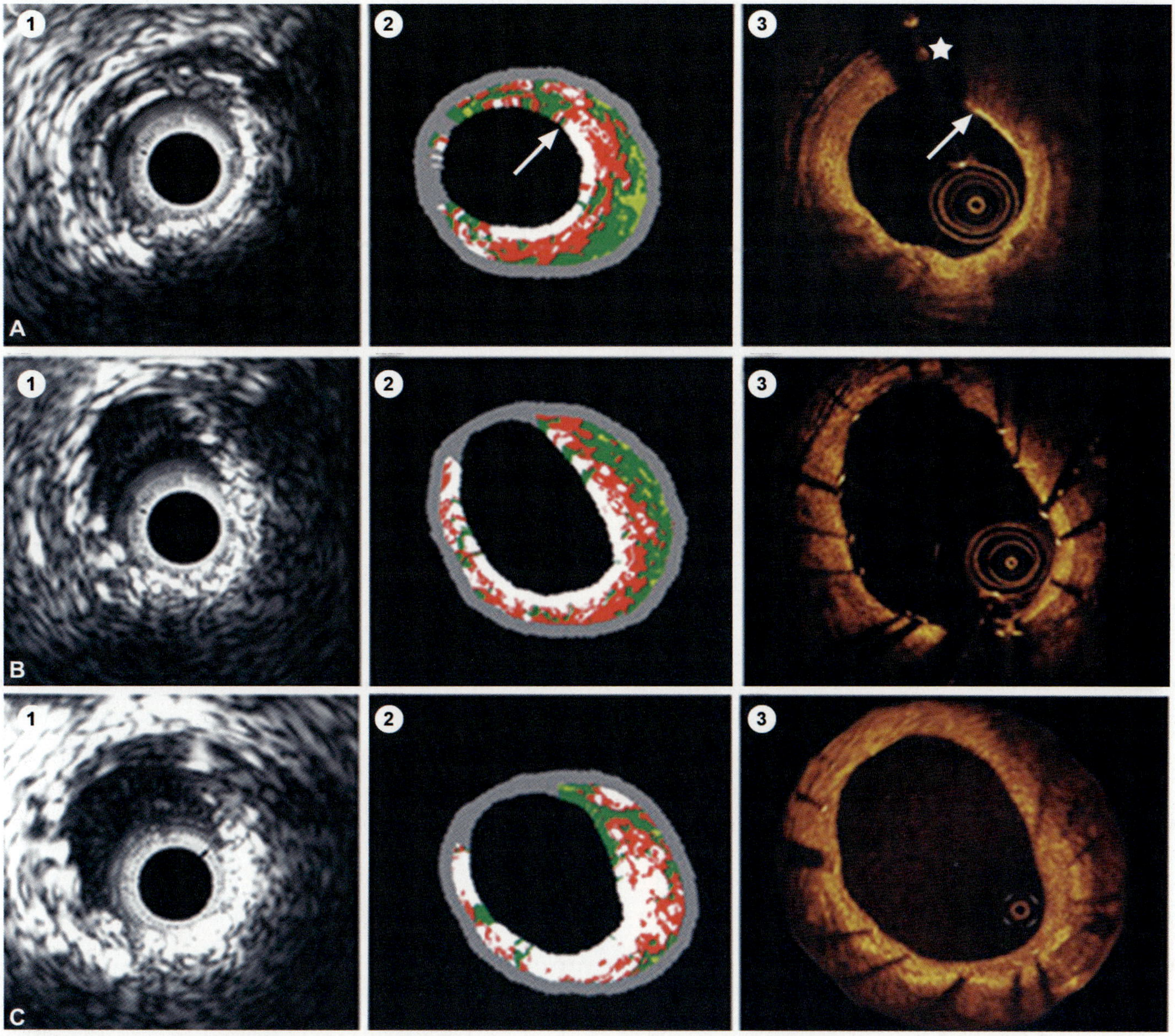


**Fig. 6.37:** Matched grayscale IVUS (1), IVUS-VH (2) and OCT (3) images of the IVUS-derived, thin-capped fibroatheroma (A) before stenting with the vProtect® Luminal Shield, (B) immediately after treatment with the vProtect® Luminal Shield and (C) at the 6-month follow-up appointment. The arrow in panel-A part 2 indicates the necrotic core in contact with the lumen. The arrow in panel-A part 3 indicates the thin fibrous cap, and the asterisk indicates a guidewire artifact. In the IVUS-VH images (parts 2): red, necrotic core; dark green, fibrotic tissue; light green, fibrofatty tissue; and white, dense calcium. IVUS=intravascular ultrasound; IVUS-VH=intravascular ultrasound virtual histology; OCT=optical coherence tomography

The system consists of a remote interventional cockpit and a multicomponent bedside unit that enables the operator to advance, retract, and rotate guidewires and rapid exchange catheters. The primary endpoint was device clinical success (30% residual stenosis) without in-hospital major adverse cardiac events. Technical success was defined as the ability of the system to complete all the planned angioplasty steps on the basis of procedural segments. Patients were followed up to 30 days after angioplasty procedure.

The retrospective evaluation study of lens injuries and dose (RELID) study revealed that interventional cardiologists have cataract-type eye opacities 3 times more often than age-matched controlled group. The mean fluoroscopy time from this study compares favorably with the results of the study of 9,650 patients undergoing single-vessel PCI (11.5 min *vs* 18.3 min) and with a subgroup of 7,242 patients whose fluoroscopy time was 23 minutes (11.5 min *vs* 12.7 min). Shorter fluoroscopy time translated into reduced radiation exposure for the patient and the

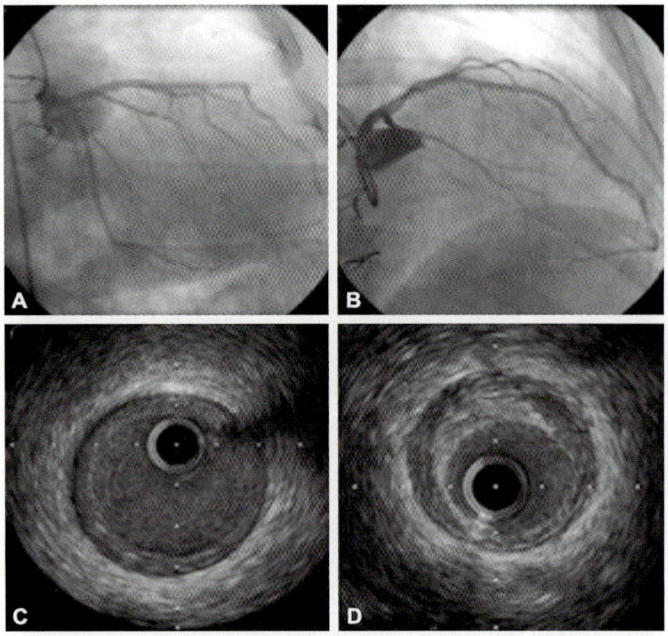


**Fig. 6.38:** (A and B) Coronary angiography did not suggest disease in this artery, (C) intravascular ultrasound images of the anterior descending artery in a patient transplanted 5 years previously, showing both the concentric intimal thickening typical of cardiac allograft vasculopathy and (D) an eccentric plaque typical of atherosclerotic coronary disease

operator and reduced contrast fluid usage. In our study, 1 of the most important findings was the significant (97.1%) reduction in radiation exposure to the operator performing the robotic PCI procedure. The patient radiation exposure was within the normal reported limits—2.1 Gy *vs* 1.9 Gy. Also, although the study was not designed to show differences in contrast volume usage, the total volume of contrast agents used in this study seemed to be less, compared with what has been reported in other clinical series. The lower contrast usage might be attributed to the complete procedure control enabled by the interventional cockpit environment. Another subjective but still important finding was the level of technical 'comfort' expressed by the operators. Although no specific measurement of this variable was used in this study, both operators perceived this system to be more comfortable compared with the typical technique used for coronary intervention. Most of the cases were performed under a controlled environment, in which the operator had the opportunity to focus on the performance of the procedure, having a close proximity of the monitors and not distracted by the physical strain of the lead apron and standing position.

In early clinical experience, the use of the robotic system seems not to reduce the overall periprocedural times compared with manual PCI of single lesions. However, we believe that, as this technology underwent initial clinical

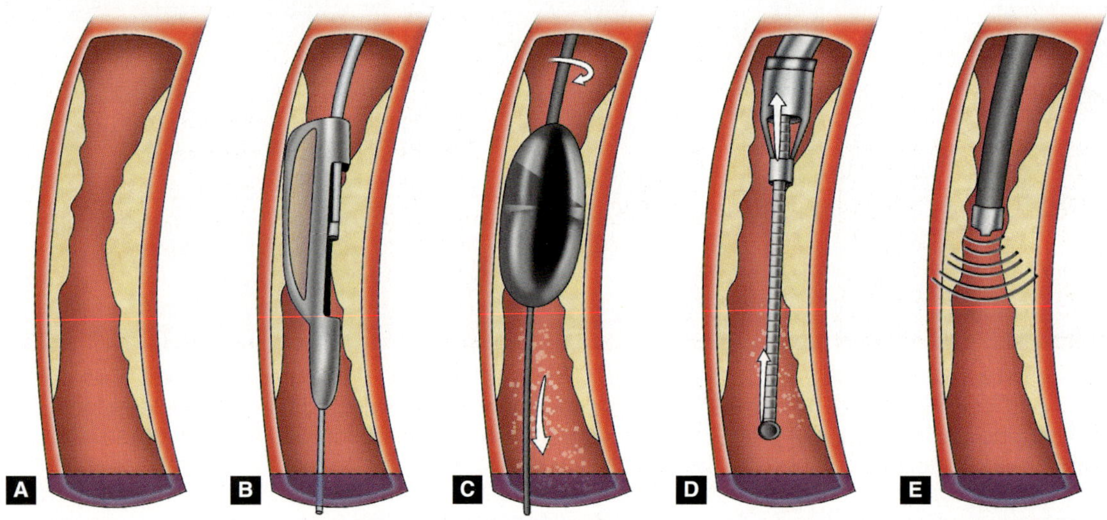


**Fig. 6.39:** (A) Atherectomy—this is a minimally invasive procedure that involves the use of specialized catheters for mechanical removal of plaque from the arterial walls. The plaque is either scraped out or pulverized with the help of tiny blades. The design and working of these devices ensures that the arterial wall remains damage-free. The catheter is inserted into an artery in the leg or arm, through an incision in the groin or wrist. It is then routed to the blockage site, and the plaque is mechanically scraped out. Depending on the type of device or catheter used, atherectomy procedures employed are: (B) Directional—here, the catheter has a scraping blade attached to it along with a low pressure balloon on the opposite side. Once at the blockage site the balloon is inflated, as a result of which the blade is pushed towards the plaque. The plaque is then scraped out, and the catheter is rotated to ensure complete plaque removal. The plaque fragments are collected in a chamber present at the tip of the device. (C) Rotational—a rotational atherectomy catheter has small, diamond-tipped, rotating edges which disintegrate the plaque into microscopic fragments. These fragments flow through the circulatory system, and are removed from the body through normal waste-removal processes. (D) Transluminal extraction—the catheter used in this procedure has two stainless steel, rotating blades attached to a hollow tube. At the site of blockage, the rotating blades grind the plaque, and the resultant fragments are collected into the hollow tube by vacuum suction. (E) Laser—in this procedure, a laser-tipped catheter is used to vaporize the plaque. The resultant molecules are removed by the body via liver and kidneys

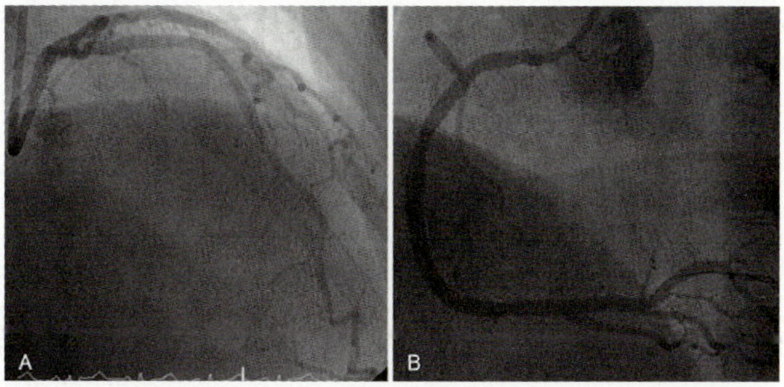


**Fig. 6.40:** CAG showed no residual stenosis in each lesion after two Cypher stents (Cordis/Johnson & Johnson, USA) were implanted in the lesions. (A) Post-PCI angiography revealed well-deployed SES in midportion of the LAD. (B) post-PCI angiography revealed well-deployed SES in mid-portion of the RCA. CAG= coronary angiography, PCI=percutaneous coronary intervention

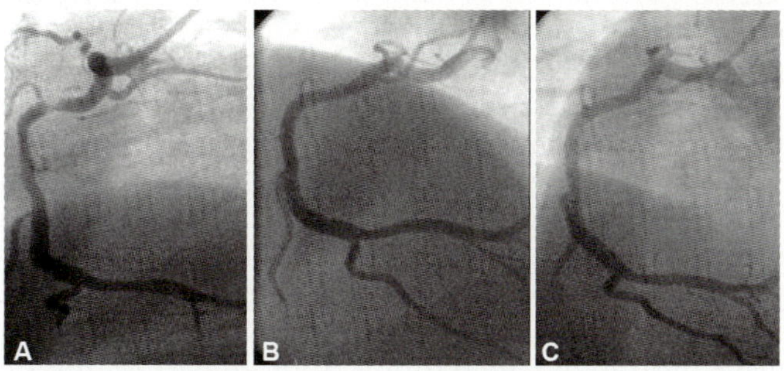


**Fig. 6.41:** (A) Severe lesion in the middle right coronary artery, (B) immediate direct postimplantation of a 4 × 15 mm driver stent, (C) angiographic control at 6 months' follow-up

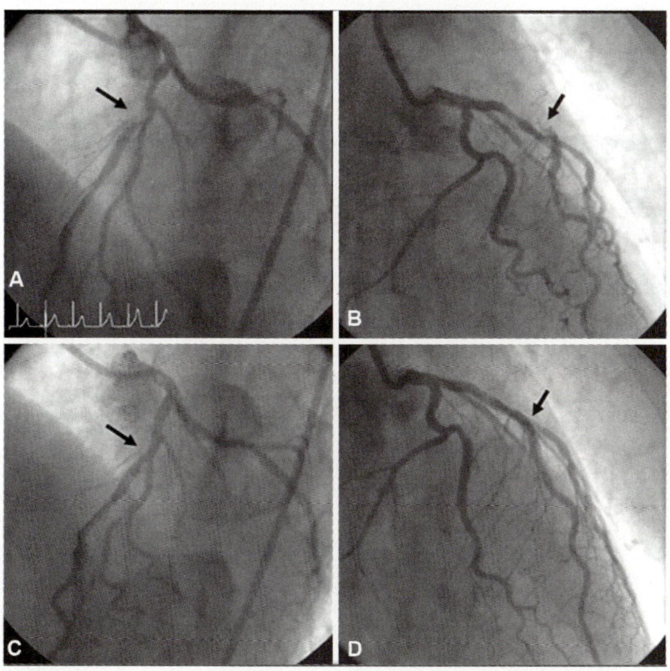


**Fig. 6.42:** (A and B) The left coronary angiography showed significant stenosis in m-LAD, (C and D) After deployment of 3.0 × 28 mm Cypher stent in this lesion, angiography showed no residual stenosis with good distal flow

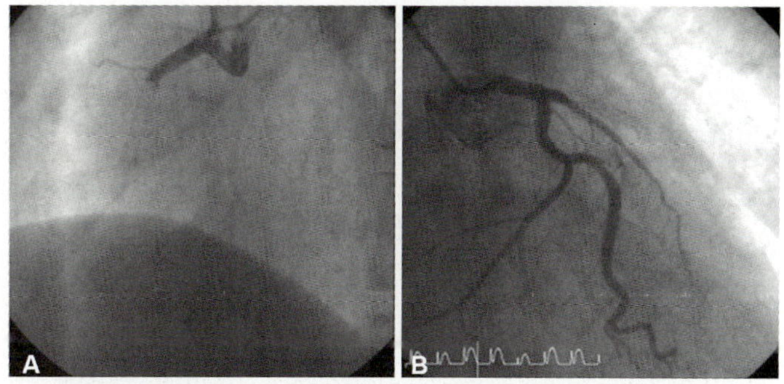


**Fig. 6.43:** The emergency coronary angiography revealed totally occluded proximal LAD and proximal RCA at the same time, the sites of the implantation of sirolimus-eluting stents. (A) LAO view of RCA, (B) RAO caudal view of LAD

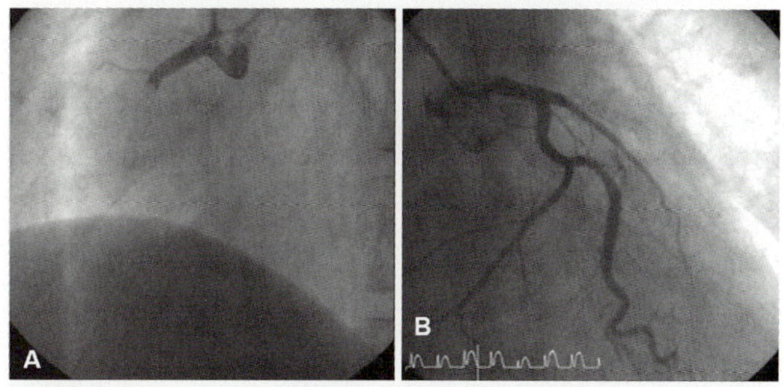


**Fig. 6.44:** A 28 mm stent deployment in a patient specific right coronary artery. The expansion is projected to the angiographic image

evaluation, the rigor of the study procedure in addition to the time required to register the data added additional procedural time. In addition, from the operator point of view, there was an initial learning and technology adaptation curve that we believe will improve over time, leading to shorter procedural times. However, this study still represents an early feasibility study in a small cohort of patients, and the use of this technology in more challenging anatomies including the presence of severe tortuosity, severe calcification, or interventions requiring multiple wires and balloons needs to be further studied. A larger, prospective, multicenter pivotal clinical trial designed to test the robotic angioplasty system in a larger number of patients is underway.

### Ancillary Devices

*Thrombus extraction catheters:* In addition to balloons, stents, and atherectomy devices, other devices such as thrombus extraction catheters and distal embolic protection devices have found roles in PCI. In the TAPAS trial (thrombus aspiration during percutaneous coronary intervention in acute myocardial infarction), which studied the use of thrombus aspiration during primary PCI for ST-elevation myocardial infarction, thrombus aspiration with an export catheter before stenting had a reduced all-cause mortality (4.7% *vs* 7.6%) and reduced cardiac death (3.6% *vs* 6.7%) at 1 year compared with conventional PCI.

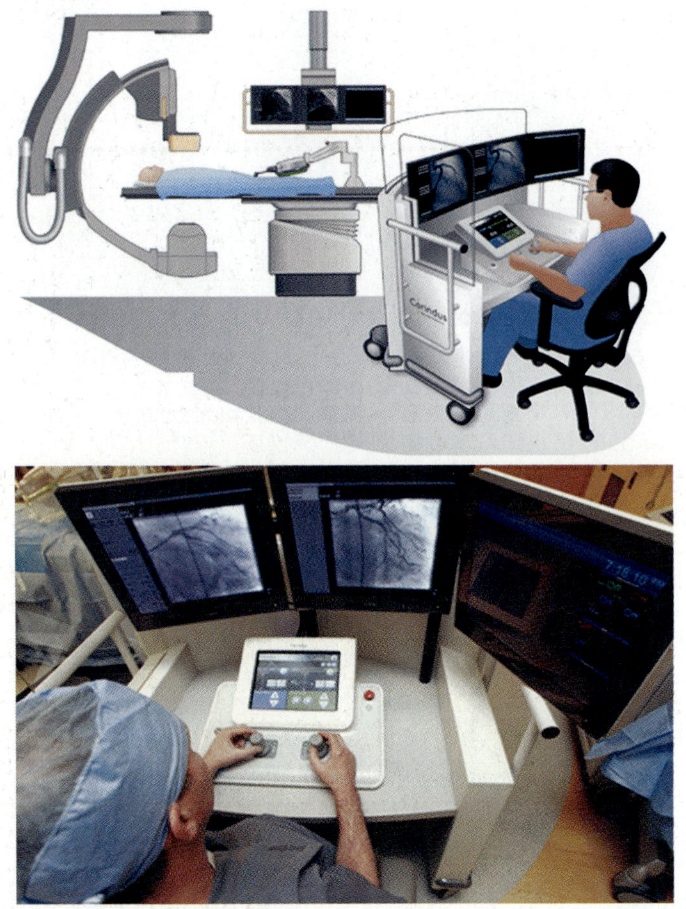

**Fig. 6.45:** Method of performing robot-assisted coronary angioplasty

In a pooled analysis of data from 3 prospective randomized trials, De Vita et al. found that although increasing time to treatment was associated with a decreased rate of optimal reperfusion in patients receiving standard PCI, this trend was not seen in patients treated with thrombus aspiration. De Vita et al. concluded that the use of thrombus aspiration limits the adverse effects that prolonged time to treatment has on myocardial reperfusion. The use of distal embolic protection during saphenous vein graft intervention has become the standard of care. The SAFER trial (saphenous vein graft angioplasty free of emboli randomized) initially proved the benefit of embolic protection in reducing 30-day rates of major adverse cardiac events (MACE) (9.6% *vs* 16.5%, P=0.004), myocardial infarction (8.6% *vs* 14.7%), and no reflow (3% *vs* 9%) (Figs 6.46–6.48).

### Stable Angina (PCI *vs* Medical Therapy)

Early trials demonstrated the benefit of percutaneous coronary intervention over medical therapy for symptomatic angina in single and multivessel coronary artery disease, with improvements in symptoms, reduction in need to take antianginal medications, improvement in exercise duration, and similar survival rates to medical therapy.

The randomized intervention in the treatment of angina (RITA-II) study demonstrated that balloon angioplasty results in better control of ischemic symptoms and greater improvement in exercise capacity than does medical therapy, but balloon angioplasty is associated with an increased incidence of the combined endpoint of death and myocardial infarction.

In RITA-II, in which 1018 patients with stable angina were randomized to balloon angioplasty or medical therapy, death or definite myocardial infarction occurred in 6.3% of the balloon angioplasty patients and in 3.3% of the medical patients; only 44% of the deaths were actually due to heart disease. Angina improved in both groups, but a 16.5% absolute excess of grade 2 or worse angina occurred in the medical group 3 months following randomization.

In the RITA-II study, 23% of the medical group required revascularization during follow-up. During follow-up, 7.9% of the angioplasty patients required bypass surgery,

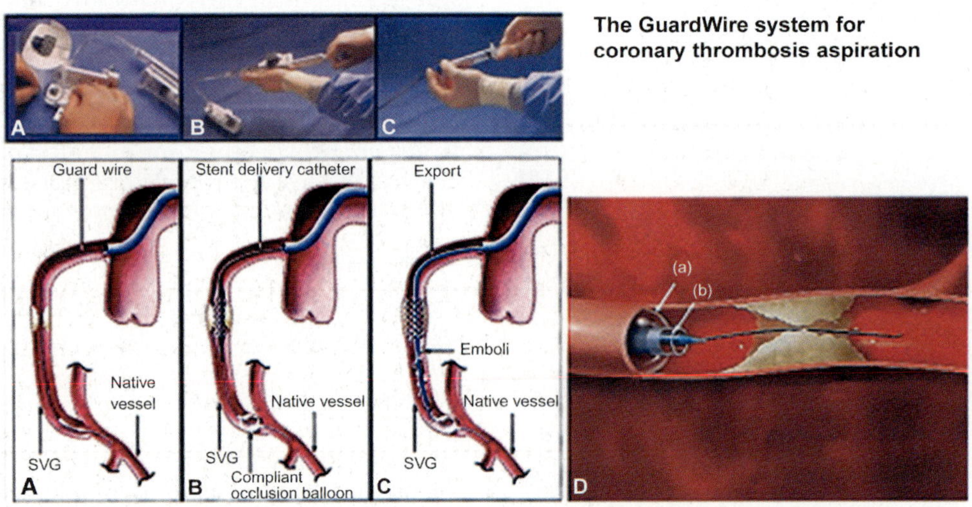


**Fig. 6.46:** The GuardWire system. Upper panel corresponds to lower panel—the GuardWire, used to cross the lesion, is inserted into the microseal adapter (A), connected to the EZ flator, which is inflated to occlude the vessel (B), debris is aspirated using the export aspiration catheter (C), SVG=saphenous vein graft (D). The Proxis system is delivered through a guiding catheter, and the sealing balloon (a) is inflated proximal to the stenosis, arresting flow, and debris aspirated through the Proxis system (b)

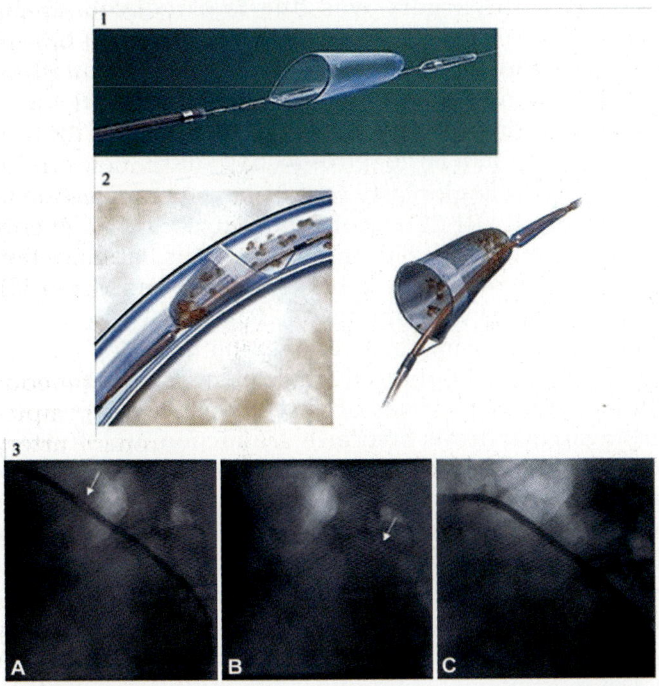


Fig. 6.47: The Filterwire system (Panel 1). The polyurethane porous membrane filter attached to a nitinol loop (Panel 2). The filter is deployed distal to the lesion, and the nitinol loop self-expands to fit the vessel upon retraction of the delivery sheath (Panel 3). (A) Saphenous vein graft containing thrombus, seen as intraluminal filling defect, (B) treated with percutaneous coronary intervention using filterwire protection, (C) achieving a good result after stenting

compared with 5.8% of the medically treated patients. Although the patients in RITA-II were asymptomatic or mildly symptomatic, it is important to emphasize that most had severe anatomic coronary artery disease; 62% had multivessel coronary artery disease, and 34% had important disease of the proximal left anterior descending artery.

In the atorvastatin versus revascularization treatment (AVERT) trial, after 18 months of follow-up, 13% of the medically treated group had ischemic events, compared with 21% of the angioplasty group, suggesting that in low-risk patients with stable coronary artery disease, aggressive lipid-lowering therapy may be as effective as balloon angioplasty in reducing ischemic events. In the study, 341 patients with stable coronary artery disease symptoms, normal left ventricle (LV) function, and class I or II angina were assigned randomly to balloon angioplasty or medical therapy with atorvastatin.

Based on the limited data available from randomized trials comparing medical therapy with balloon angioplasty, considering medical therapy seems prudent for the initial management of most patients with Canadian Cardiovascular Society Classification Class I and II symptoms, and reserving percutaneous or surgical revascularization is appropriate for patients with more severe symptoms and ischemia.

The clinical outcomes utilizing revascularization and aggressive drug evaluation (COURAGE) trial demons-

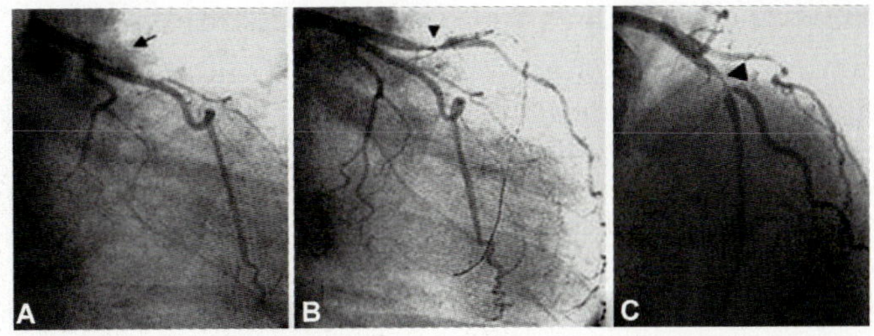


Fig. 6.48: Coronary angiogram in acute anterior myocardial infarction. The basal angiogram (A) shows total occlusion of the left anterior descending artery (LAD) with thrombus image bulging into the left main artery (arrow). After thrombus removal (B and C), the culprit lesion (arrowheads) is observed in the mid-LAD more than 20 mm distal to the original occlusion site

trated that in patients with stable angina symptoms and coronary artery stenosis, medical therapy alone may be an appropriate strategy if medical therapy can control the angina symptoms. The trial randomized the addition of percutaneous coronary intervention to intensive pharmacological therapy, with the endpoints of death from any cause and nonfatal myocardial infarction during a median follow-up period of 4.6 years. Inclusion criteria for the study included patients with a 70% or greater lesion in onr or more proximal epicardial arteries, AHA/ACC Class I or II indications for PCI, and objective evidence of myocardial ischemia on stress testing. Both primary endpoints demonstrated no statistical benefit between those patients who received PCI with medical therapy and those who received only medical therapy (19.0% *vs* 18.5%).

Teo et al. found that in older patients with stable coronary artery disease, optimal medical treatment without percutaneous coronary intervention remains an appropriate initial management strategy. Analysis of 904 patients aged 65 years or older showed that, during a median 4.6 year follow-up, clinical outcome in patients randomized to optimal medical treatment plus PCI was no better or worse than in patients who received optimal medical treatment alone. Compared with 1381 patients younger than 65 years with coronary artery disease, older patients had similar success in achieving treatment targets and similar rates of myocardial infarction, stroke, and major cardiac events, although the death rate was 2- to 3-fold higher in the older patients.

This analysis was done from patients enrolled in the COURAGE trial, and thus the limitations of that study have to be kept in mind, including the following:

- All patients had angiography prior to enrollment
- Only 1 in 12 patients who were screened were actually enrolled
- At the time of enrollment, most patients were either asymptomatic or had minimal symptoms overall, medical therapy is recommended as first-line therapy in patients with stable angina unless the following occur: a change in symptom severity, failed medical therapy, high-risk coronary anatomy, or worsening LV dysfunction, which provide an indication for cardiac catheterization and PCI of coronary artery bypass graft.

### Stable Angina (PCI *vs* Surgical Revascularization)

Two prospective clinical trials have evaluated balloon angioplasty versus surgery for revascularization of isolated left anterior descending coronary artery disease. Using a combined endpoint (cardiac death, myocardial infarction, or refractory angina requiring revascularization by surgery), the medicine, angioplasty, or surgery study (MASS) showed, after 3 years of follow-up, that endpoint events occurred in 24% of angioplasty patients, 17% of medical patients, and 3% of surgical patients. However, overall survival rates between the 3 groups were similar.

The other trial compared balloon angioplasty and bypass surgery with an internal mammary artery graft to the LAD artery and also showed no difference in survival during follow-up. Although 94% of the angioplasty patients and 95% of the bypass patients were free of limiting symptoms, those treated by angioplasty required more antianginal drugs. At median follow-up of 2.5 years, 86% of the surgery patients were free from late events, compared with 43% of angioplasty patients. This difference was primarily due to restenosis requiring a second revascularization procedure. Emphasizing that balloon angioplasty, rather than stent placement, was used in these trials is important; thus, current rates of restenosis with stenting should be lower.

Five large (>300 patients) randomized trials comparing balloon angioplasty with bypass surgery in patients with multivessel coronary artery disease all showed that in appropriately selected patients, the incidence rates of death or of myocardial infarction were similar regardless of whether balloon angioplasty or bypass surgery was used. However, more patients treated with angioplasty required a second revascularization procedure.

In the bypass angioplasty revascularization investigation (BARI), 5-year survival was 86.3% for those assigned to angioplasty versus 89.3% for those assigned to surgery, and 5-year freedom from Q-wave myocardial infarction was 78.7% and 80.4%, respectively. However, after 5 years of follow-up, 54% of those assigned to angioplasty required an additional revascularization procedure, compared with only 8% of those assigned to surgery.

In a similar manner, the 3-year follow-up of the argentine randomized trial of percutaneous transluminal coronary angioplasty versus coronary artery bypass surgery in multivessel disease (ERACI) showed that freedom from combined cardiac events was significantly better for bypass surgery (77% *vs* 47%) than for angioplasty. However, no differences occurred in overall and cardiac mortality rates or in the frequency of myocardial infarction between the 2 groups. Patients who had bypass surgery were free of angina more frequently (79% *vs* 57%) and had fewer additional revascularization procedures (6% *vs* 37%) than patients treated with angioplasty.

Patients with diabetes mellitus are an exception regarding equivalent mortality rate results of balloon angioplasty and bypass surgery in multivessel disease. Among diabetic patients in the BARI trial, 5-year survival was 65.5% in those treated by balloon angioplasty and 80.6% for those having bypass surgery. The improved survival with surgery was due to a reduced cardiac mortality rate (5.8% *vs* 20.6%) and was confined to those receiving at least 1 internal mammary artery graft. Better survival among diabetic patients with multivessel disease treated with bypass surgery rather than angioplasty also was observed in a large retrospective study.

The bypass angioplasty revascularization investigation 2 diabetes (BARI 2D) trial randomized 2364 men and women with type 2 diabetes mellitus, documented coronary artery disease, stable symptoms, and myocardial ischemia treated with optimal medical therapy to an initial strategy of coronary revascularization (REV) or watchful waiting with the option of subsequent revascularization (MED). At 5 years, rates of survival or the composite of cardiovascular death, myocardial infarction, and stroke did not differ significantly between the groups. A substudy of the BARI 2D trial reports that the REV strategy improved outcomes at the 3-year follow-up, with patients experiencing a lower rate of worsening angina, new angina, and subsequent coronary revascularizations, and a higher rate of angina-free status.

Long-term mortality rates are similar after CABG and PCI in most patient subgroups with multivessel coronary artery disease; therefore, the choice of treatment should depend on patient preferences for other outcomes. In a collaborative analysis of individual patient data from 10 randomized trials, Hlatky and colleagues found CABG to be a superior option for patients with diabetes and patients aged 65 years or older because mortality was lower in these subgroups.

### Bare Metal Stents and Coronary Artery Bypass Grafting

The major limitations of balloon angioplasty have been acute vessel closure and restenosis. Early studies with intracoronary stents showed that these devices were highly effective for treating or preventing acute or threatened vessel closure and, thus, avoiding emergency bypass surgery. Two randomized trials, STRESS and BENESTENT, demonstrated that coronary stenting of de novo lesions in native vessels reduced angiographic restenosis by approximately 30%, compared with conventional balloon angioplasty. Stenting produces a larger lumen diameter than conventional balloon angioplasty immediately following the procedure (acute gain) and at follow-up (net gain), resulting in less restenosis.

The use of stenting, instead of balloon angioplasty, was compared with bypass surgery for the treatment of multivessel coronary artery disease in the arterial revascularization therapies study (ARTS), and after 1 year of follow-up, no difference was noted between the groups in the rate of death, stroke, or myocardial infarction. Event-free survival was better in the surgery group than in the stent group (87.8% *vs* 73.8%), and only 3.5% in the surgery group required a second revascularization procedure, versus 16.8% in the stent group.

In the ERACI and BARI trials, 37% and 54%, respectively, needed a second revascularization when treated by balloon angioplasty. Overall, patients with diabetes and those who received incomplete surgical revascularization did worse. The cost of the initial revascularization procedure was $4212 less for those treated by stent placement, but because of the need for more repeat revascularization procedures in the stent group, the cost advantage for stenting was reduced to $2973 after 1 year.

The stent or surgery (SoS) trial compared base metal stents (BMS) with CABG in similar patients and reported a 21% 2 year target vessel revascularization rate in stent patients, versus 6% in CABG patients, with similar death and myocardial infarction rates in the 2 groups. However, the SoS trial had a higher noncardiac death rate in the PCI arm, thought to be attributed to a type II error that may have affected the study results. Few stent patients in the SoS trial received glycoprotein (GP) IIb/IIIa receptor inhibitors. Still, this and the ARTS study do point to the safety of PCI treatment in multivessel disease. Mortality risk is low (discounting the noncardiac deaths), and the rates for repeat target vessel revascularization have been halved.

### Drug-eluting Stents and Coronary Artery Bypass Grafting

Sirolimus-eluting stents were associated with an 8% MACE rate (13% for CABG in ARTS I) and an 8.5% target vessel revascularization rate (4% for CABG and 21% for PTCA in ARTS I), according to the ARTS II trial. The use of drug-eluting stents was compared with CABG in stable angina populations in the ARTS II trial, which was a registry comparing sirolimus-eluting stent (Cypher) with the PTCA and CABG arms of the ARTS I trial. The 1-year MACE rate was 10.5% for sirolimus-eluting stent patients.

The New York Cardiac Registry, as previously reported with data from bare metal stents, also found that patients who underwent PCI had a higher rate of target vessel revascularization than those who underwent CABG (30.6% *vs* 5.2%). They analyzed 17,400 patients who either received a drug-eluting stent (9,963) or CABG (7,437) and observed them for 18 months. Unadjusted survival curves did not demonstrate a statistical significance in survival for 2- or 3-vessel disease. However, when adjusted for several factors (age; sex; ejection fraction; hemodynamic state; history or no history of myocardial infarction before the procedure; the presence or absence of cerebrovascular disease, peripheral arterial disease, congestive heart failure, chronic obstructive pulmonary disease, diabetes, and renal failure; and involvement of the proximal LAD artery), there was statistically significant 18-month survival benefit of CABG over PCI with drug-eluting stents.

The SYNTAX study assessed differences in quality of life and angina score in 1,800 patients undergoing bypass surgery or PCI. Patients with 3-vessel or left main coronary artery disease were randomized to CABG or PCI with paclitaxel-eluting stents. Quality of life and angina scores were improved in both groups at 6 and 12 months. Angina score improved more in the CABG group, but the between-group differences were small.

The ongoing FREEDOM trial will compare drug-eluting stents and CABG in patients with diabetes and multivessel coronary artery disease.

### Acute Coronary Syndromes (Unstable Angina and NSTEMI)

The management of patients with non–Q-wave myocardial infarction and unstable angina has changed considerably over the past 5 years. Before the widespread use of stents and GP IIb/IIIa receptor inhibitors, conventional balloon angioplasty in this subgroup of patients was associated with substantial risks, including myocardial infarction (as much as 9%), restenosis (as much as 50%), need for emergency coronary bypass surgery (as much as 12%), and death (as much as 5%). The optimal strategy in patients presenting with acute coronary syndromes remains a controversial issue in contemporary cardiology. Several studies have investigated the use of a conservative strategy versus an early invasive strategy of revascularization for patients with unstable coronary syndromes.

To better assess the natural history of coronary artery disease, 697 patients with an acute coronary syndrome treated with PCI were evaluated at the time of the procedure with multivessel intravascular ultrasonography (grey scale and radiofrequency) in the PROSPECT study. The major findings included the following: In patients with ACS treated with PCI, adverse events during a median follow-up of 3.4 years were divided evenly between recurrence at the site of culprit lesions and to nonculprit lesions. Intravascular ultrasonography predictors of nonculprit lesions that will progress include a large plaque burden, small luminal area, and thin-cap fibroatheroma.

The veterans affairs non-Q-wave infarction strategies in hospital (VANQWISH) trial compared an invasive strategy with conservative medical treatment in patients with non-Q-wave myocardial infarction and found that the rates of death or nonfatal myocardial infarction were higher in the invasive strategy group than in the conservative strategy group before hospital discharge, at 1 month, and at 1 year. Criticisms of this study include the exclusion of patients at very high risk; the lack of current aggressive medical therapies; a high rate of crossover to angiography in the conservative arm; a higher surgical mortality rate than expected compared with contemporary standards; and the observation that most of the complications at 30 days occurred in patients who underwent coronary artery bypass surgery and very few occurred in patients who underwent balloon angioplasty.

In contrast to the VANQWISH trial, 3 randomized studies found that an early invasive approach in patients with acute coronary syndromes was associated with improved outcomes.

The thrombolysis in myocardial infarction (TIMI) IIIb study showed less ischemia, shorter hospital stays, fewer readmissions, and fewer symptoms in patients treated by an early invasive approach.

The fragmin and fast revascularization during instability in coronary artery disease (FRISC) II trial prospectively randomized 2457 patients to an early invasive treatment versus a noninvasive treatment strategy and used intracoronary stenting; they found that at 6 months, the composite endpoint of death or myocardial infarction was higher in the noninvasive treatment group than in patients undergoing an early invasive approach to management. Additionally, symptoms of angina and hospital readmissions in the noninvasive arm were twice that observed using the invasive treatment strategy.

The randomized intervention in the treatment of angina (RITA-III) study reported improved outcomes with early invasive therapy in 1810 patients at 5 years of follow-up. There was a statistically significant difference for all-cause mortality (15.1% *vs* 12.1%) and cardiac death/myocardial infarction (15.9% *vs* 12.2%) when comparing an interventional strategy and conservative medical therapy.

Based on various results, the American Heart Association/American College of Cardiology (AHA/ACC) guidelines recommended that an early (within 48 h) invasive approach should be used to treat patients presenting with the following higher-risk features—PCI or CABG in the past 6 months, new ST-segment depression, elevated cardiac biomarkers, recurrent angina at rest or low level of activity, left ventricular systolic function of less than 40%, or TIMI score greater than 2. In lower-risk patients (TIMI score of $\leq$2), evidence has shown that invasive therapy and medical therapy provide similar outcomes.

### Acute Myocardial Infarction (STEMI)

The recognition that intracoronary thrombosis is the primary mechanism of vessel occlusion in acute myocardial infarction and that prompt restoration of vessel patency provides significant clinical benefit has led to the development of aggressive new treatments for this disorder.

Thrombolytic therapies, such as front-loaded tissue plasminogen activator (tPA), reteplase (r-PA), and tenecteplase (TNK), open approximately 80% of infarct-related vessels within 90 minutes, but only 50% will have normal (TIMI grade 3) flow. In addition, 10% of vessels opened by thrombolysis either reocclude or are the source for recurrent symptoms of angina. Because of these limitations to thrombolytic therapy, several randomized trials have evaluated mechanical revascularization, so-called primary angioplasty, in the setting of acute myocardial infarction.

An analysis of 23 trials confirms the superiority of primary angioplasty over fibrinolytic therapy in terms of adverse events and mortality reduction in both the short term and long term. Overall, primary PCI was associated with significant reductions in death, recurrent myocardial infarction, reinfarction, and the combined endpoint of death, myocardial infarction, and stroke.

In the situation where patients are transferred from outside hospitals, primary angioplasty is often preferred to onsite fibrinolytic therapy for patients with the following—expected door-to-balloon time less than 90 minutes and symptom duration less than 3 hours, symptom duration more than 3 hours, cardiogenic shock, contraindications to fibrinolytic therapy, and age older than 75 years. The use of thrombolytic therapy and then referral for intentional PCI (facilitated PCI) has not been shown to be superior to primary PCI and may actually worsen outcomes with increased risk of stroke and bleeding (ASSENT 4).

Recent data suggest that early use of GP IIb/IIIa inhibitors may help to achieve earlier infarct vessel patency and better outcomes during PCI. Whether this is so for all of these agents is being assessed in several studies. One meta-analysis has shown that abciximab is associated with a 46% reduction in death and reinfarction in primary PCI patients and the AHA/ACC STEMI guidelines currently recommend early use of abciximab in these patients. When fibrinolytic therapy is given but fails to produce ST resolution, then immediate PCI (rescue PCI) is recommended.

Some of the most important considerations in providing effective primary PCI relate to the logistical issues and barriers that are known to exist. The PCI system or network, ambiguity of leadership and organization, protocols/care, pathways/interfacility transfer, and reimbursement issues are the main areas of contention. Studies of the US primary PCI sites that are considered the best (those sites that deliver door-to-balloon times consistently within 90 minutes, which is currently about 5% of the US myocardial infarction population) have identified the key determinants of shorter door-to-balloon times as the following—ECG being performed within 10 minutes, the emergency department independently making the decision to engage the catheterization laboratory team, and interdisciplinary teamwork.

The key factor for effective primary PCI is timely reperfusion therapy. Studies from the National Registry of Myocardial Infarction (NRMI) data have shown that shortening door-to-balloon time to less than 90 minutes is associated with a reduction in mortality. In certain situations, timely reperfusion may be best achieved with fibrinolytic therapy if delays are likely in accessing primary PCI.

From a procedural perspective, because primary PCI involves a thrombotic plaque, the potential risk of more complications exists, especially no reflow and distal embolization. These patients should achieve final TIMI 3 flow. Stenting plus GP IIb/IIIa inhibition has been shown to improve outcomes, reducing target vessel revascularization and myocardial infarction rates in comparison with balloon angioplasty. The use of adjunctive antithrombotic approaches, including early GP IIb/IIIa inhibition use and mechanical thrombectomy, has shown benefit. Important issues remain as to which type of stent to use (drug-eluting or bare metal), and timing of antiplatelet therapy (both IV and oral) might provide better outcomes for certain patients.

Stone and colleagues studied the safety and efficacy of drug-eluting stents and bare-metal stents in patients with STEMI undergoing primary PCI. Patients ($n$=3006) were assigned in a 3:1 ratio to receive paclitaxel-eluting stents or otherwise identical bare-metal stents. Paclitaxel-eluting stents significantly reduced angiographic evidence of restenosis and recurrent ischemia necessitating repeat revascularization, compared with bare-metal stents, at 12-month follow-up. Rates of death and stent thrombosis were similar for the 2 groups.

### General Comparison of PCI and CABG

A 2007 research review by the Agency for Healthcare Research and Quality (AHRQ) examined 23 randomized controlled trials of PCI versus CABG (9963 patients) and found that short-term survival was high for both procedures and did not differ significantly. However, freedom from procedural stroke was significantly higher after PCI than after CABG.

In the AHRQ study, there was no significant difference in long-term survival (1–5 years of follow-up) between the 2 procedures. However, survival was significantly better after PCI in patients with single-vessel disease that did not involve the proximal LAD and was significantly better after CABG in patients with extensive triple-vessel or left main artery disease. Long-term freedom from angina was significantly greater after CABG than after PCI, as was the need for repeat coronary revascularization procedures. The use of coronary artery stents narrowed, but did not close, the gap between PCI and CABG in repeat revascularization procedures. Although PCI initially was less costly than CABG, the cost difference narrowed substantially over time, to roughly 5%.

## Optical Coherence Tomography

The technique is based on optical technology and commercially available fiberoptic components adapted for ophthalmic use (Figs 6.49–6.51). OCT is a noninvasive technique that does not utilize ionizing radiation to provide in vivo images. OCT has numerous potential clinical applications and, in effect, creates 'optical biopsies' of tissues. It has also been used in the detection, characterization and management of skin tumors and other dermatological diseases, cardiology, and intravascular disease. OCT may be able to contribute to early diagnosis of vulnerable atherosclerotic lesions. Noninvasive imaging modalities such as magnetic resonance and computerized tomography are currently under intense investigation. Catheter-based diagnostic techniques, however, can provide structural information with higher resolution than noninvasive methods. Intravascular magnetic resonance is being actively investigated for plaque detection and characterization. Intravascular ultrasound magnetic resonance is being actively investigated for plaque detection and characterization. Intravascular ultrasound is widely used in interventional cardiology. A recent publication suggests a correlation between the presence of echolucent zones in coronary plaques on IVUS images and acute coronary events. Preliminary angioscopic studies have suggested that the presence of yellow plaques with a glistening surface correlates with acute events. More quantitative approaches which measure molecular absorption overtones of lipid or the Raman shift of cholesterol, may provide unique signals from vessel walls to identify large lipid pools. Based on the hypothesis that local inflammation within vulnerable

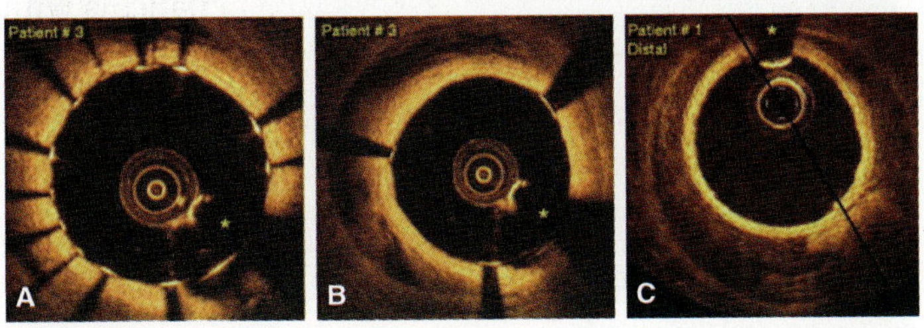


**Fig. 6.49:** OCT findings after coronary stenting. (A) Well-expanded and apposed stent. (B) Residual abluminal hematoma at the stented segment. (C) Residual intramural hematoma distal to the stented segment (*=shadow caused by the wire artifact)

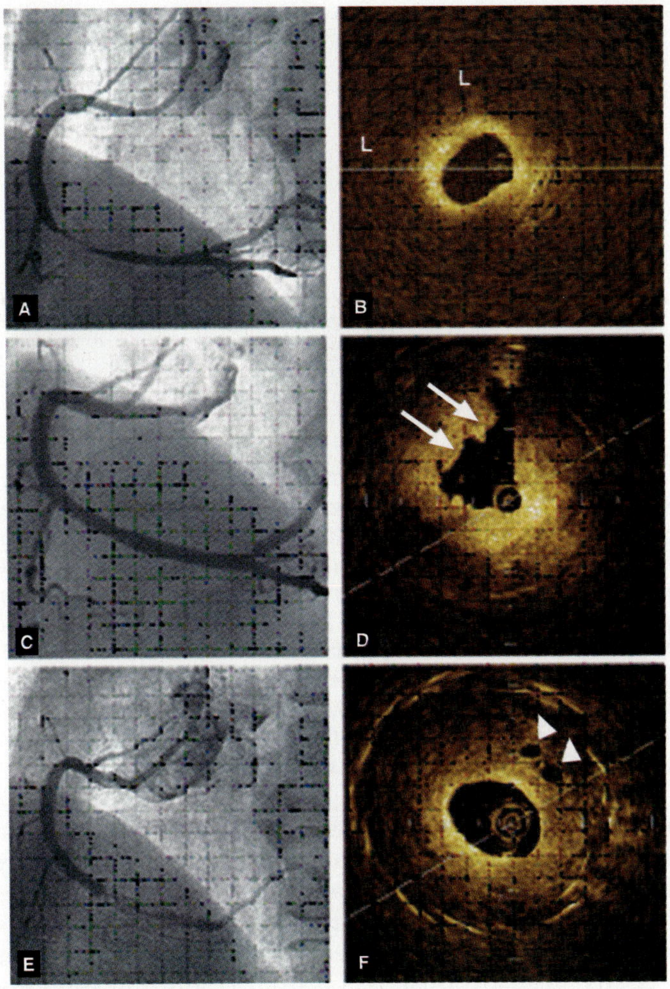


**Fig. 6.50:** Coronary angiography showed a 90%; stenosis in the mid-right coronary artery (A) and optical coherence tomography (OCT: Light Lab TM) was performed to assess plaque morphology. OCT revealed diffusely bordered signal poor region with overlying signal-rich band at the culprit site (L indicates lipid core in B). Two sirolimus-eluting stents (Cypher TM; 3.0 × 33 and 3.0 × 33 mm) were deployed in the culprit lesion and excellent angiographic results were obtained (C). The final intravascular ultrasound also demonstrated the well-expanded and apposed stents with no plaque protrusion. The patient was prescribed aspirin 100 mg and ticlopidin 200 mg orally daily for 1 year. 12 months follow-up coronary angiography showed a 99%; stenosis with contrast filling defect in the stents (Panel D). At this site, OCT revealed a low-backscattering projections irregular mass protruding into the lumen (white arrows in E) with some microchannels (white arrow heads in F). This finding may suggest that organized thrombus was the main component of restenotic tissue 12 months after sirolimus-eluting stent implantation

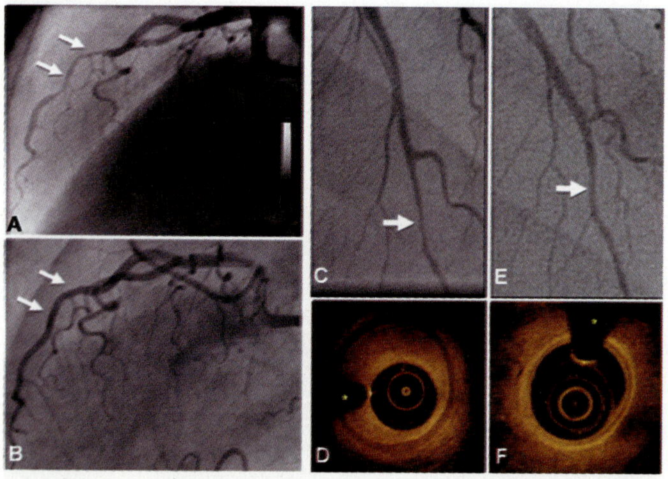


**Fig. 6.51:** Late spontaneous resolution of angiographic images corresponding to SCAD on OCT. (A) Diffuse, confined lesion in the mid-left anterior descending coronary artery (arrows) (note normal proximal and distal segments) with complete resolution at late angiographic follow-up (B). (C) Diffuse lesion (arrow) on the distal left anterior descending coronary artery where OCT revealed an intramural hematoma (D). (E) At late follow-up, the angiographic image significantly improved, and a normal vessel wall was demonstrated by OCT (F). *shadow caused by the wire artifact; SCAD=spontaneous coronary artery dissection

plaques may lead to local elevations in temperature, a temperature-sensing catheter has been used to study temperature heterogeneity and temperature differences between atherosclerotic plaque and healthy vessel walls Intravascular optical coherence tomography (OCT) has recently been proposed as a high-resolution imaging method for plaque characterization. Optical coherence tomography is an optical analog of ultrasound imaging because it measures the amplitude of backscattered light (optical echoes) returning from a sample as a function of delay. *In vitro* studies have shown that the resolution of OCT (10–20 µm) can resolve the thin fibrous caps thought to be responsible for plaque vulnerability. Additionally, the intrinsic optical properties of typical plaque constituents have provided sufficient contrast in these studies for OCT to differentiate between lipid, calcium and fibrous tissue. Recent experiments performed in vivo have demonstrated intravascular OCT imaging of normal rabbit aortas and swine coronary arteries. Here we present the first application, to our knowledge, of intracoronary OCT in living patients. The goals of this study were:

1. To demonstrate the feasibility and safety of OCT imaging in patients
2. To assess OCT images of human coronary pathology acquired in vivo by comparison with IVUS images obtained from corresponding locations

A catheter-based imaging technology called optical coherence tomography can successfully identify the characteristics of coronary plaques in patients with various cardiac symptoms. The ability to identify dangerous plaques before they rupture and produce a heart attack or sudden cardiac death will be crucial to innovative preventive therapies. Plaques are deposits of fats, cholesterol and other materials that collect in major arteries, restricting or sometimes blocking blood flow. While some plaques are relatively stable, others are vulnerable to rupture and release their contents into the bloodstream, causing a blood clot to form. Heart attacks and other acute coronary events usually result from the rupture of high-risk, vulnerable plaques in coronary arteries, and the characteristics of those plaques have been determined primarily by autopsy studies. OCT uses infrared light delivered via fiberoptic catheter to produce high-resolution, cross-sectional images of blood vessels. The OCT images showed that the heart attack and ACS patients had more lipid in their plaques and significantly thinner fibrous caps than did the stable angina patients. Overall, vulnerable plaques were identified in 72% of the heart attack patients, 50% of those with ACS and only 20% of stable angina patients. 'This is the first technique that allows to study the structural changes underlying vulnerable plaques in living patients, and it supports the conclusions of previously reported postmortem studies,' says Jang. We still need to gather more data to confirm these characteristics, and our group will carry out further studies of how plaques develop and rupture. Some day OCT may provide information that will guide treatments to prevent plaque rupture and its disastrous consequences.

## COMPLICATIONS ASSOCIATED WITH PCI

Early registries of balloon angioplasty results showed complication rates that were much higher than those typically observed today (Figs 6.52–6.59). With advancements in technique, devices, and adjuvant medical therapy, percutaneous transluminal coronary intervention is now associated with mortality and emergency bypass rates of less than 1%. The rate of nonfatal myocardial infarction following coronary angioplasty ranges from 5–15%, whereas the rate following stent placement is

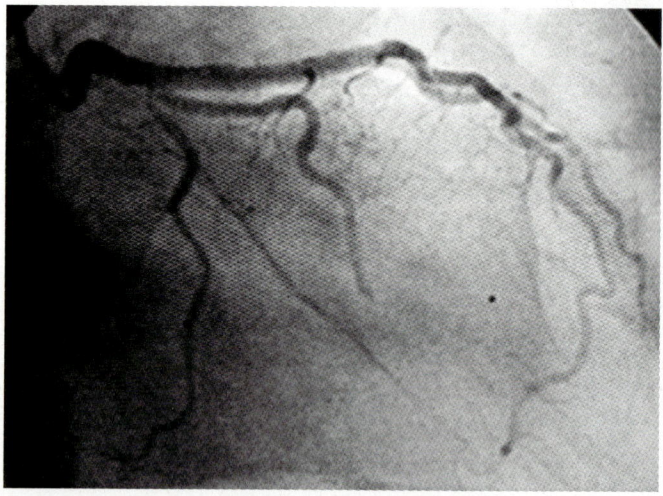

**Fig. 6.52:** One day after percutaneous transluminal coronary angioplasty with stenting, a follow-up coronary angiography revealed the patent stents of the left main coronary artery and proximal left anterior descending coronary artery with remaining thrombotic occlusion of the distal intermediate branch

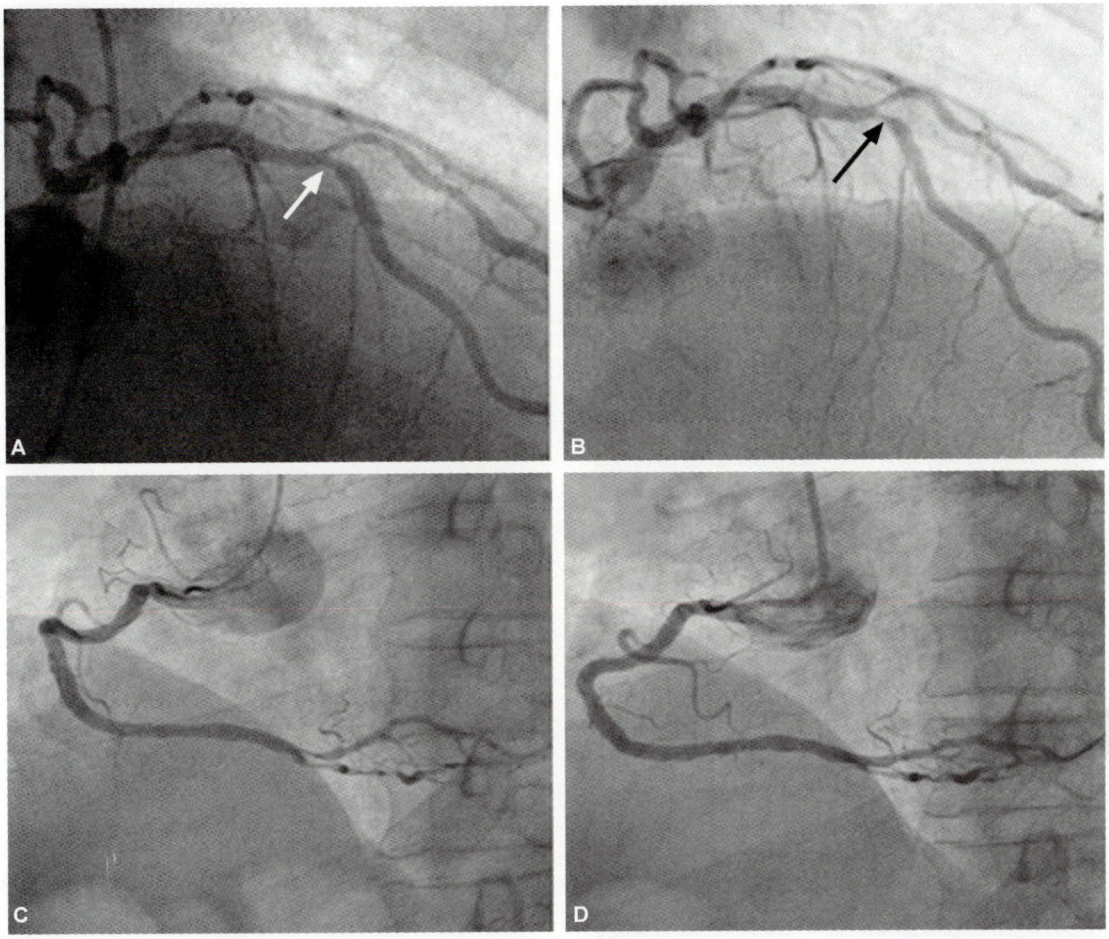


**Fig. 6.53:** (A and B) Follow-up coronary angiogram showed stent fracture with abundant movement and displacement of fractured fragment over 1 mm during cardiac cycle (type 4) was shown compared to previous coronary angiogram (A) 3 years ago, (B) severe stenosis at the fracture site. (C and D) After 2 years, his symptoms returned due to RCA obstruction, (C) he was then stented successfully (D)

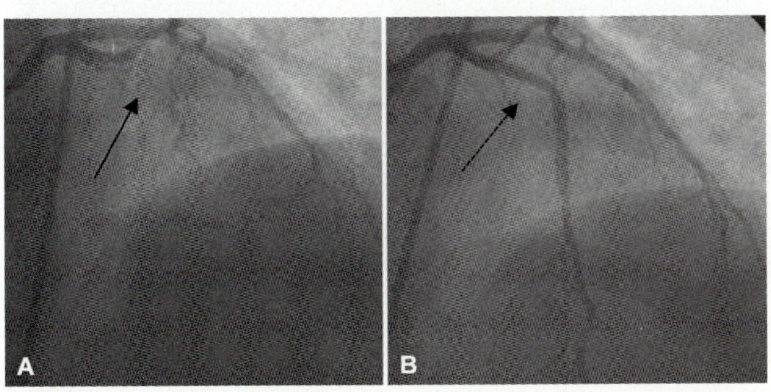


**Fig. 6.54:** Second findings of coronary angiogram. The second CAG showed total occlusion (dark arrow) in the previous stent-implanted area of the LAD (A) and restored lesion (dotted arrow) after successful PCI with ReoPro (abciximab) infusion (B). CAG= coronary angiography, LAD=left anterior descending artery, PCI= percutaneous coronary intervention

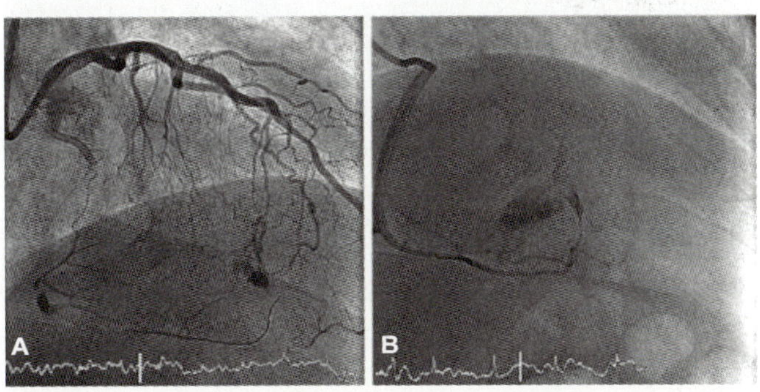


**Fig. 6.55:** (A) Passage of an angioplasty balloon has caused rupture of the septal branch used. (B) In the final angiography after the procedure, the right coronary artery is patent with several stents implanted in the region of the occlusion and a fistula from septal rupture to the right ventricle. This complication did not lead to hemodynamic deterioration and the patient was discharged 4 days later

2–5%. Restenosis after balloon angioplasty requiring a second revascularization procedure is a major limitation occurring in about 15–30% of patients, depending on the definition of restenosis applied. However, with drug-eluting stents, restenosis rates are now less than 10%.

Reduction in the complications of balloon angioplasty has been complemented by improvements in the acute success rate. Registries, such as the National Heart, Lung, and Blood Institute (NHLBI) Coronary Angioplasty

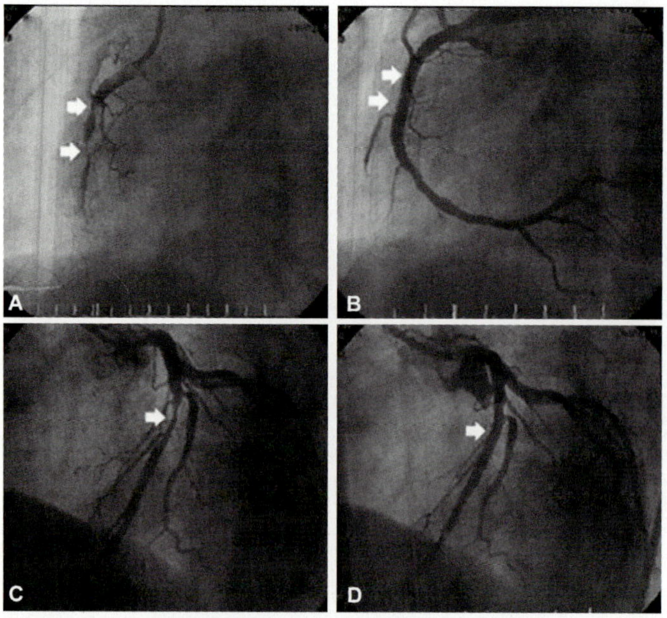


**Fig. 6.56:** Initial coronary angiography in September 2004. (A) Thrombotic near total occlusion of the mid-RCA (Type C, 99%, TIMI flow I), (B) 3.5 × 32 mm paclitaxel-eluting stent (Taxus Express[2], Boston Scientific Corporation) was deployed in RCA. (C) Critical stenosis in mid-LAD (Type B2, 90%, TIMI flow III). (D) 3.0 × 20 mm Taxus-eluting stent in the LAD. Final CAG showed good distal flow without residual stenosis

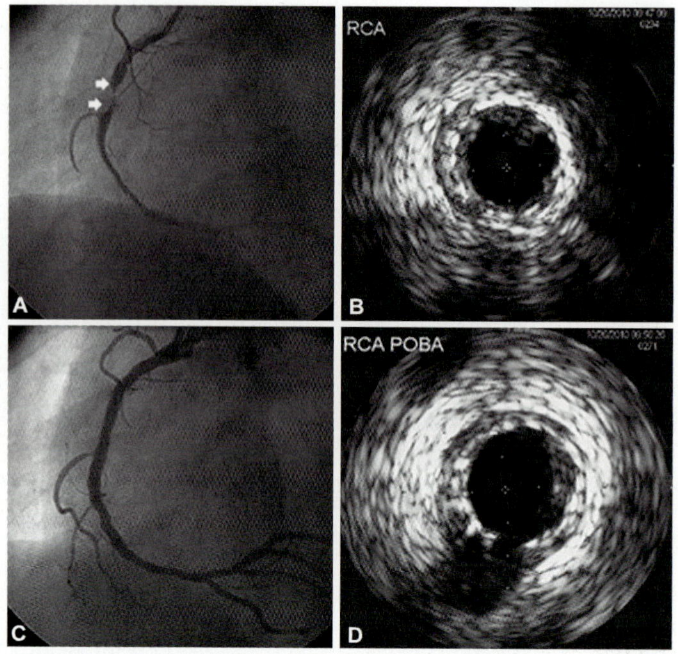


**Fig. 6.58:** (A) Right coronary angiogram showed very late stent thrombosis in RCA stent, (B) IVUS showed neointima breakdown and ruptured plaque within the RCA stent, (C) Coronary angiography after plain old balloon angioplasty (POBA). Final coronary angiogram showed good distal flow, and (D) IVUS showed markedly decreased residual stenosis

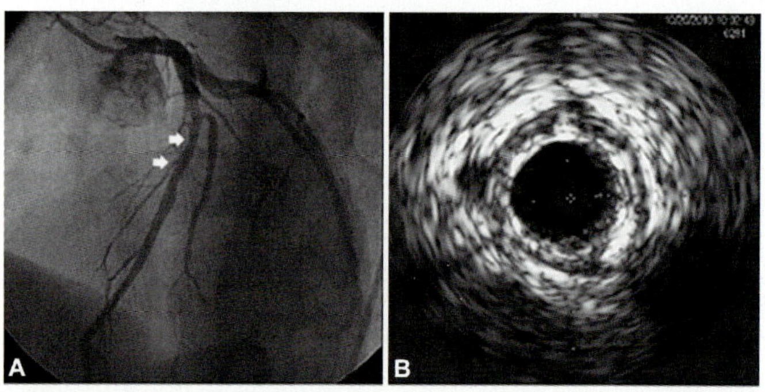


**Fig. 6.57:** (A) Left coronary angiography showed mild type II in-stent restenosis in LAD, (B) IVUS showed plaque in LAD stent

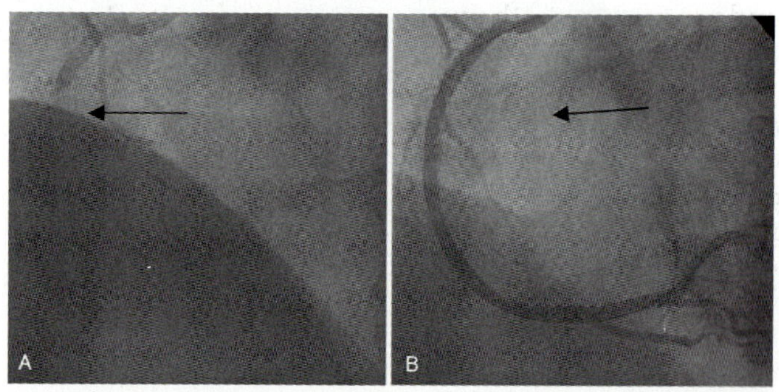


**Fig. 6.59:** The coronary angiogram. (A and B) CAG showed total occlusion (dark arrow) in the earlier stent-implanted lesion of the RCA and recanalized lesion (dotted arrow) after successful PCI. CAG=coronary angiography, RCA=right coronary artery, PCI=percutaneous coronary intervention

Registry from the early 1980s, reported primary success rates of 61%. Today, success rates are 95–99% with the use of stents and adjunctive pharmacotherapy.

The mechanism by which balloon angioplasty or stenting improves luminal diameter is associated with significant local trauma to the vessel wall, which can, in turn, lead to occlusive complications in a minority of patients. Coronary artery dissection typically results from the vessel injury secondary to balloon expansion. Animal and postmortem studies have shown that localized dissection at the site of balloon expansion is a common occurrence, detected angiographically in as many as 50% of patients immediately following the procedure. Such small dissections probably are necessary to obtain adequate lumen expansion, rarely interfere with antegrade blood flow, or are important. Angiographic follow-up typically shows no residual evidence of a dissection as early as 6 weeks after angioplasty in most of the cases studied. However, larger dissections can lead to complications.

### Abrupt Vessel Closure

It may occur in as many as 5% of balloon angioplasty cases and typically develops when there is compression of the true lumen by a large dissection flap, thrombus formation, superimposed coronary vasospasm, or a combination of these processes. The presence of large coronary dissections immediately after balloon angioplasty is associated with a 5-fold increase in the risk of abrupt closure. This underscores the importance of a good postprocedure angiographic result on clinical outcomes.

Since the introduction and use of intracoronary stents and newer antiplatelet drugs, the incidence of abrupt closure has significantly decreased (to <1%). Microembolization of plaque debris or adherent thrombus may also cause acute complications during angioplasty and may contribute to postprocedure cardiac enzyme elevation and chest pain in some patients.

In less than 1% of patients undergoing angioplasty, microembolization of the platelet-rich thrombus may cause diffuse distal arteriolar vasospasm secondary to the release of vasoactive agents, resulting in the phenomenon of no-reflow. This complication is difficult to treat but may respond to intracoronary calcium channel antagonists, adenosine, or nitroprusside. Patients undergoing balloon angioplasty of saphenous vein graft lesions and primary angioplasty in the setting of acute myocardial infarction with a large amount of adherent thrombus are at greatest risk of distal embolization.

*Coronary perforation or rupture following balloon angioplasty:* It is very rare (<1%) and is typically associated with the use of ablative devices or oversized balloons.

### Restenosis

Following balloon angioplasty or stent implantation, the vessel wall undergoes a number of changes. Platelets and fibrin adhere to the site within minutes of vessel injury. Within hours to days, inflammatory cells infiltrate the site and vascular smooth muscle cells begin to migrate toward the lumen.

The vascular smooth muscle cells then hypertrophy and excrete an extensive extracellular matrix. During this period of vascular smooth muscle cell proliferation, endothelial cells colonize the surface of the lumen and regain their normal function. Over the course of several weeks to months, multiple forces interact to cause remodeling of the vessel wall with either a decrease in lumen diameter (negative remodeling) or an increase in lumen diameter (positive remodeling). The amount of late loss in lumen diameter is dependent on the amount of neointimal proliferation and the degree of remodeling following intervention. After 6 months, the repair process stabilizes and the risk of restenosis decreases significantly.

*Mechanism of restenosis following percutaneous transluminal coronary angioplasty (PTCA):* Several studies have shown that the lumen diameter or area after treatment is one of the major predictors of restenosis. The use of coronary artery stents has decreased the rate of restenosis by improving the acute gain achieved and by minimizing negative remodeling. Depending on the definition used, angiographic restenosis has been reported in as many as 50% of patients within 6 months after balloon angioplasty, necessitating repeat target vessel revascularization (TVR) in approximately 20–30% of patients. Drug-eluting stents have reduced restenosis rates to less than 10%. Poststent lumen diameter and lesion complexity are still the major predictors of restenosis with these newer stents.

### Stent Thrombosis

While drug-eluting stents have significantly reduced restenosis events, concerns of stent thrombosis with these newer stents still exist. In fact, the rate of thrombosis with a drug-eluting stent is virtually identical to that for a bare metal stent at 1 year (0.5–0.7%). However, late stent thrombosis (>1 year) continues to occur with a drug-eluting stent, while it is exceedingly rare for a bare metal stent.

The biggest factor contributing to stent thrombosis is interruption of antiplatelet therapy. Current guidelines recommend a minimum of 1 year of dual antiplatelet therapy for drug-eluting stents and a month for bare metal stents. Drug-eluting stents take longer to endothelialize on the coronary vessel wall than bare metal stents, and discontinuing dual antiplatelet therapy may expose patients to an increased risk for stent thrombosis over time. In some clinical situations (such as before urgent noncardiac surgery where antiplatelet therapy may have to be discontinued and in patients with known or potential medicine compliance issues), implanting a bare metal stent may be preferred during PCI rather than using a drug-eluting stent. Another important factor is final stent diameter and area.

Underdeployment or incomplete apposition of the drug-eluting stent may also increase the risk for stent thrombosis. This is not to say that drug-eluting stents are unsafe. In fact, there is no difference in long-term rates of death and myocardial infarction between drug-eluting and bare metal stents; however, there is a striking reduction in restenosis. Stone and colleagues found that although stent thrombosis is infrequent, it results in higher rates of myocardial infarction and death. The more frequent target lesion revascularization results in a lower rate of myocardial infarction and death. Although late stent thrombosis is a risk with drug-eluting stents, the noticeable reduction in restenosis may offset the risk.

#### KEY POINTS

- Permanent intracoronary scents have demonstrated considerable efficacy in the treatment of PTCA-induced abrupt arterial occlusion, suboptimal dilatation, and restenosis. Despite their benefit, permanent stents have significant limitations including subacute thrombosis, need for anticoagulation with resultant vascular complications, prolonged hospitalization, and high costs.
- Temporary stem's have the potential for achieving many of the beneficial effects of permanent stenting without some of the iatrogenic complications.
- The heat activated removable temporary stent (HARTS) removable stent employs the shape memory alloy Nitinol, and has the properties of being balloon deployable, but recoverable to a preset 'memory' shape by heating it with warmed crystalloid solution.
- Preclinical experience first with a wire stent design and more recently with a slotted tubular design, has demonstrated the

*Contd...*

*Contd...*

feasibility of implanting and recovering the HARTS device. Speculative applications of this technology include treatment of acute postangioplasty occlusion and suboptimal angioplasty results; 'stentoplasty'—the application of a temporary stent for several hours at the time of a primary angioplasty; and reduction of restenosis rate by inhibition of elastic recoil following short-term (hours) stenting. Further, the HARTS device may be an important vehicle for local delivery of drugs or other biologically active agents to the arterial wall. All research to date has been preclinical and controlled clinical trials will be necessary to define the safety, efficacy, and potential applications of the HARTS removable stent.

- New generation of DES, dedicated bifurcation stents, and improvement of procedural techniques will probably improve the clinical outcome.
- The new antiplatelet agents (prasugrel and ticagrelor) could improve the safety of PCI in complex LM lesions, but they need to be evaluated in this particular setting.
- The future EXCEL trial (evaluation of Xience Prime or Xience V-eluting stent *vs* CABG for effectiveness of LM revascularization) will evaluate the safety and efficacy of PCI with Xience Prime or Xience V EES *vs* CABG in patients with ULMCA disease with a low or intermediate SYNTAX score (<33). The composite measure of all-cause mortality, MI, or stroke at an anticipated median follow-up duration of 3 years will be the primary endpoint. The need for repeat revascularization will be considered as a secondary endpoint. The results of the trial might impact the current guidelines.

## BIBLIOGRAPHY


1. Argenziano M, Katz M, Bonatti J, et al. Results of the prospective multicenter trial of robotically assisted totally endoscopic coronary artery bypass grafting Ann Thorac Surg 2006;81:1666–74, discussion: 1674–75.
2. Barlis P, Schmitt JM. Current and future developments in intracoronary optical coherence tomography imaging. Euro Intervention 2009;4:529–33.
3. Beyar R, Gruberg L, Delleanu D, et al. Remote-control percutaneous coronary interventions. Concept, validation, and first-in-humans clinical trial. J Am Coll Cardiol 2006; 47: 296–300.
4. Beyar R, Wenderow T, Lindner D, et al. Concept, design and pre-clinical studies for remote control percutaneous coronary interventions EuroIntervention 2005;1:340–345.
5. Boden WE, O'Rourke RA, et al. Optimal medical therapy with or without PCI for stable coronary disease. N Engl J Med 2007;356(15):1503–16.
6. Camenzind E, Steg PG, Wijns W. Stent thrombosis late after implantation of first-generation drug-eluting stents: a cause for concern. Circulation 2007;115:1440–55, discussion: 55.
7. Di Biase L, Wang Y, Horton R, et al. Ablation of atrial fibrillation utilizing robotic catheter navigation in comparison to manual navigation and ablation: single-center experience J Cardiovasc Electrophysiol 2009;20:1328–35.
8. Dotter CT, Judkins MP. Transluminal treatment of arteriosclerotic obstruction. Circulation 1964;30(5):654–70.
9. Duran AD, Duran GD, Ramirez RR, et al. Cataracts in interventional cardiology personnel. Retrospective evaluation study of lens injuries and dose (RELID Study). Eur Heart J 2009;30:872.
10. European Society of Cardiology Science News, 2007 Thrombosis is the price for the success of drug-eluting stents
11. Gruntzig AR, Senning A, Siegenthaler WE. Nonoperative dilatation of coronary-artery stenosis: percutaneous transluminal coronary angioplasty. N Engl J Med 1979;301:61–8.
12. Guagliumi G, Sirbu V, Costa M, et al. Long-term Strut Coverage of Paclitaxel Eluting Stents Compared to Bare-Metal Stents Implanted During Primary PCI in Acute Myocardial Infarction. A Prospective, Randomized, Controlled Study Performed with Optical Coherence Tomo-graphy. HORIZONS-OCT. Paper presented at: Late Breaking Trials, American Heart Association Annual Meeting, November 15, 2008; New Orleans, LA.
13. Guagliumi G, Sirbu V. Optical coherence tomography: high resolution intravascular imaging to evaluate vascular healing after coronary stenting. Catheter Cardiovasc Interv 2008;72: 237–47.
14. Hannan EL, Wu C, Walford G, et al. Drug-eluting stents vs coronary-artery bypass grafting in multivessel coronary disease. N Engl J Med 2008;358(4):331–41.
15. Hoffmann R, Mintz GS, Dussaillant GR, Popma JJ, et al. Patterns and mechanisms of in-stent restenosis. A serial intravascular ultrasound study. Circulation 1996;94:1247–54.
16. Joner M, Finn AV, Farb A, Mont EK, Kolodgie FD, et al. Pathology of drug-eluting stents in humans: delayed healing and late thrombotic risk. J Am Coll Cardiol 2006;48:193–202.
17. Kedhi E, Joesoef KS, McFadden E, t al. Second-generation everolimus-eluting and paclitaxel-eluting stents in real-life practice (COMPARE): a randomised trial. Lancet 2010;375: 201–9.
18. Kline LW, Miller DL, Balter S, et al. Occupational hazards in the interventional laboratory: time for a safer environment Catheter Cardiovasc Interv 2009;73:432–8.
19. Kolata, Gina. New Heart Studies Question the Value Of Opening Arteries. The New York Times, March 21, 2004. Retrieved January 29, 2011.
20. Kubo T, Imanishi T, Kitabata H. Comparison of vascular response after sirolimus-eluting stent implantation between patients with unstable and stable angina pectoris: a serial optical coherence tomography study. J Am Coll Cardiol Img. 2008;1:475–84.
21. Marescaux J, Leroy J, Gagner M, et al. Transatlantic robot-assisted telesurgery Nature 2001;413:379–80.
22. Mauri L, Hsieh WH, Massaro JM, et al. Stent thrombosis in randomized clinical trials of drug-eluting stents. The New England Journal of Medicine 2007;356(10):1020–9.
23. Meier B, Bachmann D, Lüscher T. 25 years of coronary angioplasty: almost a fairy tale. Lancet 2003;361(9356):527.
24. Mercado, N, Flather, MD, Boersna, E, et al. On Behalf of the Trial Investigators CABG vs Stenting for Multivessel Disease: a Meta-analysis of ARTS-1, SoS, ERACI-2, and MASS-2, Presentation at European Society of Cardiology Congress 2003;(23): 2093–8.
25. Michaels AD, Chatterjee K. Cardiology patient pages. Angioplasty versus bypass surgery for coronary artery disease. Circulation 2002;106(23):e187–90.

26. Morice MC, Serruys PW, Sousa JE, et al. A randomized comparison of a sirolimuseluting stent with a standard stent for coronary revascularization. N Engl J Med 2002;346: 1773–80.
27. Nordmann AJ, Briel M, Bucher HC. Mortality in randomized controlled trials comparing drug-eluting vs. bare metal stents in coronary artery disease: a meta-analysis. Eur Heart J 2006;27:2784–814.
28. Rasmussen K, Maeng M, Kaltoft A, et al. Efficacy and safety of zotarolimus-eluting and sirolimus-eluting coronary stents in routine clinical care (SORT OUT III): a randomised controlled superiority trial. Lancet 2010;375:1090–9.
29. Schaar JA, Muller JE, Falk E. Terminology for high-risk and vulnerable coronary artery plaques. Report of a meeting on the vulnerable plaque, June 17 and 18, 2003, Santorini, Greece. Eur Heart J 2004;25:1077–82.
30. Serruys PW, De Jaegere P, Kiemeneij F, Macaya C, et al. A comparison of balloon-expandable-stent implantation with balloon angioplasty in patients with coronary artery disease. Benestent Study Group. N Engl J Med 1994;331:489–95.
31. Serruys PW, Ormiston JA, Onuma Y. A bioabsorbable everolimus-eluting coronary stent system (ABSORB): 2-year out-comes and results from multiple imaging methods. Lancet. 373;2009:897–910.
32. Sigwart U, Puel J, Mirkovitch V, Joffre F, Kappenberger L. Intravascular stents to prevent occlusion and restenosis after transluminal angioplasty. N Engl J Med 1987;316:701–6.
33. Sigwart U, Urban P, Golf S, Kaufmann U, Imbert C, et al. Emergency stenting for acute occlusion after coronary balloon angioplasty. Circulation 1988;78(5 Pt 1):1121–7.
34. Solomon SB, Patriciu A, Bohlman ME, Kavoussi LR, Stoianovici D. Robotically driven interventions: a method of using CT fluoroscopy without radiation exposure to the physician Radiology 2002;225:277–82.
35. SoS Investigators. Coronary artery bypass surgery versus percutaneous coronary intervention with stent implantation in patients with multivessel coronary artery disease (the Stent or Surgery trial): a randomised controlled trial. Lancet 2004; 360;(9338):965–70.
36. Stefanini GG, Kalesan B, Serruys PW, Heg D, Buszman P, Linke A, et al. Long-term clinical outcomes of biodegradable polymer biolimus-eluting stents versus durable polymer sirolimus-eluting stents in patients with coronary artery disease (LEADERS): 4 year follow-up of a randomised non-inferiority trial. Lancet 2011;378:1940–8.
37. Stone GW, Ellis SG, Cox DA, Hermiller J, O'Shaughnessy C, Mann JT, et al. A polymer-based, paclitaxel-eluting stent in patients with coronary artery disease. N Engl J Med 2004;350: 221–31.
38. Stone GW, Rizvi A, Newman W, et al. Everolimus-eluting versus paclitaxel-eluting stents in coronary artery disease. N Engl J Med 2010;362: 1663–74.
39. Stroupe KT, Morrison DA, Hlatky MA, Barnett PG, Cao L, Lyttle C, Hynes DM, Henderson WG. Cost-effectiveness of coronary artery bypass grafts versus percutaneous coronary intervention for revascularization of high-risk patients. Circulation 2006;114(12):1251–57.
40. Subramanian VA, Patel NU, Patel NC, Loulmet DF. Robotic assisted multivessel minimally invasive direct coronary artery bypass with port-access stabilization and cardiac positioning: paving the way for outpatient coronary surgery? Ann Thorac Surg 2005;79:1590–6, discussion: 1596.
41. UK's NHS endorsed 'Best Treatments' advice on 'clinical evi-dence for patients from the BMJ' on Coronary angioplasty and its risks.
42. Virmani R, Guagliumi G, Farb A, Musumeci G, Grieco N, Motta T, et al. Localized hypersensitivity and late coronary thrombosis secondary to a sirolimus-eluting stent: should we be cautious? Circulation 2004;109:701–5.
43. Weintraub WS, Spertus JA, Kolm P, et al. Effect of PCI on quality of life in patients with stable coronary disease. The N Engl J Med 2008;359(7):677–87.
44. Yamaguchi T, Terashima M, Akasaka T. Safety and feasibility of an intravascular optical coherence tomography image wire system in the clinical setting. Am J Cardiol 2008;101:562–67.
45. Yang EH, Gumina RJ, Lennon RJ, et al. 2003 Journal of the American College of Cardiology 2005;46(11):2004–2009.

# 7 Acute Pulmonary Edema

## INTRODUCTION

Pulmonary edema is the term used when edema happens in the lungs. The immediate area outside of the small blood vessels in the lungs is occupied by very tiny air sacs called the alveoli. This is where oxygen from the air is picked up by the blood passing by, and carbon dioxide in the blood is passed into the alveoli to be exhaled out. Alveoli normally have a thin wall that allows for this air exchange, and fluids are usually kept out of the alveoli unless these walls lose their integrity (Fig. 7.1).

Pulmonary edema occurs when the alveoli fill up with excess fluid seeped out of the blood vessels in the lung instead of air. This can cause problems with the exchange of gas (oxygen and carbon dioxide), resulting in breathing difficulty and poor oxygenation of blood. Sometimes, this can be referred to as 'water in the lungs' when describing the condition to patients.

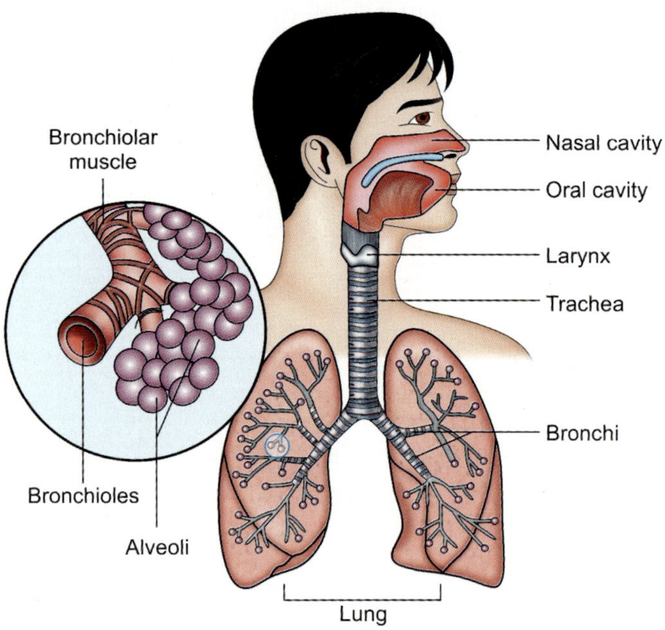


**Fig. 7.1:** Illustration showing anatomy of airway system involved in pulmonary edema

Pulmonary edema can be caused by many different factors. It can be related to heart failure, called cardiogenic pulmonary edema, or related to other causes, referred to as non-cardiogenic pulmonary edema.

## TYPES AND CAUSES OF PULMONARY EDEMA

As mentioned earlier, pulmonary edema can be broadly divided into cardiogenic and non-cardiogenic causes. Some of the common causes are listed below.

1. **Cardiogenic:** Cardiogenic causes of pulmonary edema results from high pressure in the blood vessels of the lung due to poor heart function. Congestive heart failure due to poor heart pumping function (arising from various causes such as arrhythmias and diseases or weakness of the heart muscle), heart attacks, or abnormal heart valves can lead to accumulation of more than the usual amount of blood in the blood vessels of the lungs. This can, in turn, cause the fluid from the blood vessels to be pushed out to the alveoli as the pressure builds up.
2. **Non-cardiogenic:** Non-cardiogenic pulmonary edema can be commonly caused by the following:
   - Acute respiratory distress syndrome (ARDS), a potentially serious condition caused by severe infections, trauma, lung injury, inhalation of toxins, lung infections, cocaine smoking, or radiation to the lungs. In ARDS, the integrity of the alveoli become compromised as a result of underlying inflammatory response, and this leads to leaky alveoli that can fill up with fluid from the blood vessels.
   - Kidney failure and inability to excrete fluid from the body can cause fluid build-up in the blood vessels, resulting in pulmonary edema. In people with advanced kidney disease, dialysis may be necessary to remove the excess body fluid.

- High altitude pulmonary edema, which can happen due to rapid ascent to high altitudes of more than 10,000 feet.
- Brain trauma, bleeding in the brain (intracranial hemorrhage), severe seizures, or brain surgery can sometimes result in fluid accumulation in the lungs, causing neurogenic pulmonary edema.
- A rapidly expanding lung can sometimes cause re-expansion pulmonary edema. This may happen in cases when the lung collapses (pneumothorax) or a large amount of fluid around the lung (pleural effusion) is removed, resulting in rapid expansion of the lung. This can result in pulmonary edema on the affected side only (unilateral pulmonary edema).
- Rarely, an overdose on heroin or methadone can lead to pulmonary edema.
- Aspirin overdose or chronic high dose use of aspirin can lead to aspirin intoxication, especially in the elderly, which may cause pulmonary edema.
- Other more rare causes of non-cardiogenic pulmonary edema may include pulmonary embolism (blood clot which has traveled to the lungs), transfusion-related acute lung injury (TRALI), some viral infections, or eclampsia in pregnant women.

## AETIOLOGICAL FACTORS IN PULMONARY EDEMA

Pulmonary edema is often caused by congestive heart failure. When the heart is not able to pump blood to the body efficiently, it can back up into the veins that take blood through the lungs to the left side of the heart.

As the pressure in these blood vessels increases, fluid is pushed into the air spaces (alveoli) in the lungs. This fluid reduces normal oxygen movement through the lungs. This and the increased pressure can lead to shortness of breath.

- Heart attack, or any disease of the heart that weakens or stiffens the heart muscle (*cardiomyopathy*)
- Leaking or narrowed heart valves (mitral or aortic valves)
- Sudden, severe high blood pressure (hypertension)

  Pulmonary edema may also be caused by:
  - Certain medications
  - High altitude exposure
  - Kidney failure
  - Narrowed arteries that bring blood to the kidneys
  - Lung damaged by poisonous gas or severe infection
  - Major injury

## SYMPTOMS IN PULMONARY EDEMA

Symptoms of pulmonary edema may include:

- Coughing up blood or bloody froth
- Difficulty breathing when lying down (orthopnea) — you may notice the need to sleep with your head propped up or use extra pillows.
- Feeling of 'air hunger' or 'drowning' (if this feeling wakes you from sleep and causes you to sit up and try to catch your breath, it is called 'paroxysmal nocturnal dyspnea').
- Grunting, gurgling, or wheezing sounds with breathing.
- Inability to speak in full sentences because of shortness of breath.

### Other Symptoms

- Anxiety or restlessness
- Decrease in the level of alertness (consciousness)
- Leg swelling
- Pale skin
- Sweating (excessive)

## CLINICAL EXAMINATION IN PULMONARY EDEMA

The healthcare provider will perform a physical examination and use a stethoscope to listen to your lungs and heart. The following may be detected:

- Abnormal heart sounds
- Crackles in your lungs, called rales
- Increased heart rate (tachycardia)
- Pale or blue skin color (pallor or cyanosis)
- Rapid breathing (tachypnea)

### Laboratory Tests

- Blood chemistries
- Blood oxygen levels (oximetry or arterial blood gases)
- Complete blood count (CBC)

### Imaging Studies

1. **Chest X-ray** (Figs 7.2 and 7.3).
2. **Echocardiogram (ultrasound of the heart)** (Figs 7.4–7.6) to see if there are problems with the heart muscle (such as weakness, thickness, failure to relax properly,

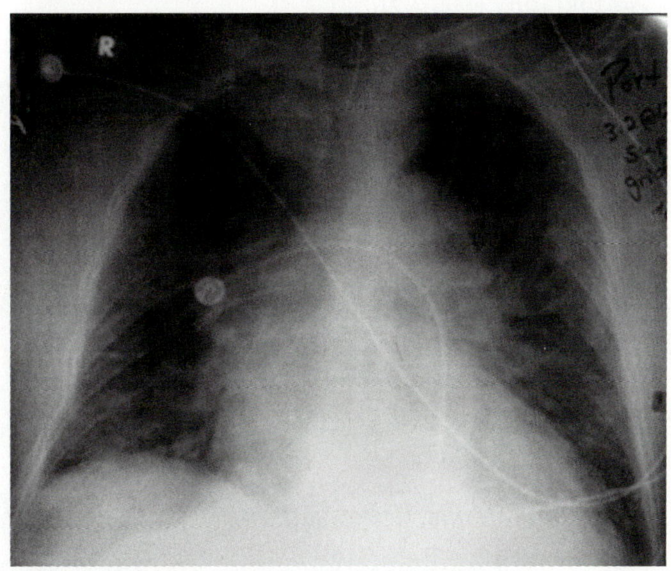

**Fig. 7.2:** Radiograph shows acute pulmonary edema in a patient known to have ischemic cardiomyopathy. Findings are Kerley B lines (1 mm thick and 1 cm long) in the lower lobes and Kerley A lines in the upper lobes

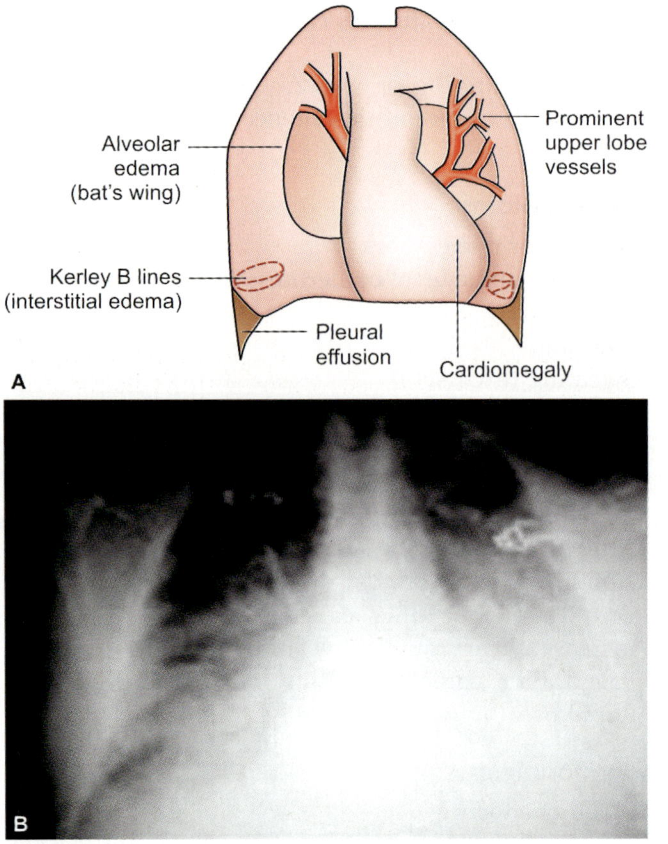


**Fig. 7.3:** (A) Classic signs of acute heart failure that can be seen on a chest X-ray of left ventricular failure, (B) pleural effusion on a chest X-ray

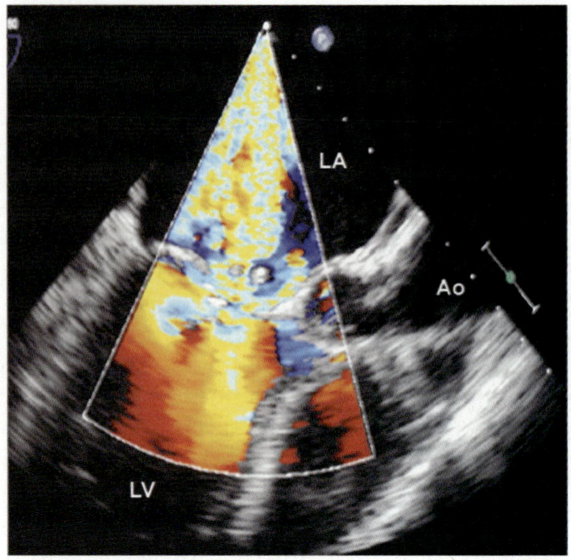


**Fig. 7.4:** Color imaging reveals severe mitral regurgitation (LA=left atrium; LV=left ventricle; Ao=aorta)

leaky or narrow heart valves, or fluid surrounding the heart).
3. **Electrocardiogram (ECG)** (Figs 7.7 and 7.8) to look for signs of a heart attack or problems with the heart rhythm
4. **Aortography** (Fig. 7.9)

## MANAGEMENT OF PULMONARY EDEMA

The initial management of patients with cardiogenic pulmonary edema (CPE) should address the ABCs of resuscitation, that is, airway, breathing, and circulation. Oxygen should be administered to all patients to keep oxygen saturation at greater than 90%. Any associated arrhythmia or MI should be treated appropriately.

Methods of oxygen delivery include the use of a face mask, noninvasive pressure-support ventilation [which includes bilevel positive airway pressure (BiPAP) and continuous positive airway pressure (CPAP)], and intubation and mechanical ventilation. Which method is used depends on the presence of hypoxemia and acidosis and on the

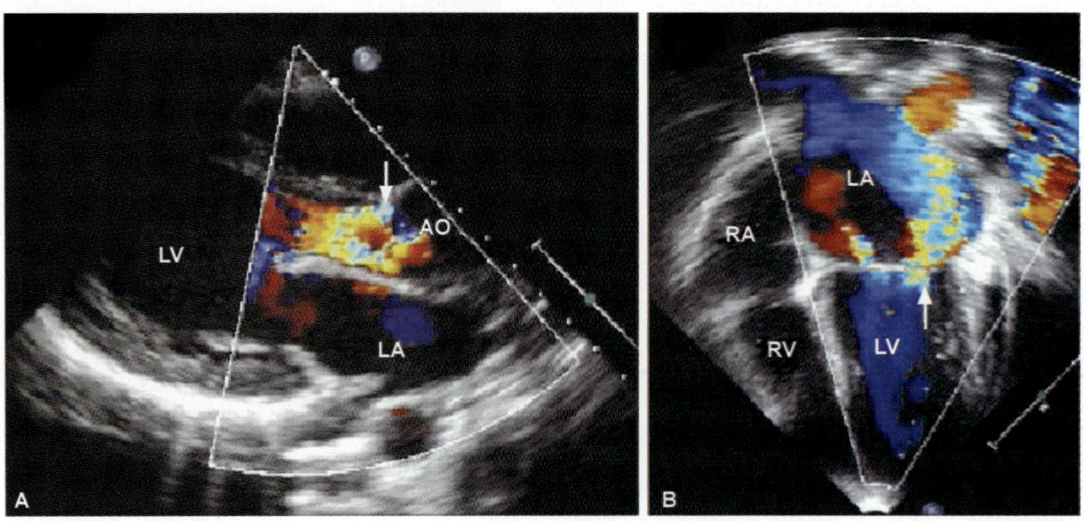


**Fig. 7.5:** (A) Two-dimensional color and spectral Doppler echocardiographic studies of patients with rheumatic heart disease show moderate to severe aortic valve insufficiency with no stenosis (A. arrow) and bowing of the anterior mitral leaflet with severe insufficiency and no stenosis (B. arrow)

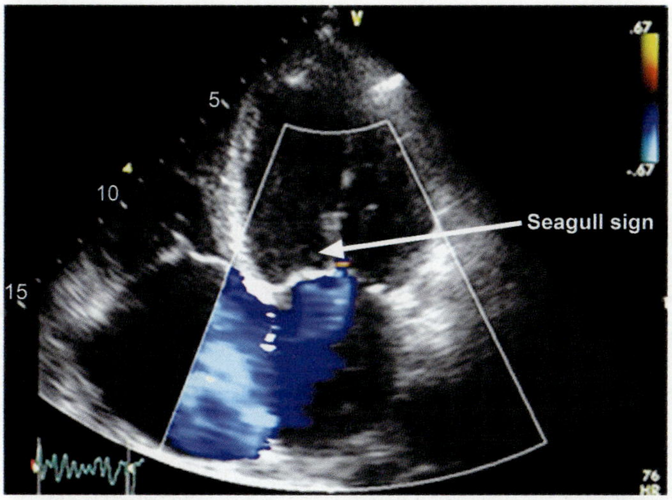


**Fig. 7.6:** 'Seagull sign' on transthoracic echocardiography of moderate-severe IMR. A transthoracic echocardiographic image demonstrating the 'seagull sign' present in moderate-severe IMR. The shape of the anterior mitral valve leaflet is distorted by tethering of secondary strut chordae tendineae. This tethering impairs leaflet coaptation resulting in MR

patient's level of consciousness. For example, intubation and mechanical ventilation may become necessary in cases of persistent hypoxemia, acidosis, or altered mental status. Following initial management, medical treatment of CPE focuses on three main goals:

1. Reduction of pulmonary venous return (preload reduction),
2. Reduction of systemic vascular resistance (afterload reduction), and, in some cases,
3. Inotropic support.

Preload reduction decreases pulmonary capillary hydrostatic pressure and reduces fluid transudation into the pulmonary interstitium and alveoli. Afterload reduction increases cardiac output and improves renal perfusion, which allows for diuresis in the patient with fluid overload.

Patients with severe LV dysfunction or acute valvular disorders may present with hypotension. These patients may not tolerate medications to reduce their preload and afterload. Therefore, inotropic support is necessary in this subset of patients to maintain adequate blood pressure.

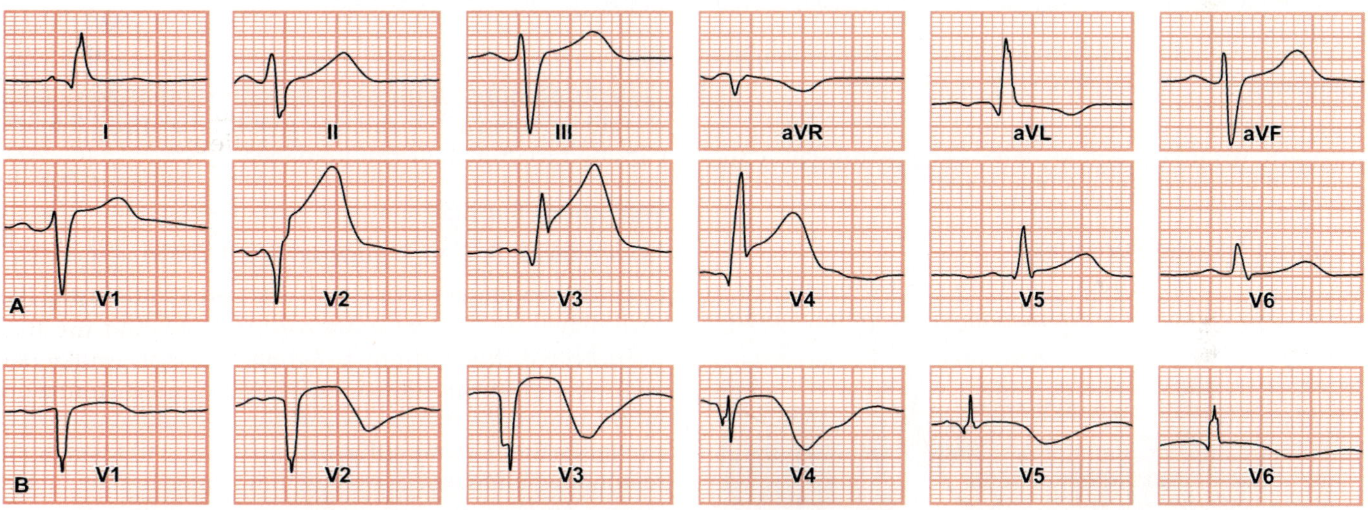


**Fig. 7.7:** Acute extensive anterior myocardial infarction—see in (A) probable LAH in the limb leads with high ST

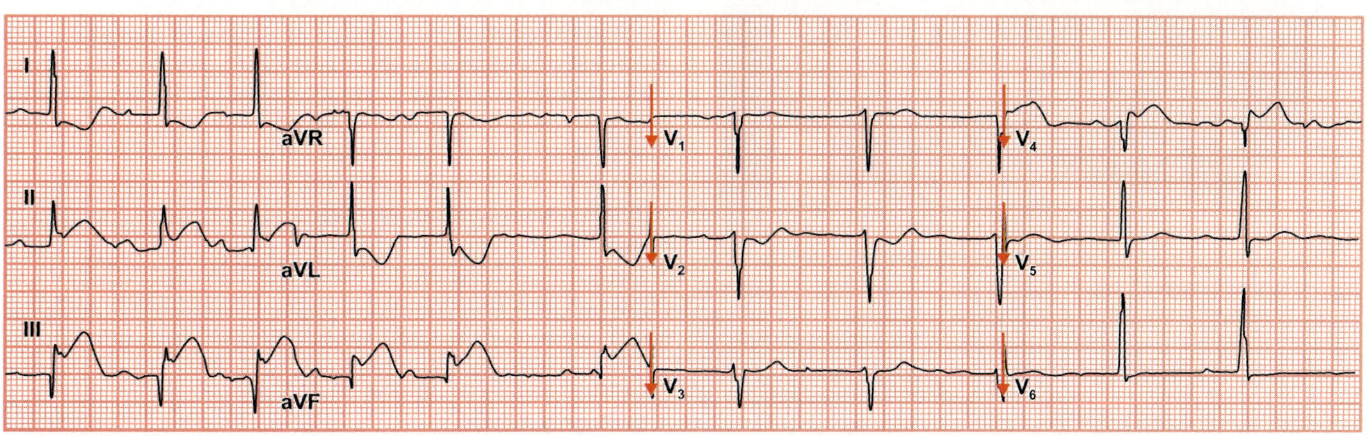


**Fig. 7.8:** ECG showing right ventricular MI. There is an inferior STEMI with ST-elevation in lead III > lead II. There is subtle ST-elevation in V1 with ST-depression in V2. There is ST-elevation in V4R

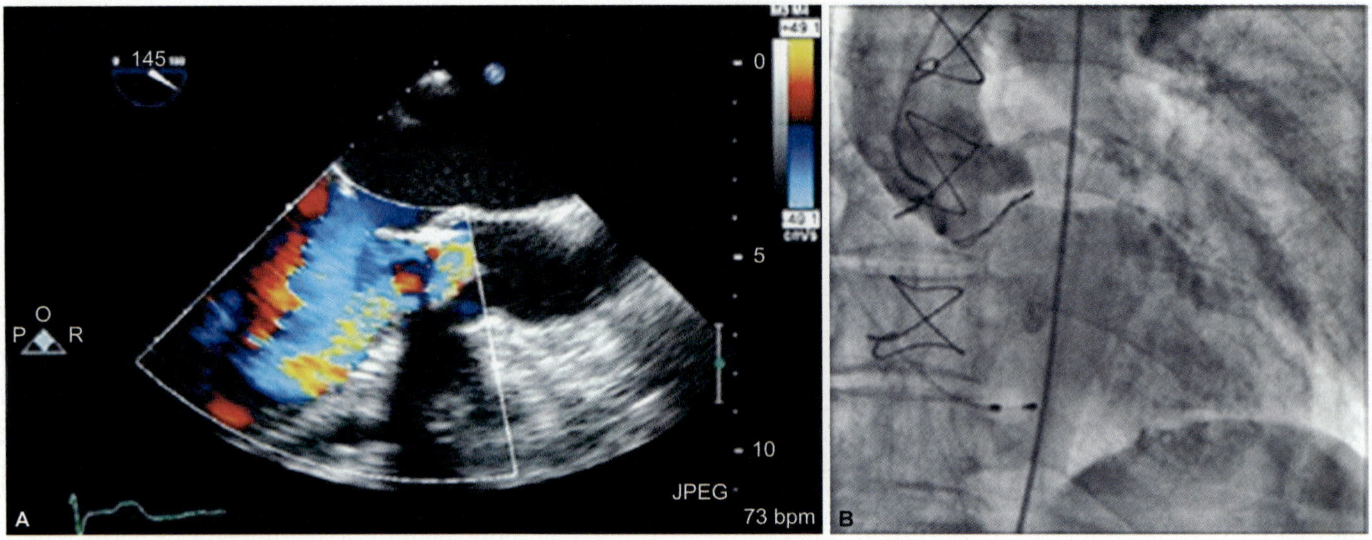


**Fig. 7.9:** Aortic regurgitation documented by transesophageal echocardiography (A) and aortography (B). The patient was referred for aortic valve replacement surgery for worsening of LV functions

Patients who remain hypoxic despite supplemental oxygenation and patients who have severe respiratory distress require ventilatory support in addition to maximal medical therapy.

## Ultrafiltration

Ultrafiltration is a fluid removal procedure that is particularly useful in patients with renal dysfunction and expected diuretic resistance (Fig. 7.10).

## Intra-aortic Balloon Pumping

Intra-aortic balloon pumping (IABP) can be employed to achieve hemodynamic stabilization in the patient before definitive therapy. The IABP decreases afterload as the pump deflates; during diastole, the pump inflates to improve coronary blood flow.

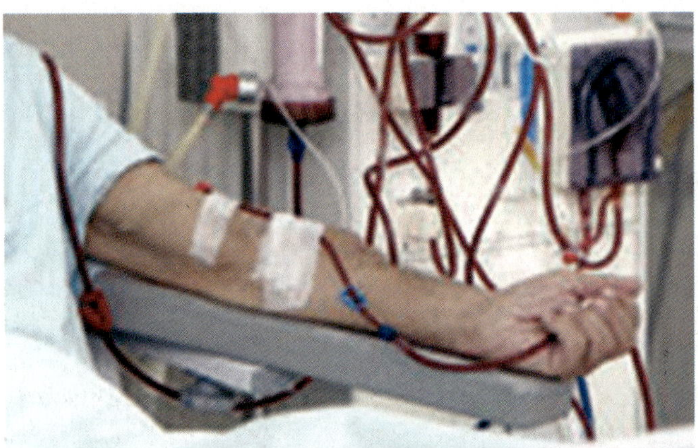

**Fig. 7.10:** Venovenous ultrafiltration technique, in patients with acute decompensated heart failure with worsening of kidney function, a condition referred to as acute cardiorenal syndrome (type 1). Diuretics are commonly used to treat persistent congestion in these patients, but these drugs might worsen kidney function. An alternative therapeutic approach is venovenous ultrafiltration, which can improve control over the rate and volume of fluid removal, increases net loss of sodium, and reduces neurohormonal activation

## Diet

Patients admitted with heart failure or pulmonary edema should be given a low-salt diet to minimize fluid retention. Closely monitor their fluid balance.

## Ventilatory Support

### *Noninvasive Pressure-support Ventilation*

Consider noninvasive pressure-support ventilation (NPSV) early when treating patients with severe CPE.

In NPSV, the patient breathes through a face mask against a continuous flow of positive airway pressure. NPSV maintains the patency of the fluid-filled alveoli and prevents them from collapsing during exhalation. As a result, the patient saves energy that would have been spent trying to reopen collapsed alveoli. NPSV improves pulmonary air exchange, and it increases intrathoracic pressure with reduction in preload and afterload.

Several studies suggest that NPSV is associated with decreased length of stay in the ICU, decreased need for mechanical ventilation, and decreased hospital costs. A few clinical trials showed that in patients with CPE—mainly defined as having severe dyspnea, oxygen saturation of less than 90%, and basal rales—early and prehospital NPSV treatment by paramedics is safe and associated with faster improvement of oxygen saturation. However, the mortality and the need for intensive care did not differ between the patients who were treated with NPSV and those who were treated with a Venturi face mask in most of those studies.

### *CPAP and BiPAP*

Two types of NPSV are CPAP and BiPAP. In CPAP, a single airway pressure is maintained throughout all phases of the respiratory cycle. In BiPAP, high pressures can be applied during inspiration and low pressures, during expiration, increasing the patient's comfort.

A randomized trial comparing CPAP, noninvasive intermittent positive pressure ventilation (NIPPV), and standard oxygen therapy in 1069 patients with acute cardiogenic pulmonary edema demonstrated no mortality benefit from noninvasive ventilation, but improvements were seen in symptomatology and oxygenation.

In one small study, researchers compared CPAP with BiPAP and found that BiPAP was associated with more rapid improvement in vital signs but also with an increased rate of MIs. Moreover, patients who received BiPAP initially had more chest pain than did patients who received CPAP. Other randomized clinical trials, however, did not show an increased rate of MI in patients who received CPAP or BiPAP compared with those who received oxygen by means of a face mask.

As of now, the data are insufficient to compare the efficacy and safety of BiPAP with those of CPAP. Therefore, the authors suggest that CPAP be the preferred method employed when NPSV is used unless the patient has obstructive airway disease (Fig. 7.11).

### Mechanical Ventilation

In general, use endotracheal intubation and mechanical ventilation when patients with CPE remain hypoxic despite maximal noninvasive supplemental oxygenation, when patients have evidence of impending respiratory failure (e.g. lethargy, fatigue, diaphoresis, worsening anxiety), or when patients are hemodynamically unstable (e.g. hypotensive, severely tachycardic).

Mechanical ventilation maximizes myocardial oxygen delivery and ventilation. Positive end-expiratory pressure is generally recommended to increase alveolar patency and to enhance oxygen delivery and carbon dioxide exchange.

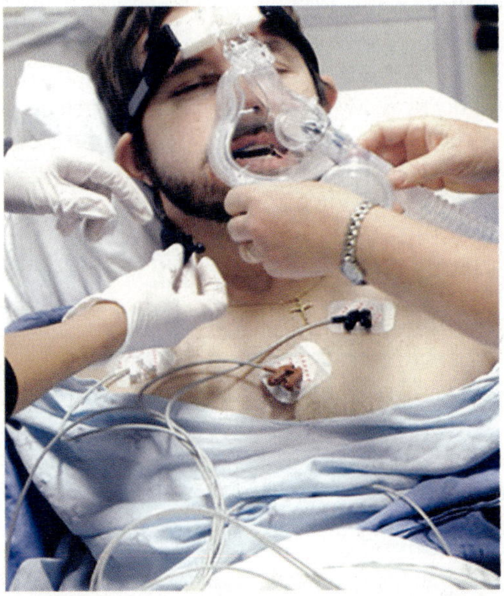

**Fig. 7.11:** A middle-aged patient with acute pulmonary edema was fitted with CPAP and got relief after its application

### Preload Reduction

*Nitroglycerin:* Nitroglycerin (NTG) is the most effective, predictable, and rapidly-acting medication available for preload reduction. Several studies demonstrated greater efficacy and safety and a faster onset of action with NTG than with furosemide or morphine sulfate. The use of sublingual NTG is associated with preload reduction within 5 minutes and with some afterload reduction.

Topical NTG may be as effective as sublingual NTG in most patients with CPE, but it should be avoided in patients with severe LV failure, because of poor skin perfusion (manifesting as skin pallor or mottling) and resultant poor absorption.

Intravenous (IV) NTG at high dosages provides rapid and titratable preload and afterload reduction and is excellent monotherapy for patients with severe CPE. IV NTG can be started with 10 mcg/min and then rapidly uptitrated to more than 100 mcg/min. The other alternative is NTG given as 3 mg IV boluses every 5 minutes.

The antianginal dose of NTG of 0.4 mg every 5 minutes has the bioequivalence of an NTG IV infusion of less than 80 mcg/min. Therefore, the dosage of NTG for patients with CPE is higher than the standard antianginal dosage would be.

Considering the short half-life of nitrates, physicians should be comfortable with the high dosage for CPE, especially in most patients with CPE, who present with a hyperadrenergic state and moderately elevated blood pressure. However, nitrates should not be used in hypotensive patients, and they should be used with extreme caution in patients with aortic stenosis and pulmonary hypertension.

*Diuretics:* Loop diuretics have been considered the cornerstone of CPE treatment for many years. Furosemide is used most commonly. Loop diuretics are presumed to decrease preload through two mechanisms—diuresis and direct vasoactivity (venodilation).

In most patients, diuresis does not occur for at least 20–90 minutes; therefore, the effect is delayed. Loop diuretics affect the ascending loop of Henle; therefore, the diminished renal perfusion in CPE may delay the onset of effects of loop diuretics.

Many patients with CPE do not have fluid overload. Continued use of diuretics in these patients after their acute symptoms have resolved may be associated with adverse outcomes, including electrolyte derangements, hypotension, and worsening renal function (GFR, glomerular filtration rate) as a result of tubuloglomerular feedback.

The presumption that these medications have a direct vasoactive (venodilating) effect has been questioned. Some studies demonstrated initial adverse hemodynamic consequences (e.g. elevations of PCWP, LV filling pressure, heart rate, and systemic vascular resistance) after the administration of IV furosemide.

Premedication with drugs that decrease preload (e.g. NTG) and afterload [e.g. angiotensin-converting enzyme (ACE) inhibitors] before the administration of loop diuretics can prevent potential adverse hemodynamic changes.

*Morphine sulfate:* The use of morphine sulfate in CPE for preload reduction has been commonplace for many years, but good evidence supporting a beneficial hemodynamic effect is lacking. Data suggest that morphine sulfate may contribute to a decrease in cardiac output and that it may be associated with an increased need for ICU admission and endotracheal intubation.

Adverse effects (e.g. nausea and vomiting, local or systemic allergic reactions, respiratory depression) may outweigh any potential benefit, especially given the availability of medications that are more effective than morphine in reducing preload (e.g. NTG).

Any beneficial hemodynamic effect from morphine is probably due to anxiolysis, with a resulting decrease in catecholamine production and a decrease in systemic vascular resistance. An alternative can be low-dose benzodiazepines (e.g. lorazepam 0.5 mg IV) in patients who are extremely anxious. This alternative reduces the risk of respiratory depression in patients whose condition responded to initial therapy.

*Nesiritide:* Nesiritide is recombinant human BNP that decreases PCWP, pulmonary artery pressure, RA pressure, and systemic vascular resistance while increasing the cardiac index and stroke volume index. Therapy with nesiritide has decreased plasma renin, aldosterone, norepinephrine, and endothelin-1 levels and has reduced ventricular ectopy and ventricular tachycardia. Heart-rate variability also improves with nesiritide.

Most of the beneficial effects of nesiritide were shown in the landmark vasodilation in the management of acute congestive heart failure (VMAC) study. Investigators compared IV nesiritide with IV NTG. IV nesiritide was associated with some hypotension but was otherwise well tolerated.

However, the VMAC study also showed a trend toward increased mortality in the IV nesiritide group compared with the patients receiving IV NTG, although the difference was not statically significant (90-day mortality, 19% for nesiritide *vs* 13% for NTG). The most important limitation of this study was the use of suboptimal dosages of IV NTG (mean 30–40 mcg/min) because the dosage was based on physician's decision and not on a protocol.

A later meta-analysis of 3 randomized trials of 485 patients receiving nesiritide and 377 patients not receiving nesiritide showed a 7.2% 30-day mortality with nesiritide versus 4% without nesiritide.

Another analysis, which included 5 randomized trials, showed that patients who received nesiritide were more likely than others to have significant renal failure.

In the largest study of nesiritide to date, the acute study of clinical effectiveness of nesiritide in decompensated heart failure (ASCEND HF), nesiritide had a neutral effect on survival and rehospitalization and a small effect on dyspnea when used in combination with other treatments. In the study, powered to show the effects of the drug on survival and renal function, no association was found between the drug and deteriorating renal function, although nesiritide was associated with a slight increase in hypotension. The authors recommended against the routine use of nesiritide in the broad population of patients with acute heart failure.

### Afterload Reduction

*ACE inhibitors:* ACE inhibitors are generally considered the cornerstones for treating CHF, and studies have demonstrated excellent results with ACE inhibitors for the treatment of acute decompensated CHF and CPE. The use of ACE inhibitors in CPE is associated with reduced admission rates to ICUs and decreased endotracheal intubation rates and length of ICU stay.

The hemodynamic effects of ACE inhibitors include reduced afterload, improved stroke volume and cardiac output, and a slight reduction in preload. The last effect happens when renal perfusion improves after cardiac output improves and diuresis occurs.

Enalapril 1.25 mg IV or captopril 25 mg, given sublingually, result in hemodynamic and subjective improvements within 10 minutes. Improvements occur much more slowly with the oral route.

*Angiotensin II receptor blockers:* Angiotensin II receptor blockers (ARBs) have comparable beneficial effects in heart failure. Studies have proposed a role for ACE inhibitors and ARBs in preventing structural and electrical remodeling of the heart, resulting in a reduced incidence of arrhythmias.

The valsartan heart failure trial (Val-HeFT) showed that valsartan reduces the incidence of atrial fibrillation (AF) by 37%. (BNP level and advanced age were the strongest independent predictors for AF occurrence.) Similarly, the candesartan in heart failure: assessment in reduction of mortality and morbidity (CHARM) trial showed a reduction in the onset of AF in patients who were treated with Candesartan compared with placebo, with a median follow-up period of 37.7 months.

*Nitroprusside:* Nitroprusside results in simultaneous preload and afterload reduction by causing direct smooth-muscle relaxation, with an increased effect on afterload. Afterload reduction is associated with increased cardiac output. The potency and rapidity of onset and offset of effect make this an ideal medication for patients who are critically ill. It may induce precipitous falls and labile fluctuations in blood pressure; intra-arterial blood pressure monitoring is often recommended.

Nitroprusside should generally be avoided in the setting of acute MI. Its use is associated with the shunting of blood away from ischemic myocardium toward healthy myocardium (i.e. coronary steal syndrome), which potentiates ischemia.

If nitroprusside is used, convert therapy to oral or alternative IV vasodilator therapy as soon as possible because prolonged use is associated with thiocyanate toxicity. Use in pregnancy is associated with fetal thiocyanate toxicity. Prolonged infusion can induce tolerance, and reflex tachycardia may occur.

*Catecholamines:* Inotropic support is usually used when preload and afterload-reduction strategies are not successful or when hypotension precludes the use of these strategies. Two main classes of inotropic agents are available—catecholamine agents and phosphodiesterase inhibitors (PDIs). Calcium-sensitizer agents are a new class of medications that have notably beneficial effects in acute decompensated heart failure; these drugs are under investigation.

*Dobutamine:* Dobutamine, a catecholamine agent, mainly serves as a beta1-receptor agonist, though it has some beta2-receptor and minimal alpha-receptor activity. IV dobutamine induces significant positive inotropic effects, with mild chronotropic effects. It also induces mild peripheral vasodilation (decrease in afterload). The combination effect of increased inotropy with decreased afterload significantly increases cardiac output. Combination use with IV NTG may be ideal for patients with MI and CPE and mild hypotension to simultaneously reduce preload and increase cardiac output. In general, avoid dobutamine in patients with moderate or severe hypotension (e.g. systolic BP <80 mmHg), because of the peripheral vasodilation.

*Dopamine:* The vascular and myocardial receptor effects of dopamine, a catecholamine agent, are dose dependent. Low dosages of 0.5–5 mcg/kg/min stimulate dopaminergic receptors in the renal and splanchnic vascular beds, causing vasodilation and increasing diuresis. Moderate dosages of 5–10 mcg/kg/min stimulate beta-receptors in the myocardium, increasing cardiac contractility and heart rate.

High dosages of 15–20 mcg/kg/min stimulate alpha-receptors, resulting in peripheral vasoconstriction (increased afterload), increased blood pressure, and no further improvement in cardiac output.

Moderate and high dosages are arrhythmogenic and increase myocardial oxygen demand (with the potential for myocardial ischemia). Therefore, use these dosages only in patients with CPE who cannot tolerate dobutamine because of severe hypotension (e.g. systolic blood pressure 60–80 mmHg).

*Norepinephrine:* Norepinephrine, a catecholamine agent, primarily stimulates alpha receptors, significantly increasing afterload (and the potential for myocardial ischemia) and reducing cardiac output. Norepinephrine is generally reserved for patients with profound hypotension (e.g. systolic blood pressure <60 mmHg). After blood pressure is restored, add other medications to maintain cardiac output.

*Phosphodiesterase inhibitors:* PDIs increase the level of intracellular cyclic adenosine monophosphate (cAMP) by preventing the breakdown of cAMP to 5'AMP. This results in a positive inotropic effect on the myocardium, in peripheral vasodilation (decreased afterload), and in a reduction in pulmonary vascular resistance (decreased preload). Unlike the catecholamine inotropes, PDIs do not depend on adrenoreceptor activity. Therefore, patients are less likely to develop tolerance to PDIs than they are to other medications (tolerance to catecholamine inotropes can rapidly develop by means of a down-regulation of adrenoreceptors.)

PDIs are less likely than catecholamine inotropes to cause the adverse effects that are typically associated with adrenoreceptor activity (e.g. increased myocardial oxygen demand, myocardial ischemia).

Several direct comparisons of PDIs (milrinone) to dobutamine in patients with CPE demonstrated that milrinone produced equal or greater improvements in stroke volume, cardiac output, PCWPs (preload), and systemic vascular resistance (afterload). However, milrinone was associated with the same or more tachycardia and with an increased incidence of tachyarrhythmias.

Furthermore, the use of milrinone in the outcomes of a prospective trial of intravenous milrinone for exacerbations of chronic heart failure (OPTIME-CHF) study did not reduce hospital length of stay and was associated with a significant increase in adverse events compared with placebo.

All known IV inotropic agents are associated with an increased long-term mortality compared with placebo and therefore should be reserved for patients with heart failure and a markedly depressed cardiac index and stroke volume.

*Calcium sensitizers:* Levosimendan is a calcium sensitizer that is used in several European countries to manage moderate to severe heart failure. It has inotropic, metabolic, and vasodilatory effects. Levosimendan increases contractility by binding to troponin C. It does not increase myocardial oxygen demand, and it is not a proarrhythmogenic agent.

Levosimendan opens potassium channels sensitive to adenosine triphosphate (ATP), causing peripheral arterial and venous dilatation. It also increases coronary flow reserve. Moreover, studies have shown levosimendan to have an anti-inflammatory effect.

Overall, levosimendan has been an effective and safe alternative to dobutamine. The most common adverse effects of levosimendan treatment are hypotension and headache. A randomized clinical study—the survival of patients with acute heart failure in need of intravenous inotropic support (SURVIVE) trial—demonstrated no mortality benefit from levosimendan in comparison with dobutamine in patients with acute decompensated CHF.

*Tolvaptan:* Tolvaptan is an oral vasopressin V2-receptor antagonist that was evaluated in a large (4133 patients), randomized, double-blind, placebo-controlled trial in patients with acute clinically decompensated CHF. This study, the efficacy of vasopressin antagonism in heart failure outcome study with tolvaptan (EVEREST), demonstrated no mortality or CHF hospitalization benefit at a median follow-up of 9.9 months. However, patients randomized to tolvaptan demonstrated early (1–7 d) improvements in body weight, dyspnea, serum sodium, and edema, as compared with placebo.

### Intra-aortic Balloon Pumping

Kantrowitz initially described intra-aortic balloon pumping in 1953, but IABP was first used clinically in 1969 in a patient with cardiogenic shock. Since the 1980s, IABP has been increasingly applied in various clinical situations as a life-saving intervention to achieve hemodynamic stabilization before definitive therapy. The IABP decreases afterload as the pump deflates, and it improves coronary blood flow as it inflates during diastole.

The intra-aortic balloon pump is inserted percutaneously through the femoral artery using a modified Seldinger technique. The distal end of the pump is placed just distal to the aortic knob and the origin of the left subclavian artery. Fluoroscopy may be used for correct positioning of the balloon, and a subsequent radiograph should be obtained to document satisfactory placement of the balloon. Helium, a low-density gas with minimal water solubility, is used to inflate the balloon.

Proper timing of counterpulsation is necessary for maximum hemodynamic support. The timings of balloon inflation and deflation are best evaluated and adjusted at a pump ratio of 1:2. Inflation of the balloon should occur in early diastole, just after the aortic valve closes, and it should correspond to the dicrotic notch of the aortic pressure waveform. Balloon deflation should occur in early systole, just before the aortic valve opens.

Proper inflation leads to an assisted peak diastolic pressure higher than the unassisted peak systolic arterial pressure. Proper deflation results in assisted aortic end-diastolic pressure of approximately 10 mmHg lower than the unassisted end-diastolic pressure.

Diastolic augmentation enhances perfusion of the coronary circulation and carotid arteries. The reduction in end-diastolic pressure decreases aortic impedance (afterload) and augments systole.

By reducing aortic impedance and systolic pressure, IABP leads to a 15–25% reduction in LV wall stress. This level of afterload reduction improves LV volume, LV emptying, and myocardial oxygen consumption.

Diastolic aortic pressure augmentation improves myocardial perfusion and coronary blood flow. The effects on coronary blood flow may be variable but generally consist of a boost of 10–20% in the ischemic territories.

IABP decreases LV filling pressures by 20–25% and improves cardiac output by 20% in patients with cardiogenic shock. Therefore, IABP substantially reduces myocardial oxygen demand, although increased oxygen supply to the myocardium may also be a beneficial effect in some clinical situations.

IABP is effective in providing temporary support to patients in cardiogenic shock and end-stage cardiomyopathy while definite therapies, such as angioplasty, cardiac bypass surgery, or cardiac transplantation, are undertaken. In this case, the use of IABP is considered a bridge to a definitive revascularization procedure or implementation of an LV-assist device.

IABP is effective in stabilizing patients with unstable angina refractory to medical therapy before a definitive revascularization procedure.

IABP may be a life-saving intervention in patients with acute mitral regurgitation secondary to papillary muscle rupture or in patients with ventricular septal defect as a complication of MI. IABP reduces afterload and thereby reduces the severity of mitral regurgitation. It enhances forward cardiac output, reduces LA pressure, and improves pulmonary edema. Furthermore, IABP decreases LV afterload and improves cardiac output.

IABP can also provide hemodynamic support in the perioperative and postoperative period in high-risk patients, such as those with severe coronary disease, severe LV dysfunction, or recent MI (Fig. 7.12).

*Contraindications:* Absolute contraindications for IABP counterpulsation are a dissecting aortic aneurysm, severe aortic regurgitation, a large arteriovenous shunt, and severe coagulopathy. Relative contraindications are severe

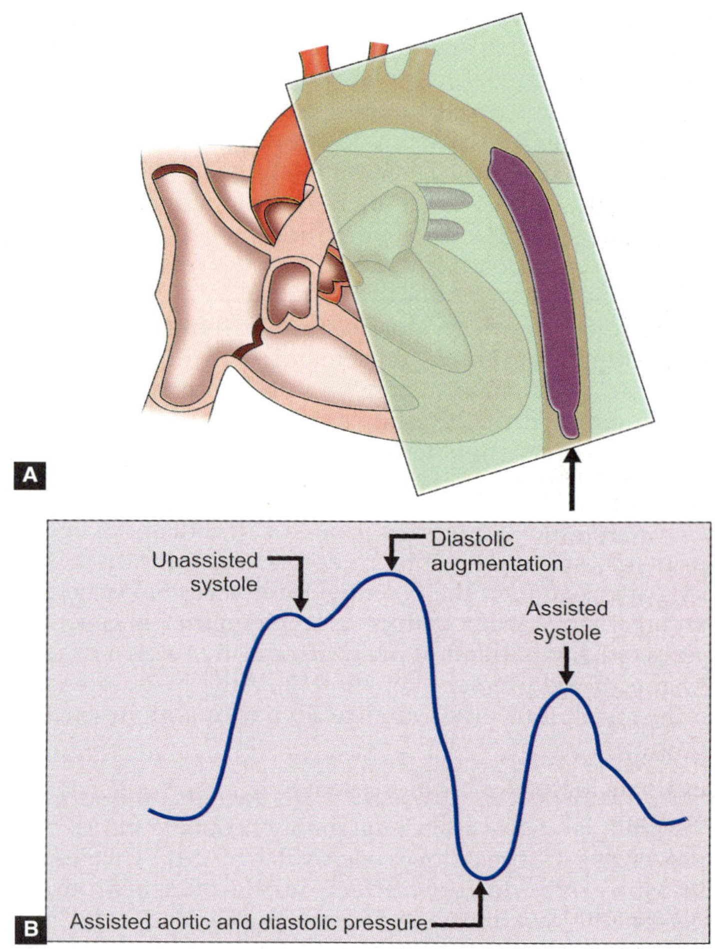


**Fig. 7.12:** (A) Showing introduction of intra-aortic balloon in aorta. (B) improvement in diastolic blood pressure in cardiogenic shock with heart failure

peripheral vascular disease, recent thrombolytic therapy, bleeding diathesis, and descending aortic and peripheral vascular grafts.

*Complications:* IABP can cause several complications, which should be monitored while the patient is receiving IABP support. In general, the patient's platelet counts are mildly reduced; however, the counts usually do not fall below $100 \times 10^9$/L.

Complications also may occur during cannulation of the femoral artery. These include perforation, laceration, or dissection of the artery (1–6%). Thrombosis of the iliofemoral artery and distal emboli may also occur (1–7%), and limb ischemia is reported in up to 40% of patients. Limb ischemia is reversible by removing the intra-aortic balloon pump, unless thrombosis develops; if thrombosis does occur, embolectomy is required to save the limb.

The other complications are localized bleeding (3–5%), infection (2–4%), thrombocytopenia (<1%), and intestinal ischemia (<1%).

*Ultrafiltration:* Ultrafiltration (UF) is a method of fluid removal that is particularly useful in patients with renal dysfunction and expected diuretic resistance.

The randomized ultrafiltration versus intravenous diuretics for patients hospitalized for acute decompensated heart failure (UNLOAD) trial demonstrated that ultrafiltration was superior to the use of IV diuretics in controlling net fluid loss and rehospitalization in hypervolemic patients with heart failure. These results indicated that UF should be considered in patients with volume overload and acute CHF who have not responded well to moderate to large doses of diuretic treatment or in whom the adverse effects of such treatment (e.g. renal dysfunction) do not allow initiation or continuation of the therapy. Broader application of UF needs further investigation with larger clinical trials to determine the efficacy and safety of this method.

*Inpatient care:* After the patient's condition has been stabilized, further inpatient care depends on the underlying cause of the episode of CPE.

Admit patients to a telemetry unit to monitor for acute dysrhythmias. Pay strict attention to the patient's fluid balance and closely monitor fluid input and output. Maintain a negative fluid balance in patients who are fluid overloaded by using diuretics or hemodialysis (in patients with renal failure).

Check cardiac enzyme levels to evaluate for MI. Stress testing can also be performed during hospitalization to evaluate for reversible ischemia as the cause of pulmonary edema.

Consider electrocardiography to evaluate for evidence of acute valvular dysfunction and wall-motion abnormalities and to assess the patient's ejection fraction. Patients with poor ejection fractions or severe dilated cardiomyopathies are often given digoxin.

In general, begin with oral vasodilator therapy, most commonly ACE inhibitors. If the patient was initially treated with inotropic medications, wean the patient off of these as soon as his or her condition is stable, to minimize adverse effects.

Patients in whom pulmonary edema is due to dietary factors or medication noncompliance need strict counseling and education to help prevent recurrences.

*Transfer of patient:* Transfer of patients to a tertiary receiving hospital is generally indicated if the initial hospital lacks adequate resources to care for the patient. Most patients with CPE can be treated well at community hospitals. However, if definitive surgery is required to stabilize the cause of CPE, transfer is often indicated.

Examples of patients who may require transfer include the following:

- Patients with CPE due to acute valvular dysfunction requiring urgent valve replacement
- Patients with acute MI that results in cardiogenic shock manifesting as CPE with hypotension (thrombolysis may be attempted at the initial hospital, but outcomes are generally poor without percutaneous coronary intervention or coronary artery bypass surgery)
- Patients with CPE who require inotropic support

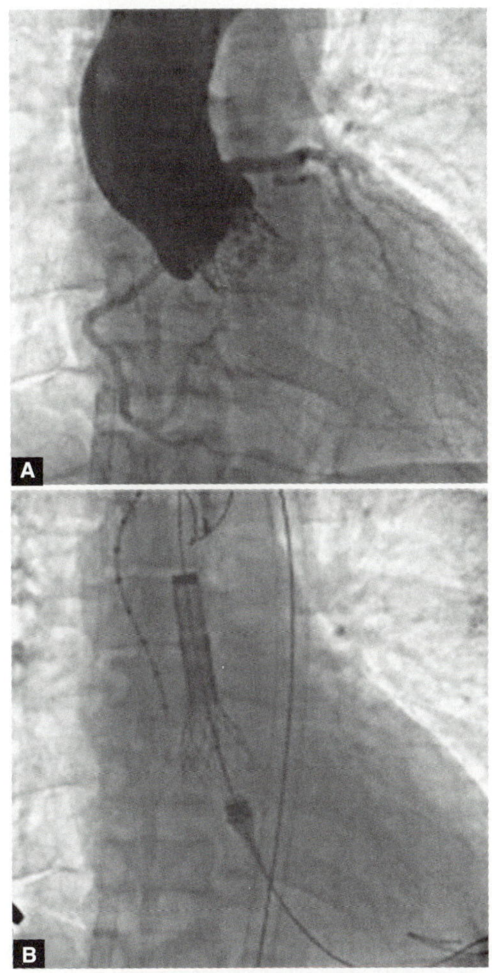


**Fig. 7.13:** (A) Controlled expansion of the aortic prosthesis. (B) Angiogram after successful implantation of aortic valve in an elderly patient with severe aortic stenosis and AR with heart failure

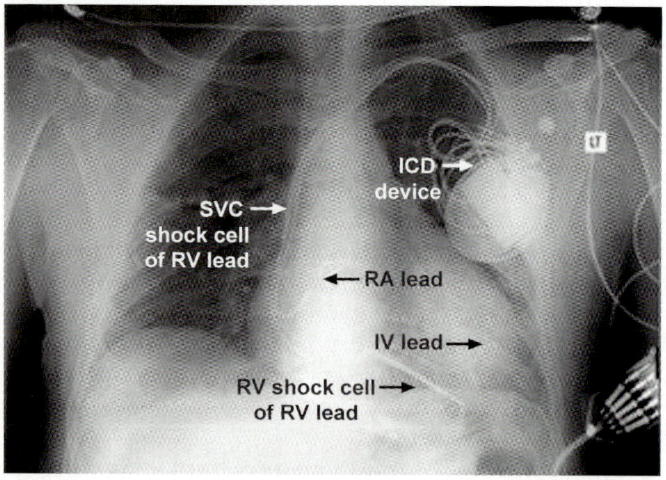


**Fig. 7.14:** X-ray chest showing ICD device fitted in a patient with cardiac arrhythmias and heart failure

*Consultations:* Consultations with subspecialists depend on the underlying cause of the episode of CPE. If the acute episode is attributed to an acute MI, acute cardiac ischemia, or an acute dysrhythmia, consultation with a cardiologist is often warranted.

If the episode is attributed to fluid overload in a patient with renal failure, consultation with a nephrologist is indicated for emergency or urgent hemodialysis.

If CPE results from acute valvular dysfunction, consultation with a cardiothoracic surgeon (including a cardiologist) for urgent valve replacement may be indicated, depending on the integrity of the valve (Figs 7.13 and 7.14).

In patients who develop cardiogenic shock, consultation with a cardiologist and/or critical care specialist is generally indicated to assist with titrating inotropic medication and, in some cases, to place an intra-aortic balloon pump as a temporizing measure before surgery (e.g. valve replacement or coronary revascularization).

## QUICK READINGS IN MANAGEMENT OF ACUTE PULMONARY EDEMA

Because of the fundamental differences between cardiogenic and non-cardiogenic pulmonary edema, each requires different management and has a different prognosis. Treatment should be directed at reversing the specific cause although this may not be possible.

Management is otherwise supportive and directed at improving oxygenation, perfusion and haemodynamics, and preventing further cardiac and/or renal damage.

### Prehospital Treatment

*Resuscitation—as necessary:* Sit the patient up; give oxygen (if available) by face mask—100% if no pre-existing lung disease (but even in patients with chronic obstructive pulmonary disease (COPD), give high oxygen flow initially but monitor with blood gases to ensure hypercapnia is avoided). Aim for oxygen saturations =95% (>90% in those with COPD).

*Judge clinical severity:* Some patients do not require hospital admission, e.g. those with mild and stable pulmonary edema with a known cause that is treatable without admission. However, most patients require urgent admission to hospital.

*Insert an intravenous cannula and give* nitrates are first-line vasodilators where systolic blood pressure is >90 mmHg and there is no serious obstructive valvular disease. Give sublingual or buccal nitrate, e.g. glyceryl trinitrate (GTN) spray two puffs sublingual, or 1–3 mg buccal isosorbide dinitrate.

*Furosemide* 20–40 mg intravenously (slowly) produces transient venodilation and subsequent diuresis. This may need to be repeated based on response of clinical symptoms—diuretic effectiveness is greatly reduced in the presence of hypotension and when patients have been taking oral diuretics for a long time.

*Opiates:* The use of opiates is controversial and opiates should not be given to patients with acute decompensated heart failure (see 'initial treatment', below). However, analgesia and sedation may be appropriate where the patient is in pain or distressed.

*Diamorphine* 2.5–5 mg intravenously slowly (or morphine 5–10 mg intravenously slowly) can be used to relieve anxiety, pain and distress.

*Persistent coughs:* Have a heart for your health.

### Acute Heart Failure with Pulmonary Congestion/Edema without Shock

#### *Initial Treatment*

An intravenous loop diuretic is recommended to improve breathlessness and relieve congestion. Symptoms, urine output, renal function and electrolytes should be monitored regularly during use of the intravenous diuretic.

*High-flow oxygen* is recommended in patients with a capillary oxygen saturation <90% or $PaO_2$ <60 mmHg (8.0 kPa) to correct hypoxaemia. Oxygen should not be used routinely in non-hypoxaemic patients, as it causes vasoconstriction and a reduction in cardiac output.

Thrombo-embolism prophylaxis [e.g. with low molecular weight heparin (LMWH)] is recommended in patients not already anticoagulated and with no contra-indication to anticoagulation, to reduce the risk of deep venous thrombosis and pulmonary embolism.

*Opiates*, e.g. *morphine* may be useful in some patients with acute pulmonary edema, as they reduce anxiety and relieve distress associated with dyspnoea.

However, opiates depress respiratory drive, potentially increasing the need for invasive ventilation. Alertness and ventilatory effort should be monitored frequently after administration.

Some studies have suggested a strong association between the use of opiates and increased mortality and morbidity (e.g. intensive care unit admissions or intubation rates) and opiates should not be used routinely in the treatment of acute pulmonary edema.

Opiates should be avoided in acute decompensated heart failure.

*Vasodilators:* An intravenous infusion of a nitrate should be considered in patients with pulmonary congestion/edema and a systolic blood pressure >110 mmHg, who do not have severe mitral or aortic stenosis, to reduce pulmonary capillary wedge pressure and systemic vascular resistance.

Nitrates may also relieve dyspnoea and congestion. Symptoms and blood pressure should be monitored frequently during administration of intravenous nitrates.

*Inotropic agents* are NOT recommended unless the patient is hypotensive (systolic blood pressure <85 mmHg), hypoperfused, or shocked because of safety concerns (atrial and ventricular arrhythmias, myocardial ischemia, and death).

Inotropes cause sinus tachycardia and may induce myocardial ischemia and arrhythmias. There is concern that inotropes may increase mortality.

Levosimendan (or a phosphodiesterase III inhibitor such as milrinone) may be used to counteract the effect of a beta-blocker.

Phosphodiesterase inhibitors (milrinone and enoximone) may be preferred to dobutamine in patients on beta-blocker therapy or with inadequate response to dobutamine. They are peripheral vasodilators and should only be used if systolic blood pressure is adequate. They may increase mortality in those with coronary artery disease.

Levosimendan is a calcium sensitiser that appears effective in patients with decompensated chronic heart failure already on beta-blockers.

*Patients with hypotension, hypoperfusion or shock:* *Electrical cardioversion* is recommended if an atrial or ventricular arrhythmia is thought to be contributing to hemodynamic compromise.

**An intravenous infusion of an inotrope (e.g. dobutamine)** should be considered in patients with hypotension (systolic blood pressure <85 mmHg). The ECG should be monitored continuously because inotropic agents can cause arrhythmias and myocardial ischemia.

Short-term mechanical circulatory support should be considered in patients remaining severely hypoperfused despite inotropic therapy and with a potentially reversible cause (e.g. viral myocarditis) or a potentially surgically correctable cause (e.g. acute interventricular septal rupture).

**An intravenous infusion of levosimendan** (or a phosphodiesterase inhibitor) may be considered to reverse the effect of beta-blockade if beta-blockade is thought to be contributing to hypoperfusion.

A vasopressor (e.g. dopamine or noradrenaline (norepinephrine) may be considered in patients who have cardiogenic shock, despite treatment with an inotrope. Intra-arterial blood pressure measurement should be considered.

Short-term mechanical circulatory support may be considered in patients deteriorating rapidly before a full diagnostic and clinical evaluation can be made.

*Monitoring:* Systolic blood pressure, heart rhythm and rate, saturation of peripheral oxygen ($SpO_2$) using a pulse oximeter, and urine output should be monitored on a regular and frequent basis until the patient is stabilised.

It is important to examine the patient repeatedly, including assessment for any new heart murmurs, e.g. a patient who has severe pulmonary edema following a myocardial infarction may go on to develop a ventricular septal defect or mitral regurgitation (confirm with an echocardiogram).

Renal function, electrolytes, serial ECGs and cardiac enzymes should also be closely monitored.

Intra-arterial line—insertion of an intra-arterial line should only be considered in patients with persistent heart failure and a low systolic blood pressure despite treatment.

*Pulmonary artery catheterisation:* *Right heart* catheterisation does not have a general role in the management of acute heart failure, but may help in the treatment of a minority of selected patients with acute heart failure.

### After Stabilisation

*Angiotensin-converting enzyme (ACE) inhibitor/angiotensin-II receptor antagonist (AIIRA):* In patients with reduced EF not already receiving an ACE inhibitor (or AIIRA), this treatment should be started as soon as possible, blood pressure and renal function permitting.

***Beta-blocker:*** In patients with reduced EF not already receiving a beta-blocker, this treatment should be started as soon as possible after stabilisation, blood pressure and heart rate permitting.

*Mineralocorticoid (aldosterone) receptor antagonist (MRA):* in patients with reduced EF not already receiving an MRA, this treatment should be started as soon as possible, renal function and potassium permitting. As the dose of MRA used to treat heart failure (HF) has a minimal effect on blood pressure, even relatively hypotensive patients may be started on this therapy during admission.

***Digoxin:*** In patients with reduced EF, digoxin may be used to control the ventricular rate in atrial fibrillation, especially if it has not been possible to up-titrate the dose of beta-blocker. Digoxin may also provide symptom benefit and reduce the risk of hospital admission for heart failure in patients with severe systolic heart failure.

It is common to restrict sodium intake to <2 g/day and fluid intake to <1.5–2.0 L/day, especially during the initial management of an acute episode of heart failure associated with volume overload, although there is no firm evidence to support this practice.

*Noninvasive ventilation:* Continuous positive airway pressure and noninvasive positive pressure ventilation relieve dyspnoea and improve certain physiological measures (e.g. oxygen saturation) in patients with acute pulmonary edema.

***Noninvasive ventilation*** should be considered in dyspnoeic patients with pulmonary edema and a respiratory rate >20 breaths/minute to improve breathlessness and reduce hypercapnia and acidosis.

Noninvasive ventilation can reduce blood pressure and should not generally be used in patients with a systolic blood pressure of <85 mmHg (and blood pressure should be monitored regularly when this treatment is used).

A recent large RCT showed that neither type of noninvasive ventilation reduced mortality or the rate of endotracheal intubation when compared with standard therapy, including nitrates and opiates.

*Endotracheal intubation and invasive ventilation:* The primary indication for endotracheal intubation and invasive ventilation is respiratory failure leading to hypoxaemia, hypercapnia, and acidosis.

Physical exhaustion, diminished consciousness, and inability to maintain or protect the airway are other reasons to consider intubation and ventilation.

*Mechanical circulatory support:* The conventional indications for an intra-aortic balloon pump are to support the circulation before surgical correction of specific acute mechanical problems, during severe acute myocarditis and in selected patients with acute myocardial ischemia or infarction before, during, and after percutaneous or surgical revascularisation. There is no good evidence that an IABP is of benefit in other causes of cardiogenic shock. More recently, balloon pumps (and other types of short-term, temporary circulatory support) have been used to bridge patients until implantation of a ventricular assist device or heart transplantation.

**Ventricular assist devices and other forms of mechanical circulatory support (MCS)** may be used as a 'bridge to decision' or longer term in selected patients.

*Ultrafiltration:* Venovenous isolated ultrafiltration is sometimes used to remove fluid in patients with heart failure, although it is usually reserved for those unresponsive or resistant to diuretics.

### Other Treatments

*Arrhythmias:* Pacing is recommended in patients hemodynamically compromised by severe bradycardia or heart block.

Renal dysfunction may limit the use of ACE inhibitors and AIIRAs; progressive acute kidney injury and volume overload may require renal replacement therapy.

*Surgical options* include coronary revascularisation, correction of anatomical lesions, valve replacement or reconstruction, mechanical assist devices for temporary circulatory support and heart transplantation.

In severe cases of refractory cardiogenic shock, consider early transfer of appropriate patients to a tertiary medical center where, if clinically indicated, more advanced treatments, such as implantation of a left ventricular assist device and or cardiac transplantation, may be performed.

## BIBLIOGRAPHY


1. Bauer JB, Randazzo MA. Nesiritide for outpatient treatment of heart failure. Am J Health Syst Pharm 2005;15;62(24): 2639–2642.
2. Binanay C, Califf RM, Hasselblad V, et al. Evaluation study of congestive heart failure and pulmonary artery catheterization effectiveness: the ESCAPE trial. JAMA 2005;294(5): 1625–33.
3. Cheng JW, Merl MY, Nguyen HM. Effect of nesiritide on renal function: a retrospective review. Curr Med Res Opin 2005;21(11):1857–63.
4. Ducharme A, Swedberg K, Pfeffer MA, et al. Prevention of atrial fibrillation in patients with symptomatic chronic heart failure by candesartan in the Candesartan in Heart failure: Assessment of Reduction in Mortality and morbidity (CHARM) program. Am Heart J 2006;152(1):86–92.
5. Earl GL, Fitzpatrick JT. Levosimendan: a novel inotropic agent for treatment of acute, decompensated heart failure. Ann Pharmacother 2005;39(11):1888–96.
6. Follath F, Franco F, Cardoso JS. European experience on the practical use of levosimendan in patients with acute heart failure syndromes. Am J Cardiol 2005;96(6A):80G–5G.
7. Frontin P, Bounes V, Houze-Cerfon CH, et al. Continuous positive airway pressure for cardiogenic pulmonary edema: a randomized study. Am J Emerg Med. 2011;29(7):775–81.
8. LHer E, Duquesne F, Girou E, de Rosiere XD, et al. Noninvasive continuous positive airway pressure in elderly cardiogenic pulmonary edema patients. Intensive Care Med 2004;30(5):882–8.
9. Maggioni AP, Latini R, Carson PE, et al. Valsartan reduces the incidence of atrial fibrillation in patients with heart failure: results from the Valsartan Heart Failure Trial (Val-HeFT). Am Heart J 2005;149(3):548–57.
10. Mehta S, Jay GD, Woolard RH. Randomized, prospective trial of bilevel versus continuous positive airway pressure in acute pulmonary edema. Crit Care Med 1997;25(4):620–8.
11. Mehta S, Nava S. Mask ventilation and cardiogenic pulmonary edema: another brick in the wall. Intensive Care Med 2005;31(6):757–9.
12. Newby D. Efficacy of non-invasive ventilation in patients with acute cardiogenic pulmonary edema: The 3CPO trial. Presented at the ESC meeting. Sept 2007.
13. O'Connor CM, Starling RC, Hernandez AF, et al. Effect of nesiritide in patients with acute decompensated heart failure. N Engl J Med 2011;365(1):32–43.
14. Parissis JT, Filippatos G, Farmakis D, et al. Levosimendan for the treatment of acute heart failure syndromes. Expert Opin.
15. Ray P, Arthaud M, Birolleau S, et al. Comparison of brain natriuretic peptide and probrain natriuretic peptide in the diagnosis of cardiogenic pulmonary edema in patients aged 65 and older. J Am Geriatr Soc 2005;53(4):643–8.
16. Scroggins N, Edwards M, Delgado R (3rd). Increased cost effectiveness with nesiritide vs. milrinone or dobutamine in the treatment of acute decompensated heart failure. Congest Heart Fail 2005;11(6):311–4.
17. Weitz G, Struck J, Zonak A, et al. Prehospital noninvasive pressure support ventilation for acute cardiogenic pulmonary edema. Eur J Emerg Med 2007;14(5):276–9.

# 8 Recognition and Management of Heart Failure

Heart failure is the pathophysiologic state in which the heart, via an abnormality of cardiac function (detectable or not), fails to pump blood at a rate commensurate with the requirements of the metabolizing tissues or is able to do so only with an elevated diastolic filling pressure. Heart failure is a common condition, affecting up to 3 per cent of the population aged 45 and older, and is associated with high mortality and poor quality of life. Major diagnostic and therapeutic advances have been made over the past three decades, but international and national audits suggest that many patients are incompletely investigated and treated.

Heart failure may be caused by myocardial failure, but may also occur in the presence of near-normal cardiac function under conditions of high demand. Heart failure always causes circulatory failure, but the converse is not necessarily the case, because various noncardiac conditions (e.g. hypovolemic shock, septic shock) can produce circulatory failure in the presence of normal, modestly impaired, or even supranormal cardiac function. To maintain the pumping function of the heart, compensatory mechanisms increase blood volume, cardiac filling pressure, heart rate, and cardiac muscle mass. However, despite these mechanisms, there is progressive decline in the ability of the heart to contract and relax, resulting in worsening heart failure.

Signs and symptoms of heart failure include tachycardia and manifestations of venous congestion (e.g. edema) and low cardiac output (e.g. fatigue). Breathlessness is a cardinal symptom of left ventricular (LV) failure that may manifest with progressively increasing severity (Figs 8.1 and 8.2).

## CLASSIFICATION IN HEART FAILURE

Heart failure can be classified according to a variety of factors (*see* heart failure criteria and classification).

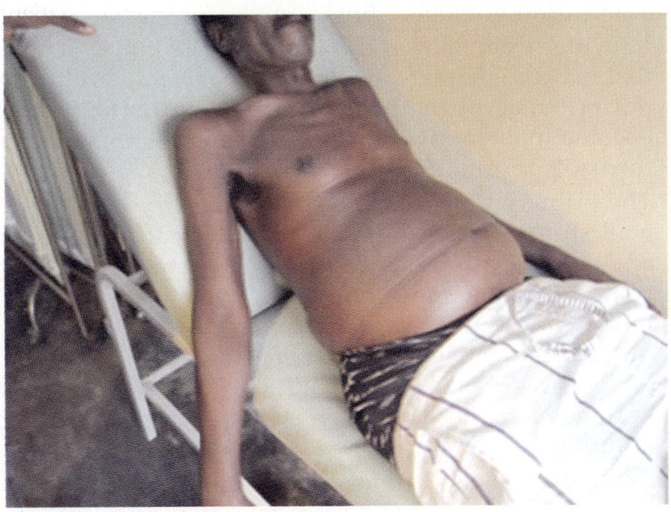

**Fig. 8.1:** A 40-year-old male patient showing generalized edema of the body, ascites and semiconscious state of mind in severe form of heart failure

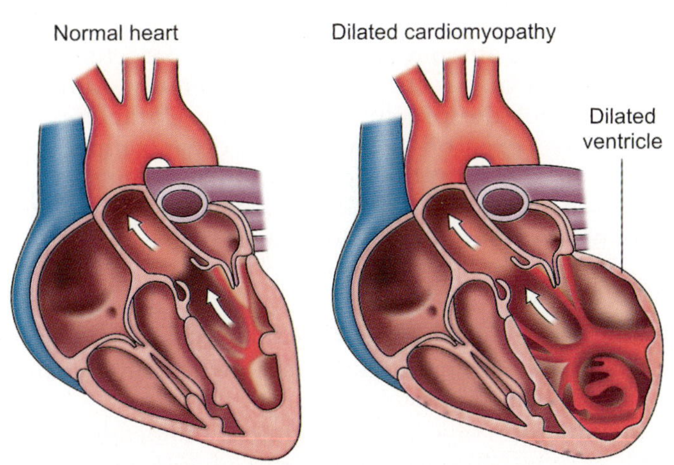


**Fig. 8.2:** Normal heart (left) and dilated cardiomyopathy as one of the causes of heart failure

**Table 8.1:** NYHA functional classification of heart failure

| Class | Functional capacity |
|---|---|
| I | Patients without limitation of physical activity |
| II | Patients with slight limitation of physical activity, in which ordinary physical activity leads to fatigue, palpitation, dyspnea, or anginal pain; they are comfortable at rest |
| III | Patients with marked limitation of physical activity, in which less than ordinary activity results in fatigue, palpitation, dyspnea, or anginal pain; they are comfortable at rest |
| IV | Patients who are not only unable to carry on any physical activity without discomfort but also have symptoms of heart failure or the anginal syndrome even at rest; the patient's discomfort increases if any physical activity is undertaken |

*Source:* American Heart Association. Classes of heart failure. Available at:http://www.heart.org/HEARTORG/Conditions/HeartFailure/AboutHeartFailure/Classes-of-Heart-Failure_UCM_306328_Article.jsp. Accessed: September 6, 2011.

The New York Heart Association (NYHA) classification for heart failure comprises four classes, based on the relationship between symptoms and the amount of effort required to provoke them, as follows (Table 8.1):

- Class I patients have no limitation of physical activity
- Class II patients have slight limitation of physical activity
- Class III patients have marked limitation of physical activity
- Class IV patients have symptoms even at rest and are unable to carry on any physical activity without discomfort

The American College of Cardiology/American Heart Association (ACC/AHA) heart failure guidelines complement the NYHA classification to reflect the progression of disease and are divided into four stages, as follows:

- **Stage A** patients are at high risk for heart failure but have no structural heart disease or symptoms of heart failure
- **Stage B** patients have structural heart disease but have no symptoms of heart failure
- **Stage C** patients have structural heart disease and have symptoms of heart failure
- **Stage D** patients have refractory heart failure requiring specialized interventions

## PATHOPHYSIOLOGY OF HEART FAILURE

The common pathophysiologic state that perpetuates the progression of heart failure is extremely complex, regardless of the precipitating event. Compensatory mechanisms exist on every level of organization, from subcellular all the way through organ-to-organ interactions. Only when this network of adaptations becomes overwhelmed does heart failure ensue (Fig. 8.3).

### Adaptations

Most important among the adaptations are the following:

- The Frank-Starling mechanism, in which an increased preload helps to sustain cardiac performance
- Alterations in myocyte regeneration and death
- Myocardial hypertrophy with or without cardiac chamber dilatation, in which the mass of contractile tissue is augmented.

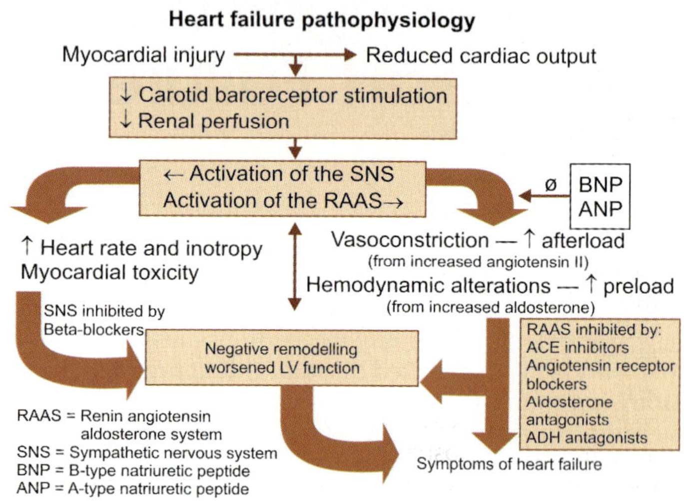


**Fig. 8.3:** Various stepts in the pathophysiology of heart failure

### Activation of Neurohumoral Systems

The release of norepinephrine by adrenergic cardiac nerves augments myocardial contractility and includes activation of the renin-angiotensin-aldosterone system (RAAS), the sympathetic nervous system (SNS), and other neurohumoral adjustments that act to maintain arterial pressure and perfusion of vital organs.

- In acute heart failure, the finite adaptive mechanisms that may be adequate to maintain the overall contractile performance of the heart at relatively normal levels become maladaptive when trying to sustain adequate cardiac performance.
- The primary myocardial response to chronic increased wall stress is myocyte hypertrophy, death/apoptosis, and regeneration. This process eventually leads to remodeling, usually the eccentric type. Eccentric remodeling further worsens the loading conditions on the remaining myocytes and perpetuates the deleterious cycle. The idea of lowering wall stress to slow the process of remodeling has long been exploited in treating heart failure patients.
- The reduction of cardiac output following myocardial injury sets into motion a cascade of hemodynamic and neurohormonal derangements that provoke activation of neuroendocrine systems, most notably the above-mentioned adrenergic systems and RAAS.

- The release of epinephrine and norepinephrine, along with the vasoactive substances endothelin-1 (ET-1) and vasopressin, causes vasoconstriction, which increases calcium afterload and, via an increase in cyclic adenosine monophosphate (cAMP), causes an increase in cytosolic calcium entry. The increased calcium entry into the myocytes augments myocardial contractility and impairs myocardial relaxation (lusitropy).
- The calcium overload may induce arrhythmias and lead to sudden death. The increase in afterload and myocardial contractility (known as inotropy) and the impairment in myocardial lusitropy lead to an increase in myocardial energy expenditure and a further decrease in cardiac output. The increase in myocardial energy expenditure leads to myocardial cell death/apoptosis, which results in heart failure and further reduction in cardiac output, perpetuating a cycle of further increased neurohumoral stimulation and further adverse hemodynamic and myocardial responses.
- In addition, the activation of the RAAS leads to salt and water retention, resulting in increased preload and further increases in myocardial energy expenditure. Increases in renin, mediated by decreased stretch of the glomerular afferent arteriole, reduce delivery of chloride to the macula densa and increase beta1-adrenergic activity as a response to decreased cardiac output. This results in an increase in angiotensin II (Ang II) levels and, in turn, aldosterone levels, causing stimulation of the release of aldosterone. Ang II, along with ET-1, is crucial in maintaining effective intravascular homeostasis mediated by vasoconstriction and aldosterone-induced salt and water retention.
- The concept of the heart as a self-renewing organ is a relatively recent development.This new paradigm for myocyte biology has created an entire field of research aimed directly at augmenting myocardial regeneration. The rate of myocyte turnover has been shown to increase during times of pathologic stress. In heart failure, this mechanism for replacement becomes overwhelmed by an even faster increase in the rate of myocyte loss. This imbalance of hypertrophy and death over regeneration is the final common pathway at the cellular level for the progression of remodeling and heart failure.

### Ang II

Research indicates that local cardiac Ang II production (which decreases lusitropy, increases inotropy, and increases afterload) leads to increased myocardial energy expenditure. Ang II has also been shown *in vitro* and *in vivo* to increase the rate of myocyte apoptosis. In this fashion, Ang II has similar actions to norepinephrine in heart failure.

Ang II also mediates myocardial cellular hypertrophy and may promote progressive loss of myocardial function. The neurohumoral factors above lead to myocyte hypertrophy and interstitial fibrosis, resulting in increased myocardial volume and increased myocardial mass, as well as myocyte loss. As a result, the cardiac architecture changes, which, in turn, leads to further increase in myocardial volume and mass.

### Myocytes and Myocardial Remodeling

In the failing heart, increased myocardial volume is characterized by larger myocytes approaching the end of their life cycle. As more myocytes drop out, an increased load is placed on the remaining myocardium, and this unfavorable environment is transmitted to the progenitor cells responsible for replacing lost myocytes.

Progenitor cells become progressively less effective as the underlying pathologic process worsens and myocardial failure accelerates. These features namely, the increased myocardial volume and mass, along with a net loss of myocytes are the hallmark of myocardial remodeling. This remodeling process leads to early adaptive mechanisms, such as augmentation of stroke volume (Frank-Starling mechanism) and decreased wall stress (Laplace's law), and, later, to maladaptive mechanisms such as increased myocardial oxygen demand, myocardial ischemia, impaired contractility, and arrhythmogenesis.

As heart failure advances, there is a relative decline in the counterregulatory effects of endogenous vasodilators, including nitric oxide (NO), prostaglandins (PGs), bradykinin (BK), atrial natriuretic peptide (ANP), and B-type natriuretic peptide (BNP). This decline occurs simultaneously with the increase in vasoconstrictor substances from the RAAS and the adrenergic system, which fosters further increases in vasoconstriction and thus preload and afterload. This results in cellular proliferation, adverse myocardial remodeling, and antinatriuresis, with total body fluid excess and worsening of heart failure symptoms.

### Systolic and Diastolic Failure

Systolic and diastolic heart failure each results in a decrease in stroke volume. This leads to activation of peripheral and central baroreflexes and chemoreflexes that are capable of eliciting marked increases in sympathetic nerve traffic (Tables 8.2–8.4).

**Table 8.2:** Causes of systolic heart failure

- Coronary artery disease
- Hypertension
- Alcohol
- Valvular heart disease
- Familial genetic cardiomyopathy
- Myocarditis
- Toxins (chemotherapy, cocaine)
- Collagen vascular disease
- Metabolic disorders
- Endocrine disorders
- Electrolyte disorders
- Acidosis
- Sepsis
- Hypoxia
- Severe sleep apnea

**Table 8.3:** Criteria for diagnosis of diastolic heart failure

*European study group*

1. Evidence of CHF
2. Normal or mildly abnormal LV systolic function
3. Evidence of abnormal LV relaxation, filling, distensibility or stiffness

*Framingham heart study*

1. Definitive diagnosis of CHF (signs and symptoms; CXR; response to diuretics)
2. LVEF greater than or equal to 50% within 72 hours of episode
3. Objective evidence of LV diastolic dysfunction (abnormal LV relaxation/filling distensibility indices by catheterization)

While there are commonalities in the neurohormonal responses to decreased stroke volume, the neurohormone-mediated events that follow have been most clearly elucidated for individuals with systolic heart failure. The ensuing elevation in plasma norepinephrine directly correlates with the degree of cardiac dysfunction and has significant prognostic implications. Norepinephrine, while directly toxic to cardiac myocytes, is also responsible for a variety of signal-transduction abnormalities, such as down-regulation of beta1-adrenergic receptors, uncoupling of beta2-adrenergic receptors, and increased activity of inhibitory G-protein. Changes in beta1-adrenergic receptors result in overexpression and promote myocardial hypertrophy.

## PATHOPHYSIOLOGY OF DIASTOLIC HEART FAILURE (DHF)

Diastole is the process by which the heart returns to its relaxed state; it is also the time for cardiac perfusion. Drastic changes occur in cardiac pressure-volume relationships during diastole. The diastolic process has four identifiable phases: isovolumetric relaxation time, the time of aortic valve closure to mitral valve opening; early rapid filling after mitral valve opening; diastasis, a period of low flow during mid-diastole and late filling of the ventricles by atrial contraction.Diastole is a complex process that is affected by a number of factors, including hypertension, ischemia, heart rate, velocity of relaxation, cardiac compliance (i.e. elastic recoil and stiffness), hypertrophy and segmental wall coordination of the heart muscle. The pathophysiology of diastolic dysfunction includes delayed relaxation, impaired LV filling and/or increased stiffness. These conditions result typically in an upward displacement of the diastolic pressure-volume relationship with increased end-diastolic, left atrial and pulmocapillary wedge pressure leading to DHF.Chronic hypertension is the most common cause of diastolic dysfunction and failure. It leads to left ventricular hypertrophy and increased connective tissue content, both of which decrease cardiac compliance.

The hypertrophied ventricle has a steeper diastolic pressure-volume relationship; therefore, a small increase

**Table 8.4:** Clues for differentiating between systolic and diastolic dysfunction in patients with heart failure

| Clues from the evaluation | Systolic dysfunction | Diastolic dysfunction |
|---|---|---|
| History | | |
| Hypertension | XX | XXX |
| Coronary artery disease* | XXX | X |
| Diabetes mellitus | XXX | XX |
| Valvular heart disease* | XXX | — |
| Physical examination | | |
| Third heard sound (S 3) gallop* | XXX | X |
| Fourth heart sound (S 4) gallop* | X | XXX |
| Rales | XX | XX |
| Jugular venous distention | XX | X |
| Edema | XX | X |
| Displaced point of maximal impulse* | XX | — |
| Mitral regurgitation* | XXX | X |
| Chest radiograph | | |
| Cardiomegaly* | XXX | X |
| Pulmonary congestion | XXX | XXX |
| Electrocardiogram Q-wave | XX | X |
| Left ventricular hypertrophy* | X | XXX |
| Echocardiogram Decreased ejection fraction* | XXX | — |
| Dilated left ventricle* | XX | — |
| Left ventricle hypertrophy* | X | XXX |

X=suggestive; the number of Xs reflects the relative weight; —=not suggestive. *=Particularly helpful in distinguishing systolic from diastolic dysfunction in heart failure. Adapted with permission from Young JB. Assessment of heart failure. In: Braunwald E. Atlas of heart disease. Vol 4. Philadelphia: Current Medicine, 1995:7.1–7.2

in left ventricular end-diastolic volume causes a marked increase in left ventricular end diastolic pressure. Another most common cardiac disease associated with abnormal LV diastolic function is myocardial ischemia. Relaxation of the ventricles involves the active transport of calcium ions into the sarcoplasmic reticulum, which allows the dissociation of myosin-actin cross bridges. Myocardial ischemia deprives the system of adequate adenosine triphosphate, which in turn inhibits the dissociation process by altering the balance of the adenosine triphosphate to adenosine diphosphate ratio, which may contribute to diastolic dysfunction. The heart rate determines the time that is available for diastolic filling, coronary perfusion and ventricular relaxation. In DHF, increase in cardiac output relatively depends upon heart rate but a rapid heart rate may further elevate abnormal LV filling pressures.

Tachycardia adversely affects diastolic function by several mechanisms; it decreases left ventricular filling and coronary perfusion times, increases myocardial oxygen consumption and causes incomplete relaxation because the stiff heart cannot increase its velocity of relaxation as heart rate increases. In effect, the ventricle may never fully relax to receive blood adequately. Similarly, atrial fibrillation completely eliminates the late diastolic atrial contribution to LV filling, upon which patients with diastolic dysfunction are dependent, often precipitating pulmonary edema.

Diastolic dysfunction is more common in elderly persons, partly because of increased collagen cross-linking, increased smooth muscle content and loss of elastic fibers. These changes tend to decrease ventricular compliance it making more susceptible to the adverse effects of hypertension, tachycardia and atrial fibrillation.

In last two decades there is a substantial increase in prevalence of diastolic heart failure from 38–54%. The prognosis of patients suffering from DHF is as ominous as prognosis of patients suffering from systolic heart failure (SHF). The various predisposing factors are old age, female gender, metabolic syndrome, diabetes, arterial hypertension and left ventricular hypertrophy. Elderly patients usually present with DHF in the setting of acute myocardial infarction. As there is epidemiological evolution towards DHF in the population all over the world, a reappraisal of original established set of criteria is necessary for diagnosis of DHF. However, newer modalities of Echo-Doppler strain techniques may help in predicting the precursors of DHF. These echo variables include left atrial (LA) strain and strain rate, LA stiffness and LA ejection fraction. Segmental left ventricular (LV) deformation analysis for calculating contractile parameters such as strain and strain rate is now possible using noninvasive echo-Doppler techniques. It has been reported that LA systolic and diastolic function can also be assessed using these Doppler strain techniques. Although LA enlargement increases with the severity of diastolic dysfunction, the ability of LA volume measurements to discriminate asymptomatic LV diastolic dysfunction from early DHF heart failure has not been possible. However, the concept that an alteration in LA function or stiffness may be the early indicators of occult diastolic dysfunction and is therefore novel and worth exploring.

## Diagnosis of Diastolic Heart Failure

The working group for the european society of cardiology proposed that diagnosis of DHF requires three obligatory diagnostic criteria to be simultaneously satisfied; signs and symptoms of congestive heart failure; normal or mildly abnormal systolic LV systolic function and evidence of LV diastolic dysfunction (abnormal LV relaxation, filling, diastolic distensibility or diastolic stiffness).

1. Signs and symptoms of congestive heart failure signs include lung crepitations, pulmonary edema, ankle swelling, hepatomegaly, dyspnea on exertion and fatigue.
2. Normal or mildly abnormal systolic left ventricular function.

The presence of normal or mildly abnormal systolic LV function constitutes the second criterion for the diagnosis of heart failure (HF) with normal left ventricular ejection fraction (LVEF)-HFNLVEF. In the present consensus document, an LVEF >50% is also considered consistent with the presence of normal or mildly abnormal systolic LV function. LVEF needs to be assessed in accordance to the recent recommendations for cardiac chamber quantification of the American Society of Echocardiography and the European Association of Echocardiography. It is of importance to note that in DHF reduced long-axis shortening is frequently compensated for by increased short-axis shortening. As already demonstrated by Frank, Starling, and Wiggers and later re-appraised, LV relaxation depends on endsystolic load and volume. The criterion of presence of normal or mildly abnormal LV function therefore needs to be implemented with measures of LV volumes. To exclude significant LV enlargement 25, LVEDVI and LV end-systolic volume index cannot exceed 97 ml/m$^2$ and 49 ml/m$^2$, respectively.

### *ANP and BNP*

ANP and BNP are endogenously generated peptides activated in response to atrial and ventricular volume/pressure expansion. ANP and BNP are released from the atria and ventricles, respectively, and both promote vasodilation and natriuresis. Their hemodynamic effects are mediated by decreases in ventricular filling pressures, owing to reductions in cardiac preload and afterload. BNP, in particular, produces selective afferent arteriolar vasodilation and inhibits sodium reabsorption in the proximal convoluted tubule. It also inhibits renin and aldosterone release and, therefore, adrenergic activation. ANP and BNP are elevated in chronic heart failure. BNP, in particular, has potentially important diagnostic, therapeutic, and prognostic implications.

### *Other Vasoactive Systems*

Other vasoactive systems that play a role in the pathogenesis of heart failure include the ET receptor system, the adenosine receptor system, vasopressin, and tumor necrosis factor-alpha (TNF-alpha). ET, a substance produced by the vascular endothelium, may contribute to the regulation of myocardial function, vascular tone, and peripheral resistance in heart failure. Elevated levels of ET-1 closely correlate with the severity of heart failure. ET-1 is a potent vasoconstrictor and has exaggerated vasoconstrictor effects in the renal vasculature, reducing renal plasma blood flow, glomerular filtration rate (GFR), and sodium excretion. TNF-alpha has been implicated in response to various infectious and inflammatory conditions. Elevations in TNF-alpha levels have been consistently observed in heart failure and seem to correlate with the degree of myocardial dysfunction. Some studies suggest that local production of TNF-alpha may have toxic effects on the myocardium, thus worsening myocardial systolic and diastolic function.

In individuals with systolic dysfunction, therefore, the neurohormonal responses to decreased stroke volume result in temporary improvement in systolic blood pressure and tissue perfusion. However, in all circumstances, the existing data support the notion that these neurohormonal responses contribute to the progression of myocardial dysfunction in the long term.

### *Heart Failure with Normal Ejection Fraction*

In diastolic heart failure [heart failure with normal ejection fraction (HFNEF)], the same pathophysiologic processes occur that lead to decreased cardiac output in systolic heart failure, but they do so in response to a different set of hemodynamic and circulatory environmental factors that depress cardiac output.

In HFNEF, altered relaxation and increased stiffness of the ventricle (due to delayed calcium uptake by the myocyte sarcoplasmic reticulum and delayed calcium efflux from the myocyte) occur in response to an increase in ventricular afterload (pressure overload). The impaired relaxation of the ventricle then leads to impaired diastolic filling of the left ventricle (LV). Morris et al. found that RV subendocardial systolic dysfunction and diastolic dysfunction, as detected by echocardiographic strain rate imaging, are common in patients with HFNEF. This dysfunction is potentially associated with the same fibrotic processes that affect the subendocardial layer of the LV and, to a lesser extent, with RV pressure overload. This may play a role in the symptomatology of patients with HFNEF.

### LV Chamber Stiffness

An increase in LV chamber stiffness occurs secondary to any one of, or any combination of, the following three mechanisms:

#### *Rise in Filling Pressure*

- Shift to a steeper ventricular pressure-volume curve
- Decrease in ventricular distensibility
- A rise in filling pressure is the movement of the ventricle up along its pressure-volume curve to a steeper portion, as may occur in conditions such as volume overload secondary to acute valvular regurgitation or acute LV failure due to myocarditis.
- A shift to a steeper ventricular pressure-volume curve results, most commonly, not only from increased ventricular mass and wall thickness (as observed in aortic stenosis and long-standing hypertension) but also from infiltrative disorders (e.g. amyloidosis), endomyocardial fibrosis, and myocardial ischemia.
- Parallel upward displacement of the diastolic pressure-volume curve is generally referred to as a decrease in ventricular distensibility. This is usually caused by extrinsic compression of the ventricles.

#### *Concentric LV Hypertrophy*

Pressure overload that leads to concentric LV hypertrophy (LVH), as occurs in aortic stenosis, hypertension, and hypertrophic cardiomyopathy, shifts the diastolic pressure-volume curve to the left along its volume axis. As a result, ventricular diastolic pressure is abnormally elevated, although chamber stiffness may or may not be altered.

Increases in diastolic pressure lead to increased myocardial energy expenditure, remodeling of the ventricle, increased myocardial oxygen demand, myocardial ischemia, and eventual progression of the maladaptive mechanisms of the heart that lead to decompensated heart failure.

### Arrhythmias

While life-threatening rhythms are more common in ischemic cardiomyopathy, arrhythmia imparts a significant burden in all forms of heart failure. In fact, some arrhythmias even perpetuate heart failure. The most significant of all rhythms associated with heart failure are the life-threatening ventricular arrhythmias. Structural substrates for ventricular arrhythmias that are common in heart failure, regardless of the underlying cause, include ventricular dilatation, myocardial hypertrophy, and myocardial fibrosis. At the cellular level, myocytes may be exposed to increased stretch, wall tension, catecholamines, ischemia, and electrolyte imbalance. The combination of these factors contributes to an increased incidence of arrhythmogenic sudden cardiac death in patients with heart failure.

## AETIOLOGICAL FACTORS

Most patients who present with significant heart failure do so because of an inability to provide adequate cardiac output in that setting. This is often a combination of the causes listed below in the setting of an abnormal myocardium. The list of causes responsible for presentation of a patient with heart failure exacerbation is very long, and searching for the proximate cause to optimize therapeutic interventions is important.

From a clinical standpoint, classifying the causes of heart failure into the following four broad categories is useful:

1. **Underlying causes:** Underlying causes of heart failure include structural abnormalities (congenital or acquired) that affect the peripheral and coronary arterial circulation, pericardium, myocardium, or cardiac valves, thus leading to increased hemodynamic burden or myocardial or coronary insufficiency.

2. **Fundamental causes:** Fundamental causes include the biochemical and physiologic mechanisms, through which either an increased hemodynamic burden or a reduction in oxygen delivery to the myocardium results in impairment of myocardial contraction.
3. **Precipitating causes:** Overt heart failure may be precipitated by progression of the underlying heart disease (e.g. further narrowing of a stenotic aortic valve or mitral valve) or various conditions (fever, anemia and infection) or medications [chemotherapy, (NSAIDs)] that alter the homeostasis of heart failure patients.
4. **Genetics of cardiomyopathy:** Dilated, arrhythmic right ventricular and restrictive cardiomyopathies are known genetic causes of heart failure.

## UNDERLYING CAUSES

Specific underlying factors cause various forms of heart failure, such as systolic heart failure (most commonly, left ventricular systolic dysfunction), heart failure with preserved LVEF, acute heart failure, high-output heart failure, and right heart failure.

*Underlying causes of systolic heart failure include the following:*
- Coronary artery disease
- Diabetes mellitus
- Hypertension
- Valvular heart disease (stenosis or regurgitant lesions)
- Arrhythmia (supraventricular or ventricular)
- Infections and inflammation (myocarditis)
- Peripartum cardiomyopathy
- Congenital heart disease
- Drugs (either recreational, such as alcohol and cocaine, or therapeutic drugs with cardiac side effects, such as doxorubicin)
- Idiopathic cardiomyopathy
- Rare conditions (endocrine abnormalities, rheumatologic disease, neuromuscular conditions).

*Underlying causes of diastolic heart failure include the following:*
- Coronary artery disease
- Diabetes mellitus
- Hypertension
- Valvular heart disease (aortic stenosis)
- Hypertrophic cardiomyopathy
- Restrictive cardiomyopathy (amyloidosis, sarcoidosis)
- Constrictive pericarditis

*Underlying causes of acute heart failure include the following:*
- Acute valvular (mitral or aortic) regurgitation
- Myocardial infarction
- Myocarditis
- Arrhythmia
- Drugs (e.g. cocaine, calcium channel blockers, or beta-blocker overdose)
- Sepsis

*Underlying causes of high-output heart failure include the following:*
- Anemia
- Systemic arteriovenous fistulas
- Hyperthyroidism
- Beriberi heart disease
- Paget disease of bone
- Albright syndrome (fibrous dysplasia)
- Multiple myeloma
- Pregnancy
- Glomerulonephritis
- Polycythemia vera
- Carcinoid syndrome.

*Underlying causes of right heart failure include the following:*
- Left ventricular failure
- Coronary artery disease (ischemia)
- Pulmonary hypertension
- Pulmonary valve stenosis
- Pulmonary embolism
- Chronic pulmonary disease
- Neuromuscular disease.

### *Precipitating Causes of Heart Failure*

A previously stable, compensated patient may develop heart failure that is clinically apparent for the first time when the intrinsic process has advanced to a critical point, such as with further narrowing of a stenotic aortic valve or mitral valve. Alternatively, decompensation may occur as a result of failure or exhaustion of the compensatory mechanisms but without any change in the load on the heart in patients with persistent, severe pressure or volume overload. In particular, consider whether the patient has underlying coronary artery disease or valvular heart disease (Table 8.5).

The most common cause of decompensation in a previously compensated patient with heart failure is

**Table 8.5:** Decompensated advanced heart failure, precipitating factors

- Poor medication or dietary compliance (sodium, fluid)
- Uncontrolled hypertension
- Cardiac arrhythmias
  - New onset sustained tachy or brady arrhythmias
  - Paroxysmal atrial fibrillation/flutter
- Envioronmental factors/stresses
- Inadequate chronic therapy
  - Inadequate ACE inhibition
- Myocardial infarction/ischemia
- Progression of underlying cardiac disease
- Superimposed new disease
  - Pulmonary infection
  - Pulmonary thromboembolism
  - Thyroid disease (amiodarone)
  - Anemia

inappropriate reduction in the intensity of treatment, such as dietary sodium restriction, physical activity reduction, or drug regimen reduction. Uncontrolled hypertension is the second most common cause of decompensation, followed closely by cardiac arrhythmias (most commonly, atrial fibrillation). Arrhythmias, particularly ventricular arrhythmias, can be life threatening. Also, patients with one form of underlying heart disease that may be well compensated can develop heart failure when a second form of heart disease ensues. For example, a patient with chronic hypertension and asymptomatic LVH may be asymptomatic until a myocardial infarction (MI) develops and precipitates heart failure.

Systemic infection or the development of unrelated illness can also lead to heart failure. Systemic infection precipitates heart failure by increasing total metabolism as a consequence of fever, discomfort, and cough, increasing the hemodynamic burden on the heart. Septic shock, in particular, can precipitate heart failure by the release of endotoxin-induced factors that can depress myocardial contractility.

Cardiac infection and inflammation can also endanger the heart. Myocarditis or infective endocarditis may directly impair myocardial function and exacerbate existing heart disease. The anemia, fever, and tachycardia that frequently accompany these processes are also deleterious. In the case of infective endocarditis, the additional valvular damage that ensues may precipitate cardiac decompensation. Patients with heart failure, particularly when confined to bed, are at high risk of developing pulmonary emboli, which can increase the hemodynamic burden on the right ventricle by further elevating right ventricular (RV) systolic pressure, possibly causing fever, tachypnea, and tachycardia. Intense, prolonged physical exertion or severe fatigue, such as may result from prolonged travel or emotional crisis, is a relatively common precipitant of cardiac decompensation. The same is true of exposure to severe climate change (i.e. the individual comes in contact with a hot, humid environment or a bitterly cold one).

Excessive intake of water and/or sodium and the administration of cardiac depressants or drugs that cause salt retention are other factors that can lead to heart failure. Because of increased myocardial oxygen consumption and demand beyond a critical level, the following high-output states can precipitate the clinical presentation of heart failure:

- Profound anemia
- Thyrotoxicosis
- Myxedema
- Paget disease of bone
- Albright syndrome
- Multiple myeloma
- Glomerulonephritis
- Cor pulmonale
- Polycythemia vera
- Obesity
- Carcinoid syndrome
- Pregnancy
- Nutritional deficiencies (e.g. thiamine deficiency, beriberi)

Longitudinal data from the Framingham Heart Study suggests that antecedent subclinical left ventricular systolic or diastolic dysfunction is associated with an increased incidence of heart failure, supporting the notion that heart failure is a progressive syndrome. Another analysis of over 36,000 patients undergoing outpatient echocardiography reported that moderate or severe diastolic dysfunction, but not mild diastolic dysfunction, is an independent predictor of mortality.

### Genetics of Cardiomyopathy

Autosomal dominant inheritance has been demonstrated in dilated cardiomyopathy and in arrhythmic right ventricular cardiomyopathy. Restrictive cardiomyopathies are usually sporadic and associated with the gene for cardiac troponin I. Genetic tests are available at major genetic centers for cardiomyopathies.

In families with a first-degree relative who has been diagnosed with a cardiomyopathy leading to heart failure, the at-risk patient should be screened and followed. The recommended screening consists of an electrocardiogram and an echocardiogram. If the patient has an asymptomatic left ventricular dysfunction, it should be treated.

The Heart Failure Society of America (HFSA) also has the following recommendations for genetic evaluation of cardiomyopathy:

- For all patients with cardiomyopathy, take a detailed family history for at least three generations [hypertrophic cardiomyopathy (HCM), dilated cardiomyopathy (DCM), arrhythmic right ventricular dysplasia (ARVD), left ventricular noncompaction (LVNC), restrictive cardiomyopathy (RCM), and cardiomyopathies associated with extra-cardiac manifestations].
- Carefully assess the patient's medical history as well as that of asymptomatic first-degree relatives, with special focus on heart failure symptoms, arrhythmias, presyncope, and syncope.
- Screen asymptomatic first-degree relatives for cardiomyopathy (HCM, DCM, ARVD, LVNC, RCM, and cardiomyopathies associated with extra-cardiac manifestations).
- Screen for cardiomyopathy at intervals in asymptomatic at-risk relatives who are known to carry the disease-causing mutation(s).
- Screen for cardiomyopathy in asymptomatic at-risk first-degree relatives who have not undergone genetic testing or in whom a disease-causing mutation has not been identified.

**Note:** Due to the complexity of genetic evaluation, testing, and counseling of patients with cardiomyopathy, it is recommended that patients be referred to centers with expertise in these matters and in family-based management.

## Medical History

In evaluating heart failure patients, the clinician should ask about the following comorbidities and/or risk factors:

- Myopathy
- Previous MI
- Valvular heart disease
- familial heart disease
- Alcohol use
- Hypertension
- Diabetes
- Dyslipidemia
- Coronary/peripheral vascular disease
- Sleep-disordered breathing
- Collagen vascular disease, rheumatic fever
- Pheochromocytoma
- Thyroid disease
- Substance abuse history
- History of chemotherapy/radiation to the chest

*The New York Heart Association (NYHA) classification of heart failure:* It is widely used in practice and in clinical studies to quantify clinical assessment of heart failure. Breathlessness, a cardinal symptom of LV failure, may manifest with progressively increasing severity as the following:

- Exertional dyspnea
- Orthopnea
- Paroxysmal nocturnal dyspnea
- Dyspnea at rest
- Acute pulmonary edema

Other cardiac symptoms of heart failure include chest pain/pressure and palpitations. Common noncardiac signs and symptoms of heart failure include anorexia, nausea, weight loss, bloating, fatigue, weakness, oliguria, nocturia, and cerebral symptoms of varying severity, ranging from anxiety to memory impairment and confusion. Findings from the Framingham Heart Study suggest that subclinical cardiac dysfunction and noncardiac comorbidities are associated with increased incidence of heart failure, supporting the idea that heart failure is a progressive syndrome and that noncardiac factors are extremely important.

### Exertional Dyspnea

The principal difference between exertional dyspnea in patients who are healthy and exertional dyspnea in patients with heart failure is the degree of activity necessary to induce the symptom. As heart failure first develops, exertional dyspnea may simply appear to be an aggravation of the breathlessness that occurs in healthy persons during activity, but as LV failure advances, the intensity of exercise resulting in breathlessness progressively declines; however, subjective exercise capacity and objective measures of LV performance at rest in patients with heart failure are not closely correlated. Exertional dyspnea, in fact, may be absent in sedentary patients.

### Orthopnea

Orthopnea is an early symptom of heart failure and may be defined as dyspnea that develops in the recumbent position and is relieved with elevation of the head with pillows. As in the case of exertional dyspnea, the change in the number of pillows required is important. In the recumbent position, decreased pooling of blood in the lower extremities and abdomen occurs. Blood is displaced from the extrathoracic compartment to the thoracic compartment. The failing LV, operating on the flat portion of the Frank-Starling curve, cannot accept and pump out the extra volume of blood delivered to it without dilating. As a result, pulmonary venous and capillary pressures rise further, causing interstitial pulmonary edema, reduced pulmonary compliance, increased airway resistance, and dyspnea. Orthopnea occurs rapidly, often within a minute or two of recumbency, and develops when the patient is awake. Orthopnea may occur in any condition in which the vital capacity is low. Marked ascites, regardless of its aetiology, is an important cause of orthopnea. In advanced LV failure, orthopnea may be so severe that the patient cannot lie down and must sleep sitting up in a chair or slumped over a table.

**Cough,** particularly during recumbency, may be an 'orthopnea equivalent.' This nonproductive cough may be caused by pulmonary congestion and is relieved by the treatment of heart failure.

### Paroxysmal Nocturnal Dyspnea

Paroxysmal nocturnal dyspnea usually occurs at night and is defined as the sudden awakening of the patient, after a couple of hours of sleep, with a feeling of severe anxiety, breathlessness, and suffocation. The patient may bolt upright in bed and gasp for breath. Bronchospasm increases ventilatory difficulty and the work of breathing and is a common complicating factor of paroxysmal nocturnal dyspnea. On chest auscultation, the bronchospasm associated with a heart failure exacerbation can be difficult to distinguish from an acute asthma exacerbation, although other clues from the cardiovascular examination should lead the examiner to the correct diagnosis. Both types of bronchospasm can be present in a single individual.

In contrast to orthopnea, which may be relieved by immediately sitting up in bed, paroxysmal nocturnal dyspnea may require 30 minutes or longer in this position for relief. Episodes may be so frightening that the patient may be afraid to resume sleeping, even after the symptoms have subsided.

### Dyspnea at Rest

Dyspnea at rest in heart failure is the result of the following mechanisms (Fig. 8.4):

- Decreased pulmonary function secondary to decreased compliance and increased airway resistance
- Increased ventilatory drive secondary to hypoxemia due to increased pulmonary capillary wedge pressure (PCWP); ventilation/perfusion (V/Q) mismatching due to increased PCWP and low cardiac output; and increased carbon dioxide production

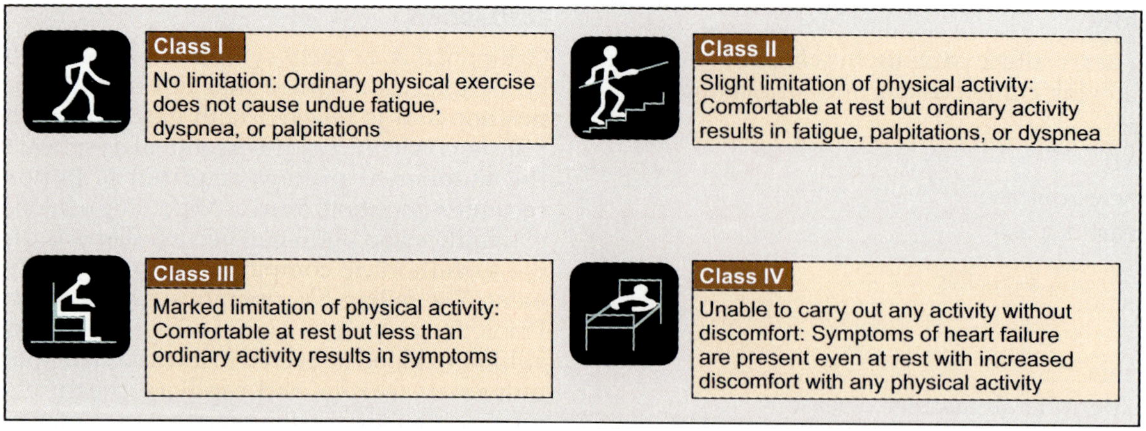


**Fig. 8.4:** Classification of heart status according to physical activity

- Respiratory muscle dysfunction, with decreased respiratory muscle strength, decreased endurance, and ischemia.

### Pulmonary Edema

Acute pulmonary edema is defined as the sudden increase in PCWP (usually more than 25 mmHg) as a result of acute and fulminant left ventricular failure. It is a medical emergency and has a very dramatic clinical presentation. The patient appears extremely ill, poorly perfused, restless, sweaty, tachypneic, tachycardic, hypoxic, and coughing, with an increased work of breathing and using respiratory accessory muscles and with frothy sputum that on occasion is blood tinged.

### Chest Pain/Pressure

Chest pain/pressure may occur as a result of either primary myocardial ischemia from coronary disease or secondary myocardial ischemia from increased filling pressure, poor cardiac output (and therefore poor coronary diastolic filling), or hypotension and hypoxemia.

**Palpitations** are the sensation a patient has when the heart is racing. It can be secondary to sinus tachycardia due to decompensated heart failure, or more commonly, it is due to atrial or ventricular tachyarrhythmias.

### Fatigue and Weakness

Fatigue and weakness are often accompanied by a feeling of heaviness in the limbs and are generally related to poor perfusion of the skeletal muscles in patients with a lowered cardiac output. Although they are generally a constant feature of advanced heart failure, episodic fatigue and weakness are also common in earlier stages.

### Nocturia and Oliguria

Nocturia may occur relatively early in the course of heart failure. Recumbency reduces the deficit in cardiac output in relation to oxygen demand, renal vasoconstriction diminishes, and urine formation increases. Nocturia may be troublesome for patients with heart failure because it may prevent them from obtaining much-needed rest. Oliguria is a late finding in heart failure and is found in patients with markedly reduced cardiac output from severely reduced LV function.

### Cerebral Symptoms

The following may occur in elderly patients with advanced heart failure, particularly in those with cerebrovascular atherosclerosis:

- Confusion
- Memory impairment
- Anxiety
- Headaches
- Insomnia
- Bad dreams or nightmares
- Rarely, psychosis with disorientation, delirium, or hallucinations.

## Physical Examination

Patients with mild heart failure appear to be in no distress after a few minutes of rest, but they may be obviously dyspneic during and immediately after moderate activity. Patients with LV failure may be dyspneic when lying flat without elevation of the head for more than a few minutes. Those with severe heart failure appear anxious and may exhibit signs of air hunger in this position (Figs 8.5–8.10).

Patients with recent onset of heart failure are generally well nourished, but those with chronic severe heart failure are often malnourished and sometimes even cachectic. Chronic marked elevation of systemic venous pressure may produce exophthalmos and severe tricuspid regurgitation and may lead to visible pulsation of the eyes and of the neck veins. Central cyanosis, icterus, and malar flush may be evident in patients with severe heart failure.

In mild or moderate heart failure, stroke volume is normal at rest; in severe heart failure, it is reduced, as reflected by a diminished pulse pressure and a dusky discoloration of the skin. With very severe heart failure, particularly if cardiac output has declined acutely, systolic arterial pressure may be reduced. The pulse may be weak, rapid, and thready; the proportional pulse pressure (pulse pressure/systolic pressure) may be markedly reduced. The

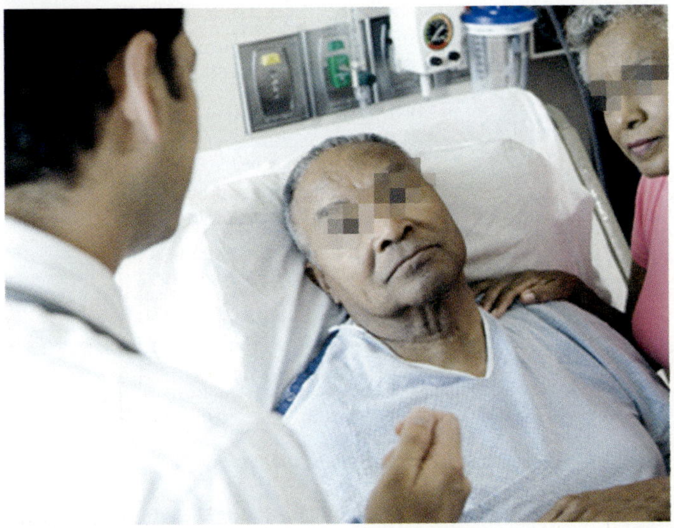

**Fig. 8.5:** A middle aged patient with dilated cardiomyopathy with class III–IV is being examined by the attending doctor

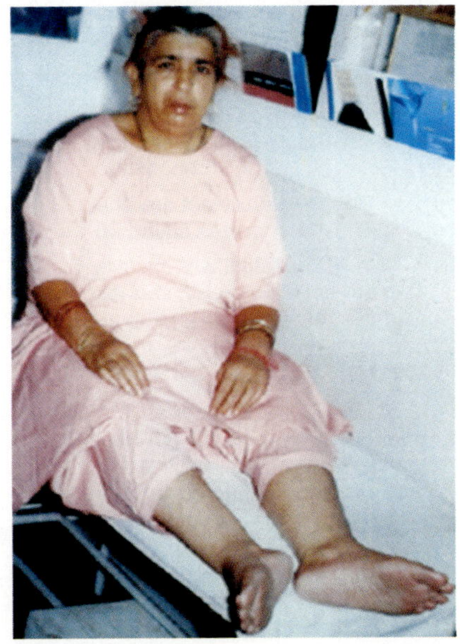

**Fig. 8.6:** Rough, dry hair, skin, facial puffiness, edema of whole body and cardiomegaly in a middle-aged lady with hypothyroidism and heart failure

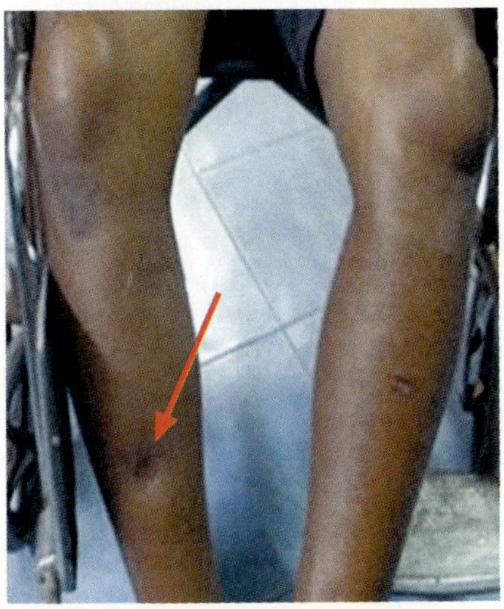

**Fig. 8.7:** Pitting edema in a patient with heart failure

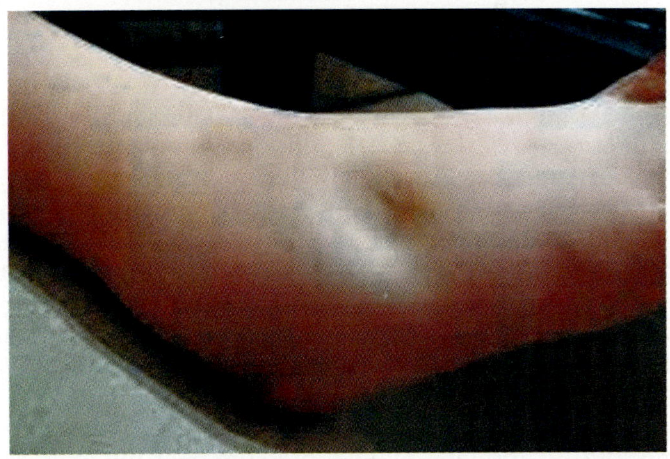

**Fig. 8.8:** Pitting edema over foot in a patient with heart failure

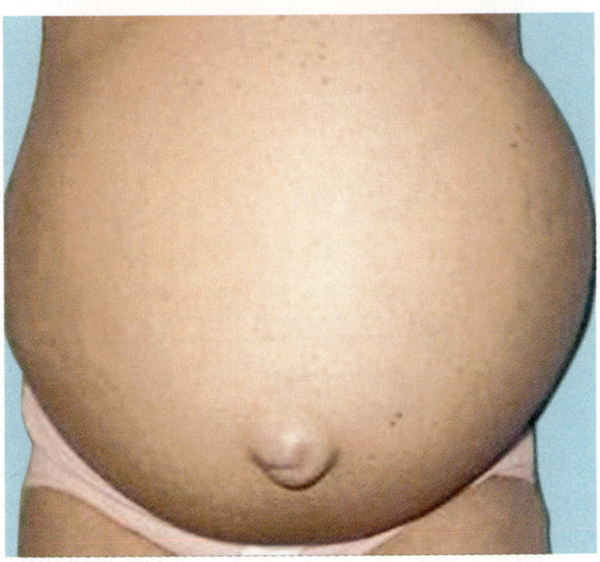

**Fig. 8.9:** Ascites in a patient with congestive heart failure

proportional pulse pressure correlates reasonably well with cardiac output. In one study, when pulse pressure was less than 25%, it usually reflected a cardiac index of less than 2.2 L/min/m$^2$.

**Ascites** occurs in patients with increased pressure in the hepatic veins and in the veins draining into the peritoneum and usually reflects long-standing systemic venous hypertension. Fever may be present in severe decompensated heart failure because of cutaneous vasoconstriction and impairment of heat loss.

**Increased adrenergic activity** is manifested by tachycardia, diaphoresis, pallor, peripheral cyanosis with pallor and coldness of the extremities, and obvious distention of the peripheral veins secondary to venoconstriction. Diastolic arterial pressure may be slightly elevated.

**Rales** heard over the lung bases are characteristic of heart failure of at least moderate severity. With acute pulmonary edema, rales are frequently accompanied by wheezing and

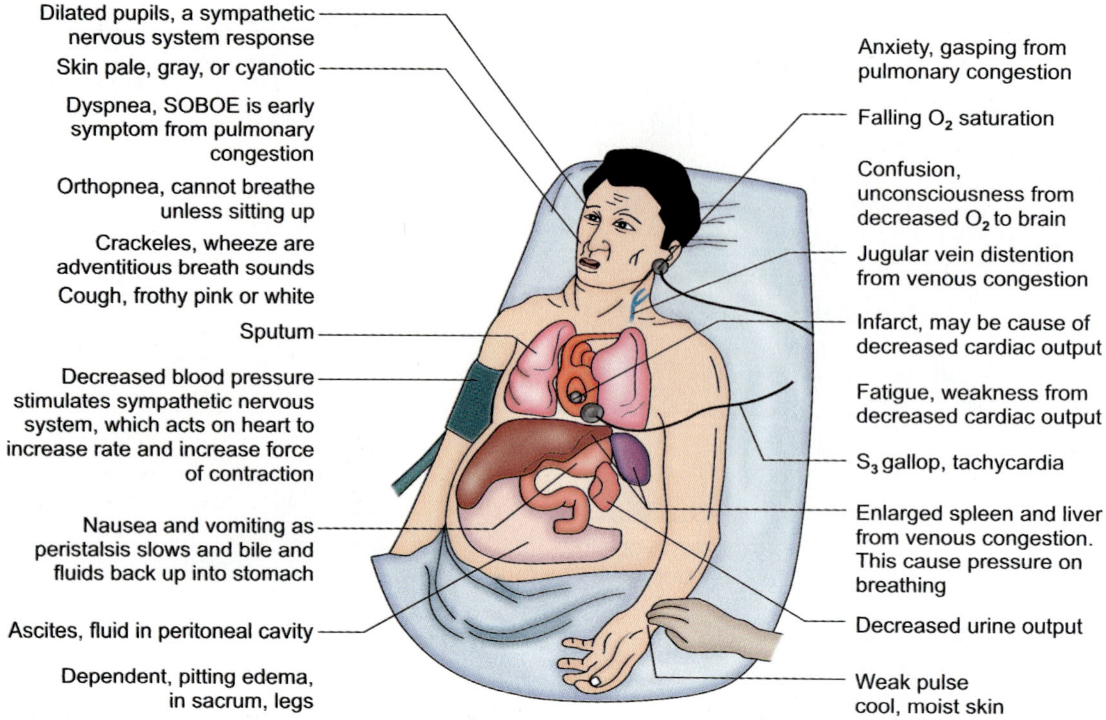


**Fig. 8.10:** Various signs and symptoms in heart failure

expectoration of frothy, blood-tinged sputum. The absence of rales certainly does not exclude elevation of pulmonary capillary pressure due to LV failure.

**Systemic venous hypertension** is manifested by jugular venous distention. Normally, jugular venous pressure declines with respiration; however, it increases in patients with heart failure, a finding known as the Kussmaul sign (also found in constrictive pericarditis). This reflects an increase in right atrial pressure and therefore right-sided heart failure.

**Hepatojugular reflux** is the distention of the jugular vein induced by applying manual pressure over the liver; the patient's torso should be positioned at a 45° angle. Hepatojugular reflux occurs in patients with elevated left-sided filling pressures and reflects elevated capillary wedge pressure and left-sided heart failure.

Although edema is a cardinal manifestation of heart failure, it does not correlate well with the level of systemic venous pressure. In patients with chronic LV failure and low cardiac output, extracellular fluid volume may be sufficiently expanded to cause edema in the presence of only slight elevations in systemic venous pressure. Usually, a substantial gain of extracellular fluid volume (i.e. a minimum of 5 L in adults) must occur before peripheral edema develops. Edema in the absence of dyspnea or other signs of LV or RV failure is not solely indicative of heart failure and can be observed in many other conditions, including chronic venous insufficiency, nephrotic syndrome, or other syndromes of hypoproteinemia or osmotic imbalance (Figs 8.12 and 8.13).

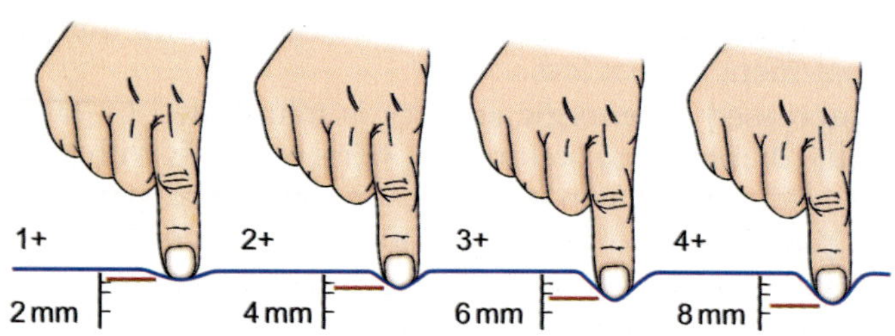


**Fig. 8.11:** Assessment of the severity of peripheral edema

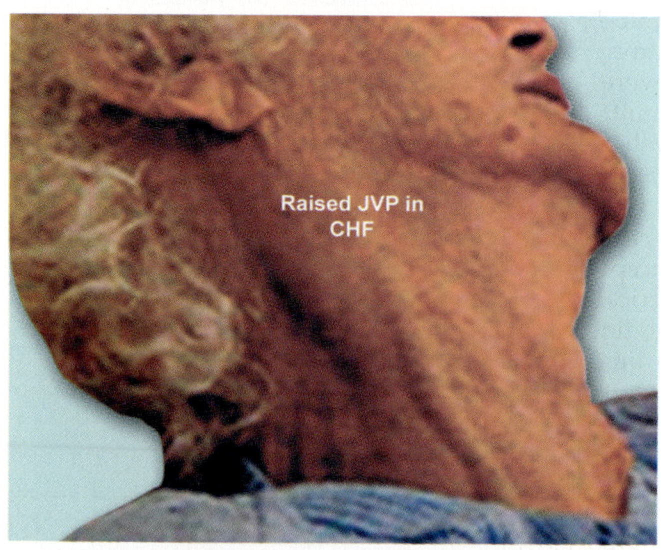


**Fig. 8.12:** Still photograph showing distended elevated jugular venous pressure with prominent V-wave in a patient with heart failure

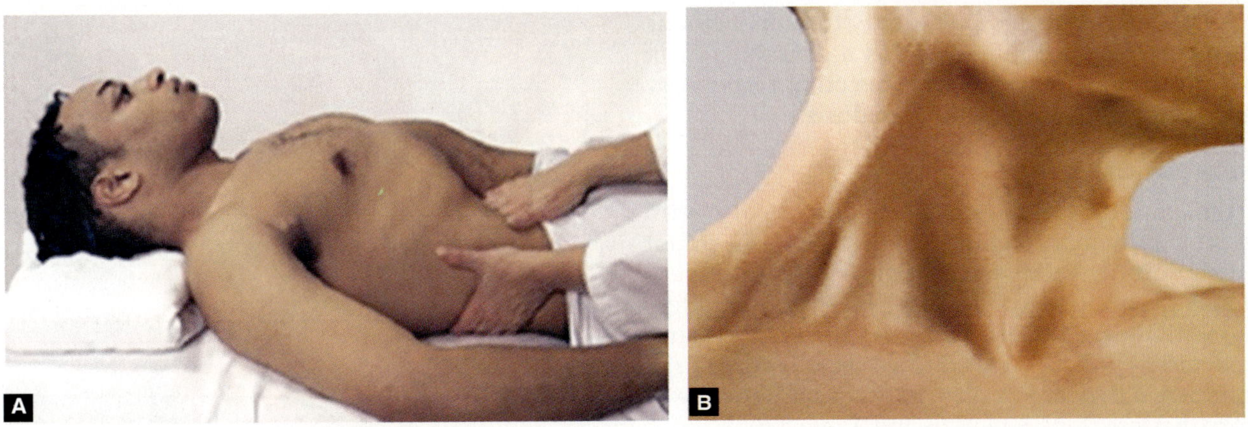


**Fig. 8.13:** (A) A patient with an elevated JVP after compressing over the liver for 30 seconds (hepatojugular reflux), (B) the JVP increases by 3 cm and remains there for >10 cardiac cycles

**Hepatomegaly** is prominent in patients with chronic right-sided heart failure, but it may occur rapidly in acute heart failure. When hepatomegaly occurs acutely, the liver is usually tender. In patients with considerable tricuspid regurgitation, a prominent systolic pulsation of the liver, attributable to an enlarged right atrial V wave, is often noted. A presystolic pulsation of the liver, attributable to an enlarged right atrial A wave, can occur in tricuspid stenosis, constrictive pericarditis, restrictive cardiomyopathy involving the right ventricle, and pulmonary hypertension (primary or secondary).

**Hydrothorax** is most commonly observed in patients with hypertension involving both the systemic and pulmonary circulation. It is usually bilateral, although when unilateral, it is usually confined to the right side of the chest. When hydrothorax develops, dyspnea usually intensifies because of further reductions in vital capacity.

### Cardiac Findings

Protodiastolic (S3) gallop is the earliest cardiac physical finding in decompensated heart failure in the absence of severe mitral or tricuspid regurgitation or left-to-right shunts. The presence of an S3 gallop in adults is important, pathologic, and often the most apparent finding on cardiac auscultation in patients with significant heart failure.

**Cardiomegaly** is a nonspecific finding that nonetheless occurs in most patients with chronic heart failure. Notable exceptions include heart failure from acute MI, constrictive pericarditis, restrictive cardiomyopathy, valve or chordae tendineae rupture, or heart failure due to tachyarrhythmias or bradyarrhythmias.

**Pulsus alternans** (during pulse palpation, this is the alternation of 1 strong and 1 weak beat without a change in the cycle length) occurs most commonly in heart failure due to increased resistance to LV ejection, as occurs in hypertension, aortic stenosis, coronary atherosclerosis, and dilated cardiomyopathy. Pulsus alternans is usually associated with an S3 gallop, signifies advanced myocardial disease, and often disappears with treatment of heart failure.

Accentuation of P2 heart sound is a cardinal sign of increased pulmonary artery pressure; it disappears or improves after treatment of heart failure. Mitral and tricuspid regurgitation murmurs are often present in patients with decompensated heart failure because of ventricular dilatation. These murmurs often disappear or diminish when compensation is restored. Note that correlation between the intensity of the murmur of mitral regurgitation and its significance in patients with heart failure is poor. Severe mitral regurgitation may be accompanied by an unimpressively soft murmur.

**Cardiac cachexia** is found in long-standing heart failure, particularly of the right ventricle, because of anorexia from hepatic and intestinal congestion and sometimes because of digitalis toxicity. Occasionally, impaired intestinal absorption of fat occurs, and rarely, protein-losing enteropathy occurs. Patients with heart failure may also exhibit increased total metabolism secondary to augmentation of myocardial oxygen consumption, excessive work of breathing, low-grade fever, and elevated levels of circulating tumor necrosis factor (TNF).

## Predominant Right-sided Heart Failure

Ascites, congestive hepatomegaly, and anasarca due to elevated right-sided heart pressures transmitted backward into the portal vein circulation may result in increased abdominal girth and epigastric and right upper quadrant (RUQ) abdominal pain. Other gastrointestinal symptoms, caused by congestion of the hepatic and gastrointestinal venous circulation, include anorexia, bloating, nausea, and constipation. In preterminal heart failure, inadequate bowel perfusion can cause abdominal pain, distention, and bloody stools. Distinguishing right-sided heart failure from hepatic failure is often clinically difficult.

Dyspnea, prominent in LV failure, becomes less prominent in isolated right-sided heart failure because of the absence of pulmonary congestion. On the other hand, when cardiac output becomes markedly reduced in patients with terminal right-sided heart failure (as may occur in isolated RV infarction and in the late stages of primary pulmonary hypertension and pulmonary thromboembolic disease), severe dyspnea may occur as a consequence of the reduced cardiac output, poor perfusion of respiratory muscles, hypoxemia, and metabolic acidosis.

### Heart Failure in Children

In children, manifestations of heart failure vary with age. Signs of pulmonary venous congestion in an infant generally include tachypnea, respiratory distress (retractions), grunting, and difficulty with feeding. Often, children with heart failure have diaphoresis during feedings, which is possibly related to a catecholamine surge that occurs when they are challenged with eating while in respiratory distress (Figs 8.14–8.16 and Table 8.6).

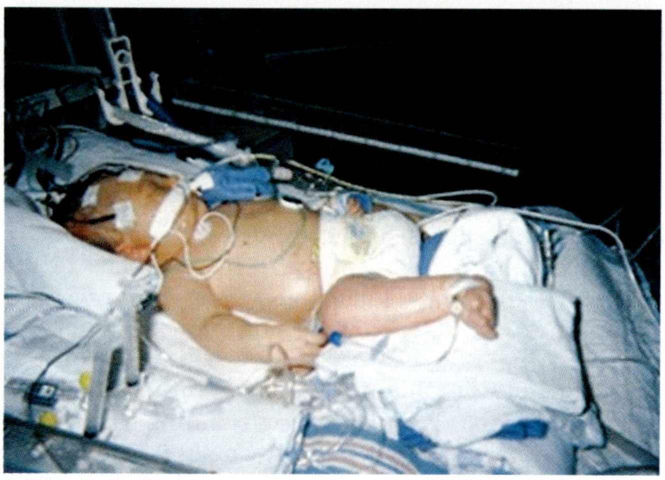

**Fig. 8.14:** Generalised edema of the an infant with heart failure

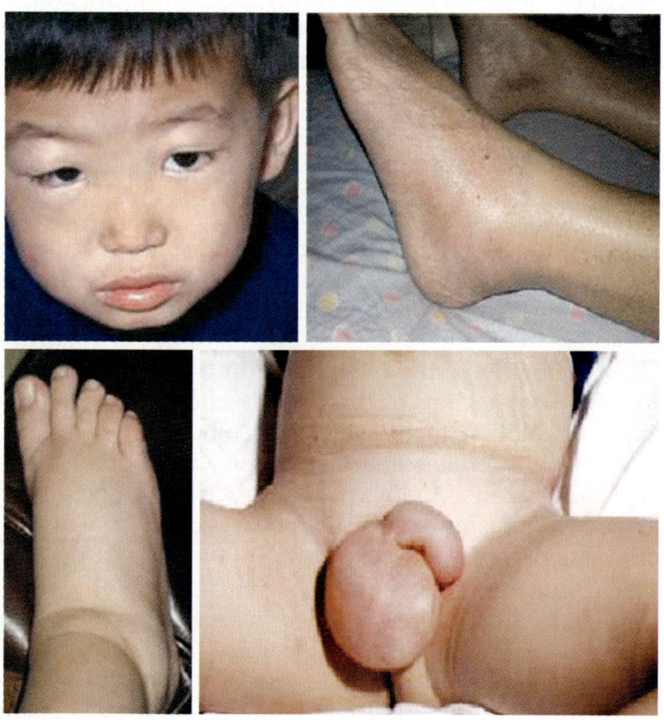

**Fig. 8.15:** Edema of various parts of the body such as face, eyelids, feet and scrotum

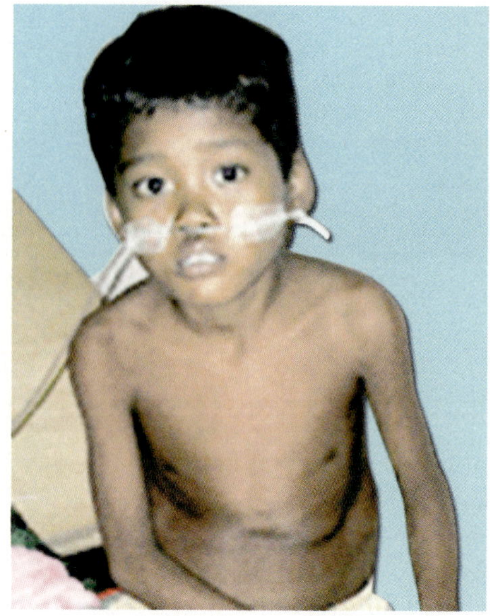

**Fig. 8.16:** Treatment of heart failure with administration of intranasal oxygen in an older child with ASD septum primum defect

| Table 8.6: Leading causes of CHF in relation to age |
|---|
| ***Birth to first week*** |
| Aoratic atresia |
| Transposition of great vessels |
| Coarctation of aorta |
| ***1 week to 1 month*** |
| Coarctation of aorta |
| TGA |
| Endocardial fibroelastosis |
| ***1 month to 2 months*** |
| TGA |
| Endocardial fibroelastosis |
| ***2 months to 3 months*** |
| Coarctation of aorta |
| Total anomalous pulmonary venous return |
| VSD |
| ***3 months to 6 months*** |
| VSD |
| ***6 months to 12 months*** |
| VSD |
| ASD (Ostium primum) |
| CHF is rarely present in utero with exception of paroxysmal surpraventricular tachycardia and anemia due to Rh incompatibility. It is often interpreted as intrauterine asphyxia and mother is subjected to cesarean section. |
| ***After first year of life, CHF is much less frequent and it is due to variety of causes*** |
| • Arrhythmias |
| • Viral myocarditis |
| • Acute rheumatic carditis |
| • Cardiomyopathy |

Right-sided venous congestion is characterized by hepatosplenomegaly and, less frequently, with edema or ascites. Jugular venous distention is not a reliable indicator of systemic venous congestion in infants, because the jugular veins are difficult to observe. Also, the distance from the right atrium to the angle of the jaw may be no more than 8–10 cm, even when the individual is sitting upright. Uncompensated heart failure in an infant primarily manifests as a failure to thrive. In severe cases, failure to thrive may be followed by signs of renal and hepatic failure. In older children, left-sided venous congestion causes tachypnea, respiratory distress, and wheezing (cardiac asthma). Right-sided congestion may result in hepatosplenomegaly, jugular venous distention, edema, ascites, and/or pleural effusions. Uncompensated heart failure in older children may cause fatigue or lower-than-usual energy levels. Patients may complain of cool extremities, exercise intolerance, dizziness, or syncope cesarean section.

## Heart Failure Criteria, Classification, and Staging

*Framingham system for diagnosis of heart failure:* In the Framingham system, the diagnosis of heart failure requires that either two major criteria or 1 major and 2 minor criteria be present concurrently, as minor criteria are accepted only if they cannot be attributed to another medical condition.

### NYHA Classification of Functional Heart Failure

The New York Heart Association (NYHA) functional classification of heart failure is based on the patient's symptom severity and the amount of exertion that is needed to provoke their symptoms.

### ACC/AHA Stages of Heart Failure

The American College of Cardiology/American Heart Association (ACC/AHA) developed a classification that described the development and progression of heart failure and that 'recognizes that there are established risk factors and structural prerequisites for the development of HF and that therapeutic interventions introduced even before the appearance of LV dysfunction or symptoms can reduce the population morbidity and mortality of HF.'

## ACC/AHA Staging

### Stage A

ACC/AHA stage A patients are at high risk for heart failure but do not have structural heart disease or symptoms of heart failure. Thus, management in these cases focuses on prevention, through reduction of risk factors. Measures include the following:

- Treat hypertension
- Encourage smoking cessation
- Treat lipid disorders
- Encourage regular exercise
- Discourage alcohol intake and illicit drug use
- Patients who have a family history of dilated cardiomyopathy should be screened with a comprehensive history and physical examination together with echocardiography and transthoracic echocardiography every 2–5 years.

### Stage B

ACC/AHA stage B patients are asymptomatic, with LV dysfunction from previous MI, LV remodeling from LV hypertrophy, and asymptomatic valvular dysfunction, which includes patients with New York Heart Association (NYHA) class I heart failure. In addition to the heart failure education and aggressive risk factor modification used for stage A, treatment with an ACEI/ARB and/or beta-blockade is indicated.

- Evaluation for coronary revascularization either percutaneously or surgically, as well as correction of valvular abnormalities, may be indicated. Treatment with an ICD for primary prevention of sudden death in patients with an LVEF of less than 30% that is more than 40 days post-MI is reasonable if expected survival is more than 1 year.
- There is less evidence for implantation of an ICD in patients with nonischemic cardiomyopathy, an LVEF less than 30%, and no heart failure symptoms. There is no evidence for use of digoxin in these populations. Aldosterone receptor blockade with eplerenone is indicated for post-MI LV dysfunction.

### Stage C

ACC/AHA stage C patients have structural heart disease and current or previous symptoms of heart failure; ACC/AHA stage C corresponds with NYHA class II and III heart failure. The preventive measures used for stage A disease are indicated, as is dietary sodium restriction.

- Drugs routinely used in these patients include ACEI/ARBs, beta-blockers, and loop diuretics for fluid retention. For selected patients, therapeutic measures include aldosterone receptor blockers, hydralazine and nitrates in combination, and cardiac resynchronization with or without an ICD (see electrophysiologic intervention).
- A meta-analysis performed by Badve et al. suggested that the survival benefit of treatment with beta-blockers extends to patients with chronic kidney disease and systolic heart failure (risk ratio 0.72).

### Stage D

ACC/AHA stage D patients have refractory heart failure (NYHA class IV) that requires specialized interventions. Treatment includes all the measures used in stages A, B, and C. Treatment considerations include heart transplantation or placement of an LV assist device in eligible patients; pulmonary catheterization; and options for end-of-life care. For palliation of symptoms, continuous intravenous infusion of a positive inotrope may be considered.

## Differential Diagnoses

- Acute renal failure
- Acute respiratory distress syndrome

**Table 8.7:** Prevalence of signs and symptoms in systolic and and diastolic heart failure

| | Diastolic HF (LVEF >50%) | Systolic HF (LVEF <50%) |
|---|---|---|
| *Symptoms* | | |
| Dyspnea on exertion | 85% | 96% |
| Paroxysmal nocturnal dyspnea | 55% | 50% |
| Orthopnea | 60% | 73% |
| *Physical examination* | | |
| Jugular venous distension | 35% | 46% |
| Rales | 72% | 70% |
| Displaced apical impulse | 50% | 60% |
| S3 | 45% | 65% |
| S4 | 45% | 66% |
| Hepatomegaly | 15% | 16% |
| Edema | 30% | 40% |
| *Chest film* | | |
| Cardiomegaly | 90% | 96% |
| Pulmonary venous hypertension | 75% | 80% |

**Table 8.8:** Abnormalities resulting in systolic dysfunction

*Myocyte compartment*

- Myocyte loss (necrosis, apoptosis and aging)
- Abnonnal force transduction (e.g. dystrophin mutations)
- Abnonnal force generation (calcium release, substrate deficiency)
- Abnonnal relaxation (abnormal calcium reuptake)
- Excessive myocyte hypertrophy

*Myocardial load*

- Volume overload (mitral or aortic regurgitation, renal or hepatic failure) Pressure overload (hypertension, increased arterial stiffness)

*Heart rate and conduction*

- Excessive tachycardia (weeks)
- Discoordinate contraction (right ventricular pacing)

*Extracellular matrix compartment*

- Fibrosis
- Altered metabolism (cardiofibroblast function, protein Synthesis and degradation, paracrine/autocrine signaling)

*Cardiac structure*

- Abnonnal myocardial fiber "wrapping" or alignment
- Focal infarction or aneurysm.
- Advanced remodeling (increased sphericity)

- Chronic obstructive pulmonary disease
- Cirrhosis
- Emphysema
- Goodpasture syndrome
- Myocardial infarction
- Nephrotic syndrome
- Pneumonia, bacterial
- Pneumonia, community-acquired
- Pneumonia, viral
- Pneumothorax
- Pulmonary edema, cardiogenic
- Pulmonary edema, neurogenic
- Pulmonary embolism
- Pulmonary fibrosis, idiopathic
- Pulmonary fibrosis, interstitial (nonidiopathic)
- Respiratory failure
- Venous insufficiency

## ROUTINE LABORATORY TESTS

Laboratory studies should include a complete blood count (CBC), serum electrolytes (including calcium and magnesium), and renal and liver function studies. Other tests may be indicated in specific patients. The CBC aids in the assessment of severe anemia, which may cause or aggravate heart failure. Leukocytosis may signal underlying infection. Otherwise, CBCs are usually of little diagnostic help.

*Serum electrolyte* values are generally within reference ranges in patients with mild to moderate heart failure before treatment. In cases of severe heart failure, however, prolonged, rigid sodium restriction, coupled with intensive diuretic therapy and the inability to excrete water, may lead to dilutional hyponatremia, which occurs because of a substantial expansion of extracellular and intravascular fluid volume and a normal or increased level of total body sodium.

Potassium levels are usually within reference ranges, although the prolonged administration of diuretics may result in hypokalemia. Hyperkalemia may occur in patients with severe heart failure who show marked reductions in glomerular filtration rate (GFR) and inadequate delivery of sodium to the distal tubular sodium-potassium exchange sites of the kidney, particularly if they are receiving potassium-sparing diuretics and/or angiotensin-converting enzyme inhibitors (ACEIs).

### Renal Function Tests

Blood urea nitrogen (BUN) and creatinine levels can be within reference ranges in patients with mild to moderate heart failure and normal renal function, although BUN levels and BUN/creatinine ratios may be elevated.

Patients with severe heart failure, particularly those on large doses of diuretics for long periods, may have elevated BUN and creatinine levels indicative of renal insufficiency because of chronic reductions of renal blood flow from reduced cardiac output. Diuresing this group of patients is complex. In some individuals, diuretics will improve renal congestion and renal function, whereas in others, over aggressive diuresis may aggravate renal insufficiency due to volume depletion.

### Liver Function Tests

Congestive hepatomegaly and cardiac cirrhosis are often associated with impaired hepatic function, which is characterized by abnormal values of aspartate aminotransferase (AST), alanine aminotransferase (ALT), lactic dehydrogenase (LDH), and other liver enzymes. Hyperbilirubinemia secondary to an increase in the directly and indirectly reacting bilirubin is common. In severe cases of acute RV or LV failure, frank jaundice may occur.

Acute hepatic venous congestion can result in severe jaundice, with a bilirubin level as high as 15–20 mg/dL, elevation of AST to more than 10 times the upper reference range limit, elevation of the serum alkaline phosphatase level, and prolongation of the prothrombin time. The clinical and laboratory pictures may resemble viral hepatitis, but the impairment of hepatic function is rapidly resolved by successful treatment of heart failure. In patients with long-standing heart failure, albumin synthesis may be impaired, leading to hypoalbuminemia and intensifying the accumulation of fluid. Fulminant hepatic failure is an uncommon, late, and sometimes terminal complication of cardiac cirrhosis.

### Natriuretic Peptides

Clinical findings and routine diagnostic tests are not always sufficient to diagnose heart failure. In such ambiguous cases, rapid measurement of B-type natriuretic peptide (BNP) or N-terminal proBNP (NT-proBNP) levels can aid clinicians in differentiating between cardiac and noncardiac causes of dyspnea. That is, BNP is mostly limited to the differentiation of heart failure versus other causes of dyspnea in patients with an atypical presentation (Table 8.9).

BNP is a 32-amino-acid polypeptide containing a 17-amino-acid ring structure common to all natriuretic peptides. The major source of plasma BNP is the cardiac ventricles, and the release of BNP appears to be in direct proportion to ventricular volume and pressure overload. BNP is an independent predictor of high LV end-diastolic pressure and is more useful than atrial natriuretic peptide (ANP) or norepinephrine levels for assessing mortality risk in patients with heart failure. Although BNP has been determined to be the strongest predictor of systolic versus nonsystolic heart failure (followed by oxygen saturation, history of myocardial infarction, and heart rate), BNP does not reliably differentiate between heart failure with preserved ejection fraction and heart failure with reduced ejection fraction. Increased NT-proBNP was found to be the strongest independent predictor of a final diagnosis of acute heart failure. Measurement of B-type natriuretic peptide (BNP) and its precursor, N-terminal proBNP (NT-proBNP), in the urgent care setting can be used to establish the diagnosis of heart failure when the clinical presentation is ambiguous or when confounding comorbidities are present BNP and NT-proBNP assays have different cutoff values for ruling in and ruling out heart failure. The American College of Cardiology/American Heart Association (ACC/AHA),the Heart Failure Society of America (HFSA), and the European Society of Cardiology (ESC) recommend measuring BNP or NT-proBNP in the workup of heart failure when the diagnosis is unclear. The HFSA recommends this test in all cases of suspected heart failure, particularly in ambiguous cases.

BNP levels correlate closely with the NYHA classification of heart failure.BNP levels greater than 100 pg/ml have a specificity greater than 95% and a sensitivity greater than 98% when comparing patients without heart failure to all patients with heart failure. Even BNP levels greater than 80 pg/ml have a specificity greater than 95% and a sensitivity greater than 98% in the diagnosis of heart failure. BNP and NT-proBNP levels are higher in older patients, women, and patients with renal dysfunction or sepsis. Atrial fibrillation has also been associated with increased BNP levels in the absence of acute heart failure. However, BNP levels may be disproportionately lower in patients who are obese due to fat metabolism or who have hypothyroidism or advanced end-stage heart failure (the latter due to increased fibrosis). NT-proBNP plasma levels are also lower in obese heart failure patients relative to nonobese patients with heart failure, regardless of whether the aetiology is ischemic or nonischaemic.

However, NT-proBNP may be elevated in severely obese patients (BMI >40 kg/$m^2$) due to an increased cardiac

**Table 8.9:** Evidence-based BNP and NT-proBNP cutoff values for diagnosing HF

| | | BNP, pg/ml | | NT-proBNP, pg/ml | |
|---|---|---|---|---|---|
| Criterion | | HF unlikely (LR-negative) | HF unlikely (LR-positive) | HF unlikely (LR-negative) | HF unlikely (LR-positive) |
| Age (year) | >17 | <100 (0.13)[*] | >500 (8.1)[*] | – | – |
| | >21 | – | – | <300 (0.2)[†] | – |
| | 21–50 | – | – | – | >450 (14)[†] |
| | 50–75 | – | – | – | >900 (5.0)[†] |
| | >75 | – | – | – | >1800 (3.1)[†] |
| Estimated GFR <60 ml/min | | <200 (0.13) | >500 (9.3) | – | – |

BNP=B-type natriuretic peptide; GRF=glomerular filtration rate; HF=heart failure; LR=likelihood ratio; NPV=negative predictive value; NT-pro-BNP=N-terminal proNBP; PPV=positive predictive value; –=not specifically defined.

[*]Derived from breathing not properly data (1586 emergency department [ED] patients, prevalence of HF=47%. [†]Derived from PRIDE data (1256 ED patients, prevalence of HF=57%).

burden in these individuals. NT-proBNP may be a better marker for detecting cardiac dysfunction than BNP, because its chemical stability is better in circulating blood than that of BNP, and it is a sensitive marker of cardiac function even in early cardiac decompensation. BNP measurement not indicated with nesiritide therapy.

Nesiritide is a synthetic BNP analogue; therefore, the measurement of BNP is not indicated in patients who are receiving nesiritide. If BNP is used as a diagnostic marker to rule in heart failure, the level must be determined before nesiritide therapy is started. In a study by Miller et al. levels of NT-proBNP and BNP decreased in patients with advanced heart failure after therapy with nesiritide, but the majority of the patients did not have biochemically significant decreases in these markers even with a clinical response. The investigators were unable to give a definitive reason for their results, and they indicated that nesiritide therapy should not be guided by the use of levels of both markers. Fitzgerald et al. also found decreased levels of both natriuretic peptides following nesiritide therapy in patients with decompensated heart failure.

## GENETIC TESTING

Cardiomyopathy phenotypes that have known genetic cause(s) include hypertrophic (HCM), dilated (DCM), restrictive (RCM), arrhythmogenic right ventricular dysplasia/cardiomyopathy (ARVD/C), and left ventricular noncompaction (LVNC). Because most cases of cardiomyopathy are treatable which is not the case in many genetic diseases and screening for genetic risk of cardiomyopathy before the onset of disease can guide the recommendations for early detection of disease and therapy, it is recommended that consideration be given for patients with cardiomyopathy to be referred to centers with expertise in these matters and in family-based management. These specialized centers will have a better understanding of the complexities involved in genetic evaluation, testing, and counseling of patients with cardiomyopathy.

To establish specific gene testing and laboratories offering tests, please visit www.genetests.org for further information and larger e–views. Genetic testing has the highest yield in three types of cardiomyopathy—DCM, HCM, and autosomal dominant ARVD/C. The diagnosis must be established using the specific criteria for each type of cardiomyopathy, as the genetic testing is different for each type.

## ASSESSMENT OF HYPOXEMIA

### Arterial and Venous Blood Gases

Although arterial blood gas (ABG) measurement is more accurate than pulse oximetry for measuring oxygen saturation, it is unclear if ABG results add any clinical utility to pulse oximetry. In the setting of acute heart failure, ABG measurement is rarely performed. Indications include severe respiratory distress, documented hypoxemia by pulse oximetry not responsive to supplemental oxygen, and evidence of acidosis by serum chemistry or elevated lactate level (Table 8.10).

In general, heart failure patients who do not have comorbid lung disease do not manifest hypoxemia except in severe acute decompensation. Patients with severe heart failure may have signs and symptoms ranging from severe hypoxemia, or even hypoxia, along with hypercapnia, to decreased vital capacity and poor ventilation.

*ABG measurement* helps assess the presence of hypercapnia, a potential early marker for impending respiratory failure. Hypoxemia and hypocapnia occur in stages 1 and 2 of pulmonary edema because of V/Q mismatch. In stage 3 of pulmonary edema, right-to-left intrapulmonary shunt develops secondary to alveolar flooding and further contributes to hypoxemia. In more severe cases, hypercapnia and respiratory acidosis are usually observed. The decision regarding intubation and the use of mechanical ventilation is frequently based on many clinical parameters, including oxygenation, ventilation, and mental status. ABG values in isolation are rarely useful, but they may add to the entire clinical picture.

Mixed venous oxygen saturation (obtained from the main pulmonary artery in the absence of an intracardiac shunt) is a good marker of the blood circulation time and therefore of cardiac output and cardiac performance. Patients who have advanced heart failure have low cardiac output and slower circulation time, which translate into an increased oxygen extraction by the tissue and therefore lower saturation of oxygen (<60% saturation).

### Pulse Oximetry

Pulse oximetry is highly accurate at assessing the presence of hypoxemia and, therefore, the severity of acute heart failure presentations. Patients with mild to moderate acute heart failure may show modest reductions in oxygen saturation, whereas patients with severe heart failure may have severe oxygen desaturation, even at rest. Pulse oximetry is also useful for monitoring the patient's response to supplemental oxygen and other therapies.

Patients with mild to moderate heart failure may have normal oxygen saturations at rest, but they may exhibit marked reductions in oxygen saturations during physical exertion or recumbency. In general, arterial desaturation during exercise is not expected in heart failure and suggests the presence of comorbid lung disease. The use of continuous oxygen may be needed until compensation returns oxygen saturation to normal during exertion and recumbency or on a permanent basis if oxygen desaturation during exertion and/or recumbency exists during compensated severe chronic heart failure.

### Chest Radiography

Chest radiographs are used in cases of heart failure to assess heart size, pulmonary congestion, pulmonary or thoracic causes of dyspnea, and the proper positioning of any implanted cardiac devices. Posterior-anterior and lateral views are recommended (Figs 8.17–8.19).

Although up to 50% of patients with heart failure and documented elevation of PCWP do not manifest typical radiographic findings of pulmonary congestion, the

**Table 8.10:** Recommendations for the evaluation of patients with heart failure

| |
|---|
| **Class I** |
| • Thorough history and physical examination<br>• Initial and ongoing assessment of ability to perform routine and desired activities of daily living. Initial and ongoing assessment of volume status<br>• Initial measurement of complete blood count, urinalysis, serum electrolytes, blood urea nitrogen, serum creatinine, blood glucose, liver function tests, thyroid-stimulating hormone<br>• Serial monitoring of serum electrolytes and renal function<br>• Initial 12-lead EKG and chest radiograph<br>• Initial 2-dimensional echocardiography with Doppler or radionuclide ventriculography to assess left ventricular systolic function<br>• Cardiac catheterization with coronary angiography in patients with angina who are candidates for revascularization |
| **Class IIa** |
| • Cardiac catheterization with coronary angiography in patients who are candidates for revascularization with chest pain who have not had evaluation of their coronary anatomy known of suspected CAD but without angina<br>• Noninvasive assessment of ischemia and viability in patients with known CAD without angina<br>• Maximal exercise testing with measurement of respiratory gas exchange to determine cause of exercise limitation candidacy for cardiac transplantation<br>• Echo cardiography in asymptomatic first-degree relatives of patients with IDCM<br>• Repeat measures of ejection fraction in patients with change in clinical status<br>• Screening for hemochromatosis<br>• Measurement of ANA, RF, urinary VMA and metanephrines in selected patients |
| **Class IIb** |
| • Noninvasive imaging to define likelihood of CAD<br>• Maximal exercise testing to prescribe exercise program<br>• Endomyocardial biopsy in patients with known or suspected inflammatory or infiltrative disorder HIV testing |
| **Class III** Endomyocardial biopsy in routine evaluation |
| • Routine Holter-monitoring or signal-averaged electrocardiography<br>• Repeat coronary angiography or noninvasive testing in patients in whom CAD has been excluded previously as the cause of left ventricular dysfunction<br>• Routine measurement of norepinephrine |

CAD=coronary artery disease; IDCM=idiopathic dilated cardiomyopathy; ANA=antinuclear antibody; RF=rheumatoid factor; VMA= vanellylmandelic acid; HIV=human im munodeficiency virus.

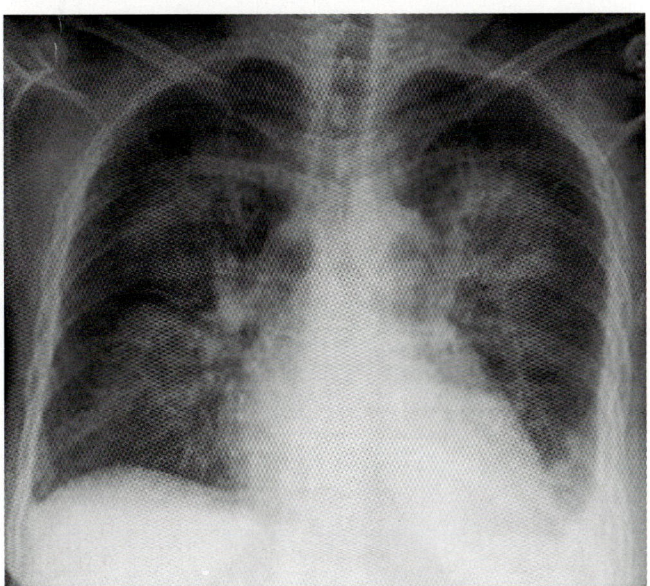

**Fig. 8.17:** Chest radiograph in PA view shows an enlarged cardiac silhouette and edema at the lung bases, signs of acute heart failure

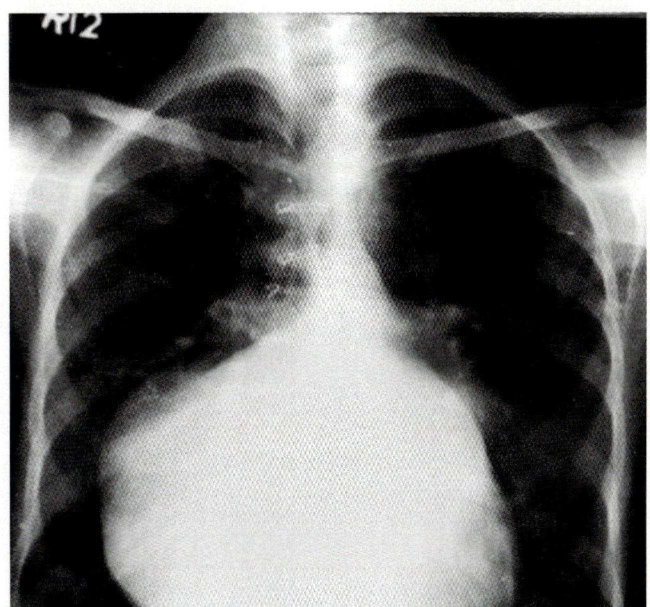


**Fig. 8.18:** Chest X-ray PA view showing globular heart in in patient with biventricular failure

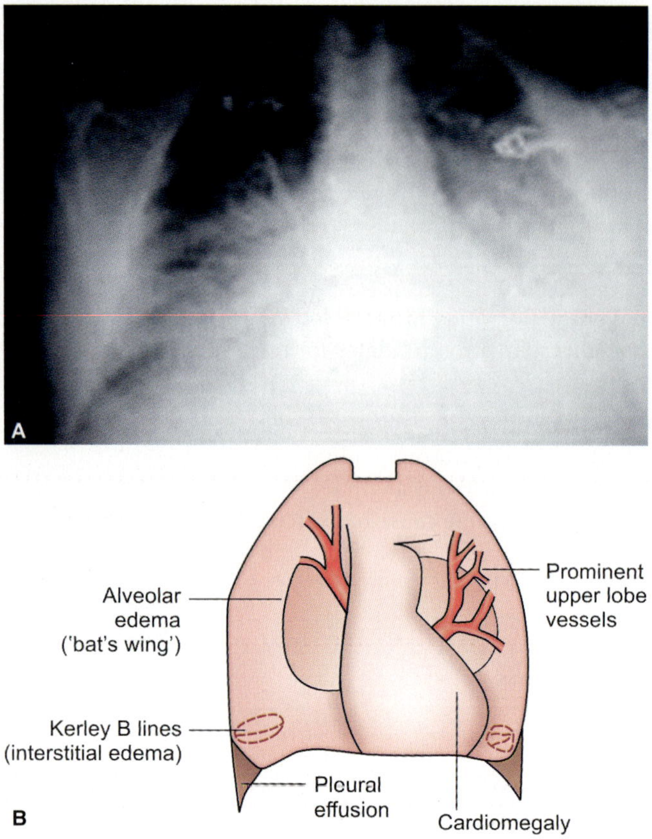


**Fig. 8.19:** (A) Classic signs of acute heart failure that can be seen on a chest X-ray of left ventricular failure. (B) Pleural effusion on a chest X-ray

following two principal features of chest radiographs are useful in the evaluation of patients with heart failure: (1) the size and shape of the cardiac silhouette and (2) edema at the lung bases.

## Electrocardiography

A screening electrocardiogram (ECG) is reasonable in patients with symptoms suggestive of heart failure. The presence of left atrial enlargement and LVH is sensitive (although nonspecific) for chronic LV dysfunction. It is unlikely that an ECG would be completely normal in the presence of heart failure; therefore, an alternative diagnosis should be sought in such cases. Electrocardiography may suggest an acute tachyarrhythmia or bradyarrhythmia as the cause of heart failure. It may also aid in the diagnosis of acute myocardial ischemia or infarction as the cause of heart failure or may suggest the likelihood of prior MI or the presence of coronary artery disease as the cause of heart failure (Figs 8.20–8.28).

## Echocardiography

Two-dimensional (2-D) echocardiography is recommended in the initial evaluation of patients with known or suspected heart failure. Ventricular function may be evaluated, and primary and secondary valvular abnormalities may be accurately assessed (Figs 8.29–8.31).

Doppler echocardiography, along with 2-D echocardiography, may play a valuable role in determining diastolic function and in establishing the diagnosis of diastolic heart failure. Approximately 30–40% of patients presenting with

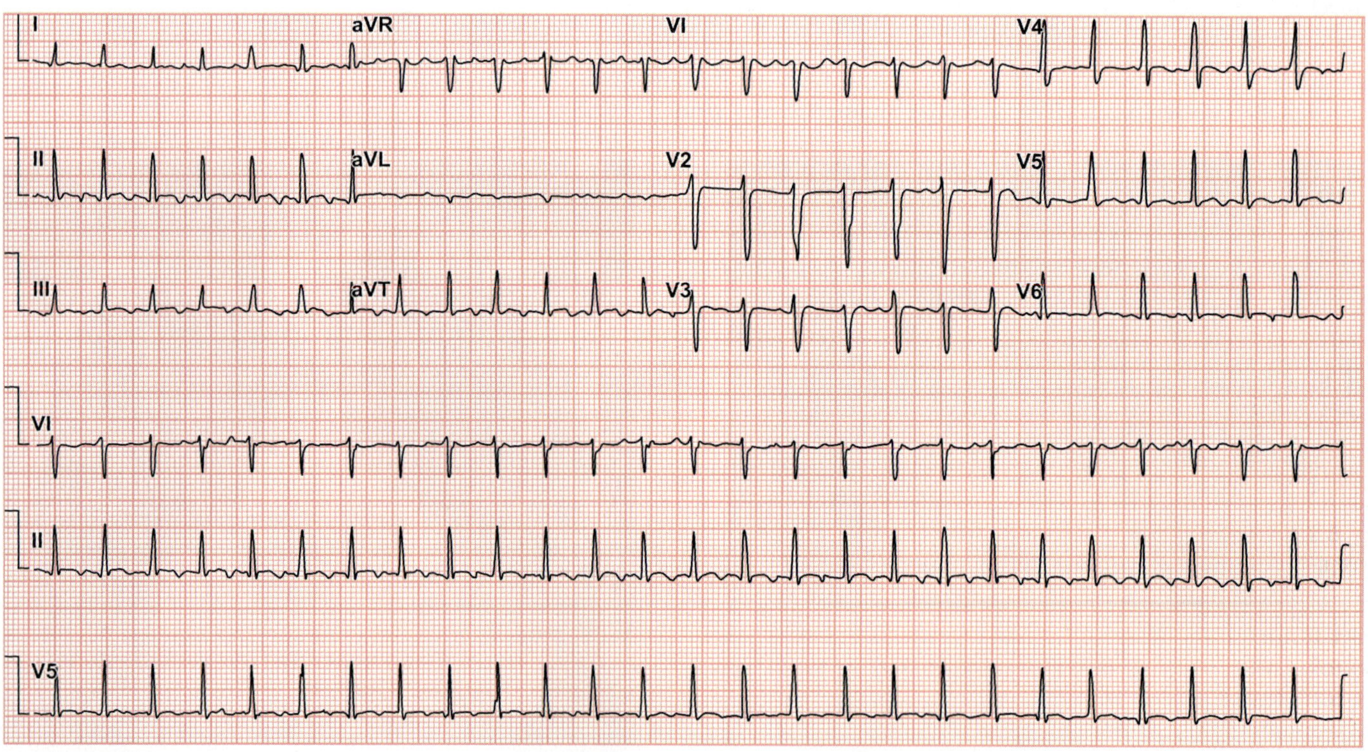


**Fig. 8.20:** ECG record of a patient with history of coronary artery disease, congestive heart failure with ejection fraction of 35%, presents to the emergency room with worsening shortness of breath and palpitations. ECG shows T-wave inversion in leads II, III, aVF, V4–V6

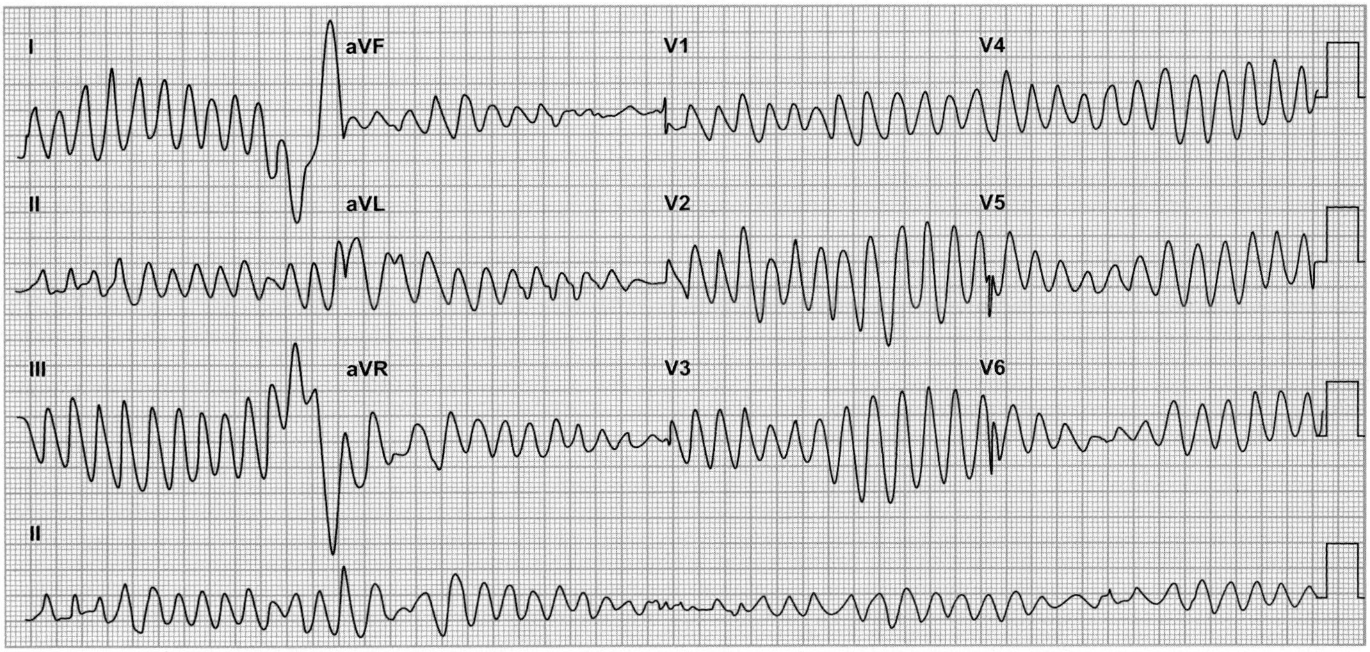


**Fig. 8.21:** ECG showing ventricular tachycardia in a case of heart failure

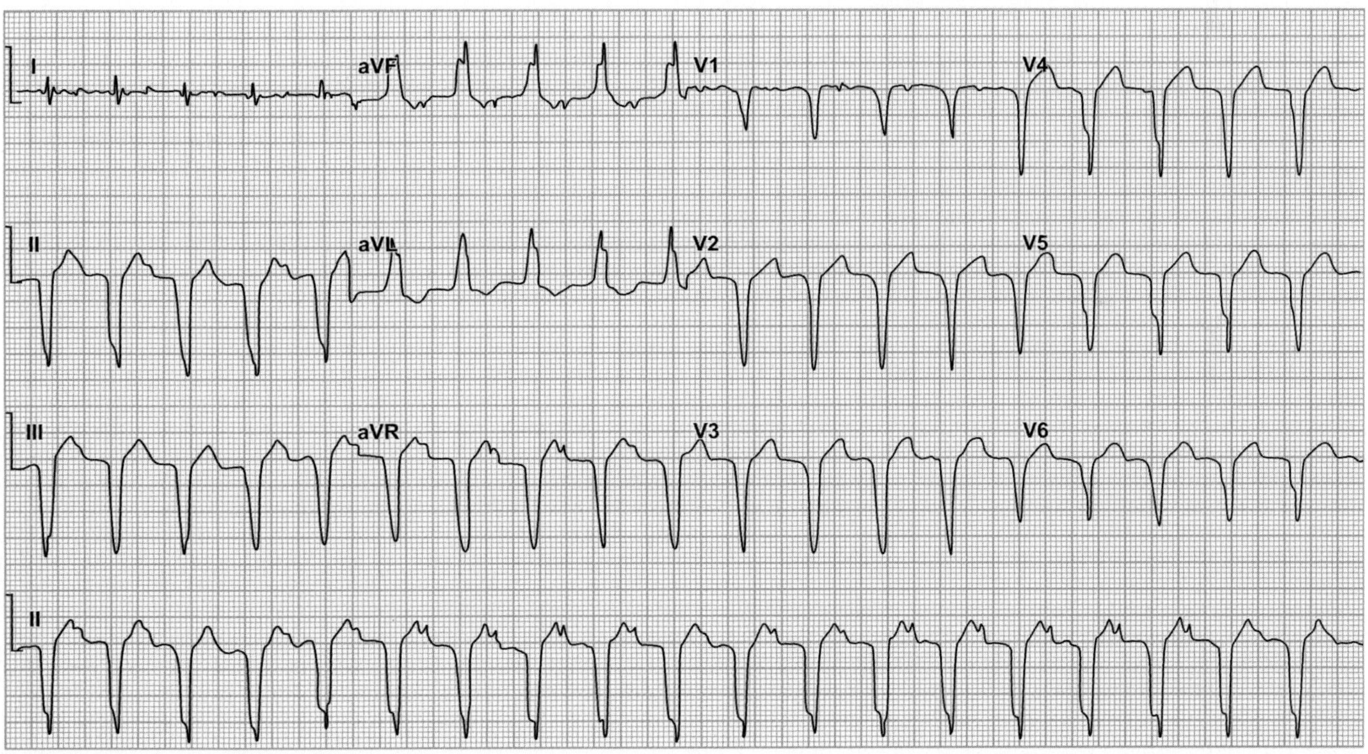


**Fig. 8.22:** Electrocardiogram (ECG) demonstrates a tachycardia with a 1:1 atrial-ventricular relationship in a 52-year-old male with recent-onset congestive heart failure and syncope

heart failure have normal systolic function but abnormal diastolic relaxation. The primary finding to differentiate diastolic heart failure is the presence of a normal ejection fraction; however, note that findings of diastolic dysfunction are common in the elderly and may not be associated with clinical heart failure. Because the therapy for this condition is distinctly different from that for systolic dysfunction, establishing the appropriate aetiology and diagnosis is essential.

Doppler and 2-D echocardiography may also be used to determine both systolic and diastolic LV performance, cardiac output (ejection fraction), and pulmonary artery and ventricular filling pressures. In addition, echocardiography may be used to identify clinically important valvular disease.

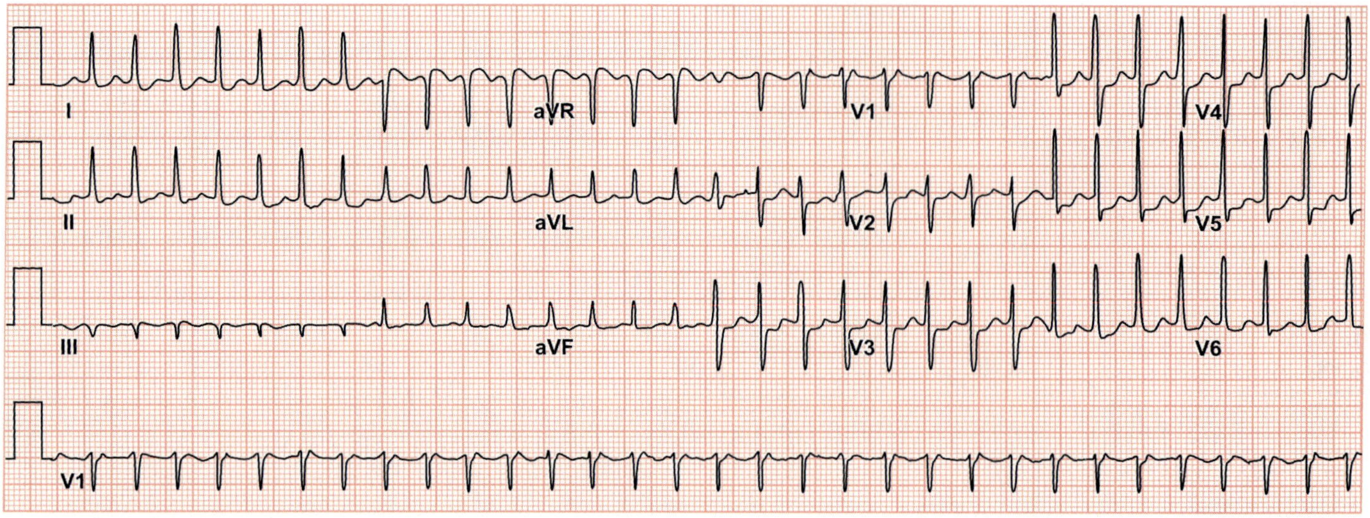


**Fig. 8.23:** ECG showing hemodynamically stable supraventricular tachycardia in a patient with heart failure

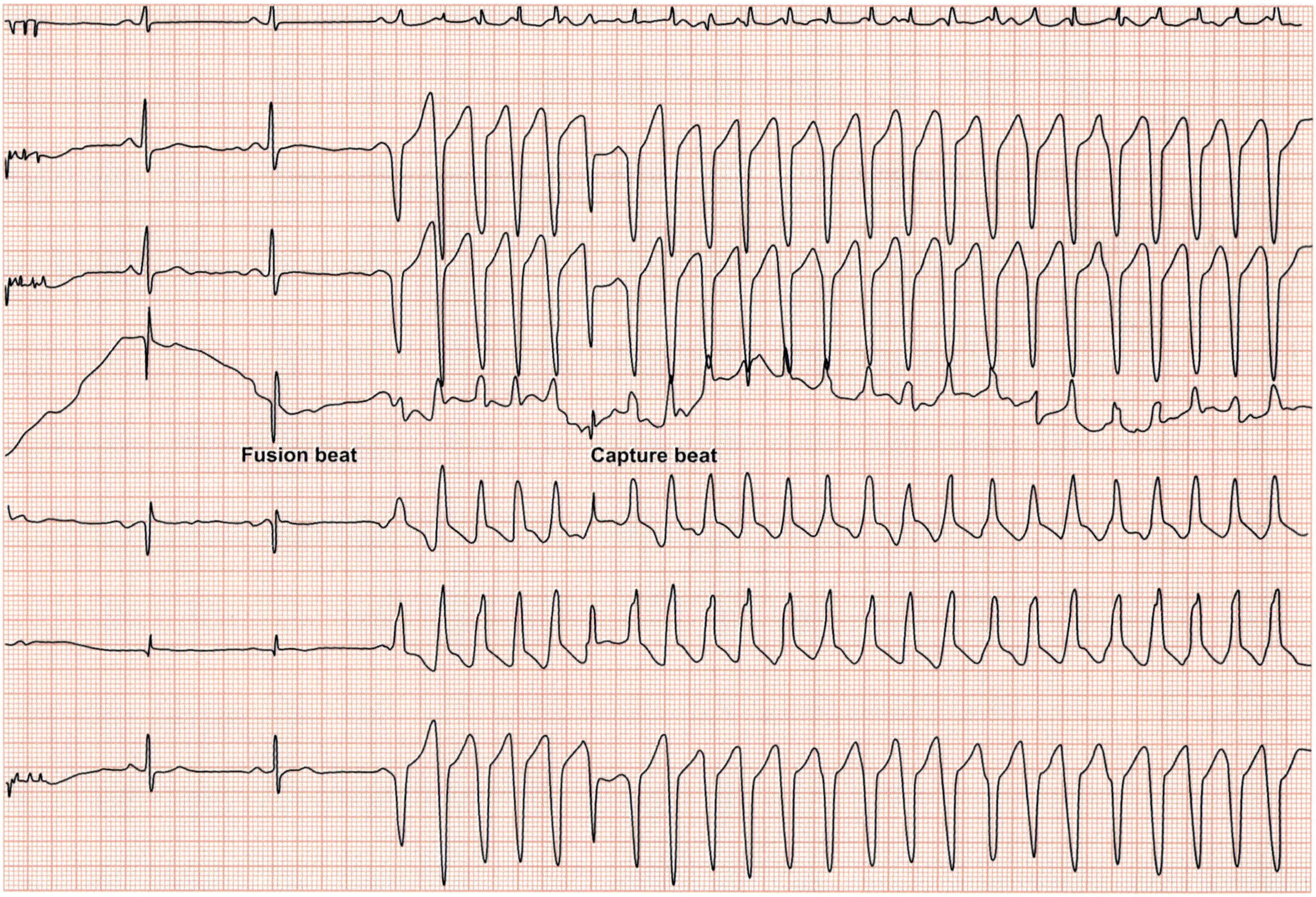


**Fig. 8.24:** ECG showing morphology of ventricular tachycardia (VT) in a patient with heart failure

### *Transesophageal Echocardiography*

Transesophageal echocardiography is particularly useful in patients who are on mechanical ventilation or are morbidly obese and in patients whose transthoracic echocardiogram is suboptimal in its imaging. It is an easy and safe alternative to conventional transthoracic echocardiography and provides better imaging quality (Fig. 8.32).

### *Stress Echocardiography*

Stress echocardiography, also known as dobutamine or exercise echocardiography, has several uses; however, in

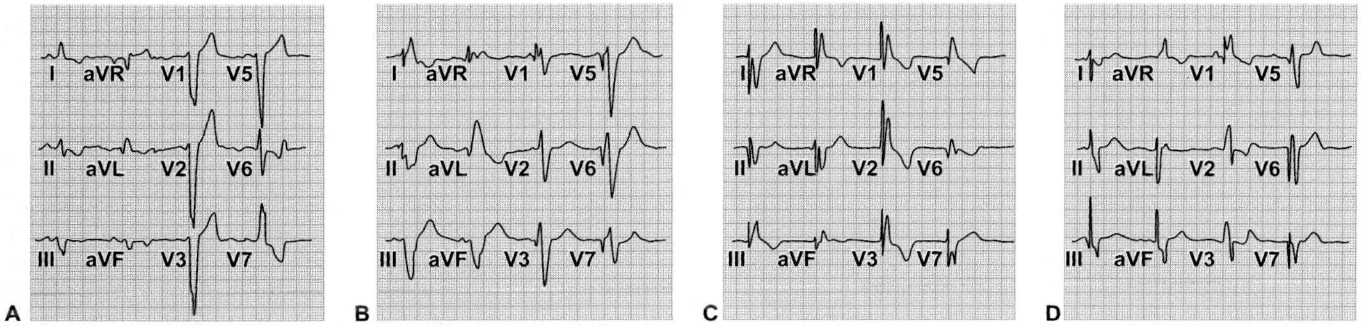


**Fig. 8.25:** Sample ECGs (average beat) during sinus rhythm, right ventricular pacing, left ventricular pacing, and biventricular pacing. (A) Subject in sinus rhythm. (B) Subject during right ventricular pacing. (C) Subject during left ventricular pacing. (D) Subject during biventricular pacing

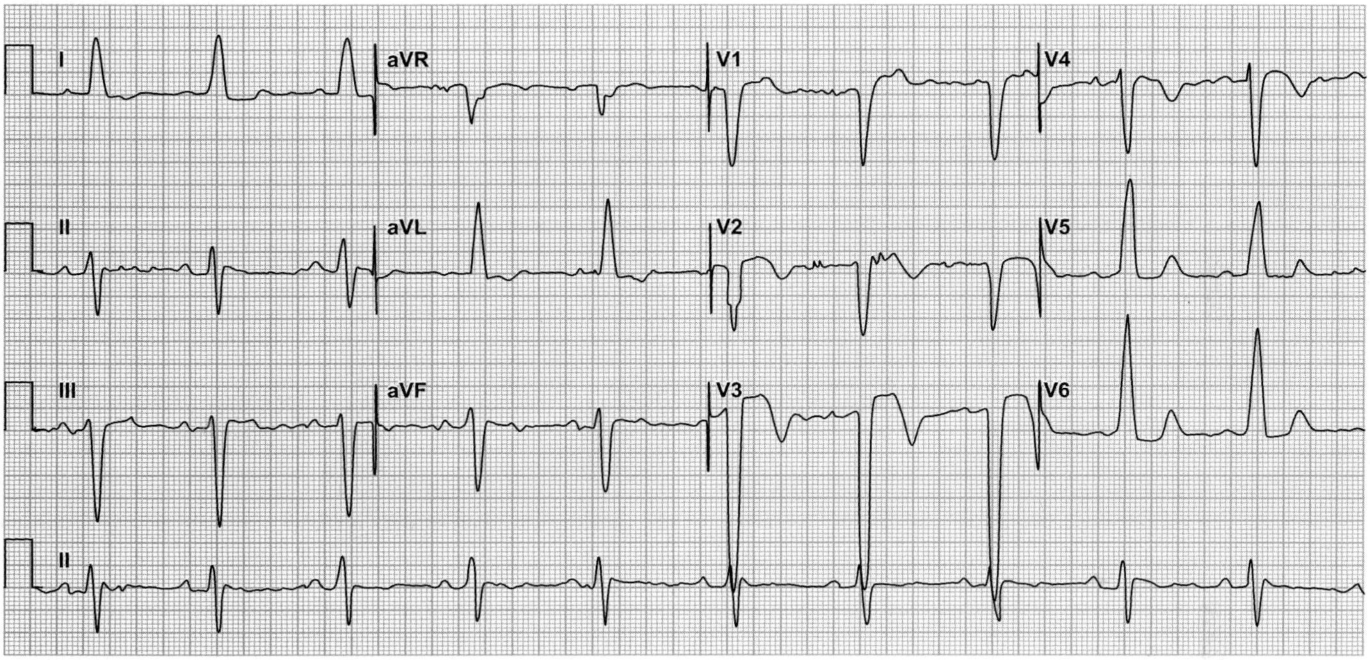


**Fig. 8.26:** The rhythm on this electrocardiogram (ECG) is sinus with borderline PR prolongation. There is evidence of an acute/evolving anterior ischemia/myocardial infarction (MI) superimposed on the left bundle branch block-like (LBBB) pattern in 75 years old man with heart failure

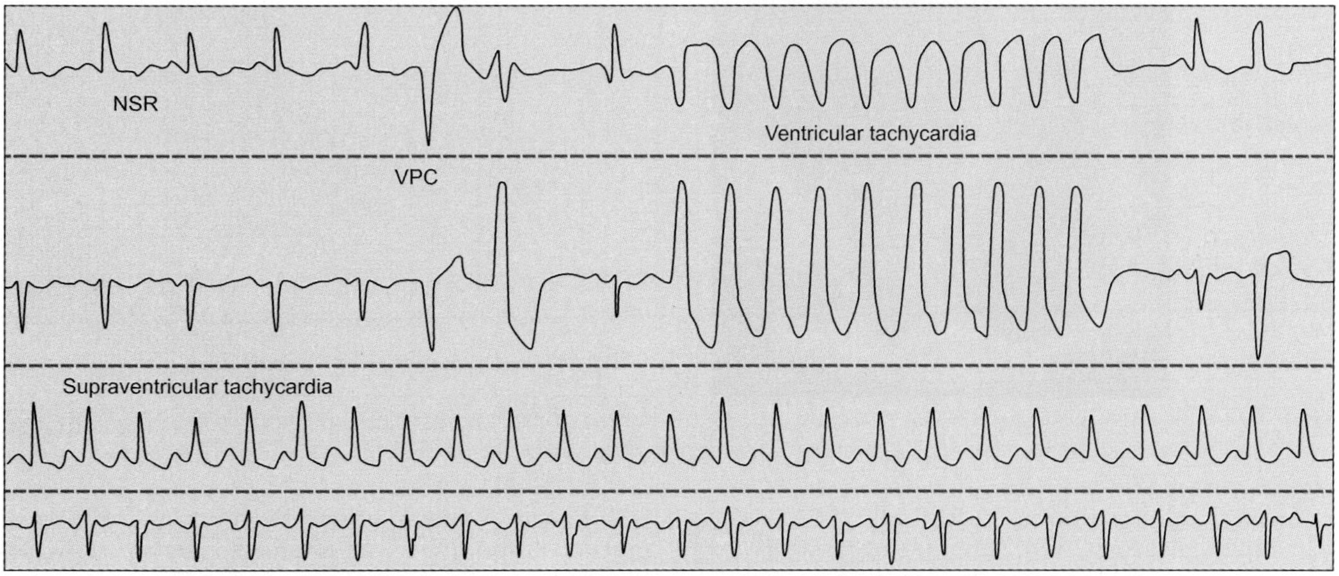


**Fig. 8.27:** Holter graph showing ventricular tachycardia in patient with ischemic heart failure

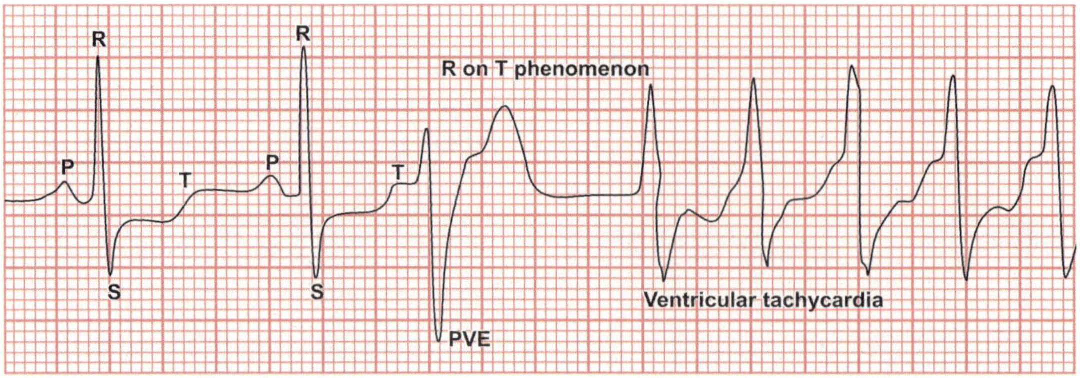


**Fig. 8.28:** ECG recorded by telemetry on a patient. The major time lines are 0.2 of a second. Note that the tachycardia is initiated with a premature ventricular beat with the retrograde P-wave sitting on the up sloping section of the T-wave. There is a long P-R interval to the next QRS with is the beginning of the tachycardia at a rate of about 160/min. With this tachycardia the patient had chest pain and a blood pressure of 70 mm systolic. A coronary angiogram found severe triple vessel coronary disease

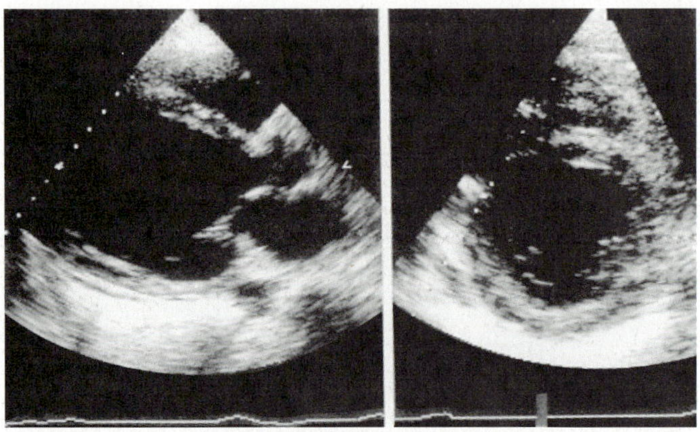

**Fig. 8.29:** Long axis and short axis 2D views of LV showing posterior wall infarction and hypokinetic anterior wall with cavity dilatation and poor LVEF =<15% in patient with breathlessness and effort angia

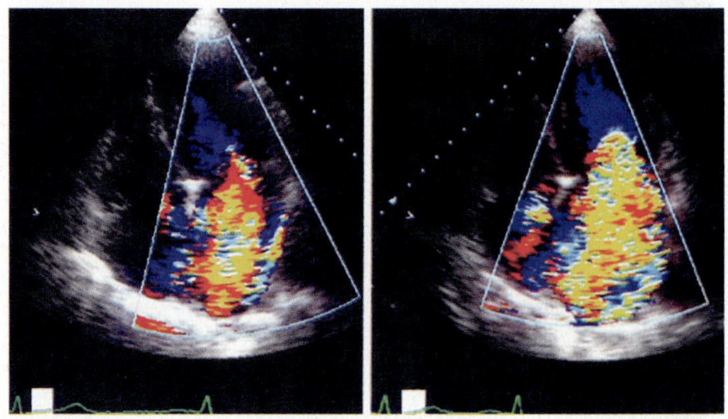

**Fig. 8.30:** Apical 4C view from a patient with ischemic cardiomyopathy and significant functional mitral regurgitation at rest (left). Note the increase in MR severity with stress, indicating development of severe ischemic dysfunction with stress

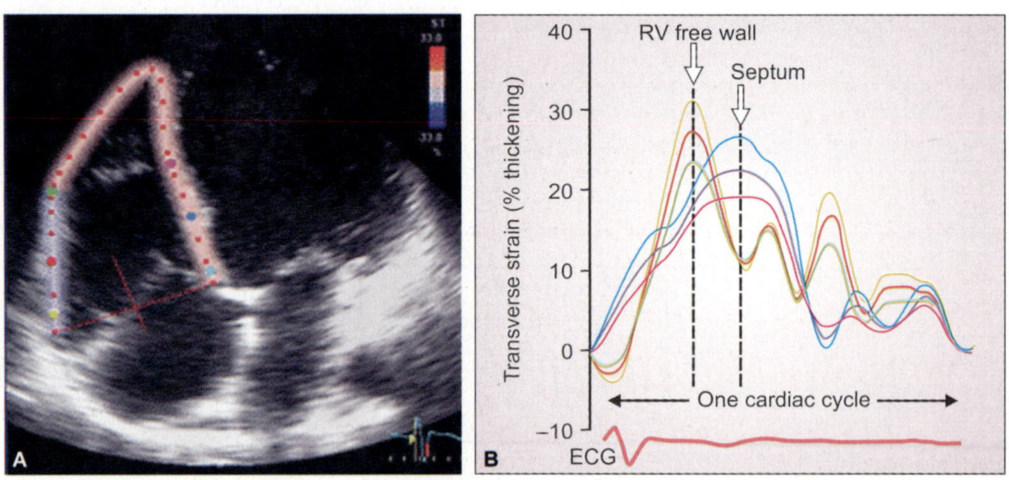


**Fig. 8.31:** RV failure. (A) Speckle tracking of 2D-echocardgraphic image of the right ventricle. (B) Strain vs time plotted for various regions of the RV. It shows delay in time to peak strain in the septum compared to the RV free wall

heart failure, this technique is used mainly to assess coronary artery disease (CAD). This imaging modality may be used to detect ventricular dysfunction caused by ischemia, evaluate myocardial viability in the presence of marked hypokinesis or akinesis, identify myocardial stunning and hibernation, and relate heart failure

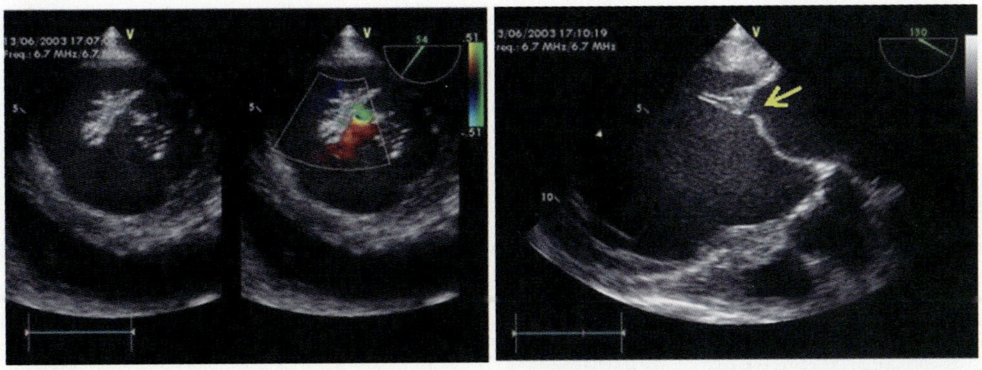

**Fig. 8.32:** Ischemic dilated cardiomyopathy with chronic mitral regurgitation due to important dilatation of the LV cavity, annular dilatation and loss of leaflet coaptation (arrow). TEE transgastric short and long axis views. Notice also the systolic restriction of the posterior leaflet (right picture)

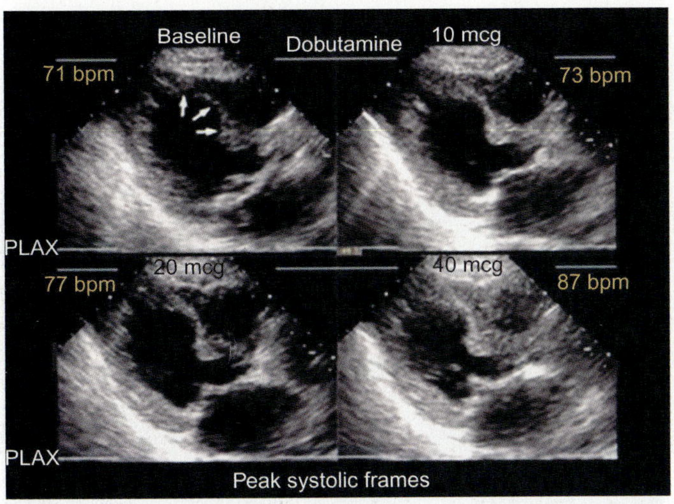


**Fig. 8.33:** A 64-years-old female with coronary artery disease and aortic valve disease underwent dobutamine stress echocardiography. Graded doses of dobutamine were infused in 3 minutes stages to a peak dose of 40 g/kg/min. Atropine (0.4 mg $\times$ 3) was given to achieve heart rate targets. Maximal heart rate achieved was 118 bpm (74% of predicted heart rate) and blood pressure was 110/82 mmHg. Patient had no symptoms. Baseline electrocardiogram showed normal sinus rhythm with ST abnormalities suggestive of a digitalis effect. Baseline echocardiogram showed dialated ventricular cavity size with estimated ejection fraction (EF) of 40–45% with akinesis and thinning of the basal-to-midanteroseptal and anterior wall. Images at peak infusion showed no increase in global systolic function (estimated EF 40%). The akinetic anteroseptal and anterior segments became progressively dyskinetic during the infusion consistent with a transmural infarct/scarring. In addition, the inferior wall, mildly hypokinetic at baseline, becomes akinetic at the high dose of dobutamine. Overall study was consistent with a large anterior and anteroseptal infarct with no significant peri-infarct ischemia. Sensitivity was limited because target heart rate was not achieved

symptoms to valvular abnormalities. However, stress echocardiography may have a lower sensitivity and specificity in heart failure patients because of LV dilatation or because of the presence of bundle branch block (Fig. 8.33).

### Conventional Doppler Assessment of LV Diastolic Dysfunction

Mitral inflow measurements which included peak early (E) and peak late (A) flow velocities, the E/A ratio, the deceleration time of early mitral flow velocity (DT), the isovolumetric relaxation time (IVRT) at rest and during the Valsalva maneuver and the pulmonary venous flow measurements, characterized by peak systolic (S), diastolic (D), and atrial reversal (Ard) velocities; the systolic filling fraction (S/D); and the time difference between A and the duration of atrial reverse flow (Ard-Ad) were originally considered to be indicative of diastolic LV dysfunction if they exceeded specific cut-off values indexed for age group. Because of the absence of pseudonormalization on tissue Doppler imaging (TDI) lengthening velocity measurements, the use of blood flow Doppler measures of diastolic LV function is no longer recommended as a first-line diagnostic approach to diastolic LV dysfunction. Only when TDI lengthening velocities are suggestive but nondiagnostic or when plasma levels of natriuretic peptides are elevated does the simultaneous presence of a low E/A ratio and a prolonged DT or a prolonged Ard-Ad index provide diagnostic evidence of diastolic LV dysfunction (Figs 8.34–8.36).

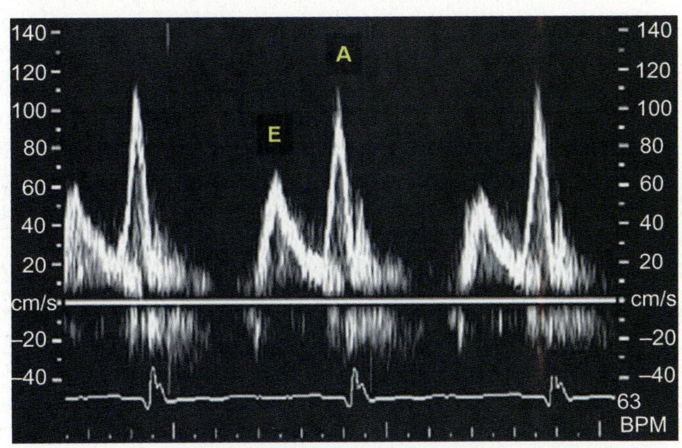


**Fig. 8.34:** Trans-mitral valve Doppler flow tracing in a patient with mild diastolic dysfunction (abnormal relaxation). The E- to A-wave ratio is <1.0

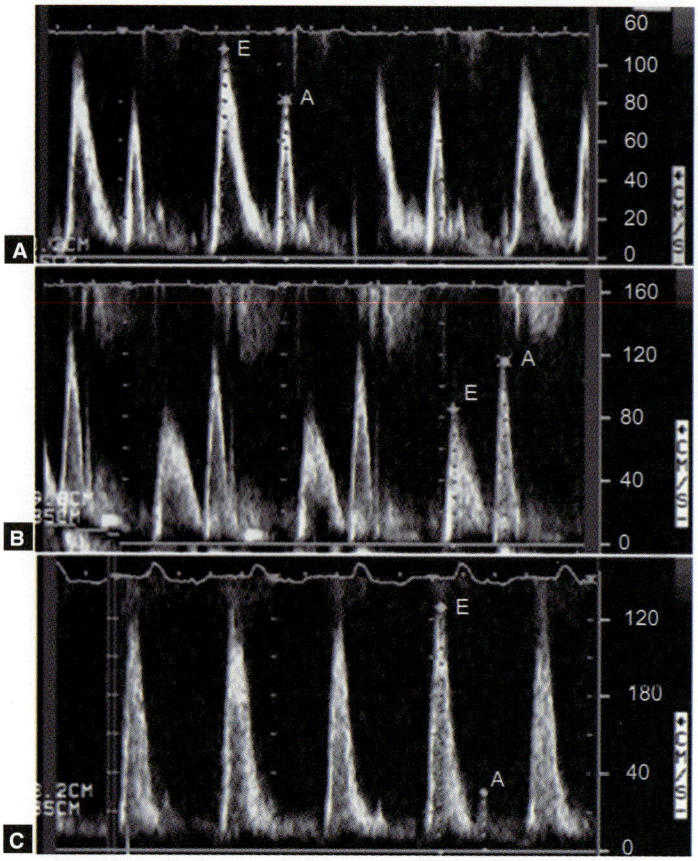


**Fig. 8.35:** Trans-mitral valve spectral Doppler flow pattern in a normal subject (A), in a patient with mild diastolic dysfunction (abnormal relaxation; B), and in a patient with severe (restrictive) diastolic dysfunction (C). In (A) the E/A wave ratio is approx. 1.5–1.0, and in (B) the E/A wave ratio is <1.0. In (C) the E/A wave ratio is abnormally high and A wave velocity is very low

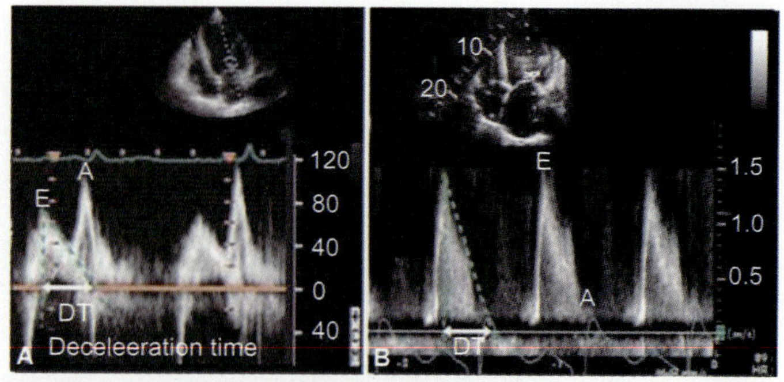


**Fig. 8.36:** Mitral inflow profiles showing evidence of diastolic dysfunction in dilated cardiomyopathy. The mitral inflow pulse Doppler profile in dilated cardiomyopathy often shows an impaired relaxation pattern (A) with prolonged deceleration time (DT >200 ms) and reversal of the normal E—a ratio during the early stages. Later worsening of diastolic dysfunction is accompanied by a compensatory increase in left atrial filling pressures (driving pressure) results in early rapid filling of the left ventricle (a tall, thin E-wave) in the setting of a dilated left atrium. The marked fall in the A-wave velocity reflects atrial systolic dysfunction owing to a poorly compliant left ventricle (B)

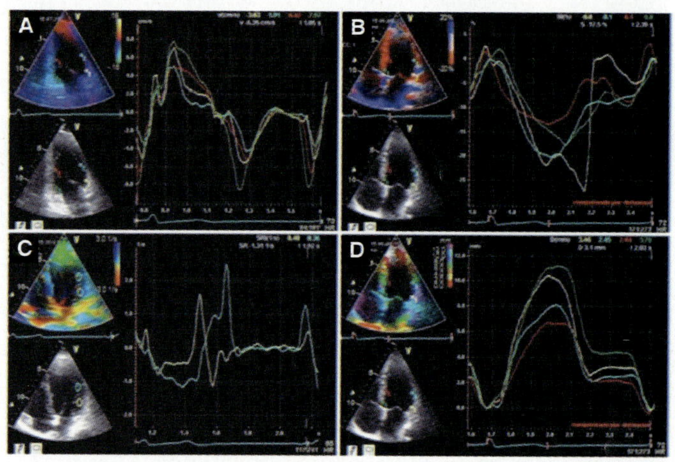


**Fig. 8.37:** Examples of tissue Doppler imaging measurements: (A) myocardial longitudinal segmental velocity in four regions of the anterior and inferior LV walls; (B) myocardial longitudinal segmental strain in lateral and septal LV walls; (C) myocardial longitudinal segmental strain rate in two regions in the lateral wall demonstrating some decrease in the velocity of deformation in the region represented by the yellow line; (D) myocardial longitudinal tissue displacement

## Tissue Doppler Assessment of LV Diastolic Dysfunctions

Tissue Doppler (TD) echocardiography helps to accurately quantify LV diastolic function (Figs 8.37–8.39). TD may be used to quantify myocardial velocities in multiple segments of the myocardium from different echocardiographic acoustic windows. The most frequently used modality of TD is measurement of LV basal (annular), longitudinal myocardial shortening, or lengthening velocity. Measurements can be obtained either at the septal or at the lateral side of the mitral annulus. The peak systolic (S) shortening velocity and the early diastolic (E2) lengthening velocities are considered to be sensitive measures of LV systolic or diastolic function. Especially, the ratio of early mitral valve flow velocity (E) divided by E2 correlates closely with LV filling pressures. E depends on left atrial driving pressure, LV relaxation kinetics, and age but E′ depends mostly on LV relaxation kinetics and age. Hence, in the ratio E/E2, effects of LV relaxation kinetics and age are eliminated and the ratio becomes a measure of left atrial driving pressure or LV filling pressure. E2 can also be conceptualized as the amount of blood entering the LV during early filling, whereas E represents the gradient necessary to make this blood enter the LV. A high E/E2 thus represents a high gradient for a low shift in volume. Information on LV filling pressures can also be derived from the time interval between the onset of E and the onset of E2 (TE-E2).

When the ratio E/E2 exceeds 15, LV filling pressures are elevated and when the ratio is lower than 8, LV filling pressures are low. E/E2 is a powerful predictor of survival after myocardial infarction and E/E2 >15 is superior as predictor of prognosis than clinical or other echocardiographic variables. The close correlation between E/E2 and LV filling pressures has been confirmed in heart failure patients with depressed (<50%) or preserved LV

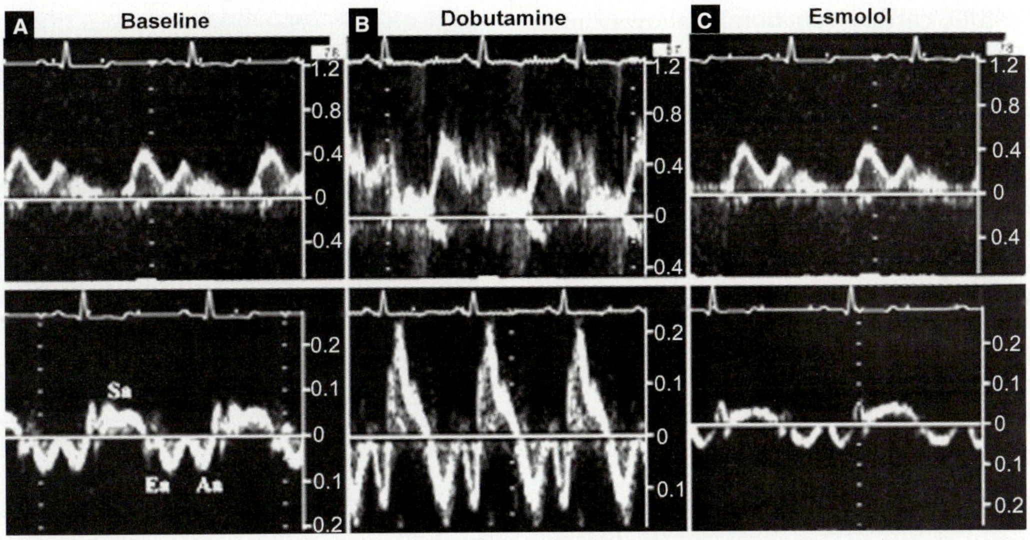


**Fig. 8.38:** Representative recordings of the lateral tricuspid annular motion velocity using tissue Doppler imaging (TDI) at baseline (A), with dobutamine (B), and with esmolol (C). Ea, ventricular early diastolic velocity; Aa, ventricular late diastolic velocity

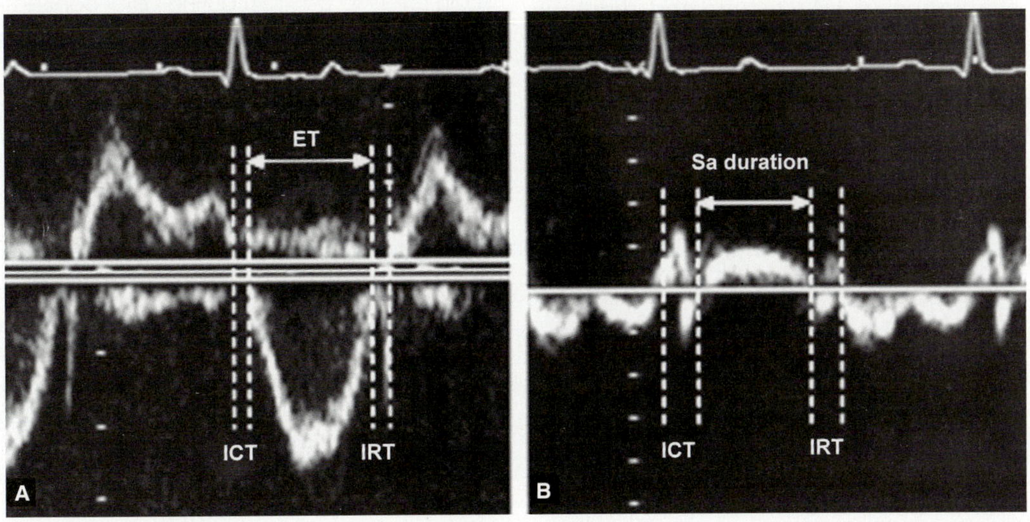


**Fig. 8.39:** Pulsed Doppler (PD)-derived myocardial performance index (MPI—A) and tissue Doppler-derived modified MPI (B). ET=ejection time; ICT=isovolumic contraction time; IRT=isovolumic relaxation time; Sa=ventricular systolic velocity

ejection fraction and in patients with slow relaxation or pseudonormal early mitral valve flow velocity filling patterns. The ratio E/E2 is considered diagnostic evidence of presence of diastolic LV dysfunction if E/E2 >15, and diagnostic evidence of absence of HFNLVEF if E/E2 <8. An E/E2 ratio ranging from 8–15 is considered suggestive but nondiagnostic evidence of diastolic LV dysfunction and needs to be implemented with other noninvasive investigations.

### Invasive Method of Assessment of LV Diastolic Dysfunction

Definite evidence of abnormal LV relaxation, filling, diastolic distensibility or diastolic stiffness can be acquired invasively during cardiac catheterization. Such evidence consists of a time constant of LV relaxation ($\tau$) > 48 ms, an LV enddiastolic pressure >16 mmHg or a mean pulmonary capillary wedge pressure >12 mmHg. A diastolic LV stiffness modulus >0.27 also provides diagnostic evidence of diastolic LV dysfunction. It has been pointed out that mitral flow Doppler alone, with its 40–70% specificity, cannot reliably detect diastolic dysfunction in HFNLVEF TDI including the transmitral flow velocity to annular velocity ratio (E/E2 index), which measures myocardial velocities during the cardiac cycle, is considered more reliable for diagnosing diastolic dysfunction. Oh et al. proposed comprehensive Doppler echocardiography with color flow or TDI as the most practical and reproducible method for either confirming or excluding diastolic dysfunction in HFNLVEF. In contrast, Maurer et al. recently argued that Doppler-derived diastolic parameters do not provide specific information on intrinsic passive diastolic properties and thus that diastolic dysfunction cannot be diagnosed by Doppler echocardiography. Invasive measurement of pressure–volume (PV) relationships with a conductance catheter system is generally considered most accurate for characterizing diastolic cardiac function. It allows direct detection of LV relaxation abnormalities and passive LV stiffness characterized by a change in diastolic LV pressure relative to diastolic LV volume. A recent study Mario Kasner et al. was the first to investigate the accuracy of several echocardiographic Doppler techniques in detecting diastolic dysfunction in HFNLVEF by direct comparison with invasive PV loop data. It was found that no diastolic index of conventional Doppler echocardiography alone was sufficient to make the correct diagnosis. These indices correlated only weakly with diastolic relaxation anomalies and not at all with the degree of LV stiffness. On the other hand, TDI investigations and the LV filling index E/E2 lat were well suited for detecting invasively proven diastolic dysfunction in HFNLVEF patients.

### Newer Techniques for Assessment of LV Dastolic Dysfunctions

Many studies have shown that atrial function is particularly important when ventricular dysfunction exists. Kurt et al. has shown that evaluation of LA systolic and diastolic function using strain Doppler echocardiography has reasonably high accuracy. This study showed that patients with DHF have a significantly reduced LA strain and strain rate during LV systole and increased LA stiffness index. Increased LA stiffness as assessed invasively and noninvasively readily identify patients with DHF from those with LV diastolic dysfunction. On the other hand, LV mass, volumes, and systolic function, LA volumes and atrial pump function were not significantly different in the patients of DHF and LVDD.

### *LA Strain and Strain Rate*

These are new emerging real time ultrasound techniques that provide a measure of wall motion or a measure of deformation. Radial and longitudinal atrial or ventricular function can be assessed by the analysis of wall deformation using the rate of deformation of a myocardial segment (strain rate) and its deformation over time (strain).

A negative strain rate corresponds to myocardial shortening or thickening, whereas a positive strain rate corresponds to myocardial lengthening or thinning. Atrial strain and strain rate measurements are usually obtained during ventricular and atrial systole using sample volumes placed in the atrial myocardium near but clearly superior to the mitral annulus. For LA 'diastolic' strain variables (during LV systole) the source of the strain is the ventricle doing external work on the atrium as the LV ejects blood into the aorta. Deformation in the atria is reciprocally related to the deformation of the ventricles, as both apex and the atrial roof are relatively immobile, the ventricle shortens while atria elongates during systole, ventricle elongates and atria shortens during the diastolic phases. In diastasis, there is no deformation. And so the amount and rate of strain measured is determined primarily by ventricular and LV afterload attributes, although it follows that passive atrial tissue properties on which the LV is also doing work. In addition, because of its thin wall, strain rate imaging in the atria is extra prone to artefacts due to low

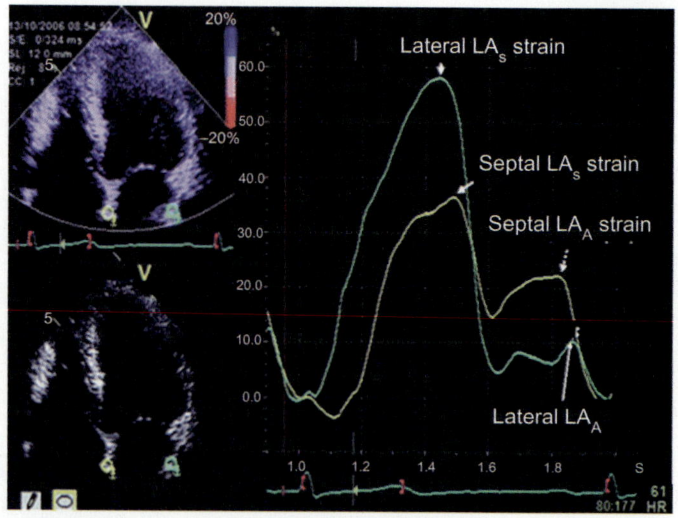


**Fig. 8.40:** Example of LA strain curves. Septal LA strain is shown in yellow, and lateral strain is shown in blue. LAS strain refers to LA strain during the systolic phase of the cardiac cycle, and LAA strain refers to LA strain during atrial contraction

lateral resolution. Kurt et al. has shown that patients with DHF had significantly a lower LA systolic strain and SR as compared to patients with LVDD alone. However, late diastolic strain and SR were similar in patients with DHF and LV diastolic dysfunction (Fig. 8.40).

### *LA Stiffness Index* (Fig. 8.41)

Stiffness is conventionally defined as the force required to displace a passive spring a unit length. Physiologically it is the change in pressure required to increase the volume of a passive container a unit amount. LA stiffness can be estimated invasively, i.e. by ratio of pulmonary wedge pressure to LA systolic strain and noninvasive LA stiffness can be calculated by ratio of E/E2 and LA strain. LA systolic strain is determined by averaging values from four sites in the

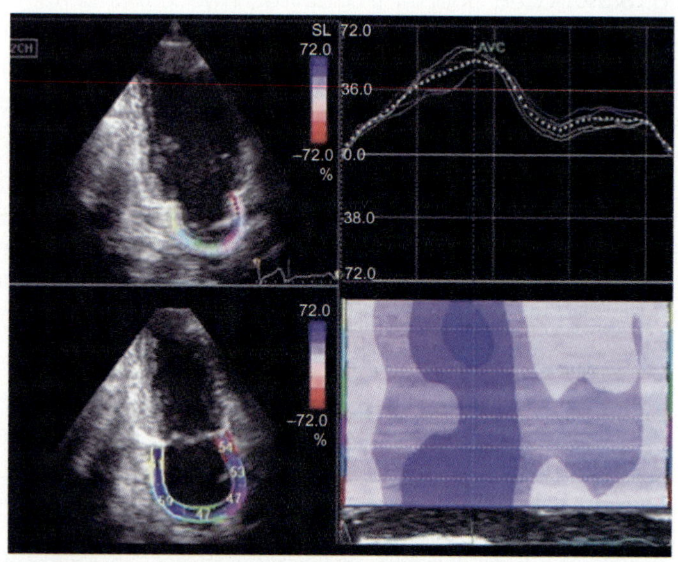

**Fig. 8.41:** Speckle echocardiographic left atrial strain and stiffness index as predictors of maintenance of sinus rhythm after cardioversion

LA myocardium. The units of LA stiffness are mmHg. Importantly, the denominator in this expression, although measured in the LA wall, is determined primarily by longitudinal apically directed displacement of the mitral annulus by the contracting ventricle, whereas the posterior aspect of the LA remains fixed. Hence this index, usually attributed to the LA as a stiffness measure, is very strongly influenced by LV properties. LA stiffness as assessed invasively and noninvasively readily identified patients with DHF from those with LV diastolic dysfunction. Kurt et al. has shown that a LA stiffness index of >1.1 mmHg had a sensitivity of 84%, and a specificity of 100% in distinguishing patients with DHF from those with LV diastolic dysfunction. Using E/E2 ratio in lieu of PCWP was also accurate in identifying DHF patients and an index of 0.99 had a sensitivity of 85% and a specificity of 78% in distinguishing patients with DHF from those with LV diastolic dysfunction.

*Left atrial volume measurements:* A left atrial volume indexed to body surface area (left atrial volume index) >32 ml/m$^2$ was first recognized in the elderly as a strong predictor (p=0.003) of a cardiovascular event with a higher predictive value than other echocardiographically derived indices such as LV mass index (p=0.014) or LV diastolic dysfunction (p=0.029). In a population-based study, left atrial volume index was also strongly associated with the severity and duration of diastolic LV dysfunction; the left atrial volume index progressively increased from a value of 23+6 ml/m$^2$ in normals to 25+8 ml/m$^2$ in mild diastolic LV dysfunction, to 31+8 ml/m$^2$ in moderate diastolic LV dysfunction, and finally to 48+12 ml/m$^2$ in severe diastolic LV dysfunction. Left atrial volume index was therefore proposed as a biomarker of both diastolic LV dysfunction and cardiovascular risk. Left atrial volume index (LAVi) is a more robust marker than left atrial area or left atrial diameter (Fig 8.42).

For these reasons, a left atrial volume index >40 ml/m$^2$ has been taken to provide sufficient evidence of diastolic LV dysfunction when the E/E2 ratio is nonconclusive

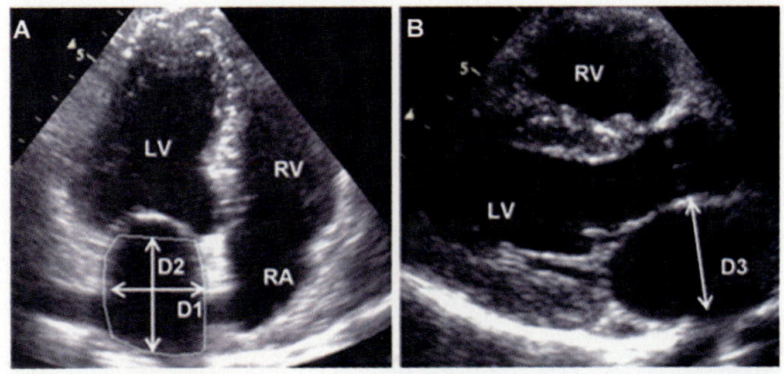


**Figs 8.42A and B:** Measurement of left atrial (LA) volume from the prolate ellipse method using apical four-chamber and parasternal long-axis views at ventricular end systole (maximum LA size). D2 is measured from the mitral annular plane to the back wall. D1 is the orthogonal short-axis dimension to D2. D3 is measured from the blood-tissue interface of the anterior and posterior walls. LA volume is (D1 × D2×D3)×(0.523). LV=left ventricle; RA=right atrium; RV=right ventricle

(i.e. 15 >E/E2 >8) or when plasma levels of natriuretic peptides are elevated. Similarly, a left atrial volume index <29 ml/m$^2$ is proposed as a prerequisite to exclude HFNLVEF. Left atrial volume index values of 29 and 40 ml/m$^2$ correspond, respectively, to the lower cut-off values of mildly abnormal and severely abnormal LA size in the recent recommendations for cardiac chamber quantification of the American Society of Echocardiography and the European Association of Echocardiography.

### LV Torsion with 2D Speckle Tracking Echocardiography

Left ventricular torsion (LVtor) and subsequent untwisting play an important role in diastolic filling. Sung-Ji et al. has shown that systolic torsion and diastolic untwisting are significantly increased in patients with mild diastolic dysfunction. However, analysis of LVtor with speckle tracking echocardiography needs to be further explored to elucidate the role of torsion in patients with LV diastolic dysfunction (Figs 8.43–8.50).

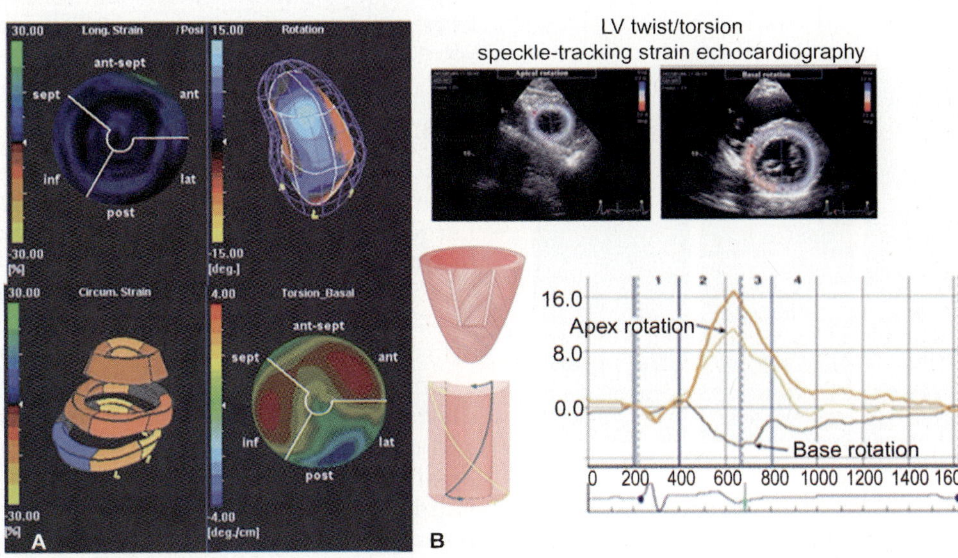


**Figs 8.43A and B:** Different parameters (longitudinal strain, rotation, circumferential strain and torsion-basal) displayed in different formats

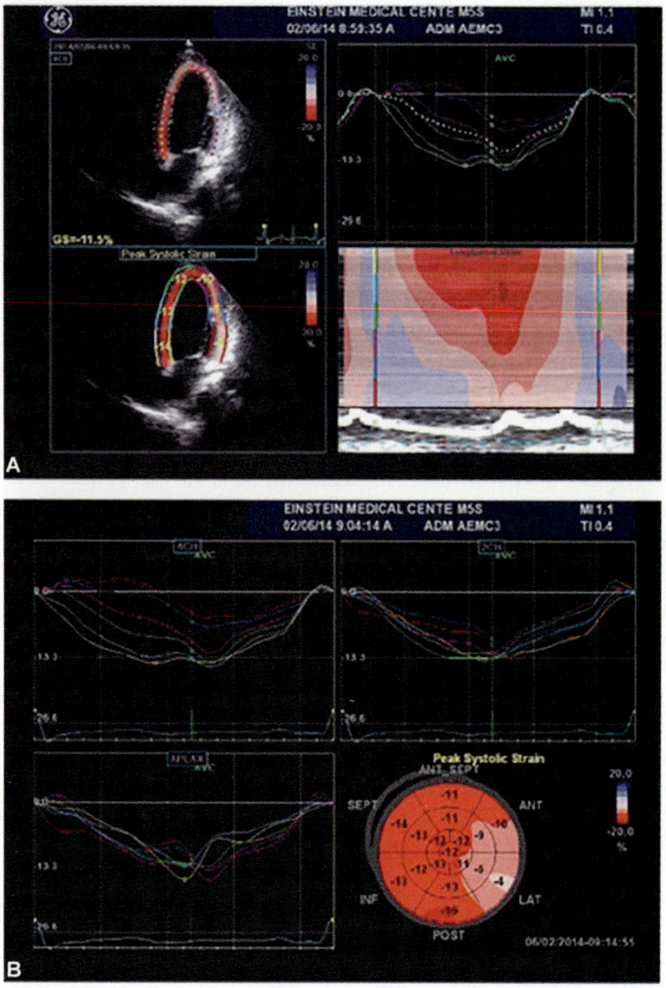


Fig. 8.44: Speckle-tracking echocardiography-derived longitudinal strain in a patient with cardiomyopathy with a left ventricular ejection fraction of 40%. (A, top left) Peak longitudinal strain in a apical four-chamber view. (A, top right) Wave form display. (A, bottom left) Quantitative parametric overlay. (A, bottom right) Color M-mode display. (B) Bull's eye presentation of strain

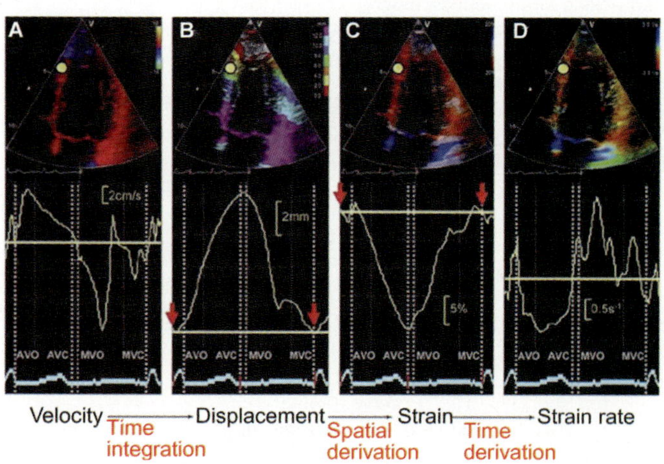


Fig. 8.45: Parameters of myocardial deformation derived from one region of interest (yellow dot) using tissue Doppler imaging. (A) Velocity, (B) displacement, (C) strain, (D) strain rate

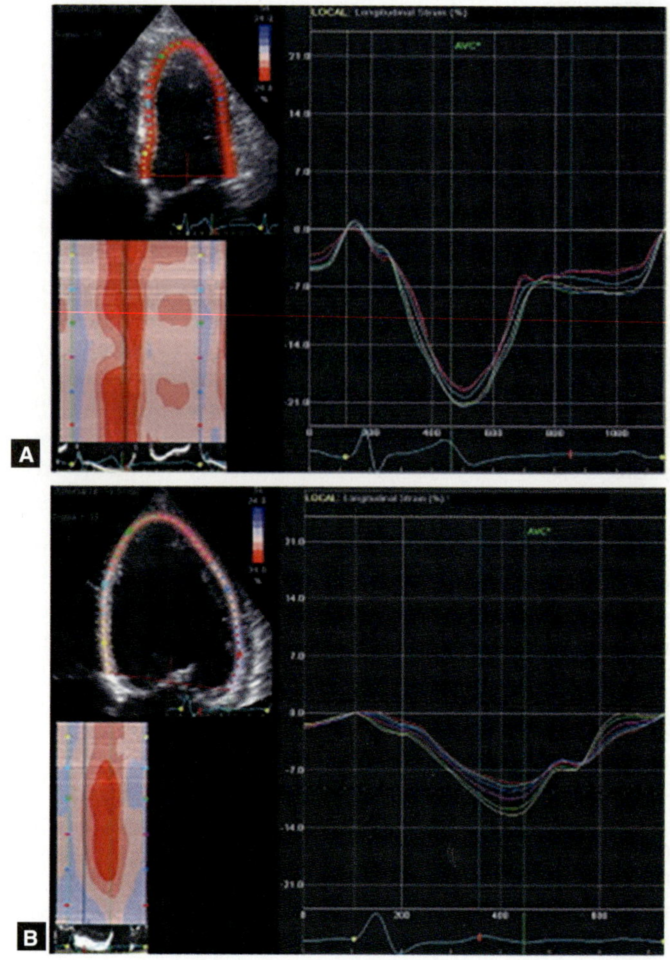


Fig. 8.46: Longitudinal strain by speckle tracking imaging in a normal subject and a heart failure patient. (A) An example of speckle tracking imaging of longitudinal strain using the apical four-chamber view in a normal subject demonstrating peak longitudinal strain of –16.5% and –21.5%, respectively. (B) An example of speckle tracking imaging of longitudinal strain using the apical four-chamber view in a heart failure patient with depressed ejection fraction demonstrating smaller peak longitudinal strain of –8.0% and –12.5%, respectively. AVC = aortic valve closure

## Role of BNP in DHF

Measurements of the levels of B-natreuretic peptide (BNP) have been used to confirm the diagnosis of heart failure. Large population-based studies using BNP to screen for heart failure demonstrate a sensitivity of 40–50% and a specificity of 95% in detecting ejection fraction of less than 40%. The diagnostic accuracy of BNP increases tremendously if we include diastolic heart-failure patients. Therefore, the same authors found that when including diastolic dysfunction on echo, BNP had a sensitivity of 91% and a specificity of 82%. Doust et al. reviewed 20 studies looking at the accuracy of BNP in the diagnosis of heart failure and found that BNP had an area under the receiver operator curve of 0.83. Using the pooled diagnostic odds ratio (DOR) [sensitivity/(1-sensitivity)]/[(1-specificity)/specificity] they demonstrated a DOR of 11.6 for studies

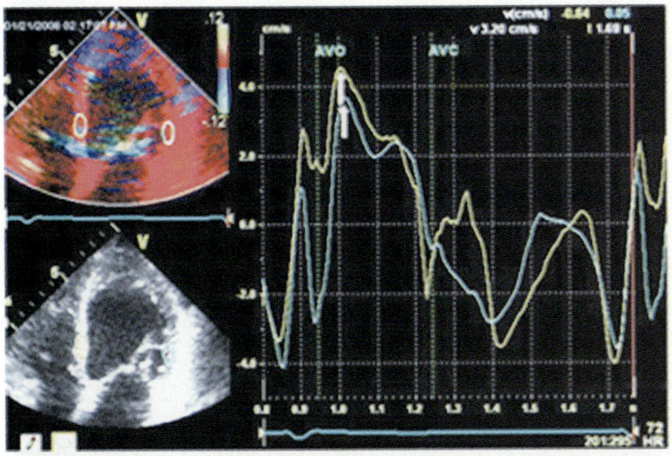


**Fig. 8.47:** Color-coded tissue Doppler image using the apical four-chamber view from a heart failure patient with widened QRS, but no significant mechanical dyssynchrony before cardiac resynchronization therapy. There was similar timing in peak velocities (arrows) from septal to lateral wall, determined between aortic valve opening (AVO) and aortic valve closure (AVC). This patient did not have a favourable clinical nor ventricular function response to resynchronization therapy

that compared BNP with impaired ejection fraction and a DOR of around 30 for studies that compared BNP with clinical heart failure including patients with diastolic heart failure. Therefore, BNP's diagnostic accuracy was increased when diastolic heart failure patients were included in the disease group. Moreover, in normal individuals, the concentration of BNP rises with age and is higher in women than in men. BNP levels can be influenced by comorbidities such as sepsis, liver failure, or kidney failure, pulmonary hypertension as a result of chronic obstructive pulmonary disease, pulmonary embolism, or mechanical ventilation and obesity. BNP levels are therefore recommended mainly for exclusion of HFNLVEF and not for diagnosis of HFNLVEF. Furthermore, when used for diagnostic purposes, BNP levels alone does not provide diagnostic standard evidence of HFNLVEF and always need to be complemented with other echocardiographic variables.

## CT Scanning and MRI

Computed tomography (CT) scanning or magnetic resonance imaging (MRI) may be useful in evaluating chamber size and ventricular mass, cardiac function, and wall motion; delineating congenital and valvular abnormalities; and demonstrating the presence of pericardial disease. However, cardiac CT scanning is usually not required in the routine diagnosis and management of heart failure, and echocardiography and MRI may provide similar information without exposing the patient to ionizing radiation (Fig. 8.51).

The benefits of cardiac MRI (cMRI) include the ability to obtain a great deal of information with a noninvasive test. This modality provides detailed functional and morphologic information; can be used to assess ischemic versus nonischemic disease, infiltrative disease, and hypertrophic disease; and can be employed to determine viability. It is used principally for the delineation of con-

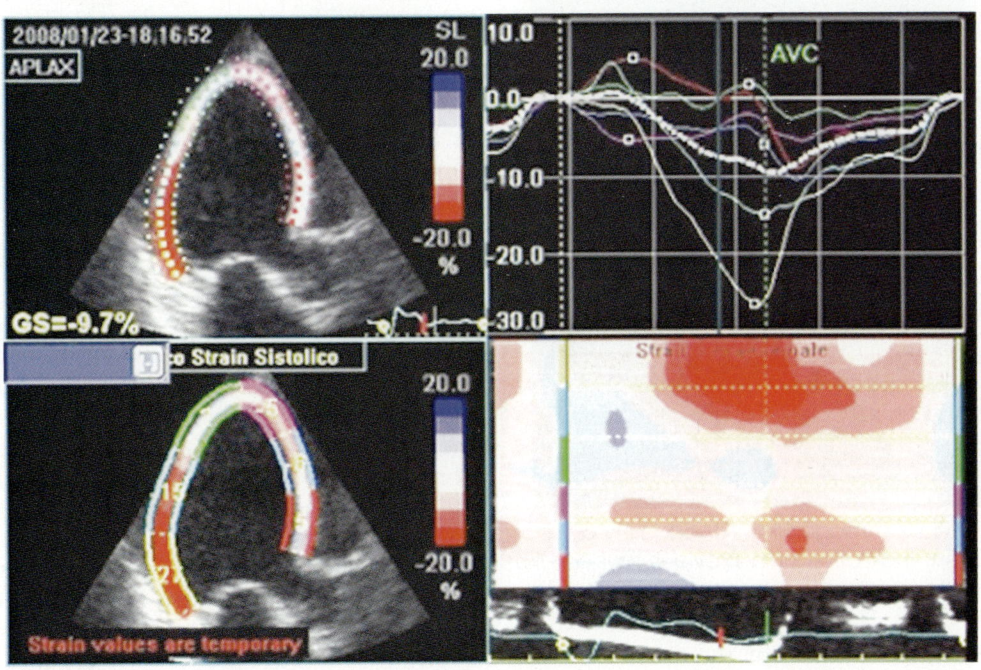


**Fig. 8.48:** Representation of 2D-strain (speckle tracking) of the left ventricle in the apical long axis view in a patient with systolic heart failure. The upper right panel depicts the strain curves sampled in each of the analyzed myocardial segments. It is also possible to calculate a global strain index (GS), which in this case is clearly diminished (GS=9,7%; see upper left panel). The lower left panel shows peak systolic strain for each segment while the lower right panel shows longitudinal strain processed according to a color map of curvilinear anatomical M-mode. From top to bottom: the basal, mid, and apical posterolateral wall, followed by the apical, mid, and basal interventricular anterior septum wall; in red the segments with higher contractility

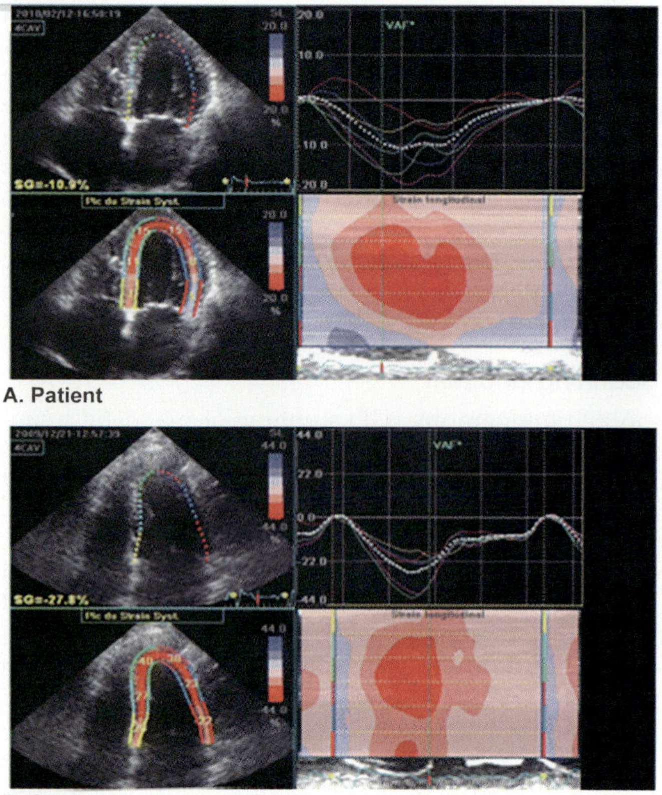


A. Patient

B. Control

**Fig. 8.49:** (A) Two-dimensional strain in an apical four-chamber view in a patient with heart failure and preserved ejection fraction and (B) in a control patient

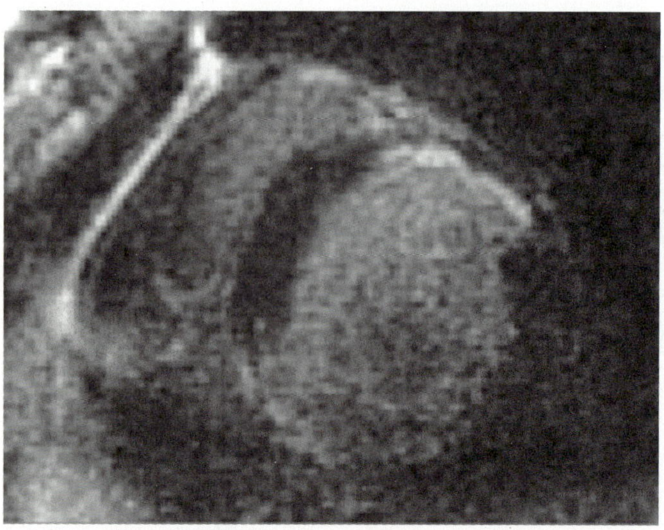

**Fig. 8.51:** Magnetic resonance image shows a scar in the anterior cardiac wall in a patient indicative of a previous myocardial infarction precipitating heart failure

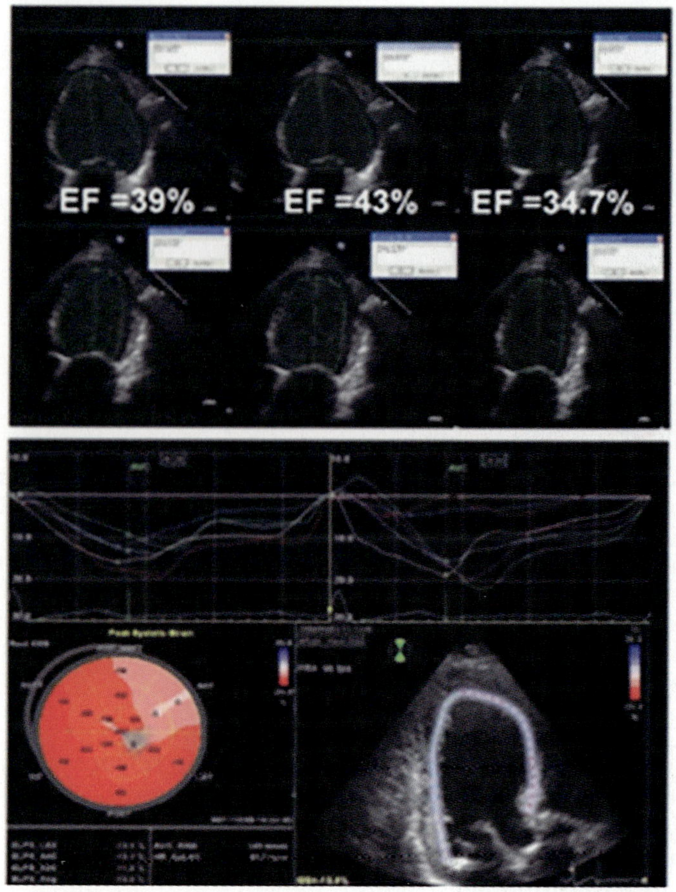


**Fig. 8.50:** (A) Left ventricular evaluation in heart failure (HF). Successive tracings may place this patient's EF above or below the threshold for device insertion, (B) Benefit of an automated approach to EF-based decision-making. Repeat measurements of global strain are highly likely to be reproducible

genital cardiac abnormalities and for the assessment of valvular heart disease, and it is the gold standard for evaluating RV function MRI has become particularly useful for evaluating abnormalities in wall motion and viable myocardium, and MRI results can help predict the success of revascularization in patients with low ejection fractions. However, the detailed information obtained by MRI must be balanced by its high costs and the fact that this imaging modality cannot be performed in patients with implantable defibrillators.

## Nuclear Imaging

The incidence of heart failure (HF) is increasing and it remains the only area in cardiovascular disease wherein hospitalization rates and mortalities have worsened in the past 25 years. This review is provided to assess the role of radionuclide imaging in HF. The focus is on three aspects—the value of nuclear imaging to distinguish ischemic from nonischemic etiologies; risk stratification of patients with HF with evaluation of candidates for specific treatment strategies; and the role of cardiac neuronal imaging in patients with HF. Distinguishing ischemic from non-ischemic cardiomyopathy is important because patients with ischemic cardiomyopathy can potentially have dramatic improvement with revascularization. Single photon emission computed tomography (SPECT) has excellent reported sensitivity and negative predictive value in the detection of coronary artery disease in HF patients. SPECT imaging is also useful in establishing treatment strategies in patients with HF, including those with new onset CHF. Cardiac neuronal imaging of mIBG is parti-

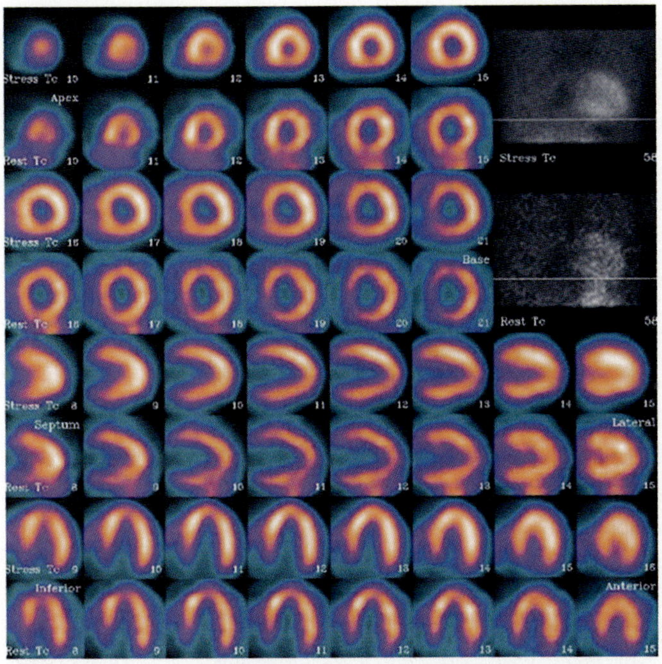

**Fig. 8.52:** Myocardial perfusion imaging was performed with dipyridamole stress test using one day Tc-99m-tetrofosmin rest-stress protocol. There were no symptoms or ECG changes to suggest dipyridamole induced myocardial ischemia. The images do not show any reversible perfusion defects to suggest presence of dipyridamole induced myocardial ischemia. Left ventricle is dilated (EDV 176 ccs) and hypertrophied. Gated images show global hypokinesis with an ejection fraction of 34%. These findings suggest nonischemic cardiomyopathy. Echocardiography showed left ventricular hypertrophy and dilatation with a globally reduced ejection fraction of 30–40%

cularly helpful in risk stratification of patients with HF. The modality can be used to monitor the response to therapy as dysfunctional mIBG uptake may show improvement with pharmacological treatment (Figs 8.52 and 8.53).

### Radionuclide Multiple-gated Acquisition Scanning

Radionuclide multiple-gated acquisition (MUGA) scan is a reliable imaging technique for evaluation of LV and RV function and wall motion abnormalities. Because of its reliability, LV ejection fraction (LVEF), as determined by MUGA scanning, is often used for serial assessment of postchemotherapy LV function (Fig. 8.54).

### Electrocardiogram-gated Myocardial Perfusion Imaging

The high photon flux of compounds labeled with technetium-99m (99m TC) makes it feasible to acquire myocardial perfusion images in an ECG-gated mode. ECG-gated single-photon emission CT (SPECT) images allow for assessment of global LVEF, regional wall motion, and regional wall thickening at rest in patients with documented stress-induced wall motion and perfusion abnormalities (Fig. 8.55).

In general, LVEF from gated SPECT agrees well with resting LVEF determined by other modalities. Quality assurance is important, however, because determinations of LVEF with gated SPECT may be less accurate, even invalidated, in the presence of an irregular heart rate, low count density, intense extracardiac radiotracer uptake adjacent to the LV, or a small LV.

*Combined interpretation of perfusion and function on ECG-gated images* substantially increases the confidence of interpretation. Taillefer and associates reported that the interpretation of stress and rest end-diastolic section, rather than summed ungated sections, may enhance the overall sensitivity for the detection of mild coronary artery disease.

ECG-gated images are useful for recognizing artifactual defects caused by attenuation (breast and diaphragm) and thus are useful in the quality control of SPECT imaging. ECG-gated SPECT imaging is currently considered the state of the art of radionuclide myocardial perfusion imaging.

There are three important practical issues that need to be addressed in the evaluation of patients with presumed ischemic dysfunction, as follows:

- Assessment of the relative regional myocardial uptake of thallium-201 (201 Tl; often after rest reinjection), 99m Tc-sestamibi, or 99m Tc-tetrofosmin (often after rest administration of nitroglycerin); when the resting uptake of radiotracer is greater than 50% of normal, expect recovery of function after revascularization.
- Assessment of the presence of demonstrable ischemia (e.g. partially reversible defect) in a myocardial segment with decreased uptake, even if the resting uptake is less than 50%.

Data reported in 2011 from a STICH viability substudy failed to demonstrate a significant impact on survival based on the extent of viable myocardium in patients with CAD and LV dysfunction treated surgically or medically.

### Equilibrium Radionuclide Angiocardiography

Equilibrium radionuclide angiocardiography (ERNA) uses ECG events to define the temporal relationship between the acquisition of nuclear data and the volumetric components of the cardiac cycle. Sampling is performed repetitively over several hundred heartbeats, with physiologic segregation of nuclear data in accordance with their occurrence within the cardiac cycle (Fig. 8.56).

Data are quantified and displayed in an endless-loop, cinegraphic format for additional qualitative visual interpretation and analysis. Equilibrium blood-pool labeling is achieved by use of 99m-Tc. Data are analyzed by use of a computer, generally with some operator interaction.

Analysis may be obtained in either the frame or list mode. Radionuclide data are collected and segregated temporally. The process generally requires 3–10 minutes for completion of each view. Following data acquisition, data from the several hundred individual beats are summed, processed, and displayed as a single representative cardiac cycle. Data from the left anterior oblique (LAO) view are also used for qualitative analysis of global LV function. On this view, overlap of the two ventricles is

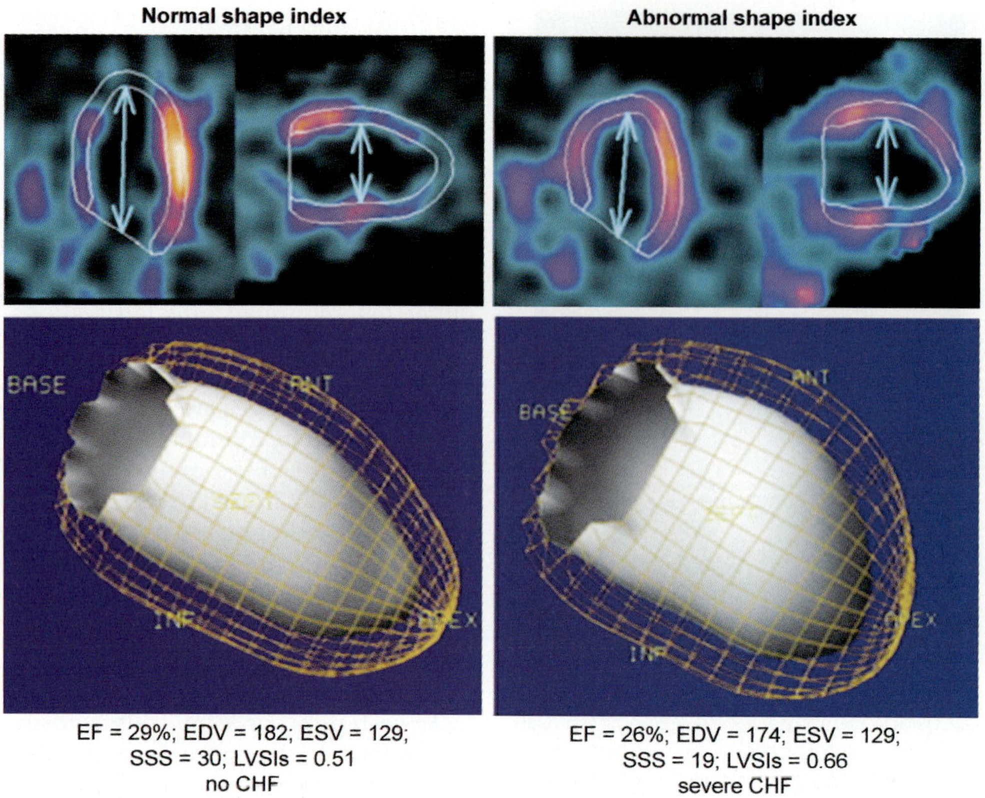


**Fig. 8.53:** Illustration of two cases with similar low LVEF but differing LV shape index. (A) The patient with no signs of congestive heart failure (CHF) has a more severe perfusion defect than the other patient but has a normal LV shape index and an elongated LV cavity. (B) The other patient, who has severe congestive heart failure, has an abnormal LV shape index and a more spherical left ventricle. ANT=Anterior; SEPT=septal; INF=inferior; LVSIs=systolic LV shape index (*reproduced with permission*)

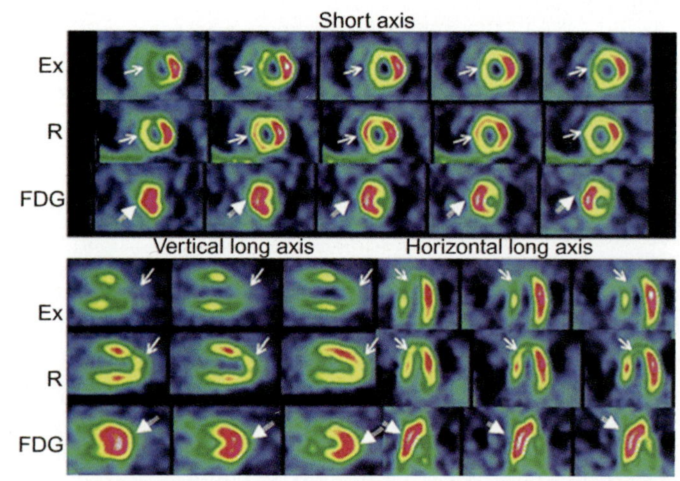


**Fig. 8.54:** Simultaneous myocardial perfusion and metabolism imaging after dual intravenous injection of 99mTc-sestamibi and 18F-FDG at peak exercise (Ex). Dual-isotope simultaneous acquisition was performed 40–60 min after exercise study was completed. Rest 99mTc-sestamibi imaging (R) was performed separately. In this patient with angina and no prior myocardial infarction, note evidence of extensive reversible perfusion defect in anterior, septal, and apical regions. Coronary angiogram showed 90% stenosis of left anterior descending and 60% of left circumflex coronary arteries. Corresponding 18F-FDG image shows intense uptake in regions with reversible sestamibi defects reflecting metabolic correlate of exercise-induced myocardial ischemia

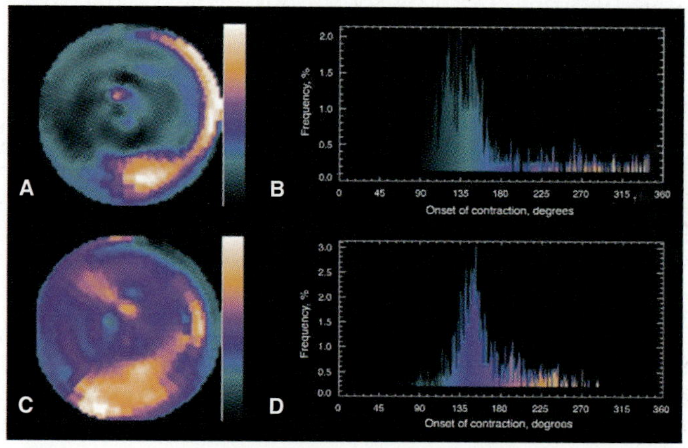


**Fig. 8.55:** Fourier analysis of a gated myocardial perfusion single-photon emission computed tomography. Before resynchronization (A), the phase histogram amplitude increases abnormally. The polar map (B) shows that the greatest delay occurs in the inferior-lateral region of the left ventricle. After cardiac resynchronization therapy (C), the histogram amplitude (D) improves significantly. The patient improved clinically and left ventricular ejection fraction improved from 18–32% lower (images courtesy of Dr. Santiago Aguadé-Bruix, Hospital Universitari Vall d'Hebron, Barcelona)

minimal. In a count-based approach, LVEF and other indices of filling and ejection are calculated from the LV radioactivity preset at various points throughout the cardiac cycle.

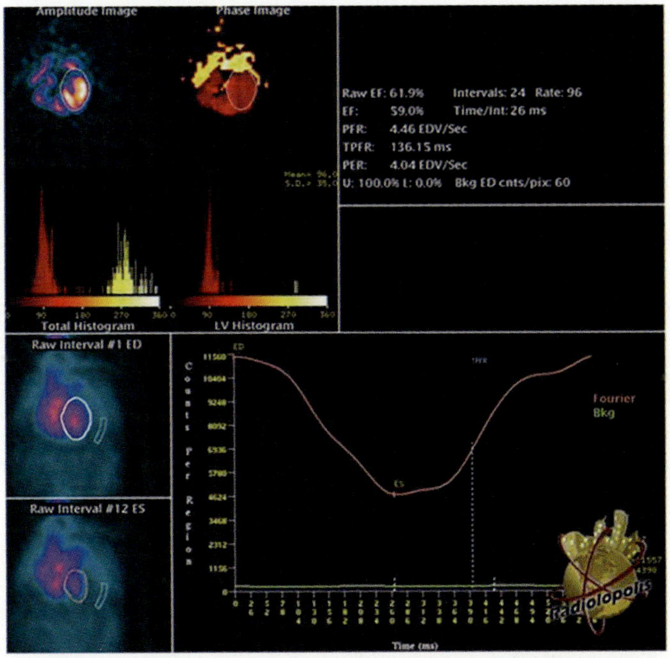


Fig. 8.56: Normal LV MUGA scan (equilibrium radionuclide angiography)

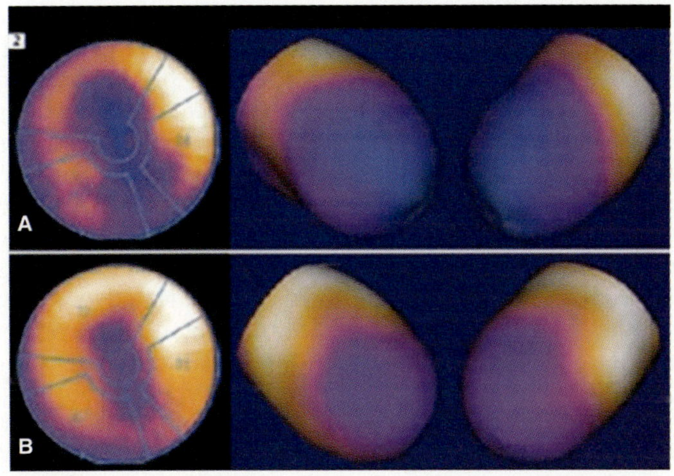


Fig. 8.57: Polar plots and volume rendering of stress (A) and rest (B) IQ•SPECT images show gross, but reversible, ischemia in the apical, anterior and anteroseptal walls and inferior and inferolateral walls. The apex and adjacent anterior wall show significant resting hypoperfusion, which may reflect hibernating myocardium. The posterolateral wall was relatively well perfused. Stress LVEF is significantly low at 39% with normal resting LVEF (56%), indicating severe stress induced LV dysfunction

RV function is best evaluated by first-pass techniques. The LAO view provides qualitative information concerning contraction of the septal, inferoapical, and lateral walls. The anterior view provides data concerning regional motion of the anterior and apical segments. The left lateral or left posterior oblique view provides optimal qualitative information concerning contraction of the inferior wall and posterobasal segment.

**ERNA may easily be combined with additional physiologic stress testing or provocation,** which may be in the form of either physiologic stress, such as exercise; pharmacologic stress, with the use of positive inotropic agents, such as dobutamine or isoproterenol; or psychological stress. The degree of confidence with ERNA is moderately high. False-positive and false-negative findings are infrequent.

### *Radionuclide Ventriculography*

Radionuclide ventriculography is most often performed as part of a myocardial perfusion scan to obtain accurate measurements of LV function and right ventricular EF, but it is unable to directly assess valvular abnormalities or cardiac hypertrophy and has limited value for assessing volumes or more subtle indices of systolic or diastolic function (Fig. 8.57).

## Catheterization and Angiography

In patients with a nonischemic cardiomyopathy, perfusion deficits and segmental wall-motion abnormalities suggestive of coronary artery disease are commonly present on noninvasive imaging. Only coronary angiography, however, can reliably demonstrate or exclude the presence of obstructed coronary vessels (Fig. 8.58).

According to the American College of Cardiology/American Heart Association (ACC/AHA), Heart Failure Society of America (HFSA) and European Society of Cardiology (ESC), cardiac catheterization and coronary angiography should be considered for patients with heart failure in the following situations; when symptoms worsen without a clear cause in patients with heart failure, no angina, and known coronary artery disease. In heart failure caused by systolic dysfunction in association with angina or regional wall-motion abnormalities and/or scintigraphic evidence of reversible myocardial ischemia when revascularization is being considered When pretest probability of underlying ischemic cardiomyopathy is high and surgical

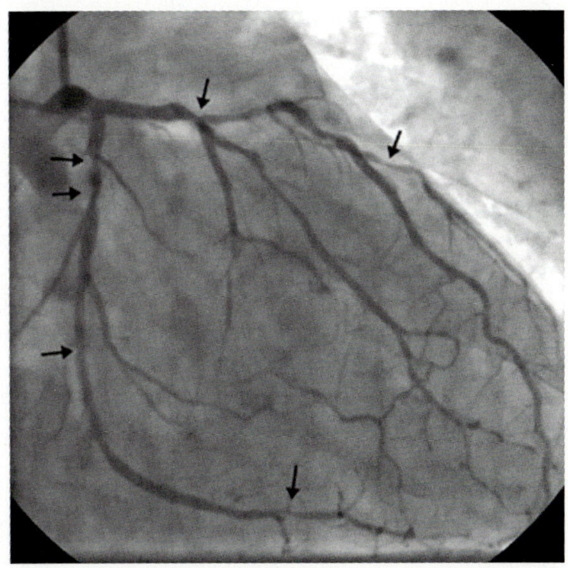

Fig. 8.58: Extensive coronary artery disease. Multiple stenoses are present; they involve the left anterior descending coronary artery and the circumflex coronary artery and their branches. in an elderly patient with heart failure

coronary procedures are being considered. Before cardiac transplantation or left ventricular assist device placement. In cases of heart failure secondary to postinfarction ventricular aneurysm or other mechanical complications of myocardial infarction For these patients, the procedures are frequently indicated when systolic dysfunction of unexplained cause is present on noninvasive testing or when normal systolic function with episodic heart failure suggests ischemically mediated LV dysfunction. However, although coronary angiography may be indicated in young patients to exclude the presence of congenital coronary anomalies, this procedure may not be as useful in older patients, because revascularization has not been shown to improve clinical outcomes in patients without angina. Despite this, because revascularization may improve LV function, some experts suggest that coronary artery disease should be excluded whenever possible, especially in patients with diabetes mellitus or other states associated with silent myocardial ischemia. The degree of confidence is moderately high.

### *Right-sided Heart Catheterization*

Right heart catheterization is useful in providing important hemodynamic information about filling pressures, vascular resistance, and cardiac output when there is doubt about the patient's fluid status; in heart failure refractory to initial therapy; in the presence of significant hypotension (systolic blood pressure typically $<90$ mmHg or symptomatic low systolic blood pressure) and/or worsening renal function during initial treatment; and when heart transplantation or placement of a mechanical circulatory support device is being considered. However, it plays a limited role in the diagnosis of heart failure, as studies evaluating right heart catheterization and overall improved outcomes have been essentially neutral. Normal right-sided hemodynamics include right atrial pressure $<7$ mmHg, RV pressure $<30/7$ mmHg, pulmonary pressure $<30/18$, pulmonary capillary wedge pressure (PCWP) $<18$ mmHg, and cardiac index (CI) $>2.2$ L/min/m$^2$.

PCWP can be measured by using a pulmonary arterial catheter (Swan-Ganz catheter). This helps differentiate cardiogenic causes of decompensated heart failure from noncardiogenic causes, such as acute respiratory distress syndrome (ARDS), which occurs secondary to injury to the alveolar-capillary membrane rather than to alteration in Starling forces. A PCWP exceeding 18 mmHg in a patient not known to have chronically elevated left atrial pressure is indicative of cardiogenic decompensated heart failure. In patients with chronic pulmonary capillary hypertension, capillary wedge pressures exceeding 25 mmHg are generally required to overcome the pumping capacity of the lymphatics and produce pulmonary edema.

Large V waves may be observed in the PCWP tracing in patients with significant mitral regurgitation because large volumes of blood regurgitate into a poorly compliant left atrium. This raises pulmonary venous pressure and may cause pulmonary edema.

### *Left-sided Heart Catheterization*

Left-sided heart catheterization and coronary angiography should be undertaken when the aetiology of heart failure cannot be determined by clinical or noninvasive imaging methods or when the aetiology is likely to be due to acute myocardial ischemia or infarction. Coronary angiography is particularly helpful in patients with LV systolic dysfunction and known or suspected coronary artery disease in whom myocardial ischemia is thought to play a dominant role in the reduction of LV systolic function and the worsening of heart failure.

### Endomyocardial Biopsy

Endomyocardial biopsy is indicated only when a specific diagnosis is suspected that would influence therapy in

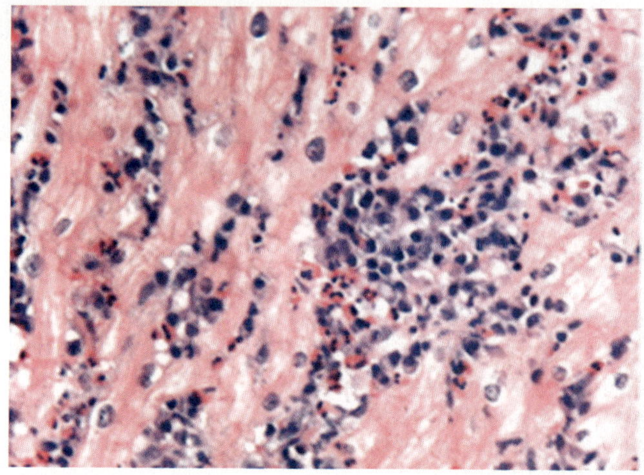

**Fig. 8.59:** Eosinophilic myocarditis. The patient had severe heart failure and peripheral eosinophilia. Immunosuppression improved her heart failure and probably primary hyper-eosinophilic syndrome (H and E; original magnification X 400)

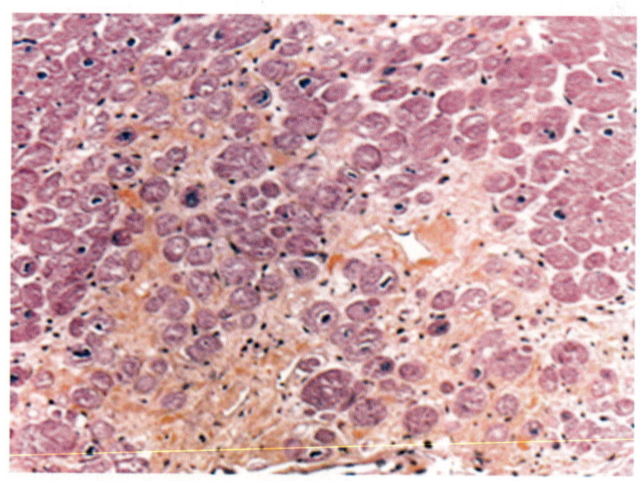

**Fig. 8.60:** Dilated cardiomyopathy. Middle-aged man with congestive heart failure. The photomicrograph shows cardiomyocytes with nuclear hypertrophy, myocytolysis and interstitial fibrosis. This is a nonspecific histological appearance that can be seen with many cardiomyopathies. Clinical information is always required (HPS; original magnification X 200)

patients presenting with heart failure (see the image below). The Heart Failure Society of America (HFSA) suggests that endomyocardial biopsy be considered in patients with rapidly progressive clinical heart failure or ventricular dysfunction, despite appropriate medical therapy, as well as in patients suspected of having myocardial infiltrative processes (e.g. sarcoidosis, amyloidosis) or in patients with malignant arrhythmias out of proportion to their LV dysfunction (e.g. sarcoidosis, giant cell myocarditis) (Figs 8.59 and 8.60).

### Assessment of Functional Capacity

The European Society of Cardiology (ESC) indicates the 6-minute walk test is a good indicator of functional status and prognosis in patients with heart failure. It evaluates distance walked, dyspnea index on a Borg scale from 0–10, oxygen saturation, and heart rate response to exercise. A normal value is walking more than 1500 feet. Patients who walk less than 600 feet have severe cardiac dysfunction and a worse short- and long-term prognosis.

*Cardiopulmonary stress testing* (Fig 8. 61) (maximal exercise stress testing with measurement of respiratory gas exchange) can help assess a patient's chance of survival within the next year, as well as determine the need for referral for either cardiac transplantation or implantation of mechanical circulatory support. The ACC/AHA and HFSA do not recommend routine maximal exercise stress testing. It may be useful in situations such as the following with measurement of gas exchange:

- To assess the disparity between symptomatic limitation and objective indicators of disease severity
- To distinguish non HF-related causes of functional limitation, specifically cardiac versus pulmonary
- To consider whether patients are candidates for cardiac transplantation or mechanical circulatory support
- To determine the prescription for cardiac rehabilitation
- Values of peak oxygen consumption of less than 50% of predicted or less than 14 cc/kg/min reflect poor cardiac performance and a likelihood of 1-year survival less than 50%, facilitating referral for cardiac transplantation or mechanical circulatory device placement.

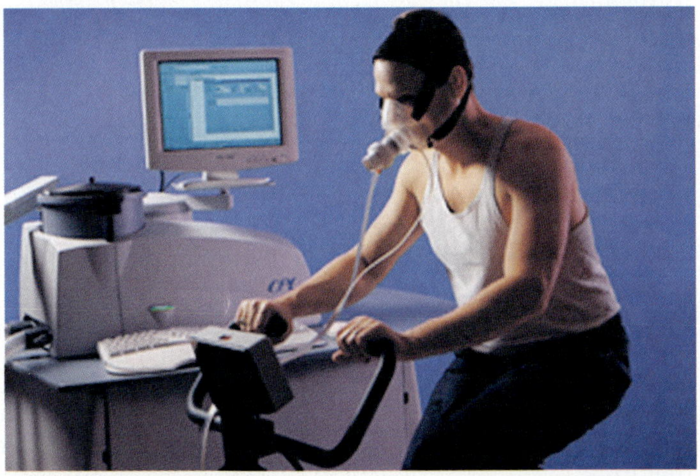

**Fig. 8.61:** Cardiopulmonary stress test. It is simply 'stress-testing' with some additional complementary measurements. Stress tests use a bicycle or treadmill to look at heart function at rest and during exercise stress

### Medical Care Approach Considerations

Medical care for heart failure (HF) includes a number of nonpharmacologic, pharmacologic, and invasive strategies to limit and reverse the manifestations of heart failure. Depending on the severity of illness, nonpharmacologic therapies include dietary sodium and fluid restriction; physical activity as appropriate; and attention to weight gain. Pharmacologic therapies include the use of diuretics, vasodilators, inotropic agents, anticoagulants, beta-blockers, and digoxin (Table 8.11).

**Table 8.11:** Initial management for AHFS

| | |
|---|---|
| 1. Treat immediate life-threatening conditions/stabilize patient | Life-saving measures may precede or parallel diagnostic evaluation (i.e. unstable arrhythmia, flash pulmonary edema, STEMI) |
| 2. Establish the diagnosis | Based on medical history, signs (JVP, S3, edema), symptoms (dyspnea), biomarkers (e.g. BNP) and CXR |
| 3. Determine clinical profile and begin initial treatment | Key components include HR, BP, JVP, presence of pulmonary congestion, ECG, CXR, renal function, troponin, BNP, pulse oximetry, history of CAD |
| 4. Determine and manage the cause or precipitant | Such as ischemia, hypertension, arrhythmias, acute valvular pathologies, worsening renal function, uncontrolled diabetes, and/or infectious etiologies is critical to ensure maximal benefits from HF management |
| 5. Alleviate symptoms (e.g. dyspnea) | Usually a diuretic with or without other vasoactive agents. Morphine may also be used for pulmonary edema |
| 6. Protect/preserve myocardium and renal function | Avoid hypotension or increase in HR, particularly in patients with CAD. Use of inotropes should be restricted to those with low-output state (low BP with organ hypoperfusion) |
| 7. Make disposition | Majority are admitted to telemetry, with a small number discharged home. Robust evidence to support risk stratification and disposition identifying the low-risk patient for safe discharge with close outpatient follow-up is lacking |

CXR=chest X-ray; ECG=electrocardiogram; HR=heart rate; JVP=jugular venous pressure; STEMI=ST-segment elevation myocardial infarction

Invasive therapies for heart failure include electrophysiologic intervention such as cardiac resynchronization therapy (CRT), pacemakers, and implantable cardioverter-defibrillators (ICDs); revascularization procedures such as coronary artery bypass grafting (CABG) and percutaneous coronary intervention (PCI); valve replacement or repair; and ventricular restoration. When progressive end-stage heart failure occurs despite maximal medical therapy, when the prognosis is poor, and when there is no viable therapeutic alternative, the criterion standard for therapy has been heart transplantation. However, mechanical circulatory devices such as ventricular assist devices (VADs) and total artificial hearts (TAHs) can bridge the patient to transplantation; in addition, VADs are increasingly being used as permanent therapy.

## Consideration of Comorbidities

### Coronary Artery Disease

Patients with heart failure should be evaluated for coronary artery disease, which can lead to heart failure (*see* aetiology). Not only may this condition be the underlying cause in up to two thirds of heart failure patients with low ejection fraction, but coronary artery disease may also play a role in the progression of heart failure through mechanisms such as endothelial dysfunction, ischemia, and infarction, among others.

Patients with coronary artery disease with modestly reduced ejection fraction and angina demonstrate symptomatic and survival improvement with coronary artery bypass grafting (CABG) in studies; however, the studies did not include individuals with heart failure or those with severely reduced ejection fractions. In patients with angina and ventricular dysfunction, evaluation with coronary angiography should not be delayed (see catheterization and angiography). Noninvasive cardiac testing is not recommended in patients with significant ischemic chest pain, as revascularization is advised in these patients independent of their degree of ischemia/viability.

Although there are no reports of controlled trials evaluating heart failure without angina and their outcomes with coronary revascularization, surgical revascularization is recommended in those with significant left main stenosis and in those with extensive noninfarcted but hypoperfused and hypocontractile myocardium on noninvasive testing. In patients with heart failure and reduced left ventricular ejection fraction but without angina, it has not yet been determined whether routine evaluation of possible myocardial ischemia/viability and coronary artery disease should be performed.

For patients with heart failure from LV dysfunction without chest pain and without a history of coronary artery disease, coronary angiography may be useful in young patients to exclude congenital coronary anomalies. However, because clinical outcomes have not been shown to improve in patients without angina, coronary angiography may not be as useful in older patients for evaluating the presence of coronary artery disease. Some experts nonetheless suggest excluding coronary artery disease whenever possible, particularly in the presence of diabetes or other states associated with silent myocardial ischemia, because LV function may show improvement with revascularization.

In general, if coronary artery disease has already been excluded as the cause of abnormalities in LV function, it is not necessary to perform repeated evaluations for ischemia (invasive or noninvasive) provided the patient's clinical status has not changed to suggest the development of ischemic disease.

For more information, *see the Medscape Reference articles Primary and Secondary Prevention of Coronary Artery Disease, Risk Factors for Coronary Artery Disease, and Risk Factors for Coronary Artery Disease.*

Valvular heart disease may be the underlying aetiology or an important aggravating factor in heart failure. For more information, *see the Medscape reference article valvular surgery.*

### Sleep Apnea

Sleep apnea has an increased prevalence in patients with heart failure and is associated with increased mortality due to further neurohormonal activation, although randomized, controlled data are lacking. Sleep apnea should be treated aggressively in heart failure patients.

A long-term study involving 283 heart failure patients who had an implanted cardiac resynchronization device with cardioverter-defibrillator concluded that obstructive sleep apnea (OSA) and/or central sleep apnea (CSA) are independently associated with an increased risk for ventricular arrhythmias requiring cardioverter-defibrillator therapies.

### Anemia

Anemia is also common in chronic heart failure. Whether anemia is a reflection of the severity of heart failure or contributes to worsening heart failure is not clear. Potential etiologies of anemia in heart failure involve poor nutrition, ACEIs, the RAAS, inflammatory cytokines, hemodilution, and renal dysfunction. Anemia in heart failure is associated with increased mortality.

The ACC/AHA, HFSA, and ESC make no recommendations regarding the administration of iron to patients with heart failure, although the ACC/AHA noted that several small studies suggested a benefit in mild anemia and heart failure. More and larger studies are needed.

### Cardiorenal Syndrome

Cardiorenal syndrome reflects advanced cardiorenal dysregulation manifested by acute heart failure, worsening renal function, and diuretic resistance. It is equally prevalent in patients with heart failure with normal ejection fraction (HFNEF) and those with LV systolic dysfunction. Worsening renal function is one of the three predictors of increased mortality in hospitalized patients with heart failure regardless of the LVEF.

Cardiorenal syndrome can be classified into the following five types:

- **CR1:** Rapid worsening of cardiac function leading to acute kidney injury (HFNEF, acute heart failure, cardiogenic shock, and RV failure)
- **CR2:** Worsening renal function due to progression of chronic heart failure
- **CR3:** Abrupt and primary worsening of kidney function leading to acute cardiac dysfunction (heart failure, arrhythmia, and ischemia)
- **CR4:** Chronic kidney disease leading to progressive cardiac dysfunction, LVH, and diastolic dysfunction
- **CR5:** Combination of cardiac and renal dysfunction due to acute and chronic systemic conditions

The pathophysiology of CR1 and CR2 is complex and multifactorial, involving neurohormonal activation (RAAS, sympathetic nervous system, arginine vasopressin, natriuretic peptides, adenosine receptor activation), low arterial pressure, and high central venous pressure, leading to lower transglomerular perfusion pressure and decreased availability of diuretics to the proximal nephron. This results in an increased reabsorption of sodium and water and poor diuretic response—hence, diuretic resistance despite escalating doses of oral or intravenous diuretics.

Treatment of cardiorenal syndrome in patients with heart failure is largely empirical, but it typically involves the use of combination diuretics, vasodilators, and inotropes as indicated ultrafiltration is recommended for symptomatic relief by the ACC/AHA guidelines for patients with heart failure that is refractory to diuretic therapy.

A sudden increase in creatinine can be seen after initiation of diuretic therapy and is often mistakenly considered evidence of overdiuresis or intravascular depletion (even in the presence of fluid overload). A common error in this situation is to decrease the dose of ACEI/ARB and/or diuretics or to even withdraw one of these agents. In fact, when diuresis or ultrafiltration is continued, patients demonstrate improved renal function, decreased total body fluid, and increased response to diuretics, as central venous pressure falls.

Low-dose dopamine has been used in combination with diuretic therapy, on the supposition that it can increase kidney perfusion. Data have been contradictory, however. In a randomized controlled study, Giamouzis et al. found that the combination of low-dose furosemide and low-dose dopamine was equally as effective as high-dose furosemide for kidney function in patients with acute decompensated heart failure. In addition, patients who received dopamine and furosemide were less likely to have worsened renal function or hypokalemia at 24 hours.

Use of nesiritide, a synthetic natriuretic peptide, to increase diuresis in these cases has not been studied. A meta-analysis of several trials using nesiritide suggests the potential of worsening renal function, although this has not been demonstrated in prospective trials. Results of the acute study of clinical effectiveness of nesiritide in decompensated heart failure (ASCEND-HF) trial suggest that, although nesiritide is safe, it does not provide additional efficacy when added to standard therapy.

The efficacy of vasopressin antagonism in heart failure outcome study with tolvaptan (EVEREST) trial showed that the addition of the vasopressin antagonist tolvaptan to diuretic therapy facilitates diuresis in acute heart failure. However, tolvaptan had no impact on mortality or hospitalizations in this setting.

Adenosine receptor antagonists have been proposed for protecting renal function in acute heart failure. However, in a double-blind, placebo-controlled trial, the adenosine A1-receptor antagonist rolofylline demonstrated no benefit for patients hospitalized for acute heart failure with impaired renal function

A meta-analysis performed by Badve et al. suggests that treatment with beta-blockers was found to reduce all-cause mortality in patients with chronic kidney disease and systolic heart failure (risk ratio, 0.72).

### *Atrial Fibrillation*

Many patients with heart failure also have atrial fibrillation, and the two conditions can adversely affect each other. However in the AFFIRM trial, there was no difference in stroke, heart failure exacerbation, or CV mortality in patients treated with rhythm control (amiodarone) and patients treated with rate control. All of these patients require anticoagulation for stroke prevention. This can be achieved by using warfarin or a direct thrombin inhibitor (no need to follow protime).

In a prospective controlled study by Hsu et al. catheter ablation for atrial fibrillation in patients with heart failure and an LVEF of less than 45% resulted in a 21% increase in LVEF and improvement in LV dimensions, exercise capacity, symptoms, and quality of life. At a mean of 12 months, 78% of patients remained in sinus rhythm without antiarrhythmic drugs.

A meta-analysis found that patients with LV systolic dysfunction who underwent catheter ablation for atrial fibrillation demonstrated significant improvements in LVEF, and their risk for recurrent atrial fibrillation or atrial tachycardia after catheter ablation was similar to that in patients with normal LV function after ablation. However, patients with LV systolic dysfunction were more likely to require repeat procedures.

In contrast, MacDonald et al. reported that in patients with advanced heart failure and severe LV systolic dysfunction, radiofrequency ablation for persistent atrial fibrillation resulted in long-term restoration of sinus rhythm in only 50% of cases. Radiofrequency ablation also failed to improve such secondary outcomes as walking distance or quality of life, and the rate of related serious complications was 15%.

## Nonpharmacologic Therapy

Patients with heart failure can benefit from attention to exercise, diet, and nutrition. Restriction of activity promotes physical deconditioning, so physical activity should be encouraged. However, limitation of activity is appropriate during acute heart failure exacerbations and in patients with suspected myocarditis. Most patients should not participate in heavy labor or exhaustive sports (Fig. 8.62).

Dietary sodium restriction to 2–3 g/day is recommended. Fluid restriction to 2 L/day is recommended for patients with evidence of hyponatremia (Na <130 mEq/dL) and for those whose fluid status is difficult to control despite sodium restriction and the use of high-dose diuretics. Caloric supplementation is recommended for patients with evidence of cardiac cachexia.

### Ultrafiltration and Refractory Heart Failure

In ultrafiltration, blood is removed from the body and run through a device that applies hydrostatic pressure across a semipermeable membrane to separate isotonic plasma water. Solutes cross the semipermeable membrane freely, so fluid can be removed without causing significant changes in the concentration of electrolytes and other solutes in serum (Fig. 8.63).

Ultrafiltration was shown to be an effective alternative to intravenous diuretics in the ultrafiltration versus intravenous (IV) diuretics for patients hospitalized for acute decompensated heart failure (UNLOAD) trial. The ACC/AHA and ESC recommend the use of ultrafiltration for fluid reduction for patients with refractory heart failure that is not responsive to medical therapy.

### Indications for Hospitalization

A patient whose condition is refractory to standard therapy will often require hospitalization to receive IV diuretics, vasodilators, and inotropic agents. The 2010 Heart Failure Society of America (HFSA) guidelines recommend hospitalization for acute heart failure in the presence of the following:

- Severe acute decompensated heart failure (low blood pressure, worsening renal dysfunction, altered mentation)
- Dyspnea at rest
- Hemodynamically significant arrhythmia

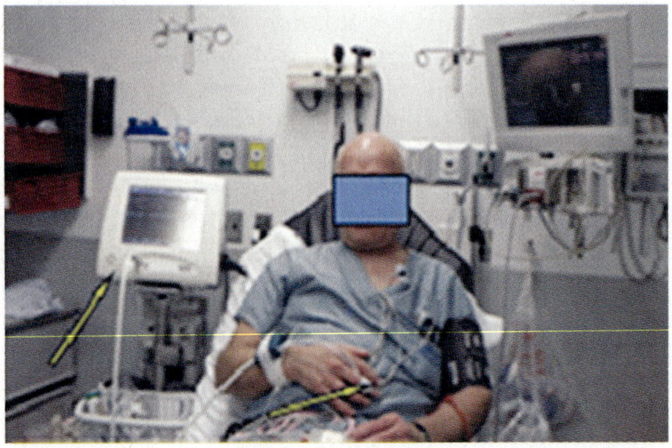

**Fig. 8.62:** Finger photoplethsmography can measure beat to beat blood pressure, pulse, stroke volume, cardiac output and left ventricular end diastolic pressure

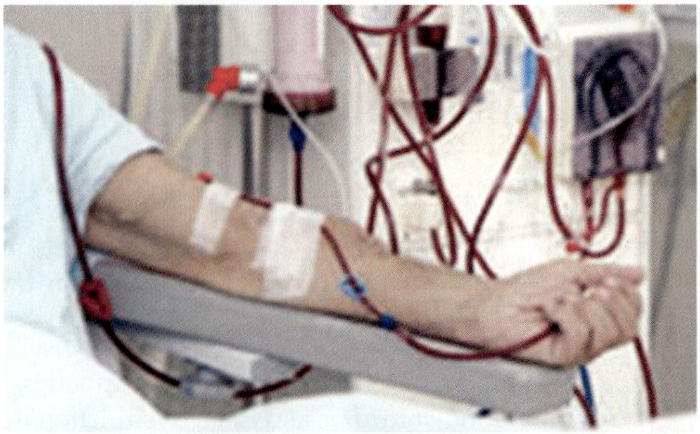

**Fig. 8.63:** Venovenous ultrafiltration technique, in patients with acute decompensated heart failure with worsening of kidney function, a condition referred to as acute cardiorenal syndrome (type 1). Diuretics are commonly used to treat persistent congestion in these patients, but these drugs might worsen kidney function. An alternative therapeutic approach is venovenous ultrafiltration, which can improve control over the rate and volume of fluid removal, increase net loss of sodium, and reduce neurohormonal activation

- Acute coronary syndrome

Hospitalization should also be considered in the presence of the following:

- Worsening congestion with or without dyspnea
- Worsening signs and symptoms of systemic or pulmonary congestion, even in the absence of weight gain
- Major electrolyte abnormalities
- Associated comorbid conditions (e.g. pneumonia, pulmonary embolism, diabetic ketoacidosis, stroke/strokelike symptoms)
- Repeat ICD firings
- New diagnosis of heart failure with signs of active systemic/pulmonary congestion.
- Most patients requiring hospitalization should be admitted to a telemetry bed or intensive care unit; a small percentage can be admitted to the floor or observation unit. The goal is to continue the diagnostic and therapeutic processes started in the office or emergency department. Treatment includes the following:
    - Volume and hemodynamic status are optimized using careful clinical monitoring, and the heart failure medical regimen is optimized.
    - Surgical intervention with a ventricular device has been considered.
    - Heart failure education, behavior modification, and exercise and diet recommendation are made.
    - Enrollment in heart failure disease management programs for patients with advanced and difficult-to-control heart failure.

*Invasive hemodynamic monitoring:* Invasive hemodynamic monitoring is not indicated for stable patients with heart failure responding appropriately to medical therapy. The evaluation study of congestive heart failure and pulmonary artery catheterization effectiveness [ESCAPE] trial showed no mortality or hospitalization benefit in such cases. In patients with acute decompensated heart failure, the following are indications for invasive hemodynamic monitoring:

- Respiratory distress
- Signs of impaired perfusion
- Inability to determine intracardiac pressures on the basis of clinical examination
- No improvement in clinical status despite maximal heart failure therapy

Clinical situations in which invasive hemodynamic monitoring is recommended to guide therapy include the following:

1. Persistent symptomatic hypotension despite initial therapy
2. Worsening renal function despite initial therapy or despite adjustment of recommended therapies
3. Need for parenteral vasoactive agents after initial clinical improvement
4. Presumed cardiogenic shock requiring escalating inotrope and/or pressor therapy and consideration of mechanical support
5. Consideration of advanced device therapy or transplantation

### Discharge

The patient must be on a stable oral regimen for at least 24 hours before discharge. Patients are ready for discharge when they meet the following criteria:

*Exacerbating factors have been addressed:*

- Volume status has been optimized
- Diuretic therapy has been successfully transitioned to oral medication, with discontinuation of IV vasodilator and inotropic therapy for at least 24 hours
- Oral chronic heart failure therapy has been achieved with stable clinical status
- Before discharge, patient and family education should be completed, and extensive postdischarge instructions and follow-up in 3–7 days should be arranged. Refractory end-stage heart failure (ACC/AHA stage D, NYHA class IV) is often difficult to manage on an outpatient basis. Therefore, these patients may be referred to a heart failure program with expertise in management of refractory heart failure
- To ensure compliance and understanding of a complex medical regimen, a follow-up phone call can be made 3 days after discharge by a nurse with training in heart failure. Ideally, the patient should be seen in clinic 7–10 days after discharge.

Different monitoring methods have been implemented by physicians in an attempt to reduce hospitalization for heart failure. The results have been equivocal, regardless of the severity of heart failure. No differences in death or hospitalization for heart failure have been found with either standard outpatient monitoring or intense telemonitoring for heart failure.

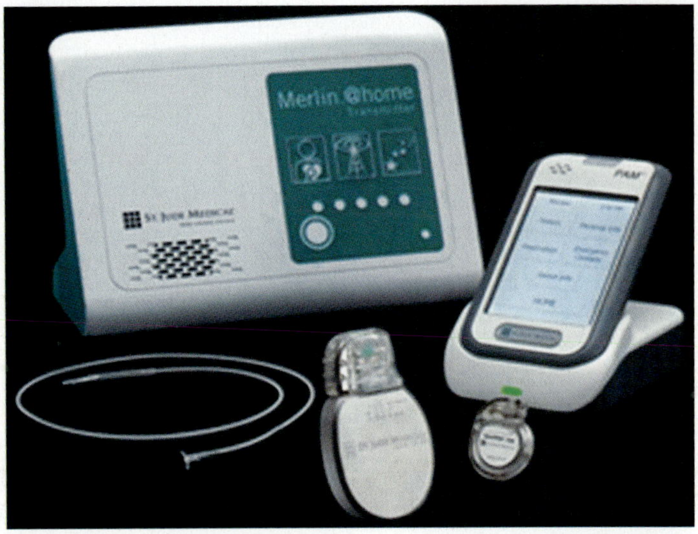


**Fig. 8.64:** Continuous left atrial pessure monitoring in CHF patients recently published study that analyzed the clinical benefits of frequent and regular left atrial pressure (LAP) monitoring in patients with heart failure, patients wore a special device, called Heart POD, that monitored their LAP and routed the data wirelessly to their cardiologist

*An investigational approach to monitoring* is the use of a wireless implanted pulmonary artery pressure sensor. This device permits ambulatory monitoring and is designed to detect early-stage elevations in pulmonary artery pressure, so that appropriate medical intervention can be provided before worsening elevation leads to congestion. In a 6-month study in patients with NYHA class III heart failure, heart failure–related hospitalizations were approximately 30% lower with use of the device (Fig. 8.64).

### Treatment of Heart Failure with Normal LVEF

Treatment of heart failure with normal left ventricular ejection fraction (HFNEF) is directed toward alleviating symptoms and addressing the underlying condition triggering HFNEF. Evaluation of cardiac ischemia or sleep apnea as potential precipitating factors should also be considered (Table 8.12).

There is a paucity of randomized, controlled studies addressing HFNEF. Control of blood pressure, volume, or other risk factors is the mainstay of therapy. Lifestyle modification in important and may include the following:

- Low-sodium diet
- Restricted fluid intake
- Daily measurement of weight
- Exercise
- Weight loss
- Diuretic therapy is recommended to reduce fluid retention. However, patients must be monitored carefully to avoid hypotension.
- ACEI/ARBs are used as indicated for patients with atherosclerotic disease, prior MI, diabetes mellitus, or hypertension. Use of candesartan, irbesartan, or perindopril has not been shown to decrease mortality but has

**Table 8.12:** Stepwise approach: evaluation and therapy of decompensated heart failure

| |
|---|
| *Stablize acute stiuation* |
| • Brief assessment/examination<br>• Oxygenation – assess, treat with $O_2$<br>• Blood pressure/peripheral perfusion |
| *Assess volume status/Diagnosis* |
| • History and physical exam<br>• noninvasive testing - (+ Review records)<br>• Invasive testing - (+ Review Records) |
| *Therapy* |
| • Correct/reverse precipitating cause<br>• Oxygen<br>• Diuretics<br>• Morphine sulphate (low dose) for central effect<br>• Vasodilators<br>• Inotropic agents<br>• Mechanical assist devices complete diagnostic evaluation if new onset heart failure |

produced a trend toward improved morbidity and decreased hospitalizations. Some evidence shows that losartan and valsartan may promote LV reverse remodeling, with improvement in diastolic function and regression of left ventricular hypertrophy (LVH).

- Beta-blockers are indicated for patients with prior MI or hypertension and for control of ventricular rate in those with atrial fibrillation. In the ADHERE registry, the subset of patients with HFNEF not treated with a beta-blocker had a higher mortality, potentially because of the higher incidence of coronary artery disease (CAD) in this population.
- Aldosterone receptor blockers are indicated for hypertension and to reduce myocardial fibrosis, although no randomized, controlled studies have been performed to evaluate their role in HFNEF. Calcium channel blockers may improve exercise tolerance via their vasodilatory properties, and nondihydropyridine calcium channel blockers are also used for ventricular rate control in patients with atrial fibrillation. Amlodipine has antianginal properties and is also indicated in hypertension.
- Restoration of sinus rhythm should be considered if the patient remains symptomatic despite the above efforts. Use of digitalis or inotropes in patients with HFNEF is not indicated.

## Electrophysiologic Intervention

Devices for electrophysiologic intervention in heart failure include pacemakers, cardiac resynchronization therapy (CRT) devices, and implantable cardioverter-defibrillators (ICDs) (Tables 8.13 and 8.14).

The 2010 Heart Failure Society of America (HFSA) guidelines indicate that device therapy is an integral part of the treatment of heart failure and that considerations such as the nature and severity of the condition and any patient comorbidities are essential in optimizing the use of this therapy. The Committee for Practice Guidelines (CPG) of the European Society of Cardiology (ESC) and the ACC/AHA/Heart Rhythm Society (HRS) emphasized the importance of medical devices in heart failure in their respective 2010 and 2012 focused updates on these interventions.

In addition, the AHA has published guidelines on heart device strategies, patient selection, and postoperative care. The guidance focuses on risk stratification and early referral of high-risk patients with heart failure to centers that can implant mechanical circulatory support devices (MCS).

**Table 8.13:** Use of implantable defibrillators in patients with heart failure

| |
|---|
| *Class I* |
| • Cardiac arrest due to ventricular fibrillation (VF) or ventricular tachycardia (VT) not due to transient or reversible cause<br>• Sportaneous sustained VT in association with structural heart disease<br>• Syncope of undetermined origin with clinically relevant sustained VT or VF induced at electrophysiological study<br>• Nonsustained VT with coronary artery disease, prior myocardial infraction and inducible<br>• Nonsuppressible VT |
| *Class IIa* |
| • Left ventricular ejection fraction less than or equal to 30%, at least 1 month following myocardial infraction and 3 months after surgical revascularization NB |
| *Class IIb* |
| • Cardiac arrest presumed to be due to VF when electrophysiologic testing is precluded by other medical conditions. Severe symptoms, such as syncope, in patients awaiting cardiac transplantation. Nonsustained VT with sustained VT at electrophysiologic study in patients with ischemic heart disease<br>• Recurrent syncope of undetermined aetiology in the presence of ventricular dysfunction. |
| *Class III-contraindicated* |
| • Increscent VT or VF (ICD may be indicated after arrhythmia control)<br>• VT or VF due to a transient or reversible condition<br>• Projected life expectancy less than 6 months<br>• Significant psychiatric illness that may be aggravated by device implantation or that may preclude device follow-up<br>• NYHA class IV heart failure in patinets who are not candidates for cardiac transplantation |

### Pacemakers

Maintaining a normal chronotropic response and AV synchrony may be particularly significant for patients with heart failure. Because RV pacing may worsen heart failure due to an increase in ventricular dysynchrony, the current 2010 HFSA practice guidelines recommend against placement of a dual-chamber pacemaker in heart failure patients in the absence of symptomatic bradycardia or high-degree AV block.

**Table 8.14:** Interventional therapies for heart failure—established and investigational

- Revascularization-percutaneous/surgical
- Correction of structural pathology
- Ablation-therapeutic
- Cardiac re-synchronization (± ICD)
- Cardiac contractility modulation through non-excitatory electrical signal*
- Ventricular wall stress reduction therapy
  - Batista (partial ventriculectomy)
  - Dor (infarct exclusion, surgical ventricular restoration)
  - Device (myosplint*, Cardioclasp*)
- Cardiomyoplasty
  - Dynamic-tissue/device *
  - Static-device (Cor Cap, Acorn)*
- Ultrafiltration-Hemofiltration
- Descending aortic flow augmentation (Orqis Cancion System)*
- Immuno-modulatory therapy (Vasogen, Inc).
- Ventricular Assist Devices
  - Balloon counterpulsation
  - Pulsatile
  - Axial flow
- Total artificial heart
- Transplantation (Allograft, Cellular*)

The ACC/AHA heart failure guidelines recommend consideration of cardiac resynchronization therapy (CRT) for patients with heart failure who have indications for permanent pacing (e.g. first implant, upgrading of a conventional pacemaker) and NYHA class III-IV symptoms or those who have an LVEF less than 35% despite being on optimal heart failure therapy and who may have a dependence on RV pacing. These recommendations now also include patients with NYHA class II symptoms and the presence of left-bundle-branch block with a QRS duration that is greater than or equal to 150 ms.

*Implantable cardioverter-defibrillators* (Fig. 8.65)

- The role of the ICD has rapidly expanded. Sudden death is 5–10 times more common in patients with heart failure than in the general population. ICD placement results in remarkable reductions in sudden death from ischemic and nonischemic sustained ventricular tachyarrhythmias in heart failure patients. Consequently, current AHA/ACC guidelines recommend an ICD in virtually all patients with an LVEF of less than 35%.

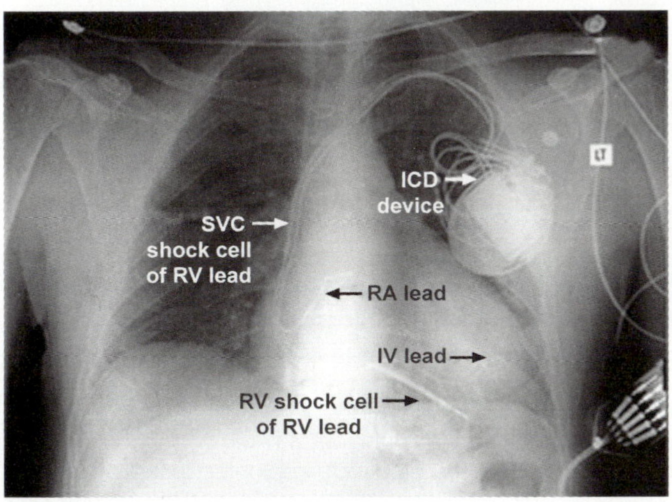


**Fig. 8.65:** X-ray chest showing ICD device fitted in a patient with cardiac arrhythmias and heart failure

- The AHA/ACC and ESC recommend ICD placement for the following categories of heart failure patients.
- Patients with LV dysfunction (LVEF=35%) from a previous MI who are at least 40 days post-MI.
- Patients with nonischemic cardiomyopathy; with an LVEF of 35% or less; in NYHA class II or III; receiving optimal medical therapy; and expected to survive longer than 1 year with good functional status.
- Patients with ischemic cardiomyopathy who are at least 40 days post-MI; have an LVEF of 30% or less; are in NYHA functional class I; are on chronic optimal medical therapy; and are expected to survive longer than 1 year with good functional status.
- Patients who have had ventricular fibrillation (VF).
- Patients with documented hemodynamically unstable ventricular tachycardia (VT) and/or VT with syncope; with an LVEF less than 40%; on optimal medical therapy; and expected to survive longer than 1 year with good functional status.
- In moderately symptomatic heart failure patients with an LVEF of 35% or less, primary prevention with an ICD provides no benefit in some cases but substantial benefit in others. A model based on routinely collected clinical variables can be used to predict the benefit of ICD treatment, according to a study by Levy et al. Using data from the placebo arm of the sudden cardiac death in heart failure trial (SCD-HeFT) with their risk prediction model, Levy et al. showed that patients could be classified into 5 groups on the basis of predicted 4-year mortality. In the treatment arm, ICD implantation decreased relative risk of sudden cardiac death by 88% in patients with the lowest baseline mortality risk but only by 24% in the highest-risk group. ICD treatment decreased relative risk of total mortality by 54% in the lowest-risk group but only by 2% in the highest-risk group.
- It is important to note that use of the SCD-HeFT model has not been prospectively validated for risk stratification in the decision for ICD implantation. More trials are needed.

*Cardiac resynchronization therapy/biventricular pacing:* Patients with heart failure and interventricular conduction abnormalities (roughly defined as those with a QRS interval >120 ms) are potential candidates for CRT by means of an inserted biventricular pacemaker. CRT aims to improve cardiac performance by restoring the heart's interventricular septal electrical and mechanical synchrony. Thus, it reduces presystolic mitral regurgitation and optimizes diastolic function by reducing the mismatch between cardiac contractility and energy expenditure (Fig 8.66).

The ACC/AHA guidelines recommend resynchronization therapy for patients in sinus rhythm or atrial

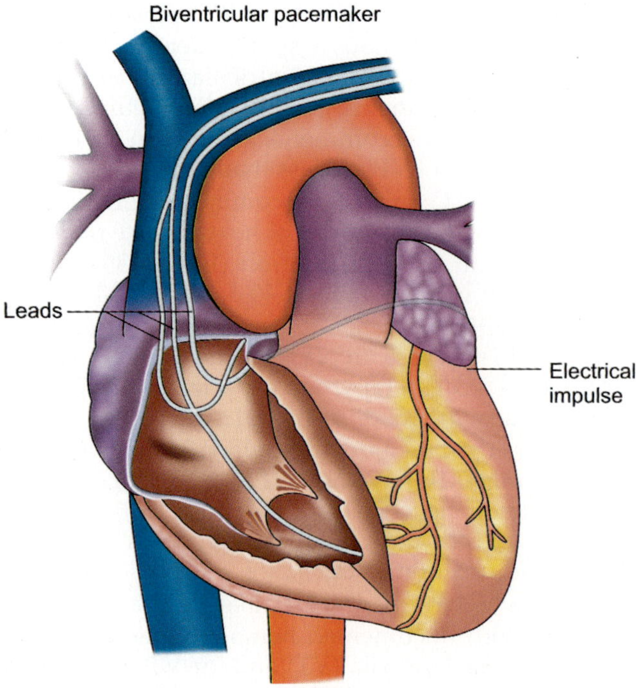


**Fig. 8.66:** Cardiac resynchronization therapy (CRT), also called biventricular pacing, uses a special kind of pacemaker, called a biventricular pacemaker, designed to help the ventricles contract more normally. It keeps the right and left ventricles pumping together by sending small electrical impulses through the leads. This therapy has been shown to improve the symptoms of heart failure and overall quality of life in certain patients with severe symptoms that are not controlled with medication

fibrillation with a QRS duration of 120 ms or longer (the greatest benefit is in patients with a QRS >150 ms) and an LVEF of 35% or less with persistent, moderate-to-severe heart failure (NYHA class III and functional NYHA class IV) despite optimal medical therapy. A 2012 update of ACC/AHA/HRS guidelines on CRT expanded Class I indications to patients with NYHA class II symptoms and left-bundle-branch block of =150 ms.

*Biventricular pacing may also be considered in the following patients* (Figs 8.68–8.70)

- Patients with reduced LVEF and a 2QRS of 150 ms or longer who have NYHA I or II symptoms.
- Patients with reduced LVEF who require chronic pacing and in whom frequent ventricular pacing is expected.

  The combination of biventricular pacing with ICD implantation (CRT-ICD) may be beneficial for patients with class II heart failure, an LVEF of 30% or less, and QRS duration of more than 150 ms. The MADIT-CRT and resynchronization/defibrillation for ambulatory heart failure trial (RAFT) investigators reported significant improvement in mortality and morbidity with CRT-ICD treatment versus ICD alone in this group of patients.
- Patients with unfavorable coronary sinus anatomy often cannot have a CRT properly placed adjacent to the posterolateral wall of the LV. A study by Giraldi et al. suggests that in such patients, a mini-thoracotomy allows for proper lead placement. These patients, when compared with patients who had typical transvenous placement (thus not allowing for preferred posterolateral

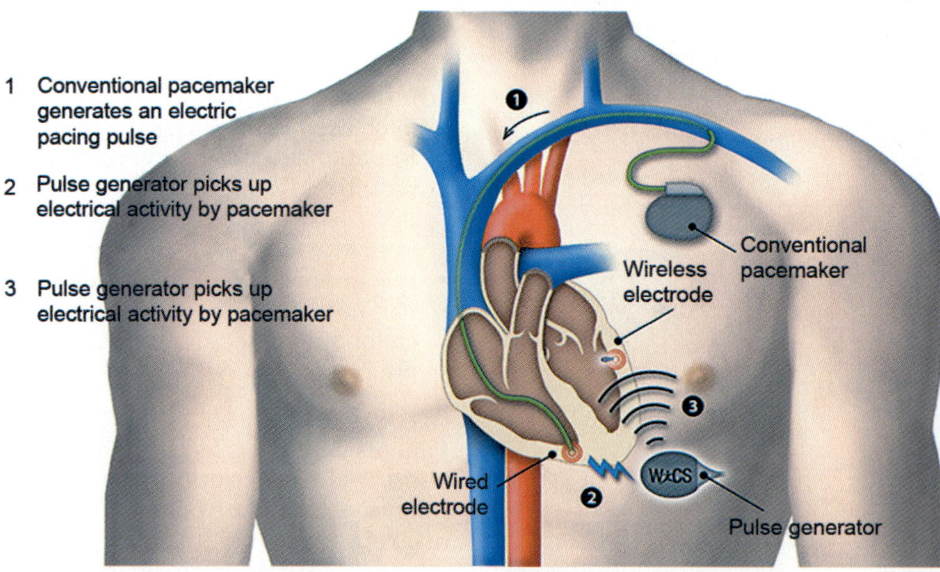


**Fig. 8.67:** Leadless pacemaker. The wireless cardiac stimulation system (WiCS) comprises two units, an implantable electrode and an external control unit. The electrode incorporates an ultrasonic, wireless receiver and delivers an electrical stimulus to the heart based on triggering signals from the external control unit. In its current iteration the WiCS system is designed to work with conventional pacemakers/defibrillators pacing the right ventricle of patients requiring biventricular pacing. The WiCS external control unit senses the pacing stimulus delivered to the right ventricle and initiates a burst of stimulus from the electrode implanted in the left ventricle. According to the company, the wireless left ventricular pacing approach removes the need for complex surgery and the complications often associated with the coronary sinus leads used to pace the left ventricle

A

B

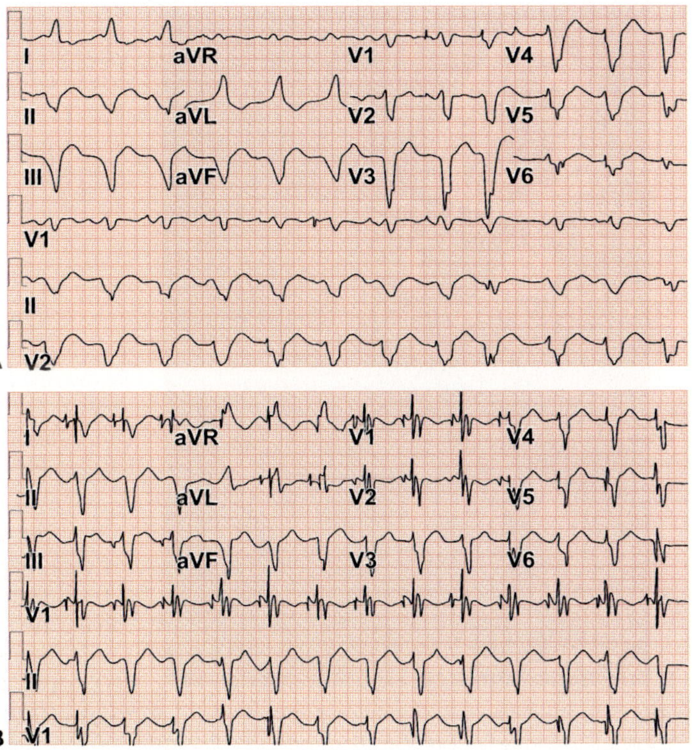


**Fig. 8.68:** Electrocardiogram (ECG) changes with (A) right ventricular (RV) and biventricular pacing 12-lead ECG from a patient with cardiomyopathy during RV apical pacing, and (B) biventricular (BiV) pacing cardiac resynchronization therapy (CRT) with alteration in the QRS duration and axis. Typically, a left bundle branch block pattern is observed in the presence of RV pacing, whereas a right bundle branch block pattern dominates when the left ventricular (LV) is also paced. Pacing from the RV apex is further identified by a superior axis in inferior leads (negative QRS in II, III, aVF)

wall lead placement), had improved outcomes in terms of improved EF and decreased end-systolic volume.

Regarding technique, three cardiac leads are placed transvenously: an atrial lead; an RV lead; and an LV lead, which is threaded through the coronary sinus and out one of its lateral wall tributaries. Surgeons have assisted difficult transvenous LV placements by epicardially inserting LV leads using a number of techniques (e.g. mini-thoracotomy, thoracoscopy, robotically assisted methods).

**Studies of medical versus surgical therapy for CAD have historically focused on patients with normal LV function.**

However, a significantly increased survival rate after coronary artery bypass surgery in a subset of patients with an LVEF of less than 50%, in comparison with the survival rate in patients who were randomly selected to receive medical therapy, was demonstrated in the veterans affairs cooperative study of surgery. This survival benefit was particularly evident at the 11-year follow-up point (50% vs 38%). Surgical revascularization prolonged survival to a greater degree than did medical therapy in most clinical and angiographic subgroups in the coronary artery surgery study (CASS) of patients with left main equivalent disease. Of importance, this study demonstrated that surgical therapy markedly improved the 5-year cumulative survival rate in patients with an EF of less than 50% (80% *vs* 47%) These early randomized trials were limited by their inclusion of patients who had what is currently considered a good EF. That is, many patients referred for coronary revascularization live with EFs of less than 35%.

### *Coronary Artery Bypass Grafting*

The role of CABG in patients with CAD and heart failure has been unclear. Clinical trials from the 1970s that established the benefit of CABG for patients with CAD excluded patients with an EF of less than 35%. In addition, major advances in medical therapy and cardiac surgery have taken place since these trials (Fig. 8.70).

Investigators from Yale and the University of Virginia, among many others, have published their results of CABG in patients with extremely poor LV function who were on the transplant waiting list. Elefteriades et al. reported that in patients with EFs of less than 30% who had CABG, the survival rate was 80% at 4.5 years. This figure approaches that of cardiac transplantation. Kron et al. reported a similar 3-year survival rate, of 83%, in patients who underwent coronary artery bypass with an EF of less than 20%.

### *STICH Trial*

The surgical treatment for ischemic heart failure (STICH) study found no significant difference between medical therapy alone and medical therapy plus CABG with respect to death from any cause (the primary study outcome). STICH included 1212 patients with an EF of 35% or less and CAD amenable to CABG. Patients were randomized to either CABG with intensive medical therapy or medical therapy alone and followed up for a median of 56 months.

There was no difference between the treatment groups for all-cause mortality. Owing to the lack of significant difference in the primary endpoint, the secondary endpoints should be viewed cautiously. Except for 30-day mortality, secondary study results favored CABG; compared with study patients assigned to medical therapy alone, patients assigned to CABG had lower rates of death from cardiovascular causes and of death from any cause or hospitalization for cardiovascular causes. Surprisingly, the presence of viable, hibernating myocardium was not predictive of improved outcomes from CABG.

Taken together, these findings suggest that in the absence of severe angina or left main disease, medical therapy alone remains a reasonable option for patients with an EF of 35% or less and CAD. Furthermore, current methods of assessing myocardial viability/hibernating myocardium may not accurately predict benefit from revascularization, although cardiac magnetic resonance imaging offers a promise of accuracy in identifying viable myocardium and predicting the success of revascularization in patients with low EFs.

The adoption of techniques on and off cardiopulmonary bypass, as well as beating-heart techniques for revascularization, highlight the aim of treating high-risk patients. The surgery in the STICH trial was performed with these

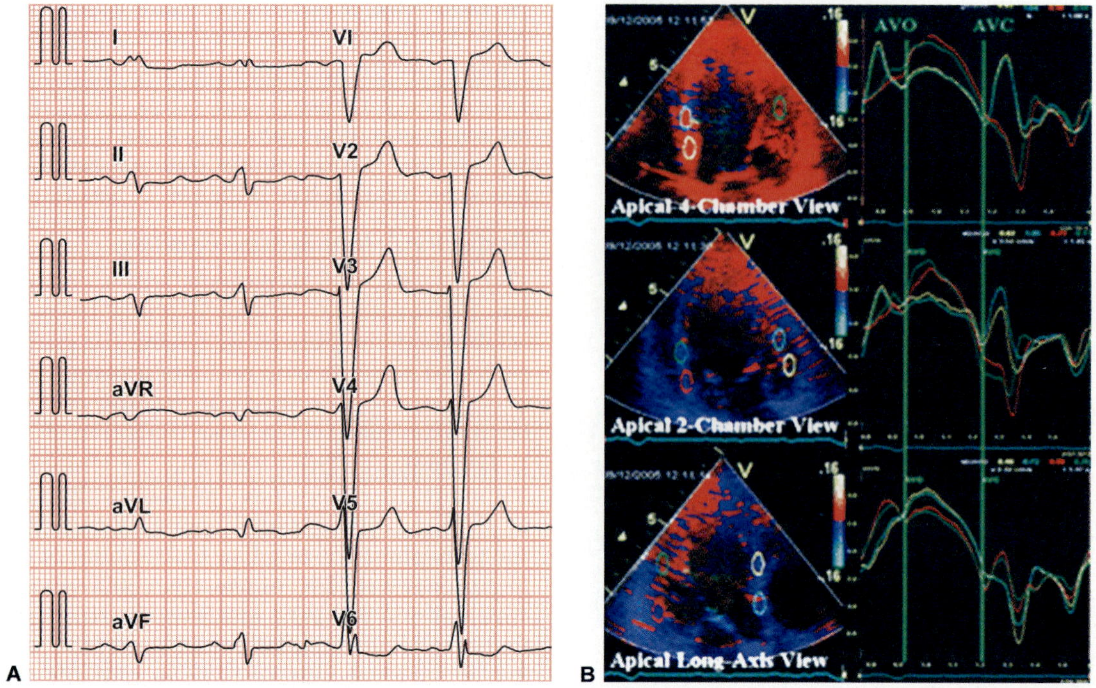


**Fig. 8.69:** (A) A 12-lead electrocardiogram before cardiac resynchronization therapy (CRT), demonstrating a QRS width of 160 ms with a left bundle branch block. (B) Longitudinal dyssynchrony by myocardial velocity before cardiac resynchronization therapy was as follows: 23 ms in Yu index and 35 ms in opposing wall delay, indicating no longitudinal dyssynchrony. AVO=aortic valve opening; AVC=aortic valve closure. Apical four-chamber view: yellow, basal-interior septum; blue, mid-inferior septum; red, basal-lateral; green, mid-lateral. Apical two-chamber view: yellow, basal-anterior; blue, mid-anterior; red, basal-inferior; green, mid-inferior. Apical long-axis view: yellow, basal-anterior septum; blue, mid-anterior septum; red, basal-posterior; green, mid-posterior

modern surgical advantages. Preventive strategies include the increased use of bilateral mammary and arterial grafting.

## Valvular Surgery

Valvular heart disease may be the underlying aetiology or an important aggravating factor in heart failure.The ACC/AHA recommends that valve repair or replacement in patients with hemodynamically significant valvular stenosis or regurgitation and asymptomatic heart failure should be based on contemporary guidelines. In addition, the ACC/AHA indicates that such surgery should be considered for patients with severe aortic or mitral valve stenosis or regurgitation, even when ventricular function is impaired (Figs 8.71 and 8.72).

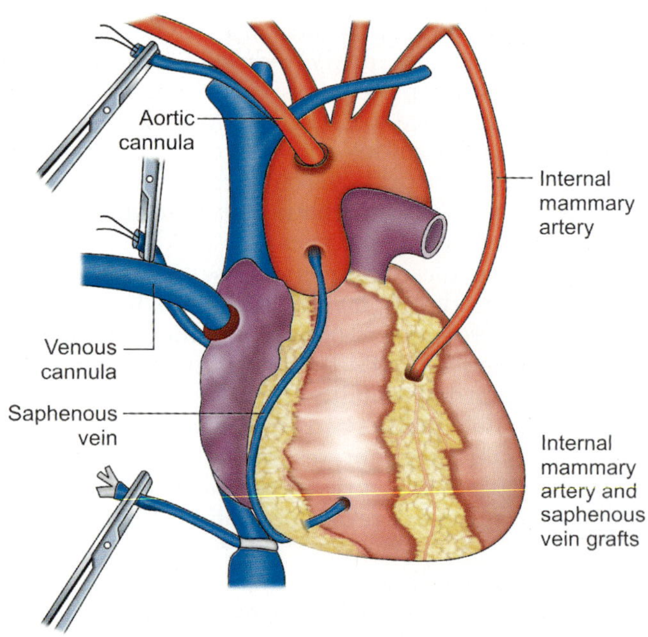


**Fig. 8.70:** Coronary artery bypass grafting in an elderly patient with severe triple vessels coronary artery disease with heart failure

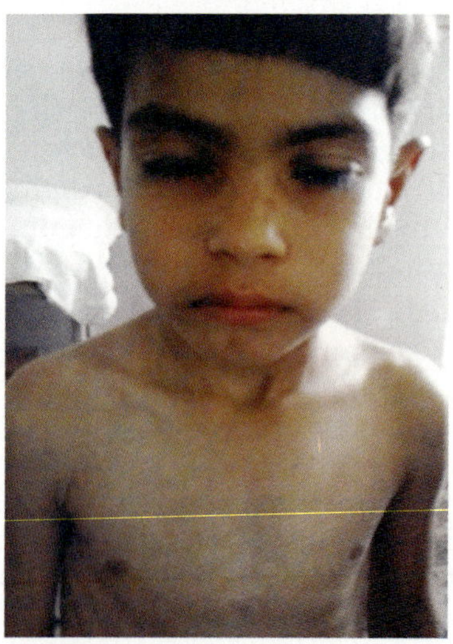

**Fig. 8.71:** A 7-year-old child who had juvenile rheumatic mitral stenosis (MVA <2.0 cm$^2$) with severe MR (grade III–IV) enlarged LA with PAH and exertional dyspnea and showed early signs of heart failure. He is advised minimal invasive surgery

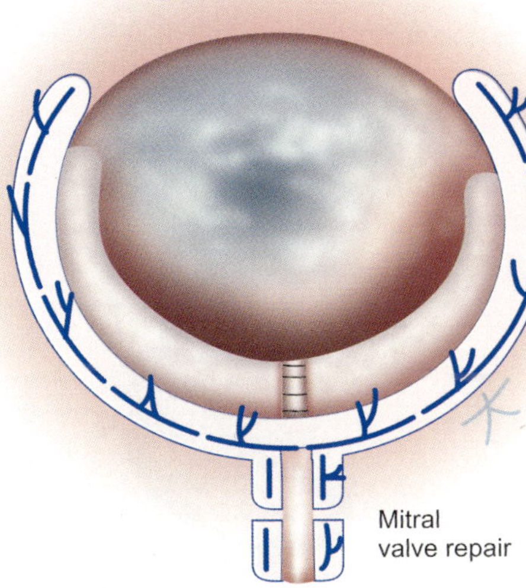


**Fig. 8.72:** Annuloplasty—complete repair of the damaged valve in the mitral valve apparatus

The ESC notes that although impaired LVEF is an important risk factor for higher perioperative and postoperative mortality, surgery may be considered in symptomatic patients with poor LV function. However, it is essential that optimal conservative management of the patient's heart failure and any comorbidities be undertaken before surgery, with a thorough clinical and echocardiographic assessment that focuses on cardiovascular and noncardiovascular comorbidities.

### Aortic Valve Replacement

Diseases of the aortic valve can frequently lead to the onset and progression of heart failure. Although the natural histories of aortic stenosis and aortic regurgitation are well known, patients are often followed up conservatively after they present with clinically significant heart failure.

Heart failure is a common indication for aortic valve replacement (AVR), but one must be cautious in patients with a low LVEF and possible aortic stenosis (Figs 8.73 and 8.74).

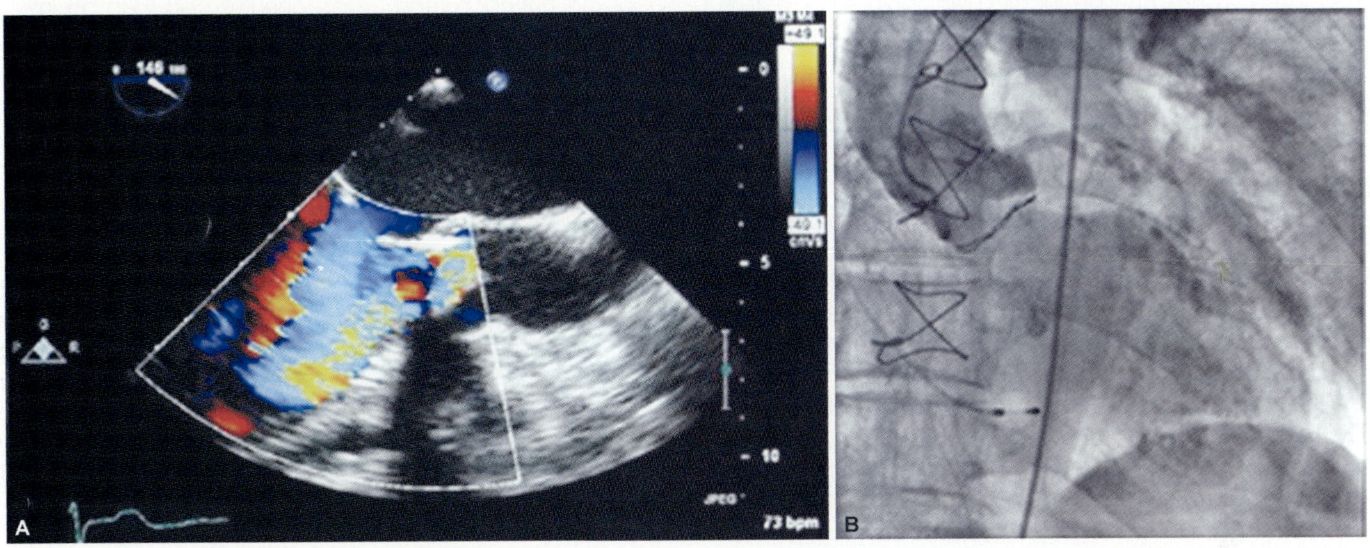


**Fig. 8.73:** (A) Aortic regurgitation documented by transesophageal echocardiography, and (B) aortography. The patient was referred for aortic valve replacement surgery for worsening of LV functions

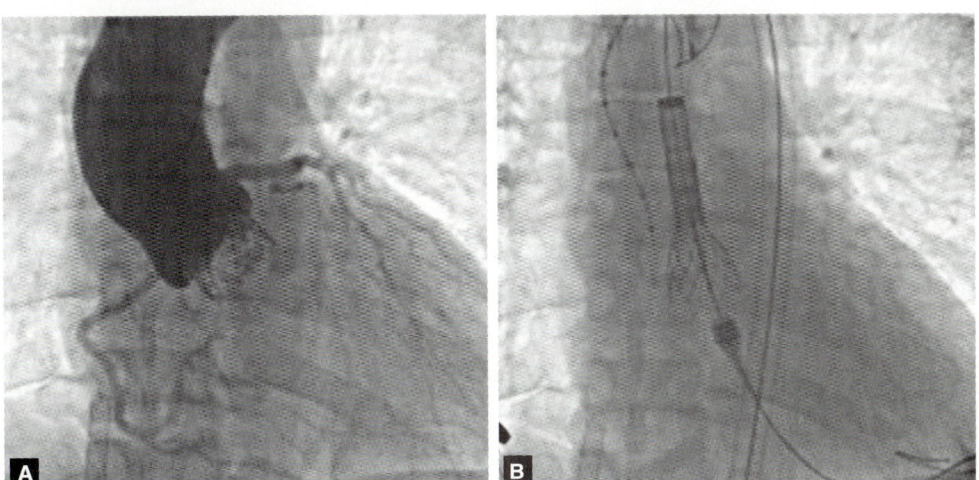


**Fig. 8.74:** (A) Controlled expansion of the aortic prosthesis. (B) Angiogram after successful implantation of aortic valve in an elderly patient with severe aortic stenosis and AR with heart failure

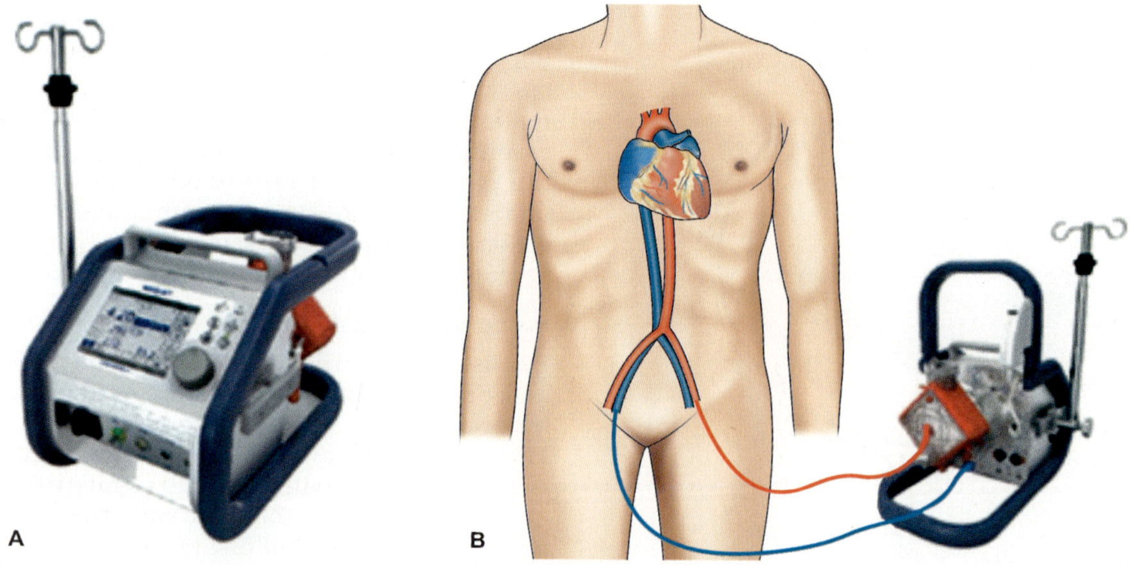


**Fig. 8.75:** (A) The device is compact and easily portable, with a total weight of only 9 kg. (B) Veno-arterial extracorporeal membrane oxygenation (ECMO) is established by cannulation of a femoral vein and artery using the Seldinger technique. To expedite interhospital transfer these vessels can be located with guidewires before arrival of the outreach team. The cannulas can then be inserted rapidly to begin ECMO before transport by air or ground ambulance. Images of the Cardiohelp® device courtesy of Maquet Cardiopulmonary AG©

## Extracorporeal Membrane Oxygenation

In some cases of extreme cardiopulmonary failure (i.e. ACC/AHA stage D), the only recourse is complete support with extracorporeal membrane oxygenation (ECMO) (Fig. 8.75). ECMO provides both oxygenation and circulation of blood, allowing the lungs and heart time to recover. Unlike cardiopulmonary bypass, whose duration of use is measured in hours, ECMO can be used for 3–10 days.

For ECMO, one cannula is placed percutaneously via the right jugular vein or femoral vein into the right atrium, or it is placed surgically into the right atrial appendage, and another cannula is placed arterially either in the femoral artery or in the aortic arch. The drained venous blood is pumped through the ECMO device, where it is oxygenated, warmed, and anticoagulated. It is then returned to the arterial circulation.

ECMO devices can be used for short-term circulatory support in patients who are expected to recover from a major cardiac insult. Despite encouraging results with ECMO for the management of cardiogenic shock, most patients requiring circulatory assistance can be helped with ventricular support alone.

## Ventricular Assist Devices

Ventricular assist devices (VADs) are invaluable tools in the treatment of heart failure. A number of these devices are available to support the acutely or chronically decompensated heart (i.e. ACC/AHA stage D). Depending on the particular device used, the right ventricle and left ventricle can be assisted with a left ventricular assist device (LVAD), a right VAD (RVAD), or a biventricular assist device (BiVAD). An alternative term for a VAD is a ventricular assist system (VAS) (Figs 8.76 and 8.77).

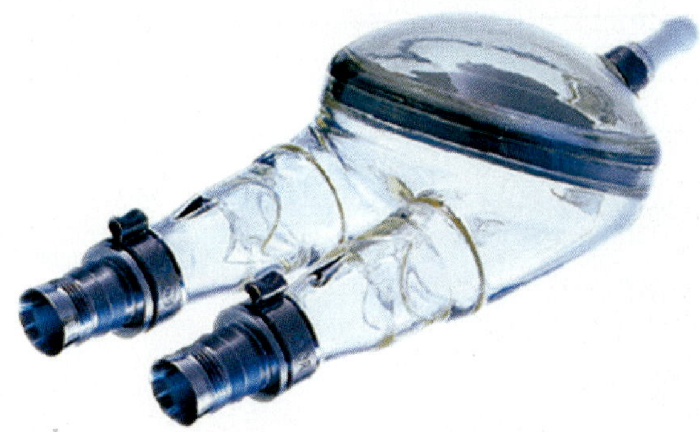

**Fig. 8.76:** Excor pediatric heart pump for treating shock conitions in children

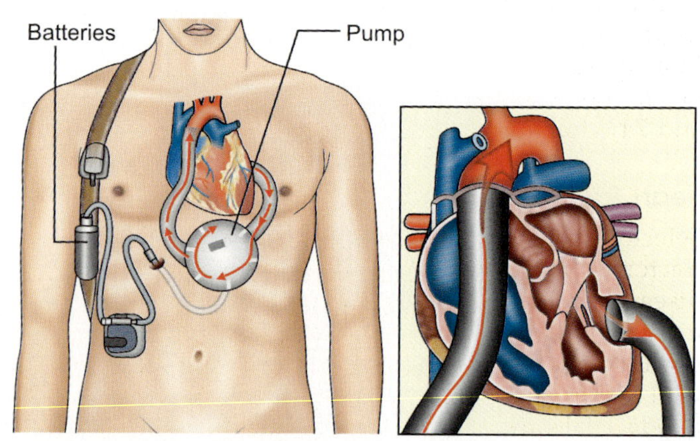


**Fig. 8.77:** VADs which are used for people with end-stage refractory congestive heart failure that has not responded to medicine. In the heart, the left ventricle does most of the work. It is usually the chamber that fails first. VADs can be used to support the left ventricle, right ventricle, or both. Getting a VAD is a way to improve the heart's ability to pump without having a heart transplant

In concept, LVADs, RVADs, and BiVADs are similar. Blood is removed from the failing ventricle and diverted into a pump that delivers blood to either the aorta (in the case of an LVAD) or the pulmonary artery (in the case of an RVAD). An exception is the Impella (Abiomed, Inc). This device is inserted percutaneously into the left ventricle; it draws blood from the left ventricle and expels it into the ascending aorta.

LVADs can often be placed temporarily. In patients with acute, severe myocarditis or those who have undergone cardiotomy, this approach can serve as a bridge to recovery, unloading the dysfunctional heart and perhaps allowing reverse remodeling; in patients with end-stage heart failure, it can serve as a bridge to heart transplantation, allowing them to undergo rehabilitation and possibly go home before transplantation.

Long-term use (i.e. destination therapy rather than bridge therapy) may be a consideration when no definitive procedure is planned. Patients with severe heart failure who are not transplant candidates and who otherwise would die without treatment are candidates for lifetime use of VADs. Destination therapy with LVADs is superior to medical therapy in terms of quantity and quality of life, according to the randomized evaluation of mechanical assistance for the treatment of congestive heart failure (REMATCH) trial and several later studies. In the United States, several Food and Drug Administration (FDA) approved options are available for bridging the patient to recovery and transplantation. These options continue to change and evolve. Some examples include are as follows.

Recommendations for clinical management of continuous-flow LVAD were published in 2010, assisting providers with standardized care for this patient population. Bleeding, infection, and stroke are postimplant complications, and death may occur due to right heart failure, sepsis, or stroke. A multidisciplinary approach to LVAD implantation is needed, as destination therapy identifies patients at high risk for complications and the need to optimize these patients medically before surgery. In a recent report from INTERMACS, 1-year survival for destination-therapy patients was 61% for pulsatile devices and 74% for continuous-flow devices.

## Heart Transplantation

Selected patients with severe heart failure, debilitating refractory angina, ventricular arrhythmia, or congenital heart disease that cannot be controlled despite pharmacologic, medical device, or alternative surgical therapy should be evaluated for heart transplantation. The patient must be well informed, motivated, and emotionally stable; have a good social support network; and be capable of complying with intensive medical treatment (Figs 8.78 and 8.79).

Since Christiaan Barnard performed the first orthotopic heart transplantation in 1967, the world has seen tremendous advancement in the field of cardiac transplantation. For patients with progressive end-stage heart failure despite maximal medical therapy who have a poor prognosis and no viable alternative form of treatment, heart transplantation has become the criterion standard for therapy.

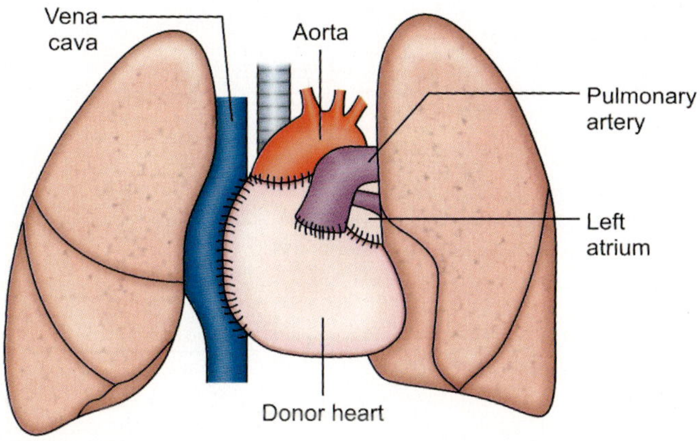


**Fig. 8.78:** Diagram illustrating the placement of a donor heart in an orthotopic procedure. Notice how the back of the patient's left atrium and great vessels are left in place

Compared with patients who receive only medical therapy, transplant recipients have fewer rehospitalizations; marked functional improvements; enhanced quality of life; more gainful employment; and longer survival, with 50% surviving 10 years postoperatively (heart transplantation is associated with a 1 year survival rate of 83%; subsequently, survival decreases in a linear manner by approximately 3.4% per year).

Careful selection of donors and recipients is critical for ensuring good outcomes. In addition, transplant teams must strive to minimize potential perioperative dangers, including ischemic times, pulmonary hypertension, mechanical support, and cardiogenic shock.

### Indications

According to the ACC/AHA, absolute indications for heart transplantation include hemodynamic compromise following heart failure, including the following scenarios:

- Refractory cardiogenic shock
- Dependence on IV inotropic support for adequacy of organ perfusion
- Peak oxygen consumption per unit time ($VO_2$) less than 10 ml/kg/min
- Severe ischemic symptoms with consistent limitations of routine activity that are not amenable to revascularization procedures (CABG, percutaneous coronary intervention)
- Recurrent symptomatic ventricular arrhythmias despite all therapeutic interventions
- Relative indications for heart transplantation include the following:
    - Peak $VO_2$ between 11 and 14 ml/kg/min (or 55% of predicted) with major limitation of routine activities
    - Recurrent unstable ischemia that is not amenable to other treatment
    - Recurrent instability of fluid balance/renal function despite patient compliance with medical therapy

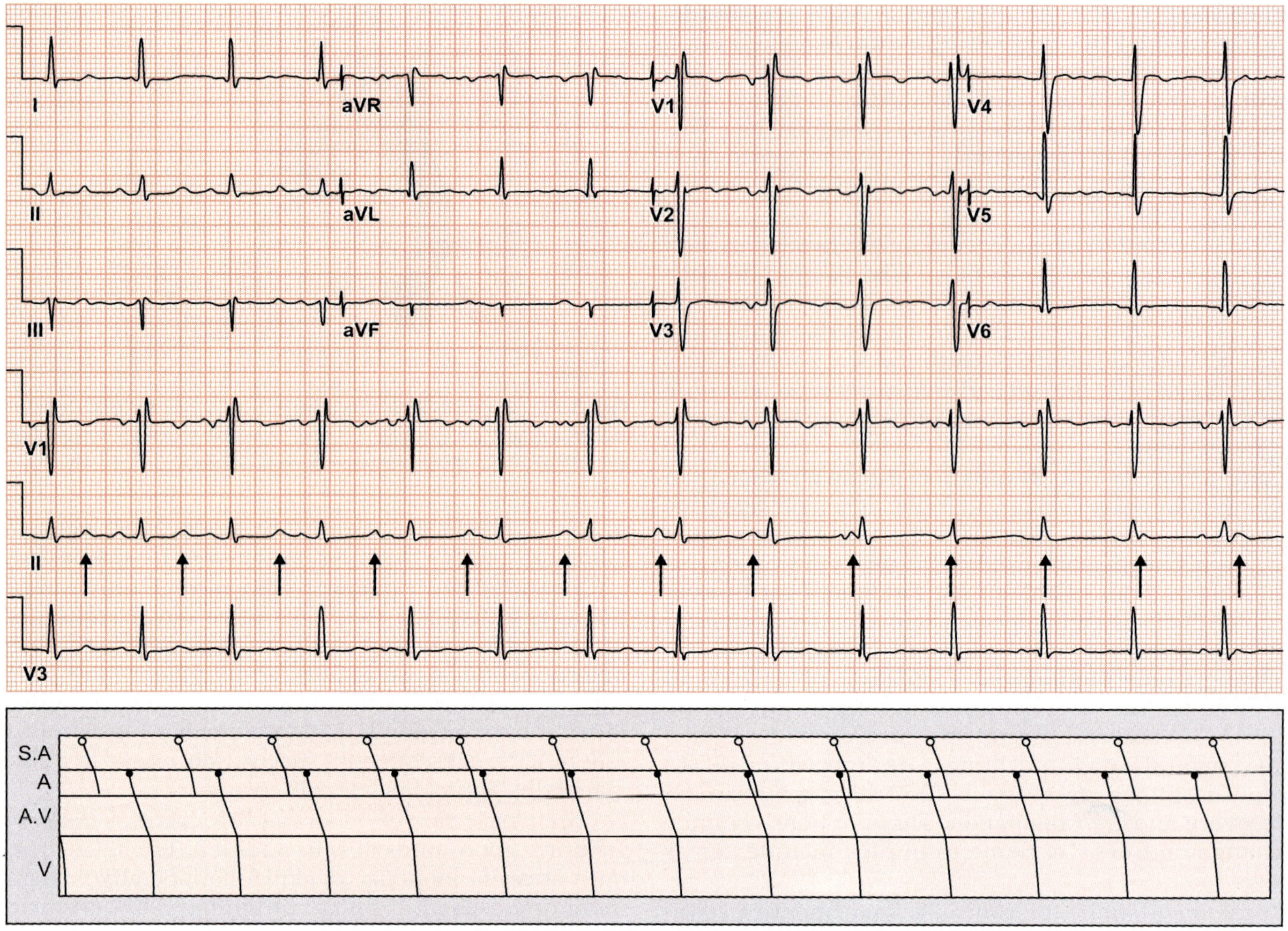


**Fig. 8.79:** ECG of orthotopic heart transplant. Recipient P-waves (arrows)

- In the absence of other indications, however, the following are not sufficient indications for heart transplantation:
  - Low LVEF
  - History of NYHA class III/IV heart failure symptoms
  - Peak $VO_2$ >15 ml/kg/min (and >55% predicted)

### Contraindications

The ESC indicates that heart transplantation is contraindicated in patients with the following conditions.

- Current alcohol and/or drug abuse
- Lack of compliance
- Uncontrolled or mental health disease
- Active malignancy
- Multiorgan systemic disease
- Active infection except for LVAD infection
- Significant renal failure (creatinine clearance <50 ml/min), significant hepatic dysfunction, or pulmonary disease (FEV1 <50% of predicted or <1 L)
- Irreversible high pulmonary vascular resistance (6–8 wood units and mean transpulmonary gradient >15 mmHg)
- Recent thromboembolic complications
- Unhealed peptic ulcer
- Other serious comorbidity with a poor prognosis
- Note that the HFSA and ESC indicate that cardiomyoplasty and partial left ventriculectomy (Batista operation) is not recommended to treat heart failure, nor should it be used as an alternative to heart transplantation.

### Coronary Graft Atherosclerosis

The Achilles heel of the long-term success of heart transplantation is the development of coronary graft atherosclerosis, the cardiac version of chronic rejection. Coronary graft atherosclerosis is uniquely different from typical coronary artery disease in that it is diffuse and is usually not amenable to revascularization.

### Shortage of Donor Hearts

In the United States, fewer than 2500 heart transplantation procedures are performed annually. Each year, an estimated 10–20% of patients die while awaiting a heart transplant. Of the 5 million people with heart failure, approximately 30,000–100,000 have such advanced disease that they would benefit from transplantation or mechanical circulatory support. This disparity between the number of patients needing transplants and the availability of heart donors has refocused efforts to find other ways to support severely failing hearts.

### Cell Replacement Strategy

Cell replacement strategy is a new era in therapy for patients with myocardial dysfunction (Fig. 8.80). It has been postulated that therapies directly targeted at replacing or regenerating damaged myocardial tissue could prevent progression to heart failure and therefore would be an important contribution to the treatment of ischemic damage to the myocardium. Many cell types have been successfully transplanted into damaged myocardium, including fetal cardiomyocytes, skeletal myoblasts, embryonic stem cells, and bone marrow-derived stem cells. The best characterized of these is skeletal myoblast, an immature muscle cell that retains the ability to proliferate. Several studies have used human autologous skeletal myoblasts transplantation to determine if engraftment of these cells leads to long-term improvements in left ventricle function. However, these exciting progresses have many unanswered questions including potential arrhythmic and oncogenic potential of these cells, which can only be resolved by larger clinical trials with long-term follow-up.

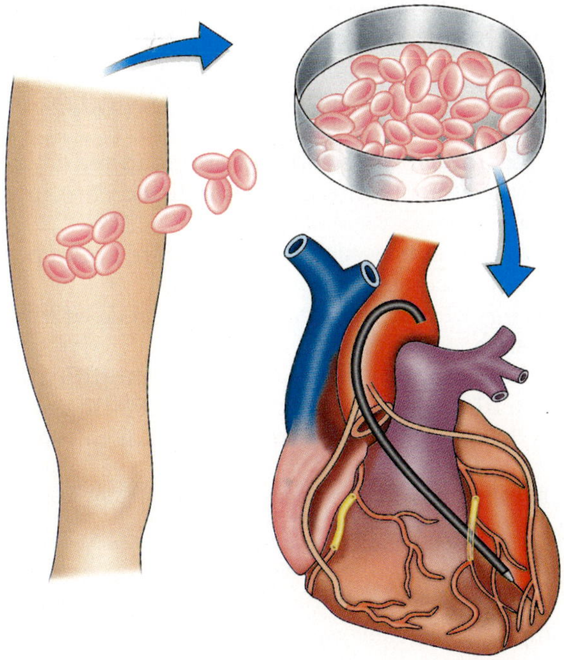

**Fig. 8.80:** Diagrammatic depiction of myogenesis in the heart muscle. Myoblasts are super powerhouse cells that originate from human body's muscle stem cells. These cells have the ability to take on the properties of the other cells such as cardiac muscle cells that make up the heart. Unlike cardiac muscle myoblasts can regenerate and repair themselves. The myoblasts can be transplanted from the skeletal muscles into heart and can stimulate myogenesis. A biopsy of muscle cells from patient thigh is taken and isolated and expanded in culture in a special cell laboratory for 3 weeks. These multiple cells are injected directly into the areas of heart where the muscle is damaged

### Other Modes of Management

#### *Maintain infant's temperature in euthermic range*

Posture: A patient in CHF has cardiomegaly and congested lungs. Both diminish the volume available for air exchange. In addition hepatomegaly will limit diaphragmatic excursion in recumbent posture so keep the patient in a suitable chair in inclined posture.

*Oxygen administration:* If there is respiratory distress, pulmonary venous desaturation is pronounced, so increase inspired oxygen concentration will benefit the patient.

*Sedation:* Restlessness is very common in patients with CHF which raises oxygen demands. Sedation with chloral hydrate is useful in infants and children. Morphine is the sedative of choice in acutely ill patient and in postoperative period when pain is an additional factor.

*In the second 24 hours:* If the patient has good diuresis, respiratory distress has lessened and heart rate has slowed down, maintenance digoxin and diuretics are switched over to the oral route. But if inotropics and preload reducers do not produce the desired effect, search for additional problem is made because digoxin has got dynamic action depending upon the pH of blood, electrolyte normality, abnormal blood sugar level and hemoglobin concentration. If child is very anemic, packed blood cells are given which increase oxygen carrying capacity. Attempt is made to maintain electrolyte balance, normal blood sugar and proper blood pH. If child has got pulmonary infection adequate antibiotic treatment is given. If inspite of above variables being normal, after load reducers are considered. Two more therapeutic principles that can be followed both in the hospital as well as at home are:

- Salt restriction should not interfere with patient's eating.
- Restriction of physical activity is not the issue in pediatrics. It may be counter productive because it increases oxygen consumption. When the baby improves, can tolerate room air and develops an appetite sufficient to gain weight-maintenance of inotropics and diuretics should be decided and further investigation for proper surgical management should be carried out.

### Vasopeptidase Inhibitors

Neutral peptidase is an enzyme that inactivates several of the peptides like atrial natriuretic peptide, brain type natriuretic peptide, bradykinin and adrenomedullin. These peptides have vasodilator, natriuretic and antiproliferative properties. Simultaneous inhibition of neutral peptidase and angiotensin converting enzyme markedly reduces vasoconstriction, improves sodium and water balance, decrease peripheral vascular resistance and blood pressure and improves local blood flow when compared with angiotensin converting enzyme inhibition alone.

The only available vasopeptidase inhibitor that has been evaluated in adults with heart failure is omapatrilat, which is not yet recommended for use at this time. Candoxatril and ecadotril are oral forms of neutral peptidase inhibitors which increase levels of natriuretic peptides and are currently in trials in adult patients with heart failure.

### *Endothelin Receptor Antagonists*

Endothelin-1 levels are increased in patients with heart failure and progressively higher plasma concentrations are found in patients with heart failure as their functional class deteriorates. Endothelin-1 plasma level also correlates with pulmonary artery pressure and pulmonary vascular resistance. Although the expression of endothelin-1 within the myocardium may initially represent an adaptive response to stress, over expression of endothelin-1 may eventually be maladaptive by producing focal vasospasm, myocyte necrosis and increased myocardial fibrosis. Nonselective endothelin receptor antagonists such as bosentan, tezosentran and enrasentran are now being evaluated in clinical trials in adults but have yet to demonstrate their clinical utility. Sitaxsentan is a selective endothelin-1A receptor antagonist and a selective pulmonary vasodilator.

## Total Artificial Heart

- The creation of a suitable total artificial heart (TAH) for orthotopic implantation has been the subject of intense investigation for decades (in 1969, Dr Denton Cooley implanted the Liotta TAH, which is no longer made) into a high-risk patient after failing to wean the patient off cardiopulmonary bypass after LV aneurysm repair. The patient was sustained until, after 3 days, a donor heart became available, but the patient subsequently died of pneumonia and multiple organ failure.
- Compared with LVADs, the TAH has several potential advantages, including the ability to assist patients with severe biventricular failure; a lack of device pocket and thus a lessened risk of infection; and the opportunity to treat patients with systemic diseases (e.g. amyloidosis, malignancy) who are not otherwise candidates for transplantation.
- At present, 2 TAHs are receiving the most attention: SynCardia (formerly CardioWest) TAH (SynCardia Systems, Inc) AbioCor TAH (Abiomed, Inc)
- The SynCardia TAH is a structural cousin of the original Jarvik-7 TAH (Jarvik Heart, Inc) that was implanted into patient Barney Clark with great publicity in 1982. In 2004, investigators reported data that allowed this device to receive FDA approval for use as a bridge to transplantation.
- The AbioCor TAH involves a novel method of transcutaneous transmission of energy, freeing the patient from external drivelines. The patient exchanges the external battery packs, which can last as long as 4 hours. This TAH is unique in that it is the first TAH to use coils to transmit power across the skin; therefore, no transcutaneous conduits are needed. This feature allows for the advantages of a closed system, which potentially reduces sources of infection, a known complication of earlier devices.
- The first clinical implantation of this TAH was performed in July 2001. Before the end of 2004, 14 patients had received this device as part of a trial in patients whose expected survival was less than 30 days. Although all subsequently died, 4 patients were ambulatory after surgery, and 2 were discharged from the hospital to a transitional-care setting. One of the discharged patients was discharged on postoperative day 209. A limitation of the AbioCor TAH is its large size, which permits its implantation in only 50% of men and 20% of women. In 2006, the FDA approved the Abiocor TAH as a permanent TAH for humanitarian uses.
- The SynCardia and AbioCor TAHs require recipient cardiectomy before implantation. The devices are similar in that they are sewn to atrial cuffs and to the great vessels after the native heart is explanted.
- Despite more than 40 years of effort, the clinical application of artificial-heart technology is still immature. However, with the approval of the SynCardia device and with new efforts to create small pumps, TAHs will ultimately be routine components of heart failure surgery for very sick patients with heart failure and biventricular failure.

## Drug Therapy

The goals of pharmacotherapy for heart failure are to reduce morbidity and to prevent complications (Table 8.15). Along with oxygen, medications assisting with symptom relief include:

- Diuretics, which reduce edema by reduction of blood volume and venous pressures,
- Vasodilators, for preload and afterload reduction,
- Digoxin, which can cause a small increase in cardiac output,
- Inotropic agents, which help to restore organ perfusion and reduce congestion,
- Anticoagulants, to decrease the risk of thromboembolism,
- Beta-blockers, for neurohormonal modification, left ventricular ejection fraction (LVEF) improvement, arrhythmia prevention, and ventricular rate control,

**Table 8.15:** Drug therapy and dosage schelule for treatment of CHF

- Initial oral digitalization dose
  (IV or IM dose is two-thirds of oral dose)
- Maintenance digoxin:
  - Premature
    - <1500 gm 0.02 mg/kg 0.005 mg/kg
    - >1500 gm 0.04 mg/kg 0.01 mg/kg
  - Newborns and upto six months 0.04 mg/kg 0.01 mg/kg
  - 6 months–2 years 0.06 mg/kg 0.015 mg/kg
  - 2 years–10 years 0.04 mg/kg 0.01 mg/kg
  - >10 years 0.04 mg/kg 0.01 mg/kg
- Dopamine 5–10 mcg/kg/min in 5% glucose
  - Morphine 0.1 mg/kg/dose
  - Chloral hydrate 20 mg/kg/dose

- Angiotensin-converting enzyme inhibitors (ACEIs), for neurohormonal modification, vasodilatation, and LVEF improvement,
- Angiotensin II receptor blockers (ARBs), also for neurohormonal modification, vasodilatation, and LVEF improvement, and
- Analgesics, for pain management.

Drugs that can exacerbate heart failure should be avoided, such as nonsteroidal anti-inflammatory drugs (NSAIDs), calcium channel blockers (CCBs), and most antiarrhythmic drugs (except class III). NSAIDs can cause sodium retention and peripheral vasoconstriction, and they can attenuate the efficacy and enhance the toxicity of diuretics and ACEIs. CCBs can worsen heart failure and may increase the risk of cardiovascular events; only the vasoselective CCBs have been shown not to adversely affect survival. Antiarrhythmic agents can have cardiodepressant effects and may promote arrhythmia; only amiodarone and dofetilide have been shown not to adversely affect survival.

### Beta-blockers, Alpha Activity

Beta-blockers inhibit the sympathomimetic nervous system and block alpha1-adrenergic vasoconstrictor activity. These agents have moderate afterload reduction properties and cause slight preload reduction. In addition to decreasing mortality rates, beta-blockers also reduce hospitalizations and the risk of sudden death; improve LV function and exercise tolerance; and reduce heart failure functional class. Although other beta-blockers with similar pharmacologic properties might hypothetically be beneficial in heart failure, the target doses have not been identified in clinical trials.

### Carvedilol (Cor, e.g. Coreg CR)

Carvedilol is a nonselective beta-and alpha1-adrenergic blocker. It does not appear to have intrinsic sympathomimetic activity. Carvedilol at the target dose of 25 mg twice daily has been shown to reduce mortality in clinical trials of heart failure patients with reduced ejection fraction.

### Beta-blockers, Beta-1 Selective

Certain beta-1 blockers are selective in blocking beta-1 adrenoreceptors. These agents are used in heart failure to reduce heart rate and blood pressure.

### Metoprolol (Lopressor, Toprol XL)

Metoprolol is a selective beta1-adrenergic blocker at lower doses. It inhibits beta2-receptors at higher doses. It does not have intrinsic sympathomimetic activity. The long-acting formulation (metoprolol succinate) at a target dose of 200 mg daily has been shown to reduce mortality in a clinical trial of patients with heart failure and low ejection fraction.

### Bisoprolol (Zebeta)

Bisoprolol is a highly selective beta1-adrenergic receptor blocker that decreases the automaticity of contractions. Bisoprolol at the target dose of 10 mg daily has been shown to reduce mortality in a clinical trial of patients with heart failure and reduced ejection fraction, but is not approved for heart failure use in the United States.

### ACE Inhibitors

Angiotensin-converting enzyme inhibitors (ACEIs) prevent conversion of angiotensin I to angiotensin II, which results in lower aldosterone secretion. Use of ACEIs increases survival, improves symptoms, and decreases repeat hospitalizations.

### Captopril

Captopril prevents conversion of angiotensin I to angiotensin II, a potent vasoconstrictor, resulting in lower aldosterone secretion. Captopril at a target dose of 25 mg three times daily has been shown to improve survival in patients with low ejection fraction after myocardial infarction.

### Enalapril (Vasotec)

Enalapril prevents conversion of angiotensin I to angiotensin II, a potent vasoconstrictor, resulting in increased levels of plasma renin and a reduction in aldosterone secretion. It helps control blood pressure and proteinuria. Enalapril decreases the pulmonary-to-systemic flow ratio in the catheterization laboratory and increases systemic blood flow in patients with relatively low pulmonary vascular resistance. It has a favorable clinical effect when administered over a long period. It helps prevent potassium loss in distal tubules. The body conserves potassium; thus, less oral potassium supplementation is needed. Enalapril at a target dose of 10 mg twice daily has been shown to improve survival in patients with heart failure and reduced ejection fraction.

### Lisinopril (Prinivil, Zestril)

Lisinopril prevents conversion of angiotensin I to angiotensin II, a potent vasoconstrictor, resulting in increased levels of plasma renin and a reduction in aldosterone secretion. Lisinopril at a target dose of 10 mg daily has been shown to reduce mortality after myocardial infarction.

### Ramipril (Altace)

Ramipril prevents conversion of angiotensin I to angiotensin II, a potent vasoconstrictor, resulting in increased levels of plasma renin and a reduction in aldosterone secretion. Ramipril at a target dose of 5 mg twice daily has been shown to reduce mortality in patients with heart failure after myocardial infarction.

### Quinapril (Accupril)

Quinapril prevents conversion of angiotensin I to angiotensin II, a potent vasoconstrictor, resulting in increased levels of plasma renin and a reduction in aldosterone secretion.

### ARBs

Angiotensin receptor blockers (ARBs) are reasonable first-line therapy for patients with mild to moderate heart failure symptoms and left ventricular (LV) dysfunction when patients are already taking these agents for other indications. ARBs block the renin-angiotensin-aldosterone system (RAAS) by competitive inhibition of the AT1 receptor, thereby decreasing afterload and preventing LV remodeling. The use of ARBs increases survival and decreases hospitalization rates, but these agents are not superior to angiotensin-converting enzyme inhibitors (ACEIs). ARBs can also be used as add-on therapy for patients who have refractory heart failure symptoms despite optimal heart failure therapy.

### Losartan (Cozaar)

Losartan blocks the vasoconstrictor and aldosterone-secreting effects of angiotensin II at tissue receptor sites. It may induce more complete inhibition of the renin-angiotensin system than ACE inhibitors, and it does not affect the response to bradykinin (less likely to be associated with cough and angioedema). These agents are used in patients unable to tolerate ACE inhibitors. Losartan has not been demonstrated to improve survival in heart failure.

### Valsartan (Diovan)

Valsartan is a prodrug that produces direct antagonism of angiotensin II receptors. It displaces angiotensin II from the AT1 receptor and may lower blood pressure by antagonizing AT1-induced vasoconstriction, aldosterone release, catecholamine release, arginine vasopressin release, water intake, and hypertrophic responses. It may induce more complete inhibition of the renin-angiotensin system than ACE inhibitors, does not affect the response to bradykinin, and is less likely to be associated with cough and angioedema. It is used in patients unable to tolerate ACE inhibitors. Valsartan at a target dose of 160 mg twice daily has been shown to improve survival in patients with heart failure and reduced ejection fraction.

### Candesartan (Atacand)

Candesartan blocks the vasoconstriction and aldosterone-secreting effects of angiotensin II. It may induce more complete inhibition of the renin-angiotensin system than ACE inhibitors, does not affect the response to bradykinin, and is less likely to be associated with cough and angioedema. Use candesartan in patients unable to tolerate ACE inhibitors. Candesartan at a target dose of 32 mg daily has been shown to improve survival in patients with heart failure and reduced ejection fraction.

### Irbesartan (Avapro)

Irbesartan blocks the vasoconstrictor and aldosterone-secreting effects of angiotensin II at tissue receptor sites. It may induce more complete inhibition of the renin-angiotensin system than ACE inhibitors, and it does not affect the response to bradykinin (less likely to be associated with cough and angioedema). Irbesartan has not been shown to improve survival in heart failure

### Azilsartan (Edarbi)

Azilsartan blocks the vasoconstrictor and aldosterone-secreting effects of angiotensin II at tissue receptor sites. It may induce more complete inhibition of the renin-angiotensin system than ACE inhibitors, and it does not affect the response to bradykinin (less likely to be associated with cough and angioedema).

### Inotropic Agents

Inotropic agents such as milrinone, digoxin, dopamine, and dobutamine are used to increase the force of cardiac contractions. Intravenous positive inotropic agents should only be used in inpatient settings—and then only in patients who manifest signs and symptoms of low cardiac output syndrome (volume overload with evidence of organ hypoperfusion).

#### *Milrinone*

Milrinone is a type 3 phosphodiesterase inhibitor that increases inotropy, chronotropy, and lusitropy, acting via cyclic guanosine monophosphate (cGMP) to increase the intramyocardial adenosine triphosphate (ATP). It is a potent vasodilator agent, being a venous and arterial vasodilator, and it is used in patients with pulmonary hypertension. Milrinone can be used in the presence of a beta-blocker. Milrinone is thought to create less tachycardia, because it does not directly stimulate beta-receptors.

#### *Digoxin (Lanoxin)*

Digoxin is a cardiac glycoside with direct inotropic effects, in addition to indirect effects, on the cardiovascular system. It acts directly on cardiac muscle, increasing myocardial systolic contractions. Indirect actions result in increased carotid sinus nerve activity and enhanced sympathetic withdrawal for any given increase in mean arterial pressure. It is used to improve symptoms associated with HF by enhancing cardiac contractility. Although digoxin does not confer a survival benefit, it has reduced the number of hospitalizations that occur as a result of worsening heart failure.

#### *Dopamine*

Dopamine is a naturally occurring catecholamine that acts as a precursor to norepinephrine. It stimulates both adrenergic and dopaminergic receptors. The hemodynamic effect is dose dependent. Low-dose use is associated with dilation within renal and splanchnic vasculature, resulting in enhanced diuresis. Moderate doses enhance cardiac contractility and the heart rate. Higher doses cause increased afterload through peripheral vasoconstriction. Administer by continuous intravenous infusion. It is usually used in severe heart failure and is reserved for patients with moderate hypotension (e.g. systolic blood pressure 70–90 mmHg). Typically, moderate or higher doses are used.

### Dobutamine

Dobutamine, a beta-receptor agonist, increases inotropy and chronotropy and decreases afterload, thereby improving end-organ perfusion. It produces vasodilation and increases the inotropic state. At higher dosages, it may cause increased heart rate, exacerbating myocardial ischemia. Careful hemodynamic and patient monitoring is required.

### Vasodilators

In addition to diuretic therapy, vasodilators are recommended as first-line therapy for patients with acute heart failure in the absence of hypotension, for relief of symptoms. Vasodilators decrease preload and/or afterload as well as reduce systemic vascular resistance (SVR).

### Nitroprusside Sodium (Nitropress)

Nitroprusside sodium is a potent balanced arterial and venous vasodilator, resulting in a very efficient decrease of intracardiac filling pressures. It requires careful hemodynamic monitoring using indwelling catheters and monitoring for cyanide toxicity, especially in the presence of renal dysfunction. It is particularly helpful for patients who present with severe pulmonary congestion in the presence of hypertension and severe mitral regurgitation. The drug should be titrated down to cessation rather than abruptly stopped, owing to the rebound potential.

### Hydralazine

Hydralazine decreases systemic resistance through direct vasodilation of arterioles. A hydralazine and nitrate combination reduces preload and afterload. Combinations of hydralazine and nitrates are recommended to improve outcomes for African Americans with moderate-to-severe symptoms of heart failure on optimal medical therapy with ACEIs/ARBs, beta-blockers, and diuretics.

### Nitrates

Nitrates improve hemodynamic effects in heart failure by decreasing left ventricular filling pressure and systemic vascular resistance. These agents also result in a slight improvement on cardiac output.

### Nitroglycerin (Nitrostat, Nitro-Dur, Nitrolingual, Nitro-Time, NitroMist, Minitran)

Nitroglycerin is first-line therapy for patients who are not hypotensive. It provides excellent and reliable preload reduction. Higher doses provide mild afterload reduction. It has rapid onset and offset (both within minutes), allowing rapid clinical effects and rapid discontinuation of effects in adverse clinical situations. It produces vasodilation and increases inotropic activity of the heart. At higher dosages, it may exacerbate myocardial ischemia by increasing the heart rate.

### Isosorbide Dinitrate (Dilatrate-SR, Isordil Titradose)

Isosorbide dinitrate relaxes vascular smooth muscle by stimulating intracellular cyclic GMP. It decreases left ventricular pressure (preload) and arterial resistance (afterload). By decreasing left ventricular pressure and dilating arteries, it reduces cardiac oxygen demand. Chronic use of isosorbide dinitrate as a sole vasodilating agent is not recommended.

### Isosorbide Dinitrate and Hydralazine

This is a fixed-dose combination of isosorbide dinitrate (20 mg/tab), a vasodilator with effects on both arteries and veins, and hydralazine (37.5 mg/tab), a predominantly arterial vasodilator. It is indicated for heart failure in black patients, based in part on results from the African American heart failure trial. Two previous trials in the general population of patients with severe heart failure found no benefit but suggested a benefit in black patients. Black patients showed a 43% reduction in mortality rate, a 39% decrease in hospitalization rate, and a decrease in symptoms from heart failure.

### Isosorbide Mononitrate (Monoket)

Isosorbide mononitrate causes relaxation of vascular smooth muscle and consequent dilatation of peripheral arteries and veins. Dilation of the veins promotes peripheral pooling of blood and decreases venous return to the heart, thereby reducing left ventricular end-diastolic pressure and pulmonary capillary wedge pressure (preload). Arteriolar relaxation reduces systemic vascular resistance, systolic arterial pressure, and mean arterial pressure (afterload).

### Other Cardiovascular Agents

Human B-type natriuretic peptides (hBNPs) such as nesiritide are used in patients with acutely decompensated heart failure. These agents reduce pulmonary capillary wedge pressure and improve dyspnea.

#### Nesiritide (Natrecor)

Nesiritide is a recombinant DNA form of hBNP that dilates veins and arteries. hBNP binds to the particulate guanylate cyclase receptor of vascular smooth muscle and endothelial cells. Binding to the receptor causes an increase in cGMP, which serves as a second messenger to dilate veins and arteries. It reduces PCWP and improves dyspnea in patients with acutely decompensated HF.

#### Diuretics, Loop

Diuretics remain the mainstay of therapy and the current standard of care for acute heart failure. First-line diuretic therapy is a loop diuretic (furosemide, bumetanide, torsemide) in the lowest effective dose, either once or twice a day, although it can be used up to 3–4 times a day, depending on the individual response and renal function. Response to diuretic therapy often depends on bioavailability of the drug (better on an empty stomach) and nutritional level (loop diuretics are bound to proteins for renal delivery).

### Furosemide (Lasix)

Furosemide increases the excretion of water by interfering with the chloride-binding cotransport system, which, in turn, inhibits sodium and chloride reabsorption in the ascending loop of Henle and distal renal tubule. The dose must be individualized to the patient. Depending on the response, administer furosemide at small dose increments (20–200 mg) until desired diuresis occurs.

### Torsemide (Demadex)

Torsemide acts from within the lumen of the thick ascending portion of the loop of Henle, where it inhibits the sodium, potassium, and chloride carrier system. It increases urinary excretion of sodium, chloride, and water, but does not significantly alter the glomerular filtration rate, renal plasma flow, or acid-base balance. Torsemide is roughly twice as potent as furosemide on a milligram basis. Depending on the response, administer furosemide at small dose increments (10–100 mg) until desired diuresis occurs.

### Bumetanide

Bumetanide increases the excretion of water by interfering with the chloride-binding cotransport system, which, in turn, inhibits sodium, potassium, and chloride reabsorption in the ascending loop of Henle. These effects increase urinary excretion of sodium, chloride, and water, resulting in profound diuresis. Renal vasodilation occurs following administration, renal vascular resistance decreases, and renal blood flow is enhanced. Bumetanide is roughly four times as potent as furosemide on a milligram basis. Depending on the response, administer bumetanide at small dose increments (0.5–5 mg) until desired diuresis occurs.

### Other Diuretics

Metolazone is a diuretic of the quinazoline class and has thiazide-like properties. This agent interferes with the renal tubular mechanism of electrolyte reabsorption.

### Metolazone (Zaroxolyn)

Metolazone increases excretion of sodium, water, potassium, and hydrogen ions by inhibiting reabsorption of sodium in the distal tubules. Metolazone may be more effective in patients with impaired renal function.

### Diuretics, Potassium-Sparing

The potassium-sparing diuretics interfere with sodium reabsorption at the distal tubules, resulting in decreased potassium secretion. These agents have a weak diuretic and antihypertensive effect when used alone. The potassium-sparing diuretics spironolactone or triamterene are usually used in addition to the loop diuretics. Note that careful monitoring of renal function and potassium is necessary for all diuretics.

### Spironolactone (Aldactone)

Spironolactone is used for the management of edema resulting from excessive aldosterone excretion. It competes with aldosterone for receptor sites in the distal renal tubules, increasing water excretion while retaining potassium and hydrogen ions. Spironolactone at a target dose of 25 mg has been shown to improve survival in patients with heart failure and reduced ejection fraction.

### Amiloride (Midamor)

Amiloride is unrelated chemically to other known antikaliuretic or diuretic agents. It is a potassium-conserving (antikaliuretic) drug that, compared with thiazide diuretics, possesses weak natriuretic, diuretic, and antihypertensive activity.

### Triamterene (Dyrenium)

Triamterene is a potassium-sparing diuretic with relatively weak natriuretic properties. It exerts its diuretic effect on the distal renal tubules by inhibiting the reabsorption of sodium in exchange for potassium and hydrogen. It increases sodium excretion and reduces excessive loss of potassium and hydrogen associated with hydrochlorothiazide.

### Alpha/Beta-adrenergic Agonists

In the presence of significant hypotension, adrenergic agonists are used to improve cardiac output and organ perfusion.

### Epinephrine (Adrenaclick, Adrenalin, EpiPen, EpiPen Jr.)

Epinephrine is an alpha-agonist and its effects include increased peripheral vascular resistance, reversed peripheral vasodilatation, systemic hypotension, and vascular permeability. Beta2-agonist effects include bronchodilatation, chronotropic cardiac activity, and positive inotropic effects.

### Norepinephrine (Levophed)

Norepinephrine is a naturally occurring catecholamine with potent alpha-receptor and mild beta-receptor activity. It stimulates beta1-and alpha-adrenergic receptors, resulting in increased cardiac muscle contractility, heart rate, and vasoconstriction. It increases blood pressure and afterload. Increased afterload may result in decreased cardiac output, increased myocardial oxygen demand, and cardiac ischemia. It is generally reserved for use in patients with severe hypotension (e.g. systolic blood pressure $<70$ mmHg) or hypotension that is unresponsive to other medications.

### Aldosterone Antagonists, Selective

Aldosterone antagonists are weak diuretics that reduce mortality and the risk of sudden death by blocking the effects of aldosterone, thereby decreasing myocardial and vascular inflammation and collagen production. This, in turn, prevents apoptosis, decreases stimulation of the renin-angiotensin-aldosterone system (RAAS) and sympathetic nervous system (SNS), and acts as a membrane stabilizer, thus preventing arrhythmia. Aldosterone antagonists are recommended for patients who have moderately severe and severe heart failure and reduced left ventricular (LV) systolic function [randomized aldactone evaluation study (RALES)] who can be carefully monitored for preserved renal function and normal potassium concentration.

### Eplerenone (Inspra)

Eplerenone selectively blocks aldosterone at the mineralocorticoid receptors in epithelial (e.g. kidney) and non-epithelial (e.g. heart, blood vessels, and brain) tissues; thus, it decreases blood pressure and sodium reabsorption. It is indicated to improve survival for heart failure or left LV dysfunction following acute MI. Compared with placebo, a significant risk reduction (15%) has been observed. The EMPHASIS-HF trial has shown that patients with systolic heart failure with mild symptoms treated with eplerenone have a significant reduction in cardiovascular death or heart failure hospitalization when compared with placebo.

### Anticoagulants, Cardiovascular

Patients with heart failure and depressed left ventricular (LV) ejection fraction are thought to have an increased risk of thrombus formation due to low cardiac output. Hospitalized patients with heart failure are at a high risk for venous thromboembolism and should receive prophylaxis. Anticoagulation with an international normalized ratio (INR) goal of 2–3 is indicated in the presence of: (1) an LV thrombus, (2) a thromboembolic event with or without evidence of an LV thrombus, and (3) paroxysmal or chronic atrial arrhythmias.

### Warfarin (Coumadin, Jantoven)

Warfarin interferes with hepatic vitamin K-dependent carboxylation. It is used for the prophylaxis and treatment of thromboembolic disorders.

### Dabigatran (Pradaxa)

Competitive, direct thrombin inhibitor. Thrombin enables fibrinogen conversion to fibrin during the coagulation cascade, thereby preventing thrombus development. Inhibits both free and clot-bound thrombin and thrombin-induced platelet aggregation.

### Calcium Channel Blockers

Generally, calcium channel blockers (CCBs) should be avoided. CCBs do not play a direct role in the management of heart failure; however, these agents may be used to treat other conditions, such as hypertension or angina in heart failure patients.

CCBs may be used in heart failure with normal left ventricular ejection fraction. These drugs may also improve exercise tolerance via their vasodilatory properties.

### Amlodipine (Norvasc)

Amlodipine has antianginal and antihypertensive effects. It blocks the postexcitation release of calcium ions into cardiac and vascular smooth muscle, thereby inhibiting the activation of ATPase on myofibril contraction. The overall effect is reduced intracellular calcium levels in cardiac and smooth muscle cells of the coronary and peripheral vasculature, resulting in dilatation of the coronary and peripheral arteries. It also increases myocardial oxygen delivery in patients with vasospastic angina.

### Nifedipine (Adalat CC, Afeditab CR, Nifediac CC, Nifedical XL, Procardia, Procardia XL)

Nifedipine relaxes coronary smooth muscle and produces coronary vasodilation, which in turn, improves myocardial oxygen delivery. Sublingual administration is generally safe, despite theoretical concerns.

### Felodipine

Felodipine is a dihydropyridine calcium channel blocker. It inhibits the influx of extracellular calcium across the myocardial and vascular smooth muscle cell membranes. The resultant decrease in intracellular calcium inhibits the contractile processes of the smooth muscle cells, resulting in dilation of coronary and systemic arteries.

### Opioid Analgesics

Opioid analgesics such as morphine sulfate may help to relieve patients' anxiety, distress, and dyspnea.

#### *Morphine Sulfate*

Morphine is the drug of choice for narcotic analgesia because of its reliable and predictable effects, safety profile, and ease of reversibility with naloxone. Morphine sulfate administered intravenously may be dosed in a number of ways and commonly is titrated until the desired effect is obtained. Morphine sulfate also decreases preload in heart failure and relieves dyspnea.

#### *Cytokine Antagonists*

The current interest in understanding the role tissue necrotizing factor alpha in heart failure, relates to the observation that many aspects of the syndrome of heart failure can be explained by the known biologic effects of this cytokine. When expressed at sufficiently high concentration, tumor necrosis factor alpha mimics some aspects of the so called heart failure phenotype, including (but not limited to) progressive left ventricular dysfunction, pulmonary edema, left ventricle remodeling, fetal gene expression, and cardiomyopathy. Elevated levels of tumor necrosis factor alpha and other inflammatory cytokines have been associated with heart failure in children with congenital heart disease. Trials with etanercept, a soluble recombinantly produced chimeric tumor necrosis factor alpha antagonist and infliximab, a monoclonal antibody against tumor necrosis factor alpha are underway for treatment of heart failure in adults.

### Coenzyme Q 10

Although coenzyme Q 10 (2, 3-dimethoxy-5-methyl-6-decaprenyl-1, 4-benzoquinone) has theoretical benefits to improve the energetics in failing myocardium by helping as an electron carrier in production of adenosine tri-phosphate, an antioxidant and free radical scavenger with membrane stabilizing properties, no beneficial effects of Coenzyme Q 10 supplementation on the left ventricular ejection fraction, peak oxygen consumption, or exercise duration are found by Khatta and co-workers. Therefore, Coenzyme Q 10 is not recommended at this time until large scale clinical trials have been performed.

### Metabolic Therapy

The heart is able to utilize a variety of substrates for energy generation, including carbohydrates (glucose and lactate), lipids (free fatty acids and triglycerides), and ketones. This allows a normal heart to maintain its functional performance in a wide range of physiological conditions without experiencing an energy debt. However, an energy deficit has been observed during the develop an energy deficit has been observed during the development of heart failure that directly relates to patient prognosis. Long-term follow-up studies in patients with idiopathic dilated cardiomyopathy demonstrate that decreased phospho-creatinine (which is the source of instant adenosine tri-phosphate) is an independent predictor of mortality, suggesting that impaired myocardial energetics play an active role in the progression of heart failure. This notion is further supported by consistent observations in clinical trials revealing that energy-costly treatment, such as positive inotropic agents (beta-receptor mimetic drugs, phosphodiesterase inhibitors) increase mortality, while energy-sparing treatments (e.g. angiotensin converting enzyme inhibitors, angiotensin II blockers, or beta-blockers) reduce mortality.

Carbohydrates are the primary substrates for fetal hearts, while fatty acids become the predominant fuel in adult hearts, supporting more than two-thirds of the total adenosine tri-phosphate synthesized. An important change in energy metabolism is observed in hypertrophied and failing heart; increasing reliance on carbohydrates while decreasing fatty acid utilization, an apparent reoccurrence of the fetal metabolic profile. Studies using animal model of heart failure reveal that this shift of substrate preference is associated with the down regulation of peroxisome proliferator-activated receptor alpha, a transcriptor factor controlling the expres.

### Prognosis in Heart Failure

Prognosis is poor on the whole, with approximately 50% of people with heart failure dying within four years of diagnosis. The mortality rate in the UK appears to be improving. A UK study found that the 6-month mortality rate for people with heart failure had improved from 26% in 1995 to 14% in 2005. The prognosis for people with heart failure and preserved left ventricular ejection fraction is a little better than the prognosis for people with heart failure and reduced ejection fraction (Table 8.16).

## MANAGEMENT OF RIGHT VENTRICULAR FAILURE

Right ventricular (RV) failure occurs when the RV fails to maintain enough blood flow through the pulmonary circulation to achieve adequate left ventricular filling (Figs 8.81–8.87). This can occur suddenly in a previously healthy heart due to massive pulmonary embolism or right-sided myocardial infarction, but many cases encountered in the intensive care unit involve worsening of compensated RV failure in the setting of chronic heart and lung disease. Management of RV failure is directed at optimizing right-sided filling pressures and reducing afterload. Due to a lower level of vascular tone, vasoactive medications have

**Table 8.16:** Prognostic indicators and potential targets of therapy in AHFS

| | |
|---|---|
| SBP | Admission and early postdischarge SBP inversely correlates with postdischarge mortality. The higher the BP, the lower both in-hospital and postdischarge mortality. However, the readmission rate of approximately 30% is independent of the SBP at time of admission |
| CAD | Extent and severity of CAD appears to be a predictor of poor prognosis |
| Troponin release | Results in a 3-fold increase in in-hospital mortality, a 2-fold increase in postdischarge mortality, and a 3-fold increase in the rehospitalization rate |
| Ventricular dyssynchrony | Increase in QRS duration occurs in approximately 40% of patients with reduced systolic function and is a strong predictor of early and late postdischarge mortality and rehospitalization |
| Renal impairment | Associated with a 2- to 3-fold increase in post-discharge mortality. Worsening renal function during hospitalization or soon after discharge is also associated with an increase in in-hospital and postdischarge mortality |
| Hyponatremia | Defined as serum sodium <135 mmol/L, occurs in approximately 25% of patients, and is associated with a 2- to 3-fold increase in postdischarge mortality |
| Clinical congestion at time of discharge | An important predictor of postdischarge mortality and morbidity. EF Similar early postdischarge event rates and mortality between reduced and preserved EF |
| BNP/NT-proBNP | Elevated natriuretic peptides associated with increased resource utilization and mortality |
| Functional capacity at time of discharge | Predischarge functional capacity, defined by the 6-min walk test, is emerging as an important predictor of postdischarge outcomes. |

Adapted and modified, with permission, from Gheorghiade et al. CAD=coronary artery disease.

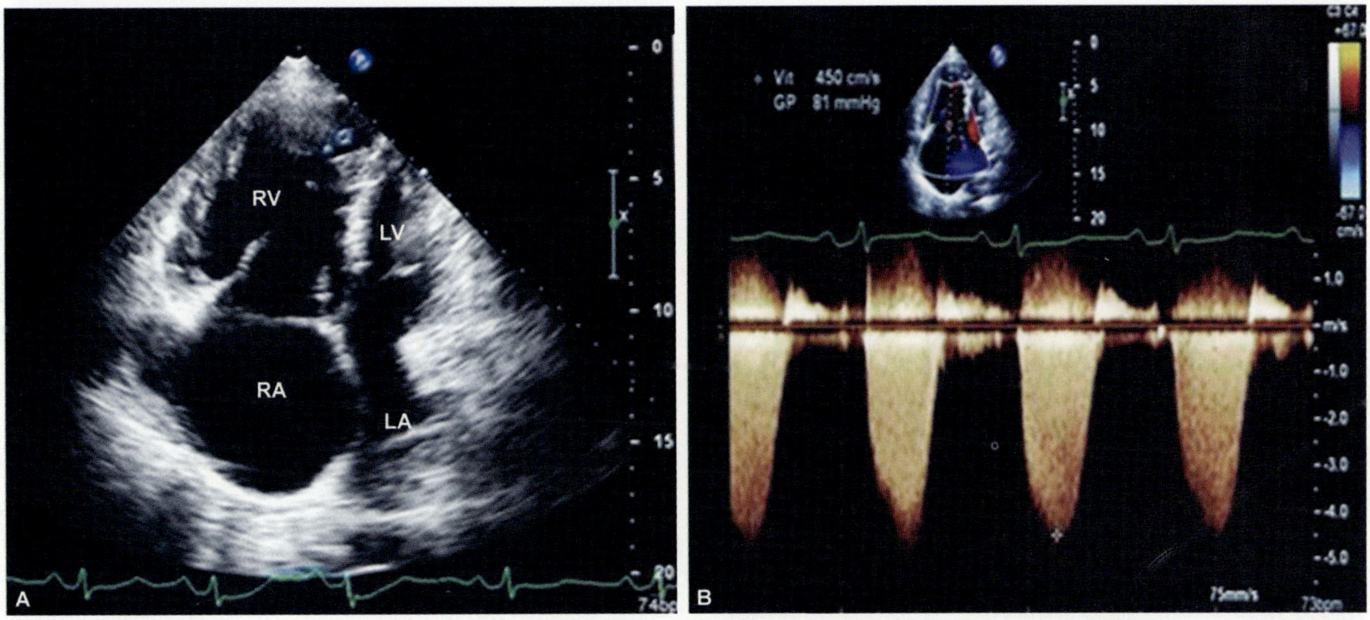


**Fig. 8.81:** Right ventricular failure. (A) Apical 4-chamber view showing gross dilatation of RA and RV. (B) Color Doppler view at tricuspid valve showing gross tricuspid regurgitation with gradient of more than 100 mmHg in a patient with primary pulmonary hypertension with CCR

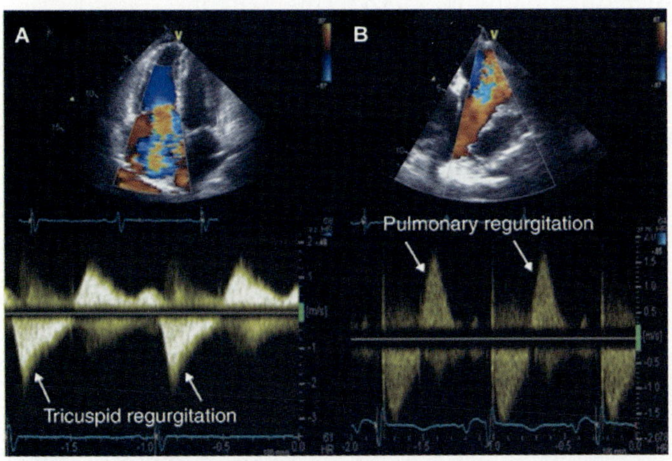


**Fig. 8.82:** Transthoracic echocardiography: Severe tricuspid (A) and pulmonary (B) regurgitation, shown by Color Doppler (top) and continuous wave Doppler (bottom)

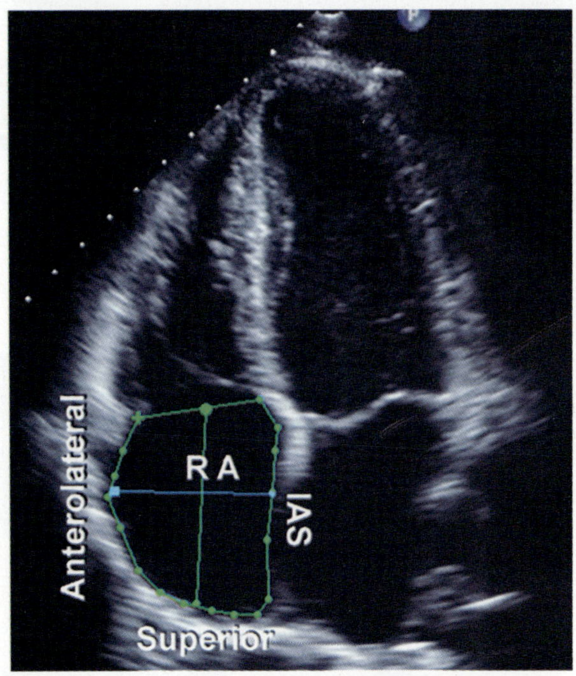


**Fig. 8.83:** Tracing of the right atrium (RA) is performed from the plane of the tricuspid annulus (TA), along the interatrial septum (IAS), superior and anterolateral walls of the RA. The right atrial major dimension is represented by the green line from the TA center to the superior right atrial wall, and the right atrial minor dimension is represented by the blue line from the anterolateral wall to the IAS

less salient effects on reducing vascular resistance in the pulmonary than in the systemic circulation. Successful management requires reversal of any conditions that heighten pulmonary vascular tone and the use of selective pulmonary vasodilators at doses that do not induce systemic hypotension or worsening of oxygenation. Systemic systolic arterial pressure should be kept close to RV systolic pressure to maintain RV perfusion. When these efforts fail, the judicious use of inotropic agents may help improve RV contractility enough to maintain cardiac output. Extracorporeal life support is increasingly being used to support patients with acute RV failure who fail to respond to medical management while the underlying cause of their RV failure is addressed.

Current therapies directed toward pulmonary vasoconstriction, cellular proliferation, and thrombotic factors have improved the quality of life and survival in many patients with severe pulmonary arterial hypertension.

Likewise, therapies with afterload-reducing agents, β-receptor antagonists, inotropes, and diuretics have improved the functional status and prognosis of patients with left ventricular failure. Moreover, acute responsiveness to pulmonary vasodilators is associated with a better prognosis and survival in patients with advanced heart failure. Afterload reduction, however, cannot be achieved in many cases, but the increased right ventricular wall thickness and reversal of a fetal gene expression program have not yet been investigated as potential targeted treatments. Chronic intravenous epoprostenol infusion therapy in patients with pulmonary arterial hypertension appears to improve right ventricular function (although dilation and hypertrophy may not reverse over a 1-year period of observation, and the effects of the endothelin receptor antagonist bosentan on echocardiographic right ventricular parameters have also suggested a similar improvement in right ventricular function. However, the specific myocardial effects of these or other therapies for pulmonary arterial hypertension remain incompletely understood. In addition, right ventricular function, right ventricular–left ventricular interaction, and right ventricular–pulmonary arterial coupling have largely been overlooked as potential targets for investigation or therapy.

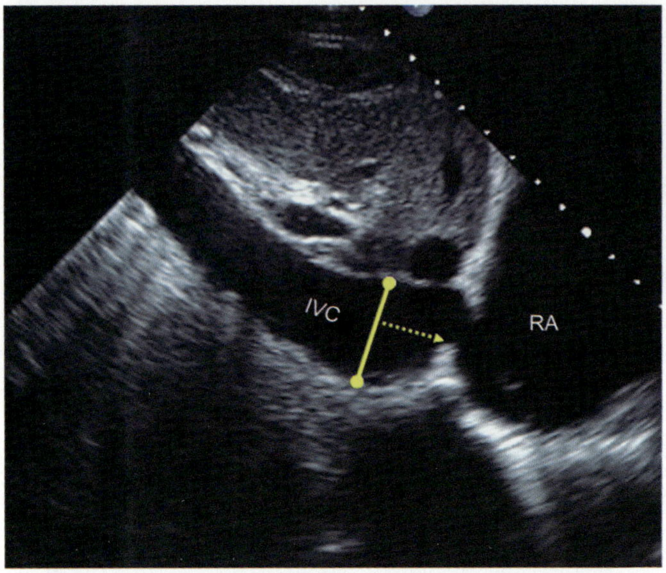


**Fig. 8.84:** Inferior vena cava (IVC) view. Measurement of the IVC. The diameter (solid line) is measured perpendicular to the long axis of the IVC at end-expiration, just proximal to the junction of the hepatic veins that lie approximately 0.5–3.0 cm proximal to the ostium of the right atrium (RA)

Continuous intravenous prostacyclin (epoprostenol) infusion therapy improves survival in idiopathic pulmonary arterial hypertension patients more than in patients with the limited variant of scleroderma-associated pulmonary arterial hypertension. Although the reasons for this discrepancy in treatment outcome are not clear, one possible explanation is the presence of a myocardial global microangiopathy in scleroderma patients.

## Diagnosis and Treatment of Right Ventricular Heart Failure

Management of right ventricular (RV) failure includes treatment of the underlying cause; optimization of preload, afterload, and RV contractility; maintenance of sinus rhythm; and atrioventricular synchrony. Hypotension should be avoided, as it can potentially lead to further RV ischemia.

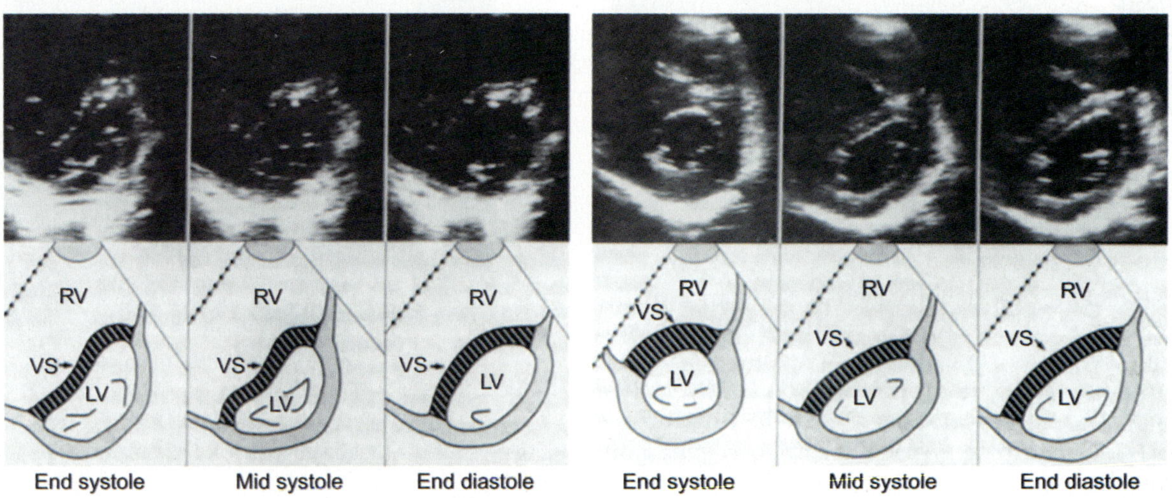


**Fig. 8.85:** Serial stop-frame short-axis two-dimensional echocardiographic images of the left ventricle at the mitral chordal level with diagrams from a patient with isolated right ventricular (RV) pressure overload due to primary pulmonary hypertension (left) and from a patient with isolated RV volume overload due to tricuspid valve resection (right). Whereas the left ventricular (LV) cavity maintains a circular profile throughout the cardiac cycle in normal subjects, in RV pressure overload there is leftward ventricular septal (VS) shift and reversal of septal curvature present throughout the cardiac cycle with most marked distortion of the left ventricle at end-systole. In the patient with RV volume overload, the septal shift and flattening of VS curvature occurs predominantly in mid to late diastole with relative sparing of LV deformation at end-systole *(reproduced with permission from J Am Coll Cardiol)*

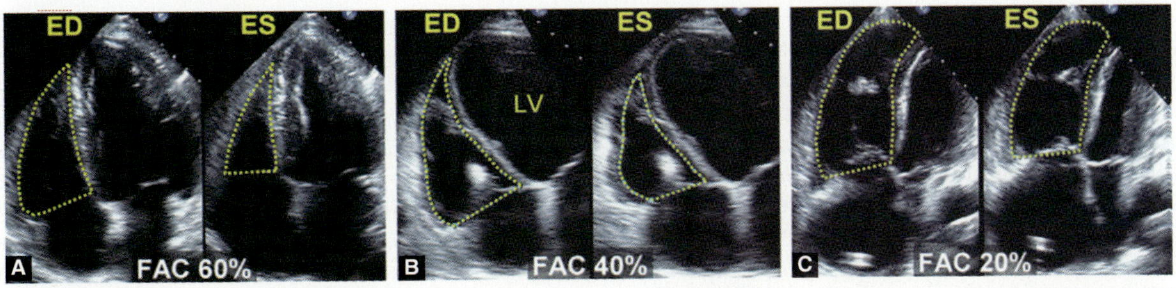


**Fig. 8.86:** Examples of right ventricular fractional area change (FAC). Percentage FAC = 100 end-diastolic area (area ED) endsystolic area (area ES)/end-diastolic area. The endocardial border is traced in apical four-chamber (A4C) views from the tricuspid annulus along the free wall to the apex, then back to the annulus, along the interventricular septum at end-diastole (ED) and end-systole (ES). Trabeculation, tricuspid leaflets, and chords are included in the chamber. (A) Normal subject, FAC 60%. (B) Moderately dilated right ventricle (RV), FAC 40%, and a markedly dilated left ventricle (LV). (C) Dilated RV, FAC 20%, and the LV is foreshortened as a result of optimizing the view for the right ventricular chamber

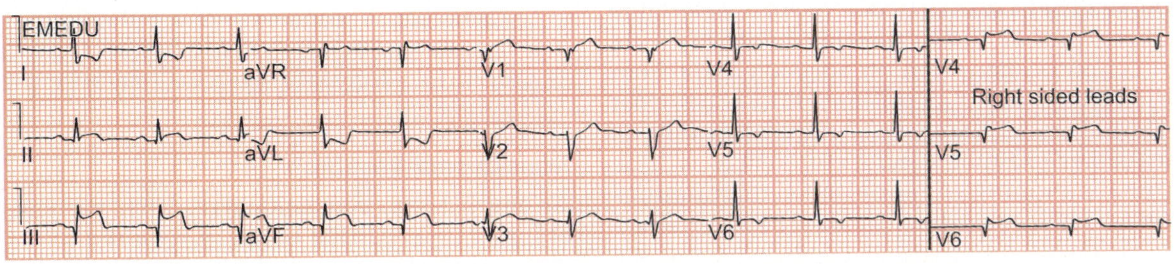


**Fig. 8.87:** ECG trace showing ST-elevation in leads II, III, AVF and V4–V6 in right sided precordial leads in acute right ventricular infarction

### Assessment of Right Ventricular Functions

Although a fair amount of study has been devoted to assessment of right ventricular function, there remains a need to understand how to better define normal parameters of right ventricular function. Critical information is required to determine the most sensitive and specific variables to describe abnormal right ventricular function. It is likely that the definition of function will include parameters of geometry, ejection volume, hypertrophy, dilation, contraction, and oxygen supply to the ventricular wall. A clear picture of these parameters would help in determining which measurements are the best predictors of early right ventricular failure (such as right ventricular wall thickness, muscle perfusion, or metabolic activity). Ideally, a combination of approaches would be used to evaluate right heart function, including imaging techniques (Doppler echocardiography, computed tomography, magnetic resonance imaging, positron emission tomography), implanted continuous monitoring devices, and electrophysiology. Collaboration with the National Institute of Biomedical Imaging and Bioengineering to promote the development of imaging methods to study right ventricular function and dysfunction should be encouraged.

### Distinguishing Characteristics of Right Heart Compared with Left Heart

Preliminary inquiry suggests that there are distinctions between the ventricles that need to be further evaluated and clarified to understand the differences, similarities, and interplay between the left and right heart. This issue can be addressed with chamber-specific studies in animal models that examine changes in gene expression, protein synthesis, histology, and geometry during development, injury, and stress (exercise and disease).

### Investigation of Mechanism and Role of Hypertrophy

Although initial right ventricular hypertrophy in response to pressure overload may be adaptive, it is also the seemingly initial step in a remodeling process that is ultimately damaging, perhaps irreversibly so. Attention should be devoted to determining whether right ventricular hypertrophy is good or bad. Research is needed to compare hypertrophy seen in athletes with that seen in patients with diseases such as pulmonary arterial hypertension. Mechanisms of right ventricular hypertrophy and remodeling need to be determined.

### Effect of Pulmonary Disease on Right Ventricular Function

Few studies address the interaction of right ventricular and pulmonary function. Research is needed to study the complex interaction of the heart and lungs and how changes in one affect the other. Examples of changes include inflammation, stress due to hypoxia or exercise, autoimmune reactions, infarction, and hypertension.

### Models of Right Ventricular Failure

Researchers must develop reliable, reproducible, and relevant animal models of right ventricular failure. Animal models would be particularly useful in determining factors that initiate right ventricular dysfunction. Models would also help to identify biomarkers and changes in gene expression and protein synthesis associated with right ventricular failure. Valuable information could be obtained from animal models through side-by-side comparisons of changes in the left and right ventricles. Parameters on which to focus would include tissue analysis; gene and protein expression; and markers of oxidative stress, apoptosis, and cell growth. When possible, such analyses should compare tissue from patients with animal models of right heart failure and pulmonary hypertension to address the question of whether data obtained from manipulated animal right ventricles can be extrapolated to right ventricular or interventricular septal biopsy material from the hearts of patients with severe pulmonary hypertension. Animal models will be a necessary component to determine whether right ventricle failure is associated with myocyte apoptosis or cytokine expression. In addition, data from animal studies suggest that significant differences exist between sexes in the development of right heart failure. Studies that further examine gender differences will be important for developing potential new therapeutics and determining whether treatment should be determined by sex.

General measures of treatment should be applied, as follows:

- Sodium and fluid restriction
- Moderate physical activity, with avoidance of isometric exercises
- Avoidance of pregnancy
- Compliance with medications

Avoidance, or rapid treatment of precipitating factors such as:

- Sleep apnea
- Pulmonary embolism
- Sepsis
- Arrhythmia
- Ischemia
- High altitude
- Anemia
- Hypoxemia
- Use of an ACEI/ARB is beneficial if RV failure is secondary to LV failure; the efficacy of these agents in isolated RV failure is not known. The same recommendation applies for use of beta-blockers. The role of nesiritide in RV failure is not well defined. Use of digoxin in RV failure associated with chronic obstructive pulmonary disease (COPD) not associated with LV dysfunction appears not to improve exercise tolerance or RV ejection fraction. Treatment of pulmonary-induced RV failure is to address the correction of a primary pulmonary aetiology and a decrease in RV afterload via specific pulmonary artery vasodilatory therapies.
- In patients with severe, hemodynamically compromising RV failure, inotropic therapy is administered, using dobutamine (2–5 mcg/kg/min), dobutamine and inhaled nitric oxide, or dopamine alone. Milrinone is preferred if the patient is tachycardic or on beta-blockers.
- Anticoagulation indications are standard for evidence of intracardiac thrombus, thromboembolic events, pulmonary arterial hypertension, paroxysmal or persistent atrial fibrillation/flutter, and mechanical right-sided valves. Hypoxemia should be corrected, and positive pressure should be avoided when mechanical ventilation is needed.
- Atrial septostomy can be considered as a palliative measure in patients with severe symptoms in whom standard therapy has failed. RV mechanical assist device is indicated only for RV failure secondary to LV failure or postcardiac transplantation.
- The prognosis in patients with RV failure depends on the aetiology. Volume overload, pulmonary stenosis, and Eisenmenger syndrome are associated with a better prognosis. Decreased exercise tolerance predicts poor survival.

### Translational Research

An emphasis on translational research, particularly studies of human myocardial tissue, is required to determine the important markers of right ventricular function and dysfunction. Studies to identify markers in plasma as well as those in tissue might facilitate prediction of early diagnosis of ventricular dysfunction and may prevent failure. Robust parameters that predict outcome for patients with right heart failure are needed.

### Right Ventricular Morphogenesis

The developmental aspects of right heart formation need to be studied to identify mechanisms involved in congenital heart disease and related pulmonary vascular disease.

### Targeted Therapy

The development of new therapeutic strategies for right heart failure should be promoted. These new strategies might include cell-based or gene therapy, new drugs, or new combinations of existing drugs.

### Awareness

Awareness should be promoted in the pulmonary and cardiology research communities about the lack of knowledge of the right ventricle with well-publicized requests for research proposals. New and established investigators should be encouraged to enter this fruitful area of research. The consensus of the working group is that the role of the right ventricle in a spectrum of cardiovascular diseases has been relatively neglected proportionate to its central importance. Advancing knowledge through research about the unique genetic, molecular, cellular, and functional characteristics of the right ventricle and their vulnerability to disease will lead to progress in the treatment of cardiomyopathy, pulmonary arterial hypertension, right ventricular ischemic syndromes, and valvular heart disease. The success in such effort requires collaborations between and among clinical and basic investigators from various disciplines, including those in respiratory/pulmonary and cardiovascular fields as well from neuroscientists, immunologists, endocrinologists, and biomedical engineers. Joint meetings of the American Heart Association and the American Thoracic Society would be appropriate venues to promote the importance of understanding the right ventricle and would help to accelerate the gathering of information leading to better treatment and preventative means to reduce morbidity and mortality associated with right heart failure and left heart failure.

### Future Directions

Given the pivotal involvement of the right ventricle in both common and rare cardiovascular diseases and the paucity of basic knowledge at all levels about its normal and pathological functions, support for further research should be a high priority for investigators and National Institutes of Health Funding. Areas of deficient understanding worthy of further exploration include the following issues.

## KEY POINTS IN HEART FAILURE

- Patients with severe acute decompensated HF (ADHF) are best managed in hospital; those with mild decompensation or chronic compensated HF are often managed as outpatients by their GPs.
- Heart failure (HF) should be considered in all older patients presenting with a new wheeze.
- Understand the importance of new onset or exacerbation of HF as a risk factor for perioperative complications, especially in the elderly.
- Use the history and physical exam to stratify the patient's risk for cardiac complications of surgery, employing one of the available risk indices. Recognize that most patients with HF will be at high risk.
- Determine if the patient has 'decompensated' HF, which is present if the patient has NYHA Class III or IV symptoms or evidence of HF on physical exam or chest X-ray. If decompensated HF is present, postpone elective surgery in order to optimize management.
- Recognize the importance of the risk associated with the surgery itself, and with various forms of anesthesia.
- Obtain the following laboratory studies:
    - ECG
    - BUN and creatinine levels
    - Results of previous cardiovascular studies (echocardiogram, stress test, catheterization data)
    - Obtain an echocardiogram for patients with a history of HF and changes in symptoms to assess ventricular function/ejection fraction and structural/valvular abnormalities.

*Contd...*

*Contd...*

- Optimize the patient's medical regimen for HF and other cardiac disease before surgery.
- Consider preoperative transfusion if the patient's baseline hematocrit level is <8 mg/dl and extensive surgery or major blood loss is anticipated.
- Consider reducing or holding ACE inhibitors and/or diuretics on the day of elective surgery depending on the patient's clinical status and proposed surgery.
- Continue beta-blockers perioperatively in patients receiving them chronically.
- Use adequate pain management to reduce the risk for postoperative cardiac complications.
- Resume the patient's usual medications as soon as possible after surgery.

## BIBLIOGRAPHY

1. American Heart Association. Classes of heart failure. Hunt SA, Abraham WT, Chin MH, et al. and the American College of Cardiology Foundation; American Heart Association. 2009 Focused update incorporated into the ACC/AHA 2005 guidelines for the diagnosis and management of heart failure in adults: a report of the American College of Cardiology Foundation/American Heart Association Task Force on practice guidelines developed in collaboration with the International Society for Heart and Lung Transplantation. J Am Coll Cardiol 2009;53(15).
2. Anversa P, Nadal-Ginard B. Myocyte renewal and ventri-cular remodelling. Nature 2002;415(6868):240–3.
3. Braunwald E, Ross J Jr, Sonnenblick EH (2nd edn). Mechanisms of Contraction of the Normal and Failing Heart. Boston: Little Brown & Co; 1976:417.
4. Braunwald E. The pathogenesis of heart failure: Then and now. Medicine 1991;70:68.
5. Bursi F, McNallan SM, Redfield MM, et al. Pulmonary pressures and death in heart failure a community study. J Am Coll Cardiol 2012;59(3):222–31.
6. Cardiovascular Diseases. Dean T. Jamison, Richard G. Feachem, Eduard R. Bos, Malegapuru W. Makgoba, Florence K. Baingana, Karen J. Hofman, Kahma O. Rogo. Disease and mortality in Sub-Saharan Africa. 2. Washington D.C: World Bank Publications. 2006:21.
7. Chen J, Normand SL, Wang Y, Krumholz HM. National and regional trends in heart failure hospitalization and mortality rates for Medicare beneficiaries, 1998–2008. JAMA 2011; 306(15):1669–78.
8. Clifford R Greyson, MD. Pathophysiology of right ventri-cular failure. Crit Care Med 2008;36(Suppl):S57–65.
9. Cody RJ. Hormonal alterations in heart failure. In: Hosenpud JB, Greenberg BH (Eds). Congestive Heart Failure: Pathophysiology, Diagnosis and Comprehensive Approach to Management. Philadelphia: Lippincott Williams & Wilkins; 2000:199–212.
10. Cohn JN. Structural basis for heart failure. Ventricular remodeling and its pharmacological inhibition. Circulation 1995;91(10):2504–7.

11. Damasceno A, Cotter G, Dzudie A, Sliwa K, Mayosi BM. Heart failure in sub-saharan Africa: time for action. J Am Coll Cardiol 2007;50(17):1688–93 [Medline].
12. Dewalt DA, Schillinger D, Ruo B, Bibbins-Domingo K, Baker DW, Holmes GM, et al. A Multisite Randomized Trial of a Single-versus Multi-Session Literacy Sensitive Self-Care Intervention for Patients with Heart Failure. Circulation 2012;[Medline].
13. Dickstein K, Cohen-Solal A, Filippatos G, et al. For the Task Force for the Diagnosis and Treatment of Acute and Chronic Heart Failure 2008 of the European Society of Cardiology. ESC Guidelines for the diagnosis and treatment of acute and chronic heart failure 2008: the Task Force for the Diagnosis and Treatment of Acute and Chronic Heart Failure 2008 of the European Society of Cardiology. Developed in collabo-ration with the Heart Failure Association of the ESC (HFA) and endorsed by the European Society of Intensive Care Medicine (ESICM). Eur Heart J 2008;29(19):2388–442.
14. Dries DL, Exner DV, Domanski MJ, Greenberg B, Stevenson LW. The prognostic implications of renal insufficiency in asymptomatic and symptomatic patients with left ventricular systolic dysfunction. J Am Coll Cardiol 2000;35(3):681–9.
15. Dunlay SM, Eveleth JM, Shah ND, McNallan SM, Roger VL. Medication adherence among community-dwelling patients with heart failure. Mayo Clin Proc 2011;86(4):273–81. [Medline] [Full Text].
16. Feldman AM, Combes A, Wagner D, et al. The role of tumor necrosis factor in the patho-physiology of heart failure. J Am Coll Cardiol 2000; 35(3):537–44.
17. Fonarow GC, Adams KF Jr, Abraham WT, Yancy CW, Boscardin WJ. Risk stratification for in-hospital mortality in acutely decompensated heart failure: classification and regression tree analysis. JAMA 2005;293(5):572–80.
18. Fonarow GC. Epidemiology and risk stratification in acute heart failure. Am Heart J 2008;155(2):200–7.
19. Gheorghiade M, Pang PS. Acute heart failure syndromes. J Am Coll Cardiol 2009;53(7):557–73.
20. Gottlieb SS, Khatta M, Friedmann E, Einbinder L, Katzen S, Baker B, et al. The influence of age, gender, and race on the prevalence of depression in heart failure patients. J Am Coll Cardiol 2004;43(9):1542–9.
21. Haddad F, Doyle R, Murphy DJ, Hunt SA. Right ventricular function in cardiovascular disease, part II: pathophysiology, clinical importance, and management of right ventricular failure. Circulation 2008;117(13):1717–31.
22. Halley CM, Houghtaling PL, et al. Mortality rate in patients with diastolic dysfunction and normal systolic function. Arch Intern Med 2011; 171(12):1082–7 [Medline].
23. He J, Ogden LG, Bazzano LA, et al. Risk factors for congestive heart failure in US men and women: NHANES I epidemio-logic follow-up study. Arch Intern Med 2001;161(7):996–1002 [Medline].
24. Ho JE, Liu C, Lyass A, Courchesne P, Pencina MJ, Vasan RS, et al. Galectin-3, a marker of cardiac fibrosis, predicts incident heart failure in the community. J Am Coll Cardiol 2012; 60(14):1249–56 [Medline].
25. Ho KK, Anderson KM, Kannel WB, Grossman W, Levy D. Survival after the onset of congestive heart failure in Framingham Heart Study subjects. Circulation 1993;88(1): 107–15 [Medline].
26. Hunt SA. For the Task Force on Practice Guidelines (Writing Committee to Update the 2001 Guidelines for the Evaluation and Management of Heart Failure). ACC/AHA 2005 guide-line update for the diagnosis and management of chronic heart failure in the adult: a report of the American College of Cardiology/American Heart Association Task Force on Practice Guidelines. J Am Coll Cardiol 20 2005; 46(6):e1–82.
27. Jencks SF, Williams MV, Coleman EA. Rehospitalizations among patients in the Medicare fee-for-service program. N Engl J Med 2009;360(14):1418–28.
28. Kajstura J, Leri A, Castaldo C, Nadal-Ginard B, Anversa P. Myocyte growth in the failing heart. Surg Clin North Am 2004;84(1):161–77
29. Kajstura J, Leri A, Finato N, Di Loreto C, Beltrami CA, Anversa P. Myocyte proliferation in end-stage cardiac failure in humans. Proc Natl Acad Sci USA 1998;95(15):8801–5.
30. Ketchum ES, Levy WC. Establishing prognosis in heart failure: a multimarker approach. Prog Cardiovasc Dis 2011; 54(2):86–96.
31. Lam CS, Lyass A, Kraigher-Krainer E, et al. Cardiac dysfunc-tion and noncardiac dysfunction as precursors of heart failure with reduced and preserved ejection fraction in the community. Circulation 2011;124(1):24–30.
32. Leri A, Claudio PP, Li Q, Wang X, Reiss K, Wang S, et al. Stretch-mediated release of angiotensin II induces myocyte apoptosis by activating p53 that enhances the local renin-angiotensin system and decreases the Bcl-2-to-Bax protein ratio in the cell. J Clin Invest 1998;101(7):1326–42.
33. Levy D, Kenchaiah S, Larson MG, et al. Long-term trends in the incidence of and sur-vival with heart failure. N Engl J Med 2002;347(18): 1397–402.
34. Lindenfeld J, Albert NM, Boehmer JP, et al. for the Heart Failure Society of America. Executive summary: HFSA 2010 comprehensive heart failure practice guideline. J Card Fail 2010;16(6):e1–194
35. Lindenfeld J, Albert NM, Boehmer JP, et al. HFSA 2010 Comprehensive Heart Failure Practice Guideline. J Card Fail 2010;16(6):e1–194. [Medline].
36. Lloyd-Jones D, Adams RJ, Brown TM, et al. Executive summary: heart disease and stroke statistics—2010 update: a report from the American Heart Association. Circulation 2010;121(7):948–54.
37. Lucas C, Johnson W, Hamilton MA, et al. Freedom from congestion predicts good survival despite previous class IV symptoms of heart failure. Am Heart J 2000;140(6):840–7.
38. MacIntyre K, Capewell S, Stewart S, et al. Evidence of improving prognosis in heart failure: trends in case fatality in 66 547 patients hospitalized between 1986 and 1995. Circulation 2000;102(10):1126–31.
39. Masoudi FA, Havranek EP, Smith G, et al. Gender, age, and heart failure with preserved left ventricular systolic function. J Am Coll Cardiol 2003; 41(2):217–23.
40. Morris DA, Gailani M, Vaz Perez A, et al. Right ventricular myocardial systolic and diastolic dysfunction in heart failure with normal left ventricular ejection fraction. J Am Soc Echocardiogr 2011;24(8):886–97.
41. Murphy RT, Starling RC. Genetics and cardiomyopathy: where are we now? Cleve Clin J Med 2005;72(6):465–6, 469–70, 472–3.

42. Onwuanyi A, Taylor M. Acute decompensated heart failure: pathophysiology and treatment. Am J Cardiol 2007; 99(6B): 25D–30D.
43. Rebecca Gary, RN, PhD, Leslie Davis, MSN, RN, et al. Diastolic heart failure. Heart & Lung 2007;37(6):405–16.
44. Roger VL, Go AS, Lloyd-Jones DM, et al. for the American Heart Association Statistics Committee and Stroke Statistics Subcommittee. Heart disease and stroke statistics—2011 update: a report from the American Heart Association. Circulation 2011;123(4):e18–e209.
45. Ross J Jr, Braunwald E. Studies on Starling's law of the heart. The effects of impeding venous return on performance of the normal and failing human left ventricle. Circulation 1954;30:719.
46. Stewart S, Wilkinson D, Hansen C, Vaghela V, Mvungi R, McMurray J, et al. Predominance of heart failure in the Heart of Soweto Study cohort: emerging challenges for urban African communities. Circulation 2008;118(23):2360–7.
47. Stiles S. FDA Approves Heart Sympathetic Activity Imaging Agent for HF Evaluation. Framingham Classification: Ho KK, Pinsky JL, Kannel WB, Levy D. The epidemiology of heart failure: the Framingham Study. J Am Coll Cardiol 1993; 22(4 Suppl A):6A–13A.
48. van Diepen S, Bakal JA, McAlister FA, Ezekowitz JA. Mortality and readmission of patients with heart failure, atrial fibrillation, or coronary artery disease undergoing non-cardiac surgery: an analysis of 38 047 patients. Circulation 2011;124(3):289–96.

# 9 Management of Heart Failure with Implantation of Newer Devices

Several new devices for the treatment of heart failure (HF) patients have been introduced and are increasingly used in clinical practice or are under clinical evaluation in either observational and/or randomized clinical trials. These devices include cardiac contractility modulation, spinal cord stimulation, carotid sinus nerve stimulation, cervical vagal stimulation, intracardiac atrioventricular nodal vagal stimulation, and implantable hemodynamic monitoring devices. This task force believes that an overview on these technologies is important. Special focus is given to patients with HF New York Heart Association Classes III and IV and narrow QRS complex, who represent the largest group in HF compared with patients with wide QRS complex. An overview on potential device options in addition to optimal medical therapy will be helpful for all physicians treating HF patients.

The Committee for Scientific Documents of the European Heart Rhythm Association felt, that several new devices for the treatment of heart failure (HF) patients have been introduced and are increasingly used in clinical practice or are under clinical evaluation in either observational and/or randomized clinical trials. So far, most of these technologies, if not all, have not been addressed in guidelines or position papers. Recently, several expert consensus documents and guidelines on device therapy in HF have been published followed by the publication of the 2012 EHRA/HRS consensus statement and new 2013 ESC guidelines on cardiac pacing and cardiac resynchronization therapy in 2013. Therefore, this position paper does not include any recommendation on cardiac resynchronization therapy (CRT) in heart failure.

Recommendations should represent evidence-based medicine. However, except for cardiac contractility modulation (CCM), no data based on randomized trials are available, and for none of the new devices clinical outcome data, in particular mortality data, are available.

Nevertheless, this task force believes that an overview on these new technologies is important and necessary. Special focus is given to patients with HF. New York Heart Association (NYHA) Classes III and IV and narrow QRS complex, who represent the largest group in HF compared with patients with wide QRS complex. Therefore, the task force believes that an overview on potential device options in addition to optimal medical therapy (OMT) would be helpful for all physicians treating HF patients (Figs 9.1– 9.3, Tables 9.1 and 9.2).

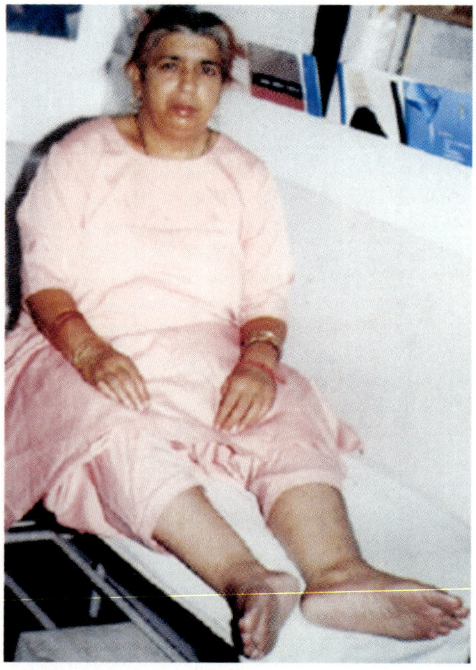

**Fig. 9.1:** Rough, dry hair, skin, facial puffiness, edema of whole body and cardiomegaly in a middle-aged lady with hypothyroidism and heart failure

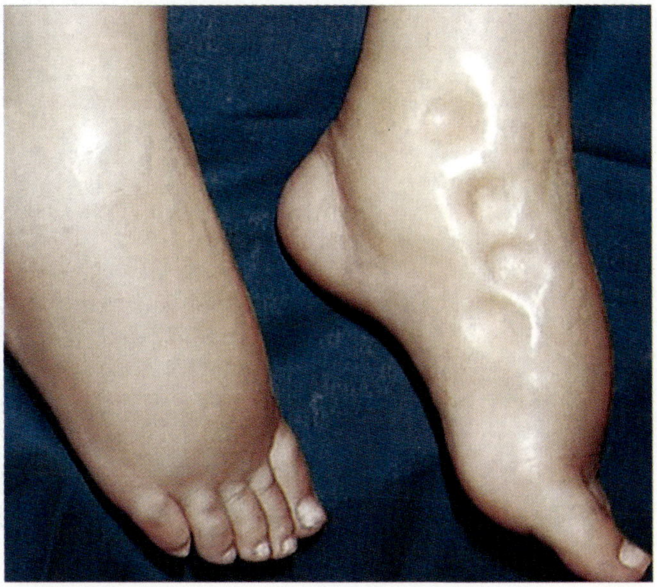

**Fig. 9.2:** Pitting edema. Bilateral, dependent pitting edema occurs with heart failure

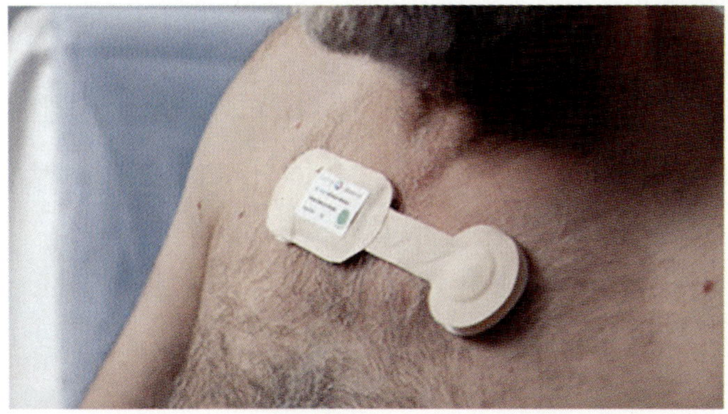

**Fig. 9.3:** Low cost wireless ECG cardiac monitor can save lives and cut healthcare costs. Developed by British Medical Services startup Isansys and based on the class-leading performance of Nordic nRF24AP2 ANT chips—the LifeTouch HRV011 cardiac monitor supports low cost yet continuous, clinical-grade ECG monitoring for the first time and can thus be used to detect post-cardiac arrest and other problems when they are usually straightforward to treat, avoiding life-threatening and costly emergency room readmissions

**Table 9.1:** New therapeutic devices in heart failure

| | Characteristics | Effects and status of trials |
|---|---|---|
| Cardiac contractility modulation (CCM) | Proteins and genes involved in Ca handling<br>• CCM signals are nonexcitatory signals delivered to the LV ~30 ms after QRS onset<br>• Effects are independent of QRS duration and additive to those of CRT<br>• CCM signals acutely affect calcium handling but also expression | • Enhances the strength of LV contraction<br>• Decreases LV volumes and increases EF<br>• Improves exercise tolerance and quality of life<br>• RCTs: FIX-HF-4, FIX-HF-5 |
| Spinal cord stimulation | • Stimulation of afferent spinal nerve fibres<br>• Increase of central vagal tone and decrease of sympathetic tone via central reflex activation<br>• Reduces risk of ischemic ventricular | • Improves cardiac output, reduces peripheral resistance<br>• Increases cardiac work efficiency, decreases myocardial oxygen demand arrhythmia<br>• SCS-HEART (ongoing non-RCT)<br>• DEFEAT-HF (ongoing RCT) |
| Carotid sinus nerve stimulation | • Stimulation of afferent fibres coupled to arterial baroreceptors<br>• Increase of central vagal tone and decrease of sympathetic tone via central reflex activation | • Improves systolic and diastolic LV function<br>• Slight decrease of heart rate and blood pressure<br>• XR-1 heart failure study; HOPE4HF study (ongoing RCTs) |
| Cervical vagal nerve stimulation | • Stimulation of cervical preganglionic parasympathetic fibres<br>• Direct activation of overall cardiac vagal tone | • Antiarrhythmic, rate slowing, antifibrotic, anti-inflammatory, and reverse remodelling effects<br>• Decreases LV volumes and increases EF<br>• Improves exercise tolerance and quality of life<br>• CardioFit study (non-RCT)<br>• INNOVATE-HF (ongoing RCT) |
| Intracardiac AV-nodal vagal stimulation | • Stimulation of postganglionic cardiac parasympathetic nerves selectively innervating AV node | • Dynamic ventricular rate control during AF<br>• AV nodal selective<br>• May avoid inappropriate shock delivery in patients with AF and ICD/CRT-D<br>• AVNS study (ongoing non-RCT) |

**Table 9.2:** Implantable hemodynamic monitoring devices

| Device | Characteristics (*Monitors*) | Clinical outcome |
|---|---|---|
| RV-pressure monitoring | • Systolic and diastolic RV pressure<br>• RV d*P*/d*t*<br>• Pulmonary artery diastolic pressure<br>• Heart rate<br>• Patient activity<br>• Core body temperature | • Nonsignificant reduction of all CHF-related events (COMPASS-HF) |
| LA-pressure monitoring (Heart-POD) | • LA pressure<br>• Intracardiac electrogram<br>• Body temperature | • Reduces death and CHF events<br>• Adequate adjustment of drug-therapy results in improvement of NYHA class and LVEF (HOMEOSTASIS study) |
| Pulmonary artery pressure (CardioMEMS) | • PAP | • Reduces significantly rate and duration of CHF-related hospitalization (CHAMPION study) |

## CARDIAC CONTRACTILITY MODULATION

### Resynchronization Therapy Device

Cardiac contractility modulation signals are nonexcitatory signals which, when applied during the absolute refractory period, enhance the strength of left ventricular (LV) contraction and improve exercise tolerance as well as QoL in patients with heart failure. As the signals influence cell function without any affecting activation sequence, the effects are independent of QRS duration and should be additive to those of CRT.

### *Concept of Cardiac Contractility Modulation*

Cardiac contractility modulation signals are electrical impulses delivered during the absolute refractory period. Cardiac contractility modulation signals used in clinical practice are delivered ≥30 ms after detection of the QRS complex onset and consist of two biphasic ±7 V pulses spanning a total duration of >20 ms. These signals do not elicit a new action potential or contraction, as is the case with extra-or postextrasystolic contractions. Moreover, they do not affect the sequence of electrical or mechanical activation, nor do they recruit additional contractile elements. On this basis, CCM signals are referred to as 'nonexcitatory'.

If your heart is not beating efficiently and you meet the eligibility criteria, you may be eligible for a cardiac resynchronization therapy (CRT) heart device (Figs 9.4 and 9.5).

A CRT device sends small, undetectable electrical impulses to both lower chambers of the heart to help them beat together in a more synchronized pattern. This improves the heart's ability to pump blood and oxygen to the body.

The heart device itself is actually a tiny computer, plus a battery, contained in a small titanium metal case that is about the size of a pocket watch. It weighs about 3 ounces.

In addition to the heart device, insulated wires called leads are implanted for two purposes—to carry information signals from your heart to the heart device, and to carry electrical impulses to your heart.

The third part of your implantable device system is a programmer, an external computer located in your doctor's

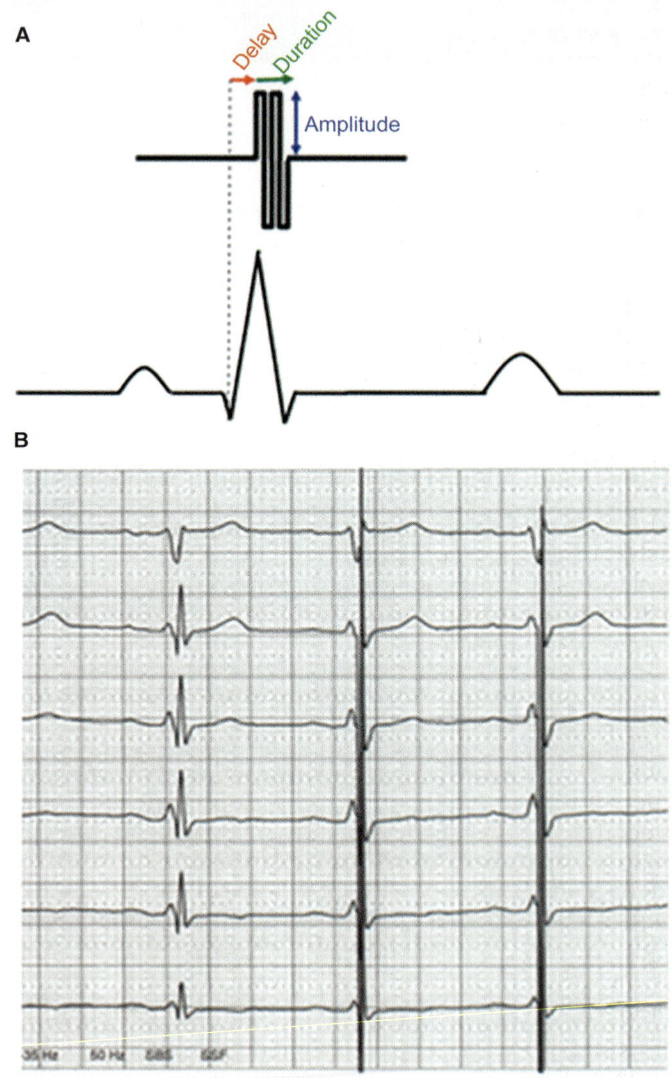


**Fig. 9.4:** (A) Top and middle—cardiac contractility modulation (CCM) signals are biphasic pulses, delivered after a defined delay from detection of local electrical activation. (B) Body surface electrocardiogram (leads V1–V6) showing one beat prior to initiating CCM signals and the first two beats of CCM signal application. Please note the stimulation artefact in beats 2 and 3 reflect CCM signals

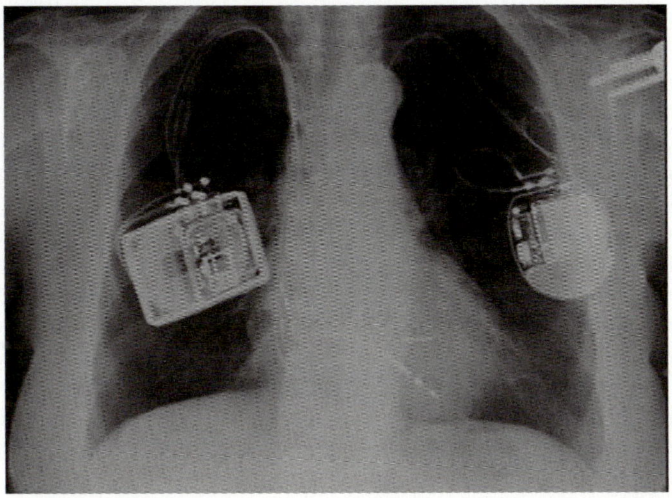

**Fig. 9.5:** Chest X-ray showing an implanted CCM system (CCM, right side) and one-chamber ICD device (left side). The CCM system consists of a can and three pace-sense electrodes. Two of them are fixed to the midseptum and the third one to the right atrium

office or clinic that is used to program the heart device and retrieve information from your heart device that will assist your doctor in your heart failure treatment.

There are two types of implantable heart failure heart devices—a CRT pacemaker and a combination CRT pacemaker with defibrillation therapy. Both of these devices help to coordinate the heart's pumping action and improve blood flow. They can also speed up a heart that is beating too slowly.

The CRT pacemaker with defibrillation therapy (CRT-D) also offers the ability to detect and treat dangerously fast heart rhythms, which some individuals with a damaged heart muscle may be at risk for developing. Your doctor will determine which CRT device is appropriate for your medical condition.

Cardiac resynchronization therapy improves symptoms, quality of life (QoL), exercise tolerance, and reduces hospitalizations in patients with advanced HF and prolonged electrical activation (i.e. increased QRS duration). The results of a recent study showed that patients with mechanical dyssynchrony detected by tissue Doppler imaging but a normal QRS duration did not benefit from CRT. While the results of outcome trials of CRT in patients with a normal QRS duration are negative including Echo-CRT, a QRS ≥120 ms remains as one of the criterion for selecting patients for CRT. Patients with a QRS duration >120 ms represent 31% of HF patients in a recent trial. The indications for CRT have been summarized in a recent update of ESC guidelines on devices in heart failure.

Although CRT is indicated in patients with a prolonged QRS duration, up to 60% of patients with HF have a normal QRS duration. According to European registries published recently, even in the broad QRS population, those cared in hospital cardiology setting and meeting the current indications to CRT therapy were 6%, and among them approximately one-third only were actually implanted with a CRT device. Therefore, although the last ESC guidelines on HF extended the indications to CRT in chronic heart failure, a substantial proportion of patients remain either not eligible for CRT or simply do not respond. At a time when pharmacological therapy for HF has made only little advances, it is appropriate to explore whether new device-based therapies have anything else to offer to patients with heart failure.

The CCM system consists of a can and three pace-sense electrodes. Two of them are fixed to the mid-septum and the third one to the right atrium. The impact of a HF therapy on myocardial energetics is an important factor to consider in long-term safety and efficacy. Therefore, the acute effects of CCM on myocardial energetics were investigated in a clinical study in which myocardial oxygen uptake ($MVO_2$) and LV $dP/dt_{max}$ were measured in 9 patients exposed to acute CCM signals. In this study, acute CCM was associated with an increase in $dP/dt_{max}$ from ~630 to ~800 mmHg/s (an ~20% increase). Despite an acute increase in contractility, there was no detectible increase in myocardial oxygen consumption. These data were compared with those of Nelson et al., who had also measured $MVO_2$ and $dP/dt_{max}$ during temporary RV and biventricular pacing (BIV) pacing. In this study, contractility was increased first by applying CRT and then dobutamine to achieve a comparable increase in $dP/dt_{max}$. As expected from its effects on calcium cycling, dobutamine increased both $dP/dt_{max}$ and $MVO_2$. In contrast, CCM increased $dP/dt_{max}$ but not $MVO_2$. Thus, like CRT, the acute, modest increase in contractility achieved by CCM does not increase energy demands. In addition to acute hemodynamic effects noted above, improvement in global ventricular function has also been reported during chronic CCM signal application. In one study, 30 patients with ejection fraction (EF) <35% and NYHA III symptoms despite OMT underwent three-dimensional echocardiography at baseline and 3 months after CCM treatment. Left ventricular ejection fraction (LVEF) increased by 4.8 ± 3.6% and LV end-systolic volumes decreased by 11.5 ± 10.5%, respectively. These findings indicate that LV reverse remodelling could be achieved by CCM in the background of optimum medical therapy.

### Combining Cardiac Contractility Modulation with Cardiac Resynchronization Therapy

As discussed above, CCM signals applied in the acute setting to HF patients simultaneously receiving CRT provide additive effects on LV contractility indexed by $dP/dt_{max}$. In view of the fact that symptoms persist in more ≥30% of patients with prolonged QRS duration receiving CRT, it can be postulated that addition of CCM treatment may provide an option for these patients. The initial experience of combining CCM in a CRT non-responders has been published.

It was demonstrated that the implantation procedure is technically feasible, that the OPTIMIZER and CRT defibrillator (CRT-D) devices can coexist without interference and that acute hemodynamic and clinical improvements can be observed. These preliminary results, however, have to be confirmed in a prospective study that is underway to systematically investigate the effects of CCM in CRT non-responders.

### Clinical Perspectives

Two large-scale studies have validated the safety and suggested the effectiveness of CCM therapy. Results of these trials show that CCM improves exercise tolerance as indexed by peak $VO_2$. Other indices of exercise tolerance (e.g. 6 min hall walk) and QoL (NYHA class and MLWHFQ) have also been shown to improve. Data from both clinical trials suggest that mortality rates are unaffected by CCM therapy. However, the aim of these studies was to demonstrate an absence of increase in mortality as a safety end-point and was not powered to show a mortality benefit. The level of recommendation would be substantially higher if a gain in mortality can be demonstrated. In this respect, a specific subgroup of HF patients (EF ≥25%) is more likely to respond favourably. Moreover, more research is probably required to determine the optimal pacing configuration (single or biphasic stimuli, optimal delay from the pacing spike, optimal duration of each phase, and optimal amplitude of the signal), the optimal daily duration of application, the optimal localization of the pacing sites, and the optimal number of pacing sites to gain the maximal benefit from this therapy. The potential interest of CCM in early stages of HF has not been investigated.

### Required Technical Improvement

Some technical limitations should be solved in the future—(i) with the last version of the device, CCM cannot be delivered in patients with AF or frequent ectopy, as it is designed to inhibit CCM delivery on arrhythmias and relies on detection of a P-wave. A future device is supposed to incorporate an algorithm that does not rely on P-wave detection and therefore could be used in patients with AF. (ii) The development of a device combining CCM with implantable cardioverter defibrillator (ICD) functions would be desirable in this population of HF patients. Future studies will be required to define whether CCM is additive to CRT pacemaker or CRT-D in patients with wide QRS. This would be facilitated by the development of a single device that incorporates pacing, antitachycardia therapies, and CCM. (iii) A simple peri-implantation method to guide lead positioning would be desirable, beyond the invasive LV $dP/dt_{max}$ measurement.

### Neuromodulation

Heart failure is associated with significant perturbances of the autonomic balance with predominant sympathetic activation over the parasympathetic system. Several indirect markers of cardiac vagal tone like heart rate variability, heart rate turbulence, baroreflex sensitivity are suppressed in CHF which in turn is predictive for a worse outcome of CHF. Likewise, an increase of cardiac vagal tone by pharmacological β-receptor blockade has substantially improved functional status and survival of HF patients. Cardiac vagal tone is controlled by preganglionic parasympathetic cardiac neurons mainly residing in the nucleus ambiguus and the dorsal motor nucleus of the brainstem. Of note, parasympathetic cardiac efferent neurons in the nucleus ambiguus are intrinsically electrically silent, thus needing presynaptic input to generate and modulate parasympathetic efferent activity and tone. Such input is likely provided by sensory afferent fibres from arterial baroreceptors or respiratory sensory neurons, but spinal cord afferent fibres may also connect to the brainstem and modulate cardiac vagal tone Thus, attempts to therapeutically increase the cardiac parasympathetic tone by electrical neural stimulation may operate at any part of this integrative circuit. This has led to four neurostimulation approaches, two of which are focusing on reflex activation of the parasympathetic tone and sympathetic inhibition via afferent fibre stimulation [spinal cord stimulation (SCS), carotid sinus nerve stimulation], while two are concentrating on efferent parasympathetic stimulation (cervical vagal and intracardiac vagal stimulation).

## Spinal Cord Stimulation

Preliminary work suggests some benefits from neuromodulation with SCS in HF patients. Spinal cord stimulation has been used for over 40 years in the management of chronic intractable pain. According to the American Association of Neurosurgical Surgeons, as many as 50,000 neurostimulators are implanted worldwide every year. Among multiple indications, the benefits have been confirmed in patients with refractory angina associated with end-stage CAD and in the absence of CAD (syndrome X) Positive effects have also been demonstrated in the peripheral vascular beds—patients with severe pain due to distal atherosclerosis, in Raynaud's disease, and at the level of cerebral vasculature.

### Mechanisms of Action

Spinal cord stimulation compared positively with surgical and laser endomyocardial revascularization in patients with severe refractory angina associated with severe CAD without any increase in adverse ischemic events. This suggests that the improvement in symptoms and the clinical condition of these patients was mediated only partially through the 'gate-control' mechanisms described by Melzack and Wall in 1965. The involved mechanisms remain incompletely understood and appear to be far more complex than just the suppression of the nociceptive influx associated with myocardial ischemia: SCS seems to affect the balance between oxygen demand and supply. Since there is little evidence that SCS improves the coronary blood flow in ischemic patients, other factors acting in the balance between oxygen requirements and supplies have to play an important role. Spinal cord stimulation applied at the low cervical (C7–C8) and/or high thoracic (T1–T6) level exerts effects through reflex activation of the vagus nerve and sympathetic.

Overall, the cumulated effects on both the sympathetic and the parasympathetic system seems to be a re-equilibrium of the balance in favour of the latter. Other positive effects via the cytokines and the NO/NOS system have been identified and there may even be some direct protective mechanisms on the myocardium during ischemia (Figs 9.6–9.9 and Table 9.3).

### Clinical Perspectives

Spinal cord stimulation, via complex mechanisms, appears promising in preclinical experiments to improve the systolic function of the LV and to decrease the ventricular arrhythmias associated with this condition. According to Clinicaltrials.org, there are at the present time two ongoing clinical studies that are directly addressing the role—and possible benefits—of SCS in severely afflicted HF patients. SCS-HEART is a nonrandomized feasibility study that aims to determine the safety of SCS in 20 patients with a LVEF between 20 and 35%, in NYHA functional class III, and who already have an ICD implanted. Results should be available in the second part of 2014. On the other hand, DEFEAT-HF (sponsored by Medtronic) is a single blind randomized study involving similar patients but that will compare SCS 'ON' *vs* 'OFF' in 250 recipients. Results are also expected for the end of 2014. Until these studies are completed, it remains impossible to recommend this therapy in HF patients outside of the current recognized indications.

### Carotid Sinus Nerve Stimulation

Baroreceptors are embedded into the wall of arterial vessels and can be preferentially found in the aortic arch at the

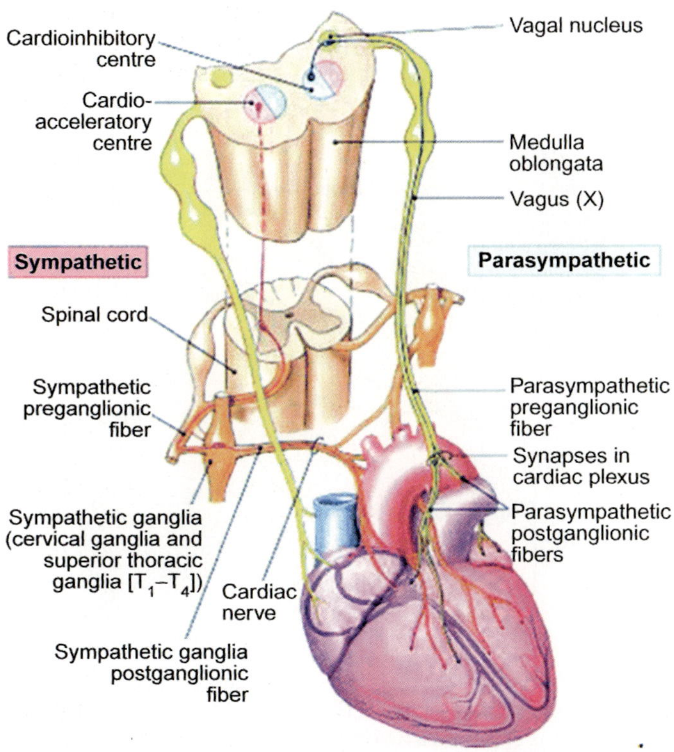


**Fig. 9.6:** Parasympathetic and sympathetic innervations of the heart. Functional anatomy—efferent preganglionic vagal nerve (parasympathetic) fibres course from the brainstem towards the heart and connect with postganglionic cells in circumscript epicardial ganglionic plexus. Sympathetic preganglionic fibres (orange color) switch to postganglionic fibres inside the stellate ganglion. Major afferent inputs to the central autonomic centres are the carotid sinus nerves and spinal cord afferents

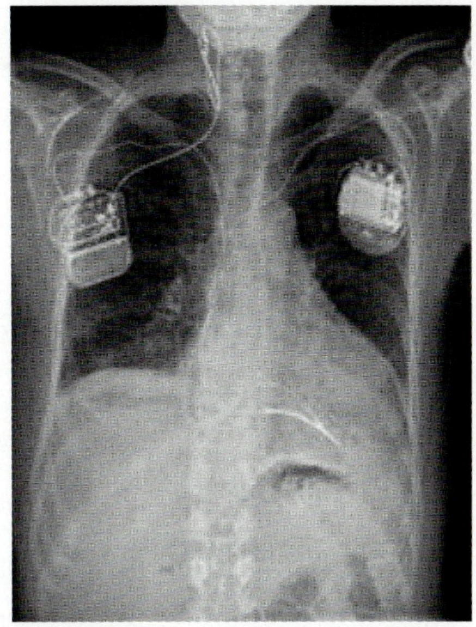

**Fig. 9.7:** CardioFit is an implantable electrical stimulation device designed to restore balance in the autonomic nervous system and improve heart function in patients with HF

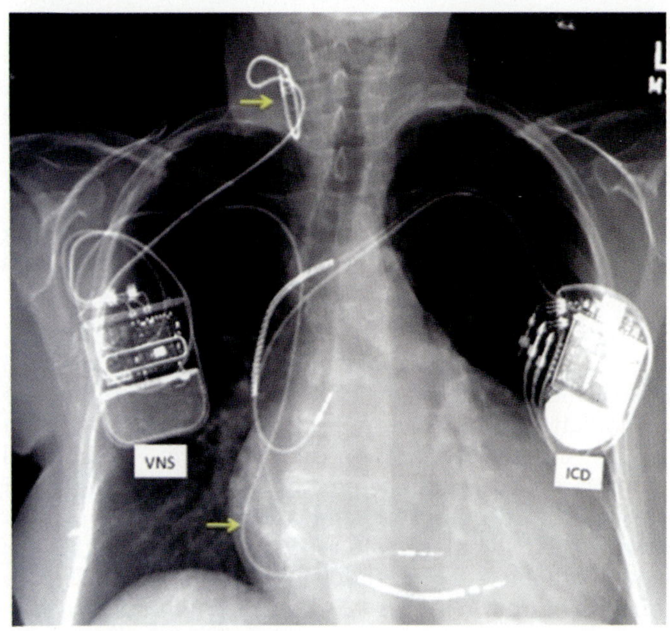


**Fig. 9.8:** X-ray of a patient with a vagal nerve stimulator with a previously implanted implantable cardioverter defibrillator. The arrows show a lead attached to the vagus nerve on the right side and an additional right ventricular sensing lead connected to the vagal nerve stimulator device

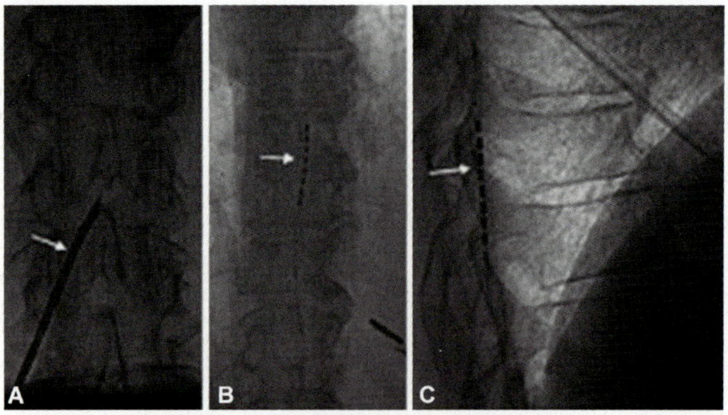


**Fig. 9.9:** Spinal cord stimulation—single-lead placement. (A) Introducer (arrow) is directed into the epidural space. (B and C) anteroposterior and lateral views demonstrate the lead in the posterior epidural space in the midthoracic region at approximately T1 (arrows)

| **Table 9.3:** Major findings reported with SCS |
|---|
| *Spinal cord stimulation has been shown to have positive impact on cardiac ischemia due to CAD* |
| 1. The mechanisms involved go beyond suppression of the nociceptive stimuli. |
| 2. SCS has limited impact on coronary blood flow, therefore the mechanisms must lie somewhere else. |
| 3. SCS has a profound positive impact on the cardiac sympathetic/parasymapathetic balance. |
| 4. SCS also affects positively the NO/NOS and cytokines system at the myocardial level. |
| *Spinal cord stimulation has shown some effects on LV function and ventricular arrhythmias* |
| 1. One preliminary report on four HF patients who improved clinically with SCS. |
| 2. SCS was associated with smaller deterioration of LVEF due to adenosine administration in patients with multivessel CAD. |
| 3. SCS was associated with better invasive hemodynamic evaluation in patients with normal LV function. |
| 4. SCS was associated with reduced risk of ventricular arrhythmias and LV function improvement in animal models of HF. |

origins of the brachiocephalic or left subclavian artery, in the brachiocephalic artery at its bifurcation into the right subclavian and right common carotid artery, in the carotid sinuses, along both common carotid arteries, and in both common carotid arteries at the origin of the superior thyroid artery. They respond to changes in arterial pressure and mediate their signals via afferent rapid conducting (2.5–60 m/s) myelinated A fibres and slow conducting (<2.5 m/s) nonmyelinated C fibres to the brainstem where they connect to efferent vagal neurons. A-type receptors respond to normal arterial pressures and are regularly discharging at high frequency (>100 Hz) synchronously to the pulsatile pressure wave. By contrast, C-type baroreceptor respond to higher threshold values of the mean arterial pressure with irregular firing at lower frequency of 20–30 Hz. Increases of arterial blood pressure elicit a reflectory activation of efferent vagal fibres resulting in a decrease of the sinus heart rate. The baroreflex activation is considered as powerful contributor to the baseline parasympathetic tone.

### Mechanisms of Action

Electrical stimulation of the baroreceptor fibres (carotid sinus nerve fibres) elicits a graded response decrease of heart rate and arterial pressure via parasympathetic efferent activation and sympathetic withdrawal and has recently been clinically introduced for treatment of resistant arterial hypertension. The potential of electrical carotid sinus nerve stimulation to shift the autonomic balance towards a higher parasympathetic tone has also been investigated in HF models. In fact, chronic low-intensity carotid sinus stimulation, which lowers blood pressure by only 10–15 mmHg and which does not critically decrease heart rate was able to improve survival in dogs with pacing-induced HF In addition, LV systolic and diastolic function improved due to reverse LV geometric and interstitial remodeling. In parallel, the downregulation of $\alpha 1$ receptor density in CHF was almost normalized to control levels and serum catecholamine levels declined which may be taken as evidence for a direct or reflectory decrease of the systemic sympathetic tone in these models (Fig. 9.10).

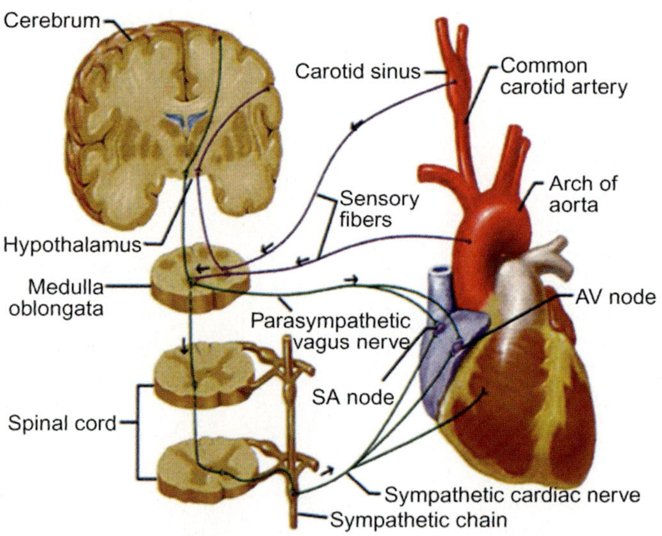


**Fig. 9.10:** Baroreceptor reflexes. Congestive heart failure is a syndrome that is usually initiated by a reduction in pump function of the heart, i.e. a decrease in cardiac output. Initially, a reduction in cardiac output leads to unloading of baroreceptor reflex that, in turn, increases heart rate through vago-sympathetic mechanisms and total peripheral resistance via an increase in sympathetic outflow to vascular beds. During human HF, this baroreflex is profoundly suppressed and worsens with deterioration of CHF. Thus, electrical stimulation of afferent carotid sinus nerves, which connect baroreceptors to the brainstem may evolve as tool for increasing cardiac vagal tone during HF

### Clinical Data

The Rheos system was the first baroreceptor stimulation system by CVRx implanted in hypertensive patients. The Rheos system was so far evaluated in three multicentre clinical studies in patients with resistant hypertension—the DEBuT-HT/DEBuT-HET in Europe and the Rheos Feasibility Trial and Rheos Pivotal Trial which mostly included patients in the USA. The Rheos Pivotal trial is in long-term follow-up by now. The randomized part of the trial with a 12-month blinded follow-up was published in 2011: 265 patients with resistant hypertension received the device and were either randomized to immediate BAT or delayed BAT following the 6-month visit. Three of the five prespecified coprimary endpoints were met—long-term sustained response to baroreceptor activation therapy, with 88% responders after 12 months of follow-up, incidence of short-term AEs (6-month follow-up), and long-term AEs (12-month follow-up). The study did not meet the endpoints for acute responders (54 *vs* 46% responders after 6-month follow-up) and procedural safety (event-free rate 74.8%). A majority of these events were related to the carotid sinus lead placement and involved transient or permanent nerve injury that occurred during the implant. The majority (76%) of procedure-related AEs resolved completely (Figs 9.10 and 9.11).

To date, there exist no randomized clinical data evaluating the effectiveness of BAT in patients with systolic HF. In addition to experimental data, several sub-studies and single-centre data indicated beneficial physiological effects of BAT beyond just blood pressure reduction.

### Cervical Vagal Nerve Stimulation

The efferent cardiac parasympathetic signalling chain comprises preganglionic parasympathetic neurons originating in the brainstem, which course inside the vagal nerve and connect via nicotinergic acetylcholine receptors to post-ganglionic neurons, which are aggregated in circumscript cardiac ganglionic plexus inside the heart. Postganglionic fibres then innervate the cardiac target cells via muscarinergic acetylcholine receptors. During CHF, the density of cardiac muscarinergic receptors is increased, which is most probably due to an adaptive upregulation secondary to a decreased efferent vagal input. However, the post-ganglionic vagal nerve transmission seems to be intact in HF; selective electrical stimulation of post-ganglionic vagal nerve fibres to the sinus node leads to a larger decrease of the sinus rate in HF dogs than in controls, which would be in line with an increased number of muscarinergic receptors in HF. By contrast, electrical stimulation of presynaptic cervical vagal fibres led to a smaller decrease of the sinus rate in CHF animals as compared with control animals. Thus, pre-to-post ganglionic parasympathetic efferent neurotransmission via nicotinergic acetylcholine receptors seems to be impaired during CHF. Importantly, these nicotinergic receptors are agonist dependent and chronic exposure to a nicotinic agonist during HF has been shown to re-establish efferent parasympathetic neural control of the sinus node. These experiments form a pathophysiological rationale to apply electrical preganglionic cervical vagal nerve stimulation to re-establish the diminished cardiac vagal tone in CHF (Figs 9.12 and 9.13).

### Mechanisms of Action

Several studies in various chronic HF animal models have shown a reduction of the progression of HF and a survival benefit with cervical vagal nerve stimulation. Major contributing mechanisms are detailed as follows:

*Antiarrhythmic effects:* Vagal nerve stimulation increases the ventricular refractory period in humans, leads to a prolongation of the epicardial action potential duration, and decreases ventricular vulnerability to ventricular fibrillation. These electrophysiological effects may contribute to its potent antifibrillatory effects as demonstrated during cervical vagal nerve stimulation experiments in postinfarction animal models. In addition, vagal nerve stimulation in HF reduces the loss of Cx43, which may prevent proarrhythmic conduction delays and dispersion of action potential duration.

*Rate slowing effects:* Vagal nerve stimulation exerts profound negative chronotropic and dromotropic effects. Since an increased heart rate is associated with adverse prognosis in CHF, a reduction of heart rate both in SR and AF might contribute beneficial therapeutic effects in CHF.

*Antifibrotic effects:* In a coronary microembolization-induced HF model, chronic cervical vagal nerve stimulation

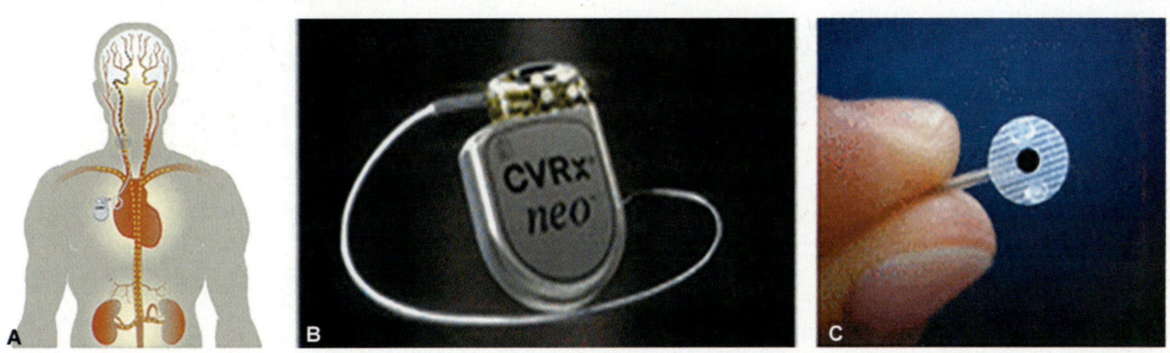


**Fig. 9.11:** (A) The principle of carotid sinus nerve stimulation. The device is implanted via the right side and is connected to a patch electrode fixed on the right-sided carotid sinus. (B) An example of a carotid sinus nerve stimulator. The device carries one electrode connected to the patch electrode. (C) Demonstrates a patch electrode which will be fixed to the carotid sinus nerve

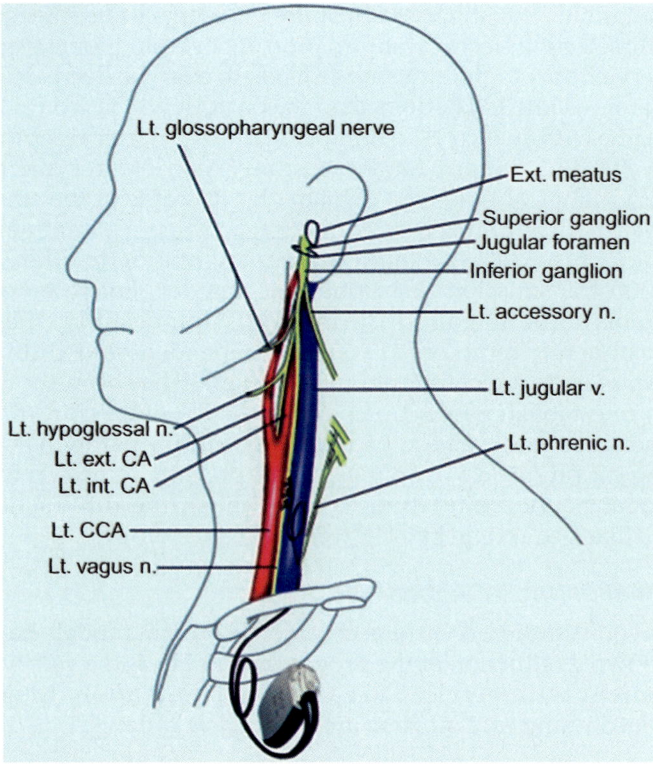


**Fig. 9.12:** Anatomical relationship between vagus nerve and surrounding structures and location of VNS

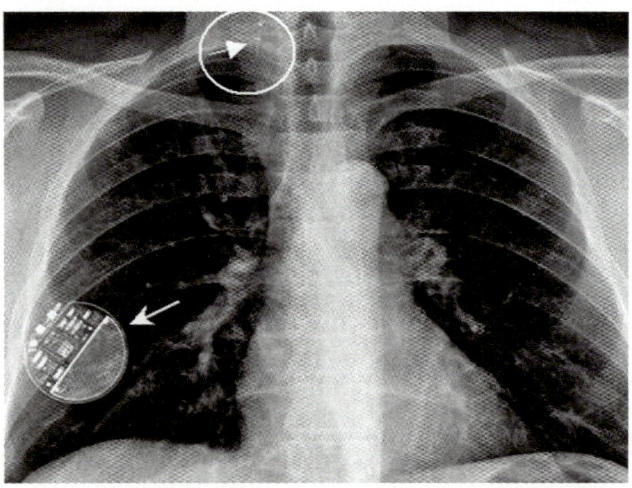

**Fig. 9.13:** Plain thoracic X-rays displaying the vagus nerve stimulator (VNS) implanted on the right side in a patient. Encircled upper arrow points to the VNS around the right vagus nerve trunk. VNS generator is positioned at the right paraaxillary region (arrow)

has been shown to decrease ventricular replacement fibrosis and to blunt the development of CHF-associated cellular hypertrophy of remaining myocytes.

*Anti-inflammatory effects:* Vagal nerve stimulation has potent anti-inflammatory effects. Recently, vagal nerve stimulation was shown to blunt HF-associated increases of tumor necrosis factor-α, interleukin-6, and C-reactive protein in two animal models of HF.

*Reverse remodelling:* Vagal nerve stimulation decreases ventricular end-systolic and end-diastolic diameters and improves LVEF. Chronic vagal stimulation has also been shown to reduce NT-proBNP levels in a dog HF model and biventricular weight in a rat HF model.

### Clinical Data

The first multicentre, open-label phase II, two-staged study (8-patient feasibility phase plus 24-patient safety and tolerability phase) enroled 32 NYHA Class II–IV patients (age 56 + 11 years, LVEF 23 + 8%). Right cervical vagal nerve stimulation (VNS) with an implantable system started 2–4 weeks after implant, slowly raising intensity; patients were followed 3 and 6 months thereafter with optional 1-year follow-up. Overall, 26 serious AEs occurred in 13 of 32 patients (40.6%), including three deaths and two clearly device-related AEs (postoperative pulmonary edema, need of surgical revision). Expected nonserious device-related AEs (cough, dysphonia, and stimulation-related pain) occurred early but were reduced and disappeared after stimulation intensity adjustment. There were significant improvements ($P = 0.001$) in NYHA Class QoL, 6 min walk test (from 411 + 76 to 471 + 111 m), LVEF (from 22 + 7 to 29 + 8%), and LV systolic volumes ($P = 0.02$). These improvements were maintained at 1 year.

Several scientific articles have summarized the use of cervical vagal nerve stimulator (CVS) in patients with CHF. Naturally, the data provided in those articles are limited, due to the small patient cohort and the nonrandomized nature of first in man and safety and feasibility studies; however important considerations can be drawn from them:

- Patients with mild-to-moderate HF can tolerate the higher current amplitudes and other parameters used in chronic vagal stimulation vs the parameters used for treatment of epilepsy.
- Vagal stimulation may generate side effects like hoarseness, voice alteration, and increased cough. The majority of side effects are related to the underlying disease or a multitude of comorbidities.
- In patients with both CVS and ICD, no interferences from vagal stimulation were recognized by the ICD nor were detectable on the intracardiac electrogram of the device.
- CVS increased parasympathetic tone of subjects with HF (as measured by heart rate variability on 24-hour Holter recordings; and as inferred by reduction of resting heart rate).
- Vagal stimulation improved subjective, as well as objective clinically relevant parameters of functional class, quality of life, submaximal exercise capacity, and cardiac structure and function in a first clinical study.

## Unresolved Issues

### Atrial Proarrhythmia

At the atrial level, an increased vagal tone substantially shortens the atrial refractory period and increases the heterogeneity of refractory periods in the atria. Whether this might promote the occurrence of AF especially in HF patients with a diseased atrial substrate is unknown. Experimental evidence in healthy dogs, however, suggests that the occurrence of AF during cervical vagal nerve stimulation depends on the intensity of vagal stimulation with no AF occurrence at lower level stimulation. Data on the occurrence of AF during vagal stimulation in HF patients need to be gathered prospectively (Fig. 9.14).

### Selectivity of Neural Stimulation

The cervical vagal nerve contains efferent and afferent fibres coursing not only to the thoracic but also to or from the abdominal viscera. So far, the issue of concomitant stimulation of efferent parasympathetic fibres to the gastrointestinal tract has not yet been thoroughly investigated. Such inadvertent stimulation might increase gastric acid secretion or increase intestinal motility. Likewise, afferent electrical stimulation or block of the vagal nerve below the diaphragm has been shown to decrease food intake and to reduce weight gain. Since these fibres potentially course through the cervical vagal nerve inadvertent stimulation or block of these fibres may occur during vagal nerve stimulation for HF possibly inducing weight loss masking as cardiac cachexia.

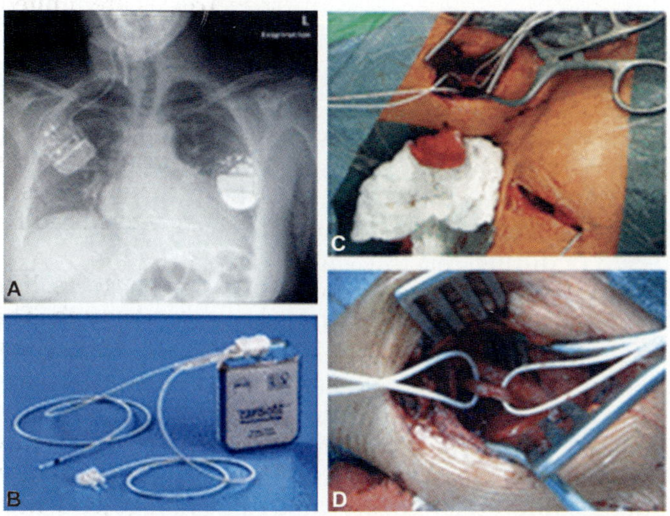


**Fig. 9.14:** (A) Chest X-ray of an implanted cervical vagal nerve stimulator in a patient with severely reduced LV systolic function. The device has been implanted via the right side and consists of a ventricular sensing lead and a cervical vagal nerve electrode. On the left side an ICD had been previously implanted. (B) Example of a cervical vagal stimulator. The device carries two electrodes—one conventional RV screw-in pace/sense electrode monitors the heart rate during vagal nerve stimulation, while the other cuff electrode is wrapped around the cervical vagal nerve. (C) Local implantation site of the CVS; there are two incisions, one for exposure of the cervical vagal nerve and a second one for implanting the RV electrode. The vagal electrode is tunnelled subcutaneously to the impulse generator, which is implanted below the collarbone. (D) Exposed cervical vagal nerve

### Intracardiac Atrioventricular Nodal Vagal Stimulation

Thirty to forty percent of patients with CHF eventually will develop AF. Rapid ventricular rates during AF may further deteriorate HF or decrease the degree of LV resynchronization in patients with cardiac resynchronization devices and may ultimately lead to inappropriate shock delivery in up to 5% of ICD recipients. Long-term selective atrioventricular (AV) nodal vagal stimulation for ventricular rate control has been developed as potential adjunctive treatment modality for these patients (Figs 9.15–9.18).

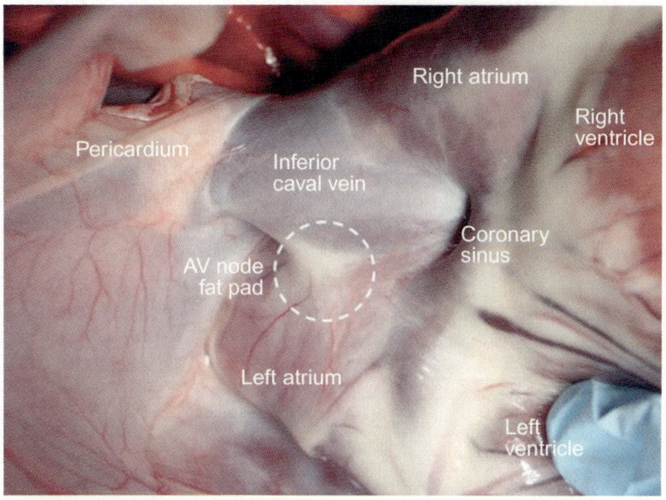


**Fig. 9.15:** Anatomical location of the atrioventricular node fat pad. The diagram uses as a background a real anatomical epicardial image of heart. The heart has been lifted up towards the head to show the anatomical position of the epicardial AV node fat pad (dashed circle)

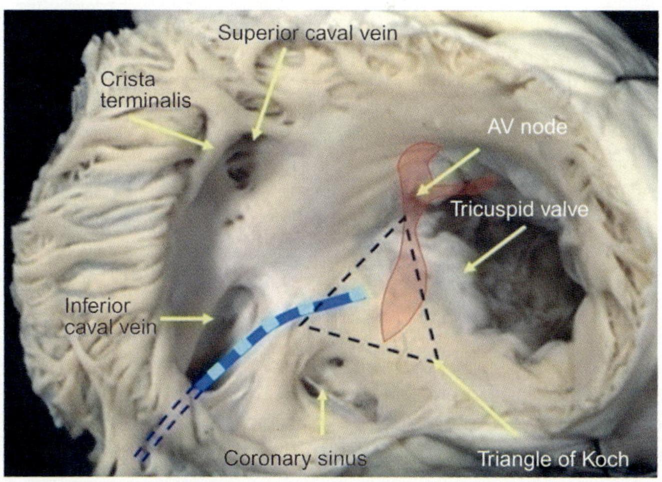


**Fig. 9.16:** Vagal stimulation site for endocardial approach in the human heart. A schematic diagram showing the site at the posterior right atrium at which optimal AV conduction delay could be achieved by electrical postganglionic vagal stimulation delivered with an endocardial catheter inserted through the inferior caval vein. Anatomical image of endocardial view of human right atrium provided by *Prof. RH Anderson*)

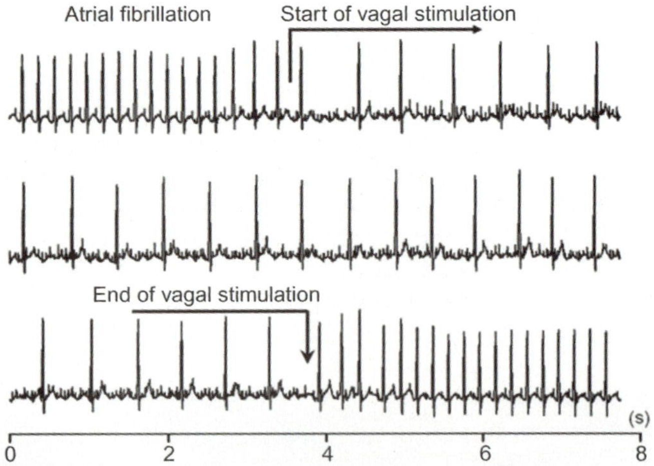


**Fig. 9.17:** Surface ECG recordings from a chronic dog implanted with an AV node vagal stimulation device. The top trace shows at the beginning a rapid ventricular rate (>240 bpm) during AF without vagal stimulation. The arrow indicates the start of vagal stimulation and the immediate resultant slowing of the ventricular rate. The middle trace shows the maintenance of slow ventricular rate (105 bpm) during continuous vagal stimulation. The bottom trace shows the prompt restoration of the initial (fast) ventricular rate after vagal stimulation was terminated (arrow)

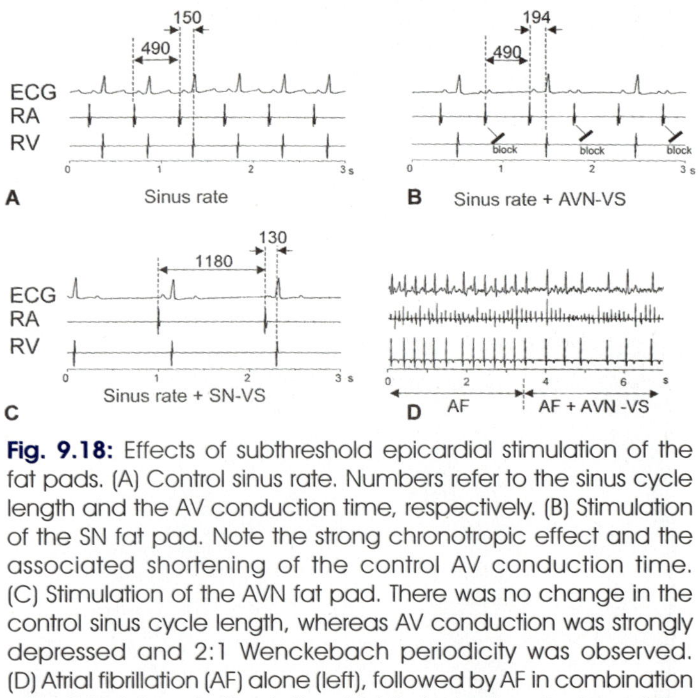


**Fig. 9.18:** Effects of subthreshold epicardial stimulation of the fat pads. (A) Control sinus rate. Numbers refer to the sinus cycle length and the AV conduction time, respectively. (B) Stimulation of the SN fat pad. Note the strong chronotropic effect and the associated shortening of the control AV conduction time. (C) Stimulation of the AVN fat pad. There was no change in the control sinus cycle length, whereas AV conduction was strongly depressed and 2:1 Wenckebach periodicity was observed. (D) Atrial fibrillation (AF) alone (left), followed by AF in combination with AVN fat-pad stimulation (right). Note the slowing of the ventricular rate during vagal stimulation. ECG=electrocardiogram; RA=right atrium; VS=vagal stimulation

## Mechanisms and Experimental Models

Postganglionic cardiac vagal fibres, which preferentially supply the AV node reside in an inferior right ganglionated plexus (IRGP) at the postero-inferior interatrial septum.This makes them amenable to stimulation from the endocardial surface, thus resulting in a graded response negative dromotropic effect. Chronic stimulation of the IRGP in animal models provides reliable and well-tolerated ventricular rate control in dogs and has been shown to be hemodynamically superior to His bundle ablation and RV pacing probably because ventricular conduction over the His–Purkinje system is maintained.

## Technology and Implant Technique

The IRGP is located at the epicardial surface of the heart between the ostium of the coronary sinus and the entrance of the inferior vena cava. For chronic electrostimulation of this plexus, atrial pacing leads of current technology can be screwed into the IRGP from the right atrial endocardial site at the posteroinferior interatrial septum either by using specifically shaped guiding catheters or manually shaped conventional mandrins.

## Clinical Data

Recently, the feasibility of such an approach was shown in a series of chronic human implants in HF patients with AF. A prospective multicentre study (AVNS: AV node stimulation study, which investigates whether short-term probatory AV nodal vagal stimulation may avoid inappropriate shock delivery in patients with resynchronization defibrillators is ongoing.

## Electrical Determinants of Neurostimulation

Electrical stimulation of parasympathetic pre- or postganglionic efferent fibres obeys the same fundamental laws as myocardial electrostimulation with the exception that the chronaxie time of 180 ms is shorter. In contrast to the myocardial action potential, the action potential of neurons is very short lasting only 10–20 ms. Thus, transmitter release and physiological effects may be elicited by electrical stimulation at higher frequencies, which typically is set to 20–50 Hz during cervical vagal stimulation for seizures or depression, 100 Hz for carotid sinus stimulation, or 4–20 Hz for cervical vagal stimulation in HF. For postganglionic efferent parasympathetic stimulation the frequency-response curve is bell-shaped with an optimum at 40 Hz. Since most stimulated nerve structures contain afferent and efferent autonomic fibres with varying fibre diameter and conduction velocities, efforts have been undertaken to preferentially stimulate efferent fibres. For example, cervical vagal nerve stimulation for treatment of HF aims to stimulate efferent parasympathetic B fibres coursing towards the heart but tries to avoid afferent A and C fibre excitation. This can be achieved by hyperpolarizing the nerve fibres at the anode thus preventing excitation and simultaneously depolarizing fibres at the cathode. Since larger afferent A fibres (diameter 520 μm) are more sensitive to hyperpolarization than smaller efferent B fibres (13 μm) inside the vagal nerve preferential efferent stimulation can be accomplished. Besides electrode configuration, the applied stimulus strength also affects differential recruitment of A–C fibres and changes the frequency dependence of afferent neural stimulation. Finally, the application of biphasic impulses may bare the benefit of decharging the membrane with the second phase of the impulse thus preventing damage to the neurocytes.

### *Implantable Hemodynamic Monitoring Devices*

Clinical management to prevent acute decompensated heart failure (ADHF) and/or hospitalization in ambulatory HF patients remains challenging. There is an urgent need to develop strategies to reduce hospitalizations and re-admission rates for HF. Frequent monitoring of physiological data is imperative in the management of HF. The development of wireless and remote technology makes it possible to frequently monitor and transfer data via telemonitoring. The concept of telemonitoring involves patient-activated automatic devices which provide physiological parameters such as weight, blood pressure, heart rate, rhythm, and activity logs. Results of studies using telemonitoring have been contradictory. A meta-analysis demonstrated that telemonitoring may provide better outcomes compared with usual care, with a reduction in mortality and HF hospitalizations. Recently, the value of telemonitoring has been challenged by two randomized clinical trials. The results of the Telemedical Interventional Monitoring in Heart Failure (TIM-HF) trial showed no significant difference in all-cause mortality (primary endpoint) or in the composite of cardiovascular death or HF hospitalization. The study of Chaudhry et al. demonstrated that telemonitoring failed to reduce HF hospital admissions, duration of hospital stay, or the frequency of admissions. One explanation might be the insensitivity of daily weight monitoring to predict HF hospitalization, which is >20%. Another strategy is the use of cardiac implantable devices (defibrillators and CRT) to stratify the risk of ADHF based on a single parameter as thoracic impedance or heart rate variability, or a combination of parameters. These parameters, single or combined, have a sensitivity of 60–70%, a positive predictive value up to 7.8%, and false-positive alarms ranging from 1.8 to 2.7 per patient-year of monitoring. Although these parameters enable physicians to identify patients at increased risk of ADHF, they do not impact patient outcomes and are not sufficiently accurate to adjust treatment. A new approach to monitor the status of ambulatory HF patients and preventing potential hospitalizations may involve implantable devices providing real-time hemodynamic data to the clinician. Device companies began to develop new implantable devices designed to collect hemodynamic data. These investigational devices include RV, left atrial pressure (LAP), and pulmonary artery pressure (PAP) sensors (Figs 9.19 and 9.20).

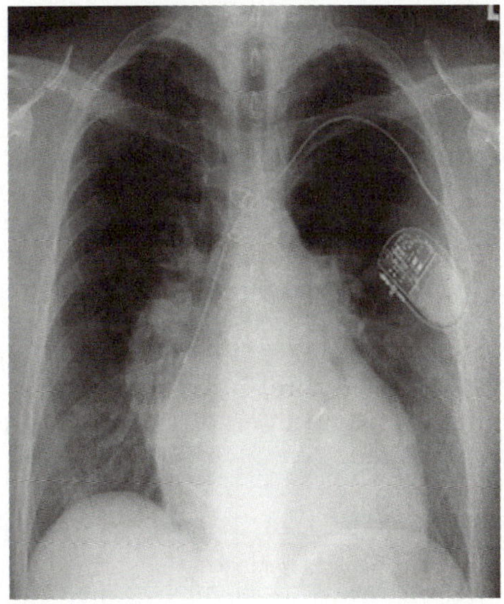

**Fig. 9.19:** The implant procedure of the Chronicle implantable hemodynamic monitoring is similar to that of a cardiac pacemaker, whereby the device is positioned subcutaneously in the pectoral area with the lead positioned transvenously in the right ventricular outflow tract. Average implant time is >1 hour

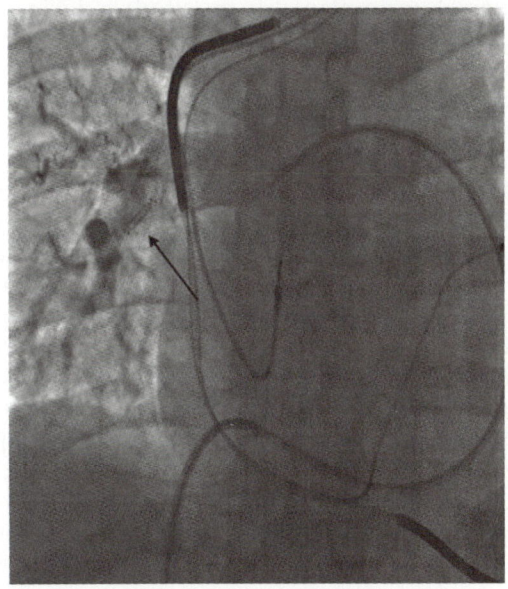

**Fig. 9.20:** Heart failure sensor implanted through right heart catheterization in the right pulmonary artery (arrow), although left is the preferred location. Flow is noted around the sensor on venogram

## Right Ventricular Pressure Monitoring

### *The Device, Implantation, and Monitored Data*

The Chronicle (model 9520, Medtronic Inc.) is an implantable hemodynamic monitor. The system consists of a specialized transvenous lead that has a sensor incorporated near the tip to measure intracardiac pressure and a programmable device similar in size and shape to a pacemaker. Details of the components have been previously described. The device is able to monitor and telemeter systolic and diastolic RV pressure, RV $dP/dt$ (positive and negative), to estimate pulmonary artery diastolic pressure, to monitor heart rate and patient's activity, and to measure core body temperature. In addition, continuous remote monitoring of data is available. The implantation procedure is similar to that of a single-lead pacemaker. The device is positioned subcutaneously in the pectoral area and the lead is placed transvenously in the RV outflow tract or septum. The patient is furnished with a small external device, which aids in correcting for barometric pressure.

The monitor capabilities includes pressure sensing circuitry and a memory to store continuous pressure trends, as well as specific triggered events such as bradyarrhythmias, tachyarrhythmias, or patient-activated episodes. The device continuously measures and stores RV systolic, diastolic, and pulse pressure, estimated pulmonary arterial diastolic pressure (ePAD), RV d*P*/d*t*, pre-ejection interval, and systolic time interval. The ePAD is defined as the RV pressure at the time of pulmonary valve opening or maximal RV d*P*/d*t* and has been shown to correlate with PA diastolic pressures ($r = 0.87$ at baseline and 1 year), thus reflecting LV filling pressure. In addition, heart rate, patient activity levels, and central venous temperature are also monitored and stored.

### Clinical Perspectives

In March 2007, FDA's circulatory system devices panel voted against the approval of Chronicle implantable hemodynamic monitor because its use was not proved to significantly improve clinical outcomes in the COMPASS-HF randomized, controlled trial. The following step has been the planning of a trial designed to test the potential usefulness of combining the hemodynamic monitoring capabilities of an implantable monitoring device with an ICD in patients at risk of sudden cardiac death. Indeed, a new trial, REDUCEhf, was designed to enrol 850 patients (then increased to 1300) with indication for an ICD (NYHA functional class II or III with reduced LVEF) to test the hypothesis that the use of RV pressure-guided patient management would reduce HF-related events (hospitalization and emergency department or urgent clinic visit requiring parenteral therapy) Because of technical complications, REDUCEhf was prematurely ended after enrolment of 400 patients. Data analysis showed no benefit from haemodynamic monitoring and a lower than expected event rate. Demonstrating the efficacy of HF disease management programmes using RV pressure monitoring was particularly difficult and many issues appear to condition the ability to demonstrate a substantial clinical benefit. These factors include the degree of HF severity in the tested population, the quality of comparative usual care (with a potential low-external validity if the trial is managed by highly specialized centres), the choice of the primary endpoint (the need for medical visits may actually increase during continuous monitoring in view of earlier detection of worsening HF, but this may imply avoidance of subsequent hospitalizations), as well as the specific characteristics of the disease management programme adopted. Moreover, it is possible that a substantial improvement in patient care will require to couple the information provided by an implantable hemodynamic sensor to an effect or capable of promptly instituting an appropriate therapy, thus 'closing the loop' and limiting the need for interventions of healthcare providers.

### Left Atrial Pressure Monitoring

Patients admitted for decompensated HF usually have elevated LAP causing pulmonary congestion and edema. The rise in LAP is usually gradual and precedes the onset of symptoms. Therefore, monitoring of LAP has the potential to forecast and abort HF decompensation by adjusting drug therapy (Figs 9.21 and 9.22).

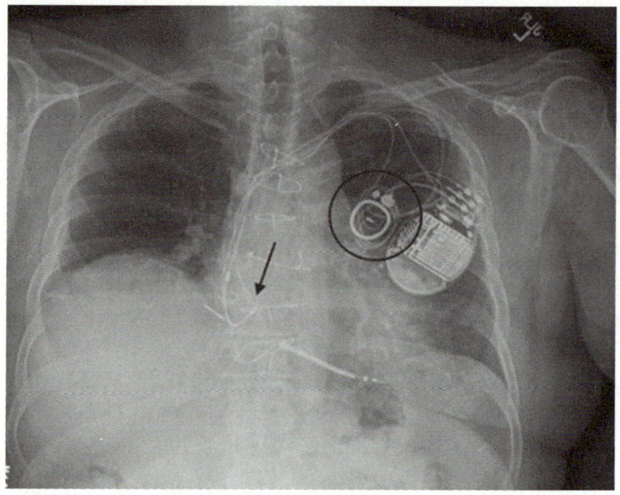

**Fig. 9.21:** Heartpod (left atrial pressure sensor, arrow) in the transseptal location attached to the coil antenna (circle) implanted in the subpectoral area. This patient also has a dual-chamber defibrillator for primary prevention with right atrial and right ventricular leads

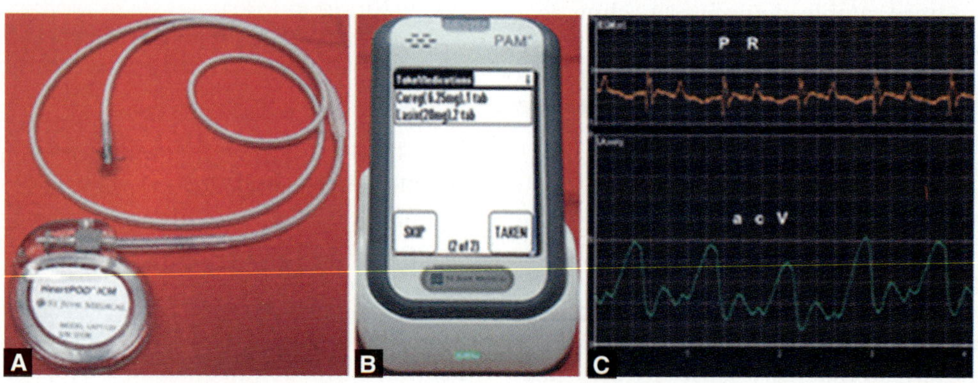


**Fig. 9.22:** (A) A standalone HeartPOD device with the communicator module connected to the sensor lead. (B) The PAM that powers the HeartPOD by telemetry, records data, and provides therapeutic advice to the patient. (C) Electrograms and LAP waveforms recorded by the HeartPOD (reproduced with kind permission by St Jude Medical)

### The Device

The HeartPOD (St Jude Medical) comprises an implantable sensor lead that measures pressure, intracardiac electrograms, and temperature, coupled to a coil antenna positioned in the subcutaneous tissue. Folding proximal and distal nitinol anchors fix the sensor lead onto the interatrial septum. The device is either standalone or coupled to a CRT-D unit. A handheld patient advisory module (PAM) powers the implanted device (which has no battery) by radiofrequency wireless transmission. The PAM also measures the atmospheric pressure, that is then subtracted from the pressure measured in the implant to obtain LAP. During interrogation, physiological waveforms of LAP and intracardiac electrograms are captured in the memory of the PAM for periods of up to 20 s. The PAM has the capacity to store ~3 months of data with six daily interrogations.

### Clinical Perspectives

Self-titration of HF therapy by patients based upon LAP readings (similar to diabetics adjusting insulin levels with glycemia) is a paradigm shift in HF management. This strategy of course requires patient participation and compliance, and may not be suitable for many individuals. Patients with diastolic HF are a therapeutic challenge, in whom volume overload may rapidly cause pulmonary congestion. Analysis of the LAPTOP-HF data in this subset of patient will clarify whether titration of diuretics based upon LAP readings improves outcome. LAP data may be of use to optimize AV delays in CRT-HeartPOD devices (as the left atrial A-wave is recorded), but has not as yet been tested.

In conclusion, preliminary data relating to the HeartPOD show good mid-term device function and hold promise for improving patient self-management in HF. These data however need to be confirmed by the ongoing randomized LAPTOP-HF trial. Device implantation requires special training, and techniques are still evolving. The presence of a lead allows extraction (contrary to PAP monitor), but further experience is required to better evaluate procedural complications (Figs 9.23 and 9.24).

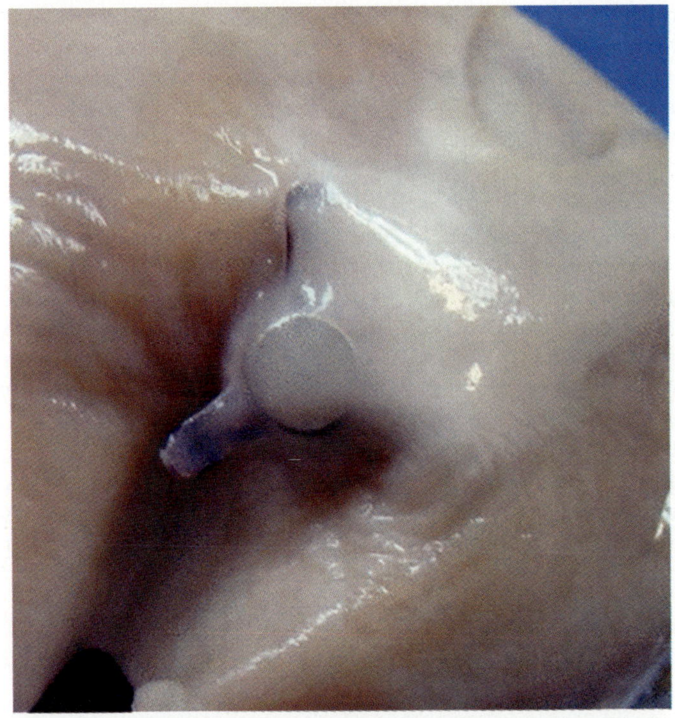

**Fig. 9.23:** Autopsy in a patient after 37 months of implantation of a HeartPOD showing endothelialisation of the pressure sensor (reproduced with kind permission by St Jude Medical)

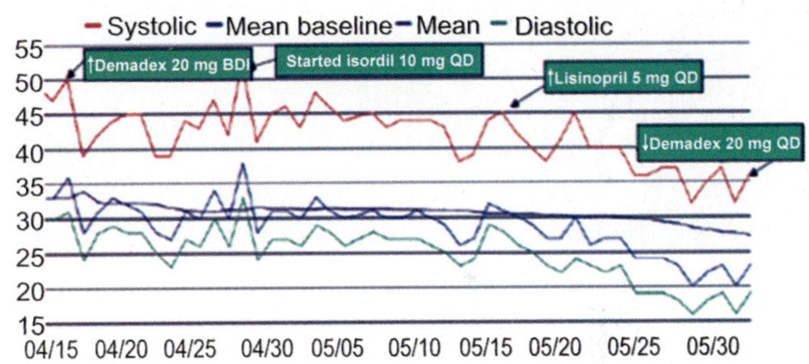


**Fig. 9.24:** Pressure-guided sensor has been used in a patient with heart failure. The patient had a history of NYHA Class III ischemic cardiomyopathy, cardiac resynchronization therapy combined with a defibrillator, atrial fibrillation, and renal insufficiency. At device implantation, the patient was on low-dose angiotensin-converting enzyme inhibitor, diuretic, and β-blocker. Vasodilating therapy and diuretic doses were titrated to maintain prespecified target pressures

## Pulmonary Artery Pressure Monitoring

### The Device

The CardioMEMS heart failure sensor (Cardio MEMS Inc.) consists of a coil and a pressure-sensitive capacitor housed in a hermetically sealed silica capsule covered in medical-grade silicone. Two wired nitinol loops at the ends of the capsule serve as anchors to prevent distal migration of the sensor. The coil and capacitor form an electrical circuit that resonates at a specific frequency. The coil allows for electromagnetic coupling to the sensor by an external antenna, which is held against the patient's body. The antenna powers the implanted device, continuously measures its resonant frequency, which is then converted to a pressure waveform. The interrogating device measures the atmospheric pressure, which is subtracted from the pressure measured by the implanted sensor. The CardioMEMS sensor is designed to measure PAP.

### Sensor Delivery System and Implantation

The CardioMEMS sensor is supplied preloaded and attached to a tether wire at the end of the delivery catheter. The sensor is implanted by using a venous femoral approach. First, a Swan–Ganz catheter is advanced into the deployment site in the pulmonary artery. After identification of the target artery, a guidewire (0.018–0.025 inch) is placed through the Swan–Ganz catheter to allow the sensor delivery catheter system to be advanced. The delivery catheter is advanced over the wire and released in the target vessel. After removal of the delivery catheter, the Swan–Ganz catheter is replaced into the pulmonary artery proximal to the sensor. Subsequently, the implanted sensor is calibrated using PAPs acquired from the Swan–Ganz catheter (Figs 9.25 and 9.26).

### Clinical Perspectives

In November 2011, FDA's circulatory system devices panel voted against the approval of the CardioMEMS implantable haemodynamic monitor because its use was not proved to significantly improve clinical outcomes in the randomized, single-blind CHAMPION trial. The greatest concern is the trial's design, which made it impossible to distinguish any treatment effect from the device itself in the single-blind trial. Physicians knew which patients had the device and specific treatment recommendations were made in the treatment group and not in the control group. Ambulatory HF patients are at high risk for hospital admission. There is an urgent need to develop strategies to reduce hospitalizations and readmission rates for HF. New technologies for invasive hemodynamic monitoring have been developed as an adjunct to clinical follow-up. The results of studies with implantable hemodynamic monitoring devices show great promise as adjunctive tools in the management of HF patients. The technology of haemodynamic monitoring is not incorporated in current defibrillators or devices with CRT. Future studies have to evaluate whether a role exists for combining impedance measurements by current cardiac devices with hemodynamic sensors.

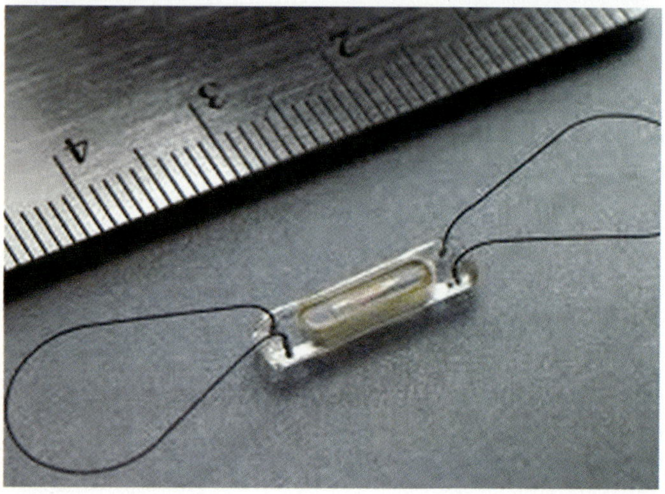

**Fig. 9.25:** The CardioMEMS sensor consists of a coil and a pressure-sensitive capacitor housed in a hermetically sealed silica capsule covered in medical-grade silicone. Two wired nitinol loops at the ends of the capsule serve as anchors to prevent distal migration of the sensor

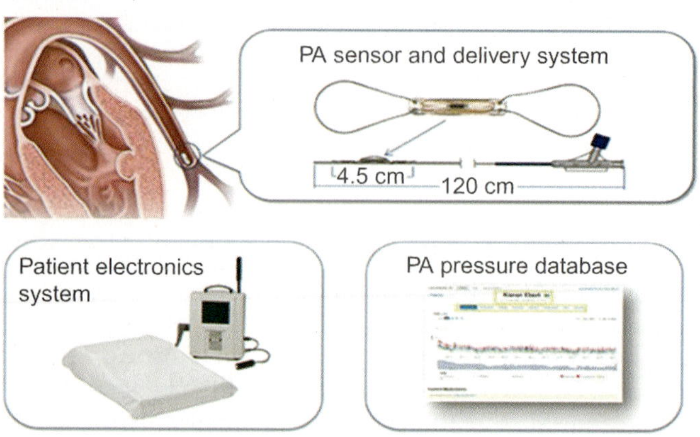


**Fig. 9.26:** FDA approves first implantable wireless device with remote monitoring to measure pulmonary artery pressure in certain heart failure patients

## BIBLIOGRAPHY

1. Abraham WT, et al Wireless pulmonary artery haemodynamic monitoring in chronic heart failure: a randomised controlled trial. Lancet 2011;377:658–66.
2. Abraham WT, et al. Cardiac resynchronization in chronic heart failure. N Engl J Med 2002;346:1845–53.
3. Abraham WT, et al. Subgroup analysis of a randomized controlled trial evaluating the safety and efficacy of cardiac contractility modulation in advanced heart failure. J Card Fail 2011;17:710–7.
4. Adamson PB, et al. Continuous hemodynamic monitoring in patients with mild to moderate heart failure: results of The Reducing Decompensation Events Utilizing Intracardiac Pressures in Patients with Chronic Heart Failure (REDUCEhf) trial. Congest Heart Fail 2011;17:248–54.
5. Andresen MC, et al. Nucleus tractussolitarius—gateway to neural circulatory control. Annu Rev Physiol 1994;56:93–116.
6. Ardell JL, et al. Dorsal spinal cord stimulation obtunds the capacity of intrathoracic extracardiac neurons to transduce myocardial ischemia. Am J Physiol Regul Integr Comp Physiol 2009;297:R470–77.
7. Armour JA, et al. Long-term modulation of the intrinsic cardiac nervous system by spinal cord neurons in normal and ischaemic hearts. Auton Neurosci 2002;95:71–9.
8. Bedder MD, et al. Spinal cord stimulation surgical technique for the nonsurgically trained. Neuromodulation 2009;12:1–19.
9. Beshai JF, et al. Cardiac-resynchronization therapy in heart failure with narrow QRS complexes. N Engl J Med 2007.
10. Bibevski S, et al. Ganglionic mechanisms contribute to diminished vagal control in heart failure. Circulation 1999;99:2958–63.
11. Bibevski S, et al. Prevention of diminished parasympathetic control of the heart in experimental heart failure. Am J Physiol Heart Circ Physiol 2004;287:H1780–5.
12. Binkley PF, et al. A polymorphism of the endothelial nitric oxide synthase promoter is associated with an increase in autonomic imbalance in patients with congestive heart failure. Am Heart J 2005;149:342–8.
13. Binkley PF, et al. Parasympathetic withdrawal is an integral component of autonomic imbalance in congestive heart failure: demonstration in human subjects and verification in a paced canine model of ventricular failure. J Am Coll Cardiol 1991;18:464–72.

14. Bisognano JD, et al. Baroreflex activation therapy lowers blood pressure in patients with resistant hypertension: results from the double-blind, randomized, placebo-controlled Rheos pivotal trial. J Am Coll Cardiol 2011; 58: 765–73.
15. Blank M, et al. Initial interactions in electromagnetic field-induced biosynthesis. J Cell Physiol 2004;199:359–63.
16. Borggrefe MM, et al. Randomized, double blind study of non-excitatory, cardiac contractility modulation electrical impulses for symptomatic heart failure. Eur Heart J 2008;29: 1019–28.
17. Bourge RC, et al. Randomized controlled trial of an implantable continuous hemodynamic monitor in patients with advanced heart failure: the COMPASS-HF study. J Am Coll Cardiol 2008;51:1073–9.
18. Brandt MC, et al. Baroreflex activation as a novel thera-peutic strategy for diastolic heart failure. Clin Res Cardiol 2011;100: 249–51.
19. Brignole M, et al. ESC guidelines on cardiac pacing and cardiac resynchronization therapy: the task force on cardiac pacing and resynchronization therapy of the European Society of Cardiology (ESC). Developed in collaboration with the European Heart Rhythm Association (EHRA). Europace 2013;15:1070–118.
20. Bristow MR, et al. Cardiac-resynchronization therapy with or without an implantable defibrillator in advanced chronic heart failure. N Engl J Med 2004;350:2140–50.
21. Bristow MR, et al. Decreased catecholamine sensitivity and beta-adrenergic-receptor density in failing human hearts. N Engl J Med 1982;307:205–11.
22. Brodison A, et al. Spinal-cord stimulation in management of angina. Lancet 1999;354:1748–9.
23. Brook AL, et al. Spinal cord stimulation: a basic approach. Tech Vasc Interv Radiol 2009;12:64–70.
24. Brunner-La Rocca HP, et al. Effect of cardiac sympathetic nervous activity on mode of death in congestive heart failure. Eur Heart J 2001;22:1136–43.
25. Burkhoff D, et al. 'Responder analysis' for assessing effectiveness of heart failure therapies based on measures of exercise tolerance. J Card Fail 2009;15:108–15.
26. Burkhoff D, et al. Nonexcitatory electrical signals for en-hancing ventricular contractility: rationale and initial investigations of an experimental treatment for heart failure. Am J Physiol Heart Circ Physiol 2005;288:H2550–6.
27. Butter C, et al. Cardiac contractility modulation electrical signals improve myocardial gene expression in patients with heart failure. J Am Coll Cardiol 2008;51:1784–9.
28. Butter C, et al. Enhanced inotropic state of the failing left ventricle by cardiac contractility modulation electrical signals is not associated with increased myocardial oxygen consumption. J Card Fail 2007;13:137–42.
29. Cameron T. Safety and efficacy of spinal cord stimulation for the treatment of chronic pain: a 20-year literature review. J Neurosurg 2004;100:254–67.
30. Cardinal R, et al. Spinal cord activation differentially modulates ischaemic electrical responses to different stressors in canine ventricles. Auton Neurosci 2004;111:37–47.
31. Cardinal R, et al. Spinal cord stimulation suppresses bradycardias and atrial tachyarrhythmias induced by mediastinal nerve stimulation in dogs. Am J Physiol Regul Integr Comp Physiol 2006;291:R1369–75.
32. Castro PF, et al. A wireless pressure sensor for monitoring pulmonary artery pressure in advanced heart failure: initial experience. J Heart Lung Transplant 2007;26:85–8.
33. Chandler MJ, et al. A mechanism of cardiac pain suppres-sion by spinal cord stimulation: implications for patients with angina pectoris. Eur Heart J 1993;14:96–105.
34. Creager MA, et al. Arterial baroreflex regulation of blood pressure in patients with congestive heart failure. J Am Coll Cardiol 1994;23:401–5.
35. Cygankiewicz I, et al. MuerteSubita en Insuficiencia Cardiaca Investigators. Heart rate turbulence predicts all-cause mortality and sudden death in congestive heart failure patients. Heart Rhythm 2008;5:1095–102.
36. Czachurski J, et al. Localization of neurons with baroreceptor input in the medial solitary nucleus by means of intracellular application of horseradish peroxidase in the cat. Neurosci Lett 1982;28:133–7.
37. Daubert JC, et al. EHRA/HRS expert consensus statement on cardiac resynchronization therapy in heart failure: implant and follow-up recommendations and management. Europace 2012;14:1236–86.
38. de Jongste MJ, et al. Stimulation characteristics, complications, and efficacy of spinal cord stimulation systems in patients with refractory angina: a prospective feasibility study. Pacing Clin Electrophysiol 1994;17:1751–60.
39. de Vries J, et al. An open label, single-centre, randomized trial of spinal cord stimulation vs. percutaneous myocardial laser revascularization in patients with refractory angina pectoris: the spirit trial. Eur Heart J 2006;27:1631–2. [Author reply 1632].
40. Dickstein K, et al; ESC Committee for Practice Guidelines. 2010 Focused Update of ESC Guidelines on device therapy in heart failure: an update of the 2008 ESC Guidelines for the diagnosis and treatment of acute and chronic heart failure and the 2007 ESC Guidelines for cardiac and resynchronization therapy. Developed with the special contribution of the Heart Failure Association and the European Heart Rhythm Association. Europace 2010;12: 1526–36.
41. Diedrichs H, et al. [Increased myocardial blood flow after spinal cord stimulation in patients with refractory angina pectoris]. Med Klin (Munich) 2003;98:146–50.
42. Diedrichs H, et al. Symptomatic relief precedes improvement of myocardial blood flow in patients under spinal cord stimulation. Curr Control Trials Cardiovasc Med 2005;6:7.
43. Eckberg DL, et al. Defective cardiac parasympathetic control in patients with heart failure. N Engl J Med 1971; 285:877–83.
44. Ekre O, et al. Feasibility of spinal cord stimulation in angina pectoris in patients with chronic pacemaker treatment for cardiac arrhythmias. Pacing Clin Electrophysiol 2003;26: 2134–41.
45. Eliasson T, et al. Myocardial turnover of endogenous opioids and calcitonin-gene-related peptide in the human heart and the effects of spinal cord stimulation on pacing-induced angina pectoris. Cardiology 1998;89:170–7.
46. Eliasson T, et al. Spinal cord stimulation in angina pectoris with normal coronary arteriograms. Coron Artery Dis 1993;4:819–27.

47. Enggaard TP, et al. Spinal cord stimulation for refractory angina in patients implanted with cardioverter defibrillators: five case reports. Europace 2010;12:1336–7.
48. Fan W, et al. Graded and dynamic reflex summation of myelinated and unmyelinated rat aortic baroreceptors. Am J Physiol 1999;277:R748–56.
49. Ferrero P, et al. Spinal cord stimulation affects T-wave alternans in patients with ischaemic cardiomyopathy: a pilot study. Europace 2008;10:506–8.
50. Foody JM, et al. Beta-blocker therapy in heart failure: scientific review. JAMA 2002;287:883–9.
51. Foreman RD, et al. Modulation of intrinsic cardiac neurons by spinal cord stimulation: Implications for its therapeutic use in angina pectoris. Cardiovasc Res 2000;47:367–75.
52. Georgakopoulos D, et al. Chronic baroreflex activation: a potential therapeutic approach to heart failure with preserved ejection fraction. J Card Fail 2011;17:167–78.
53. Gersbach PA, et al. Spinal cord stimulation treatment for angina pectoris: more than a placebo? Ann Thorac Surg 2001; 72:S1100–04.
54. Gibbons DD, et al. Neuromodulation targets intrinsic cardiac neurons to attenuate neuronally mediated atrial arrhythmias. Am J Physiol Regul Integr Comp Physiol 2012;302:R357–64.
55. Hautvast RW, et al. Effect of spinal cord stimulation on heart rate variability and myocardial ischemia in patients with chronic intractable angina pectoris—a prospective ambulatory electrocardiographic study. Clin Cardiol 1998; 21:33–8.
56. Hautvast RW, et al. Spinal cord stimulation in chronic intractable angina pectoris: a randomized, controlled efficacy study. Am Heart J 1998;136:1114–20.
57. Hegarty D. Spinal cord stimulation: the clinical application of new technology. Anesthesiol Res Pract 2012;2012: 375–691.
58. Henderson JM, et al. Nans training requirements for spinal cord stimulation devices: selection, implantation, and follow-up. Neuromodulation 2009;12:171–4.
59. Heusser K, et al. Chronic baroreflex activation: a potential therapeutic approach to heart failure with preserved ejection fraction carotid baroreceptor stimulation, sympathetic activity, baroreflex function, and blood pressure in hypertensive patients. Hypertension 2010; 55:619–26.
60. Hosobuchi Y. Electrical stimulation of the cervical spinal cord increases cerebral blood flow in humans. Appl Neurophysiol 1985;48:372–6.
61. Illig KA, et al. An implantable carotid sinus stimulator for drug-resistant hypertension: surgical technique and short-term outcome from the multicenter phase II Rheos feasibility trial. J Vasc Surg 2006;44:1213–8.
62. Imai M, et al. Therapy with cardiac contractility modulation electrical signals improves left ventricular function and remodeling in dogs with chronic heart failure. J Am Coll Cardiol 2007;49:2120–8.
63. Issa ZF, et al. Thoracic spinal cord stimulation reduces the risk of ischemic ventricular arrhythmias in a postinfarction heart failure canine model. Circulation 2005;111:3217–20.
64. Jacques F, et al. Spinal cord stimulation causes potentiation of right vagus nerve effects on atrial chronotropic function and repolarization in canines. J Cardiovasc Electrophysiol 2011;22:440–7.
65. Jesus S, et al. Initial experience with spinal cord stimulation (SCS) for the treatment of advanced heart failure. J Card Fail 2010;16:S67.
66. Kadish A, et al. A randomized controlled trial evaluating the safety and efficacy of cardiac contractility modulation in advanced heart failure. Am Heart J 2011;161:329–37.
67. Kirchheim HR. Systemic arterial baroreceptor reflexes. Physiol Rev 1976;56:100–77.
68. Klomp HM, et al. Systematic review and meta-analysis of controlled trials assessing spinal cord stimulation for inoperable critical leg ischaemia (Br J Surg 2004;91:948–55). Br J Surg 2005;92:120. author reply 120–1.
69. Kollai M, et al. Relation between baroreflex sensitivity and cardiac vagal tone in humans. Am J Phy 1994;266:H21–7.
70. Kosharskyy B, et al. Feasibility of spinal cord stimulation in a patient with a cardiac pacemaker. Pain Physician 2006; 9:249–51.
71. Kujacic V, et al. Assessment of the influence of spinal cord stimulation on left ventricular function in patients with severe angina pectoris: an echocardiographic study. Eur Heart J 1993;14:1238–44.
72. La Rovere MT, et al. ATRAMI (Autonomic Tone and Reflexes After Myocardial Infarction) Investigators. Baroreflex sensitivity and heart-rate variability in predic-tion of total cardiac mortality after myocardial infarction. Lancet 1998;351:478-84.
73. Lanza GA, et al. Effect of spinal cord stimulation on sponta-neous and stress-induced angina and 'ischemia-like' ST-segment depression in patients with cardiac syndrome X. Eur Heart J 2005;26:983–9.
74. Latif OA, et al. Spinal cord stimulation for chronic intractable angina pectoris: a unified theory on its mechanism. Clin Cardiol 2001;24:533–41.
75. Lawo T, et al. Electrical signals applied during the absolute refractory period: an investigational treatment for advanced heart failure in patients with normal QRS duration. J Am Coll Cardiol 2005;46:2229–36.
76. Li W, et al. Inflammatory cytokines and nitric oxide in heart failure and potential modulation by vagus nerve stimu-lation. Heart Fail Rev 2011;16:137–45.
77. Liu Y, et al. Thoracic spinal cord stimulation improves cardiac contractile function and myocardial oxygen consumption in a porcine model of ischemic heart failure. J Cardiovasc Electrophysiol 2011.
78. Long DM, et al. Electrical stimulation of the spinal cord and peripheral nerves for pain control. A 10-year experience. Appl Neurophysiol 1981;44:207–17.
79. Lopshire JC, et al. Spinal cord stimulation improves ventricular function and reduces ventricular arrhythmias in a canine postinfarction heart failure model. Circulation 2009;120:286–94.
80. Lund LH, et al. Prevalence, correlates, and prognostic significance of QRS prolongation in heart failure with reduced and preserved ejection fraction. Eur Heart J 2013;34:529–39.
81. Maggioni AP, et al. EURObservational Research Programme: the Heart Failure Pilot Survey (ESC-HF Pilot). Eur J Heart Fail 2010;12:1076–84.
82. Mannheimer C, et al. The problem of chronic refractory angina; report from the esc joint study group on the treatment of refractory angina. Eur Heart J 2002;23:355–70.

83. Marin-Neto JA, et al. Abnormal baroreflex control of heart rate in decompensated congestive heart failure and reversal after compensation. Am J Cardiol 1991;67:604–10.
84. Markos F, et al. Nitric oxide facilitates vagal control of heart rate via actions in the cardiac parasympathetic ganglia of the anaesthetised dog. Exp Physiol 2002;87:49–52.
85. McMurray JJ, et al. ESC guidelines for the diagnosis and treatment of acute and chronic heart failure 2012: The Task Force for the Diagnosis and Treatment of Acute and Chronic Heart Failure 2010 of the European Society of Cardiology. Developed in collaboration with the Heart Failure Association (HFA) of the ESC. Eur Heart J 2012;33:1787–847.
86. McNab D, et al. An open label, single-centre, randomized trial of spinal cord stimulation vs. percutaneous myocardial laser revascularization in patients with refractory angina pectoris: the spirit trial. Eur Heart J 2006;27:1048–53.
87. Mekhail NA, et al. Retrospective review of 707 cases of spinal cord stimulation: indications and complications.Pain Pract 2011;11:148–53.
88. Melzack R, et al. Pain mechanisms: a new theory. Science 1965;150:971–9.
89. Mendelowitz D. Firing properties of identified parasympathetic cardiac neurons in the nucleus ambiguus. Am J Physiol 1996;271:H2609–14.
90. Merchant FM, et al. Implantable sensors for heart failure. Circ Arrhythm Electrophysiol 2010;3:657–67.
91. Mohri S, et al. Cardiac contractility modulation by electric currents applied during the refractory period. Am J Physiol Heart Circ Physiol 2002;282:H1642–7.
92. Molon G, et al. ICD and neuromodulation devices: is peaceful coexistence possible? Pacing Clin Electrophysiol 2011; 34:690–3.
93. Morita H, et al. Cardiac contractility modulation with nonexcitatory electric signals improves left ventricular function in dogs with chronic heart failure. J Card Fail 2003; 9:69–75.
94. Nägele H, et al. Cardiac contractility modulation in nonresponders to cardiac resynchronization therapy. Europace 2008;10:1375–80.
95. Neelagaru SB, et al. Nonexcitatory, cardiac contractility modu-lation electrical impulses: feasibility study for advanced heart failure in patients with normal QRS duration. Heart Rhythm 2006;3:1140–7.
96. Nelson GS, et al. Left ventricular or biventricular pacing improves cardiac function at diminished energy cost in patients with dilated cardiomyopathy and left bundle-branch block [In Process Citation]. Circulation (Online) 2000;102: 3053–9.
97. Olgin JE, et al. Effects of thoracic spinal cord stimulation on cardiac autonomic regulation of the sinus and atrioventricular nodes. J Cardiovasc Electrophysiol 2002;13:475–81.
98. Olshansky B, et al. Parasympathetic nervous system and heart failure: pathophysiology and potential implications for therapy. Circulation 2008;118:863–71.
99. Ooi YC, et al. Simultaneous use of neurostimulators in patients with a preexisting cardiovascular implantable electronic device. Neuromodulation 2011;14:20–5. discussion 25–26.
100. Pappone C, et al. Cardiac contractility modulation by electric currents applied during the refractory period in patients with heart failure secondary to ischemic or idio-pathic dilated cardiomyopathy. Am J Cardiol 2002;90:1307–13.
101. Pappone C, et al. Electrical modulation of cardiac contractility: clinical aspects in congestive heart failure. Heart Fail Rev 2001;6:55–60.
102. Pappone C, et al. First human chronic experience with cardiac contractility modulation by nonexcitatory electrical currents for treating systolic heart failure: mid-term safety and efficacy results from a multicenter study. J Cardiovasc Electrophysiol 2004;15:418–27.
103. Reig E, et al. Spinal cord stimulation: a 20-year retrospective analysis in 260 patients. Neuromodulation 2009;12:232–9.
104. Ritzema J, et al. Direct left atrial pressure monitoring in ambulatory heart failure patients: initial experience with a new permanent implantable device. Circulation 2007; 116:2952–9.
105. Ritzema J, et al. Physician-directed patient self-management of left atrial pressure in advanced chronic heart failure. Circulation 2010;121:1086–95.
106. Romano M, et al. Efficacy and safety of permanent cardiac DDD pacing with contemporaneous double spinal cord stimulation. Pacing Clin Electrophysiol 1998;21:465–7.
107. Rydlewska A, et al. Changes in autonomic balance in patients with decompensated chronic heart failure. Clin Auton Res 2011;21:47–54.
108. Sabbah HN, et al. Cardiac contractilty modulation with the impulse dynamics signal: studies in dogs with chronic heart failure. Heart Fail Rev 2001;6:45–53.
109. Sabbah HN, et al. Chronic electrical stimulation of the carotid sinus baroreflex improves left ventricular function and promotes reversal of ventricular remodeling in dogs with advanced heart failure. Circ Heart Fail 2011;4:65–70.
110. Schau T, et al. Long-term outcome of cardiac contractility modulation in patients with severe congestive heart failure. Europace 2011;13:1436–44.
111. Scheffers IJM, et al. Novel baroreflex activation therapy in resistant hypertension: results of a European multi-center feasibility study. J Am Coll Cardiol 2010;56:1254–8.
112. Schimpf R, et al. Potential device interaction of a dual chamber implantable cardioverter defibrillator in a patient with continuous spinal cord stimulation. Europace 2003; 5:397–402.
113. Schwartz PJ, et al. Sympathetic-parasympathetic interaction in health and disease: abnormalities and relevance in heart failure. Heart Fail Rev 2011;16:101–7.
114. Shenkman HJ, et al. Congestive heart failure and QRS duration: establishing prognosis study. Chest 2002;122:528–34.
115. Sibell DM, et al. Successful use of spinal cord stimulation in the treatment of severe Raynaud's disease of the hands. Anesthesiology 2005;102:225–7.
116. Southerland EM, et al. Preemptive, but not reactive, spinal cord stimulation mitigates transient ischemia-induced myocardial infarction via cardiac adrenergic neurons. Am J Physiol Heart Circ Physiol 2007;292:H311–7.
117. Stix G, et al. Chronic electrical stimulation during the absolute refractory period of the myocardium improves severe heart failure. Eur Heart J 2004;25:650–5.
118. Tordoir JH, et al. An implantable carotid sinus baroreflex activating system: surgical technique and short-term

outcome from a multi-center feasibility trial for the treatment of resistant hypertension. Eur J Vasc Endovasc Surg 2007;33: 414–21.
119. Troughton RW, et al. Direct left atrial pressure monitoring in severe heart failure: long-term sensor performance. J Cardiovasc Transplant Res 2011;4:3–13.
120. Ubbink DT, et al. Spinal cord stimulation for non-reconstructable chronic critical leg ischaemia. Cochrane Database Syst Rev 2005:CD004001.
121. Vanoli E, et al. Vagal stimulation and prevention of sudden death in conscious dogs with a healed myocardial infarction. Circ Res 1991;68:1471–81.
122. Vatner DE, et al. Physiological and biochemical evidence for coordinate increases in muscarinic receptors and Gi during pacing-induced heart failure. Circulation 1996; 94:102–7.
123. Verdejo HE, et al. Comparison of a radiofrequency-based wireless pressure sensor to swan-ganz catheter and echo-cardiography for ambulatory assessment of pulmonary artery pressure in heart failure. J Am Coll Cardiol 2007; 50:2375–82.
124. Visocchi M, et al. Spinal cord stimulation and cerebral hemo-dynamics: updated mechanism and therapeutic implications. Stereotact Funct Neurosurg 2011;89:263–74.
125. Wang J, et al. Synaptic and neurotransmitter activation of cardiac vagal neurons in the nucleus ambiguus. Ann N Y Acad Sci 2001;940:237–46.
126. Wang M, et al. Long-term baroreflex activation therapy increases the threshold for the induction of lethal ventricular arrhythmias in dogs with chronic advanced heart failure. Circulation 2008;118:S721.
127. Whellan DJ, et al. Review of advanced heart failure device diagnostics examined in clinical trials and the potential benefit from monitoring capabilities. Prog Cardiovasc Dis 2011;54:107–14.
128. Wu M, et al. Putative mechanisms behind effects of spinal cord stimulation on vascular diseases: a review of experimental studies. Auton Neurosci 2008;138:9–23.
129. Wustmann K, et al. Effects of chronic baroreceptor stimulation on the autonomic cardiovascular regulation in patients with drug-resistant arterial hypertension. Hypertension 2009;54:530–6.
130. Yu CM, et al. Impact of cardiac contractility modulation on left ventricular global and regional function and remodeling. JACC Cardiovasc Imaging 2009;2:1341–9.
131. Yu CM, et al. Intrathoracic impedance monitoring in patients with heart failure: correlation with fluid status and feasibility of early warning preceding hospitalization. Circulation 2005;112:841–8.
132. Zucker IH, et al. Chronic baroreceptor activation enhances survival in dogs with pacing-induced heart failure. Hypertension 2007;50:904–10.

# 10 Recognition and Management of Syncopal Attacks

Syncope is defined as a partial or complete loss of consciousness with interruption of awareness of oneself and ones surroundings. When the loss of consciousness is temporary and there is spontaneous recovery, it is referred to as syncope or, in nonmedical quarters, fainting. Syncope accounts for one in every 30 visits to an emergency room. It is pronounced sin-ko-pea.

Syncope is due to a temporary reduction in blood flow and therefore a shortage of oxygen to the brain. This leads to lightheadedness or a 'black out' episode, a loss of consciousness. Temporary impairment of the blood supply to the brain can be caused by heart conditions and by conditions that do not directly involve the heart.

Careful and thorough evaluation of the cause of syncope is warranted in all patients. Determining that certain individuals are at 'low mortality risk' is inadequate; syncope, although often benign from a mortality perspective, tends to recur, is associated with risk of physical injury, diminishes quality-of-life, and might lead to restriction from employment or avocation. However, the diagnostic evaluation and treatment of syncope is challenging for many reasons. First, syncope is only 1 of many causes of transient loss of consciousness. Second, the patient's symptoms are fleeting, and the patient is generally fully recovered when seen in the clinic; only infrequently are there helpful physical findings. Third, spontaneous events are often unwitnessed by medical professionals; consequently, the medical history of symptom events is usually a 'second-hand' or 'third-hand' story. Finally, there is often an excessive sense of diagnostic 'urgency' that tends to result in a rush to undertake multiple poorly considered 'diagnostic' testing procedures; a deliberate approach based on initial risk stratification is more likely to reap the dual rewards of a correct diagnosis and initiation of effective treatment in a cost-effective manner (Figs 10.1–10.3).

### *How common is syncope?*

Syncope is a common condition. It affects 3% of men and 3.5% of women at some point in life. Syncope is more common as you get older and affects up to 6% of people

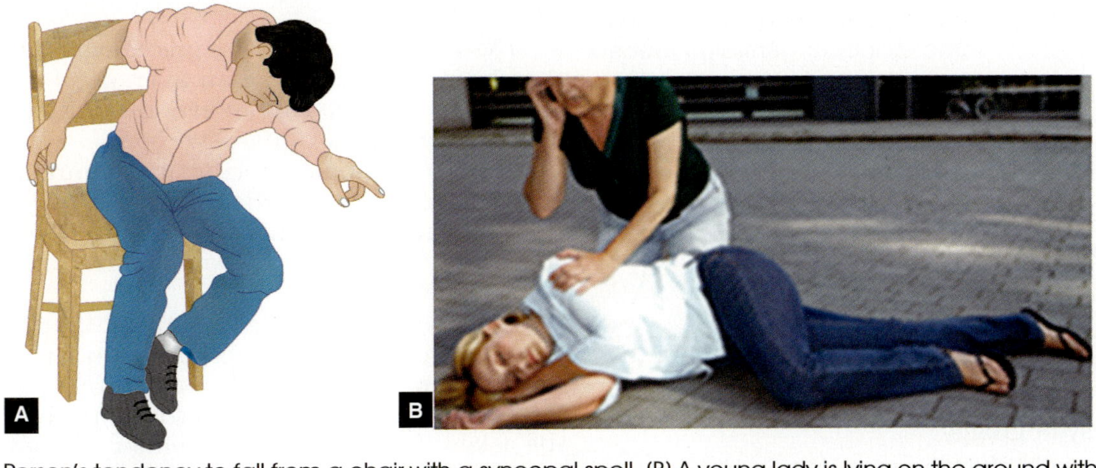

**Fig. 10.1:** (A) Person's tendency to fall from a chair with a syncopal spell. (B) A young lady is lying on the ground with syncopy and her mother is calling for medical help

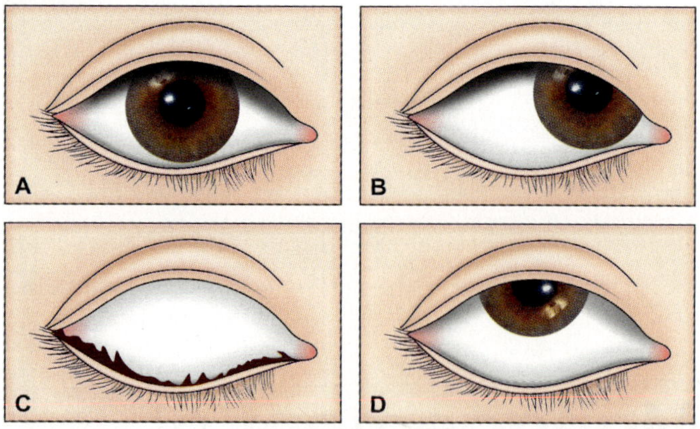


**Fig. 10.2:** Eye closure and gaze in various epileptic and non-epileptic seizures. (A) Staring during a temporal lobe seizure. (B) Lateral gaze during an extratemporal lobe seizure. (C) Closed eyes during a psychogenic; non-epileptic attack. (D) Upward gaze during a syncope

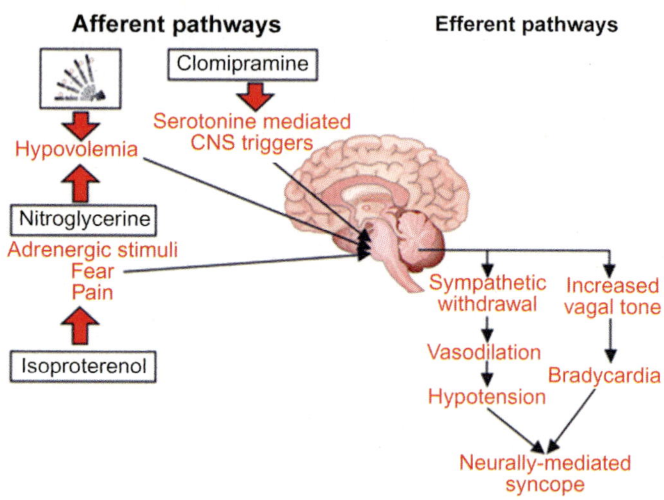


**Fig. 10.3:** This figure shows very schematically the different possible afferent pathways of neurally-mediated syncope and how tilt testing and the different drugs can act on these different triggers. Tilt testing and nitroglycerin provoke central hypovolemia by increasing venous pooling; isoproterenol, increases the adrenergic nerve tone, as happens in those cases triggered by fear or pain; clomipramine enhances central serotonergic activity as probably happens in some syncopal centrally-induced syncopal episodes

over age 75. The condition can occur at any age and happens in people with and without other medical problems.

*What are the symptoms of syncope?*

The most common symptoms of syncope include:

- Blacking out
- Feeling lightheaded
- Falling for no reason
- Feeling dizzy
- Feeling drowsy or groggy
- Fainting, especially after eating or exercising
- Feeling unsteady or weak when standing
- Changes in vision, such as seeing spots or having tunnel vision
- Headaches
- Many times, patients feel an episode of syncope coming on. They have what are called 'premonitory symptoms,' such as feeling lightheaded, nauseous, and heart palpitations (irregular heartbeats that feel like 'fluttering' in the chest). If you have syncope, you will likely be able to keep from fainting if you sit or lie down and put your legs up if you feel these symptoms.
- Syncope can be a sign of a more serious condition. So, it is important to get treatment right away after you have an episode of syncope. Most patients can prevent problems with syncope once they get an accurate diagnosis and proper treatment

*The following questions should be answered:*

- Was loss of consciousness complete?
- Was loss of consciousness with rapid onset and short duration?
- Was recovery spontaneous, complete, and without sequelae?
- Was postural tone lost?

If the answers to these questions are positive, the episode has a high likelihood of being syncope. If one or more answers are negative, consider other forms of loss of consciousness prior to proceeding with syncope evaluation. The clinician should attempt to gather all information with respect to symptoms preceding the syncope.

Prior faintness, dizziness, or light-headedness occurs in 70% of patients experiencing true syncope. Other symptoms, such as vertigo, weakness, diaphoresis, epigastric discomfort, nausea, blurred or faded vision, pallor, or paresthesias, may also occur in the presyncopal period.

Symptoms of nausea or diaphoresis prior to the event may suggest syncope rather than seizure when the episode was not witnessed, whereas an aura may suggest seizure.

Patients with true syncope do not remember actually falling to the ground. Presyncope involves the same symptoms and pathophysiology but terminates prior to loss of consciousness and can occasionally include loss of postural tone.

The duration of symptoms preceding a syncopal episode has been reported to be an average of 2.5 minutes in vasovagal syncope and an average of only 3 seconds in arrhythmia-related cardiac syncope.

Clinicians should specifically inquire as to red flag symptoms, such as exertional onset, chest pain, dyspnea, low back pain, palpitations, severe headache, focal neurologic deficits, diplopia, ataxia, or dysarthria prior to the syncopal event.

Patients should be asked to estimate the duration of their loss of consciousness. Syncope is associated with patient estimates ranging from seconds up to 1 minute in most cases. To discriminate from seizures, patients should also be asked if they remember being confused about their surroundings after the event or whether they have oral trauma, incontinence, or myalgias.

A detailed account of the event must also be obtained from any available witnesses. Witnesses can aid the clinician in differentiating among syncope, altered mental status, and seizure.

Convulsive activity, automatisms, or attempts to elicit focality can indicate seizure. Witnesses may be able to estimate the duration of unconsciousness and to assist in ascertaining whether the patient experienced postevent confusion.

Postevent confusion is the most powerful tool for discriminating between syncope and seizure. A postictal phase suggests that a seizure has occurred. Postevent confusion has been described with syncope, but the confusion should not last more than 30 seconds. Seizure-like activity can occur with syncope if the patient is held in an upright posture.

A medication history must be obtained in all patients with syncope with special emphasis placed on cardiac and antihypertensive medications. Drugs commonly implicated in syncope include the following:

- Agents that reduce blood pressure (e.g. antihypertensive drugs, diuretics, and nitrates)
- Agents that affect cardiac output (e.g. beta-blockers, digitalis, and antiarrhythmics)
- Agents that prolong the cardiac output (QT) interval (e.g. tricyclic antidepressants, phenothiazines, quinidine, and amiodarone)
- Agents that alter sensorium (including alcohol, cocaine, analgesics with sedative properties)
- Agents that alter serum electrolytes (especially diuretics)

Inquiry must be made into any personal or familial past medical history of cardiac disease. Patients with a history of myocardial infarction (MI), arrhythmia, structural cardiac defects, cardiomyopathies, or CHF have a uniformly worse prognosis than other patient groups.

Remember to consider the broad differential diagnosis of syncope. Assess whether the patient has a history of seizure disorder, diabetes, stroke (CVA), deep venous thrombosis (DVT), or abdominal aortic aneurysm or if pregnancy is a possibility.

**Table 10.1:** Causes of nonsyncopal attacks (commonly misdiagnosed as syncope)

*Disorders without any impairment of consciousness*

- Falls
- Cataplexy
- Drop attacks
- Psychogenic pseudosyncope
- Transient ischaemic attacks (TIA) of carotid origin

*Disorders with partial or complete loss of consciousness*

- Metabolic disorders, including hypoglycemia, hypoxia, hyperventilatio with hypocapnia
- Epilepsy
- Intoxications
- Vertebro-basilar TIA

## Causes

Cardiac (cardiopulmonary) syncope may be due to vascular disease, cardiomyopathy, arrhythmia, or valvular dysfunction and predicts a worse short-term and long-term prognosis. Obtaining an initial ECG is mandatory if any of these causes are possible for the differential diagnosis. Low flow states, such as those associated with advanced cardiomyopathy, CHF, and valvular insufficiency, may result in hypotension and cause transient global cerebral hypoperfusion. Often, these patients are on medications that reduce afterload, which may contribute to the cause of syncope (Tables 10.1–10.3 and Fig. 10.4 ).

*Diagnosis of syncope:* Dizzy spells or syncopal attacks can be diagnosed with different approaches because it is considered as multifactorial entity (Table 10.4).

*Ventricular arrhythmias* (Fig. 10.5), such as ventricular tachycardia and torsade de pointes, tend to occur in older patients with known cardiac disease. These patients tend to have fewer recurrences and have a more sudden onset with few, if any, presyncopal symptoms. Associated chest pain or dyspnea may be present. This type of syncope is generally unrelated to posture and can occur during lying, sitting, or standing. Often, these arrhythmias are not

**Table 10.2:** Clinical features suggestive of specific causes of syncope

*Neurally-mediated syncope*

- Absence of cardiac disease
- Long history of syncope
- After sudden unexpected unpleasant sight, sound, smell or pain
- Prolonged standing or crowded, hot places
- Nausea, vomiting associated with syncope
- During or in the absorptive state after a meal
- With head rotation, pressure on carotid sinus (as in tumors, shaving, tight collars)
- After exertion

*Syncope caused by orthostatic hypotension*

- After standing up
- Temporal relationship with start of medication leading to hypotension or changes of dosage
- Prolonged standing especially in crowded, hot places
- Presence of autonomic neuropathy or Parkinsonism
- After exertion

*Cardiac syncope*

- Presence of severe structural heart disease
- During exertion, or supine
- Preceded by palpitation or accompanied by chest pain
- Family history of sudden death

*Cerebrovascular syncope*

- With arm exercise
- Differences in blood pressure or pulse in the two arms

**Table 10.3:** Causes of syncope

*Neurally-mediated (reflex)*

- Vasovagal syncope (common faint)
  - Classical
  - Nonclassical
- Carotid sinus syncope
- Situational syncope
  - Acute hemorrhage
  - Cough, sneeze
  - Gastrointestinal stimulation (swallo, defaecation, visceral pain)
  - Micturition (post-micturition)
  - Postexercise
  - Postparandial
  - Others (e.g. brass instrument playing, weightlifting)
- Glossopharyngeal neuralgia

*Orthostatic hypotension*

- Automomic failure
  - Primary autonomic failure syndromes (e.g. pure autonomic failure, multiple system atrophy, Parkinson's disease with autonomic failure)
  - Secondary autonomic failure syndromes (e.g. diabetic neuropathy, amyloid neuropathy)
  - Drugs and alcohol
  - Postexercise
  - Postparadial
- Volume depletion
  - Hemorrhage, diarrhoea, and Addison's disease

*Cardiac arrhythmias as primary cause*

- Sinus node dysfunction (including bradycardia/tachycardia syndrome)
- Atrioventricular conduction system disease
- Paroxysmal supraventricular and ventricular tachycardias
- Inherited syndromes (e.g. long QT syndrome, Brugada syndrome)
- Implanted device (pacemaker, implantable cardioverter-defibrillator) malfunction
- Drug-induced arrhythmias

*Structural cardiac or cardiopulmonary disease*

- Obstructive cardiac valvular disease
- Acute myocardial infarction/ischemia
- Obstructive cardiomyopathy
- Atrial myxoma
- Acute aortic dissection

revealed on the initial ECG but may be captured with prolonged monitoring.

*Supraventricular tachyarrhythmias* include supraventricular tachycardia and atrial fibrillation with rapid response. These may be associated with palpitations, chest pain, or dyspnea. Patients typically have prodromal symptoms and may have syncope while attempting to stand or walk because of resultant hypotension. These symptoms may spontaneously resolve prior to evaluation but are often noted during initial triage and assessment. Be sure to scrutinize ECG findings for evidence of Wolff-Parkinson-White syndrome, Brugada syndrome, and long QT syndrome (Fig. 10.6).

*Bradyarrhythmias* (Figs 10.7) include sick sinus syndrome, sinus bradycardia, high-grade atrioventricular blocks, pacemaker malfunction, and adverse medication reactions. Generally, these patients have a history of cardiac problems and are symptomatic. Chest pain, dyspnea, decreased exercise tolerance, and fatigue may all be present. Consider cardiac ischemia and medication side-effects as additional causes.

Cardiac outflow obstruction may also result in sudden-onset syncope with little or no prodrome. One critical clue is the exertional nature, and the other is the presence of a cardiac murmur. Young athletes may present with this aetiology for syncope. Specific pathology includes aortic stenosis, hypertrophic obstructive cardiomyopathy, mitral stenosis, pulmonary stenosis, pulmonary embolus, left atrial myxoma, and pericardial tamponade.

Syncope can also result from an acute MI, acute aortic dissection, and pulmonary embolus. These conditions can have associated chest pain, neck pain, shoulder pain, dyspnea, epigastric pain, hypotension, alteration of mental status and can result in sudden death.

*Reflex* (neurally mediated) syncope may be due to vasovagal syncope, which is mediated by emotional distress such as fear or physical pain. Situational syncope describes syncope that occurs with a fixed event such as micturition, deglutition, exercise induced, and carotid sinus syncope. These causes tend to be more benign and do not predict poor outcomes (Table 10.5).

*Vasovagal syncope* is the most common type in young adults but can occur at any age. It usually occurs in a standing position and is precipitated by fear, emotional stress, or pain (e.g. after a needlestick). Autonomic symptoms are predominant. Classically, nausea, diaphoresis, fading or 'graying out' of vision, epigastric discomfort, and light-headedness precede syncope by a few minutes. Syncope is thought to occur secondary to efferent vasodepressor reflexes by a number of mechanisms, resulting in decreased peripheral vascular resistance. It is not life threatening and occurs sporadically.

*Situational syncope* is essentially a reproducible vasovagal syncope with a known precipitant. Micturition, defecation, deglutition, tussive, and carotid sinus syncope are types of situational syncope. These stimuli result in autonomic reflexes with a vasodepressor response, ultimately leading to transient cerebral hypotension. These are not life-threatening but can cause morbidity. The treatment involves avoidance of the precipitant when possible and the initiation of counter manoeuvres when anticipated.

*Syncope due to orthostatic hypotension* can occur through several mechanisms. Pure autonomic failure can be associated with Parkinson's disease or dementia. Secondary

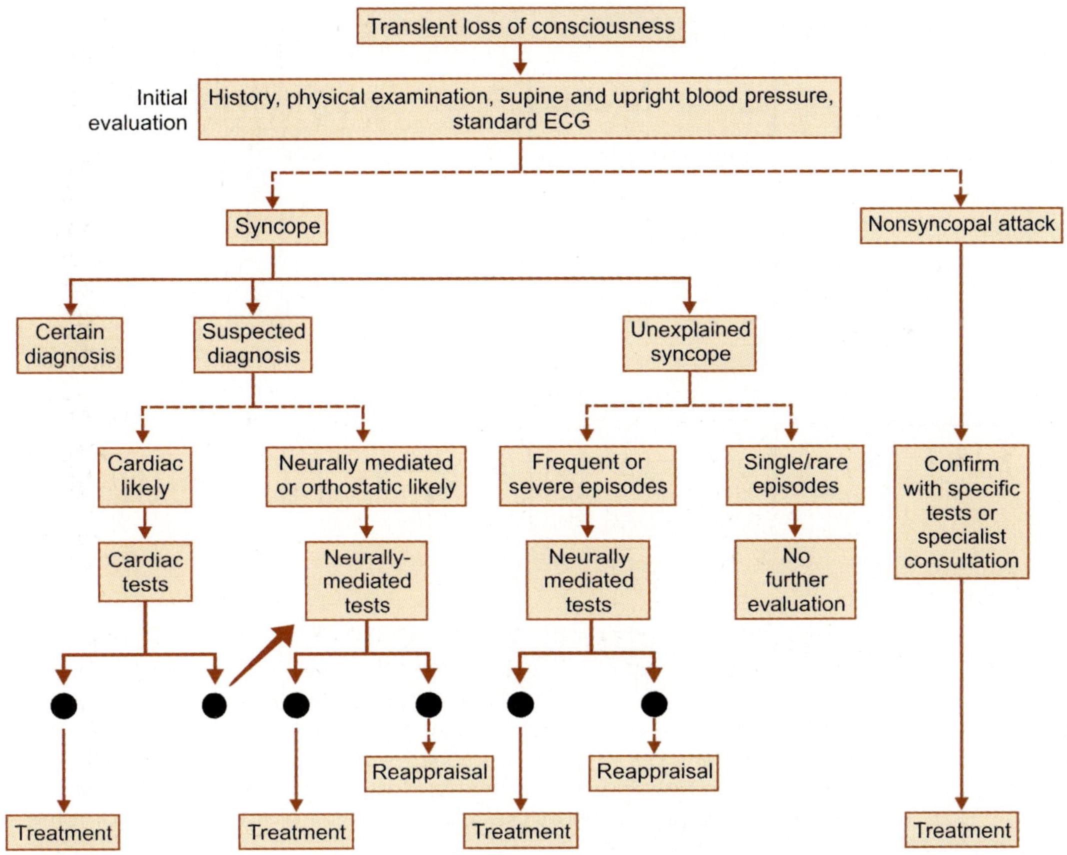


**Fig. 10.4:** Flow diagram outlining an approach to the evaluation of loss of consciousness on the basis of the initial evaluation. Differentiating true syncope from other 'nonsyncopal' spells is the first diagnostic step and affects the subsequent diagnostic strategy. Among cardiac investigations, echocardiography, prolonged electrocardiographic (ECG) monitoring, stress testing, electrophysiological study, and implantable loop recorder (ILR) are most useful. Among neurally-mediated investigations, tilt test, carotid sinus massage, and ILR are most useful. From Europace,1 with permission from the European Society of Cardiology

**Table 10.4:** Recommendations—diagnostic criteria with initial evaluation

| Recommendations | Class[a] | Class[b] |
|---|---|---|
| • VVS is diagnosed if syncope is precipitated by emotional distress or orthostatic stress and is associated with typical prodrome | I | C |
| • Situational syncope is diagnosed if syncope occurs during or immediately after specific triggers listed in Table 10.5 | I | C |
| • Orthostatic syncope is diagnosed when it occurs after standing up and there is documentation of OH | I | C |
| • Arrhythmia-related syncope is diagnosed by ECG when there is: | | |
| » Persistent sinus bradycardia <40 bpm is awake or repetitivesinoatrial block or sinus pauses ≥3s | | |
| » Mobitz II second or third degree AV block | | |
| » Alternating left and right BBB | | |
| » VT or rapid paroxysmal SVT | | |
| » Non-sustained episodes of polymorphic VT and long or short QT interval | | |
| » Pacemaker or ICD malfunction with cardiac pauses | | |
| • Cardiac ischemia-related syncope is diagnosed when syncope presents with ECG evidence of acute ischemia with or without myocardial infarction | I | C |
| • Cardiovascular syncope is diagnosed when syncope presents in patients with prolapsing atrial myxoma, severe aortic stenosis, pulmonary hypertension, pulmonary embolus, or acute aortic dissection | I | C |

[a]Class of recommendation. [b]Level of evidence. AV=atrioventricular; BBB=bundle branch block; ECG=electrocardiogram; ICD=implantable cardioverter defibrillator; OH=orthostatic hypotension; SVT=supraventricular tachycardia; VVS=vasovagal syncope; VT=ventricular tachycardia.

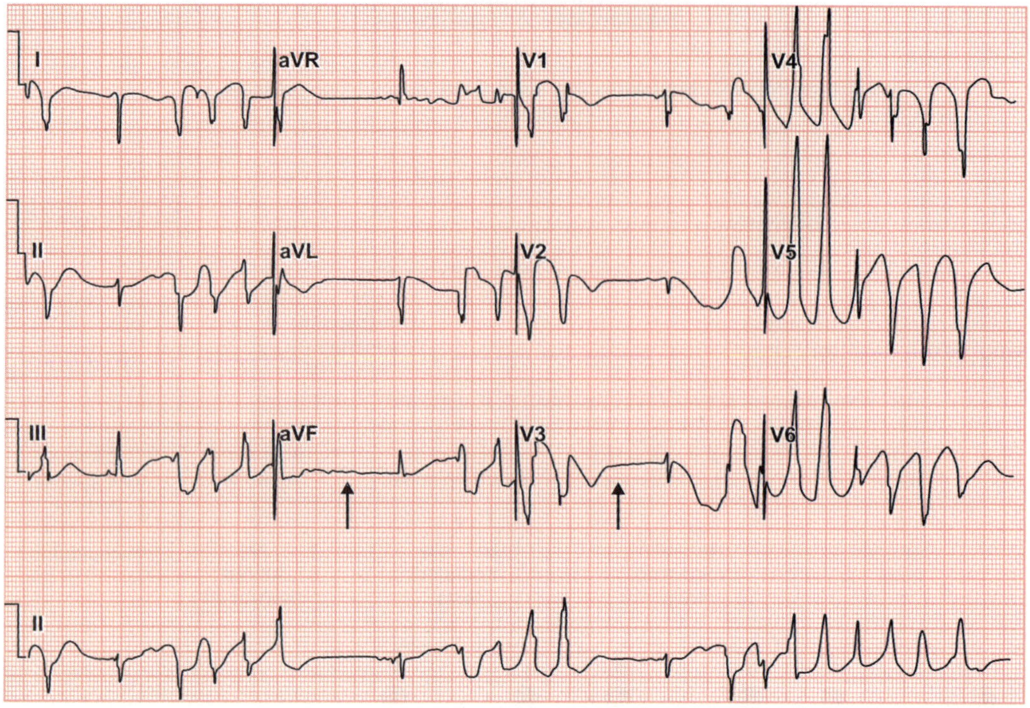


**Fig. 10.5:** 38 years of patient presented with syncope showed defects in ion channels predispose patients to episodes of torsade de pointes (TdP), which can cause cardiac arrest. TdP is a form of polymorphic ventricular tachycardia that results in a characteristic twisting of the QRS complex around the isoelectric baseline. This arrhythmia is associated with LQTS and can degenerate into more unstable rhythms. In the case of acquired LQTS, a pause usually precedes the onset of TdP. This form of TdP is said to be 'pause dependent' (arrows). Image courtesy of ECG Wave-Maven

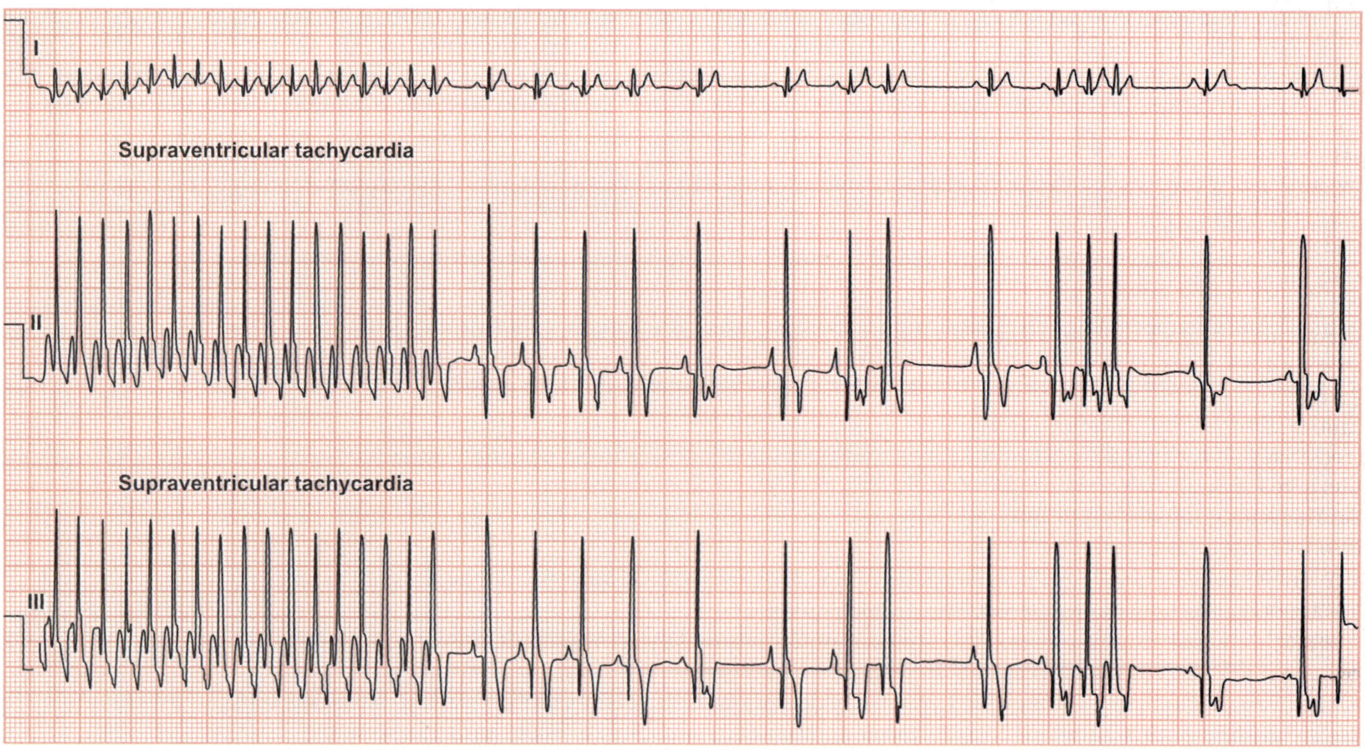


**Fig. 10.6:** 48-years-patient presented with syncope showed episodes of supraventricular tachycardia

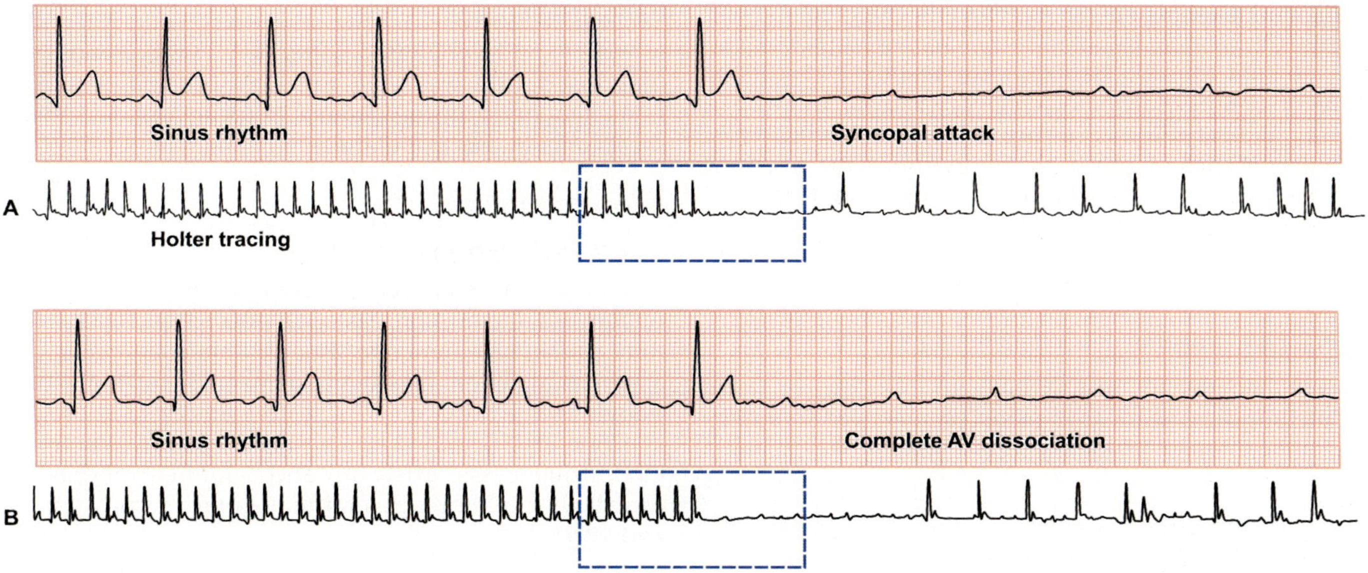


**Fig. 10.7:** Holter EC graph showing narrow QRS complex in a patient suffering from congenital complete heart block respectively presening as syncopal attacks

**Table 10.5:** Recommendations: treatment of reflex syncope

| Recommendations | Class[a] | Class[b] |
|---|---|---|
| • Explanation of the diagnosis, provision of reassurance, and explanation of risk of recurrence are indicated in all patients | I | C |
| • Isometric PCMs are indicated in patients with prodrome | I | B |
| • Cardiac pacing should be considered in patients with dominant cardioinhibitory CSS | IIa | B |
| • Cardiac pacing should be considered in patients with frequent recurrent reflex syncope, age >40 years, and documented spontaneous | IIb | B |
| • Midodrine may be indicated in patients with VVS refractory to lifestyle measures | IIb | B |
| • Tilt training may be useful for education of patients but long-term benefit depends on compliance | IIb | B |
| • Cardiac pacing may be indicated in patients with recurrent frequent unpredictable syncope and age >40 after alternative therapy has failed | IIb | C |
| • Cardiac pacing is not indicated in the absence of a documented cardioinhibitory reflex | III | C |
| • β-adrenergic blocking drugs are not indicated | III | A |

[a]Class of recommendation. [b]Level of evidence. CSS=carotid sinus syndrome; PCM=physical isometric counterpressure manouuvre; VVS=vasovagal syncope.

autonomic insufficiency can be due to diabetes, uremia, or spinal injury. Drugs such as alcohol cause orthostatic intolerance and medications such as vasodilators and antidepressants block orthostatic reflexes. Volume depletion due to blood loss, vomiting, diarrhea, poor oral intake, and diuretics also cause orthostatic syncope.

Dehydration and decreased intravascular volume contribute to orthostasis (Table 10.6).

Orthostatic syncope describes a causative relationship between orthostatic hypotension and syncope. Orthostatic hypotension increases in prevalence with age as a blunted baroreceptor response results in failure of compensatory cardioacceleration. In elderly patients, 45% of these cases are related to medications. Limited evidence suggests that polydipsia may reduce recurrences.

Orthostasis is a common cause of syncope and tends to be recurrent. Bedside orthostatics cannot exclude this as an aetiology; if suspected, patients should be referred to a primary care provider for outpatient tilt-table testing.

Dehydration and decreased intravascular volume contribute to orthostasis. Orthostatic syncope describes a

**Table 10.6:** Recommendations: treatment of orthostatic hypotension

| Recommendations | Class[a] | Class[b] |
|---|---|---|
| • Adequate hydration and salt intake must be maintained | I | C |
| • Midodrine should be administered as adjunctive therapy if needed | IIa | B |
| • Fludrocortisone should be administered as adjunctive therapy if needed | IIa | C |
| • PCMs may be indicated | IIb | C |
| • Abdominal binders and/or support stockings to reduce venous pooling may be indicated | IIb | C |
| • Head-up tilt sleeping (>10°) to increase fluid volume may be indicated | IIb | C |

[a]Class of recommendation. [b]Level of evidence. PCM=physical counter pressure manoeuvre.

causative relationship between orthostatic hypotension and syncope. Orthostatic hypotension increases in prevalence with age as a blunted baroreceptor response results in failure of compensatory cardioacceleration. In elderly patients, 45% of these cases are related to medications. Limited evidence suggests that polydipsia may reduce recurrences. Orthostasis is a common cause of syncope and tends to be recurrent. Bedside orthostatics cannot exclude this as an aetiology; if suspected, patients should be referred to a primary care provider for outpatient tilt-table testing.

## LABORATORY STUDIES

Currently, no specific testing has sufficient power to be absolutely indicated for evaluation of syncope. Research-based and consensus guideline recommendations are listed below.

*Serum glucose level:* In one study, 2 of 170 patients with syncope tested for serum glucose were found to be hypoglycemic. Despite this low yield, rapid blood glucose assessment is easy, fast, and may be diagnostic, leading to efficient intervention.

*CBC count:* If performed empirically, a CBC count has an exceedingly low yield in syncope. Some risk stratification protocols use a low hematocrit level as a poor prognostic indicator.

A prospective evaluation of syncope found that 4 of 170 patients had signs and symptoms of GI hemorrhage with a confirmatory CBC count. No occult bleeding was diagnosed based on an empiric CBC count in this study. Anemia has been shown in several studies to suggest poor short-term outcomes.

### Serum Electrolyte Levels with Renal Function

These tests if performed empirically have an exceedingly low yield in syncope. Some risk stratification protocols use electrolyte level abnormalities and renal insufficiency as poor prognostic indicators. In the study by Martin et al. 134 patients with syncope had electrolytes drawn as part of the routine workup. One patient was unexpectedly found to be hyponatremic secondary to diuretic use.

Serum electrolyte tests are indicated in patients with altered mental status or in patients in whom seizure is being considered. If arrhythmia is noted, evaluation of electrolytes may be useful.

### Cardiac Enzymes

These tests are indicated in patients who give a history of chest pain with syncope, dyspnea with syncope, or exertional syncope; those with multiple cardiac risk factors; and those in whom a cardiac origin is highly suspected.

### Total Creatine Kinase

A rise in creatine kinase (CK) levels may be associated with prolonged seizure activity or muscle damage secondary to a prolonged period of loss of consciousness.

**BNP level** >300 pg/ml is a predictor of serious outcomes at 30 days.

### Urinalysis/Dipstick

In elderly and debilitated patients, UTI is common, easily diagnosed, and treatable and may precipitate syncope. UTIs may occur in the absence of fever, leukocytosis, and symptoms in this population.

## IMAGING STUDIES

### Chest Radiography

In elderly patients and in patients who are debilitated, pneumonia is common, easily diagnosed, and treatable and may precipitate syncope. Pneumonia may occur in the absence of fever, leukocytosis, and symptoms in this population. Evaluation of a select number of etiologies of syncope may be aided by chest radiography. Pneumonia, CHF, lung mass, effusion, and widened mediastinum can all be seen if present and may guide therapy (Figs 10.8 and 10.9).

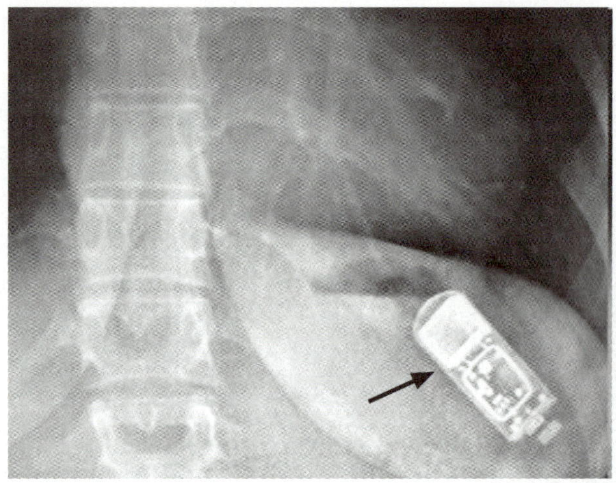

**Fig. 10.8:** Collimated frontal view of the chest shows an implantable loop recorder (arrow) in the left breast of a 25-year-old woman with syncope

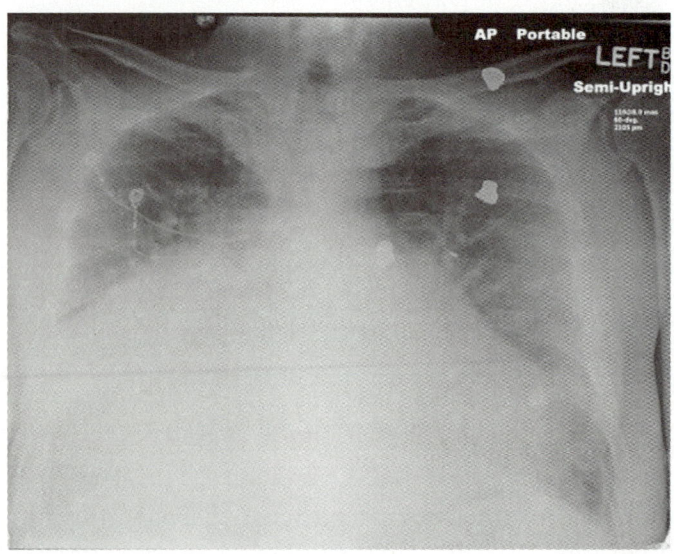


**Fig. 10.9:** Chest X-ray showing massive cardiomegaly due to CHF in elderly person with syncopal attacks

### Head CT Scanning (Noncontrast)

Head CT scanning is not indicated in a nonfocal patient after a syncopal event. This test has a low diagnostic yield in syncope.

Of 134 patients prospectively evaluated for syncope using CT scanning, 39 patients had abnormal findings on scans. Only 1 head CT scan was diagnostic in a patient not expected to have intracranial pathology. Of the remaining scans, 5 showed subdural hematomas thought to be secondary to syncope.

Head CT scanning may be clinically indicated in patients with new neurologic deficits or in patients with head trauma secondary to syncope.

*Chest/abdominal CT scanning* (Fig. 10.10): This imaging study is indicated only in select cases, such as cases in which aortic dissection, ruptured abdominal aortic aneurysm, or pulmonary embolus is suspected.

*Brain MRI/magnetic resonance arteriography (MRA)* (Fig. 10.11): These tests may be required in select cases to evaluate vertebrobasilar vasculature and are more appropriately performed on an inpatient basis in consultation with a neurologist or a neurosurgeon.

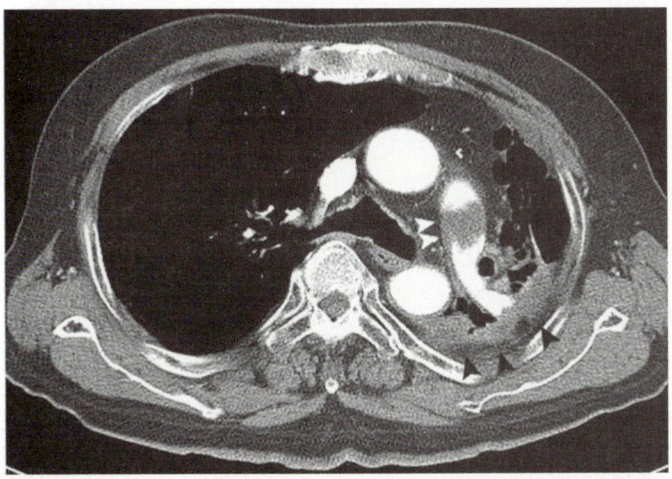

**Fig. 10.10:** Rarity of isolated pulmonary embolism and acute aortic syndrome occurring outside of the field of view of dedicated coronary CT angiography in patient with syncope

*Ventilation-perfusion (V/Q) scanning:* This test is appropriate for patients in whom pulmonary embolus is suspected.

*Echocardiography* (Figs 10.12 and 10.13): In patients with known heart disease, left ventricular function and ejection fraction have been shown to have an accurate predictive correlation with death. Echocardiography is the test of choice for evaluating suspected mechanical cardiac causes of syncope

*Electrocardiography* (Figs 10.14–10.20 and Tables 10.7–10.9): Obtain a standard 12-lead ECG in syncope. This is a level A recommendation by 2007 ACEP consensus

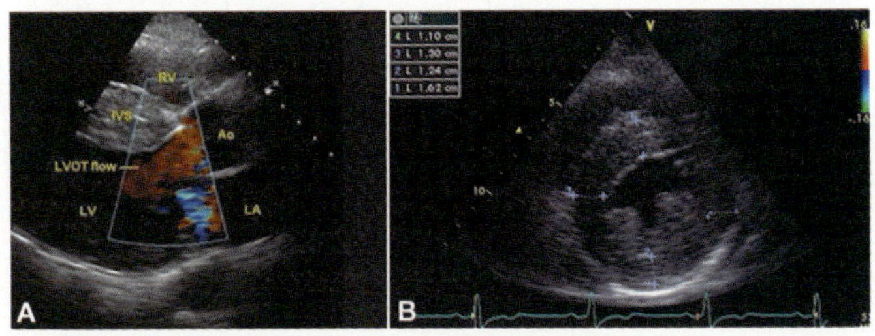


**Fig. 10.12:** Color Doppler 2-D echocardiogram in long (A) and short axis (B) views showing marked hypertrophy of interventricular septum and posterior left ventricular wall, almost approximating anterior mitral valve leaflet with hypertrophied interventricular septum producing severe left ventricular outflow tract obstruction in patient with hypertrophic cardiomyopathy presenting as syncopal attack

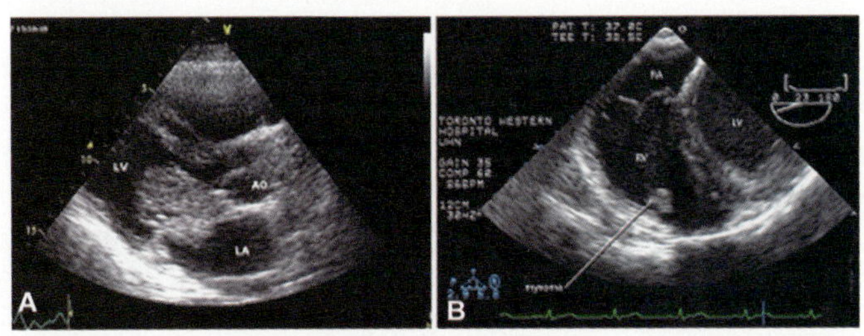


**Fig. 10.13:** (A) 2-D LAX view showing mass prolapsing across the mitral valve during diastole. (B) TEE showing myxoma in the right ventricular cavity in two different patients presenting with syncopal attacks

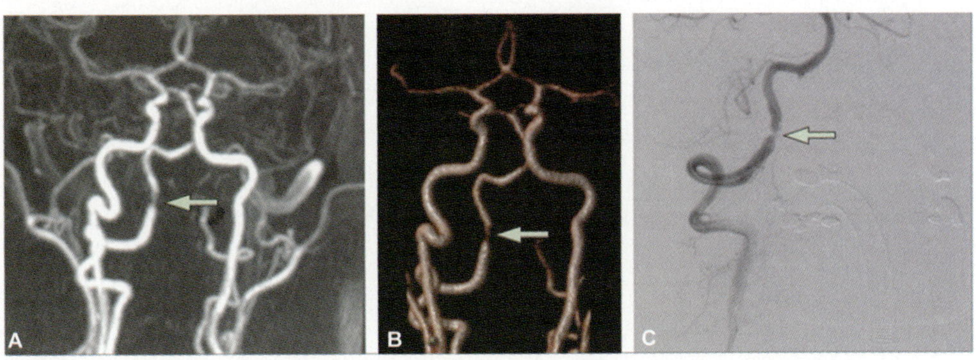


**Fig. 10.11:** MRI (A) CT angiography (B) and conventional angiography (C) of posterior circulation in an elderly patient with ischemic stroke and transient syncopal attack

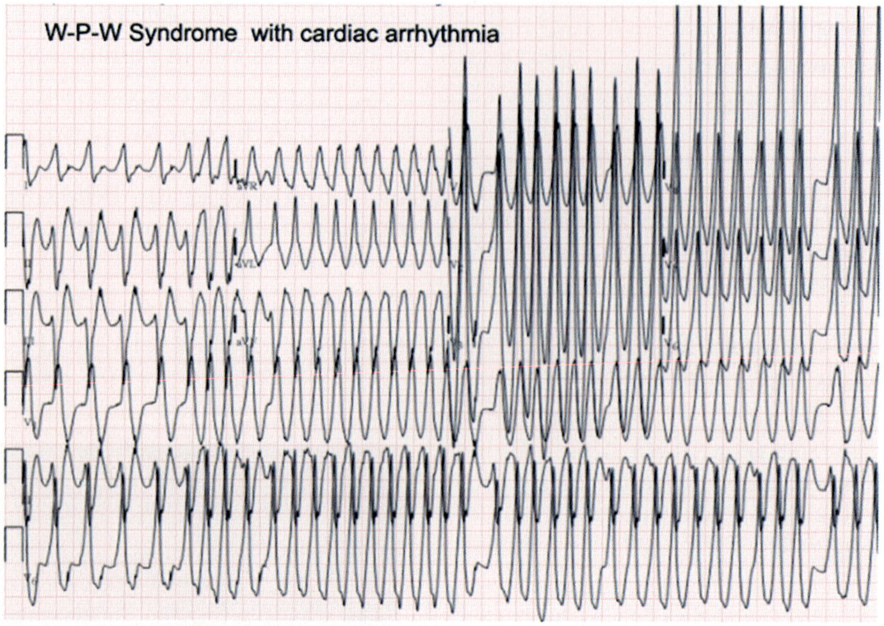


**Fig. 10.14:** ECG—supraventricular arrhythmia in W-P-W syndrome in patient with syncopal attacks

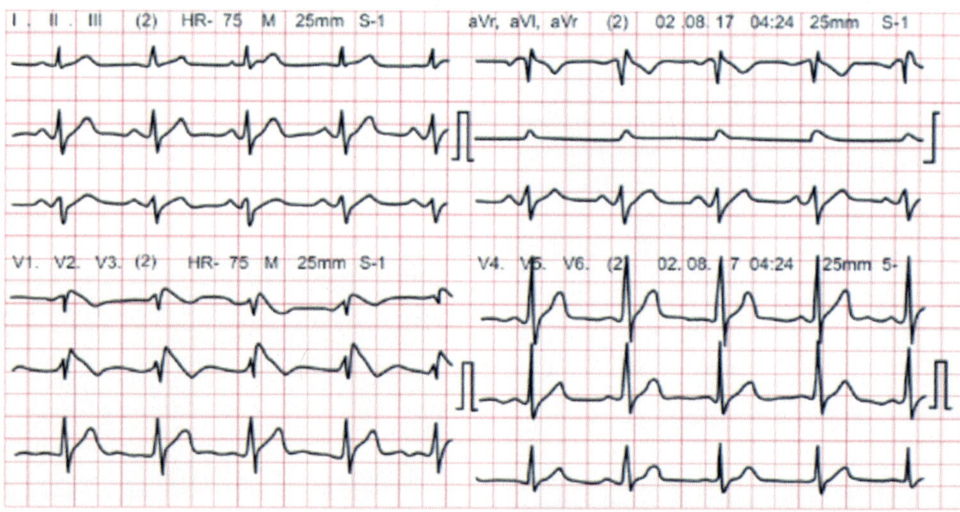


**Fig. 10.15:** Holter diagnosis of Brugada syndrome in a young male who presented with syncopal episode

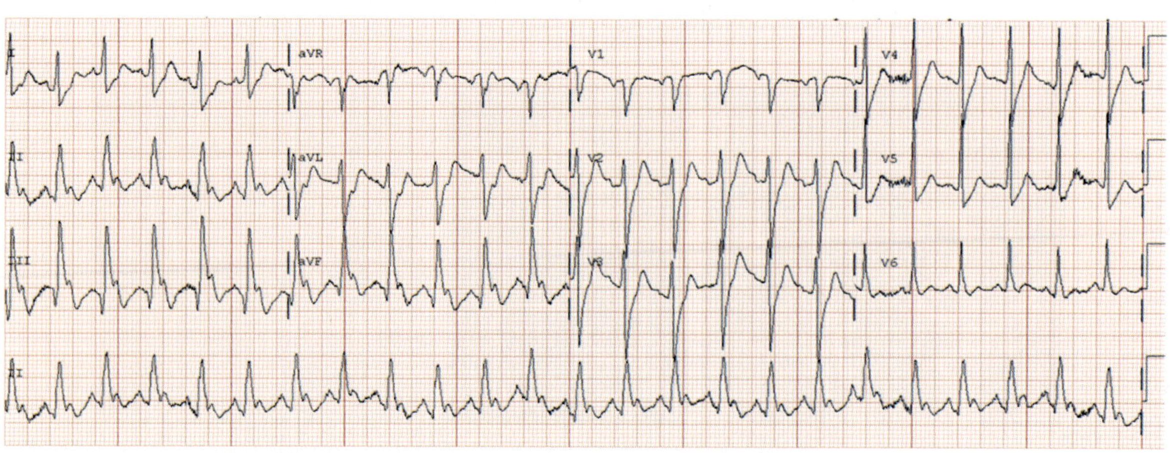


**Fig. 10.16:** ECG—atrial flutter in patient with syncopal attacks

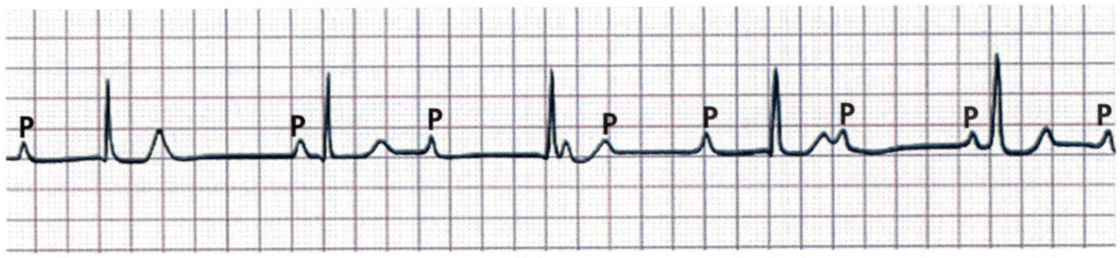


**Fig. 10.17:** ECG—complete AV dissociation in patient with syncopal attacks

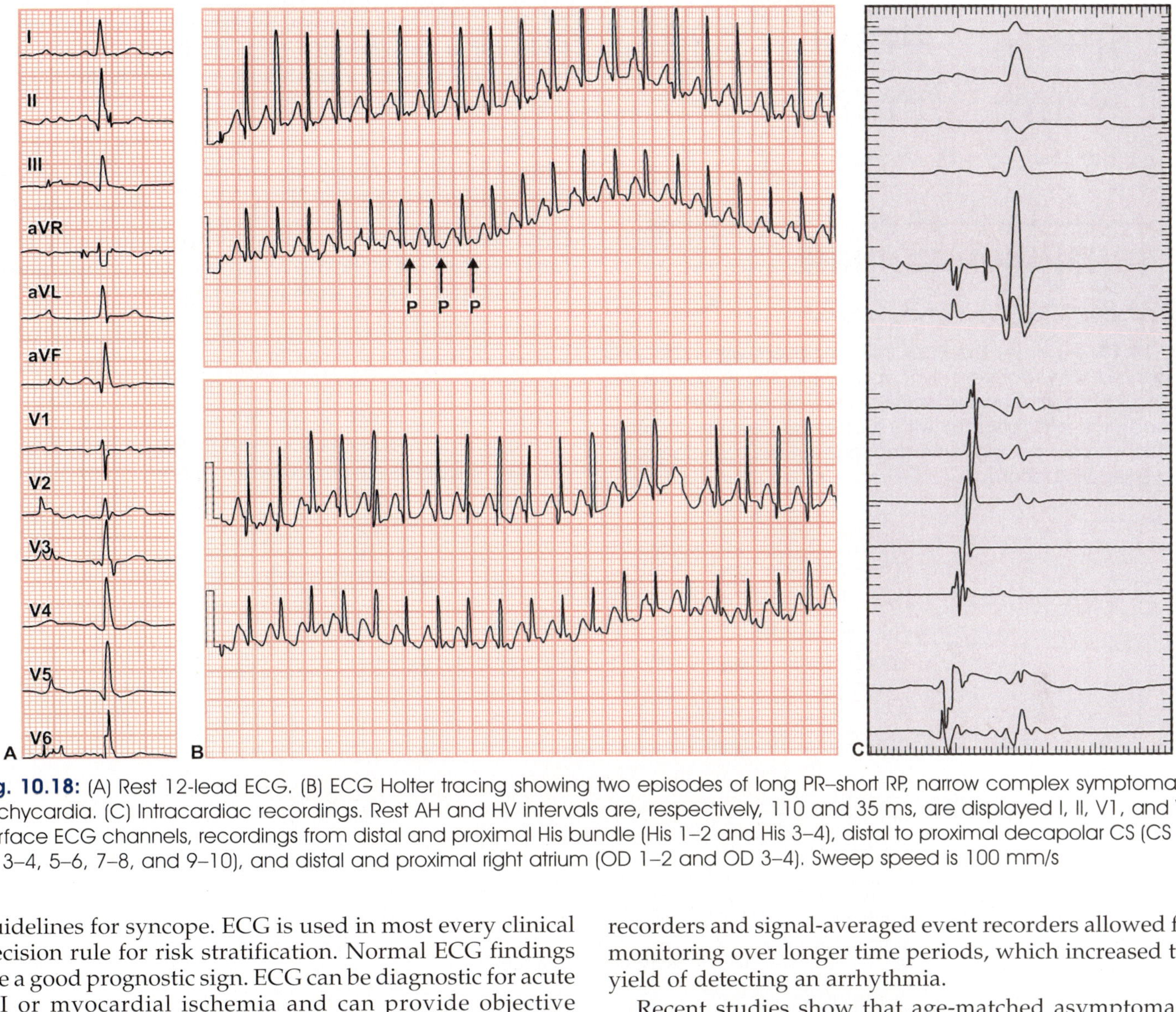


**Fig. 10.18:** (A) Rest 12-lead ECG. (B) ECG Holter tracing showing two episodes of long PR–short RP, narrow complex symptomatic tachycardia. (C) Intracardiac recordings. Rest AH and HV intervals are, respectively, 110 and 35 ms, are displayed I, II, V1, and V6 surface ECG channels, recordings from distal and proximal His bundle (His 1–2 and His 3–4), distal to proximal decapolar CS (CS 1–2, 3–4, 5–6, 7–8, and 9–10), and distal and proximal right atrium (OD 1–2 and OD 3–4). Sweep speed is 100 mm/s

guidelines for syncope. ECG is used in most every clinical decision rule for risk stratification. Normal ECG findings are a good prognostic sign. ECG can be diagnostic for acute MI or myocardial ischemia and can provide objective evidence of preexisting cardiac disease or dysrhythmia such as **Wolff-Parkinson-White syndrome, Brugada syndrome, atrial flutter, or AV blocks.**

Bradycardia, sinus pauses, nonsustained ventricular tachycardia and sustained ventricular tachycardia, and atrioventricular conduction defects occur with increasing frequency with age and are truly diagnostic only when they coincide with symptoms.

*Holter monitor/loop event recorder* (Figs 10.21–10.25): This is an outpatient test. In the past, all patients with syncope were monitored for 24 hours in a hospital. Later, loop recorders and signal-averaged event recorders allowed for monitoring over longer time periods, which increased the yield of detecting an arrhythmia.

Recent studies show that age-matched asymptomatic populations have an equivalent number of arrhythmic events recorded by ambulatory monitoring. Loop recorders have a higher diagnostic yield than Holter monitor evaluation with a marginal cost savings. A study completed through an ECG outpatient registry in Vermont by Gibson and Heitzman involving 1512 patients referred for syncope, showed that symptomatic arrhythmias were found in just 0.5% of patients. In fact, patients had symptoms without arrhythmias more often than symptoms with arrhythmias, advancing the notion that ambulatory monitoring has a higher negative than positive diagnostic yield.

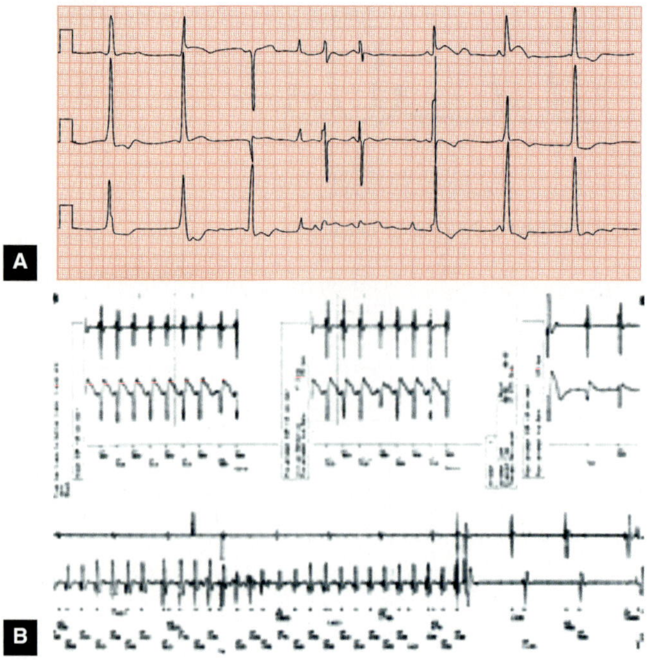


**Fig. 10.19:** HCM. (A) This ECG from a patient with HCM who presented with recurrent syncopal spells shows severe left ventricular hypertrophy and Wolff-Parkinson-White pattern. (B) ICD intracardiac electrogram with successful conversion using antitachycardia pacing for VT (top) and an appropriate shock-converting VF (bottom)

*Head-up tilt-table test* (Figs 10.26 and 10.27, Tables 10.10 and 10.11): This test is useful for confirming autonomic dysfunction and can generally be safely arranged on an outpatient basis. The test involves using a tilt table to stand a patient at 70 degrees for 45 minutes. Various modified protocols with concomitant medications, fasting, and maneuvers exist. Normally norepinephrine (NE) levels rise initially and are maintained to hold BP constant. A positive result occurs when NE levels fatigue with time and a falling BP and pulse rate produce symptoms. The head-up tilt-table test is less sensitive than electrophysiologic stress testing, and a negative result does not exclude the diagnosis of neurogenic syncope.

*Electrophysiological studies:* It may be useful in those cases where Holter ECG and other noninvasive studies are found noncontributory (Figs 10.28–10.30 and Table 10.12).

*Electroencephalography:* Electroencephalography (EEG) can be performed at the discretion of a neurologist if seizure is considered a likely alternative diagnosis.

*Stress test:* Stress test/electrophysiologic studies (EPS) have a higher diagnostic yield than the Holter monitor and should be obtained for any patient with a suspected arrhythmia as a cause of syncope.

A cardiac stress test is appropriate for patients in whom cardiac syncope is suspected and in whom have risk factors

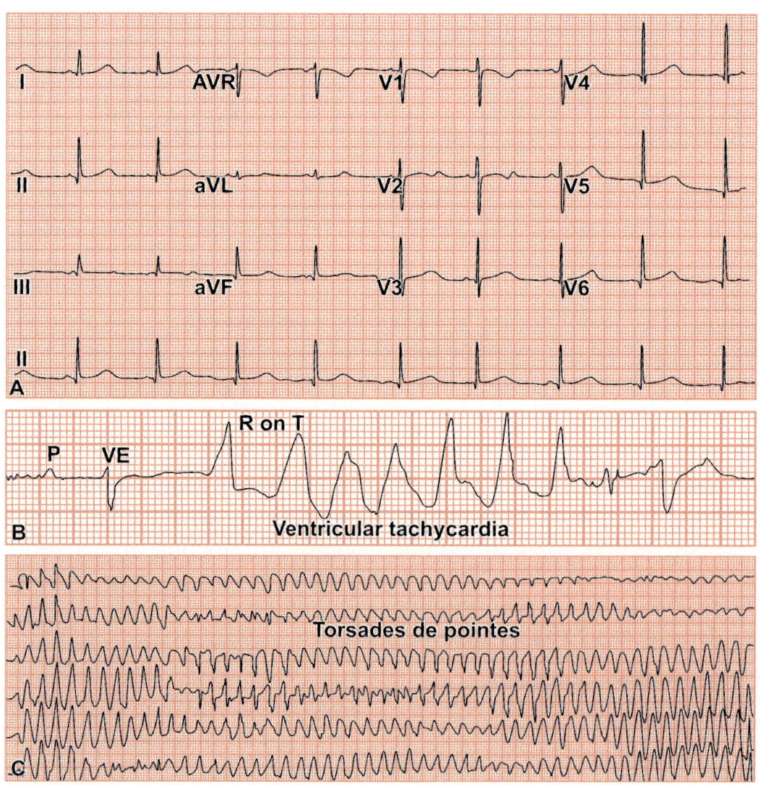


**Fig. 10.20:** ECG findings in patient with long QT syndrome type 2. (A) ECG of an 80-year-old woman with recurrent syncope. As is typical in LQTS, the QTc interval is prolonged at 500 ms. The subtype of LQTS can be predicted from a detailed examination of the T-wave (Zhang et al. 2004). In this case, the biphasic T-waves in V2 and lead III were consistent with a hERG mutation. (B) Cardiac telemetry recording showed the onset of TdP, with an 'R on T' initiation. (C) Subsequent ECG, during syncope, illustrates the characteristic appearance of TdP

**Table 10.7:** Recommendations—electrophysiological monitoring

| Recommendations | Class[a] | Class[b] |
|---|---|---|
| *Indications* | | |
| ECG monitoring is indicated in patients who have clinical or ECG features suggesting arrhythmic syncope (listed in Table 10.10). The duration (and technology) of monitoring should be selecated according the risk and the predicted recurrence rate of syncope. | I | B |
| • Immediate in-hospital monitoring (in bed or telemetric) is indicated in high risk patients defined in Table 10.11 | I | C |
| • Holter monitoring is indicated in patients who have very frequent syncope or pre-syncope (≥1 per week) | I | B |
| • ILR is indicated in: | | |
| » An early phase of evaluation in patients with recurrent syncope of uncertain orgin, abscence of high risk criteria listed in Table 10.11 and a high likehood of recurrence within battery longevity of the device | I | B |
| » High risk patients in whom a comprehensive evaluation did not demonstrate a cause of syncope or lead to a specific treatment | I | B |
| • ILR should be considered to assess the contribution of bradycardia before embarking cardiac pacing in patients with suspected or certain reflex syncope presenting with frequent or traumatic syncopal episodes | IIa | B |
| • External loop recorders should be considered in patients who have an intersymptom interval ≤4 weeks | IIa | B |
| *Diagnostic criteria* | | |
| • ECG monitoring is diagnostic when a correlation between syncope and an arrhythmia (brady- or tachyarrhythmia) is detected | I | B |
| • In the absence of such correlation, ECG monitoring is diagnostic when periods of Mobiz II or III degree AV block or a ventricular pause >3s (with the possible exception of young trained persons, during sleep, medicated patients, or rate-controlled atrial fibrilation), or rapid prolonged paroxysmal SVT or Vt are detected. The absence of arrhychmia during syncope excludes arrhythmic syncope | I | C |
| • The ECG documentation of pre-syncope without any relevant arrhythmia is not an accurate surrogate for syncope | III | C |
| • Aysmptomatic arrhythmias (other than those listed above) are not an accurate surrogate for syncope | III | C |
| • Sinus bradycardia (in the absence of syncope) is not an accurate surrogate for syncope | III | C |

[a]Class of recommendation. [b]Level of evidence. AV=atrioventricular; ECG=electrocardiogram; ILR=implantable loopr recorder; SVT=supraventriculartachyradia; VT=ventricular tachycardia.

**Table 10.8:** ECG abnormalities suggesting arrhythmic syncope

- Bifascicular block (defined as either left bundle branch block or right bundle branch block combined with left anterior or left posterior fascicular block)
- Other intraventricular conduction abnormalities (QRS duration ≥0.12 s)
- Mobitz I second degree atrioventricular block
- Asymptomatic sinus bradycardia (<50 beats/min) or sinoatrial block
- Pre-excited QRS complexes
- Prolonged QT interval
- Right bundle branch block pattern with ST-elevation in leads V1–V3 (Brugada syndrome)
- Negative T-waves in right precordial leads, epsilon waves and ventricular late potentials suggestive of arrhythmogenic right ventricular dysplasia
- Q-waves suggesting myocardial infarction

for coronary atherosclerosis. This test can assist with cardiac risk stratification and can guide future therapy.

## PROCEDURES

*Carotid sinus massage* (Figs 10.31 and Table 10.13) has been used with some success to diagnose carotid sinus syncope. Patients are placed on a cardiac monitor and beat-to-beat BP monitoring device. Atropine is kept at the bedside.

Longitudinal massage lasting 5 seconds is initiated at the point of greatest carotid pulse intensity at the level of the thyroid cartilage on one side at a time. The maximal response occurs after approximately 18 seconds, and a positive result is one that produces 3 seconds of asystole or syncope. If the result is negative, the process is repeated on the other carotid sinus. Carotid sinus massage may theoretically precipitate an embolic stroke in persons with preexisting carotid artery disease.

**Table 10.9:** Most useful and less useful tests

| | Test | Suspected diagnosis |
|---|---|---|
| Most useful | Carotid sinus massage | Neurally-mediated |
| | Tilt testing | Neurally-mediated |
| | Echocardiogram | Cardiac |
| | Holter/external loop monitoring | Cardiac |
| | Electrophysiological test | Cardiac |
| | Exercise stress testing | Cardiac |
| | Implantable loop recorder | Neurally-mediated and cardiac |
| Less useful (indicated only in selected cases) | Electroencephalography | Epilepsy and TIA |
| | Brain computed tomography | Epilepsy and TIA |
| | Brain magnetic resonance imaging | Epilepsy and TIA |
| | Carotid Doppler sonography | Epilepsy and TIA |
| | Coronary angiography | Cardiac |
| | Pulmonary computed tomography/scintigraphy | Cardiac |
| | Chest X-ray | Cardiac |
| | Abdominal ultrasound examination | Comorbidities |

TIA=transient ischemic attack

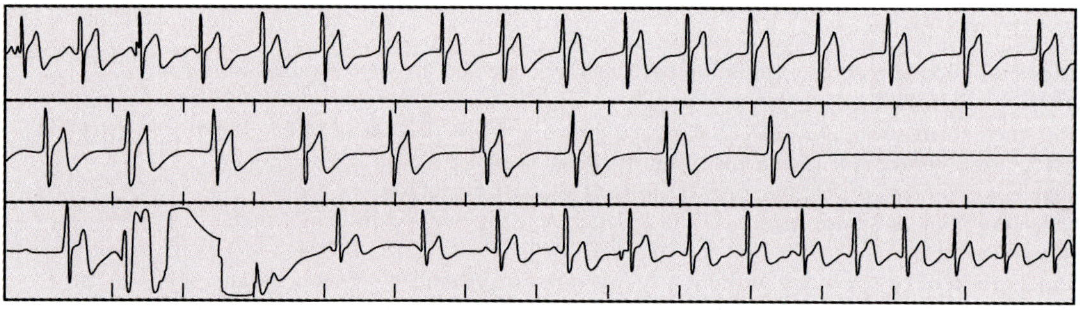

**Fig. 10.21:** Utility of implantable loop recorder in the diagnosis of unexplained syncope. Event recorder tracing showing a 4.8s asystole period in a 31-year-old subject. Time is indicated on the right scale. After a few sinus beats, there is a progressive slowing of a junctional rhythm ending into asystole. Recovery of sinus rhythm is evident in the bottom panel

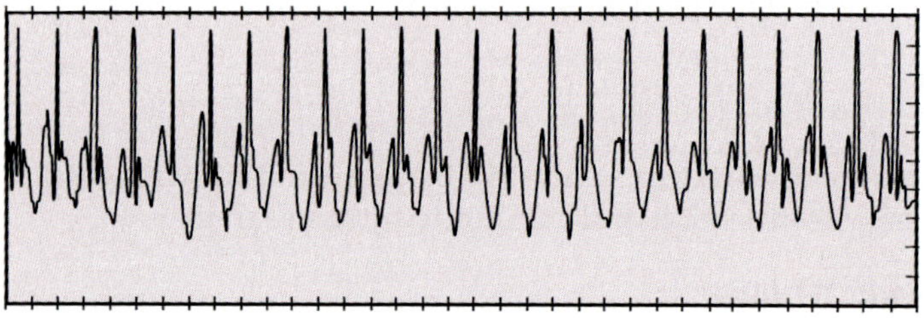

**Fig. 10.22:** The single-lead ECG tracing from ILR in patient 13 showing SVT at 214 beats per minute

## EMERGENCY DEPARTMENT CARE

In patients brought to the ED with a presumptive diagnosis of syncope, appropriate initial interventions include intravenous access, oxygen administration, and cardiac monitoring. ECG and rapid blood glucose evaluation should be promptly performed. A study to determine the sensitivity and specificity of the San Francisco Syncope Rule (SFSR) ECG criteria for determining cardiac outcomes found that when used correctly, the criteria can help predict which syncope patients are at risk of cardiac outcomes. ECG

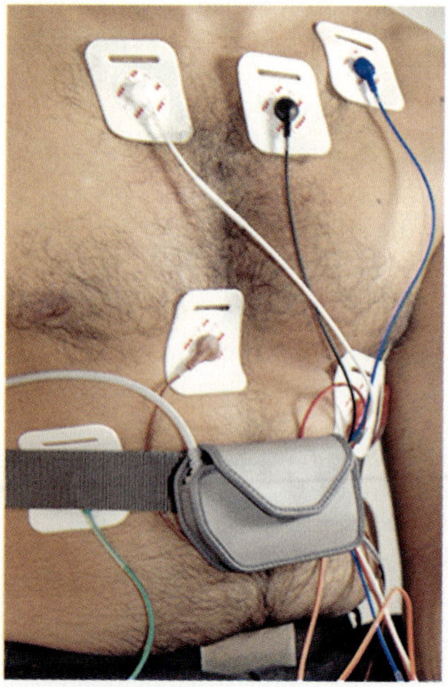

**Fig. 10.23:** Holter fitting on the chest of 30-year-old man with frequent syncopal attacks

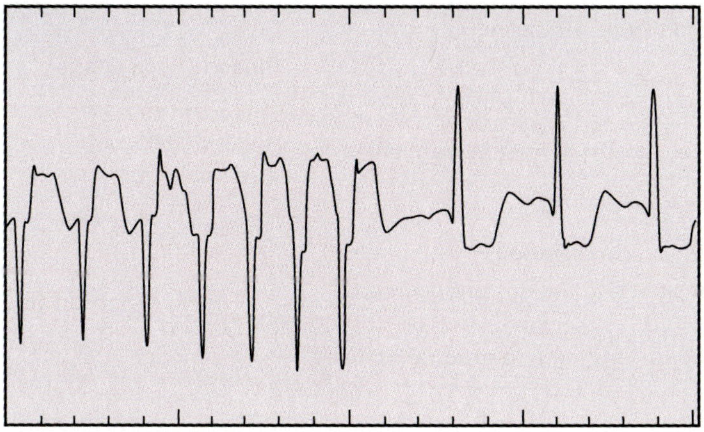

**Fig. 10.24:** The single-lead ECG tracing from ILR in patient 20 shows nonsustained VT with abrupt termination, followed by normal sinus rhythm

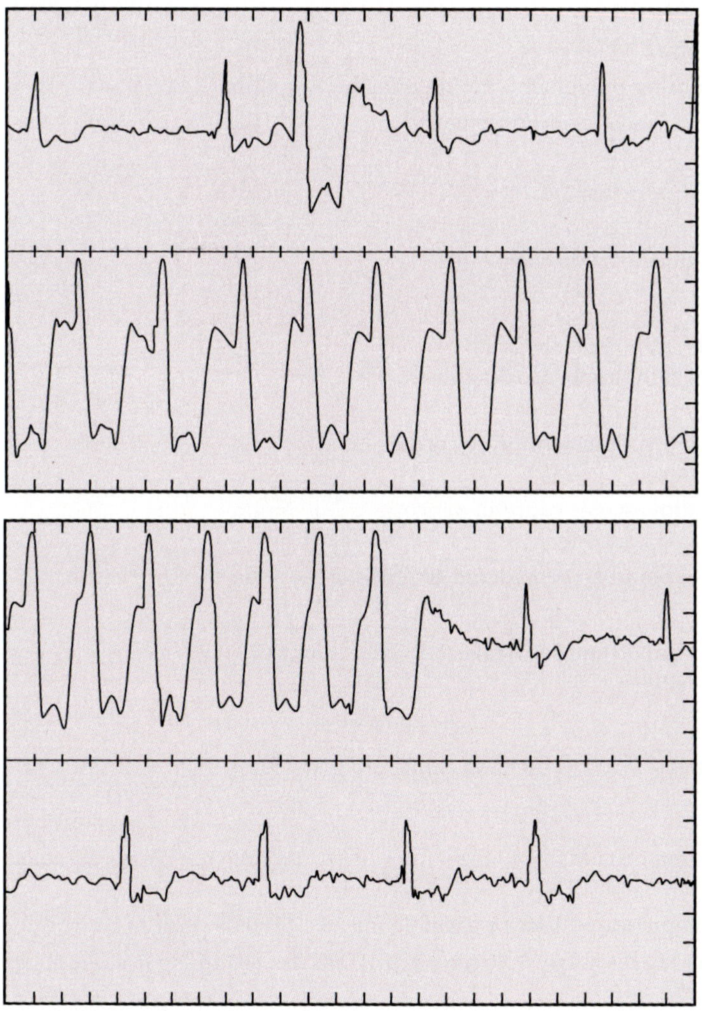

**Fig. 10.25:** Utility of implantable loop recorder in the diagnosis of unexplained syncope event recorder tracing showing a bout of wide QRS tachycardia during a syncopal episode

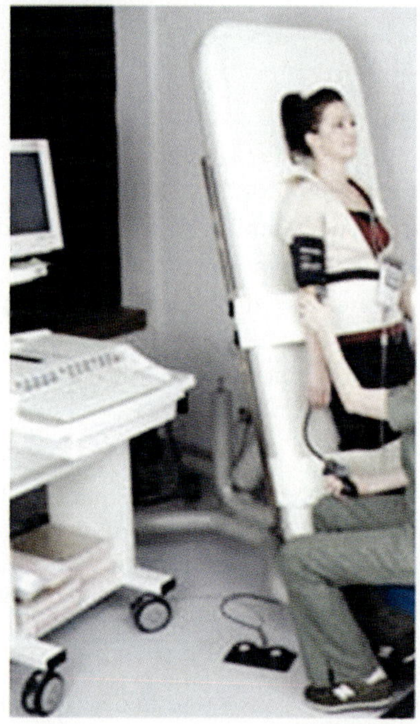

**Fig. 10.26:** Performance of HUTT Test a patient with syncopal attack

criteria predicted 36 of 42 patients with cardiac outcomes, with a sensitivity of 86%, a specificity of 70%, and a negative predictive value of 99% (Table 10.14).

Syncope may be the manifestation of an acute life-threatening process but is generally not emergent. Clinically ruling out certain processes is important. The treatment choice for syncope depends on the cause or precipitant of the syncope. Patients in whom a cause cannot be ascertained in the ED, especially if they have experienced significant trauma, warrant supportive care and monitoring.

Situational syncope treatment focuses on educating patients about the condition. For example, in carotid sinus syncope, patients should be instructed not to wear tight collars, to use a razor rather than electric shaver, and to maintain good hydration status; they should also be informed of the possibility of pacemaker placement in the future.

Orthostatic syncope treatment also focuses on educating the patient. Inform patients about avoiding postprandial dips in BP, teach them to elevate the head of their bed to prevent rapid BP fluctuations on arising from bed, and emphasize the importance of assuming an upright posture slowly. Additional therapy may include thromboembolic disease (TED) stockings, mineralocorticoids (e.g. fludrocortisone for volume expansion), and other drugs such as midodrine (an alpha1-agonist with vasopressor activity). Patients' medications must be reviewed carefully to eliminate drugs associated with hypotension. Intentional oral fluid consumption is useful in decreasing frequency and severity of symptoms in these patients.

**Table 10.10:** Recommendations—tilt testing

| **Recommendations** | **Class**[a] | **Class**[b] |
|---|---|---|
| *Methodology* | | |
| • Supine pre-tilt phase of at least 5 min. when no venous cannulation, and of at least 20 min. when cannulation is undertaken, is recommended | I | C |
| • Tilt angle between 60° and 70° is recommended | I | B |
| • Passive phase of a minimum of 20 min and a maximum of 45 min is recommended | I | B |
| • For nitroglycerine, a fixed dose of 300–400 μg sublingually administered in the upright position is recommended | I | B |
| • For isoproterenol, an incremental infusion rate from 1 mg/min up to 3 mg/min in order to increase average heart rate by ~20–25% over baseline is recommended | I | B |
| *Indications* | | |
| • Tilt testing is indicated in the case of an unexplained single syncopal episode in high risk setting (e.g. occurrence of, or potential risk of physical injury or with occupational implications) or recurrent episodes in the absence of organic heart disease, or in the presence of organic heart disease, after cardiac causes of syncope have been excluded | I | B |
| • Tilt testing is indicated when it is of clinical value to demonstrate susceptibility to reflex syncope to the patient | I | C |
| • Tilt testing should be considered to discriminate between reflex and OH syncope | IIa | C |
| • Tilt testing may be considered for differentiating syncope with jerking movements from epilepsy | IIb | C |
| • Tilt testing may be indicated for evaluating patients with frequent syncope and psychiatric disease | IIb | C |
| • Tilt testing is not recommended for assesment of treatment | IIb | C |
| • Tilt testing is not recommended for assessment of treatment | III | B |
| • Isoproterenol tilt testing is contraindicated in patients with ischemic heart disease | III | C |
| *Diagnostic criteria* | | |
| • In patients without structural heart disease the induction of reflex hypotension/bradycardia with reproduction of syncope or progessive OH (with or without symptoms) are diagnostic of reflex syncope and OH, respectively | I | B |
| • In patients without structural heart disease the induction of reflex hypotension/bradycardia without reproduction of syncope may be diagnostic of reflex syncope | IIa | B |
| • In patients with structural heart disease, arrhythmia or other cardiovascular cause of syncope should be excluded prior to considering positive tilt test results as diagnostic | IIa | C |
| • Induction of LOC in absence of hypotension and/or bradycardia should be considered diagnostic of psychogenic pseudosyncope. | IIa | C |

[a]Class of recommendation. [b]Level of evidence. BP=blood pressure; CSM=carotid sinus massage; HR=heart rate; LOC=loss of consciousness; OH=orthostatic hypotension; TIA=transient ischaemic attack; mg=micrograms.

**Table 10.11:** Classification of vasovagal syncope induced by head-up tilt table testing

| **Type** | **Classification** |
|---|---|
| Type 1 mixed | Ventricular rate during syncope 40 bpm or falls to <40 bpm for <10 sec asystole for <3 sec. BP falls prior to heart rate |
| Type 2A cardioinhibitory | Ventricular rate during syncope <40 bpm for >10 sec or asystole for >3s. BP falls prior to heart rate |
| Type 2B cardioinhibitory | Ventricular rate at syncope <40 bpm for >10s or asystole for >3s. BP falls to <80 mmHg systolic at or after rapid fall in heart rate (as above) |
| Type 3 pure vasodepressor | Heart rate does not fall more than 10% from its peak at syncope. Fall in BP precipitates syncope. |

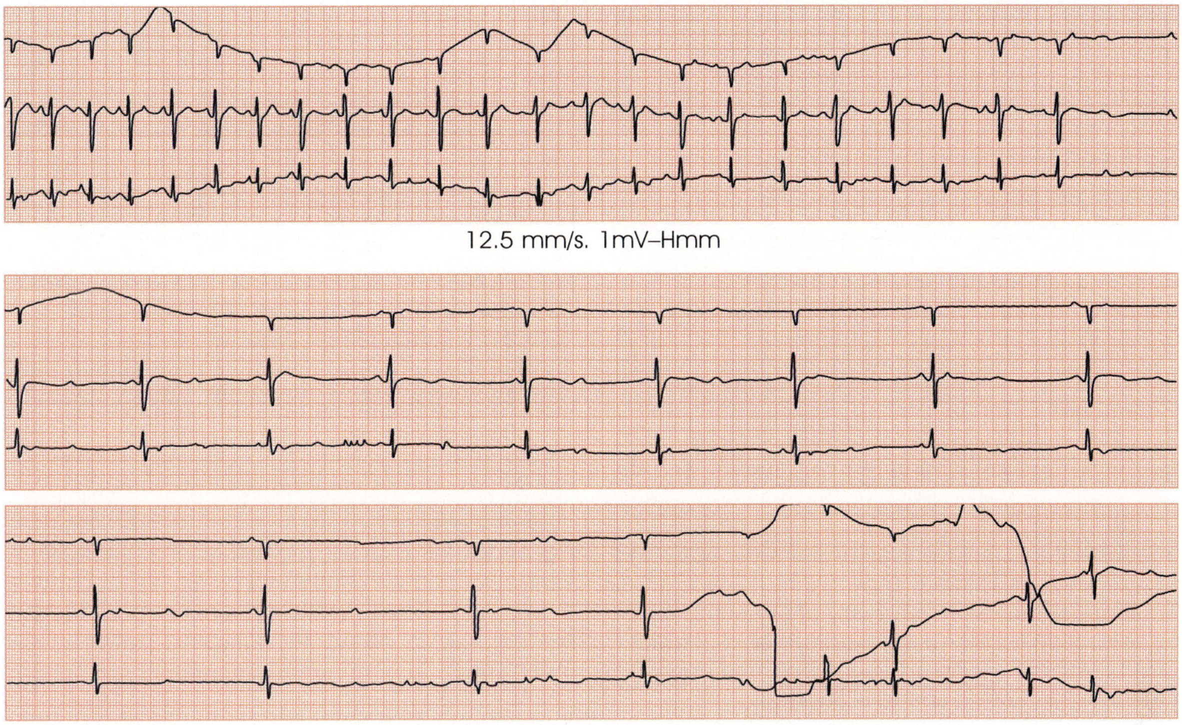


**Fig. 10.27:** Electrocardiographic characteristics of atrioventricular block induced by tilt testing. Electrocardiographic Holter recordings at 12.5 mm/s, 3 consecutive strips. The electrocardiographic tracing begins with sinus rhythm slowing, PR prolongation and then 2:1 (48.4% of patients) atrioventricular block occurs, ending with Mobitz I (35.5% of patients) second-degree atrioventricular block

**Table 10.12:** Recommendations—electrophysiological study

| Recommendations | Class[a] | Class[b] |
|---|---|---|
| *Indications* | | |
| • In patients with ischemic heart disease EPS is indicated when initial evaluation suggests an arrhythmic cause of syncope (listed in Table 10.10) unless there is already an established indication for ICD | I | B |
| • In patients with BBB, EPS should be considered when noninvasive tests have failed to make the diagnosis | IIa | B |
| • In patients with syncope proceded by sudden and brief palpitations, EPS may be performed when other non-invasive tests have failed to make the diagnosis | IIb | B |
| • In patients with Brugada syndrome, ARVC and hypertrophic cardiomyopathy an EPS may be performed in selected cases | IIb | C |
| • In patients with high-risk occupations, in whom every effort to exdude a cardiovascular cause of syncope is warranted, an EPS may be performed in selected cases | IIb | C |
| • EPS is not recommended in patients with normal ECG, no heart disease, and no palpitations | III | B |
| *Diagnostic criteria* | | |
| • EPS is diagnostic, and no additional tests are required, in the following causes: | | |
| » Sinus bradycardia and prolonged CSNRT (>525 ms) | I | B |
| » BBB and either a baseline HV interval of ≥100 ms, or second or third degree His-Purkinje block is demonstrated during incremental airtal packing or with pharmacological challenge | I | B |
| » Induction of sustained monomorphic VT in patients with previous myocardial infarction | I | B |
| » Induction of rapid SVT which reproduces hypotensive or spontanous systems | I | B |
| • An HV interval between 7 ms and 100 ms should be considered diagnostic | IIa | B |
| • The induction of polymorphic VT or ventricular fibrilation in patients with Brugada syndrome, ARVC and paitnets resuscitated from cardiac arrest may be considered diagnostic | IIb | B |
| • The induction of polymorphic VT or ventricular fibrillation in patients with ischemic cardiomyopathy or DCM cannot be considered a diagnostic finding | III | B |

[a]Class of recommendation. [b]Level of evidence. ARVC=arrhythmogenic right ventricular cardiomyopathy; BBB=bundle branch block; CSNRT=corrected sinus node recovery time; DCM=dilated cardiomyopathy; EPS=electrophysiological study; ICD=implantable cardioverter defibrillator; HV=His-ventricle; SVT=supraventricular tachycardia; VT=ventricular tachycardia.

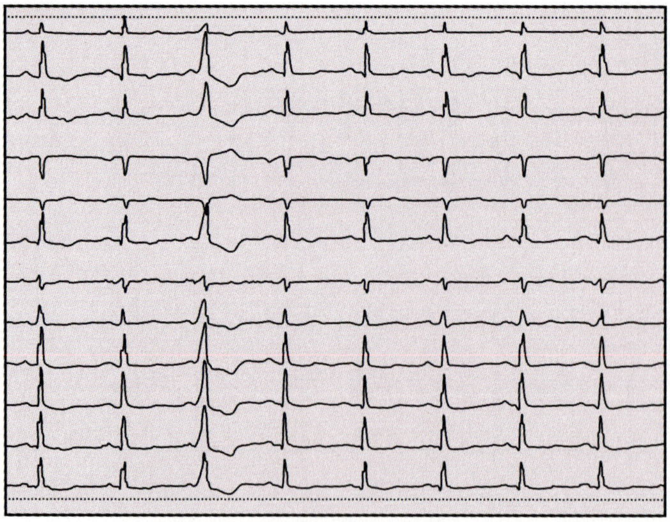

Fig. 10.28: Intermittent fasciculoventricular pathway: ECG and electrophysiologic findings, clinical implications 12-lead ECG unregistered during electrophysiologic study after resumption of sinus rate acceleration induced by isoproterenol infusion. Intermittent ventricular pre-excitation visualized (third complex from the left to the right). Sweep speed is 50 mm/s

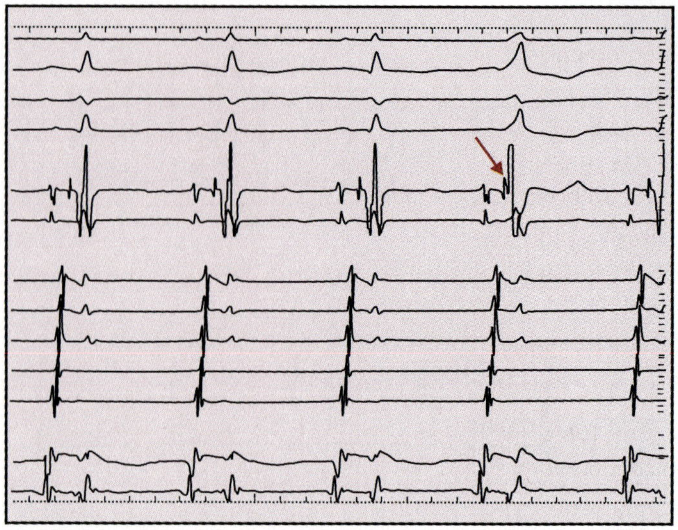

Fig. 10.29: Intracardiac recordings of an intermittent pre-excited ventricular complex (fourth complex—black arrow—from the left to the right). H and V potentials are merged. There is no change among the CS ventricular activation pattern. Sweep speed is 100 mm/s

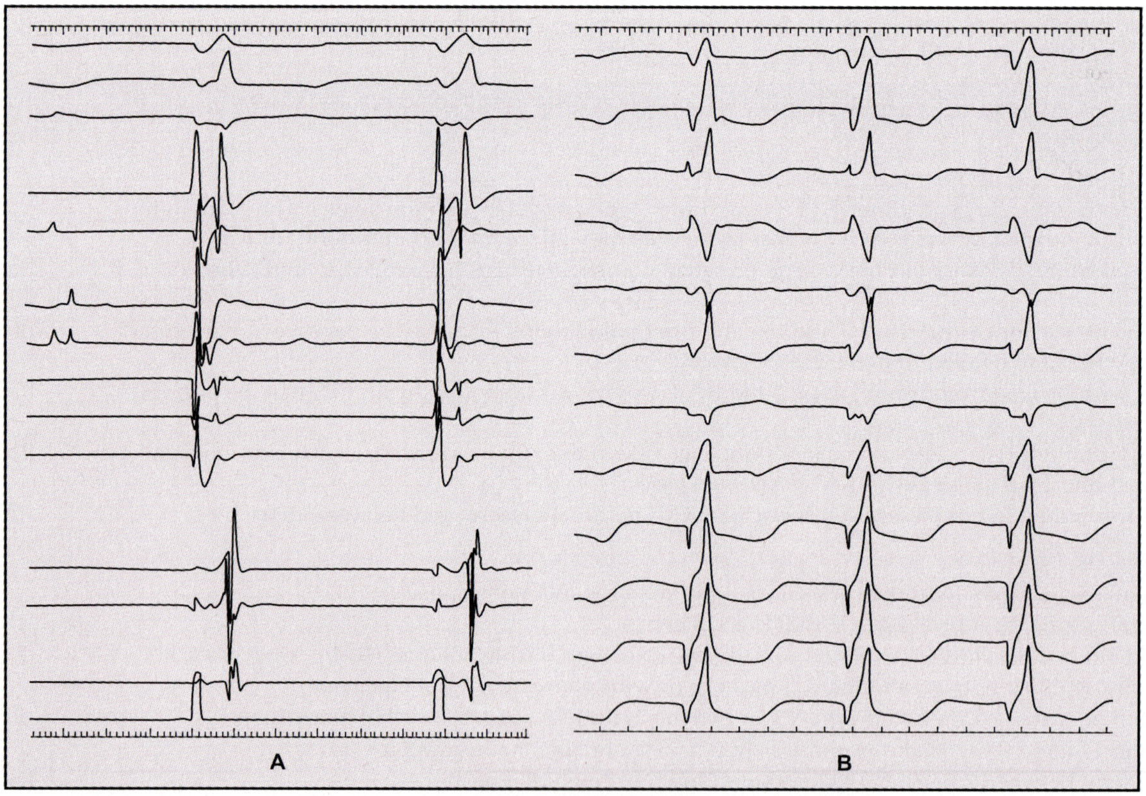


Fig. 10.30: (A) Intracardiac recordings during pacing from the para-Hisian region. Capture of the FV accessory pathway. The QRS morphology induced by pacing reproduces exactly the intermittent ventricular pre-excitation pattern visualized previously (Figs 2 and 3), are displayed leads I, aVF, and V1 surface ECG channels, recordings from the distal and proximal para-Hisian catheter (ABL d and ABL p), distal to proximal decapolar His bundle (His 1–2, 3–4, 5–6, 7–8, and 9–10), distal to proximal CS (CS 1–2 and CS 3–4), and bipolar right atrium (RA d). Sweep speed is 150 mm/s. (B) 12-lead ECG recordings during pacing from the para-Hisian region with capture of the FV accessory pathway. The QRS morphology is identical to that of the intermittent ventricular pre-excitation pattern. Sweep speed is 100 mm/s

| Table 10.13: Recommendations—carotid sinus massage | | |
|---|---|---|
| **Recommendations** | **Class**[a] | **Class**[b] |
| *Indications* | | |
| • CSM is indicated in patients >40 years with syncope of unknown aetiology after initial evaluation | I | B |
| • CSM should be avoded in patients with TIA or stroke within the past 2 months and in patients with carotid bruits (except if carotid Doppler studies) | III | C |
| *Diagnostic criteria* | | |
| • CSM is diagnostic if syncope is reproduced in the presence of asystole longer than 3s and/or a fall in systolic BP >50 mmHg | I | B |

[a]Class of recommendation. [b]Level of evidence. BP=blood pressure; CSM=carotid sinus massage; TIA=transient ischemic attack.

**Table 10.14:** Recommendations—indications for ICD in patients with unexplained syncope and a high risk of SCD

| Recommendations | Class[a] | Level[b] | Comments |
|---|---|---|---|
| • In patients with ischemic cardiomyopathy with severely depressed LVEF or HF. ICD–cardiac resynchronization therapy implantation | I | A | |
| • In patients with nonischemic cardiomyopathy with severely depressed LVEF or HF. ICD therapy is indicated according to current guidelines for ICD–cardiac resynchronization therapy implantation | I | A | |
| • In hypertrophic cardiomyopathy ICD therapy should be condisered in patients at high risk (see text) | IIa | C | In non-high risk, consider ILR |
| • In right ventricular cardiomyopathy ICD thrapy should be condisered in patients at high risk (see text) | IIa | C | In non-high risk, consider ILR |
| • In Brugada syndrome ICD therapy should be considered in patients with spontaneous type I ECG | IIa | B | In the absence of spontaneous type I pattern, consider ILR |
| • In long QT syndrome, ICD therapy, in conjunction with beta-blockers, should be consider in patients at risk | IIa | B | In non-high risk, consider ILR |
| • In patients with ischemic cardiomyopathy without severely depressed LVEF or HF and negative programmed electrical stimulation ICD therapy may be considered | IIb | C | Consider ILR to help define the nature of unexplained syncope |
| • In patients with nonischemic cardiomyopathy without severely depressed LVEF or HF ICD therapy may be considered | IIb | C | Consider ILR to help define the nature of unexplained syncope |

[a]Class of recommendation. [b]Level of evidence. HF=heart failure; ECG=electrocardiogram; ICD=implantable cardioverter defibrillator; ILR=implantable loop recorder; LVEF=left ventricular ejection fraction; SCD=sudden cardiac death

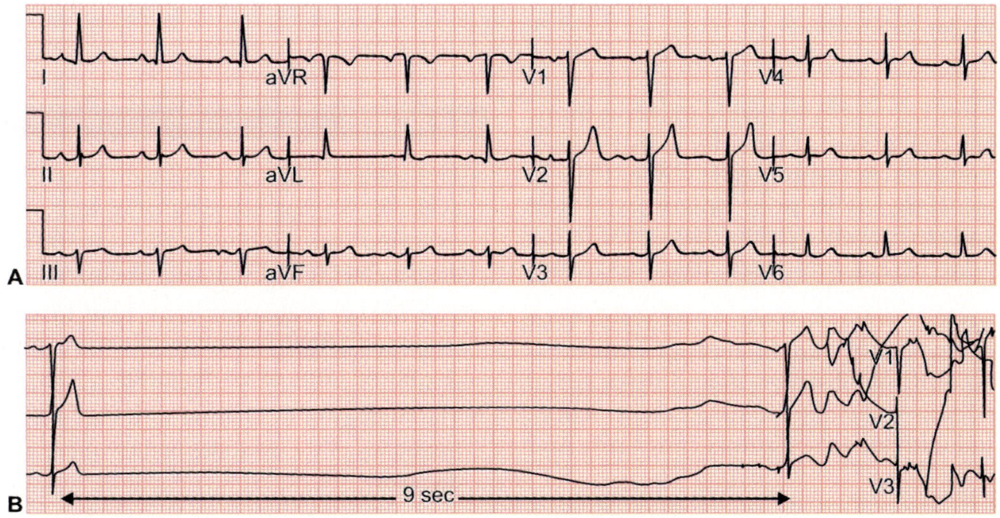


**Fig. 10.31:** Carotid sinus hypersensitivity revealed during massage manoeuvre. (A) Electrocardiographic at rest. Heart rate=72 bpm, PR interval=174 ms. (B) Electrocardiographic during carotid sinus massage resulting in syncopal attack

**Table 10.15:** Recommendations—treatment of syncope due to cardiac arrhythmias

| Recommendations | Class[a] | Level[b] |
|---|---|---|
| • Syncope due to cardiac arrhythmias must receive treatment appropriate to the cause | I | C |
| *Cardiac pacing* | | |
| • Pacing is indicated in patients with sinus node disease in whom syncope is demonstrated to be due to sinus arrest (symptom ECG correlation) without a correctable cause | I | C |
| • Pacing is indicated in sinus node disease patients with syncope and abnormal CSNRT | I | C |
| • Pacing is indicated in sinus node disease patients with syncope and asymptomatic pauses $\geq$3s (with the possible eaxceptions of yound trained persons, during sleep and in medicated patients) | I | C |
| • Pacing is indicated in patients with syncope and second degree Mobilz II, advanced or complete AV block | I | B |
| • Pacing is indicated in patients with syncope, BBB, and positive EPS | I | B |
| • Pacing should be considered in patients with unexplained syncope and BBB | IIa | C |
| • Pacind may be indicated in patients with unexplained syncope and sinus node disease with persistent sinus bradycardia itself asymptomatic | IIb | C |
| • Pacing is not indicated in patients with unexplained syncope without evidence of any conduction disturbance | III | C |
| *Catheter ablation* | | |
| • Catheter ablation is indicated in patients with symptom–arrhythmia ECG correlation in both SVT and VT in the absence of structural heart disease (with the exception of atrial fibrillation | I | C |
| • Catheter ablation may be indicated in patients with syncope due to the onset of rapid atrial fibrillation | IIb | C |
| *Antiarrhythmic drug therapy* | | |
| • Antiarrhythmic drug therapy, including rate control drugs, is indicated in patients with syncope due to onset of rapid atrial fibrillation | I | C |
| • Drug therapy should be considered in patients with symptom–arrhythmia ECG correlation in both SVT and VT when catheter ablation cannot be undertaken or has failed | IIb | C |
| *Implantable cardioverter defibrillator* | | |
| • ICD is indicated in patients with documented VT and structural heart disease | I | B |
| • ICD is indicated when sustained monomorphic VT is induced at EPS in patients with previous myocardial infarction | I | B |
| • ICD should be considered in patients with documented VT and inherited cardiomyopathies or channelopathies. | IIa | B |

[a]Class of recommendation. [b]Level of evidence. AV=atrioventricular; BBB=bundle branch block; CSNRT=corrected sinus node recovery time; ECG=electrocardiogram; EPS=electrophysiological study; ICD=implantable cardioverter defibrillator; SVT=supraventricular tachycardia; VT=ventricular tachycardia.

*Cardiac arrhythmic syncope* is treated with antiarrhythmic drugs or pacemaker placement. Consider cardiologist evaluation or inpatient management since this is more commonly associated with poor outcomes. Trials assessing beta-blockade to prevent syncope have conflicting results, but no clear effect has been demonstrated (Table 8.15).

*Cardiac mechanical syncope* may be treated with beta-blockade to decrease outflow obstruction and myocardial workload. Valvular disease may require surgical correction. This, too, is associated with increased future morbidity and mortality.

**KEY POINTS**

- The starting point for evaluation of syncope is the 'initial evaluation' that consists of history taking and physical examination, including orthostatic blood pressure measurements and standard electrocardiogram.
- The initial evaluation may lead to certain diagnosis, or suspected diagnosis that needs to be confirmed by appropriate diagnostic tests, or no diagnosis.
- The strategy of evaluation varies according to the severity and frequency of the episodes and the presence or absence of heart disease.

*Contd...*

*Contd...*

- In general, the absence of suspected or certain heart disease excludes a cardiac cause of syncope.
- Conversely, the presence of heart disease is a strong predictor of a cardiac cause of syncope and virtually includes all cardiac syncopes, but its specificity is low as about half of patients with heart disease have a noncardiac cause of syncope.
- Determining the mechanism of syncope is a prerequisite for advising patients with regard to prognosis, and to developing an effective mechanism-specific treatment.
- Most patients with syncope require only reassurance and education regarding the nature of the disease and the avoidance of triggering events.

## BIBLIOGRAPHY


1. Andrea U, Attilio DR, Franco G, et al. Early and late outcome of treated patients referred for syncope to emergency department: the EGSYS 2 follow-up study. Eur Heart J 18;2010.
2. Birnbaum A, Esses D, Bijur P, Wollowitz A, Gallagher EJ. Failure to validate the San Francisco Syncope Rule in an independent emergency department population. Ann Emerg Med 2008;52(2):151–9.
3. Calkins H, Shyr Y, Frumin H, Schork A, Morady F. The value of the clinical history in the differentiation of syncope due to ventricular tachycardia, atrioventricular block, and neurocardiogenic syncope. Am J Med 1995;98(4):365–73.
4. Chen L, Chen MH, Larson MG, Evans J, Benjamin EJ, Levy D. Risk factors for syncope in a community-based sample (the Framingham Heart Study). Am J Cardiol 2000;85(10): 1189–93.
5. Costantino G, Perego F, Dipaola F, et al. Short- and long-term prognosis of syncope, risk factors, and role of hospital admission: results from the STePS (Short-Term Prognosis of Syncope) study. J Am Coll Cardiol 2008;51(3):276–83.
6. Dipaola F, Costantino G, Perego F, Borella M, Galli A, Cantoni G. San Francisco Syncope Rule, Osservatorio Epidemiologico sulla Sincope nel Lazio risk score, and clinical judgment in the assessment of short-term outcome of syncope. Am J Emerg Med 2010;28(4):432–9.
7. Gibson TC, Heitzman MR. Diagnostic efficacy of 24-hour electrocardiographic monitoring for syncope. Am J Cardiol 1984;53(8):1013–7.
8. Huff JS, Decker WW, Quinn JV, et al. Clinical policy: critical issues in the evaluation and management of adult patients presenting to the emergency department with syncope. [Guideline] Ann Emerg Med 2007;49(4):431–44.
9. Martin GJ, Adams SL, Martin HG, et al. Prospective evaluation of syncope. Ann Emerg Med 1984;13(7):499–504.
10. Martin TP, Hanusa BH, Kapoor WN. Risk stratification of patients with syncope. Ann Emerg Med 1997;29(4):459–66.
11. Middlekauff HR, Stevenson WG, Stevenson LW, Saxon LA. Syncope in advanced heart failure: high risk of sudden death regardless of origin of syncope. J Am Coll Cardiol 1993; 21(1):110–6.
12. Moya A, Sutton R, Ammirati F, et al. Guidelines for the diagnosis and management of syncope (version 2009): the Task Force for the Diagnosis and Management of Syncope of the European Society of Cardiology (ESC). Eur Heart J 2009;30(21):2631–71.
13. Pratt JL, Fleisher GR. Syncope in children and adolescents. Pediatr Emerg Care 1989;5(2):80–2.
14. Quinn J, McDermott D. Electrocardiogram findings in emergency department patients with syncope. Acad Emerg Med 2011;18(7):714–8.
15. Quinn JV, Stiell IG, McDermott DA, et al. Derivation of the San Francisco Syncope Rule to predict patients with short-term serious outcomes. Ann Emerg Med 2004;43(2):224–32.
16. Reed MJ, Newby DE, Coull AJ, Prescott RJ, Jacques KG, Gray AJ. The ROSE (risk stratification of syncope in the emergency department) study. [Best Evidence] J Am Coll Cardiol 2010; 55(8):713–21.
17. Rockx MA, Hoch JS, Klein GJ, et al. Is ambulatory monitoring for "community-acquired" syncope economically attractive? A cost-effectiveness analysis of a randomized trial of external loop recorders versus Holter monitoring. Am Heart J 2005;150(5):1065.
18. Sarasin FP, Hanusa BH, Perneger T, Louis-Simonet M, Rajeswaran A, Kapoor WN. A risk score to predict arrhythmias in patients with unexplained syncope. Acad Emerg Med 2003;10(12):1312–7.
19. Savage DD, Corwin L, McGee DL, Kannel WB, Wolf PA. Epidemiologic features of isolated syncope: the Framingham Study. Stroke 1985;16(4):626–9.
20. Serrano LA, Hess EP, Bellolio MF, et al. Accuracy and quality of clinical decision rules for syncope in the emergency department: a systematic review and meta-analysis. Ann Emerg Med 2010;56(4):362–73.e1.
21. Shen WK, Decker WW, Smars PA, et al. Syncope Evaluation in the Emergency Department Study (SEEDS): a multidisciplinary approach to syncope management. Circulation 2004;110(24):3636–45.
22. Soteriades ES, Evans JC, Larson MG, et al. Incidence and prognosis of syncope. N Engl J Med 2002;347(12):878–85.
23. Suzuki M, Hori S, Nakamura I, Soejima K, Aikawa N. Long-term survival of Japanese patients transported to an emergency department because of syncope. Ann Emerg Med 2004;44(3):215–21.
24. Thiruganasambandamoorthy V, Hess EP, Alreesi A, et al. External validation of the San Francisco Syncope Rule in the Canadian setting. Ann Emerg Med 2010; 55(5):464–72.

# 11 Electrophysiological Study and Catheter Management of Cardiac Arrhythmia

*Historical aspects of electrophysiology (EP) study:* Clinical cardiac electrophysiologic testing has evolved rapidly since 1968, when the technique was first described. In an electrophysiologic study, electrode catheters are positioned within the heart to record electrical activity from the atrium, atrioventricular conduction tissue, and ventricle. Programmed stimulation is then performed, which involves pacing of the atrium or ventricle and introducing critically timed premature stimuli during sinus rhythm or paced rhythm. The use of programmed stimulation in conjunction with intracardiac recordings in electrophysiologic studies has facilitated the diagnosis of mechanisms of arrhythmias and the assessment of therapy.

Electrophysiologic testing (Fig. 11.1) is useful in selected patients with sinus node dysfunction, conduction system disorders, supraventricular tachycardia, ventricular tachycardia, or ventricular fibrillation and in survivors of out-of-hospital cardiac arrest and patients with symptomatic but unsubstantiated rhythm disturbances. Therapeutic approaches that can be assessed by electrophysiologic testing include serial drug testing to determine the effectiveness of antiarrhythmic agents, antitachycardia pacing, the implantable defibrillator, transcatheter ablation, and electrophysiologically guided surgical procedures. In this review, we discuss the methods of electrophysiologic testing, its clinical applications in diagnosing the various cardiac rhythm disturbances, and its use in assessing various therapeutic modalities.

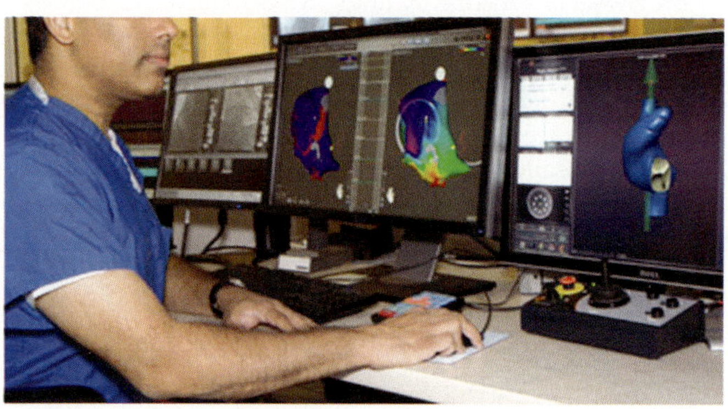

**Fig. 11.1:** The electrophysiology lab for carrying out EP studies and catheter ablation of various types in drug-resistant cardiac arrhythmias

## An Overview of the Procedure

While ECGs are noninvasive, an EP study is somewhat invasive. The study is performed after giving local anesthesia and conscious sedation (twilight sleep) to keep the patient as comfortable as possible. The procedure involves inserting a catheter—a narrow, flexible tube-attached to electricity monitoring electrodes, into a blood vessel, often through a site in the groin or neck, and winding the catheter wire up into the heart. The journey from entry point to heart muscle is navigated by images created by a fluoroscope, an X-ray-like machine that provides continuous, 'live' images of the catheter and heart muscle. Once the catheter reaches the heart, electrodes at its tip gather data and a variety of electrical measurements are made. These data pinpoint the location of the faulty electrical site. During this "electrical mapping," the cardiac arrhythmia specialist, an electrophysiologist, may instigate, through pacing (the use of tiny electrical impulses), some of the very arrhythmias that are the crux of the problem. The events are safe, given the range of experts and resources close at hand and are necessary to ensure the precise location of the problematic tissue.

Once the damaged site or sites are confirmed, the specialist may administer different medications or electrical impulses to determine their ability to halt the arrhythmia and restore normal heart rhythm. Based on this data, as well as information garnered before the study, sometimes the specialist will proceed to place an implantable cardioverter device (ICD) or a pacemaker or will perform radiofrequency ablation. In any case, the information proves useful for diagnosis and treatment.

Throughout the procedure, the patient is sedated but awake and remains still. Patients rarely report pain, more often describing what they feel as discomfort. Some watch the procedure on monitors and occasionally ask questions. The procedure usually takes about 2 hours. The patient remains still for 4–6 hours afterward to ensure the entry point incision begins to heal properly. Once mobile again, patients may feel stiff and achy from lying still for hours.

### The Importance of the Flow of Electricity

Each heart has it own normal rhythm brought about by the seamless flow of electrical impulses throughout the organ. This electrical flow begins in the heart's natural 'pacemaker' (also know as the sinoatrial node or sinus node) in the upper right heart chamber, the right atrium. The electricity flows through the upper chambers (atria), crosses the bridge between upper and lower chambers (atrioventricular node) and travels to the lower chambers (ventricles). The passage of electricity culminates in a carefully coordinated contraction of heart muscle that pushes blood through the human body. Problems in the precise flow of electricity are the cause of arrhythmias (Fig. 11.2).

### Clinical Application of EP Study

An electrophysiologic, or EP, study provides information that is key to diagnosing and treating arrhythmias. Although it is more invasive than an electrocardiogram (ECG) or echocardiogram, and involves provoking arrhythmias, the test produces data that makes it possible to:

1. Diagnose the source of arrhythmia symptoms
2. Evaluate the effectiveness of certain medications or procedures in controlling the heart rhythm disorder
3. Predict the risk of a future cardiac event, such as sudden cardiac death
4. Assess the need for an implantable device (a pacemaker or ICD) or treatment procedure (radiofrequency catheter ablation)

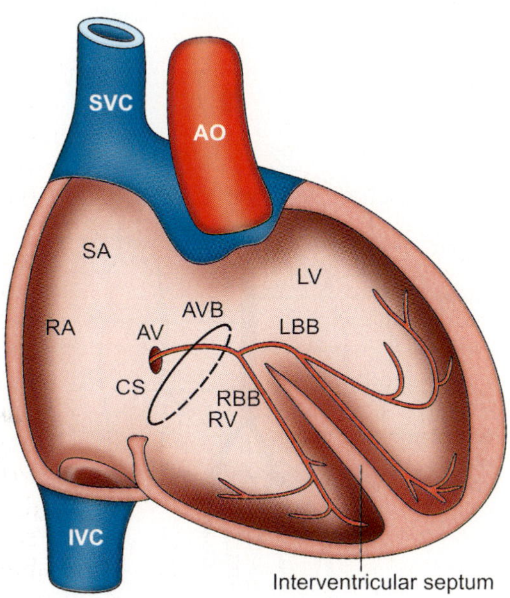


**Fig. 11.2:** Anatomical features of bundle of His as a conduction system of the heart close to tricuspid valve

#### *Who performs the test and where?*

Since potentially dangerous arrhythmias are provoked during an EP study, it is crucial that specialized staff are present to handle all situations. A physician electrophysiologist, with advanced training in the diagnosis and treatment of heart rhythm problems, performs the EP study. The electrophysiologist leads a team of specially trained health care professionals, technicians and nurses, who assist during the procedure. The team performs the EP study in an electrophysiology laboratory, or EP lab, a well-equipped, controlled clinical environment usually located within a hospital or clinic. As a result, the test is quite safe and complications are rare.

### Complications in EP study

The procedure is generally very safe. Possible risks include:

- Arrhythmias
- Bleeding
- Blood clots that lead to embolism
- Cardiac tamponade
- Heart attack
- Infection
- Injury to the vein
- Low blood pressure

## TECHNICAL CONSIDERATIONS IN PERFORMANCE OF ELECTROPHYSIOLOGICAL STUDY

### I. Before the Procedure

- Your physician will explain the procedure to you and offer you the opportunity to ask any questions that you might have about the procedure.
- You will be asked to sign a consent form that gives your permission to do the test. Read the form carefully and ask questions if something is not clear.
- Notify your physician if you are sensitive to or are allergic to any medications, iodine, latex, tape, or anesthetic agents (local and general).
- You will need to fast for a certain period of time prior to the procedure. Your physician will notify you how long to fast, usually overnight.
- If you are pregnant or suspect that you may be pregnant, you should notify your physician.
- Notify your physician if you have any body piercing on your chest and/or abdomen.
- Notify your physician of all medications (prescription and over-the-counter) and herbal supplements that you are taking.
- Notify your physician if you have heart valve disease, as you may need to receive and antibiotic prior to the procedure.

- Notify your physician if you have a history of bleeding disorders or if you are taking any anticoagulant (blood-thinning) medications, aspirin, or other medications that affect blood clotting. It may be necessary for you to stop some of these medications prior to the procedure.
- Your physician may request a blood test prior to the procedure to determine how long it takes your blood to clot. Other blood tests may be done as well.
- Notify your physician if you have a pacemaker.
- If a sedative is given before the procedure, you may need someone to drive your home afterwards.
- The area around the catheter insertion (groin area) may be shaved.
- Based upon your medical condition, your physician may request other specific preparation.

### II. During the Procedure (Figs 11.3–11.6)

An EP study may be performed on an outpatient basis or as part of your stay in a hospital. Procedures may vary depending on your condition and your physician's practices.

*Generally, an EP study follows this process:*

- You will be asked to remove any jewelry or other objects that may interfere with the procedure.
- You will be asked to remove clothing and will be given a gown to wear.
- You will be asked to empty your bladder prior to the procedure.
- An intravenous (IV) line will be started in your hand or arm prior to the procedure for injection of medication and to administer IV fluids, if needed.
- You will be placed in a supine (on your back) position on the procedure table.
- You will be connected to an ECG monitor that records the electrical activity of the heart and monitors the heart during the procedure using small, adhesive electrodes. Your vital signs (heart rate, blood pressure, breathing rate, and oxygenation level) will be monitored during the procedure.
- There may be several monitor screens, showing your vital signs and the images of the catheter being moved through the body into the heart.
- You will receive a sedative medication in your IV before the procedure to help you relax. However, you will likely remain awake during the procedure.
- Your pulses below the IV site may be checked and marked with a marker so that the circulation to the limb below the site can be checked after the procedure.
- A local anesthetic will be injected into the skin at the insertion site. You may feel some stinging at the site for a few seconds after the local anesthetic is injected.

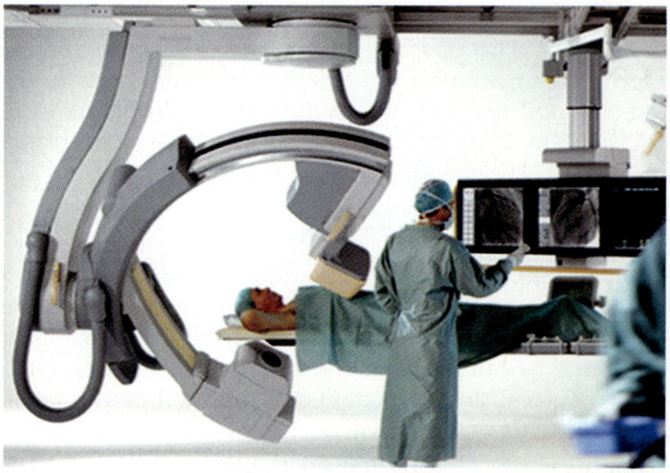

**Fig. 11.3:** Cardiac catheterization laboratory. Electrophysiologist is busy in performing electrophysiological study for diagnosis of cardiac arrhythmia

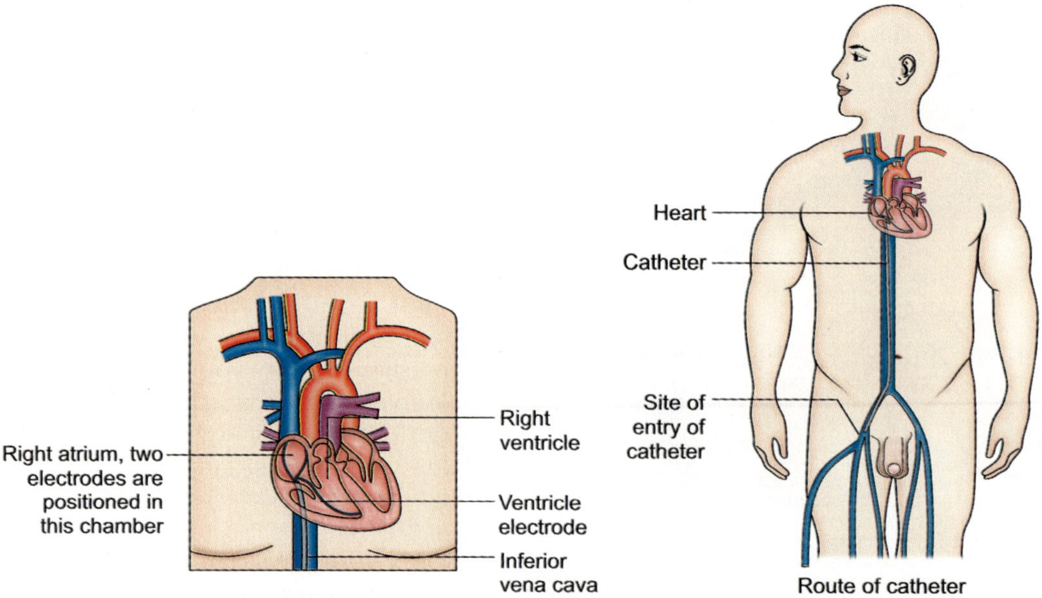


**Fig. 11.4:** Routes inserting catheter in intracardiac electrocardiographic study

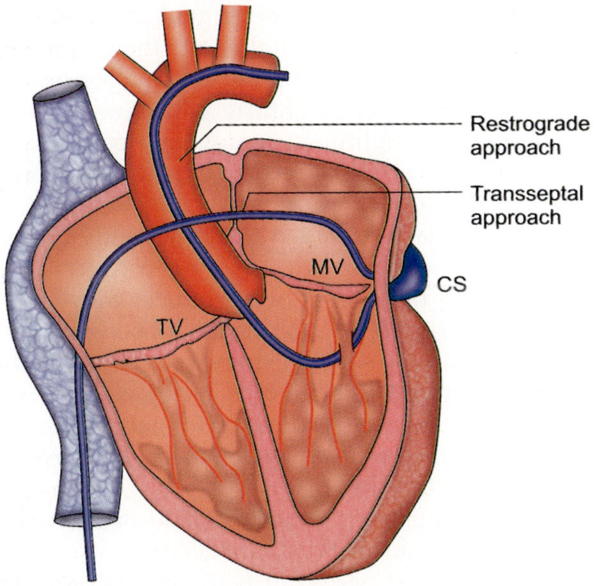


**Fig. 11.5:** Illustration showing transseptal and retrograde approaches in EP study

- Once the local anesthetic has taken effect, a sheath, or introducer, will be inserted into the blood vessel. This is a plastic tube through which the catheter will be inserted into the blood vessel and advanced into the heart.
- One or more catheters will be inserted through the sheath into the blood vessel. The physician will advance the catheter through the blood vessel into the right side of the heart. Fluoroscopy (a special type of X-ray that is displayed on a TV monitor), may be used to assist in advancing the catheter to the heart.
- Once the physician has the catheter(s) placed properly, the electrical testing will begin by sending very small electrical impulses to certain areas within the heart. If a dysrhythmia occurs, you may begin to feel lightheaded or dizzy.

***Medication will be given to you IV to treat the dysrhythmia. Alternatively, a shock will be delivered to stop the dysrhythmia. You will be sedated before this type of shock is given.***

- If a certain area of tissue is found to be causing a dysrhythmia, the physician may perform an ablation to eliminate the tissue. This is done with radio waves (radiofrequency ablation). The radio waves are delivered through the catheter to the tissue.
- If you notice any discomfort or pain, such as chest pain, neck or jaw pain, back pain, arm pain, shortness of breath, or breathing difficulty, let the physician know.
- Once the procedure has been completed, the catheter(s) will be removed from the insertion site. The physician or an assistant will hold pressure on the insertion site so that the blood can begin to form a clot at the site and stop the bleeding.
- Once the bleeding has stopped, a bandage will be placed on the site.
- You will be assisted to slide from the table onto a stretcher so that you can be taken to the recovery area.

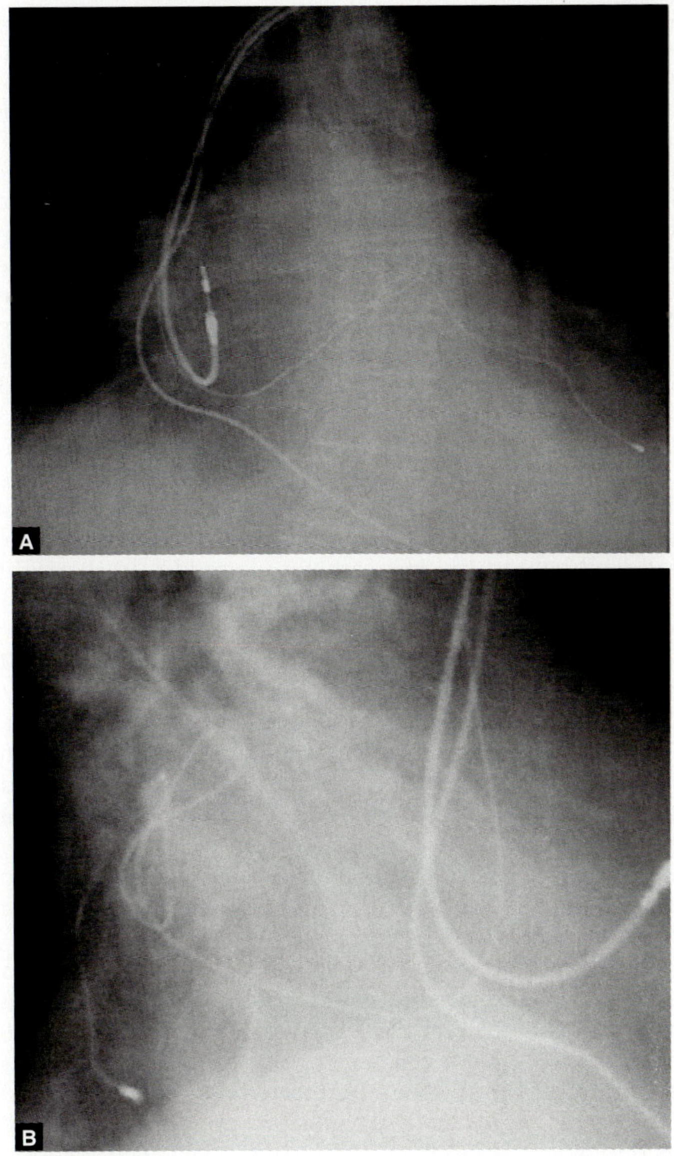


**Fig. 11.6:** (A) X-ray chest AP view showing 'granny knot' of left ventricular lead in coronary sinus (B) X-ray chest lateral view showing 'granny knot' of left ventricular lead in coronary sinus

**Note:** If the insertion was in the groin, you will not be allowed to bend your leg for a few hours.

- To help you remember to keep your leg straight, the knee of the affected leg may be covered with a sheet and the ends will be tucked under the mattress on both sides of the bed to form a type of loose restraint.

### Transseptal Approach Technique in EP Study

Throughout the diagnostic electrophysiological study and transseptal procedure the patients were kept well hydrated with a continuous infusion of normal saline, receiving at least 500 ml before the transseptal procedure. The transseptal procedures were performed using a standard Brockenborough needle and either a Mullins sheath (Bard Inc, Billerica, Massachusetts, USA) or a Swartz sheath and dilator (Daig Corporation, Minnetonka, Minnesota, USA). The needle was connected to a standard catheterisation manifold by a short length of flexible tubing, so that contrast could be injected and pressure could be displayed and recorded. Biplane fluoroscopic projections used were (right anterior oblique 45° and left anterior oblique 40°) in all cases, providing en face and longitudinal views of the interatrial septum respectively. The transseptal sheath/dilator was placed in the superior vena cava and then the dilator/sheath/needle combination was withdrawn inferiorly in the left anterior oblique projection until the tip of the dilator 'popped' into the fossa ovalis. Positioning was always checked in the right anterior oblique projection to ensure that the tip of the needle/sheath assembly was pointing directly away from the plane of vision and slightly anterior. A test injection of contrast was delivered through the dilator in the left anterior oblique projection to check for 'tenting' of the fossa at the intended puncture site. This was typically just below the level of the His recording catheter in the left anterior oblique 40° projection, and well behind the His catheter electrodes in the right anterior oblique 45°. The needle was then advanced and a second test injection was made following needle advancement to check that the needle had entered the left atrium; left atrial pressure was then recorded. The sheath/dilator were advanced over the needle into the left atrium. Once the dilator was well into the left atrium, the sheath was advanced over the dilator, but the needle remained just inside the dilator to give support for advancement of the long sheath. Once the needle is withdrawn, the tip of the dilator tends to flex. This makes it hazardous to redeploy the needle, since this may result in penetration of the wall of the dilator.

Patients then received 5000 units of heparin, with a further 2500 units being given if left sided deployment lasted more than one hour. If deployment exceeded 90 minutes, activated partial thromboplastin time was estimated. Ablations were performed using 4 mm tipped 'Steerocath' or 'Blazer-T' thermistor tipped electrodes (EP Technologies, Sunnyvale, California, USA). The ablation catheter was passed through the sheath into the left atrium and positioned on the mitral annulus. Care was always taken to flush the sheath during catheter advancement to avoid entrainment of air. Suitable ablation sites were obtained using conventional criteria. Patients remained in the laboratory with transseptal sheath in place for 30 minutes after the procedure (particularly after accessory pathway ablation) for confirmation of success. After successful ablation, transseptal sheaths were withdrawn across the interatrial septum with the ablation catheter tip protruding slightly. This technique was employed to avoid inadvertent displacement of adherent coagulum from the catheter at the sheath tip.

## III. After the Procedure

### *In the Hospital*

- After the procedure, you may be taken to the recovery room for observation or returned to your hospital room. You will remain flat in bed for a few hours after the procedure. The circulation and sensation of the limb where the catheter was inserted will be monitored. A nurse will monitor your vital signs, the insertion site, and circulation/sensation in the affected leg or arm.
- You should immediately inform your nurse if you feel any chest pain or tightness, or any other pain, as well as any feelings of warmth, bleeding, or pain at the insertion site in your leg or arm.
- Bed-rest may vary from 2–6 hours depending on your specific condition.
- In some cases, the sheath or introducer may be left in the insertion site. If so, the period of bed-rest will be prolonged until the sheath is removed. After the sheath is removed, you may be given a light meal.
- You may be given pain medication for pain or discomfort related to the insertion site or having to lie flat and still for a prolonged period.
- You may resume your usual diet after the procedure, unless your physician decides otherwise.
- After the specified period of bed-rest has been completed, you may get out of bed. The nurse will assist you the first time you get up, and will check your blood pressure while you are lying in bed, sitting, and standing. You should move slowly when getting up from the bed to avoid any dizziness from the long period of bed-rest.
- When you have completed the recovery period, you may be discharged to your home unless your physician decides otherwise. If this procedure was performed on an outpatient basis, you must have another person drive you home.

## IV. Discharge Instructions and Care

- Your heart rhythm specialist will discuss specific individualized recommendations in regard to your discharge care. The following are general recommendations:
- Limit heavy lifting or strenuous exertion for 4–5 days after your study
- You may shower after your return home the day of the procedure
- You may remove any dressing or bandages placed at the catheter site after you return home
- You may typically return to work in 1–2 day, as long as it does not involve heavy lifting or strenuous exertion
- Call your physician if your incision site (typically in the groin) appears to swell or become more painful
- It is normal to develop some bruising at the catheter site with a transition to a 'black-and-blue appearance' however, this should not become more painful or lead to increased swelling
- Follow-up with your physician in approximately 1 month for a clinic visit.

### *At Home*

Once at home, you should monitor the insertion site for bleeding, unusual pain, swelling, and abnormal discoloration or temperature change at or near the injection site.

A small bruise is normal. If you notice a constant or large amount of blood at the site that cannot be contained with a small dressing, notify your physician. It will be important to keep the insertion site clean and dry. Your physician will give you specific bathing instructions. You may be advised not to participate in any strenuous activities. Your physician will instruct you about when you can return to work and resume normal activities.

*Postprocedural Information to your physician about your physical problems such as:*

- Fever and/or chills
- Increased pain, redness, swelling, or bleeding or other drainage from the insertion site
- Coolness, numbness and/or tingling, or other changes in the affected extremity
- Chest pain/pressure, nausea and/or vomiting, profuse sweating, dizziness, and/or fainting

Your physician may give you additional or alternate instructions after the procedure, depending on your particular situation.

### Management of Cardiac Arrhythmias with Catheter Ablation

Radiofrequency catheter ablation (RFCA) has revolutionized treatment for tachyarrhythmias and has become first-line therapy for some tachycardias. Although developed in the 1980s and widely applied in the 1990s, formalized guidelines for its use in clinical practice were not developed until recently.

### Different Types of Catheters Employed in Ablation

The design and functionality of catheters is constantly evolving. Most atrial fibrillation ablations today use single point radiofrequency energy catheters, which have a success rate-freedom from atrial fibrillation-of about 70%. It's believed that different types of catheters could have higher success rates or fewer complications. Here are the different types of catheters available today for atrial fibrillation catheter ablations (Figs 11.7–11.10).

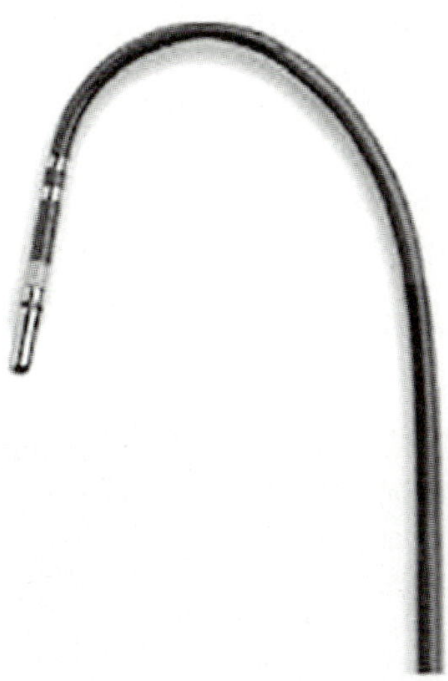

**Fig. 11.7:** A typical ablation catheter with a distal tip consisting of electrodes that can measure the electrical activity in the heart as well as deliver radiofrequency, or heat, energy to ablate cardiac arrhythmias

*Single point radiofrequency catheters* emit radiofrequency energy from a single point at the catheter tip. To make lesions, electrophysiologists ablate one spot after another,

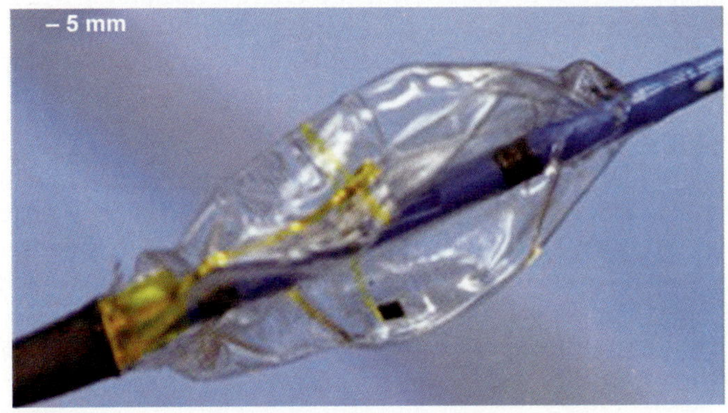


**Fig. 11.8:** Flexible electronics with multisensing cardiac ablation catheter. As an early example that was just announced, an international team of researchers built and tested a balloon ablation catheter capable of measuring intracardiac pressure, EKG, and local temperature around the device tip. All this data can be monitored in real time by the physician during ablation without having to switch devices catheters. Finally, these catheters enable the use of bipolar radiofrequency energy, which may reduce certain complications that are seen with unipolar radiofrequency energy. However, there is limited clinical data on multielectrode catheters, which means that complications arising from these procedures may not be fully known or understood

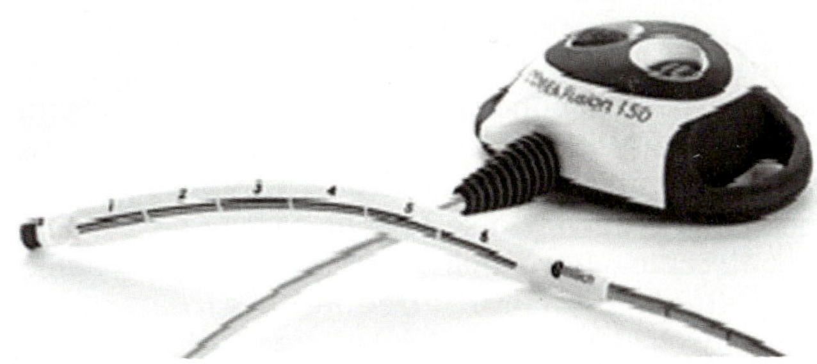

**Fig. 11.9:** An Estech Cobra ablation system

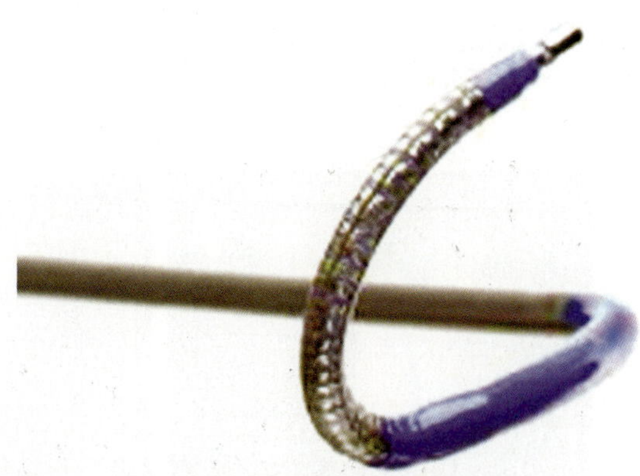

**Fig. 11.10:** Hansen Medical's robotic catheter control system for EP study

similar to drawing a line by making dots one after the other. If all the dots are not connected, afib could re-enter the heart in the unablated space (gap).

*Multielectrode radiofrequency catheters* have several electrodes, each of which can transmit radiofrequency energy. These catheters can ablate a larger area of tissue than single point radiofrequency energy catheters, which could decrease procedure times. In addition, multielectrode catheters may be better at making contiguous lesions (lesion lines without any gaps) than single point.

*Contact force sensing radiofrequency catheters:* Contact force is one of the variables that affects transmurality. If there is not enough pressure, the lesion may not fully penetrate the tissue, which would allow afib to re-enter the heart. If there is too much pressure, complications, such as steam pops, can occur. These catheters tell the electrophysiologist how much pressure is being applied to the catheter and tissue.

*Balloon catheters:* After the balloon catheter is inserted into the left atrium, the electrophysiologist inflates the balloon at the tip of the catheter. Balloon catheters can ablate a larger area of tissue than single point radiofrequency catheters, which enhances the prospects that lesions will be contiguous (without gaps) and could shorten procedure times. There are balloon catheters using cryothermy, laser energy, and even radiofrequency energy. In general, balloon catheters have difficulty reaching the right pulmonary veins.

## Robotic Catheter Navigation for Ablation

Robotic catheter ablation is performed at some centers. Robotic systems could improve navigation of the catheter, keep the catheter in a stable position, and shorten procedure times. In general, robotic catheter ablations have had similar outcomes as traditional (manual) catheter ablation, meaning that the success and complications rates aren't significantly better or worse. Robotic systems are expensive, so not all centers have them. Performing catheter ablation with a single point radiofrequency catheter can be technically challenging, particularly for doctors who have not performed many ablations. In theory, using a robot will simplify the procedure and decrease the expertise needed. However, studies that test this theory have not been performed. A robotic ablation starts the same way as a traditional catheter ablation. The doctor inserts a catheter into the groin and guides the catheter to the right side of the heart. After making a puncture in the septum, the wall that separates the right and left sides of the heart, the doctor leaves the patient's side and goes to the control system for the robotic system, which is usually located in an adjacent room.

## Leading Robotic Systems Used in Catheter Ablations

*Niobe (Stereotaxis):* Niobe is a magnetic system that only works with the CARTO electroanatomic mapping system and Biosense Webster mapping and ablation catheters. It does not look like a robot, but is considered a robotic system. The patient's bed lies between two large magnets, which track the movement in the catheter and send the information to the system. The doctor uses a joystick like those used in video games to change the position of the magnets, which then makes the catheters move. People who have a pacemaker or ICD cannot have a Niobe procedure because these devices would be affected by the magnets.

*Sensei (Hansen Medical):* Sensei has a robotic arm that is attached to the patient's bed. It works with both Ensite NaVx and CARTO as well as standard mapping and ablation catheters. Similar to the Niobe system, the doctor uses a joystick to change the catheter's location. When the doctor moves the joystick in the Sensei system, the robotic arm moves the catheter. Robotic technology is changing the paradigm for catheter ablation treatment of atrial fibrillation to read about the largest study to date comparing Sensei to traditional catheter ablations, which was presented at Boston Atrial Fibrillation Symposium 2010.

*Amigo (Catheter Robotics):* Amigo is a less expensive system than Niobe and Sensei and works with a variety of mapping and ablation catheters. It is in a clinical trial in the United States.

*Artis zeego (Siemens):* Artis zeego uses computed tomography (CT) imaging technology to guide navigation, and is also in clinical studies.

## Catheter Ablation Technology

The goal of any catheter or energy source is to create a transmural lesion while minimizing complications (Figs 11.11–11.17). A transmural lesion-scar tissue that completely

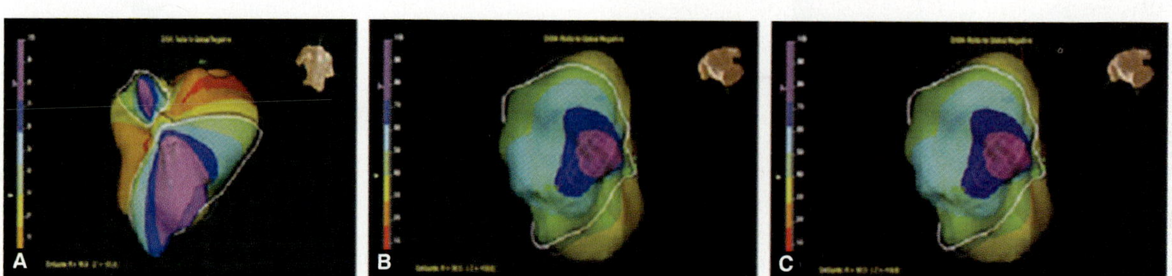


**Fig. 11.11A to C:** Three-dimensional views showing large anteroapical scars

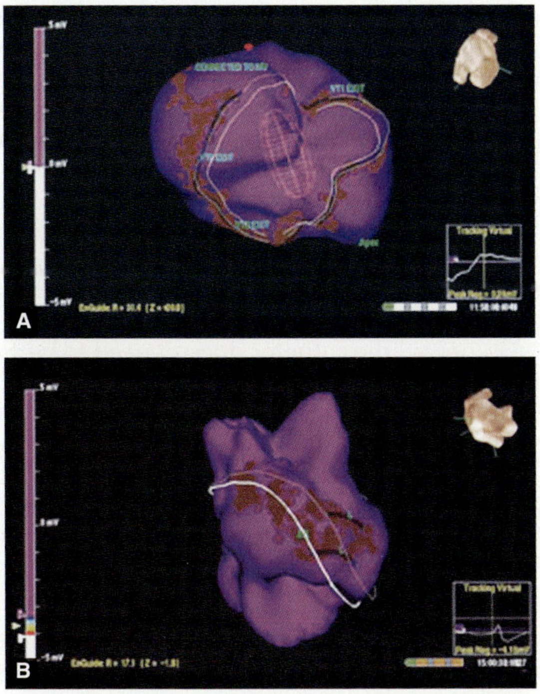


**Fig. 11.12:** (A) Three-dimensional view of multiple radiofrequency ablations in a line along the border of large anterior scar connecting it to mitral annulus, (B) three-dimensional view of multiple radiofrequency ablations in a line along the border of large posterior scar at the site of VT exit

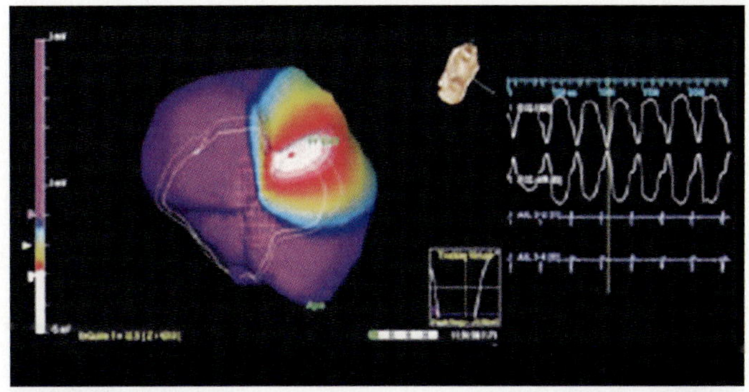

**Fig. 11.13:** Three-dimensional view showing the exit of ventricular tachycardia from the scar area

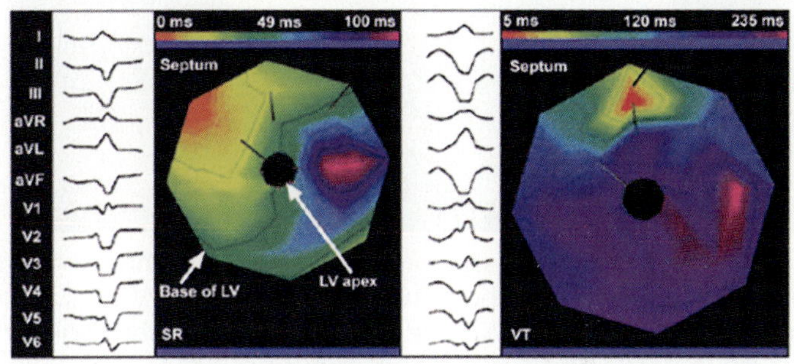


**Fig. 11.15:** 32-site bipolar mapping of ventricular tachycardia. The outer circle is located near the base of the left ventricle (LV) while the inner circle is positioned within the LV apex. Left panel—mapping during sinus rhythm (SR) shows that the earliest endocardial activation (red) is in the region near the basal septum; activation then spreads rapidly in a radial pattern over the endocarium. The area in purple/pink is activated last. Right panel—during ventricular tachycardia (VT), there is a change in the activation sequence and an increase in the activation time, indicated by the blue/purple color over the majority of the LV endocardium (reprinted by permission from Schalij MJ, van Rugge P, Siezenga M, et al. Circulation. 1998;98:2168)

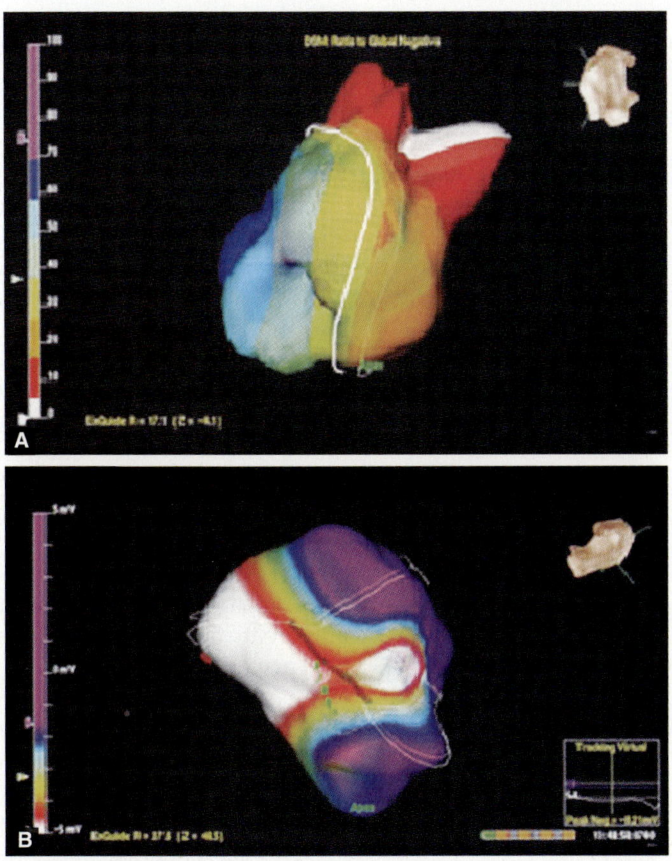


**Fig. 11.14A and B:** Three-dimensional views showing large areas of posterior scar

penetrates the heart tissue is key to a successful ablation because it keeps errant electrical signals from being transmitted. Making a transmural lesion is as much of an art as it is a science. It depends on the temperature generated by the energy source, how much pressure is applied to the catheter (contact force), and how long the catheter remains in contact with tissue. There are different energy sources that can be used in various types of catheters, and each has advantages and disadvantages, so it's important for patients to understand the different options.

## Energy Sources

Here are the energy sources being used today in atrial fibrillation catheter ablations.

*Radiofrequency (RF) energy* is radio waves that are converted to heat to ablate and create scar tissue. It reliably achieves transmurality and is the most widely used energy source in catheter ablations. In general, high temperatures are needed to make sure that all layers of tissue are ablated. Traditional catheters use unipolar radiofrequency energy,

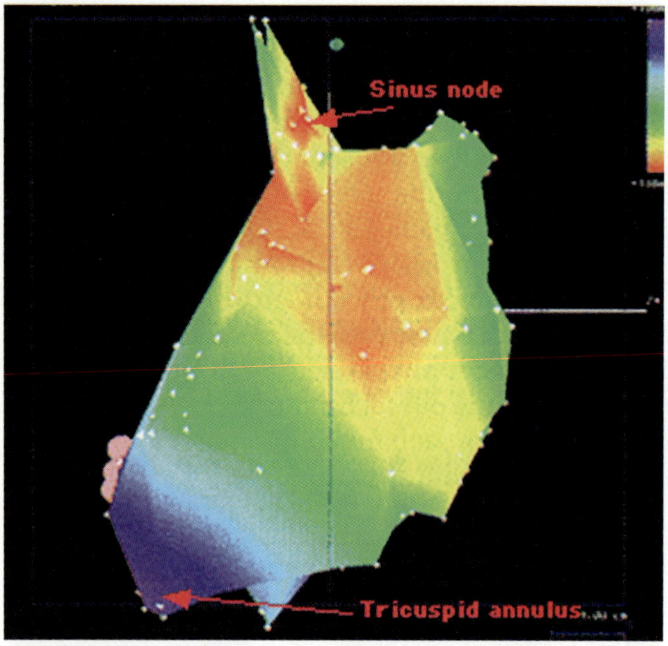


**Fig. 11.16:** Activation sequence during sinus rhythm. Electro-anatomic mapping of the right atrium with the CARTO system during sinus rhythm shows the earliest activation in the region of the sinus node (red), spreading throughout the atrium. The last part to be activated is the region of the tricuspid annulus and coronary sinus as (dark blue/purple). (Reprinted with permission from Cooke PA, Wilber DJ. Pacing Clin electrophysiol. 1998; 21:1802)

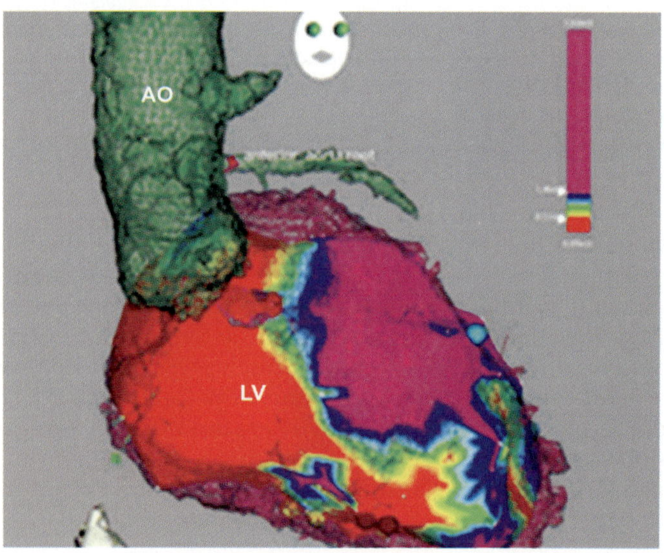


**Fig. 11.17:** The 3-D composed tomographic reconstruction of the left ventricle (LV) displayed as purple wireframe aligned with the 3-D LV endocardial voltage map (solid color map). Red areas represent dense scar and purple areas represent normal myocardium; dark brown points indicate ablation sites. AO=aorta.

which simply means that the radiofrequency energy is transmitted from a single point at the catheter's tip.

*Cryothermy, or cryo energy*, is intense cold that is used to form ice crystals within the tissue, causing the cells to die and creating scar tissue. It may be easier to make lesions using cryothermy since the cold temperatures cause tissue to stick to the catheter. In addition, cryo energy may have fewer major complications. Animal studies have shown cryo energy to have a much lower incidence of thrombus (clot) formation than radiofrequency energy, which suggests that cryothermy could lower the risk of a stroke. Cryo energy can be used in single point catheters or balloon catheters. Laser energy is light waves that are converted to heat to ablate and create scar tissue. It may be a safer heat-based energy than unipolar radiofrequency energy. With laser energy, the catheter doesn't need to be in direct contact with tissue, which could mean it will have fewer complications than radiofrequency energy. Unlike other energy sources, contact force is not a factor in whether a laser lesion is transmural. In addition, laser energy can be adjusted when ablating tissues of varying thickness, with higher energy applied to thicker tissue and lower energy applied to thinner structures in the heart.

*Other energy sources,* such as microwave and high intensity focused ultrasound (HIFU), have been studied but these energy sources aren't widely used in catheter ablation. The tools used to assist with catheter ablation are constantly evolving. Here are some of the tools that are commonly used for atrial fibrillation catheter ablations.

## Mapping and Navigation Tools for Ablation

The tools used to assist with catheter ablation are constantly evolving. Here are some of the tools that are commonly used for atrial fibrillation catheter ablations

1. *CT and MR imaging of the atrium and pulmonary veins* provides pre-ablation imaging to help doctors locate anatomic features and identify variations in anatomy of the individual heart
2. *Fluoroscopy X-ray* helps doctors guide mapping and ablation catheters in the body by generating 2D (flat) black and white images, but can't show contours in anatomy, such as the 'curve' of a pulmonary vein, and also exposes the patient and doctor to radiation
3. *Pulmonary vein venography* helps determine the location of the pulmonary vein ostia, the base of the pulmonary veins, and guide the manipulation of the catheter
4. *Intracardiac echocardiography (ICE)* provides real time information about anatomy to facilitate the transseptal puncture (from the right atrium to the left atrium) and to guide catheter ablation
5. *Electroanatomic mapping system* reduces fluoroscopy exposure to doctors and patients and allows doctors to visualize structures in 3D and create appropriate lesions, particularly with the incorporation of previously-acquired MR or CT images
6. *Robotic catheter navigation* improves navigation precision and may shorten procedures, and includes the Stereotaxis' Niobe magnetic navigation system, Hansen Medical's Sensei robot, and Catheter Robotics' Amigo robot
7. *Multielectrode circumferential mapping catheter* verifies that the pulmonary veins are electrically isolated

### Electroanatomic Mapping Systems for Ablation

Because of the shortcomings of fluoroscopy, some electrophysiologists use electroanatomic mapping systems like Ensite NaVx (St. Jude Medical) and CARTO (Biosense Webster), which provide colorful 3D images that show variations in a patient's anatomy. These systems may assist doctors in assuring that lesions are contiguous (no gaps) and in reducing complications, such as perforation of the heart or esophagus. In addition, the use of an electro-anatomic mapping system may lessen the time that doctors and patients are exposed to radiation. However, the systems are expensive, so they are not available at all facilities.

Using these systems, electrophysiologists create a real time 3D view of the heart by positioning a mapping catheter in the heart. When the doctor moves the catheter in a sweeping motion, the systems track the catheter's location. CARTO and Ensite NaVx use different methods to do this. In a CARTO procedure, the table where the patient lies has an electromagnetic pad that tracks movement of the catheter, whereas in an EnSite NaVx procedure, patches on the patient's skin track the catheter. Both systems use algorithms to translate data on the catheter's location into a 3D image. It usually takes about 20 minutes to complete this process.

Electroanatomic mapping systems are sometimes called multimodality mapping or image integration systems because they can show pictures or data from other sources. For instance, patient CT or MRI scans taken a few days or weeks before the procedure may be loaded onto Ensite NaVx or CARTO and matched with the real time 3D image of the heart. The doctor does this by moving the catheter slightly, verifying its location in the heart, and taking note of large structures like the pulmonary veins. After several common areas on the two images are identified, the system merges the real time view and pre-procedure scan into one 3D picture. It usually takes about 15 minutes to complete this process, which is called registration. However, the positioning of anatomy can even change within just a week, so if the pre-procedure scan doesn't easily correspond with the real time view of the heart, it can take much longer. Electroanatomic mapping systems also provide real time data on electrical activity within the heart, which means that electrophysiologists can see whether conduction block has been achieved. The systems also provide other real time information, such as atrial pressure and volume, so doctors can easily monitor the patient during the procedure.

### Catheter Ablation Techniques

Catheter ablation techniques are constantly evolving. Initial catheter ablations attempted to recreate the lesion set used in the open-chest Cox maze procedure by creating linear ablation lines that interrupted the atrial fibrillation wavelets (Figs 11.18–11.21). However, doctors had difficulty

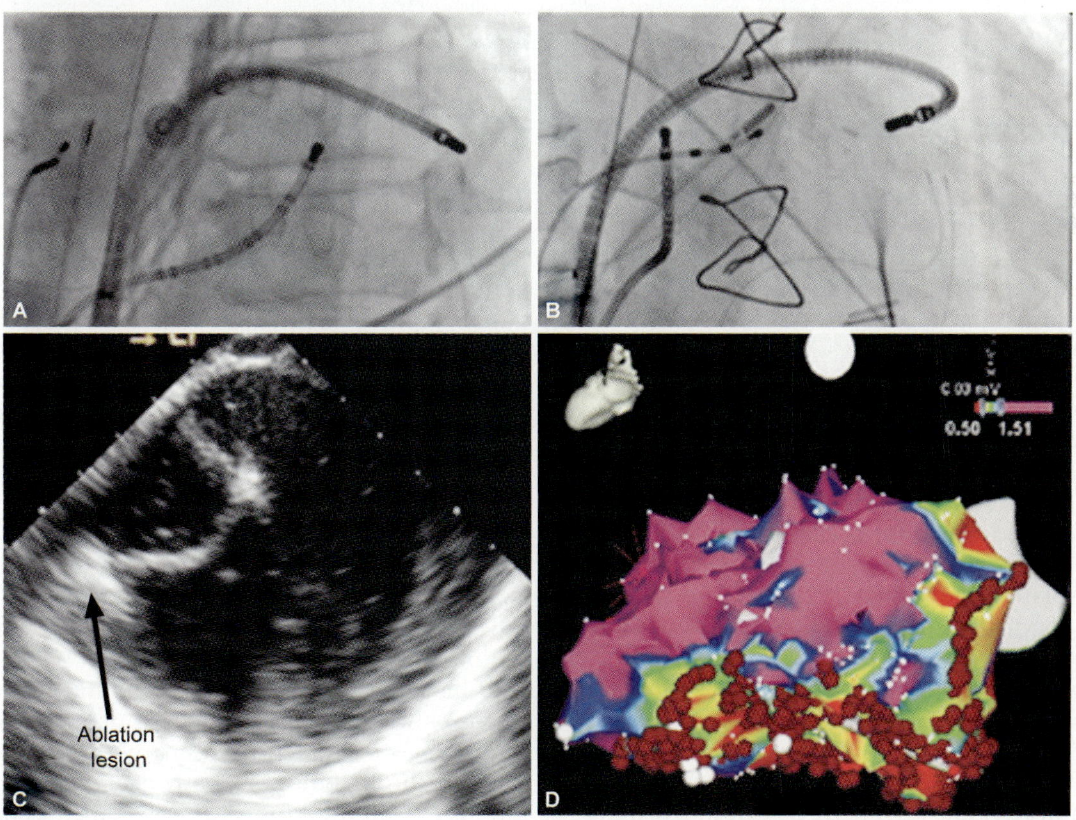


**Fig. 11.18:** Mapping and ablation of a basal lateral scar. (A, B) Robotic catheter position in left and right anterior oblique fluoroscopic views, respectively. The mid-lateral wall is being mapped, (C) intracardiac echocardiographic image showing catheter contact and lesion formation in the left ventricular lateral wall, (D) three-dimensional map of the lateral scar and the ablation lesions created

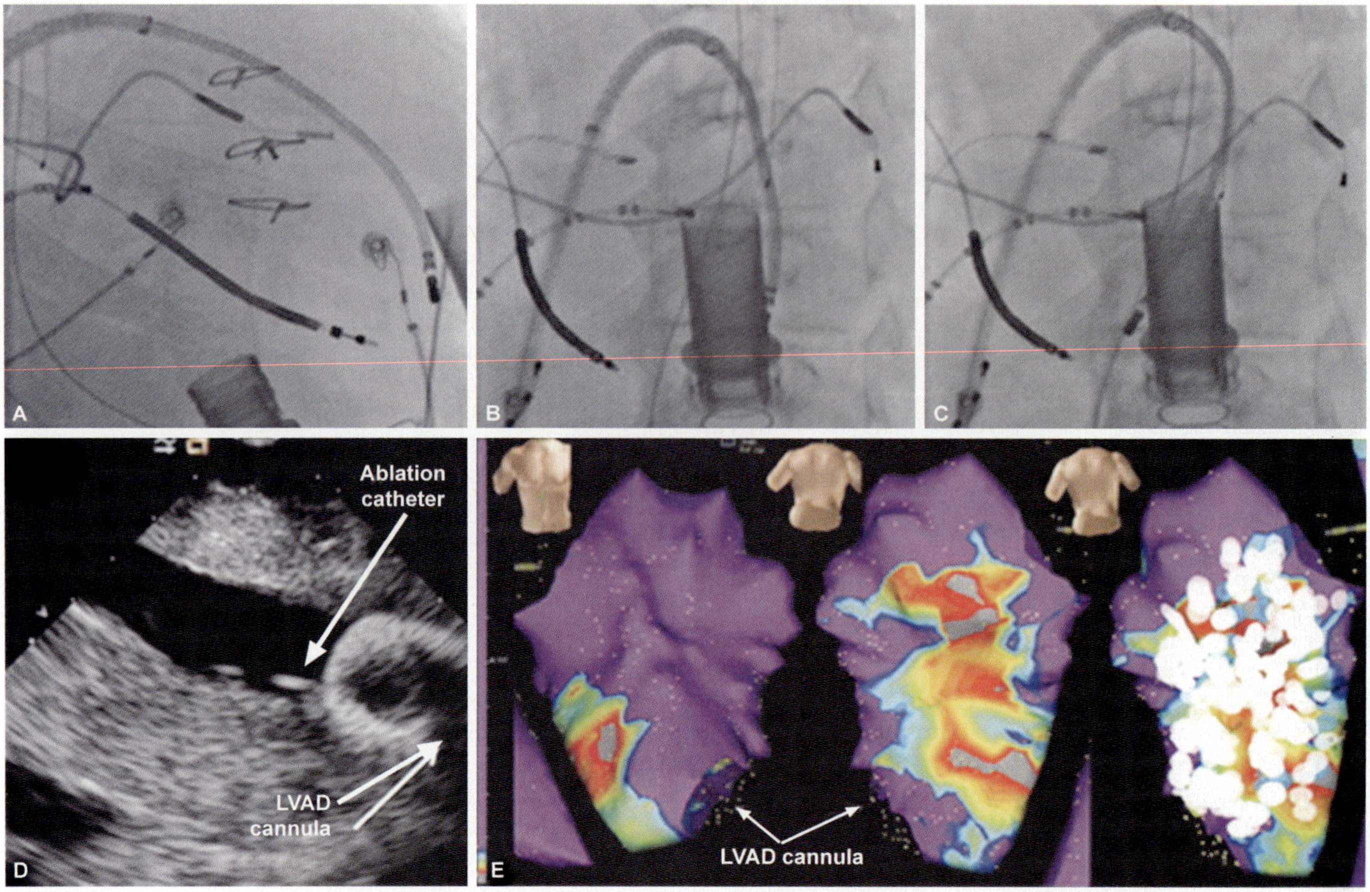


**Fig. 11.19:** Mapping and ablation of an inferior wall scar in the presence of a left ventricular assist device (LVAD). (A to C) Robotic catheter position in the right (A) and left (B, C) anterior oblique fluoroscopic views, with the catheter tip around the LVAD inflow cannula. (D) Intracardiac echocardiographic image of the LVAD cannula and the ablation catheter. (E) Three-dimensional scar maps and ablation lesions

duplicating the Cox maze lesion set during a closed-chest catheter ablation. The procedure had high complication rates and required long fluoroscopy times. Research in Bordeaux, France, by Michel Haïssaguerre, MD, and colleagues, suggested that electrophysiologists didn't need to duplicate the Cox maze lesion set. Dr. Haïssaguerre's group found that over 90% of atrial fibrillation is triggered (starts) in or near the pulmonary veins. As a result of these findings, a new type of catheter ablation technique, called segmental pulmonary vein isolation or ostial pulmonary vein isolation, was created. Dr. Haïssaguerre and his colleagues used radiofrequency energy to ablate the pulmonary vein ostium, the opening to the pulmonary veins. When 'isolated', pulmonary veins can no longer be a trigger point for atrial fibrillation. Dr. Haïssaguerre and his colleagues were able to terminate atrial fibrillation in, and stop prescribing antiarrhythmic drugs for, 62% of patients in the study.

This pulmonary vein isolation approach continues to be the cornerstone of catheter ablation strategies for the treatment of paroxysmal atrial fibrillation. However, pulmonary vein isolation can mean different things to different doctors. Indeed, it has become a catch-all term to describe any ablation of the pulmonary veins. This can lead to misunderstandings between doctors and patients, and can make a big difference in the rate of freedom from afib after ablation. Perhaps the most important difference among doctors relates to whether the pulmonary veins are isolated, or just ablated. In order for a procedure to be called a pulmonary vein isolation, the doctor must confirm that the pulmonary veins are 'blocked', in other words, that conduction block was achieved. This is done with a mapping catheter that can determine whether there is any electrical activity around the pulmonary veins. If conduction block isn't confirmed, then the procedure is an ablation, not an isolation. Thus, it is important to ask doctors what type of lesion set will be made and whether they will confirm that conduction is blocked.

There have been several updates to the segmental (ostial) pulmonary vein isolation developed by Dr. Haïssaguerre and his colleagues. First, it was found that ablating tissue in the ostia (opening) of the pulmonary veins could lead to pulmonary vein stenosis (narrowing), which is a serious complication that can obstruct oxygenated blood from flowing from the lungs into the heart. Second, it has been found that more extensive lesion sets are better at stopping afib. This is probably because the pulmonary veins aren't the only area in the heart that can trigger atrial fibrillation.

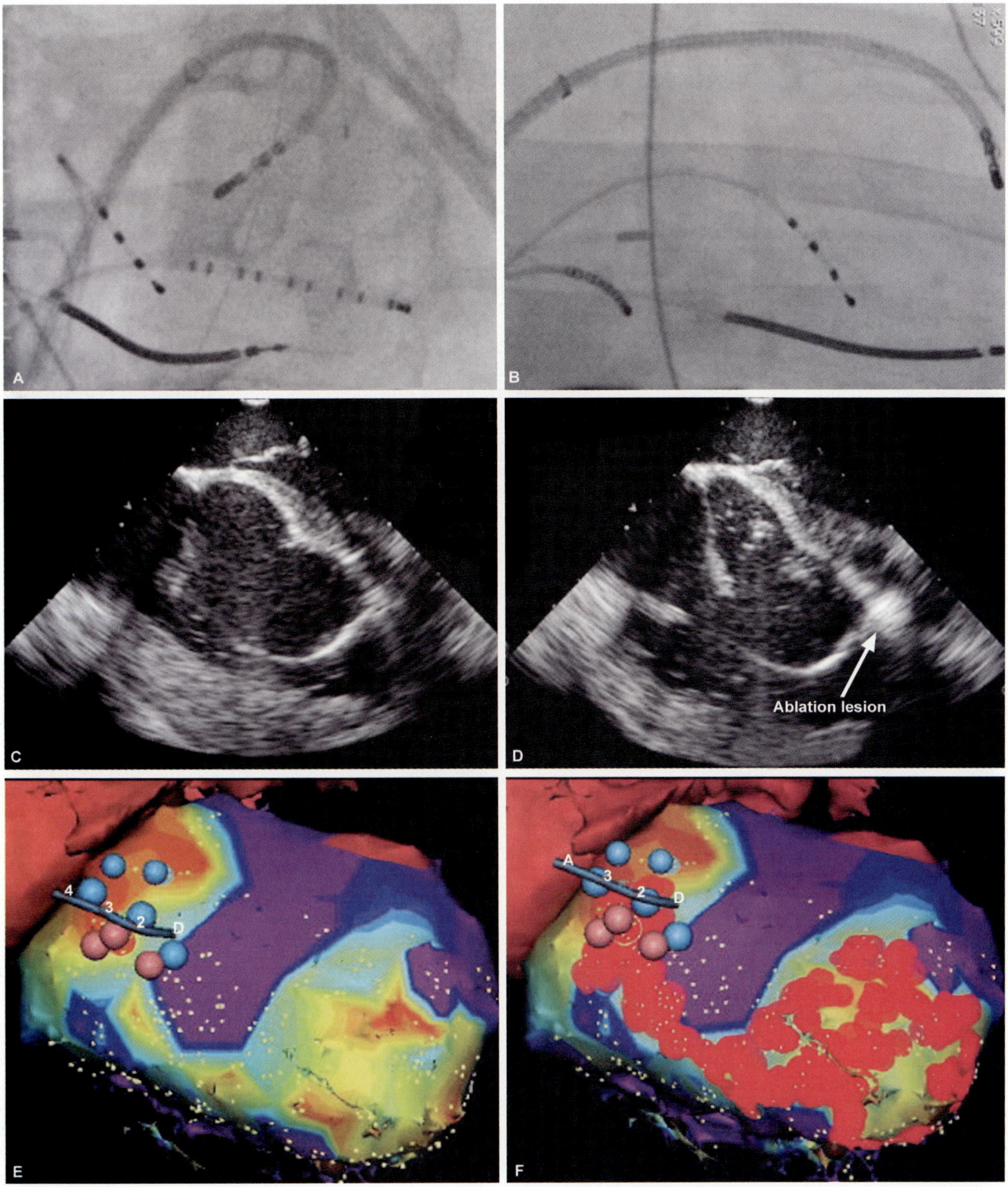


**Fig. 11.20:** Mapping and ablation of a septal scar. Stable catheter positioning allowed real-time monitoring of lesion creation on intracardiac echocardiography. (A, B) Robotic catheter position in left and right anterior oblique fluoroscopic views, respectively. The septal aspect of the apex was being mapped. (C, D) Intracardiac echocardiographic images before and 15 seconds after application of radiofrequency. The catheter tip is in the distal septum, where increased echogenicity is seen at the ablation site. (E, F) Three-dimensional maps of the large septal and apical scar and the ablation lesions, respectively

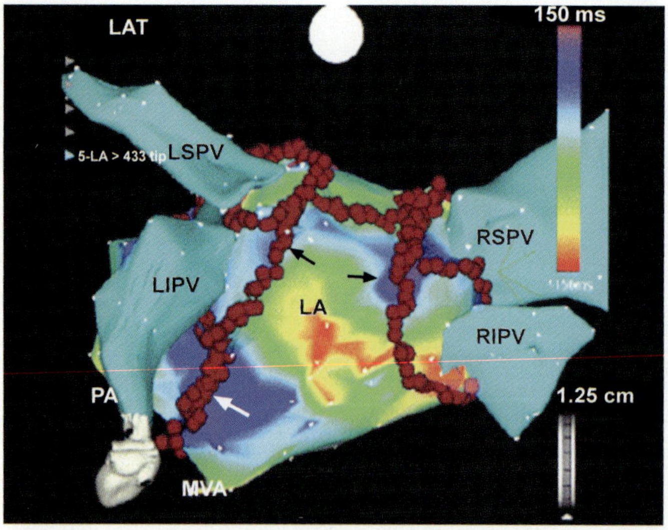


**Fig. 11.21:** Postablation electroanatomic map showing a wide area circumferential ablation in a patient with persistent atrial fibrillation. Shown are the left superior pulmonary vein (LSPV), left inferior pulmonary vein (LIPV), right superior pulmonary vein (RSPV), and right inferior pulmonary vein (RIPV). Ablative rings circumscribe the left and right pulmonary vein sets. The carinal lines between the veins, a line connecting the right to the left pulmonary vein rings, and an ablative line (white arrow) from the LIPV to the mitral valve annulus (MVA) are also shown. LA=left atrium. (With permission from Packer DL. Catheter ablation for atrial fibrillation: A promising alternative to drug therapy

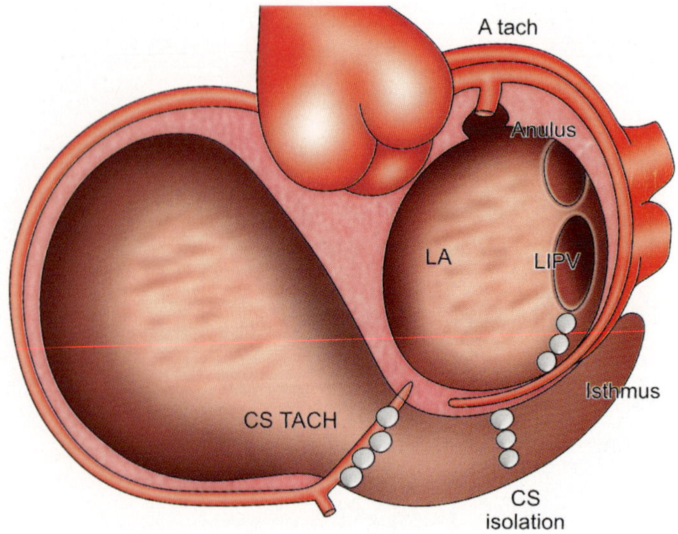


**Fig. 11.22:** Diagrammatic representation of ablation sites which may involve injury to the major coronary arterial system. Septal mitral annular tachycardias may result in injury to the proximal circumflex coronary artery, whereas the more distal portions of this artery can be injured during Ic or coronary sinus-based ablation

Over time, afib can create new pathways, called macro reentry sites, where it can 'cycle' in the heart. Macro reentry sites are different for each patient.

Ablation strategies and techniques continue to evolve, as does the terminology, as doctors learn more about areas of the heart that could act as a trigger or reentry site. Thus, the term 'segmental pulmonary vein isolation' is rarely used today, and instead we refer to the anatomic area that will be ablated or to the technical approach to ablation.

### Basic Catheter Ablation Techniques

Here are the most frequently used basic catheter ablation techniques, shown in order of the fewest to the greatest number of ablation (lesion) lines.

*Antrum pulmonary vein ablation:* Because of the issues with the ostia, as mentioned above, the antrum (base) of the pulmonary veins became the site of catheter ablations. The antrum includes the posterior (back) wall of the left atrium and extends to the anterior (front) of the right pulmonary veins. In essence, it is a wide perimeter around the pulmonary veins. Antrum pulmonary vein ablation entails lesion lines in this area, but doctors do not confirm conduction block.

1. *Pulmonary vein antrum isolation (PVAI or PVI)* (Figs 11.22 and 11. 23): Lesion lines are made in the antrum of the pulmonary veins, and doctors confirm that conduction block has been achieved. Some electrophysiologists also make additional lesion lines. These may include the superior vena cava, roof of the atrium, or the septum, the wall that separates the two sides of the heart. You can see these structures in this diagram of the heart. However, the location of the additional lesions varies by doctor. That is, there is not a standard that requires that all pulmonary vein antrum isolations include a lesion line along the superior vena cava.
2. *Circumferential ablation:* Similar to pulmonary vein antrum isolation, circumferential ablation entails lesions encircling the pulmonary veins. Some electrophysiologists also make an ablation line that connects the pulmonary veins on the posterior (back) wall of the left atrium or ablate tissue from the pulmonary veins to the mitral valve. In addition, a mapping catheter is used to identify 'potentials', which are areas that could serve as a trigger or macro reentry site for atrial fibrillation. According to the HRS Consensus Statement, there is not a single endpoint, or goal, for circumferential ablation. Some doctors confirm that conduction block has been achieved, whereas others look for elimination of 'potentials' or a reduction in electrical activity in the ablated area.

### Advanced Catheter Ablation Techniques

Atrial fibrillation leads to atrial remodeling over time, meaning that afib can change the deeper layers of heart tissue (substrate) or change the way electricity is conducted within the heart. This is also known as substrate modification. Advanced catheter ablation techniques, which are primarily used to treat persistent and long-standing persistent afib, target anomalies in the substrate or electrical conduction. However, clinical data is inconclusive, meaning that it is not clear whether these

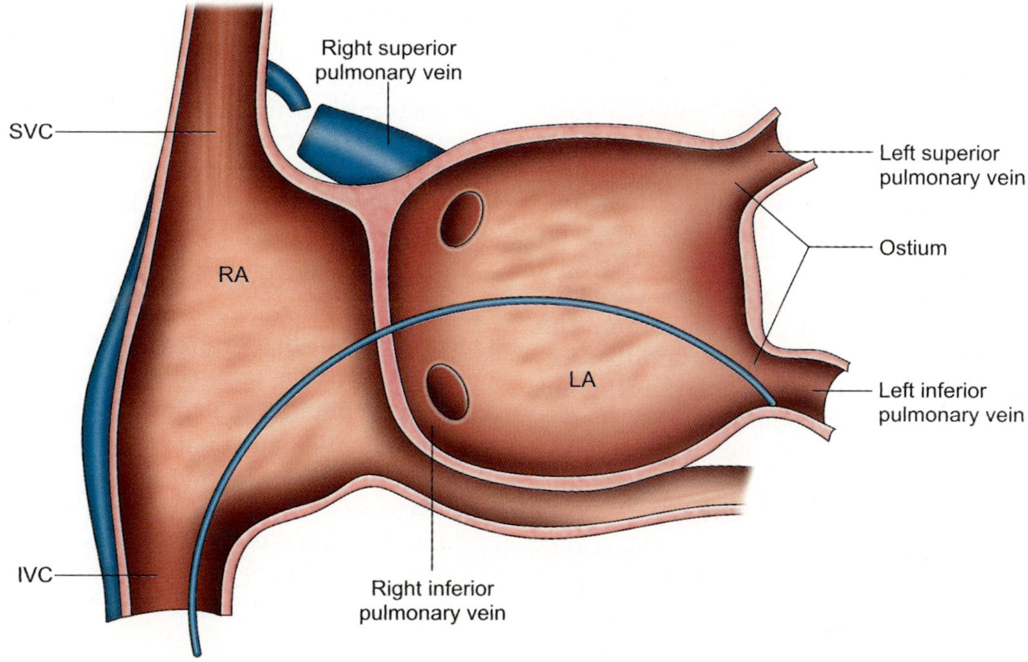


**Fig. 11.23:** Targeting the triggers in atrial fibrillation (AF) ablation

techniques can stop persistent or longstanding persistent afib for the majority of patients.

*The most commonly used advanced catheter ablation techniques are:*

1. ***Stepwise ablation:*** Stepwise ablation is the only ablation strategy with a stated goal of terminating afib. It involves isolation of the pulmonary veins and entails additional lesion lines, which differ by electrophysiologist. It is sometimes called sequential ablation because the additional ablation lines are performed in a specified order. That is, doctors may make a lesion line along the roof of the left atrium, and then pace or use a mapping catheter to determine whether conduction has been stopped. If there continues to be afib activity, the doctor will ablate the next area in the sequence. The lesion lines and sequences vary by doctor. Most electrophysiologists make a lesion on the roof of the left atrium after isolating the pulmonary veins. After this, some doctors will ablate the coronary sinus, the vessel between the left atrium and the left ventricle, whereas others might ablate the mitral isthmus, the area where the mitral valve and the left inferior pulmonary vein meet. There isn't one specific sequence that has proven to have the best results, largely because clinical trials haven't been performed on this.
2. ***Complex fractionated atrial electrograms:*** Ablation of complex fractionated atrial electrograms (CFAE, pronounced cafe) is performed by some electrophysiologists to treat persistent and longstanding persistent afib. A complex fractionated atrial electrogram is a site where there is an unusual electrical pattern, which could be due to the length of the electrical wave (long or short), the frequency of electrical activity (a lot or a little), or the speed of conduction (fast or slow). Complex fractionated atrial electrograms appear to represent macro reentry sites for atrial fibrillation, so ablation of these sites should stop afib, but that has not been proven by clinical data. In fact, CFAE ablation has been shown to be less effective in stopping afib than a pulmonary vein antral isolation with additional lesion lines at the roof of the left atrium and along the mitral isthmus. To learn more, *see* can catheter ablation successfully treat persistent atrial fibrillation, which discusses a session at the Heart Rhythm Society about ablating persistent afib.
3. ***Ganglionated plexi ablation:*** Another advanced strategy for stopping afib is to ablate the ganglionated plexi (GPs), which are 'fat pads' in the heart. Nerves that control automatic functions, such as breathing, are located in these ganglionated plexi. These nerves also initiate electrical activity at various places in the heart. It is thought that when one ganglionated plexus is activated, another ganglionated plexus located nearby will also be activated. Some doctors use mapping catheters with high frequency electrodes to identify ganglionated plexi, while others simply ablate the four primary ganglionated plexi in the left atrium. Ablation of the ganglionated plexi has not been widely adopted by electrophysiologists, which may be because there is little research data available.
4. ***Hybrid ablation:*** Hybrid ablation is an emerging treatment for patients with more severe forms of atrial fibrillation, typically persistent and longstanding persistent afib. Hybrid ablation is a dual approach in which an electrophysiologist ablates from inside the heart and a cardiac surgeon ablates on the outside of the heart. A hybrid ablation may enhance the prospects that ablation lines fully penetrate all layers of the cardiac tissue, which

is crucial to stopping afib. In addition, higher success rates and fewer complications could be possible because each specialty (electrophysiology and cardiac surgery) can ablate areas of the heart that are best suited to their different approaches. *See* hybrid procedure may offer better outcomes for persistent and longstanding persistent atrial fibrillation for Dr. James Edgerton's presentation on hybrid ablations at Boston Atrial Fibrillation Symposium in January 2011. Another dual approach, the convergent procedure, also has surgeons and electrophysiologists collaborate on ablation. The convergent procedure is different from hybrid procedures in that it uses a different entry point and a different device, in this case a unipolar radiofrequency device instead of a bipolar radiofrequency one.

## Clinical Applications of Catheter Ablation

*There are three classes of indications for catheter ablation:*

1. The first is symptomatic supraventricular tachycardia (SVT) due to atrioventricular nodal re-entrant tachycardia (AVNRT), Wolff-Parkinson-White syndrome, unifocal atrial tachycardia, or atrial flutter (especially common right atrial forms). For these conditions, catheter ablation is first-line therapy if that is the patient's preference.
2. The second indication is atrial fibrillation with lifestyle-impairing symptoms and inefficacy or intolerance of at least 1 antiarrhythmic agent. Both left atrial ablation for restoration of sinus rhythm and AV junction ablation for rate control are class I indications, depending on the circumstance.
3. The third indication is symptomatic ventricular tachycardia (VT). Catheter ablation is first-line therapy in idiopathic VT, if that is the patient's preference. In structural heart disease, catheter ablation is generally performed for drug inefficacy or intolerance, or as adjunctive therapy in patients with an implantable cardioverter-defibrillator (ICD) who are experiencing frequent ICD discharges.

*Uncommon indications for catheter ablation include the following:*

1. Symptomatic drug-refractory (inefficacy or intolerance) idiopathic sinus tachycardia
2. Lifestyle-impairing ectopic beats
3. Symptomatic junctional ectopic tachycardia
4. RFCA has been applied to most clinical tachycardias, even to polymorphic ventricular tachycardia and ventricular fibrillation in preliminary studies. Success rates are highest in patients with common forms of SVT, namely AVNRT and orthodromic reciprocating tachycardia (ORT).

## Contraindications to Radiofrequency Catheter Ablation

Few absolute contraindications to RFCA exist. Left atrial ablation and ablation for persistent atrial flutter should not be performed in the presence of known atrial thrombus. Similarly, mobile left ventricular thrombus would be a contraindication to left ventricular ablation. Mechanical prosthetic heart valves are generally not crossed with ablation catheters. Reproductive-aged women should not be exposed to fluoroscopy if any possibility exists that they are pregnant.

**Table 11.1:** Characteristics of catheter ablation for selected cardiac arrhythmias

| Arrhythmia | Ablation location | Success rate (%) | Complication rate (%) | Potential complications | Indications |
|---|---|---|---|---|---|
| Atrial tachycardia | Variable, anywhere in right or left atrium | 86–100 | 0–8 | Atrioventricular or sinus node dysfunction; cardiac perforation with tamponade; phrenic nerve injury | Incessant tachycardia; symptomatic tachycardia-mediated cardiomyopathy |
| Atrioventricular reentrant tachycardia | Right atrium, perinodal | 96 | 0.5–1 | Atrioventricular nodal block, usually requiring pacemaker implantation | First-line therapy innodal patients willing and able to undergo catheter ablation |
| Atrioventricular reciprocating tachycardia | Variable, left or right atrioventricular | Approximately 95 | 2–4 | Complete atrioventricular nodal block; cardiac perforation with tamponade | First-line therapy for symptoms, single or infrequent episodes, or with atrial fibrillation and rapid conduction |
| Atrial flutter | Right atrium, if common variety of atrial flutter | 88–100 | 2.5–3.5 | Cardiac perforation with tamponade; heart block; myocardial infarction; thromboembolic events | First-line therapy for poorly tolerated or recurrent episodes |
| Atrial fibrillation | Left atrium, pulmonary vein antra | 60–80 | 6–10 | Cardiac perforation with tamponade; phrenic nerve injury; pulmonary vein stenosis; thromboembolic events; vascular complications | Alternative to drug therapy for recurrent atrial in fibrillation in symptomatic patients with minimal or no left atrial enlargement |

## Preprocedural Considerations in Ablation Procedure

- Anesthesia for catheter ablation
- The procedure is typically performed under conscious sedation with intravenous tranquilizers and narcotics. General anesthesia is used in children and selected adults.
- Clinical examination of patient prior to ablation: The preprocedural evaluation always includes a thorough history and physical examination, as well as review of electrocardiograms (12-lead, if available) performed during the tachycardia and with the patient in sinus rhythm. At a minimum, preprocedure blood studies typically includes a complete blood cell count and an assessment of renal function and electrolyte levels.
- An echocardiogram is frequently obtained to exclude structural heart disease. Other tests that are indicated in specific situations include exercise testing with or without cardiac imaging (especially for exercise-induced tachyarrhythmias), and cardiac catheterization.
- The patient should fast overnight before the procedure. Cardiac medications with electrophysiologic effects, such as beta-blockers, calcium channel blockers, digoxin, and class I and III antiarrhythmic drugs, are often tapered and/or discontinued prior to the procedure. Warfarin is typically discontinued for at least a few doses prior to the procedure.

## Technique Employed in Catheter Ablation in Different Clinical Situations

Typically, 2–5 electrode catheters are percutaneously inserted via the femoral or internal jugular veins and are positioned within the left heart, right heart, or both. Multiple catheters are needed to induce and map various tachyarrhythmias prior to radiofrequency catheter ablation (RFCA). Cannulation of the coronary sinus is helpful to exclude left-sided accessory pathways or other left-sided tachyarrhythmia substrates. For left heart catheterization, 1 of 2 approaches may be taken: transseptal catheterization via the interatrial septum or retrograde catheterization across the aortic valve. Anticoagulation with intravenous heparin is used to reduce the risk of periprocedural thromboembolism.

## A. Ablation in Atrial Fibrillation

The simplest catheter ablation procedure performed in patients with atrial fibrillation is RFCA of the AV junction. AV nodal modification is less therapeutic than AV junction ablation and less commonly performed. Catheter ablation of atrial tissue to cure atrial fibrillation is still evolving. The procedure is technically demanding, more risky, and less successful than AV junction or AV nodal ablation. Nevertheless, the observation of Haissaguerre and others that pulmonary vein foci can trigger atrial fibrillation has stimulated much additional research, and there is considerable scientific excitement that this common tachyarrhythmia may be amenable to a curative catheter procedure. The complete surgical Maze procedure (incisions in both atria +/− transmural radiofrequency lesions) is still the most effective technique for potentially curing atrial fibrillation in all comers, regardless of chronicity or whether structural heart disease is present. The best success rates with left atrial catheter ablation are in patients with paroxysmal atrial fibrillation and hearts that are not too structurally abnormal. No consensus exists on the optimal left atrial ablation technique or what constitutes a clinically successful procedure. Nevertheless, evidence is accruing that catheter ablation for atrial fibrillation is more effective than antiarrhythmic drug therapy, especially in patients who have already failed an antiarrhythmic drug. The 2006 ACC/AHA/ESC guidelines for the management of atrial fibrillation now list catheter ablation as a reasonable strategy for patients with life-style impairing symptoms who have failed at least one antiarrhythmic agent (Figs 11.24–11.28).

RFCA of the atrioventricular (AV) junction is the simplest catheter ablation procedure performed in patients

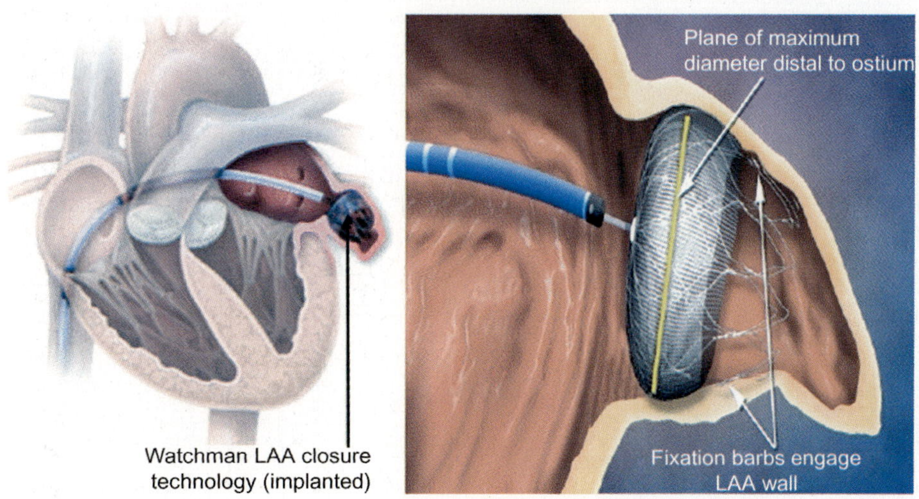


**Fig. 11.24:** A novel procedure using WATCHMAN left atrial appendage closure device implantation. Device is indicated to reduce the risk of thromboembolism from the left atrial appendage in patients with nonvalvular atrial fibrillation who are at increased risk for stroke and systemic embolism

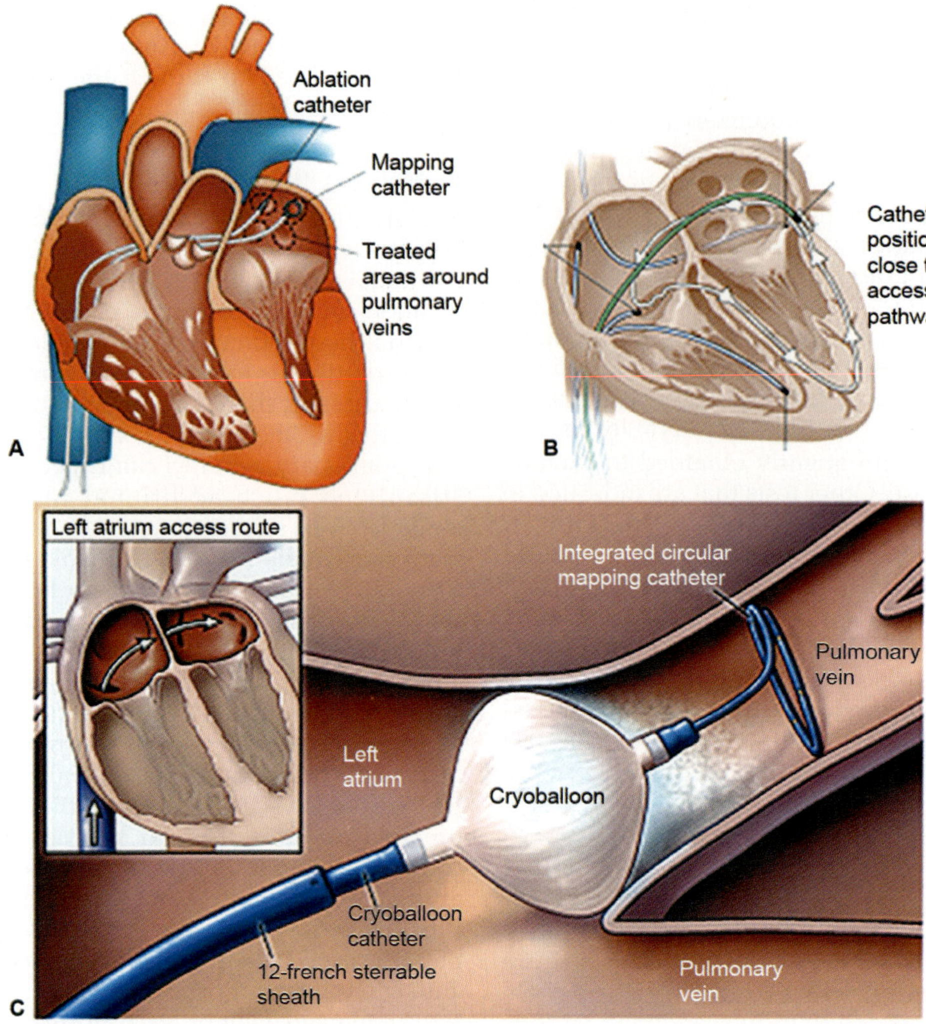


**Fig. 11.25:** (A) Shows treated area around pulmonary vein after introducing mapping and ablation catheters, (B) shows ablation catheter close to accessory pathway, (C) shows cryoablation catheter around the pulmonary vein

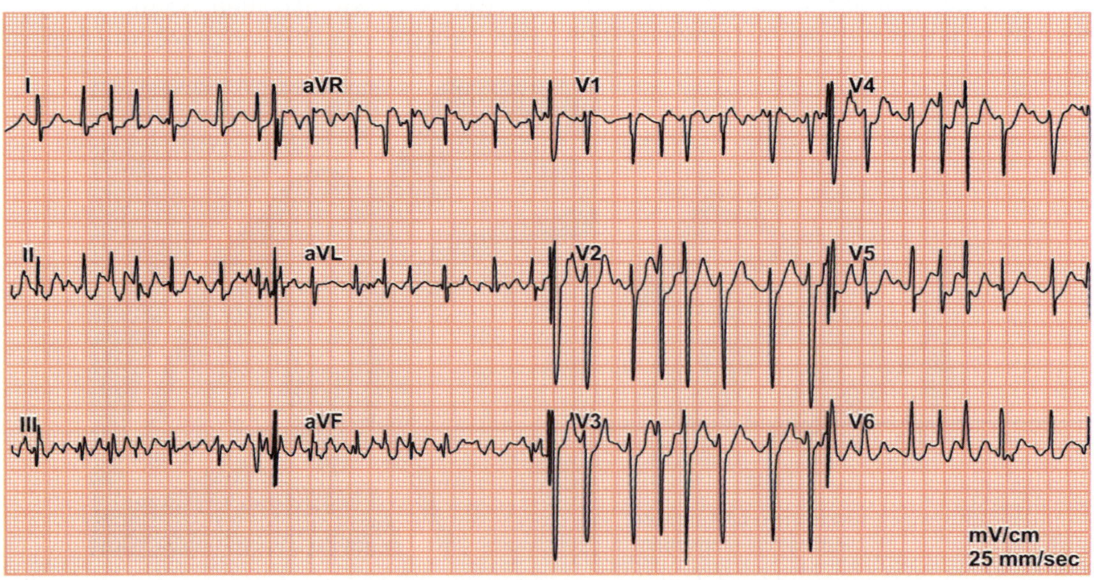


**Fig. 11.26:** Atrial fibrillation 12-lead ECG shows a rapid, irregularly irregular rhythm due to paroxysmal atrial fibrillation which was refractory to multiple medications

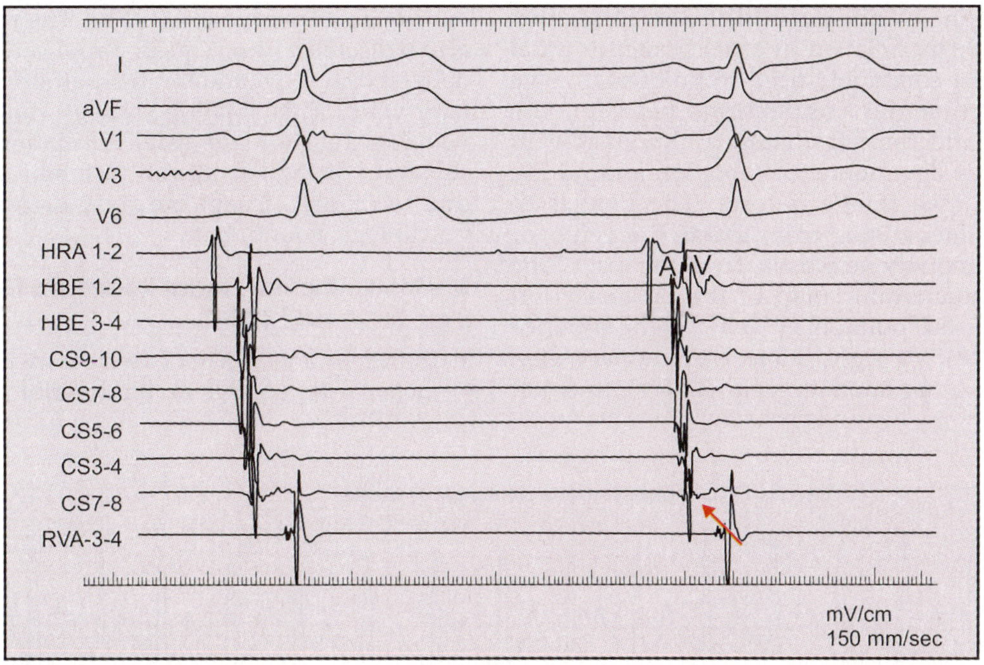


**Fig. 11.27:** Electrophysiologic mapping in Wolff-Parkinson-White syndrome. Shown are five surface ECG leads (I, aVF, V1, V3, V6) and intracardiac recordings from the high right atrium (HRA), lateral mitral annulus (HBE 1-2 and HBE 3-4), coronary sinus (proximal to distal, CS9-10, CS7-8, CS5-6, CS3-4, and CS1-2), and the right ventricular apex (RVA3-4). During the diagnostic electrophysiology study, orthodromic atrioventricular re-entrant tachycardia was induced recordings from the CS demonstrated that the earliest site of ventricular activation was at CS7-8, indicating a left lateral location of the accessory pathway (arrow). The mapping catheter (HBE1-2, 3-4) was advanced through a patient foramen ovale to the lateral mitral annulus. Activation mapping was used to select the ablation site; during sinus rhythem the ablation catheter was manoeuvreted to the site along the mitral annulus which recorded earliest ventricular activity (HBE1-2), i.e. the atrial (A) and ventricular (V) electrograms recorded from the ablation catheter tip were continuous and the local ventricular activity preceded the onset of the delta wave on the surface ECG

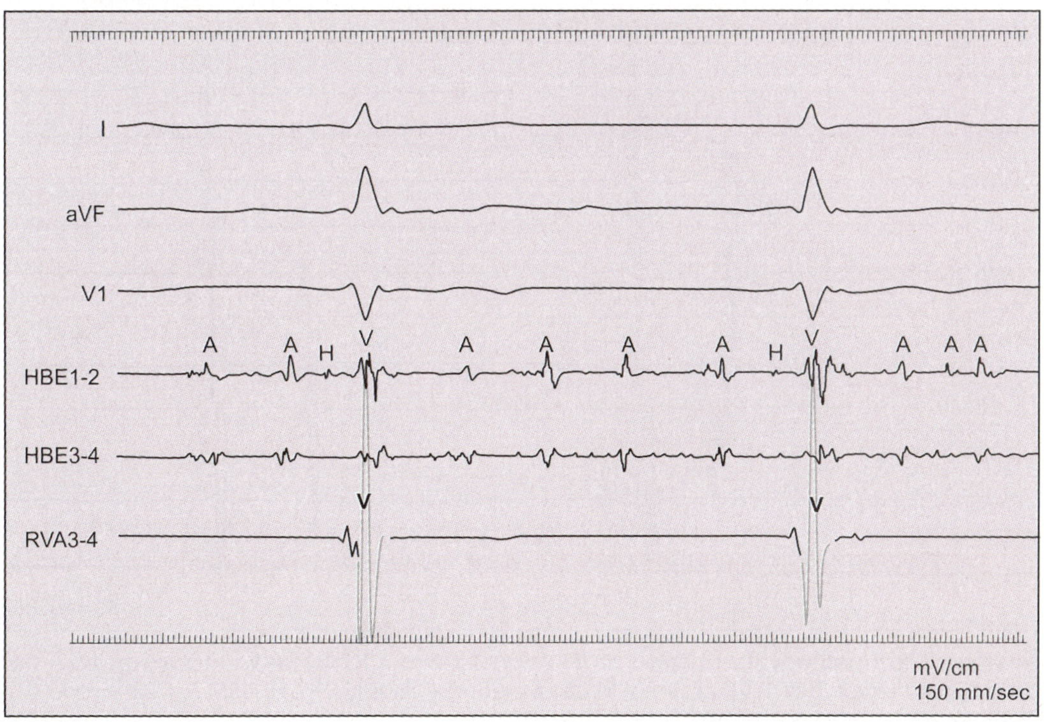


**Fig. 11.28:** Intracardiac electrograms during atrial fibrillation. Three surface ECG leads (I, aVF, V1) and intracardiac recordings from the atrioventricular (AV) junction region (HBE1–2, HBR3–4), and the right ventricular apex (RVA3–4) in a patient with atrial fibrillation. The patient has extremely symptomatic, medically refractory atrial fibrillation with rapid ventricular rates and recurrent congestive heart failure. The mapping catheter (HBE) has been manoeuvred from the area of maximal His bundle activity to a more proximal position, where a larger atrial (A) and smaller His electrogram (H) are recorded. V=ventricular electrogram

with atrial fibrillation. AV nodal modification is less often performed. For catheter ablation of atrial tissue for atrial fibrillation, the most commonly used techniques involve ablation of the muscular connections between the pulmonary veins and the left atrium (pulmonary vein isolation), or a wide circumferential ablation around the pulmonary veins (see image below). The goal is to electrically isolate foci arising from inside the veins, or adjacent to the pulmonary vein ostia, from the rest of the left atrium. Electroanatomic map of the posterior left atrium, illustrating the pulmonary veins: right superior pulmonary vein (RSPV), right inferior pulmonary vein (RIPV), left superior pulmonary vein (LSPV), and left inferior pulmonary vein (LIPV). The red circles represent actual discrete radiofrequency applications, predominantly delivered in a circumferential pattern around the pulmonary veins. This ablation strategy can isolate pulmonary vein foci that initiate atrial fibrillation, and/or alter the substrate of the left atrium to inhibit fibrillatory activity due to reentry. Image courtesy of American College of Cardiology Foundation.

### B. Atrioventricular Nodal Reentrant Tachycardia

(Figs 11.29 and 11.30)

- In the common form of atrioventricular nodal reentrant tachycardia (AVNRT), the inferior atrionodal input to

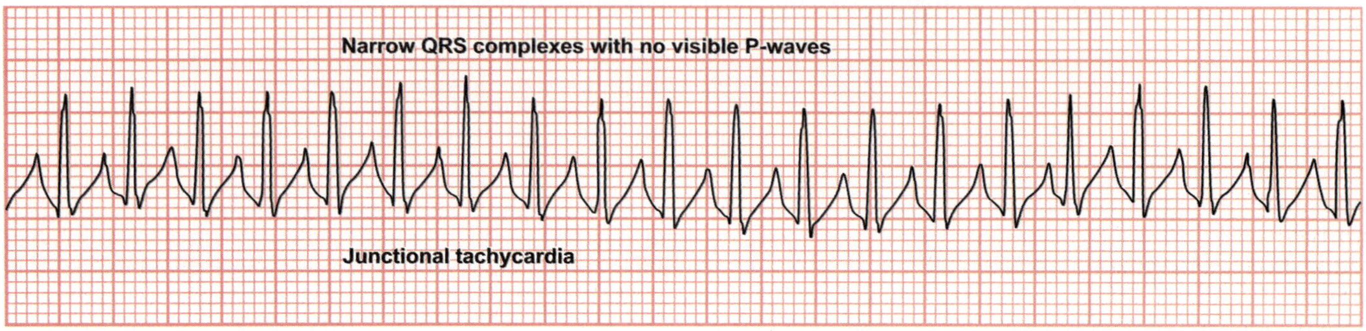


**Fig. 11.29:** Junctional tachycardia: Narrow QRS complexes with no visible P-waves

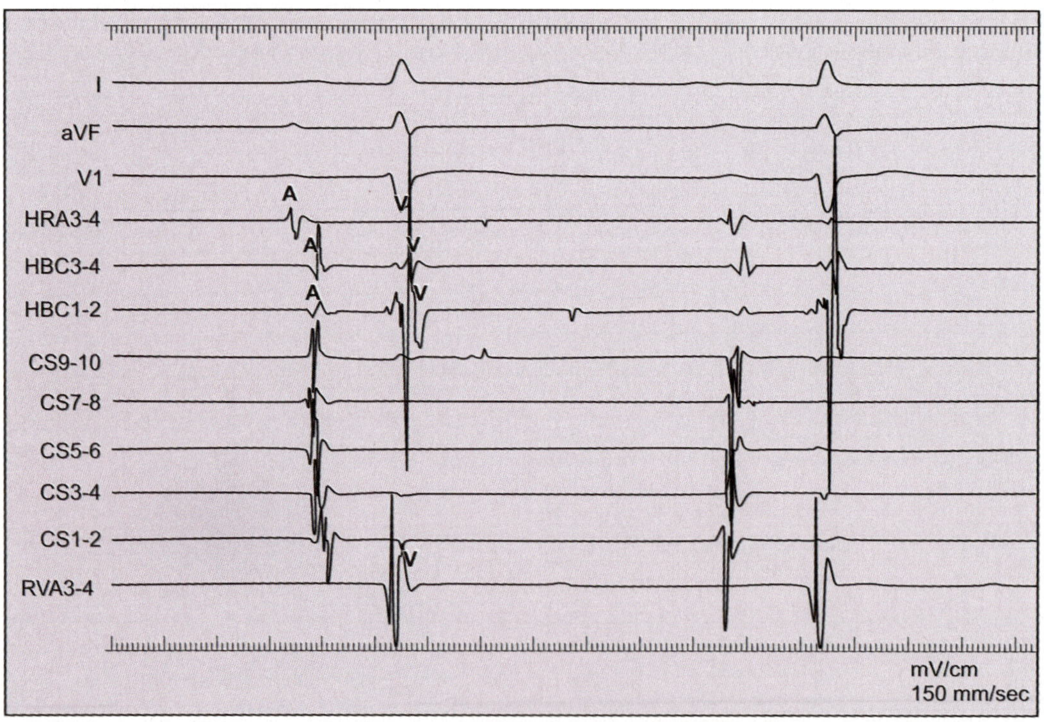


**Fig. 11.30:** Identification of slow pathway for ablation of AV nodal reentrant tachycardia recordings from the high right atrium (HRA3–4) and distal His bundle region (HBE1–2), proximal to distal coronary sinus (CS9–10, CS5–6, CS3–4, and CS1–2), and the right ventricular apex (RVA3–4). The patient had a history of medically refractory supraventricular arrhythmia and the diagnostic study revealed easily inducible, typical atrioventricular (AV) nodal reentrant tachycardia. The HBE catheter was manoeuvred from the His position to the slow pathway region, which is typically inferior and posterior to the His bundle and just anterior to the coronary sinus ostium. This is an ideal site for slow pathway ablation and has a small atrial electrogram (A) and large ventricular electrogram (V), with no evidence of His bundle activity. The tip of the HBE catheter (HBE1–2) records such a signal, and is used for ablation

the atrioventricular (AV) node serves as the anterograde limb (i.e. the slow pathway) of the reentry circuit, and the superior atrionodal input serves as the retrograde limb (i.e. the fast pathway). Typically, AVNRT can be cured by targeting the slow pathway near the inferior tricuspid valve annulus at the level of the coronary sinus os or somewhat higher.

- The risk of iatrogenic heart block with ablation in this region is quite low (1–2%). Targeting the slow pathway is safer than targeting the fast pathway, which is located closer to the compact AV node.

### C. Orthodromic Reciprocating Tachycardia

In orthodromic reciprocating tachycardia (ORT) the AV node serves as the anterograde limb and an accessory AV connection (i.e. the accessory pathway) serves as the retrograde limb (see images below). Schema of orthodromic reciprocating tachycardia (ORT). The atrioventricular node serves as the antegrade limb, whereas an accessory pathway (atrioventricular connection) serves as the retrograde limb. For ECG features of ORT, see the image below. Supraventricular tachycardia (SVT) in a patient with orthodromic reciprocating tachycardia (ORT) due to a concealed pathway. Note the retrograde P-wave, seen best in lead V2, separated from the QRS complex by an isoelectric baseline. (Compare to the first ECG above, in which the P-wave is fused to the QRS.) This pattern of 'short R-P tachycardia' (in which the interval between the QRS complex and retrograde P-wave is shorter than the subsequent P-R interval and the P-wave is in the first half of the R-R interval) suggests an SVT incorporating an accessory pathway. Typically, ORT can be cured by targeting the accessory pathway as it crosses the mitral or tricuspid valve annulus (Figs 11.31 and 11.32).

### D. Antidromic Reciprocating Tachycardia

An **antidromic tachycardia** refers to a fast heart rhythm that utilizes the *manifest accessory* pathway to preexcite the ventricles, irregardless of whether the normal *AV node* is used in a retrograde fashion. In other words, other *SVTs*, such as *atrial tachycardia* or *atrial flutter* and *fibrillation* can now conduct at fast heart rates to the ventricles in a 1 to 1 fashion (no protection to limit this conduction since the *AV node* is not in use). This is the theoretical danger of an *accessory* pathway that allows conduction to the *ventricles* in an uncontrolled, potentially fast rate, with repetitive stimulation of the *ventricles* potentially leading to *ventricular fibrillation* with hemodynamic collapse and sudden cardiac death. This situation is rare and it is estimated that this tragic event has less than a 0.1% chance (1 in a 1000) of occurring each year in patients with manifest WPW (Figs 11.33 and 11.34).

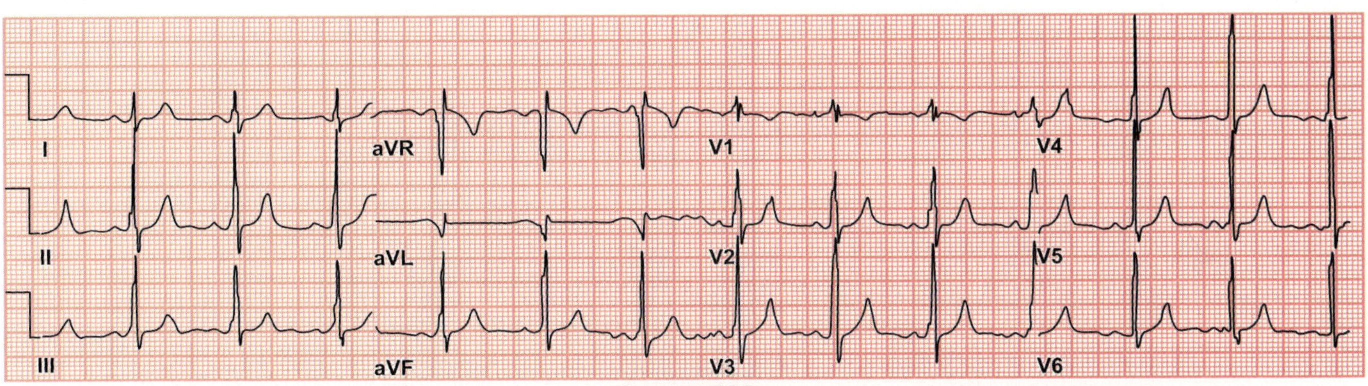


Baseline ECG

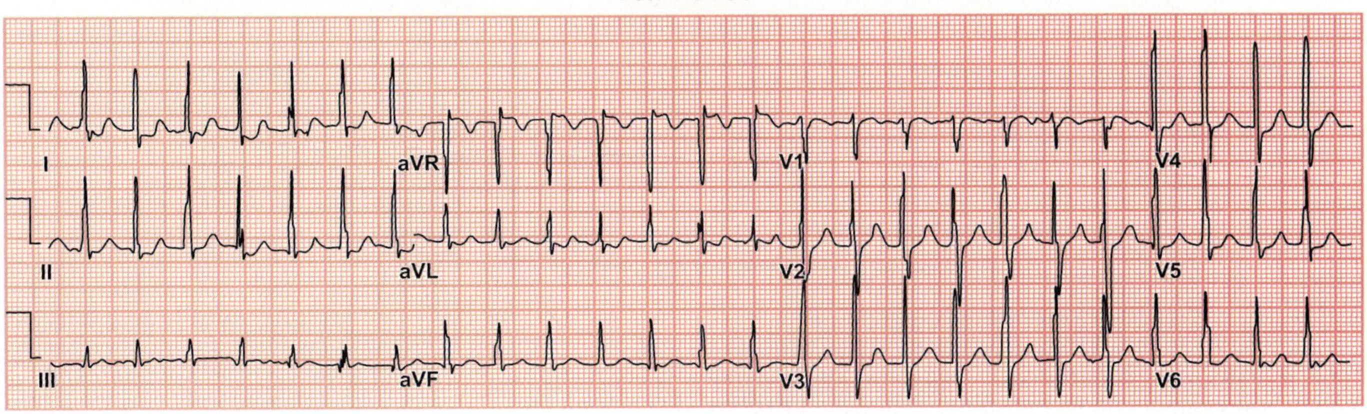


Orthodromic reciprocating tachycardia

**Fig. 11.31:** Left lateral accessory pathway (AP). It is prudent to recognise that the delta wave vector can only be determined with precision when the ECG shows maximum preexcitation. A right-sided AP with minimal preexcitation but with a posteroseptal location can not be determined with a high probability until ART occurs

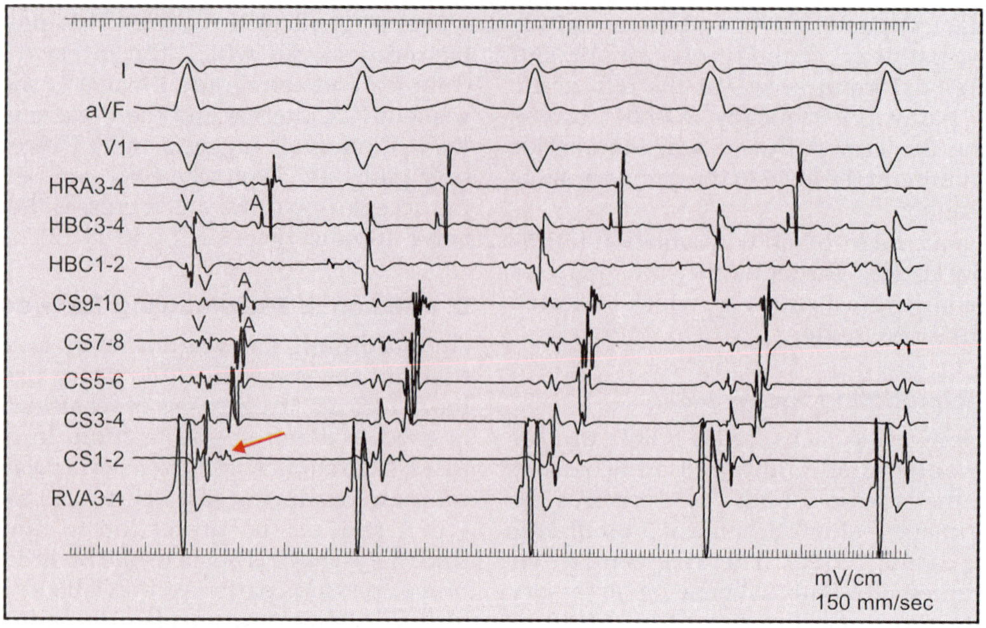


**Fig. 11.32:** Orthodromic AV reentrant tachycardia in concealed accessory pathway. Shown are three surface ECG leads (I, aVF, V1) and intracardiac recording from the high right atrium (HRA), proximal (HBE3–4) and distal His bundle region (HBE1–2), proximal to distal coronary sinus (CS9–10, CS7–8, CS5–6, CS3–4 and CS1–2), and right ventricular apex (RVA3–4) in a patient with atrioventricular reentrant tachycardia (AVRT). During an orthodromic AVRT, there is retrograde atrial (A) activation which occurs after ventricular activation (V); the earliest atrial activation (arrow) is seen in the lateral mitral annulus (CS1-2) due to a conceated left lateral accessory pathway

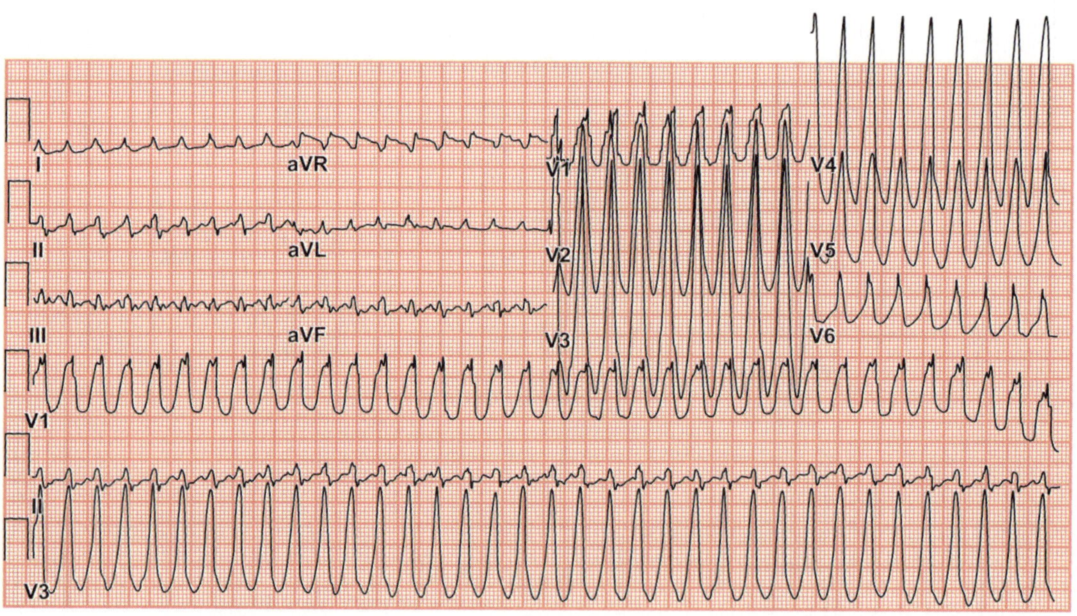


**Fig. 11.33:** Antidromic AV reciprocating tachycardia (ART)

Not all *accessory* pathways are manifest with a *delta* wave on the 12-lead EKG (no *WPW EKG pattern* seen). *Concealed* **WPW** is actually more common than *manifest WPW*. In these situations, the patient will have a normal baseline EKG but a clinical narrow-complex SVT of unclear origin. These accessory pathways are *concealed* may conduct only in the reverse, or retrograde fashion, leading to *orthodromic AVRT* as described above, but no clues to its existence with a normal baseline EKG. In addition, multiple accessory pathways are present in as many as 13% of patients referred to a heart rhythm specialist because of *WPW syndrome*.

## E. Unifocal Atrial Tachycardia

Unifocal atrial tachycardia (Fig. 11.35), which can arise from either atrium, is somewhat more challenging to ablate than the more common forms of generic SVT. For those

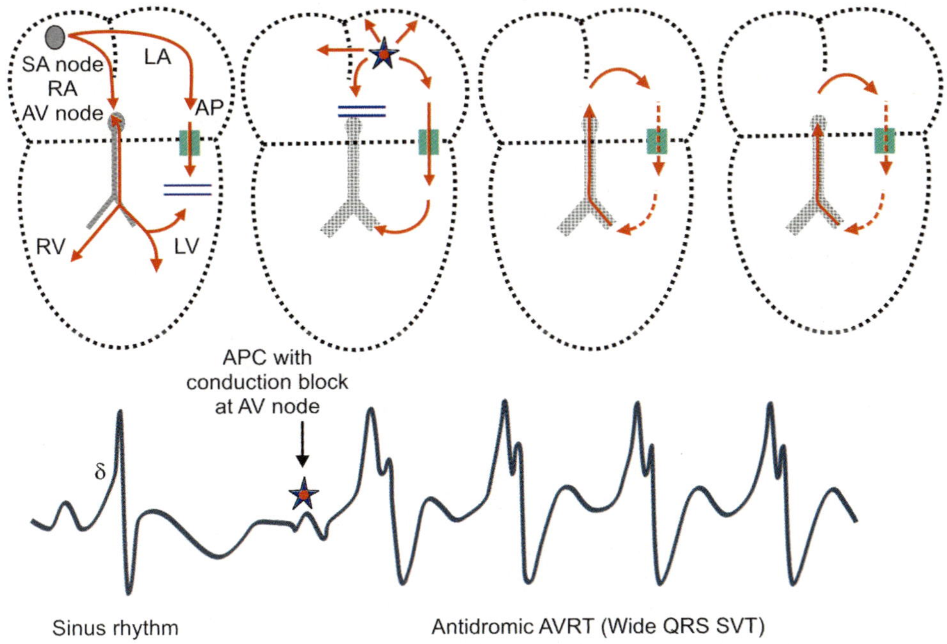


**Fig. 11.34:** Antidromic AV reciprocating tachycardia in a patient with left-sided AP

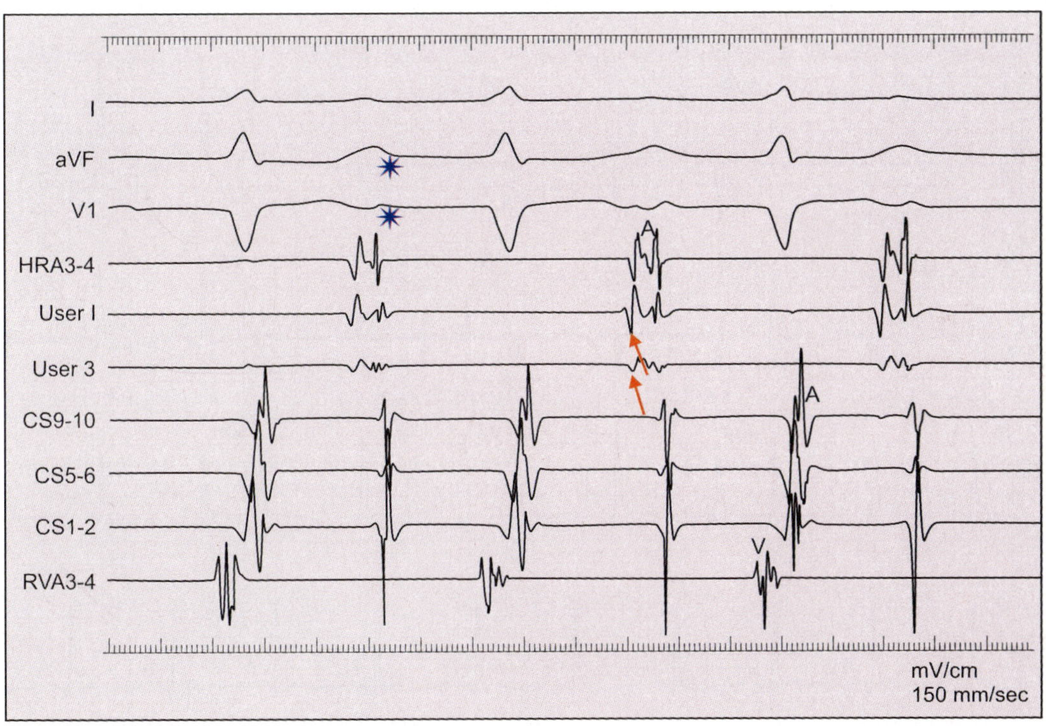


**Fig. 11.35:** Electrophysiologic mapping of atrial tachycardia. Three surface ECG leads (I, aVF, V1) and intracardiac recordings from the high posterior right atrium (HRA); posterior left atrium (USER 1 and USER 3); proximal, mid, and distal coronary sinus (CS9–10, CS5–6, CS1–2); and right ventricular apex (RVA). The patient had an incessant atrial tachycaria and dilated cardiomyopathy (left ventricular ejection fraction 9%) referred for cardiac transplant evaluation. The P-wave (*) falls at the end of the T-wave on the surface ECG; its onset is difficult to discern. However, the intracardiac electrograms demonstrate obvious atrial (A) and ventricular (V) activity. Activation mapping involves positioning the mapping catheters in the right (HRA) and left atrial (USER) to the record earliest electrical activity (arrow) than the right atrial catheter, but the timing with respect to the surface P-wave is obscured because of the T-wave of the preceding QRS complex

tachycardias originating from the left atrium, transseptal catheterization via a patent foramen ovale or transseptal puncture is usually required.

### F. Wolff-Parkinson-White syndrome

Typically, a transition from ORT to atrial fibrillation can be the cause of rapid preexcited tachycardia in Wolff-

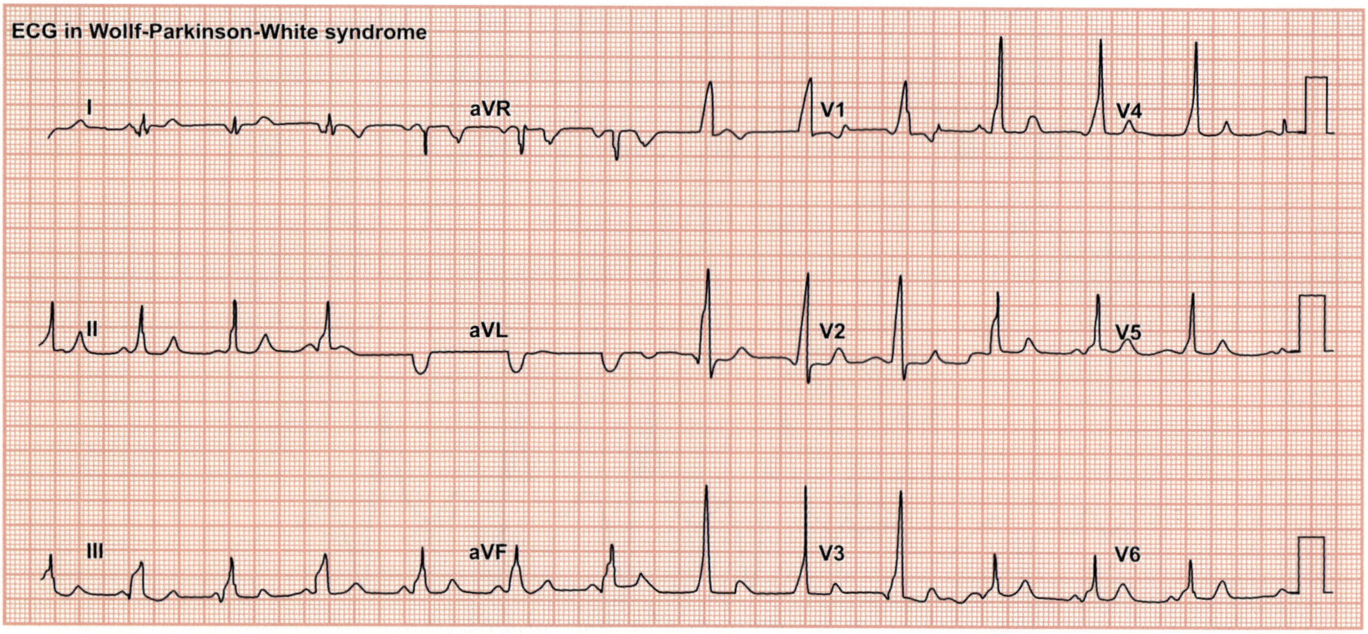


**Fig. 11.36:** ECG shows the short PR interval and slurred upstroke of the QRS (delta wave). The QRS is positive in V1 and in the inferior leads; thus, the pathway is left-sided and anterior (free wall)

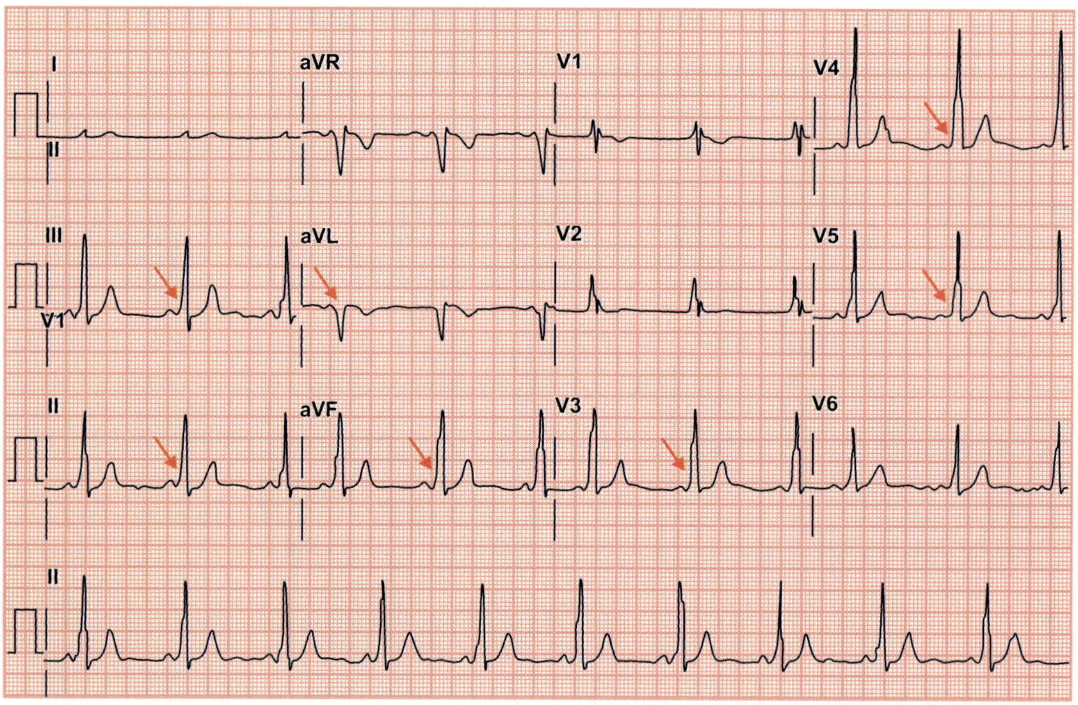


**Fig. 11.37:** Resting ECG shows delta waves (red arrows) in the inferior and lateral leads

Parkinson-White syndrome. Ablation of the accessory pathway cures the syndrome, eliminating ORT and atrial fibrillation in most instances (Figs 11.36–11.39).

### G. Atrial Flutter

Atrial flutter is most commonly due to a large reentrant circuit in the right atrium, involving an isthmus of tissue between the tricuspid valve annulus and the inferior vena cava (Figs 11.40 and 11.41). Most commonly, reentry proceeds counterclockwise up the atrial septum and down the lateral wall of the right atrium, inscribing inverted (i.e. 'sawtooth') flutter waves in the inferior leads and upright P-waves in V1 schema of the common variety of atrial flutter. The reentry circuit is confined to the right atrium and circulates as a counterclockwise macroreentrant circuit proceeding superiorly over the atrial septum and inferiorly

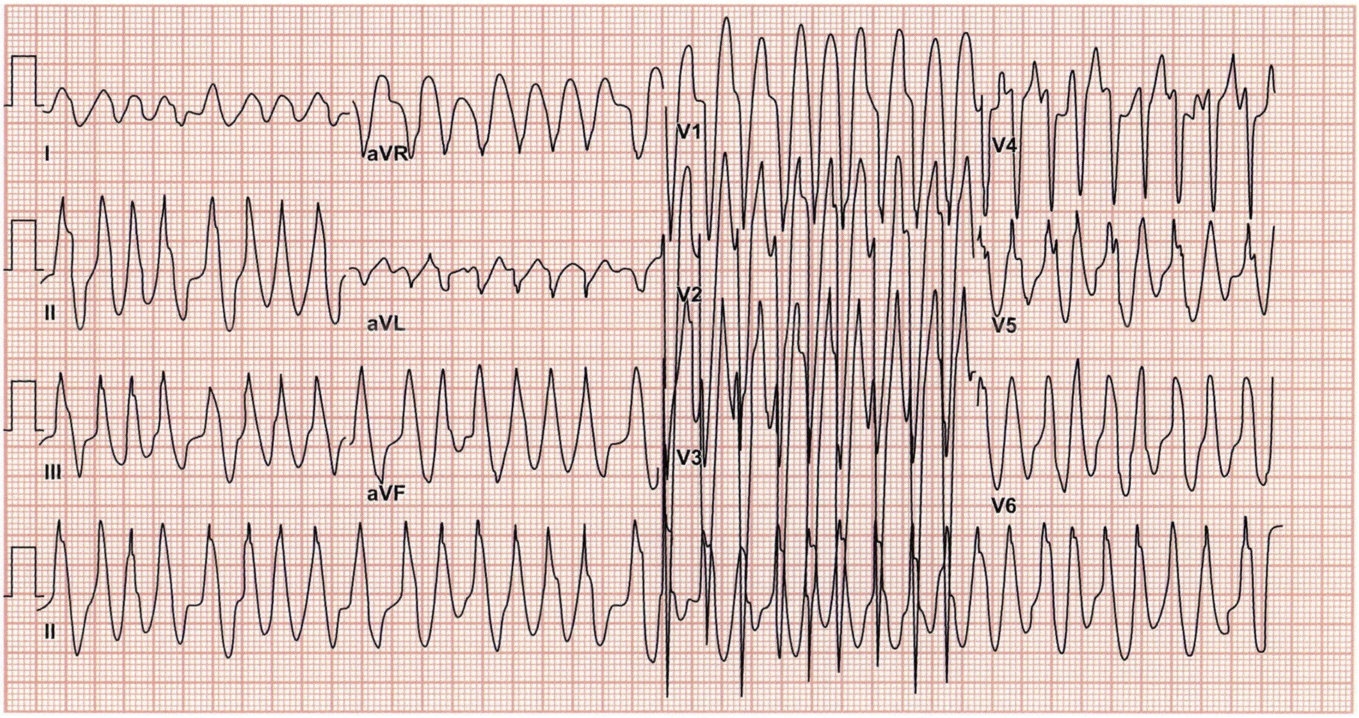


**Fig. 11.38:** ECG morphology showing preexcited atrial fibrillation

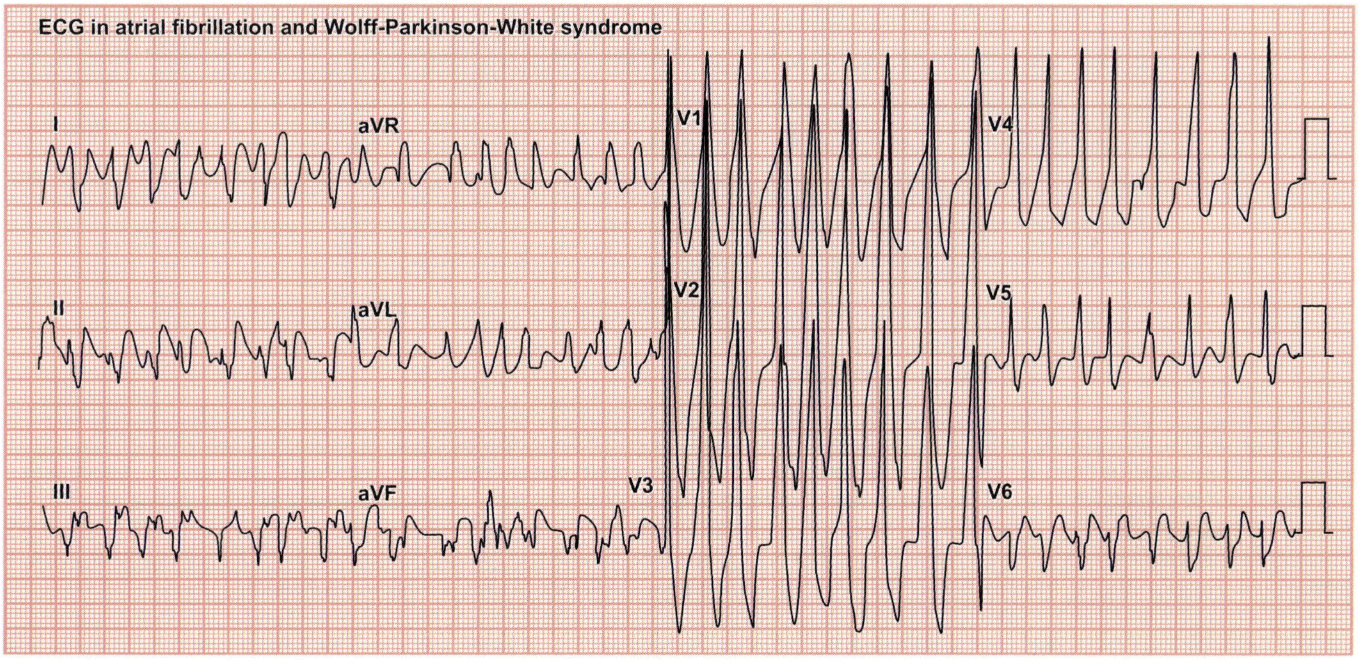


**Fig. 11.39:** ECG shows an irregular broad-complex tachycardia. Almost all irregular tachycardias are atrial fibrillation.QRS morphology varies because of the varying contributions of the atrioventricular node and the accessory pathway in atrial fibrillation to activation of the ventricle. This ECG shows preexcited atrial fibrillation. The shortest RR Interval is 200 milliseconds; intervals <260 milliseconds are associated with a risk of sudden death

over the lateral atrial wall. The wave front circulates through a narrow isthmus of tissue between the tricuspid valve annulus and the inferior vena cava. Linear ablation across this isthmus cures this common form of atrial flutter.

An example of a typical counterclockwise atrial flutter, the most common form of atrial flutter. The cardinal features are a perfectly regular atrial rhythm with inverted P-waves inferiorly that have a positive overshoot, upright P-waves in V1, and inverted P-waves in V6. Clockwise reentry using this same circuit can also occur, giving upright P-waves inferiorly and inverted P-waves in V1. Linear ablation of the cavotricuspid isthmus cures these

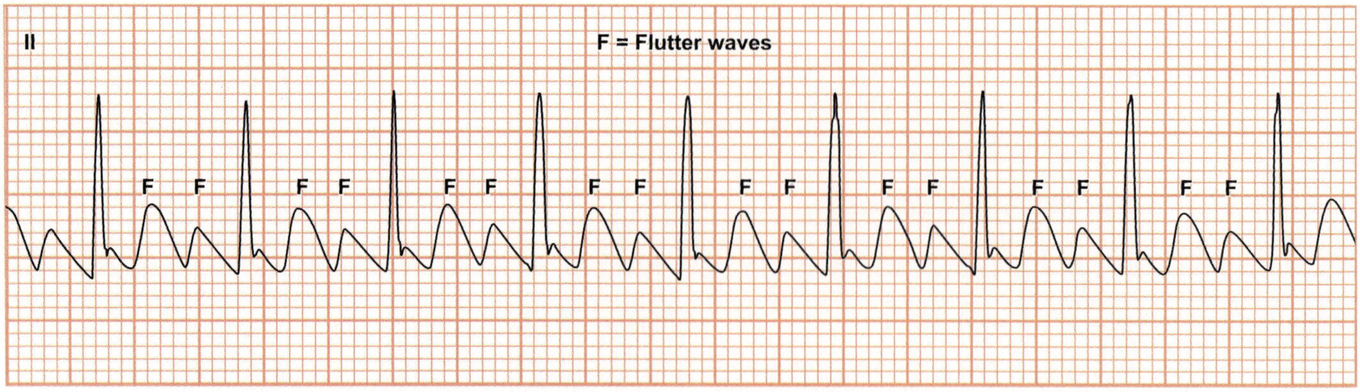


**Fig. 11.40:** Atrial flutter. Narrow QRS complexes are associated with regular flutter waves

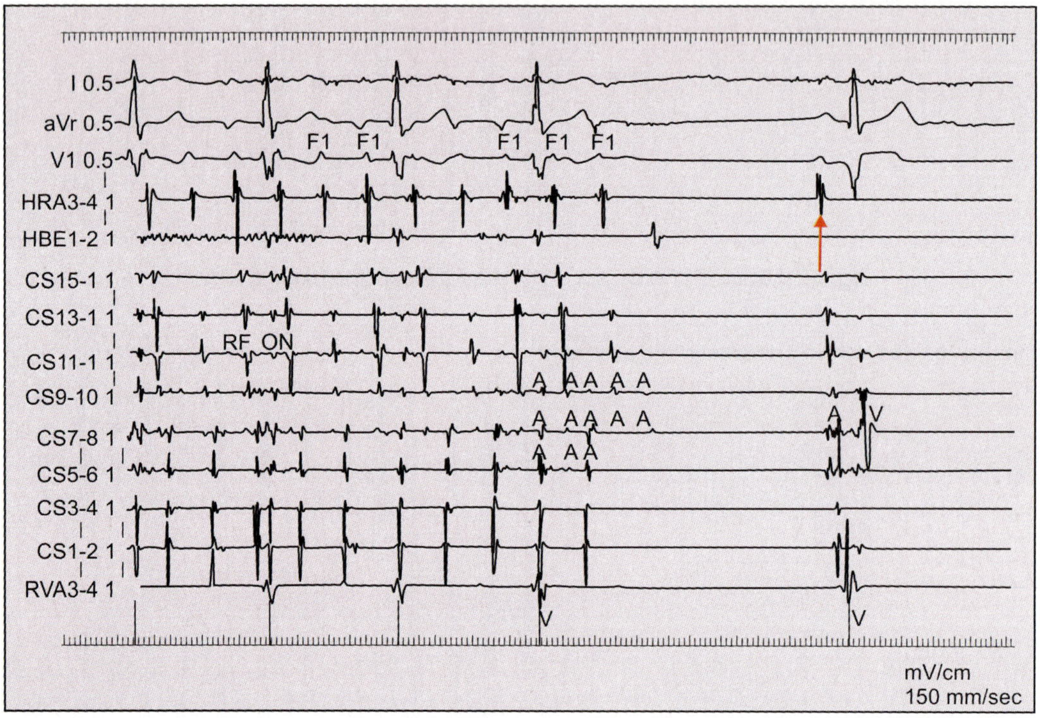


**Fig. 11.41:** Radiofrequency catheter ablation of typical atrial flutter. There surface ECG leads (I, aVF, V1) and intracardiac recordings from the high right atrium (HRA), a mapping catheter in the isthmus between the tricuspid valve and inferior vena cava (TV-IVC) (HBE1–2), eight recordings from a catheter extending from the lateral right atrial wall through the TV-IVC isthmus and into the ostium of the coronary sinus (CS15–1 to CS1–2), and right ventricular apex (RVA3–4) in a patient with typical atrial flutter. The tip of the mapping catheter was initially positioned on the tricuspid annulus, and then dragged through the TV-IVC isthmus to the ostium of the IVC during RF application; atrial flutter terminated. Note that the atrial activation (A) blocks between CS7–8 and CS5–6, which on fluoroscopy corresponded to the position of the mapping catheter. Fl=flutter waves, V=ventricular electrogram

common forms of atrial flutter.Non-isthmus-dependent flutters can occur elsewhere in the right atrium as well as in the left atrium. Left atrial flutters are uncommon, may be difficult to ablate, and generally require a 3-dimensional mapping system to facilitate the procedure. A 3-dimensional electroanatomic map of cavotricuspid isthmus flutter. The colors progress from red to purple and represent relative conduction time in the right atrium (early to late). An ablation line (red dots) has been created from the tricuspid annulus to the inferior vena cava. This interrupts the flutter circuit.

### H. Ablation in Accessory Pathways

Since first described in 1989, radiofrequency catheter ablation of accessory pathways has gained rapid and widespread acceptance as a safe and curative treatment for patients with the Wolff-Parkinson-White syndrome and/ or paroxysmal supraventricular tachycardia involving a concealed accessory pathway. Catheter ablation of accessory pathways is now considered as first line therapy for the treatment of patients with the Wolff-Parkinson-White syndrome and is considered an alternative to antiarrhythmic therapy for patients with paroxysmal supraventricular tachycardia (Figs 11.42–11.48).

### I. Ablation in Ventricular Tachycardia (Figs11.49 to 11.51)

Idiopathic ventricular tachycardia (VT) most commonly arises from the right ventricular outflow tract and less commonly originates in the inferoseptal left ventricle near the apex. These forms of VT are amenable to catheter ablation, although success rates are somewhat lower than those for the common forms of SVT. For patients with stable VT, the potential benefit of catheter ablation before implantation of an ICD was demonstrated in the Ventricular Tachycardia Ablation in Coronary Heart Disease (VTACH) study. This prospective, randomized, controlled international trial in 104 patients found that time to recurrence of VT or ventricular fibrillation (VF) was longer in the ablation group (median, 18.6 mo) than in the control group (5.9 mo). At 2 years, estimates for survival free from VT or VF were 47% in the ablation group and 29% in the control group (Figs 11.49–11.51).

## Measures to be Adopted After Ablation Procedure in the Following Clinical Situations

### Atrial Fibrillation

Radiofrequency catheter ablation (RFCA) of the atrioventricular (AV) junction results in excellent rate control, relieves palpitations, and improves functional capacity; however, patients who undergo this procedure require permanent pacemaker implantation to manage the resulting AV block and require warfarin therapy to prevent stroke because the atrial fibrillation itself is not affected. AV nodal modification is less therapeutic than AV junction ablation and may result in late heart block.

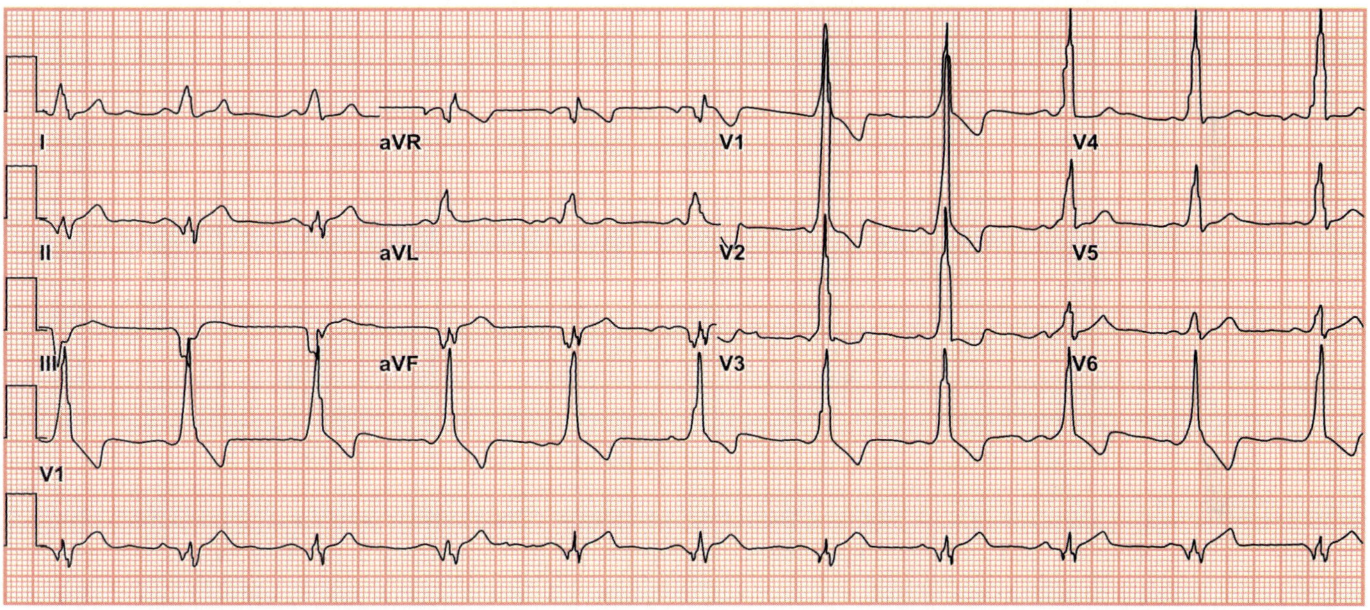


**Fig. 11.42:** Left posteroseptal accessory pathway (AP). A negative delta wave in lead I, aVL and V6 (rightward QRS axis) with a positive delta wave in lead V1 suggests a left lateral pathway

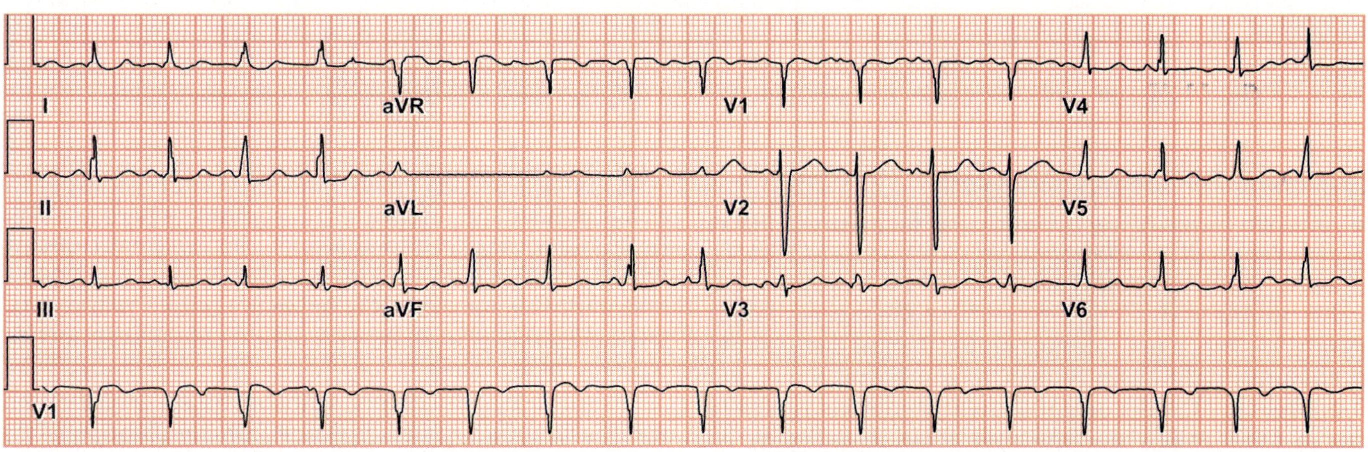


**Fig. 11.43:** Right anteroseptal accessory pathway (AP). A left axis (with a negative delta wave in lead V1) suggests a right lateral AP

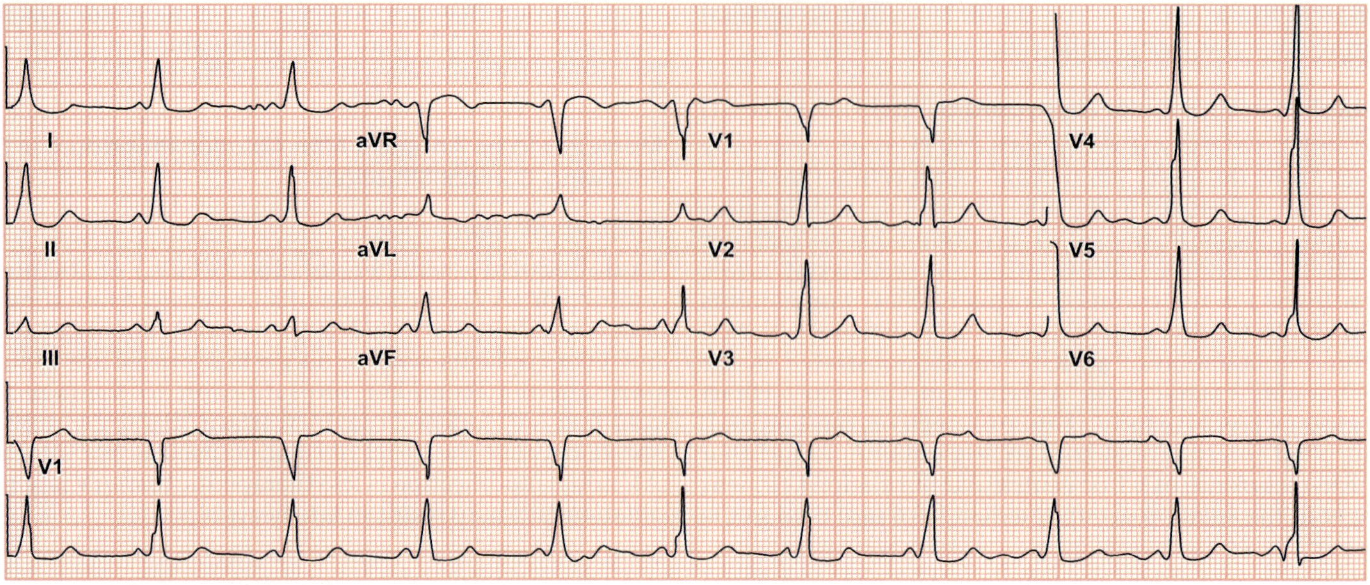


**Fig. 11.44:** Right lateral accessory pathway (AP). If the delta waves in the inferior leads are negative, then it denotes a posteroseptal AP right, or left, depending on the delta wave vector in lead V1 as described earlier

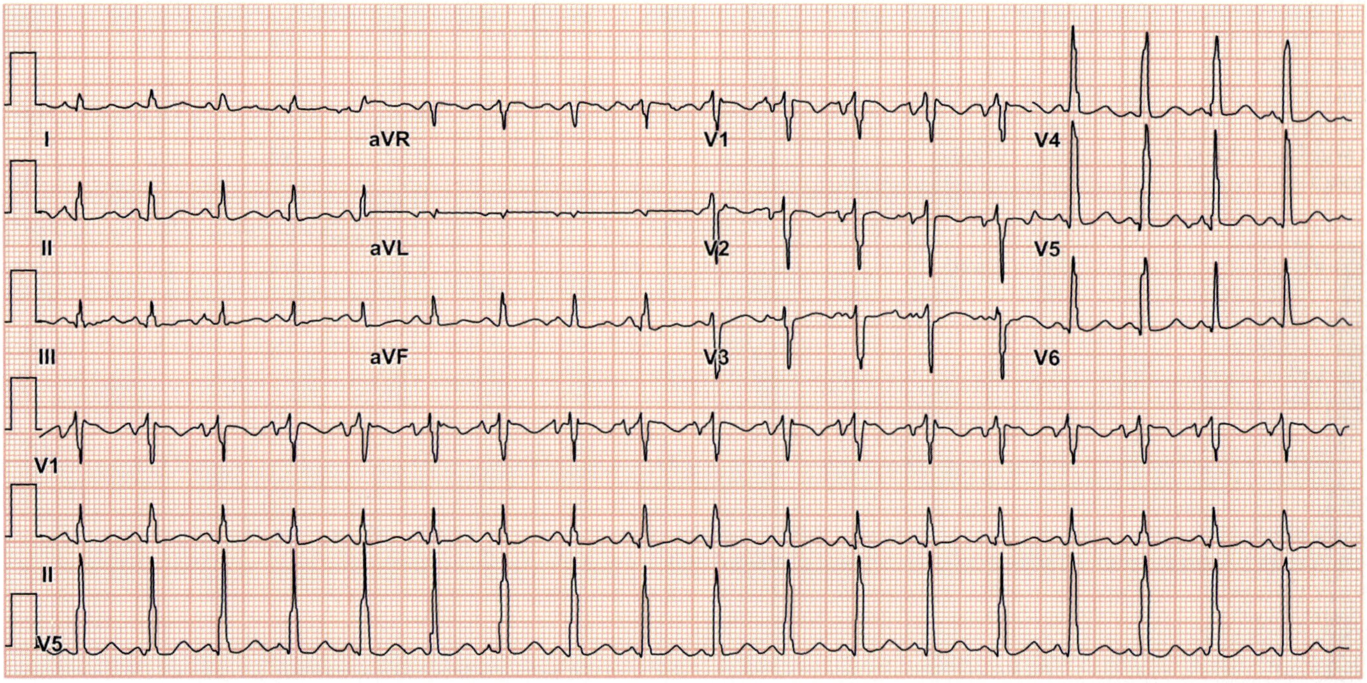


**Fig. 11.45:** Left lateral accessory pathway (AP) showing signs of minimal preexcitation in the inferior leads

### *Supraventricular Tachyarrhythmias*

The common forms of supraventricular tachycardia (SVT) (e.g. atrioventricular nodal reentrant tachycardia [AVNRT], SVT associated with Wolff-Parkinson-White syndrome) are usually curable with a single procedure; the success rate is typically 90–95%. Cure rates for unifocal atrial tachycardia and common right atrial flutter are somewhat lower but still approach 90%. Recurrent tachyarrhythmias typically occur in the first few months after ablation and may be amenable to cure with a second procedure.

AVNRT is usually amenable to cure with a slow pathway ablation near the inferior atrial septum, where the risk of heart block is 1–2%. In the uncommon circumstances in which ablation near the compact AV node is required (e.g. fast pathway for AVNRT, or an accessory pathway in a para-Hisian location), the risk of heart block may approach 5% or a little higher.

In a number of centers, catheter-based cryoablation is used rather than radiofrequency catheter ablation (RFCA) near the compact AV node to minimize the risk of heart

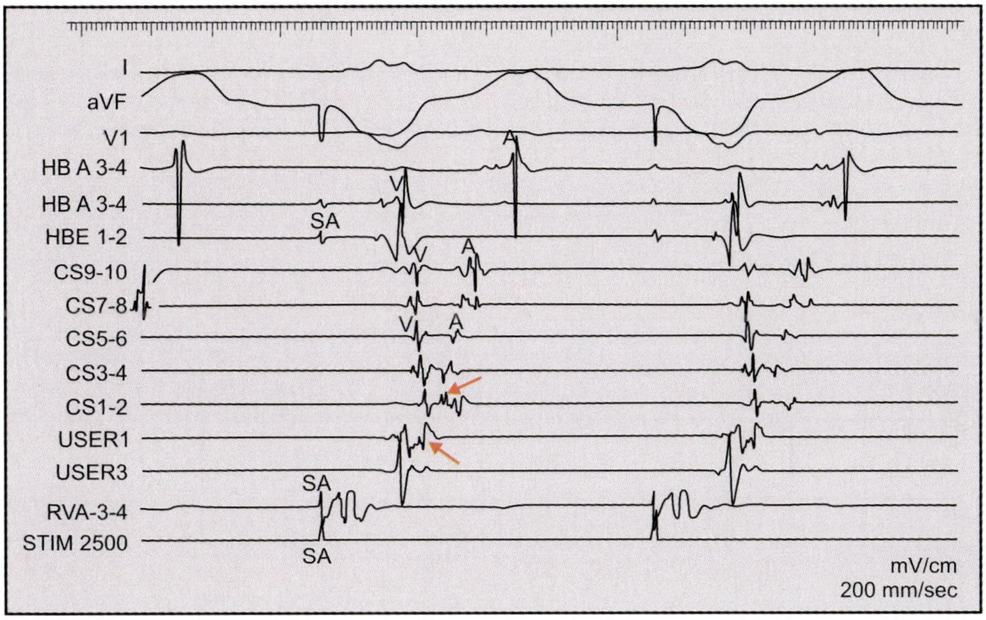


**Fig. 11.46:** Electrophysiologic mapping of concealed accessory pathway during ventricular pacing. Shown are three surface ECG leads (I, aVF, and V1) and intracardiac recording from the high right atrium (HRA), proximal (HBE3–4) and distal His bundle region (HBE1–2), proximal to distal coaronary sinus (CS9–10, CS7–8, CS5–6, CS3–4, and CS1–2), right ventricular apex (RVA3–4), from a mapping catheter's distal (USER1) and proximal (USER3) electrode pairs, and a stimulus artifact (SA) channel (STIM). The mapping catheter was advanced through the right femoral artery and retrograde across the aortic valve into the left ventricle. With each ventricular paced beat (V); there is retrograde conduction from the ventricle to atrium (A) via the left free wall accessory pathway. The mapping catheter has been manoeuvred to the site along the mitral annulus which records the earliest atrial activity (red arrow); the atrial activity recorded at the tip electrode of USER1 precedes the earliest atrial activity (black arrow) noted in the coronary sinus (CS1–2) by 25 msec

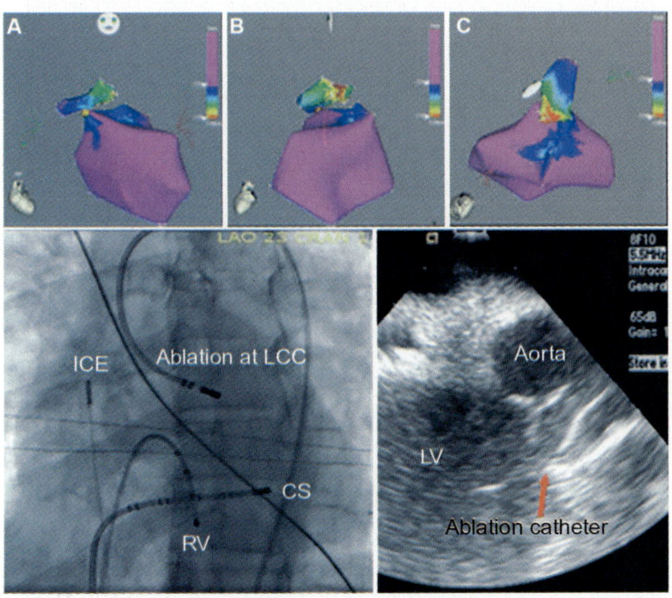


**Fig. 11.47:** Top, electroanatomic map (CARTO) showing the left ventricle relative to the site of earliest activation in the left coronary cusp (A) anterior-posterior view; (B) left lateral view; (C) superior view). Bottom left, fluoroscopic view of the successful ablation site. Bottom right, ICE image showing the ablation catheter at the site of successful ablation in the LCC. LV=left ventricle, ICE=intracardiac echocardiography catheter, RV=right ventricle, CS=coronary sinus catheter, and LCC=left coronary cusp

block. With cryoablation, heart block is generally reversible with prompt rewarming. However, cryoablation appears to be slightly less effective than radiofrequency as an energy source, especially for deep accessory pathways.

Success rates for curing atrial fibrillation with RFCA are highest (up to 87% in the 5 randomized trials reported through 2006) for paroxysmal atrial fibrillation in the absence of structural heart disease and lowest (50% or less) with persistent atrial fibrillation in the presence of structural heart disease and left atrial enlargement. Repeat procedures are typically needed in 25% or more of patients.

Success rates have historically been based on patient symptoms and periodic electrocardiographic monitoring. Success rates are lower if intensive ambulatory monitoring to detect asymptomatic atrial fibrillation recurrences is used, such as daily monitoring for a month with an auto-triggering event monitor. Some patients require the use of previously ineffective antiarrhythmic drugs to maintain success.

### *Ventricular Tachyarrhythmias*

Idiopathic ventricular tachycardia (VT) is curable (success rate approximately 80%), assuming it is readily inducible during electrophysiology studies. The most common location for these VTs is the right ventricular outflow tract. Because these VTs are usually not reentrant in nature, a significant percentage are not inducible. Some cannot be

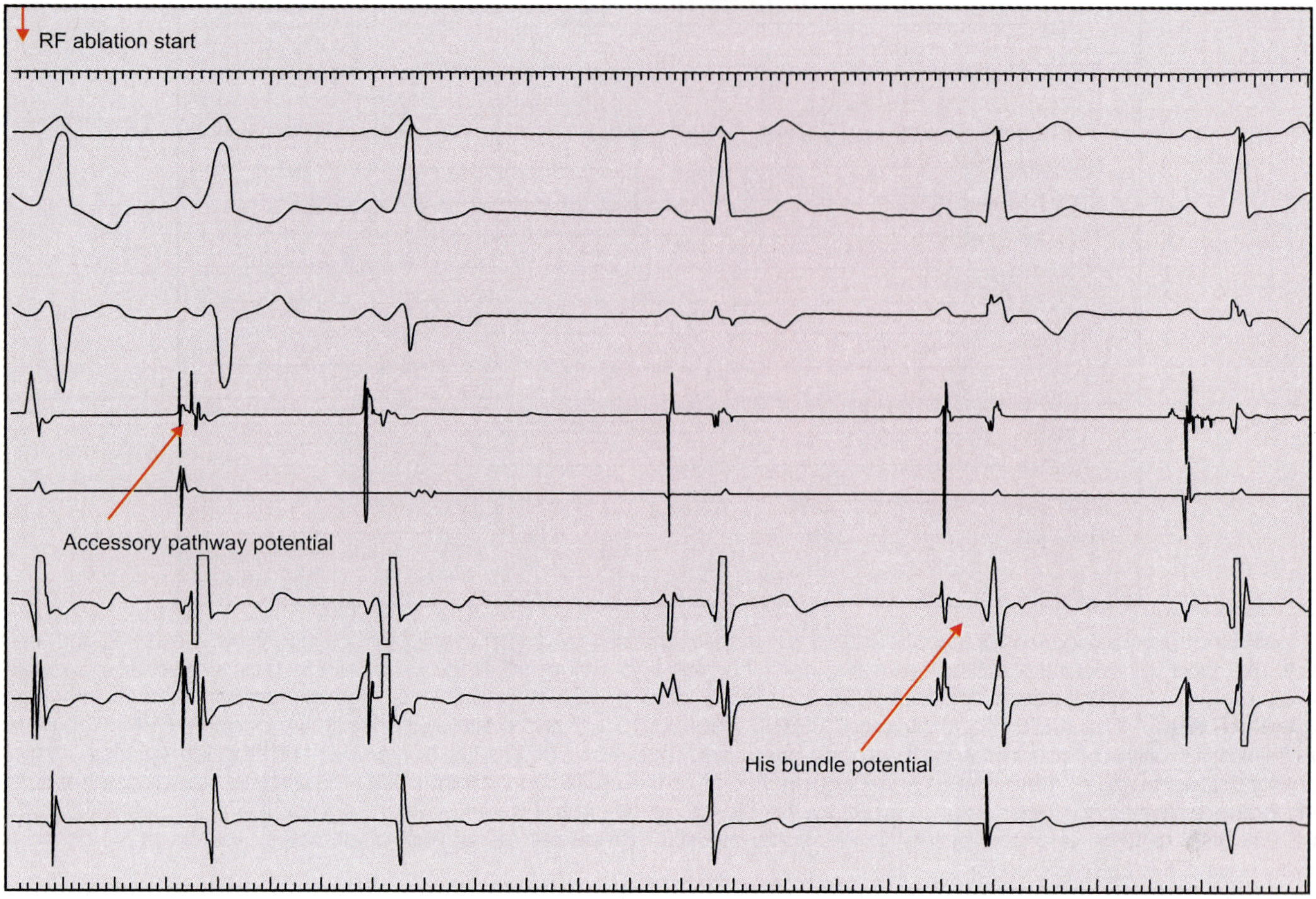


**Fig. 11.48:** Accessory pathway potential and local AV fusion at successful RF ablation site with loss of preexcitation and return of normal HV interval

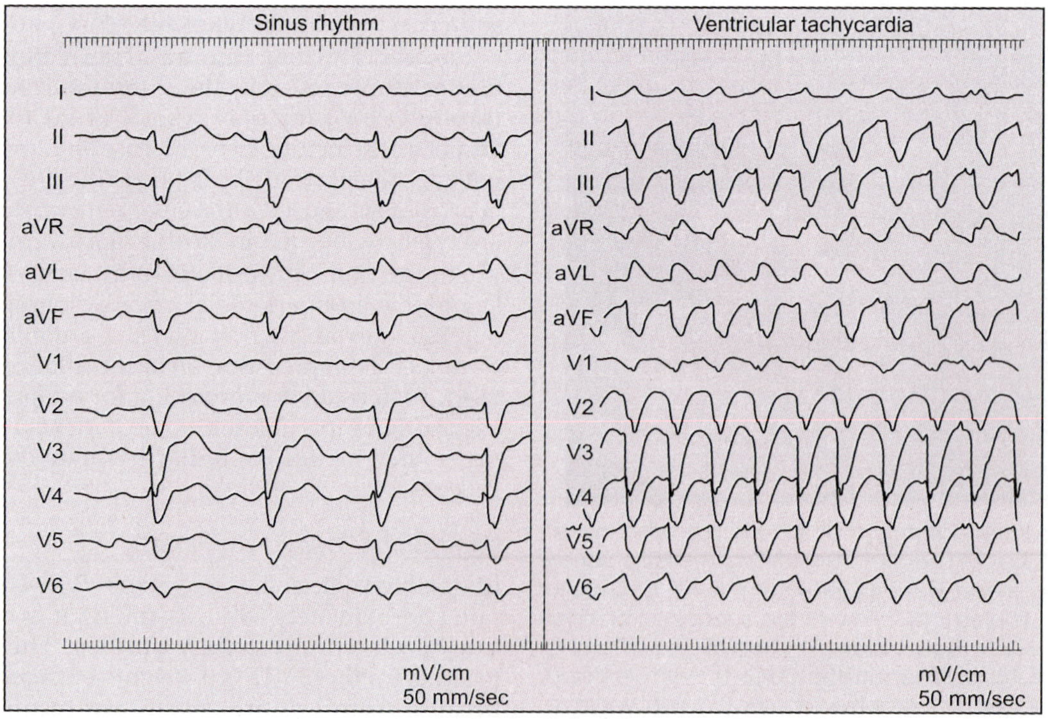


**Fig. 11.49:** Bundle branch reentrat tachcardia. Left panel—12 lead ECG during sinus rhythm; there is a left bundle type intraventricular conduction delay. Right panel—12 lead ECG during ventricular tachycardia; there is a remarkable similarity in QRS morphology during VT and sinus rhythm. The HV interval during sinus rhythm was 65 mse, suggesting underlying His-Purkinje conduction disease

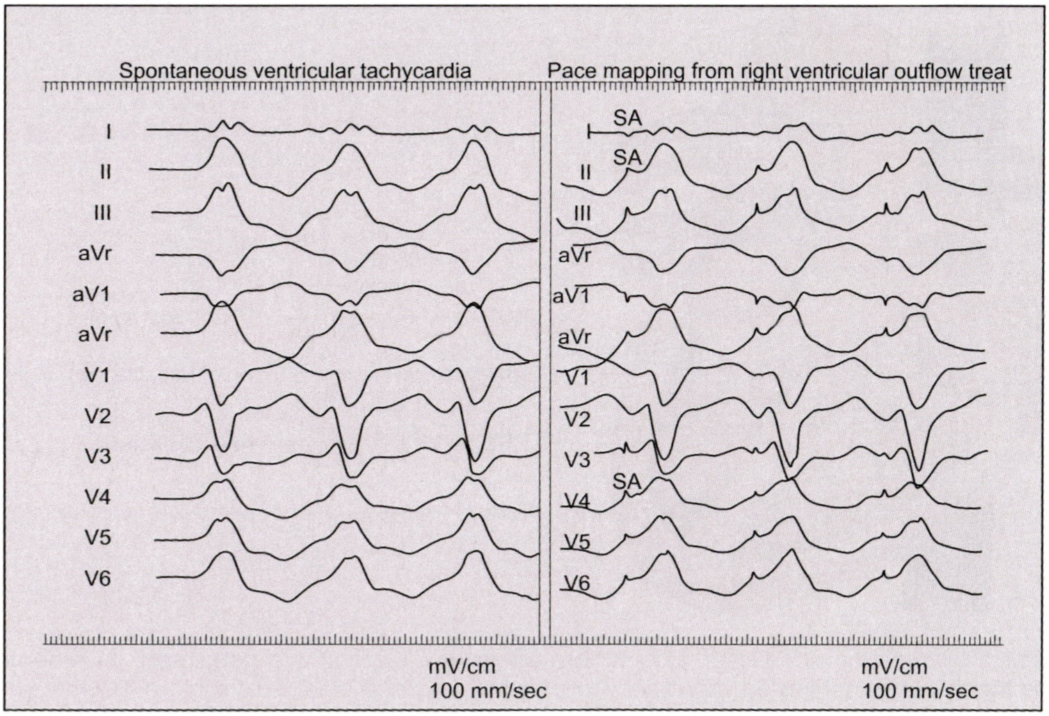


**Fig. 11.50:** Pace mapping of an idioipathic RVOT tachycardia. Left panel—12 lead ECG of spontaneous ventricular tachycardia (VT) in a patient with a structurally normal heart. The VT has a left bundle branch block (LBBB) and an inferior axis morphology, suggesting that the origin is in the right ventricular outflow tract (RVOT). Right panel—A mapping catheter has been positioned in the RVOT and pacing is performed from its tip during sinus rhythm. The 'pace map' closely approximates the QRS morphology of the spontaneous VT in all 12 leads, suggesting that the mapping catheter is at or near the VT focus. SA=pacing stimulus artifact

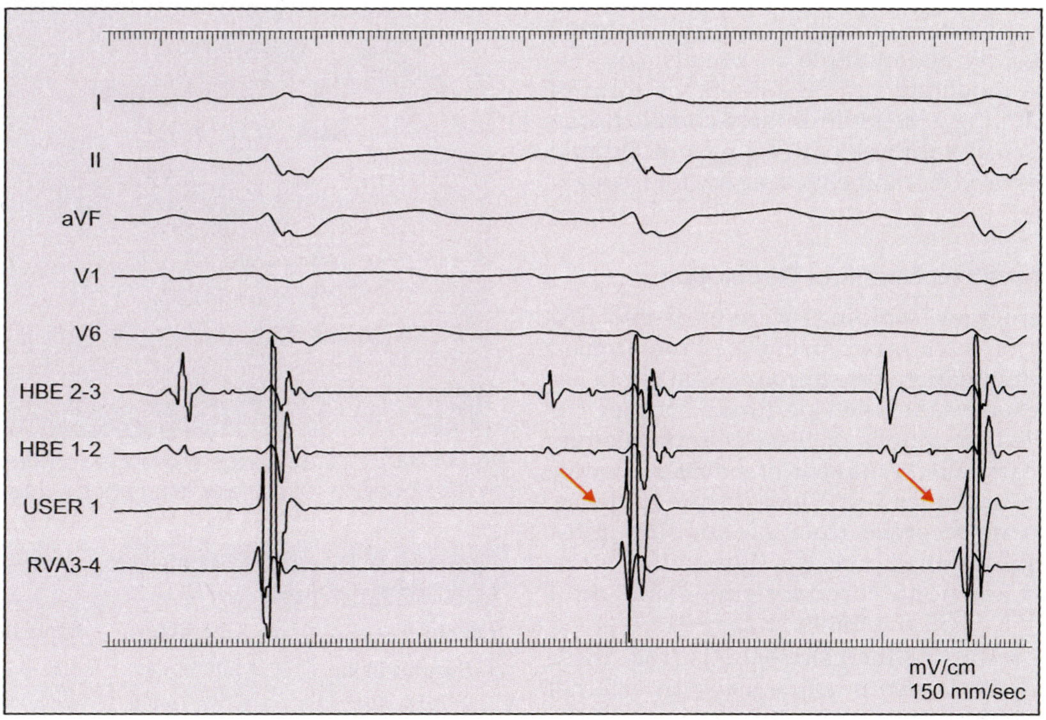


**Fig. 11.51:** Bundle branch reentrant ventricular tachcyardia. Five surface ECG leads (I, II, aVF, V1, V6) and intracardiac recordings from the His bundle region (HBE2–3, 1–2), the right ventricular apex (RVA3–4), and a mapping catheter (USER1) positioned distal to the His catheter along the RV septum to record a right bundle potential (arrow). The right bundle potential was recorded 30 ms after the His potential (HP). A=atrial electrogram, V=ventricular electrogram)

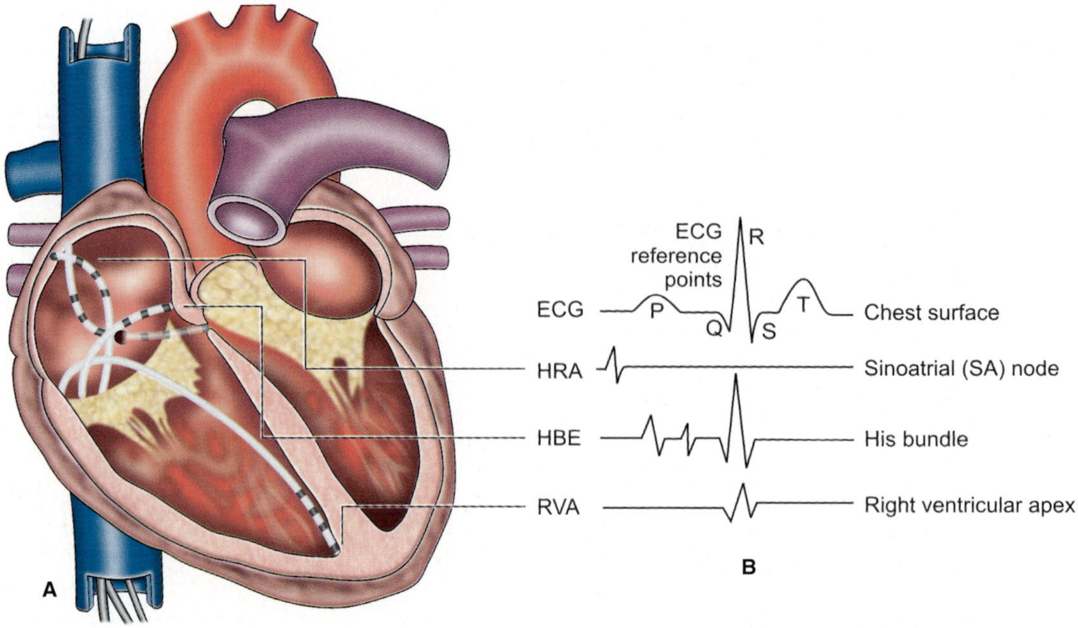


**Fig. 11.52:** (A) Different intracardiac conduction system from where electrograms are generated. (B) Schematic illustrations of several intracardiac electrograms contrasted with a conventional body-surface electrocardiogram (ECG)

ablated because of their deep septal or epicardial location. Some left ventricular VTs originate near a coronary cusp, which may preclude a successful ablation because of concern regarding coronary artery damage. Approximately half the cases of VTs associated with structural heart disease can be palliated by catheter ablation. Extensive scarring in these ventricles may limit the efficacy of the relatively small lesions made by RFCA, and multiple VT circuits may also contribute to this moderate success rate. Some form of 3-dimensional mapping is helpful for these complex ablations. In practice, many of these patients have ICDs, and catheter ablation is used as adjunctive therapy for frequent device activations.

## Diagnostic Programmed Electrical Stimulation

Intracardiac electrogram recordings were measured first in the 1960s, and the methods of diagnostic programmed electrical cardiac stimulation were introduced in the 1970s. These procedures are safe when performed under the carefully controlled conditions of the electrophysiology (EP) laboratory. Typically, a number of catheters (wires) are placed in the heart under X-ray fluoroscopic guidance, and electrograms are recorded from various sites, most frequently the high right atrium, His bundle [i.e. atrioventricular (AV) junction], coronary sinus, and right ventricle (Figs 11.52. 11.53 and Table 11.2).

In addition to recording the electrograms from these sites, pacing the heart is also possible using an external stimulator. This setup provides the ability to assess the conduction properties of the heart, as well as the ability to induce and terminate cardiac arrhythmias using various pacing protocols. Analysis of the electrogram patterns and the patient's response to pacing interventions and drugs provides an accurate diagnosis of the mechanisms and

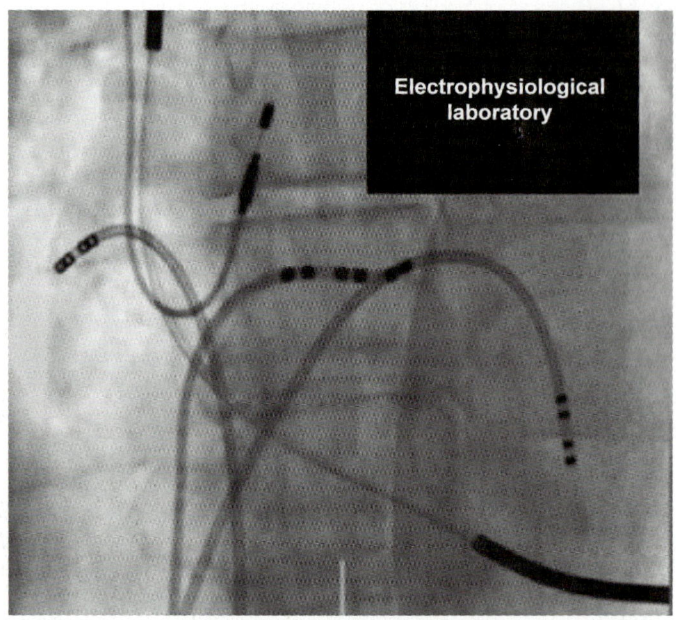


**Fig. 11.53:** An X-ray image showing three catheters introduced into the heart to record electrical signals and for circuit testing

**Table 11.2:** Diagnosis of different conduction abnormalities along the His bundle

| Location | Character | Morphology |
|---|---|---|
| 1. Supra-Hisian (above the HB) | 1st° block<br>2nd° block<br>3rd° block | Normal QRS or narrow QRS |
| 2. Intra-Hisian (inside) | –do– | Widening or Split His bundle potentials |
| 3. Infra-Hisian (below HB) | –do– | Wide QRS |

circuits for most arrhythmias. The introduction of radiofrequency catheter ablation in the 1980s provided the option for therapeutic interventions during the EP study. This has revolutionized the treatment of cardiac arrhythmias and has high success rates, particularly for reentrant supraventricular arrhythmias.

### Indications for Programmed Electrical Stimulation

- Risk stratification (regarding ventricular arrhythmias) in patients with structural heart disease
- Risk assessment in patients with Wolff-Parkinson-White (WPW) syndrome
- Evaluation of patients with syncope
- Characterization of AV conduction
- Determining the mechanism of supraventricular tachycardia
- Assessment of efficacy of catheter ablation
- Determining the mechanism of a wide QRS complex tachycardia
- Determining the mechanism of ventricular tachycardia
- Determining the impact of pacing on initiation and termination of the tachycardia

## Methods of Programmed Electrical Stimulation of the Heart

*Types of pacing protocols are used during EP testing:*

- Burst pacing or continuous pacing: The atrium or ventricle is paced at a faster fixed rate than the underlying sinus rate. For example, during measurement of sinus node function
- Decremental pacing is burst pacing but with a continuous increase in the pacing rate and hence a decrease in the cycle length (CL). For example, as in the measurement of the Wenckebach CL or the rate at which the AV node blocks a beat in conduction from the atrium to the ventricle
- *Extrastimuli:* Typically, 6–8 beats are delivered at a fixed rate (drive train), followed by 1–3 additional premature beats at a shorter CL or faster rate, for example, used particularly for induction of reentrant supraventricular or ventricular arrhythmias
- A standard electrophysiology protocol involves single premature atrial extrastimuli at two cycle lengths, and from 1 site, single, double, and triple ventricular premature extrastimuli from two right ventricular sites at two-cycle lengths. There are various ways to decrement atrial and ventricular premature extrastimuli during fixed rate pacing.
- Occasionally, isoproterenol or other drugs are given to help initiate a tachycardia.
- *Extrastimuli during tachycardias:* Premature atrial or ventricular beats may be introduced during tachycardia to help differentiate the circuit and mechanism of the arrhythmia. In addition, accelerating the rate of tachycardia by pacing at a faster rate with a catheter in or near the circuit is possible; this is called entrainment.
- *Pace termination:* Pacing at a faster rate (shorter CL) near the circuit can frequently terminate reentrant tachycardias

**Note:** A heart rate (HR) of 60 beats per minute (bpm) corresponds to a CL of 1000 milliseconds (1 second); thus, CL (in milliseconds) equals 60,000/HR.

## Measurements during Electrophysiology Testing

### Conduction Intervals

The AH interval is defined as the conduction time from the low right atrium through the AVN to the His bundle. It is measured on the His catheter electrogram. The normal range is 50–150 ms. The AH interval varies tremendously, depending on the patient's autonomic tone. The HV interval is defined as the time from the His bundle deflection to the earliest ventricular signal, measured in any intracardiac or surface recording. It represents the conduction time through the His-Purkinje system and is typically 35–55 milliseconds (Figs 11.54–11.62).

### Sinus Node Assessment

The sinus node recovery time is measured by pacing the high right atrium at a rate faster than the sinus rate for up to 1 minute and then measuring the interval from the last

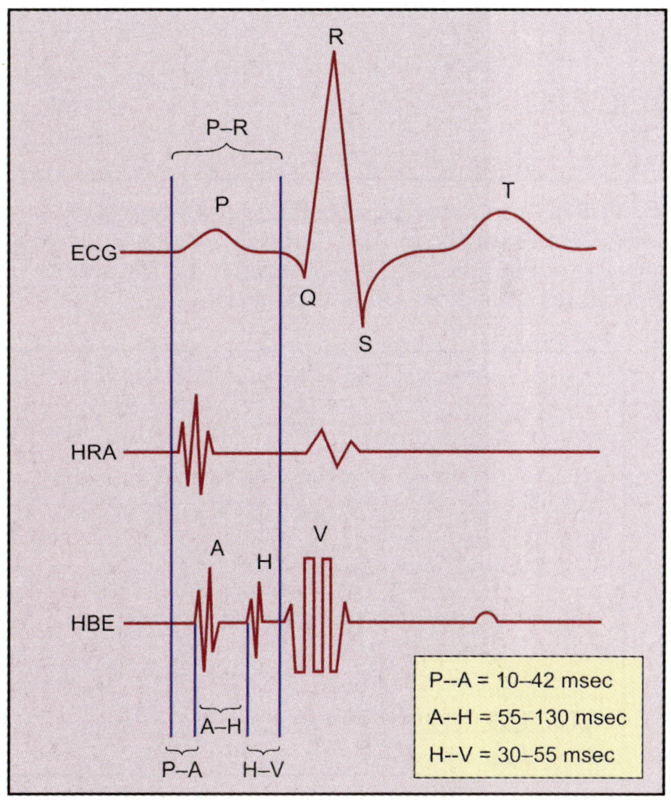


**Fig. 11.54:** Intracardiac electrograms. Schematic illustrations of several intracardiac electrograms contrasted with a conventional body-surface electrocardiogram (ECG). HRA=high right atrial electrogram; HBE=His bundle electrogram, in which A=low right atrial activity, H=His bundle activity, and V=ventricular septal activity; also shown are the P–R, P–A, A–H, and H–V intervals

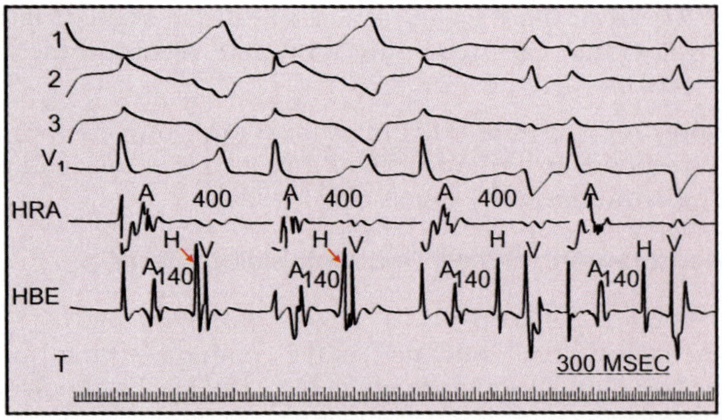


**Fig. 11.55:** Graph showing influence of atrial pacing on conduction over an AV bypass tract. In this electrophysiological study, the atrial are being paced at a cycle length of 400 msec. First two complexes show marked preexcitation with the antegrade His bundle potential (H) buried in the QRS complex. Constant AH intervals and normal QRS complex results when sudden block appears during pacing

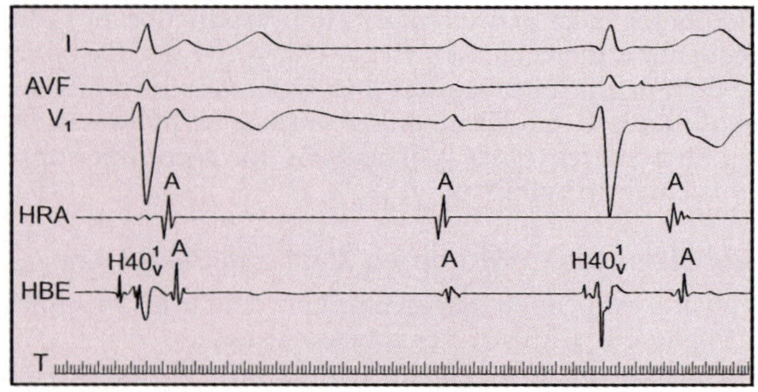


**Fig. 11.56:** Graph (upper panel) leads 1 aVF and V1 shows morphology of complete heart block in which there is no association of P-waves with QRS complex and all atrial impulses are unable to conduct due to block at AV junction. His bundle electrogram in this case reveals that each junctional escape QRS complex is preceded by a His bundle deflection (H) with a normal H–V interval (40 msec) in congenital complete heart block

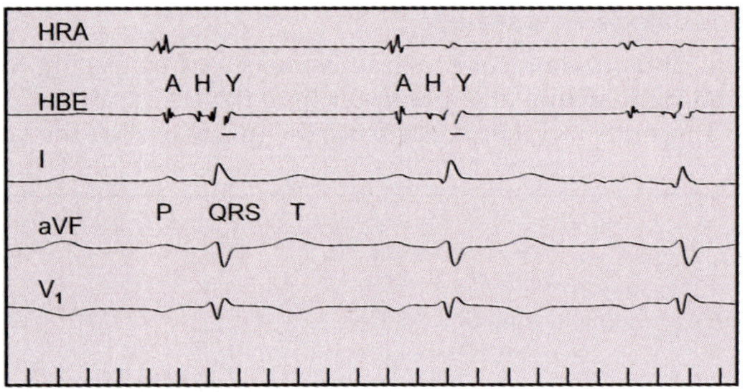


**Fig. 11.57:** Graph showing spontaneous rhythm with normal features of HBE with normal PA, AH and HV intervals. HRA=High right atrium, HBE=His bundle electrogram, 1, aVF and V1 are standard and precordial leads respectively

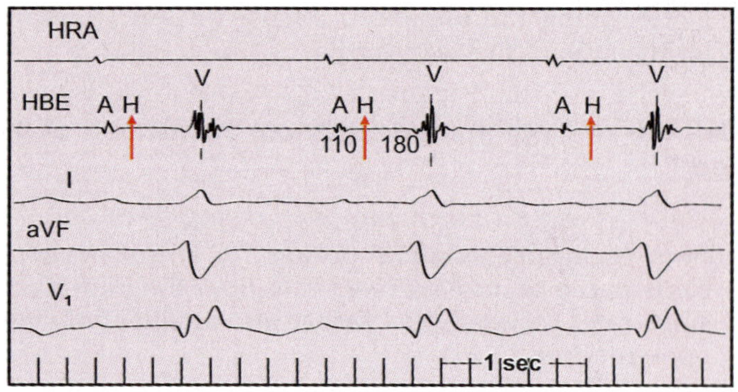


**Fig. 11.58:** Graph shows (HBE) marked prolongation of HV interval to 180 msec in a patient suffering from bifascicular block and prolonged P-R interval

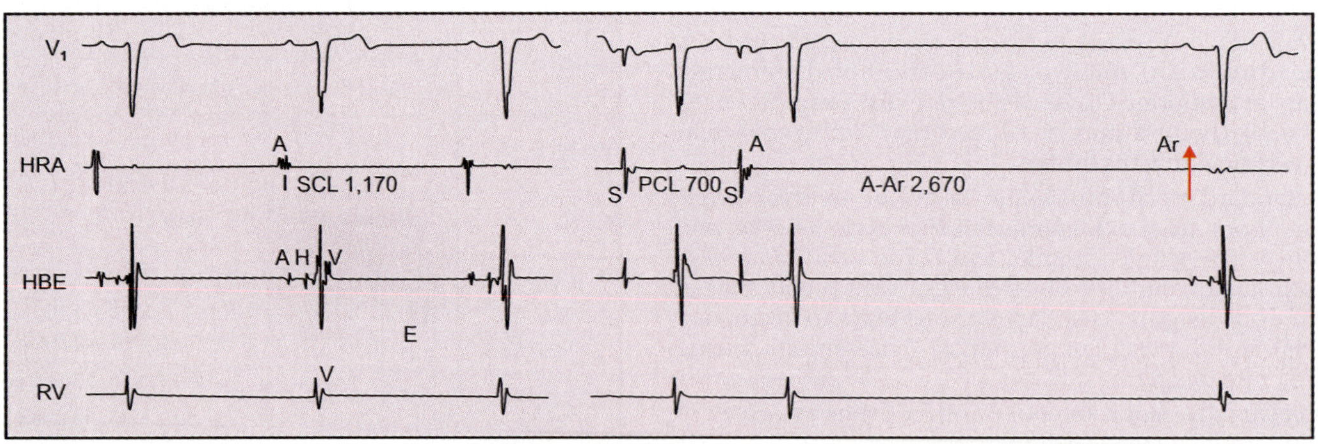


**Fig. 11.59:** Graph (upper panel) shows features of sinus bradycardia in sick sinus syndrome (V1), whereas, in HRA, there is marked delay in the sinoatrial conduction time (more than 2670 msc) with 700 pacing cycle length. His bundle electrogram shows normal HV

paced beat to the first sinus beat. The normal range is less than 1500 milliseconds. The corrected sinus node recovery time is the difference between the sinus node recovery time and the sinus cycle length; the normal value is < 550 ms. Patients with sick sinus syndrome have prolonged sinus node recovery times.

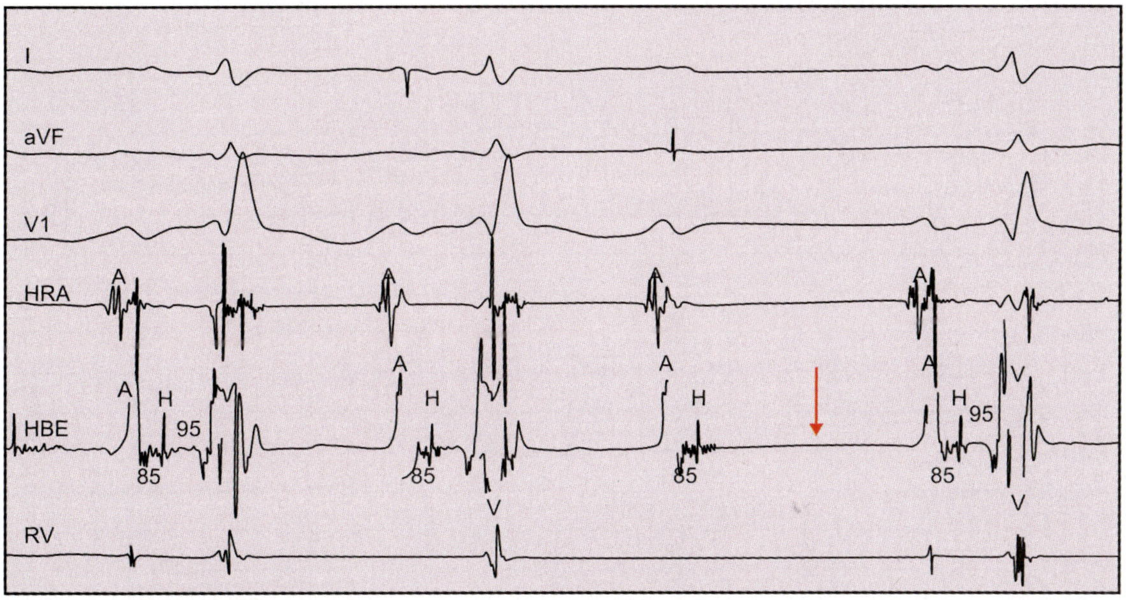


**Fig. 11.60:** Graph shows features of spontaneous type 11 second degree infra-Hisian block. Note that AH and HV intervals remain constant during conducted inpulses at 85 msec and 95 mec respectively. The third AH interval complex, however is suddenly and unexpectedly not followed by a ventricular depolarization. The complex followed by the blocked one revealed no change in the conduction intervals

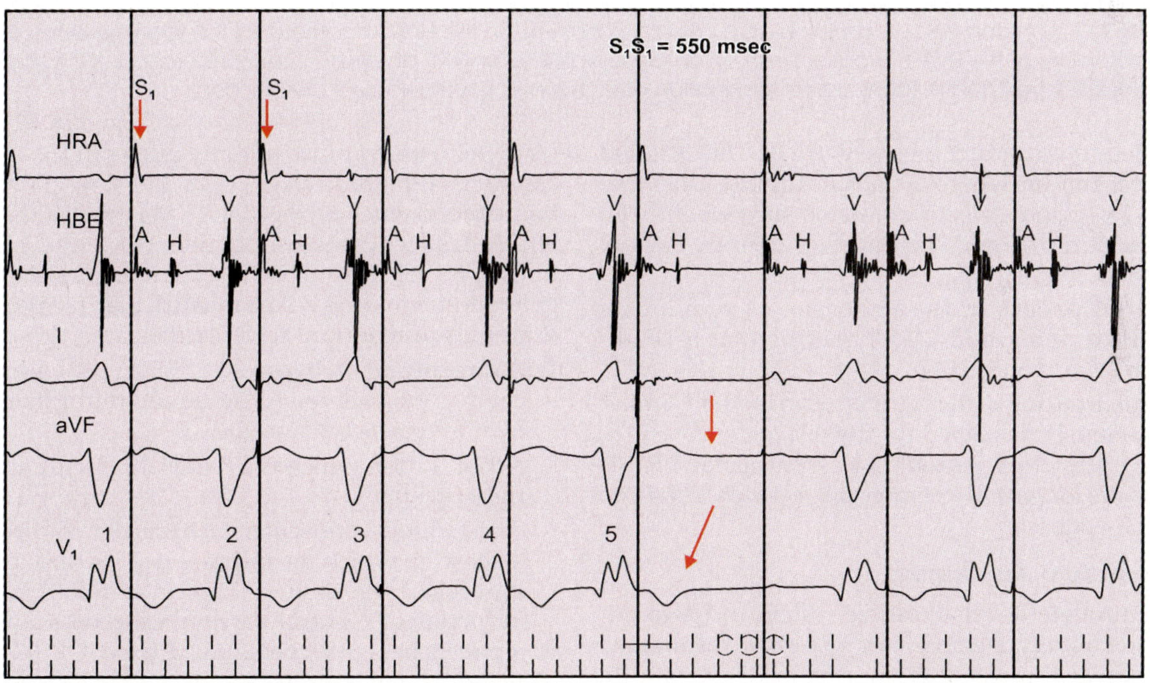


**Fig. 11.61:** Graph shows block distal to His bundle during atrial pacing Mobitz 11 second degree AV block is seen following 5th beat of atrial pacing at 550 msec (110 beats/min). There is absence of ventricular activity following His deflection in the 5th beat, clearly demonstrating Mobitz 11 AV block (second degree)

## *AV Node Assessment*

The function of the AV node is to control the rate of impulse conduction from the atria to the ventricles. When the atrial rate increases above a certain rate (typically 150–200 bpm), the AV node initially causes AV block in a Wenckebach pattern and then generates higher degrees of block if the atrial rate increases further, thus controlling the ventricular rate and preserving cardiac output.

*Two measurements of AV nodal function are as follows:*

- Wenckebach CL uses decremental pacing to measure the lowest rate (longest CL) at which a dropped
- Ventricular beat occurs
- The AV nodal effective refractory period (ERP) is measured by introducing a single extrastimulus (S2)
- After a drive train of 8 stimuli at a fixed rate (all S1), at which time the S1–S2 interval is decreased until the S2

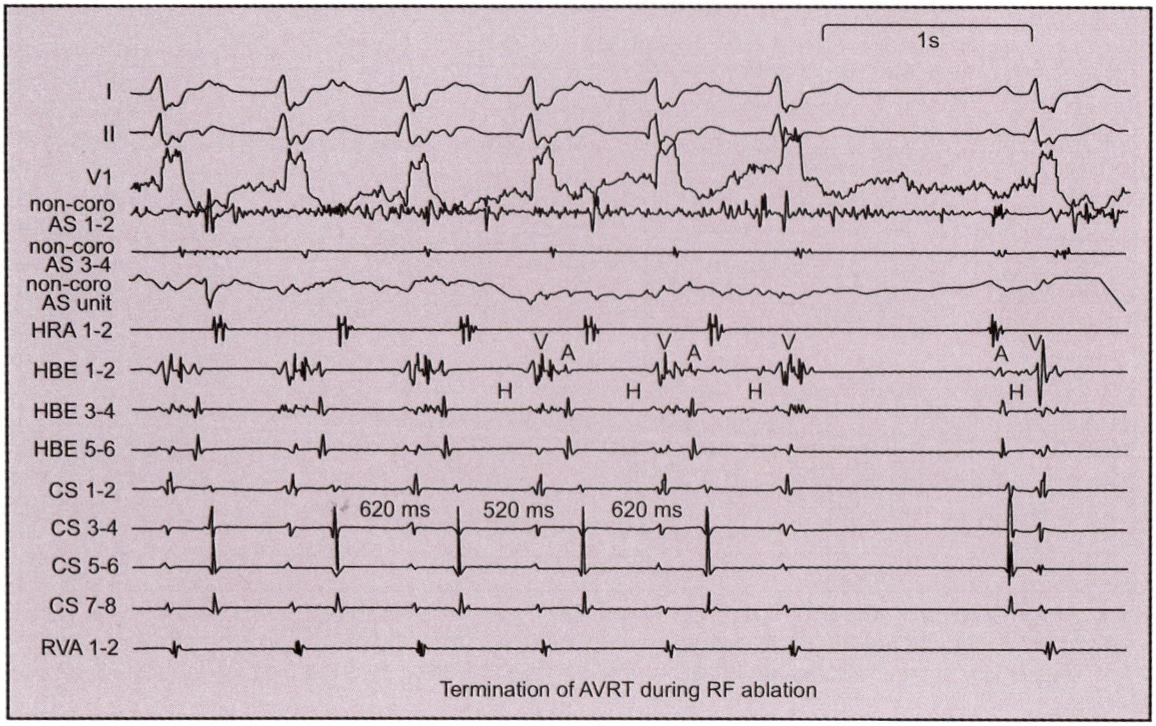


**Fig. 11.62:** Tracings are ECG leads I, II, V1, and intracardiac electrograms recorded from a mapping catheter in the noncoronary AS (non-coro AS1–2, non-coro AS3–4, and non-coro AS unit), a catheter in the HRA, a catheter at the region (HBE), a catheter within the CS, and a catheter at the RVA in a patient with an anteroseptal AP during RF ablation in the noncoronary AS. A single RF delivery at this site successfully resulted in tachycardia termination after 15s and ventriculoatrial dissociation

impulse does not conduct to the ventricle. This is noted on the electrogram where an atrial impulse does not result in a His bundle electrogram and subsequently no ventricular stimulation. This interval defines the AV nodal ERP

- Decremental pacing of the ventricle, as previously described for antegrade (A-V) conduction, assesses retrograde (V-A) conduction
- Extrastimulus pacing in the ventricle, in a method similar to that previously described for the AV node, measures ventricular refractory periods. The ventricular ERP is defined as the longest S1–S2 interval in which S2 fails to capture the ventricle.

### *His-Purkinje System Assessment*

Conduction through the His-Purkinje system and determination of refractory period can provide important information regarding conduction system disease and a need for a permanent pacemaker. The latter is especially important if infra-Hisian block is observed.

### Induction of Arrhythmias

Most arrhythmias encountered during EP testing are reentrant in nature and are therefore amenable to induction by the methods of extrastimuli. A reentrant arrhythmia requires a circuit with different limbs that have different refractory periods. When conduction blocks in one limb, the electrical impulse may travel down the other limb and then return (re-enter) via the limb that was blocked. For example, in typical AV nodal reentrant tachycardia (AVNRT), the impulse initially blocks in the fast pathway, conducts antegrade (A-V) over the slow pathway, and is then able to enter retrograde (V-A) over the fast pathway, which has recovered conduction. When the impulse continues to travel around this circuit, a reentrant arrhythmia is generated, yielding a supraventricular tachycardia. Other examples of reentrant tachycardias are:

1. AV reentrant tachycardia (AVRT), in which antegrade conduction over the AV node and retrograde conduction over a bypass tract occur.
2. Atrial flutter, which is a reentrant circuit, usually in the right atrium.
3. Scar-related ventricular tachycardia of coronary artery disease, in which the impulse travels through or around the area of scar tissue. A typical stimulation protocol for induction of reentrant arrhythmias uses a drive train of 8 paced beats (S1 beats) at a fixed CL (e.g. 500 milliseconds) with a premature beat (S2) added to the end of the drive train. The S2 stimulus is brought into atrial or ventricular refractoriness in intervals of 10 milliseconds. When S2 no longer captures, this defines the ERP of the tissue. A second extrastimulus, S3, is then added, with S2 set at a coupling interval 20 milliseconds above the ERP. The S2–S3 interval is also decremented until refractoriness is reached. If no arrhythmia is induced, the pacing sequences may be repeated using a third extrastimulus, i.e. S4. By convention, drive CLs (S1) of 500 and 400 milliseconds are used in ventricular pacing protocols. Arrhythmias with a reentrant mechanism are most often induced with this method. Another type of

pacing sequence is the continuous (or straight) burst pacing sequence, in which the atrium or ventricle is paced at a fixed rate (S1) for up to 10 seconds. In arrhythmias that have mechanisms other than reentry, this method is more likely to induce such triggered activityIn addition, burst pacing at a rate faster than the arrhythmia CL often terminates reentrant arrhythmias.

### Termination of Arrhythmias

- Programmed stimulation can also be used to terminate reentrant cardiac arrhythmias. In ventricular tachycardia, pacing at a rate faster than the tachycardia rate (overdrive pacing) can capture part of the tissue in the circuit and render it refractory, thus terminating the tachycardia. This is used clinically in the methods of overdrive pacing or antitachycardia pacing used in implantable cardioverter-defibrillator (ICD) devices
- Overdrive pacing in the right atrium can terminate atrial flutter, and either atrial or ventricular pacing can terminate AVNRT and AVRT. Pacing methods are not successful in treatment of atrial or ventricular fibrillation because these arrhythmias comprise multiple small reentrant circuits or breakdown of spiral waves

### Complications after Catheter Ablation

Radiation risk in catheter ablation is low, but it may exceed the risk from common radiologic procedures. The average risk for genetic defects has been computed at 1 case per million births. The average risk for fatal malignancies ranges from 0.3 to 2.3 deaths per 1000 cases for every 60 minutes of fluoroscopy. Many ablation procedures require less than 60 minutes of fluoroscopy. Major complications occur in approximately 3% of patients who have ablation procedures, including thromboembolism in less than 1% (higher in some atrial fibrillation ablation series) and death in 0.1–0.2% of all procedures. The incidence of cardiac complications varies, based on the site and type of ablation. Cardiac complications include the following:

- High-grade AV block
- Cardiac tamponade (highest in atrial fibrillation ablation, up to 6%)
- Coronary artery spasm/thrombosis
- Pericarditis
- Valve trauma
- Vascular complications, which occur in approximately 2–4% of procedures, include the following:
- Retroperitoneal bleeding
- Hematoma
- Vascular injury
- Transient ischemic attack/stroke
- Hypotension
- Thromboembolism or air embolism

*Pulmonary complications include the following:*

- Pulmonary hypertension with and without hemoptysis (secondary to pulmonary vein stenosis)
- Pneumothorax

*Miscellaneous complications include the following:*

1. Left atrial esophageal fistula
2. Acute pyloric spasm/gastric hypomotility
3. Phrenic nerve paralysis
4. Radiation or electrically induced skin damage
5. Infection at access site
6. Inappropriate sinus tachycardia
7. Proarrhythmia

## LONG-TERM MONITORING

Some physicians empirically treat patients with 4–12 weeks of aspirin therapy to possibly reduce the risk of thromboembolic sequelae. Echocardiography is not routinely performed unless a complication may have occurred (e.g. pericardial effusion). Postprocedure electrophysiologic testing is not performed routinely unless recurrent tachyarrhythmias are suspected.

## SURGICAL INTERVENTIONS IN THE MANAGEMENT OF CARDIAC ARRHYTHMIAS

### Maze Procedure (Surgical Ablation)

The surgical ablation maze procedure, or Cox-Maze IV, evolved from the Cox-Maze III cut-and-sew procedure (Fig. 11.63). Instead of using incisions, a surgical ablation

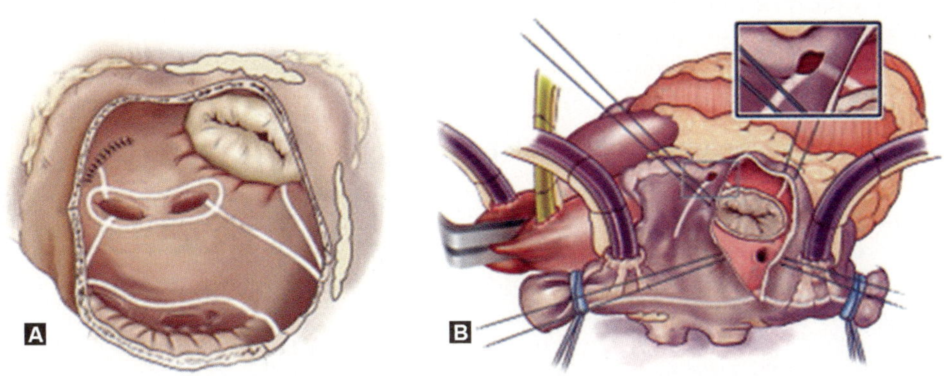


**Fig. 11.63:** Biatrial Cox-Maze IV lesion set. (A) Left atrial lesions. (B) Right atrial lesions. Irrigated radiofrequency ablation for treatment of AF during cardiac surgery was associated with a low complication rate. No device-related complications occurred. The Cox-Maze lesion set was effective at restoring sinus rhythm and had higher success rates in patients with smaller left atrial diameters and longer ablation times

energy source is used to create a conduction block of scar tissue to stop the errant electrical signals. The surgical ablation version of the maze procedure is much faster than Cox-Maze III and is considered very effective As an open-chest procedure, it is usually performed on patients needing open-heart surgery for other issues, such as valve replacement or repair or coronary artery bypass (CABG). This is called 'concomitant surgery,' meaning that it's done along with another procedure. It is performed on either a stopped or a beating heart.

### Maze Surgical Ablation (Open Chest)

While this open-chest maze surgery is sometimes done as a standalone procedure on patients with atrial fibrillation only, more often these afib-only cases are handled by the closed chest mini maze procedure.

### Maze Procedure Success Rates

The open-chest maze procedures done by surgical ablation have been found to have similar success rates to Cox-Maze III procedures, including those utilizing a variety of surgical ablation energy sources. Many centers doing this maze surgery also cite freedom from stroke in excess of 99%.

### Mini Maze Procedure Risks

The blood clots and strokes that are occassional complications with catheter ablation are rarely found in the mini maze procedure as no catheters are involved. And since the surgeon uses a thoracoscope to see the heart directly, there may be less risk of obstructing the pulmonary veins (pulmonary vein stenosis).

However, any procedure dealing with the heart has risks. While we rarely see any of the following, the risks of a mini maze procedure do include:

- Collapsed lung from deflating the lung in surgery, which is correctable with a chest tube
- Vein inflammation (phlebitis)
- Heart tissue inflammation (pericarditis)
- Blood vessel or heart damage
- Death

In most studies reviewed, there are minimal complications, though in one study there was one death very early on due to tearing of the left atrial appendage. Research has also shown that there is some risk of blood clots and a stroke following surgery.

### Abnormal Heart Rhythms and Implantable Cardioverter Defibrillators

Treatment for abnormal heart rhythms is possible with an implantable cardioverter defibrillators (ICD), or implantable cardioverter defibrillator. An ICD is an electronic device that constantly monitors your heart rate and rhythm. When it detects a very fast, abnormal heart rhythm, it delivers energy to the heart muscle. This causes the heart to beat in a normal rhythm again (Fig. 11.64).

The ICD has two parts—the lead(s) and a pulse generator. The lead(s) monitor the heart rhythm and deliver

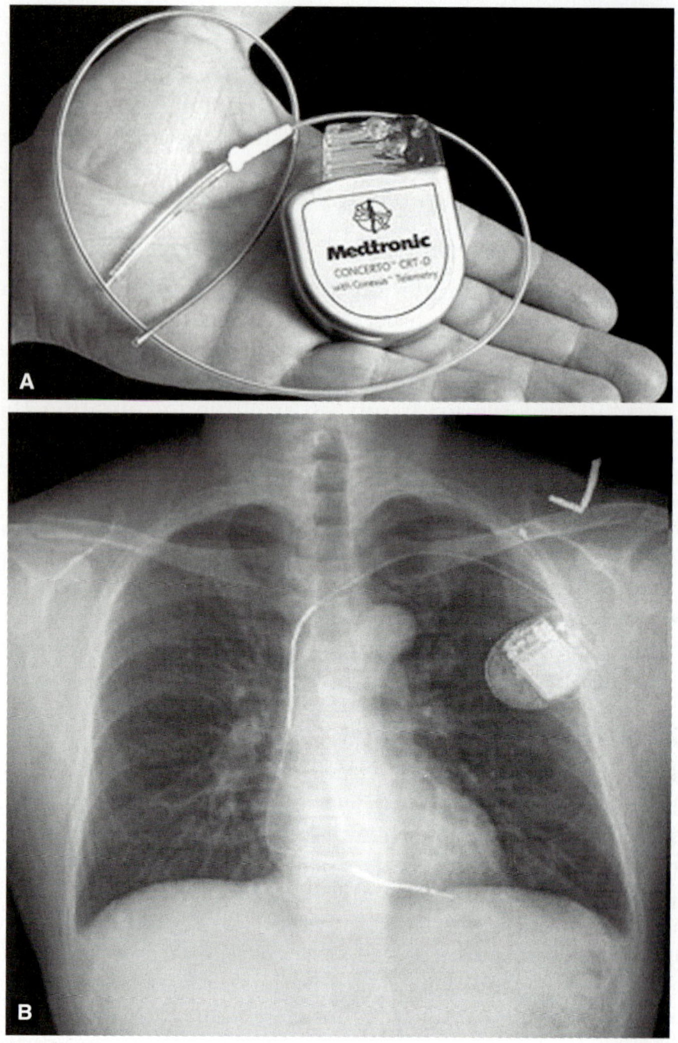


**Fig. 11.64:** (A) An implantable cardioverter-defibrillator (ICD). (B) Chest X-ray showing an implantable cardioverter-defibrillator (ICD), with its battery fixed at left subclavicular region and is connected with a wire placed in the trabecular part of the right ventricular apex

energy used for pacing and/or defibrillation (see below for definitions). The generator houses the battery and a tiny computer. Energy is stored in the battery until it is needed. The computer receives information from the leads to determine how well the heart is beating.

#### Types of ICDs, including:

- Single chamber ICD: A lead is attached in the right ventricle. If needed, energy is delivered to the ventricle to help it contract normally.
- Dual chamber ICD: Leads are attached in the right atrium and the right ventricle. Energy is delivered first to the right atrium and then to the right ventricle, helping your heart to beat in a normal sequence.
- Biventricular ICD: Leads are attached in the right atrium, the right ventricle and the left ventricle. This technique helps the heart beat in a more balanced way and is specifically used for patients with heart failure.

Your doctor will determine which type of ICD is best for you.

### How does an ICD Work?

The ICD monitors the heart rhythm, identifies abnormal heart rhythms, and determines the appropriate therapy to return your heartbeat to a normal rhythm. Your doctor programs the ICD to include one or all of the following functions:

- Anti-tachycardia Pacing (ATP): When the heart beats too fast, a series of small electrical impulses are delivered to the heart muscle to restore a normal heart rate and rhythm.
- Cardioversion: A low energy shock is delivered at the same time as your heartbeat to restore a normal heart rhythm.
- Defibrillation: When the heart is beating dangerously fast, a high-energy shock is delivered to the heart muscle to restore a normal rhythm.
- Bradycardia pacing: When the heart beats too slow, small electrical impulses stimulate the heart muscle to maintain a suitable heart rate.

### Who is a Candidate for an ICD?

- People who have had an episode of sudden cardiac arrest or ventricular fibrillation.
- People who have had a heart attack and are at high risk for sudden cardiac arrest.
- People who have hypertrophic cardiomyopathy and are at high risk for sudden arrest.
- People who have had at least one episode of ventricular tachycardia, an abnormal heart rhythm.

## BIBLIOGRAPHY

1. Blomström-Lundqvist C, Scheinman MM, Aliot EM, et al. For the European Society of Cardiology Committee, NASPE-Heart Rhythm Society. ACC/AHA/ESC guidelines for the management of patients with supraventricular arrhythmias-executive summary. J Am Coll Cardiol 2003;42(8):1493–1531.
2. Calkins H, Canby R, Weiss R, et al. For the 100W Atakr II Investigator Group. Results of catheter ablation of typical atrial flutter. Am J Cardiol 2004;94(4):437–42.
3. Calkins H, Langberg J, Sousa J, et al. Radiofrequency catheter ablation of accessory atrioventricular connections in 250 patients. Abbreviated therapeutic approach to Wolff-Parkinson-White syndrome. Circulation 1992;85(4):1337–46.
4. Calkins H, Sousa J, el-Atassi R, et al. Diagnosis and cure of the Wolff-Parkinson-White syndrome or paroxysmal supraventricular tachycardias during a single electrophysiologic test. N Engl J Med 1991;324(23):1612–18.
5. Calkins H, Yong P, Miller JM, et al. For the Atakr Multicenter Investigators Group. Catheter ablation of accessory pathways, atrioventricular nodal reentrant tachycardia, and the atrioventricular junction: Final results of a prospective, multicenter clinical trial. Circulation 1999;99(2):262–70.
6. Chen SA, Chiang CE, Wu TJ, et al. Radiofrequency catheter ablation of common atrial flutter: comparison of electrophysio-logically guided focal ablation technique and linear ablation technique. J Am Coll Cardiol 1996;27(4):860–8.
7. Hindricks G. The multicentre European radiofrequency survey (MERFS): Complications of radiofrequency catheter ablation of arrhythmias. The Multicentre European Radiofrequency Survey (MERFS) Investigators of The Working Group on Arrhythmias of the European Society of Cardiology. Eur Heart J 1993;14(12):1644–53.
8. Jackman WM, Wang XZ, Friday KJ, et al. Catheter ablation of accessory atrioventricular pathways (Wolff-Parkinson-White syndrome) by radio-frequency current. N Engl J Med 1991;324(23):1605–11.
9. Kottkamp H, Hügl B, Krauss B, et al. Electromagnetic versus fluoroscopic mapping of the inferior isthmus for ablation of typical atrial flutter: A prospective randomized study. Circulation 2000;102(17):2082–6.
10. Kuck KH, Schlüter M, Geiger M, Siebels J, Duckeck W. Radio-frequency current catheter ablation of accessory atrioventri-cular pathways. Lancet 1991;337(8757):1557–61.
11. Langberg JJ, Leon A, Borganelli M, et al. A randomized, prospective comparison of anterior and posterior approaches to radiofrequency catheter ablation of atrioventricular nodal reentry tachycardia. Circulation 1993;87(5):1551–6.
12. Lesh MD, Van Hare GF, Scheinman MM, Ports TA, Epstein LA. Comparison of the retrograde and transseptal methods for ablation of left free wall accessory pathways. J Am Coll Cardiol 1993;22(2):542–9.
13. Man KC, Knight B, Tse HF, et al. Radiofrequency catheter ablation of inappropriate sinus tachycardia guided by activation mapping. J Am Coll Cardiol 2000;35(2):451–7.
14. Paydak H, Kall JG, Burke MC, et al. Atrial fibrillation after radiofrequency ablation of type I atrial flutter: time to onset, determinants, and clinical course. Circulation 1998;98(4):315–22.
15. Pérez FJ, Schubert CM, Parvez B, Pathak V, Ellenbogen KA, Wood MA. Long-term outcomes after catheter ablation of cavotricuspid isthmus dependent atrial flutter: a meta-analysis. Circ Arrhythmia Electrophysiol 2009;2(4):393–401.
16. Scheinman M, Calkins H, Gillette P, et al. North American Society of Pacing and Electrophysiology. NASPE policy statement on catheter ablation: personnel, policy, procedures, and therapeutic recommendations. Pacing Clin Electrophysiol 2003;26(3):789–99.
17. Scheinman MM. NASPE survey on catheter ablation. Pacing Clin Electrophysiol 1995;18(8):1474–8.
18. Tsai CF, Tai CT, Yu WC, et al. Is 8-mm more effective than 4-mm tip electrode catheter for ablation of typical atrial flutter? Circulation 1999;100(7):768–71.
19. Walsh EP, Saul JP, Hulse JE, et al. Transcatheter ablation of ectopic atrial tachycardia in young patients using radiofrequency current. Circulation 1992;86(4):1138–46.
20. Willems S, Weiss C, Ventura R, et al. Catheter ablation of atrial flutter guided by electroanatomic mapping (CARTO): a randomized comparison to the conventional approach. J Cardiovasc Electrophysiol 2000;11(11):1223–30.

# 12 Recognition and Management of Infective Endocarditis

In the century and a quarter since William Osler delivered his famed lectures on endocarditis, substantial advancements have occurred in the understanding and treatment of this disease.

Streptococcus viridans is the most common microbial agent responsible for infective endocarditis in children and adults. However, currently, staphylococcal aureus endocarditis is emerging as one of the leading causes of acute infective endocarditis particularily among those patients who are found to be malnourished and have congenital or acquired type of hypogammaglobulinemia with or without associated heart ailment. Despite the decline in rheumatic heart disease world wide and the use of antibiotic prophylaxis, there is no evidence that the incidence of infective endocarditis is decreasing. In fact, some data suggest it may be increasing. Several factors explain this apparent paradox (Fig. 12.1).

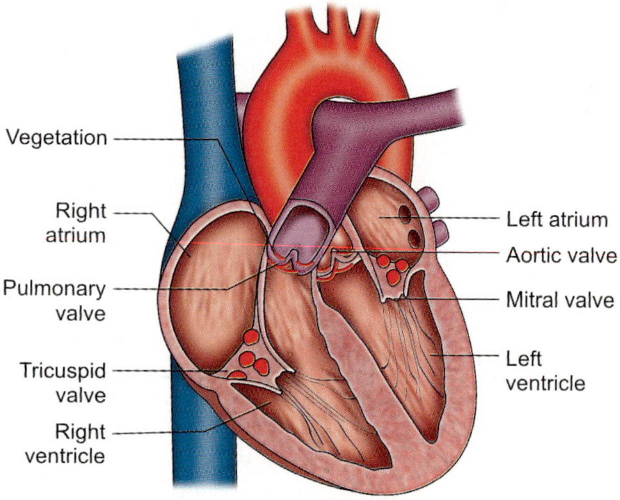


**Fig. 12.1:** This cross-sectional view shows vegetations (accumulations of bacteria and blood clots) on the four valves of the heart

- **First**, in industrialized nations, patients are living longer; this results in a higher prevalence of degenerative cardiac disease, which can serve as a nidus for endocardial infection.
- **Second** there is an increase in nosocomial infections. which are often caused by species of bacteria or yeasts associated with infective endocarditis.
- **Third** intravenous drug use has increased in industrialized societies.
- **Fourth** increasing application of cardiac surgery has provided new substrates for endocardial infection.
- **Fifth** the increased use of indwelling intravascular lines and implantable devices has resulted in many more catheter-related infections, bacteremias, and device-related infections.
- **Finally** the increased application of echocardiography has probably increased the rate at which infective endocarditis is diagnosed.

These factors have also increased the variety of ways infective endocarditis can present. The classical fever of unknown origin presentation represents a minority of infective endocarditis cases today. Thus, clinicians need to be vigilant about keeping infective endocarditis in mind with some of these more unusual presentations. Gram-negative and fungal endocarditis occur most often followig cardiac surgery or in debilitated patients. A wide variety of organisms have been implicated in the causation of infective endocarditis. Cardiac malformation is the major factor predisposing to infective endocarditis. With the better survival rate in congenital heart disease, the incidence in this group has shown rather on the increase; whereas with rheumatic heart disease it had shown upward trend in developing countries and concomitant decrease in developed countries of the world. Cardiac defects which are more prone to this infection are tetralogy of Fallot, VSD with aortic regurgitation or obstruction, MVP with MR and those with prosthetic valve. The patients who had under-

**Table 12.1:** The organisms responsible for IE

| | |
|---|---|
| *Staphylococcus aureus* | The most common cause of IE overall (acute and subacute); most common with prosthetic valves, acute IE and IE related to intravenous drug abuse. High mortality rate. Coagulase-negative *S. aureus* causes subacute disease similar to *Streptococcus viridans*. Accounts for 30% of IE associated with prosthetic valves. |
| **Streptococci** | ***S. viridans:*** 50–60% of subacute IE cases.<br>**Group D streptococci:** Usually subacute and the third most common cause of IE. |
| ***Streptococcus intermedius*** | Acute and subacute infection. Causes 15% of all cases of IE. |
| **Group A, C and G streptococci** | Acute IE is similar to that with *S. aureus*. High mortality (up to 70%). |
| **Group B streptococci** | Acute disease, high mortality often requiring valve replacement. Occurs in pregnancy and the elderly particularly. |
| *Pseudomonas aeruginosa* | Usually acute IE and requires surgery for cure. **HACEK organisms** (*Haemophilus* spp., *Aggregatibacter actinomycetemcomitans*, *Cardiobacterium* spp., *Eikenella corrodens*, *Kingella kingae*) usually subacute disease and about 5% of all IE. |
| **Fungi** | Cause subacute disease. |
| **Enterococci** | |

gone recent cardiac surgery are also more prone to infective endocarditis.

## Pathogenesis

Infective endocarditis is a disease caused by microbial infection of the endothelial lining of the heart. The characteristic lesion is a vegetation,which usually develops on a heart valve. In the pathogenesis of infectious endocarditis, local turbulence is believed to promote a sterile network of fibrin and platelets on the endocardial surface, which is colonized later by microorganisms entering the bloodstream from a distant site (Tables 12.1 and 12.2).

The infecting microorganisms are protected by the microthrombus from normal host defense mechanisms and from antibiotic penetration, requiring high dose parenteral antimicrobial agents over a long period.Whether the result of colonization of previously damaged heart endothelium or de novo infection of healthy tissues, the lesion is a vegetation whose primary features are a heavy colonization of microorganisms, a stroma consisting primarily of fibrin and a relative paucity of leukocytes. Once established, the vegetations have a tendency to enlarge with further deposition of fibrin and multiplication of the infecting organisms. The fibrin acts as a barrier to leukocytes; yet it permitis diffusion of essential nutrients from the blood.

**Table 12.2:** Localization of organisms according to the condition and site of origin

| Condition | Location of stream |
|---|---|
| Coarctation | Downstream wall |
| Patent ductus arterosus | Pulmonary artery |
| A-V fistula | Veins |
| Aortic insufficiency | Ventricular surface of valves |
| Mitral insufficiency | Atrial surface of mitral valve |
| Pulmonary insufficiency | Ventricular surface of pulmonary valve |
| Tricuspid insufficiency | Atrial surface of tricuspid valve |

The high density of infecting organisms and the difficulty for leukocytes to penetrate the nidus of infection partially explains the necessity of prolonged antimicrobials of primarily nature.

Its cure usually requires surgical excision of the infected vegetations and valve replacement. Infective endocarditis represents an endothelial infection that usually occurs at sites of endothelial damage, with the superimposed thrombus serving as the nidus. For the nidus to become infected, bacteria must enter the blood stream in sufficient numbers from a break in the epidermal or mucosal surfaces of the body. As the vegetation grows, regurgitation of the affected valve almost always occurs due to destruction, scarring, and retraction of the leaflet Occasionally, chordal involvement results in rupture, causing sudden severe atrioventricular valve regurgitation. Very large vegetations rarely can obstruct the valve orifice. Embolization of vegetations can result in damage to other organs from ischemia or remote infection. Invasion of the valve annulus by the organisms can lead to abscesses and fistulas. Infection of arterial walls due to vegetation embolization would lead to aneurysm formation and rupture, which can be devastating in the central nervous system.

*Incidence:* Osler's portentous words are as relevant now as when originally published. Despite improved preventive strategies, rational antibiotic prescribing, advances in imaging, and increasing use of early life saving cardiac surgery, the incidence of infective endocarditis remains high at 1.7–6.2 per 100,000 person years in the USA and Europe, with a one year mortality approaching 40%. The classical patient with infective endocarditis described in textbooks no longer represents the majority of cases in practice. The emergence of staphylococcal infection, often associated with indwelling devices, co-existent medical conditions and resistant to conventional antibiotic regimes, a variety of other atypical organisms, and the persistent syndrome of culture negative endocarditis make diagnosis and treatment as great a challenge as ever.

*Diagnostic criteria* (Table 12.3) The original von Reyn diagnostic criteria for infective endocarditis, based upon clinical and microbiological features, have now been surpassed by the Duke criteria which emphasise the role of echocardiography, the key imaging tool for both diagnosis and assessment of prognosis. Many studies have now demonstrated the superiority of the Duke criteria and a recent scientific statement of the American Heart Association concluded that they should be adopted as the primary diagnostic schema in the clinical evaluation of patients in whom infective endocarditis is suspected. Nevertheless, clear deficiencies remain.

*Major criteria:* Two positive blood cultures with atypical microbe, new murmur or echocardiogram finding of oscillating mass, abscess, or prosthetic valve dehiscence.

*Minor criteria:* Predisposing cardiac condition or IV drug use, fever >38°C, vascular phenomena, such as Osler's nodes, Janeway lesions. Immunologic phenomena, such as splenomegaly, echocardiogram consistent with endocarditis, but not meeting major criteria.

*Positive blood culture,* but not meeting major criteria, or positive serology for a combatable microbe.

*Definite diagnosis:* Positive histology or positive culture from vegetation. Two major criteria, one major and three minor criteria—all six minor criteria.

*Diagnosis rejected:* Alternative diagnosis established, resolution of illness after 4–5 days of antibiotics.

*Possible diagnosis* neither definite nor rejected.

## Clinical Presentation

*Symptoms and signs:* Malaise, weight loss, fatigue, night sweats, fever, chills, arthralgias, myalgias. Specific symptoms due to sites of damge, such as dyspnea with heart failure due to severe valvular regurgitation.

**Physical Examination** (Fig. 12.2)

- Osler's node, Janeway lesion, petechiae, and splinter
- Hemorrhages, Roth spots, and blue toe syndrome
- Fever
- Regurgitant heart murmurs, especially new or Worsemng
- Signs of heart failure
- Signs of stroke
- Splenomegaly

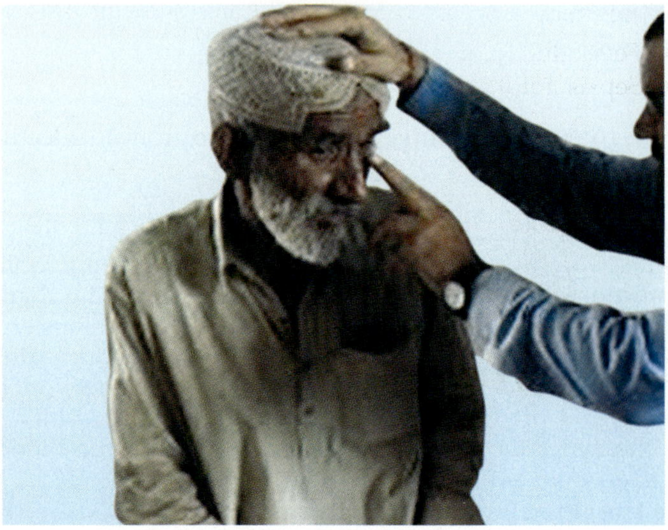

**Fig. 12.2:** Doctor is physically examining a patient with infective endocarditis

**Table 12.3:** Duke criteria for the diagnosis of infective endocarditis

| | |
|---|---|
| *Major criteria* | 1. Positive blood cultures (>2) with microbe typical for infective endocarditis, or persistently positive blood cultures with compatible microbe |
| | 2. Evidence of endocardial involvement: new regurgitant murmur or positive echocardiogram for oscillating mass, abscess, or prosthetic valve dehiscence |
| *Minor criteria* | 1. Predisposing cardiac condition or intravenous drug use |
| | 2. Fever >38.0°C (100.4°F) |
| | 3. Vascular phenomena |
| | 4. Immunologic phenomena |
| | 5. Echocardiogram consistent with endocarditis, but not meeting major criteria |
| | 6. Positive blood culture, but not meeting major criteria, or positive serology or molecular test for compatible microbe |
| *Diagnosis* | |
| Definite endocarditis | 1. Positive histology, or positive culture from vegetation, or |
| | 2. Two major criteria, or |
| | 3. One major and three minor criteria, or |
| | 4. Five minor criteria |
| *Rejected* | 1. Firm alternative diagnosis established |
| | 2. Resolution after <4 days of antibiotic treatment |
| | Possible endocarditis (neither definite nor rejected) |

*Osler's or Austrian triad?* Osler's or Austrian triad consists of endocarditis, pneumonia, and meningitis. The most common organism is *Streptococcus pneumoniae*, which is especially prevalent in alcoholic (40%), elderly, and diabetic patients. The course is fulminant, with rapid valve de struction and abscess formation. The aortic valve is most often, followed by the tricuspid valve. Infection is usually responsive to penicillin, but resistant strains that require vancomycin are becoming more common.

*Four peripheral stigmata of IE* (Figs 12.3–12.6)

1. Splinter hemorrhages (Fig. 12.3)
2. Janeway lesions (Figs 12.4 and 12.5)
3. Roth's spots
4. Osler's nodes

### Differential Diagnosis

- Fever due to other causes
- Sepsis not due to infective endocarditis
- Valvular lesions on echocardiography that resemble vegetations (e.g. myxomatous valves)

### Laboratory Tests

- Blood cultures: Three from separate venipunctures over 24 hours
- Serologic testing for organisms such as Histoplasma, Q fever, Brucella
- Rheumatoid factor may be falsely positive
- Leukocytosis, elevated gamma globulins, elevated erythrocyte sedimentation rate, anemia

### Laboratory Approach for Blood Sample Study

Optimal antiseptic skin preparation is important and at least 10 ml of blood (less in children) should be obtained for each culture. Bacteraemia is usually continuous and there is no rationale for timing blood cultures to coincide with peaks of pyrexia. If there is a history of prior antibiotic treatment, maximum diagnostic yield may be achieved by diluting the culture broth and considering the use of sodium polyanetholsulfonate or a dedicated adsorbent resin, both of which inactivate antimicrobial effects. Multiple separate blood cultures are required and most guidelines recommend at least two, and most usually three

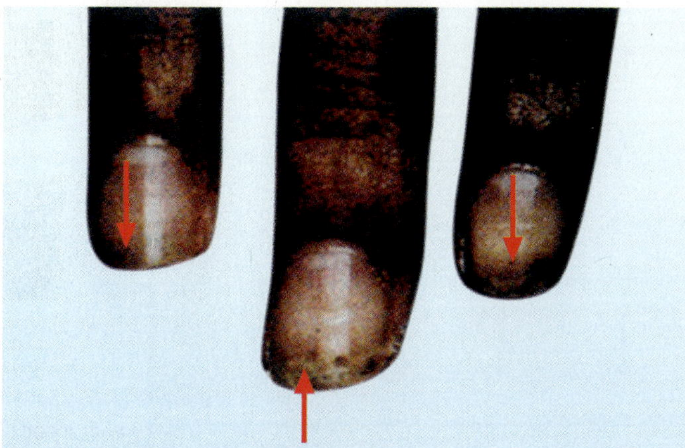

**Fig. 12.3:** Suhungual or splinter hemorrahage in patient with infective endocarditis

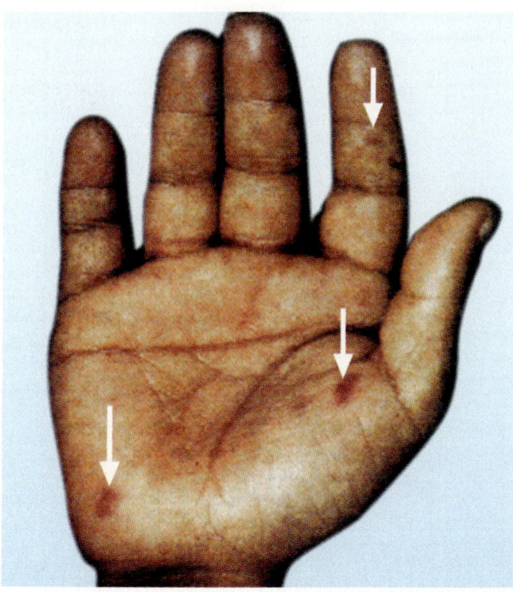

**Fig. 12.4:** Janeway lesions on the palm in the same patient

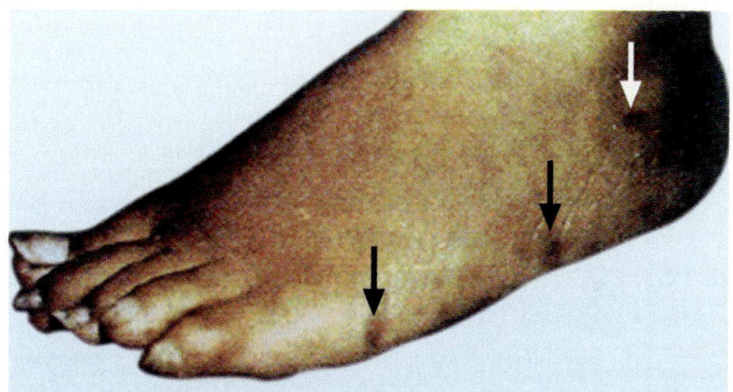

**Fig. 12.5:** Janeway lesions on the foot of the same patient

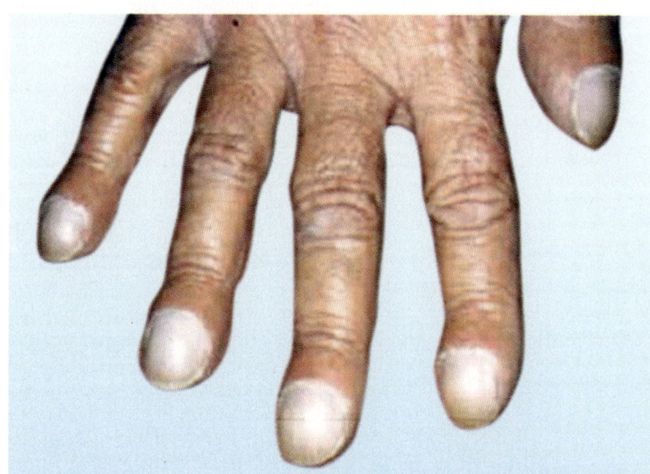

**Fig. 12.6:** Clubbing of fingers in infective endocarditis

sets. Although endocarditis caused by anaerobes is uncommon, blood cultures should be incubated in both aerobic and anaerobic atmospheres to detect organisms such as Bacteroides or Clostridium species. If all blood cultures remain negative at 5 days but infective endocarditis remains likely on clinical grounds, subculture onto chocolate agar plates may allow identification of an atypical organism, although prolonged culture for up to 2–3 weeks is associated with rising likelihood of contamination. At this stage, therefore, serum should be analysed for antibodies to organisms that cannot be cultured by routine methods, and, if available, antibodies to gram-positive bacterial cell walls. Excised valves, vegetations or other relevant material should undergo microscopy, culture, histopathology, and relevant molecular techniques (usually PCR) which can also be applied to newly acquired blood samples or the original growth negative blood culture substrate.

### Electrocardiography

Aortic valve abscess formation can lead to first second-, or third-degree heart block. Increased QRS voltage in acute aortic or mitral regurgitation owing to left ventricular volume increase (Figs 12.7 and 12.8).

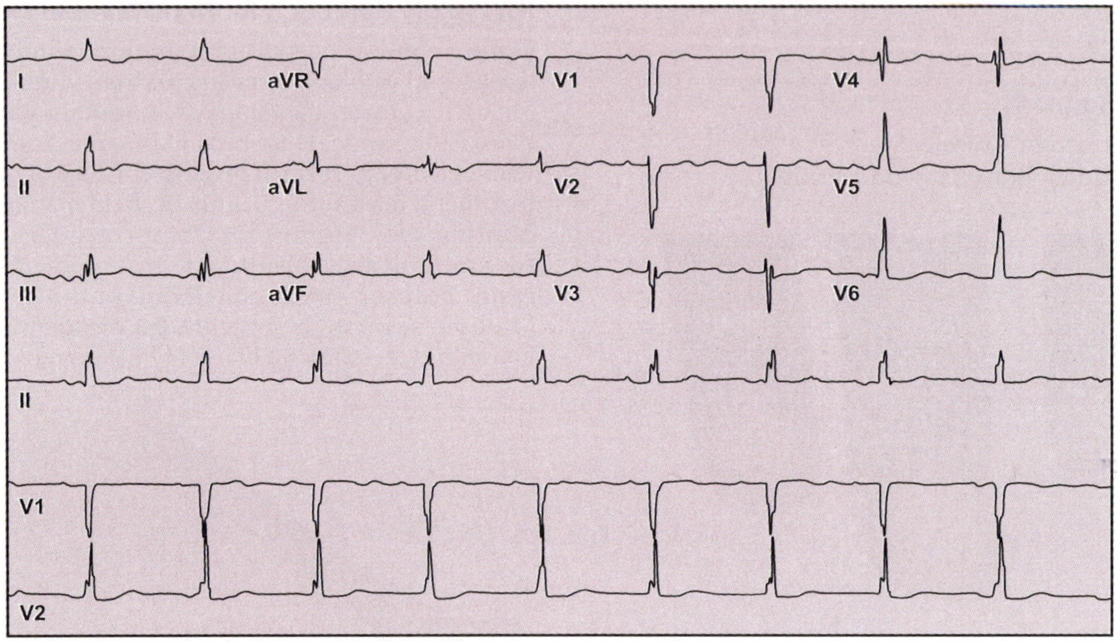


**Fig. 12.7:** ECG of a patient with infective endocarditis. Note the first-degree AV block, nonspecific intraventricular conduction delay, and nonspecific ST-T-wave abnormalities

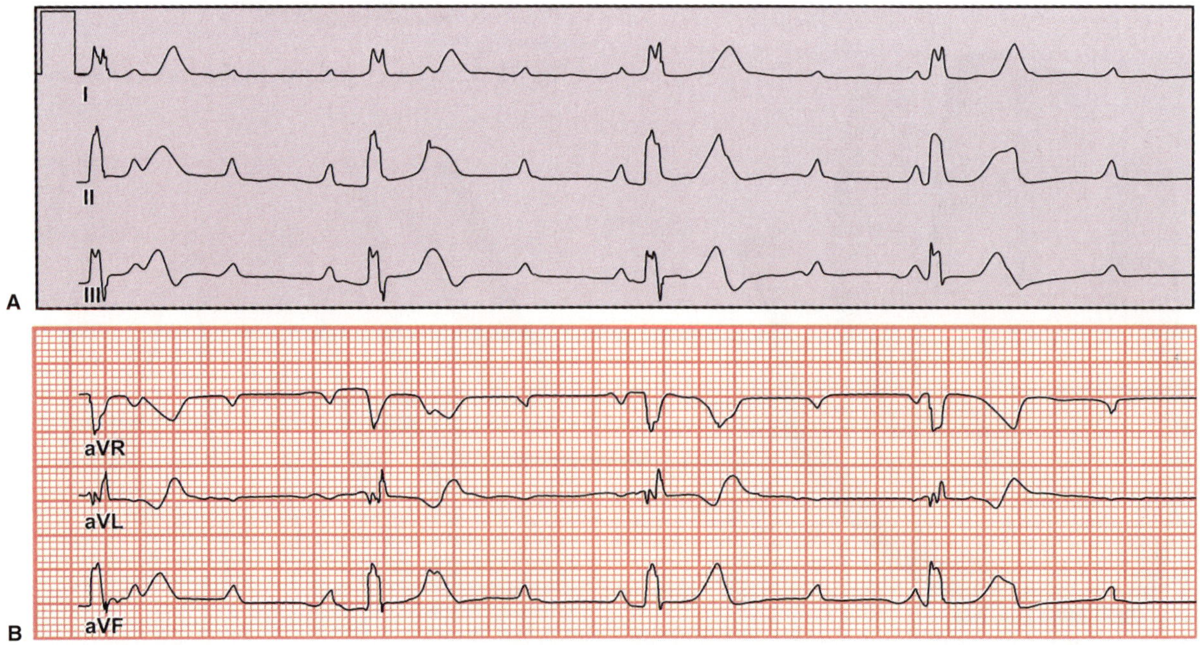


**Fig. 12.8A and B:** Electrocardiograms show complete heart block in infective endocarditis due to abcess along IVS

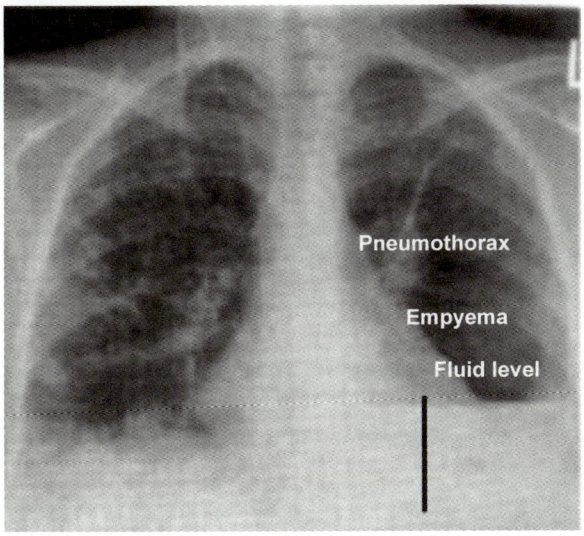


**Fig. 12.9:** X-ray chest PA view in the same patient showing multiple alveolar opacities in the right lung. Abscess formation in the left lung has caused a bronchopleural fistula, pneumothorax and emphysema,hence the air fluid level

### Imaging Studies

Chest X-ray may show cardiomegaly pulmonary edema, or septic pulmonary emboli (right-sided endocarditis) (Fig. 12.9).

### Echocardiography in Infective Endocarditis

Since Dillon and colleagues' in 1973 described valvar vegetations by M mode echocardiography, the technique has assumed an increasingly important role in the assessment and management of endocarditis. The development of two dimensional and later transesophageal echocardiography (TEE) has significantly improved the noninvasive detection of vegetations. Moreover, echo-Doppler studies provide clinically important information on the presence and degree of valvar destruction and their hemodynamic consequences, as well as on the existence of perivalvar infection. The diagnostic strategy proposed by Durack and colleagues (the Duke criteria) combined echocardiographic findings with clinical and microbiological data. Three echocardiographic findings were considered to be major criteria for the diagnosis of endocarditis. Transesophageal echocardiography is the preferred diagnostic technique because of its high sensitivity and specificity comparedwith transthoracic echocardiography (Tables 12.4, 12.5, and Box 12.1).

1. Findings that are almost certainly endocarditis include (major criteria) oscillating low-density masses, abscess, fistulas, and prosthetic valve dehiscence.
2. Probable endocarditis findings include localized leaflet thickening, nonmobile valve related masses, chordal rupture, aortic leaflet prolapse, and paraprosthetic valve regurgitation (minor criteria).
3. Possible endocarditis findings include valve lesions such as diffuse thickening, which could be a substrate for endocarditis, but specific findings are not seen.

**BOX 12.1:** Echocardiographic characteristics of infective endocarditis

| *Location* | *Findings* |
|---|---|
| Aortic valve | Shaggy nonuniform thickening in systole or diastole with unrestricted leaflet motion |
| | Dense shaggy echoes moving across valve and into LVOT |
| | Flail or ruptured cusps |
| | Fine diastolic fluttering on anterior mitral leaflet secondary to aortic insufficiency |
| Mitral valve | Thick shaggy echoes attached to or moving behind leaflets demonstrat-ingunne stricted motion |
| | Systolic flutter of prolapsing segments of mitral valve |
| | Fuzzy leaflet echoes in left atrial cavity during systole (differentiate from myxoma) |
| TV and PV | Shaggy thickening of leaflets, demonstrating unrestrictive motion. |
| | Mass of echoes moving with leaflets (dependent motion) |
| | Rupture of tricuspid chordae tendinae |
| Prosthetic valve | Thick shaggy collection located behind site of attachment of prosthesis to valve ring. |
| | Evidence of severe regurgitation. |

4. A negative echocardiographic study does not completely rule out endocarditis, but makes it less likely. If clinical suspicion remains high, a repeat study should be done in 5 days. Presence of vegetations defined as:
   - Mobile echodense masses implanted in a valve or mural endocardium in the trajectory of a regurgitant jet or implanted in prosthetic material with no alternative anatomical explanation;
   - Presence of abscess/s; or
   - Presence of a new dehiscence of a valvar prosthesis.

Abnormal echocardiographic findings not fulfilling those definitions were considered minor criteria. More recently the use of TEE has resulted in better imaging and therefore doubtful findings are not considered minor criteria any longer. Since the definite diagnosis of endocarditis requires the presence of two major criteria, or one major and three minor criteria, it is clear that echocardiography has assumed a crucial role in the diagnosis of the disease, particularly when blood cultures are negative. A negative TEE has an important clinical impact on the diagnosis of endocarditis with a high negative predictive value ranging from 86–97%. In patients with native heart valves a negative TEE virtually rules out the diagnosis of infective endocarditis. However, in the study of Sochowski and colleagues. 5 out of 65 patients (7.6%) with an initially negative TEE were finally diagnosed with endocarditis: in three of the patients a TEE performed 1–2 weeks after the initial examination showed the presence of vegetations. This study underlines the importance of recognising the

**Table 12.4:** Anatomic and echocardiographic definitions

| | *Surgery/necropsy* | *Echocardiography* |
|---|---|---|
| **Vegetation** | Infected mass attached to an endocardial structure, or on implanted intracardiac material | Oscillating or nonoscillating intracardiac mass on valve or other endocardial structures, or on implanted intracardiac material |
| **Abscess** | Perivalvular cavity with necrosis and purulent material not communicating with the cardiovascular lumen | Thickened, nonhomogeneous perivalvular area with echodense or echolucent appearance |
| **Pseudoaneurysm** | Perivalvular cavity communicating with the cardiovascular lumen | Pulsatile perivalvular echo-free space, with colour-Doppler flow detected |
| **Perforation** | Interruption of endocardial tissue continuity | Interruption of endocardial tissue continuity traversed by colour-Doppler flow |
| **Fistula** | Communication between two neighbouring cavities through a perforation | Colour-Doppler communication between two neighboring cavities through a perforation |
| **Valve aneurysm** | Saccular outpouching of valvular tissue | Saccular bulging of valvular tissue |
| **Dehiscence of a prosthetic valve** | Dehiscence of the prosthesis | Paravalvular regurgitation identified by TTE/TEE, with or without rocking motion of the prosthesis |

Anatomically, IE is characterized by a combination of vegetations and destructive lesions

phase of the disease in which the study is performed, since vegetations may not be large enough to be visualised when endocarditis is suspected very early on. In common with other diagnostic techniques, specificity of echocardiography is related to the clinical indication and the type of population studied. The technique does not permit differentiation between septic vegetations and other aseptic vegetations present in other situations such as Libman-Sacks endocarditis in systemic lupus erythematosus, and antiphospholipid syndrome or marantic endocarditis. Vegetations persisting after effective treatment must not be interpreted as a clinical recurrence of the disease unless supported by clinical features and bacteriologic evidence. Specificity is influenced mainly by the presence of valvar thickening or calcifications and also by rupture mitral chordae tendinae or Lambl's nodules which can be confused with vegetation images. The usefulness of TEE in patients with suspected endocarditis on a native valve is related to the results of the TTE. TEE is useful when TTE is negative or inconclusive.

## Detection of Vegetations

There is no better technique for noninvasive visualisation of vegetations than echocardiography. Overall the detection rate for vegetations by transthoracic echocardiography (TTE) in patients with a clinical suspicion of endocarditis averages around 50%. The diagnostic yield of the technique in the detection of vegetations is influenced by several factors, i.e. image quality, echogenicity and vegetation size, vegetation location, presence of previous valvar disease or valvar prosthesis, experience and skill of the examiner, and pretest probability of endocarditis.

### *Native valve endocarditis*

The use of harmonic imaging has improved study quality, but not the sensitivity in the visualisation of vegetations. 'Vegetation size also affects TTE sensitivity' since only 25%

**Table 12.5:** Risk of infective endocarditis associated with pre-existing cardiac disorders

**Prophylaxis for endocarditis recommended**

- *High-risk cardiac condition*
  - Prosthetic heart valves
  - Previous infective endocarditis
  - Cyanotic congenital heart disease (single ventricle states, transposition of the great arteries, tetralogy of Fallot)
  - Surgically constructed systemic—pulmonary shunts (e.g. Blalock shunt)
- *Intermediate-risk cardiac condition*
  - Mitral valve prolapse with regurgitation
  - Acquired valvular dysfunction (e.g. rheumatic heart disease)
  - Hypertrophic cardiomyopathy
  - Most congenital cardiac malformations (other than those listed above and below)

**Prophylaxis for endocarditis not recommended**

- *Low-risk cardiac condition (Risk no greater than general population)*
  - Mitral valve prolapse without regurgitation
  - Trivial valvular regurgitation on echocardiography without structural abnormality (except mitral valve prolapse)
  - Isolated atrial septal defect
  - Atherosclerotic plaque
  - Coronary disease or previous coronary artery bypass surgery
  - Cardiac pacemakers or defibrillators
  - Previous Kawasaki's disease or rheumatic fever without valvular dysfunction
  - Surgically repaired intracardiac lesions, with minimal or no hemodynamic abnormality more than 6 m after operation
  - Innocent heart murmur

Adapted from Dajani AS, Taubert KA, Wilson W, et al. Prevention of bacterial endocarditis: recommendations by the American Heart Association. Circulation. 1997;96:358–86.

of vegetations <5 mm and 70% of those between 6–10 mm are identified. Underlying valve disease may influence the diagnostic accuracy of TTE when a myxomatous mitral valve or sclerotic or calcified valves are present. These limitations have been overcome by TEE owing to its better resolution and multiple study planes. Many studies have compared the sensitivity and specificity of TTE and TEE in the diagnosis of vegetations. In the majority of these studies TTE sensitivity ranges between 40–63% and that of transesophgeal echocardiography (TEE) between 90–100% (Figs 12.10 –12.13).

A negative TEE has an important clinical impact on the diagnosis of endocarditis with a high negative predictive value ranging from 86–97%. In patients with native heart valves a negative TEE virtually rules out the diagnosis of infective endocarditis. However, in the study of Sochowski and colleagues, 5 out of 65 patients (7.6%) with an initially negative TEE were finally diagnosed with endocarditis.

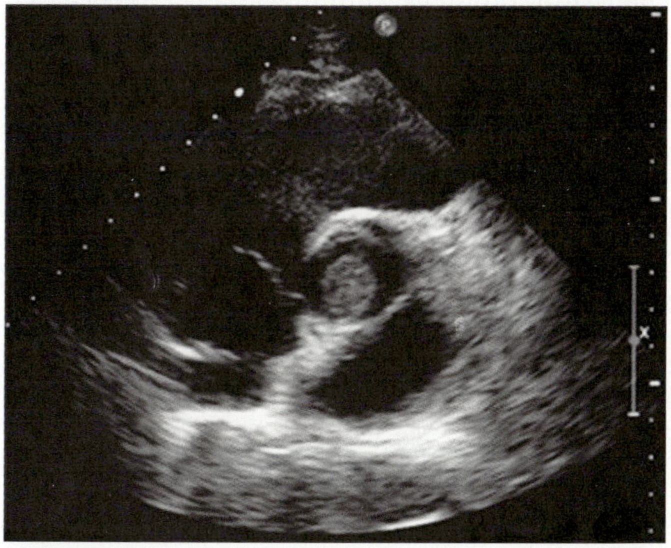

**Fig. 12.10:** Echocardiography demonstrates a large vegetation on the aortic valve

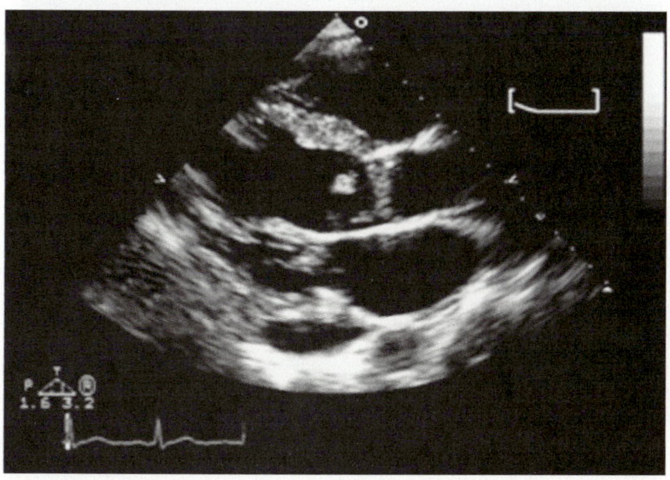

**Fig. 12.11:** Aortic valve vegetation using harmonic TTE. This demonstrates an echodense mass attached to the aortic valve leaflet consistent with a vegetation using harmonic TTE imaging

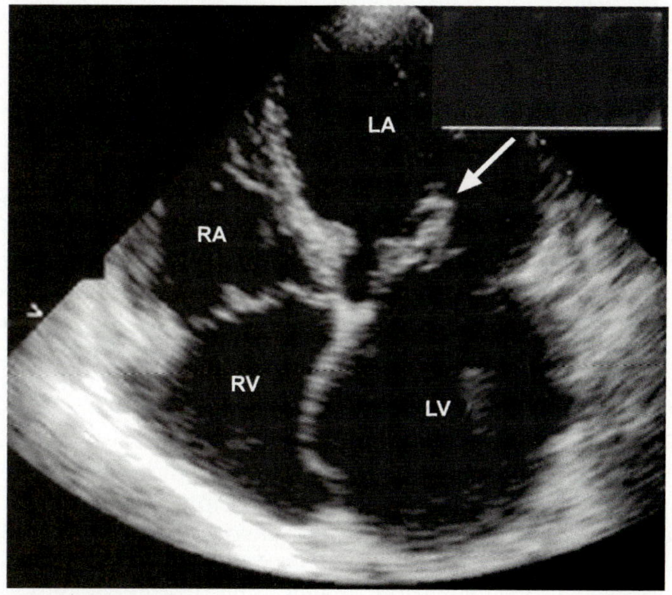


**Fig. 12.12:** Mitral valve vegetation shown (arrow) by echocardiogram. The vegetation is the mass seen in the dark space between the left atrium (LA) and left ventricle (LV). RA=indicates right atrium; RV=right ventricle

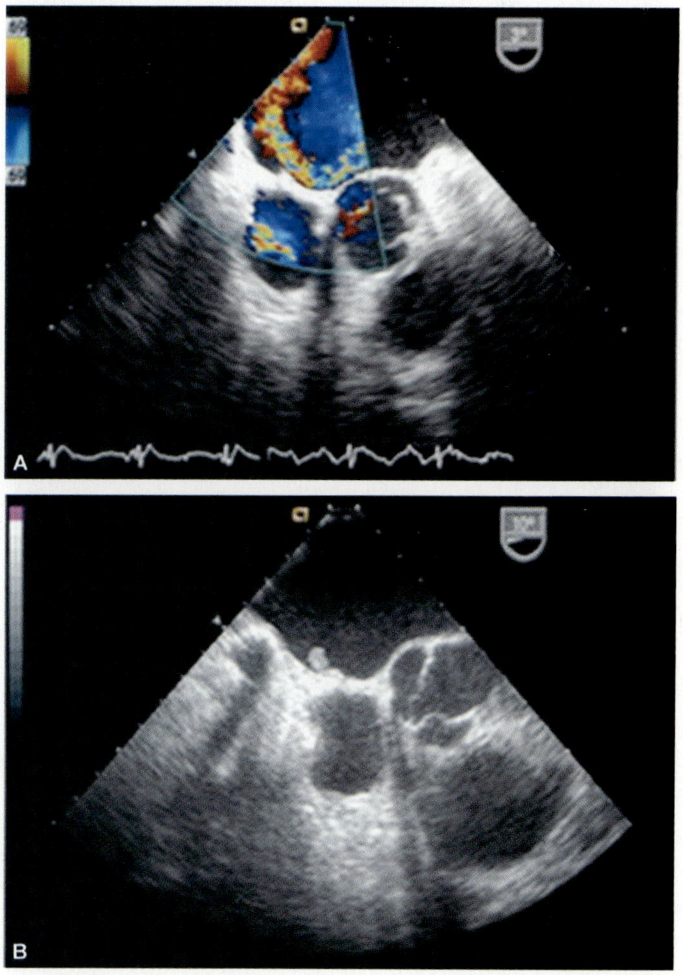


**Fig. 12.13:** (A and B) Mitral color jet on the interatrial septum and vegetation

In three of the patients a TEE performed 1–2 weeks after the initial examination showed the presence of vegetations. This study underlines the importance of recognising the phase of the disease in which the study is performed, since vegetations may not be large enough to be visualised when endocarditis is suspected very early on. In common with other diagnostic techniques, specificity of echocardiography is related to the clinical indication and the type of population studied. The technique does not permit differentiation between septic vegetations and other aseptic vegetations present in other situations such as Libman-Sacks endocarditis in systemic lupus erythematosus, and antiphospholipid syndrome or marantic endocarditis. Vegetations persisting after effective treatment must not be interpreted as a clinical recurrence of the disease unless supported by clinical features and bacteriologic evidence. Specificity is influenced mainly by the presence of valvar thickening or calcifications and also by rupture mitral chordae tendinae or Lambl's nodules which can be confused with vegetation images. The usefulness of TEE in patients with suspected endocarditis on a native valve is related to the results of the TTE. TEE is useful when TTE is negative or inconclusive.

*Prosthetic valve endocarditis:* Vegetations on prosthetic valves are more difficult to detect by TTE than those involving native valves, and therefore, TEE should always be used if the diagnosis of prosthetic endocarditis is suspected. The sewing ring and support structures of mechanical and bioprosthetic valves are strongly echogenic and may prevent vegetation detection within the valve apparatus or its shadow (Fig. 12.14).

The vegetative growth appears as thickening and irregularity of the normally smooth contour of the sewing ring. Both thrombus and pannus have a similar appearance and cannot be distinguished from vegetative material. It is also important to recognise strands to avoid false positive diagnoses. Strands are commonly observed by TEE on prosthetic valves, particularly in the early postoperative months, especially in mitral prostheses. In large series of prosthetic endocarditis TEE has shown an 86–94% sensitivity and 88–100% specificity for vegetation diagnosis, while TTE sensitivity was only 36–69%. Bioprosthetic valve leaflets may become infected with secondary destruction of leaflet tissue. The distinction between wear-and-tear degeneration of tissue valves and endocarditis is often difficult. TEE also led to an improved diagnostic accuracy in the diagnosis of endocarditis on bioprosthetic valves.

*Right-sided endocarditis and pacemaker lead infections:* Staphylococcal endocarditis in injection drug users is now the dominant form of the disease in many urban communities where there is a high incidence of injection drug use and homelessness. Right-sided endocarditis accounts for 10% of all IE in population based surveys' and a higher proportion of IE in injection drug users. Modern echocardiographic techniques have considerably augmented our ability to diagnose IE and to understand its natural history. Despite this, there are many areas in which our understanding of right-sided IE remains incomplete. Right-sided IE has a significant morbidity and mortality that adds a notable economic burden to stretched inner city health care facilities. The challenges of caring for this population of patients should not be underestimated and demands a logical and coordinated approach among care providers and physicians from a variety of specialties (Figs 12.15 and 12.16).

### Epidemiology and Predisposing Factors

Although right-sided IE may occur in association with congenital heart disease and instrumentation of the right heart, it is overwhelmingly a disease of injection drug users, at least in western populations. Among injection drug users presenting with fever, 13% will have echocardiographic

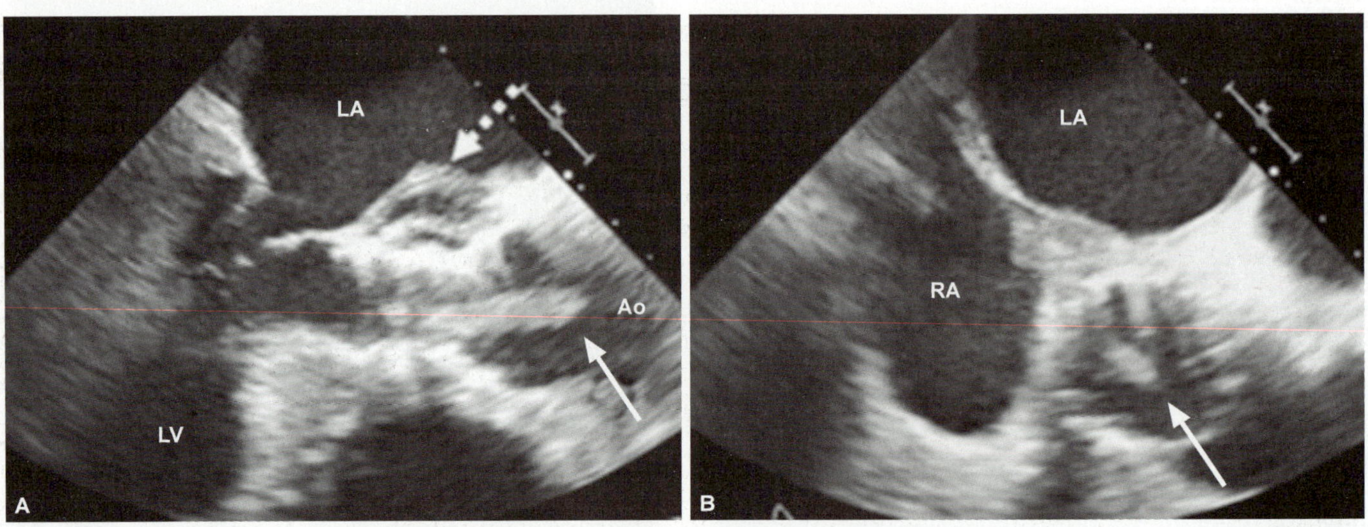


**Fig. 12.14:** Two-dimensional transesophageal echocardiogram of prosthetic valve endocarditis after transcatheter aortic valve replacement. Two-dimensional transesophageal echocardiography (A) long axis; (B) short axis) showing a 3 cm floating endocarditic lesion within the stent lumen of a prosthetic transcatheter aortic valve (solid arrow). Signs of a paravalvular abscess can be seen close to the noncoronary sinus Valsalva (dashed arrow). Transesophageal images were obtained with a Philips X7-2t transducer/ iE33 ultrasound system on admission and a Siemens Acuson Sequoia ultrasound system 3 months before. Ao=aortic root; LA=left atrium; LV=left ventricle; and RA=right atrium

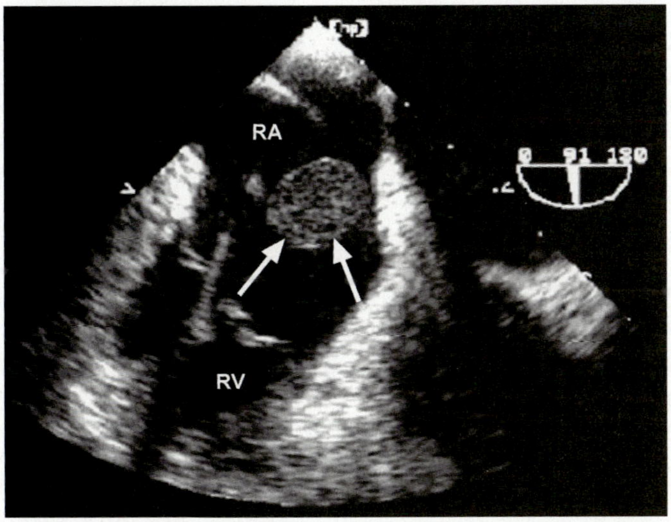


**Fig. 12.15:** Endocarditis on a pacemaker or defibrillator lead. Ball-like vegetation on pacemaker lead (vertical echoes seen in right atrium (RA). Horizontal echoes between RA and right ventricle (RV) represents the tricuspid valve (arrows)

evidence of IE.' If injection drug users with bacteraemia from an inner city demographic are considered, up to 41% will have evidence of IE.'The pathogenic mechanisms that explain the increased prevalence of right-sided IE in injection drug users are not fully elucidated. Damage to the right-sided valves from injected particulate matter in the setting of injected bacterial loads is thought to be important, while subtle abnormalities of immune function may also have a role in pathogenesis. In keeping with the demographic characteristics of injection drug use, this disease occurs most commonly in young males in their 20s and 30s. Before infection the tricuspid valve is usually structurally normal. Reinfection of a tricuspid valve that has been damaged by previous IE accounts for a significant proportion of cases and can add to the difficulty of echocardiographic interpretation. It seems logical that valves previously damaged by infection are more likely than normal valves to become infected. Earlier reports of IE in injection drug users emphasised the dominance of right-sided involvement. The tricuspid valve is most frequently involved followed by the mitral and then the aortic valve. Concurrent involvement of both left and right-sided valves is not infrequent. In right-sided IE it is almost always the tricuspid valve that is involved. One study of injection drug users found vegetations involving the tricuspid valve in 127 episodes, the pulmonary valve in four, and both valves in one instance. Involvement of other right-sided structures such as the Eustachian valve has been reported but is rare.

The dominant infective organism is *Staphylococcus aureus*, in most series accounting for around 70% of infections, with the remainder being caused mainly by streptococcal species or, less frequently, by Gram negative organisms, fungi or diphtheroids. Pseudomonal infections may have a predilection for multivalve involvement. Infections with unusual organisms and polymicrobial infections do occur, probably as the result of the injection of contaminated diluent, but are relatively unusual. Blood cultures are positive in a high proportion of cases of right-sided IE. When culture negative right-sided IE occurs, it is usually as a result of antibiotic use before the drawing of blood cultures. Bartonella infection has been described as a cause of culture negative IE in a homeless inner city population, and in right-sided IE. Although patterns of drug use in relation to IE have not been extensively studied, cocaine use may be a risk factor, presumably as a consequence of the much higher frequency of injections than in heroin users. The reported prevalence of HIV disease in patients with right-sided IE is variable. In a Spanish series of injection drug users with IE, 76% were HIV positive. In a

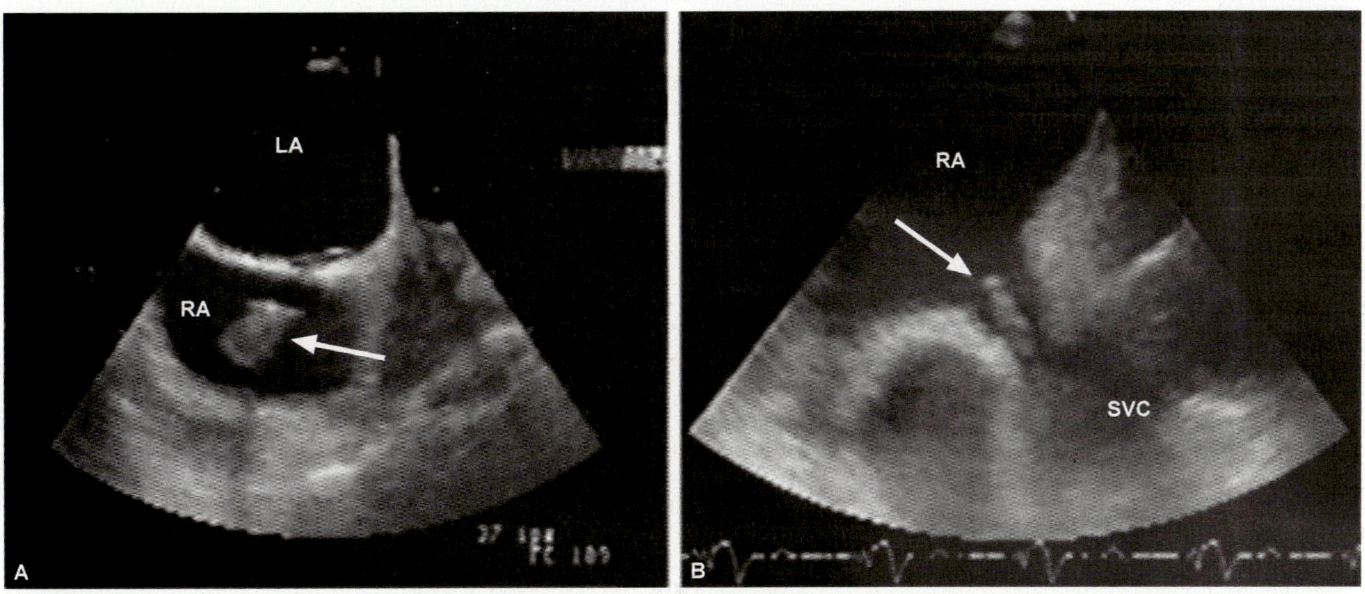


**Fig. 12.16:** Pacemaker lead infective endocarditis (transoesophageal echocardiography). (A) Typical vegetation on a pacemaker lead (arrow). (B) Thickening of the pacemaker lead with a sleeve-like appearance (arrow). RA=right atrium; LA=left atrium; SVC=superior vena cava

cohort of injection drug users with IE, those who were HIV positive were more likely to exhibit right-sided involvement. Advanced HIV infection is probably a risk factor for IE.

### Diagnostic Procedures

Rarely, cardiac catheterization is done to draw blood cultures in proximity of the valve lesions.

*Medications* (Table 12.6): Appropriate antibiotic therapy.

### Surgery

1. Cardiac surgery, usually to replace the infected valve(s) Absolute indications for valve surgery in endocarditis; Intracardiac abscess or fistula
2. Left heart failure
3. Endocarditis due to fungi or Gram-negative organisms, new prosthetic valve paravalve regurgitation, fistula, ascess, or dehiscence.

### Monitoring

ECG and blood pressure monitoring as appropriate in the hospital. Repeat blood cultures to assess response to therapy.

### Diet and Activity

Restricted activiry. Low-salt diet.

### Hospital Discharge Criteria

1. Resolution of problem
2. Sufficient IV therapy to warrant oral antibiotics
3. Successful surgery

### Follow up

After course of antibiotics, repeat blood cultures and echocardiogram in 2–4 weeks; then careful clinical follow-up at 3-, 6-, then 12-month intervals.

### Complications

- Heart failure
- Pulmonary edema
- Pericarditis
- Myocarditis
- Myocardial infarction
- Heart block
- Stroke
- Brain abscess
- Renal failure
- Sudden death

**Table 12.6:** Circumstances where short course antibiotic treatment for infective endocarditis is not appropriate

- Confirmed or suspected left-sided endocarditis
- Metastatic sites of infection or empyema
- Cardiac or extracardiac complications
- Methicillin resistant *Staphylococcus aureus* (MRSA)
- Presence of any prosthetic valve
- Vegetation size >10 mm
- Incomplete response to treatment
- HIV positive and CD4 count <200/mm$^2$

### Prognosis

Despite modern antibiotics and improved surgical techniques, mortaliry rate for patients with infective endocarditis is almost 40%.

### Prevention

Antibiotic prophylaxis for invasive procedures/surgery in naturally colonized places such as the mouth, and gastrointestinal tract in patients with the substrate for endocarditis, such as rheumatic valvular disease, audible heart murmurs, or cyanotic congenital heart disease (Table 12.7).

**Table 12.7:** Recommendations for prophylaxis in dental or surgical procedures

**Prophylaxis recommended for high- and medium-risk cardiac condition**

- Oropharyngeal Procedures
    - Dental procedures known to induce gingival or mucosal bleeding
    - Tonsillectomy and/or adenoidectomy
    - Bronchoscopy with a rigid bronchoscope
- Gastrointestinal Procedures[a]
    - Surgical operations that involve intestinal mucosa
    - Sclerotherapy for esophageal varices
    - Esophageal stricture dilatation
    - Billary surgery
    - Endoscopic biliary cannulation with biliary obstruction
- Genitourinary Procedures
    - Cystoscopy
    - Urethral dilatation
    - Prostate surgery
- Miscellaneous
    - Incision and drainage of infected tissue

**Prophylaxis not recommended**

- Oropharyngeal
    - Dental procedures not likely to induce gingival bleeding
    - Injection of local intraoral anesthetic (except intraligamentary injections)
    - Shedding of primary teeth
    - Tympanostomy tube insertion
    - Endotracheal intubation
    - Bronchoscopy with a flexible bronchoscope with or without biopsy[b]
- Gastrointestinal Procedures[b]
    - Transesophageal echocardiography
    - Endoscopy with or without gastrointestinal biopsy
- Genitournary Procedures
    - Postoperative suture removal
    - Cesarean section

*Contd...*

*Contd...*

- Vaginal hysterectomy or uncomplicated vaginal delivery[b]
- Circumcision
- Specific procedures in the absence of infectio, including:
  - Urethral catheterization
  - Dilatation and curettage
  - Therapeutic abortion
  - Sterilization procedures
  - Insertion or removal of intrauterine device
- Cardiac Procedures
  - Cardiac catheterization or balloon angioplasty
  - Implanted stents, pacemakers, or defibrillators

[a]Prophylaxis is recommended for high-risk but is optional for medium-risk cardiac conditions. [b]Prophylaxis is optional for high-risk cardiac conditions. Adapted from Dajani AS, Taubert KA, Wilson W, et al. Prevention of bacterial endocarditis: recommendations by the American Heart Association. Circulation. 1997;96:358–66.

## Culture Negative Infective Endocarditis and Atypical Organisms

Negative blood cultures occur in 2.5–31% of all cases of infective endocarditis, often delaying diagnosis and the onset of treatment with profound impact on clinical outcome. Moreover, the sensitivity of the Duke criteria, which rely heavily on microbiological indices, is diminished in this setting. Negative cultures arise most commonly as a consequence of prior antibiotic administration, but an increasingly common scenario is infection by fastidious organisms with limited proliferation under conventional culture conditions, or requiring specialised tools for identification. Such pathogens include Coxiella, Legionella, the HACEK group (Haemophilus species, *Actinobacillus actinomycetemcomitans, Cardiobacterium hominis, Eikenella corrodens, and Kingella kingae*), Chlamydia, Bartonella, *Tropheryma whippelii,* and fungi, including Candida, Histoplasma, and Aspergillus species, and *Torulopsis glabrata*. These organisms may be particularly common in cases of infective endocarditis affecting patients with prosthetic valves, indwelling venous lines, pacemakers, renal failure, and immuno-compromised states.

## Modified Criteria and New Diagnostic Techniques

In 1997, Lamas and Eykyn proposed a number of clinical modifications to the Duke criteria to include newly diagnosed splenomegaly or clubbing, elevated inflammatory markers, haematuria, and the presence of central and peripheral venous lines ('the St Thomas modifications'). Simultaneously, recognition of the role of Q fever, a worldwide zoonosis caused by *Coxiella burnetti* and a particularly frequent cause of infective endocarditis in France, increasing prevalence of staphylococcal infection, and widespread use of transoesophageal echocardiography resulted in further modifications; these involved incorporating the acceptance of positive Q fever serology or bacteraemia caused by *Staphylococcus aureus* (regardless of its source) as major criteria and the elimination of minor echocardiographic criteria A recent study compared these modifications in pathologically proven yet culture negative cases. Only 21% were classified as definite by the original Duke criteria, while 32% were definite by the modified Duke criteria, and the St Thomas modifications classified 62% correctly. Interestingly, the four additional cases identified correctly by the modified Duke criteria were upgraded on account of positive Q fever serology. Furthermore, careful scrutiny led to identification of the causative organism in almost 50% of culture negative cases, achieved by serology (*C. burnetti*, Bartonella, *Chlamydia psittaci*) in 24%, culture of the excised valve in 14%, microscopy of the excised valve in 5%, and nonvalve culture in 6%.

*Histological/immunological techniques:* Histological findings are included in the Duke and von Reyn diagnostic criteria and pathological examination of resected valvar tissue or embolic fragments remains the gold standard for the diagnosis of infective endocarditis. Pathological examination may also guide antimicrobial treatment if the causative agent can be identified by means of special stains or immuno histological techniques, and allow distinction from conditions whose echocardiographic features mimic infective endocarditis (for example, myxomas, fibroelastomas, and rheumatoid nodules). It should be noted that specimens are potentially infectious to the examiner, particularly when Q fever is suspected. The pathological hallmark of endocarditis is the demonstration of inflammatory changes in valvar tissue and/or vegetations, characteristically at the site of attachment or base of a vegetation. This finding is not specific, however, and inflammation is also a feature of degenerative and other valve pathology. Electron microscopy has high sensitivity and may help to characterise new microorganisms. However, it is time consuming and expensive and therefore reserved for cases in which other techniques fail to detect an organism. Histological criteria for the diagnosis of endocarditis have been proposed and a variety of specialised stains and immunohistological techniques (immunoperoxidase staining, enzyme linked immunosorbent (ELISA) and immunofluorescent ELIFA) assays, and direct immunofluorescence using fluorescein conjugated monoclonal antibodies) are now available to allow the identification of elusive bacteria and fungi. *C. burnetti* and Bartonella species are the most common aetiological agents in culture negative endocarditis and may be easily detected by serological testing using indirect immunofluorescence or ELISA. Immunological analysis of urine may also allow detection of microorganism degradation products and ELISA detection of Legionella species has been described using this technique. However, the incorporation of these techniques into accepted diagnostic criteria awaits prospective validation.

## Molecular Techniques

Several molecular approaches have been assessed for the detection and identification of pathogens in a wide variety of infectious diseases. The polymerase chain reaction (PCR) utilising nucleic acid target or signal amplification, alone or in combination with sequence analysis, is most widely used and allows rapid and reliable detection of fastidious and nonculturable agents in blood and surgical material of patients with infective endocarditis. It may also be of value when phenotypic characterisation is essential following isolation of two or more organisms in separate cultures (most commonly caused by contamination with skin commensals during sampling or polymicrobial infection in intravenous drug abusers). Indeed, the incorporation of such techniques as a major Duke diagnostic criterion has been proposed with widespread support. Specific primers are now available for many bacterial agents including *T. whippelii*, *C. burnetti*, and species of Bartonella, Chlamydia, Brucella, Legionella, Mycobacteria, and Mycoplasma. Future improvements include the possibility of quantitation by real time PCR eliminating the need for gel electrophoresis with faster, more accurate results, and the possibility of investigating common antimicrobial resistance genes enabling a targeted approach to antibiotic treatment.

## Indications and Optimal Timing for Surgery in Infective Endocarditis

More and more patients are operated on during theactive phase of infective endocarditis (IE) (Tables 12.8–12.10). The principal indications for cardiac surgery are:

- Heart failure,
- No control of infection,
- Embolisms,
- Large size of vegetations,

**Table 12.8:** Indications for Surgery in IE

| |
|---|
| **Congestive heart failure*** |
| • Congestive heart failure caused by severe aortic or mitral regurgitation or, more rarely, by valve obstruction caused by vegetations |
| • Severe acute aortic or mitral regurgitation with echocardiographic signs of elevated left ventricular end-diastolic pressure or significant pulmonary hypertension |
| • Congestive heart failure as a result of prosthetic dehiscence or obstruction |
| **Periannular extension** |
| • Most patients with abscess formation or fistulous tract formation |
| **Systemic embolism†** |
| • Recurrent emboli despite appropriate antibiotic therapy |
| **Large vegetations** (>10 mm) after 1 or more clinical or silent embolic events after initiation of antibiotic therapy |
| • Large vegetations and other predictors of a complicated course |
| • Very large vegetations (>15 mm) without embolic complications, especially if valve-sparing surgery is likely (remains controversial) |
| • Cerebrovascular complications‡ |
| • Silent neurological complication or transient ischemic attack and other surgical indications |
| • Ischemic stroke and other surgical indications, provided that cerebral hemorrhage has been excluded and neurological complications are not severe (e.g. coma) |
| **Persistent sepsis** |
| • Fever or positive blood cultures persisting for >5 to 7 days despite an appropriate antibiotic regimen, assuming that vegetations or other lesions requiring surgery persist and that extracardiac sources of sepsis have been excluded |
| • Relapsing IE, especially when caused by organisms other than sensitive streptococci or in patients with prosthetic valves |
| **Difficult organisms** |
| • *S. aureus* IE involving a prosthetic valve and most cases involving a left-sided native valve |
| • IE caused by other aggressive organisms (Brucella, *Staphylococcus lugdunensis*) |
| • IE caused by multiresistant organisms (e.g. methicillin-resistant *S. aureus* or vancomycin-resistant enterococci) and rare infections caused by gram-negative bacteria |
| ***Pseudomonas aeruginosa* IE** |
| • Fungal IE |
| • Q fever IE and other relative indications for intervention |
| **Prosthetic valve endocarditis** |
| • Virtually all cases of early prosthetic valve endocarditis |
| • Virtually all cases of prosthetic valve endocarditis caused by *S. aureus* |
| • Late prosthetic valve endocarditis with heart failure caused by prosthetic dehiscence or obstruction, or other indications for surgery |

Surgery should be performed immediately, irrespective of antibiotic therapy, in patients with persistent pulmonary edema or cardiogenic shock. If congestive heart failure disappears with medical therapy and there are no other surgical indications, intervention can be postponed to allow a period of days or weeks antibiotic treatment under careful clinical and echocardiographic observation. In patients with well tolerated severe valvular regurgitation or prosthetic dehiscence and no other reasons for surgery, conservative therapy under careful clinical and echocardiographic observation is recommended with consideration of deferred surgery after resolution of the infection, depending upon tolerance of the valve lesion.

**Table 12.9:** Timing of surgery

- Emergency surgery (within 24 hours)
- Native (aortic or mitral) or prosthetic valve endocarditis and severe congestive heart failure or cardiogenic shock caused by:
- Acute valvular regurgitation
- Severe prosthetic dysfunction (dehiscence or obstruction)
- Fistula into a cardiac chamber or the pericardial space
- Urgent surgery (within days)
- Native valve endocarditis with persisting congestive heart failure, signs of poor hemodynamic tolerance, or abscess
- Prosthetic valve endocarditis with persisting congestive heart failure, signs of poor hemodynamic tolerance, or abscess
- Prosthetic valve endocarditis caused by staphylococci or Gram-negative organisms
- Large vegetation (>10 mm) with an embolic event
- Large vegetation (>10 mm) with other predictors of a complicated course
- Very large vegetation (>15 mm), especially if conservative surgery is available
- Large abscess and/or periannular involvement with uncontrolled infection
- Early elective surgery (during the in-hospital stay)
- Severe aortic or mitral regurgitation with congestive heart failure and good response to medical therapy
- Prosthetic valve endocarditis with valvular dehiscence or congestive heart failure and good response to medical therapy
- Presence of abscess or periannular extension
- Persisting infection when extracardiac focus has been excluded
- Fungal or other infections resistant to medical cure

**Table 12.10:** Indications and timing of surgery in native and prosthetic valve infective endocarditis

| Indication for surgery | Timing | Class | Level of evidence |
|---|---|---|---|
| **HEART FAILURE** | | | |
| Aortic or mitral IE or PVE with severe acute regurgitation, obstruction or fistula causing refractory pulmonary edema or cardiogenic shock | Emergency | I | B |
| Aortic or mitral IE with severe acute regurgitation or obstruction and persisting heart failure or echocardiographic signs of poor hemodynamic tolerance (early mitral closure or pulmonary hypertension) | Urgent | I | B |
| Aortic or mitral IE or PVE with severe regurgitation and no HF | Elective | IIa | B |
| Right HF secondary to severe tricuspid regurgitation with poor response to diuretic therapy | Urgent/Elective | IIa | C |
| **UNCONTROLLED INFECTION** | | | |
| Locally uncontrolled infection (abscess, false aneurysm, fistula, and enlarging vegetation) | Urgent | I | B |
| Persisting fever and positive blood cultures >7–10 days | Urgent | I | B |
| Infection caused by fungi or multiresistant organisms | Urgent/Elective | I | B |
| PVE caused by staphylococci or gram negative bacteria | Urgent/Elective | IIa | C |
| **PREVENTION OF EMBOLISM** | | | |
| Aortic or mitral IE or PVE with large vegetations (>10 mm) following one or more embolic episodes despite appropriate antibiotic therapy | Urgent | I | B |
| Aortic or mitral IE or PVE with large vegetations (>10 mm) and other predictors of complicated course (heart failure, persistent infection, and abscess) | Urgent | I | C |
| Aortic or mitral IE or PVE with isolated very large vegetations (>15 mm)* | Urgent | IIb | C |
| Persistent tricuspid valve vegetations >20 mm after recurrent pulmonary emboli | Urgent/Elective | IIa | C |

*IE=infective endocarditis; PVE=prosthetic valve endocarditis *Surgery may be preferred if procedure preserving the native valve is feasible.*

- Severe valvar and perivalvar lesions, and
- Infection caused by some atypical microorganisms

### Indications for Cardiac Surgery

1. **Heart failure:** If heart failure is present, the mortality rate of native valve infective endocarditis is 55–85% in the case of medical treatment and 10–35% in operated patients. The first indication for cardiac surgery in infective endocarditis is heart failure: it represents more than half of the indications. Heart failure caused by aortic regurgitation is particularly poorly tolerated (heart failure is better tolerated in the case of mitral regurgitation because the left atrium and the pulmonary vascular bed adapt better than the left ventricle to the

regurgitant volume), and it progresses faster, thus needing rapid surgery. Not only does heart failure increase the mortality rate if there is no surgery, but it also increases the perioperative mortality rate from 5–10% in patients without heart failure to 15–35% in patients with heart failure. Moreover, delaying surgery increases the risk of perivalvar infection (Table 12.11).

2. **Resistance infection:** The first step is to make sure that there is no extracardiac infectious location. If there is no such extracardiac location, cardiac surgery should be performed if the course of fever and inflammatory syndrome is unfavourable after 1 week of appropriate antibiotic treatment.
3. **Vegetations and embolic risk:** The literature on this topic contrasts greatly. The embolism rate varies from 10–50% in different series. 'Three quarters of embolisms occur before the beginning of antibiotic treatment.' The embolic risk decreases greatly and regularly over time, from 15% after one week of treatment to 1% after 4 weeks of treatment. In mitral infective endocarditis, embolisms look to be more frequent if vegetations are located on the anterior leaflet than on the posterior leaflet. Embolisms are more frequent when vegetation size is more than 20 mm in some studies, but not in other studies. In a recent study, embolisms were more frequent when the size of the vegetations was more than 10 mm or when vegetations were very mobile.' Embolisms should always be looked for not only by clinical means but also by systematic scanners (for example, cerebral, thoracoabdominal), searching for clinically silent embolisms, especially in spleen and kidneys. Rapid surgery must be performed when there has been an embolic episode and when large and mobile vegetations remain. When there are large and/or mobile vegetations but no embolic event, the medical community is divided. The decision is easier in the case of mitral infective endocarditis when valve repair looks possible, or when there are other arguments for surgery (heart failure, no control of infection, severe valvar and perivalvar lesions, etc).
4. **Perivalvar infection:** Infective endocarditis on the aortic valve and prosthetic infective endocarditis are those most commonly associated with perivalvar infection, such as abscesses and intracardiac fistula. 10–40% of aortic valve infective endocarditis and 45–100% of prosthetic infective endocarditis. Occurrence and persistence of conduction disturbances are not very sensitive indicators of perivalvar infection, but they look very specific (85–90%). Rapid surgery is recommended in most cases since the perioperative risk increases with the delay to surgery. However, in large aortic abscesses, a large resection exposes the patient to the risk of postoperative complete atrioventricular block. Valvar obstruction—Valvar obstruction is an obvious indication for urgent surgery. Unstable prosthesis—dehiscence of an infected prosthesis means that there is perivalvar infection, and hemodynamic deterioration usually occurs quickly. Thus rapid surgery is recommended (Fig. 12.17).
5. **Prosthetic infective endocarditis:** In early prosthetic infective endocarditis >12 months after valve replacement), most often the microorganism is a Staphylococcus and lesions are severe (abscess, prosthesis dehiscence).

**Table 12.11:** Factors and complications that predispose to a poor outcome

- Congestive heart failure (leading adverse prognostic factor)
- Nonstreptococcal disease
- Aortic valve involvement
- Infection of a prosthetic valve
- Older age
- Abscess formation
- HIV with CD4 count <200
- Delayed diagnosis
- CNS or coronary embolization
- Recurrent infective endocarditis

CNS=Central nervous system; HIV=Human immunodeficiency virus

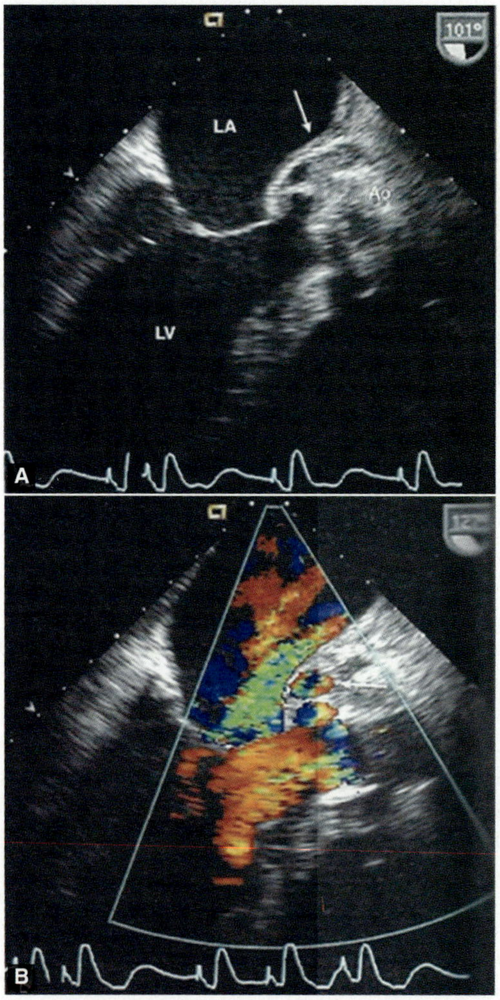


**Fig. 12.17:** Paravalvular abscess. (A) A TEE long-axis image in a patient with aortic valve endocarditis shows irregular areas of echoluency and echodensity odensity in the aortic annulus and sinuses (arrow), (B) Color-Doppler shows both mitral regurgitation and flow in the echolucent areas in the aortic annulus. At surgery, a paravalvular abscess was present

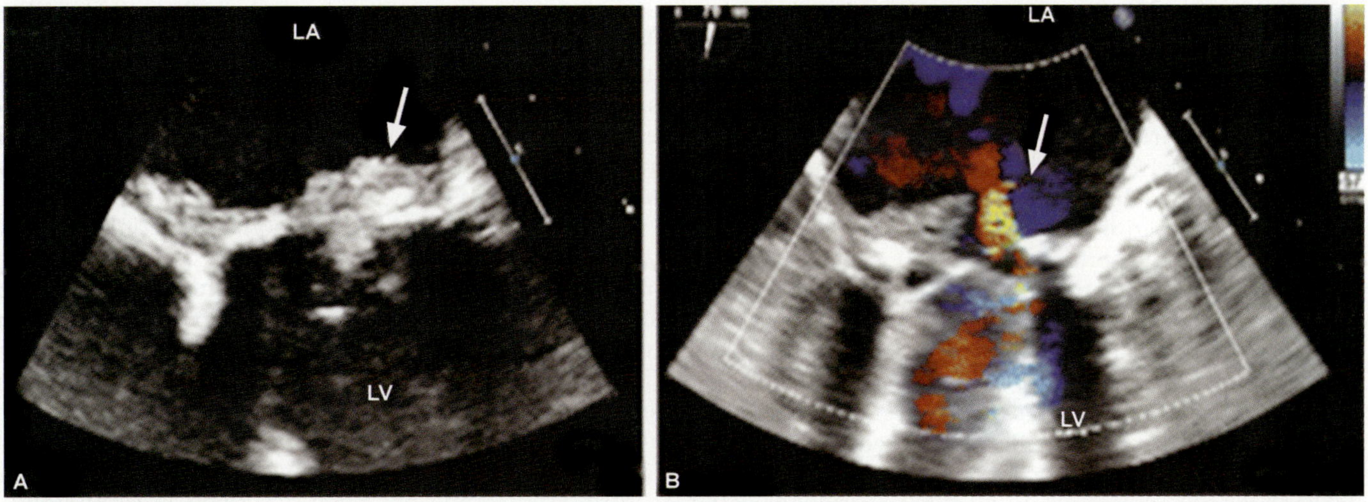


**Fig. 12.18:** Mitral prosthetic valve endocarditis with prosthetic obstruction (transoesophageal echocardiography). (A) Large vegetation prolapsing into the mitral mechanical prosthetic valve (arrow), (B) central regurgitation associated with the absence of the physiological regurgitant jets (arrow). LV=left ventricle; LA=left atrium; RV=right ventricle

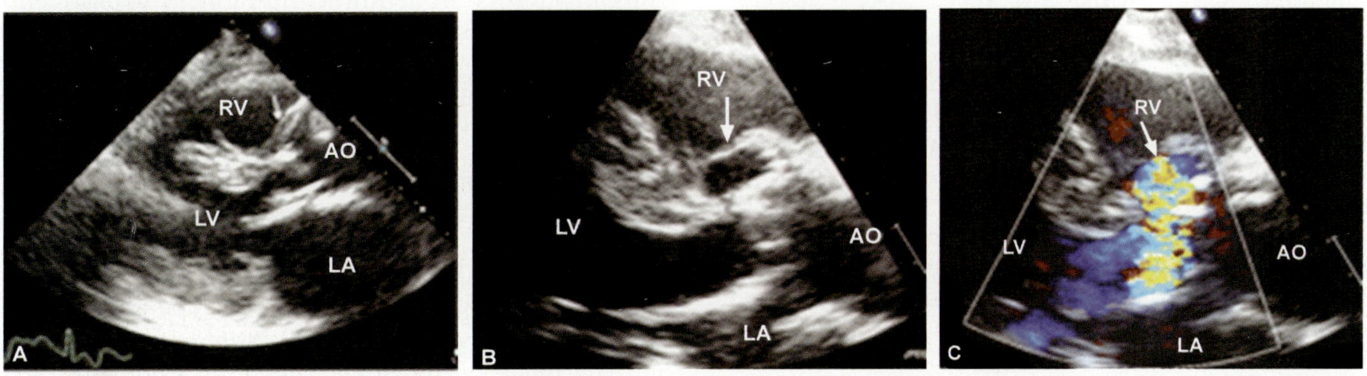


**Fig. 12.19:** Evolution of an anterior aortic bioprosthetic abscess (TTE). (A) Initial evaluation showing the absence of abscess formation, (B) second evaluation showing the presence of a new anterior free space corresponding to an abscess, (C) color-Doppler showing that the abscess communicates with the left ventricle (arrow) (pseudoaneurysm)

Redo surgery is associated with a lower mortality rate than medical treatment alone, and it is most often necessary, although it may be technically difficult. The mortality rate of prosthetic infective endocarditis caused by *Staphylococcus aureus* is about 75% in the case of medical treatment and 25% in the case of combined medical and surgical treatment. Surgery is thus recommended in prosthetic infective endocarditis caused by *S. aureus* when there is an intracardiac complication. Medical treatment only may be sufficient in cases of late infective endocarditis caused by some microorganisms (oral streptococci, organisms from the HACEK group—Haemophilus species, *Actinobacillus actinomycetemcomitans, Cardiobacterium hominis, Eikenella corrodens,* and *Kingella kingae*), if there are no signs of perivalvar infection (Figs 12.18 and 12.19).

6. **Fungal infective endocarditis**: Infective endocarditis caused by Candida or Aspergillus are often complicated with very large vegetations, infectious metastases, perivalvar infection, and embolisms. Amphotericin B poorly penetrates into vegetations. Rapid surgery is thus most often needed (Fig. 12.20).

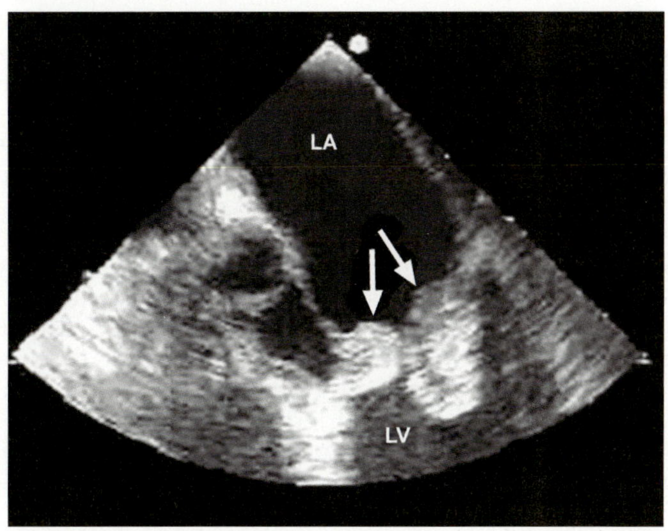


**Fig.12.20:** Large vegetations (arrows) in the mitral valve secondary to fungal endocarditis. LA=left atrium; LV=left ventricle

7. **Difficult-to-treat microorganisms**: Surgery is almost always needed in infective endocarditis caused by

certain gram-negative bacilli (for example, *Pseudomonas aeruginosa, Achromobacter xylosoxitans*), by Brucella, or by highly resistant enterococci.

8. **Neurological complications:** The rate of neurological complications varies from 15–45% in different series.' They mostly are ischemic cerebral vascular accidents, but also cerebral hemorrhages, ruptured mycotic aneurysms, meningitis, and encephalopathy. A cerebral scan must always be performed in infective endocarditis, to look for silent cerebral vascular accidents. In the case of cerebral hemorrhage, an arteriography or an angiomagnetic resonance image must be performed, to look for a mycotic aneurysm. There is a risk of cerebral hemorrhage associated with cardiac surgery because of anticoagulation during and after the procedure. The risk of cerebral hemorrhage is not increased in the case of a stroke without hemorrhage, but it is greatly increased if the stroke is hemorrhagic. In this case, cardiac surgery should be delayed 2–3 weeks.If there is a ruptured mycotic aneurysm, it must be resected, clipped or embolised before cardiac surgery.

*Timing of Cardiac Surgery:* Classically, early surgery was considered to be a greater risk than delayed surgery because of tissue inflammation and the surgery was technically more difficult. In fact,the duration of antibiotic treatment before surgery does not appear to influence the perioperative mortality, nor the rate of recurrent infective endocarditis. Surgery should be rapid in the case of hemodynamic deterioration, where there is no control of infection, or there are large and mobile vegetations. Decision as to the timing of surgery is particularly difficult when there is a neurological complication.

## RIGHT-SIDED ENDOCARDITIS

### Clinical Manifestations

The presenting clinical features of right and left-sided endocarditis are different. While most patients with right-sided endocarditis will have systolic murmurs, the murmur is clearly pathologic in a minority of cases.' Murmurs are, in fact, left-sided and nonspecific in most instances. The usual manifestations are persistent fever, bacteraemia, and multiple pulmonary emboli. Peripheral embolic manifestations are characteristically absent; rather, symptoms and complications arise from the involvement of the pulmonary vasculature by multiple septic pulmonary emboli, chest pain, dyspnea, cough, and hemoptysis may be presenting feature. When peripheral embolic or neurologic features occur, either left-sided endocarditis or paradoxical embolism should be considered. The conjunction of bacteraemia, fever, and multiple pulmonary infiltrates on chest radiography should always prompt a search for right-sided endocarditis.

### Complications of Right-sided Endocarditis

It may be thought of as either cardiac or pulmonary. A variety of complications attributed to septic pulmonary emboli have been described including pulmonary infarction, pulmonary abscesses, bilateral pneumothoraces, pleural effusions, and empyema. Mycotic aneurysms of the pulmonary arteries may be complicated by potentially fatal pulmonary hemorrhage. Multiple pulmonary emboli may result in right-sided chamber dilatation, right heart failure, and a worsening of tricuspid regurgitation. The embolisation of vegetations large enough to result in obstruction of a significant portion of the pulmonary arterial circulation has been described but is unusual. Cardiac complications may arise as a consequence of tricuspid valve destruction and severe tricuspid regurgitation with right-sided volume overload, chamber dilatation, and right heart failure. Chronic right atrial dilatation may be a substrate for supraventricular arrhythmias, including atrial flutter and fibrillation. Paravalvar abscess formation occurs infrequently. Vasculitis may complicate right-sided IE, but is not a typical feature. Hypoxemia has been described in right-sided IE when right atrial pressure is raised sufficiently to cause right to left shunting through a patent foramen ovale. Paradoxical embolism resulting from the transit of an embolus across an acquired pulmonary arteriovenous malformation has been reported. It should be recalled that a variety of coexistent medical problems such as hepatitis or HIV disease might be present in this population as a result of complications of injection drug use and poor self care.

### Diagnosis of Right-sided Endocarditis

*Duke criteria:* The Duke system defines a major echocardiographic criterion for IE as the finding of an oscillating intracardiac mass on the valve or supporting structures, in the path of a regurgitant jet. A paravalvar abscess or new dehiscence of a prosthetic valve. Although the sensitivity and specificity of tbe Duke criteria have not been 'specifically studied in the right-sided endocarditis with finding of anyone of these echocardiographic features involving right heart structures. In the presence of positive blood cultures with atypical organism should be regarded as diagnostic of right-sided endocarditis. There are nonetheless some conceptual difficulties in uncritically applying the Duke criteria to right-sided endocarditis. Right-sided murmurs are more difficult to detect. This is especially true of many patients who are injection drug users with their first episode of endocarditis, who will have normal or only slightly elevated right ventricular pressures and in whom a lower velocity, less turbulent tricuspid regurgitant jet might be anticipated. One should not allow the lack of a murmur, therefore, to preclude further investigation if the clinical suspicion is high. Immunologic and vascular phenomena, which feature as minor criteria in the Duke system, are also less common. Septic pulmonary emboli are listed as a minor criterion in the Duke scheme; it could be argued that this important diagnostic feature is somewhat underweighted in the present Duke criteria. On balance, however, it seems reasonable to continue to use the Duke criteria as a useful diagnostic framework.

*Electrocardiography*: It can help in diagnosing serious complications of right-sided endocarditis, such as pulmonary embolism (Fig 12.21).

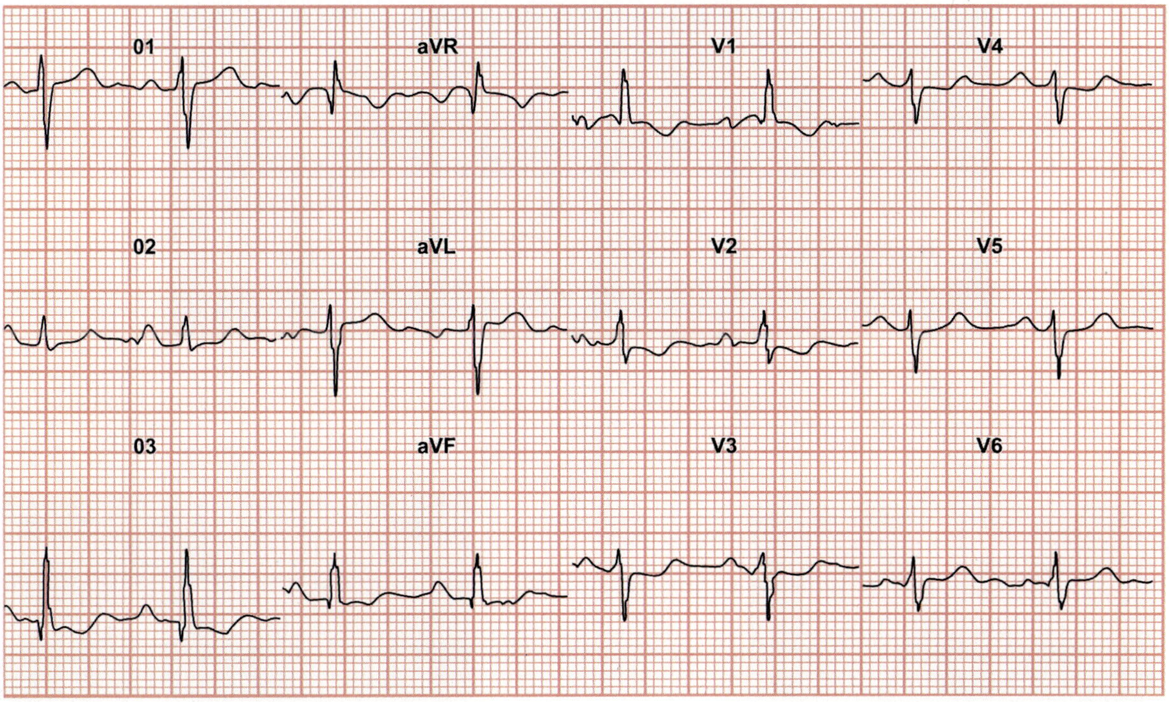


**Fig. 12.21:** Pulmonary embolism ($S_1$, $Q_3$ and $T_3$ signs) and signs of right frontal axis are shown in right-sided endocarditis

*Chest radiography*: The chest X-ray is a helpful laboratory aid in diagnosing right-sided endocarditis with 55% of radiographs at presentation showing evidence of pulmonary infiltrates compatible with pulmonary emboli (Fig. 12.22).

*Transthoracic echocardiography (TTE)*: Modern echocardiographic techniques have significantly improved our ability to diagnose right-sided endocarditis and are now the cornerstone of the diagnosis in this disease (Figs 12.23–12.30). In febrile injection drug users, standard laboratory testing and physical examination without echocardiography were ineffective in detecting the patients with endocarditis.' The key echocardiographic finding in right-sided endocarditis is that of vegetation(s) in association with the tricuspid or rarely the pulmonary valve. As with vegetations on the left-sided valves, they tend to be localised to the atrial side of the valve in the path of the regurgitant jet. Tricuspid vegetations are often large and may be in excess of 2 cm, a finding that does not necessarily suggest the presence of fungal endocarditis. On rare occasions, vegetations may be sufficiently large so as to be confused with an intracardiac tumor. Entrapment of an embolised vegetation in the tricuspid chordal apparatus is sometimes

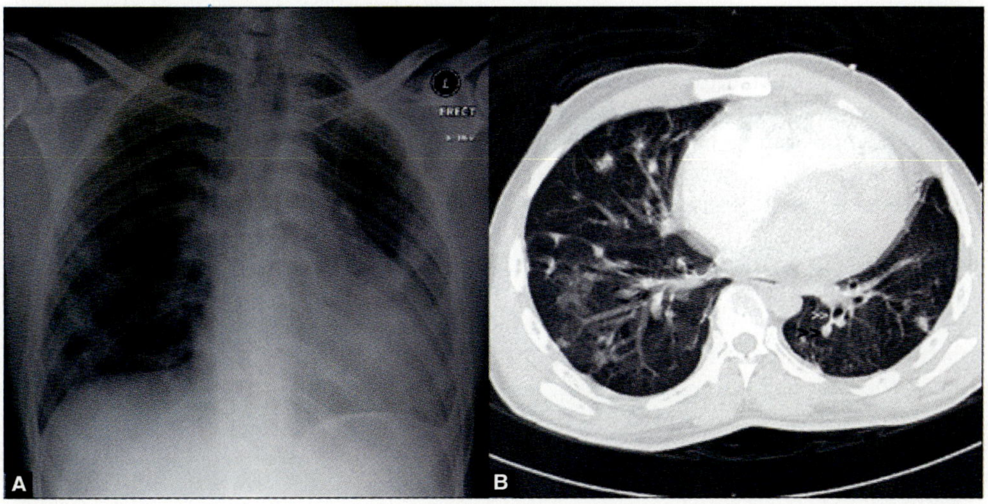


**Fig. 12.22:** (A) Chest X-ray showing cardiomegaly with bilateral lung infiltrates, and (B) CT scan of chest showing bilateral irregular pulmonary infiltrates with multiple nodules (black arrowheads) with distinct central feeding vessel (white arrowheads), consistent with septic pulmonary emboli in a patient with intravenous drug abuse and tricuspid valve endocarditis

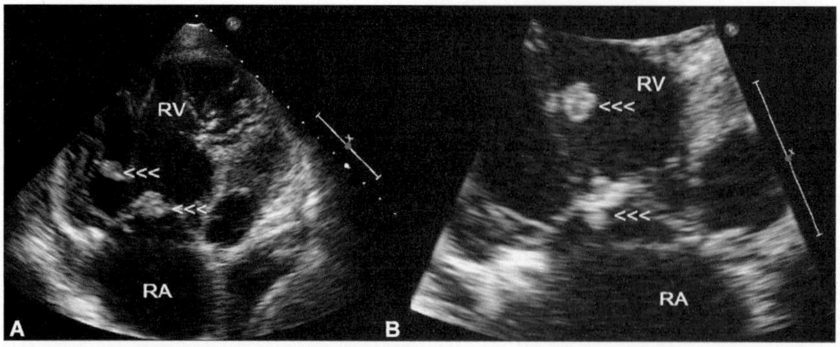


Fig. 12.23: Transthoracic echocardiography (A and B) showing multiple vegetations attached to tricuspid valve leaflets (arrowheads) and one large vegetation on the chordae of anterior tricuspid leaflet (upper arrowheads) in a patient with IV drug abuse and septic pulmonary emboli. RA=right atrium; RV=right ventricle

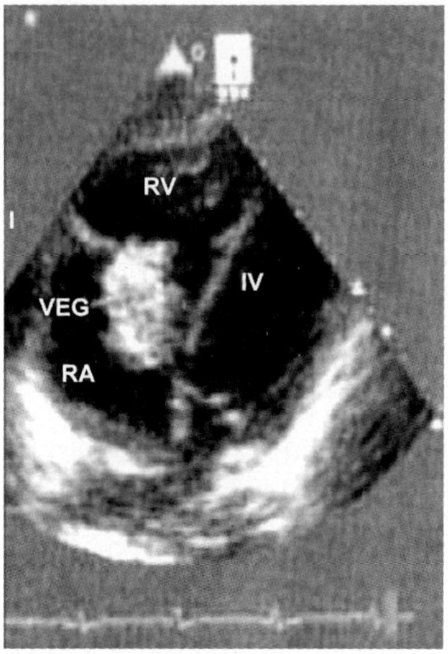


Fig. 12.24: An apical 4C view showing large vegetation attached to the tricuspid valve in patient with infective endocarditis on tricuspid valve who had been using intravenous narcotic drugs

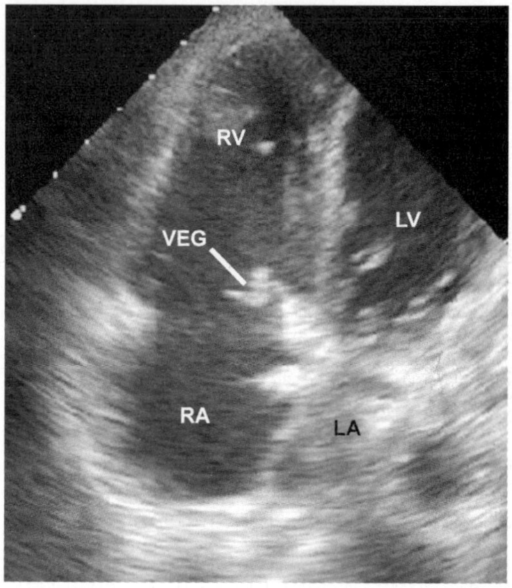


Fig. 12.25: An apical 4C view showing vegetation on tricuspid valve

seen. Similarly, embolised vegetations have been seen floating free in the right ventricle or pulmonary artery. Occasionally the presence of normal anatomic variants such as Chiari network or prominent Eustachian valve may cause diagnostic confusion, more particularly with transthoracic imaging; similarly venous catheters erroneously placed in the right atrium need to be identified and distinguished from vegetations. Right atrial thrombus may be distinguished from vegetation in that it is less likely to lie in the path of the jet and tends to layer on the right atrial wall. Past infection with damage to the tricuspid valve is commonly seen in this group, so the presence of vegetation does not in itself signify the presence of active infection. Extensive valve destruction with failure of leaflet cooptation and severe tricuspid regurgitation is a common sequel to tricuspid endocarditis. Although older or healed vegetations tend to be more echogenic and may even be calcified, this finding cannot reliably distinguish new from old infection. It should be clearly understood that echocardiographic findings need always to be taken in their clinical context. The finding of new or worsening tricuspid regurgitation, which is otherwise unexplained, should always prompt a diligent search for evidence of tricuspid endocarditis in the injection drug using patient.

*Transesophageal echocardiography (TEE)*: Many injection drug users have good thoracic ultrasound windows meaning that high resolution images can be obtained with transthoracic echocardiographic examination in many patients (Figs 12.31–12.38). This, combined with the relative proximity of the tricuspid valve to the ultrasound transducer, means that this valve is often well imaged by the transthoracic technique. Careful attention to the adjustment of sector width, depth, and focus settings will help in accurate identification of vegetations. Under some circumstances higher frequency transducers, e.g. 4 MHz or broad-band transducers switched to a 'resolution setting' may be used to improve spatial resolution. Alternatively use of the 'zoom function' (on some machines) may assist with lesion identification. The need for routine transoesophageal echocardiography (TEE) in right-sided

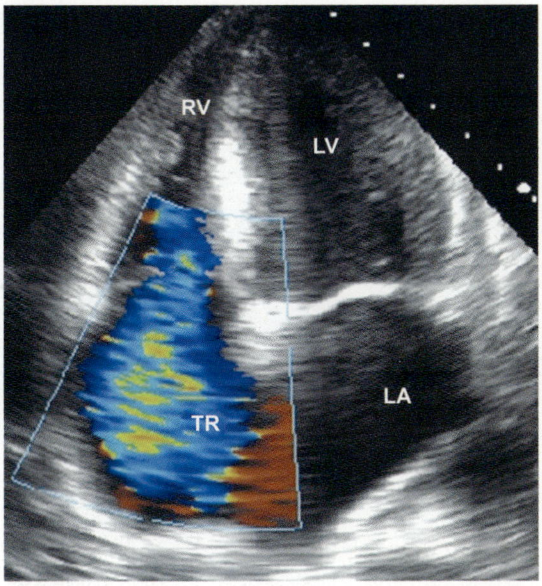


**Fig. 12.26:** Tricuspid regurgitation jet due to vegetation on the tricuspid valve

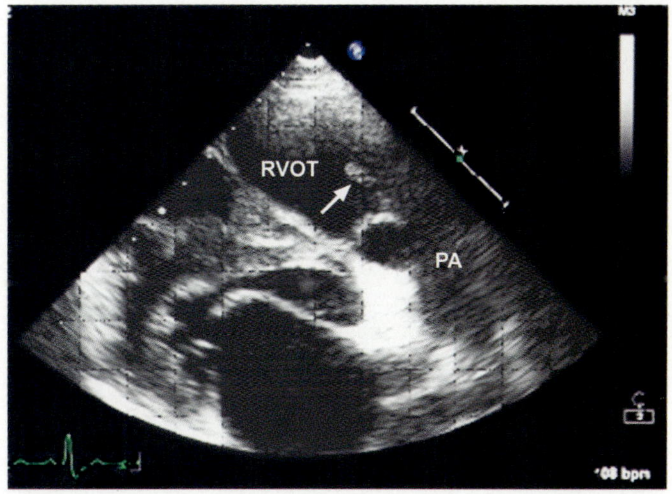


**Fig. 12.27:** Two-dimensional transthoracic echocardiography showing vegetations attached to the pulmonary valve cusps (arrow). RVOT=right ventricular outflow tract; PA=pulmonary artery

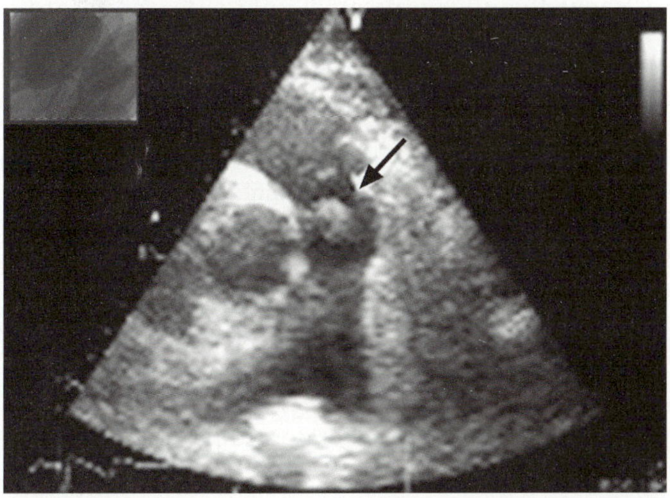

**Fig. 12.28:** Short-axis view of vegetation on pulmonary valve after 6 weeks of antibiotic therapy, indicated by the white arrow

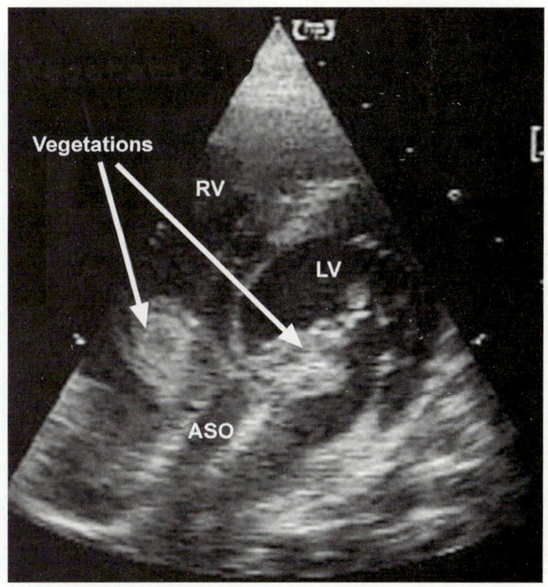


**Fig. 12.29:** Transthoracic echocardiographic image in a modified apical 4-chamber imaging plane showing a large vegetation located above the tricuspid valve. The ASO device is seen within the atrial septum, and the mitral valve vegetation is again visualized. RV=indicates right ventricle; LV=left ventricle

endocarditis is therefore questionable. TEE may be useful in detecting paravalvar abscess formation and for diagnosing unusual forms of right-sided endocarditis such as pulmonary valve involvement or infection on the Eustachian valve. The rationale for this approach is the simplicity and reduced cost of TTE and the importance of having the TTE information to direct and target a subsequent TEE examination appropriately. If there is a moderate or high suspicion of IE, and the initial TTE is negative, the TTE is repeated after an interval of about 1 week. TEE is then used in those patients in whom diagnostic quality images are not obtained with transthoracic imaging, and those who have negative TTE examinations where the suspicion of endocarditis is moderate or high (especially in the setting of staphylococcal bacteraemia). Occasionally pacing wires or right-sided prosthetic valves are encountered; where there is a suspicion of endocarditis TEE is usually indicated. Rotation of the crystal array and angulation of the probe tip in order to visualise the valves in a number of orientations is mandatory during TEE.

*HIV and right-sided endocarditis:* Significant immunosuppression (CD4 count <200/mm) is associated with a higher mortality rate in right-sided IE in HIV infected injection drug users, though it is not clear that this increased mortality is as a consequence of the IE. As in non-HIV infected patients with right-sided endocarditis, the

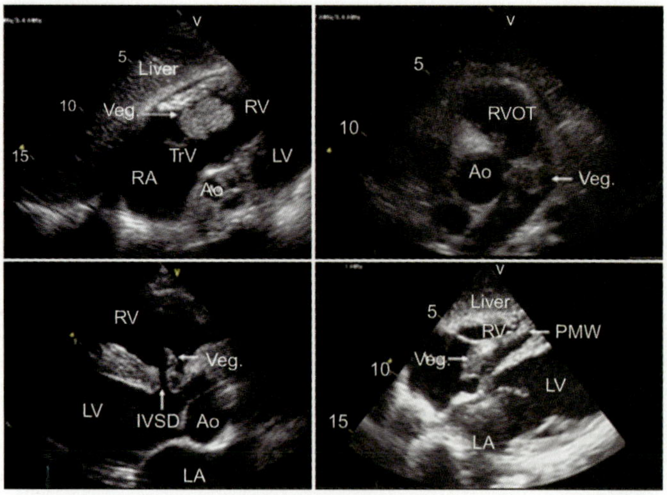


**Fig. 12.30:** Cases of right-sided infective endocarditis. AO=aorta; LV=left ventricle; LA=left atrium; RV=right ventricle; Veg= vegetation; PMW=pacemaker wire; IVSD=interventricular septal defect; TrV=tricuspid valve

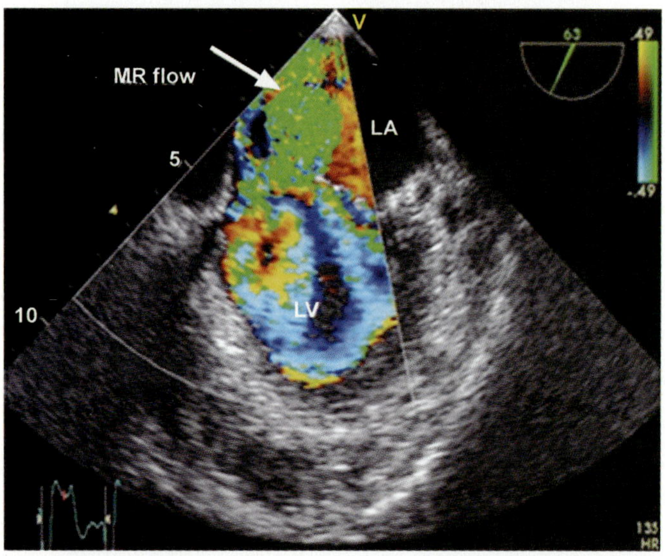


**Fig. 12.32:** Color-Doppler transesophageal study demonstrated aneurismal cavity with central perforation due to infective endocarditis in midpart of anterior mitral leaflet with severe mitral regurgitation

involvement of the left-sided valves is predictive of an increased risk of death.

*Treatment of right-sided endocarditis*: Short course antibiotic treatment for right-sided endocarditis and management of addiction. The successful management of a complicated case often requires the close cooperation of a cardiologist, an infectious disease physician, and occasionally a cardiac surgeon. The role of physicians in managing intercurrent drug withdrawal and maintaining the patient in hospital has been understated in the past methadone and/or other agents may be needed to control withdrawal symptoms. These patients may be difficult and disruptive and often engender negative attitudes in health care professionals. Their lack of adherence to in-hospital treatment is a major practical hurdle and has stimulated interest in developing shorter duration antibiotic regimens. There is reasonable evidence that short course antibiotic treatment for uncomplicated right-sided endocarditis is effective. The benefit of gentamicin in native valve endocarditis lies in earlier defervescence of fever and the sterilisation of blood cultures; there is no proven survival advantage. In the presence of a relative or absolute contraindication to gentamicin, therefore, a 2-week course of cloxacillin alone may be adequate. In the event that the patient cannot be persuaded to stay in hospital for the full two weeks, a 28-day course of oral treatment with ciprofloxacin and rifampin is prescribed, ideally with administration in a supervised setting such as a drug treatment facility. There are some situations in which short course antibiotic treatment is not appropriate In general nonstaphylococcal right-sided endocarditis is treated in a similar fashion to left-sided endocarditis (Table 12.12).

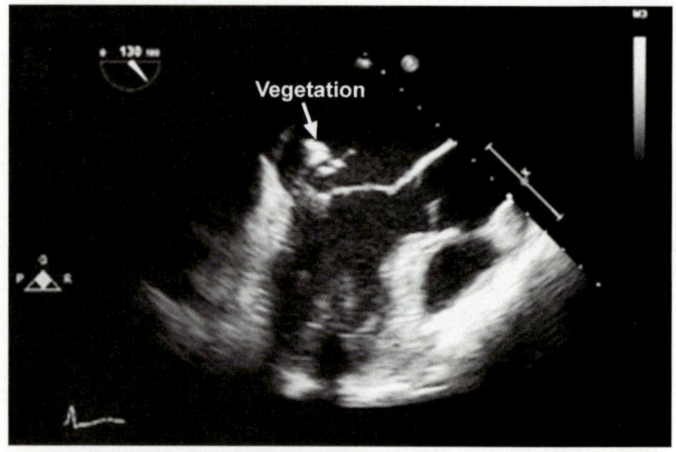


**Fig. 12.31:** Transoesophageal echocardiogram showing vegetation in the P2 scallop of the posterior mitral valve leaflet

*Prognosis and surgical treatment of right-sided endocarditis*: Right-sided endocarditis is generally regarded as having a relatively benign prognosis and inhospital mortality is less than 10% (Table 12.13). Most will survive even if they leave hospital before the full course of treatment has been completed. As follow up in the injection drug using population is notoriously difficult, few data are available on their long term outlook. It is clear that there will be a significant late mortality from causes other than IE and right heart failure, such as noncardiac infections, drug overdose, and AIDS related complications. Mortality is higher where there is left-sided involvement. Fortunately most patients can be treated medically, with surgery being necessary in only a small minority of cases. Indications for surgical treatment are better defined for left than for right-sided endocarditis. Sepsis, which is uncontrolled despite adequate antibiotic treatment, and intractable right heart failure despite appropriate medical treatment, are the most important indications for surgical intervention. The finding of a paravalvar abscess or fungal endocarditis are usually indications for surgery. Recurrent pulmonary embolism

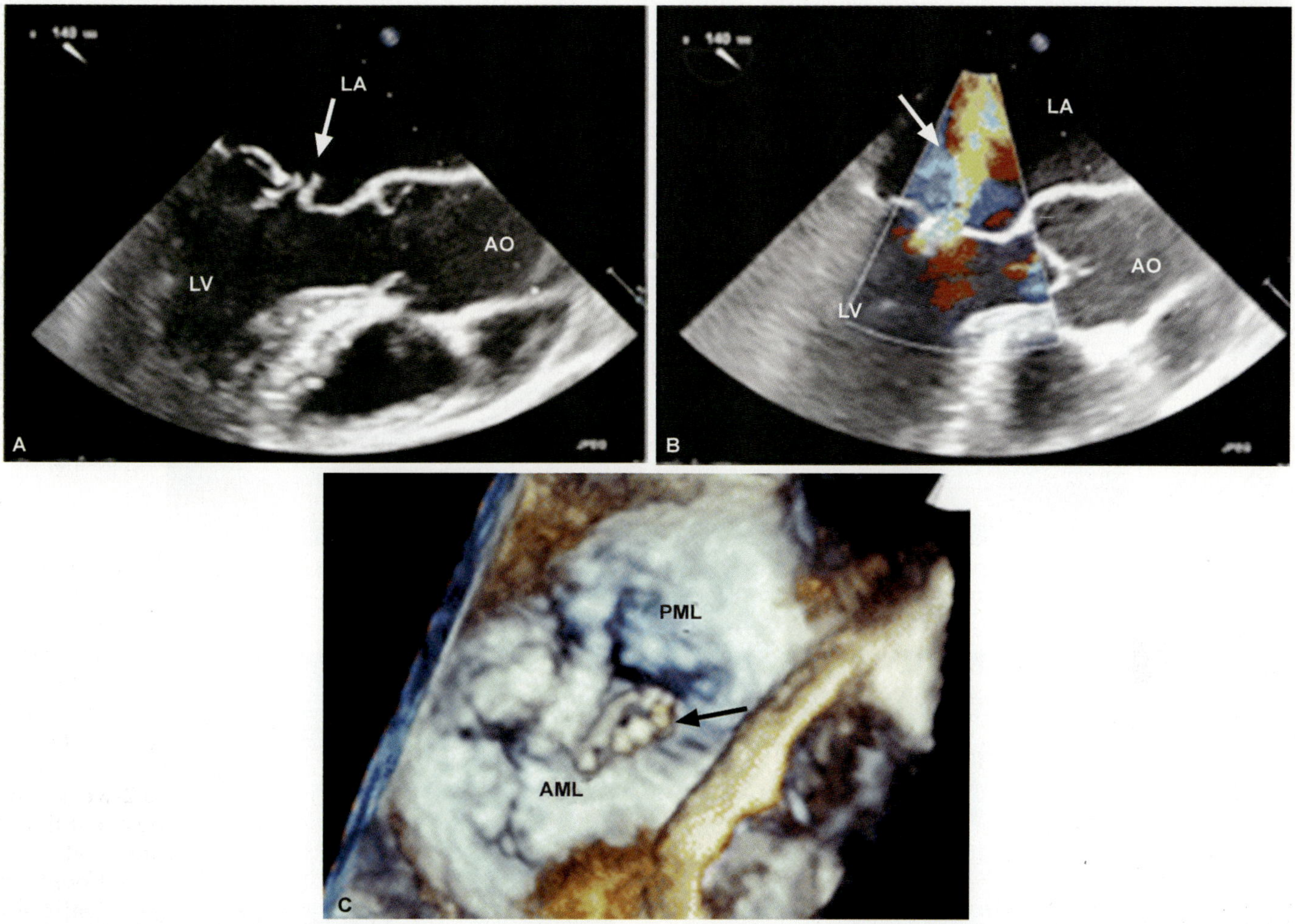


**Fig. 12.33:** Perforation of the anterior mitral leaflet (arrow). (A) TEE. (B) Color-Doppler. (C) Three-dimensional echocardiography. LA=left atrium; LV=left ventricle; AML=anterior mitral leaflet; PML=posterior mitral leaflet; Ao=aorta

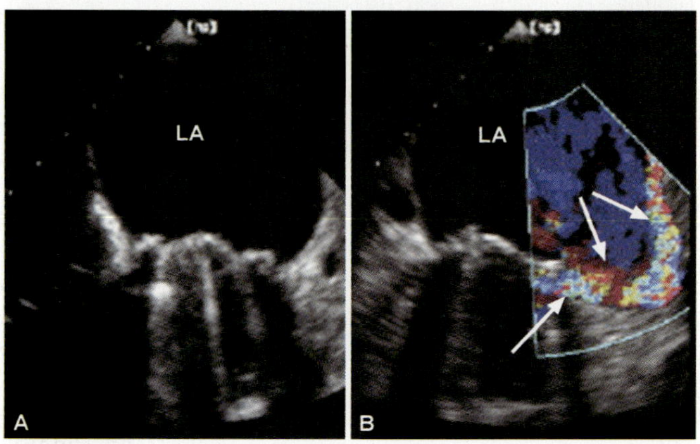


**Fig. 12.34:** TEE echocardiography showing vegetations on mitral valve prosthesis

**Table 12.12:** Injection drug use and right-sided endocarditis—key points

- In inner city communities most cases of infective endocarditis (IE) occur in injection drug users; many of these will have right-sided IE caused by staphylococci
- If injection drug users with bacteraemia from an inner city demographic are considered, up to 41% will have evidence of endocarditis
- The conjunction of bacteraemia, fever, and multiple pulmonary infiltrates on chest radiography should always prompt a search for right-sided IE
- A transoesophageal echocardiographic examination is not necessary in many cases of right-sided IE
- Coexistent medical problems such as hepatitis or HIV disease may be present
- Successful treatment of right-sided IE in injection drug users requires a multidisciplinary approach
- Most patients will recover with medical treatment: short course or rarely oral antibiotic treatment may be useful in certain situations

following the initiation of antibiotic treatment may occur and does not in itself represent an indication for surgery. Some authors have felt that large vegetation size (diameter >10 mm) in the context of persisting fever identifies a set of patients who are likely to benefit from surgery. Others have felt that many of these patients will eventually recover with medical treatment. Very large vegetations (>20 mm), however, are associated with a poor outcome. Patients may

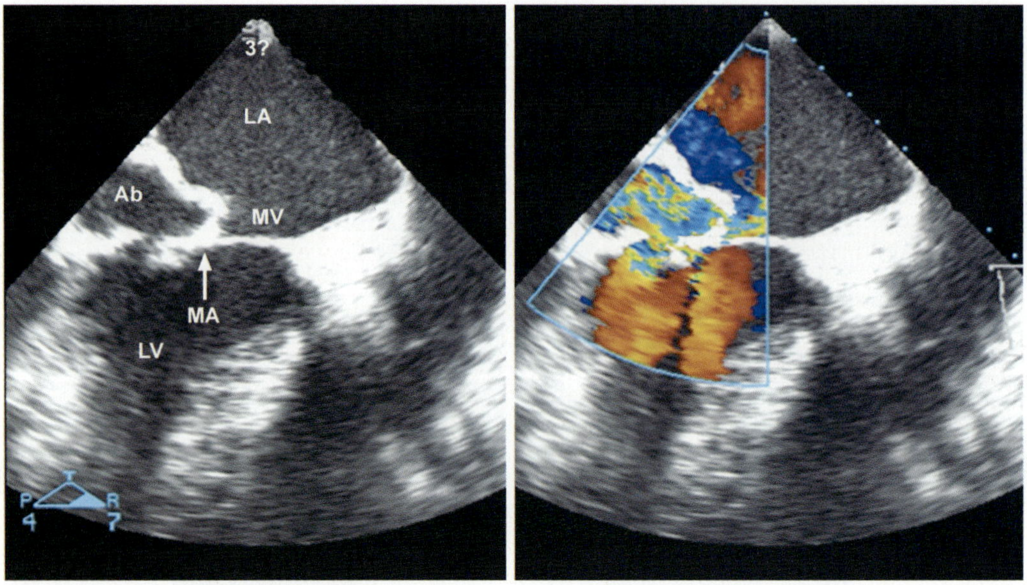


**Fig. 12.35:** Transesophageal echocardiogram showing mitral paravalvular abscess with ventriculo-atrial fistula. LA=indicates left atrium; MV=mitral valve; MA=mitral annulus; LV=left ventricle; and Ab=abscess

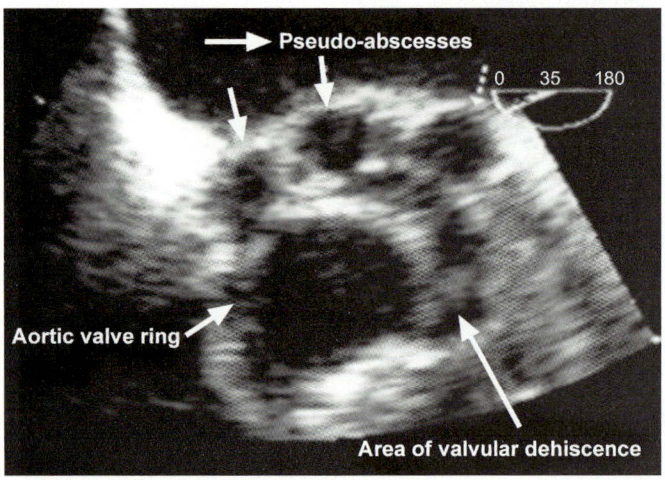


**Fig. 12.36:** Multiple pseudo-abscesses following aortic valve replacement Mid-oesophageal short-axis view magnified with zoom

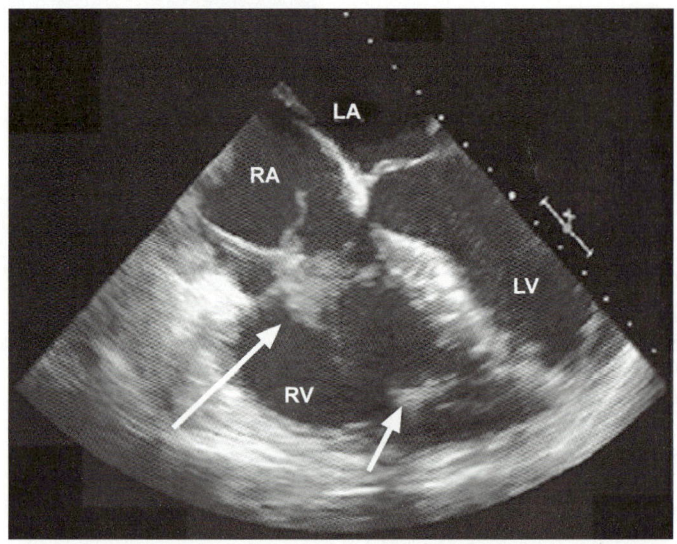


**Fig. 12.37:** Transesophageal echocardiography. Four chamber view shows multiple vegetations on the tricuspid valve (long arrow) and pacing leads (short arrow)

also require an operation to treat concomitant left-sided endocarditis. Enthusiasm for surgery is tempered by the knowledge that the majority of patients will resume injection drug use following hospital discharge. Surgical approaches vary, with valve removal or replacement being the historical, commonly recommended approaches. Both approaches are controversial and there is a lack of controlled trials in the literature upon which to base decision making. Valvectomy may result in permanent damage to the right ventricle and ultimately intractable right heart failure and death. Significant early mortality (11 %) was reported in one group where this approach was used. More recent attention has focused on tricuspid valve vegetectomy or repair. The repair has the advantage of avoiding or minimising the implantation of foreign material in the infected area while preserving the function of the valve. Several different techniques have been used, including cusp resection (rendering the valve bicuspid), commissural plication, the use of artificial chordae, and pericardial patch repair of the tricuspid leaflet (sometimes in conjunction with mobilisation of the secondary chordae and tricuspid annuloplasty). Where extensive valvar destruction has occurred, replacement of the tricuspid valve may be necessary. When valve replacement is unavoidable our current approach is to use cryopreserved mitral homografts in the tricuspid position, which usually requires the addition of a tricuspid ring to provide annular stability. Reinfection of the valve can be anticipated in some cases; when this occurs, antibiotic treatment may result in a cure of the prosthetic valve endocarditis.

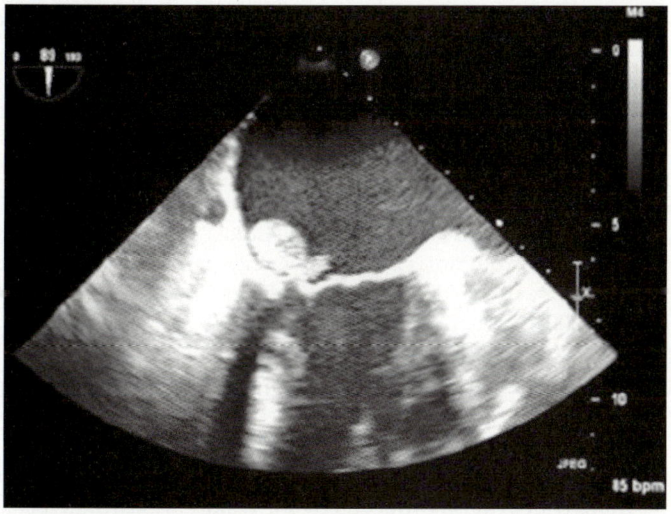

**Fig. 12.38:** Transesophageal echocardiogram showing a 2 cm mobile mass on the atrial surface of the posterior mitral valve leaflet consistent with a vegetation

### Prevention

It is possible that harm reduction strategies aimed at reducing injection frequency (such as methadone availability) or clean injection strategies (clean injection education, injection rooms, needle exchange programmes or legal heroin) may have a beneficial effect. The clinical suspicion is low. If the clinical suspicion is high TEE should be performed. TEE should also be performed if the results of the TTE are equivocal owing to underlying structural abnormalities or poor acoustic windows. If the TEE is negative, observation or reevaluation of the clinical data are warranted. If the suspicion of endocarditis is high TEE should be repeated after 7–10 days to allow potential vegetations to become more apparent. A repeated negative study should virtually rule out the diagnosis unless TEE images are of poor quality.

### Conclusion

To date, definitive studies of infective endocarditis have been difficult to perform because of its heterogenous nature. Launched in 1999, the international collaboration on endocarditis was conceived to develop a large global database of patients whose clinical, echocardiographic, and microbiological findings have been characterised using standard methodology. Modification of the original Duke criteria is now proposed to enhance diagnostic sensitivity, especially in culture negative cases. Increased emphasis on symptoms and signs coupled with improved likelihood of identification of a causative pathogen using serology, additional culture, or newer histological and molecular techniques will improve the sensitivity of the diagnosis and increase therapeutic specificity. These measures, combined with close collaboration and communication between the cardiologist, cardiac surgeon, and microbiologist, are essential to ensure optimal diagnosis and management and a favourable impact on patient outcome.

**Table 12.13:** Echocardiographic features suggesting potential need for surgical intervention

- Vegetation
- Persistent vegetation after systemic embolization
- Anterior mitral leaflet vegetation, particularly with size >10 $mm^2$
- One or more embolic events during first 2 weeks of antimicrobial therapy
- Two or more embolic events during or after antimicrobial therapy
- Increase in vegetation size after 4 weeks of antimicrobial therapy
- Valvular dysfunction
- Acute aortic or mitral insufficiency with signs of ventricular failure
- Heart failure unresponsive to medical therapy
- Valve perforation or rupture
- Perivalvular extension
- Valvular dehiscence, rupture, or fistula
- New heart block
- Large abscess, or extension of abscess despite appropriate antimicrobial therapy.

## BIBLIOGRAPHY

1. A useful contemporary snapshot of IE epidemiology. Weisse AB, Heller DR, Schimenti RJ, et al. The febrile parenteral drug user: a prospective study in 121 patients. J Am Med 1993;94: 274–80.
2. Additional references appear on the Heart website-www. heartinl.com/supplemental
3. Alestig K, Hogevik H, Olaison l. Infective endocarditis: a diagnostic and therapeutic challenge for the new millennium. Scand) Infect Dis 2000;32:343–56.
4. Alexander RW, Schlent RC, Foster V, (Eds.). Hurst's The Heart 9/ed. New York: MGraw-Hill, 1998:2205–42.
5. Arbulu A, Holmes R, Asfaw I. Surgical treatment of intractable right-sided infective endocarditis in drug addicts: 25 yrs experience.) Heart Valve Dis 1993;2:129–37; discussion 138–9.
6. Bayer AS, Bolger AF, Taubert KA, et al. Diagnosis and management of infective endocarditis and its complications. Circulation 1998;98:2936–48.
7. Blumberg EA, Karalis DA, Chandrasekaran K, et al. Endocarditis-associated paravalvular abscesses. Do clinical parameters predict the presence of abscess? Chest 1995; 107:898–903.
8. Cabell CH, Abrutyn E. Progress toward a global understanding of infective endocarditis. Early lessons from the International Collaboration on Endocarditis investigation. Infect Dis Clin North Am 2002;16:255–72.
9. Cabell CH, Jollis JG, Peterson GE, et al. Changing patient characteristics and the effect on mortality in endocarditis. Arch Intern Med 2002;162:90–4.
10. Carozza A, Renzulli A, De FM, et al. Tricuspid repair for infective endocarditis: clinical and echocardiographic results. Texas Heart Inst J 2001;28:96–101. Contemporary insight into surgical approaches to tricuspidendocarditis.

11. Case control study of a cohort of injection drug users that compares those with and without HIV infection.
12. Chastre J, Trouillet JL. Early infective endocarditis on prosthetic valves. fur Heart) 1995;16(suppl B):32–8,217.
13. Chon Kl. Early clinical course and long-term outcome of patients with infective endocarditis complicated by perivalvular abscess. Can Moo Assoc 2002;167:19–24.
14. Choussat R, Thomas D, Isnard R, et al. Perivalvular abscesses associated with endocarditis: clinical features and prognostic factors of overall survival in a series of 233 cases. Perivalvular abscess French multicenter study. for Heart 1999;20:232–41.
15. Chua JD, Wilkoff B, et al. Diagnosis and management of infections involving implantable electrophysiologic cardiac devices. Ann Intern Med 2000;133:604–8.
16. Cicalini S, Forcina G, De Rosa FG. Infective endocarditis in patients with human immunodeficiency virus infection. Infect 2001;42:267-71.Retrospective study of IE in an HIV population.
17. Correspondence to: Professor Francois Delahaye, Hopital cardiovasculaire et pneumologique, BP Lyon Montchat, 69394-Lyon Cedex 03, France; francois.delahaye@chu-lyonJr.
18. Crane LR, Levine DP, Zervos MJ, et al. Bacteremia in narcotic addicts at the Detroit Medical Center. I. Microbiology, epidemiology, risk factors, and empiric therapy. Rev Infect Dis 1986;8:364–73.
19. D'Udekem Y, David TE, Feindel CM, et al. Long-term results of surgery for active infective endocarditis. fur) Cardiothorac Surg 1997;11:46–52.
20. Dajani AS, Taubert KA, Wilson W, et al. Prevention of bacterial endocarditis: recommendations by the American Heart Association. Circulation 1997;96:358–66.
21. Daniel WG, Mogge A, Martin RP, et al. Improvement in the diagnosis of abscesses associated with endocarditis by transesophageal echocardiography. N Eng J Med 1991;324: 795–800.
22. Delahaye F, Celard M, Roth O, de Gevigney G, Hopital cardiovasculaire et pneumologique, Lyon, France.
23. Di Salvo G, Habib G, Pergola V, et al. Echocardiography predicts embolic events in infective endocarditis. J Am Col Cordial 2001;37:1069–76.
24. Dillon JC, Feigenbaum H, Konecke LL, et al. Echocardiographic manifestations of volvular vegetations. Am Heart 1973;6:698–704.
25. DiNubile MJ. Short-course antibiotic therapy for right-sided endocarditis caused by Staphylococcus aureus in injection drug users. Ann Intern Med 1994;121:873–6.Review focusing on short course antibiotic treatment in right-sided IE.
26. Dressler FA, Roberts WE. Infective endocarditis in opiate addicts:analysis of 80 cases studied at necropsy. Am Cardiol 1989;63:1240–57.
27. Durack DT, Lukes AS, Bright DK, et al. New criteria for diagnosis of infective endocarditis: utilization of specific echocardiographic findings. Am J Med 1994;96:200–9.
28. Durack DT, Lukes AS, Bright DK. New criteria for diagnosis of infective endocarditis: utilization of specific echocardiogrophic findings. Duke endocarditis service. Am J Med 1994;96:200–9. Classic paper that underscores the key role of echocardiography in the diagnosis of IE; it has formed the basis for increased accuracy in the diagnosis of IE and provided a solid basis for defining entry criteria in clinical and epidemiological studies.
29. Durack DT, Lukes AS, Bright DK. New criteria lor diagnosis of infective endocarditis: utilization of specific echocardiographic Finding: Duke Endocarditis Service. Am Moo 1994; 96:200–9.
30. Durack DT. Prevention of infective endocarditis. N Engl J Med 1995;332:38–44. Durack DT, Lukes AS, Bright DK. New criteria for diagnosis of infective endocarditis: utilization of specific echocardiographic findings. Am J Med 1994;96: 200–209.
31. Erbel R, Rohmann S, Drexler M, et al. Improved diagnostic value of echocardiography in potients with infective endocarditis by transoesophageal approach. A prospective study. Eur Heart 1988;9:43–53.
32. Fournier PE, Casalta JP, Habib G, et al. Modification of the diagnostic criteria proposed by the Duke endocarditis service to permit improved diagnosis of Q fever endocarditis. Am J Med 1996;100:629–33.
33. Gillinov AM, Shah RV, Curtis WE, et al. Valve replacement in patients with endocarditis and acute neurologic deficit. Ann Thorac Surg 1996;61:1125–30.
34. Gordon SM, Serkey JM, Longworth DL, et al. Early onset prosthetic valveendocarditis: the Cleveland Clinic experience 1992–7. Ann Thorac Surg2000;69:1388–92.
35. Grijalva M, Horvath R, Dendis M, et al. Molecular diagnosis of culture negative infective endocarditis: clinical validation in a group of surgically treated patients. Heart 2003;89:263–8.
36. Habib G, Derumeaux G, Avierinos J-F, et al. Value and limitations of the Duke criteria for the diagnosis of infective endocarditis. J Am Coll Cardiol 1999;33:2023–9.
37. Hecht S, Berger M. Right-sided endocarditis in intravenous drug users. Prognostic features in 102 episodes. Ann Intern Med 1992;117:560–6. Definitive retrospective study of right-sided IE.
38. Heiro M, Nikoskelainen J, Engblom E, et al. Neurologic manifestations of infective endocarditis: a 17-year experience in a teaching hospital in Finland. Arch Intern Mad 2000;160: 2781–7.
39. Heldman AW, Hartert TV, Ray SC, et al. Oral antibiotic treatment of right-sided staphylococcal endocarditis in iniection drug users: prospective randomized comparison with parenteral therapy. Am J Med1996;101:68–76. Oral treatment compared prospectively with intravenous treatment in right-sided IE.
40. Hoen B, Alia F, Selton-Suty C, et al. Changing profile of infective endocarditis: results of a 1-year survey in France JAMA 2002;288:75–81.
41. Hoen B, Alia F, Selton-Suty C, et al. For the AEPEI group. Changing profile of infective endocarditis. Results of a 1-year survey in France. JAMA 2002;288:75–81.
42. Houpikian P, Raoult D. Diagnostic methods. Current best practices and guidelines for identification of difficult-to-culture pathogens in infective endocarditis. Infect Dis Clin N Am 2002;16:377–92.
43. John MD, Hibberd PL, Karchmer AW, et al. Staphylococcus aureus prosthetic valve endocarditis: optimal management and risk factors for death. Infect Dis 1998;26:1302–9.

44. Karalis OO, Bansal RC, Hauck AJ, et al. Transesophageal echocardiographic recognition of subaortic complications in aortic valve endocarditis. Circulation 1992;86:353–62.
45. Karchmer AW. Infecious Endocarditis. In: Braunwald E, (Ed.) Heart disease: a textbook of cardiovascular medicine, 6th ed. Philadelphia: WB Saunders, 2002:1723–48. Otto C. The practice of clinical echocardiography, 2/e. Philadelphia: WB Saunders, 2002:451–69.
46. Khanderia BK, Seward JB, Oh JK, et al. Value and limitations of transesophageal echocardiography in assessment of mitral valve prostheses. Circulation 1991;83:1956–68.
47. Knosalla C, et al. Surgical treatment of active infective aortic valve endocarditis with associated periannular abscesses with 11 year results. Eur Heart J 2000;21:490–7.
48. Knosalla C, Weng Y, Yankah AC, et al. Surgical treatment of active infective aortic valve endocarditis with associated periannular abscess. 11 year results. Eur Heart 2000;21:490–7.
49. Lamas C, Eykyn SJ. Suggested modifications to the Duke criteria for the clinical diagnosis of native valve and prosthetic valve endocarditis: analysis of 118 pathologically proven cases. Clin Infect Dis 1997;25:713–9.
50. Lamas CC, Eykyn SJ. Blood culture negative endocarditis endocarditis: analysis of 63 cases presenting over 25 years. Eur Heart 2003;89:258–62.
51. Lengyel M. The impact of transesophageal echocardiography on management of prosthetic valve endocarditis: experience of 31 cases and review of the literature. Heart Valve Dis 1997;6:204–11.
52. Lepidi H, Durack DT, Raoult D. Diagnostic methods. Current best practices and guidelines for histologic evaluation in infective endocarditis. Infect Dis Clin N Am 2002;16:339–61.
53. Li JS, Sexton DJ, Mick N, et al. Proposed modifications to the Duke criteria for the diagnosis of infective endocarditis. Clin Infect Dis 2000;30:633–8.
54. Li JS, Suton DJ, Mick N, et al. Proposed modifications to the Duke criteria lor the diagnosis of infective endocarditis C in Infect Dis 2000;30:633–8.
55. Lisby G, Gutschik E, Durack DT. Molecular methods for diagnosis of infective endocarditis. Infect Dis Clin North Am 2002;16:393–412.
56. Manolis AS, Melita H. Echocardiographic and clinical correlates in drug addicts with infective endocarditis. Implications 01 vegetation size. Arch Intern Med 1988;148:2461–5.
57. Mathew J, Addai T, Anand A et al. Clinical features, site of involvement, bacteriologic findings, and outcome of infective endocarditis in intravenous drug users. Arch Intern Med 1995;155:1641–8. Important retrospective cohort study of intravenous drug users with native valve endocarditis.
58. Mestres CA, Miro JM, Pare JC, et al. Six-year experience with cryopreserved mitral homogralts in the treatment of tricuspid valve endocarditis in HIV-infected drug addicts. J Heart Valve Dis 1999;8:575–7.
59. Millar BC, Moore JE, Mallon P, et al. Molecular diagnosis of infective endocarditis–a new Duke's criterion. Scand J Infect Dis 2001;33:673–80.
60. Miyagishima R, Brumwell M, Eric JW, et al. Tricuspid valve replacement using a cryopreserved mitral homogralt. Surgical technique and initial results. Heart Valve Dis 2000;9:805–8; discussion 808–9.
61. Moore JE, Millar BC, Yongmin X, et al. A rapid molecular assay for the detection of antibiotic resistance determinants in cause of infective endocarditis. J Appl Microbiol 2001;90: 719–26.
62. Moyer D, Edwards JE. Fungal endocarditis. In: Kaye D, (Ed.) Infective endocarditis. New York: Raven Press, 1992:299–312.
63. Mugge A, Daniel WG, Frank G, et al. Echocardiography in infective endocarditis: reassessment of prognostic implications of vegetation size determined by the transthoracic and the transesophageal approach. Am Coli Cardio 1989;14: 631–8.
64. Olaison L, Pettersson G. Current best practice and guidelines: indications for surgi-cal intervention in infective endocarditis. Infect Dis Clin North Am 2002;16: 453–75.
65. Olaison L, Pettersson G. Current best practices and guidelines indications for surgical intervention in infective endocarditis. Infect Dis Clin North Am 2002;16:453–75.
66. Palepu A, Cheung SS, Montessori V, et al. Factors other than the Duke criteria associated with infective endocarditis among injection drug users. Cl in Invest Med 2002;25: 118–25. This study examines the usefulness of the Duke criteria in an intravenous drug user population and non-Duke clinical variables that predict a diagnosis of IE.
67. Raoult D, et al. Cultivation of the bacillus of Whipple's disease. N Engl J Med 2000; 342:620–5.
68. Reynolds HR, Jagen MA, Tunick PA, et al. Sensitivity of transthoracic versus transesophageechocardiography lor the detection of native valve vegetations in the modern era. Am So Echocardiogr 2003;16:67-70.
69. Ribera E, Miro JM, Cortes E, et al. Influence of human immunodeficiency virus 1 infection and degree of immunosuppression in the clinical characteristics and outcome of infective endocarditis in intravenous drug users. Arch Intern Med 1998;158:2043–50.
70. Robbins M, Frater R, Soeiro R, et al. Influence of vegetation size on clinicol outcome of right-sided infective endocarditis. Am J Med 1986;80:165–71.
71. Rohmann S, Erbel R, Gorge G, et al. Clinical relevance of vegetation localization by transoesophageal echocardiography in infective endocarditis. Eur Heart. 1992;13:446–52.
72. Rozich JD, Edwards WD, Hanna RD, et al. Mechanical prosthetic valve associated strands: Pathologic correlates to transesophageal echocardiography. Am Soc Echocardiogr 2003;J6:97–100.
73. San Roman JA, Vilacosta I, Zamorano J, et al. Transesophageal echocardiography in right-sided endocarditis.) Am Coli Cordial 1993;21:1226–30. This paper questions the routine role of TOE in the diagnosis of right-sided endocarditis.
74. Sanders GP, Yeon SB, Grunes J, et al. Impact of a specific echocardiographic report comment regarding endocarditis prophylaxis on compliance with American Heart Association Recommendations. Circulation 2002;106:300-303.
75. Sexton DJ, Spelman D. Current best practice and guidelines: assessment and management of complications in infective endocarditis. Infect Dis Clin North Am 2002; 16:507–21.
76. Shapiro SM, Young E, De Guzman S, et al. Transesophageal echocardiography in diagnosis of infective endocarditis. Chest 1994;105:377–82.

77. Shively BK, Gurule FT, Roldan CA, et al. Diagnostic value of transesophogeal compored with transthoracic echocordiography in infective endocarditis. Am Coli Cardio 1991;18: 391–7.
78. Sochowski RA, Chan K-I. Implicotion of negative results on a monoplane transesophageal echocardiographic study in patients with suspected infective endocarditis. Am Coli Cardio 1993;21:216–21.
79. Son Roman JA, Vilacosta I, Zamorano JL, et al. Transesophageal echocardiography in right-sided endocarditis. Am Coli Cardio 1993;21:1226–30.
80. Truninger K, Attenhofer Jost CH, et al. Long term follow up of prosthetic valve endocarditis: what characteristics identify patients who weretreated successfully with antibiotics alone? Heart 1999;82:714–20.
81. von Reyn CF, Levy BS, Arbeit RD, et al. Infective endocarditis: an analysis based on strict case definitions. Ann Intern Med 1981;94:505–17.
82. Wallace SM, et al. Mortality from infective endocarditis: clinical predictors of out-come. Heart 2002;88:53–60.
83. Wilson LE, et al. Prospective study of infective endocarditis among injection drug users. J Infect Dis 2002;1 85:1761–66.
84. Wilson LE, Thomas DL, Astemborski J, et al. Prospective study of infective endocarditis among injection drug users. Infect Dis 2002;185: 1761–6.
85. Wilson WR, Karchmer AW, Dajani AS, et al. Antibiotic treatment of adults with infective endocarditis due to streptococci, enterococci, staphylococci, and HACEK microorganisms. JAMA 1995;274:1706–13.

# 13 Recognition and Management of Acute Myocarditis

Myocarditis is an acute or chronic inflammatory disease of the myocardium which can be viral, postinfectious immune or primarily organ-specific autoimmune. Clinical manifestations of acute and chronic myocarditis are extremely varied, ranging from mild to severe. Affected patients may recover or develop (dilated) cardiomyopathy (DCM) with life-threatening symptoms including heart failure, conduction disturbances, arrhythmias, cardiogenic shock or sudden cardiac death.

The diagnosis of myocarditis is a challenging process and not only because of a diverse presentation; other problems are limited sensitivity of endomyocardial biopsies (EMB) and overlapping symptoms. Furthermore, the diagnosis is not well defined. However, early diagnosis is mandatory to address specific etiology-directed therapeutic management in myocarditis that influences patient morbidity and mortality.

## INCIDENCE AND PREVALENCE

Difficult to determine; the majority of patients are clinically silent and resolve spontaneously without treatment. Highly variable incidence owing to differences in methods used for diagnostic evaluation. One estimate has been 8–10 cases per 100,000 of the US population. The prevalence of myocarditis among unselected autopsy series is as high as 1–5%. The prevalence of viral myocarditis is variable and is related to the periodic cycle of viral epidemics. A recent study pointed out that myocarditis is a frequently underdiagnosed disorder. Viral RNA was detected in a large amount of biopsy samples obtained from patients that were initially diagnosed as idiopathic dilated cardiomyopathy (IDCM). These findings suggest that viral myocarditis is frequently the etiology of heart failure in patients who were initially identified as having IDCM using current standard diagnostic techniques.

## ETIOLOGICAL FACTORS

The most common form of myocarditis, endemic in both rural Central and South America, is Chagas' disease, caused by the parasitic protozoan *Trypanosoma cruzi*. In North America, viral infections cause most cases of myocarditis. Enteroviruses, most importantly coxsackievirus B, are the most frequently reported cause of epidemics of viral myocarditis in children. However, more recent reports indicated that adenoviral infection is as common a cause as enteroviral infection is, if not more so. Rarely, bacteria, fungi, protozoa, parasites, and rickettsiae are causative agents. Myocarditis has also been associated with immune-mediated diseases, collagen vascular diseases, and toxins (Table 13.1).

## EPIDEMIOLOGICAL FEATURES OF MYOCARDITIS

Occurrence of myocarditis can be affected by viral epidemics. An outbreak of coxsackievirus B in Europe in 1965 correlated with cardiac dysfunction in 5% of infected patients. Incidences were as high as 12% that same year in Scotland, Finland, and Austria. Seasonal viral distributions have been recognized for decades (influenza prevalent during winter months; poliovirus and coxsackievirus A and B typically isolated during summer and fall). Myocarditis has been a prominent finding during epidemics of influenza; thus, occurrence may be seasonal.

## AGE AND GENDER

Age plays a marked role in prevalence. During the neonatal period, myocarditis is usually abrupt, severe, and often fatal, with mortality as high as 75%. Infants infected with coxsackievirus B during the first year of life have a high incidence of myocarditis. Myocarditis has been linked to sudden infant death syndrome, because inflammatory infiltrates have been found on autopsies of some victims.

**Table 13.1:** Aetiology of myocarditis

| **Viruses** | **Immune-mediated diseases** | **Drugs** |
|---|---|---|
| Coxasackievirus A | Rheumatoid arthritis | Sulfonamides |
| Coxasackievirus B | Rheumatic fever | Cyclophosphamide |
| Echovirus | Ulcerative colitis | Acetazolamide |
| Adenovirus | Systemic lupus erythematosis | Amphotericin B |
| Rubella virus | | Indomethacin |
| Measles virus | **Toxins** | Tetracycline |
| Varicella virus | Ethanol | Phenytoin |
| Polio virus | Heavy metals: iron, copper, lead | Penicilin |
| Mumps virus | Arsenic | |
| Herpesvirus | Bee and wasp sting | **Fungi and yeast** |
| Epstein-Barr virus | Carbon monoxide | Aspergilus |
| Cytomegalovirus | Scorpion bites | Candida |
| Human immunodeficiency virus | Spider bites | |
| | Snake bites | **Protozoa** |
| **Bacteria** | *Toxoplasma gondii* | *Trypanosoma cruzi* |
| Meningococci | | |
| *Borrelia burgdorferi* (Lyme disease) | **Physical conditions or agents** | **Parasties** |
| Salmonellae | Hyperpyrexia | *Ascaris* |
| Mycobacteria | Electric shock | *Schistosoma* |
| Streptococci | Radiation | Trichinella spirals |

Incidence increases again during late childhood and adolescence; the myocarditis usually has a delayed onset and patients recover.

Male predominance has been noted with coxsackievirus B heart disease, particularly in adolescents and adults. In these age groups, two-thirds to three-quarters of patients with myocarditis are male. Male predominance has also been reported with coxsackievirus A myocarditis and poliomyelitis. Whether or not differences between the sexes occur in other viral infections is unknown.

## PATHOPHYSIOLOGY

Although viral infection is the most common initiator of acute myocarditis, the subsequent autoimmune response plays a lead role in myocyte injury. The principal mechanism of myocardial damage is not just viral replication; it includes cell-mediated immunological reactions.

The pathophysiology of myocarditis has been studied in mice infected with a cardiotropic virus, such as coxsackievirus B. After systemic infection, the virus enters the myocyte, where it replicates in the cytoplasm of the cell. Some replicated viruses then enter the interstitium and are phagocytized by activated macrophages. Macrophage activation is due to both viral particles in the interstitium and the release of interferon γ by natural killer (NK) cells. The release of interferon γ is followed by release of proinflammatory cytokines (interleukins 1β and 2 and tumor necrosis factor α). When activated by interleukin 2, NK-cells eliminate virally infected myocytes and inhibit virus replication The significance of the action of NK-cells in the pathogenesis of the disease is well established; in animals depleted of NK-cells before infection, a more severe myocarditis develops. As noted earlier, myocarditis after infection with coxsackievirus B occurs more often in men. This propensity may be related to differences between the sexes in the activation of NK-cells. After infection, myocarditis that develops in female mice is less severe than that in male mice. In one study, after the same infection, male mice were markedly less efficient than female mice in activating NK-cells. This decrease in NK-cell activation presumably results in decreased viral clearance with a resultant increase in illness severity. This difference in NK-cell activation may explain the male predominance for the development of clinically significant myocarditis. Unlike NK-cells, T cells may contribute to damage in both infected and noninfected myocytes. Activation of T cells results in accumulation of macrophages within the myocyte and production of cell-mediated cytotoxic effects. Although T cells can lyse virus-infected myocytes, the accumulation of macrophages and the concomitant cytotoxic effects create a fine balance between viral clearance and myocyte damage. Adding to myocyte injury, lysis by T cells is indiscriminate; it occurs in both infected and noninfected cells. The result is necrosis of healthy as well as infected myocytes. Therefore, a percentage of myocardial damage comes from 'friendly fire,' specifically the patient's own immune response.

Permanent myocardial damage can be the end result of myocarditis. Such damage is thought to be due to an overaggressive immunological activation in which persistent T-cell infiltration leads to long-term tissue destruction and subsequent dilated cardiomyopathy. Infection with enteroviruses plays a major role in chronic forms of dilated cardiomyopathy.

Myocarditis is classified as fulminant, acute, or chronic. Fulminant myocarditis is preceded by a viral prodrome that is followed by sudden onset of severe hemodynamic compromise. Acute myocarditis has a less distinct onset and, initially, less severe compromise but is followed by a worse outcome than fulminant myocarditis. McCarthy et al. found that adults with fulminant myocarditis had excellent long-term survival, whereas patients with acute myocarditis had progressive failure that led to death or the need for a heart transplant. Chronic myocarditis can be defined as persistent (lasting >3 months), recurrent, and latent.

Diagnosing myocarditis in children can be challenging. Not only can children have a wide range of nonspecific signs and symptoms, but depending on cognitive development, they may not be able to communicate their symptoms. Despite a variety of invasive and noninvasive studies, myocarditis is a presumptive diagnosis based on history and clinical features.

## CLINICAL HISTORY

Clinical features of viral myocarditis are affected by age, sex, and the child's baseline health status. These variables affect the balance between pathogen clearance and degree of inflammation. Older children may have a history of upper respiratory infection; infants may have anorexia, vomiting, and lethargy. Often, signs and symptoms are nonspecific or may resemble the signs and symptoms of relatively common diagnoses in children, including bronchiolitis, pneumonia, failure to thrive, and gastroenteritis.

Both cases described earlier had the potentially insidious manifestations of viral myocarditis. In the first case, the signs and symptoms suggested benign gastroenteritis with slight dehydration, a situation that is not unusual in toddlers and preschool children. KM, who had a history of gastroenteritis, also had syncope, wheezing, and increased work of breathing. His history of asthma confounded his clinical features. Consequently, he initially received treatment for an exacerbation of asthma.

Older children may have **chest pain** (the sole symptom in some patients). Some have abdominal pain. Atypical manifestations such as syncope (KM), seizures, and sudden death also have been reported. A more focused cardiac examination when no signs of congestive heart failure occur may be prompted by patients' reports of chest pain, dyspnea, exercise intolerance, or fatigue. Tachycardia of unknown origin in an otherwise healthy child may be an ominous sign. Newborns and infants, unlike older children, are more likely to have circulatory shock.

When myocarditis is suspected, a thorough history is imperative for identifying possible causes. Parents should be asked about exposures to potential infectious agents, pharmacological agents that can cause myocardial inflammation, and toxins, including illicit drugs (e.g. cocaine). Immunization status should be obtained because several infectious diseases of childhood (diphtheria, poliomyelitis) are potential causes.

## PHYSICAL SIGNS AND SYMPTOMS

During episodes of cardiac compromise, neurohormonal responses activate the sympathetic nervous system and the renin-angiotensin-aldosterone system, resulting in improved contractility, increase in heart rate, vasoconstriction, and fluid and sodium retention. Tachycardia out of proportion for age is common in children with myocardial compromise as the heart attempts to compensate for inadequate oxygen delivery to the tissues. Vasoconstriction occurs to improve preload and maintain blood pressure. This decrease in peripheral perfusion is manifested as cool extremities, described by level of coolness (e.g. cool to midcalf, cool to knee), quality of pulses, capillary refill time (compromise considered at >3 seconds with the extremity at the level of the heart), decreased urine output (<1 ml/kg per hour), and changes in mental status. Pulse quality is characterized by using the 0–4 pulse intensity scale (0=no pulses detected, 4=bounding). Extremities may appear mottled or pale. Despite these alterations in perfusion, it must be emphasized that vasoconstriction in children will maintain a blood pressure within a normal range for age even when tissue perfusion is inadequate. Hypotension is considered not only a late finding of cardiac failure but also an ominous one (Table 13.2).

Often, an **$S_3$ (ventricular gallop)** occurs because of rapid filling of a noncompliant, poorly contracting left ventricle. Murmurs are less common, although a soft systolic murmur may be heard if mitral or tricuspid insufficiency is present. Heart sounds may be muffled if concomitant pericarditis is present. Rhythm irregularities may be detected, especially supraventricular tachycardia or ventricular ectopic beats as with KM.

**Table 13.2:** Signs and symptoms of myocarditis in children

| | |
|---|---|
| Subjective | Chest pain |
| | Abdominal pain |
| | Dyspnea/orthopnea |
| | Exercise intolerance |
| | Fatigue |
| Objective | Tachycardia |
| | Tachypnea |
| | Wheezing, cough, increased work of breathing |
| | Alternation in peripheral perfusion |
| | • Prolonged capillary refill |
| | • Decrease in pulse quality |
| | • Extremity coolness |
| | • Painless, mottling |
| | • Decreased urine output |
| | Murmur |
| | Gallop |
| | Rhythm irregularities |
| | • Ventricular ectopy |
| | • Atrioventricular block |
| | • Sinus tachycardia or supraventricular tachycardia |
| | Hepatomegaly[a] |
| | Rales[b] |
| | Hypotension[b] |

[a]May or may not be present
[b]Late findings

Tachypnea is a common sign of myocardial failure in children. Tachypnea is the result of pulmonary edema due to left ventricular failure. Clinical findings can include wheezing, a cough, grunting, nasal flaring, and intercostal retraction. Older children may report orthopnea or inability to catch their breath. Cyanosis is rare. Rales are typically a late sign of pulmonary congestion and may not occur at all in infants.

Hepatomegaly, an indication of venous congestion, may or may not occur. Liver tenderness or absence of a firm edge on palpation below the right costal margin may indicate liver engorgement.

## NONINVASIVE DIAGNOSTIC STUDIES

The diagnostic approach for a child with suspected myocarditis includes strategies to both aid in establishing the diagnosis and rule out disease processes that may mimic myocarditis (e.g. a structural cardiac defect or pericardial effusion). In addition, many of these interventions provide an estimate of myocardial function and can help in establishing clinical interventions (Table 13.3).

### X-ray Chest

Evidence of cardiomegaly on a chest radiograph is an important clinical finding in myocarditis; however, the degree of heart enlargement depends on the stage of the disease. Subacute or chronic myocarditis is characterized by cardiomegaly; cardiomegaly may or may not occur in children with fulminant myocarditis.In fact, the possibility of myocarditis is often not considered until late, when cardiomegaly is evident on chest radiographs. Myocarditis should not be ruled out in infants or children with marked cardiovascular compromise or collapse of unknown cause who do not have evidence of heart enlargement on radiographs (Fig. 13.1).

### Electrocardiography

Although not diagnostic, findings on an electrocardiogram are rarely normal in patients with myocarditis (Fig. 13.2). Some children have such mild illness that a conduction disturbance on an electrocardiogram is the only abnormal finding. Sinus tachycardia is a common finding with

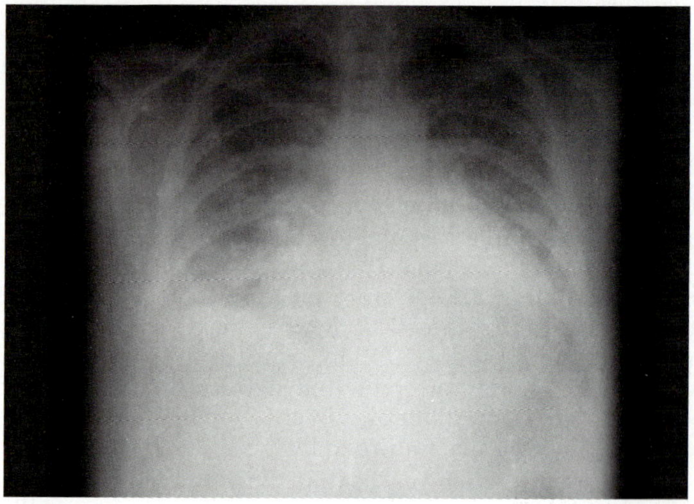

**Fig.13.1:** X-ray chest frontal view showing pulmonary edema in a patient with cardiogenic shock as a result of acute myocarditis in a 12 years old child

**Table 13.3:** Diagnosis of myocarditis

| Assessment | Findings |
|---|---|
| **Chest radiography** | Cardiomegaly |
| **Electrocardiography** | Tachycardia—sinus or supraventricular |
| | Atrioventricular block |
| | Low-voltage ORS complexes |
| | ST-T-wave abnormalities (elevation or depression) |
| | Prolonged QT interval |
| | Ventricular ectopy |
| **Echocardiography** | Impared ventricular function (left > right) |
| | Ventricular dilation |
| | Atrioventricular valve regurgitation |
| | Left ventricular thrombi |
| **Laboratory studies** | |
| *Serological tests* | Increased levels of creatine kinase and its MB isoenzyme |
| | Increased level of cardiac troponin C |
| | Elevated sedimentation rate |
| | Increased level of C reactive protein |
| | Increased level of white blood cells, with lymphocytes predominating viral titers |
| | Increased level of immunoglobulin G |
| *Cultures:* Blood, stool, cerebro, spinal fluid, nasopharyngeal, secretions | Presence of virus |
| **Myocardiat biopsy** | Myocyte destruction, fibrosis, inflammatory cells, and lymphocytic infiltrates |

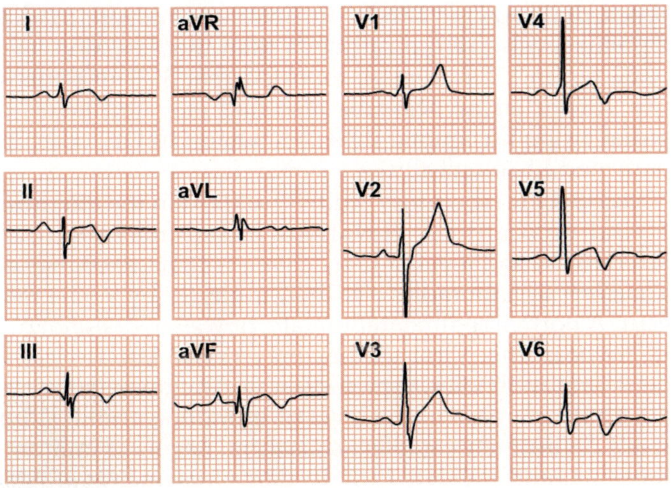


**Fig. 13.2:** The T-waves are deeply and symmetrically inverted in I, II, III, and V4–6, suggesting a diffuse myocardial process in a young patient with acute viral myocarditis

myocarditis. Low-voltage QRS complexes, ST-T-wave abnormalities, or prolonged QT interval may be apparent. Left ventricular hypertrophy with repolarization changes (strain) is typical. Complete atrioventricular block has also been described. Occasionally, evidence of myocardial infarction is seen.

## Echocardiography

Findings on echocardiograms are rarely normal in patients with myocarditis. As with KM, impaired left ventricular function with dilatation of 1 or more chambers is typical. KM's echocardiogram showed poor left ventricular systolic function, with dilatation and slightly diminished right ventricular function. In the absence of any structural abnormalities, these findings help establish the diagnosis. Generally, right ventricular function is less compromised than is left ventricular function; atrioventricular valve regurgitation may occur. Occasionally, left ventricular thrombi are found (Figs 13.3 amd 13.4).

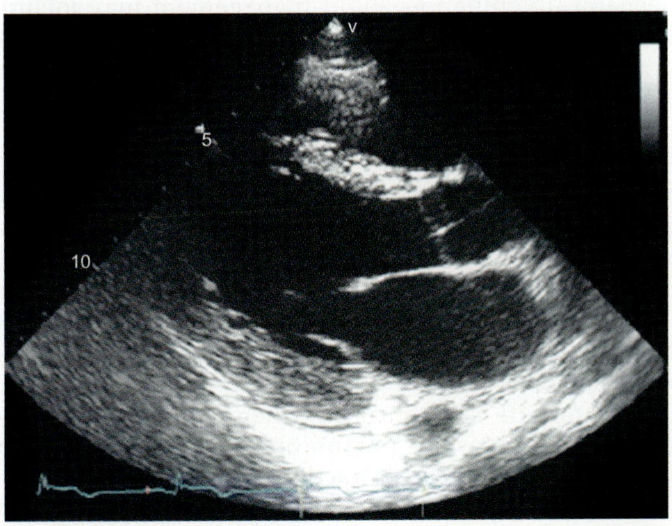


**Fig. 13.3:** Two-dimensional parasternal long-axis view depicting disproportionate thickening, increased echogenicity, and dyskinesis of the inferolateral wall relative to the septum; findings are consistent with tissue edema

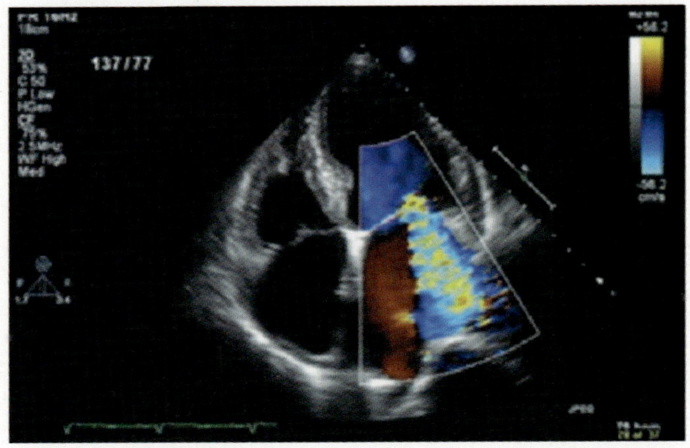


**Fig. 13.4:** Color-Doppler echocardiography shows MR appears as a systolic regurgitation from the left ventricle to the left atriumin a young patient with acute myocarditis

*CMR imaging:* Recent studies have demonstrated that CMR has shown promising results in the early diagnosis and the follow-up of AM and its subsequent stages. CMR includes several techniques that can be used in various combinations to assess left ventricular (LV) functional parameters, morphology, myocardial perfusion, and myocardial disorders within one examination (Fig.13.5).

# LABORATORY TESTS

## Endomyocardial Biopsy

Historically, despite its limited sensitivity and specificity and its inherent risks, endomyocardial biopsy has been the reference standard for diagnosing viral myocarditis (Fig. 13.6).

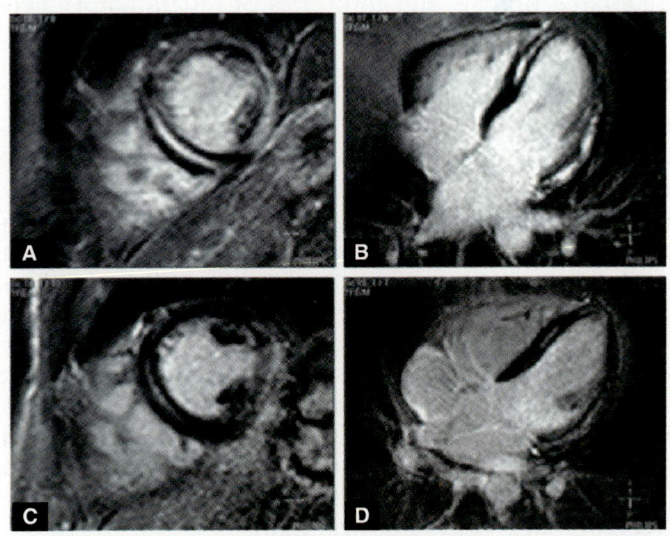


**Fig. 13.5:** Acute and chronic phase of myocarditis in a patient. (A, B) Acute myocarditis—short-axis view and 4-chamber view showing an extensive pattern of midwall contrast enhancement. Only the basal septal wall and distal anterolateral wall are spared. (C, D) Chronic myocarditis—short-axis and 4-chamber view showing the same pattern of midwall delayed contrast enhancement with lower signal intensity

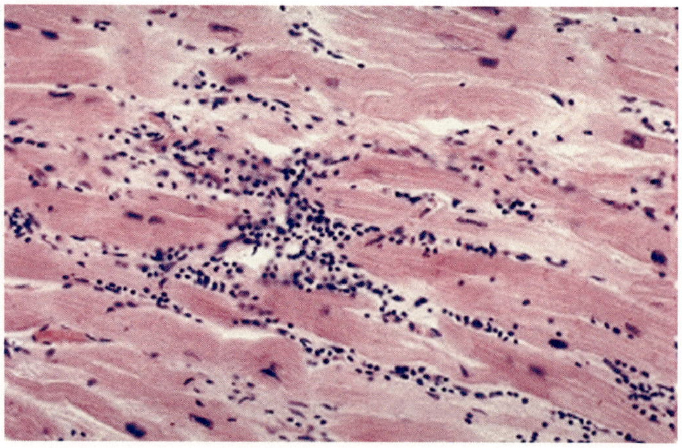

**Fig. 13.6:** Histo-photograph H/E stain showing interstitial inflammatory infiltrates mostly lymphocytes in acute viral myocarditis

Nevertheless, for several reasons, endomyocardial biopsy is used less often in children than in adults. First, biopsy can be associated with significant sampling error. Several tissue specimens (5 or more) are needed because of the focal nature of the disease; many clinicians think that biopsy leads to underestimation of the presence of the disease. Second, borderline myocarditis can result in little to no evidence of myocyte destruction. Third, expert interpretation can vary, including variance with other markers of viral infection. Because of the possibility of false-negative results, lack of an endomyocardial biopsy positive for myocarditis does not rule out this disease. For KM, findings on endomyocardial biopsy on hospital day 8 confirmed the diagnosis. Tissue specimens from the right ventricle had intact myocytes with small foci of lymphocytic infiltrates and extensive areas of myocyte destruction with organizing fibrosis and infiltrates of inflammatory cells most consistent with myocarditis.

### Polymerase Chain Reaction

Recently, use of less invasive means of diagnosing myocarditis in children has been emphasized.Use of polymerase chain reaction (PCR) and in situ hybridization has increased the sensitivity for diagnosing viral myocarditis. Tracheal aspirates for PCR analysis in intubated children are useful for detecting viral genomes in children with or without myocarditis. Akhtar et al. reported that PCR of tracheal aspirates had a sensitivity of 100% for predicting the results of PCR of endomyocardial biopsy specimens, albeit for a small (n=10) sample size. Although a tracheal aspirate positive for virus is not diagnostic for myocarditis itself, PCR of tracheal aspirates may provide a safer means of identifying a viral cause for illness in children with cardiac decompensation of unknown origin.

*Serological studies* may reveal an elevation in myocardial enzyme levels (creatine kinase, normal value 25–190 IU/L [to convert to microkatals, multiply by 0.0167]; MB isoenzyme of creatine kinase, normal value <12% of creatine kinase). In children, the level of cardiac troponin T is a more sensitive indicator of myocardial damage than are myocardial enzyme levels. In healthy children, cardiac troponin levels are typically less than the detection level (<0.02 ng/ml). Lauer et al. reported that 35% of patients with suspected myocarditis also had elevated levels of cardiac troponin; among those, 98% had viral myocarditis confirmed histologically.

Nonspecific laboratory studies may aid in the diagnosis of viral myocarditis. Elevations in sedimentation rate (>20 mm/h) and level of C-reactive protein (>0.05 mg/dl; to convert to nanomoles per liter, multiply by 9.524) may occur. A normal sedimentation rate, however, does not rule out myocarditis. Viral studies may reveal enteroviral or adenoviral antibodies, Esptein-Barr virus, cytomegalovirus, or a 4-fold increase in the level of immunoglobulin G but do not definitively establish causation. Levels of immunoglobulin G antibodies to Epstein-Barr virus nuclear antigen were elevated in KM. PCR may also be used to detect viral genomes.

Elevation in white blood cell count with predominance of lymphocytes may suggest viral causes of myocarditis. Cultures of blood, stool, cerebrospinal fluid, or nasopharyngeal secretions are less specific than cultures of tracheal aspirates; Martin et al. found that cultures showed growth in only 27% of children with viral myocarditis.

## MANAGEMENT IN MYOCARDITIS (Tables 13.4 and 13.5)

### *Critical Care*

Care of children with clinical features consistent with myocarditis depends on the severity of myocardial dysfunction. Management is designed around supportive measures rather than being aimed at a causative agent. Maintenance of cardiac output with aggressive support of cardiac function is essential. Such support includes initiation and monitoring of inotropic therapy, afterload reduction, arrhythmia management, and adequate tissue oxygenation. Respiratory support may require intubation and mechanical ventilation. Fluid management may include both administration of fluid boluses and diuretic therapy. Monitoring of and interventions to prevent complications should be ongoing.

### *Inotropic Support*

When cardiac output is inadequate, a rapid acting inotropic agent is administered. Inotropic agents are administered cautiously because the myocardium is irritable and use of inotropic agents can instigate and/or worsen arrhythmias. One inotropic agent or a combination of such agents, including dopamine, dobutamine, and milrinone, can be administered .

Dobutamine is often used when the primary cause of inadequate tissue perfusion is cardiac in origin. Dobutamine improves contractility and decreases systemic vascular resistance, providing afterload reduction in addition to improving cardiac output. A mild increase in heart rate can occur, although significant tachycardia is unusual. Although dobutamine increases myocardial oxygen demand in adults with congestive heart failure, in

**Table 13.4:** Contiouns infusion inotropic support

| Drug | Classification | Dose, µg/kg per minute | Action | Adverse effect |
|---|---|---|---|---|
| Dopamine | Sympathomimetic | 0.5–2 | Dopaminergic—renal vasodilatation<br>Promotion of sodium excertion | Tachyarhythmias<br>Reduced renal blood flow at >5 mg kg per minute |
| | | 5–10 | beta-1adrengic effect | |
| | | 10–15 | Mixed alpha1-beta1 adrenergic effect | Increased myocardial oxygen demand |
| | | >20 | Predominantly alpha1-adrenergic effect | Ectopy |
| Dobutamine | Sympathomimetic | 2–20 | Pure beta1-adrenergic effect | Tachycardia<br>Tachyarhythmias<br>Hypotension |
| Epinephrine | Sympathomimetic | 0.1–1.0 | Adrenergic agoinst effect, predominatly alpha1-adrenergic effect | Tachyarrhythmias<br>Ventricular ectopy<br>Hypertension<br>Myocardial ischemia |
| Milrinone | Phosphodiesterase enzyme inhibitor | May use loading dose of 50–75 µg/kg before infusion | Improves contractility<br>Alterload reduction | Hypotension<br>Thrombocytopenia<br>Ventricular ectopy |

**Table 13.5:** Intravenous antiarrhythmic agents

| Drug | Classification | Dose | Action | Adverse effect |
|---|---|---|---|---|
| Adenosine | Antiarrhythmic | 0.05–0.1 mg/kg rapid intravenous bolus<br>Repeated to a maximum of 0.3 mg/kg total<br>Can give 12 mg maximum dose for children who weigh > 50 kg | Slows conduction time through the atriventricular node, interrupting reentry pathways | Arhythmias<br>Bradycardia<br>Heart block<br>Hypotension |
| Digoxin | Cardiac glycoside<br>*Rapid:* 0.4–0.6 mg IV<br>*Contineously:* 0.1–0.3 mg/ 6–8 hourly | | Positive inotropic effects<br>Decreases conduction through the sinoatrial and atrioventricular nodes | Sinus bradycardia<br>Atrioventricular block, sinoalrial block<br>Ventricular arrhythmias<br>Hyperkalemia with toxic effects |
| Amiodarone | Antriarrhythmic | Loading: 1 mg/kg given over 5–10 minutes, can be repeated 5 times | Inhibits adrenergic stimulation | Bradycardia, heart block, sinus arrest, paroxysmal ventricular tachycardia stimulation |
| | | Continuous intravenous infusion at 10–15 mg/kg per day | Decreases atrioventricular node conduction and sinus function | Congestive heart failure, cardiogemic shock, hypotension<br>Pulmonary toxic effect (pneumonitis, fibrosis, acute respiratory distress syndrome) |
| Lidocaine | Antiarrhythmic | Loading: 1 mg/kg followed by a continous infusion of 20–50 ug/kg per minute | Suppressess automatically of the conduction system | Bradycardia, heart block arrhythmias, hypotension, seizures |

children with patent coronary arteries, coronary blood flow, and oxygen supply to the heart actually increase.

Dopamine has both inotropic and vasopressor properties and is useful in patients who are in shock with cardiac dysfunction and associated mild-to-moderate hypotension. Dopamine is not routinely used to tidal volume (pressure ventilation), a decrease in oxygen saturation, and asymmetric chest rise. If the tube migrates into the right main bronchus, the child should immediately be placed back in the previous position and reassessed. Breath sounds should be assessed after any change in body position.

Neck extension increases airway length, potentially causing unintentional extubation because the uncuffed tube can easily pass upward through the vocal cords. Immediate respiratory distress, decrease in oxygen saturation, marked decrease in or undetectable end-tidal carbon dioxide levels, grunting, or vocalization can indicate possible inadvertent extubation. If dislodgement of the endotracheal tube into the esophagus is suspected, the tube should be removed and bag-valve-mask ventilation performed until reintubation or effective spontaneous breathing occurs.

Although a common practice in intensive care units, endotracheal suctioning should not be performed routinely. Suctioning can be associated with complications, including hypoxemia, bradycardia, atelectasis, and dysrhythmias. Suctioning should be done on an as-needed basis rather than routinely. Indications for suctioning include increase in airway pressure, decrease in tidal volume, decrease in oxygen saturation, visualization of secretions in the tube, development of rhonchi, and coughing. Hyperoxygenation may or may not be required before suctioning, depending on the child's arterial oxygenation and tolerance to the procedure. The catheter should not be deeper than the end of the endotracheal tube. Catheters inserted to the point of resistance (carina) cause tissue inflammation and damage. Instillation of normal saline for lavage should be avoided because that practice is not supported by research and may actually be harmful.

Routine bedside nursing interventions such as dressing changes, bathing, weighing, and repositioning all significantly increase tissue oxygen consumption. Delay in carrying out these procedures may be necessary. Conversely, some or all of these activities may be clustered if tolerated in order to allow longer periods of rest.

Fever increases oxygen consumption 10% for each 1°C elevation in body temperature. Although not all fever is 'bad,' treatment of fever is recommended in children with cardiopulmonary disease. Attempts should be made to maintain normothermia. Unless contraindicated, antipyretics (acetaminophen, ibuprofen) should be administered. Fever reduction can also be attempted with external cooling, usually by sponging with tepid water.

Pain and anxiety significantly increase oxygen demand and consumption and cause considerable distress for children in the PICU. Assessment and management of pain and anxiety should be ongoing.

### Arrhythmias

Heart rate and rhythm require monitoring. Arrhythmias are a significant life-threatening complication of myocarditis. Development of bradycardia or tachyarrhythmias is unlikely to be tolerated and requires immediate recognition and treatment (Figs 13.7–13.9).

Infants and small children depend on heart rate for adequate cardiac output because stroke volume is relatively fixed; in young children, bradycardia can rapidly diminish cardiac output. Because chronotropic drugs can induce ventricular tachycardia in patients with viral myocarditis,

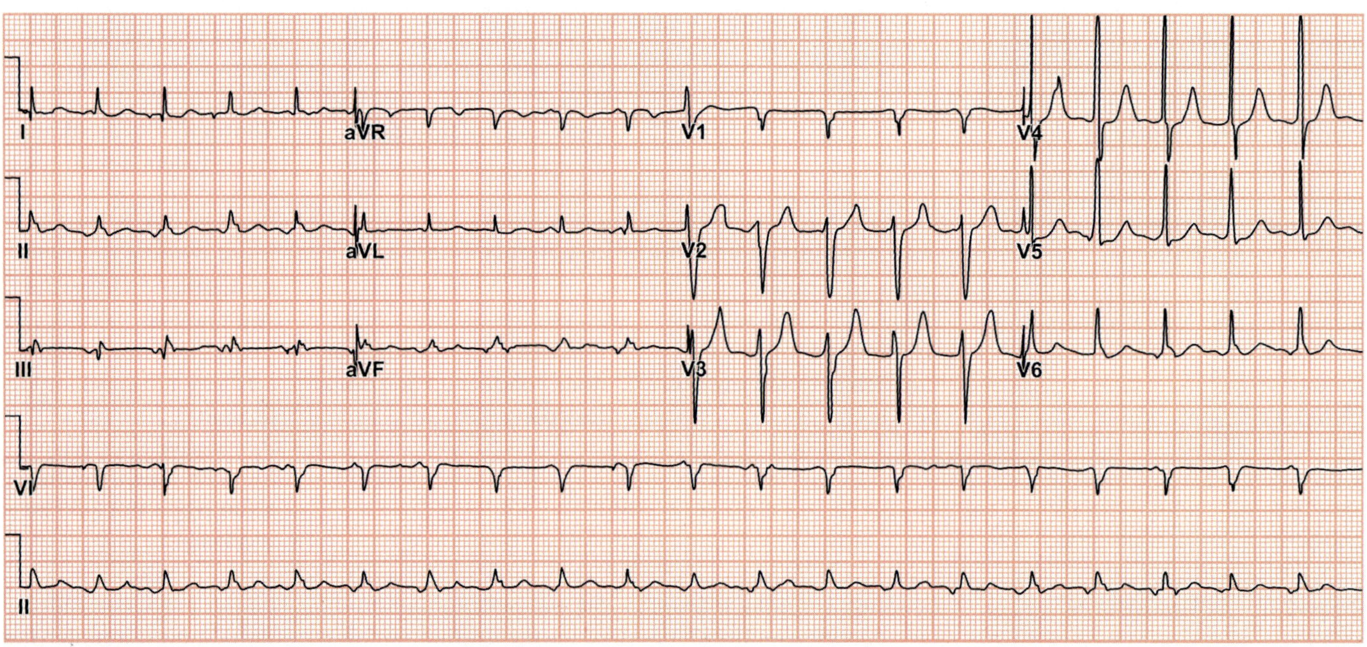


**Fig. 13.7:** Ectopic atrial tachycardia. There is a narrow complex tachycardia at 120 bpm. Each QRS complex is preceded by an abnormal P-wave—upright in V1, inverted in the inferior leads II, III and aVF

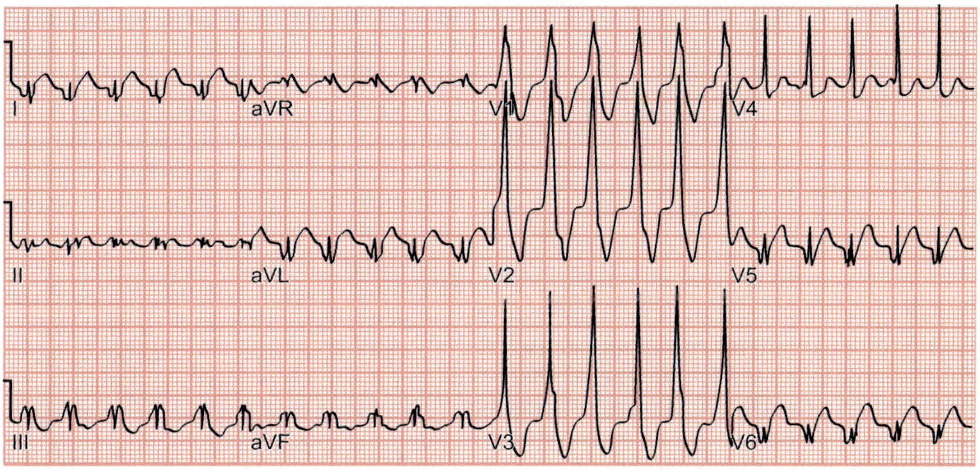


**Fig. 13.8:** ECG demonstrating ventricular tachycardia with right bundle branch block morphology in a patient with myocarditis

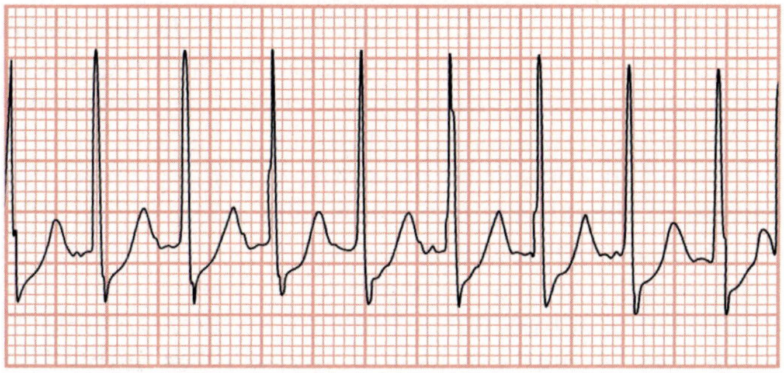

**Fig. 13.9:** ECG showing features of supraventricular tachycardia in a patient with myocarditis

cardiac pacing is the preferred treatment for life-threatening bradyarrhythmias, including atrioventricular block.

Transcutaneous or transthoracic pacing is a noninvasive procedure that can be done rapidly. Two electrodes are placed on the patient with the anterior electrode in the $V_2$ to $V_5$ position and the posterior electrode under the scapula to the left of the spine. Electrode adherence should be checked frequently, especially if the child is diaphoretic. If needed for prolonged periods, electrodes should be changed a minimum of every 24 hours to maintain effectiveness of the contact gel.

For ongoing bradyarrhythmias, invasive pacing should be considered. Transvenous leads are placed percutaneously via a large vessel into the right atrium or ventricle. Leads are stiff; nurses must be alert for indications of ventricular perforation, including cardiac tamponade. An extra battery should be kept at the bedside of any patient who is pacemaker dependent. Hospital policy should be followed when caring for the insertion site and catheter.

Conversely, an excessively rapid heart rate will decrease ventricular filling time, resulting in inadequate preload and subsequent cardiac output. Tachycardias also result in inadequate coronary artery filling time. Coronary arteries fill and perfuse the myocardium during diastole; the faster the heart rate, the shorter is diastole, leading to a decrease in myocardial oxygen supply during a time of increasing consumption.

Differentiation between sinus tachycardia and supraventricular tachycardia is critical. Typically, sinus tachycardia is heart rate greater than 140/min in children, greater than 160/min in infants, and varies from beat to beat. Heart rate generally remains less than 200/min. Sinus tachycardia can be the result of a variety of factors, including fear, anxiety, fever, pain, intravascular dehydration, and marked vasodilatation. Sinus tachycardia will resolve, or partially resolve, with resolution of the inciting factor.

Supraventricular tachycardia is an extremely rapid heart rate (200–280/min); is unresponsive to resolution of fever, pain, hypovolemia, and so on; and has no beat-to-beat variability. Rates of sinus tachycardia and supraventricular tachycardia can overlap, making determination of the type of tachycardia difficult. A 12-lead electrocardiogram may be necessary to differentiate between the two. Once supraventricular tachycardia has been established, rapid treatment with adenosine in the patients with stable hemodynamic status or cardioversion in patients with unstable hemodynamic status is performed. A defibrillator should remain near any child who has myocarditis or recurring supraventricular tachycardia.

### Hemodynamic Monitoring

With invasive hemodynamic monitoring, physiological variables specific to cardiovascular function can be monitored and, when coupled with clinical examination, the results provide data for sound clinical decision making.

### Arterial Pressure

Continuous blood pressure monitoring via an arterial catheter is preferred in children with severe cardiac dysfunction, particularly those who require infusions of vasoactive agents (Fig. 13.10). Noninvasive measurements may be inaccurate or impossible to obtain because of impaired peripheral perfusion and vasoconstriction. Arterial catheters can be placed peripherally (radial artery) or centrally (femoral artery) and provide a dynamic picture of systolic, diastolic, and mean blood pressures. Because evaluations of interventions and their effectiveness will be

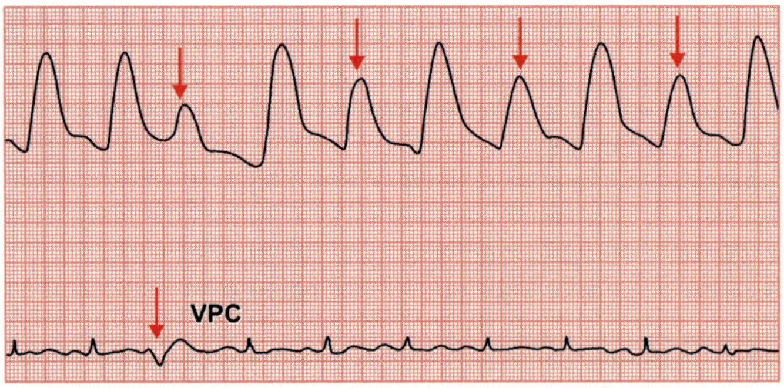


**Fig. 13.10:** Hemodynamic study shows an alternating pulse-arterial pressure recording in severe left ventricular failure. After the second beat a ventricular premature beat triggers an episode of alternating pulse

based partly on invasive measurement of blood pressure, care must be taken to ensure accuracy of readings. Routinely inspecting for proper transducer placement (phlebostatic axis), zeroing the transducer a minimum of once a shift, inspecting for and eliminating air bubbles in the system, and using noncompliant pressure tubing will help ensure accurate measurements.

Normal blood pressure in children is dependent on age and size. As previously noted, however, children with myocarditis can maintain a blood pressure within normal limits for age until very late in the disease. No single clinical parameter should determine critical care interventions, and this rule is particularly true for blood pressure, unless hypotension is present. Adequacy of tissue perfusion is determined by analysis of clinical findings on bedside examination along with blood pressure. The extremity distal to the arterial catheter should be assessed at least once a shift to monitor for any compromise in perfusion related to catheter placement. Extremity coolness, color changes, delayed capillary refill, and diminishing pulse quality can indicate inadequate perfusion. Numbness, tingling, and motor deficit can also be indicators of impaired circulation. Development or change in any one or more of these variables requires immediate attention and potentially removal of the catheter.

### Central Venous Pressure

Central venous pressure (CVP) or right atrial monitoring provides a continual reflection of intravascular volume status and is a good determinant of right ventricular end-diastolic volume, or preload. CVP should be interpreted along with other measures of cardiac function (heart rate, peripheral perfusion, urine output). In critically ill children, the absolute value is not as important as serial measurements and changes in response to interventions.

CVP monitoring should be done via the distal lumen of the catheter. Monitoring can be continual or intermittent, depending on availability of intravenous access. If the distal lumen is being used for continuous intravenous administration of fluids and/or drugs, CVP should be assessed a minimum of once an hour and after any administration of fluid boluses or diuresis. When inter mittent CVP monitoring is used, care must be taken to ensure that no cardiotonic medications are infused through the distal port. If such infusions are used, turning the stopcock for pressure readings causes a disruption in the delivery of medication and potential hemodynamic compromise. Ideally, infusions of inotropic or vasoactive agents should be given through the medial or proximal lumen only.

Normal CVP values can vary widely in infants and children, depending on age, disease, concomitant conditions, and critical care therapies. In healthy infants, normal values can range from –2 to +4 mmHg, from 4 to 8 mmHg in those with congenital heart disease, and from 2 to 6 mmHg in those with respiratory disease requiring mechanical ventilation. In this age group, measurements above 8 mmHg are generally indicative of myocardial dysfunction or high intrathoracic pressure. In older children without underlying disease, a CVP range of 2 to 6 mmHg is considered normal. Values can vary markedly and should be interpreted along with the child's underlying disease state, concomitant conditions, and critical care therapies.

CVP measurements do not stand alone and must be considered in context of the entire clinical picture. Any changes in intrathoracic pressure will affect CVP values; spontaneous respirations decrease CVP, whereas increased intrathoracic pressure increases CVP. Values lower than expected may or may not indicate hypovolemia; high CVP values may or may not indicate hypervolemia. Elevated CVP values may also occur in patients receiving positive pressure ventilation and with the addition of positive end-expiratory pressure. Conditions that increase pulmonary vascular resistance (hypothermia, hypoxemia, acidosis, severe respiratory disease, underlying pulmonary hypertension) also increase CVP. High CVP values do not necessarily reflect cardiac disease but may be an indication of elevated right ventricular end-diastolic pressure, suggesting right ventricular dysfunction. Variables that affect interpretation of CVP values must be considered when therapies are determined.

*Complications of central venous catheters* include bloodstream infection (increased risk with multilumen catheters), venous thrombosis, thrombophlebitis, and catheter occlusion. Routine maintenance of the catheter and insertion site should be done per hospital policy.

### Pulmonary Artery Pressure

Pulmonary artery catheters can provide valuable information in children with cardiopulmonary failure. The ability to measure pulmonary artery pressures, cardiac output/index, and systemic and pulmonary vascular resistance can provide important data for directing therapies. However, because of potential complications, pulmonary artery catheters tend to be used less often in children than in adults. Pulmonary artery catheters are therefore indicated only when the additional data obtained will enhance clinical decision making.

### Hospital-acquired Infections

Hospital-acquired infections are a constant threat for any critically ill child in the PICU. Acquired nosocomial infection coupled with extreme severity of illness in a child with myocarditis significantly increases morbidity and mortality. Nurses' diligence in preventing and monitoring for infection is essential. Within hours of admission, hospital-associated bacteria can be detected on skin and in the respiratory and genitourinary tracts. Invasive devices, antibiotic use, and/or critical care procedures increase the risk of bacterial invasion. Some of the highest rates of hospital-acquired infection occur in PICUs; bloodstream infection and ventilator-associated pneumonia are the most common.

Fever is often the first sign of infection in children; however, infants often have decreases in body temperature because of the immaturity of the brain's temperature-regulating center. Monitoring of temperature changes in this age group can be complicated by the use of radiant warmers, designed to maintain normothermia. Radiant warmer temperature is adjusted according to an infant's skin temperature; consequently, decreases in body temperature related to infection may be masked. Although skin temperature is continuously monitored in infants under a radiant warmer, core body temperature should be monitored a minimum of once an hour, if not continuously, in all age groups. White blood cell count with a differential count should be assessed closely. Leukocytosis (elevation) or leukopenia (decrease) develop in children with infection, depending on age. A normal total white blood cell count is 5000–10 000 cells/µL but varies depending on the age of the child; the younger the child, the higher the upper range limit. Monitoring trends is as important as getting absolute counts.

The differential count provides the percentage of each subset of white blood cells (eosinophils, neutrophils, basophils, monocytes, and lymphocytes) and can aid in differentiating the type of infection. In older infants and children, a 'shift to the left,' or an excess of immature neutrophils (bands), usually indicates bacterial infection. An increase in the number or percentage of bands along with fever may warrant further workup (e.g. blood cultures for detection of secondary bacterial infection). Coagulase-negative staphylococci are the most common cause of nosocomial bloodstream infections in the PICU. Unlike older children, young infants commonly have neutropenia when infected because of their small storage pools and inability to produce white blood cells at a fast rate.

Pulmonary secretions should be monitored for changes in viscosity, color, and amount. Changes in the character of the secretions along with evidence of new pulmonary infiltrates may indicate the development of ventilator-associated pneumonia (the second most common hospital-acquired infection in PICUs) in intubated patients. Although nosocomial urinary tract infections occur less often than do acquired bloodstream or pulmonary infections in children, urine should be routinely examined for color, odor, and changes in opacity, particularly if a child has a urinary catheter in place.

Any invasive catheter is a potential source of infection. Insertion sites should be routinely inspected for edema, redness, and drainage. Although central venous catheters are not routinely changed in children, signs of infection at the site may warrant removal of the catheter. Factors increasing the risk for bloodstream infection include multilumen catheters, repeated catheterizations, and certain types of dressing. In order to minimize risk of infection, catheters should be manipulated as little as possible and should be removed as soon as they are no longer needed.

Immobility and alteration in tissue perfusion increase the potential for skin breakdown. Skin should be kept free from exposure to moisture and secretions; moisture-barrier products can be applied to the perineal area. Application of topical moisturizers, with avoidance of products containing perfume or alcohol, aids in maintaining skin hydration. Mouth care, a minimum of every 8 hours, helps keep oral mucosa clean and moist. In children without a blink response (chemically paralyzed) or with incomplete lid closure, the eyes should be kept moist with artificial tears and/or lubricant as needed. Frequent turning (as tolerated), alleviation of pressure points on bony prominences (use of pillows, stuffed animals), and alternating pressure points related to mechanical devices (oxygen saturation probes, blood pressure cuffs, and electrodes) should be performed on a routine basis. Air mattresses or rotating beds can also be used to prevent skin breakdown. Any evidence of altered skin integrity should be immediately addressed.

### Prognosis in Myocarditis

The survival rate in children and adults with myocarditis is approximately 80%. Lee et al. found that patients who died almost always did so within the first few hospital days. Survival after 72 hours in patients not requiring ECMO is as high as 97%. Some centers have had a 1-year survival rate of 80% in children who required mechanical circulatory support.

Unfortunately, survival to discharge does not imply full recovery. Although Lee et al. found that recovery of ventricular function without the need for ongoing cardiac medications or restrictions in physical activity was the norm, some evidence suggests that myocarditis can progress to dilated cardiomyopathy. Viral persistence in the myocardium has been associated with progressive impairment of left ventricular function and is predictive of adverse outcomes. Progression from myocarditis to dilated cardiomyopathy is further supported by the finding of a coxsackie virus B—adenovirus receptor gene present in larger amounts in the myocardium of patients with dilated cardiomyopathy than in healthy hearts. The discovery of this receptor also suggests a role in not only the viral origin of myocarditis but also the occasional 'familial' case of myocarditis. Survival in children with dilated cardiomyopathy ranges from 60% to 70% at 1 year to 34–56% at 5 years. Gagliardi et al. reported that in children with dilated cardiomyopathy, the first 2 years after diagnosis are the most crucial. Favorable events (nearly complete recovery) and worse outcomes (death or need for a transplant) occur during this period. For children with residual myocardial dysfunction at discharge, diuretics and afterload reducers are considered first-line agents. Diuretics are used for congestive heart failure of any cause because they reduce respiratory signs and symptoms associated with heart failure. Thiazides (diuril, hydrochlorothiazide) are often used; the addition of spironolactone may obviate potassium supplementation. Angiotensin-converting enzyme inhibitors (captopril and enalapril) may also improve chronic signs and symptoms

*The use of digoxin in patients with chronic congestive heart failure as a result of myocarditis remains controversial.* The poor diastolic function associated with myocarditis is not improved with digoxin. Digoxin also increases the risk of ventricular arrhythmias if myocardial inflammation is still present. If digoxin is used, digitalization should be accomplished during a 24–36-hour period with 75% of the usual total loading dose to minimize the possibility of arrhythmia development.

Beta-blockade may improve outcome in children with dilated cardiomyopathy. Carvedilol, a nonselective beta-blocker used in adults, has been examined as an adjunct therapy for management of heart failure in children. Carvedilol may improve congestive heart failure through several mechanisms, including decreased heart rate leading to improved myocardial oxygen consumption and enhanced coronary artery blood flow, improvement in left ventricular ejection fraction, and reduction in neurohormonal vasoconstrictor systems. Carvedilol may also prevent ventricular arrhythmias and sudden death.

*Use of carvedilol* in children remains controversial. Bruns et al. studied the use of carvedilol in 46 children with heart failure in 6 different centers and found improvement in left ventricular function and overall signs and symptoms in 67%. Schwartz and Wessel also examined use of carvedilol in children with heart failure and found no statistically significant effect; left ventricular ejection fraction improved in both the carvedilol and the placebo groups. Although carvedilol is effective in reducing mortality in adults, more research into the use of carvedilol is needed in children with heart failure.

*Transplantation* is sometimes the only option for children with significant cardiac failure or dilated cardiomyopathy due to myocarditis. Preferably, children are not put on a list for transplantation until they have progressed to the chronic phase of the disease, because recovery is possible in even the most severe cases. Transplantation may, however, be considered an option for a child who requires ECMO for more than 10 days and has no clinical signs of improvement.

## SUMMARY

Viral myocarditis remains an uncommon but challenging illness. In children, the initial signs and symptoms are often those of common pediatric illnesses and without any obvious cardiac signs. Adding to the challenge is the potential inability of the child to convey precise symptoms or describe location or intensity of pain or discomfort. A history of asthma or congenital heart disease can skew the clinical picture. Although few children actually have viral myocarditis diagnosed and require admission to the PICU, practitioners must maintain a heightened sense of awareness for the 'zebra in the herd of horses.' Concomitantly, for any previously healthy child with sudden cardiogenic shock, myocarditis must be included in the differential diagnosis.

Most children with myocarditis recover without requiring admission to the PICU; only a small percentage progress to development of significant cardiopulmonary compromise that requires intensive cardiopulmonary support and monitoring. Critical care management is aimed at supportive rather than curative measures and depends on the severity of myocardial dysfunction. The most common techniques used in the PICU for children with cardiovascular compromise or collapse include invasive hemodynamic monitoring, infusions of inotropic agents, antiarrhythmics, afterload reducers, mechanical ventilation, prevention of complications, and, when a child is unresponsive to ordinary PICU therapies, extracorporeal life support.

### KEY POINTS IN ACUTE MYOCARDITIS

Myocarditis, an inflammation of the myocardium, is classified as idiopathic in more than 50% of patients. Other causes include viruses or bacteria, various toxins including alcohol, or those causes secondary to a coexisting systematic disease such as HIV or lupus erythematosus.

Although myocarditis often resolves spontaneously without treatment, some patients present with heart failure, cardiogenic shock, or cardiac arrhythmias, all of which require urgent treatment as appropriate.

Diagnosis is complicated owing to the highly variable clinical presentation of myocarditis and the difficulty in providing laboratory confirmation of the diagnosis and etiology. Blood troponin I (TnI) and creatine kinase (CK)-MB cardiac enzyme levels and imaging studies such as echocardiography or magnetic resonance imaging (MRI) may be helpful, but a myocardial biopsy remains the gold standard.

Treatment includes therapy targeted at the cause of myocarditis if an infectious agent or toxic substance, and supportive therapy aimed at the clinical manifestations such as congestive heart failure and arrhythmias. Multiple treatment approaches for viral myocarditis are currently under evaluation. In particular, immunoglobulin and immunosuppressive therapy have shown promise in selected small clinical trials.

*Contd...*

*Contd...*

Prognosis depends on both the individual patient and the causative agent. Overall mortality rates vary. The Myocarditis Treatment trial, currently the largest clinical study to evaluate long-term prognosis of myocarditis, showed a 20% mortality rate at 1.0 year and a 56% mortality rate at 4.3 years

Urgent antitoxin treatment may be indicated in cases in which myocarditis is caused by the *Corynebacterium diphtheriae* bacteria.

## BIBLIOGRAPHY


1. Adhoot J, Galindo A, Alejos JC, et al. Use of OKT3 for acute myocarditis in infants and children. J Heart Lung Transplant 2000;19(11):1118–21.
2. Akhtar N, Ni J, Stromberg D, Rosenthal GL, Bowles NE, Towbin JA. Tracheal aspirate as a substrate for polymerase chain reaction detection of viral genome in childhood pneumonia and myocarditis. Circulation 1999;99(15): 2011–8.
3. American Heart Association 2006.
4. Archard LC, Khan MA, Soteriou BA, Why HJ, Robinson NM, Richardson PJ. Characterization of coxsackie B virus RNA in myocardium from patients with dilated cardiomyopathy by nucleotide sequencing of reverse transcription-nested polymerase chain reaction products. Hum Pathol 1998; 29(6):578–84.
5. Aretz HT, Billingham ME, Edwards WD, et al. Myocarditis: a histopathologic definition and classification. Am J Cardiovasc Pathol 1987;1(1):3–14.
6. Baboonian C, McKenna W. Eradication of viral myocarditis: is there hope? J Am Coll Cardiol 2003;42(3):473–6.
7. Batra AS, Lewis AB. Acute myocarditis. Curr Opin Pediatr 2001;13(3):234–9.
8. Baughman KL. Diagnosis of myocarditis: death of Dallas criteria. Circulation 2006;113(4):593–5.
9. Bohn D, Macrae D, Chang AC. Acute viral myocarditis: mechanical circulatory support. Pediatr Crit Care Med 2006;7(6)(Suppl):S21–S24.
10. Bowles NE, Towbin JA. Molecular aspects of myocarditis. Curr Infect Dis Rep 2000;2(4):308–14.
11. Calabrese F, Rigo E, Milanesi O, et al. Molecular diagnosis of myocarditis and dilated cardiomyopathy in children: clinicopathologic features and prognostic implications. Diagn Mol Pathol 2002;11(4):212–21.
12. Chavda KK, Dhuper S, Makhok A, Chowdjury D. Seizures secondary to a high-grade atrioventricular block as a presentation of acute myocarditis. Pediatr Emerg Care 2004; 20(6):387–90.
13. Craig J, Fineman LD, Moynihan P, Baker AL. Cardiovascular critical care problems.In: Curley MAQ, Moloney-Harmon PA, eds. Critical Care Nursing of Infants and Children, 2nd ed. Philadelphia, PA: WB Saunders Co, 2001;629–31.
14. Curley MAQ, Meyer EC. Caring practices: the impact of the critical care experience on the family. In: Curley MAQ, Moloney-Harmon PA. Critical Care Nursing of Infants and Children. 2nd ed. Philadelphia, PA: WB Saunders Co, 2001;47–67.
15. Curley MAQ, Thompson JE. Oxygenation and ventilation. In: Curley MAQ, Moloney-Harmon, PA. Critical Care Nursing of Infants and Children. 2nd ed. Philadelphia, PA: WB Saunders Co, 2001;233–308.
16. Drucker NA, Colan SD, Lewis AB, et al. Gamma-globulin treatment of acute myocarditis in the pediatric population. Circulation 1994;89(1):252–7.
17. Drucker NA, Newburger JW. Viral myocarditis: diagnosis and management. Adv Pediatr 1997;44:141–69.
18. Feldman AM, McNamara D. Medical progress: myocarditis. N Engl J Med 2000;343(19):1388–98.
19. Friedman RA. Myocarditis. In: Garson A, Bricher JT, McNamara DG, eds. The Science and Practice of Pediatric Cardiology. Philadelphia, PA: Lea & Febiger 1990;1577–89.
20. Fujioka S, Kitaura Y, Ukimara A, et al. Evaluation of viral infection in the myocardium of patients with idiopathic dilated cardiomyopathy. J Am Coll Cardiol 2000;36(6):1920–6.
21. Gagliardi MG, Bevilacqua M, Bassano C, et al. Long-term follow-up of children with myocarditis treated by immuno-suppression and of children with dilated cardiomyopathy. Heart 2004;90(10):1167–71
22. Hastings LA, Heitmiller ES, Nyhan D. Peri-operative monitoring. In: Nichols DG, Ungerleider RM, Spevak PJ, et al. Critical Heart Disease in Infants and Children. 2nd ed. Philadelphia, PA: Mosby 2006;479–506.
23. Hazinski MF. Children are different. In: Hazinski MF. Nursing Care of the Critically Ill Child. 2nd ed. St Louis, MO: Mosby, 1992;1–17.
24. Hoffman TM, Wernovsky G, Atz AM, et al. Efficacy and safety of milrinone in preventing low cardiac output syndrome in infants and children after corrective surgery for congenital heart disease. Circulation 2003;107(7):996–1002.
25. Kawai C. From myocarditis to cardiomyopathy: mechanisms of inflammation and cell death. Circulation 1999;99(8):1091–1100.
26. Kühl U, Pauschinger M, Noutsias, M, Kapp JF, Schultheiss HP. Diagnosis and treatment of patients with virus induced inflammatory cardiomyopathy. Eur Heart J Suppl 2002; 4(Suppl I):I73–I80.
27. Lauer B, Neiderau C, Kuhl U, et al. Cardiac troponin T in patients with clinically suspected myocarditis. J Am Coll Cardiol 1997;30(5):1354–9
28. Lee KJ, McCrindle BW, Bohn DJ, et al. Clinical outcomes of acute myocarditis in childhood. Heart 1999;82(2):226–33.
29. Leonard EG. Viral myocarditis. Pediatr Infect Dis J 2004; 23(7):665–66.
30. Levi D, Alejos J. Diagnosis and treatment of pediatric viral myocarditis. Curr Opin Cardiol 2001;16:77–83.
31. Macrae D, Chang AC. Pediatric cardiac intensive care consensus: myocarditis. Paper presented at: Pediatric Cardiac Intensive Care Symposium; December 11, 2005; Miami, FL.
32. Martin AB, Webber S, Fricker FJ, et al. Congenital cardiovascular disease/diabetes: acute myocarditis: rapid diagnosis by PCR in children. Circulation 1994;90(1):330–9.
33. Matsumori A, Igata H, Ono K, et al. High doses of digitalis increase the myocardial production of proinflammatory cytokines and worsen myocardial injury in viral myocarditis: a possible mechanism of digitalis toxicity. Jpn Circ J 1999;63(12):934–40.

34. McCarthy RE, Boehmer JP, Hruban RH, et al. Long-term outcome of fulminant myocarditis as compared with acute (non-fulminant) myocarditis. N Engl J Med 2000; 342(10):690–5.
35. Mecham N. Acute viral myocarditis in the ED pediatric patient: three case presentations. J Emerg Nurs 2004;30(2): 179–82.
36. Nguyen QV. Hospital-acquired infections. http://www.emedicine.com/ped/topic1619.htm. Updated August 21, 2007. Accessed November 27, 2007.
37. Park MK, Troxler RG. Pediatric Cardiology for Practitioners. 4th ed. St Louis, MO: Mosby 2002;289–90.
38. Pophal SG, Sigfusson G, Booth KL, et al. Complications of endomyocardial biopsy in children. J Am Coll Cardiol 1999; 34(7): 2105–10.
39. Pres S, Lipkind RS. Acute myocarditis in infants: initial presentation. Clin Pediatr. 1990;29(2):73–6.
40. Schwartz SM, Wessel DM. Medical cardiovascular support in acute viral myocarditis in children. Pediatr Crit Care Med 2006;7(6)(Suppl):S12–S16.
41. Slota MC. Clinical assessment of cardiovascular function. In: Slota MC (Ed.). Core Curriculum for Pediatric Critical Care Nursing. 2nd ed. Philadelphia, PA: WB Saunders Co, 2006; 176–85.
42. Thompson A. Pediatric emergency airway management. In: Dieckmann RA, Fiser DH, Selbst SM (Eds.) Illustrated Textbook of Pediatric Emergency and Critical Care Procedures. Louis, MO: Mosby-Yearbook Inc, 1997;104–15.
43. Throckmorton AL, Lim DS, McCulloch MA, et al. Computational design and experimental performance testing of an axial-flow pediatric ventricular assist device. ASAIO J 2005; 51(5):629–35.
44. Tobias JD, Deshpande JK, Johns JA, Nichols DG. Inflammatory heart disease. In: Nichols DG, Ungerleider RM, Spevak PJ, et al. (Eds.) 2nd ed. Critical Heart Disease in Infants and Children. Philadelphia, PA: Mosby, 2006:899–925.
45. Weiss WJ. Pulsatile pediatric ventricular assist devices. ASAIO J 2005;51(5):540–5.
46. Woodruff JF. Viral myocarditis. Am J Pathol 1980;101(2): 427–84.
47. Yong ES, Timmons OD, Uhl MW, et al. Reduction of blood gases in a pediatric ICU (PICU): a process improvement. Paper presented at: 11th Annual Pediatric Critical Care Colloquium; September 1998; Chicago, IL.

# 14 Cardiac Tamponade

Cardiac tamponade is a clinical syndrome caused by the accumulation of fluid in the pericardial space, resulting in reduced ventricular filling and subsequent hemodynamic compromise. Cardiac tamponade is a medical emergency. The overall risk of death depends on the speed of diagnosis, the treatment provided, and the underlying cause of the tamponade.

## PATHOPHYSIOLOGY

The pericardium, which is the membrane surrounding the heart, is composed of 2 layers. The thicker parietal pericardium is the outer fibrous layer; the thinner visceral pericardium is the inner serous layer. The pericardial space normally contains 20–50 ml of fluid. Pericardial effusions can be serous, serosanguineous, hemorrhagic, or chylous (Fig. 14.1).

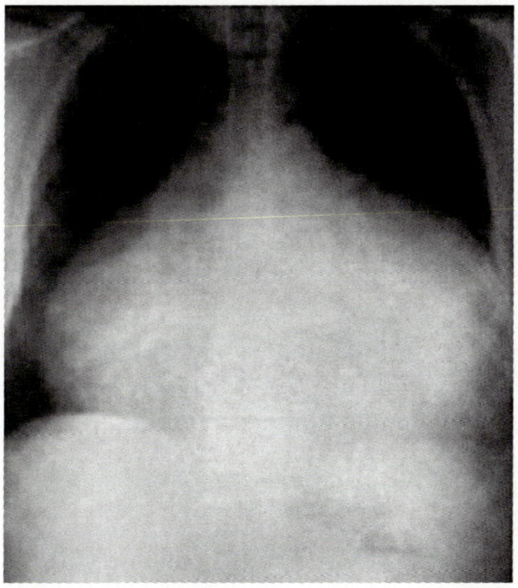

**Fig. 14.1:** This anteroposterior view chest radiograph shows a massive bottle-shaped heart and conspicuous absence of pulmonary vascular congestion

### Stages of Hemodynamic Changes in Tamponade

- **Phase I:** The accumulation of pericardial fluid causes increased stiffness of the ventricle, requiring a higher filling pressure. During this phase, the left and right ventricular filling pressures are higher than the intrapericardial pressure.
- **Phase II:** With further fluid accumulation, the pericardial pressure increases above the ventricular filling pressure, resulting in reduced cardiac output.
- **Phase III:** A further decrease in cardiac output occurs, which is due to equilibration of pericardial and left ventricular (LV) filling pressures.

The underlying pathophysiologic process for the development of tamponade is markedly diminished diastolic filling because transmural distending pressures are insufficient to overcome the increased intrapericardial pressures. Tachycardia is the initial cardiac response to these changes to maintain the cardiac output. Systemic venous return is also altered during tamponade. Because the heart is compressed throughout the cardiac cycle due to the increased intrapericardial pressure, systemic venous return is impaired and right atrial and right ventricular collapse occurs. Because the pulmonary vascular bed is a vast and compliant circuit, blood preferentially accumulates in the venous circulation, at the expense of LV filling. This results in reduced cardiac output and venous return. The amount of pericardial fluid needed to impair the diastolic filling of the heart depends on the rate of fluid accumulation and the compliance of the pericardium. Rapid accumulation of as little as 150 ml of fluid can result in a marked increase in pericardial pressure and can severely impede cardiac output, whereas 1000 ml of fluid may accumulate over a longer period without any significant effect on diastolic filling of the heart. This is due to adaptive stretching of the pericardium over time. A more compliant pericardium can allow considerable fluid accumulation over a longer period without hemodynamic insult.

### Mortality/Morbidity

Cardiac tamponade is a medical emergency. Early diagnosis and treatment are crucial to reduce morbidity and mortality. Untreated, it is rapidly and universally fatal.

### Sex

In children, cardiac tamponade is more common in boys than in girls, with a male-to-female ratio of 7:3. In adults, cardiac tamponade appears to be slightly more common in men than in women. The male-to-female ratio of 1.25:1 observed at author's referral center based on the international classification of diseases (ICD) code 423.9. However, a male-to-female ratio of 1.7:1 is observed at another level 1 trauma center.

### Age

Cardiac tamponade related to trauma or HIV is more common in young adults, whereas tamponade due to malignancy and/or renal failure occurs more frequently in elderly individuals.

### Clinical History

Symptoms vary with the underlying cause and the acuteness of the tamponade. Patients with acute tamponade may present with dyspnea, tachycardia, and tachypnea. Cold and clammy extremities from hypoperfusion are also observed in some patients.

A comprehensive review of the patient's history usually helps identify the probable etiology of a pericardial effusion, which may result in cardiac tamponade.

- Patients with systemic or malignant disease present with weight loss, fatigue, or anorexia.
- Chest pain may be the presenting symptom in patients with pericarditis or myocardial infarction.
- Musculoskeletal pain or fever may be present in patients with an underlying connective tissue disorder.
- A history of renal failure can lead to a consideration of uremia as a cause of pericardial effusion.
- Careful review of a patient's medications may indicate drug-related lupus leading to a pericardial effusion.
- Recent cardiovascular surgery, coronary intervention, or trauma can lead to the rapid accumulation of pericardial fluid and tamponade.
- Recent pacemaker lead implantation or central venous catheter insertion can lead to the rapid accumulation of pericardial fluid and tamponade.
- Consider HIV-related pericardial effusion and tamponade if the patient has a history of intravenous drug abuse or opportunistic infections.
- Inquire about chest wall radiation (i.e. for lung, mediastinal, or esophageal cancer).
- Inquire about symptoms of night sweats, fever, and weight loss, which may be indicative of tuberculosis.

## PHYSICAL EXAMINATION

In a retrospective study, the most common symptoms noted by Roy et al are dyspnea, tachycardia, and elevated jugular venous pressure. Evidence of chest wall injury may be present in trauma patients. Tachycardia, tachypnea, and hepatomegaly are observed in more than 50% of patients with cardiac tamponade, and diminished heart sounds and a pericardial friction rub are present in approximately one third of patients. Some patients may present with dizziness, drowsiness, or palpitations. Cold, clammy skin and weak pulse due to hypotension are also observed in patients with tamponade.

- The **Beck triad** or acute compression triad
  - Described in 1935, this complex of physical findings refers to increased jugular venous pressure, hypotension, and diminished heart sounds.
  - These findings result from a rapid accumulation of pericardial fluid. However, this classic triad is usually observed in patients with acute cardiac tamponade.
- **Pulsus paradoxus or paradoxical pulse**
  - This is an exaggeration (>12 mmHg or 9%) of the normal inspiratory decrease in systemic blood pressure.
  - To measure the pulsus paradoxus, patients are often placed in a semirecumbent position; respirations should be normal. The blood pressure cuff is inflated to at least 20 mmHg above the systolic pressure and slowly deflated until the first Korotkoff sounds are heard only during expiration. At this pressure reading, if the cuff is not further deflated and a pulsus paradoxus is present, the first Korotkoff sound is not audible during inspiration. As the cuff is further deflated, the point at which the first Korotkoff sound is audible during both inspiration and expiration is recorded. If the difference between the first and second measurement is greater than 12 mmHg, an abnormal pulsus paradoxus is present.
  - The paradox is that while listening to the heart sounds during inspiration, the pulse weakens or may not be palpated with certain heartbeats, while S1 is heard with all heartbeats.
  - A pulsus paradoxus can be observed in patients with other conditions, such as constrictive pericarditis, severe obstructive pulmonary disease, restrictive cardiomyopathy, pulmonary embolism, rapid and labored breathing, and right ventricular infarction with shock.
  - A pulsus paradoxus may be absent in patients with markedly elevated LV diastolic pressures, atrial septal defect, pulmonary hypertension, and aortic regurgitation.
- **Kussmaul sign**
  - This was described by Adolph Kussmaul as a paradoxical increase in venous distention and pressure during inspiration.

  - This sign is usually observed in patients with constrictive pericarditis but occasionally is observed in patients with effusive-constrictive pericarditis and cardiac tamponade.
- **Ewart sign**
  - Also known as the Pins sign, this is observed in patients with large pericardial effusions.
  - It is described as an area of dullness, with bronchial breath sounds and bronchophony below the angle of the left scapula.
- **The y descent**
  - The y descent is abolished in the jugular venous or right atrial waveform.
  - This is due to an increase in intrapericardial pressure, preventing diastolic filling of the ventricles.
- **Dysphoria:** Behavioral traits such as restless body movements, unusual facial expressions, restlessness, sense of impending death were reported by Ikematsu in about 26% patients with cardiac tamponade.
- **Low-pressure tamponade:** In severely hypovolemic patients, classical physical findings such as tachycardia, pulsus paradoxus, and jugular venous distension were infrequent. Sagrista-Sauleda et al. identified low-pressure tamponade in 20% of patients with cardiac tamponade. They also reported low-pressure tamponade in 10% of large pericardial effusions.

## AETIOLOGICAL FACTORS

For all patients, malignant diseases are the most common cause of pericardial tamponade. Among etiology of tamponade, Merce et al. reported malignant diseases in 30–60% of cases, uremia in 10–15% of cases, idiopathic pericarditis in 5–15%, infectious diseases in 5–10%, anticoagulation in 5–10%, connective tissue diseases in 2–6%, and Dressler or postpericardiotomy syndrome in 1–2%. Tamponade can occur as a result of any type of pericarditis.

- HIV infection
- Infection—viral, bacterial (tuberculosis), fungal
- Drugs—hydralazine, procainamide, isoniazid, and minoxidil
- Postcoronary intervention (i.e. coronary dissection and perforation)
- Trauma to the chest
- Cardiovascular surgery (postoperative pericarditis)
- Postmyocardial infarction (free wall ventricular rupture, Dressler syndrome)
- Connective tissue diseases—systemic lupus erythematosus, rheumatoid arthritis, and dermatomyositis
- Radiation therapy to the chest
- Iatrogenic—after sternal biopsy, transvenous pacemaker lead implantation, pericardiocentesis, or central line insertion
- Uremia
- Anticoagulation treatment
- Idiopathic pericarditis
- Complication of surgery at the esophagogastric junction such as antireflux surgery
- Pneumopericardium (due to mechanical ventilation or gastropericardial fistula)
- Other causes include hypothyroidism, acupuncture, Still disease, and Duchenne muscular dystrophy
- Type A aortic dissection

## DIFFERENTIAL DIAGNOSES

- Cardiogenic shock
- Pericarditis, constrictive
- Pericarditis, constrictive-effusive
- Pulmonary embolism
- Tension pneumothorax

### Other Problems may Cause Concern

*Large pleural effusion:* Cases of cardiac tamponade have been reported with large pleural effusions. The increased intrapleural pressure resulting from large pleural effusions can be transmitted to the pericardial space and impair ventricular filling, thus simulating the hemodynamic equivalent of cardiac tamponade.

*Tension pneumopericardium:* The hemodynamic changes simulate acute cardiac tamponade. Clinically, distant heart sounds, bradycardia, and shifting tympany occur over the precordium and a characteristic murmur is heard, termed bruit de la roue de moulin. This is usually observed in infants with mechanical ventilation but is also observed after sternal bone marrow aspiration, penetrating chest wall injury, esophageal rupture, and bronchopericardial fistula.

*Rapid and labored breathing:* Large decreases in intrathoracic pressure with deep inspirations, often observed during respiratory failure, can accentuate the pulsus paradoxus, simulating pericardial tamponade.

## LABORATORY STUDIES

- *Creatine kinase and isoenzymes:* Levels are elevated in patients with myocardial infarction and cardiac trauma.
- *Renal profile and CBC count with differential:* These tests are useful in the diagnosis of uremia and certain infectious diseases associated with pericarditis.
- *Coagulation panel:* The prothrombin time and activated partial thromboplastin time are useful for determining bleeding risk during interventions, such as pericardial drainage, the placement of pericardial windows, or both.
- *Antinuclear antibody assay, erythrocyte sedimentation rate, and rheumatoid factor:* Although nonspecific, results from these tests may give clues to a connective tissue disease predisposing to the development of pericardial effusion.
- *HIV testing:* Approximately 24% of all pericardial effusions are reported to be associated with HIV infection.
- *Purified protein derivative testing:* This is used to diagnose tuberculosis, which is an important and not uncommon cause of pericardial effusion and tamponade.

## Imaging

Chest radiography findings may show cardiomegaly, water bottle-shaped heart, pericardial calcifications, or evidence of chest wall trauma. This anteroposterior-view chest radiograph shows a massive bottle-shaped heart and conspicuous absence of pulmonary vascular congestion.

- Bowed catheter sign on chest radiograph in children after central venous catheter insertion may be suggestive of tamponade.

  **Echocardiography** provides useful information, cardiac tamponade is a clinical. The following may be observed with 2-dimensional echocardiography (Figs 14.2–14.5):

  - An echo-free space posterior and anterior to the left ventricle and behind the left atrium: After cardiac surgery, a localized posterior fluid collection without significant anterior effusion may occur and may readily compromise cardiac output.
  - Early diastolic collapse of the right ventricular free wall
  - Early diastolic collapse of right ventricular free wall (subcostal view)
  - Early diastolic collapse of right ventricular free wall (parasternal short-axis view at aortic valve)
  - Late diastolic compression/collapse of the right atrium
  - Late diastolic collapse of right atrium (subcostal view)
  - Swinging of the heart in its sac
  - LV pseudohypertrophy
  - Inferior vena cava plethora with minimal or no collapse with inspiration
  - Dilated inferior vena cava
  - A greater than 40% relative inspiratory augmentation of right-side flow
  - A greater than 25% relative decrease in inspiratory flow across the mitral valve

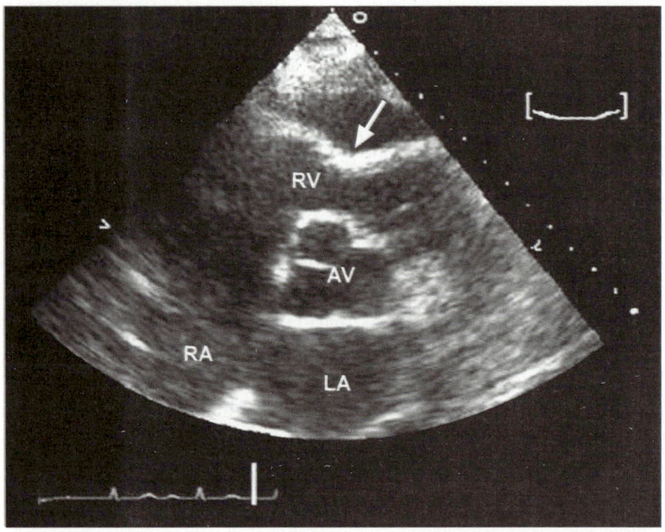


**Fig. 14.2:** Early diastolic collapse of right ventricular free wall (parasternal short-axis view at aortic valve)

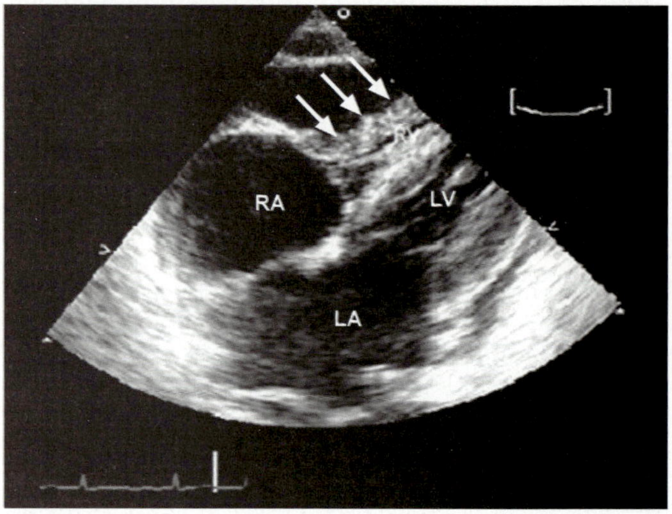


**Fig.14.4:** Early diastolic collapse of right ventricular free wall (subcostal view)

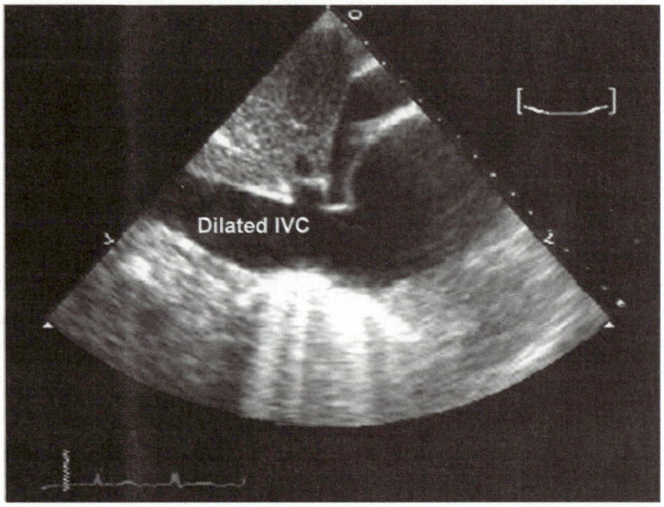


**Fig.14.3:** Dilated inferior vena cava in cardiac tamopnade

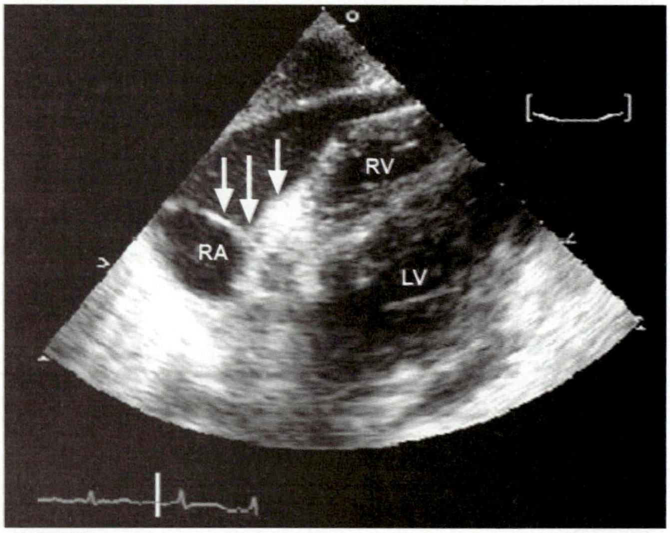


**Fig. 14.5:** Late diastolic collapse of right atrium (subcostal view)

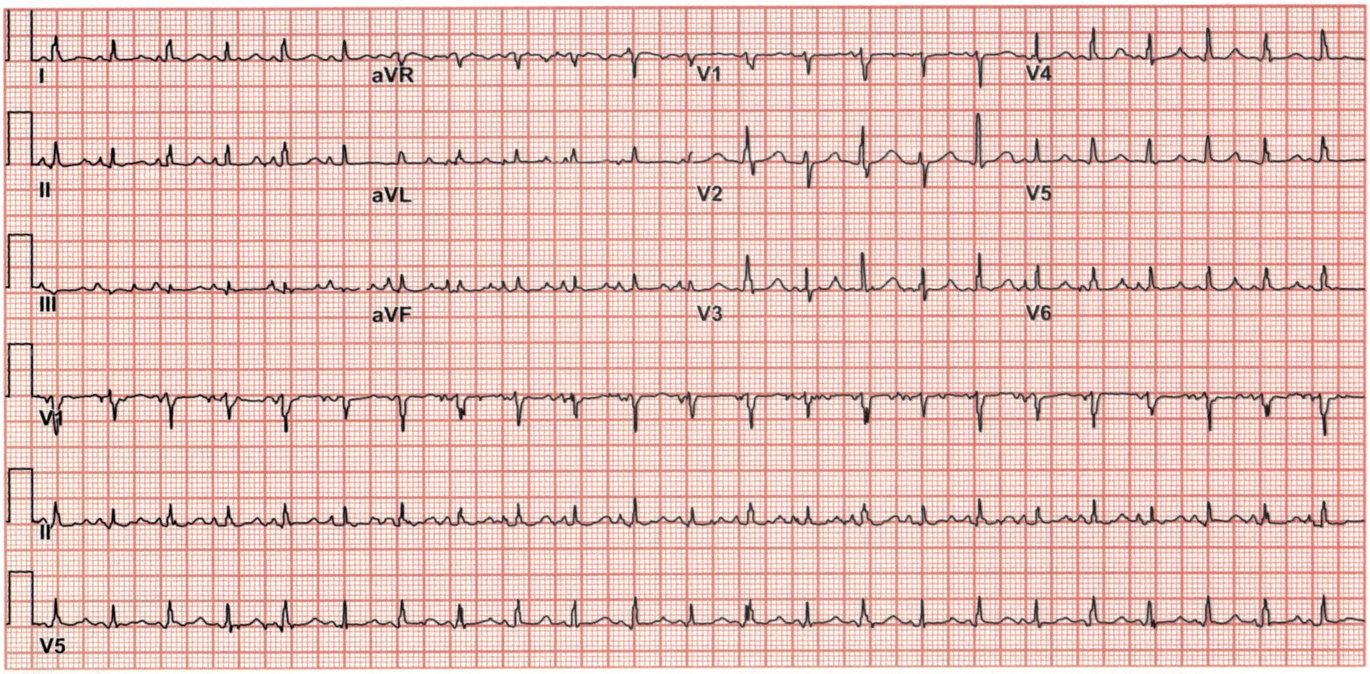


**Fig. 14.6:** ECG shows low voltage graph, QRS alterans and sinus tachycardia in cardiac tamponade

- Conditions that may simulate pericardial effusion on 2-dimensional echocardiography include the following:
  - A large left pleural effusion
  - Any tumor surrounding the heart
  - Mitral annular calcification
  - A descending thoracic aorta
  - A catheter in the right ventricle
  - An enlarged left atrium
  - An annular subvalvular LV aneurysm
  - A bronchogenic cyst

### Other Sective Tests

**12-lead electrocardiogram:** The following findings are suggestive but not diagnostic of pericardial tamponade.

- Sinus tachycardia (Figs 14.6)
- Low-voltage QRS complexes
- Electrical alternans (also observed during supraventricular and ventricular tachycardia): Alternation of QRS complexes, usually in a 2:1 ratio, on electrocardiogram findings is called electrical alternans. This is due to movement of the heart in the pericardial space. Electrical alternans is also observed in patients with myocardial ischemia, acute pulmonary embolism, and tachyarrhythmias.
- PR segment depression
- A 12-lead electrocardiogram showing sinus tachycardia with electrical alternans.

*Computed tomography (CT) imaging of the heart:* Gold et al. reported compression of the coronary sinus as observed by CT imaging as an earlier marker for cardiac tamponade in 46% of patients (Figs 14.7, 14.9 and 14.10).

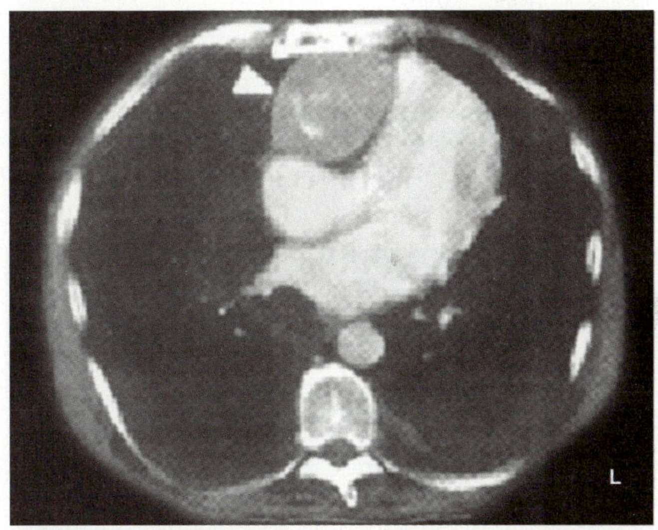


**Fig.14.7:** CAT scan showing localised cardiac tamponad caused by intrapericardial hematoma after 10 years of open heart surgery

*Pulse-oximetry:* Respiratory variability in pulse-oximetry waveform noted in patients with pulsus paradoxus. In a small group of patients with tamponade, Stone et al. noted increased respiratory variability in pulse-oximetry waveform in all patients. This should raise the suspicion for hemodynamic compromise. In patients with atrial fibrillation, pulse-oximetry may aid to detect the presence of pulsus paradoxus.

### Procedures

- Before or after insertion of the Swan-Ganz catheter, the system must be zeroed after positioning the transducer

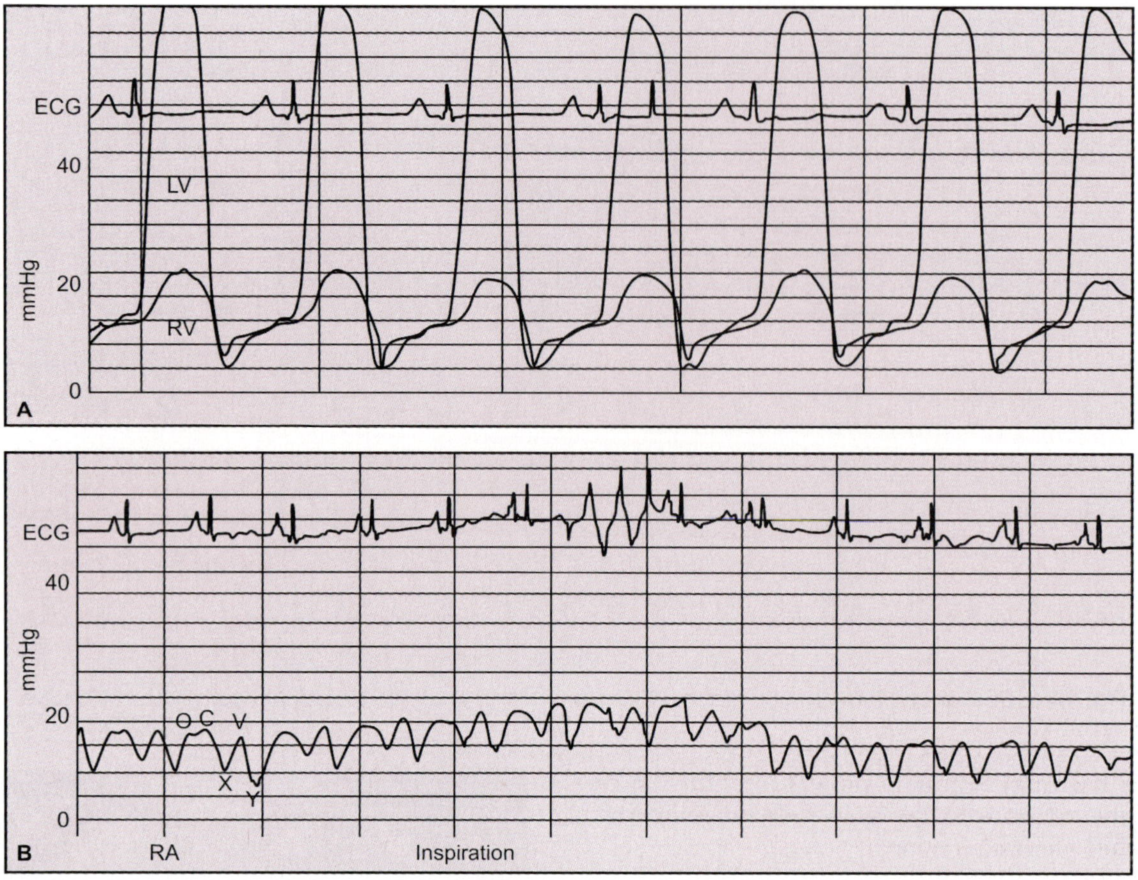


**Fig. 14.8:** Hemodynamic monitoring can confirm the diagnosis of pericardial tamponade. Equalization of diastolic pressures on the left and right sides of the heart, elevated right atrial pressure, and Kussmaul sign (i.e. increase in right atrial pressure with inspiration) are noted

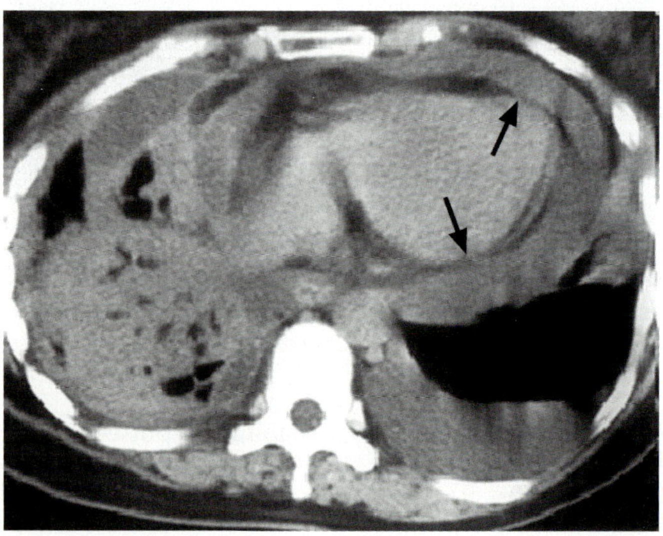

**Fig. 14.9:** Cardiac tamponade. CT scan shows a large pericardial effusion (arrows), which was positive for ovarian cancer. There are also malignant pleural effusions with consolidation of the right lung base

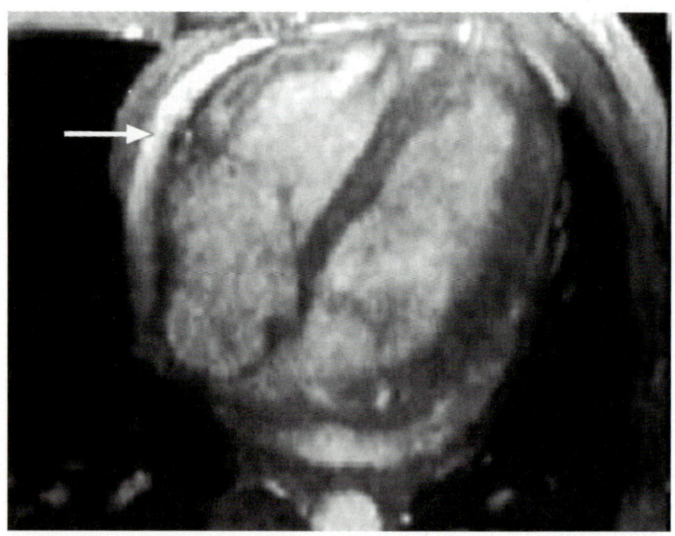

**Fig. 14.10:** This two chamber long axis gradient echo image shows a bright fluid collection in the pericardial space (arrowhead). If this fluid accumulated quickly, the patient may experience symptoms of cardiac tamponade

at the midpoint of the left atrium. Then calibrate the monitoring system. Prior to insertion, test the balloon and flush all the ports. Then insert the catheter into one of the major veins. At a depth of 20 cm, inflate the balloon and slowly advance the catheter, while continuously monitoring the pressure from the distal lumen. Always deflate the balloon before withdrawing the Swan-Ganz catheter. The waveforms help indicate the position of the catheter tip if fluoroscopy is not readily accessible. At approximately the 40–50 cm mark, the wedge pressure is usually recorded. Secure the catheter position, and obtain a chest radiograph to confirm the position (Fig. 14.8).

- In tamponade, near equalization (within 5 mmHg) of the right atrial, right ventricular diastolic, pulmonary arterial diastolic, and pulmonary capillary wedge pressure (reflecting left atrial pressure) occurs. The right atrial pressure tracings display a prominent systolic x descent and abolished systolic y descent.
- Boltwood et al. described the diastolic equalization of pulmonary capillary and right atrial pressures as predominantly inspiratory, known as the inspiratory traction sign. This is due to inspiratory traction of the taut pericardium by the diaphragm.

## HISTOLOGIC FINDINGS

Occasionally, a pericardial biopsy is performed when the etiology of the pericardial effusion that caused the tamponade is unclear. This is especially useful in cases of tuberculous pericardial effusions because cultures of the pericardial fluid in these cases rarely yield a positive result for mycobacteria. However, granulomas seen on pericardial biopsy specimens are often seen in patients with tuberculous pericarditis. In general, cytopathologic findings from pericardial fluid and histologic findings from pericardial biopsy specimens depend on the underlying pathology. Cytological examination identifies etiopathological cause of tamponade in about 75% of cases.

## MANAGEMENT

### Medical Care

Cardiac tamponade is a medical emergency. Preferably, patients should be monitored in an intensive care unit.

- All patients should receive the following:
  - Oxygen
  - Volume expansion with blood, plasma, dextran, or isotonic sodium chloride solution, as necessary to maintain adequate intravascular volume: Sagrista-Saauleda et al. noted significant increase in cardiac output after volume expansion.
  - Bed rest with leg elevation: This may help increase venous return.
  - *Inotropic drugs (e.g. dobutamine):* These can be useful because they do not increase systemic vascular resistance while increasing cardiac output.
- Positive-pressure mechanical ventilation should be avoided because it may decrease venous return and aggravate signs and symptoms of tamponade.
- Further medical care includes pericardiocentesis. Removal of pericardial fluid is the definitive therapy for tamponade and can be done by the following methods.

### Emergency Subxiphoid Percutaneous Drainage

This is a life-saving bedside procedure. The subxiphoid approach is extrapleural; hence, it is the safest for blind pericardiocentesis. A 16- or 18-gauge needle is inserted at an angle of 30–45° to the skin, near the left xiphocostal angle, aiming towards the left shoulder. When performed emergently, this procedure is associated with a reported mortality rate of approximately 4% and a complication rate of 17% (Fig. 14.11).

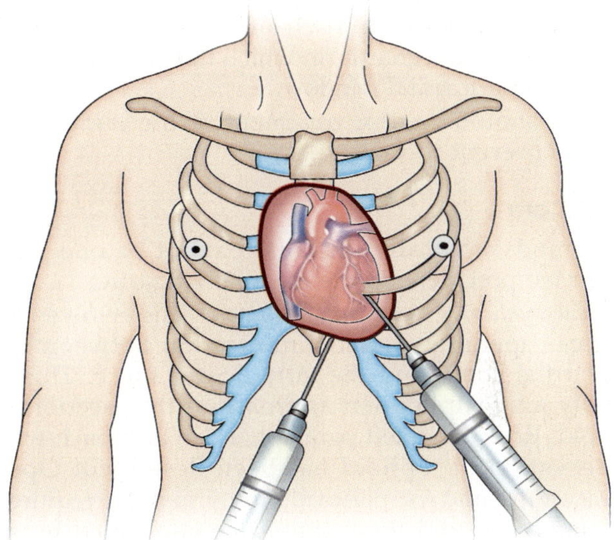

**Fig. 14.11:** Cardiac tamponade pericardiocentesis, a potentially lethal procedure, should be done using echocardiographic guidance in a cardiac catheterization laboratory and should be supervised by a cardiologist or thoracic surgeon if possible. Resuscitation equipment must be at hand. IV sedation (e.g. morphine 0.1 mg/kg or meperidine 1 mg/kg plus midazolam 3 to 5 mg) is desirable. The patient should be recumbent, with the head elevated 30° from the horizontal. Under aseptic conditions, the skin and subcutaneous tissues are infiltrated with lidocaine A 75 mm short-beveled, 16-gauge needle is attached via a 3-way stopcock to a 30 or 50 ml syringe. The pericardium may be entered via the right or left xiphocostal angle or from the tip of the xiphoid process with the needle directed inward, upward, and close to the chest wall. The needle is advanced with constant suction applied to the syringe. Echocardiography may be used to guide the needle as agitated saline is injected through it. Echocardiography is also increasingly used to identify the optimal puncture site and the needle trajectory. Once in place, the needle should be clamped next to the skin to prevent it from entering further than necessary and possibly puncturing the heart or injuring a coronary vessel. ECG monitoring is essential for detecting arrhythmias produced when the myocardium is touched or punctured. As a rule, right atrial pressure and pulmonary artery occlusion pressure (pulmonary capillary wedge pressure) are monitored. Fluid is withdrawn until intrapericardial pressure falls below right atrial pressure, usually to subatmospheric levels. If continued drainage is needed, a plastic catheter may be passed through the needle into the pericardium and the needle withdrawn. The catheter may be left in place for 2–4 days

### Echocardiographically Guided Pericardiocentesis

This is usually performed from the left intercostal space. First, mark the site of entry based on the area of maximal fluid accumulation closest to the transducer. Then, measure the distance from the skin to the pericardial space. The angle of the transducer should be the trajectory of the needle during the procedure. Avoid the inferior rib margin while advancing the needle to prevent neurovascular injury. Leave a 16-gauge catheter in place for continuous drainage (Figs 14.12–14.15).

- **Percutaneous balloon pericardiotomy:** This can be performed using an approach similar to that for echo-guided pericardiocentesis, in which the balloon is used to create a pericardial window.
- Patients should receive treatment of the underlying cause to prevent recurrence.

### Surgical Care

For a hemodynamically unstable patient or one with recurrent tamponade, provide the following care:

- *Surgical creation of a pericardial window:* This involves the surgical opening of a communication between the pericardial space and the intrapleural space. This is usually a subxiphoidian approach with resection of xiphoid. Recently, a left paraxiphoidian approach with preservation of xiphoid has been described. Open thoracotomy and/or pericardiotomy may be required in some cases, and these should be performed by an experienced surgeon.
- *Pericardiocentesis or sclerosing the pericardium:* This is a therapeutic option for patients with recurrent pericardial effusion or tamponade. Through the intrapericardial catheter, corticosteroids, tetracycline, or antineoplastic drugs (e.g. anthracyclines, bleomycin) can be instilled into the pericardial space.
- *Pericardio-peritoneal shunt:* In some patients with malignant pericardial effusions, creation of a pericardio-peritoneal shunt helps prevent recurrent tamponade.
- *Pericardiectomy:* Resection of the pericardium (pericardiectomy) through a median sternotomy or left thoracotomy is rarely required to prevent recurrent pericardial effusion and tamponade. Monaco et al. investigated the efficacy of a modified, video-assisted thoracoscopic procedure in the treatment of 15 patients with cardiac tamponade. Using a right hemithoracic approach, a 15-mm trocar was employed on the fourth right intercostal space on the anterior axillary, and a 10-mm trocar was used on the seventh right intercostal space on the median axillary line. Utilization of a 5-mm optic allowed 2 instruments, for the optic and for the endoscopic forceps, to be employed simultaneously

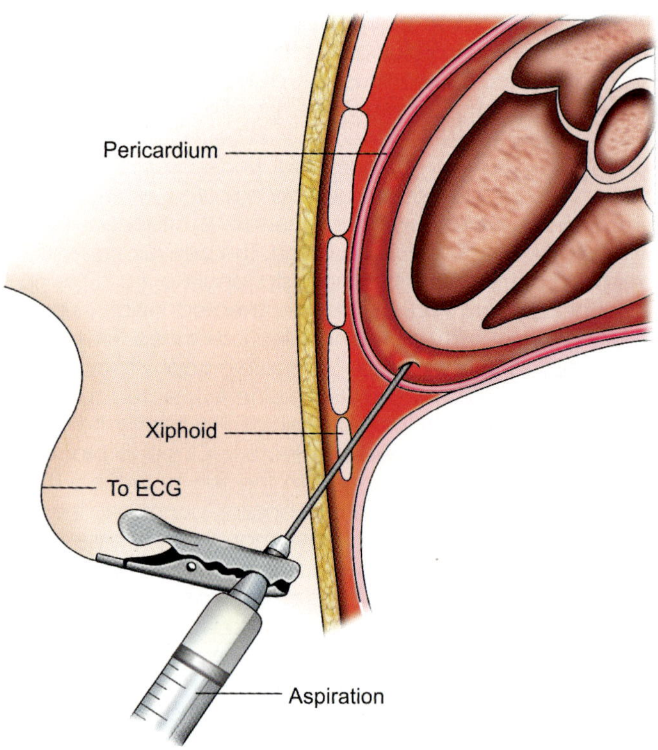


**Fig. 14.12:** Steps and proper positioning of pericardiocentesis needle

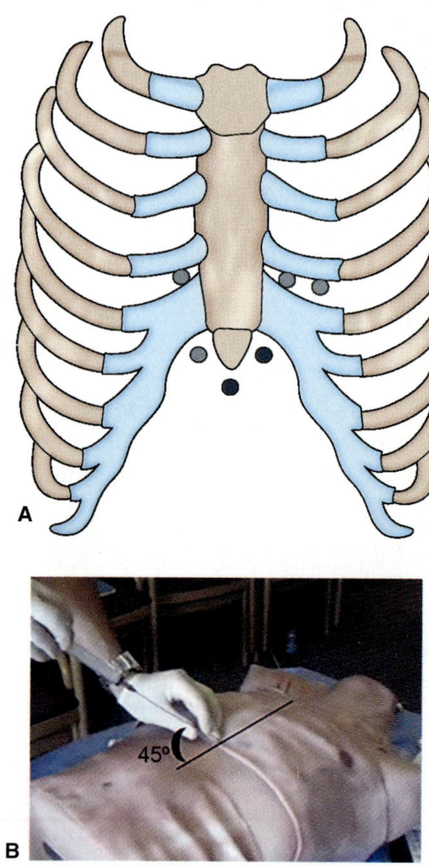


**Fig. 14.13:** (A) Pericardiocentesis needle insertion sites. The subxiphoid and the left sternocostal margin are the most commonly used sites (black dots). (B) Needle insertion—insert the spinal needle through the skin incision directed toward the left shoulder at a 45-degree angle to the abdominal wall and 45 degrees off the midline sagittal plane

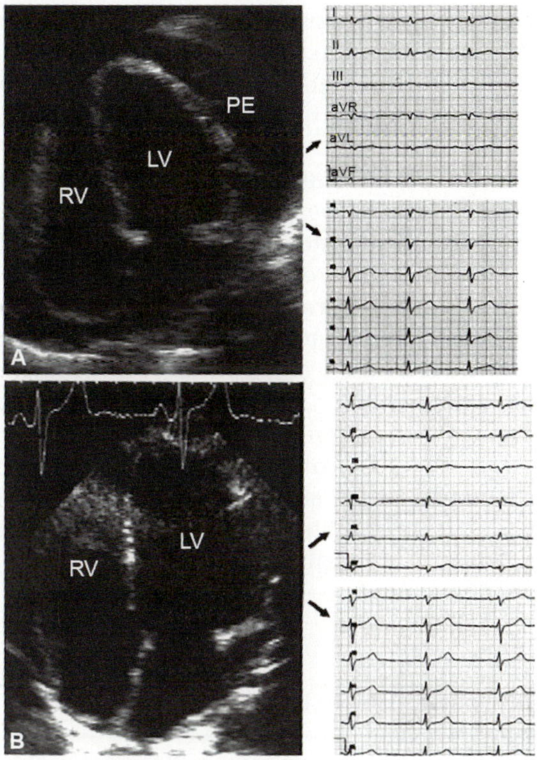


**Fig.14.14:** (A) A 23-year-old man with acute lymphatic leukemia who was treated with prednisolone due to recurrent malignant pericardial effusion. Note low QRS voltage in the limb leads before initiation of medical treatment. (B) Same patient as in (A) 6 days after initiation of anti-inflammatory treatment. Note the change of the QRS axis and the significant increase of maximum QRS amplitude in the limb leads. LV=left ventricle; RV=right ventricle

using 1 trocar; this left the second trocar available for dissecting scissors. All patients underwent a pericardial resection equal to those achieved via anterolateral thoracotomy.

The pericardial effusion was effectively drained in all patients, with no intraoperative mortality or perioperative morbidity encountered. The investigators concluded, therefore, that the modified, video-assisted procedure employed in the study seems to be a feasible treatment for cardiac tamponade.

### Consultations

- Hemodynamically stable patients—cardiologist
- Hemodynamically unstable patient—cardiologist, cardiothoracic surgeon

### Activity

Initially, the patient should be on bed rest with leg elevation to increase the venous return. Once signs and symptoms of tamponade resolve, activity can be increased as tolerated.

### Medication

The role of medication therapy in cardiac tamponade is limited. Occasionally, inotropic agents that do not increase the peripheral vascular resistance, such as dobutamine, may be used.

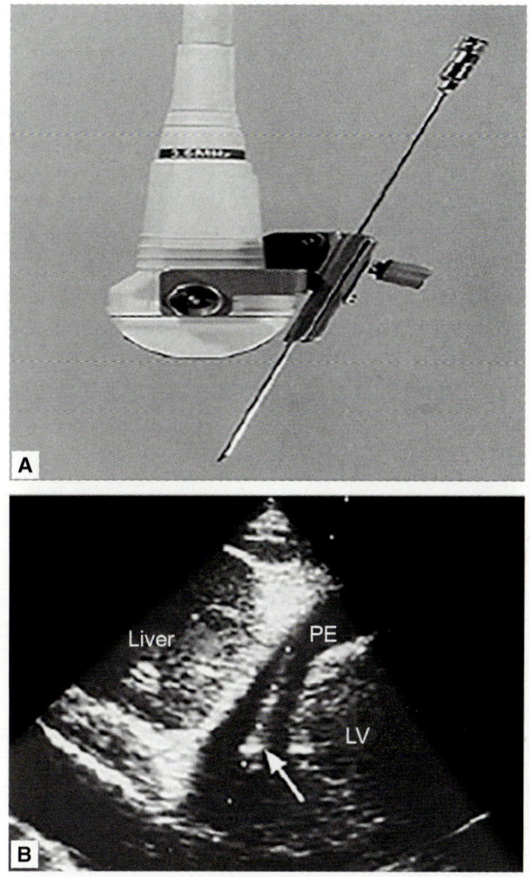


**Fig.14.15:** (A) Echocardiographic probe (UST-944B) with needle attached. The needle is held at an invariable angle with respect to the probe. (B) Two-dimensional echocardiographic image obtained during pericardiocentesis before introduction of the guidewire. The line of dots shows the direction of the puncture

### Adrenergic Agonist Agents

By stimulating beta-1 receptors in the heart, stroke volume and cardiac output are increased.

### Dobutamine (Dobutrex)

Synthetic catecholamine and a direct inotropic agent that stimulates cardiac beta-receptors with minimal increase in systemic vascular resistance.

#### *Adult*

0.5–1 mcg/kg/min IV initially; titrate until desired therapeutic effect attained

#### *Pediatric*

Follow-up.

### Further Inpatient Care

- After pericardiocentesis, leave the intrapericardial catheter in place after securing it to the skin using sterile procedure and attaching it to a closed drainage system via a 3-way stopcock. Periodically check for reaccumulation of fluid, and drain as needed. The catheter can be left in place for 1–2 days and can be used for pericardiocentesis. Serial fluid cell counts can be useful for helping discover an impending bacterial catheter infection, which could be catastrophic. If the WBC count rises significantly, the pericardial catheter must be removed immediately.

- A Swan-Ganz catheter can be left in place for continuous monitoring of hemodynamics and to assess the effect of reaccumulation of pericardial fluid.
- A repeat echocardiogram should be performed within 24 hours.
- A repeat chest radiograph should be performed within 24 hours.

## FURTHER OUTPATIENT CARE

A follow-up echocardiogram and chest radiograph should be performed at a monthly follow-up examination to check for recurrent fluid accumulation.

### Complications

- Pulmonary edema
- Shock
- Death

### Prognosis

Prognosis depends on prompt recognition and management of the condition and the underlying cause of the tamponade. Cornily et al. reported 1-year mortality of 76.5% in patients with malignant disease compared with 13.3% in patients without malignant disease. They also noted a median survival of 150 days in patients with malignant disease.

### Medicolegal Pitfalls

- Be aware of clinical conditions that may simulate tamponade or pericardial effusion on two-dimensional echocardiography findings.
- Pulsus paradoxus may be absent in patients with low-pressure tamponade, right heart tamponade, or atrial septal defects.
- Pulsus paradoxus can be observed in patients with nontamponade conditions involving labored breathing (e.g. asthma, severe chronic obstructive pulmonary disease) and in those with right ventricular infarction.
- Tension pneumothorax may clinically simulate cardiac tamponade.
- Early diagnosis with a high index of suspicion is necessary to minimize the morbidity and mortality from tamponade.

## QUICK READINGS IN CARDIAC TAMPONADE

Cardiac tamponade is accumulation of blood in the pericardial sac of sufficient volume and pressure to impair cardiac filling. Patients typically have hypotension, muffled heart tones, and distended neck veins. Diagnosis is made clinically and often with bedside echocardiography. Treatment is immediate pericardiocentesis or pericardiotomy.

Fluid in the pericardial sac can impair cardiac filling, leading to low cardiac output and sometimes shock and death. If fluid accumulates slowly (e.g. due to chronic inflammation), the pericardium can stretch to accommodate up to 1–1.5 L of fluid before cardiac output is compromised. However, with rapid fluid accumulation, as occurs with traumatic hemorrhage, as little as 150 ml may cause tamponade.

In trauma, the cause is more often penetrating than blunt trauma. The wound is often medial to the nipples (for anterior wounds) or the scapulae (for posterior wounds). Tamponade due to blunt trauma involves cardiac chamber rupture, which is typically fatal before patients can be brought for treatment.

### Symptoms and Signs

Classically, patients have Beck triad, which consists of the following:

- Hypotension
- Muffled heart tones
- Venous pressure increase (e.g. neck vein distention)

However, hypotension has multiple potential causes in trauma patients, muffled heart tones can be difficult to assess during a noisy trauma resuscitation, and neck vein distention can be absent due to hypovolemia. Pulsus paradoxus (*see* pulsus paradoxus), a decrease in systolic BP during inspiration of >10 mmHg, is also suggestive, but again not easy to assess in a noisy setting.

### Diagnosis

- Clinical evaluation
- Often bedside echocardiography

Diagnosis can be difficult. Beck triad is considered diagnostic but may not be present or easy to recognize. In addition, tension pneumothorax (*see* pneumothorax (tension) also should be considered in patients with hypotension and neck vein distention, although this disorder typically causes markedly decreased breath sounds and hyperresonance on the affected hemithorax. Bedside transthoracic echocardiography can be diagnostic and can be done during the initial evaluation and resuscitation but may be falsely negative. The diagnosis sometimes is suggested by unexplained failure to respond to volume resuscitation.

### Treatment

#### *Pericardiocentesis*

Sometimes pericardiotomy or creation of a pericardial window.

Subxiphoidal pericardiocentesis is done in unstable patients when cardiac tamponade is suspected. Electrocardiographic monitoring during the insertion needle for ST-segment elevation (indicating contact with the epicardium and the need to withdraw the needle) is done if possible. Pericardiocentesis is a temporizing measure. Removal of as little as 10 ml of blood may normalize BP. However, failure to aspirate blood does not exclude the diagnosis; fresh blood in the pericardium is often clotted. Thoracotomy with pericardiotomy or establishment of a subxiphoidal pericardial window are more definitive treatments, which are indicated in patients in whom the diagnosis is confirmed or strongly suspected. If adequately trained personnel are available and the patient is unstable and fails to respond to other resuscitative measures, one of these procedures can be done at the bedside in the emergency setting. Otherwise, the procedure is done in the operating room as soon as feasible.

## KEY POINTS

1. Cardiac tamponade is most often caused by a penetrating wound medial to the nipples (for anterior wounds) or the scapulae (for posterior wounds).
2. The triad of muffled heart tones, hypotension, and neck vein distention is diagnostic but not always present; in their absence, bedside echocardiography should be done if the diagnosis is suspected.
3. Subxiphoidal pericardiocentesis is a temporizing measure and may be falsely negative; a pericardial window or pericardiotomy are more definitive.

## BIBLIOGRAPHY


1. Aikat S, Ghaffari S. A review of pericardial diseases: clinical, ECG and hemodynamic features and management. Cleve Clin J Med 2000;67(12):903–14.
2. Alam HB, Levitt A, Molyneaux R, et al. Can pleural effusions cause cardiac tamponade. Chest 1999;116(6):1820–2.
3. Allen KB, Faber LP, Warren WH, Shaar CJ. Pericardial effusion: subxiphoid pericardiostomy versus percutaneous catheter drainage. Ann Thorac Surg 1999;67(2):437–40.
4. Beauchamp KA. Pericardial tamponade: an oncologic emergency. Clin J Oncol Nurs 1998;2(3):85–95.
5. Best Evidence] Roy CL, Minor MA, Brookhart MA, Choudhry NK. Does this patient with a pericardial effusion have cardiac tamponade. JAMA 2007;297(16):9.
6. Boltwood C, Rieders D, Gregory KW. Inspiratory tracking sign in pericardial disease. Circulation 1984;70(Suppl II):103.
7. Chen Y, Brennessel D, Walters J, et al. Human immunodeficiency virus-associated pericardial effusion: report of 40 cases and review of the literature. Am Heart J 1999; 137(3): 516–21.
8. Cornily JC, Pennec PY, Castellant P, et al. Cardiac tamponade in medical patients: a 10-year follow-up survey. Cardiology 2008;111(3):197–201.
9. Eisenberg MJ, de Romeral LM, Heidenreich PA, et al. The diagnosis of pericardial effusion and cardiac tamponade by 12-lead ECG. A technology assessment. Chest 1996;110(2): 318–24.
10. Gold MM, Spindola-Franco H, Jain VR, et al. Coronary sinus compression: an early computed tomographic sign of cardiac tamponade. J Comput Assist Tomogr 2008;32(1):72–7.
11. Goldstein JA. Cardiac tamponade, constrictive pericarditis, and restrictive cardiomyopathy. Curr Probl Cardiol 2004; 29(9):503–67.
12. Griffin S, Fountain W. Pericardio-peritoneal shunt for malignant pericardial effusion. J Thorac Cardiovasc Surg 1989; 98(6):1153–4.
13. Guberman BA, Fowler NO, Engel PJ, et al. Cardiac tamponade in medical patients. Circulation. 1981;64(3):633–40.
14. Holmes DR Jr, Nishimura R, Fountain R, et al. Iatrogenic pericardial effusion and tamponade in the percutaneous intracardiac intervention era. JACC Cardiovasc Interv 2009; 2(8):705–17.
15. Ikematsu Y. Incidence and characteristics of dysphoria in patients with cardiac tamponade. Heart Lung 2007;36(6): 440–9.
16. Kaplan LM, Epstein SK, Schwartz SL, et al. Clinical, echocardiographic, and hemodynamic evidence of cardiac tamponade caused by large pleural effusions. Am J Respir Crit Care Med 1995;151(3 Pt 1):904–8.
17. Lee YM, Kim HJ, Lee JE, et al. Cardiac tamponade following insertion of an internal jugular vein catheter for hemodialysis. Clin Nephrol 2009;72(3):220–3.
18. Medary I, Steinherz LJ, Aronson DC, La Quaglia MP. Cardiac tamponade in the pediatric oncology population: treatment by percutaneous catheter drainage. J Pediatr Surg 1996;31(1): 197–9; discussion 199–200.
19. Monaco F, Barone M, David A, et al. [Cardiac tamponade: a modified video-assisted thoracoscopic approach]. Chir Ital 2009;61(3):321–6.
20. Motas C, Motas N, Rus O, Horvat T. Left paraxiphoidian approach for drainage of pericardial effusions. Interact Cardiovasc Thorac Surg 2010;10(1):4–5.
21. Müller-Stich BP, Linke G, Leemann B, Lange J, Zerz A. Cardiac tamponade as a life-threatening complication in antireflux surgery. Am J Surg 2006;191(1):139–41.
22. Parvez N, Carpenter JL. Cardiac tamponade in Still disease: a review of the literature. South Med J 2009;102(8):832–7.
23. Patel MR, Meine TJ, Lindblad L, Griffin J, Granger CB, Becker RC. Cardiac tamponade in the fibrinolytic era: analysis of >100,000 patients with ST-segment elevation myocardial infarction. Am Heart J 2006;151(2):316–22.
24. Paunovic B, Sharma S, Miller A. Swan-Ganz Catheterization. eMedicine Journal [serial online]. 2005.
25. Petcu DP, Petcu C, Popescu CF, Bataiosu C, Alexandru D. Clinical and cytological correlations in pericardial effusions with cardiac tamponade. Rom J Morphol Embryol 2009; 50(2):251–6.
26. Reddy PS, Curtiss EI, Uretsky BF. Spectrum of hemodynamic changes in cardiac tamponade. Am J Cardiol 1990; 66(20): 1487–91.
27. Reddy PS, Curtiss EI. Cardiac tamponade. Cardiol Clin 1990; 8(4):627–37.

28. Rylski B, Siepe M, Schoellhorn J, et al. Endoscopic treatment for delayed cardiac tamponade. Eur J Cardiothorac Surg 2009.
29. Sagristà-Sauleda J, Angel J, Sambola A, et al. Low-pressure cardiac tamponade: clinical and hemodynamic profile. Circulation 2006;114(9):945–52.
30. Sagristà-Sauleda J, Angel J, Sambola A, et al. Hemodynamic effects of volume expansion in patients with cardiac tamponade. Circulation 2008;117(12): 1545–9.
31. Saito Y, Donohue A, Attai S, et al. The syndrome of cardiac tamponade with 'small' pericardial effusion. Echocardiography 2008;25(3):321–7.
32. Spodick DH. Diseases of the pericardium. In: Chatterjee K, (Ed.) Cardiology: An Illustrated Text/Reference. Vol 2. New York, NY: Gower Medical. 1991:10.38–10.64.
33. Spodick DH. Pericarditis, pericardial effusion, cardiac tamponade, and constriction. Crit Care Clin 1989;5(3): 455–76.
34. Stone MK, Bauch TD, Rubal BJ. Respiratory changes in the pulse-oximetry waveform associated with pericardial tamponade. Clin Cardiol 2006;29(9):411–4.
35. Towbin R. The bowed catheter sign: a risk for pericardial tamponade. Pediatr Radiol 2008;38(3):331–5.

# 15 Recognition and Management of Cardiomyopathies

Cardiomyopathy, or heart muscle disease, is a type of progressive heart disease in which the heart is abnormally enlarged, thickened, and/or stiffened. As a result, the heart muscle's ability to pump blood is weakened, often causing heart failure and the backup of blood into the lungs or rest of the body. The disease can also cause abnormal heart rhythms.

Usually, cardiomyopathy begins in the heart's lower chambers (the ventricles), but in severe cases can affect the upper chambers or atria as well.

## DEFINITION AND CLASSIFICATION

Cardiomyopathies are defined as diseases of the myocardium associated with cardiac dysfunction. They are classified as dilated cardiomyopathy, hypertrophic cardiomyopathy, restrictive cardiomyopathy, and arrhythmogenic right ventricular cardiomyopathy (Figs 15.1, 15.2 and Table 15.1).

### Dilated Cardiomyopathy

Dilated cardiomyopathy is characterized by dilatation and impaired contraction of the left ventricle or both ventricles. It may be idiopathic, familial/genetic, viral and/or immune, alcoholic/toxic, or associated with recognized cardiovascular disease in which the degree of myocardial dysfunction is not explained by the abnormal loading conditions or the extent of ischemic damage. Histology is nonspecific. Presentation is usually with heart failure, which is often progressive. Arrhythmias, thromboembolism, and sudden death are common and may occur at any stage.

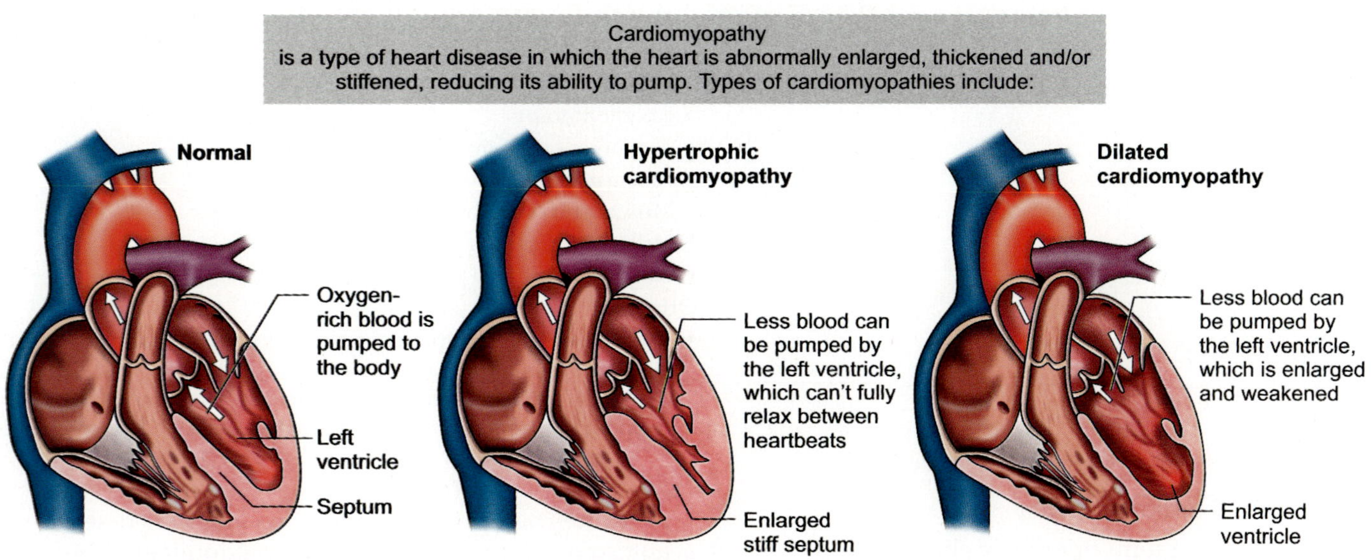


**Fig. 15.1:** Comparative description of normal heart functioning with two common types of cardiomyopathies

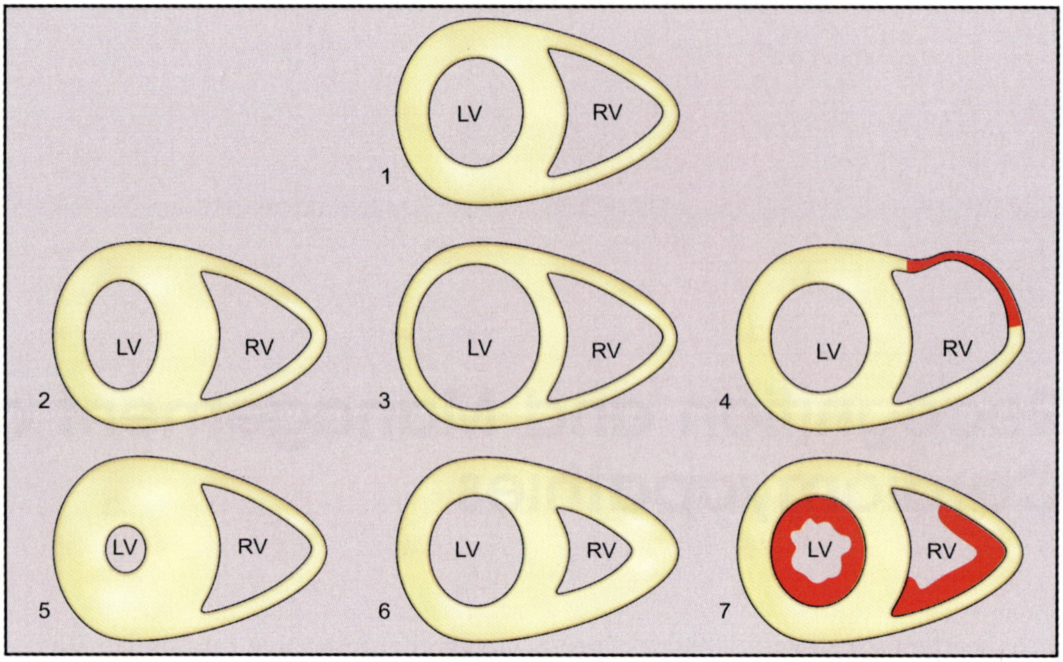


**Fig. 15.2:** Diagrammatic representation of different types of cardiomyopathies at short axis views and right and left ventricles at mid-septal levels. (1) Normal, (2) HCM, nonobstructive hypertrophic cardiomyopathy, (3) DCM, dilated cardiomyopathy, (4) ARVD, arrhythmogenic right ventricular dysplasia, (5) HOCM, hypertrophic obstructive cardiomyopathy, (6) RCM, restrictive cardiomyopathy, (7) EMF, endomyocardial fibrosis or obliterative cardiomyopathy

**Table 15.1:** Classification of cardiomyopathies

| Primary/intrinsic cardiomyopathies | Secondary/extrinsic cardiomyopathies |
|---|---|
| **Genetic**<br>• Hypertrophic cardiomyopathy (HCM or HOCM)<br>• Arrhythmogenic right ventricular cardiomyopathy (ARVC)<br>• Isolated ventricular noncompaction<br>• Mitochondrial myopathy<br>**Mixedc**<br>• Dilated cardiomyopathy (DCM)<br>• Restrictive cardiomyopathy (RCM)<br>**Acquired**<br>• Takotsubo cardiomyopathy<br>• Loeffler endocarditis | **Metabolic/storage**<br>• Amyloidosis<br>• Hemochromatosis<br>**Inflammatory**<br>• Chagas disease<br>**Endocrine**<br>• Diabetic cardiomyopathy<br>• Hyperthyroidism<br>• Acromegaly<br>**Toxicity**<br>• Chemotherapy<br>• Alcoholic cardiomyopathy<br>**Neuromuscular**<br>• Muscular dystrophy<br>**Nutritional diseases**<br>• Obesity-associated cardiomyopathy<br>**Other**<br>• 'Ischemic cardiomyopathy' is a weakness in the muscle of the heart due to inadequate oxygen delivery to the myocardium with coronary artery disease being the most common cause. Not supported by caurent cardiomyopathies classification schemes. |

## Hypertrophic Cardiomyopathy

Hypertrophic cardiomyopathy is characterized by left and/or right ventricular hypertrophy, which is usually asymmetric and involves the interventricular septum. Typically, the left ventricular volume is normal or reduced. Systolic gradients are common. Familial disease with autosomal dominant inheritance predominates. Mutations in sarcomeric contractile protein genes cause disease. Typical morphological changes include myocyte hypertrophy and disarray surrounding areas of increased loose connective tissue. Arrhythmias and premature sudden death are common.

### Restrictive Cardiomyopathy

Restrictive cardiomyopathy is characterized by restrictive filling and reduced diastolic volume of either or both ventricles with normal or near-normal systolic function and wall thickness. Increased interstitial fibrosis may be present. It may be idiopathic or associated with other disease (e.g. amyloidosis; endomyocardial disease with or without hypereosinophilia).

### Arrhythmogenic Right Ventricular Cardiomyopathy

Arrhythmogenic right ventricular cardiomyopathy is characterized by progressive fibrofatty replacement of right ventricular myocardium, initially with typical regional and later global right and some left ventricular involvement, with relative sparing of the septum. Familial disease is common, with autosomal dominant inheritance and incomplete penetrance; a recessive form is described. Presentation with arrhythmias and sudden death is common, particularly in the young.

### Unclassified Cardiomyopathies

Unclassified cardiomyopathies include a few cases that do not fit readily into any group (e.g. fibroelastosis, non-compacted myocardium, systolic dysfunction with minimal dilatation, and mitochondrial involvement).

Some diseases may present with features of more than one type of cardiomyopathy (i.e. amyloidosis, systemic hypertension). It is recognized that arrhythmias and conduction disease may be primary myocardial disorders. At this time, however, it was elected not to include them as cardiomyopathies.

### Specific Cardiomyopathies

The term specific cardiomyopathies is now used to describe heart muscle diseases that are associated with specific cardiac or systemic disorders. These were previously defined as specific heart muscle diseases.

**Ischemic cardiomyopathy** presents as a dilated cardiomyopathy with impaired contractile performance not explained by the extent of coronary artery disease or ischemic damage.

**Valvular cardiomyopathy** presents with ventricular dysfunction that is out of proportion to the abnormal loading conditions.

**Hypertensive cardiomyopathy** often presents with left ventricular hypertrophy in association with features of dilated or restrictive cardiomyopathy with cardiac failure.

**Inflammatory cardiomyopathy** is defined by myocarditis in association with cardiac dysfunction. Myocarditis is an inflammatory disease of the myocardium and is diagnosed by established histological, immunological, and immunohistochemical criteria. Idiopathic, autoimmune, and infectious forms of inflammatory cardiomyopathy are recognized. Inflammatory myocardial disease is involved in the pathogenesis of dilated cardiomyopathy and other cardiomyopathies, e.g. Chagas' disease, HIV, enterovirus, adenovirus, and cytomegalovirus.

**Metabolic cardiomyopathy** includes the following categories: Endocrine, e.g. thyrotoxicosis, hypothyroidism, adrenal cortical insufficiency, pheochromocytoma, acromegaly, and diabetes mellitus; familial storage disease and infiltrations, e.g. hemochromatosis, glycogen storage disease, Hurler's syndrome, Refsum's syndrome, Niemann-Pick disease, Hand-Schüller-Christian disease, Fabry-Anderson disease, and Morquio-Ullrich disease; deficiency, e.g. disturbances of potassium metabolism, magnesium deficiency, and nutritional disorders such as kwashiorkor, anemia, beri-beri, and selenium deficiency; amyloid, e.g. primary, secondary, familial, and hereditary cardiac amyloidoses, familial mediterranean fever, and senile amyloidosis.

**General system disease** includes connective tissue disorders, e.g. systemic lupus erythematosus, polyarteritis nodosa, rheumatoid arthritis, scleroderma, and dermatomyositis. Infiltrations and granulomas include sarcoidosis and leukemia.

**Muscular dystrophies** include Duchenne, Becker-type, and myotonic dystrophies.

**Neuromuscular disorders** include Friedreich's ataxia, Noonan's syndrome, and lentiginosis.

Sensitivity and toxic reactions include reactions to alcohol, catecholamines, anthracyclines, irradiation, and miscellaneous. Alcoholic cardiomyopathy may be associated with a heavy alcohol intake. At present we cannot define a causal versus a conditioning role of alcohol or apply precise diagnostic criteria.

Peripartal cardiomyopathy may first manifest in the peripartum period. This is probably a heterogeneous group.

## DILATED CARDIOMYOPATHY

Dilated cardiomyopathy (DCM) is a condition in which the heart becomes weakened and enlarged, and it cannot pump blood efficiently. The decreased heart function can affect the lungs, liver, and other body systems.

There are several different types of cardiomyopathy. Dilated cardiomyopathy is the most common form.

### Aetiological Factors

There are many causes of dilated cardiomyopathy. Some of these are:

- Alcohol (alcoholic cardiomyopathy) or cocaine abuse
- Atrial fibrillation, supraventricular tachycardia, or other heart rhythm problems in which the heart beats very fast for a long period of time (called tachycardia-mediated cardiomyopathy)
- Autoimmune illnesses that involve the heart, such as systemic lupus erythematosus and rheumatoid arthritis
- Catecholamine excess from a tumor that releases catecholamines (pheochromocytoma)

- Coronary artery disease (*see* ischemic cardiomyopathy)
- Deficiencies of certain vitamins and minerals (thiamine, calcium, and magnesium)
- End-stage kidney disease
- Family history of cardiomyopathy (some cardiomyopathies run in families and have a genetic component)
- Infections that involve the heart muscle, such as viruses, HIV infection, Chagas disease, and Lyme disease
- Inherited disorders such as muscular dystroph
- Medications that can be toxic to the heart (such as some chemotherapy drugs used to treat cancer)
- Poorly controlled high blood pressure
- Pregnancy
- Stress-induced cardiomyopathy
- Trace elements, such as lead, arsenic, or mercury

This condition can affect anyone at any age. However, it is most common in adult men.

The most common causes of dilated cardiomyopathy in children are:

- Heart (coronary) disease
- Myocarditis
- Some infections
- Unknown cause (idiopathic dilated cardiomyopathy)

### Symptoms in Dilated Cardiomyopathy

Symptoms of heart failure are most common. Usually, they develop slowly over time. However, sometimes symptoms start very suddenly and are severe. Common symptoms are:

- Shortness of breath with activity or after lying down (or being asleep) for a while
- Swelling of feet and ankles (in adults)
- Irregular or rapid pulse
- Fatigue, weakness, and faintness
- Swollen liver
- Loss of appetite
- Cough

*Other symptoms may include:*

- Failure to thrive (in children)
- Need to urinate at night (in adults)

### Physical Exams and Laboratory Tests

Cardiomyopathy is usually discovered when the doctor is examining and testing you for the cause of heart failure.

- Tapping over the heart with the fingers and feeling the area may indicate that the heart is enlarged.
- Listening to the chest with a stethoscope reveals lung crackles, heart murmur, or other abnormal sounds.
- The liver may be enlarged.
- Neck veins may be bulging.

A number of laboratory tests may be done to determine the cause:

- Antinuclear antibody (ANA), erythrocyte sedimentation rate (ESR), and other tests to diagnose autoimmune illnesses
- Antibody test to identify infections such as Lyme disease and HIV
- Serum TSH and T4 test to identify thyroid problems

*Children will have:*

- Poor growth
- Pale skin
- Difficulty feeding
- Weak pulses in the legs and arms

Heart enlargement, congestion of the lungs, decreased movement/functioning of the heart, or heart failure may show on these tests:

- **Echocardiogram (ultrasound of the heart** (Figs 15.3–15.6)
- **Cardiac stress tests**
- **Cardiac catheterization and coronary angiography**

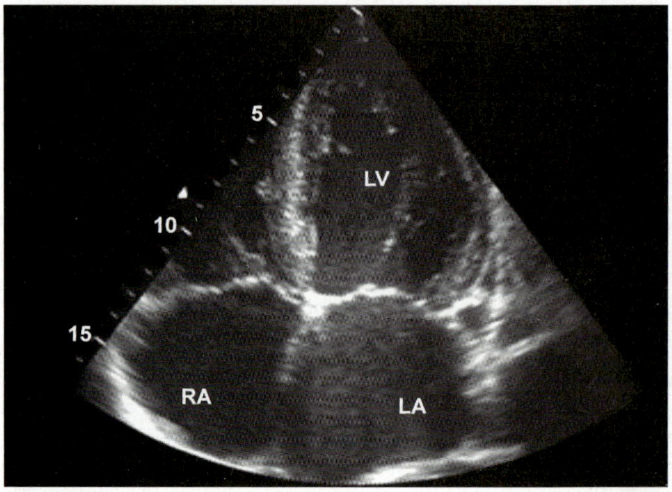


**Fig. 15.3:** Dilated cardiomyopathy in a 45-year-old woman with AIDS. Apical 4-chamber echocardiographic view shows marked enlargement of all four chambers, as well as spontaneous echo contrast ('smoke') in the left-sided chambers because of a very low ejection fraction and sluggish flow. LA=left atrium, LV=left ventricle, RA=right atrium, RV=right ventricle

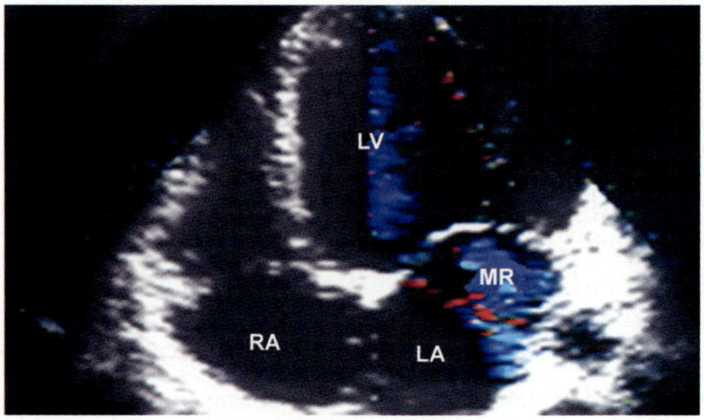


**Fig. 15.4:** Apical two-dimensional echocardiogram with color Doppler display (systolic image) in a patient with dilated cardiomyopathy shows a jet of mitral regurgitation (MR) into a large left atrium (LA) (Doppler encoded blue). Note the dilatation of the left ventricle (LV) compared with the right ventricle

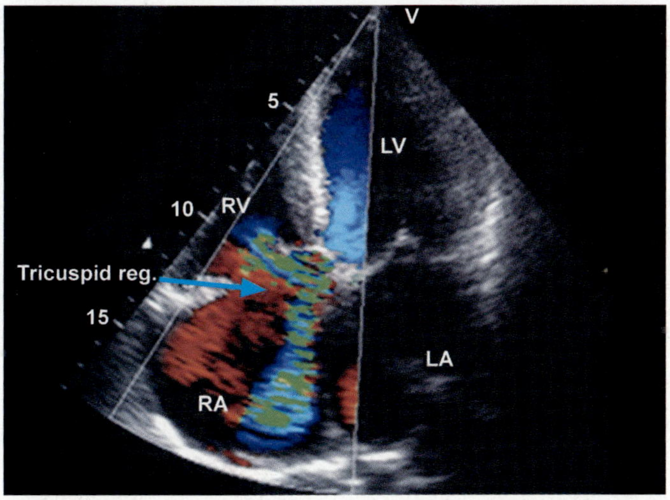


**Fig. 15.5:** Dilated cardiomyopathy in a 45-year-old woman with AIDS. Apical four-chamber view obtained with color-Doppler flow imaging shows an eccentric jet of severe regurgitation through the tricuspid valve. LA=left atrium, LV=left ventricle, RA=right atrium, RV=right ventricle

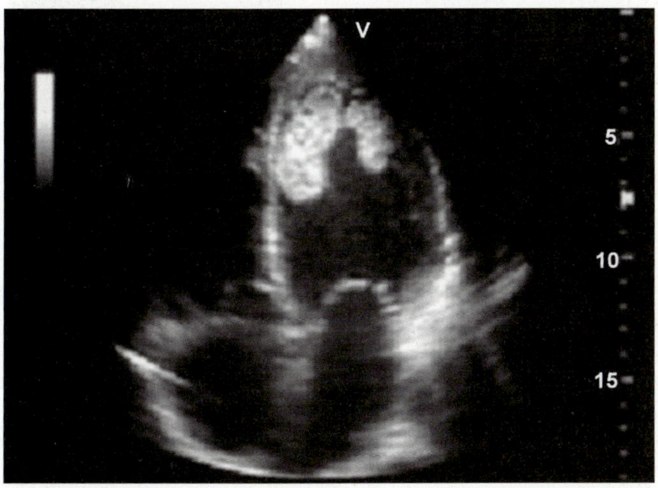


**Fig. 15.6:** Peripartum cardiomyopathy with left ventricular thrombus

- **Chest CT scan or MRI of the heart** (Figs 15.7 and 15.8)
- **Chest X-ray** (Fig. 15.9)
- **Nuclear heart scan (MUGA, RNV)** (Fig. 15.10)

*Other tests may include:*
- **ECG** (Fig. 15.11)
- **Heart biopsy**

Lab tests vary depending on the suspected cause.

### Treatment in DCM

Treatment for cardiomyopathies focuses on treating heart failure. They include (Fig. 15.12):
- Making important changes in your lifestyle
- Knowing your body and the symptoms of heart failure
- Taking medicines for heart failure
- A pacemaker to help treat slow heart rates or help your heart contract in a more coordinated fashion.

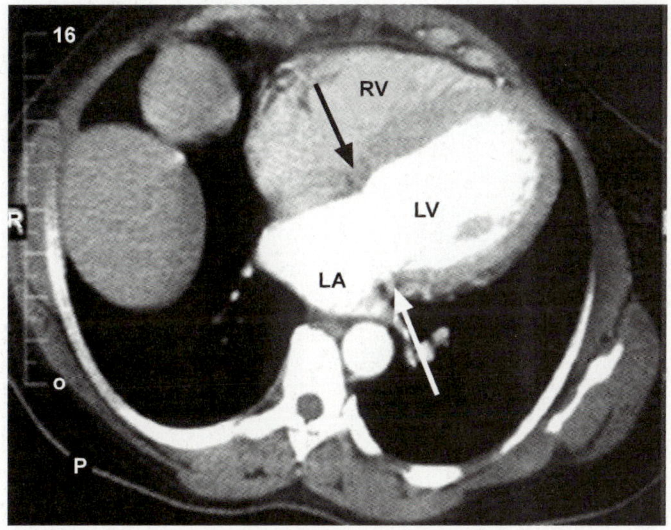


**Fig. 15.7:** Spiral computed tomography (CT) scan obtained with intravenous contrast enhancement at the level of the center of the mitral valve (between arrows) and tricuspid valve in a patient with dilated cardiomyopathy. Left ventricle (LV) is dilated compared with the right ventricle (RV)

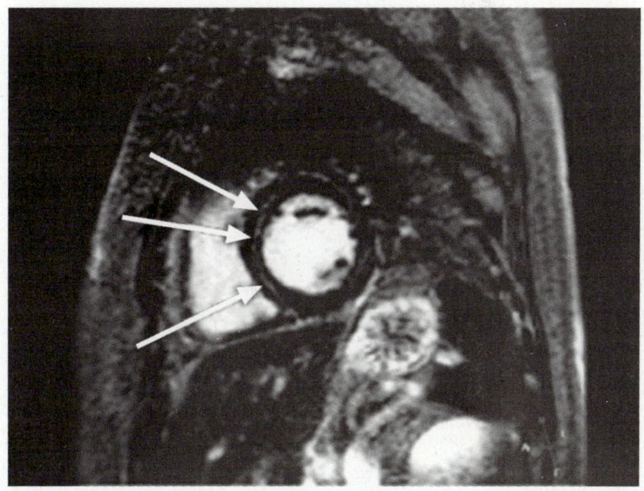

**Fig.15.8:** Typical mid-septal rim of nonischemic hyperenhancement in a patient with dilated cardiomyopathy

- A defibrillator that recognizes life-threatening, abnormal heart rhythms and sends an electrical pulse to stop them.

Cardiac catheterization might be done to see if you may benefit from coronary artery bypass (CABG) surgery or a balloon procedure (angioplasty), which could improve blood flow to the damaged or weakened heart muscle.

A heart transplant may be recommended for patients who have failed all the standard treatments and still have very severe symptoms.

### Prognosis in DCM

The outcome varies. Some people remain in a stable condition for long periods of time, some continue to gradually get sicker, and others quickly get worse. Cardiomyopathy can only be corrected if the disease that caused it can be cured.

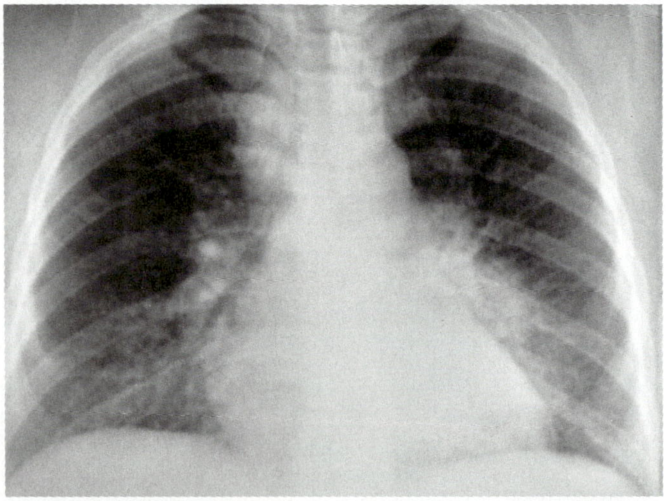

**Fig. 15.9:** Chest radiograph in a patient presenting with heart failure, which was subsequently found to be the result of dilated cardiomyopathy. Although cardiac size is at the upper limit of normal, left ventricular function is poor, causing severe pulmonary edema with bilateral alveolar edema and marked dilatation of the superior vena cava

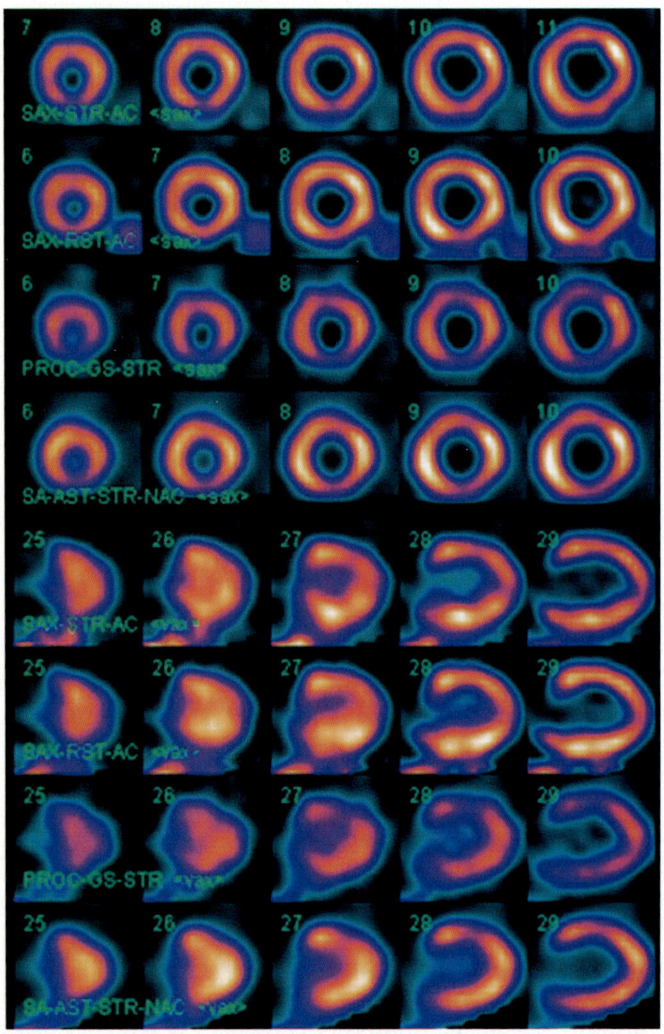

**Fig. 15.10:** Tec99 Sestamibi cardiac perfusion study demonstrates dilated left ventricular cavity

About one-third of children recover completely, one-third recover but continue to have some heart problems, and one-third die.

### *Possible Complications*

- Arrhythmias (Fig. 15.13)
- Congestive heart failure
- Pulmonary edema
- Side effects of medications, including:
  - » Headache
  - » Gastrointestinal upset
  - » Light-headedness and fainting
  - » Low blood pressure
  - » Lupus reaction (a group of symptoms including a skin rash and arthritis)

#### *When to contact a medical professional*

- Call your health care provider if you have symptoms of cardiomyopathy.
- If chest pain, palpitations, or faintness develop seek emergency medical treatment immediately.

#### *Prevention in DCM*

- Eat a well-balanced and nutritious diet
- Exercise to improve heart fitness
- Stop smoking
- Minimize alcohol consumption

## HYPERTROPHIC CARDIOMYOPATHY

Hypertrophic cardiomyopathy (HCM) is a condition in which the heart muscle becomes thick. The thickening makes it harder for blood to leave the heart, forcing the heart to work harder to pump blood.

### Aetiological Factors

Hypertrophic cardiomyopathy is often asymmetrical, meaning one part of the heart is thicker than the other parts. The condition is usually passed down through families (inherited). It is believed to be a result of several problems (defects) with the genes that control heart muscle growth. Younger people are likely to have a more severe form of hypertrophic cardiomyopathy. However, the condition is seen in people of all ages.

### Symptoms in HCM

- Chest pain
- Dizziness
- Fainting, especially during exercise
- Heart failure (in some patients)
- High blood pressure (hypertension)
- Light-headedness, especially with or after activity or exercise
- Sensation of feeling the heart beat (palpitations)
- Shortness of breath

Other symptoms that may occur are:

- Fatigue, reduced activity tolerance
- Shortness of breath when lying down

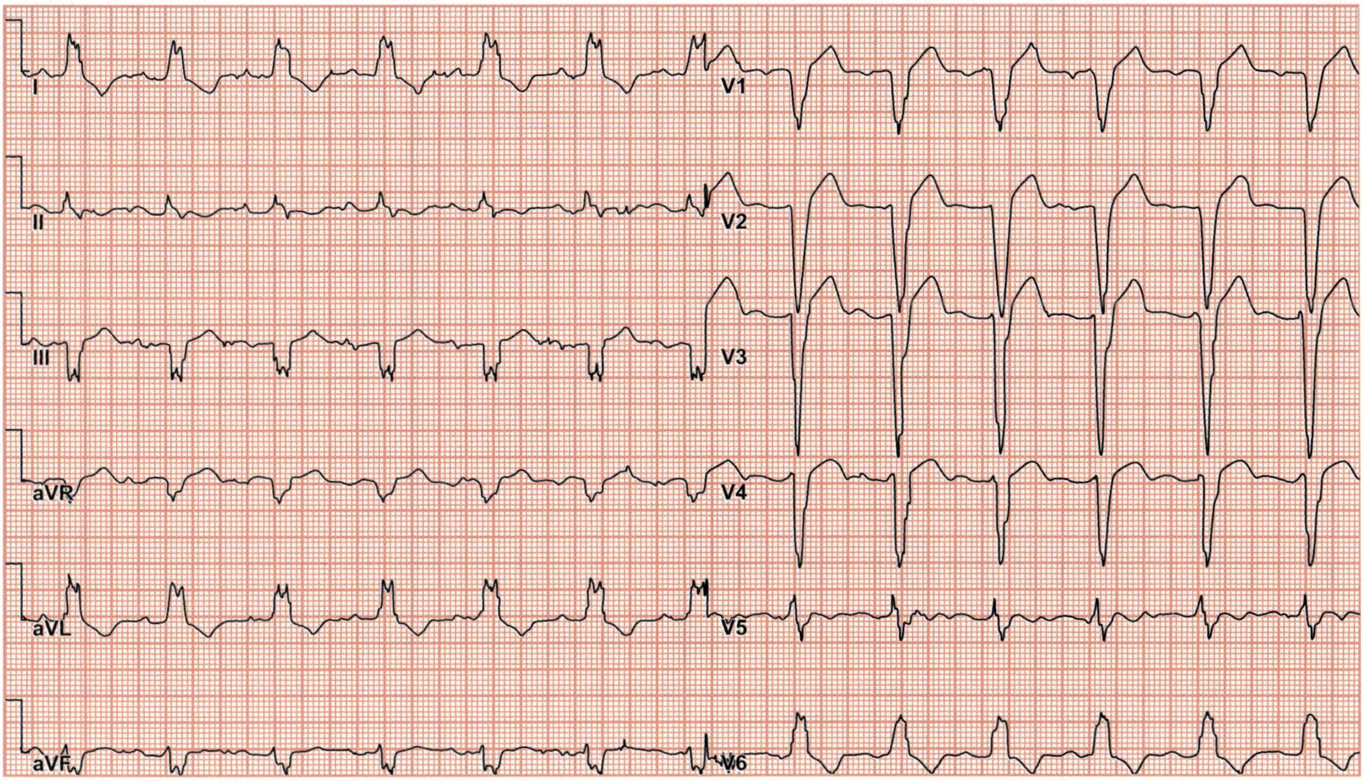


**Fig. 15.11:** LBBB in dialated cardiomyopathy

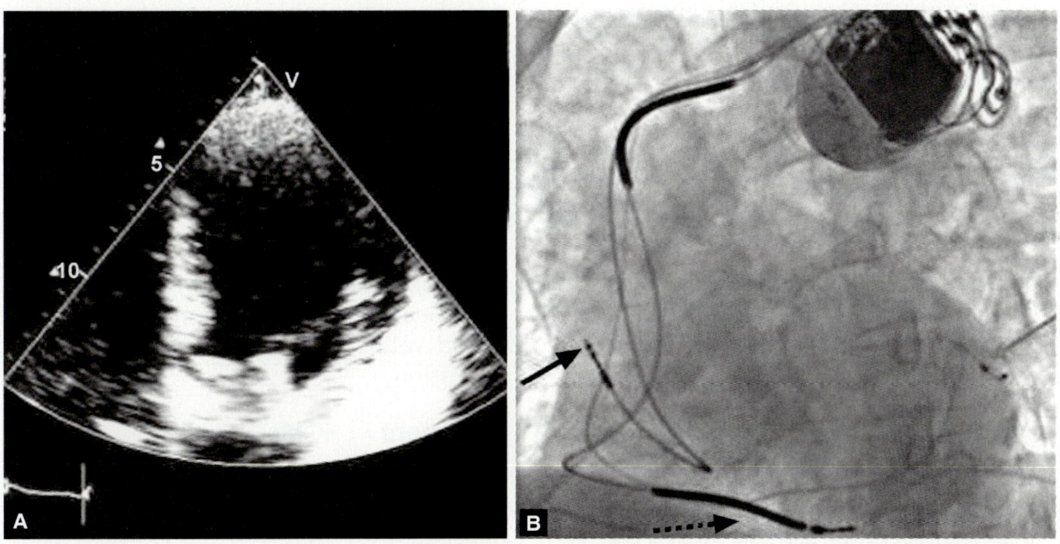


**Fig. 15.12:** (A) Echocardiography showing diastolic wall motion defect in cardiac failure. (B) CRT in dilated cardiomyopathy

Some patients have no symptoms. They may not even realize they have the condition until it is found during a routine medical exam.

The first symptom of hypertrophic cardiomyopathy among many young patients is sudden collapse and possible death. This is caused by very abnormal heart rhythms (arrhythmias), or from the blockage of blood leaving the heart to the rest of the body.

Hypertrophic cardiomyopathy is a major cause of death in young athletes who seem completely healthy but die during heavy exercise. However, certain normal changes in athletes' hearts can confuse the diagnosis.

### Physical Examination

The health care provider will perform a physical exam and listen to the heart and lungs with a stethoscope. Listening with a stethoscope may reveal abnormal heart sounds or a murmur. These sounds may change with different body positions.

The pulse in your arms and neck will also be checked. The doctor may feel an abnormal heartbeat in the chest.

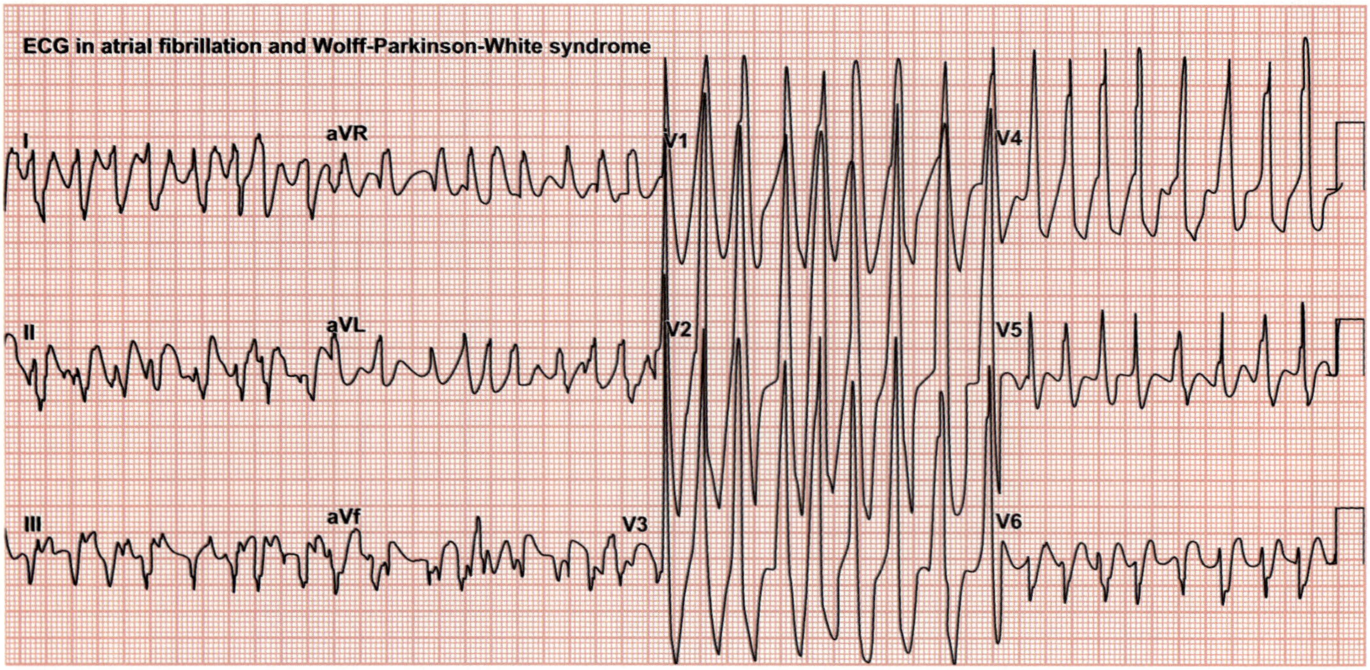


**Fig. 15.13:** This ECG shows preexcited atrial fibrillation. The shortest RR interval is 200 milliseconds; intervals <260 milliseconds are associated with a risk of sudden death in patient with DCM

## Laboratory and Imaging Studies

Tests used to diagnose heart muscle thickness, problems with blood flow, or leaky heart valves (mitral valve regurgitation) may include:

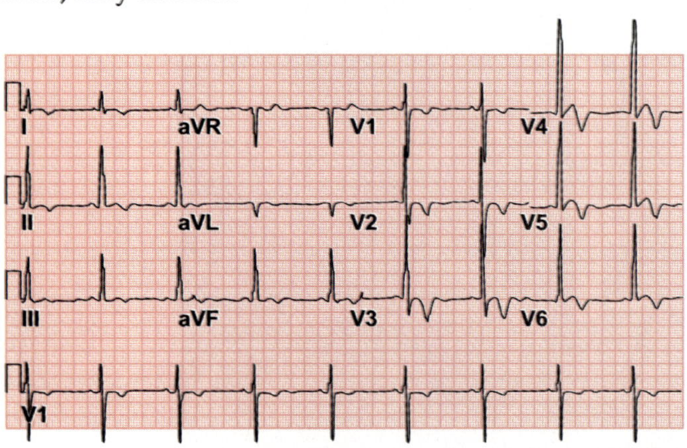


**Fig. 15.14:** ECG from a 53-year-old man with apical hypertrophic cardiomyopathy. Note elevated QRS voltages associated with left ventricular hypertrophy and inverted T-waves in all precordial leads

- ECG (Fig. 15.14)
- 24-hour Holter monitor (heart monitor) (Fig. 15.15)
- Echocardiography (the most common test) with Doppler ultrasound (Figs 15.16–15.19)

***MRI/CT Scan*** (Fig. 15.20)

*Cardiac catheterization* (Figs 15.21 and 15.22)

Not all of these tests are useful for evaluating all of these conditions.

*Blood tests* may be done to rule out other possible diseases. If you are diagnosed with hypertrophic cardiomyopathy, your health care provider may recommend that your close blood relatives (family members) be screened for the condition.

## Treatment in HCM

The goal of treatment is to control symptoms and prevent complications. Some patients may need to stay in the hospital until the condition is under control (stabilized).

If you have symptoms, you may need medication to help the heart contract and relax correctly. Some medications

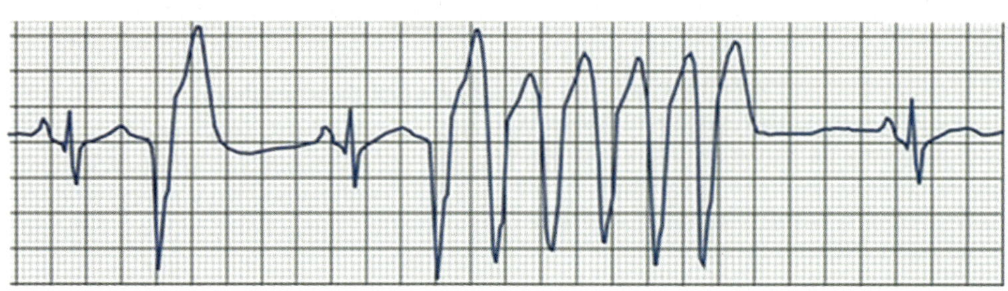

**Fig. 15.15:** Nonsustained ventricular tachycardia in a patient with hypertrophic cardiomyopathy

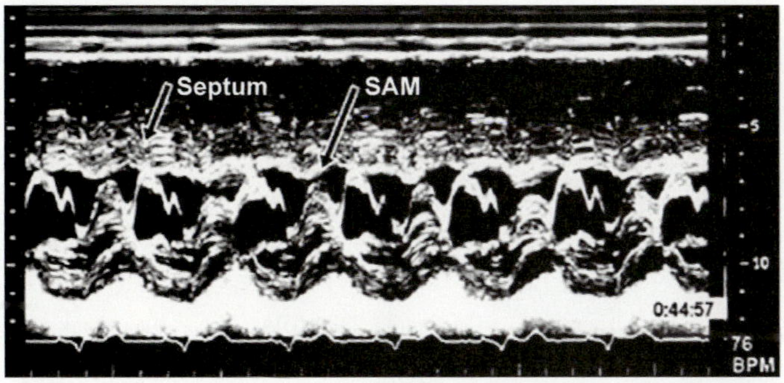


**Fig. 15.16:** M-mode echocardiogram in obstructive hypertrophic cardiomyopathy showing systolic anterior motion of the mitral valve (SAM) (arrows indicating septum and mitral valve leaflet contact)

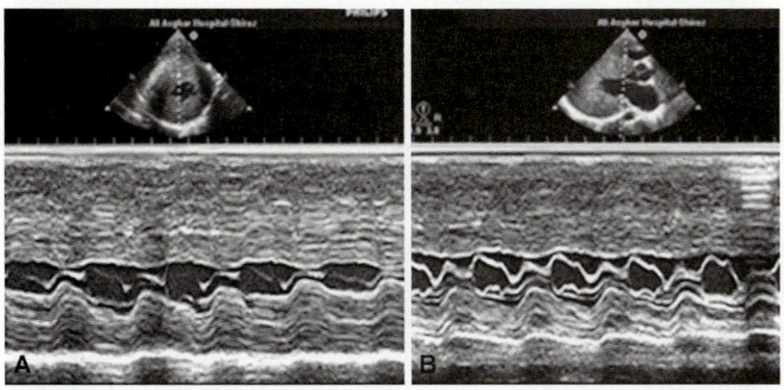


**Fig. 15.17:** M-mode echocardiography in parasternal window of a patient presented with recurrent episodes of syncope. (A) Short axis view of the left ventricle at the level of papillary muscle which shows severe hypertrophy of the left ventricle more prominently in the septum. (B) M-mode echocardiography of the mitral valve in long axis view demonstrates systolic anterior motion of the mitral valve leaflets

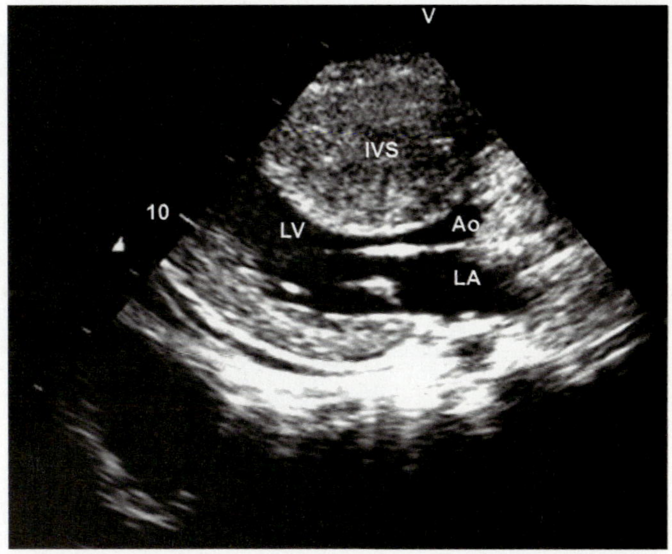


**Fig. 15.19:** Diffuse hypertrophy variant of hypertrophic cardiomyopathy (HCM). This pattern of hypertrophy is classically seen in younger patients. Ao, aorta; IVS, interventricular septum; LA, left atrium; LV, left ventricle

used include beta-blockers and calcium channel blockers, which may reduce chest pain and other symptoms, particularly with exercise. Medications will often relieve symptoms so patients do not need more invasive treatments.

Some people with arrhythmias may need anti-arrhythmic medications. If the arrhythmia is due to atrial fibrillation, blood thinners may also be used to reduce the risk of blood clots.

Some patients may have a permanent pacemaker placed. However, pacemakers are used less often today than they were in the past.

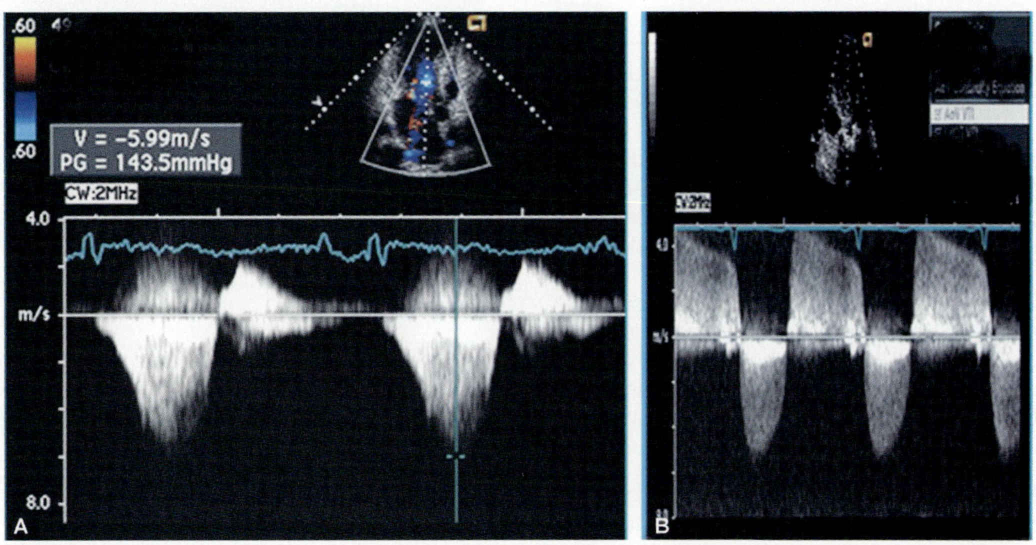


**Fig. 15.18:** Comparison of Doppler profiles of hypertrophic cardiomyopathy (HCM) (A), and aortic stenosis (B). Because aortic stenosis is a fixed obstruction, a contour of the aortic valve gradient can be seen. In contrast, the Doppler profile of HCM is seen as the classic dagger shape, reflecting the dynamic obstruction

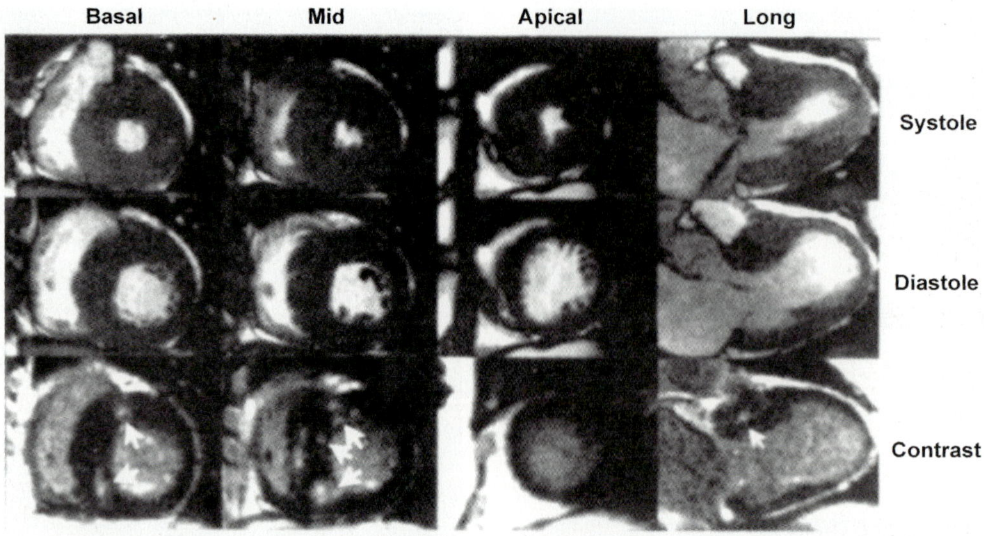


**Fig. 15.20:** Scans showing hypertrophy (maximum wall thickness, 27 mm) and scarring. There are multiple foci of scar tissue, which are located predominantly in the mid-myocardial region *(Mid)* and are not present in the lateral free wall. The long-axis *(Long)* cine images demonstrate systolic anterior motion of the mitral valve, systolic flow turbulence in the left ventricular outflow tract, and mitral regurgitation in patient with myocardial scarring in asymptomatic or mildly symptomatic hypertrophic cardiomyopathy

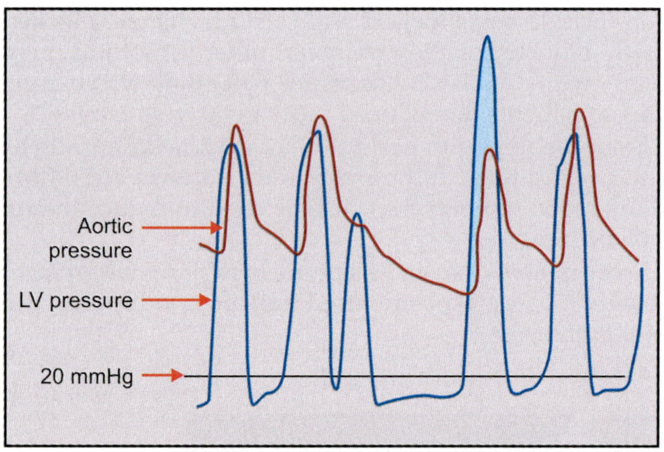


**Fig. 15.21:** Brockenbrough's response. The Brockenbrough's response in the postpremature ventricular contraction (PVC) is classic for hypertrophic cardiomyopathy (HCM). Post-PVC, there is increased preload secondary to a compensatory pause. The increased contractility associated with the post-PVC beat results in increased left ventricular outflow tract (LVOT) obstruction in HCM patients and a subsequent increase in the left ventricular-aortic gradient and decreased aortic pulse pressure during the post-PVC beat. In contrast, in subjects with no LVOT obstruction, a PVC results in increased cardiac contractility, but there is no left ventricle aortic gradient, either at rest or in the post-PVC beat. The aortic pulse pressure in the post-PVC beat usually increases because of the increased contractility. LV=left ventricular

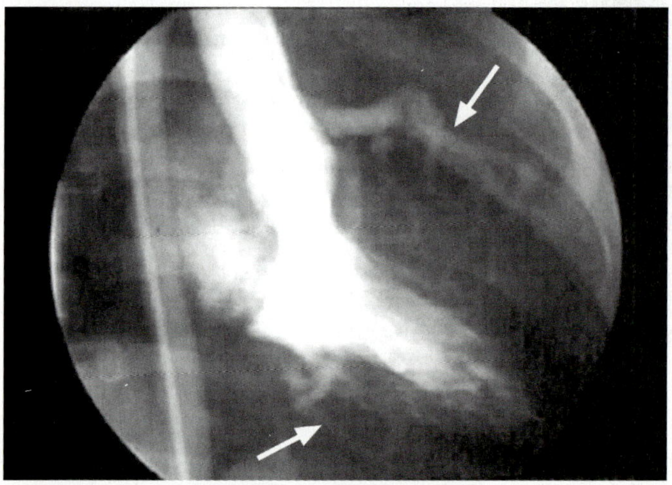

**Fig. 15.22:** Cardiomyopathy, hypertrophic. Conventional end-systolic right anterior oblique left ventriculogram acquired during the same cardiac catheterization study as in the previous image shows a small left-ventricular cavity with mild-mitral regurgitation (M). Note the increased distance between the ventricular cavity and the coronary arteries (arrows), which define the epicardial surface of the heart as the myocardium becomes thickened in systole

When blood flow out of the heart is severely blocked, an operation called surgical myectomy may be done. This procedure cuts and removes a portion of the thickened part of the heart. Patients who have this procedure often show significant improvement. If the heart's mitral valve is leaking, surgery may be done to repair or replace the valve.

In some cases, patients may be given an injection of alcohol into the arteries that feed the thickened part of the heart (alcohol septal ablation), essentially causing a controlled heart attack (Figs 15.23–15. 25).

An implantable-cardioverter defibrillator (ICD) may be needed to prevent sudden death. ICDs are used in high-risk patients. High risks include (Fig. 15.26):

- Drop in blood pressure during exercise
- Family history of cardiac arrest
- History of cardiac arrest or ventricular tachycardia
- History of unexplained fainting

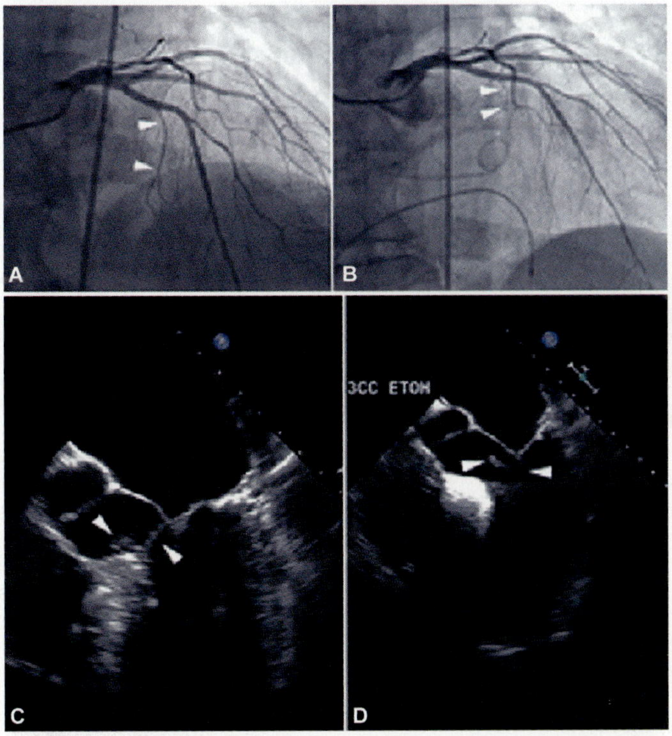

**Fig.15.23:** (A) Pre-alcohol septal ablation left coronary angiography highlighting the first septal perforator (arrowheads), (B) post-alcohol septal ablation left coronary angiography demonstrating subtotal occlusion of the first septal perforator (arrowheads). Echo scan shows change in systolic anterior motion of the accessory mitral valve tissue (arrowheads) following alcohol septal ablation, (C) pre-alcohol septal ablation; (D) post-alcohol septal ablation

- Life-threatening heart rhythms on a Holter monitor
- Severe heart muscle thickness

### Prognosis In HCM

Some people with hypertrophic cardiomyopathy may not have symptoms and live a normal lifespan. Others may get worse gradually or rapidly. The condition may develop into a dilated cardiomyopathy in some patients.

People with hypertrophic cardiomyopathy are at higher risk for sudden death than the normal population. Sudden death can occur at a young age.

Hypertrophic cardiomyopathy is a well-known cause of sudden death in athletes. Almost half of deaths in hypertrophic cardiomyopathy happen during or just after the patient has done some type of physical activity.

If you have hypertrophic cardiomyopathy, always follow your doctor's advice concerning exercise and medical appointments. Patients are sometimes advised to avoid strenuous exercise.

### Possible Complications in HCM

- Dilated cardiomyopathy
- Heart failure
- Life-threatening heart rhythm problems (arrhythmias)
- Severe injury from fainting

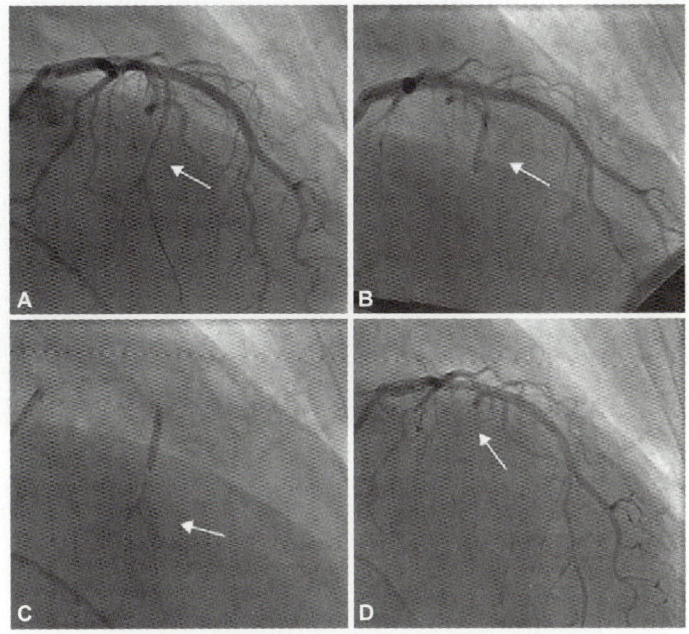

**Fig. 15.24:** Angiographic demonstration of alcohol septal ablation technique. Left coronary angiography shows the target septal branch (arrow); an angioplasty guidewire is already inserted inside the septal branch (A); optimal positioning of the balloon catheter (arrow) in the proximal part of the septal artery without compromise of the left anterior descending artery (B); injection of angiographic contrast dye through the central lumen of the inflated balloon catheter (arrow) determines the supply area of the septal branch and excludes leakage into the left anterior descending artery or other coronary vessels (C); final demonstration of the septal artery stump (arrow) after alcohol-induced occlusion (D)

#### *When to Contact a Medical Professional*

Call for an appointment with your health care provider if:

- You have any symptoms of hypertrophic cardiomyopathy
- You develop chest pain, palpitations, faintness, or other new or unexplained symptoms

### Prevention in HCM

If you are diagnosed with hypertrophic cardiomyopathy, your health care provider may recommend that your close blood relatives (family members) be screened for the condition.

Some patients with mild forms of hypertrophic cardiomyopathy are only diagnosed by screening echocardiograms because of their known family history.

If you have high blood pressure, make sure you take your medication and follow your doctor's recommendations.

## ISCHEMIC CARDIOMYOPATHY

Ischemic cardiomyopathy is a term used to describe patients whose heart can no longer pump enough blood to the rest of their body due to coronary artery disease.

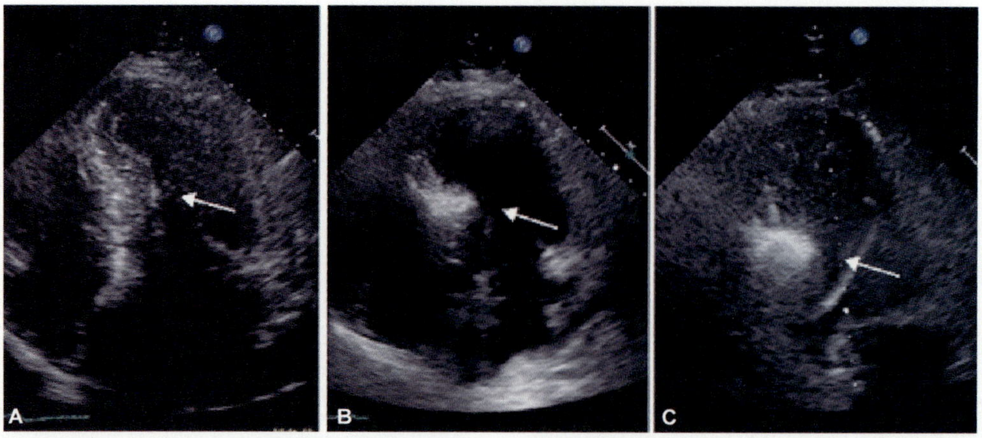


**Fig.15.25:** Myocardial contrast echocardiography during alcohol septal ablation. (A) First, the anatomy of the heart is presented and the target septal area is identified. (B) Injection of echocardiographic contrast into the target septal branch opacifies the basal part of the septum, verifying the optimal choice of septal branch. (C) A more sustained opacification of the basal septum after alcohol injection signifies a good alcohol depot

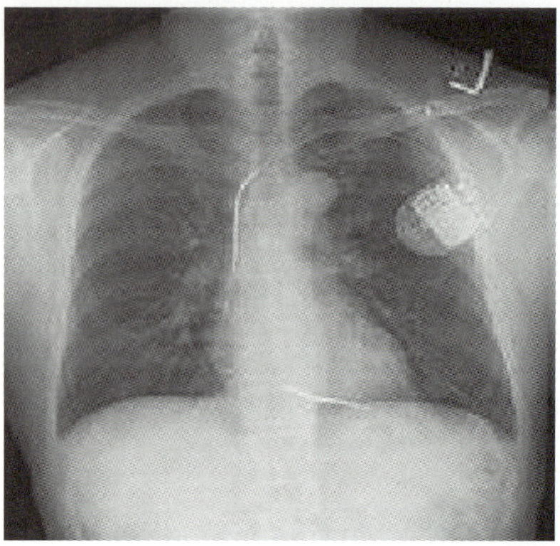

**Fig. 15.26:** Chest X-ray showing an implantable cardioverter-defibrillator in patient with hypertrophic obstructive cardiomyopathy

Coronary artery disease is a narrowing of the small blood vessels that supply blood and oxygen to the heart.

These patients often have heart failure.

## Aetiological Factors

Ischemic cardiomyopathy is caused by coronary heart disease—the buildup of a hard substance called plaque in the arteries to the heart. This may also be called hardening of the arteries.

When the arteries that bring blood and oxygen to the heart are blocked or very narrowed, over time, the heart muscle does not work as well. It becomes harder for the heart to fill and pump blood to the body. Patients with this condition usually have a history of heart attacks or angina (chest pain).

Ischemic cardiomyopathy is a common cause of heart failure. It is the most common type of cardiomyopathy in the United States. It most often affects middle-aged and elderly people

Patients with this condition often have had symptoms of angina or a heart attack. Sometimes, patients do not notice any symptoms

## Symptoms in ICM

Symptoms of heart failure usually develop slowly over time. Common symptoms include:

- Cough
- Fatigue, weakness, and faintness
- Irregular or fast pulse, or a sensation of feeling the heart beat (palpitations)
- Loss of appetite
- Shortness of breath, especially with activity
- Shortness of breath that occurs after lying down
- Swelling of feet and ankles (in adults)
- Swelling of the abdomen (in adults)
- Waking up from sleep after a couple of hours due to shortness of breath

## Physical Exams and Lab Tests

The physical exam may be normal, or there may be signs that fluid is building up in the body:

- 'Crackles' in the lungs (heard with a stethoscope)
- Enlarged liver
- Extra heart sounds
- Leg swelling
- Raised pressure in the neck vein

There may be other signs of heart failure.

This condition is usually diagnosed if a test shows that the heart is not pumping as well as it should. This is called a decreased ejection fraction. A normal ejection fraction is around 55–65%. Many patients with this disorder have ejection fractions much less than this.

People with ischemic heart disease can have the symptoms and signs of ischemic cardiomyopathy even when their ejection fraction is normal or near normal. This is

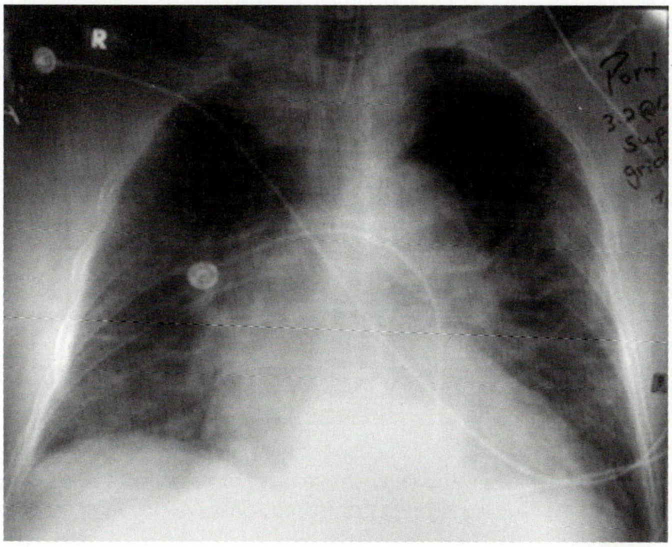


**Fig. 15.27:** Chest X-ray showing gross cardiomegaly with bilateral congestion due to congestive heart failure in ischemic cardiomyopathy

because the heart does not fully relax (impaired filling). It is sometimes called 'diastolic heart failure' or 'heart failure with preserved ejection fraction.'

Tests used to measure ejection fraction include:

- Chest X-ray (Fig. 15.27)
- Electrogardiogram (Figs 15.28 and 15.29)
- Echocardiogram (Fig. 15.30)
- Gated SPECT (Fig. 15.31)
- MRI of heart/CT angiography (Fig.15.32)
- Ventriculogram or cardiac blood pooling imaging (Fig. 15.33)

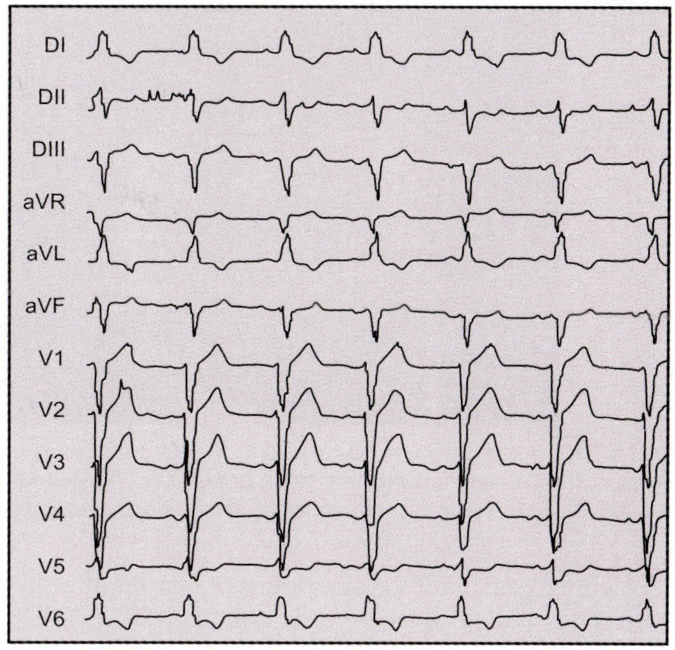


**Fig. 15.29:** Resynchronization therapy in a man of 57 years old with ischemic cardiomyopathy, ejection fraction 20%-NYHA Class III-optimal medical therapy-QRS 145 ms aspect of left bundle branch

*Biopsy of the heart* is needed in rare cases to rule out other conditions.

### Treatment in ICM

To treat ischemic cardiomyopathy, your doctor will treat and manage your heart failure by

- Showing you how to make important changes in your lifestyle

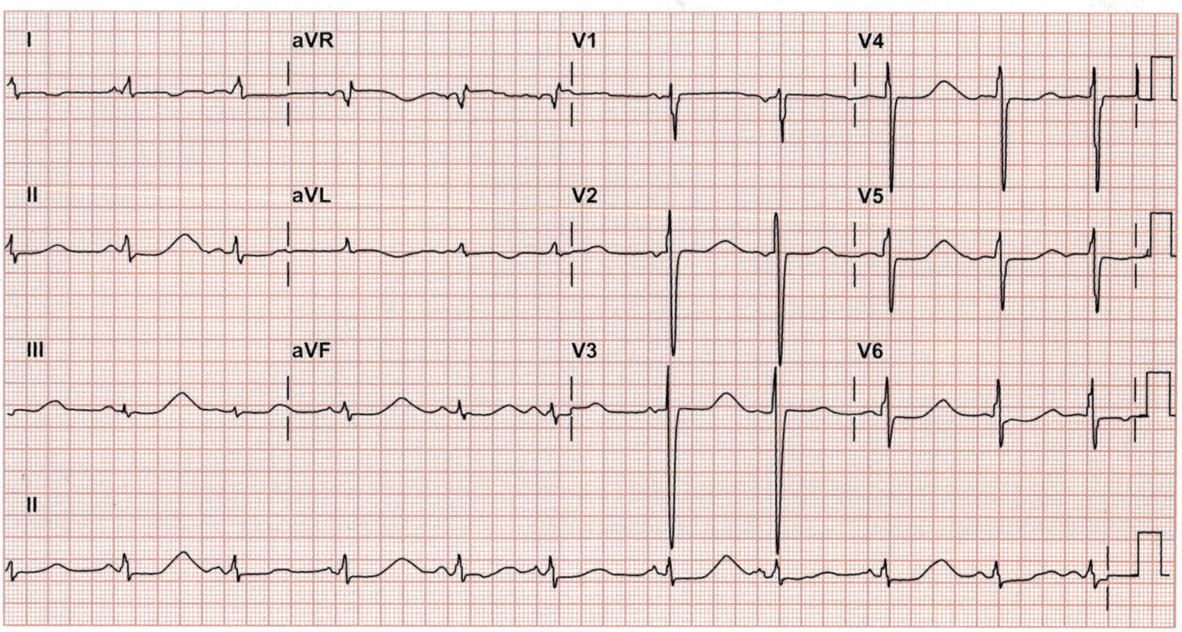


**Fig.15.28:** ECG morphology of a 83-year-old man with known ischemic cardiomyopathy with prolonged Qt interval, had an out-of-hospital cardiac arrest. He is rushed to the ED by paramedics

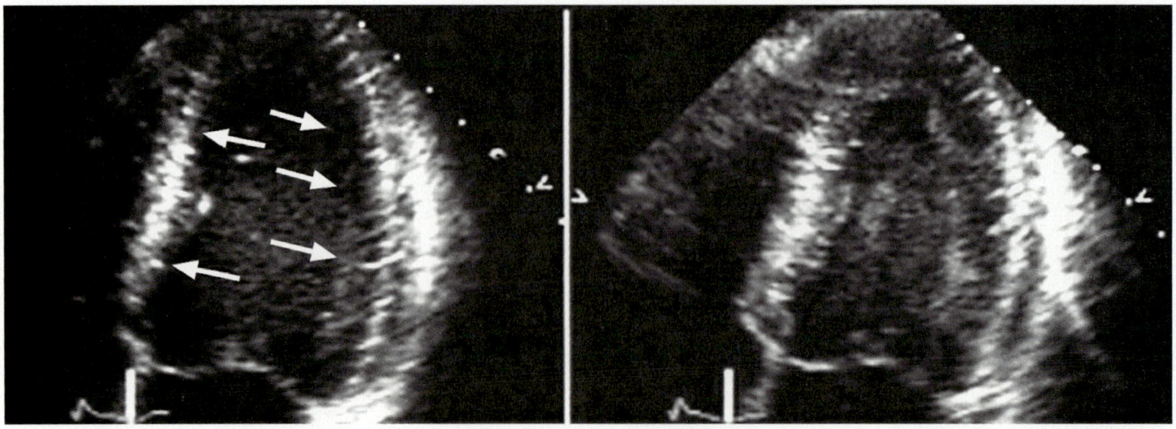

**Fig. 15.30:** Transthoracic two-dimensional echocardiogram (apical four chamber view, end systolic) at rest (left panel) and during infusion of low dose dobutamine (right panel) in a patient with ischemic cardiomyopathy and severe hypokinesia of the septum and lateral wall. During low dose dobutamine, improved contraction of the dysfunctional segments indicates myocardial viability

- Teaching you about the symptoms of heart failure
- Giving you medicines for heart failure
- Giving you a pacemaker to help treat a slow heart rate or help the heart beat in a more normal way
- Implanting a defibrilator, which recognizes abnormal heart rhythms and sends an electrical pulse to stop them.

A cardiac catheterization might be done to see if you need coronary artery bypass (CABG) surgery or a balloon procedure (angioplasty). These procedures can improve blood flow to the damaged or weakened heart muscle.

You may need a heart transplant if you have tried all the standard treatments and still have very severe symptoms. Implantable, artificial heart pumps are now available. However, very few patients are able to have these advanced treatments (Fig. 15.34).

## Prognosis in ICM

Often, heart failure can be controlled with medicine, lifestyle changes, and by treating the disease that caused it.

Heart failure may suddenly become worse due to angina, heart attack, infections, other illnesses, eating foods that high in salt, and not taking medicines correctly.

Heart failure is usually a long-term (chronic) illness. It may get worse over time.

Some people develop severe heart failure. Medicines, surgery, and other treatments no longer help. They are at risk for dangerous heart rhythm problems.

### *When to Contact a Medical Professional*

- You have symptoms of ischemic cardiomyopathy

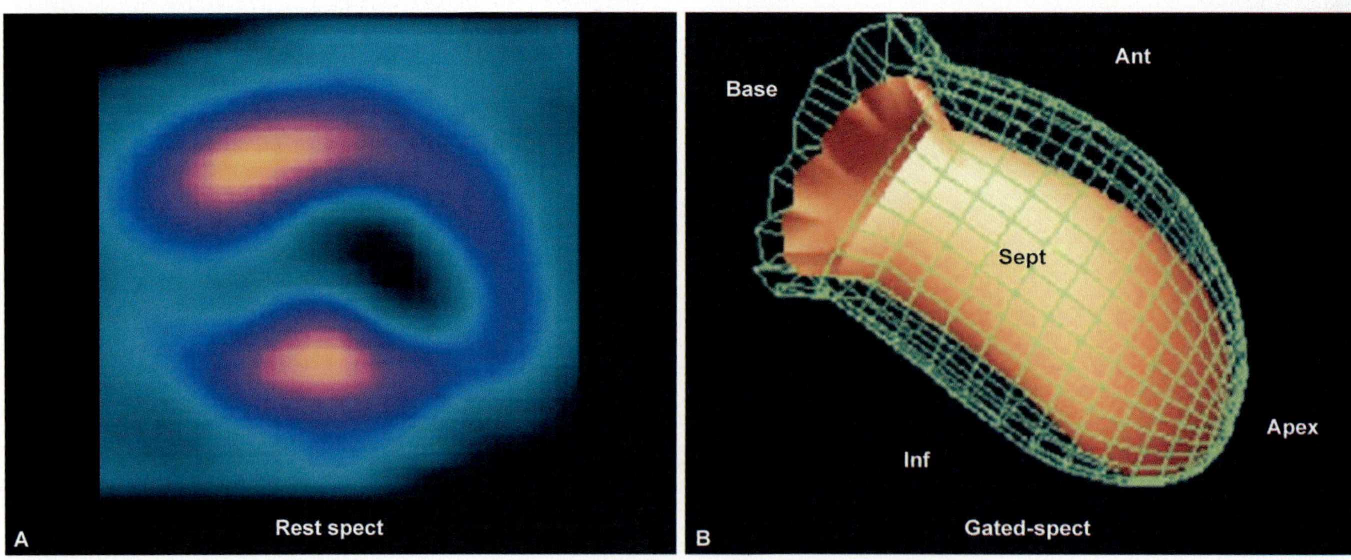


**Fig. 15.31:** Ischemic cardiomyopathy. (A) Divergent left ventricular pattern (transversal diameter at the apical level > transversal diameter at the basal level in vertical long-axis view) and absence of anteroapical uptake in myocardial perfusion SPECT at rest in a patient with anterior infarction. These criteria are highly specific for myocardial nonviability. (B) Gated-SPECT of the same patient in whom anterior akinesia and septal and apical dyskinesia can be observed. End-diastolic volume, 248 ml; end-systolic volume, 203 ml; ejection fraction, 18%. Ant=anterior; Inf=inferior; SPECT=single-photon emission computed tomography

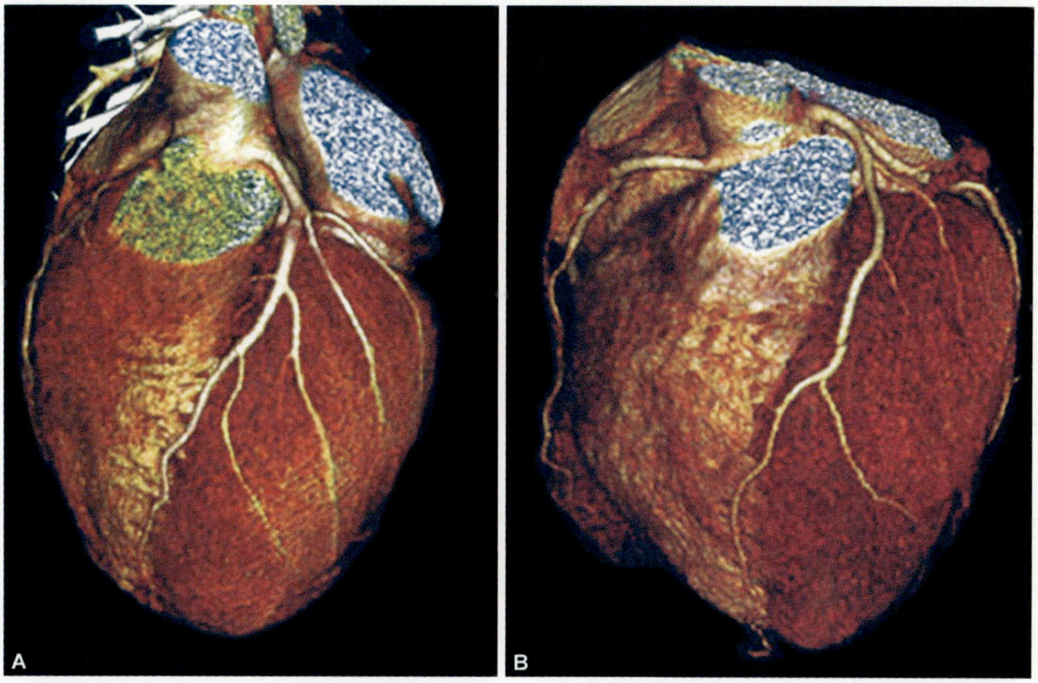


**Fig. 15.32:** Multislice CT reconstructions of (A) control heart and (B) a heart affected by IDCM, showing marked epicardial coronary artery mismatch for left ventricular mass and side-branch reduction. IDCM=idiopathic dilated cardiomyopathy

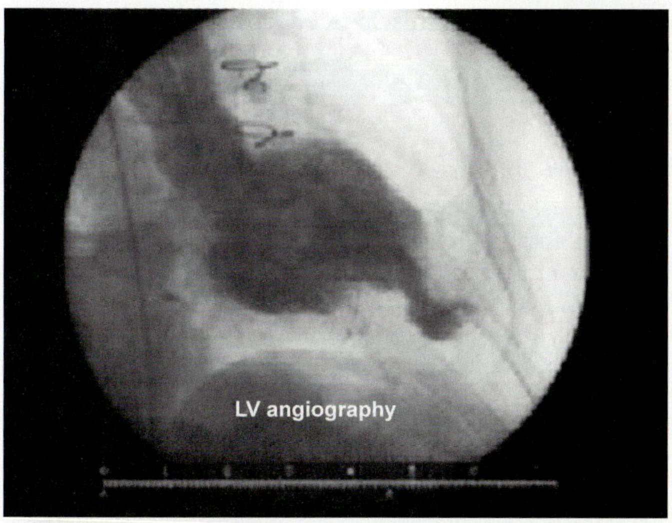


**Fig. 15.33:** LV angiography showing apical left ventricular dyskinesis (ventricular aneurysm) after an anterior myocardial infarction

- You have chest pain that is not relieved by rest or nitroglycerin
- You pass out (syncope)

### Prevention in ICM

Some of the risks for heart disease that you CAN change are:

- Do not smoke or use tobacco.
- Get plenty of exercise—at least 30 minutes a day, at least 5 days a week (talk to your doctor first)
- Stay at a healthy weight. Try for a body mass index (BMI) of between 18.5 and 24.9.

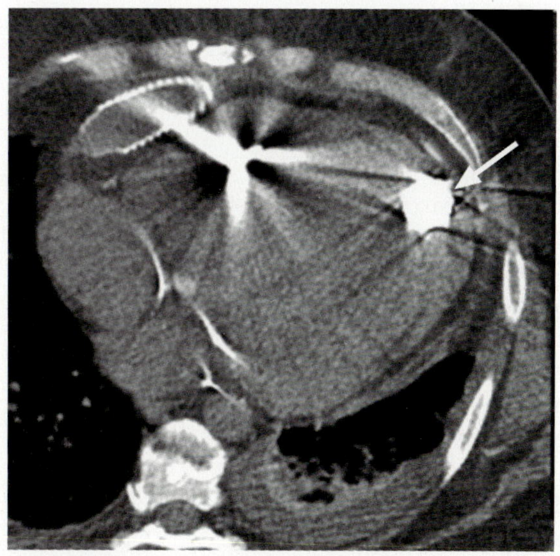

**Fig. 15.34:** 67-year-old man with HeartMate II (Thoratec) that was implanted for ischemic cardiomyopathy and ejection fraction of 10%

- Get checked and treated for depression.
- Women at high risk for heart disease should take omega-3 fatty acid supplements.

If you drink alcohol, limit yourself to no more than one drink a day for women, and no more than two drinks a day for men. Because alcohol in large amounts can be toxic to the heart, you may be asked to limit your alcohol even more, or stop drinking it completely.

Good nutrition is important for your heart health and will control some of your risk factors. See also heart disease and diet.

## RESTRICTIVE CARDIOMYOPATHY

Restrictive cardiomyopathy (RCM) refers to a group of disorders in which the heart chambers are unable to properly fill with blood because of stiffness in the heart.

### Aetiological Factors

In restrictive cardiomyopathy, the heart is of normal size or only slightly enlarged. However, it cannot relax normally during the time between heartbeats when the blood returns from the body to the heart (diastole).

Later in the disease, the heart may not pump blood efficiently. The abnormal heart function can affect the lungs, liver, and other body systems. Restrictive cardiomyopathy may affect either or both ventricles. It may be associated with a disease of the heart muscle.

The most common causes of restrictive cardiomyopathy are amyloidosis and scarring of the heart from an unknown cause (idiopathic myocardial fibrosis). It frequently occurs after a heart transplant.

*Other causes of restrictive cardiomyopathy include:*

- Carcinoid heart disease
- Diseases of the heart lining (endocardium), such as endomyocardial fibrosis and Loeffler's syndrome (rare)
- Iron overload (hemochromatosis)
- Radiation fibrosis
- Sarcoidosis
- Scleroderma
- Tumors of the heart

### Symptoms in RCM

Symptoms of heart failure are most common. Usually, these symptoms develop slowly over time. However, sometimes symptoms start very suddenly and are severe.

*Common symptoms are:*

- Cough
- Difficulty breathing
  - at night
  - especially with exertion
  - when lying flat
- Fatigue, poor exercise tolerance
- Irregular or rapid pulse
- Loss of appetite
- Swelling of the abdomen
- Swelling of the feet and ankles

*Other symptoms may include:*

- Chest pain
- Decreased alertness or concentration
- Failure to thrive (in children)
- Low urine production
- Need to urinate at night (in adults)
- Shock (low blood pressure)

### Physical Examination and Laboratory Tests

An examination may show:

- Enlarged (distended) or bulging neck veins
- Enlarged liver
- Lung crackles and abnormal or distant heart sounds when listening to the chest with a stethoscope (auscultation)
- Fluid backup into the hands and feet
- Signs of heart failure

*Children will have:*

- Difficulty feeding
- Pale skin
- Poor growth
- Weak pulses in the legs and arms

*Laboratory and Imaging studies in restrictive cardiomyopathy include:*

- Chest X-ray (Fig. 15.35)
- ECG (electrocardiogram) (Fig. 15.36)
- Echocardiogram and Doppler study (Figs 15.37–15.42)
- Chest CT scan (Fig. 15.43)
- Cardiac catheterization and coronary angiography
- MRI of the heart (Fig. 15.44)

### Nuclear Heart Scan (MUGA, RNV)

Occasionally, patients with dilated or restrictive cardiomyopathy may have a nuclear cardiac stress test to evaluate how well the heart muscle is being supplied with blood and how well the ventricles or chambers are working. This information is used to determine the best way to treat their symptoms.

### Serum Iron Studies

The term iron overload cardiomyopathy describes the different forms of cardiac dysfunction secondary to myocardial iron deposition. Besides being a major cause of morbidity, IOC accounts for one-third of deaths in hereditary hemochromatosis, especially in young male patients; it is the leading cause of mortality in thalassemia

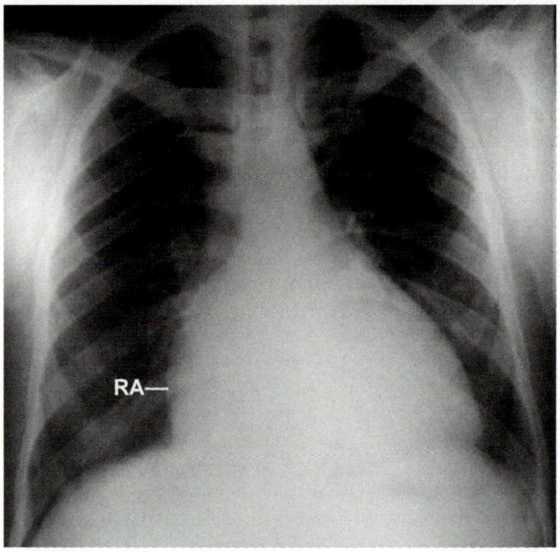


**Fig. 15.35:** X-ray chest PA view showing cardiomegaly with right atrial enlargement in restrictive cardiomyopathy

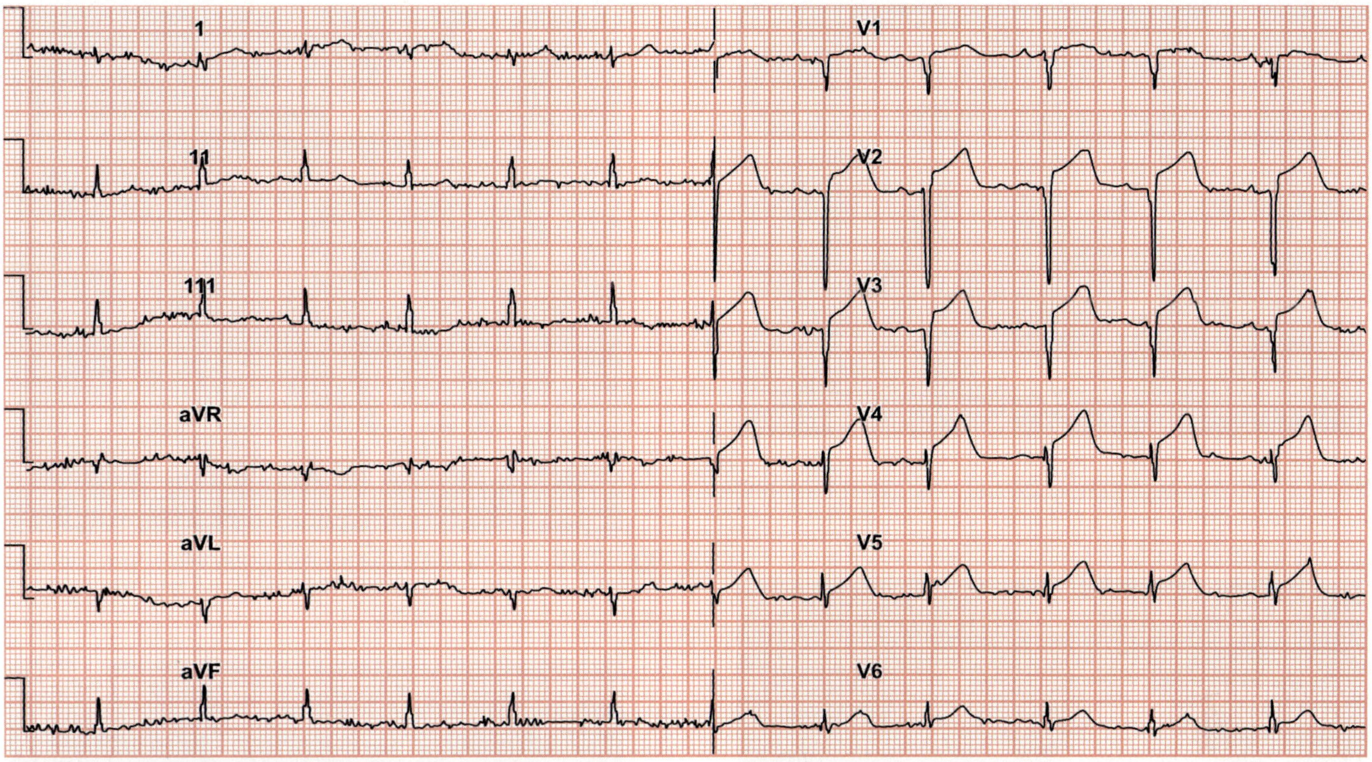


**Fig. 15.36:** Mixed constrictive-restrictive cardiomyopathy. ECG shows sinus rhythm (79/min) with absent progression of R-wave (V1–V4) and ST-elevation in precardial leads (V1–V6)

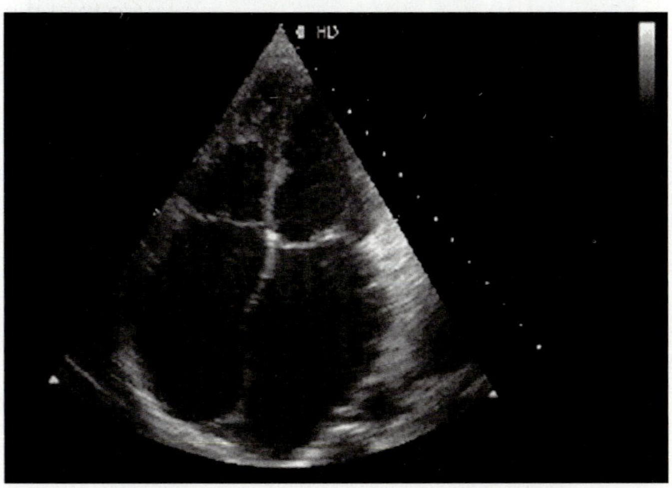

**Fig. 15.37:** A classical restrictive cardiomyopathy. Both atria balloon out as they face stiff resistance from the ventricles

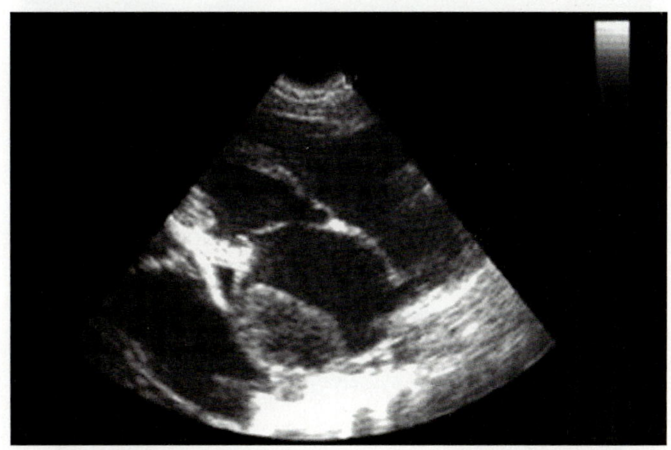

**Fig. 15.38:** Real-time ultrasound from a 5-year-old boy with restrictive cardiomyopathy showing pleural effusion and a thrombus in the left atrium

major; and it is also a major cause of death in other conditions associated with secondary iron overload.

Restrictive cardiomyopathy may be hard to tell apart from constrictive pericarditis. A biopsy of the heart muscle or cardiac catheterization may help confirm the diagnosis.

### Treatment in RCM

When the cause of any cardiomyopathy can be found, that condition is treated.

Few treatments are known to be effective for restrictive cardiomyopathy. The main goal of treatment is to control symptoms and improve quality of life.

The following treatments may be used to control symptoms or prevent problems:

- Blood thinning medications, either aspirin or warfarin
- Chemotherapy (in some situations)
- Diuretics to remove fluid and help improve breathing
- Medications to prevent or control irregular or abnormal heart rhythms
- Steroids for specific causes

A heart transplant may be considered if the heart function is very poor and the patient has many symptoms.

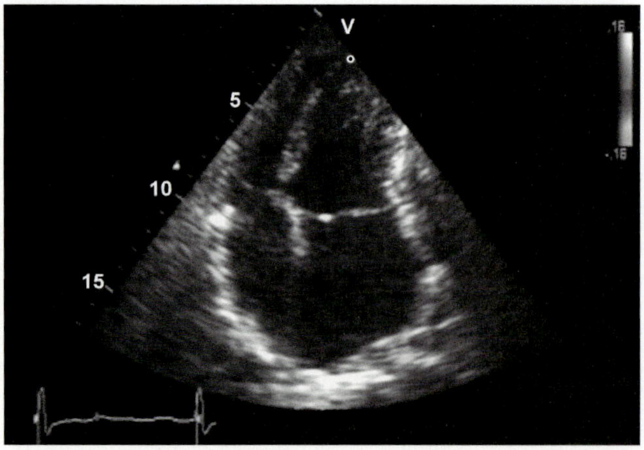


**Fig. 15.39:** Two-dimensional apical four-chamber image showing moderate to severe bi-atrial enlargement in a patient with restrictive cardiomyopathy

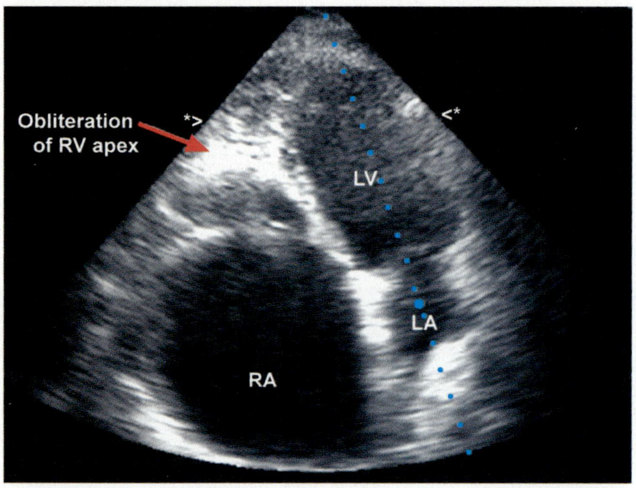


**Fig. 15.42:** Echocardiogram in right ventricular endomyocardial fibrosis

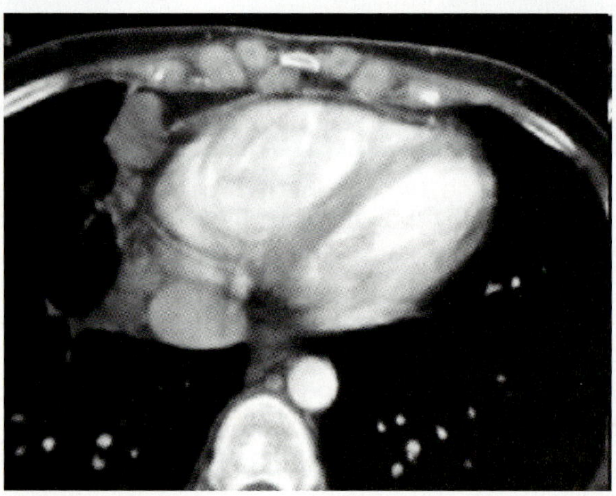

**Fig. 15.43:** Restrictive cardiomyopathy. Axial contrast-enhanced CT image through the heart (same patient as in previous image) shows a thin pericardium without calcification. Note the cardiophrenic and internal mammary lymph nodes. The patient had extensive mediastinal and hilar adenopathy, as well as interstitial lung changes

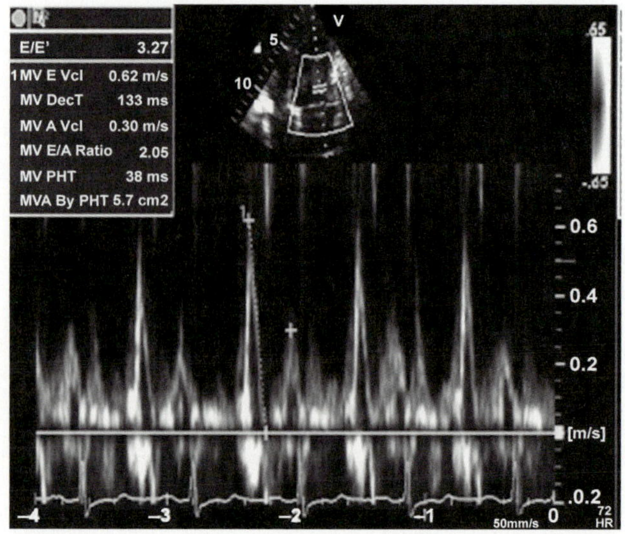


**Fig. 15.40:** Pulsed wave Doppler of transmitral flow; mitral valve E and A velocity measured 0.74 and 0.36 m/s, respectively. in restrictive cardiomyopathy

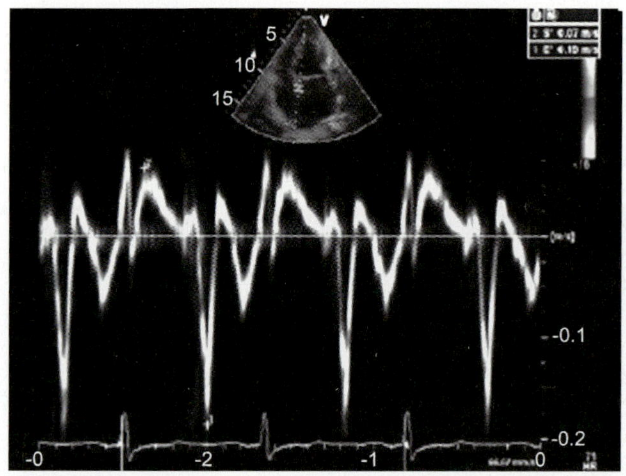


**Fig. 15.41:** Tissue Doppler imaging; E and S measured 19 and 7 cm/s, respectively, E/E ratio was 3 in case of a restrictive cardiomyopathy

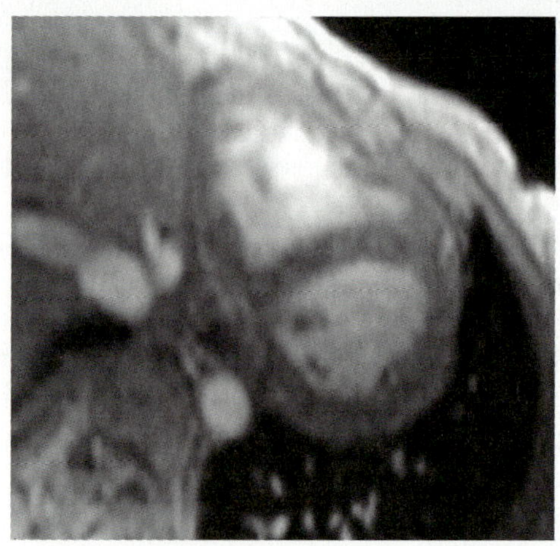

**Fig. 15.44:** Restrictive cardiomyopathy. Axial double inversion-recovery MRI of the heart in a 30-year-old woman with sarcoid demonstrates a normal pericardium

### Prognosis in RCM

People with restrictive cardiomyopathy may be heart transplant candidates. The outlook depends on the cause of the condition, but it is usually poor. Average survival after diagnosis is 9 years.

#### *Possible complications*

- Arrhythmias
- Mitral regurgitation
- Progressive heart failure
- Tricuspid regurgitation

### *When to Contact a Medical Professional*

Call your health care provider if you have symptoms of restrictive cardiomyopathy.

## NONCOMPACTION CARDIOMYOPATHY

Noncompaction cardiomyopathy (NCC), also called spongiform cardiomyopathy, is a rare congenital cardiomyopathy that affects both children and adults. It results from the failure of myocardial development during embryogenesis.

During development, the majority of the heart muscle is a sponge-like meshwork of interwoven myocardial fibers. As normal development progresses, these trabeculated structures undergo significant compaction that transforms them from spongy to solid. This process is particularly apparent in the ventricles, and particularly so in the left ventricle. Noncompaction cardiomyopathy results when there is failure of this process of compaction. Because the consequence of noncompaction is particularly evident in the left ventricle, the condition is also called left ventricular noncompaction. Other hypotheses and models have been proposed, none of which is as widely accepted as the noncompaction model.

Symptoms can range however are often a result of a poor pumping performance by the heart. The disease can be associated with other problems with the heart and the body.

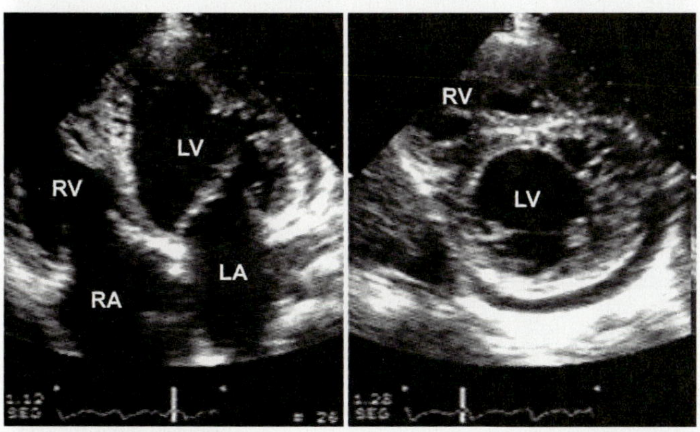


**Fig. 15.45:** Two-dimensional apical four chamber and parasternal short axis images at the level of the ventricles show dilatation of both ventricles, multiple trabeculae and intertrabecular recesses in inferior, lateral, anterior walls, middle and apical portions of the septum and apex of the left ventricle in a case with noncompacted cardiomyopathy

### Diagnosis

Trabeculation of the ventricles is normal, as are prominent, discrete muscular bundles greater than 2 mm. In noncompaction there is excessively prominent trabeculations. Chin et al. described echocardiographic method to distinguish noncompaction for normal trabeculation. They described a ratio of the distance from the trough and peak, of the trabeculations, to the epicardial surface. Noncompaction is diagnosed when the trabeculations are more than twice the thickness of the underlying ventricular wall.

### Imaging Studies

- Echocardiography (Figs 15.45–15.50)
- MRI (Fig. 15.51)

### *Genetics*

The American Heart Association's 2006 classification of cardiomyopathies considers noncompaction cardiomyopathy a genetic cardiomyopathy. Mutations in LDB3 (also known as 'Cypher/ZASP') have been described in patients with the condition. There is recent information in which

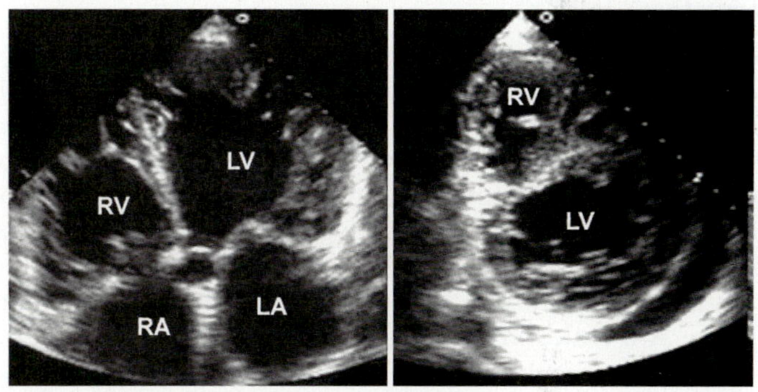


**Fig. 15.46:** Transthoracic two-dimensional echocardiogram in apical four chamber and parasternal short axis at the level of both ventricles demonstrate dilatation, deep trabeculae and intertrabecular recesses in the inferior, lateral, anterior walls, middle and apical portions of the septum and apex of the left ventricle in a case with noncompacted cardiomyopathy

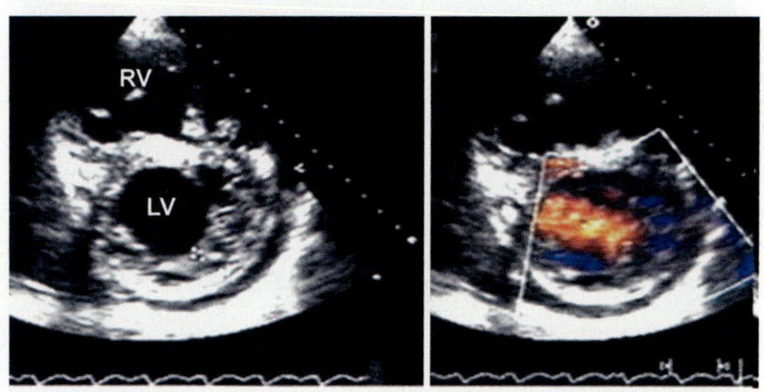


**Fig. 15.47:** Two-dimensional parasternal and color-Doppler images at the level of both ventricles that show the noncompacted-compacted wall ratio and how the color enters the intertrabecular recesses in a case with noncompacted cardiomyopathy

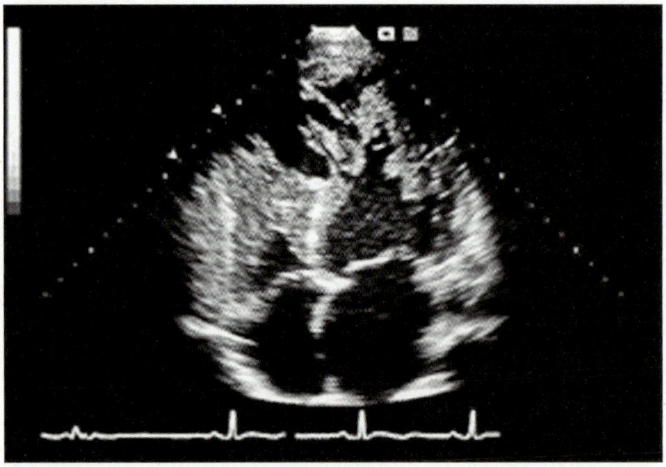

**Fig. 15.48:** Apical four chamber view on transthoracic echocardiogram (apex up) revealing a left ventricle with a thick spongy endocardial surface that is severely trabeculated at the apex characteristic of left ventricular noncompaction

NCC has been seen in combination with 1q21.1 deletion syndrome.

## Symptoms in NCC

Subjects' symptoms from noncompaction cardiomyopathy range widely. It is possible to be diagnosed with the condition, yet not to suffer from any of the symptoms associated with heart disease. Likewise it possible to suffer from severe heart failure, which even though the condition is present from birth, may only manifest itself later in life. Differences in symptoms between adults and children are also prevalent with adults more likely to suffer from heart failure and children from depression of systolic function.

Common symptoms associated with a reduced pumping performance of the heart include:

- Breathlessness

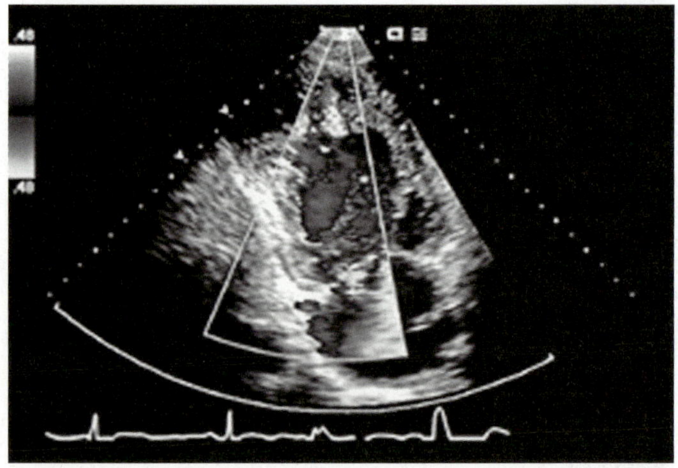

**Fig. 15.50:** Apical two chamber view on transthoracic echocardiogram (apex up) with low-scale color-Doppler showing multiple large recesses in the left ventricular apex being perfused from the left ventricular cavity

- Fatigue
- Swelling of the ankles
- Limited physical capacity and exercise intolerance

Two conditions though that are more prevalent in noncompaction cardiomyopathy are: tachyarrhythmia which can lead to sudden cardiac death and clotting of the blood in the heart.

### *Complications*

The presence of NCC can also lead to other complications around the heart and elsewhere in the body. These are not necessarily common complications and no paper has yet commented on how frequently these complications occur with NCC as well.

- Cardiac

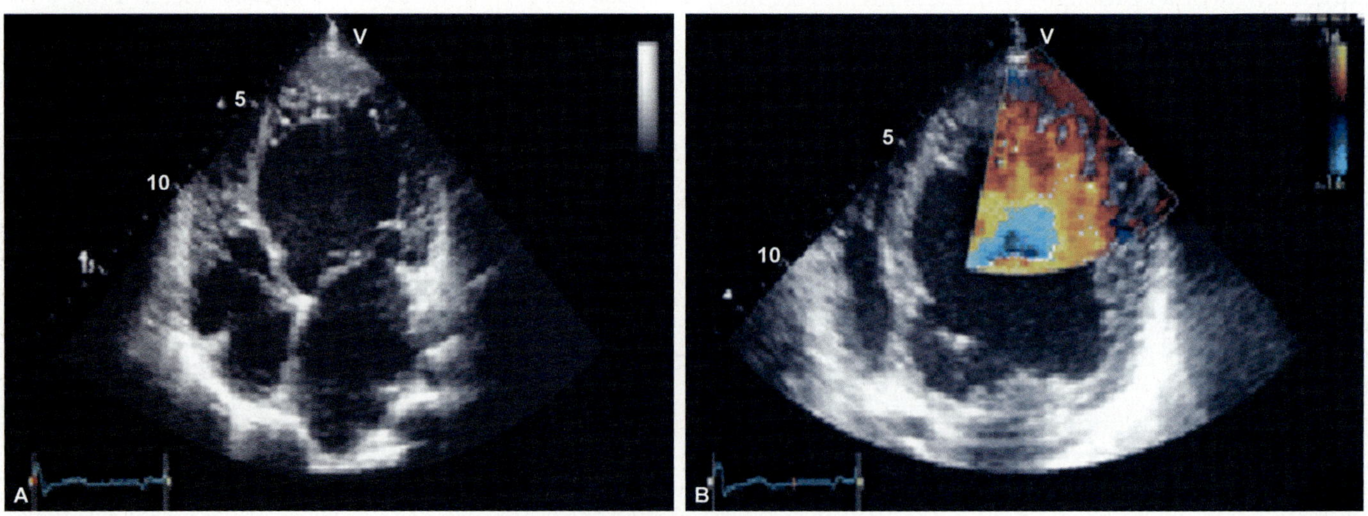


**Fig. 15.49:** Left ventricular noncompaction. (A) There is marked LV dilatation and dysfunction, thinning of the septum and hypertrophy, excessive trabeculation of the lateral wall and apex. (B) Color flow mapping shows flow within deep recesses, extending to the epicardium at the apex

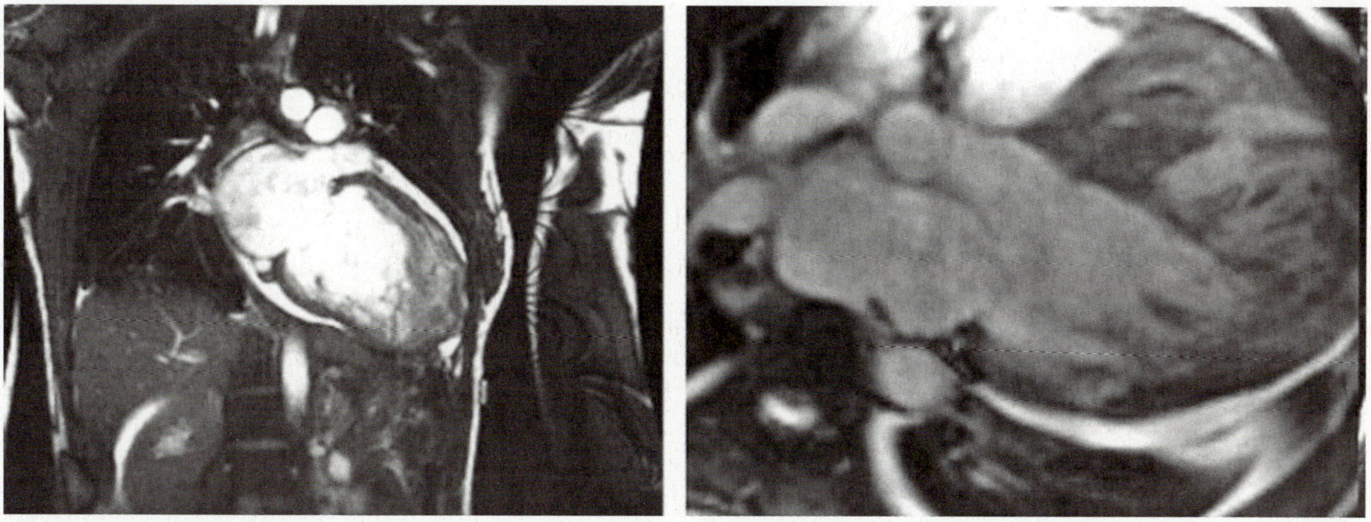

**Fig. 15.51:** Images from cardiac MRI showing a markedly dilated left ventricle and left atrium. The left ventricle shows prominent trabeculation particularly along the apex. A small pericardial effusion and a small pleural effusion are also noted in a case with non-compacted cardiomyopathy

- Abnormalities of the origin of the left coronary artery
- Pulmonary atresia
- Stenosis
- Right or left ventricle obstruction
- Hypoplastic left ventricle
- Mitral regurgitation
- Neuromuscular (pertaining to both nerves and muscles)
  - Becker's muscular dystrophy
  - Mitochondrial myopathy
  - Polyneuropathy and metabolic myopathy
- Genetic related
  - Emery-dreifuss muscular dystrophy
  - Myotubular cardiomyopathy
  - Barth syndrome

### Prognosis in NCC

Due to noncompaction cardiomyopathy being a relatively new disease, its impact on human life expectancy is not very well understood. In a 2005 study which documented the long term follow up of 34 patients with NCC, 35% had died at the age of 42 +/– 40 months with a further 12% having to undergo a heart transplant due to heart failure. However, this study was based upon symptomatic patients referred to a tertiary care center, and so were suffering from more severe forms of NCC than might be found typically in the population. As NCC is a genetic disease, immediate family members are being tested as a precaution which is turning up more supposedly healthy people with NCC who are asymptomatic. The long term prognosis for these people is currently unknown.

### Management in NCC

These are similar to management programs for other types of cardiomyopathies which include the use of ACE inhibitors, beta-blockers and aspirin therapy to relieve the pressure on the heart, surgical options such as the installation of pacemaker is also an option for those thought to be at a high risk of arrhythmia problems.

In severe cases, where NCC has led to heart failure, with resulting surgical treatment including a heart valve operation, or a heart transplant.

## ARRHYTHMOGENIC RIGHT VENTRICULAR CARDIOMYOPATHY

Arrhythmogenic right ventricular cardiomyopathy (ARVC) is a primary disease of heart muscle that results in fibrofatty replacement of the right ventricle and the subepicardial region of the left ventricle. Patients are at high risk for ventricular tachyarrhythmias and sudden death (see the image below).

Arrhythmogenic right ventricular cardiomyopathy, biventricular, autopsy heart in a young man who died suddenly playing basketball. Top left demonstrates increased fat in the outer walls of the right ventricle and left ventricular posterolateral walls. A higher magnification of the right ventricle is seen at the top right image; the anterior wall is nearly completely replaced with fat, and fibrofatty irregular posterior wall involvement is seen. Note that no actual thinning of the wall itself exists, although the muscular portion is in some areas completely missing. The bottom left image demonstrates a full thickness of the right ventricle stained with Masson trichrome. The residual muscle is present only in a band like area of scarring, and subepicardial scarring is present as well. The characteristic myocyte vacuolization, depicted in the bottom right image, is seen in nearly all areas of ARVC within the scarred areas.

Although ARVC was initially described in the right ventricle, examination of the heart in autopsy cases of ARVC, microscopically or with sensitive imaging techniques, has established that most patients with ARVC have biventricular involvement.

The left ventricular involvement is typically subepicardial, and the changes are related more to fibrosis than to fat or fibrofatty infiltration, although at times the changes are probably similar to those seen in the right ventricle. However, because the right ventricle is relatively thin, the subepicardial nature of disease is difficult to appreciate in imaging studies and has only infrequently been investigated at autopsy. Atrial involvement appears not to have been adequately investigated.

Previously, investigators postulated that ARVC begins in the right ventricle and progresses to biventricular involvement and heart failure. However, newer imaging techniques have revealed that left ventricular involvement is typical from the onset.

Some patients with ARVC develop heart failure and intractable arrhythmias and are treated with heart transplantation. A subset of these patients carries the clinical diagnosis of idiopathic dilated cardiomyopathy. In such patients, the pathologic diagnosis of ARVC is made initially on finding fibrofatty replacement on histologic sections of the recipient's explanted heart.

### Aetiological Factors

The aetiology of arrhythmogenic right ventricular cardiomyopathy is unknown. The presence of inflammatory infiltrates in most cases that have been seen at autopsy has led to the theory that it is a resolving myocarditis. Families have been described with phenotypic alterations ranging from myocarditis to fibrofatty cardiac infiltrates, and imaging studies have demonstrated a progression from myocarditis to ARVC.

Family studies have suggested that ARVC is caused by genetic alterations in desmosomal proteins, especially plakoglobin and desmoplakin. One family study demonstrated desmosomal mutations in just fewer than 20% of patients. ARVC is possibly an inflammatory process that is modulated by genetic influences in desmosome-related proteins.

### Prognosis in ARVC

Because autopsy studies are skewed toward fatal arrhythmogenic right ventricular cardiomyopathy and by consent for autopsy, it has been assumed that ARVC is uniformly lethal. The clinical diagnosis has been hampered by the nonspecificity of electrocardiographic and imaging findings. However, with improvements in cardiac MRI and computed tomography scanning, the clinical diagnosis has become more precise.

Studies of families with ARVC have suggested that with antiarrhythmic treatment, including the implantation of defibrillators, the prognosis may be improved. Young age, a family history of juvenile sudden death, QRS dispersion greater than or equal to 40 ms, T-wave inversion, left ventricular involvement, ventricular tachycardia, syncope, and previous cardiac arrest are the major risk factors for adverse prognosis. Preparticipation screening for sport eligibility has been proven to be effective in detecting asymptomatic patients and sport disqualification has saved lives; sudden death in young athletes has substantially declined.

### Diagnosis in ARVC

Laboratory and imaging studies

Electrocardiogram (Fig. 15.52 and 15.53)

Electrophysiological study (Fig. 15.54)

### MRI Studies

The primary symptoms of arrhythmogenic right ventricular cardiomyopathy are related to arrhythmias and conduction

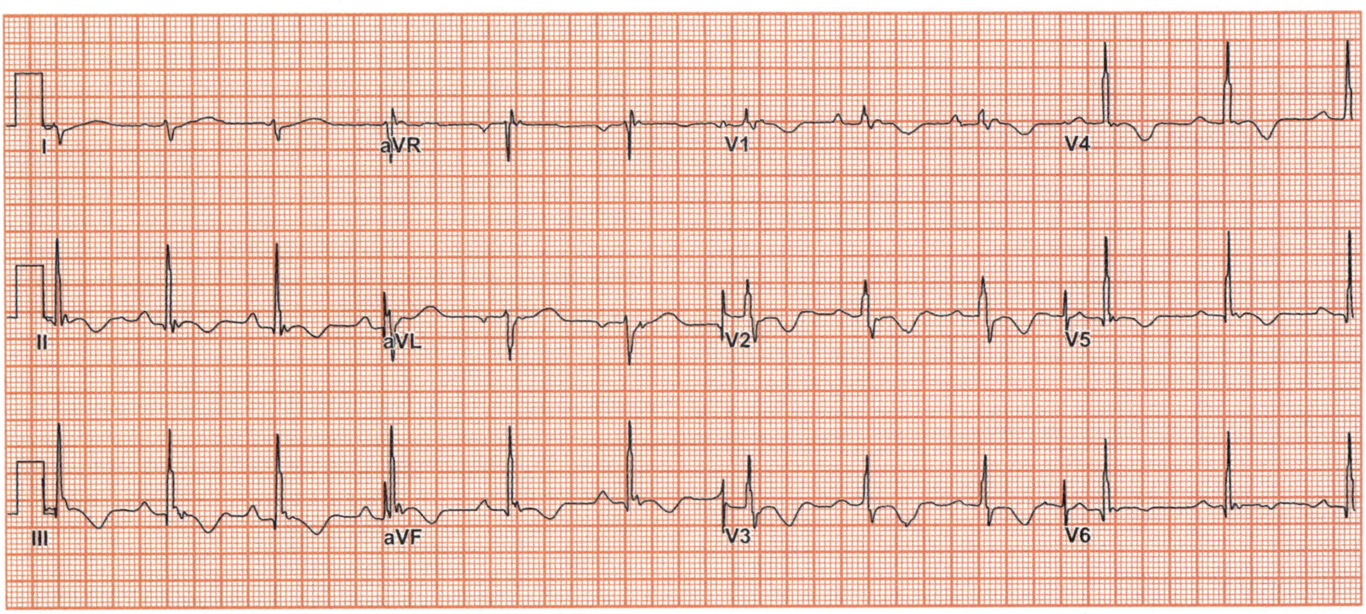


**Fig. 15.52:** Right ventricular hypertrophy in a patient with arrhythmogenic right ventricular cardiomyopathy—right axis deviation. R/S ratio in V1 > 1 Right ventricular strain pattern with T-wave inversion and ST-depression in the right precordial (V1–3) and inferior (II, III, aVF) leads

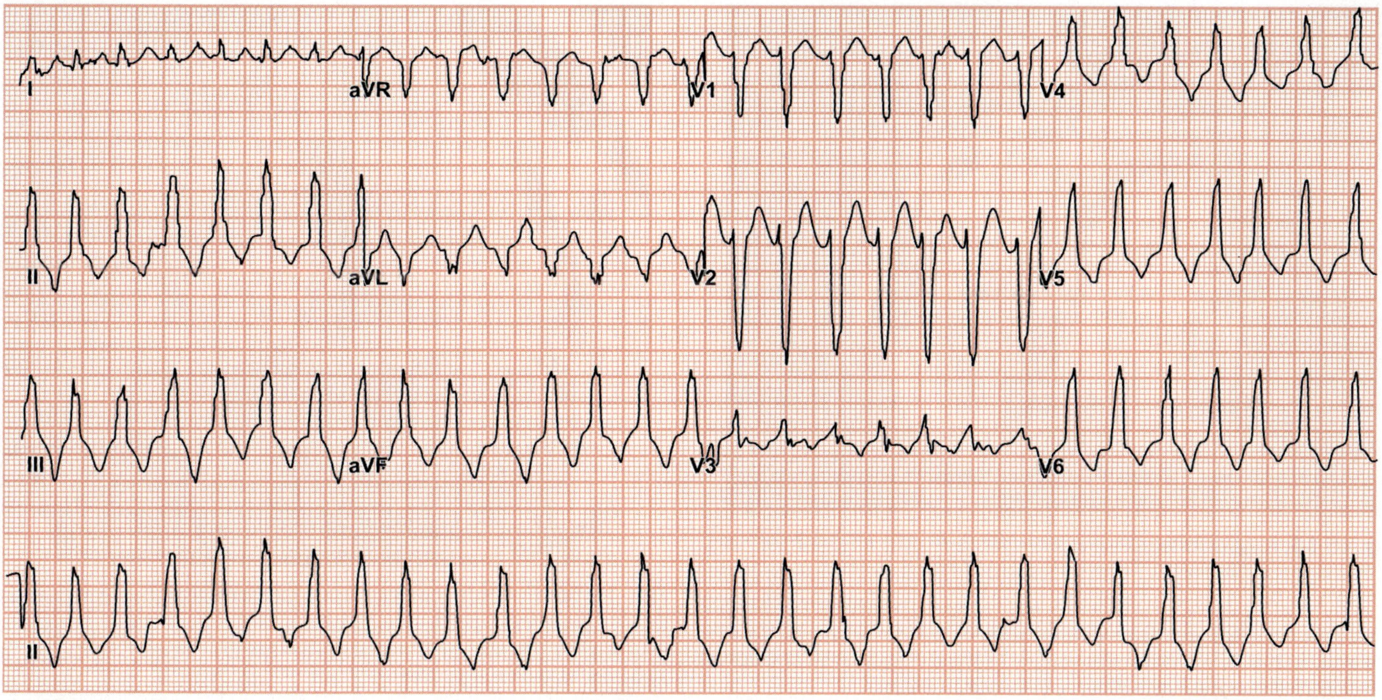


**Fig. 15.53:** Arrhythmogenic right ventricular cardiomyopathy with evidence of biventricular involvement. Electrocardiogram obtained on admission showing monomorphic ventricular tachycardia with left superior axis and left bundle branch block type configuration, indicating origin in the right ventricle

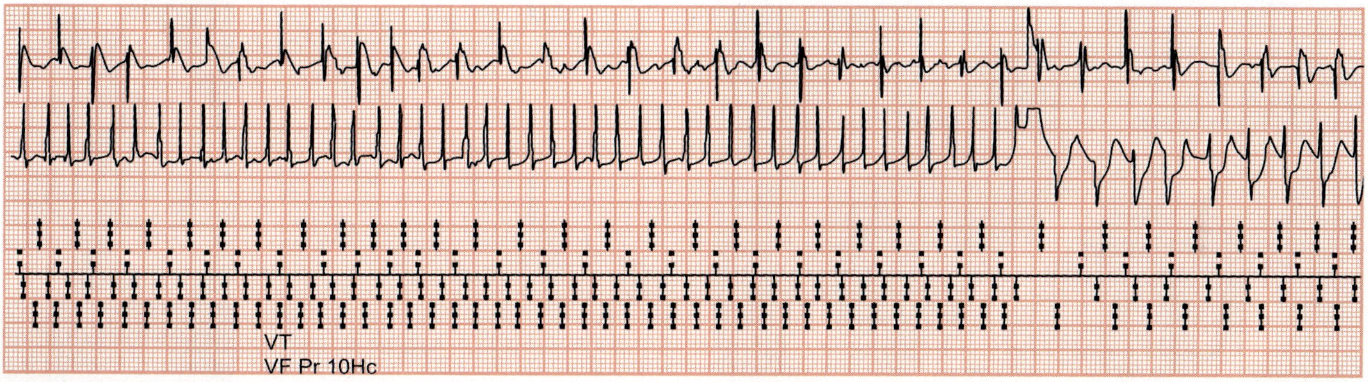


**Fig. 15.54:** Electrophysiological study—it showed caffeine-induced malignant ventricular arrhythmia in a young patient with arrhythmogenic cardiomyopathy. At electrophysiological study, long runs of self-terminating atrial and ventricular tachycardia were inducible from the right-ventricular upper lateral regions of RV

disturbances. However, the condition is frequently symptomless, with the first manifestation being sudden, unexpected death. Moreover, symptoms, hemodynamics, and electrocardiographic findings are relatively non-specific, although advances in cardiac imaging, especially magnetic resonance imaging (MRI), have increased the reproducibility of clinical diagnosis (Figs 15.55–15.59).

The diagnosis of ARVC is generally made pathologically at autopsy or at examination of explanted hearts at orthotopic heart transplantation. Endomyocardial biopsy is unreliable, as sampling the apical septum does not typically reveal diagnostic material, and biopsies of the septal endomyocardium may not show the characteristic lesions.

At autopsy, the major differential diagnosis includes normal fat deposits in the right ventricle, and subepicardial scars of ischemic origin. Adipose tissue is normally present in the right ventricle, especially in the anterior wall toward the apex, but no associated fibrosis or myocyte changes exist. In the left ventricle, subepicardial scars can be associated with ischemic heart disease, especially if there is embolization of thromboembolic material from epicardial coronary lesions.

In cases of unexplained exertional death in young adults, submitting multiple sections of ventricular septum and right ventricle to exclude arrhythmogenic forms of cardiomyopathy is reasonable, as ARVC most typically involves

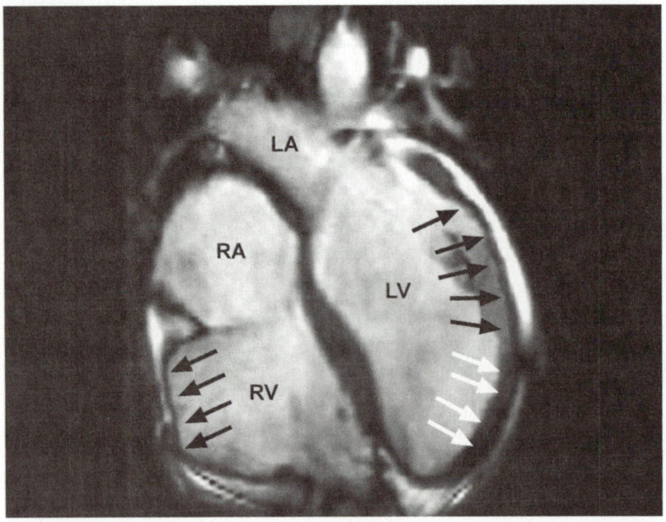


**Fig. 15.55:** Four chamber view shows severe global enlargement of the right ventricle (RV) with localised dilation at the inflow tract (black arrows). The left ventricle (LV) is also moderately dilated. Regional thinning of the posterolateral LV wall is observed (black arrows). Normal LV wall thickness is highlighted by white arrows for comparison. LA=left atrium; RA=right atrium

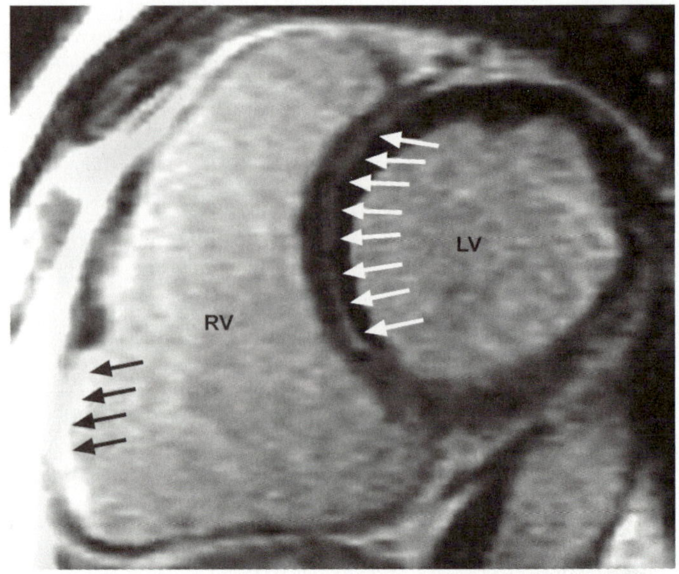


**Fig. 15.56:** Following intravenous administration of gadolinium-DTPA, late enhancement was observed in both the right ventricle (RV) (black arrows) and the septum (white arrows). Since fat was absent from these regions on corresponding T1 weighted turbospin images, the appearances are consistent with myocardial fibrosis. The mid-myocardial distribution is typical of fibrosis secondary to cardiomyopathy

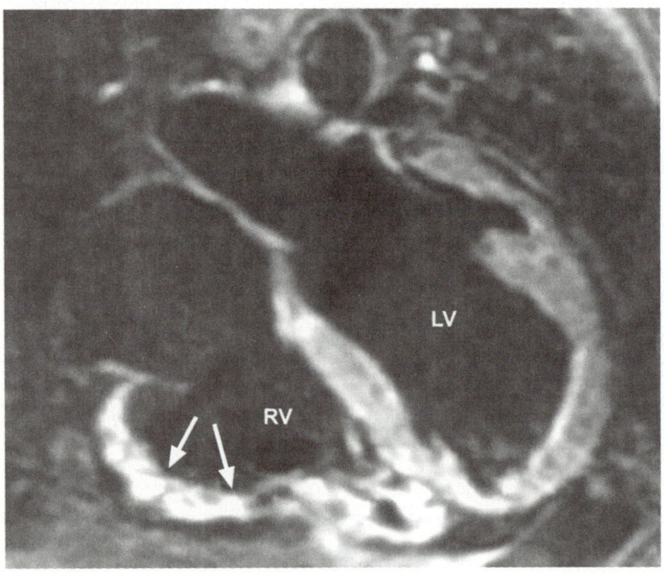


**Fig. 15.57:** T2 weighted spin echo image in the four chamber view with fat suppression. The bright areas within the grey myocardium (white arrows) are likely to represent edema, suggesting the presence of patchy inflammatory infiltrates

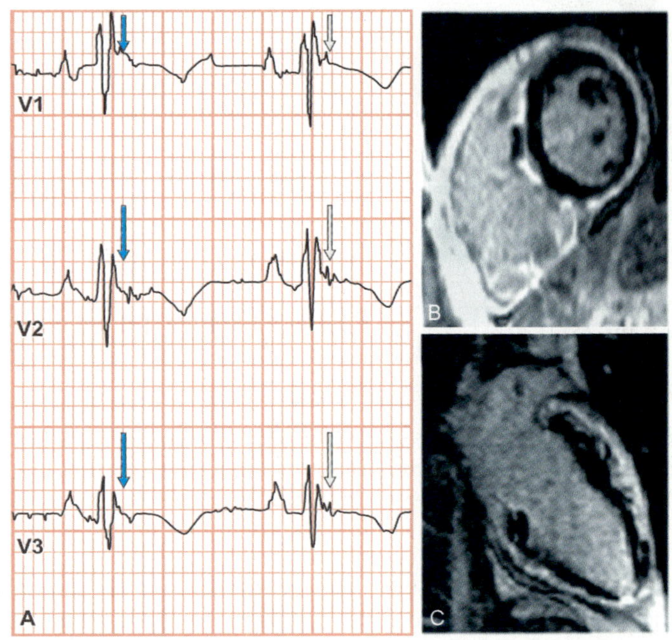


**Fig. 15.58:** A 48-year-old man presented with syncope due to ventricular tachycardia of left ventricular origin and was electrically cardioverted to sinus rhythm. Resting electrocardiography displayed epsilon waves. (A) Coronary angiography revealed unobstructed arteries. Cardiac magnetic resonance (CMR) demonstrated a severely dilated right ventricle and biventricular systolic dysfunction. Short axis imaging following gadolinium at mid-ventricular level. (B) Identified patchy late enhancement of the right ventricular border of the septum, extending into the subepicardium of the anterior and inferior walls. A two chamber view of the left ventricle. (C) Demonstrated extensive mid-myocardial and subepicardial enhancement

the right ventricle and may be difficult to see grossly; additionally, hypertrophic cardiomyopathy may involve the interventricular septum without obvious grossly abnormalities. Because both of these entities often cause exertional death, taking multiple sections of right ventricle and ventricular septum in cases of exertional deaths is prudent.

Several clinical criteria for the diagnosis of ARVC have been proposed, including those of the working groups on Myocardial and Pericardial Disease and Arrhythmias of the European Society of Cardiology and of the Scientific

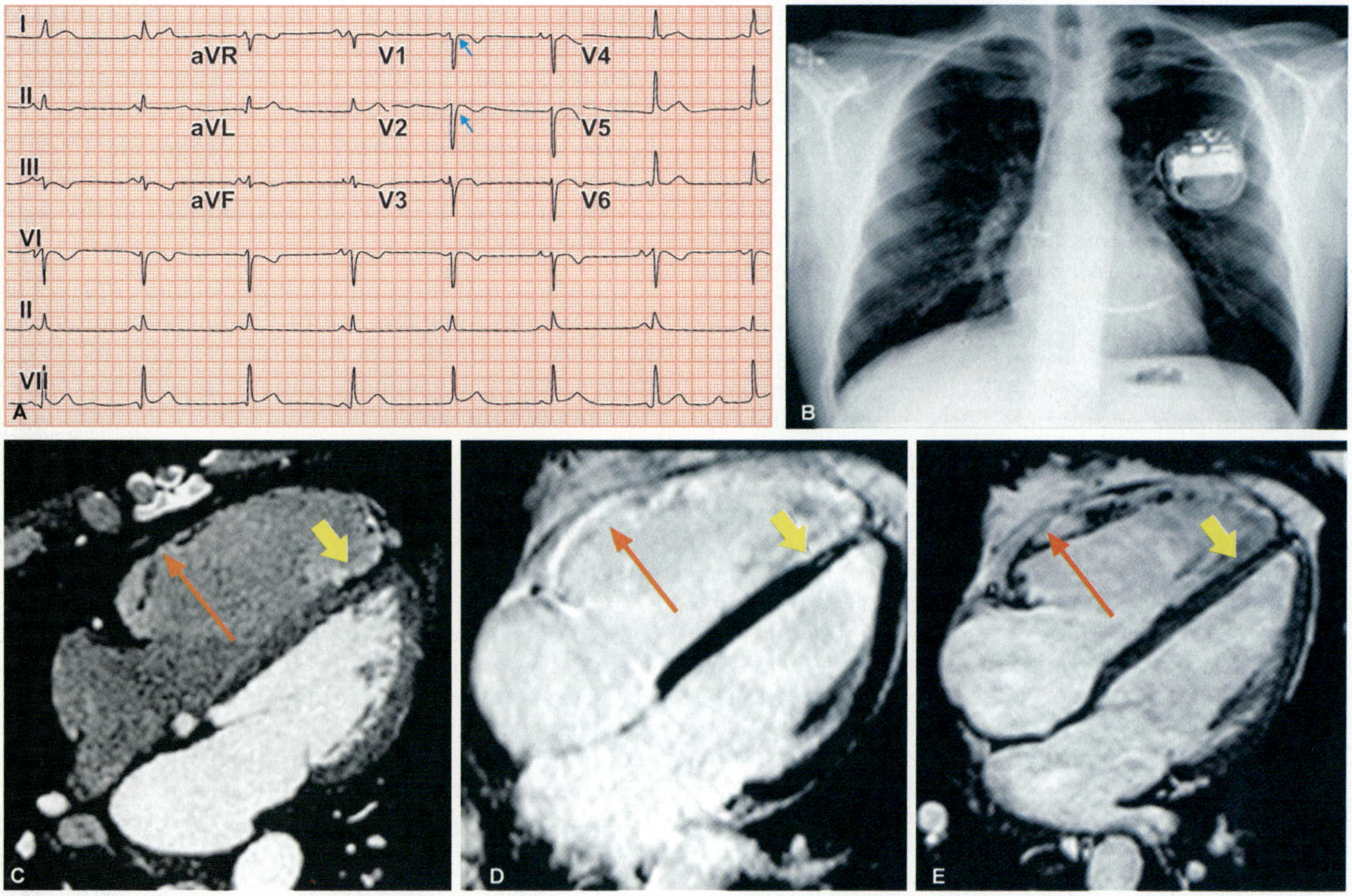


**Fig. 15.59:** (A) ECG with typical signs for ARVC; negative T-waves and epsilon waves in the precordial leads (arrow). (B) Chest X-ray after ICD implantation. Both the atrial and ventricular leads are visible. (C through E) signal attenuation in RV septum on MDCT. (D) Increased signal intensity on delayed enhancement images. (E) Decreased signal intensity on steady-state free precession images

Council on Cardiomyopathies of the World Heart Federation in 2000, with a revision in 2002).

### Immunohistochemistry

In general, immunohistochemistry (IHC) is not useful in the diagnosis arrhythmogenic right ventricular cardiomyopathy. Some investigators have postulated that diffuse loss of desmosomal proteins, as seen immunohistochemically, is suggestive of the diagnosis of ARVC. These proteins include connexin-43 and plakoglobi.

## TAKOTSUBO CARDIOMYOPATHY

Takotsubo cardiomyopathy, also known as transient apical ballooning syndrome, apical ballooning cardiomyopathy stress-induced cardiomyopathy, Gebrochenes-Herz-syndrom, and simply stress cardiomyopathy, is a type of nonischemic cardiomyopathy in which there is a sudden temporary weakening of the myocardium (the muscle of the heart). Because this weakening can be triggered by emotional stress, such as the death of a loved one, a break-up, or constant anxiety, the condition is also known as broken heart syndrome. Stress cardiomyopathy is a well-recognized cause of acute heart failure, lethal ventricular arrhythmias, and ventricular rupture.

### Clinical Presentation

The typical presentation of someone with takotsubo cardiomyopathy is a sudden onset of congestive heart failure associated with ECG changes suggestive of an anterior wall myocardial infarction. During the course of evaluation of the patient, a bulging out of the left ventricular apex with a hypercontractile base of the left ventricle is often noted. It is the hallmark bulging out of the apex of the heart with preserved function of the base that earned the syndrome its name 'takotsubo', or octopus trap in Japan, where it was first described. The cause appears to involve high circulating levels of catecholamines (mainly adrenaline/epinephrine). Evaluation of individuals with takotsubo cardiomyopathy typically includes a coronary angiogram, which will not reveal any significant blockages that would cause the left ventricular dysfunction. Provided that the individual survives their initial presentation, the left ventricular function improves within 2 months. Takotsubo cardiomyopathy is more commonly seen in post-menopausal women. Often there is a history of a recent severe emotional or physical stress.

## Aetiological Factors

The aetiology of takotsubo cardiomyopathy is not fully understood, but several mechanisms have been proposed.

1. *Wraparound LAD:* The left anterior descending artery (LAD) supplies the anterior wall of the left ventricle in the majority of patients. If this artery also wraps around the apex of the heart, it may be responsible for blood supply to the apex and the inferior wall of the heart. Some researchers have noted a correlation between takotsubo and this type of LAD. Other researchers have shown that this anatomical variant is not common enough to explain takotsubo cardiomyopathy. This theory would also not explain documented variants where the midventricular walls or base of the heart does not contract (akinesis).
2. *Transient vasospasm:* Some of the original researchers of takotsubo suggested that multiple simultaneous spasms of coronary arteries could cause enough loss of blood flow to cause transient stunning of the myocardium. Other researchers have shown that vasospasm is much less common than initially thought. It has also been noted that when there are vasospasms, even in multiple arteries, that they do not correlate with the areas of myocardium that are not contracting.
3. *Microvascular dysfunction:* The theory gaining the most traction is that there is dysfunction of the coronary arteries at the level where they are no longer visible by coronary angiography. This could include microvascular vasospasm, however it may well also have some similarities to the diseases such as diabetes mellitus. In such disease conditions the microvascular arteries fail to provide adequate oxygen to the myocardium.
4. *Mid-ventricular obstruction,* apical stunning It has also been suggested that a mid-ventricular wall thickening with outflow obstruction is important in the pathophysiology.

It is likely that there are multiple factors at play which could include some amount of vasospasm, failure of the microvasculature, and an abnormal response to catecholamines (such as epinephrine and norepinephrine, released in response to stress).

Case series looking at large groups of patients report that some patients develop takotsubo cardiomyopathy after an emotional stress, while others have a preceding clinical stressor (such as an asthma attack or sudden illness). Roughly one-third of patients have no preceding stressful event. A recent large case series from Europe found that takotsubo was slightly more frequent during the winter season. This may be related to two different possible/suspected pathophysiological causes coronary spasms of microvessels, which are more prevalent in cold weather, and viral infections such as parvovirus B19, which occur more frequently during the winter season.

- Laboratory and imaging studies
- Electrocardiogram (Fig. 15.60)
- Echocardiogram (Fig. 15.61)
- MRI (Fig. 15.62)

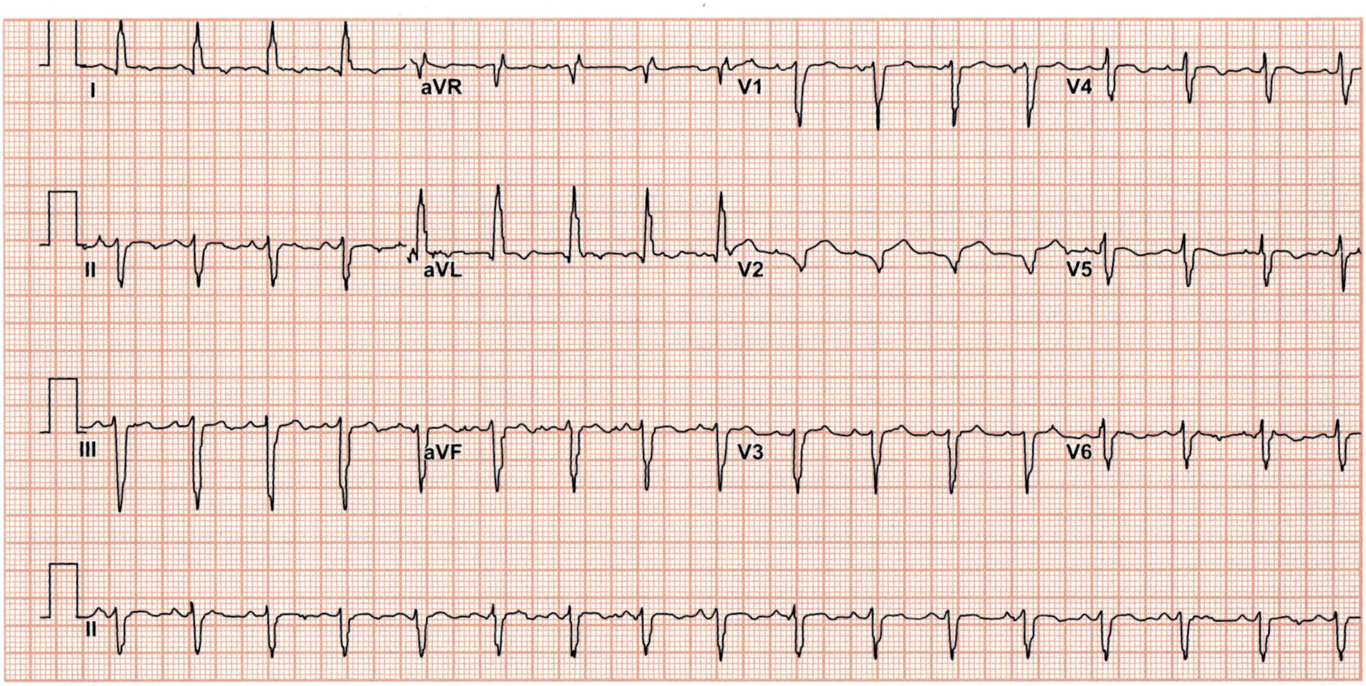


**Fig. 15.60:** ECG showing sinus tachycardia and nonspecific ST- and T-wave changes from a patient with confirmed takotsubo cardiomyopathy

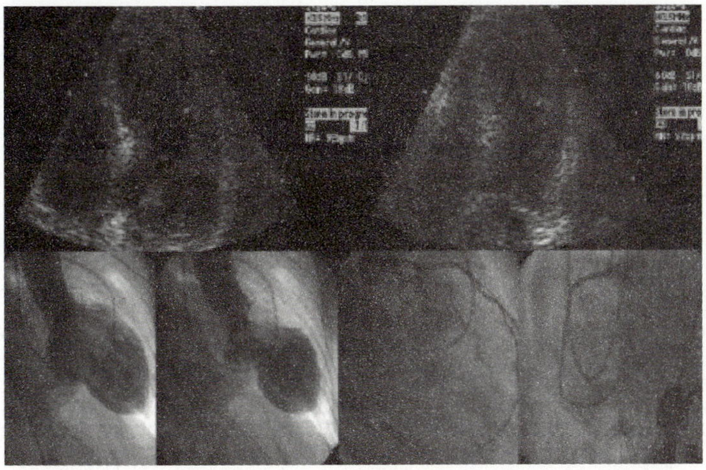

**Fig. 15.61:** Classic echocardiographic feature of apical ballooning, as can be seen in systole and diastole by echocardiography (upper panel), apical ballooning involving all left ventricular walls not limited to any single coronary territory, confirmed by ventriculography with normal angiogram (lower panel)

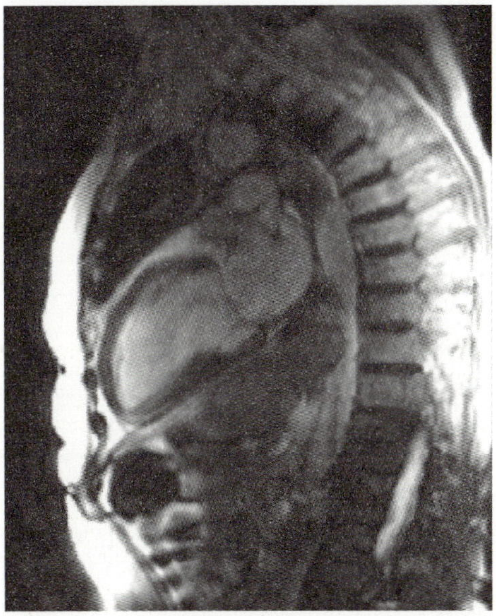

**Fig.15.62:** MRI scan shows dilated left ventricle with apical ballooning is demonstrated with slightly reduced left ventricular function (left ventricular ejection fraction 46%, normalized end diastolic volume 87 ml/m$^2$, normalized end systolic volume 47 ml/m$^2$, normalized stroke volume 40 ml/m$^2$). No myocardial hypertrophy (SWT 6 mm, PWT 9 mm, normalized myocardial mass 35 g/m$^2$) or myocardial scar formation was found. These findings are compatible with a Takotsubo-cardiomyopathy. Accompanying pleural effusions were also noted (not illustrated) I /CT scan

### Cardiac Catheterization Procedure

Transient apical ballooning syndrome or takótsubo cardiomyopathy is found in 1.7–2.2% of patients presenting with acute coronary syndrome. While the original case reports reported on individuals in Japan, takotsubo cardiomyopathy has been noted more recently in the United States and Western Europe. It is likely that the syndrome went previously undiagnosed before it was described in detail in the Japanese literature (Figs 15.63 and 15.64).

The diagnosis of takotsubo cardiomyopathy may be difficult upon presentation. The ECG findings are often confused with those found during an acute anterior wall myocardial infarction. It classically mimics ST-segment elevation myocardial infarction, and is characterised by acute onset of transient ventricular apical wall motion abnormalities (ballooning) accompanied by chest pain, dyspnea, ST-segment elevation, T-wave inversion or QT-interval prolongation on ECG. Elevation of myocardial enzymes is moderate at worst and there is absence of significant coronary artery disease. The diagnosis is made by the pathognomonic wall motion abnormalities, in which the base of the left ventricle is contracting normally or is hyperkinetic while the remainder of the left ventricle is akinetic or dyskinetic. This is accompanied by the lack of significant coronary artery disease that would explain the wall motion abnormalities. Although, apical ballooning has been classically described as the angiographic manifestation of takotsubo, it has been shown that left ventricular dysfunction in this syndrome includes not only the classic apical ballooning, but also different angiographic morphologies such as mid-ventricular ballooning and rarely local ballooning of other segments.

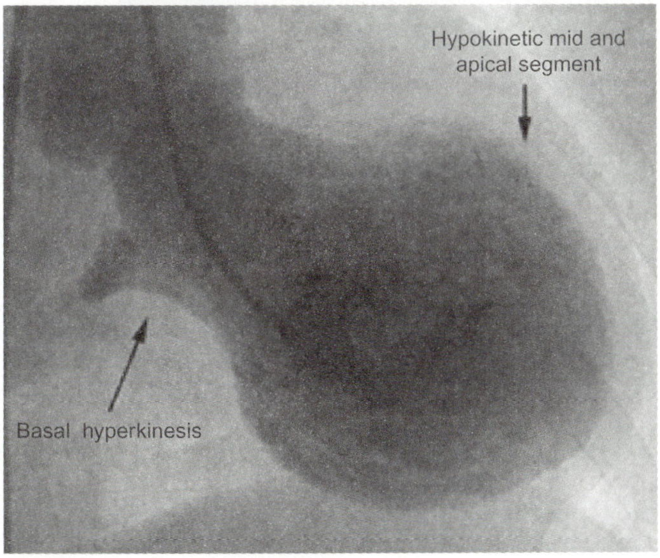


**Fig. 15.63:** Cardiac catheterization shows hypokinesia of basal, mid and apical segments of LV with ballooning features in takotsubo cardiomyopathy

The ballooning patterns were classified by Shimizu et al. as takotsubo type for apical akinesia and basal hyperkinesia, reverse takotsubo for basal akinesia and apical hyperkinesia, mid-ventricular type for mid-ventricular ballooning accompanied by basal and apical hyperkinesia and localised type for any other segmental left ventricular ballooning with clinical characteristics of takotsubo-like left ventricular dysfunction.

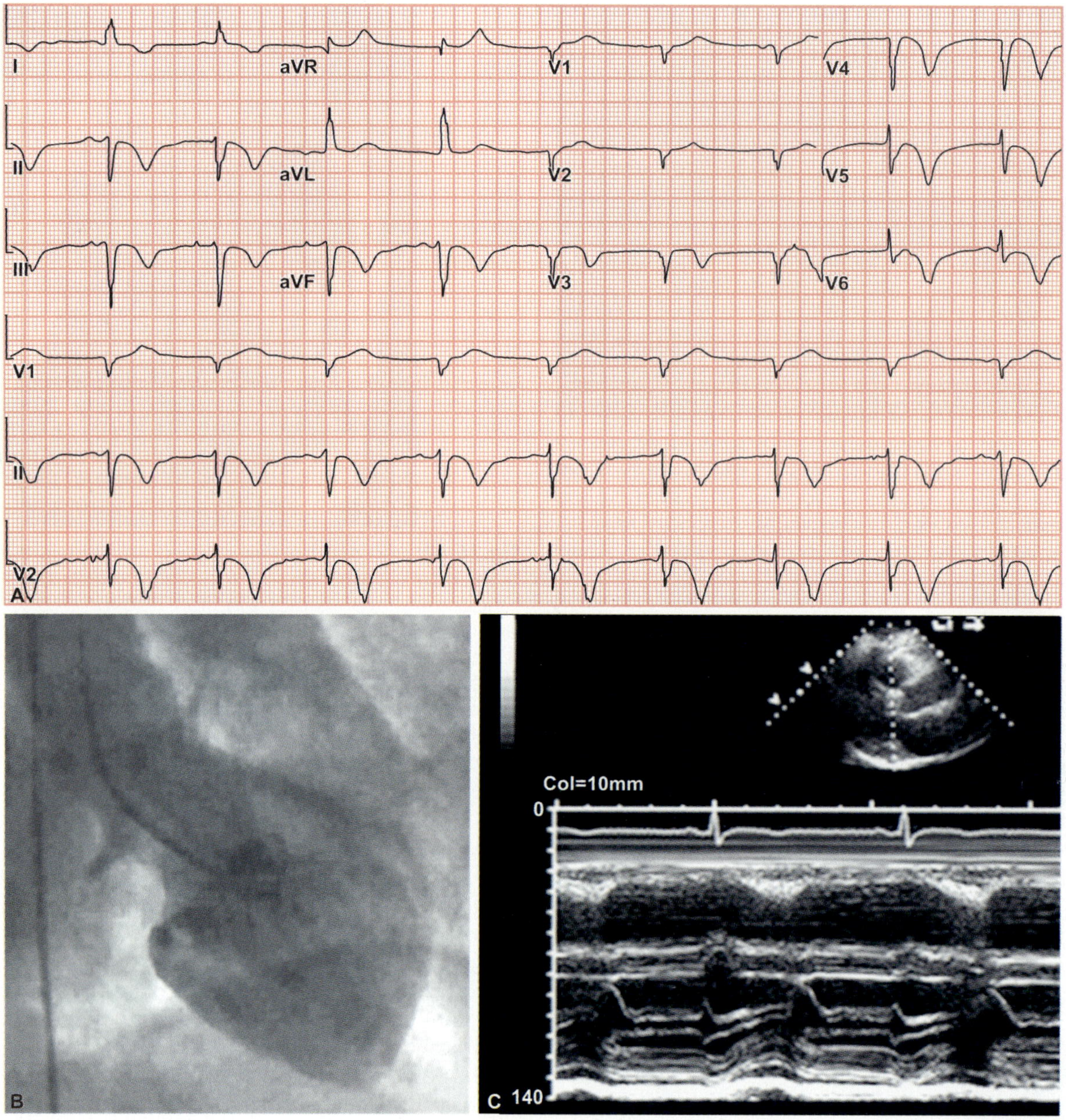


**Fig.15.64:** First episode of takotsubo cardiomyopathy. (A) ECG at time of admission consistent with ischemia, (B) left ventriculography during first episode of takotsubo cardiomyopathy 6 years earlier at end-systolic phase showing similar features as the second presentation, (C) M-mode 2D echocardiography 4 years after the initial episode revealing normal function of the left ventricle and complete recovery

## Prognosis

Despite the grave initial presentation in some of the patients, most of the patients survive the initial acute event, with a very low rate of in-hospital mortality or complications. The patients are expecting a favorable outcome once recovering from the acute stage of the syndrome, and the long-term prognosis is excellent. Even when ventricular systolic function is heavily compromised at presentation, it typically improves within the first few days and normalises within the first few months. Although infrequent, recurrence of the syndrome has been reported and seems to be associated with the nature of the trigger.

## Treatment

The treatment of takotsubo cardiomyopathy is generally supportive in nature. Although patients with takotsubo heart disease may be hypotensive, treatment with inotropes will usually exacerbate the disease. Since the disease is due to a high catecholamine state, patients should not be given inotropes. Treatment recommendations include intra-aortic balloon pump, fluids, and negative inotropes such as beta-blockers or calcium channel blockers. In many individuals, left ventricular function normalizes within 2 months. Aspirin and other heart drugs also appear to help in the treatment of this disease, even in extreme cases.

## BIBLIOGRAPHY


1. Basso C, Thiene G, Corrado D, Angelini A, Nava A, Valente M. Arrhythmogenic right ventricular cardiomyopathy. Dysplasia, dystrophy, or myocarditis? Circulation 1996; 94(5):983-91.
2. Bauce B, Basso C, Rampazzo A, et al. Clinical profile of four families with arrhythmogenic right ventricular cardiomyopathy caused by dominant desmoplakin mutations. Eur Heart J 2005;26(16):1666–75.
3. Bernstein D. Diseases of the myocardium. In: Kliegman RM, Behrman RE, Jenson HB, Stanton BF, (Eds.) Nelson Textbook of Pediatrics. 18th ed. Philadelphia, Pa: Saunders Elsevier; 2007:chap 439.
4. Burke AP, Farb A, Tashko G, Virmani R. Arrhythmogenic right ventricular cardiomyopathy and fatty replacement of the right ventricular myocardium: are they different diseases? Circulation 1998;97(16):1571–80.
5. Chin TK, Perloff JK, Williams RG, et al. Isolated noncompaction of left ventricular myocardium. A study of eight cases. Circulation 1990;82(2):507–13.
6. Dokuparti MV, Pamuru PR, Thakkar B, et al. Etiopathogenesis of arrhythmogenic right ventricular cardiomyopathy. J Hum Genet 2005;50(8):375–81.
7. Engberding R, Bender F. Identification of a rare congenital anomaly of the myocardium by two-dimensional echocardiography: Persistence of isolated myocardial sinusoids. Am J Cardiol 1984;53(11):1733–4.
8. Espinola-Zavaleta Nilda, Soto Elena, Castellanos Luis Munoz, Játiva-Chávez Silvio, Keirns Candace (2006). "Non-compacted Cardiomyopathy: Clinical-Echocardiographic Study". Cardiovasc Ultrasound 4 (1): 35. doi:10.1186/1476-7120-4-35.
9. Ferreira AC, Garcia SA, Pasquale MA, Canoniero MJ, Peter A. Arrhythmogenic right ventricular dysplasia in the elderly. Heart Dis 2003;5(6):393–6.
10. Fidler LM, Wilson GJ, Liu F, et al. Abnormal connexin in arrhythmogenic right ventricular cardiomyopathy caused by plakophilin-2 mutations. J Cell Mol Med 2009;13(10): 4219–28.
11. Francés RJ. Arrhythmogenic right ventricular dysplasia/cardiomyopathy. A review and update. Int J Cardiol 2006; 110(3):279–87.
12. Hare JM. The dilated, restrictive, and infiltrative cardiomyopathies. Bonow RO, Mann DL, Zipes DP, Libby P, (Eds.) In: Braunwald's Heart Disease: A Textbook of Cardiovascular Medicine. 9th ed. Philadelphia, Pa: Saunders Elsevier; 2011:chap 68.
13. Hare JM. The dilated, restrictive, and infiltrative cardiomyopathies. Libby P, Bonow RO, Mann DL, Zipes DP. In: Braunwald's Heart Disease: A Textbook of Cardiovascular Medicine, 8th ed. Philadelphia, Pa: Saunders Elsevier; 2007:chap 64.
14. Lobo FV, Silver MD, Butany J, Heggtveit HA. Left ventricular involvement in right ventricular dysplasia/cardiomyopathy. Can J Cardiol 1999;15(11):1239–47.
15. Maron BJ. Hypertrophic cardiomyopathy. Zipes DP, Libby P, Bonow RO, Braunwald E, (Eds.) Braunwald's Heart Disease: A Textbook of Cardiovascular Medicine. 8th ed. St. Louis, Mo: WB Saunders; 2007:chap 65.
16. Maron B, Towbin J, Thiene G, Antzelevitch C, Corrado D, Arnett D, Moss AJ, Seidman CE, et al. Contemporary Definitions and Classification of the Cardiomyopathies (webpage). American Heart Association Journals (American Heart Association) 2006;113(14):1807.
17. Morrow DA, Boden WE. Stable ischemic heart disease. In: Bonow RO, Mann DL, Zipes DP, Libby P, (Eds.) Braunwald's Heart Disease: A Textbook of Cardiovascular Medicine. 9th ed. Philadelphia, Pa; Saunders Elsevier; 2011:chap 57.
18. Oechslin, Erwin; Jenni, Rolf (2005). Non-compaction of the Left Ventricular Myocardium—From Clinical Observation to the Discovery of a New Disease. Archived from the original on 2007-09-29.
19. Pignatelli RH, McMahon CJ, Dreyer WJ, et al. Clinical characterization of left ventricular non-compaction in children: a relatively common form of cardiomyopathy. Circulation 2003;108(21):2672–8.
20. Rampazzo A, Nava A, Malacrida S, et al. Mutation in human desmoplakin domain binding to plakoglobin causes a dominant form of arrhythmogenic right ventricular cardiomyopathy. Am J Hum Genet 2002;71(5):1200–6.
21. Sen-Chowdhry S, Syrris P, Ward D, Asimaki A, Sevdalis E, McKenna WJ. Clinical and genetic characterization of families with arrhythmogenic right ventricular dysplasia/cardio-myopathy provides novel insights into patterns of disease expression. Circulation 2007;115(13):1710–20.
22. Syrris P, Ward D, Evans A, et al. Arrhythmogenic right ventricular dysplasia/cardiomyopathy associated with mutations in the desmosomal gene desmocollin-2. Am J Hum Genet 2006;79(5):978–84.
23. Thiene G, Corrado D, Basso C. Arrhythmogenic right ventricular cardiomyopathy/dysplasia. Orphanet J Rare Dis 2007; 2:45.
24. Vatta M, Mohapatra B, Jimenez S, et al. Mutations in Cypher/ZASP in patients with dilated cardiomyopathy and left ventricular non-compaction. J Am Coll Cardiol 2003;42(11): 2014–27.
25. Weiford BC, Subbarao VD, Mulhern KM. Noncompaction of the ventricular myocardium. Circulation 2004;109(24): 2965–71.
26. Wexler RK, Elton T, Pleister A, Feldman D. Cardiomyopathy: An overview. Am Fam Physician 2009;79:778–784.

# 16 Recognition and Management of Cardiac Valvular Emergencies

Chronic rheumatic valvular dysfunctions can lead to very high morbidity and mortality among patients unless they are helped with either reconstructive surgery or replacement of an artificial valve. Two types of artificial valves which are available today have their own limitations and till date there is no ideal valve which could closely resemble with natural valve in terms of cost and postoperative long term outcome. Recently attempts have been made in constructing artificial heart valves with the help of stem cell modification and genetic engineering techniques though long term follow up is still awaited. Synthetic valve do give rise to bleeding disorders due to anticoagulants and predispose to thromboembolic phenomenon and infection leading to vital organ dysfunctions.

Although tissue valves do not need anticoagulants but still it could be the seat of infections and are often rejected in mismatched cases. Undoubtedly, tissue valve is preferable in pregnant women and younger children where anticoagulants may pose life-threatening complications. The life span of this valve is shorter than the synthetic valve due to its rapid degeneration.

In developing countries, rheumatic process is so extensive that often more than one valves (multivalvular) are affected which further complicates the final management of the patients besides the cost implications among poor patients (Fig. 16.1).

Sincere efforts are still continued to manufacture such a valve which could satisfy all the properties of an ideal valve and come within the reach of low socioeconomic strata of people where a large segment of population is affected every year particularly in developing countries of South-East Asia. Valvular heart disease is an important cause of cardiac morbidity in developed countries despite a decline in the prevalence of rheumatic disease in those countries. Valvular heart disease can give rise to stenosis, regurgitation or a combination of lesions at one or more valves. The more common significant anomalies currently encountered are mitral regurgitation, caused by mitral valve prolapse; aortic stenosis, caused by a congenital bicuspid valve or by senile valvular calcification; and aortic regurgitation, caused by a bicuspid aortic valve or dilatation of the aorta. Valvular lesions can occur as a result of pathologic changes in the valve leaflets or supporting structures (i.e. the chordae or papillary muscles). Ventricular or aortic enlargement can also produce valvular regurgitation as a result of annular dilatation and inadequate leaflet coaptation in the absence of any specific valve pathology. Valvular heart disease tends to progress over time as degenerative changes are superimposed on the primary pathology. Iatrogenic causes of valvular disease are increasingly recognized.

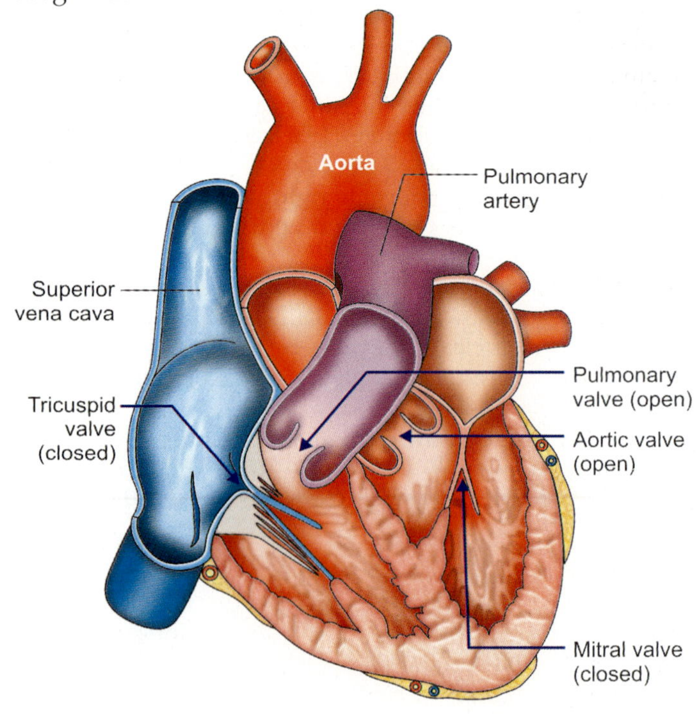


**Fig. 16.1:** Anatomical placement of four native valves in human body

Valvular problems may be caused by infection, heart disease, trauma or congenital valvular conditions and may be isolated to a single valve or effect multiple valves. Right sided (tricuspid, pulmonary) valvular disease is much less common than left sided (aortic, mitral) valvular disease. Roughly 90% of valvular disease is chronic, having developed gradually over many years. Complications of rheumatic fever, congenital disorders and aging cause the vast majority of chronic valvular disease. The remaining 10% of valvular disease that develops acutely (over days to weeks) is often due to complications of recent heart attack or infections.

## AETIOLOGICAL FACTORS IN VALVULAR DYSFUNCTIONS

### Congenital Disorders

Anomalies in the development of valve cusps are common at the aortic or pulmonary positions. The normal configuration of these valves is tricuspid. Stenosis is the rule when only one cusp develops, whereas bicuspid valves may be stenotic or regurgitant. Congenital anomalies of the atrioventricular valves are uncommon; the most common abnormality is congenital cleft mitral valve. Valvular abnormalities can be seen in specific developmental syndromes, such as pulmonary stenosis in rubella syndrome and supravalvular aortic stenosis in Williams syndrome.

### Myxomatous Degeneration

Myxomatous degeneration most often involves the mitral or tricuspid valve. In this condition, leaflet tissue, particularly chordal tissue, is abnormally extensible and weak. The affected valves are therefore more likely to prolapse, leading to significant regurgitation. Chordal rupture is common and may precipitate a rapid clinical deterioration from sudden severe regurgitation. The precise abnormality in valvular tissue is unknown but is thought to involve the structural proteins, such as collagen. A familial tendency is often noted in this disease. Inherited connective tissue diseases such as Marfan syndrome produce valvular abnormalities similar to those found in myxomatous degeneration.

### Rheumatic Heart Disease

Rheumatic heart disease remains the most common cause of mitral stenosis and a frequent cause of aortic regurgitation. It is the most common cause of multivalvular heart disease. Isolated outbreaks of rheumatic fever continue to be reported in the United States, even in affluent communities. Rheumatic heart disease remains a significant problem in immigrants, especially those from Latin America and Southeast Asia. Rheumatic fever appears to cause valvular heart disease by an autoimmune phenomenon whereby antibodies against streptococcal antigens cross-react with valvular tissue. Valvular involvement can present acutely as a result of edema of valvular tissue. Progressive fibrosis, superimposed calcification, and scarring with retraction of leaflet tissue lead to valvular stenosis, incompetence, or both. The interval between the occurrence of rheumatic fever and clinical manifestations varies, as does the degree of involvement. Both mitral and aortic valves are usually involved.

### Degenerative Disease

Degenerative calcification can occur in aortic stenosis among the elderly and in patients with renal dysfunction; it results from calcium deposition on the body of the valvular leaflets rather than on the commissures. Factors found to promote degenerative valvular changes are increasing age, a low body mass index, hypertension, and hyperlipidemia. Histologic changes that simulate atheroma and involve lipid deposition and inflammatory cell infiltration of the leaflets have been described in patients with early degenerative changes in the aortic leaflets. Even mild degenerative changes in the aortic valve have been reported to be adverse prognostic factors. Calcification of the mitral annulus is common in the elderly; it is more common in women than in men and can produce mitral regurgitation. Occasionally, mitral annular calcification extends onto the valvular leaflets, causing stenosis.

### Endocarditis

Endocarditis usually occurs on previously abnormal valves, although overwhelming sepsis can infect normal valves. The predominant hemodynamic manifestation of endocarditis is valvular regurgitation. Contributory causes of endocarditis include leaflet prolapse (resulting from a large vegetation), leaflet perforation, and chronic scarring of infected tissue. In rare cases, large vegetations lead to valvular stenosis.

### Coronary Artery Disease

Mitral regurgitation is common in coronary artery disease; it has a number of causal mechanisms. Acute ischemia or infarction of a papillary muscle or of the wall to which the papillary muscle is attached leads to impaired leaflet coaptation and mitral regurgitation. Regurgitation can be severe and can vary with the severity of the ischemia. Papillary head rupture or, more rarely, muscle rupture, leads to catastrophic regurgitation that is often fatal.

### Connective Tissue Disease

Libman-Sacks endocarditis consists of noninfected warty vegetations involving predominantly the mitral valve; it is characteristic of systemic lupus erythematosus (SLE). Significant regurgitation and stenosis rarely occur acutely but are seen with scarring from chronic disease. Valvular involvement in rheumatoid arthritis is common and leads to valvular thickening but is usually not of hemodynamic significance. Aortitis in ankylosing spondylitis may produce significant aortic regurgitation.

### Iatrogenic Causes of Valvular Heart Disease

Iatrogenic causes include radiation therapy, the use of serotonin agonists such as methysergide, and the use of anorexiants such as fenfluramine and phentermine in combination. Radiation leads to scarring and calcification of valvular leaflets many years after the initiating radiation. The effects of both methysergide and anorexiant agents on valvular tissue often simulate rheumatic disease, but regurgitation rather than stenosis predominates as the hemodynamically severe lesion. Serotonin is also thought to play a role in the valvulopathy produced by anorexiants; the precise mechanism by which this occurs remains to be established.

### Other Causes of Valvular Heart Disease

Amyloid disease causes valvular thickening but rarely causes significant stenosis. The carcinoid syndrome most often involves the valves on the right side of the heart and leads to stenosis or incompetence of the tricuspid or pulmonary valve.

### Secondary Involvement

Left ventricular dilatation can cause dilatation of the mitral annulus and, thereby, mitral regurgitation. Common secondary causes of mitral regurgitation include coronary artery disease, aortic valvular disease, and dilated cardiomyopathy. Similarly, tricuspid regurgitation results from right ventricular enlargement secondary to pulmonary hypertension or an atrial septal defect. Dilatation of the ascending aorta, especially involving the annulus of the aortic valve, can lead to aortic regurgitation. This condition is seen in hypertension and in aneurysms of the ascending aorta.

### Assessment and Management

Valvular heart disease often remains asymptomatic for many years, but once symptoms develop, survival is reduced if the lesion is not corrected. The evaluation of symptoms can require a stress test or stress echocardiogram in addition to a careful history. Characterization of the lesions and assessment of hemodynamic severity are often possible on physical examination but are aided by additional testing, such as Doppler echocardiography and cardiac catheterization. Doppler echocardiography measures the flow velocity across a narrowed valve. By use of the modified Bernoulli equation, the pressure gradient (P), measured in mmHg, may be estimated from the flow velocity (v), which is measured in m/sec: $P = 4v^2$. Therefore, if the peak velocity recorded across the aortic valve by Doppler echocardiography is 4 m/sec, then the peak pressure gradient will be estimated as $4(4^2)$ or 64 mmHg. The effects of valvular heart disease on chamber size and function are best assessed serially by echocardiography or, at the time of cardiac catheterization, by ventriculography. In cases of stenotic lesions, intervention is rarely required until symptoms occur. Indications for intervention in regurgitant lesions are more complex; such indications include significant symptoms or, in the absence of symptoms, increasing ventricular size, overt ventricular contractile dysfunction, or both.

All patients with even mild valvular heart disease require prophylaxis against endocarditis at the time of dental procedures or other procedures that can produce significant bacteremia. The prophylactic regimens recommended by the American Heart Association have been revised despite the increase in intravascular volume, pregnancy is usually well tolerated in previously asymptomatic patients with valvular heart disease. Patients with hemodynamically significant valvular heart disease should generally avoid participation in competitive sports. Reference should be made to the recommendations of the American College of Cardiology for more information about specific lesions. Valvular heart disease is a chronic disease requiring periodic examination and follow-up, even in asymptomatic patients and in those who have had corrective surgical or other procedures. Patients with prosthetic valves should be seen at least yearly.

## VALVULAR EMERGENCIES

Common valvular emergencies found in emergency department are as follows:

- Mitral stenosis
- Mitral regurgitation
- Mitral valve prolapse
- Aortic stenosis
- Aortic regurgitation
- Right-sided valvular heart disease

### Newely Discovered Heart Murmur (Fig. 16.2)

#### *Ruptured Sinus of Valsalva Aneurysm*

Sinus of Valsalva aneurysms are rare congenital or acquired cardiac anomalies, most commonly involving the right or noncoronary sinuses. (1) Congenital sinuses of Valsalva aneurysm account for ~0.5% to 3% of all congenital cardiac defects. In addition, inflammatory diseases, such as syphilis, tuberculosis, endocarditis, and Behçet disease, as well as traumatic events and connective tissue disorders,

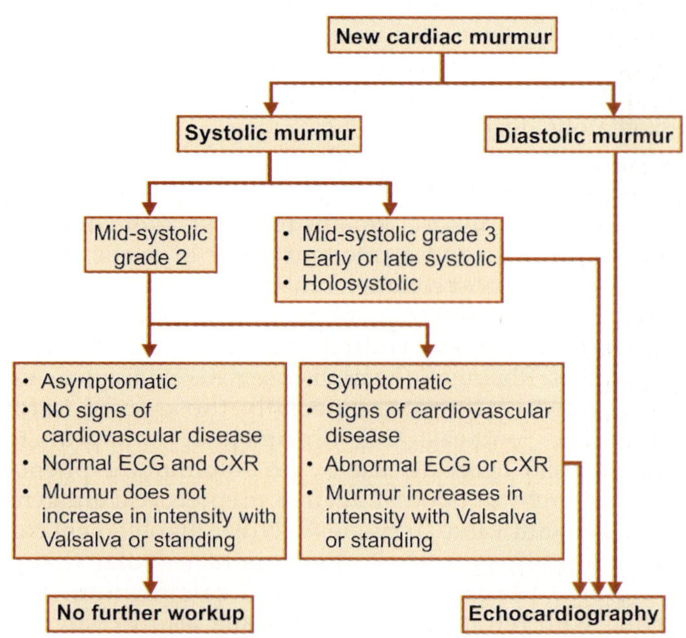


**Fig. 16.2:** Evaluation of newely discovered murmur

such as Marfan syndrome, can be the cause of this anomaly. (2) Rupture of a sinus of Valsalva aneurysm requires definitive repair because of progressive right heart failure. Magnetic resonance imaging with the phase-contrast method is a reliable noninvasive way to assess the cardiac shunt ratio, thereby helping to guide therapy. The treatment of choice is a surgical approach, although transcatheter occlusion has occasionally been shown to be an alternative. Sudden onset of a cardiac murmur should always include the differential diagnosis of a ruptured sinus of Valsalva aneurysm.

BOX 16.1: Grading of murmurs

Murmurs are graded on a four point or, more commonly, a six-point scale. A common six-point scale is:

Grade 1—audible with difficulty

Grade 2—faint but recognizable

Grade 3—moderate intensity

Grade 4—loud

Grade 5—louder, but still needing a stethoscope

Grade 6—audible without a stethoscope.

## SPECIFIC VALVULAR LESIONS

### MITRAL VALVE DISORDERS

The mitral valve normally allows one way flow of blood from the left atrium to the left ventricle. Disorders of the mitral valve may cause mitral valve stenosis, mitral valve regurgitation or mitral valve prolapse (previously discussed).

### 1. Mitral Valvular Stenosis

It is narrowing of the mitral valve opening that usually gradually occurs over time due chronic scarring. Rheumatic fever is still the most common cause of mitral valve stenosis.

As the mitral opening narrows the left atrium enlarges (dilates) over time because it must work harder to pump blood into the left ventricle. Many people (up to 50%) eventually develop atrial fibrillation because of progressive dilatation of the left atrium. In atrial fibrillation the left atrium quivers instead of effectively pumping blood to the left ventricle causing a decreased amount of blood to the left ventricle.

Severe stenosis may also cause pressure to built up in the lung blood vessels (pulmonary veins) that supply blood to the left atrium. The lung blood vessels are normally under much lower pressure (as is the right side of the heart that pumps blood to the lungs) than the left ventricle, aorta and its arterial branches. Increased blood pressure in the lungs is called pulmonary hypertension.

#### *Aetiology of Mitral Stenosis*

1. Rheumatic fever
2. Cardiac tumors
3. Rheumatologic disorders (lupus, rheumatoid arthritis)
4. Myxoma
5. Congenital defects: Parachute valve

#### *Clinical Manifestations*

*A. Symptoms:*

1. **Dyspnea** on exertion is usually the first symptom. It may progress from grade 1 to 4 in severe cases in which case it may be accompanied by orthopnea or paroxysmal nocturnal dyspnea. Acute pulmonary edema is a grave and dreaded complication of mitral stenosis.
2. **Palpitation** on exertion is also a frequent symptom, representing an increased awareness by the patient of her precordial impulse, which in turn may be due to the hypertrophied right ventricle. At times, when the onset of a palpitation is sudden, it may be a manifestation of a transient paroxysmal atrial tachycardia or atrial fibrillation.
3. **Cough** is usually brought on by exertion. Some patients develop a chronic bronchitis precipitated by chilly weather, which is very similar to the usual idiopathic chronic bronchitis.
4. **Chest pain:** Noncardiac localised in left inframammary region is common in neurotic individuals. True angina pectoris can also occur, especially in patients with severe pulmonary hypertension or associated with coronary artery disease in elderly group of patients.
5. **Hemoptysis** is frequent, and often the presenting complaint. It is usually the result of rupture of congested veins in the bronchial mucosa, but occasionally it may be the presenting symptom of pulmonary infarction.
6. **Embolic phenomenon** results in blocking of a cerebral artery presenting as a sudden stroke, of the splenic or renal artery manifesting with acute abdominal pain, or of a peripheral limb artery with acute pain and other manifestations of ischemia. Obstruction of the aortic bifurcation by a large embolus is a particularly serious complication.
7. Due to compression of the left recurrent laryngeal nerve by a dilated and tense main pulmonary artery, it may lead to paralysis of left vocal cord presenting as hoarseness of the voice (Ortner's syndrome).

*B. Physical examination:*

1. The patients may have a typical mitral facies with pinkish purple patches on the cheeks.
2. The pulse is usually normal, but may be weak if stroke volume is reduced (Fig 16.3).
3. A prominent 'a' wave may be present in the jugular venous pulse of patients in sinus rhythm with pulmonary hypertension.
4. A palpable first heart sound (S1) suggests a pliable anterior mitral valve leaflet. A right ventricular heave and a palpable pulmonic component of the second heart sound (P2) suggests pulmonary hypertension.
5. Aloud first heart sound (S1) occurs because the valve is fibrotic but pliable and higher than normal left ventricular systolic pressure is required to close it.

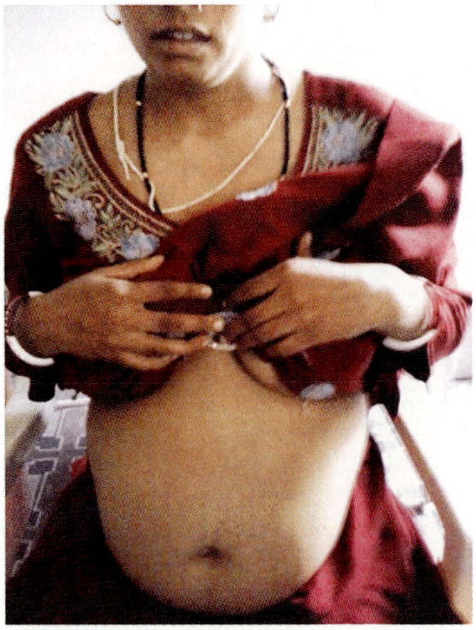

**Fig 16.3:** Photograph of a young lady with 8 months pregnancy with tight mitral valvular stenosis

6. The opening snap (OS) is best heard at the apex and is as a result of the sudden tensing and deceleration of the mitral valve leaflets when they are fully open. It usually suggests that the valve is still pliable and not rigidly calcified. The duration of the interval between the aortic component of the second heart sound and the opening snap correlates inversely with left atrial pressure.
7. A low-pitched diastolic rumble which is produced by blood flow across the narrowed mitral valve can be best heard at the apical region, often best heard with the patient in the left lateral decubitus position. The duration of the rumble roughly correlates with increasing severity of mitral stenosis. It may be masked by noisy respirations or by low cardiac output and may be accentuated by increasing cardiac output with exercise. One may encounter a palpable diastolic thrill at the apex.
8. There may be an apical holosystolic murmur of associated rheumatic mitral regurgitation.
9. There may be a holosystolic murmur of tricuspid regurgitation from right ventricular dilatation along the lower left sternal border.
10. There could be a mixture of murmurs produced as a result of involvement of their respective valves, such as aortic, tricuspid and pulmonary inorigion. Normally, the cross-sectional area of the mitral valve is at least 4 $cm^2$. Mitral stenosis leads to a reduction in valve area and is considered severe when the valve area is less than 1 $cm^2$. To maintain flow through the valve, leftatrial pressure rises, leading to an increase in the pressure gradient across the valve and to increased pulmonary venous and capillary pressures, with resultant dyspnea. Flow through the stenotic valve is dependent on the duration of diastole. Tachycardia shortens diastole disproportionately and causes a further elevation in left atrial pressure and can precipitate symptoms even in patients with relatively mild stenosis. Elevated left atrial pressure contributes to left atrial enlargement, which in turn predisposes the patient to atrial fibrillation, atrial thrombus formation, and thromboembolism, all of which are common complications of mitral stenosis. Severe mitral stenosis is often associated with an increase in pulmonary arterial pressure, leading to right-sided heart failure and secondary tricuspid and pulmonary incompetence. In patients with severe pulmonary hypertension, cardiac output at rest is reduced; this output reduction can cause a relatively low pressure gradient across the mitral valve even in patients with severe stenosis.

### Diagnosis of Mitral Stenosis

It is suspected in a person with a history of congestive heart failure, findings of a specific type of mitral heart murmur on physical exam, and confirmed with the following set of examination.

### Chest Radiography

For patients with mitral stenosis, the chest radiograph may exhibit certain specific and nonspecific findings that are generally a consequence of left atrial enlargement, mitral calcification, pulmonary hypertension, and congestive heart failure (CHF). The degree of confidence is reasonably good for mitral stenosis. Findings are sometimes nonspecific (Figs 16.4–16.7).

***Electrocardiography:*** If the patient is in sinus rhythm, the electrocardiogram shows abnormality of the LA. LA abnormality is manifested by prolongation of the P-wave, with a double-saddleback contour (p mitrale) in limb lead II. This contour represents a right atrial P-wave followed by delayed LA P-wave associated with an enlarged left atrium. LA abnormality is seen as a terminal negative deflection following the initial upright P-wave in

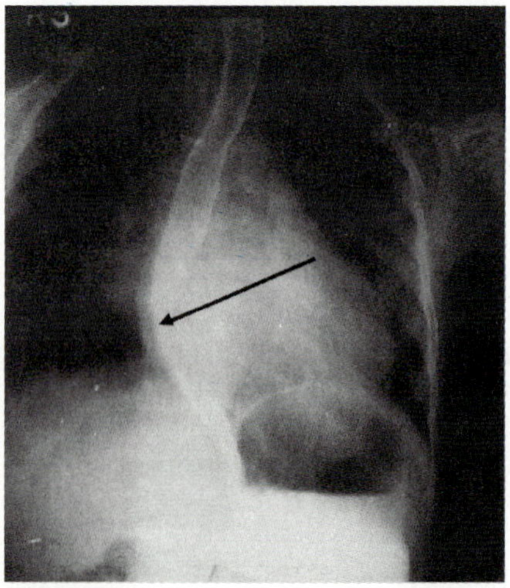

**Fig. 16.4:** Photograph of barium meal study (arrow) showing indentation of barium filled esophagus in moderate enlargement of LA in rheumatic MS

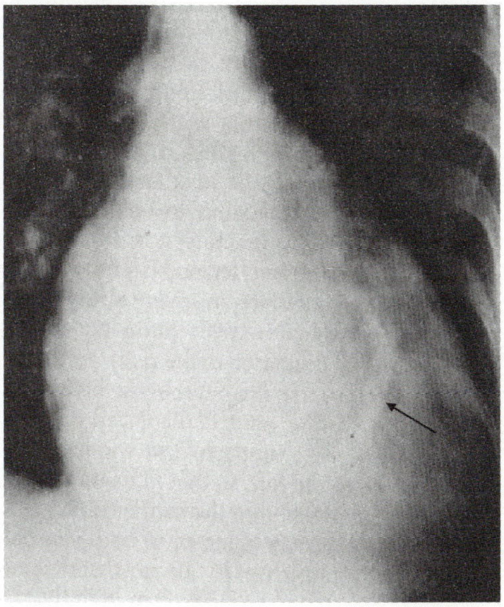

**Fig. 16.5:** Calcification of mitral annulus as indicated by broad and curved density (arrow) in chronic mitral valve disease

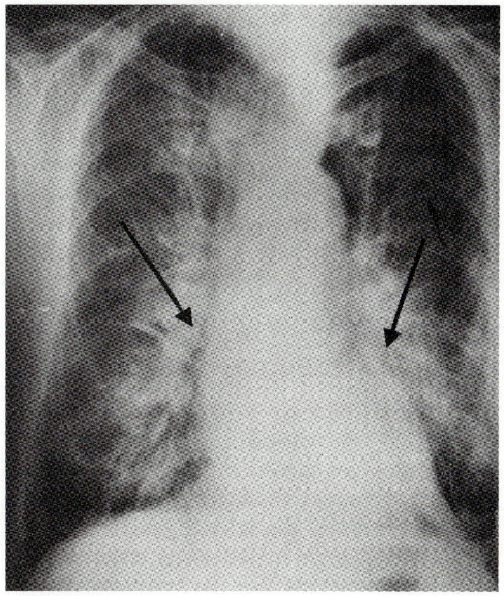

**Fig. 16.6:** Interstitial pulmonary edema as indicated by indistinct haze in the perihilar region (arrow) in a patient with critical mitral stenosis

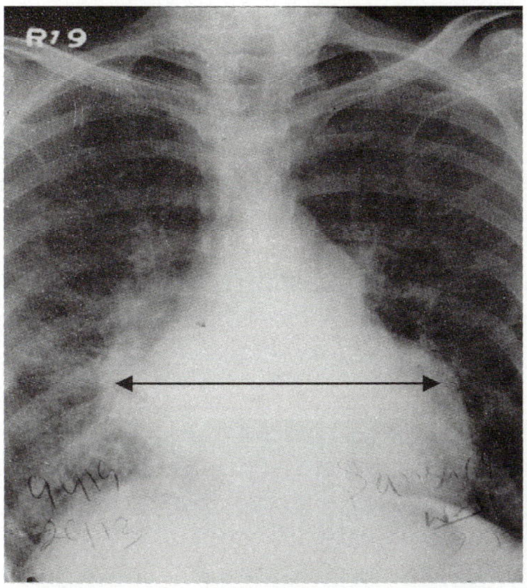

**Fig. 16.7:** X-ray chest PA view (arrow) showing moderate enlargement of RA in patient with rheumatic MS, TR and PAH

the chest lead V1. The main rhythm is usually sinus in the beginning. However, atrial fibrillation increases in frequency as mitral stenosis advances. If pulmonary arterial hypertension has developed, electrocardiography may show signs of RV hypertrophy (Fig. 16.8).

***Echocardiography:*** Definitive diagnosis is made using of echocardiography when entire valve can be visualized Echocardiography, especially Doppler echocardiography, is the procedure of choice for evaluating the degree of mitral stenosis; in most of the patients, echocardiography may be adequate for the planning of therapeutic interventions. Echocardiography generally provides sufficiently detailed images of the mitral valve and is the most important diagnostic tool in establishing the diagnosis. Doppler echocardiography is used to accurately depict the severity of mitral stenosis. Typical two-dimensional (2D) echocardiographic findings include thickening of the mitral valve cusps; enlargement of the LA, with a normal or small LV; and a reduction in the size of the mitral valve orifice in diastole. A diminished E-F slope is noted on M-mode images. Doppler studies demonstrate an increase in the mean pressure gradient across the mitral orifice; Doppler studies are also helpful in quantifying the severity of mitral stenosis (Figs 16.9–16.14).

### Computed Tomography

CT scans occasionally depict calcification in the enlarged LA in patients with mitral stenosis. It may be seen to occupy the wall of the atrium, or it may appear within a thrombus attached to the wall.

Whenever calcification is observed in the atrial appendage, it generally indicates associated mitral stenosis. Calcification in the wall of the atrium or in the appendage is usually considered an unfavorable prognostic sign.

When calcification in the atrium is suspected but is not positively identified on the chest radiograph, fluoroscopy or CT may be used to confirm the diagnosis. In the current era, CT scanning is rarely performed; rather, echocardiography has gained widespread use, owing to its portability and the fact that there is none of the risk associated with the use of radiation (Fig. 16.15).

### Magnetic Resonance Imaging

For patients with mitral stenosis, MRI may be helpful if Doppler echocardiographic findings are insufficient or are inconsistent with clinical data. This problem occurs in

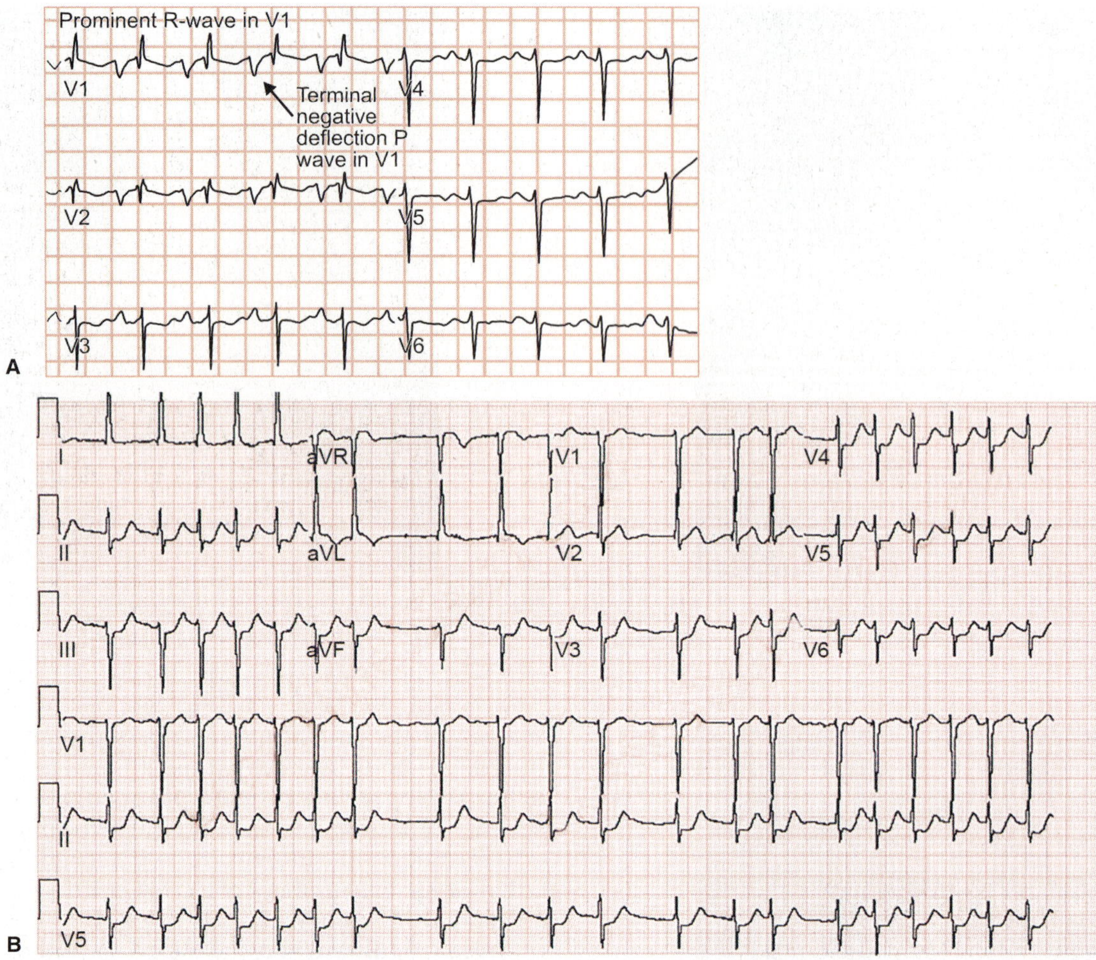


**Fig. 16.8:** (A) ECG trace shows terminal negative deflection of P-wave in V1 due to LA enlargement and right ventricular hypertrophy in a young patient with chronic mitral valvular stenosis. (B) Shows atrial fibrillation with rapid ventricular response in a pregnant women with severe type of mitral stenosis

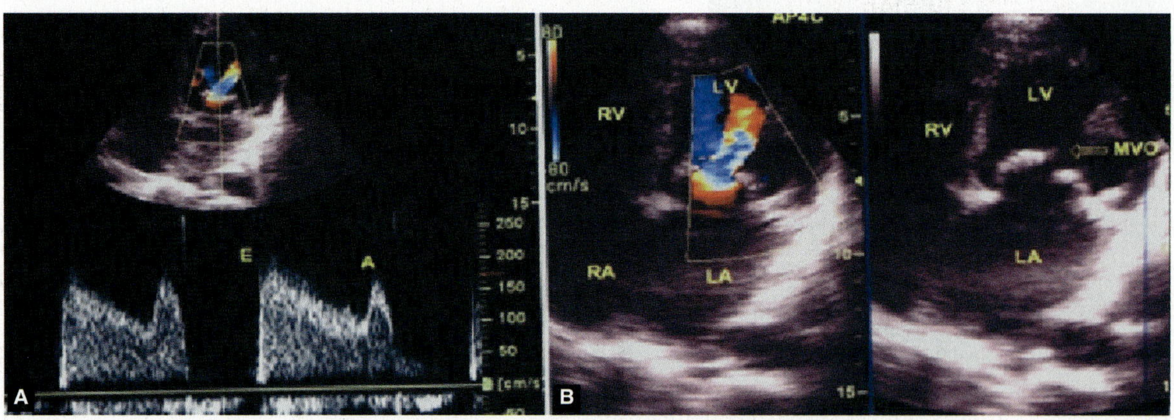


**Fig. 16.9:** (A) Pulse Doppler tracing with an early diastolic E-wave and a late diastolic A-wave (during atrial systole). In normal persons, there will be a gap between the two waves, when the atrial and ventricular diastolic pressures are equal (diastasis). Diastasis is absent in mitral stenosis as the pressures do not equalise—left atrial pressure is always higher and there is a gradient throughout diastole. Mitral valve area can be estimated from the downward slope of the E-wave. The slope becomes more flat as the severity of the mitral stenosis increases. The A-wave is absent in atrial fibrillation. (B) Two pictures, one with colour flow mapping and another without the color flow mapping. The colour flow mapping shows the turbulent flow from left atrium to left ventricle through the stenosed mitral valve. The domed mitral leaflets in the open position with a narrow orifice is visible in the frame without colour flow mapping. Both images are in the apical four chamber view. RA=right atrium; LA=left atrium; LV=left ventricle; RV=right ventricle; MVO=mitral valve orifice

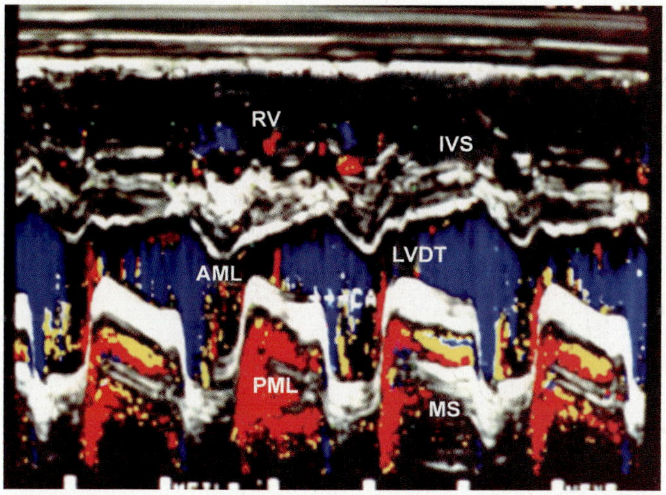


**Fig. 16.10:** Color flow M-mode showing markedly thickened anterior and posterior mitral leaflets with paradoxical movement of posterior leaflet in patient with rheumatic mitral native valvular stenosis alongwith dilated and hypertrophied RV

approximately 10% of patients because of air-tissue attenuation of ultrasound. MRI is often used in cases in which there is associated complex congenital heart disease because of its three-dimensional (3D) capabilities and high resolution (Fig. 16.16).

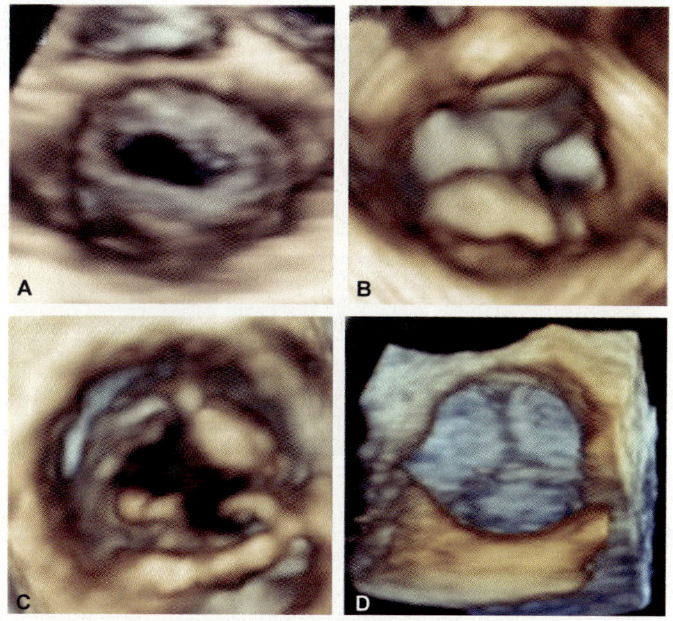


**Fig. 16.11:** Valvular anatomic features displayed by 3D TTE. Three-dimensional (3D) transthoracic echocardiography (TTE) images of (A) a stenotic rheumatic mitral valve from the left atrial perspective, (B) a mitral valve with P2 segmental prolapse from the left atrial perspective, (C) a normal tricuspid valve from the right ventricular perspective, and (D) a normal aortic valve as viewed from the aorta

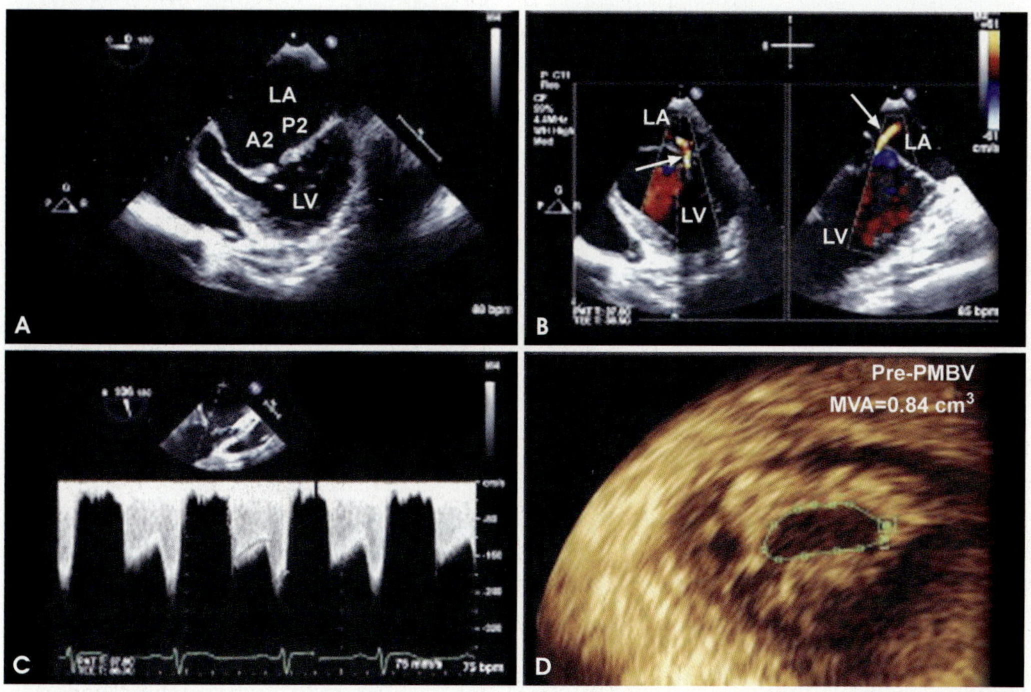


**Fig. 16.12:** Pre-procedural assessment of a stenotic MV by TEE. (A) Transesophageal echocardiography (TEE) at mid-esophageal level at 0° (4-chamber view). Note moderate bileaflet thickening involving the mid-distal segments of the mitral valve (MV) with reduced opening. (B) Simultaneous biplane imaging of the MV at the mid-esophageal level at 0° and 90° (right) with color-Doppler showing mild mitral regurgitation (arrow) at baseline. (C) Continuous-wave Doppler indicating increased transmitral gradients. (D) Real-time three-dimensional imaging with multiplanar reformatting showing a severely stenotic MV with important commissural fusion (MVA=0.84 $cm^2$). A2=middle anterior scallop; LA=left atrium; LV=left ventricle; MVA=mitral valve area; P2=middle posterior scallop; PMBV=percutaneous mitral balloon valvuloplasty

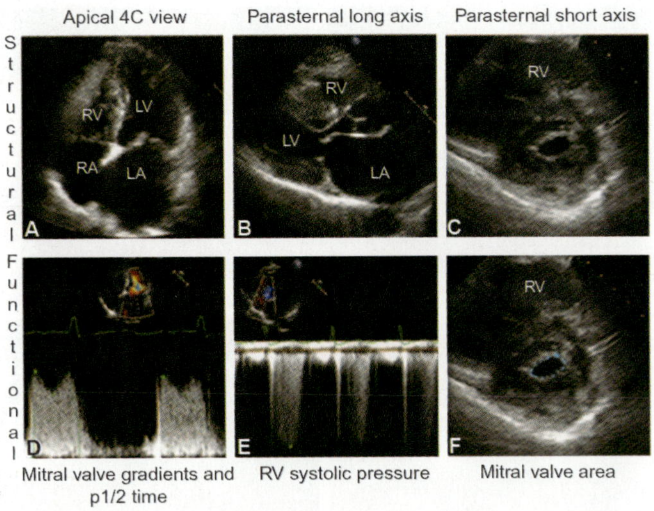


**Fig. 16.13:** Two-dimensional and Doppler echocardiography in mitral stenosis. Traditionally 2D echocardiography has provided structural information regarding the morphology of the mitral valve in mitral stenosis. In addition chamber size, and ventricular function is assessed by echocardiography. Doppler methods provide hemodynamic functional information regarding the mitral valve in mitral stenosis. Peak and mean mitral valve gradients, pressure half time derived mitral valve area and systolic pulmonary pressure are usually recorded in these patients. RV=right ventricle; LV=left ventricle; RA=right atrium; LA=left atrium

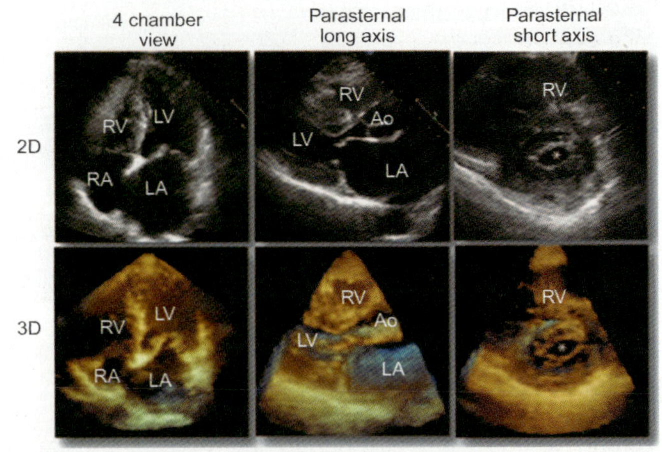


**Fig. 16.14:** Comparison of 2D and 3D transthoracic echocardiography in mitral stenosis. The most useful views to evaluate patients with mitral stenosis include the apical 4 chamber view as well as the parasternal long and short axis views. This figure illustrates the added value of 3D imaging in better characterizing the mitral valve apparatus. The third dimension increases the anatomic detail of the leaflets, commissures and subvalvular tissue. RV=right ventricle; LV=left ventricle; RA=right atrium; LA=left atrium; Ao=aorta

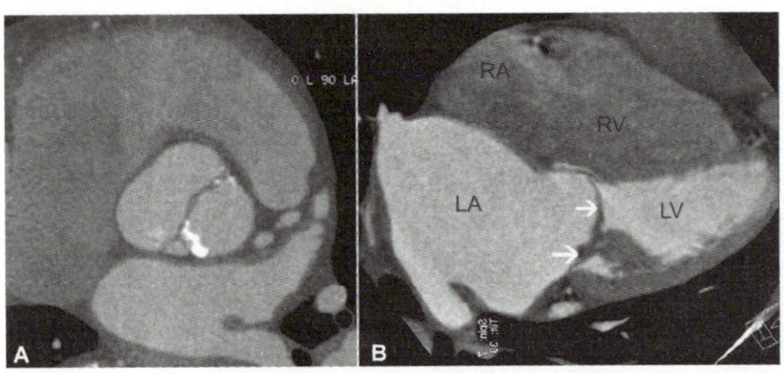


**Fig. 16.15:** Valvular lesions. Short-axis CT image (A) through the aortic valve shows a bicuspid valve, with calcification of the leaflet. Four-chamber reconstructed CT image. (B) Shows severe thickening of the mitral leaflets (arrows) in a patient with mitral stenosis with associated severe left atrial enlargement

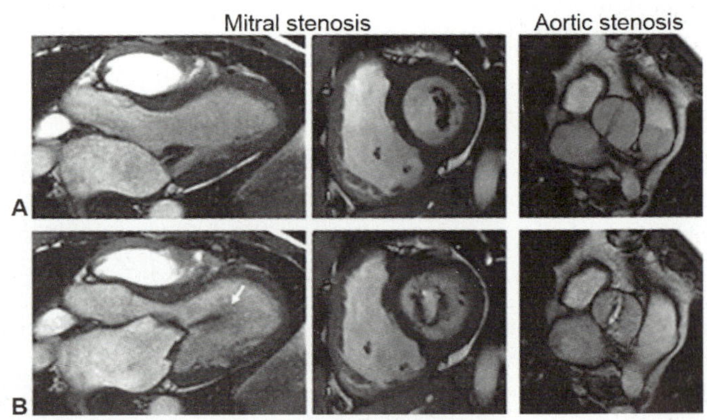


**Fig. 16.16:** SSFP images of abnormal mitral and aortic valves with the abnormal valve leaflets (A) closed and (B) at maximal opening. Rheumatic mitral stenosis is shown in the 3-chamber and short-axis image plane. Note significant thickening and calcification of both the mitral valve leaflets and chordae tendineae, along with chordal fusion, as well as severe left atrial enlargement. At maximal opening of the mitral valve leaflets, the signal void seen within the left ventricle represents turbulent diastolic filling of the left ventricle (arrow). A bicuspid aortic valve with significant aortic stenosis is shown in a short-axis image plane (MR images courtesy of Raymond J. Kim, MD, Duke Cardiovascular Magnetic Resonance Center, Durham, NC)

MRI is of limited use in patients with atrial fibrillation, a common finding in mitral stenosis. Irregular rhythm may be a potential source of error in the measurements.

## Cardiac Catheterization

Cardiac catheterization is usually unnecessary for assessing the severity of mitral stenosis. Nonetheless, coronary arteriography is performed in many patients with mitral stenosis who are in an age group in which there is a relatively high incidence of coronary disease and for whom heart surgery is anticipated or who have coexistent angina. In such cases, left- and right-sided heart catheterizations are performed to evaluate the coronary arteries, to confirm the transmitral gradient, and to determine the valve area. The valve area is determined by use of the Gorlin equation: Mitral valve area = [CO(DFP × HR)]/37.6 × $h$½), where CO is cardiac output (in milliliters per minute), DFP is the diastolic filling period, HR is the heart rate, and $h$ is the mean gradient.

### Management

Once symptoms develop in mitral stenosis, the chance of survival decreases without surgical or balloon dilatation or valve replacement. In the absence of symptoms, management is directed at preventing recurrence of rheumatic fever.

#### *Medical Therapy*

Patients in atrial fibrillation require heart-rate control with a beta-blocker (e.g. atenolol, 50 mg q.d.), digoxin (0.125–0.25 mg q.d.), or both. Systemic anticoagulation with warfarin is definitely indicated to prevent thromboembolism under the following situations when

1. Atrial fibrillation is present
2. There is a history of embolism, or
3. A thrombus is detected in the atrium.

Anticoagulation should be considered for patients with paroxysmal atrial fibrillation, a dilated left atrium (>50 mm in diameter on echocardiography), or severe atrial stasis (as evidenced by swirling echoes or smoke in the left atrium on echocardiography). Regarding symptomatic patients for whom surgical intervention poses a relatively high risk, the judicious use of diuretics and drugs to control heart rate (i.e. digoxin, calcium channel blockers, or beta-blockers) may allow symptomatic relief without the need for surgical intervention.

### SURGICAL INTERVENTION

Intervention to increase valve area is indicated before the onset of symptoms of dyspnea in the following patients—women with severe stenosis who wish to become pregnant but are unlikely to tolerate the volume load of pregnancy, patients who experience recurrent thromboembolic events, and patients who have severe pulmonary hypertension. A number of interventions are currently available to increase the valve area in mitral stenosis. These interventions include:

1. Percutaneous balloon valvuloplasty performed in the cardiac catheterization laboratory
2. Surgical commissurotomy
3. Replacement of the mitral valve with a prosthesis.

#### *1. Percutaneous Balloon Valvuloplasty*

- Percutaneous balloon mitral valvulotomy—a balloon tipped catheter is threaded through an artery into the heart. The balloon is inflated to expand the mitral valve. This technique has been very effective in younger patients with valves that are not calcified (excessively stiff) (Figs 16.17–16.18).
- It is now usually performed under direct vision after cardiopulmonary bypass. Surgical commissurotomy may be feasible when balloon valvuloplasty is impossible, such as in patients with significant mitral regurgitation, subvalvular stenosis, or atrial thrombus. A number of studies comparing surgical commissurotomy with balloon commissurotomy have shown equivalent immediate and medium-term (3–4 years) results regarding increase in valve area, improvement in symptoms, and freedom from repeat intervention in appropriately selected patients. However, commissurotomy, whether effected by a balloon or surgically, is a palliative procedure, and in most cases further intervention is eventually required.
- Repeat commissurotomy is sometimes feasible; but most often, mitral valve replacement is also necessary is heavily scarred or calcified or if severe mitral regurgitation is present. Morbidity and mortality are higher with

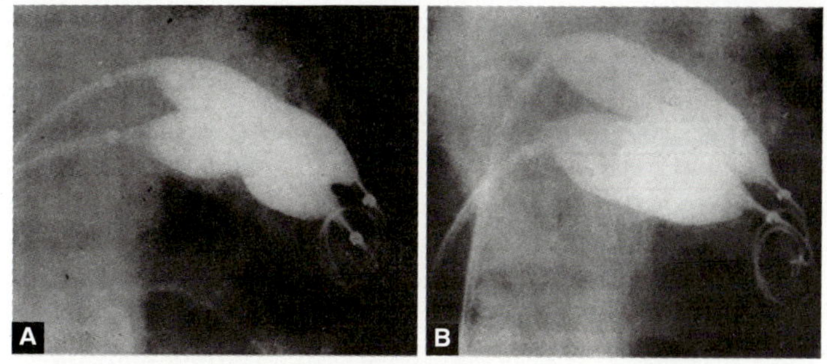


**Fig. 16.17:** (A) Double balloon across the mitral valve indicating the waist found by the stenotic valve. (B) Fully inflated balloon with disappearance of the waist as seen in (A)

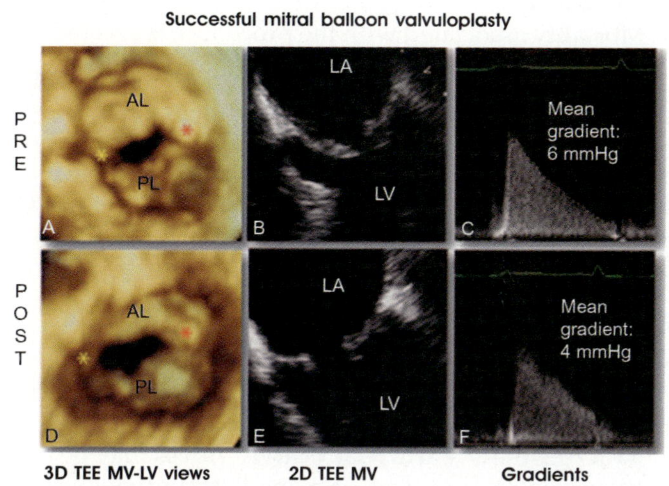


**Fig. 16.18:** (A) and (D) depict the mitral valve orifice as seen from the LV. Note the commissural fusion and the small mitral orifice in the pre-procedure image (A). In (D) the commissures are now split and the area of the mitral orifice has increased. (B) and (E) illustrate the 2D TEE views of the mitral valve pre- and post-procedure. Note the increased leaflet distance post-procedure. (C) and (F) illustrate the transmitral Doppler gradients pre- and post-procedure. The pre-procedure gradients had already diminished under general anesthesia and the post-procedure gradients showed only a mild drop despite good bi-commissural splitting. This is not uncommon to see in the immediate post-procedure studies and is probably related to decreased left atrial compliance, therefore to gauge procedural success; we rely mostly on the 3D visualization of the mitral orifice size and commissural splitting.Yellow asterisk-lateral commissure; red asterisk-medial commissure

prosthetic replacement than with either surgical or balloon commissurotomy.

- It is performed by inflating a specially designed balloon catheter in the mitral orifice to split the fused commissures. Excellent symptomatic relief is obtained in suitable patients. This intervention is currently the initial choice in mitral stenosis. Typically, the mitral valve area doubles in size from 1.0 to 2.0 $cm^2$, with a concomitant reduction in the pressure gradient.

*Complications of balloon mitral valvuloplasty* include:

1. Severe mitral regurgitation (3%)
2. Thromboembolism (3%),
3. Residual atrial septal defect with significant shunting (10–20%).
4. Mortality associated with the procedure is less than 1%.

*Contraindications to balloon mitral valvuloplasty* include significant mitral regurgitation, which will likely increase after balloon inflation; left atrial thrombus, which can be dislodged at the time of the procedure; and significant subvalvular involvement or leaflet calcification, each of which increases the risk of complications and limits the degree of dilatation produced.

### 2. Surgical Intervention

A. **Mitral valvulotomy (commissurotomy)** the natural valve is widened by making a cut in the mitral valve.

B. **Total valve replacement—the mitral valve is replaced by a prosthetic ('artificial') valve.** Valves may be either bioprosthetic (pig, cow, or human) or synthetic (usually metal alloys). Valvular replacement is usually required in older patients with heavily calcified (stiff) mitral valves (Fig. 16.19).

C. **Mitral valve repair:** Mitral valve repair is an open heart procedure performed by cardiothoracic surgeons to treat stenosis (narrowing) or regurgitation (leakage) of the mitral valve. The mitral valve is the 'inflow valve' for the left side of the heart. Blood flows from the lungs, where it picks up oxygen, and into the left atrium (Fig. 16.20).

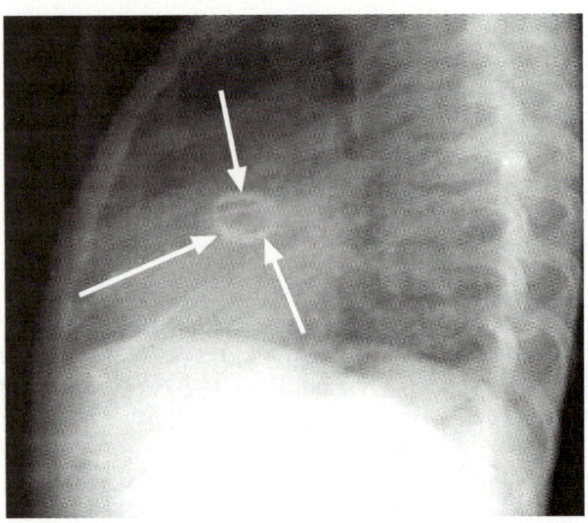

**Fig. 16.19:** Anatomical location of Bjork Shilley mitral valve visualised in lateral position of X-ray chest PA view with mitral valve replacement in a patient with calcified native mitral valve

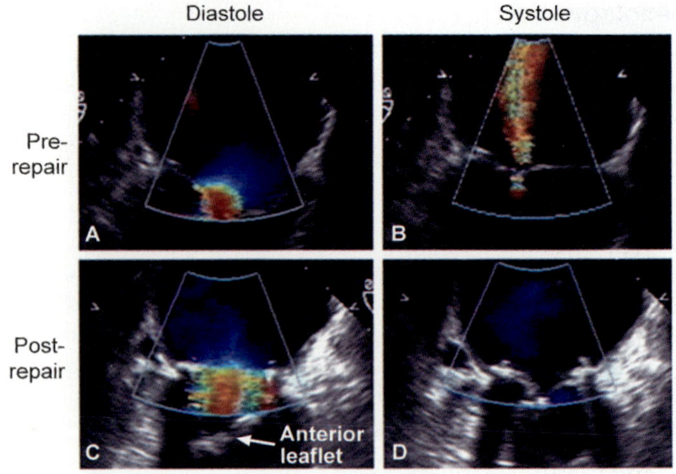


**Fig. 16.20:** A patient with long-standing rheumatic mitral stenosis and regurgitation undergoing a rheumatic repair. (A and B) on pre-bypass echo, the stenotic and insufficient mitral valve is demonstrated. (C and D) after insertion of an autologous pericardial patch into the posterior leaflet, decalcifying commissurotomy, resection of the submitral apparatus to the anterior leaflet, and re-attachment of the mobile anterior leaflet to both papillary muscles with adjustable ACR, the valve is fully competent with insignificant gradient. A full rigid ring also is placed (AnnuloFlow, Sorin Group). These types of more comprehensive ACR repairs for rheumatic valves have been quite stable in the intermediate term

### Prognosis

Most people have no symptoms for the first 10 years, increasing shortness of breath on exertion for the next 10 years followed by worsening symptoms that may begin to occur at rest during the next decade.

All people having mitral stenosis of any degree require antibiotic prophylaxis to prevent infective endocarditis prior to dental or surgical procedures.

## MITRAL REGURGITATION

It occurs when blood flows back into the left atrium from the left ventricle during left ventricular contraction because of a 'leaky' mitral valve. Mitral regurgitation can occur acutely (suddenly) with infective endocarditis or with a heart attack that causes rupture of the papillary muscles or chordae tendineae. Symptoms of severe congestive heart failure (severe shortness of breath, fast heart rate, and fluid in the lungs) requiring urgent surgical intervention usually occur with acute mitral valve rupture.

Rheumatic fever is the most common cause of chronic (gradual over many years) mitral regurgitation. Chronic regurgitation, even with large regurgitant blood flow, is often tolerated for years due to compensatory changes in the heart. The left atrium dilates over time to handle the increased blood volume.

### Aetiology

- Mitral regurgitation (acute)
- Ruptured papillary muscle (infarction, trauma)
- Papillary muscle dysfunction (ischemia)
- Ruptured chordae tendineae (trauma, endocarditis and myxomatous)
- Valve perforation (endocarditis)
- Weight-loss medications (fenfluramine, dexfenfluramine)

### Signs and Symptoms

Signs and symptoms of mitral regurgitation are as follows:

- Acute pulmonary edema
- Jugular venous pressure (JVP) exhibits cannon A waves and giant V-waves.
- Harsh blowing apical crescendo-decrescendo murmur radiating to the axilla
- Palpable thrill at apex
- S3 and S4
- Palpitations
- Atrial fibrillation
- Dyspnea
- Orthopnea
- Nocturnal paroxysmal dyspnea
- Peripheral edema
- Systemic emboli
- Normal JVP
- Left ventricular hypertrophy (LVH)
- Apical high-pitched pansystolic murmur
- Decreased or obscured S1
- Widely split S2 sound
- S3 sound

### Diagnosis of Mitral Regurgitation

#### *Clinical Manifestations*

In most patients, mitral regurgitation remains asymptomatic for many years. Dyspnea, fatigue from low cardiac output, and edema occur late in the course of the disease. Mitral regurgitation is recognized clinically by a systolic murmur at the apex, radiating to the axilla and increasing on expiration. In patients with a posteriorly directed jet of mitral regurgitation, the murmur is heard well at the back. In more severe cases, the murmur lasts throughout systole, the first and second heart sounds are soft or difficult to hear, and a third heart sound is present. A midsystolic click can be present in myxomatous disease; in less severe cases, this click can precede the murmur. The murmur can also be confined to late systole, with papillary muscle dysfunction. Mitral regurgitant murmurs caused by ischemia can be variable in duration and intensity, depending on the degree of ischemia and the loading conditions.

#### *Imaging Studies*

1. **2D and 2D Doppler echocardiography:** Doppler echocardiography is the noninvasive method of choice in confirming the presence of mitral regurgitation. Echocardiography is used to diagnose the mechanism of the regurgitation (e.g. prolapse or annular dilatation); color-flow mapping is used to provide a semi-quantitative assessment of severity based on the size and penetration of the left atrium by the regurgitant jet. Additionally, echocardiography can be used to assess the effects of the regurgitation on left ventricular size and function. Quantitative measurements of regurgitation, such as the regurgitant volume, regurgitant fraction [(regurgitant volume) plus stroke volume) divided by regurgitant volume)], and regurgitant orifice area (the area through which the valve leaks), are now possible with newer Doppler techniques. These techniques are useful in determining the true severity of the lesion and following it over time. Left ventricular size and volume, as well as contractile function assessed by the ejection fraction, are used to determine the need for surgical intervention (Figs 16.21–16.23).

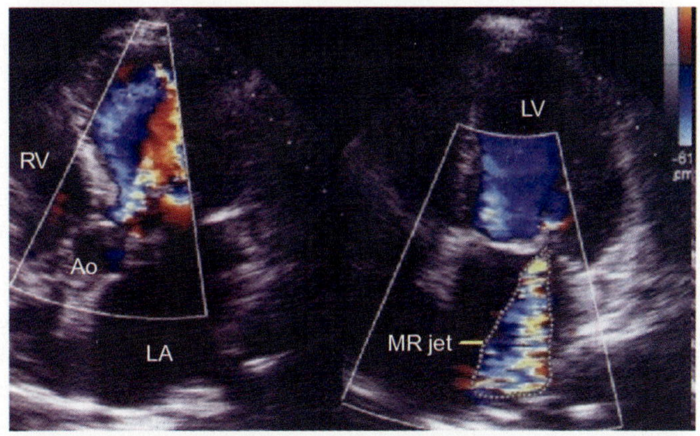


**Fig. 16.21:** 2D color-Doppler echocardiogram in RHD, showing moderate mitral regurgitation

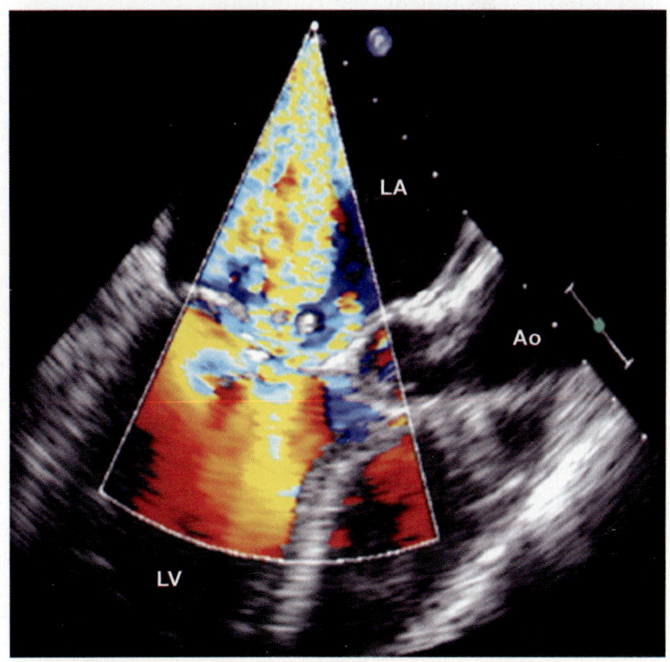


**Fig. 16.22:** Color-Doppler imaging in 4C view reveals severe mitral regurgitation. LA=left atrium; LV=left ventricle; Ao=aorta

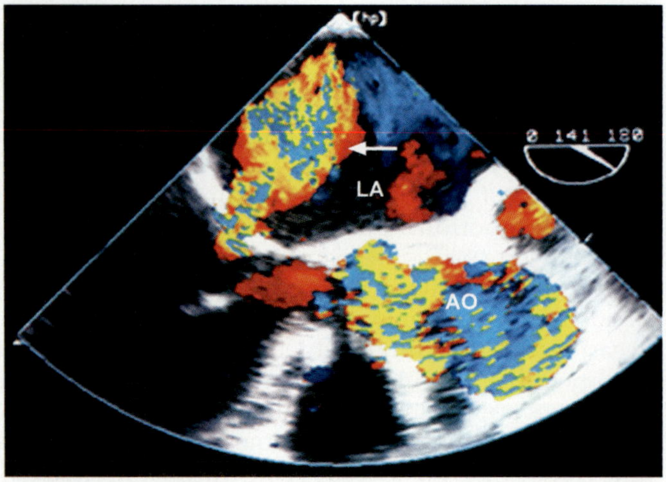


**Fig. 16.23:** Transesophageal echocardiography image (three-chamber plane) demonstrating a jet of mitral regurgitation (arrow) in the left atrium (LA). Ao=aorta; LV=left ventricle

However, asymptomatic mitral regurgitation is more difficult to assess and manage than other valvular lesions because in this condition, the true contractile function of the left ventricle is difficult to determine with conventional measures such as the ejection fraction. These measurements of contractility are confounded by the increase in ventricular preload caused by the extra volume of blood in the left atrium and the variable effect on afterload. Afterload is increased by left ventricular dilatation, but this effect is offset as the ventricle ejects much of its blood into a relatively low pressure system (the left atrium). The left ventricular ejection fraction can appear falsely elevated in mitral regurgitation and usually falls after surgical correction. An ejection fraction of less than 60% should be considered abnormally low in patients with mitral regurgitation.

2. **Transesophageal echocardiography** is very sensitive in the detection of mitral regurgitation and is used mainly in those patients who are difficult to evaluate by the transthoracic approach. Contrast ventriculography is used to determine the severity of mitral regurgitation in patients undergoing cardiac catheterization. This procedure involves injecting radiopaque contrast medium into the left ventricle and assessing the extent and duration of opacification of the left atrium. In patients undergoing hemodynamic monitoring, large systolic V waves on the pulmonary arterial wedge tracing raise the suspicion of acute severe mitral regurgitation, as can occur in acute ischemia, but such V waves can occur in the absence of severe regurgitation.
3. **Stress echocardiography** is useful in detecting latent left ventricular dysfunction not evident on a resting study. Failure of the left ventricular ejection fraction to increase on exercise or of the left ventricular end-systolic volume to decrease on exercise is predictive of incipient left ventricular dysfunction and should be considered an indication for early surgery.
4. **Other echocardiographic indices** that have been associated with a less favorable surgical outcome include an absolute end-systolic dimension that is greater than 4.5 cm or that is greater than 2.6 cm/m$^2$ when indexed for body surface area; an end-systolic volume of greater than 50 ml/m$^2$; and a resting ejection fraction of less than 60%. Surgical referral should be considered if ventricular size and function approach these indices. Serial echocardiographic evaluation should be performed at least yearly and should be performed more frequently as ventricular dilatation progresses in patients with severe asymptomatic mitral regurgitation. Studies indicate a better long-term survival rate in patients with severe mitral regurgitation when surgery is performed early. Symptomatic severe mitral regurgitation is considered an indication for surgical intervention if the valve is primarily involved.

*Management of mitral regurgitation*: In the management of asymptomatic mitral regurgitation, it should be borne in mind that left ventricular dysfunction is often latent and that, once present, the dysfunction cannot be corrected by operative intervention. Therefore, it is important to refer patients for surgery before the onset of true left ventricular dysfunction even in the absence of symptoms. Unfortunately, no load-independent measure of contractile function is readily available. In order to manage mitral regurgitation, one should always differentiate between acute and chronic MR.

*Acute:*

- Afterload reduction (nitroglycerin, morphine, or sodium nitroprusside)
- Diuresis
- Intra-aortic balloon pump (temporizing for urgent surgery)

*Chronic:*

- Diuresis
- Nitrates
- Hydralazine
- ACE inhibitor
- Digoxin
- Adrenergic blocker (ventricular rate control)
- Calcium antagonist (ventricular rate control)
- Heparin (if atrial fibrillation)
- Endocarditis
- Endocarditis prophylaxis/education

### Surgical Intervention

- Decisions in regard to the treatment of acute mitral regurgitation are strongly influenced by the cause of the regurgitation. In 1 series, the causes were acute MI in 45% of cases, degenerative valvular disease in 26%, and infective endocarditis in 28%. Although the technical treatment of the mitral valve may be similar, each cause requires a different approach and has a different outcome. Furthermore, unlike aortic regurgitation—wherein repair is rarely possible—mitral regurgitation can be treated by means of repair or replacement.

- Adequate surgical exposure of the mitral valve is crucial. Exposure is often difficult when regurgitation is acute and the left atrium is not dilated; therefore, surgery must be approached carefully. Expeditious use of CPB, optimal myocardial protection, and excellent valve exposure yield the best results. The intraoperative approach to the mitral valve is also crucial, a variety of techniques should be considered, particularly when endocarditis affects multiple structures or the annulus, or when extensive annular reconstruction is needed. Approaches include a lateral Sondergaard incision in the groove in the left atrium, transatrial incisions, left atrial dome incisions, or transection of the superior vena cava with a more anterolateral approach to the left atrium. This last is particularly useful when endocarditis is noticeably destructive and more extensive annular reconstruction is required. Although median sternotomy is typical, experienced surgeons can execute less invasive approaches.
- Symptomatic patients with ischemic mitral regurgitation often require mitral valve surgery in addition to revascularization. Mitral regurgitation secondary to left ventricular dilatation often improves with afterload reduction, and surgical intervention is not usually indicated. Patients with moderately severe left ventricular dysfunction (ejection fraction <35%) and significant mitral regurgitation were thought in the past to be poor surgical candidates because of high operative risk. However, recent research has shown that there is acceptable risk associated with operations in these patients. Symptoms usually improve, but a survival benefit associated with surgery in this group has not yet been shown. Patients who are not considered suitable for surgery because of left ventricular dysfunction often benefit from afterload reduction and diuretics. However, in patients who have primary asymptomatic mitral regurgitation with preserved left ventricular function, afterload reduction has not been shown to delay surgery or improve left ventricular function in the few small studies that have addressed this issue; afterload reduction is not currently recommended to treat such patients. Afterload reduction is beneficial for stabilizing patients with hemodynamically significant acute mitral regurgitation in preparation for surgery. Mitral valve repair is currently the technique of choice in the surgical management of mitral regurgitation because the operative mortality is lower, ventricular function is better preserved, and long-term complications such as thromboembolism and infection are lower with repair than with replacement. Valve repair is most likely to be feasible in patients with myxomatous disease, especially if such disease involves the posterior leaflet, and is least likely to be successful in patients with rheumatic disease and endocarditis. Valve repair is accomplished by use of a variety of techniques, depending on the mechanism and aetiology of the regurgitation. Such techniques include partial leaflet resection, chordal shortening or transfer, and insertion of an annuloplasty ring to reduce the size of the annulus. Long-term failure of repair occurs at a rate of 1–2% a year, but is higher in patients with rheumatic disease. If mitral valve repair is not possible, a mitral prosthesis is implanted. Chordal and papillary muscle preservation is increasingly being employed when a mitral prosthesis is inserted, because preserving the muscles has been shown to help conserve left ventricular function after surgery.
- Organic causes of mitral regurgitation are managed similarly to those of acute aortic regurgitation. Supportive therapy can provide patients with stability and resuscitation en route to the operating room. The use of IABPs can be beneficial. In organic mitral regurgitation, the fundamental abnormality is structural and therefore requires surgical intervention. In functional mitral regurgitation, medical therapy may be sufficient to avoid immediate operative intervention; however, surgery should be considered if therapy fails.
- In patients with acute functional mitral regurgitation, therapy is directed at restoring blood flow to the territory at risk. Severe mitral regurgitation affects 7% of patients who experience cardiogenic shock. Acute mitral regurgitation in these patients is a sign of a poor prognosis: an observed mortality rate of 55% improved to only 39% in patients who were selected for emergency surgery. The SHOCK trial determined that early revascularization improved outcomes at 6 months in patients with cardiogenic shock and acute MI. Upon further analysis, the prognostic importance of mitral regurgitation to the short- and long-term survival of such patients was inversely related to the degree of regurgitation. This suggests that aggressive treatment with early revascularization may improve survival in patients with severe mitral regurgitation after acute MI. Therefore, if revascularization is needed, the presence of severe mitral regurgitation should prompt surgical intervention.
- Acute mitral regurgitation in the presence of acute cardiomyopathy or decompensated heart failure can respond to aggressive heart-failure therapy. The use of IABPs is effective in patients with acute functional mitral regurgitation of any cause, and IABPs are particularly useful in patients with underlying myocardial ischemia or cardiomyopathy. Although the role of LV assist devices has not been well studied in acute mitral regurgitation, these devices may be used in cases of decompensated heart failure that does not respond to medical therapy.
- Valvular thrombosis that results in acute regurgitation sometimes responds to thrombolytic therapy. However, in patients whose prosthetic valve dysfunction is severe and symptomatic, the ACC/AHA and ESC guidelines recommend surgery first. Thrombolytic agents should be reserved to treat patients who have confirmed valvular thrombosis when surgery is risky or unavailable, or when the thrombus burden is small and the patient has few symptoms.

### *Anesthetic Considerations*

Patients with acute mitral regurgitation can experience acute cardiopulmonary collapse at any time; however, the instability of their condition may not be as clear as it is in patients with acute aortic regurgitation. The surgical team should be present during the induction of anesthesia, in case CPB is urgently needed. Acute mitral regurgitation from profound, ongoing myocardial ischemia often requires additional anesthetic techniques that will optimize myocardial oxygen supply and demand, preload and afterload, and coronary perfusion pressure. The preoperative placement of an IABP can improve coronary perfusion and mitigate the effects of anesthetic induction

*Mitral valve repair:* It is almost always preferable to replacement. Therapeutic options, technical feasibility, and surgical priorities depend upon cause, acute pathophysiology, underlying pathology, and comorbidities. If the initial repair is unsatisfactory, further CPB and either repeat repair or valve replacement is necessary. Repair should therefore be undertaken when procedural success is likely, because a hemodynamically unstable patient might not be able to tolerate additional CPB. Influential factors include papillary muscle rupture; chordal rupture; annular dilation; hibernating, stunned, or infarcted myocardium; and the severity of coronary artery disease. Repair techniques include ring annuloplasty, annular reconstruction with pericardium, leaflet resection, leaflet reconstruction with pericardium, chordal replacement, vegetation excision, and edge-to-edge (Alfieri) approximation. Valve repair is more usual when acute annular dilation is the cause, such as in ischemia, or when the pathology involves the posterior leaflet only, such as in myxomatous valve disease or endocarditis with or without annular dilation. In annular involvement with infection or in anterior leaflet involvement with degenerative disease, the ability to repair the mitral valve dramatically decreases (Figs 16.24–16.28).

- Having to replace a mitral valve after an unsuccessful repair should not be viewed as a failure. Patients with acute regurgitation are less likely to tolerate repeat exploration and repair. The loss of tolerance is more pronounced after a complex, time-consuming repair attempt, as in cases involving tissue destruction due to endocarditis. Frequently, annular involvement precludes simple repair with predictably good initial results.
- In valve replacement, adequate débridement can avoid periprosthetic leaks due to inadequate visualization, poor tissue quality, or an undrained abscess. Preservation of the posterior and anterior chordae tendineae is ideal, because the LV has not adapted as in chronic regurgitation. Either a mechanical valve or a bioprosthesis can be used in cases of degenerative, ischemic, or infectious disease. Mechanical prostheses are

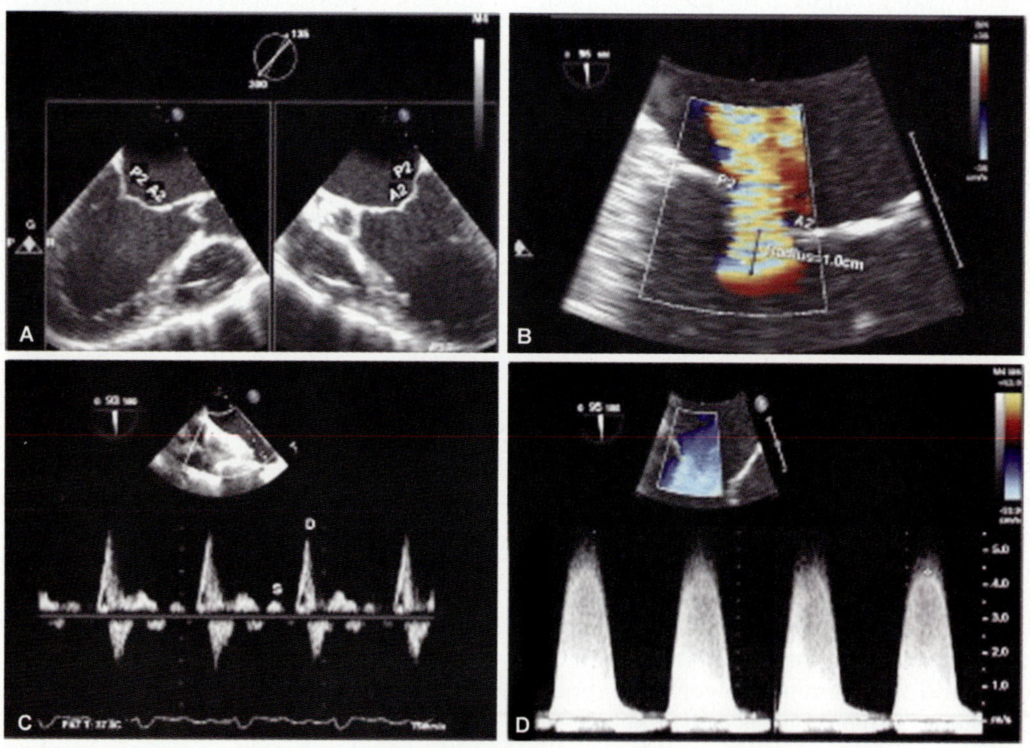


**Fig. 16.24:** TEE assessment of MV morphology, regurgitation mechanism, and quantification. (A) Two-dimensional TEE at mid-esophageal level 0° using real-time biplane imaging with orthogonal planes showing functional MR with MV annular dilation and leaflet tethering leading to central malcoaptation between A2 and P2 scallops, (B) Mid-esophageal zoomed view at 95° of the MV with color-Doppler showing systolic frame representing severe central mitral regurgitation jet. Note the proximal flow convergence zone with large radius (1.0 cm). (C) Pulse-wave Doppler interrogation of the right upper pulmonary vein flow showing marked systolic blunting (S) indicative of elevated LA pressures. (D) Continuous-wave Doppler through the MV, which demonstrates a dense holosystolic regurgitant jet with high peak velocity. All these features are consistent with severe MR

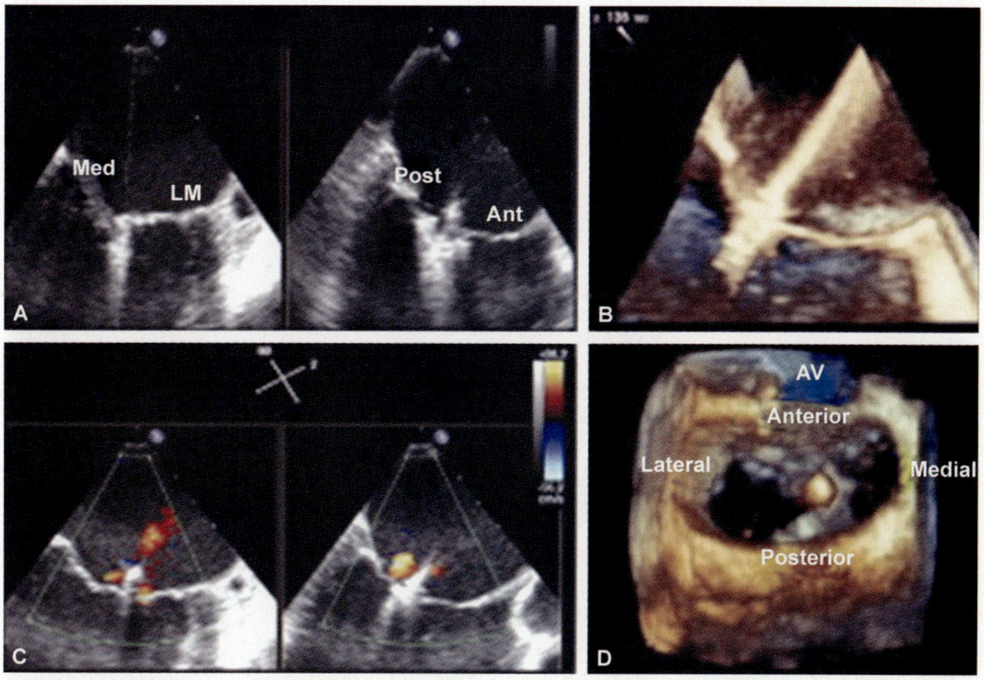


**Fig. 16.25:** Sequence of events in the deployment of edge-to-edge MV repair technique (MitraClip). (A) Simultaneous biplane imaging at 60° and 150° demonstrates the exact location of the MitraClip within the MV structure. Once the position is confirmed, grasping of the MV leaflet occurs, (B) live 3D zoomed view of the delivery catheter and MitraClip grasping the A2 and P2 scallops of the MV, (C) similar to A, simultaneous biplane imaging at 60° and 150° demonstrates trivial to mild (1+) MR after MitraClip grasps the MV leaflets, (D) MitraClip system is finally released from the delivery system and seen (arrow) in the center of the new 'figure-of-8' MV. Ant=anterior; Post=posterior

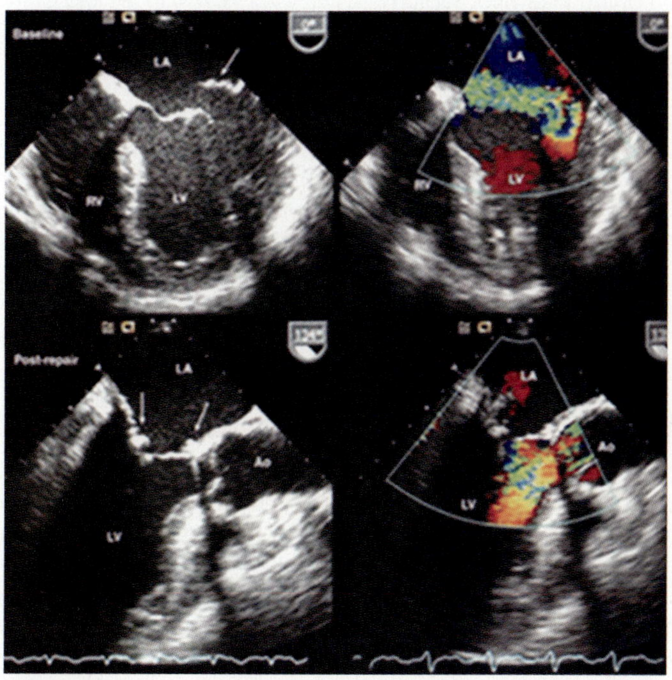


**Fig. 16.26:** Mitral valve repair. 2D (left) and color-Doppler (right) intraoperative TEE images were taken in a patient with myxomatous mitral valve defect before (top) and after (bottom) mitral valve repair, before repair severe mitral prolapse with partial flail leaflet segment and moderate to severe MR in the four chamber view. After repair, the long axis view shows the annuloplasty ring (arrows). Regurgitation was not detected after successful repair

often preferred because of their durability, low profile, and ease of insertion.

## Ischemic Mitral Regurgitation

Ischemic mitral regurgitation is caused by wall-motion abnormalities that in turn cause tethering, papillary muscle dysfunction, or annular dilation. In myocardial ischemia, revascularization is mandatory. Cardiac catheterization is important in the evaluation and stabilization of patients who present with an acute coronary syndrome, with or without cardiogenic shock (Fig. 16.29).

Careful review of the preoperative coronary angiograms is essential during preparation for coronary artery bypass grafting (CABG). In patients who are hemodynamically unstable, too much time may be needed to prepare the internal mammary artery, and CABG might be best completed with the use of venous conduits. In addition, myocardial protection in the presence of acute MI is challenging. Either antegrade or retrograde delivery of cardioplegic solution is feasible; antegrade delivery through the newly placed venous conduits can increase myocardial protection. In contrast, particularly when ischemia is acute, the metabolically enhanced, slow induction of warm-blood cardioplegic solution can avoid systolic contracture of the LV ('stone heart' syndrome).

- Controlled and potentially prolonged reperfusion at the conclusion of the operation may enable the recovery of myocardial function. For the same purpose, intra-aortic balloon counterpulsation is typically maintained for at

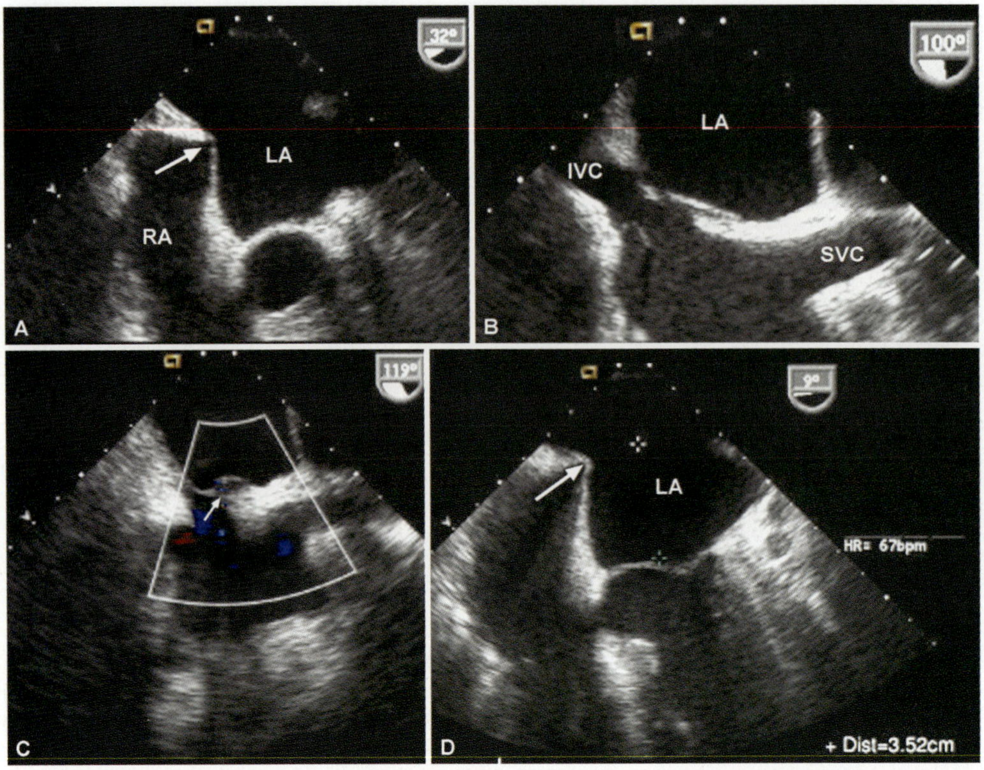


**Fig. 16.27:** TEE during initial stages of percutaneous MV repair by Evalve clip mid-esophageal transesophageal views used for guided transseptal puncture during percutaneous edge to edge MV repair. (A) Short-axis view at the base (showing the anterior–posterior portion of the interatrial septum with tenting (white arrow) at the junction of septum primum with septum secundum or the edge of the fossa, (B) Bicaval view showing the superior–inferior portion of the interatrial septum, (C) Bicaval view with tenting at the junction of ostium primum with ostium secundum (white arrow), (D) Mid-esophageal 4-chamber view (for assessing height of the tenting site above the MV plane) to allow perpendicular approach of the guide and device catheter towards the MV. IVC=inferior vena cava; SVC=superior vena cava

least 24 hours postoperatively. Papillary muscle rupture, a rare complication of MI, occurs in 1–3% of MIs and is associated with a mortality rate of 80% with medical therapy alone. Historically, operative mortality rates were as high as 67%, and patients were frequently denied surgery for this reason. With the addition of CABG to mitral valve replacement or repair, the operative mortality rate is now less than 10%.

### Mitral Valve Endocarditis

- Acute mitral valve regurgitation consequent to endocarditis requires operative debridement and reconstruction. The therapeutic approach is driven by the principle that all sites of active infection must be excised. The decision to repair the leaflet, to replace the chordae or the entire valve, or to reconstruct the annulus is best made after debridement. It can be especially challenging to reconstruct the fibrous trigone of the heart, which involves the annular support of both the aortic and mitral valves. The tissues are edematous and friable, and even the most experienced surgeon may find it difficult to achieve a 3-dimensional view. The use of aortic homografts may be optimal when both the mitral and aortic annuli show active infection or abscess. Repeat mitral valve surgery, such as in prosthetic valve endocarditis, poses a unique challenge. Even gentle manipulation of the mitral annulus, coupled with ongoing infection and previous scarring, can result in atrioventricular disruption. This catastrophic event is high-risk and must be anticipated. All people having mitral regurgitation require antibiotic prophylaxis to prevent infective endocarditis prior to dental or surgical procedures.

## MITRAL VALVE PROLAPSE (CLICK MURMUR SYNDROME)

It is a condition that has caused much debate and controversy in the medical community. Mitral valve prolapse (MVP) occurs when one or both of the mitral valve leaflets push back (bow) into the left atrium during contraction of the left ventricle. MVP is probably only important if a person has both excess bowing of the mitral leaflets into the atrium and actual regurgitation of blood from the left ventricle to the left atrium when the heart contracts (Figs 16.30–16.32).

People, particularly women, with heart palpitations due to anxiety often see a doctor and have heart evaluation (including ultrasound) performed. Many persons with a panic (anxiety) disorder were found to have mild mitral valve bowing on ultrasound. It was believed that panic attacks were more common in people with mitral valve

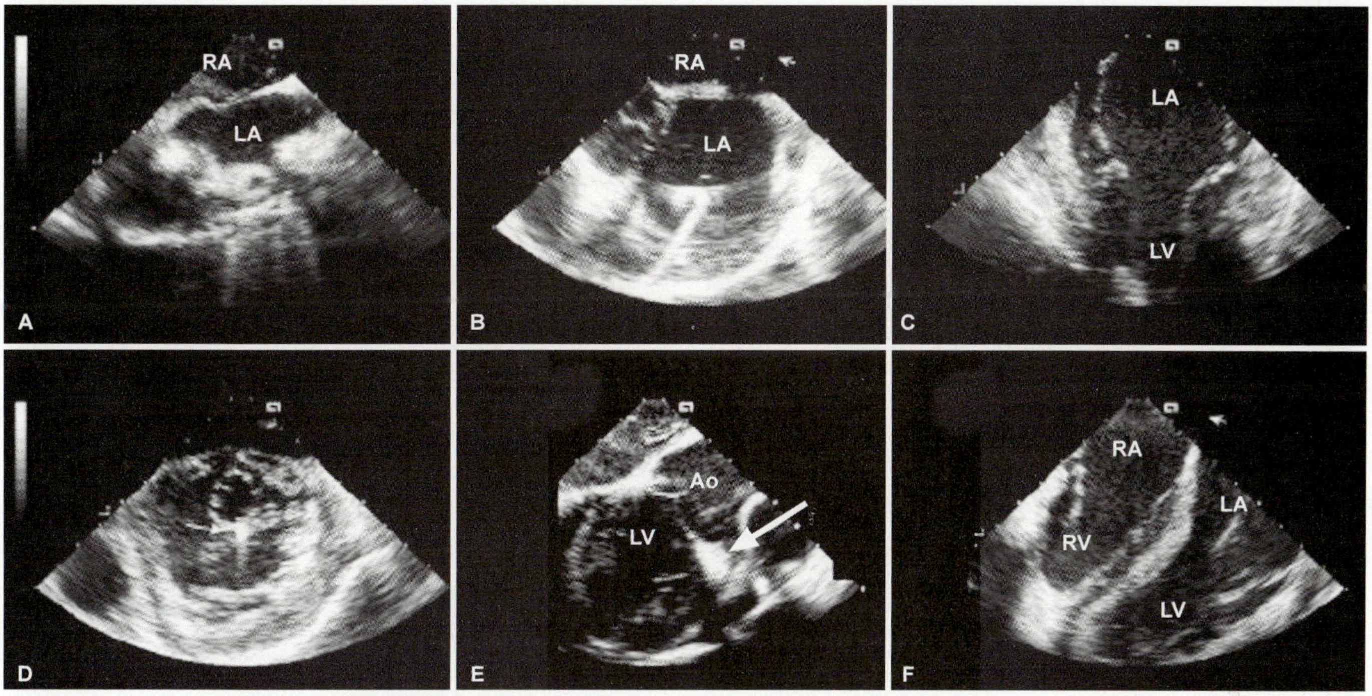


**Fig. 16.28:** Intracardiac echocardiography during percutaneous MV therapy. Intracardiac views obtained by Acunav catheter in the right atrium of a swine. (A) Tenting of the interatrial septum (white arrow) by the Brockenbrough needle. (B) J-shaped tip of guidewire in the LA after transseptal puncture. (C) Anterior and posterior leaflets of the MV with the ICE catheter advanced across the interatrial septum into the LA and the transducer facing down. (D) A short-axis view of the MV at the base with a central suture and clip (white arrow) and a double orifice MV created after the deployment of suture and clip (Edwards Lifesciences, Irvine, California). The SAX view was obtained by advancing the ICE catheter across the tricuspid and pulmonic valves. (E) Aortic root, left main coronary artery (white arrow), and LV, and F is a 4-chamber view obtained by advancing the ICE catheter tip into the right ventricle

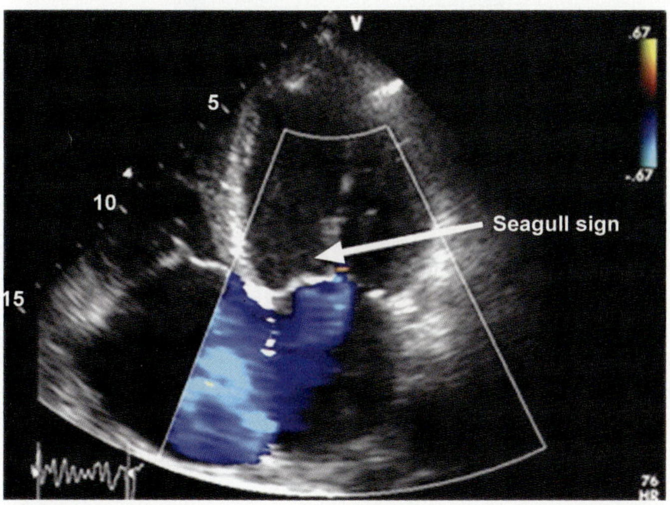


**Fig. 16.29:** 'Seagull sign' on transthoracic echocardiography of moderate-severe ischemic mitral regurgitation (IMR). A transthoracic echocardiographic image demonstrating the 'seagull sign' present in moderate-severe IMR. The shape of the anterior mitral valve leaflet is distorted by tethering of secondary strut chordae tendineae. This tethering impairs leaflet coaptation resulting in MR

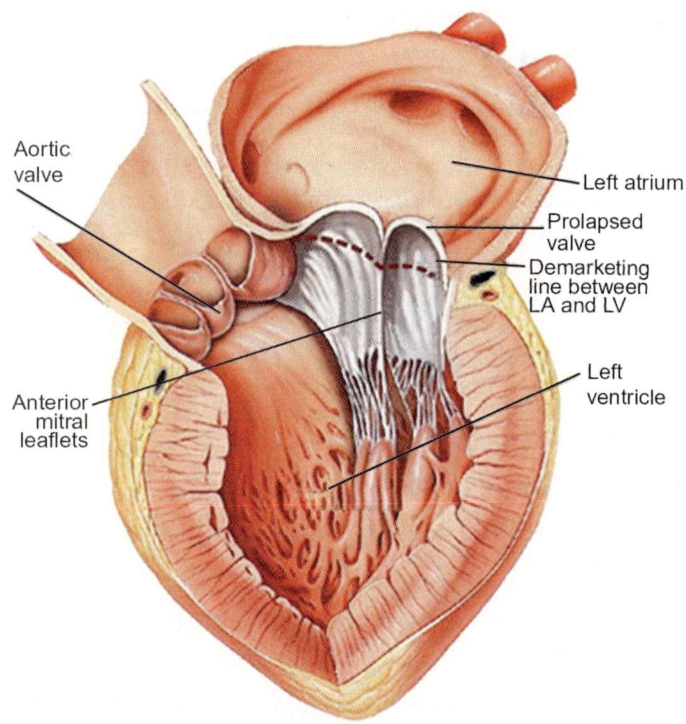


**Fig. 16.30:** A normal demarkating line between LA and LV with mitral valve that separates the left atrium from the left ventricle. It also shows mitral valve prolapsing into the LA

prolapse. Newer studies suggest there is no correlation between panic attacks and mitral valve prolapse. Most patients who had ultrasounds and were diagnosed with

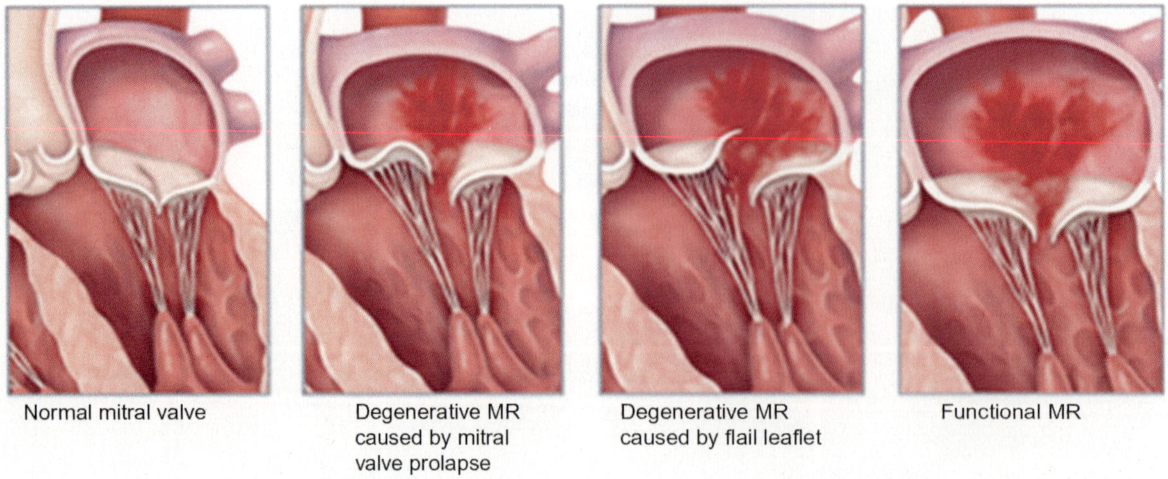


**Fig. 16.31:** Valvular positions in normal MV and comparing with mitral regurgitation of MVP and other common causes of MR

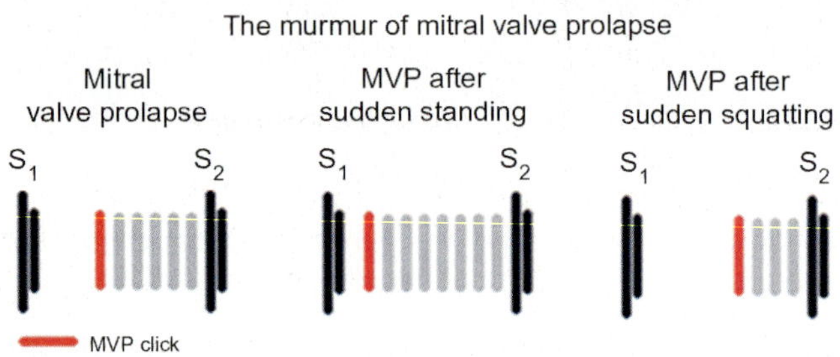


**Fig. 16.32:** Mitral valve prolapse responds to dynamic auscultation. MVP click and murmur varies after sudden standing and sudden squatting as demonstrated in this illustration. It therefore helps in differentiating other conditions with click and murmur

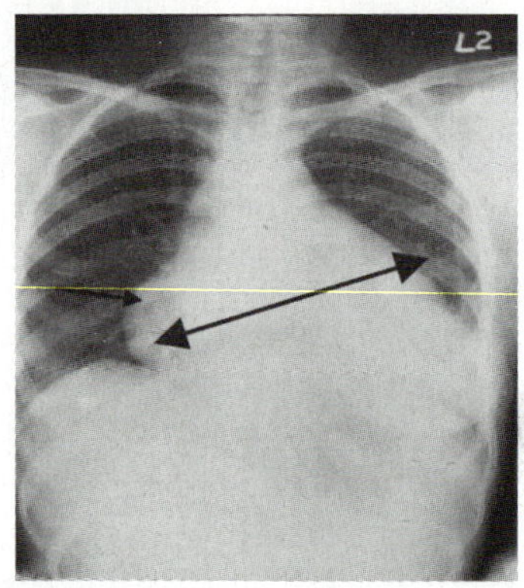


**Fig. 16.33:** X-ray chest (PA view) shows cardomegaly (LV type) in mitral valve prolapse with MR

MVP did not have true MVP but simply normal variation in the shape of their mitral valve. For many patients and physicians it may have been easier to accept that a physical condition was responsible for panic attacks. Most people have no symptoms of MVP.

Persons with MVP having demonstrated regurgitation are at slightly increased risk of developing endocarditis during dental/surgical procedures and should receive antibiotic prophylaxis. A very small number are at increased risk of sudden death.

## Invasive and Noninvasive Procedures

### *Chest Radiography*

Radiographs may demonstrate the progression from asymptomatic to chronic, severe mitral regurgitation with the development of cardiomegaly secondary to left atrial and left ventricular dilatation and evidence of heart failure (Fig. 16.33).

### *Electrocardiography*

The ECG usually is normal, but can show nonspecific ST-segment and T-wave abnormalities especially in leads II, III, Avf (Fig. 16.34).

### *Echocardiography*

The use of echocardiogram (ultrasound of the heart) over the past 20 years has revolutionized examination of the heart. Using earlier ultrasound criteria it was estimated 5–10% of the population has MVP. However, recent studies suggest that slight bowing of the mitral valve (not accompanied by regurgitation) is normal for many people and that MVP was likely over diagnosed because of the ability of ultrasound to see extremely small variations in the mitral valve shape. Using revised criteria it is believed that MVP is present in less than 1% of the general population (Figs 16.35–16.41).

*Diagnostic criteria:* Perloff et al. set the stage for accurately diagnosing mitral valve prolapse (MVP) by expanding the diagnostic standards to include clinical and echocardiographic criteria. In a Framingham Heart Study, Freed et al. historically described echocardiographic criteria for MVP as classic versus nonclassic. Use of the parasternal long-axis view reduce the over diagnosis of MVP.

*Findings are as follows:*

1. Classic MVP: The parasternal long-axis view shows >2 mm superior displacement of the mitral leaflets into

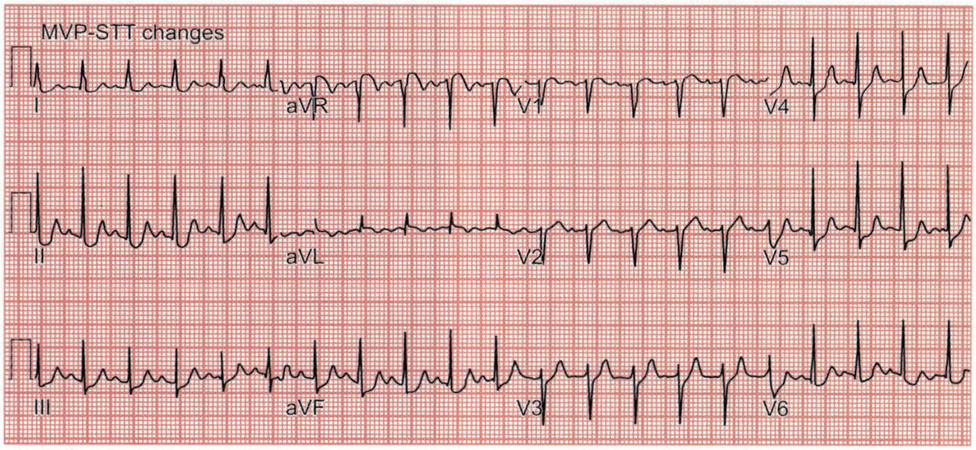


**Fig. 16.34:** ECG shows nonspecific ST-segment and T-wave depression in inferior leads II, III, aVF

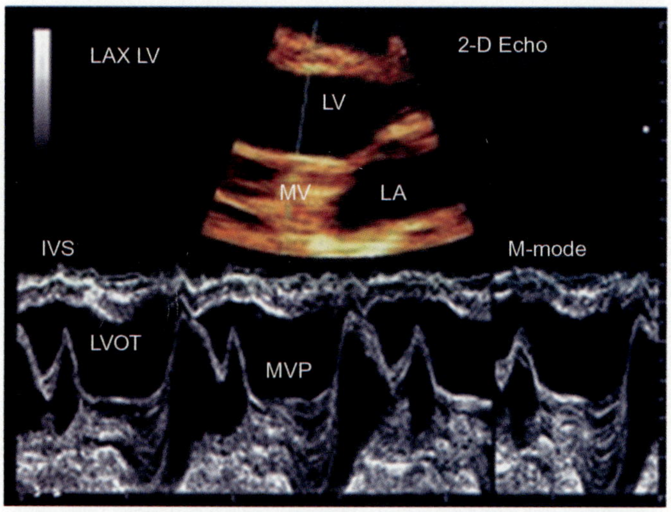


**Fig. 16.35:** M-mode study shows abrupt posterior displacement in midsystole (MVP) of the anterior and posterior mitral leaflets

the left atrium during systole, with a leaflet thickness of at least 5 mm.

2. Nonclassic MVP: Displacement is >2 mm, with a maximal leaflet thickness of <5 mm.
3. Other: Other echocardiographic findings that should be considered as criteria are leaflet thickening, redundancy, annular dilatation, and chordal elongation.

### *Ambulatory 24-hour Electrocardiogram*

A Holter monitor may help identify the nature and frequency of arrhythmic activity. Premature ventricular beats (38%), multiform couplets, and tachyarrhythmias (8%) are usual findings (Fig. 16.42).

*Exercise testing:* This is useful in patients with palpitations and exercise-related symptoms.

Premature ventricular beats (16%), ventricular tachycardia (4%), and supraventricular ectopy are common findings. Ventricular fibrillation is a rare finding.

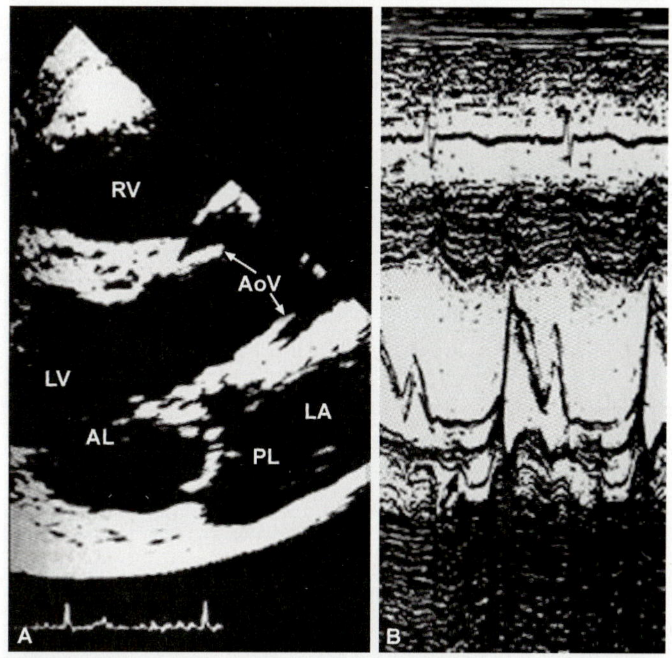


**Fig. 16.36:** Echocardiogram from a patient with mitral valve prolapse. (A) Parasternal long-axis view in systole show the posterior leaflet (PL) of the mitral valve with superior displacement (bowing) into the left atrium (LA), i.e. arching posteriorly above the level of the atrioventricular groove and behind the normal coaptation point of the left atrium. (B) M-mode study shows abrupt posterior displacement in midsystole (arrow) of the posterior mitral leaflet. There are multiple echoes arising in the area of the valve during systole as a result of the redundancy of the leaflets. These findings are characteristic of mitral valve proplapse. LV=left ventricle; AL=anterior leaflet of mitral valve; RV=right ventricle; AoV=aortic valve

### Cardiovascular Magnetic Resonance Imaging

(Fig. 16.43)

Cardiovascular magnetic resonance (CMR) has the potential to visualize all parts of the valve (leaflets, chordae tendineae, and papillary muscles) throughout the entire cardiac cycle. Congenitally abnormal valve leaflets

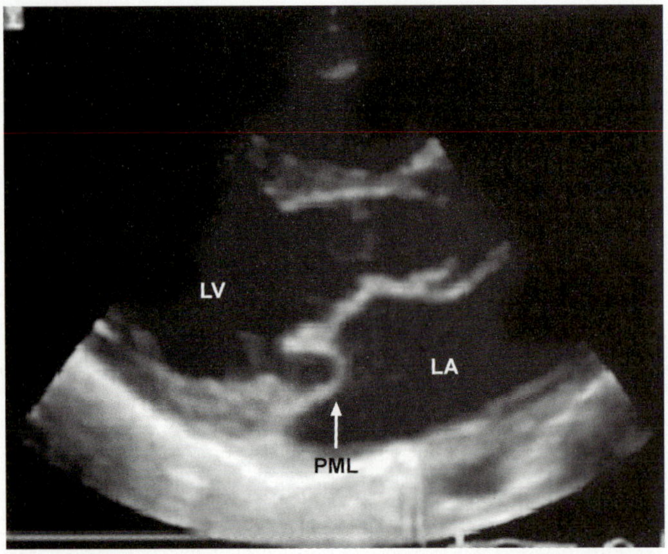


**Fig. 16.37:** Two-dimensional echocardiographic long axis parasternal view of mitral valve prolapse (arrow). MV=mitral valve, LV=left ventricle, LA=left atrium, RV=right ventricle, Ao=aorta

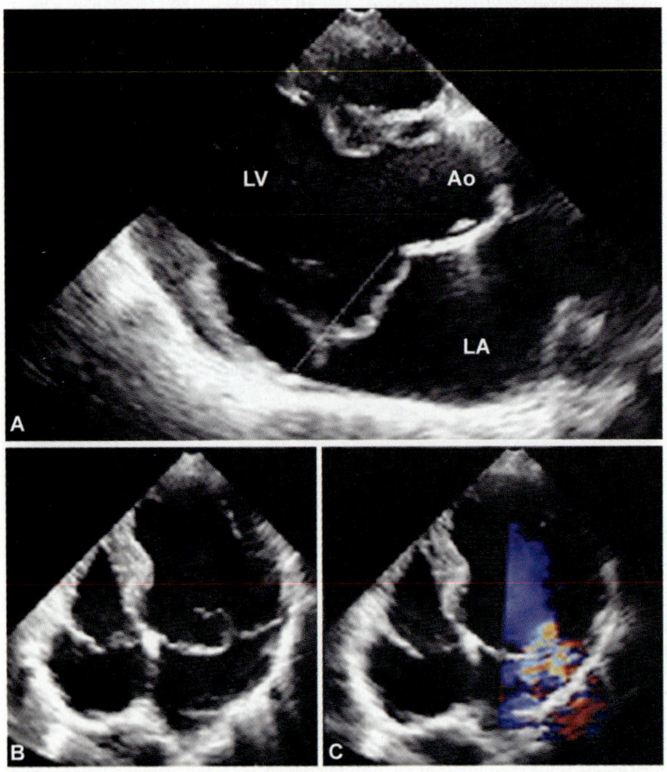


**Fig. 16.38:** Mitral valve prolapse. (A) Echocardiographic parasternal long-axis view showing the mitral leaflets prolapsing more than 2 mm above the plane of the mitral annulus (dotted line) during systole in a child with Marfan syndrome. (B) Echocardiographic apical four-chamber view showing bileaflet prolapse in the same patient. (C) Color-Doppler view showing moderate mitral regurgitation. Ao=aorta; LA=left atrium; LV=left ventricle

(bicuspid), aberrant papillary muscles or aberrant chordal attachments (parachute mitral valve), leaflet thickening, presence and extent of calcification, leaflet redundancy and

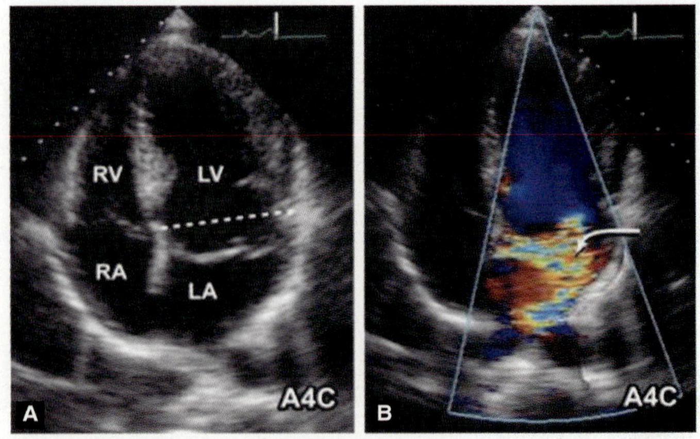


**Fig. 16.39:** Bileaflet prolapse is easily visualized in the apical four-chamber (A4C) view. However the mitral valve profile is normally exaggerated in this view and may lead to overdiagnosis of mitral valve prolapse (A). Severe mitral regurgitation was present (B)

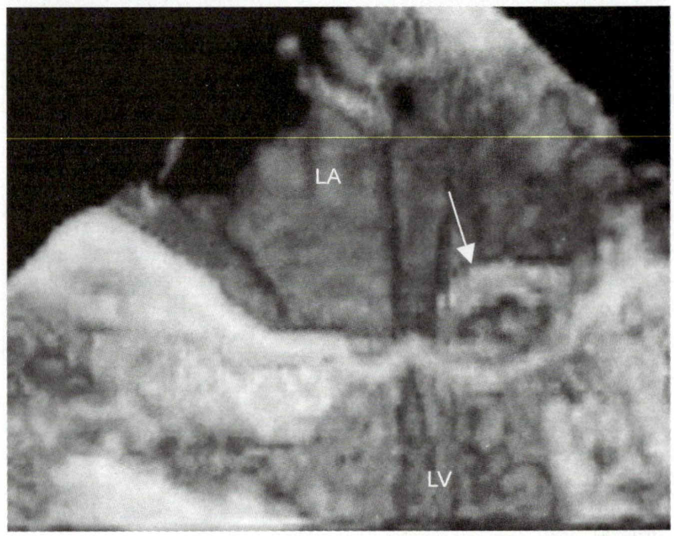


**Fig. 16.40:** Three-dimensional reconstruction obtained from the TEE in a patient with prolapse posterior mitral valve leaflet (arrow)

prolapse, and commissural fusion are all anatomic descriptions that have been reported by CMR. However, two-dimensional (2D) echocardiography is superior for imaging structures that are thin and highly mobile owing to its greater temporal resolution and the absence of partial volume effects. Although 2D echocardiography remains the primary approach for visualization of valve anatomy, CMR is a reasonable alternative if ultrasound windows are poor.

## Cardiac Catheterization and Angiography

These tests are generally restricted to patients with MVP and severe MR who may require valve repair or replacement. Associated coronary artery disease can also be confirmed or excluded. A left ventricular angiogram, taken in the right anterior oblique view, best shows the posterior leaflet. A left anterior oblique projection shows the anterior leaflet. Other abnormalities that may be revealed include

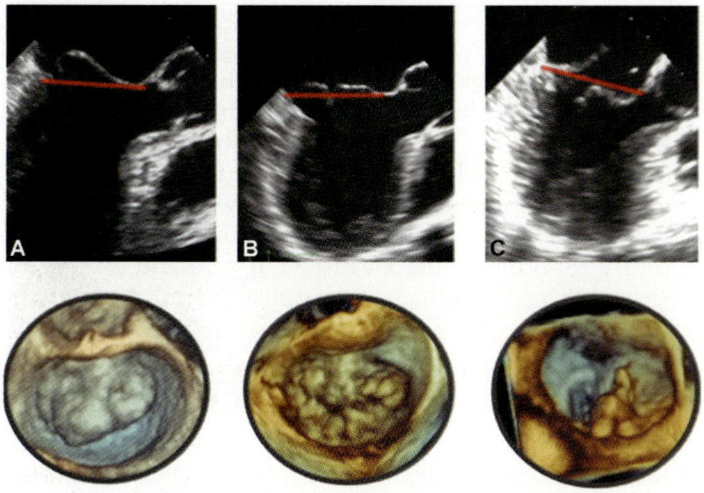


**Fig. 16.41:** Differential diagnoses of mitral leaflet prolapse. 2D TEE long-axis view demonstrating anterior leaflet prolapse (A, top) with a 3D transesophageal example as seen from the left atrium (A, bottom). Leaflet prolapse should be diagnosed when the free edge of the leaflet overrides the plane of the mitral annulus during systole. 2D TEE long-axis view demonstrating bileaflet billowing of the mitral valve with prolapse due to chordae elongation (B, top) with 3D transesophageal example as seen from the left atrium (B, bottom). Leaflet billowing is diagnosed when there is systolic excursion of the leaflet body into the left atrium due to excess leaflet tissue, with the leaflet free edge remaining below the plane of the mitral annulus. 2D TEE long-axis view demonstrating flail valve due to chordae rupture (C, top) with a 3D transesophageal example of P2 flail as viewed from the left atrium

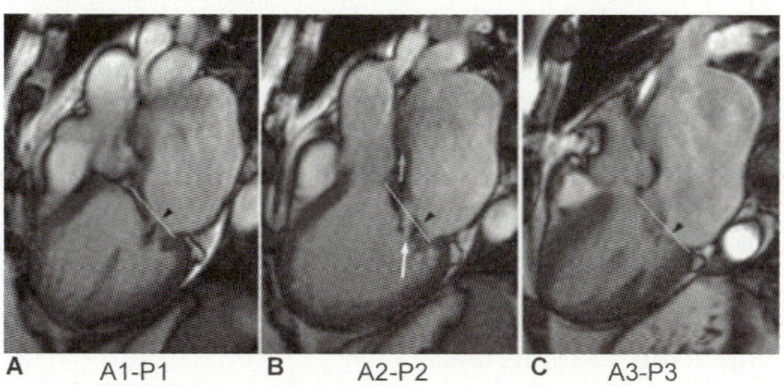


**Fig. 16.43:** Prolapse of P2 causing mitral regurgitation. (A) A1-P1, (B) A2-P2, (C) A3-P3. Arrowhead shows the posterior leaflet. This can be seen to be prolapsed at (B) P2. The yellow line shows the mitral annular plane. The arrows show the eccentric jet of mitral regurgitation which results from failure of coaptation of A2-P2 and is anteriorly directed along the wall of the left atrium. The white arrow points to a central bright jet core in the A2-P2 bSSFP image, with a dark streak of signal loss beyond (grey arrow). This is in accord with relatively severe regurgitation

dilatation, decreased systolic contraction, calcification of the mitral annulus, and poor contraction of the basal portion of the left ventricle (Fig. 16.44).

### *Electrophysiology*

**Indications for electrophysiology** (EPS) are similar to those in general clinical practice. EPS is useful in the presence of

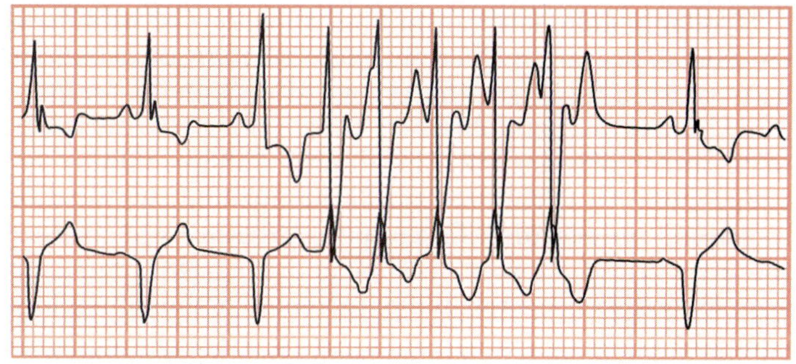

**Fig. 16.42:** Two channel Holter recording strip with 5 beats run of ventricular tachycardia in patient with mitral valve prolapse with mitral regurgitation

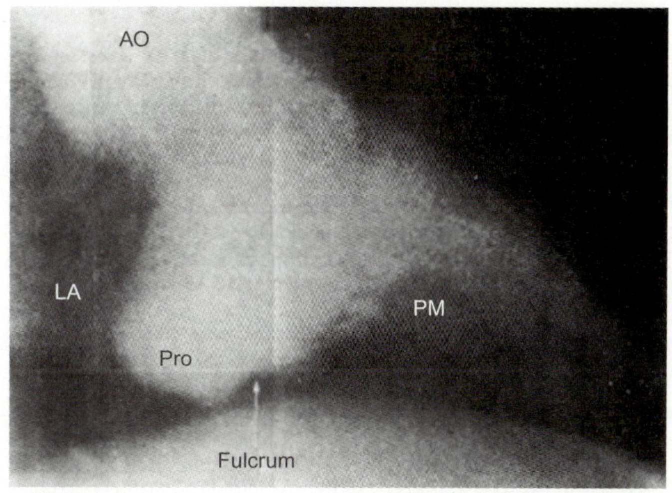


**Fig. 16.44:** Left ventricular angiogram during systole demonstrating prolapse of mitral valve (Pro). The posteromedial commissural scallop of the posterior mitral leaflet extends posteriorly and inferiorly to the fulcrum (arrow)

supraventricular tachycardia because accessory atrioventricular pathways are common in patients with MVP. In this subset of patients, EPS is important because radiofrequency ablation can be performed during the same procedure, with a very high curative success rate.

**Tilt test:** Upright tilt studies with blood pressure and cardiac rhythm monitoring may be valuable in patients with light-headedness or syncope when vasodepressor-vasovagal reaction is suspected and confirmation of clinical symptoms is desired.

## Histologic Findings

Mitral valves excised from patients with severe MR secondary to MVP have large leaflets and show various alterations. The most specific, fundamental, and characteristic histologic changes are (1) collagen dissolution and disruption in the pars fibrosa of the mitral valve leaflet and (2) replacement of the dense collagenous fibrosa by loose myxomatous connective tissue with high acid mucopolysaccharide content.

Similar histologic abnormalities are observed in chordae tendineae. Scanning electron photomicrographs demonstrate surface folds and focal loss of endothelial cells on mitral valve leaflets obtained from patients with severe MVP and significant MR. These surface abnormalities may predispose to thromboembolic complications and/or infectious endocarditis. Continuous pressure and stress on the leaflets and chordae tendineae during left ventricular systole contribute to gradual progression of these histologic changes.

### Medical Treatment

In childhood, the condition is not progressive, and specific therapy is not indicated for the vast majority. Asymptomatic patients with isolated mitral systolic clicks need only counseling and reassurance. Avoid excessive use of caffeine, cigarettes, alcohol, and prescription or over-the-counter drugs that contain stimulants such as epinephrine or ephedrine to minimize catecholamine and cyclic adenosine monophosphate (AMP) stimulation. Prevention of volume depletion before, during, and immediately after exercise may help. Subacute bacterial endocarditis antibiotic prophylaxis coverage for at-risk procedures is indicated in patients with mitral valve prolapse (MVP) and MR.

*Additional dental care recommended for patients at risk for infective endocarditis includes the following:*

- Regular toothbrushing after eating. No cookies, sweets, or sweet drinks between meals.
- Regular dental checks every 6 months. Fluoride supplements in locations where the fluoride in drinking water is less than 0.3 ppm for children younger than 2 years or less than 0.7 ppm for children younger than 2 years. Dental treatments (more than 2) scheduled at an interval of 14 days or longer.

*Surgical intervention:* Recent advances have made reconstructive mitral valve surgery feasible in patients with congestive heart failure, severe MR secondary to MVP, or both (Fig. 16.45).

*Robotic mitral valve repair*: Robotic mitral valve repair (Fig. 16.46) allows complete anatomic correction of all categories of leaflet prolapse using techniques identical to open approaches. Robotic repair effectively corrects mitral regurgitation, offers excellent freedom from adverse events, and facilitates rapid weaning from ventilation, translating into earlier hospital dismissal. Safety and efficacy after both open and robotic mitral valve repair are higher than recently reported in the EVEREST II trial and establish a benchmark against which nonsurgical therapies should be evaluated.

*Group consultations:* A multidisciplinary approach is preferable, with a team from the following specialties:

- Pediatrics
- Pediatric cardiology
- Radiology
- Genetics
- Cardiothoracics
- Physiotherapy
- Family medicine
- Orthopedics

*Advice for physical activity:* A gradual return to exercise may be tolerated. In the absence of studies on the effect of exercise on the progression of MVP, the best approach at present is based on common sense and good clinical judgment.

- Patients with symptoms of syncope, presyncope, or palpitations upon exertion should undergo thorough evaluations and avoid competitive sports for at least 6 months after the last significant episode.
- In the presence of significant MR, limitations apply as for any other cause of MR.
- Coexisting aortic root dilatation and aortic regurgitation can further limit activity.
- Patients with cardiac arrhythmia should have periodic exercise tests performed and ambulatory ECG recordings obtained while doing the type of exercise they are likely to undertake.
- Sudden death is extremely uncommon in MVP.

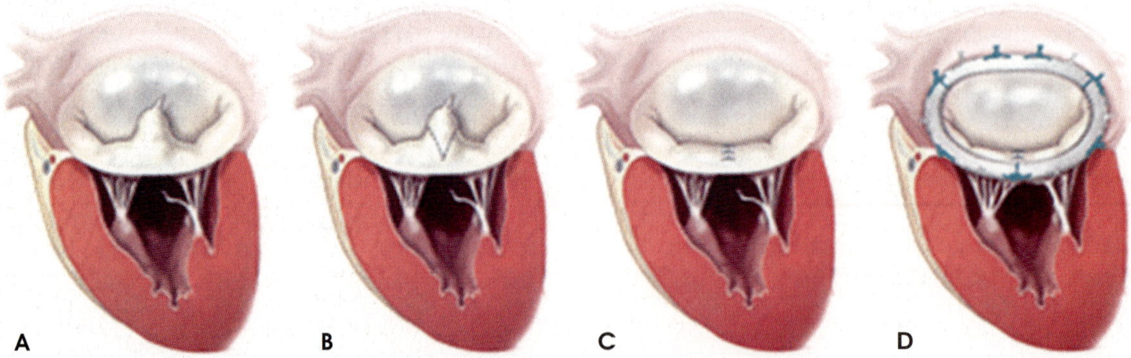


**Fig. 16.45:** Triangular resection and ring annuloplasty. (A) Fibroelastic deficiency with P2 (posterior middle scallop) prolapse. (B) Dashed lines represent area of leaflet to be excised. (C) Reconstructed leaflet after triangular resection. (D) Completed repair after ring annuloplasty

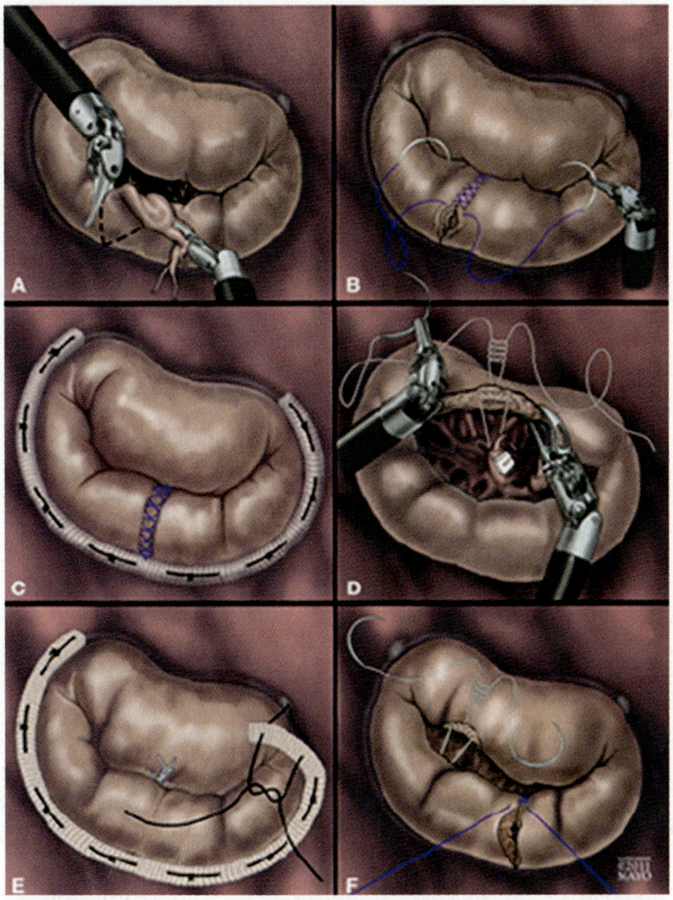

**Fig. 16.46:** Robotic mitral valve repair for all prolapse subsets using techniques identical to open valvuloplasty. Standard Mayo Clinic mitral valve repair techniques using robotic instrumentation. (A) The extent of posterior leaflet prolapse is determined and a triangular-shaped resection performed to eliminate redundancy predominating at the leading edge, restoring the position of the coapting margin to the annular plane and decreasing leaflet height. (B) The remaining leaflet edges are reapposed using a 2-layer prolene stitch, restoring normal leaflet coaptation. (C) After posterior leaflet correction, a standard-length 63-mm flexible posterior annuloplasty band is inserted using interrupted Ethibond sutures from right to left fibrous trigones. (D) Anterior leaflet prolapse is corrected by placing two 5–0 Gore-Tex (WL Gore and Associates, Inc. Flagstaff, Ariz) neochords between the subtending papillary muscle to the unsupported leaflet edge using a double-armed Gore-Tex pledget-backed mattress stitch. (E) After anterior leaflet correction, a 63-mm flexible posterior annuloplasty band is inserted using interrupted Ethibond sutures from right to left fibrous trigones. (F) Bileaflet repair is performed using a combination of posterior leaflet resection/reconstruction, anterior leaflet neochord resuspension, and standard-length 63-mm flexible posterior annuloplasty band

## AORTIC VALVE DISORDERS

The aortic valve normally allows one way flow of blood from the left ventricle to the aorta. Disorders of the aortic valve may cause aortic valve stenosis or aortic valve regurgitation.

### 1. AORTIC STENOSIS

It is defined as narrowing of the aortic valve from its normal diameter due to numerous conditions as follows:

#### Aetiological Factors

- Congenital aortic stenosis: Male > Female (4:1)
- Congenital bicuspid valve (1–2%)
- Rheumatic aortic stenosis
- Calcific aortic stenosis

#### Signs and Symptoms

- Exertional angina
- Syncope (during exercise)
- CHF (initially diastolic failure, then systolic)
- Sudden death secondary to ventricular fibrillation
- Harsh crescendo-decrescendo (diamond-shaped) systolic murmur at aortic focus radiating to carotids
- Absent aortic component of S2
- Delayed upstroke in peripheral pulse (pulsus parvus et tardus)
- S4 gallop
- Ejection click

#### Aetiology of Aortic Stenosis?

Most people do not develop symptoms until late in the course of aortic stenosis. Age at onset of symptoms (clinically apparent aortic stenosis) usually indicates the cause of aortic stenosis. Symptoms in people younger than 30 years is almost always due to congenital causes (usually bicuspid aortic valve). Symptoms in people 30–70 years may be due to either bicuspid valve or rheumatic heart disease. Aortic stenosis caused by rheumatic fever occurs 10–15 years later than mitral stenosis caused by rheumatic fever. Symptoms developing in the elderly are usually due to calcific degenerative changes of a normal aortic valve (wear and tear of aging).

#### Clinical Diagnosis of Aortic Stenosis

People may see their doctor concerning symptoms of aortic stenosis. Chest pain or passing out during exertion is very concerning and may prompt a doctor into examining the heart in detail. If aortic stenosis is present a certain type of heart murmur may be detected when a doctor listens with a stethoscope. The doctor may order further tests. Aortic stenosis can be definitively diagnosed using echocardiogram (heart ultrasound). Atrial fibrillation and traveling emboli are less common in isolated aortic stenosis (Fig. 16.47).

#### Laboratory Studies

*Chest radiography:* Chest radiographs may show several significant findings consistent with aortic stenosis. The aortic valve may appear calcified. With plain images, calcification is best detected on the lateral view. Calcification of the aortic valve is found in almost all adults with hemodynamically significant aortic stenosis. The LV

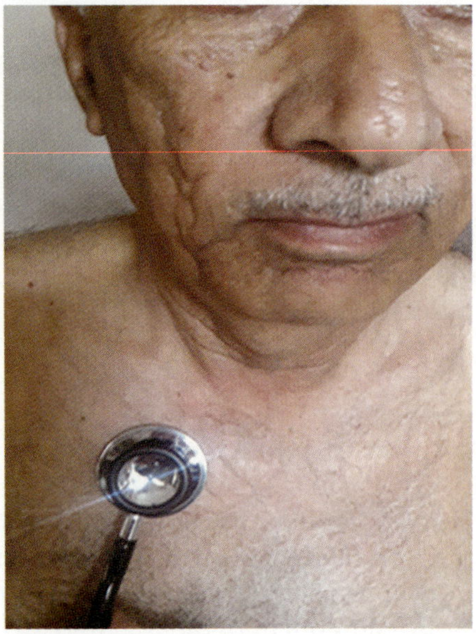

**Fig. 16.47:** A 68-year-old person sought consultation of a cardiologist for syncopal attack who was found to be suffering from degenerative type of valvular aortic stenosis

may be slightly enlarged, with a rounded apex; this is a nonspecific finding. The left atrium may be enlarged as well. Visible calcification on plain chest films usually indicates a gradient of 50 mmHg or more across the valve, which is severe enough to require surgery (Fig. 16.48).

### Electrocardiography

Generally, ECG is not a reliable test for aortic stenosis. The results vary widely in patients with this disorder and overlap with other cardiac conditions (Fig. 16.49).

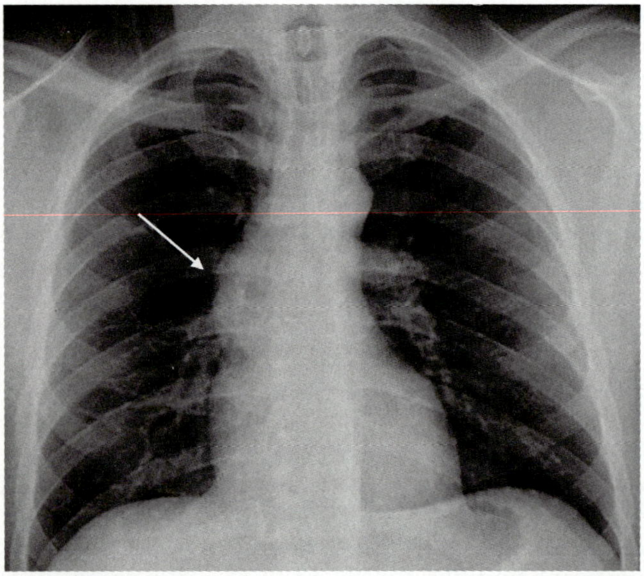

**Fig. 16.48:** Frontal chest radiograph in another patient with aortic stenosis shows a dilated ascending aorta 9 (white arrow) that abnormally projects farther to the right than the right heart border. This is caused by poststenotic dilatation of the aorta

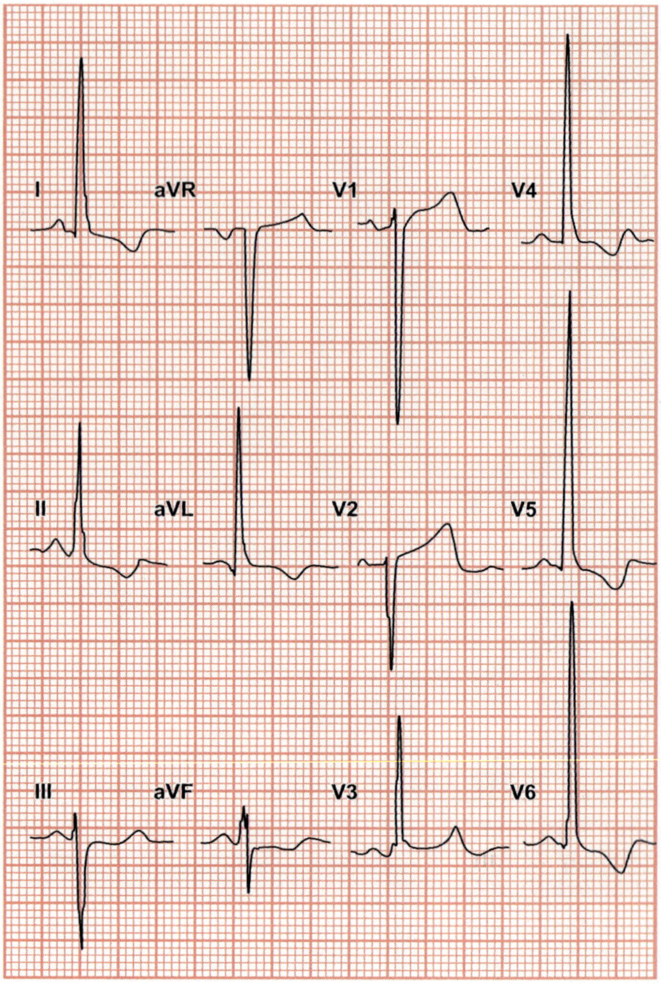


**Fig. 16.49:** ECG showing deep S-waves in V1–V2 and tall R-waves in V4–V6 as voltage criteria of LVH in patient with aortic stenosis

Although the ECG findings may be entirely normal, the principal finding is left ventricular hypertrophy (LVH), which is found in 85% of patients with severe aortic stenosis; however, its absence does not preclude critical aortic stenosis. Patients with significant aortic stenosis who may not show clear ECG evidence of ventricular hypertrophy include elderly persons with significant myocardial fibrosis and adolescents, who may experience ST-segment changes before QRS changes.

T-wave inversion and ST-segment depression in leads with predominantly positive QRS complexes are common. ST-depression exceeding 0.3 mV in patients with aortic stenosis indicates LV strain and suggests severe LVH. Occasionally, a septal pseudoinfarct pattern can be seen. Left atrial enlargement with a preterminal negative P-wave in lead V1 is noted in 80% of cases of severe isolated aortic stenosis. The presence of left atrial enlargement suggests an associated mitral valve process.

The correlation between absolute voltages in precordial leads and the severity of obstruction, unlike in children with congenital aortic stenosis, is poor in adults.

The rhythm usually is normal sinus. Atrial fibrillation can be seen at late stages or as a consequence of coexistent MV disease or hyperthyroidism.

Extension of calcification into the conduction system can cause atrioventricular or intraventricular block in 5% of cases of aortic stenosis. Approximately 10% of all cases of left anterior fascicular block are secondary to calcific aortic valve disease. Ambulatory ECG monitoring frequently shows complex ventricular arrhythmias, particularly in cases with myocardial dysfunction.

While the degree of severity of changes on a single ECG does not correlate well with the degree of hemodynamic compromise, serial ECGs performed over time (months to years) can be valuable in demonstrating the progression of the disease.

### Echocardiography

Echocardiography is the preferred imaging test for aortic stenosis. Echocardiography is indispensable to the assessment of the extent of LV hypertrophy, systolic ejection performance, and anatomy of the aortic valve. Doppler interrogation of the aortic valve makes use of the modified Bernoulli equation (gradient = 4 × velocity$^2$) to assess the severity of the stenosis. As blood flows from the body of the LV across the stenotic valve, the flow rate must accelerate for the volume to remain constant. Doppler interrogation of the valve detects this increase in velocity and helps estimate the valvular gradient. In summary, echocardiography may demonstrate the following findings (Figs 16.50–16.53):

- Concentric LV hypertrophy
- Reduced separation of the cusp of the aortic valve
- Mean gradients greater than 50 mmHg in patients with severe aortic stenosis on Doppler echocardiography.

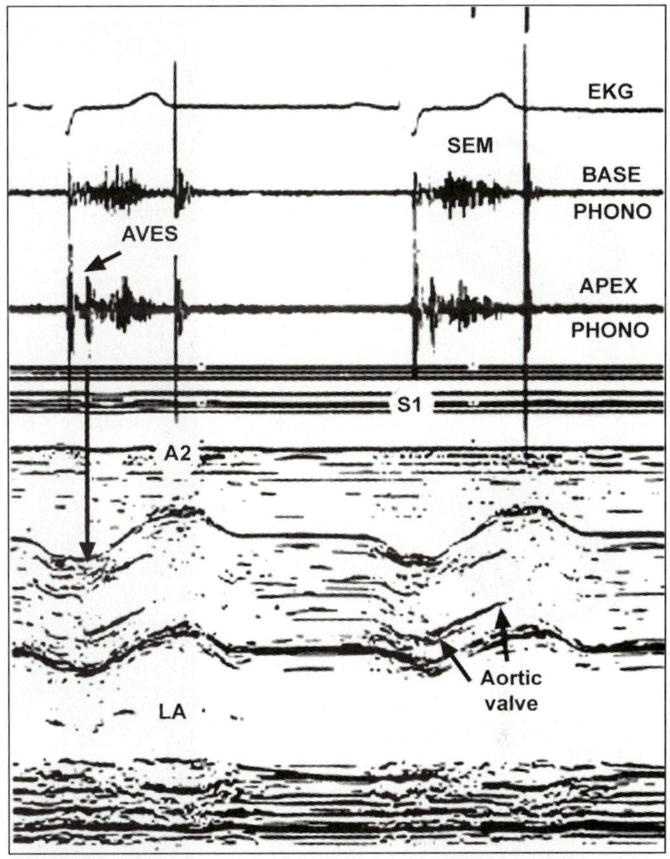


**Fig. 16.51:** Simultaneous recordings of base, apexcardiograms and aortic valve echocardiogram showing a prominent aortic valvular ejection click (AVES) is recorded at the apex and is coincident with the maximal excursion of the aortic valve in early systole. It is followed by a crescendo-decrescendo SEM that ends well before a loud A2 in young patient with valvular aortic stenosis

### CT Scanning

CT scans may exhibit chamber enlargement and calcification of the aortic valve. This calcification is a reliable indicator of severe stenosis, particularly when it is present in a young patient (Fig. 16.54).

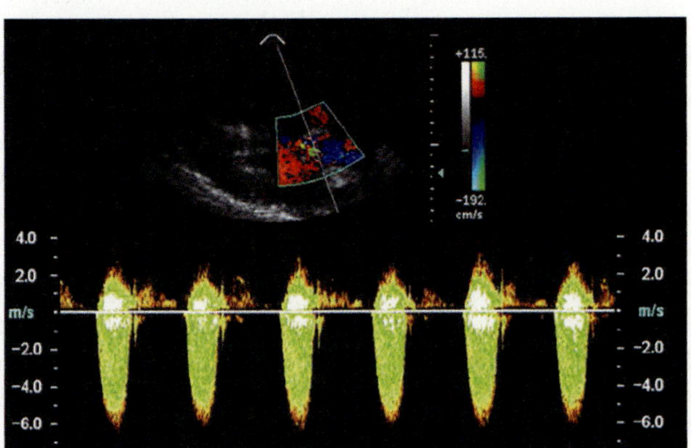


**Fig. 16.50:** Color flow guided evaluation of aortic stenosis jet from apical five chamber view with continuous wave Doppler interrogation

### Magnetic Resonance Imaging

Cine MRI may be used to depict the signal void caused by high-velocity jet flow across a narrow valvular orifice associated with the opened valve in aortic stenosis. The signal void is projected into the ascending aorta in systole. Despite the good anatomic detail obtainable with MRI, echocardiography has superseded MRI because of its improved portability (Fig. 16.55).

### Cardiac Catheterization and Angiography

During catheterization, the transvalvular pressure gradient across the aortic valve is measured by use of a catheter in the LV and another in the proximal aorta or femoral artery. A mean pressure gradient greater than 30 mmHg usually represents clinically significant aortic stenosis. As a result of the dire consequences of missing the diagnosis of symptomatic aortic stenosis, the physician must have a low threshold for obtaining an echocardiogram whenever the possibility of aortic stenosis cannot be excluded during physical examination (Figs 16.56 and 16.57).

Asymptomatic patients with suggestive murmurs benefit from early diagnosis, which allows both the patient

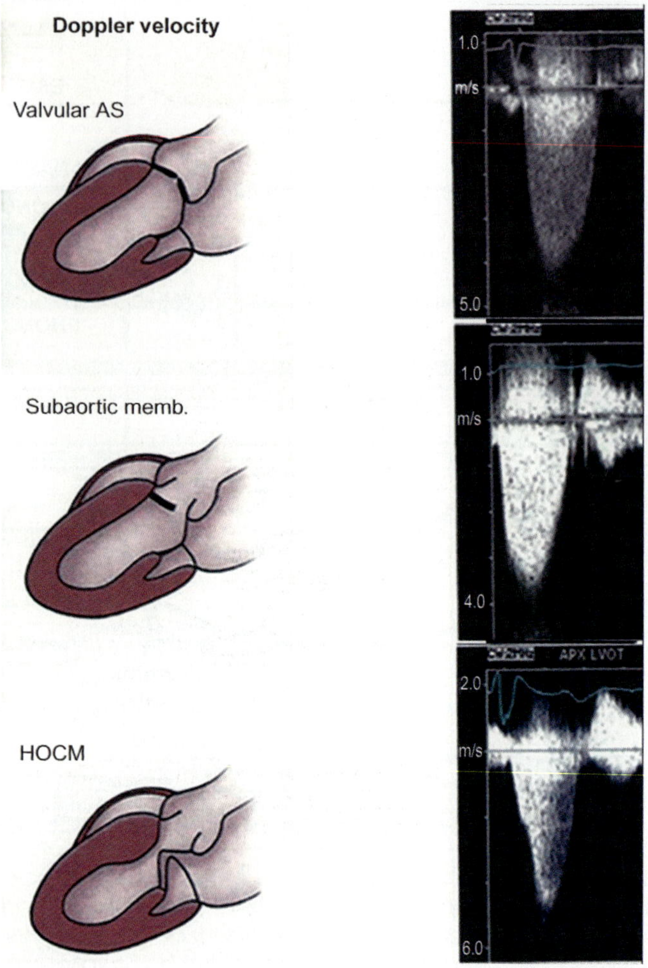


**Fig. 16.52:** CW Doppler study in different types of LV outflow obstructions

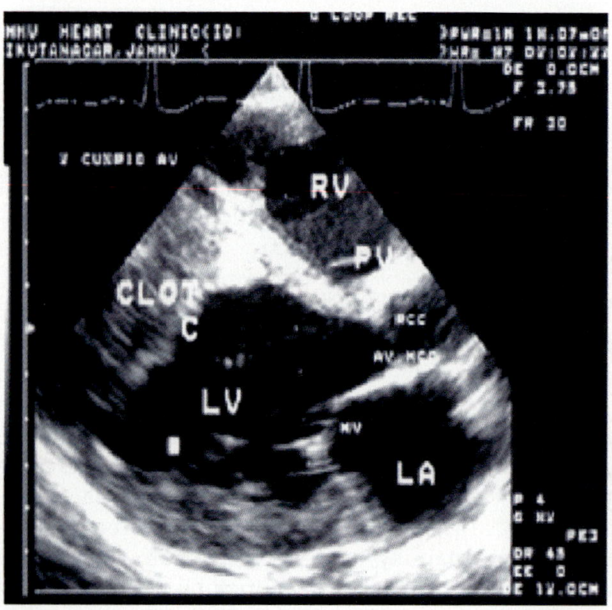


**Fig. 16.53:** 2D LAX view of LV showing dilated LV cavity with apical clot in patient with severe type of aortic stenosis

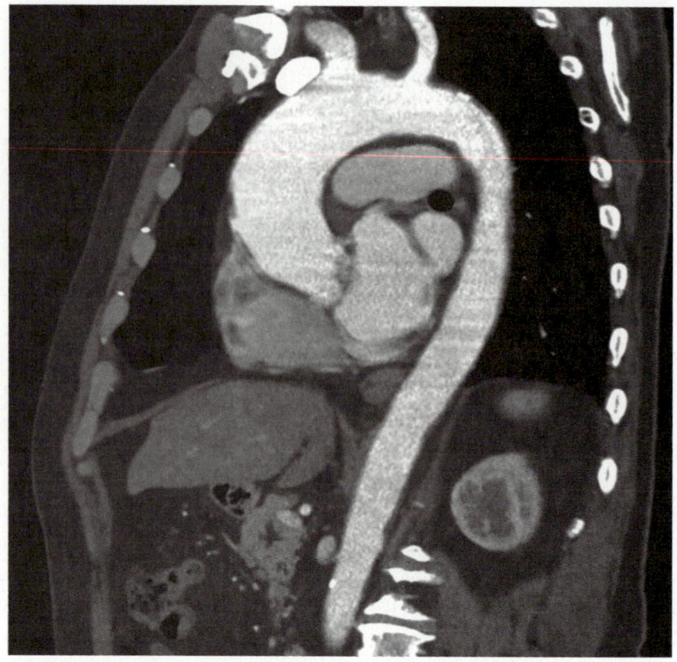

**Fig. 16.54:** CTA of the thorax confirms enlargement of the ascending aorta with a normal caliber descending aorta. Non-contrast CT image depicts aortic valve calcification

and the physician to be most vigilant regarding possible early signs and symptoms and to guide the use of prophylactic regimens to prevent bacterial endocarditis.

### Treatment of Aortic Stenosis

- Gentle diuresis if CHF
- Mild hydration if hypotensive and not in CHF
- Avoid nitrates and afterload reduction
- Digoxin
- Intra-aortic balloon pump (temporize for surgery)
- Endocarditis prophylaxis/education
- Asymptomatic persons with mild stenosis do not have to limit physical activity.
- Periodic monitoring should be done because rapid narrowing can occur over as little as a few years.
- Persons with more severe stenosis should be evaluated by a cardiologist whether or not they have symptoms.
- Persons with symptoms of passing out on exertion, angina or congestive heart failure due to aortic stenosis require immediate evaluation by a cardiologist and may be considered for valve repair or replacement.
- Your doctor may treat symptoms of either angina or congestive heart failure with medications as they occur. If these symptoms are caused by aortic stenosis definitive treatment is valve repair or replacement. Very old age (80s) is not a contraindication to valve replacement as long heart function and overall health are reasonable. Persons requiring treatment for this disorder must be under the care of a physician (Figs 16.58–16.60).

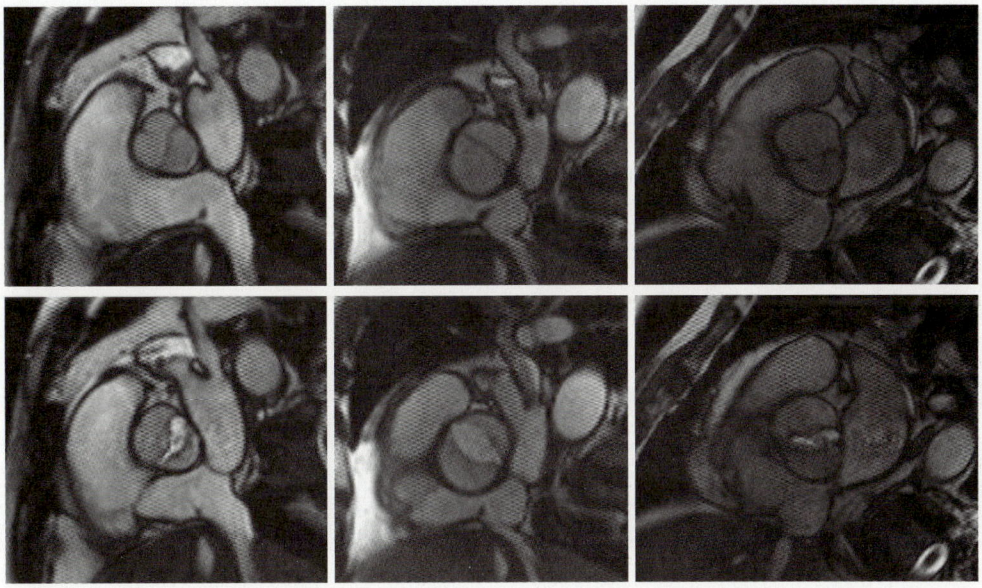

**Fig. 16.55:** Typical SSFP cine CMR still frames of BAV. An oblique orientation is given through the aortic valve. The perspective is from the left-anterior side of the LV towards the aorta. CMR visualizes different types of BAV in diastole (top row) and systole (bottom row). Type 1 LR (left), type 0-lateral (centre), and type 0-AP (right)

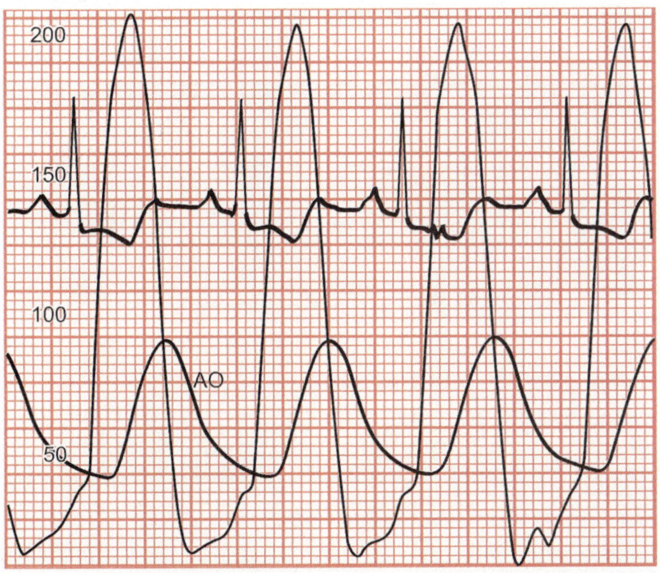


**Fig. 16.56:** Simultaneous tracing of ECG and hemodynamic pressure recording across aorta and LV showing marked gradient between LV and aorta in patient with moderately severe AS

### Prognosis in Aortic Stenosis

Once symptoms develop aortic stenosis is very serious. The presence of symptoms almost always means that the aortic valve is extremely narrow and will not tolerate further narrowing. Once symptoms occur with aortic stenosis, particularly angina or shortness of breath with minimal exertion or congestive heart failure, many people die within several years if not treated. Sudden death, due to cardiac arrhythmias, may occur in up to 20% of people with aortic stenosis. The cause of sudden death is speculative (unknown).

## 2. AORTIC REGURGITATION

It is defined as leakage of blood from either malformed aortic valve or damaged due to number of conditions as follows:

### Aetiology

- Infective endocarditis
- Rupture of sinus of Valsalva
- Acute aortic dissection
- Chest trauma
- Following valve surgery
- Bicuspid aortic valve
- Rheumatic fever
- Weight-loss medications (fenfluramine, dexfenfluramine)
- Collagen vascular or connective-tissue diseases
- Systematic lupus erythematosus
- Marfan syndrome
- Pseudoxanthoma elasticum
- Ankylosing spondylitis
- Ehlers-Danlos syndrome
- Polymyalgia rheumatic

### Signs and Symptoms (Tables 16.1 and 16.2)

- Fatigue
- Dyspnea on exertion
- Paroxysmal nocturnal dyspnea
- Orthopnea
- Syncope
- Acute pulmonary edema

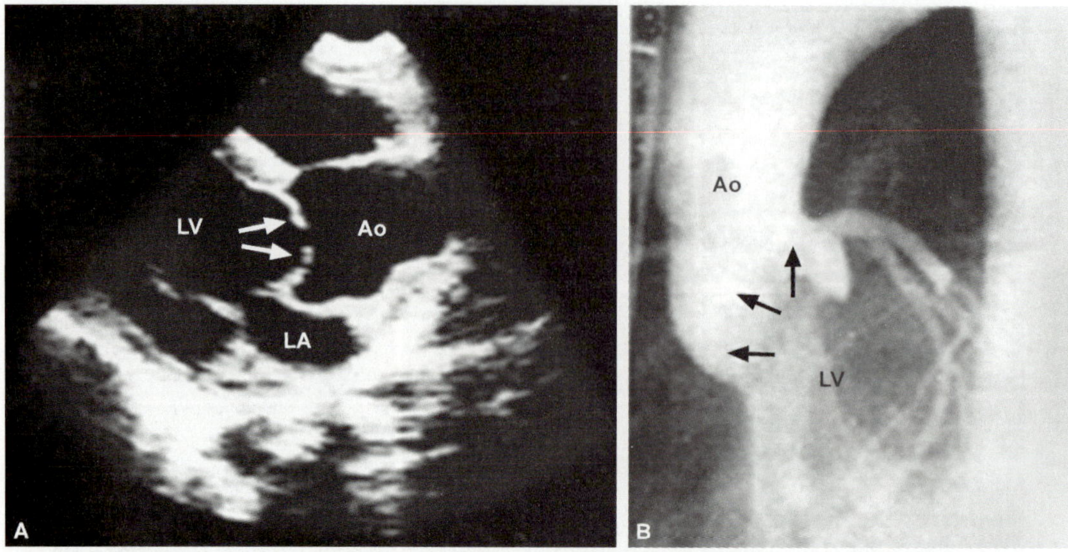


**Fig. 16.57:** (A) 2D echocardiographic study with the transducer in the long-axis parasternal position demonstrating leaflet doming and thickening. (B) Aortogram from the same patient showing doming of the aortic valve leaflets. The negative shadow in the proximal aortic root (Ao) is caused by a jet of non-opacified blood from the left ventricle (LV) as it exits through the stenotic aortic valve

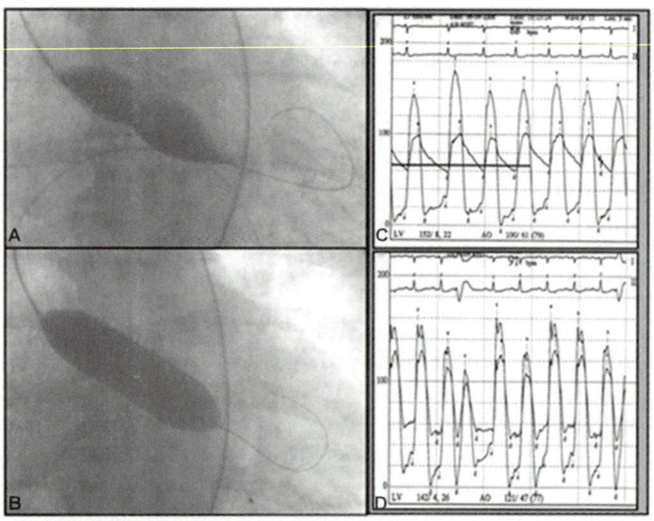


**Fig. 16.58:** (A) Preinflated balloon catheter across aortic valve (B) Fully inflated aortic valve. Aortic and left ventricular traces pre-(C) and post-(D) valvuloplasty. The mean aortic pressure gradient has reduced significantly from 50 mmHg to 25 mmHg

- High-pitched blowing decrescendo diastolic murmur at aortic area
- Accentuated A2 heart sound
- Wide pulse pressure
- Corrigan pulse (collapsing pulse)
- Duroziez sign (to and fro murmur)
- De Musset sign (head bobbing with systole)
- Quincke pulse (nail bed pulsations)
- Austin Flint murmur (soft diastolic rumble)

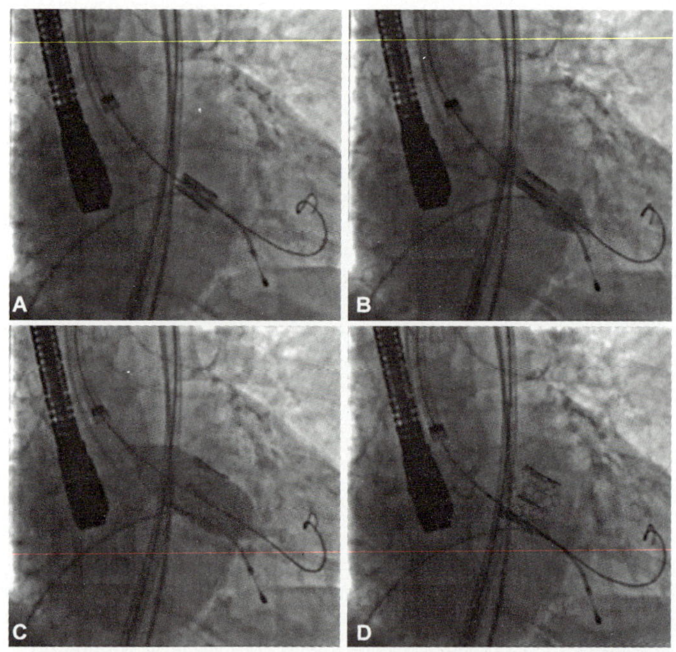


**Fig. 16.59:** Phases of percutaneous heart valve replacement (TAVI). (A) Edwards heart valve is guided under fluoroscopy imaging into the correct position. (B) Balloon is inflated to expand the prosthetic valve. (C) Maximal balloon inflation for valve delivery; (D) Definitive valve positioning

## Diagnosis in Aortic Regurgitation

All patients in whom acute valvular regurgitation is suspected should undergo electrocardiography and chest radiography. Electrocardiograms typically reveal sinus tachycardia with nonspecific ST- and T-wave abnormalities. Ischemic ST changes can indicate regurgitation mediated by ischemia—coronary artery disease, or aortic dissection

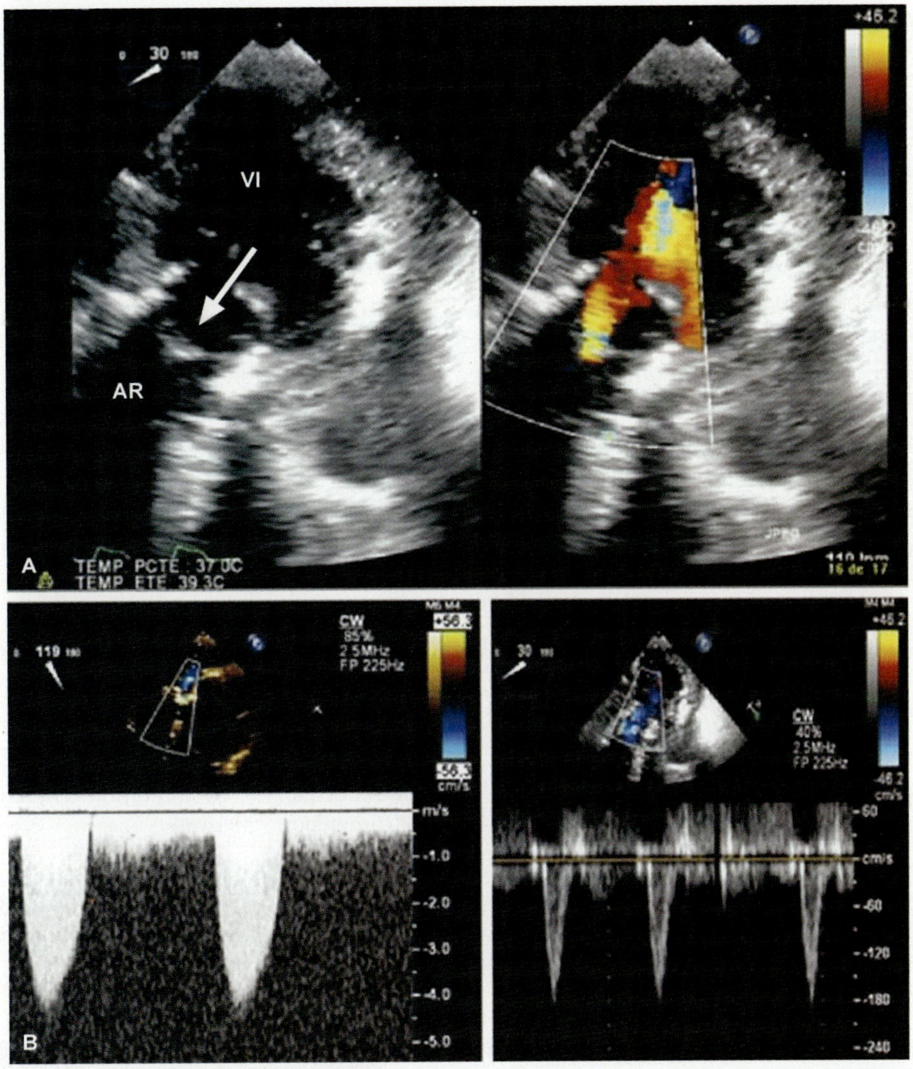


**Fig. 16.60:** Aortic valve hemodynamic assessment before and after transthoracic implantation of the aortic valve prosthesis. (A) Two-dimensional deep transgastric transesophageal view (left) and color-Doppler (right); the prosthesis is well-positioned, the leaflets show coaptation, and there is mild central regurgitation. (B) Spectral Doppler data obtained continuously during intraoperative transesophageal echocardiography before (left) and after (right) transthoracic implantation of the aortic valve prosthesis; note the normalization of the transvalvular flow velocity. AR=aortic root; LV=left ventricle

**Table 16.1:** Physical signs associated with hyperdynamic pulse in chronic aortic regurgitation

| Physical sign | Description |
|---|---|
| Water-hammer or Corrigan's pulse | Rapid upstroke followed by quick collapse |
| DeMusset's sign | Head bob with each heartbeat |
| Traube's sign | Pistol shot sound heard over the femoral arteries in both systole and diastole |
| Muller's sign | Systolic pulsation of the uvula |
| Duroziez's sign | Systolic murmur over the femoral artery with compressed proximally ad diastolic murmur when compressed distally or systolic-diastolic murmur with increasing compression over femoral artery |
| Quincke's sign | Capillary pulsations visible in the lunula of the nailbed |
| Hill's sign | Popliteal cuff systolic pressure exceeding brachial cuff systolic pressure by >60 mmHg |
| Becker's sign | Arterial pulsations visible in the retinal arteries and pupils |

**Table 16.2:** Indications for aortic valve replacement in severe chronic aortic regurtitation

| Indication | Class |
|---|---|
| Patients with NYHA functional class III or IV symptoms and preserved left ventricular (LV) systolic function, defined as normal ejection fractinal rest (ejection fraction ≥0.50) | I |
| Patients with NYHA functional class II symptoms and preserved LV systolic function (ejection fraction ≥0.50) but with progressive LV dilatation or declining ejection fraction at rest on serial studies or declining effort tolerance on exercise testing | I |
| Patients with Canadian Heart Association functional class II or greater angina with or without coronary artery disease | I |
| Asymptomatic or symptomatic patients with mild to moderate LV dysfunction at rest (ejection fraction 0.25–0.49). Patients undergoing coronary artery bypass surgery or surgery on the aorta or other heart values | I |
| Patients with HYHA functional class II symptoms and preserved LV systolic function (ejection fraction ≥0.50 at rest) with stable LV size and systolic function on serial studies and stable exercise tolerance | IIa |
| Asymptomatic patients with normal LV systolic function (ejection fraction >0.50) but with severe LV dilation (end-diastolic dimension >75 mm or end-systolic dimension >55 mm) | IIa |
| Patients with severe LV dysfunction (ejection fraction <0.25) | IIb |
| Asymptomatic patients with normal systolic function at rest (ejection fraction >0.50) and progressive LV dilatation when the drgree of dilatation is moderalelly severe (end-diastolic dimension 70–75 mm, end-systolic dimension 50–55 mm) | IIb |
| Asymptomatic patients with normal systolic function at rest (ejection fraction >0.50) but with a decline in ejection fraction during | III |
| Exercise radionuclide angiography | IIb |
| Stress echocardiography | III |
| Asymptomatic patients with normal systolic function at rest (ejection fraction >0.50). LV dilatation when degree of dilatation is not severe (end-diastolic dimension <70 mm, end-systolic dimension <50 mm) | III |

NYHA, New York Heart Association.

Adapted from Bonow HO, Carabello B, de leon AC Jr, et al. Guidelines for the management of patients with valvular heart disease; a report of the American College of Cardiology/Americal Heart Association Task Force on Practice Guidelines (Committee on Management of Patients with Valvular Heart Disease). J AM Coll Cardiol 1998;32:1496.

that affects the coronary ostia. Hemodynamic disturbances, such as very high LVEDP, can exacerbate coronary insufficiency. Chest radiographs typically show pulmonary edema and a left heart of normal size. Cardiomegaly can indicate the worsening of an existing valvular condition, and a widened mediastinum suggests aortic dissection. This may be mistaken for pneumonia, particularly if the patient has endocarditis or is not severely ill. Measuring cardiac biomarkers aids the diagnosis of acute coronary syndromes and ischemia; determining the level of B-type natriuretic peptide can help distinguish cardiac causes from non-cardiac causes of dyspnea and shock

### Chest Radiography

Standard chest radiography may show evidence of structural abnormalities (aortic dilation, prosthetic valve dislodgement, and aortic valvular calcification) or functional compromise (pulmonary edema, cardiomegaly). In acute aortic regurgitation, the following may be seen (Fig. 16.61):

- Minimal cardiac enlargement
- Normal aortic root/arch
- Pulmonary venous pattern increased
- In chronic aortic regurgitation, the following may be seen:

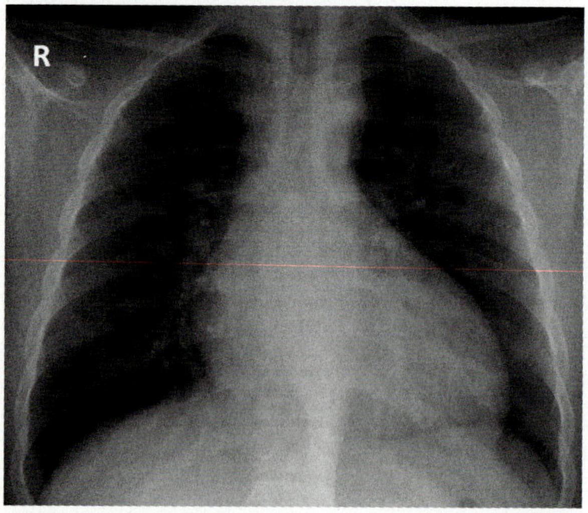


**Fig. 16.61:** Chest radiograph demonstrating *left ventricular enlargement* secondary to chronic aortic regurgitation as a result of increased left ventricular systolic pressure and volume overload

- Marked cardiac enlargement
- Prominent aortic root/arch
- Normal pulmonary venous pattern

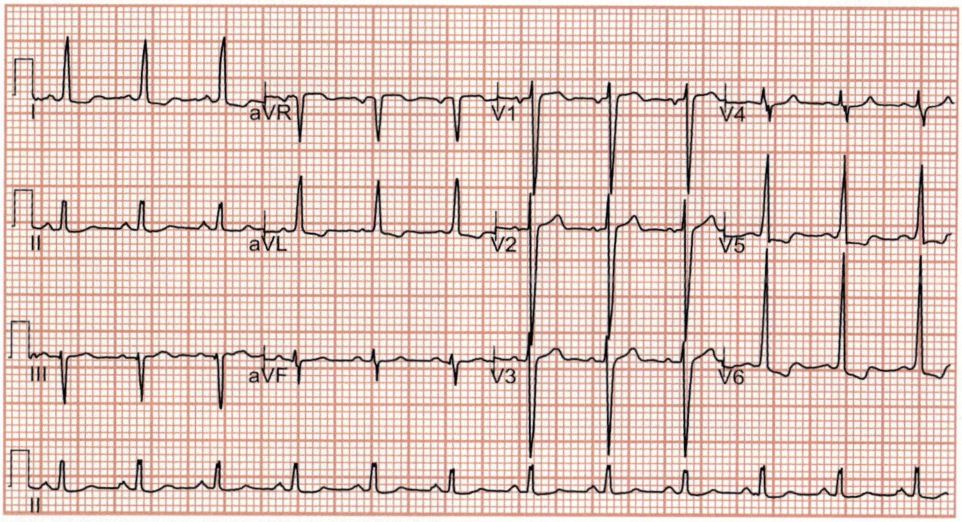


**Fig. 16.62:** ECG demonstrates many of the features of LV hypertrophy—markedly increased LV voltages; S wave in V1+R wave in V6 >35 mm; R wave in aVL >11 mm. Increased R wave peak time—the upstroke of the QRS complex is slurred in V5-6, resulting in minor QRS broadening. Left ventricular strain pattern—T-wave inversion in the lateral leads V5-6, I and aVL. Left axis deviation. Signs of *left atrial enlargement*

**Electrocardiography** (Fig. 16.62)

Electrocardiographic findings are nonspecific but may include evidence of the following:

- LV hypertrophy
- Left axis deviation
- Left atrial enlargement
- LV volume overload pattern—prominent Q-waves in leads I, aVL, and $V_3$ to $V_6$ and relatively small r waves in $V_1$
- LV conduction defects—typically late in the disease process

*Echocardiography* is essential in the diagnosis of acute valvular dysfunction. Severe aortic or mitral regurgitation, normal LV size, and normal or hyperdynamic ventricular function all point to an acute process. Quantitative measures are more useful in chronic regurgitation than in acute regurgitation. The estimation of effective regurgitant orifice area and regurgitant volume can be inaccurate in acute regurgitation (particularly in the presence of tachycardia) and depends upon dynamic loading conditions. Echocardiography typically reveals the mechanism of regurgitation, such as aortic dissection or ruptured mitral chordae tendineae. In patients whose chronic regurgitation has led to ventricular enlargement, the acuteness of regurgitation is difficult to evaluate unless a clinical examination is performed and comparisons with prior studies are made (Figs 16.63–16.66).

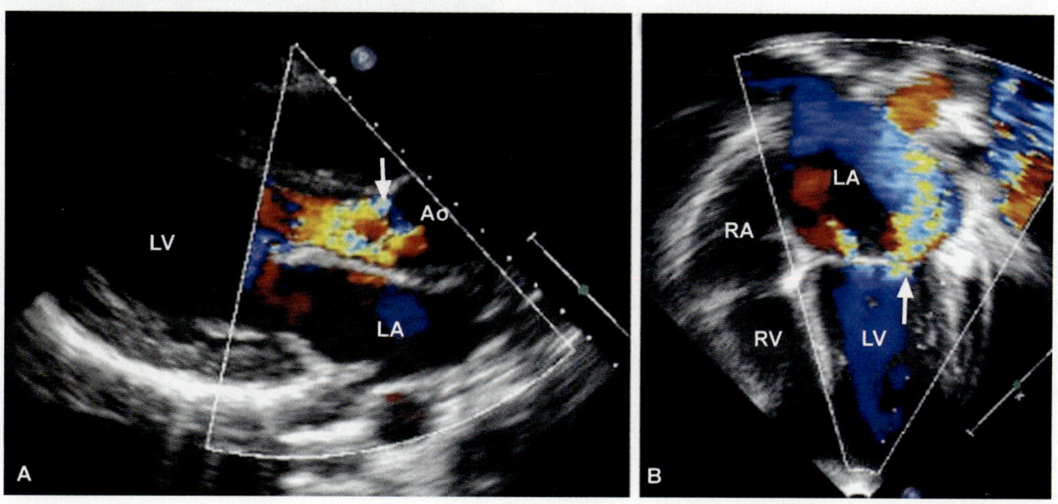


**Fig. 16.63:** Two-dimensional color and spectral Doppler echocardiographic studies of patients with rheumatic heart disease show moderate to severe aortic valve insufficiency with no stenosis (A, arrow) and bowing of the anterior mitral leaflet with severe insufficiency and no stenosis (B, arrow)

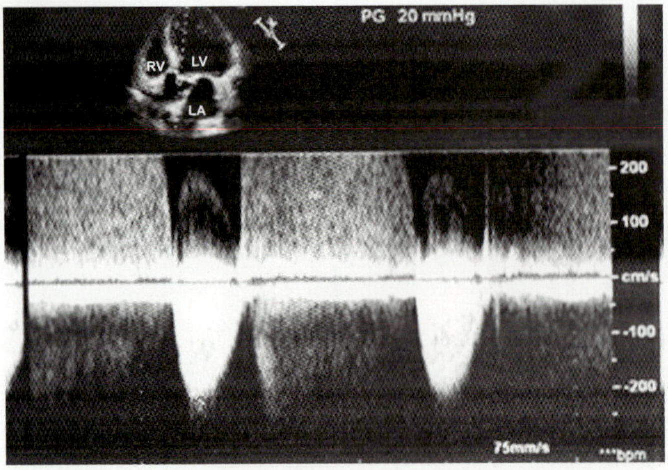


**Fig. 16.64:** Doppler tracing in aortic regurgitation (bottom) in apical five chamber view (top)

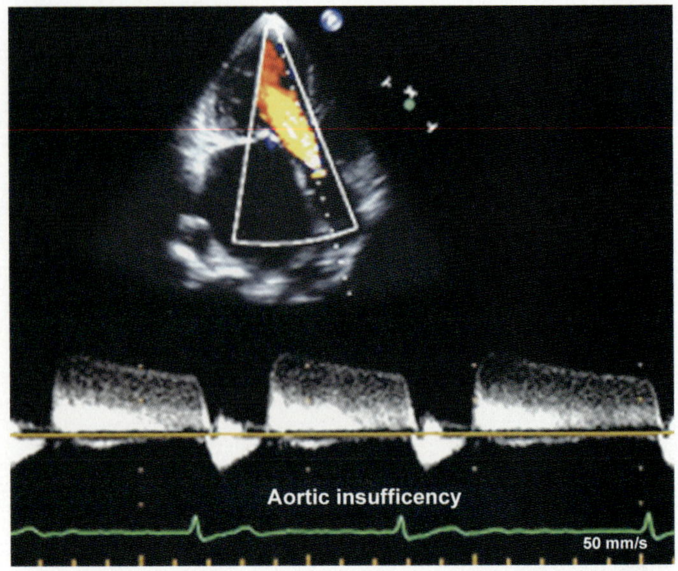


**Fig. 16.65:** Color-Doppler tracing in aortic regurgitation

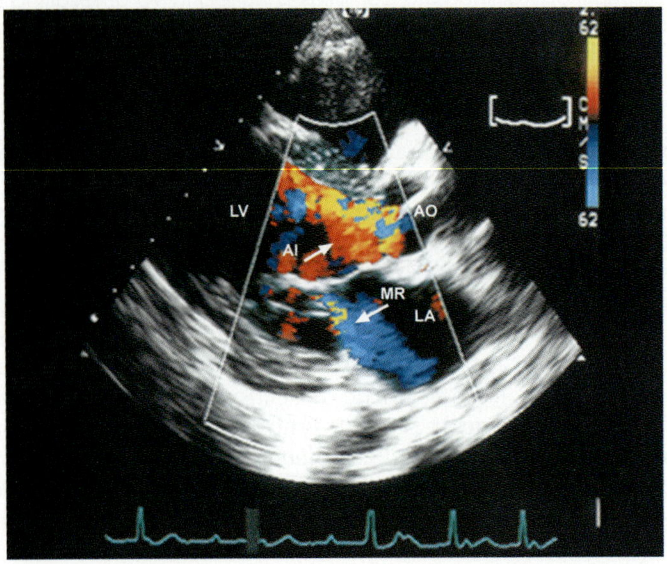


**Fig. 16.66:** Parasternal long-axis image of acute severe aortic regurgitation (AR). The accompanying marked elevation of LV diastolic pressure causes diastolic mitral regurgitation (MR). Ao=aorta; LA=left atrium; LV=left ventricle

*Doppler echocardiography* can lead to an underestimation of the severity of regurgitation, particularly if the regurgitant jet is eccentric. If a transthoracic study is not conclusive, transesophageal echocardiography (TEE) can reveal the mechanism and severity of the regurgitation. In prosthetic valve dysfunction, TEE can also show artifacts. Interpreting the results of TEE is often crucial to the planning of operative repair, such as the identification of leaflet or annular involvement. During planning for the use of aortic homografts or a Ross repair, TEE data on annular size are indispensable. However, if TEE results will not change the decision to perform surgery, the images can be obtained in the operating room.

## Cardiac CT Scanning and Magnetic Resonance Imaging

Cardiac computed tomography (CT) scanning and magnetic resonance imaging (MRI) have not yet achieved widespread adoption in the management of AR, although support in the literature is increasing for the potential clinical use of these imaging techniques (Figs 16.67 and 16.68).

## Radionuclide Imaging

Radionuclide imaging may provide complementary clinical information, including the AR regurgitant fraction and the LV/right ventricular (RV) stroke volume ratio. In the absence of mitral regurgitation and tricuspid regurgitation,

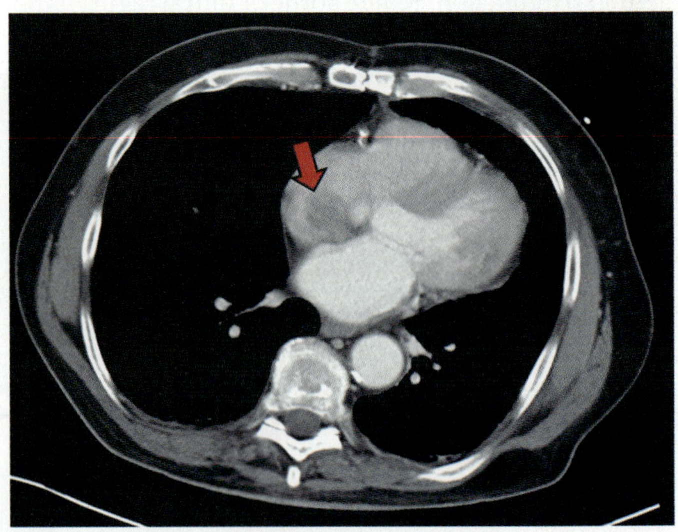

**Fig. 16.67:** Chamber view on CT scan showing the aortic regurgitation

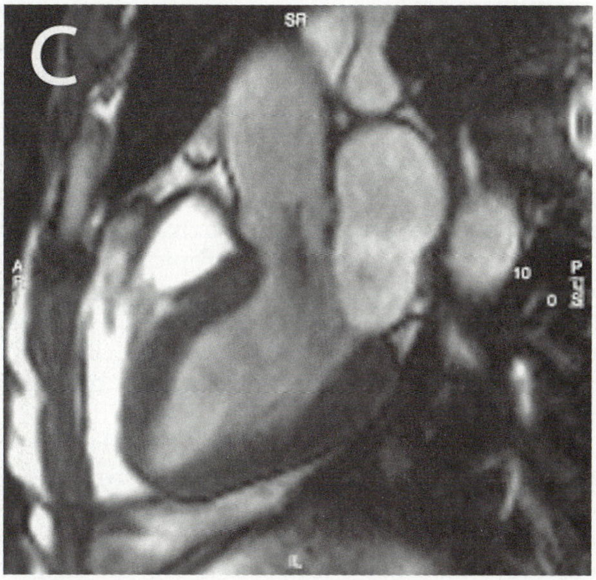

**Fig. 16.68:** Chamber view showing the aortic regurgitation. Cardiac magnetic resonance (CMR) imaging confirmed a quadricuspid valve with four equal and fully separated cusps (Hurwitz and Roberts type A) and a central regurgitation orifice

an LV/RV stroke volume ratio of 2.5 or more denotes severe aortic regurgitation. Demonstration of a fall in the EF with exercise is one of the most important indications for surgery in patients who are asymptomatic (Fig. 16.69).

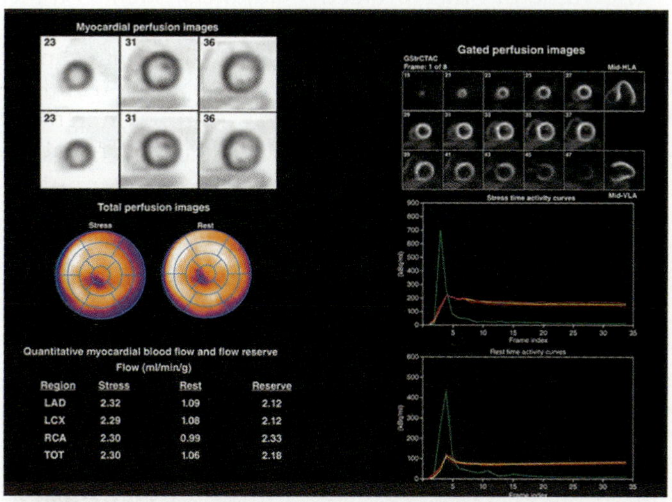


**Fig. 16.69:** Multidimensional cardiac imaging protocol with positron emission tomography. The *left upper panel* demonstrates stress and rest short-axis images of the left and right ventricles demonstrating normal regional myocardial perfusion. The middle panel demonstrates the quantitative bull's-eye display to evaluate the extent and severity of perfusion defects. The *lower right panel* illustrates the time-activity curves for quantification of myocardial blood flow. The *right upper panel* demonstrates electrocardiogram-gated myocardial perfusion images from which one can determine the presence of regional wall motion abnormalities and calculate left ventricular volumes and ejection fraction. LAD=left anterior descending artery; LCX=left circumflex artery; RCA=right coronary artery; TOT=total left ventricle

## Left-heart Catheterization

It is not routinely indicated in the preoperative evaluation of patients with acute valvular regurgitation. Catheterization can be considered when electrocardiographic changes suggest acute ischemia. Patients with acute mitral regurgitation from ischemia or papillary muscle rupture may benefit from revascularization along with mitral valve repair or replacement. Conversely, patients whose mechanisms of regurgitation are nonischemic (such as mitral regurgitation due to chordal rupture or aortic regurgitation) may poorly tolerate the contrast medium and the time needed for catheterization. Patients with aortic dissection rarely require cardiac catheterization, and the procedure may worsen the dissection. When the aortic dissection is diagnosed by use of echocardiography, cross-sectional imaging can fully reveal the dissection anatomy; however, in most instances, cross-sectional imaging leads to the diagnosis before echocardiography does. Because the morbidity and mortality rates of acute severe regurgitation are high if it is untreated, rapid diagnosis is crucial. Definitive treatment should not be delayed (Fig. 16.70).

## Aortic Angiography

Aortic angiography, which may be performed during a cardiac catheterization procedure, may provide useful information regarding the severity of the patient's AR (Fig. 16.71). Traditional angiographic grading is as follows:

- Mild (1+): A small amount of contrast enters the LV during diastole and clears with each systole.
- Moderate AR (2+): Contrast enters the LV with each diastole, but the LV chamber is less dense than the aorta.
- Moderately severe AR (3+): The LV chamber is equal in density to the ascending aorta.
- Severe AR (4+): Complete, dense opacification of the LV chamber occurs on the first beat, and the LV is more densely opacified than the ascending aorta.

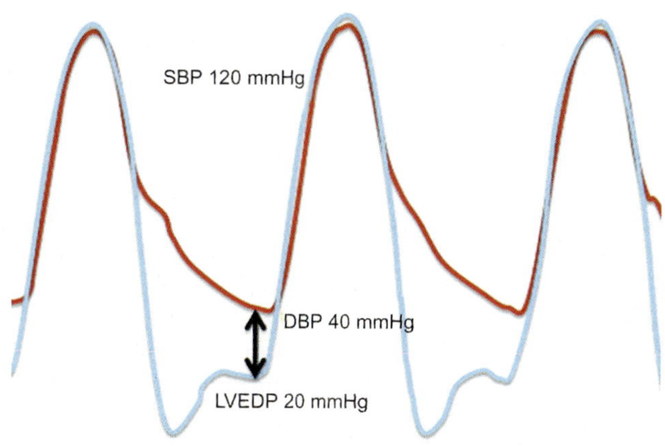


=[(DBP – LVEDP)/SBP]×100

=[(40–20)/120]×100 = 16.7

**Fig. 16.70:** The AR index is strongly associated with the severity of peri-AR and independently predicts 1-year mortality after TAVI. It provides prognostic information that is complementary to the degree of peri-AR and can be used to guide periprocedural clinical decisions

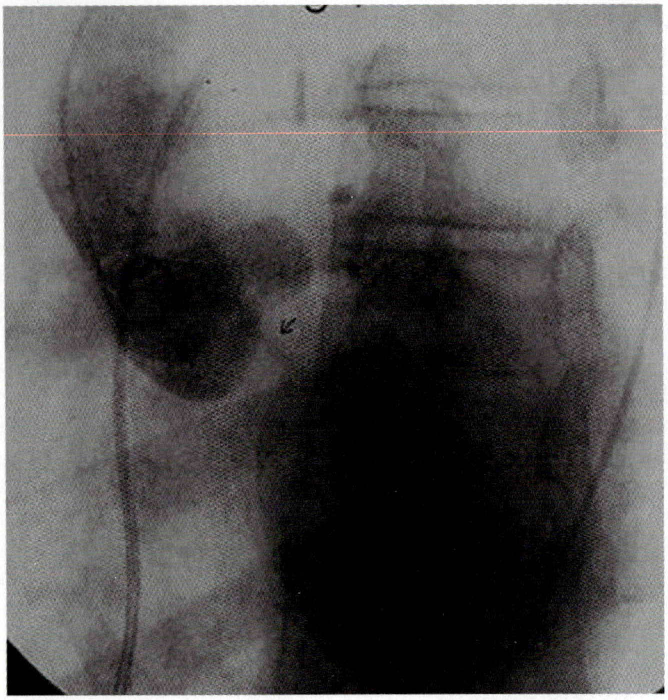

**Fig. 16.71:** Aortic regurgitation. Aortic-root angiography shows regurgitation of contrast material into the left ventricle (LV)

Assessment of the anatomy of the aorta and coronary ostia usually produces normal findings, except for the visible reflux of dye from the aortic root into the ventricle.

### Medical Therapy

Chronic:

- Preload and afterload reduction
- Digoxin
- Diuretics
- Endocarditis prophylaxis/education

#### *Acute*

- Preload and afterload reduction
- Intra-aortic balloon pump
- Urgent surgery

The treatment for acute aortic regurgitation is aortic valve repair or replacement. Medical therapy can stabilize the patient's condition before surgery, but it is not a substitute for surgery. Vasodilators such as sodium nitroprusside can be used to improve forward flow, and inotropic agents such as dobutamine can improve the patient's cardiac output. Intra-aortic balloon pumps (IABPs) tend to be contraindicated in acute aortic regurgitation, because balloon inflation during diastole may impair LV hemodynamics. Balloon use is specifically contraindicated in cases of aortic dissection.

### Surgical Treatment of Acute Aortic Valve Regurgitation

- *Anesthetic Considerations:* Inducing anesthesia in a critically ill patient who has acute aortic regurgitation can be a challenge. Low diastolic pressure, tachycardia, and increased wall stress can impair coronary flow. If anesthesia further reduces blood pressure, coronary ischemia can exacerbate the patient's unstable condition. Therefore, the anesthesiologist should try to prevent tachycardia or hypotension during intubation and the induction of anesthesia. Hemodynamic monitoring is also crucial, and in many cases monitoring lines will have been placed before the patient's arrival in the operating room. The appropriate use of inotropic drugs, vasoconstrictors, sedatives, and anesthetic agents can increase the chances of optimal outcomes. The surgical team should be present during induction, ready to initiate support if the patient experiences cardiopulmonary collapse.
- *Surgical Considerations:* Surgical options depend upon the pathophysiology and anatomy of the valve and the expected long-term outcome of correcting the acute aortic regurgitation. Myocardial protection is crucial, because the incompetent aortic valve and any associated aortic root disorder makes the antegrade delivery of cardioplegic solution ineffective or even dangerous. The reliable placement of a coronary sinus cannula for retrograde delivery of cardioplegic solution is essential. Necessity may justify placing bicaval cannulae and directly intubating the coronary sinus. Then, after the aortic valve and root have been properly evaluated, adjuvant cardioplegic solution can be delivered from a handheld apparatus through the coronary ostia. A LV vent placed through the right superior pulmonary vein may aid ventricular decompression and diastolic arrest. The value of other protective adjuncts, such as topical cooling or systemic hypothermia on cardiopulmonary bypass (CPB), is unclear (Fig. 16.72).

### Aortic Valve Endocarditis

- Aortic valve endocarditis can prevent leaflet coaptation, lead to leaflet erosion, or affect the aortic annulus—singly or in combination. During planning for surgery, directly evaluating the aortic annulus by use of intraoperative TEE is important. Annular integrity can be compromised by abscess formation and endocarditic

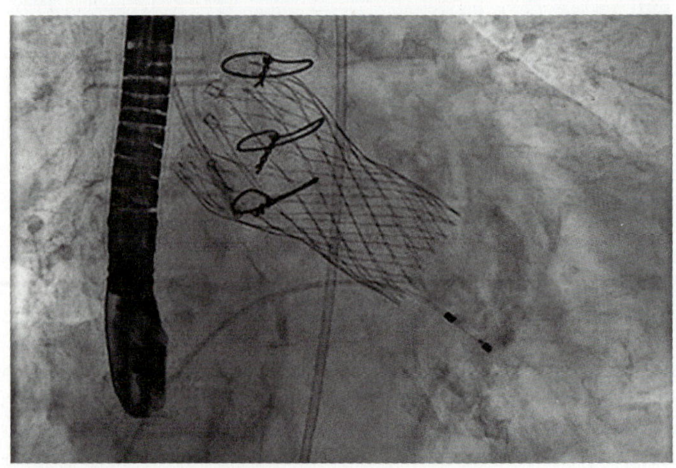

**Fig. 16.72:** Self-expanding replacement aortic valve placed during TAVR procedure

erosion. In cases of annular involvement, the use of a homograft is typically recommended. Although aortic homografts are susceptible to prosthetic valve endocarditis, the additional tissue included with the homograft (the LV outflow tract and the anterior leaflet of the mitral valve) is sometimes essential for successful aortic root reconstruction. When endocarditis is limited to the valve leaflets, procedures beyond leaflet excision and aortic valve replacement are not indicated. Because the rates of infection are similar between mechanical and bioprosthetic replacement valves, after native-valve endocarditis, either type is suitable.

- Some centers use a pulmonary autograft (the Ross procedure), particularly in children. However, as in elective aortic valve surgery, the benefits and risks of the Ross repair are debatable. In theory, a durable aortic valve replacement will grow with a child and not require future intervention. On the other hand, 'single-valve disease' becomes 'double-valve disease,' and data suggest that the new aortic valve requires replacement in 10–20% of patients within 10 years of the operation. Thus, the long-term outcomes may offset the theoretical benefit. Some patients cannot tolerate additional CPB time, so Ross repair is limited to a specific patient population in centers that have had extensive surgical experience. Finally, depending upon the clinical status of the patient and the condition of the aortic root, a 2-staged approach may be beneficial; simple valve replacement, followed by root reconstruction after the patient has recovered from multisystem organ failure.

### Aortic Dissection

- Stanford type A dissection can lead to aortic insufficiency through various pathophysiologic processes, and the cause dictates the treatment. When an aortic valve is trileaflet, reconstructing the aortic root with valve resuspension and replacing the ascending aorta with an interpositional graft can frequently correct valvular regurgitation. This is accomplished by reestablishing the commissural heights at the sinotubular junction and reattaching the sinuses of Valsalva to the aortic wall. When an aortic valve is bicuspid or when there is an aneurysm of the ascending aorta, correction can be achieved by performing a modified Bentall procedure, using a valved conduit with direct coronary reimplantation. A study of aortic root replacement with the use of mechanical conduits and aortic allografts revealed no significant difference in 1-and 5-year survival rates on the basis of conduit choice, including in patients with aortic dissection. Aortic root remodeling surgery (the Yacoub procedure) and aortic root reimplantation (the David procedures) have also been used successfully in aortic dissection. However, coronary ischemia can occur due to coronary artery involvement from aortic dissection or technical problems with coronary artery reimplantation, and surgical expertise is necessary for optimal outcomes.

### Trauma or Ruptured Fenestration

- Leaflet disruption can occur consequent to trauma or ruptured fenestration. Anatomy permitting, the leaflets can be successfully repaired most commonly by patching with autologous pericardium. Other pericardial substitutes have also been used. Nonetheless, valve replacement is the safest choice for most surgeons. In blunt chest trauma, aortic valve regurgitation most often occurs because of leaflet perforation, dissection, or loss of commissural suspension. The choice of repair, replacement, or reconstruction depends upon the surgical anatomy.

## TRICUSPID VALVE DISORDERS

Isolated valvular disorders of the right side of the heart (receiving and pumping venous blood to the lungs for oxygenation) are much less common than left sided valvular disease. Combined left (mitral and/or aortic) and right (tricuspid and/or pulmonic) heart valvular disease is more common.

### 1. TRICUSPID VALVE STENOSIS

It is defined as narrowing of valvular area from its normal range due to many causes as follows:

### Aetiology

At least four conditions can cause obstruction of the native tricuspid valve. These include (1) rheumatic heart disease, (2) congenital abnormalities, (3) metabolic or enzymatic abnormalities, (4) active infective endocarditis.

- **Rheumatic tricuspid stenosis:** In this entity, diffuse thickening of the leaflets occurs, with or without fusion of the commissures. The chordae tendineae may be thickened and shortened. Calcification of the valve rarely occurs. The leaflet tissue is composed of dense collagen and elastic fibers that produce a major distortion of the normal leaflet layers.
- **Carcinoid heart disease:** Carcinoid valve lesions characteristically manifest as fibrous white plaques located on the valvular and mural endocardium. The valve leaflets are thickened, rigid, and reduced in area. Fibrous tissue proliferation is present on the atrial and ventricular surfaces of the valve structure.
- **Congenital tricuspid stenosis:** These lesions are observed more commonly in infants. They may manifest as incompletely developed leaflets, shortened or malformed chordae, small annuli, abnormal size and number of the papillary muscles, or any combination of these defects.
- **Infective endocarditis:** Large infected vegetations obstructing the orifice of the tricuspid valve may produce stenosis. This condition is relatively uncommon, even in those who abuse intravenous drugs.
- **Unusual causes:** Rare causes of tricuspid stenosis include Fabry disease and giant blood cysts.

- **Mimickers of tricuspid stenosis:** Several conditions may mimic tricuspid stenosis by obstructing flow through the valve. These conditions include supravalvular obstruction from congenital diaphragms, intracardiac or extracardiac tumors, thrombosis or emboli, or large endocarditis vegetations. In addition, conditions that impair right-sided filling can produce similar symptoms and physical findings. These conditions include *constrictive pericarditis* and *restrictive cardiomyopathy*.

### Symptoms and Signs

- Fatigue, due to limited cardiac output, may be present.
- Systemic venous congestion leads to abdominal discomfort and swelling. The onset is usually gradual, but it may be rapid if atrial fibrillation or flutter develops.
- Dyspnea may be present but is not severe unless concomitant mitral valve disease is present.
- Patients may complain about prominent pulsations in the neck.
- When tricuspid stenosis occurs concomitantly with mitral stenosis, the decrement of cardiac output to the pulmonary bed may paradoxically diminish the dyspnea, hemoptysis, and orthopnea typically seen with mitral stenosis.
- Obtain information regarding preceding rheumatic fever, symptoms of the carcinoid syndrome, and possible congenital abnormalities.

### Physical Examination

- With sinus rhythm (more common with tricuspid stenosis than with mitral stenosis), the jugular venous pulse increases and the A wave is prominent (may be confused with an arterial pulse).
- If atrial fibrillation occurs, the A wave is lost.
- Peripheral edema and ascites are frequent.
- Without significant mitral pathology, the patient should not be dyspneic and can probably lie flat without symptoms.
- A prominent right atrium may be palpable to the right of the sternum. If not obscured by mitral stenosis sounds, a tricuspid opening snap may be heard. A diastolic murmur is audible along the left sternal border or at the xiphoid, which increases with inspiration. Often, *tricuspid regurgitation* is also present, represented by a holosystolic murmur in a similar location.
- The first heart sound may be split widely. The second heart sound may be single. This single sound is due to the inaudible closure of the pulmonary valve from the decrease in blood flow through the stenotic tricuspid valve.

**Chest radiography:** Cardiac size may range from normal to enlarged, (i.e. cardiomegaly). Right atrial enlargement may be prominent. Findings specific to a particular associated congenital heart disease may also be seen (Fig. 16.73).

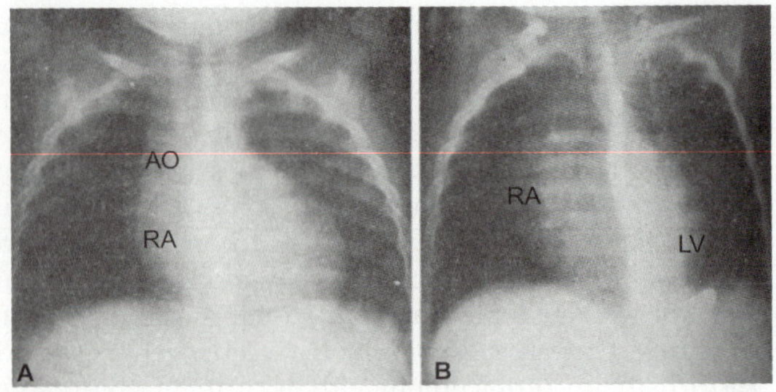


**Fig. 16.73:** Chest X-ray in a patient withsevere form of *tricuspid stenosis* demonstrating the following features: (A) reduced pulmonary blood flow, prominent *aortic root* (AO) and *right atrium* (RA), (B) the left anterior oblique projection on the right side shows distinctive humped appearance of the anterior cardiac silhouette due to *right atrial* (RA) enlargement in the absence of a *right ventricle*. The *left ventricle* (LV) is enlarged

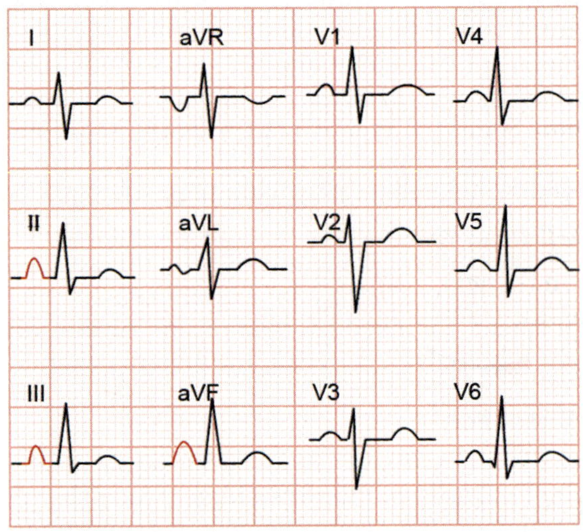


**Fig. 16.74:** Right atrial enlargement produces a peaked P-wave (P pulmonale) with amplitude >2.5 mm in the inferior leads (II, III and AVF) >1.5 mm in V1 and V2 in a patient with tricuspid stenosis

**Electrocardiogram:** Arrhythmias are frequent in this patient population. Because of the enlargement of the right atrium, the presence of atrial flutter and/or fibrillation should not be surprising. In sinus rhythm, right atrial enlargement or abnormality (tall P-waves on inferior leads) may be noted (Fig. 16.74).

**Echocardiography:** This test has become the procedure of choice for the diagnosis of valvular disorders. The test results help delineate the structure of the tricuspid valve and any other intracardiac pathology that may contribute to the pathophysiology of the process (Fig. 16.75).

### Procedures

**Cardiac catheterization:** This may be required prior to surgery in older patients to assess for concomitant coronary artery disease. Right heart catheterization can be used to determine the gradient across the valve and valve area (i.e.

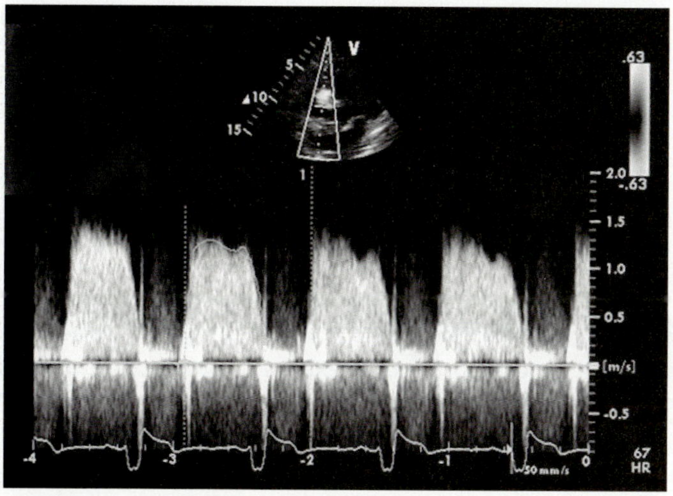


**Fig. 16.75:** CW Doppler echocardiogram of a patient showing tricuspid valve stenosis

severity of stenosis) and assess the presence of associated congenital defects (e.g. septal defects, intracardiac shunts, anomalous veins) if present. Assessment of aortic and mitral valves via left heart catheterization is useful in patients with rheumatic disease (Fig 16.76).

## Management of Tricuspid Stenosis

### *Medical Treatment*

**Digoxin (Lanoxin):** Used for prophylaxis and treatment of venous thrombosis, pulmonary embolism, and thromboembolic disorders. Cardiac glycoside with direct inotropic effects and indirect effects on the cardiovascular system. Acts directly on cardiac muscle and increases myocardial systolic contractions. Indirect actions result in increased carotid sinus nerve activity and enhanced sympathetic withdrawal for any given increase in mean arterial pressure.

**Warfarin (Coumadin):** Interferes with hepatic synthesis of vitamin K-dependent coagulation factors. Tailor dose to maintain an INR in the range of 2–3.

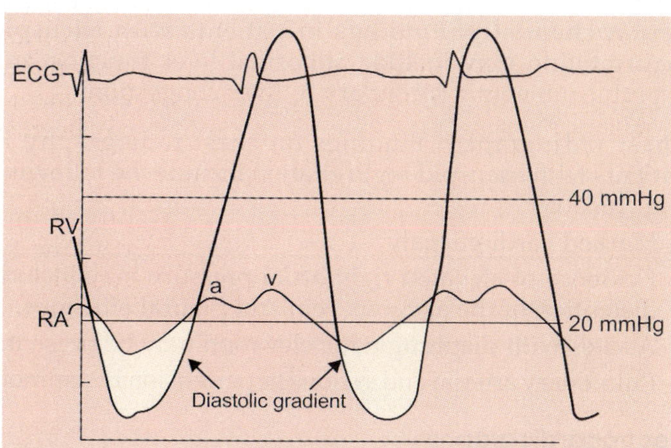


**Fig 16.76:** Tracings of simultaneous right atrial (RA) and right ventricular (RV) pressure waveforms in a patient with tricuspid stenosis

### Surgical Care (Fig. 16.77)

- Tricuspid stenosis remains a surgical disease and requires either commissurotomy or replacement of the valve if right heart failure or low cardiac output has resulted. Surgery is rarely performed solely on the tricuspid valve; it is usually performed in combination with mitral and/or aortic valve disease repair.
- With tricuspid valve replacement, the risk of thrombosis is significant and many surgeons advise warfarin therapy for either mechanical or bioprosthetic valve placement.
- Percutaneous balloon valvuloplasty has been used successfully, as long as concomitant regurgitation is not significant.
- The therapy chosen depends on the structure of the valve and the degree of deformity encountered.
- When possible, excise intracavitary pathology, whether it be tumors or other structural abnormalities.
- Redundant portions of the dilated right atrium can be excised during the same procedure for restoring the atrium back to normal size.

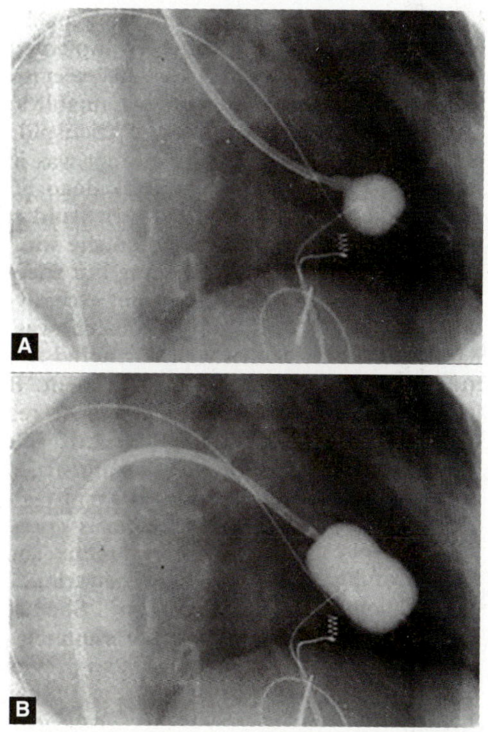


**Fig. 16.77:** The Inoue balloon was used for dilatation of tricuspid stenosis in an adolescent. The valve was reached by an over-the-wire approach with a 0.025 exchange length guide wire. The Inoue stylet would not reach the tricuspid orifice because the right atrium was so large. The Inoue balloon's special dilatation characteristics allowed good positioning at the tricuspid orifice. After dilatation to 27.5 mm, the pressure drop across the valve was reduced from 12–5 mmHg. Further dilatation at 30 mm, however, created moderately severe tricuspid reflux without a further reduction of gradient. The Inoue balloon is suitable for dilatation of tricuspid stenosis but small increments in dilatation size may be required for optimal reduction in gradient without creating significant reflux

- In selected patients with prior tricuspid valve surgery and significant stenosis of a bioprosthetic tricuspid valve or a right atrium to right ventricle (RA-to-RV) conduit, percutaneous tricuspid valve replacement may be an option.
- Transcatheter valve-in-valve implantation with either the Melody or Edwards SAPIEN valve may be a potential procedure for patients with significant tricuspid stenosis, significant tricuspid regurgitation, or a mixed lesion and a failing bioprosthesis.

### Complications

Complications that can be encountered after tricuspid valve replacement include infection of the prosthetic valve, particularly in those instances when endocarditis was present preoperatively. Tricuspid insufficiency and thromboembolization can also occur.

### Prognosis

The prognosis is generally good if therapy is provided for tricuspid stenosis. For those cases in which tumors are the cause of the stenosis, the prognosis is directly related to the prognosis of the underlying disease. In those cases of precipitating infection, if the behavior that caused the initial infection (e.g. intravenous drug use) can be modified, prognosis for the patient is good.

*Further inpatient care:* Inpatient care consists of treating the underlying precipitating condition. For acute bacterial endocarditis or rheumatic causes, antibiotic therapy is indicated until the acute phase has resolved. Then, valve surgery can be considered, if indicated. After valve replacement, inpatient care consists of regulating the anticoagulation and treating postoperative arrhythmias until stability has been achieved. After valve replacement, adjust anticoagulation to an international normalized ratio (INR) of 3–4 because of the low-pressure and low-flow state of the right side. Because of the high risk of thrombosis in this low-pressure system, some authors recommend warfarin therapy for bioprosthetic or mechanical valves.

## 2. TRICUSPID VALVE REGURGITATION

It is defined as leakage of blood into the right atrium during systole of right ventricle.

### Clinical History

Patients with tricuspid regurgitation present with the signs and symptoms of right-sided heart failure. The spectrum of presenting symptoms depends on whether the condition is secondary to left ventricular (LV) dysfunction.

Common presenting complaints in patients with LV dysfunction include the following:

- Dyspnea on exertion
- Orthopnea
- Paroxysmal nocturnal dyspnea
- Ascites
- Peripheral edema
- Exercise intolerance may also be observed. Rarely, patients report angina, which may result from RV overload and strain, even in the absence of coronary artery disease
- These patients, especially those experiencing febrile episodes, must be questioned regarding risk factors for *infective endocarditis*, which is a common cause of tricuspid valvular disease. Risk factors include intravenous drug use, alcoholism, and a history of *rheumatic fever*.

### Physical Examination

Findings on cardiovascular examination in patients with tricuspid regurgitation include the following:

- $S_3$ gallop
- Jugular venous distention with a prominent V wave
- In some patients, a pansystolic murmur
- Diminished peripheral pulse volume secondary to impaired forward blood flow; patients with this sign may have relative hypotension secondary to therapeutic interventions used to decrease volume overload
- Pulmonary rales, if the tricuspid regurgitation is associated with left ventricular dysfunction or *mitral stenosis*
- Right ventricular heave and $S_4$ gallop that increases with inspiration
- Ascites
- Peripheral edema
- Cachexia and jaundice
- Atrial fibrillation
- The pansystolic murmur associated with tricuspid regurgitation is high pitched and is loudest in the fourth intercostal space in the parasternal region. The murmur is usually augmented during inspiration and is reduced in intensity and duration in the standing position and during a Valsalva manoeuvre. A short, early diastolic flow rumble may be present due to increased flow across the tricuspid valve.

### Laboratory Studies

**Serum chemistry:** Findings in patients with tricuspid regurgitation may include abnormal liver function and hyperbilirubinemia secondary to liver congestion.

**Chest radiography:** Findings on chest radiography in patients with tricuspid regurgitation include the following (Fig. 16.78):

- Marked cardiomegaly
- Evidence of elevated right atrial pressure may include distention of the azygous vein and pleural effusions.
- Ascites with diaphragmatic elevation may be present.
- Pulmonary arterial and venous hypertension is common.

### Electrocardiography

ECG findings are usually nonspecific. Typical abnormalities are incomplete right bundle-branch block, Q-waves in lead V1, and atrial fibrillation (Fig. 16.79).

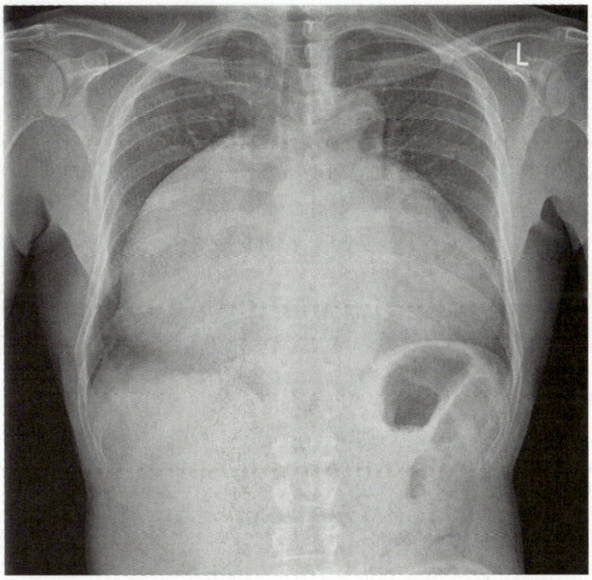


**Fig. 16.78:** Chest X-ray (PA view) showing cardiomegaly with dilatation of RV which was severely impaired, a gigantic RA with free TR and a normal sized LV

### Echocardiography

Color flow Doppler echocardiography is a mainstay for evaluating tricuspid regurgitation. Doppler techniques are used to directly visualize regurgitant jets, measure the flow velocities of the regurgitant jets, and accurately estimate right ventricular systolic pressure (Figs 16.80–16.83).

In trivial-to-mild tricuspid regurgitation, the jet is central and narrow. In moderate-to-severe pulmonic regurgitation, the width of the jet increases, as does the penetration of the jet into the right atrium.

European Society of Cardiology (ESC)/European Association for Cardio-Thoracic Surgery (EACTS) echocardiographic criteria for severe tricuspid regurgitation include the following:

- Abnormal/flail/large coaptation defect
- Very large color flow central jet or eccentric wall impinging jet
- Dense/triangular continuous-wave signal of regurgitant jet with early peaking

Echocardiography is also extremely useful in determining whether the incompetence of the valve is from primary

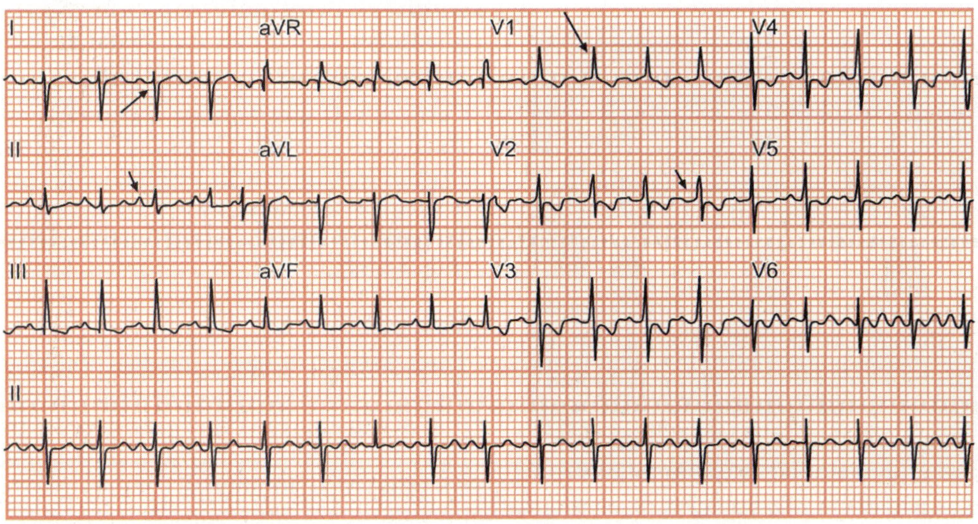


**Fig. 16.79:** Electrocardiogram demonstrating the changes of right ventricular hypertrophy (long arrow) with strain in a patient with primary pulmonary hypertension. Right axis deviation (short arrow), increased P-wave amplitude in lead II (black arrowhead), and incomplete right bundle branch block (white arrowhead) are highly specific but lack sensitivity for the detection of right ventricular hypertrophy

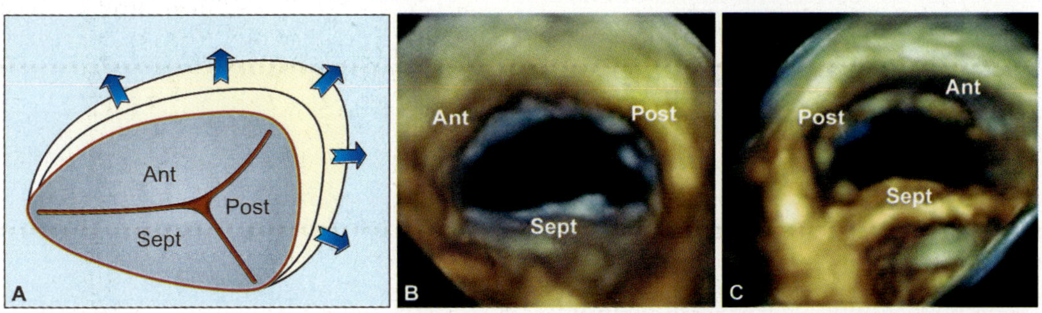


**Fig. 16.80:** 3D TTE assessment of the tricuspid valve. (A) Schematic of the tricuspid valve annulus as it becomes more dilated and circular with tricuspid regurgitation. 3D TTE zoomed view of a normal tricuspid valve from the (B) right atrial and (C) right ventricular perspectives. Ant=anterior; Post=posterior; Sept=septum

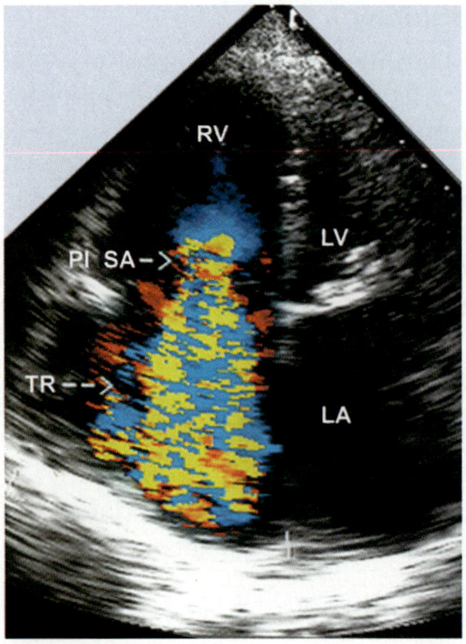


**Fig. 16.81:** Apical four-chamber view of severe tricuspid regurgitation. The Doppler color jet fills the tricuspid regurgitation. LA=left atrium; LV=left ventricle; PISA=proximal isovelocity surface area; RV=right ventricle; TR=tricuspid regurgitation

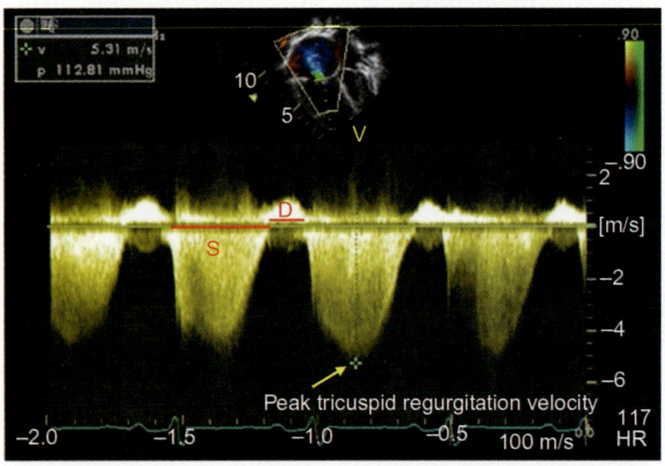


**Fig. 16.83:** Tricuspid regurgitation estimating right ventricular pressure in a patient with pulmonary hypertension. Systolic (S) to diastolic (D) ratio from tricuspid regurgitation velocity can be measured

structural abnormalities of the leaflets and chordae or from secondary myocardial dysfunction and dilatation.

Other possible findings on echocardiography include the following:

- Prolapse of the tricuspid valve, endocarditis, rheumatic heart disease, or Ebstein anomaly may be evident
- The right ventricle is dilated
- Paradoxical motion of the ventricular septum is observed and is similar to that found in an *atrial septal defect*

Using pulsed wave and continuous wave Doppler, right ventricular and pulmonary arterial systolic pressure can be estimated (using continuous wave Doppler) by measuring the peak regurgitant flow velocity across the

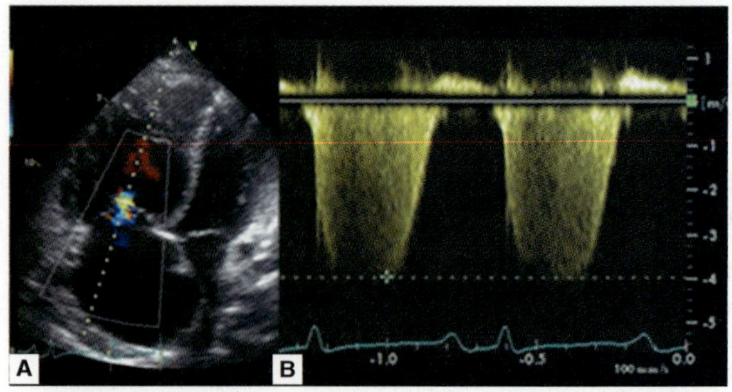


**Fig. 16.82:** (A) 2D Apical 4C view showing tricuspid regurgitation jet into right atrium. (B) Continuous wave (CW)-color Doppler showing tricuspid regurgitant jet

tricuspid valve, converting it to a pressure gradient (by use of the modified Bernoulli equation), and then adding the gradient to an estimate of the right atrial pressure Yang and colleagues proposed that quantification of tricuspid regurgitation by Doppler echocardiography is crucial for estimating prognosis. Their study in patients with severe isolated tricuspid regurgitation found that vena contracta width (VCW) of more than 7 mm is a powerful independent predictor of worsening heart failure, tricuspid valve surgery, and cardiovascular death.

**Cardiac catheterization:** On cardiac catheterization, right atrial pressure and right ventricular end-diastolic pressure are elevated. A rise or no change in right atrial pressure on deep inspiration is characteristic of tricuspid regurgitation. The use of angiography in this setting is controversial (Fig. 16.84).

### Medical Therapy

The medical therapy used in the treatment of tricuspid regurgitation is directed toward the control of heart failure that is causing or contributing to the problem. Drugs used include diuretics, digoxin, and angiotensin-converting enzyme (ACE) inhibitors. Patients who have atrial fibrillation

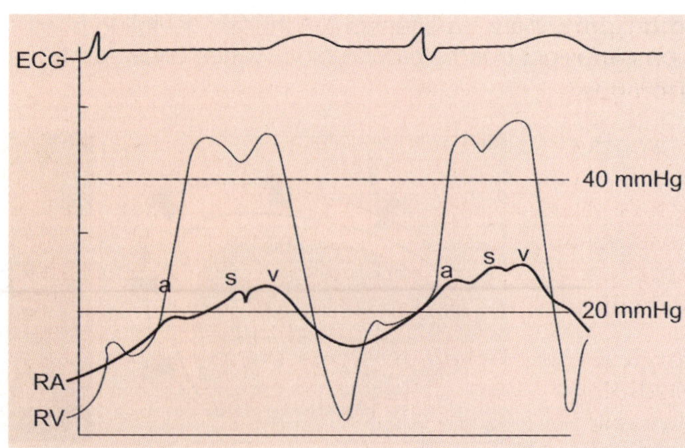


**Fig. 16.84:** Tracings of simultaneous right atrial (RA) and right ventricular (RV) pressure waveforms in a patient with tricuspid regurgitation

or who have received a prosthetic valve require anticoagulation. For patients in whom tricuspid regurgitation is secondary to left-sided heart failure, treatment centers on adequate control of fluid overload and failure symptoms (e.g. diuretic therapy). Patients should be instructed to reduce their intake of salt. Elevation of the head of the bed may improve symptoms of shortness of breath.

**Furosemide (Lasix):** Furosemide increases excretion of water by interfering with the chloride-binding cotransport system, which in turn inhibits sodium and chloride reabsorption in the ascending loop of Henle and distal renal tubule. The dose must be individualized to the patient. Depending on response, administer at increments of 20–40 mg, no sooner than 6–8 h after the previous dose, until desired diuresis occurs. When treating infants, titrate with 1 mg/kg/dose increments until a satisfactory effect is achieved.

**Digoxin (Lanoxin, Digox):** Digoxin is a cardiac glycoside with direct inotropic effects in addition to indirect effects on the cardiovascular system. This agent acts directly on cardiac muscle, increasing myocardial systolic contractions. Its indirect actions result in increased carotid sinus nerve activity and enhanced sympathetic withdrawal for any given increase in mean arterial pressure.

**ACE inhibitors** are used to provide afterload reduction, thereby decreasing the volume load on the right ventricle.

**Captopril:** Captopril prevents conversion of angiotensin I to angiotensin II, a potent vasoconstrictor, resulting in increased levels of plasma renin and a reduction in aldosterone secretion.

**Enalapril (Vasotec):** Enalapril is a competitive ACE inhibitor that reduces angiotensin II levels and decreases aldosterone secretion.

**Lisinopril (Zestril, Prinivil):** Lisinopril prevents conversion of angiotensin I to angiotensin II, resulting in decreased aldosterone secretion.

**Anticoagulants, Cardiovascular:** In patients who have undergone valve replacement for treatment of severe tricuspid regurgitation, anticoagulants are used to prevent thrombosis and embolization from the prosthetic valve.

**Warfarin (Coumadin, Jantoven):** Warfarin interferes with hepatic synthesis of vitamin K-dependent coagulation factors. It is used for prophylaxis and treatment of venous thrombosis, pulmonary embolism, and thromboembolic disorders. Tailor the dose to maintain an international normalized ratio (INR) in the range of 2–3.

**Surgical Care:** Guidelines from the European Society of Cardiology and the European Association for Cardio-Thoracic Surgery (ESC/EACTS) note that the need for correction of tricuspid regurgitation is usually considered at the time of surgical correction of left-sided valve lesions (Fig. 16.85).

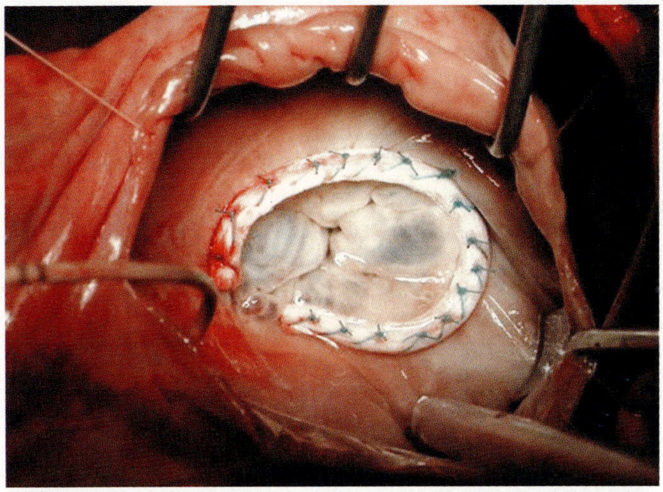

**Fig. 16.85:** Tricuspid valve annuloplasty using semiflexible ring (provided Doc. Petr Nimec, M.D., PhD., Center of Cardiovascular and Transplant Surgery, Brno, Czech Republic)

*Class I ESC/EACTS indications for tricuspid valve surgery are as follows:*
- Symptomatic patients with severe tricuspid stenosis
- Patients with severe tricuspid stenosis undergoing left-sided valve intervention
- Patients with severe primary or secondary tricuspid regurgitation undergoing left-sided valve surgery
- Symptomatic patients with severe isolated primary tricuspid regurgitation without severe right ventricular (RV) dysfunction

*Class IIa ESC/EACTS indications for tricuspid valve surgery are as follows:*
- Patients with moderate primary tricuspid regurgitation undergoing left-sided valve surgery
- Patients with mild or moderate secondary tricuspid regurgitation with dilated annulus undergoing left-sided valve surgery
- Asymptomatic or mildly symptomatic patients with severe isolated primary tricuspid regurgitation and progressive RV dilatation or deterioration of RV function

The ESC/EACTS guidelines also recommend that after left-sided valve surgery, isolated tricuspid valve surgery should be considered in patients with severe tricuspid regurgitation who are symptomatic or who have progressive RV dilatation/dysfunction, provided that they do not have left-sided valve dysfunction, severe right or left ventricular dysfunction, or severe pulmonary vascular disease.

Severe regurgitation has been successfully treated with tricuspid annuloplasty. Long-term results with prosthetic rings are superior to those achieved with suture annuloplasty.

## Long-term Monitoring

Patients with a history of tricuspid regurgitation should be carefully monitored for control of any heart failure. Repeat echocardiography is indicated at 6-month intervals for patients in whom the valve has been removed. Annual echocardiography should be considered in patients whose valve has been replaced.

## PULMONARY VALVULAR DISORDERS

Diseases of the pulmonary valve are most often congenital, and only rarely do acquired disorders such as carcinoid and *rheumatic fever* affect the pulmonary valve. The pulmonary valve may be stenotic or atretic, or the leaflets of the valve may be absent. Pulmonary stenosis may be valvar, supravalvar, or subvalvar (i.e. *double-chambered right ventricle*); it may also be in the branch pulmonary arteries. These lesions are collectively described as right ventricular outflow tract obstructions.

### 1. PULMONIC STENOSIS

A stenotic pulmonary valve usually occurs without associated congenital abnormalities, although it may be associated with other structural abnormalities of the heart. To distinguish the former from the latter, terms such as pulmonary stenosis with a normal aortic root or pulmonary stenosis with an intact ventricular septum have been used. However, the term isolated pulmonary valve stenosis is preferred. The term isolated may be used even when a patent foramen ovale or a small atrial septal defect is present. The term congenital need not be used because most are congenital.

#### Pathologic Anatomy

Pathologic features of the stenotic pulmonary valve vary. The most common pathology is a dome-shaped pulmonary valve. The fused leaflets of the pulmonary valve protrude from their attachment into the pulmonary artery as a conical, windsock-like structure. The size of the pulmonary valve orifice varies from a pinhole to several millimeters. The orifice is most usually central but can be eccentric. Raphae, presumably fused commissures of the valve, extend from the stenotic orifice to a variable distance down lmonary valve stenosis into the base of the dome-shaped valve. The number of the raphe may vary from 0–7. Relatively uncommon variants are unicommissural, bicuspid, and tricuspid valves. The valve annulus is abnormal in most cases, and the fibrous back bone is partially or completely lacking; therefore, a true annulus may not be present.

Hypoplasia of the pulmonary valve ring and dysplastic pulmonary valves may be present in a few of patients. Pulmonary valve dysplasia is characterized by thickened, nodular, and redundant valvular leaflets with minimal or no commissural fusion; hypoplasia of the valve ring; and lack of poststenotic dilatation of the pulmonary artery. The obstruction is mainly related to thickened, myxomatous, immobile pulmonary valve cusps and hypoplasia of the valve ring.

Changes secondary to pulmonary valve obstruction occur in the right ventricle and pulmonary artery. Hypertrophy of the right ventricular muscle is proportional to the degree (and perhaps the duration) of obstruction. The muscle hypertrophy is particularly prominent in the infundibular region and may become physiologically important; this appears to be related to the degree and duration of obstruction. Mild dilatation of the right ventricular cavity is present. In extremely severe or critical obstruction, the right ventricular cavity may be markedly dilated. In rare cases, the right ventricle may be hypoplastic.

The main pulmonary artery is dilated in almost all cases. This dilatation is independent of the severity of the pulmonary valve obstruction and presumably related to a high-velocity jet across the stenotic valve. As noted above, such poststenotic dilatation is remarkably absent in patients with dysplastic pulmonary valves. An interatrial communication, a *patent foramen ovale* or an *atrial septal defect* may be present and may be the seat for right-to-left shunt in patients with severe or long-standing pulmonary stenosis.

Pulmonary valve stenosis is the most common cardiac lesion in *Noonan syndrome* [phenotypically *Turner syndrome* and genotypically normal (XX or XY)]. Supravalvar pulmonary stenosis is often associated with rubella syndrome and Williams syndrome (i.e. elfin facies, supravalvar aortic stenosis, and hypercalcemia with or without mental retardation). Isolated infundibular or subvalvar pulmonary stenosis is uncommon and usually associated with a *ventricular septal defect (VSD)*, such as in tetralogy of Fallot. Peripheral pulmonary stenosis is frequently observed in newborns. It is related to relative narrowing of the branch pulmonary arteries and the acute angle of the origin of the branch pulmonary arteries at this age. This represents fetal pattern and, in most cases, resolves over time.

#### Clinical History

Most children with pulmonic stenosis, particularly those with trivial and mild pulmonary stenosis, present with asymptomatic cardiac murmurs that are detected during routine examination.

Patients with moderate or severe pulmonary stenosis may have mild exertional dyspnea. Adults may be asymptomatic irrespective of the severity of their obstruction.

Patients with severe or critical obstruction may present with signs of systemic venous congestion, which are usually interpreted as signs of congestive heart failure (CHF). The signs are due to severe right ventricular dysfunction or to cyanosis secondary to a right-to-left shunt across a patent foramen ovale or an atrial septal defect.

Lightheadedness, *syncope*, and chest pain that resembles angina pectoris are rare, even in patients with severe obstruction.

Of note, many patients with moderate or severe pulmonary stenosis remain asymptomatic.

#### Physical Examination

##### *Degree of Obstruction*

Physical findings depend on the degree of obstruction. Most patients with pulmonary stenosis appear healthy and are well developed. Indeed, the chubby and rounded faces, described as moon facies, were initially thought to be characteristic for this anomaly, but this facial appearance is not a helpful diagnostic tool. Most patients with trivial, mild, or moderate stenosis, and many with severe stenosis, are acyanotic. However, some may have cyanosis secondary to an interatrial right-to-left shunt.

**The jugular venous pulse** is normal. However, in patients with decreased right ventricular compliance (i.e. severe stenosis), a prominent α wave may be visualized in the neck pulsation. Patients may have a concomitant presystolic pulsation in the liver as well.

In patients with trivial or mild obstruction, the right ventricular impulse is normal. When the pulmonary stenosis is moderate to severe, a sustained and forceful right ventricular impulse and a right ventricular heave are felt.

**A thrill** may be felt in the suprasternal notch and at the left upper sternal border (pulmonic area). The precordial thrill is most likely to be associated with severe obstruction, although no consistent relationship is observed between the thrill and the degree of obstruction.

**Upon auscultation,** the first heart sound may be normal in intensity or may be loud. The second heart sound is widely split. The width of the split increases with worsening stenosis. The intensity of pulmonary component of the second heart sound may be loud (in mild stenosis) or may be soft, diminished, or absent, depending on the severity of obstruction. A fourth heart sound may be heard at the left lower sternal border in patients with severe obstruction and is usually associated with prominent α wave in the jugular pulse.

**An ejection systolic click** is heard along the left sternal border and varies with respiration (decreases or disappears during inspiration). With increasing severity, the click comes closer to the first heart sound.

**An ejection systolic murmur** of grade II/VI to V/VI is best heard at the left upper sternal border with radiation into infraclavicular regions, axillae, or back. The intensity of the murmur is not necessarily related to the severity of pulmonary valve obstruction, but the duration and timing of peaking of the murmur are related to the severity of stenosis.

**An early diastolic decrescendo murmur** of pulmonary regurgitation is not usually heard in the typical case of pulmonary stenosis. Previous surgical or balloon intervention or valvar calcification may result in such a murmur.

**A holosystolic murmur** at the left lower sternal border, which indicates *tricuspid regurgitation,* may be audible in some patients with extremely severe pulmonary stenosis.

**Hepatosplenomegaly** is not usually present and may develop in cases of CHF.

**Peripheral pulmonary stenosis (commonly encountered in the neonate)** is usually associated with a grade II/VI ejection systolic murmur that radiates into the posterior lung fields and axillae. The pathology of peripheral pulmonary stenosis is related to branch pulmonary arteries that are relatively small compared with the large main pulmonary artery, as well as to the acute angular takeoff of the branch pulmonary arteries from the main pulmonary artery specific to a neonate's anatomy. This condition and the associated murmur usually resolve spontaneously in the first month of life.

### *Clinical Assessment of Severity*

The severity of the obstruction of the pulmonary valve can often be estimated by carefully analyzing the ausculatory findings. The timing of the ejection click, the extent of splitting of the second heart sound, the intensity of the pulmonary component of the second sound, the duration of the systolic murmur, and the timing of the peaking of the ejection murmur usually indicate the severity of pulmonary valve stenosis.

**In valvar pulmonic stenosis**, the severity of obstruction may be judged by auscultatory findings. In mild stenosis, the ejection click (EC) is clearly separated from the first heart sound (S1). The murmur starts with the click, peaks in early systole, and ends way before the aortic component of the second heart sound (A2) The pulmonary component of the second heart sound (P2) is normal to increased in intensity. In moderate pulmonic stenosis, the click is closer to the first heart sound, the ejection murmur peaks later in the systole and the murmur reaches the A2, and the second heart sound is widely split with soft pulmonary component. In severe valvar obstruction, the click is either absent or occurs so close to S1 that it cannot be heard separately, and the murmur peaks late in systole and extends beyond the A2. The second heart sound is widely split with an extremely soft or inaudible P2.

1. **With trivial and mild cases of pulmonary valve obstruction**, the click is clearly separated from the first heart sound. Almost normal splitting of the second heart sound with normal or slightly increased pulmonary component of the second heart sound is heard. An ejection systolic, diamond-shaped murmur that peaks early in systole and that ends much before the aortic component of the second heart sound is appreciated.
2. **Findings in moderate pulmonary valve stenosis** include an ejection systolic click that is closer to the first heart sound than it is in mild forms, a widely split second sound with a diminished pulmonary component, and an ejection systolic murmur that peaks in mid-to-late systole and that ends just before the aortic component of the second heart sound.
3. **In severe narrowing of the pulmonary valve**, ausculatory features are an ejection systolic click that is absent or that occurs so close to the first heart sound that it becomes inseparable from it, markedly increased splitting with a soft or inaudible pulmonary component of the second heart sound, and a long ejection systolic murmur that peaks late in systole and that extends beyond the aortic component of the second heart sound so that the latter cannot be heard. The duration and time of peaking of the ejection systolic murmur, and not its intensity, indicate the severity of the pulmonary valve obstruction. The longer the murmur and the later it

peaks, the more severe the obstruction. Likewise, the shorter the interval between the first heart sound and ejection click, the wider the splitting of the second heart sound, and the softer the pulmonary component, the more severe the stenosis of the pulmonary valve.

### Aetiological Factors

Pulmonary valve stenosis is primarily due to maldevelopment of the pulmonary valve tissue and the distal portion of the bulbus cordis, which is characterized by fusion of leaflet commissures, resulting in a thickened and domed appearance of the valve. Although familial forms of pulmonary stenosis are described, it is generally considered to be multifactorial in origin. Rates of recurrence in siblings are on the order of 2–3%. The prevalence of pulmonary stenosis in the offspring of a parent with pulmonary stenosis is 3.6%. Aberrant flow patterns in utero may also be partly associated with maldevelopment of the pulmonary valve.

### Laboratory Studies

Laboratory evaluation is usually not helpful in pulmonary valve stenosis.

**Hemoglobin and hematocrit measurements** in patients with cyanosis may be helpful in that they are increased in patients with right-to-left shunt. The degree of polycythemia is proportional to the degree and duration of right to left shunt. Microcytosis and hypochromia suggest iron deficiency and warrant treatment with iron supplement.

**Oximetry** provides information of potential right-to-left shunting in borderline cyanotic lesions but does not help in identifying the cause of the shunt (pulmonary, interatrial, interventricular, and great arterial).

Although arterial blood gas (*ABG*) analysis is usually not needed, one notable exception is the hyperoxia test in the newborn with cyanosis of undetermined origin.

**The fraction of inspired oxygen (FIO2)** of 1 (100% oxygen) generally does not increase the partial pressure of oxygen to more than 100 mmHg in patients with a cyanotic congenital heart defect (right-to-left intracardiac shunt).

### Chest Radiography

Chest radiographs reveal a prominent main pulmonary artery segment, but the size of the heart is usually normal posteroanterior chest roentgenogram in a patient with valvar pulmonic stenosis shows normal-sized heart with normal pulmonary vascular markingswith prominent main pulmonary (Fig. 16.86).

Pulmonary vascular markings are usually normal, but they may be decreased in severe pulmonary stenosis with associated right-to-left shunt. Cardiomegaly with right ventricular and right atrial enlargement may be seen in severe valvar pulmonary stenosis, with or without tricuspid insufficiency.

### Electrocardiography

Electrocardiographic (ECG) findings are usually normal in mild pulmonary stenosis. Right-axis deviation and right ventricular hypertrophy occur in moderate and severe valvar pulmonary stenosis. The degree of right ventricular hypertrophy is well correlated with the severity of pulmonary stenosis. Some studies demonstrated good correlation between the height of the R wave in lead V1 and right ventricular peak systolic pressure; the height of the R wave in V1 in mm multiplied by 5 is predictive of right ventricular peak systolic pressure. While the electrocardiogram is a useful noninvasive tool in the evaluation of severity of pulmonary stenosis, Doppler echocardiography provides a more direct indication of the severity of obstruction. Right atrial hypertrophy and right ventricular hypertrophy with strain pattern are observed when pulmonary stenosis is severe. A superior QRS axis (left-axis deviation) is seen with dysplastic pulmonary valves and Noonan syndrome (Fig. 16.87).

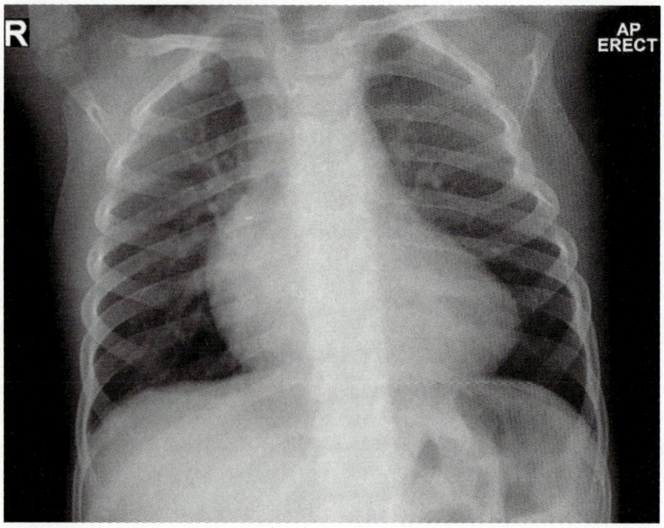


**Fig. 16.86:** Elevation of the cardiac apex and cardiomegaly with peripheral pruning of the pulmonary vasculature

### Echocardiography

The sine qua non of diagnosis is two-dimensional and Doppler echocardiography. A thickened pulmonary valve with restricted systolic motion (doming) in the parasternal short axis and subcostal views is demonstrated. Multiple views are used to confirm the absence of coexistent congenital cardiac disease. Dilatation of the main pulmonary artery distal to the stenotic orifice commonly occurs. Markedly thickened, nodular, and immobile pulmonary valve leaflets may be recognized easily and suggest dysplastic pulmonary valves (Figs 16.88 and 16.89).

The pulmonary valve annulus can also be visualized and measured. Measurements can be compared with normal values to determine if the annulus is hypoplastic. Such measurements are also useful in selecting the diameter of the balloon to be used during balloon valvuloplasty.

**Pulsed, continuous-wave (or high-frequency pulsed), and color-Doppler evaluation,** in conjunction with two-dimensional echocardiography, is most useful in confirming the clinical diagnosis and in quantitating the degree of obstruction.

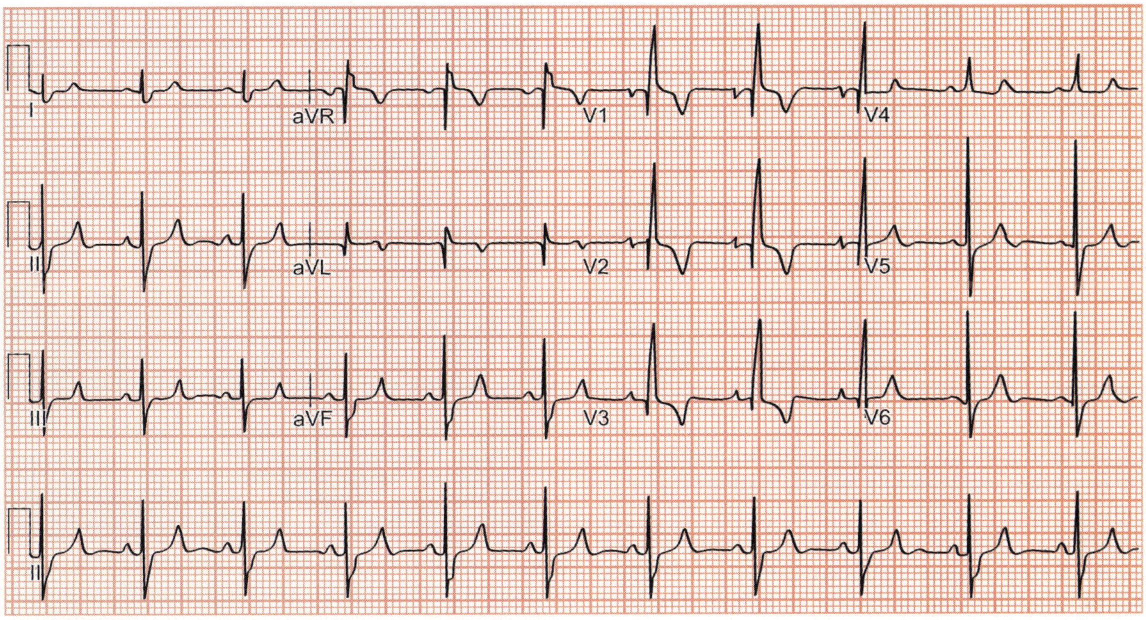


Fig. 16.87: Patient with severe pulmonary stenosis. The ECG shows right bundle branch block with right ventricular hypertrophy

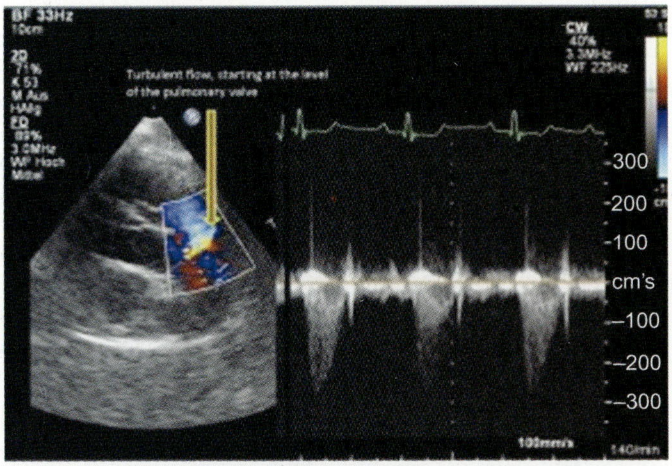


Fig. 16.88: Color flow Doppler—systolic turbulence starting at the pulmonic valve and extending into the pulmonary artery. Mild pulmonic insufficiency. Mild tricuspid regurgitation

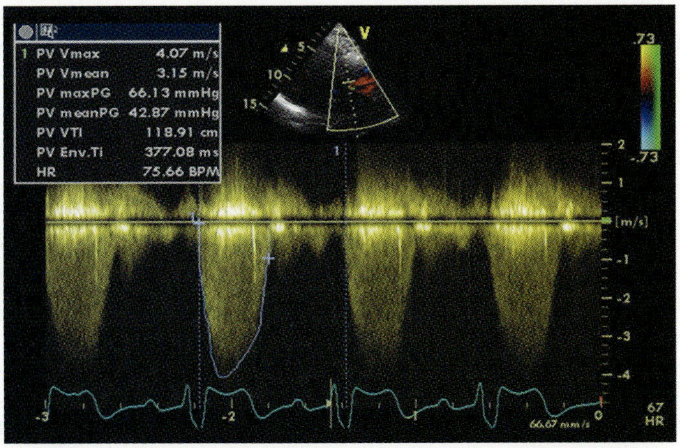


Fig. 16.89: Continuous-wave Doppler signal of transpulmonary flow in pulmonic stenosis

**Pulsed Doppler interrogation of the right ventricular outflow tract** with sample volume moved across the pulmonary valve demonstrates an abrupt increase in peak Doppler flow velocity, which suggests pulmonary valve obstruction. In addition, the flow pattern in the main pulmonary artery is turbulent instead of laminar. Color-Doppler imaging also shows smooth, laminar sub-pulmonary flow (blue) and some flow acceleration (red) immediately beneath the pulmonary valve, with turbulent (mosaic) flow beginning immediately distal to the pulmonary valve leaflets.

Doppler studies can be used to accurately determine the velocity of flow at single or multiple levels, which then can be converted to reproducible pressure gradients by applying the modified Bernoulli equation, as follows: pressure gradient (in millimeters of mercury) = 4 × (velocity in meters/second) 2.

The use of several views and measurements increases the accuracy of the predicted gradient of peak systolic pressure.

Doppler study should be performed when the patient is quiet and in a resting state. Young children and patients who are extremely anxious may have to be mildly sedated.

Severe pulmonary stenosis with gradients of more than 50 mmHg, as diagnosed using a continuous-wave Doppler recording through the pulmonary valve, should be treated with balloon valvuloplasty or surgery. However, Doppler measurements represent peak instantaneous gradients, whereas catheterization gradients are peak-to-peak gradients; recognition of this concept is more important with aortic-valve gradients than with pulmonary-valve gradients. The peak instantaneous gradient was initially thought to reflect the peak-to-peak systolic gradient measured during cardiac catheterization. However, this peak instantaneous gradient overestimates the peak-to-peak gradient, presumably because of a pressure-recovery phenomenon. In the authors' experience, the catheter peak-to-peak gradient is somewhere in between the Doppler peak instantaneous and mean gradients.

Infundibular gradients secondary to severe right ventricular hypertrophy may be present, but these are not usually observed because severe obstruction of the distal pulmonary valve masks infundibular gradients. However, the infundibular gradients do appear after balloon pulmonary valvuloplasty. A triangular pattern of Doppler signal, similar to that described in subaortic obstruction, is characteristic of infundibular obstruction.

Pulmonary insufficiency is easily seen during pulsed, continuous-wave, or color-Doppler imaging, but is unlikely to be present without previous surgical or balloon pulmonary valvuloplasty.

**Color-Doppler and pulsed Doppler interrogation** of the atrial septum is useful and may reveal a left-to-right or right-to-left shunt. Because of high sensitivity of color-Doppler imaging, contrast echocardiography is not routinely used to document right-to-left shunt. Most children with pulmonary stenosis do not require evaluation beyond echocardiograph.

### Computed Tomography Scanning and Magnetic Resonance Imaging

Computed tomography (CT) scanning and magnetic resonance imaging (MRI) may reveal pulmonary valve stenosis, but the state-of-the-art echocardiography and Doppler studies are more useful than CT or MRI in diagnosing and quantitating pulmonary valve obstruction (Fig. 16.90).

### Nuclear Studies

Myocardial energy demands and perfusion may be evaluated by performing magnetic resonance spectroscopy and positron emission tomography (PET), respectively. However, the clinical use of these techniques in the management of pulmonic stenosis has not been established.

### Cardiac Catheterization and Selective Cineangiography

Catheterization is not indicated in mild pulmonary stenosis but is essential in severe stenosis and is an integral part of balloon pulmonary valvuloplasty. This procedure is used to confirm the diagnosis; to discern the degree of obstruction; to assess the morphology of the right ventricle, pulmonary outflow tract, and pulmonary arteries; and to exclude other associated cardiac abnormalities.

### Staging

The severity of pulmonary valve obstruction may be categorized (staged) as follows, based on peak-to-peak catheter-measured pulmonary valvar gradient:

- Trivial: Gradient of less than 25 mmHg
- Mild: Gradient of 25–49 mmHg
- Moderate: Gradient of 50–79 mmHg
- Severe: Gradient of more than 80 mmHg

This severity classification is useful in categorizing patients as per the natural history studies and in formulating treatment algorithms.

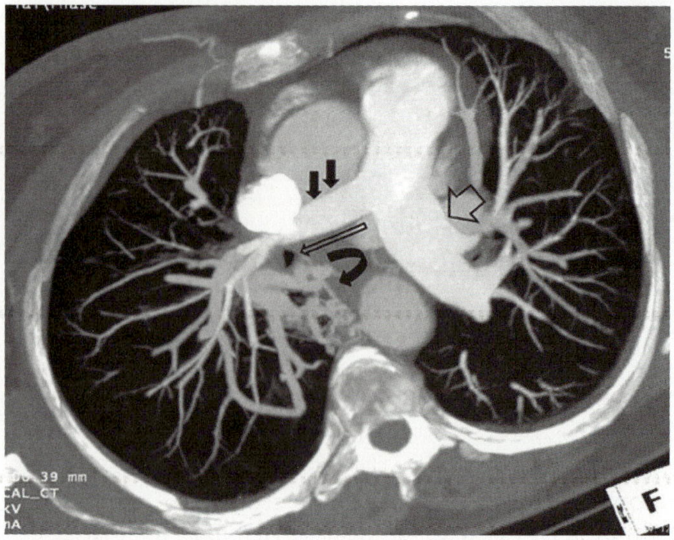

**Fig. 16.90:** On axial MIP CT image; at the upper and lower branches of the right main pulmonary artery (black arrows) diffuse hypoplasia, left main pulmonary artery (open thick arrow), hypoplasia of the right intermediate and middle lobe bronchus (open long arrow) was detected

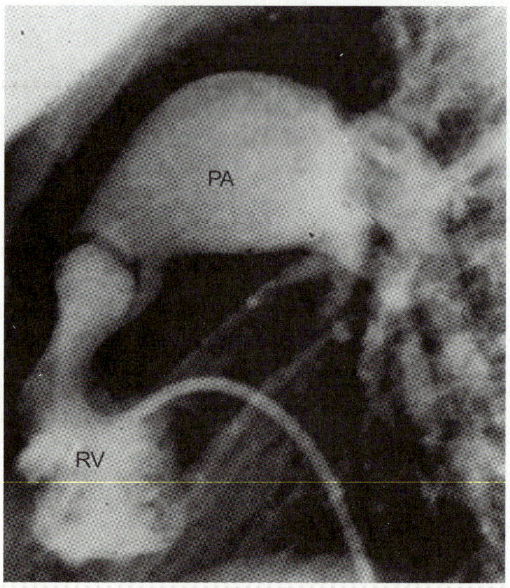


**Fig. 16.91:** Right ventricular (RV) cineangiogram in lateral view in a child with valvar pulmonary stenosis demonstrating thickened and domed pulmonary valve leaflets and poststenotic dilatation of the pulmonary artery (PA). Reproduced with permission from Rao PS. Diagnosis and management of acyanotic heart disease: Part I–obstructive lesions. Indian J Pediatr 2005;72:495–502

Patients with echocardiographic evidence of clinically significant pulmonary stenosis (50–60 mmHg) should undergo diagnostic and therapeutic cardiac catheterization with preparation for balloon dilatation of the pulmonary valve.

Oxygen-saturation data usually do not show evidence of left-to-right shunts. A right-to-left shunt across the patent foramen ovale (or an atrial defect) may be present in moderate-to-severe obstruction of the pulmonary valve.

### Pressure Measurements

Note the following:

- Right atrial pressure (particularly a wave) may be increased.
- Right-ventricular peak systolic pressure is increased; the magnitude of the pressure is proportional to the degree of obstruction.
- The transpulmonary valve peak-to-peak gradient also indicate the severity of obstruction. A peak-to-peak gradient in excess of 50 mmHg is usually considered an indication for therapeutic intervention. Some workers use 40 mmHg as an indication for intervention.

### Cine-Angiography

Right ventricular angiography usually reveals thickened and domed leaflets of the pulmonary valve (see the image below) with a thin jet of contrast material across the pulmonary valve. Enlargement and hypertrophy of the right ventricle and a dilated main pulmonary artery are also seen. In patients with severe or long-standing pulmonary valve obstruction, infundibular constriction may be seen.Additional cineangiograms at other locations are not necessary unless the echocardiographic and hemodynamic data suggest other abnormalities (Fig. 16.91).

### Medical Care

#### *Prehospital Care in Patients with Pulmonary Valve Stenosis*

Collect essential information about vital signs, including the patient's pulse, respiratory rate, work of breathing, and blood pressure (BP) in the upper and lower extremities. Note the presence or absence of cyanosis.

Associated congenital cardiac anomalies should be anticipated until proven otherwise.

If the patient has a known large left-to-right shunt, such as *patent ductus arteriosus (PDA)* or ventricular septal defect (VSD), and if the patient is in respiratory distress, diuresis should be attempted. Diuresis is effective in reducing the cyanosis secondary to pulmonary edema, which is unusual in patients with isolated pulmonary valve stenosis.

Use of oxygen may reduce pulmonary artery pressure in patients with a reactive pulmonary vasculature, increasing pulmonary blood flow, which is also unusual in patients with isolated pulmonary valve stenosis.

Administer oxygen to any patient with cyanosis and respiratory distress. However, cyanosis-related intracardiac right-to-left shunting does not resolve hypoxemia.

#### *Emergency Department Care*

Limited diagnostic tests are needed after the structural diagnosis is made. Workup performed for the cyanotic infant with respiratory distress and hypotension or shock is often the same as that performed in a septic patient.

If a neonate or young infant presents to the emergency room with severe cyanosis, ductal dependent lesions should be considered. Prostaglandin infusion may open the ductus, augment pulmonary blood flow, and improve oxygen saturation.

#### *Therapeutic Approach*

Patients with trivial (gradient <25 mmHg) or mild (gradient <50 mmHg) pulmonary stenosis do not need intervention to relieve the obstruction of the pulmonary valve. They should be clinically followed up at periodic intervals, perhaps on a yearly basis. During the period of rapid growth (infancy and adolescence), follow-up more frequent than this may be indicated. Routine well-child care, including immunizations by the primary physician, should be provided. Patients with pulmonary stenosis are candidates for infective endocarditis prophylaxis before they undergo any *bacteremia*-producing procedures and surgery, as indicated in the recommendations of the American Heart Association. Limitations in exercise or activity levels are not needed. Patients with moderate (gradient, 50–79 mmHg) and severe (gradient, >80 mmHg) obstruction should undergo intervention to relieve the stenosis of the pulmonary valve. After the obstruction is relieved, recommended routine care, endocarditis prophylaxis, and exercise limitations are the same as those described for trivial and mild stenosis.

Patients with signs of right ventricular failure should be promptly treated with anticongestive measures, including digitalis and diuretics. However, the problem does not resolve until the obstruction is relieved. Therefore, prompt balloon or surgical intervention should be undertaken. Right ventricular function may not recover completely if intervention is withheld for too long and if myocardial damage sets in.

A fetus with critical pulmonary stenosis or atresia with intact ventricular septum may benefit from pulmonary balloon valvuloplasty in utero, which promotes growth of the right ventricle.

Although the consensus is to offer relief of pulmonary valve obstruction in children with moderate or severe stenoses, this approach is somewhat controversial in adults because of reported lack of progression and the lack of complications in 1 group of adults monitored for 5–24 years in the 1970s. However, a prudent strategy may be to relieve pulmonary valve obstruction in adults with moderate-to-severe pulmonary stenosis, irrespective of their symptoms, because of the potential (1) for myocardial damage associated with long-term pressure overload of the right ventricle, (2) for generally lowered cardiac indices both before and after exercise in adults compared with children, and (3) for exercise-induced hemodynamic abnormalities in adults.

### Surgical Care

#### *Balloon Pulmonary Valvuloplasty*

Rubio-Alverez et al. first attempted to relieve pulmonary valve obstruction with transcatheter methods in the early 1950s. They used a ureteral catheter with a wire to cut open the stenotic pulmonary valve.

In 1979, Semb et al. used a balloon-tipped angiographic (Berman) catheter to rupture pulmonary valve commissures by rapidly withdrawing the inflated balloon across the valve. More recently, Kan et al. applied the techniques of Dotter and Judkin and Gruntzig et al. to relieve

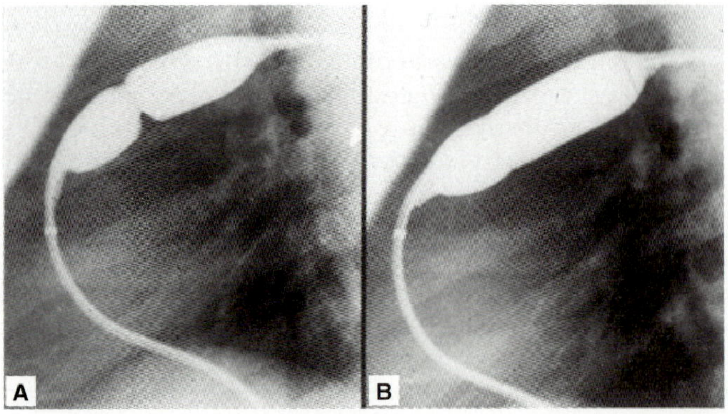

**Fig. 16.92:** Selected cineradiographic frames of a balloon dilatation catheter placed across a stenotic pulmonary valve. Note 'waisting' of the balloon during the initial phases of the balloon inflation (A), which was almost completely abolished during the later phases of balloon inflation (B) (reproduced from Rao PS. Balloon pulmonary valvuloplasty for isolated pulmonic stenosis. In: Rao PS, ed: Transcatheter Therapy in Pediatric Cardiology New York, NY: Wiley-Liss. 1993;59–104)

pulmonary valve obstruction by using the radial forces of balloon inflation of a balloon catheter positioned across the pulmonic valve. This static balloon-dilation technique is currently performed worldwide to relieve pulmonary valve obstruction.

The general consensus based on current data is that balloon valvuloplasty is the treatment of choice for managing isolated pulmonary valve stenosis (Fig. 16.92).

*Indications:* In general, indications for balloon pulmonary valvuloplasty are similar to those used in surgical pulmonary valvotomy (i.e. moderate pulmonary valve stenosis with a peak-to-peak gradient >50 mmHg with a normal cardiac index). Some cardiologists change this criterion to a gradient of 40 mmHg or right ventricular pressure of 50 mmHg. Careful evaluation of the available data suggests that (1) right ventricular pressure is only marginally reduced if mildly stenotic valves are dilated, (2) trivial and mild stenoses (gradient <50 mmHg) are likely to remain mild at follow-up (as shown in natural-history studies) and (3) an increase in gradient is easily quantitated on follow-up Doppler echocardiography. If an increased gradient is documented, the patient can then undergo balloon dilatation. Given these observations, balloon dilation should be performed only in patients with peak-to-peak gradient of more than 50 mmHg.

More recently, the interventional procedures are increasingly performed under general anesthesia and the gradients are usually lower with general anesthesia than with conscious sedation. Consequently, the same criteria should not be applied. Therefore, the Doppler gradients (discussed in echocardiography) should be used in making the decision regarding balloon pulmonary valvuloplasty.

*Technique:* The technique of balloon pulmonary valvuloplasty involves positioning a balloon catheter across the stenotic valve, usually over an extra-stiff exchange-length guide wire and inflating the balloon with diluted contrast material to accomplish valvotomy. The initially recommended balloon-to-annulus ratio was 1.2–1; subsequent data suggested a ratio of 1.2–1.25. When the pulmonary valve annulus is too large to dilate with a single balloon (about 20 mm), valvuloplasty with simultaneous inflation of 2 balloons across the pulmonary valve may be performed, although the current availability of large-diameter balloons make this technique unnecessary. However, the double balloon technique may be more effective and stable in some cases. The Inoue balloon has been used in adults with success. The major advantage of the Inoue balloon over conventional balloons is its adjustable diameter that makes stepwise dilation possible. Nucleus balloons with a waist in the middle have been approved by FDA. They do have theoretical advantage; however, these balloons require large sheaths and not a lot of clinical experience has been accumulated so far. The results of balloon pulmonary valvuloplasty for patients with dysplastic pulmonary valves are generally poor with the use of conventional balloon pulmonary valvuloplasty techniques. Use of large balloons, up to 150% of pulmonary valve annulus, or high-pressure balloons may increase the effectiveness of balloon therapy and avoid the need for surgery.

*Mechanism of valvuloplasty:* Inflation of a balloon placed across an obstructive lesion exerts radial forces on the stenotic lesion without any axial component. The mechanism of valvuloplasty is assessed by directly visualizing the valvar mechanism during surgeryand postmortem examination and by indirect means, such as angiography and echocardiography. Splitting of the valve commissures and tearing and avulsion of the valve leaflets have been observed and are conceivably the mechanism by which balloon dilation relieves pulmonary valve obstruction. The circumferential dilating force that balloon inflation exerts is likely to rupture (tear) the weakest part of the valve mechanism. The fused commissures are the likely weakest links that can be broken with balloon dilation. However, when fused commissures are strong and cannot be torn, the valve cusps can be torn or the valve leaflet avulse. These events are likely to worsen pulmonary insufficiency.

Pulmonary valve dysplasia, if severe, may preclude successful balloon valvuloplasty unless an associated commissural fusion is present.

*Immediate results:* Results observed immediately after balloon valvuloplasty include reduced peak-to-peak gradients and right ventricular-to-left ventricular pressure ratios and increased pulmonary artery pressures, jet widths, and free motion of the pulmonary valve leaflets with decreased doming. Improvement of right ventricular function, tricuspid insufficiency, and right-to-left shunt, if present before dilation, are also documented.

*Infundibular stenosis:* Infundibular gradients occur in nearly 30% patients. The older the patient's age and the greater the severity of obstruction, the greater the prevalence of infundibular reaction. When residual infundibular gradient is >50 mmHg beta-blockade is generally recommended. Infundibular obstruction greatly regresses at follow-up (see the image below), as demonstrated for infundibular reactions after surgical valvotomy. Rare patients require surgical intervention.

*Follow-up evaluation:* Clinical, ECG, and Doppler echocardiographic evaluations are generally recommended at 1 month, 6 months, and 12 months after the procedure and yearly thereafter. Regression of right ventricular hypertrophy, as shown on ECG after balloon dilatation, is well documented. ECG is a useful adjunct in the evaluation of follow-up results. However, ECG evidence of hemodynamic improvement does not become apparent until 6 months after valvuloplasty. The Doppler gradient generally reflects residual obstruction and is a useful and reliable noninvasive monitoring tool.

*Intermediate-term results:* At intermediate-term follow-up (usually <2 years), both catheterization-measured peak-to-peak and Doppler-measured peak instantaneous gradients remain improved as a whole. However, restenosis (gradient >50 mmHg) is observed in nearly 10% patients.

Predictors of restenosis include a balloon-to-annulus ratio of less than 1.2 and a gradient of more than 30 mmHg immediately after valvuloplasty. In addition, early in the study period, a small valve annulus, and a postsurgical or complex pulmonary stenosis were also predictive of restenosis.

Patients with restenosis have been successfully treated with redilatation with balloons larger than those used for initial balloon valvuloplasty. Redilatation is the procedure of choice for managing restenosis after previous balloon dilatation. However, if the pulmonary valve annulus is hypoplastic, if the pulmonary valve leaflets are dysplastic, or if clinically significant supravalvar pulmonary artery stenosis is the major reason for the restenosis, surgery is recommended.

*Long-term follow-up results:* Although immediate and short-term results have been documented, data on long-term results are scarce. Published studies reveal generally low residual peak instantaneous Doppler gradients with minimal (1–2%) late recurrence of pulmonary stenosis (beyond that seen at intermediate follow-up).

In one study, approximately 5% of patients needed surgical intervention to relieve fixed subvalvar or **supravalvar stenosis**. Actuarial freedom for reintervention was 88% and 84%, respectively, at 5 and 10 years. Pulmonary valve insufficiency was noted in 80–90% patients, but right ventricular volume overloading did not develop, and none of the patients required surgical intervention because of pulmonary insufficiency. Based on these data, the authors concluded that balloon pulmonary valvuloplasty may continue to be the treatment of choice for moderate-to-severe valvar pulmonary stenosis, and 10-year to 20-year follow-up studies to evaluate the clinical significance of residual pulmonary insufficiency should be undertaken.

*Clinically significant pulmonary insufficiency:* One report documented the development of clinically significant pulmonary insufficiency in 6 (6%) of 107 patients at late follow-up. Some of these patients required pulmonary valve replacement. In a recent report, 53 patients with pulmonary valve stenosis who had percutaneous balloon valvuloplasty were followed for 10–24 years (median, 15 years); there was only 2% prevalence of restenosis, but late pulmonary regurgitation developed in 89% patients.

### Comparison with Surgical Valvotomy

Comparison of balloon therapy with surgical valvotomy has limitations, but the mortality and morbidity rates are generally higher after surgery. Greater reduction of the gradient is observed after surgery, but the degree and frequency of pulmonary insufficiency may be higher after surgery than after balloon therapy.

*Critical pulmonary stenosis in the neonate:* The term critical pulmonary stenosis with intact ventricular septum is applied to severe pulmonary valvar obstruction resulting in suprasystemic right ventricular systolic pressure with resultant tricuspid insufficiency, a right-to-left shunt across the atrial septum, and often a ductal-dependent pulmonary circulation.

Although the surgical approach to relieve the obstruction with or without aorta-pulmonary shunt was standard treatment in the past, transcatheter treatment is now first-line therapy.

Prostaglandin E1 is infused to augment pulmonary blood flow and improve systemic arterial desaturation, followed by cardiac catheterization and biplane (sitting-up and lateral views) right ventricular cineangiography. A right coronary artery, angled glide, balloon wedge, or cobra catheter (according to the operator's preference) is placed in the right ventricular outflow tract, and a floppy-tipped coronary guidewire is advanced across the pulmonary valve and into the right or left pulmonary artery or into the descending aorta through the ductus. The catheter is advanced across the pulmonary valve into a distal pulmonary artery or the descending aorta. The guidewire is then exchanged for a guidewire that is suited to position the balloon-dilation catheter. Then, balloon pulmonary valvuloplasty is performed in manner described earlier.

In some cases, the balloon catheter cannot be advanced across a severely stenotic pulmonary valve, and balloon catheters 3–6 mm in diameter may be used for initial predilation and then replaced with larger, more appropriately sized balloon catheters (Fig. 16.93).

Although the results of this approach are reasonably good, the need for reintervention to address the complications associated with the procedure, residual obstruction, or associated defects is 25% in neonates compared with older children 8–10%.

### Other Catheter Interventions

Numerous other catheter interventions may become necessary in patients with pulmonary stenosis.

*Transcatheter occlusion of a patent ductus arteriosus (PDA):* Some patients with pulmonary stenosis may have a PDA of significant size. In such patients, transcatheter occlusion of the PDA performed with a coil (for small PDAs) or with an Amplatzer duct occluder (for medium or large PDAs)

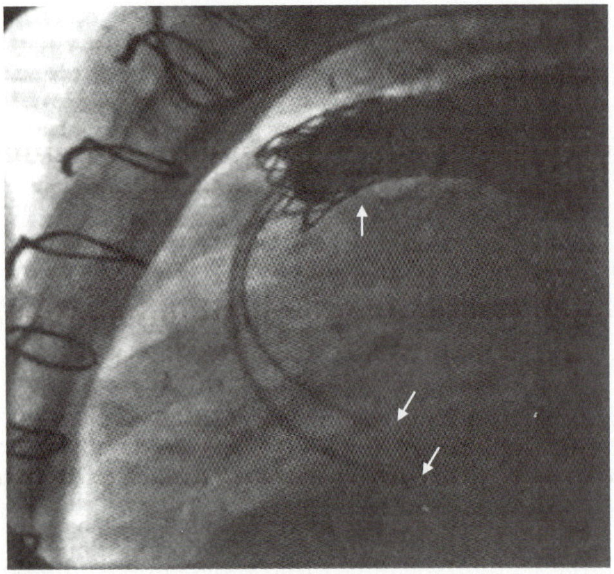

**Fig. 16.93:** Double balloon (arrows) across PV for dilatation of valve in patient with pulmonic stenosis

is recommended immediately after balloon pulmonary valvuloplasty.

*Occlusion of a patent foramen ovale or atrial septal defect:* A patent foramen ovale or atrial septal defect may occur in association with pulmonary stenosis. If these atrial defects do not spontaneously close during follow-up after balloon valvuloplasty, they may be closed with an Amplatzer septal occluder or Helex device, if the criteria for their closure are met. Sometimes, the defects may need to be closed to prevent recurrent paradoxical embolisms.

*Balloon atrial septostomy:* In neonates with a severely hypoplastic right ventricle, balloon atrial septostomy may be necessary to provide adequate egress to the systemic venous return. Indications are clinical signs of systemic venous congestion, restrictive patent foramen ovale on Doppler echocardiography, markedly elevated right atrial pressure with tall a waves, and/or a mean atrial pressure difference of more than 5 mmHg.

In neonates, Rashkind balloon septostomy is effective. Beyond the neonatal period, Park blade septostomy or surgical septostomy may be necessary. In patients with only mild or moderate right ventricular hypoplasia, balloon septostomy should be avoided so that forward flow through the right ventricle is encouraged with a consequent opportunity for its growth.

*Cardiac catheterization with balloon valvuloplasty:* This is the preferred therapy for severe or critical valvar pulmonary stenosis. In neonates with critical valvar pulmonary stenosis, mortality rates related to balloon dilation are lower than those related to surgery mortality, and balloon dilation is the treatment of choice.

### Other Surgical Techniques

Since the first description of surgical relief of pulmonary stenosis by closed pulmonary valvotomy in the late 1940s, various techniques were developed and include valvotomy with inflow occlusion, hypothermia and cardiopulmonary bypass. The currently preferred approach is transpulmonary arterial valvotomy under cardiopulmonary bypass.

*Results:* Results of surgery are generally good with low mortality rate (3–7%) and decreased right ventricular pressures and pulmonary valve gradients. In a natural-history study in the United States, only 3% of 294 operated patients had gradients of more than 50 mmHg at 4–8 years after surgery. The incidence of pulmonary insufficiency at follow-up was 60–90%. Despite these good results, transluminal balloon pulmonary valvuloplasty (discussed above) has replaced surgical pulmonary valvotomy.

*Indications:* Surgery is reserved for cases in which balloon valvuloplasty is not feasible or not successful. One example is dysplastic pulmonary valve with valve ring hypoplasia. The treatment of this disorder is to excise the obstructive valve leaflets and enlarge the annulus by a transannular patch. Other examples are fixed infundibular and supravalvar stenosis after successful balloon valvuloplasty.

*Blalock-Taussig shunt:* Patients with critical pulmonary stenosis and marked hypoplasia of the right ventricle may need a Blalock-Taussig shunt in addition to or instead of balloon or surgical valvotomy.

*Right ventricular repair/bypass:* Right ventricular hypoplasia, as alluded to above, occurs in some patients with pulmonary stenosis, although this hypoplasia is most common in patients with pulmonary atresia and an intact ventricular septum. The right ventricle may enlarge after right ventricular outflow obstruction is relieved, particularly in tripartite right ventricles. If the right ventricle does not grow adequately to support the pulmonary circulation, 1.5 or single ventricular repair should be considered. In 1.5-ventricular repair, a bidirectional Glenn procedure (superior vena cava-to-right pulmonary artery anastomosis, end to side) is performed to divert the blood from the upper part of the body directly into the pulmonary artery, and the atrial septal defect is closed to allow the blood from the lower part of the body to go into the lungs through the right ventricle. In the single ventricle repair, the right ventricle is bypassed by the Fontan procedure. In the Fontan procedure, staged total cavopulmonary connection is performed by bidirectional Glenn initially and then extra conduit diversion of the inferior cava into the pulmonary artery.

## 2. PULMONIC REGURGITATION

The pulmonic valve is normally a thin tricuspid structure that prevents blood from regurgitating into the right ventricle once ejected into the low-pressure pulmonary circulation. Pulmonic regurgitation refers to retrograde flow from the pulmonary artery into the right ventricle during diastole. Physiologic (trace-to-mild) pulmonic regurgitation is present in nearly all individuals, particularly in those with advanced age. However, pathologic conditions that produce excessive and clinically significant regurgitation can result in impairment of right ventricular function and eventual clinical manifestations of right-sided volume overload and heart failure. Often, pulmonic regurgitation is not the primary process but a finding secondary to an underlying process such as pulmonary hypertension or dilated cardiomyopathy.

### Clinical History

Pulmonic regurgitation is seldom clinically significant. However, symptoms of right-sided *heart failure* can occur when the severity and duration of the regurgitation result in right ventricular enlargement and decompensation. Dyspnea on exertion is the most common complaint. Easy fatigability, light-headedness, peripheral edema, chest pain, palpitations, and frank syncope may occur in patients with any cause of right-sided heart failure and do little to elucidate the aetiology of the right-sided failure. Patients who experience these symptoms may attribute them to poor physical fitness or anxiety, delaying evaluation until their condition worsens. In more advanced presentations of right-sided heart failure, abdominal distension secondary to ascites, right upper quadrant pain secondary to hepatic distension, and early satiety may occur.

Other symptoms specific to the underlying disease process causing pulmonic regurgitation may occur. Such disease processes include connective-tissue disease, infective endocarditis, carcinoid heart disease, rheumatic heart disease, and primary or secondary pulmonary hypertension. For example, hemoptysis is generally not associated with pulmonic regurgitation *perse*, but, in severe pulmonary hypertension causing pulmonic regurgitation, it may occur as a result of the associated pulmonary arteriole rupture and hemorrhage and/or parenchymal inflammation.

### Physical Examination

Jugular venous pressure (JVP) is usually increased. Often, an increased A wave is present, but this may be less apparent when significant tricuspid regurgitation with a dominant V wave is also present. When right ventricular enlargement is present, a palpable impulse (lift or heave) is usually present at the left lower sternal border. Palpable pulmonary artery pulsation at the left upper sternal border may be present in the setting of significant pulmonary artery dilatation. With significant pulmonary hypertension, pulmonic valve closure can be palpated.

The pulmonic component of the second heart sound ($P_2$) is inaudible in the absence of a pulmonic valve, whether congenital or secondary to surgical resection. In pulmonic regurgitation due to pulmonary hypertension, $P_2$ is accentuated; with increased right ventricular end-diastolic volume, the ejection time is increased, $P_2$ is delayed, and the $S_2$ split is widened.

A low-pressure regurgitant flow across the pulmonic valve, as occurs when the pulmonary arterial pressure is normal, is heard as a brief, decrescendo early diastolic murmur at the upper left sternal border. It is made louder by squatting or inspiration and softer by Valsalva manoeuvres or expiration. An $S_3$ or $S_4$ may be noted at the left mid-to-lower sternal border because of the presence of right ventricular hypertrophy or failure and is augmented by inspiration.

The Graham Steell murmur of pulmonary hypertension is a high-pitched, early diastolic decrescendo murmur noted over the left upper-to-left midsternal area and is a result of high-velocity regurgitant flow across an incompetent pulmonic valve. The regurgitant flow murmur may be present during the whole of diastole because there is a pulmonary-to-right ventricular pressure gradient throughout this time period. Typically, the murmur occurs in severe pulmonary hypertension when the pulmonary artery systolic pressure is more than 60 mmHg. The quality of this high-pitched early decrescendo diastolic murmur is identical to that of aortic insufficiency. However, the peripheral manifestations of aortic insufficiency are absent. The associated findings of tricuspid regurgitation are frequently present, that is, prominent JVP with surging V waves, holosystolic murmur at the lower left sternal border (louder with inspiration), and enlarged, pulsatile liver.

### Aetiological Factors

Significant pulmonic regurgitation occurs variably as a complication of various conditions.

#### *Primary and Pulmonary Hypertension*

*Primary pulmonary hypertension* occurs in approximately 1 instance per 500,000 cases. This diagnosis can be made only after all other causes have been excluded.

**Secondary pulmonary hypertension (multiple causes)** is the most common cause of pulmonic regurgitation in adults.

#### *Tetralogy of Fallot*

*Tetralogy of Fallot*, especially with congenital absence of the pulmonary valve or postoperative following surgical repair of this condition (e.g. pulmonary valvotomy), may cause significant pulmonic regurgitation.

**Infective endocarditis:** In rare cases, *infective endocarditis* results in significant pulmonic regurgitation. It may occur in an intravenous drug user or an individual with an atrial septal defect and a large left-to-right intracardiac shunt.

#### *Rheumatic and Carcinoid Heart Diseases*

In *rheumatic heart disease* leading to significant pulmonic regurgitation, the pulmonary valve is affected following mitral, aortic, and tricuspid valve involvement.

#### *Medications*

- Medications that act via serotoninergic pathways may result in significant pulmonic regurgitation (e.g. methysergide, pergolide and fenfluramine).
- Disorders that dilate the pulmonic valve ring to create valvular incompetence.

These are the most common cause of pulmonic regurgitation and include primary or secondary pulmonary hypertension, dilatation of the pulmonary trunk in Marfan syndrome or Takayasu arteritis, and idiopathic causes.

*Acquired disorders that alter pulmonic valve morphology:* These conditions include the following:

- ***Rheumatic heart disease:*** In most cases, the other valves (i.e. mitral, aortic, and tricuspid) are also substantially affected.
- ***Trauma from a Swan-Ganz catheter:*** This cause is unusual, but it can result if the catheter tip is withdrawn across the pulmonic valve with the balloon inflated.
- ***Complications related to therapeutic balloon catheter dilatation of a stenotic pulmonic valve*** (e.g. pulmonary balloon valvuloplasty). Such complications are not uncommon; however, in most cases, the degree of regurgitation is clinically insignificant, rendering pulmonic valve balloon catheter dilation a safe and effective treatment for moderate-to-severe pulmonic stenosis in adult and pediatric patients.
- ***Complications of surgical repair of pulmonic stenosis or congenital heart disease,*** such as:
  1. Tetralogy of Fallot
  2. Syphilis infection
  3. *Carcinoid heart disease:* The heart is affected in up to 60% of patients in whom carcinoid has metastasized to the liver, most commonly manifesting as valvular disease. In Pellikka and colleagues' 1993 series of 74 patients, the pulmonic valve was involved in 88%. Of those, 49% exhibited significant pulmonic stenosis, and 81% had significant pulmonic regurgitation.
- ***Congenital disorders that produce an incompetent pulmonic valve:*** These include complete absence of the pulmonic valve and valvular abnormalities (e.g. fenestrations or redundant leaflets).

## Laboratory Studies

Japanese investigators suggest that evels of plasma brain natriuretic peptide (BNP) have the potential to be useful for postsurgical long-term monitoring of patients with tetralogy of Fallot who are under consideration for pulmonary valve replacement to correct pulmonary regurgitation or right-ventricular dysfunction. In their study of 33 patients who underwent repair of tetralogy of Fallot, significantly higher plasma BNP levels were found not only in patients with moderate-severe pulmonary regurgitation compared to those with insignificant or mild pulmonary regurgitation ($P = 0.013$.) but also in patients with cardiac symptoms compared to asymptomatic patients ($P = 0.005$). Following pulmonary valve replacement, there was a significant reduction in mean BNP levels, and the plasma BNP level correlated with the right-ventricular end-diastolic pressure. The investigators reported 32.15 pg/ml was the optimal BNP cut-off level for considering pulmonary valve replacement.

## Chest Radiography

Plain radiographs change little with pulmonic regurgitation unless tricuspid regurgitation also occurs, in which case

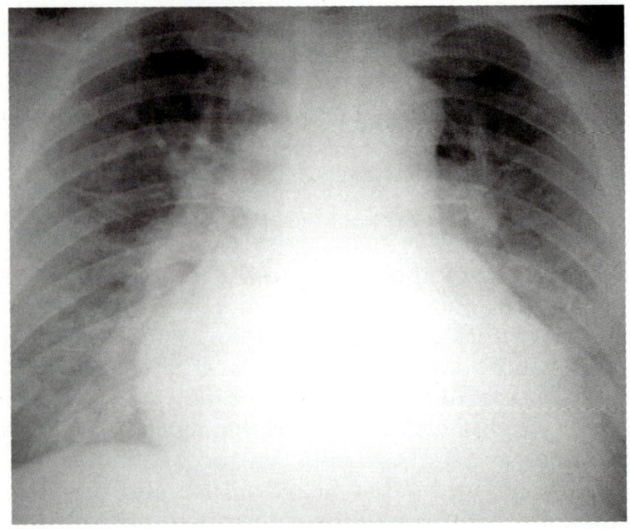

**Fig. 16.94:** Prominent central pulmonary arteries with enlarged hilar vessels and loss of vascularity in the peripheral lung fields ('pruning') suggests severe pulmonary hypertension with valvular regurgitation

cardiomegaly and enlargement of the right-sided heart contour are observed.

Prominent central pulmonary arteries with enlarged hilar vessels and loss of vascularity in the peripheral lung fields ('pruning') suggests severe pulmonary hypertension (Fig. 16.94).

## Electrocardiography

ECG may demonstrate findings of right ventricular dilatation (occurs either while in a compensated volume overload state or in a decompensated pressure overload state), including incomplete right bundle branch block and right axis deviation. Right ventricular hypertrophy may be present by ECG criteria (Fig. 16.95).

In the presence of right ventricular hypertrophy (representing a compensated state of pressure overload), the following may be present:

- Tall R wave in $V_1$ or qR in $V_1$
- R wave greater than S wave in $V_1$
- R wave progression reversal in the precordial leads
- Inverted T-wave in the anterior precordial leads
- Right axis deviation
- Right atrial enlargement

## Echocardiography

Two-dimensional echocardiography (2DE) and M-mode echocardiography can reveal right ventricular hypertrophy and dilatation. Right ventricular volume overload may induce a characteristic abnormal septal wall motion, which appears as flattening of the septum during diastole. Conversely, right ventricular pressure overload usually appears as flattening of the septum during systole. The lack of a pulmonic valve or valve deformities can be noted with 2DE, but the pulmonic valve apparatus typically appears unremarkable. In some cases, pulmonic ring dilatation with poor valve leaflet coaptation may be observed (Figs 16.96–16.98).

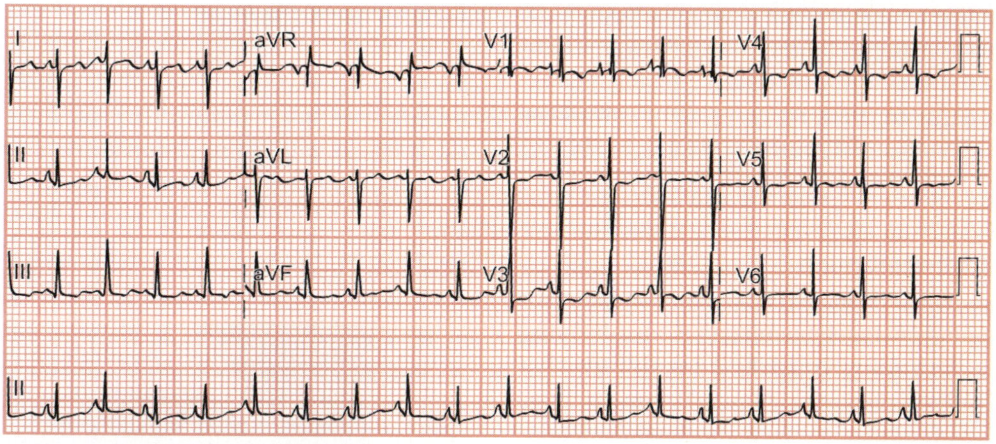


**Fig. 16.95:** ECG showing tall R-wave in V1 or qR in V1, R-wave progression reversal in the precordial leads right axis deviation and right atrial enlargement in pulmonary regurgitation

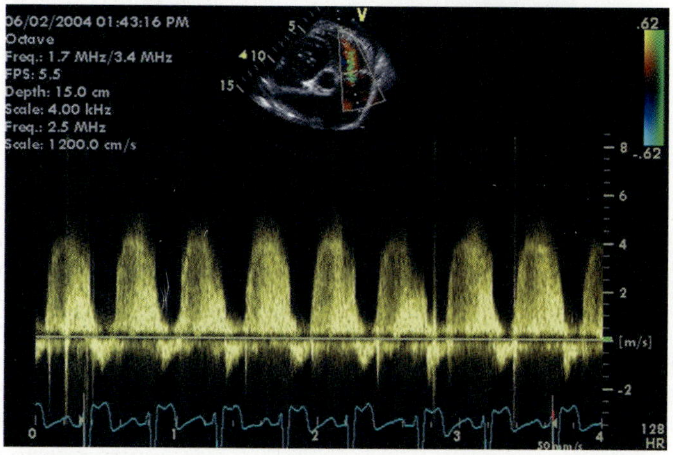


**Fig. 16.96:** Doppler echo scan showing severe type of pulmonary regurgitation in patient with pulmonary valvular insufficiency. Note the positive wave which is consistent with pulmonary insufficiency (positive signals are directed toward the transducer while negative signals are away from the trasducer

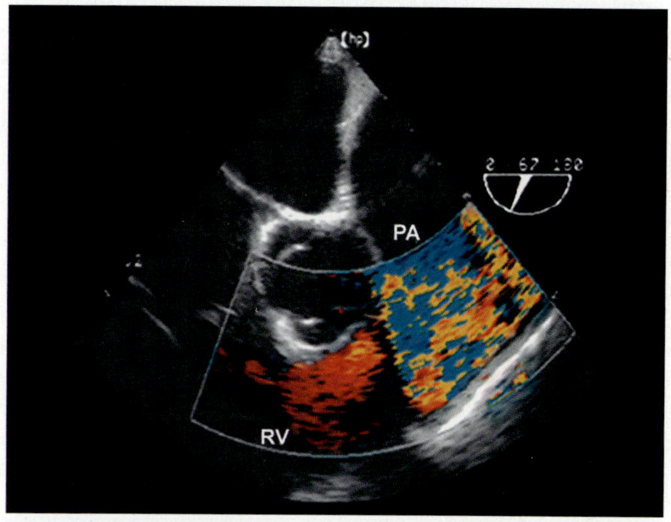


**Fig. 16.97:** Transesophageal echocardiography image with color-Doppler, showing high-velocity, turbulent flow in the main pulmonary artery. Ao=aorta; LA=left atrium; PA=pulmonary artery; RA=right atrium; RV=right ventricle

Doppler techniques are used to visualize the regurgitant flow. These techniques are useful to directly visualize regurgitant jets, measure the flow velocities of the regurgitant jets, and accurately estimate pulmonary pressures. Regurgitation that persists throughout diastole suggests the presence of pulmonary hypertension, whereas regurgitation that diminishes earlier in diastole suggests more normal pulmonary arterial pressures. Normally, peak flow velocity across the pulmonic valve is achieved within 140 milliseconds of systole. With pulmonary hypertension, the peak flow velocity is reached faster. The shortening of the interval within which the peak velocity is reached (acceleration time) is linearly inversely proportional to the severity of the pulmonary hypertension.

Color flow Doppler echocardiography is the mainstay for recognizing pulmonic regurgitation. In trivial-to-mild pulmonic regurgitation, the jet is central and narrow. In moderate-to-severe pulmonic regurgitation, the width of the jet increases, as does the penetration of the jet into the right ventricular outflow tract. In free or open pulmonic regurgitation (usually due to congenitally absent pulmonic valve), color-Doppler can miss the jet altogether due to the brisk and laminar regurgitant flow.

Using pulsed wave and continuous wave Doppler, pulmonary artery systolic and diastolic pressures can be calculated. Pulmonary artery systolic pressure can be estimated (using continuous wave Doppler) in the presence of tricuspid regurgitation by measuring the peak regurgitant flow velocity across the tricuspid valve, converting it to a pressure gradient (by use of the modified Bernoulli equation), and then adding the gradient to an estimate of the right atrial pressure.

Pulmonary artery diastolic pressure can be estimated by measuring the end-diastolic regurgitant flow velocity across the pulmonic valve (at the QRS complex on the ECG), converting it to a pressure gradient, and then adding the gradient to the estimated right atrial pressure. Both pulmonary artery systolic pressure and diastolic pressure are predictors of cardiac status and outcome.

Pulmonary arterial mean pressure can also be estimated by converting the early diastolic regurgitation velocity to a pressure gradient, and then adding it to the estimated right atrial pressure.

### Fluoroscopy and Catheterization

Cardiac catheterization is usually not necessary for diagnosis but may be helpful in determining the underlying aetiology and for determining coexisting conditions that may influence treatment and/or repair decisions (Fig. 16.99).

Pulmonary artery angiography may reveal evidence of multiple pulmonary emboli as a cause of pulmonary hypertension when the degree of clinical suspicion is high. Ventilation/perfusion scanning or CT angiography is now more commonly performed in most hospitals. Pulmonary emboli must be excluded before the diagnosis of primary pulmonary hypertension is possible.

If pressure measurements are performed, the pulmonary artery and right ventricular pressure curves equalize in late diastole in individuals with severe pulmonary regurgitation.

### Cardiac Magnetic Resonance Imaging

Cardiac magnetic resonance imaging (CMRI) has shown promise based on recent studies of pulmonary regurgitation. CMR has excellent temporal and spacial resolution and can provide accurate estimation of the severity of regurgitation, mechanism of regurgitation, and right ventricular size and function. However, size and time constraints limit the use of CMR in clinical practice (Fig. 16.100).

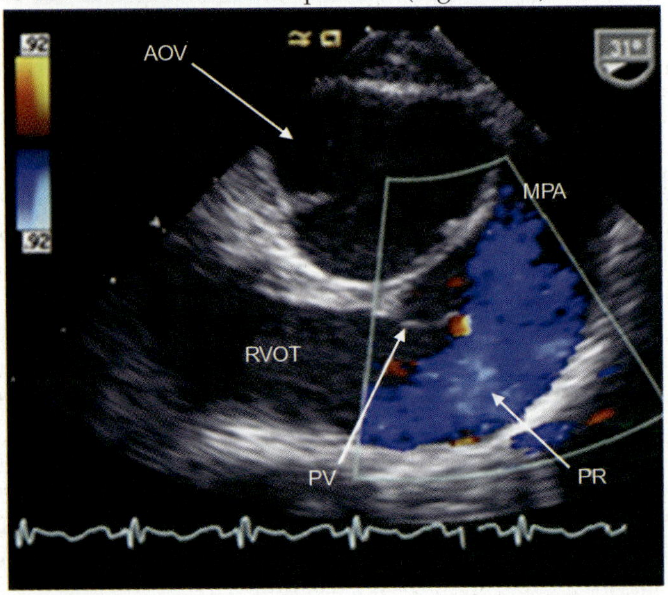


**Fig. 16.98:** Preoperative echocardiogram demonstrating severe pulmonary valve regurgitation located anteriorly through the gap created by the transannular patch. AOV=aortic valve; MPA=main pulmonary artery; PR=pulmonary regurgitation; PV=pulmonary valve; RVOT=right ventricular outflow tract

### Medical Management

Medications are directed according to the specific aetiology resulting in pulmonic regurgitation in addition to the treatment of heart failure (if present). Complete infective endocarditis antibiotic prophylaxis should be considered for patients whose pulmonic regurgitation is due to valve leaflet abnormalities. Pulmonic regurgitation is seldom severe enough to warrant special treatment because the right ventricle normally adapts to low-pressure volume

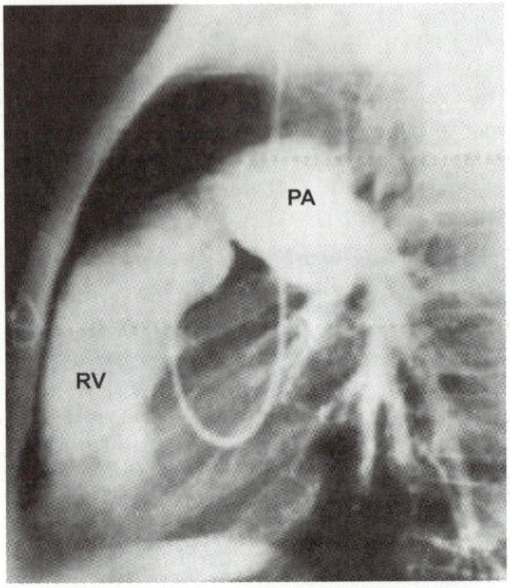


**Fig. 16.99:** Contrast medium has been injected into the main pulmonary artery (PA) and regurgitation back into an enlarged right ventricle (RV) in patient with pulmonic valvular regurgitation

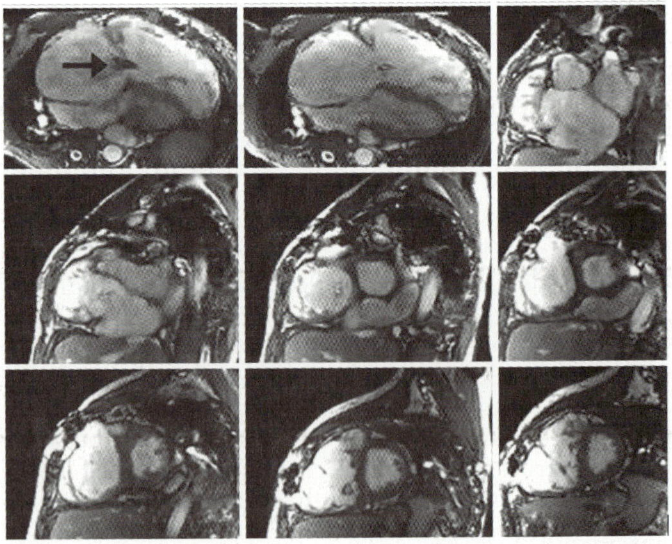

**Fig. 16.100:** CMR imaging in a 37-year-old patient with repaired TOF, severe pulmonary regurgitation, moderate tricuspid regurgitation (arrow), and severe right ventricular dilatation (end-diastolic volume index 386 ml/m$^2$) and dysfunction (ejection fraction 15%). This patient who also exhibited severe heart failure symptoms had only modest decrease in RV size and no improvement in RV function after pulmonary valve replacement. Geva Journal of Cardiovascular Magnetic Resonance 2011;13:9

overload without difficulty. High-pressure volume overload leads to right-sided heart strain and, ultimately, heart failure. Underlying etiologies causing severe pulmonic regurgitation, whether congenital or acquired, must be treated to prevent or reverse right-sided heart strain and failure that may further complicate the clinical picture. A discussion of therapeutic interventions in pulmonary hypertension by aetiology is beyond the scope of this article. Refer to the articles for each entity under differentials for a detailed discussion of treatment options.

If pulmonary hypertension is identified with pulmonic regurgitation, determining the aetiology is essential to institute appropriate therapy as expeditiously as possible. For instance, primary pulmonary hypertension, secondary pulmonary hypertension due to thromboembolism, severe mitral stenosis, and pulmonary carcinomatosis can all manifest as severe pulmonary hypertension with pulmonic regurgitation.

No aspect of medical management of heart failure is uniquely applicable to pulmonic regurgitation, and the discussion of management of right-sided heart failure is beyond the scope of this article. In general, similar approaches to those used in the treatment of patients with left-sided congestive heart failure can be useful. In some circumstances, such as in patients with pulmonary hypertension, vasodilator therapies must be very carefully considered and monitored. In addition, therapies aimed toward the underlying aetiology may also reduce pulmonic regurgitation. The American Heart Association and the American College of Cardiology have published guidelines on the management of patients with valvular heart disease.

### Surgical Care

When right-sided heart failure due to pulmonic regurgitation from an abnormal pulmonic valve cannot be ameliorated by medical management, appropriate options include surgical reconstruction or replacement of the pulmonic valve, preferably with a bioprosthetic valve. Although congenital pulmonic regurgitation is usually well tolerated, the much more rare congenital absence of the pulmonic valve usually requires valve replacement.

#### *Percutaneous Intervention*

More recently, percutaneous intervention for dysfunctional right ventricular outflow tract conduits has become available. The intermediate-term results have shown that percutaneous bioprosthetic valve implantation is a reasonable option for patients with dysfunctional right ventricular outflow tract conduits, especially those with high surgical risk. Freedom from valve dysfunction or reintervention following percutaneous bioprosthetic valve placement was 93.5% at 1 year (Figs 16.101 and 16.102).

### Complications

Right-sided heart failure is a complication of volume overload of the right ventricle due to severe pulmonic regurgitation. Other complications are related to the underlying disease processes resulting in pulmonic regurgitation.

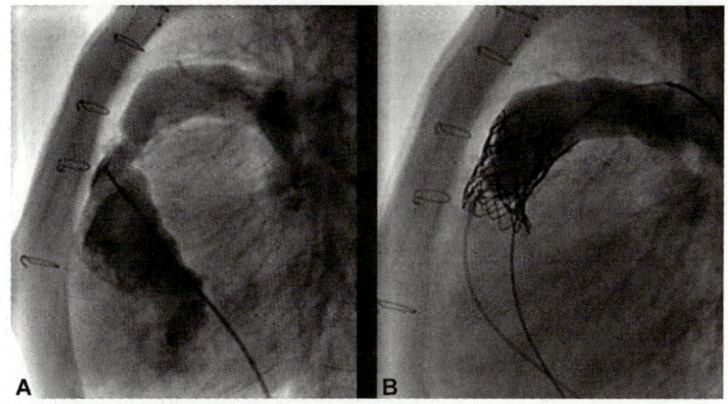

**Fig. 16.101:** The implantation of the percutaneous pulmonary valve was performed with excellent results. (A) Severe stenosis of the homograft. (B) Resolution of the stenosis, no regurgitation

### Prognosis

In general, survival is not significantly affected by mild-to-moderate pulmonic regurgitation. If pulmonic regurgitation is severe, the right ventricle is initially able to compensate for the volume overload state, and the state may remain well compensated for years. Persistently elevated right ventricular volumes may eventually cause right ventricular dilatation, and, finally, failure. As previously stated, the various disorders causing pulmonary hypertension are the most common causes of clinically significant pulmonic regurgitation. The principal prognostic indicators of mortality in pulmonic regurgitation associated with pulmonary hypertension are (1) the severity and duration of the pulmonary hypertension at the time of diagnosis and (2) the right ventricular response to the state of volume overload. In all etiologies of pulmonary hypertension, early diagnosis that allows for intervention to slow or reverse the cause of pulmonary hypertension is essential, although, in many cases, diagnosis is difficult and requires a high degree of clinical suspicion. In primary pulmonary hypertension, the pathologic process is often insidious, and symptoms manifest at an advanced disease state, resulting in an average survival period of 2.5 years from the time of diagnosis. In congenital regurgitation of the pulmonic valve, the prognosis depends upon the initial severity, progression of the regurgitation, and the ability of the right ventricle to adapt to volume overload. Usually, the degree of regurgitation in this condition is no more than moderate, so no clinical sequelae occur. Congenital absence of the pulmonic valve, a much rarer condition, confers an increased risk of morbidity and mortality because of more severe regurgitation and usually warrants pulmonic valve replacement for improved prognosis.

### Activity

Since pulmonic regurgitation is usually of a mild-to-moderate degree, restriction of athletic activities is unnecessary. Follow-up echocardiographic studies can provide data to assess for changes in pulmonic regurgitation and right ventricular functional status in order to more objectively base activity limitation recommendations.

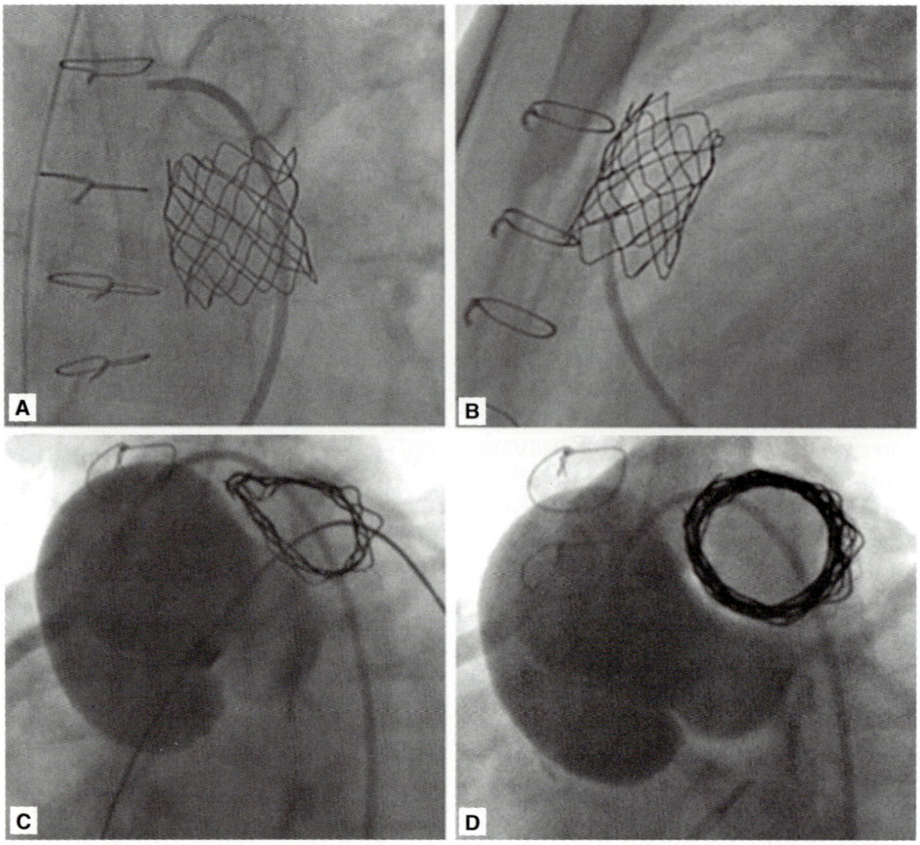

**Fig. 16.102:** (A and B) Anteroposterior and lateral fluoroscopic images demonstrating compression of the implanted Melody valve stent in a patient with a heavily calcified right ventricular outflow tract homograft conduit that is directly apposed to the anterior chest wall. (C) Aortic root angiogram in a caudal left anterior oblique projection demonstrates distortion and compression of the Melody valve from the rightward posterior aspect by a dilated neoaortic root in a patient with conduit obstruction after a Ross procedure. (D) After placement of 2 bare metal stents and a second transcatheter pulmonary valve within the fractured Melody valve, the cylindrical valve can be seen to indent the dilated neoaortic root

### Further Outpatient Care

Regurgitation may worsen with time. Therefore, periodic echocardiographic reassessment with Doppler color flow studies provides a longitudinal comparison of the progression of both the regurgitation and right ventricular size and function. In cases of significant pulmonic regurgitation, exercise capacity should be assessed and quantitated serially, observing for a change or decrease in function, the goal being to accurately assess the need and potential timing for surgical repair.

### Further Inpatient Care

Aspects of inpatient care are primarily governed by the treatment indicated for the particular disorder that causes pulmonic regurgitation. As previously mentioned, if heart failure is present that is due to or exacerbated by pulmonic regurgitation, usual heart failure management applies.

## EMERGENCY PROSTHETIC VALVULAR HEART DISEASES

Replacement of diseased valves with prosthetic heart valves reduces the morbidity and mortality associated with native valvular disease, but it comes at the expense of risking complications related to the implanted prosthetic device. Emergency physicians must be able to rapidly identify patients at risk and begin appropriate diagnostic testing, stabilization, and treatment. Even when promptly recognized and treated, acute prosthetic valve failure is associated with a high mortality rate (Figs 16.103–16.113). FDA approves CoreValve self-expanding transcatheter aortic valve.

In January 2014, the FDA approved the self-expanding transcatheter aortic valve CoreValve (Medtronic, Minneapolis, MN) for patients unable to undergo aortic-valve surgery. Approval included the 23 mm, 26 mm, 29 mm, and 31 mm valves. The approval was based on a study of patients too sick or frail to be treated with conventional aortic-valve replacement surgery; the study demonstrated CoreValve to be safe and effective, with low rates of stroke and paravalvular leak. The rate of all-cause death and stroke among patients who received CoreValve in the study was 25.5%.

### Signs and Symptoms

Signs and symptoms of prosthetic heart valve malfunction depend on the type of valve, its location, and the

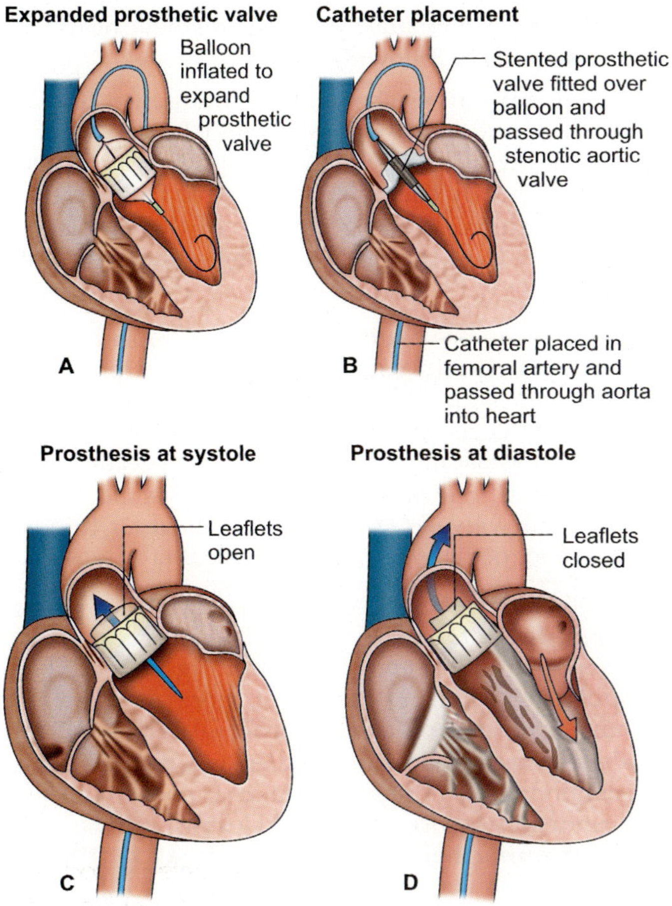


Fig. 16.103: (A) Expanded prosthetic aortic valve. (B) Catheter placement of aortic valve. (C) Aortic valve prosthesis during systole and (D) in diastole

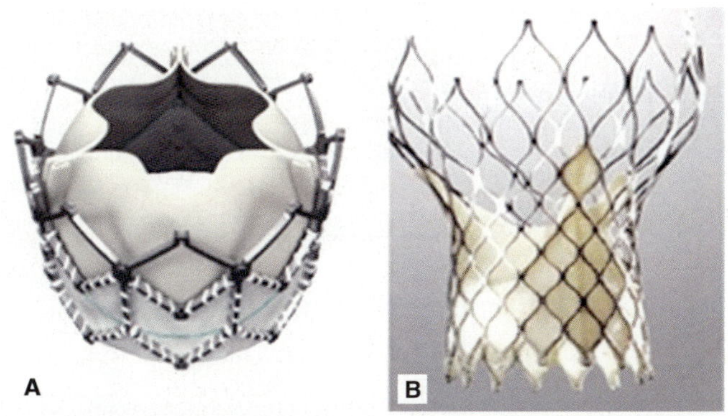


Fig. 16.104: Biological aortic valve prothesis with stent. (A) SAPIEN XT™, Edwards make (B) CoreValve™ medtronic make

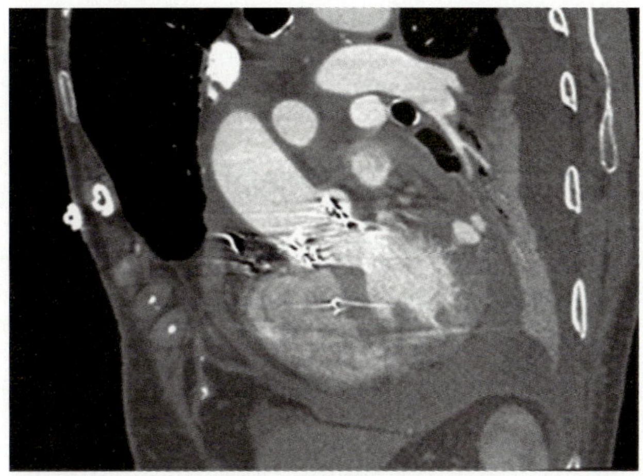

Fig. 16.105: Sagittal CT reconstruction of the thorax showing the implanted aortic valve. The left ventricle free wall defect with small pseudoaneurysm is also again noted

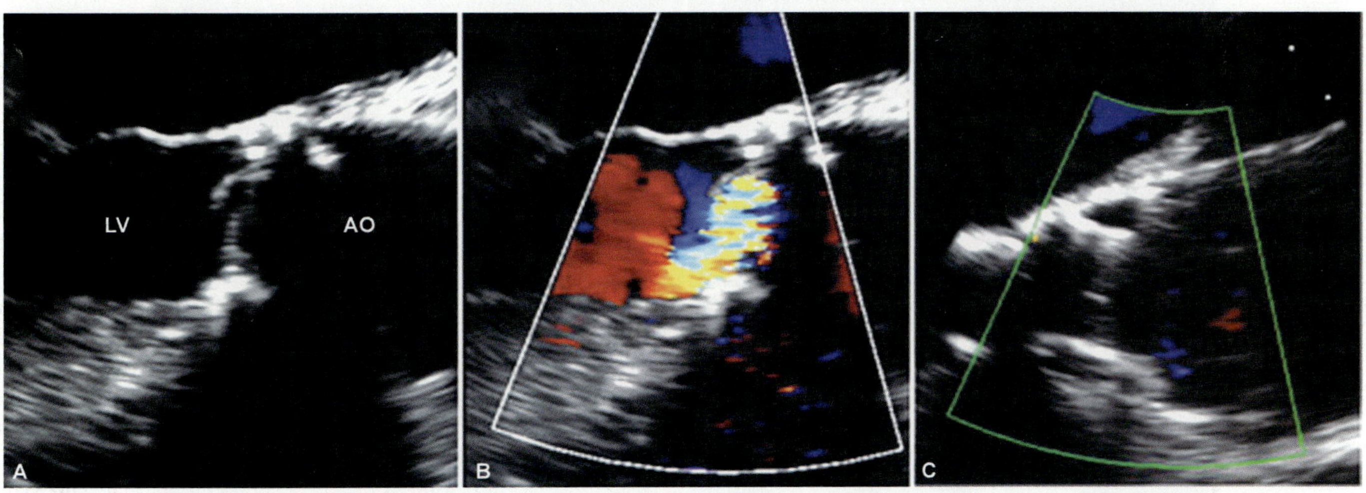


Fig.16.106: Echocardiographic results of 'valve-in-valve' implantation in a patient with degenerated aortic bioprosthesis. (A) and (B)—Carpentier-Edwards bioprosthesis with severe aortic regurgitation. (C) Absence of residuel regurgitation after Medtronic CoreValve implantation. AO=aorta, LV=left ventricle

nature of the complication. Presentations may include the following:

- **Acute prosthetic valve failure:** Sudden onset of dyspnea, syncope, or precordial pain
- **Acute aortic valve failure:** Sudden death; survivors have acute severe dyspnea, sometimes accompanied by precordial pain, or syncope
- **Subacute valvular failure:** Symptoms of gradually worsening congestive heart failure; they also may present

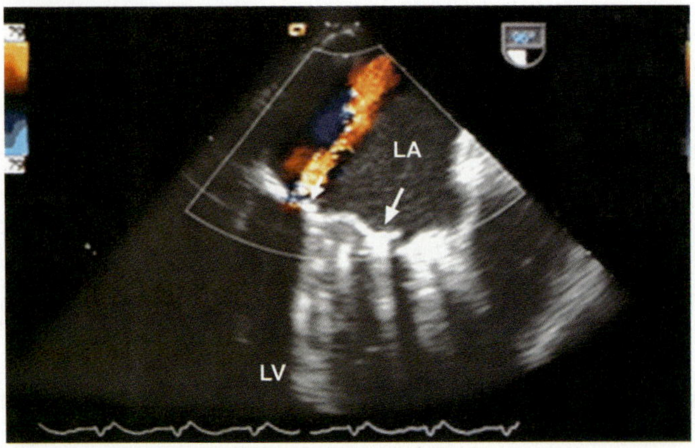


**Fig. 16.107:** Paravalvar leak. Transoesophageal, two-dimensional, color-Doppler image (longitudinal section) of the left atrium (LA) and left ventricle (LV) showing a bileaflet mitral prosthesis with the sewing ring marked by arrows and a posteriorly located paravalvar leak causing mild mitral regurgitation

with unstable angina or, at times, may be entirely asymptomatic
- **Embolic complications:** Symptoms related to the site of embolization [e.g. stroke, myocardial infarction (MI), sudden death, or symptoms of visceral or peripheral embolization].
- **Anticoagulant-related hemorrhage**: Symptoms related to the site of hemorrhage

A history of fever should raise the possibility of prosthetic valve endocarditis (PVE).

On physical examination, normal prosthetic heart valve sounds include the following:

- **Mechanical valves**: Loud, high-frequency, metallic closing sound; soft opening sound (tilting disc and bileaflet valves); low-frequency opening and closing sounds of nearly equal intensity (caged ball valves).
- **Tissue valves:** Closing similar to those of native valves, low-frequency early opening sound in the mitral position.

*Prosthetic heart valve murmurs noted include the following:*
- **Aortic prosthetic valves:** Some degree of outflow obstruction with a resultant systolic ejection murmur (loudest in caged ball and small porcine valves); low-intensity diastolic murmur (tilting disc and bileaflet valves).
- **Mitral prosthetic valves:** Low-grade systolic murmur (caged ball valves); short diastolic murmur (bioprostheses and, occasionally, St. Jude bileaflet valves).

*Additional findings may include the following:*
- ***Acute valvular failure:*** Evidence of poor tissue perfusion; hyperdynamic precordium and right ventricular impulse (50% of cases); absence of a normal valve closure sound or presence of an abnormal regurgitant murmur.
- ***Subacute valvular failure:*** Rales and jugular venous distention; signs of right-side failure; a new regurgitant murmur or absence of normal closing sounds; a new or worsening hemolytic anemia (may be the only presenting abnormality)
- ***PVE (often obscure):*** Fever (97% of cases); a new or changing murmur (56% of cases); classic signs of native

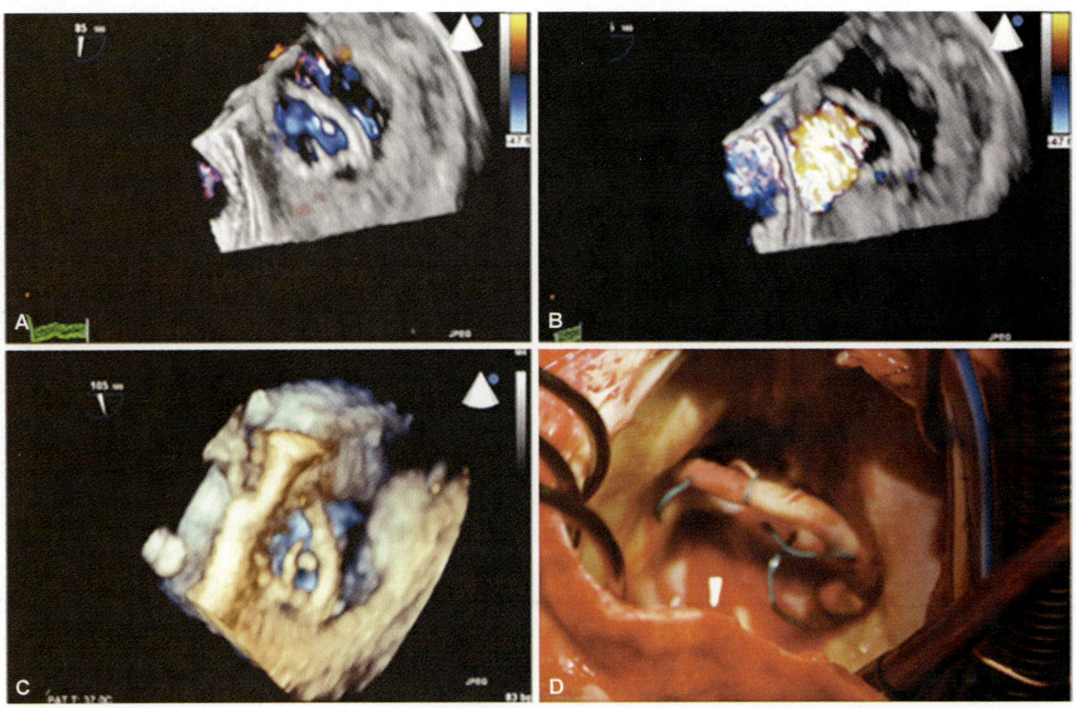


**Fig. 16.108:** A real-time three-dimensional (3D) transesophageal echocardiography zoom image demonstrates a peri-ring tissue defect (arrow) of the mitral posterior ring (arrow) on surgeon's view in end-systole (A) and mid-diastole (B). A full-volume 3D color image reveals the regurgitant jet from the peri-ring defect (arrow), differentiated from valvular regurgitation (C); this view is similar to what the surgeon saw (D)

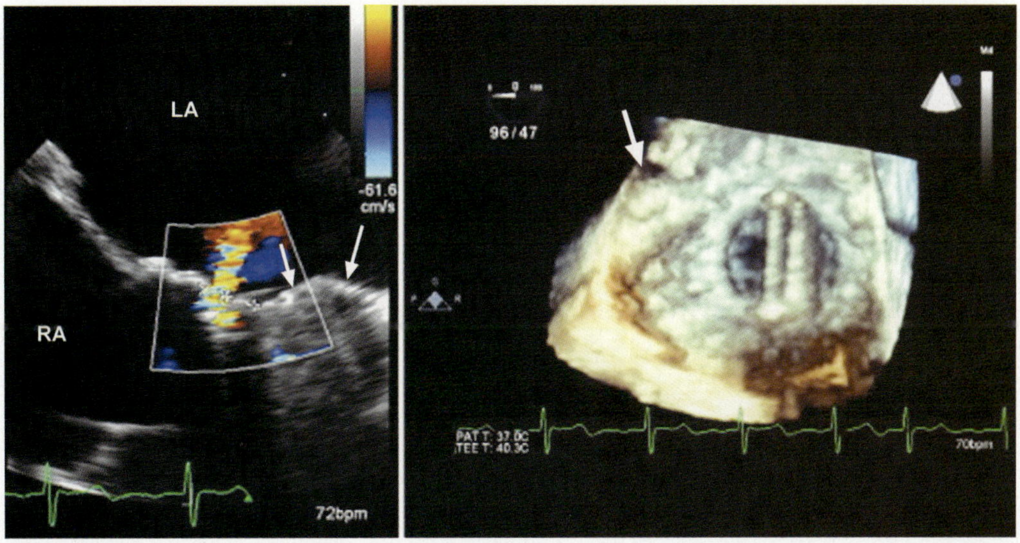


**Fig. 16.109:** 2D and 3D TEE in PV leak. Mid-esophageal 2D TEE view at 0° showing paravalvular (PV) leak located anteromedially between St. Jude's aortic and mitral prostheses. St. Jude's mitral valve disks in the closed position are shown by white arrows in A. (B) is the 3D TEE view showing St. Jude's mitral valve disks in the open position from the atrial aspect. A PV hole is seen at the 10 o'clock position (white arrow). The location of the PV leak made percutaneous repair nonfeasible. LA=left atrium; RA=right atrium

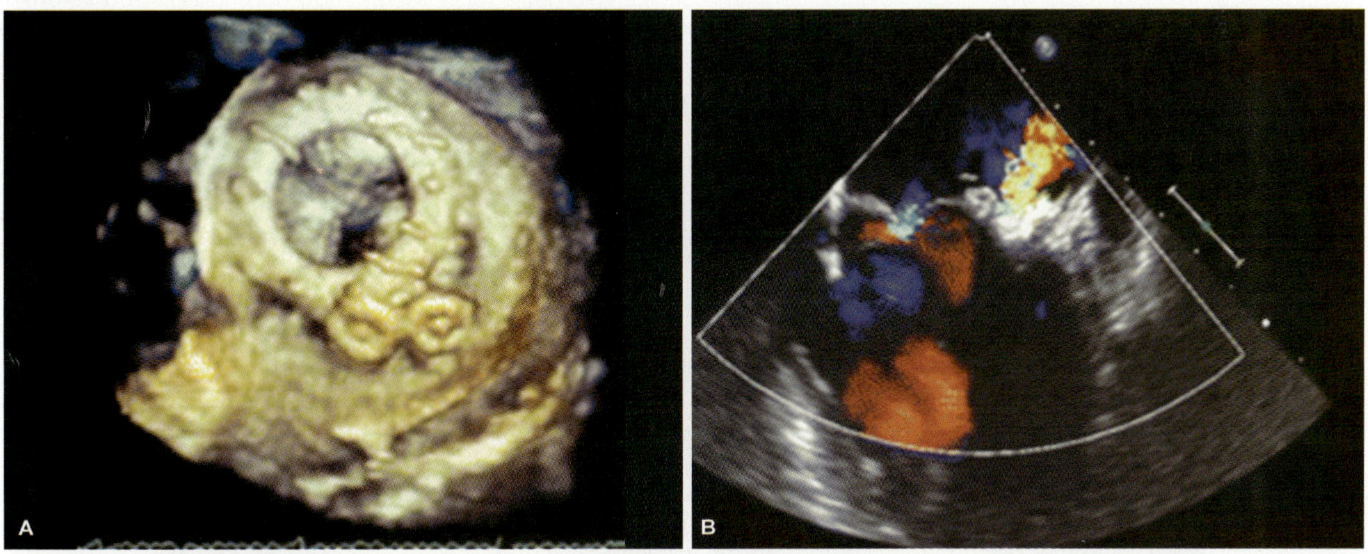


**Fig. 16.110:** (A) Two-dimensional TEE image with colour of mitral bioprosthesis demonstrating a significant reduction in the paravalvular leak after placement of two Amplatzer occluder devices. The degree of paravalvular regurgitation is significantly reduced after device placement (compare with figure prior to device placement). (B) Real-time 3D TEE assisted in the placement of this second Amplatzer Duct Occluder device (10/8 mm) deployed posterior to the first device occluding the majority of the paravalvular defect

valve endocarditis; splenomegaly; congestive heart failure, septic shock, or primary valvular failure; systemic emboli

## Diagnosis

A. Laboratory studies that may be useful include the following:
- Complete blood count
- Blood urea nitrogen (BUN) and creatinine levels
- Urinalysis
- Blood culture
- Prothrombin time (PT) or international normalized ratio (INR)

B. Imaging studies that may be helpful include the following:
- **Chest radiography:** This can help in delineating the valvular morphology and determining whether the valve and occluder are intact; each of the most commonly used valve types has its own characteristic radiographic appearance

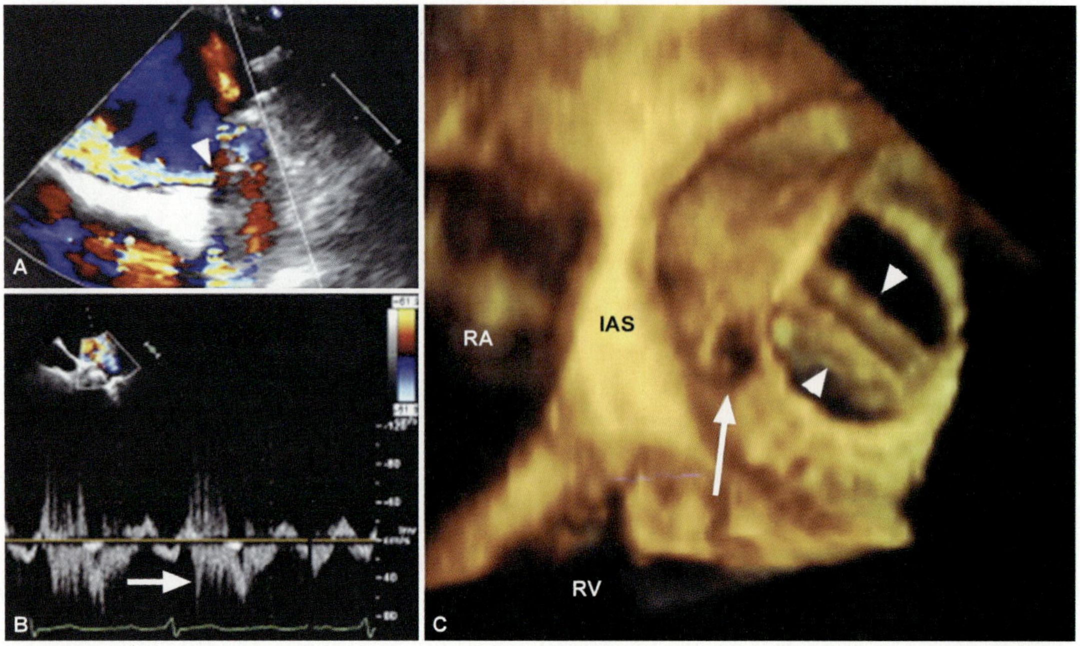


**Fig. 16.111:** Multidimensional echocardiographic evaluation of a prosthetic mitral PVL. (A) A 2D TEE demonstrating the paravalvular defect (arrowhead) with severe paravalvular regurgitation. (B) A 2D TEE pulse wave Doppler demonstrating marked systolic flow reversal (arrow) in the right upper pulmonary vein. (C) Real-time 3D TEE volumetric reconstruction demonstrating the anteromedial location of the paravalvular defect (arrow) and mechanical mitral valve leaflets (arrowheads). IAS=interatrial septum; PVL=paravalvular leak; RA=right atrium; RV=right ventricle; TEE=transesophageal echocardiography; 2D=2-dimensional; 3D=3-dimensional

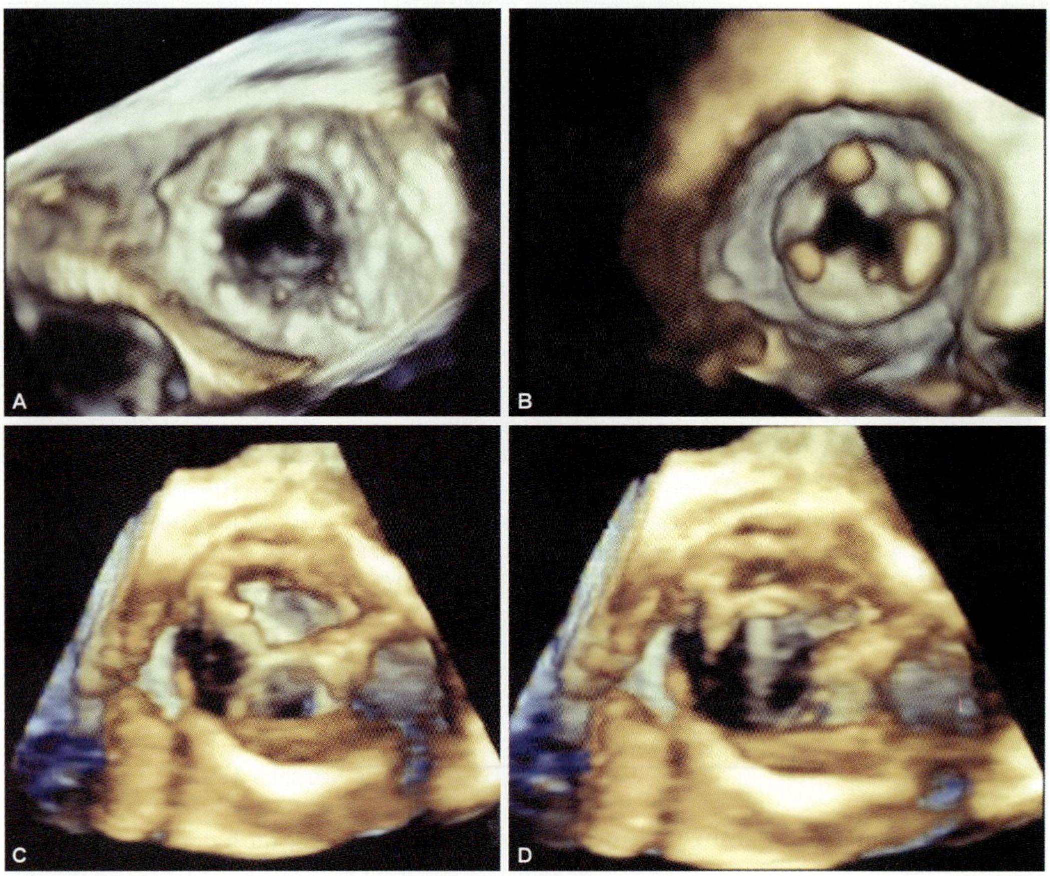


**Fig. 16.112:** Real-time three-dimensional transesophageal echocardiography (RT3D TEE) of a normal bioprosthetic tricuspid valve during diastole oriented as seen from the right atrium (A) and the right ventricle (B). The tricuspid ring is easily visualized but the leaflets are poorly seen. RT3D TEE of a normal bioprosthetic aortic valve oriented as seen from the aorta (C) and the left ventricular outflow tract (D). Again, the aortic leaflets, in contrast to the ring, are poorly visualized

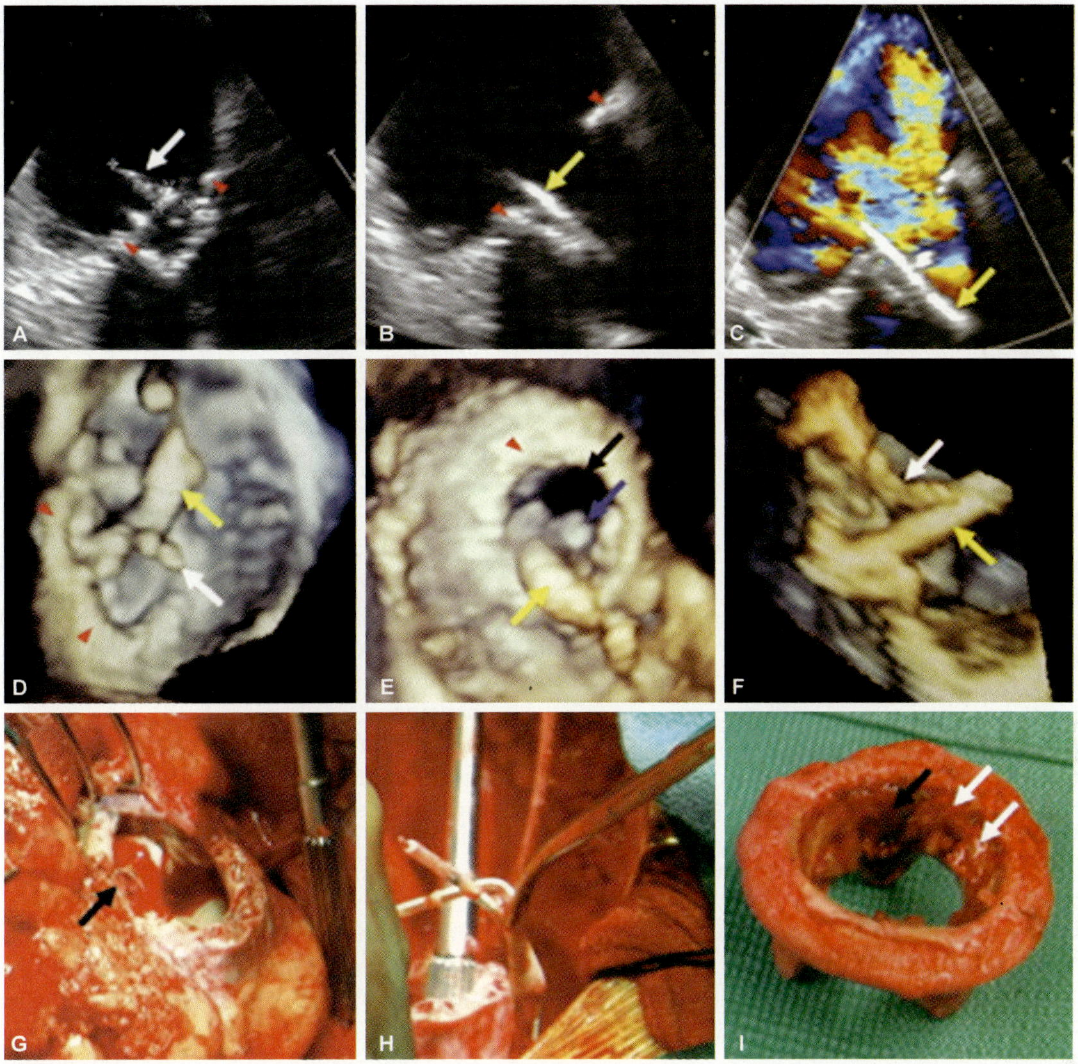

**Fig. 16.113:** Bioprosthetic tricuspid valve vegetation visualization by TEE and RT3D TEE and at valve explantation patient is a 53-year-old man with a history of intravenous drug abuse, hepatitis C infection, end-stage renal disease on hemodialysis, porcine tricuspid valve replacement, and a pacemaker placement 6 years ago. He had two episodes of infective endocarditis with enterococcus treated with vancomycin. Loud systolic murmur of tricuspid regurgitation and chest pain prompted echocardiographic evaluation. 2D TEE at mid-esophageal views of tricuspid inflow (A and B) demonstrate a vegetation (white arrows) protruding into the right atrium in proximity to the bioprosthetic tricuspid valve ring (red arrowheads) and an ICD lead (yellow arrows) that is traversing the tricuspid valve apparatus. Color-Doppler in the same plane (C) shows severe transvalvular tricuspid valve regurgitation. RT3D TEE full volume data sets show the tricuspid valve from the right atrial aspect (D and E) and in a longitudinal view (F). The entire profile of the bioprosthetic tricuspid valve ring is seen and can be distinguished from the ICD lead. A large perforation (black arrow) in the bioprosthetic tricuspid valve leaflet is seen in E. A large vegetation is seen in D and F (white arrows), originating from the tricuspid valve leaflet and sliding along the ICD lead. Intraoperative view of the bioprosthetic tricuspid valve (G) shows bioprosthetic tricuspid valve leaflet tear (black arrow). No vegetation is seen involving the atrial or ventricular pacemaker leads (H). The patient underwent tricuspid valve replacement. Leaflet tear is shown adjacent to the vegetation on the explanted tricuspid valve bioprosthesis (I)

- **Echocardiography** [two-dimensional, Doppler, transesophageal (the study of choice for a suspected prosthetic valve complication), transthoracic]
- **Cinefluorography:** This may detect impaired occluder movement but often cannot readily determine the aetiology
- **Computed tomography:** A consensus statement from the Society of Cardiovascular Computed Tomography (SCCT) states that CT should be performed as part of the evaluation of all patients being considered for transcatheter aortic valve implantation (TAVI)/transcatheter aortic valve replacement (TAVR), except those in whom CT is contraindicated, and that the CT images should be interpreted with a member of the TAVI/TAVR team or reviewed with the operator before the procedure.

## Management

In patients with acute valvular failure, diagnostic studies must be performed simultaneously with resuscitative efforts.

*Treatment approaches to primary valve failure include the following:*

- Emergency valve replacement
- Concomitant adjunctive therapy
- Afterload reduction and inotropic support
- In selected cases, intra-aortic balloon counterpulsation

*Treatment approaches to PVE include the following:*

- Intravenous antibiotics administered as soon as two sets of blood cultures are drawn
- Cessation of warfarin until central nervous system involvement is ruled out and invasive procedures are determined to be unnecessary
- **Consideration of anticoagulation**
- Consideration of emergency surgery in patients with moderate to severe heart failure or with an unstable prosthesis noted on echocardiography or fluoroscopy

*Treatment approaches to thromboembolic complications include the following:*

- Anticoagulation (if it has not already been initiated or if the patient has a subtherapeutic INR)
- Assessment of valve function

*Treatment approaches to prosthetic valve thrombosis include the following:*

- Surgery (historically the mainstay of treatment but associated with a high mortality)
- Thrombolytic therapy (appropriate for selected patients with thrombosed prosthetic valves)—should always be performed in conjunction with cardiovascular surgical consultation
- In cases of major anticoagulant-related hemorrhage, reversal of anticoagulation

## KEY POINTS

- In patients evaluated in the emergency department for chest pain, dyspnea, syncope, arrhythmia, or shock, the possibility of valvular heart disease should be considered.
- Emergency echocardiography is essential in elucidating whether acute valvular pathology is responsible for hemodynamic collapse in a patient with cardiogenic shock.
- An asymptomatic patient with a grade 2/6 systolic murmur needs no further work-up.
- Diastolic murmurs are always pathologic and require echocardiography.
- Endocarditis prophylaxis is recommended only for dental procedures and no longer needed for gastrointestinal or genitourinary procedures.

### Medication in Valvular Heart Diseases

- *Atenolol:* 0.3–2 mg/kg/d PO, max. 2 mg/kg/d (peds: 1–2 mg/kg/dose PO daily suggested)
- *Digoxin:* 0.5 mg bolus IV, then 0.25 mg IV q2h up to 1 mg; 0.125–0.375 mg/d PO
- *Diltiazem:* 0.25 mg/kg IV over 2 min (repeat in 15 min PRN with 0.35 mg/kg) then 5–15 mg/h
- *Enalapril:* 1.25 mg IV q6h; PO 2.5–10 mg b.i.d. (peds: 0.1–0.5 mg/kg/d PO div. q12–24h; max: 0.58 mg/kg/d or 40 mg/d
- *Esmolol:* IV: 500 ¼g bolus, then 50–400 ¼g/kg/min
- *Furosemide:* 20–80 mg/d PO/IV/IM; titrate up to 600 mg/d for severe edematous states (peds: 1 mg/kg IV/IM slowly under close supervision; not to exceed 6 mg/kg)
- *Heparin:* 80 IU/kg IV bolus, then 18 IU/kg/hr drip, adjust to maintain partial thromboplastin time 1.5–2 × control (INR 2–3)
- *Hydralazine:* 10–25 mg IV q2–4h (peds: 0.1–0.5 mg/kg IM/IV q4–6h; max. 20 mg/dose)
- *Metoprolol:* 5 mg IV q2min × 3 doses; then 50 mg PO q6h × 48 hr
- *Nitroglycerin:* Start at 20 mcg/min IV and titrate to effect (up to 300 mcg/min); SL 0.3–0.6 mg p.r.n.; Topical 1–2 inches of 2% q6h (peds: 0.25–0.5 ¼ g/kg/min IV, increase by 0.5–1 mg/kg/min; max. 20¼g/kg/min)
- *Phentolamine:* 5 mg bolus IV, then 1–2 mg/min IV infusion
- *Propranolol IV:* 1–3 mg at 1 mg/min
- *Sodium nitroprusside IV:* 0.5 ¼g/kg/min; increase in increments of 0.5 to 1.0 ¼g/kg/min q5–10 min up to 10¼g/kg/min
- *Amoxicillin:* 2 g PO 1h before the procedure; alternatively, 3 g PO 1h before the procedure, followed by 1.5 g PO 6h after the initial dose:
- *Pediatric dose:* 50 mg/kg PO 1h before procedure
- *Ampicillin:* 2 g IV/IM 30 min before the procedure (peds: 50 mg/kg IV/IM 30 min before the procedure)
- *Clindamycin:* 600 mg PO 1h before procedure (peds: 20 mg/kg PO 1h before procedure; not to exceed 600 mg).

## BIBLIOGRAPHY

1. Acikel M, Erol MK, Yekeler I, Ozyazicioglu A. A case of free-floating ball thrombus in right atrium with tricuspid stenosis. Int J Cardiol 2004;94(2–3):329–30.
2. Acker MA, Parides MK, Perrault LP, et al, for The Cardiothoracic Surgical Trials Network. Mitral-valve repair versus replacement for severe ischemic mitral regurgitation. N Engl J Med 2013.
3. Adachi O, Saiki Y, Akasaka J, Oda K, Iguchi A, Tabayashi K. Surgical management of aortic regurgitation associated with takayasu arteritis and other forms of aortitis. Ann Thorac Surg 2007;84(6):1950–3.
4. Aggarwal A, Raghuvir R, Eryazici P, Macaluso G, Sharma P, Blair C, et al. The development of aortic insufficiency in continuous-flow left ventricular assist device-supported patients. Ann Thorac Surg 2013;95(2):493–8.
5. Aggarwal A, Raghuvir R, Eryazici P, Macaluso G, Sharma P, Blair C, et al. The development of aortic insufficiency in continuous-flow left ventricular assist device-supported patients. Ann Thorac Surg 2013;95(2):493–8.

6. Alpert MA, Mukerji V, Sabeti M, et al. Mitral valve prolapse, panic disorder, and chest pain. Med Clin North Am 1991; 75(5):1119–33.
7. American College of Cardiology/American Heart Association. ACC/AHA 2006 guidelines for the management of patients with valvular heart disease. A report of the American College of Cardiology/American Heart Association Task Force on Practice Guidelines (writing committee to revise the 1998 guidelines for the Manag. J Am Coll Cardiol 2006;48:1–148.
8. American College of Cardiology/American Heart Association. ACC/AHA guidelines for the management of patients with valvular heart disease. A report of the American College of Cardiology/American Heart Association. Task Force on Practice Guidelines (Committee on Management of Patients with Valvular Heart Disease. J Am Coll Cardiol 1998;32(5):1486–588.
9. Anderson C, Filsoufi F, Farivar RS, Adams DH. Optimal management of severe tricuspid regurgitation in cardiac transplant recipients. J Heart Lung Transplant. 2001; 20(2):247.
10. Antonini-Canterin F, Moura LM, Enache R, Leiballi E, Pavan D, Piazza R. Effect of hydroxymethylglutaryl coenzyme-a reductase inhibitors on the long-term progres-sion of rheumatic mitral valve disease. Circulation 2010; 121(19):2130–6.
11. Atalar E, Yorgun H, Canpolat U, Sunman H, Kepez A, Kocabas U, et al. Prevalence of coronary artery disease before valvular surgery in patients with rheumatic valvular disease. Coron Artery Dis 2012;23(8):533–7.
12. Avierinos JF, Gersh BJ, Melton LJ 3rd, Bailey KR, Shub C, Nishimura RA, et al. Natural history of asymptomatic mitral valve prolapse in the community. Circulation 2002; 106(11):1355–61.
13. Babu AN, Kymes SM, Carpenter Fryer SM. Eponyms and the diagnosis of aortic regurgitation: what says the evidence?. Ann Intern Med 2003;138(9):736–42.
14. Badheka AO, Shah N, Ghatak A, Patel NJ, Chothani A, Mehta K, et al. Balloon Mitral Valvuloplasty in United States: A 13 year perspective. Am J Med 2014.
15. Barbieri A, Bursi F, Grigioni F, Tribouilloy C, Avierinos JF, Michelena HI, et al. Prognostic and therapeutic implications of pulmonary hypertension complicating degenerative mitral regurgitation due to flail leaflet: A Multicenter Long-term International Study. Eur Heart J 2011;32(6):751–759.
16. Barnett HJ, Boughner DR, Taylor DW, Cooper PE, Kostuk WJ, Nichol PM. Further evidence relating mitral-valve prolapse to cerebral ischemic events. N Engl J Med 1980; 302(3):139–44.
17. Bekeredjian R, Grayburn PA. Valvular heart disease: aortic regurgitation. Circulation 2005;112(1):125–34.
18. Bhudia SK, McCarthy PM, Kumpati GS, Helou J, Hoercher KJ, Rajeswaran J, et al. Improved outcomes after aortic valve surgery for chronic aortic regurgitation with severe left ventricular dysfunction. J Am Coll Cardiol 2007;49(13): 1465–71.
19. Bonow RO, Carabello BA, Chatterjee K, de Leon AC Jr, Faxon DP, Freed MD. 2008 focused update incorporated into the ACC/AHA 2006 guidelines for the management of patients with valvular heart disease: a report of the American College of Cardiology/American Heart Association Task Force on Practice Guidelines (Writing Committee to revise the 1998 guidelines for the management of patients with valvular heart disease). Endorsed by the Society of Cardiovascular Anesthesiologists, Society for Cardiovascular Angiography and Interventions, and Society of Thoracic Surgeons. J Am Coll Cardiol 2008;52(13):e1–142.
20. Bonow RO, Carabello BA, Chatterjee K, et al. 2008 focused update incorporated into the ACC/AHA 2006 guidelines for the management of patients with valvular heart disease: a report of the American College of Cardio-logy/American Heart Association Task Force on Practice Guidelines (Writing Committee to revise the 1998 guidelines for the management of patients with valvular heart disease). Endorsed by the Society of Cardiovascular Anesthesiologists, Society for Cardiovascular Angiography and Interventions, and Society of Thoracic Surgeons. J Am Coll Cardiol 2008; 52(13):e1–142.
21. Bonow RO, Carabello BA, Kanu C, et al. ACC/AHA 2006 guidelines for the management of patients with valvular heart disease: a report of the American College of Cardio-logy/American Heart Association Task Force on Practice Guidelines (writing committee to revise the 1998 Guidelines for the Management of Patients With Valvular Heart Disease): developed in collaboration with the Society of Cardiovascular Anesthesiologists: endorsed by the Society for Cardiovascular Angiography and Interventions and the Society of Thoracic Surgeons. Circulation 2006; 114(5): e84–231.
22. Bonow RO, Cheitlin MD, Crawford MH, Douglas PS. Task Force 3: valvular heart disease. J Am Coll Cardiol 2005; 45(8):1334–40.
23. Braunwald E. Heart Disease: A Textbook of Cardiovascular Medicine. 3rd ed. Philadelphia, Pa: Saunders; 1988.
24. Bruce CJ, Nishimura RA. Newer advances in the diagnosis and treatment of mitral stenosis. Curr Probl Cardiol 1998; 23(3):125–92.
25. Bryhn M, Persson S. The prevalence of mitral valve prolapse in healthy men and women in Sweden. An echocardiographic study. Acta Med Scand 1984;215(2): 157–60.
26. Carabello BA, Paulus WJ. Aortic stenosis. Lancet 2009; 373(9667):956–66.
27. Carabello BA. Progress in mitral and aortic regurgitation. Prog Cardiovasc Dis 2001;43(6):457–75.
28. Chambers JB. Aortic stenosis. Eur J Echocardiogr 2009; 10(1):i11–9.
29. Chand EM, Freant LJ, Rubin JW. Aortic valve rheumatoid nodules producing clinical aortic regurgitation and a review of the literature. Cardiovasc Pathol 1999;8(6): 333–8.
30. Christ T, Grubitzsch H, Claus B, Konertz W. Long-term follow-up after aortic valve replacement with Edwards Prima Plus stentless bioprostheses in patients younger than 60 years of age. J Thorac Cardiovasc Surg 2012.
31. Ciancamerla F, Paglia I, Catuzzo B, Morello M, Mangiardi L. Sudden death in mitral valve prolapse and severe mitral regurgitation. Is chordal rupture an indication to early surgery? J Cardiovasc Surg (Torino) 2003;44(2):283–6.
32. Collins MJ, Butany J, Borger MA, Strauss BH, David TE. Implications of a congenitally abnormal valve: a study of

1025 consecutively excised aortic valves. J Clin Pathol 2008; 61(4):530–6.
33. DeLeon MA, Gidding SS, Gotteiner N, Backer CL, Mavroudis C. Successful palliation of Ebstein's malformation on the first day of life following fetal diagnosis. Cardiol Young 2000; 10(4):384–7.
34. Ducharme V, Guauque-Olarte S, Gaudreault N, Pibarot P, Mathieu P, Bossé Y. NOTCH1 genetic variants in patients with tricuspid calcific aortic valve stenosis. J Heart Valve Dis 2013;22(2):142–9.
35. Dujardin KS, Enriquez-Sarano M, Schaff HV, Bailey KR, Seward JB, Tajik AJ. Mortality and morbidity of aortic regurgitation in clinical practice. A long-term follow-up study. Circulation 1999;99(14):1851–7.
36. Duncan AI, Lin J, Koch CG, Gillinov AM, Xu M, Starr NJ. The impact of gender on in-hospital mortality and morbidity after isolated aortic valve replacement. Anesth Analg 2006; 103(4):800–8.
37. Eberhardt RT, Dhadly M. Giant cell arteritis: diagnosis, management, and cardiovascular implications. Cardiol Rev 2007;15(2):55–61.
38. Ennezat PV, Marechaux S, Iung B, Chauvel C, LeJemtel TH, Pibarot P. Exercise testing and exercise stress echocardio-graphy in asymptomatic aortic valve stenosis. Heart 2009; 95(11):877–84.
39. Enriquez-Sarano M, Avierinos JF, Messika-Zeitoun D, Detaint D, Capps M, Nkomo V, et al. Quantitative determinants of the outcome of asymptomatic mitral regurgitation. N Engl J Med 2005;352(9):875–83.
40. Etchells E, Bell C, Robb K. Does this patient have an abnormal systolic murmur? JAMA 1997;277(7):564–71.
41. Faletra F, La Marchesina U, Bragato R, De Chiara F. Three dimensional transthoracic echocardiography images of tricuspid stenosis. Heart 2005;91(4):499.
42. Fann JI, Ingels NB, Miller DC. Pathophysiology of Mitral Valve Disease. Cardiac Surgery in the Adult. 3rd ed. New York, NY: McGraw-Hill; 2008. chap 41.
43. Fedak PW, Verma S, David TE, Leask RL, Weisel RD, Butany J. Clinical and pathophysiological implications of a bicuspid aortic valve. Circulation 2002;106(8):900–4.
44. Feldman T, Cilingiroglu M. Percutaneous leaflet repair and annuloplasty for mitral regurgitation. J Am Coll Cardiol 2011; 57(5):529–37.
45. Feldman T, Foster E, Glower DG, et al. Percutaneous repair or surgery for mitral regurgitation. N Engl J Med 2011; 364(15):1395–406.
46. Feldman T. Rheumatic heart disease. Curr Opin Cardiol 1996; 11(2):126–30.
47. Feldman T. Rheumatic Mitral Stenosis. Curr Treat Options Cardiovasc Med 2000;2(2):93–104.
48. Filsoufi F, Anyanwu AC, Salzberg SP, et al. Long-term outcomes of tricuspid valve replacement in the current era. Ann Thorac Surg 2005;80(3):845–50.
49. Frater R. Tricuspid insufficiency. J Thorac Cardiovasc Surg 2001;122(3):427–9.
50. Freed LA, Levy D, Levine RA, et al. Prevalence and clinical outcome of mitral-valve prolapse. N Engl J Med 1999; 341(1):1–7.
51. Friedman T, Mani A, Elefteriades JA. Bicuspid aortic valve: clinical approach and scientific review of a common clinical entity. Expert Rev Cardiovasc Ther 2008;6(2):235–48.
52. Gatti G, Maffei G, Lusa AM, Pugliese P. Tricuspid valve repair with the Cosgrove-Edwards annuloplasty system: early clinical and echocardiographic results. Ann Thorac Surg 2001;72(3):764–7.
53. Gaztanaga J, Pizarro G, Sanz J. Evaluation of cardiac valves using multidetector CT. Cardiol Clin 2009;27(4): 633–44.
54. Gerber IL, Stewart RA, Legget ME, et al. Increased plasma natriuretic peptide levels reflect symptom onset in aortic stenosis. Circulation 2003;107(14):1884–90.
55. Gerber MA, Baltimore RS, Eaton CB, Gewitz M, Rowley AH, Shulman ST, et al. Prevention of rheumatic fever and diagnosis and treatment of acute Streptococcal pharyngitis: a scientific statement from the American Heart Association Rheumatic Fever, Endocarditis, and Kawasaki Disease Committee of the Council on Cardiovascular Disease in the Young, the Interdisciplinary Council on Functional Genomics and Translational Biology, and the Interdisciplinary Council on Quality of Care and Outcomes Research: endorsed by the American Academy of Pediatrics. Circulation 2009;119(11): 1541–51.
56. Giuliani E. Cardiology: Fundamentals and Practice. 2nd ed. Philadelphia, Pa: Mosby Year Book; 1991.
57. Godart F, Baruteau AE, Petit J, et al. Transcatheter tricuspid valve implantation: A multicentre French study. Arch Cardiovasc Dis 2014;107(11):583–91.
58. Gorlin R, Gorlin SG. Hydraulic formula for calculation of the area of the stenotic mitral valve, other cardiac valves, and central circulatory shunts. Am Heart J 1951;41(1): 1–29.
59. Gould KL, Carabello BA. Why angina in aortic stenosis with normal coronary arteriograms?. Circulation 2003; 107(25):3121–3.
60. Gould ST, Srigunapalan S, Simmons CA, Anseth KS. Hemodynamic and cellular response feedback in calcific aortic valve disease. Circ Res 2013;113(2):186–97.
61. Ha JW, Chung N, Jang Y, Rim SJ. Tricuspid stenosis and regurgitation: Doppler and color flow echocardiography and cardiac catheterization findings. Clin Cardiol 2000; 23(1): 51–2.
62. Henri C, Pierard LA, Lancellotti P, Mongeon FP, Pibarot P, Basmadjian AJ. Exercise Testing and Stress Imaging in Valvular Heart Disease. Can J Cardiol 2014;30(9): 1012–26.
63. Holmes DR Jr, Mack MJ. Transcatheter valve therapy a professional society overview from the american college of cardiology foundation and the society of thoracic surgeons. J Am Coll Cardiol 2011;58(4):445–55.
64. Horstkotte D, Niehues R, Strauer BE. Pathomorphological aspects, aetiology and natural history of acquired mitral valve stenosis. Eur Heart J. 1991; Suppl B:55–60.
65. Iwataki M, Takeuchi M, Otani K, et al. Calcific extension towards the mitral valve causes non-rheumatic mitral stenosis in degenerative aortic stenosis: real-time 3D transoesophageal echocardiography study. Open Heart 2014; 1(1):e000136.

66. Jain D, Halushka MK. Cardiac pathology of systemic lupus erythematosus. J Clin Pathol 2009;62(7):584–92.
67. Jeserich M, Ihling C, Holubarsch C. Aortic valve endocarditis with Whipple disease. Ann Intern Med 1997;126(11): 920.
68. Kaden JJ, Eckert JP, Poerner T, et al. Prevalence of atherosclerosis of the coronary and extracranial cerebral arteries in patients undergoing aortic valve replacement for calcified stenosis. J Heart Valve Dis 2006;15(2):165–8.
69. Keane MG, Pyeritz RE. Medical management of Marfan syndrome. Circulation 2008;117(21):2802–13.
70. Khan IA. Ebstein's anomaly of the tricuspid valve with associated mitral valve prolapse. Tex Heart Inst J 2001; 28(1):72.
71. Khanna D, Miller AP, Nanda NC, et al. Transthoracic and transesophageal echocardiographic assessment of mitral regur-gi-tation severity: usefulness of qualitative and semi-quantitative techniques. Echocardiography 2005;22(9): 748–69.
72. Kloner R. The Guide to Cardiology. 2nd ed. New York: Le Jacq Communications; 1990.
73. Kulbertus HE. Ventricular arrhythmias, syncope and sudden death in aortic stenosis. Eur Heart J 1988; Suppl E: 51–2.
74. Lancellotti P, Tribouilloy C, Hagendorff A, Moura L, Popescu BA, Agricola E, et al. European Association of Echocardiography recommendations for the assessment of valvular regurgitation. Part 1: aortic and pulmonary regurgitation (native valve disease). Eur J Echocardiogr 2010;11(3): 223–44.
75. Leach RM, McBrien DJ. Brachioradial delay: a new clinical indicator of the severity of aortic stenosis. Lancet 1990; 335(8699):1199–201.
76. Lee JL, Naguwa SM, Cheema GS, Gershwin ME. Acute rheumatic fever and its consequences: a persistent threat to developing nations in the 21st century. Autoimmun Rev 2009;9(2):117–23.
77. Lee JL, Naguwa SM, Cheema GS, Gershwin ME. Revisiting Libman-Sacks endocarditis: a historical review and update. Clin Rev Allergy Immunol 2009;36(2–3):126–30.
78. Lev M, Liberthson RR, Joseph RH, Seten CE, Eckner FA, Kunske RD, et al. The pathologic anatomy of Ebstein's disease. Arch Pathol 1970;90(4):334–43.
79. Levine RA, Triulzi MO, Harrigan P, Weyman AE. The relationship of mitral annular shape to the diagnosis of mitral valve prolapse. Circulation 1987;75(4):756–67.
80. Libby P, Bonow RO, MD, Zipes DP, Mann DL. Valvular Heart Disease. Braunwald's Heart Disease. 8th ed. Philadelphia, PA: Saunders Elsevier; 2008. chap. 62.
81. Luo GH, Ma WG, Sun HS, et al. Correction of traumatic tricuspid insufficiency using the double orifice technique. Asian Cardiovasc Thorac Ann 2005;13(3):238–40.
82. Magne J, Lancellotti P, O'Connor K, et al. Prediction of exer-cise pulmonary hypertension in asymptomatic degenerative mitral regurgitation. J Am Soc Echocardiogr 2011;24(9): 1004–12.
83. Marcus RH, Sareli P, Pocock WA, et al. The spectrum of severe rheumatic mitral valve disease in a developing country. Correlations among clinical presentation, surgical pathologic findings, and hemodynamic sequelae. Ann Intern Med 1994;120(3):177–83.
84. Matsunaga A, Duran CM. Progression of tricuspid regurgitation after repaired functional ischemic mitral regurgitation. Circulation 2005;112(9 Suppl):I453–7.
85. Maurer G. Aortic regurgitation. Heart 2006;92(7):994–1000.
86. Mehta RH, Eagle KA, Coombs LP, Peterson ED, Edwards FH, Pagani FD, et al. Influence of age on outcomes in patients undergoing mitral valve replacement. Ann Thorac Surg. 2002;74(5):1459–67.
87. Mehta Y, Singh R. Quantification of AS and AR. Ann Card Anaesth 2009;12(2):166.
88. Minners J, Allgeier M, Gohlke-Baerwolf C, Kienzle RP, Neumann FJ, Jander N. Inconsistencies of echocardiographic criteria for the grading of aortic valve stenosis. Eur Heart J 2008;29(8):1043–8.
89. Morello A, Gelfand EV. Cardiovascular magnetic resonance imaging for valvular heart disease. Curr Heart Fail Rep 2009; 6(3):160–6.
90. Moyssakis I, Tektonidou MG, Vasilliou VA, Samarkos M, Votteas V, Moutsopoulos HM. Libman-Sacks endocarditis in systemic lupus erythematosus: prevalence, associations, and evolution. Am J Med 2007;120(7):636–42.
91. Myerson SG. Valvular and hemodynamic assessment with CMR. Heart Fail Clin 2009;5(3):389–400.
92. Nishimura RA, Carabello BA, Faxon DP, et al. ACC/AHA 2008 Guideline update on valvular heart disease: focused update on infective endocarditis: a report of the American College of Cardiology/American Heart Asso-ciation Task Force on Practice Guidelines endorsed by the Society of Cardiovascular Anesthesiologists, Society for Cardiovascular Angiography and Interventions, and Society of Thoracic Surgeons. J Am Coll Cardiol 2008;52(8):676–85.
93. Nishimura RA, Otto CM, Bonow RO, Carabello BA, Erwin JP 3rd, Guyton RA, et al. 2014 AHA/ACC guideline for the management of patients with valvular heart disease: a report of the American College of Cardiology/American Heart Association Task Force on Practice Guidelines. J Am Coll Cardiol 2014;63(22):e57–185.
94. Nishimura RA, Otto CM, Bonow RO, et al. AHA/ACC guideline for the management of patients with valvular heart disease: a report of the American College of Cardiology/American Heart Association Task Force on Practice Guidelines. J Am Coll Cardiol 2014;63(22):e57–185.
95. Normand J, Loire R, Zambartas C. The anatomical aspects of adult aortic stenosis. Eur Heart J 1988; Suppl E: 31–6.
96. O'Brien KD, Reichenbach DD, Marcovina SM, et al. Apolipo-proteins B, (a), and E accumulate in the morphologically early lesion of 'degenerative' valvular aortic stenosis. Arterioscler Thromb Vasc Biol 1996;16(4): 523–32.
97. O'Riordan M. Early surgery bests "watchful waiting" in severe MR patients without symptoms. Medscape Medical News. Accessed August 19, 2013.
98. O'Riordan M. FDA approves MitraClip for degenerative MR. Oct. 25, 2013. Abbott. Abbott's first-in-class MitraClip device now available for U.S. patients [press release]. 2013.
99. O'Riordan M. Repair and surgery fare equally well in ischemic MR. Heartwire 2013.
100. Ortiz JT, Shin DD, Rajamannan NM. Approach to the patient with bicuspid aortic valve and ascending aorta

aneurysm. Curr Treat Options Cardiovasc Med 2006;8(6): 461–7.

101. Otto CM, Kuusisto J, Reichenbach DD, Gown AM, O'Brien KD. Characterization of the early lesion of 'degenerative' valvular aortic stenosis. Histological and immunohistochemical studies. Circulation 1994;90(2):844–53.
102. Otto CM. Surgery for mitral regurgitation: sooner or later?. JAMA 2013;310(6):587–8.
103. Palazzi C, D'Angelo S, Lubrano E, Olivieri I. Aortic involvement in ankylosing spondylitis. Clin Exp Rheumatol 2008; 26(3 Suppl 49):S131–4.
104. Palta S, Pai AM, Gill KS, Pai RG. New insights into the progression of aortic stenosis: implications for secondary prevention. Circulation 2000;101(21):2497–502.
105. Perloff JK, Child JS, Edwards JE. New guidelines for the clinical diagnosis of mitral valve prolapse. Am J Cardiol 1986;57(13):1124–9.
106. Perloff JK, Child JS. Mitral valve prolapse. Evolution and refinement of diagnostic techniques. Circulation 1989; 80(3):710–1.
107. Picano E, Pibarot P, Lancellotti P, Monin JL, Bonow RO. The emerging role of exercise testing and stress echocardiography in valvular heart disease. J Am Coll Cardiol 2009;54(24):2251–60.
108. Pizarro R, Bazzino OO, Oberti PF, Falconi M, Achilli F, Arias A, et al. Prospective validation of the prognostic usefulness of brain natriuretic peptide in asymptomatic patients with chronic severe mitral regurgitation. J Am Coll Cardiol 2009; 54(12):1099–106.
109. Quere JP, Monin JL, Levy F, et al. Influence of preoperative left ventricular contractile reserve on postoperative ejection fraction in low-gradient aortic stenosis. Circulation. 2006; 113(14):1738–44.
110. Rahimtoola SH. Choice of prosthetic heart valve in adults an update. J Am Coll Cardiol 2010;55(22):2413–26.
111. Rahimtoola SH. Choice of Prosthetic Heart Valve in Adults An Update. J Am Coll Cardiol. 2010;55(22):2413–26.
112. Rajamannan NM, Bonow RO, Rahimtoola SH. Calcific aortic stenosis: an update. Nat Clin Pract Cardiovasc Med 2007; 4(5):254–62.
113. Roberts PA, Boudjemline Y, Cheatham JP, et al. Percutaneous Tricuspid Valve Replacement in Congenital and Acquired Heart Disease. JACC 2011;58:117–22.
114. Roberts PA, Boudjemline Y, Cheatham JP. Percutaneous Tricuspid Valve Replacement in Congenital and Acquired Heart Disease. JACC 2011;58:117–22.
115. Roberts WC, Vowels TJ, Ko JM. Natural history of adults with congenitally malformed aortic valves (unicuspid or bicuspid). Medicine (Baltimore) 2012;91(6):287–308.
116. Rosenhek R, Rader F, Klaar U, Gabriel H, Krejc M, Kalbeck D, et al. Outcome of watchful waiting in asymptomatic severe mitral regurgitation. Circulation 2006;113(18): 2238–44.
117. Rossi A, Dini FL, Faggiano P, et al. Independent prognostic value of functional mitral regurgitation in patients with heart failure. A quantitative analysis of 1256 patients with ischaemic and non-ischaemic dilated cardiomyopathy. Heart 2011;97(20):1675–80.
118. Sambola A, Tornos P, Ferreira-Gonzalez I, Evangelista A. Prognostic value of preoperative indexed end-systolic left ventricle diameter in the outcome after surgery in patients with chronic aortic regurgitation. Am Heart J 2008; 155(6):1114–20.
119. Sampat U, Varadarajan P, Turk R, Kamath A, Khandhar S, Pai RG. Effect of beta-blocker therapy on survival in patients with severe aortic regurgitation results from a cohort of 756 patients. J Am Coll Cardiol 2009;54(5):452–7.
120. Saura D, Peñafiel P, Martínez J, de la Morena G, García-Alberola A, Soria F, et al. [The frequency of systolic aortic regurgitation and its relationship to heart failure in a consecutive series of patients]. Rev Esp Cardiol 2008; 61(7):771–4.
121. Schirmer M, Weidinger F, Sandhofer A, Gschwendtner A, Wiedermann C. Valvular disease and myocardial infarctions in a patient with Behçet disease. J Clin Rheumatol 2003; 9(5):316–20.
122. Schlosshan D, Aggarwal G, Mathur G, Allan R, Cranney G. Real-time 3D transesophageal echocardiography for the evaluation of rheumatic mitral stenosis. JACC Cardiovasc Imaging 2011;4(6):580–8.
123. Shah PM, Raney AA. Tricuspid valve disease. Curr Probl Cardiol 2008;33(2):47–84.
124. Simula DV, Edwards WD, Tazelaar HD, et al. Surgical pathology of carcinoid heart disease: a study of 139 valves from 75 patients spanning 20 years. Mayo Clin Proc 2002; 77(2):139–47.
125. Singh JP, Evans JC, Levy D, et al. Prevalence and clinical determinants of mitral, tricuspid, and aortic regurgitation (the Framingham Heart Study). Am J Cardiol 1999; 83(6): 897–902.
126. Sinning JM, Vasa-Nicotera M, Chin D, Hammerstingl C, Ghanem A, Bence J, et al. Evaluation and management of paravalvular aortic regurgitation after transcatheter aortic valve replacement. J Am Coll Cardiol 2013;62(1): 11–20.
127. Sugimoto T, Okada M, Ozaki N, et al. Long-term evaluation of treatment for functional tricuspid regurgitation with regurgitant volume: characteristic differences based on primary cardiac lesion. J Thorac Cardiovasc Surg 1999; 117(3):463–71.
128. Suri RM, Vanoverschelde JL, Grigioni F, Schaff HV, Tribouilloy C, Avierinos JF, et al. Association between early surgical intervention vs watchful waiting and outcomes for mitral regurgitation due to flail mitral valve leaflets. JAMA 2013;310(6):609–16.
129. Thourani VH, Weintraub WS, Guyton RA, Jones EL, Williams WH, Elkabbani S, et al. Outcomes and long-term survival for patients undergoing mitral valve repair versus replacement: effect of age and concomitant coronary artery bypass grafting. Circulation 2003;108(3):298–304.
130. Topilsky Y, Khanna AD, Oh JK, et al. Preoperative factors associated with adverse outcome after tricuspid valve replacement. Circulation 2011;123(18):1929–39.
131. Topilsky Y, Tribouilloy C, Michelena HI, Pislaru S, Mahoney DW, Enriquez-Sarano M. Pathophysiology of tricuspid regurgitation: quantitative Doppler echocardiographic assessment of respiratory dependence.Circulation. 2010; 122(15):1505–13.
132. Towler DA. Molecular and cellular aspects of calcific aortic valve disease. Circ Res 2013;113(2):198–208.

133. Tribouilloy C, Grigioni F, Avierinos JF, Barbieri A, Rusinaru D, Szymanski C, et al. Survival implication of left ventricular end-systolic diameter in mitral regurgitation due to flail leaflets a long-term follow-up multicenter study. J Am Coll Cardiol 2009;54(21):1961–8.
134. Vahanian A, Alfieri O, Andreotti F, Antunes MJ, Barón-Esquivias G, Baumgartner H, et al. Guidelines on the management of valvular heart disease (version 2012): The Joint Task Force on the Management of Valvular Heart Disease of the European Society of Cardiology (ESC) and the European Association for Cardio-Thoracic Surgery (EACTS). Eur Heart J 2012;33(19):2451–96.
135. Vahanian A, Alfieri O, Andreotti F, Antunes MJ, Barón-Esquivias G, Baumgartner H, et al. Guidelines on the management of valvular heart disease (version 2012). Eur Heart J 2012;33(19):2451–96.
136. Vahanian A, Alfieri O, Andreotti F, Antunes MJ, Barón-Esquivias G, Baumgartner H, et al. Guidelines on the management of valvular heart disease (version 2012): The Joint Task Force on the Management of Valvular Heart Disease of the European Society of Cardiology (ESC) and the European Association for Cardio-Thoracic Surgery (EACTS). Eur Heart J 2012;33(19):2451–96.
137. Vahanian A, Alfieri O, Andreotti F, Antunes MJ, Barón-Esquivias G, Baumgartner H, et al. Guidelines on the management of valvular heart disease (version 2012): The Joint Task Force on the Management of Valvular Heart Disease of the European Society of Cardiology (ESC) and the European Association for Cardio-Thoracic Surgery (EACTS). Eur Heart J 2012;33(19):2451–96.
138. Vahanian A, Alfieri O, Andreotti F, et al. Guide-lines on the management of valvular heart disease (version 2012): The Joint Task Force on the Management of Valvular Heart Disease of the European Society of Cardiology (ESC) and the European Association for Cardio-Thoracic Surgery (EACTS).Eur Heart J 2012;33(19):2451–96.
139. Vahanian A, Baumgartner H, Bax J, et al. Guidelines on the management of valvular heart disease: The Task Force on the Management of Valvular Heart Disease of the European Society of Cardiology. Eur Heart J 2007;28(2): 230–68.
140. Vlahos AP, Feinstein JA, Schiller NB, Silverman NH. Extension of Doppler-derived Echocardiographic Measures of Pulmonary Vascular Resistance to Patients with Moderate or Severe Pulmonary Vascular Disease. J Am Soc Echocardiogr 2008.
141. Waller BF. Morphological aspects of valvular heart disease: Part I. Curr Probl Cardiol 1984;9(7):1–66.
142. Waller BF. Morphological aspects of valvular heart disease: Part II. Curr Probl Cardiol 1984;9(8):1–74.
143. Wann LS, Curtis AB, Ellenbogen KA, et al. 2011 ACCF/AHA/HRS focused update on the management of patients with atrial fibrillation (update on dabigatran): a report of the American College of Cardiology Foundation/American Heart Association Task Force on practice guidelines. J Am Coll Cardiol 2011;57(11):1330–7.
144. Warnes CA, Williams RG, Bashore TM, Child JS, Connolly HM, Dearani JA, et al. ACC/AHA 2008 Guide-lines for the Management of Adults with Congenital Heart Disease: a report of the American College of Cardiology/American Heart Association Task Force on Practice Guidelines (writing committee to develop guidelines on the management of adults with congenital heart disease). Circulation 2008; 118(23):e714–833.
145. Wilson W, Taubert KA, Gewitz M, Lockhart PB, Baddour LM, Levison M, et al. Prevention of infective endocarditis: guidelines from the American Heart Asso-ciation: a guideline from the American Heart Association Rheu-matic Fever, Endocarditis, and Kawasaki Disease Com-mittee, Council on Cardiovascular Disease in the Young, and the Council on Clinical Cardiology, Council on Cardio-vascular Surgery and Anesthesia, and the Quality of Care and Outcomes Research Interdisciplinary Working Group. Circulation 2007;116(15):1736–54.
146. Wunderlich NC, Beigel R, Siegel RJ. Management of mitral stenosis using 2D and 3D echo-Doppler imaging. JACC Cardiovasc Imaging 2013;6(11):1191–205.
147. Yang WI, Shim CY, Kang MK, et al. Vena contracta width as a predictor of adverse outcomes in patients with severe isolated tricuspid regurgitation. J Am Soc Echocardiogr 2011; 24(9):1013–9.
148. Yeow WL, Roberts-Thomson P, Shetty S, Yong G. Expanding Role for Transcatheter Aortic Valve Replacement: Successful Transfemoral Implantation of a Medtronic CoreValve for Severe Aortic Regurgitation. Heart Lung Circ 2012;21(11): 754–8.

# 17 Deep Vein Thrombosis and Pulmonary Embolism

Pulmonary embolism (PE) is a blockage of the main artery of the lung or one of its branches by a substance that has travelled from elsewhere in the body through the bloodstream (embolism). PE most commonly results from deep vein thrombosis (a blood clot in the deep veins of the legs or pelvis) that breaks off and migrates to the lung, a process termed venous thromboembolism (VTE). A small proportion of cases are caused by the embolization of air, fat, or talc in drugs of intravenous drug abusers or amniotic fluid. The obstruction of the blood flow through the lungs and the resultant pressure on the right ventricle of the heart lead to the symptoms and signs of PE. The risk of PE is increased in various situations, such as cancer or prolonged bed rest (Fig. 17.1).

A pulmonary embolus is one of the life-threatening causes of chest pain and should always be considered when a patient presents to a healthcare provider with complaints of chest pain and shortness of breath. There are special types of pulmonary embolus that are not due to blood clots, but instead are due to other body materials. These are rare occurrences and include:

1. Fat emboli from a broken femur,
2. An amniotic fluid embolus in pregnancy, and
3. In some cases, tumor tissue from cancer.

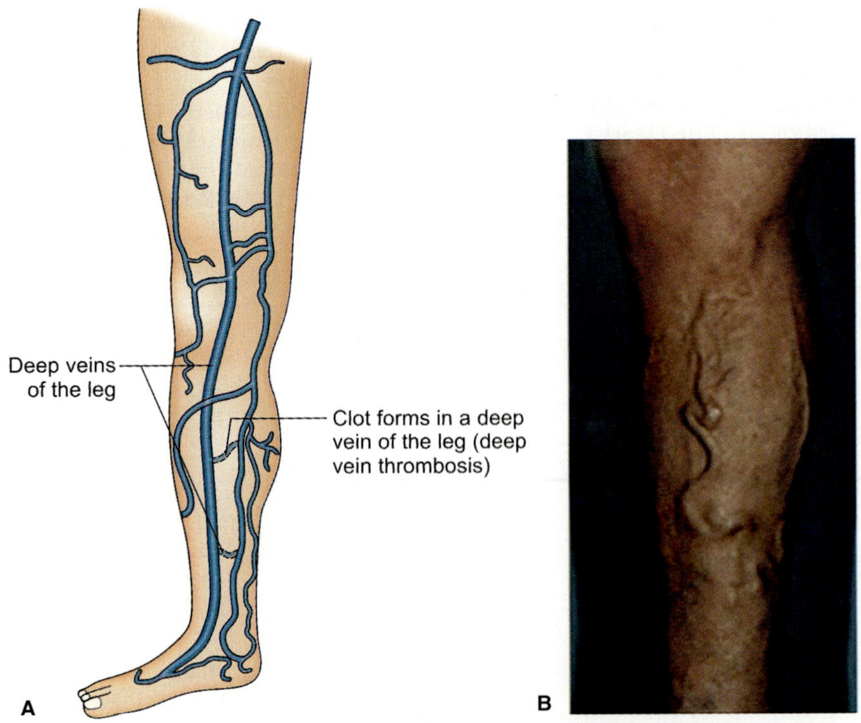


**Fig. 17.1:** (A) Anatomy of vein thrombosis. (B) Thrombosis of the varicose veins

The signs and symptoms are the same as that of a blood clot, and is caused by blockage of part of the arterial tree of the lung, and prevents the bloods ability to reach all parts of the lung tissue. Pulmonary embolus is the end result of a deep vein thrombosis or blood clot elsewhere in the body. Most commonly, the DVT begins in the leg, but they also can occur in veins within the abdominal cavity or in the arms. Symptoms of pulmonary embolism include difficulty breathing, chest pain on inspiration, and palpitations. Clinical signs include low blood oxygen saturation and cyanosis, rapid breathing, and a rapid heart rate. Severe cases of PE can lead to collapse, abnormally low blood pressure, and sudden death. Diagnosis is based on these clinical findings in combination with laboratory tests (such as the D-dimer test) and imaging studies, usually CT pulmonary angiography. Treatment is typically with anticoagulant medication, including heparin and warfarin. Severe cases may require thrombolysis ("clot busting") with drugs such as tissue plasminogen activator (tPA) or may require surgical intervention via pulmonary thrombectomy.

## EPIDEMIOLOGY

Pulmonary embolism occur in more than 0.6 million people in the United States each year. It results in between 50,000 and 200,000 deaths per year in the United States. The risk in those who are hospitalized is around 1%. The rate of fatal pulmonary emboli has declined from 6–2% over the last 25 years in the United States.

## MEDICAL HISTORY

The challenge in dealing with pulmonary embolism is that patients rarely display the classic presentation of this problem, that is, the abrupt onset of pleuritic chest pain, shortness of breath, and hypoxia. Studies of patients who died unexpectedly from pulmonary embolism have revealed that often these individuals complained of nagging symptoms for weeks before death. Forty percent of these patients had been seen by a physician in the weeks prior to their death (Fig. 17.2).

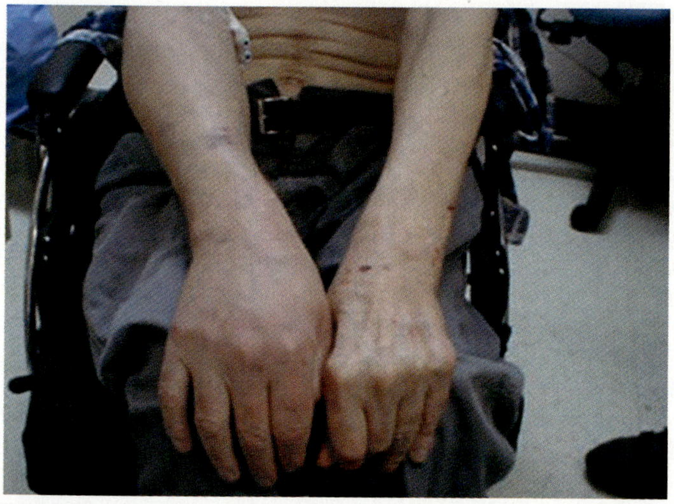

**Fig. 17.2:** A patient with deep vein thrombosis in the right arm developed in ICU

The following risk factors can be indications for the presence of pulmonary embolism:
- Venous stasis
- Hypercoagulable states
- Immobilization
- Surgery and trauma
- Pregnancy
- Oral contraceptives and estrogen replacement
- Malignancy
- Hereditary factors resulting in a hypercoagulable state
- Acute medical illness
- Drug abuse [intravenous (IV) drugs]
- Drug-induced lupus anticoagulant
- Hemolytic anemias
- Heparin-associated thrombocytopenia
- Homocystinemia
- Homocystinuria
- Hyperlipidemias
- Phenothiazines
- Thrombocytosis
- Varicose veins
- Venography
- Venous pacemakers
- Venous stasis
- Warfarin (first few days of therapy)
- Inflammatory bowel disease

The PIOPED II study listed the following indicators for pulmonary embolism:
1. Travel of 4 hours or more in the past month
2. Surgery within the last 3 months
3. Malignancy, especially lung cancer
4. Current or past history of thrombophlebitis
5. Trauma to the lower extremities and pelvis during the past 3 months
6. Smoking
7. Central venous instrumentation within the past 3 months
8. Stroke, paresis, or paralysis
9. Prior pulmonary embolism
10. Heart failure
11. Chronic obstructive pulmonary disease

## PATHOPHYSIOLOGY

Pulmonary emboli most often arise from the deep veins of the lower extremity and pelvis. Thrombi dislodge from these veins and embolize to the pulmonary arteries, where they cause abnormalities in hemodynamics and gas exchange (Fig. 17.3).

The hemodynamic response to PE is determined by the size of the embolus, the patient's underlying cardiopulmonary status, and compensatory neurohumoral adaptations. In addition to physical obstruction, acute PE leads to the release of pulmonary artery vasoconstrictors and hypoxemia, with a subsequent increase in pulmonary vascular resistance and right ventricular (RV) afterload. The

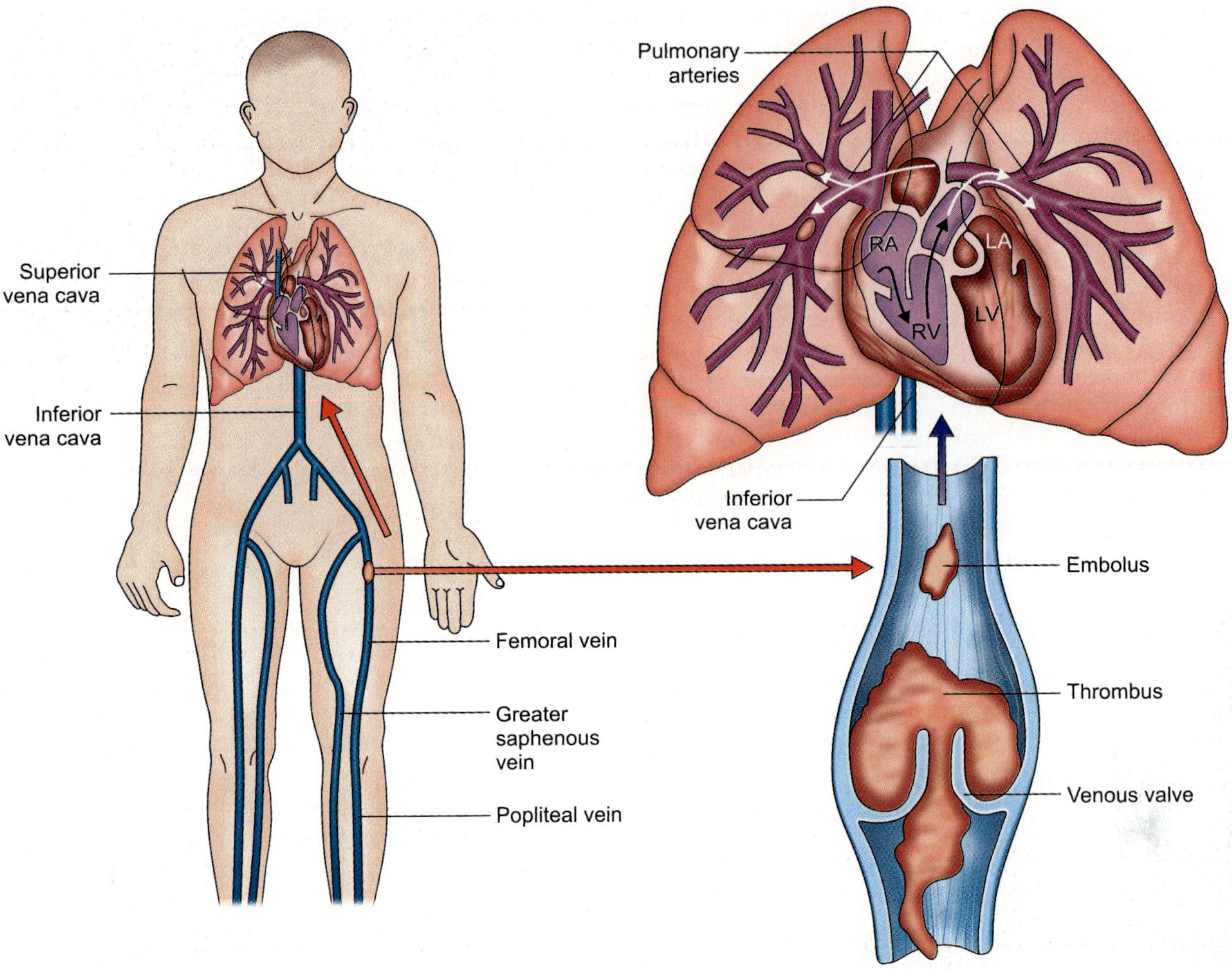


**Fig. 17.3:** The pathophysiology of pulmonary embolism. Although pulmonary embolism can arise from anywhere in the body, most commonly it arises from the calf veins. The venous thrombi predominately originate in venous valve pockets (inset) and at other sites of presumed venous stasis. To reach the lungs, thromboemboli travel through the right side of the heart. RA=right atrium; RV=right ventricle; LA=left atrium; LV=left ventricle

abrupt increase in RV afterload can cause RV dilatation and hypokinesis, tricuspid regurgitation, and ultimately RV failure. Patients with RV failure may rapidly progress to systemic arterial hypotension and cardiac arrest. RV pressure overload can also lead to interventricular septal flattening and deviation toward the left ventricle (LV) in diastole, thereby impairing LV filling. This manifestation of interventricular dependence also leads to an alteration of normal transmitral flow with left atrial contraction, represented by the A wave on Doppler echocardiography, making a greater contribution to LV diastole than passive filling, represented by the E wave. RV pressure overload also increases wall stress and leads to ischemia by increasing myocardial oxygen demand while limiting supply. Mechanisms leading to impaired gas exchange include ventilation-to-perfusion mismatch, increases in total dead space, and right-to-left shunting. Arterial hypoxemia and an increased alveolar-arterial oxygen gradient are the two most common abnormalities of gas exchange. Hyperventilation may contribute to hypocapnia and respiratory alkalosis. The presence of hypercapnia suggests massive PE leading to increased anatomic and physiological dead space and impaired minute ventilation.

## SIGNS AND SYMPTOMS

Symptoms of PE are typically sudden in onset and include dyspnea (shortness of breath), tachypnea (rapid breathing), chest pain of a "pleuritic" nature (worsened by breathing), cough and hemoptysis (coughing up blood). More severe cases can include signs such as cyanosis (blue discoloration, usually of the lips and fingers), collapse, and circulatory instability because of decreased blood flow through the lungs and into the left side of the heart. About 15% of all cases of sudden death are attributable to PE.

On physical examination, the lungs are usually normal. Occasionally, a pleural friction rub may be audible over the affected area of the lung (mostly in PE with infarct). A pleural effusion is sometimes present that is exudative, detectable by decreased percussion note, audible breath sounds and vocal resonance. Strain on the right ventricle may be detected as a left parasternal heave, a loud pulmonary component of the second heart sound, and raised jugular venous pressure. A low-grade fever may be present, particularly if there is associated pulmonary hemorrhage or infarction.

More rarely, inability of the right ventricle to remove fluid from the tissues leads to fluid accumulation in the legs (peripheral edema), congestion of the liver with mild jaundice and tenderness, and ascites (fluid in the abdominal cavity).

## PHYSICAL EXAMINATION

Physical examination findings (Fig. 17.4 and Tables 17.1–17.3) are quite variable in pulmonary embolism and, for convenience, may be grouped into four categories as follows:
- Massive pulmonary embolism
- Acute pulmonary infarction
- Acute embolism without infarction
- Multiple pulmonary emboli or thrombi

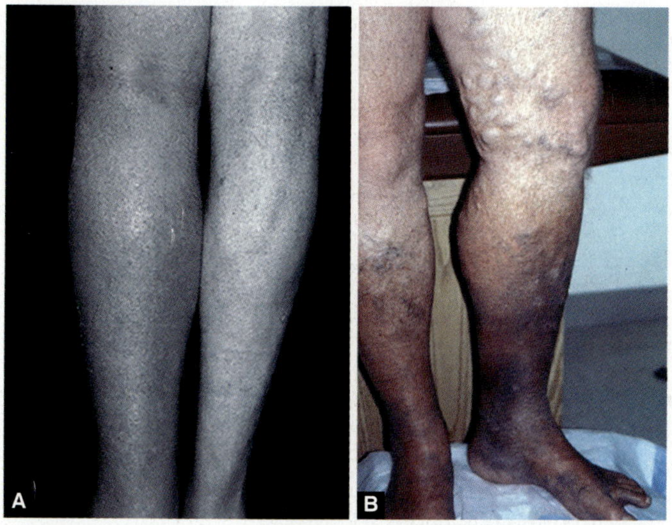

**Fig. 17.4:** (A) Deep vein thrombosis in the left leg, (B) Skin ulceration in the lateral malleolus from postthrombotic syndrome of the leg

The presentation of pulmonary embolism may vary from sudden catastrophic hemodynamic collapse to gradually progressive dyspnea (prior poor cardiopulmonary status of the patient is an important factor leading to hemodynamic collapse.) Most patients with pulmonary embolism have no obvious symptoms at presentation. In contrast, patients with symptomatic DVT commonly have pulmonary embolism confirmed on diagnostic studies in the absence of pulmonary symptoms. Sickle cell disease often creates a diagnostic difficulty with regard to pulmonary embolism. A chest infection is often the presenting symptom.

Patients with pulmonary embolism may present with atypical symptoms. In such cases, strong suspicion of pulmonary embolism based on the presence of risk factors can lead to consideration of pulmonary embolism in the differential diagnosis. These symptoms include the following:
- Seizures
- Syncope
- Abdominal pain
- Fever
- Productive cough
- Wheezing
- Decreasing level of consciousness
- New onset of atrial fibrillation
- Flank pain
- Delirium (in elderly patients)

The diagnosis of pulmonary embolism should be sought actively in patients with respiratory symptoms unexplained by an alternative diagnosis. The symptoms of pulmonary embolism are nonspecific therefore, a high index of suspicion is required, particularly when a patient has risk factors for the condition.

*Acute respiratory consequences of pulmonary embolism include the following:*
1. Increased alveolar dead space
2. Hypoxemia
3. Hyperventilation

**Table 17.1:** Clinical feautres/Risk factors in DVT

| | Score |
|---|---|
| • Active cancer within 6 months (ongoing treatment or palliative) | 1 |
| • Immobilization by paralysis or plaster dressings | 1 |
| • Recent surgery (within 4 weeks) or bed rest longer than 3 days | 1 |
| • Localized tenderness along distribution of the deep venous system | 1 |
| • Calf swelling (>3 cm increase in calf circumference compared to asymptomatic leg) measured 10 cm below tibial tuberosity | 1 |
| • Thigh and calf swelling (entire swollen leg) | 1 |
| • Pitting edema confined to symptomatic leg | 1 |
| • Collateral superficial veins (nonvaricosed) | 1 |
| • Alternative diagnosis as likely or greater than that of DVT | –2 |

Pretest probability calculated as the total score—low 0; moderate 1 or 2; high 3. In the newer scoring system proposed by Wells et al. the probability of having a DVT is likely if a score of two or higher is obtained; a score of less than two indicates that the probability of acute DVT is unlikely. The more symptomatic leg is used if patients have symptoms in both legs.

**Table 17.2:** Quick Assessment of Deep vein thrombosis

**Physical:** Massive pulmonary embolism (PE) causes hypotension due to acute cor pulmonale, but the physical examination findings early in submassive PE may be completely normal.

- After 24–72 hours, loss of pulmonary surfactant often causes atelectasis and alveolar infiltrates that are indistinguishable from pneumonia on clinical examination and by radiography.
- New wheezing may be appreciated. If pleural lung surfaces are affected, a pulmonary rub may be heard.
- In patients with recognized PE, the incidence of physical signs has been reported as follows:
  - 96% have tachypnea (respiratory rate >16/min)
  - 53% have an accentuated second heart sound
  - 43% have fever (temperature >37.8°C)
  - 34% have an S3 or S4 gallop
  - 24% have lower extremity edema
  - 23% have a cardiac murmur
  - 58% develop rales
  - 44% have tachycardia (heart rate >100/min)
  - 36% have diaphoresis
  - 32% have clinical signs and symptoms suggesting thrombophlebitis
  - 19% have cyanosis

**Causes:** As stated in the pathophysiology section, the aetiology of venous thrombosis and subsequent thromboembolism results from a distortion in Virchow's triad by venostasis, hypercoagulability, or vessel wall inflammation. These risk factors for venous thrombosis and pulmonary embolism can be broken down into hereditary factors and acquired factors.

- Hereditary factors (most result in a hypercoagulable state)
  - Antithrombin III deficiency
  - Protein S deficiency
  - Plasminogen abnormality
  - Plasminogen activator abnormality
  - Resistance to activated protein C
  - Protein C deficiency
  - Factor V Leiden (most common genetic risk factor for thrombophilia)
  - Fibrinogen abnormality
- Acquired factors (the most important clinically identifiable risk factors for DVT and PE are a prior history of DVT or PE, recent surgery or pregnancy, prolonged immobilization, or underlying malignancy.)
  - Reduced mobility
    - Fractures
    - Immobilization
    - Burns
    - Obesity
  - Acute medical illness
    - AIDS (lupus anticoagulant)
    - Behçet disease
    - Congestive heart failure (CHF)
    - Myocardial infarction
    - Polycythemia
    - Systemic lupus erythematosus
    - Ulcerative colitis
  - Hemolytic anemias
  - Homocysteinemia
  - Hyperlipidemias
  - Thrombocytosis
  - Venography
  - Venous stasis
  - Old age
  - Malignancy
    - Chemotherapy
  - Trauma/major surgery
    - Spinal cord injury
    - Catheters (indwelling venous infusion catheters)
    - Postoperative
  - Pregnancy
    - Postpartum period
    - Oral contraceptives
    - Estrogen replacements (high dose only)
  - Drug abuse [intravenous (IV) drugs]
  - Drug-induced lupus anticoagulant
  - Heparin-associated thrombocytopenia
  - Homocystinuria
  - Phenothiazines
  - Varicose veins
  - Venous pacemakers
  - Warfarin (first few days of therapy)

In patients with recognized pulmonary embolism, the incidence of physical signs has been reported as follows:

- Tachypnea (respiratory rate >16/min)—96%
- Rales—58%
- Accentuated second heart sound—53%
- Tachycardia (heart rate >100/min)—44%
- Fever (temperature >37.8°C)—43%
- Diaphoresis—36%
- S3 or S4 gallop—34%
- Clinical signs and symptoms suggesting thrombophlebitis—32%
- Lower extremity edema—24%
- Cardiac murmur—23%
- Cyanosis—19%
- The PIOPED study reported the following incidence of common symptoms of pulmonary embolism:
- Dyspnea (73%)
- Pleuritic chest pain (66%)
- Cough (37%)
- Hemoptysis (13%)
- Fever of less than 39°C may be present in 14% of patients; however, temperature higher than 39.5°C is not from pulmonary embolism.
- Chest wall tenderness upon palpation, without a history of trauma, may be the sole physical finding in rare cases.

**Table 17.3:** Wells clinical score for DVT

| Clinical parameter score | Score |
|---|---|
| Active cancer (treatement ongoing, or within 6 months or palliative | +1 |
| Paralysis or recent plaster immobile | +1 |
| Recently bedridden for >3 days or major surgery 4 weeks | +1 |
| Localized tenderness along the distribution of the deep venous system | +1 |
| Entire leg swelling | +1 |
| Calf swelling >3 cm compared with the asymptomatic leg | +1 |
| Pitting edema (greater in the symptomatic leg) | +1 |
| Previous DVT documented | +1 |
| Collateral superficial veins (non varicose) | +1 |
| Alternative diagnosis (as likely or greater than that of DVT) | –2 |
| **Total of above score** | |
| High probability | ≥3 |
| Moderate probability | 1 or 2 |
| Low probability | ? 0 |
| **Clinical parameter score** | |
| Active cancer (treatment ongoing, or within 6 months or paliative) | +1 |
| Paralysis or recent plaster immobilization of the lower extremities | +1 |
| Recently bedridden for >3 days or major surgery 4 weeks | +1 |
| Localized tenderness along the distribution of the deep venous system | +1 |
| Entire leg swelling | +1 |
| Calf swelling >3 cm compared with the asymptomatic leg | +1 |
| Pitting edema (greater in the symptomatic leg) | +1 |
| Previous DVT documented | +1 |
| Collateral superfacial venis (nonvaricose) | +1 |
| Alternative diagnosis (as likely or greater than that of DVT) | –2 |
| **Total of above score** | |
| High probability | ≥3 |
| Moderate probability | 1 or 2 |
| Low probability | ? 0 |

- **Pleuritic chest** pain without other symptoms or risk factors may be a presentation of pulmonary embolism. Pleuritic or respirophasic chest pain is a particularly worrisome symptom. Pleuritic chest pain is reported to occur in as many as 84% of patients with pulmonary emboli. Its presence suggests that the embolus is located more peripherally and thus may be smaller. Pulmonary embolism has been diagnosed in 21% of young, active patients who come to emergency departments (EDs) complaining only of pleuritic chest pain. These patients usually lack any other classical signs, symptoms, or known risk factors for pulmonary thromboembolism. Such patients often are dismissed inappropriately with an inadequate workup and a nonspecific diagnosis, such as musculoskeletal chest pain or pleurisy.

### Massive Pulmonary Embolism

Patients with massive pulmonary embolism are in shock. They have systemic hypotension, poor perfusion of the extremities, tachycardia, and tachypnea. In addition, patients appear weak, pale, sweaty, and oliguric and develop impaired mentation. Signs of pulmonary hypertension, such as palpable impulse over the second left intercostal space, loud P2, right ventricular S3 gallop, and a systolic murmur louder on inspiration at left sternal border (tricuspid regurgitation), may be present.

Massive pulmonary embolism has been defined by hemodynamic parameters and evidence of myocardial injury rather than anatomic findings because the former is associated with adverse outcomes. Although previous studies of CT scans in the diagnosis of pulmonary embolus suggested that central obstruction was not associated with adverse outcomes, a new multicenter study clarifies this observation. Vedovati et al. found no association between central obstruction and death or clinical deterioration in 579 patients with pulmonary embolus. However, when a subset of 516 patients who were hemodynamically stable was assessed, central localization of emboli was found to be an independent mortality risk factor while distal localization was inversely associated with adverse events. Thus, anatomic findings by CT scan may be important in assessing risk in hemodynamically stable patients with pulmonary embolus.

### Acute Pulmonary Infarction

Approximately 10% of patients have peripheral occlusion of a pulmonary artery, causing parenchymal infarction. These patients present with acute onset of pleuritic chest pain, breathlessness, and hemoptysis. Although the chest pain may be clinically indistinguishable from ischemic myocardial pain, normal ECG findings and no response to nitroglycerin rules out myocardial pain. Patients with acute pulmonary infarction have decreased excursion of the involved hemithorax, palpable or audible pleural friction rub, and even localized tenderness. Signs of pleural effusion, such as dullness to percussion and diminished breath sounds, may be present.

### Acute Embolism without Infarction

Patients with acute embolism without infarction have nonspecific physical signs that may easily be secondary to another disease process. Tachypnea and tachycardia frequently are detected, pleuritic pain sometimes may be present, crackles may be heard in the area of embolization, and local wheeze may be heard rarely.

### Multiple Pulmonary Emboli or Thrombi

Patients with pulmonary emboli and thrombi have physical signs of pulmonary hypertension and cor pulmonale. Patients may have elevated jugular venous pressure, right ventricular heave, palpable impulse in the left second intercostal space, right ventricular S3 gallop, systolic murmur over the left sternal border that is louder during inspiration, hepatomegaly, ascites, and dependent pitting edema. These findings are not specific for pulmonary embolism and require a high index of suspicion for pursuing appropriate diagnostic studies.

### Pulmonary Emboli in Children

Many physical findings are typically less marked in children than they are in adults, presumably because children have greater hemodynamic reserve and, thus, are better able to tolerate the significant hemodynamic and pulmonary changes. Because of the rarity of pulmonary emboli in children, these patients are probably underdiagnosed. For the same reason, much of the information pertaining to diagnosis and management of pulmonary embolism has been derived from adult practice.

1. Cough is present in approximately 50% of children with pulmonary emboli.
2. Tachypnea occurs with the same frequency. Hemoptysis is a feature in a minority of children with pulmonary emboli, occurring in about 30% of cases.
3. Crackles are heard in a minority of cases.
4. Cyanosis and hypoxemia are not prominent features of pulmonary embolism. If present, cyanosis suggests a massive embolism leading to a marked ventilation-perfusion (V/Q) mismatch and systemic hypoxemia. Some case reports have described massive pediatric pulmonary embolism with normal saturation.
5. A pleural rub is often associated with pleuritic chest pain and indicates an embolism in a peripheral location in the pulmonary vasculature. Signs that indicate pulmonary hypertension and right ventricular failure include a loud pulmonary component of the second heart sound, right ventricular lift, distended neck veins, and hypotension. An increase in pulmonary artery pressure is reportedly not evident until at least 60% of the vascular bed has been occluded.
6. A gallop rhythm signifies ventricular failure, while peripheral edema is a sign of congestive heart failure. Various heart murmurs may be audible, including a tricuspid regurgitant murmur signifying pulmonary hypertension.
7. Fever is an unusual sign that is nonspecific, and diaphoresis is a manifestation of sympathetic arousal. Signs of other organ involvement in patients with sickle cell disease would be elicited, such as sequestration crisis, priapism, anemia, and stroke.

## Blood Testing

### Clinical Scoring Systems

Evidence-based literature supports the practice of determining the clinical probability of pulmonary embolism before proceeding with testing. A clinical practice guideline from the American Academy of Family Physicians (AAFP) and the American College of Physicians (ACP) recommends that validated clinical prediction rules be used to estimate pretest probability of pulmonary embolism and to interpret test results. The guideline, current diagnosis of venous thromboembolism in primary care, advocates use of the Wells prediction rule for this purpose but notes that the Wells rule performs better in younger patients without comorbidities or a history of venous thromboembolism than in other patients.

One study assessed the performance of four clinical decision rules in addition to D-dimer testing to exclude acute PE. All four rules, Wells rule, simplified Wells rule, revised Geneva score, and simplified revised Geneva score, showed similar performance for excluding acute PE when combined with a normal D-dimer result.

### D-Dimer Follow-Up on Low-to-Moderate Pretest Probability

When clinical prediction rule results indicate that the patient has a low or moderate pretest probability of pulmonary embolism, D-dimer testing is the usual next step.

D-Dimer, a degradation product produced by plasmin-mediated proteases of cross-linked fibrin, is measured by a variety of assay types, including quantitative, semiquantitative, and qualitative rapid enzyme-linked immunosorbent assays (ELISAs); quantitative and semiquantitative latex; and whole-blood assays. A systematic review of prospective studies of high methodologic quality concluded that the ELISAs—especially the quantitative rapid ELISA—dominate the comparative ranking among the D-dimer assays for sensitivity and negative likelihood ratio. The quantitative rapid ELISA has a sensitivity of 0.95 and negative likelihood ratio of 0.13; the latter is similar to that for a normal to near-normal lung scan in patients with suspected pulmonary embolism. Negative results on a high-sensitivity D-dimer test in a patient with a low pretest probability of pulmonary embolism indicate a low likelihood of venous thromboembolism and reliably exclude pulmonary embolism. A large, prospective, randomized trial found that in patients with a low probability of pulmonary embolism who had negative D-dimer results, forgoing additional diagnostic testing was not associated with an increased frequency of symptomatic venous thromboembolism during the subsequent 6 months. D-dimer testing is most reliable for excluding pulmonary embolism in younger patients who have no associated comorbidity or history of venous thromboembolism and whose symptoms are of short duration. However, it is of questionable value in patients who are older than 80 years, who are hospitalized, who have cancer, or who are pregnant, because nonspecific elevation of D-dimer concentrations is common in such patients.

D-dimer testing should not be used when the clinical probability of pulmonary embolism is high, because the test has low negative predictive value in such cases. Combining D-dimer results with measurement of the exhaled end-tidal ratio of carbon dioxide to oxygen ($etCO_2/O_2$) can be useful for diagnosis of pulmonary embolism. Kline et al found that, in moderate-risk patients with a positive D-dimer (>499 ng/ml), an $etCO_2/O_2$ <0.28 significantly increased the probability of finding segmental or larger pulmonary embolism on computed tomography multidetector-row pulmonary angiography, while an $etCO_2/O_2$) >0.45 predicted the absence of segmental or larger pulmonary embolism. Because of the poor specificity, positive D-dimer measurements are generally not helpful in diagnosis. In addition, the use of D-dimers in children is not well studied. A small pediatric series reported that D-dimers findings are negative in 40% of patients.A retrospective series reported an elevated D-dimer in 86% of patients at presentation.

### Ischemia-modified Albumin Levels

A potential alternative to D-dimer testing is assessment of the ischemia-modified albumin (IMA) level, which data suggest is 93% sensitive and 75% specific for pulmonary embolism. Notably, in a study comparing the prognostic value of IMA to D-dimer testing, IMA assessment in combination with Wells and Geneva probability scores appeared to positively impact overall sensitivity and negative predictive value. The positive predictive value of IMA, in particular, is better than D-dimer. However, it should not be used alone.

### White Blood Cell Count

The white blood cell (WBC) count may be normal or elevated in patients with pulmonary embolism, with a WBC count as high as 20,000 being not uncommon in patients with this condition.

### Arterial Blood Gases

Arterial blood gas determinations characteristically reveal hypoxemia, hypocapnia, and respiratory alkalosis; however, the predictive value of hypoxemia is quite low. The $PaO_2$ and the calculation of alveolar-arterial oxygen gradient contribute to the diagnosis in a general population thought to have pulmonary embolism. Nonetheless, in high-risk settings such as patients in postoperative states in whom other respiratory conditions can be ruled out, a low $PaO_2$ in conjunction with dyspnea may have a strong positive predictive value.

The $PO_2$ on arterial blood gases analysis (ABG) has a zero or even negative predictive value in a typical population of patients in whom pulmonary embolism is suspected clinically. This is contrary to what has been taught in many textbooks, and even though it seems counterintuitive, it is demonstrably true. This is because other etiologies that masquerade as pulmonary embolism are more likely to lower the $PO_2$ than pulmonary embolism. In fact, because other diseases that may masquerade as pulmonary embolism [e.g. chronic obstructive pulmonary disease (COPD), pneumonia, CHF] affect oxygen exchange more than does pulmonary embolism, the blood oxygen level often has an inverse predictive value for pulmonary embolism.

In most settings, fewer than half of all patients with symptoms suggestive of pulmonary embolism actually turn out to have pulmonary embolism as their diagnosis. In such a population, if any reasonable level of $PaO_2$ is chosen as a dividing line, the incidence of pulmonary embolism will be higher in the group with a $PaO_2$ above the dividing line than in the group whose $PaO_2$ is below the divider. This is a specific example of a general truth that may be demonstrated mathematically for any test finding with a Gaussian distribution and a population incidence of less than 50%. Conversely, in a patient population with a very high incidence of pulmonary embolismand a lower incidence of other respiratory ailments (e.g. postoperative orthopedic patients with sudden onset of shortness of breath), a low $PO_2$ has a strongly positive predictive value for pulmonary embolism.

The discussion above holds true not only for arterial $PO_2$ but also for the alveolar-arterial oxygen gradient and for the oxygen saturation level as measured by pulse oximetry. In particular, pulse oximetry is extremely insensitive, is normal in the majority of patients with pulmonary embolism, and should not be used to direct a diagnostic workup.

### Troponin Levels

**Serum troponin** levels can be elevated in up to 50% of patients with a moderate to large pulmonary embolism, presumptively due to acute right ventricular myocardial stretch.

Although troponin assessment is not currently recommended as part of the diagnostic workup, studies have shown that elevated troponin levels in the setting of pulmonary embolism correlate with increased mortality.

However, further studies need to be performed to identify subsets of patients with pulmonary embolism who might benefit from this testing. Serum troponin, although seemingly marginal for purposes of diagnosis of pulmonary embolism, may contribute significantly to the ability to stratify patients by risk for short-term death or adverse outcome events when they reach the ED. In patients with pulmonary embolism and normal blood pressure specifically, elevated serum troponin level has been associated with right ventricular overload.

**Leptin:** It is another cardiovascular risk factor that may be associated with outcome in acute pulmonary embolism. Dellas et al conducted a prospective analysis of 264 patients with acute pulmonary embolus and found that serum leptin levels were inversely associated with the risk of adverse outcomes. Further study will be needed to confirm these findings and determine the clinical utility of leptin measurement.

### Brain Natriuretic Peptide

Although brain natriuretic peptide (BNP) tests are neither sensitive nor specific, patients with pulmonary embolism tend to have higher BNP levels. BNP testing had a sensitivity and specificity of only 60% and 62%, respectively, in a case-control study of 2213 hemodynamically stable patients with suspected acute pulmonary embolism. Elevated levels of BNP or of its precursor, N-terminal pro-brain natriuretic peptide (NT-proBNP), do correlate with an increased risk of subsequent complications and mortality in patients with acute pulmonary embolism. One meta-analysis revealed that patients with a BNP level greater than 100 pg/ml or an NT-proBNP level greater than 600 ng/L had an all-cause in-hospital mortality rate 6- and 16-fold higher than those below these cutoffs, respectively. In a second smaller observational study, serum BNP levels greater than 90 pg/ml were associated with a higher rate of complications, such as the need for cardiopulmonary resuscitation, need for mechanical ventilation, need for vasopressor therapy, and death.

BNP testing is not currently recommended as part of the standard evaluation of acute pulmonary embolism, and future studies may aid in defining its role in this setting.

Elevated levels of brain-type natriuretic peptides (BNP) may also provide prognostic information. A meta-analysis demonstrated a significant association between elevated N-terminal-pro-BNP (NT-pro-BNP) and right ventricular function in patients with pulmonary embolism (P <.001), leading to an increased risk for complicated in-hospital course [odds ratio (OR) 6.8; 95% confidence interval [CI], 9.0–13] and 30-day mortality (OR 7.6; 95% CI, 3.4–17). Importantly, increased NT-pro-BNP alone does not justify more invasive treatment. A recent study by Scherz et al. analyzed a large sample of patients hospitalized with acute pulmonary embolism.

**Hyponatremia** at presentation was common and was associated with a higher risk of 30-day mortality and readmission.

## INVASIVE LABORATORY STUDIES

### Venography

Venography is the criterion standard for diagnosing DVT. With the advent of noninvasive imaging, it has become less common in pediatric and adult practice (Figs 17.5–17.8).

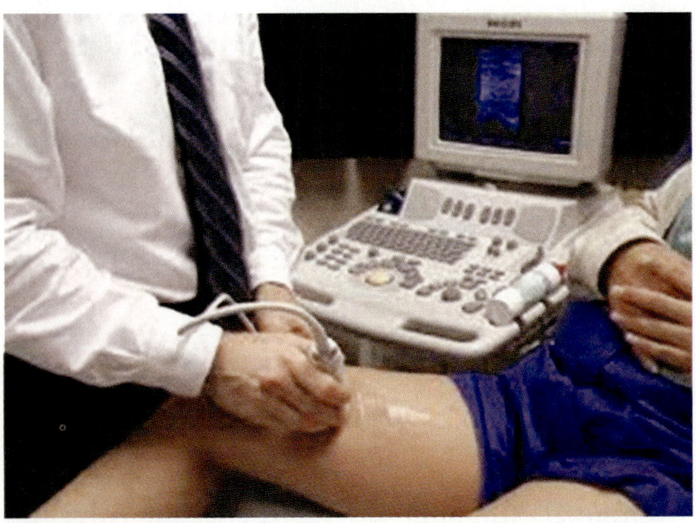

**Fig. 17.5:** Operator performing dual venous ultrasound examination for deep venous thrombosis and venous insuffiency in a young boy

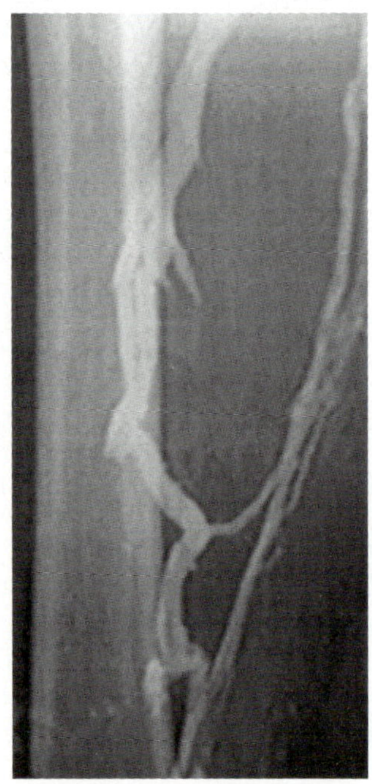

**Fig. 17.6:** Lower-extremity venogram shows a nonocclusive chronic thrombus. The superficial femoral vein (lateral vein) has the appearance of 2 parallel veins, when in fact, it is 1 lumen containing a chronic linear thrombus. Although the chronic clot is not obstructive after it recanalizes, it effectively causes the venous valves to adhere in an open position, predisposing the patient to reflux in the involved segment

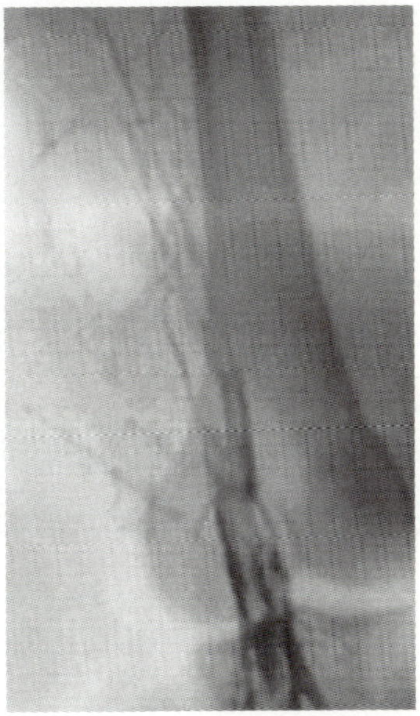

**Fig. 17.7:** Lower-extremity venogram shows outlining of an acute deep venous thrombosis in the popliteal vein with contrast enhancement

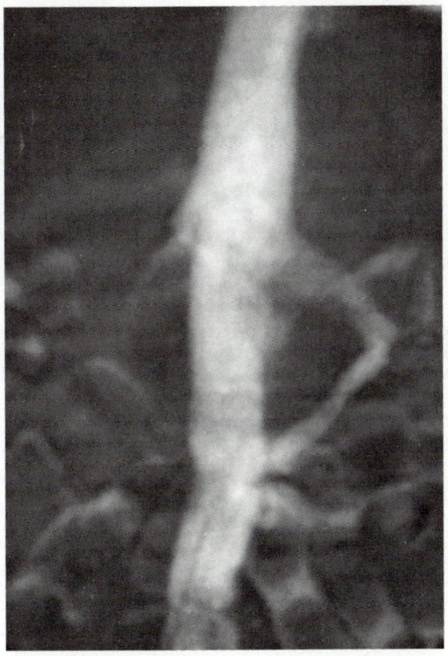

**Fig. 17.8:** Anteroposterior image from an inferior venacavographic examination demonstrates an inferior vena cava of normal diameter without thrombus. In addition, the inflow from the renal veins can be seen at the level of the L1 vertebral body

## NONINVASIVE LABORATORY STUDIES

### Chest Radiography

Chest radiographs are abnormal in most cases of pulmonary embolism, but the findings are nonspecific. Common radiographic abnormalities include atelectasis, pleural effusion, parenchymal opacities, and elevation of a hemidiaphragm. The classic radiographic findings of pulmonary infarction include a wedge-shaped, pleura-based triangular opacity with an apex pointing toward the hilus (Hampton hump) or decreased vascularity (Westermark sign). These findings are suggestive of pulmonary embolism but are infrequently observed. A prominent central pulmonary artery (knuckle sign), cardiomegaly (especially on the right side of the heart), and pulmonary edema are other findings. In the appropriate clinical setting, these findings could be consistent with acute cor pulmonale (Fig. 17.9).

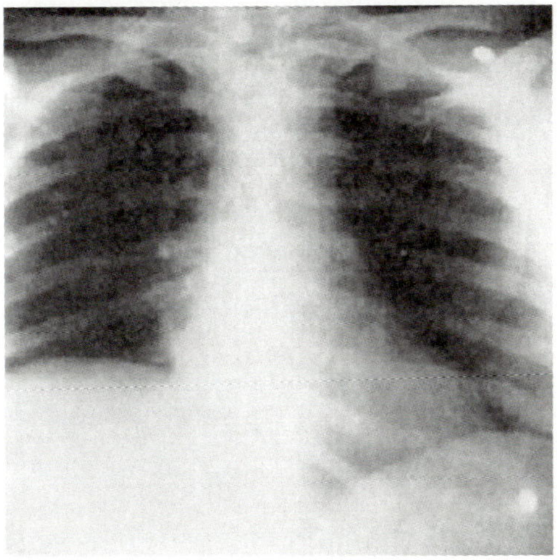

**Fig. 17.9:** Photograph X-ray chest PA view shows elevation of hemidiaphragm on right side is significant of deep vein thromboembolism

A normal-appearing chest radiograph in a patient with severe dyspnea and hypoxemia, but without evidence of bronchospasm or a cardiac shunt, is strongly suggestive of pulmonary embolism. The ACR recommends chest radiography as the most appropriate study for ruling out other causes of chest pain in patients with suspected pulmonary embolism. Initially, the chest radiographic findings are normal in most cases of pulmonary embolism. However, in later stages, radiographic signs may include a Westermark sign (dilatation of pulmonary vessels and a sharp cutoff), atelectasis, a small pleural effusion, and an elevated diaphragm. Generally, chest radiographs cannot be used to conclusively prove or exclude pulmonary embolism; however, radiography and electrocardiography may be useful for establishing alternative diagnoses.

### Electrocardiography

The most common ECG abnormalities in the setting of pulmonary embolism are tachycardia and nonspecific ST-T-wave abnormalities (Figs 17.10 and 17.11). The finding of S1 Q3 T3 is nonspecific and insensitive in the absence of clinical suspicion for pulmonary embolism. The classic findings of right heart strain and acute cor pulmonale are tall, peaked P-waves in lead II (P pulmonale); right axis deviation; right bundle-branch block; an S1 Q3 T3 pattern; or atrial fibrillation.

Unfortunately, only 20% of patients with proven pulmonary embolism have any of these classic electrocardiographic abnormalities. If electrocardiographic abnor-

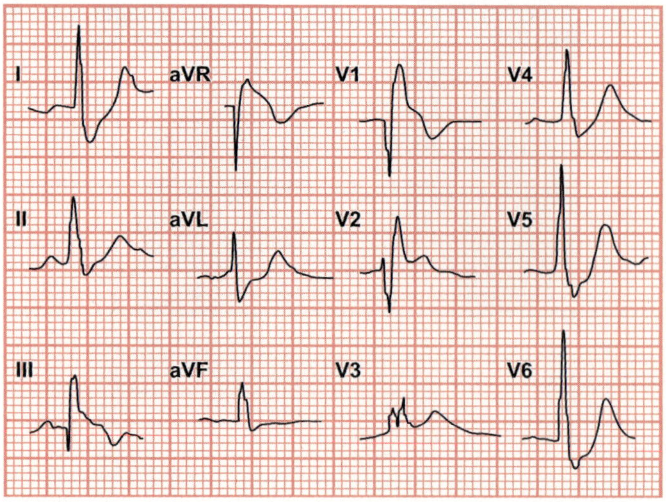


**Fig. 17.10:** SI, Q3, T3 pattern right bundle branch block (incomplete or complete). T-wave inversion in the right precordial leads P pulmonale. Right axis deviation in a patient with acute pulmonary embolism

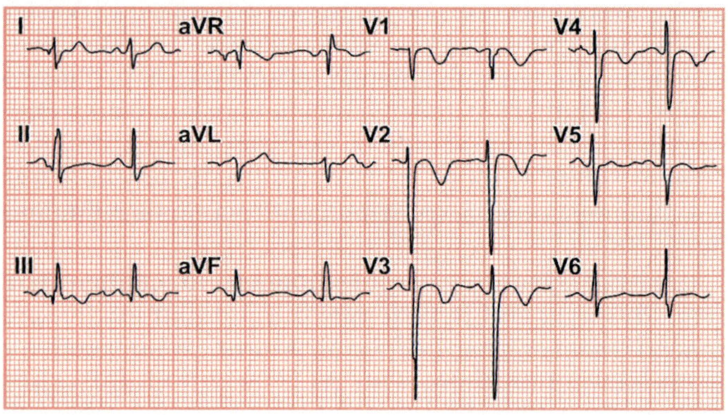


**Fig. 17. 11:** Acute pulmonary embolism—10 days postoperatively the patient developed acute dyspnea and hypotension (note the T-wave inversion in the right precordial leads and limb lead III)

malities are present, they may be suggestive of pulmonary embolism, but the absence of such abnormalities has no significant predictive value.

## Echocardiography

This modality generally has limited accuracy in the diagnosis of pulmonary embolism. Transesophageal echocardiography may identify central pulmonary embolism, and the sensitivity for central pulmonary embolism is reported to be 82%. Overall sensitivity and specificity for central and peripheral pulmonary embolism is 59% and 77%. Echocardiography (ECHO) provides useful information (Figs 17.12–17.14).

It may allow diagnosis of other conditions that may be confused with pulmonary embolism, such as pericardial effusion. ECHO allows visualization of the right ventricle and assessment of the pulmonary artery pressure. ECHO serves a prognostic function; the mortality rate is almost 10% in the presence of right ventricular dysfunction and 0% in the absence of right ventricular dysfunction. (Vanni

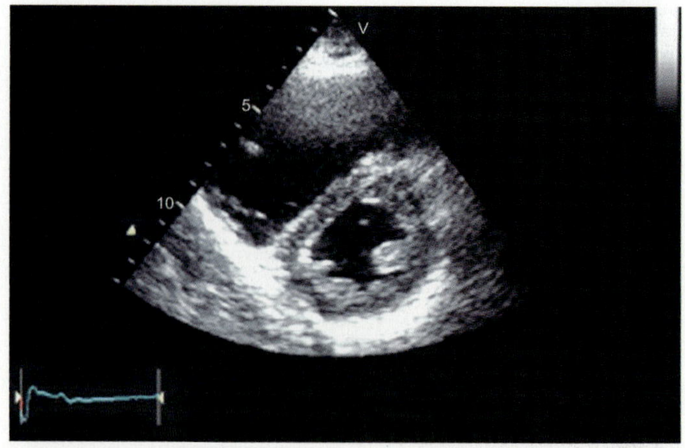


**Fig. 17.12:** 2D echocardiography parasternal short axis view at the level of papillary muscles—shows right ventricular dilatation, leftward shift of the interventricular septum as seen in pulmonary embolism

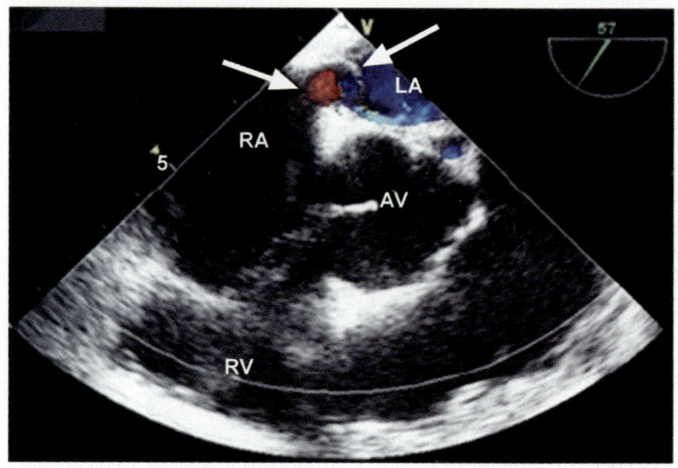


**Fig. 17.13:** A transesophageal echo was done intraoperatively which revealed normal left ventricle with mildly depressed systolic function, with an estimated ejection fraction of 50%. There was flattening of the interventricular septum consistent with right ventricular pressure overload. The interatrial septum was mobile with a large PFO and a large right to left shunt identified by color-Doppler analysis and agitated saline injection. The right ventricle was severely enlarged and hypokinetic. The right atrium was moderately enlarged. RV systolic pressure is 58 mmHg and the IVC was also dilated. There was mild-to-moderate tricuspid regurgitation with pulmonary hypertension. No other cardiac thrombi were noted

et al. reported that a right ventricular strain pattern is associated with a worse short-term outcome.) ECHO may be used to identify the presence of right-chamber emboli. The subcostal view is preferred at initial screening for mechanical activity and pericardial fluid and for gross assessment of global and regional abnormalities. To obtain a subcostal view, place the transducer on the left subcostal margin with the beam aimed at the left shoulder. The parasternal view allows visualization of the aortic valve, proximal ascending aorta, and posterior pericardium and permits determination of left ventricular size. It is

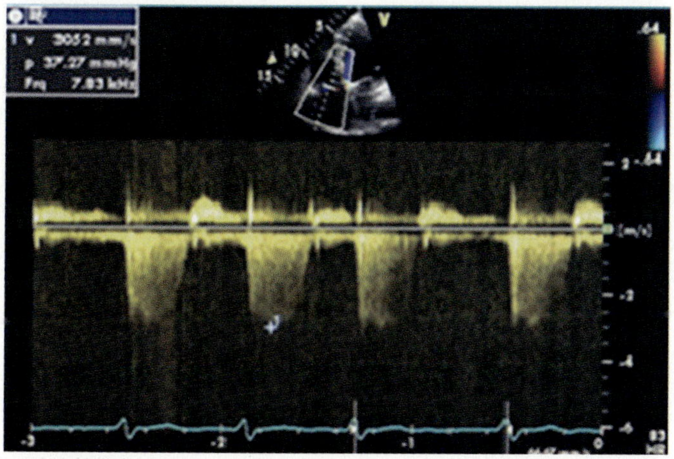

**Fig. 17.14:** Continuous Doppler echocardiography at the tricuspid valve—Doppler recording indicating tricuspid regurgitation, with an estimated RV-RA gradient of 37 mmHg in a patient with pulmonary embolism

particularly helpful when the subcostal view is difficult to obtain. To obtain a parasternal view, place the transducer in the left parasternal area between the second and fourth intercostal spaces. The plane of the beam is parallel to a line drawn from the right shoulder to the left hip. Several echocardiographic findings have been proposed for noninvasive diagnosis of right ventricular dysfunction at the bedside, including right ventricular enlargement and/ or hypokinesis of the free wall, leftward septal shift, and evidence of pulmonary hypertension. If right ventricular dysfunction is seen on cardiac ultrasonography, the diagnosis of acute submassive or massive pulmonary embolism is supported. While the presence of right ventricular dysfunction can be used to support the clinical suspicion of pulmonary embolism, prognostic information can be obtained by assessing the severity of right ventricular dysfunction.

### Computed Tomography Scanning

Technical advances in CT scanning, including the development of multidetector-array scanners, have led to the emergence of CT scanning as an important diagnostic technique in suspected pulmonary embolism (Fig. 17.15). Contrast-enhanced CT scanning is increasingly used as the initial radiologic study in the diagnosis of pulmonary embolism, especially in patients with abnormal chest radiographs in whom scintigraphic results are more likely to be nondiagnostic. Computed tomography angiography (CTA) is the initial imaging modality of choice for stable patients with suspected pulmonary embolism. The American College of Radiology (ACR) considers chest CTA to be the current standard of care for the detection of pulmonary embolism. A study by Ward et al. determined that a selective strategy in which CTA is used after compression ultrasonography is cost-effective for patients with a high pretest probability of pulmonary embolism. This strategy may reduce the need for CTA and help eliminate adverse effects associated with CTA.

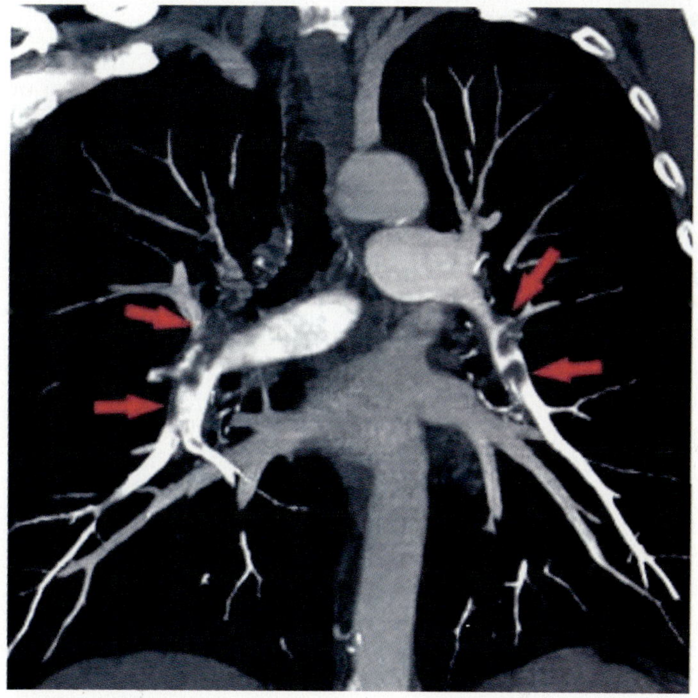

**Fig. 17.15:** Coronal maximum intensity projection reconstruction of a computed tomography pulmonary angiogram in a patient with multiple, bilateral pulmonary embolisms (arrows)

Toward a goal of reducing unnecessary CTA and associated radiation exposure, Drescher et al. studied the effect of implementing a computerized decision support system for pulmonary embolism evaluation in the ED. Before implementation, the rate of positive pulmonary embolism diagnosis for CTAs performed was 8.3%; after, the positivity rate rose to 12.7%. The positive yield would have been higher (16.7%) had emergency physicians adhered in all cases to the outcome of the decision support system; in 27% of cases they did not.

Like pulmonary angiography, CT scanning shows emboli directly, but it is noninvasive, cheaper than pulmonary angiography, and widely available. CT scanning is the only test that can provide significant additional information related to alternate diagnoses; spiral (helical) CT scanning results may suggest an alternative diagnosis in up to 57% of patients. This is a clear advantage of CT scanning over pulmonary angiography or scintigraphy.

A study of multidetector computed tomography (MDCTA) for detection of right ventricular dysfunction in 457 patients with acute pulmonary embolism found reasonable correlation with echocardiography, the reference standard. The criterion selected, a right-to-left ventricular dimensional ratio of 0.9 or more at MDCTA, had 92% sensitivity for right ventricular dysfunction. The combination of quantatative assessment of ventricular dimensions by CT and measurement of biomarkers may provide additional diagnostic accuracy for the presence of right ventricular dysfunction.

### Magnetic Resonance Imaging

With magnetic resonance imaging (MRI), evidence of pulmonary emboli may be detected by using standard or gated spin-echo techniques (Fig. 17.16). Pulmonary emboli demonstrate increased signal intensity within the pulmonary artery. By obtaining a sequence of images, this signal that is originating from slow blood flow may be distinguished from pulmonary embolism. However, this remains a problem in pulmonary hypertension.

Magnetic resonance angiography is performed following intravenous administration of gadolinium. Gadolinium-based contrast agents [gadopentetate dimeglumine (Magnevist), gadobenate dimeglumine (MultiHance), gadodiamide (Omniscan), gadoversetamide (OptiMARK), gadoteridol (ProHance)] have been linked to the development of nephrogenic systemic fibrosis (NSF) or nephrogenic fibrosing dermopathy (NFD). The disease has occurred in patients with moderate to end-stage renal disease after being given a gadolinium-based contrast agent to enhance MRI or magnetic resonance angiography scans. NSF/NFD is a debilitating and sometimes fatal disease. Characteristics include red or dark patches on the skin; burning, itching, swelling, hardening, and tightening of the skin; yellow spots on the whites of the eyes; joint stiffness with trouble moving or straightening the arms, hands, legs, or feet; pain deep in the hip bones or ribs; and muscle weakness. MRI has a sensitivity of 85% and specificity of 96% for central, lobar, and segmental emboli; MRI is inadequate for the diagnosis of subsegmental emboli. Few data are available regarding the use of MRI in children suspected of having a pulmonary embolism. Its use in these patients should be considered investigational at this time. Few investigators have reported the feasibility of MRI in the evaluation of pulmonary embolism. However, the role of MRI is mostly limited to the evaluation of patients who have impaired renal function or other contraindications for the use of iodinated contrast material. Newer blood-pool contrast agents and respiratory navigators may enhance the role of MRI in the diagnosis of pulmonary embolism.

### Ventilation-Perfusion Scanning

V/Q scanning of the lungs is an important modality for establishing the diagnosis of pulmonary embolism. However, V/Q scanning should be used only when CT scanning is not available or if the patient has a contraindication to CT scanning or intravenous contrast material. Children generally have a more homogenous perfusion scan; thus, deficits in perfusion are more likely to represent real or significant pulmonary embolism than they are in adults (Figs 17.17 and 17.18).

*A. The high-probability criteria are as follows:*
- Two large (>75% of a segment) segmental perfusion defects without corresponding ventilation or chest radiographic abnormalities
- One large segmental perfusion defect and two moderate (25–75% of a segment) segmental perfusion defects

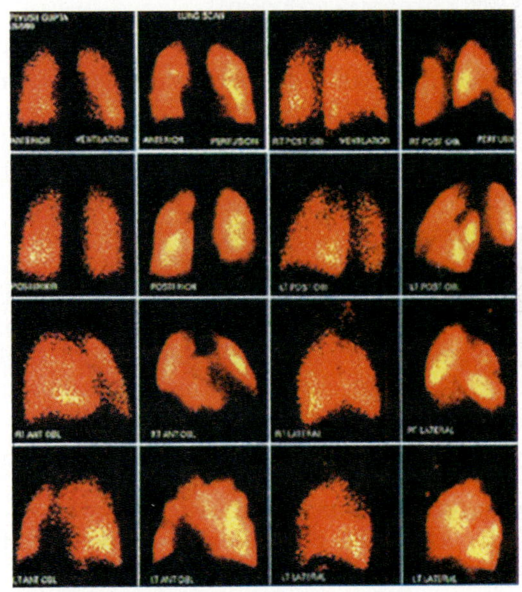

**Fig. 17.17:** Ventilation-perfusion scan of the patient showing reduced perfusion in right inferior and left upper lobes

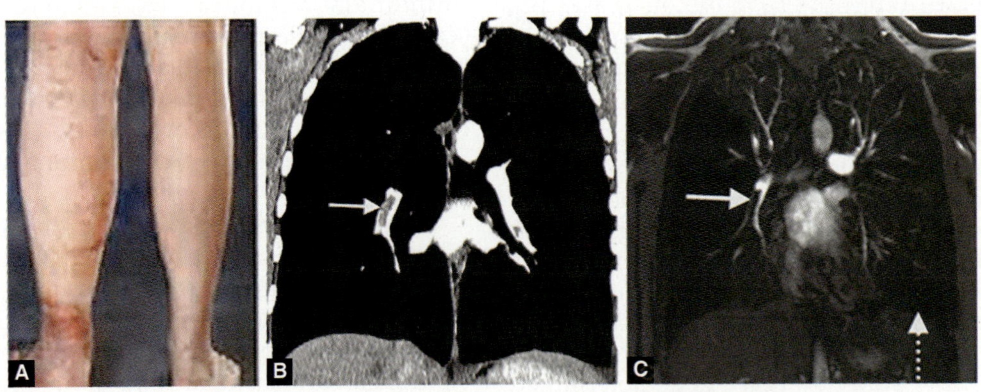


**Fig. 17.16:** A young female patient with swelling of the left leg. (A) CT angiography demonstrates thromboembolic material in the right (arrow) and left lower pulmonary artery. (B) High spatial resolution MR angiography performed using an intravascular contrast media. Both emboli were visualised; the image shows the thrombus in the right lower lobe (arrow). Also note the perfusion defect on right lower lobe. On the left side, the subsequent perfusion defect (dotted arrow) can be seen as an indirect sign of central vascular obstruction (C)

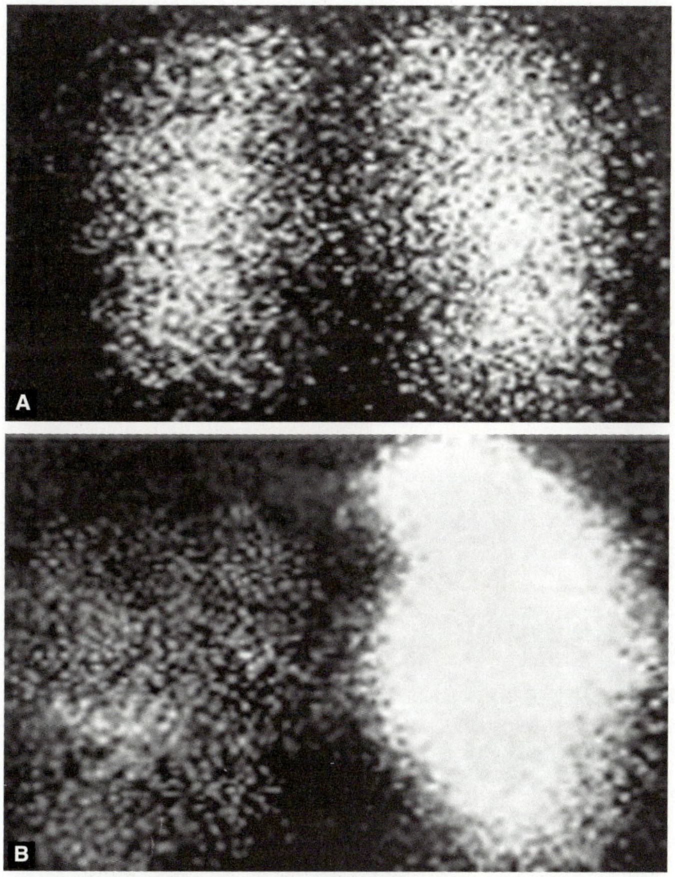


**Fig. 17.18:** (A) Normal ventilation scan. (B) Scan reveals defect in the right lung. Emboli in left lung not visualised

without corresponding ventilation or radiographic abnormalities
- Four moderate segmental perfusion defects without corresponding ventilation or chest radiographic abnormalities

*B. The intermediate-probability criteria are as follows:*
- One moderate to fewer than two large segmental perfusion defects without corresponding ventilation or chest radiographic abnormalities
- Corresponding V/Q defects and radiographic parenchymal opacity in lower lung zone
- Single moderate matched V/Q defects with normal chest radiographic findings
- Corresponding V/Q and chest radiography small pleural effusion
- Difficult to categorize as normal, low, or high probability

*C. Low probability criteria are as follows:*
- Multiple matched V/Q defects, regardless of size, with normal chest radiographic findings
- Corresponding V/Q defects and radiographic parenchymal opacity in upper or middle lung zone
- Corresponding V/Q defects and large pleural effusion
- Any perfusion defects with substantially larger radiographic abnormality
- Defects surrounded by normally perfused lung (**stripe sign**)
- More than three small (<25% of a segment) segmental perfusion defects with normal chest radiographic findings
- Nonsegmental perfusion defects (cardiomegaly, aortic impression, and enlarged hila)
- The normal finding is the presence of no perfusion defects and perfusion outlines the shape of the lung seen on a chest radiograph.
- The very low–probability criterion is the presence of three small (<25% of a segment) segmental perfusion defects with normal chest radiographic findings.

### *Pulmonary Angiography*

Pulmonary angiography (Fig. 17.19) remains the criterion standard for the diagnosis of pulmonary embolism. Following injection of iodinated contrast, anteroposterior, lateral, and oblique studies are performed on each lung. Positive results consist of a filling defect or sharp cutoff of the affected artery (as shown in the image below). Nonocclusive emboli are described as having a tram-track appearance. Abnormal findings on V/Q scans performed prior to angiography guide the operator to focus on abnormal areas. Angiography generally is a safe procedure. The mortality rate for patients undergoing this procedure is less than 0.5%, and the morbidity rate is less than 5%. Patients who have long-standing pulmonary arterial hypertension and right ventricular failure are considered high-risk patients. Negative pulmonary angiogram findings, even if false negative, exclude clinically relevant pulmonary embolism.

A pulmonary angiogram shows the abrupt termination of the ascending branch of the right upper-lobe artery, confirming the diagnosis of pulmonary embolism.

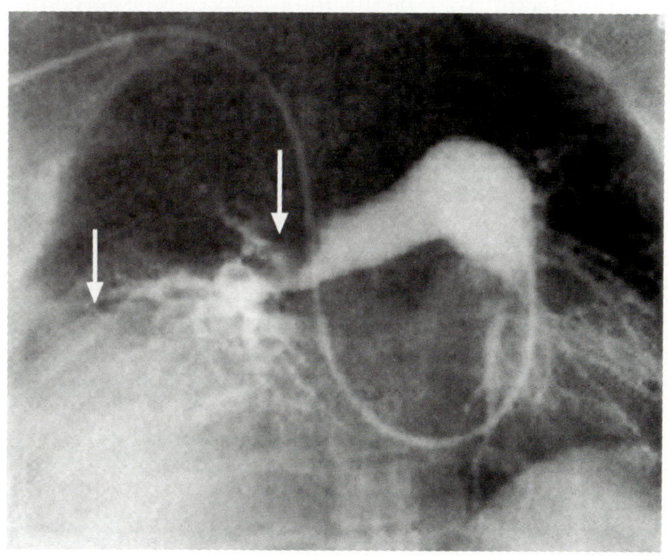

**Fig. 17.19:** Pulmonary angiography showing massive thrombus in the right pulmonary artery with almost complete obstruction to the blood flow (arrow). Note also the elevation of right hemidiaphragm (arrow)

If multidetector-row computed tomography angiography (MDCTA) is unavailable, conduct pulmonary angiography. Long the criterion standard for pulmonary embolism diagnosis, pulmonary angiography is nevertheless more invasive and harder to perform than MDCTA, and for these reasons, it is rapidly being replaced. However, pulmonary angiography remains a useful diagnostic modality when MDCTA cannot be performed.

When pulmonary angiography has been performed carefully and completely, a positive result provides virtually a 100% certainty that an obstruction to pulmonary arterial blood flow exists. A negative pulmonary angiogram provides a greater than 90% certainty for the exclusion of pulmonary embolism.

A positive angiogram is an acceptable endpoint no matter how abbreviated the study. However, a complete negative study requires the visualization of the entire pulmonary tree bilaterally. This is accomplished via selective cannulation of each branch of the pulmonary artery and injection of contrast material into each branch, with multiple views of each area. Even then, emboli in vessels smaller than third order or lobular arteries are not seen. Small emboli cannot be seen angiographically, yet embolic obstruction of these smaller pulmonary vessels is very common when postmortem examination follows a negative angiogram. These small emboli can produce pleuritic chest pain and a small sterile effusion even though the patient has a normal V/Q scan and a normal pulmonary angiogram. In most patients, however, pulmonary embolism is a disease of multiple recurrences, with large and small emboli already present by the time the diagnosis is suspected. Under these circumstances, the V/Q scan and the angiogram are likely to detect at least some of the emboli. Pulmonary angiography demonstrates subsegmental vessels in more detail than does CT scanning, although the superimposition of the small vessels remains a limiting factor. As a result, the interobserver agreement rate for isolated subsegmental pulmonary embolism is only 45%.

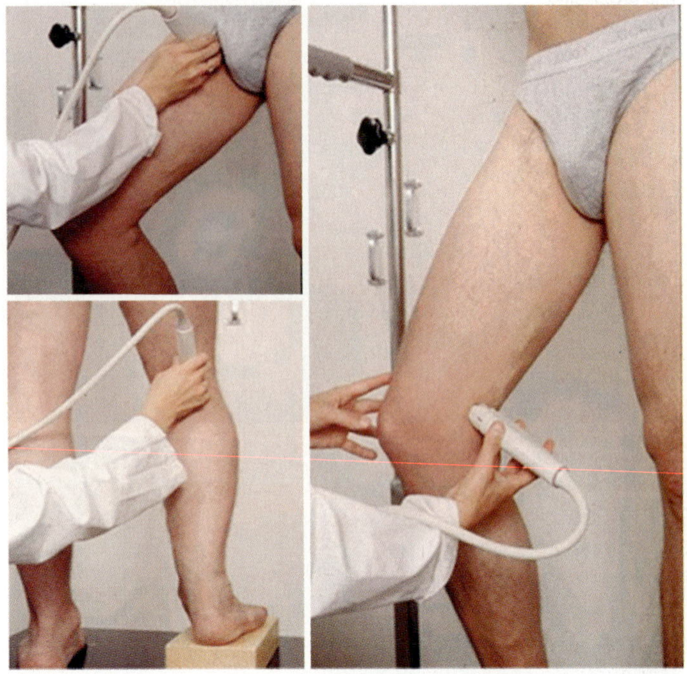

**Fig. 17.20:** Duplex ultrasound investigation of the veins in chronic venous disease of the lower limbs

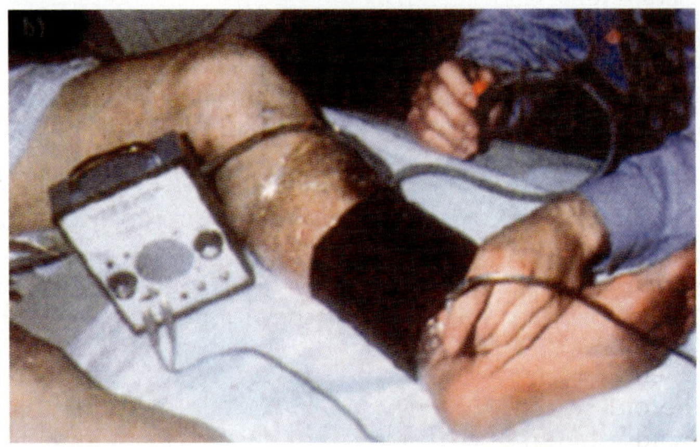

**Fig. 17.21:** Hand held Doppler and pneumatic cuff for determining the ankle brachial index in a diabetic patient with venu-arterial disease

### Duplex Ultrasonography and Plethysmography

The diagnosis of pulmonary embolism can be proven by demonstrating the presence of a DVT at any site. This may sometimes be accomplished noninvasively by using duplex ultrasonography. To look for DVT using ultrasonography, the ultrasonographic transducer is placed against the skin and pressed inward firmly enough to compress the vein being examined. In an area of normal veins, the veins are easily compressed completely closed, while the muscular arteries are extremely resistant to compression. Where DVT is present, the veins do not collapse completely when pressure is applied using the ultrasonographic probe. A negative ultrasonographic scan does not rule out DVT, because many DVTs occur in areas that are inaccessible to ultrasonographic examination. Before an ultrasonographic scan can be considered negative, the entire deep venous system must be interrogated using centimeter-by-centimeter compression testing of every vessel. In two-thirds of patients with pulmonary embolism, the site of DVT cannot be visualized with ultrasonography, so a negative duplex ultrasonographic scan does not markedly reduce the likelihood of pulmonary embolism (Figs 17.20–17.27).

### Probability Testing

Recent recommendations for a diagnostic algorithm have been published by the PIOPED investigators; however, these recommendations do not reflect research using 64 slice MDCT.

*These investigators recommended:* Low clinical probability. If negative D-dimer, PE is excluded. If positive D-dimer, obtain MDCT and based treatment on results.

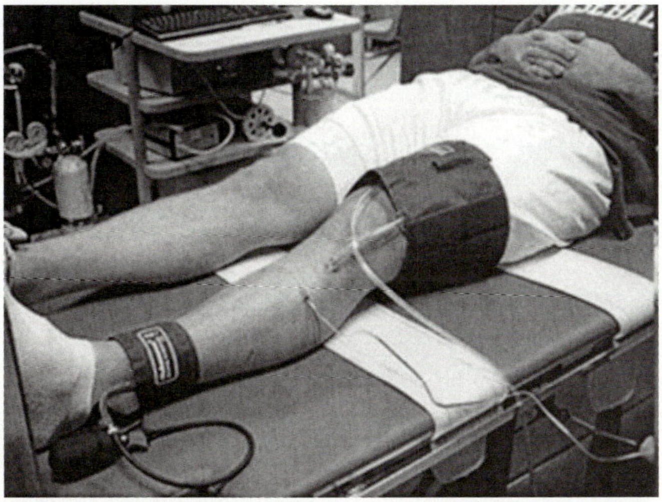

Fig. 17.22: Laboratory setup showing the thigh and ankle cuffs of the plethysmograph with the mercury-in-rubber strain gauge secured to the midcalf region

- ***Moderate clinical probability:*** If negative D-dimer, PE is excluded. However, the authors were not concerned that a negative MDCT with negative D-dimer in this setting has an 5% probability of being false. Presumably, the 5% error rate will fall as 64 slice MDCT is more commonly used. If positive D-dimer, obtain MDCT and based treatment on results.
- ***High clinical probability:*** Proceed to MDCT. If positive, treat, if negative, additional tests are needed to exclude PE.

### Pulmonary Embolism Rule-out Criteria

The pulmonary embolism rule-out criteria (PERC) help assess people in whom pulmonary embolism is suspected, but unlikely. Unlike the Wells Score and Geneva score, which are clinical prediction rules intended to risk stratify patients with suspected PE, the PERC rule is designed to rule out risk of PE in patients when the physician has already stratified them into a low-risk category.

Patients in this low risk category without any of these criteria may undergo no further diagnostic testing for PE:

- Hypoxia — $SaO_2$ <95%,
- Unilateral leg swelling,
- Hemoptysis,
- Prior DVT or PE,
- Recent surgery or trauma,
- Age >50,
- Hormone use,
- Tachycardia.

The rationale behind this decision is that further testing (specifically CT angiogram of the chest) may cause more harm (from radiation exposure and contrast dye) than the risk of PE. The PERC rule has a sensitivity of 97.4% and specificity of 21.9% with a false negative rate of 1.0%.

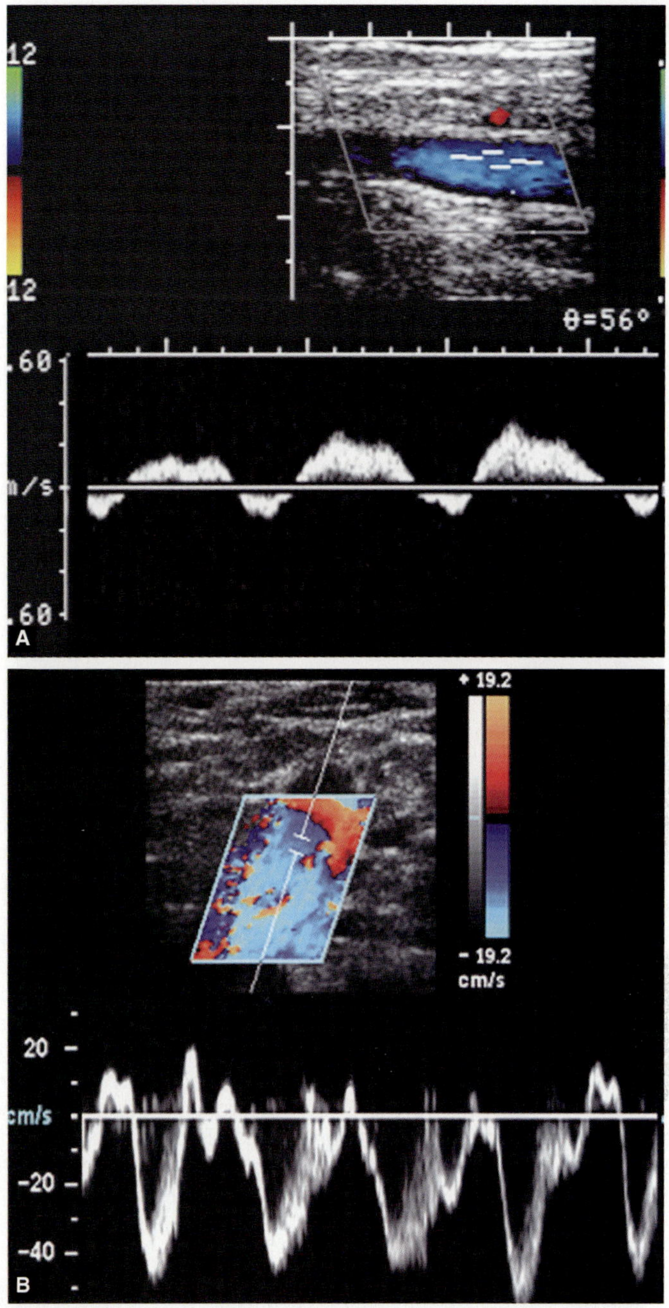


Fig. 17.23: (A) normal peripheral vein. (B) Duplex Doppler demonstrating nonphasic flow in a peripheral vein with thrombosis

### Risk Factors in PE

A deep vein thrombosis as seen in the right leg is a risk factor for PE. The most common sources of embolism are proximal leg deep venous thrombosis (DVTs) or pelvic vein thromboses. Any risk factor for DVT also increases the risk that the venous clot will dislodge and migrate to the lung circulation, which may happen in as many as 15% of all DVTs. The conditions are generally regarded as a continuum termed venous thromboembolism (VTE) (Table 17.4).

The development of thrombosis is classically due to a group of causes named Virchow's triad (alterations in blood

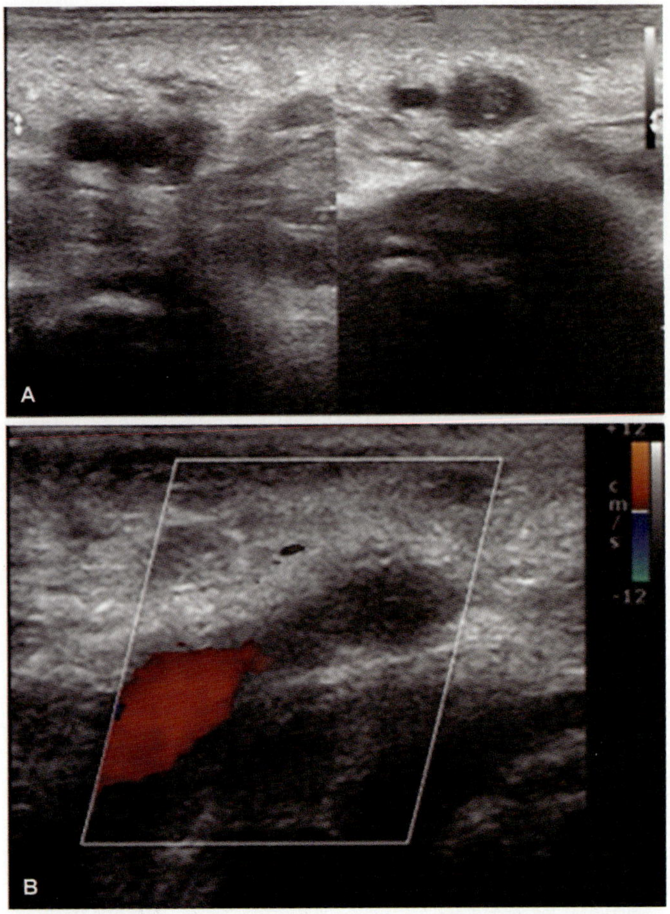


**Fig. 17.24:** Acute thrombosis of the common femoral vein in 2-year-old boy is demonstrated by cross-sectional imaging of the femoral vessels. (A) The left panel shows a dilated common femoral vein with echolucent luminal material. The right panel shows that the common femoral vein is not compressible, despite the use pressure that reduced the common femoral artery diameter by half. (B) The common femoral vein from the same patient is viewed with color imaging. The vein is dilated, contains echolucent material, and has absence of flow in contrast to normal flow in the adjacent common femoral artery

**Table 17.4:** Risk factors for DVT have been identified in many different epidemiologic studies

| | |
|---|---|
| **General** | • Age<br>• Immobilization longer than 3 days<br>• Pregnancy and the postpartum period<br>• Major surgery in previous 4 weeks<br>• Long plane or car trips (>4 h) in previous 4 weeks |
| **Medical** | • Cancer<br>• Previous DVT<br>• Stroke<br>• Acute myocardial infarction (AMI)<br>• Congestive heart failure (CHF)<br>• Sepsis<br>• Nephrotic syndrome<br>• Ulcerative colitis |
| **Trauma** | • Multiple trauma<br>• CNS/spinal cord injury<br>• Burns<br>• Lower extremity fractures |
| **Vasculitis** | • Systemic lupus erythematosus (SLE) and the lupus anticoagulant<br>• Behçet syndrome<br>• Homocystinuria |
| **Hematologic** | • Polycythemia rubra vera<br>• Thrombocytosis<br>• Inherited disorders of coagulation/fibrinolysis<br>• Antithrombin III deficiency<br>• Protein C deficiency<br>• Protein S deficiency<br>• Prothrombin 20210A mutation<br>• Factor V Leiden<br>• Dysfibrinogenemias and disorders of plasminogen activation |

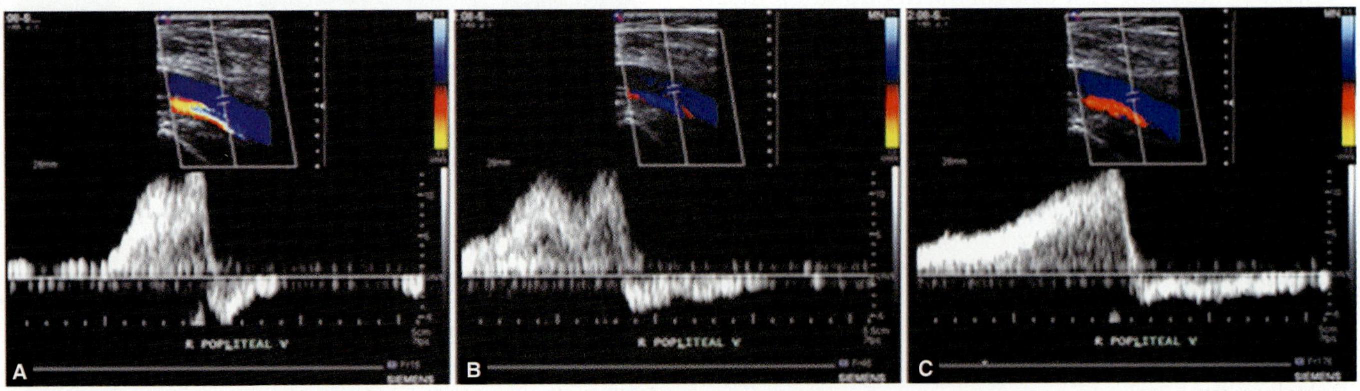


**Fig. 17.25:** Variability of reflux response. The effect of the length of augmentation on the tendency of lower extremity veins to reflux. All images are obtained from the same sample site in the popliteal vein of the same patient. (A) Short augmentation resulting in reflux time of only 0.7 seconds. (B) Longer augmentation resulting in reflux time of 1.5 seconds. (C) Prolonged augmentation resulting in continuous reflux for many seconds

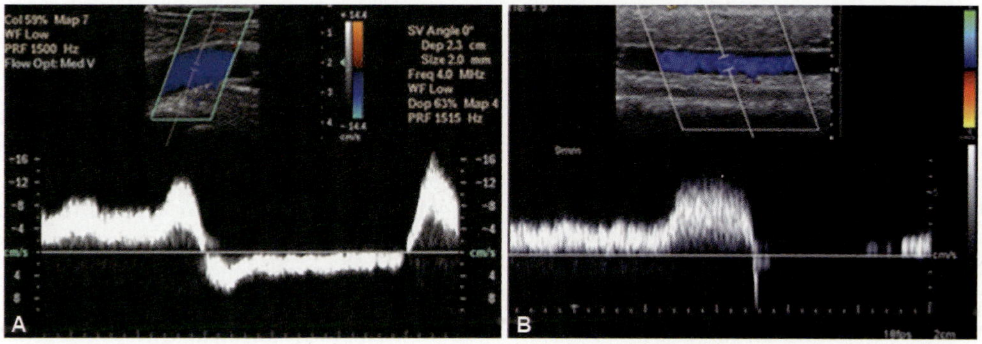

**Fig. 17.26:** (A) Refluxing deep vein. Reflux in the femoral vein elicited with a sustained Valsalva or simulated Valsalva manoeuvre lasting three seconds. (B) Competent superficial vein. Well-optimised duplex image of flow in a competent superficial vein. Wide color box was used in order for a long segment of the vein to be visualised. Spectral waveform is large and clear. Spontaneous venous flow is seen in the left side of the spectral trace, followed by manual augmentation. There is a sharp 'click' or 'snap' of venous valve closure followed by a period of absent flow. Once arterial inflow refills the peripheral vascular bed, normal antegrade flow resumes again on the right side of the spectral Doppler trace

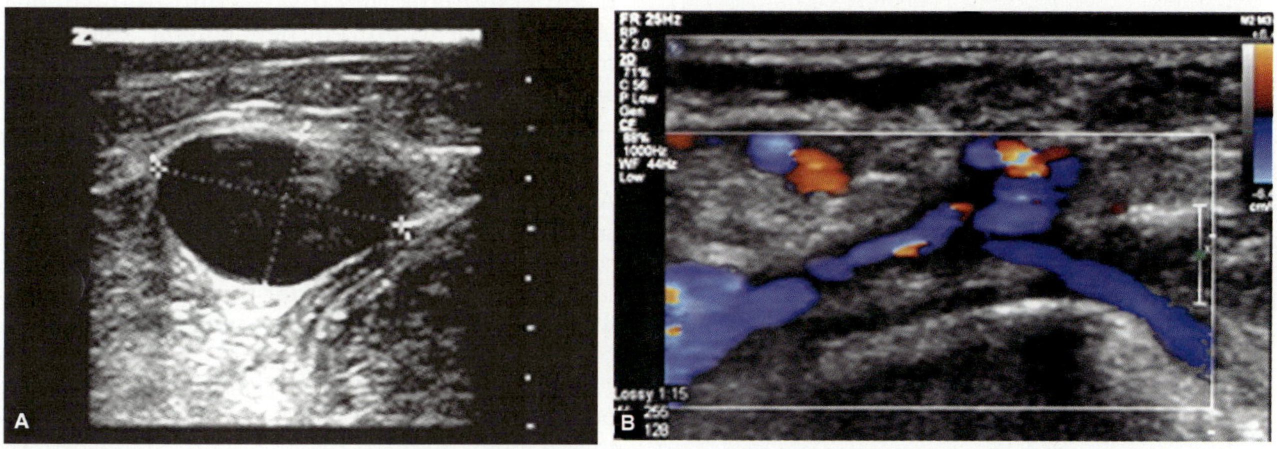

**Fig. 17.27:** (A) Patient is a 19-year adolescent that presented with swelling and aching of both lower extremities. He had bilateral varicose veins especially on the right with discoloration and stasis changes however no ulceration or previous ulceration was reported. He denied previous deep venous thrombosis or phlebitis. The patient was finally diagnosed as venous aneurysm of inferior vena cava. (B) Chronic thrombosis of the common femoral vein is seen a year after it was diagnosed in a 4-month-old girl. Echogenic material is seen in the lumen of the partially recanalized vein. Irregular flow channels are seen through the old thrombus in the common femoral vein

flow, factors in the vessel wall and factors affecting the properties of the blood). Often, more than one risk factor is present.

Alterations in blood flow—immobilization (after surgery, injury, pregnancy (also procoagulant), obesity (also procoagulant), and cancer (also procoagulant).

Factors in the vessel wall—surgery, catheterizations causing direct injury ('endothelial injury').

*Complications of pulmonary embolism* include the following:

- Sudden cardiac death
- Obstructive shock
- Pulseless electrical activity
- Atrial or ventricular arrhythmias
- Secondary pulmonary arterial hypertension
- Cor pulmonale
- Severe hypoxemia
- Right-to-left intracardiac shunt
- Lung infarction
- Pleural effusion
- Paradoxical embolism
- Heparin-induced thrombocytopenia
- Thrombophlebitis

## PREVENTION OF PULMONARY EMBOLISM

Preventing idiopathic outpatient pulmonary embolism is difficult, if not impossible. That said, the majority of pulmonary embolisms occur in hospitalized patients. The incidence in these cases can be reduced through appropriate prophylaxis, achieved mechanically or via the administration of heparin, LMWH, or warfarin. The incidence of venous thrombosis, pulmonary embolism, and death can be significantly reduced by embracing a prophylactic strategy in high-risk patients.

Prevention of DVT in the lower extremities inevitably reduces the frequency of pulmonary embolism; therefore, populations at risk must be identified, and safe and efficacious prophylactic modalities should be used. The Q-thrombosis algorithm is intended to identify currently asymptomatic adults at greatest future risk of venous thrombosis based on established risk factors. According to the study in which it was developed and validated, Q-thrombosis estimates the absolute risk of venous thrombosis at 1 year and 5 years into the future, information that can be used to guide prophylaxis and medication decisions.

## TREATMENT

Anticoagulant therapy is typically the mainstay of treatment. Acutely, supportive treatments, such as oxygen or analgesia, may be required. People are often admitted to hospital in the early stages of treatment, and tend to remain under inpatient care until the INR has reached therapeutic levels. Increasingly, however low-risk cases are managed at home in a fashion already common in the treatment of DVT.

### Anticoagulation

In most cases, anticoagulant therapy is the mainstay of treatment. Unfractionated heparin, low molecular weight heparin (LMWH), or fondaparinux is administered initially, while warfarin, acenocoumarol, or phenprocoumon therapy is commenced (this may take several days, usually while the patient is in the hospital). LMWH may reduce bleeding among patients with pulmonary embolism as compared to heparin according to a systematic review of randomized controlled trials by the Cochrane collaboration. The relative risk reduction was 40%. For patients at similar risk to those in this study (2.0% had bleeding when not treated with low molecular weight heparin), this leads to an absolute risk reduction of 0.8%. 125 patients must be treated for one to benefit.

Warfarin therapy often requires frequent dose adjustment and monitoring of the international normalized ratio (INR). In PE, INRs between 2.0 and 3.0 are generally considered ideal. If another episode of PE occurs under warfarin treatment, the INR window may be increased to e.g. 2.5–3.5 (unless there are contraindications) or anticoagulation may be changed to a different anticoagulant, e.g. LMWH. In patients with an underlying malignancy, therapy with a course of LMWH may be favored over warfarin based on the results of the CLOT trial. Similarly, pregnant women are often maintained on low molecular weight heparin until at least 6 weeks after delivery to avoid the known teratogenic effects of warfarin, especially in the early stages of pregnancy. Warfarin therapy is usually continued for 3–6 months, or 'lifelong' if there have been previous DVTs or PEs, or none of the usual risk factors is present. An abnormal D-dimer level at the end of treatment might signal the need for continued treatment among patients with a first unprovoked pulmonary embolus.

### Thrombolysis

Massive PE causing hemodynamic instability (shock and/or hypotension, defined as a systolic blood pressure <90 mmHg or a pressure drop of 40 mmHg for >15 min if not caused by new-onset arrhythmia, hypovolemia or sepsis) is an indication for thrombolysis, the enzymatic destruction of the clot with medication. It is the best available medical treatment in this situation and is supported by clinical guidelines. The use of thrombolysis in nonmassive PEs is still debated. The aim of the therapy is to dissolve the clot, but there is an attendant risk of bleeding or stroke. The main indication for thrombolysis is in submassive PE where right ventricular dysfunction can be demonstrated on echocardiography, and the presence of visible thrombus in the atrium.

#### *Inferior vena cava filter in the prevention of thromboembolism*

If anticoagulant therapy is contraindicated and/or ineffective, or to prevent new emboli from entering the pulmonary artery and combining with an existing blockage, an inferior vena cava filter may be implanted (Fig. 17.28).

#### *Catheter-based endovascular therapies in deep venous thrombosis*

Acute DVT should be viewed as a chronic disease by treating physicians, because the associated long-term patient disability is quite substantial (Figs 17.29–17.31). Catheter-based endovascular therapies offer the potential to preserve life and limb (for severely affected patients), prevent PTS, and improve quality of life in patients with proximal DVT. Multicenter randomized clinical trials are ongoing to determine which patients should be treated in this manner. Selected patients with established The post-thrombotic syndrome (PTS) may also now have a reasonable chance of experiencing symptom alleviation

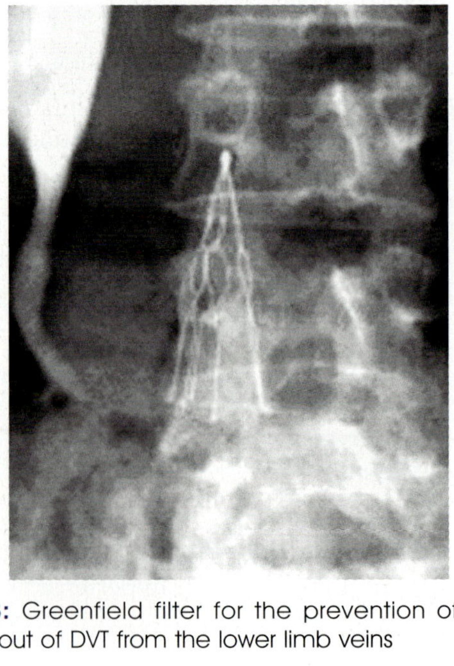

**Fig. 17.28:** Greenfield filter for the prevention of thromboembolism out of DVT from the lower limb veins

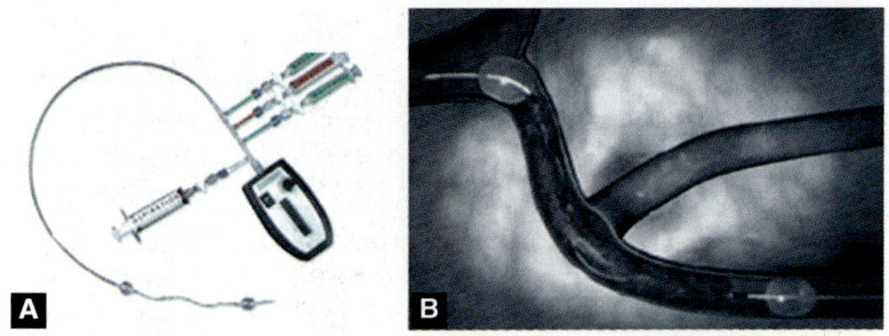

**Fig. 17.29:** (A) The Trellis-8 system (Bacchus Vascular, Santa Clara, CA) consists of proximal and distal balloons, with balloon inflation syringes, a thrombolysis infusion port, the thrombus aspiration syringe, and a drive unit for mechanical dispersion of the thrombolytic agent. (B) Trellis catheter ablation treatment for deep vein thrombosis

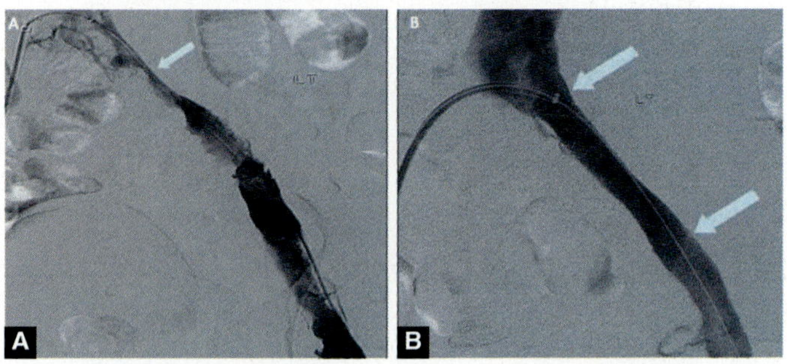

**Fig. 17.31:** (A) A left iliac vein angiogram reveals stenosis of the proximal left common iliac vein (arrow), suggestive of May-Thurner syndrome. (B) Final angiogram of the left iliac vein after stent deployment reveals complete resolution of thrombus and stenosis (arrows)

with the use of endovascular therapies. Hematologists and other thrombosis physicians should be aware of these options and consult their endovascular colleagues for patients in need of salvage therapy.

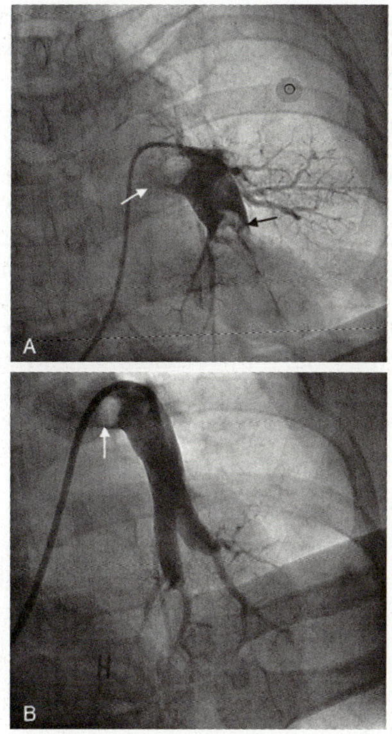

**Fig. 17.30:** Pulmonary artery angiogram. (A) The pulmonary artery angiogram showed massive thromboembolism at the left main pulmonary artery (arrow) without distal flow. (B) After percutaneous catheter thrombectomy, the opacity and distal flow was improved, but a large thrombus (arrow) remained at the left main pulmonary artery

## Stentoplasty in SVC Stenosis

**Superior vena cava (SVC) obstruction** can occur from extrinsic compression, intrinsic stenosis or thrombosis (Fig. 17.32). Malignancies are the main cause and is

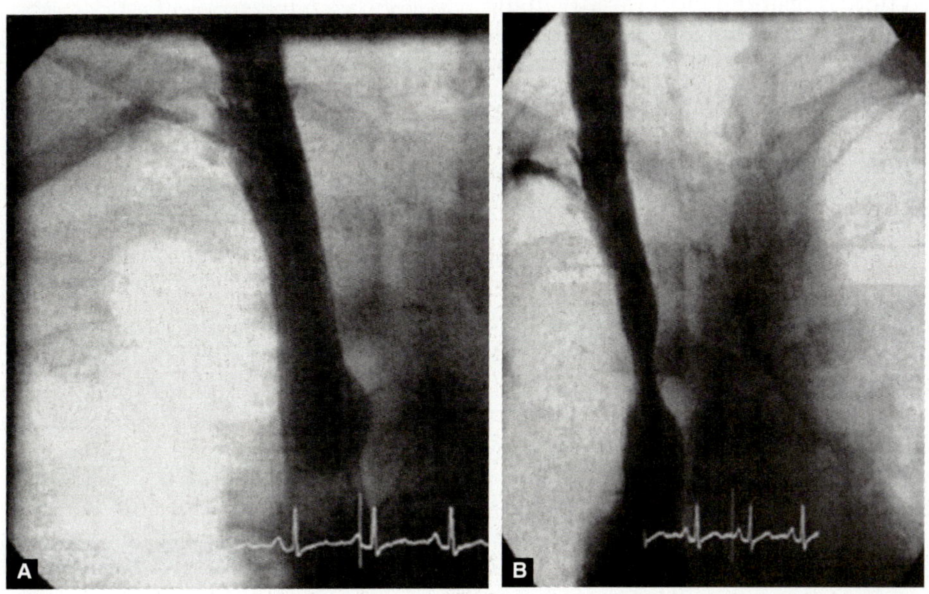

**Fig. 17.32:** (A) Superior venogram before stent deployment shows narrowing of the SVC. (B) Check angiogram showing no residual stenosis and good antegrade flow in the SVC

considered an oncologic emergency. **Superior vena cava syndrome (SVCS)** refers to the clinical syndrome with symptoms that results from this obstruction.

### Surgical Intervention

Surgical management of acute pulmonary embolism (pulmonary thrombectomy) is uncommon and has largely been abandoned because of poor long-term outcomes. However, recently, it has gone through a resurgence with the revision of the surgical technique and is thought to benefit certain people. Chronic pulmonary embolism leading to pulmonary hypertension (known as chronic thromboembolic hypertension) is treated with a surgical procedure known as a pulmonary thromboendarterectomy (Fig. 17.33).

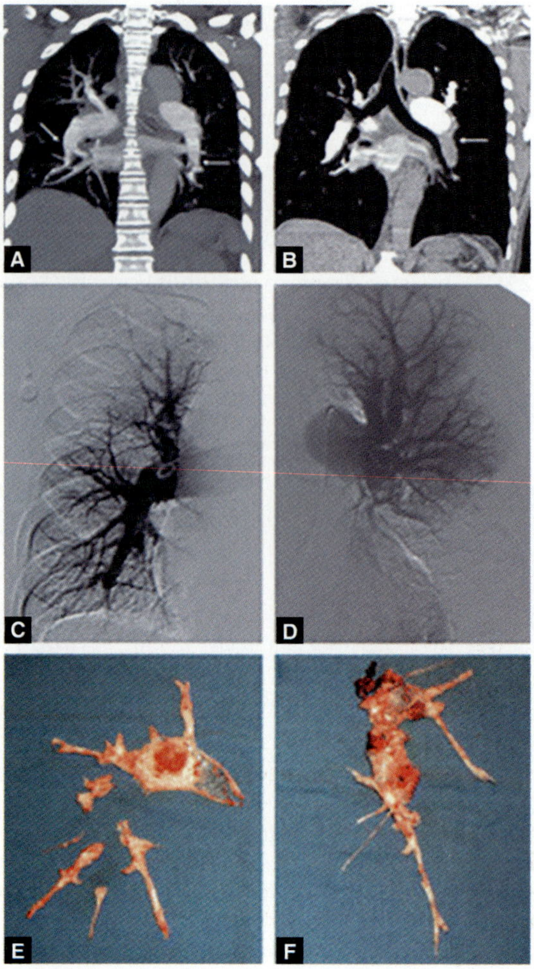

**Fig. 17.33.** (A) Computed tomography (CT) pulmonary angiogram showing evidence of webs in the descending branch of the right and left pulmonary artery (arrows). (B) CT pulmonary angiogram performed 1 year later after referral to our centre, demonstrating the presence of new large thrombi in the left pulmonary artery (arrow) that occurred despite treatment with low molecular weight heparin. (C) Pulmonary angiogram of the right pulmonary artery showing evidence of segmental defects in the right upper and lower lobes. (D) Pulmonary angiogram of the left pulmonary artery showing an occlusion of the descending branch to the left lower lobe. (E) Pulmonary endarterectomy specimen of the right lung. (F) Pulmonary endarterectomy specimen of the left lung

### Prognosis

Mortality from untreated PE is said to be 26%. This figure comes from a trial published in 1960 by Barrit and Jordan, which compared anticoagulation against placebo for the management of PE. Barritt and Jordan performed their study in the Bristol Royal Infirmary in 1957. This study is the only placebo controlled trial ever to examine the place of anticoagulants in the treatment of PE, the results of which were so convincing that the trial has never been repeated as to do so would be considered unethical. That said, the reported mortality rate of 26% in the placebo group is probably an overstatement, given that the technology of the day may have detected only severe PEs.

Prognosis depends on the amount of lung that is affected and on the coexistence of other medical conditions; chronic embolisation to the lung can lead to pulmonary hypertension. After a massive PE, the embolus must be resolved somehow if the patient is to survive. In thrombotic PE, the blood clot may be broken down by fibrinolysis, or it may be organized and recanalized so that a new channel forms through the clot. Blood flow is restored most rapidly in the first day or two after a PE. Improvement slows thereafter and some deficits may be permanent. There is controversy over whether or not small subsegmental PEs need to be treated at all and some evidence exists that patients with subsegmental PEs may do well without treatment. Once anticoagulation is stopped, the risk of a fatal pulmonary embolism is 0.5% per year.

## LONG-TERM MONITORING

PT should be measured on a regular basis; the goal is an INR of 2–3. The length of treatment depends on the presence of risk factors. If no underlying risk factors are present, therapy can be stopped within 1–2 months. If risk factors are present, especially anticardiolipin antibodies, therapy should continue for at least 4–6 months. Long-term anticoagulation is essential for patients who survive an initial DVT or pulmonary embolism. The optimum total duration of anticoagulation is controversial, but general consensus holds that at least 6 months of anticoagulation is associated with significant reduction in recurrences and a net positive benefit. Patients may have treatment initiated using concomitant warfarin and unfractionated heparin for 5 days in the hospital, with discharge on warfarin alone when the international normalized ratio (INR) is 2. Alternatively, patients may be discharged on concomitant therapy with a LMWH and warfarin for at least 5 days. The LMWH is then discontinued in the outpatient setting when the INR reaches 2.

## BIBLIOGRAPHY

1. Aklog L, Williams CS, Byrne JG, Goldhaber SZ. Acute pulmonary embolectomy: a contemporary approach. Circulation 2002;105:1416–9.

2. Bauer KA. The thrombophilias: well-defined risk factors with uncertain therapeutic implications. Ann Intern Med 2001; 135:367–73.
3. Brandjes DP, Buller HR, Heijboer H, Huisman MV, de Rijk M, Jagt H, et al. Randomised trial of effect of compression stockings in patients with symptomatic proximal-vein thrombosis. Lancet 1997;349:759–62.
4. Crowther MA, Harrison L, Hirsh J. Reply. Warfarin: less may be better. Ann Intern Med 1997:127:333.
5. Decousus H, Leizorovicz A, Parent F, Page Y, Tardy B, Girard P, et al. A clinical trial of vena caval filters in the prevention of pulmonary embolism in patients with proximal deep-vein thrombosis. N Engl J Med 1998;338:409–15.
6. Geerts WH, Heit JA, Clagett GP, Pineo GF, Colwell CW, Anderson FA Jr, et al. Prevention of venous thromboembolism. Chest 2001;119(1 Suppl):132S–75S.
7. Hull RD, Raskob GE, Brant RF, Pineo GF, Elliott G, Stein PD, et al. Low-molecular-weight heparin vs heparin in the treatment of patients with pulmonary embolism. American-Canadian Thrombosis Study Group. Arch Intern Med 2000;160:229–36.
8. Hull RD, Raskob GE, Rosenbloom D, Panju AA, Brill-Edwards P, Ginsberg JS, et al. Heparin for 5 days as compared with 10 days in the initial treatment of proximal venous thrombosis. N Engl J Med 1990;322:1260–4.
9. Hyers TM, Agnelli G, Hull RD, Morris TA, Samama M, Tapson V, et al. Antithrombotic therapy for venous thromboembolic disease. Chest 2001;119(1 suppl): 176S–93S.
10. Juergens CP, Semsarian C, Keech AC, Beller EM, Harris PJ. Hemorrhagic complications of intravenous heparin use. Am J Cardiol 1997;80:150–4.
11. Kearon C, Ginsberg JS, Kovacs MJ, Anderson DR, Wells P, Julian JA, et al. Comparison of low-intensity warfarin therapy with conventional-intensity warfarin therapy for long-term prevention of recurrent venous thrombo-embolism. N Engl J Med 2003;349:631–9.
12. Konstantinides S, Geibel A, Heusel G, Heinrich F, Kasper W. Heparin plus alteplase compared with heparin alone in patients with submassive pulmonary embolism. N Engl J Med 2002;347:1143–50.
13. Kovacs MJ, Anderson D, Morrow B, Gray L, Touchie D, Wells PS. Outpatient treatment of pulmonary embolism with dalteparin. Thromb Haemost 2000;83:209–11.
14. Kovacs MJ, Rodger M, Anderson DR, Morrow B, Kells G, Kovacs J, et al. Comparison of 10-mg and 5-mg warfarin initiation nomograms together with low-molecular-weight heparin for outpatient treatment of acute venous thromboembolism. A randomized, double-blind, controlled trial. Ann Intern Med 2003;138:714–9.
15. Lee AY, Levine MN, Baker RI, Bowden C, Kakkar AK, Prins M, et al. Low-molecular-weight heparin versus a coumarin for the prevention of recurrent venous thromboembolism in patients with cancer. N Engl J Med 2003;349:146–53.
16. Levine M, Gent M, Hirsh J, Leclerc J, Anderson D, Weitz J, et al. A comparison of low-molecular-weight heparin administered primarily at home with unfractionated heparin administered in the hospital for proximal deep-vein thrombosis. N Engl J Med 1996;334:677–81.
17. Lilienfeld DE. Decreasing mortality from pulmonary embolism in the United States, 1979–1996. Int J Epidemiol 2000;29:465–9.
18. Pinede L, Ninet J, Duhaut P, Chabaud S, Demolombe-Rague S, Durieu I, et al. Comparison of 3 and 6 months of oral anticoagulant therapy after a first episode of proximal deep vein thrombosis or pulmonary embolism and comparison of 6 and 12 weeks of therapy after isolated calf deep vein thrombosis. Circulation 2001;103:2453–60.
19. Ramzi DW, Leeper KV. DVT and pulmonary embolism: part I. Diagnosis. Am Fam Physician 2004;69:2829–36.
20. Raschke RA, Reilly BM, Guidry JR, Fontana JR, Srinivas S. The weight-based heparin dosing nomogram compared with a "standard care" nomogram. A randomized controlled trial. Ann Intern Med 1993;119:874–81.
21. Ridker PM, Goldhaber SZ, Danielson E, Rosenberg Y, Eby CS, Deitcher SR, et al. Long-term, low-intensity warfarin therapy for the prevention of recurrent venous thromboembolism. N Engl J Med 2003;348:1425–34.
22. Savage KJ, Wells PS, Schulz V, Goudie D, Morrow B, Cruickshank M, et al. Out-patient use of low molecular weight heparin (dalteparin) for the treatment of deep vein thrombosis of the upper extremity. Thromb Haemost 1999;82:1008–10.

# 18 Aortic Dissection

Aortic dissection is defined as separation of the layers within the aortic wall. Tears in the intimal layer result in the propagation of dissection (proximally or distally) secondary to blood entering the intima-media space. Much has been written on the subject of aortic dissections, from the first well-documented case of aortic dissection, when King George II of England died while straining on the commode, to the first successful operative repairs by DeBakey in 1955, to modern techniques of diagnosing and repairing thoracic aortic dissections.

Aortic dissection is the most common catastrophe of the aorta, 2–3 times more common than rupture of the abdominal aorta. When left untreated, about 33% of patients die within the first 24 hours, and 50% die within 48 hours. The 2-week mortality rate approaches 75% in patients with undiagnosed ascending aortic dissection.

## CLASSIFICATION

Dissections of the thoracic aorta have been classified anatomically by two different methods. The more commonly used system is the Stanford classification, which is based on involvement of the ascending aorta and simplifies the DeBakey classification (Figs 18.1 and 18.2).

*The Stanford classification divides dissections into two types, type A and type B:*

- **Type A** involves the ascending aorta (DeBakey types I and II).
- **Type B** descending aorta is involved (DeBakey type III).
- This system also helps delineate treatment. Usually, type A dissections require surgery, while type B dissections may be managed medically under most conditions.

*The DeBakey classification divides dissections into three types:*

- **Type I** involves the ascending aorta, aortic arch, and descending aorta.
- **Type II** is confined to the ascending aorta.
- **Type III** is confined to the descending aorta distal to the left subclavian artery. Type III dissections are further divided into **IIIa and IIIb.**

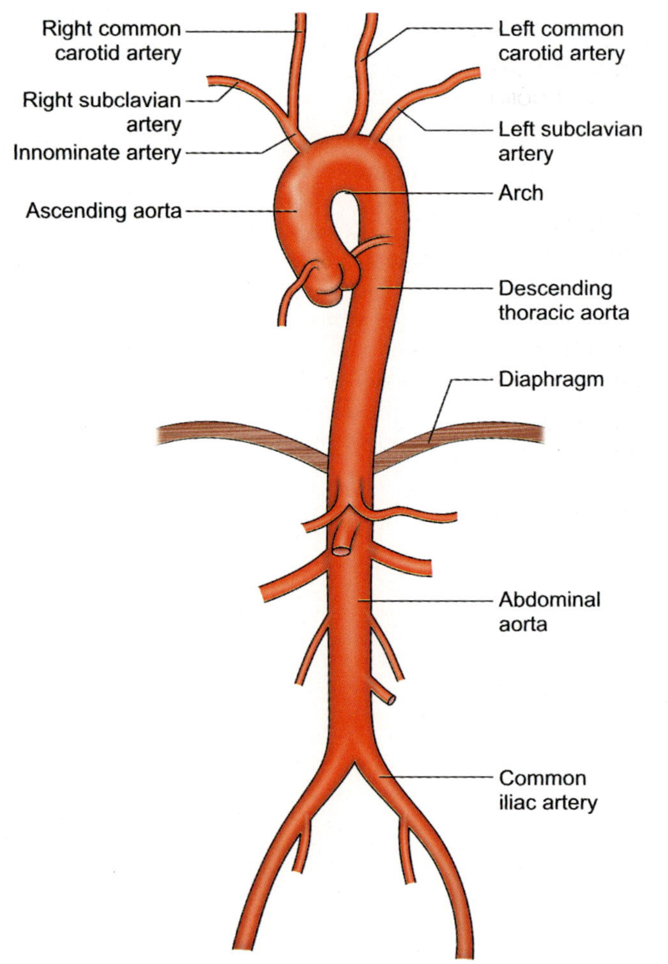


**Fig.18.1:** Anatomy of human normal aorta showing different branches arising out of ascending, arch, thoracic and abdominal aorta

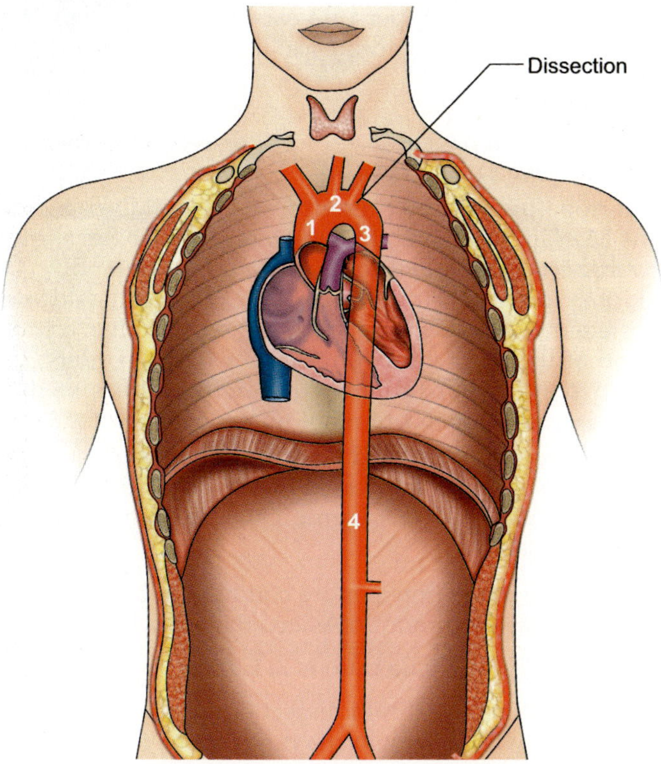


**Fig. 18.2:** Dissection of the descending part of the aorta (3), which starts from the left subclavian artery and extends to the abdominal aorta (4). The ascending aorta (1) and aortic arch (2) are not involved

- **Type IIIa** refers to dissections that originate distal to the left subclavian artery but extend both proximally and distally, mostly above the diaphragm.
- **Type IIIb** refers to dissections that originate distal to the left subclavian artery, extend only distally and may extend below the diaphragm.

Thoracic aortic dissections should be distinguished from aneurysms (i.e. localized abnormal dilation of the aorta) and transections, which are caused most commonly by high-energy trauma.

*Pathophysiology:* The essential feature of aortic dissection is a tear in the intimal layer, followed by formation and propagation of a subintimal hematoma. The dissecting hematoma commonly occupies about half and occasionally the entire circumference of the aorta. This produces a false lumen or double-barreled aorta, which can reduce blood flow to the major arteries arising from the aorta. If the dissection involves the pericardial space, cardiac tamponade may result.

### Cystic Medial Necrosis

The normal aorta contains collagen, elastin, and smooth muscle cells that contribute the intima, media, and adventitia, which are the layers of the aorta. With aging, degenerative changes lead to breakdown of the collagen, elastin, and smooth muscle and an increase in basophilic ground substance. This condition is termed cystic medial necrosis. Atherosclerosis that causes occlusion of the vasa vasorum also produces this disorder. Cystic medial necrosis is the hallmark histologic change associated with dissection in those with Marfan syndrome.

Cystic medial necrosis was first described by Erdheim in 1929. Sources disagree over the accuracy of this term in elderly patients because the true histopathologic changes are neither cystic nor necrotic. Researchers have used the term cystic medial degeneration. Early on, cystic medial necrosis described an accumulation of basophilic ground substance in the media with the formation of cystlike pools. The media in these focal areas may show loss of cells (i.e. necrosis). This term still is used commonly to describe the histopathologic changes that occur.

## DISSECTION SITES

The most common site of dissection is the first few centimeters of the ascending aorta, with 90% occurring within 10 centimeters of the aortic valve (Fig. 18.3). The

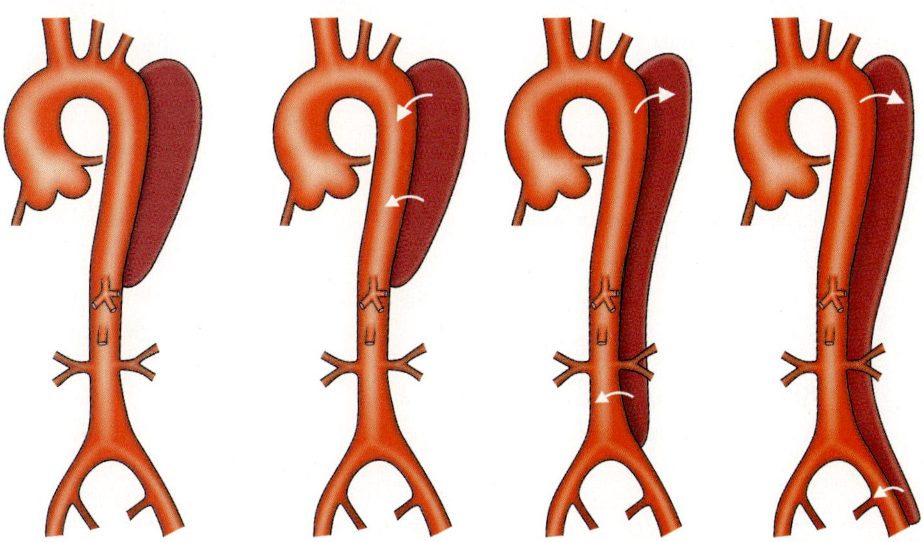

**Fig. 18.3:** Descending aortic dissections (Stanford type B or DeBakey type III) are divided in four types for endovascular purposes

second most common site is just distal to the left subclavian artery. Between 5% and 10% of dissections do not have an obvious intimal tear. These often are attributed to rupture of the aortic vasa vasorum as first described by Krukenberg in 1920.

## DESCENDING AORTIC DISSECTIONS

Descending aortic dissections (Stanford type B or DeBakey type III) are divided in four types for endovascular purposes:

- Type 1 has no identifiable intimomedial tears in the descending thoracic aorta
- Type 2 has one or more intimomedial tears in the descending thoracic aorta and there is no tear at or distal to the level of the celiac artery
- Type 3 has intimomedial tears involving the abdominal aorta (with or without concomitant tears in the descending thoracic aorta)
- Type 4 has intimomedial tears distal to the aortic bifurcation (with or without concomitant tears in the descending thoracic and abdominal aorta

## DISEASES LEADING TO AORTIC DISSECTION

Certain diseases, such as Marfan, Ehlers-Danlos, and other connective tissue diseases, affect the media of the aorta and make it prone to dissection. Pulsatile flow and high blood pressure contribute to propagation of the dissection.

Diseases that weaken the aortic wall predispose the patient to aortic dissection. Shearing forces separate the layers in the media of the aorta. Intimal rupture occurs at points of fixation along the aorta where hydraulic stress is maximal (Table 18.1).

## INCIDENCE

The true incidence of dissection is difficult to estimate. Most estimates are based on autopsy studies. One population-based study estimated the incidence at roughly 6 new aneurysms per 100,000 person-years. Evidence of dissection is found in 1–3% of all autopsies.

### Mortality/Morbidity

- From 1–2% of patients with aortic dissection die per hour for the first 24–48 hours.
- Aortopathy may be present in heritable diseases such as Marfan syndrome, Ehlers-Danlossyndrome, annulo-aortic ectasia, familial aortic dissections, adult polycystic kidney disease, Turner syndrome, Noonan syndrome, osteogenesis imperfecta, bicuspid aortic valve, coarctation of the aorta, and connective tissue disorders. It is also seen in heritable metabolic disorders such as homocystinuria and familial hypercholesterolemia.
- Incidence is increased in pregnancy and syphilis. Thoracic aortic dissection also is associated with **crack cocaine use** and iatrogenic causes, such as cardiac catheterization.

*Race:* Aortic dissection is more common in blacks than in whites and less common in Asians than in whites.

*Sex:* The male-to-female ratio is 3:1.

*Age:* Approximately 75% of dissections occur in those aged 40–70 years, with a peak in the range of 50–65 years.

*History:* 'Spontaneous tear of the arterial coats is associated with atrocious pain, with symptoms, indeed, in the case of the aorta of angina pectoris and many instances have been mistaken for it' William Osler, 1910.

*Chest pain* is the most common presenting symptom in patients with an aortic dissection. Consider thoracic aortic dissection in the differential diagnosis of all patients presenting with chest pain.

The pain usually is described as ripping or tearing. The description of ripping or tearing has been shown to have a likelihood ratio for aortic dissection of 1.2 and 10.8.

The sudden onset of chest pain has been shown to have a sensitivity of 84%.

**Table 18.1:** Causes of thoracic aortic aneurysm

| Aetiology | Aortic segment | Pathophysiology |
|---|---|---|
| Marfan syndrome | Ascending aorta and root, aortic arch | Defective fibrillin: secondary cystic medial degeneration |
| Ehlers-Danios syndarome | Ascending aorta, predominantly aortic arch | Defective collagen: secondary cystic medial degeneration |
| Cystic medial degeneration | Ascending aorta, aortic arch | *De novo* cystic medial degeneration |
| Atherosclerotic | Descending aorta | Atherosclerotic plaques, weakening vessel walls |
| Traumatic | Aortic isthmus, proximal descending aorta | Damaged vessel wall, intramural hematoma |
| Inflammatory | Variable | Takayasu's arteritis, giant cell arteritis, HLA-B27-associated spondyloarthropathies |
| Infectious | Aortic root (syphilis), variable (mycolic) | CMD (syphilis), inflammatory changes (mycotic) |
| Posistenotic | Ascending (aortic stenosis), descending (coarctation) | Hemodynamic insult |
| Postsurgical | Aortic valve replacement, s/p aortic | Weakening of the anastamotic walls |

HLA=human leukocyte antigen

This description is not universal, and some patients present with only mild pain, often mistaken for musculoskeletal conditions, located in the thorax, groin, or back.

The pain of aortic dissection typically is distinguished from the pain of acute myocardial infarction (AMI) by its abrupt onset.

Aortic dissection should be considered strongly in all patients reporting acute, sudden, and severe chest pain that is maximal at onset.

The truly sudden onset of chest pain is seen in few other conditions. In 1926, Spiegel and Wassermann found that acute stretching of the aortic wall produces pain.

**The nervi vascularis**, bundles of nerve fibers found in the aortic adventitia, are involved in the production of pain. Remember to cover the **P, Q, R, S, and T** (pain, quality, radiation, severity, and timing) of pain in all able patients. Assess the following characteristics of pain.

## SEVERITY

### Character

- **Timing,** including rate of onset, duration, and frequency of episodes
- **Migration,** including aggravating or alleviating factors and associated symptoms

The description of the pain may indicate where the dissection arises.

Anterior chest pain and chest pain that mimics AMI usually are associated with anterior arch or aortic root dissection. This is caused by the dissection interrupting flow to the coronary arteries, resulting in myocardial ischemia.

Pain that is described in the neck or jaw indicates that the dissection involves the aortic arch and extends into the great vessels of the arch.

Tearing or ripping pain that is felt in the intrascapular area may indicate that the dissection involves the descending aorta. The pain typically changes as the dissection evolves.

Aortic dissection is painless in about 10% of patients. Painless dissection is more common in those with neurologic complications from the dissection and those with Marfan syndrome.

*Presenting signs and symptoms in acute thoracic aortic dissection include the following:*

- Anterior chest pain—ascending aortic dissection
- Neck or jaw pain—aortic arch dissection
- Interscapular tearing or ripping pain; descending aortic dissection

*Chest pain myocardial infarction*

- Neurologic symptoms
- Syncope
- Stroke symptoms
- Altered mental status
- Limb paresthesias, pain, or weakness
- Hemiparesis or hemiplegia
- Horner syndrome
- Dyspnea
- Dysphagia
- Orthopnea
- Anxiety and premonitions of death
- Flank pain if renal artery is involved
- Dyspnea and hemoptysis if dissection ruptures into the pleura

### Physical

- Blood pressure may increase or decrease. Hypertension may result from a catecholamine surge or underlying essential hypertension.

  Hypotension is an ominous finding and may be the result of excessive vagal tone, cardiac tamponade, or hypovolemia from rupture of the dissection.
- A blood pressure differential of greater than 20 mmHg was an independent predictor of aortic dissection. A pressure differential of greater than 20 mmHg should increase the suspicion of aortic dissection. Significant interarm blood pressure differentials may be found in 20% of people without aortic dissection.

Neurologic deficits are a presenting sign in up to 20% of cases.

The most common neurologic findings are syncope and altered mental status.

Syncope is part of the early course of aortic dissection in about 5% of patients and may be the result of increased vagal tone, hypovolemia, or dysrhythmia.

Other causes of syncope or altered mental status include strokes from compromised blood flow to the brain or spinal cord and ischemia from interruption of blood flow to the spinal arteries. Peripheral nerve ischemia can manifest with numbness and tingling in the extremities.

Hoarseness from recurrent laryngeal nerve compression also has been described.

Horner syndrome is caused by interruption in the cervical sympathetic ganglia and presents with ptosis, miosis, and anhidrosis.

**Superior vena cava syndrome**, caused by compression of the superior vena cava from a large distorted aorta, may occur.

Dyspnea may be caused by congestive heart failure or tracheal or bronchial compression.

Dysphagia from compression of the esophagus may be present.

Findings suggestive of cardiac tamponade, such as muffled heart sounds, hypotension, pulsus paradoxus, jugular venous distension, and Kussmaul sign, must be recognized quickly.

**Other diagnostic clues include** a new diastolic murmur, asymmetrical pulses, and asymmetrical blood pressure measurements. Pay careful attention to carotid, brachial, and femoral pulses on initial examination and look for progression of bruits or development of bruits on re-examination.

Physical findings of a hemothorax may be found if the dissection ruptures into the pleura.

**Causes:** Aortic dissection is more common in patients with hypertension, connective tissue disorders, congenital aortic stenosis or bicuspid aortic valve, and in those with first-degree relatives with history of thoracic dissections. These diseases affect the media of the aorta and predispose it to dissection.

*Aortopathy may be due to the following heritable diseases:*

- Marfan syndrome
  - Ehlers-Danlos syndrome
  - Annuloaortic ectasia
  - Familial aortic dissections
  - Adult polycystic kidney disease
  - Turner syndrome
  - Noonan syndrome
  - Osteogenesis imperfecta
  - Bicuspid aortic valve
  - Coarctation of the aorta
  - Connective tissue disorders
  - Metabolic disorders (e.g. homocystinuria, familial hypercholesterolemia)
  - Hypertension or pulsatile blood flow can propagate the dissection.
  - An estimated 50% of all cases of aortic dissection that occur in women younger than 40 years are associated with pregnancy.
- Syphilis may cause aortic dissection.
  - Crack cocaine use may precipitate aortic dissection.
  - Iatrogenic causes of aortic dissection include cardiac catheterization.

### Other Problems to be Considered

Musculoskeletal chest pain

## LAB STUDIES

- **Blood studies**
- Usually, the diagnosis is made before the blood work is returned; however, leukocytosis may be present.

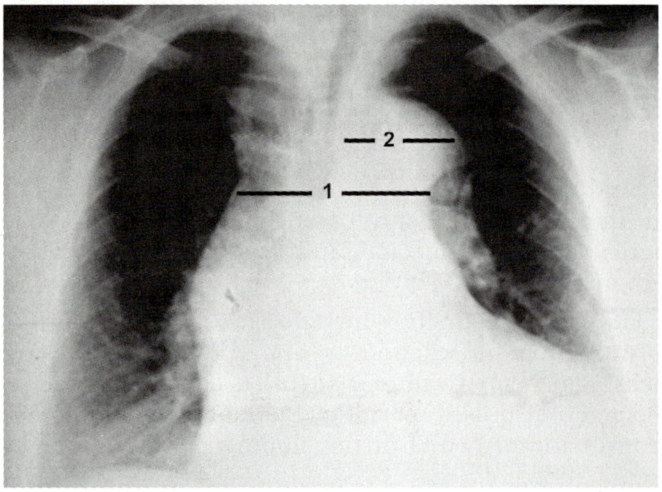


**Fig. 18.4:** Skiagram of chest PA view showing aortic dissection as wider diameter of aortic knob

- BUN and creatinine are elevated if the dissection involves the renal arteries.
- Troponin and creatine kinase (CK) can be elevated if the dissection has caused myocardial ischemia.
- Decreases in the hemoglobin and hematocrit are ominous findings suggesting the dissection either is leaking or has ruptured.

  Some studies suggest that **D-dimer** should be a part of the initial workup if aortic dissection is suspected. A negative result makes the presence of the disease unlikely.
- Hematuria, oliguria, and even anuria (<50 ml/d) may occur if the dissection involves the renal arteries.

## IMAGING STUDIES

### Chest Radiography

Findings are abnormal in 80% of patients and are more commonly abnormal in ascending aortic dissections. Findings suggesting hemothorax may be found if the dissection ruptures into the pleura (Figs 18.4 and 18.5).

*Radiographic findings* in acute thoracic dissection include a widened mediastinum in many cases In 2000, the international registry of acute aortic dissection published data on 464 patients that showed only 25% presenting with this finding. A widened mediastinum is sometimes difficult to identify on a portable anteroposterior (AP) radiograph. If the patient is hemodynamically stable and cooperative, an AP radiograph can be obtained at bedside. Look for a mediastinal width greater than 8 cm on AP chest radiograph.

- A tortuous aorta, common in hypertensive patients, may be hard to distinguish from a widened mediastinum. If in doubt, a good posterior-anterior radiograph is recommended.
- The differential diagnosis of a widened mediastinum includes tumor, adenopathy, lymphoma, and enlarged

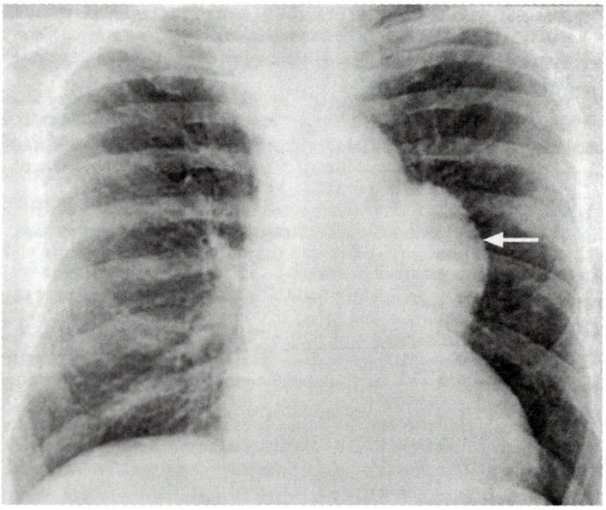

**Fig. 18.5:** Anteroposterior chest X-ray showing a mediastinal shadow (arrow) extending to the left beyond the cardiac silhouette, in the region of the descending thoracic aorta

thyroid. Abnormal (i.e. blunted) aortic knob was observed in 66% of patients in one study.

- **Ring sign** (displacement of the aorta >5 mm past the calcified aortic intima) is considered a specific radiographic sign. Other radiologic abnormalities seen on chest radiography include the following:

**Left apical cap**
- Tracheal deviation
- Depression of left main stem bronchus

**Esophageal deviation**
- Loss of the paratracheal stripe

The international registry for aortic dissection revealed that over 12% of the chest radiographs of patients with aortic dissection were read as normal. Several studies concluded that the overall diagnosis of aortic dissection is not determined by any one sign, rather a combination of all findings leads to suspicion of dissection.

*Angiography:* Still considered by some as the diagnostic criterion standard test for aortic dissection, it is being replaced by newer imaging modalities.

Angiography leads to accurate diagnosis of aortic dissection in over 95% of patients and aids the surgeon in planning the repair operation because blood vessels of the arch can be assessed easily. Benefits include visualization of the true and false lumens, intimal flap, aortic regurgitation, and coronary arteries

*Drawbacks include the following:* The procedure is invasive. The patient must be transported to the radiology department, leaving the ED. The use of contrast media may be harmful to patients who have renal insufficiency or an allergy to iodine. Misdiagnoses can occur if the false channel is thrombosed. In this instance, the false lumen and intimal flap may not be visualized. Possible simultaneous opacification of the true and false lumens may make discerning the presence of a dissection difficult.

### Computed Tomography Scanning

The accepted diagnostic criterion standard, angiography, is being challenged by state-of-the-art CT angiography. With the advent of helical CT with multiplanar and 3D reconstruction and CT angiography, CT scanning is quickly replacing angiography as the diagnostic test of choice in many institutions.Prospective studies have shown a sensitivity of 83–94% with a specificity of 87–100% (Figs 18.6–18.9).

Spiral CT scanning is associated with a higher rate of detection and better resolution than incremental CT scanning. High-quality 2D and 3D reconstructions are possible with spiral CT scanning, which greatly adds to the usefulness of this imaging modality.

More importantly, imaging information, including the type of lesion, location of the pathologic lesion, extent of the disease, and evaluation of the true and false lumen can be assessed quickly and help the surgeon plan the operation.

- This information helps determine if hypothermic circulatory arrest is necessary for surgery; this procedure increases the complexity, length, morbidity, and mortality associated with surgery.
- Faster scanners have decreased the acquisition time to the range of a breath hold, resulting in less motion artifact from breathing.

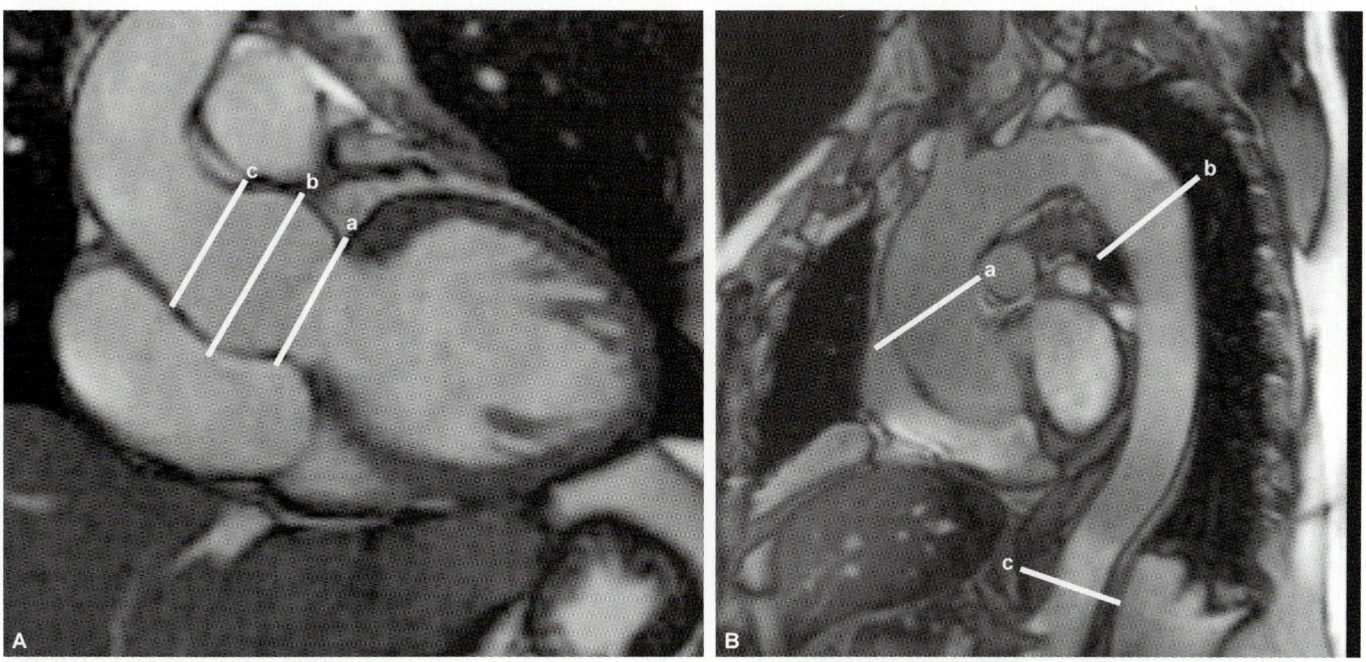


**Fig. 18.6:** (A) Coronal slice of the aortic root in which the following can be observed—(a) aortic ring; (b) sinuses of Valsalva; and (c) sinotubular junction. (B) oblique sagittal slice of the aorta in which the following are observed—(a) ascending aorta; (b) descending aorta, and (c) abdominal aorta

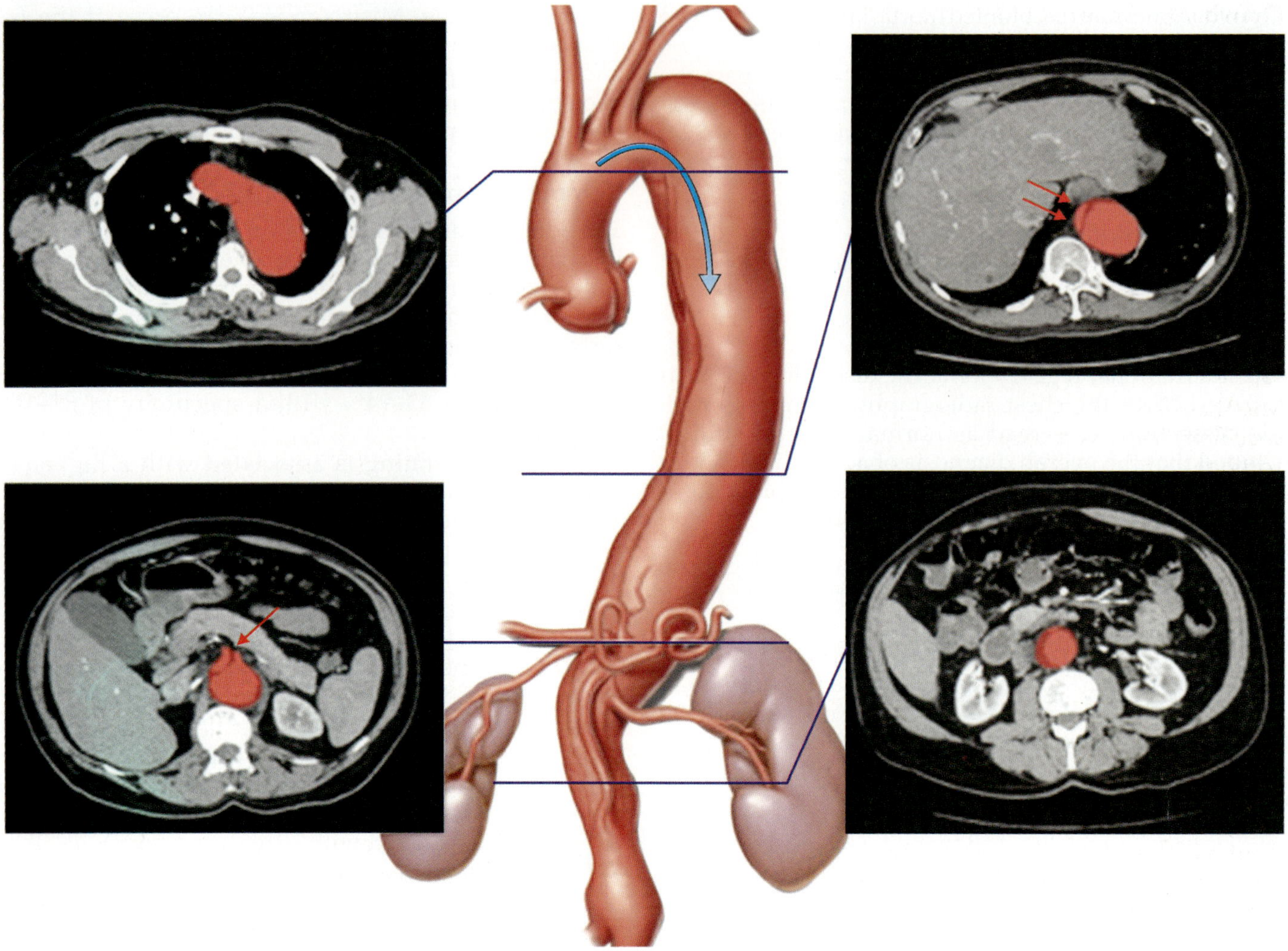

**Fig. 18.7:** Preoperative anatomy. Illustration and sections from a computed tomography scan showing the patient's thoracoabdominal aortic aneurysm, which was associated with chronic aortic dissection. Note the narrow true lumen (double arrows) and the extension of the dissection into the celiac axis (single white arrow). The aneurysm begins to taper in the infrarenal region

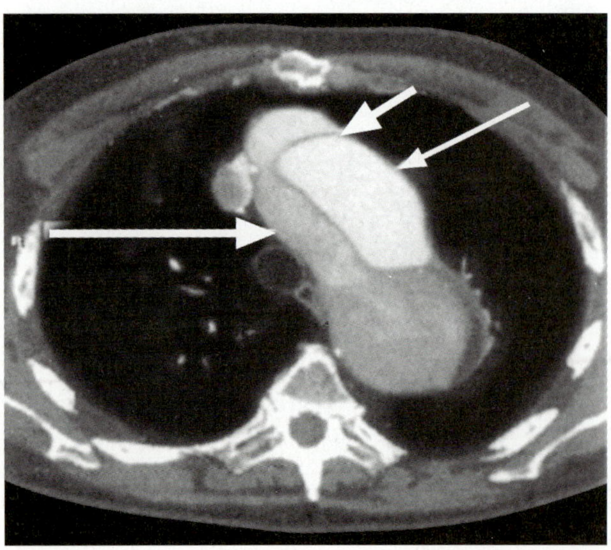

**Fig. 18.8:** MDCT axial planar view. Dissection flap (arrowhead) separating true lumen (short arrow) and false lumen (long arrow)

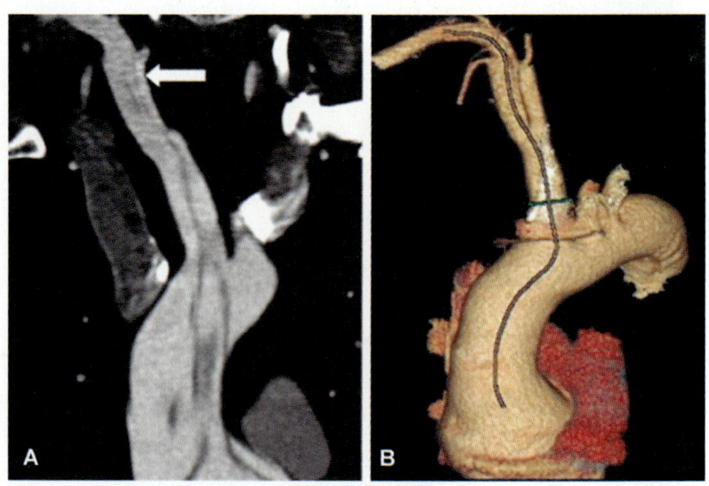


**Fig. 18.9:** (A) Contrast-enhanced CT scan showing the intimal flap due to dissection from the aortic root to the ascending aorta, innominate artery and subclavian artery. (B) Enhanced reconstructed CT scan image showing the path of dissection

- **Drawbacks include the following:**
  - Transportation of a patient in potentially unstable condition from the ED, even for the relatively short time needed for this procedure, places the patient at risk.
  - CT angiography requires the injection of iodinated contrast.
  - The use of contrast material may harm a patient who has impaired renal function or an allergy to contrast media.
  - CT scanning provides no information on aortic regurgitation.

### Magnetic Resonance Imaging (Figs 18.10 and 18.11)

- MRI has over 90% sensitivity and greater than 95% specificity. It is the most sensitive method for diagnosing aortic dissection and has similar specificity to CT scanning.
- MRI shows the site of intimal tear, type and extent of dissection, and presence of aortic insufficiency, as well as the surrounding mediastinal structures.
- Other benefits are that MRI requires no contrast medium and no ionizing radiation. It is the preferred modality for patients with renal failure and those with an allergy to iodine.
- Contrast-enhanced magnetic resonance angiography (CE-MRA) is a principle technique for evaluating the thoracic aorta.
- MRI is the preferred tool for imaging chronic dissections and postsurgical follow-up.
- Contrast 3D MRA is an accurate noninvasive imaging modality. It has the advantage of being able to evaluate the aortic valve more effectively than CT angiography.

*Drawbacks include the following:* MRI is not readily available at most institutions, requiring transportation of patients in unstable condition away from the ED. MRI requires much more time to acquire images than CT scanning.

Patients with permanent pacemakers cannot undergo MRI. Most patients with prosthetic heart valves or coronary stents can safely have an MRI.

- **Echocardiography** (Figs 18.12–18.23)
- With its increasing acceptance and use in the ED, ultrasonography is becoming a valuable diagnostic aid, although transthoracic echocardiography (TTE) has a much lower sensitivity (80%) and lower specificity (90%) than angiography.
- TTE is most useful in ascending aortic dissections, especially those closest to the aortic root and within a few centimeters of the aortic valve. Sensitivity is highest in this location.
- Echocardiography also is useful in diagnosing cardiac tamponade and aortic regurgitation.
- Benefits include its rapid simple bedside use in the ED and its noninvasive nature.
- Drawbacks include the lack of sensitivity and specificity, especially with arch and descending aortic dissections, and dependence on operator experience.

**Transesophageal echocardiography (TEE)** has greater sensitivity and specificity than TTE (in the range of 97–99% and 97–100%, respectively).

- Advantages include its quick and easy bedside use in the ED, which makes it ideal for patients in unstable condition. TEE detects involvement of the coronary arteries, aortic insufficiency, and cardiac tamponade.
- It is a relatively quick study to perform and relatively noninvasive. The main drawback of TEE is its strong dependence on operator experience.
- Other drawbacks are that false-positive results can occur from reverberations in the ascending aorta and that the

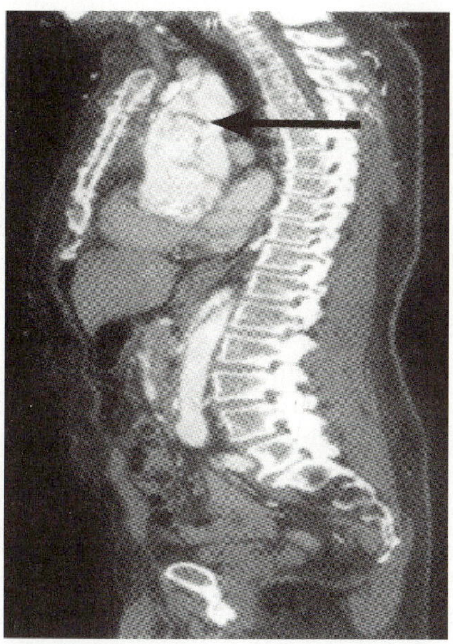

**Fig. 18.10:** MDCT MPR. Complex type A dissection flap (arrow)

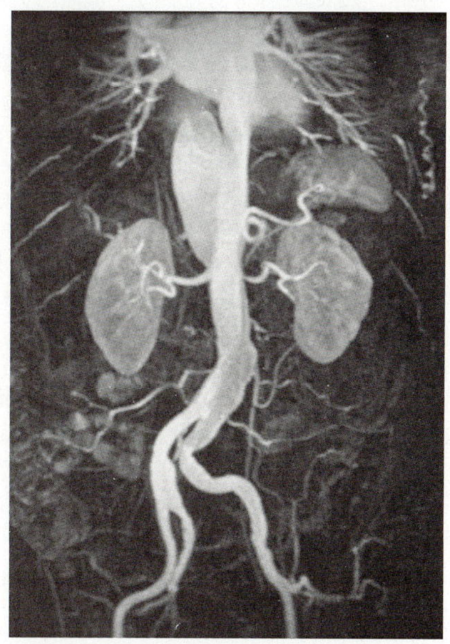

**Fig. 18.11:** MRI (MRA) AP MIP stanford type B thoracoabdominal dissecting aneurysm

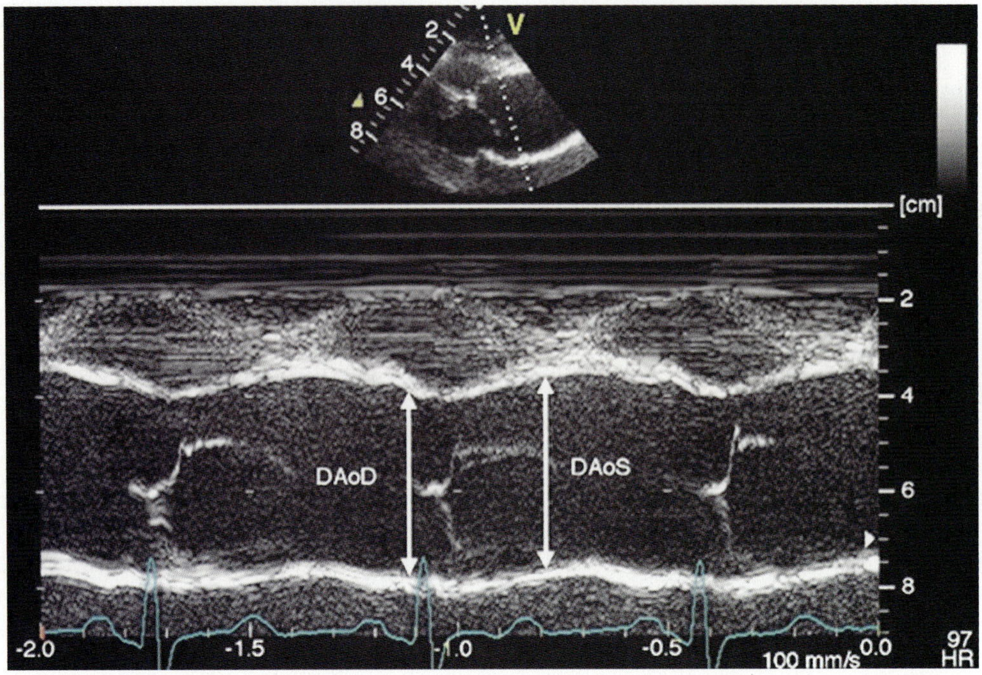


**Fig. 18.12:** Measurement of aortic diameters using M-mode ultrasound in the aortic sinuses of Valsalva in systolic and diastolic phases. DAoD, diameter of the aorta in diastole; DAoS, diameter of the aorta in systole

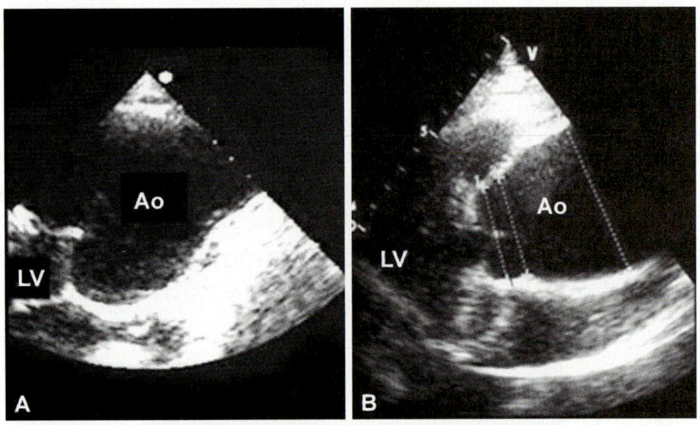


**Fig. 18.13:** Parasternal long-axis view by transthoracic echocardiography. (A) Annuloaortic ectasia with pyriform morphology. (B) Ascending aorta aneurysm located in the upper part of the sinotubular junction

upper ascending aorta and arch may not be visualized well, leading to false-negative results.

- TEE cannot be performed in patients with esophageal varicosities or stenosis. If the findings are negative and clinical suspicion remains high, a second diagnostic test is recommended.

### Other Tests

*Electrocardiogram:* All patients with suspected thoracic aortic dissection should have an ECG.

- In acute thoracic dissection, ECG can mimic the changes seen in acute cardiac ischemia. In the presence of chest pain, these signs can make distinguishing dissection from AMI very difficult. Keep this in mind when administering thrombolytics to patients with chest pain.
- ST-elevation can be seen in Stanford type A dissections because the dissection interrupts blood flow to the coronary arteries.
- The incidence of abnormal ECG findings is greater in Stanford type A dissections than in other types of dissections.
- In one study, 8% of patients with type A dissections had ST-elevation, while no patients with type B dissections had ST-elevation.
- More commonly, the ECG abnormality is ST-depression.
- If the dissection involves the coronary ostia, it is the right coronary artery that is most commonly involved, leading to inferior ST-segment elevation pattern.

## MANAGEMENT

*Medical therapy:* Initiate medical therapy as soon as the diagnosis is considered. The goal is to decrease the blood pressure and the shearing forces of myocardial contractility in order to decrease the intimal tear and propagation of the dissection.

Admit the patient to the intensive care unit or coronary care unit for hemodynamic studies, as follows:

- Arterial blood pressure monitoring with an arterial line

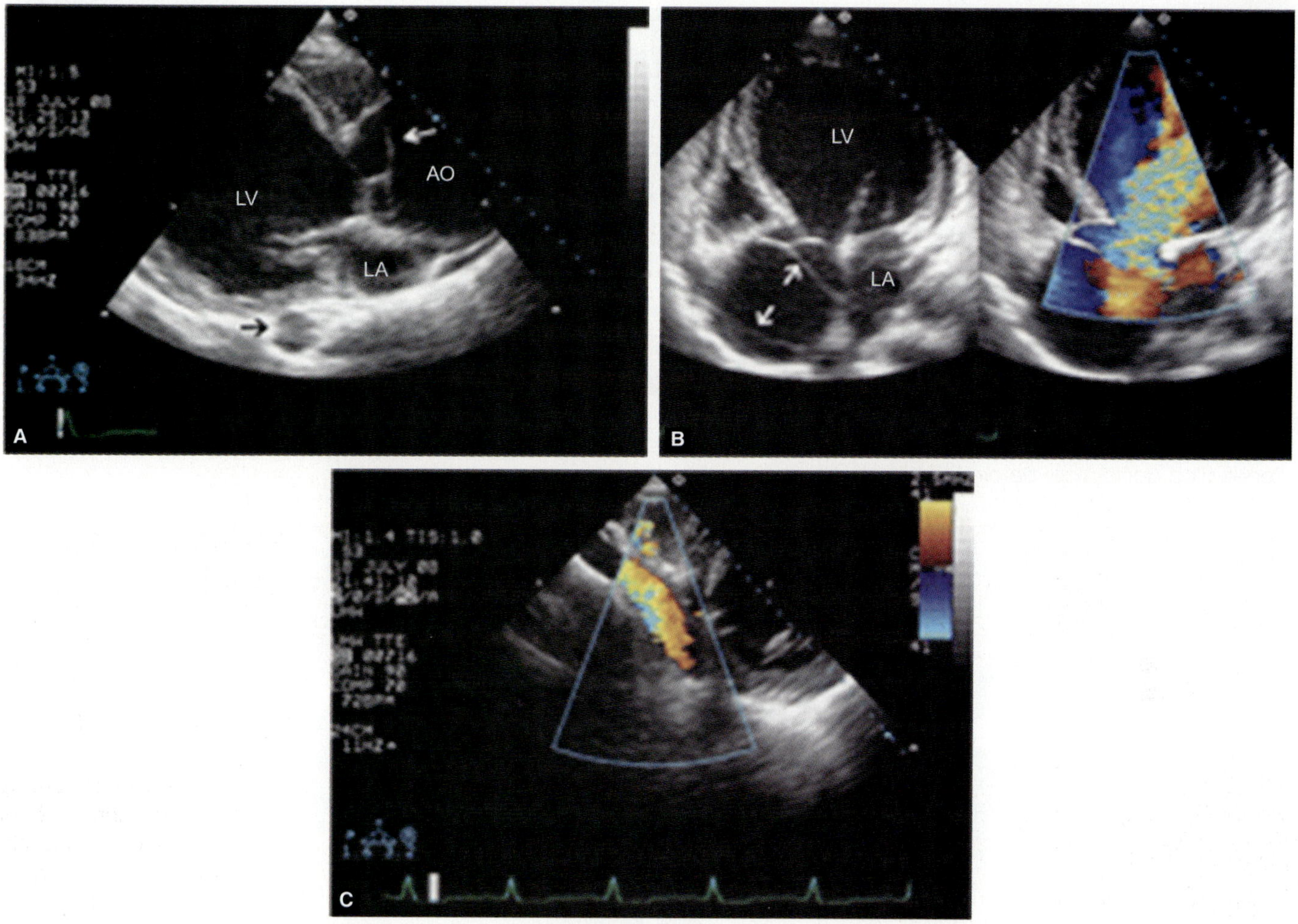


**Fig. 18.14:** Transthoracic echocardiography in a patient with Marfan's syndrome and type A dissection. (A) Parasternal long-axis view. There is severe dilatation of the aorta and a linear echo is seen just above the aortic valve (white arrow). Note the normal caliber and appearance of the descending thoracic aorta, posterior to the left atrium (black arrow). LV=left ventricle; LA=left atrium; AO=aorta, (B) Apical five-chamber view. The dilated aortic root, with two reflections of the intimal flap, (white arrows) is seen. Severe aortic regurgitation (right panel) is seen with color flow mapping, (C) Subcostal view. Normal caliber, no dissection flap and normal flow are seen

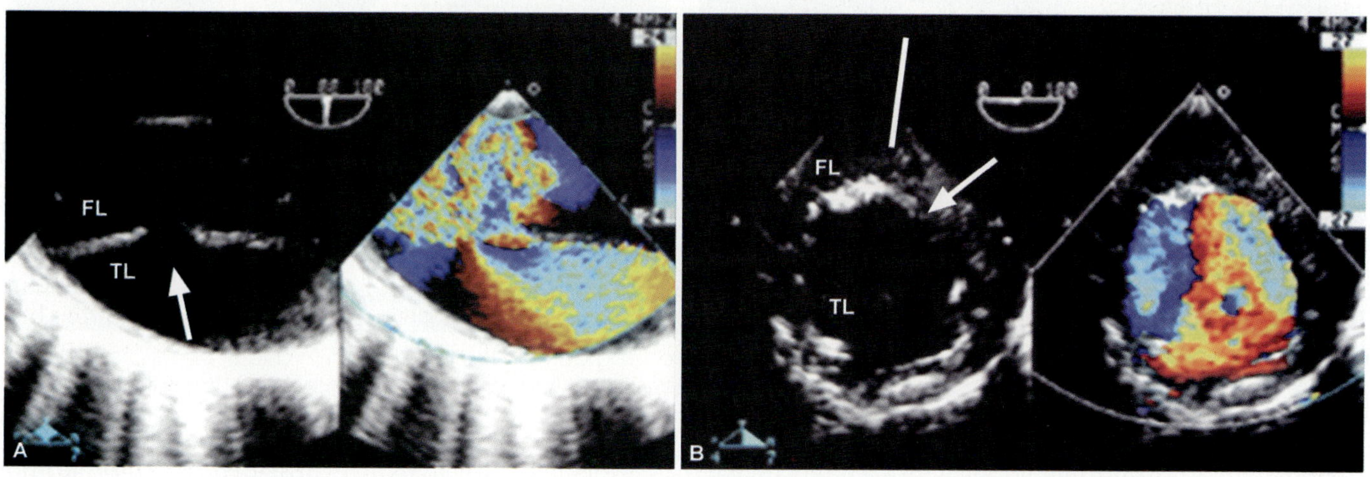


**Fig. 18.15:** A 53-year-old male, 5 weeks after acute thoracic pain and diagnosis of aortic type-B dissection. (A) long axis view of the entry site of a type-B aortic dissection in 2D and color-Doppler TEE before stent-graft implantation. Arrow marks the entry. TL=true lumen; FL=false lumen. (B) post-stent-graft implantation. Arrow indicates the bright echo of the stent graft; white line points to the beginning formation of clot in the false lumen

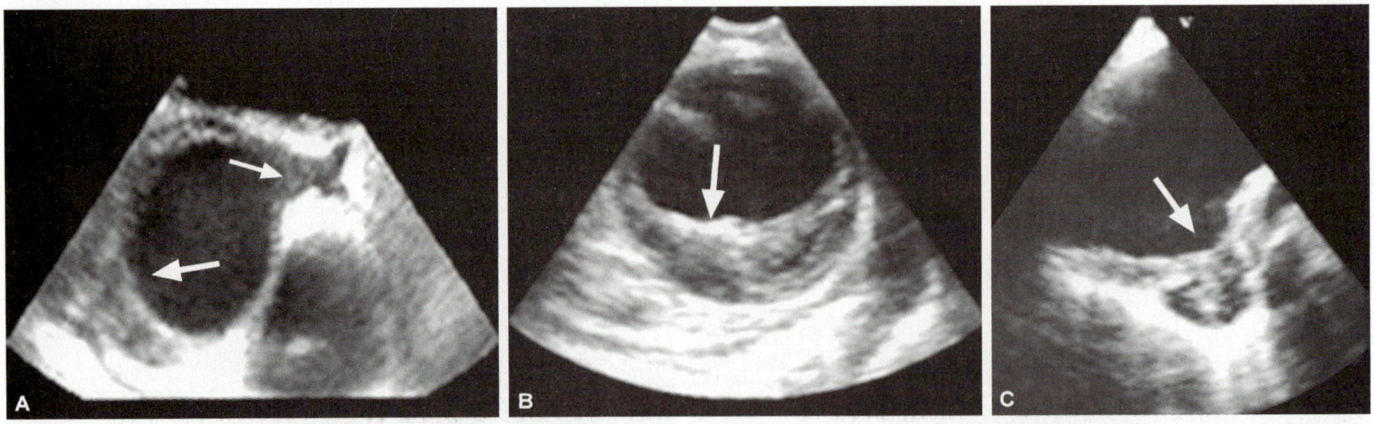


**Fig. 18.16:** Transoesophageal echocardiography. (A) Crescentic intramural hematoma in ascending aorta (large arrow) adjacent to the left main coronary ostium (small arrow). (B) Intramural hematoma in descending aorta. Arrow shows intima calcification. (C) Penetrating aortic ulcer deforming the adventitia (arrow)

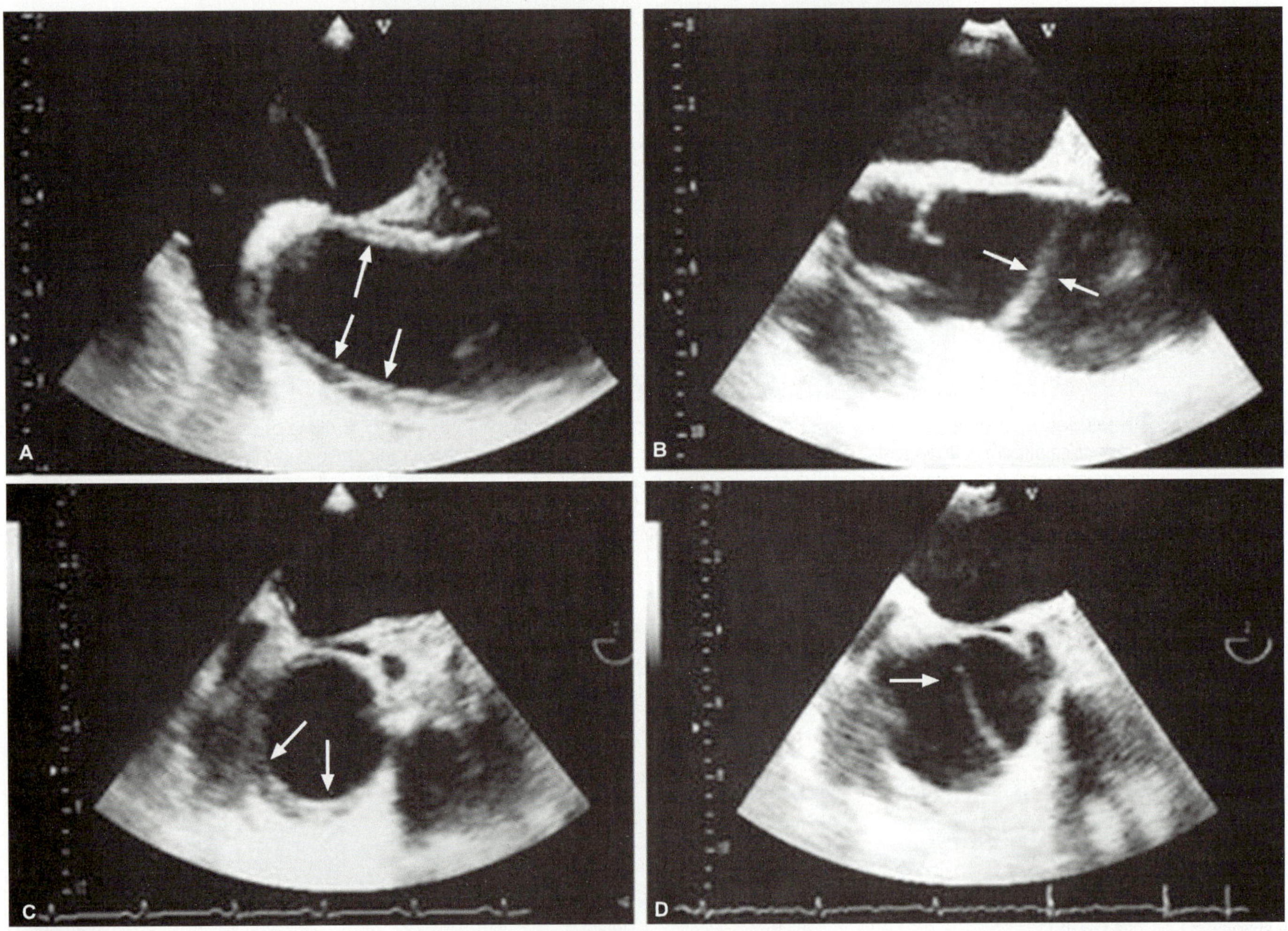


**Fig. 18.17:** Transesophageal echocardiography visualizing the ascending aorta in the longitudinal (A and B) and transverse (C and D) planes. Intramural hematoma (A) in the ascending aorta (arrows) evolving into dissection at 3 months (B). The arrows indicate the intimal dissection

- Central venous pressure monitoring with a central catheter
- Cardiac performance and filling pressures with Swan-Ganz catheterization
- Urine output monitoring with a Foley catheter and bag.

Initiate therapy to reduce cardiac contractility. Administer drugs with negative inotropic effects, such as beta-blockers (the agents of choice); administer calcium channel blockers if beta-blockers are contraindicated. The following beta-blockers are commonly used:

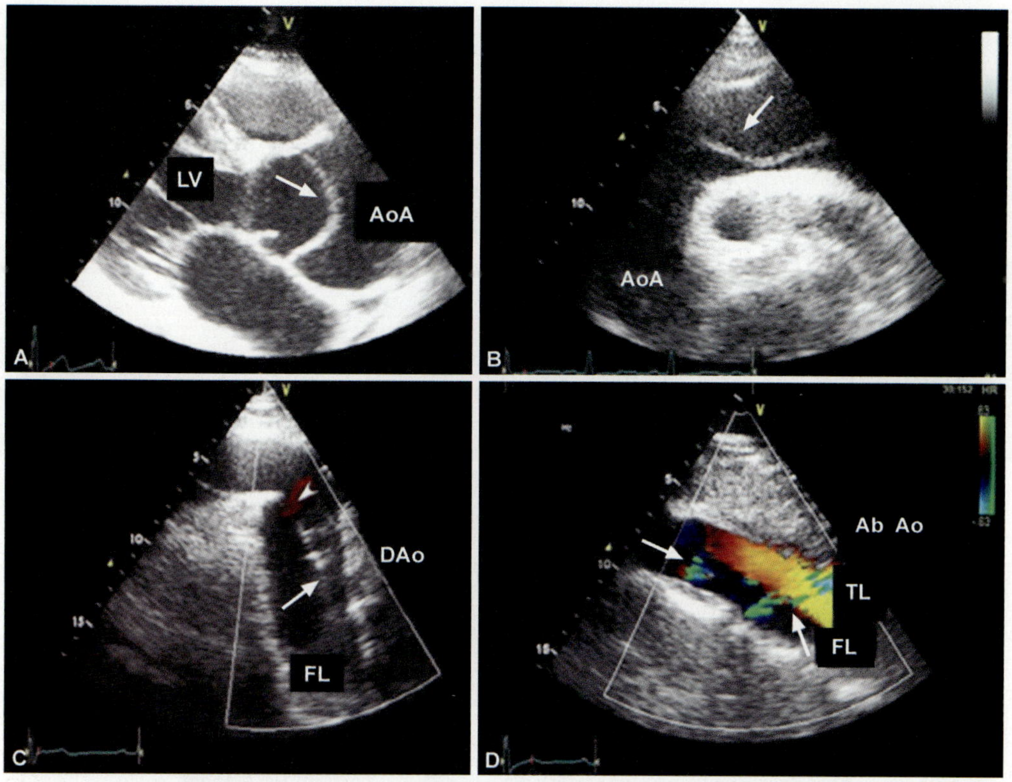


**Fig. 18.18:** Aortic dissection diagnosis by transthoracic echocardiography. Intimal flap (arrows) and two lumina are visualized in—(A) aortic root, (B) aortic arch and distal ascending aorta, (C) proximal descending aorta (arrowhead shows the entry tear), and (D) dissection of abdominal aorta. Color-Doppler helps to identify the true lumen (TL). Arrowheads signal secondary communications

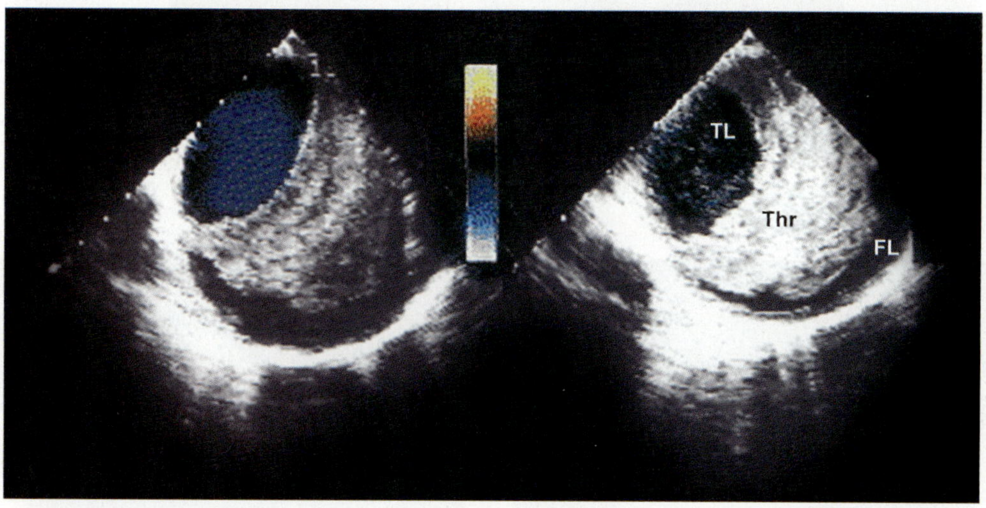


**Fig. 18.19:** Dissection of the ascending thoracic aorta. A dissecting aneurysm of the ascending segment of the thoracic aorta was diagnosed by two-dimensional transesophageal echocardiography. The horizontal imaging plane is approximately 3 cm above the aortic valve and shows a separation of the true lumen (TL) and the false lumen (FL) of the dissecting aneurysm. A color-coded flow signal in blue identifies flow away from the aortic valve in the true lumen. An echogenic crescent-shaped thrombus (Thr) almost completely fills the false lumen and leaves only a narrow unobstructed mural rim. Two images, taken at slightly different gray-scale gain settings, are shown side by side; the lower setting in the image on the left allows better visualization of the color-coded flow signal. Blue denotes flow away from and red or yellow flow toward the transducer

- Intravenous or oral labetalol
- Intravenous or oral propranolol
- Intravenous or oral esmolol

Initiate therapy to reduce systemic arterial pressure and shear stress if the patient's blood pressure allows for this type of intervention. The following agents are commonly used.

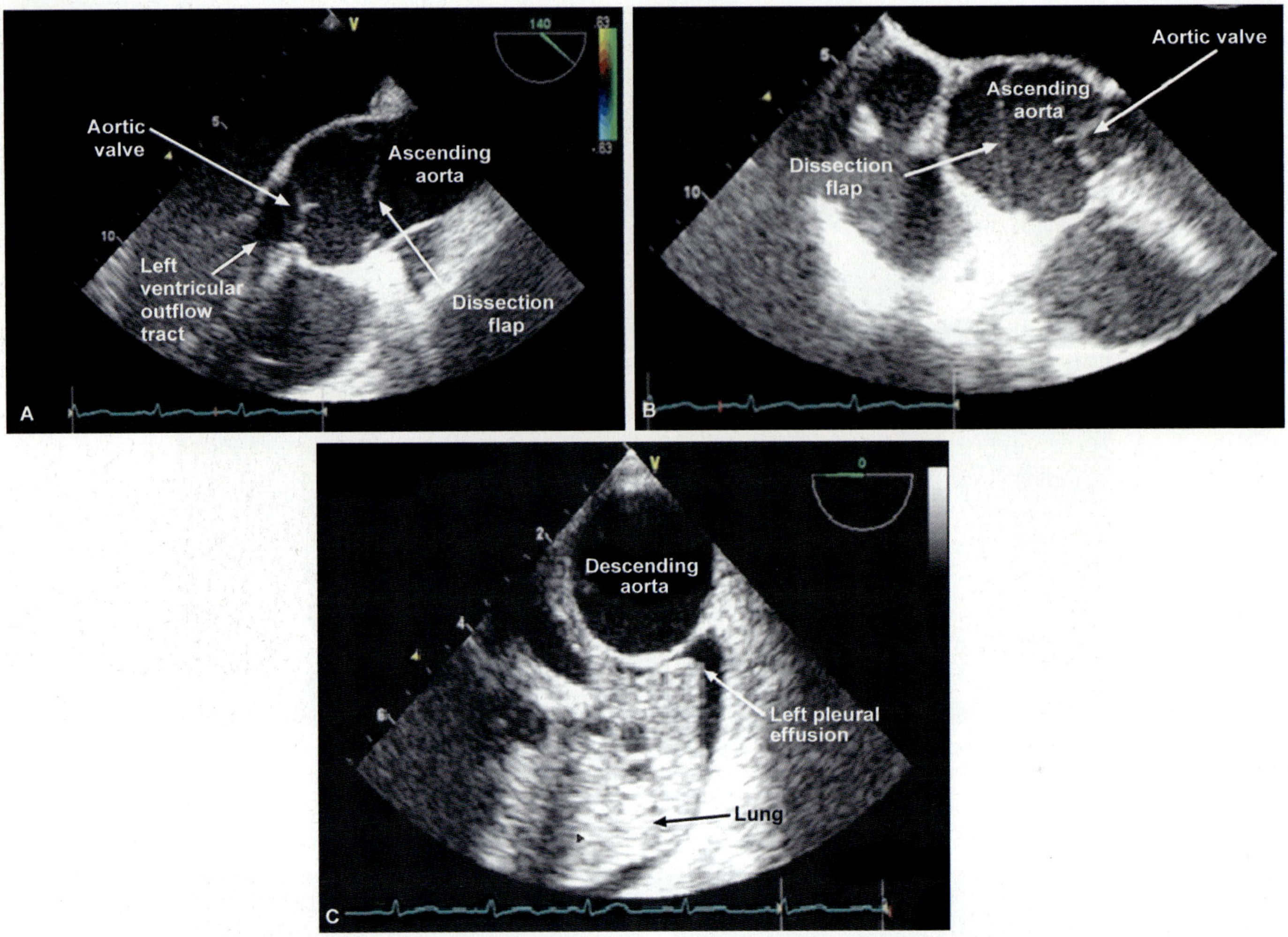


**Fig. 18.20:** (A, B and C) The TEE confirmed a 5.5 cm aortic aneurysm with a dissection flap in the sinuses of Valsalva extending distally to the sinotubular junction. The dissection did not involve the coronary arteries, but did extend into the aortic arch and further into the thoracic aorta. There was minimal aortic insufficiency but a left pleural effusion (assumed to be a hemothorax) was present. It was also noted that the aortic arch and descending aorta were dilated and aneurismal

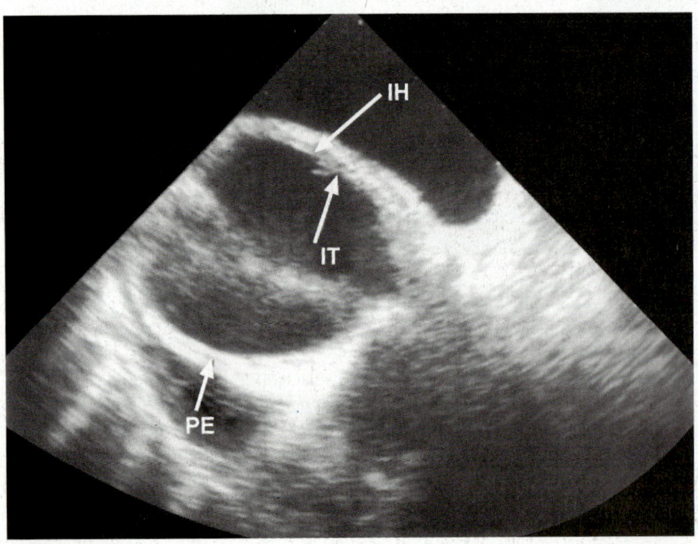


**Fig. 18.21:** TEE imaging shows subtle typical signs of discrete dissection of the proximal ascending aorta

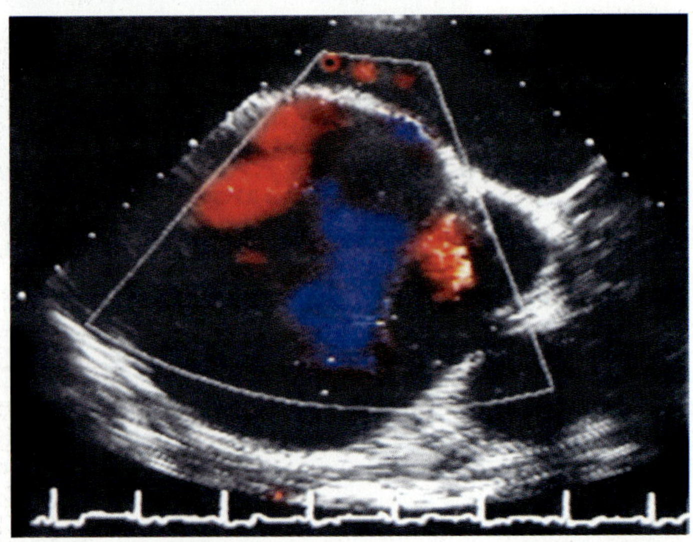

**Fig. 18.22:** TEE scan showing dissection of ascending aorta in patient with hypertension admitted in emergency department with acute chest pain

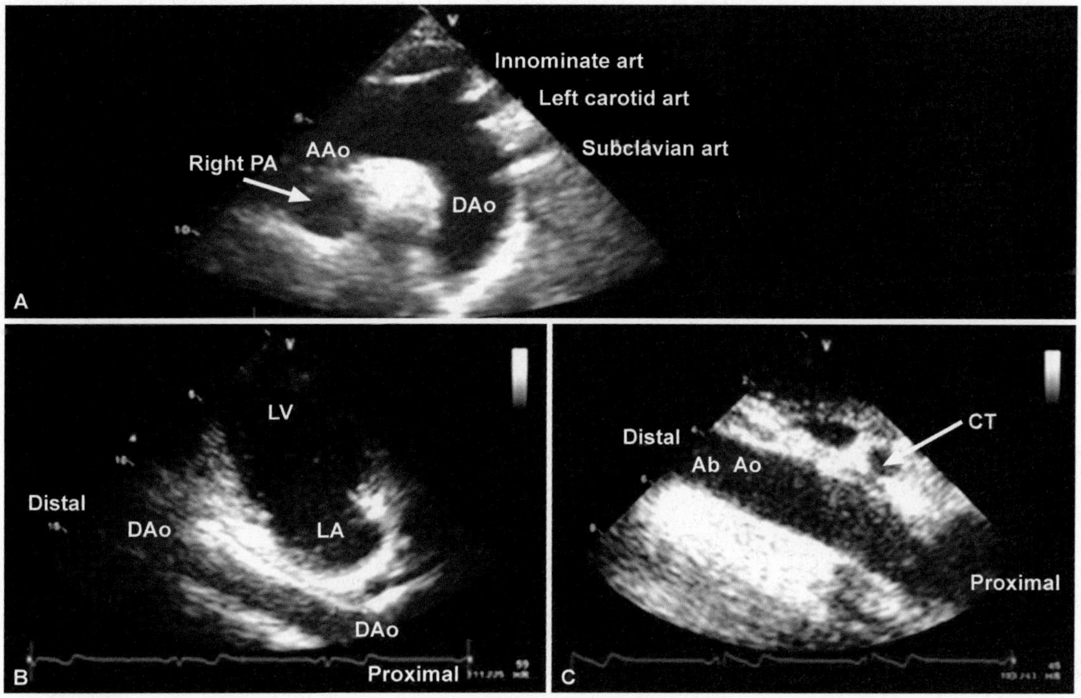


**Fig. 18.23:** (A) Suprasternal view of aortic arch and supraaortic great arteries. (B) Mid part of the descending thoracic aorta visualized by long-axis view from apical window, (C) Abdominal aorta visualized by subcostal view. In nonobese patients, it is not difficult to visualize distal abdominal aorta. (art=artery; PA= pulmonary artery; AAo=ascending aorta; DAo=descending aorta; CT=coeliac trunk)

- Intravenous nitroprusside drip
- Intravenous labetalol has a dual effect by decreasing blood pressure and cardiac contractility alcium channel blockers (e.g. diltiazem) lower blood pressure and cardiac contractility.

*The following conditions contraindicate beta-blocker therapy:*

- Hypersensitivity to drug/class
- Severe asthma

Heart block uncompensated heart failure, bradycardia (heart rate <60 beats/min), severe chronic obstructive pulmonary disease, and hypotension.

*The following conditions contraindicate calcium channel blocker therapy:*

- Hypersensitivity to drug/class
- Second- or third-degree atrioventricular block, sick sinus syndrome, and hypotension
- Left ventricular dysfunction
- Pulmonary congestion

*The following conditions contraindicate nitroprusside infusion:*

- Hypersensitivity to drug/class
- Poor cerebral perfusion
- Poor coronary perfusion

Pain management is always difficult in persons with aortic dissection. Narcotics and opiates are the preferred agents. Medical therapy is also administered to surgical patients preoperatively, intraoperatively, and postoperatively to prevent progression or recurrence of aortic dissection.

*Surgical therapy:* The major objectives of surgery for aortic dissection are to alleviate the symptoms, decrease the frequency of complications, prevent aortic rupture and death. Improved cardiopulmonary bypass circuits have decreased the prevalence of injury to blood elements. A decrease in complications such as brain injury has resulted from a more detailed understanding of the physiology and limitations of hypothermic circulatory arrest (Figs 18.24–18.28) (Table 18.2).

**Aortic arch repair and reconstruction** can be partial or complete. A number of advances have resulted in a decreased frequency of complications associated with surgery on the aorta. Dacron grafts with impregnated collagen or gelatin have been developed that are impervious to blood. Adjunct procedures, including distal aortic perfusion, profound hypothermia, cerebrospinal fluid drainage, and monitoring of somatosensory and motor evoked potentials in the brain and spinal cord, have decreased the frequency of procedure-related spinal cord injury during descending aorta and thoracoabdominal surgeries. Percutaneous fenestrations and stent placements are peformed. The area of the aorta with the intimal tear is usually resected and replaced with a Dacron graft. The operative mortality rate is usually less than 10%; serious complications are rare with ascending aortic dissections. The development of more impermeable grafts, such as

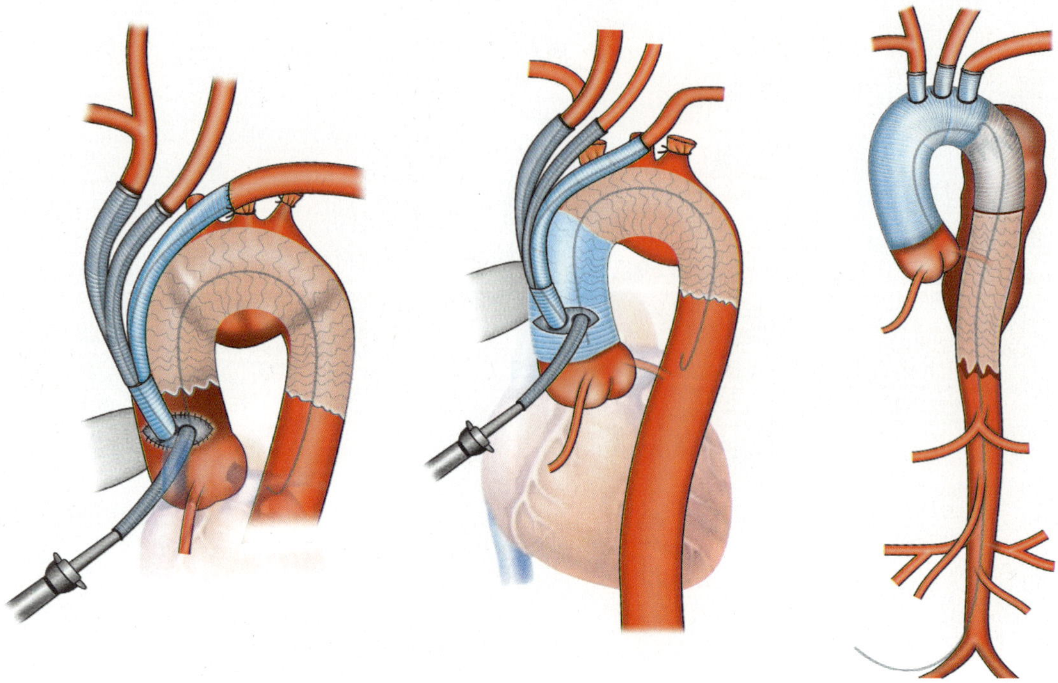


**Fig. 18.24:** Hybrid aortic arch repair. Types I, II and III

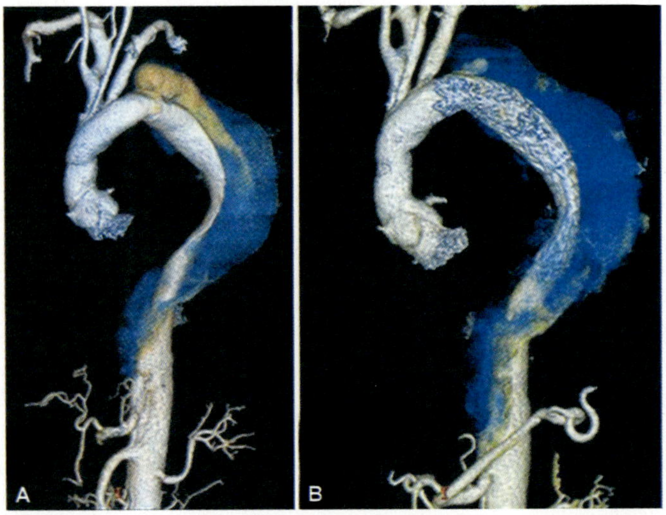


**Fig. 18.25:** (A) Preoperative three-dimensional reconstruction of computed tomography scan of the chest in a patient with a 5 cm aneurysm of the descending thoracic aorta associated with a chronic type B aortic dissection. (B) Postoperative three-dimensional computed tomography scan of the chest following endovascular repair of a 5 cm aneurysm of the descending thoracic aorta associated with a chronic type B aortic dissection which demonstrates a proximal type I endoleak and a small retrograde type I endoleak in the false lumen

woven Dacron, collagen-impregnated Hemashield (Meadox Medicals; Oakland, NJ), aortic grafts, and gel-coated Carbo-Seal Ascending Aortic Prothesis (Sulzer CarboMedics; Autin, Tex), has greatly enhanced the surgical repair of thoracic aortic dissections. Morbidity and mortality rates associated with this highly invasive surgery have decreased with the introduction of profound hypothermic circulatory arrest and retrograde cerebral perfusion.

Dissections involving the arch are more complicated than those involving only the ascending aorta because the innominate, carotid, and subclavian vessels branch from the arch. Deep hypothermic arrest is usually required. If the arrest time is less than 45 minutes, the rate of central nervous system complications is less than 10%.

Retrograde cerebral perfusion may improve the protection of the CNS during the arrest period. The mortality rate associated with aortic arch dissections is approximately 10–15%, with significant neurologic complications occurring in an additional 10% of patients.

**Preoperative details:** A number of factors may increase mortality and morbidity rates for surgical intervention on the aorta, including a history of myocardial infarction, respiratory failure, renal failure, and/or stroke.

Preoperative evaluation is therefore essential in patients with these histories. Because aortic dissection is more common in elderly patients (i.e. aged 70–80 years), this group of patients has different comorbidities.

Patients older than 50 years have a high prevalence of atherosclerotic heart disease and may require a thorough cardiac workup. Symptoms of aortic dissection are always difficult to differentiate from those of myocardial infarction.

Patients with ECG changes suggestive of myocardial infarction or ischemia undergo workups with emergency cardiac catheterization and angiography, followed by

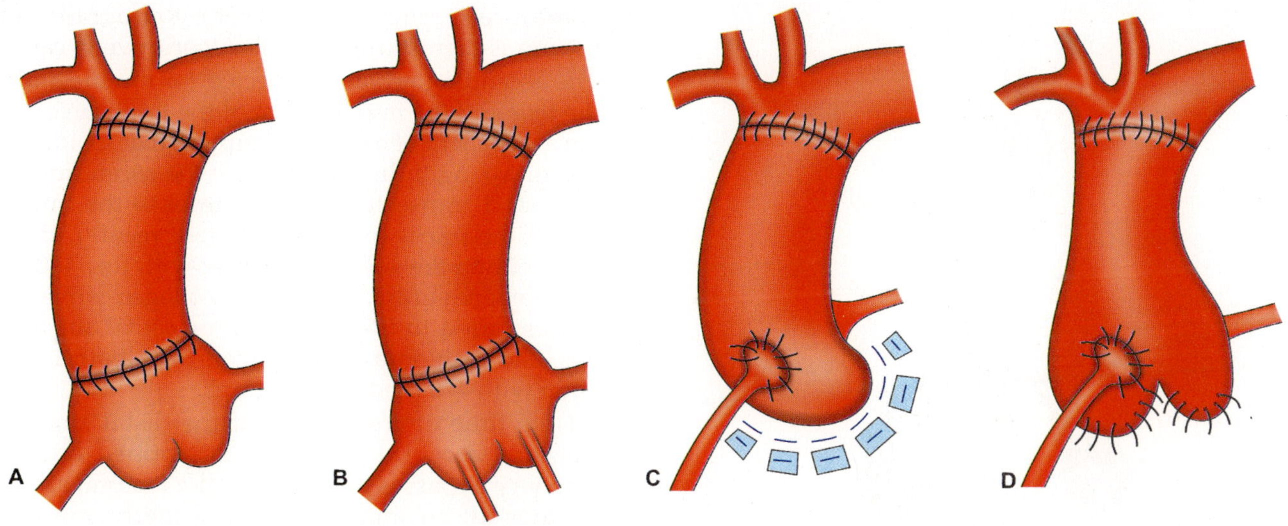


**Fig. 18.26:** Operations for aortic dissection or ascending aortic replacement. (A) Simple tube replacement of the aorta for the sinotubular junction to the brachiocephalic origin. (B) Tube graft replacement and aortic valve replacement as separate components of the operation. (C) Composite graft replacement. (D) Leaflet sparing aortic root replacement

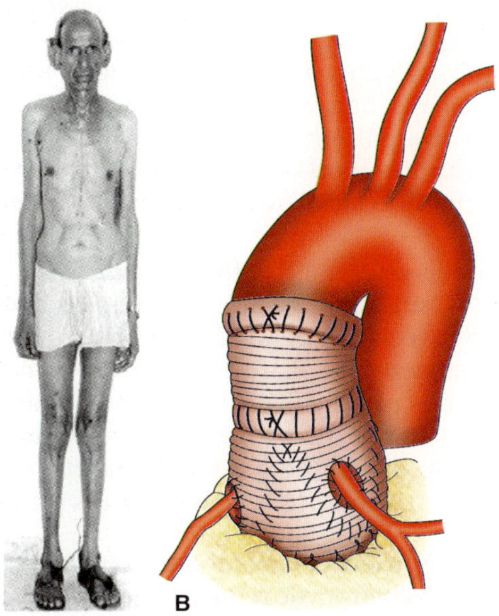


**Fig. 18.27:** (A) Middle-aged patient operated for annuloaortic ectasia in Marfan syndrome (see midsternal scar). (B) Valve-sparing aortic root repair

percutaneous transluminal coronary angioplasty or coronary artery bypass grafting concomitant with aortic repair or construction.

Patients with valvular heart disease undergo workups with echocardiography or coronary angiography. If any valvular abnormalities are found, then appropriate surgical correction (valve replacement or commissurotomy) is performed prior to or simultaneous with aortic repair.

Surgeries involving the descending or thoracoabdominal aorta require a lateral thoracotomy. A history of smoking or chronic obstructive pulmonary disease is of significant concern; perform pulmonary function testing on such patients. Additionally, arterial blood gas testing may be required. In elective cases, treat reversible restrictive diseases and excessive sputum production with antibiotics and bronchodilators.

Preoperative renal dysfunction is considered the most important predictor of postoperative acute renal failure (ARF). Preoperative management involves adequate hydration and avoidance of hypotension, a low cardiac output state, and hypovolemia in order to decrease the frequency of ARF.

**Table 18.2:** Surgical versus medical therapy for aortic dissection

| Medical therapy | Surgical therapy |
|---|---|
| Uncomplicated type III dissection | Acute: Type I or II dissection |
| Stable: Lone arch dissection | Acute: Complicated type III dissection<br>End-organ dystunction<br>Rupture/impending rupture<br>Aortic insufficiency<br>Associated with Marfan syndrome<br>Retrograde extension into the ascending aorta |
| Stable: Chronic dissection (more than 2 weeks after onset of symptoms) | |

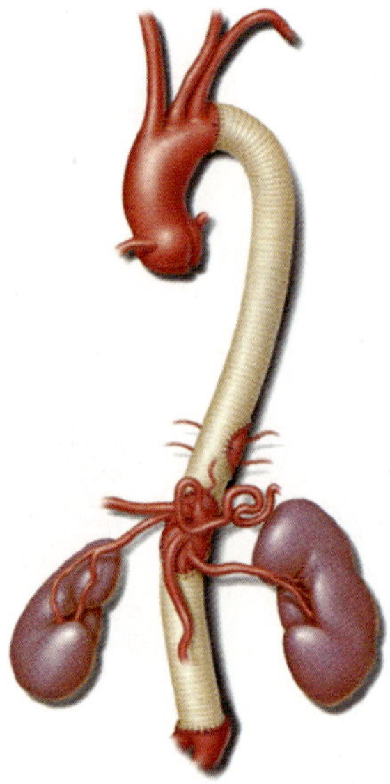

**Fig. 18.28:** Completed aortic reconstruction. The completed extent II repair. Note the proximal anastomosis located just distal to the left subclavian artery; the intercostal patch incorporating two pairs of intercostal arteries; the single visceral patch incorporating the celiac axis, superior mesenteric artery, and both renal arteries; and the distal anastomosis at the aortic bifurcation

Perform appropriate workups for patients presenting with any neurological signs suggestive of CNS pathology (e.g. stroke). This usually consists of Doppler imaging of the carotid arteries and, if needed, angiography of brachiocephalic and intracranial arteries. If the study findings are positive, perform a carotid endarterectomy before the aortic surgery.

**Intraoperative details:** The objectives of surgical therapy for aortic dissection are to resect the damaged segment, excise the intimal tear, and obliterate the entry into in the false lumen. Suturing the edges of the dissected aorta both proximally and distally obliterates the entry into the false lumen. The desirability of obliterating the entrance to the false lumen is controversial because of multiple portals. Aortic continuity after dissection of a diseased segment is reestablished by means of a prosthetic sleeve graft between the two ends of the aorta.

Patients with type A dissections are treated with immediate surgical correction. This involves transfer to the operating room, where median sternotomy is performed. Profound hypothermia is initiated after the patient is placed on cardiopulmonary bypass. Cardiopulmonary bypass is performed by femoral-femoral cannulation and through the superior vena cava for retrograde cerebral perfusion. Myocardial temperature is kept below 15°C (59°F) by cardioplegic perfusion via the coronary sinus. This provides myocardial protection throughout the procedure.

Ventricular distension is avoided by decompressing the left ventricle by venting through the left superior pulmonary vein or artery. The pump is stopped when the electroencephalogram is isoelectric and the nasopharyngeal temperature reaches 12°C (53.6°F). Retrograde cerebral perfusion is then started via the superior vena cava.

The ascending aorta is inspected for the site and extent of the tear and the involvement of the transverse arch and for an assessment of intimal disruption that requires repair. Through a longitudinal approach, the ascending aorta is opened and transected just proximal to the innominate artery. If the transverse arch is free of reentry, the intima and adventitia are sutured together with fine 4–0 and 5–0 polypropylene suture. A gelatin-or collagen-woven Dacron graft is sutured to the reinforced proximal aortic arch in end-to-end fashion and reinforced from both inside and outside with 4–0 pledgeted sutures.

At the time of completion of the distal anastomosis, retrograde cerebral perfusion is stopped and cardiopulmonary bypass is restarted via the femoral artery. This evacuates all air and debris from the brachiocephalic vessels. The graft is clamped proximal to the origin of the innominate artery. Flow to the cerebral and systemic circulation is restored after clamping the graft proximal to the origin of the innominate artery.

Hypothermic circulatory arrest is a valuable tool in aortic dissection repair. Emptying the major vessels allows ingress of air, which causes complications related to air embolism, a major hazard associated with this procedure. Ensure that the patient's head is not elevated; rather, depress it and allow blood to gravitate into the head vessels, thus displacing the air (upward) to the periphery. This is essential.

The patient is rewarmed with restoration of anterograde flow through a side arm line inserted in the ascending aorta. The aortic valve is suspended with 4–0 polypropylene pledgeted sutures if it is normal and no evidence of aortic root dilatation is present. The intima and adventitia of the aorta superior to the coronaries are sutured together and reinforced from inside the graft. If the aortic valve or the root is dilatated, a composite valve graft is placed.

**A button or modified Cabrol technique** is used to reattach the coronaries. When aortic regurgitation is present, simple decompression of the false lumen may be all that is required to allow resuspension of the aortic leaflets and restoration of valvular competence. More often, however, the two layers of the dissected aortic wall are approximated, and resuspension of the commissures is accomplished with pledgeted sutures. Prosthetic aortic valve replacement also may be necessary in certain situations. After the procedure is completed and the patient is brought to sinus rhythm by defibrillation, the patient is weaned from cardiopulmonary bypass. In patients with involvement of the transverse aortic arch, either the proximal arch or the total arch is replaced. If the intima is fragmented or shows evidence of rupture, then the whole arch is replaced.

**Surgical management of acute type B aortic dissections** is undertaken only in the presence of indications such as persistent pain, aneurysmal dilatation greater than 5 cm, end organ or limb ischemia, or evidence of retrograde dissection to the ascending aorta. The remaining patients are treated with intense medical therapy.

The operation involves transection of the proximal descending aorta distal to the left subclavian artery. Similar to operation on the ascending aorta, the proximal and distal intima and adventitia of the transected aorta are reinforced in the same manner as that for the ascending aorta, with a 4–0 polypropylene suture. A gelatin-or collagen-woven Dacron graft is sewn directly to the reinforced acutely dissected proximal thoracic aorta, with the posterior row reinforced using interrupted polypropylene sutures. Blood is rechanneled into the true lumen of the distal aorta by cutting the descending thoracic graft and suturing it to the reinforced distal aorta.

Adjunct procedures are used to minimize complications. The entire thoracoabdominal aorta is opened if extensive involvement of the descending and abdominal aorta is present that requires replacement. The septum between the false and true lumen is excised, and the visceral vessels and renal arteries are reattached to the graft directly or via a Dacron graft.

**In chronic dissections, the intercostal arteries (T9–T12) are reimplanted by side graft or a side hole.** This is in contrast to acute dissections, in which the intercostals and lumbar arteries are ligated. Newer surgical techniques have been developed that use fibrin sealant or gelatin-resorcin-formaldehyde glue. Glue replaces the use of pledgeted sutures to seal the false lumen of the aortic stumps after resection of the diseased aortic segment and before the implantation of the Dacron prosthesis. The glue hardens and reinforces the dissected aortic tissue. Other advantages include simplification of the operation, facilitation of the resuspension of the aortic valve, and, possibly, reduction in the frequency of late aortic root aneurysm formation.

Because of high operative mortality rates in people with renal or visceral artery compromise from dissection, endovascular techniques are under investigation. Several endovascular techniques are available. One involves the formation of a site of reentry to allow blood to pass from the false lumen to the true lumen. This requires passing a wire past the intact intimal flap, passing a balloon-tipped catheter over the wire, and tearing a hole in the intimal flap by inflating the balloon. Another technique involves percutaneous stenting to decrease the ischemic complications of aortic dissection. This is performed on arteries that have compromised flow from the dissection. Sutureless intraluminal prostheses placed during cardiopulmonary bypass are also being used. Another technique involves **percutaneously placed intraluminal stent-grafts using a transfemoral catheter technique**. This procedure results in the closure of the site of entry into the false lumen and decompresses and promotes thrombosis of the false lumen. It also alleviates obstruction of the branch vessels complicating a dissection.

**Intramural hematomas** and penetrating atherosclerotic ulcers of the aorta are conditions that result in aortic dissection or rupture. Both are more common in the descending aorta; medical therapy is the first-line treatment. When either affects the ascending aorta or the arch, the need for surgery is more likely. Intramural hematomas are hemorrhage into the medial layer of the aortic wall without an intimal tear. Because these hematomas have a natural history similar to aortic dissection and aneurysm, they are treated similarly.

Surgical therapy is initiated for patients with proximal hematomas; medical therapy is reserved for patients with distal hematomas. Medical therapy consists of optimizing blood pressure control, decreasing aortic pulse pressure, controlling risk factors for atherosclerosis, and maintaining close long-term follow-up care. Penetrating atherosclerotic ulcers penetrate the internal elastic lamina, causing hematoma formation within the media of the aortic wall. Almost all are in the descending aorta. Because the natural history of these ulcers is undefined, a definitive treatment strategy has not been formulated.

Consider surgery in patients with penetrating atherosclerotic ulcers who are hemodynamically unstable or who have evidence of pseudoaneurysm formation or transmural rupture. Other indications for surgery include recurrent pain, distal embolization, and progressive aneurysmal dilatation from the ulcer. If patients do not present with these complications, they are treated with antihypertensive medications and close monitoring.

**Postoperative details:** Postoperative complications for extensive disease involving the thoracoabdominal aorta include myocardial infarction, respiratory failure, renal failure, stroke, and paraparesis or paraplegia.

**Follow-up care:** Provide the following long-term care for patients with aortic dissection, whether treated medically or surgically:

- One-month follow-up check for any new symptoms, such as chest or back pain, and signs suggestive of progression of the aortic dissection.
- Adequate blood pressure control, with the systolic blood pressure maintained at 90–120 mmHg
- Routine chest radiographs, CT scans with contrast, and MRIs, at 3-, 6-, and 12-month intervals, respectively, in an outpatient setting to evaluate any progression of the condition

**Complications** are diverse and numerous; anatomic-related complications are deducible and include the following (Fig. 18.29 and Table 18.3):

- Hypotension and shock as a result of aortic rupture and eventual death from exsanguination. Pericardial tamponade secondary to hemopericardium—complicates type A aortic dissection
- Acute aortic regurgitation as a complication of proximal aortic dissection propagating into a sinus of Valsalva with resultant aortic valve insufficiency
- Pulmonary edema secondary to acute aortic valve regurgitation
- Rare occurrence of right or left coronary ostium involvement leading to myocardial ischemia

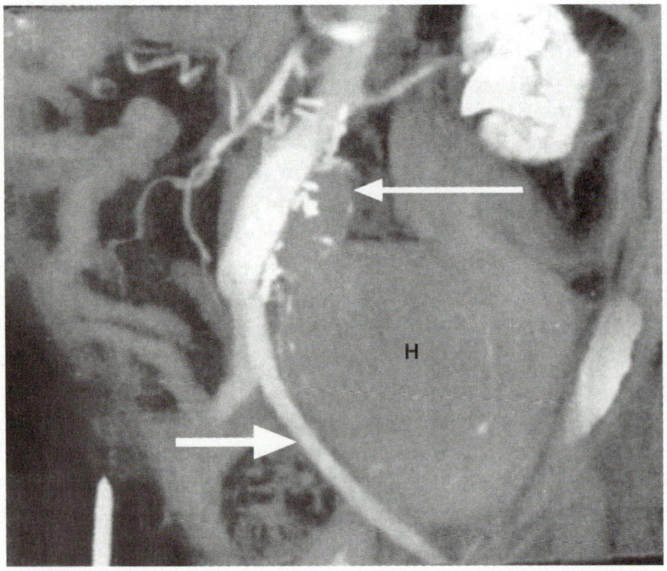


**Fig. 18.29:** 3-D VR MDCT. Large hematoma (H) post AAA surgical repair (arrow) displacing left iliac arteries (arrowhead)

**Table 18.3:** Complications in patients undergoing abdominal aortic aneurysm repair

| Complication | Incidence (%) |
|---|---|
| Death | 9.6 |
| Myocardial infarction | 7.2 |
| Cerebrovascular accident | 4.8 |
| Paralysis/paresis | 6.0 |
| Non-Q-wave mycardial infarction | 8.4 |
| Distal emboli/thrombosis | 6.0 |

- Neurologic findings due to carotid artery obstruction—ischemic CVA, hemiplegia, hemianesthesia (aortic branch involvement can lead to spinal cord ischemia, ischemic paraparesis, and paraplegia)
- Mesenteric and renal ischemia—can lead to bowel or visceral ischemia, renal infarction, hematuria, or ARF.

**Compressive symptoms,** such as superior vena cava syndrome, Horner syndrome (when it affects the superior cervical ganglia), dysphagia (when it involves the esophagus), airway compromise, and hemoptysis (when it compresses the bronchus)

- Other compressive symptoms—can be associated with vocal cord paralysis and hoarseness
- Claudication—can develop from extension of the dissection into the iliac arteries.

**Redissection and progressive aortic diameter enlargement**

- Aneurysmal dilatation and saccular aneurysm also can complicate aortic dissection
- Hospital-based mortality rates for aortic dissection are approximately 30%
- Patients with type A aortic dissection who undergo surgical treatment have a 30% mortality rate; patients who receive medical treatment have a mortality rate of 60%. Comorbidities and advanced aged can pose a contraindication to surgery in selected patients.

Medically treated patients with type B dissection have a 10% mortality rate; surgically treated patients with type B dissection have a 30% mortality rate.

Treated aortic dissection patients have a 60% 10-year survival rate. The mortality rate is influenced by the patient's clinical condition. The aortic dissection mortality rate is still high despite advancements in diagnostic and therapeutic modalities. Ideally, researchers will devise a test that detects aortic dissection before severe complications develop, thus allowing early intervention and eventually reducing mortality rates.

The findings of the smooth muscle myosin heavy-chain assay are not elevated in persons with acute myocardial infarction or other nonaortic conditions of chest pain syndromes. The test's sensitivity and specificity are promising, and, in the future, a battery of tests will help determine a genetic predisposition to aortic dissection, including conditions such as Ehlers-Danlos syndrome and Marfan syndrome.

*Emergent surgical correction is the preferred treatment for the following classifications of aortic dissection:*

- Stanford type A (DeBakey type I and II) ascending aortic dissection
- Complicated Stanford type B (DeBakey type III) aortic dissections with clinical or radiological evidence of the following conditions:
  - Propagation (increasing aortic diameter)
  - Increasing size of hematoma
  - Compromise of major branches of the aorta
  - Impending rupture
  - Persistent pain despite adequate pain management
  - Bleeding into the pleural cavity
  - Development of saccular aneurysm

### *Prehospital Care*

- Assure adequate breathing, maintain oxygenation, treat shock, and obtain useful historic information.
- Establishing the diagnosis in the field is usually difficult or impossible, but certain salient features of aortic dissection may be observed. It is life threatening if not quickly recognized and treated.
- Radio communication with the receiving hospital permits the medical control physician to direct care and select a capable destination hospital while permitting the ED to mobilize appropriate resources.
- In the rare event that the diagnosis can be made based on prehospital information, the physician directing prehospital care should request transport to a facility capable of operative treatment of an aortic dissection.

### *Emergency Department Care*

- The mortality rate of patients with aortic dissection is 1–2% per hour for the first 24–48 hours. Initial therapy should begin when the diagnosis is suspected. This includes two large-bore intravenous lines (IVs), oxygen, respiratory monitoring, and monitoring of cardiac rhythm, blood pressure, and urine output.

- Clinically, the physician should reassess the patient frequently for hemodynamic compromise, mental status changes, neurologic or peripheral vascular changes, and development or progression of carotid, brachial, and femoral bruits.
- Aggressive management of heart rate and blood pressure should be initiated.
- Beta-blockers should be given initially to reduce the rate of change of blood pressure (dP/dt) and the shear forces on the aortic wall.
- The target heart rate should be 60–80 beats per minute.
- The target systolic blood pressure should be 100–120 mm-Hg.
- End organ perfusion should be evaluated. Balancing the risks of dP/dt on the aortic wall versus the benefits of acceptable end organ perfusion may be a difficult clinical decision.
- Urgent surgical intervention is required in type A dissections.
- The area of the aorta with the intimal tear usually is resected and replaced with a Dacron graft.
- The operative mortality rate is usually less than 10%, and serious complications are rare with ascending aortic dissections.
- The development of more impermeable grafts, such as woven Dacron, collagen-impregnated Hemashield (Meadox Medicals, Oakland, NJ), aortic grafts, and gel-coated Carbo-Seal Ascending Aortic Prothesis (Sulzer CarboMedics, Austin, TX) has greatly enhanced the surgical repair of thoracic aortic dissections.
- With the introduction of profound hypothermic circulatory arrest and retrograde cerebral perfusion, the morbidity and mortality rates associated with this highly invasive surgery have decreased.
- Dissections involving the arch are more complicated that those involving only the ascending aorta because the innominate, carotid, and subclavian vessels branch from the arch. Deep hypothermic arrest usually is required. If the arrest time is less than 45 minutes, the incidence of central nervous system complications is less than 10%.
- Aortic stent grafting is a challenging technique. It may prove feasible and has offered good results in a small series of patients. It may be a reasonable alternative in high-risk patients in the near future.
- Retrograde cerebral perfusion may increase the protection of the central nervous system during the arrest period.
- The mortality rate of aortic arch dissections is about 10–15%, with significant neurologic complications occurring in another 10%.
- The mortality rate is influenced by the patient's clinical condition.
- The definitive treatment for type B dissections is less clear.
- Uncomplicated distal dissections may be treated medically to control blood pressure.
- Distal dissections treated medically have the same or a lower mortality rate as those treated surgically.
- Surgery is reserved for distal dissections that are leaking, ruptured, or compromising blood flow to a vital organ.
- Acute distal dissections in patients with Marfan syndrome usually are treated surgically.
- Inability to control hypertension with medication is also an indication for surgery in those with a distal thoracic aortic dissection.
- Patients with a distal dissection are usually hypertensive, emphysematous, or older.

**Long-term medical therapy** involves a beta-adrenergic blocker combined with other antihypertensive medications. Avoid antihypertensives (e.g. hydralazine, minoxidil) that produce a hyperdynamic response that would increase dP/dt (i.e. alter the duration of P or T-waves).

- Survivors of surgical therapy also should receive beta-adrenergic blockers.
- A recent series of patients with type B dissections demonstrates that aggressive use of distal perfusion, CSF drainage, and hypothermia with circulatory arrest improves early mortality and long-term survival rates.
- Aortic stent grafting may play a role in how type B dissections are treated in the near future.
- Definitive treatment involves segmental resection of the dissection with interposition of a synthetic graft.
- When thoracic dissections are associated with aortic valvular disease, replace the defective valve.
- With combined reconstruction—valve replacement, the operative mortality rate is approximately 5% with a late mortality rate of less than 10%.
- Operative repair of the transverse aortic arch is technically difficult, with an operative mortality rate of 10% despite induction of hypothermic cardiocirculatory arrest.
- Repair of the descending aorta is associated with a higher incidence of paraplegia than repair of other types of dissections because of interruption of segmental blood supply to the spinal cord.
- The operative mortality rate is approximately 5%.

## Consultations

- Once a thoracic dissection is suspected, consult a thoracic surgeon.
- Because many patients with this disorder have concomitant medical illness, consult the patient's primary care physician to expedite preoperative preparation.
- Early consultation is encouraged when ordering further imaging studies if the patient requires rapid operative intervention.
- Consult a radiologist prior to obtaining aortography.

Initial therapeutic goals include elimination of pain and reduction of systolic blood pressure to 100–120 mmHg or to the lowest level commensurate with adequate vital organ (i.e. cardiac, cerebral, and renal) perfusion.

Whether systolic hypertension or pain is present, beta-blockers are used to reduce arterial dP/dt.

To prevent exacerbations of tachycardia and hypertension, treat patients with IV morphine sulfate. This reduces the force of cardiac contraction and the rate of rise of the aortic pressure (dP/dt). It then retards the propagation of the dissection and delays rupture

## Pharmacology of Dissection of Aorta

### Drug Category

*Antihypertensives:* These agents are used to reduce arterial dP/dt. For acute reduction of arterial pressure, the potent vasodilator sodium nitroprusside is effective. To reduce dP/dt acutely, administer an IV beta-blocker in incremental doses until a heart rate of 60–80 beats/min is attained.

When beta-blockers are contraindicated, such as in second-or third-degree atrioventricular block, consider using calcium channel blockers. Sublingual nifedipine successfully treats refractory hypertension associated with aortic dissection.

*Drug name:* Esmolol (brevibloc)—ultrashort-acting beta2-blocker, particularly useful in patients with labile arterial pressure, especially if surgery is planned, because it can be discontinued abruptly if necessary. Normally used in conjunction with nitroprusside. May be useful as a means to test beta-blocker safety and tolerance in patients with history of obstructive pulmonary disease who are at uncertain risk of bronchospasm from beta-blockade. Elimination half-life is 9 min.

*Adult dose:* 250–500 mcg/kg/min for 1 min as loading dose, followed by a 4-min maintenance infusion of 50 mcg/kg/min; repeat loading dose and follow with maintenance infusion using increments of 50 mcg/kg/min for 4 min; if therapeutic effects not observed in 5 min, repeat sequence up to 4 times prn. As desired BP is approached, omit loading infusion and reduce incremental dose of maintenance infusion from 50 mcg/kg/min to 25 mcg/kg/min or lower; may increase interval between titration steps to 5–10 min if desired.

*Pediatric dose:* Not established

*Contraindications:* Documented hypersensitivity; uncompensated CHF; bradycardia; cardiogenic shock; AV conduction abnormalities

*Interactions:* Aluminum salts, barbiturates, NSAIDs, penicillins, calcium salts, cholestyramine, and rifampin may decrease bioavailability and plasma levels, possibly resulting in decreased pharmacologic effect; sparfloxacin, astemizole **(recalled from US market)**, calcium channel blockers, quinidine, flecainide, and contraceptives may increase cardiotoxicity; digoxin, flecainide, acetaminophen, clonidine, epinephrine, nifedipine, prazosin, haloperidol, phenothiazines, and catecholamine-depleting agents may increase toxicity

*Pregnancy:* C-Safety for use during pregnancy has not been established.

*Precautions:* Beta-adrenergic blockers may mask signs and symptoms of acute hypoglycemia and clinical signs of hyperthyroidism; symptoms of hyperthyroidism, including thyroid storm, may worsen when medication is withdrawn abruptly; withdraw drug slowly and monitor patient closely

*Drug name:* Labetalol (normodyne, trandate)—blocks alpha-, beta1-, and beta2-adrenergic receptor sites, decreasing BP.

*Adult dose:* Initial dose—20 mg (0.25 mg/kg for 80 kg patient) IV over 2 min; follow with 20–80 mg q10–15 min until BP controlled. Maintenance dose—2 mg/min continuous IV infusion; titrate up to 5–20 mg/min; not to exceed a total dose of 300 mg

*Pediatric dose:* Not established

*Contraindications:* Documented hypersensitivity; cardiogenic shock; AV block; uncompensated CHF; pulmonary edema; bradycardia; reactive airway disease

*Interactions:* Decreases effects of diuretics and increases toxicity of methotrexate, lithium, and salicylates; may diminish reflex tachycardia associated with nitroglycerin use without interfering with hypotensive effects; cimetidine may increase blood levels; glutethimide may decrease effects by inducing microsomal enzymes

*Pregnancy:* C-Safety for use during pregnancy has not been established.

*Precautions:* Caution in impaired hepatic function; discontinue therapy with signs of liver dysfunction; in elderly patients, lower response rate and higher incidence of toxicity may be observed.

*Drug name:* Propranolol (inderal, betachron E-R)—class II antiarrhythmic nonselective beta-adrenergic receptor blocker. Has membrane-stabilizing activity and decreases automaticity of contractions. Not suitable for emergency treatment of hypertension. Do not administer IV in hypertensive emergencies.

*Adult dose:* 40–80 mg PO bid initially; increase to usual range of 160-320 mg/d prn; up to 640 mg/d may be required

*Pediatric dose:* 0.5 mg/kg/d PO divided bid/qid; increase gradually q3–7d; usual dosage range is 2–4 mg/kg/d divided bid; not to exceed 16 mg/kg/d

*Contraindications:* Documented hypersensitivity; uncompensated CHF; bradycardia; cardiogenic shock; AV conduction abnormalities

*Interactions:* Aluminum salts, barbiturates, NSAIDs, penicillins, calcium salts, cholestyramine, and rifampin may decrease effects; calcium channel blockers, cimetidine, loop diuretics, and MAOIs may increase toxicity; may increase toxicity of hydralazine, haloperidol, benzodiazepines, and phenothiazines

*Pregnancy:* B-Usually safe but benefits must outweigh the risks.

*Precautions:* Beta-adrenergic blockade may decrease signs of acute hypoglycemia and hyperthyroidism; abrupt withdrawal may exacerbate symptoms of hyperthyroidism, including thyroid storm; withdraw drug slowly and monitor closely.

*Drug name:* Metoprolol (lopressor)—selective beta1-adrenergic receptor blocker that decreases automaticity of contractions. During IV administration, carefully monitor BP, heart rate, and ECG. When considering conversion from IV to PO dosage forms, use ratio of 2.5 mg PO to 1 mg IV metoprolol.

*Adult dose:* 100 mg/d PO qd or divided bid/tid initially; increase at 1-week intervals prn; not to exceed 450 mg/d prn

*Pediatric dose:* Not established

*Contraindications:* Documented hypersensitivity; uncompensated CHF; cardiogenic shock; bradycardia; AV conduction abnormalities

*Interactions:* Aluminum salts, barbiturates, NSAIDs, penicillins, calcium salts, cholestyramine, and rifampin may decrease bioavailability and plasma levels, possibly resulting in decreased pharmacologic effects; sparfloxacin, phenothiazines, astemizole **(recalled from US market)**, calcium channel blockers, quinidine, flecainide, and contraceptives may increase toxicity; may increase toxicity of digoxin, flecainide, clonidine, epinephrine, nifedipine, prazosin, verapamil, and lidocaine

*Pregnancy:* B-Usually safe but benefits must outweigh the risks.

*Precautions:* Beta-adrenergic blockade may reduce signs and symptoms of acute hypoglycemia and may decrease clinical signs of hyperthyroidism; abrupt withdrawal may exacerbate symptoms of hyperthyroidism, including thyroid storm; monitor patient closely and withdraw drug slowly; during IV administration, carefully monitor BP, heart rate, and ECG

*Drug name:* Nitroprusside (nitropress) causes peripheral vasodilation by direct action on venous and arteriolar smooth muscle, thus reducing peripheral resistance. Commonly used IV because of rapid onset and short duration of action. Easily titratable to reach desired effect. Light sensitive; both bottle and tubing should be wrapped in aluminum foil. Prior to initiating nitroprusside, administer beta-blocker to counteract physiologic response of reflex tachycardia that occurs when nitroprusside used alone. This physiologic response increases shear forces against aortic wall, thus increasing dP/dt. Objective is to keep heart rate at 60–80 bpm.

*Adult dose:* 0.5–3 mcg/kg/min IV; rates >4 mcg/kg/min may lead to cyanide toxicity

*Pediatric dose:* Administer as in adults

*Contraindications:* Documented hypersensitivity; subaortic stenosis; idiopathic hypertrophic subaortic stenosis; atrial fibrillation or flutter

*Interactions:* None reported

*Pregnancy:* C-Safety for use during pregnancy has not been established.

*Precautions:* Caution in increased intracranial pressure, hepatic failure, severe renal impairment, and hypothyroidism; in renal or hepatic insufficiency, levels may increase and can cause cyanide toxicity; sodium nitroprusside has ability to lower BP and thus should be used only in patients with mean arterial pressures >70 mmHg

*Drug category:* Analgesics—pain control is essential to quality patient care. It ensures patient comfort, promotes pulmonary toilet, and prevent exacerbations of tachycardia and hypertension.

*Drug name:* Morphine sulfate (astramorph, infumorph)—DOC for narcotic analgesia because of reliable and predictable effects, safety profile, and ease of reversibility with naloxone. Similar to fentanyl, morphine sulfate easily titrated to desired level of pain control. If administered IV, may be dosed in a number of ways; commonly titrated until desired effect obtained.

*Adult dose:* Initial dose—0.1 mg/kg IV/IM/SC. Maintenance dose: 5–20 mg/70 kg q4h IV/IM/SC.

*Pediatric dose:* 0.1–0.2 mg/kg IV/IM/SC q2-4h prn.

*Contraindications:* Documented hypersensitivity; hypotension; potentially compromised airway in which establishing rapid airway control would be difficult.

*Interactions:* Phenothiazines may antagonize analgesic effects; tricyclic antidepressants, MAOIs, and other CNS depressants may potentiate adverse effects.

*Pregnancy:* C-Safety for use during pregnancy has not been established.

*Precautions:* Avoid in hypotension, respiratory depression, nausea, emesis, constipation, and urinary retention; caution in atrial flutter and other supraventricular tachycardias; has vagolytic action and may increase ventricular response rate.

### Further Inpatient Care

- Patients with symptomatic dissection should undergo immediate repair, especially if it is leaking or expanding.
- Symptomatic patients require admission to a center experienced in cardiopulmonary bypass and operative care.
- Completely asymptomatic patients may have their repair performed electively but may require admission to

expedite their evaluation or for preoperative stabilization of their condition.
- Patients with chest pain should undergo serial ECGs and CK determinations if AMI is indicated.

### Further Outpatient Care

- Follow-up examinations with radiologic studies are recommended at 3-month intervals for the first year and every 6 months for the next 2 years.
- After this, follow up annually.

### Transfer

- Symptomatic patients require care at a facility equipped to perform cardiopulmonary bypass with aortic and/or valvular repair.
- Contact the receiving physician as soon as possible to transfer patients before their condition deteriorates.
- Early airway management is indicated in the presence of hemoptysis or stridor.
- If coronary insufficiency is suspected, nitrates may be used, but therapy with thrombolytic agents and aspirin should be avoided.
- Patients should be monitored and accompanied by personnel capable of resuscitation.
- If a prolonged ground transport time is anticipated, consider air transport.

### Prognosis

- On the basis of his experience, Crawford has stated that 'no patient should be considered cured of the disease.'
- The 5-year survival rate is about 75% whether the patient is treated medically or surgically.

The 10-year survival rate is between 40% and 69% for both surgically and medically treated dissections.

In the pretreatment era, the 1-year survival rate was 5–10%.

Reoperation may be necessary for late complications.

### Medical/Legal Pitfalls

- Failure to diagnose (especially in patients presenting with chest pain). Use of thrombolytics in the patient presenting with chest pain and ECG changes
- Multiple case reports describe patients who received thrombolytics and were found later to have a dissection. The diagnosis of aortic dissection can be subtle.

The diagnosis depends on clinical suspicion, with contributory findings on history, physical examination, and imaging studies.

Obtaining a chest radiograph prior to administering thrombolytics is considered prudent.

Checking blood pressures in both arms and listening for carotid bruits also can help diagnose aortic dissection prior to administering thrombolytics. The entire clinical picture must be taken into account knowledgement.

## KEY POINTS

1. Aortic dissection may originate anywhere along the aorta but is most common at the proximal ascending aorta (within 5 cm of the aortic valve) or the descending thoracic aorta just beyond the origin of the left subclavian artery.
2. Dissection requires preexisting degeneration of the aortic media (e.g. caused by connective tissue disorders, injury) but hypertension is commonly also involved.
3. Patients typically have excruciating, tearing precordial or interscapular pain.
4. Other manifestations depend on whether the aortic root and/or branches of the aorta are affected, and the presence and location of any rupture; heart failure, organ ischemia and hemorrhagic shock may occur.
5. Diagnose using TEE, CTA, or MRA.
6. Immediately give beta-blockers and other drugs as needed to control BP.
7. Drug therapy alone is appropriate for uncomplicated, stable dissection confined to the descending aorta or the aortic arch; other cases require surgery.

## BIBLIOGRAPHY


1. Bickerstaff LK, Pairolero PC, Hollier LH, et al. Thoracic aortic aneurysms: a population-based study. Surgery 1982; 92(6):1103-8.
2. Chen K, Varon J, Wenker OC, et al. Acute thoracic aortic dissection: the basics. J Emerg Med 1997;15(6): 859–67.
3. Cigarroa J, Isselbacher E, DeSanctis R. Diagnostic Imaging in the Evaluation of Suspected Aortic Dissection. N Engl J Med 1993;328(1):35–43.
4. De Bakey ME, Cooley DA, Creech O. Surgical considerations of dissecting aneurysm of the aorta. Ann Surg 1955; 142(4): 586–610;(discussion),611–2.
5. De Bakey ME, Cooley DA. Successful resection of aneurysm of thoracic aorta and replacement by graft. J Am Med Assoc 1953;152(8):673–6.
6. DeSanctis R, Doroghazi R, Austen G. Aortic Dissection. N Engl J Med 1987;317(17):1060–66.
7. Erbel R, Engberding R, Daniel W, et al. Echocardiography in diagnosis of aortic dissection. Lancet 1989;1(8636):457–61.
8. Erdheim J. Medionecrosis Aorte Idiopathica Apitca. Virchows Arch Pathol Anat 1930;276:187–229.
9. Goldman L, Ausiello D. Cecil Textbook of Medicine, 22nd ed. Philadelphia, Pa: WB Saunders Co; 2004.
10. Hagan PG, Nienaber CA, Isselbacher EM, et al. The International Registry of Acute Aortic Dissection (IRAD): new insights into an old disease. JAMA 2000;283(7): 897–903.
11. Hasham SN, Lewin MR, Tran VT, et al. Nonsyndromic genetic predisposition to aortic dissection: a newly recog-nized, diagnosable, and preventable occurrence in families. Ann Emerg Med 2004;43(1):79–82.
12. Jagannath AS, Sos TA, Lockhart SH, et al. Aortic dissection: a statistical analysis of the usefulness of plain chest radiographic findings. AJR Am J Roentgenol 1986; 147(6): 1123–6.

13. Januzzi JL, Marayati F, Mehta RH, et al. Comparison of aortic dissection in patients with and without Marfan's syndrome (results from the International Registry of Aortic Dissection). Am J Cardiol 2004;94(3):400–2.
14. Knaut AL, Cleveland JC. Aortic emergencies. Emerg Med Clin North Am 2003;21(4):817–45.
15. Krukenberg E. Beitrage zur Frage des Aneurysma Dissecans. Beitr Pathol Anat Allerg Pathol 1920;67:329–51.
16. Lee JT, White RA. Current status of thoracic aortic endograft repair. Surg Clin North Am 2004;84(5):1295–318,
17. Nichols F. Observations Concerning the Body of His Late Majesty. Philos Trans Lond 1762;52:265–75.
18. Pansini S, Gagliardotto PV, Pompei E, et al. Early and late risk factors in surgical treatment of acute type A aortic dissection. Ann Thorac Surg 1998; 66(3):779–84.
19. Ponraj P, Pepper J. Aortic dissection. Br J Clin Pract 1992 Summer; 46(2):127–31.
20. Prokop EK, Palmer RF, Wheat MW Jr. Hydrodynamic forces in dissecting aneurysms. In-vitro studies in a Tygon model and in dog aortas. Circ Res 1970; 27(1):121–7.
21. Rogers RL, McCormack R. Aortic disasters. Emerg Med Clin North Am 2004; 22(4):887–908.
22. Safi HJ, Miller CC, Reardon MJ, et al. Operation for acute and chronic aortic dissection: recent outcome with regard to neurologic deficit and early death. Ann Thorac Surg 1998; 66(2):402–11.
23. Sarasin FP, Louis-Simonet M, Gaspoz JM, et al. Detecting acute thoracic aortic dissection in the emergency department: time constraints and choice of the optimal diagnostic test. Ann Emerg Med 1996;28(3):278–88.
24. Spiegel EA, Wassreman S. Experimentalstudien uber die Entsehungdes Aortenschmerzes und seine Leitung zum zentralnervensystem. Ztschr F. d. ges. Exper Med 1926;52: 180–96.
25. Svensson LG, Crawford ES, Hess KR, et al. Experience with 1509 patients undergoing thoracoabdominal aortic operations. J Vasc Surg 1993;17(2):357–68;(discussion) 368–70.
26. Tatli S, Yucel EK, Lipton MJ. CT and MR imaging of the thoracic aorta: current techniques and clinical applications. Radiol Clin North Am 2004; 42(3):565–85.

# 19 Peripheral Vascular Disease and Endovascular Therapy

## ANATOMICAL BASIS OF PERIPHERAL VASCULAR SYSTEM

Peripheral vascular diseases (PVDs) are circulation disorders that affect blood vessels outside of the heart and brain. PVD typically strikes the veins and arteries that supply the arms, legs, and organs located below your stomach. These are the blood vessels that are distant from the heart. They are known as peripheral vessels. In PVD, blood vessels are narrowed. Narrowing is usually caused by arteriosclerosis. Arteriosclerosis is a condition where plaque builds up inside a vessel. It is also called 'hardening of the arteries.' Plaque decreases the amount of blood and oxygen supplied to the arms and legs. As plaque growth progresses, clots may develop. This further restricts the affected vessel. Eventually, arteries can become obstructed.

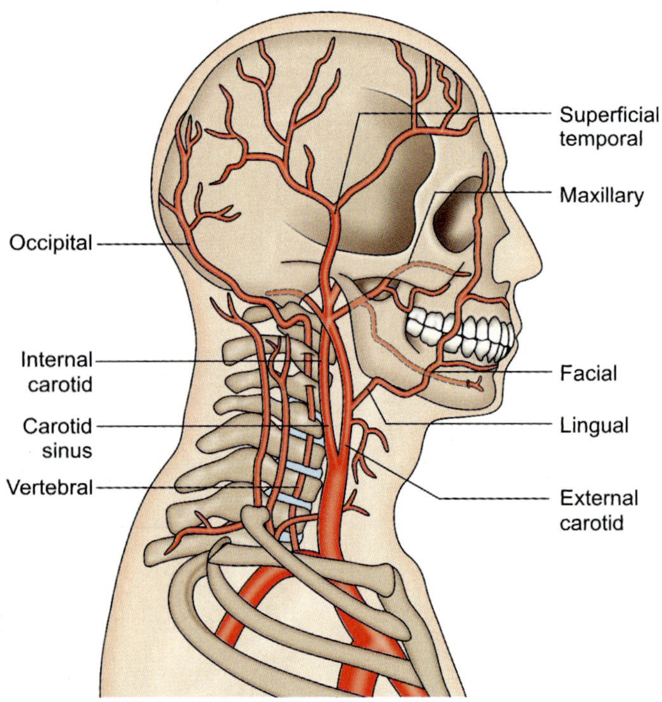


**Fig. 19.1:** Anatomical localization of arterial system of head and neck

PVD that develops only in the arteries is called peripheral arterial disease (PAD). This is the most common form of PVD. Approximately 12–20% of people over age 65 have PAD. PVD that develops in the deep veins in the body is usually caused from claudication and is called deep vein thrombosis (DVT) (Figs 19.1–19.6).

PVD and PAD are often used to mean the same condition that affects the arteries. PVD may also be referred to as:

- Arteriosclerosis obliterans
- Arterial insufficiency of the legs
- Claudication
- Intermittent claudication

### Types of PVD

There are two main types of PVD (Tables 19.1 and 19.2):

1. **Functional PVD:** This does not involve physical problems in the blood vessels. It causes incidental or short-term symptoms. Usually these spasms occur erratically.
2. **Organic PVD:** This involves changes in blood vessel structure. This type of PVD causes inflammation, tissue damage, and blockages.

### Causes of PVD

**Functional PVD:** The body responds to certain external stimuli by restricting blood flow to the peripheral vessels. The most common causes of functional PVDs are:

- Emotional stress
- Smoking
- Cold temperatures
- Operating vibrating machinery or tools

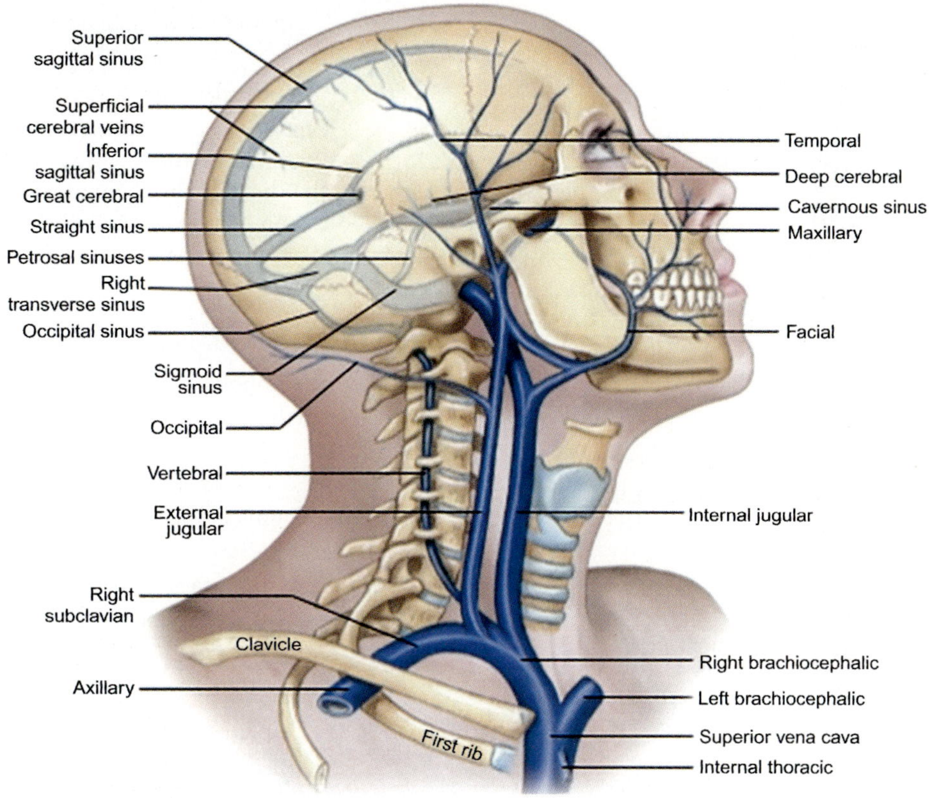


**Fig. 19.2:** Anatomical localization of venous system of head and neck

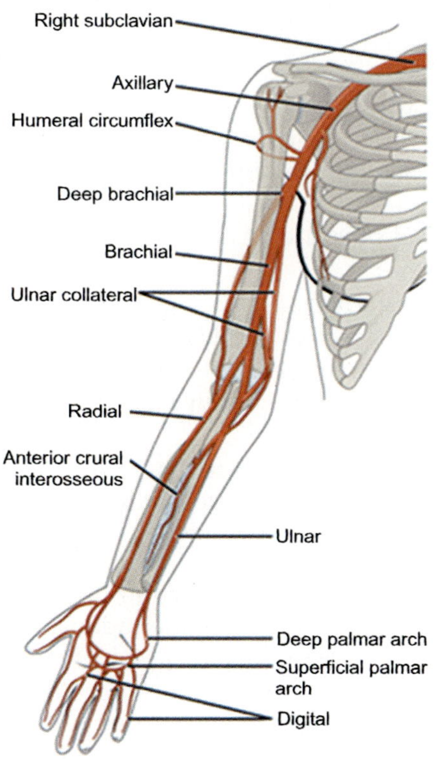


**Fig. 19.3:** Anatomy of various arteries of upper limbs

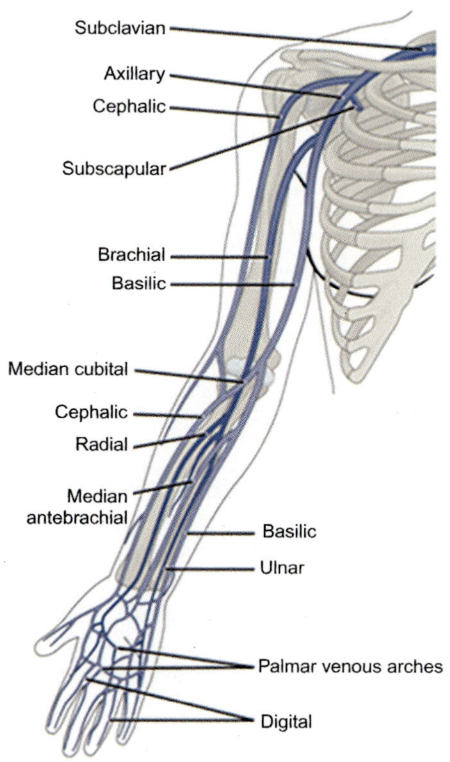


**Fig. 19.4:** Anatomical localization of various veins of upper limbs

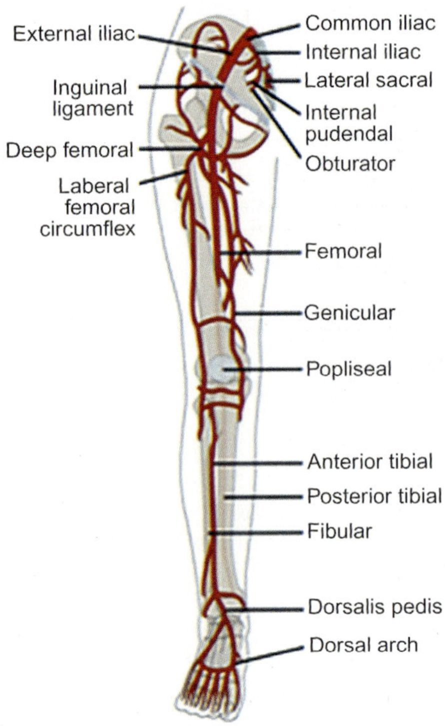


**Fig. 19.5:** Anatomical localization of various arteries of lower limbs

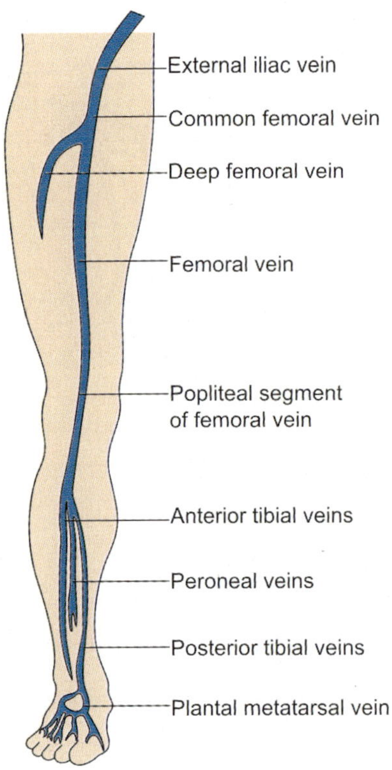


**Fig. 19.6:** Anatomical localization of various veins of lower limbs

**Table 19.1:** Fontaine classification of peripheral arterial disease (PAD)

| Stage | Characteristic symptoms |
|---|---|
| 1 | Clinically symptom-free vascular occlusion |
| 2 | Exercise-induced ischemia causing intermittent claudication. No pain at rest |
| 3 | Ischemia at rest, causing rest pain |
| 4 | Ulceration and ischemic gangrene |

**Table 19.2:** Non-atherosclerotic causes of PAD

- Peripheral emboli
- Aneurysm thrombosis or thromboembolism (aortic, popliteal)
- Arteritis
- Takayasu's disease
- Thromboangitis obliterans (Buerger's disease)
- Giant cell arteritis
- Polyarteritis nodosa
- Fibromuscular dysplasia
- Prior trauma or irradiation injury
- Aortic coarctation
- Endofibrosis of the external iliac artery syndrome in cyslists)
- Primary vascular tumors
- Pseudoxanthoma elasticum
- Young patients
- Adventitial cyst of the popliteal artery
- Popliteal entrapment
- Persistent sciatic artery

## Organic PVD

Physical changes can affect the structure of blood vessels. For example, arteriosclerosis can cause plaque buildup. The primary causes of such organic PVDs are:

- Smoking
- High blood pressure
- Diabetes
- High cholesterol
- Additional causes of organic PVDs include:
  - injury to extremities
  - muscles or ligaments with abnormal structures
  - infection
  - coronary artery disease There are numerous risk factors for PVD. Some are due to underlying medical conditions, age, and gender while others are due to lifestyle choices.
- You are at a higher risk for acquiring PVD if you are a man over age 50 or a postmenopausal woman. The likelihood of developing PVD also increases if you have:
  - abnormal cholesterol
  - cerebrovascular disease (stroke)
  - heart disease

- diabetes mellitus (type 1 diabetes)
- family history of high cholesterol, high blood pressure, or PVD
- high blood pressure
- kidney disease on hemodialysis

• The lifestyle choices that can increase your risk of developing PVD are:
  - being overweight
  - being sedentary and not engaging in physical exercise
  - smoking

## CLINICAL EXAMINATION

Examination of the pulse can provide clues to the presence of systemic diseases. Ancient physicians would diagnose heart, liver, renal, and gastrointestinal problems from assessment of the pulse. Today, other tests have been developed to assist in the work-up of systemic illness, but examination of the pulse is still an important part of patient assessment (Figs 19.7–19.56 and Table 19.3).

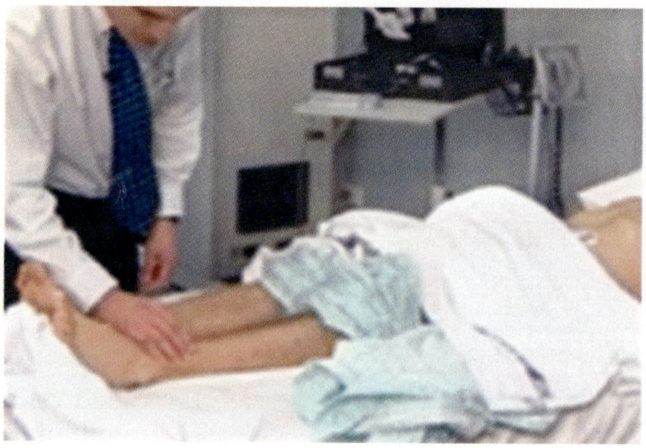

**Fig. 19.7:** A doctor conducting clinical examination of a patient with vascular disease of the leg

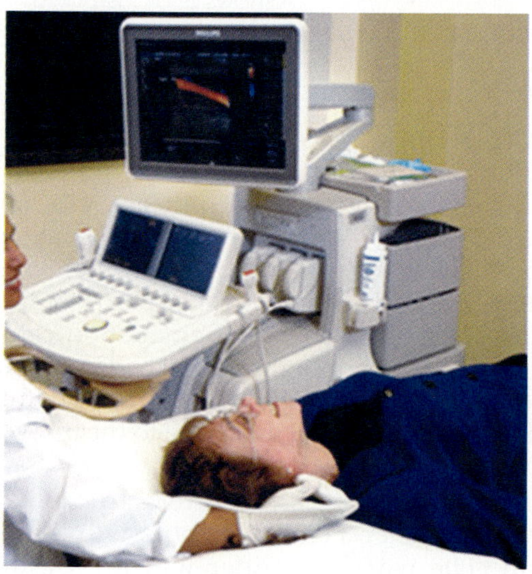

**Fig. 19.8:** Duplex ultrasonography transducer is being placed in the neck by a doctor on young patient

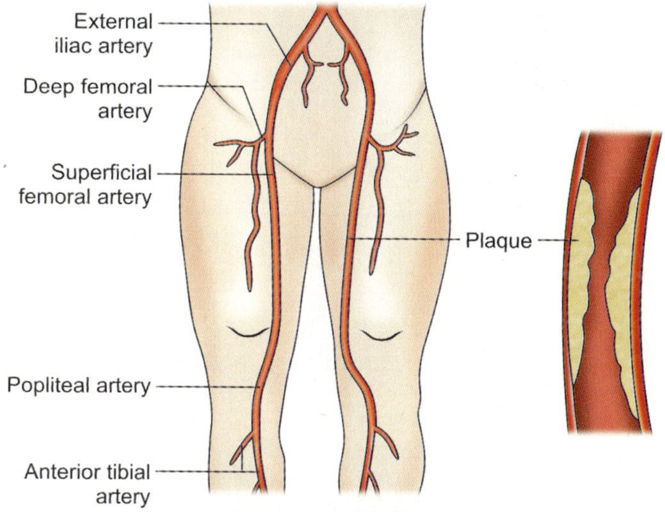


**Fig. 19.9:** Different arteries of lower limbs with atherosclerotic occlusion of left superficial femoral artery

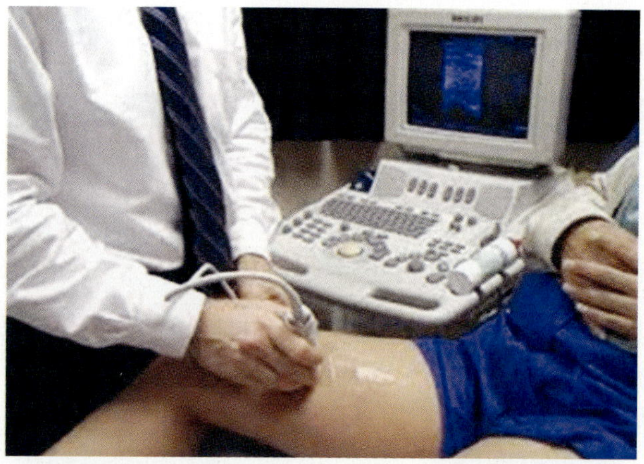

**Fig. 19.10:** A doctor examining lower limb artery with Doppler ultrasonography

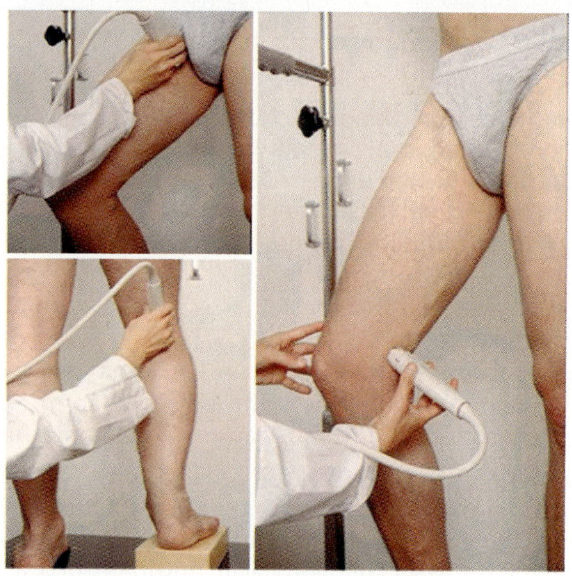

**Fig. 19.11:** A doctor examining lower limb arteries with Doppler ultrasonography

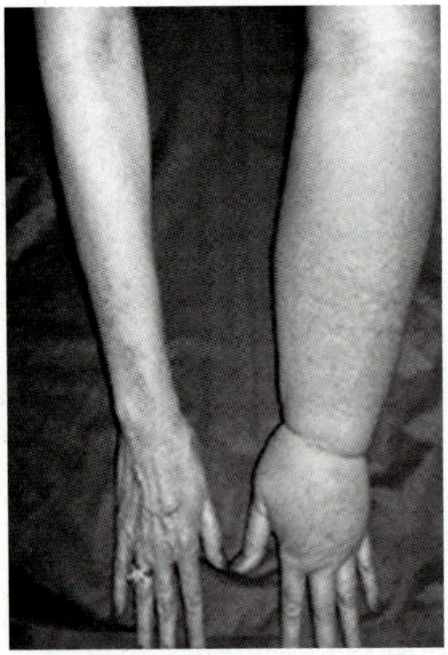

**Fig. 19.12:** Secondary lymphedema—left upper extremity lymphedema 2 years after mastectomy, radiation, and lymphadenectomy for breast cancer

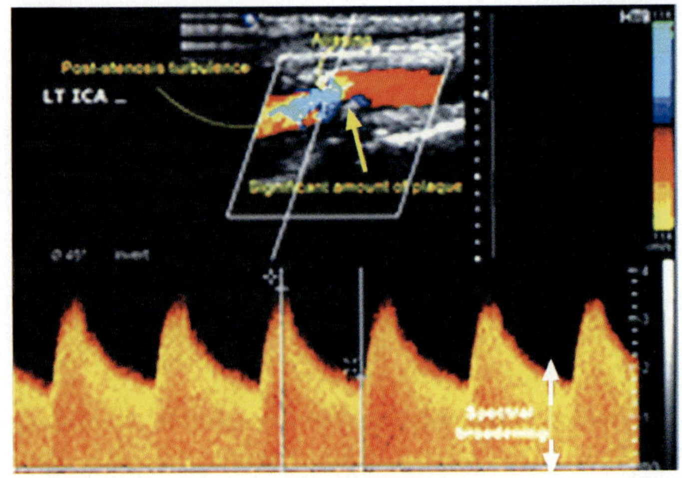


**Fig. 19.14:** Severe stenosis (70% to near occlusion) of the ICA. Duplex US image of the left ICA shows a high PSV (366 cm/sec), a significant amount of visible plaque, the presence of aliasing despite a high color scale setting (114 cm/sec), color flow turbulence immediately distal to the stenotic segment, broadening of the PW Doppler spectrum, and a high end-diastolic velocity (182 cm/sec)

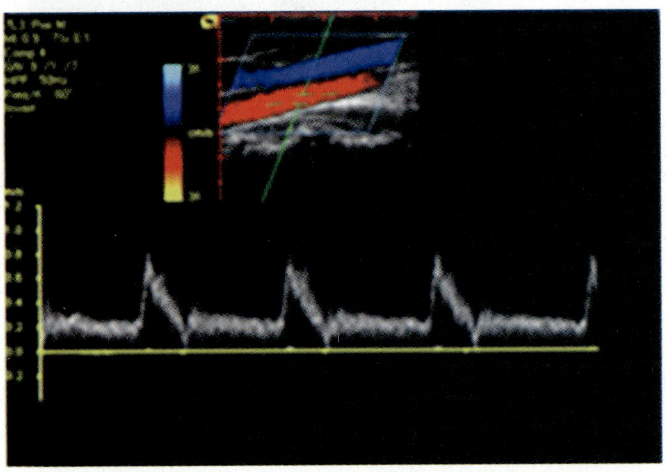

**Fig. 19.13:** Normal common carotid artery (CCA)—PW Doppler

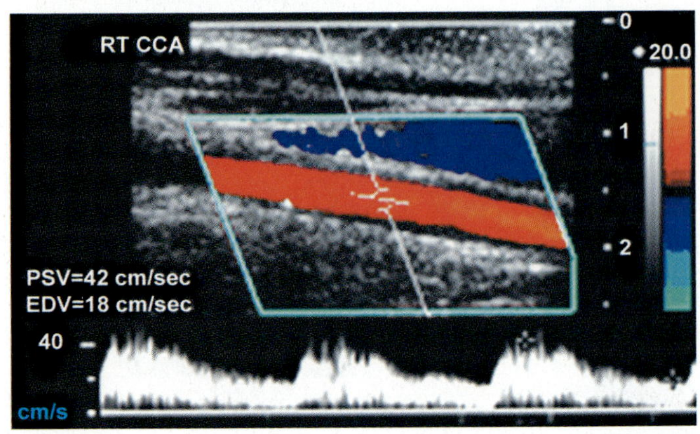


**Fig. 19.15:** Severe stenosis of the innominate artery. PW Doppler spectral image of the right CCA shows a tardus-parvus waveform, which is suggestive of a severe stenosis proximal to the point of sampling

Conditions associated with tachycardia or bradycardia have been discussed, as have the causes of a pulse irregularity. Reduced or absent arterial pulses are a sign of impaired blood flow. The causes include:

1. Congenital abnormalities (coarctation of the aorta, anomalous peripheral arteries);
2. Intrinsic arterial disease (atherosclerosis, thrombosis, and arteritis);
3. Vasospastic disorders (Raynaud's phenomenon); or
4. Involvement of the vessel by extrinsic compression (thoracic outlet syndrome, trauma, and neoplasms).

The resultant alteration of pulses, with or without accompanying bruits, may be indicative of either acute or chronic changes in a given patient. The vascular history, together with associated physical findings such as skin color, temperature, and neuromotor status of the extremity, should help to elucidate these points. More refined diagnostic techniques such as Doppler ultrasound examination and arteriography may be required to evaluate abnormalities suspected from the physical examination. In this regard, it is important to understand that significant arterial occlusive disease of the lower extremities may exist in a patient who has almost normal peripheral pulses in the resting state, since collateral circulation can produce pulsatile flow in the peripheral arterial bed in some patients. If such an individual is instructed to exercise to the point of claudication, however, pulse distal to the major vascular occlusion will diminish or disappear.

Significant widening of an artery to the examining fingers may be the best clue to an otherwise silent arterial aneurysm. The wary examiner will not be misled by tortuosity of the vessel giving a false impression of increased diameter. Careful palpation may also reveal the

**Table 19.3:** Clinical tests used in the diagnosis of peripheral arterial diseases (PAD)

| Test modality | Diagnostic indicators |
|---|---|
| Medical history | • Evidence of atherosclerosis, such as ischemic heart disease, cerebrovascular disease<br>• Risk of atherosclerosis, such as cigarette smoking, diabetes mellitus |
| Pulses in the lower limb | Popliteal, posterior tibial, dorsalis pedis and peroneal pulses<br>• Pulse quality (bounding, full, normal, weak, and absent)<br>• Rate (beats/minute)<br>• Regularity (regular, irregular, irregular, and irregularly irregular) |
| Presenting symptoms | • Cold, numb feet<br>• Intermittent claudication<br>• Rest pain<br>• Painful ulceration |
| Ankle-branchial index (ABI) | • 0.9–1.1 = normal<br>• 0.7–0.9 = PAD, some compromise of tissue viability<br>• 0.5–0.7 = severe PAD, compromised tissue viability<br>• <0.5 = threat of ischaemic gangrene/very poor tissue viability<br>• >1.2 = calcification of tunica media of leg/foot artery, compromised tissue viability |
| Segmental systolic pressure | Serial measurement of systolic blood pressure along length of limb<br>• A sudden decrease indicates the location of the vascular obstruction |
| Venous filling time<br>Note: This test is not valid if the patient has venous incompetence | • The time it takes for veins to refill in a limb that has been drained of venous blood (with the patient supine, the leg is elevated to 45° for 1 minute, then the leg placed in a dependent position and the timetaken for the dorsal foot veins to refil)<br>• <15 seconds = normal<br>• 20–30 seconds = moderate ischemia<br>• >40 second = severe ischemia |
| Buerger's test | • The observation of the change in skin color in response to limbe elevation and dependency (with the patient supine, the leg is elevated to 45° for 1 minute, then the leg is placed in a dependent position and the time taken for normal skin color to return is noted)<br>• <10 seconds = normal response<br>• Patchy persistent rubor indicates limb ischemia<br>• Persistent pallor (>10 seconds) indicates limb ischemia<br>• Presistent cyanosis indicates limb ischemia |
| Buerger's angle | • The color response of the sole of the foot to limb elevation (with the patient supine, the leg is elevated and the angle of limb elevation is noted when the skin of medial longitudinal arch shows pallor)<br>• 60–70° = normal arterial supply to foot<br>• <45° = compromised arterial supply to foot<br>• <30° = severe compromised arterial supply to foot |
| Capillary refill time<br>Note: This test is not valid if the patient has signs of current Raynaud's disease | • The time taken for normal skin tone of a horizontal limb to retum after the nail bed or digital pulp has been compressed by thumb pressure<br>• <5 seconds = normal response<br>• >5 seconds = some ischaemia<br>• >15 seconds = marked ischemia |
| Doppler sounds | • Triphasic = normal<br>• Biphasic = normal/some loss of arterial elasticity<br>• Monophasic = loss of arterial elasticity/arterial stenosis<br>• Loud = high rate of blood flow<br>• Quiet = slow rate of blood flow<br>• No sound = no blood flow (proximal arterial occlusion) |
| Skin temperature<br>Note: This test is not vaild if the patient has signs of current Raynaud's disease | • ~31°C = normal foot skin temperature<br>• <29°C = possible poor skin perfusion |

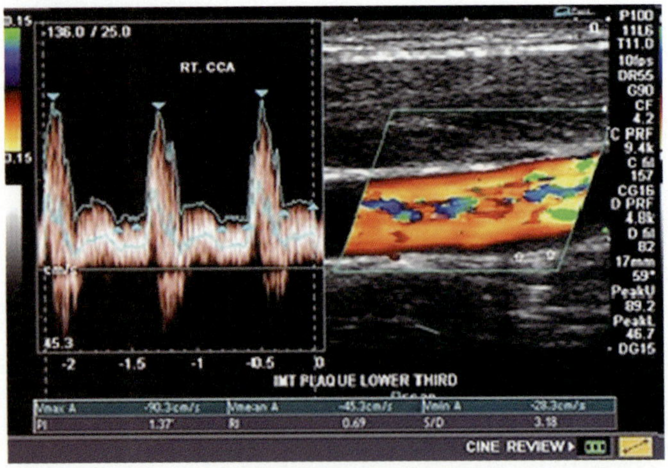


**Fig. 19.16:** This middle-aged male patient had a recent partial stroke affecting the left side of face and left upper limb. The B-mode ultrasound images of the right common carotid artery show an atheromatous plaque of the lower third of the vessel. This plaque is noncalcific and shows no evidence of ulceration. The color-Doppler images of the common carotid artery show no significant obstruction to blood flow in this artery. Possibly, there might have been a small embolic episode some time ago resulting in cerebral ischemia on this side

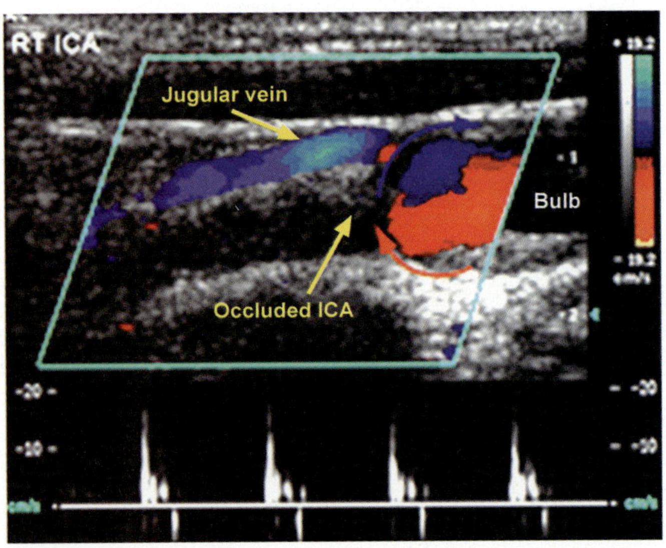


**Fig. 19.17:** Thud flow. Color-Doppler image of the right ICA and carotid bulb shows no flow in the ICA lumen and reversed flow in the bulb at the point of occlusion

rock-hard vessel wall of calcified atherosclerosis, the harsh systolic thrill of a tight arterial stenosis, or the continuous thrill of a peripheral arteriovenous fistula. In the latter condition, auscultation should confirm a continuous, or machinery-like, murmur with systolic accentuation. Much valuable information can be gained from examination of the peripheral pulses in addition to the status of the arterial system itself. The attentive examiner may detect variations in the rate, rhythmicity, intensity, and contour of the pulse wave that yield insight into a variety of disease states. The rapid, thready pulse of hypovolemic shock is a well-known clinical sign, as is the rapid, snapping pulse characteristic of thyrotoxicosis, and the collapsing, 'water-hammer' pulse of aortic insufficiency.

There are at least four reasons why it is important to determine if a patient does or does not have thrombophlebitis. These include the threat and prophylaxis of pulmonary embolism, the risk of septicemia, the use of certain drugs other than anticoagulants, and the occasional detection of any other primary disease processes.

Deep vein thrombophlebitis requires hospitalization and anticoagulation to prevent morbidity and mortality from associated pulmonary embolism. The efficacy of anticoagulant therapy in this setting was clearly demonstrated in control studies done many years ago. Evidence is not convincing that anticoagulant therapy is of benefit in phlebitis clearly isolated to superficial veins of the arm or saphenous system of the leg. However, there are communicating leg veins between the superficial and deep venous system, and the examiner bears the responsibility for determining that the aforementioned signs of deep phlebitis are absent.

Pelvic thrombophlebitis and thrombophlebitis associated with indwelling intravenous catheters are a surprisingly frequent source of septicemia. Recognition of either requires careful evaluation of the patient for evidence of bloodstream infection. Thrombophlebitis and pulmonary embolism are more frequent in recently diuresed patients. One should therefore use therapeutic discretion in planning diuretic therapy for patients who belong to any of the previously described 'suspicious clinical settings.' In addition, patients receiving corticosteroid therapy are more susceptible to phlebitis. The same is true for women taking estrogen-containing oral contraceptives; other family planning measures should be substituted for such therapy in the presence of spontaneous thrombophlebitis. Thrombophlebitis that is either recurrent, located in unusual veins (subclavian, jugular), or migratory to various superficial veins may be the first sign of an underlying disease process such as occult malignancy or systemic lupus erythematosus.

### Brachiocephalic Artery or Trunk

The brachiocephalic artery or trunk is the first and largest artery that branches to form the right common carotid artery and the right subclavian artery. This artery provides blood to the right upper chest, right arm, neck, and head, through a branch called right vertebral artery. The right and left vertebral artery feed into the basilar artery and upward to the posterior cerebral artery, which provides most of the brain with oxygenated blood. The posterior cerebral artery and the posterior communicating artery are within the circle of Willis.

*The left common carotid artery* divides to form the internal carotid artery (ICA) and an external carotid artery (ECA). The ICA supplies the brain. The ECA supplies the neck and face. The left subclavian artery and the right subclavian artery, one on each side of the body form the internal thoracic artery, the vertebral artery, the thyrocervical trunk, and the costocervical trunk. The subclavian becomes the axiliary artery at the lateral border of the first rib. The left subclavian artery also provides blood to the left upper chest and left arm.

### *Subclavian Artery*

The subclavian arteries are a pair of large arteries in the thorax that supply blood to the thorax, head, neck, shoulder and arms.

*Course:* On the left side of the body the subclavian comes directly from the aortic arch whereas on the right side it arises from the brachiocephalic trunk. Both course above the cervical pleura towards the anterior scalene muscle and through the posterior scalene gap (between the anterior and medial scalene muscles). It enters the axilla between the first rib and the clavicle and becomes the axillary artery. During its course it gives off numerous branches:

*The Thoracic Region:* The following branches arise medial to the scalenus anterior muscle:

- The first artery is the vertebral artery which ascends until it reaches the vertebral column at the transverse foramen of the sixth or seventh cervical vertebra.
- Second is the internal thoracic artery which runs in the opposite direction to the vertebral artery behind the sternum and costal cage. It branches off into three smaller arteries.
- The superior epigastric artery arises and runs below the costal margin, entering the rectus sheath. The pericardiophrenic artery accompanies the phrenic artery at the level of the fourth cervical vertebra and helps supply the pericardium.
- The musculophrenic artery supplies the upper musculature of the diaphragm.
- The third artery is the **thyrocervical trunk** which gives off four branches as it ascends.
- The inferior thyroid artery ascends, makes a loop behind the common carotid artery and courses towards the backside of the thyroid crossing the recurrent laryngeal nerve. It branches off arteries to the larynx (inferior laryngeal artery), infrahyoid and prevertebral muscles and many more smaller ones to the surrounding structures.
- The ascending cervical artery is next and ascends along the phrenic nerve at the level of the fourth cervical vertebra.
- The **transverse cervical artery** divides into a superficial and deep branch. The superficial branch runs superficially in the lateral cervical region and then under the trapezius muscle (together with the accessory nerve). The deep branch branches off into two smaller arteries, one of which follows the dorsal scapular nerve along the medial border of the scapula.
- The **suprascapular artery** courses above the scapula in front of the anterior scalene muscle and behind the clavicle. It anastomoses with the scapular circumflex and thoracoacromial arteries (via the acromial branches).
- **The costocervical trunk** arises behind the anterior scalene muscle and divides into two main branches.
- The supreme intercostal artery is the highest of all intercostal arteries and supplies the upper two intercostal spaces, the deep neck and back muscles, the skin of the back and the vertebral canal.
- As the trunk descends it gives rise to the deep cervical artery between the first rib and the seventh cervical vertebra which supplies the deep neck musculature.

### Cervical Region

Very often the deep branch of the transverse cervical artery arises directly from the subclavian artery lateral to the anterior scalene muscle. It is then referred to as the dorsal scapular artery. In this case it passes through the brachial plexus, usually through the upper and superior trunk.

### *Brachial Artery*

The brachial artery stems from the axillary artery and moves along the humerus (upper arm bone) down to the elbow. It gives rise to the deep brachial artery, which curves around the back of the humerus to supply blood to the triceps muscles (Fig. 19.18).

Shorter branches pass into various other muscles on the front of the upper arm, and others descend down each side of the elbow to join arteries in the forearms.To examine the *brachial artery* in the right arm, the examiner supports the patient's forearm in his left hand, with the subject's upper arm abducted, the elbow slightly flexed, and the forearm externally rotated. The examiner's right hand is then curled over the anterior aspect of the elbow to palpate along the course of the artery just medial to the biceps tendon and lateral to the medial epicondyle of the humerus. The position of the hands should be switched when examining the opposite limb.

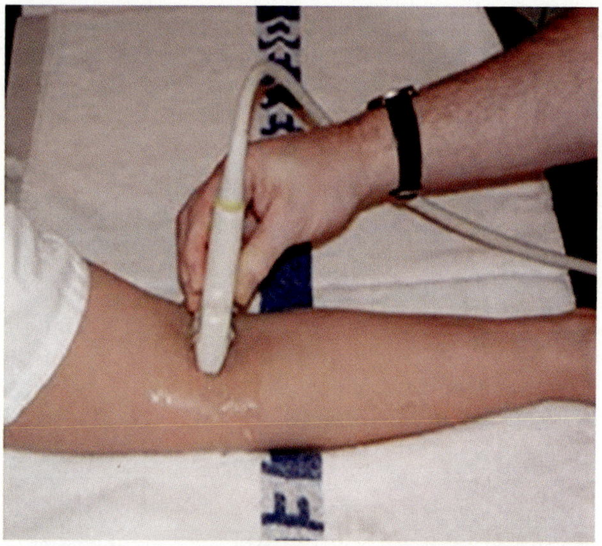

**Fig. 19.18:** Study of brachial artery with vascular Doppler which communicates by way of its neck (arrow) with the radial artery (RA)

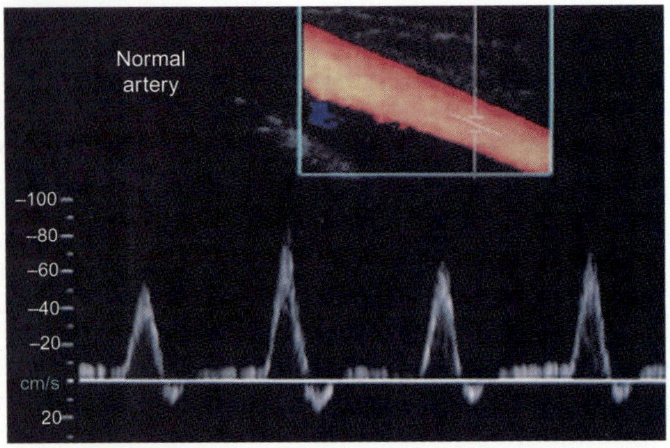


**Fig. 19.19:** Doppler flow of brachial artery showing normal velocity of this vessel

### *Radial Artery*

For the radial artery the patient's forearm should be supported in one of the examiner's hands and his other hand used to palpate along the radialvolar aspect of the subject's forearm at the wrist.

This can best be done by curling the fingers around the distal radius from the dorsal toward the volar aspect, with the tips of the first, second, and third fingers aligned longitudinally over the course of the artery (Fig. 19.20).

### *Aorta*

The aorta is the largest artery of your body, and it is a strong and sturdy vessel. In this lesson, you will learn about its downward path through the chest and abdomen and discover the organs and structures supplied by its branches (Figs 19.21 and 19.22).

### *Descending Aorta*

The largest artery in your body is called the aorta (Figs 19.23–19.31). We previously learned that it originates at the left ventricle of the heart and ascends a short distance before making a U-turn at the aortic arch and plunging downward through your chest, which is referred to as the thorax, and into your abdomen. In this lesson, you will learn about the descending aorta, which begins at the aortic arch and is divided into two sections, the thoracic and the abdominal aorta.

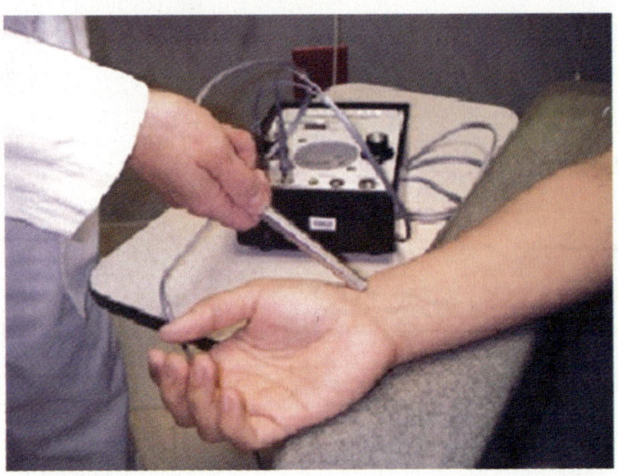

**Fig. 19.20:** Study of radial artery with vascular Doppler

The main thing to note about the descending aorta is that it has a number of branches coming off of it, much like back roads would come off of a highway. These branches

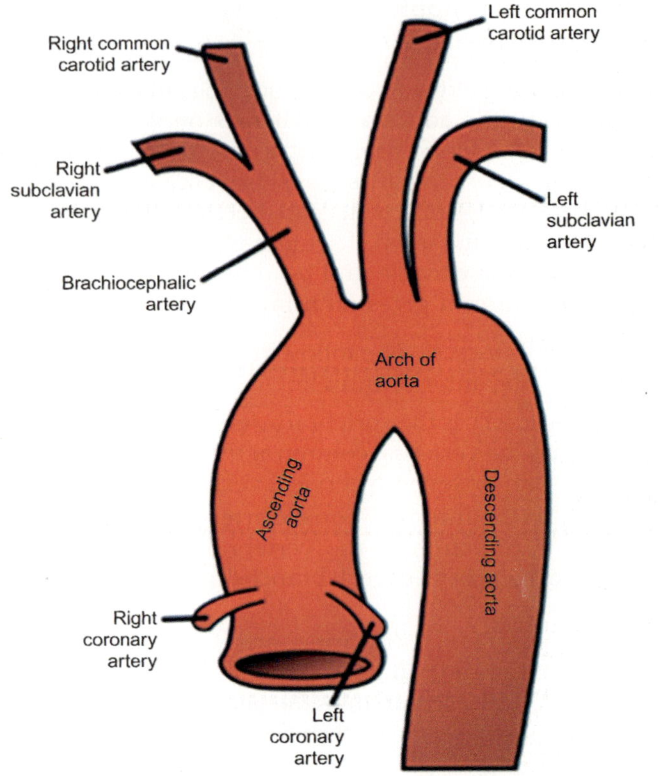


**Fig. 19.21:** Ascending aorta, emerging left and right coronary arteries, arch of aorta with its branches and descending aorta

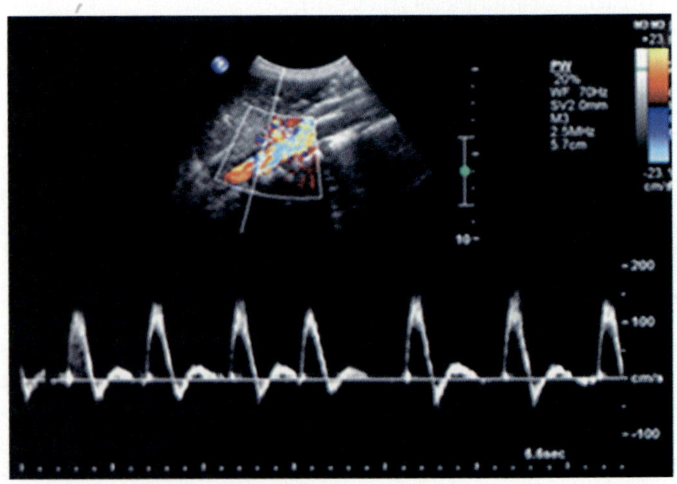

**Fig. 19.22:** Normal Doppler spectrum from the upper abdominal aorta in a 20-year-old boy shows a typical waveform characterized by a sharp increase in antegrade flow velocity during systole, followed by a reversal of flow in early diastole and then low-velocity antegrade flow in the remainder of diastole

feed the organs and structures within the thorax and abdomen before terminating into two final branches that eventually supply the legs.

The aorta is a very large artery and where it originates, right off of the left ventricle of the heart, it's about the size of a garden hose. It maintains this large size and decreases only slightly in size as it runs down through your body to its end. The different sections of the aorta are named for their location.

### Thoracic Aorta

Therefore, we see that the section that runs through your thorax is named the thoracic aorta. This portion of the aorta spans from the aortic arch to the level of the diaphragm. The thoracic aorta has a number of paired blood vessels that branch off like back roads off of a highway. If you think about the organs and structures that are found in your chest, you will easily be able to tell where these branches travel (Fig. 19.23).

For instance, there's a paired branch of arteries that come off of the thoracic aorta that feed the lungs, there are branches that feed your esophagus, which lies deep and runs through your thoracic cavity. There are also branches that feed the surrounding structures, including the diaphragm, which lies at the bottom of the thoracic region, just below the lungs and just above the liver.

### Abdominal Aorta

The abdominal aorta is the next section of the aorta, and it travels from the diaphragm through the abdominal cavity. It travels just anterior to your spinal column. In fact, it travels so close to your spine that it traces the natural curve of your lumbar spine (Fig. 19.23).

The first branch off of the abdominal aorta is called the **celiac trunk**. You can recall this term by remembering that the word 'celiac' is the anatomical term that refers to the abdomen.

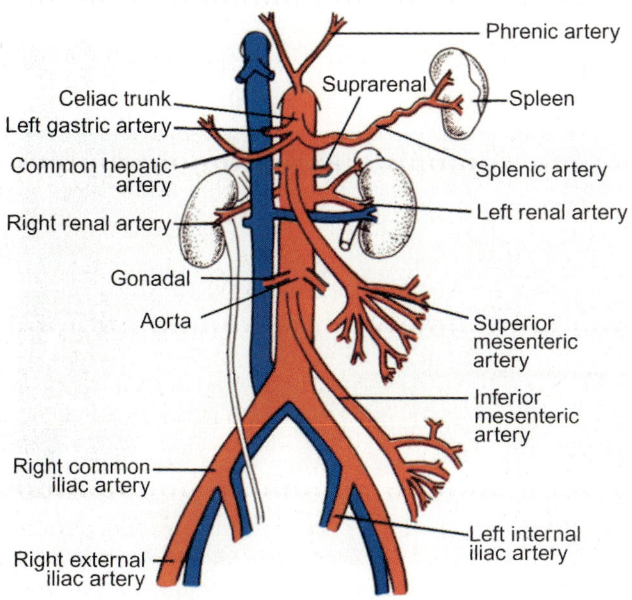


**Fig. 19.23:** Arterial system of the abdomen

The celiac trunk is a single vessel, but it has three branches. If you think about the abdominal aorta as a major highway, then the celiac trunk can be thought of as an exit ramp that leads to three back roads. Here again, if you think abut the organs and structures that are found in the top portion of your abdomen, then you will have a good idea of what these back roads, or branches, feed. What we find is that the branches supply blood to the stomach, the spleen, the pancreas, and the liver.

Additional branches off of the abdominal aorta supply the remaining organs and structures of the abdomen, including the intestines, kidneys, reproductive organs, and muscles of the region. These branches are not simply named branch 1, branch 2, branch 3, but their naming system is still pretty easy to remember. The reason that it's easy to remember is because these branches are often named for the organs or area that they supply. For instance, the term 'renal' stands for 'kidneys,' and the renal arteries come directly off of the abdominal aorta and serve the kidneys.

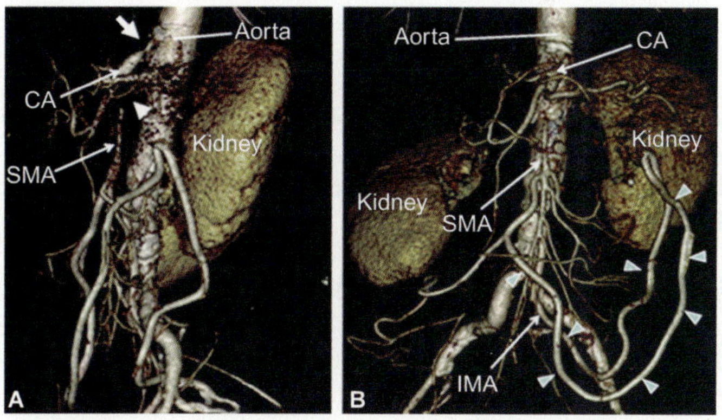


**Fig. 19.24:** Volume-rendered CT angiograms demonstrate the normal anatomy of the celiac axis. The left gastric artery (arrow) is seen to arise from the celiac axis

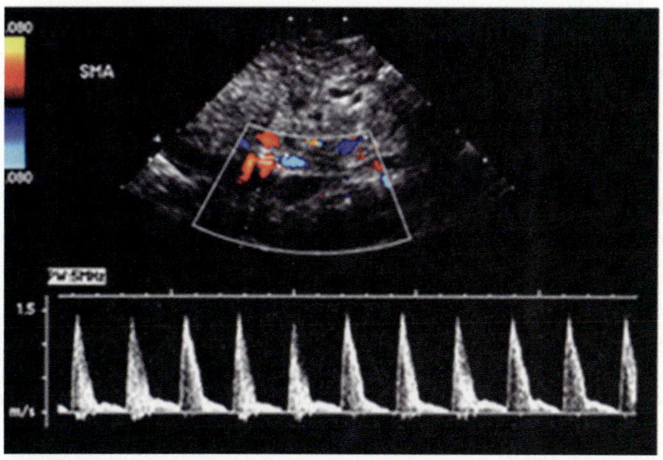


**Fig. 19.25:** Normal spectral waveforms in the superior mesenteric artery. Fasting waveform from a person showing a high-resistance flow pattern

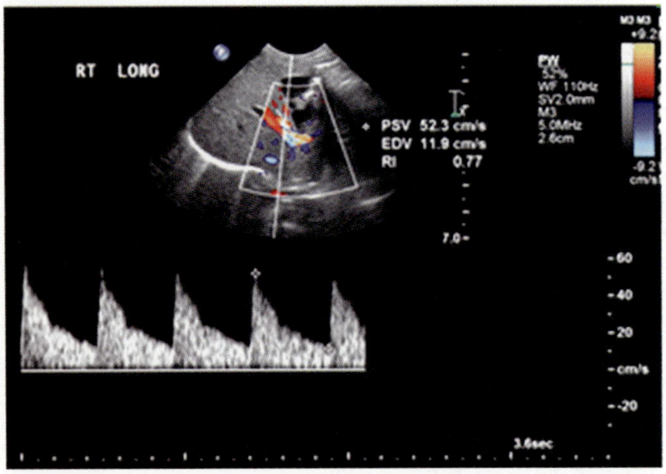


**Fig. 19.26:** Normal spectral waveforms from different segments of the hepatic artery. Spectrum from the hepatic artery at the porta hepatis in a patient with low-resistance and high-velocity diastolic flow

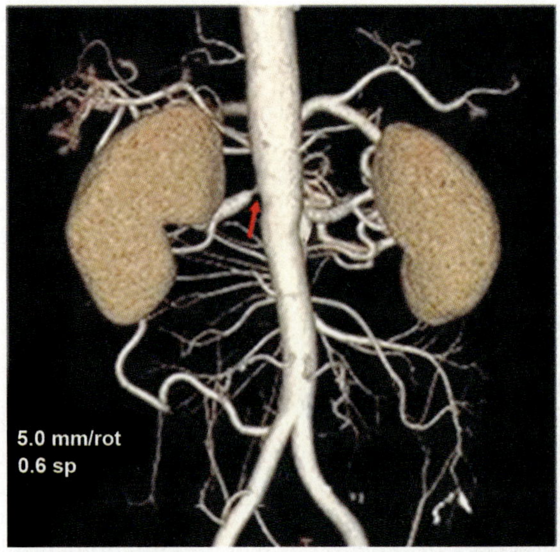


**Fig. 19.27:** A MD computed tomographic renal angiogram with right sided renal artery stenosis (arrow)

At this point, there is the end of the abdominal aorta as it splits into two final branches called the right and left common iliac arteries. The term 'iliac' comes from the fact that the vessels are situated near the large pelvic bone called the ilium. These arteries split at the level of the pelvis and travel down toward each leg. Therefore, they supply blood to the pelvic organs and legs. This would include the bladder, rectum, reproductive organs, and muscles of the lower extremities.

## Branches of the Abdominal Aorta Mnemonic

Here's a mnemonic which can help the readers to remember the branches of the abdominal aorta from superior to inferior—Canned Soup Really Good In Cups.

- Celiac trunk
- Superior mesenteric artery
- Renal arteries
- Gonadal arteries
- Inferior mesenteric artery
- Common Iliacs

The branches of the celiac trunk are common hepatic, left gastric, and splenic artery. The branches of the splenic artery are left gastroepiploic artery and short gastric arteries.

## Middle Suprarenal Artery

- These arise level with the superior mesenteric artery.
- The right passes behind the IVC.
- Both are related to the coeliac ganglion of the respective sides.
- These anastomose with the suprarenal branches of the inferior phrenic and renal arteries.

### *Renal Vessels*

- These two larger arteries branch from the aorta, just inferior to the level of the superior mesenteric artery (Figs 19.27–19.30).

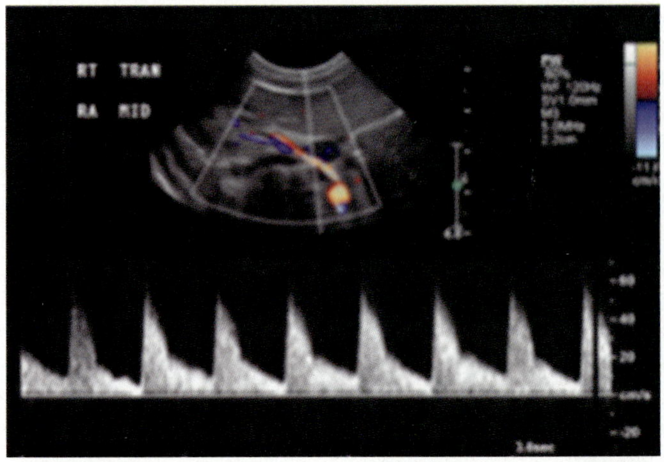


**Fig. 19.28:** Normal spectral waveforms from renal arteries. Spectrum from the midportion of the right renal artery in a person with a prominent systolic peak, with antegrade flow throughout diastole

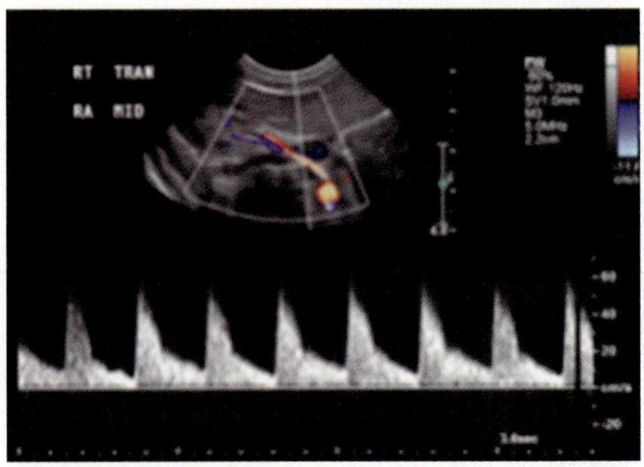


**Fig. 19.29:** Normal spectral waveforms from renal arteries. Spectrum from an intraparenchymal renal artery in a preterm 6-day-old girl

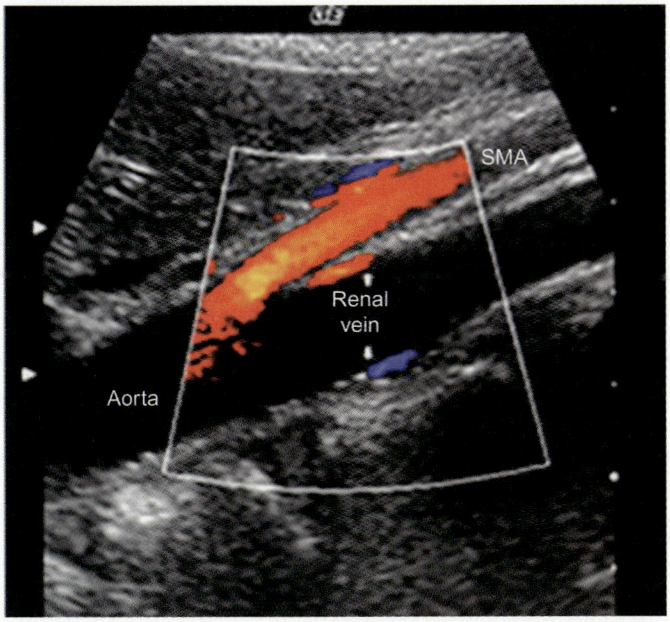


**Fig. 19.30:** Anomalous left renal vein. The patient has a retroaortic left renal vein. A sagittal color-Doppler image captured in diastole shows the renal vein in cross section on each side of the abdominal aorta

- The right is longer and passes posterior to the IVC, right renal vein, body of the pancreas and descending part of the duodenum.
- The left passes posterior to the left renal vein, body of the pancreas and splenic vein.
- Each of these divides into 4 or 5 branches.
- Each renal artery gives off an inferior suprarenal branch and supplies the ureter in its upper extent.

### *Testicular Artery* (Fig. 19.31)

- These two arise anteriorly from the aorta, slightly inferior to the renal artery.
- Each passes anterior to the psoas major behind the parietal peritoneum.

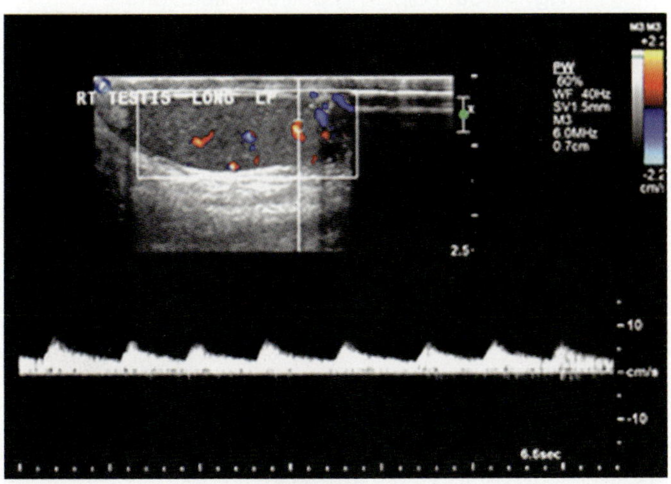

**Fig. 19.31:** Spectra from intratesticular arteries. Waveform shows a normal low-resistance flow pattern

- They then pass to the deep inguinal ring and enter.
- The testicular artery supplies the testis, perirenal fat, ureter, iliac lymph nodes and cremaster.

### *Ovarian Artery* (Fig. 19.32)

- These correspond to the testicular arteries, but are obviously in the female.
- They enter the pelvis to supply the ovaries.
- After entering the suspensory ligament of the ovary, they continue into the broad ligament of the uterus.
- Branches are given off to the ovary, ureter, uterine tubes and one branch passes to the side of the uterus to anastomose with the uterine artery. Other branches follow the round ligament of the uterus to the inguinal ligament and supply the skin of the labium majus.

### *Common Femoral Artery*

The *common femoral artery* (Figs 19.33 and 19.34) emerges into the upper thigh from beneath the inguinal ligament one-third of the distance from the pubis to the anterior

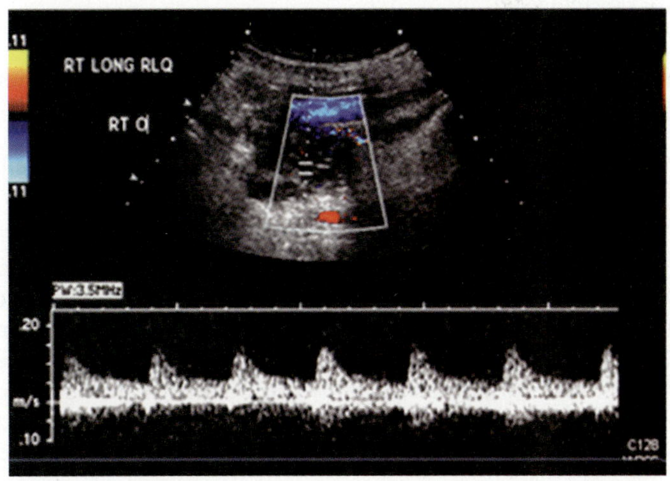


**Fig. 19.32:** Spectrum from a normal intra-ovarian artery in a person with low-resistance flow and a low PSV

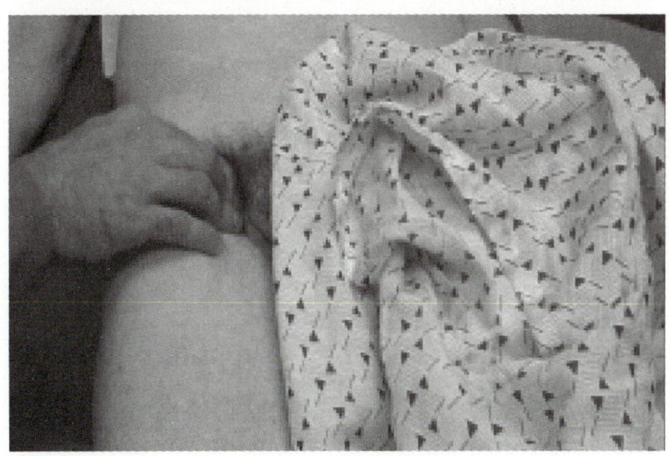

**Fig. 19.33:** Palpation of right common femoral artery in inguinal region

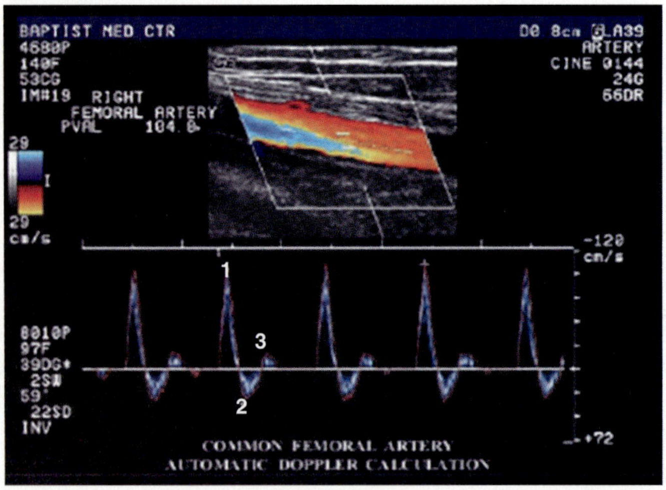


**Fig. 19.34:** A Doppler spectral waveform from a normal right femoral artery. The Doppler signal was obtained from a longitudinal view and with the Doppler sample volume placed in middle of the lumen. The characteristic triphasic Doppler signal shows a fast upstroke to peak systole (1), reversal of blood flow during early diastole (2), and a forward flow component during late diastole (3)

superior iliac spine. It is best palpated with the examiner standing on the ipsilateral side of the patient and the fingertips of the examining hand pressed firmly into the groin. Auscultation should be performed in this area, as well.

### Popliteal Artery

The popliteal artery passes vertically through the deep portion of the popliteal space just lateral to the midplane (Fig. 19.35). It may be difficult or impossible to palpate in obese or very muscular individuals. Generally this pulse is felt most conveniently with the patient in the supine position and the examiner's hands encircling and supporting the knee from each side. The pulse is detected

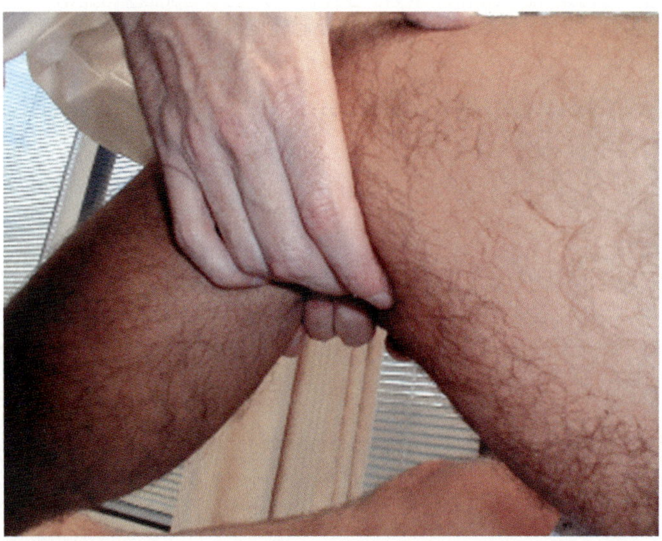

**Fig. 19.35:** Doctor palpating popliteal artery in popliteal fossa with application of fingers of both of his two hands

by pressing deeply into the popliteal space with the supporting fingertips. Since complete relaxation of the muscles is essential to this examination, the patient should be instructed to let the leg 'go limp' and to allow the examiner to provide all the support needed.

### Posterior Tibial Artery

The *posterior tibial artery* lies just posterior to the medial malleolus. It can be felt most readily by curling the fingers of the examining hand anteriorly around the ankle, indenting the soft tissues in the space between the medial malleolus and the Achilles tendon, above the calcaneus. The thumb is applied to the opposite side of the ankle in a grasping fashion to provide stability. Again, obesity or edema may prevent successful detection of the pulse (Fig. 19.36).

### Dorsalis Pedis Artery

The *dorsalis pedis artery* (Fig. 19.37) is examined with the patient in the recumbent position and the ankle relaxed. The examiner stands at the foot of the examining table and places the fingertips transversely across the dorsum of the forefoot near the ankle. The artery usually lies near the

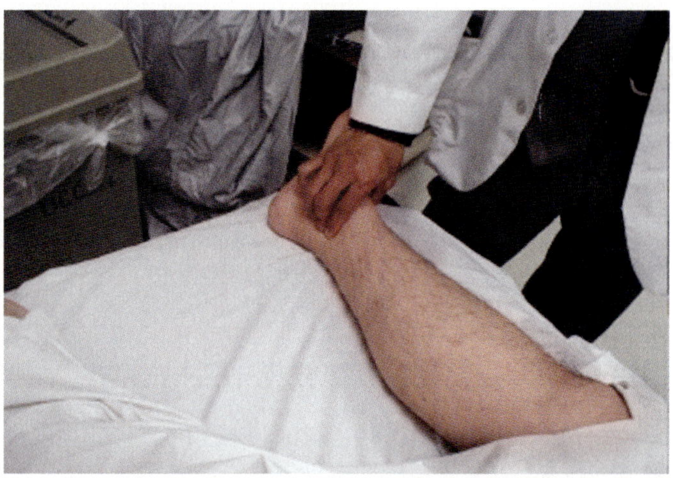

**Fig. 19.36:** Palpating posterior tibial artery

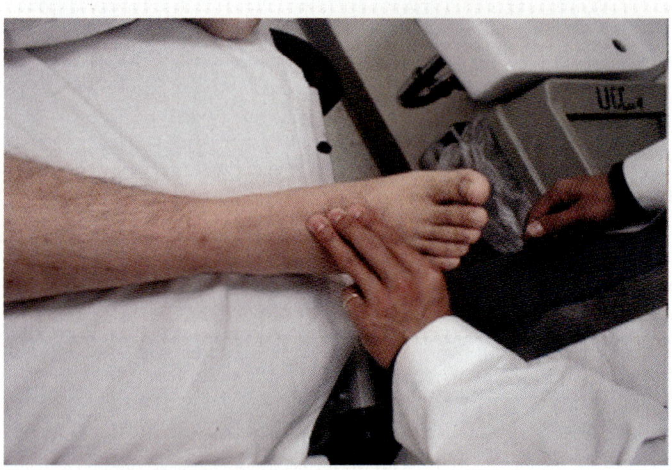

**Fig. 19.37:** Palpating dorsalis pedis artery

center of the long axis of the foot, lateral to the extensor hallucis tendon but it may be aberrant in location and often requires some searching. This pulse is congenitally absent in approximately 10% of individuals.

### Bruits

After palpating the artery, auscultation for a bruit should be performed. Bruits are detected by auscultation over the large and medium-sized arteries (e.g. carotid, brachial, abdominal aorta, femoral) with the diaphragm of the stethoscope using light to moderate pressure. Excessive pressure may produce, intensify, or prevent a bruit from being detected by indenting the vessel wall or occluding blood flow in the artery.

One should listen over the artery after palpation of the artery to avoid overlooking a significant lesion. Occasionally, bruits are audible over the upper abdomen in young, healthy individuals. These sounds apparently originate from tortuous vessels and are of no clinical significance; if the subject has a normal blood pressure and is free of abdominal symptoms, such findings may be disregarded. Frequently the examiner will detect a "thrill" or palpable vibratory sensation over a vessel in which a loud bruit is audible. The thrill is indicative of marked turbulence in local blood flow and suggests significant vascular pathology. If a thrill is noted during examination of the pulses, it should be recorded in the appropriate space on the data base (Figs 19.38 and 19.39).

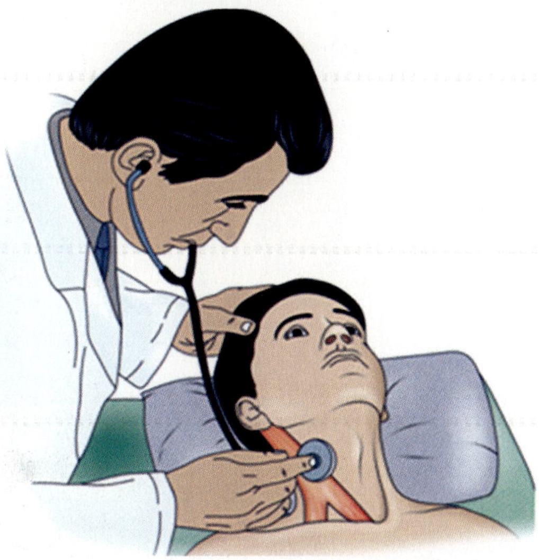

**Fig. 19.38:** Auscultation over the carotid artery

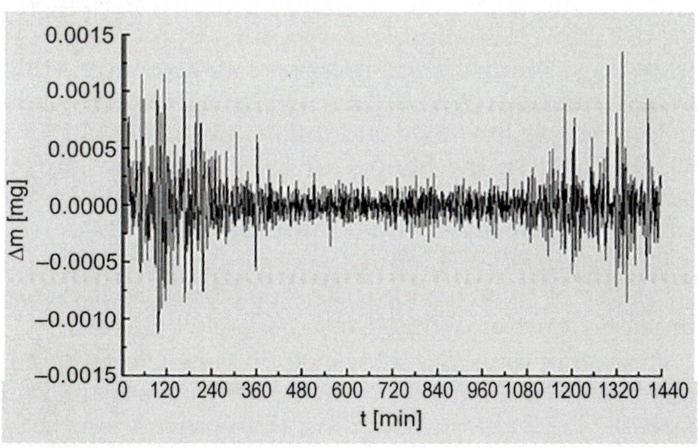


**Fig. 19.39:** A carotid bruit is an abnormal sound from the heart. The sound is in synchronization with the heartbeat. It is generally caused by turbulent blood flow, caused by irregularities in the wall of the blood vessel or by an abnormal connection (fistula) between an artery and vein. A bruit that is normally heard over the carotid artery is a sign that there are fats in the wall of the vessel. The bruit can be heard by using a stethoscope to listen to blood flow in the carotid artery. The carotid artery is the main artery in the neck region and is responsible for bringing blood to the head. A bruit indicates a fatty buildup (atherosclerosis) in the artery. Carotid bruit is a sign of the person's higher stroke risk

### Venous System of the Abdomen

Peripheral venous disease is a term describing damage, defects or blockage in the veins that carry blood from the hands and feet to the heart. Peripheral venous disease can occur almost anywhere in the body but is mostly seen in the arms and legs (Fig. 19.40).

### Phlebitis

With the patient supine, the veins of the extremities usually cannot be palpated but can be examined by inspection. Phlebitis most commonly occurs in the superficial arm veins and the deep veins of the lower extremity (Figs 19.41 and 19.43).

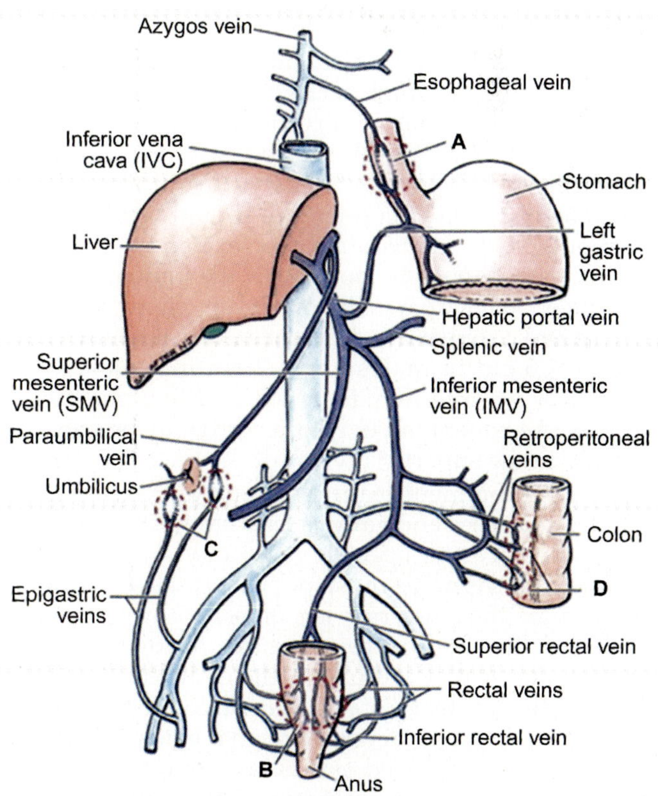


**Fig. 19.40:** Venous system of the body

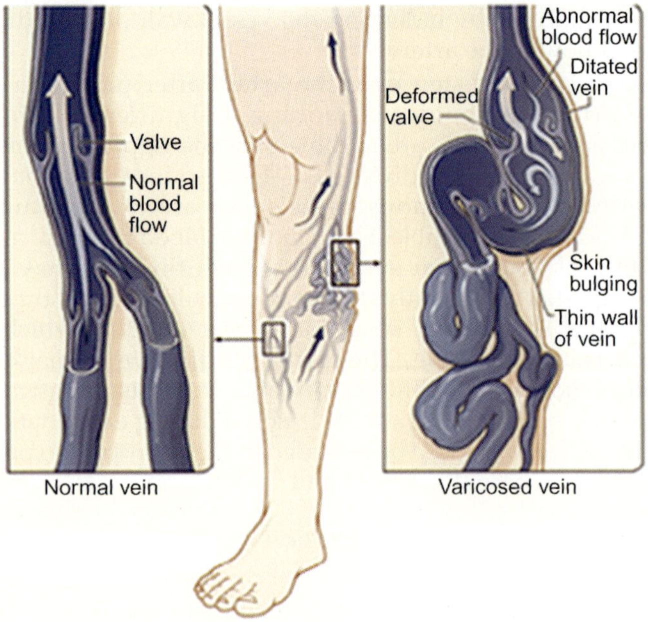


**Fig. 19.41:** The illustration shows how a varicose vein forms in a leg. (A) shows a normal vein with a working valve and normal blood flow, (B) shows a varicose vein with a deformed valve, abnormal blood flow, and thin, stretched walls. The middle image shows where varicose veins might appear in a leg

Arm vein phlebitis is suggested by noting erythema occurring along the course of the vein, which may be tender to palpation if secondary venous thrombosis has occurred; this may be palpable (i.e. a 'cord'). Lower extremity thrombophlebitis can be clinically silent and may be very difficult to detect by physical examination. Changes secondary to the venous obstruction may develop and be observed as increased thigh or calf girth, erythema, warmth, tenderness, or palpation of a cord. Numerous laboratory techniques have been developed to assist the physician in the search for lower extremity thrombophlebitis. Measurement of calf circumference should be obtained in all patients with suspected lower extremity thrombophlebitis. This should be done with the patient standing and the feet 30 cm apart. The maximum circumference is recorded and a significant difference exists if the two sides differ by 1.5 cm in males and 1.2 cm in females. Skin erythema or warmth may be noted in active phlebitis. A thrombosed segment of vein (i.e. a cord) may be palpable, especially in the superficial veins of the lower extremity.

Pain is a prominent feature of muscular, synovial, or vascular leg disease and various tests have been suggested to help identify the specific aetiology. Homan's test **(dorsiflexion sign)** is most popularly used to detect irritability of the posterior leg muscles through which inflamed or thrombosed veins course. A popular clinical misconception is that calf pain is the endpoint of the test; however, Homan clearly stated that 'discomfort need have no part in this reaction.' A positive sign is when dorsiflexion of the foot on the affected side is less complete or is met with more resistance than on the unaffected side. Resistance to dorsiflexion may also be manifested by involuntary

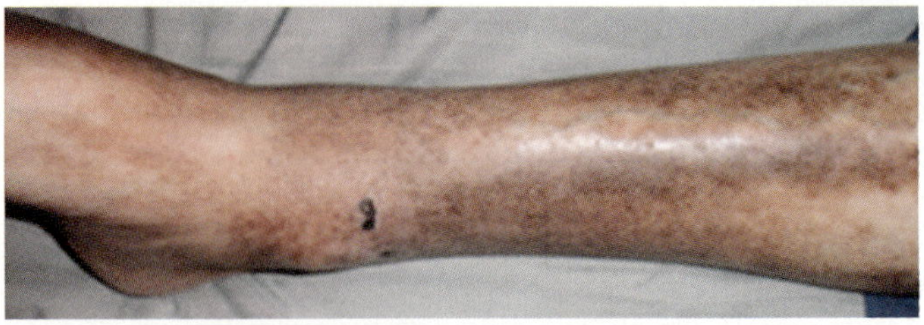

**Fig. 19.42:** Arterial obstruction in the leg with swelling, redness and skin discoloration

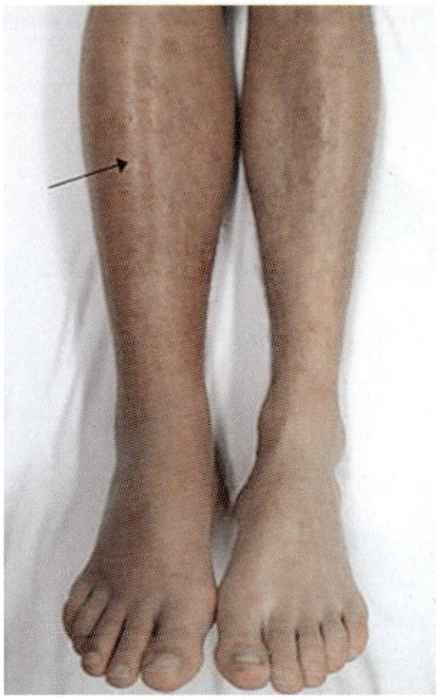

**Fig.19.43:** DVT in the right leg with swelling and redness

flexion of the knee. The **Lowenberg cuff test** is another helpful clinical manoeuvre for detection of calf vein thrombosis. Wrap a blood pressure cuff around the thigh just above the knee, taking care not to pinch the skin behind the knee. Close the valve and inflate the cuff gradually to 180 mmHg. Ask the patient to tell you of any unusual discomfort. Minimal discomfort immediately under the cuff is common. Spontaneous complaint of calf pain at 20–80 mmHg (that is, above venous pressure) is highly suggestive of local venous disease, particularly if 150–180 mmHg contralateral thigh pressure is well tolerated.

Other symptoms and signs include Moses' test (calf pain greater with anteroposterior than side-to-side palpation), localized leg pain on coughing (**Lawrence's sign**), and tenderness to touch in the sole of the foot **(Owane's sign).**

*Classification:* Peripheral artery occlusive disease. It is commonly divided in the Fontaine stages, introduced by René Fontaine in 1954 for ischemia:

- **Stage I**: Asymptomatic, incomplete blood vessel obstruction
- **Stage II**: Mild claudication
- **Stage IIA**: Claudication at a distance of greater than 200 metres
- **Stage IIB**: Claudication distance of less than 200 metres

- **Stage III**: Rest pain, mostly in the feet
- **Stage IV**: Necrosis and/or gangrene of the limb

A more recent classification by Rutherford consists of three grades and six categories.

- **Category 0**: Asymptomatic
- **Category 1**: Mild claudication
- **Category 2**: Moderate claudication
- **Category 3**: Severe claudication
- **Category 4**: Rest pain
- **Category 5**: Minor tissue loss; ischemic ulceration not exceeding ulcer of the digits of the foot
- **Category 6**: Major tissue loss; severe ischemic ulcers or frank gangrene

## EPIDEMIOLOGICAL FEATURES

The prevalence of peripheral vascular disease in the general population is 12–14%, affecting up to 20% of those over 70; 70–80% of affected individuals are asymptomatic; only a minority ever require revascularisation or amputation. Peripheral vascular disease affects 1 in 3 diabetics over the age of 50.

In the USA peripheral arterial disease affects 12–20 percent of Americans age 65 and older. Approximately 10 million Americans have PVD. Despite its prevalence and cardiovascular risk implications, only 25% of PAD patients are undergoing treatment.

The incidence of symptomatic PVD increases with age, from about 0.3% per year for men aged 40–55 years to about 1% per year for men aged over 75 years. The prevalence of PVD varies considerably depending on how PAD is defined, and the age of the population being studied. Diagnosis is critical, as people with PAD have 4–5 times higher risk of heart attack or stroke.

The Diabetes Control and Complications Trial and The United Kingdom prospective diabetes study trials in people with type 1 and type 2 diabetes, respectively, demonstrated that glycemic control is more strongly associated with microvascular disease than macrovascular disease. It may be that pathologic changes occurring in small vessels are more sensitive to chronically elevated glucose levels than is atherosclerosis occurring in larger arteries.

For many people, there are no symptoms of PVD. For others, the first signs of PVD begin slowly and irregularly. You may feel discomfort in your legs and feet. You may experience:

- Painful cramping
- Achiness
- Fatigue
- Burning

Typically, you will feel these sensations when you walk. You may first notice them when walking quicker, with more exertion, or for long distances. The pain will intensify with activity and subside when you rest. This is called intermittent claudication. Intermittent claudication occurs because your muscles need more blood flow during activity. In PVD, the vessels are narrowed with plaque. They can only supply a limited amount of blood. This causes more problems during activity than at rest. Lack of blood causes pain and discomfort. As your PVD progresses, symptoms will occur more frequently. It will require less exertion to bring them on. Eventually, you will experience leg pain and fatigue even at rest.

Additional symptoms may occur as a result of reduced blood supply. With PVD, you may have:

- Skin changes on your legs and feet (thinning, shiny, or paleness may occur)
- Weak pulses in your legs and feet
- Gangrene—tissue death caused by lack of blood flow
- Wounds or ulcers on the legs and feet that won't heal
- Reduced hair growth on your legs
- Toes that turn blue
- Severe burning pain in your toes
- Leg cramps and pain when you are lying in bed
- Muscles that feel numb or heavy
- Arms and legs that are reddish blue
- Toenails that are thick and opaque

It is important to tell your doctor if you experience any symptoms of PVD. Do not assume that the symptoms are simply the results of aging. Delaying diagnosis and treatment could allow the disease to progress further.

## COMPLICATIONS OF PVD

Complications from undiagnosed and untreated PVD can be serious and even fatal (Figs 19.44–19.56). The restricted blood flow of PVD can be a warning sign of other forms of vascular disease. When arteries leading to the heart and brain become clogged with plaque, it can cause:

- Heart attack
- Stroke
- Death

Complications of PVD can include:

- Bood clots that obstruct small arteries
- Coronary artery disease
- Limb amputation due to tissue death in the limb
- Heart attack
- Impotence
- Pallor or paleness
- Pain when the legs are elevated
- Severe pain that restricts mobility
- Stroke
- Wounds that don't heal

If you have any of the classic symptoms of PVD, it is important to tell your doctor. Early diagnosis is crucial to successful treatment. It can prevent life-threatening complications, such as heart attack and stroke. To diagnose PVD, your physician will begin with a complete medical history and physical exam. Several tests may be used to diagnose PVD.

Your physician can check the pulses in your legs and feet with a stethoscope. A whooshing sound called a bruit indicates a narrowed area in the vessel.

**Table 19.4:** Risk factors for the development of peripheral arterial disease (PAD)

| Risk factor | Feature of the risk factor |
|---|---|
| ***Modifiable factor*** | |
| Smoking | Cigarette smoking is the most powerful risk factor for the development of PAD. It is dose-dependent and the risk declines within 6 months of quiting. A non-smoker is 10 times less likely to develop PAD than a smoker |
| Blood lipid disorders | Plasma cholesterol levels of >5.2 mmol/L<br>Increased plasma concentrations of low-density lipoprotein (LDL) cholesterol, low plasma concentrations of high-density lipoproteins (HDLs), and higher concentrations of plasma triglycerides all correlate with incraeased incidence of PAD<br>Familial hyper cholesterolaemia (affecting 1:500 in UK)<br>Familial combined hyperlipidaemia (affecting 1:250 in UK) |
| Diabetes mellitus (DM) | Type 2 DM increases risk of PAD by 1.5–4.0, due to the associated hypertension, hyperlipidaemia and altered vascular reactivity |
| Hypertension | Raised systolic blood pressure (BP) incareases the risk of PAD and atherosclerosis by 4 due to endothelial injury caused by increased intra-arterial shear stresses at the blood-endothelium interface (raised systolic pressure are more predictive than raised diastolic pressures) |
| Obesity | Central obesity is an independent risk for PAD, but also predisposesto other risk factors for PAD, such as type 2 DM, hypertension |
| Homocysteine | Homocyteine is an amino acid that in high levels is associated with thromboembolism |
| Haemostatic variables | Increased levels of clotting factors FXII, FXI, FIX prothrombin and fibrinogen are associated with increased risk of atherosclerosis |
| Sedentary lifestyle | Low levels of regular activity are associated with increased risk of PAD (higher levels of activity are associated with higher levels of plasma HDL-cholesterol and reduced blood pressures and facilitate the development of the collateral circulation. |
| Dietary deficiencies | Low levels of antioxidant vitamins (vitamins C and E) and polyunsaturated fatty acids facilitate the formation of oxidized LDLs and thus predispose to the risk of atherosclerosis. |
| Type A behaviours (TABs) | People who tend to aggression, ambitiousness, restlessness, time urgency and high anxietytend to an increased incidence of PAD, possibly due to increased levels of circulating catecholamines |
| ***Non-modifiable or fixed factor*** | |
| Age and sex | Atherosclerosis is more common in males, and in postmenopausal women |
| Family history | Atherosclerosis shows familial patterns of incidence, possibly due to genetic factors and/or lifestyle choices and patterns |
| Early environment | Fetal origins hypothesis—adverse conditions in utero or infancy pedispose to the risk of cardiovascular disease in later life (e.g. statistically, small-birth-weight babies have a higher incidence in adult life of hypertension, type 2 DM, altered plasma lipids, altered bone densities, altered stress responses, less elastic arteries, thicker-walled ventricles and 'age' quicker) |

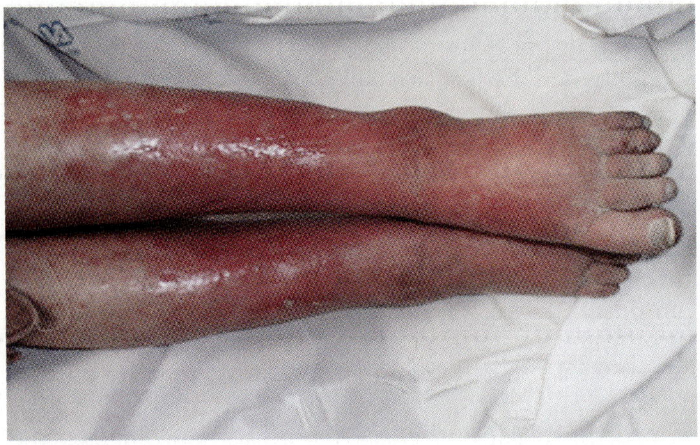

**Fig. 19.44:** Swelling of both legs in patient with cellulitis

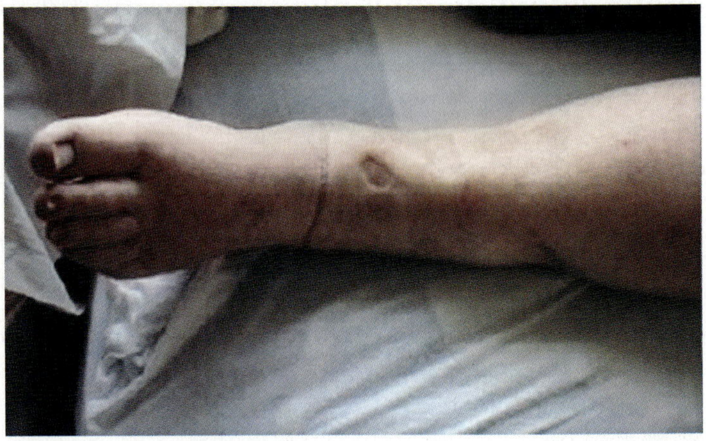

**Fig. 19.45:** Massive edema. Note: Remaining imprint of fingers

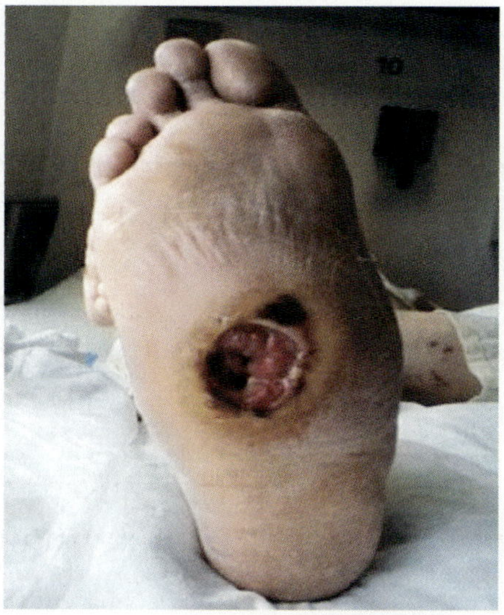

**Fig.19.46:** Neuropathic ulcer in a patient with diabetic neuropathy

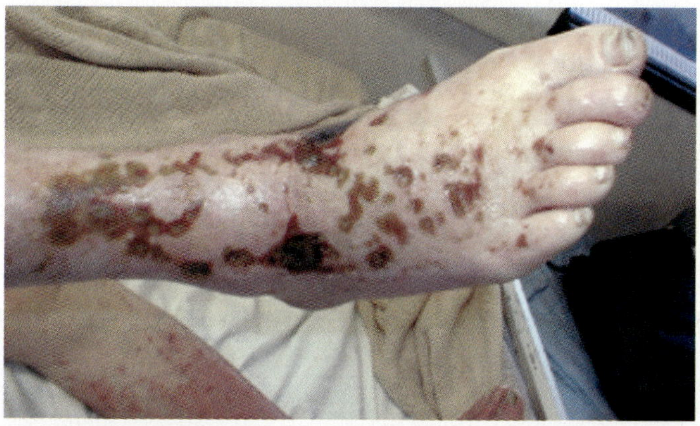

**Fig. 19.47:** Swelling and discoloration of right leg in patient with chronic arterial insufficiency with ulcers

## INVASIVE AND NONINVASIVE TECHNIQUES IN PVD

*Doppler ultrasound:* This test shows the blood flow in your vessels. Ultrasound is not invasive. It uses sound waves to take images (Figs 19.44–19.56).

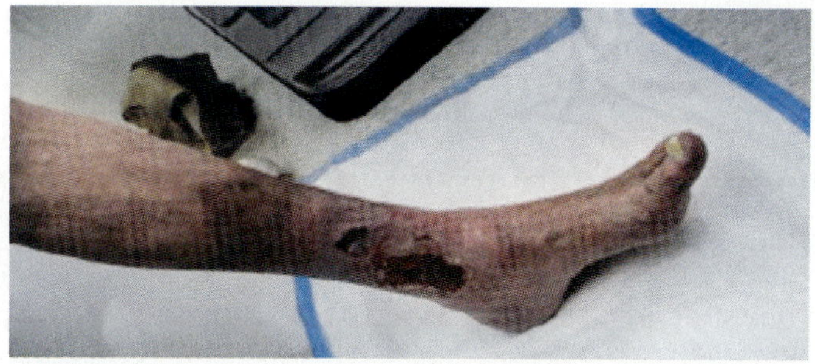

**Fig. 19.48:** Swelling and discoloration of left leg in a patient with venous stasis ulcer

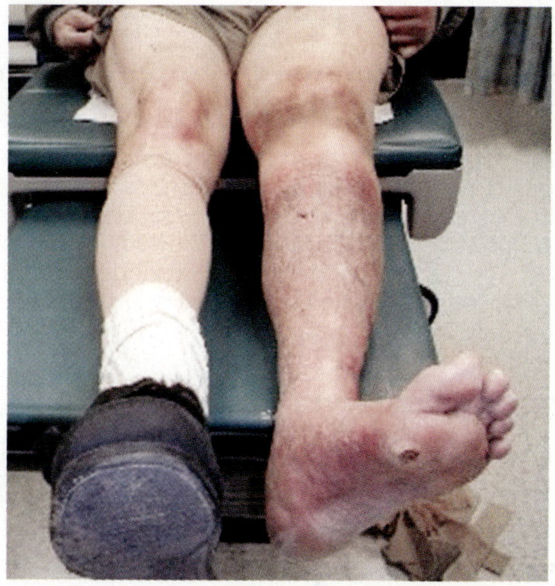

**Fig. 19.49:** Ischemic changes with ulcer over left foot in patient with peripheral occlusive arterial disease

*Ankle-brachial index (ABI)* (Fig. 19.57 and Table 19.5): This is the most common test used to diagnose PVD. A blood pressure cuff and ultrasound assess blood pressure and flow. The blood pressure in your ankle is compared to the blood pressure in your arm. In some cases, readings will be taken before and after you walk on a treadmill. This helps demonstrate how the arteries react to exercise.

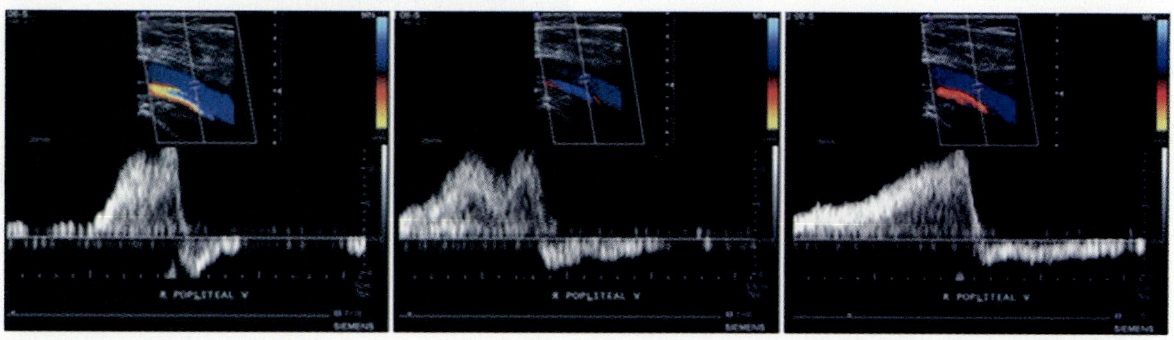

**Fig. 19.50:** Variability of reflux response. The effect of the length of augmentation on the tendency of lower extremity veins to reflux. All images are obtained from the same sample site in the popliteal vein of the same patient. Left image—short augmentation resulting in reflux time of only 0.7 seconds. Middle image—longer augmentation resulting in reflux time of 1.5 seconds. Right image—prolonged augmentation resulting in continuous reflux for many seconds

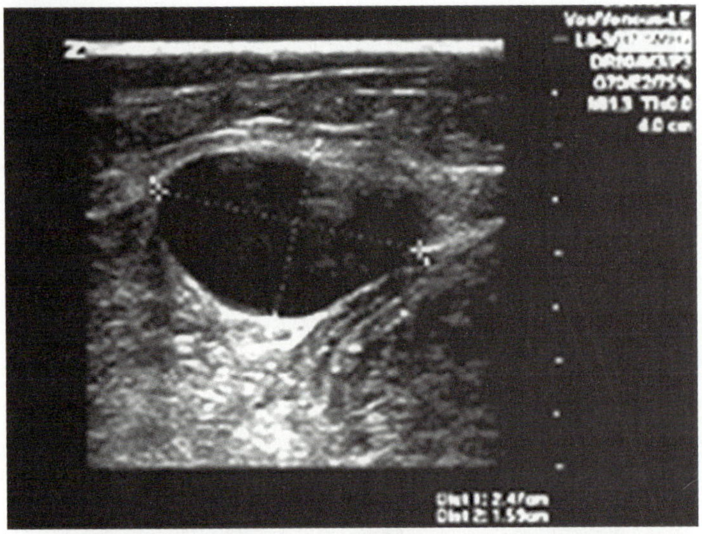

**Fig. 19.51:** Patient is a 59-years-old male that presented with swelling and aching of both lower extremities. He had bilateral varicose veins especially on the right with discoloration and stasis changes however no ulceration or previous ulceration was reported. He denied previous deep venous thrombosis or phlebitis. The patient was finally diagnosed as venous aneurysm of inferior vena cava

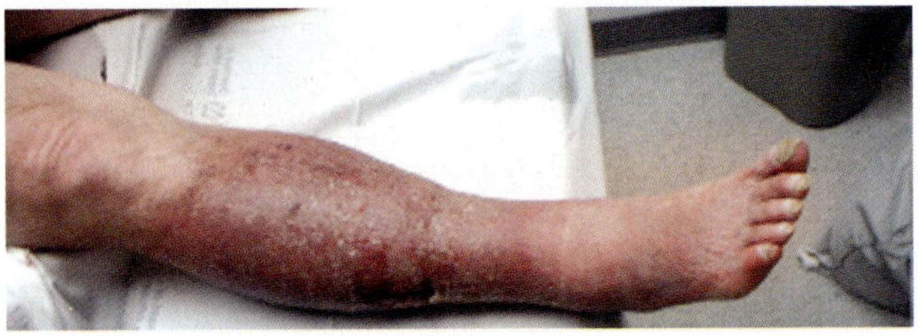

**Fig. 19.52:** Swelling and discoloration of right leg in patient with venous insufficiency

*Pulse volume recording (PVR):* This test checks the blood flow in your legs. Blood pressure cuffs are wrapped around one arm and leg as you are lying down. The cuffs are inflated slightly. As blood flows through the arteries, a device records the ability of the vessels to expand (Fig. 19.57).

*Angiography:* A catheter is guided through an artery in your groin. It is passed to the targeted area. Contrast dye is injected. An X-ray can then diagnose the clogged artery. By inflating a balloon at the end of the catheter, the artery can be opened in the same procedure (Figs 19.58–19.63).

*Noninvasive imaging studies:* These are noninvasive imaging techniques that allow doctors to view blood flow and diagnose blockages (Figs 19.65–19.69).

- Treat conditions such as diabetes, high blood pressure, or high cholesterol

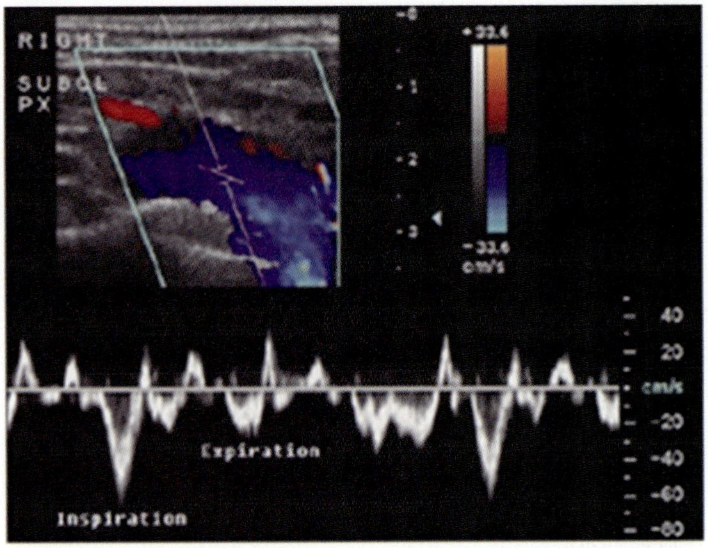


**Fig. 19.53:** Doppler spectra of the right subclavian vein from a healthy volunteer, which is characterized by two phasic variations in amplitude. The action of the right atrium is reflected back into the vessel and manifests as a choppy and sometimes biphasic flow pattern, otherwise known as cardiac pulsatility. Also notice the respiratory phasicity reflected in the spectral waveform. Considerable flow is seen with inspiration, whereas there is decrease in flow during expiration. Of note, there is increased pulsatility of the upper extremity spectral waveforms when compared with those of the lower extremity veins because of their proximity to the heart

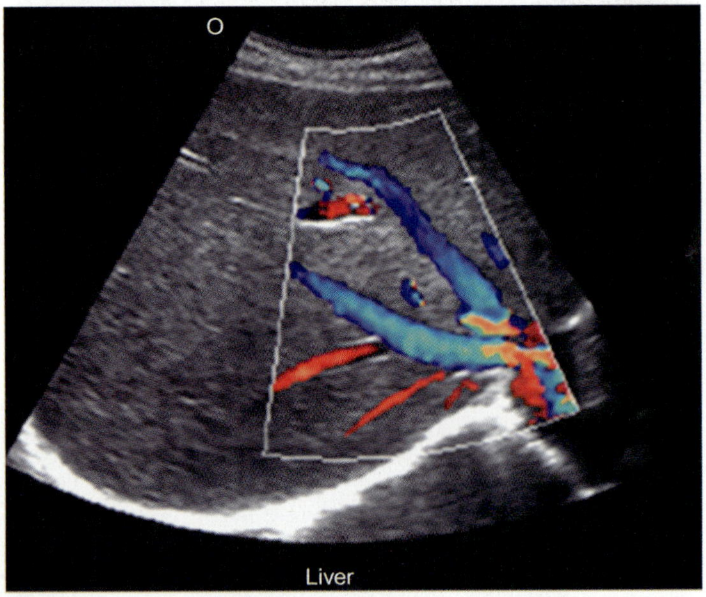


**Fig. 19.54:** Color-Doppler ultrasonography showing normal vasculature of the liver

- Smoking cessation is one of the most important ways to treat PVD. Smoking directly causes reduced blood flow in vessels.

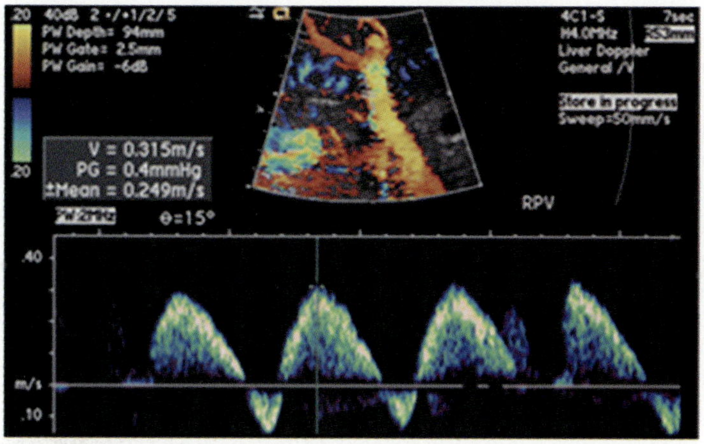


**Fig. 19.55:** Spectral Doppler ultrasound image shows a pulsatile waveform with flow reversal in the right portal vein. The waveform may be systematically characterized as predominantly antegrade, pulsatile, biphasic-bidirectional, and di-inflectional

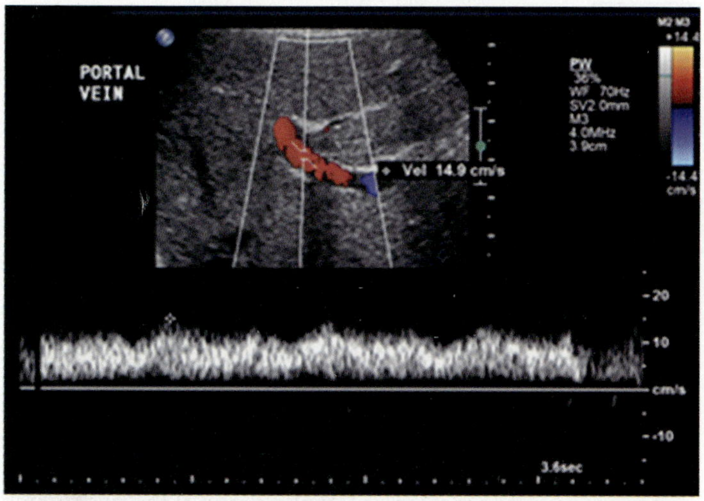


**Fig. 19.56:** Spectral waveform from the portal vein in a patient who shows a typical flow pattern, with fairly uniform velocity and slight phasic variations due to respiration and cardiac motion

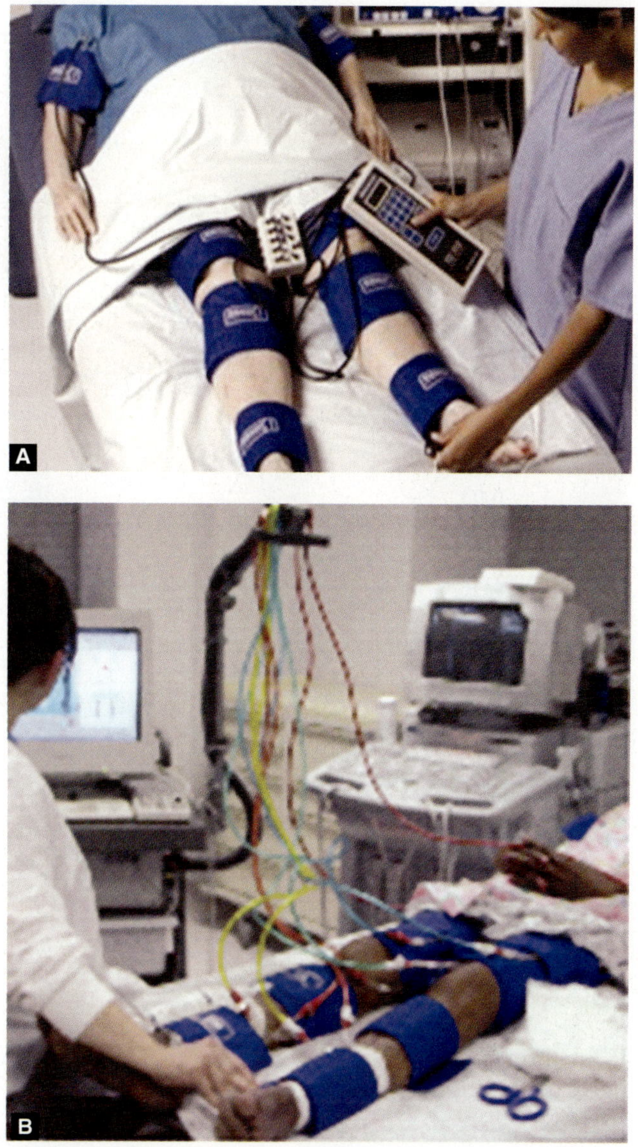

**Fig. 19.57:** (A) Pulse volume recording with plethysmography to various levels of legs, (B) pulse volume recording and segmental pressures measurements in patient with PVD

**Table 19.5:** Ankle-brachial index (ABI) results

| ABI number | Diagnosis | What it means |
|---|---|---|
| 1.00 to 1.29 | Normal | Your ABI is in the normal range and you are not likely to have PAD |
| 0.91–0.99 | Borderline | Your ABI is slightly lower than normal, but not low enough to diagnose PAD. Your doctor may want to measure your ABI again soon to make sure it is not getting worst, or measure your ABI after exercise. |
| 0.41–0.90 | Mild-to-moderate PAD | You have PAD. Working with your doctor to get your risk factors under control can prevent the disease from getting worse, and treatments are available to help relieve your PAD symptoms. |
| 0.40 to less | Severe PAD | The blood flow in your legs is severely obstructed, and you may need immediate treatment to relieve your symptoms and prevent serious complications. |

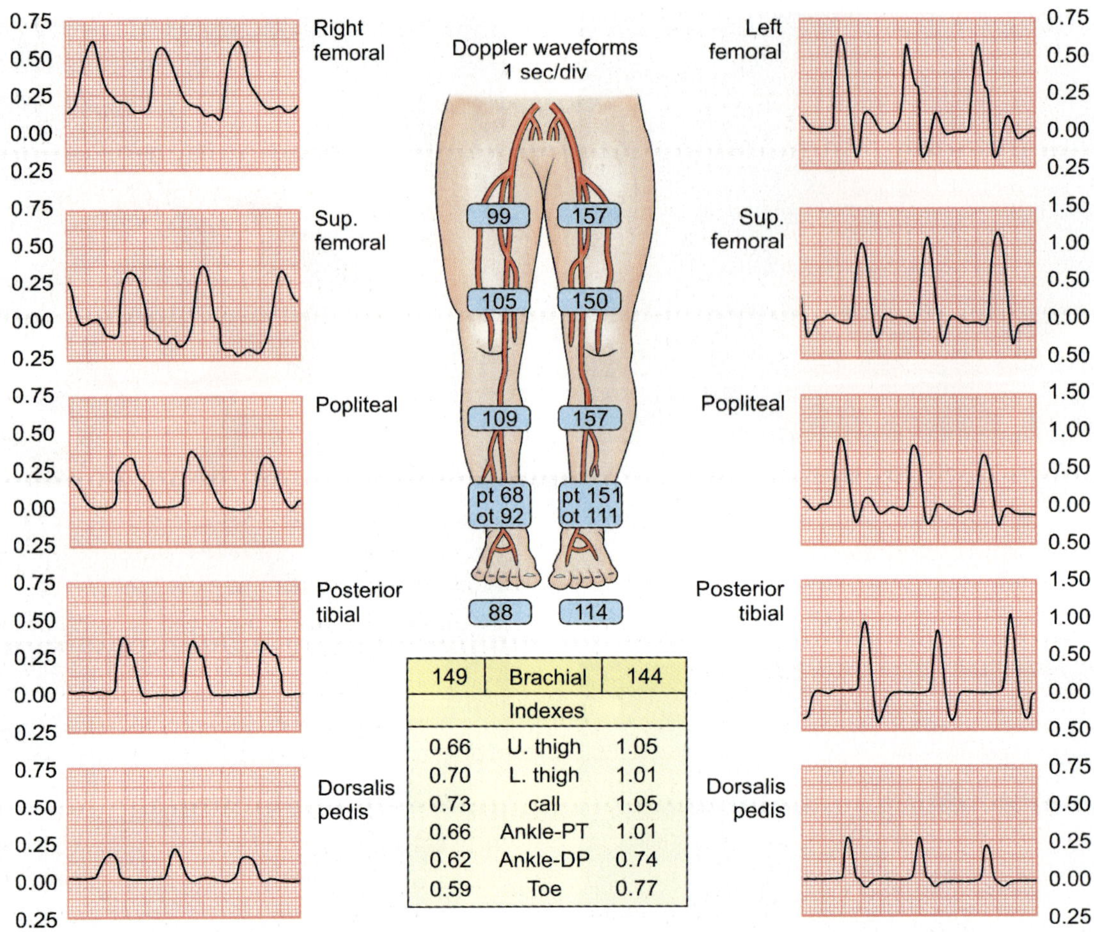


**Fig. 19.57C:** Typical report of peripheral vascular study with arterial segmental pressure measurement plus Doppler evaluation of the lower extremity

- If lifestyle changes do not control your PVD, you may need medication.

*Treatment for peripheral vascular disease:* There are two main goals for treatment of peripheral artery/vascular disease—control the symptoms and halt the progression of the disease to lower the risk for heart attack, stroke, and other complications. Specific treatment will be determined by your physician based on:

- Age, overall health, and medical history
- Extent of the disease
- Signs and symptoms
- Tolerance for specific medications, procedures, or therapies
- Expectations for the course of the disease
- Lifestyle modifications to control risk factors, including regular exercise, proper nutrition, and smoking cessation
- Aggressive treatment of existing conditions that may aggravate PVD, such as diabetes, hypertension, and hyperlipidemia (elevated blood cholesterol)
- Medications for improving blood flow, such as antiplatelet agents (blood thinners) and medications that relax the blood vessel walls Whether medication is a good choice for you depends on the underlying cause of your peripheral vascular disease. Medications used to treat peripheral vascular disease and intermittent claudication include those that aim to lower the risk and progression of atherosclerosis throughout the body, such as those to help stop smoking, lower blood pressure, lower cholesterol, and optimize the bloodsugar in people with diabetes.

## MEDICATIONS

*Pentoxifylline (trental):* How this drug helps in intermittent claudication is not completely understood. It is believed to improve blood flow by decreasing the viscosity of blood and making red blood cells more flexible. With these alterations, the blood can move more easily past-obstructions in the blood vessel.

*Cilostazol (pletal):* This drug keeps platelets from clumping together. This clumping promotes formation of clots and slows down blood flow. The drug also helps dilate, or expand, the blood vessels, encouraging the flow of blood. Sudden blockage of an artery by a blood clot (thrombus) has been treated with medication for many years. Choices include antiplatelet agents, anticoagulants, and 'clot-busters' (thrombolytics).

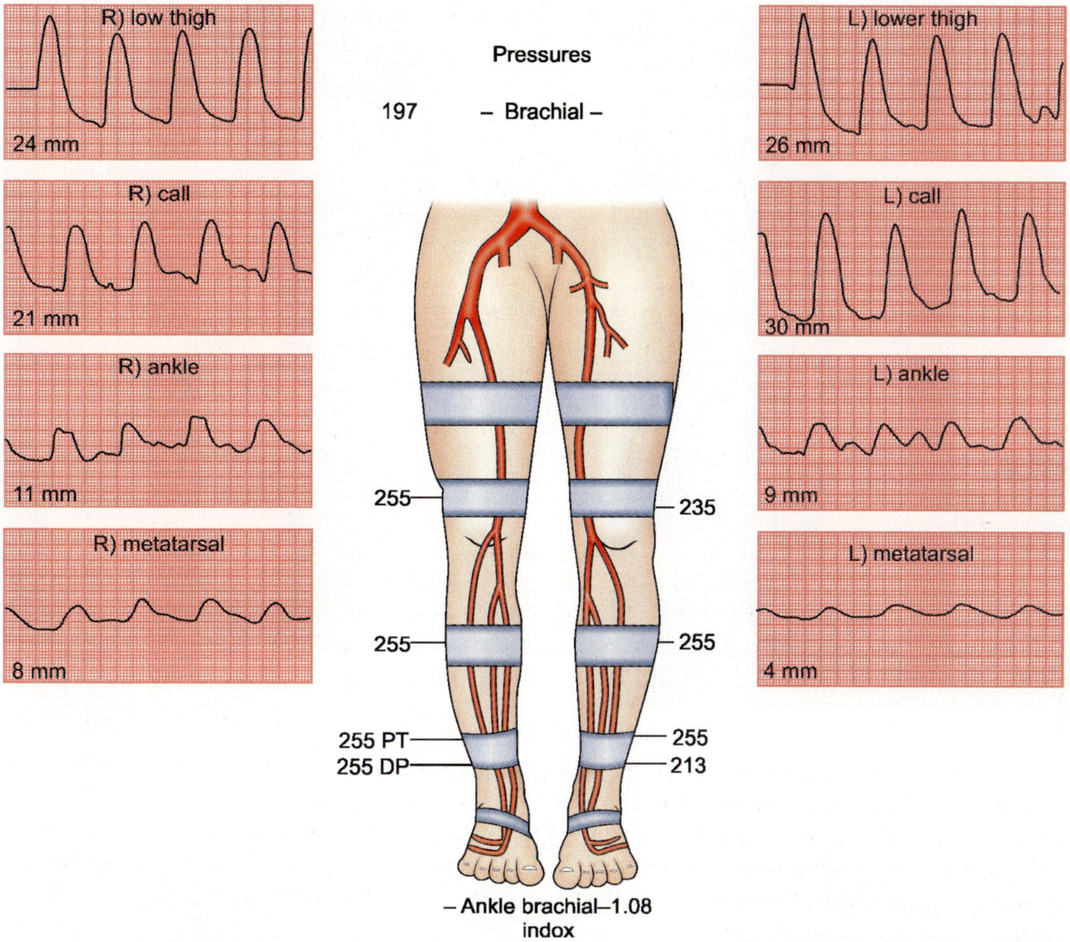


**Fig. 19.57D:** Segmental blood pressure, ABI, and PVRs at rest and after exercise. The tracings display PVRs taken at the thigh, calf, ankle, metatarsal, and toe. The lowest diagram depicts an ankle PVR after exercise. The ABIs at rest are 0.80 on the right and 1.16 on the left. The patient walked on a treadmill for 3 min 20 sec. The exercise was ended because of right calf pain. The ABIs after exercise are 0.45 on the right and 0.76 on the left. The right ankle pressure is 98 mmHg at rest and decreases to 65 mmHg with exercise. The left ankle pressure is 141 mmHg at rest and decreases to 108 mmHg with exercise. The brachial artery systolic pressure is 122 mmHg at rest and augments to 143 mmHg with exercise. Note the pressure drop between the right thigh and the right calf, and the lack of augmentation of the right calf pulse volume waveform, which are consistent with right superficial femoral artery or popliteal artery disease. The left side was normal at rest but the decrease in ankle pressure after exercise indicates that there is peripheral artery disease in the left leg as well. The location of disease cannot be determined on the left. ABI=ankle-brachial index; DP=dorsalis pedis; PT=posterior tibial; PVRs=pulse volume recordings

*Antiplatelet agents:* These include aspirin, ticlopidine, and clopidogrel. These agents do not get rid of an existing clot. They prevent further clots from forming by keeping blood cells and platelets from clumping together.

Anticoagulant agents include heparin, warfarin (coumadin), enoxaparin (lovenox), and low-molecular-weight heparin. These agents also do not remove an existing clot. They interfere with the sequence of blood clotting factors that causes a clot to form.

*Thrombolytics:* These are powerful drugs that can actually dissolve an existing clot. They can be used only under certain circumstances and are given only in the hospital. They can be injected directly into the blocked artery under angiographic guidance. To be effective, they have to be administered intravenously within the first 4–8 hours after a patient develops symptoms. The most effective medications are those that help prevent the development and progression of atherosclerosis.

### Invasive and Minimal Invasive Treatment of Peripheral Vascular Disease (Figs 19.71–19.90)

*Angioplasty:* A catheter (long hollow tube) is used to create a larger opening in an artery to increase blood flow. Angioplasty may be performed in many of the arteries in the body. There are several types of angioplasty procedures, including:

- **Balloon angioplasty**—a small balloon is inflated inside the blocked artery to open the blocked area

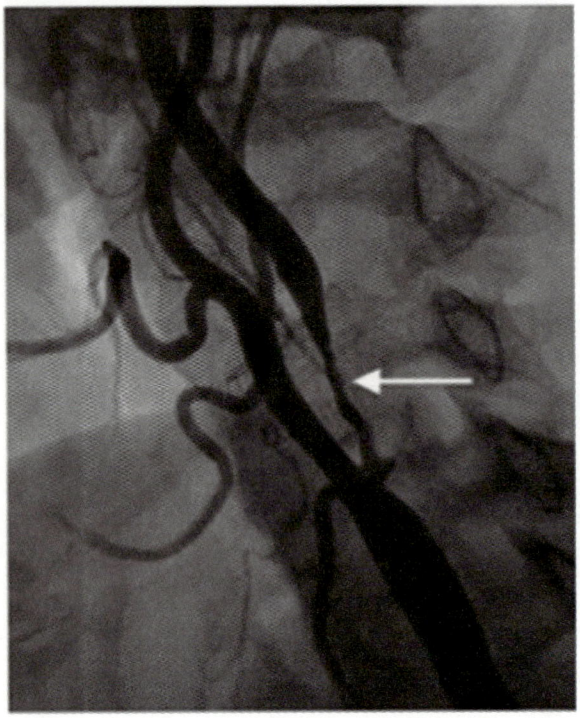

**Fig. 19.58:** Angiogram of carotid artery showing more than 90% of stenosis of left internal carotid artery (arrow)

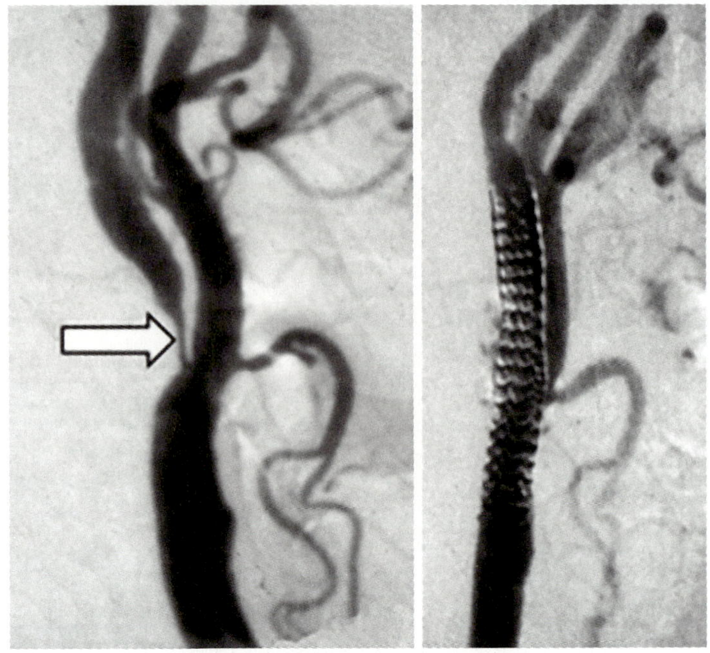

**Fig. 19.60:** Carotid angiography after injection of dye into the carotid artery showing severe carotid artery narrowing in the left hand figure (arrow). The right hand figure shows the appearances after the insertion of a metallic stent across the narrowing

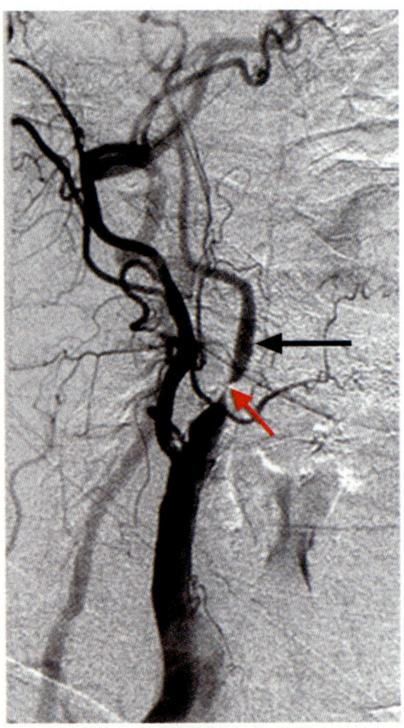

**Fig. 19.59:** Red arrow points to site of occlusion. Arrow points to collateral filling of the distal portion of the internal carotid artery on delayed film

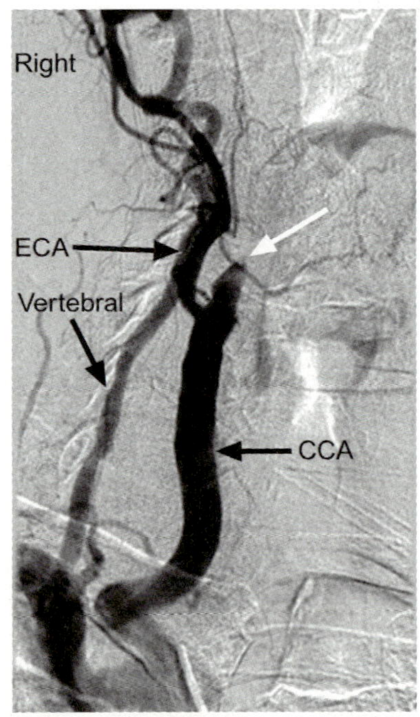


**Fig. 19.61:** Internal carotid artery stenosis white arrow—occlusion of internal carotid artery. ECA=external carotid artery; CCA= common carotid artery

- **Atherectomy**—the blocked area inside the artery is 'shaved' away by a tiny device on the end of a catheter
- **Laser angioplasty**—a laser is used to 'vaporize' the blockage in the artery

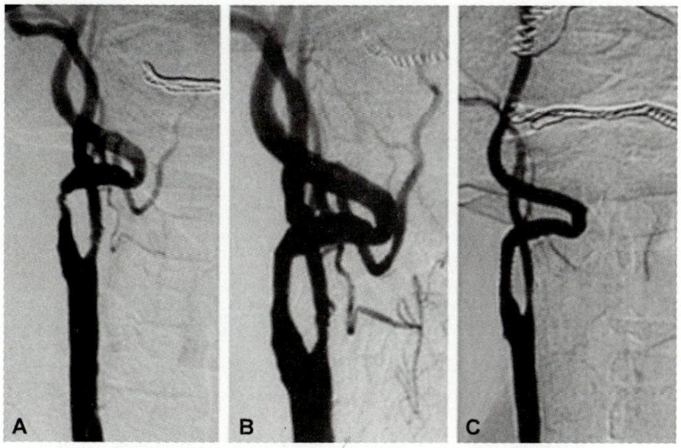


**Fig. 19.62:** (A) Right common carotid angiogram shows severe stenosis and tortuosity of the right ICA. (B) Control angiogram after stent placement. (C) Follow-up angiogram obtained at 6 months demonstrates a patent stent without stenosis

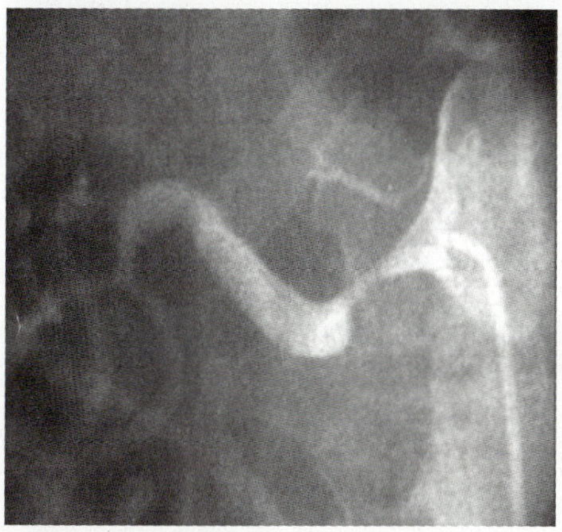

**Fig. 19.63:** Renal angiography showing renal artery stenosis in chronic persistent hypertension

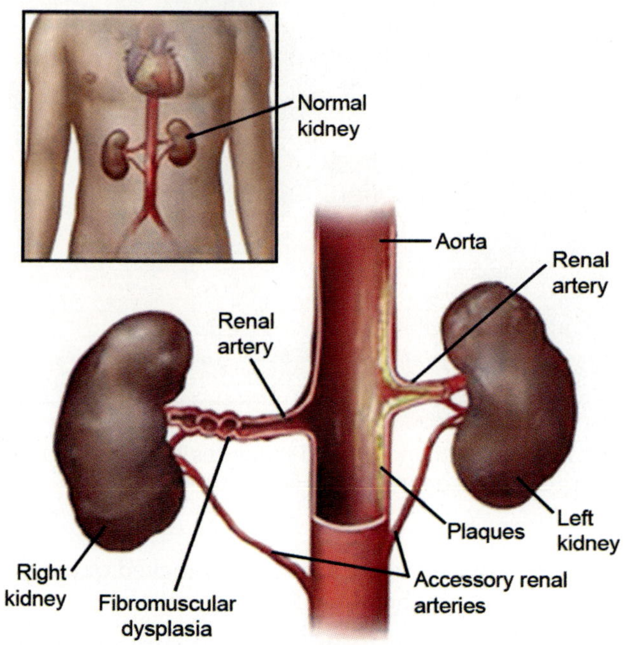


**Fig. 19.64:** Fibromuscular dysplasia in chronic persistent hypertension

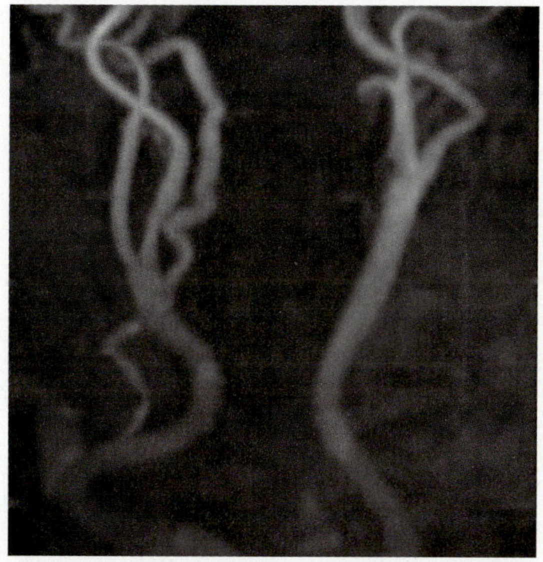

**Fig. 19.65:** High grade left proximal subclavian artery stenosis with signal loss of the left VA on time-of-flight images due to flow reversal. The normal antegrade flow signal of the left VA is missing in the 3D TOF images. On time-resolved 3D CE-MRA, the vessel shows delayed, retrograde contrast filling

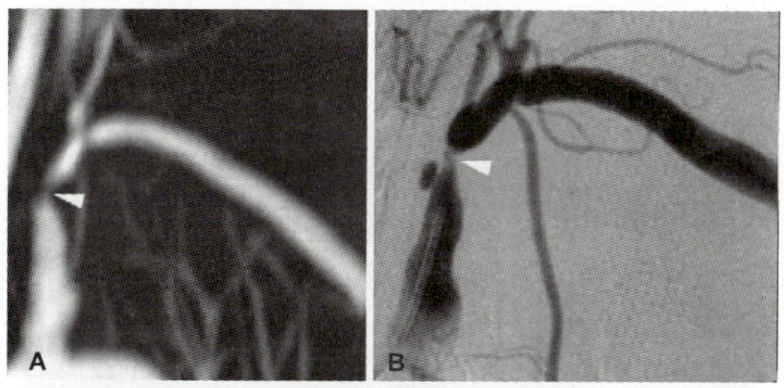


**Fig. 19.66:** (A) Typical example of a subclavian artery stenosis, initially detected by CE-MRA and (B) confirmed by DSA. The arrow indicates the location of the stenosis

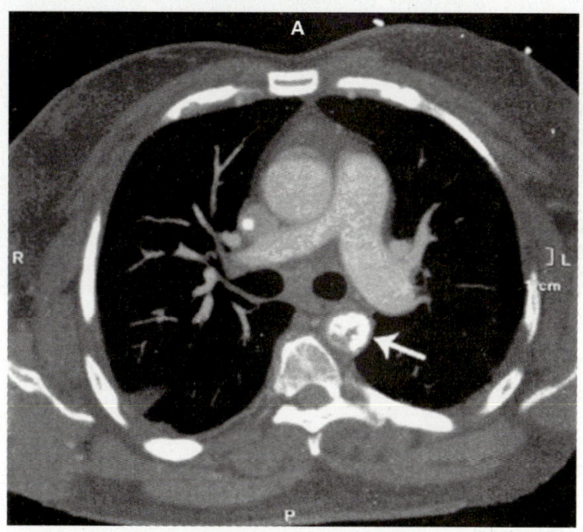


**Fig. 19.67:** 64 slice sagital section at the level of calcific plaque revealed nondilated descending thoracic aorta, densely calcific and lumen filled with superadded thrombus (white arrow)

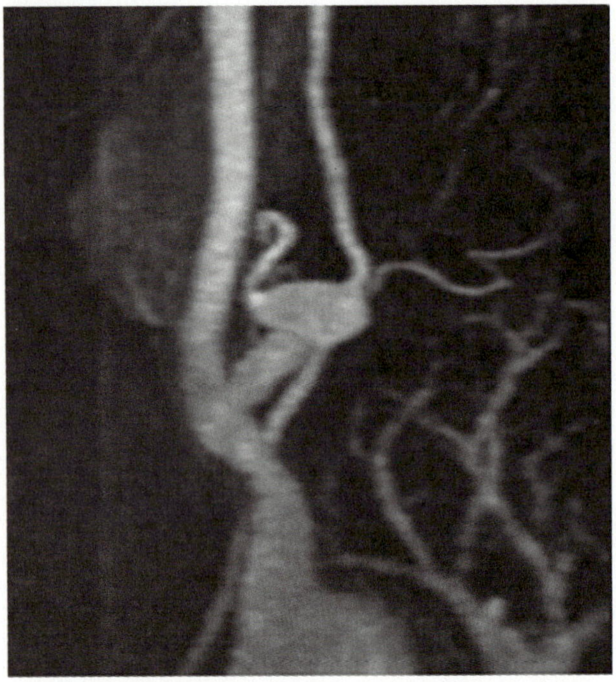

**Fig. 19.68:** CE-MRA thin-slab MIP A. Max 3 cm aneurysm of the right subclavian artery giving rise to the vertebral artery, the thyrocervical trunk, and the internal thoracic artery

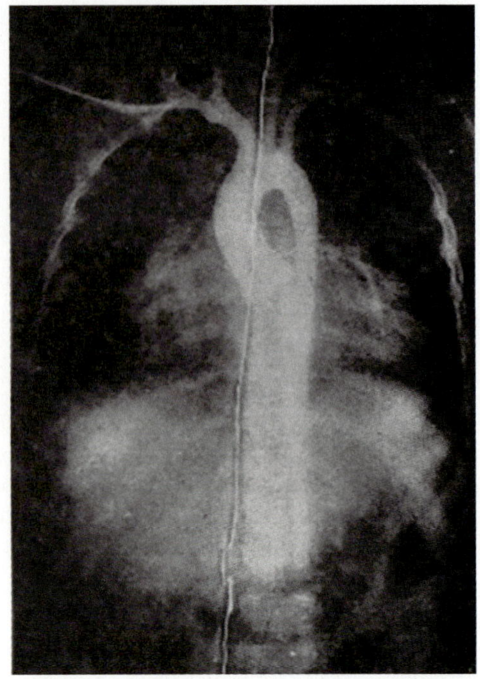

**Fig. 19.70:** Aortography showlng narrowlng of descending aorta in nonspecific aorto-arteritis syndrome

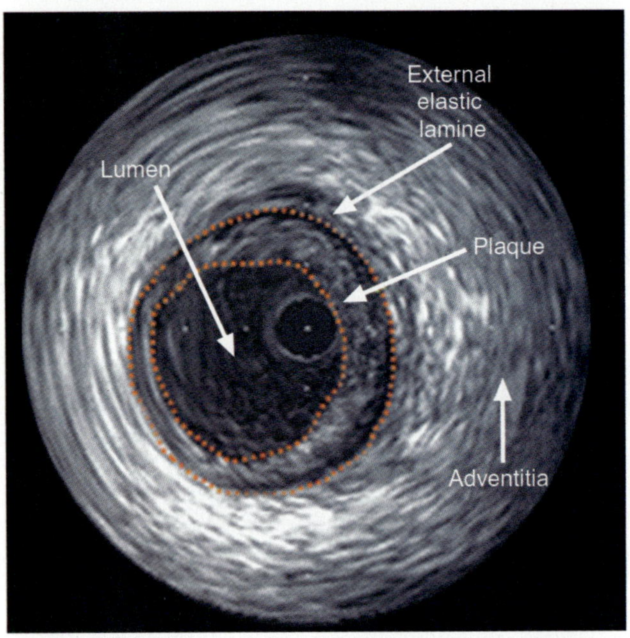


**Fig. 19.69:** IUVS scan of an artery showing all the three layers and plaque inside two circles

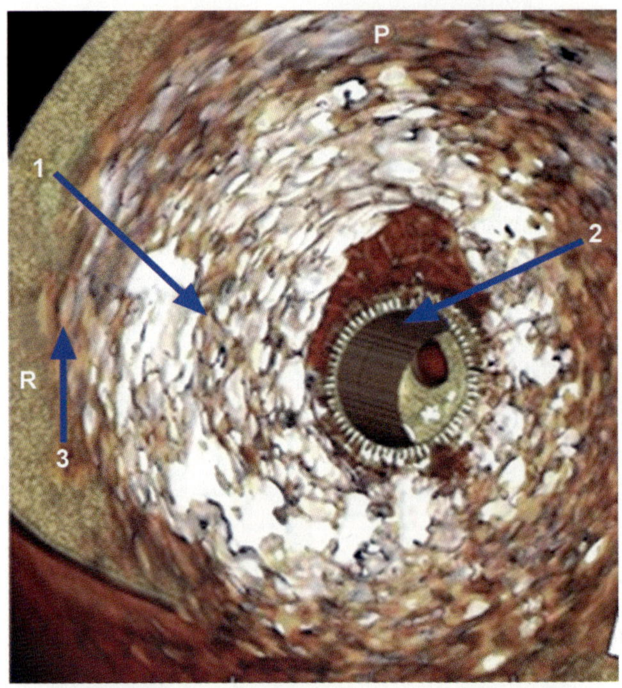


**Fig. 19.71:** Sectional anatomical structutes in superficial femoral artery. 1=stent, 2=artery and 3=IUVS catheter

- **Stent**—a tiny coil is expanded inside the blocked artery to open the blocked area and is left in place to keep the artery open
- **Vascular surgery**—a bypass graft using a blood vessel from another part of the body or a tube made of synthetic material is placed in the area of the blocked or narrowed artery to reroute the blood flow.

With both angioplasty and vascular surgery, an angiogram is often performed prior to the procedure.

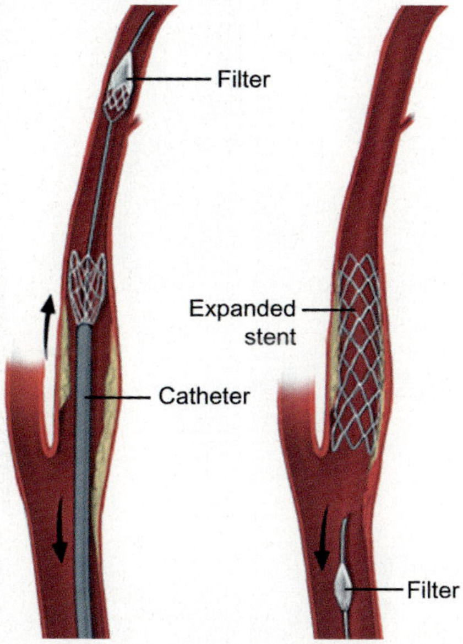


**Fig. 19.72:** Diagrammatic representation of placement of stents in the management of occluded carotid arteries

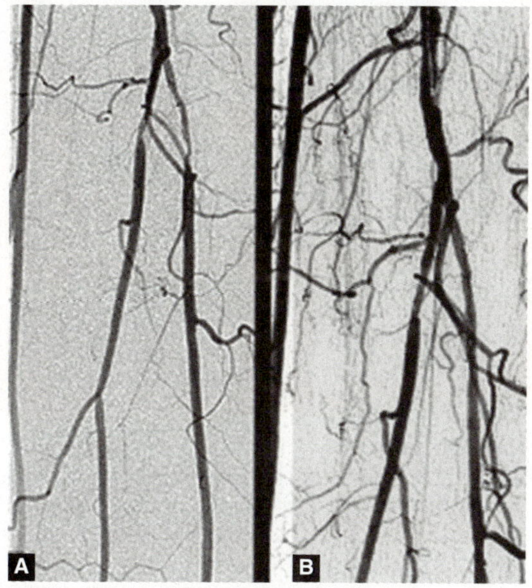


**Fig. 19.74:** Angiography. (A) Occluded femoral artery. (B) Fully revascularized after laser angioplasty

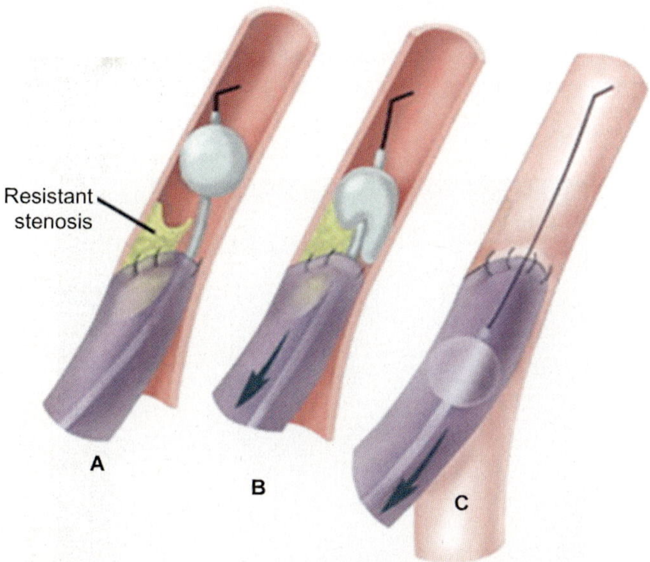


**Fig. 19.73:** Fogarty thrombectomy of resistant thrombus. (A) A 4-F over-the-wire Fogarty catheter is advanced into the brachial artery beyond the resistant inflow stenosis, and the balloon is inflated. (B) The catheter is forcefully withdrawn. (C) Dislodging the resistant thrombus

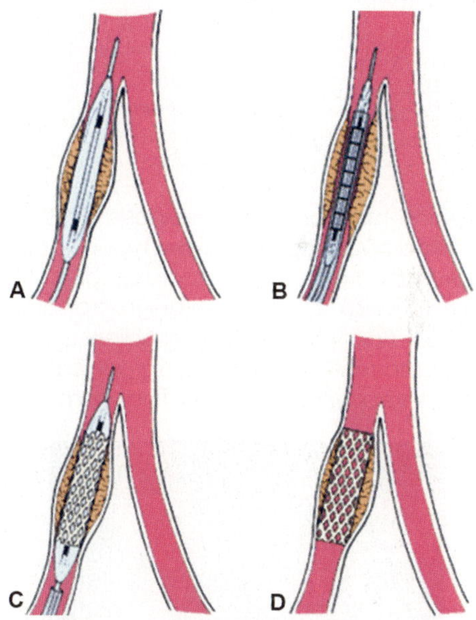


**Fig. 19.75:** Schematic diagram of a peripheral artery being treated with angioplasty and stenting. (A) Balloon angioplasty of the blockage. (B) Positioning of a balloon-expandable stent, (C) Deployment of the stent. (D) Final result with the stent in place

## HOW TO PREVENT PVD

You can reduce your risk of developing PVD by having a healthy lifestyle. This includes (Fig. 19.91).

- avoiding smoking
- controlling your blood sugar, if you have diabetes
- setting an exercise goal of 30 minutes a day, 3 times a week
- working to lower cholesterol and blood pressure
- eating a healthy diet that is low in saturated fat

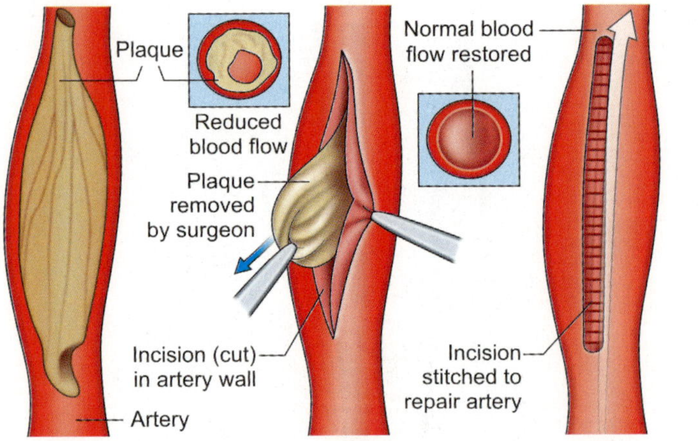


**Fig. 19.76:** Endarterectomy. This surgical procedure involves the manual removal of plaque from the affected artery. It is generally used in case of arteries that are easily accessible, and is more commonly used in the treatment of carotid artery blockages

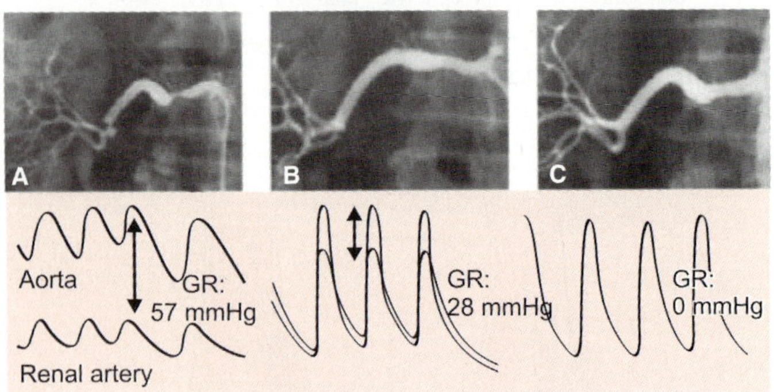


**Fig. 19.77:** Treatment of renal artery stenosis with balloon angioplasty and stenting. (A) Angiogram showing substantial narrowing of the renal artery and a systolic pressure gradient of 57 mmHg. (B) After balloon angioplasty, the angiographic stenosis is improved with a residual translesional gradient of 28 mmHg. (C) Following stent placement, minor angiographic improvement is evident, but the hemodynamic gradient has completely resolved

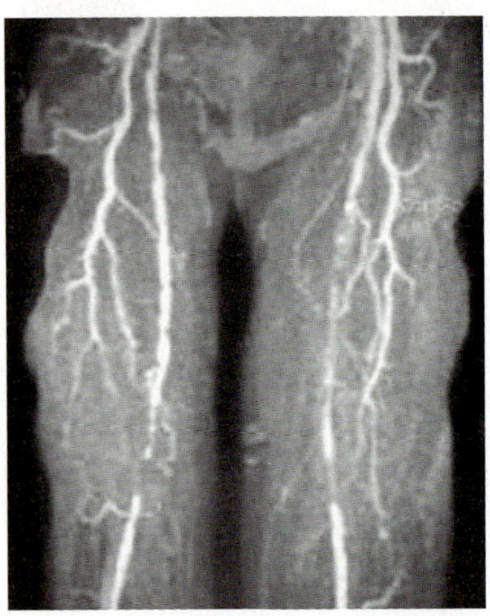

**Fig. 19.78:** This magnetic resonance angiogram (MRA) of the lower extremities was obtained by using the bolus-chase technique. Atherosclerotic disease involves the bilateral superficial femoral arteries. Note the multiple lesions, which are primarily in the middle portions, and the large collateral arterial supply

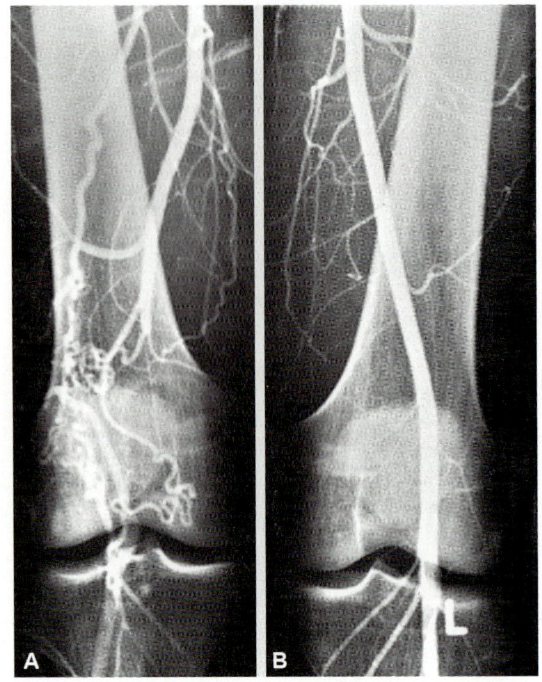


**Fig. 19.79:** Angiograms of acute arterial occlusion. (A) Acute embolic occlusion at the typical location of the trifurcation just below the knee joint. There is a typical cut-off of the contrast column and only a few collaterals are seen. (B) Acute thrombotic occlusion of the superficial femoral artery secondary to atherosclerotic stenosis. Note contrast around fresh thrombus (arrows) and tortuous collaterals as seen in preexisting stenosis

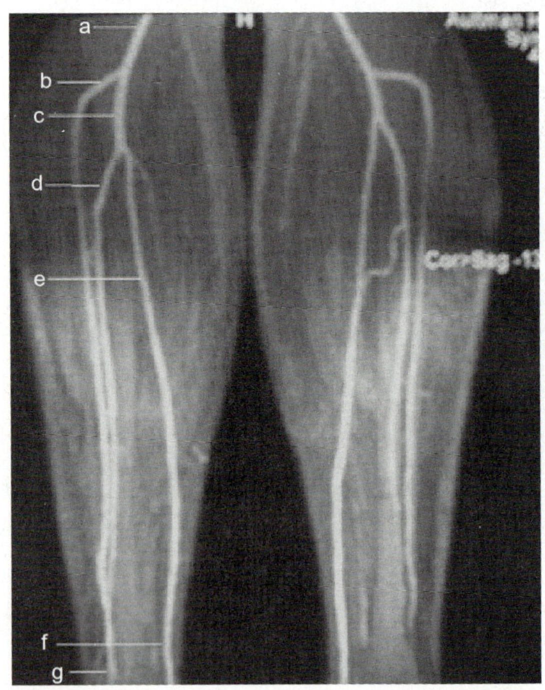


**Fig. 19.80:** Magnetic resonance angiogram (MRA) obtained by using the bolus-chase technique shows the normal anatomy of the lower-extremity arterial vasculature, including the popliteal artery (a), the anterior tibial artery (b), the tibioperoneal trunk (c), the peroneal artery (d), and the posterior tibial artery (e)

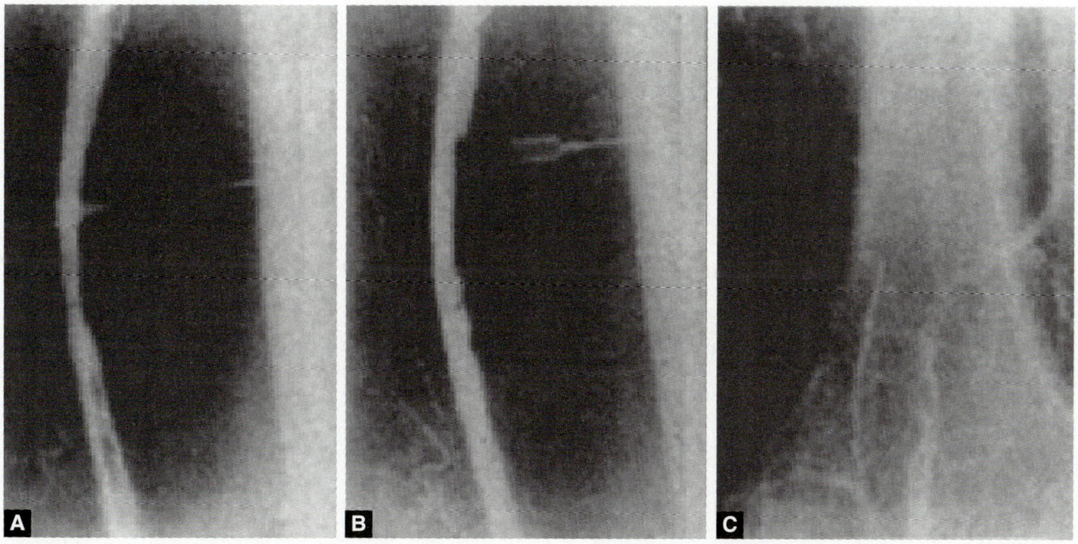


**Fig. 19. 81:** (A) Filling defect probably representing thrombus that partly occludes the superficial femoral artery. (B) Disappreance of the filling defect after balloon angioplasty. (C) Laser evidence of distal thrombus migration,resulting in occlusion of the trifurcation vessels

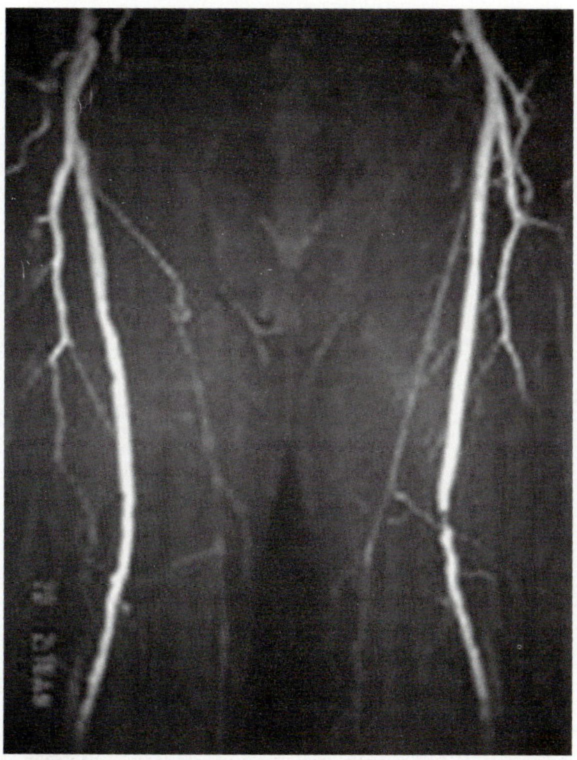

**Fig. 19.82:** This magnetic resonance angiogram (MRA) of the lower extremities was obtained by using the bolus-chase technique. A short-segment high-grade stenosis is present in the middle of the left superficial femoral artery. Note the collateral arterial supply

- keeping your weight at a healthy level
- if you experience symptoms of PVD, talk to your doctor. Your doctor may also recommend testing if you are at risk for the disease.

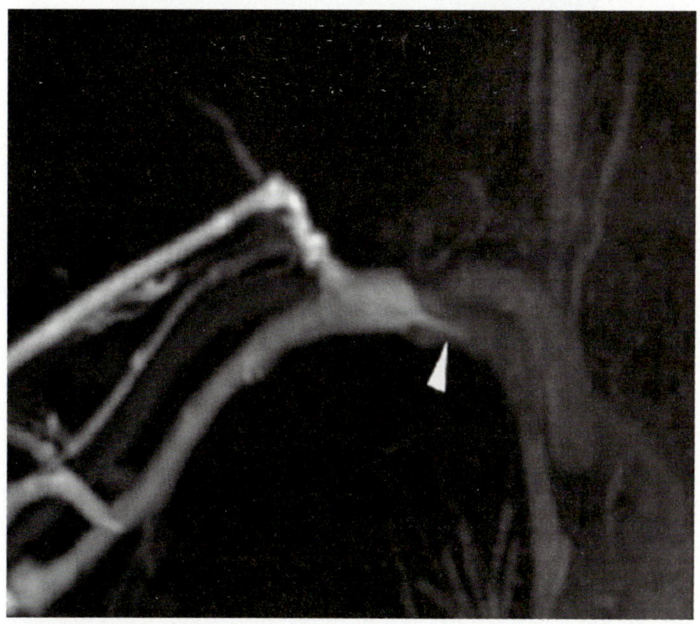

**Fig. 19.83:** Example of a direct MR venogram of a patient with a central venous stenosis. The arrowhead points at the venous outflow stenosis

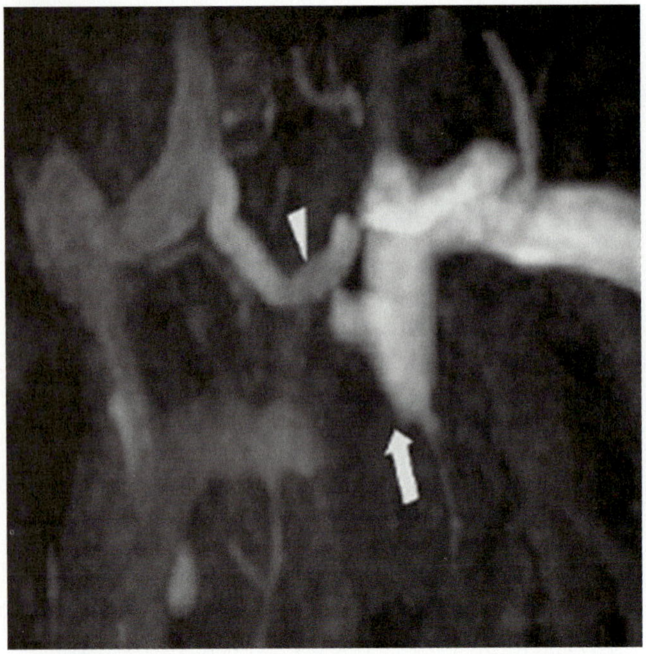

**Fig. 19.84:** Brachiocephalic vein occlusion in a patient who had multiple central venous catheters. The arrow points at the obstructed brachiocephalic vein in the direct CE-MR venogram. The arrowhead indicates a draining collateral vein

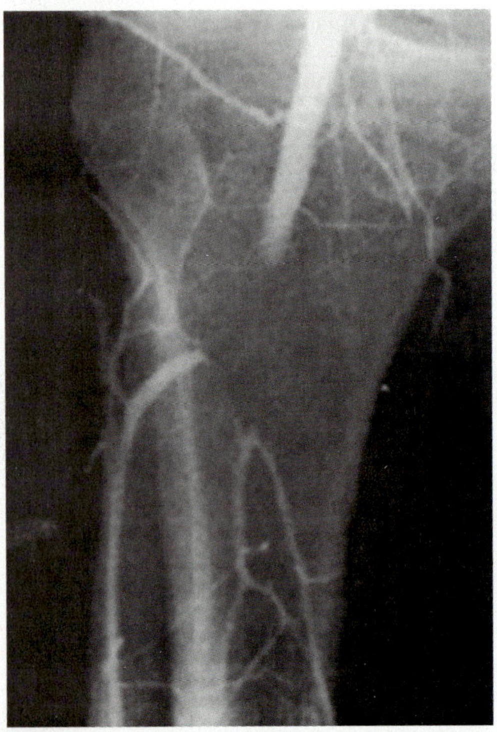

**Fig. 19.85:** A newly formed thrombolic occlusion of the poplitial and trifurcation vessels and successfully treated with urokinase infusion

- early diagnosis and treatment can keep symptoms to a minimum. They can also increase the effectiveness of your treatment.

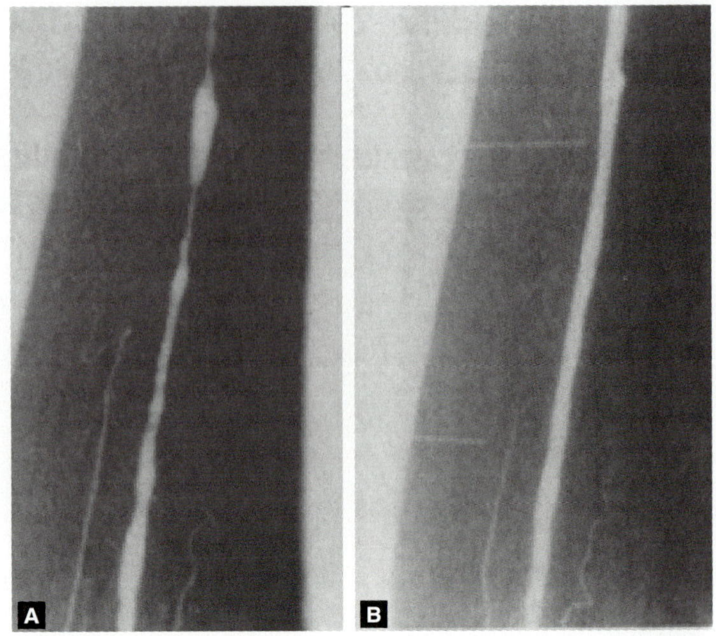


**Fig. 19.86:** (A) Angiographic picture showing diffusely diseased segment of the superficial femoral artery, (B) treated successfully with the atherectomy catheter

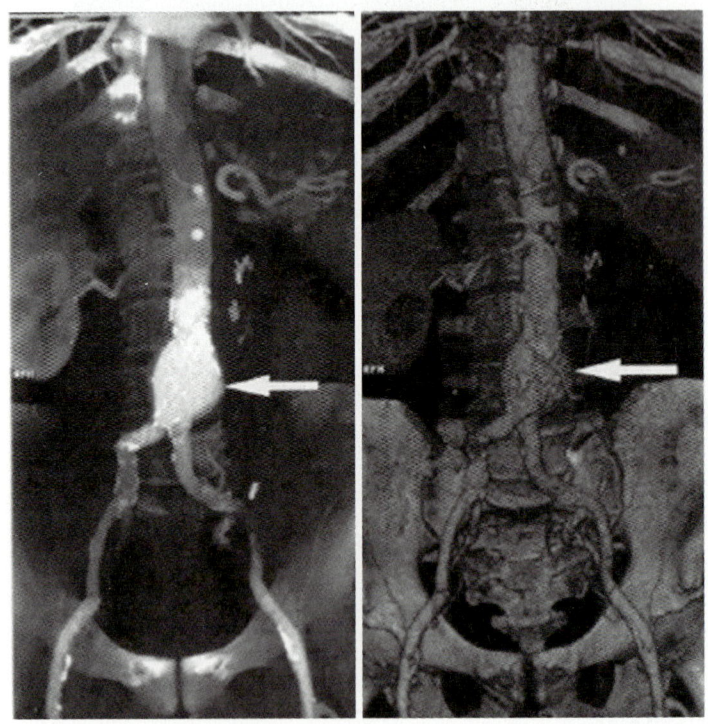

**Fig. 19.87:** 3-D VR MDCT. Abdominal fusiform aneurysm (arrow)

## Prognosis for PVD

If diagnosed early, most cases of PVD will respond to lifestyle treatments. One way to measure improvement is to determine how far you can walk without pain.

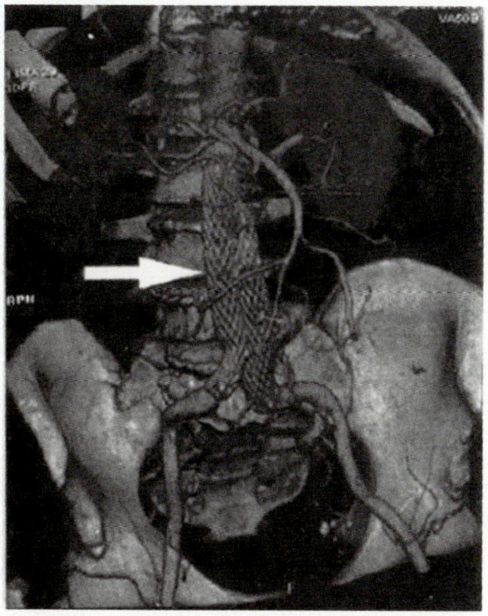

**Fig. 19.88:** 3-D VR MDCT. Endovascular aortic stent (arrow)

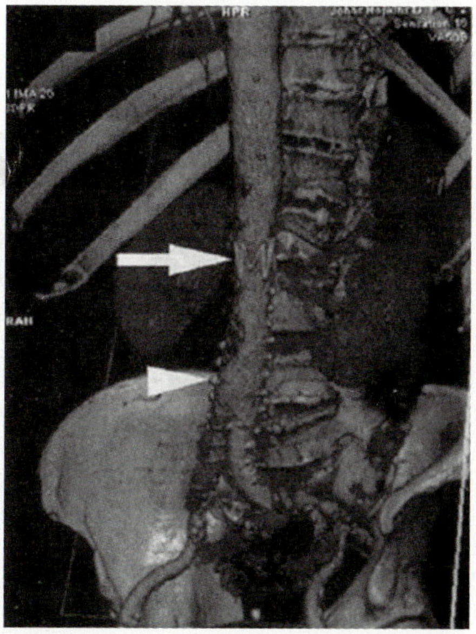

**Fig. 19.89:** VR MDCT. Endovascular stent. Stent neck (arrow) and stent body (arrowhead) components

With effective treatment, you should be able to gradually increase the distance.

Contact your doctor if your symptoms get worse or you experience any of the following:

- Your leg looks pale or blue
- Your leg becomes cold
- Chest pain accompanies leg pain
- Your leg becomes red, swollen, or hot
- New sores or ulcers develop and do no heal
- You experience fever, chills, weakness, or other signs of infection.

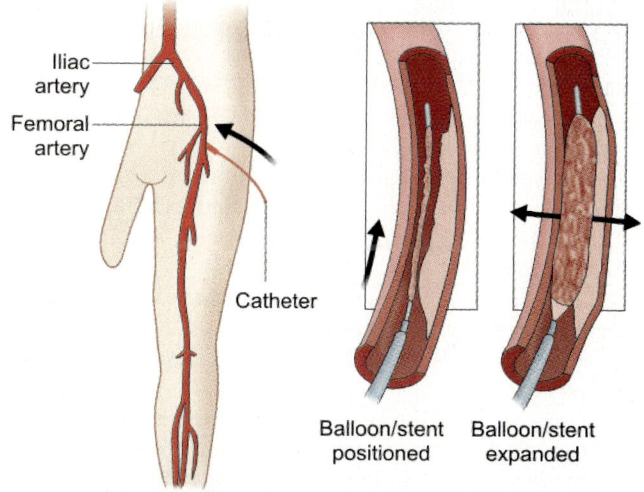


**Fig. 19.90:** Management of iliac artery by stentoplasty

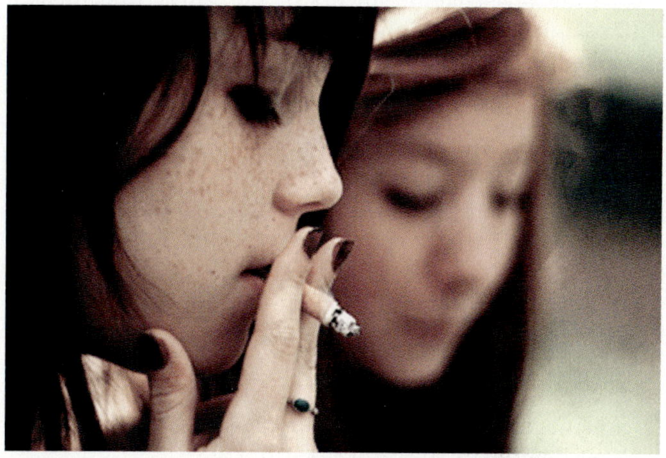

**Fig. 19.91:** Stopping cigarette smoking not only prevents PAD but it can significantly regress the process of atherosclerosis

## BIBLIOGRAPHY

1. Albers M, Fratezi AC, De Luccia N. Assessment of quality of life of patients with severe ischemia as a result of infrainguinal arterial occlusive disease. J Vasc Surg 1992; 16:54–9.
2. Aronow WS. Office management of peripheral arterial disease. Am J Med 2010;123(9):790–2.
3. Bergamini TM, Towne JB, Bandyk DF, Seabrook GR, Schmitt DD. Experience with in situ saphenous vein bypasses during 1981 to 1989: determinant factors of long-term patency. J Vasc Surg 1991;13:137–47.
4. Brown AL, Juergens JL. Arteriosclerosis and atherosclerosis. In: Allen EV, et al. Peripheral vascular disease. Philadelphia: Saunders, 1972;57–66.
5. Burns P, Gough S, Bradbury AW. Management of peripheral arterial disease in primary care. BMJ 2003; 326(7389):584–8.
6. Cheshire NJ, Wolfe JH, Noone MA, Davies L, Drummond M. The economics of femorocrural reconstruction for critical leg ischemia with and without autologous vein. J Vasc Surg 1992;15:167–74.

7. Cutajar CL, Marston A, Newcombe JF. Value of cuff occlusion pressures in assessment of peripheral vascular disease. Br Med J 1973;2(863):392–5.
8. DeBakey ME, Crawford ES, Garrett E, et al. Occlusive disease of the lower extremities in patients 16 to 37 years of age. Ann Surg 1964;159:873–90.
9. Diagnosis and management of peripheral arterial disease, Scottish Intercollegiate Guidelines Network-SIGN (2006).
10. Diagnosis and Treatment of Peripheral Artery Diseases, European Society of Cardiology (2011).
11. Donaldson MC, Mannick JA, Whittemore AD. Femoral-distal bypass with in situ greater saphenous vein. Long-term results using the Mills valvulotome. Ann Surg 1991;213: 457–64.
12. Dormandy J, Verstraete M, Andreani D, et al. Second European consensus document on chronic critical leg ischemia. Circulation 1991;84(suppl 4):1–26.
13. Eklund AE, Eriksson G, Olsson AG. A controlled study showing significant short term effect of prostaglandin E1 in healing of ischaemic ulcers of the lower limb in man. Prostaglandins Leukot Med 1982;8:265–71.
14. Golledge J. Lower-limb arterial disease. Lancet 1997;350: 1459–65.
15. Gordon T, Kannel WB. Predisposition to atherosclerosis in the head, heart, and legs. The Framingham study. JAMA 1972;221:661–6.
16. Haid SP, Conn J Jr, Bergan JJ. Cystic adventitial disease of the popliteal artery. Arch Surg 1970;101:765–70.
17. Haimovici H. Patterns of arteriosclerotic lesions of the lower extremity. Arch Surg 1967;95:918–33.
18. Lower limb peripheral arterial disease, NICE Clinical Guideline (August 2012).
19. Mangiafico RA, Fiore CE. Current management of intermittent claudication: the role of pharmacological and Curr Vasc Pharmacol 2009;7(3):394–413.
20. Mavor GE. The pattern of occlusion in atheroma of the lower limb arteries. The correlation of clinical and arteriographic findings. Br J Surg 1956;43:352–64.
21. Mazari FA, Gulati S, Rahman MN, et al. Early outcomes from a randomized, controlled trial of supervised exercise, Ann Vasc Surg 2010;24(1):69–79. Epub 2009 Sep 17.
22. No authors listed. MRC/BHF Heart Protection Study of cholesterol lowering with simvastatin in 20, 536 high-risk individuals: a randomised placebo-controlled trial; Lancet 2002;360(9326):7–22.
23. Ouriel K, McDonnell AE, Metz CE, Zarins CK. Critical evaluation of stress testing in the diagnosis of peripheral vascular disease. Surgery 1982;91:686–93.
24. Peach G, Griffin M, Jones KG, et al. Diagnosis and management of peripheral arterial disease. BMJ 2012;345: e5208. doi:10.1136/bmj.e5208.
25. Percutaneous atherectomy of femoropopliteal arterial lesions with plaque excision devices, NICE Interventional Procedure Guideline (February 2011).
26. Peripheral arterial disease-cilostazol, naftidrofyryl oxalate, pentoxifylline and inositol nicotinate; NICE Technology Appraisal Guideline (May 2011).
27. Quinones-Baldrich WJ, Prego AA, Ucelay-Gomez R, Freischlag JA, Ahn SS, Baker JD. Long-term results of infrainguinal revascularization with polytetrafluoroethylene: a ten-year experience. J Vasc Surg 1992;16:209–17.
28. Robless P, Mikhailidis DP, Stansby GP. Cilostazol for peripheral arterial disease. Cochrane Database Syst Rev 2008;(1):CD003748.
29. Ruffolo AJ, Romano M, Ciapponi A. Prostanoids for critical limb ischaemia. Cochrane Database Syst Rev 2010;(1): CD006544.
30. Santilli JD, Rodnick JE, Santilli SM. Claudication: diagnosis and treatment. Am Fam Physician 1996;53:1245–53.
31. Schuler JJ, Flanigan DP, Holcroft JW, Ursprung JJ, Mohrland JS, Pyke J. Efficacy of prostaglandin E1 in the treatment of lower extremity ischemic ulcers secondary to peripheral vascular occlusive disease: results of a prospective randomized, double-blind, multicenter clinical trial. J Vasc Surg 1984;1:160–70.
32. Taylor LM Jr, Edwards JM, Porter JM. Present status of reversed vein bypass grafting: five-year results of a modern series. J Vasc Surg 1990;11:193–205.
33. Taylor LM Jr, Porter JM. Current status of the reversed saphenous vein graft. In: Bergan JJ, Yao J, eds. Arterial surgery. New York: Grune and Stratton, 1987:494–501.
34. The Edinburgh Claudication Questionnaire.
35. Vascular disease-clopidogrel and dipyridamole, NICE Technology Appraisal Guideline (December 2010).
36. Watson L, Ellis B, Leng GC. Exercise for intermittent claudication. Cochrane Database Syst Rev 2008;(4):CD000990.
37. Weiss N, Hilge R, Hoffmann U. Mild hyperhomocysteinemia: risk factor or just risk predictor for cardiovascular diseases? Vasa 2004;33(4):191–203.
38. Welch HJ. Chronic lower extremity ischemia. Compr Ther 1997;23:534–8.
39. Yusuf S, Sleight P, Pogue J, et al. Effects of an angiotensin-converting-enzyme inhibitor, ramipril, on cardiovascular events in high-risk patients. The Heart Outcomes Prevention Evaluation Study Investigators. N Engl J Med 2000; 342(3): 145–53.

# 20 Recognition and Management of Cardiac Arrhythmia

Arrhythmias may be defined as a disturbance in either the formation of impulse or its transmission through various pathways of conduction or through both the combinations. The term sinus arrhythmia is a misnomer as the phenomenon is only an exaggeration of the normal and the impulse arises normally at the S-A node. Similarly, the term nodal rhythm is misleading as this does not mean that the impulse arises at the S-A node. It has now been replaced by the term A-V junctional rhythm.

## GENESIS OF CARDIAC DYSARRHYTHMIA

### The Heart's Electrical System

The atria (the heart's upper chambers) and ventricles (the heart's lower chambers) work together, alternately contracting and relaxing to pump blood through the heart. The electrical system of the heart is the power source that makes this possible (Figs 20.1–20.3).

#### *What Happens during a Normal Heartbeat*

Irregular heart rhythms can also occur in normal, healthy hearts. Arrhythmias can also be caused by certain

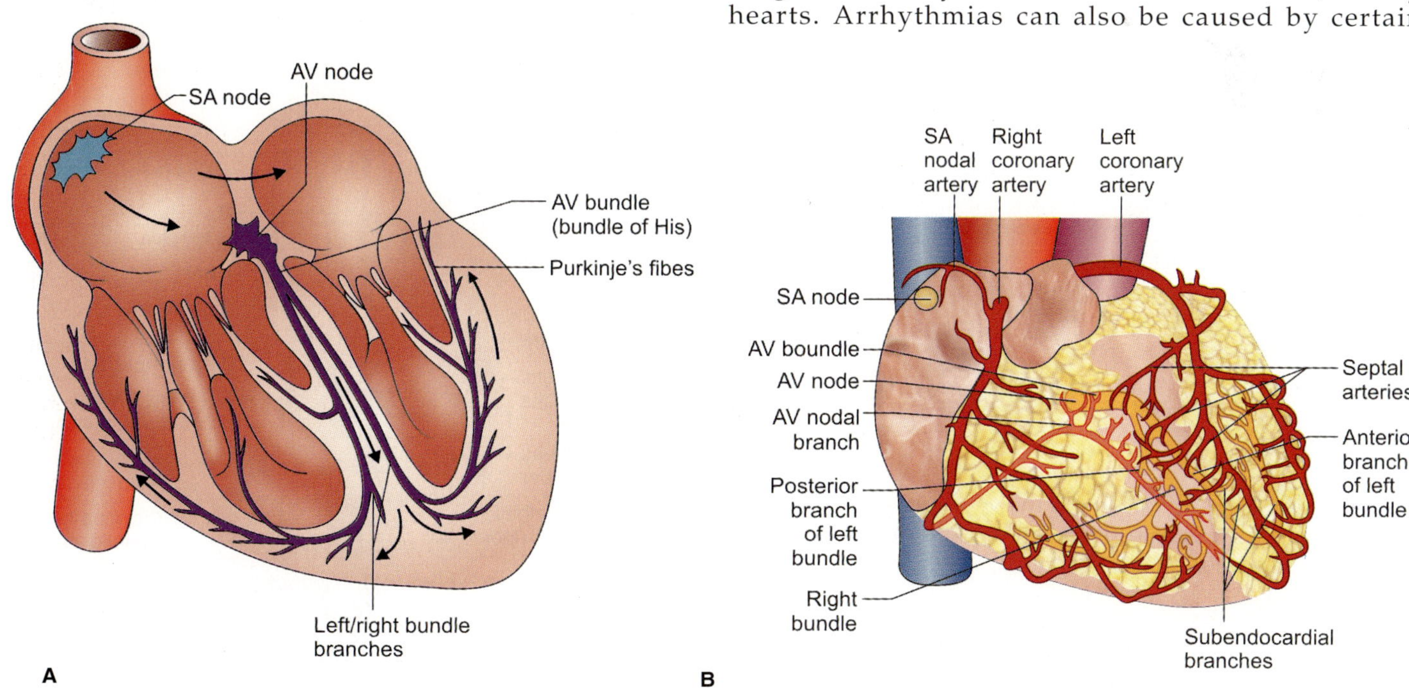


**Fig. 20.1:** (A) Diagrammatic representation of anatomical structures of conduction system of the heart. (B) Shows blood supply of conduction system of the heart

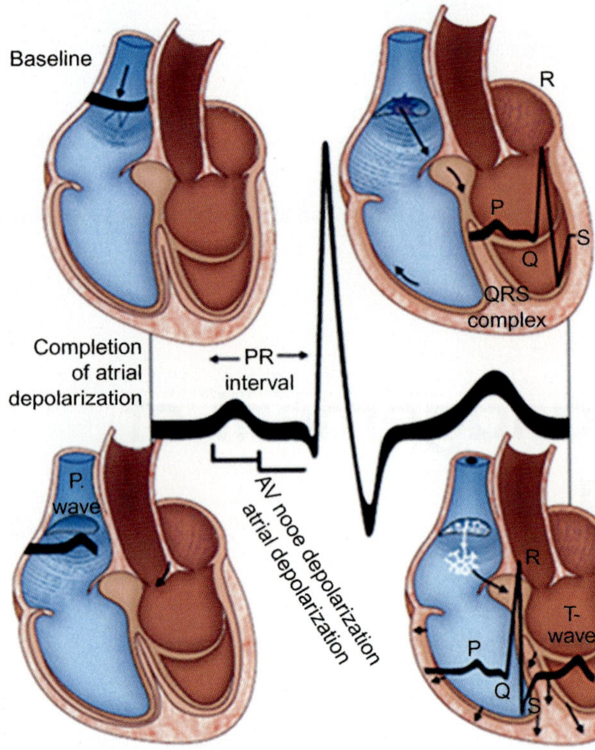


Fig. 20.2: The formation and conduction of cardiac impulse by the process of depolarization along the conducting system

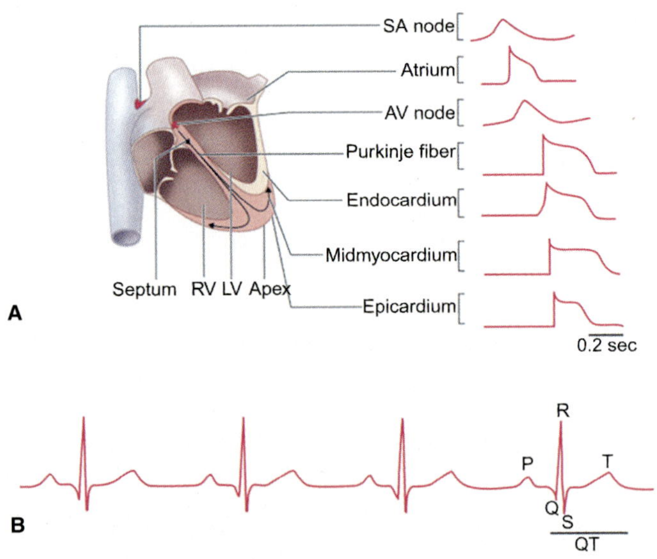


Fig. 20.3: Electrical activity in the myocardium. (A) Schematic of a human heart with illustration of typical action potential waveforms recorded in different regions. (B) Schematic of a surface

substances or medications, such as caffeine, nicotine, alcohol, cocaine, inhaled aerosols, diet pills, and cough and cold remedies. Emotional states such as shock, fright or stress can also cause irregular heart rhythms. Arrhythmias that are recurrent or related to an underlying heart condition are more concerning and should always be evaluated by a doctor. In most cases, treating the underlying condition will take care of the arrhythmia. If not, many medications and procedures are available to eliminate or control the abnormal heart rhythm. It can be caused either by the disturbance of impulse formation or impulse conduction or both.

*Disturbance of impulse formation:* Disturbance of cardiac impulse formation may lead to the common type of cardiac arrhythmia, called ectopic rhythm.

*Ectopic rhythms:* These are of two types, either escape beats and escape rhythms or extra systoles and ectopic tachycardias. An escape beat appears when there is a pause in the existing rhythm, and it is, thus always late in appearance and never premature. If the sinus node fails for a long period, repeated escape beats will occur, giving a characteristically slow escape rhythm. The commonest site of escape rhythm is the A-V junction. Extrasystoles and ectopic rhythms arise from foci in the specialized electrocardiogram; three sequential beats are displayed (Figs 20.1–20.4) (From Nerbonne J, Kass R. Molecular physiology of cardiac repolarization. Physiol Rev. 2005; 85:1206) conducting tissue, which have been well-defined in the intranodal tracts of the atria. If the extra-systole or tachycardia is above the bifurcation of the bundle of His, it is termed as A-V junctional tachycardia.

## CLASSIFICATION OF CARDIAC ARRHYTHMIAS

Anatomically, the dysrhythmias may be classified according to the site of origin of the impulse. Given below is a simple and workable classification of cardiac arrhythmias (Tables 20.1 and 20.2).

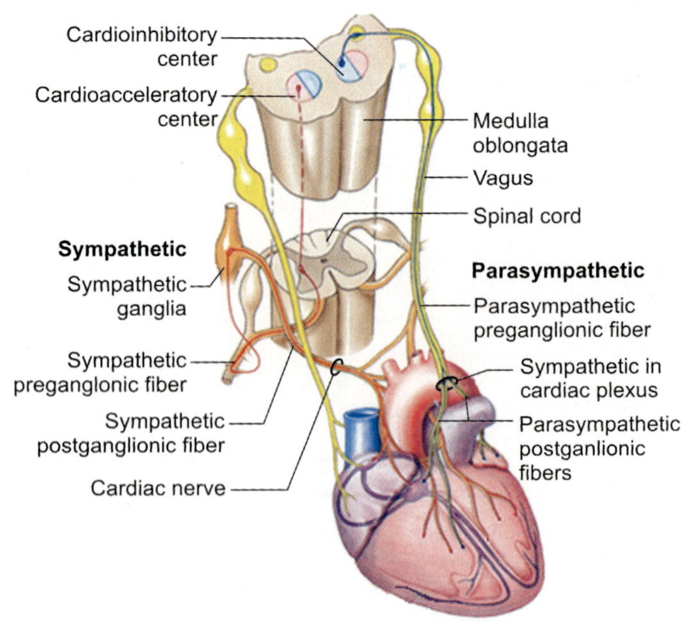


Fig. 20.4: Diagrammatic representation of sympathetic and parasympathetic nerve innervation of the heart influencing cardiac rhythm

**Table 20.1:** ECG features of supraventricular tachycardias

| | R-R regularity | P-wave morphology |
|---|---|---|
| **Atrial tachycardias** | | |
| Sinus tachycardia | Regular | Positive in II, III, aVF |
| Sinus node re-entry | Regular | Positive in II, III, aVF |
| Atrial tachycardia, unifocal | Regular | P different from sinus |
| Atrial tachycardia, multifocal | Irregular | ≥3 different P-wave morphologies |
| Atrial flutter, common, counter- AV block | Regular, irregular if variable negative in II, III, aVF | Sawtooth flutter waves; regular waveform; clockwise |
| Atrial flutter, uncommon, clockwise | Regular, irregular if variable AV block | Upright flutter waves; positive waveform II, III, aVF |
| Atrial fibrillation | Irregularly irregular | Irregular fibrillation waves |
| **AV junctional tachycardias** | | |
| ***AV re-entry (using accessory pathways)*** | | |
| Orthodromic | Regular | Retrograde P in ST-T-wave |
| Antidromic | Regular preexcited | Retrograde P, short RP |
| Slow conducting | Regular | Retrograde P at end of T-wave or later (long RP) |
| Atriofascicular (antidromic) | Regular preexcited | Retrograde P, short RP |
| ***AV nodal re-entry*** | | |
| Common (slow-fast) | Regular | Retrograde P obscured by QRS or alters the end of QRS (short RP) |
| Uncommon (fast-slow) | Regular | Retrograde P at end of T-wave or later (long RP) |
| Others (slow-slow) | Regular | PR-RP approximately equal |
| Nonparoxysmal junctional tachycardia | Regular, slow rate | AV dissociation |
| Automatic junctional tachycardia | Regular | AV dissociation |

**Table 20.2:** P-wave morphology in atrial tachycardia—general principles

| Location | | P-wave polarity during atrial tachycardia | |
|---|---|---|---|
| Right atrium | + or ± in aVL and – in VI | Crista terminalis (CT) | May be +, ±, or – in II, III, aVF in the high, mid and inferior CT, respectively; – or ± inVI; – in aVR |
| | | Tricuspid annulus | – in V1–V2; + in a VL and frequently in 1 |
| | | Right atrial appendage | Insufficient data |
| Left atrium | – in aVL and + in VI | Right pulmonary veins | + in V1–V6; + in 1: narrow P-wave in VI |
| | | Left pulmonary veins | + in V1–V6; –/isoelectric in aVL; broad or notched P-wave in VI |
| | | Mitral annulus | ± with initially narrow negative deflection in V1; –/isoelectric in 1 aVL; slightly +/isoelectric in II, III, aVF |
| Interatrial spetum and adjacent structures | Specific to location | Coronary sinus ostium | + in V1; isoelectric in I: – in II, III, aVF; + in aVL, aVR |
| | | Snteroseptum | –/± in V1; +/± in II, III, aVF |
| | | Mid septum | –/± in V1; in two of three inferior leads (II, III, aVF) |
| | | Left septum | Uncommon; variable findings |

+ positive; – negative; ± biphasic

Site of origin and type of dysrhythmia:

1. **Sinu-atrial node**
   i. Sinus tachycardia
   ii. Sinus bradycardia
   iii. Sinus arrhythmia
   iv. S-A arrest of block
   v. Wandering pacemaker
   vi. Sinu extrasystoles
2. **Atria**
   i. Atrial extrasystoles
   ii. Atrial tachycardia
   iii. Atrial flutter
   iv. Atrial fibrillation
   v. Chaotic atrial rhythm
   vi. Atrial standstill

3. **Atrio-ventricular junction**
   i. A-V junctional extrasystoles
   ii. A-V junctional tachycardia
   iii. A-V junctional rhythm
   iv. Heart block-first, second and third degree
4. **Ventricles**
   i. Bundle branch block
   ii. Ventricular extrasystoles
   iii. Ventricular tachycardia
   iv. Ventricular flutter and fibrillation
   v. Ventricular standstill.

It has been, frequently, observed that most of the arrhythmias are transient and may be of only a few seconds duration. It is in that brief period, if the ECG is taken, that a particular type of arrhythmia could be found out, otherwise, in majority of the patients, it could be missed. This problem has been overcome by frequent use of the Holter monitoring system which can detect cardiac arrhythmia, not only being present for a shorter period, but can also provide useful therapeutic guidelines for its final management. The arrhythmias, which originate in the sinus (or sinoatrial SA) node, are classified as sinus tachycardia, sinus bradycardia, sinus arrhythmia, SA block, SA nodal re-entry, sick sinus syndrome, and sinus arrest. In all these conditions, the sinus node is the pacemaker of the heart, though its rate may be too fast, too slow, irregular, or inconsistent.

## SINUS TACHYCARDIA

In a patient with sinus tachycardia, there is regular sinus rhythm of more than 100 beats/min. It can be considered as one of the first signs of congestive heart failure, cardiogenic shock, pulmonary embolism, or infarct extension (Figs 20.5–20.7).

### ECG Characteristics

1. Rate : >100 beats/min
2. Rhythm : Regular
3. PR interval : Normal, although the PR may be too long or too short because of other conditions. All the P-waves have the same shape and are upright in leads I, II, aVF, and V4 to V6
4. QRS complex : Normal but may be prolonged due to other associated conditions

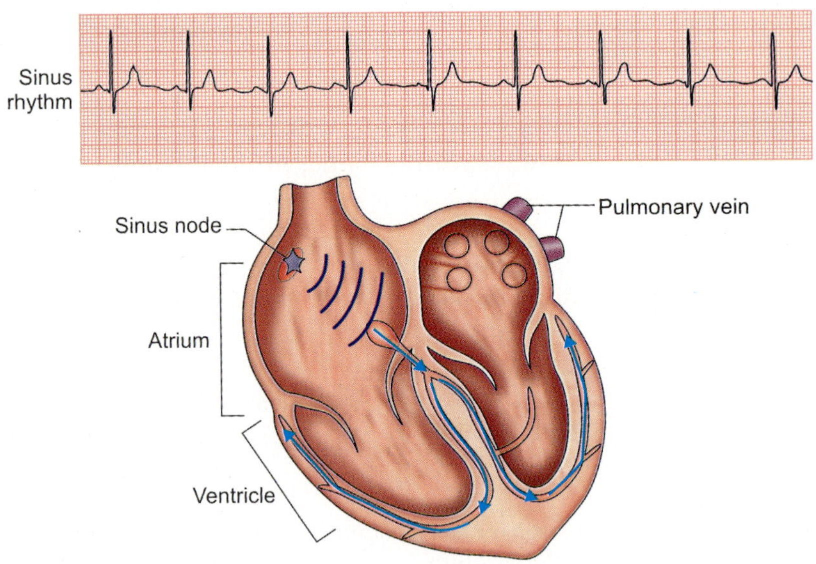


**Fig. 20.5:** This illustration shows the normal pathway through which electric activities needed for cardiac excitation (impulse conduction pathway) are transmitted. First generated at the site called the sinus node in the atrium, the electric impulse is transmitted via the atrioventricular node to the ventricle, which causes the ventricular contraction to pump blood to the entire body

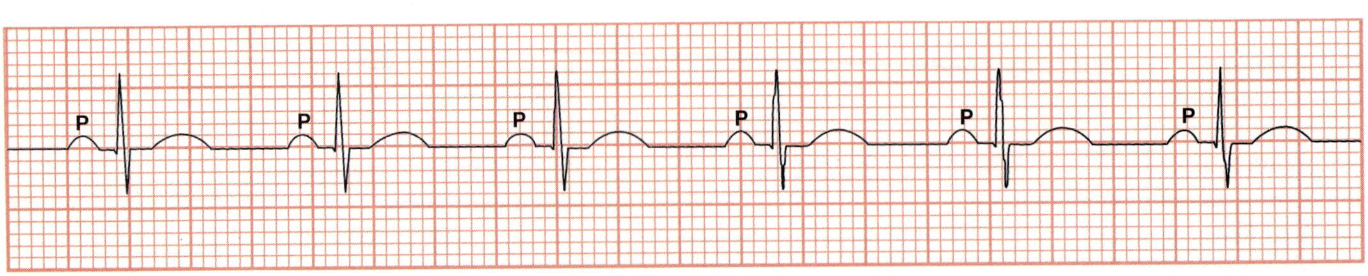


**Fig. 20.6:** ECG trace showing normal sinus rhythm. Each narrow complex is preceded by a normal P-wave

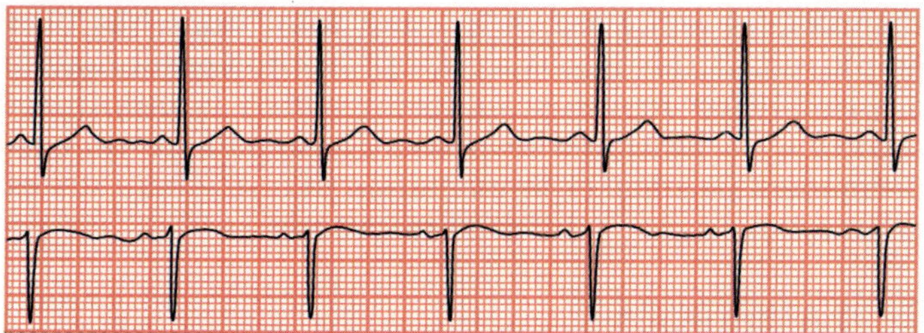

| Heart rate | Rhythm | P-wave | PR interval (in seconds) | QRS (in seconds) |
|---|---|---|---|---|
| 60–100 bpm | Regular | Before each QRS, identical | .12 to .20 | <.12 |

**Fig. 20.7:** ECG trace showing sinus tachycardia above and its markers at bottom end

### Causes

1. Drug
   i. Atropine,
   ii. Isoproterenol (isuprel),
   iii. Quinidine,
   iv. Epinephrine (adrenalin)
2. Exercise, emotions, fever or pain
3. Hyperthyroidism
4. Conditions involving increased sympathetic stimulation.

Sinus tachycardias vary only if they are part of a bradycardia-tachycardia syndrome or because of associated conditions, such as AV block, bundle-branch block, PVCs, or PACs.

The diagnosis of sinus tachycardia is always made by identifying uniform P-wave with regular rhythm.

### Treatment of Sinus Tachycardia

The basic treatment is of the underlying cause. Beta-blockers will slow down the rate. Sinus tachycardia caused by thyrotoxicosis will respond to beta-blockers; on the other hand. Sinus tachycardia resulting from left ventricular dysfunction, usually, should not be treated with beta-blockers as these drugs may precipitate heart failure.

## SINUS BRADYCARDIA

Sinus bradycardia can be diagnosed both clinically and electrocardiographically when the peripheral pulse is of regular rhythm with heart rate less than 60 beats/min, and has regular sinus rhythm character (Fig. 20.8 and Table 20.3).

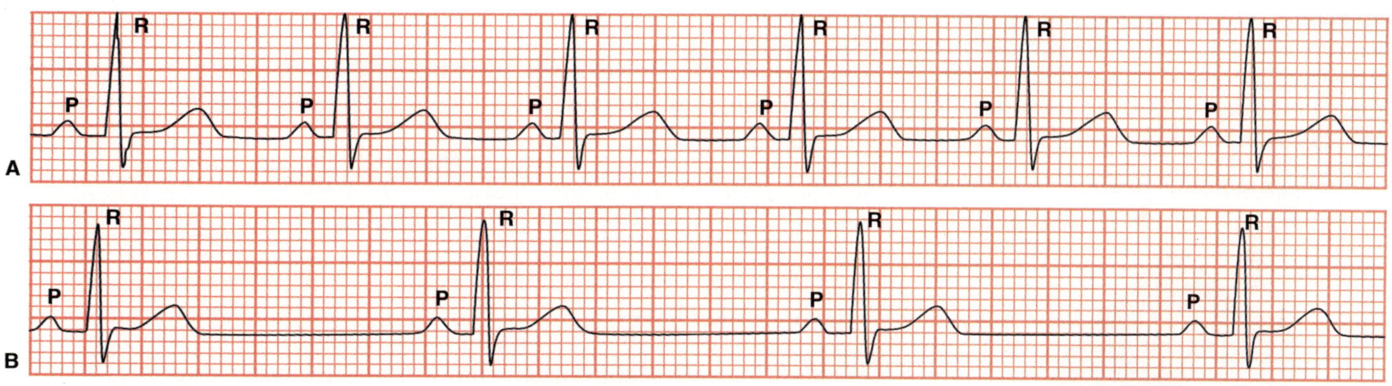


**Fig. 20.8:** The EKG shows normal sinus rhythm (A) and sinus bradycardia (B) with heart rate less than 60 beats/min

**Table 20.3:** Differential diagnosis in bradyarrhythmias (ventricular rate less than 60)

| Nature of defect | Ventricular | A-V relationship | Atrial rate | Additional clues |
|---|---|---|---|---|
| 1. Sinus bradycardia | Less than 60 | Normal (1:1) | Less than 60 | May be sinus arrhythmia |
| 2. Sinus arrest | Less than 60 | May be nodal or ventricular | Less than 60; abrupt | none halving of atrial rate |
| 3. AV-nodal rhythm | Less than 60 | Short P-R or P-wave buried in QRS or superimposed on S-T segment | Less than 60 | Normal QRS complexes-P waves may be hard to see |
| 4. Wenekebach block | Less than atrial rate | P-R interval lengthens with successive beats until QRS is is dropped. The cycle is repeated | Normal; usually over 60 | QRS complexes often in pairs or triplets |
| 5. Second degreee block | Usually 30–50; (1/2, 1/3) | 2:1 AV block or greater (3:1, 4:1, etc.) | Normal; usually over 60 | P-waves never occur in QRS complexes |
| 6. Third degree (complete block) | Regular 30–50 (no P-QRS relationship) | A-V dissociation | Normal; usually over 60 | P-waves from time to time in QRS complexes |

### ECG Characteristics

1. Rate : <60 beats/min
2. Rhythm : Regular
3. PR interval : Normal, although the PR may be too long or too short because of other conditions. All the P-waves have the same shape and are upright in leads I, II, aVF, and V4 to V6
4. QRS complex : Normal, although the QRS may be prolonged as a result of other associated conditions.

### Causes

1. During fast sleep
2. Cardiac response in atheletes
3. Increased vagal tone
4. Therapy with beta-adrenergic drugs

Sinus bradycardias vary only if they are part of a bradycardia-tachycardia or because of associated conditions, such as AV block, bundle-branch block, PVCs, or PACs. The diagnosis of sinus bradycardia is always established by looking at the underlying rhythm.

### Treatment of Sinus Bradycardia

It is treated only if the patient is symptomatic or if the condition is associated with hemodynamic deterioration and marked decrease in cardiac output. Acute treatment in the sick sinus syndrome includes 0.5 mg of atropine sulfate IV, administered every 5 minutes until the desired response is achieved or a 2 mg total does has been employed. If this is unsuccessful, isoproterenol may be administered in infusion form, which is monitored according to heart and response. These patients do need permanent pacemaker implantation in case where stokes-adams attacks are manifested frequently.

## SINUS ARRHYTHMIA

Sinus arrhythmia can be diagnosed by an irregular sinus rhythm in which the cycles lengths vary so that the difference between the shortest PP interval and the longest PP interval is 0.12 sec (Fig. 20.9).

### ECG Characteristics

1. Rate : It varies with respiration: faster with inspiration-slower with expiration
2. Rhythm : Irregular
3. PR interval : Normal, although the PR may be too long or too short because of other conditions. All the P-waves have the same shape and are upright in leads. I, II, aVF, and V4 to V 6
4. QRS complex : Normal, although the QRS may be prolonged as a result of other conditions.

It can be isolated from other conditions by the presence of varying rate, cyclical, irregular rhythm, and uniform shape of the P-waves.

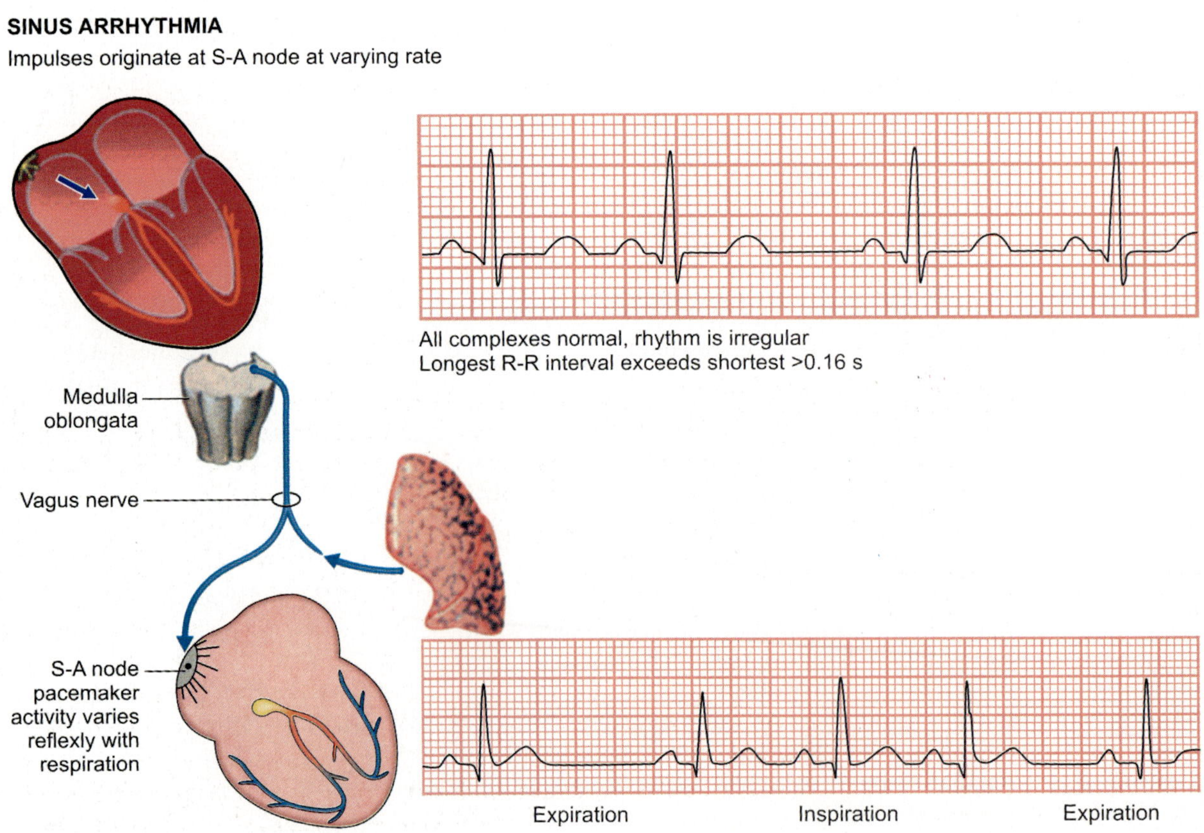


**Fig. 20.9:** Lead II showing normal sinus rhythm with sinus arrhythmia in a healthy person. Note the marked variation in the P-P intervals induced by respiration

### Causes

**Normal respiratory pattern:** Sinus arrhythmia can be differentiated from SA nodal re-entry due to the presence of transition with abrupt faster rate which is, usually, not related to respiration although P-waves may remain of similar morphology in both the conditions.

## SA BLOCK

SA block is characterized by the absence of P-waves, intermittently, due to incomplete conduction of sinus P-waves as they emerge from the sinus pacemaker (Fig. 20.10).

### ECG Characteristics

1. Rate : Normal, but varies because of pauses.
2. Rhythm : Irregular
3. PR interval : Normal, although the PR may too long or too short because of other conditions. All the P-waves have the same shape and upright in leads I,II, aVF, and V4 to V6
4. QRS complex : Normal, although the QRS may be prolonged as a result of other conditions.

### Causes

1. Acute infection
2. Digitalis, quinidine, or salicylates
3. Carotid sinus sensitivity and increased vagal tone.
4. Coronary artery disease.

### Distinguishing Features

**Type-I (wenchebach) SA block:** PP intervals shorten until a P-wave is dropped; pauses are less than twice the shortest cycle.

**Type-II SA block:** PP intervals are an exact multiple of the sinus cycle and are regular, before and after the dropped P-wave.

*Differential Diagnosis:* Nonconducted PACs are far more common and should be suspected first. Usually, the P-wave can be seen distorting the T-wave before the pause. The diagnosis of sinus arrest can be made after ruling out nonconducted PACs and SA block.

## SINUS ARREST

Sinus arrest may be defined as that condition in which the sinus impulses are not generated, with the result that one

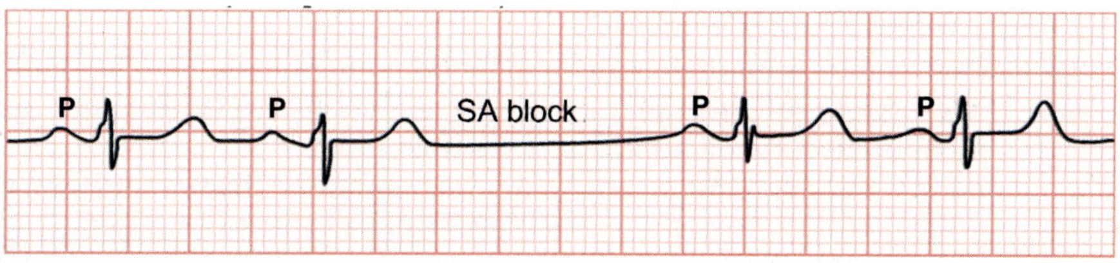


**Fig. 20.10:** SA block. The basic rhythm is regular. The length of the pause is not a multiple of the sinus interval

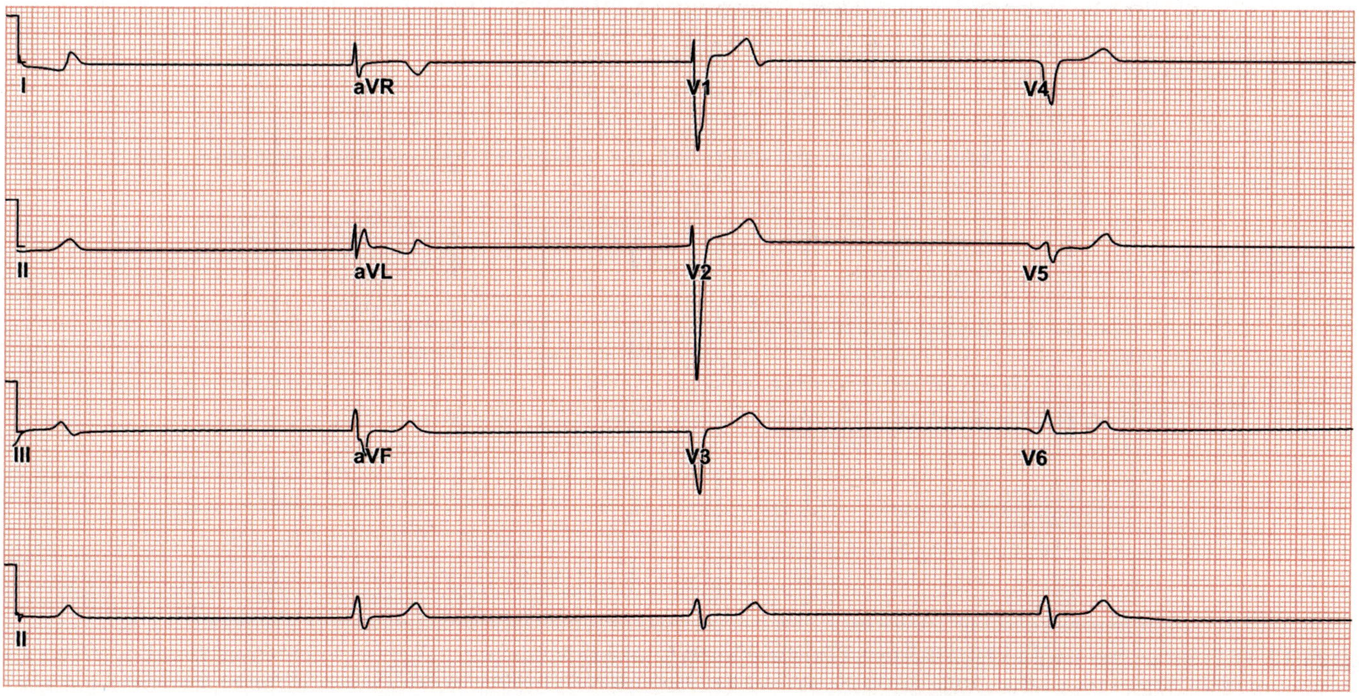


**Fig. 20.11:** Sinus arrest with a ventricular escape rhythm

may find occasional absent P-waves. In case this type of rhythm persists, it may lead to atrial standstill (Fig. 20.11).

### ECG Characteristics

1. Rate : Normal, but varies because of pauses.
2. Rhythm : Irregular
3. PR interval : Normal, althought the PR may be too long or too short as a result of other conditions. All the P-waves have the same shape and are upright in leads I, II, aVF, and V4 to V6.
4. QRS complex : Normal, although the QRS may be prolonged. Because of other conditions.
5. Distinguishing features : Abrupt interruption of the sinus rhythm. PP interval of the pause is not a multiple of the sinus cycle.

### Causes

1. Digitalis, quinidine, or salicylates
2. Coronary artery disease
3. Acute infection
4. Carotid sinus sensitivity and increased vagal tone.

### Differential Diagnosis

Nonconducted PACs are far common and are always suspected first. Usually, the P-wave can be seen distorting the T-wave before the pause.The diagnosis of sinus arrest can be made after ruling out nonconducted PACs and SA block.

## SICK SINUS SYNDROME

Sick sinus syndrome may be defined clinically by the presence of near syncope, syncope, convulsions, fatigue, angina pectoris and other symptoms of hypoperfusion of the brain and electrocardiographic manifestations of bradycardia and tachycardia along with other features of cardiac arrhythmia due to sinus node dysfunction and failure of an adequate escape pacemaker (Fig. 20.12).

### ECG Characteristics

1. Rate : Too fast or too slow
2. Rhythm : Irregular
3. PR interval : May be abnormal
4. QRS complex : Normal, although the QRS may be prolonged because of other conditions.

### Distinguishing Features

Any of the following arrhythmias may be present and associated with syncope:

1. Severe sinus bradycardia
2. Sinu arrest
3. Atrial stand still
4. SA block
5. Sinus bradycardia with recurring atrial fibrillation
6. Bradycardia-tachycardia
7. Temporary asystole following tachycardia or following electrical cardioversion of atrial tachyarrhythmia
8. Paroxysmal atrial fibrillation
9. Failure of the sinus node to accelerate in response to fever or exercise.

### Causes

1. Ischemic disease due to obstructive blood supply to the sinus node
2. Inflammatory disease of sinus node
3. Amyloidosis: Infilteration of the sinus node with amlyoid material
4. Collagen disease
5. Metastatic disease
6. Surgical injury
7. Idiopathic

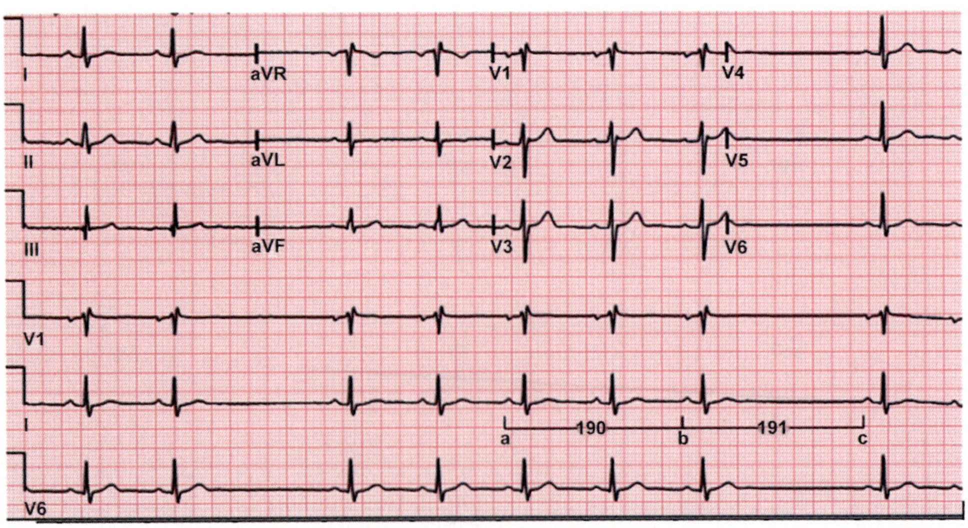


**Fig. 20.12:** ECG shows the irregularity of the QRS complexes with changing rates and the changing P-waves in sick sinus syndrome, a pattern of atrial dysbalance, which can be of the slow or the fast type. The conduction velocity is different from beat-to-beat and there are blocked actions with sinus pauses

### Variations

There are many variations among which are:

1. SSS with type II second-degree SA block
2. SSS in the form of a bradycardia- tachycardia syndrome
3. SSS with inappropriate overdrive suppression following an early PAC (in the T-wave before the pause)

### Treatment

Before a pacemaker is inserted, ensure that no drugs have been given at all for several days; the arrhythmia may be drug related.

## PAROXYSMAL SINUS TACHYCARDIA RESULTING FROM NODAL RE-ENTRY

Paroxysmal sinus tachycardia is the sudden onset of the sinus tachycardia (Fig. 20.13).

### ECG Characteristics

1. Rate : Too fast
2. Rhythm : Irregular
3. PR interval : Normal although the PR may be too long or too short because of other conditions. All the P-waves have the same shape and are upright in leads I, II, aVF, and V4 to V6
4. QRS complex : Normal, although the QRS may be prolonged as a result of other conditions.
5. Distinguishing features :
   a. Heart rate suddenly accelerates; tachycardia ends abruptly
   b. Rhythm of the tachycardia, usually, regular
   c. Normal sinus P-waves.

### Causes

1. Ischemia
2. Cardiomyopathy.

### Differential Diagnosis

Sinus arrhythmia

### Treatment

Short paroxysms may require no treatment.

1. Termination may, often be achieved by vagal manoeuvres, but carotra artery message should not be advised in patients with or at risk for carotid artery disease
2. Intravenous verapamil is considered by some to be treatment of choice, but should be used cautiously in those patients who had poor left ventricular functions.
3. Digitalis and beta-blockers, which prolong AV nodal conduction and refractoriness in both alpha and beta-pathways are usually, effective.
4. Type IA antiarrhythmic agents may be useful.
5. Oral diltizaem, 90 mg 3 times a day, may be effective in preventing recurrence.

In situations where one can find severe hemodynamic disturbances, direct synchronous cardioversion, using 40/w/s, is, often, quite contributory.

## SUPRAVENTRICULAR ARRHYTHMIA (Figs 20.14–20.23 and Table 20.4)

1. Premature atrial contraction (PAC)
2. Atrial flutter
3. Atrial fibrillation
4. Atrial tachycardia

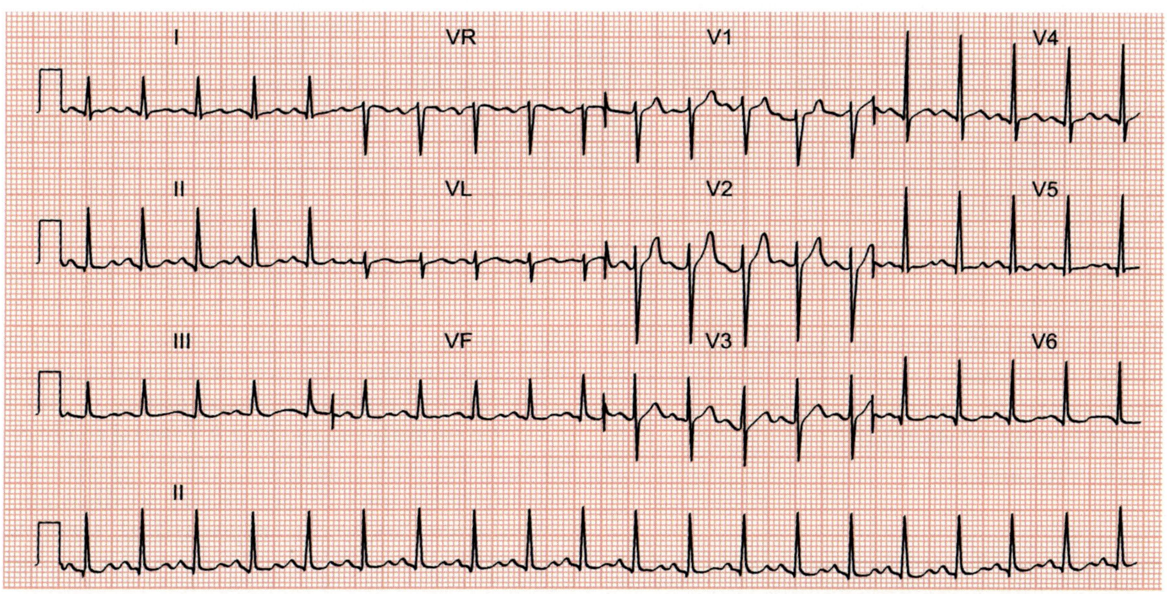


**Fig. 20.13:** ECG trace showing features of sinus tachycardia with heart rate more than 150 beat/min

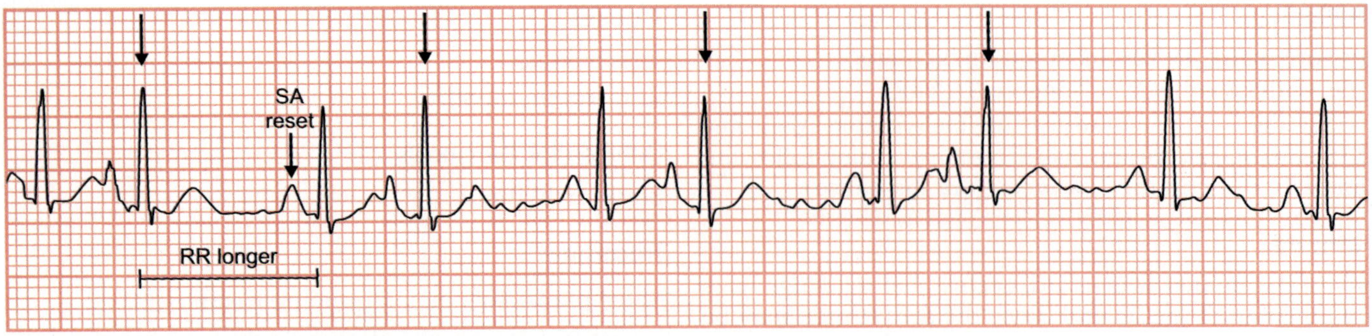


**Fig. 20.14:** This rhythm strip displays the typical pattern of frequent PACs (arrows) separated by postextrasystolic pauses

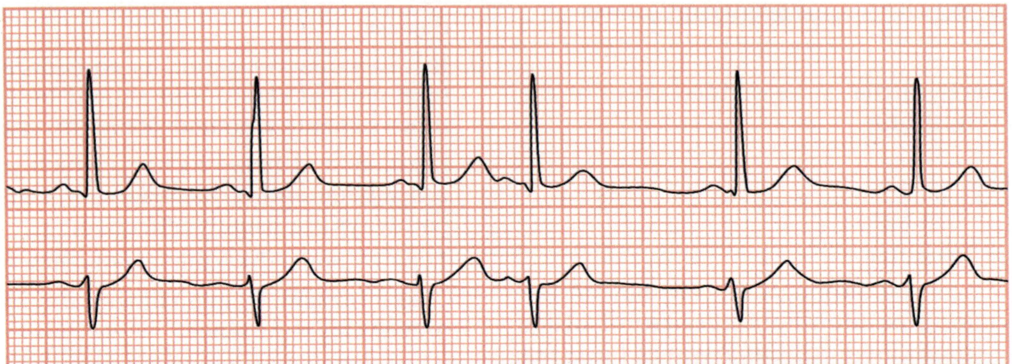

| Heart rate | Rhythm | P-wave | PR interval (in seconds) | QRS (in seconds) |
|---|---|---|---|---|
| N/A | Irregular | Premature and abnormal or hidden | <.20 | <.12 |

**Fig. 20.15:** Premature atrial contraction with pause

**Table 20.4:** Differential diagnosis in atrial ectopic tachycardia and PSVT

| | Atrial ectopic tachycardia | PSVT (AV nodal re-entry) | Sinus tachycardia |
|---|---|---|---|
| 1. P-waves | Visible | Usually, buried within QRS complex; may distort V1 patterns (pseudo RBBB) | Visible |
| | + in II, III and aVF (digitalis toxicity) | Retrograde (negative in II, III and aVF) | Normal |
| 2. Rate | Gradually incareases (warm-up) | Begins abruptly and remains the same; ends abruptly | Gradually incareases; gradually decreases |
| 3. P-R interval | Normal | Long (first one) | |

5. Atrial fusion
6. Atrial parasystole
7. Paraxysmal supraventricular tachycardia (PSVT)
8. Wandering pacemaker
9. Premature junctional contraction (PJC).
10. Accelerated junctional rhythm.
11. Junctional tachycardia.

## Mechanism

Cardiac arrhythmia, which usually, has it origin outside the sinus node and above the branching portion of the bundle of His, can be called as supraventricular arrhythmia, manifesting, initially, as ectopic(s). They may be either abnormal premature mechanisms or normal escape mechanisms, occurring in response to an abnormality in the sinus node. The two most common mechanisms involved are enhanced automaticity in the atria or AV junction (bundle of His) and AV nodal re-entry or re-entry, using an accessory pathway (WPW syndrome). Enhanced automaticity may be secondary to digitalis, electrolyte imbalance, hypoxia, myocardial stretch, or acute myocardial infarction, and may result in single PACs or PJCs, ectopic atrial tachycardia, accelerated junctional rhythm, or junctional tachycardia.

**Premature atrial contraction: aberrantly conducted PAC: QRS is Bizarre**

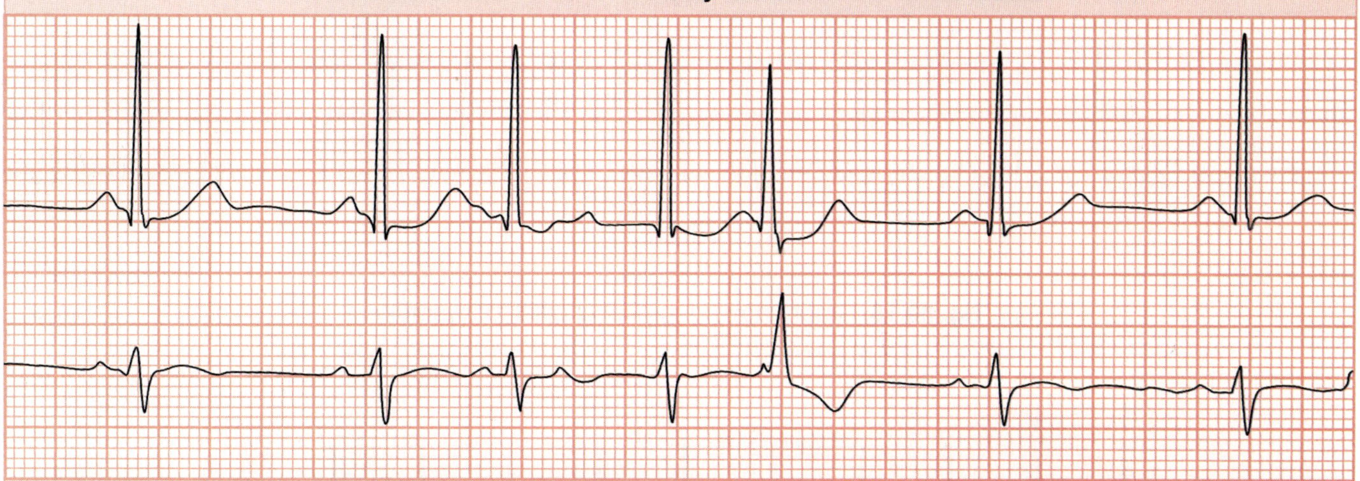

| Heart rate | Rhythm | P-wave | PR interval (in seconds) | QRS (in seconds) |
|---|---|---|---|---|
| N/A | Irregular | Premature and abnormal or hidden | <.20 | <.12 abnormal shape |

**Fig. 20.16:** PAC with RBBB aberrant conduction

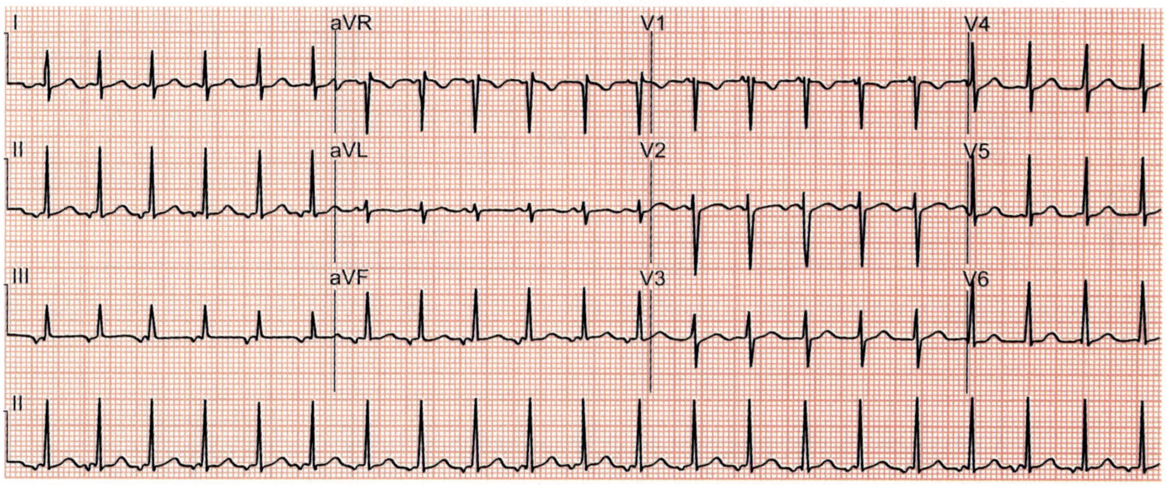


**Fig. 20.17:** ECG trace showing atrial tachycardia with 2.1 conduction with heart rate more than 120 bpm. Each QRS complex is preceded by an abnormal P-wave, upright in V1, inverted in the inferior leads II, III and aVF

An AV nodal re-entry mechanism may be initiated by a single premature atrial, junctional, or ventricular complex, resulting in paroxysmal supraventricular tachycardia (PSVT).

## PREMATURE ATRIAL ECTOPICS (PAC)

PACs are premature atrial beats that originate outside the sinus node. The resulting ECG deflection is called a P′ (P prime) wave.

### Pathophysiology and Mechanism

PACs are a result of enhanced automaticity or after depolarizations. The mechanisms of AV conduction and compensatory pauses, following PACs are described here.

**AV conduction.** The PAC may be so premature that it is not conducted at all, because both bundle branches are refractory or, it may be conducted down only one bundle branch and be blocked in the other (aberrant ventricular conduction).

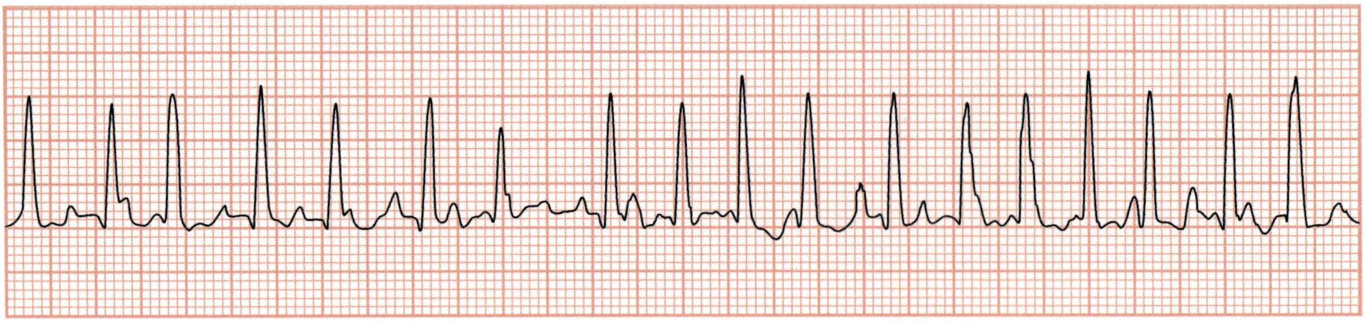

**Fig. 20.18:** Graph showing multifocal atrial tachycardia

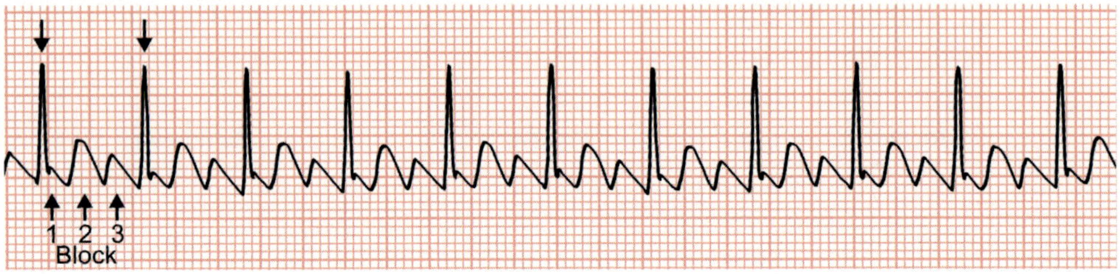


**Fig. 20.19:** Atrial flutter. Narrow QRS complexes are associated with regular flutter waves (arrows)

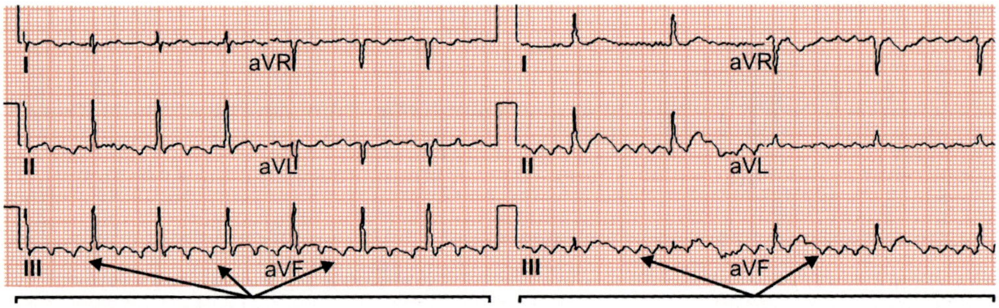


**Fig. 20.20:** Atrial flutter with negative flutter waves in leads II and III (left panel) and positive flutter waves (right panel)

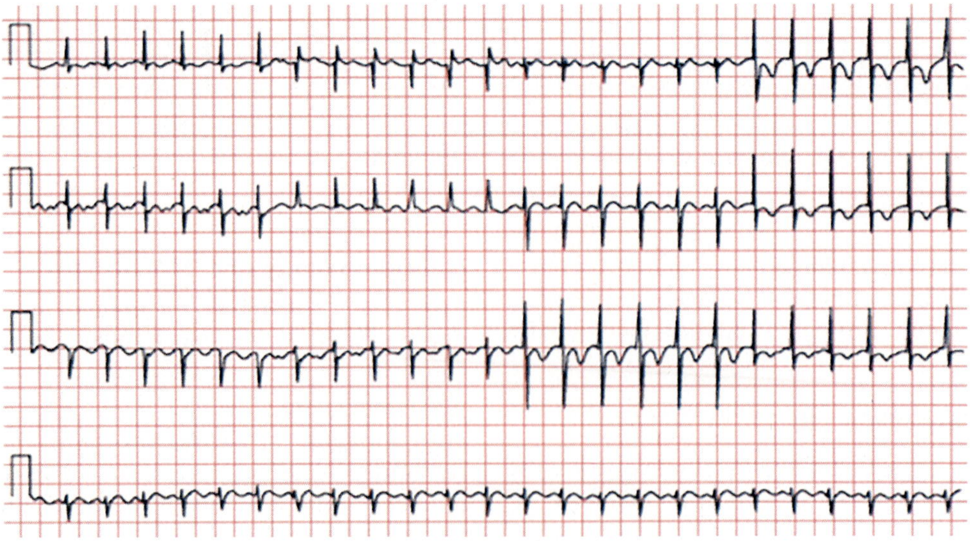

**Fig. 20.21:** Atrial flutter (heart rate >300 bpm) with regular R-R interval

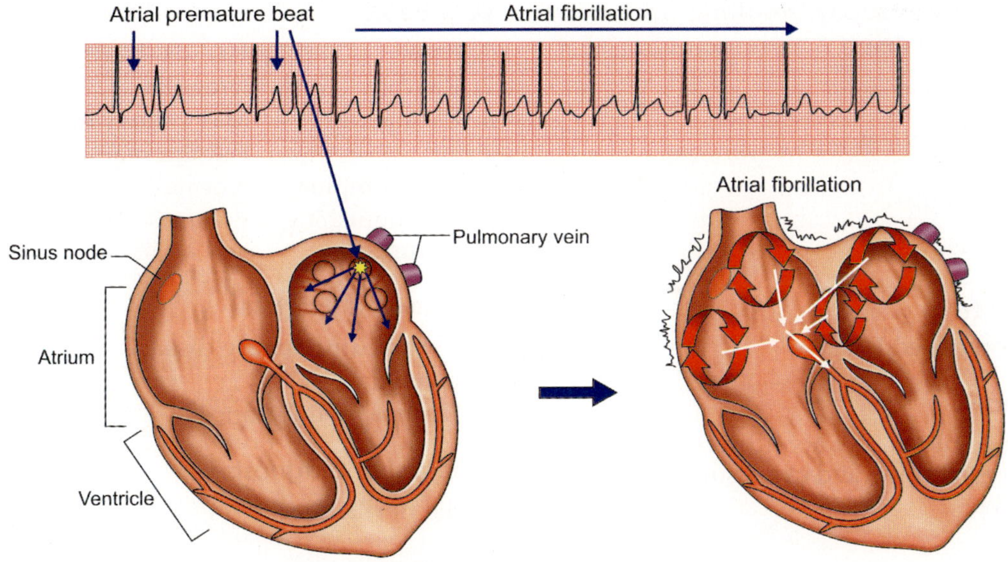


**Fig. 20.22:** Mechanism of onset of atrial fibrillation

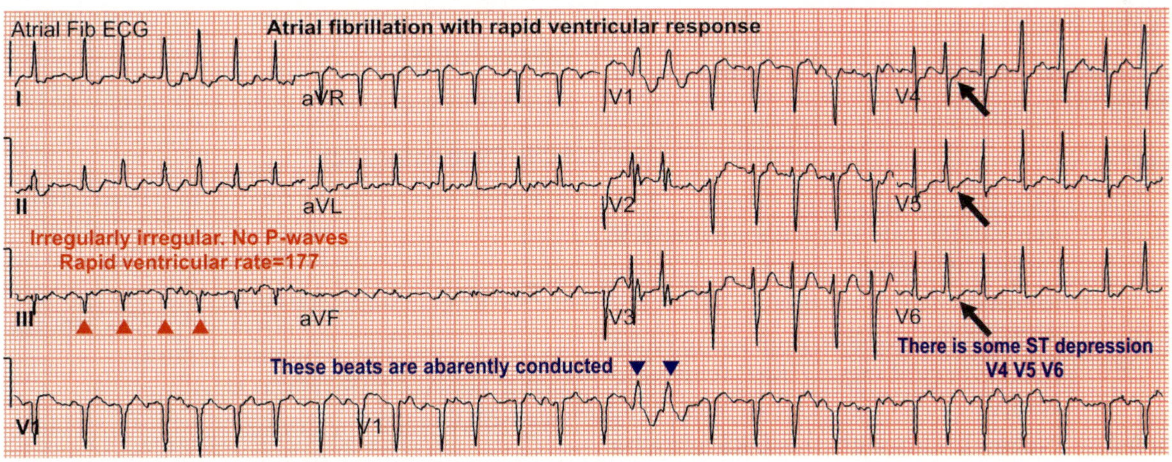


**Fig. 20.23:** Various ECG diagnostic features of atrial fibrillation

**Less-than-full compensatory pause.** The PAC resets the SA node, causing the next expected sinus P-wave to be on time if measured from the PAC, but earlier than it would have if the sinus node had not been disturbed.

**Full or more-than- full compensatory pause.** The PAC may suppress the SA node (overdrive suppression) and cause the next few sinus cycles to lengthen.

### ECG Characteristics

1. Rate : That of the underlying rhythm
2. Rhythm : Irregular, resulting from PACs (underlying rhythm may be regular)
3. PR interval : Normal, although the PR interval may be too long or too short because of other conditions. All the P-waves have the same shape and upright in leads I,II, aVF, and V4 to V6 (the P-R interval may be the same, longer, or shorter than the PR interval, or the P-wave may not be conducted to the ventricles (a blocked PAC).
4. QRS complex : Normal, although the QRS may be prolonged as a result of aberrancy or other conditions
5. Distinguishing features : Normal QRS and a P-wave that is premature and different in shape from the sinus P-wave.

### Aetiological Factors

1. Various stimuli—emotion, tobacco, or coffee
2. Congestive heart failure (in the setting of myocardial infarction).

3. Atrial dilation or hypertrophy, resulting from mitral stenosis or atrial septal defect
4. Electrolyte imbalance
5. Hypoxia
6. Digitalis toxicity

### Variations

1. PACs hidden in T-waves
2. Bigeminal PACs
3. Nonconducted PACs
4. Bigeminal nonconducted PACs.

### Differential Diagnosis

Sinus arrest or SA block. Nonconducted PACs are statistically far more common and can, usually, be stotted distorting the T-wave.

### Treatment

PACs are not treated, but in association with acute myocardial infarction, their cause is identified and treated.

## ATRIAL TACHYCARDIA

Atrial tachycardia is an ectopic atrial rhythm with a rate of 140–250 beats/min.

### ECG Features

| | | |
|---|---|---|
| 1. Rate | : | 140–250 beats/min (atrial). The ventricular rate depends on the AV conduction ratio |
| 2. Rhythm | : | Regular |
| 3. PR interval | : | Not applicable; P-R interval may be normal or prolonged. The P-waves are ectopic. |
| 4. QRS complex | : | Normal, although the QRS may be prolonged because of other conditions. |
| 5. Distinguishing features | : | Rate and AV conduction ratio, which is, usually, 2:1. In digitalis toxicity, the P-wave axis is, often, superior-inferior (positive in inferior leads), and often, in 2:1 block. The PP interval, across the QRS, is shorter than the one without a QRS (ventriculo-Phasic PP interval) |

### Causes

1. Digitalis toxicity
2. Heart disease.

### Variations

Atrial tachycardia with 4:1 AV conduction (other conduction ratios are also possible).

## CHAOTIC ATRIAL TACHYCARDIA (CAT)

Chaotic atrial tachycardia is a multifocal atrial tachycardia.

### ECG Features

| | | |
|---|---|---|
| 1. Rate | : | 100–250 beats/min. |
| 2. Rhythm | : | Irregular |
| 3. PR interval | : | May or may not be normal. P-R intervals may vary. |
| 4. QRS complex | : | Normal |
| 5. Distinguishing features | : | P-waves of several different shapes and an irregular rhythm. |

### Aetiological Factors

1. Chronic pulmonary disease
2. Hypoxia
3. Electrolyte imbalance

### Differential Diagnosis

Atrial fibrillation.

### Treatment

Verapamil is found to be effective but basic underlying cause/s, leading to such abnormality, is important to manage first.

## ATRIAL FLUTTER

Atrial flutter is a rapid atrial tachycardia of two types.

### ECG Characteristics

| | | |
|---|---|---|
| 1. Rate | : | Type-1 (classical). The atrial rate ranges from 230–250 beats/min Type-II. The range is 340–430 beats/min. |
| 2. Rhythm | : | Atrial rhythm is regular, ventricular rhythm depends on the AV conduction pattern. |
| 3. P-R interval | : | 0.26–0.46 sec |
| 4. QRS complex | : | Normal |
| 5. Distinguishing features | : | Regular sawtooth pattern in II, III, aVF sharp positive P-waves in V1. Normal QRS complexes AV conduction in 2:1 to 8:1 ratios. T-wave may distort the flutter pattern. |

### Causes

1. Any form of heart disease such as rheumatic heart disease, coronary artery disease, preexcitation syndrome etc.
2. Acute illness

### Variations

1. Varying degrees of AV conduction ratios
2. Atrial flutter with AV dissociation (an accelerated idioventricular rhythm).

### Differential Diagnosis

When the conduction ratio is 2:1, atrial flutter is, often, mistaken for sinus tachycardia of 140–175 beats/min. The ventricular rate makes one suspicious of a hidden flutter wave, and, usually, the onset of the R wave is distorted by the flutter wave.

### Treatment

1. The hemodynamic compromise is present due to a fast ventricular rate, direct synchronous cardioversion with 40–50 w/s should be administered.
2. Fast ventricular response rate can be controlled with digitalis. Propranolol or verapamil can also be used but are less effective. Normal rhythm can be achieved, usually, by the administration of these drugs.
3. Digoxin and verapamil should not be prescribed to patients with flutter associated with Wolff-Parkinson-White syndrome.
4. Reversion to sinus rhythm may also be, often, achieved with the use of a type IA antiarrhythmic agents.
5. A patient should not be administered quinidine until digitalization is achieved since quinidine may facilitate AV conduction. Procainamide may rarely increase the ventricular response to atrial flutter by slowing the flutter rate; the AV node may conduct every second atrial depolarization instead of every third, producing an increased ventricular rate.
6. Atrial flutter can be converted to sinus rhythm with temporary overdrive pacing. It is done by pacing 115–125% of the spontaneous atrial rate at a critical duration. Overdrive pacing can also be successful, utilizing a special esophageal electrode.
7. If an artial thrombus has been diagnosed by echocardiography, the patient should be given warfarin with the prothrombin time, 1.2–1.5 times of control, for 3 weeks. If there is an abnormal slow atrial flutter rate or a high degree of AV block when the patient is receiving no antiarrythmic agents, disease of the AV node should be suspected, and backup temporary pacing should be done till the rhythm is converted to normal rate response.

## ATRIAL FIBRILLATION

Atrial fibrillation (AF) is an ectopic atrial arrhythmia characterized by erratic depolarization of the atrial.

### Newer Classification of AF

Some of the workers have classified atrial fibrillation into three different types on electrophysiological studies. They observed that all patients had uniform conduction in the free wall of the right atrium, during sinus rhythm, rapid atrial pacing procedure.

**Type-I** seen in 40% of patients in whom there are uniform, single broad wave fronts that propagate through the atrial wall without significant conduction delay. There may be short areas of conduction block, small areas of slow conduction, that do not interfere with the main course of propagation. The cycle length is somewhat slow (median 174 ms), there is almost no re-entry, and no source of activation waves is visible, despite the persistence of atrial fibrillation.

**Type-II,** found in 32% of patients in which there is intermediate pattern, which describes either a single wave associated with major areas of conduction block and/or slow conduction or two wavelets, separated by a line of functional conduction block.

**Type-III** which manifests with a highly fragmented and complex pattern, seen in 28% of cases, and characterized by three or more wavelets, associated with lines of functional conduction block under the mapping electrode. This type of fibrillation is associated with a shorter cycle length (median interval, 136 ms) than type I and with a wide 100 ms variation in cycle length spanning very short and very long cycles. It may also be kept in mind that the three types of atrial fibrillation do not constitute three separate entities, but rather a continuous spectrum of increasing complexity.

### ECG Characteristics

1. Rate : Uncontrolled, 110–180 beats/min. controlled, 70–80 beats/min.
2. Rhythm : Irregular
3. PR interval : Absent P-waves
4. QRS complex : Normal
5. Distinguishing features : Absent P-waves and irregular ventricular response.

### Causes

i. Mitral valve disease
ii. Ischemic disease, particularly acute myocardial infarction.
iii. Hypertension
iv. Thyrotoxicosis
v. Increasing left-atrial size in elderly patients.
vi. Idiopathic (lone) type of atrial fibrillations.

### Variations

1. Coarse atrial fibrillation with signs of digitalis toxicity (regularization of the ventricular response)
2. Fine atrial fibrillation with uncontrolled ventricular response.
3. Atrial fibrillation with complete AV block
4. Atrial fibrillation with conduction over an accessory pathway.

### Treatment

1. Therapy with digoxin still remains the basic method of treatment of atrial fibrillation in controlling the ventricular response. Depending upon the clinical urgency and the ventricular rate, it may be given orally or intravenously. Digoxin is strongly contraindicated in atrial fibrillation with antegrade pre-excitation by an accessory pathway. Verapamil is also contraindicated in this situation
2. If severe hemodynamic compromise is present due to atrial fibrillation with a rapid ventricular response, synchronous cardioversion is considered. After cardio-

version, it may be helpful to administer digitalis and/or to start procainamide or quinidine to help maintain the patient in sinus rhythm.

3. In a stable patient, one should determine if the rhythm is acute or chronic and whether electrical cardioversion is required. The patient should be anticoagulated with warfrain for 3 weeks if the rhythm has been present for more than 2 days or if the duration is uncertain, prior to cardioversion. The prothrombin time should be 1.2 to 1.5 times of the control. While the patient is being anticoagulated, the ventricular response should be controlled with digitalis, at times, adding either beta-blockers or verapamil. The digoxin may be initated intravenously, and, when the ventricular rate is brought under check, it should be switched over to the oral medication. Acute short-term heparinization does not exclude the possibility of embolic episode, following cardioversion, and should not be employed. Quinidine or procainamide is, usually, started 24–48 hours to elective cardioversion. Occasionally, this will produce cardioversion, and usually, the medication should be continued after successful electrical cardioversion to prevent recurrence.
4. Long term administration of anticoagulation be considered in patients with chronic atrial fibrillation.
5. If atrial fibrillation is as short as 2–3 days' duration, medical cardioversion may be considered by administering 1–2 mg of digoxin over 24 hours. If the patient fails to achieve normal rhythm, procainamide or quinidine is added. A patient should be fully digitalized prior to starting quinidine which may increase the ventricular response.
6. Electrical cardioversion is usually, successful, but atrial fibrillation may return if the underlying cause is not removed. Quinidine or procainamide should be given, after cardioversion, to check further reoccurrence of atrial fibrillation.
7. Electrical or medical cardioversion should be avoided in sick sinus syndrome, if the ventricular rate is less than 80 beats per minute, or if digitalis toxicity is suspected. If necessary, such patients may be electively cardioverted, after a temporary pacing catheter is inserted, to avoid a bout of asystole.
8. Beta-blockers and diltiazem may show some therapeutic response on rare occasions when added to the therapeutic does of digioxin to control the ventricular rate in chronic atrial fibrillation.

## WANDERING PACEMAKER

It may be defined as that of atrial arrhythmia in which there is shifting of impulse formation from focus to focus within the atrial tissue virtually with every beat. Sinus beats may be interspersed throughout. P-waves are of many forms, and the cadence tends to be somewhat irregular. Ventricular complexes are without alteration (Fig. 20.24).

### ECG Characteristics

1. Rate : Normal or 50 beats/min
2. Rhythm : Slightly irregular
3. PR interval : Normal
4. QRS complex : Normal
5. Distinguishing features : A sinus rhythm that gives way to an ectopic atrial or junctional rhythm, often, with atrial beats at the transitions; there is retrograde conduction to the atria from junctional focus.

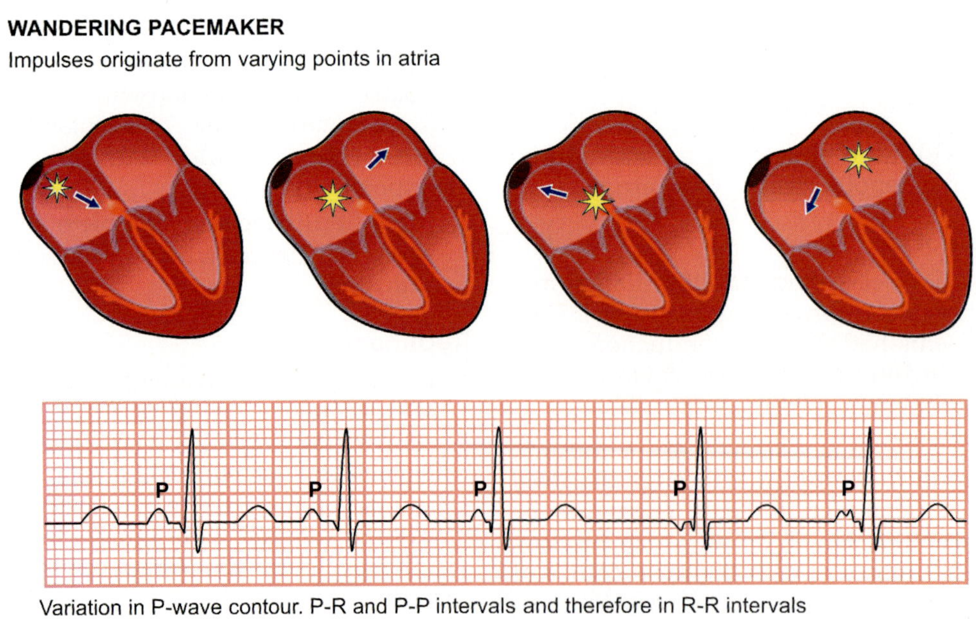


**Fig. 20.24:** Graph showing changing P-wave morphology between sinus node and atrioventricular junction in wandering pacemaker rhythm

Junctional rhythm

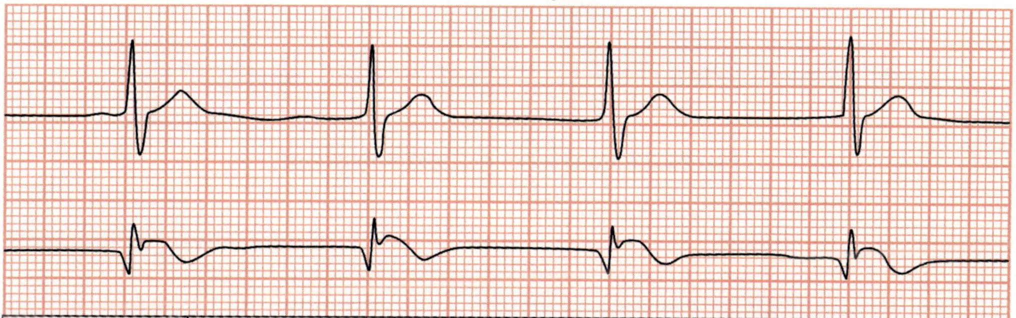

| Heart rate | Rhythm | P-wave | PR interval (in seconds) | QRS (in seconds) |
|---|---|---|---|---|
| 40–60 bpm | Regular | Inverted, absent or after QRS | <.12 | <.12 |

**Fig. 20.25:** Junctional escape rhythm. This is a sequence of 3 or more junctional escapes occurring by default at a rate of 40–60 bpm. There may be AV dissociation or the atria may be captured retrogradely by the junctional pacemaker. In the ECG example below the retrograde P-waves are not seen and must be hidden in the QRS the significant Q-wave with ST-elevation in the bottom strip suggests an acute MI

### Causes

1. It is associated with ischemic heart disease, involving the sinus node.
2. Acute rheumatic fever
3. Digitalis toxicity enhancing vagal tone.
4. Normal heart due to vagotonia.

### Variations

Normal sinus rhythm with an accelerated junctional or atrial rhythm.

### Treatment

If there is a normal escape mechanism, no treatment is indicated unless there is haemodynamic deterioration, and then, IV atropine may be appropriate, Ask the patient to cough; coughing decreases vagal tone and promotes the reappearance of the sinus rhythm. If the ectopic rhythm is enhanced, then the cause should be sought and treated.

## JUNCTIONAL ECTOPIC MECHANISMS: PREMATURE AND ESCAPE JUNCTIONAL BEATS

A junctional beat takes its origin from the bundle of His and may be either premature or escape, and it may or may not follow retrograde conduction to the atria (Figs 20.25–20.35).

### ECG Characteristics

1. Rate : It is of the underlying rhythm
2. Rhythm : Irregular as a result of the premature and escape junctional beats (PJCs) (underlying rhythm may be regular)
3. PR interval : Normal in the underlying sinus rhythm. The P-wave associated with the junctional beat may be absent if there is no retrograde conduction to the atria. If present, it is negative in II, III and aVF, and may appear before, during or after the QRS complex.
4. QRS complex : It is normal although it may be prolonged due to other conditions.

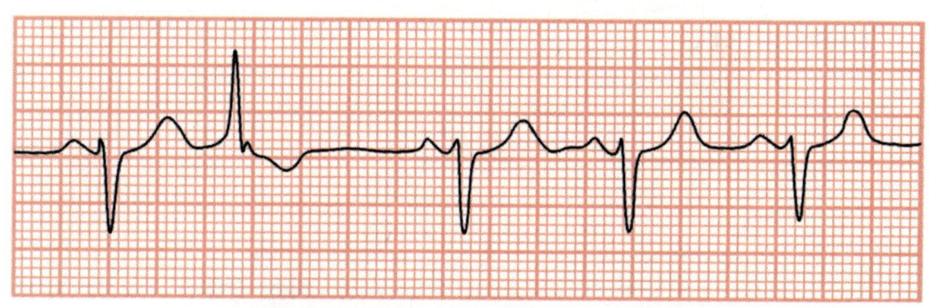

**Fig. 20.26:** Junctional ectopic

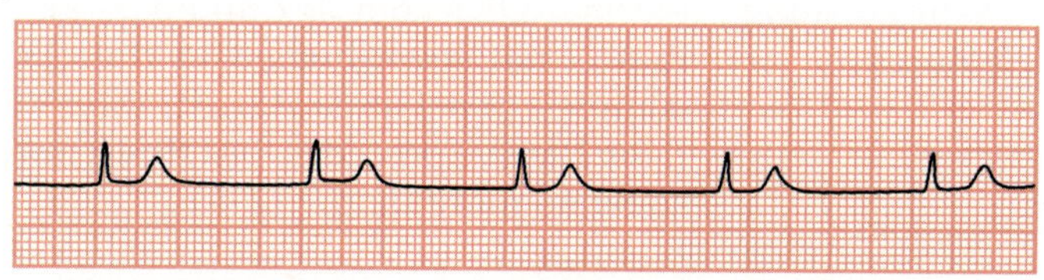

**Fig. 20.27:** Atrioventricular junctional rhythm with P-waves buried in QRST complex

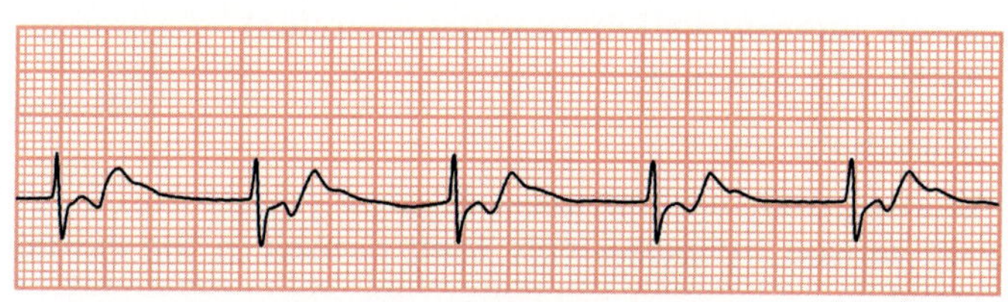

**Fig. 20.28:** Atrioventricular junctional rhythm with P-waves follow the QRS complexes and distorts ST-segment

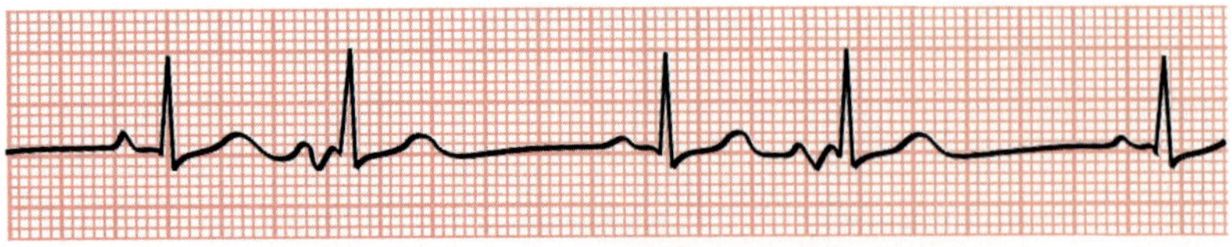

Fig. 20.29: Junctional ectopic with pause

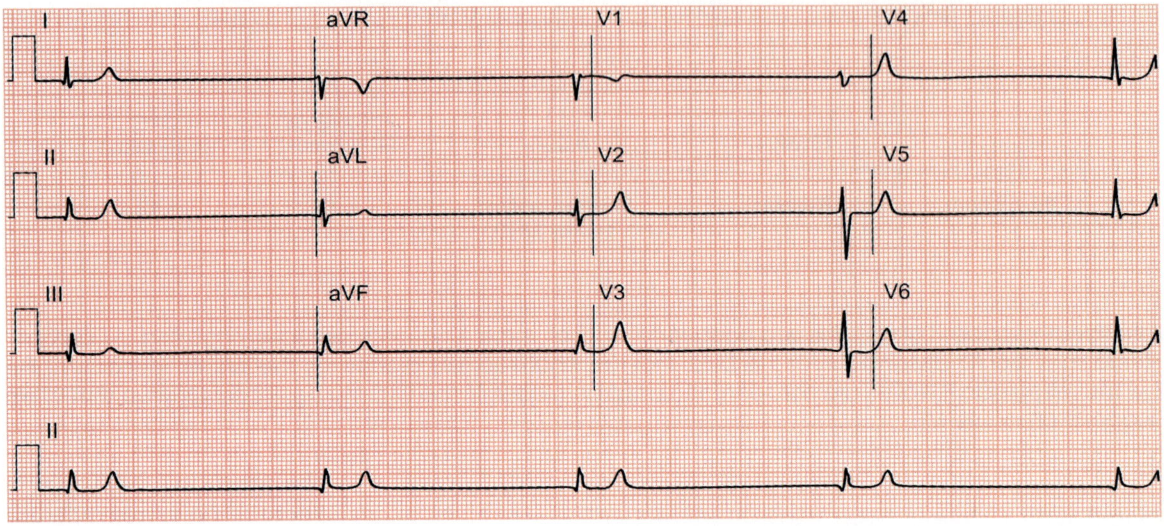


Fig. 20.30: ECG showing a junctional bradycardia with wide QRS, deep anterior Q-waves and tall anterior T-waves

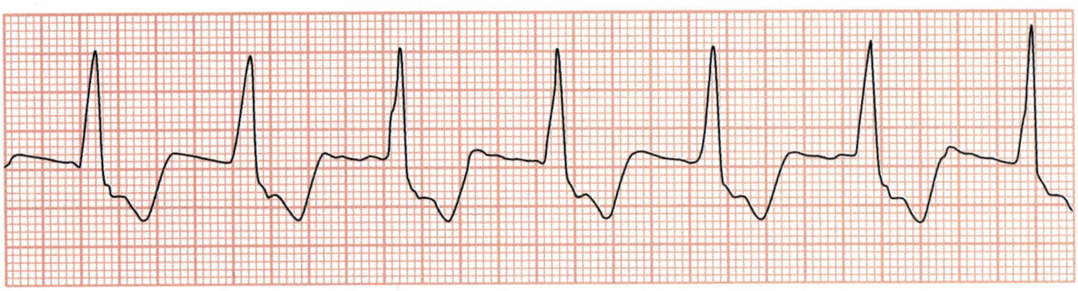

Fig. 20.31: Accelerated Idiojunctional rhythm

5. Distinguishing features : Normal QRS complex and a P-wave that is not seen, buried in the QRS complex, or negative in II, III, and aVF. If the P-wave precedes the QRS, it does so by no more than 0.12 sec.

### Aetiological Factors

1. Digitalis
2. Acute inferior-wall myocardial infarction
3. Tricuspid prosthesis
4. Rheumatic fever
5. Distinguishing features: Escape junctional beats are caused by excessively long pauses in the cardiac cycle.

### Variations

1. Premature junctional contraction (PJC) with the P receding the QRS complex
2. PJC with the P hidden in the QRS complex.
3. PJC with the P following the QRS complex.

### Treatment

Normally, PJCs are not treated, but if their cause is identified, these should be, appropriately treated.

## ACCELERATED IDIOJUNCTIONAL RHYTHM

It may be defined as that ectopic rhythm which originates from the bundle of His and monitors the ventricles at a rate of 60–100 beats/min. when the rate exceeds 100 beats/min, it is called junctional tachycardia.

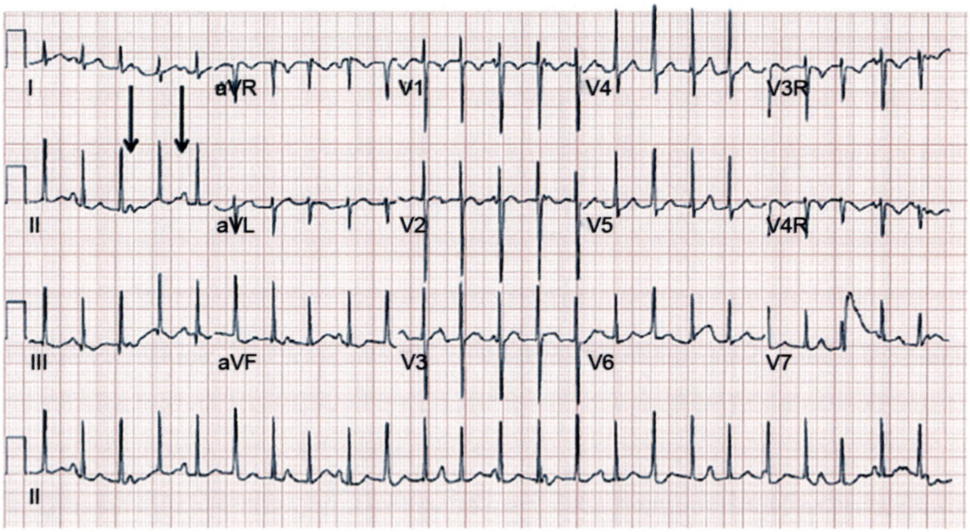


**Fig. 20.32:** Junctional ectopic tachycardia. ECG of 5-year-old girl with junctional ectopic tachycardia. Arrows denote P-waves with atrial rate of 100 bpm. Narrow QRS complexes originating from the AV junction occur at the rate of 144 bpm. There is AV dissociation with a faster junctional than atrial rate

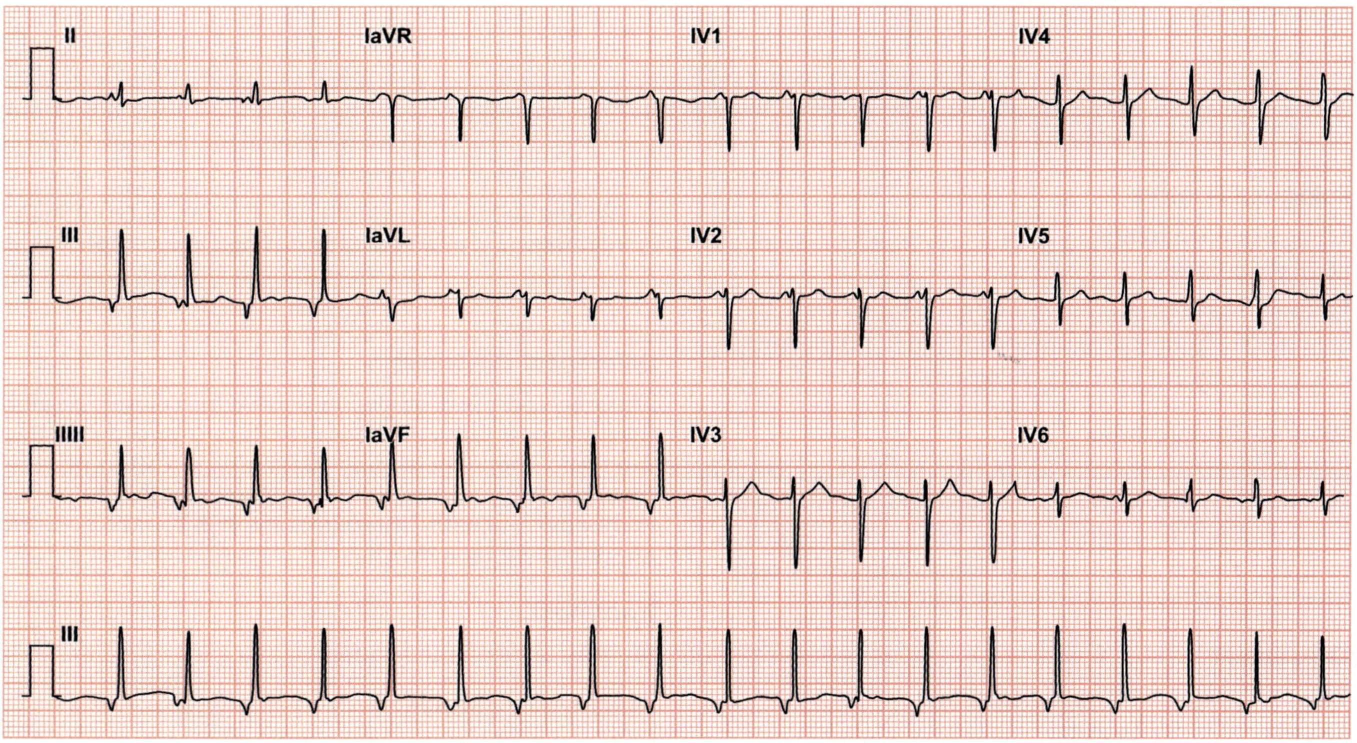


**Fig. 20.33:** Accelerated junctional rhythm. Narrow complex tachycardia at 115 bpm. Retrograde P-waves, inverted in II, III and aVF; upright in V1 and aVR. Short PR interval (<120 ms) indicates a junctional rather than atrial focus

## ECG Features

1. Rate : 60–100 beats/min
2. Rhythm : Regular
3. PR interval : Normal in the underlying sinus rhythm. When the junctional focus begins to take over. The PR interval may appear to shorten. However. When this happens, there is no relationship between the P-wave and the QRS complex (AV dissociation).
4. QRS complex : Normal, although the QRS complex may be prolonged as a result of other conditions.
5. Distinguish features : A junctional rhythm reveals itself when its rate is about the same as that of the sinus node. Resulting in AV

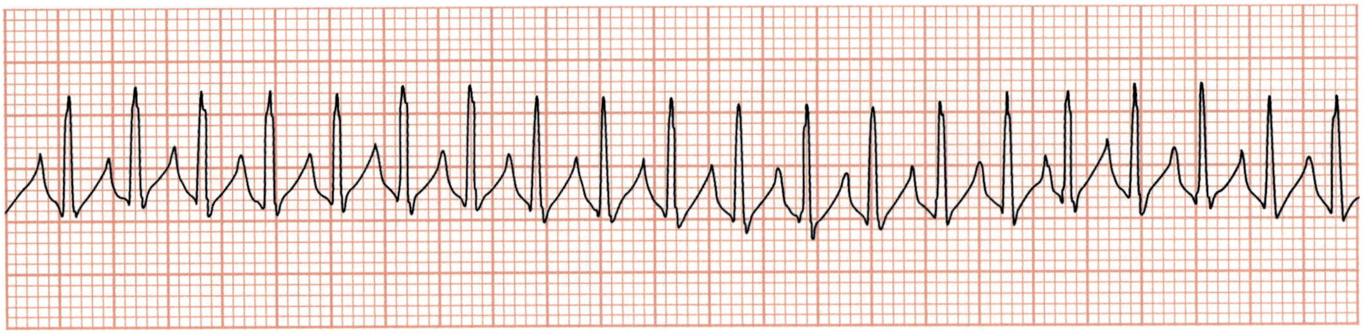

**Fig. 20.34:** ECG trace showing junctional tachycardia. Narrow QRS complexes with no visible P-waves

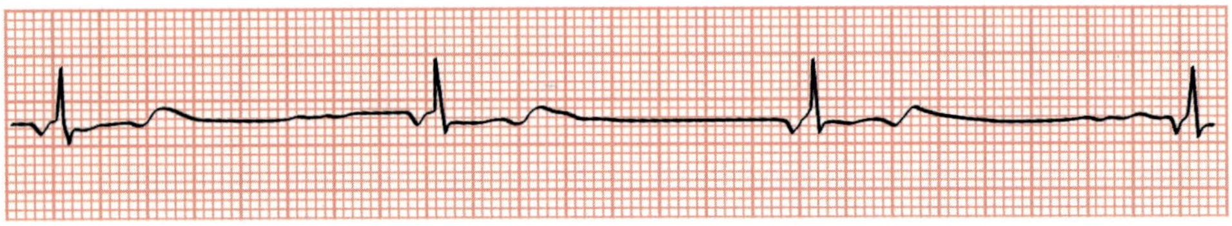

**Fig. 20.35:** ECG trace showing features of junctional escape rhythm

dissociation. P-waves get closer and closer to the QRS complex as the rate of the junctional focus exceeds that of the sinus node.

### Aetiological Factors

1. Myocardial infarction
2. Digitalis toxicity.

**Treatment:** No treatment is advisable unless it is associated with hemodynamic disturbances when 0.5–1.0 mg atropine I/V may be required for the treatment.

### Junctional Tachycardia

This kind of ectopic rhythm is produced as a result of focus, with enhanced automaticity, lying in the bundle of His, and controlling the ventricles at a rate of 100–130 beats/min. if the rate is less than 100 beats/min, it is termed accelerated junctional or idiojunctional rhythm.

### ECG Features

1. Rate : 100–130 beats/min
2. Rhythm : Regular
3. PR interval : When the junctional focus begins to take over. The PR interval may appear to shorten; however, when this happens, there is no relationship between the P and the QRS complex (AV dissociation). The P-wave will be absent if there is no retrograde conduction to the atria; if present, it is negative in II, III, and aVF and may be before. During, or after the QRS complex depending on the relative speed of anterograde and retrograde conduction and the location of the ectopic focus in the bundle of His.
4. QRS complex : Normal, although the QRS complex may be prolonged as a result of other conditions.
5. Distinguishing features : A junctional rhythm of more than 100 beats/min. The QRS complex will be narrow if there is no associated intraventricular conduction problem.

### Differential Diagnosis

There is hardly any other condition which closely resembles the junctional tachycardia unless its rate exceeds 130 beats/min, and then, there may difficulty in differentiating it from an AV node re-entry mechanism (PSVT). A vagal manoeuvre, usually, interrupts the PSVT and has no effect on junctional tachycardia.

### Treatment

Identify and treat the cause.

## JUNCTIONAL ESCAPE

In junctional (AV junctional) beat or rhythm the atrial depolarization current points cephalad and to the right, away from lead II and toward lead aVR. Therefore, the P-wave, if seen, would be negative in lead II and positive in lead aVR. However this P-wave is usually buried by the QRS complex and not visible. On less common occasions when the P-wave is visible, it may be either immediately before or immediately after the QRS complex. Since the impulse is conducted to the ventricles via the His bundle and bundle branches, the QRS complex of junctional beats is narrow and looks exactly like the QRS complex of the sinus beat. The inherent rate of junctional escape rhythm is 40–60 beats/min.

## PAROXYSMAL SUPRAVENTRICULAR TACHYCARDIA RESULTING FROM AV NODAL RE-ENTRY

It has it supraventricular origin, and, usually, comes in recurrent episodes, and, hence, termed as paroxysmal supraventricular tachycardia (PSVT). It is characterized by spontaneous and abrupt termination. It may be, further, supported by either an AV nodal re-entry or by an AV re-entry circuit and achieves rates of 170–250 beats/min (Figs 20.36–20.38).

### ECG Characteristics

1. Rate : 170–250 beats/min
2. Rhythm : Regular
3. PR interval : It may be normal in the sinus rhythm. The P-R interval at the onset of the tachycardia is, abnormally, long
4. QRS complex : Identical features of the sinus conducted QRS complex. It may be aberrantly, conducted at times.
5. Distinguishing features : A narrow QRS tachycardia that, usually, exceeds 170 beats/min and begins, abruptly, with a prolonged P-R interval. This is necessary to accommodate the refractoriness, and establish the re-entry circuit. The rest of the P-waves will either not be seen or they will distort the end of the QRS (P-waves just barely showing). There is no alternans of the QRS after the first 5–6 seconds: may be interrupted by a vagal manoeuvre.

### Aetiological Factors

1. One early PAC
2. Rarely, a PJC

### Variations

1. AV nodal re-entry, using a slow anterograde intranodal pathway and a fast retrograde pathway, causing simultaneous atrial and ventricular activation (P buried within or peeking out at the end of the QRS).
2. AV nodal re-entry, using a fast anterograde intranodal pathway and a slow retrograde pathway, causing atrial activation to follow ventricular activation with a long PR interval.

### Treatment

Short paroxysms may require no treatment.

1. Termination may, often, be achieved by vagal manoeuvres, but carotid artery massage should not be advised in patients having or likely to have carotid artery disease.
2. Intravenous verapamil is considered by some to the treatment of choice, but should be used cautiously in those patients who had poor left ventricular functions.
3. Digitalis and beta-blockers, which prolong AV nodal conduction and refractoriness in both alpha and beta pathways, are usually, effective.
4. Type IA anti-arrhythmic agents may be useful.
5. Oral diltiazem, 90 mg, 3 times a day, may be effective in preventing recurrence.

In situations, where one can find severe hemodynamic disturbances, direct synchronous cardioversion, using 40 w/s, is often, quite contributory.

## VAGOTONIC MANOEUVRES FOR PSV

1. **Carotid sinus stimulation:** Out of vagotonic manoeuvres, carotid sinus stimulation is, commonly, practised by physicians and quite reliable test when done by an experienced health worker. The main purpose of this test is to create an elevation of blood pressure in the

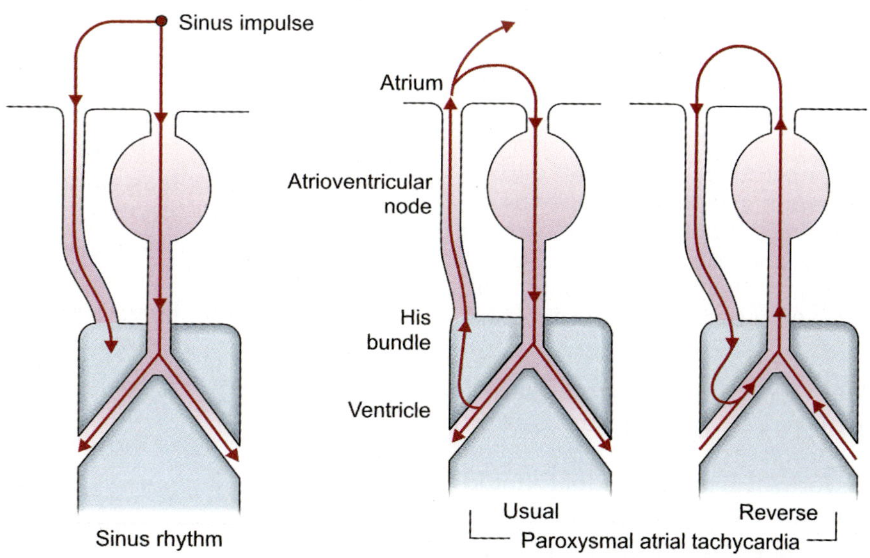


**Fig. 20.36:** Normal conduction system and the accessary atrioventricular connection showing the conduction sequence during sinus rhythm in the left hand panel and during tachycardia in the middle and right hand panels

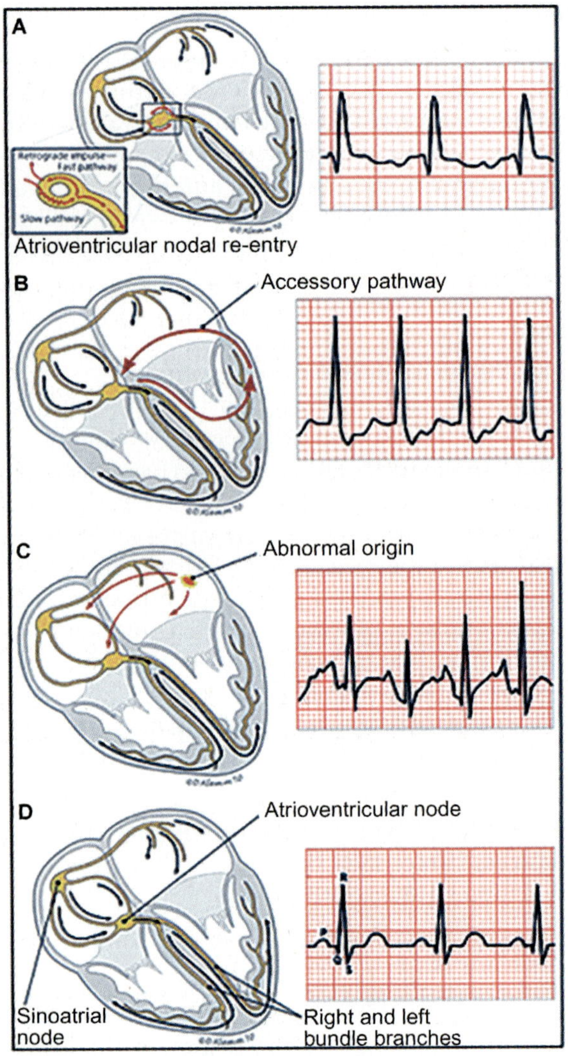


**Fig. 20.37:** (A) In typical atrioventricular nodal re-entrant tachycardia (antegrade conduction down the slow atrioventricular nodal pathway and retrograde conduction up the fast pathway), the retrograde P-wave may not be seen or may be visible early after the QRS complex. When visible, it often appears as a pseudo R wave in lead V1. (B) In atrioventricular reciprocating tachycardia, there is typically a short RP interval, with the timing and morphology of the P-wave dependent on the site and conduction velocity of the accessory pathway. (C) Atrial tachycardia typically produces variable RP and PR intervals because atrioventricular conduction depends on atrioventricular nodal properties and the tachycardia rate. In atrial tachycardia, the morphology and axis of the P-wave are influenced by atrial site of origin and tachycardia mechanism. Short- and long-term therapies are discussed in the text. (D) Normal sinus rhythm

carotid sinus so that there will be reflex slowing of AV conduction. This is achieved by pressing the carotid sinus against the lateral processes of the vertebra. It will cause pain for a seconds for which the individual should be educated before performing this manoeuvre.

2. **Technical aspects:** To start with, grip the patient's chin, with your right palm, and swing your right thumb around; you will find that it, automatically, falls at the angle of the jaw, the location of the carotid bifurcation. This area, then, is pressed with tolerable force with the thumb for not more than 3 seconds as a longer duration of pressure, with greater force, may lead to dangerous complications. Prior to the performance of this manoeuvre, one should always record the history of transient ischemic attacks and listen to the carotid bruit. One should never perform sinus stimulation test without ECG monitoring so that the results can be observed and acted upon, if required. This manoeuvre is relatively safe and effective.
3. **Gagging:** This is a good vegotonic manoeuvre. If the episodes of PSVT occur, instruct the patient to try to vomit.
4. **Trendelenburg position:** The patient can be instructed to perform this at home.
5. **Valsalva manoeuvre:** Blowing against a closed glottis is an effective vegotonic manoeuvre.
6. **Squatting:** Squatting with hands, gripped across the belly and pulling in, is a fairly easy thing to do and is very effective. This is obvious not for the older patient who cannot squat. It is, usually, prescribed for a younger patient. It is not only ineffective, but it is also dangerous as it may lead to retinal detachment in a few elderly patients.

## ATRIAL FUSION COMPLEXES

The collision of two atrial impulses, within atria, leads to the formation of a new complex, which is termed as atrial fusion complex (Fig. 20.39).

### ECG Characteristics

| | |
|---|---|
| 1. Rate | : That of the underlying rhythm |
| 2. Rhythm | : Regular |
| 3. PR interval | : The PR interval of the fusion beat is the same as that of the sinus rhythm. The P-wave of the fusion beat is, sometimes, isoelectric or intermediate between the P-waves of the fusing impulses. |
| 4. QRS complex | : It is same as that of the underlying rhythm. |
| 5. Distinguishing features | : There are other atrial ectopic beats in the tracing, and there is reason to believe that one beat was due at the same time as the sinus P-wave. |

### Causative Factors

These are the same as those of the atrial ectopics or atrial rhythm.

### Variations

1. Atrial parasystole
2. Wandering pacemaker

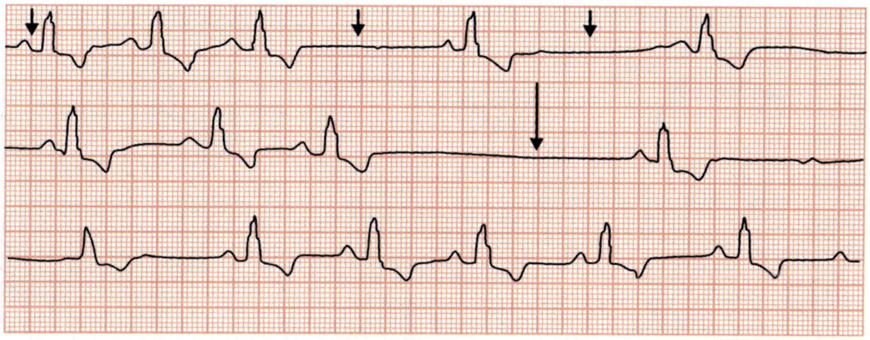

**Fig. 20.38:** Graph explaining as to how pressure on carotid sinus produces sinus arrest or sinus block

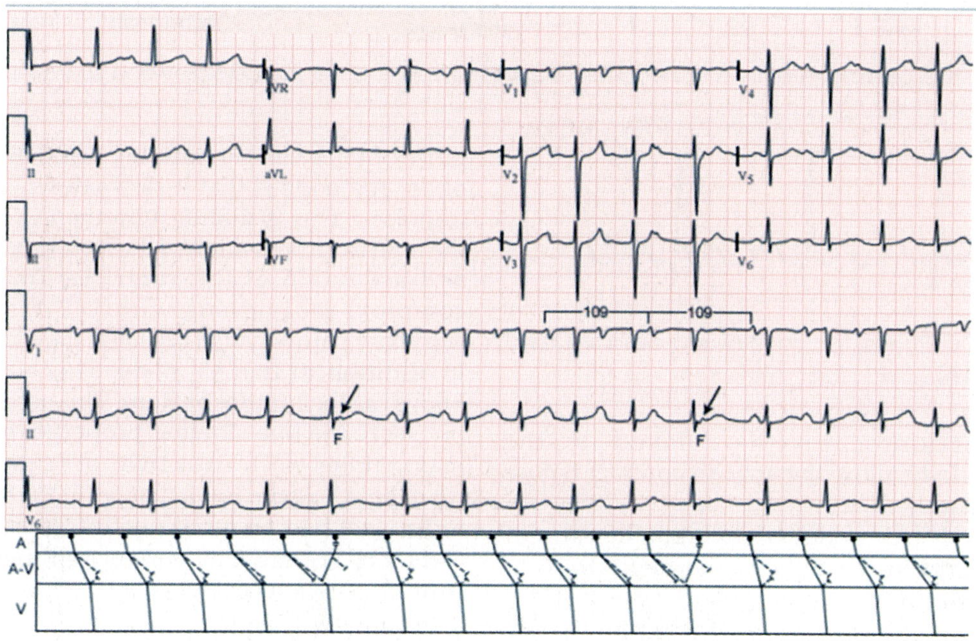


**Fig. 20.39:** ECG showing atrial fusion beats (F)

## Atrial Parasystole

Atrial parasystole is an independent and undisturbable ectopic rhythm whose pacemaker cannot be discharged by impulses of the dominant (usually, sinus) rhythm. It is far less common than the ventricular parasystole (Fig. 20.40).

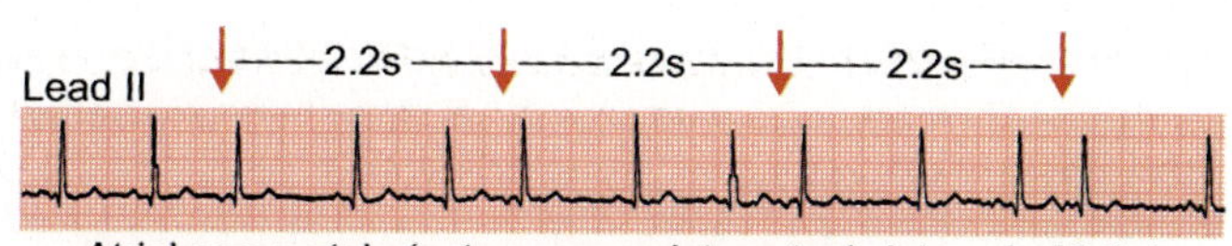


Atrial parasystole (note common interectopic interval of 2.2s)

**Fig. 20.40:** Parasystolic rhythms involve an independent ectopic pacemaker resulting in nonfixed coupled premature beats. Parasystole may occur in the atria, as seen in this example, in the AV junction, and in the ventricles. Note the common interectopic interval separating the parasystolic PACs

### ECG Characteristics

1. Rate : That of the underlying rhythm.
2. Rhythm : Irregular, because of atrial premature beats
3. PR interval : Normal
4. QRS complex : Normal
5. Distinguishing features : Atrial ectopic with no fixed coupling Interectopic intervals that are multiples of a common denominator

### Cause

Myocardial infarction.

### Differential Diagnosis

PACs and fusion beats

## Pre-excitation Syndromes and Accessary Pathways

**Pre-excitation syndrome** is a condition where the ventricles of the heart become depolarized too early, which leads to their partial premature contraction (Figs 20.41–20.58 and Table 20.5). Normally, the atria (chambers taking venous blood) and the ventricles (chambers pumping blood towards organs) are electrically isolated, and electrical contact between them exists only at the 'atrioventricular node'. In all pre-excitation syndromes, at least one more conductive pathway is present. Physiologically, the normal

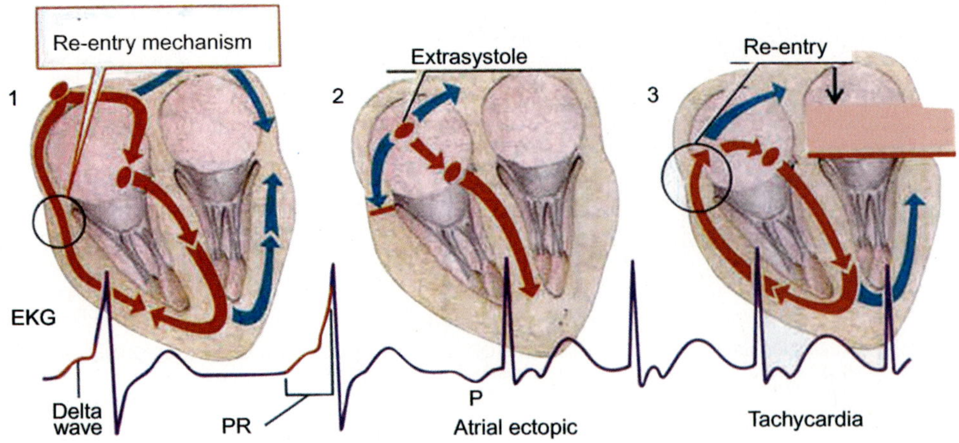


**Fig. 20.41:** Diagrams explaining re-entry mechanism in the WPW syndrome, i.e. extrasystoles and supraventricular tachycardia

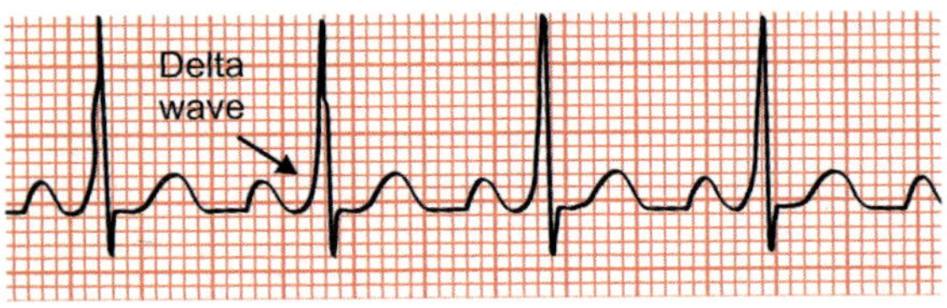


**Fig. 20.42:** Short PR (<120 ms), broad QRS and delta waves in WPW syndrome (arrows)

electrical depolarization wave is delayed' at the atrioventricular node to allow the atria to contract before the ventricles contract.

This function of the AV node is important, be cause if the signals generated in the atria of the heart were to increase in rate (as they do during atrial fibrillation or atrial flutter), the AV node will limit the electrical activity that conducts to the ventricles. For instance, if the atria are electrically activated at 300 beats per minute, half those electrical impulses are blocked by the AV node, so that the ventricles are activated at 150 beats per minute (giving a pulse of 150 beats per minute). Another important property of the AV node is that it slows down individual electrical impulses. This is manifest on the ECG as the PR interval, the time from activation of the atria (manifest as the P-wave) and activation of the ventricles (manifest as the QRS complex) individuals with WPW syndrome have an accessory pathway that connects the atria and the ventricles, in addition to the AV node. This accessory pathway is known as the **bundle of Kent.** This accessory pathway does not share the rate-slowing properties of the AV node, and may conduct electrical activity at a significantly higher rate than the AV node. For instance, in the example above, if an individual had an atrial rate of 300 beats per minute, the accessory bundle may conduct all the electrical impulses from the atria to the ventricles, causing the ventricles to activate at 300 beats per minute. Extremely fast heart rates are potentially dangerous, and cause hemodynamic instability. In some cases, the combination of an accessory pathway and cardiac arrhythmias can trigger ventricular fibrillation, a leading cause of sudden cardiac death.

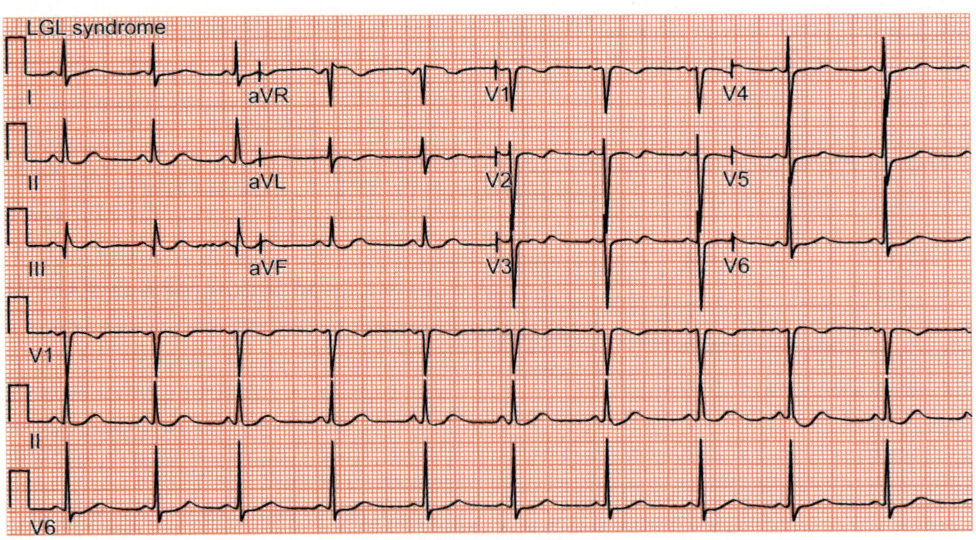


**Fig. 20.43:** ECG trace showing LGL syndrome. Very short PR interval, narrow QRS complexes and no evidence of delta waves

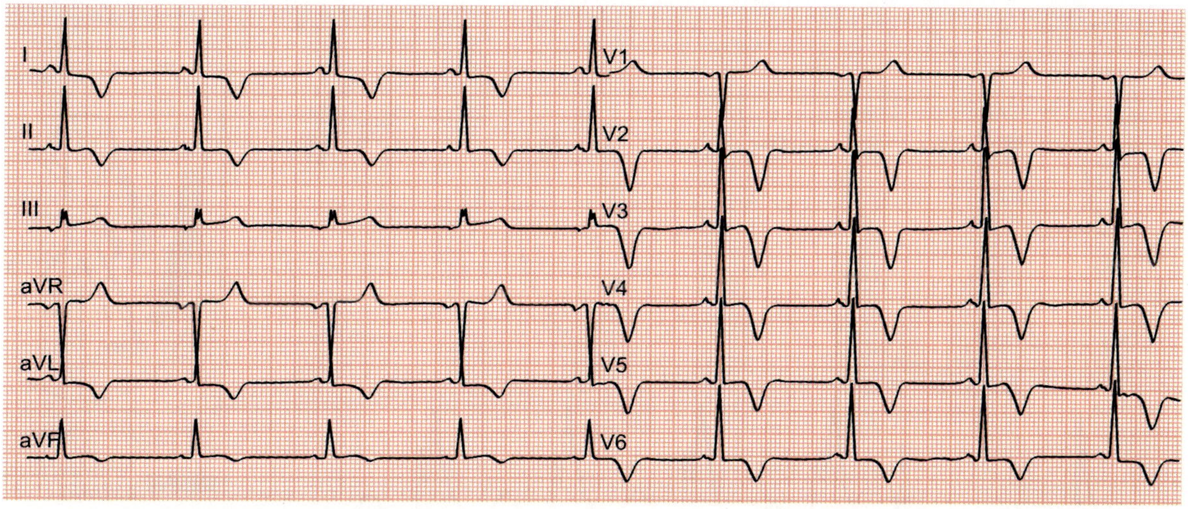


**Fig. 20.44:** ECG showing type A WPW pattern with dominant R-wave in V1 and right precordial T-wave inversions simulating RVH. Sinus rhythm with short PR interval and large delta waves seen best in precordial leads, and confirming Wolff-Parkinson-White (WPW) syndrome of pre-excitation down an accessory pathway. There are large upright R-waves in right precordial leads because the accessory pathway is left lateral, depolarizing the ventricle from left to right) and repolarization

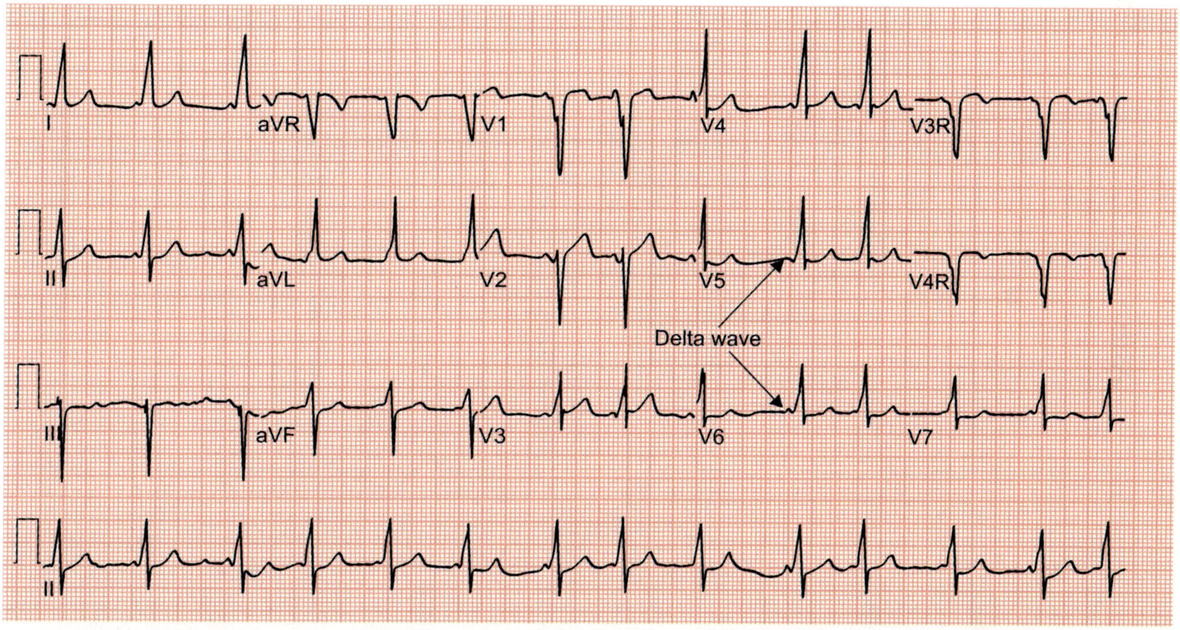


**Fig. 20.45:** Sinus rhythm with very short PR interval (<120 ms). Broad QRS complexes with a slurred upstroke to the QRS complexes—the *delta* wave. Dominant S-wave in V1—this pattern is known as 'Type B' WPW and indicates a right-sided accessory pathway. Tall R-waves and inverted T-waves in the inferior leads and V4–V6 mimic the appearance of left ventricular hypertrophy—again, this is due to WPW and does not indicate underlying LVH

**Table 20.5:** Showing conduction pathways in various types of pre-excitations

| Type | Conduction pathway | PR interval | QRS interval | Delta wave |
|---|---|---|---|---|
| Wolff-Parkinson-White syndrome | Bundle of Kent (atria to ventricles) | Short | Long | Yes |
| Lown-Ganong-Levine syndrome | James bundle (atria to bundle of His) | Short | Normal | No |
| Mahaim-type | Mahaim fibers | Normal | Long | Yes |

## Diagnosis

One beat from a rhythm strip in V2 demonstrating characteristic findings in WPW syndrome. Note the characteristic delta wave (subtler here than in some cases), the short PR interval of 0.08 seconds, and the long QRS complex at 0.12 seconds. WPW syndrome is commonly

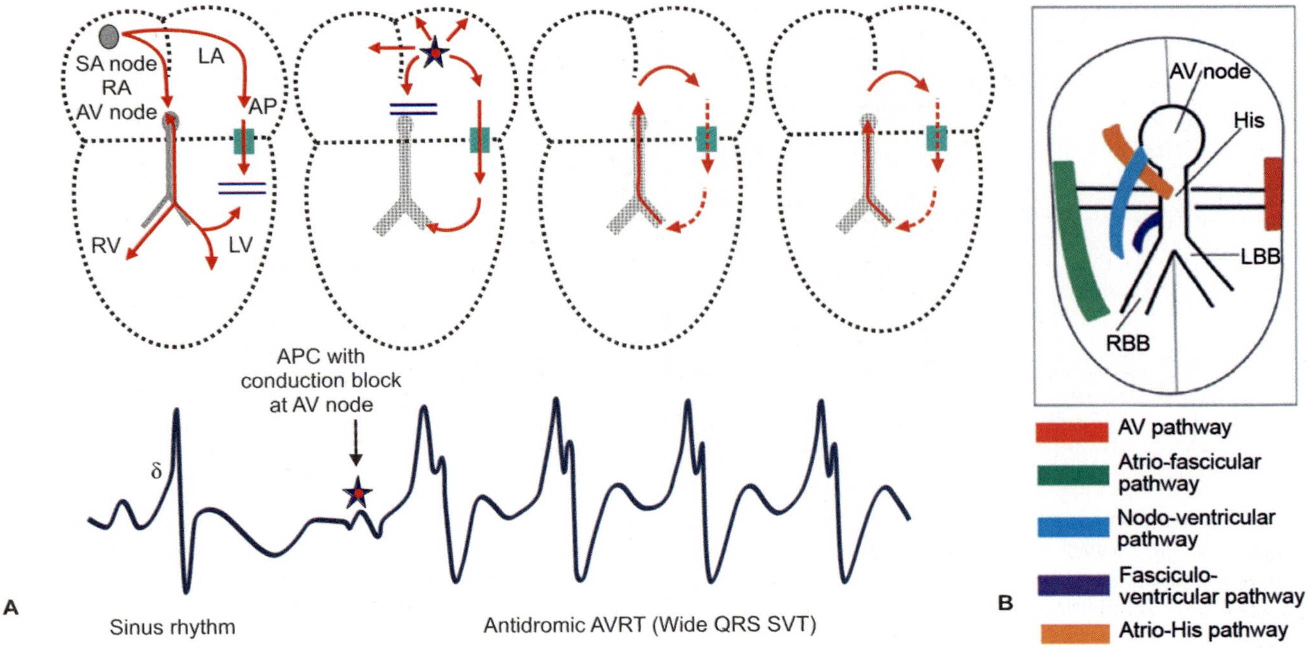


**Fig. 20.46:** (A) Conduction of cardiac impulse through aberrant pathways. (B) Schema of type of accessory pathways

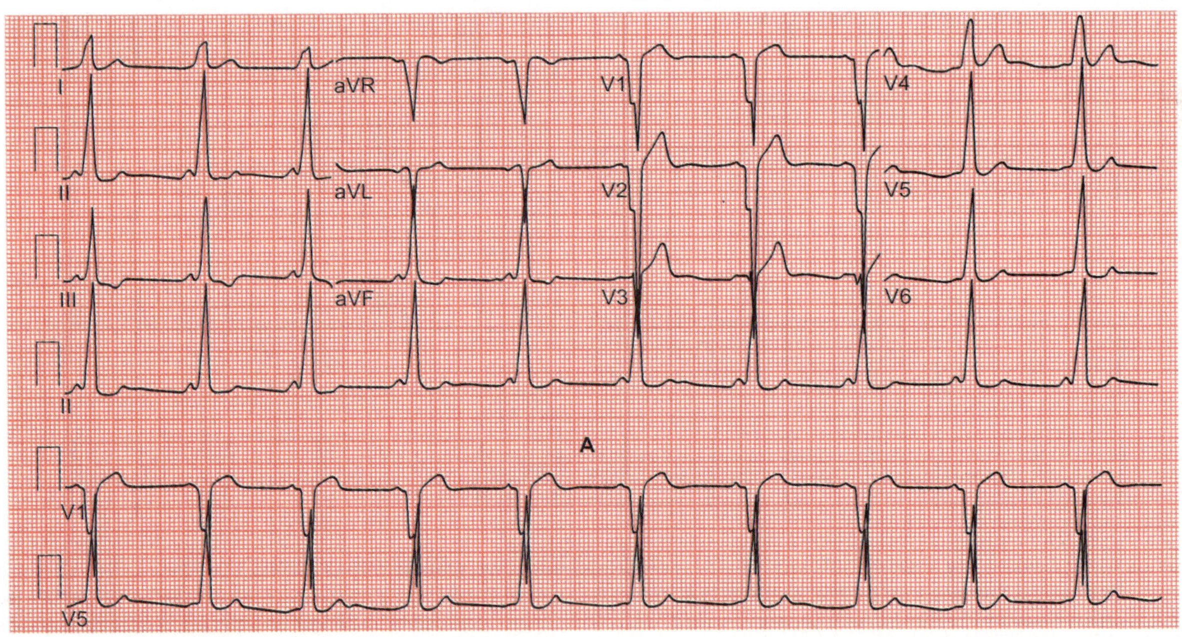


**Fig. 20.47:** Right anteroseptal accessory pathway (AP). A left axis (with a negative delta wave in lead V1) suggests a right lateral AP

diagnosed on the basis of the surface ECG in anasymptomatic individual. In this case it is manifested as a **delta wave**, which is a slurred upstroke in the QRS complex that is associated with a short PR interval.

The short PR interval and slurring of the QRS complex is actually the impulse making it through to the ventricles prematurely (across the accessory pathway) without the usual delay experienced in the AV node. If the patient experiences episodes of atrial fibrillation, the ECG will show a rapid polymorphic wide-complex tachycardia (without torsades de pointes). This combination of atrialfibrillation and WPW is considered dangerous, and most antiarrhythmic drugs are contraindicated. When an individual is in normal sinus rhythm, the ECG characteristics of WPW syndrome are a short PR interval, widened QRS complex (greater than 120 ms in length) with slurred upstroke of the QRS complex, and secondary repolarization changes reflected in ST-segment-T-wave changes. In individuals with WPW syndrome, electrical activity that is initiated in the SA node travels through the accessory pathway *as well as* through the AV node to activate the ventricles via both pathways. Since the accessory pathway

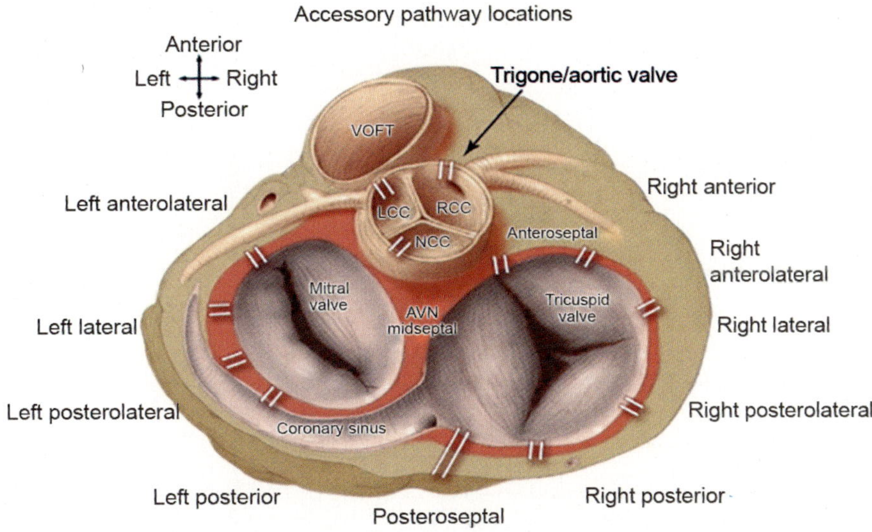


**Fig. 20.48A:** Atrial ventricular accessory pathways may occur anywhere along the atrial ventricular annulus. Note the posteroseptal region is not a part of the true septum. Note also the position of the aortic annulus interspersed between the right and left anteroseptal regions. Midseptal pathways are among the most difficult to ablate because of the proximity of the AV node. VOFT=ventricular outflow tract; LCC=left coronary cusp; RCC=right coronary cusp; NCC=noncoronary cusp; AVN=AV node

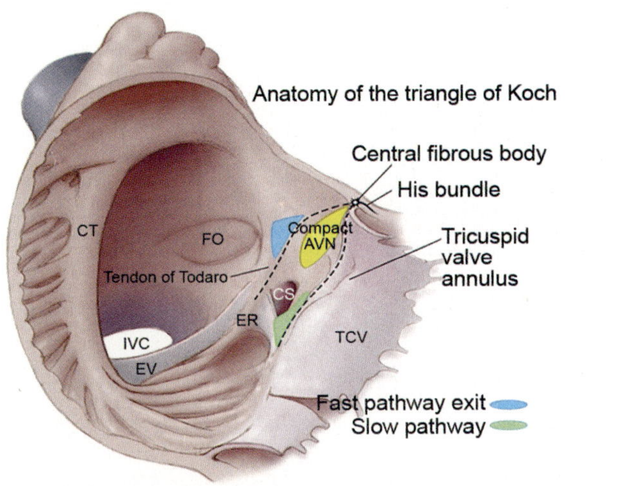


**Fig. 20.48B:** The true interatrial septum near the tricuspid annulus consists of the anterior and midseptal regions. Midseptal pathways are inserted into the triangle of Koch region, close to the compact AV node. Accurate assessment of pathway slant and ablation preferably of the ventricular insertion site along with the use of cryoenergy may all be required to minimize the risk of AV block when ablating pathways in this region. CT=cristo-terminalis; FO=Forman ovale; EV=Eustachian valve; IVC=inferior vena cava; TCV=tricuspid valve; CS=coronary sinus; ER=Eustachian ridge; AVN=AV node

does not have the impulse slowing properties of the AV node, the electrical impulse first activates the ventricles via the accessory pathway, and immediately afterwards via the AV node. This gives the short PR interval and slurred upstroke to the QRS complex known as the delta wave. Patients with WPW often exhibit more than one accessory pathway, and in some patients as many as eight additional abnormal pathways can be found. This has been seen in individuals with Ebstein's anomaly. Wolff-Parkinson-White syndrome is sometimes associated with Leber's hereditary optic neuropathy (LHON), a form of mitochondrial disease. WPW syndrome is, basically, a type of pre-excitation characterized by narrow P-R interval, delta wave, wide QRS complex and normal PQRST duration on electrocardiographic recording. It was first described by three workers, Wolff, Parkinson and White, in 1930. However, ECG parameters of the syndrome were clearly demonstrated by Wilson in 1915, and, later, by Wedd in 1921. The WPW syndrome is considered as a benign entity and no subjective symptoms or hemodynamic changes are recorded unless associated with ecotopic tachyarrhythmias. The tachyarrhythmias may be recorded at birth or during infancy, childhood or adult life. The individuals, already, disgnosed as having WPW syndrome are, usually, found to be in sinus rhythm suffering from no organic heart ailment in about 60.70% of the cases. The true incidence of the WPW syndrome is difficult to assess, but it is estimated to be 0.15–0.2% in the general population. The syndrome occurs more frequently in men than in women, with an incidence of 54–70% in males.

## Diagnosis in WPW Syndrome

It can be disgnosed by the following methods.

### *Clinical Manifestations*

The clinical manifestations of the WPW syndrome are mainly dependent up the physiologic properties of the accessory pathways. The dominant symptom which these patients mostly manifest is the recurrent palpitation due to underlying paroxysmal regular supraventricular tachycardia and/or atrial fibrillation which may be, at times, so severe as to cause sudden death. The other symptoms in such patients are, dyspnea, anginal pain, perspiration, fatigue, anxiety, dizziness and oliguria.

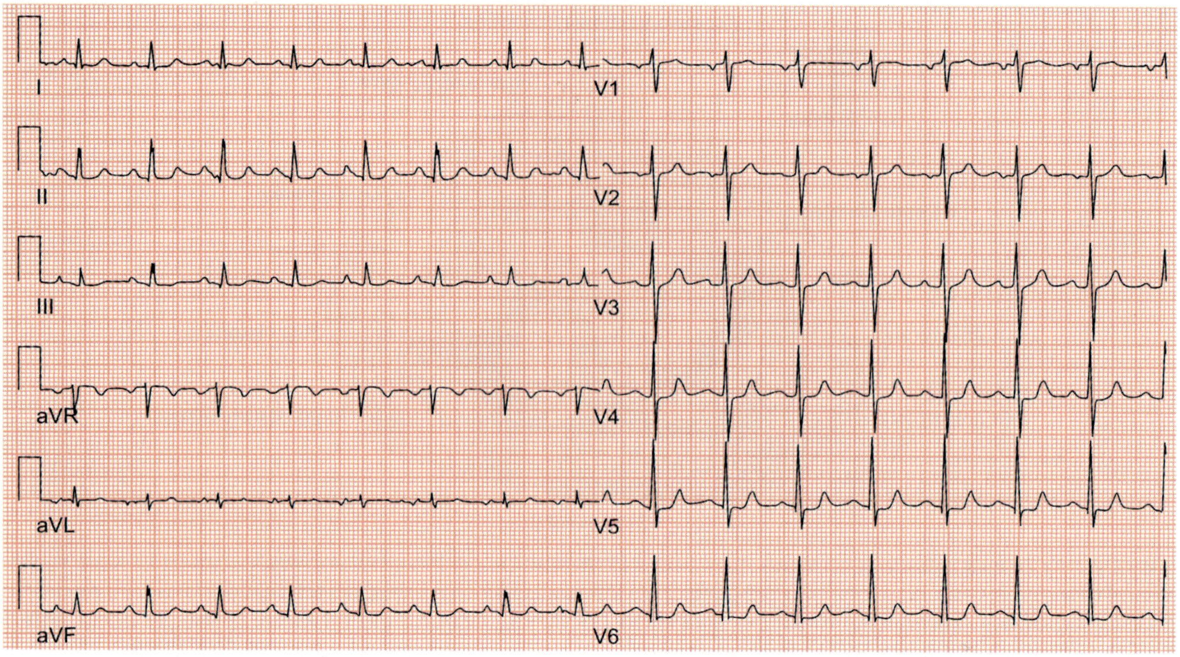


**Fig. 20.49:** Right lateral accessory pathway (AP). If the delta waves in the inferior leads are negative, then it denotes a posteroseptal AP right, or left, depending on the delta wave vector in lead V1 as described above

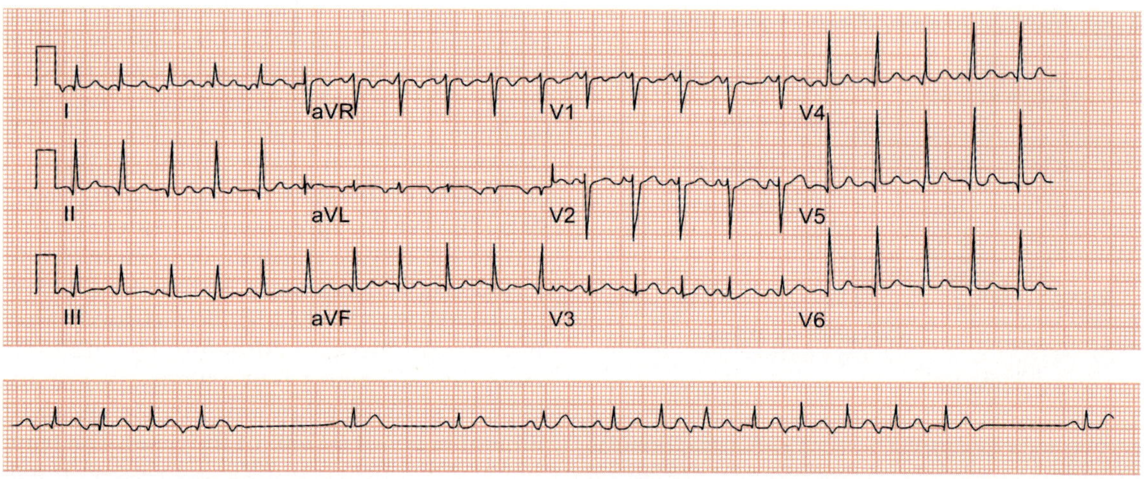


**Fig. 20.50:** Permanent from of junctional reciprocating tachycardia (PJRT) in a patient with a left-sided accessory pathway. The 12-lead electrocardiogram demonstrates a long RP interval-short PR interval tachycardia, which in contrast to the usual form of PJRT, exhibits negative P-waves in leads I and aVL. The rhythm strips below (lead I) indicate that whenever a nonconducted P-wave occurs, the tachycardia always terminates, only to begin again after several sinus beats

### Parameters

The typical ECG findings include a short P-R interval and a prolonged QRS interval due to a delta wave (initial slurring of the QRS complex). Recoginition of the delta wave is a key point in the diagnosis of the syndrome. In some patients who have WPW syndrome, however, the delta wave may *not* be obvious. However, the P-R interval may be longer than 0.12 see, whereas the QRS interval may be narrower than 0.10 see in the proven WPW syndrome. The P-R and the QRS intervals in the WPW syndrome are greatly influenced by the pre-existing values of these intervals.

The term **'Lown-Ganong-Levine (LGL) syndrome'** is used when the ECG shows a short P.R interval and narrow QRS complex, without a clear-cut delta wave, associated with recurrent tachyarrhythmias. In reality, the LGL syndrome is considered to be a variant of the WPW syndrome. It is very well known that many normal individuals may have a short P-R interval, particularly during stressful situations. Obviously, this isolated ECG finding, usually, does not have any clinical significance in WPW syndrome: In a doubtful case of WPW syndrome, the His bundle ECG may be necessary to confirm the diagnosis. The H-V interval is shorter than normal; the His

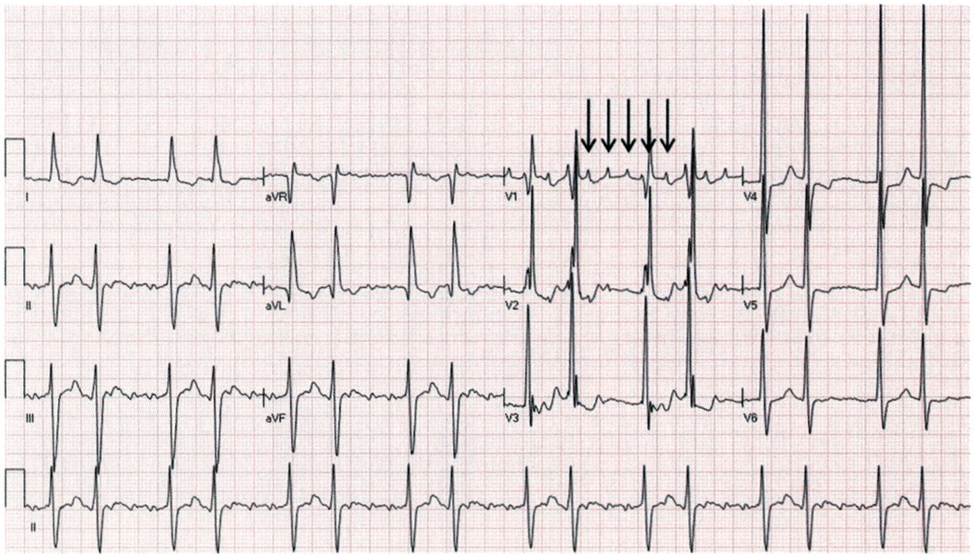


**Fig. 20.51:** ECG is suggestive of an atypical atrial flutter with variable atrioventricular conduction. An electrophysiology study demonstrated a macro-reentrant atrial tachycardia around the mitral annulus with an area of slow conduction medial to the left atrial appendage on the anterior mitral annulus. Solid arrows point to the atrial tachycardia waves in lead V1

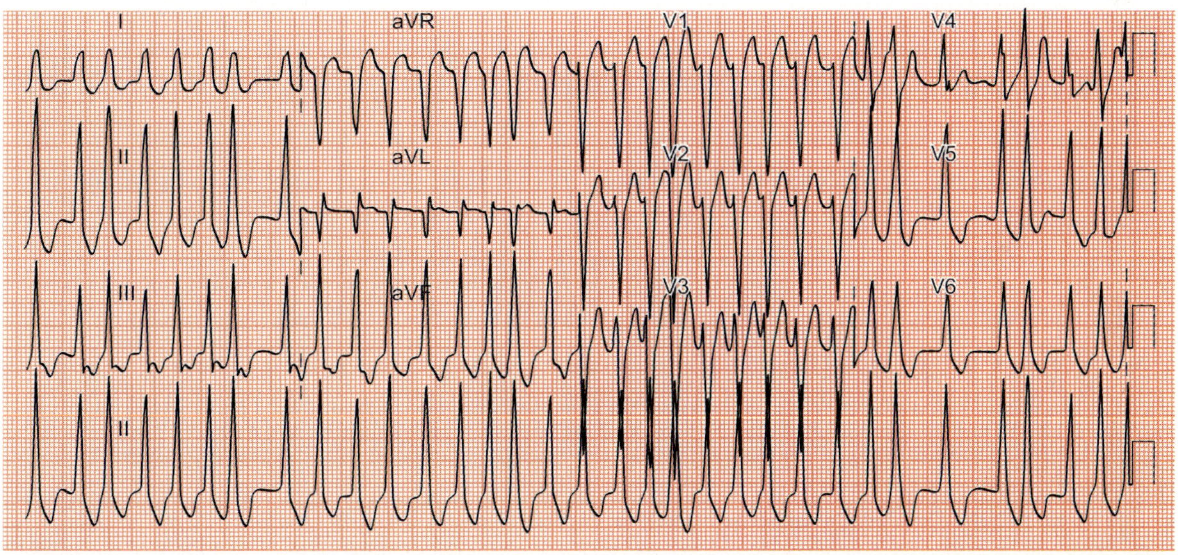


**Fig. 20.52:** Pre-excited wide complex tachycardia in a patient with Wolff-Parkinson-White (WPW) and atrial fibrillation

bundle potential may occur simultaneously with the ventricular deflection, or the His bundle potential may occur even later than the onset of the ventricular deflection. These findings occur because of a premature activation of a portion of the ventricles by way of anomalous conduction.

## Classification of WPW Syndrome

The WPW syndrome is traditionally classified into two types, A and B, depending upon the direction in the delta wave. This classification, however, is an over simplification because many cases with WP syndrome do not belong either to type A or B. The direction of the delta wave is primarily influenced by the location of the accessory pathway.

### *Type A WPW Syndrome*

i. In type A, the delta wave is directed anteriorly (commonly to the right and less commonly to the left).
ii. In general, lead VI shows R. RS, Rs, RSr′ and Rsr′ patterns, whereas leads V5 and V6 show Rs or R deflection.
iii. Superficially, type A WPW syndrome resembles the right bundle branch block (RBBB), right ventricular hypertrophy, and posterior myocardial infarction (MI).
iv. When the QRS complexes, in all precordial leads, are upright, a type A WPW syndrome should be considered as the first diagnostic possibility.
v. In type A, a premature activation occurs in the left ventricle.

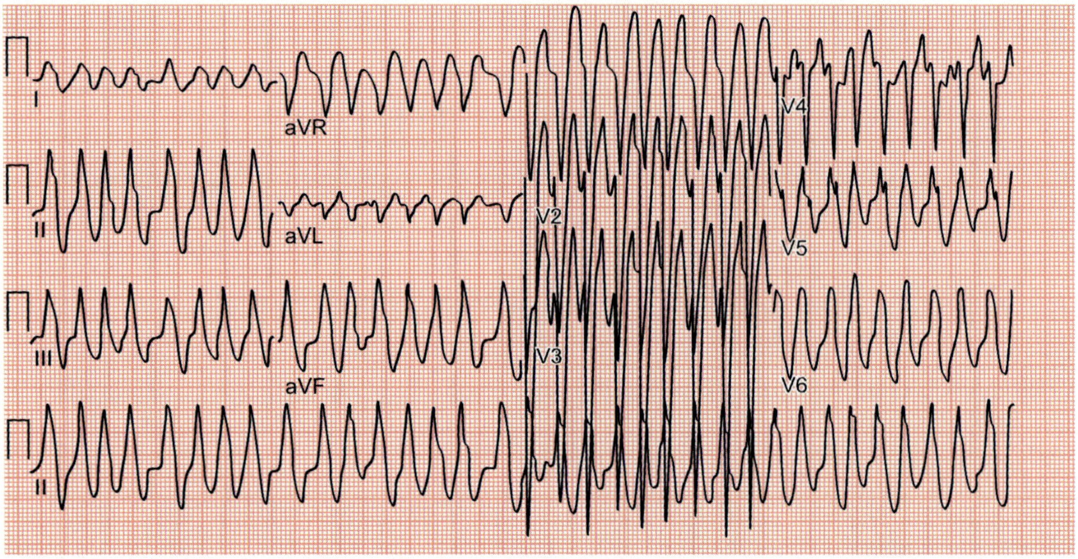


**Fig. 20.53:** ECG shows atrial fibrillation in a patient with WPW; rapid, irregular, broad complex tachycardia (overall rate >200 bpm) with a LBBB morphology (dominant S-wave in V1). This could easily be mistaken for AF with LBBB. However, the morphology is not typical of LBBB, the rate is too rapid (up to 300 bpm in places, i.e. too rapid to be conducted via the AV node) and there is a subtle beat-to-beat variation in the QRS width which is more typical of WPW (LBBB usually has fixed width QRS complexes)

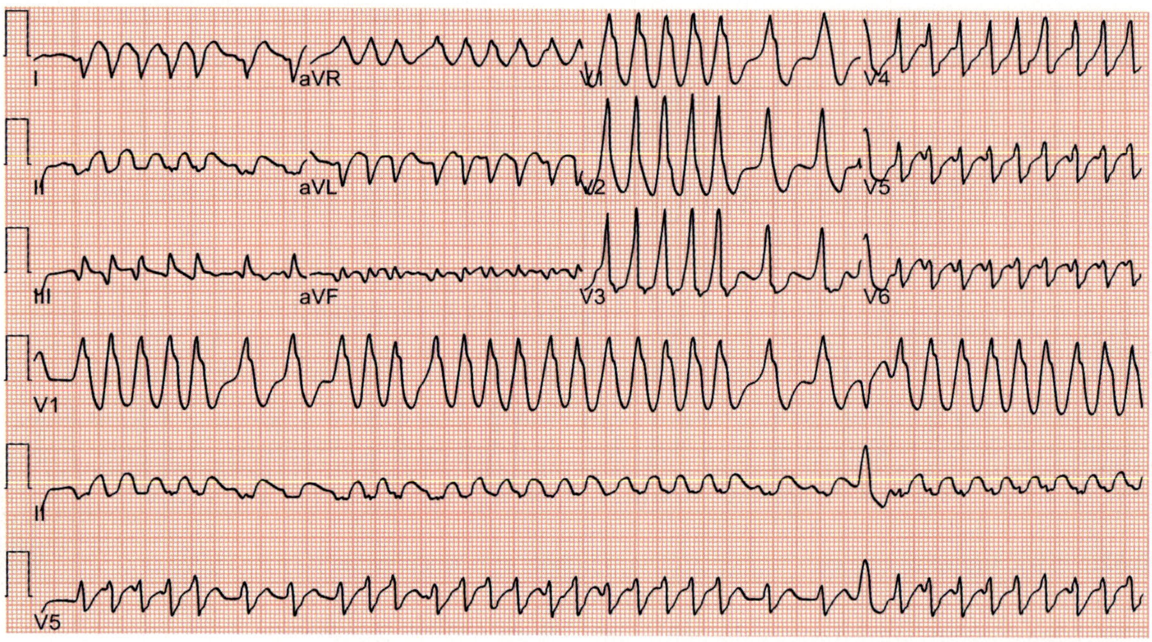


**Fig. 20.54:** ECG of a patient with atrial fibrillation and WPW syndrome. Note the wide-complex, irregularly irregular rhythm with delta waves. This ECG can be mistaken for polymorphic ventricular tachycardia (Tosades de Pointes), however the QRS axis remains stable in the setting of atrial fibrillation with WPW

### *Type B WPW Syndrome*

i. In type B, the delta wave is directed posteriorly (commonly to the left and less commonly to the (right).
ii. Thus, the left precordial leads (leads I, aVL and V4) show tall R waves with delta waves, whereas leads V1-V2 show negative QRS complexes (Q-S waves) with delta waves.
iii. The ECG findings in type B WPW syndrome may closely resemble left bundle branch block (LBBB) and left ventricular hypertrophy.
iv. At times, a pseudoanteroseptal myocardial infarction is produced in WPW syndrome, type B.
v. In type B, a premature activation takes place in the right ventricle. In both type A and type B WPW syndromes, the delta wave is, often, directed

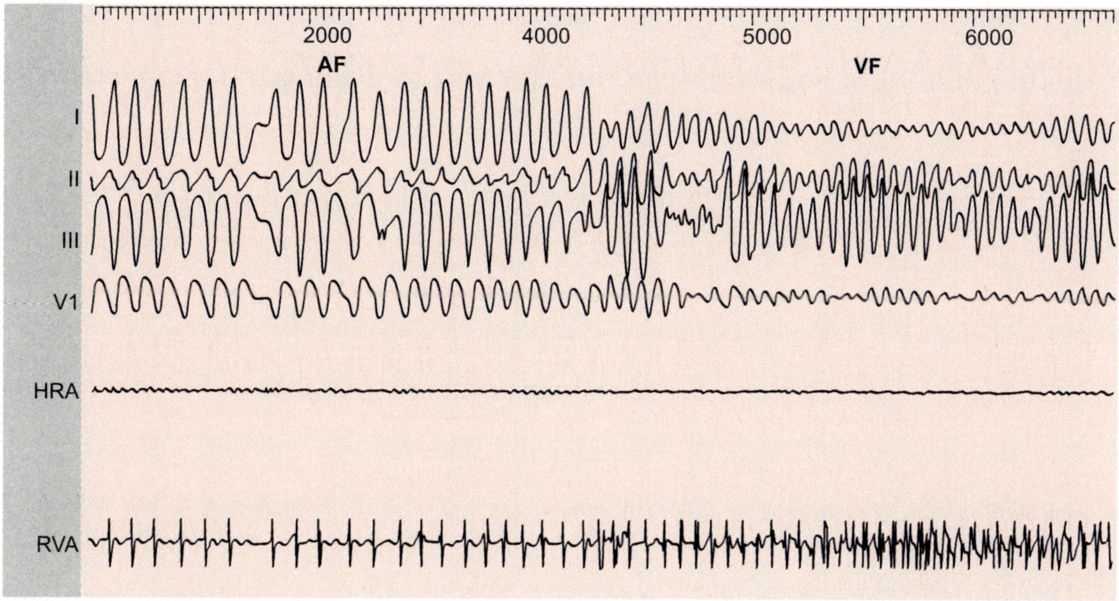


**Fig. 20.55:** ECG showing atrial fibrillation (AF) becoming ventricular fibrillation (VF)

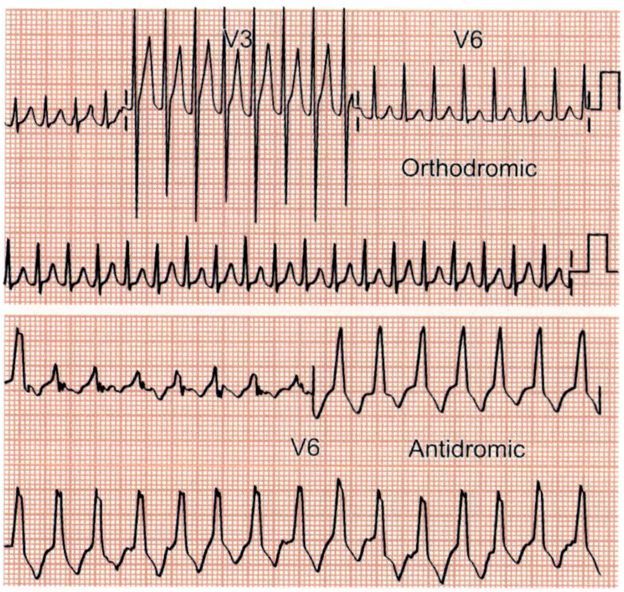


**Fig. 20.56:** ECG showing difference between the two conduction pathways. In orthodromic the normal 'Fast' conduction pathway of the ventricles is 'borrowed' by the arrhythmia, so the complexes on an ECG are narrow. In antidromic AVRT the conduction of the signal through the ventricles travels from cell to cell (more slowly) and therefor the complexes on an ECG are broad

superiorly. This ECG) finding, commonly, produces Q-S or Q-waves in leads II, III and aVF, that closely.

## SIMULATE DIAPHRAGMATIC (INFERIOR) MI

### Types of Cardiac Arrhythmias in WPW Sydrome

The most clinically significant feature of the WPW syndrome is the frequent occurrence of supraventricular tachyarrhythmias. The incidence of tachyarrhythmias in WPW syndrome is 40–80%.

### Reciprocating Tachycardia

Reciprocating tachycardia (the usual rate 140–250 beats/min) is found in most cases (75–80% of all tachyarrhythmias). This type of tachycardia is also called **'paroxysmal atrial tachycardia'**. The term 'reciprocating' or 're-entrant tachycardia' is, more commonly used because the tachycardia is considered to be due to a re-entry phenomenon. On the other hand, the term 'circus movement tachycardia' is used frequently by other workers. In reciprocating tachycardia, the QRS complex is, usually, normal (narrow); the broad QRS complex due to anomalous conduction is much less common.

Atrial flutter or fibrillation is rather uncommon in the WPW syndrome, the incidence rates constituting only 20–25% of all tachyatrhythmias. Of these two rhythm disorders, atrial flutter is rare. The QRS complexes during

**Key points:** *Supraventricular tachycardias*

- The following groups of patients may benefit from referral to a cardiac electrophysiologists
  1. All patients with regular SVT on antiarrhythmic drugs
  2. All patients with recurrent regular SVT
  3. Patients with established AF in whom control of the ventricular response is suboptimal
  4. Patients with lone paroxysmal AF in whom maintenance of sinus rhythm cannot be achieved with class Ic antiarrhythmics
- It is likely that an effective curative catheter ablation procedure for established AF will be established within the next 10 years

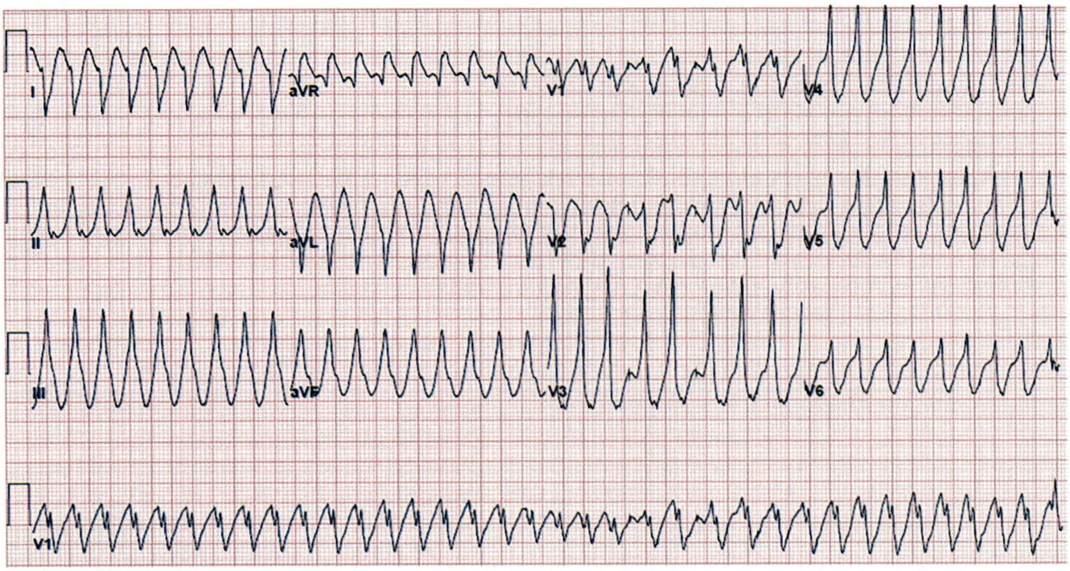


**Fig. 20.57:** ECG of a patient with atrial fibrillation and WPW syndrome. Note the wide-complex, irregularly irregular rhythm with 'delta waves.' This ECG can be mistaken for polymorphic ventricular tachycardia (Torsades de pointes), however the QRS axis remains stable in the setting of atrial fibrillation with WPW

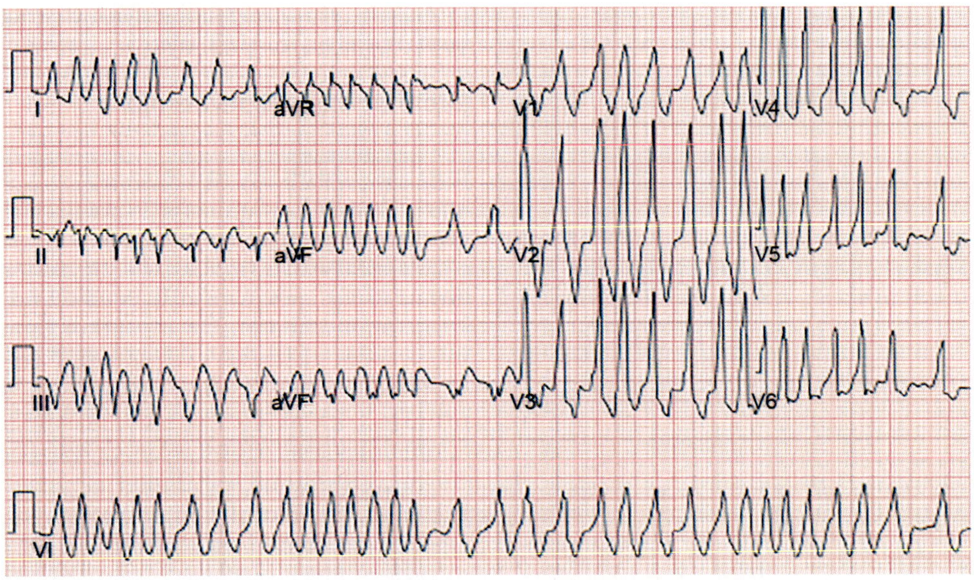


**Fig. 20.58:** Aberrant conduction

atrial fibrillation or flutter in the WPW syndrome are extremely bizarre and broad in most cases, because of anomalous A-V conduction due to the nature of the WPW syndrome itself plus aberrant ventricular conduction due to very rapid ventricular rate. Ventricular tachycardia (Vf) or even ventricular fibrillation (VF) is closely.

## VENTRICULAR ARRHYTHMIAS (Figs 20.59–20.81)

1. Premature ventricular contractions (PVC)
2. Ventricular tachycardia
3. Ventricular fibrillation
4. Torsades de points
5. Accelerated idioventricular rhythm

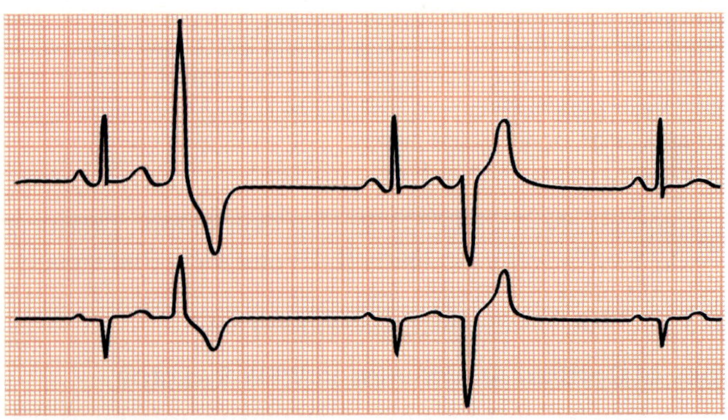

**Fig. 20.59:** Multifocal PVCs—more than one shape.

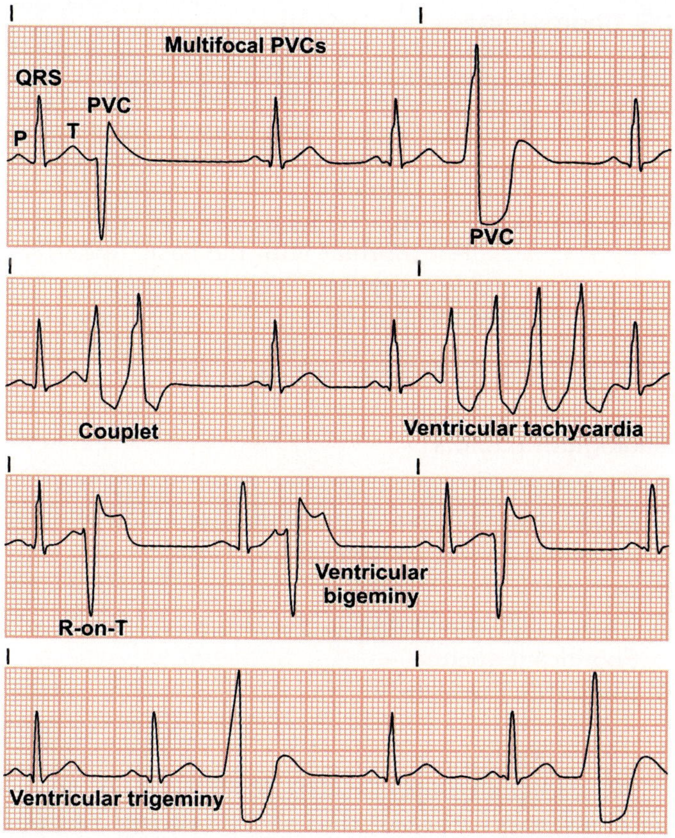


**Fig. 20.60:** Different types of ventricular ectopic activity

6. Ventricular parasystole
7. Ventricular fusion
8. Ventricular flutter.

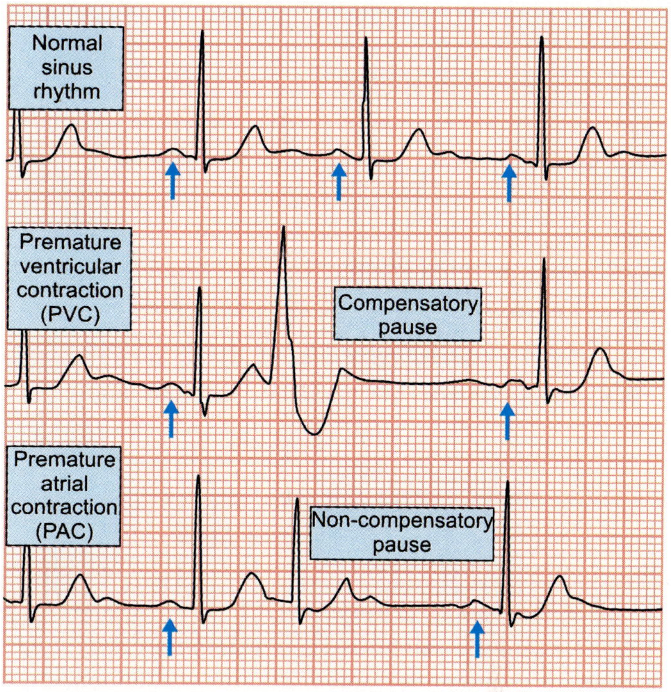


**Fig. 20.62:** Atrial and ventricular premature beats with compensatory and noncompensatory pauses

## PREMATURE VENTRICULAR COMPLEXES

Premature ventricular complexes (PVCS) are premature ectopics, which are generated in the ventricles below the branching of the bundle of His (Table 20.6). Ventricular ectopics are produced as a result of enhanced automaticity

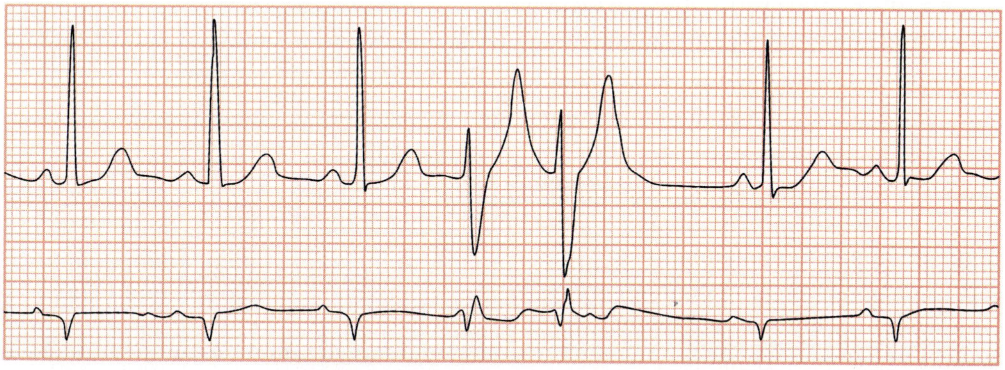

**Fig. 20.61:** Coupled PVCs—occurs in pairs

**Table 20.6:** Modified lown classification for ventricular ectopy and common synonyms used for description of ventricular arrhythmias on long-term monitoring

| | | | |
|---|---|---|---|
| 0 | No ectopy | | |
| 1 | Occasional VPBs (30/hours) | 'Isolated' | |
| 2 | Frequent VPBs (>30/hours) | | Low grade |
| 3 | Multiform VPBs | | Moderate grade |
| 4a | Couplets | | |
| 4b | VT or VF | 'Repetitive' | High grade |
| 5 | Early VPB (R on T) | | |

VPB, ventricular premature beta; VT, ventricular tachycardia (≥3 consecutive beats): and VF, ventricular fibrillation

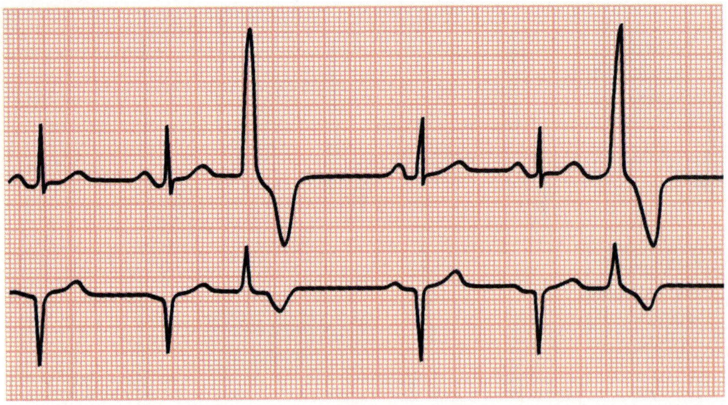

**Fig. 20.63:** Trigeminal PVCs—every third beat is a VPC

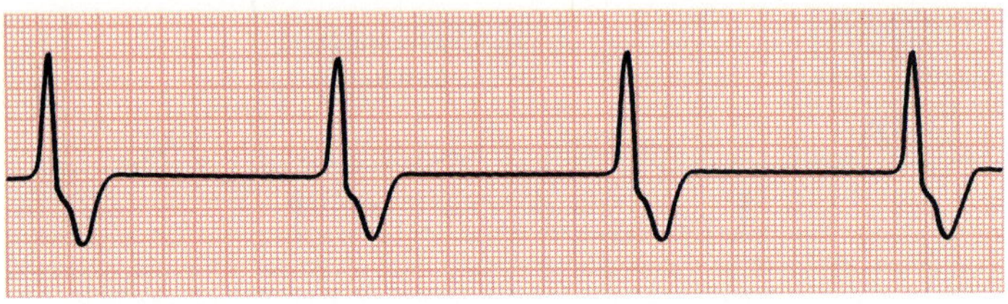

**Fig. 20.64:** ECG trace showing features of ventricular escape rhythm

re-entry, or altered depolarizations. These manifest as premature beats, ventricular tachycardia, ventricular fibrillation, accelerated idioventricular rhythm, or parasystole. Premature ventricular complexes (PVCs) may be right or left ventricular, unifocal, multifocal, bigeminal, interpolated, R-on-T, end- diastolic, or fusion beats; in the setting of acute myocardial infarction, they produce dangerous consequences and are treated on emergency basis.

## ECG Characteristics

1. Rate : It is of the underlying rhythm
2. Rhythm : It is irregular, due to PVC
3. PR interval : It is of the underlying rhythm. There is no P-wave associated with the PVC.
4. QRS complex : It is wider due to PVC and may be normal with the basic underlying rhythm
5. Distinguishing : No related P-wave: premature, broad QRS complex; T-wave of opposite polarity.

## Aetiological Factors

1. Digitalis
2. Drugs (epinephrine, isoproterenol, or aminophylline)
3. Hypoxia
4. Ischemia
5. Myocardial infarction
6. Significant anemia
7. Myocardial stretch

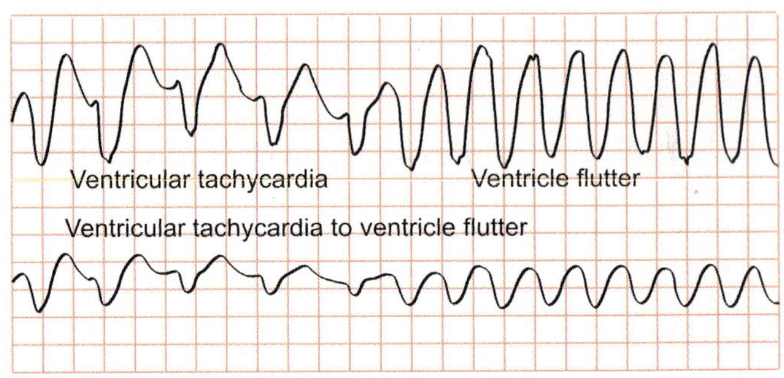


**Fig. 20.66:** Episodes of sustained ventricular tachycardia, ventricular flutter, and ventricular fibrillation

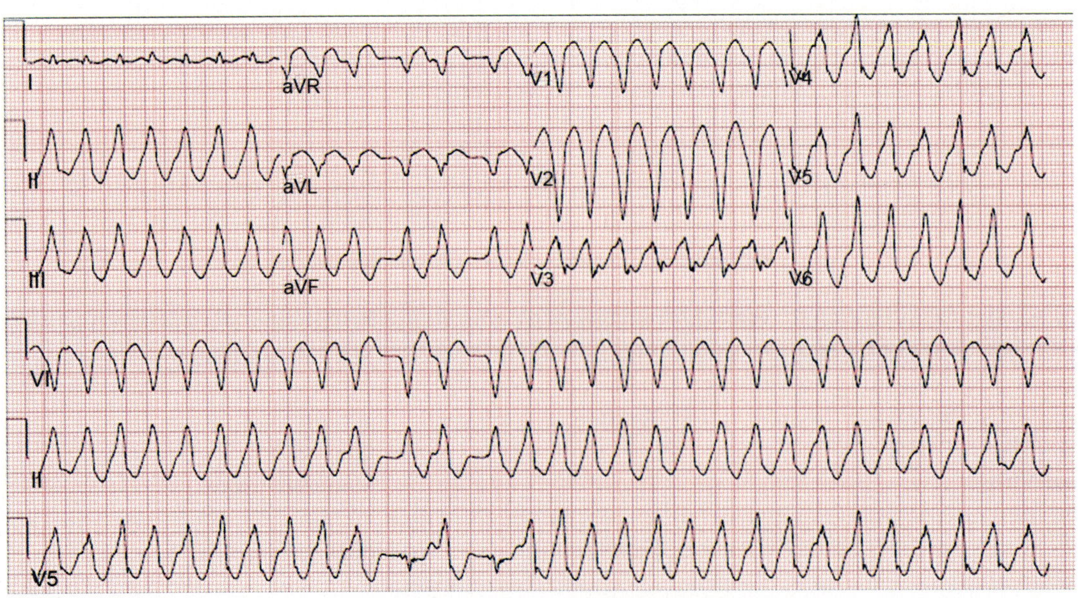


**Fig. 20.65:** Ventricular tachycardia

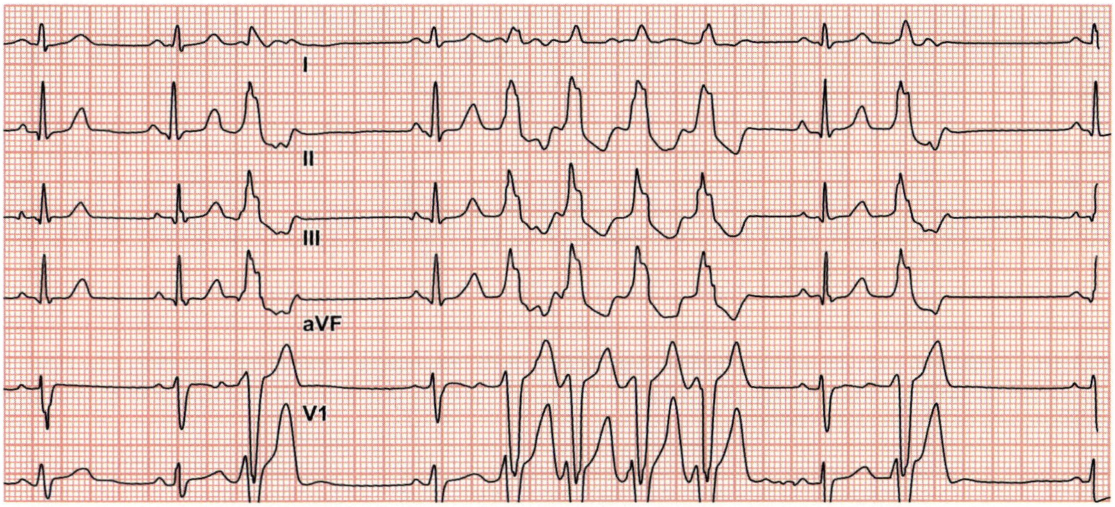


**Fig. 20.67:** ECG showing nonsustained ventricular tachycardia

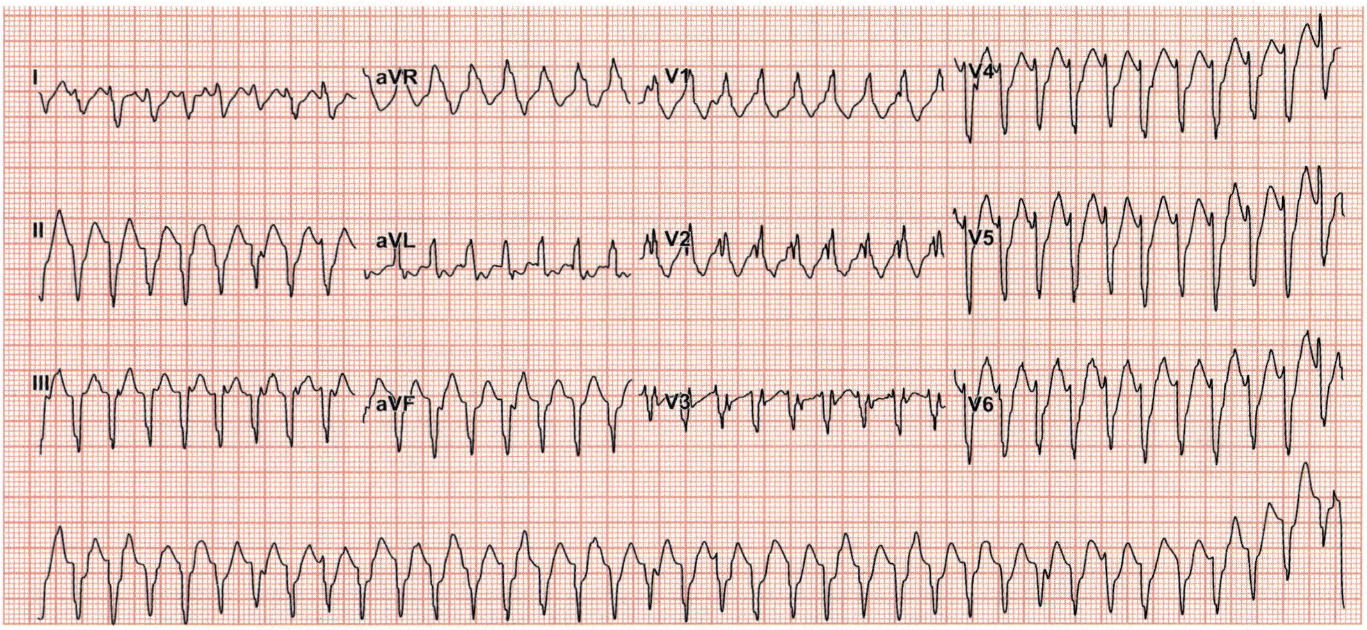


**Fig. 20.68:** Monomorphic VT. Although there is a broad complex tachycardia (HR >100, QRS >120), the appearance in V1 is more suggestive of SVT with aberrancy, given that the complexes are not that broad (<160 ms) and the right rabbit ear is taller than the left. However, on closer inspection there are signs of AV dissociation, with superimposed P-waves visible in V1. Also, the presence of a northwest axis and an rS complex in V6 (tiny R-wave, deep S-wave) indicate that this is VT

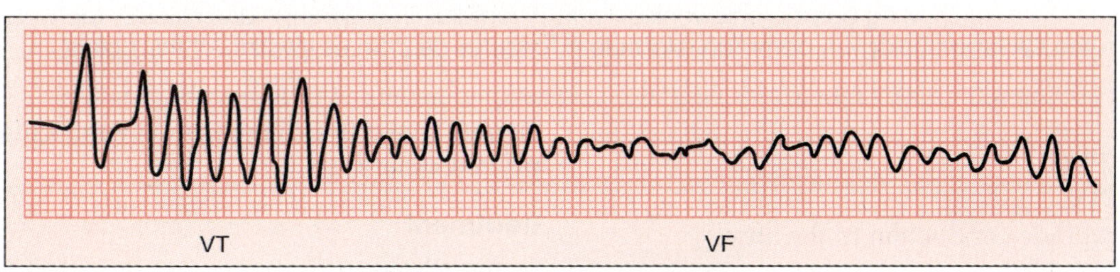


**Fig. 20.69:** Ventricular fibrillation

8. Catecholamines
9. Caffeine
10. Hypokalemia
11. Hypomagnesemia

### Variations

1. Unifocal PVCs and ventricular bigeminy
2. Ventricular trigeminy (one normal and two PVCs)
3. Paired PVCs

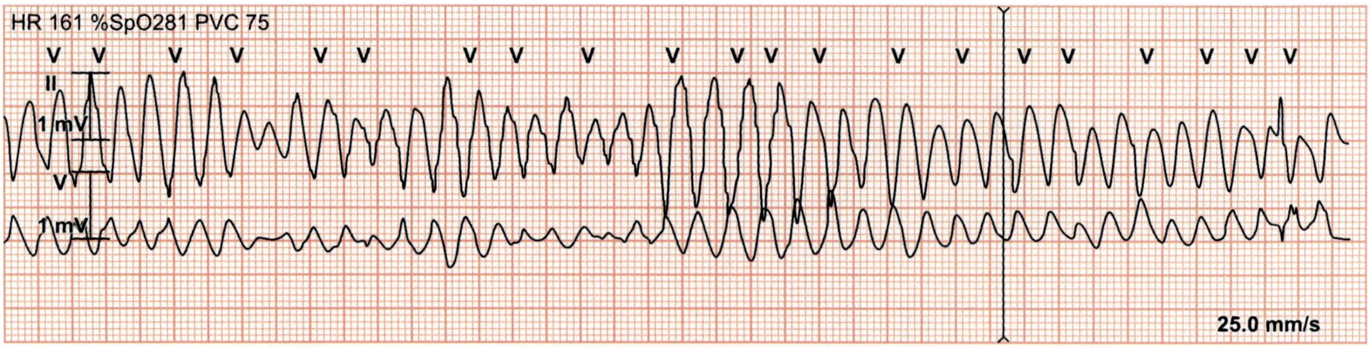


**Fig. 20.70:** Ventricular fibrillation occurs when multiple ventricular foci discharge rapidly and chaotically. The ventricles twitch asynchronously and are not effective as pumps. No organized QRS complexes are seen—just disorganized oscillatory waves which can be coarse (as shown) or fine in appearance

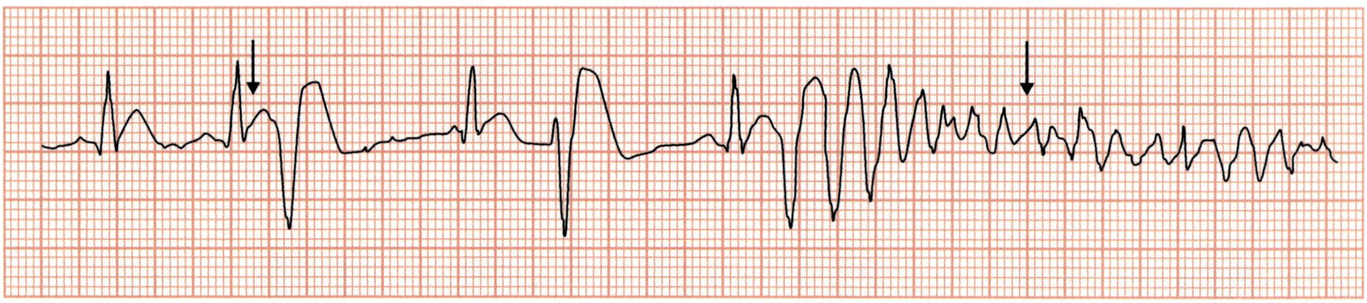

**Fig. 20.71:** ECG trace showing R on T phenomenon (arrow) giving rise to ventricular fibrillation (arrow)

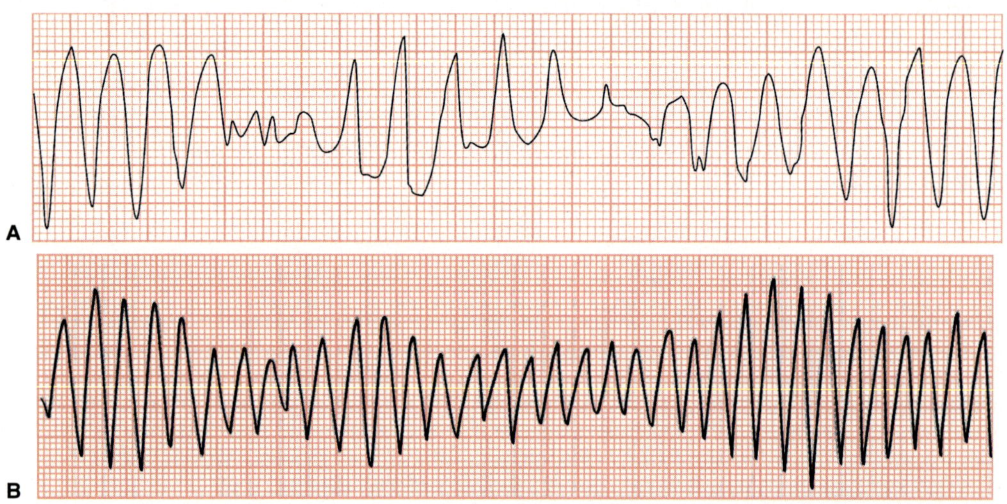

**Fig. 20.72A and B:** ECG traces showing polymorphic ventricular tachycardia. In polymorphic ventricular tachycardia, there is beat-to-beat variation in the QRS morphology. A common example is Torsades de pointes (twisting of the points)

4. R-on-T PVCs
5. End-diastolic PVC
6. Interpolated PVC
7. PVC with retrograde conduction to the atria
8. Right-ventricular PVC
9. Left-ventricular PVC

### Differential Diagnosis

Premature atrial contraction with aberrant ventricular unless a P-wave comes in front of the broad beat or there is morphological proof of ventricular aberrancy. One should always make the diagnosis of ventricular ectopy unless proved otherwise.

### Treatment

In the diseased, ischemic, or infracted heart, antiarrhythmics (lidocaine or procainamide) are given.

### Ventricular Escape

In ventricular escape beat or rhythm, the depolarization wave spreads slowly via abnormal pathway in the ventricular myocardium and not via the His bundle and bundle

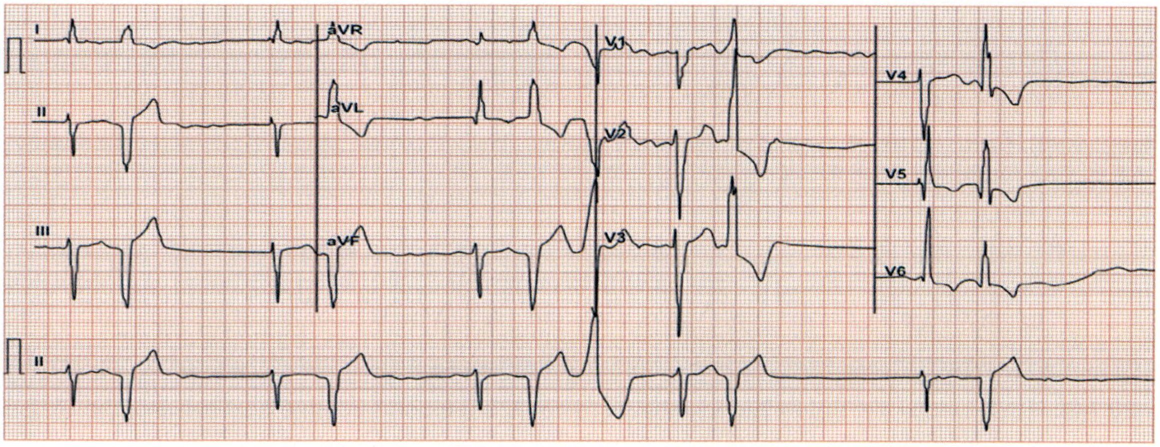


**Fig. 20.73:** Bidirectional ventricular tachycardia due to severe digoxin toxicity

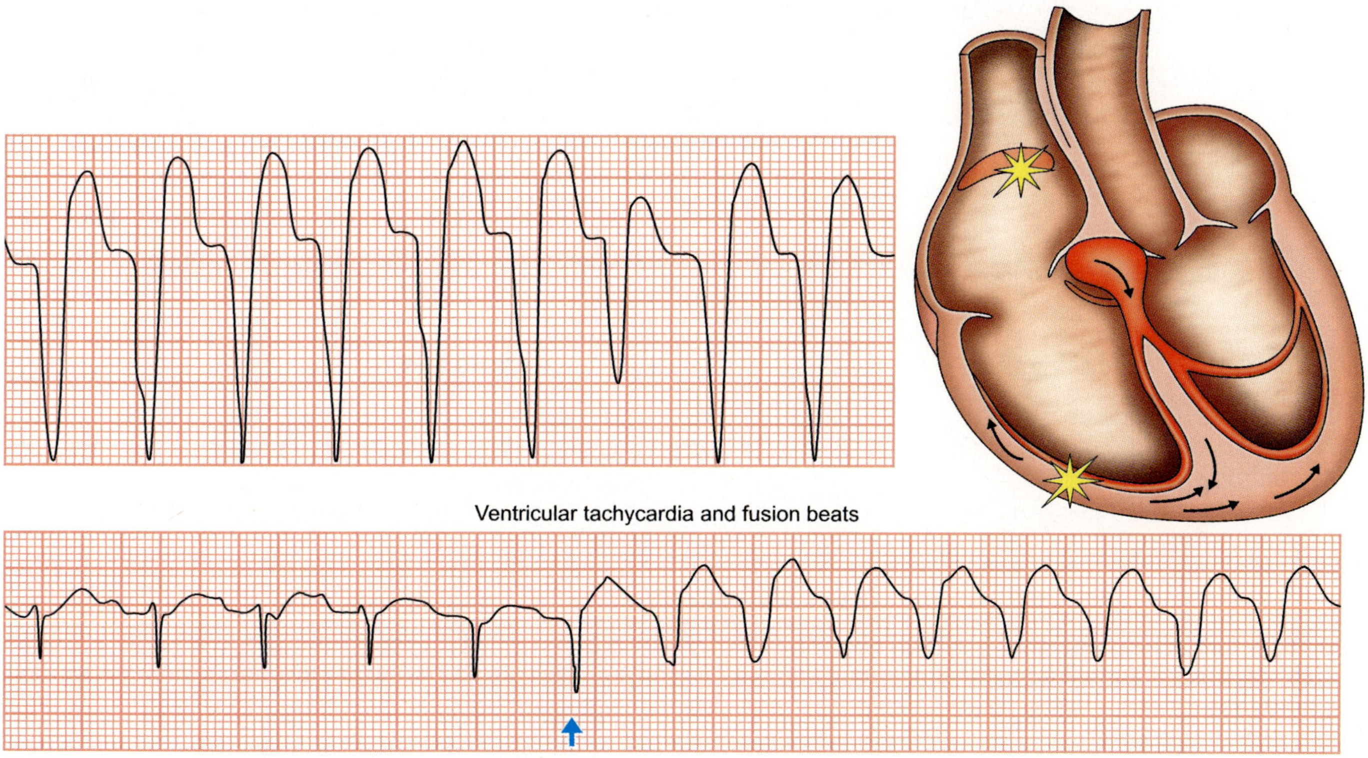


**Fig. 20.74A:** Electrocardiographic signs of AV dissociation. A fusion beat occurs when a sinus beat conducts to the ventricles via the AV node concurrent with a beat arising from the ventricles. The resulting QRS complex has an intermediate appearance between a normal beat and a VT beat. A capture beat occurs when the ventricle is depolarized via the AV node resulting in a narrow (normal-appearing) QRS (The presence of capture and/or fusion beats indicates AV dissociation and if present points to a diagnosis of VT. Their absence, however, does not exclude VT.)

branches. Therefore, the QRS complex is wide (>120 ms) and has a shape different from that of the sinus beat. If the ventricular escape rhythm is the result of sinus node failure, no P-wave of atrial contraction is seen as in the tracing above. If the ventricular escape rhythm is the result of 3rd degree (complete) heart block, the sinus node paces the atria independently and regular P-waves unrelated to the ventricular escape beats can be seen. The inherent rate of ventricular escape rhythm is between 20 and 40 beats/min.

## VENTRICULAR TACHYCARDIA

When ventricular ectopics takes the shape of a rhythm, with a rate of 100–170 beats/min, it is called as ventricular tachycardia.

### ECG Characteristics

1. Rate : 100–170 beats/min
2. Rhythm : Regular 75% of the time
3. PR interval : Not applicable

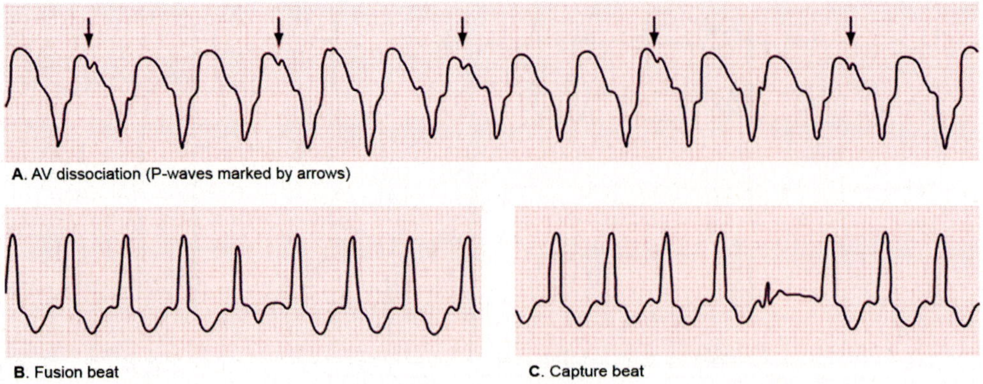


**Fig. 20.74B:** Fusion beats—the first of the narrower complexes is a fusion beat (the next two are capture beats)

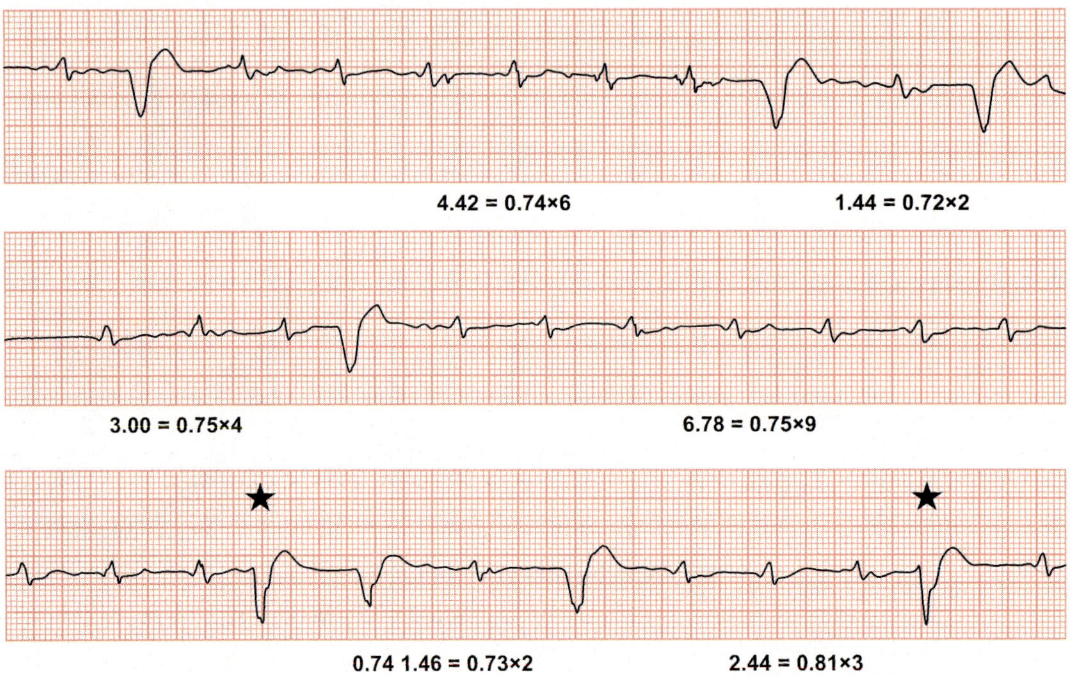


**Fig. 20.75:** In ventricular parasystole, non-fixed coupled PVCs occur at a common interectopic interval. Fusion beats, indicated by arrows, are often seen. Fusions occur when the sinus impulse entering the ventricles find the ventricles already partially depolarized by the parasystolic focus

4. QRS complex : 0.12 sec and most often 0.14 sec
5. Distinguishing features : Broad QRS complex with a regular rhythm and a rate between 100 beats/min and 170 beats/min left axis deviation, and, in VI, a monophasic R, QR, qR, RS, or a 'rabbit ear' configuration (that is, two peaks, the first being the tallest). In slower rates, AV dissociation may be seen; however, in 40% cases, there is retrograde conduction to the atria.

## Aetiological Factors

1. Drugs (digitalis, isoproterenol)
2. Coronary artery disease
3. Acute myocardial infarction
4. Significant underlying cardiac disease
5. May occur in the absence of structural heart disease.

## Variations

1. Ventricular tachycardia with retrograde conduction to the atria
2. Bidirectional ventricular tachycardia
3. Torsades de pointes
4. Ventricular flutter.

## Treatment

If there is hemodynamic deterioration, cardioversion is indicated; otherwise, lidocaine or procainamide may be given. Cardioversion attempts with 10 watt-seconds should be started and increments increased until results are obtained.

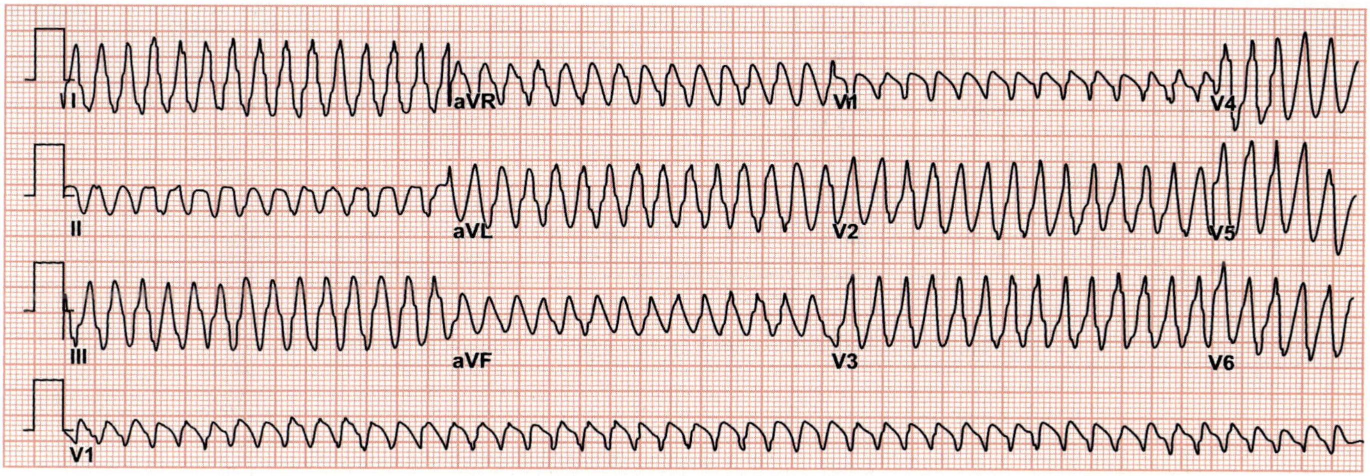


**Fig. 20.76:** Ventricular flutter

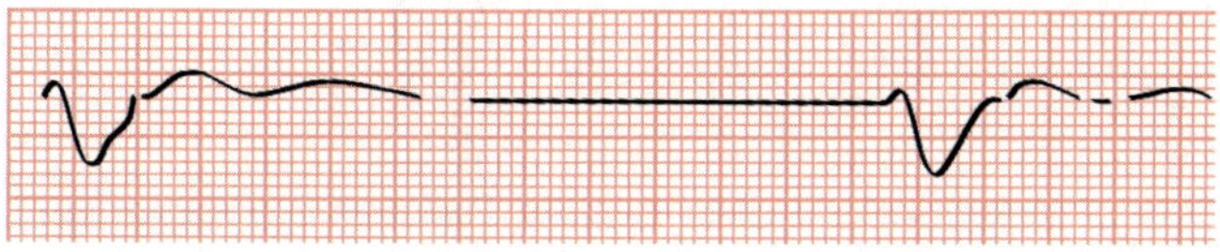

**Fig. 20.77:** ECG showing broad and slow rhythm in association with release electrical activity

## VENTRICULAR FIBRILLATION

It may be defined as disorganized electrical activity in the ventricles, resulting into inadequate contraction of the ventricle, incapable of maintaining sufficient cardiac output.

*Differential Diagnosis:* Ventricular fibrillation should always be distinguished from that of an erratic fibrillatory line within QRS complex.

### Aetiological Factors

1. Myocardial infarction
2. Myocardial ischemia
3. R-on-T, frequent, paired, or multifocal PVCs in the setting of acute myocardial infarction

### Variations

1. Coarse ventricular fibrillation
2. Fine ventricular fibrillation.

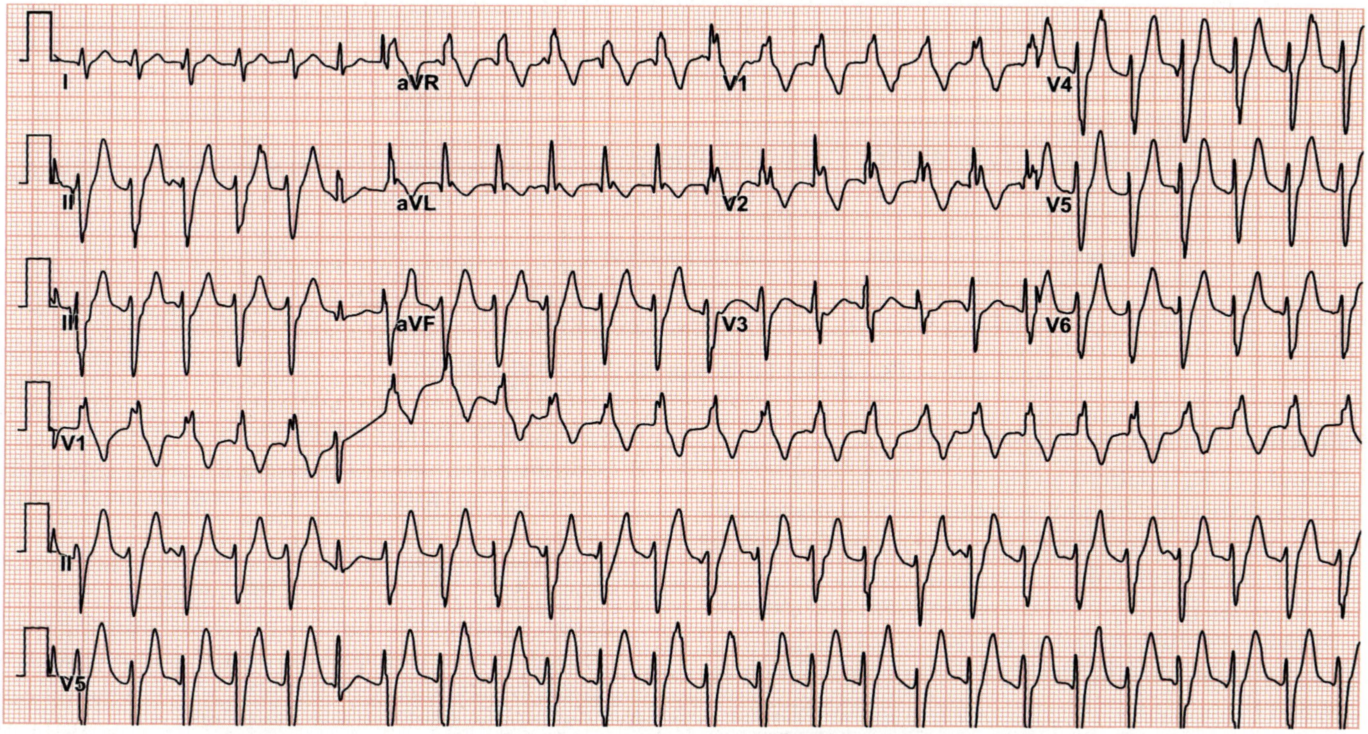


**Fig. 20.78:** Ventricular tachycardia. Broad QRS complexes with RBBB no visible P-waves

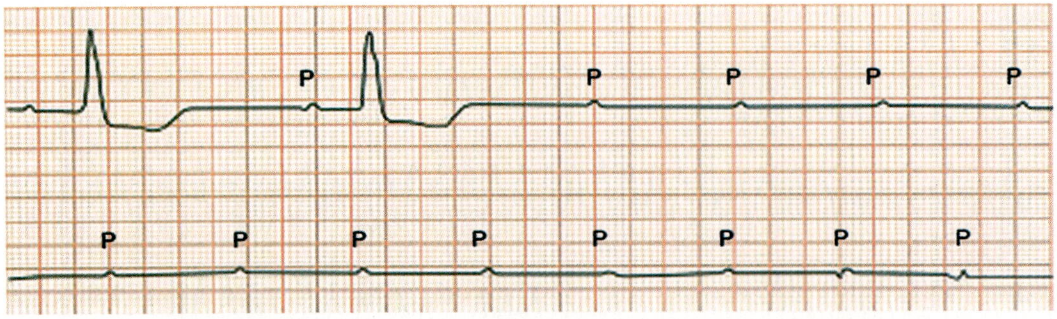


**Fig. 20.79:** ECG records a straight-line pattern indicating asystole

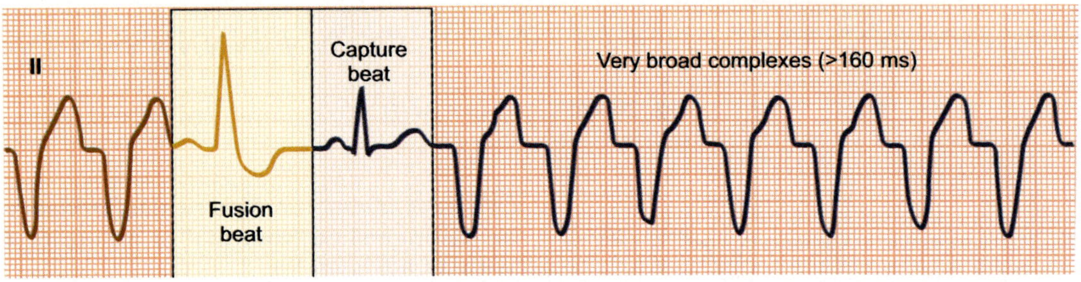


**Fig. 20.80:** Graph showing ventricular tachycardia with direct evidence of independent atrial activity. P-waves are separated by intervals of 0.75 s, and can clearly be seen after the first, third, sixth, eighth, tenth, thirteenth, fifteenth and seventeenth ventricular complexes

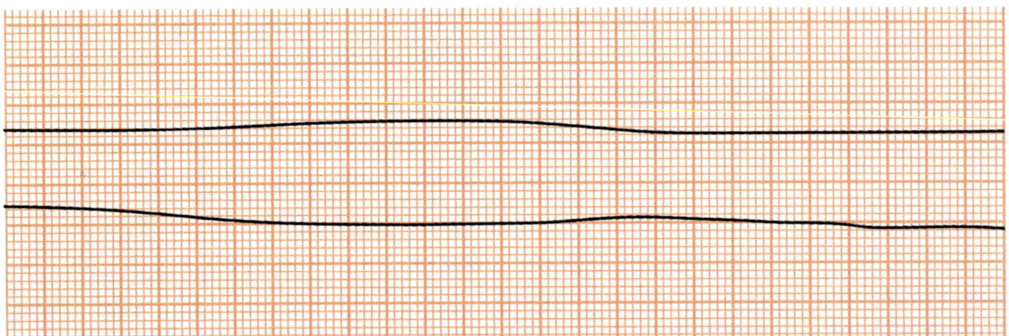

| Heart rate | Rhythm | P-wave | PR interval (in seconds) | QRS (in seconds) |
|---|---|---|---|---|
| Absent | Absent | Absent or present | N/A | Absent |

**Fig. 20.81:** Ventricular asystole (standstill)

## Treatment of Ventricular Fibrillation (VF)

1. Cough, CPR, if patient awake and able to cough
2. Defibrillate with 200 joules; repeat once, if necessary
3. If successful, administer lidocaine, a bolus and an infusion per protocol.
4. If VF persists initiate chest compression and positive pressure ventilation. Start IV line.
5. Epinephrine 1:10,000, 5 to 10 ml (0.5 to 1 mg) IV or intra-tracheal.
6. After 30–60 sec of ventilation and chest compression, defibrillate with 300–400 joules; may repeat once.
7. Bretylium 5 mg-kg IV bolus.
8. Sodium bicarbonate 1 mEq.kg IV push, especially if metabolic acidosis is documented by arterial blood gases.
9. If VF persists, attempt improvement of ventilation and oxygenation, continuous CPR, obtain arterial blood gases. Further sodium bicarbonate administration guided by arterial blood gas results, if available, if not, repeat one-half dose in 10 min.
10. Repeat epinephrine 0.5–1 mg IV stat.
11. Repeat defibrillation 300–400 joules.

12. Consider other drugs—magnesium, nitroglycerine, or additional bretylium.
13. Consider methods of 'new CPR'.

## TORSADES DE POINTES

Torsades de points (twists of points) is a polymorphous ventricular tachycardia, associated with a prolonged Q-T interval.

### ECG Characteristics

1. Rate : 150–250 beats/min
2. Rhythm : May be regular or irregular
3. PR interval : Not applicable
4. QRS complex : 0.12sec; usually, 0.14 sec
5. Distinguishing features : In sinus rhythm, the QT interval is too long (0.46–0.50 sec or 33% of baseline). This measurement is absolute as opposed to the corrected. A ventricular tachycardia, with phasic variation in the electrical polarity of the QRS complex. The tachycardia may be paroxysmal, repetitive, the patient remaining fully conscious.

*Aetiological Factors:* Any of the factors, which leads to the lengthening of the Q-T interval, as mentioned below, can lead to this disorder:

1. Antiarrhythmic drugs such as quinidine, procainamide, disopyramide, or amiodarone
2. Hypokalemia
3. Hypomagnesemia
4. Psychotropic drugs
5. Unilateral alteration of sympathetic tone
6. Profound bradycardia
7. Intracerebral pathology

### Differential Diagnosis

Coarse ventricular fibrillation, without preceding QT lengthening; ventricular flutter.

### Treatment

It consists of removing any predisposing cause and suppressing the rapid ventricular rhythm. The antiarrhythmic drugs such as quinidine, procainamide, disopyramide, and most others that may prolong the QT interval should be avoided. Magnesium may be effective, especially when the rhythm is related to an anti-arrhythmic drug. For acute management, isoproterenol infusion may be useful, particularly if there is underlying bradycardia. Atrial or ventricular overdrive pacing is also frequently very effective in acutely suppressing the rhythm. It should, usually, be continued for 24 hours. Prolonged episodes may require electrical defibrillation. If the rhythm recurs after all possible predisposing causes have been excluded, the patient should be treated with a beta-adrenergic blocking agent, which, usually, is successful. Occasionally refractory patient need operation in which a left stellate ganglion sympathectomy or implantation of an automatic, defibrillation device is considered.

Temporary overdrive ventricular or atrial pacing IV magnesium sulfate (IV push 2 g over 1–2 min IV infusion 1–2 g/h for 4–6 h)

## ACCELERATED IDIOVENTRICULAR RHYTHM

The accelerated idioventricular rhythm (AIVR) is an ectopic ventricular rhythm with a rate of 40–100 beats/min.

### ECG Characteristics

1. Rate : 40–100 beats/min
2. Rhythm : Regular
3. PR interval : Not applicable, but that of the underlying rhythm may be normal.
4. QRS complex : 0.12 sec; usually, 0.14 sec
5. Distinguishing features : A ventricular ectopic rhythm that, often, begins and ends with fusion beats and misifests itself when its rate is approximately that of the sinus node.

### Cause

Acute myocardial infarction

### Variations

Accelerated idioventricular rhythm with atrial flutter.

## VENTRICULAR FUSION COMPLEXES

It may be defined as the type of resultant complex, when two impulses collide with each other in the ventricles, like the one, seen in atrial fusion beats in atria.

### ECG Characteristics

1. Rate : That of the underlying rhythm
2. Rhythm : Regular
3. PR interval : PR interval of the fusion beat may be the same as or shorter than that of the sinus rhythm, but is never more than 0.06 sec shorter than the dominant PR interval.
4. QRS complex : Normal in the underlying rhythm, but may be variable in the fusion beats.
5. Distinguishing features : It should be differentiated from other ventricular ectopic beats by critically analyzing the basic rhythm. QRS of the fusion beat has a contour intermediate between that of the fusing impulses.

### Causes

That of the ventricular ectopic beat or rhythm.

### Variations

1. Ventricular parasystole
2. Accelerated idioventricular rhythm

3. Electronic pacemaker fusion beat
4. End-diastolic PVCs
5. Bigeminal end-diastolic PVCs

### Differential Diagnosis

Electrical alternans vs bigeminal end-diastolic PVCs.

## VENTRICULAR PARASYSTOLE

These are, usually, unifocal premature ventricular contractions which have varying coupling intervals at regular cadence. Such a constantly recurring ectopic beat is termed as parasystole. Parasystole is diagnosed by observing on active focus of automaticity, usually, in the region of ventricle, which operates independently of the dominant pacemaker. The rhythmic discharges are, somewhat, not affected by the propagation of the primary impulse. In this condition, both the dominant and the parasystolic rhythms have separate and independent cadences.

In classical ventricular parasystole, the rate of impulses from the ectopic focus is considerably slower than that of the sinus node, because the sinus node and the ventricular ectopic focus are firing independently of one another and at different rates. Premature ventricular contractions produced by this mechanism, usually, will show marked variation in coupling (R-V) intervals. Electrocardiographic analysis will reveal that the intervals, between successive premature ventricular contractions, are all multiples of a manifest or calculated minimum V-V interval. Clinically, it seems to be benign condition. The parasystolic arrhythmia is, frequently, resistant to anti-arrhythmic drug therapy.

### ECG Characteristics

1. Rate : That of the underlying rhythm
2. Rhythm : Irregular, as a result of extrasytoles
3. PR interval : Normal is the underlying rhythm
4. QRS complex : Normal in the underlying rhythm; broad in the parasystolic beats
5. Distinguishing features :
   a. No fixed coupling
   b. Interectopic intervals that have a common denominator
   c. Fusion beats

### Variations

Fixed coupling in parasystole if the rates of the two pacemaker happen to be mathematically related. No fixed coupling, but interectopic intervals are not exact multiples, because the ectopic focus is influenced, but not reset, by the sinus impulses.

### Differential Diagnosis

Accelerated idioventricular rhythm.

## VENTRICULAR FLUTTER AND FIBRILLATION

The electrocardiographic diagraphic of ventricular flutter is made, the ventricular tachyarrhythmias is greater than 200 beats/min, and large sinusoidal or zigzag waves are observed. The rate is frequently, between 240–280 beats/min. In ventricular flutter, QRS complex cannot be clearly distinguished from ST-T-waves. The diagnosis of ventricular flutter may be applied when the rate is less than 200 beats/min if the ECG morphology is absolutely typical.

Ventricular fibrillation is recognized on ECG tracing by the absence of QRS complex and T-waves and the presence of low-amplitude base-line undulations which are quite variable, both in amplitude and periodicity. Clinically, ventricular flutter is, rarely, recorded, perhaps, due to its highly unstable rhythm that tends to convert to sinus-rhythm or, more often, to ventricular fibrillation. Ventricular flutter, nearly always, leads to severe and symptomatic hemodynamic impairment.

Ventricular fibrillation on the other hand is the most catastrophic cardiac arrhythmia. It is usually, observed in myocardial infarction, hypokalamia marked hypothermia, electrocution and drug toxicity, i.e. with digitalis, quinidine, procainamide or tricyclic antidepressants. Ventricular fibrillation can lead to death, within a short period, due to cardiogenic collapse if such a rhythm is not converted to hemodynamically effective rhythm.

### ECG Characteristics

1. Rate : 150–300 beats/min
2. Rhythm : Regular or irregular
3. PR interval : Not applicable
4. QRS complex : Broad and poorly defined
5. Distinguishing features : A zig-zag, almost a sine wave configuration, instead of clearly defined QRS complex.

### Aetiological Factors

1. Myocardial infarction
2. Myocardial ischemia
3. R-on-T frequent, paired, or multifocal PVCs in the setting of acute myocardial infarction.
4. An interim arrhythmia between ventricular tachycardia and fibrillation.
5. Drugs (digitalis, procainamide, quinidine and tricyclic antidepressants).
6. Electrolyte imbalance, i.e. hypokalaemia.

### Differential Diagnosis

Torsades de pointes.

## PULSELESS ELECTRICAL ACTIVITY

Pulseless electrical activity is defined as the absence of a pulse or blood pressure measured by usual methods with the continued presence of electrical activity of the heart (Table 20.7).

### *A. Aetiology*

1. Pulseless electrical activity may result from a variety of rhythm disturbances, such as electrical mechanical

**Table 20.7:** Conditions that cause pulseless electrical activity

| Condition | Clues | Management |
|---|---|---|
| Hypovolemia | History, flat neck veins | Volume infusion |
| Hypoxia | Cyanosis, blood gases, airway problems | Ventilation |
| Cardiac temponade | History (trauma, renal failure, and thoracic malignancy), no pulse with CPR, vein distention; impending tamponade—tachycardia, hypotension, low pulse pressure—changing to sudden bradycardia as terminal event | Pericardiocentesis |
| Tension pneumothorax | History (asthma, ventilator, chronic obstructive pulmonary disease, and trauma), no pulse with CPR, neck vein distention, and tracheal deviation | Needle decompression |
| Hypothermia | History of exposure to cold, central body temperature | Warming |
| Massive pulmonary embolism | History, no pulse felt with CPR | Pulmonary arteriogram surgical embolectomy, thrombolytics |
| Drug overdose (tricyclics, digoxin, β-blockers, calcium channel blockers) | Bradycardia, history of ingestion, empty bottles at the scene, pupils, and neurologic exam | Drug screens, intubation, lavage, activated charcoal, lactulose per local protocols |
| Hyperkalemia | History of renal failure, diabetes, recent dialysis, dialysis fistulas, medications | Calcium chloride (immediate); then combination of insulin, glucose, sodium polystyrene sulfonate/sorbitol; dialysis (long term) |
| Pre-existing acidosis | History of bicarbonate-responsive pre-existing acidosis, renal failure | Sodium bicarbonate, hyperventillation |
| Acute massive MI | History, ECG, and enzymes | Treat for cardiogenic shock |

CPR=cardiopulmonary resuscitation; ECG=electrocardiography; MI=myocardial infarction from Brainard CA, 1997.

dissociation, idioventricular rhythms, and ventricular tachycardias. When the electrical activity is organized and within the physiologic range, the term electrical mechanical dissociation is used.

2. A variety of clinical situations are also associated with pulseless electrical activity, a potentially manageable condition if certain actions are undertaken rapidly.

### B. Therapy

1. Specific management of the underlying cause is most likely to result in a successful outcome
2. Emergency intervention should be initiated at once, including:
   a. Cardiopulmonary resuscitation and airway management with intubation to treat any possible hypoxia
   b. Epinephrine, 1 mg intravenous push every 3–5 minutes
   c. Atropine, 1 mg intravenously, if the rate is more than 60 beats/min; may be repeated every 3–5 minutes to a total dose of 0.03–0.04 mg/kg
   d. Empiric intravenous volume infusion

## Asystole

1. **Clinical presentation:** Asystole is defined as the absence of myocardial electrical activity. It should be confirmed by switching between several leads or changing the position of the defibrillation paddles.
   a. Most patients with asystole present in a code situation. Persons outside of the hospital who are found to have asystole by the initial responding team usually have it as a result of profound myocardial ischemia. The possibility of a successful outcome in this situation is extremely small.
   b. Hospital in patients monitored by telemetry, on the other hand, may have a favorable outcome.
2. **Aetiology:** Asystole may be due to profound parasympathetic suppression of both atrial and ventricular activity, stunning of the myocardium due to electrical defibrillation, complete heart block, or prolonged myocardial ischemia.
3. **Therapy:** Management consists of cardiopulmonary resuscitation, intubation, and atropine to unmask the possibility of profound parasympathetic suppression of both atrial and ventricular activity.
   a. Routine shocking is strongly discouraged. Electrical shocks have not been demonstrated to have any benefit in the management of asystole and may in fact produce a stunned myocardium, leading to a delay in the return of a rhythm.
   b. Pacing for asystole is controversial. If pacing is to have any effect, it must be initiated early. Patients with asystole due to myocardial ischemia are unlikely to respond to pacing, but those with asystole due to other causes might respond.

### Cardiac Conduction Abnormalities

Heart block can occur anywhere in the specialized conduction system beginning with the sinoatrial connections, the AV junction, the bundle branches and their fascicles, and ending in the distal ventricular Purkinje fibers. Disorders of conduction may manifest as slowed conduction **(1st degree)**, intermittent conduction failure **(2nd degree)**, or complete conduction failure **(3rd degree)**. In addition, 2nd degree heart block occurs in two varieties: Type I **(Wenckebach)** and Type II **(Mobitz)**. In Type I block there is **decremental conduction** which means that conduction velocity progressively slows down until failure of conduction occurs. Type II block is all or none. The term *exit block* is used to identify conduction delay or failure immediately distal to a pacemaker site. Sino-atrial (SA) block is an exit block. This section considers conduction disorders in the anatomical sequence that defines the cardiac conduction system (Figs 20.82–20.91).

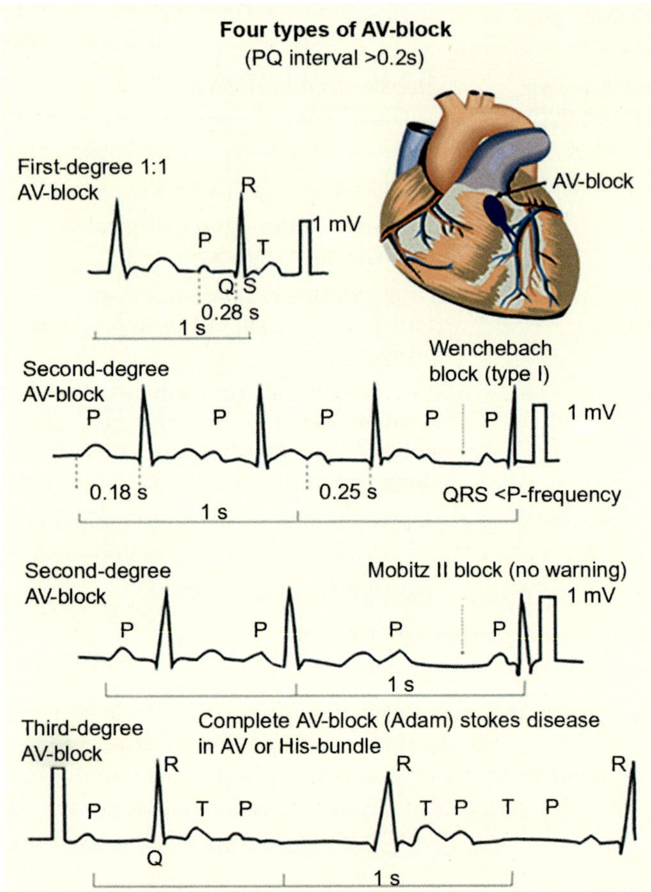


**Fig. 20.82:** ECG morphology explaining four common types of AV blocks

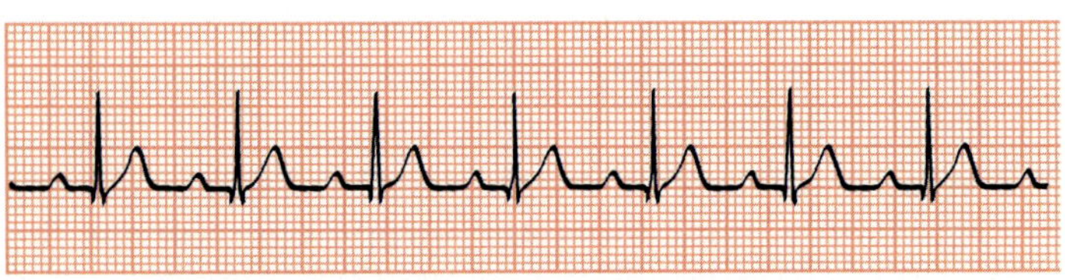

**Fig. 20.83:** First degree AV block (PR=280 ms)

## INTRAVENTRICULAR BLOCKS

### Right Bundle Branch Block

- 'Complete' right bundle branch block (RBBB) has a QRS duration ≥0.12s
- Close examination of QRS complex in various leads reveals that the terminal forces (i.e. second half of QRS) are oriented *rightward* and *anteriorly* because the right ventricle is depolarized *after* the left ventricle. This means the following:
  - Terminal R′ wave in lead V1 (usually see rSR′ complex) indicating late *anterior* forces
  - Terminal S waves in leads I, aVL, V6 indicating late *rightward* forces
  - Terminal R wave in lead aVR indicating late *rightward* forces
  - The frontal plane QRS axis in RBBB should be in the normal range (i.e. -30 to +90 degrees). If left axis deviation is present, think about *left anterior fascicular block*, and if right axis deviation is present, think about *left posterior fascicular block* in addition to the RBBB.
- 'Incomplete' RBBB has a QRS duration of 0.10–0.12s with the same terminal QRS features. This is often a normal variant.
- The 'normal' ST-T-waves in RBBB should be oriented opposite to the direction of the terminal QRS forces, i.e. in leads with terminal R or R′ forces the ST-T should be negative or downward; in leads with terminal S forces the ST-T should be positive or upward. If the ST-T-waves are in the *same direction* as the terminal QRS forces, they should be labeled primary *ST-T-wave abnormalities.*

### Left Bundle Branch Block

- 'Complete' left bundle branch block (LBBB) has a QRS duration ≥0.12s

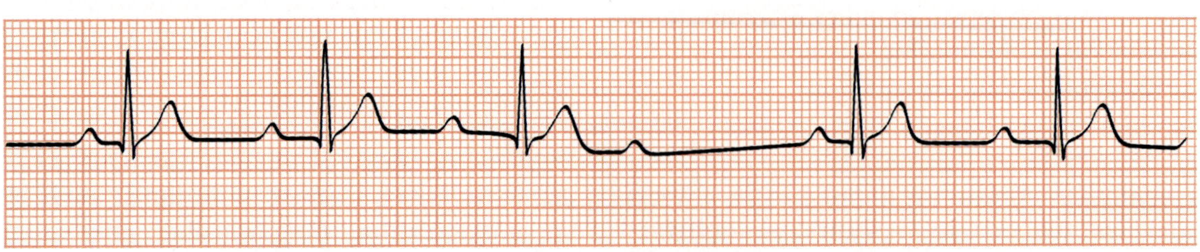

**Fig. 20.84:** Classic Wenckebach phenomenon in which there is progressive lengthening of PR interval till there is dropping of cardiac cycle

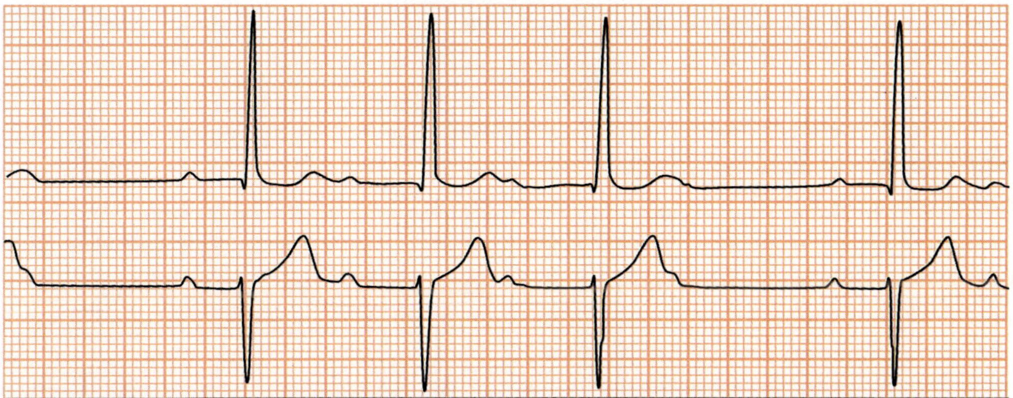

| P-wave | PR interval (in seconds) | QRS (in seconds) | Characteristics |
|---|---|---|---|
| Conduction intermittant | Increasingly prolonged | Before each QRS, identical | QRS dropped in a repreating pattern |

**Fig. 20.85:** Second degree AV block-Mobitz (Wenckebach)

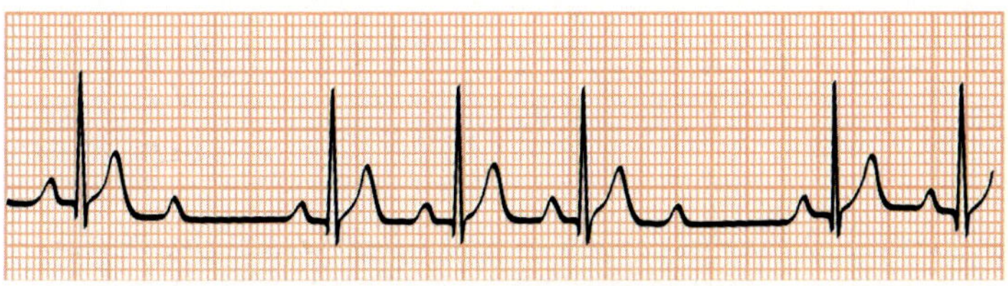

**Fig. 20.86:** AV block (Mobiz type II)

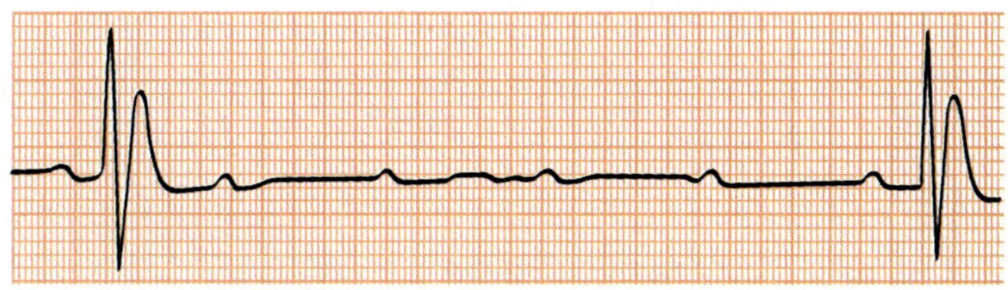

**Fig. 20.87:** High grade AV block (Mobiz type III)

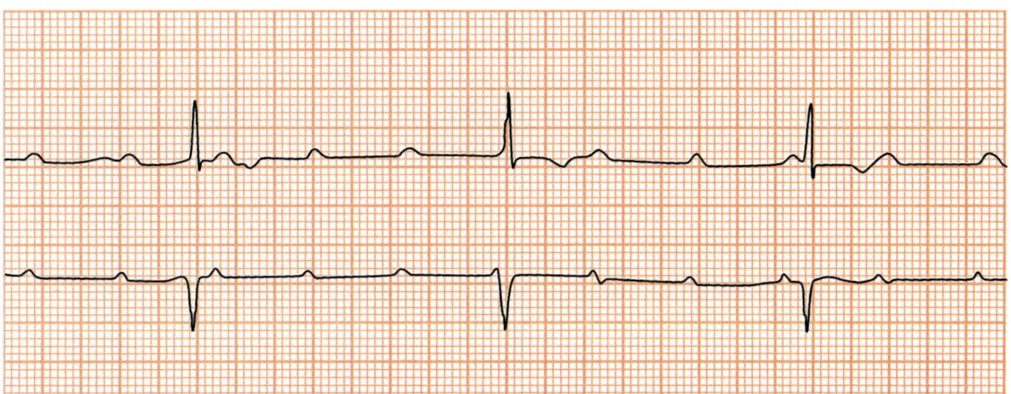

| P-wave | PR interval (in seconds) | QRS (in seconds) | Characteristics |
|---|---|---|---|
| Normal but not related to QRS | None | N/A | No relationship between P and RS |

**Fig. 20.88:** Third degree (complete) AV block

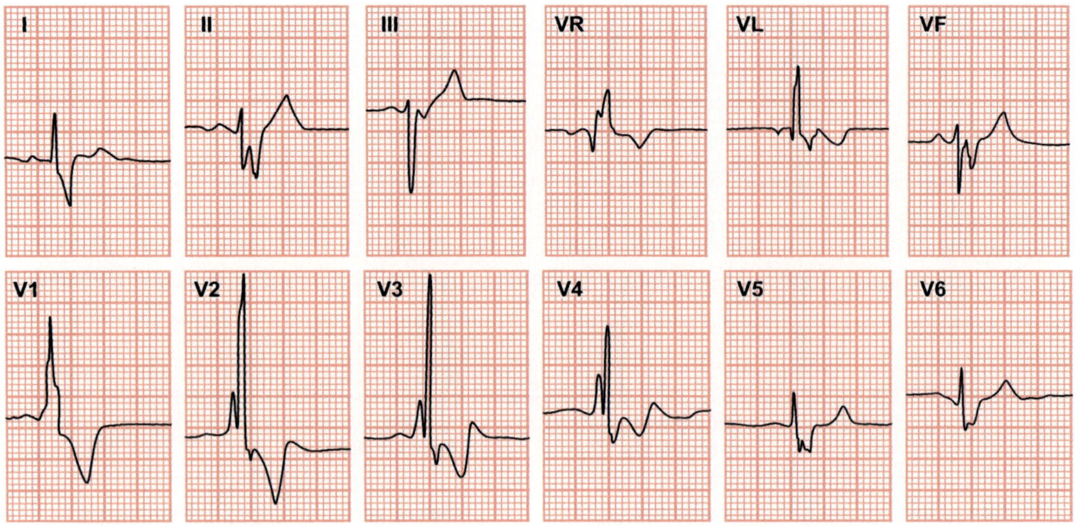


**Fig. 20.89:** Left axis deviation and RBBB in bifascicular block

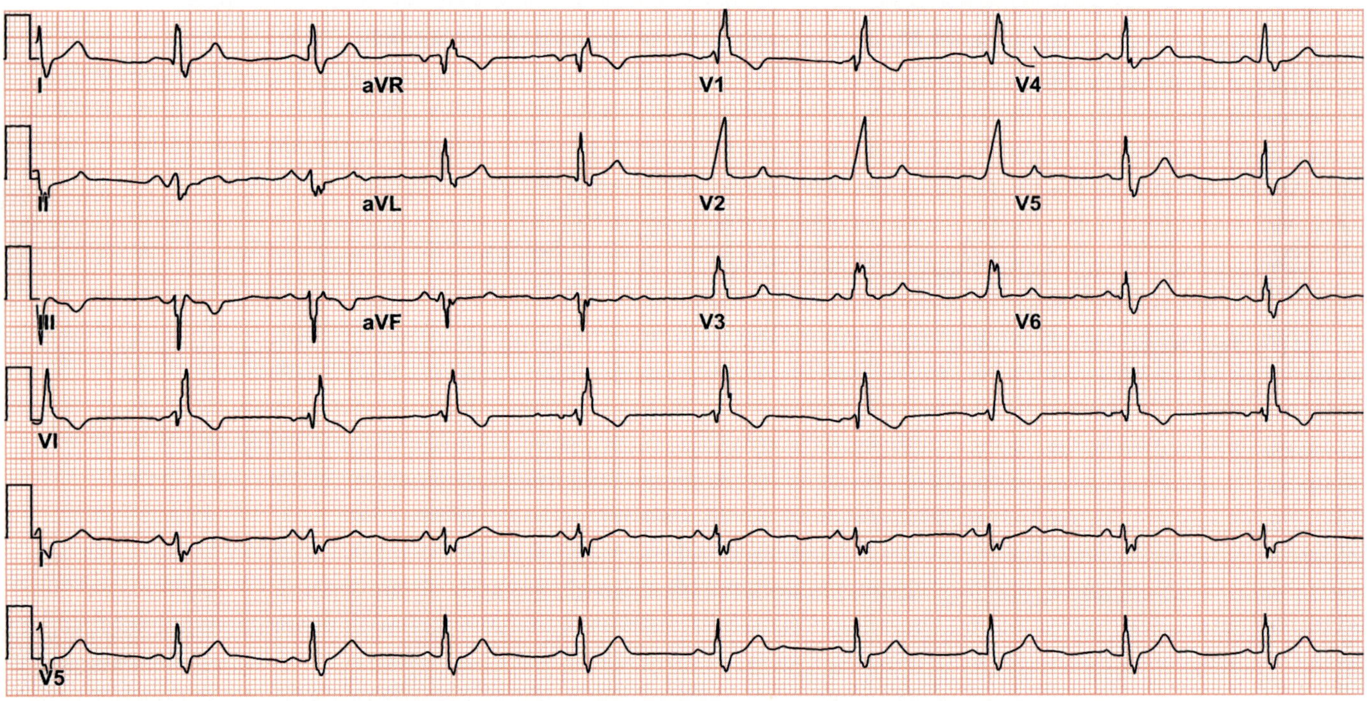


**Fig. 20.90:** Bifascicular blocks RBBB + LAFB, i.e. RBBB + LAD

- Close examination of QRS complex in various leads reveals that the terminal forces (i.e. second half of QRS) are oriented *leftward* and *posteriorly* because the left ventricle is depolarized *after* the right ventricle.
- Terminal S waves in lead V1 indicating late *posterior* forces
- Terminal R waves in lead I, aVL, V6 indicating late *leftward* forces; usually broad, monophasic R-waves are seen in these leads as illustrated in the ECG below; in addition, poor R progression from V1 to V3 is common.
- The 'normal' ST-T-waves in LBBB should be oriented opposite to the direction of the terminal QRS forces, i.e. in leads with terminal R or R′ forces the ST-T should be downward; in leads with terminal S forces the ST-T should be upward. If the ST-T-waves are in the *same direction* as the terminal QRS forces, they should be labeled *primary ST-T-wave abnormalities*. In the above ECG the ST-T-waves are 'normal' for LBBB, i.e. they are *secondary* to the change in the ventricular depolarization sequence.

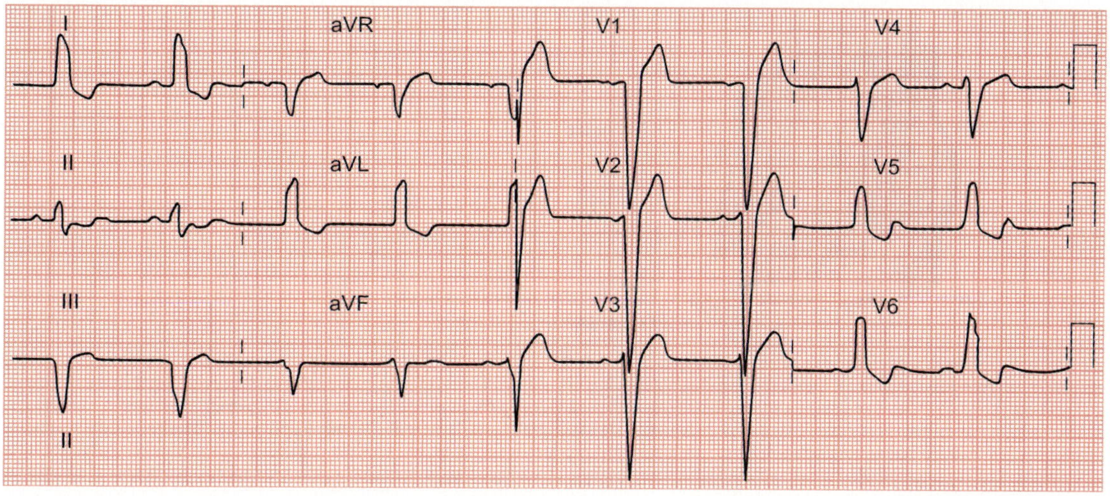


**Fig. 20.91:** In LBBB, the normal direction of septal depolarisation is reversed (become right to left), as the impulse spreads first to the RV via the right bundle branch and then to the LV via the septum. This sequence of activation extends the QRS duration to >120 ms and eliminates the normal septal Q-waves in the lateral leads

- 'Incomplete' LBBB looks like LBBB but QRS duration = 0.10–0.12s, with less ST-T change. This is often a progression of LVH.
- **Left anterior fascicular block (LAFB):** The most common intraventricular conduction defect
- Left axis deviation in frontal plane, usually –45 to –90 degrees
- rS complexes in leads II, III, aVF
- Small q-wave in leads I *and/or* aVL
- R-peak time in lead aVL >0.04s, often with slurred R wave downstroke
- QRS duration usually <0.12s unless coexisting RBBB
- Usually see poor R progression in leads V1-V3 and deeper S waves in leads V5 and V6
- May *mimic* LVH voltage in lead aVL, and *mask* LVH voltage in leads V5 and V6.
- **Left posterior fascicular block (LPFB):** Very rare intraventricular defect
- Right axis deviation in the frontal plane (usually >+100 degrees)
- rS complex in lead I
- qR complexes in leads II, III, aVF, with R in lead III>R in lead II
- QRS duration usually <0.12s unless coexisting RBBB
- **Must first exclude** (on clinical grounds) other causes of right axis deviation such as cor pulmonale, pulmonary heart disease, pulmonary hypertension, etc. because these conditions can result in the identical ECG picture.

### Bifascicular Blocks

- RBBB plus either LAFB (common) or LPFB (uncommon)
- Features of RBBB plus frontal plane features of the fascicular block (axis deviation, etc.)

## LONG QT SYNDROME

Patients with a prolonged QT interval are more prone to the risk of recurrent syncope and sudden death due to ventricular tachycardia or ventricular fibrillation. The idiopathic long QT syndrome ventricular fibrillation. The idiopathic long QT syndrome may be either autosomal recessive or autosomal dominant (Figs 20.92 and 20.93).

Prolongation of the QT interval may be:

- Acquired by patients having electrolyte imbalance,
- Taking antiarrhythmic drugs,
- Taking psychotropic drugs,
- Having myocarditis,
- Myocardial ischemia,
- Sinus node disease or
- Central nervous system disease consuming liquid protein diets

It is associated with a specific type of ventricular arrhythmia, Torsade de pointes, which is characterized by the cycles of alternating electrical polarity of the QRS complex peaks that oscillate or twist around the isoelectric line. The alternating cycles may be interrupted by periods of rapid tachycardia and polarity. The rhythm rate varies from 160 to 280 beats per minute and most often is between 200 beats and 250 beats per minute. Assessment and treatment of ventricular tachyarrhythmias present extraordinary challenges to the clinician. Moreover, the prognosis for patients is quite variable with these characteristically sudden-onset, unpredictable, and transitory arrhythmias. In some patients, ventricular ectopic activity may be benign and without sequelae, but in other patients, comparable ectopy is a harbinger of ventricular fibrillation and sudden cardiac death.

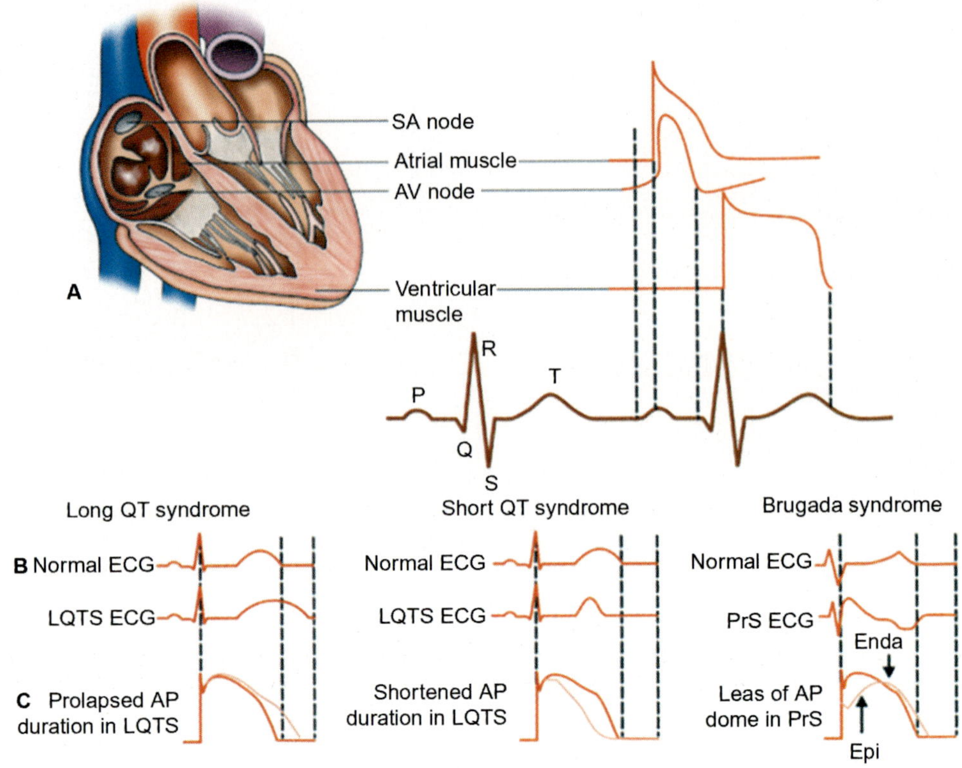


**Fig. 20.92:** The genesis of long and short QT interval

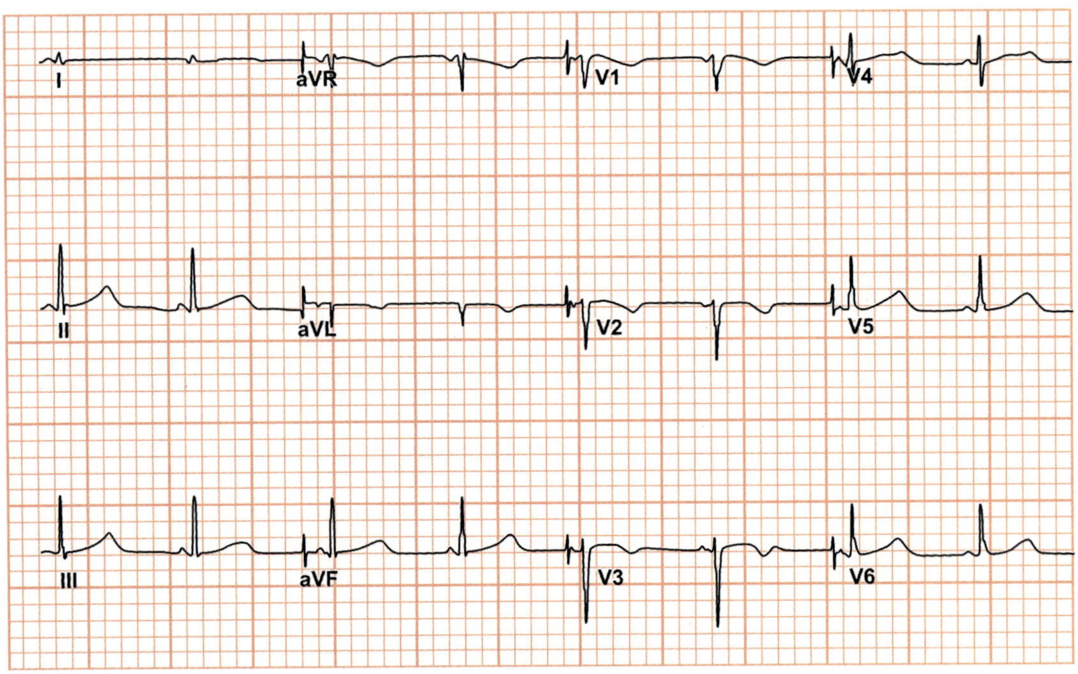


**Fig. 20.93:** ECG showing long QTc (620 mc) due to severe hypothermia

## SHORT QT SYNDROME

Short QT syndrome (Fig. 20.94) is a genetic disease of the electrical system of the heart. It consists of a constellation of signs and symptoms, consisting of a short QT interval interval on EKG (? 300 ms) that doesn't significantly change with heart rate, tall and peaked T-waves, and a structurally normal heart. Short QT syndrome appears to be inherited in an autosomal dominant pattern, and a few affected families have been identified.

Short QT syndrome is inherited in an autosmal dominant pattern. Individuals with short QT syndrome frequently complain of palpitations and may have syncope (loss of

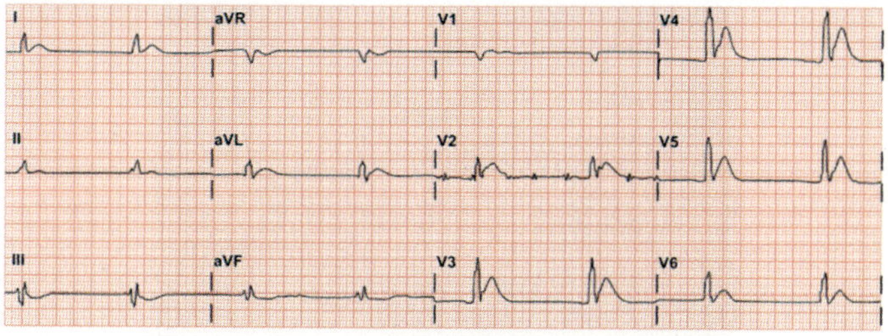


**Fig. 20.94:** ECG showing very short QTc (280 mc) with tall peaked T-waves due to congenital short QT interval

consciousness) that is unexplained. Mutations in the KCNH2, KCNJ2, and KCNQ1 genes cause short QT syndrome. These genes provide instructions for making proteins that act as channels across the cell membrane. These channels transport positively charged atoms (ions) of potassium into and out of cells. In cardiac muscle, these ion channels play critical roles in maintaining the heart's normal rhythm. Mutations in the KCNH2, KCNJ2, or KCNQ1 gene increase the activity of the channels, which changes the flow of potassium ions between cells. This disruption in ion transport alters the way the heart beats, leading to the abnormal heart rhythm characteristic of short QT syndrome. Short QT syndrome appears to have an autosomal dominant pattern of inheritance. Due to the autosomal dominant inheritance pattern, most individuals will have family members with a history of unexplained or sudden death at a young age (even in infancy), palpitations, or atrial fibrillation. Short QT syndrome is associated with an increased risk of sudden cardiac death, most likely due to ventricular fibrillation.

### Diagnosis

The diagnosis of short QT syndrome consists of characteristic history and findings on EKG and electrophysiologic testing. There are currently no set guidelines for the diagnosis of short QT syndrome.

### Electrocardiogram

The characteristic findings of short QT syndrome on EKG are a short QT interval, typically 300 ms, that doesn't significantly change with the heart rate. Tall peaked T-waves may also be noted. Individuals may also have an underlying atrial rhythm of atrial fibrillation.

## BRUGADA SYNDROME

In 1992, Brugada and colleagues described a clinical syndrome consisting of apparently healthy adults presenting with syncope or sudden death (Fig. 20.95). Their ECGs showed coved ST-segment elevation and negative T-waves in leads V1 and V2 (V3) in the absence of RBBB pattern. This ECG pattern has become to be known as the 'Brugada-ECG.' These patients were thought to have no evidence of structural heart disease, and were at high risk for recurrent syncope or sudden death. In 15–20% of patients a genetic defect in the cardiac sodium channel was

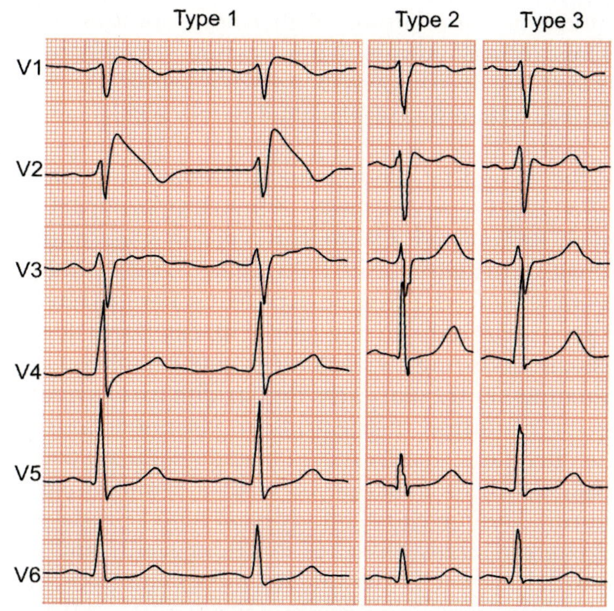


**Fig. 20.95:** ECG abnormality diagnostic or suspected of Brugada syndrome. Type 1 ECG (coved-type ST-segment elevation) is the only diagnostic ECG in Brugada syndrome and is defined as a J-wave amplitude or an ST-segment elevation of >2 mm or 0.2 mV at its peak (followed by a negative T-wave with little or no isoelectric separation). Type 2 ECG (saddle-back type ST-segment elevation), defined as a J-wave amplitude of >2 mm, gives rise to a gradually descending ST-segment elevation (remaining >1 mm above the baseline) followed by a positive or biphasic T-wave that results in a saddle-back configuration. Type 3 ECG is a right precordial ST-segment elevation (saddle-back type, coved type, or both) without meeting the aforementioned criteria

found. It has been proposed that there is a premature termination of the epicardial action potential with loss of the phase-2 dome pattern. The ECG changes are believed to be due to regional epicardial, endocardial voltage gradient during the plateau phase of the action potential. This voltage gradient may give rise to VT due to phase-2 re-entry caused by inhomogeneity of the voltage in adjacent areas of the myocardium. In patients with the Brugada syndrome, syncope and sudden death are due to polymorphic VT. Since the original description, it has been observed that the 'Brugada-ECG' type ST-segment elevation in V1 in the right precordial leads can be:

- Cove shaped,
- Saddle shaped,
- Transient, and be present in a multitude of clinical-conditions.

There has been a recent attempt to standardize this diagnostic ECG feature as follows:

- **Type I**: Coved-shaped right precordial ST-elevation, in more than one right precordial lead (V1–V3), of >2 mm followed by a negative T-wave
- **Type II**: Saddle-shaped ST-elevation, and
- **Type III**: ST-elevation of <2 mm.

Only type I is said to be diagnostic of Brugada syndrome. These ST-elevations are sensitive to heart rate and the effects of autonomic stimulation. Furthermore, sodium channel-blocking antiarrhythmic drugs such as procainamide or lecainide have been shown to 'provoke' these ECG changes in patients with otherwise normal baseline ECG, and have been proposed as a screening tool in patients suspected to have the Brugada syndrome. However, the sensitive, specificity and reproducibility of this drug provocation are not well established. Of interest, certain gene mutations are sensitive to temperature with regard to their phenotypic expression. Indeed, Brugada-type ECG changes have been seen in patients only during febrile illness. Some speculate that seizures during febrile illness may be related to self-terminating ventricular arrhythmias due to a temperature sensitive mutation in the sodium channel, giving rise to the 'Brugada syndrome.' Patients with resuscitated sudden death or syncope or with a family history of premature sudden death and typical type I Brudaga ECG changes are at increased risk of recurrent events, and should be considered for ICD therapy. Asymptomatic patients who have an unprovoked typical Brudaga ECG (type I) are also at increased risk for arrhythmic events, but the magnitude of the risk is unclear. In one study the event rate over a mean of 24 months follow up was 8% in these patients. Those presenting with typical Brugada ECG (type I) only after drug exposure or those presenting with nondiagnostic right precordial ECG abnormalities (type II, type III) are believed to be at low risk. The role of electrophysiologic study and prognostic value of inducible VF remain controversial.

## HOW ARE ARRHYTHMIAS DIAGNOSED?

Arrhythmias can be hard to diagnose, especially the types that only cause symptoms every once in a while. Doctors diagnose arrhythmias based on medical and family histories, a physical exam, and the results from tests and procedures (Figs 20.96–20.99).

### Specialists Involved

Doctors who specialize in the diagnosis and treatment of heart diseases include:

- Cardiologists: These doctors diagnose and treat adults who have heart problems.
- Pediatric cardiologists: These doctors diagnose and treat babies, children, and youth who have heart problems.
- Electrophysiologists: These doctors are cardiologists or pediatric cardiologists who specialize in arrhythmias (Table 20.8).

### Medical and Family Histories

To diagnose an arrhythmia, your doctor may ask you to describe your symptoms. He or she may ask whether you feel fluttering in your chest and whether you feel dizzy or light-headed (Table 20.9).

Your doctor also may ask whether you have other health problems, such as a history of heart disease, high blood pressure, diabetes, or thyroid problems. He or she may ask about your family's medical history, including whether anyone in your family:

- Has a history of arrhythmias
- Has ever had heart disease or high blood pressure
- Has died suddenly
- Has other illnesses or health problems

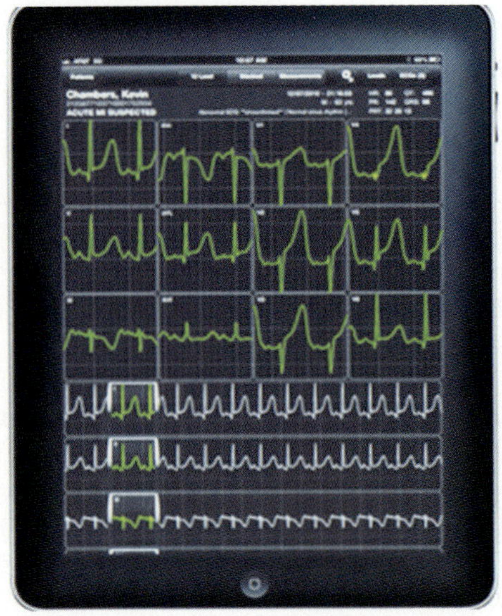

**Fig. 20.96:** ECG measurements are challenging because changes as small as 0.5 millimeters can indicate the presence of a serious or emergency heart condition. AirStrip cardiology's high resolution can detect such small differences through completely interactive iPad or iPhone views. Unlike traditional remote diagnostics, zooming in on waveforms does not affect visual clarity. With AirStrip cardiology, clinical information is available from 12- and 15-lead ECGs, supporting high precision levels. Clinicians can view current data and historical tests conducted up to 1 year ago, in 10-second increments. Regardless of where remote cardiologists are when a critical decision is needed, they can leverage AirStrip cardiology to quickly determine the best treatment paths for their patients. This may reduce the need to return to the hospital or access a computer connected to the hospital network. A remote cardiologist can now use AirStrip cardiology to precisely measure ECG waveforms, helping on-site ED clinicians determine, for example, if a patient requires Cath lab intervention

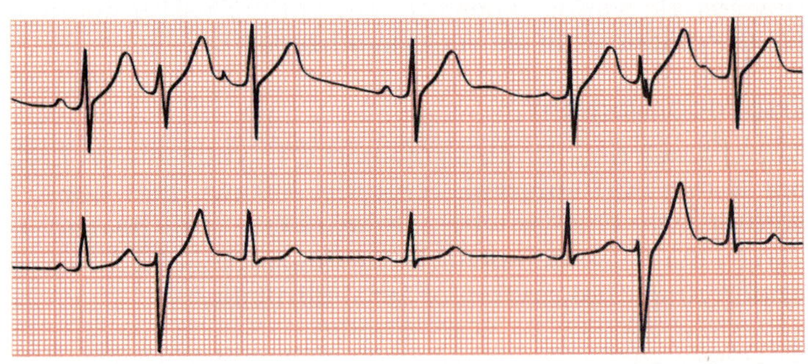

**Fig. 20.97:** Interpolated VPCs. There is no pause after the premature contractions

**Table 20.8:** Ventricular arrhythmias: who to refer and who not to refer to an electrophysiologist

| Do not refer | Do refer |
|---|---|
| • Patients with mildly symptomatic or asymptomatic ventricular ectopic activity | • Patients with highly symptomatic ventricular ectopic activity |
| • Asymptomatic patients with 'benign' ventricular tachycardia on or off antiarrhythmic drug treatment | • Symptomatic patients with 'benign' ventricular tachycardia or controlled only with unacceptable side effects from antiarrhythmic drugs |
| • Patients who are candidates for prophylactic ICD implantation but without symptomatic arrhythmia | • Patients who are candidates for prophylactic ICD implantation but with symptomatic arrhythmia |
| | • Any patient with symptomatic ventricular tachycardia with or without prophylactic ICD indication |
| | • Any patient suspected of having a 'sudden cardiac death syndrome' |
| | • Any patient in whom arrhythmia mechanism is uncertain |

ICD=implantable cardioverter-defibrillator.

**Table 20.9:** Specific arrhythmias and associated defects in adults with congenital heart disease

| Arrhythmias | Do associated defects |
|---|---|
| **Tachycardias** | |
| Accessory pathways | Ebstein's anomaly, L-TGA |
| Twin AV nodes | Heterotaxy syndrome |
| Intra-atrial re-entrant tachycardia (atrial flutter) | Postoperative mustard, postoperative senning, postoperative fontan, and others |
| Atrial fibrillation | Mitral valve disease, aortic stenosis, and unrepaired single ventricle |
| Ventricular tachycardia | Tetralogy of fallot, congenital aortic stenosis, and others |
| **Bradycardias** | |
| Congenital sinus node dysfunction | Heterotaxy syndrome |
| Acquired sinus node dysfunction | Postoperative mustard, postoperative senning, postoperative fontan, posterative glenn, and others |
| Congenital AV block | Endocardial cushion defects, L-TGA |
| Acquired AV block | VSD closure, subaortic stenosis relief, and AV valve replacement |

VSD=ventricular septal defect

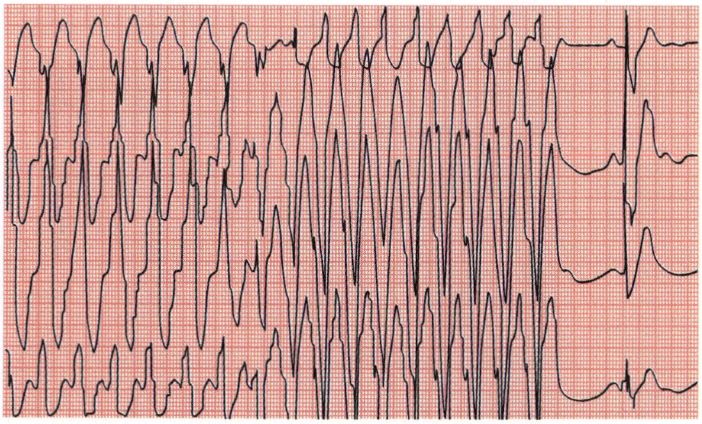

**Fig. 20.98:** Contineous Holter monitoring ECG shows ventricular tachycardia is terminated with ventricular burst pacing from the ICD

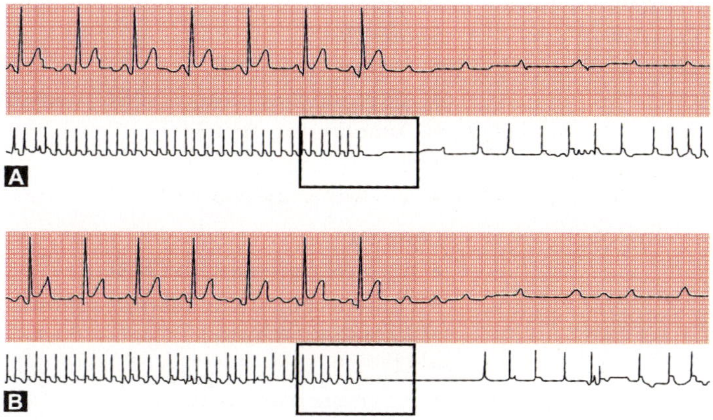

**Fig. 20.99:** Holter recording showing complete heart block in a woman who complained of attacks of palpitations and syncope

- Your doctor will likely want to know what medicines you're taking, including over-the-counter medicines and supplements.
- Your doctor may ask about your health habits, such as physical activity, smoking, or using alcohol or drugs (for example, cocaine). He or she also may want to know whether you have had emotional stress or anger.

### Physical Exam

During a physical exam, your doctor may:
- Listen to the rate and rhythm of your heartbeat
- Listen to your heart for a heart murmur (an extra or unusual sound heard during your heartbeat)
- Check your pulse to find out how fast your heart is beating
- Check for swelling in your legs or feet, which could be a sign of an enlarged heart or heart failure
- Look for signs of other diseases, such as thyroid disease, that could be causing the problem

## DIAGNOSTIC TESTS AND PROCEDURES

### Electrocardiogram

An electrocardiogram (EKG) is a simple, painless test that detects and records the heart's electrical activity. It's the most common test used to diagnose arrhythmias (Table 20.10).

An EKG shows how fast the heart is beating and its rhythm (steady or irregular). It also records the strength and timing of electrical signals as they pass through the heart.

A standard EKG only records the heartbeat for a few seconds. It won't detect arrhythmias that don't happen during the test.

To diagnose arrhythmias that come and go, your doctor may have you wear a portable EKG monitor. The two most common types of portable EKGs are Holter and event monitors.

### Holter and Event Monitors

A Holter monitor records the heart's electrical signals for a full 24- or 48-hour period. You wear one while you do your normal daily activities. This allows the monitor to record your heart for a longer time than a standard EKG.
- An event monitor is similar to a Holter monitor. You wear an event monitor while doing your normal activities. However, an event monitor only records your heart's electrical activity at certain times while you're wearing it.
- For many event monitors, you push a button to start the monitor when you feel symptoms. Other event monitors start automatically when they sense abnormal heart rhythms.
- Some event monitors are able to send data about your heart's electrical activity to a central monitoring station. Technicians at the station review the information and send it to your doctor. You also can use the device to report any symptoms you are having.
- You can wear an event monitor for weeks or until symptoms occur.

### Other Tests

Other tests also are used to help diagnose arrhythmias.

**Blood tests:** Blood tests check the level of substances in the blood, such as potassium and thyroid hormone. Abnormal levels of these substances can increase your chances of having an arrhythmia.

**Chest X-ray:** A chest X-ray is a painless test that creates pictures of the structures in your chest, such as your heart and lungs. This test can show whether your heart is enlarged.

**Table 20.10:** Initial categorization of tachycardiac rhythms using the 12-lead electrocardiogram

| Rhythm | Narrow | Wide |
|---|---|---|
| Regular | **Short-RP**<br>• Typical (slow-fast)<br>• Atypical (slow-slow) AVNRT (usually)<br>• Orthodromic, AVRT<br>• JT<br>• AT (less commonly)<br>**Long-RP**<br>• Atypical (fast-slow) AVNRT<br>• Orthodromic AVRT (slowly conducting accessory pathway)<br>• ST<br>• AT (more commonly)<br>• PJRT<br>**Flutter waves**<br>• AFI (fixed AV block) | AVNRT ST, JT, AT, AVNRT, orthodromic AVRT, or AFI with aberrancy<br>Antidromic AVRT<br>Monomorphic ventricular tachycardia |
| Irregular | AF<br>AFI (variable AV block)<br>MAT | AF, AFI or MAT with aberrancy<br>AF, AFI with pre-excitation<br>Polymorphic ventricular tachycardia |

AF=atrial fibrillation: AFI=atrial flutter; AT=atrial tachycardia; AVNRT=antriventricular node re-entrant tachycardia; AVRT=atrioventricular re-entrant tachycardia; JT=junction tachycardia; MAT=multifocal atrial tachycardia; PJRT=permanent junctinoal reciprocating tachycardia; ST=sinus tachycardia

**Echocardiography:** This test uses sound waves to create a moving picture of your heart. Echocardiography (echo) provides information about the size and shape of your heart and how well your heart chambers and valves are working.

The test also can identify areas of poor blood flow to the heart, areas of heart muscle that aren't contracting normally, and previous injury to the heart muscle caused by poor blood flow.

There are several types of echo, including stress echo. This test is done both before and after a stress test. A stress echo usually is done to find out whether you have decreased blood flow to your heart, a sign of coronary heart disease (CHD).

A transesophageal (tranz-ih-sof-uh-JEE-ul) echo, or *TEE*, is a special type of echo that takes pictures of the heart through the esophagus. The esophagus is the passage leading from your mouth to your stomach.

**Stress test:** Some heart problems are easier to diagnose when your heart is working hard and beating fast. During stress testing, you exercise to make your heart work hard and beat fast while heart tests are done. If you can't exercise, you may be given medicine to make your heart work hard and beat fast.

The heart tests done during stress testing may include nuclear heart scanning, echo, and positron emission tomography (PET) scanning of the heart.

**Electrophysiology study (EPS):** This test is used to assess serious arrhythmias. During an EPS, a thin, flexible wire is passed through a vein in your groin (upper thigh) or arm to your heart. The wire records your heart's electrical signals (Figs 20.100–20.107).

Your doctor can use the wire to electrically stimulate your heart and trigger an arrhythmia. This allows your doctor to see whether an antiarrhythmia medicine can stop the problem.

Catheter ablation, a procedure used to treat some arrhythmias, may be done during an EPS.

**Tilt table testing:** This test sometimes is used to help find the cause of fainting spells. You lie on a table that moves from a lying down to an upright position. The change in position may cause you to faint.

Your doctor watches your symptoms, heart rate, EKG reading, and blood pressure throughout the test. He or she

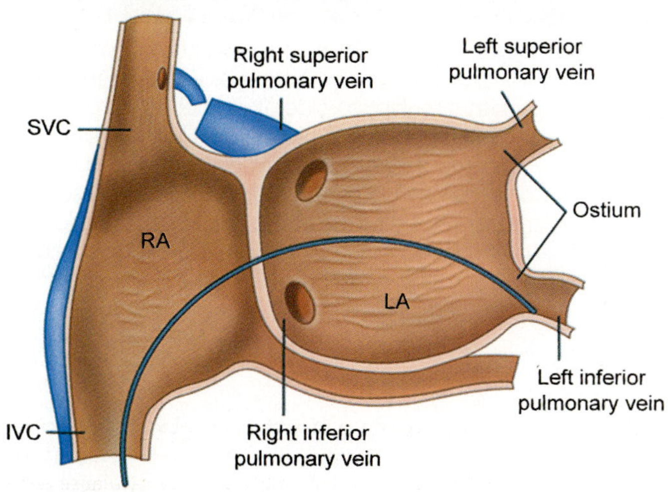


**Fig. 20.100:** Targeting the triggers in atrial fibrillation (AF) ablation

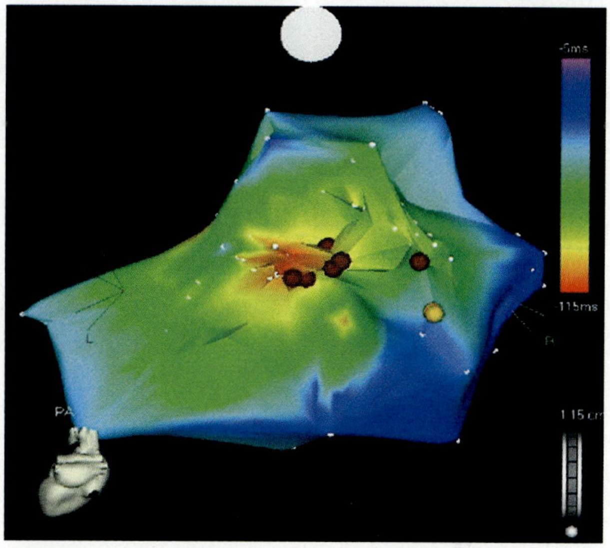

**Fig. 20.101:** A posteroanterior view of a right ventricular endocardial activation map during ventricular tachycardia in a patient with a prior septal myocardial infarction. Earliest activation is recorded in red; late activation shows as blue to magenta. Fragmented low amplitude diastolic local electrograms were recorded adjacent to the earliest (red) breakout area, and local ablation in this scared zone (red dots) resulted in termination and noninducibility of this previously incessant arrhythmia

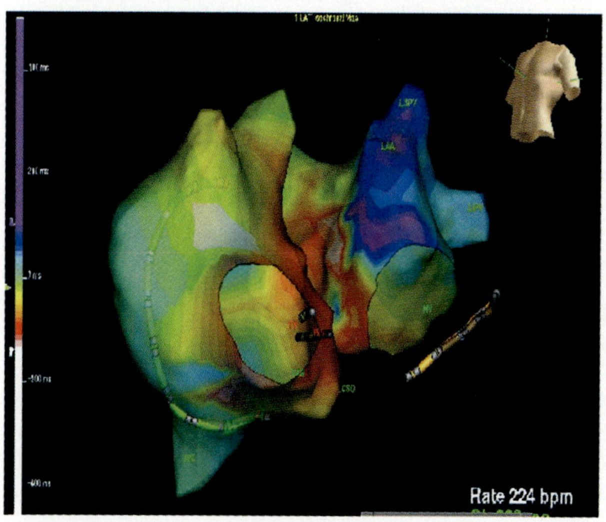


**Fig. 20.102:** Three-dimensinal mapping. This is a specialized mapping technique which utilizes a computer to delineate the source of complex arrhythmias. It works by projecting a virtual 3-D image of the heart in the computer to help the cardiac electrophysiologist navigate his catheters, in ways very similar to what GPS does for driving a car or flying an airplane. For many types of ablation, such as those for atrial fibrillation, 3-D mapping is essential to ensure optimal success rates and safety for the patients

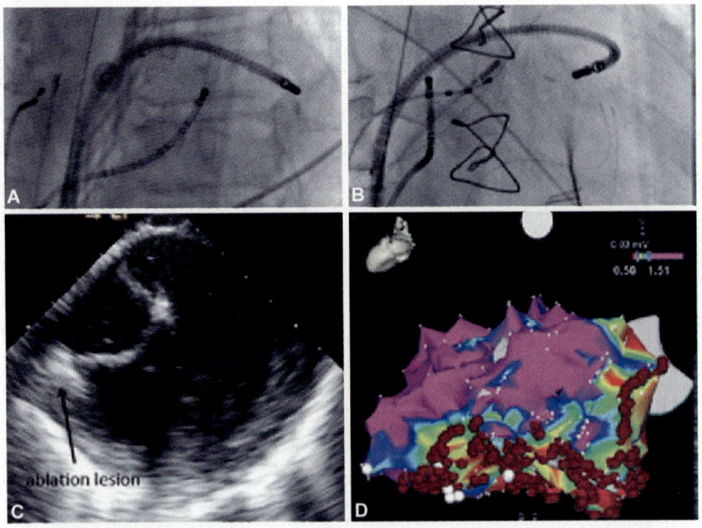


**Fig. 20.103:** Mapping and ablation of a basal lateral scar. (A and B) Robotic catheter position in left and right anterior oblique fluoroscopic views, respectively. The mid-lateral wall is being mapped. (C) Intracardiac echocardiographic image showing catheter contact and lesion formation in the left ventricular lateral wall. (D) Three-dimensional map of the lateral scar and the ablation lesions created

may give you medicine and then check your response to the medicine.

**Coronary angiography:** Coronary angiography uses dye and special X-rays to show the inside of your coronary arteries. To get the dye into your coronary arteries, your doctor will use a procedure called cardiac catheterization (KATH-e-ter-ih-ZA-shun).

A thin, flexible tube called a catheter is put into a blood vessel in your arm, groin (upper thigh), or neck. The tube is threaded into your coronary arteries, and the dye is released into your bloodstream.

Special X-rays are taken while the dye is flowing through your coronary arteries. The dye lets your doctor study the flow of blood through your heart and blood vessels. This helps your doctor find blockages that can cause a heart attack.

**Implantable loop recorder:** This device detects abnormal heart rhythms. Minor surgery is used to place this device under the skin in the chest area.

An implantable loop recorder helps doctors figure out why a person may be having *palpitations* or fainting spells, especially if these symptoms do not happen very often. The device can be used for as long as 12–24 months.

## HOW ARE ARRHYTHMIAS TREATED?

Common arrhythmia treatments include medicines, medical procedures, and surgery. Your doctor may recommend treatment if your arrhythmia causes serious symptoms, such as dizziness, chest pain, or fainting. Your doctor also may recommend treatment if the arrhythmia increases your risk for problems such as heart failure, stroke, or sudden cardiac arrest.

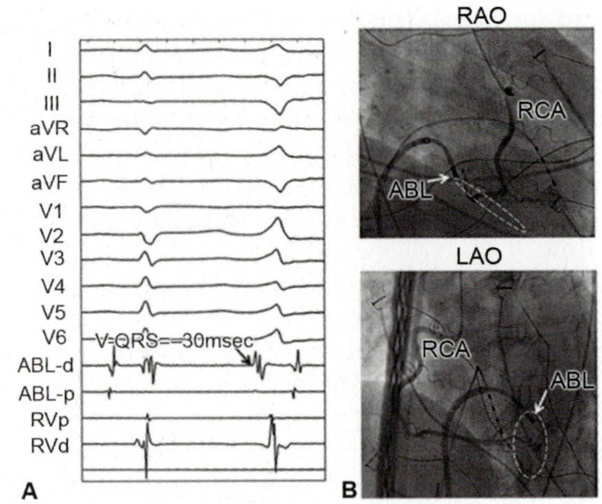


**Fig. 20.104:** (A) The intracardiac ECG at a successful middle cardiac vein (MCV) ablation site. (B) RAO (top) and LAO (bottom) fluoroscopic views at the site of successful ablation of a basal crux ventricular tachycardia within the MCV. ABL=ablation catheter; LOA=left anterior oblique; RAO=right anterior oblique; RCA=right coronary artery

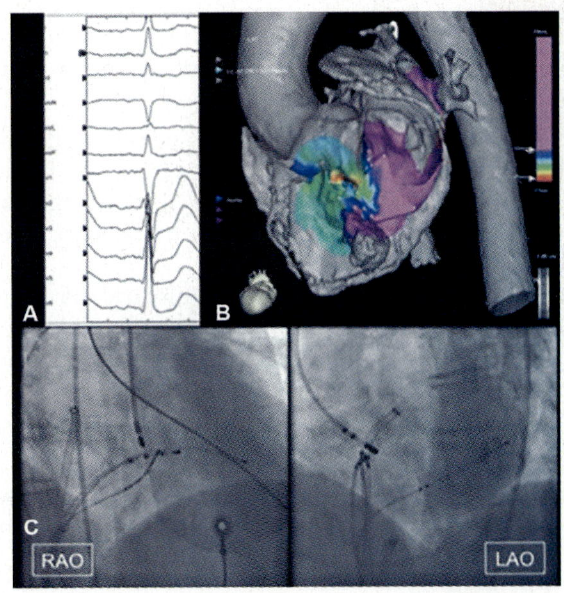


**Fig. 20.105:** Graph ablation of a focal parahisian atrial tachycardia from the noncoronary aortic sinus of Valsalva. The P-wave morphology (A) with a multiphasic configuration in V1. (B) displays an electroanatomic activation map merged into a preacquired CT geometry with the segmented ventricle removed. The red zone in the noncoronary aortic sinus of Valsalva represents the earliest breakthrough of the tachycardia with later activation seen on either side of the interatrial septum. The fluoroscopic catheter position at the successful ablation site, and (C) close proximity to the His catheter

### Medicines

Medicines can slow down a heart that's beating too fast. They also can change an abnormal heart rhythm to a normal, steady rhythm. Medicines that do this are called antiarrhythmics (Tables 20.11–20.13).

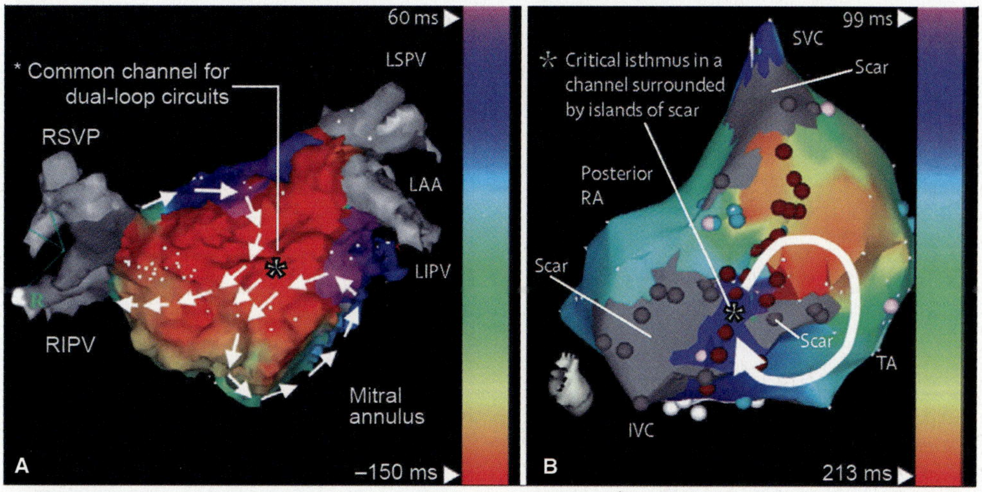


**Fig. 20.106A:** Catheter ablation of atrial arrhythmias. (A) Dual-loopleft atrial flutter (anterioposterior view), (B) Rightatrial flutter after ASD repair (right lateral view)

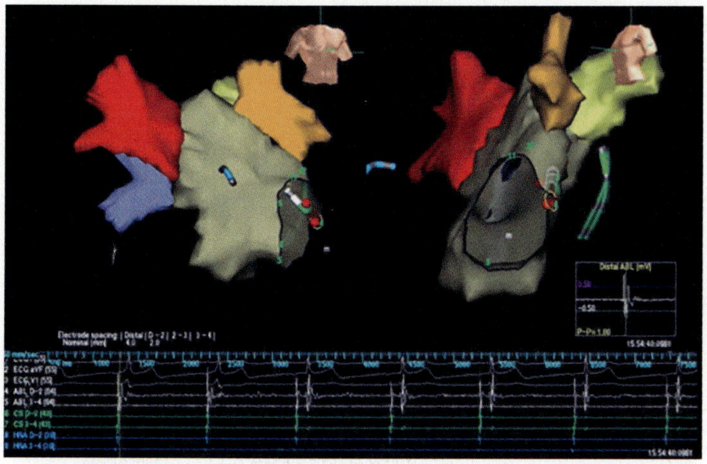

**Fig. 20.106B:** Accessory pathway ablation; palpitations and syncope found to have delta wave. Please note the near continuous activation of AV at 0300 mitral annulus. After application of RF at 25 watts, AV separate (with loss of delta wave) during the third beat

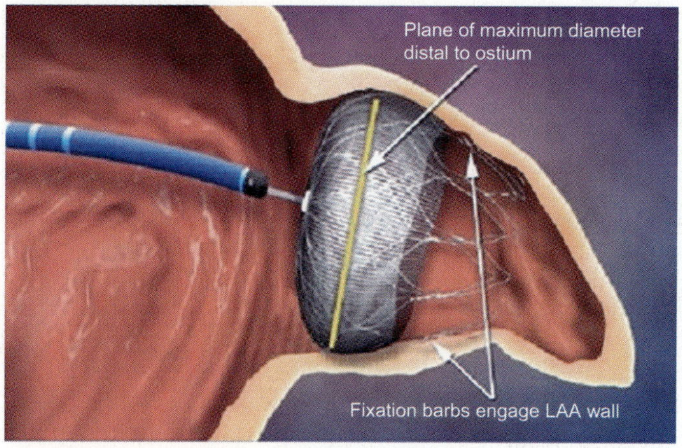


**Fig. 20.107:** Left atrial appendage closure device. Patients with atrial fibrillation (AF) are at an increased risk of stroke that can originate in the left atrial appendage (LAA). WATCHMAN device from Boston Scientific was developed to fill the space of the LAA and capture any clots that form within. Now the company received expanded indication approval in Europe to offer this treatment to AF patients that have a contraindication to the currently available anticoagulants

Some of the medicines used to slow a fast heart rate are beta-blockers (such as metoprolol and atenolol), calcium channel blockers (such as diltiazem and verapamil), and digoxin (digitalis). These medicines often are used to treat atrial fibrillation (AF).

Some of the medicines used to restore a normal heart rhythm are amiodarone, sotalol, flecainide, propafenone, dofetilide, ibutilide, quinidine, procainamide, and disopyramide. These medicines often have side effects. Some side effects can make an arrhythmia worse or even cause a different kind of arrhythmia.

Currently, no medicine can reliably speed up a slow heart rate. Abnormally slow heart rates are treated with pacemakers.

People who have AF and some other arrhythmias may be treated with blood-thinning medicines. These medicines reduce the risk of blood clots forming. Warfarin (Coumadin®), dabigatran, heparin, and aspirin are examples of blood-thinning medicines.

Medicines also can control an underlying medical condition that might be causing an arrhythmia, such as heart disease or a thyroid condition.

### Medical Procedures

Some arrhythmias are treated with pacemakers. A pacemaker is a small device that's placed under the skin of your chest or abdomen to help control abnormal heart rhythms (Figs 21.108–21.110).

Pacemakers have sensors that detect the heart's electrical activity. When the device senses an abnormal heart rhythm, it sends electrical pulses to prompt the heart to beat at a normal rate.

**Table 20.11:** Classwise antiarrhythmic drugs

| Class | Known as | Examples | Mechanism | Clinical uses in cardiology |
|---|---|---|---|---|
| Ia | Fast-channel blockers-affect QRS complex | • Quinidine<br>• Procainamide<br>• Disopyramide | $Na^+$ channel block (intermediate association/dissociation) | • Ventricular arrhythmias<br>• Prevention of paroxysmal recurrent atrial fibrillation (triggered by vagal overactivity)<br>• Procainamide in Wolff-Parkinson-White syndrome |
| Ib- | Do not affect QRS complex | • Lidocaine<br>• Phenytoin<br>• Mexiletine<br>• Tocainide | $Na^+$ channel block (fast association/dissociation) | • Treatment and prevention during and immediately after myocardial infarction, though this practice is now discouraged given the increased risk of asystole<br>• Ventricular tachycardia<br>• Atrial fibrillation |
| Ic | — | • Flecainide<br>• Propafenone<br>• Moricizine | $Na^+$ channel block (slow association/dissociation) | • Prevents paroxysmal atrial fibrillation<br>• Treats recurrent tachyarrhythmias of abnormal conduction system.<br>• Contraindicated immediately post-myocardial infarction |
| II | Beta-blockers | • Propranolol<br>• Esmolol<br>• Timolol<br>• Metoprolol<br>• Atenolol<br>• Bisoprolol | Beta blocking<br>Propranolol also shows some class I action | • Decrease myocardial infarction mortality<br>• Prevent recurrence of tachyarrhythmias |
| III | — | • Amiodarone<br>• Sotalol<br>• Ibutilide<br>• Dofetilide<br>• Dronedarone<br>• E-4031 | $K^+$ channel blocker<br>Sotalol is also a beta-blocker<br>Amiodarone has class I, II, III and IV activity | • In Wolff-Parkinson-White syndrome<br>• Sotalol: Ventricular tachycardias and atrial fibrillation<br>• Ibutilide: Atrial flutter and atrial fibrillation |
| IV | Slow-channel blockers | • Verapamil<br>• Diltiazem | $Ca^{2+}$ channel blocker | • Prevent recurrence of paroxysmal supraventricular tachycardia<br>• Reduce ventricular rate in patients with atrial fibrillation |
| V | — | • Adenosine<br>• Digoxin<br>• Magnesium sulfate | Work by other or unknown mechanisms (direct nodal inhibition). | Used in supraventricular arrhythmias, especially in heart failure with atrial fibrillation, contraindicated in ventricular arrhythmias. Or in the case of magnesium sulfate, used in torsades de pointes |

**Table 20.12:** Drugs commonly used to control ventricular rate in patients with atrial fibrillation

| Drugs | Initial dosing | Maintenance dosing | Comments |
|---|---|---|---|
| **Calcium channel blockers** | | | |
| Diltiazem (cardizem) | 15–20 mg IV over 2 minutes; may repeat in 15 minutes | 5–15 mg per hour by continuous IV infusion | Convenient; easy to titrate to heart rate goal |
| Verapamil (calan, isoptin) | 5–10 mg IV over 2 minutes; may repeat in 30 minutes | Not standardized | More myocardial depression and hypotension than with diltiazem |
| **Beta-blockers** | | | |
| Esmolol (brevibloc) | Bolus of 500 mcg per kg IV over 1 minute; may repeat in 5 minutes | 50–300 mcg per kg per minute by continuous IV infusion | Very short-acting; easy to titrate to heart rate goal |
| Propranolol (inderal) | 1 mg IV over 2 minutes 5 minutes to maximum of 5 mg | 1–3 mg IV every 4 hours may repeat every | Short duration of action; hence, need for repeat dosing |
| Digoxin (lanoxin) | 0.25–0.5 mg IV; then 0.25 mg IV every 4–6 hours to maximum of 1 mg | 0.125–0.25 mg per day IV or orally | Adjunctive therapy; less effective for rate control than beta-blockers or calcium channel blockers |

IV=intravenous.

*Adapted with permission from Li H, Easley A, Barrington W, Windle J. Evaluation and management of atrial fibrillation in the emergency department. Emerg Med Clin North Am 1998;16:389–403.*

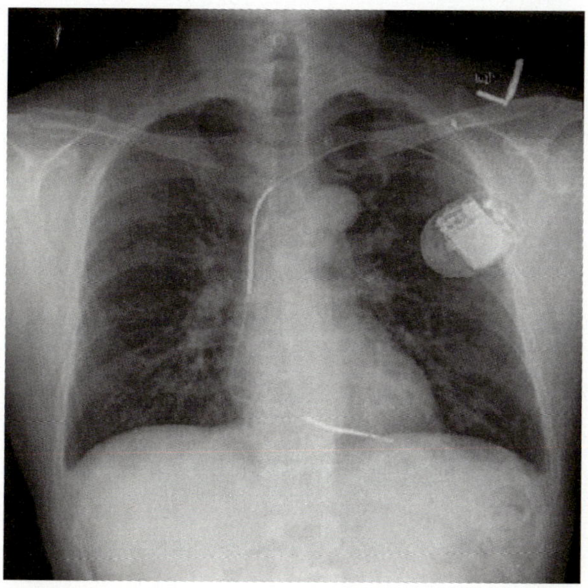

**Fig. 20.108:** Chest X-ray showing an implantable cardioverter-defibrillator (ICD), with its battery fixed at left subclavicular region and is connected with a wire placed in the trabecular part of the right ventricular apex

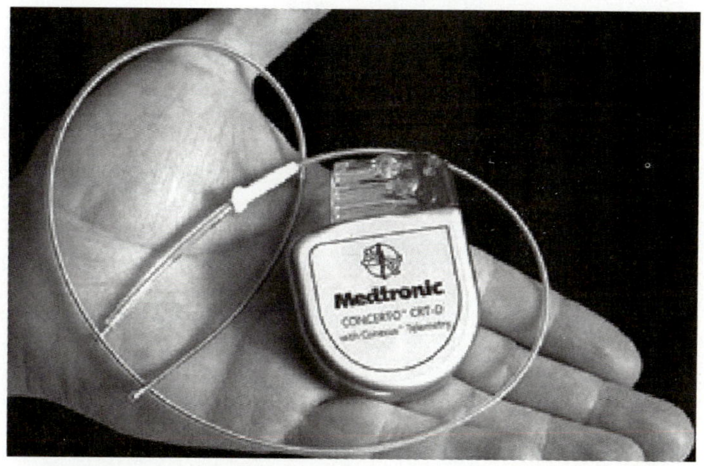


**Fig. 20.109:** An implantable cardioverter-defibrillator (ICD)

Some arrhythmias are treated with a jolt of electricity to the heart. This type of treatment is called cardioversion or defibrillation, depending on which type of arrhythmia is being treated.

Some people who are at risk for ventricular fibrillation are treated with a device called *an implantable cardioverter defibrillator (ICD)*. Like a pacemaker, an ICD is a small device that's placed under the skin in the chest. This device uses electrical pulses or shocks to help control life-threatening arrhythmias.

- An ICD continuously monitors the heartbeat. If it senses a dangerous ventricular arrhythmia, it sends an electric shock to the heart to restore a normal heartbeat.
- A procedure called catheter ablation is used to treat some arrhythmias if medicines don't work. During this procedure, a thin, flexible tube is put into a blood vessel in your arm, groin (upper thigh), or neck. Then, the tube is guided to your heart.
- A special machine sends energy through the tube to your heart. The energy finds and destroys small areas of heart

**Table 20.13:** Summarizes drugs used in the emergency management of life-threatening ventricular arrhythmias

| Medication | VF pulseless VT | Stable monomorphic VT | Stable wide complex tachycardia aetiology uncertain | Unstable monomorphic VT | Torsades de pointes |
|---|---|---|---|---|---|
| Amiodarone | Initial:300 mg<br>Recurrent/persistent: 150 mg diluted in 100 ml D5W over 10 min | 150 mg diluted in 100 mL D5W over 10 min. Follow with continuous infusion 1 mg/min for 6 h, then 0.5 mg/min for 18 h | 150 mg diluted in 100 ml D5W over with continuous infusion 1 mg/min for 6 h, then 0.5 mg/min for 18 h | Not first treatment of choice | Not treatment of choice |
| Lidocaine | Recurrent/persistent: 1–1.5 mg/kg IV push. May follow with repeat bolus every 5–10 mins. Maximum total dose: 3 mg/kg | 1.5 mg/kg IV push. May follow with repeat bolus of 0.5–0.75 mg/kg every 5 to 10 mins to max total dose of 3 mg/kg or maintenance infusion of 2–4 mg/min (30–50 mcg/kg/min) | Not treatment of choice | Not first treatment of choice | Not treatment of choice |
| Magnesium sulfate | Only indicated if hypomagnesemia is suspected or known | Only indicated if hypomagnesemia is suspected or known | Only indicated if hypomagnesemia is suspected | Only indicated if hypomagesemia is suspected | For cardiac arrest: 1–2 grams over a maximum of 15 mins given IV push |
| Procainamide | Persistent/recurrent<br>Loading dose: 20–50 mg/min (or 100 mg every 5 mins) IV infusion | Loading dose: 20–50 mg/min (or 100 mg every 5 mins) IV infusion<br>Maintenance infusion: 1–4 mg/min<br>Maximum dose: 17 mg/kg<br>Not drug of choice for persons with reduced ventricular function | Loading dose: 20–50 mg/min (or 100 mg every 5<br>Maintenance infusion: 1–4 mg/min<br>Not drug of choice for persons with reduced ventricular function | Not first treatment of choice | Not treatment of choice |

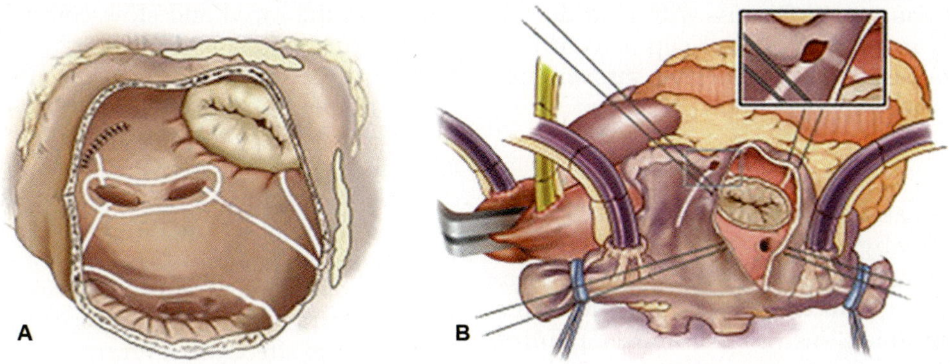


**Fig. 20.110:** Cox-Maze procedure for atrial fibrillation. Showing right atrial lesion set and left atrial lesion set. The surgeon can use small incisions, radio waves, freezing, or microwave or ultrasound energy to create scar tissue. The scar tissue, which does not conduct electrical activity, blocks the abnormal electrical signals causing the arrhythmia. The scar tissue directs electric signals through a controlled path, or maze, to the lower heart chambers (ventricles)

tissue where abnormal heart rhythms may start. Catheter ablation usually is done in a hospital as part of an electrophysiology study.

- Your doctor may recommend transesophageal echocardiography before catheter ablation to make sure no blood clots are present in the atria (the heart's upper chambers).

### Surgery

Doctors treat some arrhythmias with surgery. This may occur if surgery is already being done for another reason, such as repair of a heart valve. One type of surgery for AF is called maze surgery. During this surgery, a surgeon makes small cuts or burns in the atria. These cuts or burns prevent the spread of disorganized electrical signals. If coronary heart disease is the cause of your arrhythmia, your doctor may recommend coronary artery bypass grafting. This surgery improves blood flow to the heart muscle.

### Other Treatments

Vagal maneuvers are another type of treatment for arrhythmia. These simple exercises sometimes can stop or slow down certain types of supraventricular arrhythmias. They do this by affecting the vagus nerve, which helps control the heart rate.

Some vagal maneuvers include:

- Gagging
- Holding your breath and bearing down (Valsalva maneuver)
- Immersing your face in ice-cold water
- Coughing
- Putting your fingers on your eyelids and pressing down gently
- Vagal maneuvers aren't an appropriate treatment for everyone. Discuss with your doctor whether vagal maneuvers are an option for you.

### Living with an Arrhythmia

Many arrhythmias are harmless. It's common to have an occasional extra heartbeat or mild palpitations. People who have harmless arrhythmias can live healthy lives. They usually don't need treatment for their arrhythmias.

Even people who have serious arrhythmias often can be successfully treated and lead normal lives.

## ONGOING CARE

If you have an arrhythmia that requires treatment, you should:

- Keep all of your medical appointments. Bring a list of all the medicines you are taking to every doctor and emergency room visit. This will help your doctors know exactly what medicines you're taking, which can help prevent medication errors.
- Take your medicines as prescribed. Check with your doctor before taking over-the-counter medicines, nutritional supplements, or cold and allergy medicines. Some of these products can trigger rapid heart rhythms or interact poorly with heart rhythm medicines.
- Tell your doctor if you are having side effects from your medicines. Side effects might include depression and palpitations. These side effects often can be treated.
- Tell your doctor if arrhythmia symptoms are getting worse or if you have new symptoms.
- See your doctor for regular checkups if you are taking blood-thinning medicines. You may need routine blood tests to check how the medicines are working.
- If you have an arrhythmia, taking care of yourself is important. If you feel dizzy or faint, you should lie down. Do not try to walk or drive. Let your doctor know about these symptoms.
- Ask your doctor whether vagal manoeuvres are an option for you. These exercises can help stop a rapid heartbeat, but they are not appropriate for everyone.

- Learn how to take your pulse. Discuss with your doctor what pulse rate is normal for you. Keep a record of changes in your pulse rate and share this information with your doctor.

## LIFESTYLE CHANGES

Many arrhythmias are caused by underlying heart disease. Keep your heart healthy by following a healthy diet.

A healthy diet includes a variety of fruits and vegetables. It also includes whole grains, fat-free or low-fat dairy products, and protein foods, such as lean meats, poultry without skin, seafood, processed soy products, nuts, seeds, and beans and peas.

A healthy diet is low in sodium (salt), added sugars, solid fats, and refined grains. Solid fats are saturated fat and *trans* fatty acids. Refined grains come from processing whole grains, which results in a loss of nutrients (such as dietary fiber).

For more information about following a healthy diet, go to the national heart, lung, and blood institute's 'your guide to lowering your blood pressure with DASH' and the United States Department of Agriculture's Choose MyPlate.gov website. Both resources provide general information about healthy eating.

A healthy lifestyle also includes being physically active, quitting smoking, maintaining a healthy weight, and keeping your blood cholesterol and blood pressure at healthy levels.

Strong emotional stress or anger can lead to arrhythmias. Try to manage stress and anger through activities such as yoga, quiet time, meditation, and relaxation techniques. Getting support from friends and family also can help you manage stress.

Your doctor may want you to avoid certain substances if they make your heart beat too fast. These substances may include alcohol and cold and cough medicines.

## NEWER ANTIARRHYTHMIC DRUGS

### Dronedarone

Amiodarone is generally accepted to be a valuable antiarrhythmic drug, but it accumulates in tissues during long-term therapy, which may result in significant toxicity in several organ systems. Several compounds that were designed to be similar in structure and electrophysiological effects to amiodarone have completed or are now in clinical trials.

Dronedarone is, like amiodarone, a benzofuranyl compound with iodine removed and a methane sulfonyl group added. Removing iodine from the molecule was intended to eliminate or reduce iodine-related organ toxicity. The side chain modification decreased lipophilicity, resulting in a shorter elimination half-life with less potential for tissue accumulation. The basic and clinical pharmacology of dronedarone has been recently reviewed.

Dronedarone retains many of amiodarone's electrophysiological effects. It is a multichannel blocker with effects on the rapid and slow components of the delayed rectifier current (IKr and IKs), L-type calcium currents, (ICa-L), the inward sodium current (INa), and the inward rectifier potassium current (IK1). Dronedarone also inhibits the acetylcholine receptor-dependent $K^+$ current (IKAch) and the pacemaker current (If) and is a noncompetitive a- and β-adrenergic antagonist. Dronedarone reduces sinus rate and prolongs AV nodal conduction and refractoriness. Effects on the QT and QTc intervals have been variable when studied in different species. In several animal models of ischemia or reperfusion-induced arrhythmias, dronedarone effectively prevents spontaneous and induced ventricular fibrillation.

### Budiodarone

Unlike dronedarone, **budiodarone** (AT1-2042), another compound that structurally resembles amiodarone, retains iodine atoms in its molecular structure. A sec-butyl acetate side chain has been added at position 2 of the benzofuranyl ring. This ester modification changes the compound's metabolic pathways such that budiodarone undergoes rapid degradation by plasma and tissue esterases, not by CYP3A-mediated oxidation, to an inactive compound. During *in-vitro* studies, budiodarone has shown electrophysiological properties similar to amiodarone.

Only limited clinical data on budiodarone are available. One study assessed twice-daily placebo or doses of 200, 400, 600, and 800 mg during sequential 2-week periods in a very small group of patients with paroxysmal atrial fibrillation and implanted pacemakers. Atrial fibrillation burden (defined as percent time in atrial fibrillation) was calculated during each period. Budiodarone reduced total atrial fibrillation burden by reducing the duration but not the number of atrial fibrillation episodes. Preliminary data from a similar but a larger phase 2 trial compared placebo and budiodarone (200, 400, and 600 mg twice daily) in 72 patients with pacemakers and paroxysmal atrial fibrillation. There were 54.4% and 75% reductions in AF burden in the 400 mg and 600 mg groups. Some patients manifested a rise in thyroid-stimulating hormone, but clinical symptoms of thyroid disease did not appear.

### Celivarone

Celivarone (SSR149744C) is another noniodinated benzofuran derivative with electrophysiological effects similar to amiodarone. Few clinical data have been published in manuscript form, but a phase 2 trial tested celivarone's efficacy at 300- or 600-mg daily doses for conversion of atrial fibrillation and flutter (CORYFEE, NCT00232310) and a dose ranging study compared celivarone at 50, 100, 200, or 300 mg once daily with amiodarone for maintenance of sinus rhythm (MAIA, NCT00233441) have been completed but not yet published. A preliminary report from the dose-ranging study showed the lowest rate of atrial fibrillation recurrence at the 50 mg dose with no enhanced efficacy at the higher doses. In another study in patients with ICDs, 2 doses of celivarone (100 and 300 mg daily) were compared with placebo over 6 months of therapy. A 46% reduction in the number of sustained ventricular arrhythmia episodes requiring ICD therapy was noted in the 300 mg daily group, but this reduction did not achieve statistical significance (P=0.172). Additional trials in patients with ventricular arrhythmias and ICDs are planned.

### Vernakalant

Vernakalant is an atrial-selective, multiple ion channel blocker that is in the advanced stages of investigation for the treatment of atrial fibrillation. Both intravenous and oral forms of vernakalant have undergone clinical trials. The intravenous form has been recommended for approval by the Cardiorenal Advisory Committee of the Food and Drug Administration, but a formal letter of approval has not been issued. Vernakalant is an atrial repolarization-delaying agent with its major target IKur. Vernakalant also blocks Ito and INa, although there is little effect on IKr or IKs. As IKur is present in higher density in the atria, vernakalant is relatively atrial selective. The INa inhibition is rate- and voltage-dependent. Vernakalant has, therefore, a much greater effect in fibrillating atria than in the ventricle and is less likely to be proarrhythmic.

Vernakalant is hepatically metabolized by CYP2D6. It is not clear what effect abnormal liver function has on the metabolism of the drug. In a study of intravenous vernakalant, coadministration of CYP2D6 inhibitors did not appear to decrease clearance, and little difference was seen in maximum plasma concentrations between CYP2D6 poor and extensive metabolizers. Differences in renal function, age, sex, race, blood pressure, and heart failure status have not been shown to affect the pharmacokinetics of vernakalant. Vernakalant demonstrates 2-compartment elimination pharmacokinetics, and its half-life after intravenous administration is 2–5 hours. The oral bioavailability of vernakalant is approximately 20%. During oral therapy in the dose range of 300 to 600 mg twice daily, steady-state concentrations are achieved in 4 days. It remains to be seen whether CYP2D6 poor and extensive metabolizers will require different doses during chronic oral therapy.

Phase 3 trials have not been completed for oral vernakalant, although phase 2 trials have been promising for the long-term maintenance of sinus rhythm. The phase 2a trial was double-blinded, randomized, and compared a 300-mg dosage, a 600-mg dosage, and placebo for 25 days after cardioversion. Electrical cardioversion was permitted for patients who did not convert within 3 days after initiation of the medication. Significantly more patients remained in sinus rhythm at the end of the trial period in the 300-mg dosing group and in the combined 300- and 600-mg groups, when compared with placebo. The phase 2b trial compared 150-, 300-, and 500-mg dosages with placebo, and the trial duration was 90 days. The 500-mg dosage group showed durable maintenance of sinus rhythm at 90 days compared with placebo, with low incidence of side effects. There were no reported cases of torsades de pointes.

In summary, intravenous vernakalant for cardioversion of recent onset AF is moderately effective for rapid termination of atrial fibrillation with durable maintenance of sinus rhythm up to 24 hours. The side effect profile shows relatively modest potential for toxicity. Age, sex, ethnicity, and concomitant illnesses do not appear to alter efficacy. Of course, drugs used only for the acute conversion of atrial fibrillation must also be compared with electrical cardioversion as well as other agents. Oral vernakalant may prove useful for maintenance of sinus rhythm, but phase 3 trials have yet to be completed. If these trials show efficacy, vernakalant probably will be more widely used in conversion attempts as a step to long-term therapy. There are no clinical data on the effects of vernakalant in ventricular arrhythmias, and its mechanisms of action suggest it would not be useful.

### Ranolazine

Ranolazine is currently approved for the treatment of chronic angina pectoris. Ranolazine reduces myocardial ischemia by its effects on the late inward $Na^+$ current (INaL). During myocardial ischemia and heart failure, INaL is augmented. This results in increased sodium entry and, via sodiumcalcium exchange, increased cytosolic calcium concentrations. These changes produce action potential prolongation and increased susceptibility to early afterdepolarizations. Ranolazine is an inactivated sodium channel blocker. At concentrations near its therapeutic range for angina (2–6 µmol/L, IC50 60 µmol/L), ranolazine inhibits INaL. In the same concentration range, ranolazine inhibits peak INa in the atrium but not the ventricle. This effect results in reduced atrial excitability and a rate-dependent increase in postrepolarization atrial refractoriness. In experiments using an isolated canine ventricular wedge preparation, ranolazine results in either no change or a decrease in transmural ventricular dispersion of refractoriness and does not produce early after depolarizations, triggered activity, or polymorphic ventricular tachycardia. In other experiments, ranolazine has been shown to suppress excitability and triggered activity in an isolated canine pulmonary vein sleeve preparation, terminate acetylcholine- and isoproterenol-induced atrial fibrillation, and prevent its reinitiation.

Ranolazine has variable systemic availability after oral administration due to its extensive first-pass metabolism in the gut and liver. Metabolism is mainly via CYP3A4 and, to a lesser extent, CYP2D6. The terminal elimination half-life is 7 hours. The recommended dosage in patients with angina is 500–1000 mg twice daily. Ranolazine should not be used as concurrent therapy with strong CYP3A4 inhibitors (e.g. ketoconazole), and dose reduction is recommended with moderate CYP3A4 inhibitors (e.g. diltiazem) or P-glycoprotein inhibitors. Ranolazine is a weak inhibitor of CYP3A4 and a moderate inhibitor of CYP2D6 and P-glycoprotein.

Ranolazine's effects on ECG intervals underwent extensive study during its development for its current indication of chronic angina. Ranolazine results in a 2- to 6-ms mean increase in the QTc interval, but drug-induced polymorphic ventricular tachycardia has not been observed. The MERLIN-TIMI trial enrolled 6560 patients with a non-ST-elevation acute coronary syndrome who were randomly assigned to either ranolazine (intravenous initiation, then 1000 mg twice daily) or matched placebo, in addition to standard medical therapy. No significant improvement was shown in the primary end point of death and recurrent ischemic events with ranolazine in MERLIN-TIMI, but data from continuous ambulatory ECG recordings during the first 7 days of therapy were recently reported. Significant decreases in the frequency of nonsustained ventricular and supraventricular tachycardia were noted. A trend toward less frequent new-onset atrial fibrillation was also seen. A single case report on the successful use of ranolazine to suppress high-density ventricular tachycardia has been reported. An uncontrolled case series has also described control of recurrent atrial fibrillation in 4 of 7 patients with drug-resistant arrhythmia. Controlled trials with ranolazine as an antiarrhythmic drug in patients with atrial fibrillation are in the planning stages.

One form of the long-QT syndrome (LQT3) is caused by mutations in the SCN5A sodium channel that lead to enhanced and sustained activity of late INa. Moss et al. administered intravenous ranolazine to 5 patients with LQT3. During the infusion, ranolazine shortened QTcf by 26±3 ms. Diastolic function on echocardiography was also improved. Ranolazine may also prove useful in another form of the long-QT syndrome. The Timothy syndrome (LQT8) is a multisystem disorder characterized by facial dysmorphism, syndactyly, QT prolongation, and premature sudden death. The syndrome is caused by a missense mutation in Cav1.2, the gene that encodes the a-subunit of the L-type calcium channel, resulting in a gain in function of the L-type calcium current. In an animal model of the Timothy syndrome, ranolazine suppressed polymorphic ventricular tachycardia induced by the calcium channel agonist BayK8644. Clinical data on the chronic treatment of arrhythmias in LQT3 and Timothy syndrome patients are not available.

At present, the only approved indication for ranolazine is the treatment of angina. It remains to be proven whether it will also be useful as an antiarrhythmic agent.

### Ivabradine

Ivabradine selectively inhibits the spontaneous pacemaker activity of the sinus node by blocking the $I_f$ current. This reduces the heart rate without altering myocardial contractility or other hemodynamics. Ivabradine has been approved for use as an antianginal in Europe. It has also been used off-label in Europe as a treatment for inappropriate sinus tachycardia. It has not yet been approved for any use in the United States. The blockage of the If current is dose-dependent and heart rate-dependent. There is a greater efficiency in blocking $I_f$ at faster heart rates, limiting the risks of symptomatic bradycardia. Electrophysiological studies of ivabradine in humans have shown little effect on the conduction system or on atrial and ventricular refractoriness. Some remodeling of the sinus node appears to occur in response to ivabradine, but no rebound tachycardia has been seen after discontinuing the drug.

Ivabradine is 80% hepatically metabolized by the CYP3A4 enzyme and cannot be used concomitantly with drugs that inhibit this enzyme, such as azoles and macrolide antibiotics. There does not appear to be a difference in heart rate response between patients who are CYP3A4 rapid metabolizers and those who are slow metabolizers. It is 20% renally cleared. The oral bioavailability is approximately 40% and it takes 60 to 90 minutes to reach maximal plasma concentrations. The half-life is approximately 2 hours.

The major trial that evaluated ivabradine is the BEAUTIFUL study. This randomized, double-blind, placebo-controlled trial enrolled 10917 patients with ischemic cardiomyopathy to receive ivabradine versus placebo. There was no difference in the primary end point of cardiovascular death or admissions for acute infarction or heart failure. In patients with baseline heart rates >70 bpm, however, the secondary end points of admission for fatal and nonfatal infarction and the need for revascularization were significantly reduced. The heart rate reduction due to ivabradine was 6±2 bpm. A previous study compared ivabradine with atenolol for treatment of patients with stable angina and found that ivabradine was as effective as atenolol. It is on this basis that it was approved for use in Europe.

Composite data from phase 2 and phase 3 trials suggest that most side effects are dose-related. Ion channels in the retina that generate the $I_h$ current are also affected by ivabradine. This is the mechanism for ivabradine's major side effect, visual luminous phenomena, also known as phosphenes (14.5%). Phosphenes usually resolve with continued treatment and are a rare cause of drug discontinuation. Severe bradycardia is seen in 3.3% of patients. Other less common side effects include palpitations, nausea, headaches, vertigo, muscle cramps, hypereosinophilia, and hyperuricemia.

Little trial data exists regarding the treatment of atrial tachyarrhythmias with ivabradine. The mechanism of action suggests that ivabradine may benefit patients with inappropriate sinus tachycardia. In Europe, where the drug is being marketed, it is used off-label in the treatment of inappropriate sinus tachycardia. Further data will be needed as to its effectiveness in treating this condition.

### Adenosine A1 Receptor Agonists

Adenosine is frequently used for termination of supraventricular tachycardias (SVT). Adenosine terminates SVT in patient with AV nodal or AV re-entry by stimulating the A1 adenosine receptor to produce transient AV block. However, adenosine induces atrial fibrillation in up to 15% of patients by decreasing the refractory period of the atrium. In addition, adenosine also stimulates the A2A, A2B, and A3 adenosine receptor subtypes, which contribute to its adverse effect profile. Stimulation of these receptors leads to a variety of systemic side effects, including flushing (18%), dyspnea (12%), and chest pain (7%). Efforts have been made to identify A1 receptor-selective agonists for both the termination of SVT and rate control for atrial fibrillation. Several are under investigation currently, including tecadenoson, selodenoson, and PJ-875. Tecadenoson is the furthest along in the development process. A phase 3 trial has been completed evaluating tecadenoson for the termination of SVT, and preclinical data are promising for rate control of atrial fibrillation. Selodenoson and PJ-875 are both in the early stages of evaluation for treatment of atrial fibrillation.

Preclinical trials indicate that tecadenoson is a potent and selective agonist of the A1 receptor. Studies in animal models showed that it caused significant prolongation of AV nodal conduction and refractoriness without causing hypotension or negative inotropic effects. In addition, those effects were dose-dependent and persistent with chronic administration of the drug. A phase 1 dose-escalation trial in 32 patients showed a dose-dependent prolongation of the AH interval. There was no effect on the HV interval. The peak effect on AH interval was at 1 minute, and resolution occurred at 20 minutes. Four patients had significant heart block and 3 patients had atrial fibrillation (two after atrial pacing). Two patients had neurological effects. There is incomplete published information regarding the pharmacokinetics tecadenoson. It appears to follow a 2-compartment model and has a longer half-life than adenosine (20–30 minutes).

The most significant trial to evaluate tecadenoson to date is the phase 3 TEMPEST trial. This study was a multicenter, double-blinded, placebo-controlled trial that randomly assigned 181 patients to receive placebo versus 1 of several dose-escalating regimens of tecadenoson for termination of SVT. Overall, the conversion rates were 73.5% in the tecadenoson-treated patients and 6.7% in the placebo group. The rates of conversion did improve with dose escalation. Side effects were relatively mild and increased with dose escalation. Twelve patients had second-degree heart block. Two patients had complete heart block, and both of those patients were in the highest dose treatment group. Five patients in the 2 highest dose treatment groups developed transient atrial fibrillation or atrial flutter. The rates of flushing, dyspnea, and chest pain were 4%, 2.6%, and 3%, respectively. No patients in this study had alterations in blood pressure.

An animal study of tecadenoson for rate control of atrial fibrillation has shown promising results. In combination with metoprolol, rate control was improved with tecadenoson compared with either agent alone. Improved rate control was seen with exercise and with rest. A phase 2 clinical trial to evaluate the safety of tecadenoson to treat atrial fibrillation has been completed. Results have not yet been released.

In summary, the available data regarding adenosine A1 receptor agonists, particularly tecadenoson, is promising for the conversion of SVT and for short-term rate-control of atrial fibrillation. The rate of conversion for SVT is similar to that of adenosine, but the systemic side effects are milder. In addition, although adenosine A1 receptor stimulation is the presumed mechanism for the induction of atrial fibrillation, tecadenoson appears less likely to cause atrial fibrillation, perhaps because the maximal action potential shortening seen with a bolus of adenosine is not observed with longer-acting agents.

It is now recognized that atrial fibrillation originates from atrial tissue that has altered structure or function. Fibrosis within the atrium is one of the major mechanisms of atrial remodeling, which provides the substrate for atrial fibrillation generation and maintenance. Efforts have been made to develop 'upstream' therapies for atrial fibrillation. The renin-angiotensin-aldosterone system has been implicated in the fibrotic process. Therapies that alter renin-angiotensin-aldosterone system, as well as antiinflammatory and antioxidative drugs, are being investigated both alone and in combination with traditional antiarrhythmic drugs. For some newer drugs, data have only been generated in animal models. Further studies will be needed to delineate the full potential benefits of these and other therapies.

### KEY POINTS

- Some arrhythmias are life-threatening medical emergencies that can result in cardiac arrest. Others cause symptoms such as an abnormal awareness of heart beat (palpitations), and may be merely uncomfortable.
- The term cardiac *arrhythmia* covers a very large number of very different conditions. The most common symptom of arrhythmia is an abnormal awareness of heartbeat, called palpitations.
- *Automaticity* refers to a *cardiac muscle* cell firing off an impulse on its own. All of the cells in the heart have the ability to initiate an action potential; however, only some are designed to routinely trigger heart beats. These cells are found in the conduction system of the heart.
- Ventricular fibrillation is imminently life-threatening. Atrial fibrillation is not typically a medical emergency.
- Arrhythmia may be classified by rate (normal, *tachycardia*, bradycardia), or mechanism (automaticity, re-entry, and fibrillation). It is also appropriate to classify by site of *origin*.
- Causes of SADS in young people include viral myocarditis, *long QT syndrome*, Brugada syndrome, catecholaminergic polymorphic ventricular tachycardia, hypertrophic cardiomyopathy, and arrhythmogenic right ventricular dysplasia.
- Atrial fibrillation is an irregular atrial rhythm that may be episodic or continuous; paroxysms of tachycardia may occur.
- QRS complexes should be narrow; a wide complex occurs with intraventricular conduction defects or Wolff-Parkinson-White syndrome.
- Patients should have echocardiography and thyroid function testing.
- Heart rate is controlled (typically to <100 beats/min at rest); first-line drugs include beta-blockers and nondihydropyridine calcium channel blockers (e.g. verapamil, diltiazem).

*Contd...*

*Contd...*

- Restoration of sinus rhythm is not as important as rate control and does not eliminate the need for anticoagulation but may help patients with continuing symptoms or hemodynamic compromise (e.g. heart failure); synchronized cardioversion or drugs can be used.
- Anticoagulation is usually necessary before cardioversion.
- Long-term oral anticoagulation to prevent stroke is required for patients with risk factors for thromboembolism; aspirin is used for those with no risk factors.

## BIBLIOGRAPHY


1. A randomized, placebo-controlled trial of propafenone in the prophylaxis of paroxysmal supraventricular tachycardia and paroxysmal atrial fibrillation. UK Propafenone PSVT Study Group: Circulation 1995;92:2550.
2. Akhtar M, Jazayeri MR, Sra J, et al. Atrioventricular nodal re-entry: clinical, electrophysiological, and therapeutic considerations. Circulation 1993;88:282.
3. Amsterdam EA, Kulcyski J, Ridgeway MG. Efficacy of cardioselective beta-adrenergic blockade with intravenously administered metoprolol in the treatment of supraventri-cular tachyarrhythmias. J Clin Pharmacol 1991;31:714.
4. Blomstöm-Lundqvist C, Scheinman MM, Aliot EM, et al. ACC/AHA/ESC Guidelines for the management of patients with supraventricular arrhythmias—executive.
5. Brugada P, Brugada J, Mont L, et al. A new approach to the differential diagnosis of a regular tachycardia with a wide QRS complex. Circulation 1991;83:1649.
6. Campbell RW, Smith RA, Gallagher JJ, et al. Atrial fibrillation in the preexcitation syndrome. Am J Cardiol 1977;40:514.
7. Clague JR, Dagres N, Kottkamp H, et al. Targeting the slow pathway for atrioventricular nodal re-entrant tachycardia: initial results and long-term follow-up in 379 consecutive patients. Eur Heart J 2001;22:82.
8. Clinical Investigator's Brochure: SR33589B Dronedarone. Bridgewater, NJ, Sanofi-Syntholabe Recherche. Edition: E07, 2006.
9. Dale KM, White CM. Dronedarone: an amiodarone analog for the treatment of atrial fibrillation and atrial flutter. Ann Pharmacother. 2007;41:599–605.
10. Dreifus LS, Haiat R, Watanabe Y, et al. Ventricular fibrillation: a possible mechanism of sudden death in patients and Wolff-Parkinson-White syndrome. Circulation 1971;43:520.
11. Ehrlich JR, Biliczki P, Hohnloser SH, Nattel S. Atrial-selective approaches for the treatment of atrial fibrillation. J Am Coll Cardiol. 2008; 51:787–92.
12. Flecainide acetate prevents recurrence of symptomatic paroxysmal supraventricular tachycardia. The Flecainide Supraventricular Tachycardia Study Group: Circulation 1991;83:119. Long-term safety and efficacy of flecainide in the treatment of supraventricular tachyarrhythmias: the United States experience. The Flecainide Supraventricular Tachy arrhythmia Investigators: Am J Cardiol 1992;70:11A.
13. Kay GN, Pressley JC, Packer DL, et al. Value of the 12-lead electro-cardiogram in discriminating atrioventricular nodal reciprocating tachycardia from circus movement atrioventricular tachycardia utilizing a retrograde accessory pathway. Am J Cardiol 1987;59:296.
14. Klein GJ, Bashore TM, Sellers TD, et al. Ventricular fibrillation in the Wolff-Parkinson-White syndrome. N Engl J Med. 1979;301:1080.
15. Kottkamp H, Hügl B, Krauss B, et al. Electromagnetic versus fluoroscopic mapping of the inferior isthmus for ablation of typical atrial flutter: A prospective randomized study. Circulation 2000;102(17):2082–6.
16. Lee KL, Chun HM, Liem LB, et al. Effect of adenosine and verapamil in catecholamine-induced accelerated atrio-ventricular junctional rhythm: insights into the underlying mechanism. Pacing Clin Electrophysiol 1999;22:866.
17. Mauritson DR, Winniford MD, Walker WS, et al. Oral verapamil for paroxysmal supraventricular tachycardia: a long-term, double-blind randomized trial. Ann Intern Med 1982;96:409.
18. Mehta D, Wafa S, Ward DE, et al. Relative efficacy of various physical manoeuvres in the termination of junctional tachycardia. Lancet 1988;1:1181.
19. Overholt ED, Rheuban KS, Gutgesell HP, et al. Usefulness of adenosine for arrhythmias in infants and children. Am J Cardiol 1988;61:336.
20. Paydak H, Kall JG, Burke MC, et al. Atrial fibrillation after radiofrequency ablation of type I atrial flutter: time to onset, determinants, and clinical course. Circulation. 1998;98(4): 315–22.
21. Pérez FJ, Schubert CM, Parvez B, Pathak V, Ellenbogen KA, Wood MA. Long-term outcomes after catheter ablation of cavotricuspid isthmus dependent atrial flutter: a meta-analysis. Circ Arrhythmia Electrophysiol. 2009;2(4):393–401.
22. Ross DL, Uther JB. Diagnosis of concealed accessory path-ways in supraventricular tachycardia. Pacing Clin Electro-physiol 1984;7:1069.
23. Savelieva I, Camm AJ. Anti-arrhythmic drug therapy for atrial fibrillation: current anti-arrhythmic drugs, investigational agents, and innovative approaches. Europace. 2008; 10:647–65.
24. Scheinman MM, Huang S. The 1998 NASPE prospective catheter ablation registry. Pacing Clin Electrophysiol 2000;23:1020.
25. Singh BN, Connolly SJ, Crijns HJGM, Roy D, Kowey PR, Cappucci A, Radzik D, Aliot EM, Hohnloser SH, for the EURIDIS and ADONIS Investigators. Dronedarone for maintenance of sinus rhythm in atrial fibrillation or flutter. N Engl J Med. 2007;357:23–35.
26. Summary: a report of the American College of Cardiology/ American Heart Association Task Force on Practice Guide-lines and the European Society of Cardiology Committee for Practice Guidelines (Writing Committee to Develop Guidelines for the Management of Patients with Supraventri-cular Arrhythmias). Circulation 2003; 108:1871.
27. Sung RJ, Waxman HL, Saksena S, et al. Sequence of retrograde atrial activation in patients with dual

atrioventricular nodal pathways. Circulation 1981;64: 1059.

28. Tafreshi MJ, Rowles J. A review of the investigational antiarrhythmic agent dronedarone. J Cardiovasc Phamacol Ther. 2007;12:15–26.
29. Timmermans C, Smeets JL, Rodriguez LM, et al. Aborted sudden death in the Wolff-Parkinson-White syndrome. Am J Cardiol 1995;76:492.
30. Touboul P, Brugada J, Cappucci A, Crijns HJGM, Edvardsso N, Hohnloser SH. Dronedarone for prevention of atrial fibrillation: a dose-ranging study. Eur Heart J. 2003;24:1481–7.
31. Tsai CF, Tai CT, Yu WC, et al. Is 8-mm more effective than 4-mm tip electrode catheter for ablation of typical atrial flutter? Circulation. 1999;100(7):768–71.
32. Tschuppert Y, Buclin T, Rothuizen LE, Decosterd LA, Galleyrand J, Gaud C, Bioffaz J. Effect of dronedarone on renal function in healthy subjects. Br J Clin Pharmacol. 2007; 64:785–791.
33. Wellens HJ, Bar FW, Lie KI. The value of the electrocardiogram in the differential diagnosis of a tachycardia with a widened QRS complex. Am J Med 1978;64:27.
34. Willems S, Weiss C, Ventura R, et al. Catheter ablation of atrial flutter guided by electroanatomic mapping (CARTO): a randomized comparison to the conventional approach. J Cardiovasc Electrophysiol. 2000;11(11): 1223–30.
35. Winniford MD, Fulton KL, Hillis LD. Long-term therapy of paroxysmal supraventricular tachycardia: arandomized, double-blind comparison of digoxin, propranolol and verapamil. Am J Cardiol 1984;54:1138.
36. Yeh SJ, Lin FC, Chou YY, et al. Termination of paroxysmal supraventricular tachycardia with a single oral dose of diltiazem and propranolol. Circulation 1985;71:104.

# 21 Cardiogenic Shock

Cardiogenic shock is a major, and frequently fatal, complication of a variety of acute and chronic disorders that impair the ability of the heart to maintain adequate tissue perfusion. Cardiac failure with cardiogenic shock continues to be a frustrating clinical problem; the management of this condition requires a rapid and well-organized approach.

Cardiogenic shock is a physiologic state in which inadequate tissue perfusion results from cardiac dysfunction, most commonly following acute myocardial infarction (MI). Although, ST-elevation MI (STEM, previously termed Q-wave MI) is encountered in most patients, cardiogenic shock may also develop in patients with non–ST-elevation acute coronary syndrome (NSTEMI, NSTACS, or unstable angina). The clinical definition of cardiogenic shock is decreased cardiac output and evidence of tissue hypoxia in the presence of adequate intravascular volume. Hemodynamic criteria for cardiogenic shock are sustained hypotension (systolic blood pressure <90 mmHg for at least 30 min) and a reduced cardiac index (<2.2 L/min/$m^2$) in the presence of elevated pulmonary capillary occlusion pressure (>15 mmHg).

The diagnosis of cardiogenic shock can sometimes be made at the bedside by observing hypotension and clinical signs of poor tissue perfusion, which include oliguria, cyanosis, cool extremities, and altered mentation. These signs usually persist after attempts have been made to correct hypovolemia, arrhythmia, hypoxia, and acidosis.

## HISTORICAL BACKGROUND

Cardiogenic shock is a medical emergency. A complete clinical assessment is critical to understanding the cause of the shock and to targeting therapy for correcting the cause (Figs 21.1 and 21.2).

Cardiogenic shock following acute MI generally develops after admission to the hospital, although a small number of patients are in shock at presentation. Patients demonstrate clinical evidence of hypoperfusion (low cardiac output), which is manifested by sinus tachycardia,

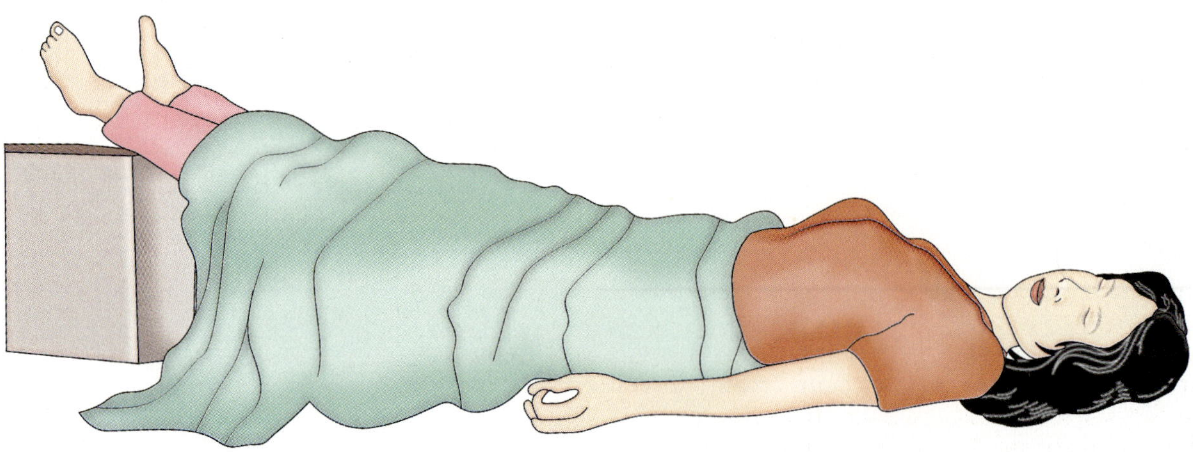

**Fig. 21.1:** Illustration showing a women patient lying unconcious with cardiogenic shock with raised legs as first step in her resuscitation by a rescue team

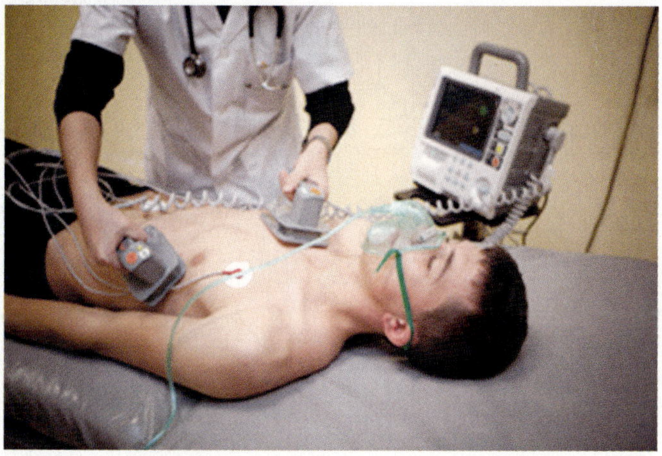

**Fig. 21.2:** A young patient with cardiac arrest being managed with cardioverter defibrillator. Electric paddles have been applied over the chest for imparting electric shock

low urine output, and cool extremities. Systemic hypotension, defined as systolic blood pressure below 90 mmHg or a decrease in mean blood pressure by 30 mm Hg, ultimately develops and further propagates tissue hypoperfusion.

Most patients who develop acute MI present with an abrupt onset of squeezing or heavy substernal chest pain; the pain may radiate to the left arm or the neck. The chest pain may be atypical, the location being epigastric or only in the neck or arm. The pain quality may be burning, sharp, or stabbing. Pain may be absent in persons with diabetes or in elderly individuals.

Patients also may report associated autonomic symptoms, including nausea, vomiting, and sweating.

A history of previous cardiac disease, use of cocaine, previous myocardial infarction (MI), or previous cardiac surgery should be obtained. A patient thought to have myocardial ischemia should be assessed for cardiac risk factors. The evaluation should reveal a history of hyperlipidemia, left ventricular hypertrophy, hypertension, or cigarette smoking or a family history of premature coronary artery disease. The presence of 2 or more risk factors increases the likelihood of acute MI.

Other associated symptoms are diaphoresis, exertional dyspnea, or dyspnea at rest. Presyncope or syncope, palpitations, generalized anxiety, and depression are other features indicative of poor cardiac function.

## PHYSICAL EXAMINATION

Cardiogenic shock is diagnosed after documentation of myocardial dysfunction and exclusion of alternative causes of hypotension, such as hypovolemia, hemorrhage, sepsis, pulmonary embolism, pericardial tamponade, aortic dissection, or pre-existing valvular disease. Shock is present if evidence of multisystem organ hypoperfusion is detected upon physical examination (Fig. 21.3 and Table 21.1).

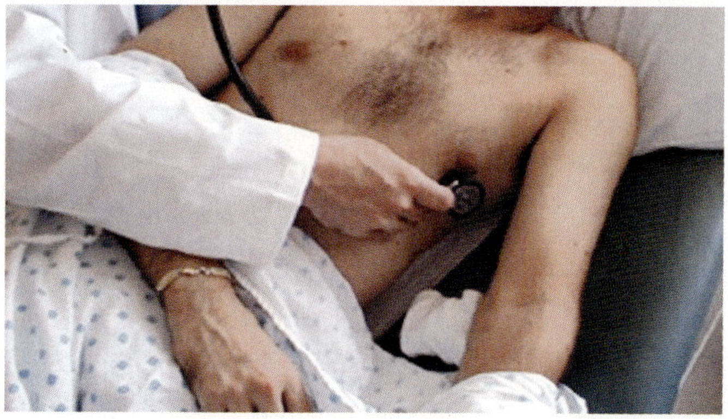

**Fig. 21.3:** A doctor conducting thorough clinical examination in a patient with cardiogenic shock

| Table 21.1: Clinical findings associated with right ventricular infarction |
|---|
| Hypotension |
| Elevated jugular venous pressure |
| Kussmaul's sign |
| Abnormal jugular venous pressure pattern (Y ≥ X descent) |
| Tricuspid regurgitation |
| Right sided S3 and S4 |
| Pulsus paradoxus |
| High-grade atrioventricular block |

*Characteristics of patients with cardiogenic shock include the following:*

- Patients in shock usually appear ashen or cyanotic and have cool skin and mottled extremities
- Peripheral pulses are rapid and faint and may be irregular if arrhythmias are present
- Jugular venous distention and crackles in the lungs are usually (but not always) present; peripheral edema also may be present.
- Heart sounds are usually distant, and third and fourth heart sounds may be present.
- The pulse pressure may be low, and patients are usually tachycardic.
- Patients show signs of hypoperfusion, such as altered mental status and decreased urine output.
- A systolic murmur is generally heard in patients with acute mitral regurgitation or ventricular septal rupture. The associated parasternal thrill indicates the presence of a ventricular septal defect, whereas the murmur of mitral regurgitation may be limited to early systole.
- The systolic murmur, which becomes louder upon Valsalva and prompt standing, suggests hypertrophic obstructive cardiomyopathy (idiopathic hypertropic subaortic stenosis).

## PREDISPOSING FACTORS IN CARDIOGENIC SHOCK

Various predisposing conditions development of cardiogenic shock include the following (Fig. 21.4 and Table 21.2).

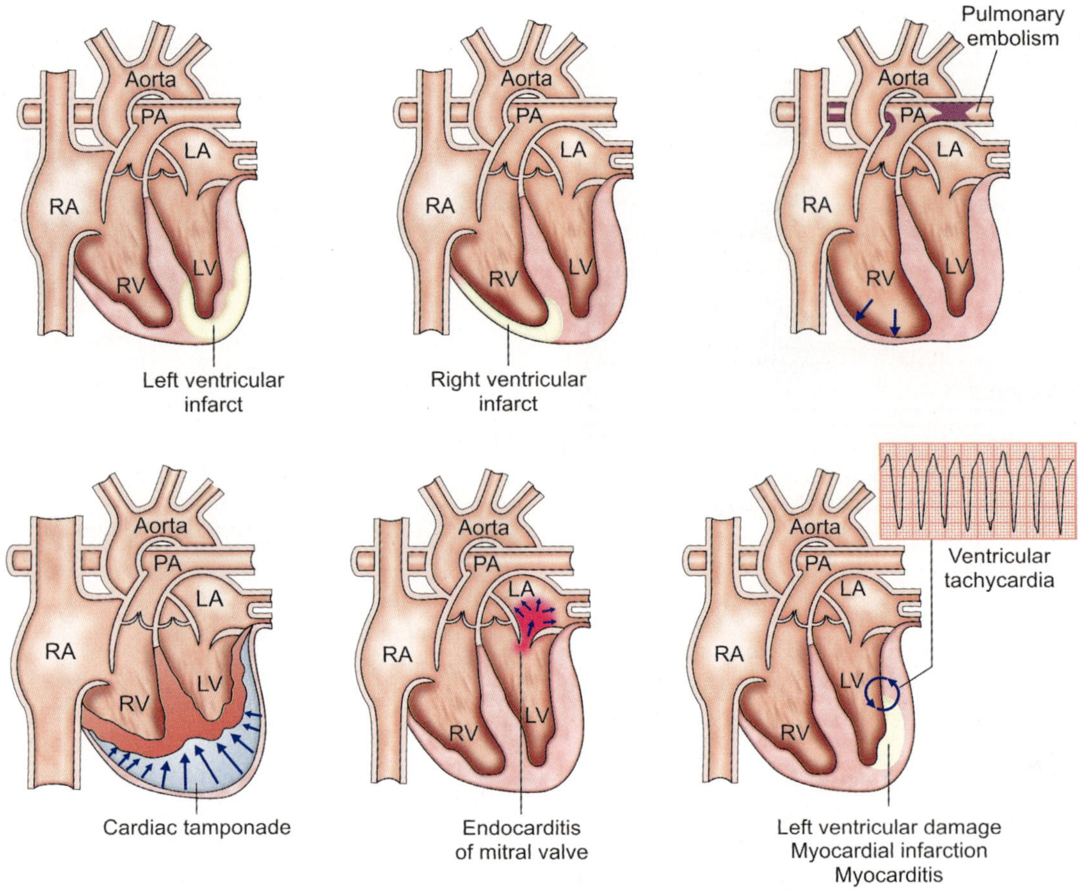


**Fig. 21.4:** Various causes of cardiogenic shock

| **Table 21.2:** Causes of hypotension among patients with inferior myocardial infarction |
|---|
| Severe right ventricular infarction |
| Bradyarrythmia |
| Acute severe mitral regurgitation |
| Prior myocardial infarction |
| Left ventricular septal rupture |
| Bezold-Jarisch reflex |

### Systemic Inflammatory Response Syndrome

- Acute coronary syndrome
- Aortic regurgitation
- Dilated cardiomyopathy
- Restrictive cardiomyopathy
- Congestive heart failure and pulmonary edema
- Mitral regurgitation
- Pericarditis and cardiac tamponade
- Hypovolemic shock
- Papillary muscle rupture
- Acute valvular dysfunction

### Right Ventricular Infarction

Right ventricular infarction occurs in up to 30% of patients with inferior myocardial infarction (MI) and becomes hemodynamically unstable in 10% of these patients. The diagnosis is made by identifying an ST-segment elevation in the right precordial leads (V3 or V4 R) and/or typical hemodynamic findings after right heart catheterization. These are elevated right atrial and right ventricular end-diastolic pressures with normal to low pulmonary artery wedge pressure and low cardiac output.

Echocardiography findings can also be very helpful in the diagnosis of right ventricular infarction. Patients with cardiogenic shock due to this condition have a better prognosis than do patients when compared to those with cardiogenic shock due to left ventricular systolic failure.

Regarding the management of cardiogenic shock due to right ventricular infarction, supportive therapy begins with the restoration and maintenance of right ventricular preload with fluid administration. However, excessive fluid resuscitation may compromise left ventricular filling by introducing an interventricular septal shift.

Inotropic therapy with dobutamine may be effective in increasing cardiac output in patients with right ventricular infarction. Maintenance of systemic arterial pressure in order to maintain adequate coronary artery perfusion may require vasoconstricting agents, such as norepinephrine. In unstable patients, an intra-aortic balloon pump (IABP) may be useful for ensuring adequate blood supply to the already compromised right ventricle.

*Revascularization of the occluded coronary artery, preferably by percutaneous transluminal coronary angioplasty (PTCA), is crucial for management and has shown to dramatically improve outcome.*

### Acute Mitral Regurgitation

Acute mitral regurgitation (Fig. 21.5) is usually associated with inferior MI due to ischemia or infarction of the papillary muscle. It occurs in approximately 1% of MIs, and posteromedial papillary muscle is involved more frequently than anterolateral muscle. Acute mitral regurgitation usually happens 2–7 days following acute MI and manifests with an abrupt onset of pulmonary edema, hypotension, and cardiogenic shock.

Echocardiography findings are extremely useful in making a diagnosis. The two-dimensional (2-D) echocardiographic image shows the malfunctioning mitral valve, and findings from a Doppler study can be used to document the severity of mitral regurgitation. Right heart catheterization is often required for stabilizing the patient. Tall V waves identified on pulmonary arterial and wedge pressure waveforms indicate acute mitral regurgitation. However, the diagnosis must be confirmed based on echocardiography or left ventriculography findings before definitive therapy or surgery is initiated.

Hemodynamic stabilization by reducing afterload, either with nitroprusside or an IABP, is often instituted. Definitive therapy requires revascularization, if ischemia is present, and/or surgical valve repair or replacement, if a structural valvular lesion is present. The mortality rate in the presurgical era was 50% in the first 24 hours, with a 2-month survival rate of 6%.

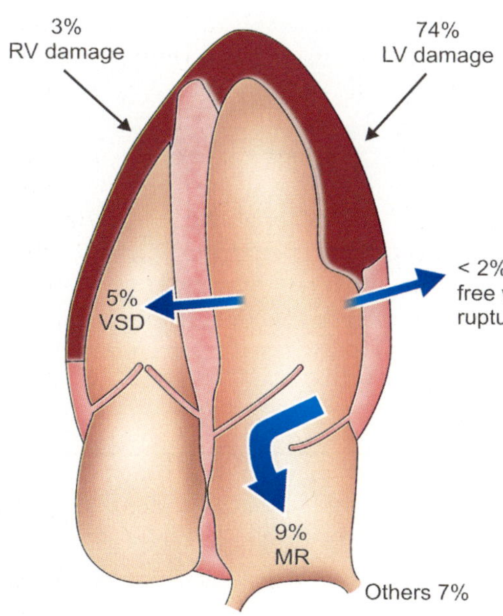


**Fig. 21.5:** Apical four-chamber echo view with relative incidence of the mechanisms responsible for cardiogenic shock in the SHOCK 8 and MILIS 4 registeries (MR=mitral regurgitation; VSD= ventricular septal defect)

### Cardiac Rupture

Rupture of the free wall of the left ventricle occurs within 2 weeks of the MI and may occur within the first 24 hours. The rupture may involve the anterior, posterior, or lateral wall of the ventricle.

Cardiac rupture often presents as sudden cardiac death. Premortem symptoms include chest pain, agitation, tachycardia, and hypotension. This diagnosis should be considered in patients with electromechanical dissociation who have a history of anginal pain. Patients rarely, if ever, survive cardiac rupture.

### Ventricular Septal Rupture

Approximately 1–3% of acute MIs are associated with ventricular septal rupture. Most septal ruptures occur within the week following MI. Patients with acute ventricular septal rupture develop acute heart failure and/or cardiogenic shock, with physical findings of a harsh holosystolic murmur and left parasternal thrill.

A left-to-right intracardiac shunt, as demonstrated by a step-up (>5% increase in oxygen saturation) between the right atrium and right ventricle, confirms the diagnosis. Alternatively, 2-D and Doppler echocardiographic findings can be used to identify the location and severity of the left-to-right shunt.

Rapid stabilization using an IABP and pharmacologic measures, followed by emergent surgical repair, is lifesaving. The timing of surgical intervention is controversial, but most experts suggest operative repair within 48 hours of the rupture.

Ventricular septal rupture portends a poor prognosis unless management is aggressive. Immediate surgical repair of patients with ventricular septal rupture is reported to be associated with survival rates of 42–75%; therefore, prompt surgical therapy is imperative as soon as possible after the diagnosis of ventricular septal rupture is confirmed.

### Reversible Myocardial Dysfunction

Other causes of severe, reversible myocardial dysfunction are sepsis-associated myocardial depression, myocardial depression following cardiopulmonary bypass, and inflammatory myocarditis. In older literature, this presentation is often referred to as cold septic shock. In these situations, myocardial dysfunction occurs from the effects of inflammatory cytokines, such as tumor necrosis factor and interleukin 1.

Myocardial dysfunction may vary from mild to severe and may lead to cardiogenic shock. For patients in cardiogenic shock, cardiovascular support with inotropic agents may be required until recovery, which generally occurs after the underlying disease process resolves.

## DIFFERENTIAL DIAGNOSES

- Myocardial infarction
- Myocardial ischemia
- Myocardial rupture

- Myocarditis
- Pulmonary edema, cardiogenic
- Pulmonary embolism
- Sepsis, bacterial
- Septic shock
- Shock, distributive
- Shock, hemorrhagic

## LABORATORY STUDIES

### Biochemical Profile

Measurement of routine biochemical parameters, such as electrolytes, renal function (e.g. urea and creatinine), and liver function tests, [e.g. bilirubin, aspartate aminotransferase, alanine aminotransferase, lactate dehydrogenase (LDH)], are useful for assessing proper functioning of vital organs.

### CBC Count

A complete blood count (CBC) is generally helpful to exclude anemia. A high white blood cell (WBC) count may indicate an underlying infection, and the platelet count may be low because of coagulopathy related to sepsis.

### Cardiac Enzymes

The diagnosis of acute myocardial infarction (MI) is aided by a variety of serum markers, which include creatine kinase and its subclasses, troponin, myoglobin, and LDH. The value for the isoenzyme of creatine kinase with muscle and blood subunits is most specific but may be falsely elevated in persons with myopathy, hypothyroidism, renal failure, or skeletal muscle injury.

The rapid release and metabolism of myoglobin occurs in persons with MI. A 4-fold rise of myoglobin over 2 hours appears to be a test result that is sensitive for MI. The serum LDH value increases approximately 10 hours after the onset of MI, peaks at 24–48 hours, and gradually returns to normal in 6–8 days. The LDH fraction 1 isoenzyme is primarily released by the heart but also may come from the kidneys, stomach, pancreas, and red blood cells.

### Troponins

Cardiac troponins T and I are widely used for the diagnosis of myocardial injury. Troponin elevation in the absence of clinical evidence of ischemia should prompt a search for other causes of cardiac damage, such as myocarditis.

Troponin I and T can be detected in serum within the first few hours after onset of acute MI. Troponin levels peak at 14 hours after acute MI, peak again several days later (biphasic peak), and remain abnormal for 10 days. This characteristic could make troponin T (in combination with CK-MB) useful for retrospective diagnosis of acute MI in patients who seek care very late. Troponin T is an independent prognostic indicator of adverse outcomes and can be used as a patient risk-stratifying tool in patients with unstable angina or non-Q-wave MI.

### Arterial Blood Gases

Arterial blood gas values indicate overall acid-base homeostasis and the level of arterial blood oxygenation. (Acidosis can have a particularly deleterious effect on myocardial function.) A base deficit elevation (reference range is +3 to –3 mmol/L) correlates with the occurrence and severity of shock. A base deficit is also an important marker to follow during resuscitation of a patient from shock.

### Lactate

An elevated serum lactate level is an indicator of shock. Serial lactate measurements are useful markers of hypoperfusion and are also used as indicators of prognosis. Elevated lactate values in a patient with signs of hypoperfusion indicate a poor prognosis; rising lactate values during resuscitation portend a very high mortality rate.

### Brain Natriuretic Peptide

Brain natriuretic peptide (BNP) may be useful as an indicator of congestive heart failure and as an independent prognostic indicator of survival. A low BNP level may effectively rule out cardiogenic shock in the setting of hypotension; however, an elevated BNP level does not rule in the disease.

## IMAGING STUDIES

### Chest Radiography

Chest radiographic findings (Figs 21.6 and 21.7) are useful for excluding other causes of shock or chest pain. A widened mediastinum may indicate aortic dissection. Tension pneumothorax or pneumomediastinum readily

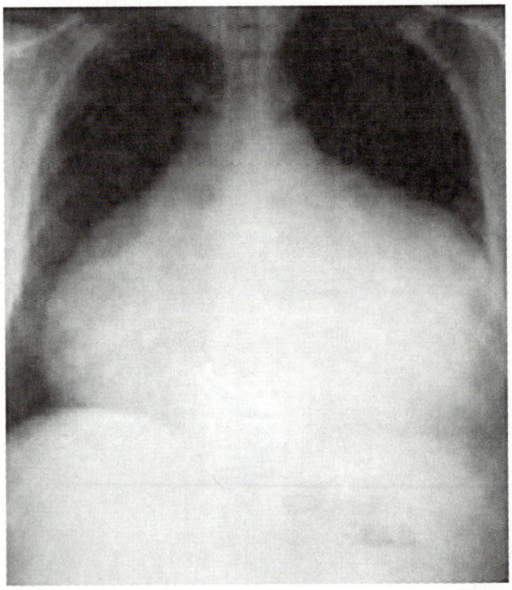

**Fig. 21.6:** This anteroposterior view chest radiograph shows a massive bottle-shaped heart and conspicuous absence of pulmonary vascular congestion in patient with cardiac tamponade

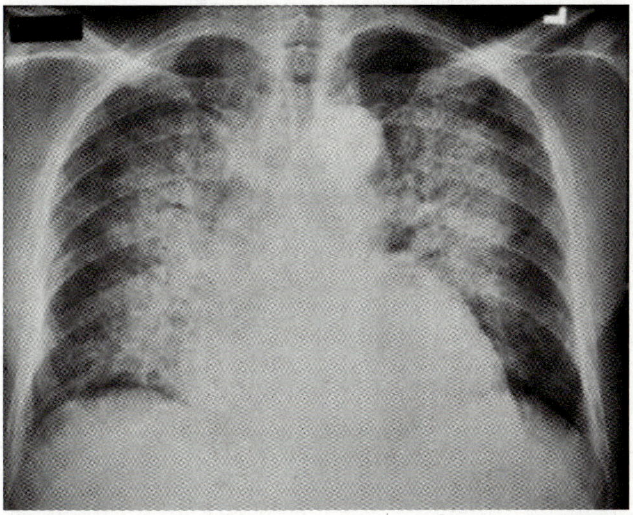

**Fig. 21.7:** Chest X-ray PA view showing cardiogenic pulmonary edema in a butterfly distribution due to left ventricular failure. It also shows large perihilar opacities in patient with enlarged cardiac silhouette

detected on radiographic films may manifest as low-output shock.

Most patients with established cardiogenic shock exhibit findings of left ventricular failure, the radiologic features of which include pulmonary vascular redistribution, interstitial pulmonary edema, enlarged hilar shadows, the presence of Kerley B lines, cardiomegaly, and bilateral pleural effusions. Alveolar edema manifests as bilateral perihilar opacities in a so-called butterfly distribution.

### Electrocardiography

Acute myocardial ischemia is diagnosed based on the presence of ST-segment elevation, ST-segment depression, or Q-waves. T-wave inversion, although a less sensitive finding, may also be seen in persons with myocardial ischemia. An ECG with right-sided chest leads may document right ventricular infarction and may be prognostically, as well as diagnostically, useful.

Perform electrocardiography immediately to help diagnose myocardial infarction (MI) and/or myocardial ischemia. A normal ECG, however, does not rule out the possibility of acute MI (Figs 21.8–21.15).

### Ultrasonography

Ultrasonography can be used to guide fluid management. In the spontaneously breathing patient, inferior vena cava (IVC) collapse with respiration suggests dehydration, whereas a lack of IVC collapse suggests intravascular euvolemia.

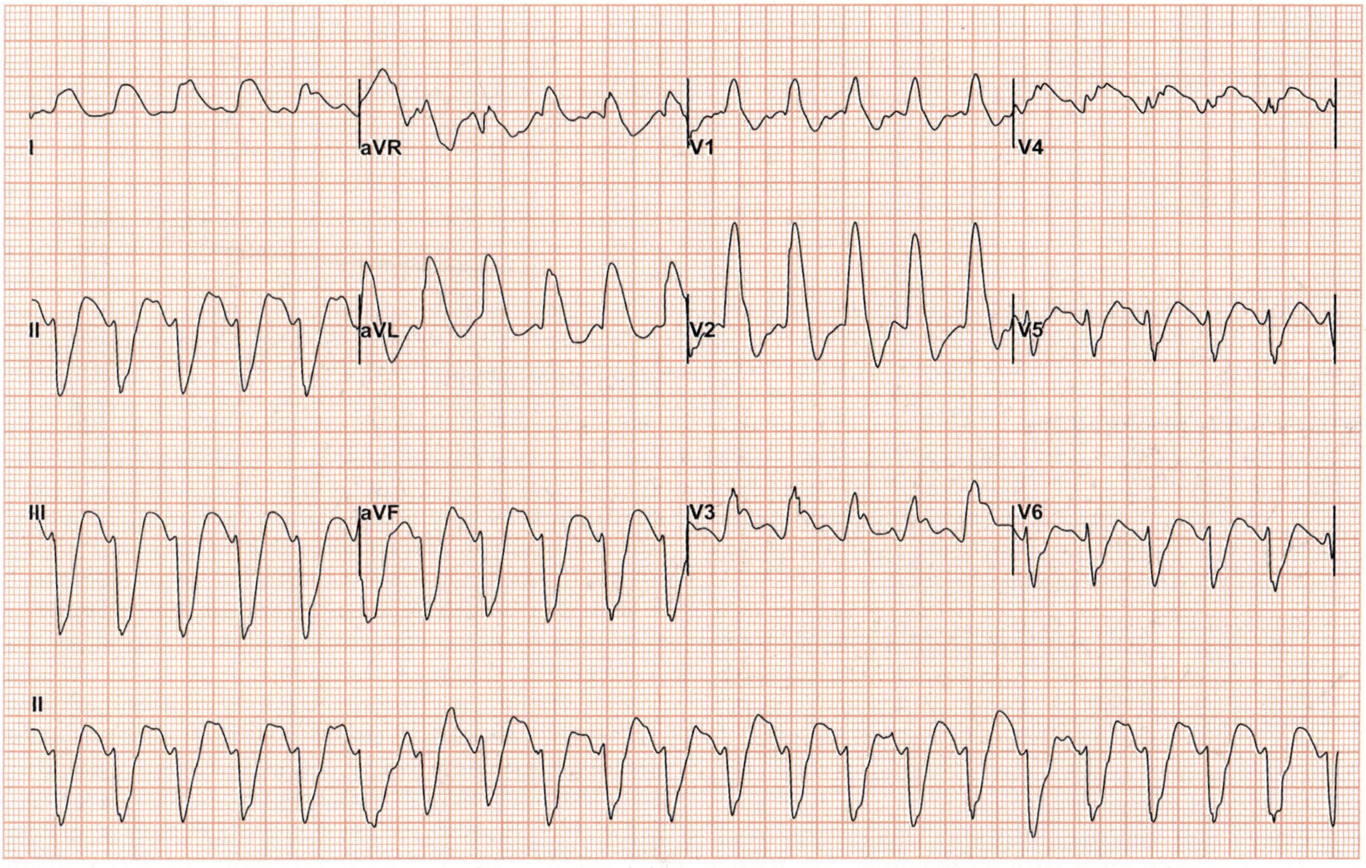


**Fig. 21.8:** A 51-year-male complained of chest pain, followed by cardiac arrest. He was resuscitated and brought to the ED where his ECG showed wide complex tachycardia, RBBB + LAFB, and massive ST elevation. He was in cardiogenic shock

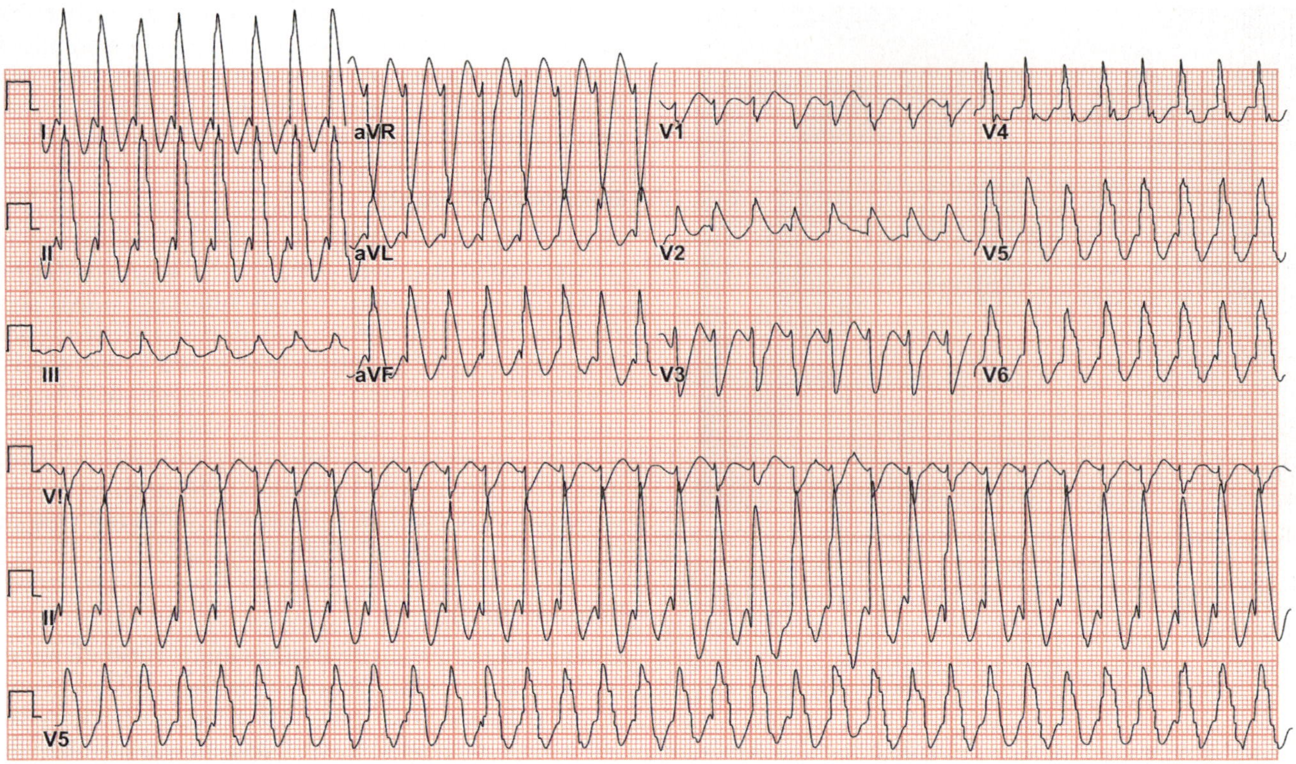


**Fig. 21.9:** ECG showed ventricular tachycardia in a 70-year-old man, admitted into emergency department with cardiogenic preshocked condition

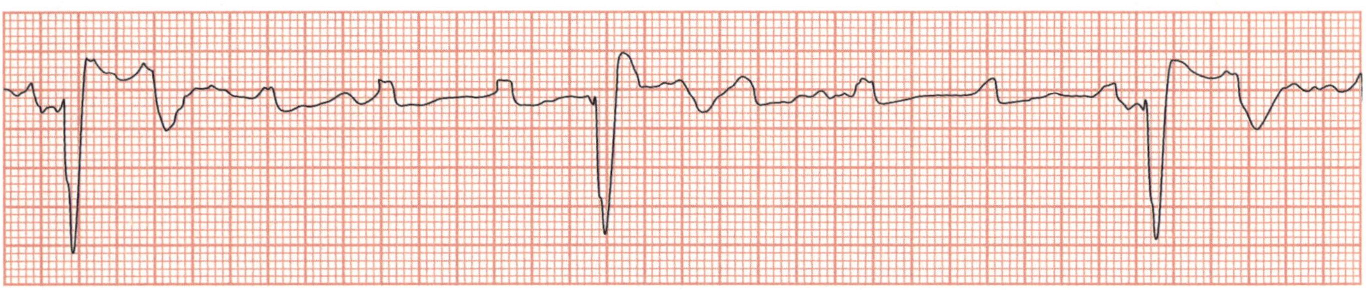

**Fig. 21.10:** ECG trace showing acute myocardial infarction with complete heart block

## MRI/CT SCANS (Fig. 21.16)

### Coronary Artery Angiography

Coronary angiography is urgently indicated in patients with myocardial ischemia or myocardial infarction (MI) who also develop cardiogenic shock. Angiography is required to help assess the anatomy of the coronary arteries and the need for urgent revascularization.

Coronary angiography findings often demonstrate multivessel coronary artery disease in persons with cardiogenic shock. In these patients, a compensatory hyperkinesis cannot occur in the noninfarct territory, because of the severe coronary artery atherosclerosis.

The most common cause of cardiogenic shock is extensive MI, although a smaller infarction in a previously compromised left ventricle also may precipitate shock. Following MI, large areas of nonfunctional, but viable, myocardium (hibernating myocardium) can also cause or contribute to cardiogenic shock.

### Echocardiography

Echocardiography should be performed early to establish the cause of cardiogenic shock. Echocardiography provides information on global and regional systolic function and on diastolic dysfunction. Echocardiography findings can also lead to a rapid diagnosis of mechanical causes of shock, such as acute ventricular septal defect, free myocardial wall rupture, pericardial tamponade, and papillary muscle rupture causing acute myocardial regurgitation (Figs. 21.17–21.26).

In addition, an echocardiogram may reveal akinetic or dyskinetic areas of ventricular wall motion or may demonstrate valvular dysfunction. Ejection fraction may be estimated as well (although results from the SHOCK trial indicated that left ventricular ejection fraction is not always depressed in the setting of cardiogenic shock). If a hyperdynamic left ventricle is found, the echocardiogram may suggest other causes of shock such as sepsis or anemia.

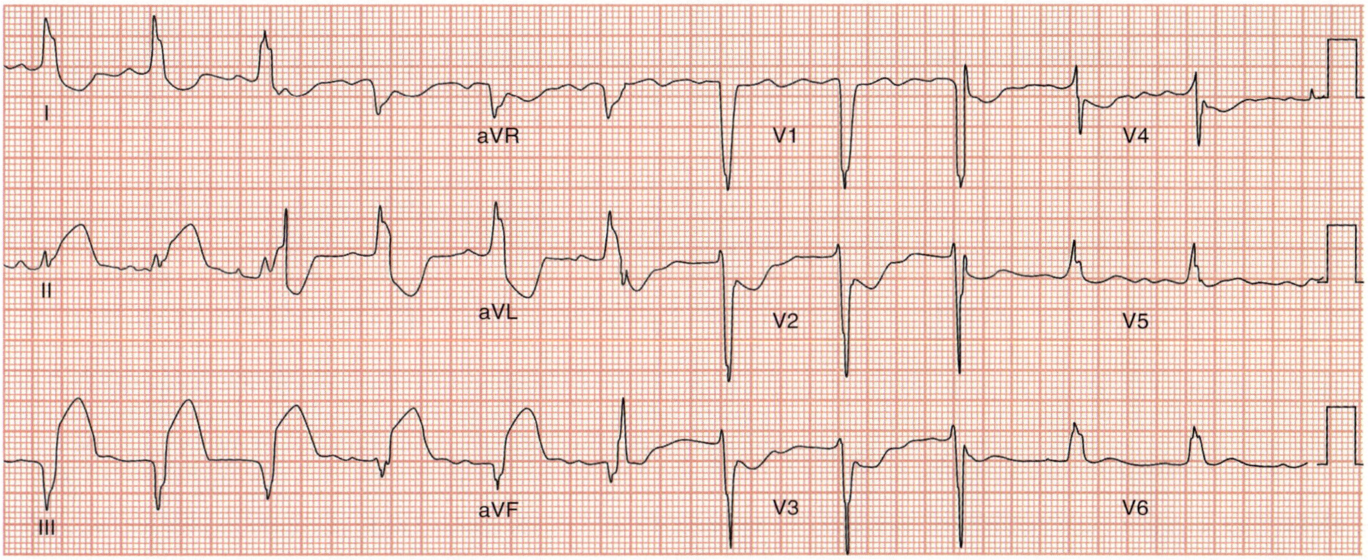


**Fig. 21.11:** Electrocardiogram displays all of the criteria for the diagnosis of acute myocardial infarction (MI) in the setting of LBBB. ST-segment elevation greater than 1 mm, concordant with QRS in lead II (5 points); ST-segment depression greater than 1 mm in lead V2 and V3 (3 points); and ST-segment elevation greater than 5 mm, discordant with QRS in leads III and VF (2 points). A score of 10 points indicates an extremely high likelihood of inferior MI (From Sgarbossa EB, Wagfier G, 1997, with permission)

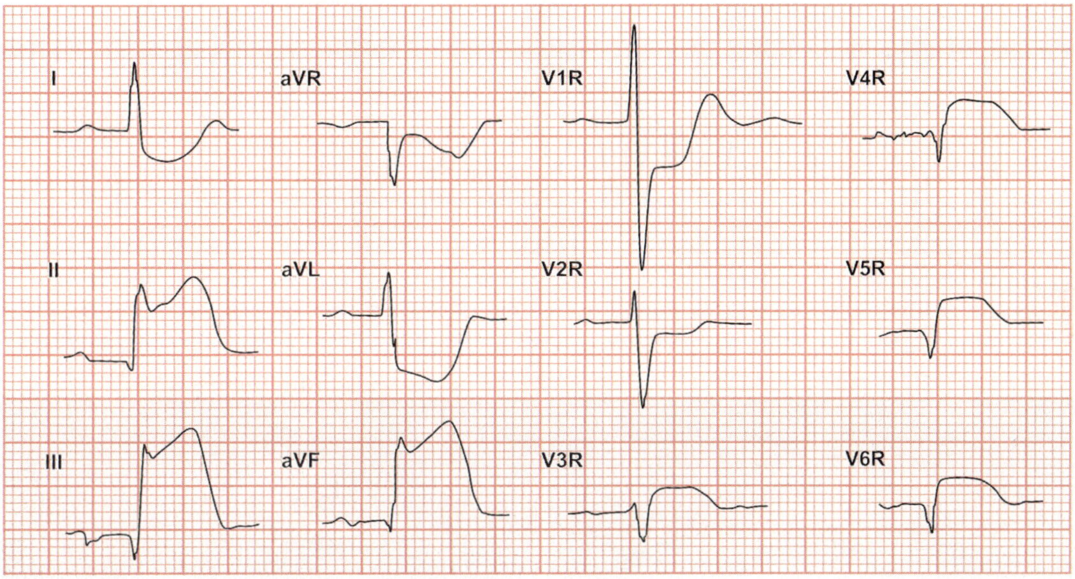


**Fig. 21.12:** Standard 12-lead electrocardiogram. (A) Showed marked ST-segment elevation in leads V4R, V5R, V6R, and ST-segment elevation in leads II, III, and aVF in right ventricular infarction

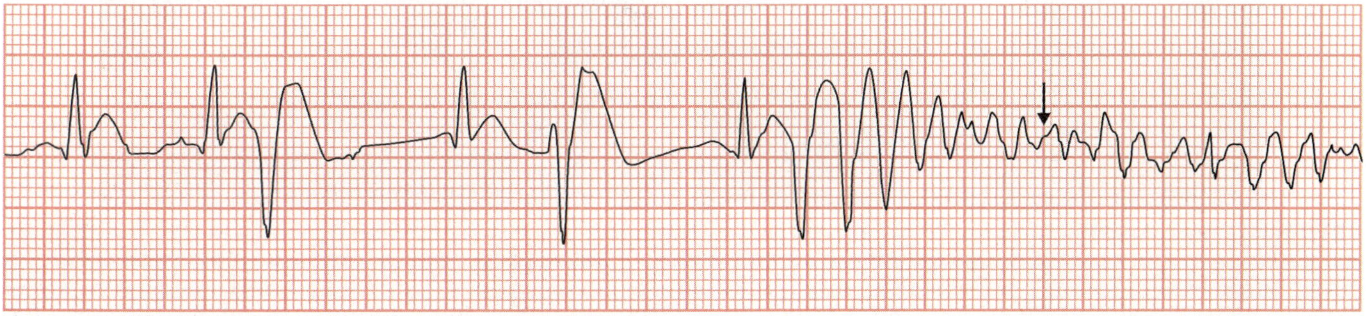

**Fig. 21.13:** ECG trace showing R on T phenomenon (arrow) giving rise to ventricular fibrillation (arrow)

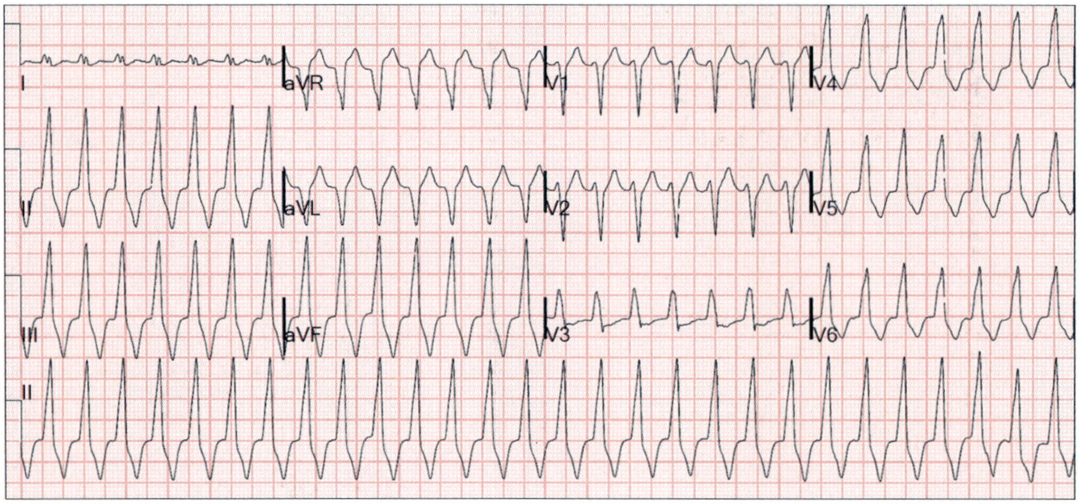


**Fig. 21.14:** Middle-aged male patient who was brought into hospital with shock showed wide complex regular tachycardia at a rate of 170

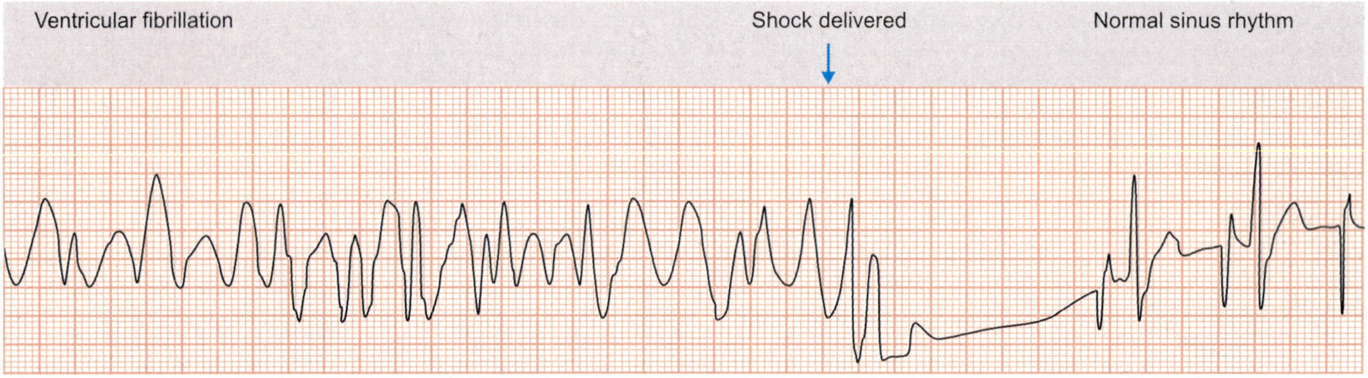


**Fig. 21.15:** An example of delivery of implantable cardioverter-defibrillator (ICD) shock therapy. The device senses ventricular electrograms. This sensed electrical activity satisfies the criteria of the device's detection algorithm and a 34 J shock is delivered (thick arrow). This returns the patient to (initially) a ventricular paced rhythm with normal sinus rhythm following shortly

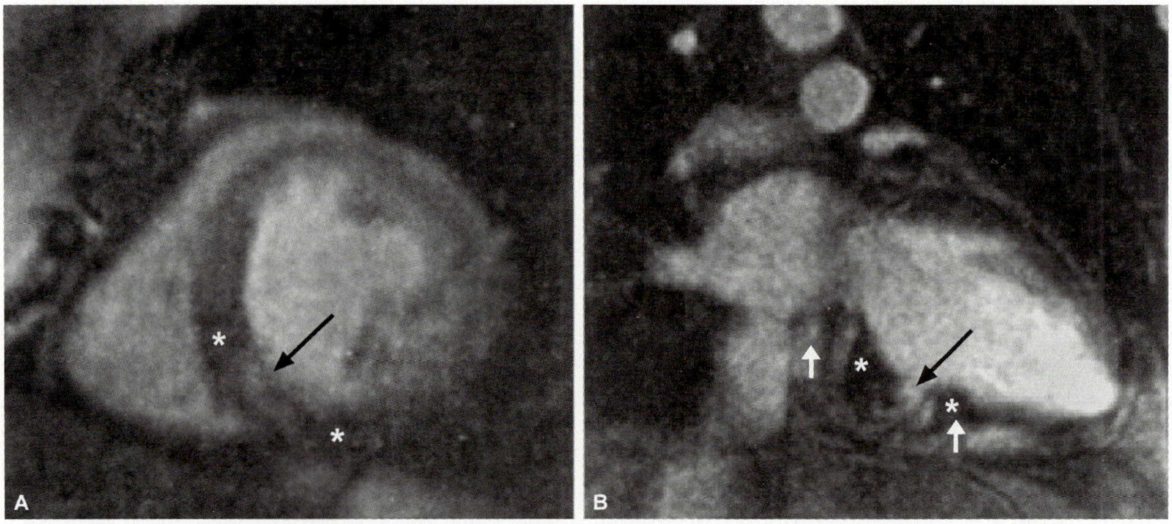


**Fig. 21.16:** (A) Contrast enhanced dynamic myocardial perfusion imaging at rest demonstrated contrast flow from the cavity of the LV into the myocardium near the basal septum (arrows). The contrast material penetrated about three quarters of the myocardial thickness, thus showing impending myocardial rupture (using late enhancement technique 10 minutes after application of contrast agent,an extended transmural inferior infarction could be seen in the long axis view. (B) Left ventricular angiogram in a LAO 60° position demonstrated an inferiorly located ventricular septal defect (white arrow)

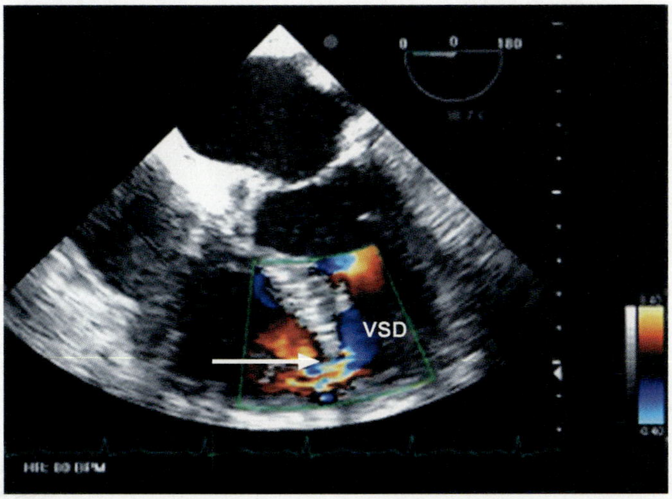


**Fig. 21.17:** TEE color scan in four-chamber view showing post-MI VSD (arrow). The defect was repaired surgically

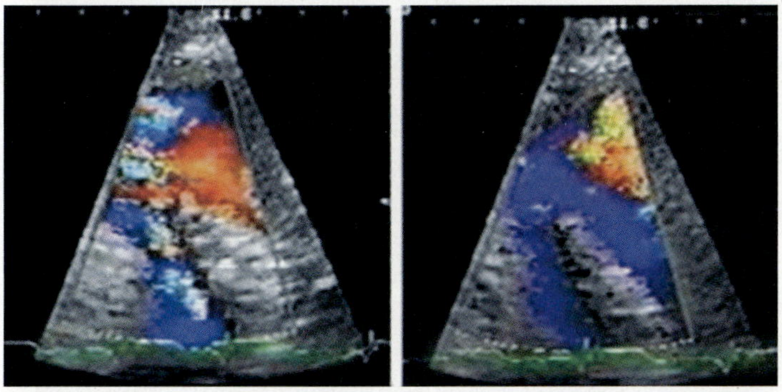

**Fig. 21.18:** An 80-year-old woman presented with chest pain and anterior AMI. An apical holosystolic murmur was heard and color doppler examination showed systolic/diastolic left to right shunt. The patient developed cardiogenic shock and died before cardiac catheterization

Pleural sliding in an intercostal space demonstrating increased lung comet artifacts suggestive of pulmonary edema.

### Invasive Hemodynamic Monitoring

Invasive hemodynamic monitoring (**Swan-Ganz catheterization)** (Figs 21.27 and 21.28) is very useful for helping exclude other causes and types of shock, e.g. volume depletion, obstructive shock, and septic shock.

The hemodynamic measurements of cardiogenic shock are a pulmonary capillary wedge pressure (PCWP) of greater than 15 mmHg and a cardiac index of less than 2.2 L/min/$m^2$.

The presence of large V waves on the PCWP tracing suggests severe mitral regurgitation, while a step-up in oxygen saturation between the right atrium and the right ventricle is diagnostic of ventricular septal rupture.

High right-sided filling pressures in the absence of an elevated PCWP, when accompanied by electrocardiographic criteria, indicate right ventricular infarction.

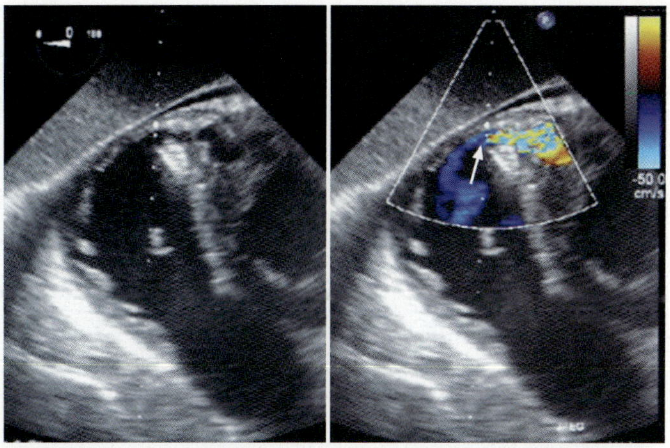

**Fig. 21.19:** The transgastric view after the first closure device implantation with significant residual VSD blood flow (arrow)

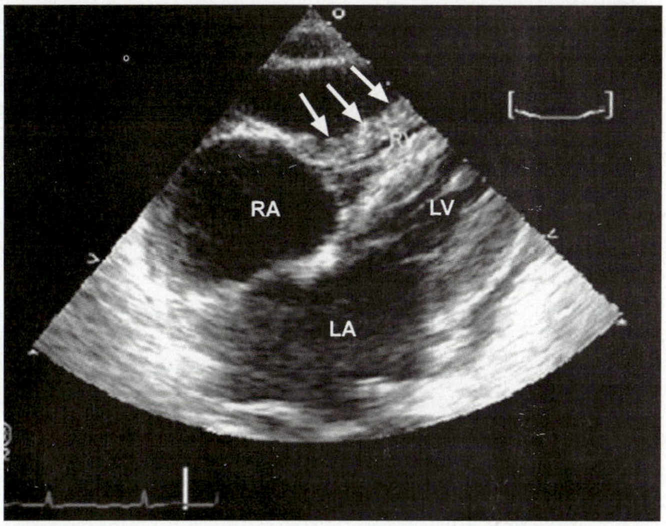


**Fig. 21.20:** Early diastolic collapse of right ventricular free wall (subcostal view) in cardiac tamponade (white arrows)

## APPROACH CONSIDERATIONS

Cardiogenic shock is an emergency requiring immediate resuscitative therapy before shock irreversibly damages vital organs. The key to a good outcome in patients with cardiogenic shock is an organized approach, with rapid diagnosis and prompt initiation of pharmacologic therapy to maintain blood pressure and cardiac output.

All patients require admission to an intensive care setting, which may involve emergent transfer to the cardiac catheterization suite, critical care transport to a tertiary care center, or internal transfer to the intensive care unit (ICU).

Early and definitive restoration of coronary blood flow is the most important intervention for achieving an improved survival rate. At present, it represents standard therapy for patients with cardiogenic shock due to myocardial ischemia.

Correction of electrolyte and acid-base abnormalities, such as hypokalemia, hypomagnesemia, and acidosis, is essential in cardiogenic shock.

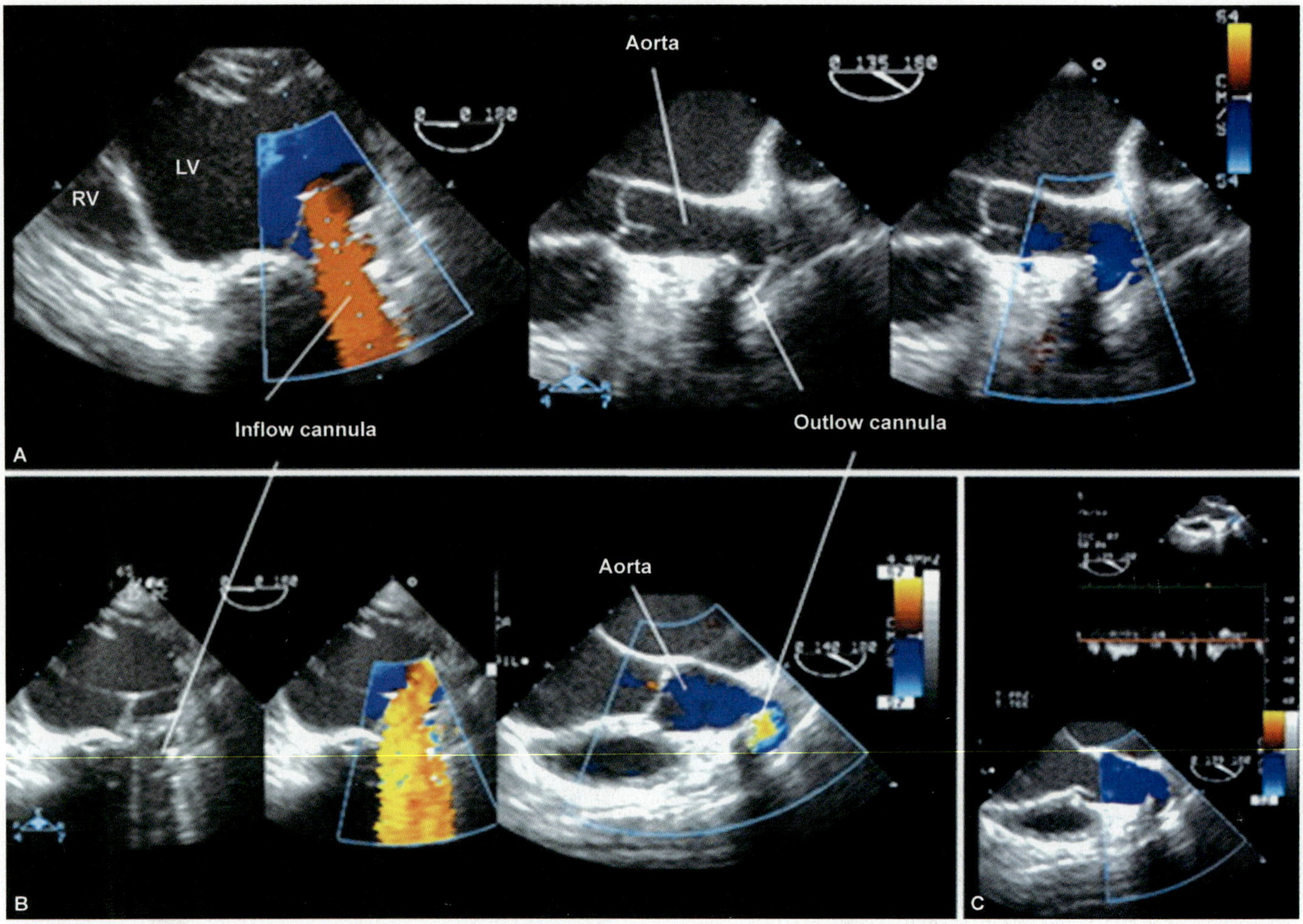


**Fig. 21.21:** Echocardiography documents a case of pump arrest. (A) Color-Doppler shows a retrograde flow from the outflow cannula visualized by midoesophageal longitudinal view at 135° (right)-through pump-to inflow cannula and left ventricle visualized by midoesophageal four-chamber view (left). (B) In the same patient color-Doppler documents high retrograde flow after v-a ECMO activation with severe LV distension. (C) Color-Doppler and pulsed wave Doppler show the interruption of aorta-to-LV shunt after LVAD outflow cannula clamping. LV=left ventricle; RV=right ventricle

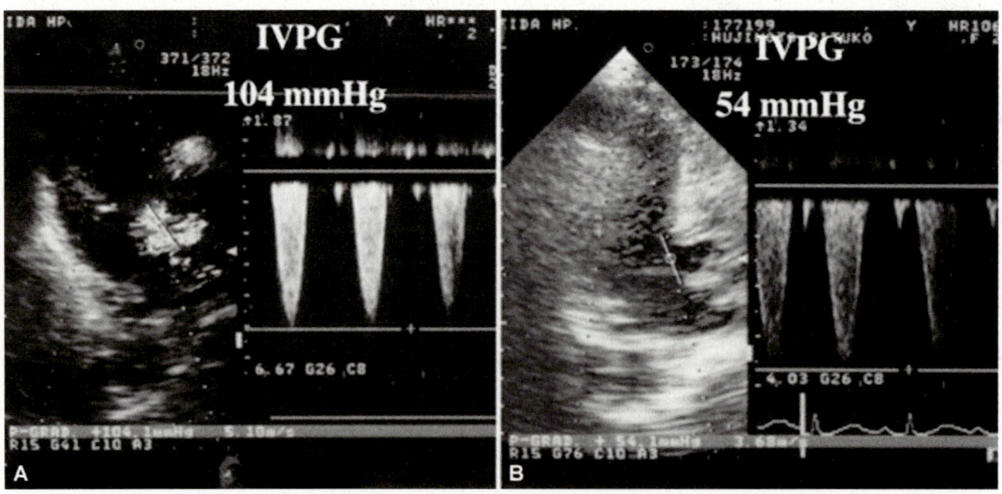


**Fig. 21.22:** (A) A Doppler echocardiogram on admission showed an intraventricular pressure gradient (IVPG) of 104 mmHg. (B) After cessation of an intravenous administration of dopamine, the IVPG decreased to 54 mmHg

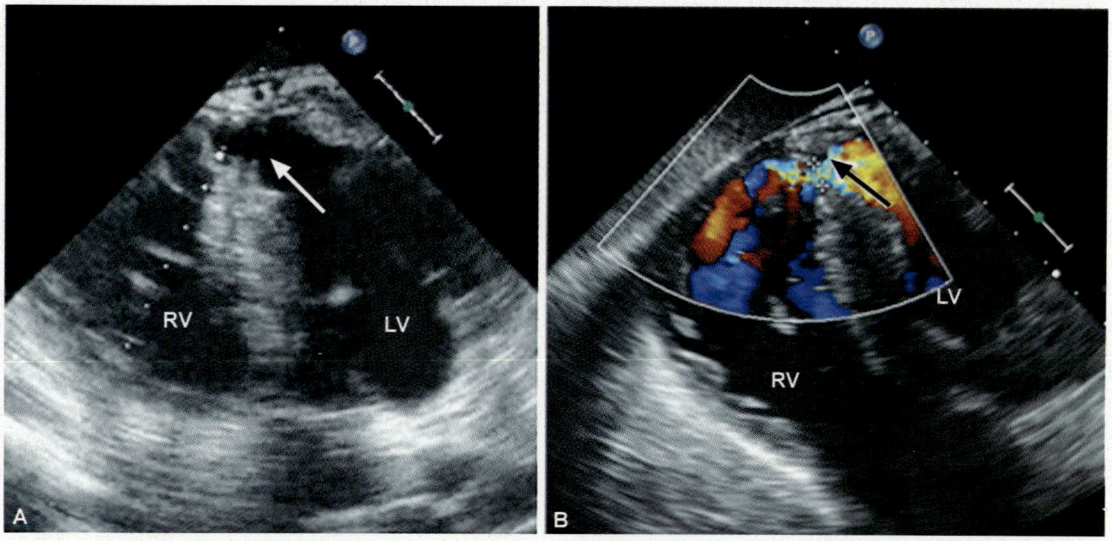


**Fig. 21.23:** Transgastric transesophageal echocardiographic images showing (A) left ventricular aneurysm (arrow) with (B) the VSD (arrow) after MI. RV=right ventricle; LV=left ventricle

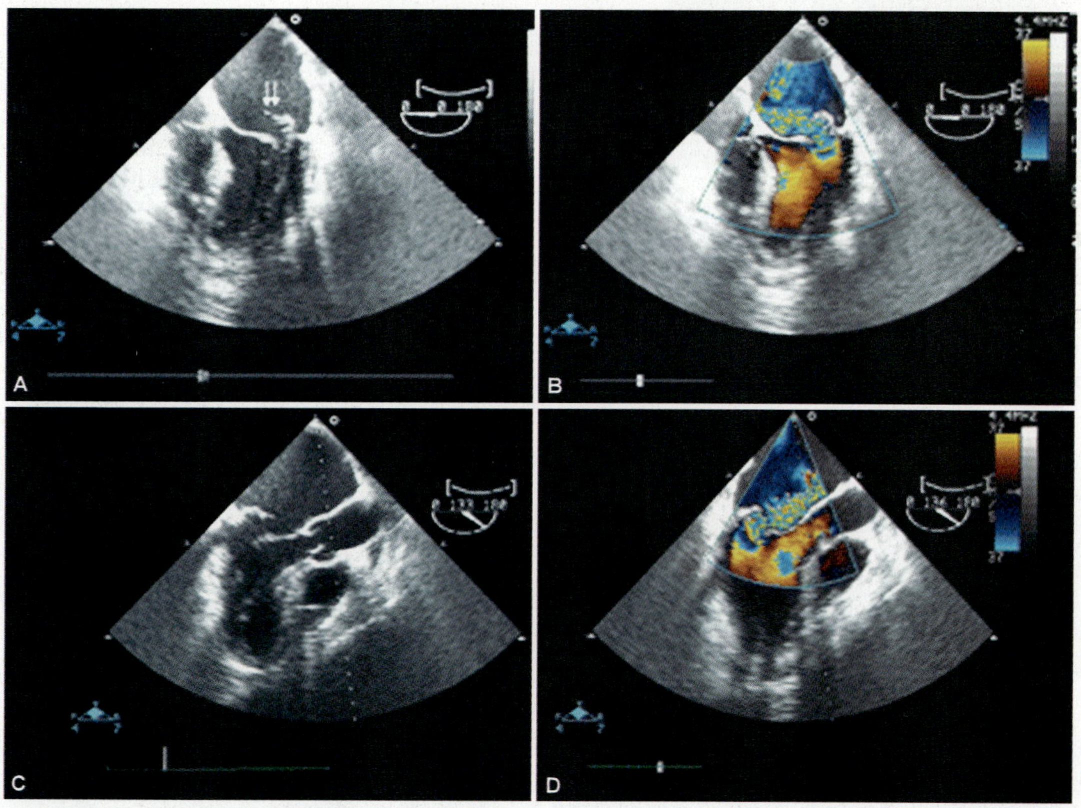


**Fig. 21.24:** (A) Four-chamber transoesophageal echocardiography (TOE) view showing the presence of chordal rupture (arrows) with a mitral leaflet prolapsing into the left atrium. (B) Four-chamber view with color-Doppler. An eccentric jet of mitral regurgitation can be observed. (C, D) Long axis TOE view showing the jet of severe mitral insufficiency directed towards the anterior portion of the left atrium

Cardiogenic shock may be prevented with early revascularization in patients with myocardial infarction (MI) and with required intervention in patients with structural heart disease.

## PROCEDURES

Placement of a central line may facilitate volume resuscitation, provide vascular access for multiple infusions, and allow invasive monitoring of central venous pressure.

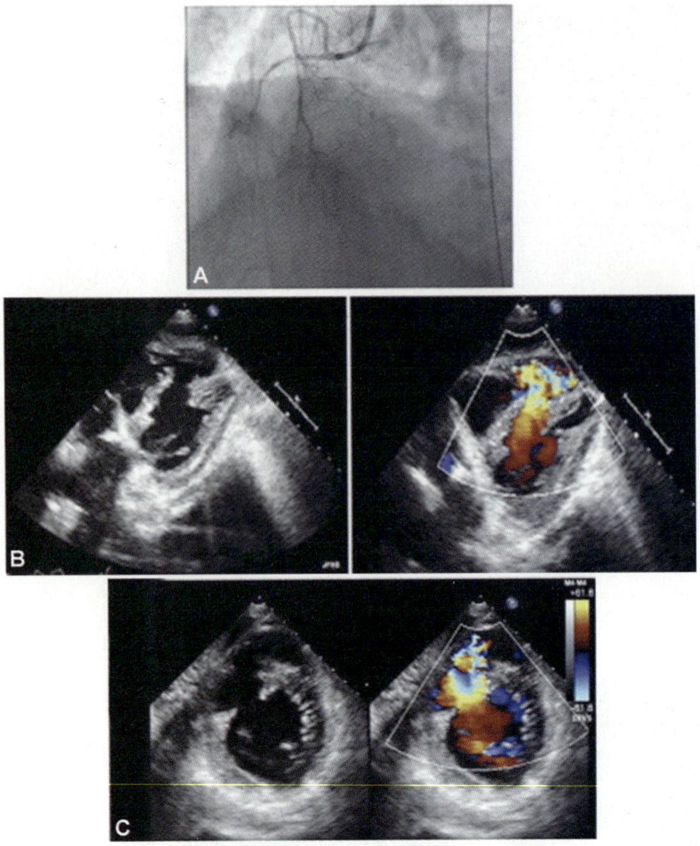


**Fig. 21.25:** Coronary angiography of RCA and echocardiogram in an elderly female ex-smoker with ventricular septal rupture. (A) Coronary angiogram of right coronary artery (RCA) showing proximal total occlusion. (B) Subcostal view on 2-dimensional electrocardiography. (C) Short axis view of the left ventricle on 2-dimensional echocardiogram, with and without color Doppler, showing large direct ventricular septal rupture

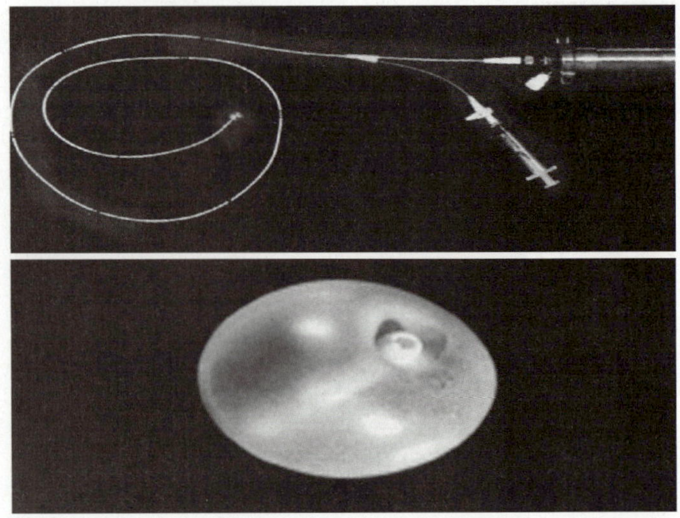

**Fig. 21.27:** Standard balloon-tipped flow-directed catheter with inflated balloon, closed inflation lumen and a pressure transducer attached to the large lumen. Close-up view of the inflated balloon

Central venous pressure may also be used to guide fluid resuscitation (Figs 21.29–21.33).

Although not necessary for the diagnosis of cardiogenic shock, invasive monitoring with a pulmonary artery catheter may be helpful in guiding fluid resuscitation in situations in which left ventricular preload is difficult to determine.

**Pulmonary artery catheter pressure measurements** may also be useful in prognosis. Retrospective evaluation of these measurements from the SHOCK trial demonstrated that stroke volume index (SVI) and stroke work index (SWI) vary inversely with mortality.

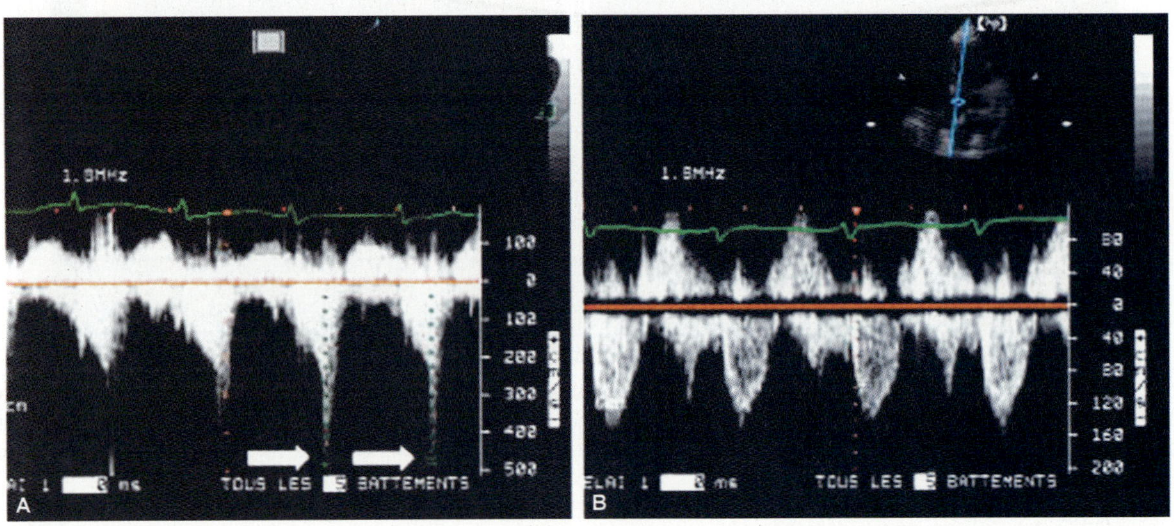


**Fig. 21.26:** Continuous-wave Doppler findings obtained with a full-feature echocardiographic platform from a ventilated patient receiving high doses of inotropes for a suspected cardiogenic shock after cardiac surgery. (A) Conventional transthoracic echocardiography revealed a systolic left ventricular obstruction with a dynamic pressure gradient up to 94 mmHg, whereas hand-held echocardiography only showed a hyperkinetic left ventricle. (B) The hemodynamics improved after repeated fluid challenges and rapid tapering of positive inotrope doses, as reflected by the absence of Doppler detectable dynamic obstruction

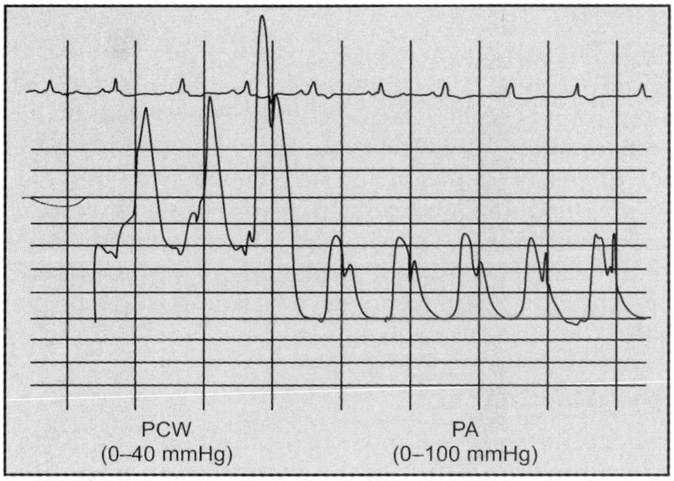


**Fig. 21.28:** Pressures recorded during insertion of a balloon-tipped flow-directed catheter. RA=right atrial pressure, RV=right ventricular pressure, PA=pulmonary arterial pressure, PCW=pulmonary capillary wedge pressure. The scale at the left calibrates pressure from 0 to 50 mmHg

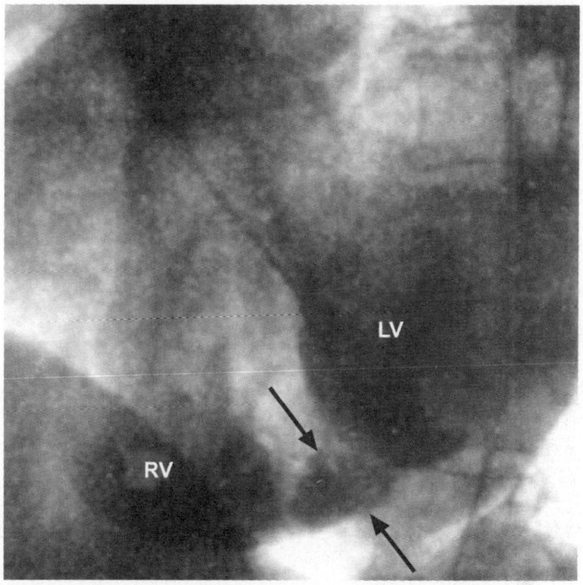


**Fig. 21.30:** A 63-year-old patient with impending septal ruptue in myocardial infarction by Left ventricular angiogram in a LAO 60° position demonstrated an inferiorly located ventricular septal defect (arrows)

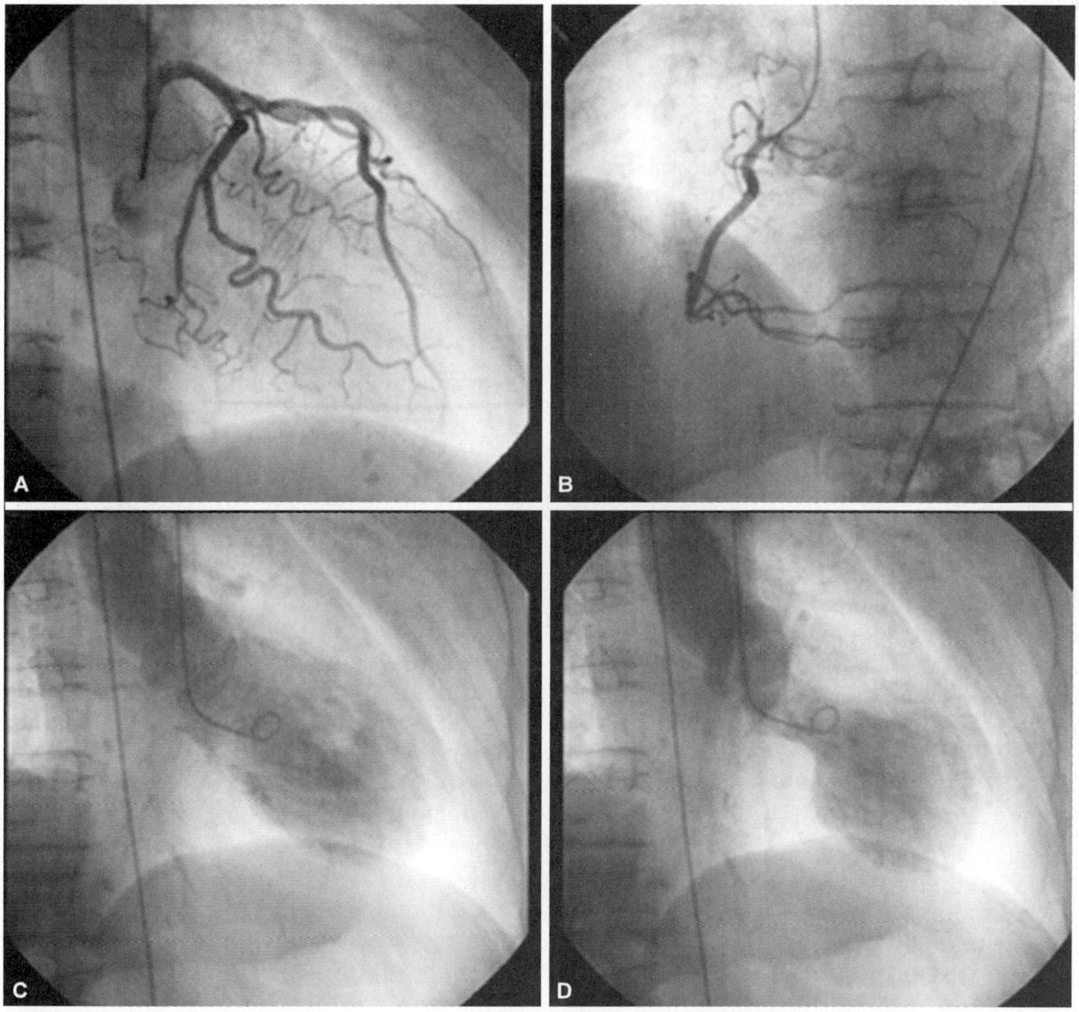


**Fig. 21.29:** Coronary angiograms showed the intact coronary arteries (A and B), and left ventriculograms showed apical ballooning and excessive hypercontraction of the basal region (C and D) in a 54-years-old male with severe hypotension

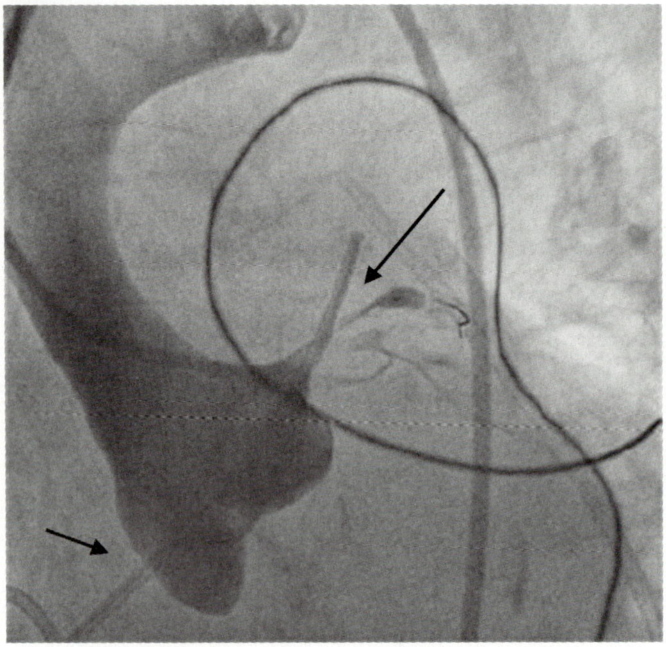

**Fig. 21.31:** An angiogram showing rupture of left main coronary artery in a 74-year-old male with cardiogenic shock

An arterial line may be placed to provide continuous blood pressure monitoring. This is particularly useful if the patient requires inotropic medications.

**An intra-aortic balloon pump** may be placed in the emergency department as a bridge to percutaneous coronary intervention (PCI) or coronary artery bypass graft (CABG), to decrease myocardial workload and to improve end-organ perfusion.

### *PCI and Coronary Artery Bypass*

Clinicians should be alert to the fact that the SHOCK trial demonstrated that either PCI or coronary artery bypass is the treatment of choice for cardiogenic shock and that each has been shown to markedly decrease mortality rates at 1 year. PCI should be initiated within 90 minutes of presentation; however, it remains helpful, as an acute intervention, within 12 hours of presentation.

If such a facility is not immediately available, thrombolytics should be considered. However, this treatment is second best. An increased mortality is seen in situations in which thrombolytics are used instead of PCI. This is due to the relative ineffectiveness of the thrombolytic medications to lyse clots in low-blood pressure situations.

## Consultations

Consult a cardiologist at the earliest opportunity because his or her insight and expertise may be invaluable for facilitating echocardiographic support, placement of an intra-aortic balloon pump (IABP), and transfer to more definitive care (e.g. cardiac catheterization suite, ICU, operating room). In severe cases, also consider discussing the case with a cardiothoracic surgeon.

## Prevention

Although cardiogenic shock is not entirely preventable, measures can be taken to minimize the risk of occurrence, recognize it at earlier stages, and begin corrective therapy more expeditiously. Deterrence and prevention require a high degree of suspicion and heightened awareness.

Care is required in treating patients with acute coronary syndromes who are not yet in cardiogenic shock. Careful use of beta-blockers and ACE inhibitors in these patients is essential to avoid hypotension leading to cardiogenic shock.

## Prehospital Care

Prehospital care is aimed at minimizing any further ischemia and shock. All patients require intravenous access, high-flow oxygen administered by mask, and cardiac monitoring.

Twelve-lead electrocardiography performed in the field by appropriately trained paramedics may be useful in decreasing door-to-PCI times and/or time to the administration of thrombolytics because acute ST-segment elevation myocardial infarctions (STEMIs) can be identified earlier. The emergency department (ED) can thus be alerted and may mobilize the appropriate resources.

Inotropic medications should be considered in systems with appropriately trained paramedical personnel.

When clinically necessary, positive pressure ventilation and endotracheal intubation should be performed. Continuous positive airway pressure (CPAP) or bilevel positive airway pressure (BiPAP) support can be considered in appropriately equipped systems.

## Resuscitation, Ventilation, and Pharmacologic Intervention

Initial management includes fluid resuscitation to correct hypovolemia and hypotension, unless pulmonary edema is present. Central venous and arterial lines are often required. Swan-Ganz catheterization and continuous percutaneous oximetry are routine.

Oxygenation and airway protection are critical; intubation and mechanical ventilation are commonly required. However, although positive pressure ventilation may improve oxygenation, it may also compromise venous return, preload, to the heart. In any event, the patient should be treated with high-flow oxygen. Studies in patients with acute cardiogenic pulmonary edema have shown noninvasive ventilation to improve hemodynamics and reduce the intubation rate. Mortality is, however, unaffected.

A study by Shin et al. suggested that patients who receive extracorporeal cardiopulmonary resuscitation (CPR) versus conventional CPR for longer than 10 minutes following in-hospital arrest have a greater chance of survival.

All patients with cardiogenic shock require close hemodynamic monitoring, volume support to ensure adequate sufficient preload, and ventilatory support.

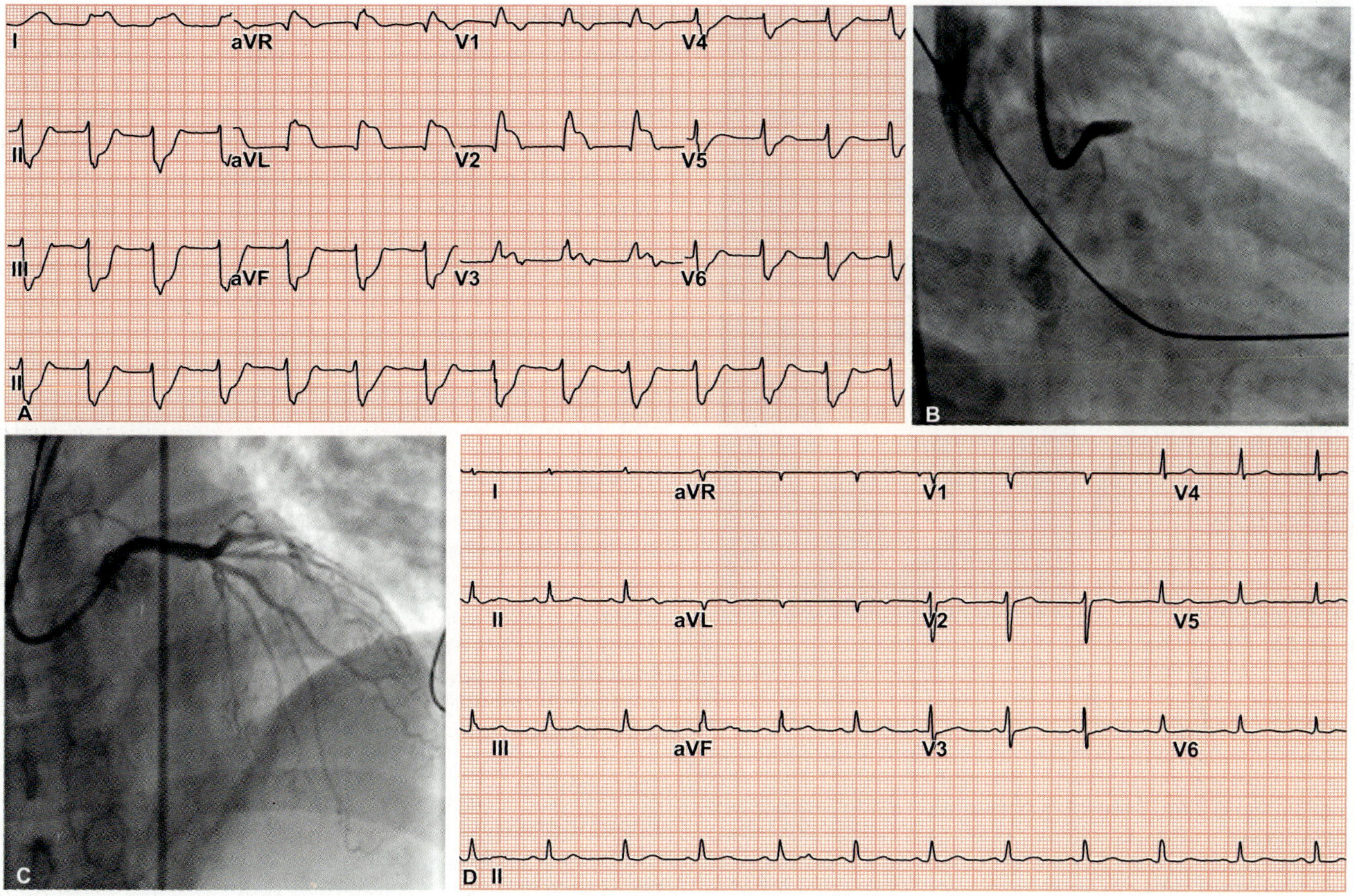


**Fig. 21.32:** A previously healthy 57-year-old man presented with chest pain that had been ongoing for 50 minutes and had begun while he was playing racquetball. He was conscious and alert, although he was in cardiogenic shock. A 12-lead electrocardiogram showed ST-segment elevation in leads V1, V2, V3, I, aVL, and aVR and ST-segment depression in leads V4, V5, V6, II, III, and aVF, findings suggestive of occlusion of the left main stem of the coronary artery (A). This was confirmed during coronary angiography (B). Prompt revascularization with a stent restored normal anterograde coronary perfusion within 110 minutes after the onset of pain (C) and led to a normal electrocardiogram (D). The creatine kinase level peaked at 1400 U per liter. Hemodynamic support was provided by a percutaneously inserted microaxial-flow pump. The severely impaired left ventricular systolic function and the extensive anterolateral akinesis returned to normal within 4 days. One year later, the patient has had no further ischemic events and remains active

### *Pharmacologic Therapy*

Patients with myocardial infarction (MI) or acute coronary syndrome are given aspirin and heparin. Both of these medications have been shown to be effective in reducing mortality in separate studies. Before initiating therapy, however, care should be taken to ensure that the patient does not have a myocardial wall rupture that is amenable to surgery.

There is no need to start clopidogrel until after angiography, since angiography may demonstrate that there is a need for urgent coronary bypass.

The glycoprotein IIb/IIIa inhibitors improve the outcome of patients with non-ST-segment elevation acute coronary syndrome (NSTACS). They have been found to reduce recurrent MI following percutaneous coronary intervention (PCI) and in cardiogenic shock.

### Hemodynamic Support

Dopamine, norepinephrine, and epinephrine are vasoconstricting drugs that help to maintain adequate blood pressure during life-threatening hypotension and help to preserve perfusion pressure for optimizing flow in various organs. The mean blood pressure required for adequate splanchnic and renal perfusion [mean arterial pressure (MAP) of 60 or 65 mmHg] is based on clinical indices of organ function.

In patients with inadequate tissue perfusion and adequate intravascular volume, initiation of inotropic and/or vasopressor drug therapy may be necessary. Dopamine increases myocardial contractility and supports the blood pressure; however, it may increase myocardial oxygen demand. Dobutamine may be preferable if the systolic blood pressure is higher than 80 mmHg; it has the

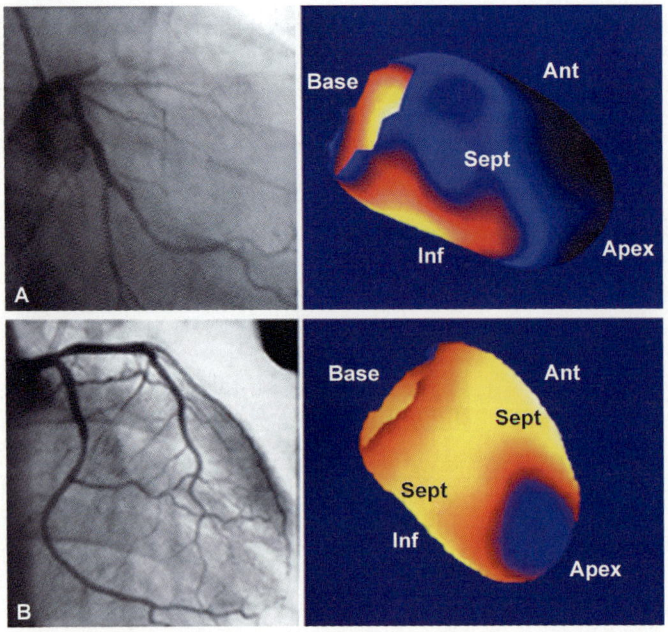


**Fig. 21.33:** After coronary reperfusion the area of myocardial infarction can be limited, but a much larger territory remains stunned with impaired contractility and compliance through reperfusion injury. (A) A coronary angiogram from a patient with an anterior myocardial infarction and proximally occluded left anterior descending artery (left panel). A 3D MPS that demonstrates a large area of hypoperfusion in the anterior wall, anterior septum, and apex (right panel, blue areas). The inferior wall is perfused normally (yellow/red areas), which corresponds to the area at risk. (B) A coronary angiogram after percutaneous intervention, with stent deployment in the proximal left anterior descending artery (left panel). A 3D MPS that demonstrates a small area of hypoperfusion at the apex (right panel, blue area). All other territories have normal perfusion (yellow/red areas), which corresponds to the final infarct size. Angiograms and MPSs courtesy of Professor Hans Erik Bøtker. ANT=anterior; INF=inferior; MPS=myocardial perfusion scintigram; PPCI=primary percutaneous coronary intervention; SEPT=septum

advantage of not affecting myocardial oxygen demand as much as dopamine does. However, the resulting tachycardia may preclude the use of this inotropic agent in some patients.

Dopamine is usually initiated at a rate of 5–10 mcg/kg/min intravenously, and the infusion rate is adjusted according to the blood pressure and other hemodynamic parameters. Often, patients may require high doses of dopamine (as much as 20 mcg/kg/min).

If the patient remains hypotensive despite moderate doses of dopamine, a direct vasoconstrictor (e.g. norepinephrine) should be started at a dose of 0.5 mcg/kg/min and titrated to maintain a MAP of 60 mmHg. The potent vasoconstrictors (e.g. norepinephrine) have traditionally been avoided because of their adverse effects on cardiac output and renal perfusion.

## Vasopressor Supportive Therapy

The following is a brief review of the mechanism of action and indications for drugs used for hemodynamic support of cardiogenic shock.

### Dopamine

Dopamine is a precursor of norepinephrine and epinephrine and has varying effects according to the doses infused. A dose of less than 5 mcg/kg/min causes vasodilation of renal, mesenteric, and coronary beds. At a dose of 5–10 mcg/kg/min, beta 1-adrenergic effects induce an increase in cardiac contractility and heart rate.

At doses of approximately 10 mcg/kg/min, alpha-adrenergic effects lead to arterial vasoconstriction and an elevation in blood pressure. The blood pressure increases primarily as a result of the inotropic effect. The undesirable effects are tachycardia and increased pulmonary shunting, as well as the potential for decreased splanchnic perfusion and increased pulmonary arterial wedge pressure.

### Norepinephrine

Norepinephrine is a potent alpha-adrenergic agonist with minimal beta-adrenergic agonist effects. Norepinephrine can increase blood pressure successfully in patients who remain hypotensive following dopamine. The dose of norepinephrine may vary from 0.2–1.5 mcg/kg/min, and large doses, as high as 3.3 mcg/kg/min, have been used because of the alpha-receptor down-regulation in persons with sepsis.

### Epinephrine

Epinephrine can increase the MAP by increasing the cardiac index and stroke volume, as well as systemic vascular resistance (SVR) and heart rate. Epinephrine decreases the splanchnic blood flow and may increase oxygen delivery and consumption.

Administration of this agent is associated with an increase in systemic and regional lactate concentrations. The use of epinephrine is recommended only in patients who are unresponsive to traditional agents. The undesirable effects are an increase in lactate concentration, a potential to produce myocardial ischemia, the development of arrhythmias, and a reduction in splanchnic flow.

### Levosimendan

Levosimendan, though not approved for use in the United States, can be considered for use in conjunction with vasopressors. It should be used with caution, however, as it can cause hypotension. Used with vasopressors, levosimendan may improve hemodynamics and improve coronary blood flow.

## Inotropic Supportive Therapy

### *Dobutamine*

Dobutamine (sympathomimetic agent) is a beta1-receptor agonist, although it has some beta2-receptor and minimal alpha-receptor activity. Intravenous dobutamine induces significant positive inotropic effects, with mild chronotropic effects. It also induces mild peripheral vasodilation (decrease in afterload). The combined effect of increased inotropy and decreased afterload induces a significant increase in cardiac output.

In the setting of acute myocardial infarction (MI), dobutamine use could increase the size of the infarct because of the increase in myocardial oxygen consumption that may ensue. In general, avoid dobutamine in patients with moderate or severe hypotension (e.g. systolic blood pressure < 80 mmHg) because of the peripheral vasodilation.

### *Phosphodiesterase Inhibitors*

Phosphodiesterase inhibitors (PDIs), which include inamrinone (formerly amrinone) and milrinone, are inotropic agents with vasodilating properties and long half-lives. The hemodynamic properties of PDIs are—(1) a positive inotropic effect on the myocardium and peripheral vasodilation (decreased afterload) and (2) a reduction in pulmonary vascular resistance (decreased preload).

PDIs are beneficial in persons with cardiac pump failure, but they may require concomitant vasopressor administration. Unlike catecholamine inotropes, these drugs are not dependent on adrenoreceptor activity; therefore, patients are less likely to develop tolerance to these medications.

PDIs are less likely than catecholamines to cause adverse effects known to be associated with adrenoreceptor activity (e.g. increased myocardial oxygen demand, myocardial ischemia). They are also associated with less tachycardia and myocardial oxygen consumption. However, the incidence of tachyarrhythmias is greater with PDIs than with dobutamine.

### Thrombolytic Therapy

Although thrombolytic therapy (TT) reduces mortality rates in patients with acute myocardial infarction (MI), its benefits for patients with cardiogenic shock secondary to MI are disappointing. When used early in the course of MI, TT reduces the likelihood of subsequent development of cardiogenic shock after the initial event.

Similarly, other studies employing a tissue plasminogen activator did not show reductions in mortality rates from cardiogenic shock. Lower rates of reperfusion of the infarct-related artery in patients with cardiogenic shock may help to explain the disappointing results from TT. Other reasons for the decreased efficacy of TT are the existence of hemodynamic, mechanical, and metabolic causes of cardiogenic shock that are unaffected by TT.

### Thrombolytic Therapy Plus IABP

A prospective cohort study demonstrated the potential survival benefit of combining TT with IABP counterpulsation in patients with MI complicated by cardiogenic shock.

Patients in cardiogenic shock who were treated with TT had lower in-hospital mortality rates than did those who did not receive TT (54% vs 64%), and patients selected for IABP counterpulsation had lower in-hospital mortality rates than did those who did not receive IABP counterpulsation (50% vs 72%).

Furthermore, a significant difference was noted in inhospital mortality rates among the four treatment groups, i.e. TT plus IABP counterpulsation (47%), IABP counterpulsation only (52%), TT only (63%), no TT and no IABP counterpulsation (77%).

Revascularization influenced in-hospital mortality rates significantly (39% with revascularization vs 78% without revascularization).

Patients who are unsuitable for invasive therapy should be treated with a thrombolytic agent in the absence of contraindications. This is a class I recommendation by American College of Cardiology (ACC)/American Heart Association (AHA) guidelines.

### Different Techniques of Resuscitation in Cardiogenic Shock (Figs 21.34–21.37)

- Intra-aortic balloon pump
- Enhanced external counterpulsation (EECP) therapy
- Venoarterial extracorporeal membrane oxygenation (ECMO)

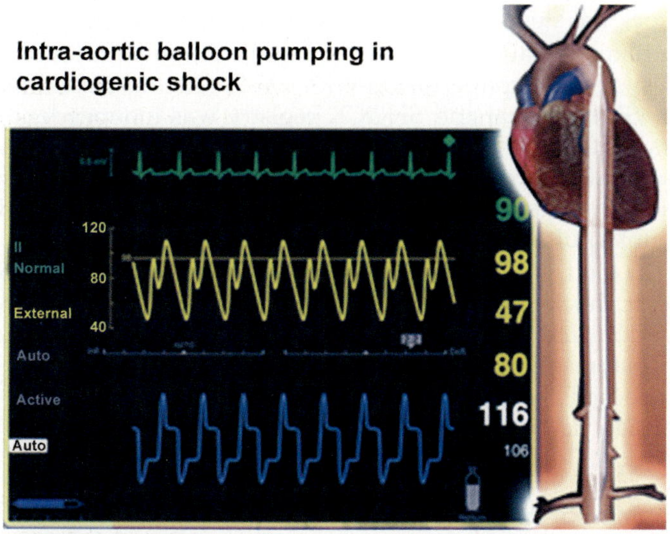


**Fig. 21.34:** Simultaneous ECG and aortic systolic and diastolic pulsations seen on the monitor screen in a patient before PCI

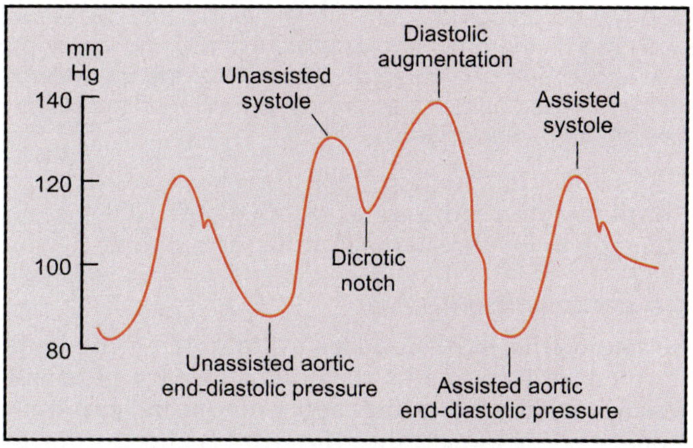


**Fig. 21.35:** Aortic systolic and diastolic pulsations after insertion of intra-aortic balloon pump

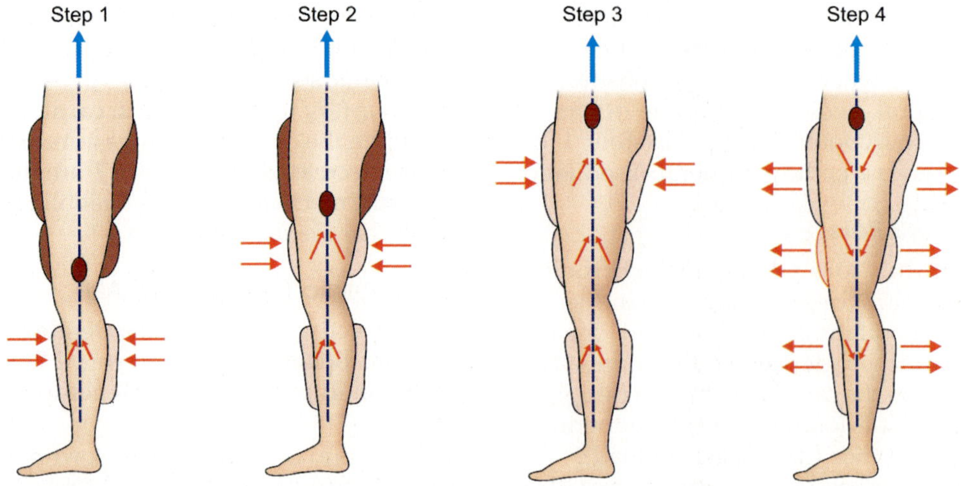


**Fig. 21.36:** Technique of EECP. Three pairs of pneumatic cuffs are applied to the calves, lower thighs, and upper thighs. The cuffs are inflated sequentially during diastole, distal to proximal. The compression of the lower-extremity vascular bed increases diastolic pressure and flow and increases venous return. The pressure is then released at the onset of systole. Inflation and deflation are timed according to the R-wave on the patient's cardiac monitor. The pressures applied and the inflation-deflation timing can be altered by using the pressure waveforms and electrocardiogram on the enhanced external counterpulsation (EECP) therapy monitor

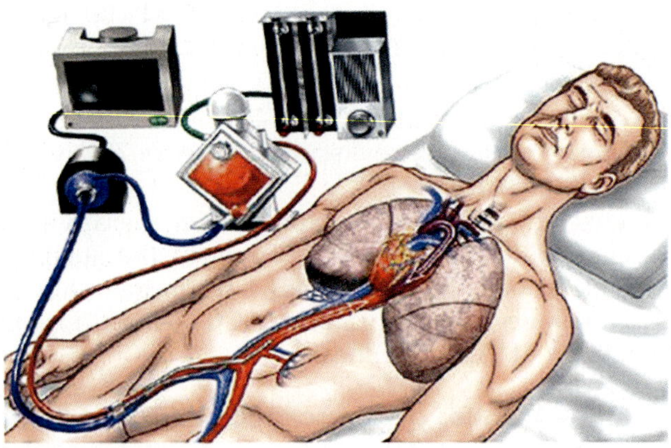

**Fig. 21.37:** Femoral venoarterial ECMO. When extracorporeal membrane oxygenation (ECMO) is implemented via femoral venous drainage and femoral arterial return in patients with residual native cardiac function and impaired lung function, reinfused oxygenated blood (red arrow), flowing retrograde through the aorta, may meet resistance from poorly oxygenated blood flowing antegrade from the left ventricle (purple arrow). Depending on the amount of cardiac function, the location of the interface between antegrade and retrograde flow will vary, and the reinfused oxygenated blood may not reach the cerebral and coronary vascular beds

- Implantable cardioverter-defibrillator (ICD) shock therapy in life-threatening cardiac arrhythmia

### Intra-aortic Balloon Pump

The use of the IABP reduces systolic left ventricular afterload and augments diastolic coronary perfusion pressure, thereby increasing cardiac output and improving coronary artery blood flow. The IABP is effective for the initial stabilization of patients with cardiogenic shock. However, an IABP is not definitive therapy; the IABP stabilizes patients so that definitive diagnostic and therapeutic interventions can be performed.

The IABP also may be a useful adjunct to thrombolysis for initial stabilization and transfer of patients to a tertiary care facility. Some studies have shown lower mortality rates in patients with myocardial infarction (MI) and cardiogenic shock treated with an IABP and subsequent revascularization, as previously mentioned.

Complications may be documented in up to 30% of patients who undergo IABP therapy; these relate primarily to local vascular problems, embolism, infection, and hemolysis.

The impact of treatment with an IABP on long-term survival is controversial and depends on the patient's hemodynamic status and the aetiology of the cardiogenic shock. Patient selection is the key issue; inserting the IABP early, rather than waiting until full-blown cardiogenic shock has developed, may result in clinical benefit.

Ramanathan et al. found that rapid and complete reversal of systemic hypoperfusion with IABP counterpulsation in the SHOCK trial and SHOCK registry was independently associated with improved inhospital, 30-day, and 1-year survival, regardless of early revascularization. This suggests that complete reversal of systemic hypoperfusion with IABP counterpulsation is an important early prognostic feature.

In the IABP-SHOCK II study, 600 patients with cardiogenic shock complicating acute myocardial infarction were randomized to intraaortic balloon counterpulsation or no intraaortic balloon counterpulsation. All patients were expected to undergo early revascularization. Use of intraaortic balloon counterpulsation did not significantly reduce 30-day mortality in these patients.

### Ventricular Assist Devices

In recent years, left ventricular assist devices (LVADs) capable of providing complete short-term hemodynamic

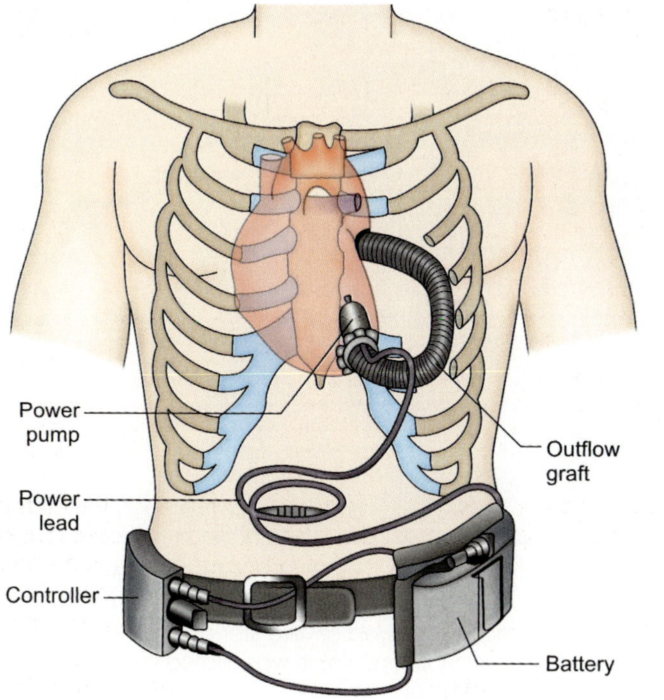


**Fig. 21.38:** Intracorporeal left ventricular assist device and its components

support have been developed. The application of LVAD during reperfusion, after acute coronary occlusion, causes reduction of the left ventricular preload, increases regional myocardial blood flow and lactate extraction, and improves general cardiac function. The LVAD makes it possible to maintain the collateral blood flow as a result of maintaining the cardiac output and aortic pressure, keeping wall tension low and reducing the extent of microvascular reperfusion injury (Figs 21.38 and 21.39).

A pooled analysis from 17 studies showed that the mean age of this group of patients with LVADs was 59.5 ± 4.5 years and that mean support duration was 146.2 ± 60.2 hours. In 78.5% of patients (range, 53.8–100%), adjunctive reperfusion therapy, mainly percutaneous transluminal coronary angioplasty (PTCA), was used. Mean weaning and survival rates were 58.5% (range, 46–75%) and 40% (range, 29–58%), respectively

In any case, comparing studies is difficult because important data are usually missing, mean age of patients were different, and time to treatment is not standardized.

Hemodynamic presentation seems to be worse compared with data reported in the SHOCK trial, with lower cardiac index, lower systolic aortic pressure, and higher serum lactates. Taking these considerations into account, LVAD support seems to give no survival improvement in patients with cardiogenic shock complicating acute myocardial infarction (MI), compared with early reperfusion alone or in combination with IABP.

In a randomized, controlled trial in which 129 patients with end-stage heart failure who were ineligible for cardiac transplantation were assigned either to receive an LVAD (68 patients) or to undergo optimal medical management, survival rates were higher in the LVAD group. The rates of survival at 1 year were 52% in the device group and 25% in the medical therapy group, while the rates at 2 years were 23% and 8%, respectively. In addition, the quality of life was significantly improved at 1 year in the device group.

**Implantable LVADs** are being used as a bridge to heart transplantation for patients with acute MI and cardiogenic shock. According to the HeartMate Data Registry, from 1986–1998, 41 patients (5% of the total number of HeartMate IP patients) were supported with this implantable pneumatic device for acute MI, and 25 (61%) were successfully bridged to heart transplantation.

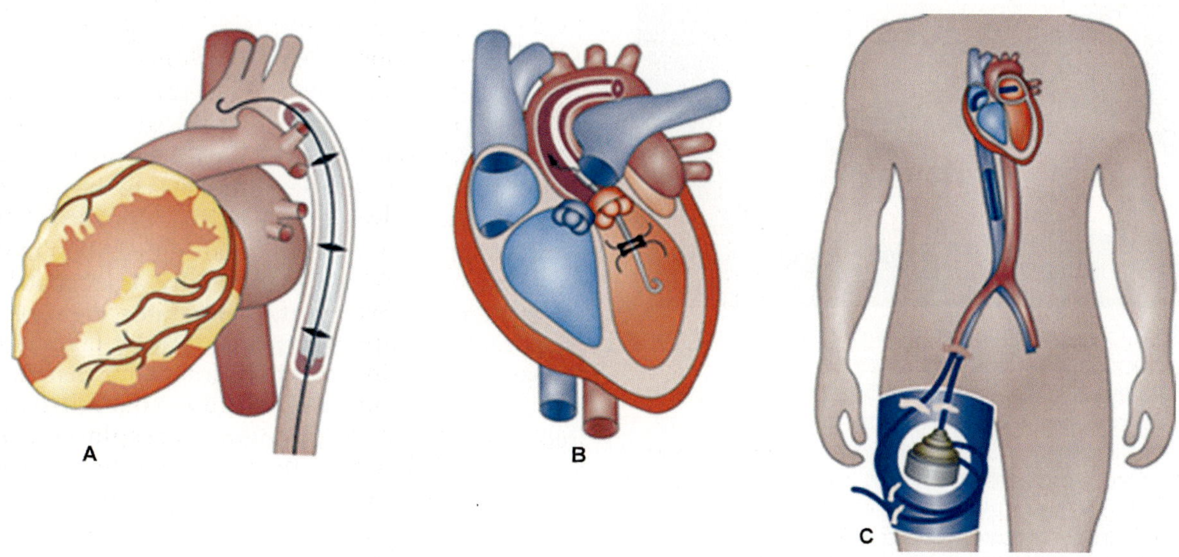


**Fig. 21.39:** These illustrations (a, b and c) are used either early and long-term accordingly in the management of cardiogenic shock

However, LVADs as a bridging option for patients with cardiogenic shock must be considered cautiously and must be avoided in patients who are unlikely to survive or are not likely to be transplant candidates. Further investigations are required to better define indications, support modalities, and outcomes (Fig. 21.40).

The indications for insertion of a ventricular assist device are controversial. Such an aggressive approach to support the circulatory system in cardiogenic shock is appropriate (1) after the failure of medical treatment and an IABP, (2) when the cause of cardiogenic shock is potentially reversible, or (3) if the device can be used as a support measure.

### Percutaneous Transluminal Coronary Angioplasty

The retrospective and prospective data favor aggressive mechanical revascularization in patients with cardiogenic shock secondary to myocardial infarction (MI) (Fig. 21.41).

Re-establishing blood flow in the infarct-related artery may improve left ventricular function and survival following MI. In acute MI, studies show that percutaneous transluminal coronary angioplasty (PTCA) can achieve adequate flow in 80–90% of patients, compared with 50–60% of patients after thrombolytic therapy (TT).

Several retrospective clinical trials have shown that patients with cardiogenic shock due to myocardial ischemia benefitted (reduction in 30d mortality rates) when treated with angioplasty. A study of direct (primary) PTCA in patients with cardiogenic shock reported lower mortality rates in patients treated with angioplasty combined with the use of stents than in patients treat with medical therapy.

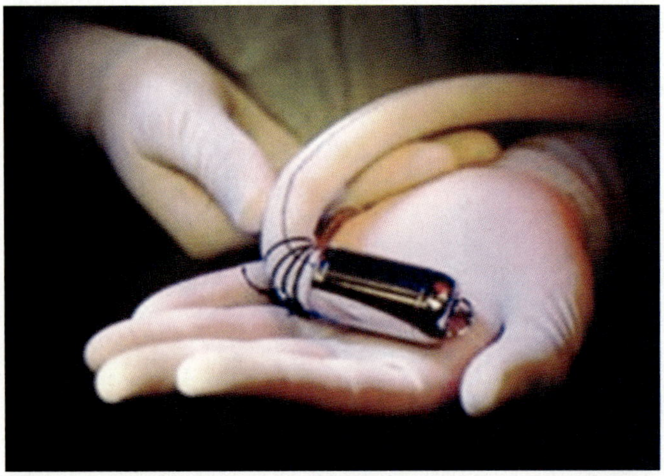

**Fig. 21.40:** The Jarvik 2000. Heart is an axial flow blood pump that uses electrical power to rotate a vaned impeller—it's only moving part. The device is 2.5 cm wide, 5.5 cm long, and weighs 85 grams. The impeller is a neodymium-iron-boron magnet, which is housed inside a welded titanium shell. The impeller is supported by ceramic bearings. A small cable, which exits the body through the abdominal wall, delivers power to the impeller. All of the blood-contacting surfaces are made of highly polished titanium. The normal operating range for the control system is 8,000–12,000 revolutions per minute, which will generate an average pump flow rate of 5 liters per minute

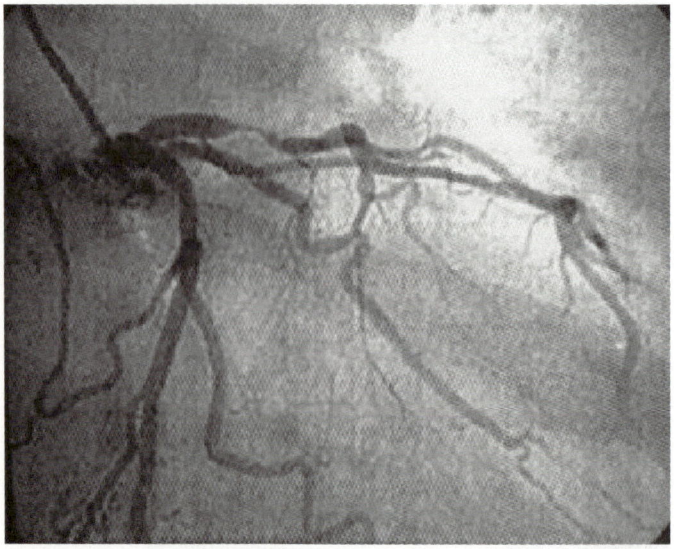

**Fig. 21.41:** A patient with an acute anterolateral myocardial infarction who developed cardiogenic shock. Coronary angiography images showed severe stenosis of the left anterior descending coronary artery, which was dilated by percutaneous transluminal coronary angioplasty

A study by Antoniucci et al. found that mortality rates increase in relation to the length of time to treatment in patients with acute MI who are not considered to be at low risk. To study the relationship of time to treatment and mortality in patients with acute MI, a series of 1336 patients who underwent successful primary PTCA were stratified into low-risk and not–low risk patient groups. The 6-month mortality rate was 9.3% for not low risk patients and 1.3% for the low-risk patients. An increase in the mortality rate from 4.8–12.9% with increasing time to reperfusion was observed in the not low-risk group. A delay from symptom onset to treatment resulted in higher mortality rates for the not low-risk patients.

## CORONARY ARTERY BYPASS GRAFTING

Critical left main artery disease and 3-vessel coronary artery disease are common findings in patients who develop cardiogenic shock. The potential contribution of ischemia in the noninfarcted zone contributes to the deterioration of already compromised myocardial function (Fig. 21.42).

Coronary artery bypass grafting (CABG) in the setting of cardiogenic shock is generally associated with high surgical morbidity and mortality rates. Because the results of percutaneous interventions can be favorable, routine bypass surgery is often discouraged for these patients.

A 2004 task force of the ACC and the AHA gave a class I recommendation to the performance of primary PCI or emergent CABG in patients younger than 75 years who have STEMI who develop shock within 36 hours of myocardial infarction (MI) and can be treated within 18 hours of shock onset. Performance of primary PCI or emergent CABG was considered reasonable in patients older than 75 years (class IIa recommendation).

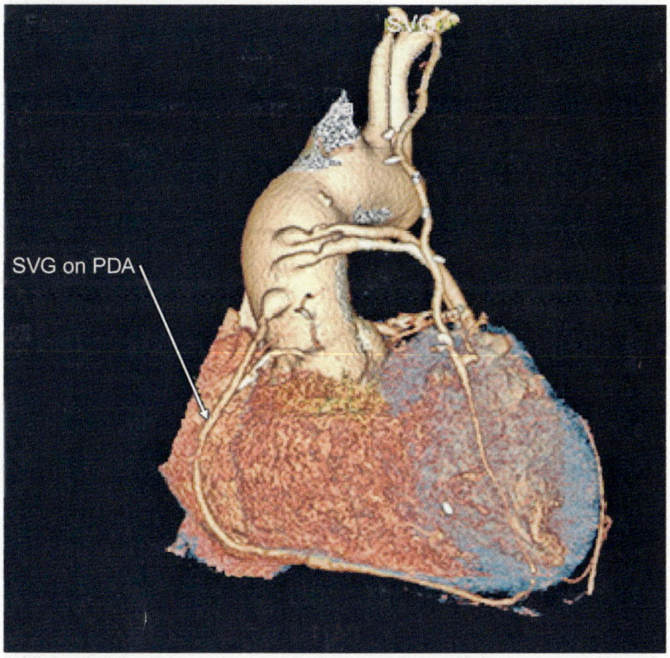


**Fig. 21.42:** Four grafts from LIMA to LAD, and SVG to diagonal, obtuse marginal and posterior descending artery with short segment stenosis of diagonal and obtuse marginal grafts

## REVASCULARIZATION IN THE SHOCK TRIAL

Results from the SHOCK trial supported the superiority of a strategy that combines early revascularization with medical management in patients with cardiogenic shock. In the study, patients were assigned to receive either optimal medical management, including an IABP and TT, or cardiac catheterization followed by revascularization using PTCA or CABG.

The mortality rates at 30 days were 46.7% in the early intervention group and 56% in patients treated with optimal medical management. Although these 30-day results did not reach statistical significance, the mortality rate at 6 months was significantly lower in the early intervention group (50.3% vs 63.1%)

The 1-year survival rates were also reported from the SHOCK trial. The survival rate at 1-year was 46.7% for patients in the early revascularization group and 33.6% in the conservative management group. The treatment benefit was apparent only for patients younger than 75 years (51.6% survival rate in early revascularization group vs 33.3% in patients treated with optimal medical management).

Based on the outcome of this study, the recommendation is that patients with acute myocardial infarction (MI) complicated by cardiogenic shock, particularly those younger than 75 years, should be rapidly transferred to a center with personnel capable of performing early angiography and revascularization procedures.

## PATIENT TRANSFER

Immediately transfer a patient who develops cardiogenic shock to an institution at which invasive monitoring, coronary revascularization, and skilled personnel are available to provide expert care.

Patients with cardiogenic shock who are admitted to a hospital without facilities for revascularization should be immediately transferred to a tertiary care center with such facilities. If time to PCI is more than 1 hour and onset of symptoms has been within 3 hours, rapid administration of TT is recommended.

It should be kept in mind, however, that attempts to transfer a patient with cardiogenic shock must be made only when everything possible has been done to stabilize his or her condition and when the level of care during the transfer will not significantly decrease.

## SUMMARY

Cardiogenic shock continues to be the most common cause of death in patients hospitalized with acute myocardial infarction. It has also been frequently associated with ST-segment elevation myocardial infarction (STEMI) and patients with comorbidities. Cardiogenic shock presents with low systolic blood pressure and clinical signs of hypoperfusion. Rapid diagnosis and supportive therapy in the form of medications, airway support and intra-aortic balloon counterpulsation is required. Initial stabilization can be followed by reperfusion by fibrinolytic therapy, emergent percutaneous intervention (PCI) or coronary artery bypass grafting (CABG). The latter two have been found to decrease mortality in the long term. Research is being carried out on the role of inflammatory mediators in the clinical manifestation of cardiogenic shock. Mechanical support devices also show promise in the future.

## KEY POINTS

1. Cardiogenic shock due to AMI continues to be the main cause of death in these patients.
2. Immediate diagnosis and management is required.
3. There are two strategies in treating cardiogenic shock: medical versus invasive.
4. If institutions lack revascularization facilities, fibrinolytic therapy and IABP should be used while provisions are made for invasive treatment.
5. However, current guidelines favor an invasive approach.
6. Prognosis is established by the outcome of revascularization regardless of the procedure used, such as PCI or surgery.
7. Newer devices are being developed for mechanical support. Inhibitors of nitric oxide have also shown favorable outcomes. These newer therapies may help in decreasing the significant mortality of cardiogenic shock in the future.

## BIBLIOGRAPHY

1. Al-Reesi A, Al-Zadjali N, Perry J, Fergusson D, Al-Shamsi M, Al-Thagafi M, et al. Do beta-blockers reduce short-term mortality following acute myocardial infarction? A systematic review and meta-analysis. CJEM. 2008; 10(3): 215–23.

2. Babaev A, Frederick PD, Pasta DJ, Every N, Sichrovsky T, Hochman JS. Trends in management and outcomes of patients with acute myocardial infarction complicated by cardiogenic shock. JAMA 2005;294(4):448–54.
3. Chen ZM, Pan HC, Chen YP, Peto R, Collins R, Jiang LX, et al. Early intravenous then oral metoprolol in 45,852 patients with acute myocardial infarction: randomised placebo-controlled trial. Lancet 2005;366(9497):1622–32.
4. Cheng JM, den Uil CA, Hoeks SE, van der Ent M, Jewbali LS, van Domburg RT, et al. Percutaneous left ventricular assist devices vs. intra-aortic balloon pump counterpulsation for treatment of cardiogenic shock: a meta-analysis of controlled trials. Eur Heart J 2009;30(17):2102–8.
5. De Luca L, Colucci WS, Nieminen MS, Massie BM, Gheorghiade M. Evidence-based use of levosimendan in different clinical settings. Eur Heart J 2006;27(16):1908–20.
6. Ellender TJ, Skinner JC. The use of vasopressors and inotropes in the emergency medical treatment of shock. Emerg Med Clin North Am 2008;26(3):759–86.
7. Fox KA, Steg PG, Eagle KA, Goodman SG, Anderson FA Jr, Granger CB, et al. Decline in rates of death and heart failure in acute coronary syndromes, 1999–2006. JAMA 2007; 297(17):1892–900.
8. Fuhrmann JT, Schmeisser A, Schulze MR, Wunderlich C, Schoen SP, Rauwolf T, et al. Levosimendan is superior to enoximone in refractory cardiogenic shock complicating acute myocardial infarction. Crit Care Med 2008; 36(8): 2257–66.
9. Garatti A, Russo C, Lanfranconi M, Colombo T, Bruschi G, Trunfio S, et al. Mechanical circulatory support for cardiogenic shock complicating acute myocardial infarction: an experimental and clinical review. ASAIO J 2007;53(3): 278–87.
10. Goldberg RJ, Samad NA, Yarzebski J, Gurwitz J, Bigelow C, Gore JM. Temporal trends in cardiogenic shock complicating acute myocardial infarction. N Engl J Med 1999; 340(15): 1162–8.
11. Hamon M, Agostini D, Le Page O, Riddell JW, Hamon M. Prognostic impact of right ventricular involvement in patients with acute myocardial infarction: meta-analysis. Crit Care Med 2008;36(7):2023–33.
12. Hasdai D, Califf RM, Thompson TD, Hochman JS, Ohman EM, Pfisterer M, et al. Predictors of cardiogenic shock after thrombolytic therapy for acute myocardial infarction. J Am Coll Cardiol 2000;35(1):136–43.
13. Hochman JS, Sleeper LA, White HD, Dzavik V, Wong SC, Menon V, et al. One-year survival following early revascularization for cardiogenic shock. JAMA 2001; 285(2):190–2.
14. Jeger RV, Lowe AM, Buller CE, Pfisterer ME, Dzavik V, Webb JG, et al. Hemodynamic parameters are prognostically important in cardiogenic shock but similar following early revascularization or initial medical stabilization: a report from the SHOCK Trial. Chest 2007;132(6):1794–803.
15. Jeger RV, Radovanovic D, Hunziker PR, Pfisterer ME, Stauffer JC, Erne P, et al. Ten-year trends in the incidence and treatment of cardiogenic shock. Ann Intern Med 2008; 149(9):618–26.
16. Naples RM, Harris JW, Ghaemmaghami CA. Critical care aspects in the management of patients with acute coronary syndromes. Emerg Med Clin North Am 2008;26(3):685–702.
17. Ramanathan K, Farkouh ME, Cosmi JE, French JK, Harkness SM, D•avík V, et al. Rapid complete reversal of systemic hypo-per-fusion after intra-aortic balloon pump counterpulsation and survival in cardiogenic shock compli-cating an acute myocardial infarction. Am Heart J 2011; 162(2):268–75.
18. Reynolds HR, Hochman JS. Cardiogenic shock: current concepts and improving outcomes. Circulation 2008; 117(5):686–97.
19. Sanborn TA, Sleeper LA, Bates ER, et al. Impact of thrombolysis, intra-aortic balloon pump counterpulsation, and their combination in cardiogenic shock complicating acute myocardial infarction: a report from the SHOCK Trial Registry. SHould we emergently revascularize Occluded Coronaries for cardiogenic shocK?. J Am Coll Cardiol 2000;36(3 Suppl A):1123–9.
20. Shin TG, Choi JH, Jo IJ, Sim MS, Song HG, Jeong YK, et al. Extracorporeal cardiopulmonary resuscitation in patients with inhospital cardiac arrest: A comparison with conventional cardiopulmonary resuscitation. Crit Care Med 2011;39(1):1–7.

# Cardiovascular Emergencies

## Recognition and Management

### Volume 2

# Cardiovascular Emergencies

## Recognition and Management

## Volume 2

**K C Verma**
MBBS, DCH, MD, DM (Cardiology)
FICP (USA), FRST M&H (Lond.), FCSI (India)
Senior Consulting Heart Specialist and
Former Professor in Cardiovascular and Thoracic Unit
Government Medical College
Jammu (J&K)

CBS

**CBS Publishers & Distributors** Pvt Ltd

New Delhi • Bengaluru • Chennai • Kochi • Kolkata • Mumbai
Bhopal • Bhubaneswar • Hyderabad • Jharkhand • Nagpur • Patna • Pune • Uttarakhand • Dhaka (Bangladesh)

**Cardiovascular Emergencies**

**Recognition and Management**

**Volume 2**

ISBN: 978-93-88725-61-3



**First Edition:** 2019



Published by Satish Kumar Jain and produced by Varun Jain for
**CBS Publishers & Distributors** Pvt Ltd
4819/XI Prahlad Street, 24 Ansari Road, Daryaganj, New Delhi 110 002, India
Ph: 23289259, 23266861, 23266867 Website: www.cbspd.com
Fax: 011-23243014 e-mail: delhi@cbspd.com; cbspubs@airtelmail.in

*Corporate Office:* 204 FIE, Industrial Area, Patparganj, Delhi 110 092
Ph: 4934 4934 Fax: 4934 4935 e-mail: publishing@cbspd.com; publicity@cbspd.com

***Branches***

- **Bengaluru:** Seema House 2975, 17th Cross, K.R. Road, Banasankari 2nd Stage, Bengaluru 560 070, Karnataka
  Ph: +91-80-26771678/79 Fax: +91-80-26771680 e-mail: bangalore@cbspd.com
- **Chennai:** 7, Subbaraya Street, Shenoy Nagar, Chennai 600 030, Tamil Nadu
  Ph: +91-44-26680620/26681266 Fax: +91-44-42032115 e-mail: chennai@cbspd.com
- **Kochi:** 42/1325, 1326, Power House Road, Opp KSEB, Power House, Ernakulam 682 018, Kochi, Kerala
  Ph: +91-484-4059061-65 Fax: +91-484-4059065 e-mail: kochi@cbspd.com
- **Kolkata:** 6/B, Ground Floor, Rameswar Shaw Road, Kolkata 700 014, West Bengal
  Ph: +91-33-22891126, 22891127, 22891128 e-mail: kolkata@cbspd.com
- **Mumbai:** 83-C, Dr E Moses Road, Worli, Mumbai 400018, Maharashtra
  Ph: +91-22-24902340/41 Fax: +91-22-24902342 e-mail: mumbai@cbspd.com

*Representatives*

- **Bhopal** 0-8319310552
- **Bhubaneswar** 0-9911037372
- **Hyderabad** 0-9885175004
- **Jharkhand** 0-9811541605
- **Nagpur** 0-9421945513
- **Patna** 0-9334159340
- **Pune** 0-9623451994
- **Uttarakhand** 0-9716462459
- **Dhaka (Bangladesh)** 01912-003485

*Printed at:* Nutech Print Services, Faridabad, Haryana, India

*to*

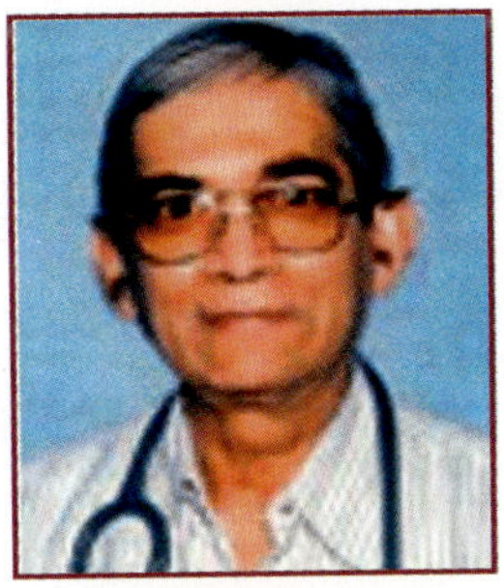

**Prof. T K Lahri**

*Eminent cardiothoracic surgeon and a great teacher*

Tapan Kumar Lahri is an Indian cardiothoracic surgeon, medical and academic writer. He is ex-Professor and Head, Department of Cardiothoracic Surgery, Institute of Medical Sciences, Banaras Hindu University, Varanasi. Born in Varanasi, Uttar Pradesh, he secured MS in general surgery in 1969 from All India Institute of Medical Sciences, New Delhi, and MCh in thoracic surgery in 1972 from the same institution before starting his career as a member of the faculty at Institute of Medical Sciences, Banaras Hindu University, where he held the posts of reader, assistant professor, professor and head of the department of cardiothoracic surgery. After his retirement in 2003, he was made professor emeritus of the institution. Government of India awarded him the fourth highest civilian honour of Padma Shri in 2016 for his contributions to medicine.

# Foreword

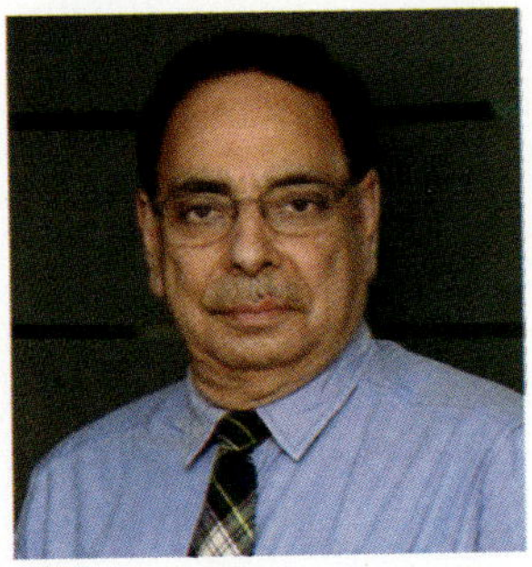

Dr KC Verma, an eminent cardiologist practising in Jammu (J&K), has done a commendable job in writing this book *Cardiovascular Emergencies: Recognition and Management*. The book is an exhaustive work covering all aspects of the management. It starts from basics like history and clinical evaluation and goes on in depth of all varieties of cardiopulmonary emergencies. I find it a very lucid and comprehensive work.

I know Dr Verma for more than 3 decades and always found him a very inquisitive person very well read and always practising ethical medicine. He has been an excellent teacher for his younger colleagues.

The book should be a great help for practising physicians as a day-to-day reference book while handling medical emergencies with cardiac issues. Many such patients would eventually need referral to higher centres for management. The initial management, however, is very important and a working knowledge of starting the correct treatment early can make all the difference in the final outcomes.

I recommend this very well written book for all the busy physicians and cardiologists who want evidence-based guidance for treating their patients.

**Prof. Upendra Kaul**

MD DM FCSI FSCAI FAPSIC FACC FAMS

Awarded Padma Shri and Dr BC Roy Award

*Chairman*

Batra Heart Centre

*Dean*

Academics and Research, Batra Hospital and Medical Research Centre, New Delhi

# Preface

Cardiac emergencies pose a special challenge to the physician both at tehsil and district headquarters and to the cardiologist in any of the established ICUs of the country and are a leading cause for emergent visits in any emergency department. Failure to quickly recognize them with rapid and appropriate therapy and delay in referring to an appropriate emergency medical care centre can have devastating results. This subject of cardiac emergencies, is therefore, an important curriculum in training ICU nurse, ICU health workers, and both undergraduate and postgraduate medical students in the field of cardiovascular emegency situations. With these objectives in mind, I have chosen most common topics in cardiac emergencies to publish it as a ready guide for the learners.

This book on cardiac emergencies begins with a brief overview of history taking, physical examination, and investigative techniques just as in any other book in discipline of medicine. Most frequently and day-to-day encountered emergencies include acute coronary syndrome, angina pectoris, myocardial infarction, venus thrombosis and pulmonary embolism, complete heart block and accelerated hypertensive vascular emergencies. These chapters have been written with easily understandable text supported with lucid graphs, line diagrams, photographs, latest noninvasive and invasive investigative techniques supported with bibliography for individual chapter for further readings.

'Percutaneous coronary interventions' remain the cornerstone in the management of both acute and chronic coronary obstructions, congenital anomalies, optical coherence tomography, IVUS and fractional flow reserve (FFR) in any of the cardiac catheterization laboratories, but till recently coronary angioplasty has also been performed with robotic interventions. A brief description of these procedures has been recorded in this book. The heart failure which is often the terminal event of many congenital and acquired heart disorders is yet another cardiac emergency which attracts physician, cardiologist, or cardiac surgeon's attention in emergency department all over the world. This subject has been written with utmost care giving details of its recognition with international recommendations and medical and surgical interventions in its management.

Cardiac arrhythmias both in children and adults are not only difficult to diagnose but also to manage these rhythm disturbances with emergent treatment. This book, therefore, describes details of investigations and pharmacological and catheter-based technologies of their respective management.

A brief description of infections leading to varying cardiac complications such as myocarditis, endocarditis, pericarditis, cardiac tamponade, and additionally DCM, valvular and vascular emergencies, hypothermia and cardiogenic shock, have been included in this book. I felt that I could do injustice to this subject of cardiac emergencies if I do not include the description of invasive procedures and noninvasive cardiovascular imaging techniques which are most essential in any emergency department.

Cardiac resuscitation is the most essential part of management of cardiac emergencies both on road side and inside ICU, hence I have been able to describe in detail the techniques of cardiopulmonary resuscitation, non-invasive ventilation, 'ECMO therapy' in acute cardiopulmonary failure.

Radiotherapy and chemotherapy are most important modes of treatment of systemic malignancy disorders and lead to varying grades of cardiac complications. This book includes the brief account of side effects and their respective management.

In emergency department the attending physician or on-duty medical officer may find young children and adolescents admitted with either heart failure, cardiac arrhythmias, intoxicated with frequently prescribed drugs such as digitalis, calcium channel blockers, β-blockers and other antiarrhythmics for their respective treatment or other addictions such as alcohol and cocaine. This book, therefore, records their brief account under separate chapters of 'cardiac emergencies in children and adolescents' and toxicological emergencies in general. Subject of 'telemedicine in emergency cardiology' is quite newer in India, where a patient with fresh cardiac problem and those with operative interventions can contact their cardiologist and cardiac surgeon immediately for remedy. With this view, a chapter on telemedicine with possible inputs including technique of setting and operating has been introduced among the list of other chapters.

In view of the abovementioned chapters included in this book of cardiac emergencies, I am very confident that readers would find it a most valuable and perfect guide and ready-reckoner in obtaining knowledge for the day-to-day management of cardiac emergencies at any level of posting in their service. Besides, it would be very useful book for ICU nurse, ICU technical officers, undergraduate and postgraduate medical students, cardiac fellows, during DM examination, and physicians posted at tehsil and district headquarter medical services.

**KC Verma**

# Acknowledgements

I am very grateful to my wife Dr (Mrs) Urmil Kanta Verma, former professor in department of blood transfusion medicine and pathology, for providing me a perfect congenital atmosphere and all material and moral support needed for writing such a basic book on *Cardiovascular Emergencies: Recognition and Management* which I am sure would prove very helpful in the workup of a heart patient.

To my lovely grandchildren — Adwita, Sidhant, Deven, Leena and Meera. I also appreciate the support of concerned staff of CBS Publishers & Distributors Pvt. Ltd., New Delhi, for their timely guidance in its perfect designing, typesetting, preparation of lucid figures and line diagrams, which itself was a big challenging task and is, therefore, joyfully acknowledged.

**K C Verma**

# Contents

# 22 Cardiopulmonary Resuscitative Procedures in Emergency Department

## AHA OFFICIAL GUIDELINES FOR CPR—LATEST 2014/2015

The American Heart Association (AHA) is a non-profit organization committed to fighting cardiovascular disease and the effects of it including cardiac arrest. Through an ongoing process the AHA reviews all available research regarding cardiopulmonary resuscitation (CPR), first aid, and advanced life support efforts utilized by healthcare providers. The result of this process is a series of patient care guidelines and improved curriculums for the courses they offer. Although the recommendations are coming from a United States based organization they are based on research from across the world. The most recent report is from 2010 and there will likely be an updated one in 2015. Here are some of the key points from the 2010 updates, with a focus on the recommendations for the average rescuer, not healthcare providers.

### Immediate Recognition and Reaction to Cardiac Arrest

Time is critical when someone's heart has stopped and any delay in starting resuscitation efforts could cost that person their life. History has shown that sometimes an individual in or nearing cardiac arrest may gasp or exhibit significantly abnormal breathing either of which is insufficient to sustain them. That breathing has been mistaken by bystanders as sufficient and CPR was delayed until professional responders arrived. The new guidelines stress the importance of recognizing the signs of cardiac arrest and taking action rapidly.

### The ABCs Becomes CAB

In the past the process of assessing and rendering aid started with addressing the patient's airway, then their breathing, and finally their circulation giving rise to the ABC approach (Figs 22.1–22.25). The current process still incorporates those

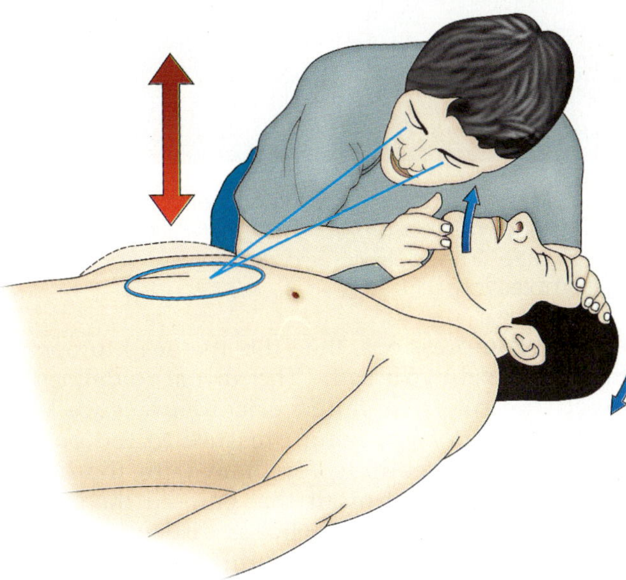

**Fig. 22.1:** Check breathing look, listen and feel

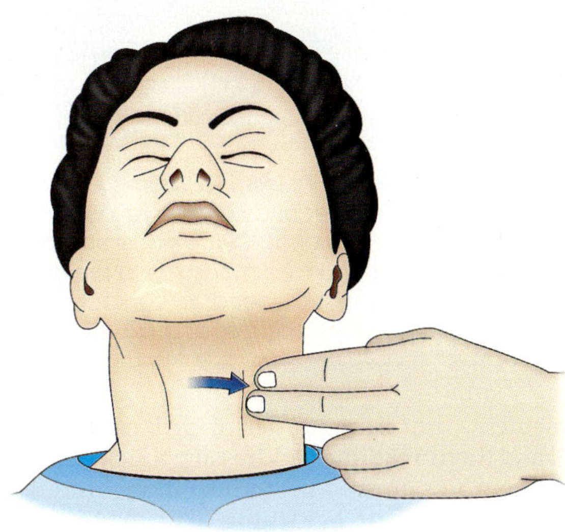

**Fig. 22.2:** Feel for carotid pulse which may indicate the conscious level of the victim and blood pressure as well

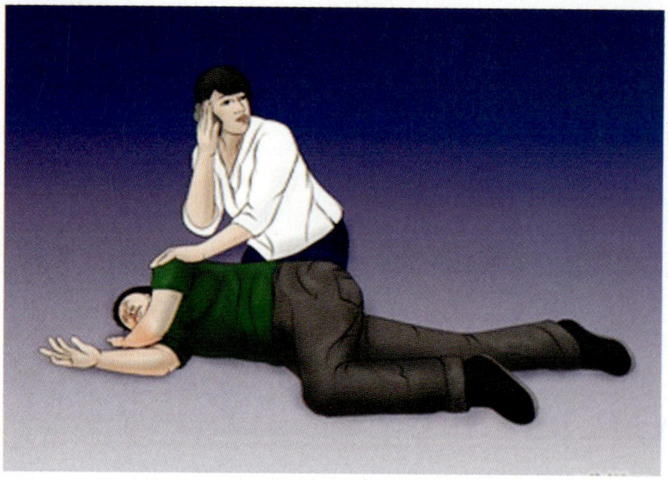

**Fig. 22.3: Method 1 step 1.** Taking vitals—check the scene for immediate danger. Make sure you're not putting yourself in harm's way by administering CPR to someone unconscious. Is there a fire? Is the person lying on a roadway? Do whatever is necessary to move yourself and the other person to safety. If there is anything that could endanger you or the victim, see if there is something you can do to counteract it. Open a window, turn off the stove, or put out the fire if possible. However, if there is nothing you can do to counteract the danger, move the victim. The best way to move the victim is by placing a blanket or coat underneath his/her back and dragging it

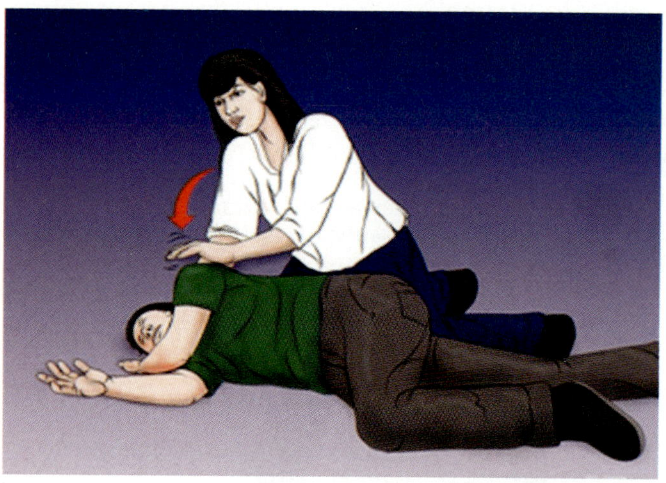

**Fig. 22.4: Method 1 step 2.** Assess the victim's consciousness. Gently tap his or her shoulder and ask 'Are you OK?' in a loud, clear voice. If he or she responds, CPR is not required. Instead, undertake basic first aid and take measures to prevent or treat shock, and assess whether you need to contact emergency services. If the victim does not respond, continue with the following steps

three elements, but in the order of CAB circulation, then airway, and then breathing. Addressing a lack of circulation through compressions is more important initially than addressing airway or breathing. The AHA estimates that the change only delays breathing for a patient by 18 seconds, but dramatically improves how soon compressions start. Now someone immediately provides

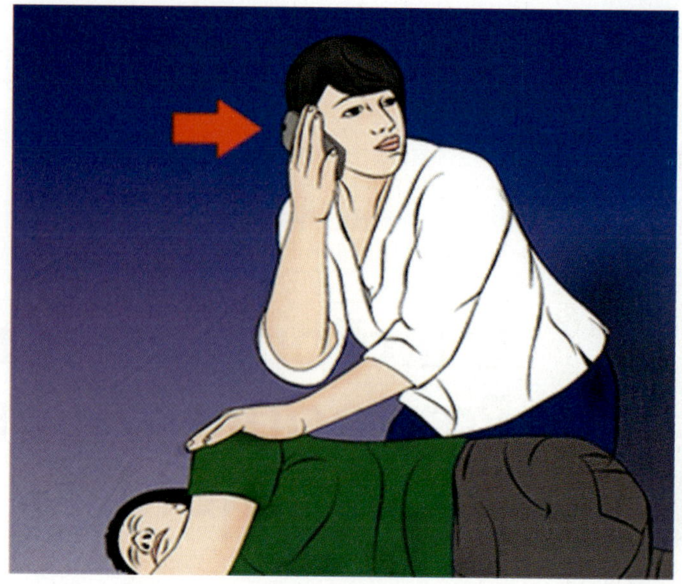

**Fig. 22.5: Method 1 step 3.** Send for help. The more people available for this step, the better. However, it can be done alone. Send someone to call for emergency medical services (EMS). Give the dispatcher your location, and notify him or her that you are going to perform CPR. If you are alone, get off the phone and start compressions after that. If you have someone else with you, have him or her stay on the line while you do CPR on the victim

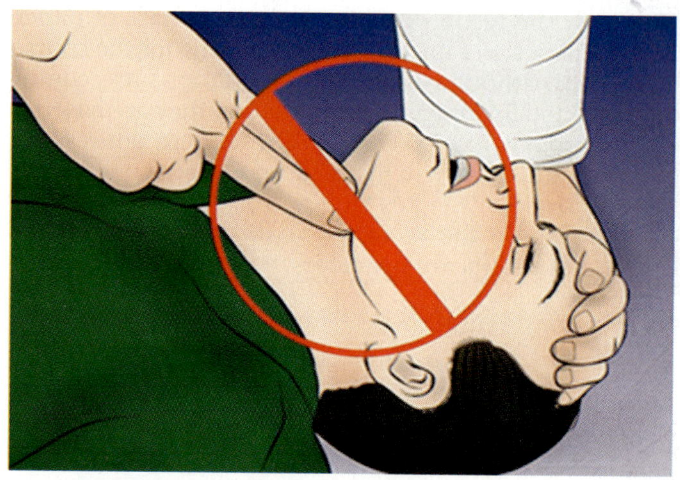

**Fig. 22.6: Method 1 step 4.** Do not check for a pulse. Unless you're a trained medical professional, odds are you'll spend too much valuable time looking for a pulse when you should be doing compressions

thirty chest compressions, then tilts the head to open the airway, then gives two breaths. The current guidelines have removed the practice called cricoid pressure which involved a rescuer applying pressure to the patient's windpipe while breathing for them with the hope of decreasing the amount of air that entered the stomach. Research has shown this practice is difficult to teach to rescuers and may not make the difference it was once thought to. For those reasons cricoid pressure is no longer recommended.

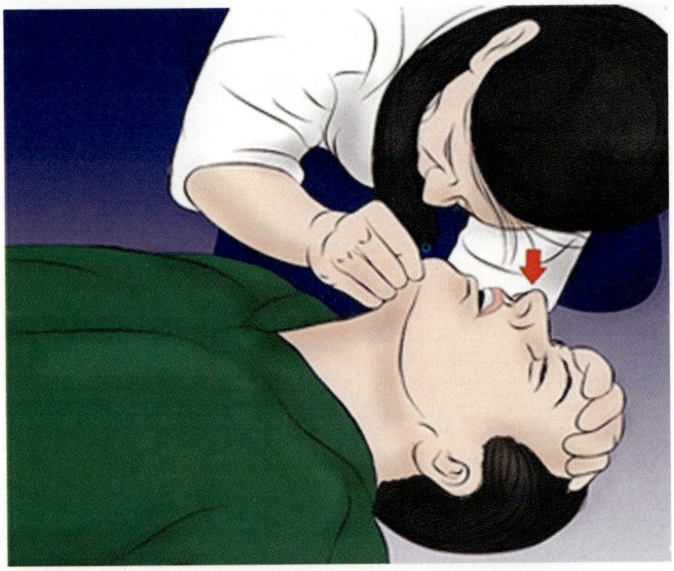

**Fig. 22.7: Method 1 step 5.** Check for breathing. Put your ear close to the victim's nose and mouth, and listen for slight breathing. If the victim is coughing or breathing normally, do not perform CPR. Doing so could cause the heart to stop beating

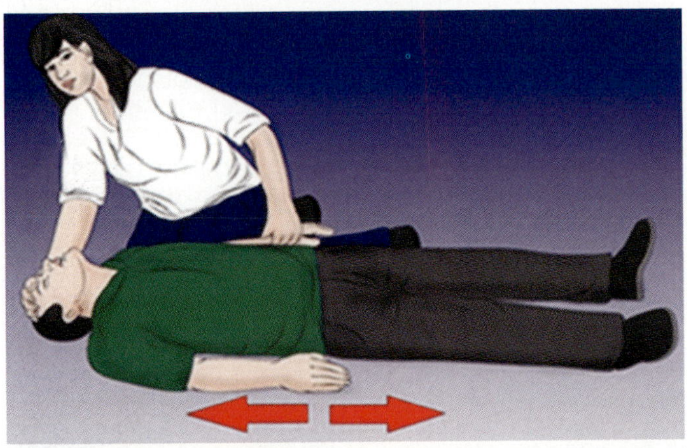

**Fig. 22.8: Method 2 step 1.** Place the victim on his or her back. Make sure he or she is lying as flat as possible, this will prevent injury while you're doing chest compressions

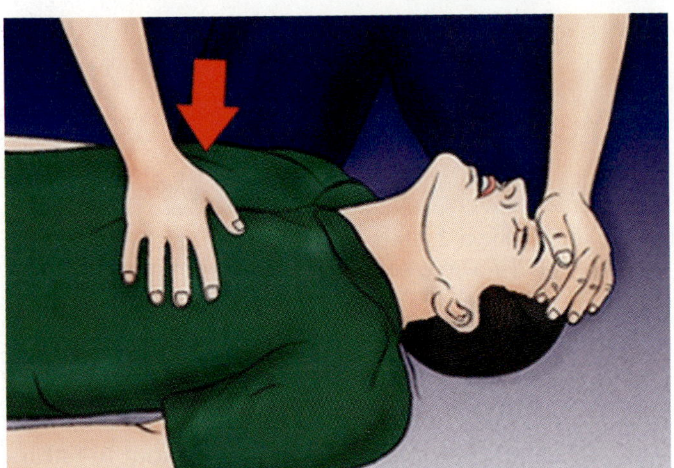

**Fig. 22.9: Method 2 step 2.** Place the heel of one hand on the victim's breastbone, exactly between the nipples

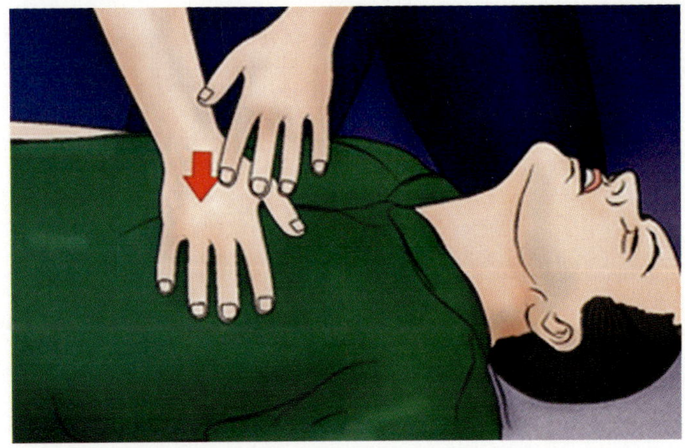

**Fig. 22.10: Method 2 step 3.** Place your second hand on top of the first hand, palm-down

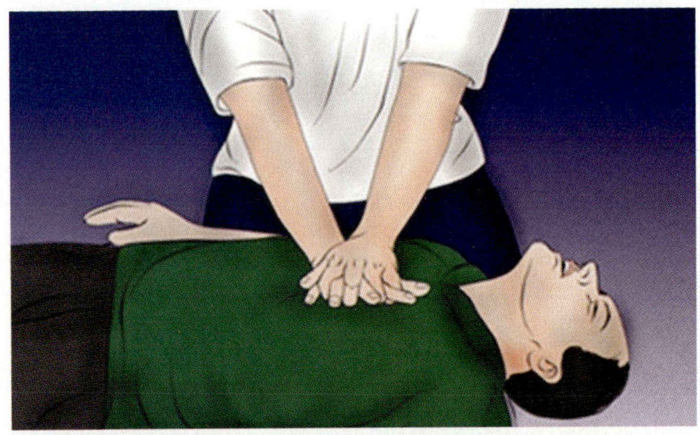

**Fig. 22.11: Method 2 step 4.** Position your body directly over your hands, so that your arms are straight and somewhat rigid

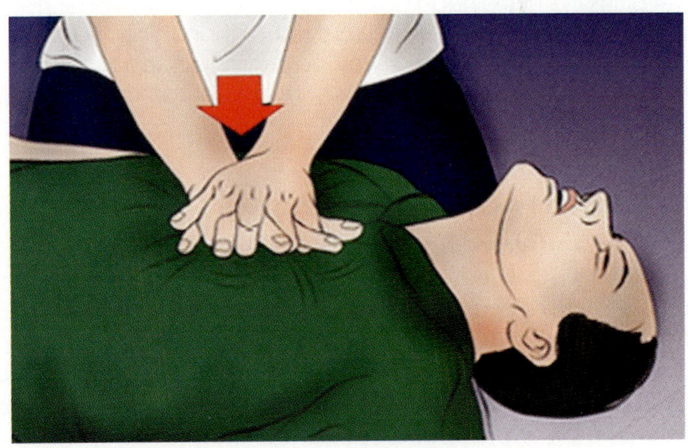

**Fig. 22.12: Method 2 step 5.** Perform 30 chest compressions. Press down with both hands directly over the breastbone to perform a compression, which helps the heart beat. Chest compressions are more critical for correcting abnormal heart rhythms (ventricular fibrillation or pulseless ventricular tachycardia). You should press down by about 2 inches (5 cm). Do the compressions in a relatively fast rhythm. Some agencies recommend doing compressions to the beat of the chorus of disco hit, or at roughly 103 beats per minute

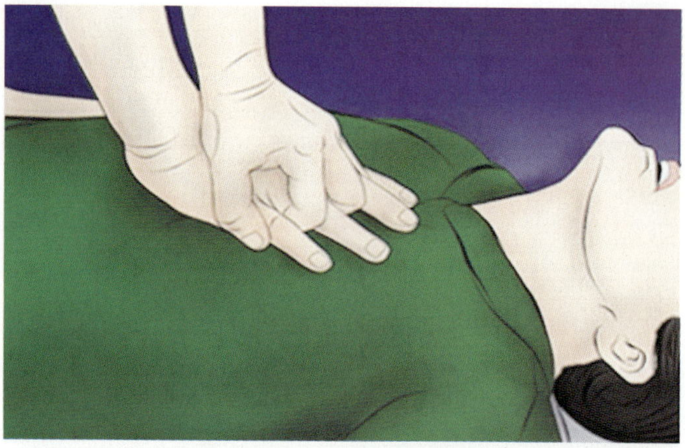

**Fig. 22.13: Method 3 Step 1.** Continuing the process until help arrives minimize pauses in chest compression that occur when changing providers or preparing for a shock. Attempt to limit interruptions to less than 10 seconds

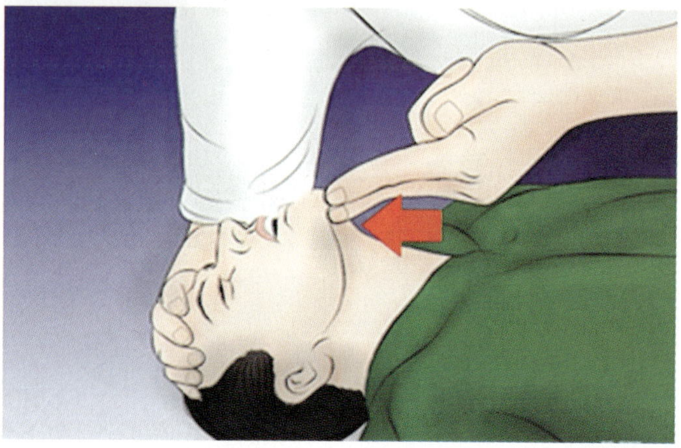

**Fig. 22.14: Method 3 Step 2.** Make sure the airway is open. Place your hand on the victim's forehead and two fingers on their chin and tilt the head back to open the airway. If you suspect a neck injury, pull the jaw forward rather than lifting the chin. If jaw thrust fails to open the airway, do a careful head tilt and chin lift. If there are no signs of life, place a breathing barrier (if available) over the victim's mouth

### Streamlined Process for Providing CPR

Barriers and complications to starting CPR have been removed with the hope of encouraging bystanders to act more quickly. One of the changes was removing the old 'Look, Listen, and Feel' process and continuing to insist that lay rescuers do not check for a pulse. Lay rescuers and even experienced healthcare providers may have a hard time finding a pulse and spend too long looking for one before starting CPR. It is far better for someone to have CPR and not need it than go without CPR when it is desperately needed.

### Continued Emphasis on High Quality CPR

Not only must CPR be started quickly it must also be good enough to benefit the patient. For untrained rescuers or those unwilling/unable to provide breaths excellent

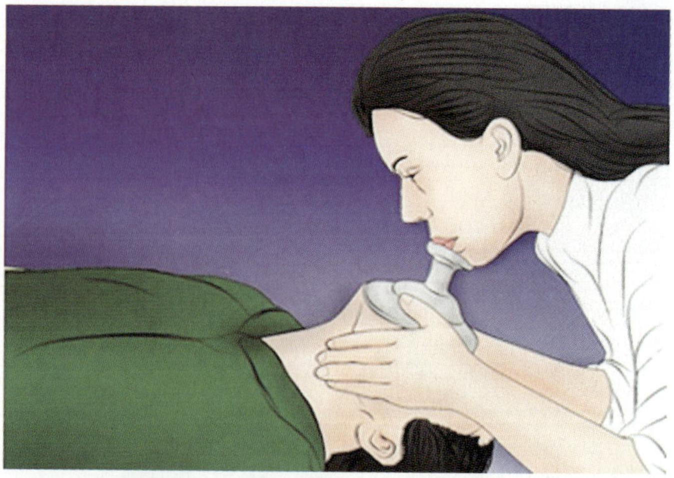

**Fig. 22.15: Method 3 Step 3.** Give two rescue breaths (optional). The American Heart Association no longer considers rescue breaths necessary for CPR, as the chest compressions are more important. If you are trained in CPR and totally confident, give two rescue breaths after your 30 chest compressions. If you've never done CPR before, or you're trained but rusty, stick with only chest compressions. Keeping the airway open, take the fingers that were on the forehead and pinch the victim's nose closed. Make a seal with your mouth over the victim's mouth and breathe out for about one second. Make sure you breathe slowly, as this will make sure the air goes in the lungs and not the stomach. If the breath goes in, you should see the chest slightly rise and also feel it go in. Give a second rescue breath. If the breath does not go in, re-position the head and try again. If it does not go in again, the victim may be choking. Do abdominal thrusts (the Heimlich manoeuvre) to remove the obstruction

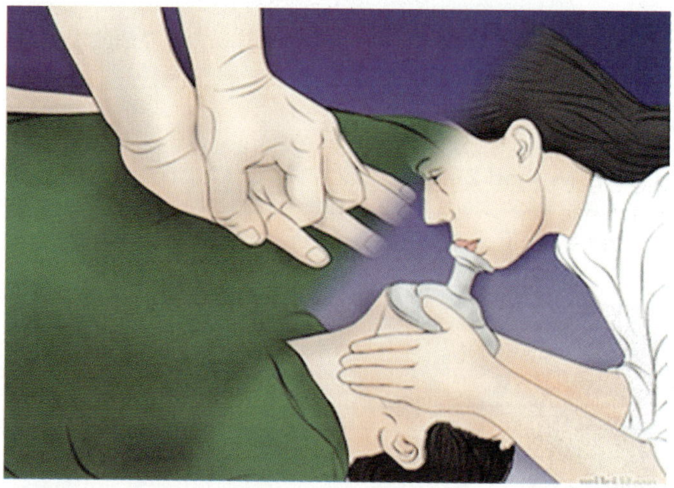

**Fig. 22.16: Method 3 Step 4.** Repeat the cycle of 30 chest compressions. If you're also doing rescue breaths, keep doing a cycle of 30 chest compressions and 2 rescue breaths. You should do CPR for 2 minutes (5 cycles of compressions to breath) before checking for signs of life

compressions provided continuously without breaths is highly desired. Compressions, with or without breathing, should be hard and fast and done in the middle of the chest. They should be at a rate of at least 100/min and the depth

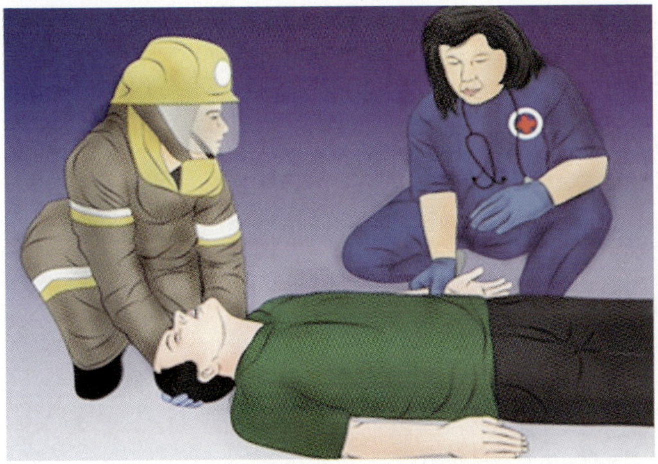

**Fig. 22.17: Method 3 Step 5.** Continue CPR until someone takes over for you, emergency personnel arrive, you are too exhausted to continue, an AED is available for immediate use, or signs of life return

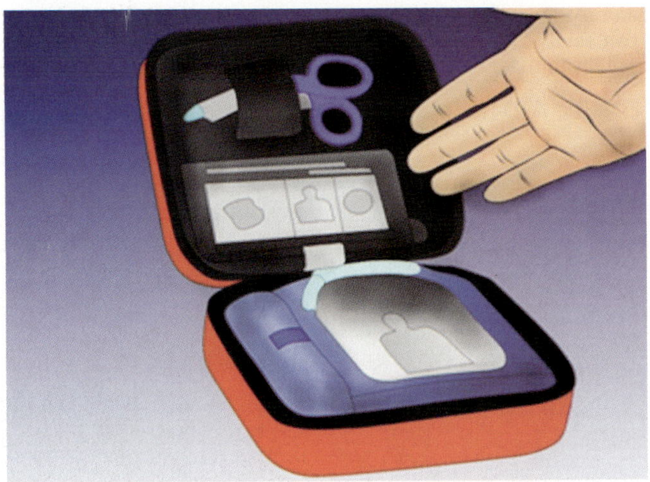

**Fig. 22.18: Method 4 Step 1.** Using an AED. Use an AED (automated external defibrillator). If an AED is available in the immediate area, use it as soon as possible to jump-start the victim's heart. Make sure there are no puddles or standing water in the immediate area

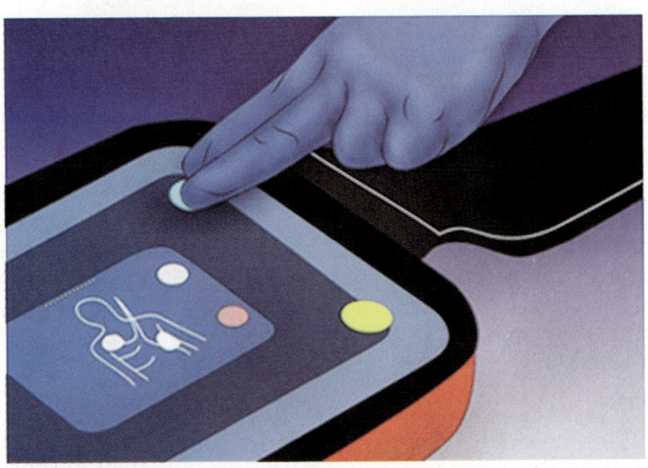

**Fig. 22.19: Method 4 Step 2.** Turn on the AED. It should have voice prompts that tell you what to do

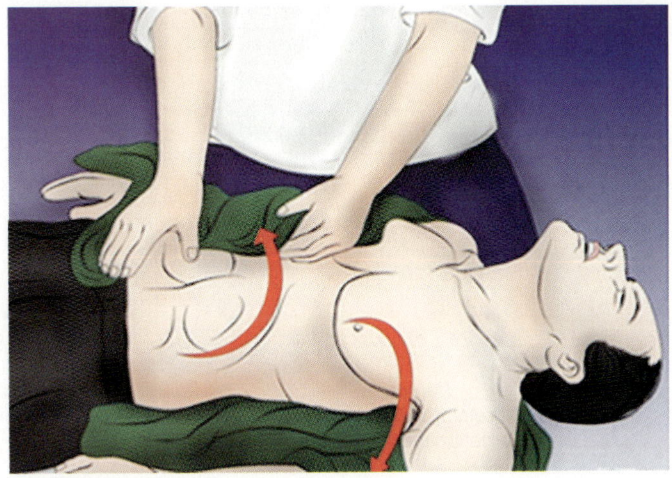

**Fig. 22.20: Method 4 Step 3.** Fully expose the victim's chest. Remove any metal necklaces or underwire bras. Check for any body piercings, or evidence that the victim has a pacemaker or implantable cardioverter defibrillator (should be indicated by a medical bracelet). Make sure the chest is absolutely dry. Note that if the person has a lot of chest hair, you may need to shave it. Some AED kits come with razors for this purpose

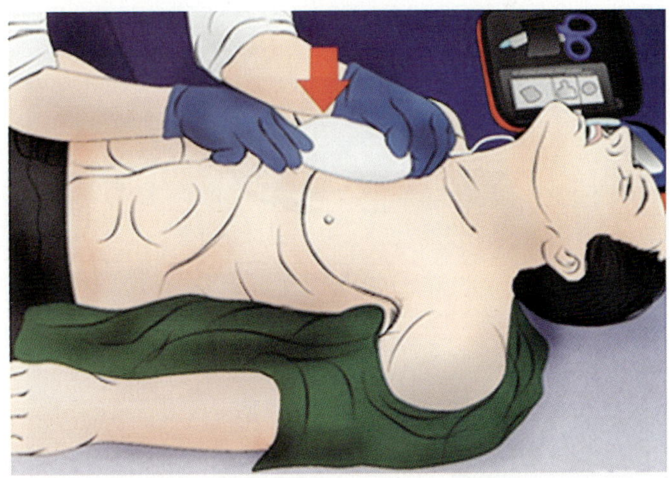

**Fig. 22.21: Method 4 Step 4.** Attach the sticky pads with electrodes to the victim's chest. Follow the instructions on the AED for placement. Move the pads at least 1 inch (2.5 cm) away from any metal piercings or implanted devices. Make sure no one is touching the person

of them must be at least 2 inches. The new depth is only a slight change from the previous 1 ½–2 inches but by encouraging people to compress the chest at least 2 inches. There is a greater likelihood that each compression will pump more blood to the brain, heart, and other organs. Providing one number to work towards is part of the AHA's effort to simplify the process and in turn improve the overall outcome for patients. The new overall process is this:

- As soon as an emergency is recognized someone should call for help and get an AED.
- If the victim is not responding to rescuers and does not appear to be breathing normally, CPR should be started.

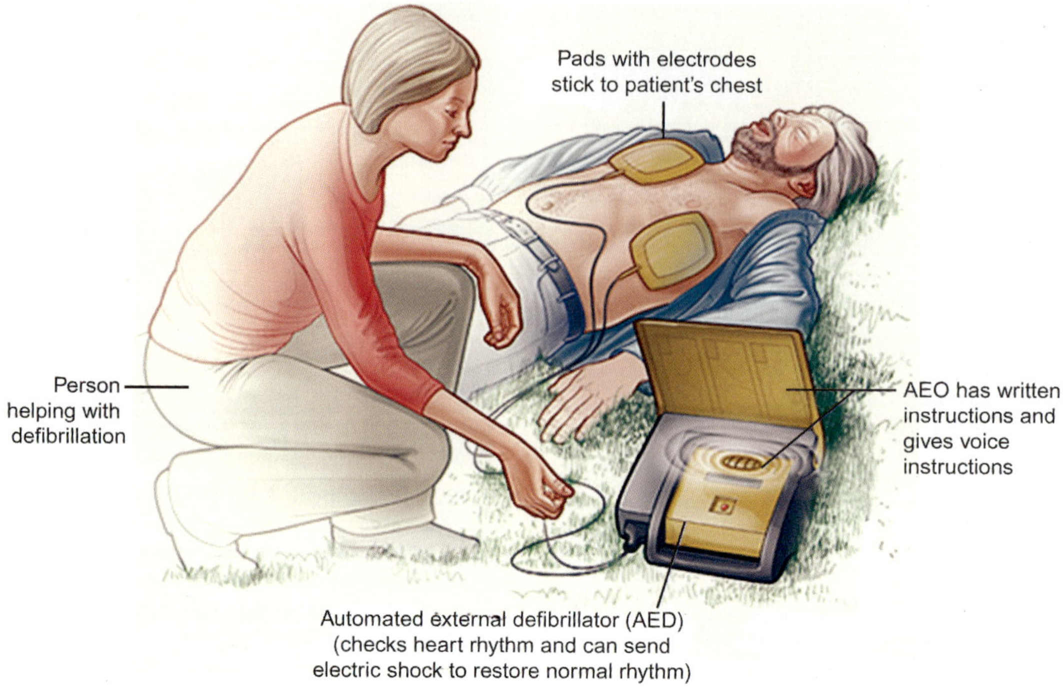


**Fig. 22.22:** A typical setup using an automated external defibrillator (AED). The AED has step-by-step instructions and voice prompts that enable an untrained bystander to correctly use the machine

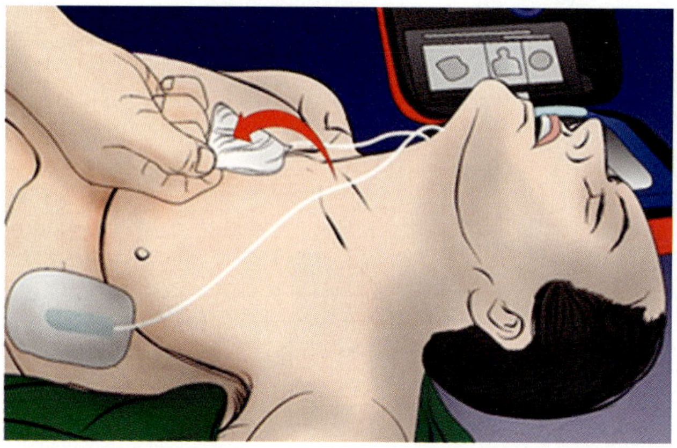

**Fig. 22.23: Method 4 Step 5.** Remove the electrode pads and resume CPR for another 5 cycles before using the AED again

- CPR begins with compressions delivered hard and fast in the middle of the victims chest. The rescuer should place the heel of one hand on the center of the victim's chest and the other hand right on top of the first with fingers intertwined.
- Each compression should be at least 2 inches deep and delivered at a rate of at least 100/minute. After giving 30 compressions a rescuer who is able to breathe for the victim should do so. If a rescuer is unable to breathe for the victim they should provide continuous high quality compressions until professional rescuers arrive.
- Breaths for the victim start by adjusting their airway. Tilt the victim's head by the forehead back and lifting the chin to open the airway. Pinch shut the victim's nose using the forefinger and thumb.

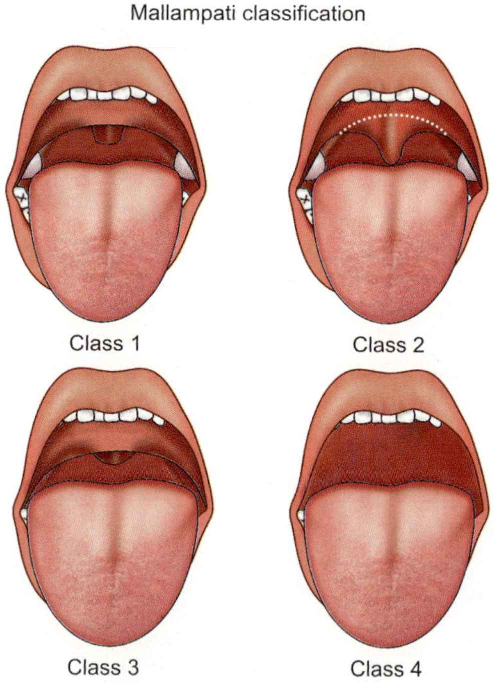


**Fig. 22.24:** The Mallampati score is as follows—class 1, full visibility of tonsils, uvula and soft palate; class 2, visibility of hard and soft palate, upper portion of tonsils and uvula; class 3, soft and hard palate and base of the uvula are visible; and class 4, only hard palate visible

- Each breath given to the victim should be a normal breath for the rescuer and delivered over 1 second while looking for the victims chest to rise.

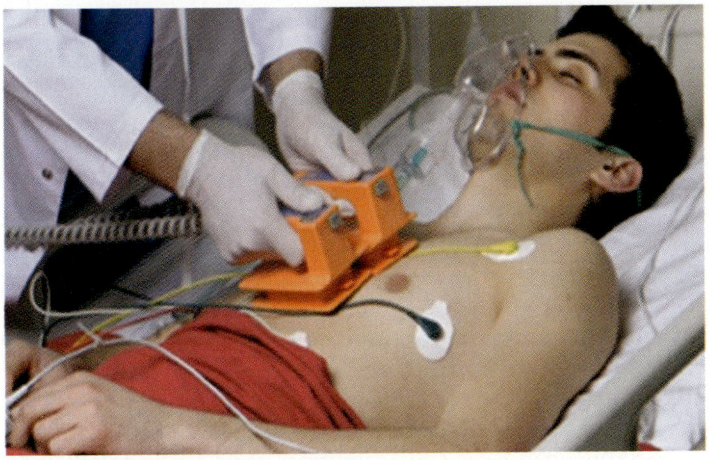

**Fig. 22.25:** Procedure of defibrillation in a patient with sudden unwitnessed, nontraumatic arrest in ventricular fibrillation

- A total of two breaths should be given to the patient and then the rescuer should immediately start chest compressions again.
- The cycle of 30 compressions and 2 breaths should be continued until the rescuer is physically unable to do so or professional rescuers arrive.
- As soon as an AED becomes available it should be turned on and its instructions followed to connect it to the patient. An AED will only work on someone who will benefit from it and will not harm someone who will not benefit from it.

As more research is conducted about the human body and the ways we treat problems associated with it the CPR standards will likely continue to evolve. It is important for individuals to stay current by renewing their CPR certification every 2–3 years as recommended by the organization issuing the CPR certification. Taking a class on a regular basis also helps to develop the skills and knowledge that must be immediately used during an emergency. At least 88% of cardiac arrests happen outside of hospitals so there is a high likelihood that an average citizen will be the first one on scene and may even be able to save that person's life. Encourage your friends and family to get certified because the life they save may be yours!

## A. CARDIOPULMONARY RESUSCITATION

Basic life support (BLS) incorporates (1) prompt recognition and action for myocardial infarction and stroke, (2) rescue breathing for victims of respiratory arrest, (3) chest compressions for victims in cardiopulmonary arrest, (4) initiation of automatic external defibrillation (AED), and (5) recognition and relief of foreign body airway obstruction. BLS is the first three links in the chain of survival—early access, early cardiopulmonary resuscitation (CPR), and early defibrillation.

CPR provides ventilatory support via forced ventilations and circulatory support via chest compressions. In BLS the term 'infant' includes the neonatal period and extends to the age of 12 months, a 'child' refers to ages 1–8 years, and anyone older than 8 years old is considered an 'adult.'

### Emergency Procedures in General

The medical professional may be called upon to render care outside the standard work area. In this situation, the rescuer should consider the following basic emergency concepts.

### Rescuer Personal Safety

The rescuer's safety is critical, because if the rescuer becomes incapacitated, he/she will not only fail in assisting the victim but will also split the resources of the response team by becoming an additional victim.

### On Spot Assessment

Upon arriving on the scene, the rescuer should, without spending excess time, survey the scene for threats to self and to the victim. Environmental threats such as power lines, fires, carbon monoxide, and traffic should be considered. Bystanders should be evaluated for threats, especially if the injury involves weapons.

### Initiation of Emergency Medical System

Guidelines recommend a 'phone first' approach for victims older than 8 years of age and 'phone first' approach for victims younger than 8 years of age (most are respiratory in nature). A nonresponsive adult victim can be assumed to be having a lethal cardiac arrhythmia. Defibrillation is the most critical action in these patients. Survival from cardiac arrest declines 7–10% each minute without defibrillation. If over 12 min have passed before defibrillation, the survival rate is 2–5%. For a lone rescuer upon discovering a nonresponsive adult, it is imperative to activate MS before proceeding with any other intervention. The 911 number should be used, if available, or the local EMS number or In-house 'code' number can be used when applicable. The provider can instruct untrained bystanders to activate EMS. The following information should be offered:

1. Location with cross streets and landmarks;
2. Call-back phone number;
3. Nature of the event, for example, medical emergency or trauma;
4. Number of victims;
5. Conditions of victims;
6. Rsources already on the scene. The need for defibrillation should be emphasized to ensure that the appropriate resources are dispatched. Excepions to the 'phone first/fast' rule include the following:
   a. Submersion/near drowning (*phone first* all ages),
   b. Trauma arrest (*phone first* all ages),
   c. Drug overdoses (*phone first* all ages),
   d. Cardiac arrests in high-risk children (*phone first* all ages), and
   e. The victim has an exsanguinating hemorrhage that needs immediate treatment. The newest AHA guidelines stress two medical conditions that are very important for BLS providers to recognize.

1. **Acute coronary syndromes (ACS).** Early recognition, early intervention, and early transport of victims with suspected ACS from the scene to the hospital could substantially reduce morbidity and mortality.
2. **Cerebral-vascular emergencies (stroke).** Each year, millions of adults suffer or die from acute stroke. New advances have made it imperative for BLS providers to be able to recognize signs and symptoms of stroke. Treatment is based on time of onset of symptoms. Options include IV fibrinolytic therapy within 3 h of presentation and intra-arterial fibrinolytic therapy within 6 h. Aetiology is disruption of blood supply to the brain. Seventy-five percent will be ischemic in nature caused by cerebral thrombosis or embolism. Hemorrhagic strokes are cause by a disruption of a cerebral artery with bleeding into the surface of the brain (subarachnoid hemorrhage) or into the tissue of the brain (intracerebral hemorrhage).
   a. **Stroke presentation.** Range of findings from mild facial paralysis or difficulty speaking to alteration of consciousness, sudden weakness or numbness affecting one side of the body, unsteadiness, unexplained dizziness, sudden falls, or loss of vision. Resolution of these symptoms in 24 h represents a transient ischemic attack (TIA). Most TIAs will last only 15 min. TIAs are significant indicators of impeding stroke with a quarter of stroke victims having suffered a TIA and 5% having a TIA within 1 month of stroke.
   b. **Management of stroke:** Rapid activation of EMS is essential once a stroke victim is identified. There are 7 Ds of management:

Detection, dispatch, delivery, door, data, decision, and drug. BLS responders are responsible for the first three Ds. Only half of stroke victims use the EMS system. Therefore initiating EMS by BLS providers is critical to ensure rapid delivery and treatment. The last four Ds are the responsibility of the hospital setting. Goals of out-of-hospital management by BLS is (1) priority of dispatch, (2) initial assessment and management, including airway support, oxygenation, ventilation, and circulation, (3) rapid identification of stroke by standardized stroke scale, (4) rapid transport of victim to stroke center capable of intervention and, (5) prearrival notification of hospital. It is very important for the BLS providers to establish the time of onset of the symptoms.

### Patient Positioning

When CPR is performed, the victim must be supine on a firm surface. A trauma victim normally should not be moved except for safety reasons, unless spontaneous respirations cannot be detected. When a rescuer evaluates a scene, she/he should quickly consider the physical consraints of performing advanced cardlac life support (ACLS) including CPR, intubation, IV access, and cardiac monitoring and if possible, position the patient to make best use of available space before the victim becomes 'fixed' at a location.

### Legal Considerations

Good Samaritan laws are intended to protect those engaged in emergency care outside a medical facility from civil liability. Although these laws vary among jurisdictions, they generally cover those who have no duty to respond, who perform in good faith, and who are not grossly negligent in their response.

### Patient Disposition

BLS continues until one of the following conditions occurs: (1) the patient regains a spontaneous pulse and respirations; (2) ACLS is initiated; (3) the rescuer is too exhausted to continue; or (4) the patient is declared dead by appropriate personnel. The emotional needs of the victim's family, especially with a pediatric victim, need to be taken into consideration before the resuscitation effort is terminated.

### Adult Cardiac Arrest

One million deaths per year can be attributed to cardiovascular disease, with approximately half of those due to coronary artery disease, most of whom present with sudden death. Two-thirds of the sudden death victims suffer arrest outside the home within 2 h after the onset of symptoms. Drowning, electrocution, drug intoxication, and trauma are other etiologies of sudden death. The time from onset of cardiorespiratory arrest to the initiation of CPR. and subsequent administration of ACLS is critical to patient outcome. Since the earliest possible time to start CPR is in the field by lay rescuers, BLS training should be available to as many persons within a community as possible in addition to those most likely to encounter a cardiac emergency.

A. **The ABCs and D of adult CPR.** In each step of the BLS process, the rescuer must perform an adequate assessment before proceeding to the next, more invasive, step. In the initial assessment, the victim is assessed for unresponsiveness. Tapping or gently shaking the victim while asking, 'Are you OK?' is appropriate. If the victim gives no response, EMS should be activated. The patient should then be positioned supine on a firm surface so that the rescuer can proceed with the following ABCs and D of CPR.

   1. **Airway:** The victim's tongue and epiglottis are elevated from the posterior pharynx by the head tilt-chin lift manoeuvre. One hand is used to lift the chin upward while the other hand is used to tilt the head backward by placing pressure on the forehead. In the case of suspected trauma, the rescuer should establish the airway while maintaining cervical spine precautions by using the modified jaw thrust technique. This is performed by using the rescuer's hands to lift up on the angle of the mandible to open the victim's mouth and establish an airway. The victim's nose or mouth can then be occluded with the rescuer's mouth for ventilations
   2. **Breathing:** After kneeling next to the victim, the rescuer places his/her ear next to the victim's mouth

and looks toward the victim's chest. Respirations are detected by listening for air exchange, feeling for airflow, and looking for chest rise and fall. This evaluation should last no more than 10s. If the victim is breathing adequately, helshe should be placed in the 'recovery' position. If no spontaneous respirations are detected, two effective ventilations must be supplied via rescue breathing. If no chest rise is visible, reposition the airway and reattempt ventilation. If ventilation is still not possible, the rescuer must assume a foreign body airway obstruction (FBAO). The patient should be ventilated 10–12 times a minute (one breath every 4–5s) in cases of respiratory arrest,when chest compressions are not being performed. Each breath should be given slowly over 1.5–2s to help prevent gastric inflation. The volume of each breath should be 10 cc/kg (700–1,000 cc). This new recommendation is meant to minimize gastric inflation. Cricoid pressure may also be used by health care professionals to reduce gastric inflation and help decrease the risk of regurgitation and aspiration. This technique applies pressure to the patient's cricoid cartilage, which subsequently pushes the trachea posteriorly compressing the esophagus. This technique should be used only when an *extra* rescuer is present. It is performed as follows:

- Locate the thyroid cartilage (Adam's apple) with your index finger,
- Slide your finger to the base of the thyroid cartilage and palpate the prominent horizontal ring below (cricoid cartilage), and
- Using the tips of your thumb and index finger, apply firm backward pressure to the cricoid cartilage.

*Different techniques of ventilation include the following:*

a. **Mouth-to-mouth ventilation.** This technique is very safe and effective. While maintaining the head tilt-chin lift position, the rescuer pinches the victim's nose while placing his/her mouth over the victim's mouth and giving two slow rescue breaths, verifying that the chest rises and falls with each respiration

b. **Mouth-to-mask ventilation.** The use of a mask provides a sanitary seal to the rescuer while allowing for adjunctive oxygen application and enhanced cervical spine control. The key to mask use is to make a complete seal on the victim's face. The mask is placed with the point of the tear over the victim's nose. Two techniques are utilized. The cephalic technique positions the rescuer above the victim's head. It is useful during respiratory arrest or during two-rescuer CPR. The lateral technique places the rescuer at the victim's side and uses a head tilt/chin-lift position. This technique is ideal for lone rescuer CPR. The rescuer should be able to maintain cervical spine precautions during the resuscitation. The tidal volumes should be identical to mouth to mouth breathing unless supplemental oxygen in present. If available, 10 L/min of $O_2$ can provide an inspired oxygen of more than 40%, and smaller volumes can be used to further reduce the risk of gastric inflation.

c. **Mouth-to-nose, mouth-to-stoma ventilation.** In situations where the mouth is not an effective entry into the respiratory tract (trauma, trismus, submersion injuries where there is difficulty in maintaining a tight mouth-to-mouth seal). The rescuer may try mouth-to-nose ventilation by closing the victim's mouth and placing his or her mouth over the victim's nose. If a patient has a tracheostomy stoma as an airway, it can also be an appropriate entry point.

d. **Mouth-to-face shield.** A clear plastic/silicone sheet separates rescuer and victim. The opening of the face shield is placed over victim's mouth. Pinch victim's nose closed and seal your mouth over center opening maintaining jaw thrust/chin-lift position. Provide slow breaths through one-way valve allowing victim's exhaled air to escape between shield and victim's face. This method is used as a substitute for mouth-to-mouth and should be converted to mouth-to-mask as soon as possible.

e. **Bag-mask ventilation.** Consists of a self-inflating bag and a nonrebreathing valve attached to a face mask.

Use of this technique is best utilizing a two-person rescue to ensure a good seal of the mask to the victim's face. Supplemental oxygen should be used with this technique, 8–12 L/min. The use of smaller tidal volumes will reduce gastric inflation.

The key is maintaining a good seal to assure successful ventilation. The one-rescuer technique is performed by using the index and thumb on the edge of the mask while the remaining fingers maintain the jaw-thrust position. This technique requires considerable skill and should be practiced frequently to ensure effective ventilation.

3. **Circulation.** After two effective ventilations are completed, the patient is no longer assessed for a palpable carotid pulse by lay rescuers. This was considered the 'gold standard' method for assessing cardiac function since the guidelines were first published in 1968. Studies since have shown serious variability in detecting a carotid pulse and delay in initiating chest compressions. The lay rescuer should be instructed on assessing signs of circulation. The layperson will (1) provide rescue breaths, (2) look for any evidence of spontaneous circulation such as normal breathing, coughing or any movement, (3) immediately begin compressions and attach an AED if no signs of spontaneous circulation are present. The overall assessment should take no longer than 10s. The health-care professional should continue to include a carotid pulse check as part of his/her assessment. This effort should be limited to 5–10s. If an adequate pulse is palpated, then rescue breathing is continued until spontaneous breathing begins. The pulse should be reassessed every few minutes. If no signs of circulation are present, circulation must be established by using external chest compressions as follows.

a. The rescuer kneels with his/her knees next to the chest of the victim exposing the chest to assist with the location of landmarks and to reduce restriction of movement.
b. Two fingers are run up the lower sternal border to the substernal notch. Using this point as a guide, the rescuer moves up the sternum two finger widths. The heel of the rescuer's other hand is placed against the finger guide along the sternum.
c. The rescuer's other hand is placed on top of the first and the fingers are interlocked. Fingers should be kept off the ribs to reduce breakaged. The rescuer should align his/her shoulder, the heels of his/her hands, and the victim's sternum and spinal cord in a single line. Bending at the hips and keeping the elbows locked, the rescuer can then compress the sternum one and a half to two inches deep at a rate of 100 compressions a minute for 15 compressions.

4. **Coordination of compression and rescue breathing:** After 15 compressions, the rescuer can move to the victim's head to deliver two rescue breaths of 1½–2s each. This is followed by another 15 chest compressions. After four cycles of two rescue breaths and 15 chest compressions, the victim is reevaluated for any evidence of return of spontaneous circulation. If there are no signs of circulation, resume CPR, beginning with chest compressions. If signs of circulation are present, check breathing status. If breathing is present, place victim in the recovery position and continue to monitor breathing and circulation. If the victim is not breathing, provide rescue breathing at 10–12 times per minute and monitor for signs of circulation every few minutes.
5. **Defibrillation:** Most adults with sudden unwitnessed, nontraumatic arrest are in ventricular fibrillation. Early defibrillation is essential to improving survival. Early defibrillation in the community is defined as within 5 min of EMS call. BLS providers must be trained to use AEDs to improve patient outcomes.

### Two-rescuer CPR

When two rescuers are available, one manages the head and airway while performing ventilations. The second rescuer performs chest compressions, pausing now and then to allow for ventilations. In two-rescuer CPR, a 15:2 ratio of compressions to ventilations is still used until the airway is secured. When the person doing chest compressions tires, she/he may call for a switch of positions. At this time the patient should be reevaluated for pulse and spontaneous respirations.

### Compression-only CPR

This method can be employed by providers who are unwilling to attempt rescue breathing for fear of disease transmission. Current evidence shows that compression-only CPR is significantly better than no attempt at CPR in adult arrest. It is recommended in the following circumstances: (1) rescuer unwilling or unable to provide mouth-to-mouth breathing or (2) use in dispatcher assisted CPR instructions where simplicity of technique allows untrained bystanders to provide intervention circulation. EMS should be activated at this time if not already done, stridor, or the victim becomes unconscious.

### Management of the pregnant or obese patient with an FBAO

When abdominal thrusts are inappropriate or ineffective because of excess abdominal mass, chest thrusts should be attempted. For the standing victim, the rescuer stands behind the victim and places his/her arms under the victim's armpits. The lateral side of the fist is placed on the sternum well above the xiphoid process. The fist is grasped with the other handand thrust into the sternum until the object is ejected or the victim becomes unconscious. For the victim who is lying down or unconscious, the rescuer kneels at the victim's side and places his/her hands in the same position as for doing CPR chest compressions. Slow and distinct thrusts are applied to dislodge the object.

## B. AIRWAY MANAGEMENT

### Assessment of the Unstable Airway

In all medical emergencies, patient care starts with the very basic ABCs. Accordingly, establishing and/or maintaining an airway must take utmost priority. Unfortunately, there is little time to contemplate one's options or seek assistance, and 'looking stuff up' is usually out of the question. Thus, proper airway management requires thorough prior familiarization with equipment, drugs, and proper techniques.

Respiratory compromise is frequently associated with cardiovascular emergencies, whether as a sequelae (as frequently occurs in adults) or as a cause (as is common in children). Regardless of the aetiology, once the ABCs have been assessed, constant vigilance is needed to manage the airway.

### Indications for Intubation

Definitive airway management may be indicated in the patients with any of the following indications:

- **Oxygenation failure.** $PO_2$ less than 60 on $FiO_2$ greater than 40%.

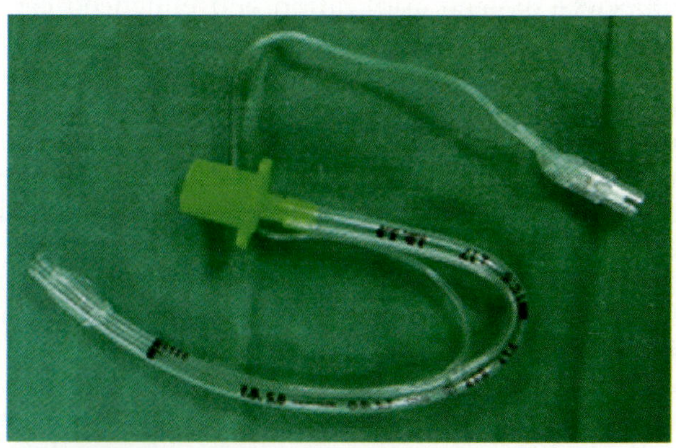

**Fig. 22.26:** Endotracheal tube showing inflated cuff

- **Ventilation failure.** $PCO_2$ greater than 55 (with previously normal $PCO_2$) or acute rise in $PCO_2$ of greater than 10 (in chronic obstructive pulmonary disorder). Need for hyperventilation, as might occur in head injury.
- **Profound shock.** Artificial ventilation reduces the work of breathing and thus minimizes energy expenditure. Need for paralysis.
- **Airway protection.** Failure to maintain normal airway reflexes in the unconscious patient.
- **Mechanical obstruction.** Present or impending compromise, e.g. edema or hematoma (apnea is included in multiple categories above).

### Signs of Impending Respiratory Failure

Mental status changes. Patients with hypoxia will often present with restlessness and agitation. Hypercapnea may manifest itself as drowsiness or unresponsiveness.

### Respiratory Mechanics

Tachypnea can be a very early sign of respiratory compromise. The inability of patients to speak in full sentences (or to even say one or two words at all) may demonstrate minimal to absent respiratory reserve. Caveats bradypnea from respiratory fatigue may be a late and ominous sign. Alternately, bradypnea and altered respiratory patterns (e.g. Kussmaul's respirations) may also demonstrate impaired CNS function.

### Heart Rate

Tachycardia can also be an early, albeit nonspecific, finding. Caveat in young children, bradycardia is a frequent response to hypoxia.

### Brief, Focused Physical Exam

The patients should undergo a quick inspection of the airway for immediate or potential compromise (e.g. obstruction from blood, teeth or most often the tongue). Auscultation for hints (e.g. crackles, unequal breath sounds, prolonged inspiration and/or expiration, etc.) to the cause of respiratory compromise can be useful as well. Cyanosis may be evident in mucous membranes. If an obvious source of respiratory compromise is identified (e.g. congestive heart failure exacerbation or pneumothorax), appropriate and timely intervention may greatly improve a patient's overall condition and possibly obviate the need for intubation. Oxygen saturation ($SaO_2$) measurement is of obvious utility. Caveats respiratory compromise often occurs in the setting of normal $SaO_2$ levels. Levels are also frequently inaccurate in shock due to abnormal peripheral perfusion. The patient's color may be a better indication of the need for airway management. Cyanosis, whether from shock or hypoxia, is an ominous sign.

### Arterial Blood Gases

A declining $PaO_2$ and/or a rising $PCO_2$/declining pH are the best objective assessments of respiratory function available. Drawbacks requires a finite period of time to obtain and transport the sample as well as the necessary analytical equipment.

### *Warnings in CPR*

Remember, if some one is not in your care, you must ask permission of the responsive victim if you can help. If they are unresponsive, you have implied consent.

1. Do not move the patient unless he or she is in immediate danger or are in a place that is life-threatening.
2. If the person has normal breathing, coughing, or movement, do not begin chest compressions. Doing so may cause the heart to stop beating.
3. If possible, wear gloves and use a breathing barrier when possible to make transmission of diseases less likely.
4. Remember that CPR is different for adults, children and infants; this CPR is meant to be administered to an adult.
5. Do not practice CPR on someone whose heart is beating and who is breathing. Doing so can stop the heart and can damage the lungs. Always use a dummy to practice.

### *Chest X-ray*

Frequently informative but time consuming and not always available. It should be mentioned that assessment and intervention are usually concurrent rather than consecutive actions. Hypoxic patients deserve immediate oxygen even if the cause is unclear. Patients with sonorous respirations may need a basic manual airway opening while other actions are being performed.

### Airway Management Equipment (Figs 22.27–22.33)

#### *Airway Adjuncts*

1. **Oral airway.** The oral airway is a question-mark shaped plastic device that lifts the tongue off the posterior pharynx to maintain a patent airway. It may also be used as a bite block once intubation has been performed.

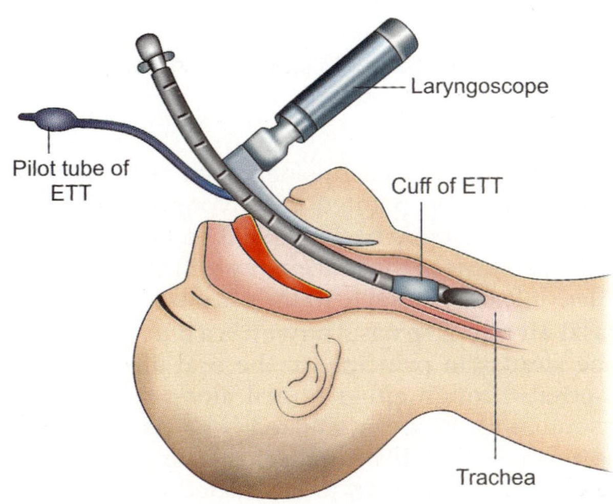


**Fig. 22.27:** The insertion of a long breathing tube or artificial airway (endotracheal tube, ETT) into the trachea (windpipe) via the mouth is called intubation. On occasion the tube may be inserted through the nose down into the trachea

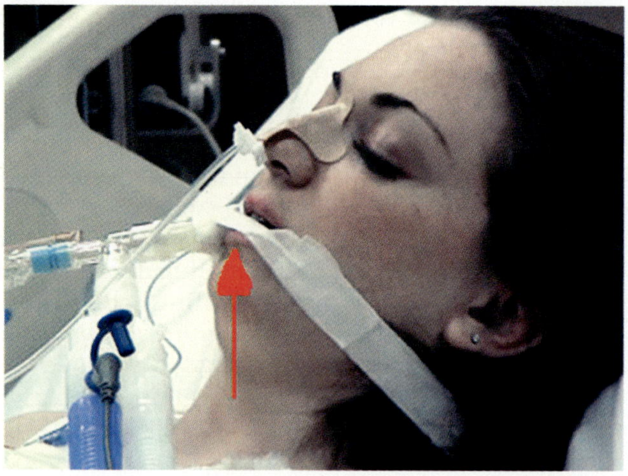

Fig. 22.28: Patient with an oral endotracheal tube

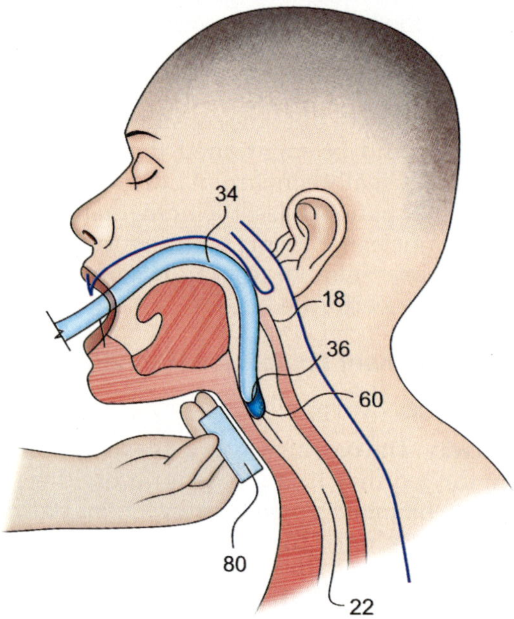


Fig. 22.29: A magnetic guide system for intubation of a tube into a patient's passage way

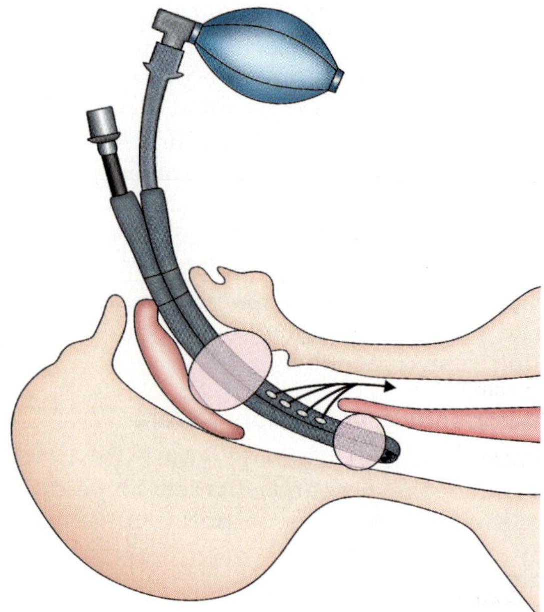

Fig. 22.30: Oesophageal tracheal combitube—ventilation when tip positioned in the oesophagus

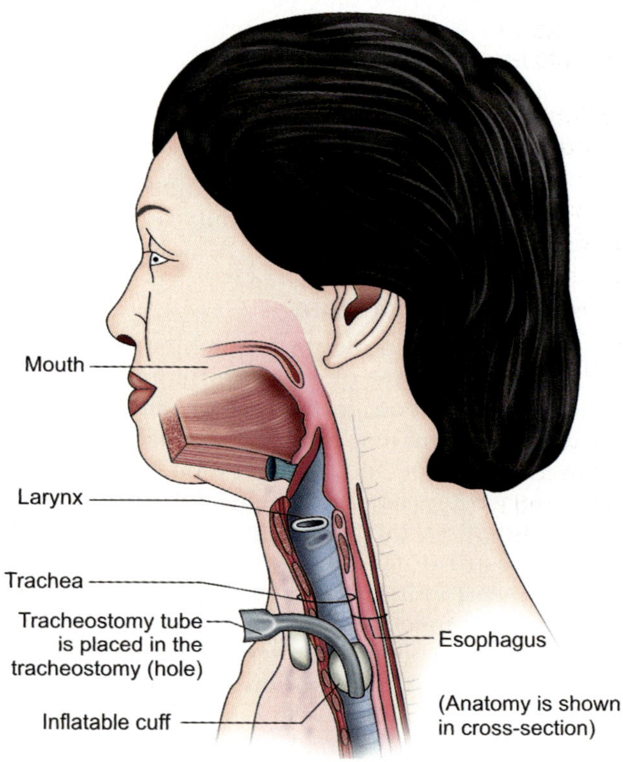


Fig. 22.31: A side view of the neck and the correct placement of a tracheostomy tube in the trachea or windpipe

Initially it is inserted upside down and rotated 180° into position (tip pointed into hypopharynx) to avoid pushing the tongue backwards, thereby worsening the obstruction. Since the oral airway will stimulate the gag reflex, it is only suitable in the unconscious patient.

2. **Nasal airway.** The nasal airway is a curved, soft rubber tube similar in principle to the oral airway, but it is inserted through either nostril along the floor of the nasopharynx. Properly situated (with the flange against the nose), its tip will be in the posterior pharynx behind the tongue, creating an unobstructed airway. Insertion is facilitated through tip lubrication, although bleeding still frequently occurs.
3. **PTL/Combitube.** The PTL and combitube are similar devices that share a basic dual purpose function. They are double lumen tubes with two cuffs—a small distal cuff (similar to an endotracheal tube) and a large proximal pharyngeal cuff. The device is inserted blindly, after which both cuffs are inflated. Ventilation is then attempted through one lumen, after which the rescuer subsequently determines its location. If the tube is found to be in the trachea, it may then be used as an

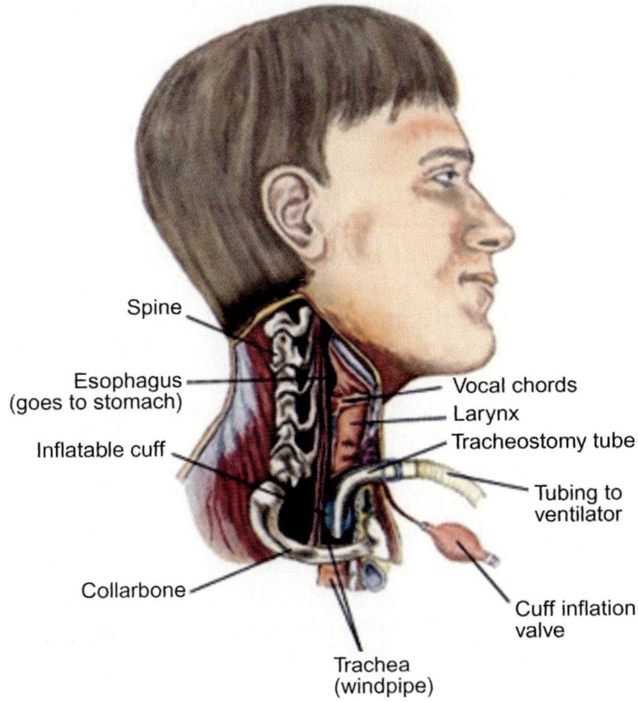


**Fig. 22.32:** The tracheotomy tube is inserted through the cricothyroid membrane. The tracheal hook can be redirected to facilitate entry of the tracheotomy tube into position

endotracheal tube. In the case of esophageal intubation, the device acts as a modified esophageal obturator airway, and ventilation is performed through the other lumen.

4. **Endotracheal tube (ET).** The ET is the gold standard for establishing a secured airway. It can be placed orally, nasally, or percutaneously through the cricothyroid membrane (CTM). It consists of a plastic tube with an inflatable balloon on the distal end. It can also protect the airway from aspiration.
5. **Laryngeal mask airway (LMA).** The LMA is a short tube (akin to a large bore ET tube) attached to a cuffed mask designed to sit snugly over the glottic opening. It can be placed blindly and is thus useful in management of difficult airways. Additionally, an ET tube can be passed through its tube (the orifice of which is directed into the trachea), providing an alternate means of orotracheal intubation.

## Airway Management Tools

1. **Laryngoscope.** It is used to lift the anterior airway upwards and forwards (from the intubator's perspective) to better align the airway axes and facilitate intubation. Two major types of blades are used. The tip of the straight Miller blade is placed posterior to the epiglottis so that it may be lifted upwards to expose the vocal cords. In contrast, the tip of the curved Macintosh blade is situated in the vallecula, where the epiglottis may be displaced via traction from upward blade movement.
2. **Lighted stylet** (a.k.a. 'light wand'). The light wand is a special stylet with a handle and a lighted tip. It is inserted blindly, and tip location is determined through transtracheal light visualization. The ET tube can then be advanced over the stylet into the trachea.
3. **Macgill forceps.** Macgill's are large curved forceps with ring tips used to guide tube placement or remove foreign bodies (e.g. teeth) from the pharynx.

## Airway Management Techniques

After determining that some form of airway management is necessary, a rescuer must decide what interventions are most appropriate for a particular situation. Endotracheal intubation is the preferred technique for airway management of any significant duration. In the emergency setting, surgical alternatives may be used following a failure to intubate, while less advanced techniques are suitable only for lesser trained personnel or for short-term airway management. Though the rescuer should anticipate the need for a definitive airway, oxygenation and ventilation should never be delayed while such preparations are undertaken.

## Manual Airway Opening

A patent airway must be ensured, either by the patient (if conscious and breathing) or by the rescuer (for unconscious

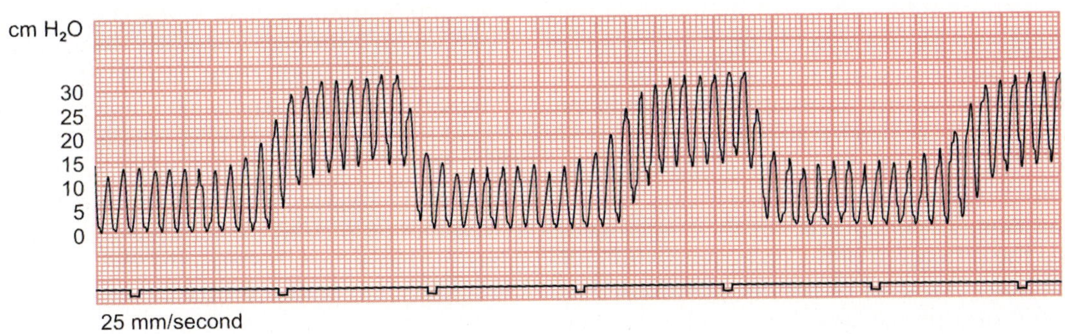


**Fig. 22.33:** A sinusoidal wave format (modified by existing pulmonary compliance) demonstrating automatic biphasic scheduling with a modulated higher frequency percussive sinusoidal respiration. Sinusoidal scheduling will ventilate neonates through pediatrics to large adult lungs with low pulmonary compliance. This provides for a balanced diffusive/convective intrapulmonary gas exchange

patients with obstructed airways). If intubation cannot be performed immediately, the airway must be opened manually to allow ventilation and oxygenation. While very simple in principle, these techniques can be deceptively difficult. The head tilt with the chin lift or jaw thrust maneuvers prevent obstruction of the airway by the tongue, which can occlude the airway at the level of the pharynx. The head tilt (contraindicated with suspected cervical spine fracture) places the patient in the 'sniffing' position with the neck flexed in relation to the thorax and the head extended in relation to the neck. The chin lift is performed by placing fingers under the symphysis of the mandible and lifting forward. The jaw thrust is the method of choice when a C-spine fracture is suspected and involves grasping the angles of the mandible and lifting forward without tilting the head.

After airway opening, bag-valve-mask ventilation can be initiated while the need for further intervention is assessed. If the patient is expected to quickly regain the ability to self manage their airway (transient loss of consciousness), no additional intervention may be necessary. Otherwise, preparations for intubation should begin while a brief preintubation exam is performed to rapidly assess airway anatomy and choose the appropriate method of intubation. Limited neck or jaw motion (less than three finger widths between teeth) and the inability to view posterior pharyngeal structures may suggest a difficult intubation, however, such findings should not delay attempts at intubation if indicated. All dentures, partial plates, and foreign bodies can be removed prior to intubation as well.

### Oral Endotracheal Intubation

There are few relative contraindications to orotracheal intubation. Severe maxillofacial trauma, continuous bleeding/excessive pharyngeal secretions, mechanical obstruction, and unusual anatomic features may hinder attempts at intubation, but the overriding need for a secure airway and the lack of better alternatives usually make it the management technique of choice. Cervical spine immobilization is not a contraindication, but the need for inline head stabilization during the procedure will make the attempt more difficult.

1. **Equipment preparation.** Preparation is imperative. The operator should check tube cuff inflation, lubricate the tip of the ET tube, and place a stylet in the tube (or have available at the user's discretion). Suction must be present and working. The laryngoscope light should be tested, and availability of proper sized blades insured (ideally of both varieties). Most adults will require a no. 3 Macintosh or a no. 2 or no. 3 Miller blade.
2. **Patient preparation.** Although frequently overlooked, this may make the difference between a successful and a failed intubation. The goal of proper positioning is alignment of the oral-pharyngeal-laryngeal axes. The patient should be placed in a 'sniffing' position with the head slightly extended. A rolled towel placed beneath the head may facilitate such alignment. Dentures should be removed, and any loose/chipped teeth noted. If the patient is apneic, intubation may proceed immediately. Otherwise, rapid sequence intubation (RSI) or an appropriate modification thereof may be necessary.
3. **Intubation procedure.** The laryngoscope is grasped in the left hand and inserted into the right side of the patient's mouth. While advancing, it is simultaneously 'swept' towards the midline, permitting airway visualization through leftward displacement of the tongue. The tip of the blade should be observed during advancement to monitor its location relative tothe vallecula/epiglottis and esophagus. Properly employed, the laryngoscope permits the user to 'lift' the anterior airway structures upward to expose the vocal cords. Despite the instinctive temptation, a 'prying' force is never used, for this does not align the airway axes correctly, and risks teeth fracture. The only force applied should be parallel to the handle (as if sliding it along an imaginary pole). Visualization of the vocal cords may be facilitated through the 'BURP' technique, when an assistant provides posterior (backward), superior (upward), and rightward pressure on the cricoid ring. A modification of the Sellick maneuver, this also reduces the risk of aspiration. Once the cords are exposed, the ET is held like a pencil and inserted from the right corner of the mouth (to allow constant visualization of placement) and passed until the cuff is below the cords. Each attempt at intubation should generally not last more than 30 s, with periods of bag-valve-mask ventilation between attempts. Once proper tube placement has occurred, the depth of the tube in relationship to the incisors should be noted. This facilitates both easy recognition of inadvertent displacement as well as adjustment in tube position based on the subsequent chest X-ray. In the average-size adult, the patient's incisors are generally at about the 22-cm mark for men and the 20-cm mark for women.
4. **Complications.** Several potential complications, such as fractured teeth and soft tissue trauma/bleeding, are minimized through proper technique. Vomiting may occur during any attempt, although proper technique (especially in manual ventilation) may lessen the risks. Systemic responses, such as hypertension, tachycardia, and arrhythmias may be blunted through proper premedication. Mainstem (usually right) intubation may occur but should normally be quickly discovered. Esophageal intubation can be fatal unless promptly discovered and remedied.

### *LMA Intubation*

Since the LMA does not provide protection from aspiration, it does not replace an ET in the establishment of a definitive airway. However, because of the relative ease of LMA placement, it is quite useful in the difficult airway, either as a temporizing measure after failed intubation or as a means to facilitate tracheal intubation. Size 3 and 4 LMAs are used in smaller and larger adults, respectively. Placement is accomplished through complete deflation of the LMA cuff and insertion along the roof ofthe oropharynx.

Care is taken to ensure the deflated cuff remains flat against the superior and then posterior pharynx as it makes the bend towards the hypopharynx. Advancement continues blindly until resistance is met, at which time the cuff is inflated. (This frequently produces a minimal protrusion of the tube from cuff movement.) Ventilation is then performed in a fashion similar to when an ET tube is used. Chest rise and an ability to provide positive pressure ventilation are indications of proper placement. However, an air leak is common with pressures over 15–20 cm $H_2O$. When used to facilitate intubation, the LMA is first inserted and the ability to ventilate is established. A 6 mm ET tube can then be passed through the specially designed fast-track intubating LMA or a standard no. 3 or no. 4 LMA. The position of the LMA orifice directs the tube into the trachea as it protrudes' beyond the mask. Once placement is confirmed through the usual methods, the ET tube BVM adapter must be temporarily removed to permit removal ofthe LMA.

### Retrograde Translaryngeal Intubation

This technique may be useful for many cases of difficult intubations. Briefly, the Seldinger technique is employed to puncture the CTM with a large-bore needle directed cephalad, through which a guidewire is passed into the oropharynx. An ET then is guided blindly over the wire into the larynx and the wire is subsequently removed. Care is taken to place the wire through the side port of the ET tube, as this permits the tube to be advanced farther into the trachea before stopping at the site of wire entry. Although specially designed kits are available, in an emergency, many over-the-wire type kits, including central line and epidural catheters, can be used.

### Lighted Stylet Intubation

In contrast to normal ET tube stylets, the tip of the lighted stylet extends beyond the tip of the ET tube and contains a bright light. Initial placement of the stylet (upon which the ET tube is placed) is blind, but subsequent observation of where the light appears permits localization of the tip. A relatively bright glow located in the midline at the level of the cricoid cartilage suggests tracheal intubation, at which point the ET tube may be inserted to the proper depth and the stylet removed. In contrast, a soft,'diffuse light, especially when seen on either or both sides ofthe midline (but less in the middle, due to tracheal obstruction) may indicate improper placement. Darkening the room and forward traction on the tongue can help facilitate this procedure.

### Surgical Airway Alternatives

There will always be situations in which rescuers cannot establish an airway in an expedient method through standard methods. Although proper training and preparation can greatly minimize such instances, a surgical airway may on occasion be the only practical method of airway management. The use of RSI has made the use of surgical airway techniques much less common.

1. **Cricothyroidotomy.** Cricothyroidotomy is used when alternative procedures are ineffective, including in patients with severe facial trauma, hemorrhage, or upper airway obstruction as well as a baseline distorted airway anatomy. Cricothyrotomy is obviously complicated by difficult anatomy. Thus, it should be avoided with major neck trauma as well as in children less than 10 years of age. Additionally, coagulopathy can make this procedure quite difficult (the speed and relative ease of this procedure make it the technique of choice over the tracheostomy in emergent situations).
   a. **Technique.** The skin is rapidly prepped with an aseptic solution, after which the CTM is located between the thyroid cartilage superiorly and cricoid ring inferiorly. The larynx is then immobilized with the left hand (if right-handed) by grasping the thyroid cartilage with the thumb and long fingers and letting the index finger rest on the CTM. A short longitudinal incision (about 3 cm) is made in the skin superficial to the CTM, and the CTM is incised with a transverse stab incision. The scalpel handle is inserted into the incision and rotated 90° to open the airway. (Alternately, hemostats or a dilator may accomplish this task.) The endotracheal or tracheostomy tube is inserted, directing caudally, and the balloon is inflated. Securing the tube in place completes the procedure.
   b. **Complications.** Bleeding is common, and damage to underlying structures may occur. Additionally, creation of a false passage may occur along with obstruction of the airway with blood and/or secretions.
2. Percutaneous transtracheal needle ventilation (PTNV) is a temporary means of establishing ventilation through a large-bore catheter. Such access may be adequate for oxygenation, but it is insufficient to maintain prolonged ventilation and should be used for only 30–45 min while a definitive airway is being secured. It may be useful in selected pediatric patients, but it cannot be routinely recommended. Indications are essentially identical to those of surgical cricothyrotomy. It should be used with caution in patients with complete upper airway obstruction, as rapid increases in intrapulmonary pressure may cause barotrauma. Additionally, in the very young child, PTNV may be harmful because of the difficulty in localizing the CTM and the lack of airway support.
   a. **Technique.** The skin is rapidly prepared with betadine prep. A 12–16-gauge angiocath is inserted through the midline of the CTM angled 30–45° caudally. As the needle is advanced, a negative syringe pressure is maintained through constant aspiration; a rush of air into the syringe will then indicate entry into the trachea. The catheter is advanced to its hub while the needle is withdrawn. It is connected to a high-pressure oxygen source (50 psi) that is linked by an apparatus to control oxygen delivery. Ventilation is performed with 1–2s breaths and a 4–5s exhalation time. (An Ambu bag does not provide adequate ventilation and should not be used.)

**b. Complications.** Barotrauma from high pressures and flow is most common, aside from the usual bleeding. (However, pneumothorax and pneumomediastinum are uncommon.) Catheter kinking and aspiration (from an unprotected airway) may also occur.

### Rapid-sequence Intubation (RSI)

Rapid-sequence intubation, or RSI, is a technique in which transient unconsciousness and paralysis is induced to facilitate rapid endotracheal intubation, reducing the chance of airway trauma and increasing the ease of the procedure. RSI utilizes the patient's spontaneous respirations (avoiding BVM ventilation) to establish an oxygen reservoir within the lungs during intubation, thereby avoiding the risk of iatrogenic gastric insufflation and minimizing the chance of subsequent aspiration (the completely unresponsive/apneic patient does not require RSI). Furthermore, RSI, when used appropriately, blunts adverse cardiovascular and intracranial responses to intubation.

However, extreme caution must be used, as drug-induced temporary paralysis eliminates the patient's ability to maintain an airway. If a rescuer cannot establish a definitive airway, rapid intervention with surgical airway techniques may be indicated.

#### A. RSI Timetable (T = 5 min)

*Prepare-ensure equipment availability and function.*

This includes the establishment of a secure IV access. Evaluate the patient to select proper tube size and to ascertain the possibility of difficult intubation.

- **Position.** Maintain inline stabilization with possible C-spine trauma. In absence of trauma, extend the neck in adults. Avoid hyperextension in children. Consider a towel roll placed between shoulders. Raise the bed to a comfortable height.
- **Plan B.** Ensure immediate availability of a backup plan (surgical or BVM) and a second person to help (T = 3–5 min).
- **Preoxygenate.** With 100% $O_2$, breaths should not be augmented with BVM unless absolutely necessary, to aviod gastric insufflation. (T = 2–5 min).
- **Pretreat.** Consider a defasciculation agent to be given prior to succinylcholine. Intracranial pressure (ICP) is often elevated during intubation but may be blunted with lidocaine (especially in head injury). Consider atropine in children to blunt the frequent vagal bradycardic response to intubation (T = 0).
- **Put down.** With induction agent.
- **Paralyze.** With succinylcholine or nondepolarizing agent (simultaneously with induction).
- **Pressure.** Apply to cricothyroid using Sellick's/BURP maneuver after loss of consciousness (T = +45 s).
- **Place.** The tube (after).
- **Placement.** Verify tube placement.

Any time paralytics are used, one must ensure that the patient begins or continues to receive proper sedatives and possibly long acting paralytics. Be especially aware of the duration of action of the sedative versus the paralytic. Do not under any circumstances permit a sedative to wear off while the effects of a paralytic are still present.

#### B. Pretreatment Drugs

- **Lidocaine.** *Dose*—1–1.5 mg/kg. May blunt rise in ICP.
- **Vecuronium.** *Dose*—0.01 mg/kg. May minimize/eliminate succinylcholine-induced fasciculations.
- **Atropine.** *Dose*—0.01 mg/kg (minimum of 0.01 mg). Minimizes bradycardia and reduces airway secretions.

#### C. Induction Drugs

Induction drugs (all doses rapid IV push unless indicated). Etomidate (amidate). *Dose*—0.1–0.4 mg/kg. *Onset*—less than 1 min; *Duration*—3–10 min.

Agent of choice for most RSI. Nonbarbiturate, non-narcotic sedative hypnotic induction agent. No analgesic properties, minimal cardiovascular/respiratory effect. No clear contraindications, but emesis and transient adrenal suppression can occur. Myoclonic movements are often seen but do not represent seizure activity.

- **Ketamine** (Ketolar). *Dose*—1–2.5 mg/kg IV. *Onset*—30–60 secs. *Duration*—5–15 min.

Agent of choice-in status asthmaticus. Dissociatiative anesthetic with multiple effects—sedation, hypnosis, analgesia, and amnesia. Sympathomimetic (making it ideal in asthma) with bronchodilation and BP/ICP elevation. Contraindicated in ischemia or CAP from increased myocardial oxygen demand. Elevates ICP/intraocular pressures, stimulates airway secretions, and may trigger laryngospasm. Benzodiazepines can attenuate unpleasant emergence phenomena. Control secretions with glycopyrrolate/atropine.

Thiopental (pentothal). *Dose*—3–5 mg/kg (5–6 mg/kg peds). *Onset*—30–60 s. *Duration*—5–15 min.

Thiopental is a short-acting barbiturate that demonstrates cerebroprotection through a reduction in ICP. It is a poor analgesic and has a cardiovascular/respiratory depressive effect. It is contraindicated in the presence of myocardial dysfunction, hypotension, and status asthmaticus (from histamine release).

#### D. Paralytics

- **Succinylcholine** (anectine). *Dose*—1.5 mg/kg IV. *Onset*—30–60 s. *Duration*—4–6 min.
- **Usual drug of choice for RSI** because of rapid onset and short duration of action. Neuromuscular junction depolarization during onset produces generalized fasciculations that may be minimized by pretreatment with a nondepolarizer at 1/10th normal dose.
- **Contraindications.** Increases ICP and serum potas-. sium; thus, contraindicated with increased ICP, hyperkalemia (e.g. renal failure), penetrating ocular trauma, and patients with neuromuscular disease. In practice, major trauma or burns of less than 48-hour old are not absolute contraindications, as hyperkalemia (crush injury not with standing) generally does not occur for several hours to days following injury.

- **Rocuronium (zemuron):** *Dose*—0.6–1.2 mg/kg. *Onset*—45–90s. *Duration*—15–40 min. Good second choice when succinycholine is contraindicated.
- **A nondepolarizing neuromuscular blocker,** it does not trigger histamine release and has little cardiovascular impact.
- **Vecuronium (norcuron):** *Dose*—0.1 mg/kg. *Onset*—2–3 min. *Duration*—25–30 min. Longer onset and duration than rocuronium. Onset can be short-ened with 2 × dose but duration is prolonged. Like rocuronium, has little histamine release.
- **Mivacurium (mivacron).** *Dose*—0.15–0.2 mg/kg. *Onset*—less than 2 min. *Duration*—6–16 min. Rapid onset similar to rocuronium but may cause histamine release and hypotension.
- **Confirming ET placement.** No technique is 100% reliable. It is best to verify placement through use of multiple methods.
- **Direct visualization.** Watching the tube enter the trachea is still a very reliable method to check tube placement.
- **Auscultation.** Listen in each hemithorax and over the epigastrum. This can be somewhat unreliable due to faint sounds in the obese and transmission of sounds in the small/thin patient.

  Color capnography: A small $CO_2$ measuring device can be placed in line between the tube and the Ambu bag. A yellow disc changes to purple upon exposure to the relatively high $CO_2$ concentrations of the lung. Color should be monitored for several breaths, as a significant amount of $CO_2$ may also be found in stomach gas.
- **End-tidal capnometry.** The waveform from an electronic $CO_2$ detector can permit quantitative monitoring of expired $CO_2$. Its utility is obvious, but its availability is limited (commonly in the ED and ICU).
- **Endotracheal intubation detector.** A large (e.g. 30 cc) syringe is connected to the end of the ET and filled rapidly by drawing air from the tube. The semirigid structure of the trachea will permit quick filling with air, whereas the soft muscular esophagus will collapse, quickly producing obstruction to filling. A variation utilizes a rubber bulb on the syringe end, resembling the turkey baster of its namesake.
- **Ultrasonic devices.** Devices exist that utilize ultrasound probes to analyze the passage distal to the tip ofthe ET (i.e. open trachea *vs* collapsed esophagus). Not commonly used at present.
- **Chest X-ray.** A standard allows tube adjustment to an ideal position, about 1–2 inches above the carina.

## C. VASCULAR ACCESS

### Principles of Vascular Access

Indications for vascular access are volume replacement and delivery of medications into the central circulation. It is needed before an emergency requiring access occurs, as a prerequisite for many monitoring techniques, and is a route for nutritional supplementation. Vascular access is always performed using aseptic technique and with universal precautions for bloodborne pathogens.

### Intravenous Catheters

Fluid dynamics determine catheter selection. Flow through a catheter is related directly to lumen diameter and inversely to length. For maximal flow rates, catheters should be as short and fat as the vessel allows. The simplest device, a butterfly, is a needle on a piece of tubing. After insertion into the vein, a flashback of blood into the tubing indicates correct placement. The needle is then taped in place. Because movement easily dislodges the needle, these are difficult to maintain for long periods.

**Over-the-needle catheters** consist of a needle with an overlying plastic catheter. After the needle is introduced into the vessel, a flashback of blood is seen in the proximal chamber. The catheter is slipped over the needle into the lumen, and the needle withdrawn. To prevent catheter embolus, the needle should not be reinserted once it is removed. Lastly, the catheter is attached to the IV line. Because of their short length, these catheters are not suitable for central access.

Through-the-needle catheters consist of a large needle inserted into a vessel, with a plastic catheter advanced through the needle. The catheter is never withdrawn through the needle, lest catheter disruption and embolization occur. The needle is withdrawn partially, and a plastic guard is snapped over the needle.

**The Seldinger technique** requires a needle on a syringe that is inserted into the vessel. After blood flashback, the syringe is removed, and a J wire is advanced through the needle. The J wire should not be forced if it does not pass easily. A constant grip should be kept on the wire to prevent its embolization. The needle is removed, and the catheter is advanced over the wire. It is sometimes necessary to enlarge the skin puncture with a scalpel prior to advancing the catheter. Once the catheter is passed, the J wire is removed. Some systems require an introducer-dilator, to be inserted over the wire before catheter placement. The introducer is advanced over the wire, followed by catheter placement over the introducer.

All IV lines should be checked for correct placement prior to use. IV fluid should run freely, without extravasation (swelling at the site), or leakage. When the line is properly placed, lowering the IV bag below the patient should result in a flow of blood downhill. This is easily visualized in the IV tubing and confirms correct placement. Antibiotic ointment can be placed at the insertion site. The catheter should be taped in place in such a manner that extravasation can be detected. Central venous catheters should be sutured in place. A gauze or film barrier dressing should cover the insertion site. Sites should be checked daily and changed every 48 h.

### Complications of Vascular Access

Complications are divided into immediate and delayed. Immediate complications include pain, bleeding, hematoma, local infiltration of IV fluids, catheter embolization, and air embolus. Delayed complications are infection, phlebitis, and tissue damage from subcutaneous infiltration of sclerosing agents. Fluid overload can complicate vascular access. Other problems are site dependent, based on the anatomic structures at risk. Air embolism is preventable. Whenever accessing the circulation, a finger should be kept over the open end of the catheter to avoid air being 'sucked' into the venous circulation. Gloves should always be worn. Infection of the physician/ancillary staff by blood-borne pathogens is a complication of vascular access.

### *Prioritization of Vascular Access Methods*

When selecting a route of access, the decision is based on the clinical state. Critically ill patients require immediate access. The time needed to perform a procedure is weighed against its risks and success rate. A simple peripheral IV line, placed rapidly with minimal complications, is of more value than a venous cutdown that has greater risks and a longer performance time. Central circulation delivery times in hemodynamically stable patients are similar for peripheral and central access techniques. During cardiopulmonary resuscitation (CPR) with a peripheral line, a 20 ml flush (5 ml in children) insures prompt delivery of medication to the central circulation.

Most patients should have an initial attempt at a peripheral line. The progression for access procedures begins with the peripheral line and advances to increasingly more invasive and risky procedures. If a peripheral attempt fails, the external jugular vein may be attempted followed by the femoral vein, the neck/chest vessels (internal jugular or subclavian veins), arid lastly a venous cutdown. In critical emergencies of young children, an intraosseous line should be considered early. Multiple attempts may be performed simultaneously.

### *Vascular Access Techniques*

*Peripheral venous cannulation and catheter lock:* Peripheral venous cannulation is the simplest method and has the lowest complication risk.

1. **Indications.** This is the first choice for most patients. Indications include volume replacement and drug delivery. A catheter lock is used when IV fluids are unnecessary but there is a potential need for access. Examples include patients who require monitoring for arrhythmias, IV medications, and if IV fluids are contraindicated (renal failure and heart failure). A catheter lock is cost-effective and requires much less monitoring.
2. **Contraindications.** Since peripheral access traverses the skin and utilizes the venous circulation, these two structures must be intact and not infected. Major extremity trauma, massive edema, overlying cellulitis, and thrombophlebitis may preclude use of the affected extremity. Line placement in the lower extremities of diabetics is a relative contraindication due to difficulties with healing and infection.
3. **Equipment needed.** Gloves, tourniquet, povidone-iodine or isopropyl alcohol swabs for skin preparation, gauze sponges, antibiotic ointment, tape, and an IV catheter are needed.
4. **Method of insertion.** Vein selection is the most important determinant of success. A large straight vein, not at a joint, in the nondominant upper extremity, is ideal. Some prefer inserting the catheter into the fork of two veins. Adjuncts for vein localization include tourniquet placement, muscular pumping of the extremity by the patient, tapping lightly over the vein, placing the extremity in a dependent position, or putting warm towels over the potential site. In the adult patient, 1/4 inch of 2% nitroglycerin paste, spread over 1 inch, at the anticipated insertion site, may help cannulate small veins.

Nitroglycerin paste should be removed after a few minutes, prior to catheter insertion. A tourniquet (Penrose drain, sphygomomanometer cuff) is placed 5 cm proximal to the planned site of insertion. It should be of sufficient tightness to occlude the veins, but not to exceed arterial pressure. Skin is prepared with either isopropyl alcohol or povidone-iodine. For most peripheral catheter insertions, anesthesia is not required. Xylocaine, 1%, is an effective anesthetic, but it should be used in volumes that do not distort the insertion site (0.1–0.2 cc). To insert an over-the-needle catheter, the skin is pulled taut and the needle introduced at approximately 30°. Once through the skin, the needle is advanced parallel with the vein until a pop is felt, or until the catheter chamber fills with blood. The catheter is advanced over the needle. If the catheter is felt to be in the lumen but fails to advance, the needle can be removed, an IV line attached, and IV fluid run in slowly while cautiously advancing the catheter. After the catheter is placed, it can be capped and flushed with saline to convert it to a catheter lock. A heparin flush does not improve the patency rate of a catheter lock.

### External Jugular Vascular Access

1. **Indications.** External jugular (EJ) cannulation is needed after peripheral attempts failed or were contraindicated. This technique's advantages include a success rate of greater than 75%, easily visualized landmarks, and a site amenable to direct pressure if the attempt fails. This procedure also avoids the complications of central access.
2. **Contraindications.** Contraindications are similar to those for peripheral access, since the EJ is essentially an anatomically constant peripheral vein. If the vessel is not visualized, another site should be chosen. Because of EJ tortuosity and valves, direct access to the central circulation is difficult without a guidewire. The anticipated need for central pressure monitoring suggests an alternative procedure. Finally, EJ access can be difficult to keep in place. In the agitated, violent, or uncooperative, another more secure method may be required. Also turning the patient's head often kinks the line, making the site positional.
3. **Equipment needed.** The same equipment is needed as for peripheral access.

4. **Method of insertion.** The patient is placed in Trendelenburg to distend the EJ and decrease the risk of air embolus. The site is prepared as for a peripheral line. Distention of the vein is aided by applying pressure with a finger just above the ipsilateral clavicle. If the patient is able, a Valsalva maneuver may cause EJ distention. The head is turned away from the insertion site and the skin is pulled taut. The catheter is introduced until vessel entry is felt. Blood flashback is not always noted in the catheter chamber. Lowering the IV bag below the level of the patient will demonstrate immediate back blood flow if the catheter is in the lumen. The catheter should be taped in place and treated in the same fashion as a peripheral IV. Looping the tubing over the ear before taping it down, will help to prevent dislodging the catheter.
5. **Complications.** The complications of EJ cannulation are similar to those of peripheral access

### Infraclavicular and Supraclavicular Subclavian Vein Access

1. **Indications.** The infraclavicular and supraclavicular routes are common approaches to the subclavian vein. The infraclavicular route is the more utilized, despite a slightly higher complication rate compared to the supraclavicular method. The indications for subclavian catheter placement include failed peripheral placement, or a specific need to access the central circulation. This procedure is one of several where fixed anatomic landmarks allow 'blind' placement. The choice of cannulation method should be strongly biased by operator experience. The supraclavicular approach is easier to perform during CPR, since it does not interfere with chest compression.
2. **Contraindications.** Contraindications to subclavian cannulation are anatomic deformity of the chest wall or clavicle, trauma to these structures, a history of radiation therapy to the region, a history of long-term subclavian catheterization, extremes of weight, and vasculitis. Because bleeding from the subclavian vessels cannot be directly compressed, this route is not used in patients with suspected coagulopathies, on anticoagulants, or if thrombolytics are anticipated. Finally, this procedure is risky in agitated patients.
3. **Equipment needed.** The choice of catheter systems determines the supplies needed. Proprietary kits may contain all that is required. This includes drapes, povidone-iodine, gauze sponges, 1% lidocaine, 25-gauge needle, 10 ml locking syringe, catheter, 4-0 suture material, needle driver, suture scissors, antibiotic ointment, and tape. Various combinations of through-the-needle, over-the-needle, and Seldinger-technique. systems are available.
4. **Method of insertion.** A thorough knowledge of the anatomic landmarks is a prerequisite for subclavian puncture. The patient is placed in the supine Trendelenburg position to decrease the risk of air embolism. To prevent injury to the thoracic duct, the right subclavian vein is most frequently used. Since pneumothorax is a complication of the procedure, if the patient is known to have one, the catheter should be placed ipsilaterally. If the attempt follows a previous failed attempt, the same side should be used, thereby preventing bilateral complications. The site is prepared in sterile fashion, with povidone-iodine, and draped. Local anesthesia with 1% xylocaine is placed in the skin and subcutaneous tissues of the conscious patient. With the infraclavicular approach, anesthesia is injected to the clavicular periosteum.
   a. **Infraclavicular approach.** The thumb and forefinger are placed, as indicated. A syringe makes needle control easier and provides the opportunity to obtain blood samples. The needle-catheter system is introduced at the junction of the middle and medial thirds of the clavicle. Care should be taken to maintain control of the needle tip. The needle is advanced, maintaining constant suction, aimed immediately above and posterior to the forefinger. A blood flashback indicates vessel lumen penetration. Do not penetrate the posterior vessel wall. Arterial cannulation is indicated by bright red or pulsatile flow. When removing the syringe from the needle, a finger is kept over the hub to prevent an air embolism.
   b. **Supraclavicular approach.** A 3 cm, 22-gauge needle may be used as a 'locator' to assist in finding the vessel before the larger catheter-needle system is introduced. The needle is placed at a point 1 cm lateral to the clavicular head of the sternocleidomastoid, and 1 cm posterior to the clavicle, in the supraclavicular fossa. It is aimed just caudal to the contralateral nipple (the axis of the needle should be approximately *10–15°* above horizontal). The needle is then advanced along a course that bisects the angle fonned by the clavicle and the sternocleidomastoid. Suction is maintained throughout the attempt. A flashback of blood, indicating vessel entry, should be seen at a depth of 2–3 cm.
5. **Complications.** Complications from subclavian placement are are as pneumothorax which is most common acutely. Even if insertion is unsuccessful, the chest should be auscultated after the procedure. A chest radiograph should be obtained to exclude pneumothorax and assure correct line placement. To prevent arrhythmias, the catheter tip should not extend into the right ventricle. If after several attempts the vessel is not cannulated, consider a different route or have a colleague attempt the procedure.

### Internal Jugular Vein Vascular Access

1. **Indications.** Internal jugular (IJ) access indications are similar to those of the subclavian. The IJ may be accessed during CPR. The choice of technique should be strongly biased by the operator experience. Since the vascular structures of the neck are easily compressed, this route is preferred over the subclavian in patients with coagulopathies.

2. **Contraindications.** Cervical trauma and anatomic distortions are contraindications. If carotid puncture occurs, contralateral attempts should be avoided. This limits the possibility of bilateral neck hematomas and associated airway compromise. Finally, carotid disease is a relative contraindication, since its puncture can cause plaque emboli.
3. **Equipment needed.** The same as for subclavian placement.
4. **Method of insertion.** The IJ is accessed by the anterior, central, or posterior approaches. A thorough anatomic knowledge prefaces any attempts at line placement. The IJ is located anterolaterally to the carotid, within the carotid sheath. In all approaches, the patient should be in Trendelenburg. If possible, a Valsalva maneuver facilitates vein distention and helps prevent air embolism. The head is turned slightly away from the insertion site. The right IJ is preferred, since the course to the superior vena cava is straighter and thoracic duct injury is prevented. The area is prepped with povidone-iodine, and in the conscious patient, local anesthesia may be obtained with 1 % xylocaine. If time permits, a 22-gauge 'locator needle' is used to preface the attempt with the larger catheter needle.

   This aids in finding the vein while minimizing damage to deep neck structures. Once the IJ is located, the procedure is repeated with the catheter needle. Carotid puncture is indicated by bright red or pulsatile blood flow. If this occurs, the attempt is terminated, the needle withdrawn, and direct pressure applied.

   a. **Anterior approach** (Fig. 22.34). After carotid identification, the needle enters the skin at the midpoint of the medial border of the sternocleidomastoid, angled at *30–45°*, and aimed at the ipsilateral nipple cannulation, without carotid puncture, may be difficult.
   b. **Central approach** (Fig. 22.35). Enter just lateral to the carotid, within a triangle fonned by the heads of the sternocleido-mastoid and clavicle, the needle is advanced caudally, at an angle of *30°*, parallel to the carotid. Constant suction is maintained. Penetration should be limited to 5 cm. With multiple attempts to prevent lacerating deep structures, withdraw the needle to the subcutaneous tissue before reinserting. Directing the needle toward the ipsilateral nipple may be used if the initial attempt fails.
   c. **Posterior approach** (Fig. 22.36). The needle enters the skin one-third of the way from the clavicle to the mastoid, just lateral to the posterior border of the sternocleidomastoid muscle.

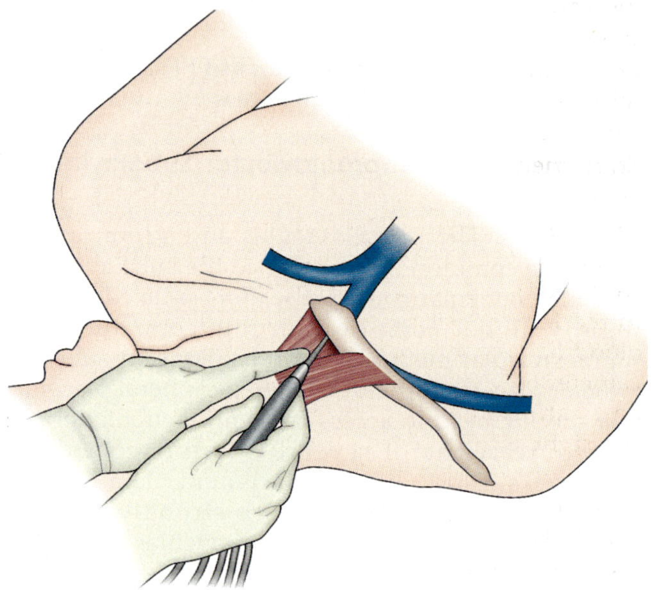

**Fig. 22.35:** Central approach to the internal jugular vein

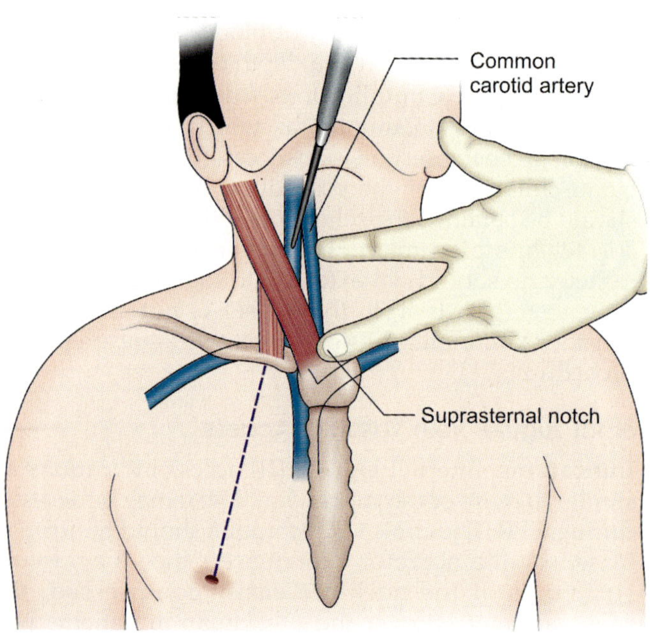


**Fig. 22.34:** Anterior approach to the internal jugular vein

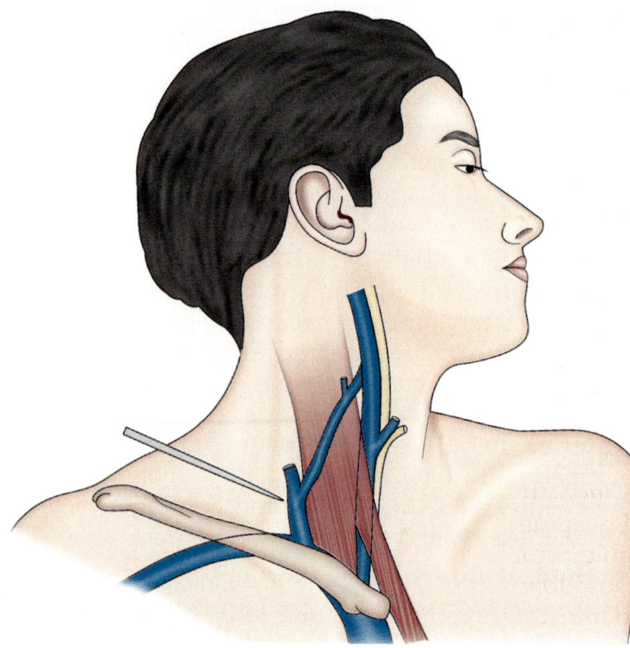

**Fig. 22.36:** Posterior approach to the internal jugular vein

While maintaining suction, the needle is directed medially and caudally, just under the sternocleidomastoid, aiming for the sternal notch, until blood is aspirated

5. **Complications.** Similar to those of the subclavian, with the addition of neck hematoma and carotid perforation. An isolated carotid puncture is treated by pressure and rarely results in dysfunction unless there is severe carotid atherosclerosis. As with any chest or neck catheterization, a chest X-ray is required to exclude pneumothorax and verify line placement. Lastly, arteriovenous fistula at the insertion site have been reported.

### Femoral Vein Vascular Access

1. **Indications.** The indication is failure to obtain peripheral access.
2. **Contraindications.** Similar to those of peripheral access, with the addition of intra-abdominal trauma. A concurrent femoral hernia is a relative contraindication.
3. **Equipment needed.** The same as needed for subclavian vein access.
4. **Method of insertion.** The site is prepared with povidone-iodine, and 1% xylocaine local anesthesia is used in the conscious patient. The needle is inserted 5–15 mm medial to the femoral pulse, while maintaining suction, until blood flashback is seen. If central access is desired, the catheter may be presized by comparing it to the patient and estimating the distance from skin entrance to the right atrium. If the catheter accesses the chest, a postprocedure X-ray should verify position. If the femoral pulse is absent (e.g. during cardiac arrest), a blind attempt may be necessary. The femoral artery crosses the midpoint of a line connecting the pubic symphysis with the anterior superior iliac crest. Punctures should be distal to this line so that, in the event of arterial laceration, direct pressure can be applied. During chest compressions of CPR, the femoral vein may pulsate. If an initial attempt aiming medial to the pulse fails, aiming at the pulsations may result in success.
5. **Complications.** Similar to those of peripheral access. In addition, femoral arterial puncture, arteriovenous fistula, femoral nerve injury, retroperitoneal hemorrhage, psoas abscess, and bowel or bladder puncture are reported.

### Saphenous Vein Cutdown Vascular Access

1. **Indications.** There are no absolute indications for saphenous vein cutdown. Because it is time-consuming, it is considered only after other methods have failed. It may be required in the chronically ill, a history of multiple recent IV lines, morbid obesity or intravenous drug users.
2. **Contraindications.** Similar to those of peripheral access.
3. **Equipment needed.** Sterile instruments should be available prior to the procedure. Materials needed include povidone-iodine, 1% xylocaine, Kelly and mosquito hemostats, scalpel with blade, 4–0 silk suture, iris scissors, catheter, 4–0 nylon skin sutures, antibiotic ointment, gauze sponges, and tape.
4. **Method of insertion.** The site is prepped with povidone-indine and draped. 1% local xylocaine is needed if conscious. If nonemergent, both exsanguination of the extremity, by raising it above the level of the heart for 5 minutes, then placement of a tourniquet proximal to the cutdown; site can limit bleeding. The greater saphenous vein runs subcutaneously anteromedially up the leg. A common site for cutdown is 1 cm anterior to the medial malleolus, where the vessel is adjacent to the tibial periosteum. It is accompanied by the saphenous nerve supplying sensation to the medial foot. A transverse skin incision is made over the vessel. Using the curved hemostat, blunt dissection parallel to the course of the vessel will free it from the surrounding tissue. Approximately, 1–3 cm of vein is mobilized and isolated. Proximal and distal silk ties are passed under the vein. The distal ligature may be tied. If a through-the-needle catheter is to be used, it may be placed into the vein under direct visualization. If using a cannula, the vessel is elevated and transversely incised 30–50% of its diameter. The cannula is passed into the vein. Once the catheter/cannula is in place, the proximal ligature is tied tightly around the vessel wall and intraluminal device. The catheter is sutured in place, and the skin closed. The extremity is immobilized to prevent accidentally dislodging the line.
5. **Complications.** Bleeding, infection, sepsis, hematoma, phlebitis, embolization, and saphenous nerve injury complicate saphenous cutdown.

### *Pediatric Vascular Access Techniques*

Many of IV access techniques in the child are similar to those in the adult; however, correctly sized equipment is required. Generally, the largest catheter that can be inserted into the vessel is used.

### *Scalp Vein Vascular Access* (Fig. 22.37)

1. **Indications, contraindications, and complications.** In the young pediatric age group, scalp veins are easily cannulated peripheral veins. Their use has the same indications, contraindications, and complications as any other peripheral IV.
2. **Equipment needed.** The same as required for peripheral IV access, as well as a razor to shave the site, and a rubber band to serve as a tourniquet.
3. **Method of insertion.** A rubber band can be placed around the head as a tourniquet, and a vein is selected. Veins are less tortuous than arteries, and their flow is toward. the heart. Shave and prepare the site. Insert the catheter as described in peripheral venous access, directed toward the heart. The rubber band is carefully removed, and the catheter is secured. A cup may be taped over the site to prevent displacement.

### *Saphenous Vein Cutdown* (Fig. 22.38)

1. **Indications, contraindications, and equipment needed.** A cutdown has the same indications, contraindications, and equipment needs as in the adult.

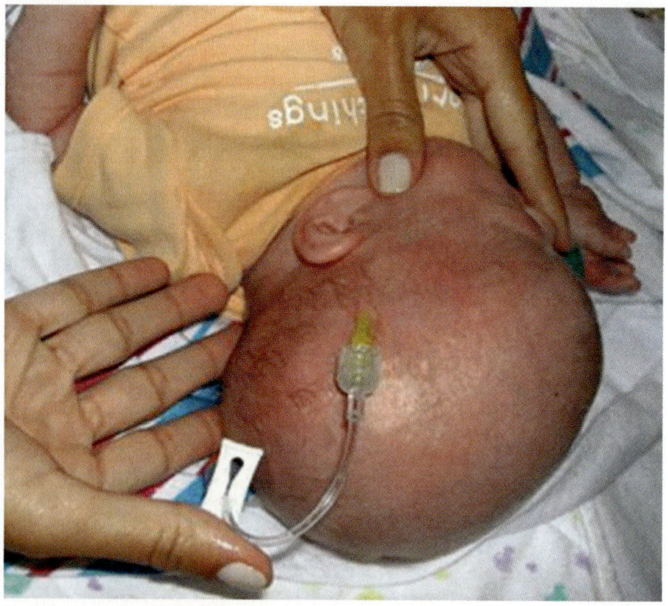

**Fig. 22.37:** Scalp vein cutdown as one the techniques for vascular access in newborn and infants

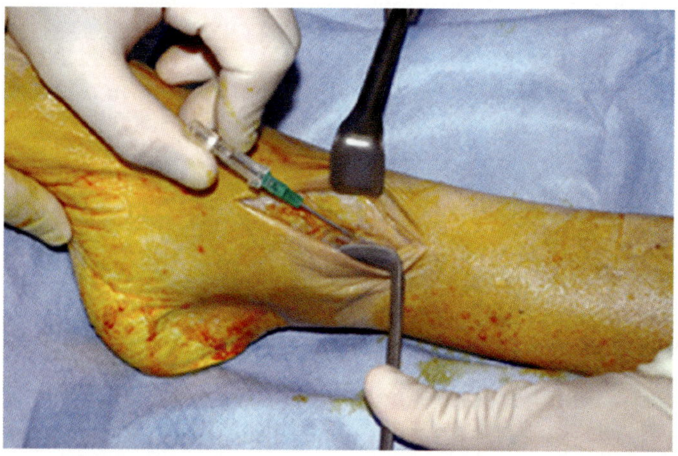

**Fig. 22.38:** Cutdown for vascular access—locate the saphenous vein along the anteromedial distal tibia. Incise skin overlying the vein and insert 18-G catheter

2. **Method of insertion**. The saphenous vein may be used for cutdown anywhere along its course. The common location is at the ankle, although the knee and groin are also used. The ankle is accessed 1–2 cm anterior and proximal to the medial malleolus. The groin site is just distal to a line joining the anterior superior iliac spine and the pubic tubercle, along the medial edge of the middle one-third of the thigh. The knee site is 1–4 cm (5–10 cm in the adult) below the joint line, along the medial ridge of the tibia. The technique is the same as in the adult. The patient may require restraint. In conscious or uncooperative patients, the extremity should be immobilized prior to the cutdown attempt. Due to smaller vessel size, a vein introducer or an 18-gauge needle with the tip bent to 90° may be used as an aid to pass the catheter into the lumen.
3. **Complications.** Bleeding, infection, sepsis, hematoma, phlebitis, embolization, and saphenous nerve injury are complications of saphenous vein cutdown (Table 22.1).

### *Intraosseous Infusion* (Fig. 22.39)

1. **Indications.** Any IV drug or solution can be given 10. The bone marrow is a noncollapsible vascular plexus with direct communication to the circulation. It is particularly useful in situations where vascular access is difficult (e.g. cardiac arrest, shock). In an emergency, only a few minutes should be given to attempt a peripheral IV before moving to the 10 route. It is considered even earlier in cardiac arrest, particularly in children less than 6 years old.
2. **Contraindications.** There is no role for 10 access in routine or elective IV placement. Other contraindications include penetrating bony trauma (inclusive of multiple

**Table 22.1:** Complications of central venous access

| |
|---|
| **General** |
| • Vascular |
| • Air embolus |
| • Adjacent artery puncture |
| • Pericardial temponade |
| • Catheter embolus |
| • Arterivenous fistula |
| • Mural thrombus formation |
| • Large vein obstruction |
| • Local hemotoma |
| • Infectious |
| • Generalized sepsis |
| • Local cellulites |
| • Osteomyelitis |
| • Septic arthritis |
| **Miscellaneous** |
| • Dysrhythmias |
| • Catheter knotting |
| • Catheter malposition |
| **Subclavian and internal jugular approaches** |
| • Pulmonary |
| • Pneumothorax |
| • Hemothorax |
| • Hydrothorax |
| • Chylothorax |
| • Hemomediastinum |
| • Hydromediastinum |
| • Neck hematoma and tracheal obstruction |
| • Tracheal perforation |
| • Endotracheal cuff perforation |
| **Neurologic** |
| • Phrenic nerve injury |
| • Brachial plexus injury |
| • Cerebral infarct |

*Source:* From Roberts JR, Hedges JR, Clinical procedures in emergency medicine, 3rd ed. Philadephia WE Saunders, 1998:376 with permission.

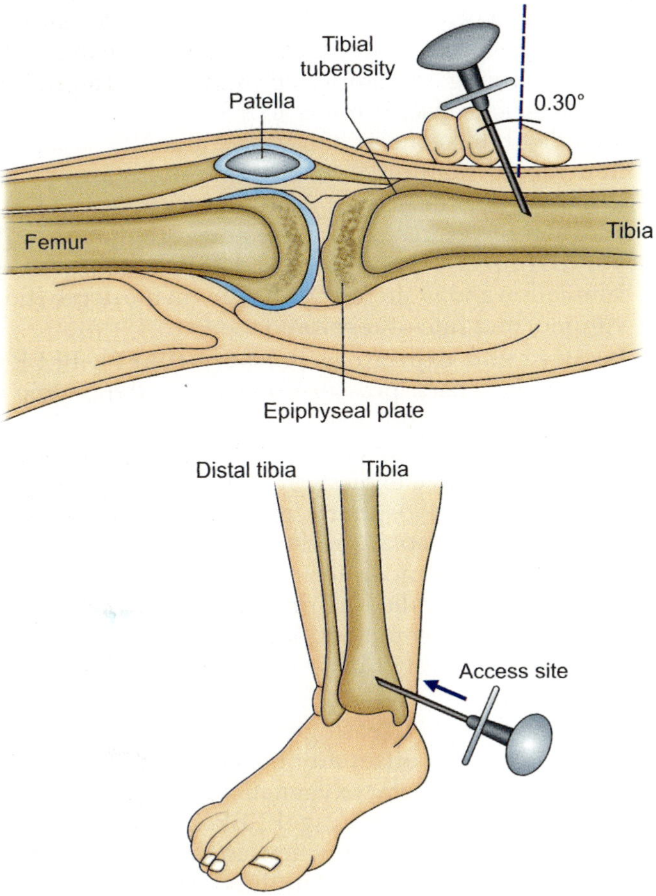


**Fig. 22.39:** Inserting the intraosseous needle

intraosseous attempts) or concurrent extremity fracture. Areas of overlying cellulitis, or osteomyelitis at the desired site, preclude 10 access. Although there is no well-defined cutoff, 10 access is more difficult with older age.

3. **Equipment needed.** Povidone-iodine, gauze sponges, hemostat, tape, and a needle are required. Commercially available 10 needles are easiest; however, bone marrow biopsy and spinal needles are alternatives. In premature infants or neonates, a 19- or 21-gauge butterfly may suffice. However, with-out a stylet, the lumen may plug with bone.
4. **Method of insertion.** The most common site for infusion is the proximal tibia 1 cm below the tibial tuberosity, medially, on the tibial plateau. The ankle malleoli, the midline distal femur 1 cm above the patella, and the iliac crests at the inferior aspect of the iliac spine are alternatives. The area is prepped with povidone-iodine. Reasonable force is required to place the needle (practice with a chicken bone is an excellent simulation). As the needle is advanced, a back and forth twisting motion eases insertion. The needle is angled away from the growth plate. A distinctive pop is felt when the marrow cavity is entered. Correctly placed, the needle should stand unsupported. To verify position, bone marrow can be aspirated and IV fluid should flow easily without extravasation. Flushing the needle may be needed if bone marrow results in obstruction. A hemostat, perpendicularly grasping the needle where it enters the skin, may be taped to the leg to help hold the needle in place. A paper cup, taped over the needle, may serve as a guard. A dressing is placed and the extremity immobilized. Alternative access should be obtained as soon as possible, since many of the complications can be avoided by the temporally short usage of this method.
5. **Complications.** Infusion fails for a number of reasons including incomplete penetration, through and through penetration of the bone, extravasation, and leakage from a previous puncture attempt. Compartment syndrome, iatrogenic fracture, and osteomyelitis are reported. Bone marrow and fat emboli may occur following intraosseous placement, but there is little effect clinically. There may be a risk of embolism in patients with right-to-left shunts

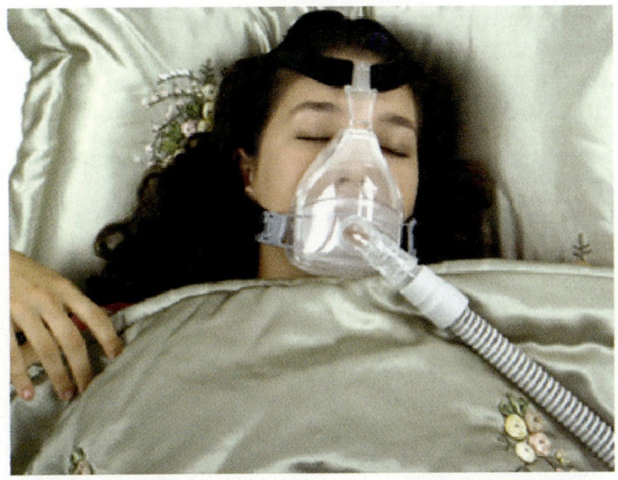

**Fig. 22.40:** A patient is sleeping with a bedside machine, which supplies continuous positive airway pressure (CPAP)

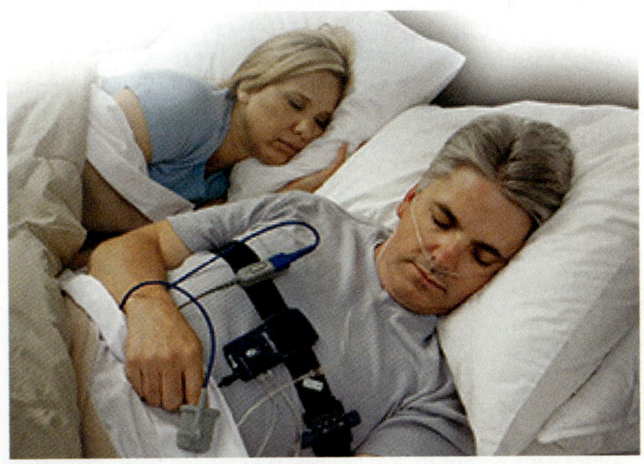

**Fig. 22.41:** At home sleep studies are most commonly recommended for people suspected of having the most common of apnea classifications, obstructive sleep apnea. This type of apnea is a blockage or partial blockage that occurs in a person's airway caused by excess tissue that collapse once muscles have relaxed during sleep (usually in people with necks size greater than 17 inches). An enlarged tongue or uvula can also be a culprit if it fall back causing restricted air to the lungs

## D. MANAGEMENT OF VENTILATION

For critically ill patients, application of contemporary lung-protective ventilator strategies can significantly impact morbidity. Additionally, noninvasive augmentation of ventilation (NIV) with devices such as continuous positive airway pressure masks and nasal bilevel positive airway pressure, has been shown to play an important role in certain, rapidly reversible causes of respiratory distress. This chapter provides a basic overview of concepts and considerations in the decision to ventilate, selection of ventilator methods, and management of the various settings (Figs 22.40 and 22.41).

### Basic Concepts and Considerations in the Decision to Assist Ventilation

#### *Respiratory Terms and Concepts*

1. **Oxygenation and ventilation** (Figs 22.42 and 22.43). Oxygenation can be thought of as the delivery of oxygen to the body. It is reflected in a number of measures including the degree to which blood is saturated with oxygen ($SaO_2$) and the partial pressure of oxygen in the blood ($PaO_2$). Ventilation generally refers to filling and emptying of the lungs with a gas. In the strict sense, it refers to the removal of carbon dioxide. In the context of invasive and NIV, oxygenation can be manipulated through alterations in the inspired concentration of oxygen ($FiO_2$) and the addition of positive end expiratory pressure (PEEP). Ventilation ($CO_2$ removal) is a function of minute ventilation and is altered by changes in the depth (tidal volume) and rate of respiration.

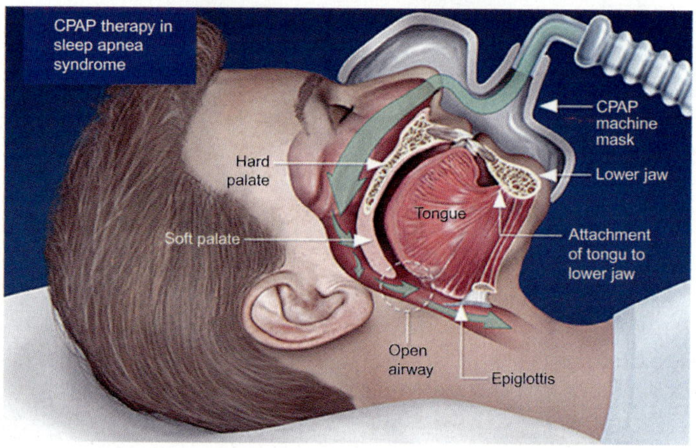


**Fig. 22.42:** Continuous positive airway pressure (CPAP) is pressurized air generated from a bedside machine. The air is delivered through a tube, connected to a mask, covering the nose. The force of the pressurized air splints the airway open. The CPAP opens the airway like air into a balloon; when air is blown into the balloon, it opens and gets wider. This is exactly how CPAP clears the airway

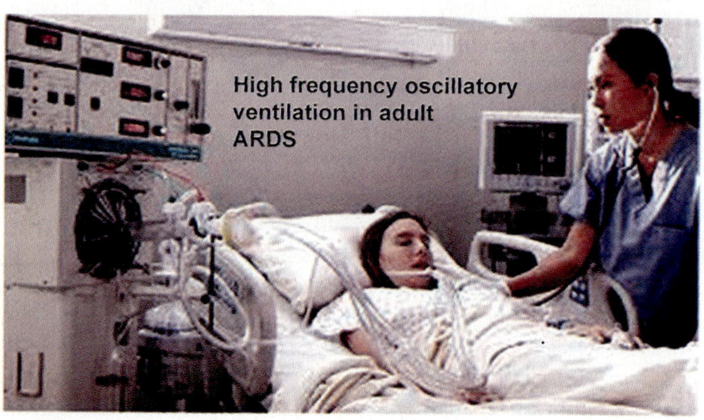


**Fig. 22.43:** High-frequency oscillatory ventilation in adult acute respiratory distress syndrome management in ED

2. **Positive end expiratory pressure (PEEP).** PEEP is essentially a back-pressure that limits the degree of expiratory flow and serves to open collapsed alveoli and prevent other alveoli from collapsing. At the end of normal passive expiration, the alveolar pressure is equal to the atmospheric pressure (zero reference point). If the alveolar pressure is intentionally maintained above atmospheric pressure at the end of expiration, it is called extrinsic PEEP. This decreases intrapulmonary shunt and increases lung compliance with the end effect of improving oxygenation.

   On the negative side, PEEP can also decrease cardiac performance by decreasing cardiac filling and cardiac output. This can offset any beneficial effects created by improving alveolar oxygenation. Caution should be observed when applying PEEP in the setting of significant cardiac dysfunction. In order to determine the optimal level of PEEP in these patients, measurement of the cardiac output must be performed and the PEEP must be titrated to balance oxygenation ($PaO_2$) and cardiac performance. The routine application of '5 cm of $H_2O$ of physiologic PEEP' to all ventilated patients hasnot been shown to be beneficial whereas small babies and children in respiratory distress generate PEEP by grunting, adults to not routinely generate 'physiologic PEEP' by forced exhalation against glottic closure. The settings in which PEEP is potentially beneficial are as follows:

   a. ***Obstructive lung disease.*** The collapse of small airways in asthma and COPD can promote air trapping. The application of PEEP can help to keep airways open, reducing the effects of this process and improving oxygenation and ventilation. The PEEP must be delivered at a level lower than the patient's COPD-related auto-PEEP.

   b. ***Enhanced oxygenation.*** In cases where inadequate oxygenation occurs despite high $FiO_2$ or where oxygen toxicity is a potential complication, the application of PEEP can improve alveolar oxygenation by the above mechanisms and allow for the use of a lower $FiO_2$. Remember that a trade-off occurs if the PEEP retards cardiac output and thereby reduces the delivery of oxygen to end organs and tissues.

3. **Intrinsic PEEP (Auto-PEEP)**. Intrinsic PEEP can be generated during rapid ventilation with high title volumes by causing incomplete exhalation of

inspired air. Auto-PEEP also occurs in patients with COPD (and during severe asthma exacerbations) due to air trapping in the alveoli. This positive pressure must be overcome during normal inspiration to move air into the lungs. This adds significantly to the work of breathing. During mechanical ventilation, failure to recognize auto-PEEP can lead to progressive air trapping until alveolar positive pressure becomes greater than proximal airway pressure. This decreases the effect of further ventilation, compromises hemodynamics and can induce pulmonary barotrauma (also called 'volutrauma'). Maintaining the inspiratory/expiratory ratio greater than 2:1 can significantly lessen the amount of auto-PEEP generated during ventilation. Auto-PEEP can be measured on a ventilator by occluding the expiratory port just before the next breath is given. When the pressures in the lungs and the ventilatory circuit equilibrate, the auto-PEEP is displayed on a pressure gauge.

4. **Continuous positive airway pressure (CPAP).** CPAP is PEEP that is applied in the setting of the spontaneously breathing patient. It can be delivered by face maskor to a spontaneously breathing patient on the ventilator.
5. **Pressure support.** *IPAP-EPAP = Pressure support.* Pressure support is a constant pressure delivered to a patient during spontaneous inspiration. By reducing the work of breathing, it serves to enhance the patient's tidal volume (TV), and improve comfort. It can be applied to a spontaneously breathing patient on a ventilator or by face mask during NIV.
6. **Peak inspiratory pressure (PIP).** Measured at the end of inspiration, the PIP is directly proportional to the resistance to airflow (airway resistance) and to the elastance of the lungs and chest wall. In lung protective ventilator strategies, monitoring the PIP has become less important than control of the plateau pressure.
7. **Plateau pressure (Pplat).** Plateau pressure reflects the pressure which causes distension of the alveoli. Plateau pressure refers to a plateau that forms in the pressure-volume curve. If the inspired volume of air is held in the lungs at the end of inspiration by occluding the ET tube or ventilator circuit for 1–2s, the pressure in the pulmonary system equilibrates such that the proximal airway pressure approximates the peak alveolar pressure. This forms the pressure-volume curve plateau. During this breath hold maneuver, there is no air flowing, therefore airflow resistance can not contribute the measurement of Pplat. Plateau pressure is then proportional only to elastance.
8. **Airflow resistance (AR).** AR occurs during bronchospasm, or by obstruction of the ETT (secretions or kinking) or of the airway by secretions or mucus plugs. AR is calculated as follows: PIP-Pplat-airflow Resistance. If peak inspiratory pressure is proportional to airflow resistance and to elastance and plateau pressure is proportional to elastance, then the difference between peak and plateau pressure approximates airflow resistance.
9. **Lung compliance.** Compliance can be thought of as distensibility or the change in volume of the lung divided by the change in pressure required to generate that volume, when the compliance is increased, the lungs are more easily distended and the same volume of air is delivered with less pressure required.
10. **Permissive hypercapnea**. By adjusting the tidal volume to less than 5–8 ml/kg, the minute ventilation falls (a product of tidal volume and respiratory rate) and the retention of $CO_2$ occurs. When this strategy of limiting pressure or volume is initiated to protect the lung from ventilation-induced injury, it is called permissive hypercapnea. Some authors advocate correction of acidosis with supplemental bicarbonate, others advocate permissive acidemia. Arterial pH of less than 7.2 has be maintained without significant complications.

### Making the Decision to Control or Assist Respiration

1. **Indications for respiratory intervention.** The primary goals of intervention in a patient's respirations are to improve gas exchange and relieve respiratory distress (by decreasing the work of breathing). Secondary goals include protection of the patient's lungs from aspiration-induced injury when airway protective reflexes, are altered; intentional hyperventilation (to manage increased intracranial pressure) and the delivery of heated humidified oxygen in hypothermic patients.
   a. **Respiratory failure.** Respiratory failure occurs when a patient is unable to oxygenate or ventilate adequately to meet their physiologic needs. The decision to intervene is based on abnormalities found on blood gas analysis and often more importantly, the clinician's observation of the patient who appears to be in respiratory distress. Generally accepted criteria for the initiation include the following.
   b. **Oxygenation failure.** $PaO_2$ less than 60 on $FiO_2$ greater than 40%.
2. **Ventilation failure**
   a. The best indicator of hypo ventilation is an abnormal pH. A pH of less than 7.3 resulting from hypoventilation should prompt intervention. Intervention at a higher pH may be necessary if the patient appears fatigued or has significant comorbidity. Chronic compensated elevation in $PaCO_2$ does not require support. Based on abnormal blood gas analysis, carbon dioxide retention with a $PaCO_2$ greater than 55 with previously normal $PaCO_2$ or rise in $PaCO_2$ by 10 acutely in COPD is an indication for assistance.
   b. **Respiratory muscle fatigue.** The increased work of breathing seen with decreases in lung compliance (pulmonary edema, consolidation, pneumothorax, atelectasis) and increases in airway resistance (bronchospasm, excessive airway secretions) can

contribute to early fatigue of respiratory muscles. This can be seen clinically by agitation, diaphoresis, nasal flaring, the use accessory muscles, and abdominal (seesaw motion) breathing.

c. **Cardiovascular support.** Under normal physiologic conditions, energy expenditure for breathing is low. During states of physiologic stress, such as cardiogenic, hypovolemic or septic shock, the oxygen demand of the pulmonary mechanism rises significantly. Early intervention with endotracheal intubation (ETI) or NIV in patients with significant hemodynamic compromise can improve oxygenation to the ischemic myocardium and lessen its workload.

d. **Aspiration protection.** When a patient appears obtunded or lacks a gag reflex, ETI becomes vital to decrease the risk of aspiration and its attendant complications.

## Invasive Ventilation

A. **Endotracheal intubation (ETI).** Unless specific contra-indications exist, virtually all intubations should be performed using rapid sequence intubation (RSn as this has become the standard of care for airway management.

B. **Ventilator mechanisms.** Ventilators can be either volume cycled or pressure cycled. In pressure cycled ventilation, inspiration ceases when a set pressure limit is reached, delivering a variable tidal volume depending on airway resistance and the compliance of the patient's lungs. Volume cycled machines deliver a preset tidal volume with each breath, irrespective of the amount of pressure required. They can also have a limit set, which will terminate inspiration after a certain maximum pressure is reached. Although both types of cycling can be used for the common ventilation modes, volume cycled ventilators have become the standard in the adult patient setting.

C. **Choosing the mode of ventilation.** Modern ventilators allow the clinician a number of choices for the mode of ventilation. The most frequently utilized modes are assist-control ventilation and intermittent mandatory ventilation. With the exception of certain specific circumstances, there is no proven advantage of one type over another. A third important, but less commonly employed mode called pressure-controlled ventilation will be briefly discussed.

1. **Assist-control ventilation (ACV or A/C).** ACV combines.

2. **Forms of ventilatory support.** In the absence of inspiratory effort, the control mode delivers a preset tidal volume to the patient at a predetermined number of times per minute. If the patient begins to take a breath spontaneously, the ventilator senses the negative pressure generated during the attempt and provides the patient an additional positive pressure breath at the preset tidal volume.

a. **Advantages of A/C.** Spontaneous breaths are assisted and less work is needed to breathe.

b. **Complications of A/C.** The delivery of a full tidal volume breath with each inspiratory effort may cause the hyperventilating patient to 'breath stack,' inducing barotrauma. Severe alkalosis can also result. These patients may benefit from IMV mode.

c. **Intermittent mandatory ventilation (IMV).** IMV, used almost exclusively in the synchronized mode (SIMV), provides a set tidal volume at a predetermined rate. If a patient initiates a spontaneous breath through the high resistance ventilator circuit, no additional assistance is provided and tidal volumes are often less than the preset volumes. The mandatory breaths are synchronized to the spontaneous ones to avoid delivery of a full tidal volume to a partially or fully inflated lung. This avoids 'breath stacking' and minimizes the risk of barotrauma.

d. **Advantages of SIMV.** Severe hyperventilation and breath stacking are less likely to occur in this mode.

e. **Complications of SIMV.** In the absence of ventila. tory assist, excessive spontaneous effort through the high-resistance ventilator circuit can lead to early respiratory muscle fatigue. Excessive work of breathing can complicate cardiac dysfunction.

3. **Pressure-controlled ventilation (PCY).** By utilizing a pressure-cycling strategy, an inspiratory breath is delivered until a preset pressure is reached, at which time passive expiration occurs. With this 'lung-protective' strategy, overdistension of alveoli is prevented and the risk of barotrauma is decreased. To be effective, the patient must be passive with little or no intrinsic inspiratory effort. The tidal volume generated depends on the patient's airway resistance and pulmonary compliance.

D. **Choosing inspired oxygen percentage ($FiO_2$).** The initial $FiO_2$ should be 100%. After evaluating the patient's oxygenation with a 20 min postintubation ABG, the percentage can be lowered to nontoxic levels (less than 60%) and titrated to keep the saturation above 90% and/or the $PaO_2$ adequate. Careful addition of PEEP can help to augment oxygenation.

E. **Choosing the tidal volume (Vt).** Traditional tidal volumes of 10–15 ml/kg were recommended to prevent alveolar collapse. Newer, lung-protective strategies recommend Vt of 5–10 ml/kg to help reduce ventilator-induced lung injury. If alveolar collapse, evidenced by hypoxemia occurs, small amounts of PEEP can be added. With Vt of less than 8 ml/kg, hypercarbia may result. In circumstances where it is well tolerated, a permissive hypercapnea strategy can be employed to lessen complications of ventilation.

F. **Choosing the rate.** Although the typical starting adult respiratory rate is 12–14 breaths per minute (BPM), it can vary considerably (6–20 BPM) depending on the goal of the ventilatory support. Since alveolar ventilation (removal of $CO_2$) is a product of the respiratory rate and tidal volume, the rate can be titrated to keep the $pCO_2$ in the desired range. Patients who benefit from hyperventilation may have respiratory rates as high as 20 BPM. In patients who have air trapping diseases (COPD, asthma), intentional hypoventilation with decreased respiratory rates can provide a longer time for air to be released from the lungs, avoiding barotrauma. A concomitant rise in $pCO_2$ is expected with lower rates, and when this strategy is employed to protect the lungs, it is called permissive hypercapnea.

**G. Additional settings**

1. **Positive end expiratory pressure (PEEP).** The routine application of '5 cm $H_2O$ of physiologic PEEP' has not proven to be physiologic or routinely beneficial. PEEP is generally added to enhance oxygenation by recruitment of alveoli and should be used in the ED when saturation is not maintained by a high $FiO_2$. Beginning with 2.5 cm $H_2O$ of PEEP, additional support can be added in 2.5 cm $H_2O$ increments every 15 min, rarely to exceed 10 cm $H_2O$. At levels above 12–15 cm $H_2O$, most patients experience a drop in cardiac output, in part as a result of decreased venous return. Caution should be used when utilizing PEEP in patients with potentially high levels of autoPEEP (COPD, asthma).
2. **Pressure support.** The addition of pressure support helps overcome the intrinsic resistance of the ET tube and the ventilator circuit in patients who are taking spontaneous breaths while in the ventilator. As the patient inspires, the ventilator delivers the preset amount of positive pressure to help the patient take a breath. This lowers the patient's respiratory rate, improves comfort and decreases the work of breathing. A typical setting is 10 cm $H_2O$.
3. **Inspiratory/expiratory ratio (IiE ratio).** The IiE ratio refers to the proportion of time allotted for inspiration and expiration. In the absence of lung disease, the typical IiE ratio is 1–2. In obstructive conditions (COPD, asthma) more time is required to complete expiration. Adjustment of the IiE ratio to 1: 3 or 1: 4 in these patients can decrease breath stacking and auto-PEEP. In volume-cycled ventilators the IiE ratio is determined by adjustment of the flow rate and respiratory rate. Higher flow rates produce shorter inspiratory times and longer expiratory times but can also increase peak inspiratory pressures. A concomitant decrease in respiratory rate will allow for smaller increases in flow rate.

## Supportive Care After the Initiation of Mechanical Ventilation

**Sedation/analgesia and paralysis.** Although inherently uncomfortable and stressful, mechanical ventilation is usually well tolerated by most patients after an initial adjustment period. When a patient continues to have problems with coughing, 'bucking,' and breathing out of sync with the ventilator, a complication or mechanical problem must first be ruled out. If intolerance still occurs, sedation and or paralysis is indicated to avoid potential patient injury. Other indications for deep sedation and paralysis include conditions such as asthma or COPD where high airway resistance can lead to injury with continued fighting of the ventilator.

1. **Sedation/analgesia.** Sedation should be titrated to keep the patient calm and relaxed. Most sedative agents do not have pain relief properties so the addition of opiates is beneficial.
   a. **Benzodiazepines.** Lorazepam (1–2 mg IV q 1–2 h), diazepam (5–10 mg IV q 1–2 h) and midazolam (1–5 mg q 2h) are all effective sedatives and anxiolytics.
   b. **Opiates.** Opiates produce analgesia and some sedation. They are best used with a benzodiazepine. Fentanyl (0.5–1 mcg/kg bolus q 30 min or by infusion of 2 mcg/kg/h) is a rapid-acting, short duration synthetic opiate that does not cause myocardial depression even in high doses. Other effective opiates include morphine (2–10 mg IV q 1h) and hydromorphone (dilaudid 1–2 mg q 2h).
   c. **Butyrophenones.** Haloperidol and droperidol (2–5 mg IV up to q 30 min) are excellent for acute agitation and delirium.
   d. **Propofol.** Propofol (diprivan) is an extremely effective sedative/amnestic with no analgesic properties. Because it can cause significant hypotension by vasodilatation, propofol should be used carefully in hypotensive or hypovolemic patients. Bolus (2 mg/kg over 2 min) followed by a continuous infusion (25–75 mcg/kg/min).
2. **Paralysis.** When appropriate sedation doses not abolish bucking and fighting the ventilator, paralysis is indicated. Remember that paralyzed patients are awake and require sedation. Nondepolarizing agents are preferable over depolarizers (such as succinylcholine).
   a. **Vecuronium.** *Dosage*—0.1 mg/kg bolus with repeat doses as needed or continuous infusion of 0.1 mcg/kg/min. Duration of bolus dose is 30–40 min.
   b. **Pancuronium.** *Dosage*—0.1 mg/kg bolus with repeat doses as needed or continuous infusion of 0.1 mcg/kg/min. Duration of bolus dose is 40–60 min. Vagolytic effects occur (increased HR and BP).

## Monitoring the Ventilated Patient

1. **Vital signs.** Acute changes in vital signs can indicate a change in the patient's underlying condition or a problem with mechanical ventilation (see below).
2. **Arterial blood gases (ABGs).** ABGs should be obtained 20 min after intubation. Changes in $pCO_2$ can be effected by altering the minute ventilation (tidal volume or respiratory rate). When permissive hypercapnea is employed, accumulation of $CO_2$ to 50–60 mmHg is acceptable and arterial pH is monitored. Acute deterioration in oxygenation can result from worsening underlying disease or from complications of mechanical ventilation.
3. **Peak inspiratory pressure (PIP) and plateau pressure (Pplat).** These values should be monitored as abrupt

changes in their values can indicate significant complications. In general, the Pplat should remain less than 35 cm $H_2O$ and the PIP less than 50 cm $H_2O$. Understanding the significance of the changes can lead one to the correct element in the differential diagnosis of the problem.

### Crises in the Ventilated Patient

The sudden, unexpected deterioration in clinical condition of a ventilated patient can be heralded by changes in objective measures or by apparent acute intolerance of mechanical ventilation. Frequently encountered abnormalities include increased airway pressures, acute reduction in oxygen saturation, abrupt rise in $PaCO_2$, or patient distress usually manifesting as acute agitation, bucking of the ventilator or an increased respiratory rate.

In any case of acute hemodynamic or respiratory deterioration, immediately remove the patient from the ventilator and hand-bag with 100% oxygen. Abrupt resolution of the problem can localize the problem to the ventilator.

#### *1. Ventilator Mechanical Problems*

Check the ventilator for mechanical dysfunction or disconnection from its oxygen source. If the ventilator is functioning properly, consider a problem with the chosen ventilator settings.

#### *2. Airway Problems*

If problems persist, the next place to look is at the airway. Evaluate the ET tube for cuff leak, or kinking. Next, suction the airway to remove any mucus plugging. Finally, evaluate for correct positioning of the ETT and rule out main stem intubation or dislodging of the ET tube and subsequent esophageal migration.

#### *3. Patient Problems*

If a source is not yet obvious, look for problems with the patient. Evaluate for mechanical problems such as pneumothorax, bronchospasm (wheezing), excessive abdominal distension or new pulmonary edema. Measure PIP, Pplat, and auto-PEEP levels. Consider the use of these values to help diagnose the specific problem. Next, consider the possibility of worsening of the patient's underlying condition or development of a new primary problem such as pulmonary embolism, acute MI or acute drop in hemoglobin.

#### *4. Sedation Problems*

Finally, after potentially life-threatening problems are ruled out, consider inadequate sedation, untreated painful condition and alcohol/drug withdrawal as causes of potential ventilator intolerance.

*ECMO (extra corporeal membrane oxygenation) support in critically ill*

The term extracorporeal membrane oxygenation (ECMO) was initially used to describe long-term extracorporeal support that focused on the function of oxygenation

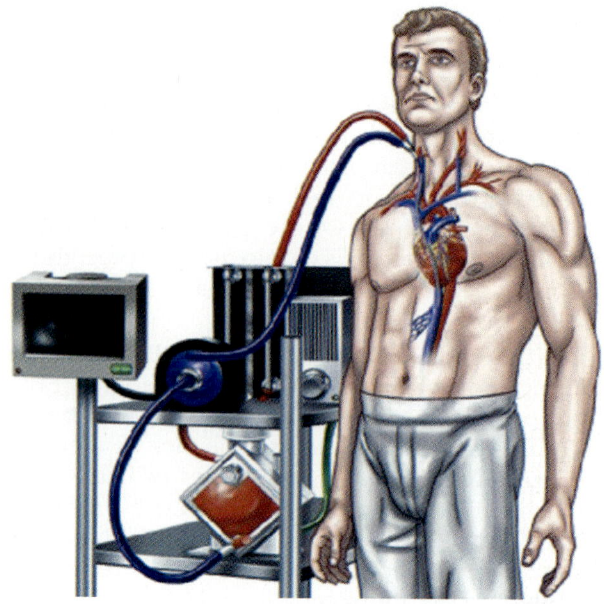

**Fig. 22.44:** ECMO in the ambulatory patient. Upper-body configurations and compact circuits facilitate mobilization in patients with respiratory failure requiring extracorporeal membrane oxygenation (ECMO)

(Fig. 22.44). Subsequently, in some patients, the emphasis shifted to carbon dioxide removal, and the term extracorporeal carbon dioxide removal was coined. Extracorporeal support was later used for postoperative support in patients following cardiac surgery. Other variations of its capabilities have been tested and used over the last few years, making it an important tool in the armamentarium of life and organ support measures for clinicians. With all of these uses for extracorporeal circuitry, a new term, extracorporeal life support (ECLS), has come into vogue to describe this technology.

In emergency medicine, extracorporeal membrane oxygenation (ECMO) is an extracorporeal technique of providing both cardiac and respiratory support oxygen to patients whose heart and lungs are so severely diseased or damaged that they can no longer serve their function. Initial cannulation of a patient receiving ECMO is performed by a surgeon and maintenance of the patient is the responsibility of the ECMO specialist and gives 24/7 monitoring care for the duration of the ECMO treatment.

*The differences between ECMO and cardiopulmonary bypass:*

- ECMO is frequently instituted using only cervical cannulation, which can be performed under local anesthesia; standard cardiopulmonary bypass is usually instituted by transthoracic cannulation under general anesthesia.
- Unlike standard cardiopulmonary bypass, which is used for short-term support measured in hours, ECMO is used for longer-term support ranging from 3–10 days.
- The purpose of ECMO is to allow time for intrinsic recovery of the lungs and heart; a standard cardiopulmonary bypass provides support during various types of cardiac surgical procedures.

### Indications for ECMO

*Patients with the following two major neonatal diagnoses require the use of ECMO:*

- Primary diagnoses associated with primary pulmonary hypertension of the newborn (PPHN), including idiopathic PPHN, meconium aspiration syndrome, respiratory distress syndrome, group B streptococcal sepsis, and asphyxia
- Congenital diaphragmatic hernia (CDH)

*Selection criteria for neonates include the following:*

- Gestational age of 34 weeks or more
- Birth weight of 2000 g or higher
- No significant coagulopathy or uncontrolled bleeding
- No major intracranial hemorrhage (grade 1 intracranial hemorrhage)
- Mechanical ventilation for 10–14 days or less
- Reversible lung injury
- No lethal malformations
- No major untreatable cardiac malformation
- Failure of maximal medical therapy

*Failure to meet these criteria is a relative contraindication for ECMO*

Qualifying patient criteria for ECMO are applied only when the infant has reached maximal ventilatory support of 100% oxygen [fraction of inspired oxygen ($FiO_2$) equals 1] with peak inspiratory pressures (PIP) often as high as 35 cm water. They include the alveolar-arterial gradient, the oxygenation index and acute deterioration.

The alveolar-arterial (A-a) gradient of 600–624 mmHg for 4–12 hours at sea level may be computed as follows (where 47=partial pressure of water vapor):

*Pediatric ECMO is indicated or considered in the following situations:*

- Low cardiac output resulting from right, left, and biventricular failure following repair of congenital heart defect
- Pulmonary vasoreactive crisis following repair of congenital heart defect leading to severe hypoxemia, low cardiac output, or both
- Rarely, as a bridge to cardiac surgery in patients with serious end-organ damage resulting from profound low cardiac output related to congenital heart disease
- As a bridge to cardiac transplant
- Possibly, as a bridge to recovery in temporary cardiomyopathy secondary to renal failure, myocarditis, and burns.

Today, other indications or less strict selection of patients in certain institutions have made the use of this technology more diverse, not only in acute cardiac problems but also in primary pulmonary diseases.

The clinical outcomes of patients undergoing ECMO can be categorized according to the indication for the ECMO—severe acute respiratory failure or cardiac failure.

#### Acute Respiratory Failure

With acute respiratory failure use of ECMO has been shown to improve survival rates. Survival rates from 50–70% have been reported in observational and uncontrolled clinical trials. The survival rates reported are better than historical survival rates.

#### Cardiac Failure

Venoarterial (VA) ECMO can provide acute support in cardiogenic shock or cardiac arrest in adults. Assuming that the brain function is normal or only minimally impaired, ECMO is provided until the patient recovers or receives a long-term ventricular assist device as a bridge to cardiac transplantation.

### Indications of ECMO in Adults

Guidelines that describe the indications and practice of ECMO are published by the extracorporeal life support organization (ELSO). Criteria for the initiation of ECMO include acute severe cardiac or pulmonary failure that is potentially reversible and unresponsive to conventional management. Examples of clinical situations that may prompt the initiation of ECMO include the following:

## BIBLIOGRAPHY


1. Advanced cardiac life support. Dallas: American Heart Association, 1997.
2. Benumoff JL. Management of the difficult adult airway. Anesthesiology 1991;75:1087–110.
3. Blackstock D. Respiratory failure. Baldwin GA (Eds). In: Handbook of pediatric emergencies. Boston: Little, Brown, 1994.
4. Bogdonoff DL, Stone DJ. Emergency management of the airway out-side the operating room. Can J Anaesth 1992;39: 1069–89.
5. Chandra NC, Hazinski MF (Eds). Textbook of basic life support for healthcare providers. Dallas: American Heart Association, 1994.
6. Cummins RO, ed. Textbook of advanced cardiac life support. Dallas: American Heart Association, 1994.
7. Guidelines 2000 for Cardiopulmonary Resuscitation and Emergency Cardiovascular Care. An International Consensus on Science. Circulation 2000;102(suppl 1–22):1–59.
8. Hurfurd WE, Bailin MT, Dvison JK, et al (Eds). Clinical anesthesia procedures of the Massachusetts General Hospital, 5th ed. Philadelphia: Lippincott-Raven Publishers, 1998.
9. Kauer S, Herd SO. Airway management and endotracheal intubation. Ripp JM, Irwin RS, Fink MP, et al (Eds). In: Procedures and techniques in intensive care medicine. Boston: Little, Brown, 1995.
10. Pediatric advanced life support. Dallas: American Heart Association, 1997–99.
11. Reisdorff EJ, Roberts MR; Wigenstein JG (Eds). Pediatric emergency medicine. Philadelphia: Saunders, 1993.
12. Roberts JR, Hedges JR (Eds). Clinical procedures in emergency medicine. Philadelphia: Saunders, 1998.

# 23 Recognition and Management of Hypertensive Emergencies

Hypertensive emergencies include both accelerated hypertension and malignant hypertension. In both cases, a recent increase in blood pressure to very high levels (≥180 mmHg systolic and ≥110 mmHg diastolic) results in target organ damage-usually seen as neurological (e.g. encephalopathy), cardiovascular or renal damage. The term malignant hypertension is usually reserved for cases, where papilloedema is present. Where there is no evidence of target organ damage (TOD), the condition is a hypertensive 'urgency' rather than 'emergency' and treatment may be more gradual. Finding accelerated hypertension or malignant hypertension in a patient demands urgent admission for assessment and treatment to lower blood pressure within hours in order to minimise further end-organ damage and reduce the risk of life-threatening events, such as myocardial infarction, encephalopathy and intracerebral or subarachnoid haemorrhage. The National Institute for Health and Care Excellence (NICE) recommends same day referral for accelerated hypertension with papilloedema and/or retinal haemorrhages, or for patients suspected of having a phaeochromocytoma (labile or postural hypotension, headache, palpitations, pallor and sweating.

*What are hypertensive emergencies ?*

Hypertensive emergencies represent severe hypertension (HTN) with acute impairment of an organ system (e.g. central nervous system [CNS], cardiovascular and renal). In these conditions, the blood pressure (BP) should be lowered aggressively over minutes to hours (Table 23.1).

**Table 23.1:** Hypertensive emergencies

- In general, diastolic blood pressure exceeds 120 mmHg
- Malignant hypertension with papilledema
- Hypertensive encephatopathy
- Severe hypertension in the setting of stroke, subarachnoid hemorrhage, and head trauma
- Acute aortic dissection[a]
- Hypertension and left ventricular failure[a]
- Hypertension and myocardial ischemia and infarction[a]
- Hypertension after coronary artery bypass operation
- Pheochromocytoma crisis[b]
- Food or Drug interactions with monoamine oxidase inhibitors[b]
- Cocaine abuse[b]
- Rebound hypertension after sudden drug withdrawal (clonidine)[b]
- Idiosyncratic drug reactions (e.g. atropine)[b]
- Eclampsia

[a]Exceptions include cardiovascular dysfusion in which low blood pressure may represent an emergency.
[b]Considered emergencies when associated with end-organ damage; otherwise treated as urgencies.

*Pathophysiology:* The pathophysiology of hypertensive emergencies is not well understood. However, an abrupt rise in vascular resistance seems to be a necessary initial step. The three major organ systems affected by high BP are the CNS , cardiovascular system, and renal system. An appreciation of the mechanisms underlying normal blood pressure regulation is vital for the correct interpretation of the many forms of hypertensive crisis and may guide the clinician in selecting the most appropriate therapy. BP is the product of cardiac output (CO) and peripheral vascular resistance (PVR), where **BP = CO × PVR.** Cardiac output is itself determined by heart rate and stroke volume, in which the latter is dependent on intrinsic myocardial contractility and the preload of the heart. For any increase in BP to occur, an imbalance in these variables is required. Most commonly, either a disproportionate increase in peripheral vascular resistance or intravascular volume is responsible, which is offset inadequately by feedback mechanisms that regulate blood pressure homeostasis. These fundamental principles apply equally to uncomplicated chronic hypertension and to a hypertensive crisis. Markedly elevated blood pressure is a cause for concern in any clinical context. However, the single most important factor leading to the development of a hypertensive crisis is not the absolute change in BP, but the rate at which mean arterial pressure (MAP) rises.

Patients with chronically elevated blood pressure undergo adaptive vascular changes, which, although in the long-term may be detrimental, may serve to protect end organs from acute increases in blood pressure. In contrast, patients who develop acutely elevated blood pressure without pre-existing hypertension suffer end-organ damage even at relatively lower blood pressure levels. When blood pressure rises, it exerts a mechanical stress on the vessel wall. Under normal circumstances, the blood vessel will respond by vasoconstriction, supporting the vascular endothelium and minimizing acute injury. This phenomenon is known as autoregulation. In severe rapidly evolving hypertensive states, this ability to autoregulate is overwhelmed, local vasodilation ensues, and the shear forces are transmitted to the endothelium. Endothelial damage leads to enhanced vascular permeability and leakage, with deposition of plasma proteins and fibrinogen in vessel walls. Mediators of coagulation and cell proliferation also are activated, with adverse short- and long-term consequences. Fibrinoid necrosis is the pathologic lesion characteristic of this type of arteriolar injury. This disruption of the arteriolar wall causes obstruction of the vessel and downstream ischemia. These changes are visible directly in the retina as linear hemorrhages dissecting along nerve fibers associated with cotton-wool spots of swollen, ischemic axons.

An important driver of many acute hypertensive emergencies is the renin-angiotensin-aldosterone system. Under normal circumstances, this system plays a valuable role in the regulation of BP and sodium homeostasis. Renin produced by the kidney stimulates the formation of angiotensin II, a potent vasoconstrictor. This in turn promotes aldosterone release and consequently the avid retention of salt and water. Significant increases in both peripheral vascular resistance and intravascular volume combine to produce an elevation in BP. In situations, such as acute intravascular volume depletion, this may be a life-saving system. However, when it is dysregulated, this system may play a central role in exacerbating hypertensive crises. Regardless of the cause of the initial abrupt rise in BP, if renovascular injury and ischemia ensue, this system will be activated, generating a feedback loop of further rises in BP, which result in yet more renovascular insult. This vicious cycle will lead inevitably to progressive end-organ damage if left unchecked.

## HYPERTENSIVE URGENCIES

Hypertensive urgencies have traditionally been described as situations, where severe elevations in BP are not causing immediate end-organ damage, but should be controlled within 24 hours (Table 23.2). However, there have been no clinical trials to clearly define which patients are at greatest risk of developing complications, if left untreated over this time period. Accordingly, this is probably the most difficult category of patient to identify within the emergency department (ED). It has been well documented that long-term treatment of HTN reduces cardiovascular morbidity and mortality. Over the years, the threshold for treatment and the targets sought have steadily fallen. The recent hypertension optimal treatment (HOT) randomized trial demonstrated a treatment benefit all the way down to a diastolic blood pressure (DBP) of 82 mmHg.

**Table 23.2:** Hypertensive urgencies

- Diastolic blood pressure exceeds 120 mmHg, but patients have no symptoms, and there are no signs of tissue damage
- Severe hypertension, accelerated hypertension
- Pheochromocytoma cirisis
- Food or drug interactions with monoamine axidase inhibitors
- Rebound hypertension after sudden drug withdrawal
- Idiosyncratic drug reactions
- Preoperative hypertension
- Postoperative hypertension

There is very little evidence however to support a significant short-term benefit of BP control. A landmark study of hypertension published in the 1960's provides useful insights in this context. It compared placebo with drug treatment in patients who have severe hypertension, defined as DBPs between 115 and 130 mmHg. No difference in adverse events within the first 3 months was demonstrated. Furthermore, there is a growing body of evidence to suggest the practice of urgently lowering blood pressure in patients who have uncontrolled severe hypertension may actually be associated with increased risk to the patient. Shayne and Pitts, in a recent review of this topic, have suggested that patients who have evidence of previous end-organ damage, but who are not acutely compromised should be defined as having a hypertensive urgency and merit closer monitoring and follow-up. Other investigators have argued for a simpler classification of just two categories, hypertensive emergency and uncontrolled severe hypertension, with all patients in the latter class receiving close follow-up until a gradual reduction in blood pressure to target levels has been achieved.

Most antihypertensive drugs with a relatively short onset of action have been shown to be effective in the treatment of severely elevated BP. Captopril is the fastest acting oral angiotensin-converting enzyme (ACE) inhibitor. At low doses, it rarely causes marked hypotension, although this potential exists particularly among those who are volume-depleted or who have renal artery stenosis. Clonidine also is widely used in this setting, and the dose can be repeated hourly to safely and effectively reduce very high blood pressure. Clonidine has similar efficacy to nifedipine but a more favorable safety profile. Side effects include rebound hypertension and sedation. Short-acting nifedipine is not recommended because patients are subjected to possible uncontrolled hypotension. Labetalol is available in an oral preparation, which can be given in hourly doses and has been shown to be highly effective in the acute reduction of blood pressure.

## EPIDEMIOLOGY

Accelerated hypertension may be seen in association with renal disease or may occur as a discrete entity and will occur in approximately 1% of patients with essential hypertension. Average age at presentation is 40 years. Men are more commonly affected than women.

## AETIOLOGY

Some conditions that can precipitate in hypertension crisis are listed in Table 23.3.

- Accelerated or Malignant hypertension may be associated with any cause of secondary hypertension
- Unilateral renovascular hypertension, e.g. renal artery stenosis
- Renin-secreting neoplasms
- Trauma to the kidneys
- Renal vasculitis, e.g. scleroderma, polyarteritis and systemic lupus erythematosus (SLE)
- Phaeochromocytoma
- Cocaine abuse
- Drugs such as monoamine-oxidase inhibitors, combined oral contraceptives or the withdrawal of alcohol, alpha stimulants, such as clonidine or beta-blockers
- Sodium-volume overload and low renin levels, e.g. acute glomerulonephritis and primary aldosteronism
- Pre-eclampsia/Eclampsia
- Hyperthyroidism or Hypothyroidism.

### Clinical Signs and Symptoms

Hypertensive emergencies may be asymptomatic or may present with any of the many symptoms and/or signs of end-organ damage:

- Headache
- Fits
- Nausea and vomiting
- Visual disturbance
- Chest pain
- Neurological deficit, e.g. cerebrovascular event (CVE)
- Bleeding due to disseminated intravascular coagulopathy (DIC)
- Microangiopathic haemolytic anemia

**Table 23.3:** Conditions that may precipitate a hypertensive crisis

- Essential hypertension (most common)
- Renovascular hypertension
- Parenchymal renal diseases
- Drug-included causes (e.g. interactions, idiosyncratic reactions exaggerated effects and abrupt withdrawal)
- Head injuries and central nervous system events (e.g. stroke and hemorrhage)
- Vascuilitis
- Collagen vascular disease

## DIAGNOSIS

The assessment and investigation of any patient thought to have accelerated hypertension should be undertaken urgently and by doctors with expertise in this field. This should include the following information:

*Full history:* It includes:

- Past medical history
- Full systems review
- Drug history including over-the-counter, herbal remedies and recreational drugs
- Full examination with blood pressure measurements—lying, standing and in both arms (looking for coarctation or aortic dissection).

*Fundoscopy:* Retinopathy, e.g. grade III (flame haemorrhages, dot and blot haemorrhages, hard and soft exudates) to grade IV (papilloedema).

*Cardiovascular examination:* Lying and standing blood pressure; look for signs of cardiac failure or pulmonary edema, carotid or renal bruits, left ventricular heave, cardiac murmurs, third or fourth heart sounds.

### Neurological Examination

### Blood Tests

- Full blood count (FBC) ± clotting screen
- Urea and electrocytes (U and Es), creatinine
- Liver and thyroid function tests (TFTs)
- Blood sugar measurement
- ± Cardiac enzymes and fasting blood lipids
- ± Ambulatory blood pressure monitoring
- Urine dip testing for protein and blood
- Plasma renin activity
- Plasma aldosterone level
- 24-hour urine for vanillylmandelic acid (VMA) and metanephrine levels
- Autoantibody levels, e.g. antinuclear factor.

## IMAGING STUDIES

1. **Chest radiography:** It is indicated in patients with chest pain or shortness of breath. Cardiac enlargement pulmonary edema widened mediastinum (Fig. 23.1).
2. **Head CT scans:** These are indicated in patients with abnormal neurologic examinations, intracranial bleeding cerebral edema (Fig. 23.2).
3. **Chest CT scan:** It can help in diagnosing dissection of aorta, dilatation and cardiomegaly (Fig. 23.3).
4. **Transesophageal echocardiography:** It can rule out aortic dissection and dilatation of aorta (Fig. 23.4).
5. **Aortic angiogram:** It is indicated in cases where aortic dissection is suspected (Figs 23.5 and 23.6).
6. **Electrocardiogram:** To assess for evidence of myocardial ischemia or left ventricular hypertrophy (Figs 23.7–23.10).

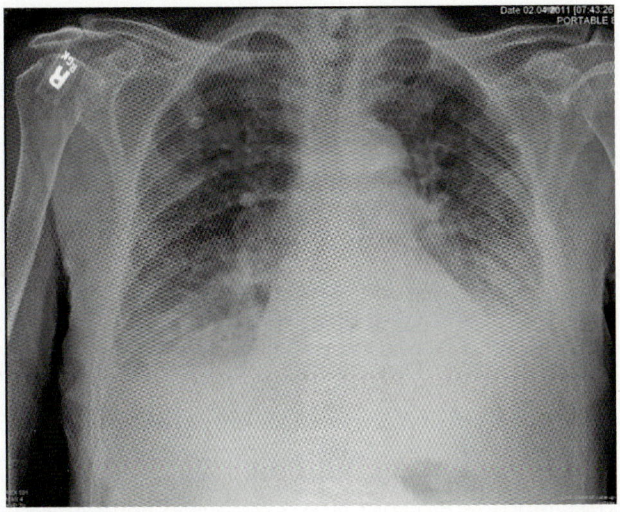

**Fig. 23.1:** This patient presented with hypoxia has larger bilateral pleural effusions and pulmonary edema. Note the vascular markings extending out to the peripheray of the lung fields and the 'cephalization' of the vascular markings (prominent vascular markings extending to the apical regions) in a patient with hypertensive crisis

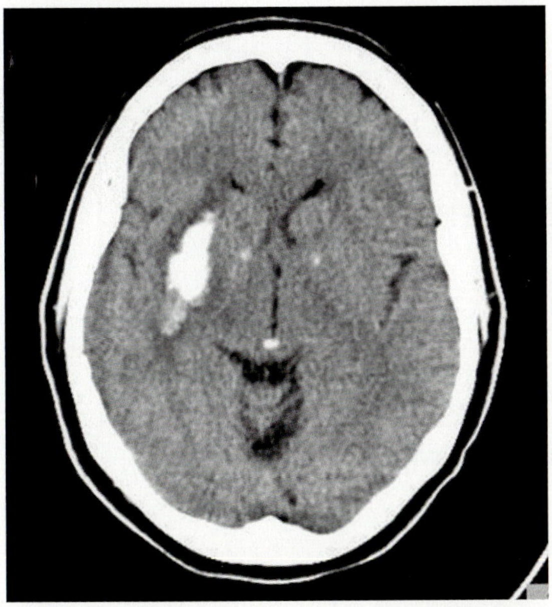

**Fig. 23.2:** A 59-year-old female with hypertension who presented with left-sided weakness demonstrated a right putaminal hemorrhage on noncontrast CT examination of the head. Tiny hyperdense foci in the basal ganglia and pineal gland represent calcifications

## MANAGEMENT

### General Measures

The aim is to reduce the blood pressure over 24–48 hours. Patients usually have altered blood pressure autoregulation and if the blood pressure is reduced too fast, there may be organ hypoperfusion.

Initially, try to reduce the mean arterial pressure by approximately 25% over the first 24–48 hours.

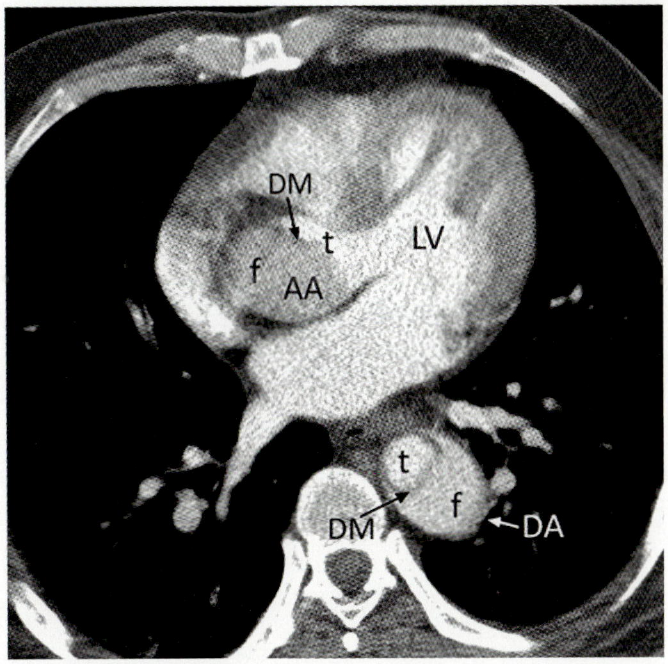


**Fig. 23.3:** A 39-year-old previously healthy man arrived with terrible chest pain and a history of transient ischemic attack. CT scanning showed DeBakey type I aortic dissection. (1) Axial CT shows the aortic dissection rising from the very beginning of the aorta ranging to the descending thoracic aorta. AA=ascending aorta; DA=descending thoracic aorta; DM=dissection membrane; f=false lumen; LV=left ventricle; t=true lumen

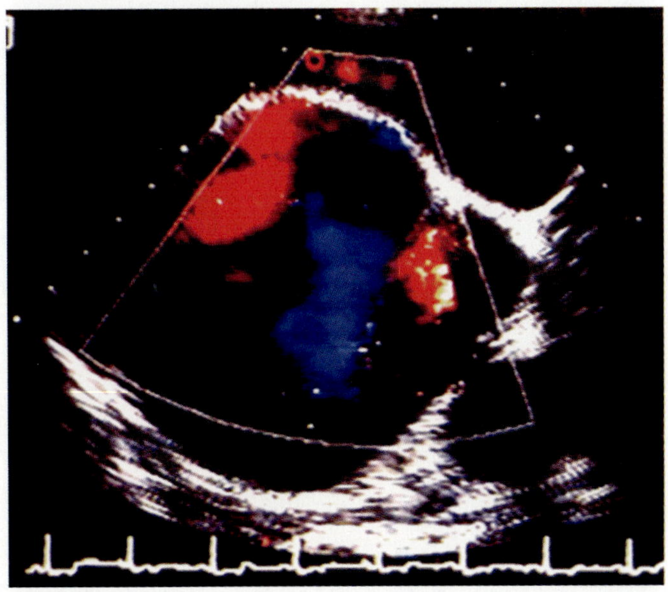

**Fig. 23.4:** Transesophageal echocardiographic view at great vessel level showing typical signs of dissection of aorta, in patient with long standing stage 11 partially treated hypertension

An arterial line is helpful for continuous blood pressure monitoring.

There may be severe sodium and volume depletion; volume expansion with isotonic sodium chloride solution may be required.

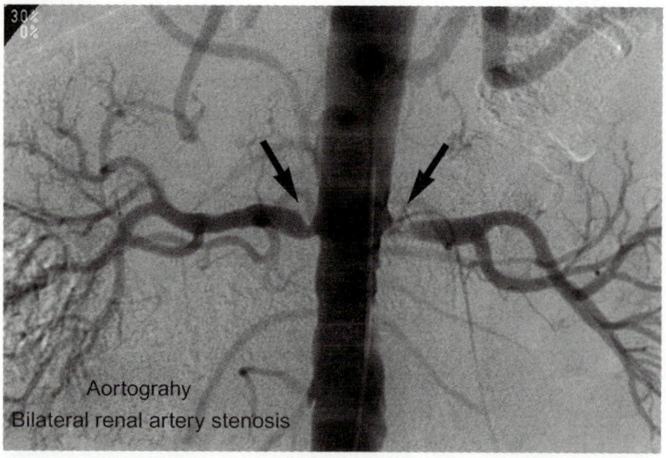


**Fig. 23.5:** Aortography shows bilateral renal artery stenosis in a patient with hypertensive crisis

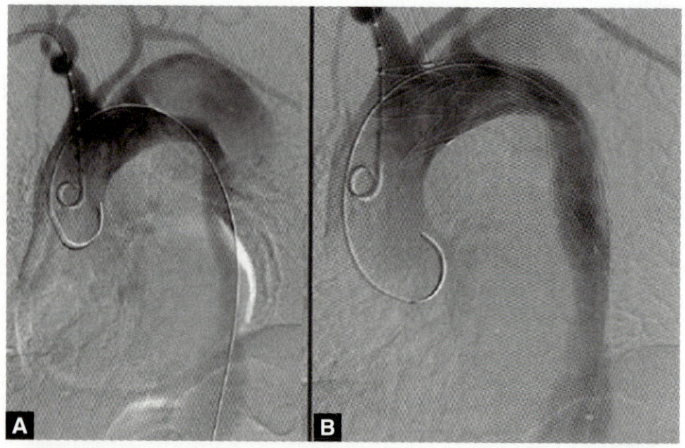


**Fig. 23.6:** (A) Intraoperative aortography demonstrating Stanford type B aortic dissection in bovine type II aortic arc. (B) Endovascular repair of Stanford type B dissection with presence of type Ia leakage

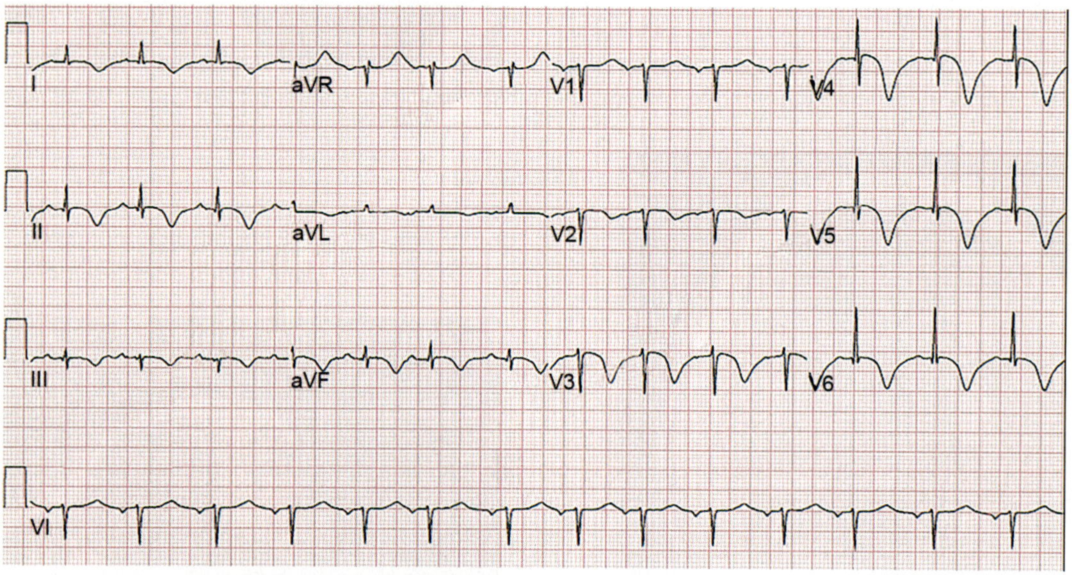


**Fig. 23.7:** Widespread deep T-wave inversion due to subarachnoid hemorrhage

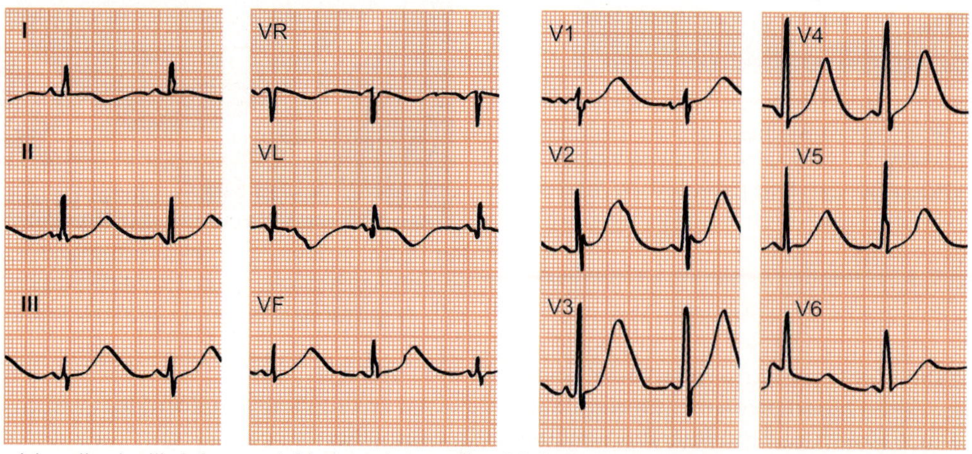


**Fig. 23.8:** A 30-year-old patient with intracranial hemorrhage. The ECG shows quite significant repolarization changes, with a very long QT-interval mainly at the expense of a very wide T-wave, positive in some leads (precordial and inferior leads) and negative in others (I, VL)

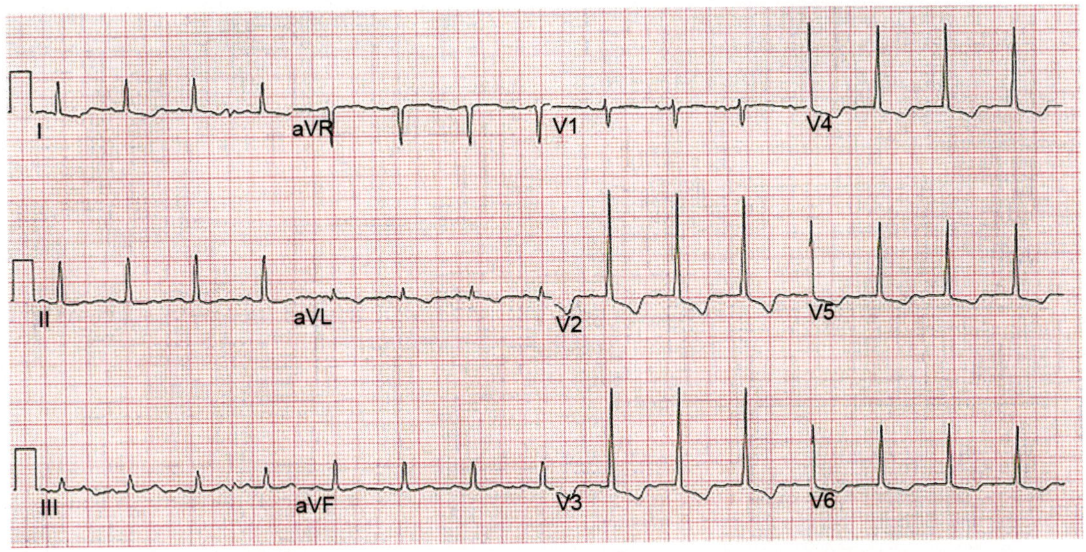


**Fig. 23.9:** Electrocardiogram ST-depression in leads 1, aVL, V2–V6 due to myocardial ischemia in severe hypertension

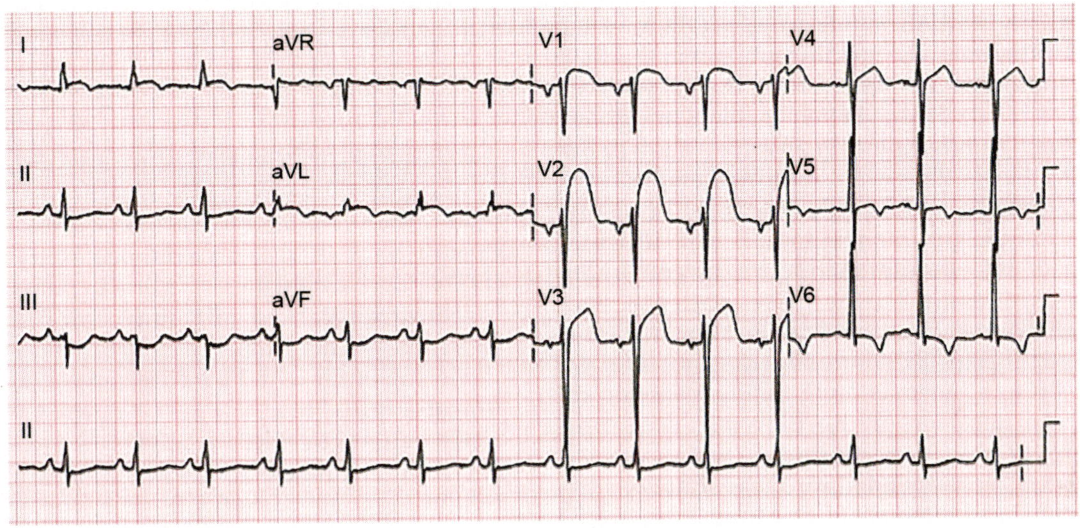


**Fig. 23.10:** Electrocardiogram showing ST-elevation and T-wave inversion in leads 1, aVL, V1 and V6 in anteroseptal myocardial infarction in elderly patient with severe hypertension

## Management of Hypertensive Emergencies

*Autoregulation:* The safe management of hypertensive emergencies requires an understanding of vascular autoregulation of vital organs. The brain, kidneys and heart exhibit mechanisms that protect from ischemic damage when blood pressure drops abruptly, a mechanism that has been described most extensively in the brain. When aortic blood pressure rises, cerebral vasoconstriction occurs. Conversely, when blood pressure falls, intracerebral vessels dilate. This ensures that cerebral blood flow remains constant over a wide range of mean arterial pressures. Although, individuals with normal cerebral vasculature can tolerate rapid reductions in blood pressure, this is not true of the majority that suffers hypertensive crises. Chronic hypertension, cerebral vascular disease and aging tend to impair normal cerebral autoregulation. When antihypertensive drugs lower the blood pressure too quickly, chronically hypertensive individuals may not tolerate the reduction and experience cerebral hypoperfusion. Symptoms include weakness and dizziness, but if this relative hypotension is sustained, there is a risk of ischemia and infarction. Strandgaard has reported that the lower limit of autoregulation occurred at an average MAP of 113 mmHg in chronic hypertensive subjects, compared with 73 mmHg in normotensive controls. A reduction in MAP of 15–20% is felt to be safe when treating most hypertensive emergencies. In the setting of stroke, greater caution is warranted as acute cerebral ischemia is associated with further impairment of cerebral autoregulation. A reduction of less than 2% in this setting may lead to an extension of the infarcted area.

*Prehospital Care:* Address the manifestations of a hypertensive emergency, such as chest pain or heart failure. Reduction of BP may not be indicated in the prehospital setting. Oxygen, furosemide (Lasix), and nitrates may all be appropriate. Under most circumstances, attempting to treat HTN directly in the prehospital setting is unwise. In particular, rapid lowering of BP can critically decrease target organ perfusion.

### Emergency Department Care

The fundamental principle in determining the necessary ED care of the hypertensive patient is the presence or absence of TOD. Initial considerations (if the patient is not in distress)—place the patient who is not in distress in a quiet room and reevaluate after an initial interview. In one study, 27% of patients with an initial DBP >130 mmHg had their DBP fall below critical levels after relaxation without specific treatment. Consider the context of the elevated BP (e.g. severe pain often causes increase in BP).

*Screen for target organ damage (TOD):* The patient's history, physical examination, laboratory studies and diagnostic tests, as outlined should be used to determine if TOD exists. Patients without evidence of TOD may be discharged with follow-up. The misconception remains that a patient never should be discharged from the ED with an elevated BP. As a result of this belief, patients are given oral medicines, such as nifedipine, in an effort to lower BP rapidly before discharge. This is not indicated and may be dangerous. Attempts to temporarily lower BP by using these medicines may result in a precipitous and difficult-to-correct drop in BP. Should this occur, target organ hypoperfusion may result. Furthermore, patients who present with high BP, may have had this elevation for some time and may need chronic BP control but may not tolerate rapid return of BP to a 'normal' level. Acute lowering of BP in the narrow window of the ED visit, does not necessarily improve long-term morbidity and mortality rates. The follow-up recommended for these situations by the Joint National Committee on High Blood Pressure is outlined in patients with TOD usually require admission and rapid lowering of BP using intravenous (IV) medications. Suggested medication depends on the affected organ system. Even in cases of hypertensive emergencies, the BP should not be lowered to normal levels. Rapid reduction in BP below the cerebral, renal, and/or coronary autoregulatory range will result in marked reduction in organ blood flow, possibly leading to ischemia and infarction. In general, the MAP should be lowered by no more than 20–25% in the first hour of treatment. If the patient remains stable, the BP should then be lowered to 160/100–110 mmHg in the next 2–6 hours. Please note the exceptions to this general rule listed below. These BP goals are best achieved by a continuous infusion of a short-acting, titratable, parenteral antihypertensive agent along with constant and intensive patient monitoring. Rapid BP reduction is indicated in the following circumstances:

1. **Acute myocardial ischemia**
   - Nitroglycerin IV
   - Beta-blockers IV
2. **Congestive heart failure with pulmonary edema**
   - Nitroglycerin IV
   - Lasix IV
   - Nitroprusside IV
3. **Acute aortic dissection:** In cases of acute aortic dissection, the systolic blood pressure (SBP) should be decreased as rapidly as possible to a goal of 100–110 mmHg or lower.
   - Labetalol IV
   - Alternative nitroprusside IV with beta-blocker IV (e.g. esmolol)
4. **Cerebral vascular accident:** Evidence exists that patients who have acute strokes have better outcomes with higher BPs. Antihypertensive therapy is not routinely recommended for patients with acute stroke and HTN. BP control affects the use of thrombolytic agents in ischemic stroke. SBP >185 mmHg or diastolic pressures >110 mmHg are contraindications to the use of tissue plasminogen activator (tPA) within the first 3 hours of an ischemic stroke. The current recommendation by the American Stroke Association states that a patient with a recent ischemic stroke and a SBP >220 mmHg or a DBP >120–140 mmHg can undergo cautious reduction of BP by about 10–15% (with IV nitroprusside or IV labetalol), if the patient is carefully monitored for neurologic deterioration related to the lower pressure. Intracranial hemorrhage (ICH)—no evidence exists to suggest that HTN provokes further bleeding in patients with ICH. A precipitous fall in SBP may compromise cerebral perfusion and increase mortality. The controlled lowering of BP with IV nitroprusside or IV labetalol (in the absence of bradycardia) is currently recommended only when the SBP is >200 mmHg or the DBP is >110. Monoamine oxidase (MAO)-tyramine interactions with:
   - *Acute hypertension*
     - Phentolamine IV
     - Labetalol IV
   - *Hypertensive encephalopathy*
     - Nitroprusside IV
     - Labetalol IV
     - Fenoldopam IV
   - *Acute renal failure*
     - Fenoldopam IV
     - Nicardipine IV
     - Beta-blockers IV
   - *Eclampsia*
     - Hydralazine IV
     - Labetalol IV
     - Magnesium IV

Lowering of BP acutely in the ED in clinical situations other than those listed here is controversial and generally should be avoided.

## Complications of Hypertension and their Management

These include:

- Hypertensive encephalopathy
- Intracerebral hemorrhage
- Subarachnoid hemorrhage
- Acute ischemic stroke
- Aortic dissection
- Myocardial ischemia or infarction
- Acute left ventricular failure
- Renal insufficiency.

### Hypertensive Encephalopathy

Hypertensive encephalopathy results from hyperperfusion of the brain when the upper limit of cerebral autoperfusion is exceeded, resulting in cerebral edema, petechial hemorrhages and microinfarcts. Today, this reaction is uncommon because even a minor reduction in blood pressure with antihypertensive therapy seems to be protective. Hypertensive encephalopathy is more likely to occur in normotensive individuals who experience a rapid rise in blood pressure, such as a child with acute renal failure caused by acute glomerulonephritis. The symptoms include severe headache, nausea, vomiting, visual disturbances, confusion and focal or generalized weakness. Signs include disorientation, seizures and focal neurologic signs. Neuroimaging is important to rule out other intracranial pathology, such as intracerebral or subarachnoid bleeding. Hypertensive encephalopathy is reversible with the reduction of blood pressure, but if it is left untreated, it may result in coma and even death. The goal of therapy is to reduce the mean arterial pressure by not more than 25% or the DBP to 100 mmHg (whichever represents the lesser reduction) in the first hour of treatment. Deterioration in neurologic function with blood pressure reduction should prompt consideration of stopping or lowering the dose of the infusion. Sodium nitroprusside has been the mainstay of treatment for hypertensive encephalopathy in the past. However, because nitroprusside is a powerful arteriolar dilator, a rise in intracerebral pressure (ICP) may rarely be precipitated. Therefore, other parenteral agents, such as labetalol, fenoldopam, and nicardipine are now used more widely.

### Intracerebral Hemorrhage

Hypertension is the most important risk factor for intracerebral hemorrhage (ICH) and is seen commonly in the acute post-hemorrhage period. This blood pressure rise tends to be more severe and less likely to resolve spontaneously compared with hypertension following cerebral infarction. An elevated blood pressure immediately after ICH is associated with hematoma expansion and poorer outcomes. However, it remains unclear whether the elevated blood pressure is primarily a cause or consequence of this association. Cerebral perfusion pressure (CPP) depends on the mean arterial pressure and intracranial pressure, where CPP = MAP – ICP. As the intracranial pressure rises, the MAP also must rise if sufficient cerebral perfusion pressure is to be maintained. However, as the MAP rises so too, theoretically, does the risk of rebleeding from ruptured small arteries and arterioles. A prospective observational study that measured baseline blood pressure and growth in the volume of ICH has not confirmed such concerns, but the frequent early use of antihypertensive agents in this series may have obscured the true nature of this relationship. This issue is further complicated by recognizing that the cerebral autoregulation curve of patients who have chronic hypertension is in many cases permanently altered, making these patients less likely to tolerate aggressive lowering of blood pressure.

Controversy remains, and the current guidelines from the American Heart Association (AHA) recommend decreasing the blood pressure when, the MAP >130 mmHg or when the SBP >220 mmHg.

### Subarachnoid Hemorrhage

Severe hypertension also is a common feature in the acute phase of subarachnoid hemorrhage (SAH). In common with ICH, the management of blood pressure must balance the risk of rebleeding with the risk of cerebral ischemia. Nimodipine has been shown to significantly improve outcomes following SAH. This is likely because of a reduction in vasospasm caused by chemical irritation of arteries by blood in the subarachnoid space. It is not recommended, however, for routine blood pressure reduction because of a high incidence in transient hypotension. The patient's cognitive status may be a useful guide to the state of cerebral perfusion pressure. If the patient is alert, then CPP probably is adequate, and careful blood pressure lowering could be considered. The management of patients who have a severely impaired level of consciousness should be more circumspect. Direct ICP monitoring allows MAP to be titrated with greater precision in these cases. If blood pressure reduction is required in the acute phase of ICH or SAH, IV esmolol or labetalol is the agent of choice because it allows rapid and safe titration. Intravenous nitroprusside should be considered to be a second-line agent because of the risk of increasing ICP.

### Acute Ischemic Stroke

The elevation in arterial blood pressure occurs in over 80% of all acute ischemic strokes (AIS). This elevation may be caused by an acute sympathetic response or by chronic hypertension, which is a major risk factor for AIS. A similar basic physiology in respect to cerebral perfusion applies, as discussed above in the context of intracranial bleeding. However, in the setting of an acute cerebral infarct, specific considerations are a little different. On the one hand, high blood pressure may be associated with an increased risk of cerebral edema and hemorrhagic transformation of the infarct. On the other hand, the elevation in ICP not matched with an increased MAP, risks extension of the infarct to involve the so-called ischemic penumbra. Furthermore, in patients who have AIS, the cerebral perfusion pressure beyond the acute obstruction is low. The distal vessels become dilated, and with ongoing ischemia, their ability to autoregulate is diminished. An abrupt restoration of brisk perfusion in this setting may run an increased risk of vascular compromise and hemorrhage and has been a significant factor limiting the overall success of reperfusion therapy in this context.

Blood pressure reduction after a stroke tends to be challenging, with even minimal intervention often leading to precipitous drops in pressure. Expectant management may be most appropriate because blood pressure often declines spontaneously in the first few hours. A decline to prestroke values within 4 days of the acute event is documented frequently. In the literature, high blood pressure after a stroke has been associated with both good and poor outcomes. Recent observational studies also demonstrate low blood pressure to be associated with poor outcome. A Cochrane review that examines 65 randomized controlled trials comprising 11,500 patients concludes that there is insufficient evidence to evaluate the effect of altering blood pressure on outcome after an acute stroke. Consequently, current AIS guidelines from the AHA recommend that BP be reduced, only if the SBP exceeds 220 mmHg, or the DBP exceeds 120 mmHg, or if there is evidence of end-organ damage believed to be related to the elevation in blood pressure. If blood pressure must be reduced after an AIS, labetolol or sodium nitroprusside is the agent suggested by both the AHA and the European stroke initiative. Patients who are being considered for thrombolysis must have a blood pressure less than 185/110 mmHg, and labetolol is the agent recommended to achieve and maintain this goal.

### Aortic Dissection

Acute aortic dissection is a rare but potentially catastrophic illness. In the ED, the immediate reduction in blood pressure and, particularly, in shear stress (the ratio of change in blood pressure [~p] with change in time [M]) is essential to limit the extent of dissection while surgical treatment is being considered or arranged. Initial therapeutic goals should include the elimination of pain and reduction of systolic blood pressure to 100–120 mmHg or the lowest level commensurate with adequate vital organ perfusion. Blood pressure reduction should proceed in tandem with reduction in the force of left ventricular contraction (~p/M). Sodium nitroprusside used in combination with a beta-blocker, such as propranolol is a good first-line therapy. Labetalol is an excellent alternative because it combines aipha- and beta-adrenergic receptor blocking properties, achieving reductions in both shear stress and arterial pressure with a single agent.

### Myocardial Ischemia or Infarction

Acute myocardial ischemia (MI) may be complicated by hypertension because of pain, anxiety and increased sympathetic tone. An elevation in blood pressure increases afterload, resulting in greater myocardial work and oxygen requirements. In addition, increased wall stress is associated with impairment of subendocardial tissue perfusion, leading to further imbalance in myocardial oxygen supply and demand. Combined with reperfusion and antithrombotic therapies, the reduction in blood pressure and heart rate can serve to minimize the extent of myocardial injury sustained. Beta-blockers are the anti-hypertensive of choice because they reduce heart rate and blood pressure while also elevating the threshold for ventricular fibrillation. Nitroglycerin is a useful adjunct for patients who have ongoing pain, especially if blood pressure remains elevated. Beta-blockers and ACE inhibitors have been shown to reduce mortality in patients who have myocardial infarction. Pure vasodilators (such as nitroprusside) should be used with caution because they can induce reflex tachycardia and hence aggravate myocardial ischemia. BP should be aggressively controlled in patients who have ST-elevation MI who are being considered for thrombolytic therapy.

### Acute Left Ventricular Failure

Patients who present with acute pulmonary edema often have marked hypertension. After treatment, many of these patients are found to have a normal ejection fraction on echocardiogram. Long-standing hypertension frequently results in myocardial hypertrophy, which leads to impaired left ventricular filling and consequent elevation in pulmonary venous pressures. Further acute rise in blood pressure in this setting may be enough to precipitate an episode of pulmonary edema or diastolic heart failure. These patients require a rapid reduction in blood pressure. Intravenous nitroprusside or nitroglycerin is very useful in this situation. Titrate the dose until the blood pressure is controlled and the signs of heart failure are alleviated. Left ventricular systolic dysfunction may also be associated with hypertension because of markedly increased sympathetic tone. Reduction in afterload and preload of the heart with nitroprusside or nitroglycine is again the mainstay of therapy in this context.

### Renal Insufficiency

Renal insufficiency is both an important cause and consequence of rapidly progressive hypertension. Both primary renal diseases (glomerulonephritis, renal artery stenosis and vasculitis) and the medications used to treat them (steroids, cyclosporin), can cause severe elevations in BP. Conversely, chronic hypertension accounts for 30% of cases of end-stage renal disease.

The primary goal in treating patients who have new onset renal disease is prevention of further renal damage through blood pressure control. Therapy should be directed toward reducing systemic blood pressure while maintaining adequate renal blood flow. Sodium nitroprusside is effective, as are IV calcium antagonists such as nicarpidine.

## Pharmacotherapy in Cardiac Emergencies

### Beta-adrenergic Blockers

These agents are used for hypertensive emergencies, especially with aortic dissection and myocardial infarction. They may be used alone or in combination with sodium nitroprusside. Pure beta-blockers should not be used alone in cases that are the result primarily of alpha stimulation (e.g. pheochromocytoma, monoamine-oxidase inhibitors (MAOIs)-tyramine interaction).

### Labetalol (Normodyne)

Alpha-, beta1-, and beta2-blocker, especially useful with aortic dissection. Lowers BP, reduces incidence of myocardial infarctions and death. Concurrent use of beta-blockers and either verapamil or diltiazem; bradycardia or heart block can occur; avoid concurrent IV use of both agents; use beta-blockers cautiously in patients with bronchospastic disease. Beta-blockers can mask prominent hypoglycemic symptoms and mask signs of thyrotoxicosis; can cause fetal bradycardia when administered in third trimester of pregnancy or at delivery; use caution in patients with renal dysfunction (active metabolite retained); do not use in treatment of hypertension associated with vasoconstriction related to hypothermia; concentrations >10 mg/ml or infusion into small veins or through a butterfly catheter should be avoided (can cause thrombophlebitis); extravasation can lead to skin necrosis and sloughing.

*Adult dose:* 20 mg (0.25 mg/kg for an 80 kg patient) intravenous push (IVP) over 2 minutes; may administer 40–80 mg at 10 minutes intervals, up to 300 mg total dose. Alternatively, IV infusion—initially, 2 mg/min; titrate to response up to 300 mg total dose, if needed.

*Pediatric dose:* 0.4–1 mg/kg/h IV; maximum dose 3 mg/kg/h.

*Contraindications:* Documented hypersensitivity to labetalol or any component of formulation, sinus bradycardia, heart block, cardiogenic shock, bronchial asthma, uncompensated cardiac failure and pregnancy (second and third trimesters).

*Interactions:* Concurrent use with alpha-blockers (prazosin, terazosin) may increase risk of orthostasis; decreases effects of sulfonylureas; may have synergistic effects when administered concurrently with verapamil or diltiazem (avoid concurrent IV use; cimetidine increases bioavailability of labetalol; CYP2D6 inhibitors, e.g. fluoxetine, miconazole, paroxetine, pergolide, quinidine and quinine) may increase levels/effects of labetalol; nonsteroidal anti-inflammatory drugs (NSAIDs) may reduce antihypertensive efficacy of labetalol; salicylates may reduce antihypertensive effects of beta-blockers.

*Pregnancy:* Safety for use during pregnancy has not been established.

*Precautions:* Caution in impaired hepatic function; discontinue therapy, if signs of liver dysfunction are present; in elderly patients, a lower response rate and higher incidence of toxicity may be observed; avoid concurrent IV use with diltiazem or verapamil; caution in compensated heart failure and monitor for worsening of condition; not for administration to patients with bronchospastic disease; may mask prominent hypoglycemic symptoms and signs of thyrotoxicosis; may cause fetal harm when administered in pregnancy.

### Esmolol (Brevibloc)

Ideal for use in patients at risk for complications from beta-blockers, especially patients with mild to moderately severe left ventricular (LV) dysfunction or peripheral vascular disease. Has short half-life of 8 minutes; thus, easily titratable to desired effect. In addition, therapy may be stopped quickly if necessary.

*Adult dose:* Loading dose—250–500 mcg/kg infused over 1–3 minutes IV. Maintenance infusion—50 mcg/kg/min IV over 4 minutes; if adequate effect not observed within 5 minutes, repeat loading dose and follow with maintenance infusion using increments of 50 mcg/kg/min IV (for 4 minutes); this regimen may be repeated up to 4 times if necessary. As desired BP approached, skip loading infusion and reduce dose increments in maintenance infusion from 50 mcg/kg/min IV to 25 mcg/kg/min; if necessary, may increase interval between titration steps from 5–10 minutes.

*Pediatric dose:* Suggested dose—100–500 mcg/kg IV over 1 minutes, then 25–200 mcg/kg/min IV; increase by 25–50 mcg/kg/min IV q5–10 minutes. Maximum dose—50–250 mcg/kg/min IV.

*Contraindications:* Documented hypersensitivity to esmolol or any component of formulation, sinus bradycardia, heart block, cardiogenic shock, bronchial asthma (relative), uncompensated cardiac failure, hypotension and pregnancy (second and third trimesters).

*Interactions:* Aluminum salts, barbiturates, NSAIDs, penicillins, calcium salts, cholestyramine and rifampin may decrease bioavailability and plasma levels of esmolol, possibly resulting in decreased pharmacologic effect; cardiotoxicity of esmolol may increase when administered concurrently with sparfloxacin, astemizole, calcium channel blockers, quinidine, flecainide and contraceptives; toxicity of esmolol increases when administered concurrently with digoxin, flecainide, acetaminophen, clonidine, epinephrine, nifedipine, prazosin, haloperidol, phenothiazines and catecholamine-depleting agents. Acetylcholinesterase inhibitors may enhance the bradycardic effect of beta-blockers; beta-blockers may enhance the vasopressor effect of alpha/beta-agonists (direct acting); beta-blockers may enhance the orthostatic effect of alpha1-blockers; beta-blockers may enhance the rebound hypertensive effect of alpha2-agonists (effect can occur when alpha2-agonist is abruptly withdrawn). Amiodarone may enhance the bradycardic effect of beta-blockers (possibly to the point of cardiac arrest); beta2-agonists may diminish bradycardic effect of beta-blockers (beta1 selective); calcium channel blockers (nondihydropyridine) may enhance the hypotensive effect of beta-blockers (bradycardia and signs of heart failure have also been reported); beta-blockers may enhance the bradycardic effect of cardiac glycosides; disopyramide may enhance the bradycardic effect of beta-blockers (use caution if coadministering disopyramide and a beta-blocker, especially if both are IV); beta-blockers may enhance hypoglycemic effect of insulin preparations; NSAIDs may diminish antihypertensive effect of beta-blockers; beta-blockers may enhance hypoglycemic effect of sulfonylureas; cardioselective beta-blockers (e.g. esmolol) may be safer than nonselective beta-blockers; and all beta-blockers appear to mask tachycardia as an initial symptom of hypoglycemia.

*Pregnancy:* Safety for use during pregnancy has not been established.

*Precautions:* Hypotension is common; patients need close BP monitoring; administer cautiously in compensated heart failure and monitor for a worsening of the condition; use caution in patients with peripheral vascular diseases (PVD) (can aggravate arterial insufficiency); use caution with sulfites.

### Alpha-adrenergic Blockers

At low doses, alpha-adrenergic receptor blockers may be used as monotherapy in treatment of hypertension. At higher does not need immediate treatment in the ED. The patient requires proper follow-up.

### Phentolamine (Regitine)

Alpha1- and alpha2-adrenergic blocking agent, effective for pheochromocytoma and hypercatecholaminergic-induced hypertension.

*Adult dose:* Load 5–20 mg IV q5min or infuse 0.2–0.5 mg/min

*Pediatric dose:* 0.05–0.1 mg/kg/dose IV; 5 mg maximum single dose

*Contraindications:* Documented hypersensitivity to phentolamine or any component of the formulation; renal impairment; coronary or cerebral arteriosclerosis; concurrent use with phosphodiesterase-5 (PDE-5) inhibitors including sildenafil (>25 mg), tadalafil or vardenafil.

*Interactions:* Concurrent administration of epinephrine or ephedrine may decrease phentolamine effects; ethanol increases phentolamine toxicity; concurrent administration with sildenafil, tadalafil, vardenafil, cause additive blood pressure-lowering effects.

*Pregnancy:* Safety for use during pregnancy has not been established.

*Precautions:* Myocardial infarction, cerebrovascular spasm and cerebrovascular occlusion have occurred following administration; caution in patients with gastritis or peptic ulcer, tachycardia, or history of cardiac arrhythmias; may use sildenafil with extreme caution.

### Antihypertensive Agents

Sodium nitroprusside is drug of choice (DOC) for most hypertensive emergencies. It is potent, rapid in onset and has a relatively short duration.

### Nitroglycerin (Nitro-Bid)

Decreases coronary vasospasm, which increases coronary blood flow. Also induces vessel dilatation, decreasing cardiac workload.

*Adult dose:* Continuous infusion—start 5 mcg/min, increase by 5 mcg/min q3-5min to 20 mcg/min; if no response at 20 mcg/min increase by 10 mcg/min q3–5min, up to 200 mcg/min.

*Pediatric dose:* Not established; suggested dose start with 0.25–0.5 mcg/kg/min continuous infusion and titrate by 1 mcg/kg/min at 20–60 minutes intervals to desired effect; 1–3 mcg/kg/min usual dose; 5 mcg/kg/min maximum.

*Contraindications:* Documented hypersensitivity to organic nitrates, isosorbide, nitroglycerin or anycomponent of formulation; concurrent use with PDE-5 inhibitors (sildenafil, tadalafil or vardenafil); angle-closure glaucoma (intraocular pressure may be increased); head trauma or cerebral hemorrhage (increase intracranial pressure); severe anemia. Additional contraindications for IV product include hypotension; uncorrected hypovolemia; inadequate cerebral circulation, constrictive pericarditis and pericardial tamponade.

*Interactions:* Reduces effect of alteplase (tissue plasminogen activator) when used with IV nitroglycerin (avoid concurrent use); antianginal effects reduced with ergot (avoid concurrent use); ethanol can cause hypotension when nitrates taken 1 hour or more after ethanol ingestion; heparin's effect may be reduced by IV nitroglycerin (may affect only a minority of patients); sildenafil, tadalafil and vardenafil cause significant reduction of systolic and diastolic BP with concurrent use (contraindicated; do not administer sildenafil, tadalafil or vardenafil within 24 hours of a nitrate preparation).

*Pregnancy:* Safety for use during pregnancy has not been established.

*Precautions:* Severe hypotension can occur; caution in volume depletion, hypotension and right ventricular infarctions; paradoxical bradycardia and increased angina pectoris can accompany hypotension (orthostatic hypotension can also occur and ethanol can accentuate this); tolerance develops to nitrates and appropriate dosing is needed to minimize this (drug-free interval).

### Sodium Nitroprusside (Nitropress)

Reduces peripheral resistance by acting directly on arteriolar and venous smooth muscle.

*Adult dose:* 0.3–0.5 mcg/kg/min IV initial infusion, increase in increments of 0.5 mcg/kg/min and titrate to desired effect. Average dose—1–6 mcg/kg/min; rates >10 mcg/kg/min may lead to cyanide toxicity.

*Pediatric dose:* 1 mcg/kg/min by continuous IV infusion; increase in increments of 1 mcg/kg/min at intervals of 20–60 minutes; titrate to desired response; 3 mcg/kg/min usual dose and 5 mcg/kg/min maximum.

*Contraindications:* Documented hypersensitivity to nitroprusside or any component of formulation; treatment of compensatory hypertension (aortic coarctation and arteriovenous shunting); high output failure and congenital optic atrophy or tobacco amblyopia.

*Interactions:* None reported.

*Pregnancy:* Safety for use during pregnancy has not been established.

*Precautions:* Except when used briefly or at low (<2 mcg/kg/min) infusion rates, nitroprusside gives rise to large cyanide quantities; do not use maximum dose for >10 minutes; use extreme caution in patients with elevated intracranial pressure and patients with hepatic or renal dysfunction (watch for cyanide toxicity in patients with impaired hepatic function); use lowest end of dosage range with renal impairment; thiocyanate toxicity occurs in patients with renal impairment or on prolonged infusions (continuous BP monitoring needed).

### Hydralazine (Apresoline)

Principal indication is treatment of eclampsia. Decreases systemic resistance through direct vasodilation of arterioles.

*Adult dose:* Initial—10–20 mg/dose PO q4–6h as needed, may increase to 40 mg/dose; change to oral therapy as soon as possible.

*Pediatric dose:* 0.1–0.2 mg/kg/dose (not to exceed 20 mg) PO q4–6h as needed, up to 1.7–3.5 mg/kg/d in 4–6 divided doses.

*Contraindications:* Documented hypersensitivity to hydralazine or any component of formulation; mitral valve rheumatic heart disease.

*Interactions:* Beta-blockers (metoprolol and propranolol) serum concentrations and pharmacologic effects may be increased (monitor cardiovascular status); propranolol increases hydralazine's serum concentrations; NSAIDs may decrease hemodynamic effects of hydralazine (avoid use if possible or closely monitor cardiovascular status).

*Pregnancy:* Safety for use during pregnancy has not been established.

*Precautions:* May cause a drug-induced lupuslike syndrome; adjust dose in severe renal dysfunction; use with caution in CAD and pulmonary HTN; monitor BP closely following IV administration; response may be delayed and unpredictable in some patients; titrate cautiously to response; hydralazine-induced fluid and sodium retention may require addition or increased dosage of diuretics.

### Fenoldopam (Corlopam)

Short-acting dopamine agonist 1 (DA1) recently approved for management of severe HTN. Increases renal blood flow and sodium excretion. It is 10X more potent than dopamine as renal vasodilator.

*Adult dose:* Initial—0.1–0.3 mcg/kg/min IV (lower initial doses may be associated with less reflex tachycardia); may be increased in increments of 0.05–0.1 mcg/kg/min IV q15-min until target blood pressure reached; maximal infusion rate reported in clinical studies was 1.6 mcg/kg/min.

*Pediatric dose:* 0.2 mcg/kg/min IV initial; may be increased to dosages of 0.3–0.5 mcg/kg/min IV q20–30min (0.8 mcg/kg/min maximum); limited to short-term (4 h) use.

*Contraindications:* Documented hypersensitivity to fenoldopam or any component of formulation.

*Interactions:* Acetaminophen may increase levels (30–70%) when administered concurrently; beta-blockers increase risk of hypotension; avoid concurrent use (it must use concurrently, close monitoring recommended).

*Pregnancy:* Usually safe but benefits must outweigh the risks.

*Precautions:* Use caution in patients with glaucoma or intraocular hypertension; dose-related tachycardia can occur, especially at infusion rates >0.1 mcg/kg/min; caution in angina patients; close monitoring of BP necessary (hypotension can occur); monitor for hypokalemia at intervals of 6 hours during infusion; continuous infusion only (not for bolus doses); effects of hemodialysis on pharmacokinetics of fenoldopam not evaluated; caution with increased intracranial pressure; may cause allergic reaction in susceptible individuals.

## Consultations

Consultations may be indicated for comorbid conditions and their definitive treatment. Because HTN is usually a chronic problem, access to a primary care physician and long-term follow-up are essential for all patients. Once, the diagnosis of a true hypertensive emergency is established and TOD is confirmed, BP should be lowered by up to 20–25% of the MAP or the DBP should be decreased to 100–110 mmHg over minutes to hours. More rapid reduction in BP should be avoided, since it may worsen target organ function.

### Further Inpatient Care

Patients with a true hypertensive emergency require the careful titration of IV medications for good control and a smooth reduction of their BP. Close monitoring is required; therefore, an intensive care unit (ICU) is the most suitable place for admission. Other problems or comorbid conditions need to be addressed appropriately (i.e. surgery for aortic dissection).

### Further Outpatient Care

Hypertension is a chronic problem. The most important factor in a patient's overall risks of morbidity and mortality is appropriate long-term care. If a patient presents with a high BP but ED evaluation reveals no evidence of TOD, the patient does not need immediate treatment in the ED. The patient does require proper follow-up.

*Transfer:* Transfer requirements are based on the ability of the institution to care for the patient and the patient's associated comorbid conditions. A patient with uncomplicated hypertensive emergency needs an ICU setting. Patients with comorbid conditions, such as aortic dissection or subarachnoid hemorrhage, may require transfer to a higher level of care.

*Deterrence/Prevention:* Good long-term control of HTN is the best method for prevention of acute hypertensive emergencies.

Patient education and close follow-up in patients who have had a hypertensive crisis are essential to prevent recurrent hypertensive emergencies. Proper use of antihypertensive medications by primary care physicians is the major tool in avoiding development of hypertensive emergencies.

*Prognosis:* Without treatment, accelerated hypertension may result in death within a year in over 90% of patients as a result of end-organ damage, e.g. myocardial infarction, CVE or renal failure. The prognosis has improved dramatically over the period of a few decades and with optimal treatment the 5-year survival rate is >80%. The 1-year mortality rate is higher than 90% for patients with untreated hypertensive emergencies. Median survival duration is 144 months for all patients presenting to the ED with a hypertensive emergency. 5-year survival rate among all patients presenting with hypertensive crisis is 74%.

*Patient education:* Patients need to continue education about antihypertensive medications and complications arising from inadequate BP control. Dangers of uncontrolled HTN must be stressed, including associated serious morbidity and death. Education and maintenance of BP control are important to help prevent further complications.

*Medical/Legal pitfalls:* Administering long-acting oral/sublingual medications to acutely lower nonurgent elevations in BP. Failure to arrange timely and appropriate follow-up. Failure to recognize the serious complications of severe HTN.

## BIBLIOGRAPHY


1. Adams RE, Powers WJ. Management of hypertension in acute intracerebral hemorrhage. Crit Care Clin 1997;13(1):131–61.
2. Aggarwal M, Khan IA. Hypertensive crisis: hypertensive emergencies and urgencies. Cardiol Clin 2006;24:135–46.
3. American Heart Association [and] the International Liaison Committee on Resuscitation. Guidelines 2000 for cardiopulmonary resuscitation and emergency cardiovascular care: part 7: the era of reperfusion: acute stroke [section 2]. Circulation 2000;102(Suppl 8):1204–16.
4. Baer L, Parra-Carrilo JZ, Radichevich I, et al. Detection of renovascular hypertension with angiotensin II blockade. Ann Intern Med 1977;86(3):257–60.
5. Bennett NM, Shea S. Hypertensive emergency: case criteria, sociodemographic profile, and previous care of 100 cases. Am J Public Health 1988;78(6):636–4.
6. Bennett NM, Shea S. Hypertensive emergency: case criteria, sociodemographic profile, and previous care of 100 cases. Am J Public Health 1988;78(6):636–40.
7. Blumenfeld JD, Laragh JH. Management of hypertensive crises: the scientific basis for treatment decisions. Am J Hypertens 2001;14(11 Pt 1):1154–67.
8. Brott T, Thalinger K, Hertzberg V. Hypertension as a risk factor for spontaneous intracerebral hemorrhage. Stroke 1986;17(6):1078–83.
9. Calhoun DA, Oparil S. Treatment of hypertensive crisis [see comments]. N Engl J Med 1990;323(17):1177–83.
10. Chobanian AV, Bakris GL, Black HR, et al. The seventh report of the Joint National Committee on Prevention, Detection, Evaluation, and Treatment of High Blood Pressure: the JNC 7 report. JAMA 2003;289(19):2560–72.
11. Colhoun HM, Dong W, Poulter NR. Blood pressure screening, management and control in England: results from the health survey for England 1994. J Hypertens 1998;16(6):747–52.
12. Finnerty FA Jr. Hypertensive encephalopathy. Am J Med 1972;52(5):672–8.
13. Frohlich ED. Target organ involvement in hypertension: a realistic promise of prevention and reversal. Med Clin N Am 2004;88(1):209–21.
14. Gallagher EJ. Hypertensive urgencies: treating the mercury? Ann Emerg Med 2003;41(4):530–1.
15. Garcia JY Jr, Vidt DG. Current management of hypertensive emergencies. Drugs 1987;34(2):263–78.
16. Gifford RW Jr, Westbrook E. Hypertensive encephalopathy: mechanisms, clinical features and treatment. Prog Cardiovasc Dis 1974;17(2):115–24.
17. Gifford RW Jr. Management of hypertensive crises. JAMA 1991;266(6):829–35.
18. Grossman E, Messerli FH, Grodzicki T, et al. Should a moratorium be placed on sublingual nifedipine capsules given for hypertensive emergencies and pseudoemergencies? JAMA 1996;276(16):1328–31.
19. Hall WD. Resistant hypertension, secondary hypertension, and hypertensive crises. Cardiol Clin 2002; 20(2):281–9.
20. Impey L. Severe hypotension and fetal distress following sublingual administration or nifedipine to a patient with severe pregnancy induced hypertension at 33 weeks. Br J Obstet Gynaecol 1993;100(10):959–61.
21. JNC 7. The seventh report of the Joint National Committee on Detection, Evaluation, and Treatment of High Blood Pressure. Hypertension 2003;42:1206–52.
22. Kaplan N, Norman M, Lieberman E. Hypertensive crises. In: Kaplan's clinical hypertension. Philadelphia: Lippincott and Wilkins, 2002;pp 339–56.
23. Kaplan NM. Treatment of hypertensive emergencies and urgencies. Heart Dis Stroke 1992;1(6):373–8.
24. Kincaid-Smith P. Management of severe hypertension. Am J Cardiol 1973;32(4):575–81.
25. Kitiyakara C, Guzman NJ. Malignant hypertension and hypertensive emergencies. J Am Sac Nephrol 1998;9(1):133–42.

26. Laragh JH. Laragh's 25 lessons in pathophysiology and 12 clinical pearls for treating hypertension [abstract, closing summary, and table of contents]. Am J Hypertens 2001; 14(12):1173–7.
27. Lassen NA, Agnoli A. The upper limit of autoregulation of cerebral blood flow on the pathogenesis of hypertensive encepholopathy. Scand J Clin Lab Invest 1972;30(2):113–6.
28. Lip GY, Beevers M, Beevers DG. Complications and survival of 315 patients with malignant-phase hypertension. J Hypertens 1995;13(8):915–24.
29. LipGY, Beevers M, Beevers G. The failure of malignant hypertension to decline: a survey of 24 years' experience in a multiracial population in England. J Hypertens 1994; 12(11):1297–305.
30. LipGY, Beevers M, Potter JF, et al. Malignant hypertension in the elderly. QJM 1995;88(9):641–7.
31. Mancia G, Sega R, Milesi C, et al. Blood-pressure control in the hypertensive population. Lancet 1997;349(9050):454–7.
32. Murphy C. Hypertensive emergencies. Emerg Med Clin North Am 1995;13(4):973–1007.
33. Murphy MB, Murray C, Shorten GD. Fenoldopam-a selective peripheral dopamine-receptor agonist for the treatment of severe hypertension. N Engl J Med 2001.
34. Neutel JM, Smith DH, Wallin O, et al. A comparison of intra-venous nicardipine and sodium nitroprusside in the immediate treatment of severe hypertension. Am J Hypertens 1994:7(7 Pt 1):623–8.
35. O'Mailia JJ, Sander GE, Giles TO. Nifedipine-associated myocardial ischemia or infarction in the treatment of hypertensive urgencies. Ann Intern Med 1987;107(2):185–6.
36. Qureshi AI, Tuhrim S, Broderick JP, et al. Spontaneous intra-cerebral hemorrhage. N Engl J Med 2001;344(19):1450–60.
37. Schwartz M, Naschitz JE, Yeshurun O, et al. Oral nifedipine in the treatment of hypertensive surgency: cerebrovascular accident following a single dose. Arch Intern Med 1990; 150(J):686–7.
38. Shayne PH, Pitts SR. Severely increased blood pressure in the emergency department. Ann Emerg Med 2003;41(4):513-29 [comment] 530–1.
39. Strandgaard S, Olesen J, Skinhoj E, et al. Autoregulation of brain circulation in severe arterial hypertension. BMJ 1973; 1(5852):507–10.
40. Strandgaard S. Autoregulation of cerebral blood flow in hypertensive patients: the modifying influence of prolonged antihypertensive treatment on the tolerance to acute, drug-induced hypotension. Circulation 1976;53(4):720–7. pressure changes induced by sodium nitroprusside in patients with intracranial mass lesions. J Neurosurg 1978; 48(3):329–31.
41. The sixth report of the Joint National Committee on preven-tion, detection, evaluation, and treatment of high blood pressure. Arch Intern Med 1997;157(21):2413–46.
42. Varon J, Marik PE. The diagnosis and management of hypertensive crises. Chest 2000;118(1):214–27.
43. Vasan RS, Beiser A, Seshadri S, et al. Residual lifetime risk for developing hypertension in middle-aged women and men: the Framingham Heart Study. JAMA 2002;287(8): 1003–10.
44. Vaughan CJ, Delanty N. Hypertensive emergencies. Lancet 2000;356(9227):411–7.
45. Wachter RM. Symptomatic hypotension induced by nifedi-pine in the acute treatment or severe hypertension. Arch Intern Med 1987;147(3):556–8.
46. Wallace JD, Levy LL. Blood pressure after stroke. JAMA 1981;246(19):2177–80.
47. Zampaglione B, Pascale C, Marchisio M, et al. Hypertensive urgencies and emergencies: prevalence and clinical presentation. Hypertension 1996;27(1):144–7.

# 24 Noninvasive Ventilation in Acute Cardiopulmonary Failure

Noninvasive ventilation (NIV) is the delivery of assisted mechanical ventilation to the lungs, without the use of an invasive endotracheal airway. NIV has revolutionised the management of patients with various forms of respiratory failure. It has decreased the need for invasive mechanical ventilation and its attendant complications. Cardiogenic pulmonary edema (CPO) is a common medical emergency, and NIV has been shown to improve both physiological and clinical outcomes. From the data presented herein, it is clear that there is sufficiently high level evidence to favour the use of continuous positive airway pressure (CPAP), and that the use of CPAP in patients with CPO, decreases intubation rate and improves survival (number needed to treat seven and eight respectively). However, there is insufficient evidence to recommend the use of bilevel positive airway pressure (BiPAP), probably the exception being patients with hypercapnic CPO. More trials are required to conclusively define the role of BiPAP in CPO (Figs 24.1, 24.2 and Tables 24.1–24.3).

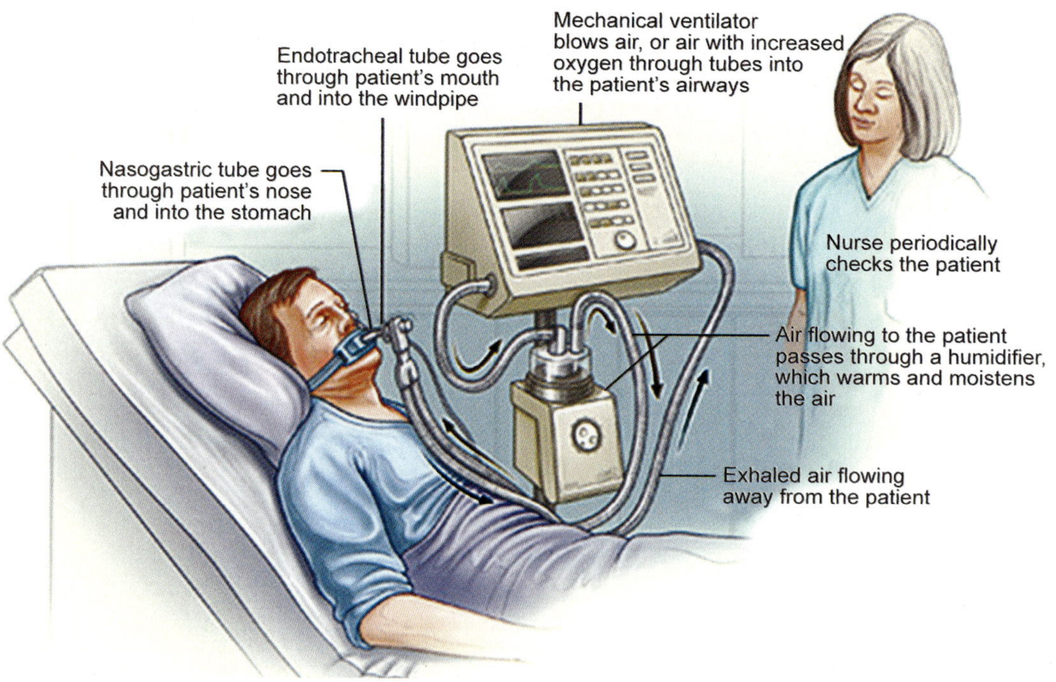


**Fig. 24.1:** A standard setup for a ventilator in a hospital room. The ventilator pushes warm, moist air (or air with increased oxygen) to the patient. Exhaled air flows away from the patient

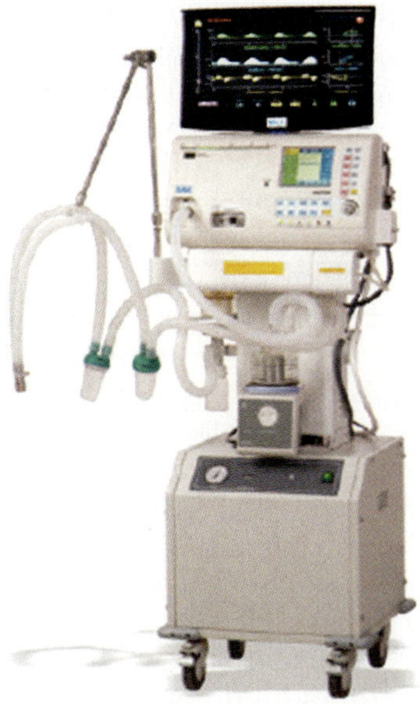

**Fig. 24.2:** Noninvasive ventilation machine with large external color LCD monitor (top) with comprehensive monitoring fitted with inbuilt nebulizer having provision of multiple unit monitoring connectivity

| **Table 24.1:** Selection criteria (at least two should be present) |
|---|
| • Moderate to severe dyspnea with use of accessory muscles and paradoxical abdominal motion |
| • Moderate to severe acidosis (pH 7.30–7.35) and hypercapnia ($PaCO_2$ 6.0–8.0 kPa, 45–60 mmHg) |
| • Respiratory frequency >25 breaths/min |

| **Table 24.2:** Predictors of success during acute applications of NPPV |
|---|
| • Younger age |
| • Lower acuty of illness (APACHE score) |
| • Able to cooperate; better neurologic score |
| • Able to coordinate breathing with ventilator |
| • Less air leaking, intact denitition |
| • Hypercarbia, but no too severe ($PaCO_2$ > 45 mmHg, < 92 mmHg) |
| • Acidernia, but not too severe (pH < 7.35, > 7.10) |
| • Improvements in gas exchange and heat and respiratory rates within first 2 hours |

NPPV=noninvasive positive pressure ventilation; APACHE=acute physiology and chronic health evaluation

| **Table 24.3:** Exclusion criteria (any may be present) |
|---|
| *Respiratory arrest* |
| • Cardiovascular instability (hypotension, arrhythmias and myocardial infarction) |
| • Somnolence, impaired mental status and uncooperative patient |
| • High aspiration risk; viscous or copious secretions |
| • Recent facial or gastroesophageal surgery |
| • Cranofacial trauma and fixed nasopharyngeal abnormalities |
| • Extreme obesity |

It has emerged as an important tool in the treatment of diverse forms of acute respiratory failure. It not only reduces the need for invasive mechanical ventilation and its associated complications, but also reduces the complications associated with stay in the intensive care unit (ICU), length of hospital stay, and mortality in selected patients. Cardiogenic pulmonary edema (CPO) is a common medical emergency and NIV in addition to conventional medical treatment is beneficial for patients with CPO, as it augments cardiac output, results in rapid improvement in gas exchange, decreases the need for endotracheal intubation and there is a trend towards decreased in-hospital mortality.

## PATHOPHYSIOLOGY OF CARDIOGENIC PULMONARY EDEMA

Cardiogenic pulmonary edema is defined as an episode of acute heart failure accompanied by severe respiratory distress and oxygen saturation <90% on room air before all treatment. The pathogenesis of CPO is related to a critical interaction between progressive decrease in left ventricular systolic function and acute increase in systemic vascular resistance with resultant exudation of fluid from the intravascular compartment into the lung interstitium and alveoli.

This leads to a vicious cycle amplified by three important processes. Firstly, as pulmonary congestion increases, oxygen saturation decreases, resulting in decreased myocardial oxygen supply. This leads to ischaemia in regions with already borderline blood supply, further impairing cardiac performance. Secondly, hypoxemia and increased fluid content in the lungs induces pulmonary vasoconstriction increasing the right ventricular pressure. This compromises left ventricular function through the ventricular interdependence mechanism. Finally, profound circulatory insufficiency results in metabolic acidosis, which further jeopardises cardiac performance.

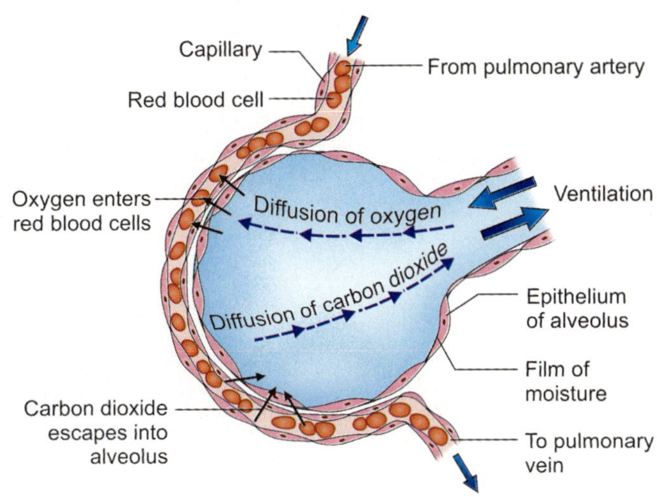


**Fig. 24.3:** Breathing has two discrete components. Ventilation—the movement of gas; and gas exchange at the alveolar-endothelial surface

Cardiogenic pulmonary edema (CPO) is characterised by an increase in extravascular lung water, which causes a decrease in respiratory system compliance, increased airway resistance, air trapping, arterial hypoxaemia and decreased diffusing capacity. Retention of carbon dioxide not previously associated with chronic obstructive pulmonary disease is a common finding in patients presenting with CPO and is associated with a poor prognosis. This hypercapnia is probably attributable to respiratory muscle fatigue, as a result of increased work of breathing from both reduced lung compliance and increased airway resistance secondary to interstitial and bronchial edema. Moreover, the respiratory muscles have to generate large negative swings in pleural pressure to start inspiratory flow and maintain adequate tidal volumes. This increase in negative intrathoracic pressure aggravates pulmonary edema by increasing both preload and afterload. Another important point to remember while managing these patients is that respiratory distress and dyspnea are not directly related to hypoxaemia, and thus can not be reversed with oxygen administration alone.

### How does Continuous Positive Airway Pressure Work?

The immediate goals in the treatment of acute CPO are to improve systemic oxygen saturation by giving oxygen with a high flow facemask, reduction of preload and afterload of both the ventricles by a combination of morphine, diuretics and nitrates. As early as 1936, continuous positive airway pressure (CPAP) had been shown to be an effective therapy for CPO unresponsive to medical treatment. CPAP therapy in patients with CPO is associated with immediate and pronounced improvements in respiratory and haemodynamic variables. CPAP augments the inspiratory and expiratory flow and pressure thereby increasing the tidal volume and unloading the inspiratory muscles. It decreases dead space ventilation and improves alveolar ventilation, re-expands flooded alveoli, and counteracts intrinsic positive end-expiratory pressure (PEEP). CPAP prevents microatelectasis and places the respiratory pressure volume characteristics in a more favourable position.

The effective filling and emptying of the heart is determined in part by the pressure difference between the inside of the heart and the intrathoracic pressure, known as the cardiac transmural pressure (PTM). The amplitude of inspiratory swings is greater in patients with CPO and leads to an increase in PTM in patients with CPO.

The more positive the PTM is during diastole, the greater the filling of the heart (preload). The more positive the PTM is during systole, the higher the workload is for the heart (afterload). During systole, CPAP induced increase in intrathoracic pressure reduces the venous return, decreasing the right and left ventricular preload, thereby improving mechanics in an overloaded ventricle, whereas in diastole, CPAP increases pericardial pressure, reduces transmural pressure, and thus decreases afterload. Although, CPAP can decrease cardiac index in normal people, it increases cardiac index in patients with CPO.

Continuous positive airway pressure also causes a significant decrease in the heart rate, resulting from increased parasympathetic tone in response to CPAP induced lung inflation. However, treatment with NIV in CPO is beneficial only in patients who have systolic dysfunction. In patients with diastolic dysfunction who require a comparatively high filling pressure, the effects of positive pressure therapy compromises venous return, resulting in deterioration of haemodynamics (Figs 24.4–24.10).

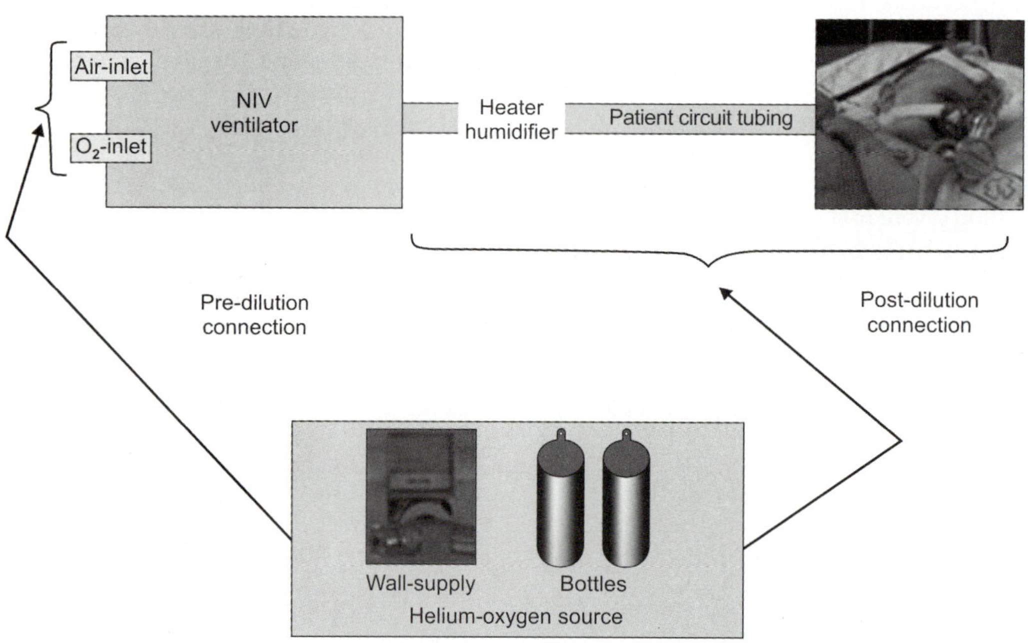


**Fig. 24.4:** Modes of adaptation of standard NIV equipment for delivery of HELIOX. Both predilution connection and postdilution connection modes are detailed in the text

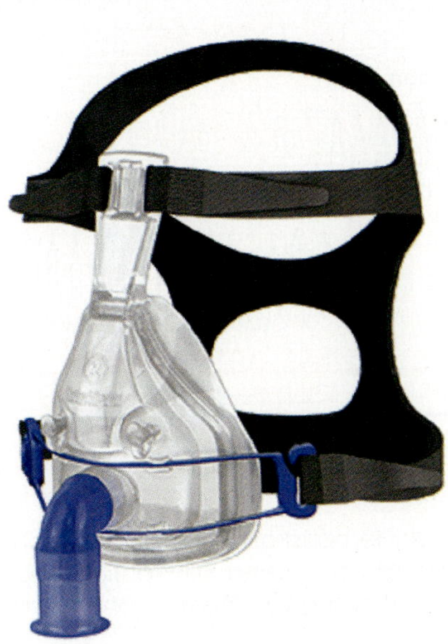

Fig. 24.5: Showing features of noninvasive ventilation mask

## How Does Bilevel Positive Airway Pressure Work?

Bilevel positive airway pressure (BiPAP) in contrast with CPAP delivers two different pressures, inspiratory positive airway pressure (IPAP) and expiratory positive airway pressure (EPAP). BiPAP decreases inspiratory work of breathing, and can improve diaphragmatic function better than CPAP alone. Recently, it has been shown that BiPAP has similar cardiac and haemodynamic benefits as CPAP in patients with CPO. In addition, BiPAP unloads the respiratory muscles, reduces respiratory effort, and increases tidal volume before any changes in pulmonary mechanics. This is in contrast with CPAP, which requires the pulmonary mechanics to change before any benefits of respiratory muscle unloading are seen.

## Continuous Positive Airway Pressure Compared with Conventional Medical Therapy

Almost 6 decades ago, Poulton and Oxon described the use of CPAP delivered by the 'pulmonary plus pressure

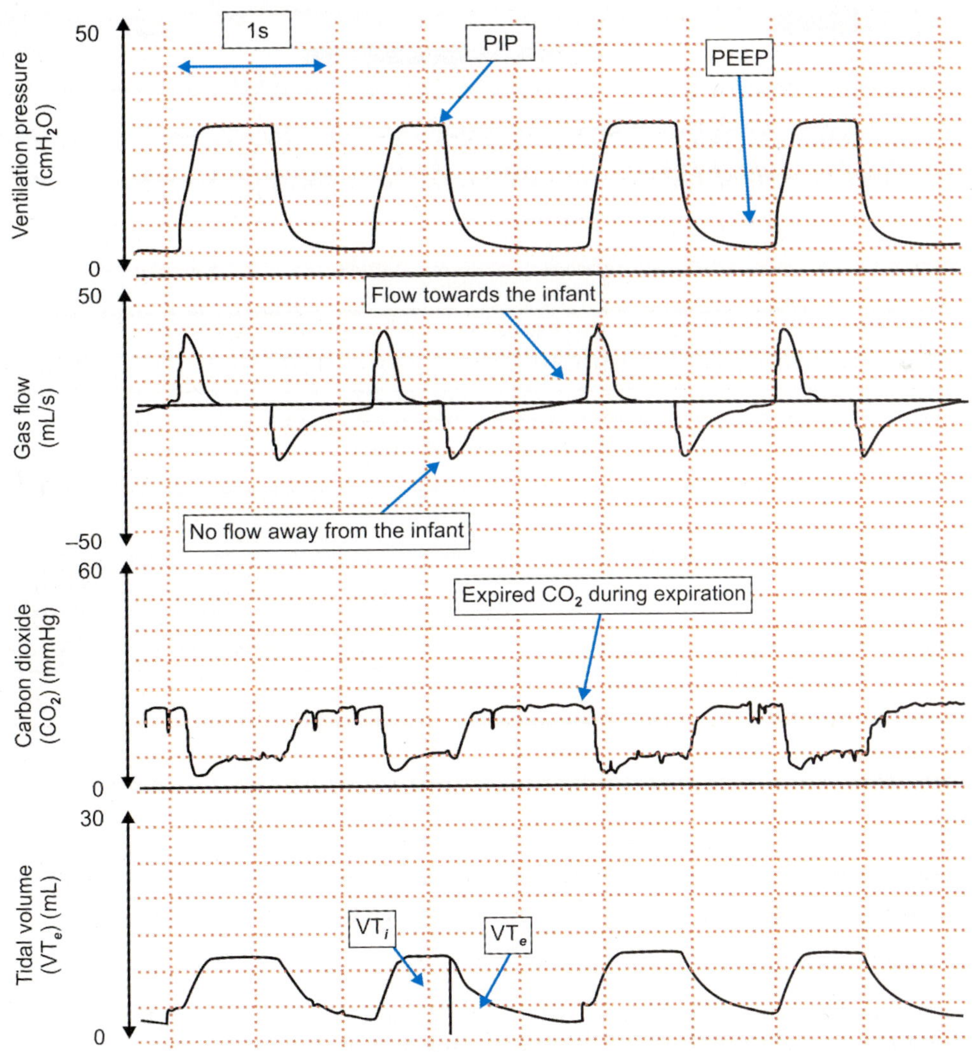


Fig. 24.6: During positive pressure ventilation (PPV), the airway pressures rise to set PIP. At the end of inspiration, PIP decreases to baseline (PEEP). The area underneath the gas flow waves during inflation and expiration is similar, which is reflected in the VT wave returning to the baseline after expiration. No leak is displayed. PIP=peak inspiratory pressure

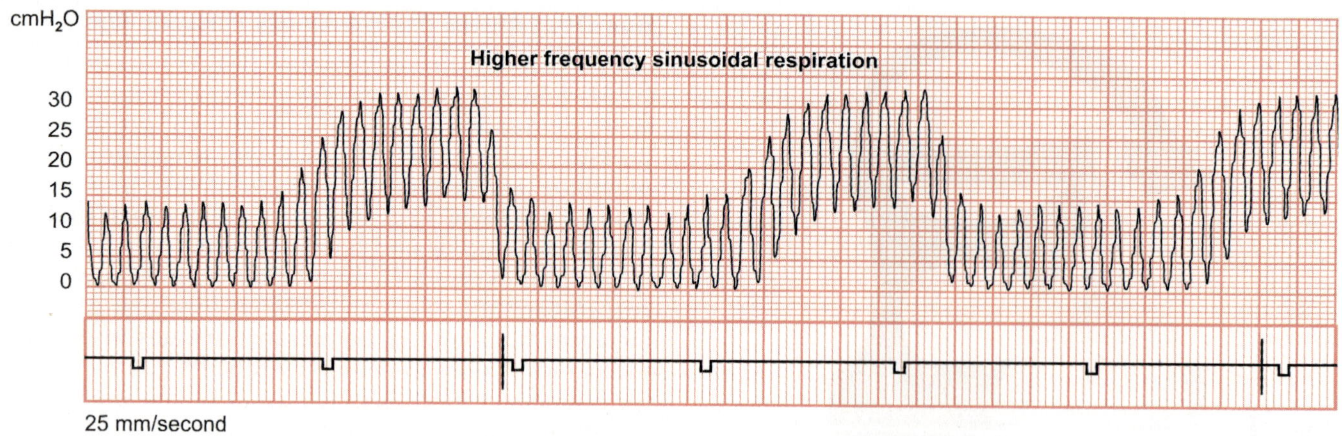


**Fig. 24.7:** A sinusoidal wave format (modified by existing pulmonary compliance) demonstrating automatic biphasic scheduling with a modulated 'higher frequency percussive sinusoidal respiration'. Sinusoidal scheduling will ventilate neonates through pediatrics to large adult lungs with low pulmonary compliance. This provides for a balanced diffusive/convective intrapulmonary gas exchange

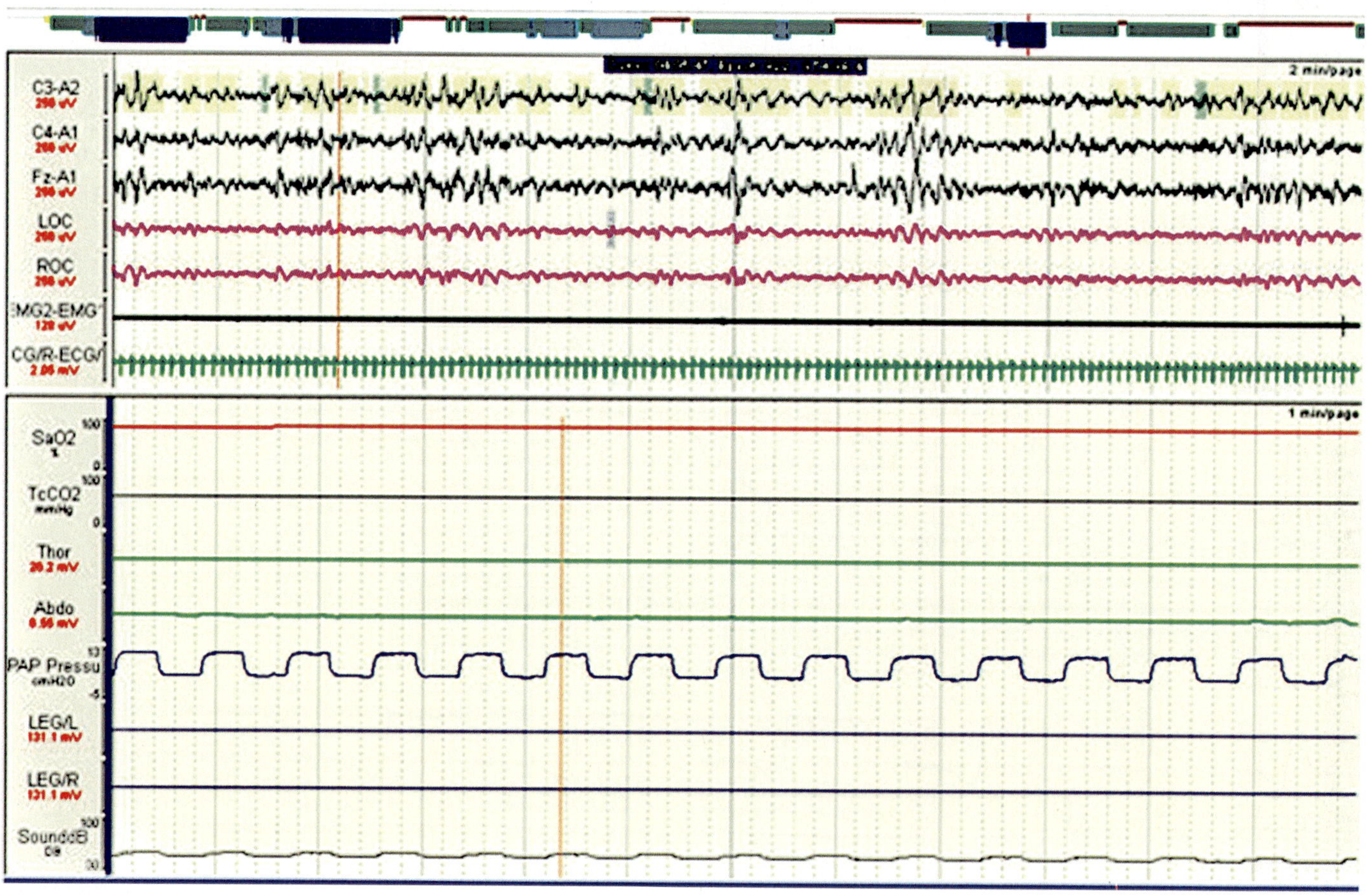


**Fig. 24.8:** Polysomnogram on ST-mode BiPAP showing regular nasal flow (CPAP pressure) and correction of patient-ventilator dyssynchrony

machine' through a facemask to patients with 'cardiac asthma.' Several studies have shown that CPAP is effective in patients with CPO, as it rapidly improves gas exchange and cardiac haemodynamics, and can decrease intubation rates and in-hospital mortality. However, most studies on CPO have not been adequately powered to detect these differences.

Rasanen et al., randomised 40 patients with CPO to either facemask CPAP (10 cmH$_2$O) or standard medical therapy, and showed improvement in gas exchange, decrease in

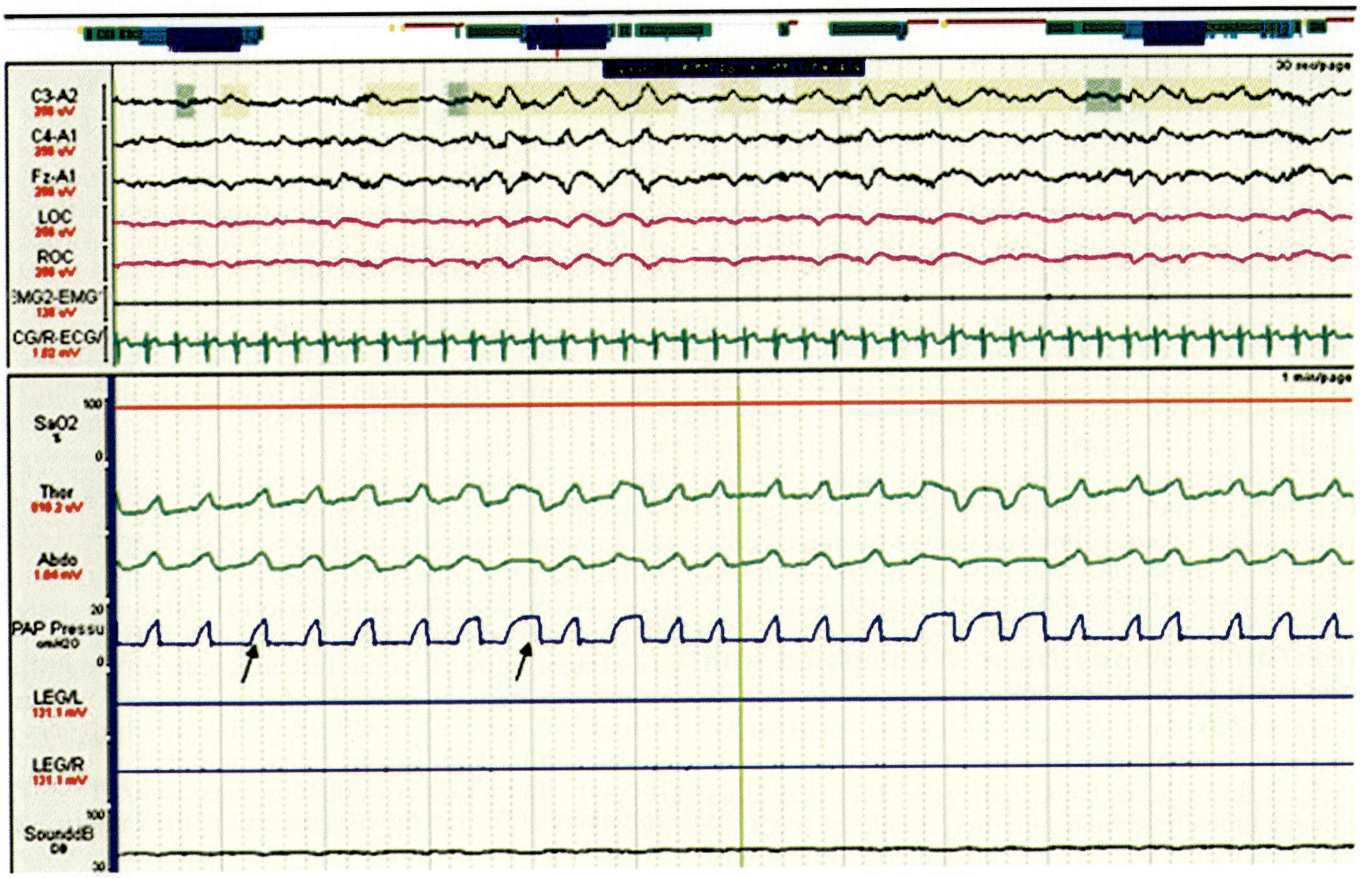

**Fig. 24.9:** Polysomnogram on S-mode BiPAP showing irregular nasal flow (CPAP pressure) due to patient-ventilator dyssynchrony (arrows)

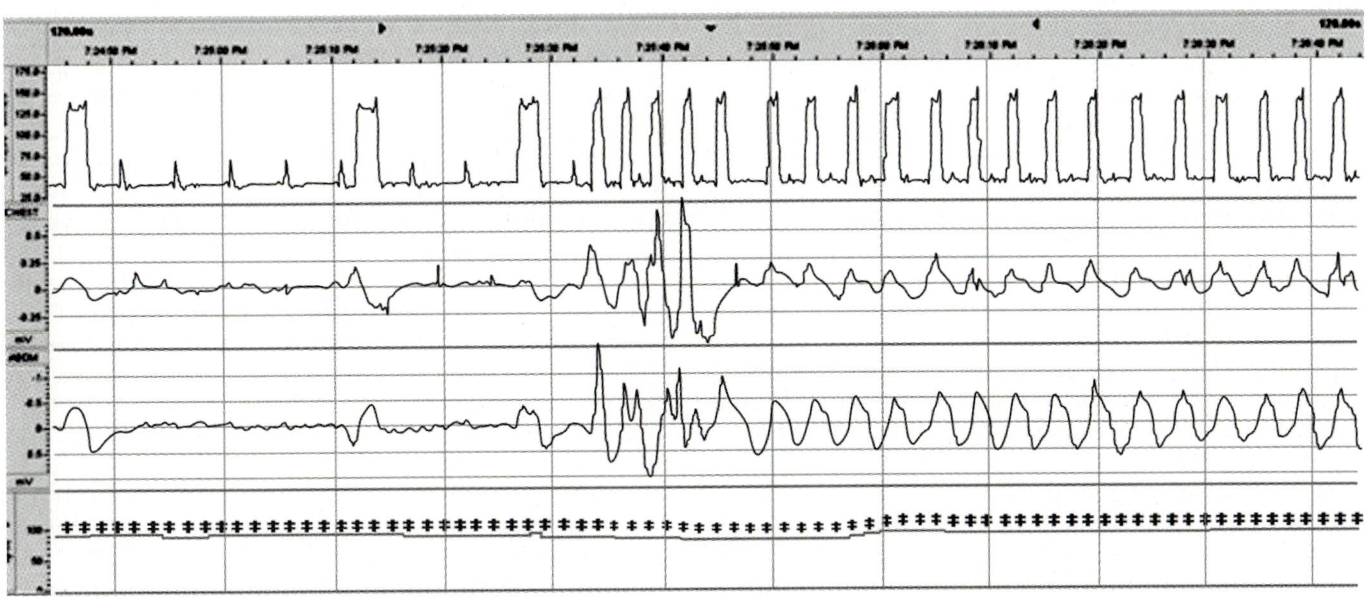

**Fig. 24.10:** Patient-ventilator asynchrony during nocturnal dyspnea

respiratory work, and reduced need for intubation. Lin et al., randomised 55 patients to CPAP or high flow oxygen therapy, and showed significant decrease in the intubation rates in the CPAP group compared with controls (28% *v* 60% respectively). Bersten et al., compared the efficacy of CPAP (10 $cmH_2O$) with that of conventional treatment in 39 patients with CPO and found a significant and rapid improvement in arterial oxygen tension and a significant decrease in arterial carbon dioxide tension in patients treated with CPAP compared with those treated conventionally. Whereas no patient required endotracheal intubation in the CPAP group, 35% of the patients in the oxygen group were intubated within 3 hours of study entry. Although, the final death rate was similar in both groups, patients receiving CPAP showed a significant reduction in ICU length of stay. Lin et al., in another study randomised 100 patients with CPO, and showed favourable effects of incremental CPAP (2.5–12.5 $cmH_2O$) on oxygenation, respiratory rates, and the need for intubation. Although, statistically not significant, the study showed trend towards improved hospital survival. Takeda et al. showed beneficial results of CPAP in CPO in the setting of acute myocardial infarction. Recently, L'Her et al., randomised 89 elderly patients with CPO to standard medical therapy or CPAP (7.5 $cmH_2O$) plus standard medical therapy, and showed that CPAP decreased intubation rates, and promoted early clinical improvement in patients attending emergency departments for severe pulmonary edema. However, only the early 48-hour mortality was reduced and no sustained benefits were seen during the overall hospital stay.

### Bilevel Positive Airway Pressure Compared with Conventional Medical Therapy

Fewer controlled trials have been performed to see if BiPAP is an effective therapy for patients with CPO.

Physiological studies have shown that BiPAP is more effective at unloading the respiratory muscles than CPAP alone in patients with chronic obstructive pulmonary disease (COPD) and in patients with acute CPO. Several open clinical studies have reported rapid improvements in gas exchange in patients with CPO treated with BiPAP. Rusterholtz et al., applied BiPAP [IPAP 20.5 (4.7) $cmH_2O$, EPAP 3.5 (2.3) $cmH_2O$] in 26 patients with CPO and found improvement in gas exchange with only 5 patients requiring endotracheal intubation. In a randomised, prospective trial of 40 patients, Masip et al. found a significantly lower rate of intubation in patients treated with BiPAP [IPAP 15.2 (2.4) $cmH_2O$, EPAP 5 $cmH_2O$] compared with oxygen treated control subjects (5% *v* 33% respectively; $p < 0.037$). Although, resolution time (oxygen saturation 96% and respiratory rate 30 breaths/min) was significantly shorter in the BiPAP group ($p < 0.002$), hospital lengths of stay and death rates were similar in the two groups. Importantly, 4 of the 6 patients (66%) requiring intubation in the conventional therapy group were hypercapnic, whereas no hypercapnic patients in the BiPAP group required intubation. The small sample size however did not permit a subgroup analysis of the impact of hypercapnia on the outcome. Three other randomised trials have also described improvement in physiological parameters but no decrease in intubation rates or mortality. On the other hand, Sharon et al., in a randomised trial of BiPAP (IPAP 8–12 $cmH_2O$, EPAP 3–5 $cmH_2O$) plus low dose nitroglycerin compared with high dose nitroglycerin in 40 patients with acute pulmonary edema showed that patients treated with BiPAP had a higher rates of intubation, myocardial infarction, and death compared with control subjects. The combined primary end point (death, mechanical ventilation or myocardial infarction) was seen in 85% of BiPAP group compared with 25% of control ($p < 0.0003$). However, the findings of this study are controversial and the 80% intubation rate in the BiPAP group is inordinately high, and may reflect the use of low inspired oxygen concentration and low airway pressures. Moreover, the classification of myocardial infarction cannot be taken as a valid end point and can probably be the cause of the emergency presentation with pulmonary edema. On the other hand, Nava et al., in a multicentre study randomised 130 patients to medical therapy or BiPAP [IPAP 14.5 (21.1) $cmH_2O$, EPAP 6.1 (3.2) $cmH_2O$]. BiPAP improved hypoxaemia, respiratory rate and dyspnea significantly faster than did oxygen therapy, but the intubation rate, hospital mortality and the duration of hospital stay were similar in the two groups. However, in the subgroup of hypercapnic patients, intubation rates were lower in the BiPAP group than oxygen therapy (2 of 33 compared with 9 of 31; $p < 0.015$). Adverse events, including myocardial infarction, were equally distributed in the two groups. Recently, Park et al., randomly assigned 80 patients with acute CPO to oxygen, CPAP and BiPAP. Treatment with CPAP or BiPAP resulted in significant improvement in the pressure of aterial oxygen/fraction of inspiral oxygen ($PaO_2/FiO_2$) ratio, subjective dyspnea score, and respiratory and heart rates compared with oxygen therapy. Endotracheal intubation was necessary in 11 of 26 patients (42%) in the oxygen group, but only in 2 of 27 patients (7%) in each NIV group ($p = 0.001$). There was no increase in the incidence of acute myocardial infarction in the CPAP or BiPAP groups. Mortality at 15 days was higher in the oxygen than in the NIV groups ($p < 0.05$).

### Continuous Positive Airway Pressure Compared with Bilevel Positive Airway Pressure

The superiority of BiPAP over standard therapy for acute CPO is not surprising, but the question of interest is whether BiPAP is superior to CPAP alone. There have been four randomised trials that have attempted to answer this question. Mehta et al., randomised patients to receive either nasal CPAP (10 $cmH_2O$) or BiPAP (IPAP 15 $cmH_2O$/EPAP 5 $cmH_2O$). Although the BiPAP group had greater reductions in partial pressure of carbon dioxide ($PaCO_2$), systolic blood pressure, mean arterial pressure, and hypercapnia than did the CPAP group, myocardial infarction rates were higher in the BiPAP group (71%) than in the CPAP group (31%) and the study was stopped prematurely after the enrolment of 27 patients. While this difference could have been attributable to unequal randomisation as more patients in the BiPAP group presented with chest pain, the results none the less raised concerns about the safety of the ventilatory techniques used to treat CPO. On the other hand, Park et al., and Bellone et al. showed that BiPAP was as effective as CPAP in the treatment of CPO and both methods improved ventilation and vital signs in patients with acute CPO. No significant differences were found in hospital mortality and acute myocardial infarction rates in patients with acute CPO in comparison with CPAP alone. Recently, Crane et al., randomised 60 patients presenting with acute CPO to receive conventional oxygen therapy, CPAP (10 $cmH_2O$), or bilevel ventilation (IPAP 15 $cmH_2O$, EPAP 5 $cmH_2O$). Although, treatment success (respiratory rate < 23 breaths per minute (bpm) oxygen saturation >90%, pH >7.35 occurred in 3 patients in the control group, seven in the CPAP group, and nine in the BiPAP group (p = 0.116), 14 of the control group patients survived to hospital discharge, compared with 20 in the CPAP group and 15 in the bilevel group (p = 0.029).

However, again like BiPAP compared with standard medical therapy group, this is not statistically significant, and more studies are required to settle this issue.

## PRACTICAL ASPECTS OF NONINVASIVE VENTILATION IN CARDIOGENIC PULMONARY EDEMA

### Where are these Patients Best Treated?

While most patients with CPO present to the emergency department, practical issues, including hospital setup and staff determine where NIV is actually performed. It is important to realise that the workload in the first 6–8 hours may be greater than that required for a conventionally managed patient. Consequently, patients with severe CPO requiring NIV need to be triaged to an environment with round the clock medical care, adequate nurse-patient ratio, and continuous electrocardiographic and pulse oximetry monitoring facilities. Many patients with CPO would be as a consequence of myocardial infarction and unlike many investigators who have excluded such patients; many centres concurrently provide support with NIV while proceeding to thrombolysis or percutaneous revascularisation (Figs 24.11–24.19 and Table 24.4).

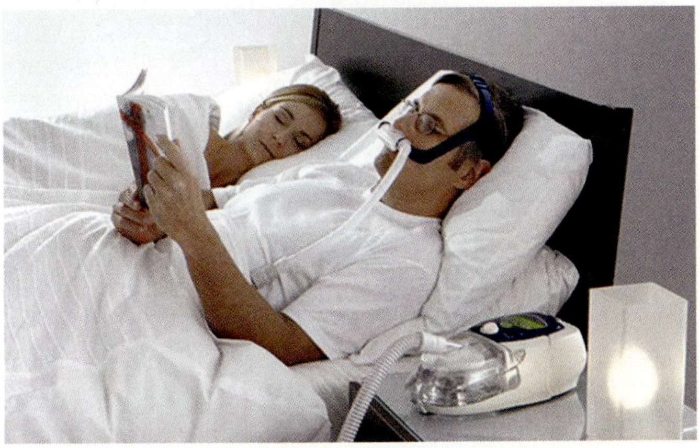

**Fig. 24.11:** Couple sleeping on the same bed fitted with PAP machine in patient with acute respiratory failure

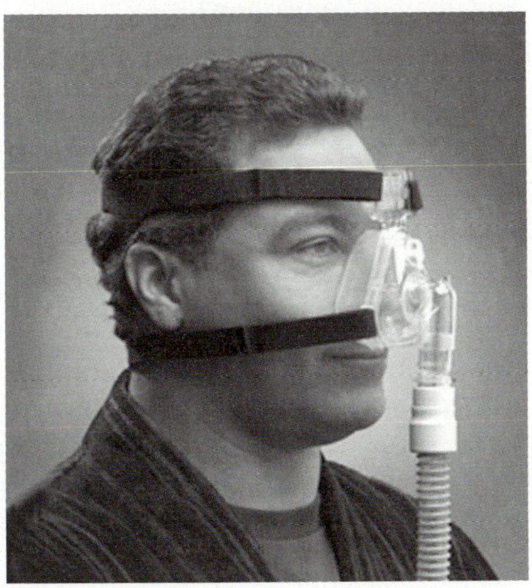

**Fig. 24.12:** Patient is fitted with noninvasive ventilation mask

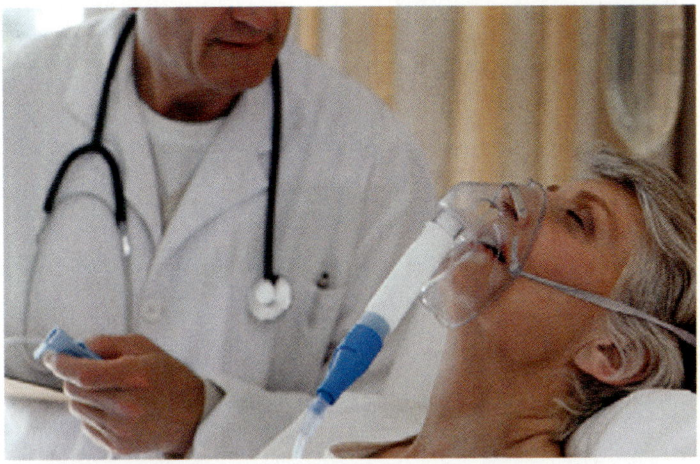

**Fig. 24.13:** An awake patient being put on NIV. He is wearing a full face mask. There are also smaller masks for patients who feel claustrophobic

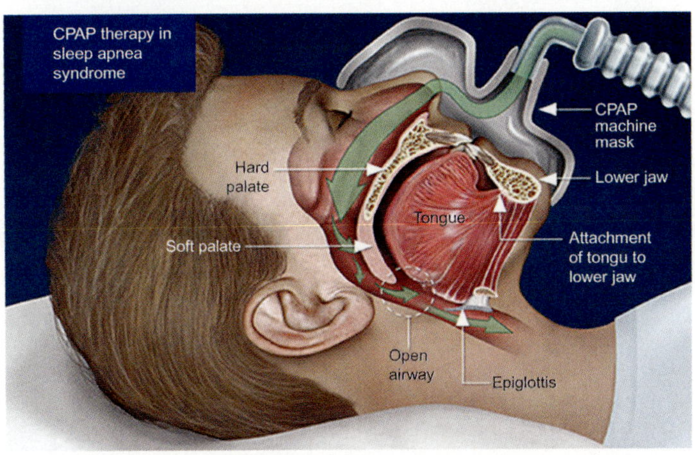


**Fig. 24.14:** Continuous positive airway pressure (CPAP) is pressurized air generated from a bedside machine. The air is delivered through a tube, connected to a mask, covering the nose. The force of the pressurized air splints the airway open. The CPAP opens the airway like air into a balloon; when air is blown into the balloon, it opens and gets wider. This is exactly how CPAP clears the airway

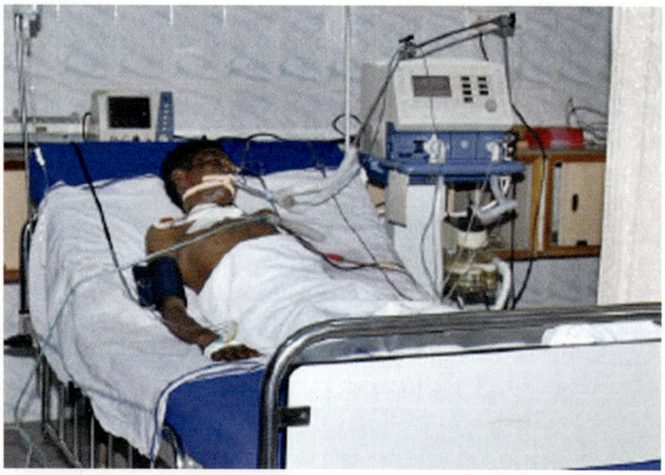

**Fig. 24.15:** Inside view of the noninvasive ventilation laboratory and ventilatory support to a patient with respiratory failure

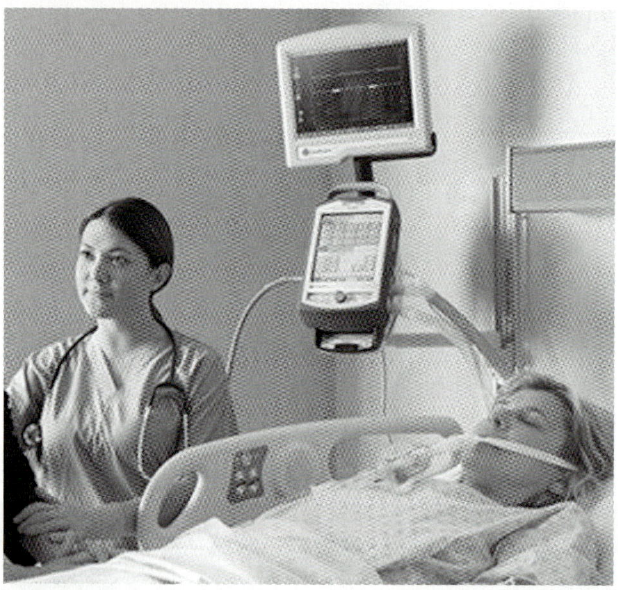

**Fig. 24.16:** Respiratory technologist fitting the face mask for non-invasive ventilation

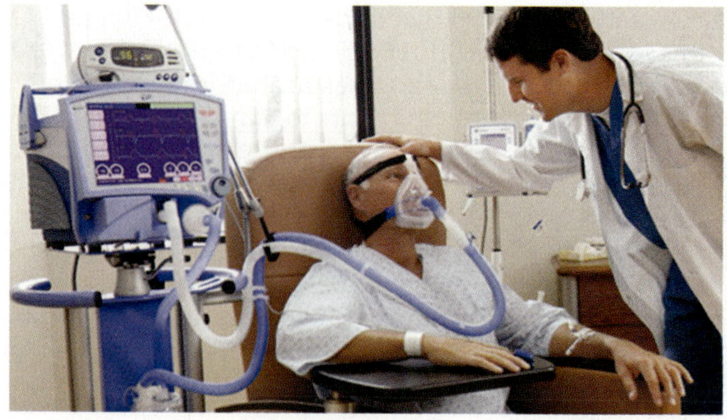

**Fig. 24.17:** Patient undergoing noninvasive positive pressure ventilation

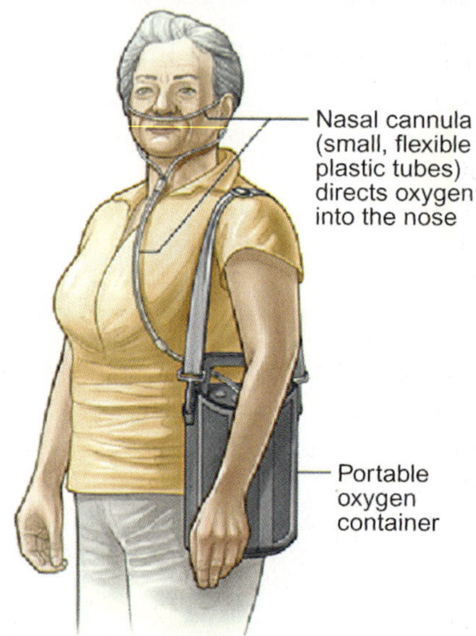


**Fig. 24.18:** The image shows how a nasal cannula and portable oxygen container are attached to a patient

### Do All Patients with Cardiogenic Pulmonary Edema Require Noninvasive Ventilation?

Not all patients with CPO require NIV. In fact, a large number of patients rapidly respond to medical treatment

**Table 24.4:** Troubleshooting of crucial issues of pressure support ventilation

| Problem | Potential cause | Corrective measure |
|---|---|---|
| Inspiratory trigger failure | Air leak | Adjust mask or Change type |
| | Autocycling | Reduce trigger sensitivity |
| | Increased work of breathing | Adjust trigger sensitivity or change to a flow trigger if pressure trigger used |
| Inadequate pressurization | Pressure rise time too long | Reduction of pressure rise time |
| | Pressure support too low | Increase inspiratory pressure |
| Failure to cycle into expiration | Air leak leading to inspiratory hang up | Adjust mask or consider switch from nasal to face mask |
| | High respiratory flow | Increase end-inspiratory flow threshold and set time limit for inspiration |
| $CO_2$ rebreathing | Single circuit with no true exhalation valve | Use low lines and use non-breathe valve |
| | High respiratory rate | Lower respiratory rate |
| | No PEEP | Add PEEP to leavage mask |
| | Large mask dead space | Reduce dead space with padding |

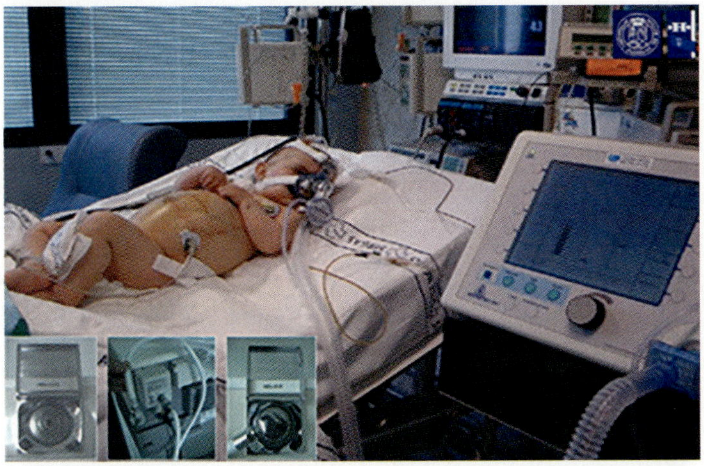

**Fig. 24.19:** Infant on BiPAP vision noninvasive ventilator adapted for HELIOX delivery; the HELIOX is introduced through the device's pressurized-oxygen inlet

and do not need additional intervention. NIV is likely to be beneficial in patients with more severe forms of CPO, especially those who present with a pH <7.25 or systolic blood pressure <180 mmHg. A potential use for NIV is to support patients who are not candidates for intubation, either because of a previous directive or as a result of poor prognosis related to an underlying disease. Another approach is to give a trial of NIV in all patients with CPO who do not respond to initial medical therapy. However, patients should be carefully monitored and failure to improve after 30 minutes on NIV should be an indication for its withdrawal, with facilities for immediate endotracheal intubation and mechanical ventilation being readily available.

### How should Noninvasive Ventilation be Applied Initially?

The application of NIV is an art of medicine. All physicians using NIV should personally apply NIV to actually understand what the patient is experiencing. You should not order a specific pressure level for a given patient without first applying NIV and assessing the patient's tolerance to the device. Initial application of NIV requires careful instruction of the patient, with a goal to gain the patient's confidence and acceptance of NIV. You must start with low pressures and the mask should be held and not strapped to the patient's face. As the patient accepts the NIV, pressures are increased to reach the gas exchange goal, but generally should not exceed 20–25 $cmH_2O$ to minimise gastric distension and the risk of vomiting. Although, time consuming, the cost savings are large compared with the alternative that is, invasive ventilation.

### What should be the Interface?

The masks most commonly used for short term applications of NIV include nasal or oronasal (also called full face) masks. Although, the nasal mask is theoretically more comfortable for the patient as it is less claustrophobic, has lower dead space volume, permits speech and eating, and better mobilisation of secretions; oronasal masks achieve better control of mouth leak in mouth breathers (common feature during acute respiratory failure) and result in better quality of ventilation, in terms of improved minute ventilation and blood gas pressures. In a study of 70 patients with acute respiratory failure randomised to receive a nasal or oronasal mask, both the masks performed similarly with regard to improvements in gas exchange and avoidance of intubation, however the nasal mask was less well tolerated because of excessive mouth leaks; probably because mouth leaks with nasal CPAP lead to high unidirectional nasal airflow and increased nasal resistance. In another study, however, no significant differences were noted irrespective of the type of mask used. From the available evidence it cannot be said that any interface is clearly superior to another in terms of important outcomes, such as intubation rate or mortality. An oronasal interface may be more effective and better tolerated than the nasal interface for patients with acute respiratory failure. Thus, a sensible approach would be to start with an oronasal mask for most patients with acute respiratory failure, and switch to a nasal mask if prolonged use is contemplated. Whichever mask is chosen, a comfortable fit is of paramount importance, and thus using a mask of proper size, not strapping the headgear too tightly, and using wound care tape on the bridge of the nose are important considerations to avoid pressure ulcers.

### Does the Type of Ventilator Make Any Difference?

Noninvasive ventilator can be delivered through ventilators designed for invasive mechanical ventilation (critical care ventilators), and portable devices. Critical care ventilators are less leak tolerant and are thus likely to sound alarms more inappropriately. But the monitoring capabilities and presence of oxygen blenders make it superior to portable devices. On the other hand, the portable ventilators are more leak tolerant and less likely to sound alarms inappropriately than the critical care ventilators. However, they may promote rebreathing by virtue of their single inspiratory and expiratory tubing (minimised by assuring adequate expiratory pressure and expiratory ports over the nasal bridge). Also, most of the portable ventilators do not have an oxygen blender and supplemental oxygen is usually given by adding it into the mask or the circuit. Thus, continuous pulse oximetry is required to monitor oxygenation when using this device in patients with CPO. However, comparisons of the two devices show that the portable device performs as well as the critical care ventilators. *Recently, ventilators that deliver either invasive ventilation or NIV have been designed.* When in the noninvasive mode, they are more leak tolerant and use only the alarms essential for the operation of NIV. On the other hand, newer portable devices with graphic monitors, oxygen blenders, and sophisticated alarms have also become available for use in the acute setting.

## CONCLUSION

There is a strong evidence for the use of CPAP by facemask in patients with CPO, and CPAP decreases the need for endotracheal intubation and improves survival. However, there is insufficient evidence to recommend the use of BiPAP, probably the exception being patients with hypercapnic CPO. Although, evidence suggests that patients presenting with CPO are more likely to survive to hospital discharge if treated with CPAP, rather than with BiPAP, and probably there is no relation between early physiological changes and hospital survival, the evidence is not strong so as to completely exclude BiPAP, and more studies are required to elucidate the role of BiPAP in CPO.

## BIBLIOGRAPHY


1. Aberman A, Fulop M. The metabolic and respiratory acidosis of acute pulmonary edema. Ann Intern Med 1972;76: 173–84.
2. Anton A, Tarrega J, Giner J, et al. Acute physiologic effects of nasal and full-face masks during noninvasive positive pressure ventilation in patients with acute exacerbations of chronic obstructive pulmonary disease. Respir Care 2003;48:922–5.
3. Appendini L, Patessio A, Zanaboni S, et al. Physiologic effects of positive end-expiratory pressure and mask pressure support during exacerbations of chronic obstructive pulmonary disease. Am J Respir Crit Care Med 1994; 149: 1069–76.
4. Atherton JJ, Moore TD, Lele SS, et al. Diastolic ventricular interaction in chronic heart failure. Lancet 1997;349:1720–4.
5. Aubier M, Trippenbach T, Roussos C. Respiratory muscle fatigue during cardiogenic shock. J Appl Physiol 1981;51: 499–508.
6. Baratz DM, Westbrooke PR, Shah PK, et al. Effect of nasal continuous positive airway pressure on cardiac output and oxygen delivery in patients with congestive heart failure. Chest 1992;102:1397–401.
7. Bellone A, Monari A, Cortellaro F, et al. Myocardial infarction rate in acute pulmonary edema: Noninvasive pressure support ventilation versus continuous positive airway pressure. Crit Care Med 2004;32:1860–5.
8. Bersten AD, Holt AW, Vedig AE, et al. Treatment of severe cardiogenic pulmonary edema with continuous positive airway pressure delivered by face mask. N Engl J Med 1991;325:1825–30.
9. Bersten AD. Noninvasive ventilation for cardiogenic pulmonary edema. Froth and bubbles? Am J Respir Crit Care Med 2003;168:1406–8.
10. Bradley TD, Holloway RM, McLaughlin PR, et al. Cardiac output responses to continuous positive airway pressure in congestive heart failure. Am Rev Respir Dis 1992;145: 377–82.
11. Brochard L, Mancebo J, Elliott MW. Noninvasive ventilation for acute respiratory failure. Eur Respir J 2002;19:712–21.
12. Brochard L. Noninvasive ventilation for acute respiratory failure. JAMA 2002;288:932–5.
13. Broseghini C, Brandolese R, Poggi R, et al. Respiratory mechanics during the first day of mechanical ventilation in patients with pulmonary edema and chronic airway obstruction. Am Rev Respir Dis 1988;138:355–61.
14. Buda AJ, Pinsky MR, Ingels NB Jr, et al. Effect of intrathoracic pressure on left ventricular performance. N Engl J Med 1979;301:453–9.
15. Chadda K, Annane D, Hart N, et al. Cardiac and respiratory effects of continuous positive airway pressure and noninvasive ventilation in acute cardiogenic pulmonary edema. Crit Care Med 2002;30:2457–61.
16. Cotter G, Metzkor E, Kaluski E, et al. Randomized trial of high-dose isosorbide dinitrate plus low-dose furosemide versus high-dose furosemide plus low-dose isosorbide dinitrate in severe pulmonary edema. Lancet 1998;351: 389–93.
17. Cotter G, Moshkovitz Y, Milovanov O, et al. Acute heart failure: a novel approach to its pathogenesis and treatment. Eur J Heart Fail 2002;4:227–34.
18. Crane SD, Elliott MW, Gilligan P, et al. Randomized controlled comparison of continuous positive airways pressure, bilevel noninvasive ventilation, and standard treatment in emergency department patients with acute cardiogenic pulmonary edema. Emerg Med J 2004;21: 155–61.
19. Ferguson GT, Gilmartin M. CO2 rebreathing during BiPAP ventilatory assistance. Am J Respir Crit Care Med 1995;151: 1126–35.
20. Fessler HE, Brower RG, Wise RA, et al. Effects of systolic and diastolic positive pleural pressure pulses with altered cardiac contractility. J Appl Physiol 1992;73:498–505.
21. Fessler HE, Brower RG, Wise RA, et al. Mechanism of reduced LV afterload by systolic and diastolic pleural pressure. J Appl Physiol 1988;65:1244–50.
22. Field S, Kelly SM, Macklem PT. The oxygen cost of breathing in patients with cardiorespiratory disease. Am Rev Respir Dis 1982;126:9–13.
23. Gehlbach BK, Geppert E. The pulmonary manifestations of left heart failure. Chest 2004;125:669–82.
24. Hess DR. The evidence for noninvasive positive-pressure ventilation in the care of patients in acute respiratory failure: a systematic review of the literature. Respir Care 2004;49: 810–29.
25. Katz J, Kraemer R, Gjerde G. Inspiratory work and airway pressure with continuous positive airway pressure delivery systems. Chest 1985;88:519–26.
26. Kelly CA, Newby DE, McDonagh TA, et al. Randomized controlled trial of continuous positive airway pressure and standard oxygen therapy in acute pulmonary edema; effects on plasma brain natriuretic peptide concentrations. Eur Heart J 2002;23:1379–86.
27. Kwok H, McCormack J, Cece R, et al. Controlled trial of oronasal versus nasal mask ventilation in the treatment of acute respiratory failure. Crit Care Med 2003;31:468–73.
28. L'Her E, Duquesne F, Girou E, et al. Noninvasive continuous positive airway pressure in elderly cardiogenic pulmonary edema patients. Intensive Care Med 2004;30:882–8.
29. Lapinsky SE, Mount DB, Mackey D, et al. Management of acute respiratory failure due to pulmonary edema with nasal positive pressure support. Chest 1994;105:229–31.
30. Lenique F, Habis M, Lofaso F, et al. Ventilatory and hemo-dynamic effects of continuous positive airway pressure in left heart failure. Am J Respir Crit Care Med 1997;155:500–5.

31. Levitt MA. A prospective, randomized trial of BiPAP in severe acute congestive heart failure. J Emerg Med 2001; 21:363–9.
32. Lin M, Chiang HT. The efficacy of early continuous positive airway pressure therapy in patients with acute cardiogenic pulmonary edema. J Formos Med Assoc 1991; 90:736–43
33. Lin M, Yang YF, Chiang HT, et al. Reappraisal of continuous positive airway pressure therapy in acute cardiogenic pulmonary edema: short-term results and long-term follow-up. Chest 1995;107:1379–86.
34. Lofaso F, Brochard L, Hang T, et al. Home versus intensive care pressure support devices. Experimental and clinical comparison. Am J Respir Crit Care Med 1996;153:1591–9.
35. Masip J, Betbese AJ, Paez J, et al. Noninvasive pressure support ventilation versus conventional oxygen therapy in acute cardiogenic pulmonary edema: a randomized trial. Lancet 2000;356:2126–32.
36. Masip J, Paez J, Merino M, et al. Risk factors for intubation as a guide for noninvasive ventilation in patients with severe acute cardiogenic pulmonary edema. Intensive Care Med 2003;29:1921–8.
37. Mehta S, Hill NS. Noninvasive ventilation. Am J Respir Crit Care Med 2001;163:540–77.
38. Mehta S, Jay GD, Woolard RH, et al. Randomized, prospective trial of bilevel versus continuous positive airway pressure in acute pulmonary edema. Crit Care Med 1997; 25:620–8.
39. Naughton MT, Rahman MA, Hara K, et al. Effect of continuous positive airway pressure on intrathoracic and left ventricular transmural pressures in patients with congestive heart failure. Circulation 1995;9:1725–31.

# 25 Cardiovascular Emergencies in Children and Adolescents

Compared with adults, cardiac emergencies are infrequent in children and clinical presentation is often quite variable. In adults, cardiac emergencies are most commonly related to complications of coronary artery disease; however, in pediatric cases, the coronaries are only rarely the underlying problem. Pediatric cardiac emergencies comprise a range of pathology including but not limited to undiagnosed congenital heart disease in the infant; complications of palliated congenital heart disease in children; arrhythmias related to underlying cardiac pathology in the teenager and acquired heart disease. The emergency room physician and pediatric intensivist will usually be the first and second lines of care for pediatric cardiac emergencies and thus it is imperative that they have knowledge of the diverse presentations of cardiac disease in order to increase the likelihood of delivering early appropriate therapy and referral. The objective of this review is to outline cardiac emergencies in the pediatric population and contrast the presentation with adults (Figs 25.1 and 25.2).

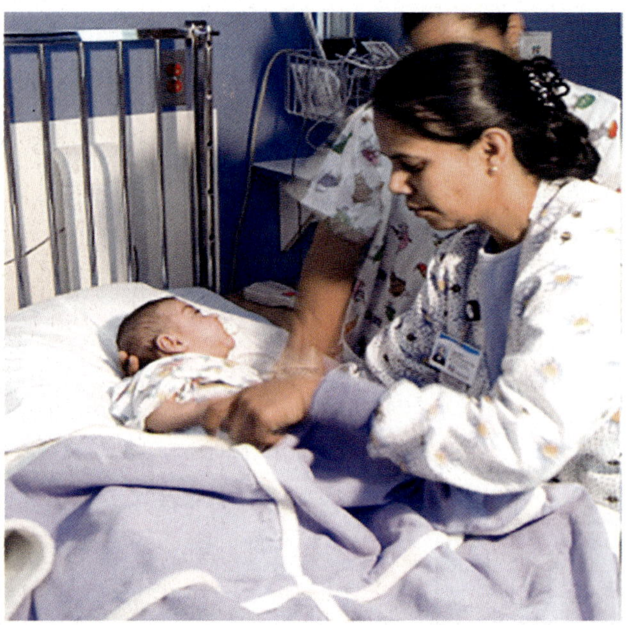

**Fig. 25.1:** Cardiologist and attending nurse are connecting life supports to a child admitted in emergency department with intractable heart failure

In adults, cardiac disease is not uncommon and the majority of causes of sudden cardiac death are due to atherosclerotic coronary artery disease. However, cardiac death in children is a rare occurrence and the cause differs based on the age of the child. For infants less than one year of age, ductal dependent congenital heart disease is the most common cause, and after the first year and into early adulthood acquired heart conditions, such as myocarditis, cardiomyopathy and aortic dissection in patients with Marfan's syndrome. The objective of this review is to outline cardiac emergencies in the pediatric population and contrast the presentation with adults. The emergency room

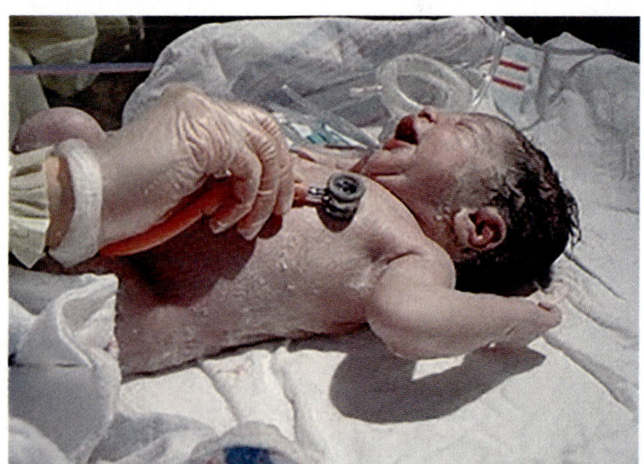

**Fig. 25.2:** Emergency physician is attending a child admitted in emergency department

**Table 25.1:** Common cardiovascular emergencies in children and adolescents

1. Congenital heart diseases
   A. Acyanotic
      - Left sided obstructive disorders HLHS
      - Dissection of aorta, Marfan syndrome
   B. Cyanotic heart diseases
      - Tetrology of Fallot
      - D-TGV
      - TAPVC
      - Abstein anomaly
2. Acquired heart disease
   - Rheumatic heart disease
   - Hypertensive heart disease
   - Myocarditis
   - Infective endocarditis
   - Kawasaki's disease
   - Pulmonary embolism
3. Coronary artery anomalies, i.e. ALCAPA
4. Heart failure
5. Cardiac arrhythmia
6. Cardiac tamponade
7. Postoperative cardiac emergencies
8. Cardiomyopathies
9. Toxicological emergencies
10. Electrolyte imbalance

HLHS=hypoplastic left-heart syndrome;D-TGV=dextro-transposition of the great vessels; TAPVC=total anomalous pulmonary venous connection; ALCAPA=anomalous origin of left coronary artery from the pulmonary artery

physician and pediatric intensivist will usually be the first and second lines of care for pediatric cardiac emergencies and thus it is imperative that they have knowledge of the diverse presentations of cardiac disease in order to increase the likelihood of delivering early appropriate therapy and referral (Table 25.1).

### Ductal Dependent Lesions

Congenital heart diseases (CHDs) are rare conditions, and the mortality is highest among infants and children and among the severe cardiac defects, such as hypoplastic left heart syndrome (HLHS). In the majority of the cases, mortality can be attributed to the underlying heart defect. Infants with severe CHD can initially be asymptomatic, with a relatively benign physical exam prior to discharge from the newborn nursery, due to the patency of the ductus arteriosus. The ductus arteriosus usually closes within the first 2 weeks of life, but some take up to 6. However, in infants with heart disease dependent on ductal patency, closure of the ductus can lead infants to become abruptly critically ill. It is important to realize then that any infant less than or equal to 6 weeks who presents in shock or profoundly cyanotic might be secondary to closure of the ductus arteriosus in conjunction with a right or left sided obstructive cardiac lesion.

### Left-sided Obstructive Lesions

These include HLHS, critical aortic stenosis, and coarctation of the aorta represent 12.4% of CHD. In HLHS, for example as the patent ductus arteriosus (PDA) closes, pulmonary overcirculation develops and systemic hypoperfusion, circulatory collapse and shock ensue (Figs 25.3 and 25.4).

The patient will present with respiratory distress, hepatomegaly, tachycardia and signs of poor perfusion. Additionally, in critical coarctation of the aorta femoral pulses are weak or absent and there is a blood pressure differential between the upper and lower extremities reflecting the gradient across the stenotic aortic segment. Prostaglandin infusion is necessary to reopen the PDA and basic resuscitative measures (ABCs) should be initiated. Oxygen therapy can either help or hurt the patient and

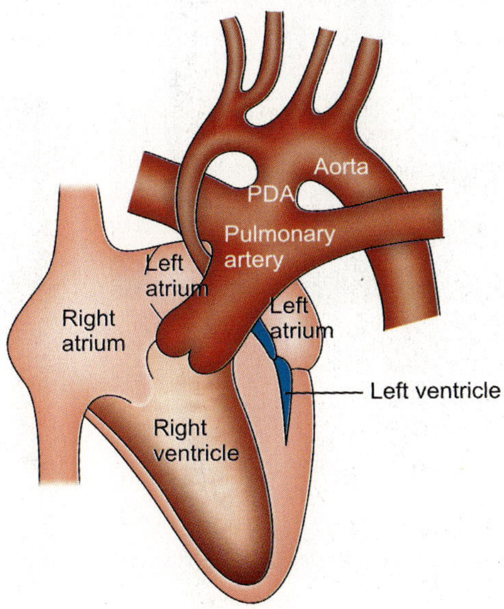


**Fig. 25.3:** Anatomical features of hypoplastic left heart right ventricle and hypoplastic left ventricle are seen

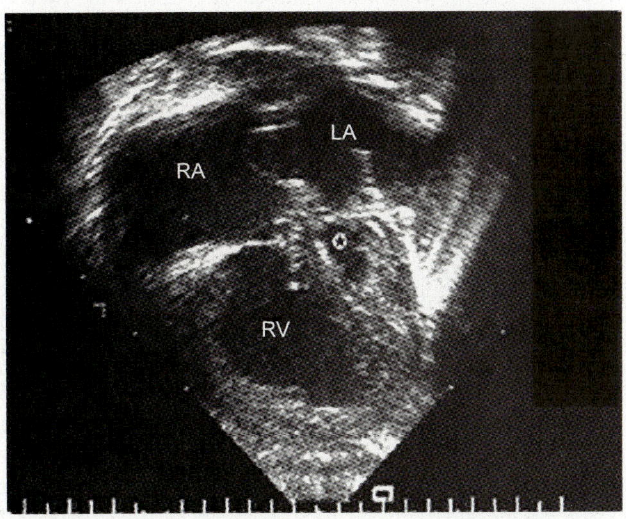


**Fig. 25.4:** This echocardiographic still frame shows chamber view of the heart in a patient with hypoplastic left heart syndrome (HLHS). RA=right atrium; LA=left atrium; RV=right ventricle

should be used judiciously, directed by the underlying anatomy and anticipated oxygen saturation for the heart defect. For example, to achieve a pulmonary circulation to systemic circulation flow ratio of 1:1, an oxygen saturation of 75–80% may be desired (such as in HLHS). In this lesion, administration of oxygen to obtain a 'normal' saturation of 100% would be detrimental, as the oxygen effect of reduced pulmonary vascular resistance compromises systemic perfusion. Of note, in patients with critical coarctation, blood supply to the lower extremities will be extremely compromised such that an intraosseous infusion (IO) in the tibia may not be adequate and a right upper extremity or scalp IV may provide better access until a surgical cut down can be obtained.

## 1. APPROACH TO THE PEDIATRIC PATIENT WITH CYANOSIS

The presentation of a child who is cyanotic can be dramatic. Appropriate management requires a logical approach to reach a general division of the various diagnoses that can be associated with cyanosis. Differentiation must be made to determine if the aetiology of the hypoxemia is secondary to respiratory or cardiac disease. Pneumothorax, airway obstruction, and severe bronchospasm are examples of the most common respiratory causes for cyanosis.

### General Approach to the Cyanotic Child with Suspected Cardiac Disease

Understanding some general concepts of cardiac physiology in each of the cyanotic heart lesions will guide the emergency physician to the appropriate management plan. Children with a cyanotic heart defect are hypoxic because systemic venous blood bypasses the alveolar capillary bed and enters the systemic circulation. The degree of cyanosis is partly determined by the amount of pulmonary venous blood that mixes with the desaturated systemic return. This mixing can occur at various levels, in the atrium, in the ventricles or across the ductus arteriosus. For most of the lesions with decreased pulmonary blood flow, the major determinant to the degree of desaturation is the severity of obstruction of flow to the pulmonary circulation. For the other lesions, the amount of mixing of saturated and desaturated blood will dictate the degree of cyanosis.

### *A. Patient Presentation*

As with acyanotic and obstructive lesions, the age of the child at the time of presentation with previously unrecognized cyanosis is helpful in narrowing the list of differential diagnoses. Children with cyanotic congenital heart disease usually present within the first few months after birth. Infants with complete transposition of the great arteries, tricuspid atresia, or pulmonary atresia with intact ven-tricular septum will usually present in the first week after birth, if not shortly after delivery. Associated lesions, such as large ventricular septal defects may lessen the degree of cyanosis and thus delay presentation. The timing of presentation for some lesions is determined by the development of obstruction to pulmonary blood flow. In tetralogy of Fallot, the initial degree of pulmonary stenosis may be quite mild and the patient may experience signs and symptoms related to a large left-to-right shunt. The infundibular stenosis, however, can be progressive leading to decrease in pulmonary blood flow and greater right-to-left shunting. In an older previously healthy child, new onset cyanosis is extremely unlikely to be the result of undiagnosed cyanotic heart lesion.

a. *Patient history:* In the newborn, there may not be much history apart from the cyanosis. Obviously, any respiratory symptoms should suggest a pulmonary process; however, this does not exclude cardiac disease. In the child who has known congenital heart disease information regarding the underlying cardiac defect, current medications, and most importantly previous surgeries altering the physiology can be crucial in guiding the emergency physician to the appropriate treatment. If the child is chronically cyanotic, most families will know the 'baseline' oxygen saturation for their child. Comparing this information with the current measured saturation will help determine if there is any acute disease process or interval change. Specific problems seen in children who have undergone corrective or palliative surgery will be discussed separately.
b. *Physical examination:* The examination should always include an accurate documentation of the patient's vital signs. Shock can present with cyanosis because of poor

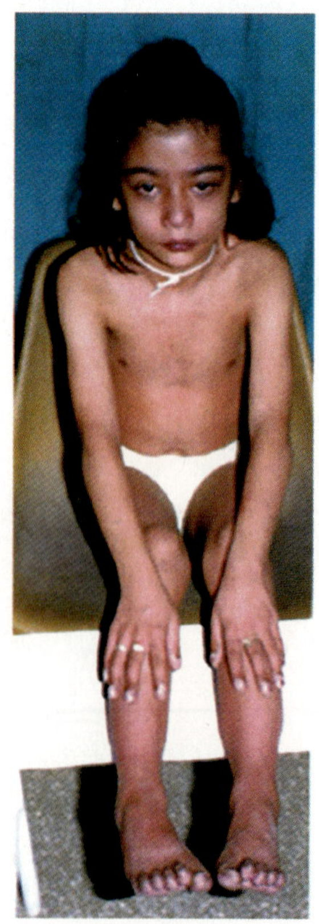

**Fig. 25.5:** Central cyanosis and digital clubbing in a child with R-L shunt

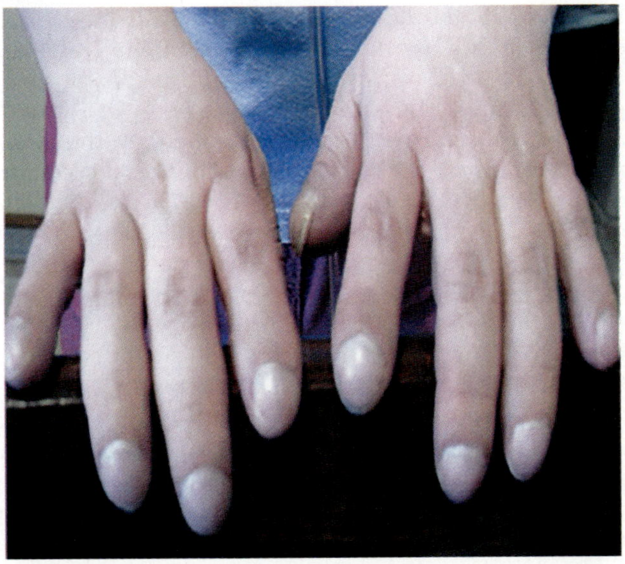

**Fig. 25.6:** Clubbing in the fingers of a 18-year-old female with Eisenmenger's syndrome (VSD, R-L shunt)

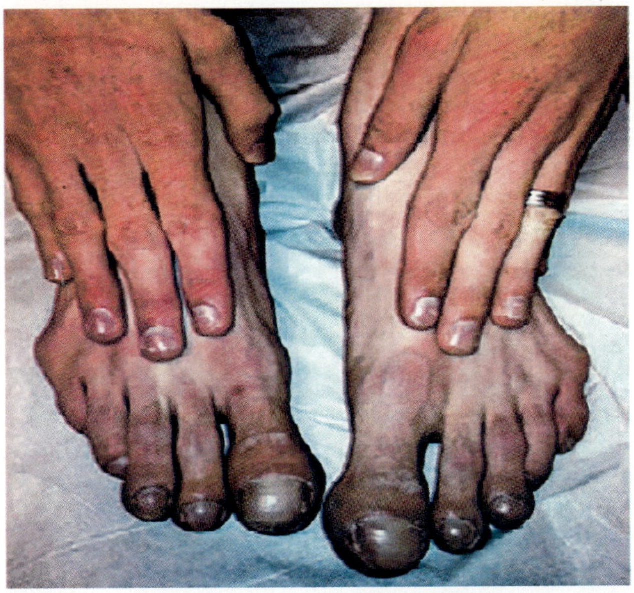

**Fig. 25.7:** A 12-year-old boy with unrepaired large PDA, Eisenmenger's syndrome, and right-to-left shunting at the ductal level producing differential cyanosis. The transcutaneous oxygen saturation in the fingers was 92% and in the toes 84%. The central hematocrit was 65%. Clubbing is more apparent in the toes than in the fingers

perfusion and venous stasis. Examination of the oral mucosa will usually determine the presence or absence of central cyanosis. It should be noted that central cyanosis can be masked by the presence of significant anemia.

Auscultation of the lung fields will determine if there is evidence of pulmonary disease (Figs 25.5–25.7 and Table 25.2).

Children with cyanotic heart defects most often have clear lung fields, with the possible exception of total anomalous pulmonary venous connection, when rales may be present. Many infants with significant cyanosis will also have an increased respiratory rate without signs of distress, so-called happy tachypnea-caused by the CNS response to hypoxemia. The absence of a heart murmur does not exclude the presence of congenital heart disease. The presence of a specific type or location of a murmur simply may indicate an associated defect and not the primary anomaly. In the majority of cyanotic defects, the second heart sound is single and loud; total anomalous pulmonary venous connection and Ebstein's malformation of the tricuspid valve are the exceptions, where the second heart sound is usually widely split.

**Table 25.2:** Pulmonary blood flow in cyanotic congenital heart defects

**Decreased pulmonary blood flow**
- Tetralogy of Fallot
- Tetralogy of Fallot with pulmonary atresia
- Pulmonary atresia with intact ventricular septum
- Critical pulmonary stenosis
- Ebstein's malformation of the tricuspid valve Tricuspid atresia with pulmonary stenosis

**Normal to slightly increased pulmonary blood flow**
- Transposition of the great arteries

**Increased pulmonary blood flow**
- Total anomalous pulmonary venous connection
- Truncus arteriosus

### B. Patient Assessment

a. *Pulse-oximetry and arterial blood gas measurement:* Transcutaneous pulse-oximetry is usually readily available and accurate to determine the level of hypoxia. In some situations, a transcutaneous saturation can not be obtained or the accuracy of the measurement is doubtful, such as in a poorly perfused child. In these situations, an arterial blood gas analysis is essential to determine the oxygenation, ventilation and acid-base status of the patient.

b. *Radiographic findings:* A chest X-ray (CXR) is important to differentiate the varied cyanotic congenital heart defects as well as to exclude the presence of pulmonary disease. It should be obtained on all patients with the initial presentation of cyanosis.

The importance of comparing the present study to any previous CXRs, if available, cannot be more strongly emphasized. Chronic pulmonary changes may mimic an infiltrate, and progressive changes in cardiac size and pulmonary vascularity in the patient with known heart disease may be diagnostic of the underlying pathology (Figs 25.8 and 25.9).

The presence ofthe stomach on the opposite side of the cardiac silhouette, as in left-sided stomach bubble with dextrocardia, suggests a high probability of a complex heart defect. The shape of the cardiac silhouette may guide the physician to the correct cardiac diagnosis.

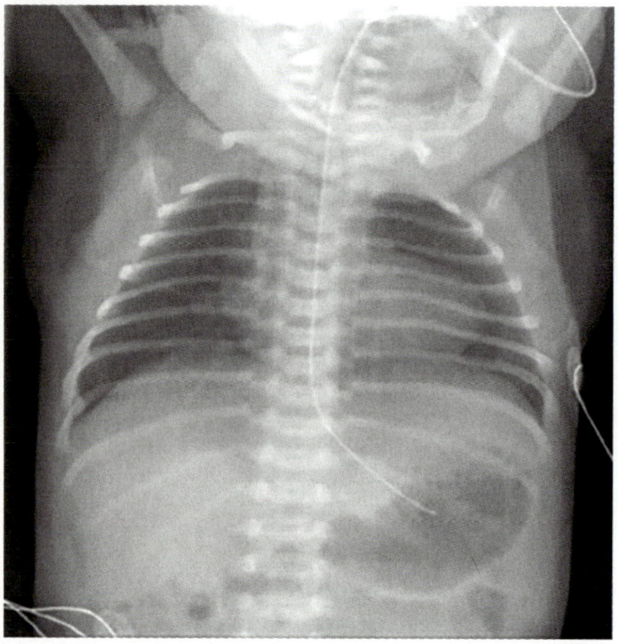

**Fig. 25.8:** Radiologically, the heart size is usually normal. There is elevation of the cardiac apex, secondary to right-ventricular hypertrophy. The cardiac silhouette is often described as 'boot-shaped'. The lung fields are usually clear and in cases of severe outflow tract obstruction may appear oligaemic. There may be a concavity of the left border of the heart usually occupied by the pulmonary artery. The radiological appearances can vary depending on other associated cardiac lesions. For example, if collateral vessels are present between the aorta and pulmonary circulations, there may be pulmonary plethora

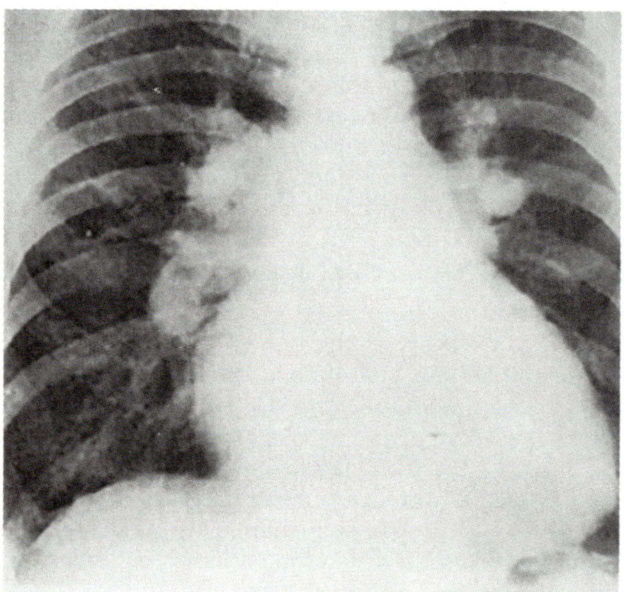

**Fig. 25.9:** Atrial septal defect, with elevated pulmonary vascular resistance. Secundum atrial septal defect. There is a larked disparity between the size of the hilar arteries and the eripheral pulmonary vessels, indicating an increase in pulmonary vascular resistance. The right ventricular pressure was almost at systemic levels

Patients with tetralogy of Fallot classically have a 'boot-shaped' heart because of absence of the pulmonary artery knob and upturned apex. In transposition of the great arteries, the silhouette has been described as an 'egg on a string,' a shape caused by the narrow mediastinum resulting from the abnormal orientation of the aorta and pulmonary artery. The cardiac shape on the CXR should be used only to collaborate the physical findings and history of the patient. Unlike the anomalies presenting with congestive heart failure (CHF), the pulmonary vascularity in cyanotic lesions can be normal, increased, or decreased. The appearance of the **right-sided obstructive lesions.**

Such as severe tetralogy of Fallot and pulmonary atresia with intact ventricular septum depend on ductal patency to provide blood flow to the pulmonary artery. As the ductus closes, infants develop progressive and rapid cyanosis not improved with oxygen administration and respiratory distress.

Prostaglandins should be started immediately to reopen the ductus arteriosus in order to provide pulmonary blood flow through left to right shunting (aorta across the PDA to pulmonary artery), as opposed to the right to left shunt on left-sided obstructive lesions. In these lesions, 100% oxygen is useful to improve pulmonary blood flow and increase dissolved $O_2$ content. pulmonary vascular markings will reflect the physiology of the patient (Figs 25.10 and 25.11).

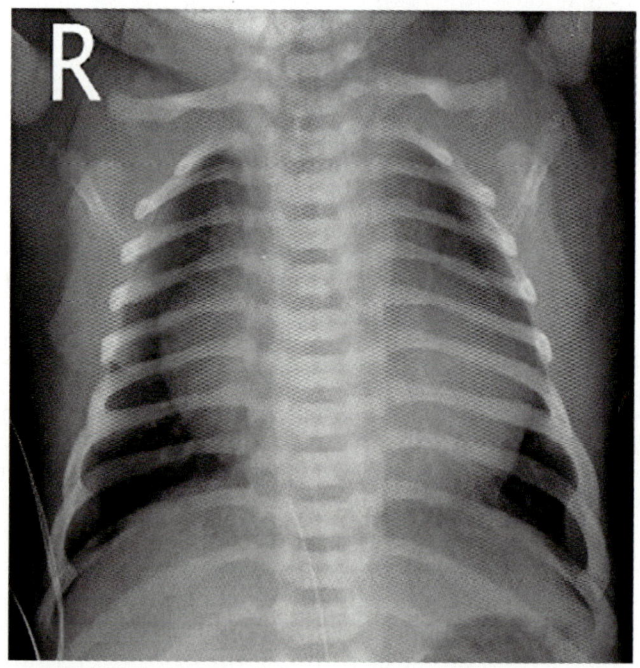


**Fig. 25.10:** X-ray chest PA view pulmonary atresia. The cardiac silhouette may be normal size, or enlarged (in the case shown to the left, this was from right atrial enlargement due to poor communication between right and left atria via a restricted foramen ovale). Fistulae from the right ventricle to the coronary circulation may be present, particularly if the right ventricle and tricuspid valve are small

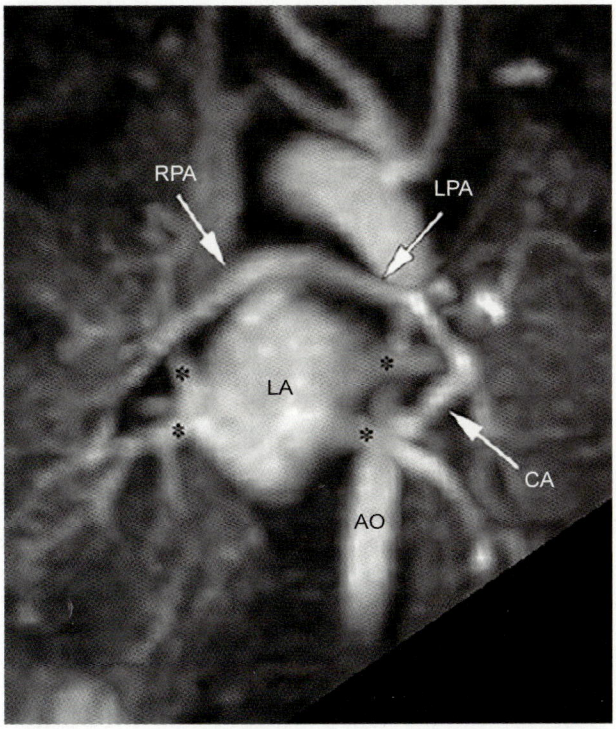


**Fig. 25.11:** Pulmonary atresia with intact ventricular septum in a 1-day-old girl. MR angiographic images demonstrate that the pulmonary arteries (LPA, RPA) are hypoplastic, confluent, and supplied by a single collateral artery (CA) from the descending aorta (AO). LA=left atrium, *=pulmonary veins. A right ventricle–pulmonary artery conduit was planned, but the patient died before surgery could be performed

c. *Electrocardiogram:* As in the patient with acyanotic heart disease with CHF, the ECG is usually not

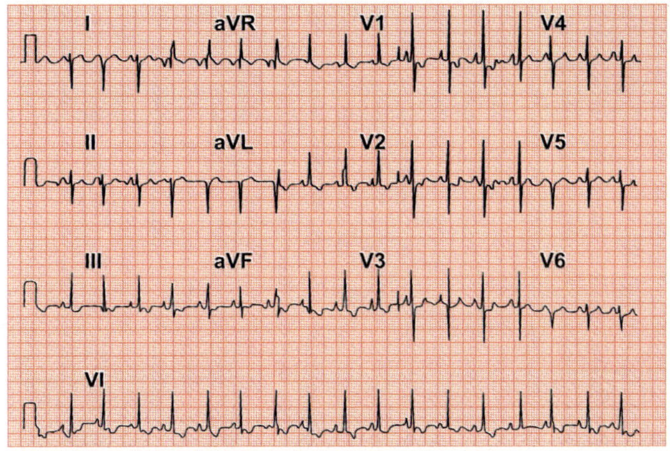


**Fig. 25.12:** A 15-year-old patient with large conoventricular ventricular septal defect and Eisenmenger's syndrome. The aortic oxygen saturation was 72% and hematocrit 74%. The tracing shows right axis deviation, right atrial enlargement, right ventricular hypertrophy, and right ventricular strain (inverted T-waves in the anterior leads)

diagnostic. The presence or absence of sinus rhythm should be determined. Any ventricular hypertrophy, atrial enlargement, and axis deviation should be noted. It should be emphasized that the age of the patient will determine the normal criteria in interpreting any ECG from a child.

Tachyarrhythmias do not typically present with cyanosis (Figs 25.12–25.15).

d. *Oxygen challenge test:* The patient who presents to the emergency department with cyanosis should be treated with oxygen supplementation. However, a few caveats should be noted.

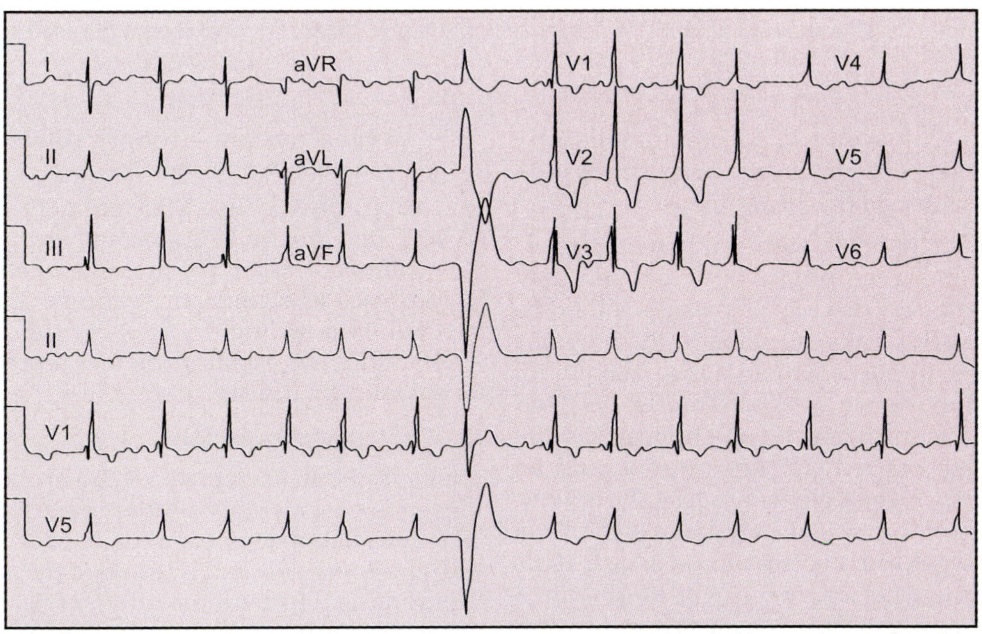


**Fig. 25.13:** Electrocardiogram of a 18-year-old girl with Eisenmenger complex, demonstrating atrial fibrillation with right axis deviation, right ventricular hypertrophy, right bundle-branch block, and premature ventricular beat

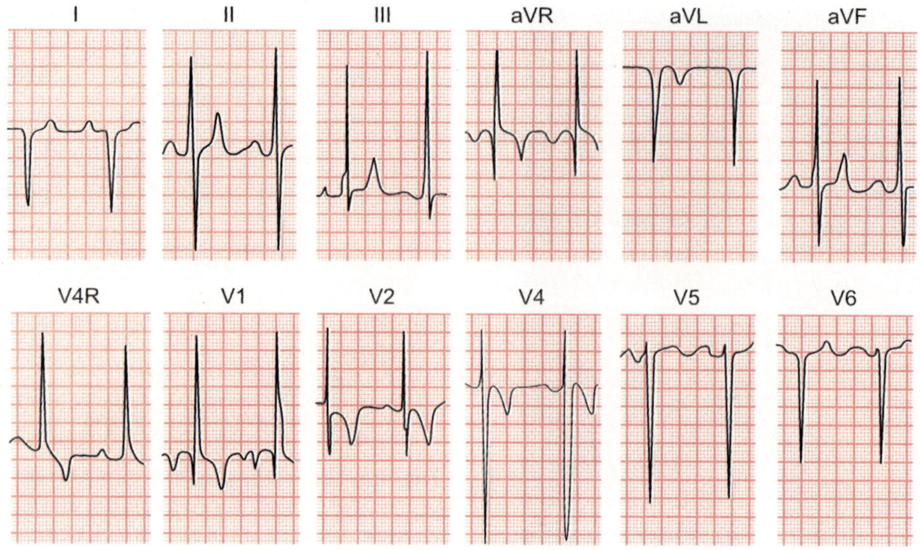


**Fig. 25.14:** Electrocardiograms showing right axis showing right axis deviation, right ventricular hypertrophy, almost QS pattern in leads 1, aVL V5 and V6 in a patient with D-transposition of great arteries

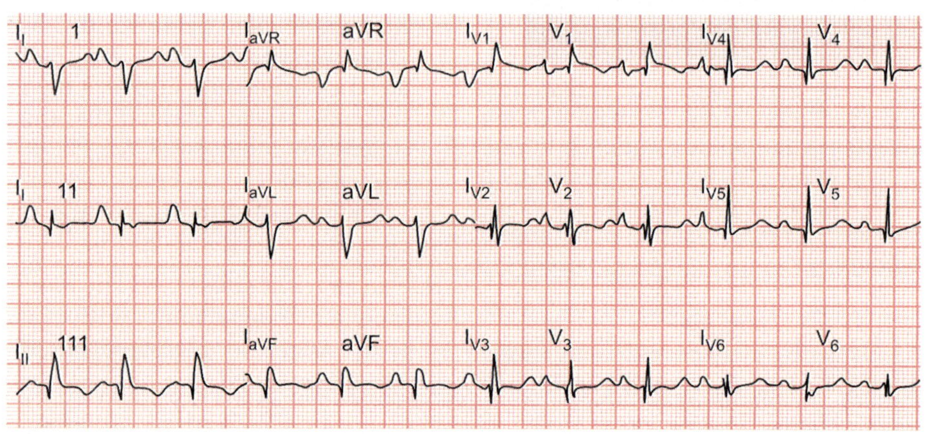


**Fig. 25.15:** The electrocardiogram showed sinus rhythm, signs of right atrial hypertrophy, and a right bundle branch block in Ebstein anomaly

- **First**, children with pulmonary pathology usually have a greater response to oxygen supplementation than children with cyanotic heart disease.
- **Second**, in older patients with pulmonary hypertension (Eisenmenger's physiology), oxygen may blunt their respiratory drive. Such patients should be closely monitored. Finally, as noted in the previous section, oxygen supplementation in the patient with cyanosis and evidence of CHF should be used cautiously. In a young infant, if cyanotic heart disease is suspected, an oxygen challenge test should be performed. The oxygen challenge test starts with documentation of the patient's arterial oxygen level in room air. Oxygen at a concentration at or near 100% is then delivered. Mter approximately 10–20 min, a repeat $PO_2$ is measured. If the $PO_2$ increases to greater than 100 mmHg, the most likely cause of the cyanosis is pulmonary disease. The lack of a significant rise in oxygen tension strongly suggests an underlying cyanotic heart lesion.

e. *Laboratory studies:* Measurement of the hemoglobin and hematocrit is important for several reasons. As mentioned earlier, the presence of anemia can mask the presence of significant cyanosis. The finding of polycythemia strongly supports the presence of long-standing hypoxemia, whether secondary to cardiac or pulmonary disease.

### C. Patient Management

The specific management of the cyanotic infant or child depends considerably on the underlying pathology. For example, in tetralogy of Fallot, the degree of obstruction is extremely variable and is the key determinant of the degree of cyanosis. Furthermore, any surgical intervention may markedly change the expected physiology of the individual lesion. The general approach to these defects will be based on the underlying pathophysiology (Fig. 25.16).

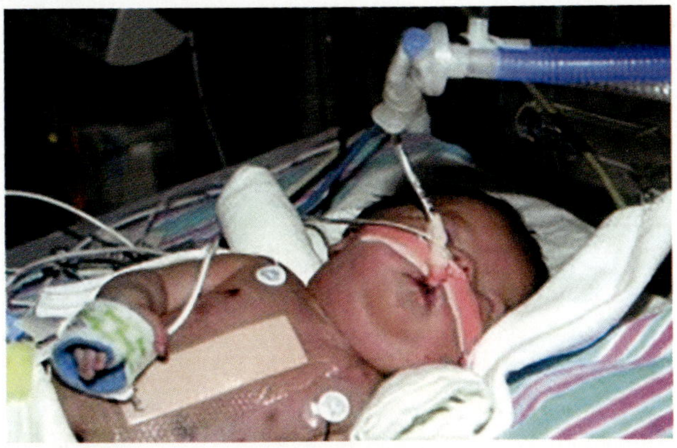

**Fig. 25.16:** An amazing Tennessee baby has become one of the smallest babies in the world to have heart bypass surgery. Tiny 4 pound Cole Latch underwent surgery at Le Bonheur Children's Medical Center in Memphis, Tenn., to repair a congenital heart defect. The 1-month-old was born prematurely on Nov. 25 and had a cardiopulmonary bypass less than a week later. 'He was born at 35 weeks with a knot in his umbilical cord'

a. *Cyanotic lesions with decreased pulmonary blood flow:* The general pathophysiologic aberration in this group is a decrease in blood flow to the lungs for oxygenation. This results in a relatively smaller amount of oxygenated pulmonary venous return mixing with the desaturated systemic venous blood. The ratio of the two will determine the oxygen level in the systemic circulation. The most common lesions in this category include tetralogy of fallot, tricuspid atresia with pulmonary stenosis, pulmonary atresia with intact ventricular septum and critical pulmonary stenosis. Therapy for this group of patients should enhance the pulmonary blood flow either by decreasing the degree of obstruction or by augmenting the pulmonary blood flow. The former effect is usually difficult to achieve on an acute medical basis and requires an interventional catheter or surgical procedure. Augmentation of pulmonary blood flow may also be quite difficult medically in the older infant and child, with the possible exception of tetralogy of Fallot, which will be discussed separately. Newborn infants presenting with severe cyanosis and decreased pulmonary blood flow often can benefit greatly from opening or dilation of the ductus arteriosus with prostaglandin E (PGE). The patent ductus can supply an alternative source offlow to the pulmonary circulation, bypassing any existing central obstruction. As in the critical left-sided obstructive lesions discussed earlier, PGE, is administered by continuous intravenous infusion at a rate of 0.1 mcg/kg/min. The major side effects of PGE1 administration are hypotension secondary to vasodilation, apnea and irritability. All patients receiving PGE, should be carefully monitored for these adverse effects. The medical staff should be prepared to intervene in anticipation of potential apnea or hypotension. Again, any patient who will require transfer to another hospital should be electively intubated and ventilated prior to transport.

i. **Tetralogy of Fallot:** Patients with unrepaired tetralogy of Fallot can be at risk for a hypercyanotic or 'tet' spell. Hypercyanotic episodes usually occur in the early waking hours. With agitation, the infant may become tachycardic and cyanotic (Table 25.3).

   As a result of the hypoxemia, the infant may become more agitated and thus more cyanotic. Accompanying respiratory distress is usually present. Some clinicians hypothesize that there is constriction of the right ventricular outflow tract (RVOT), which causes further compromise in pulmonary blood flow. Regardless of the mechanism, the relative amount of blood that exits in the heart consists of a progressively smaller proportion of oxygenated blood. With continued agitation, this cycle can perpetuate and may lead to death. The presence of a hypercyanotic episode is truly a medical emergency. The approach to the management of the patient with a hypercyanotic spell is given in. After an initial episode, the child is at marked risk for having recurrent episodes. Therefore, the occurrence of a hypercyanotic spell is an indication for surgical intervention, and appropriate arrangement for admission to a tertiary center should be made.

ii. **Ebstein's malformation of the tricuspid valve:** Most patients are diagnosed with this condition in the newborn period because of cyanosis and the presence of a murmur. The cyanosis tends to improve in the first few days of life as pulmonary vascular resistance decreases. The CXR will typically demonstrate marked cardiomegaly even in a newborn infant because of severe insufficiency of the abnormal tricuspid valve and right atrial dilation. Cyanosis, particularly associated with exercise, can return when the child is older. Treatment is limited and most often involves anticongestive therapy with diuretics and digoxin if CHF exists. There is a 5–20% incidence of

**Table 25.3:** Treatment of hypercyanotic spells in tetralogy of Fallot

- Knee to chest position
- Supplemental oxygen (100%)
- Morphine sulfate (0.1 mg/kg IM or SC)

*If not responding to above:*

- Obtain IV access
- Repeat morphine sulfate if agitated
- IV fluid bolus (10–20 ml/kg)
- Phenylephrine infusion (0.02 mg/kg IV, is used to increase SVR)
- $NaHCO_3$ (1 mEq/kg IV)
- Esmolol 500 mcg/kg over one minute IV, then maintenance of 50 mcg/kg/min can be increased in steps of 50 mcg/kg/min to maximum dose of 300 mcg/kg/min)

*If remains critical:*

- Consider general anethesia and paralytic agent.
- Urgent consultation with cardiothoracic surgery is needed for correction of basic defect.

SVR=systemic vascular resistance

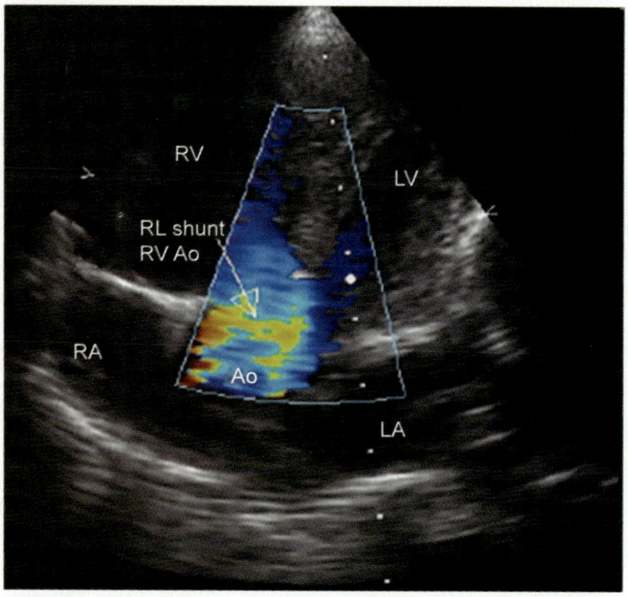


**Fig. 25.17:** Apical five chamber view in tetralogy of Fallot in systole with right to left shunt

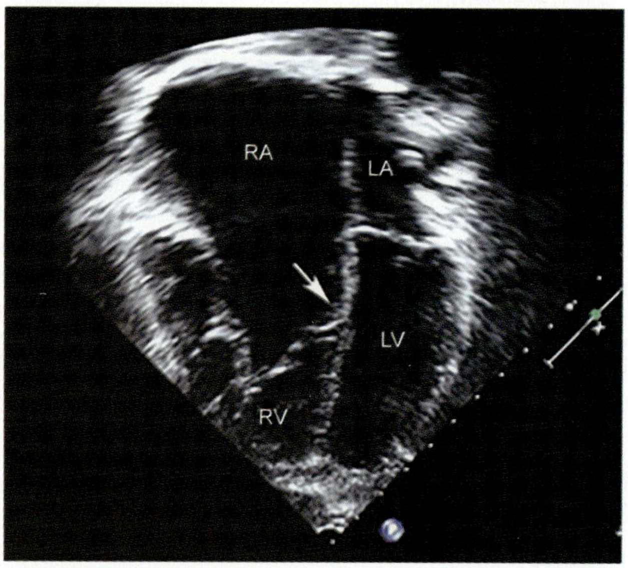


**Fig. 25.18:** Ebstein anomaly of the tricuspid valve. Apical four-chamber echocardiogram in a patient with Ebstein anomaly demonstrates severe apical displacement of the septal leaflet of the tricuspid valve (arrow), with resulting 'atrialization' of a large portion of the right ventricular sinus. The anterior leaflet of the tricuspid valve is large (often described as 'sail-like') and has multiple attachments to the apex and anterior right ventricular wall (RV). LA=left atrium; LV=left ventricle, RA=right atrium

an accessory bypass tract resulting in Wolff-Parkinson-White (WPW) syndrome in patients with Ebstein's anomaly. These patients can present with peripheral cyanosis if tachyarrhythmias are present. As in all patients with WPW, the presence of atrial flutter/fibrillation secondary to the stretched atrium is especially concerning. Rapid antegrade conduction

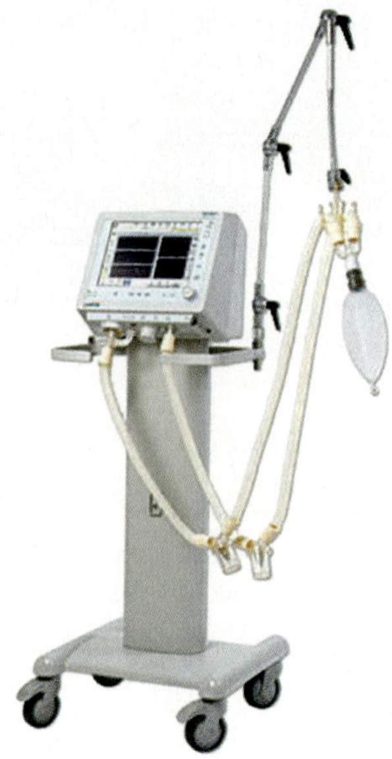

**Fig. 25.19:** Invasive and noninvasive ventilation for adult, pediatric and neonate (including premature) patients. Designed and developed for the intensive respiratory care of neonatal and pediatric patient

via the bypass tract can result in ventricular fibrillation. A patient with Ebstein's anomaly and hemodynamic instability should have an ECG to evaluate for any evidence of WPW and tachyarrhythmias (Figs 25.17 to 25.19).

b. *Cyanotic lesions with normal to slightly increased pulmonary vascularity:* Complete transposition of the great arteries (TGA) is the primary congenital heart defect in this category. The primary reason for the cyanosis in the newborn is the presence of parallel circulatory pathways instead of the pulmonary and systemic circulations functioning in series. The systemic venous blood flows through the right atrium and through the right ventricle, and then is ejected back into the systemic circulation. Parallel to this, the pulmonary venous blood circulates through the left atrium, the left ventricle, and then the pulmonary artery. The degree of mixing between the circulations across the foramen ovale, ductus arteriosus, and/or ventricular septal defect, if present, will determine the level of cyanosis. Almost all patients with simple TGA will present as newborns with intense cyanosis. Children with complicated forms of TGA can present at a later age from a lesser degree of cyanosis.

The lack of mixing of blood between the parallel circulation can lead to death. The immediate therapy should be oriented at improving the mixing of blood. Again, prostaglandin E1 (PGE1) infusion represents the major therapeutic advance that can be life-saving. In this situation the patent ductus is not necessary to augment diminished pulmonary or systemic blood flow, but serves as a site to allow oxygenated blood to reach the systemic circulation and vice versa. The dosage and side effects are similar to those previously outlined. Rarely, the administration of PGE1 does not result in a rise in oxygen levels. In these patients, immediate transfer to a center with expertise in pediatric cardiology for balloon atrial septostomy is needed. Administration of fluid boluses and aggressive correction of metabolic acidosis are intermediate palliative resuscitative maneuvers (Figs 25.20 and 25.21).

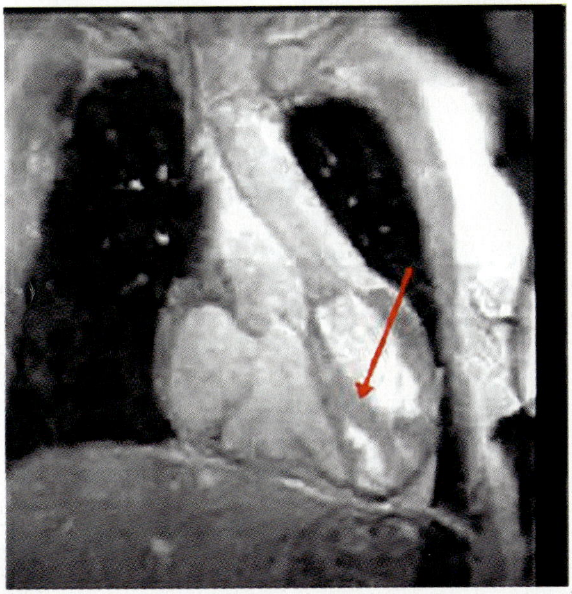

**Fig. 25.20:** This gradient echo cine image in the coronal plane shows the great vessels arising in a parallel fashion, a finding that represents transposition of the great arteries (TGA). Notice that the ventricle on the patients left is markedly trabeculated and a moderator band (arrow) is present; this therefore represents the morphologic right ventricle. In L-TGA, the morphological right ventricle is located in the usual location of the left ventricle and gives rise to the aorta. This configuration is also known as congenitally corrected transposition

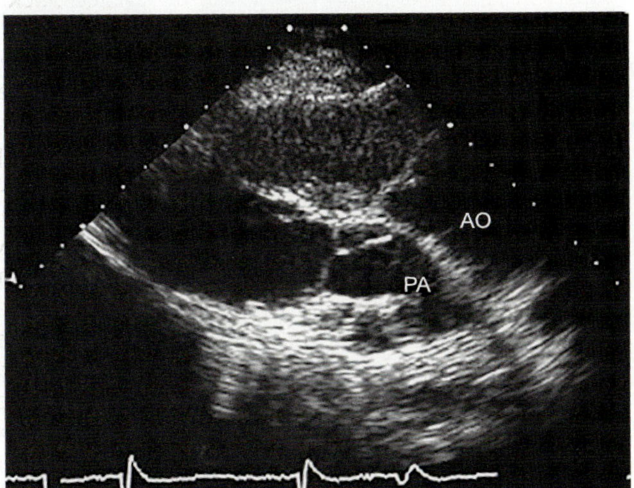



**Fig. 25.21:** D-TGV echo shows parallel position of aorta and pulmonary artery. Aorta is placed anteriorly

c. *Cyanotic lesions with increased pulmonary vascularity:* In this group of defects, the cyanosis is often variable and could be quite mild, depending on the amount of pulmonary blood flow. CHF often develops in those patients with unrestricted pulmonary blood flow. This category includes (Figs 25.22–25.27):

- Persistent truncus arteriosus
- Tricuspid atresia without pulmonary stenosis
- Total anomalous pulmonary venous return

In patients presenting with mild cyanosis, CHF and increased pulmonary vascularity on CXR, treating with high-concentration oxygen may result in a rapid decompensation caused by worsening of the CHF. This is similar to the infant or child with a large left-to-right shunt lesion without cyanosis. The hypoxemia is usually mild in this situation and not life-threatening. Immediate management should be directed toward improving the CHF, primarily with diuretics.

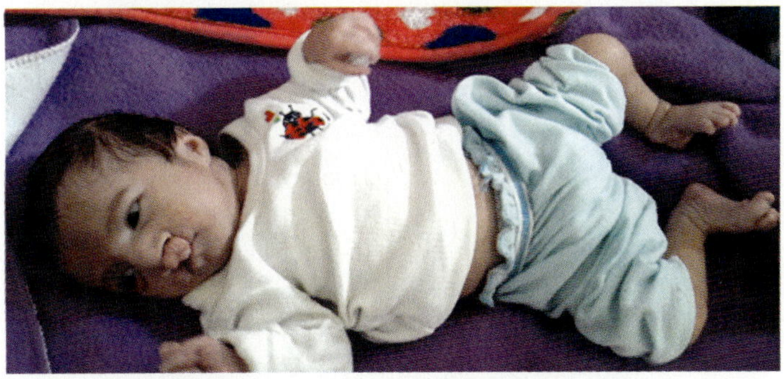

**Fig. 25.22:** 3-month-old infant who had cleft lip, syndactly of left hand, hypoplasia of left lower limb and truncus arteriosus

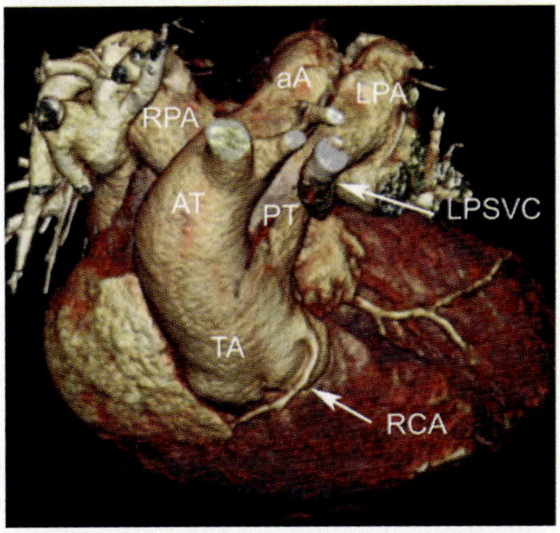



**Fig. 25.23:** A 3-month-old infant with unrepaired truncus arteriosus (TA). The three-dimensional volume-rendered cardiac computed tomography angiogram. (a) Oblique superior-inferior-maximum intensity projection view shows an anatomical pattern consistent with TA type 1A with persistent left superior vena cava. The right coronary artery branches from the noncoronary sinus at the left side of the truncus

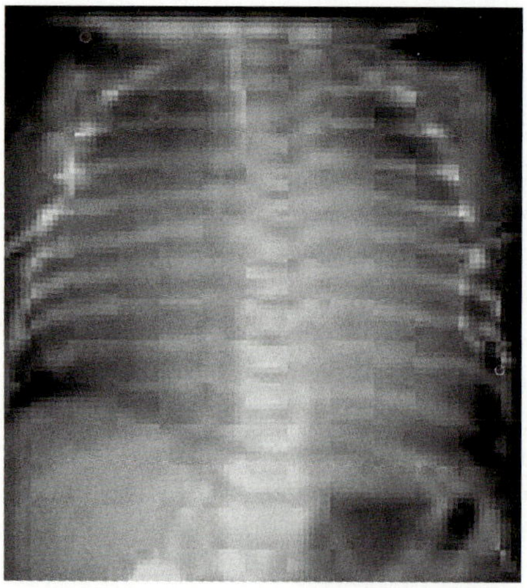

Fig. 25.24: The radiograph demonstrates marked cardiac enlargement (a carpet heart) in patient with TAPV

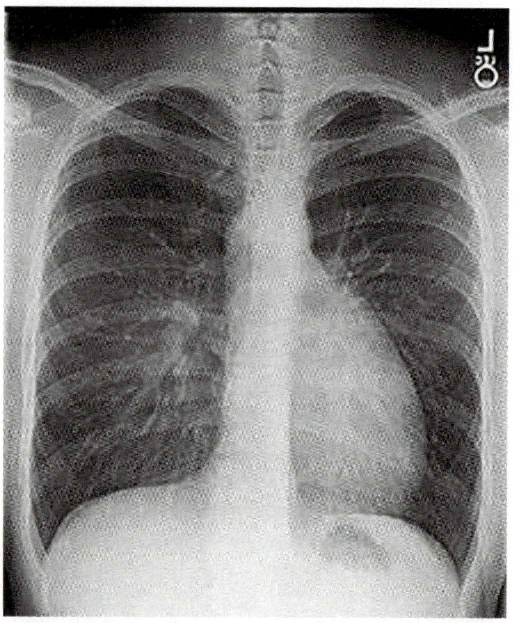


Fig. 25.25: X-ray showing characteristic finding in case of transposition of the great vessels which is called egg on side sign

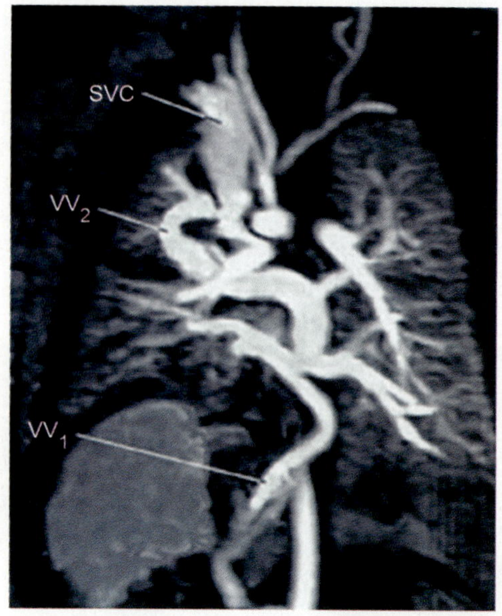


Fig. 25.26: Maximal-intensity projection coronal plane image of gadolinium-enhanced three-dimensional magnetic resonance angiogram in a newborn with obstructed mixed-type total anomalous venous connection. There is infradiaphragmatic connection by means of a vertical vein (V V-1) to the portal vein, as well as supracardiac stenotic connection to the right superior vena cava (SVC) via an additional vertical vein (V V-2)

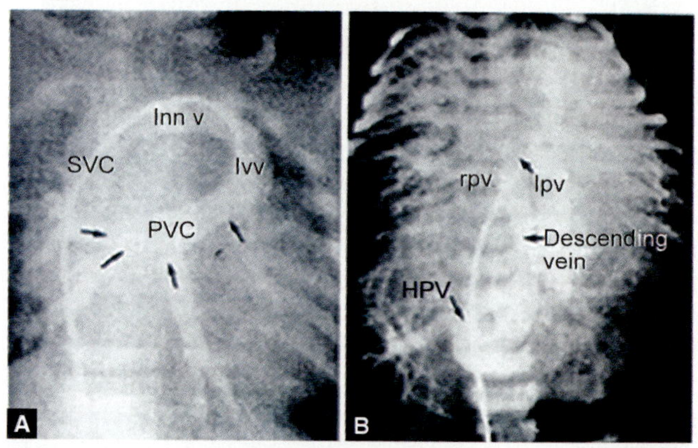


Fig. 25.27: (A) Contrast angiography showing contrast material entering into pulmonary artery (PA) showing return of pulmonary venous blood. (B) Left sided vertical vein with subsequent opacification of the right SVC (RSVC) in patient with total anomalous pulmonary venous connection

## CONGESTIVE HEART FAILURE

### Approach to the Pediatric Patient with Congestive Heart Failure

Heart failure is a pathophysiologic condition that results when the pump function of the myocardium is unable to meet the metabolic demands of the body. In infancy and childhood, this condition usually occurs from abnormal work imposed on a normal myocardium from excessive volume or pressure loads. However, intrinsic alterations in myocardial contractile performance can also exist. Both physiologic states can exist as a result of congenital or acquired diseases (Table 25.4).

A. *Patient presentation:* The age at presentation can provide important information regarding the specific aetiology of the CHF. The timing of key events in the transition from fetal to postpartum circulation has a significant influence on the onset of heart failure when certain underlying structural defects exist. Closure of the ductus arteriosus typically occurs in the first few days of life; however, it may remain patent for several weeks. In left sided obstructive lesions, such as coarctation of the aorta and hypoplastic left heart syndrome, as in the fetus, the

**Table 25.4:** Aetiological factors in heart failure in infants and children

| | | |
|---|---|---|
| **1. Common causes of heart failure in the structurally normal heart** | | |
| ***Prenatal*** | ***Neonates and infants*** | ***Childhood*** |
| Anemia | Anemia | Acquired valve disorders |
| Arrhythmia | Arrhythmia | Anemia |
| Arteriovenous fistula | Arteriovenous fistula | Arrhythmia |
| Cardiomyopathy | Dilated cardiomyopathy | Dilated cardiomyopathy |
| Twin-twin transfusion | Endocrionpathies | Hypertension |
| | Hypoglycemia | Renal failure |
| | Hypothyroidism | Restrictive cardiomyopathy |
| | Hypoxic ischemic injury | |
| | Hypertension | |
| | Infection/Sepsis | |
| | Kawasaki syndrome | |
| **2. Common causes of heart failure in patients with congenital heart disease** | | |
| ***Prenatal*** | ***Neonates and infants*** | ***Children*** |
| Atrioventricular valve regurgitation | Systemic outflow obstruction | Aortic regurgitation |
| Mitral stenosis with intact atrial septum | Aortic valve stenosis | Mitral regurgitation |
| | Coarctation of the aorta | Mitral stenosis |
| | Subaortic stenosis | Pulmonary vein stenosis |
| | Systemic inflow obstruction | |
| | Pulmonary venous stenosis | |
| | Systemic ventricular volume overload | |
| | Aortic or Mitral regurgitation | |
| | Atrial/ventricular septal defect | |
| | Mitral stenosis | |
| | Patent ductus arteriosus | |

ductus arteriosus permits perfusion of the systemic circulation by output from the right ventricle. Constriction of the ductus results in decreased systemic perfusion to all or portions of the body, with resultant CHF. In isolated coarctation, the left ventricle may experience a severe, acute rise in afterload as the result of an increase in the degree of obstruction caused by closure of ductal tissue in the juxtaductal aorta. Development of signs and symptoms of heart failure follow closely. Another major alteration in transitional circulation is the progressive decrease in pulmonary vascular resistance that occurs over the first few weeks to months of life. In cardiac anomalies characterized by left-to-right shunts, the degree of shunting is directly related to the relaxation of the pulmonary vascular bed. It is unusual for heart failure to develop in patients even with large defects before the third week of life. The presence of associated lesions, atrioventricular valve regurgitation, and anemia may hasten the development of symptoms. Another congenital anomaly that may present with the fall in pulmonary vascular resistance is anomalous left coronary artery from the pulmonary artery.

Older infants and children rarely present with CHF secondary to undiagnosed congenital heart disease. Diagnoses such as new-onset cardiomyopathy, myocarditis or pericarditis are more likely.

The clinical manifestations of heart failure in infants and children may be quite different from those of adolescents and adults. The specific signs and symptoms that result from failure of these adaptive mechanisms vary with the underlying pathologic process.

1. **History:** A careful, detailed history can often be the most useful information in helping the clinician determine the presence of CHF. Many of the physical findings, particularly in infants, can mimic those of more common pediatric ailments such as bronchiolitis. Specific areas of investigation should be the patient's feeding habits and intake, the presence of significant sweating, the breathing pattern and growth. Feeding represents the most significant form of exercise and energy expenditure for an infant. The earliest sign of CHF is increased respiratory effort during feeding that may or may not exist during rest. The increased respiratory demands often result in the need for frequent breaks between sucking and thus prolong the time required for feeding. The act of feeding may also be accompanied by significant diaphoresis caused by the increased energy expenditure and increased adrenergic state. Older children and adolescents in CHF often complain of anorexia.

   Somatic growth, particularly weight, is often affected. Infants with chronic CHF typically are underweight and undernourished. There are several underlying causes of this phenomenon. The alterations in feeding usually result in decreased caloric intake, while the increased work of the heart and respiratory muscles creates a state of increased metabolic demand. Congestion of the gastrointestinal tract results in malabsorption of nutrients. Finally, the redistribution of egional blood flow seen in severe heart failure results in decreased flow and perfusion to organs, such as the skin and skeletal muscle. In older children and adolescents, there may be weight loss due to anorexia or weight gain secondary to fluid retention.

2. **Physical examination:** Tachypnea is one of the most consistent physical findings in infants with CHF regardless of the underlying aetiology. the degree of CHF increases, alveolar and bronchiolar edema result in more labored respiratory effort, accompanied by the development of retractions, nasal flaring and grunting.

It is extremely important to note that wheezing can be a sign of heart failure in infants and should not be simply excused as bronchiolitis or virals, syndrome in this age group. The presence ofrales is rare in infants and becomes more common with advancing age. Chronic cough may also be present at any age. Central cyanosis can be seen as the result of impaired gas exchange (Fig. 25.28 and Table 25.5).

This is typically an indicator of moderately severe CHF. Peripheral cyanosis can also be seen secondary to poor peripheral perfusion. Sinus tachycardia represents a compensatory mechanism resulting from increased adrenergic tone. In pathologic conditions where there is diminished stroke volume (i.e. dilated cardiomyopathy) or congenital defects with large left-to-right shunts, systemic cardiac output is maintained by increased heart rate. Caution should be taken not to confuse a compensatory sinus tachycardia with a

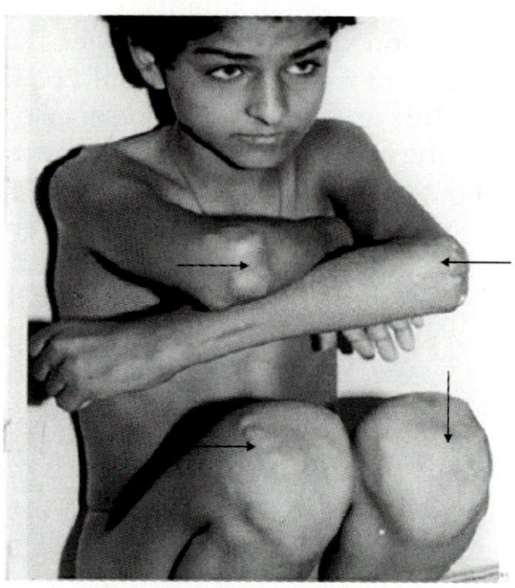

**Fig. 25.28:** Subcutaneous nodules (arrows) in a young child with acute rheumatic fever with carditis with failure

**Table 25.5:** Signs and symptoms of heart failure in infants and children

- History
  - Infants
    - Take longer to feed with frequent breaks
    - Fall asleep shortly after beginning to feed
    - Sweat excessively with feeds, cry
    - Breathe harder and faster than normal
    - Not gaining weight well
  - Older children
    - Anorexia
    - Decreased exercise tolerance
    - Orthopnea
    - Chronic nonproductive cough
- Physical findings
  - Infants
    - Tachypnea
    - Retrations, grunting, nasal flaring
    - Wheezing
    - Tachycardia
    - Gallop rhythm
    - Hepatomegaly
    - Cool extremities
    - Decreased capillary refill
    - Diminished peripheral pulses
    - Mottled skin
    - Peripheral cyanosis
    - Central cyanosis (if congestive heart failure is severe)
  - Older children and adolescents
    - Rales
    - Peripheral edema
    - Ascites
    - Systemic venous distention

supraventricular tachyarrhythmia presenting with heart failure. In general, infants with sustained heart rates of more than 230 bpm should be strongly suspected of having a tachyarrhythmia.

- **Cardiac murmurs** can be highly variable depending on the underlying lesion and are typically nondiagnostic. The absence of these findings in no way excludes heart disease, because infants and children with significant dilated cardiomyopathy may have few to no auscultatory abnormalities.
- **Palpation of the chest** may demonstrate a hyperactive precordium with displacement of the left ventricular (LV) impulse or the presence of a right ventricular (RV) heave or tap. These findings are also nonspecific and can be found in numerous cardiac etiologies. Peripheral pulses may be diminished to some degree in all infants and children with CHF. In infants less than 1 month of age, the finding of markedly diminished, absent, or differential pulses between upper and lower

extremities should strongly suggest obstructive lesions of left ventricular outflow. In lesions such as patent ductus arteriosus and arteriovenous malformations, peripheral pulses may be bounding. There is a wide pulse pressure because of the large diastolic runoff into the low-resistance pulmonary or venous circulations. Other findings of low systemic perfusion include cool extremities, mottled skin and delayed capillary refill.

- **Peripheral edema**, venous distention, and ascites in older children, as in adults, are signs of systemic venous congestion associated with significant right heart failure. These findings are extremely unusual in infants. Enlargement of the liver due to passive congestion is the most common finding in infancy and can be seen in both right and left heart failure (Fig. 25.29).
- **Hepatomegaly** should be distinguished from liver displacement secondary to lung hyperinflation and flattening of the diaphragm seen with bronchiolitis. In addition to an increased span, the liver may be pulsatile in the presence of significant right atrioventricular valve regurgitation. In newborns with severe CHF, jaundice may be secondary to liver congestion and impaired bilirubin metabolism.

B. *Patient assessment:*

1. **Radiologic studies.** Any patient suspected of having CHF should have a routine chest X-ray performed, including any infant presenting with wheezing for the first time (Figs 25.30 and 25.31).

   With the exception of obstructed total anomalous pulmonary and a variable degree of pulmonary vascular congestion depending on the severity of the heart failure and the underlying pathology.

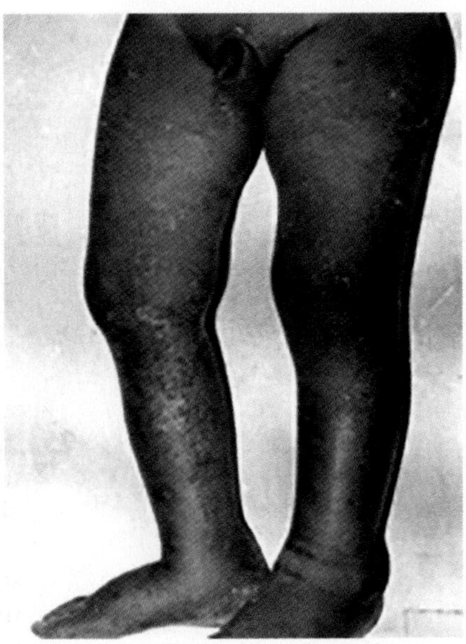

**Fig. 25.29:** Edema of ankles and lower legs in patient with congestive cardiac failure

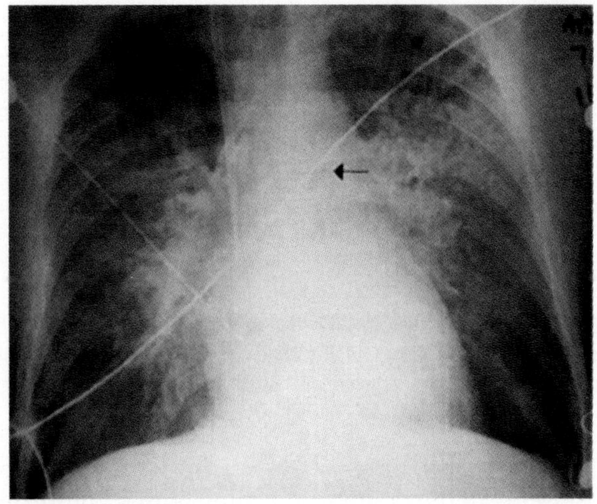

**Fig. 25.30:** Cardiogenic alveolar edema. Symmetrical airspace opacity with perihilar predominance is one characteristic pattern produced by cardiogenic edema

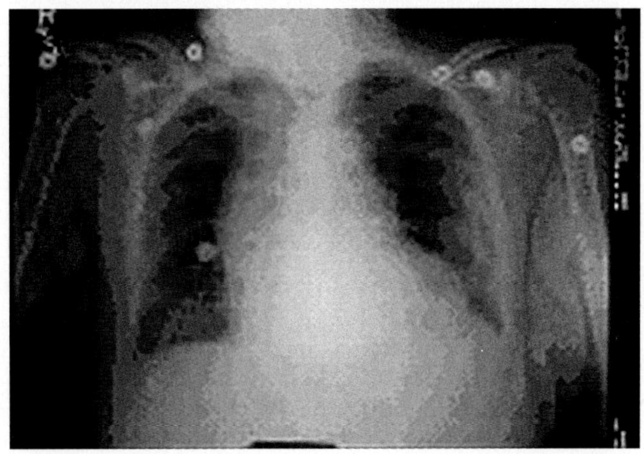

**Fig. 25.31:** Chest radiograph shows signs of congestive heart failure (CHF)

   Significant cardiomegaly in the absence of pulmonary vascular congestion should raise the possibility of a large pericardial effusion. Other findings may include hyperinflated lung fields and pleural effusions.

2. **Electrocardiogram:** There are no specific ECG findings that are diagnostic of CHF. Ventricular hypertrophy, atrial enlargement, axis deviation, and T-wave changes are relatively nonspecific indicators of the underlying aetiology. An exception would be the presence of significant left axis deviation with a mean frontal-plane QRS axis between –60 and –150 degrees, which strongly suggests the presence of an atrioventricular septal defect, either as an isolated defect or as part of a more complex condition. The ECG can be extremely helpful in determining the presence of an underlying arrhythmia or myocardial ischemia, which can be seen in anomalous left coronary artery from the pulmonary artery or Kawasaki disease (Fig. 25.32).

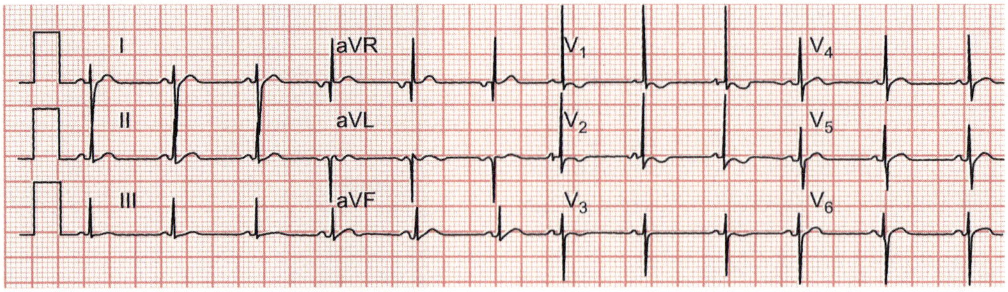


**Fig. 25.32:** Electrocardiogram. There is typically right ventricular hypertrophy with right axis deviation. Superior axis deviation is seen in patients with tetralogy of Fallot and AV canal defect. Right ventricular hypertrophy and left ventricular hypertrophy is seen in acyanotic infants with left-to-right shunting causing congestive heart failure

3. **Laboratory studies:** In patients with evidence of significant respiratory or cardiovascular compromise, an arterial blood gas (ABC) analysis can detect the presence and degree of metabolic or respiratory acidosis, hypoxemia and the presence of impending respiratory failure. Serum electrolytes may reveal underlying life-threatening derangements, especially hypokalemia in patients already receiving chronic therapies such as furosemide and digoxin. Hyponatremia may be present secondary to excessive water retention. A complete blood count with differential analysis can demonstrate evidence of severe anemia or infection as an underlying cause. It should be noted that patients in CHF can have a leukocytosis with a slight left shift.

   **Echocardiography:** It would be very helpful in the diagnosis of anatomical placement of chambers and their relationship with great vessels, cardiac hypertrophy, origin of coronary arteries and inflammation of myocardium and aneurysms of coronary arteries as seen in Kawasaki disease (Figs 25.33–25.36).

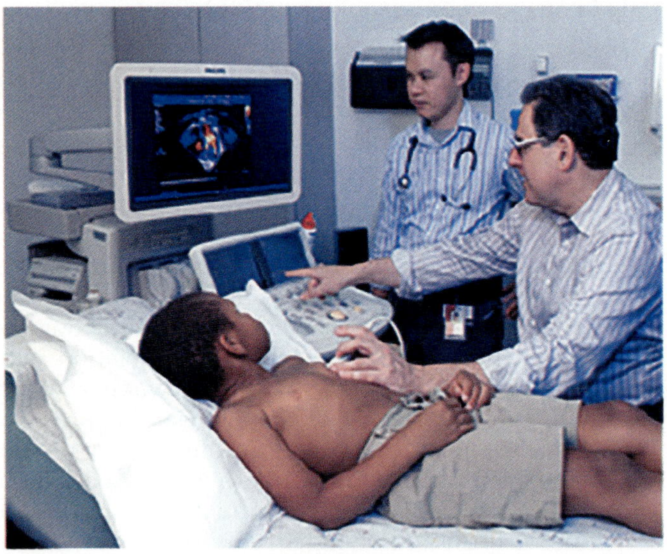

**Fig 25.33:** Echocardiographic evaluation of heart disease in a young child who was admitted into emergency department with cyanosis and heart failure

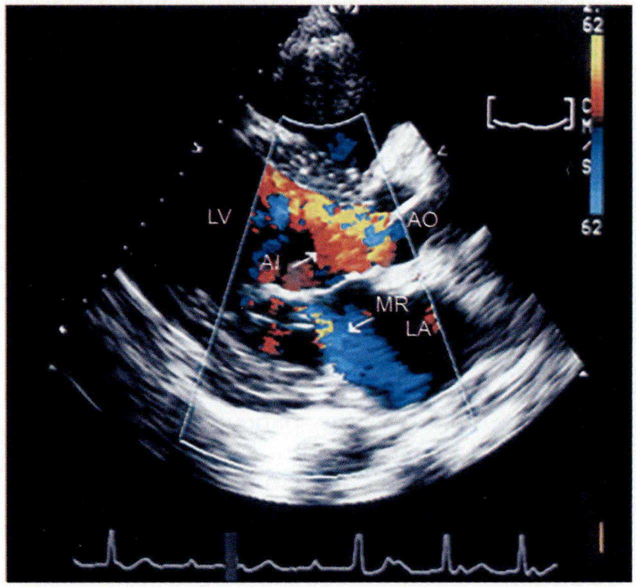


**Fig. 25.34:** Parasternal long-axis image of acute severe aortic regurgitation (AR). The accompanying marked elevation of LV diastolic pressure causes diastolic mitral regurgitation (MR). AO=aorta; LA=left atrium; LV=left ventricle

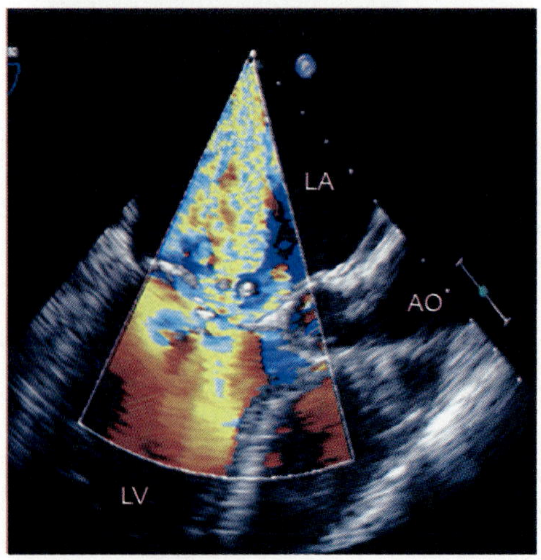


**Fig. 25.35:** Color imaging reveals severe mitral regurgitation. LA=left atrium; LV=left ventricle; AO=aorta

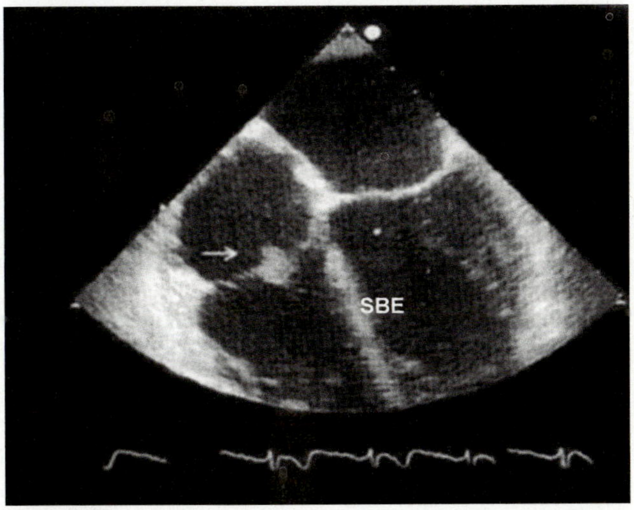


**Fig. 25.36:** Transesophageal echocardiography (TEE) four chamber view showing large mobile vegetation on tricuspid valve (arrow)

**Table 25.6:** Medical management strategies of congestive heart failure in pediatric patients

1. Remove any precipitating or aggravating factors:
   - Transfuse for severe anemia
   - Treat arrhythmias
   - Restrict fluid and salt
2. Reduce metabolic demands:
   - Reduce fever
   - Bed rest
   - Sedate agitated patient
   - Endotracheal intubation and ventilation
3. Relieve pulmonary congestion:
   - Diuresis (furosemide 1 mg/kg IV/PO)
   - Mechanical ventilation with positive end expiratory pressure
   - Morphine sulfate (0.05–0.10 mg/kg IV/IM).
4. Improve myocardial performance and oxygen delivery:
   - Inotropes (debutamine and dopamine)
   - Afterload reduction (nitroprusside)
   - Preload reduction (nitroprusside and nitroglycerin)
   - Oxygen (use cautiously in suspected left-to-right shunt lesions)
   - Prostaglandin El (0.1 (~g/kg/min) for left heart obstructive lesions. Correct metabolic acidosis with $NaHCO_3$ (1–2 mEq/kg).

C. *Patient management:* Because of the large number of potential underlying etiologies, CHF cannot be treated uniformly in all pediatric patients. After the diagnosis of 'heart failure has been established, therapeutic interventions should be aimed at removing any precipitating or aggravating causes, decreasing metabolic demands, relieving pulmonary congestion, and improving systemic perfusion and oxygen delivery require identification of the specific diagnosis and often surgical intervention, both of which may not be readily available in the emergency setting (Tables 25.6–25.8).

1. **Remove precipitating or aggravating causes:** Treat any underlying arrhythmias when present. Tachyarrhythmias should be converted to normal sinus rhythm by medical therapy, electrical cardioversion or defibrillation. The specitic treatment for various arrhythmias is discussed later in the chapter. Life-threatening bradyarrhythmias should be treated with an external pacemaker, isoproterenol infusion, or with temporary transvenous pacing when available. Significant anemia should be corrected.
2. **Decrease metabolic demands.** Endotracheal intubation with mechanical ventilation is crucial. Patients who are not in need of intubation should be oxygenated by whatever means possible, guided by blood gases or pulse-oximetry. In cases of severe pulmonary edema, endotracheal intubation with the use of positive end-expiratory pressure (PEEP) may help control the pulmonary edema and improve gas exchange. Reduce fever if present using antipyretics.

**Table 25.7:** Medications to maintain cardiac output and for postresuscitation stabilization

| Medication | Dose range | Comment |
|---|---|---|
| Amrinone | 0.75–1 mg/kg IV/IO over 5 minutes; may repeat × 2; then 2–20 µg/kg per minute | Inodilator |
| Dobutamine | 2–20 µg/kg per minute IV/IO | Inotrope; vasodilator |
| Dopamine | 2–20 µg/kg per minute IV/IO | Inotrope; chronotrope; renal and splanchnic vasodilator in low doses; pressor in high doses |
| Epinephrine | 0.1–1 µg/kg per minute IV/IO | Intrope; chronotrope; vasodilator in low doses; pressor in higher doses |
| Milrinone | 50–75 µg/kg IV/IO over 10–60 minutes then 0.5–0.75 µg/kg per minute | Inodilator |
| Norepinephrine | 0.1–2 µg/kg per minute | Inotrope; vasopressor |
| Sodium nitroprusside | 1–8 µg/kg per minute | Vasodilator; prepare only in D5W |

IV indicates intravenous; and IO, intraosseous.
Alternative formula for calculating an infusion:
Infusion rate (ml/h) = [weight (kg) × dose (µg/kg/min) × 60 (min/h)]/concentration µg/ml.

**Table 25.8:** Medications for pediatric resuscitation and arrhythmias

| Medication | Dose | Remarks |
|---|---|---|
| Adenosine | 0.1 mg/kg (maximum 6 mg)<br>Repeat: 0.2 mg/kg (maximum 12 mg) | Monitor ECG<br>Rapid IV/IO bolus |
| Amiodarone | 5 mg/kg IV/IO; repeat up to 15 mg/kg<br>Maximum: 300 mg | Monitor ECG and blood pressure<br>Adjust administration rate to urgency (give more slowly when perfusing rhythm present)<br>Use caution when administering with other drugs that prolong QT (consider expert consultation) |
| Atropine<br>0.03 mg/kg ET* | 0.02 mg/kg IV/IO<br>poisoning<br>Repeat once if needed<br>Minimum dose: 0.1 mg<br>Maximum single dose:<br>• Child 0.5 mg<br>• Adolescent 1 mg | Higher doses may be used with organophosphate |
| Calcium chloride (10%) | 20 mg/kg IV/IO (0.2 ml/kg) | Slowly<br>Adult dose: 5–10 ml |
| Epinephrine | 0.01 mg/kg (0.1 ml/kg 1:10,000) IV/IO<br>0.1 mg/kg (0.1 ml/kg 1:1,000) ET*<br>Maximum dose: 1 mg IV/IO; 10 mg ET | May repeat: q 3–5 min |
| Glucose | 0.5–1 g/kg IV/IO | D10W: 5–10 ml/kg<br>D25W: 2–4 ml/kg<br>D50W: 1–2 ml/kg |
| Lidocaine | Bolus: 1 mg/kg IV/IO<br>Maximum dose: 100 mg<br>Infusion: 20–50½ g/kg per minute<br>ET*: 2–3 mg | |
| Magnesium sulfate | 25–50 mg/kg IV/IO over 10–20 minutes; faster in torsades<br>Maximum dose: 2 g | |
| Naloxone<br>5 years or >20 kg: 2 mg IV/IO/ET* | <5 years or 20 kg: 0.1 mg/kg IV/IO/ET* | Use lower doses to reverse respiratory depression associated with therapeutic opioid use (1–15½ g/kg) |
| Procainamide | 15 mg/kg IV/IO over 30–60 minutes<br>Adult dose: 20 mg/min IV infusion up to total maximum dose 17 mg/kg | Monitor ECG and blood pressure<br>Use caution when administering with other drugs that prolong QT (consider expert consulation) |
| Sodium bicarbonate | 1 mEq/kg per dose IV/IO slowly | After adequate ventilation |

IV indicates intravenous; IO= intraosseous; and ET=via endotracheal tube
*Flush with 5 ml of normal saline and follow with 5 ventilations

Agitated patients should be sedated. Morphine sulfate administered in doses of 0.05–0.10 mg/kg IV or IM can be used for patients who, are particularly restless. Apnea can develop with narcotics administration especially in infants.

3. **Relieve pulmonary congestion:** Diuresis should be initiated by pharmacologic therapy. Loop diuretics, such as furosemide, are usually effective. Doses starting at 1 mg/kg given IV or IM should be used in cases of severe CHF with pulmonary edema. In less severe failure, oral dosing at 1–2 mg/kg 2–4 times daily should be adequate. Other diuretics, such as thiazide diuretics and aldosterone antagonists, should be reserved for chronic therapy. Aggressive treatment with loop diuretics will increase potassium loss and may result in significant hypokalemia. Electrolytes should be monitored closely. Morphine therapy can be used to improve pulmonary hemodynamics. In addition to the previously mentioned sedative effects, morphine both reduces systemic arterial resistance and increases systemic venous capacitance. This will decrease both the afterload and preload imposed on the myocardium and may improve pulmonary edema.
4. **Improve systemic perfusion and oxygen delivery:** Systemic perfusion or cardiac output is determined by the physiologic principles of preload, afterload, contractility and heart rate. Therapy aimed at improving cardiac output should address these determinants.
   a. **Inotropic agents:** In the acute setting, parenteral agents are most efficacious in augmenting myocardial performance. Betal-adrenergic receptor agonists are the inotropic agents of choice.

Dobutamine infused at rates of 10–20 mcg/kg/min produces a positive inotropic effect with minimal chronotropic changes. Stimulation of beta-adrenergic receptors produces peripheral vascular dilatation, reducing left ventricular afterload and further augmenting cardiac output. Other agents, such as isoproterenol, have similar effects, but their potent chronotropic effects often limit their use. Low-dose dopamine (3–6 mcg/kg/min) also produces vasodilation through stimulation of dopaminergic receptors with selectivity for the renal, mesenteric, cerebral and coronary vascular beds. Higher-dose dopamine should be avoided because of the potential negative effects on intracardiac shunting and increased afterload placed on the ventricular myocardium. Digoxin should be reserved for more stable patients and long-term therapy.

b. **Vasodilator therapy:** Vasodilators can influence afterload and/or preload, depending on their site of action. AB with inotropic agents, N vasodilators that are titratable and short-acting are preferable. Sodium nitroprusside affects both the arterial and venous vascular beds. Nitroglycerin has primarily venodilatory properties. The major adverse reaction to initiation of any vasodilator is hypotension. Hypotension can be avoided by initiating low-dose therapy and titrating as tolerated. An initial infusion of nitroprusside at 0.25–0.5 mcg/kg/min can be used safely in most patients. If hypotension occurs, treating with volume expansion and concurrently decreasing or discontinuing therapy is usually adequate. In rare situations, vasoconstrictors may be necessary.

c. **Oxygen therapy:** As CHF worsens, gas exchange at the alveoli becomes progressively impaired. Administration of humidified oxygen may improve oxygen delivery to the peripheral tissues. It should be emphasized strongly that oxygen therapy in patients with large left-to-right shunt lesions, such as ventricular septal defect, PDA or atrioventricular septal defect may actually result in acute worsening of their condition. This occurs as a result of oxygen's ability to lower pulmonary vascular resistance and raise systemic vascular resistance, both serving to increase the amount of left-to-right shunting.

d. **Prostaglandin therapy:** When there is evidence from the history and clinical findings to suggest a ductal-dependent circulation, such as in coarctation, interrupted aortic arch, critical aortic stenosis, or hypoplastic left heart syndrome in a newborn infant, PGE1 is often life-saving. Ductal dilation permits improved systemic perfusion via the right ventricle while decreasing pulmonary congestion. PGE1 should be administered by continuous N infusion at a rate of 0.1 mcg/kg/min.

The major side effects of PGE1 administration are hypotension secondary to vasodilation, respiratory depression with apnea, and irritability, with the latter two symptoms related to CNS effects. If the patient is not already intubated prior to initiation of therapy, the patient should be placed on cardiorespiratory monitors and equipment and personnel should be readily available in anticipation of potential apnea. Any patient who will require transfer to another hospital should be electively intubated and ventilated before transport.

5. **Correct metabolic derangements:** Many infants with left-sided obstructive lesions present with metabolic acidosis due to poor tissue perfusion and lactic acid production. Often, reestablishing distal perfusion with prostaglandin will have a major influence on correcting this problem. In the setting of severe acidosis, however, myocardial performance is greatly diminished and correction of the acidosis with sodium bicarbonate in 1–2 mEq/kg aliquots is necessary.

D. *Patient disposition:* The prognosis for an infant or child presenting with CHF is highly variable and depends a great deal on the underlying pathology. The long-term outlook, therefore, relies upon a specific and accurate diagnosis. This may not always be available in the emergency setting because of the need for specialized diagnostic testing such as two-dimensional echocardiography and cardiac catheterization, and the need for trained physicians, including pediatric cardiologists and cardiothoracic surgeons, to interpret and implement more diagnosis-specific interventions. Unfortunately, these personnel and technologies are typically available only at regional tertiary care pediatric centers. Regardless of the aetiology, the morbidity and mortality of CHF can be significantly altered by appropriate recognition and initial management in the emergency department. Whereas ductal dependent lesions typically present early after ductal closure within the first two weeks of life, other CHD usually present in 4–6 weeks after birth when the pulmonary vascular resistance has fallen, such as a large ventricular septal defect. CHF ensues from the significant left to right shunt and pulmonary congestion. Infants typically present with poor feeding, failure to thrive, tachypnea, and diaphoresis. Symptoms of older children are more typical adult symptoms of decreased exercise tolerance and dyspnea. Of note, dependent edema in children is very difficult to assess and more often a very late finding. Increased jugular venous pressure is difficult to assess in infants secondary to their short necks and liver size is used as a surrogate marker. CHF is usually related to one of the following conditions: anomalous left coronary artery arising from the pulmonary artery (ALCAPA), congenital cardiomyopathy, myocarditis, lesions resulting from a large intracardiac shunt (e.g. ventricular sepal defect) or extracardiac shunt (vein of Galen malformation), or arrhythmias.

## Anomalous Origin of Left Coronary Artery from Pulmonary Artery

ALCAPA is a type of CHD that typically presents at 2–3 months of age when pulmonary artery (PA) pressure decreases. ALCAPA is one of the most common causes of myocardial ischemia and infarction in children, specifically anterolateral infarct pattern and is associated with high mortality, where 90% of untreated patients die within the first year of life. Infants typically present with episodes of irritability (angina pain) and diaphoresis particularly during feeding (when myocardial oxygen consumption increases), signs of CHF, and a murmur of mitral regurgitation. Although, mortality is high without treatment, prompt diagnosis and surgical treatment have excellent results with improvement in myocardial function overtime. Some patients with ALCAPA may survive undetected through adolescence and adulthood due to the development of significant collateral circulation from the right coronary artery to the LCA. However, these collaterals may not be sufficient to perfuse the left ventricle, and these patients are at risk of chronic mitral regurgitation, ischemic cardiomyopathy, and sudden cardiac death from malignant ventricular arrhythmias in 80–90% of cases. Surgical intervention is recommended, even in asymptomatic adult patients with ALCAPA and preserved left ventricular function discovered incidentally, due to the potential for progressive LV dysfunction and sudden death (Figs 25.37– 25.42).

## Myocarditis

Myocarditis is an often insidious, inflammatory disease of the myocardium preceded by a non-specific flu-like illness. Myocarditis may have a fulminant presentation characterized by acute severe hemodynamic compromise with severe congestive heart failure or cardiogenic shock. It is the most common cause of dilated cardiomyopathy in children. The symptoms can range from being

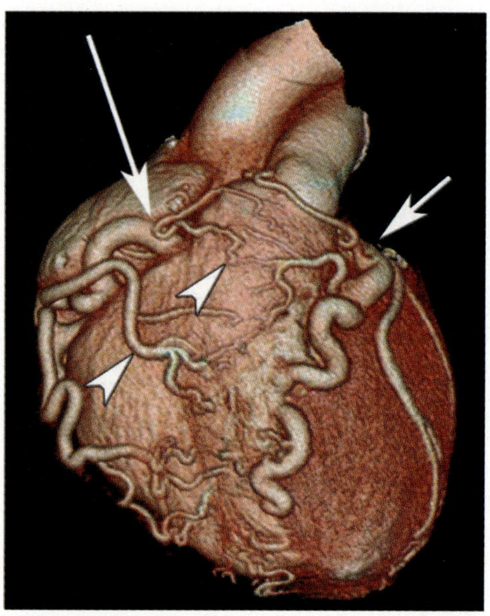

**Fig. 25.37:** Three-dimensional volume-rendered multidetector CT angiogram shows dilated intercoronary collateral arteries (arrowheads), which connect the tortuous RCA (long arrow) to the LCA (short arrow)

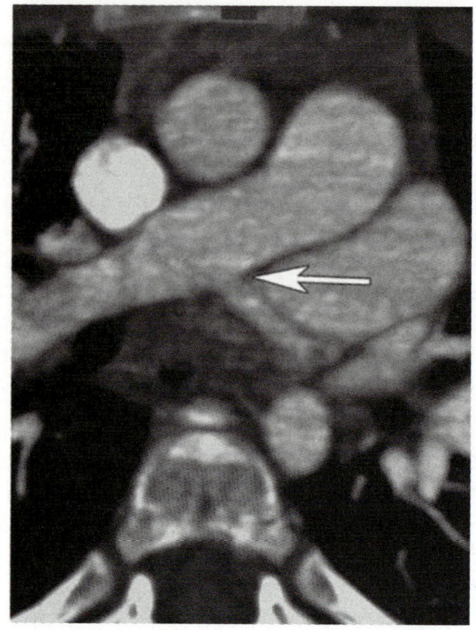

**Fig. 25.38:** ALCAPA syndrome variant in a 3-year-old boy. CT angiogram shows the left circumflex artery (arrow) arising from the posterior wall of the right pulmonary artery and coursing above the left atrial appendage to reach the atrioventricular groove

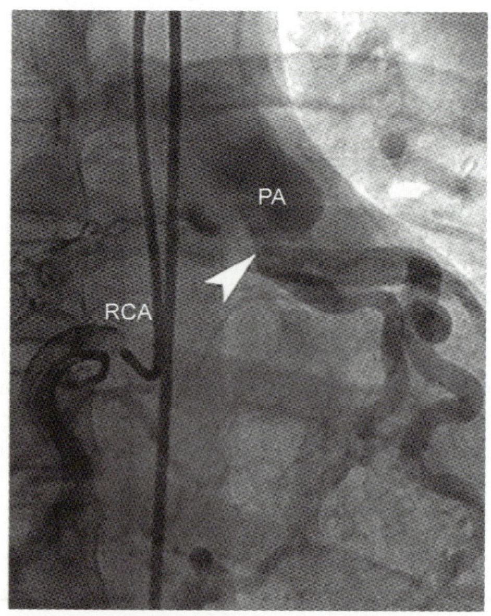


**Fig. 25.39:** ALCAPA syndrome in an adolescent. Coronary angiogram obtained with a single RCA injection shows a tortuous and dilated RCA as well as an equally tortuous and dilated LCA. The LCA opacifies the main pulmonary artery (PA). The connection of the LCA with the main pulmonary artery (arrowhead) and the resultant steal phenomenon are the main diagnostic features of ALCAPA syndrome

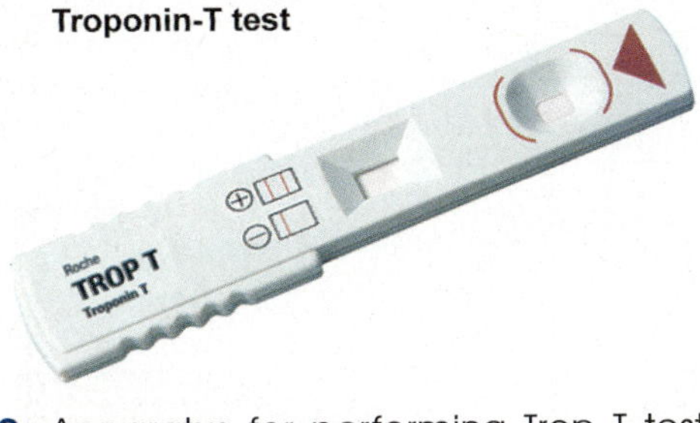


**Fig. 25.40:** Apparatus for performing Trop T test for acute myocardial injury as a result of ALCAPA in emergency department

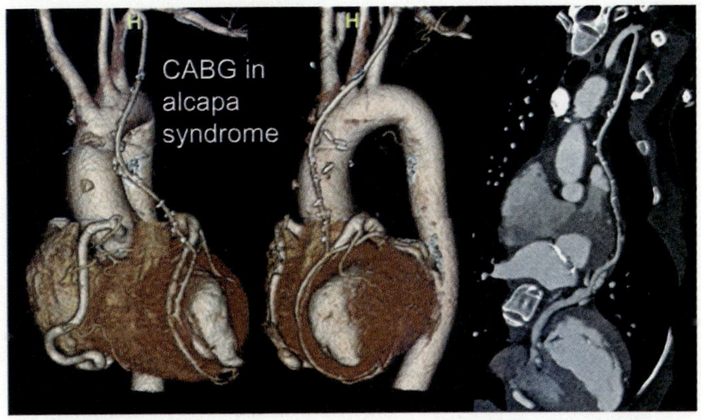


**Fig. 25.42:** MDCT (left) and volume rendering image (right) showing LM to PA closure with CABG (LIMA to LAD) due to ALCAPA

asymptomatic to cardiovascular collapse and death. It is a potentially fatal disease, accounting for 22% of unexpected deaths in persons less than 20 years, with more staggering statistics for infants and children as high as 75 and 25% respectively. Recognition and diagnosis is imperative, but may prove challenging since the clinical presentation is varied and can be similar to other common conditions, such as gastroenteritis, asthma and pneumonia. In one series, the initial evaluating physician diagnosed asthma or pneumonia in more than 50% of patients who actually had myocarditis. In contrast, cardiac symptoms of chest pain are more common in adults. In the European Study of Epidemiology and Treatment of Cardiac Inflammatory Diseases, 526 adults diagnosed with acute or chronic myocarditis of the 3,055 patients screened by endomyocardial biopsy, 32% presented with chest pain, 72% with dyspnea, and 18% had an arrhythmia. In adults, myocarditis should be considered as a possible diagnosis among many cardiac syndromes, whereas in children the clinician needs to consider myocarditis among cardiac and noncardiac presentations. ALCAPA, for example, should be on the differential in a 2–3-month-old infant with presentations, such as colic or respiratory distress, although EKG findings should help to differentiate them. The long-term prognosis is favorable if recognized quickly and managed aggressively with a heart failure regimen and possibly mechanical circulatory support as a bridge to transplantation or recovery (Figs 25.43–25.46).

## CARDIOMYOPATHIES

Cardiomyopathies are a heterogeneous group of myocardial diseases that causes significant disability and death. They are characterized by inappropriate ventricular hypertrophy or dilatation and are associated with electrical dysfunction or systolic and/or diastolic ventricular dysfunction (Figs 25.47–25.51, Tables 25.9 and 25.10).

### Dilated Cardiomyopathy

Dilated cardiomyopathy (DCM) is a heart muscle disease characterized by dilation of the left ventricle and systolic dysfunction. Progressive heart failure ensues with resultant sudden and heart failure related death. DCM is the most common reason for heart transplantation in children and adults. In children, myocarditis is the most frequently identified cause followed by neuromuscular diseases, whereas in adults the most common causes are idiopathic DCM, idiopathic myocarditis and coronary artery disease. The long-term prognosis regardless of the cause may be progressive with approximately 54% of affected individuals

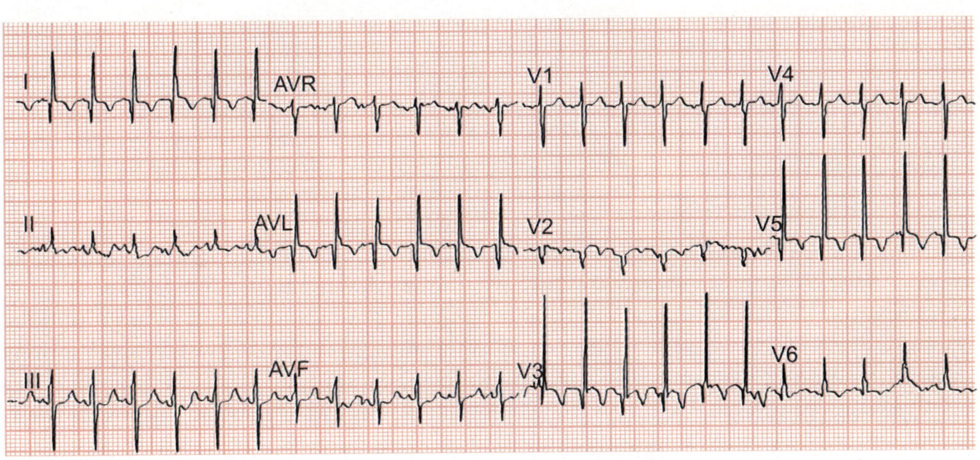


**Fig. 25.41:** ECG of a 4-month-old child who presented with congestive cardiac failure had deep Q-waves in lead 1, AVL V5 and V6 with T invertion as anterio-lateral myocardial infarction due to ALCAPA syndrome

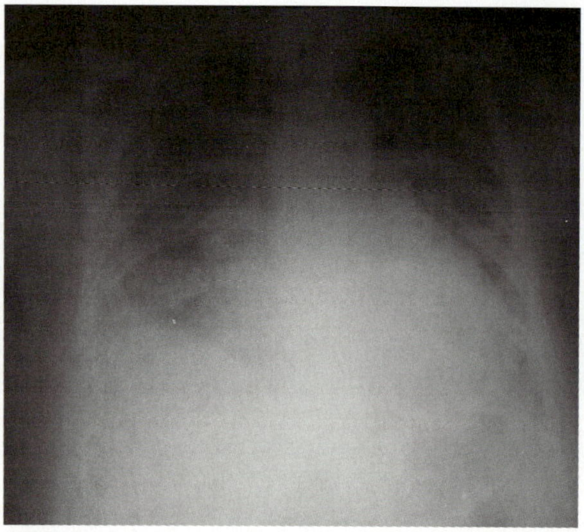

**Fig. 25.43** X-ray chest frontal view showing pulmonary edema in a patient with cardiogenic shock as a result of acute myocarditis in a 12 years old child

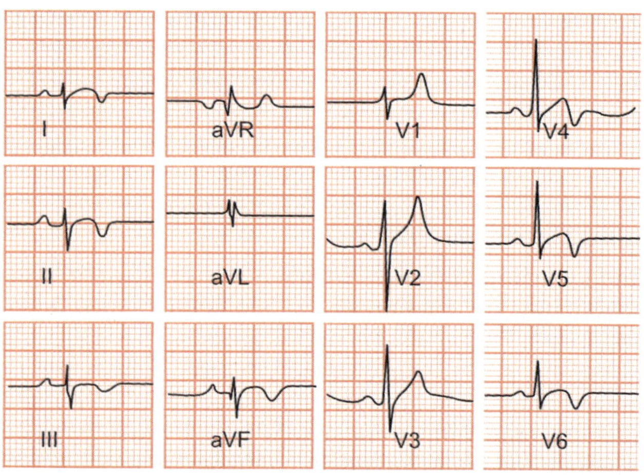


**Fig. 25.44:** The T-waves are deeply and symmetrically inverted in I, II, III and V4–6, suggesting a diffuse myocardial damage in a young patient with acute viral myocarditis

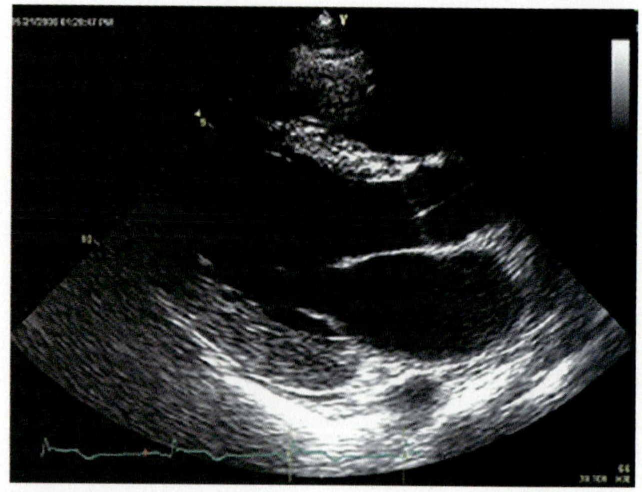

**Fig. 25.45:** Two-dimensional parasternal long-axis view depicting disproportionate thickening, increased echogenicity, and dyskinesis of the inferolateral wall relative to the septum; findings are consistent with tissue edema

within 5 years of diagnosis die or require a heart transplant. The worst outcomes were found among older children, children who had CHF symptoms, and LV dysfunction at the time of presentation. Almost two-thirds of children present with congestive heart failure. Infants may present with failure to thrive, colic, or a conglomeration of symptoms of low cardiac output, such as poor perfusion, decreased distal pulses, pallor, and tachypnea, and on exam a diffuse or displaced cardiac apex, soft heart sounds, a gallop rhythm, hepatomegaly and a mitral regurgitant murmur may be present. Adolescents may experience syncopal events, fatigue, exercise intolerance, dyspnea, pallor and tachycardia. GI symptoms of nausea, vomiting and abdominal pain are also frequently noted.

## Hypertrophic Cardiomyopathy

Unfortunately cardiac arrest and sudden death may be the first presentation of hypertrophic cardiomyopathy (HCM).

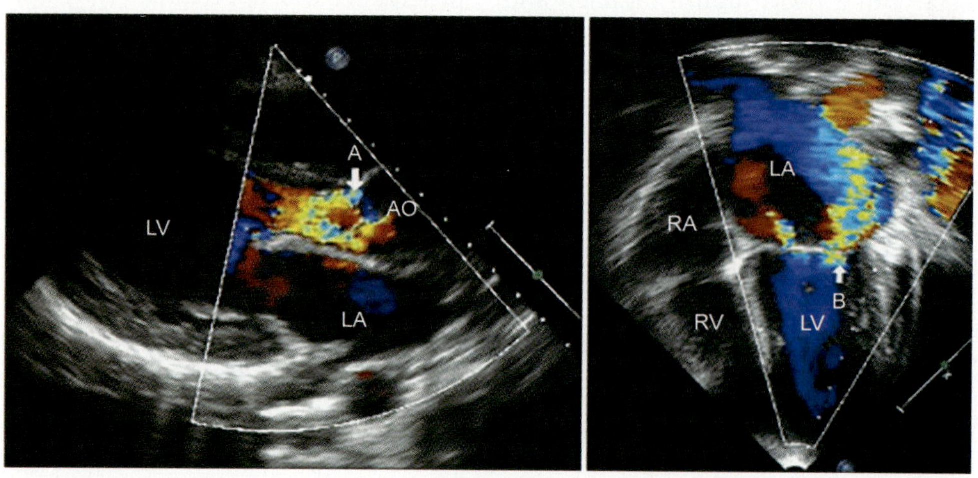


**Fig. 25.46:** Two-dimensional color and spectral Doppler echocardiographic studies of patients with acute myocarditis show moderate to severe aortic valve insufficiency without stenosis (A, arrow) and bowing of the anterior mitral leaflet with severe insufficiency without stenosis (B, arrow)

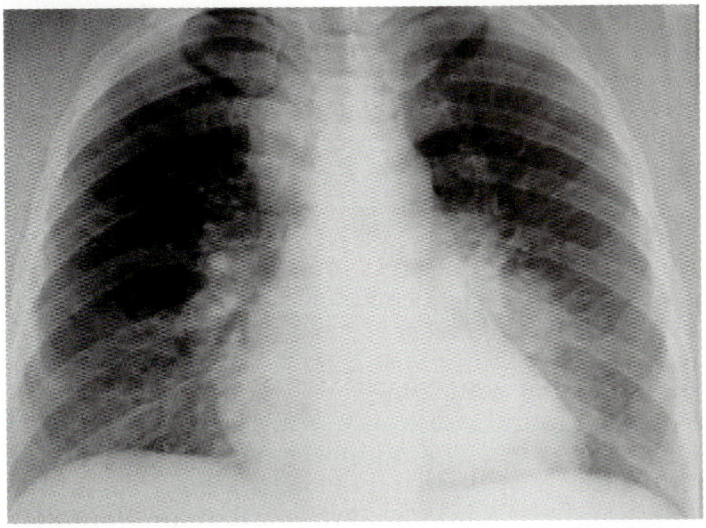

**Fig. 25.47:** Chest radiograph in a patient presenting with heart failure, which was subsequently found to be the result of dilated cardiomyopathy. Although, cardiac size is at the upper limit of normal, left ventricular function is poor, causing severe pulmonary edema with bilateral alveolar edema and marked dilatation of the superior vena cava

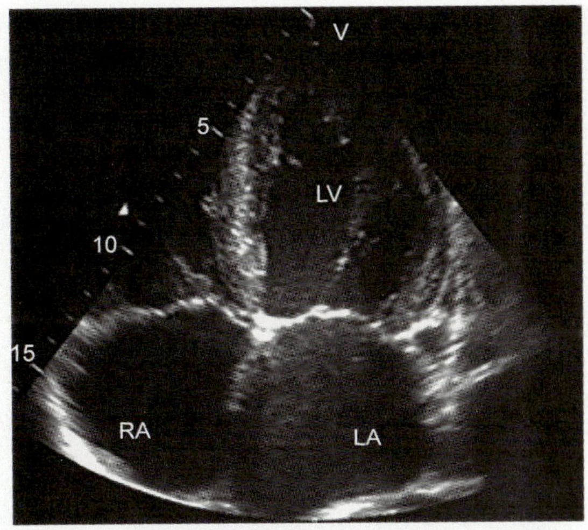


**Fig. 25.48:** In a 20-year-old adolescent instead of 45-year-old women dilated cardiomyopathy in a 45-year-old woman with AIDS. (A) Apical four-chamber echocardiographic view shows marked enlargement of all four chambers, as well as spontaneous echo contrast (smoke) in the left-sided chambers because of a very low ejection fraction and sluggish flow. (B) Apical four-chamber view obtained with color-Doppler flow imaging shows an eccentric jet of severe regurgitation through the tricuspid valve. LA=left atrium, LV=left ventricle, RA=right atrium, RV=right ventricle

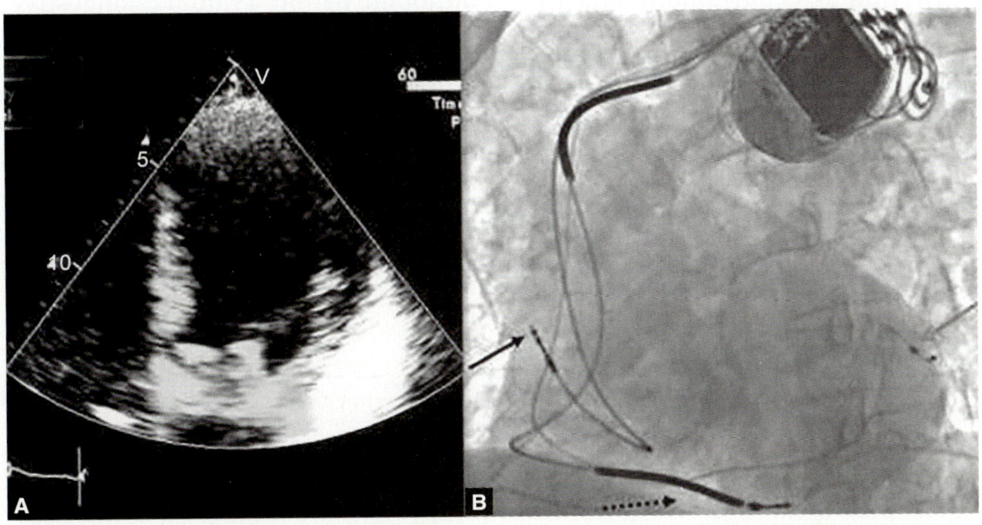


**Fig. 25.49:** (A) Echo cardiography showing diastolic wall motion defect in cardiac failure, (B) shows CRT in dilated cardiomyopathy

It is the most common cause of sudden cardiac death in the young and can lead to progressive heart failure across all ages.

The clinical presentation is varied. Young people, typically athletes aged 10–35 years old are the most common group to experience a cardiac arrest or sudden cardiac death. Evidence has shown that sudden death is primarily due to complex ventricular tachyarrhythmias, bradyarrhythmias, and supraventricular arrhythmias that lead to ventricular fibrillation or hypotension, and these events are exacerbated when there is left ventricular outflow tract obstruction or ischemia. Additionally, patients can present with symptoms related to poor diastolic function with preserved systolic function that include exertional chest pain and dyspnea, palpitations, presyncope, or syncope. The disease can then progress to end stage congestive heart failure heralded by systolic dysfunction, or patients can have atrial fibrillation associated complications, particularly embolic stroke.

## CARDIAC ARRHYTHMIAS

Arrhythmias are far more common among adults than children, but are equally as important for the clinician be able to recognize the abnormal rhythm, respond immediately and treat appropriately.

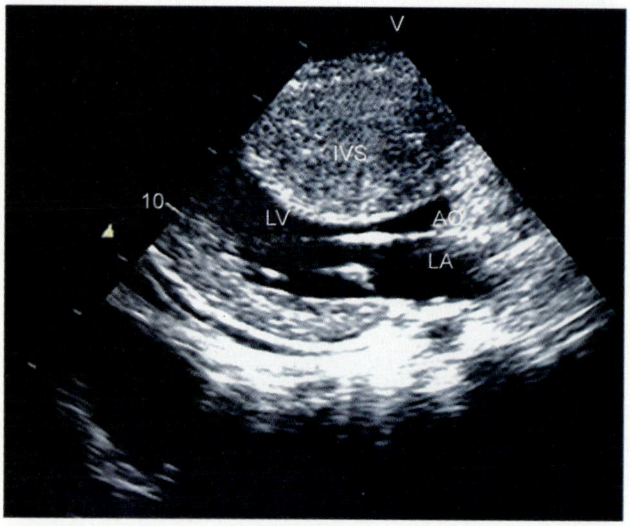


**Fig. 25.50:** 2D LAX. LPS echo view showing diffuse hypertrophy variant of hypertrophic cardiomyopathy (HCM). This pattern of hypertrophy is classically seen in younger patients. AO=aorta; IVS=interventricular septum; LA=left atrium; LV=left ventricle

Of adults presenting to the emergency room with an acute myocardial infarction, 90% have a rhythm abnormality and 25% have a conduction disturbance.

Most pediatric arrhythmias occur among children with congenital and acquired heart disease, and symptoms of congestive heart failure or cyanosis precede the dysrhythmia. In children whose initial presentation is an arrhythmia, the underlying problem is a primary conduction disorder in a structurally normal heart. Children admitted to the cardiac intensive care unit (ICU) for the medical management of heart disease, and particularly after cardiac surgery, certain catheterization procedures, and pre and post transplantation are at high risk for arrhythmias due to the underlying pathophysiology and medical and surgical interventions involved (Figs 25.52–25.70) .

### Tachyarrhythmias

These can be characterized as supraventricular or ventricular. The most common symptomatic pediatric arrhythmia is supraventricular tachycardia (SVT) with an incidence of 1 in every 250–1000 children. In infants, half are due to idiopathic causes, a quarter caused by congenital heart disease such as Ebstein's anomaly and 10–20% due to WPW syndrome, a type of AV re-entrant tachycardia characterized on EKG by a delta wave, wide QRS, and short PR interval. It should be suspected if there is a regular and rapid heart rate usually greater than 180 breath per minute (bpm) in older children and greater than 220 bpm in infants.

On the electrocardiogram, the QRS is considered narrow complex with indiscernible P-waves or retrograde P-waves due to an accessory AV pathway. Patients with bundle branch block may be confused with ventricular tachycardia (VT). Most infants are hemodynamically stable in SVT, although within 48 hours congestive heart failure may develop with rapid deterioration occurring in 50%. The infant may appear lethargic, tachypneic, fussy and mottled with signs of poor perfusion including cool extremities and hypotension. Older children rarely present in CHF and are usually able to articulate their symptoms of racing heart beat, chest pain, dizziness and lightheadedness. A 12 lead

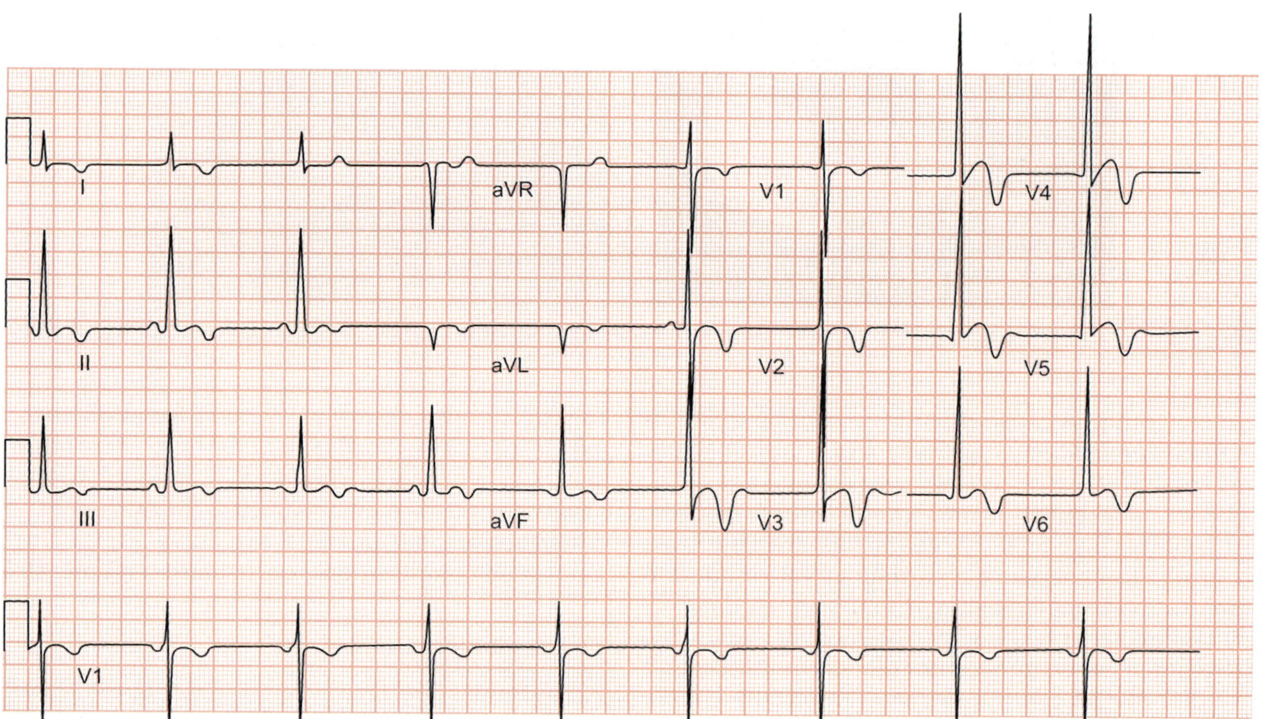


**Fig. 25.51:** ECG from a 20-year-adolescent with apical hypertrophic cardiomyopathy. Note elevated QRS voltages associated with left ventricular hypertrophy and inverted T-waves in all precordial leads

**Table 25.9:** Aetiological classification of cardiomyopathy

**Dilated cardiomyopathy**
- Idiopathic cardiomyopathy
- Noncompacted myocardium
- Postpartum cardiomyopathy
- Hemachromatosis
- Infectious
- Postviral myocarditis
- Human immunodeficiency
- Legionella infection
- Sepsis (gram negative)
- Toxic cardiomyopathy
- Adriamycin
- Alcohol
- Carbon monoxide poisoning
- Other chemotherapy

**High-output cardiomyopathy**
- Tachycardia-mediated cardiomyopathy
- Thyrotoxicosis
- Nutritional (beriberi, thiamine deficiency)
- Peripheral left to right shunt lesions
- Anemia

**Hypertrophic cardiomyopathy**
- Asymmetric septal hypertrophy
- Idiopathic hypertrophic cardiomyopathy)
- Atypical hypertrophic cardiomyopathy

**Restrictive cardiomyopathy**
- Idiopathic
- Infiltrative
- Amyloidosis
- Glycogen storage diseases
- Hemachromatosis
- Postradiation therapy
- Endocardial fibroelastosis
- Arrhythmogenic right ventricular dysplasia

**Other**
- Friederich ataxia
- Muscular dystrophies

EKG and rhythm strip should be obtained and an immediate clinical assessment should be made to determine if the patient is cardiovascularly stable or unstable. For hemodynamically unstable SVT with poor perfusion and severe heart failure, adenosine (0.1 mg/kg/dose maximum 6 mg increased to 0.2 mg/kg/dose, maximum 12 mg), pushed and flushed quickly, can be given and/or immediate synchronized cardioversion (0.5 J/kg then increased up to 1 J/kg) if IV access is not immediately available. For stable SVT, vagal manoeuvres, such as Valsalva or ice to the face may be attempted first. Adenosine can then be used if those maneuvers are unsuccessful.

### Ventricular Fibrillation and Pulseless Ventricular Tachycardia

These are the common causes of cardiac arrest in adults and often due to coronary artery disease. Fourteen percent of children compared to 23% of adults had ventricular fibrillation (VF) or pulseless VT as the first documented rhythm during in-hospital cardiac arrest. However, this is still much higher than many clinicians would have thought as the cause of cardiac arrest in children and demonstrates that those caring for children need to be capable of administering rapid defibrillation. The incidence of VF/VT as the first recorded rhythm in and out of hospital arrest in children varies by age, from 4–5% in infants and children to 15% in adolescents. In children, there is a cardiac origin in 21–71% of cases, such as in palliated congenital heart disease and cardiomyopathies. The incidence of VT after congenital heart surgery is low but can lead to a fatal outcome in an already hemodynamically unstable period. Intractable VT in the postoperative period, particularly after surgery involving manipulation of the coronary arteries, (i.e. arterial switch operation for d-transposition of the great arteries) should raise suspicion for myocardial ischemia and the possible need for surgical revision. In conduction disorders, such as in Long QT syndrome, torsades de pointes (a polymorphic VT) is characteristic and can degenerate into VF and sudden death. WPW also can rarely

**Table 25.10:** World Health Organization/International Society and Federation Cardiology classification of nonischemic cardiomyopathies

| Cardiomyopathy | Characteristics |
|---|---|
| Dilated | Dilatation and impared constraction of the left ventricle or both ventriles, nonspecification histology. Arrhythmias thromboembolism and sudden deadth are common. |
| Hypertrophic | Left and/or right ventricular hypertrophy, which is usually asymmetric and involves the interventricular septum with left ventricular volume is normal or reduced includes myocyte hypertrophy and disarry surrounding areas of increased loose connective tissue. Arrhythmias and premature sudden death are common. |
| Restrictive | Restrictive filling and reduced diastolic volume of either or both ventricles with normal or near normal systolic function and wall thickness, increased interstitial fibrosis may be present, it may be idiopathic or assocaited with other disease (e.g. amyloidosis) |
| ARVC | Progressive fibrofatty replacement of right ventricular myocardium, initially with typical regional and later global right and some left ventricular involvement, with relative sparing of the septum. Presentation with arrhythmias and sudden death is common, particularly in the young. |
| Unclassified | Unclassified cardiomyopathies includes a few cases that do not fit readily into any group. Some disease may present with features of more than one type of cardiomyopathy. |
| Specific | The term specific cardiomyopathies is not used to described heart muscle disease that are associated with specific cardiac or systemic disorders (e.g. hypertensive, cardiomyopathy) |

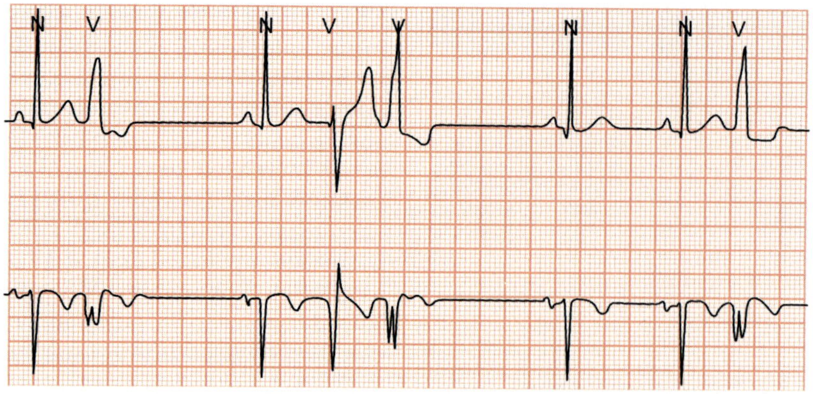


**Fig. 25.52:** Polymorphic VPC on Holter after mustard operation

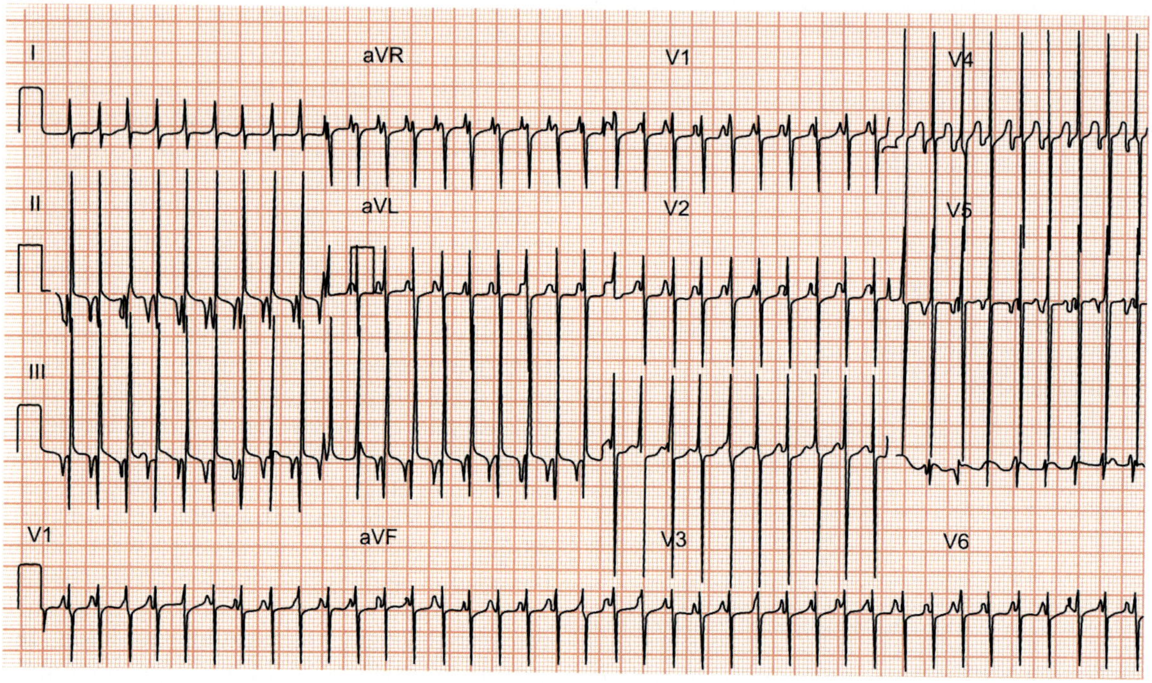


**Fig. 25.53:** Permanent junctional reciprocating tachycardia. An incessant arrhythmia with a characteristic appearance. Note the very long RP interval and the deeply inverted P-waves in leads II, III and aVF. This is a type of orthodromic atrioventricular (AV) re-entry over a relatively slowly conducting concealed right posteroseptal pathway

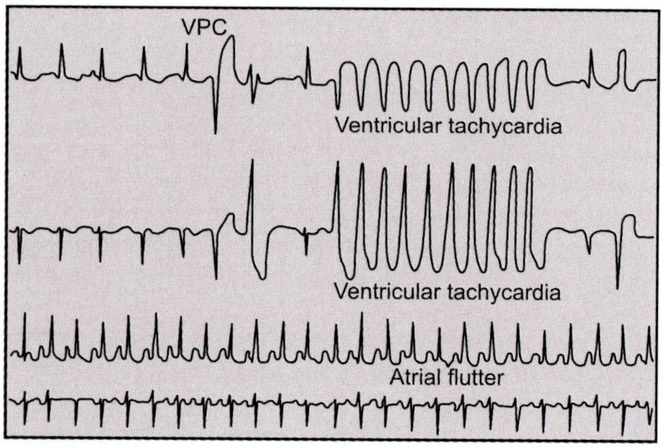


**Fig. 25.54:** Holter recording from a 15-year-old boy with dilated cardiomyopathy. The upper tracing shows non-sustained ventricular tachycardia; the lower shows sustained atrial flutter. The patient asymptomatic throughout

lead to sudden death in high-risk patients after pre-excited atrial fibrillation with a rapid ventricular response that leads to VF. On EKG, VT is a wide QRS complex tachycardia that can be monomorphic or polymorphic, and VF has a fine or coarse chaotic rhythm with no discernible QRS complexes. Defibrillation is the treatment for VT/VF along with prompt and effective cardiopulmonary resuscitation (CPR). There is clear evidence in adult cardiac arrest caused by ventricular arrhythmia that the rates of survival decreases with increasing time to defibrillation, and mortality increases by 7–10% every minute defibrillation is delayed.

## KAWASAKI DISEASE

Kawasaki disease does not usually present as a critical emergency; however, timely recognition and treatment can prevent the leading cause of acquired heart disease in children in the United States and fatal cardiac events in

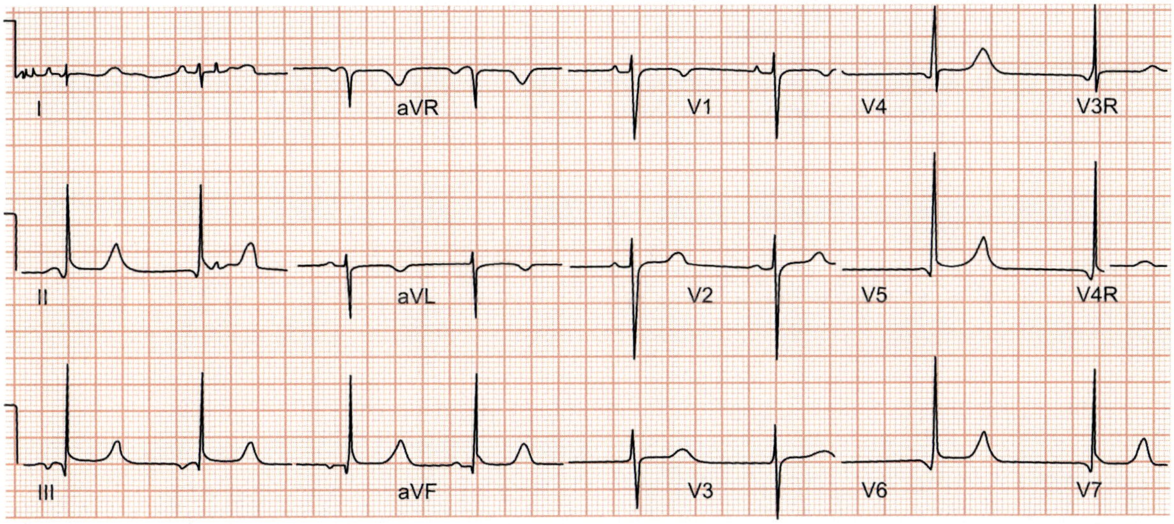


**Fig. 25.55:** Exercise in a young athlete. The QTc prolonged with exercise stress testing in the recovery period to 520 milliseconds, confirming the impression of long QT syndrome (LQTS)

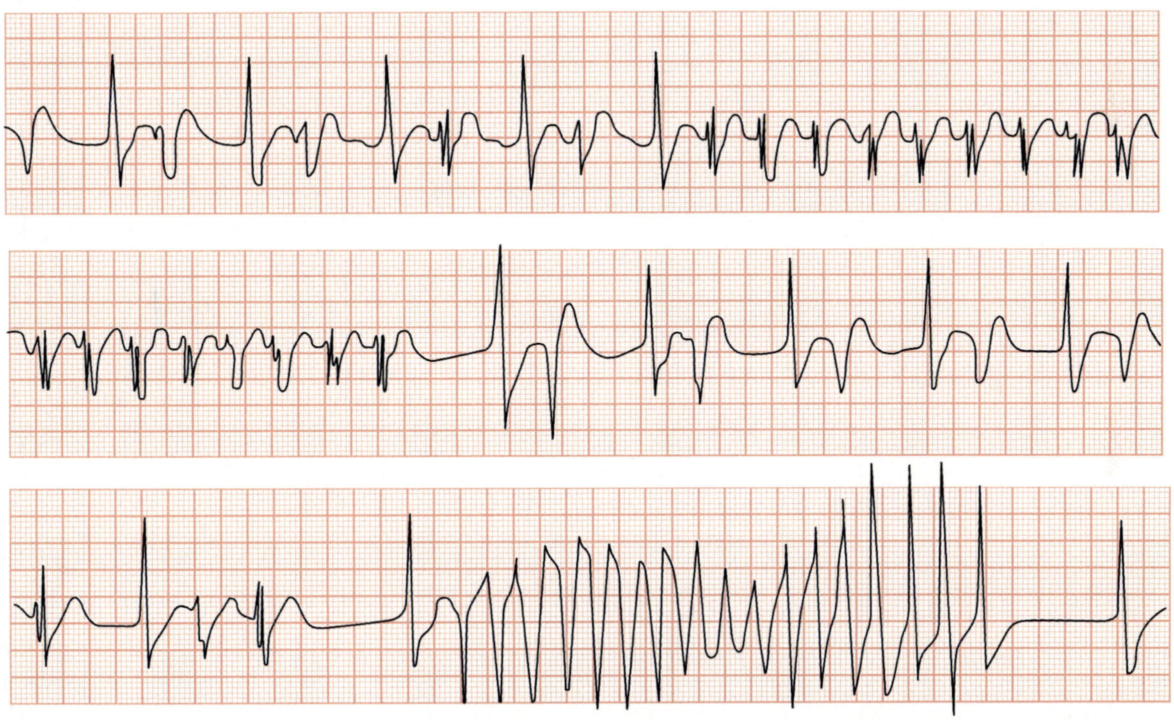

**Fig. 25.56:** A continuous rhythm strip from a 14-year-old girl who had undergone repair of tetralogy of Fallot but who had persistently elevated right ventricular pressure due to multiple peripheral pulmonary artery stenoses. She had been placed on quinidine for asymptomatic non-sustained ventricular tachycardia by Holter monitoring. Illustrated is monomorphic ventricular bigeminy, non-sustained monomorphic ventricular tachycardia, and a 4-second episode of polymorphic ventricular tachycardia (Torsade de pointes). The latter was a proarrhythmic response to the quinidine

adults. Kawasaki disease is an acute vasculitis of unknown cause that predominantly affects children under 5 years of age. In 15–25% of untreated children, coronary artery aneurysms and progressive stenosis develop, which can lead to significant morbidity and mortality from ischemic heart disease, myocardial infarction or sudden death.

The disease is diagnosed based on clinical criteria of at least 5 days of fever and at least four of the main clinical features including polymorphous rash; limbic sparing non-exudative conjunctivitis; mucocutaneous changes (e.g. strawberry tongue, dry cracked lips); cervical lymphadenopathy; and extremity changes with acute edema of the hands and feet or palmar erythema and after 2–3 weeks of illness periungual desquamation of the fingers and toes. There are also other supplemental laboratory and other clinical findings that are characteristic of the disease.

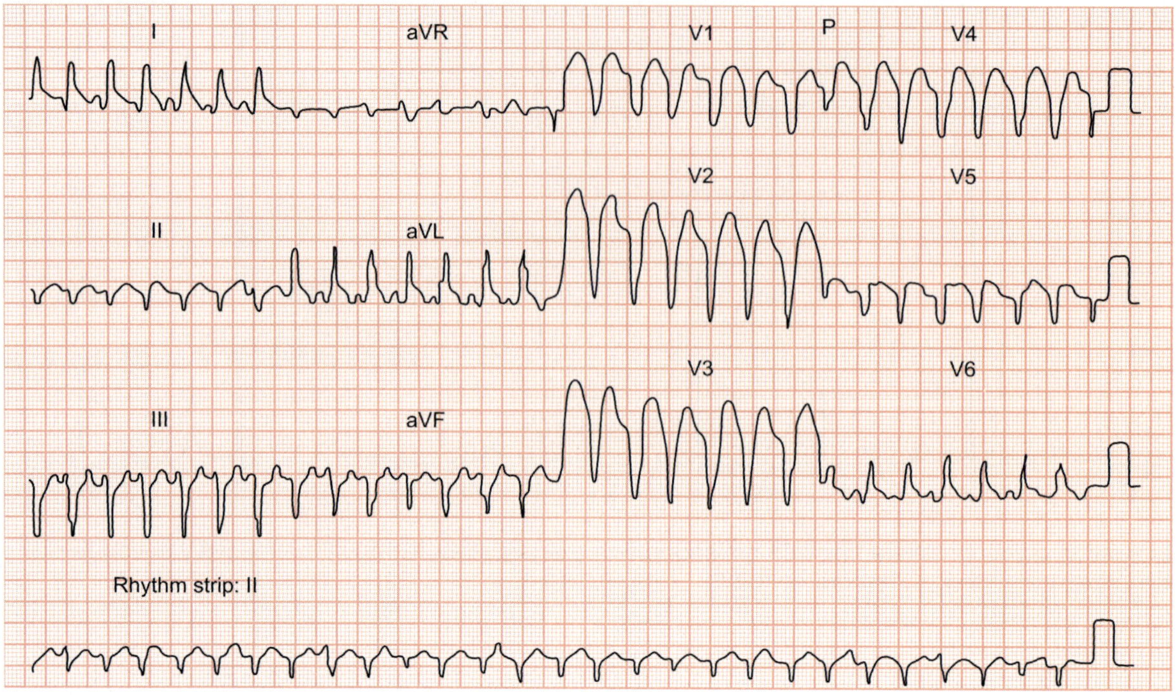


**Fig. 25.57:** ECG showing broad QRS ventricular tachycardia. The QRS duration is 160 msec. An independent P-wave can be seen in V1 (arrow). There is a leftward mean frontal axis shift

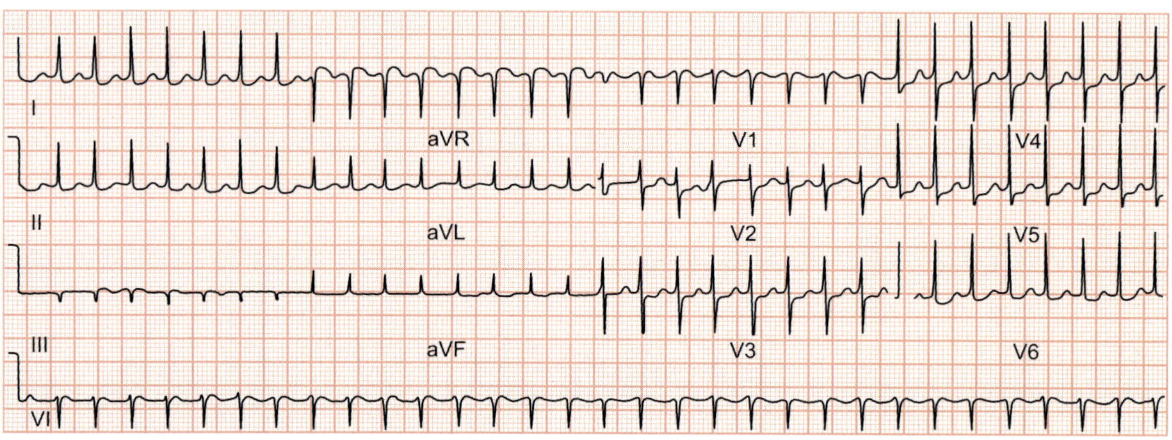


**Fig. 25.58:** ECG showing hemodynamically stable supraventricular tachycardia

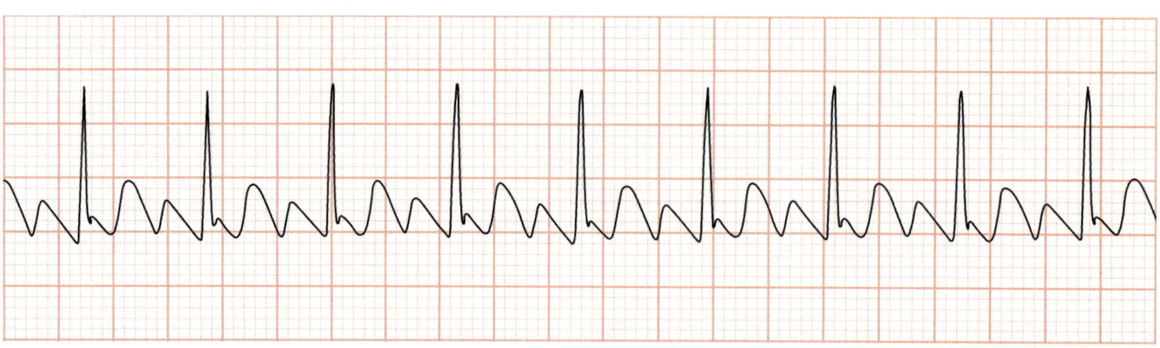

**Fig. 25.59:** ECG atrial flutter. Narrow QRS complexes are associated with regular flutter waves

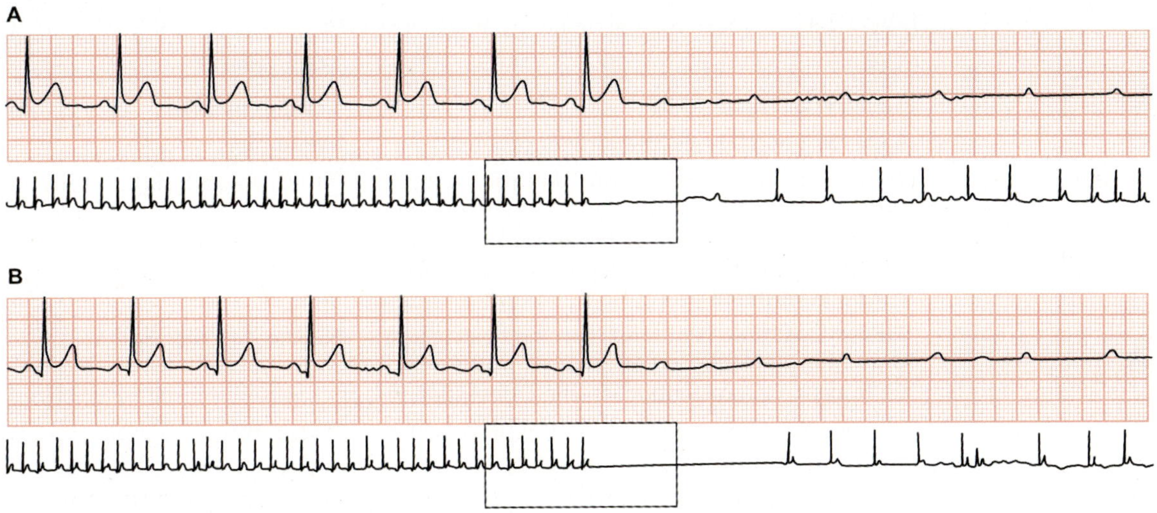


**Fig. 25.60:** (A, B) Holter recording of 2 episodes of spontaneous syncope that occurred a few minutes apart. The two episodes were very similar and were characterized by sudden-onset complete atrioventricular (AV) block without changes in P-P cycle length, which constantly remained 720 ms and long ventricular asystole of 7 and 11 s (top and bottom, compressed traces, respectively)

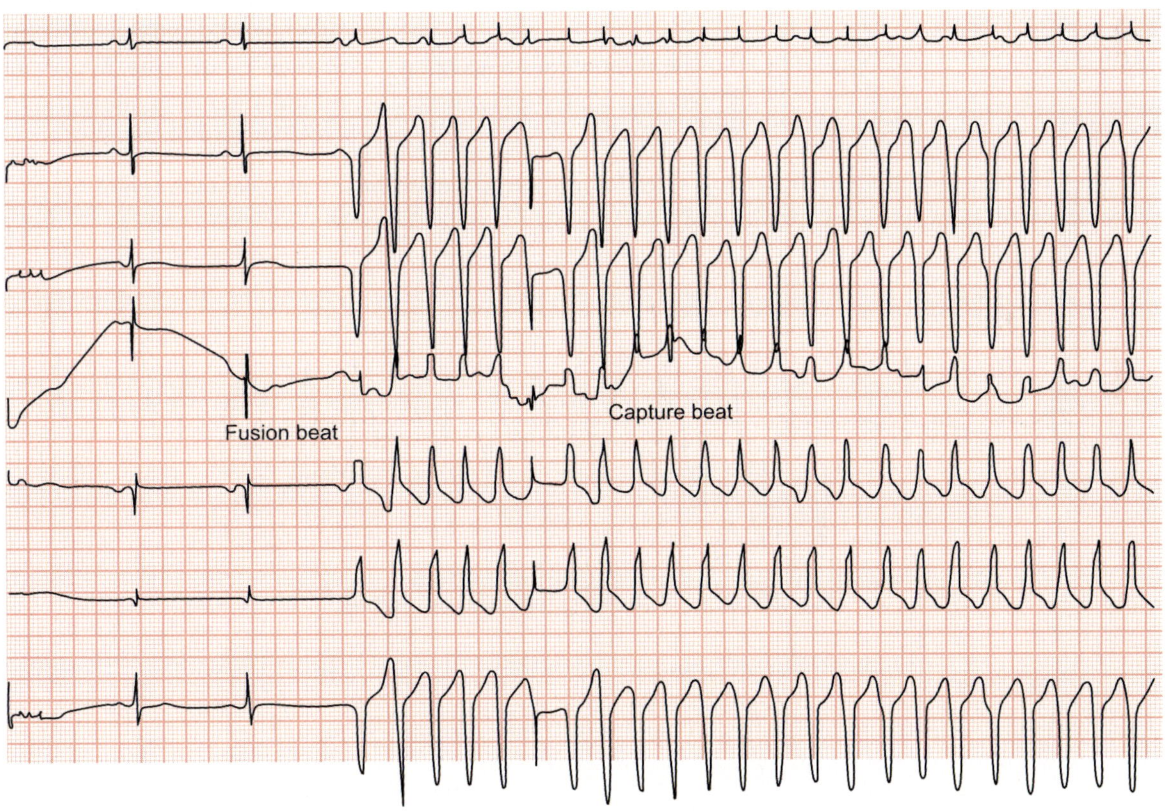


**Fig. 25.61:** ECG showing morphology of ventricular tachycardia (VT)

Children with a protracted febrile illness > 5 days with two to three of the clinical features of Kawasaki, incomplete Kawasaki should be considered. Moreover, the American Heart Association (AHA) recommends that an infant less than 6 months with fever greater than seven days and laboratory signs of systemic inflammation even without clinical features should have an echocardiogram. Mortality is principally due to the cardiac sequelae. During the acute phase of the disease, in addition to coronary arteritis, pericarditis, myocarditis and valvar heart disease can develop. Myocarditis can lead to myocardial dysfunction and children can present hypotensive and in

**Table 25.11:** Conditions that cause pulseless electrical activity

| Condition | Clues | Management |
|---|---|---|
| Hypovolemia | History, flat nedc veins | Volume infusion |
| Hypoxia | Cyanosis, bood gases and airway problems | Ventilation |
| Cardiac tamponade | History (trauma, renal failure, thoracic malignancy) and no pulse with CPR. Vein distention; impending tamponade-tachycardia, hypotension low pulse pressure-changing to sudden bradycardia as terminal event | Pericardiocentesis |
| Tension pneumothorax | History (asthma, ventilator, chronic obstructive pulmonary disease and trauma) no pulse with CPR, neck vein distention, tracheal deviation | Needle decompression |
| Hypothermia | History of exposure to cold, central body temperature | Warming |
| Massive pulmonary embolism | History, no pulse felt with CPR | Pulmonary arteriogram and surgical embolectomy thrombolytics |
| Drug overdose (tricyclics, diagoxin, b-blockers calcium) | Bradycardia, history of ingestion, empty bottles at the scene, pupils and neurologic examination | Drug screens, intubation, lavage, activated charcoal and lactulose per local protocols |
| Hyperkalemia | History of renal failure diabetes, recent dialysis dialysis fistulas and medications | Calcium chloride (immediate), then combination of insulin glucose sodium bicarbonate; then sodium polystyrene sulfonate and sorbitol; dialysis (long term) |
| Pre-existing acidosis | History of bicarbonate responsive pre-existing acidosis renal failure | Sodium bicarbonate, hyperventilation |
| Acure massive MI | History, ECG, enzymes | Treat for cardiogenic shock |

CPR=cardiopulmonary resuscitation; ECG=electrocardiography; MI=myocardial infarction. From Wnard CA, 1997.

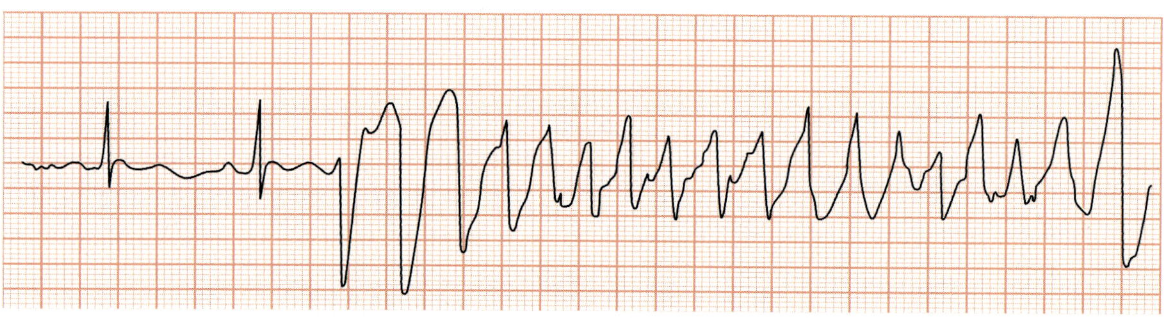

**Fig. 25.62:** ECG showing torsades de pointes

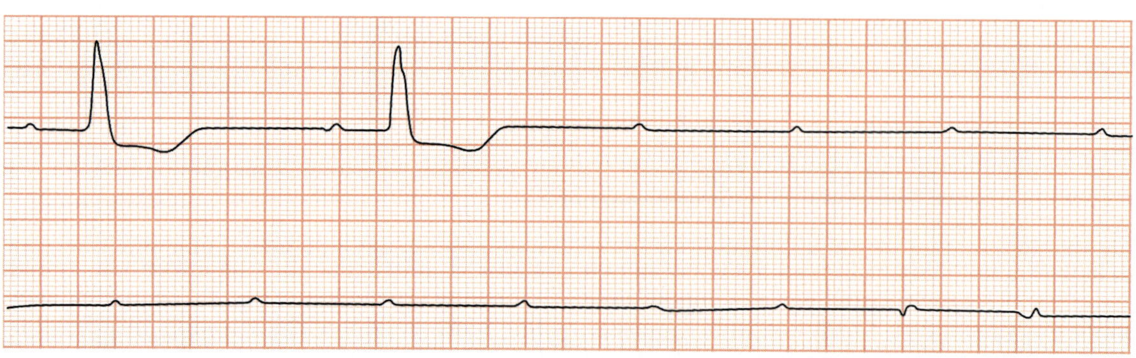

**Fig. 25.63:** ECG showing complete A-V dissociation in patient with Stokes-Adam attack

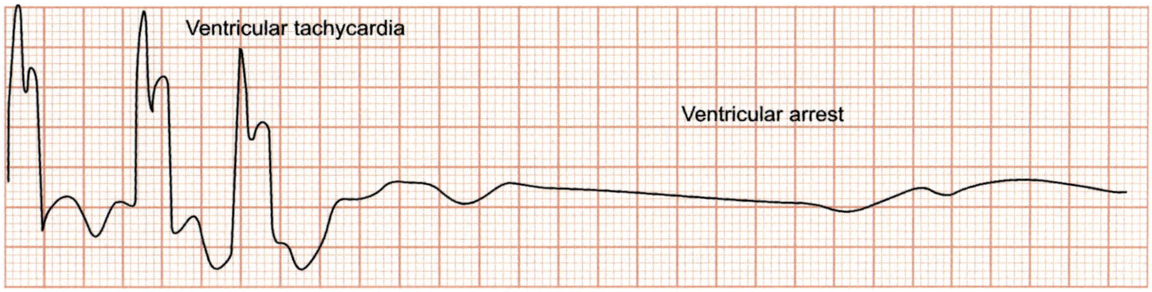


**Fig. 25.64:** Graph showing the features of ventricular tachycardia ending in a long asystole (cardiac arrest)

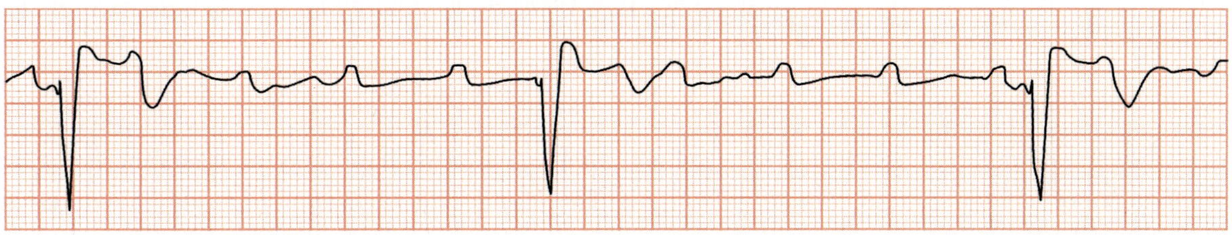

**Fig. 25.65:** ECG trace showing acute myocardial infarction with complete heart block

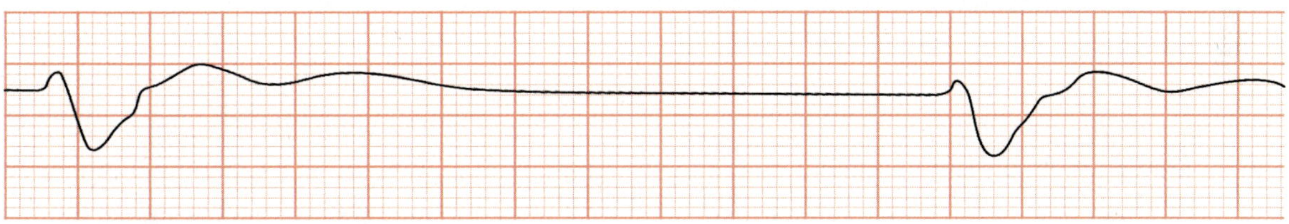

**Fig. 25.66:** ECG showing broad and slow rhythm in association with pulseless electrical activity

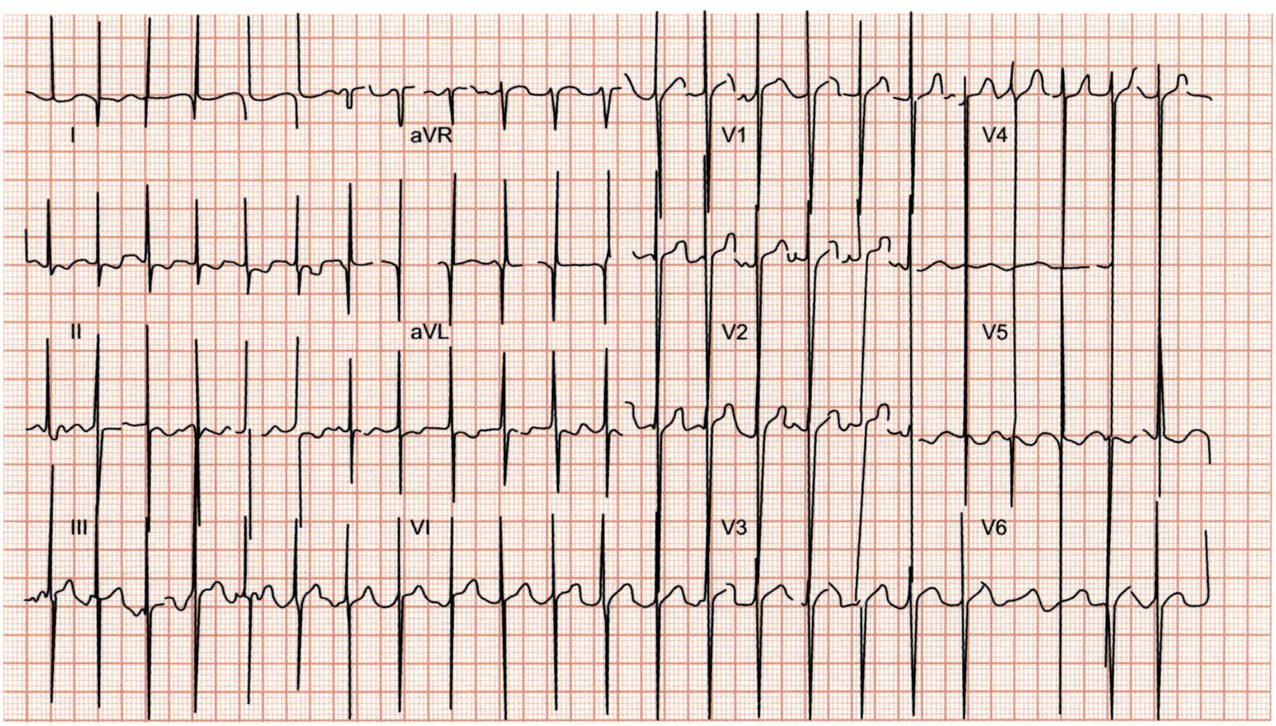


**Fig. 25.67:** EKG of an 8-month-old who initially presented to the ER with respiratory distress and wheezing and echocardiogram confirmed ALCAPA. EKG shows deep (3 mm) and wide (30 ms) Q-waves in I, aVL, V6, absent Q-waves in II, III, aVF and ST-segment changes

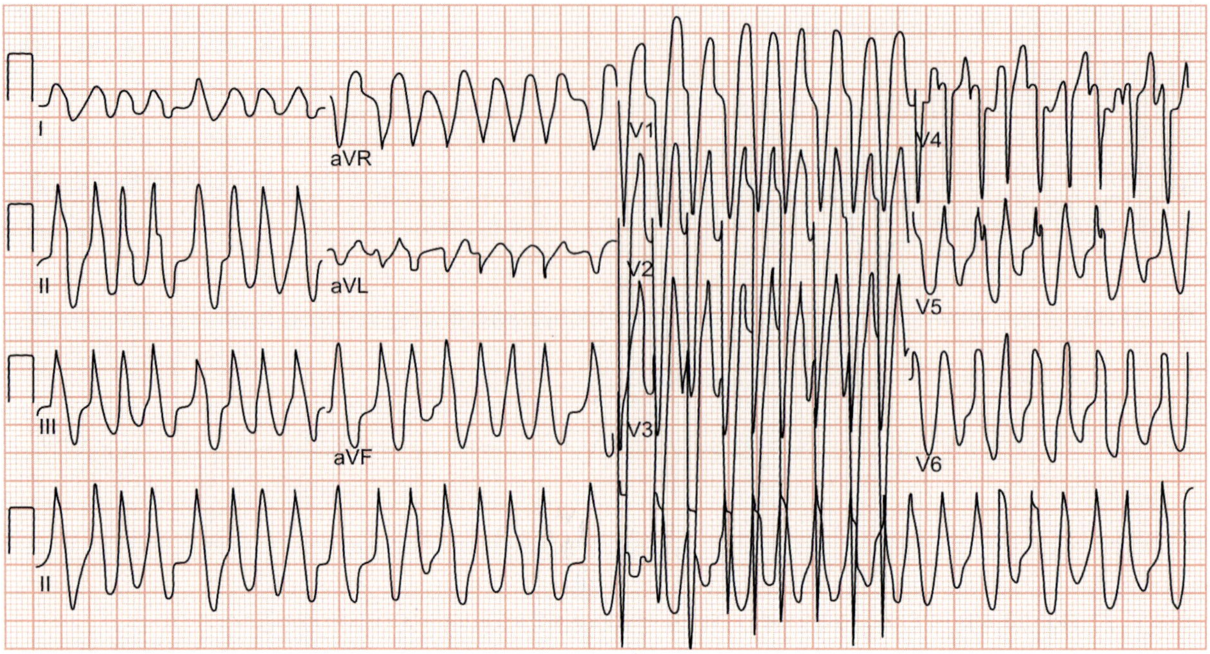


**Fig. 25.68:** ECG morphology showing pre-excited atrial fibrillation

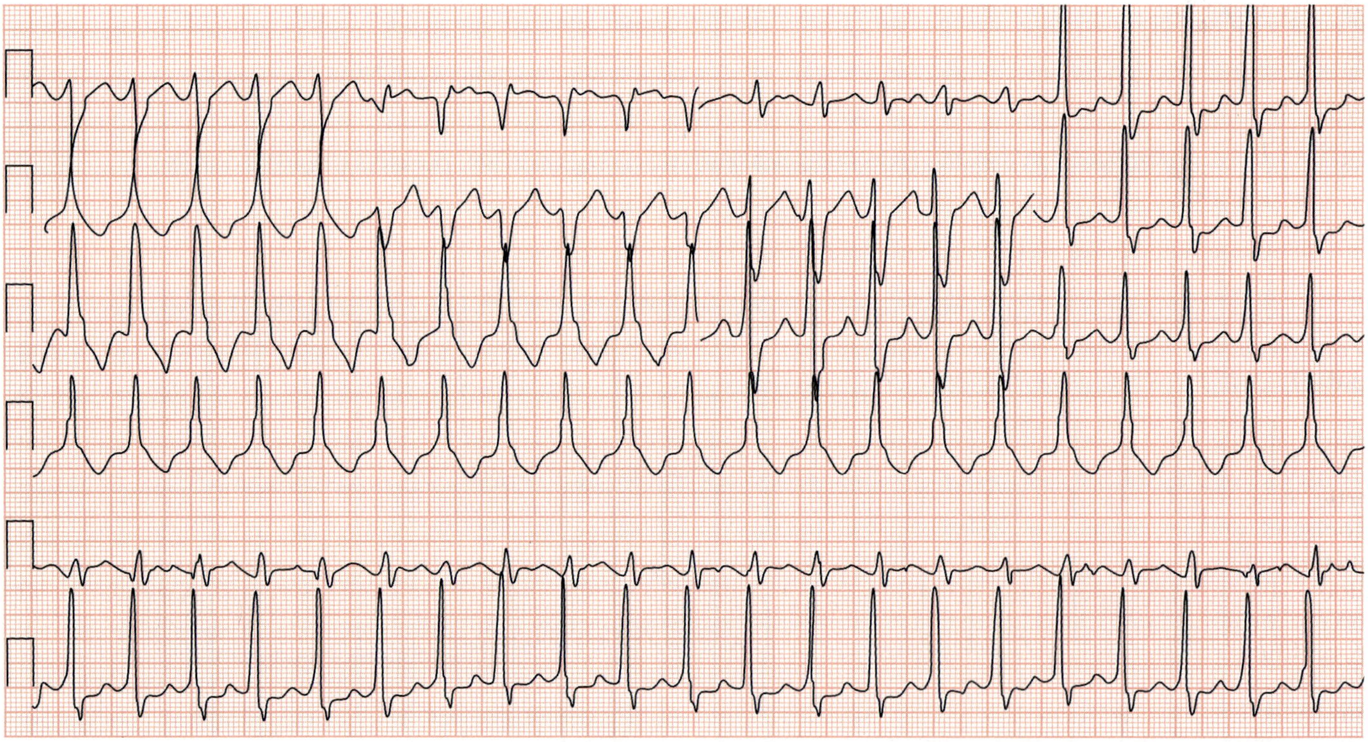

**Fig. 25.69:** Electrocardiogram illustrating left ventricular outflow tract ventricular tachycardia (LVOT VT). The S-wave in LI and R-wave transition in V1 suggest LVOT VT. In addition, an R:S amplitude ratio of 30% and an R:QRS duration ratio of 50% are seen. Presence of an S-wave in leads V5 and V6 suggests an infravalvular origin of the tachycardia

cardiogenic shock. Arrhythmias can be associated as well as PR prolongation, and non-specific ST and T-wave changes noted on electrocardiogram. There are specific guidelines associated with the acute and long-term management of Kawasaki disease. Treatment consists of IVIG 2g/kg over 12 hours and high dose aspirin 80–100 mg/kg/day in 4 doses for 48–72 hours after fever defervescence, then low dose 3–5 mg/kg/day. Patients with persistent fever (more than 36 hours after initial IVIG) or recurrent fever should be retreated with IVIG. The long-

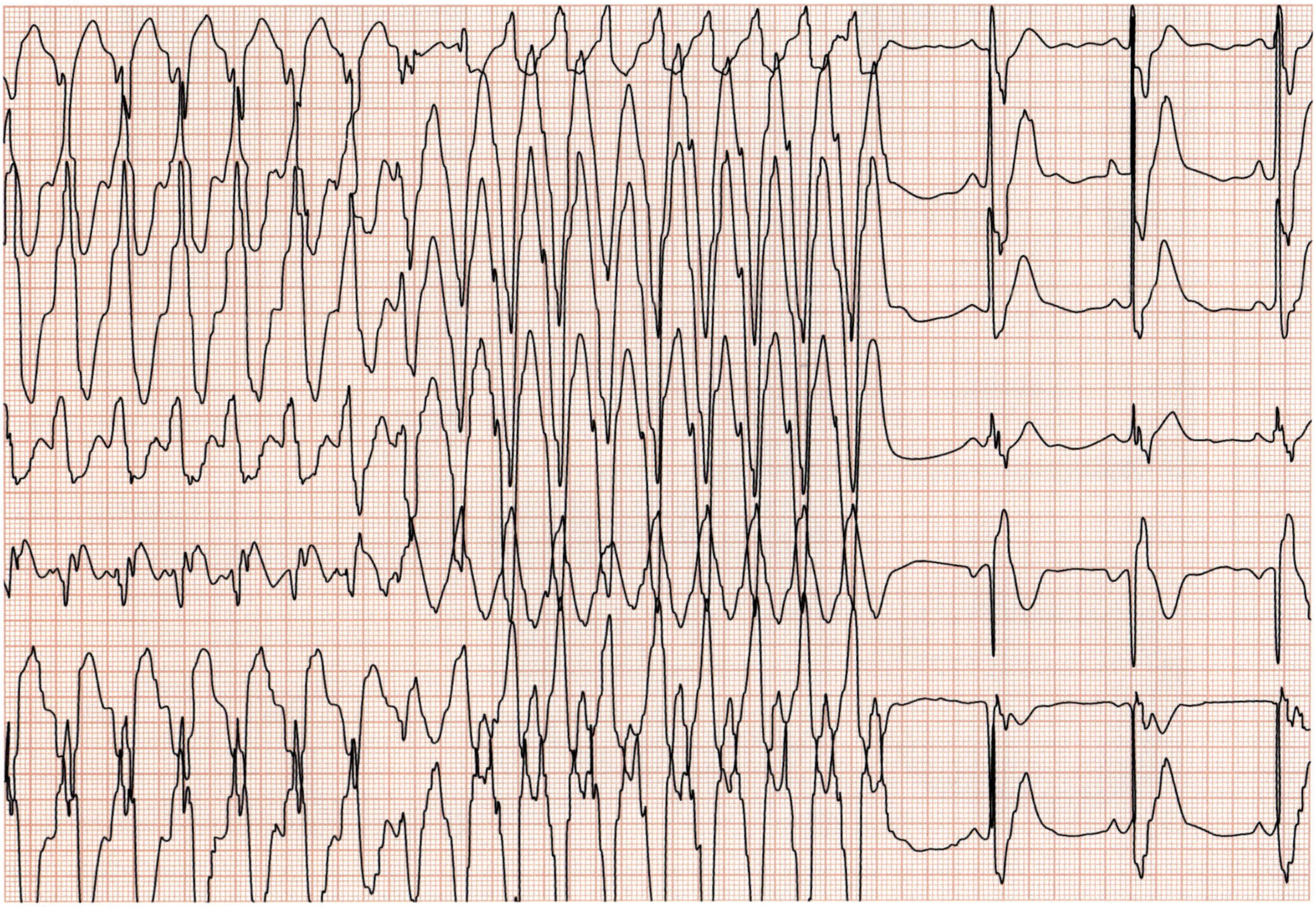

**Fig. 25.70:** ECG showing ventricular tachycardia is terminated with ventricular burst pacing from the ICD

term management should be tailored based on the degree of coronary artery involvement and the risk for ischemic events (Figs 25.71 and 25.72) .

## AORTIC DISEASE AND DISSECTION

Aortic dissection is rare in infants and children, and is associated with inherited disorders, such as Marfan syndrome and other connective tissue disorders, and after balloon dilation of coarctation and re-coarctation, complication of cardiopulmonary bypass at the aortic cannulation site, and in young adults with a bicuspid aortic valve and ascending aortic dilation. In contrast, atherosclerosis is the main cause of aortic aneurysms and dissection in adults, with hypertension being the main risk factor.

The clinical presentation in aortic dissection will vary based on the origin and extension of the dissection. Typically, there is abrupt onset of sharp pain that may change in location, followed by congestive cardiac failure due to severe aortic regurgitation. Patients may present with syncope, cardiac tamponade, stroke, limb ischemia with pulse deficits, paraplegia, and if renal or mesenteric arteries are involved may result in oliguria/anuria or have persistent abdominal pain. A diastolic murmur of aortic regurgitation and the typical wide pulse pressure is present in half of patients with proximal dissection. Aortic rupture into the pericardium with cardiac tamponade (i.e. friction rub, muffled heart sounds, hypotension, jugular venous distention, pulsus paradoxus) or the pleural space are indications for surgical emergencies. A detailed history and physical exam should be performed; a patient with stigmata of Marfan syndrome or other connective tissue disease would raise the index of suspicion for dissection compared to other possible diagnoses (such as acute coronary syndrome, pericarditis, pulmonary embolism and cholecystitis). An EKG is important to differentiate acute myocardial infarction to prevent the administration of thrombolytic therapy that would be detrimental in aortic dissection. Although, 20% of patients with dissection involving the ascending aorta have evidence of ischemia or infarction as the dissection extends into the coronary ostium, and in this situation, additional imaging studies should be performed to confirm the dissection if the index of suspicion is high. Diverse imaging modalities can be used to detect aortic dissection. Transthoracic and transesophageal echocardiography can be useful in the emergency room and operating room for emergent decision making. CT scans are the most often used technique in

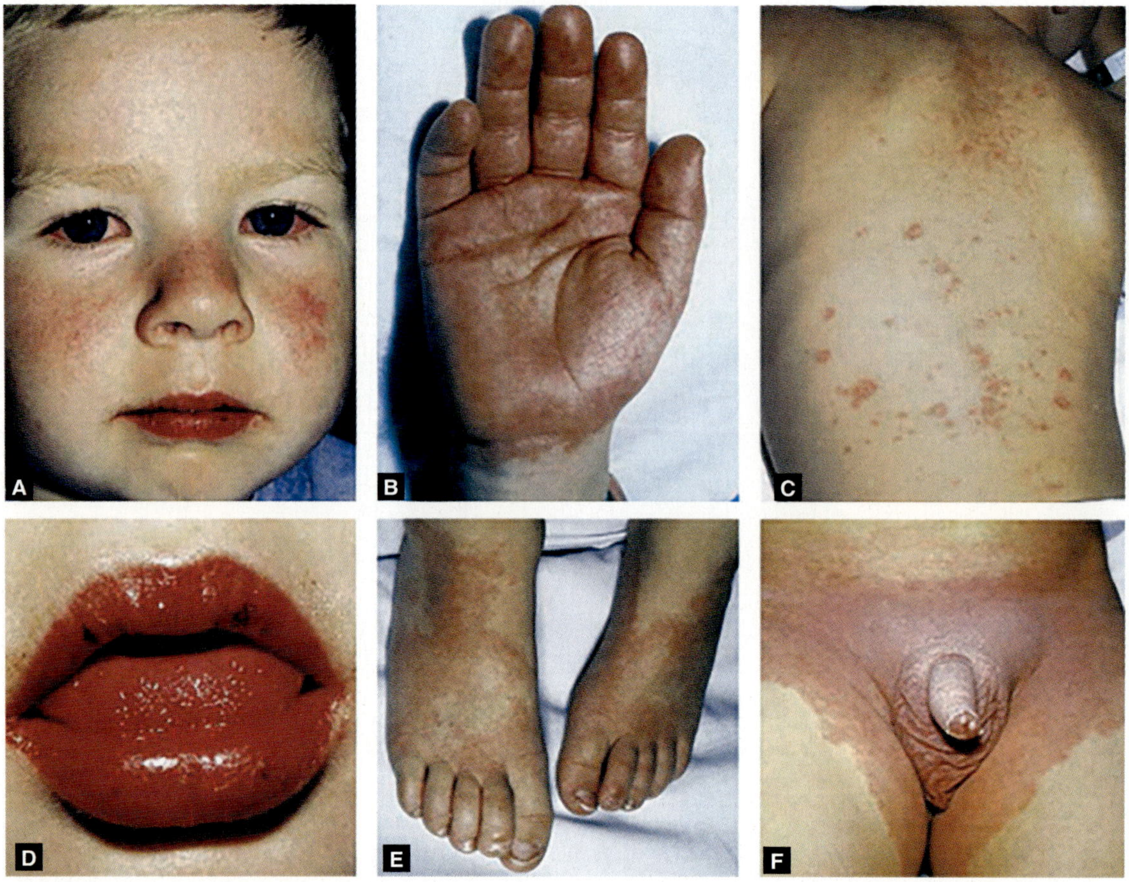

**Fig. 25.71:** Photographs of a four-year-old boy show the typical features of Kawasaki's disease. These features include bilateral nonexudative conjunctivitis (A); dry, fissured, erythematous lips and a 'strawberry' tongue (D); erythematous and edematous hands and feet (B and E); an erythematous truncal rash (C); and a desquamating perineal rash (F). The patient also had anterior cervical lymphadenopathy and sterile pyuria but none of the other complications of the disease. The child recovered uneventfully after receiving treatment with intravenous immune globulin and aspirin

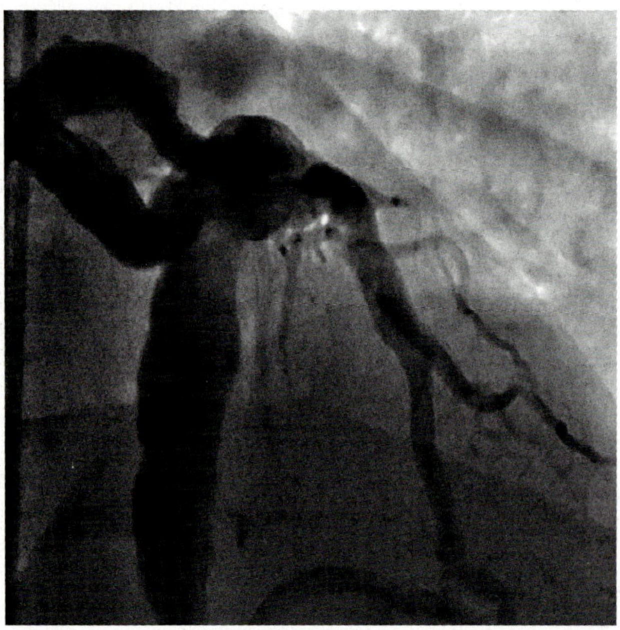

**Fig. 25.72:** Cine-angiogram image showing severe diffuse coronary artery aneurysm with left circumflex dominant circulation in Kawasaki disease

patients with suspected aortic dissection and have a high sensitivity and specificity. Branch vessel involvement can be accurately identified with contrast angiography, and should be used in patients with neurological symptoms, acute renal failure, and limb and mesenteric ischemia. Patients should be in an intensive care unit with blood pressure and heart rate monitoring. Fluid repletion, pain relief (e.g. morphine) and blood pressure lowering drugs, starting with a beta blocker and adding intravenous sodium nitroprusside for severe hypertension are important initial therapies. Surgical management in children is guided by similar principles as adults, with the emphasis on prophylactic intervention in patients with underlying dilation to prevent dissection (Figs 25.73–25.76).

## PULMONARY EMBOLISM

Pulmonary embolism (PE) is an uncommon cardiovascular emergency in children, although relatively common in adults (Figs 25.77–25.79). However, adolescent females with collagen vascular diseases or on birth control increase the risk as well as the increasing population of obese teenagers. Acute but often reversible right ventricular failure can result from pulmonary arterial occlusion by thromboemboli. The

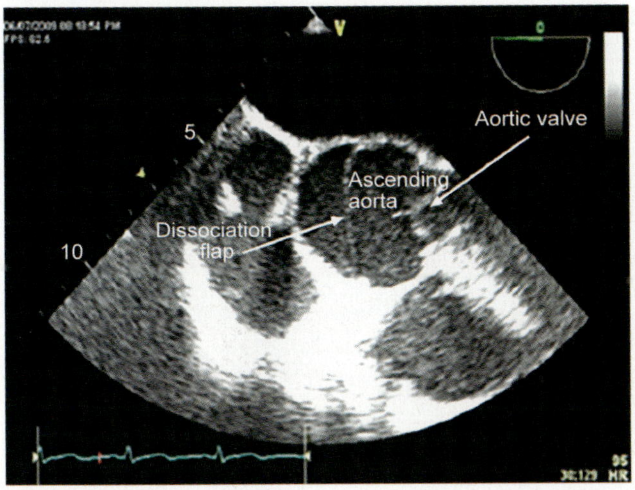


**Fig. 25.73:** Transesophegeal (TEE) echocardiogram was performed. The TEE confirmed a 5.5 cm aortic aneurysm with a dissection flap in the sinuses of Valsalva extending distally to the sino-tubular junction. The dissection did not involve the coronary arteries, but did extend into the aortic arch and further into the thoracic aorta. There was minimal aortic insufficiency but a left pleural effusion (assumed to be a hemothorax) was present. It was also noted that the aortic arch and descending aorta were dilated and aneurismal

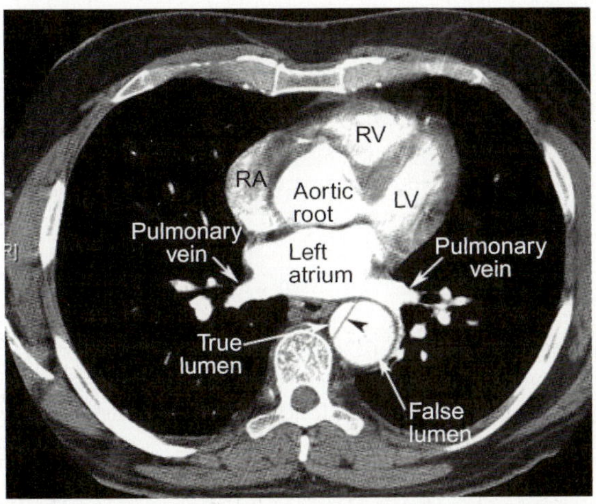


**Fig. 25.74:** CT angiography revealed aneurysmal dilatation of aorta

hemodynamic consequences of PE results when large and/or multiple emboli (occluding >30–50% of pulmonary arterial bed) acutely increase pulmonary vascular resistance, and the afterload that the right ventricular has to pump against is too high leading to right ventricle (RV) failure. This can lead to sudden death or syncope with systemic hypotension that might progress to shock and death from acute RV collapse. The mortality rate is higher in children and they are more likely to be diagnosed at autopsy, where approximately 60% presented with sudden death. The most common predisposing factors were central venous catheters, malignancy, cardiac or other major surgery, and infection/sepsis. Furthermore, thrombosis in children is more likely to originate in the upper extremity veins. Children typically present with dyspnea and

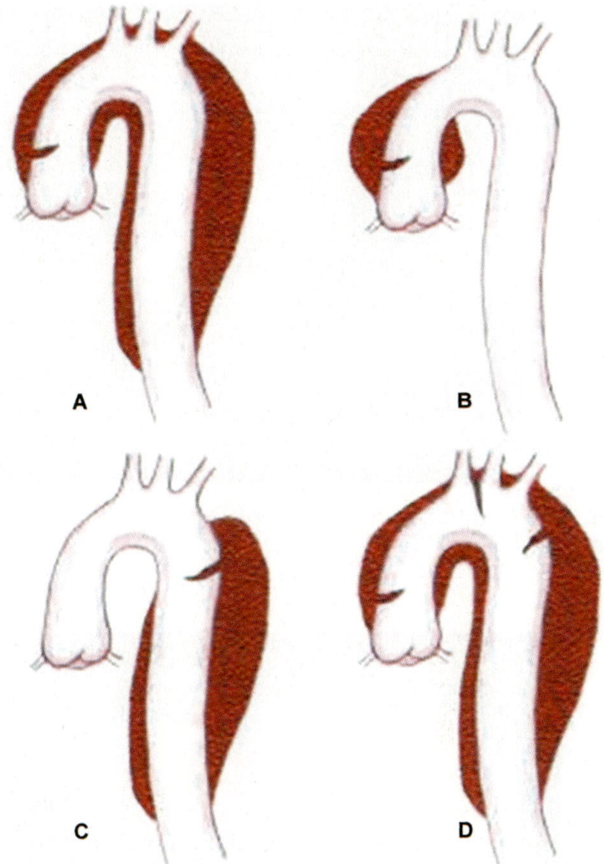


**Fig. 25.75:** Image A represents a Stanford A or a DeBakey type I dissection. Image B represents a Stanford A or DeBakey type II dissection. Image C represents a Stanford type B or a DeBakey type III dissection. Image D is classified in a manner similar to A but contains an additional entry tear in the descending thoracic aorta. Note that a primary arch dissection does not fit neatly into either classification

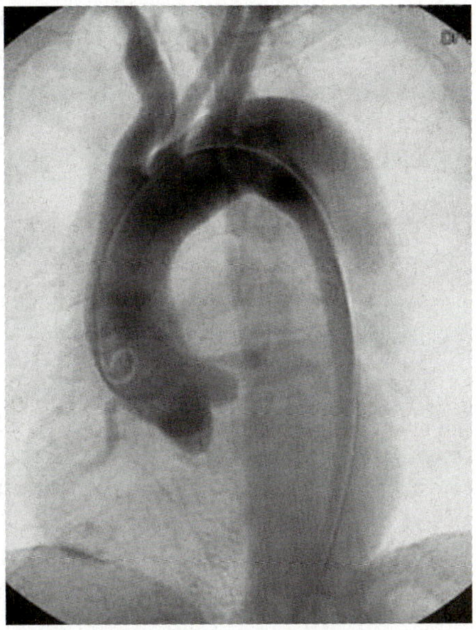

**Fig. 25.76:** Oblique arteriogram of the thoracic aorta demonstrates the double-barrel aorta sign of aortic dissection. Both the true and false lumina are opacified

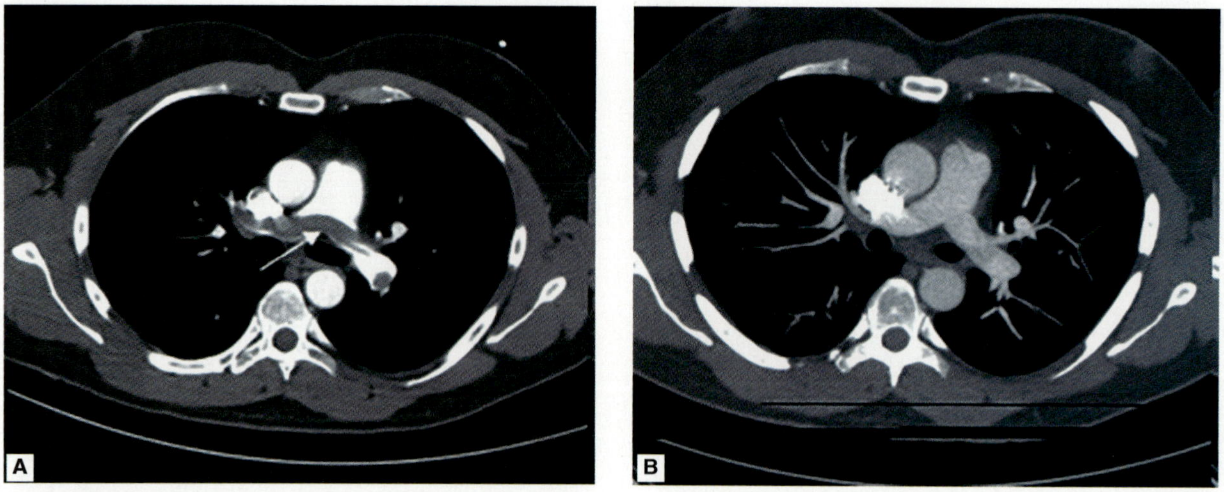


**Fig. 25.77:** (A) CT pulmonary angiogram (axial slice) revealing thrombus (arrowed) in the main pulmonary artery at the saddle extending across the origin of both right and left pulmonary arteries. (B) Repeat CTPA at 3 months confirming complete resolution of the thrombus

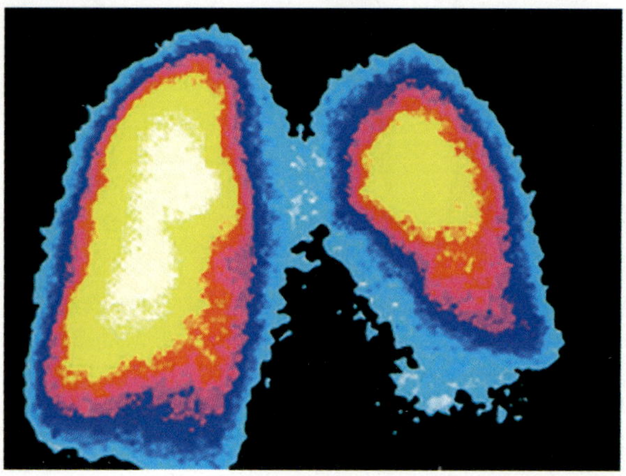

**Fig. 25.78:** Pulmonary embolism. Colored frontal chest scintigram (gamma scan) of a pulmonary embolism in the right lower lung. An embolism occurs when an abnormal blood clot (thrombus) blocks a blood vessel, in this case a pulmonary vein. Smaller emboli may cause shortness of breath, dizziness and chest pain. Larger clots can be fatal, as the blood is quickly starved of oxygen. Thrombolytic drugs can be used to break up a thrombus, and anti-coagulant drugs may help prevent the formation of others. If a thrombus is large, it may have to be surgically removed. A scintigram is a recording of the position and accumulation of a radioactive tracer in a tissue or organ

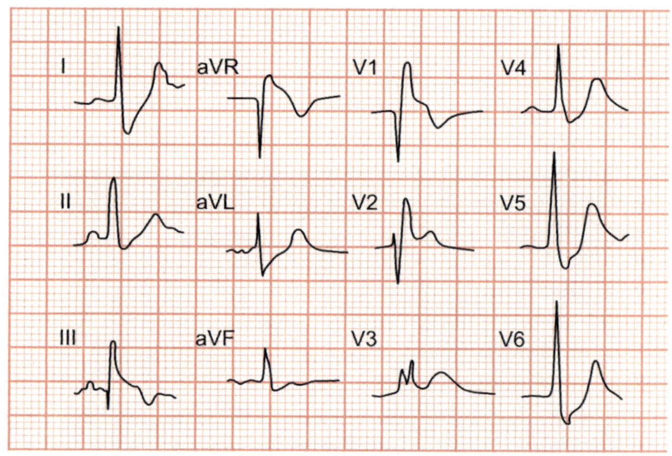


**Fig. 25.79:** ECGs show SI, Q3 and T3 pattern. Right bundle branch block (incomplete or complete). T-wave inversion in the right precordial leads P pulmonal, R-right axis deviation in patient with acute pulmonary embolism

hypoxemia, findings which are non-specific and often difficult to differentiate from symptoms attributable to the underlying disease. Adolescents have similar presenting complaints to adults including pleuritic chest pain, dyspnea, cough and hemoptysis, although there is often a delay in the diagnosis in adolescents.

The goal of diagnosis and appropriate treatment is to decrease mortality by preventing potentially lethal recurrent large thrombi. Clinical signs, symptoms and laboratory studies are not sensitive or specific to confirm or exclude PE, but should increase the index of suspicion to proceed with additional imaging. Such as, an electrocardiogram may show RV strain (classic S1, Q3, T3, new onset incomplete or complete RBBB), but this finding is not specific to PE and may be present in other causes of RV strain.

### Diagnostic Imaging in Pulmonary Embolism

These include venous ultrasonography to detect deep vein thrombosis (DVT); echocardiography to detect right heart thrombi, a right to left shunt through a patent foramen ovale (an indication of elevated right sided pressures), and right ventricular dysfunction (RV dilation, hypokinesis, increased velocity of the tricuspid regurgitation jet) findings which were associated with greater than two-fold increased risk of PE-related mortality; ventilation/perfusion (V/Q) lung scan is useful, when the scan is normal or indicates high probability, but most patients do not have findings that are definitive; pulmonary angiography is the gold standard, although it is an invasive specialized technique with associated risks that should be reserved for the small subgroup of patients in whom the diagnosis of PE can not be made by other noninvasive imaging modalities.

Heparin followed by oral anticoagulation therapy is the standard treatment for PE. In children, the use of thrombolytic therapy, such as tissue plasminogen activator (tPA), and surgical or transvenous catheter embolectomy may be considered in hemodynamically unstable patients at high risk of death due to RV failure. This can quickly reduce the RV afterload by recanalization of the occluded pulmonary arterial bed.

### Hypertensive Emergencies in Children

Hypertensive emergencies, though uncommon in children, are potentially life-threatening. While targeting blood pressure reduction to below the 90th percentile for age, gender and height, mean arterial blood pressure should be gradually lowered by one-fourth of the planned reduction over 8–12 hours, a further fourth over the next 8–12 hours, and the final 50% over the 24 hours after that. Frequent invasive or non-invasive blood pressure monitoring is essential, as is monitoring for sensorial alteration and loss of papillary reflexes. Few antihypertensive agents have been examined in children. Continuous intravenous infusions of short acting drugs, such as nitroprusside, labetalol and nicardipine are preferred to intravenous boluses of hydralazine or diazoxide. If severe symptoms are absent, oral agents such as nifedipine, clonidine, minoxidil, hydralazine, labetalol, captopril and prazosin may be used. Nicardipine and labetalol are particularly suited in emergencies with intracranial bleeding or ischemic stroke, while furosemide, sodium nitroprusside and nitroglycerine are useful in congestive cardiac failure. Therapy with oral antihypertensive drugs should be instituted within 6–12 h of parenteral therapy, and the latter gradually withdrawn over the next 12–48 hours. Oral agents have limited application as primary therapy, except when administration of intravenous infusion is likely to be delayed. This article provides a summary of the clinical approach to evaluation and management of severe symptomatic hypertension in children.

## CARDIAC TAMPONADE

Cardiac tamponade occurs when fluid builds up between the heart muscle and the surrounding tissue (called the pericardium). This fluid compresses the heart. Because of this, enough blood cannot be pumped in and out of the heart (Figs 25.80–25.86).

This condition can be life-threatening. With proper treatment, prognosis is good. Cardiac tamponade can recur after treatment, though.

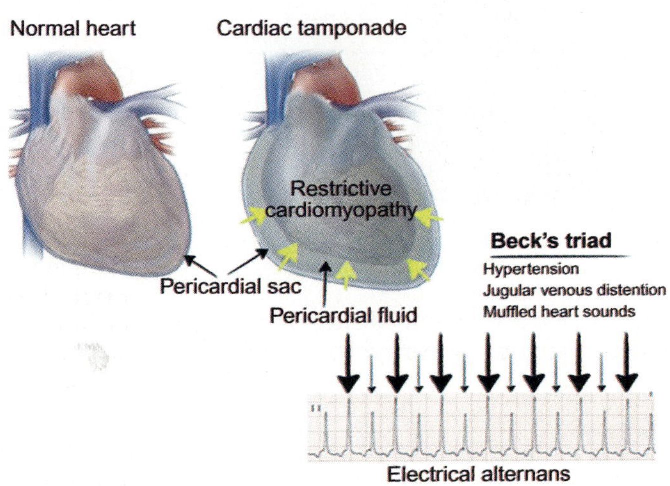


**Fig. 25.80:** Illustrations showing Beck's triad of hypotension, jugular venous distension muffled heart sounds. Pericardiocentesis should be performed emergently on patients with signs and symptoms of cardiac tamponade

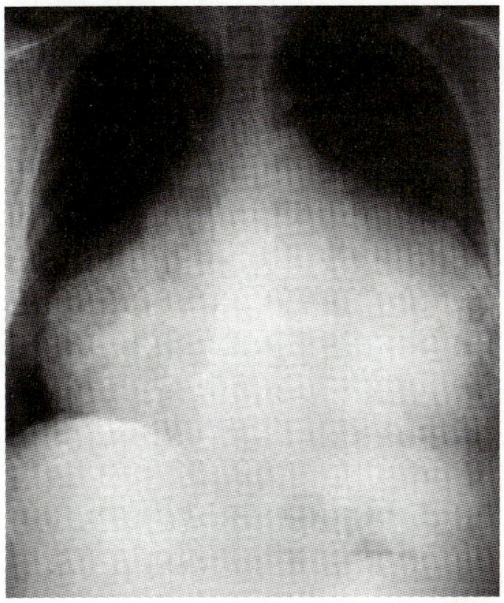

**Fig. 25.81:** This anteroposterior-view chest radiograph shows a massive, bottle-shaped heart and conspicuous absence of pulmonary vascular congestion in patient with massive pericardial effusion

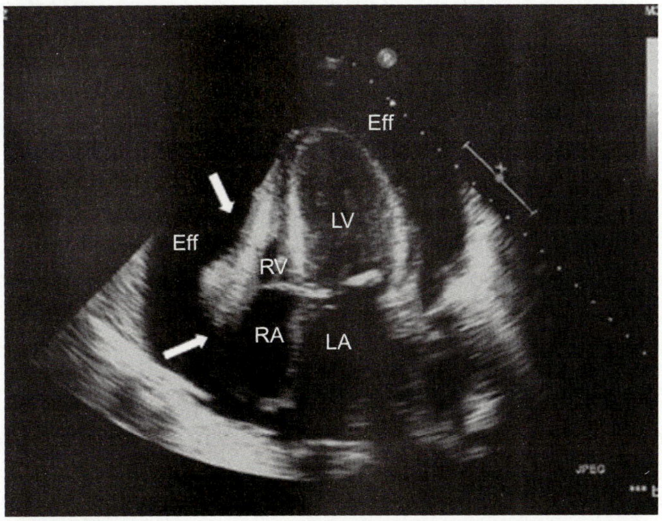


**Fig. 25.82:** Pericardial tamponade with right-sided collapse echocardiographic image showing pericardial tamponade with right-sided collapse. Reprinted, with permission, from Priscilla Peters, Cooper University Hospital, Camden, New Jersey. Eff=effusion; LA=left atrium; LV=left ventricle; RA=right atrium; RV=right ventricle

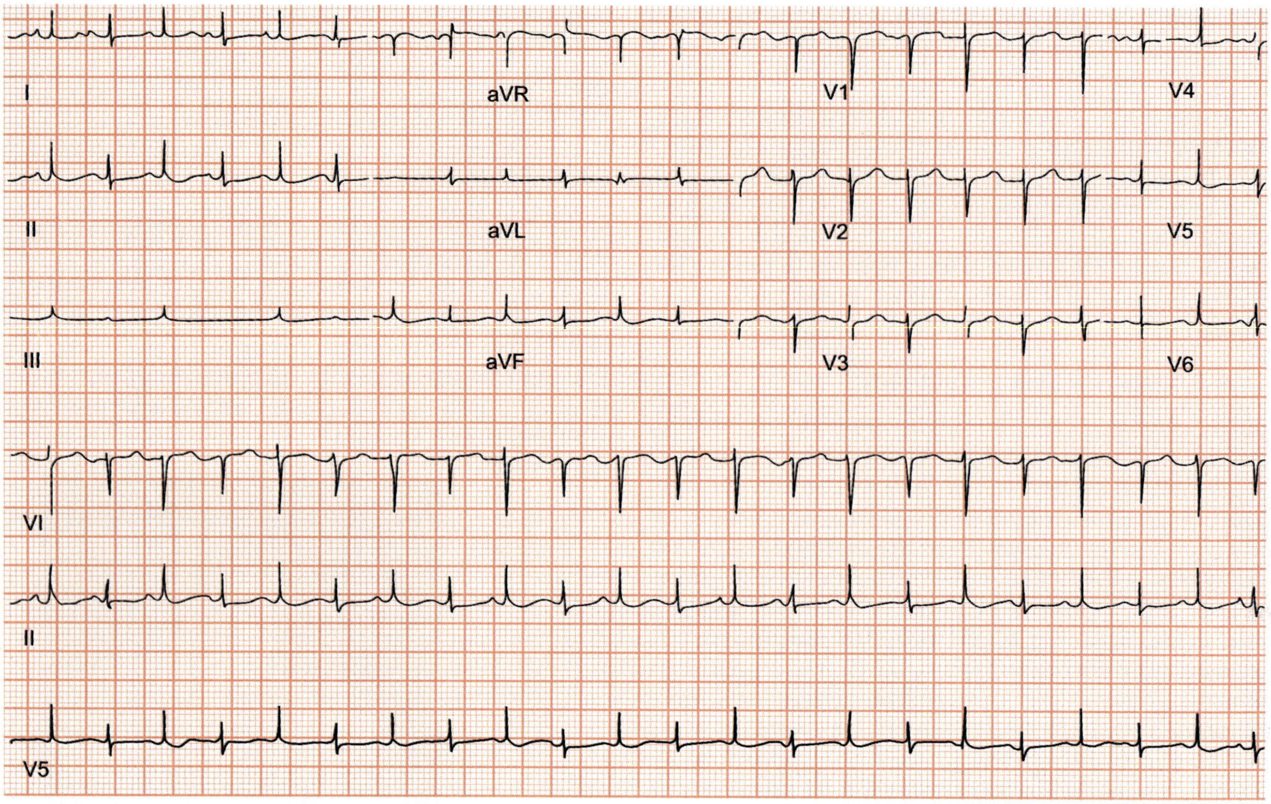


**Fig. 25.83:** Massive pericardial effusion produces a triad of low voltage tachycardia electrical alternans

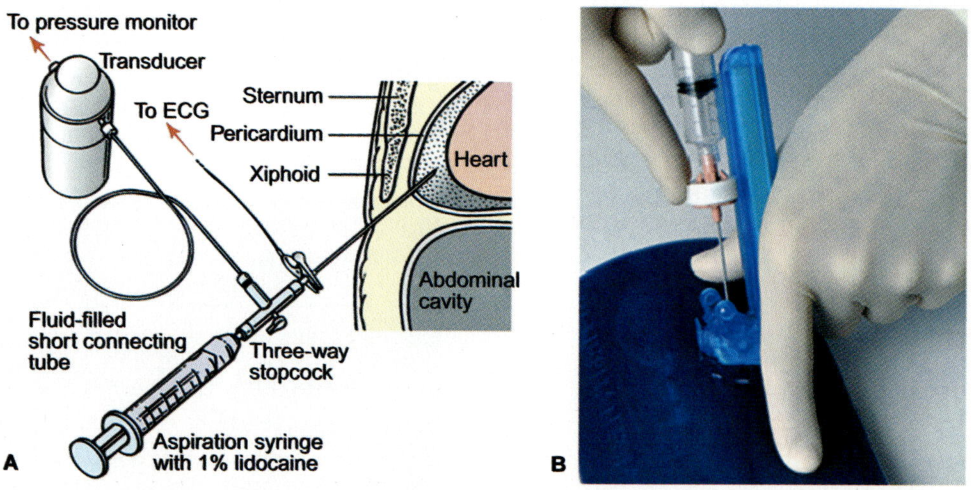


**Fig. 25.84:** (A and B) AxoTrack needle guidance ultrasound probe

The widespread use of central venous catheters in the treatment of pediatric patients has caused an increased incidence of complications. A rare, but potentially fatal complication occurs when the heart is perforated by the catheter tip causing a cardiactamponade. This perforation of the heart generally is associated with the insertion procedure, but may also occur after some time because of displacement of the catheter tip. Proper positioning of the catheter tip in the superior vena cava and a high index of suspicion are essential in preventing this serious complication. Contrast-enhanced chest X-ray after insertion of the catheter must be performed to ascertain a correct position of the tip.

### Causes

Cardiac tamponade can be caused by a variety of factors and conditions, including:

- Pericarditis (an inflammation of the sac that surrounds the heart) caused by bacterial or viral infections
- Bleeding into the pericardium, caused by injury

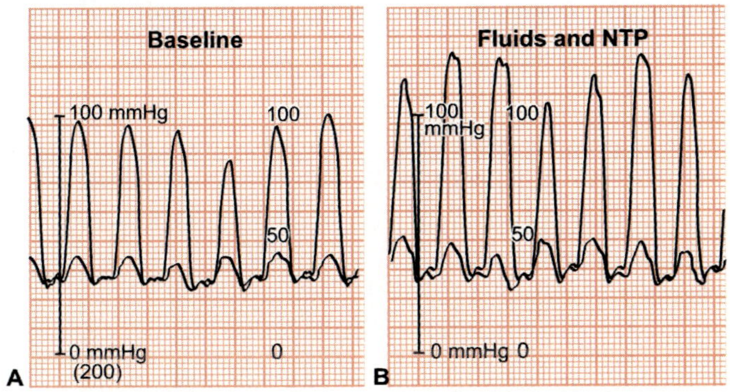


**Fig. 25.85:** High-fidelity pressure traces before and after intravenous fluids and NTP treatment in a patient who has developed pericardial tamponade. (A) High-fidelity left and right ventricular pressure traces in a patient with pericardial tamponade. There is marked elevation and equalization of diastolic pressures with loss of early diastolic filling. The left ventricular end-diastolic pressure is 32 mmHg. During the fourth beat, there is a marked drop in left ventricular systolic pressure and a rise in right ventricular systolic pressure, indicating enhancement of ventricular interaction. Overall, the systolic pressure is less than 100 mmHg. (B) The same patient after receiving emergency treatment with intravenous fluids and nitroprusside (NTP). Although, there is still evidence of enhancement of ventricular interaction and a pulsus paradoxus, the systolic pressure of the left ventricle has significantly increased to 120 mmHg. These medical treatments are a 'temporizing' approach to stabilize hemodynamics before emergency pericardiocentesis is performed

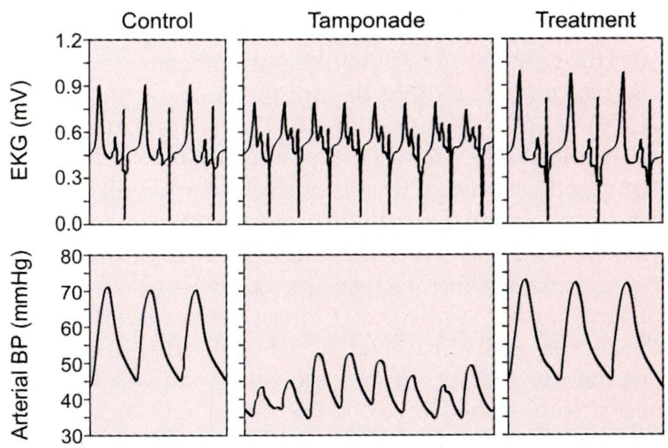


**Fig. 25.86:** Representative example of precordial ECG response to tamponade produced by infusion of 170 ml isotonic saline into pericardial space. During tamponade, there was marked elevation in heart rate (from 84 to 126 bpm), with pulsus paradoxus and reduction in arterial pressure. Tamponade was alleviated in 5 minutes with aspiration catheter, and ECG morphology and hemodynamics returned to baseline

- Ruptured heart muscle
- Cancer in or near the heart

### *Risk Factors*

These factors increase your chance of developing this condition. Tell your doctor if you have any of these risk factors:

- Heart surgery
- Tumors in the heart
- Heart attack
- Injury to the heart
- End-stage lung cancer
- Kidney failure
- Radiation therapy to the chest
- Hypothyroidism
- Systemic lupus erythematosus

### *Symptoms*

Symptoms vary from mild to severe. They typically include one or more of the following:

- Fatigue or Drowsiness
- Shortness of breath, rapid breathing, or difficulty breathing
- Dizziness or Light-headedness
- Chest pai
- That extends to the neck, shoulders, or abdomen
- Sharp or Stabbing pain
- Pain that is worsened by coughing or deep breathing
- Discomfort that can be relieved by sitting upright or leaning forward
- Swelling of the abdomen, veins in the arms or legs, or other areas
- Pale skin, or skin that is blue-or gray-tinted
- Rapid heartbeat
- Anxiety or Restlessness
- Low blood pressure
- Fainting
- Feeling of weakness
- General malaise

### *Diagnosis*

Your doctor will ask about your symptoms and medical history. You will also be examined. If you have a significant change in blood pressure between breaths, this is one way your doctor will diagnose this condition.

The following tests are also used for diagnosis:

*Echocardiogram:* A test that uses high-frequency sound waves (ultrasound) to examine the size, shape and motion of the heart. This is the primary test used to diagnose and manage cardiac tamponade.

*Cardiac catheterization:* A tube-like instrument inserted into the heart through a vein or artery (usually in the arm or leg) to detect problems with the heart and its blood supply.

*Chest X-ray:* A test that uses radiation to take a picture of structures inside the body, especially bones.

*CT scan:* A type of X-ray that uses a computer to make pictures of structures inside the chest.

*MRI scan:* A test that uses magnetic waves to make pictures of structures inside the chest.

*Coronary angiography:* X-rays taken after a dye is injected into the arteries; allows the doctor to look for abnormalities in the arteries.

*Electrocardiogram (ECG, EKG):* A test that records the heart's activity by measuring electrical currents through the heart muscle.

### Treatment of Cardiac Temponade

This is a serious condition. It can be life-threatening and requires immediate hospitalization and treatment.

Treatments are administered to:

- Save the patient's life
- Improve heart function
- Relieve symptoms

Treatments that are administered for cardiac tamponade include:

- Pericardiocentesis—a procedure to drain the fluid around the heart
- Fluids to maintain normal blood pressure
- Antibiotics
- Medications to help increase blood pressure to normal levels
- Oxygen to reduce workload on the heart
- Surgery to remove or cut part of the pericardium

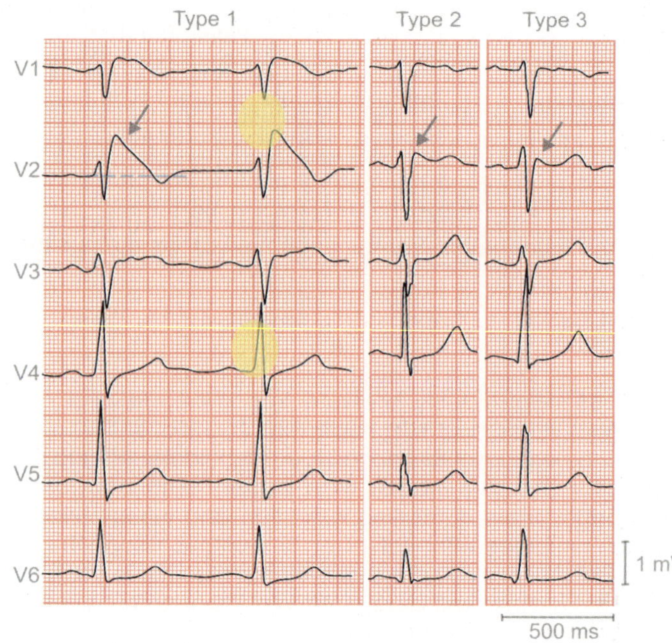


**Fig. 25.87:** Three types of ST-segment elevation in Brugada syndrome, as shown in the precordial leads on ECG in the same patient at different times. Left panel shows a type 1 ECG pattern with pronounced elevation of the J point (arrow), a coved-type ST-segment, and an inverted T-wave in V1 and V2. The middle panel illustrates a type 2 pattern with a saddleback ST-segment elevated by greater than 1 mm. The right panel shows a type 3 pattern in which the ST-segment is elevated less than1 mm. According to a consensus report (Antzelevitch, 2005), the type 1 ECG pattern is diagnostic of BrS. Modified from Wilde, 2002

## BRUGADA SYNDROME

Brugada syndrome (BrS) is a *genetic disease* that is characterised by abnormal electrocardiogram (ECG) findings and an increased risk of sudden cardiac death. It is named by the Spanish cardiologists Pedro Brugada and Josep Brugada. It is the major cause of sudden unexplained death syndrome (SUDS), also known as sudden adult death syndrome (SADS), and is the most common cause of sudden death in young men without known underlying cardiac disease in Thailand and Laos. Although, the ECG findings of Brugada syndrome were first reported among survivors of cardiac arrest in 1989, it was only in 1992 that the Brugada brothers recognized it as a distinct clinical entity, causing sudden death by causing ventricular fibrillation (a lethal arrhythmia) in the heart (Fig. 25.87).

### Treatment

The cause of sudden death in BrS is ventricular fibrillation (VF). The average age of death is 41. According to clinical reports, sudden death in people with Brugada syndrome most often happens during sleep.The episodes of syncope (fainting) and sudden death (aborted or not) are caused by fast polymorphic ventricular tachycardias or ventricular fibrillation. These arrhythmias appear with no warning. While there is no exact treatment modality that reliably and totally prevents ventricular fibrillation from occurring in this syndrome, treatment lies in termination of this lethal arrhythmia before it causes death. This is done via insertion of an implantable cardioverter-defibrillator (ICD), which continuously monitors the heart rhythm and will shock the wearer if ventricular fibrillation is sensed.

Recent studies have evaluated the role of *quinidine*, a Class Ia antiarrhythmic drug, for decreasing VF episodes occurring in this syndrome. Quinidine has been found to both decrease the number of VF episodes and correct spontaneous ECG changes, possibly via inhibiting *Ito channels*. Some drugs have been reported to induce the type-1 ECG and/or (fatal) arrhythmias in BrS patients. Patients with BrS can prevent arrhythmias by avoiding these drugs or using them only in controlled conditions. Those with risk factors for coronary artery disease may require an angiogram before ICD implantation.

### Long QT Syndrome

Patients with a prolonged QT interval are more prone to the risk of recurrent syncope and sudden death due to VT or VF. The idiopathic long QT syndrome ventricular fibrillation. The idiopathic long QT syndrome may be either autosomal recessive or autosomal dominant.

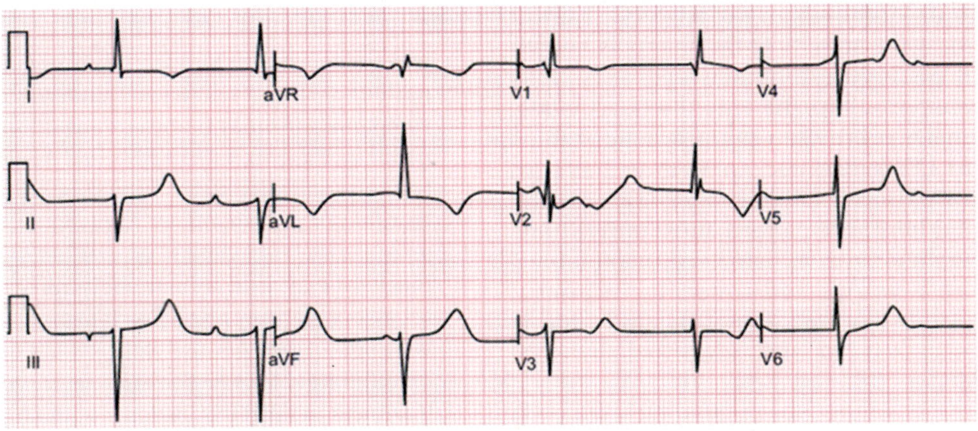


**Fig. 25.88:** Long QTc (620 ms) due to severe hypothermia

Prolongation of the QT interval may be:

- Acquired by patients having electrolyte imbalance,
- Taking antiarrhythmic drugs,
- Taking psychotropic drugs,
- Having myocarditis,
- Myocardial ischemia,
- Sinus node disease,
- Central nervous system disease,
- Consuming liquid protein diets.

It is associated with a specific type of ventricular arrhythmia, torsade de pointes, which is characterized by the cycles of alternating electrical polarity of the QRS complex peaks that oscillate or twist around the isoelectric line. The alternating cycles may be interrupted by periods of rapid tachycardia and polarity. The rhythm rate varies from 160 to 280 beats per minute and most often is between 200 and 250 beats per minute. Assessment and treatment of ventricular tachyarrhythmias present extraordinary challenges to the clinician. Moreover, the prognosis for patients is quite variable with these characteristically sudden-onset, unpredictable, and transitory arrhythmias. In some patients, ventricular ectopic activity may be benign and without sequelae, but in other patients, comparable ectopy is a harbinger of ventricular fibrillation and sudden cardiac death (Fig. 25.88).

### Short QT Syndrome

Short QT syndrome is a genetic disease of the electrical system of the heart. It consists of a constellation of signs and symptoms, consisting of a short QT interval on EKG (? 300 ms) that doesn't significantly change with heart rate, tall and peaked T-waves, and a structurally normal heart. Short QT syndrome appears to be inherited in an autosomal dominant pattern, and a few affected families have been identified (Fig. 25.89).

Short QT syndrome is inherited in an autosmal dominant patterns. Individuals with short QT syndrome frequently complain of palpitations and may have syncope (loss of consciousness) that is unexplained. Mutations in the KCNH2, KCNJ2 and KCNQ1 genes cause short QT syndrome. These genes provide instructions for making proteins that act as channels across the cell membrane. These channels transport positively charged atoms (ions) of potassium into and out of the cells. In cardiac muscle, these ion channels play critical roles in maintaining the

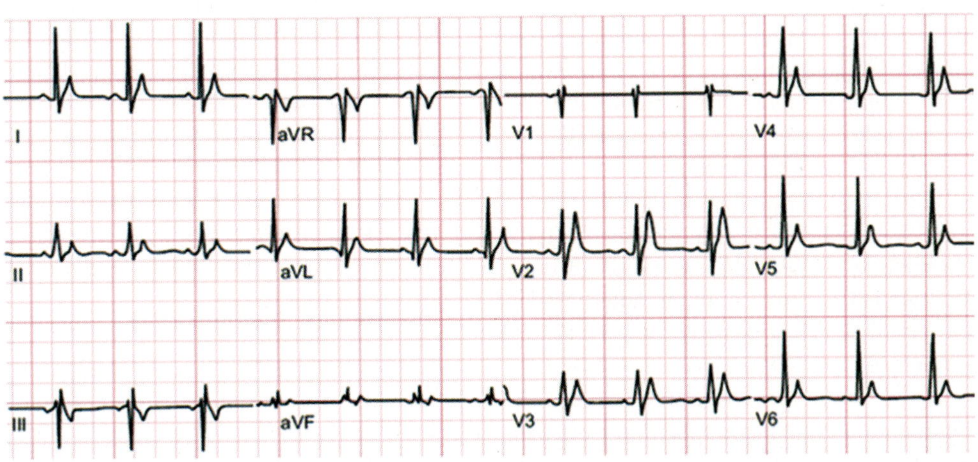


**Fig. 25.89:** Very short QTc (280 ms) with tall, peaked T-waves due to congenital short QT syndrome

heart's normal rhythm. Mutations in the KCNH2, KCNJ2 or KCNQ1 gene increase the activity of the channels, which changes the flow of potassium ions between cells. This disruption in ion transport alters the way the heart beats, leading to the abnormal heart rhythm characteristic of short QT syndrome. Short QT syndrome appears to have an autosomal dominant pattern of inheritance. Due to the autosomal dominant inheritance pattern, most individuals will have family members with a history of unexplained or sudden death at a young age (even in infancy), palpitations, or atrial fibrillation. Short QT syndrome is associated with an increased risk of sudden cardiac death, most likely due to VF.

*Diagnosis:* The diagnosis of short QT syndrome consists of characteristic history and findings on EKG and electrophysiologic testing. There are currently no set guidelines for the diagnosis of short QT syndrome.

*Electrocardiogram:* The characteristic findings of short QT syndrome on EKG are a short QT interval, typically 300 ms, that does not significantly change with the heart rate. Tall, peaked T-waves may also be noted. Individuals may also have an underlying atrial rhythm of atrial fibrillation.

## KEY POINTS

### CARDIAC EMERGENCIES IN CHILDREN

These include management of:

#### 1. Supraventricular Tachycardia

The following are key points to remember about the 2015 guideline for the management of adult patients with supraventricular tachycardia (SVT):

a. For the purposes of this document, the term 'supraventricular tachycardia' includes any arrhythmia originating above and including the bundle of His, and specifically excludes atrial fibrillation (AF).
b. Paroxysmal SVT is a regular, and typically narrow complex tachycardia that is characterized by sudden onset and termination. Its causes include atrioventricular nodal re-entrant tachycardia (AVNRT), orthodromic atrioventricular re-entrant tachycardia (AVRT) utilizing an accessory pathway and atrial tachycardia (AT). Patients with recurrent bouts of symptomatic paroxysmal SVT should be considered for electrophysiologic study and catheter ablation.
c. The most common tachycardia in patients with the Wolff-Parkinson-White (WPW) syndrome is orthodromic AVRT. AVRT can occur in patients without pre-excitation on the resting electrocardiogram (ECG). In these cases, anterograde conduction over the pathway is not possible or very slow, and the pathway is referred to as 'concealed' (as opposed to 'manifest').
d. Atrial fibrillation with extremely rapid conduction over the accessory pathway ('pre-excited AF') can lead to syncope

*Contd...*

*Contd...*

and sudden death. Sudden death is more likely to occur in patients with a history of tachycardia (i.e. with prior symptoms), but may be the first manifestation of the accessory pathway. Patients with pre-excited AF and who are otherwise hemodynamically stable should be treated with intravenous ibutilide or procainamide. Intravenous digoxin, intravenous amiodarone, intravenous or oral beta- and calcium-channel blockers may lead to extremely rapid conduction over the accessory pathway and hemodynamic compromise in patients with pre-excited AF, and thus, should be avoided. Oral beta- or calcium-blocker therapy is reasonable for ongoing treatment of AVRT in patients without pre-excitation on the resting ECG.
e. Patients with asymptomatic pre-excitation on a 12-lead ECG are said to have a 'WPW pattern.' Patients with intermittent pre-excitation on the resting ECG or abrupt loss of pre-excitation during exercise testing are considered to be at low risk for life-threatening arrhythmias. Other patients may be considered for electrophysiologic (EP) study for risk stratification. Catheter ablation of the accessory pathway should be performed if high-risk features are found on EP testing. It is also reasonable to observe patients with a WPW pattern without further evaluation. It is reasonable to consider catheter ablation in individuals who are unable to secure employment (e.g. pilots) because of a WPW pattern.
f. Catheter ablation of the cavo-tricuspid isthmus (CTI) should be considered in patients with symptomatic atrial flutter or those in whom the rate cannot be controlled with medical therapy. Patients undergoing catheter ablation of the CTI should be counseled that there is a reasonable chance that they may develop AF during follow-up. Oral anticoagulation for stroke prevention in patients with atrial flutter should be prescribed according to the patient's risk factors using the common risk stratification schemes for patients with AF.
g. The resting heart rate in patients with inappropriate sinus tachycardia (IST) is typically >100 bpm. A diagnosis of IST is made after excluding conditions associated with a heightened sympathetic tone. It is also important to evaluate the possibility of postural orthostatic tachycardia syndrome (POTS) in patients with IST, as the use of beta-blockers may exacerbate the symptoms in the former and may be helpful in the latter. Ivabradine, an inhibitor of the If channel, reduces sinus node automaticity and is useful in patients with IST.
h. Patients with adult congenital heart disease and atrial tachycardia/flutter should be treated with oral anticoagulation using the same risk stratification schemes as for AF.

#### 2. Ventricular Tachycardia

Ventricular tachycardia should be treated as an emergency unless the patient is haemodynamically stable.

In the acute situation, synchronized cardioversion at 0.5–1.0 J/kg should be the first response. Do not delay.

*Contd...*

*Contd...*

Intravenous lignocaine:
- Loading: 1 mg/kg. May repeat in 10–15 minutes for 2 doses
- Infusion: 20–50 μg/kg/min; Maintenance level: 1.5–5.0 mg/L
- Intravenous amiodarone is an alternative
- Slow bolus 5 mg/kg
- May repeat 5 mg/kg/dose up to a total of 15 mg/kg/day
- Watch for hypotension. Have $CaCl_2$ ready.

### 3. Hypercyanotic Spells ('Tet Spells')

Episodes of hyperpnoea (i.e. rapid and deep respiration), worsening cyanosis, and disappearance or attenuation of cardiac murmur in a child with tetralogy of Fallot.

It usually occurs in patients less than 2 years of age.

**Acute Management**
- A hypercyanotic attack is a medical emergency and requires prompt management to break the hypoxic cycle.
- Call for help early and inform the cardiologist in charge.
- Depending on the severity of attack, institute one or more of the following:
  - Try to calm the infant.
  - Have the parent hold the infant over the parent's shoulder or place the child in a knee-chest position.
  - Administration of oxygen (although this will not reverse cyanosis due to intracardiac shunting). Avoid if such attempts further aggravate the child.
  - Drugs (in order or preference, unless contraindicated)
    - IV sodium bicarbonate is necessary to correct metabolic acidosis. The dosage is 1–2 meq/kg as 1–2 ml/kg of 8.4% $NaHCO_3$ slow IV bolus. For infants less than 3 months of age, administer as 4.2% $NaHCO_3$ (dilute the 8.4% $NaHCO_3$ 1:1 with normal saline). Ensure the intravenous access is secure before administration as extravasation can lead to severe tissue injury.
    - b-adrenergic blockade with intravenous propranolol (0.15–0.25 mg/kg given slowly over 5–10 minutes; dose can be repeated once). In the acute attack, propranolol slows the heart rate and reduces the right ventricular outflow obstruction; it also has a sedative effect. IV esmolol (0.5 mg/kg over 1 minute and can be given as an infusion at 50 mcg/kg/min) is an alternative.
    - a-agonists: phenylephrine (0.1 mg/kg SC or IM, 0.01 mg/kg IV, or as an infusion 0.1–0.5 mcg/kg/min) or metaraminol (Aramine®) (0.01 mg/kg IV and repeated PRN, can be given as an infusion 0.1–1.0 mcg/kg/min), increases systemic vascular resistance (SVR) and reduces right to left shunting.
    - Ketamine (1–2 mg/kg IV or 5–10 mg/kg IM) is a drug, which simultaneously increases the SVR, sedates the patient. Both effects are known to terminate the spell.
    - Morphine (0.1 mg/kg IV or SC): Mechanism of action is via suppression of the respiratory centre and abolishing

*Contd...*

*Contd...*

hyperpnoea. However, its disadvantages include slow onset and respiratory depression. Be ready to intubate.
    - Ventilatory support if necessary.
    - General anaesthesia or emergency Blalock-Taussig shunt in intractable cases.
    - Maintenance therapy
    - Propranolol and sedation as required.
    - Propranolol acts by its peripheral actions of stabilizing the reactivity of the systemic arteries, thereby preventing a sudden decrease in the systemic vascular resistance. Oral dose is 0.2–0.5 mg/kg/dose 6–12 hourly, and can be slowly increased to maximum of 1 mg/kg/dose 6 hourly as needed.
    - Sedation may be with chloral hydrate or diazepam. However, avoid midazolam, which reduces systemic vascular resistance further.
- Treat fever aggressively and ensure adequate hydration.
- Avoid epinephrine, dopamine, dobutamine, digitalis and digoxin, which have positive inotropic effects and may therefore, worsen 'Tet spells'.
- Advice to parents
- Recognition of hypercyanotic spells. Parents should know that such spells can be serious and potentially life-threatening.
- Minimize triggers, which can agitate the child and calm the child down as soon as possible.
- Fever is a common trigger; so give antipyretics round the clock when the child has fever.
- Always keep the child well hydrated. See a doctor early if the child is not feeding well.
- If the child has a spell, attempt to calm the child and put in the knee chest position.
- If above measures are unable to terminate spell after 5 minutes, bring to the nearest emergency department urgently.

**Pediatric Resuscitation**
- Metronome use during chest compressions in children (October 2015).
- The 2010 American Heart Association and International Liaison Committee on Resuscitation Cardiopulmonary Resuscitation guidelines emphasize the importance of hard, fast chest compression at an optimal rate of 100 compressions per minute. Health care providers who use a metronome are more likely to achieve this rate. In a crossover trial of 155 medical personnel who performed compressions on a pediatric manikin with or without a metronome, the mean percentage of compressions delivered at an optimal rate was achieved more often when a metronome was used (72 versus 50%). The rescuers tended to perform compressions too fast when a metronome was not used).
- Timely administration of epinephrine improves survival following pediatric arrest (August 2015).
- Epinephrine is recommended during cardiopulmonary resuscitation for children with asystole or pulseless electrical

*Contd...*

*Contd...*

activity without ventricular fibrillation or tachycardia. In a retrospective review of registry data on 1558 children with inpatient arrest and a documented nonshockable initial rhythm, adjusted survival to discharge occurred in up to 37 % of patients who received epinephrine one minute or less after arrest and decreased 5 % for every additional minute delay in epinephrine administration. Survival with favorable neurologic outcome at discharge occurred in approximately 16% of all patients and in adjusted analysis also decreased 5 % for every additional minute of delay in epinephrine administration. Thus, timely administration of epinephrine is associated with improved outcomes after pediatric arrests with nonshockable cardiac rhythms.

- Oxyhemoglobin desaturation during rapid sequence intubation in children (June 2015).
- Timing the laryngoscopy duration during a pediatric endotracheal intubation attempt and discontinuing it, if intubation is unsuccessful within a specific time period (e.g. 30 seconds) may prevent oxyhemoglobin desaturation. In an observational study that used video review of 114 children undergoing rapid sequence intubation in a pediatric emergency department, at least one episode of oxyhemoglobin desaturation (pulse oximetry <90%) occurred in 33% of patients. Oxyhemoglobin desaturation was more common in children 2 years of age or younger compared with older children (59 versus 10%) and was strongly associated with the duration of laryngoscopy; 82% of patients experiencing desaturations had laryngoscopy durations of 30 seconds or longer. There was no association between the number of intubation attempts and episodes of desaturation (see Emergency endotracheal intubation in children, section on 'during laryngoscopy/intubation').
- Post-resuscitation therapeutic hypothermia not better than targeted normothermia in children (May 2015).
- Therapeutic hypothermia to maintain core body temperature below normal (typically 32–34°C) has been proposed after resuscitation from pediatric cardiac arrest based upon evidence for improved neurologic outcome in neonates and selected adults. In a multicenter trial involving children who were resuscitated from an out-of-hospital cardiac arrest, 260 patients (48 hours to 18 years of age) were randomized to either therapeutic hypothermia with a target core body temperature of 33°C or therapeutic normothermia to maintain a temperature of 36.8°C. One-year survival with good neurologic function was not significantly different in patients undergoing therapeutic hypothermia compared with therapeutic normothermia [20 versus 12%, respectively, relative likelihood 1.54, 95% confidence interval (CI) 0.86–2.76]. Of note, the number of patients randomized was insufficient to exclude an important benefit or harm from therapeutic hypothermia. Further study is needed to determine the role of therapeutic hypothermia after resuscitation from pediatric cardiac arrest; current practice is to provide targeted temperature management to prevent fever (core body temperature >38°C).

## BIBLIOGRAPHY


1. Alexi-Meskishvilla V, Berger F, Weng Y, Lange PE, Hetzer R. Anomalous origin of the left coronary artery from the pulmonary artery in adults. J Card Surg 1995;10:309–15.
2. Amabile N, Fraisse A, Bouvenot J, Chetaille P, Ovaert C. Outcome of acute fulminant myocarditis in children. Heart 2006;92:1269–73.
3. Atkins DL, Everson-Stewart S, Sears GK, Daya M, Osmond MH, Warden CR, et al. Epidemiology and outcomes from out-of-hospital cardiac arrest in children: the resuscitation outcomes consortium epistry cardiac arrest. Circulation 2009;119:1484–91.
4. Boneva RS, Botto, LD, Moore CA, Yang Q, Correa A, Erickson JD. Mortality associated with congenital heart defects in the United States: trends and racial disparities, 1979–1997. Circulation 2001;103:2376–81.
5. Caglar S, Leffler S. Prevalence of life-threatening arrhythmias in ED patients transported to the radiology suite while monitored by telemetry. Am J Emerg Med 2006;24:655–7.
6. Chang Y, Chao, H, Hsia S, Yan D. Myocarditis presenting as gastritis in children. Pediatr Emerg Care 2006;22:439–40.
7. Chau EM, Chow W, Chiu CS, Wang E. Treatment and outcome of biopsy-proven fulminant myocarditis in adults. Int J Cardiol 2006;110:405–6.
8. Codd MB, Sugrue DD, Gersh BJ, Melton LJ. Epidemiology of idiopathic dilated and hypertrophic cardiomyopathy: A population-based study in Olmsted County, Minnesota, 1975–1984. Circulation 1989;80:564–72.
9. Colletti JE, Homme JL, Woodridge DP. Unsuspected neonatal killers in emergency medicine. Emerg Med Clin North Am 2004;22:929–60.
10. Cooper LT. Myocarditis. N Engl J Med 2009;360:1526–38.
11. Decker JA, Rossano JW, O'Brian Smith E, Cannon B, Clunie SK, Gates C, et al. Risk factors and mode of death in isolated hypertrophic cardiomyopathy in children. J Am Coll Cardiol 2009;54:250–4.
12. Doniger SJ, Sharieff GQ. Pediatric dysrrhythmias. Pediatr Clin North Am 2006;53:85–105.
13. Drory Y, Turetz Y, Hiss Y, Lev B, Fisman EZ, Pines A, Kramer MR. Sudden unexpected death in persons <40 years of age. Am J Cardiol 1991;68:1388–92.
14. Freedman SB, Haladyn JK, Floh A, Kirsh JA, Taylor G. Thull-Freedman J. Pediatric myocarditis: emergency department clinical findings and diagnostic evaluation. Pediatrics 2007; 120:1278–85.
15. Gupta S, Markman DW, Drazner MH, Mammen P. Fulminant myocarditis. Nat Clin Pract Cardiovasc Med 2008; 5:693–706.
16. Hoffmam TM, Wernovsky G, Wieand TS, Cohen MI, Jennings AC, Vetter VL, et al. The incidence of arrhythmias in a pediatric cardiac intensive care unit. Ped Cardiol 2002;23: 598-604.
17. Hufnagel G, Pankuweit S, Richter A, Schonian U, Maisch B. The European Study of Epidemiology and Treatment of Cardiac Inflammatory Diseases (ESETCID): First Epidemiological Results. Herz 2000;25:279–85.
18. Johnsrude CL, Perry JC, Cecchin F, Smith EO, Fraley K, Friedman RA, et al. Differentiating anomalous left main coronary artery from the pulmonary artery in infants from

myocarditis and dilated cardiomyopathy by electrogram. Am J Cardiol 1995;75:71–4.

19. Kantor PF, Mertens LL. Clinical practice: Heart failure in children. Part I: clinical evaluation, diagnostics testing, and initial medical management. Eur J Pediatr 2010;169:269–79.
20. Kapser EK, Agema W, Hutchins GM, Deckers JW, Hare JM, Baughman KL. The causes of dilated cardiomyopathy: a clinicopathologic review of 673 consecutive patients. J Am Coll Cardiol 1994;23:586–90.
21. Litherthson RR. Sudden death from cardiac causes in children and young adults. N Engl J Med 1996;334:1039–44.
22. Mahrholdt H, Wagner A, Deluigi CC, Kispert E, Hager S, Meinhardt G, et al. Presentation, patterns of myocardial damage, and clinical course of viral myocarditis. Circulation 2006;114:1581–90.
23. Manole MD, Saladino RA. Emergency department manage-ment of the pediatric patient with supraventricular tachy-cardia. Pediatr Emerg Care 2007;23:176–85.
24. Maron BJ, Fananapazir L. Sudden cardiac death in hyper-trophic cardiomyopathy. Circulation 1992;85:I-57–I-63.
25. Maron BJ, McKenna WJ, Danielson GK, Kappenberger LJ, Kuhn HJ, Seidman CE, et al. American College of Cardio-logy/European Society of Cardiology Expert Consensus Document on Hypertrophic Cardiomyopathy: A Report of the American College of Cardiology Foundation Task Force on Clinical Expert Consensus Documents and the European Society of Cardiology Committee for Practice Guidelines. J Am Coll Cardiol 2003;42:1687–713.
26. Massin MM, Malekzadeh-Milani SG, Van Aerschot I, Dessy H. Management of cardiac emergencies in children. Minerva Pediatr 2009;61:163–73.
27. McCarthy RE, Boehmer JP, Hruban RH, Hutchins GM, Kasper EK, Hare JM, et al. Long-term outcome of fulminant myocarditis as compared with acute (Nonfulminant) myocarditis. N Engl J Med 2000;342:690–5.
28. Monserrat L, Elliott PM, Gimeno JR, Sharma S, Penas-Lado M, McKenna WJ. Non-sustained ventricular tachycardia in hypertrophic cardiomyopathy: an in dependent marker of sudden death in young patients. J Am Coll Cardiol 2003; 42:873–9.
29. Moodie DS, Fyfe D, Gill CC, Cook SA, Lytle BW, Taylor PA, et al. Anomalous origin of the left coronary artery from the pulmonary artery (Bland-White-Garland syndrome) in adult patients: long term follow up after surgery. Am Heart J 1983;106:381–8.
30. Nadkarni VM, Larkin GL, Peberdy MA, Carey SM, Kaye W, Mancini ME, et al. First documented rhythm and clinical outcome from in-hospital cardiac arrest among children and adults. JAMA 2006;295:50–7.
31. Park MK. Pediatric cardiology for practitioners. 5th ed. Missouri: Mosby; 2008;62–4, pp.314–5.
32. Samson RA, Atkins DL. Tachyarrhythmias and defibrillation. Pediatr Clin North Am 2008;55:887–907.
33. Schamberger MS. Cardiac emergencies in children. Pediatr Ann 1996;25:339–44.
34. Selzman CH, Zimmerman MA, Campbell DN. ALCAPA in an adult with preserved left ventricular function. J Card Surg 2003;18:25–8.
35. Towbin JA, Bowles NE. The failing heart. Nature 2002;415: 227–33.
36. Towbin JA, Lowe AM, Colan SD, Sleeper, LA, Orav EJ, Clunie S, et al. Incidence, causes, and outcomes of dilated cardiomyopathy in children. JAMA 2006;296:1867–76.
37. Towbin JA, Lowe AM, Colan SD. Incidence, causes, and out-comes of dilated cardiomyopathy in children. JAMA 2006; 296:1867–76.

# 26 Extracorporeal Membrane Oxygenation Support in Critically Ill Patients

## EXTRACORPOREAL MEMBRANE OXYGENATION

The term extracorporeal membrane oxygenation (ECMO) was initially used to describe long-term extracorporeal support that focused on the function of oxygenation. Subsequently, in some patients, the emphasis shifted to carbon dioxide removal, and the term extracorporeal carbon dioxide removal was coined. Extracorporeal support was later used for postoperative support in patients following cardiac surgery. Other variations of its capabilities have been tested and used over the last few years, making it an important tool in the armamentarium of life and organ support measures for clinicians. With all of these uses for extracorporeal circuitry, a new term, extracorporeal life support (ECLS), has come into vogue to describe this technology.

In emergency medicine, extracorporeal membrane oxygenation (ECMO) is an extracorporeal technique of providing both cardiac and respiratory support oxygen to patients whose heart and lungs are so severely diseased or damaged that they can no longer serve their function. Initial cannulation of a patient receiving ECMO is performed by a surgeon and maintenance of the patient is the responsibility of the ECMO specialist and gives 24/7 monitoring care for the duration of the ECMO treatment (Fig. 26.1).

*The differences between extracorporeal membrane oxygenation and cardiopulmonary bypass are as follows:*

- ECMO is frequently instituted using only cervical cannulation, which can be performed under local anesthesia; standard cardiopulmonary bypass is usually instituted by transthoracic cannulation under general anesthesia
- Unlike standard cardiopulmonary bypass, which is used for short-term support measured in hours, ECMO is used for longer-term support ranging from 3–10 days
- The purpose of ECMO is to allow time for intrinsic recovery of the lungs and heart; a standard cardiopulmonary bypass provides support during various types of cardiac surgical procedures.

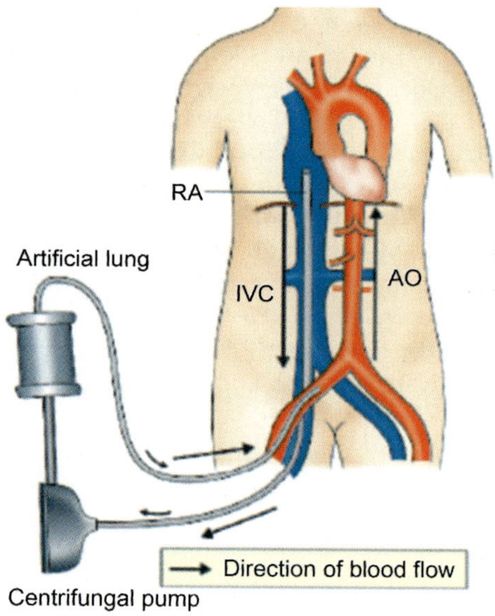


**Fig. 26.1:** ECMO system. RA=right atrium; IVC=inferior venacava; AO=aorta

## TYPES OF EXTRACORPOREAL MEMBRANE OXYGENATION

1. Single site veno-venous (VV) ECMO for respiratory failure (Fig. 26.2).
2. Two-site veno-venous extracorporeal membrane oxygenation (Fig. 26.3).
3. Veno-arterial (VA) ECMO for cardiac or respiratory failure (Fig. 26.4).
4. Extracorporeal membrane oxygenation in the ambulatory patient (Fig. 26.5).

There are several forms of ECMO, the two most common of which are veno-arterial (VA) and veno-venous (VV). In both modalities, blood drained from the venous system is oxygenated outside of the body. In VA ECMO, this blood is returned to the arterial system and in VV ECMO the blood is returned to the venous system. In VV ECMO, no cardiac support is provided.

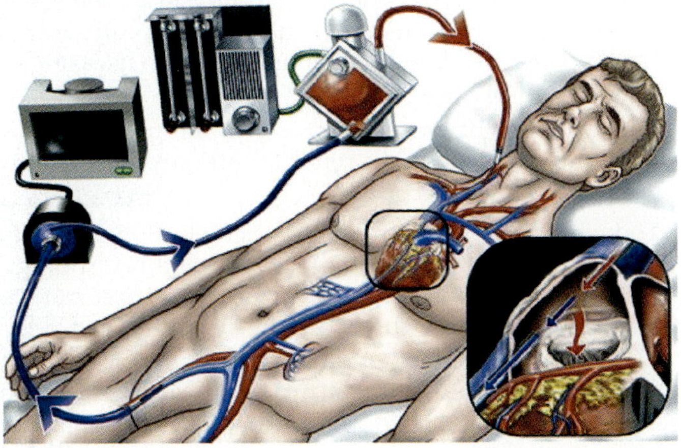

**Fig. 26.2:** Two-site venovenous extracorporeal membrane oxygenation venous blood is withdrawn from a central vein, pumped through an oxygenator, and reinfused into a central vein. (**Inset**) Drainage and reinfusion ports in close proximity may lead to oxygenated blood being drawn back into the circuit without having entered the systemic circulation, known as recirculation (**purple arrow**)

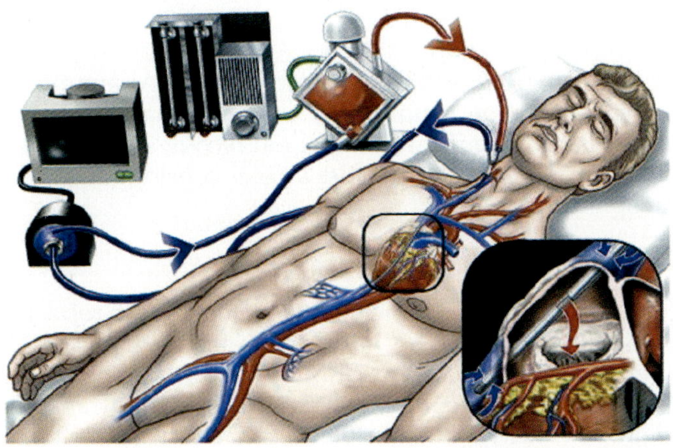

**Fig. 26.3:** Single-site venovenous extracorporeal membrane oxygenation. A dual-lumen cannula in the internal jugular vein permits both venous drainage and reinfusion without the need for femoral cannulation. (**Inset**) Deoxygenated blood is withdrawn through ports in the superior and inferior vena cavae. The reinfusion port is oriented such that oxygenated blood is directed toward the tricuspid valve

## Veno-arterial

In veno-arterial (VA) ECMO, a venous cannula is usually placed in the right common femoral vein for extraction and an arterial cannula is usually placed into the right femoral artery for infusion. The tip of the femoral venous cannula should be maintained near the junction of the inferior vena cava and right atrium, while the tip of the femoral arterial cannula is maintained in the iliac artery. In adults accessing the femoral artery is preferred because the insertion is simpler.

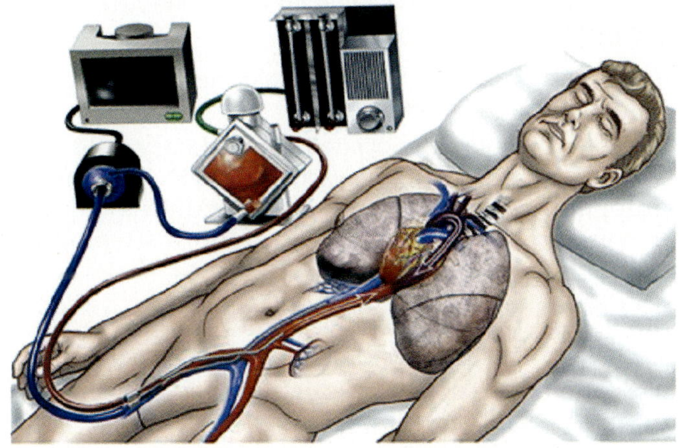

**Fig. 26.4:** Femoral veno-arterial ECMO—when extracorporeal membrane oxygenation (ECMO) is implemented via femoral venous drainage and femoral arterial return in patients with residual native cardiac function and impaired lung function, reinfused oxygenated blood (**red arrow**), flowing retrograde through the aorta, may meet resistance from poorly oxygenated blood flowing antegrade from the left ventricle (purple arrow). Depending on the amount of cardiac function, the location of the interface between antegrade and retrograde flow will vary, and the reinfused oxygenated blood may not reach the cerebral and coronary vascular beds

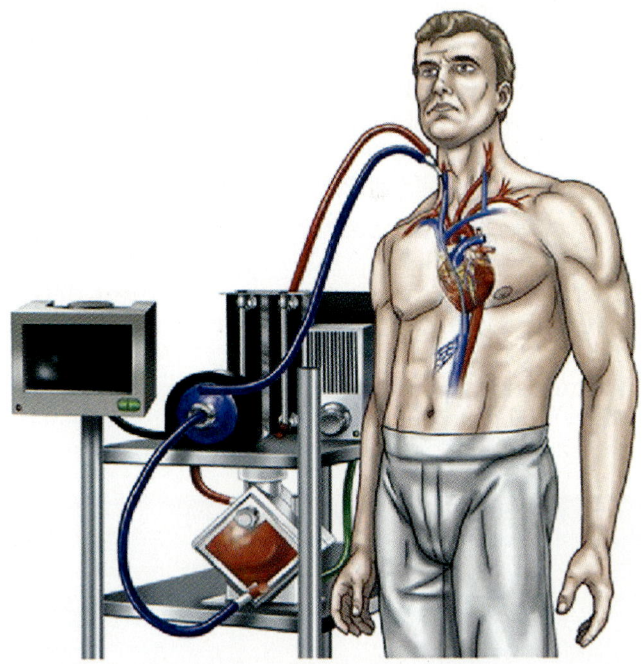

**Fig. 26.5:** ECMO in the ambulatory patient upper-body configurations and compact circuits facilitate mobilization in patients with respiratory failure requiring extracorporeal membrane oxygenation (ECMO)

## Veno-venous

In veno-venous (VV) ECMO, venous cannulae are usually placed in the right common femoral vein for drainage and right internal jugular vein for infusion.

## INDICATIONS FOR EXTRACORPOREAL MEMBRANE OXYGENATION

Patients with the following two major neonatal diagnoses require the use of ECMO:

- Primary diagnoses associated with primary pulmonary hypertension of the newborn (PPHN), including idiopathic PPHN, meconium aspiration syndrome, respiratory distress syndrome, group B streptococcal sepsis, and asphyxia (Fig. 26.6).
- Congenital diaphragmatic hernia (CDH)

*Selection criteria for neonates include the following:*

- Gestational age of 34 weeks or more
- Birth weight of 2000 g or higher
- No significant coagulopathy or uncontrolled bleeding
- No major intracranial hemorrhage (grade 1 intracranial hemorrhage)
- Mechanical ventilation for 10–14 days or less
- Reversible lung injury
- No lethal malformations
- No major untreatable cardiac malformation
- Failure of maximal medical therapy

Failure to meet these criteria is a relative contraindication for ECMO.

Qualifying patient criteria for ECMO are applied only when the infant has reached maximal ventilatory support of 100% oxygen (fraction of inspired oxygen [$FiO_2$] equals 1) with peak inspiratory pressures (PIP) often as high as 35 cm water. They include the alveolar-arterial gradient, the oxygenation index and acute deterioration.

*Pediatric ECMO is indicated or considered in the following situations:*

- Low cardiac output resulting from right, left and biventricular failure following repair of congenital heart defect
- Pulmonary vasoreactive crisis following repair of congenital heart defect leading to severe hypoxemia, low cardiac output, or both

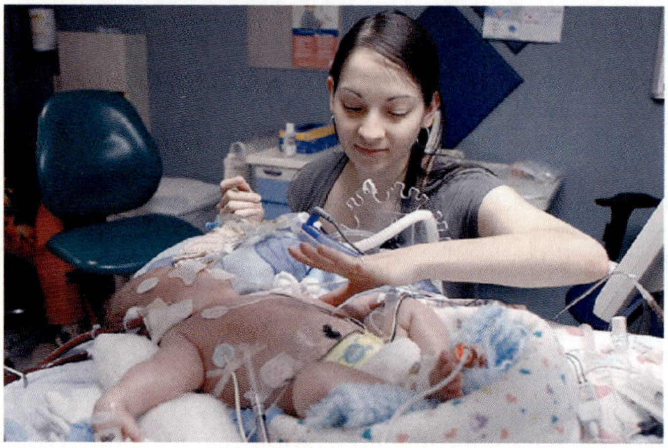

**Fig. 26.6:** A newborn baby with cardiorespiratory failure is being treated with ECMO in neonatal ICU

- Rarely, as a bridge to cardiac surgery in patients with serious end-organ damage resulting from profound low cardiac output related to congenital heart disease
- As a bridge to cardiac transplant
- Possibly, as a bridge to recovery in temporary cardiomyopathy secondary to renal failure, myocarditis and burns.

Today, other indications or less strict selection of patients in certain institutions have made the use of this technology more diverse, not only in acute cardiac problems, but also in primary pulmonary diseases.

The clinical outcomes of patients undergoing ECMO can be categorized according to the indication for the ECMO; severe acute respiratory failure or cardiac failure.

### Acute Respiratory Failure

With acute respiratory failure use of ECMO has been shown to improve survival rates. Survival rates from 50–70% have been reported in observational and uncontrolled clinical trials. The survival rates reported are better than historical survival rates.

### Cardiac Failure

Veno-arterial ECMO can provide acute support in cardiogenic shock or cardiac arrest in adults. Assuming that the brain function is normal or only minimally impaired, ECMO is provided until the patient recovers or receives a long-term ventricular assist device as a bridge to cardiac transplantation.

## INDICATIONS OF ECMO IN ADULTS

Veno-arterial-ECMO is indicated in patients with refractory cardiogenic shock who have an underlying potentially reversible heart condition, although it can also be used as a bridge to a ventricular assist device or cardiac transplantation. VA-ECMO can also be used as a salvage technique during cardiac arrest, and the current data support its use after 10 minutes of adequate but unsuccessful advanced life support (ALS) (Fig. 26.7).

In-hospital survival rate of patients with VA-ECMO varies from 30–50% according to the cause of the cardiac dysfunction. VA-ECMO can be considered in patients with systolic arterial pressure lower than 85 mmHg, cardiac index lower than 1.2 litre $min^{-1}$ $m^{-2}$, despite adequate preload, more than two inotropes in use, intra-aortic balloon counterpulsation and systemic signs of low cardiac output. The paucity of data in the literature makes it difficult to determine which patients will benefit from VA-ECMO and when ECMO support will be futile. Thus, it is strongly recommended to discuss all possible cases with the nearest ECMO centre in these circumstances.

The aim of VV-ECMO in adult patients is to provide oxygenation and rest the lungs, decreasing the insult caused by mechanical ventilation. Hence, VV-ECMO should be considered as an alternative to conventional therapy for

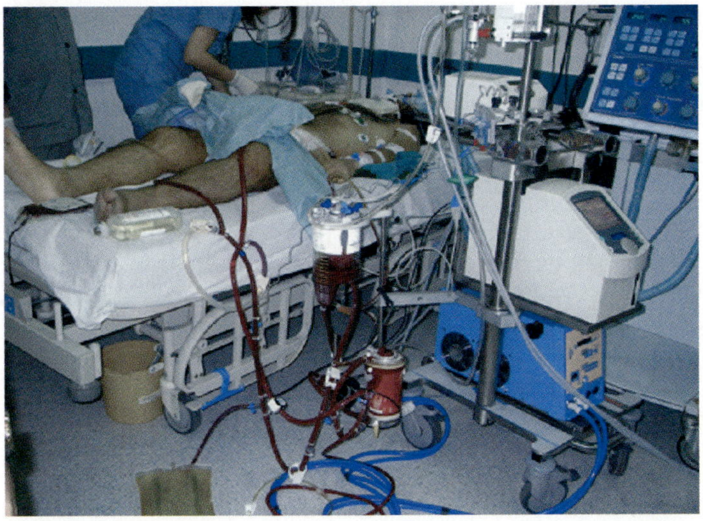

**Fig. 26.7:** An adult patient with refractory cardiogenic shock is being treated with ECMO system in ICU

adults with acute respiratory distress syndrome (ARDS) and patients with graft dysfunction after lung transplantation. VV-ECMO has a lower risk of thromboembolic complications and lung perfusion allows endocrine pulmonary function in comparison with VA-ECMO. It is sometimes necessary to use VA-ECMO, if significant haemodynamic compromise becomes apparent or if oxygenation that is provided is not sufficient; this may require changes of the cannulae position.

Extracorporeal membrane oxygenation is associated with significant inherent risks, and benefit compared with conventional therapies is still unclear. ECMO gained popularity during the H1N1/2009 pandemic, when clinicians were confronted with severe, refractory, and rapidly progressive hypoxaemia in young and fit patients. It made clinical sense to use the new generation of safer ECMO circuits in this situation. This was substantiated by the release of the Cesar trial results and no doubt catalysed by the media, influencing political choices. The Cesar trial is the third randomized controlled trial evaluating the benefits of ECMO in ARDS. The endpoint of the trial was to compare the survival at 6 months in the absence of severe disability, in patients who had developed ARDS and been randomized to be treated either in their original centre or in the treatment centre. The trial demonstrated that patients transferred to a centre with ECMO available had a better outcome than those treated at the original hospital with conventional therapy, and that this approach was cost-effective.

Whether ECMO can really replace conventional treatment of adult ARDS is still unknown. Studies to determine the group that may benefit most are still lacking but patients mechanically ventilated for longer than 7 days or in multiorgan failure are considered poor candidates as underlying lung damage might then be irreversible, and ECMO is generally not offered. ECMO therapy in ARDS allows a decrease in the stress imposed on the lung by ventilation at high airway pressure that may eventually damage the lung, and should be offered to patients with refractory hypoxaemia or hypercapnia despite optimal ventilation.

The best survival rates are observed in patients with non-necrotizing viral pneumonia and associated respiratory failure, probably because (i) these are often younger patients, (ii) they have fewer comorbidities, and (iii) the associated lung injury is often reversible.

Arteriovenous-ECMO is particularly useful in patients with severe hypercapnia, respiratory acidosis and moderate hypoxaemia. The absence of a pump makes this device simpler to use, but it means that cardiac function must be preserved for the blood to be effectively pumped. However, mortality has been reported to be high in patients with ARDS, who had AV-ECMO, and some patients may require conversion from AV-ECMO to VV- or even VA-ECMO. It does allow however easier transportation than other ECMO modes as no source of energy is required and it is smaller in size and weight.

## TECHNIQUES EMPLOYED IN ECMO

ECMO currently comes in two varieties—venoarterial (VA), and venovenous (VV) (Figs 26.8–26.10). VA-ECMO takes deoxygenated blood from a central vein or the right atrium, pumps it past the oxygenator, and then returns the oxygenated blood, under pressure, to the arterial side of the circulation (typically to the aorta). This form of ECMO partially supports the cardiac output as the flow through the ECMO circuit is in addition to the normal cardiac output. VV-ECMO takes blood from a large vein and returns oxygenated blood back to a large vein. VV-ECMO does not support the circulation. VA-ECMO helps support the cardiac output and delivers higher levels of oxygenation support than does VV-ECMO. VA-ECMO carries a higher risk of systemic emboli than does VV. VV-ECMO systems may actually recirculate previously oxygenated blood depending on the placement of the inflow and outflow catheters. Another variant of VV-ECMO is extracorporeal $CO_2$ removal (ECCO2R). With this mode of support, oxygenation is provided by slow ventilation of the native

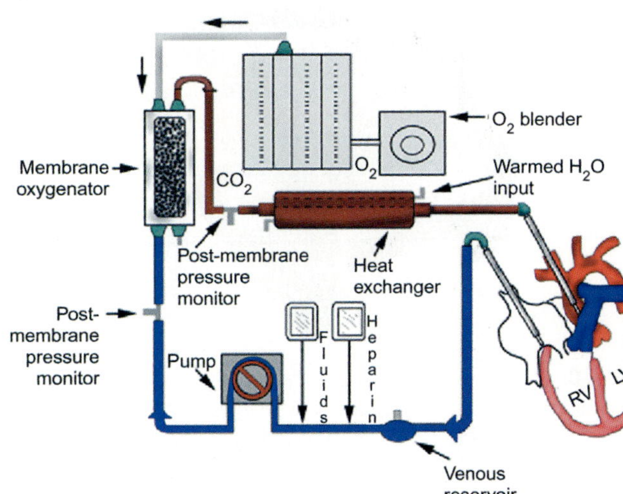


**Fig. 26.8:** Extracorporeal membrane oxygenation (ECMO) system

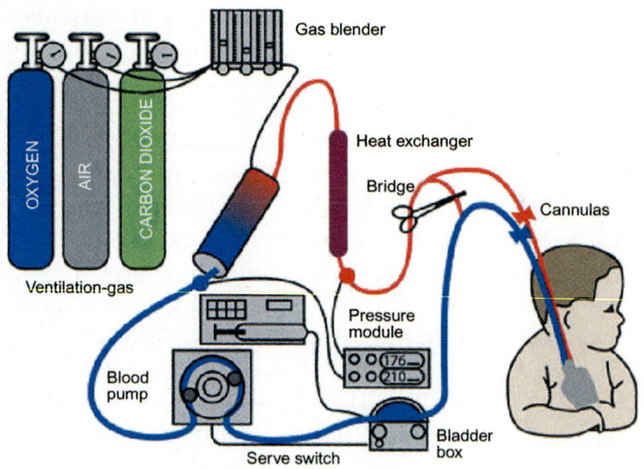


**Fig. 26.9:** Application of ECMO in neonatal cardiorespiratory failure

lungs while $CO_2$ removal is accomplished by the ECMO circuit. In all forms of ECMO, $CO_2$ removal is more efficient than $O_2$ addition because of the solubility and diffusion properties of $CO_2$ relative to $O_2$. In fact, $CO_2$ normally has to be added to ECMO circuits to offset this efficiency at $CO_2$ removal. The flow through the ECMO circuit is typically on the order of 100 ml/kg/minute. This would be from 25–75% of the cardiac output. This high flow requires the placement of large catheters into the circulation. For adults, the intravascular catheters may be 20 Fr or larger while 14 Fr catheters might be used in infants. These are generally placed by cut-down. Current circuits require the use of systemic anticoagulation with heparin to keep the systems patent. This anticoagulation is, in large part, responsible for bleeding complications that can be seen with the use of ECMO. Bleeding may occur either at the site of catheter insertion or at remote sites, such as intracranial or the gastrointestinal tract. Future catheters with inpregnated heparin may obviate the need for systemic anticoagulation and would be expected to reduce bleeding complications. Once blood leaves the patient, it comes in contact with a gas-permeable membrane that allows gas exchange to occur between the blood and the gasses (oxygen and carbon dioxide) that are run into the oxygenator. Carbon dioxide levels leaving the oxygenator can be adjusted about as low as the physician wants while oxygen levels typically reach the 400–500 mmHg level. Note that $CO_2$ content varies fairly directly with partial pressure while $O_2$ content follows the shape of the oxyhemoglobin dissociation curve. Under normobaric conditions, this limits the amount of oxygen that can be loaded into blood. If you were to try to predict the final mixed arterial oxygen content or partial pressure during VA-ECMO, you would need to know the pulmonary venous oxygen content, the ECMO effluent oxygen content, and the percentage of cardiac output flowing through the ECMO circuit:

$$CaO_2 = (EO \times EF + NO \times NF)/(EF + NF)$$

where EO = ECMO oxygen content

EF = ECMO flow

NO = non-ECMO oxygen content

NF = non-ECMO flow

Predicting final arterial content during VV-ECMO is more complex and cannot be easily calculated. During VV ECMO, the lungs may actually excrete oxygen rather than remove it from the inspired gas. Once ECMO has been

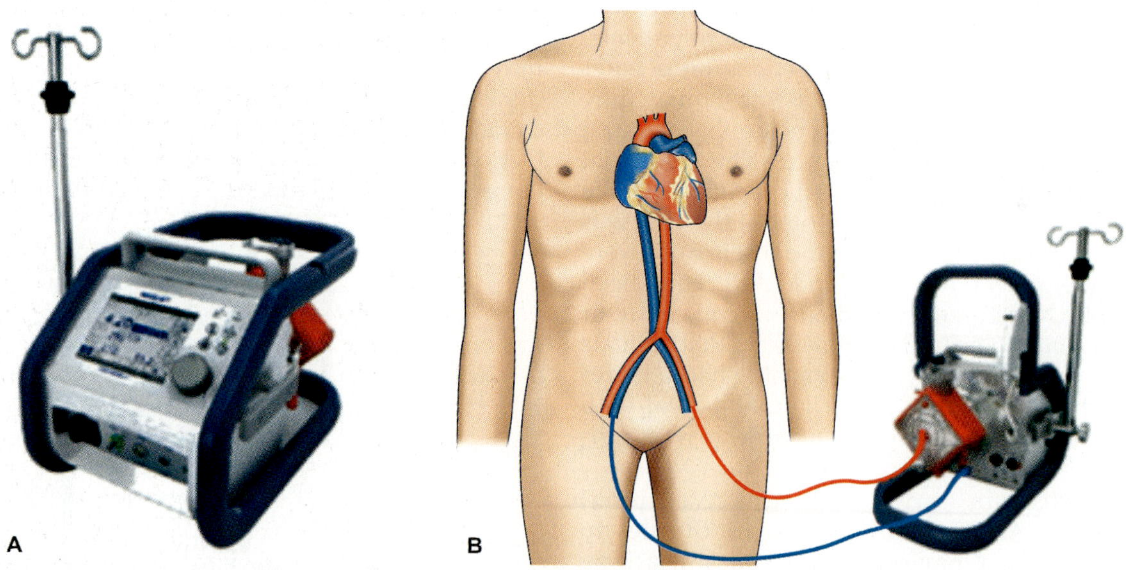


**Fig. 26.10:** The device is compact and easily portable, with a total weight of only 9 kg. Veno-arterial extracorporeal membrane oxygenation (ECMO) is established by cannulation of a femoral vein and artery using the Seldinger technique. To expedite interhospital transfer these vessels can be located with guidewires before arrival of the outreach team. The cannulas can then be inserted rapidly to begin ECMO before transport by air or ground ambulance. Images of the cardio help device courtesy of ©Maquet cardiopulmonary AG

started, the ventilator is typically reduced to minimal settings to prevent atelectasis and barotrauma. The $FiO_2$ is lowered as much as possible, perhaps to room air. The ECMO flow rate is adjusted to the minimum needed to provide for adequate gas exchange and/or circulation support in the case of VA-ECMO. ECMO is typically used for 7–12 days and is weaned when there is evidence of pulmonary improvement as indicated by compliance or radiologic appearance. ECMO can also be stopped if there are major complications or if the patient's condition is determined to be hopeless.

## TYPES OF PATIENT SELECTED FOR APPLICATION OF ECMO

As mentioned previously, usual ECMO criteria include patients with a severe reversible process that would result in a very high predicted mortality with conventional ventilatory support. The best candidates are those without multi-system organ failure that are otherwise considered to be salvageable. It would be expected, that once ECMO becomes safer and more accepted by physicians, that these criteria would be revised to eliminate the requirement for a very high predicted pretreatment mortality. There are several ways to evaluate patients to determine if they are 'sick enough' for ECMO. APACHE and other scoring systems could be used to predict mortality. More frequently, indexes to assess refractory hypoxemia are used. The a:A ratio or A-a gradient can be used, but the oxygenation index (OI) is currently in more common use—OI = ($FiO_2$) (MAP, mean arterial pressure)/$PaO_2$ An OI greater than 0.40–0.55 is thought to predict an 80% predicted mortality. Unfortunately, mortality predictors have been notoriously pessimistic since they are derived by looking at retrospective data and tend to do a poor job of predicting prospective results.

## CONTRAINDICATIONS

Most contraindications are relative, balancing the risks of the procedure (including the risk of using valuable resources which could be used for others) versus the potential benefits. The relative contraindications are:

1. Conditions incompatible with normal life if the patient recovers
2. Pre-existing conditions which affect the quality of life (CNS status, end stage malignancy, risk of systemic bleeding with anticoagulation)
3. Age and size of patient
4. Futility: Patients who are too sick, have been on conventional therapy too long, or have a fatal diagnosis.

## MAINTENANCE

Once the initial respiratory and hemodynamic goals have been achieved, the blood flow is maintained at that rate. Frequent assessment and adjustments are facilitated by continuous venous oximetry, which directly measures the oxyhemoglobin saturation of the blood in the venous limb of the ECMO circuit.

### Special Considerations

VV-ECMO is typically used for respiratory failure, while VA-ECMO is used for cardiac failure. There are unique considerations for each type of ECMO, which influence management.

#### *Blood Flow*

Near maximum flow rates are usually desired during VV-ECMO to optimize oxygen delivery. In contrast, the flow rate used during VA-ECMO must be high enough to provide adequate perfusion pressure and venous oxyhemoglobin saturation (measured on drainage blood), but low enough to provide sufficient preload to maintain left ventricular output.

#### *Diuresis*

Since most patients are fluid overloaded when ECMO is initiated, aggressive diuresis is warranted once the patient is stable on ECMO. Ultrafiltration can be easily added to the ECMO circuit, if patients are unable to produce sufficient urine for diuresis.

#### *Left Ventricular Monitoring*

Left ventricular output is rigorously monitored during VA ECMO because left ventricular output can become worse.

#### *Weaning and Discontinuing*

For patients with respiratory failure, improvements in radiographic appearance, pulmonary compliance, and arterial oxyhemoglobin saturation indicate that the patient may be ready to be taken off of ECMO support. For patients with cardiac failure, enhanced aortic pulsatility correlates with improved left ventricular output and indicates that the patient may be ready to be taken off of ECMO support. Once the decision has been made to discontinue ECMO, the cannulae are removed.

## COMPLICATIONS

ECMO complications are those associated with cannulation (pneumothorax, vascular disruptions, bleeding, infection and emboli), those associated with systemic anticoagulation (GI bleeding, intracranial bleeding, etc.), and exsanguination resulting from circuit disruptions. These potential complications require that a trained ECMO technician be present at the bedside 24 hours per day in addition to the patient's usual nursing presence. As many as 30% of ECMO treated infants reported to the Extracorporeal Life Support Organization (ELSO) registry suffer some degree of CNS injury (Fig. 26.11).

A common consequence in ECMO-treated adults is neurological injury, which may include subarachnoid hemorrhage, ischemic watershed infarctions, hypoxic-ischemic encephalopathy, unexplained coma and brain death. Fatal sepsis may occur when the large catheters inserted in the neck provide fertile field for infection Additional risks include bleeding. In adults, ECMO survival rates are around 60%. ECMO has yet to have

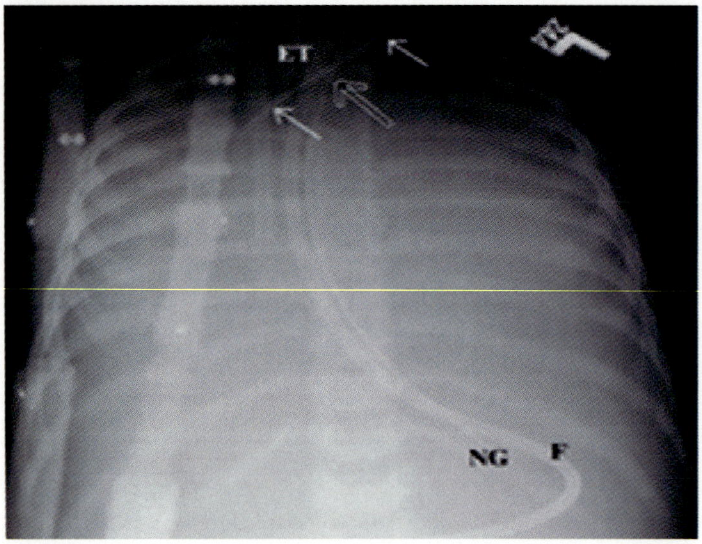


**Fig. 26.11:** Portable chest radiograph of a patient undergoing extracorporeal membrane oxygenation shows pulmonary edema in the lungs and the tubing going to the patient's right carotid artery and right jugular vein. Also seen are an endotracheal tube (ET), a right internal jugular vein catheter (black arrow), a left internal jugular vein catheter (white arrows), a nasogastric tube (NG) and a feeding tube (F)

proven survival benefit in adults with ARDS. In VA-ECMO, patients whose cardiac function does not recover sufficiently to be weaned from ECMO may be bridged to a ventricular assist device (VAD) or transplant.

In infants aged less than 34 weeks of gestation several physiologic systems are not well-developed, especially the cerebral vasculature and germinal matrix, resulting in high sensitivity to slight changes in pH, $PaO_2$ and intracranial pressure. Preterm infants are at unacceptably high risk for intraventricular hemorrhage (IVH) if administered ECMO at a gestational age less than 32 weeks. Also later, given the risk of IVH, it has become standard practice to ultrasound the brain prior to administering ECMO.

### *Bleeding*

Bleeding occurs in 30–40% of patients who receive ECMO and can be life-threatening. It is due to both the necessary continuous heparin infusion and platelet dysfunction. Meticulous surgical technique, maintaining platelet counts greater than 100,000/$mm^3$, and maintaining the target ACT reduce the likelihood of bleeding.

### *Thromboembolism*

Systemic thromboembolism due to thrombus formation within the extracorporeal circuit is an infrequent complication that can be devastating. Its impact is greater with VA-ECMO than VV-ECMO because infusion is into- the systemic circulation. Heparin infusion that achieves its target ACT and vigilant observation of the circuit for signs of clot formation successfully prevents thromboembolism in most patients.

### *Cannulation-related*

A variety of complications can occur during cannulation, including vessel perforation with hemorrhage, arterial dissection, distal ischemia and incorrect location (e.g. venous cannula within the artery). These complications are rare (<5 %). A skilled and experienced surgeon is important to avoid or address such complications.

### *Heparin-induced Thrombocytopenia*

Heparin-induced thrombocytopenia (HIT) is increasingly common among patients receiving ECMO. When HIT is suspected, the heparin infusion is usually replaced by a non-heparin anticoagulant.

## Veno-arterial Specific Complications

### *Pulmonary Hemorrhage*

Pulmonary hemorrhage can occur in patients who receive VA-ECMO.

### *Cardiac Thrombosis*

There is retrograde blood flow in the ascending aorta whenever the femoral artery and vein are used for VA-ECMO. Stasis of the blood can occur if left ventricular output is not maintained, which may result in thrombosis.

### *Coronary or Cerebral Hypoxia*

During VA-ECMO, fully saturated blood infused into the femoral artery from the ECMO circuit will preferentially perfuse the lower extremities and the abdominal viscera. Blood ejected from the heart will selectively perfuse the heart, brain and upper extremities.

### *Future*

Applications for ECMO may expand in the future to include percutaneous temporary left ventricular assistance and low flow ECMO for $CO_2$ removal (ECOOR). In addition, new technologies will improve the simplicity and safety of ECMO, including new oxygenators, pumps, and surface coatings.

### *Other Uses*

ECMO use on cadavers can increase the viability rate of transplanted organs.

## BIBLIOGRAPHY

1. Abrams D, Brodie D, Combes A. What is new in extracorporeal membrane oxygenation for ARDS in adults? Intensive Care Med 2013;39:2028–30.
2. Abrams DC, Prager K, Blinderman C, Burkart K, Brodie D. Ethical dilemmas encountered with the use of ECMO in adults. Chest 2014;145:876–82.
3. Abrams DC, Prager K, Blinderman CD, Burkart KM, Brodie D. The appropriate use of increasingly sophisticated life-sustaining technology. Virtual Mentor 2013;15:1050–55.
4. Alan H Jobe. Post-conceptional age and IVH in ECMO patients. Radiology 2004;145(2):A2.

5. Ann Arbor, MI: Extracorporeal Life Support Organization; 2013.
6. Barth E, Durand M, Heylbroeck C, et al. Extracorporeal life support as a bridge to high-urgency heart transplantation. Clin Transplant 2012;26:484–8.
7. Bermudez CA, Rocha RV, Toyoda Y, et al. Extracorporeal membrane oxygenation for advanced refractory shock in acute and chronic cardiomyopathy. Ann Thorac Surg 2011;92: 2125–31.
8. Brogan TV, Thiagarajan RR, Rycus PT, Bartlett RH, Bratton SL (2009). Extracorporeal membrane oxygenation in adults with severe respiratory failure: a multi-center database. Intensive Care Med 2009;35(12):2105–14.
9. Cave DM, Gazmuri RJ, Otto CW, et al. Part 7: CPR techniques and devices: 2010 American Heart Association guidelines for cardiopulmonary resuscitation and emergency cardiovascular care. Circulation 2010;122: S720–S728.
10. Chen YS, Lin JW, Yu HY, et al. Cardiopulmonary resusci-ta-tion with assisted extracorporeal life-support versus conventional cardiopulmonary resuscitation in adults with in-hospital cardiac arrest: an observational study and propensity analysis. Lancet 2008;372:554–61.
11. Cheng R, Hachamovitch R, Kittleson M, et al. Complications of extracorporeal membrane oxygenation for treatment of cardiogenic shock and cardiac arrest: a meta-analysis of 1,866 adult patients. Ann Thorac Surg 2014;97:610–16.
12. Chung JC, Tsai PR, Chou NK, Chi NH, Wang SS, Ko WJ; Extracorporeal membrane oxygenation bridge to adult heart transplantation. Clin Transplant 2010;24:375–80.
13. Cohen G, Permut L. Decision making for mechanical cardiac assist in pediatric cardiac surgery. Seminars in Thoracic and Cardiovascular Surgery. Pediatric Cardiac Surgery Annual: 2005;41–50.
14. Concepts of Neonatal ECMO. The Internet Journal of Per-fusionists. Last modified on Feb 13, 9 14:01:21–0600
15. Cornell T, Wyrick P, Fleming G, Pasko D, Han Y, Custer J et al. A case series describing the use of argatroban in patients on extracorporeal circulation. ASAIO J 2007;53 (4): 460–3.
16. D'Alessandro C, Aubert S, Golmard JL, et al. Extra-corporeal membrane oxygenation temporary support for early graft failure after cardiac transplantation. Eur J Cardio-thorac Surg 2010;37:343–349.
17. D'Alessandro C, Golmard JL, Barreda E, et al. Predictive risk factors for primary graft failure requiring temporary extra-corporeal membrane oxygenation support after cardiac transplantation in adults. Eur J Cardiothorac Surg 2011; 40:962–9.
18. Doll N, Kiaii B, Borger M, et al. Five-year results of 219 consecutive patients treated with extracorporeal membrane oxygenation for refractory postoperative cardiogenic shock. Ann Thorac Surg 2004;77:151–7.
19. Groopman, Jerome. How Doctors Think. Houghton Mifflin Harcourt 2007. ISBN 978-0-618-61003-7.
20. Haley MJ, Fisher JC, Ruiz-Elizalde AR, Stolar CJ, Morrissey NJ, Middlesworth W. Percutaneous distal perfusion of the lower extremity after femoral cannulation for venoarterial extracorporeal membrane oxygenation in a small child. J Pediatr Surg. 2009;44:437–40.
21. Heilmann C, Geisen U, Beyersdorf F, et al. Acquired von Willebrand syndrome in patients with extracorporeal life support ECLS. Intensive Care Med 2012;38:62–68.
22. Hemmila MR, Rowe SA, Boules TN, Miskulin J, McGillicuddy JW, Schuerer DJ, et al. Extracorporeal life support for severe acute respiratory distress syndrome in adults. Ann Surg 2004;240(4):595–605;.
23. Jackson KW, Timpa J, McIlwain RB, et al. Side-arm grafts for femoral extracorporeal membrane oxygenation cannu-lation. Ann Thorac Surg 2012;94:e111–e112.
24. Johnson SM, Itoga N, Garnett GM, Kilcommons M, Puapong DP, Woo RK. Increased risk of cardiovascular perforation during ECMO with a bicaval, wire-reinforced cannula. J Pediatr Surg 2014;49:46–50.
25. Kagawa E, Dote K, Kato M, et al. Should we emergently revascu-larize occluded coronaries for cardiac arrest? Rapid-response extracorporeal membrane oxygenation and intra-arrest percutaneous coronary intervention. Circulation 2012;126:1605–1613.
26. Kolla S, Awad SS, Rich PB, Schreiner RJ, Hirschl RB, Bartlett RH. Extracorporeal life support for 100 adult patients with severe respiratory failure. Ann Surg 1997;226(4):544–64.
27. Lebreton G, Nicolescu M, Leger P, Leprince P. Implantation of left ventricular support under extracorporeal membrane oxygenation. Eur J Cardiothorac Surg 2011;40:e165–e167.
28. Lewandowski K, Rossaint R, Pappert D, Gerlach H, Slama KJ, Weidemann H, et al. High survival rate in 122 ARDS patients managed according to a clinical algorithm including extracorporeal membrane oxygenation. Intensive Care Med 1997;23(8):819–35.
29. Madershahian N, Nagib R, Wippermann J, Strauch J, Wahlers T (2006). A simple technique of distal limb perfusion during prolonged femoro-femoral cannulation. J Card Surg 2006; 21(2):168–9.
30. Maekawa K, Tanno K, Hase M, Mori K, Asai Y. Extra-corporeal cardiopulmonary resuscitation for patients with out-of-hospital cardiac arrest of cardiac origin: a propensity-matched study and predictor analysis. Crit Care Med 2013;41:1186–1196.
31. Maggio P, Hemmila M, Haft J, Bartlett R. Extracorporeal life support for massive pulmonary embolism. J Trauma 2007;62:570–6.
32. Marasco SF, Vale M, Pellegrino V, et al. Extracorporeal membrane oxygenation in primary graft failure after heart transplantation. Ann Thorac Surg 2010;90:1541–6.
33. Mateen FJ, Muralidharan R, Shinohara RT, et al. Neurological Injury in Adults Treated With Extracorporeal Membrane Oxygenation Archives of Neurology, 2011.
34. Munakata R, Yamamoto T, Hosokawa Y, et al. Massive pulmonary embolism requiring extracorporeal life support treated with catheter-based interventions. International Heart Journal 2012;53:370–4.
35. Needham DM, Korupolu R, Zanni JM, et al. Early physical medicine and rehabilitation for patients with acute respi-ratory failure: a quality improvement project. Arch Phys Med Rehabil 2010;91:536–42.
36. Peek GJ, Moore HM, Moore N, Sosnowski AW, Firmin RK. Extracorporeal membrane oxygenation for adult respiratory failure. Chest 1997;112(3):759–64.

37. Rahimi RA, Skrzat J, Reddy DR, et al. Physical rehabilitation of patients in the intensive care unit requiring extra-corporeal membrane oxygenation: a small case series. Phys Ther 2013; 93:248–55.
38. Rastan AJ, Dege A, Mohr M, et al. Early and late outcomes of 517 consecutive adult patients treated with extracorporeal membrane oxygenation for refractory postcardiotomy cardiogenic shock. J Thorac Cardiovasc Surg 2010;139: 302–11.
39. Rehder KJ, Turner DA, Hartwig MG, et al. Active rehabilitation during extracorporeal membrane oxygenation as a bridge to lung transplantation. Respir Care 2013;58: 1291–8.
40. Rich PB, Awad SS, Kolla S, Annich G, Schreiner RJ, Hirschl RB et al. An approach to the treatment of severe adult respiratory failure. J Crit Care 1998;13(1):26–36.
41. Rosenzweig E, Brodie D, Abrams D, Agerstrand C, Bacchetta M. Extracorporeal membrane oxygenation as a novel bridging strategy for acute right heart failure in group 1 PAH. ASAIO J 2014;60:129–133.
42. Russo CF, Cannata A, Lanfranconi M, et al. Veno-arterial extracorporeal membrane oxygenation using Levitronix centrifugal pump as bridge to decision for refractory cardio-genic shock. J Thorac Cardiovasc Surg 2010;140: 1416–21.
43. Schmidt M, Brechot N, Hariri S, et al. Nosocomial infections in adult cardiogenic shock patients supported by venoarterial extracorporeal membrane oxygenation. Clin Infect Dis 2012;55:1633–41.
44. Shin TG, Choi JH, Jo IJ, et al. Extracorporeal cardiopulmonary resuscitation in patients with inhospital cardiac arrest: a comparison with conventional cardiopulmonary resuscitation. Crit Care Med 2011;39:1–7.
45. Shin TG, Jo IJ, Sim MS, et al. Two-year survival and neuro-logical outcome of in-hospital cardiac arrest patients rescued by extracorporeal cardiopulmonary resuscitation. Int J Cardiol 2013;168:3424–30.
46. Takayama H, Naka Y, Kodali SK, et al. A novel approach to percutaneous right-ventricular mechanical support. Eur J Cardiothorac Surg 2012;41:423–6.
47. Takayama H, Truby L, Koekort M, et al. Clinical outcome of mechanical circulatory support for refractory cardiogenic shock in the current era. J Heart Lung Transplant 2013;32:106–11.
48. Turner DA, Cheifetz IM, Rehder KJ, et al. Active rehabilitation and physical therapy during extracorporeal membrane oxygenation while awaiting lung transplantation: a practical approach. Crit Care Med 2011;39:2593–8.
49. Ullrich R, Lorber C, Röder G, Urak G, Faryniak B, Sladen RN et al. Controlled airway pressure therapy, nitric oxide inhalation, prone position, and extracorporeal membrane oxygenation (ECMO) as components of an integrated approach to ARDS. Anesthesiology 1999;91(6):1577–86.
50. Van Meurs K, Lally KP, Peek G, Zwischenberger JB. ECMO: Extracorporeal Cardiopulmonary Support in critical care, Extracorporeal Life Support Organization, Ann Arbor 2005.
51. Vural KM. Ventricular assist device applications. Anadolu Kardiyoloji Dergisi: AKD=the Anatolian Journal of Cardiology 2008;8(Suppl 2):117–30.
52. Wang D, Zhou X, Liu X, Sidor B, Lynch J, Zwischenberger JB. Wang-Zwische double lumen cannula-toward a percutaneous and ambulatory paracorporeal artificial lung. ASAIO J 2008;54(6):606–11.

# 27 Pulmonary Artery (Swan-Ganz) Catheterization for Hemodynamic Monitoring in Emergency Department

## PULMONARY ARTERY CATHETERIZATION

The pulmonary artery catheter is frequently referred to as a Swan-Ganz catheter, in honor of its inventors Jeremy Swan and William Ganz, from Cedars-Sinai Medical Center. The idea for a sail or balloon tip modification of Ronald Bradley's simple portex tubing method came about from Dr Swan's observation from the Santa Monica shore of sail boats on the water on relatively calm day. Boats with conventional slot sails were still; one with a spinnaker was able to make reasonable headway. Ganz added the thermistor after Swan showed him the initial balloon design, which was fabricated by Edwards Laboratories, which had previously contracted with Swan as a consultant.

The flow-directed balloon-tipped pulmonary artery catheter (PAC) (also known as the Swan-Ganz or right heart catheter) has been in clinical use for more than 30 years. Initially developed for the management of acute myocardial infarction (AMI), it gained widespread use in the management of a variety of critical illnesses and surgical procedures. This chapter covers both the clinical and technical aspects of its use (Figs 27.1 and 27.2).

### Indications

Despite widespread use of the PAC for more than 3 decades, no validated indications exist for its general use. Some publications present only authors' suggestions for indications and contraindications for the use of the PAC. Various association and subspecialty guidelines exist as consensus statements. For example, in 1998 the American College of Cardiology published a consensus statement regarding the use of the PAC in patients with cardiac disease.

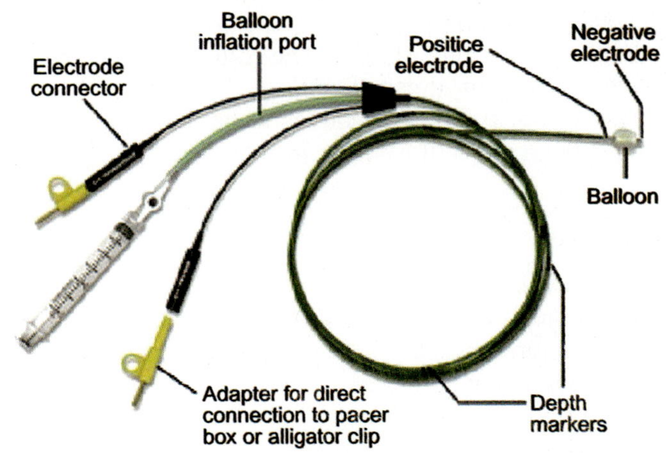


**Fig. 27.1:** Standard balloon-tipped flow-directed catheter with inflated balloon, closed inflation lumen and a pressure transducer attached to the large lumen. Close-up view of the inflated balloon

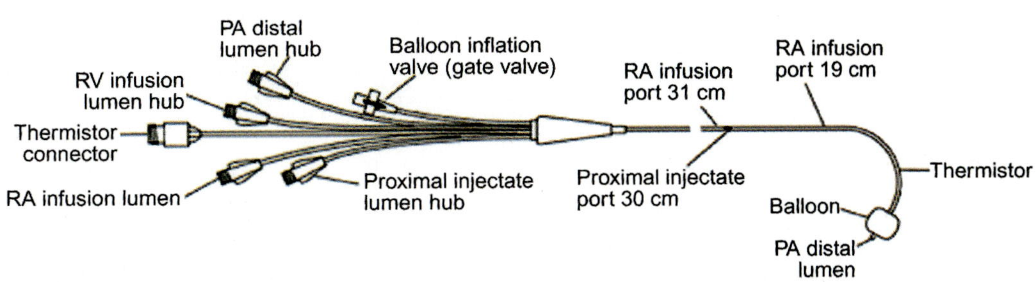


**Fig. 27.2:** Different components of Swan-Ganz catheter

Pulmonary artery catheterization is necessary for the diagnosis of pulmonary hypertension.

The following are general guidelines for clinical use of PAC:

### Diagnostic

- Diagnosis of shock states
- Differentiation of high versus low-pressure pulmonary edema
- Diagnosis of idiopathic pulmonary hypertension
- Diagnosis of valvular disease, intracardiac shunts, cardiac tamponade, and pulmonary embolus (PE)
- Monitoring and management of complicated AMI
- Assessing hemodynamic response to therapies
- Management of multiorgan system failure and/or severe burns
- Management of hemodynamic instability after cardiac surgery
- Assessment of response to treatment in patients with idiopathic pulmonary hypertension

### Therapeutic

- Aspiration of air emboli

### Contraindications

According to the 1998 the American College of Cardiology consensus statement regarding the use of the PAC in patients with cardiac disease. The following are general guidelines for clinical use of PAC:

- Tricuspid or pulmonary valve mechanical prosthesis
- Right heart mass (thrombus and/or tumor)
- Tricuspid or pulmonary valve endocarditis

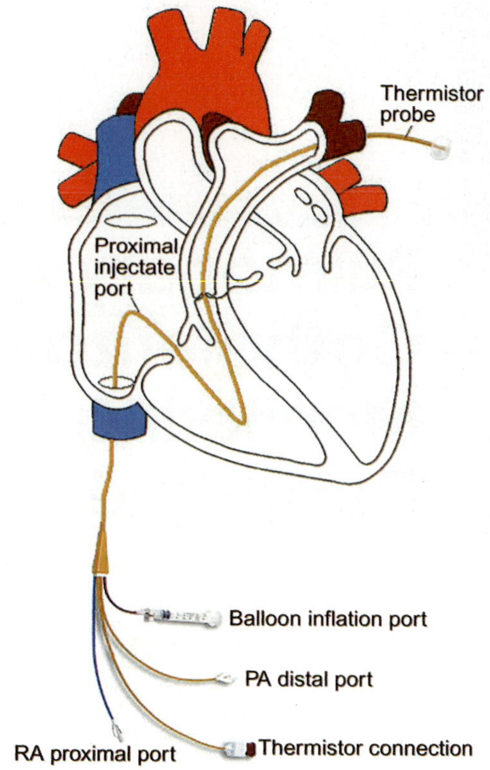


**Fig. 27.3:** The technique of insertion of Swan-Ganz catheter at different positions. Swan-Ganz Catheter also called a pulmonary artery catheter. It is inserted into the right side of the heart via a large central vein. This catheter is used when the team requires detailed information about heart function. The tip of the catheter sits in the artery just before the lungs. A Swan-Ganz catheter looks at different blood pressures and is used to guide the medical staff to choose certain treatments for those critically ill patients

### Procedure

- Swan-Ganz catheter insertion routes (Fig. 27.3)
- Internal jugular vein (Fig. 27.4 )
- External jugular vein
- Subclavian vein
- Femoral vein

Installation is performed percutaneously reaching a central vein with the aid of a dilator and the modified Seldinger technique. The catheter is preferably inserted in the internal jugular vein, advanced through the lumen of the superior vena cava, where the small ball bearing is inflated and the tip passes through the heart chambers in the direction of blood flow. When the catheter is placed in a large caliber intrathoracic vein, it reaches the right atrium through the tricuspid valve into the right ventricle and through the pulmonary valve into the pulmonary artery where it finally latches into the arterial portion of smaller diameter (Figs 27.3 to 27.9 and Table 27.1).

**Table 27.1:** Normal ranges for haemodynamic variables

| | | mmHg | Comment |
|---|---|---|---|
| Right atrial pressure | Mean | 0–5 | Same as CVP |
| Right ventricular pressure | Systolic | 20–30 | To force blood into lungs |
| | Diastolic | 0–5 | To allow flow from RA in diastole |
| Pulmonary artery pressure | Systolic | 20–30 | Continuous with RV |
| | End-diastolic | 10–15 | Pulmonary valve closed |
| | Mean | 10–20 | |
| Pulmonary artery wedge pressure (PAWP) = occlusion pressure (PAOP) | Mean | 6–12 | Roughly equals LA pressure |

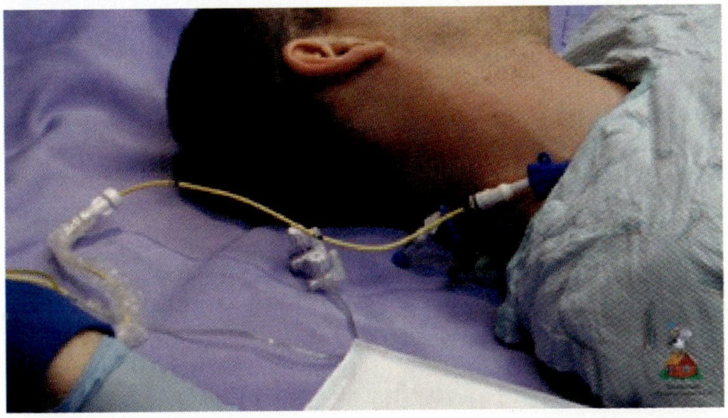

Fig. 27.4: A young patient in whom Swan-Ganz catheter is being inserted through internal jugular vein

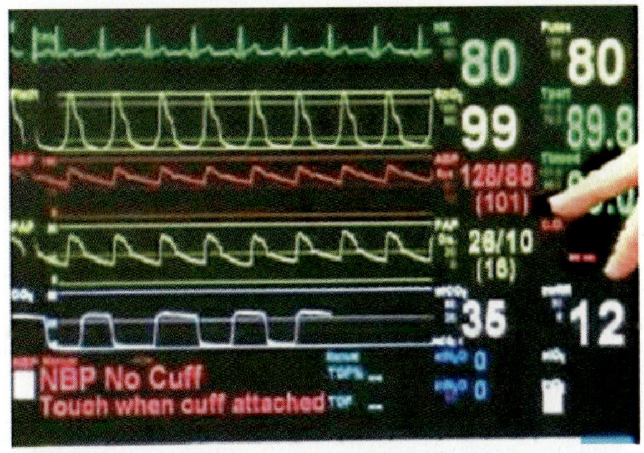


Fig. 27.5: Hemodynamic monitoring of pressure values and waves on monitor screen during catheterization

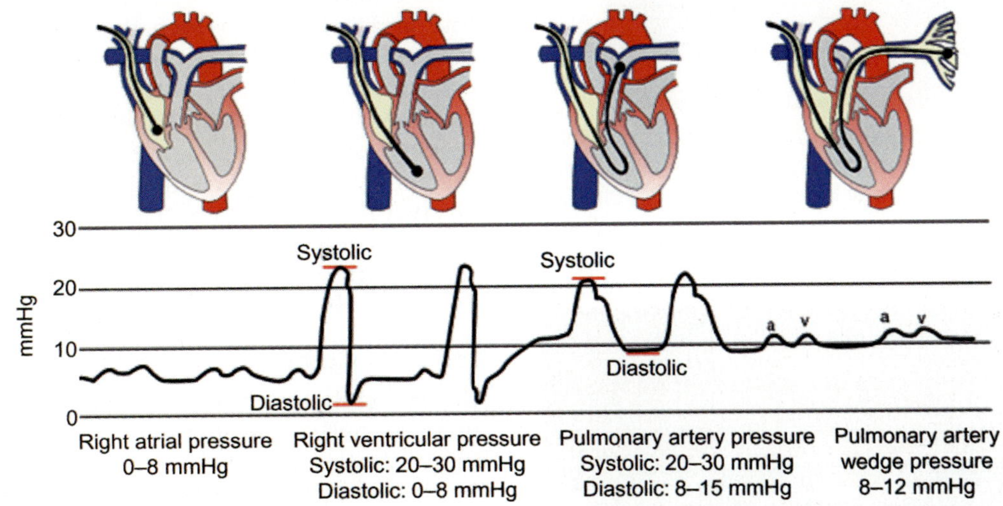


Fig. 27.6: Catheter passing through different sites of right heart measuring pressures with identification of waveforms

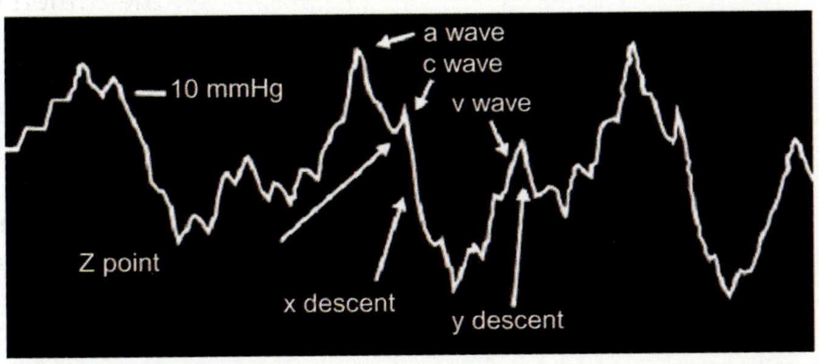


Fig. 27.7: Various waveforms of central venous pressure (CVP) monitoring

In general, no fluoroscopy is needed for inserting the Swan-Ganz catheter for two main reasons. First, the catheter is designed to be directed by the blood flow when the balloon is inflated. During insertion, the inflated balloon makes the catheter follow the flow of venous blood from the right heart to the pulmonary artery.

*Factors to consider in evaluating the patient:*

- Clinical appearance
- Hemodynamics and evolution (Figs 27.6 and 27.7)

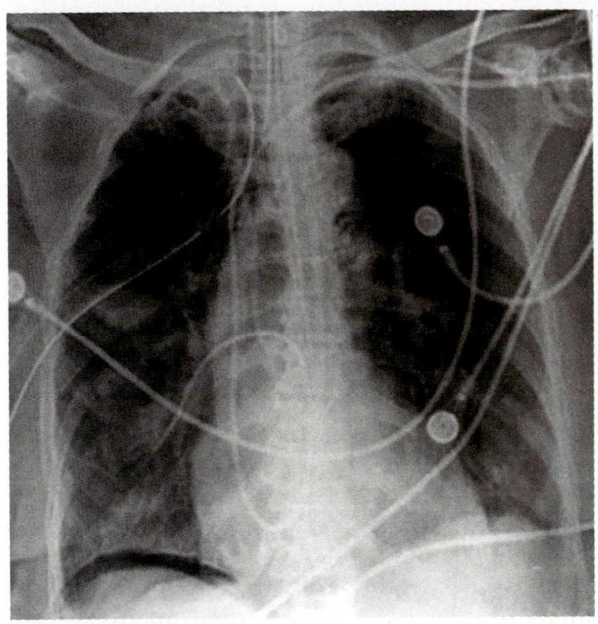

Fig. 27.8: Chest radiograph. Right Swan-Ganz catheter, with its tip within the right lower lobe pulmonary artery branch

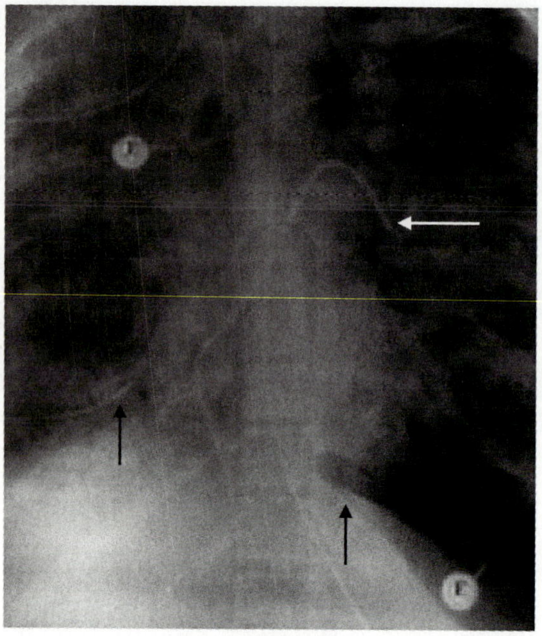

**Fig. 27.9:** Frontal chest radiograph shows a Swan-Ganz catheter (white arrow) in the left pulmonary artery via the inferior vena cava. Note also the bilateral chest tubes (black arrows) and ECG leads (E)

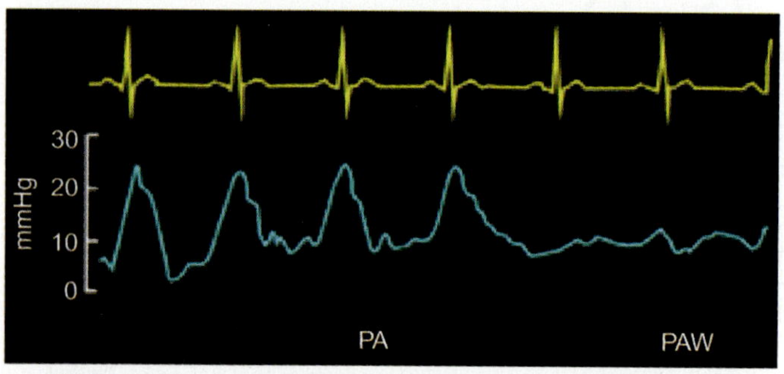


**Fig. 27.10:** Pulmonary artery catheter being introduced from pulmonary artery into wedge position

- Controlled tests
- Drugs administered
- Medicines taken
- Condition of seriousness
- Pressure curves observed on the monitor screen
- Right atrial pressure (Table 27.1)
- Right ventricular pressure (Table 27.1)
- Pulmonary pressure (Table 27.1)
- Wedge pressure (Fig. 27.10)

## TECHNICAL DEVELOPMENTS

### Thermal Dilution

After Swan developed the initial balloon tip, Ganz added a small thermistor (temperature probe) about 3 cm behind the tip. Either cold 10 mL of saline (0.9% NaCl) under 10° Celsius or room temperature (not as accurate) is injected into an opening in the right atrium. As this cooler fluid passes the tip thermistor, a very brief drop in the blood temperature is recorded. A recent variation in design is the incorporation of a heating coil on the catheter (30 cms from the tip, residing in the atrium area), which eliminates the cold fluid bolus, a major factor in human technique variation.

By attaching both the injector site and the ventricular thermistor to a small computer, the thermodilution curve can be plotted. If details about the patient's body mass index (size); core temp, systolic, diastolic, central venous pressure (CVP) (measured from the atrium by the third lumen simultaneously) and pulmonary artery pressure are input, a comprehensive flow vs pressure map can be calculated.

In crude terms, this measurement compares left and right cardiac activity and calculates preload and afterload flow and pressures which theoretically if stabilized or adjusted with drugs to either constrict or dilate the vessels to raise or lower the pressure of blood flow to the lungs, respectively, in order to maximize oxygen for delivery to the body tissues.

The ability to record results is not a guarantee of patient survivability. The true art remains with the consultant physician or intensivist in balancing fluid load, so much so that the introduction of a balloon catheter, which is usually yellow, has been nicknamed 'the kiss of the yellow snake'.

### Design of Catheter for Pharmacotherapy

Modern catheters have multiple lumens five or six are common and have openings along the length to allow administration of inotropes and other drugs directly into the atrium. Drugs to achieve these changes can be delivered into the atrium via the fourth lumen, usually dedicated to medication. Common drugs used are various inotropes, nor-adrenaline or even atropine. A further set of calculations can be made by measuring the arterial blood and central venous (from the third lumen) and inputting these figures into a spreadsheet or the cardiac output computer, if so equipped and plotting an oxygen delivery profile.

#### *$SvO_2$ Measurement*

One further development in recent years has been the invention of a catheter with a fiber-optic based probe which is extended and lodged into the ventricle wall providing instant readings of $SvO_2$ or oxygen saturation of the ventricle tissues. This technique has a finite life as the sensor becomes coated with protein and it can irritate the ventricle via the contact area.

#### *Alternatives*

Various other techniques have largely relegated the PA catheter to history, e.g. the lithium dilution technique; the external bio-resistance monitor or the very simple and reliable technique of esophageal Doppler measurements of the descending aorta.

### Complications

The procedure is not without risk and complications can be life-threatening. It can lead to arrhythmias, rupture of the pulmonary artery, thrombosis, infection, pneumothorax, bleeding and other problems.

### Controversy

The benefit of the use of this type of catheter has been controversial. Therefore, many clinicians minimize its use.

#### Evidence of Benefit

Several studies in the 1980s seemed to show a benefit of the increase in physiological information. Many reports showing benefit of the PA catheter are from anaesthetic, and intensive care settings. In these settings cardiovascular performance was optimized thinking patients would have supra-normal metabolic requirements (Figs 27.6, 27.8 and 27.10).

#### Evidence of Harm or Lack of Benefit

Contrary to earlier studies, there is growing evidence the use of a PA catheter (PAC) does not necessarily lead to improved outcome. The following explanations have been advanced. One explanation could be that nurses and physicians were insufficiently knowledgeable to adequately interpret the PVC measurements. Also, the benefits might be reduced by the complications from the use of the PAC. Furthermore, using information from the PAC might result in a more aggressive therapy causing the detrimental effect. Or, it could give rise to more harmful therapies (i.e. achieving supra-normal values could be associated with increased mortality).

#### Utility of Pulmonary Artery Catheterization

Doctors Swan and Ganz should be recognized further for this important and unique advance from the 1970s. This interpretation of Adolph Ficks' formulation for cardiac output by time/temperature curves is an expedient but limited and invasive model of right heart performance. It remains an exceptional method of monitoring volume overload leading to pulmonary edema in an intensive care unit (ICU) setting. Noninvasive echocardiography and pulse-wave cardiac output monitoring are concordant with (and much safer), if not better than invasive methods defining right and left heart performance. The advent of methicillin resistant *Staphylococcus aureus* (MRSA) and similar hospital based catheter infections now clearly limits the utility of this type of invasive cardiac ICU intervention.

## BIBLIOGRAPHY


1. Bayliss J, Norell M, Ryan A, Thurston M, Sutton GC. Bedside haemodynamic monitoring: experience in a general hospital. Br Med J (Clin Res Ed) 1983;287(6386):187–90.
2. Bernard GR, Sopko G, Cerra F, et al. Pulmonary artery catheterization and clinical outcomes: National Heart, Lung, and Blood Institute and Food and Drug Administration Workshop Report. Consensus Statement. JAMA 2000; 283(19):2568–72.
3. Binanay C, Califf RM, Hasselblad V, et al. Evaluation study of congestive heart failure and pulmonary artery catheterization effectiveness: the ESCAPE trial. JAMA 2005;294(13): 1625–33.
4. Chatterjee K. The Swan-Ganz catheters: past, present, and future. A viewpoint. Circulation 2009;119(1):147–52.
5. Chittock DR, Dhingra VK, Ronco JJ, et al. Severity of illness and risk of death associated with pulmonary artery catheter use. Crit Care Med 2004;32(4):911–5.
6. Connors AF Jr, McCaffree DR, Gray BA. Evaluation of right-heart catheterization in the critically ill patient without acute myocardial infarction. N Engl J Med 1983;308(5):263–7.
7. Connors AF Jr, Speroff T, Dawson NV, et al. The effectiveness of right heart catheterization in the initial care of critically ill patients. SUPPORT Investigators. JAMA 1996;276(11): 889–97.
8. Corcoran TB, Grape S, Duff O, Perry PL, Murray R. The pulmonary artery catheter sleeve—protective or infective? Anaesth Intensive Care 2009;37(2):290–5.
9. Djaiani G, Karski J, Yudin M, et al. Clinical outcomes in patients undergoing elective coronary artery bypass graft surgery with and without utilization of pulmonary artery catheter-generated data. J Cardiothorac Vasc Anesth 2006; 20(3):307–10.
10. Eisenberg PR, Jaffe AS, Schuster DP. Clinical evaluation compared to pulmonary artery catheterization in the hemodynamic assessment of critically ill patients. Crit Care Med 1984;12(7):549–53.
11. Fein AM, Goldberg SK, Walkenstein MD, Dershaw B, Braitman L, Lippmann ML. Is pulmonary artery catheterization necessary for the diagnosis of pulmonary edema? Am Rev Respir Dis 1984;129(6):1006–9.
12. Greenberg SB, Murphy GS, Vender JS. Current use of the pulmonary artery catheter. Curr Opin Crit Care 2009;15(3): 249–53.
13. Harvey S, Harrison DA, Singer M, et al. Assessment of the clinical effectiveness of pulmonary artery catheters in management of patients in intensive care (PAC-Man): a randomised controlled trial. Lancet 2005;366(9484):472–7.
14. Harvey S, Young D, Brampton W, et al. Pulmonary artery catheters for adult patients in intensive care. Cochrane Database Syst Rev 2006;3:CD003408.
15. Hoar PF, Wilson RM, Mangano DT, Avery GJ 2nd, Szarnicki RJ, Hill JD. Heparin bonding reduces thrombogenicity of pulmonary-artery catheters. N Engl J Med 1981;305(17): 993–5.
16. Iberti TJ, Fischer EP, Leibowitz AB, Panacek EA, Silverstein JH, Albertson TE. A multicenter study of physicians' knowledge of the pulmonary artery catheter. Pulmonary Artery Catheter Study Group. JAMA 1990;264(22):2928–32.
17. Kahwash R, Leier CV, Miller L. Role of the pulmonary artery catheter in diagnosis and management of heart failure. Heart Fail Clin 2009;5(2):241–8.
18. Kearney TJ, Shabot MM. Pulmonary artery rupture asso-ciated with the Swan-Ganz catheter. Chest 1995;108(5): 1349–52.

19. Matthay MA, Chatterjee K. Bedside catheterization of the pulmonary artery: risks compared with benefits. Ann Intern Med 1988;109(10):826–34.
20. Mermel LA, Maki DG. Infectious complications of Swan-Ganz pulmonary artery catheters. Pathogenesis, epidemiology, prevention, and management. Am J Respir Crit Care Med 1994;149(4 Pt 1):1020–36.
21. Mueller HS, Chatterjee K, Davis KB, et al. ACC expert consensus document. Present use of bedside right heart catheterization in patients with cardiac disease. American College of Cardiology. J Am Coll Cardiol 1998; 32(3): 840–64.
22. Pinsky MR, Vincent JL. Let us use the pulmonary artery catheter correctly and only when we need it. Crit Care Med 2005;33(5):1119–22.
23. Rhodes A, Cusack RJ, Newman PJ, Grounds RM, Bennett ED. A randomised, controlled trial of the pulmonary artery catheter in critically ill patients. Intensive Care Med 2002;28(3):256–64.
24. Richard C, Warszawski J, Anguel N, et al. Early use of the pulmonary artery catheter and outcomes in patients with shock and acute respiratory distress syndrome: a randomized controlled trial. JAMA 2003;290(20):2713–20.
25. Ruisi CP, Goldberg RJ, Kennelly BM, Goodman SG, Lopez-Sendon J, Granger CB, et al. Pulmonary artery catheterization in patients with acute coronary syndromes. Am Heart J 2009; 158(2):170–6.
26. Sandham JD, Hull RD, Brant RF, et al. A randomized, controlled trial of the use of pulmonary-artery catheters in high-risk surgical patients. N Engl J Med 2003;348(1):5–14.
27. Shah MR, Hasselblad V, Stevenson LW, et al. Impact of the pulmonary artery catheter in critically ill patients: meta-analysis of randomized clinical trials. JAMA 2005;294(13): 1664–70.
28. van Lelyveld-Haas LE, van Zanten AR, Borm GF, Tjan DH. Clinical validation of the non-invasive cardiac output monitor USCOM-1A in critically ill patients. Eur J Anaesthesiol. 2008;25(11):917–24.
29. Vincent JL, Pinsky MR, Sprung CL, et al. The pulmonary artery catheter: in medio virtus. Crit Care Med 2008;36(11): 3093–6.
30. West JB, Dollery CT, Naimark A. Distribution of blood flow in isolated lung; relation to vascular and alveolar pressures. J Appl Physiol 1964;19:713–24.
31. Wheeler AP, Bernard GR, Thompson BT, et al. Pulmonary-artery versus central venous catheter to guide treatment of acute lung injury. N Engl J Med 2006;354(21): 2213–24.
32. Wiener RS, Welch HG. Trends in the use of the pulmonary artery catheter in the United States, 1993-2004. JAMA 2007; 298(4):423–9.

# 28 Direct Current Cardioversion (DC Shock) in Emergency Care

## DEFIBRILLATION

Defibrillation was first demonstrated by Prevost and Batelli, from the University of Geneva, Switzerland, in 1899. They discovered that small electrical shocks could induce ventricular fibrillation in dogs and that larger charges would reverse the condition. Transthoracic defibrillation was first used in humans using alternating current (AC) in 1956.

Lown and his coworkers introduced direct current (DC) defibrillators into clinical practice. Electrical cardioversion has now become a routine procedure and is used electively or emergently to terminate cardiac arrhythmias.

Defibrillation is a nonsynchronized delivery of energy during any phase of the cardiac cycle, whereas cardioversion is the delivery of energy that is synchronized to the large R waves or QRS complex. The delivered shock in both defibrillation and cardioversion causes electric current to go from the negative to the positive electrode of the defibrillator, passing the heart on its way. It causes all the heart cells to contract simultaneously, thereby interrupting and terminating the abnormal electrical rhythm without damaging the heart, and thus allowing the sinus node to resume normal pacemaker activity. This article illustrates the basic principles and techniques of these procedures and clinical indications for their use (Figs 28.1 and 28.2).

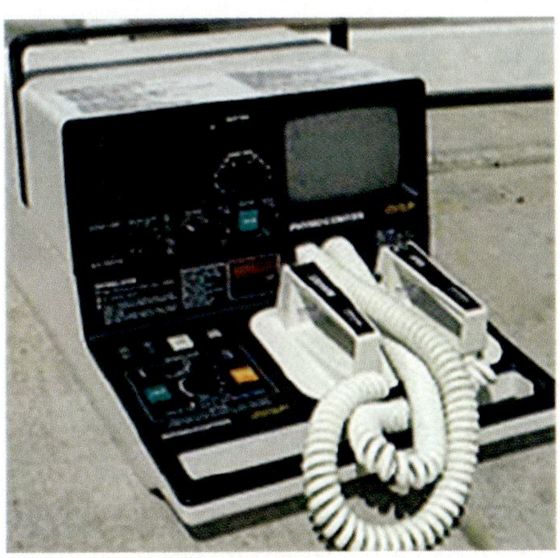

**Fig. 28.1:** A defibrillator is used to 'shock' the heart from an abnormal rhythm pattern back into a normal rhythm. Every neonatal ICU has one of these devices, but they are rarely used there. Abnormal heart rhythms are quite unusual in babies, even those babies with several cardiac abnormalities—arrhythmias are more typical of aged patients with damaged heart muscle or conduction pathways

### Indications

Indications are shown in Figures 28.3–28.5.

- Synchronized electrical cardioversion
  - Supraventricular tachycardia
  - Atrial fibrillation
  - Atrial flutter
  - Ventricular tachycardia
  - Any patient with reentrant tachycardia with narrow or wide QRS complex (ventricular rate >150), who is unstable (e.g. chest pain, pulmonary edema and hypotension)

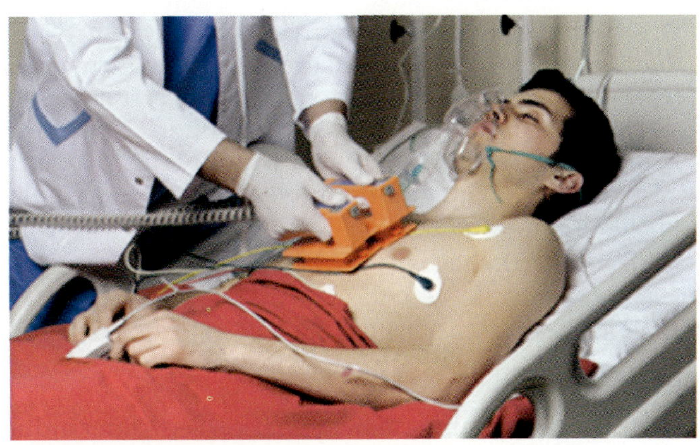

**Fig. 28.2:** Placement of pedals for the application of DC shock in a patient with cardiac arrest

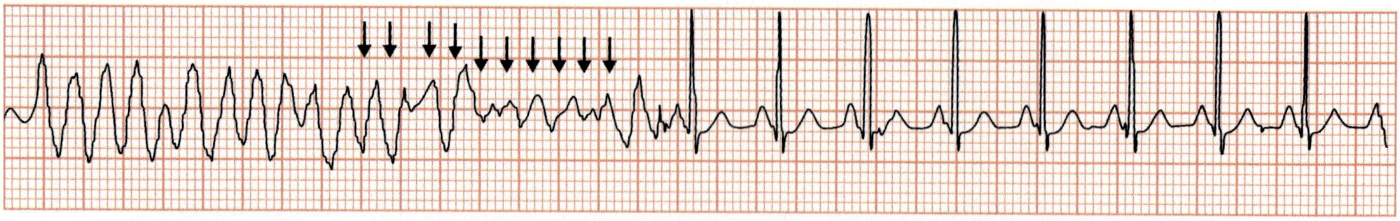

**Fig. 28.3:** Ventricular fibrillation terminated by an unsynchronized shock (arrows) to normal sinus rhythm

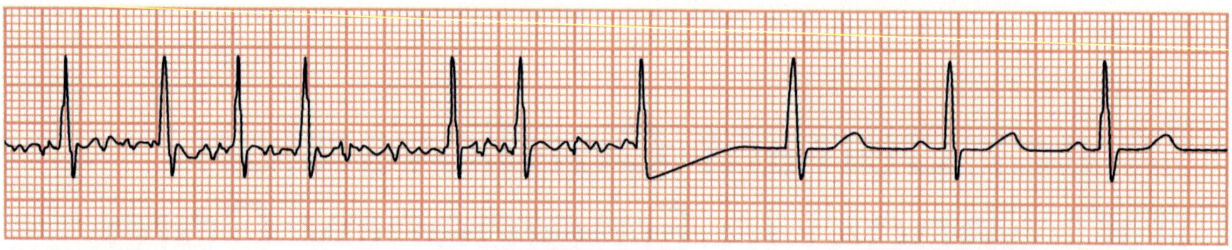


**Fig. 28.4:** Electrocardiograph strip shows a atrial fibrillation terminated by a cardioversion shock [synchronization marks (arrows) in the apex of the QRS complex] to normal sinus rhythm

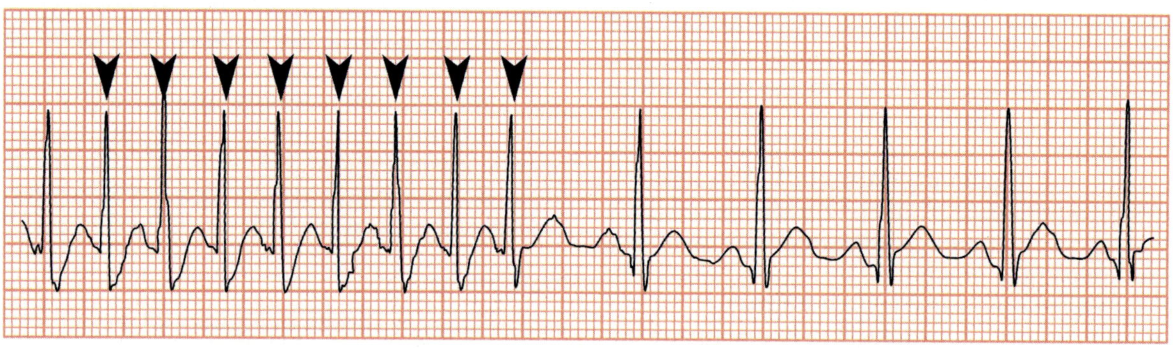

**Fig 28.5:** Electrocardiograph strip shows SVT terminated by a synchronized shock [synchronization marks (arrows) in the apex of the QRS complex] to normal sinus rhythm

- Defibrillation
  - Pulseless ventricular tachycardia (VT)
  - Ventricular fibrillation (VF)
  - Cardiac arrest due to or resulting in VF

### Contraindications

- Dysrhythmias due to enhanced automaticity, such as in digitalis toxicity and catecholamine-induced arrhythmia (in these conditions, a homogeneous depolarization state already exists. Therefore, cardioversion is not only ineffective but is also associated with a higher incidence of postshock ventricular tachycardia/ventricular fibrillation [VT/VF].)
- Multifocal atrial tachycardia

## MORE ON DEFIBRILLATION OR CARDIOVERSION

### Anesthesia

- Cardioversion is almost always performed under induction or sedation (short-acting agent such as midazolam). The only exceptions are if the patient is hemodynamically unstable or if cardiovascular collapse is imminent. For more information, *see* procedural sedation.
- Defibrillation is an emergent maneuver and when necessary should be promptly performed in conjunction with or prior to administration of induction or sedative agents.

### Equipment

Equipment are shown in Figure 28.6.

- Defibrillators
  - Automated external defibrillators (AEDs)
  - Semi-automated AED
  - Standard defibrillators with monitors
- Paddle vs adhesive patch
  - The use of hand-held paddle electrodes may be more effective than self-adhesive patch electrodes.
  - The success rates are slightly higher for patients assigned to paddled electrodes because these hand-held electrodes improve electrode-to-skin contact and reduce the transthoracic impedance.
- Conductive gel or paste
- Electrocardiography (ECG) monitor with recorder

- Oxygen equipment
- Intubation kit
- Emergency pacing equipment

### Positioning

**Paddle placement** on the chest wall has two conventional positions–anterolateral and anteroposterior (Fig. 28.6).

- *Anterolateral position:* A single paddle is placed on the left fourth or fifth intercostal space on the midaxillary line. The second paddle is placed just to the right of the sternal edge on the second or third intercostal space.
- *Anteroposterior position:* A single paddle is placed to the right of the sternum, as above, and the other paddle is placed between the tip of the left scapula and the spine. An anteroposterior electrode position is more effective than the anterolateral position for external cardioversion of persistent atrial fibrillation. The anteroposterior approach is also preferred in patients with implantable devices, to avoid shunting current to the implantable device and damaging its system.

### Technique

- Emergent application, which may be life-saving, and elective cardioversion should be used cautiously, with attention to patient selection and proper techniques. Repetitive, futile attempts at direct current cardioversion should be avoided.
- Advanced cardiac life support (ACLS) measures should be instituted in preparing the patient, such as obtaining intravenous access and preparing airway management equipment, sedative drugs and a monitoring device.

### Monophasic vs Biphasic Waveforms

- Defibrillators can deliver energy in various waveforms that are broadly characterized as monophasic or biphasic.
- Monophasic defibrillation delivers a charge in only one direction, while biphasic defibrillation delivers a charge in one direction for half of the shock and in the electrically opposite direction for the second half.
- Biphasic waveforms defibrillate more effectively and at lower energies than monophasic waveforms.

### Energy Selection for Defibrillation or Cardioversion

- Synchronized electrical cardioversion begins with 25–50 J (or the biphasic equivalent, which is generally one half of that required with monophasic waveforms) to treat atrial flutter and 50–100 J (or the biphasic equivalent) to treat atrial fibrillation for patients in stable condition, as shown below.

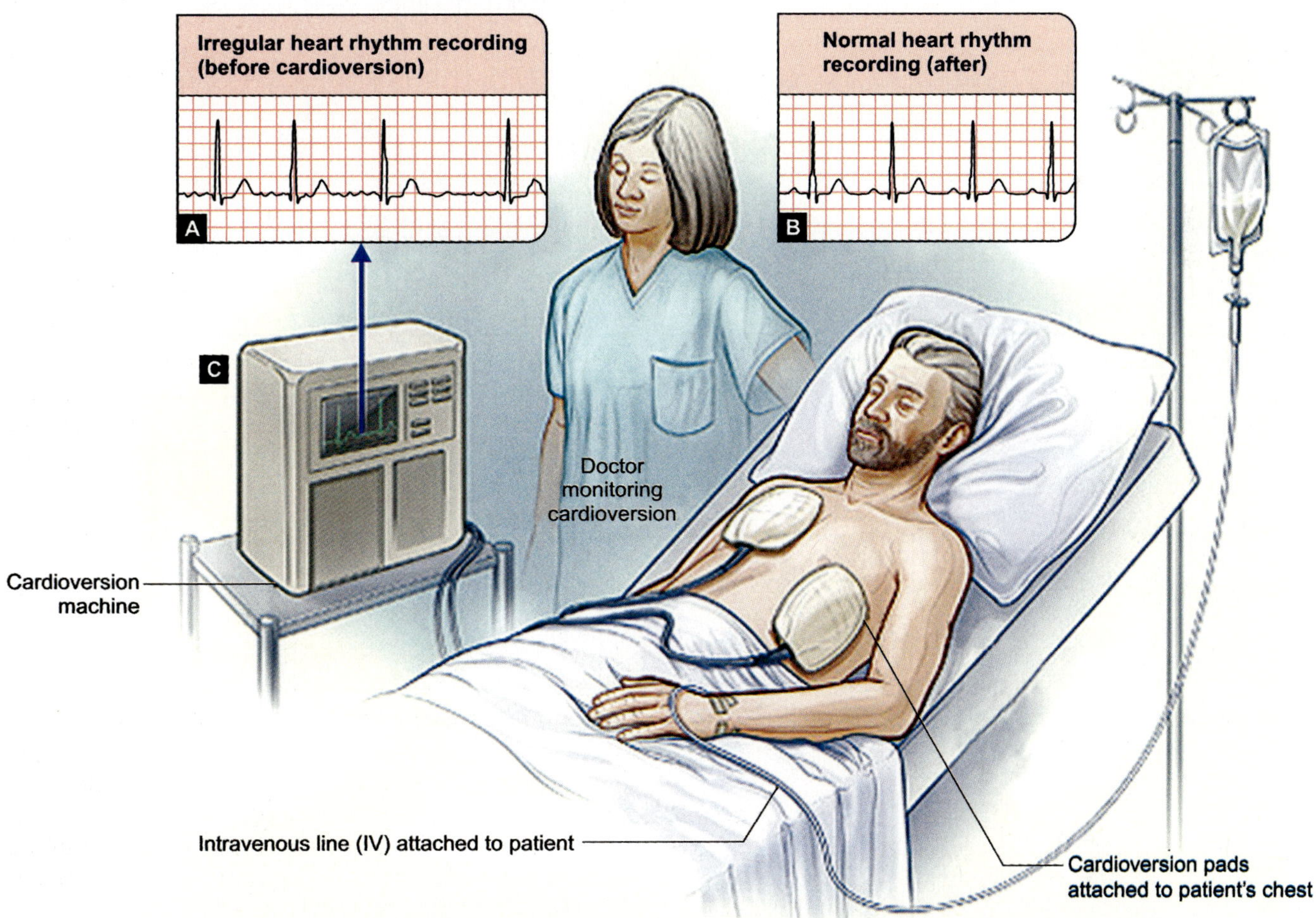


**Fig. 28.6:** Application of paddles over the chest in patient with atrial fibrillation

- Rapid polymorphic ventricular tachycardia [rate >150 (breath per minute) bpm] associated with hemodynamic instability should be treated with immediate, direct-current, nonsynchronized defibrillation with energies of 200–360 J (or biphasic equivalent [100–200 J]).
- Monomorphic ventricular tachycardia should be treated with a synchronized discharge of 100–200 J (or biphasic equivalent [50–100 J]).
- Ventricular fibrillation should be treated with unsynchronized electrical countershock with at least 200–360 J (or biphasic equivalent [100–200 J]) administered as rapidly as possible, as shown below.

## Complications

Complications are shown in Figures 28.7 and 28.8.

- The most common complications are harmless arrhythmias, such as atrial, ventricular, and junctional premature beats.
- Serious complications include VF resulting from high amounts of electrical energy, digitalis toxicity, severe heart disease or improper synchronization of the shock with the R wave.
- Thromboembolization is associated with cardioversion in 1–3% of patients, especially in patients with atrial fibrillation who have not been anticoagulated prior to cardioversion.
- Myocardial necrosis can result from high-energy shocks. ST segment elevation can be seen immediately and usually lasts for 1–2 minutes. ST segment elevation that lasts longer than 2 minutes usually indicates myocardial injury unrelated to the shock.
- Pulmonary edema is a rare complication of cardioversion and is probably due to left ventricular dysfunction or transient left atrial standstill.
- Painful skin burns can occur after cardioversion or defibrillation; they are moderate to severe in 20–25%

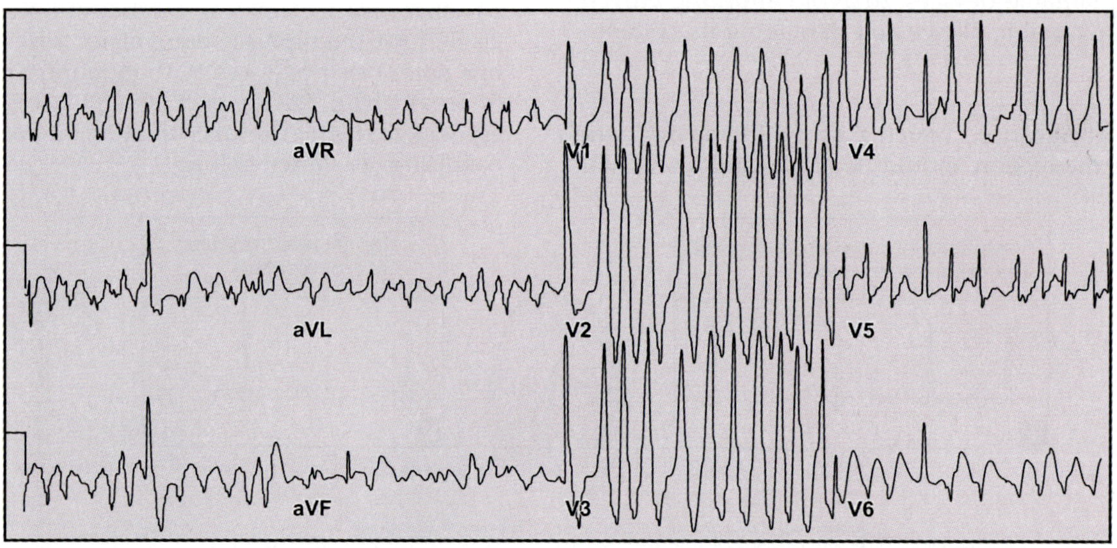


**Fig. 28.7:** Ventricular fibrillation during electrical cardioversion of pre-excited atrial fibrillation

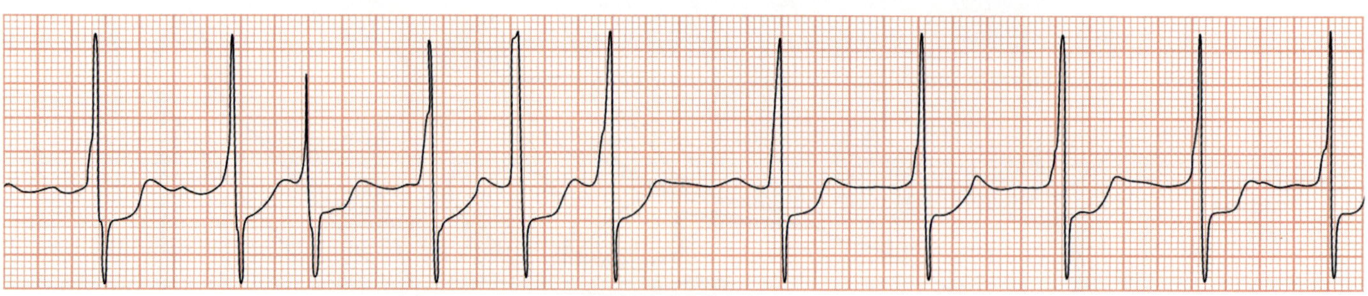

**Fig. 28.8A:** Graph strip shows marked ST-depression in precordial leads along with frequent premature atrial beat (arrow) simulating atrial fibrillation after the application of DC shock

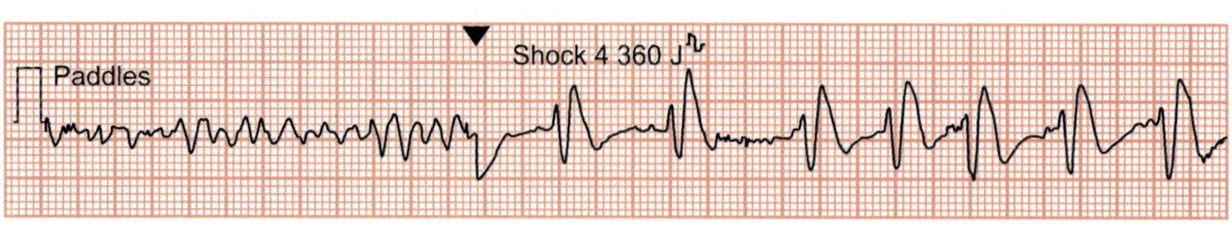


**Fig. 28.8B:** Graph strip shows transient ST-elevation after DC cardioversion from VF

of patients. They most likely are due to improper technique and electrode placement.

## BIBLIOGRAPHY

1. Ambler JJ, Sado DM, Zideman DA, Deakin CD. The incidence and severity of cutaneous burns following external DC cardioversion. Resuscitation 2004;61(3):281–8 [Medline].
2. Botto GL, Politi A, Bonini W, Broffoni T, Bonatti R. External cardioversion of atrial fibrillation: role of paddle position on technical efficacy and energy requirements. Heart 1999; 82(6):726-30 [Medline].
3. DeSilva RA, Graboys TB, Podrid PJ, Lown B. Cardioversion and defibrillation. Am Heart J 1980;100(6Pt1):881–95 [Medline].
4. Kirchhof P, Eckardt L, Loh P, Weber K, Fischer RJ, Seidl KH, et al. Anterior-posterior versus anterior-lateral electrode positions for external cardioversion of atrial fibrillation: a randomised trial. Lancet 2002;360(9342):1275–9.
5. Kirchhof P, Monnig G, Wasmer K, Heinecke A, Breithardt G, Eckardt L, et al. A trial of self-adhesive patch electrodes and hand-held paddle electrodes for external cardioversion of atrial fibrillation (MOBIPAPA). Eur Heart J 2005;26(13):1292–7 [Medline].
6. Lown B, Amarasingham R, Neuman J. New method for termi-nating cardiac arrhythmias. Use of synchronized capacitor discharge. JAMA 1962;182:548–55 [Medline].
7. Niebauer MJ, Brewer JE, Chung MK, Tchou PJ. Comparison of the rectilinear biphasic waveform with the monophasic damped sine waveform for external cardioversion of atrial fibrillation and flutter. Am J Cardiol 2004;93(12):1495–9 [Medline].
8. Schneider T, Martens PR, Paschen H, Kuisma M, Wolcke B, Gliner BE, et al. Multicenter, randomized, controlled trial of 150-J biphasic shocks compared with 200- to 360-J mono-phasic shocks in the resuscitation of out-of-hospital cardiac arrest victims. Optimized Response to Cardiac Arrest (ORCA) Investigators. Circulation 2000;102(15):1780–7 [Medline].
9. Zoll PM, Linenthal AJ, Gibson W, Paul MH, Norman LR. Termi-nation of ventricular fibrillation in man by externally applied electric countershock. N Engl J Med 1956;254(16): 727–32 [Medline].

# 29 Artificial Cardiac Pacemaker Therapy

A pacemaker (or artificial pacemaker, so as not to be confused with the heart's natural pacemaker) is a medical device which uses electrical impulses, delivered by electrodes contacting the heart muscles, to regulate the beating of the heart. The primary purpose of a pacemaker is to maintain an adequate heart rate, either because the heart's native pacemaker is not fast enough, or there is a block in the heart's electrical conduction system. Modern pacemakers are externally programmable and allow the cardiologist to select the optimum pacing modes for individual patients. Some combine a pacemaker and defibrillator in a single implantable device. Others have multiple electrodes stimulating differing positions within the heart to improve synchronisation of the lower chambers of the heart (Fig. 29.1).

## HISTORY IN PACEMAKER IMPLANTATION

### The First Implantable Pacemaker

In 1958, Arne Larsson (1915–2001) became the first to receive an implantable pacemaker. He had a total of 26 devices during his life and campaigned for other patients needing pacemakers.

The first clinical implantation into a human of a fully implantable pacemaker was in 1958 at the Karolinska Institute in Solna, Sweden, using a pacemaker designed by Rune Elmqvist and surgeon Åke Senning, connected to electrodes attached to the myocardium of the heart by thoracotomy. The device failed after 3 hours. A second device was then implanted which lasted for 2 days. The world's first implantable pacemaker patient, Arne Larsson,

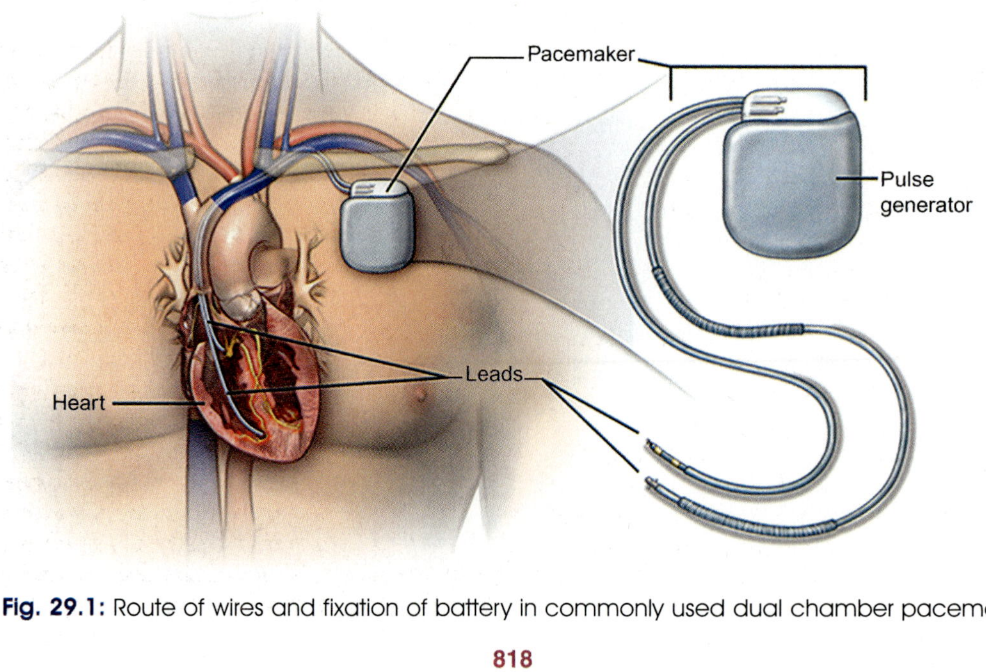


**Fig. 29.1:** Route of wires and fixation of battery in commonly used dual chamber pacemaker

went on to receive 26 different pacemakers during his lifetime. He died in 2001, at the age of 86.

In 1959, temporary transvenous pacing was first demonstrated by Furman et al., in which the catheter electrode was inserted via the patient's basilic vein.

In February 1960, an improved version of the Swedish Elmqvist design was implanted in Montevideo, Uruguay in the Casmu Hospital by Doctors Fiandra and Rubio. That device lasted until the patient died of other ailments, 9 months later. The early Swedish-designed devices used rechargeable batteries, which were charged by an induction coil from the outside.

Implantable pacemakers constructed by engineer Wilson Greatbatch entered use in humans from April 1960 following extensive animal testing. The Greatbatch innovation varied from the earlier Swedish devices in using primary cells (mercury battery) as the energy source. The first patient lived for a further 18 months.

The first use of transvenous pacing in conjunction with an implanted pacemaker was by Parsonnet in the United States of America, Lagergren in Sweden and Jean-Jaques Welti in France in 1962–63. The transvenous or pervenous procedure involved incision of a vein into which it was inserted, the catheter electrode lead under fluoroscopic guidance, until it was lodged within the trabeculae of the right ventricle. This method was to become the method of choice by the mid-1960s.

*World's first lithium-iodide cell powered pacemaker. Cardiac Pacemakers Inc. 1972*

The preceding implantable devices all suffered from the unreliability and short lifetime of the available primary cell technology which was mainly that of the mercury battery.

In the late 1960s, several companies, including ARCO in the United States of America, developed isotope powered pacemakers, but this development was overtaken by the development in 1971 of the lithium-iodide cell by Wilson Greatbatch. Lithium-iodide or lithium anode cells became the standard for future pacemaker designs.

A further impediment to reliability of the early devices was the diffusion of water vapour from the body fluids through the epoxy resin encapsulation affecting the electronic circuitry. This phenomenon was overcome by encasing the pacemaker generator in an hermetically sealed metal case, initially by Telectronics of Australia in 1969 followed by Cardiac Pacemakers Inc of Minneapolis in 1972. This technology, using titanium as the encasing metal, became the standard by the mid-1970s (Fig. 29.2).

Others who contributed significantly to the technological development of the pacemaker in the pioneering years were Bob Anderson of Medtronic Minneapolis, J.G. (Geoffrey) Davies of St George's Hospital London, Barouh Berkovits and Sheldon Thaler of American Optical, Geoffrey Wickham of Telectronics Australia, Walter Keller of Cordis Corp. of Miami, Hans Thornander who joined previously mentioned Rune Elmquist of Elema-Schonander in Sweden, Janwillem van den Berg of Holland and Anthony Adducci of Cardiac Pacema.

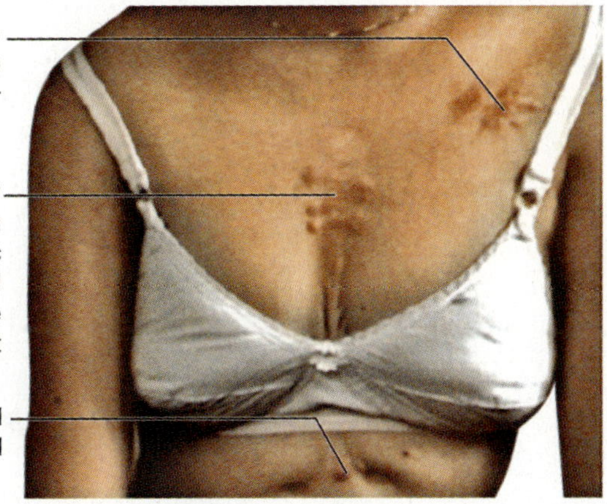


**Fig. 29.2:** A patient at the age of 20 years, her epicardial pacemaker and prosthetic tricuspid valve completely failed to work satisfactorily after 16 years. She was managed with implantation of DDD pacemaker for cardiac arrhythmia and prosthetic tricuspid valve was also replaced with synthetic tissue valve for severe type of primary tricuspid regurgitation

## BASIC PACEMAKER COMPONENTS

Permanent pacemaker systems are composed of several main parts—the pacemaker generator, the power source, the electronic circuitry, the pacemaker lead(s) and the external programmer.

### Pacemaker Generator

The pacemaker generator is a small titanium case that contains the electronic circuitry and a power source for the pacemaker. Most generators are small and lightweight. They may range in weight from 1–1¾ ounces with average dimensions of 2 inches × 2 inches × ¼ inch. To protect the pacemaker's electronic circuitry from outside interference and to protect the patient from the risk of battery leakage, the components of the generator are sealed in layers of airtight materials (Figs 29.3–29.7).

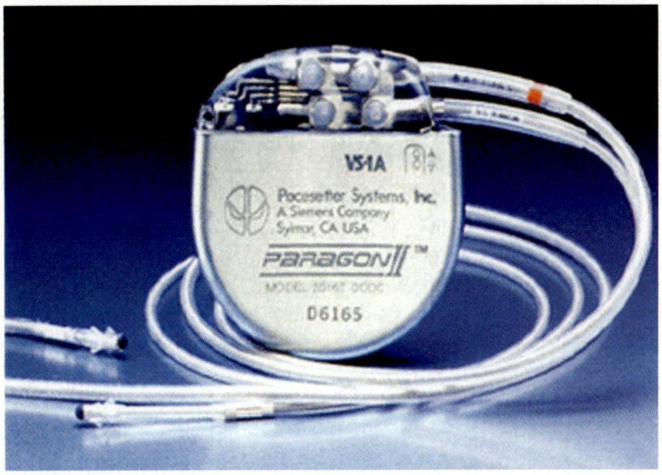


**Fig. 29.3:** Revo MRITM SureScan® pacing system, the first MR-conditional pacing system designed, tested and FDA

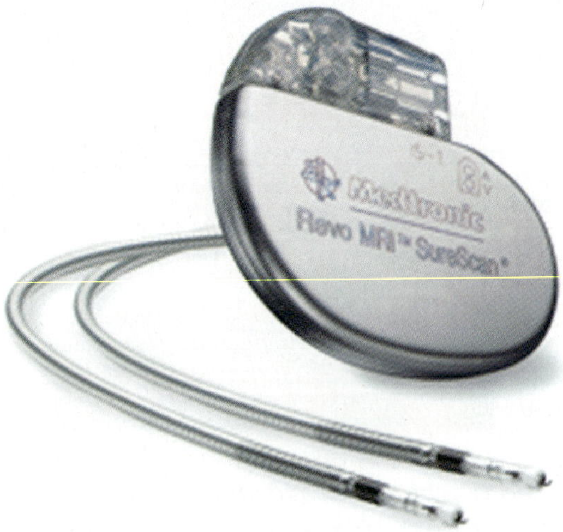


**Fig. 29.4:** DDDC type of pacemaker model approved for use in the magnetic resonance imaging (MRI) environment

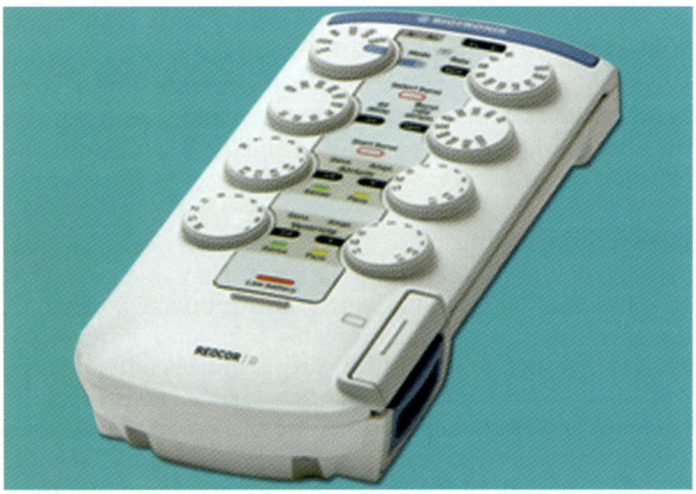


**Fig. 29.5:** BIOTRONIK's reocor external pacemaker, that is available in two models for dual- and single-chamber pacing. 'Reocor combines intuitive design with unprecedented longevity for simplified use.' 'Extended longevity increases reliability and reduces costs over time.' 'Function dials display selectable parameter values and visualize programmed settings at a glance.' 'Easy handling is guaranteed without any specific training requirements.' 'Up to 25 days of permanent pacing therapy and backup power supply during battery replacement.' 'High pacing outputs and high pacing rates for a broad range of patients.' 'Continuous status monitoring for patient safety at any time'

## Pacemaker Power Source

The power source for pacemaker generators is usually a lithium-iodide battery. Depending on use, a lithium battery typically lasts from 5 to 10 years. As lithium batteries near the end of their battery life, they show predictable, identifiable characteristics that serve as an early warning that the battery is becoming depleted. The early warning allows the physician to schedule the battery change procedure in a timely (as opposed to urgent or emergent) fashion.

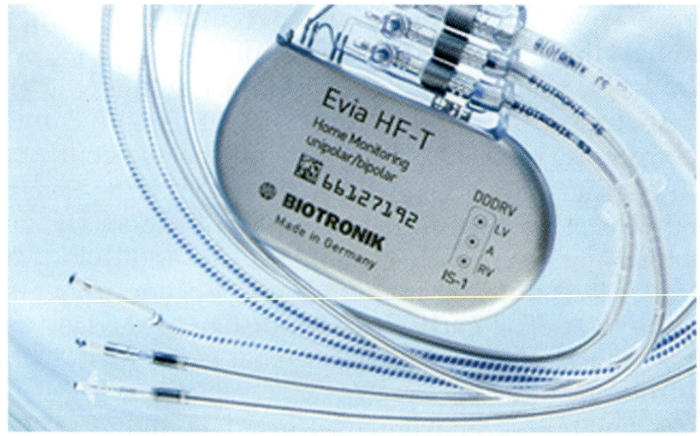


**Fig. 29.6:** BIOTRONIK's Evia HF-T, World's first MR conditional CRT-P system. Main features of this device are 'World's first MR Conditional CRT-P system.' Wide choice of MR conditional leads for RA, RV and LV application with excellent; handling and optimal electrical performance. 'Capture control (RA, RV and LV) and 6 MultiSelect LV pacing polarities as part of a range of solutions for continuous, effective biventricular pacing without complications.' Closed loop stimulation (CLS) to optimize individual rate regulation for patient with chronotropic incompetence (CI). CI is a common comorbidity present in 70% of the advanced HF patients. (1) CLS is the most physiological rate adapting system and is the only sensor to react on both physical and mental stress. Timely intervention using BIOTRONIK Home Monitoring. The results of the COMPAS study show a median gain of 122 days for medical intervention through early detection of clinically relevant events in pacemaker patients. (2) Clinical trend data with heart failure monitor offer a daily updated view on the patients HF status and the effectiveness of the CRT therapy

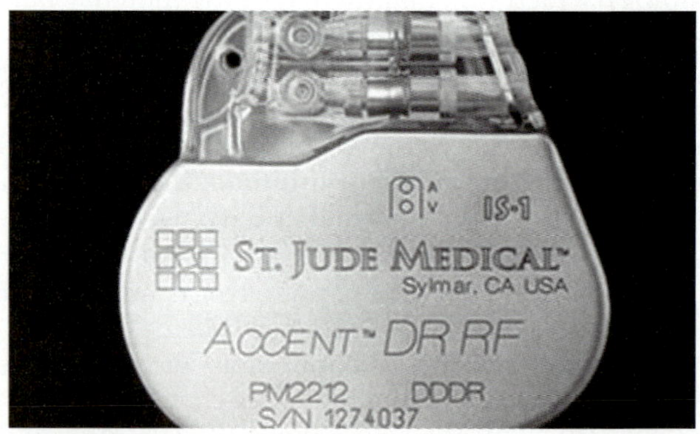


**Fig. 29.7:** The Accent RF pacemaker is the first to simplify patient management—from implant through follow-up—with wireless monitoring. With the intelligence to sense and automatically adjust device parameters, the Accent RF device, a wireless monitoring pacemaker, is designed to maintain effective therapy and enhance patient safety. The Accent RF pacemaker provides intelligent sensing and adjustment of selected device parameters and remote monitoring to help streamline follow-ups, simplify therapy optimization and enhance clinic efficiency

## Electronic Circuitry

The electronic circuitry that controls the functioning of the pacemaker is also housed in the generator. The circuitry is programmed by the physician when the pacemaker is initially implanted. The programming may be non-invasively changed at later intervals as needed. Four different types of circuits are present—a sensing circuit, a pacing or output circuit, a timing circuit, and a transceiver. The sensing circuit monitors the electrical activity in the heart. The output circuit transforms the electrical energy generated by the pacemaker battery into an electrical pulse that is delivered to the heart to initiate a heartbeat. The strength (or voltage) of the electrical impulse is carefully programmed to provide the proper amount of stimulus to the heart to stimulate depolarization. The timing circuit controls the timing of the artificial electrical impulses that are delivered to the heart by the pacemaker. It is programmed at the time that the pacemaker is implanted; its programming may be adjusted noninvasively as needed to maximize pacemaker function for the individual patient. The transceiver is an electronic device that allows the attending or monitoring physician to 'talk' to the electronic circuitry in the pacemaker by way of a specialized programmer. This permits the physician to retrieve data about the pacemaker's current settings and stored data about the pacemaker's functioning. It also allows one to change the programmed settings in the generator noninvasively.

### Pacemaker Leads

The pacemaker lead connects the pacemaker generator to the heart. A pacemaker lead serves two main functions—to deliver the pacing impulse created by the pacemaker generator directly to the heart muscle (pacing function), and to relay information about the heart's electrical activity back to the electronic circuitry in the generator (sensing function) (Figs 29.8 and 29.9).

A pacemaker lead consists of an extremely thin, flexible wire that is coated with suitable insulation, usually either silicone or polyurethane. The extreme flexibility of the wire allows the lead to withstand normal body movements without breaking. On one end of the pacemaker lead is a connector pin; this pin attaches the pacemaker lead firmly to the connector block that is located on the outside of the generator. On the other end of the pacemaker's lead is the pacing electrode that is used to deliver the electrical impulse directly to the heart. To work effectively, this electrode must be in direct contact with the heart. A second electrode is also located on the pacemaker lead. It is a sensing electrode designed to monitor and relay information about electrical activity back to the generator. Pacemaker leads may be attached to the epicardial (outer) or endocardial (inner) surface of the heart. Most permanent pacemaker leads are attached to the endocardium. To hold the pacemaker lead in position inside the heart, the pacemaker lead has a small fixation device at the tip. There are two major types of fixation devices—active fixation and passive fixation. Active fixation devices have a small screw that extends from the end of the pacemaker lead into the endocardium to hold the lead in place. Passive fixation devices have tines (like the tines of a fork) on the end; these tines are designed to become entangled in the trabeculae inside the atria or ventricle to hold the lead in place. In addition to a fixation device, pacemaker leads have a small amount of steroids in a reservoir at the tip of the lead. When the lead is positioned and attached, the steroid is released. The steroid, through its anti-inflammatory action, reduces the amount of inflammation and scar tissue that develop around the tip of the lead. Minimizing scar tissue allows

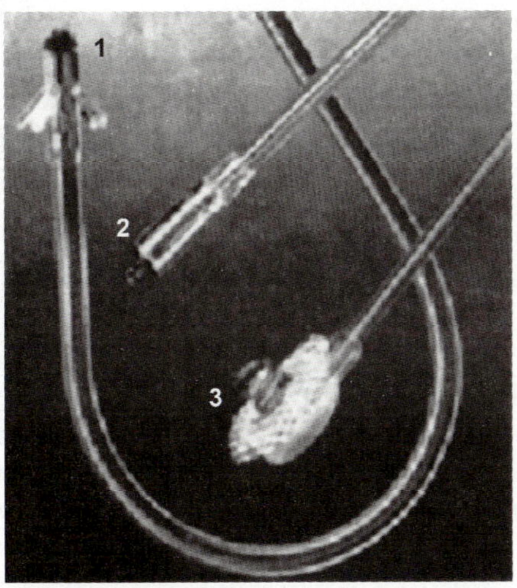


**Fig. 29.8:** Different types of tips of pacing electrode in current use (1—steroid impregnated porous transvenous lead, 2 and 3—screw type of tip for epicardial pacing)

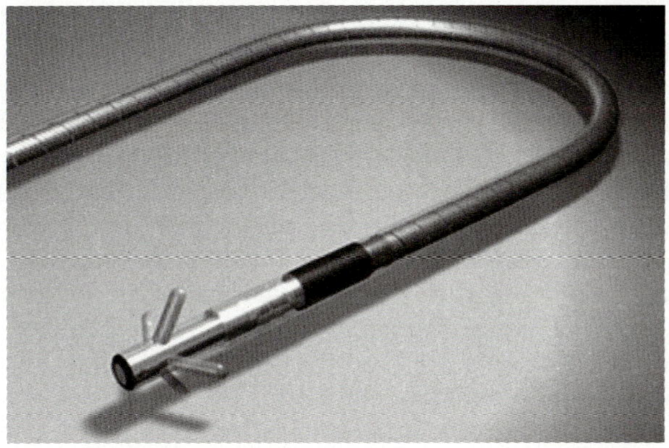

**Fig. 29.9:** Medtronic's MR-Conditional CapSure Sense MRI SureScan pacing leads received EU clearance. The passive fixation leads are the smallest MR-Conditional leads on the market, and provide physicians another option in addition to the previously approved active fixation leads that are anchored right in the heart. 'The CapSure Sense MRI SureScan(R) leads address an unmet clinical need for thoroughly tested MRI conditional passive fixation leads,' said Gianluca Botto, M.D., director of EPS Unit at St. Anna Hospital in Como, Italy. 'With this new lead, there is now a full portfolio of options available for physicians and their patients, when this lead is combined with an MR-Conditional device.' To assure the safety of patients and the effectiveness of the patients' pacing therapy, the CapSure Sense MRI leads were tested in more than 400,000 scenarios that evaluated different patient body types, scanning locations, MRI scanner types and lead lengths

the pacing electrode at the end of the lead to deliver electrical impulses more effectively.

In order for the pacemaker to deliver an effective electrical impulse to the heart, a complete electrical circuit must be present. A complete circuit requires both a positive electrode (anode) and a negative electrode (cathode). To provide the complete circuit, pacemaker leads may be designed as either unipolar or bipolar. A unipolar lead contains only a negative electrode, located on the lead tip. The metal casing of the generator acts as the positive pole or anode. A bipolar lead, on the other hand, contains both a positive and a negative electrode. The negative electrode again is located on the tip of the lead; the positive electrode is located several centimeters behind the negative electrode. Because the electrodes are relatively close together on a bipolar lead, the electrical circuit is smaller and is less likely to be disturbed or disrupted by outside electrical interference than a unipolar lead. However, some sources suggest that bipolar leads are more fragile than unipolar leads and more likely to break.

Depending on the type of pacemaker, one or more pacemaker leads may be used. Single chamber pacemakers, which pace and sense only in the ventricle or only in the atrium, use a single pacemaker lead. Dual chamber systems that are capable of sensing and pacing in both atria and ventricles use two leads. The newer biventricular pacemakers may use three leads: one positioned in the right atrium, a second in the right ventricle, and a third in the left ventricle.

### Pacemaker Programmer

In addition to the generator and pacemaker leads, which are implanted inside the person's body, the proper functioning of a permanent pacemaker requires the intermittent use of an external device called a programmer (Fig. 29.10). A pacemaker programmer consists of a relatively portable specialized computer. The technology in the programmer allows the computer to communicate with the pacemaker

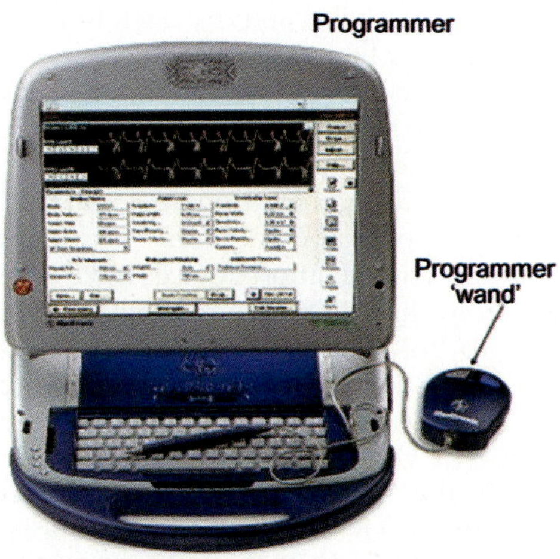


**Fig. 29.10:** Image of one device manufacturers 'programmer', the programmer 'wand' is placed over your device and uses radio waves to collect stored data and to check the integrity and functioning of your device and its intracardiac leads

via the transceiver housed in the pacemaker generator. This process of noninvasive communication is called 'interrogation' of the pacemaker. To interrogate an implanted pacemaker, a physician or other person trained in the use of pacemaker programmers holds a wand directly over the generator site. Using remote telemetric communication technology, the wand can transmit data from the pacemaker generator to the programmer. The information retrieved usually includes the current pacemaker settings and some information about past pacemaker function. In addition, data about the status of the battery and remaining battery life may also be obtained. The retrieved data may be printed for later analysis and/or documentation in the patient's medical record. Changes in pacemaker settings may also be transmitted from the pacemaker programmer through the wand to the generator. This permits the physician to adjust settings based on analysis of the pacemaker's past functioning and the assessment of the patient's current status.

## UNDERSTANDING PACEMAKER FUNCTIONS

For a permanent pacemaker to act effectively to initiate a heartbeat when the heart's own conduction system fails to do so requires the interaction of three basic functions, i.e. pacing, sensing and timing.

### Pacing Function

When the heart's normal rhythm is interrupted, the pacemaker can initiate a heartbeat by pacing the heart. Using power from its battery, the pacemaker generator creates a tiny electrical signal or impulse. This impulse is sometimes called a pacing pulse, pacing impulse or pace. The impulse is conducted through the pacing lead to the electrode on the tip. The impulse is discharged through the electrode directly into the surrounding cells of the heart. If delivered at the right time and the proper voltage, the impulse causes the surrounding cells to depolarize, thus initiating a heartbeat. As discussed, the output circuit in the pulse generator is responsible for generating an impulse that has enough voltage to trigger depolarization. At the time of implantation, the amount of electrical energy needed to depolarize the heart is carefully determined. This is sometimes referred to as the pacing threshold or the stimulation threshold. Once the pacing threshold has been established and programmed into the pacemaker generator, the pacemaker pacing function is tested to ensure that the amount of voltage delivered in each pacing impulse can successfully trigger depolarization. If the pacing impulse successfully triggers depolarization and initiates a heartbeat, the pacemaker is said to have effectively achieved 'capture.' Depending on the patient's specific conduction abnormality, pacing impulses may be delivered to the atria, the ventricles, or both. The rate and timing of the pacing impulses will vary with the pacemaker's programmed settings. The frequency of paced beats depends on the patient's underlying rhythm. In some instances, when the patient has a severe conduction abnormality, the pacemaker will pace the heart 100% of the time. If the patient's conduction problem is only intermittent, the pacemaker will fire only when needed. The ability of the pacemaker to pace the heart only when needed is referred to as 'demand' pacing. Demand pacing prevents the pacemaker from competing with the heart's own intrinsic rhythm and reduces the risk that the pacing impulse will fall at a vulnerable point in the cardiac cycle and throw the heart into a chaotic rhythm. Demand pacing enables the heart to maintain a minimum rate and prevents long pauses without an effective heartbeat, maintaining cardiac output and cerebral circulation.

### Sensing Function

For the pacemaker to deliver a pacing impulse on demand, the generator must recognize or sense when the beat is needed. Sensing occurs when the pacemaker monitors and recognizes electrical activity in the heart. As previously noted, the pacemaker lead is equipped with both a sensing function and a pacing function (Figs 29.11–29.13).

### Ventricular Oversensing and Undersensing

Ventricular sensing may result in abnormalities in the ventricular timing cycles. The pacemaker senses an event that does not represent ventricular depolarization. Parts of the QRS complex, the T-wave, after depolarizations, atrial activity, noise from lead abnormalities, myopotentials and electromagnetic interference (EMI) are possible causes of ventricular oversensing. In ventricular oversensing the additional sensed event will reset the ventricular escape interval, resulting in longer intervals than the programmed pacing cycle length. In ventricular undersensing the pacemaker does not sense an intrinsic ventricular depolarization (R wave). The ventricular escape interval is not reset by this R wave, but instead is created by the previous sensed or paced event. The pacing interval will be shorter than the pacing cycle length.

The sensing function monitors for depolarization in a specific region of the heart; if depolarization occurs, the sensing electrode transmits that information back through the pacemaker lead to the sensing circuit in the generator.

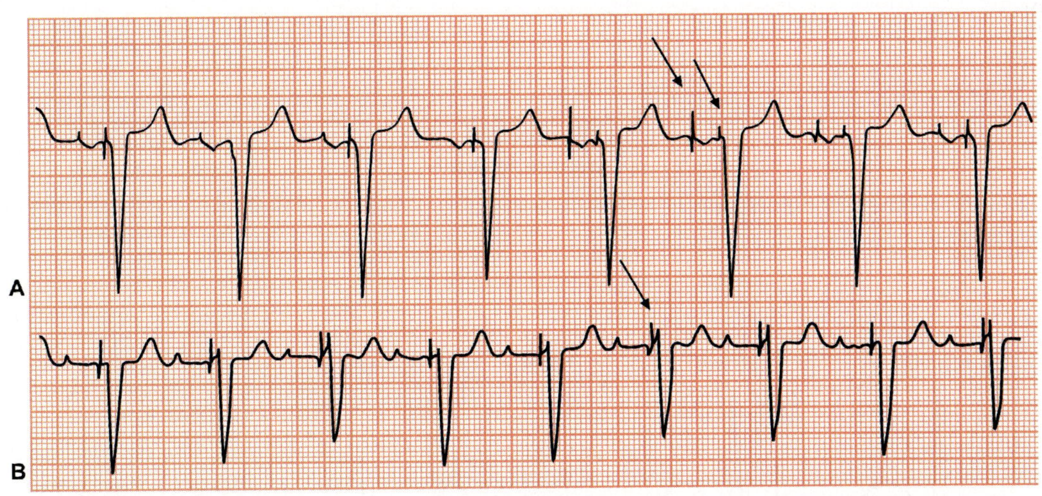


**Fig. 29.11:** Pacing ECG showing (A) single chamber pacekaker rhythm, and (B) dual chamber pacemaker rhythm

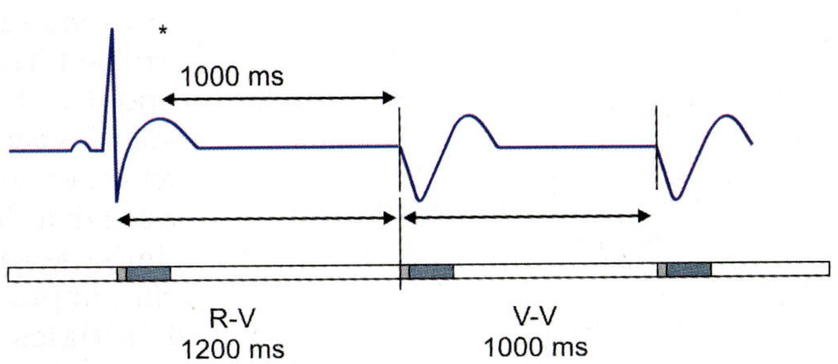


**Fig. 29.12:** V-VI ventricular oversensing. The T-wave of the first beat (indicated by asterisk) is sensed outside the ventricular refractory period. The ventricular escape interval is 1000 msec. Because of the T-wave of the first beat is sensed, the R-V interval is 1200 msec instead of 1000 msec. The following V-V interval is the expected 1000 msec

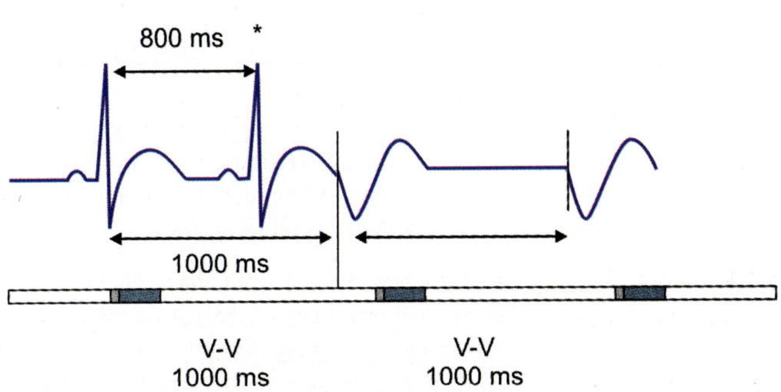


**Fig. 29.13:** V-VI ventricular undersensing. The second R-wave (indicated by asterisk) is not sensed. The next event is a ventricular paced event after a ventricular escape interval of 1000 msec. The subsequent V-V interval is also 1000 msec

The generator processes the information and responds according to its programmed parameters. For the pacemaker to recognize electrical activity in the heart correctly, the sensing threshold must be carefully established and programmed. The sensing threshold is defined as the largest electrical signal (ventricular or atrial) that can be consistently recognized by the sensing circuit. Sensing thresholds that are set too high or too low will result in improper functioning of the pacemaker's pacing function. Depending on the type of pacemaker, sensing may occur only in the atria, only in the ventricles, or in both the atria and the ventricles. The sensing function prevents the pacemaker from competing with the heart's own rhythm. It also permits the pacemaker to perform the more complex functions required by dual chamber and rate responsive pacemakers.

## Timing Function

The timing function works interactively with the pacing and sensing functions of the pacemaker to ensure that a pacing impulse is delivered to the heart when it is needed, according to the pacemaker's programmed parameters (Figs 29.14 and 29.15). The timing function is very complex; it controls a variety of intervals that are involved in a pacing cycle. The specific intervals that are programmed depend on the type of pacemaker and its parameters. The timing function common to all types of demand pacemakers is the low rate limit setting. The low rate limit setting is the rate at which the pacemaker will pace the heart when the heart fails to initiate its own beat. This setting is usually expressed in terms of beats per minute (bpm) and is often set at a rate of 50–70 bpm. To program the low rate setting limit, a low

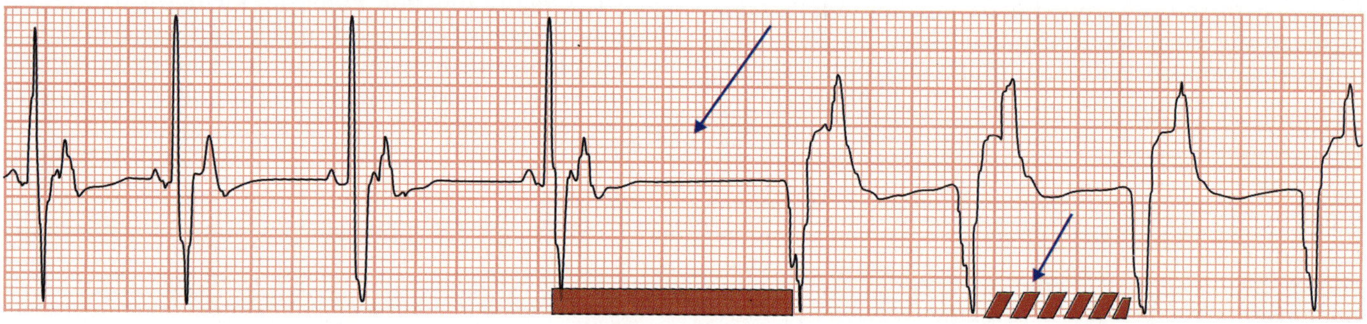


**Fig. 29.14:** Graph showing method of calculation of hysteresis and pacing intervals in hysteresis programming in the evaluation of pacemaker function (arrows)

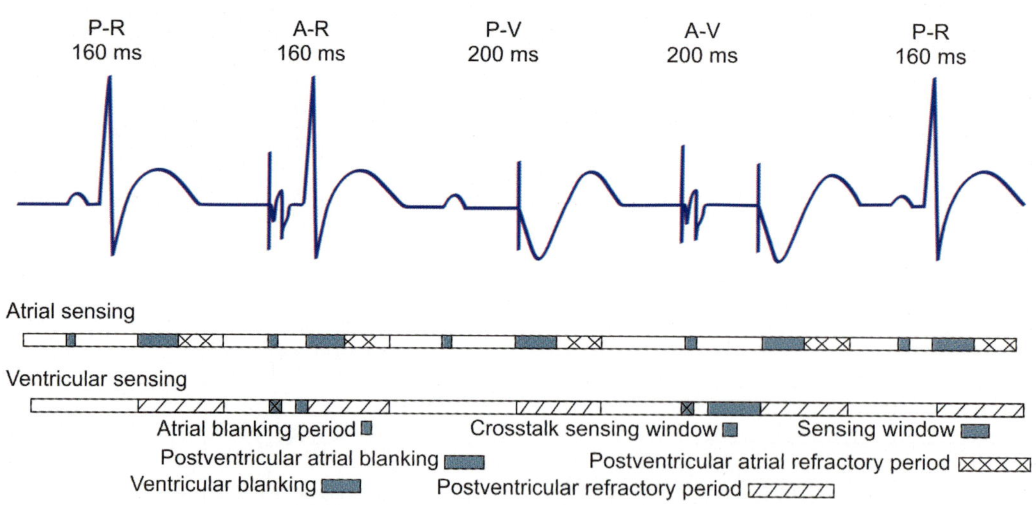


**Fig. 29.15:** DDD refractory periods. The lower rate is 60 beats per minute or 1000 ms in this example of ventricular-based timing. The atrial escape interval, the time from the R-A or V-A, is 800 msec, equal to 1000 msec minus the A-V interval of 200 msec. A=paced atrial event; P=sensed atrial event; R=sensed ventricular event; V=paced ventricular event. The refractory periods and sensing windows are given on the atrial and ventricular sensing channels. On the atrial channel, the atrial blanking period is after an atrial paced or sensed (usually) event. After a sensed or paced ventricular event, on the atrial channel, there may be a postventricular atrial blanking period followed by a postventricular atrial refractory period. On the ventricular channel, the ventricular sensed or paced event creates a ventricular refractory period. On the ventricular channel after an atrial paced event, there is a cross-channel ventricular blanking period, usually followed by a crosstalk safety pacing window and an alert period

rate setting timing interval is used. This timing interval defines the maximum length of time that may occur between two paced beats, an intrinsic beat and a paced beat, or two intrinsic beats. The interval is based on the low rate limit; if the low rate limit is set at 60 bpm, a heartbeat (either paced or intrinsic) should occur approximately every second. If the low rate limit is set at 50 bpm, a heartbeat should occur approximately every 1.2–1.3 seconds. If the end of the timing interval is reached and no heartbeat occurs, the generator sends a pacing impulse to the heart. The sequence of events is:

- The timing circuit in the generator is activated.
- The sensing circuit monitors for a heartbeat to occur before the end of the programmed low rate limit timing interval.
- If a heartbeat occurs before the end of the programmed interval, the pacing function is inhibited, and the pacemaker generator does not deliver a pacing impulse to the heart.
- The timing circuit resets.
- Following a brief refractory period, the sensing circuit monitors for the occurrence of another heartbeat within the programmed interval.
- If another normal heartbeat does not occur before the end of the programmed interval, the pacing function is not inhibited, and the pacemaker delivers a pacing impulse through the pacemaker lead to the heart.
- The timing circuit again resets.
- Following a brief refractory period, the sensing circuit monitors to determine if another heartbeat occurs before the end of the programmed interval.
- This cycle repeats continuously.

## ADVANCED PACEMAKER FUNCTIONS

In addition to the basic functions required by demand pacing, modern pacemakers may be equipped with advanced features and programmable options. These include a rate adaptive or rate responsive feature and magnet mode.

### Rate Responsive Pacing

In the past, a drawback of many permanent pacemakers was the inability of the devices to increase the rate of pacing to meet increased metabolic demands of the body. Only one pacemaker, the dual chamber pacemaker (coded DDD), had the ability to vary pacing rates (Fig. 29.16). However, in order for the dual chamber pacemaker to increase its rate, the patient's SA node had to be functioning normally. Because many people who required pacemaker therapy did not have intact SA node function, this DDD capability was of limited value.

To provide an artificial substitute for the chemical, neural, and hormonal factors that normally increase the heart rate by stimulating the SA node, researchers developed a rate adaptive or rate responsive feature for permanent pacemakers. With the rate responsive feature, the pacemaker can increase or decrease its pacing rate in response to an identifiable parameter that reflects increased activity or increased metabolic demands. In an attempt to identify the most accurate and stable indicator for rate changes, researchers initially explored a wide variety of indicators, including minute ventilation, body temperature, changes in pH, changes in venous oxygen saturation in the body, increased stroke volume, changes in force of contraction, changes in respiratory rate, changes in skeletal muscle activity and increased body motion. Activity is the most commonly employed rate indicator. The activity

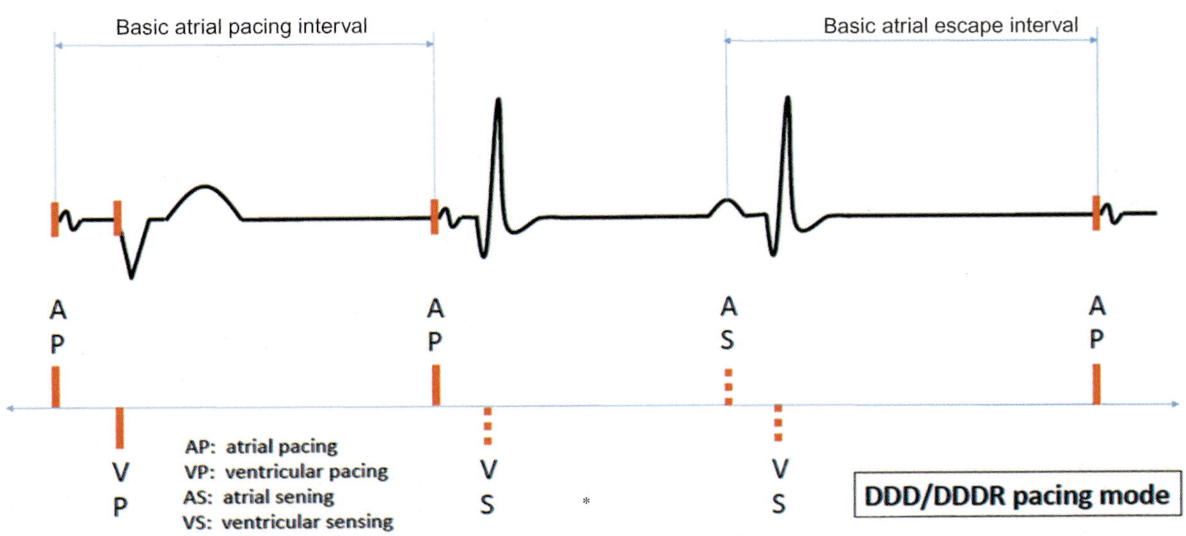


*Typical electrocardiographic feature: The DDD mode can pace or sense both atria and ventricles. Atrial pacing occurs if there is no native atrial activity for set time. Ventricular pacing occurs if there is no native ventricular activity for set tiem. Spontaneous atrial activity or atrial pacing is synchronized to the ventricular activity by using a programmable AV delay.

**Fig. 29.16:** Diagram explains the rate responsive pacing in DDD type of pacemaker sensor is a piezoelectric crystal (i.e. vibration sensor) or accelerometer (i.e. acceleration sensor) that senses vibration from motion. When the activity sensor detects increased activity, the generator responds by increasing the pacing rate according to programmed parameters. When the activity sensor detects that activity has decreased, the generator is programmed to respond by lowering the rate to a preset level. Careful programming is a critical task to ensure that the rate responsive feature functions appropriately. To facilitate optimal programming, the software in newer generators allows for initial programming of the rate response along with subsequent automatic adjustments of the parameters. These generators also have the capability for physicians to retrieve data from the pacemaker to assess the adequacy/functioning of the rate responsive programming. In addition to a low rate limit and a low rate interval setting, a rate responsive pacemaker is programmed with a high rate limit setting. This high rate limit is the highest or fastest rate at which the pacemaker will pace the heart in response to data from the rate responsive sensor that an increase in heart rate is needed. In addition, the rate responsive feature is programmed with tiered rates correlated to activity levels. This often includes the resting rate and the average daily living rate. The rate responsive feature can be included in most types of demand pacemakers (single or dual chamber). Inclusion of the rate responsive feature involves additional costs, both for the sensor and for the programming. However, the benefits of rate responsive pacing as compared to nonrate responsive function include an improved ability to complete activities of daily living, provision of a heart rate that is appropriate (i.e. neither too fast nor too slow) for a given activity level, increased quality of life for the person who requires permanent pacing and increased activity tolerance.

## Magnet Mode

Pacemakers are now available with a programmable feature referred to as the 'magnet mode.' When programmed 'on,' the magnet mode allows the programmed functioning of the pacemaker to be altered temporarily by the direct, noninvasive application of a magnet over the pacemaker generator. A pacemaker's specific response to the application of a magnet is established by the pacemaker manufacturer and will vary among different pacemaker types and brands (Fig. 29.17 and Table 29.1).

Generally, the expected response of a given pacemaker to application of a magnet should be known before the magnet is applied. Application of a magnet to a single chamber pacemaker always results in a change in pacing mode from demand to asynchronous pacing. In asynchronous mode, the sensing function is temporarily turned off, and the pacemaker generator is programmed to deliver a pacing impulse through the pacing lead at a regular interval and rate that do not vary. The term 'magnet rate' is sometimes used to describe the rate at which the

**Table 29.1:** Clinical applications of magnet on implanted cardiac device

| **Permanent pacemaker** |
|---|
| • Break pacemaker-mediated tachycardia |
| • Prevent pacing inhibition from electromagnetic interference |
| • Demonstrate ability to pace |
| • Electrocardiograph storage (electrogram mode) |
| **Implantable cardioverter-defibrillator** |
| • Cessation of inappropriate shocks |
| • Inhibit antitachycardia therapy during procedures with electromagnetic interference |

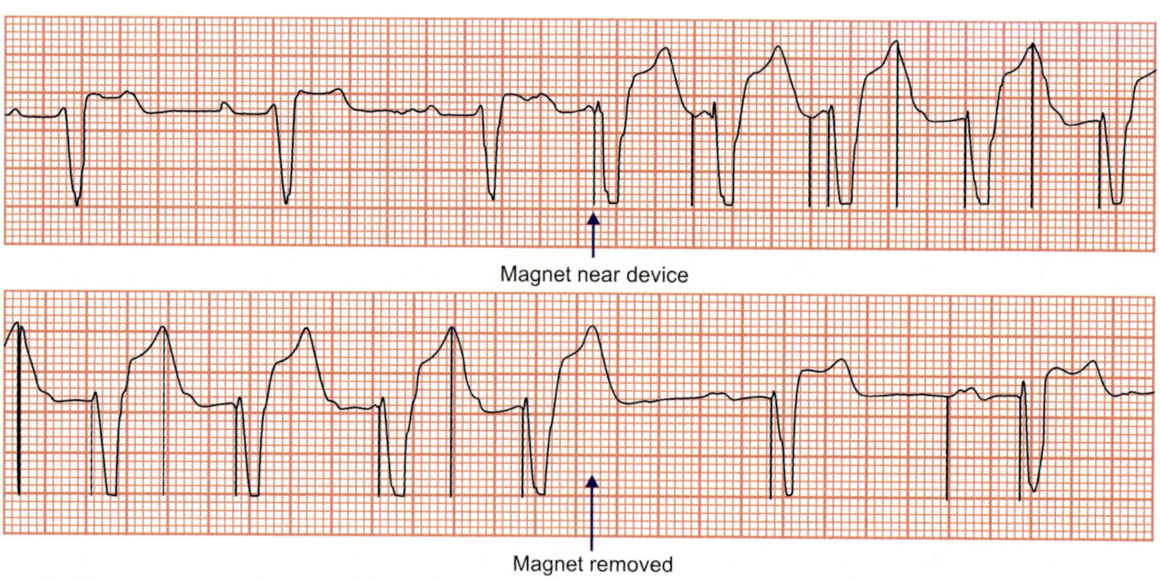


**Fig. 29.17:** Example of asynchronous pacing induced when a portable headphone was placed on a patient's chest overlying the pacemaker (top arrow 'magnet near device'). Removal of the headphone (bottom arrow 'magnet removed') resulted in an immediate return of normal pacemaker function

pacemaker paces the heart during the application of the magnet. The magnet rate may be used to evaluate the status of the pacemaker battery. As the battery voltage declines, the magnet rate will change. It is important to know the magnet rate for each specific pacemaker, as magnet rates vary greatly from manufacturer to manufacturer and even from one device to another produced by the same manufacturer.

## PACEMAKER CODING

Many types of permanent pacemakers are available. To facilitate and standardize communication about the types of pacemakers and pacemaker functions, a standardized coding system was developed through the work of the North American Society of Pacing and Electrophysiology (NASPE) and the British Pacing and Electrophysiology Group (BPEG) (Table 29.2).

The NASPE/BPEG system, commonly referred to as the NBG code, consists of up to 5 letter positions. The first three letter positions describe the antibradycardic functions of a pacemaker, the fourth addresses the rate responsive feature, and the fifth letter position designates the presence and location of multisite pacing. In the clinical setting, the first three letters are commonly used alone to describe anti-bradycardia pacemakers. If the pacemaker has additional features, the fourth and fifth letters are added.

### First Letter

The first letter in the pacemaker code (i.e. the 'first position') identifies which chamber(s) of the heart are paced by the pacemaker. 'A' refers to atrium, 'V' to ventricle, 'D' to both atrium and ventricle (or 'dual'), and 'O' if no pacing occurs.

### Second Letter

The second letter refers to which chamber, if any, the pacemaker can sense electrical activity. The same notation applies—'A' for atrial sensing, 'V' for ventricular sensing, 'D' for dual sensing in both atrium and ventricle, and 'O' to indicate no sensing if the pacemaker does not sense in any chamber of the heart.

### Third Letter

The third letter of the code describes the pacemaker's response to sensed electrical activity in the heart—'O' for no response, 'I' for inhibited, 'T' for triggered, and 'D' for dual triggered and inhibited response. These modes of response will be explained in more detail in the sections on specific types of pacemakers.

### Fourth Letter

The fourth letter is commonly used to indicate the presence of a rate modulation or rate responsive feature in the pacemaker. If the pacemaker is capable of increasing heart rate based on the body's metabolic demands, the fourth letter is coded 'R' for rate responsive. If the pacemaker is not capable of increasing the paced heart rate in response to the body's demands, the fourth letter may be omitted or coded 'O'.

### Fifth Letter

In its 2002 update of the NBG code, the task force changed the fifth letter position to designate the location or the absence of multisite pacing. The notation is:

- 'O' if the pacemaker does not have multisite pacing
- 'A' if there is
  - a pacing stimulation site present in both right and left atrium
  - more than one pacing stimulation site present in either the right or left atrium
  - pacing stimulation sites present in both atria with more than one pacing stimulation site present in either the right or left atrium or both
- 'V' if there is
  - a pacing stimulation site present in both right and left ventricles
  - more than one pacing stimulation site present in either the right or left ventricle
  - pacing stimulation sites present in both ventricles with more than one pacing stimulation site present in either the right or left ventricle or both
- 'D' if multisite pacing is present in both the atria and ventricles in any combination of A and V multi-site pacing.

### *Pacing Sites*

The pacing sites are shown in Figures 29.18–29.23.

- **Transvenous:** The most common site. Pacing wire passed into RA, RV or rarely into coronary sinus (to pace LA).
- **Epicardial:** Mainly used following cardiac surgery. Leads attached directly to epicardial surface of atrium and/or ventricle.
- **Transcutaneous:** Use of larger electrodes. improved patient tolerance can sense and deliver adequate

**Table 29.2:** The revised NASPE/BPEG generic code for antibradycardia pacing

| I | II | III | IV | V |
|---|---|---|---|---|
| Chamber(s) paced pacing | Chamber(s) sensed | Response to sensing | Rate modulation | Multisite |
| O = None | O = None | O = None | O = None | O = None |
| A = Atrium | A = Atrium | T = Triggered | R = Rate modulation | A = Atrium |
| V = Ventricle | V = Ventricle | I = Inhibited | | V = Ventricle |
| D = Dual (A+V) | D = Dual (A+V) | D = Dual (T+I) | | D = Dual (A+V) |

NASPE=North American Society of Pacing Electrophysiology; BPEG=British Pacing and Electrophysiology Group

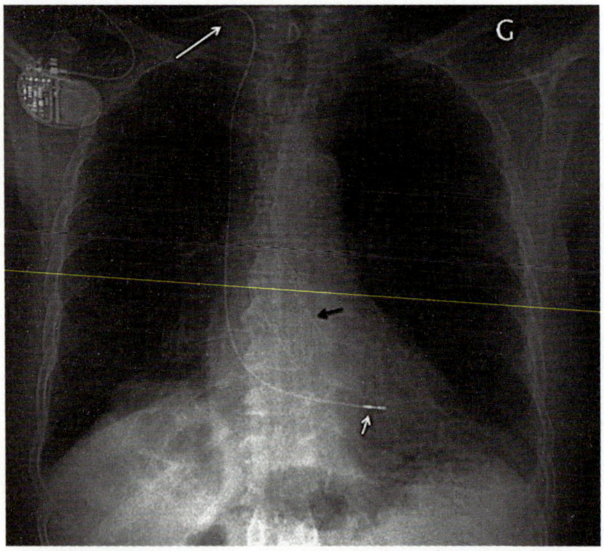


**Fig. 29.18:** X-ray chest PA view showing pacing lead in the right ventricular apex in transvenous pacing mode

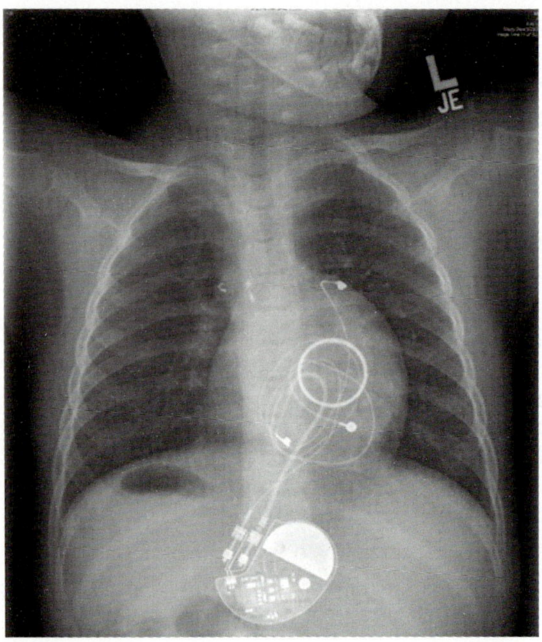


**Fig. 29.19:** Epicardial pacemaker in a patient with complex congenital heart disease

adjustable current outputs (50–150 mA) and stimuli of long duration (10–40 msec) some patients still experience significant paintemporary measure has rendered

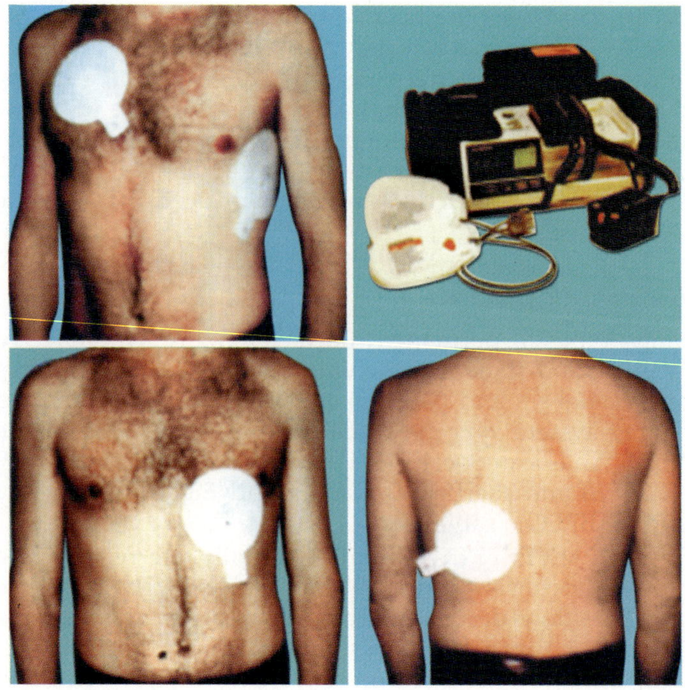

**Fig. 29.20:** Photographs showing the equipment (right upper) and placement of leads in the application of transcutaneous external temporary pacemaker

prophylactic temporary transvenous pacing redundant in most situations transcutaneous pacing (TCP), also called external pacing, is recommended for the initial stabilization of hemodynamically significant bradycardias of all types. The procedure is performed by placing two pacing pads on the patient's chest, either in the anterior/lateral position or the anterior/posterior position. The rescuer selects the pacing rate, and gradually increases the pacing current (measured in mA) until electrical capture (characterized by a wide QRS complex with a tall, broad T-wave on the ECG) is achieved, with a corresponding pulse. Pacing artifact on the ECG and severe muscle twitching may make this determination difficult. External pacing should not be relied upon for an extended period of time. It is an emergency procedure that acts as a bridge until transvenous pacing or other therapies can be applied.

- **Transthoracic myocardial puncture:** Dangerous and unreliable.
- **Transoesophageal atrial pacing:** Safe and effective in refractory atrial flutter. Probably be replaced by TCP in most situations.

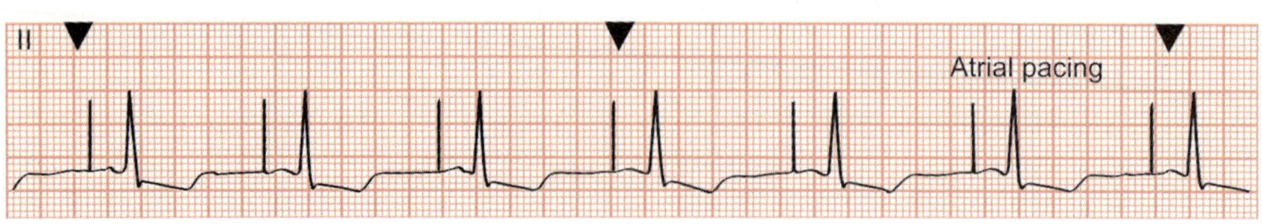


**Fig. 29.21:** This ECG strip is of atrial pacing in a patient with an intact interventricular conduction system. Generally, the pacemaker will behave in this way when the sinus node is not functioning well enough to provide adequate rate for the patient, and the conduction system from the AV node down is functioning properly

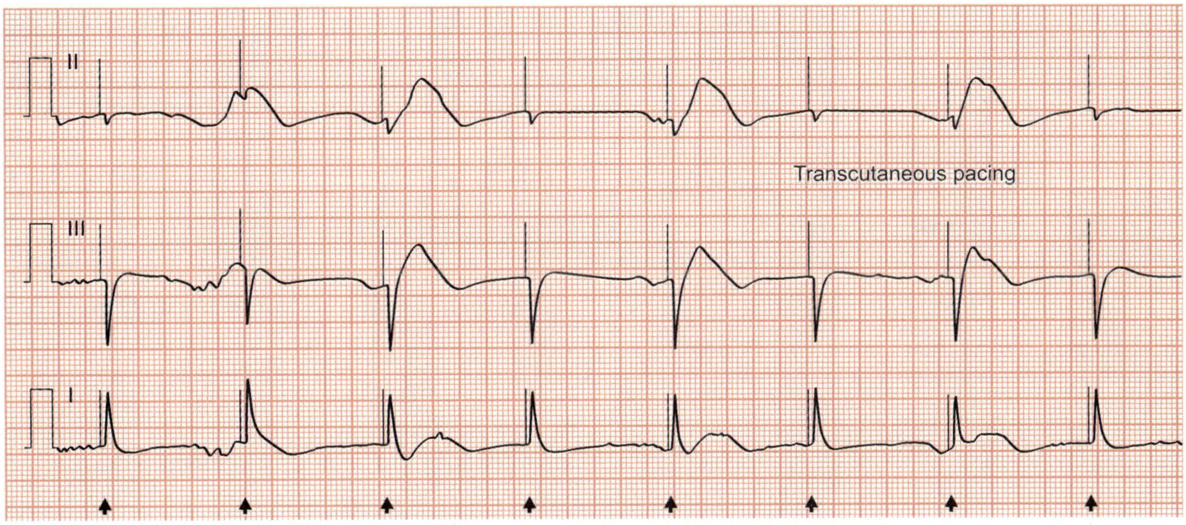


**Fig. 29.22:** Transcutaneous pacing (TCP) with true electrical capture as evidenced by tall, broad T-waves. Capture was achieved at 110 mA. Transcutaneous cardiac pacing is an effective procedure for patients with bradycardia unresponsive to drug therapy third-degree heart block, Mobitz type II second-degree heart block, when hemodynamically unstable or operation planned, overdrive pacing and asystole

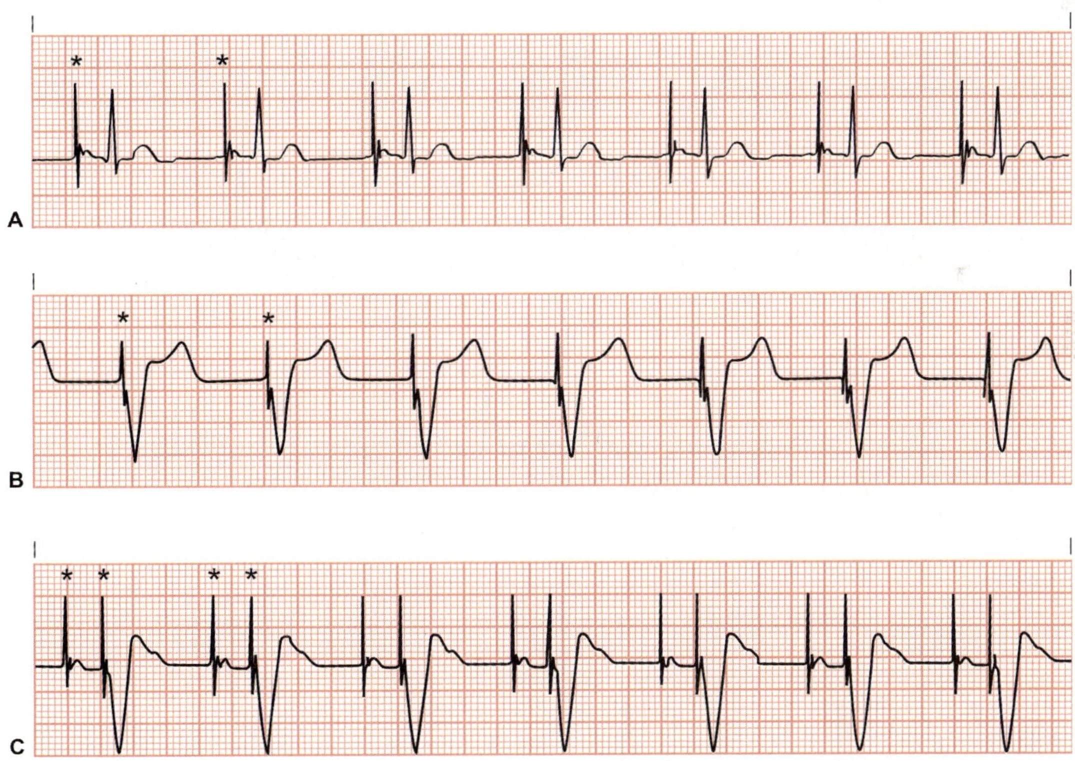


**Fig. 29.23:** Pacing examples. (A) Atrial pacing; (B) ventricular pacing; (C) dual-chamber pacing. Each asterisk represents a pacemaker impulse

## TYPES OF ANTIBRADYCARDIA PACEMAKERS

The most common types of antibradycardia pacemakers in use are atrial demand pacemakers, ventricular demand pacemakers, dual chamber pacemakers and ventricular-paced/dual-sensing single chamber pacemakers.

### Pacing Modes

Pacing modes are shown in Figures 29.24–29.30.

- **AAI:** Indicated for sinus bradycardia provided AV conduction is intact. It has the advantage of maintaining AV synchrony.

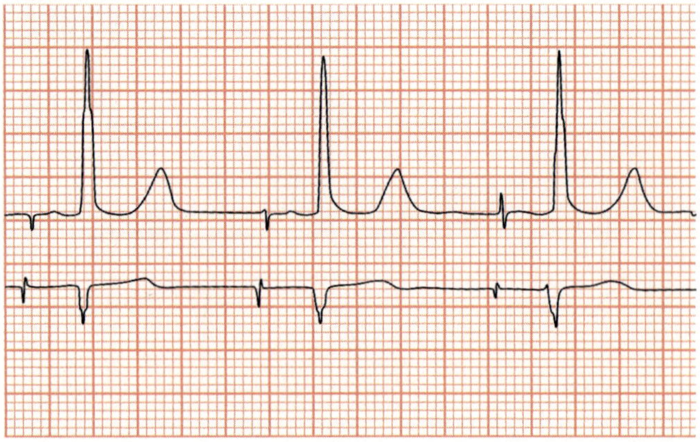

**Fig. 29.24:** VVI—most commonly used mode of choice in life-threatening bradyarrhythmias

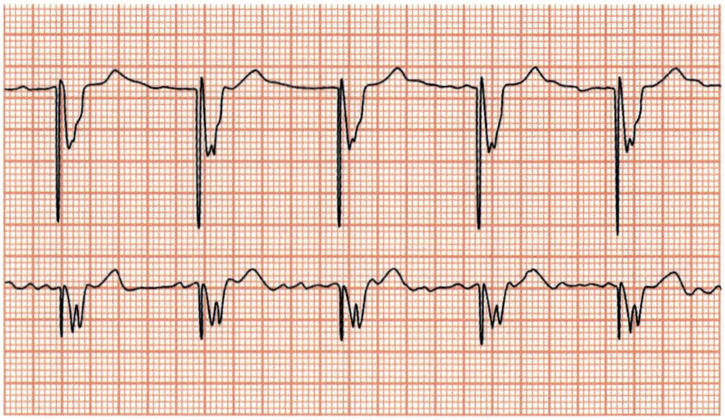

**Fig. 29.25:** Ventricular pacing in atrial fibrillation showing one spike producing a wide QRS (ventricular capture)

- **DDD:** P-wave inhibits atrial output. If it is conducted normally then ventricular output is also inhibited. If not, then ventricle is paced after a delay If there is no P-wave atrium is paced with ventricular pacing occurring after a delay if the atrial pacing impulse is not conducted to the ventricle upper rate limit needs to be set to prevent the pacemaker from following excessive atrial activity with paced ventricular responses self-inhibition can be prevented by introducing a ventricular blank (refractory) period coinciding with atrial pacing stimulus re-entry pacemaker mediated tachycardia possible (*see* above).
- **DDI:** Recently introduced and is available in some external pacemakers useful in patients with SA node dysfunction and episodes of atrial tachyarrhythmias. During atrial tachyarrhythmias pacemaker paces ventricle at back-up rate and will not track tachyarrhy-

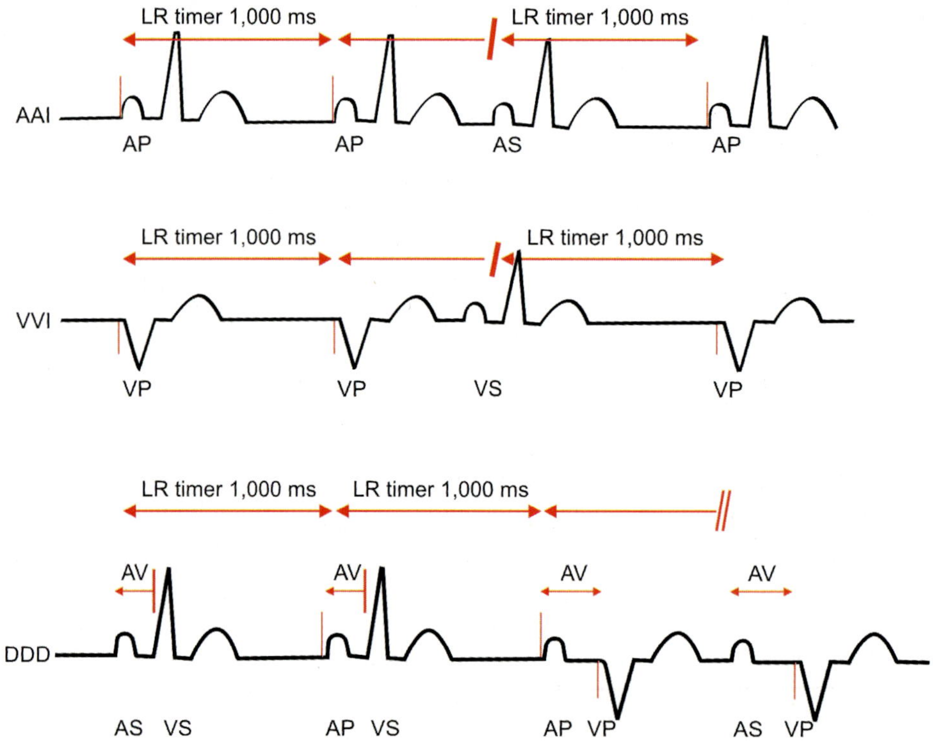


**Fig. 29.26:** Timing of events in various pacing modes. AAI is an atrial nontracking mode of pacing that provides backup atrial pacing at the programmed lower rate limit. Similarly, VVI is a ventricular nontracking mode of pacing that provides backup ventricular pacing at the programmed lower rate limit. DDD is a dual-chamber mode of pacing that can both inhibit and trigger events in both the atrium and the ventricle. AS=atrial-sensed event; AP=atrial-paced event; VS=ventricular-sensed event; VP=ventricular-paced event; LR=lower rate limit

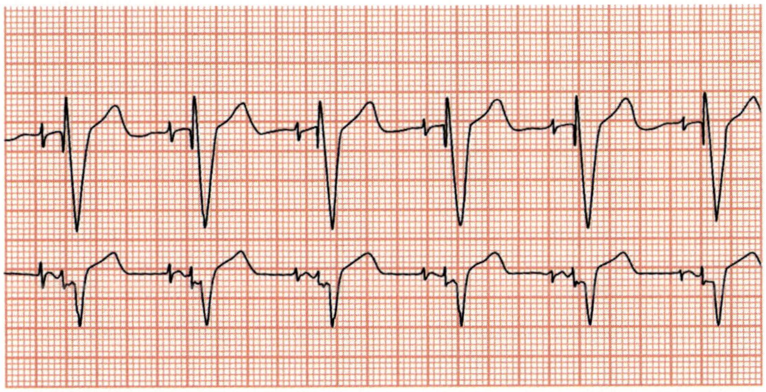

**Fig. 29.27:** VDD–atrial synchronous ventricular inhibited sensed P-wave triggers ventricular pacing indicated for high degree AV block with normal sinus rhythm re-entry pacemaker mediated tachycardias possible. Commonly initiated by a ventricular premature beat which is conducted retrogradely to the atria. Here it is sensed by the atrial channel and ventricle is paced. This impulse in turn is conducted to the atria. Conversion to asynchronous (non-sensing) mode or increasing the pacemaker atrial refractory period will prevent this problem

thmia re-entry pacemaker mediated tachycardia not possible

- **Rate modulation:** Designed so that pacemaker can mimic response of normal heart rate to increased metabolic need most commonly used systems incorporate sensors of respiratory rate (changes in thoracic impedance) or movement and therefore in many cases will not increase rate appropriately in response to critical illness.

## SINGLE CHAMBER ATRIAL DEMAND PACEMAKERS

Coded AAI or AAIR, a single chamber atrial pacemaker consists of a generator and one pacing/sensing lead. The lead is positioned in the right atrium. A single chamber atrial pacer is used when the SA node is not firing properly

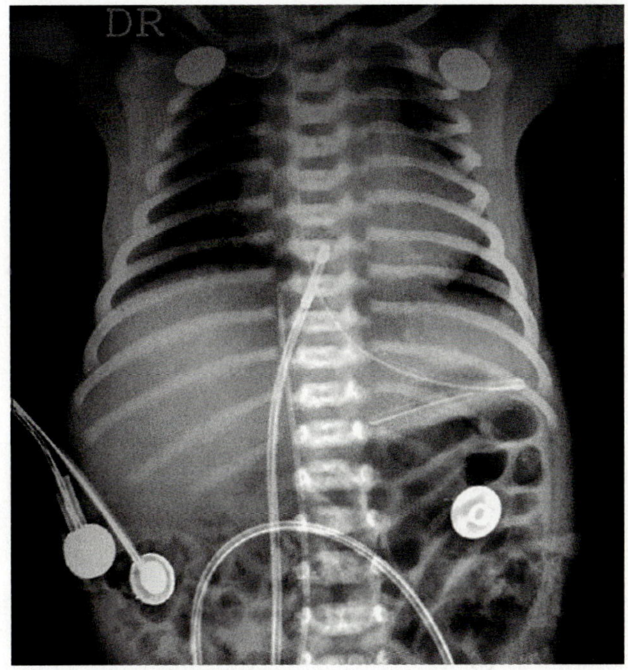


**Fig. 29.29:** Radiograph depicting the pacing wire with the tip correctly positioned in the right atrium with French pacing wire inserted through umbilical venous route

but the rest of the heart's conduction system is working correctly. Single chamber atrial demand pacemakers are capable of sensing and responding to electrical activity in the atrium. The single lead positioned in the atrium is capable of sensing the heart's electrical activity and delivering a pacing shock to the muscle of the right atrium to trigger depolarization. The AAI/AAIR pacemaker is programmed to sense when the heartbeat drops to less than the programmed low rate setting. When needed, the pacing lead delivers a pacing impulse to the right atrium; the right atrium depolarizes, and the wave of depolarization spreads to the left atrium and down to the AV node, just above the

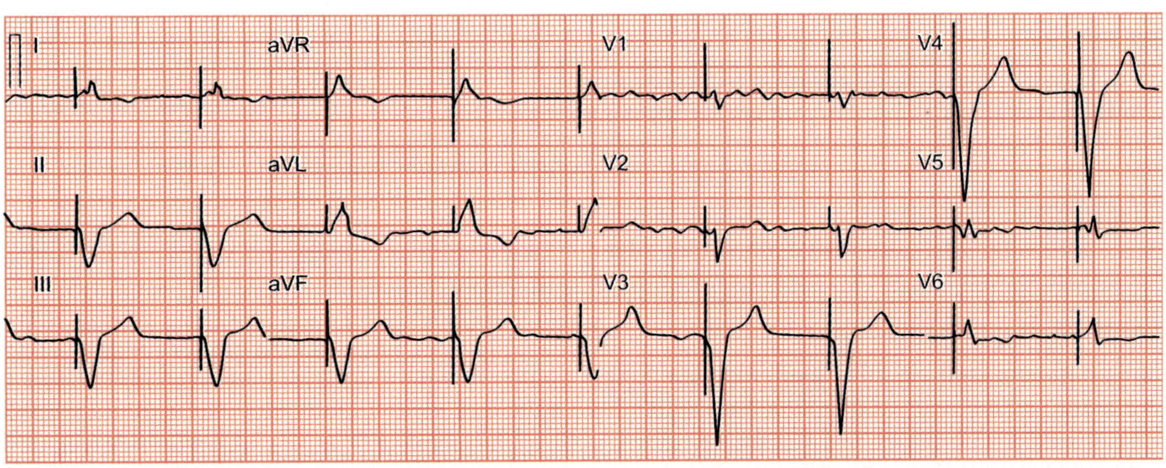


**Fig. 29.28:** The ventricular (QRS) rhythm is completely regular because of ventricular pacing. However, the underlying rhythm is atrial fibrillation. Fibrillatory waves are small in amplitude in most leads and best seen in lead V1. Most computer ECG interpretations will read this as 'ventricular pacing' without noting atrial fibrillation

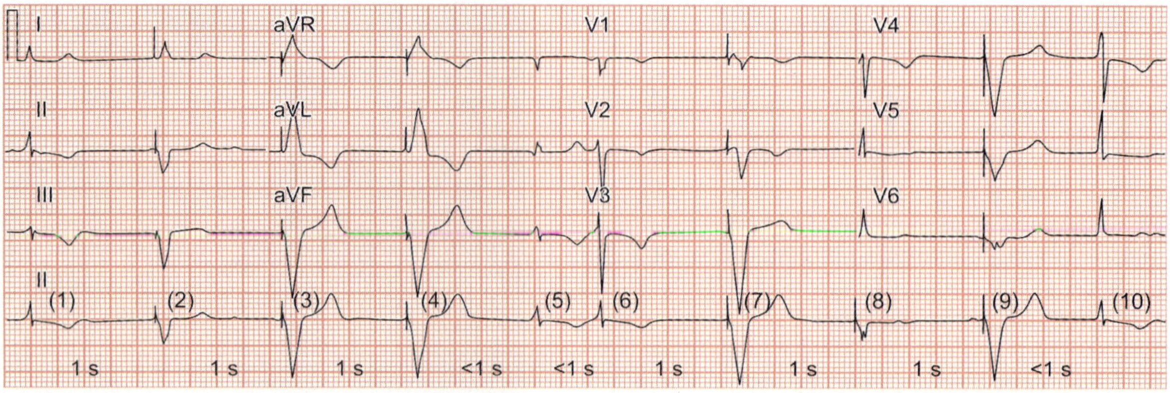


**Fig. 29.30:** As noted, modern pacemakers are programmed in the on-demand mode providing pacing support only when needed. In the case of a single-chamber pacemaker this function is accomplished by specifying the lower rate limit (For example 60 beats/min). The pacemaker constantly monitors the patient's heart rate in the implanted chamber on a beat to beat basis. Any time the rate drops below the lower rate limit (in the case of 60/min, the critical pause after aspontaneous QRS complex will be >1 sec), the pacemaker will deliver a pacing stimulus

ventricles. The impulse is conducted normally through the AV node and the remainder of the conducting system; depolarization of the ventricles occurs, followed by normal contraction. When the AAI/AAIR pacemaker senses a normal atrial impulse initiated by the SA node, the generator is inhibited and refrains from delivering an atrial pacing impulse. Because the atrial demand pacemaker does sense electrical activity in the atria, it is not an appropriate choice to use for persons with chaotic atrial rhythms, such as atrial fibrillation and atrial flutter. Chaotic atrial activity confuses the pacemaker's sensor and results in either inappropriate pacing or inappropriate inhibition of pacing. A single chamber atrial pacemaker also cannot be used if the patient's AV node is functioning abnormally. The pacemaker will stimulate the atrium to depolarize; however, if there is impaired conduction in, around, or below the AV node, the impulse will not be conducted through the AV node and bundle branches. The ventricles will not depolarize and no effective contraction will occur The atrial demand pacemaker may include the rate responsive feature.

### Programmed Settings

In addition to the pacing and sensing thresholds, there are several key settings that must be programmed appropriately for an AAI pacemaker to work correctly. These include:

- Low rate limit setting
- Upper rate limit setting for rate adaptive response if rate responsive feature present.

### Normal AAI/AAIR Pacing Patterns

Normal pacing patterns that may be seen with an AAI pacemaker include:

- *Absence of paced beats:* The patient's CG tracing reflects the patient's intrinsic rhythm. The patient's heart rate remains at or above the low rate setting.
- *Intermittent paced beats:* The patient's ECG tracing shows a mixture of the patient's beats and paced beats. All paced beats come at the correct time, as determined by the low rate setting. No intervals (or pauses) occur that are longer than the low rate interval setting limit.
- *Completely paced (100%) rhythm:* The ECG tracing shows that all beats are atrially paced. For an AAI pacemaker, the patient's heart rate remains at the low rate setting. For AAIR pacemakers, the paced rate may vary between the low rate setting and the upper rate limit for rate adaptation. The paced rate does not exceed the upper rate limit.

## SINGLE CHAMBER VENTRICULAR DEMAND PACEMAKERS

A single chamber ventricular pacemaker consists of a generator and a single pacing/sensing lead. The pacemaker lead is usually passed transvenously into and through the right atrium into the right ventricle, where it is attached to the wall of the right ventricle. VVI/VVIR pacemakers are capable of sensing and responding to electrical activity in the ventricles. The single lead positioned in the right ventricle is capable of sensing the heart's electrical activity and of delivering a pacing shock to the muscle of the right ventricle to trigger depolarization. The VVI/VVIR pacemaker is programmed to sense when the heartbeat drops to less than the programmed low rate setting. When needed, the pacing lead delivers a pacing impulse to the right ventricle; the right ventricle depolarizes and the wave of depolarization spreads to the left ventricle. Depolarization of the ventricles is followed by normal contraction. When the VVI/VVIR pacemaker senses a normal ventricular depolarization impulse, the generator is inhibited and refrains from delivering a pacing impulse to the ventricles. Because a VVI/VVIR pacemaker neither paces nor senses in the atrium of the heart, there can be a loss of the normal AV synchrony. Remember that in normal conduction, the impulse coming from the SA node is slowed at the AV node to permit the atria to contract and complete ventricular filling. With a VVI/VVIR pacemaker, atrial contraction is not synchronized with ventricular contraction, and active ventricular filling may not occur. Cardiac output can drop.

For persons with congestive heart failure, the loss of AV synchrony can increase signs of reduced cardiac output and heart failure. Because VVI/VVIR pacemakers do not sense or pace in the atrium, they are often the pacemaker of choice for persons with atrial fibrillation or atrial flutter (i.e. chaotic atrial arrhythmias), which could confuse the pacemaker. VVI/VVIR pacemakers are rarely used if the patient's SA node is functioning due to loss of AV synchrony. The rate responsive feature may be included in a ventricular demand pacemaker.

### Programmed Settings

In addition to the pacing and sensing thresholds, programmable settings for VVI/VVIR pacemaker include:

- Low rate setting
- Timing interval for the low rate setting
- Upper rate limit for rate adaptation if rate responsive feature is present

### Normal VVI/VVIR Pacing Patterns

Normal pacing patterns that the patient may have with VVI/VVIR pacemaker include:

- *Total absence of paced beats:* The ECG tracing reflects the patient's intrinsic rhythm. The patient's heart rate remains at or above the low rate limit setting of the pacemaker.
- *Intermittent paced beats:* The patient's ECG tracing shows a mixture of the patient's beats and paced beats. All paced beats come at the correct time (as determined by the low rate setting). No pauses occur that are longer than the low rate interval setting limit.
- *Completely paced (100%) rhythm:* The ECG tracing shows that all beats are ventricularly paced. For a VVI pacemaker, the patient's heart rate remains at the low rate setting. For VVIR pacemakers, the paced rate may vary between the low rate setting and the upper rate limit for rate adaptation. The paced rate does not exceed the upper rate limit.

## DUAL CHAMBER PACEMAKERS

Dual chamber pacemakers are capable of pacing and sensing in both the atria and the ventricles (Figs 29.31 and 29.32). Designed to more closely mimic the normal electrical activity of the heart, the dual chamber pacemaker

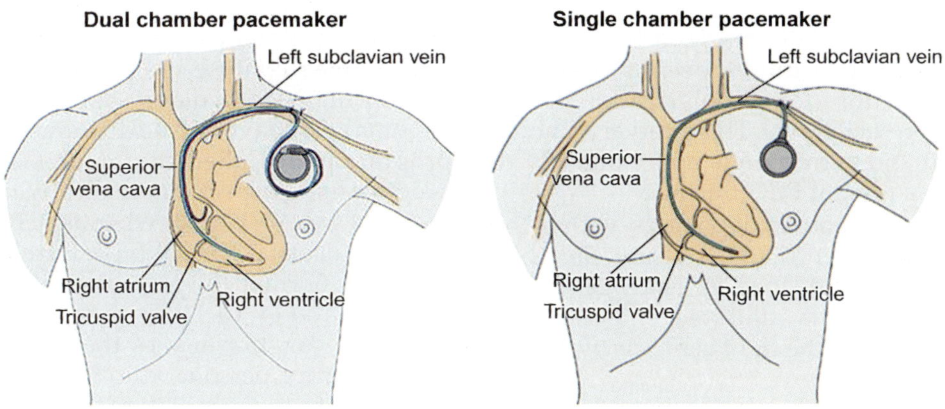


**Fig. 29.31:** Connecting leads, battery placement and ventricle paced in single and dual chamber pacemakers

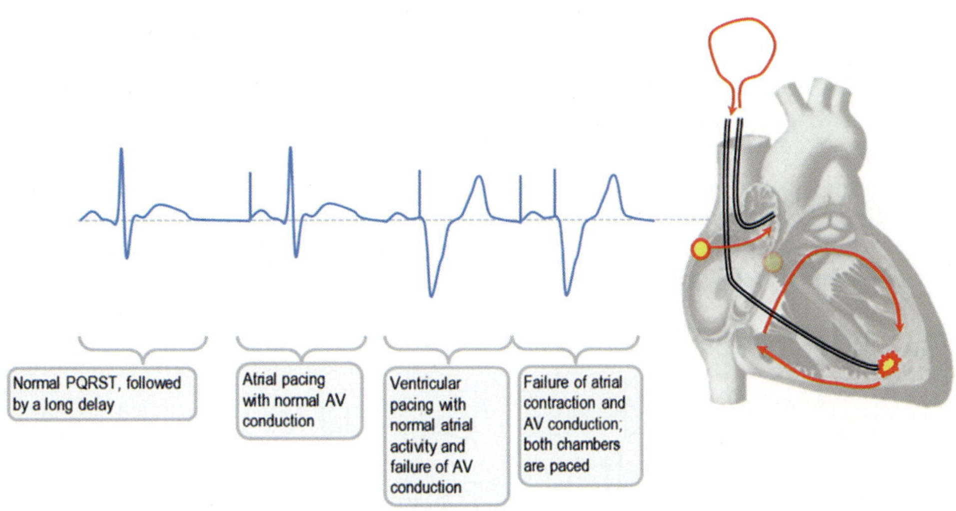


**Fig. 29.32:** An example of an AV pacemaker pacing 'on demand'

preserves the synchrony between atrial and ventricular depolarization, permitting the atria to contract and finish ventricular filling before the ventricles contract.

Coded DDD, the dual chamber pacemaker consists of a generator and two pacing leads. The electronic circuitry in the generator is more complex than the circuitry in a single chamber pacemaker. Two complete sets of circuitry are included—one for pacing and sensing in the atria and one for pacing and sensing in the ventricles. One pacing lead is positioned in the right atrium, and one in the right ventricle. The functioning of the DDD pacemaker is also more complex. The normal sequence of events in dual chamber pacing is:

- The sensing electrode in the atrium monitors for normal atrial electrical activity.
- If it senses normal electrical activity, it relays that information to the generator. The atrial pacing circuit is inhibited, and the pacemaker does not deliver a pacing impulse through the atrial pacing lead.
- If the atrial sensing electrode does not sense normal electrical activity within the preprogrammed interval, the generator delivers a pacing shock through the atrial pacing lead to the right atrium to stimulate depolarization.
- Once the atrium has been depolarized by a pacing impulse or a normal SA node firing, the sensing electrode in the ventricle monitors for depolarization of the ventricles within a preset interval. This interval is known as the AV interval and corresponds approximately to the P-R interval on a normal ECG tracing.
- If the ventricles spontaneously depolarize within the preset AV interval, the ventricular sensing electrode relays that information back to the pacemaker generator; the pacemaker generator is inhibited and does not deliver a pacing impulse to the right ventricle by way of the ventricular pacing lead.
- If the ventricles do not spontaneously depolarize within the preset AV interval, the pacemaker generator is triggered to deliver a pacing impulse through the ventricular pacing lead to the right ventricle to initiate timely depolarization of the ventricles. The ECG tracing shows a pacer spike in front of the QRS complex.

If the patient's SA node is functioning properly, a DDD pacemaker has the capability to track the SA node firing and pace the ventricles at the same rate. This capability allows the pacemaker to increase or decrease the ventricular pacing rate in response to changes in the SA node firing rate. For persons whose SA node is not working properly, a DDD pacemaker may come with the rate responsive feature. The rate responsive version is capable of increasing the atrial-pacing rate when indicated.

Dual chamber pacemakers are more expensive to implant than single chamber pacemakers. The additional cost is related to the need for a second pacing lead and the additional time needed to program the circuitry properly. However, it provides the most flexible options and has become the most common type of pacemaker implanted. Dual chamber pacemakers have several advantages as compared to single chamber pacemakers.

- As discussed earlier, the DDD pacemaker permits sequential pacing of the atria and ventricles, thereby preserving AV synchrony.
- For persons whose SA nodes are intact, the DDD pacemaker permits the pacemaker to track the patient's intrinsic SA node firing and pace the ventricles in response. This permits a 'natural' rate responsive feature very similar to the heart's normal conducting system.

As DDD pacemakers track electrical activity in the atria, they traditionally had not been implanted in persons with chronic chaotic atrial rhythms, such as atrial fibrillation or atrial flutter. Because the pacemaker can track atrial activity and pace the ventricles in response, the chaotic atrial activity may confuse the pacemaker or lead to inappropriately high ventricular responses. However, newer DDD pacemakers have an additional feature that may be programmed. Called the mode-switching feature, this programming aspect automatically causes the pacemaker to revert to a VVI mode when the circuitry recognizes the presence of atrial fibrillation or flutter. When atrial rhythm returns to normal, the programming automatically returns the pacemaker to DDD mode. The automatic mode switching function makes the DDD pacemaker a useful pacemaker for persons, who have paroxysmal, infrequent episodes of atrial fibrillation.

### Normal Pacing Patterns

Normal pacing patterns (Fig. 29.33) seen with a DDD pacemaker include:

- *Total absence of paced beats:* The patient's heart rate remains at or above the low atrial rate limit setting.
- *Intermittent paced beats:* The patient's ECG tracing shows a combination of paced beats and intrinsic beats. The precise configuration of the paced beats may vary depending on what chamber of the heart is being paced. The patient's heart rate remains at or above the low rate

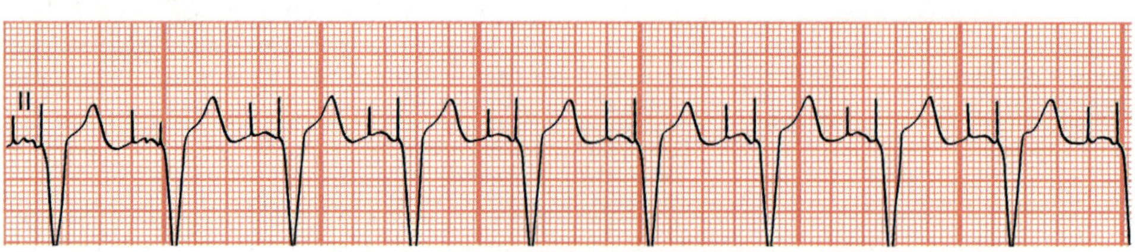


**Fig. 29.33:** ECG trace showing normal pacing in dual chamber pacing system

limit setting. No pauses occur that exceed the timing interval for the low rate limit setting.
- *Completely paced (100%) rhythm:* The ECG shows all beats paced; the precise configuration of paced rhythm may vary depending on which chamber(s) are paced. The heart rate should not drop to less than low atrial rate limit setting. If the patient's SA node is functioning, the heart rate may vary between the low and upper rate limit settings. If the rate adaptation is present, the rate may vary between the low rate limit setting and upper limit for rate adaptation.

### Programmed Settings for DDD/DDDR Pacemakers

Settings that are programmed for the DDD/DDDR pacemaker include:
- Low rate setting for atrial pacing
- Low rate setting interval (i.e. length of time permitted between one atrial depolarization and the next)
- The AV interval (i.e. length of time permitted between atrial depolarization and initiation of ventricular depolarization)
- Upper rate limit setting for ventricular tracking of SA node firing
- If rate adaptive feature is present, high rate limit for rate responsive pacing.

## ATRIAL SENSING VENTRICULAR PACEMAKERS

The single-lead, atrial-sensing ventricular pacemaker is a relatively recent development in pacemaker technology. Coded VDD, it is capable of pacing the ventricles only, but it can sense electrical activity in both the atrium and the ventricle. Like other single chamber pacemakers, it consists of a generator and one pacing/sensing pacemaker lead. It is appropriate for use in people whose sinus node is intact and who do not have atrial hypertrophy. Atrial hypertrophy is a significant risk factor for the eventual development of atrial fibrillation or atrial flutter. A VDD pacemaker provides AV synchrony. The tip of the pacing lead is positioned in the right ventricle; it has the ability to sense electrical activity in the ventricle and to deliver a pacing impulse to the ventricular wall. The pacing lead also contains a pair of electrodes that are capable only of sensing electrical activity. When the tip of the pacing lead is properly positioned in the right ventricle, these sensing electrodes fall within the right atrium. They sense atrial depolarization but cannot fire a pacing impulse to the atrium. The response of the VDD to sensed electrical events is both triggered and inhibited. When the sensing electrodes in the atrium sense atrial depolarization, they relay that information to the generator. The generator is programmed to wait a preprogrammed interval to determine if the atrial impulse triggers ventricular response. If the sensing electrode in the ventricle does not pick up a ventricular response within the defined interval, the generator triggers the discharge of a pacing impulse back through the pacing lead to the right ventricle. If the sensing electrode in the ventricle picks up a ventricular response to the atrial impulse, the generator is inhibited and no pacing impulse is fired. A VDD pacemaker provides for a physiological rate increase. Because it senses in the atrium, it can increase the rate of ventricular pacing as needed to keep up with an increase in SA node depolarizations. If the patient's own SA node firing fails to occur, the VDD pacemaker will pace the ventricles at the low rate setting. Because it only contains a single lead, it is easier to implant than a dual chamber device. VDD pacemakers do not come with a rate responsive feature. Because the VDD pacemaker does sense and respond to atrial activity, it is not an appropriate pacemaker to implant for a patient with chaotic atrial electrical activity, such as atrial fibrillation or atrial flutter (Fig. 29.34).

### Normal Pacing Patterns

Normal pacing patterns seen with a VDD pacemaker include:
- *Total absence of paced beats:* The patient's ECG reflects the patient's intrinsic heart rhythm, and the patient's

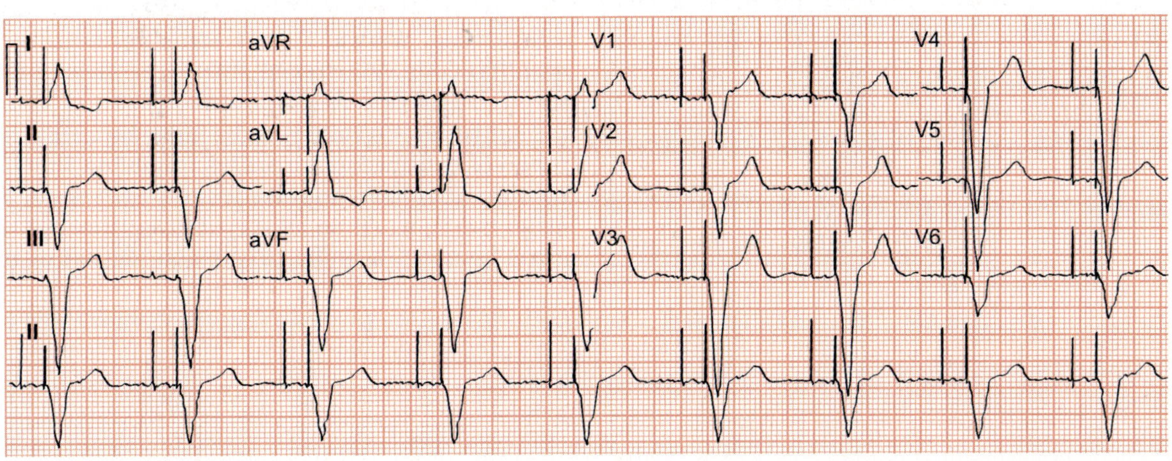


**Fig. 29.34:** Paced beat morphology in dual-chamber pacemaking. Both atrial and ventricular pacing spikes are present. The atrial pacing spike is followed by a P-wave with very low amplitude. The ventricular pacing spike is followed by a wide QRS complex with T-wave pointing in the opposite direction (discordant). The QRS after the pacing spike resembles a left bundle branch block (LBBB), with a leftward axis, consistent with pacing from the right ventricular apex

heart rate remains at or above the pacemaker's low rate setting.

- *Intermittent paced beats:* The patient's ECG tracing reflects a combination of paced beats and intrinsic rhythm. No pause occurs that lasts longer than the programmed timing interval set determined by the low rate limit setting. The patient's heart rate remains at or above the low rate setting.
- *Complete paced (100%) rhythm:* The ECG tracing reflects all paced beats. The heart rate may vary but should not drop to less than the low rate limit setting. The heart rate should not exceed the upper rate limit.

### Programmed Settings

Programmed settings (Table 29.3) for a VDD pacemaker include:

- Low rate setting for ventricular pacing
- Timing interval for the low rate setting
- Atrioventricular interval (i.e. length of time permitted between atrial depolarization and initiation of ventricular depolarization)
- Upper rate limit setting for ventricular tracking of patient's SA node firing.

## MEDICAL INDICATIONS OF ANTIBRADYCARDIA PACING

The American Heart Association (AHA) and the American College of Cardiology (ACC) have published guidelines for the implantation of cardiac pacemakers. These guidelines are based on a review of clinical findings from large, multicenter randomized clinical trials; well-designed analysis of data from smaller, nonrandomized studies or observational data registries; and the consensus opinion of experts. The guidelines address the issues of medical indications for pacing and selection of the appropriate type of pacemaker. As stated in the published guidelines, the information is reviewed annually for currency and revised (or withdrawn) as indicated. The task force that developed the guidelines separated the recommendations into categories based on the strength of the supporting evidence available. In brief, indications listed as class I are supported by evidence or general agreement that the use of pacemaker therapy for these patients is beneficial, useful and effective. Class II indications are those that have conflicting evidence and/or a difference in expert opinion about the usefulness and efficacy of permanent pacemaker therapy. Class III lists conditions that, according to available evidence and/or expert opinion, would not benefit from implantation of a permanent pacemaker. The focus of the task force's work was on the appropriate use of permanent pacemakers, not the overall management of cardiac arrhythmias (Table 29.4).

**Table 29.3:** Programmable parameters

| Basic parameters | Desirable programmability |
|---|---|
| • Stimulation mode | • AV-interval hysteresis |
| • Stimulation rate | • Atrial refractory time extension |
| • Hysteretic | • Semi-commited mode |
| • Pulse amplitude and width | • Nonphysiologic AV interval |
| • Sensitivity | • Diagnostic functions |
| • Refractory period | • Event marker |
| • AV interval | • Interval marker |
| • URL | • Stimulus threshold detection test |
| • Blanking period | • Event counter |
| • Polarity | • Intracavitary electrogram |

## SYMPTOMATIC BRADYCARDIA

The most common class I indication for implantation of a permanent pacemaker is symptomatic bradycardia. Symptomatic bradycardia (Fig. 29.35) is defined as a documented bradyarrhythmia that significantly reduces cerebral flow and results in symptoms of syncope, near syncope, light-headedness, dizziness or confusion. Patients with symptomatic bradycardia are often diagnosed after they seek medical attention following a fall, 'black-out' spell, or recurrent episodes of dizziness or near fainting.

As noted, the major signs and symptoms of symptomatic bradycardia are syncope, near syncope, confusion, light-headedness and/or dizziness during a bradyarrhythmia. In addition to the major definitive symptoms of cerebral hypoperfusion, persons with symptomatic bradycardia may also experience hypotension, fatigue, signs of congestive heart failure, shortness of breath and exercise intolerance. Specific diagnosis of symptomatic bradycardia can be challenging. The bradyarrhythmia and the symptoms should occur simultaneously and their simultaneous occurrence should be clearly documented through appropriate diagnostic tests.

Symptomatic bradycardia may be caused by a wide range of conduction disorders involving the SA node, the conduction of the impulse from the SA node through the atria, the conduction of the impulse through the various areas of the AV node, or the conduction of the impulse

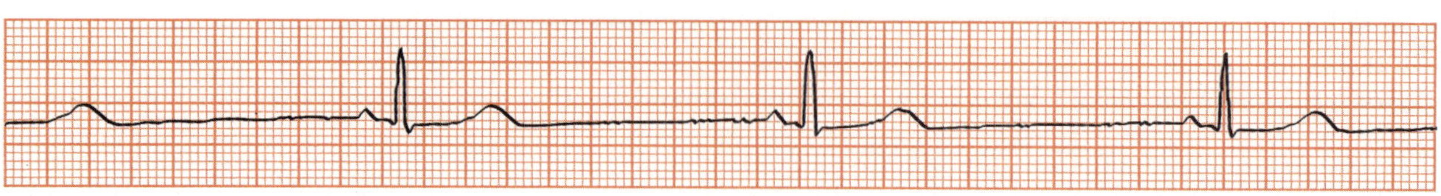

**Fig. 29.35:** An elderly patient with symptomatic bradycardia with a h/o a fall, 'black-out' spell, and recurrent episodes of dizziness or near fainting

| **Table 29.4:** Indications for permanent pacing (modified from ACC/AHA guidelines) | | |
|---|---|---|
| Acquired AV block | Class I | Third-degree AV block associated with symptoms due to bradycardia, asystole of >3s or escape rate <40 bpm |
| | | Second-degree block with symptomatic bradycardia |
| | Class II | Asymptomatic third degree AV block or type II second degree block |
| | | Asymptomatic type I second degree block with infra-His block |
| | Class III | Asymptomatic first-degree block |
| | | AV block expected to resolve, e.g. drug toxicity |
| Chronic bifascicular and trifascicular block | Class I | Intermittent third degree AV block |
| | | Type II second degree AV block |
| | Class II | Syncope not proved to be due to AV block, e.g. VT |
| | | Incidental finding of infra-His block |
| | Class III | Asymptomatic with or without first degree AV block |
| After acute phase of myocardial infarction | Class I | Persistent third degree AV block |
| | | Persistent second degree AV block with bundle branch block or symptoms |
| | | Transient second or third degree AV block with bundle branch block |
| | Class II | Persistent second degree AV block at nodal level |
| | | Transient AV block without bundle branch block |
| | Class III | Persistent first-degree AV block |
| Sinus node dysfunction | Class I | Documented bradycardia with symptoms |
| | | Chronotropic incompetence with symptoms |
| | Class II | Symptoms and bradycardia <40 bpm but not correlated |
| | Class III | Asymptomatic bradycardia |
| | | Symptoms documented not due to bradycardia |
| | | Symptoms from non-essential drug therapy |
| Carotid sinus syndrome | Class I | Syncope caused by carotid stimulation with > 3S asystole |
| | Class II | Syncope with cardioinhibitory response without clear precipitants |
| | | Syncope with cardioinhibitory response in tilt table testing |
| | Class III | Cardioinhibitory response without severe symptoms |

ACC=American College of Cardiology; AHA=American Heart Association

through the Bundle of His and the bundle branches. The major arrhythmias responsible for symptomatic bradycardia are sick sinus syndrome and second- and third-degree AV block.

### Sinus Node Dysfunction

Sinus node dysfunction occurs when the sinoatrial (SA) node is unable to pace the heart normally. Referred to as sick sinus syndrome, sinus node dysfunction encompasses a group of disorders that include:

- Chronotropic incompetence, or the inability of the sinus node to increase the rate of firing in response to increased metabolic demands or activity
- Reduced ability of the SA node to generate an action potential and depolarize
- Slowed or Blocked conduction of the electrical impulse from the SA node to the specialized conducting pathways in the atria
- Slowed or Blocked conduction of the sinus impulse through the atria to the AV node

*Signs and symptoms of sinus node dysfunction include:*

- *Sinus bradycardia:* Sinus bradycardia in sinus node dysfunction can become quite severe; the heart rate may drop to less than 40–50 bpm and create symptoms of decreased cardiac output and decreased cerebral perfusion. Sinus bradycardia in sick sinus syndrome is refractory to any kind of medication therapy.
- *Tachy-brady syndrome:* In addition to sinus bradycardia, persons with sinus node dysfunction syndrome often experience periods of atrial tachycardia that alternate with periods of profound bradycardia. Persons with tachy-brady syndrome experience signs and symptoms of decreased cardiac output during both the episodes of tachycardia and the bradycardic periods. The most common cause of the tachycardia in sinus node dysfunction is atrial fibrillation with a rapid ventricular response. The heart rate may range as high as 160 bpm during tachycardic episodes and drop to less than 40 bpm during bradycardic periods.
- *Sinus pauses:* A sinus pause occurs when the sinus node fails to depolarize (sinus arrest) or when the impulse from the SA node fails to activate the atrial conduction system so that the impulse does not depolarize the atria and is not conducted to the AV node (SA block). Short pauses of less than 3 seconds rarely cause symptoms; however, longer pauses can cause symptoms associated with decreased cardiac output and reduced cerebral blood flow. If the patient's SA node stops functioning altogether, the patient may develop an escape rhythm

in an attempt to maintain cardiac output. If conduction both at the level of the AV node and below is normal, the patient will develop a junctional escape rhythm; the AV node acts as the pacemaker for the heart and paces the heart at approximately 60 bpm. If, in addition to sick sinus syndrome, the patient also has some conduction abnormalities of the AV node, the patient may develop an escape rhythm that is paced by a site somewhere lower in the ventricles. This is called a ventricular escape rhythm; it is characterized by a rate of less than 40 bpm and a widened, bizarre-appearing QRS complex.

*Associated clinical signs and symptoms include:*

- Palpitations, angina, new or worsening congestive heart failure, muscle aches and disturbed sleep, in addition to the symptoms frequently associated with symptomatic bradycardia (i.e. syncope, heart rate <60 bpm, dizziness, light-headedness and confusion)
- Failure to increase heart rate during exertion or stress
- A heart rate that either stays relatively fixed or fails to rise during an exercise treadmill test
- Failure of the sinus node to respond to the administration of intravenous atropine. With normal sinus node function, a person's heart rate should increase to approximately 100 bpm following the administration of atropine. With sinus node dysfunction, the sinus node does not respond to the administration of atropine; the heart rate rarely increases to greater than 90 bpm.

According to the American College of Cardiology/American Heart Association permanent pacemaker implantation is indicated for sinus node dysfunction with documented symptomatic bradycardia, including frequent sinus pauses that produce symptoms.

*Level of evidence:* C (expert opinion, case studies or standard-of-care)

One of the most common causes of sinus node dysfunction is the normal aging process. As a person ages, a decrease occurs in the number of specialized cells that are present in the SA node and able to depolarize spontaneously and initiate a heartbeat. At the same time, an increase occurs in the amount of collagen tissue that is unable to generate or conduct an electrical impulse in the SA node. As a result, the ability of the SA node to act effectively as the pacemaker of the heart decreases. Another major cause of sinus node dysfunction is inferior wall myocardial infarction (MI). Cardiomyopathy, a condition in which the heart's ability to pump blood adequately is impaired, may also lead to sinus node dysfunction. Other cardiovascular diseases associated with sinus node dysfunction include hypertension, valvular heart disease and coronary artery disease. Noncardiac causes of sinus node function include hypothyroidism, sleep apnea and electrolyte imbalances. More rarely, conditions such as muscular dystrophy and amyloidosis may cause sinus node dysfunction.

### Class I Indications for Pacemaker Implantation in Sinus Node Dysfunction

For persons with sinus node dysfunction, class I indications for permanent pacemaker implantation according to ACC/AHA guidelines include:

- Sinus node dysfunction with symptomatic bradycardia
- Symptomatic chronotropic incompetence with sinus node dysfunction

### Third-degree Atrioventricular Block/Complete Heart Block

Another common cause of symptomatic bradycardia is third-degree (or complete) AV block (Fig. 29.36). Third-degree AV block occurs when none of the impulses generated by the SA node are conducted through the AV node. Sinus node function is often normal; however, conduction abnormalities at the level of AV junction or below the AV junction in the bundle of His/bundle branch region prevent the sinus impulse from reaching

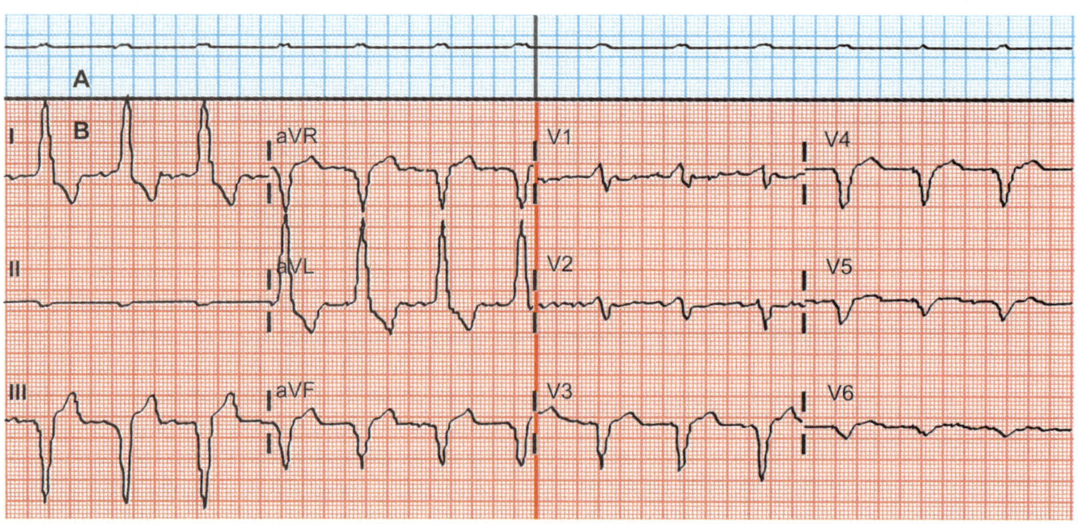


**Fig. 29.36:** Rhythm strip suggestive of complete heart block and absence of pacing (A). Simultaneous 12 lead ECG shows appropriate ventricular stimulation; the vector of the myocardial activation is close to isoelectric in II

the ventricles. The ventricles are paced by an escape rhythm.

The type and effectiveness of the escape rhythm depends on the location of the conduction abnormality. If the problem occurs high in the AV node, a junctional escape rhythm may pace the ventricles. The junctional escape rhythms are characterized by a normally configured QRS complex and a heart rate of 45–60 bpm. Junctional escape rhythms are often effective in maintaining an adequate cardiac output. If the conduction abnormality occurs lower in the ventricular conducting system (i.e. at the level of the bundle branches or below), a ventricular escape rhythm may emerge as the pacemaker of the heart. Ventricular escape rhythms are characterized by a widened, bizarre-appearing QRS complex and a heart rate of 30–40 bpm. Persons frequently develop symptoms of decreased cardiac output and diminished cerebral blood flow with a ventricular escape rhythm. The defining ECG characteristics of complete AV block include:

- A regular atrial rate, indicated by a P-P-wave interval that is constant (or almost constant) when measured
- A regular ventricular rate, as evidenced by a constant (or almost constant) R-R interval
- A complete absence of relationship between P-waves and QRS complexes

In addition to identifiable ECG changes, signs and symptoms associated with complete heart block include:

- Exacerbation of underlying cardiovascular problems, including increased angina and increased signs of congestive heart failure
- Activity intolerance
- Shortness of breath
- Signs associated with symptomatic bradycardia, including syncope, near syncope, light-headedness, and confusion

The American College of Cardiology, American Heart Association and European Society of Cardiology assert that pharmacological therapy is not recommended for maintenance of sinus rhythm in patients with atrioventricular node dysfunction unless they have a functioning electronic cardiac pacemaker.

*Level of evidence:* C (consensus opinion of experts, case studies or standard-of-care).

A major cause of complete AV block is MI. A branch of the right coronary artery usually provides the blood supply for the AV node and the bundle of His. An inferior wall MI can result in damage and impaired conduction through the node and the bundle of His. A branch of the left anterior descending (LAD) artery provides blood supply to the right and left bundle branches; an anterior wall MI may result in blocked conduction through this part of the ventricular conducting system. The development of chronic AV block has been linked with other cardiac causes, including valvular heart disease, congenital heart disease, coronary artery disease, myocarditis and cardiomyopathies. Complete heart block may develop following cardiac surgery. Antiarrhythmic medications, such as digoxin, calcium channel blockers, beta blockers and amiodarone, may also cause complete heart block. The elderly have an increased risk of developing heart block. Although, the AV node is relatively unaffected by the aging process, both the bundle of His and the bundle branches gradually lose the ability to conduct impulses effectively as a person ages. In addition, elderly individuals are often more susceptible to the effects of antiarrhythmic medications and other medications known to influence cardiac rhythm. Finally, complete heart block may be caused by radiofrequency ablation (RFA). RFA of the AV node is an interventional procedure performed to manage a variety of tachyarrhythmias that are refractory to pharmacological therapy. With RFA, the conducting cells in the AV node are destroyed and complete heart block results.

### Class I Indications

According to the ACC/AHA guidelines, the indications for permanent pacemaker implantation for the person with third-degree heart block include:

- Complete heart block associated with symptomatic bradycardia, periods of asystole that last 3 or more seconds, or an escape rhythm of less than 40 bpm
- Complete heart block in patients with atrial fibrillation and bradycardia with one or more pauses that last 5 or more seconds
- Complete heart block caused by radiofrequency ablation of the AV node for management of tachyarrhythmias
- Complete heart block caused by the necessary use of medications required to manage other arrhythmias or medical conditions
- Complete heart block caused by impaired conduction within or below the His-Purkinje system with bundle branch block that persists after the acute phase of an MI resolves
- Heart block caused by neuromuscular diseases, such as myotonic muscular dystrophy
- Heart block that occurs following surgery and is not expected to resolve.

### Second-degree Atrioventricular Block

Second-degree heart block (Fig. 29.37) occurs when impulses from the SA node are intermittently blocked at the level of the AV node or below. Some atrial impulses are conducted, and some are not. There are two types of second-degree heart block—Mobitz type I and Mobitz type II. Mobitz type I, also known as Wenckebach, is characterized by a P-R interval that gradually lengthens until a P-wave is blocked.

The pattern of gradual lengthening of the P-R interval then repeats. Mobitz type I is associated with inferior wall MIs, digitalis toxicity, and administration of calcium channel blockers or beta blockers. It may also occur for a period of time following cardiac surgery. Mobitz type II is characterized by an intermittent block of the atrial impulse; however, unlike the pattern seen in Mobitz type I, the P-R interval for conducted beats remains the same. In Mobitz type II, the conduction block occurs in or below the bundle

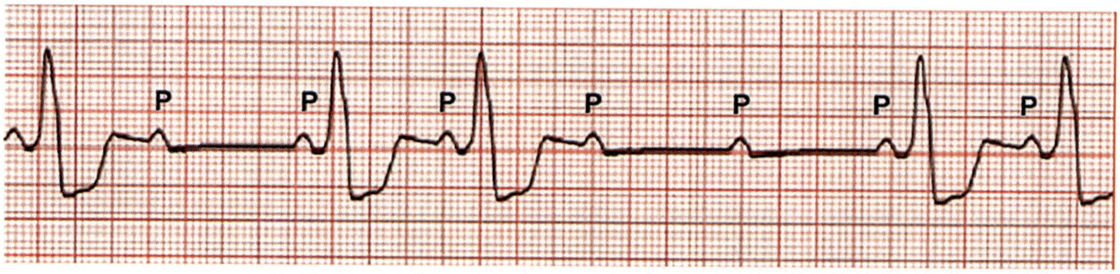


**Fig. 29.37:** ECG in Mobitz type II block, a non-conducted P-wave not followed by a QRS complex occurs suddenly without progressive prolongation of the PR interval. That is, the PR interval, which can be normal or prolonged, is constant before the non-conducted beat materializes. Mobitz type II second-degree heart block indicates more serious disease of the conduction system in regions below the AV node and can progress to total failure of AV conduction (third degree-heart block) without warning

of His. It is associated with anterior wall MIs. When it occurs after an MI, it is often an indication of a poor long-term prognosis for the patient. Mobitz type II may progress to the development of complete heart block.

### Signs and Symptoms

Clinical signs and symptoms depend in large part on how often the atrial impulses fail to be conducted to the ventricles. Blocked P-waves that occur every second or third beat can result in a severe bradycardia, with resulting symptoms of decreased cardiac output and diminished cerebral circulation.

### Class I Indications

According to the ACC/AHA guidelines, for persons with second-degree AV block, permanent pacemaker implantation is indicated for AV block

- Caused by impaired conduction in the His-Purkinje system with bundle branch block that persists following resolution of the acute phase of an MI
- That occurs with symptomatic bradycardia

## ATRIAL FIBRILLATION WITH A SLOW VENTRICULAR RESPONSE

Atrial fibrillation is an atrial arrhythmia characterized by an absence of normal P-waves and an irregularly irregular ventricular response (Fig. 29.38). In atrial fibrillation, the heartbeat is not initiated by the depolarization of the SA node. Instead, chaotic electrical activity is present in the atria. This chaotic electrical activity is reflected by fibrillation waves on the ECG tracing; they occur at excess of 400 bpm and are ineffective in depolarizing the atria. Some fibrillation waves are conducted to the AV node; some are conducted through the AV node, while others are blocked.

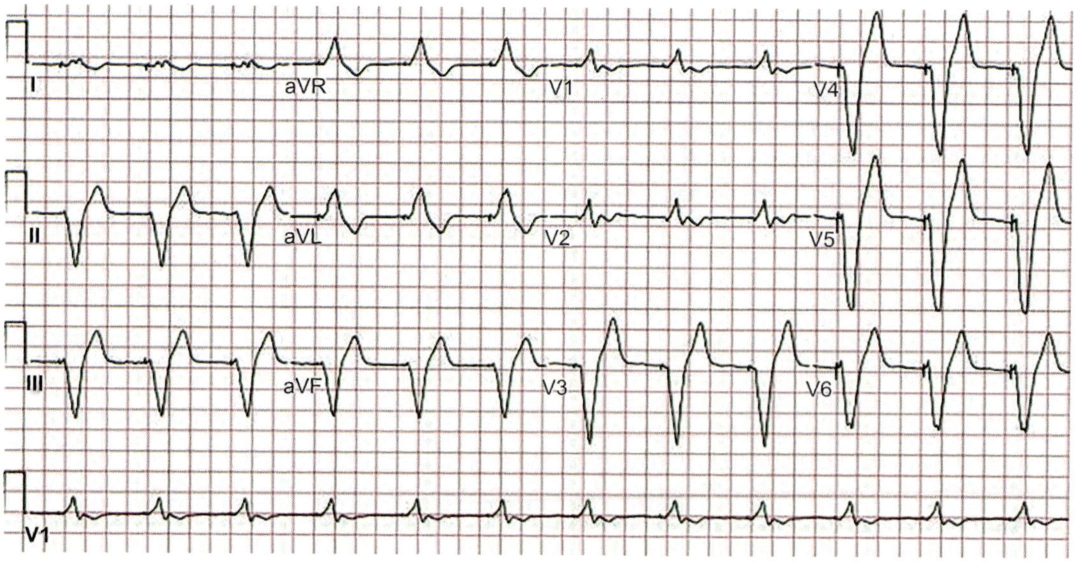


**Fig. 29.38:** The ventricular (QRS) rhythm is completely regular because of ventricular pacing. However, the underlying rhythm is atrial fibrillation. Fibrillatory waves are small in amplitude in most leads and best seen in lead V1. Most computer ECG interpretations will read this as 'ventricular pacing' without noting atrial fibrillation. Unless the reader specifies 'atrial fibrillation' in the report, this important diagnosis, which carries risk of stroke, will go unnoticed. Furthermore, on physical examination, the clinician may be 'tricked' into thinking the regular rhythm is sinus

Atrial fibrillation with slow ventricular response is defined as atrial fibrillation with an average ventricular response of less than 60 bpm. It may be induced by medications (e.g. antiarrhythmics) used to control tachyarrhythmia.

### Class I Indications

According to ACC/AHA guidelines, atrial fibrillation is an indication for permanent pacemaker implantation when it is coupled with

- Symptomatic bradycardia caused by a slow ventricular response. The slow ventricular rate may be caused by AV block or induced by necessary pharmacological therapy.
- Documented periods of asystole >3 seconds

## HYPERSENSITIVE CAROTID SINUS SYNDROME

Hypersensitive carotid sinus syndrome (Fig. 29.39) is a noncardiovascular, neurogenic cause of syncope. It is an extreme reflex that occurs in response to carotid sinus baroreceptor stimulation. To understand the pathophysiology of the syndrome, it is important to understand the normal physiology related to carotid stimulation. Normally, when pressure is exerted on the carotid sinus, the baro-receptors in the wall of the carotid sinus are stimulated. Stimulation of the baro-receptors results in vagal stimulation and a subsequent slowing of the heart. This response is normal; however, some individuals may have an exaggerated response. There are three types of hypersensitive carotid sinus syndrome. The first, called the cardioinhibitor reflex, results from increased parasympathetic tone and decreased sympathetic tone; the person may experience significant bradycardia and hypotension. The second type, vasodepressor carotid hypotension, is characterized by reduced peripheral vascular resistance caused by a decrease in sympathetic tone, resulting in hypotension. The heart rate may or may not drop. The third and most common type is a mix of the first two. Patients with the mixed type may experience hypotension caused both by a drop in peripheral vascular resistance and by significant bradycardia. Only the first and third types of hypersensitive carotid sinus syndrome may effectively be managed with the implantation of a permanent pacemaker. Aging is a major risk factor for the development of hypersensitive carotid sinus syndrome.

### Clinical Signs and Symptoms

The National Clinical Guideline Centre recommends offering carotid sinus massage as a first-line investigation for people with suspected carotid sinus syncope and for people with unexplained syncope who are aged 60 years or older. This should be conducted in a controlled environment, with ECG recording, and with resuscitation equipment available.

*Level of evidence:* Expert opinion/Consensus statement massage, which may cause/precipitate the patient's symptoms. More definitive testing is done using a tilt-table test

*Class I indications:* Permanent pacemaker implantation for persons with hypersensitive carotid syndrome include panied by recurrent syncope induced by carotid sinus stimulation.

- Presence of asystole greater than 3 seconds

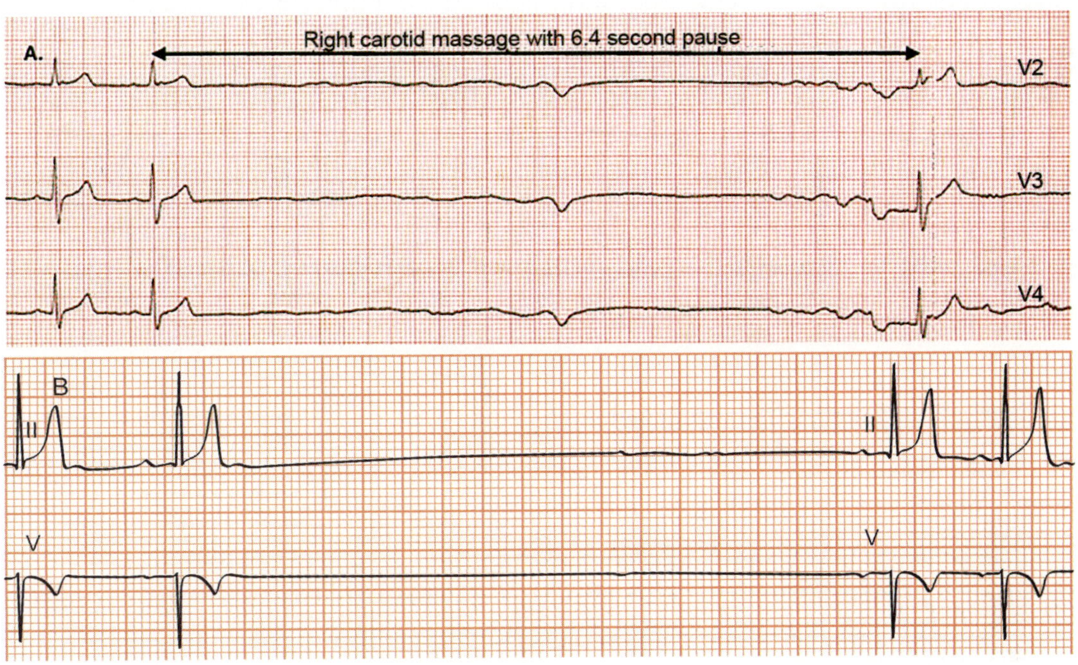


**Fig. 29.39:** ECG trace carotid sinus hypersensitivity revealed during massage manoeuvre. (A) Electrocardiographic at rest. Heart rate = 72 bpm, PR interval = 174 ms. (B) Sinus rhythm and pauses on the electrocardiogram is recorded during sleep in a young patient without heart disease. The heart rate before the pause is slow, and the PR interval is prolonged, consistent with an increase in vagal tone

## DRUG-INDUCED CONDUCTION ABNORMALITIES

Antiarrhythmic medications are commonly prescribed for the management of a wide variety of tachyarrhythen used in appropriate dosage, may cause additional conduction abnormalities. When an antiarrhythmic medication causes new or worsened arrhythmias, it is said to be **proarrhythmic**. Proarrhythmic abnormalities such as sinus node dysfunction or AV block may occur. These abnormalities may result in symptomatic bradycardia (Figs 29.40–29.42).

Medications with proarrhythmic effects the patient's arrhythmia and does not cause additional conduction problems and significant bradycardia. Use of a permanent pacemaker is often indicated in these patients to counteract the bradycardia caused by the antiarrhythmic therapy. Other noncardiovascular medications, especially when given in conjunction with cardiovascular medications, may cause arrhythmias. Cardiovascular medications given in management of coronary artery disease or hypertension may also have proarrhythmic side effects.

### Class I Indications

Indications for permanent pacemaker implantation for the management of persons who have drug-induced conduction abnormalities include:

- Sinus node dysfunction with symptomatic bradycardia induced by necessary long-term pharmacological therapy for which there is no acceptable alternative
- Third-degree AV block associated with bradycardia caused by necessary pharmacological therapy used to manage tachyarrhythmias or other medical conditions.

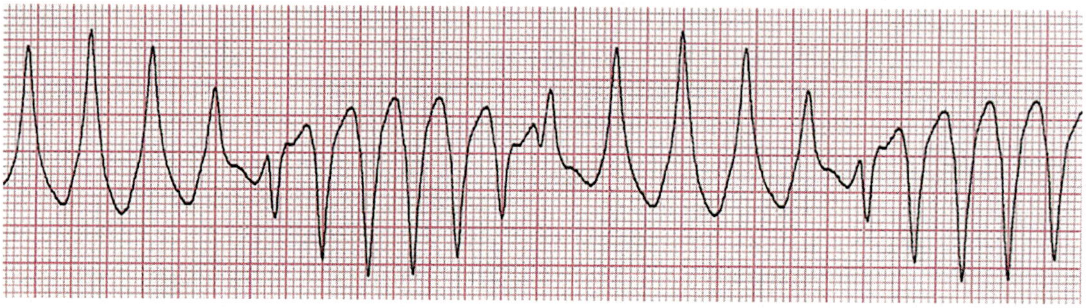

**Fig. 29.40:** ECG showing torsades de pointes is a very rapid type of ventricular tachycardia that is characterized by 'twisting' of the QRS complexes around the ECG baseline. Occurring at a rate of 250–350 bmp, these complexes change from upward to a downward deflection. The amplitude of each successive complex increases gradually, then decreases gradually, leading to aspindle shape pattern—the major risk factor for the development of torsades de pointes is excessive prolongation of the QT interval. Antiarrhythmic medications that prolong the action potential duration (and the refractory period of ventricles) may prolong the QT interval. Contributing factors to torsades de pointes also include hypomagnesemia, hypokalemia, or pre-existing bradycardia. The emergency measures to treat include use of overdrive pacing to terminate the arrhythmia, electrical cardioversion and defibrillation

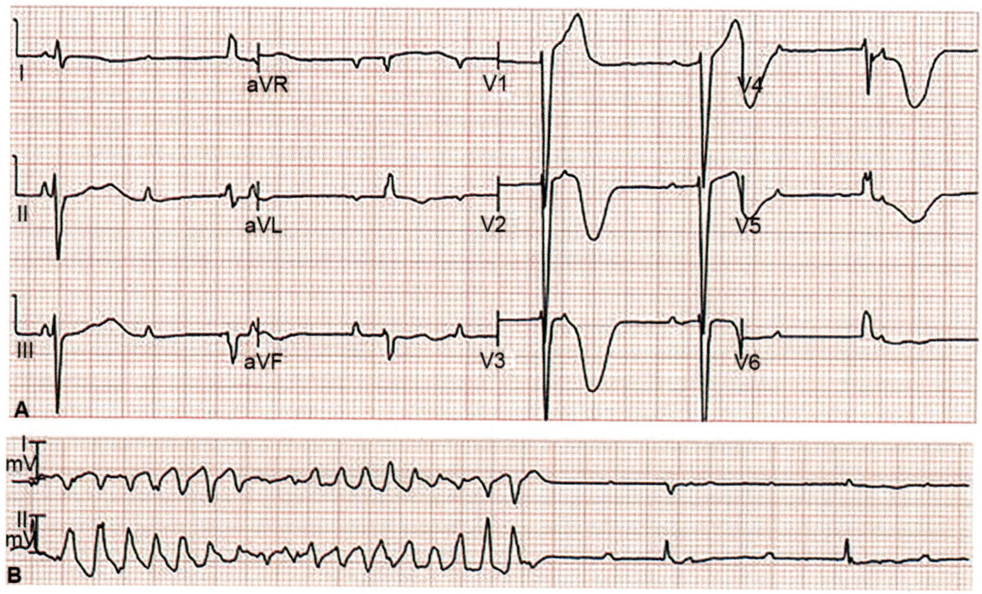


**Fig. 29.41:** Complete AV block leading to (A) a very long QT interval, with (B) episodes of torsade de pointes tachycardia

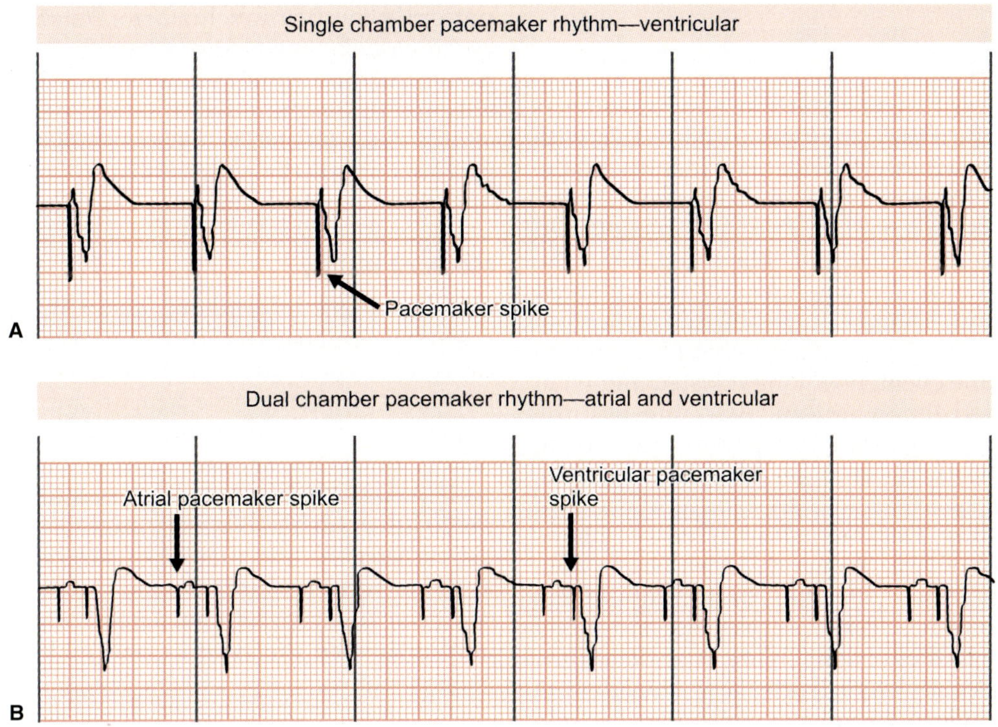


**Fig. 29.42:** ECG. (A) Single chamber ventricle pacemaker morphology. Whereas (B) demonstrates both atrial and ventricular pacing

## REMAINING ACC/AHA RECOMMENDATIONS

### Class II

As pacemaker technology continues to advance, and as medical research continues to refine knowledge of the link between normal cardiac conduction and the successful management of cardiovascular disease and its symptoms, the indications for permanent pacemaker implantation will also continue to advance. The ACC/AHA note that there are certain conditions that permanent pacemaker implantation may benefit; however, the guidelines caution that expert opinion and strength of clinical evidence to support the use of permanent pacemakers in the management of these conditions are controversial. Medical conditions that may benefit from permanent pacemaker implantation include:

- Asymptomatic third-degree heart block accompanied by a heart rate of 40 bpm or higher when the patient is not sleeping
- Asymptomatic Mobitz type II second- degree AV block
- Marked first-degree AV block in persons with known left ventricular dysfunction and symptoms of congestive heart failure
- Spontaneous or drug-induced sinus node dysfunction that results in a heart rate of <40 bpm in the absence of clear correlation between the bradyarrhythmia and the patient's symptoms

### Class III

The ACC/AHA guidelines note that implantation of a permanent pacemaker is not indicated for the management of some medical conditions. Conditions for which pacemaker therapy has not been found to be beneficial, useful, or effective include:

- Asymptomatic first-degree block. First-degree block indicates that conduction from the SA node through the atria and through AV node takes longer than normal; however, it is rarely associated with a bradycardic rate.
- Atrioventricular block that is temporary and expected to resolve. For example, with digitalis toxicity, second- or third-degree heart block may develop. When the digitalis level returns to normal, the heart block also resolves, and the person's heart rhythm returns to its usual pattern.
- Asymptomatic sinus node dysfunction
- Sinus node dysfunction that is caused by nonessential drug therapy
- Patients whose episodes of sinus node dysfunction have not been clearly and directly correlated with symptoms of cerebral blood flow
- Hypersensitive carotid syndrome either in the absence of symptoms or accompanied by vague symptoms
- Syncope that occurs from a vasovagal response precipitated by specific identifiable stimuli that can be readily avoided.

## DIAGNOSIS AND EVALUATION FOR ANTIBRADYCARDIA PACEMAKER IMPLANTATION

The decision to implant a permanent pacemaker and the selection of the specific type of pacemaker device are based on a thorough assessment and evaluation of the patient's status. Two key components of the evaluation process are the patient history and selected diagnostic tests.

## PATIENT HISTORY

### Assessing Symptoms

Thorough assessment of the patient's symptoms is necessary to determine if the symptoms are correlated with the occurrence of the arrhythmia. Begin by identifying the primary reason that the patient has sought medical care. Listen for a history of a recent fall, recurrent unexplained falls, fainting spells, or periods of 'black-out.' Ask the patient's family if he or she has had any unexplained periods of confusion. Determine when the symptom occurred, what the person was doing, what (if anything) appeared to trigger the event, how long it lasted and what (if anything) relieved the symptom. Also question the patient about any associated symptoms, including increased fatigue with no change in daily activities, shortness of breath, activity intolerance, or other signs of congestive heart failure. Determine how often symptoms occur: daily, weekly or less frequently. Also obtain data about the patient's 'usual' lifestyle; inquire about the patient's normal activity level, exercise tolerance and ability to perform normal activities of daily living. Also determine if the patient has recently experienced any exacerbation or worsening of previous symptoms; examples include increasing frequency of angina attacks in a patient with coronary artery disease or decreasing activity tolerance in a person with congestive heart failure.

### Drug-taking History

Specifically question the patient about the current medications that he or she is taking, with special attention to any cardiovascular medications. As noted, many antiarrhythmic medications prescribed to control tachyarrhythmias may cause a symptomatic bradycardia. In addition, medications that are prescribed to manage other cardiovascular conditions, such as hypertension and coronary artery disease, can affect the electrical conducting system in the heart and cause symptomatic bradycardia. Also inquire about any other medications the patient may be taking. A wide variety of medications, such as tricyclic antidepressants, lithium and phenothiazines, can interact with cardiovascular medications or antiarrhythmic medications to create bradyarrhythmias. Also assess the patient's medication history. Determine if any other cardiovascular medications have been prescribed for the patient at one time and why those medications were changed or discontinued. If indicated, consider obtaining serum drug levels for medications, such as digoxin or procainamide to determine if toxicity is present. Toxic levels of some antiarrhythmics may result in bradycardia.

### Medical History

Finally, obtain information about the patient's medical history. Specifically inquire about any history of cardiovascular diseases, including coronary artery disease, previous MI, congestive heart failure, cardiomyopathy, hypertension, valvular heart disease, and any previous history of cardiac conduction problems. Determine if the patient has any history of interventional cardiovascular procedures, such as coronary angioplasty, coronary artery bypass surgery, valvular heart surgery, or electrophysiology interventions such as radiofrequency ablation. The presence and type of concurrent cardiovascular disease may influence the type of pacemaker selected and its programming.

## DIAGNOSTIC TESTS

Generally, in order for a patient to meet criteria for the implantation of a permanent pacemaker, the patient's symptoms should be clearly correlated with episodes of bradycardia. Commonly used diagnostic tools include an ECG (12-lead or rhythm strip) and ambulatory electrocardiographic monitoring (AECG).

### 12-Lead ECG Recording

The traditional method of assessing a patient's heart rhythm is a 12-lead ECG (Fig. 29.43). It is inexpensive, noninvasive and readily performed in any healthcare setting or physician's office. Unfortunately, for persons with symptomatic bradycardia, this diagnostic tool has limited value. Typically, an ECG only records about 12 seconds of data.

Because symptoms may be transient and occur intermittently, the ECG may not capture the patient's heart rhythm at the time that the symptoms are occurring. The

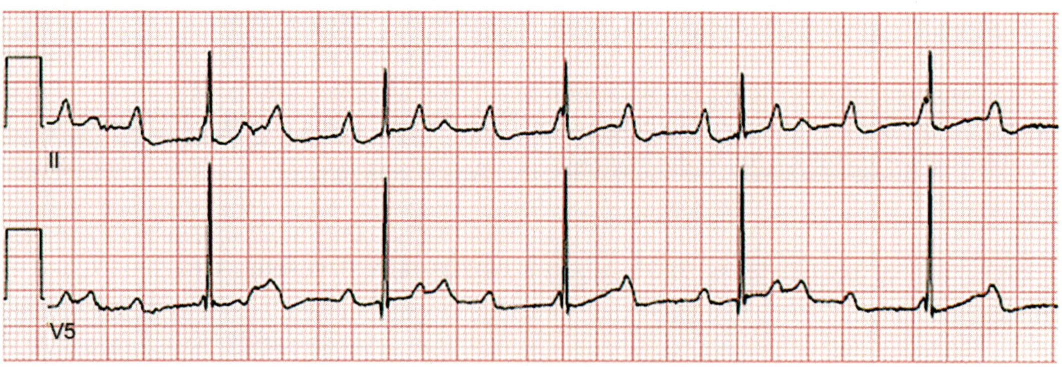


**Fig. 29.43:** ECG trace shows complete heart block with junctional escape. presenting with symptomatic bradycardia in patients who needed permanent pacemaker

patient may or may not have symptoms during an office or clinical visit. The ECG is considered a passive diagnostic tool; it only records the rhythm occurring at the time the tracing is done. It does nothing to actively precipitate an occurrence of arrhythmia.

### Ambulatory Electrocardiography

To facilitate documentation of the patient's heart rhythm at the exact time that the patient is experiencing symptoms, researchers have developed another type of ECG monitoring called ambulatory electrocardiography, or AECG (Figs 29.44–29.47). Holter monitoring is a noninvasive procedure with little to no associated risk to the patient. The device may be applied in a physician's office, outpatient clinic or inpatient hospital unit. A Holter monitor may be useful for persons who experience symptoms on a daily (or more frequent) basis; it is also useful for persons whose symptoms are severe enough to cause loss of consciousness or severe disorientation. Persons with these severe symptoms would not be able to operate some of the more complex forms of AECG. The disadvantage to Holter monitoring is that it may fail to capture a symptomatic period or a period of bradyarrhythmia.

### Outcomes from Ambulatory Electrocardiography Monitoring

Optimally, the data from AECG monitoring would clearly confirm the need for a pacemaker or definitively rule it out. In reality, several different outcomes may occur:

- The ECG recording shows the presence of a bradyarrhythmia during the precise time that the patient is experiencing one or more of the cardinal symptoms associated with symptomatic bradycardia. This finding supports the need for implantation of a permanent pacemaker and may provide data to guide the selection of the most appropriate type of pacemaker.

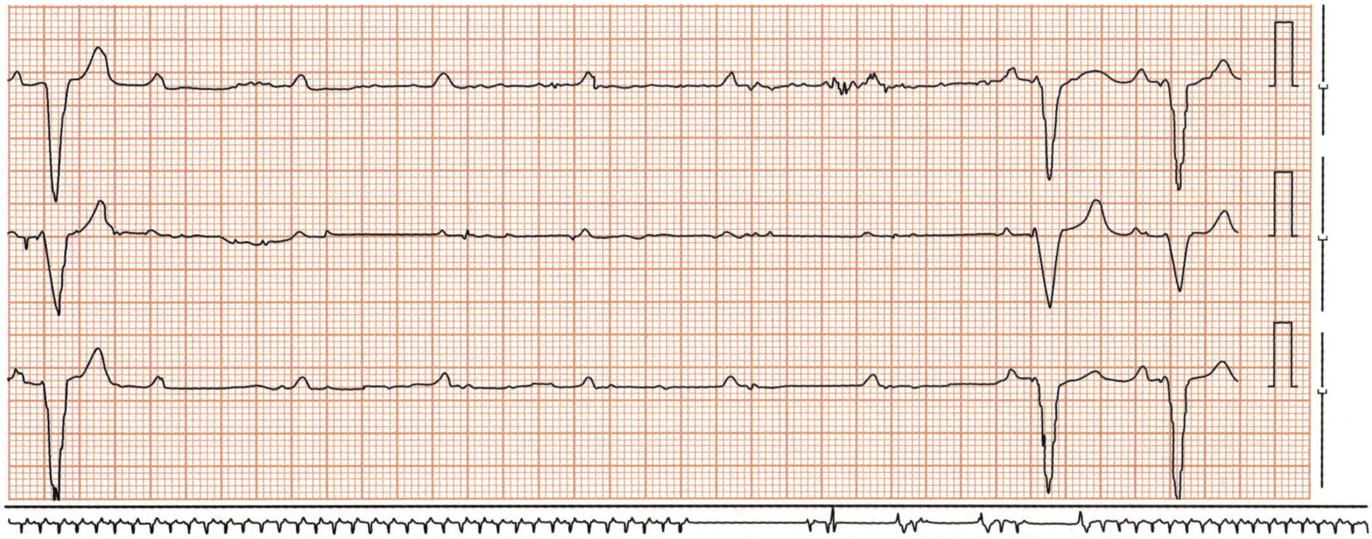

**Fig. 29.44:** Holter monitoring showing paced rhythm with a pacemaker malfunction/ventricular standstill (ventricular asystole) approximately (5.6 seconds pause)

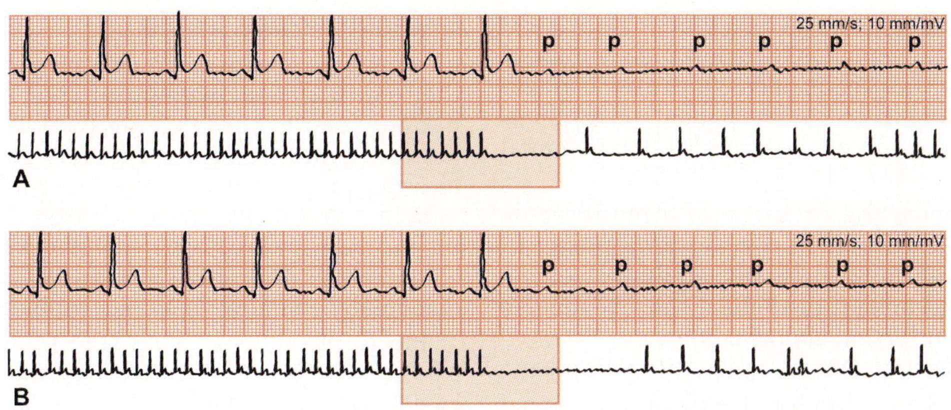


**Fig. 29.45:** Holter recording of two episodes of spontaneous syncope that occurred a few minutes apart. The two episodes were very similar and were characterized by sudden-onset complete atrioventricular (AV) block without changes in P-P cycle length, which constantly remained 720 ms and long ventricular asystole of 7 and 11 s (A and B, compressed traces, respectively)

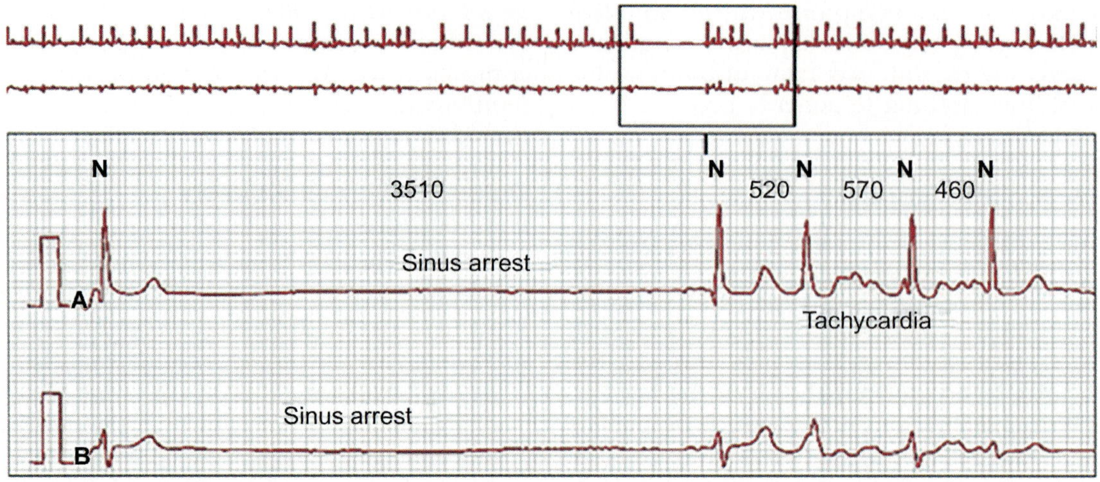


**Fig. 29.46:** An example of a patient with typical bradycardia-tachycardia syndrome—atrial fibrillation suddenly terminates and is followed by a pause until the first sinus beat due to a prolonged sinus node recovery time

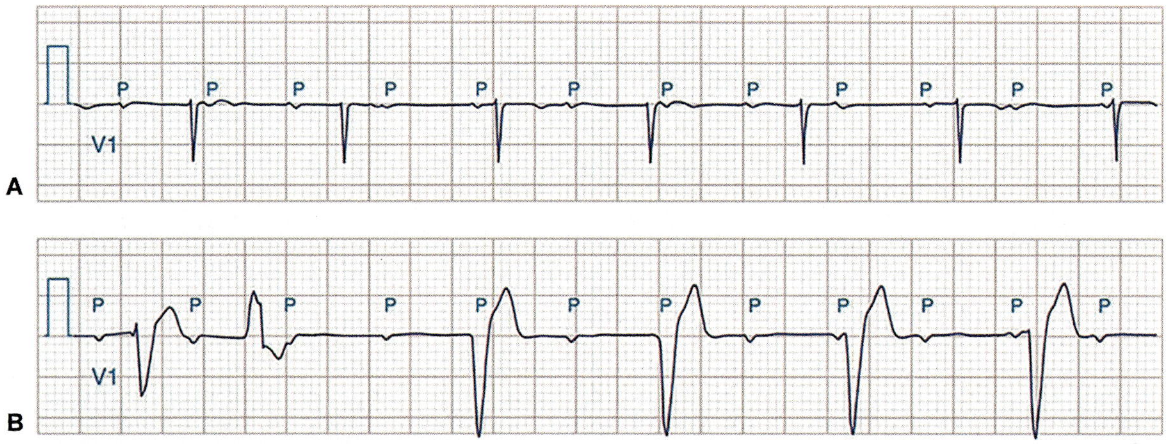


**Fig. 29.47:** Intermittent third-degree atrioventricular block with asystole in a patient who was admitted due to recurrent syncopes. The upper panel initially shows sudden onset of a third-degree atrioventricular block with no ventricular escape rhythm followed by an atrioventricular junctional escape rhythm with narrow QRS complexes in the lower panel (first 4 beats) as well as two conducted P-waves at the end of the lower panel

- The ECG recording shows no arrhythmias during the precise time that the patient is experiencing symptoms. This finding is also helpful; it rules out cardiac conduction abnormalities as a cause for the patient's symptoms. Evaluation of the patient can then turn to other potential causes.
- The ECG documents the presence of a bradycardia during a time that the patient remains asymptomatic. This is an equivocal finding; usually, additional testing is indicated to determine if the patient's symptoms are actually due to conduction abnormalities.
- The ECG shows no episodes of arrhythmias, and the patient experiences no symptoms during the period that the event monitor is used. This finding is the least helpful; it neither supports nor refutes the presence of conduction abnormalities or the need for a permanent pacemaker.

### Electrophysiology Testing

Electrophysiology testing (EPS) (Fig. 29.48) is not generally the first diagnostic method of choice when evaluating a patient for the presence of symptomatic bradycardia. However, under certain conditions, EPS may be performed in order to aid in the management of the patient, such as patients with tachy-brady syndrome; EPS can document the mechanism and location of the tachyarrhythmia. It can also determine if ablation of some area involved in the tachyarrhythmia can help control the rapid heart rate.

Electrophysiology testing (EPS) may be used to evaluate a patient for the presence of retrograde conduction. As will be discussed further, retrograde conduction (i.e. conduction that spreads from the AV node back into the atria) can interfere with optimal pacemaker functioning, and certain types of pacemakers are contraindicated in the presence of retrograde conduction. EPS may also be used

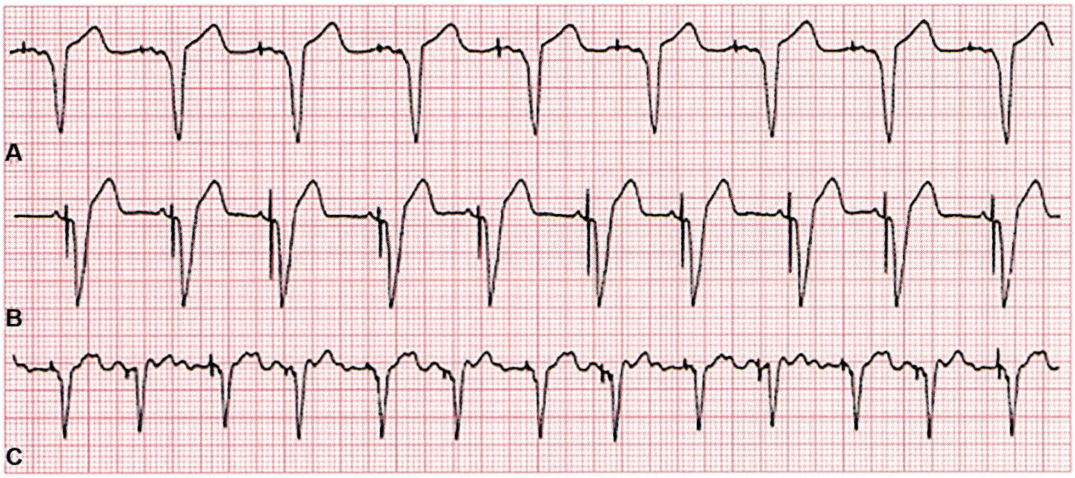


**Fig. 29.48:** Selective His bundle pacing. (A) The 12-lead electrocardiogram of a patient with complete heart block with narrow QRS escape rhythm. (B) Intracardiac electrogram recorded from the permanent His bundle pacing lead at the time of implantation. Note the His bundle electrogram (H) with injury current (arrow) followed by ventricular electrogram (V). (C) His bundle pacing. The pacing spike (circle) is followed by an isoelectric interval of 40 ms and QRS complexes identical to the intrinsic rhythm

to evaluate the extent of bundle branch block present in selected patients.

### Tilt-Table Test

When hypersensitive carotid sinus syndrome is thought to be responsible for syncopal episodes, a tilt-table test may be used to confirm the diagnosis (Fig. 29.49). Tilt-table tests are often performed in the cardiac catheterization laboratory. The patient is placed on a table that can tilt up to 80 degrees upright; safety straps are applied to prevent the patient from slipping and injuring him/herself during the test.

An IV access is started to permit the rapid administration of IV medications or fluids should those be indicated during

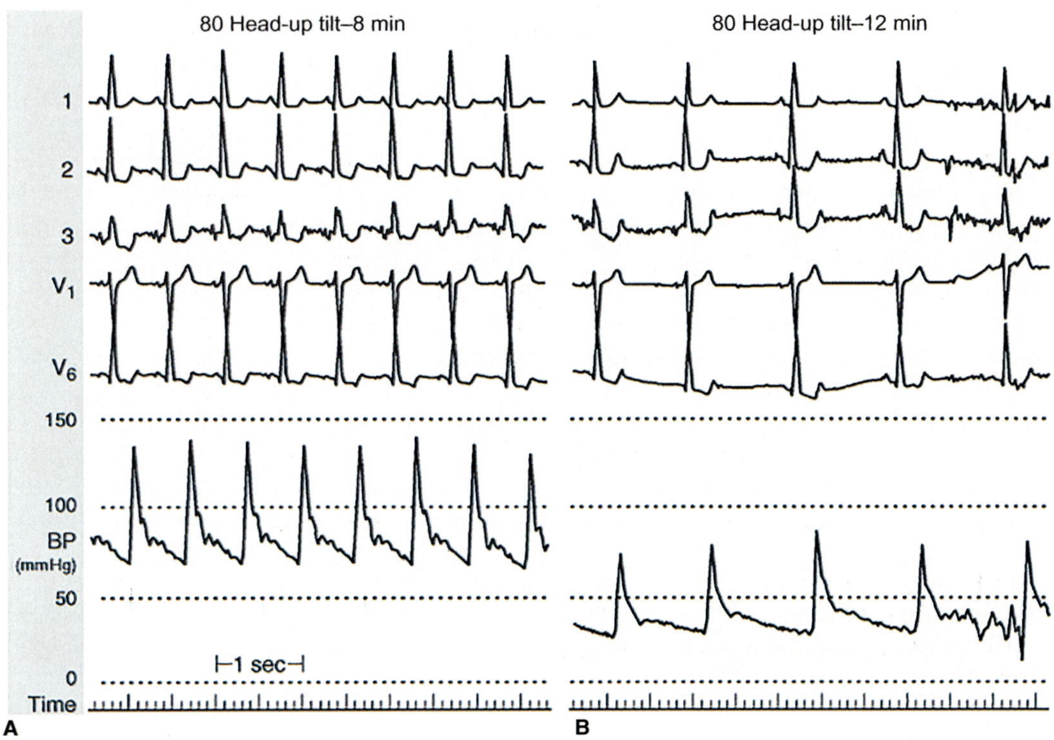


**Fig. 29.49:** Head-up tilt-table testing. Surface electrocardiogram (ECG) leads and an arterial blood pressure (BP) tracing are shown. After 8 minutes of head-up tilt at 80 degrees (A), heart rate and BP were normal and the patient was asymptomatic. Four minutes later (B), systolic BP dropped precipitously to 80 mmHg, the heart rate fell to 50 beats/min, and the patient lost consciousness. ECG artifact at right is seizure activity. This patient needed pacemaker therapy

the test. Continuous ECG and blood pressure monitoring are performed, and the use of continuous intra-arterial blood pressure monitoring via placement of an arterial line is recommended. The purpose of the tilt test is to create the physiological environment required to trigger vasovagal syncope. The patient is tilted from a supine position to a 70° angle. Patients who suffer from vasovagal syncope experience a decrease in venous return followed by a decrease in the left ventricular filling pressure when they are tilted to an upright position. The sequelae can include hypotension, bradycardia, and syncope. In addition to confirming the presence of a vasovagal syncope, a tilt-table test can also help to differentiate the major contributing cause. Permanent pacemaker implantation is indicated for syncope due to a mixed cardioinhibitory/vasodepressor response

## SELECTING PACEMAKER DEVICE TYPE

After determining that permanent pacemaker implantation is indicated, it should then be determined which type of pacemaker system will be the most effective. A number of factors should be considered in the decision, including patient factors, technical aspects and procedural issues (Table 29.5). Patient factors include:

- What is the patient's specific medical indication for pacemaker implantation? Some types of pacemakers are contraindicated for certain conduction abnormalities, and some pacemakers are significantly more effective in managing a specific type of problem than other pacemaker types.
- Does the patient require the rate responsive feature? How active is the patient's lifestyle? Is chronotropic incompetence present? Does (or will) an inability to increase the heart rate in response to increased activity create a problem for this patient?
- Is the patient likely to develop increasing conduction problems that may require additional or more complex pacing functions? If so, a pacemaker that has the capability to be reprogrammed for more complex pacing functions when needed is indicated.
- What is the patient's clinical status? Does the patient have a functioning SA node? A functioning AV node? Does the patient require AV synchrony to maintain adequate cardiac output? Does the patient have a history of chronic or paroxysmal atrial tachyarrhythmias?
- What is the cost of the pacemaker system? Initial costs include the cost of the generator and leads, implantation costs, and the cost of the initial programming. Subsequent costs include the cost of follow-up and generator replacement, when needed. In general, dual chamber pacemakers are more expensive to implant and maintain. Use of the rate responsive feature also increases implantation and programming costs.

**Table 29.5:** Matching pacemaker type to medical indication

| Clinical indication | AAI | AAIR | VVI | VVIR | VDD | DDD | DDDR |
|---|---|---|---|---|---|---|---|
| Sinus node dysfunction with symptomatic bradycardia; AV node function normal | Yes | Yes | Yes | Yes | No | Yes | Yes |
| Sinus node dysfunction with symptomatic bradycardia; AV node function normal; AV synchrony needed | Yes | Yes | No | No | No | Yes | Yes |
| Sinus node dysfunction with symptomatic bradycardia; AV node function normal; AV synchrony needed; chronotropic incompetence present | No | Yes | No | Yes | No | Yes | Yes |
| Sinus node dysfunction with symptomatic bradycardia; AV node function abnormal; AV synchrony needed | No | No | No | No | No | Yes | Yes |
| Sinus node dysfunction with symptomatic bradycardia; AV node function abnormal; AV synchrony needed; chronotropic incompetence present | No | No | No | No | No | No | Yes |
| Symptomatic sinus node chronotropic incompetence; AV node function normal | No | Yes | No | Yes | No | No | Yes |
| Symptomatic sinus node chronotripic incompetence; AV node function abnormal | No | Yes | No | Yes | No | No | Yes |
| Third-degree AV block with symptomatic bradycardia; intact sinus node | No | No | Yes | Yes | Yes | Yes | Yes |
| Third-degree AV block induced by AV node ablation; underlying atrial flutter present | No | No | Yes | Yes | No | No | No |
| Third-degree AV block induced by AV node ablation; absence of underlying atrial fibrillation or atrial flutter | No | No | Yes | Yes | Yes | Yes | Yes |
| Second-degree type II AV block with symptomatic bradycardia; intact sinus node function | No | No | Yes | Yes | Yes | Yes | Yes |
| Chronic atrial fibrillation/atrial flutter with slow ventricular response | No | No | Yes | Yes | No | No | No |
| Hypersensitive carotid sinus syndrome (mixed aetiology) with intact sinus node function; AV synchrony required | No | No | No | No | Yes | Yes | Yes |
| Hypersensitive carotid sinus syndrome (mixed aetiology) with chronic atrial fibrillation | No | No | Yes | Yes | No | No | No |

## PREPROCEDURE CARE IN PACEMAKER IMPLANTATION

### Preoperative Assessment and Preparation

After the decision is made to implant the pacemaker, the specific type of pacemaker is selected, and the patient is scheduled for pacemaker implantation. The length of stay for pacemaker implantation is generally very short and often involves only an overnight stay in an acute care facility. Some institutions are exploring the option of implanting pacemakers on an outpatient basis; however, this practice is not yet widespread. Pacemaker implantation may be safely performed in either the cardiac catheterization laboratory or the operating room. The selection of the specific site is based on an evaluation of which site will provide the best outcome and most cost-effective method for the individual patient. Some patients, such as patients who are confused, uncooperative, or have special medical needs, require the use of general anesthesia; pacemaker implantation for these patients should occur in the operating room. Implantation for patients who do not require general anesthesia, but who can be managed with moderate sedation/analgesia may be performed in the cardiac catheterization lab.

Unless the patient's medical status requires hospital admission for management prior to pacemaker implantation, the patient may be admitted to the hospital on the morning of the procedure. The patient should be nil per OS (NPO) for 6–8 hours prior to the procedure. Basic preimplantation lab work is obtained, including a complete blood count, serum electrolytes, blood urea nitrogen (BUN), creatinine, prothrombin time (PT), partial thromboplastin time, and a urinalysis. A baseline 12-lead ECG, alveolar pressure (PA), and lateral chest X-ray are also obtained. Baseline vital signs and physical assessment are performed and documented. If the patient has been taking warfarin or similar anticoagulant drugs, the patient will be instructed to discontinue taking them for several days in advance of the procedure. This will permit the patient's PT and international normalized ratio (INT) to return close to normal values in order to reduce the risk of excessive bleeding during the implantation. If it is determined that the patient is at high risk for thromboembolic events, he/she may be admitted to the hospital for temporary IV heparin therapy during the period that the other anticoagulant has been stopped. Patients who are at high risk for thromboembolism include persons with artificial heart valves. IV heparin infusions are generally discontinued 4–6 hours before the pacemaker implantation is performed. Depending on physician preference, the heparin may be restarted 12 hours after completion of the pacemaker implantation and the original anticoagulant resumed the night of the procedure. The planned site for the pacemaker generator (usually the right or left subclavicular area) is scrubbed and shaved according to institutional protocol. The patient's dominant arm is identified; generally, pacemaker generators are implanted on the nondominant side. Informed consent should always be obtained. The patient may receive a mild sedative prior to leaving for the catheterization lab or operating room. Additional sedation and/or analgesics will be administered during the procedure. Generally, the patient is instructed to continue taking his/her routine medications prior to implantation. Due to the patient's NPO status, doses of insulin or oral hypoglycemic agents may need to be temporarily reduced or held.

### Preoperative Education for Patients and Families

Education for the patient and his or her family begins in the preoperative period and continues throughout the patient's life. The focus of patient education in the preoperative period is on addressing the patient's immediate questions and concerns and providing the patient and family with information about what to expect during implantation and in the period immediately following implantation. Many patients are very anxious about undergoing pacemaker implantation. They may express fears of 'being dependent on a machine' to stay alive. Some may have heard a variety of 'old wives' tales' about pacemakers from friends or relatives. Or, they may have known of a family member 'years ago' who had a pacemaker implanted that did not work 'right,' and the person died. Some people have specific concerns about how a permanent pacemaker may interfere with their normal activities or ability to use certain types of equipment. Responding to any concerns or questions that the patient has during the preoperative period is very important. Providing specific information about what the patient can expect before, during, and immediately after pacemaker implantation can also help to reduce the patient's anxiety. The following topics are often helpful to cover in the preoperative period:

- A brief explanation of why the patient needs a pacemaker (consider the use of a diagram or model to illustrate a brief explanation of normal conduction, the patient's specific conduction problem, and how the implantation of a pacemaker will correct that problem).
- What a pacemaker generator and pacemaker leads look like. (Pacemaker manufacturers are a good source of illustrations and diagrams of their products)
- Where the pacemaker generator will be implanted
- How leads will be attached
- Use of general anesthesia or moderate sedation during the procedure to minimize discomfort
- Details of the usual preoperative preparation

Allow time for the patient and family to ask questions and clarify concerns. The AHA, the Heart Rhythm Society (HRS), and various patient education sites provided by pacemaker manufacturers may be recommended as helpful educational sources.

## PACEMAKER IMPLANTATION PROCEDURE OVERVIEW

After informed consent is obtained and the preoperative preparation is complete, the patient is taken to the operating room or cardiac catheterization lab. IV access is obtained, and continuous monitoring of ECG rhythm, oxygen saturation, and blood pressure is initiated. Depending on the implantation site and the physician's judgment, the patient

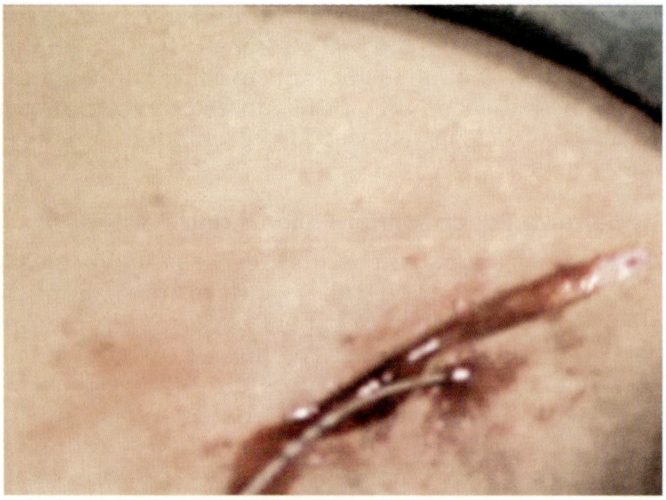

**Step 1.** To make skin incision under left collar bone

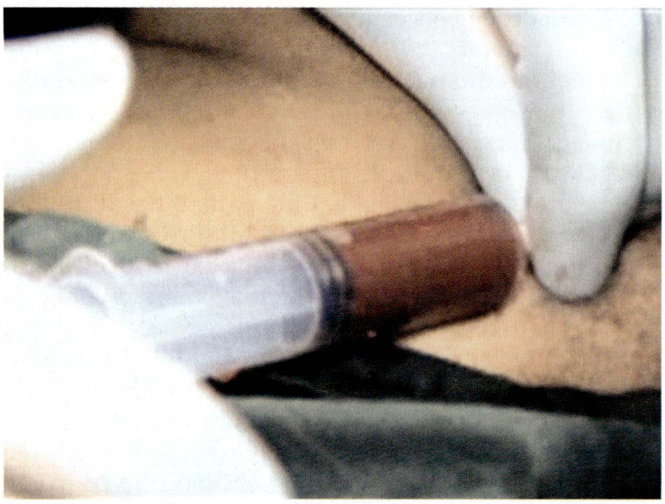

**Step 2.** Left subclavian vein accessed

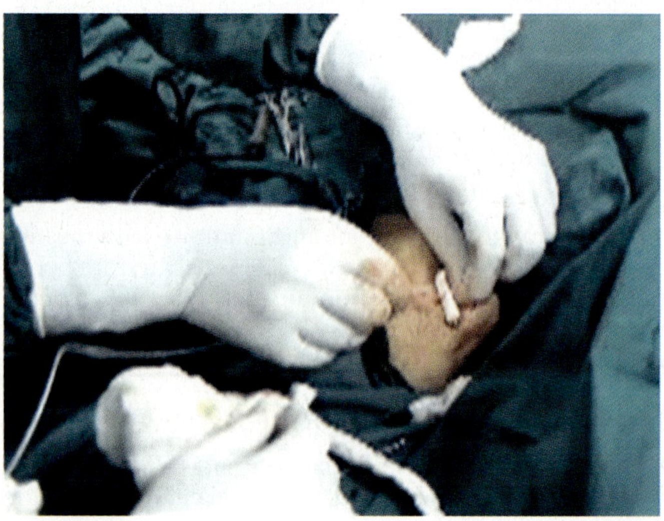

**Step 3.** Guidewire being inserted

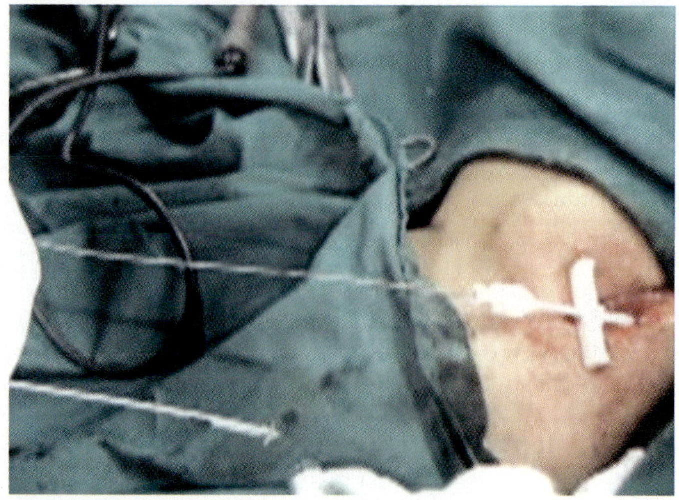

**Step 4.** Left subclavian vein catheterised

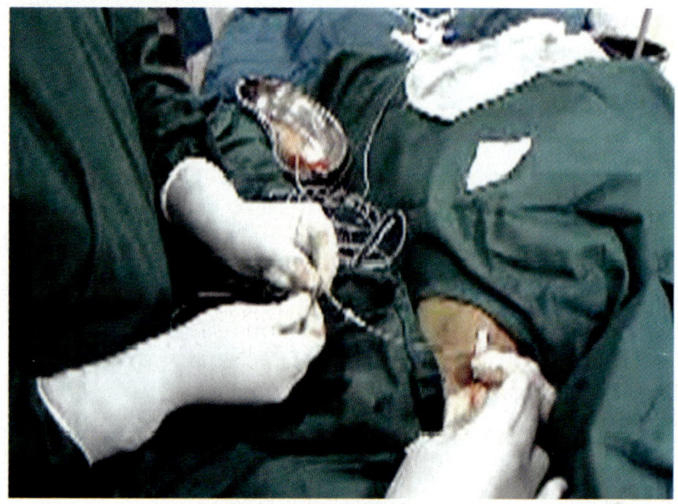

**Step 5.** External pacing done to check the leads

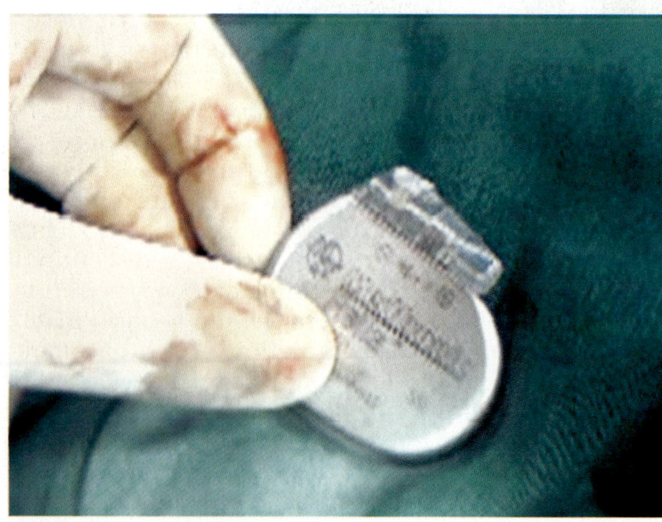

**Step 6.** Depiction of smaller size pacemaker (recent)

**Fig. 29.50A:** (Steps 1–6) stepwise minimal surgical intervention in the implantation of intracardiac pacemaker

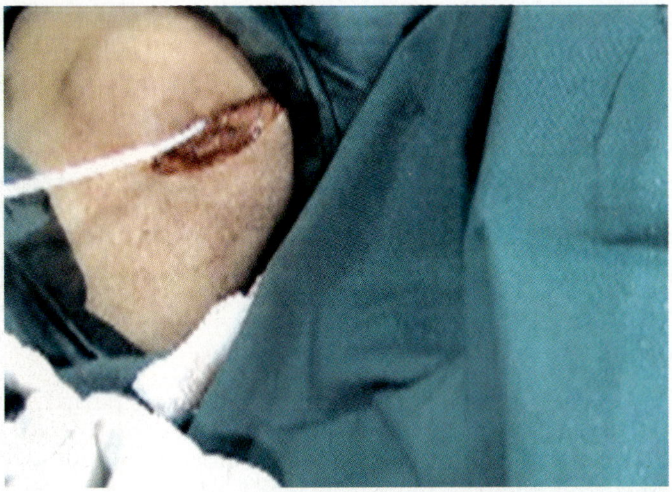

**Step 7.** Pocket prepared under the left collar bone

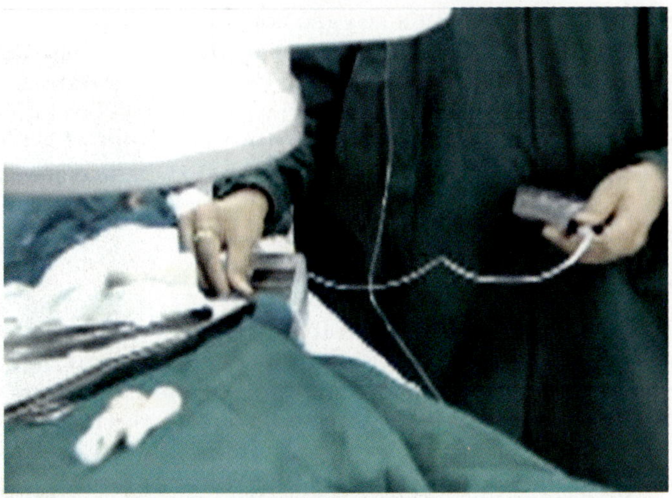

**Step 8.** Pacemaker pulse rate being set

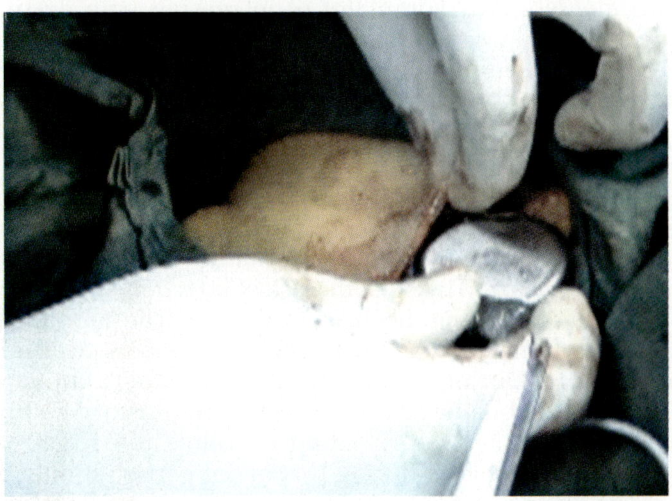

**Step 9.** Pacemaker being inserted in the skin pocket

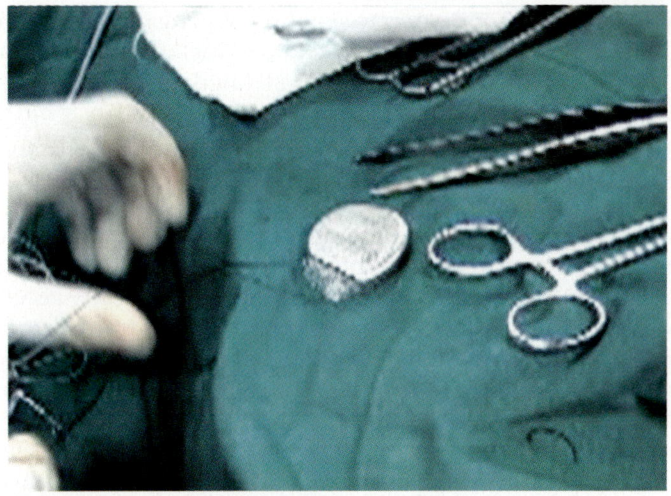

**Step 10.** Pacemaker connected with leads

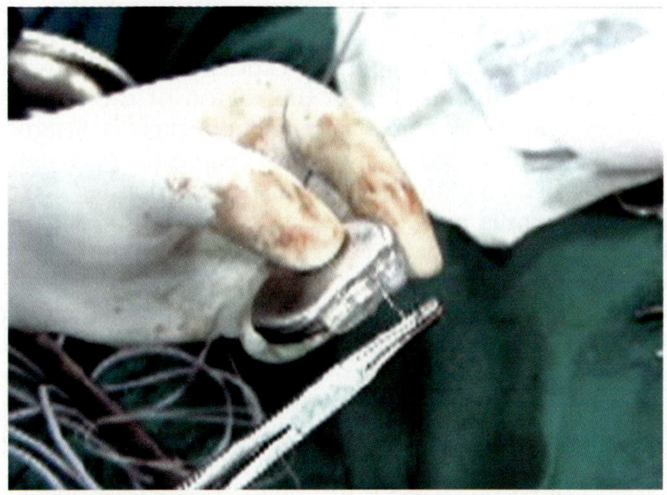

**Step 11.** Pacemaker applied stay sutured

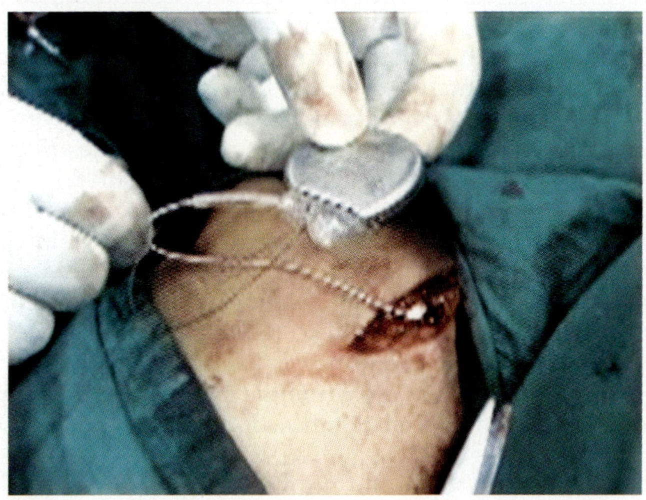

**Step 12.** Pacemaker ready to be kept in pocket already prepared under subclavicular region

**Fig. 29.50B:** (Steps 7–12) Stepwise minimal surgical intervention in the implantation of intracardiac pacemaker will receive either moderate sedation or general anesthesia. Commonly used agents for sedation include midazolam and fentanyl. Once the patient is sedated, a small surgical incision is made, approximately 2–3 inches in length, beneath the patient's clavicle. Preferably, the patient's nondominant side is chosen for placement of the incision and pacemaker generator; use of the nondominant side lessens the risk that the pacemaker leads will be dislodged by repetitive arm and shoulder movements. The incision site is positioned to provide the physician with ready access to either the subclavian or cephalic vein for transvenous insertion. Depending on the type of pacemaker, one or two pacemaker leads are inserted transvenously and passed through the vessels into the heart. Fluoroscopy is used to monitor the passage of the pacing lead through the vessels. Generally, an atrial pacemaker lead will be positioned inside the right atrial appendage; a ventricular pacemaker lead is positioned in the apex of the right ventricle. Once, it is determined that the lead is in the correct position, the lead tip is attached to the endocardial surface of the heart. When the leads are properly positioned, a small area is opened beneath the skin in the region of the original incision. This area, called a 'pacemaker pocket,' is designed to hold the pulse generator. In most people, the pacemaker pocket is created in the subcutaneous tissue located on top of the pectoralis muscle. For extremely thin individuals, the pacemaker pocket may be created beneath the pectoral muscle to provide adequate support and stability for the pacemaker generator. The connector end of the leads is firmly attached to the connector block on the outside of the pulse generator and the screw tightened to ensure good contact and stable position. The pacemaker generator is then inserted into the pacemaker pocket, and the skin is sutured shut. A dressing is applied. In some institutions, a pressure dressing may be applied. Antibiotics are frequently administered to reduce the risk of infection. The exact routine varies from institution-to-institution; some administer a single dose before or during the procedure, while others administer IV antibiotics for a 24-hour period following implantation. Extreme care is taken throughout placement of the generator and leads to avoid impairing the range of motion of the upper extremity on the affected side. Care is also taken to make sure that the generator and leads are well protected by body tissue to prevent the accidental erosion of either the leads or pacemaker generator through the skin. As previously noted, most pacemakers contain a small amount of steroid at the endocardial end of the lead to reduce the probability of inflammation causing abnormalities in function soon after implantation. Finally, the initial pacemaker settingsare programmed and pacemaker function is tested (Fig. 29.50A and B).

## IMMEDIATE POSTPROCEDURE CARE

After the procedure is completed, the patient is generally moved to a recovery area until he/she has recovered from the general anesthesia or moderate sedation. Once the patient is awake and stable, he/she is transferred back to the general unit. The goals of care in the immediate 24- to 48-hour postoperative period are to:

- Monitor the patient for signs of postoperative complications
- Manage the patient's postprocedure pain
- Monitor both the patient and the pacemaker for proper pacemaker functioning and efficacy of pacemaker therapy in relieving preimplantation symptoms
- Begin patient discharge education and address patient/family concerns

### Patient Monitoring

Complications that may develop following permanent pacemaker implantation include bleeding into the pacemaker generator pocket, hemothorax, pneumothorax and dislodgment of the pacemaker leads. Upon return to the floor, the patient's vital signs are monitored periodically. Continuous ECG monitoring is initiated. Spot checks of the patient's oxygen saturation level may be performed as needed. The pacemaker pocket site is assessed frequently for signs of excessive bleeding or swelling; if these are present, the physician should be notified immediately. A posterioanterior (PA) and lateral chest X-ray is taken to evaluate the positioning of the pacemaker leads as well as to rule out the presence of either a hemothorax or a pneumothorax.

### Pain Management

Patients often experience pain at the pacemaker implantation site. Depending on multiple factors, patients may describe pain as mild to very severe. The patient's pain level should be routinely assessed using a 10-point pain scale (1 for least, 10 for worst). The physician's orders should include analgesic medications; prescribed medications may range from acetaminophen to stronger narcotic analgesics. The effectiveness of pain medication should be assessed and documented. Any complaint of increasing pain despite adequate analgesic medication should be carefully investigated; increased pain in the pacemaker pocket may be an indication that bleeding is occurring into the pocket.

### Cautions and Precautions

Early complications associated with permanent pacemaker implantation include infection of either the incision site or the pacemaker pocket and accidental dislodgment of the pacemaker leads. To lessen the risk of infection, the patient should avoid getting the incision site wet. The site should also be routinely inspected for signs of redness, warmth, or drainage. During the patient's hospital stay, a dressing should be maintained over the incision site as ordered by the physician; if the dressing becomes dislodged or saturated with blood during this initial period, it may be changed using sterile technique. To lessen the risk of lead dislodgment, the patient should be instructed to limit movement of the affected arm and cautioned to avoid extending the arm above the level of the shoulder. Use of a sling on the affected arm can serve to promote comfort and remind the patient to limit use of that arm.

## MONITORING PACEMAKER FUNCTION

Monitoring pacemaker function is an important part of initial postimplantation care. Comprehensive evaluation of pacemaker function requires the specialized skills of a physician trained in pacemaker therapy. However, nurses working directly with the patient are in an excellent position to identify early clues indicative of potential pacemaker problems. Monitoring pacemaker function involves two key areas:

- Assessment of pacemaker performance
- Assessment of the patient's response to the pacemaker therapy.

## ASSESSMENT OF PACEMAKER PERFORMANCE

To assess the performance of a specific pacemaker, begin by obtaining information about the type of pacemaker that was implanted and its settings. Specific details to determine include:

- What type of pacemaker was implanted? Is it dual chamber, single chamber atrial or single chamber ventricular?
- Does the pacemaker have rate responsive capability? Is the rate responsive feature turned on? If so, what is the upper rate limit?
- What is the low rate setting?
- If the pacemaker is a dual chamber, what is the high rate setting? What is the programmed AV interval?

This information may be obtained from the pacemaker data documented in the progress notes in the chart. Knowing the type of pacemaker and the applicable programmed settings is critical to an accurate evaluation of the pacemaker's function

### Monitoring Heart Rate

Assessing the patient's heart rate is a basic method for screening for proper pacemaker function that can be readily performed and requires no specialized ECG interpretation skills. If a permanent pacemaker is functioning correctly, the patient's heart rate should never drop to significantly less than the low rate setting on the pacemaker. A drop of 1–2 beats per minute is not considered 'significant' and may occur normally following pacemaker implantation; however, a rate that drops significantly may indicate a pacemaker malfunction.

### Upper Rate Limit Assessment

When a patient has a pacemaker that is capable of increasing the heart rate in response to changes in activity or metabolic demands, the assessment of the patient's heart rate as an indicator of pacemaker function becomes more complex. Appropriate assessment involves both counting a pulse rate and analyzing the patient's ECG image. General guidelines to follow when evaluating a heart rate for proper upper rate limit functioning include:

- The patient's heart rate should never drop more than 1–2 beats less than the low rate setting of the pacemaker.
- When the patient's rhythm is 100% paced, the paced rate should not exceed the upper rate limit setting.
- When the patient's rhythm is a combination of paced beats and intrinsic rhythm, the patient's heart rate may exceed the upper rate limit setting.

Pacemakers that have the capability of increasing the pacing rate in response to the body's needs include any pacemaker with the rate responsive feature as well as dual chamber pacemakers in persons with intact sinus node function.

## ASSESSMENT OF PATIENT RESPONSE TO ANTIBRADYCARDIA PACING

Assessment of the patient's response to pacemaker therapy is a crucial component in the evaluation of pacemaker function. The patient's response may be the first clue that the pacemaker is not functioning properly or that the programmed settings require adjustment to optimize pacemaker function. Additionally, assessment of the patient's response may provide clues about how well the type of pacemaker and its programmed settings 'match' the patient's symptoms and needs. A pacemaker may be functioning normally according to its programmed parameters but fail to meet desired clinical goals, such as increasing the patient's ability to perform routine activities of daily living, improving the patient's quality of life, or resolving the patient's troublesome symptoms. In some instances, the patient may actually develop new or worsening symptoms following the implantation of a permanent pacemaker. Patient assessment includes:

- Questioning and monitoring the patient for any recurrence of preimplantation symptoms. A recurrence of preimplantation symptoms may indicate a pacemaker malfunction.
- Questioning and monitoring the patient for the development of new symptoms, including hypotension, dyspnea, increased fatigue, decreased activity tolerance, palpitations, or other symptoms that the patient did not have prior to pacemaker implantation. The development of new symptoms may indicate a problem known as 'pacemaker syndrome,' which occurs when the patient loses AV synchrony during pacing and will be discussed in detail later in this course. New or worsening symptoms indicate that the programmed settings need to be adjusted.
- Observing the patient's activity tolerance and ability to perform activities of daily living without symptoms. The patient's response to activity or exercise is especially important for persons whose pacemaker has a rate responsive feature. Symptoms of activity intolerance may indicate that the rate responsive programming should be adjusted. For persons who cannot increase their heart rate when needed and who do not have a rate responsive pacemaker, signs of activity intolerance may indicate the need to revise the pacemaker to one with rate responsive capabilities.

### A Clinical Conundrum

In some cases, unraveling an apparent pacemaker malfunction requires skills and great attention. For example, Patient O is admitted for overnight monitoring following a percutaneous coronary angioplasty (PTCA) with stent placement. Patient O has a history of previous coronary artery bypass surgery and radiofrequency ablation with permanent pacemaker placement for management of atrial fibrillation refractory to medications. According to patient O's medical records, his pacemaker is a VVIR. Following his admission to the hospital, patient O's vital signs remain stable and he shows no signs of complications from the PTCA. Telemetry monitoring shows his heart rhythm is 100% paced at a rate that varies from 70–100 bpm depending on his activity. That evening, patient O complains of chest pain and shortness of breath. His heart rate is 50 bpm, but his blood pressure is unchanged. The telemetry monitor indicates that patient O's rhythm is 100% paced at a rate of 50 bpm. There is no evidence of pacemaker malfunction; there are no random pacemaker spikes or long pauses. Because patient O is symptomatic, the physician is notified. By the time the physician arrives, the patient's paced rate has increased to 98 bpm. The physician interrogates the pacemaker generator to determine the programmed settings. The interrogation confirms that the pacemaker is programmed for a low rate limit setting of 70 bpm and a high rate responsive limit of 110 bpm. However, the interrogation produces an additional piece of information; at the time of insertion, the pacemaker had been programmed with a 'sleep mode.' With a sleep mode setting, the pacemaker was programmed to reduce the paced rate at a specific time in the evening and resume the more rapid rate at a preset time in the morning. The sleep mode rate is 50 bpm, and its programmed time of onset is 8:30 pm. Because the patient experienced symptoms of decreased cardiac output at a heart rate of 50 bpm, the physician programs the sleep mode to 'off.' The patient experiences no further problems. What is the lesson? Not all apparent pacemaker malfunctions are due to problems with the generator or the pacing leads. Sometimes, the 'problem' is not a pacemaker malfunction, but a mismatch between the patient's needs and the programmed settings.

## DISCHARGE EDUCATION

Discharge education begins prior to the implantation of a permanent pacemaker and continues through the patient's brief hospital stay, the initial follow-up appointment following discharge, and the long-term follow-up period. The major emphases of patient education during the patient's hospitalization include:

- Measures to prevent infection in the incision or pacemaker pocket
- Precautions to reduce the risk of injury to the pacemaker's leads or generator
- Signs and symptoms that should be reported to the physician or nurse
- Answers to any specific concerns or questions that the patient or family may have

During the immediate and long-term follow-up, the focus of patient education is on:

- Assessment of the patient's/family's understanding of pacemaker function and management
- Correction of any misperceptions, reinforcement of previously taught material, and additional explanations as indicated by patient/family assessment
- Addressing specific patient/family questions and concerns that have arisen since the last follow-up appointment.

## INCISION CARE AND TEMPORARY RESTRICTIONS

Because the hospital stay following pacemaker implantation is often very short, patients need careful instructions on incision care and prevention of infection. The following points should be covered

- Avoid getting the incision wet for the first 5–7 days after you get home. You may sponge bathe but not shower during this time or until your first follow-up visit.
- Keep the incision clean and dry.
- After bathing, carefully pat the incision line dry. Do not rub. Do not apply creams, lotions, ointments or powders to the incision line.
- Look at the incision line every day, using a mirror if necessary. Examine the area for any signs of redness, drainage, or swelling around the incision line. Notify a nurse or physician immediately if any of these signs are present or if you develop a fever (>101°F or 38°C).

During the 4–6 weeks following pacemaker implantation, dislodgment of the pacemaker leads is a common complication. To reduce the risk of accidental dislodgment of the pacemaker leads, instruct the patient to follow these precautions.

- Avoid excessive arm movement on the side that pacemaker was implanted for at least 4 weeks.
- Avoid vigorous activities (including golf and tennis) for 4–6 weeks.
- Do not lift, push, or pull more than 10 pounds for the first 4 weeks. Activities that should be restricted include carrying groceries in from the car, carrying laundry baskets and pushing vacuum cleaners.
- Do not put pressure on the pacemaker generator site. Patients who hunt should be instructed to avoid placing the rifle stock on the same shoulder as the pacemaker pocket.

## BASIC SAFETY MEASURES

Three basic safety measures to cover with the patient and family include the pacemaker identification card, notification of other physicians and healthcare providers, and monitoring pulse rate.

### Pacemaker Identification Card

At the time that a pacemaker is implanted, a temporary identification card is issued. This card lists specific information about the patient's pacemaker, including the type of pacemaker, manufacturer, date of insertion, and healthcare provider information. All patients should receive the card before discharge. Explain that the device manufacturer will mail a permanent card to the patient within a few weeks following discharge. Instruct the patient to always carry the pacemaker identification card, and encourage a family member to keep and carry an additional copy. Explain that the card contains vital information that a physician would need to know to accurately assess the patient and the pacemaker function in the event of a problem.

### Notification of Other Healthcare Providers

Instruct the patient and family to let all other medical healthcare providers, including dentists, know that the patient has a permanent pacemaker Some medical and dental procedures may temporarily affect the functioning of the pacemaker and will need to be modified. Other procedures, such as magnetic resonance imaging (MRI), are contraindicated for a person with a permanent pacemaker.

### Counting the Pulse

The patient or a family member should be taught how to check the patient's pulse. When teaching a patient to check his/her pulse, consider covering these points:

- Check your pulse regularly, at least once a week (or more often as directed by your physician).
- Count your pulse for a full minute.
- Each time that you count your heart rate, record the rate and the date in a notebook. Bring this notebook to your follow-up appointments.
- Find out from your physician what your lowest acceptable heart rate is. Notify the physician if your heart rate abruptly drops to significantly less than that level.
- If your pacemaker has an upper rate limit, determine what your highest acceptable heart rate is. If your heart rate dramatically increases beyond that limit, call your physician.

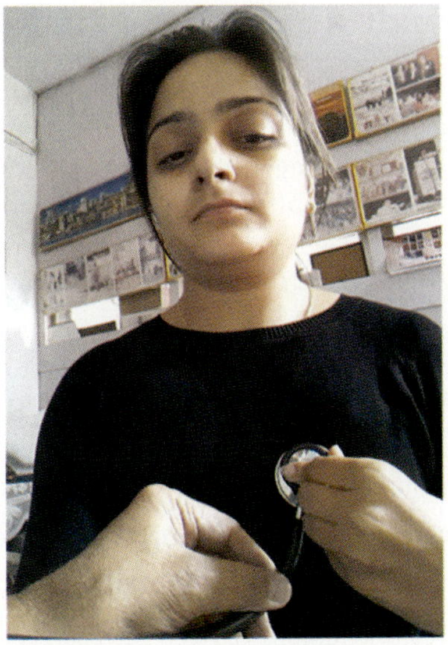

**Fig. 29.51:** Doctor examining an adolescent girl who was fitted with DDD type of pacemaker and tricuspid prosthetic tissue valve

- Your pulse might feel a little irregular. As long as your pulse rate falls within the acceptable range established by your physician, do not worry about an occasional irregularity.

## NOTIFYING THE PHYSICIAN

Instruct the patient to notify the physician if there are any signs of infection or any other symptoms that may indicate a problem with the pacemaker's functioning (Figs 29.51, 29.52 and Tables 29.6–29.8), including:

- Fever or signs of infection at the pacemaker pocket site (i.e. warmth, redness, drainage, excessive swelling, or pain not relieved with pain medications)

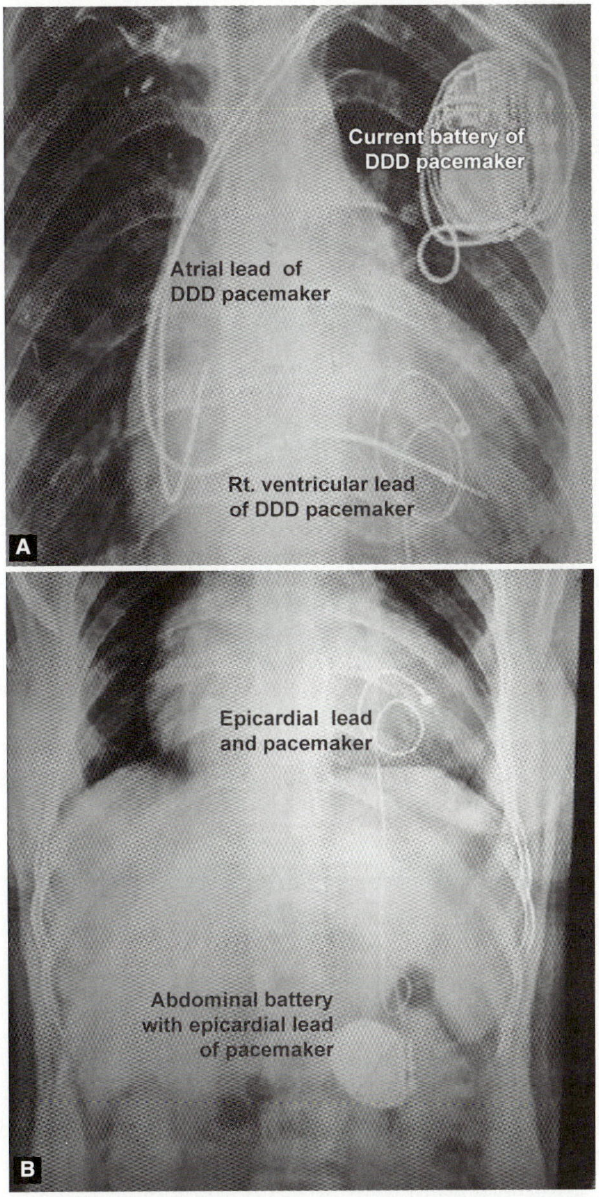


**Fig. 29.52:** (A) X-ray chest PA view showing battery, atrial and ventricular leads of DDD pacemaker with tricuspid prosthetic valve at tricuspid annulus. (B) X-ray chest PA view shows battery in the abdominal area, leads of epicardial pacemaker and tricuspid prosthetic valve

**Table 29.6:** Clinical problems faced by the physician after PPI

| Abnormality | Time of appearance after pacemaker implant | Possible fault | Management |
|---|---|---|---|
| 1. Dizziness and missed beats; recurrence of initial symptoms | Hours to days | Lead displacement or penetration resulting in the loss of capture | Reposition lead; occasionally |
| 2. Frequint and irregular beats | Hours to days | Lead displacement resuling in the loss of sensing | Reprogramming is possible |
| 3. Painful pacer site with or withour pyrexia | Usually days or weeks | Infected pacer pocket | Reomval of pacing system and resetting |
| 4. Dizziness and syncope | Often monts or years | Myoinhibition | Programme to R wave triggered or change to bipolar system |
| 5. Dizziness and heavy palpitations | Variable | Retrograde conduction pacemaker syndrome | Change to dual chamber system if symptoms sever |
| 6. Recurrence of initial symptoms | Years | Lead fracture or pacemaker failure | Replace faulty part |
| 7. Tachycardia with dual chamber pacemaker | Variable | Pacemaker mediated techycardia | Reprogramme pacemaker |

PPI=permanent pacemaker implantation

**Table 29.7:** Electromagnetic interference and medical/dental procedures

| Does not affect pacemaker | Cautions needed | Generally contraindicated |
|---|---|---|
| | Bone density test (check on type)† | |
| | Diagnostic ultrasound | |
| | Therapeutic ultrasound | |
| | Electrolysis | |
| Dental X-rays | Mechanical ventilation‡ | |
| Dental drills | Use of electrocautery during surgery | |
| Dental ultrasonic probes used for cleaning | Planned external defibrillation or cardioversion | MRI |
| Chest X-rays | Use of hearing aid with coil around the neck | |
| CT scans | Litho tripsy | |
| Mammograms* | Radiofrequency ablation | |
| | Radiation therapy | |
| | Transcutaneous electrical nerve stimulation | |

*Let technician know which side generator is on; mammogram equipment may be adjusted to decrease pressure on the pacemaker generator and increase patient comfort.

†Ionizing radiation on wrist or heel does not present a problem; most type will not intertere with the pacemaker.

‡Applies to pacemakers with a rate responsive sensor that responds to changes in breathing; in certain circumstances (such as surgery), the rate sensor may need to be turned off.

**Table 29.8:** Result of intraoperative measurements

| Parameter | Desirable | Acceptable | Unacceptable |
|---|---|---|---|
| Pacing threshold V | ≤0.5 V | ≤1.0 V | >1.0 V |
| R wave | >8.0 mV | >4.0 mV | ≤4.0 mV |
| Pacing threshold A | ≤1.0 V | ≤1.5 V | >1.5 V |
| P-wave | >4.0 mV | >2.0 mV | ≤2.0 mV |

- Occurrence (or recurrence) of dizziness or fainting spells
- Development or increase in shortness of breath
- A sudden weight gain of 3–5 pounds over 24–48 hours
- Swelling in fingers, ankles or feet
- Swelling that occurs in the arm on the same side as the pacemaker generator
- Continuous rhythmic hiccoughing
- Pulse rate that falls significantly outside the acceptable heart rate range established by the physician.

## SAFETY MEASURES: ELECTRICAL EQUIPMENT AND DEVICES

American Society of Anesthesiologists recommends the use of continuous electrocardiographic rhythm monitoring in addition to pulse oximetry during endoscopic procedures performed on patients with implanted cardiac devices due to the risk of electromagnetic interference.

### Level of Evidence: Expert Opinion/Consensus Statement

Patients with permanent pacemakers and their families have many concerns and questions about what type of equipment they can use and what devices might interfere with the proper functioning of the patient's pacemaker.

### Electromagnetic Interference

Many tools and electronic devices use both electricity and magnets. The combination creates an electromagnetic field around the device. The size and strength of the field varies with the device. A large piece of equipment, such as an MRI machine or an arc-welding device, generates a very strong, powerful electromagnetic field. Household items, such as microwave ovens, mixers and electric blankets, generate a very weak electromagnetic field. When the functioning of one electronic device disrupts or interferes with the normal functioning of another device, electromagnetic interference is said to occur. A strong electromagnetic field can disrupt the functioning of a permanent pacemaker. When electromagnetic interference occurs, the settings on the pacemaker may be altered. Sensing function may be lost, and the pacing rate may revert to the magnet mode rate. The patient may experience signs and symptoms, such as dizziness, light-headedness or a rapid heart rate. Electromagnetic interference does not permanently damage pacemaker function. To relieve the symptoms and restore normal pacemaker function, persons with pacemakers may simply move away from the offending equipment and sit down and rest until symptoms disappear.

Many patients and their families have heard a mix of accurate and inaccurate information about the impact of electromagnetic interference on the functioning of a pacemaker. Others may be unaware of the potential risk of electromagnetic interference from the use of relatively common items. Careful, precise instructions can both help relieve the patient's anxiety and prevent unnecessary disruption of pacemaker function from electromagnetic interference.

Three major areas to cover with the patient and the family are: use of cell phones, use of normal household equipment, and airport security and commercial antitheft screening devices.

### Cell Phones

Some studies have shown that cell phones may not adversely affect pacemaker functioning. However, as technology continues to advance and the use of digital technology grows, it is prudent to instruct patients to use some precautions when using or carrying a cell phone. Consider covering the following points:

- Use the ear on the opposite side from the pacemaker generator when talking on a cell phone.
- Carry the cell phone in a pocket away from the pacemaker pulse generator; avoid carrying the phone in the pocket right over pacemaker generator site.
- Cordless household telephones are not the same as cellular telephones and should not interfere with pacemaker function.

### Use of Common Household Equipment

Generally, a person with a permanent pacemaker can safely use normal household electrical devices as long as those devices are in good repair and properly grounded. Devices that are safe to use include household microwaves. Pacemaker and microwave technology have advanced enough that pacemaker functioning is not usually disrupted by microwaves.

- Cordless household telephones
- Personal computers
- Electrical hand tools
- Electrical home appliances
- Electric blankets
- Electric razors
- Amplitude modulation/Frequency modulation (AM/FM radios)
- Televisions
- Office electrical equipment, such as copy machines
- Citizen band radios

In 2007, a high-school student's report regarding potential interference as a result of portable music devices gained national attention. The study, which focused on only one brand of music device, found that 50% of patients were affected by electrical interference when the device was held 2 inches from the patients' chests for 5–10 seconds. More research is required to determine the safety measures that may ameliorate adverse effects.

### Airport Security

With the heightened emphasis on security checks at airports, patients and families may have concerns about getting through airport security. Studies have shown that while airport security devices do not damage pacemakers, the security devices will detect the implanted metal and trigger the alarm. To facilitate clearance through airport security, instruct patients to:

- Always carry their pacemaker identification card.
- Present the pacemaker identification card to the security agent before walking through a security screening device.
- Request a hand search. Ask the security guard to avoid holding the hand held screening device directly over the pacemaker generator for a prolonged period. Handheld screening devices contain a magnet and may interact with pacemaker if held directly over pacemaker generator pocket for more than a brief period.

### Antitheft Devices

Commercial antitheft devices are commonly used in many department stores in the United States. As noted, these devices have the potential to temporarily disrupt the functioning of the pacemaker. Instruct the patient to walk through the security-screening device at a reasonable pace; also instruct the patient to avoid lingering in the area around the antitheft devices.

## MEDICAL AND DENTAL PROCEDURES

Many medical and dental diagnostic procedures will not interfere with the proper functioning of a person's pacemaker; however, some procedures have the potential to disrupt normal pacemaker functioning. Instruct the patient to be sure that all healthcare providers know that he/she has a pacemaker before a procedure is performed. If the procedure has a risk of disrupting the pacemaker's functioning, the patient should discuss the risks and benefits of having that procedure done with the healthcare providers. In some instances, specific precautions may be taken to reduce the risk that a given procedure will disrupt the pacemaker's function. Pacemaker manufacturers also recommend that the pacemaker be interrogated to verify proper programming following performance of some procedures that are functioning (*see* Table 29.7).

## FOLLOW-UP CARE AFTER ANTIBRADYCARDIA PACEMAKER IMPLANTATION

The evolution of pacemaker technology has led to the development of specialized follow-up clinics staffed by trained physicians, nurses and allied health professionals. The ideal follow-up regimen should be determined by the physician and based on the patient's needs. Factors to consider may include the patient's preferences, underlying medical conditions, geographic isolation from direct follow-up and costs.

## INITIAL FOLLOW-UP

Initial follow-up goals are to:

- Evaluate thoroughly the status of the pacemaker generator pocket
- Assess basic pacemaker function and adjust pacing and sensing thresholds as needed
- Obtain and document required patient and pacemaker data
- Establish the schedule for transtelephone monitoring (TTM) and direct evaluation

### Appointments

Refer Table 29.8.

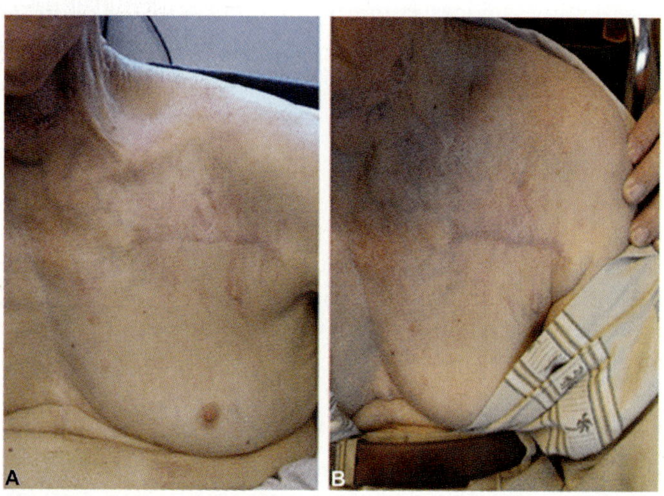


**Fig. 29.53:** The operative site at 3-month (A) and 9-month (B) follow-up examination

### Wound Assessment

The pacemaker pocket site should be carefully assessed for indications of impaired healing or signs of complications (Figs 29.53–29.57). Complications that may occur include infection in the pacemaker pocket, development of a hematoma in the pocket site, or erosion of the generator or the pacemaker lead through the tissue and skin. Persons with diabetes are more at risk to develop an infection in the pacemaker pocket. Persons taking anticoagulants are at risk to form a hematoma in the pacemaker pocket. Signs of impaired healing may include:

- Subjective complaint of increased pain at generator site
- Increased swelling present in pacemaker pocket area
- Elevated temperature or other signs of systemic infection
- Purulent drainage from incision
- Failure of incision line to heal
- Warmth or redness around the incision line or pacemaker pocket

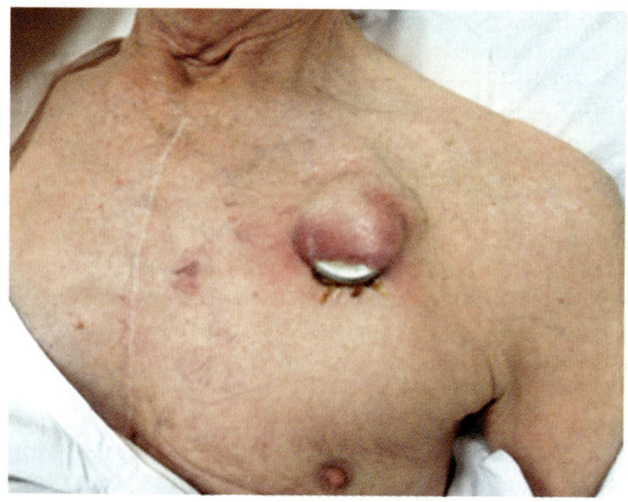

**Fig. 29.54:** A 78-year-old man presents with a pacemaker eroding through the subcutaneous tissue and skin, with redness and purulent exudate

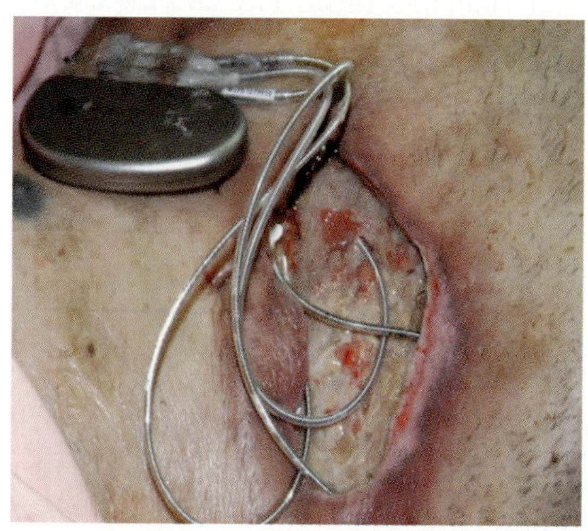

**Fig. 29.55:** An unusual treatment of pacemaker pocket infection

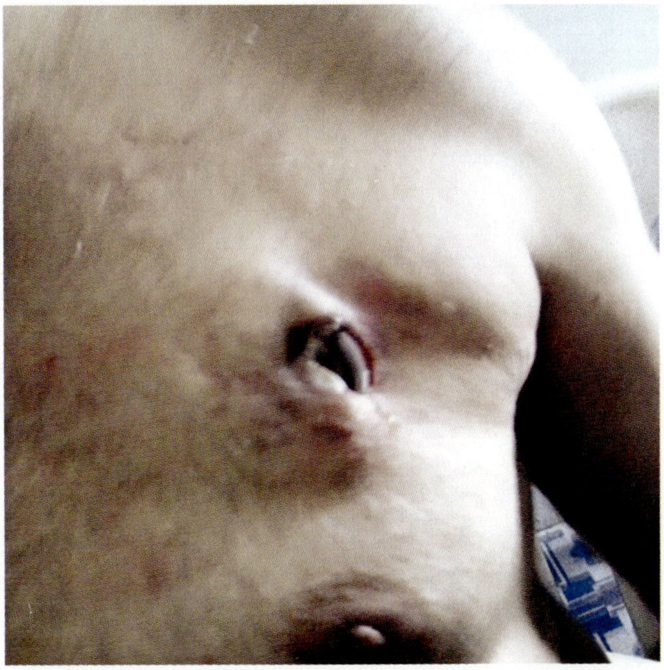

**Fig. 29.56:** Suppurative wound with visible pacemaker leads. Ablation of all material was necessary

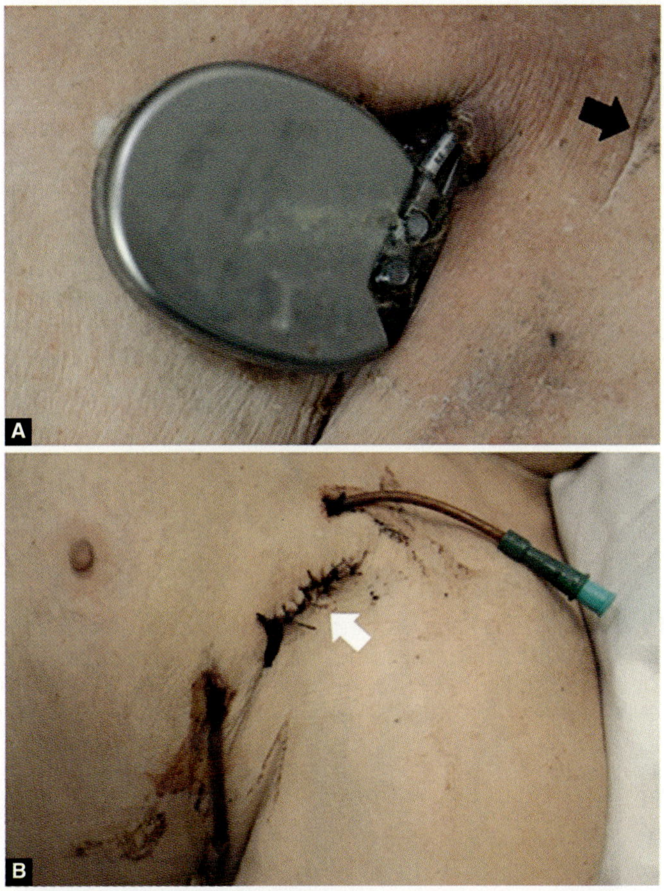


**Fig. 29.57:** (A) A photograph of the extruded ICD generator, showing encrustation adjacent to the exposed leads. Black arrow indicates the incision scar from the original implantation procedure. (B) Photograph demonstrating the Z-incision (white arrow) created for the purpose of wound debridement and the irrigation (top)-drainage (bottom) tubes *in situ* for closed system povidone-iodine irrigation

While not common, infection, hematoma and erosion are serious complications that may require surgical revision or removal of the pacemaker.

## Pacemaker Assessment

*Chest X-ray:* It is performed to verify that the pacemaker leads remain correctly positioned (Figs 29.58–29.74).

*Electrocardiography*: It is done with and without a magnet to evaluate pacemaker function (Figs 29.75 and 29.76). The pacemaker generator may be interrogated and data

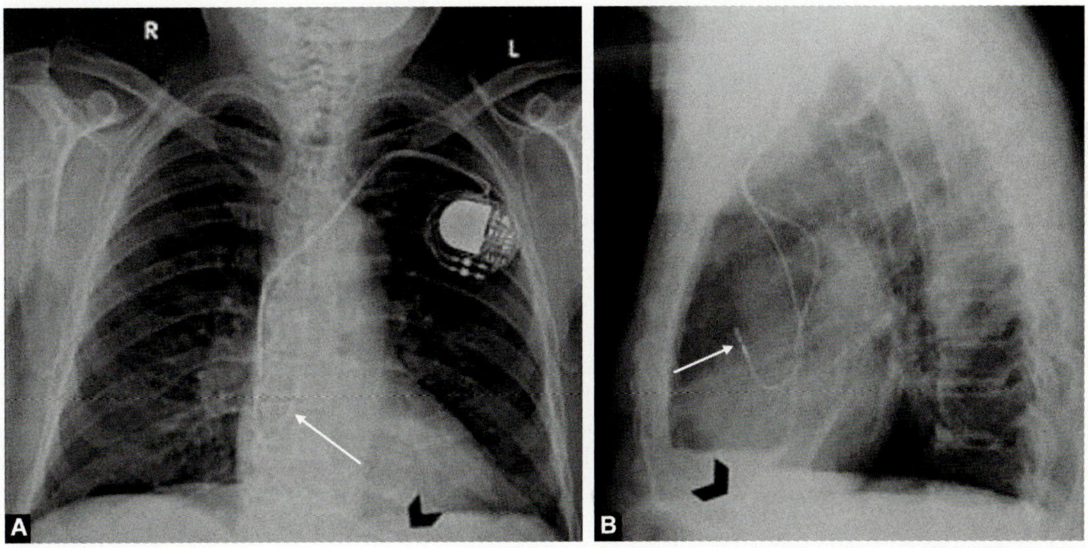


**Fig. 29.58:** A dual chamber pacemaker. (A) 89-year-old male with a dual chamber pacemaker placed via the left subclavian vein with the generator in the subcutaneous left infraclavicular fossa. Chest X-ray (A) PA view and (B) LAT view shows the right atrial lead is inferiorly directed and takes a 'J loop' curve with tip pacing the right atrial appendage (white arrow). Right ventricle lead directed inferiorly through the right atrium and tricuspid valve, then courses anteriorly and inferiorly with the tip at the right ventricular apex (black arrowhead). In single chamber pacemakers, only the right atrial or ventricular lead is present

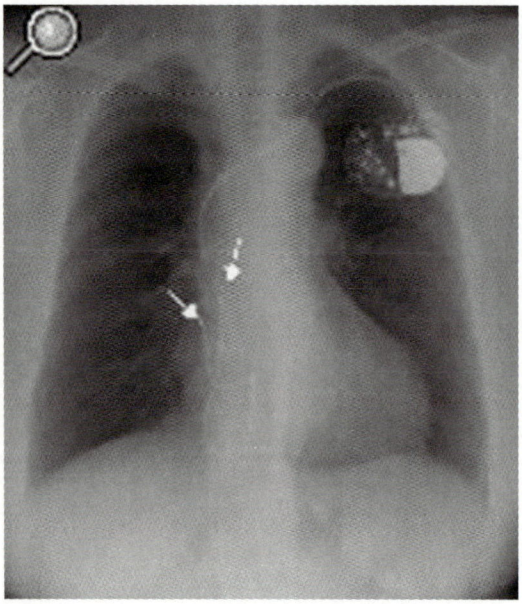

**Fig. 29.59:** Chest X-ray showing two pacemaker leads fixed on the right atrial appendage, one of them belonging to a previous pacemaker system, sectioned and abandoned in the atrial cavity (arrows)

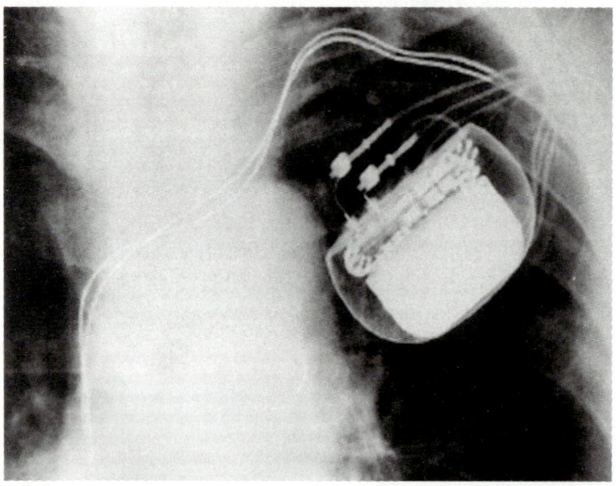

**Fig. 29.60:** DDD pacemaker implanted on the left. The leads have been introduced through the subclavian vein. The changes of direction at the junctions with the brachiocephalic vein and superior vena cava put the leads under tension, which makes it more difficult to insert a curved stylet and, in particular, to manipulate the atrial lead

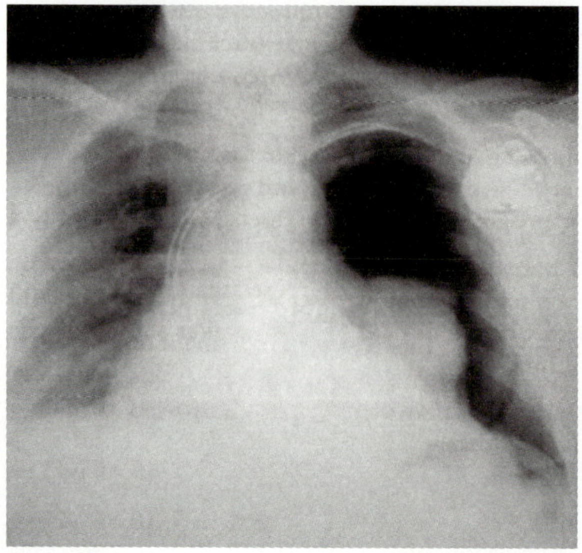

**Fig. 29.61:** X-ray image showing large pneumothorax following permanent pacemaker implantation

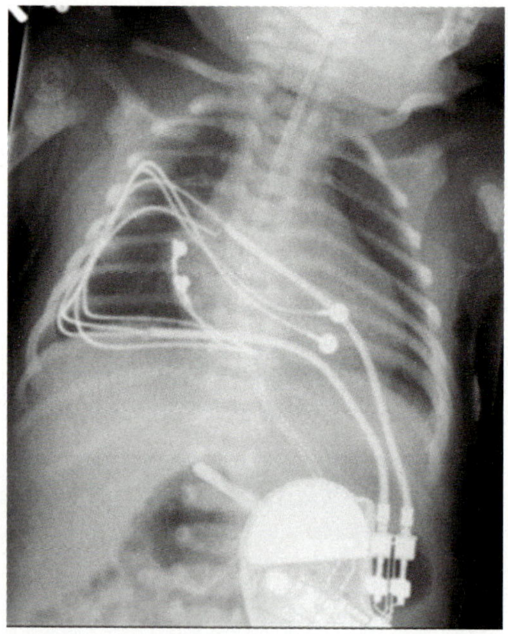

**Fig. 29.62:** X-ray chest PA and frontal abdominal views showing epicardial pacemaker leads attached proximally with heart and is supported with external battery fitted in the abdomen distally in a 4-year-old boy

obtained. Often, the sensing and pacing thresholds are tested. By the time of the first follow-up visit, the inflammation associated with implantation of the leads has resolved, and the programmed thresholds may need to be revised.

### Pacemaker Dependence

During either the initial follow-up visit or a subsequent visit, the patient's underlying rhythm should be determined and the extent of the patient's dependence on the pacemaker should be assessed. A person is considered 'pacemaker dependent' if he/she requires the proper functioning of the pacemaker in order to perform activities of daily living. Persons who are pacemaker dependent often have very little effective underlying or intrinsic heart rhythm. Abrupt cessation of pacing often results in significant hemodynamic compromise. Persons who are pacemaker dependent may require more frequent follow-up, as pacemaker failure would have severe consequences requiring emergency intervention.

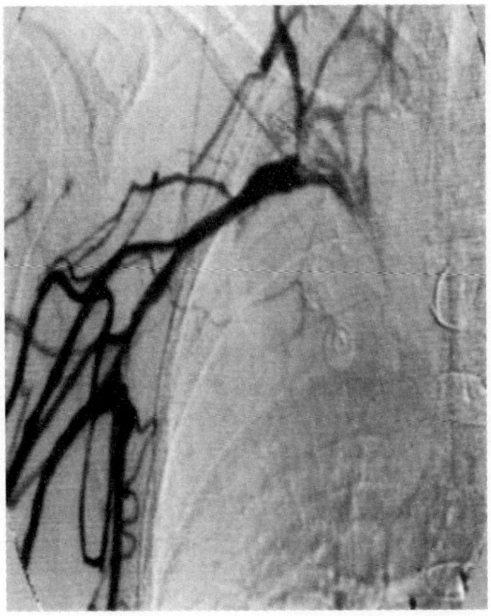

**Fig. 29.63:** Subclavian thrombosis, DSA image, early venous phase after pacer implantation

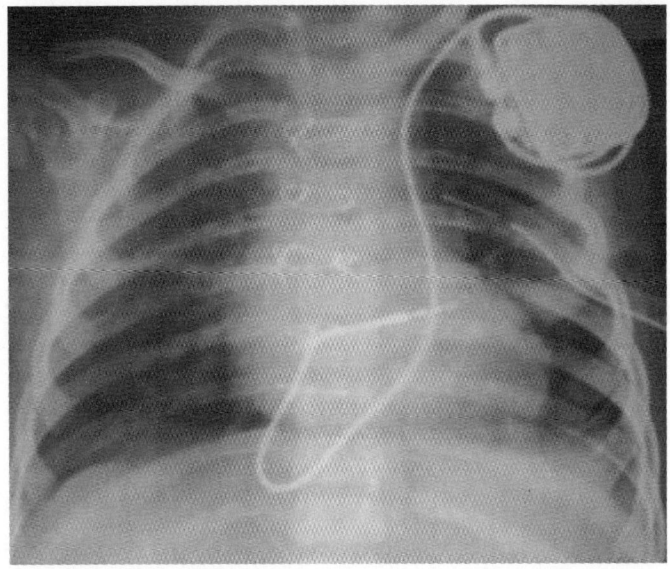

**Fig. 29.65:** Chest X-ray shows endocardial pacemaker implantation via the persistent left superior vena cava and coronary sinus

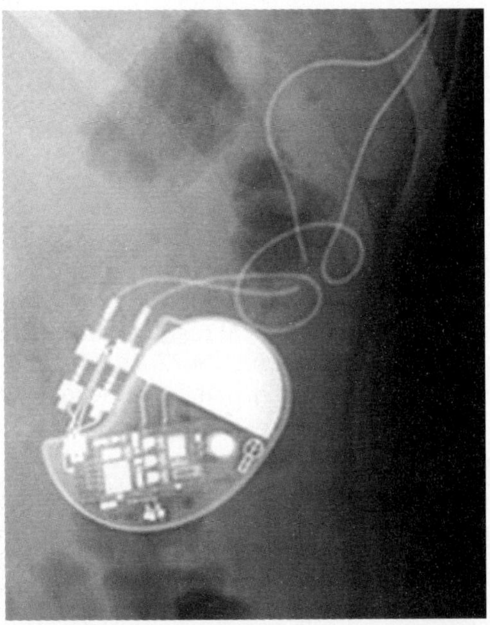

**Fig. 29.64:** Abdominal flat plate film of a patient with an atrial lead fracture several years after the Fontan procedure. This lead fracture is at the most common site, immediately below the left costal margin, which is a site of repetitive flexion. The patient was relatively asymptomatic, as pacing in the VVI mode occurred by default in the absence of atrial sensing

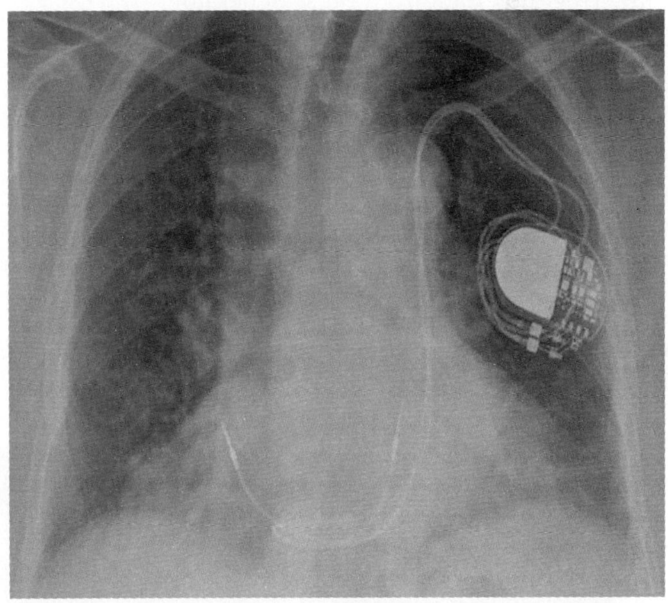

**Fig. 29.66:** Lateral chest radiograph, with distal ventricular electrode in the right ventricular outflow tract

## Follow-up Clinical Documentation

Adequate clinical documentation is vital for the effective long-term management of a person with a permanent pacemaker. Accurate evaluation of the pacemaker's function can only occur when the pacemaker type and programming are known. Current patient demographics are needed in the event that a device recall occurs and patient notification is required. Recommended information to document in the patient's file includes:

- *Demographic data:* Name, age, address, telephone number and email address (update with each visit)
- *Pacemaker data:* Generator model and serial number; pacemaker lead(s) model and serial number
- Operative note with implant data
- Examination of incision
- Chest X-ray findings
- 12-lead ECG

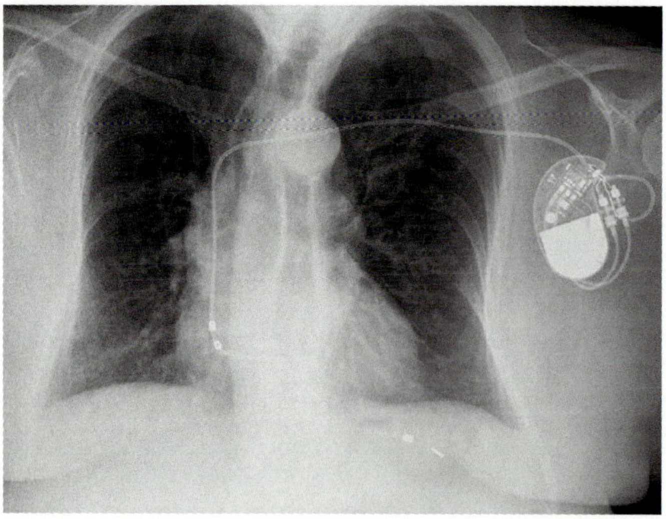

**Fig. 29.67:** Posteroanterior chest X-ray, showing the pacemaker lead tip outside the heart, below the contour of the left hemidiaphragm

- Rhythm strips
- Interrogation data from pulse generator
- Measurement of sensing and pacing thresholds
- Measurement of sensor related data
- Printout of final values/current programming

### Schedule for Future Evaluation

Before the end of the first follow-up visit, the patient and family should receive detailed instructions about long-term follow-up. This should include the schedule for both TTM and direct evaluation visits. The patient should receive the equipment required to perform TTM at home. In addition, the patient and a family member should be instructed in the procedures for contacting the TTM facility and performing the monitoring. Written instructions should supplement verbal instructions and demonstration of the equipment. Contact numbers for both the TTM center and the follow-up pacemaker clinic should be provided.

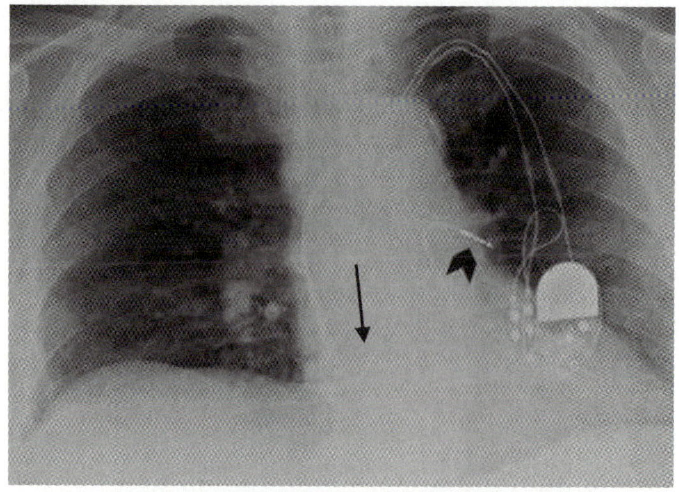

**Fig. 29.68:** Right ventricle lead in left main pulmonary artery. A 73-year-old male with a dual chamber pacemaker. Chest X-ray PA view shows the right ventricle lead is misplaced (black arrowhead), taking a 'Swan-Ganz'-like course and ending in the left main pulmonary artery instead of the right ventricle apex. Right atrium lead is correctly placed at the right atrial appendage (black arrow)

## LONG-TERM FOLLOW-UP

Ongoing follow-up of the patient after permanent pacemaker implantation is crucial to the achievement and maintenance of optimal clinical results for the patient from the pacemaker therapy (Figs 29.77–29.82). The focus of postimplantation follow-up is not merely on device

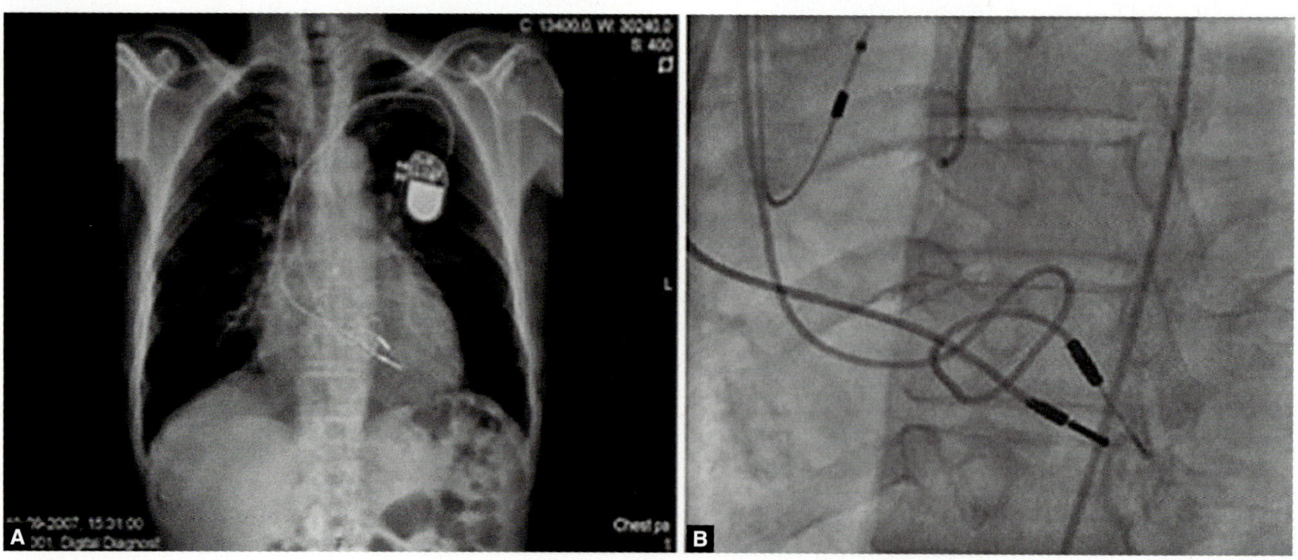


**Fig. 29.69:** (A) Chest X-ray showing two leads crossing the tricuspid valve, one forming a redundant loop; (B) improved visualization of pacemaker leads in left anterior oblique view during right heart catheterization

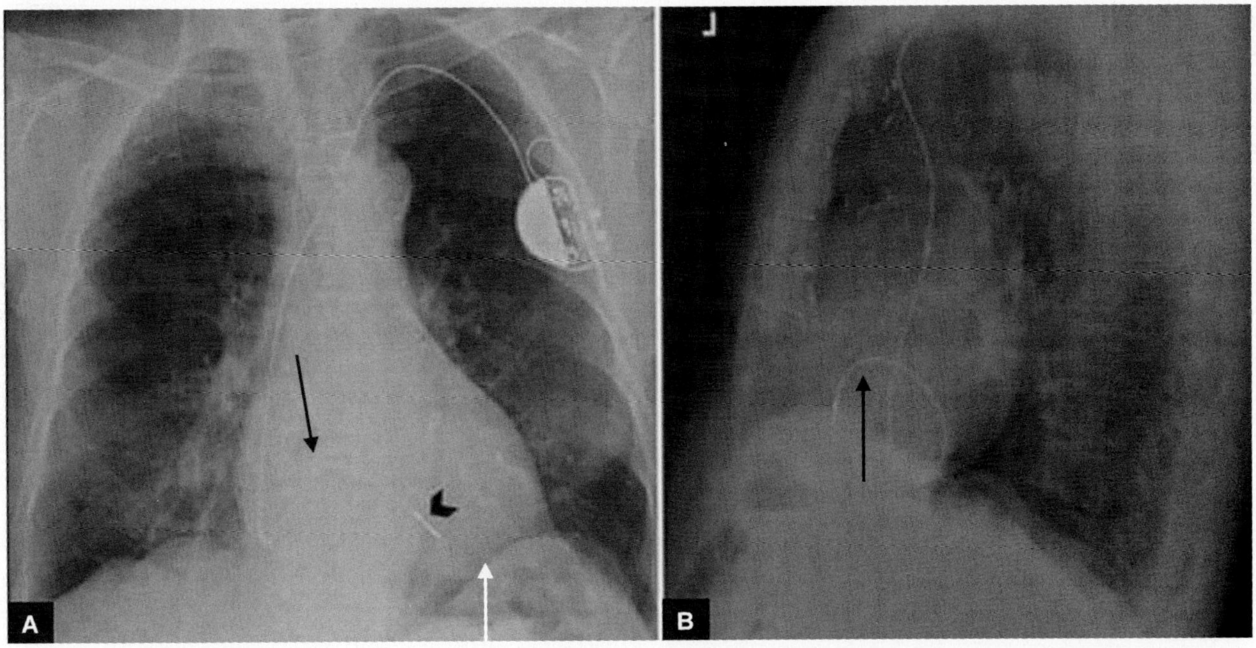


**Fig. 29.70:** Single chamber pacemaker with abnormal position of the lead. A 73-year-old male with a single chamber pacemaker placed using the subclavian transvenous approach with an abnormally positioned lead. Chest X-ray (A) PA view shows the lead is directed inferiorly through the right atrium taking a serpentine course (black arrow) through the coronary sinus with lead tip misplaced in an epicardial vein (black arrowhead) instead of the right ventricular apex (white arrow). Lead tip is passively fixed and pulse generator is placed in a subcutaneous pocket in the infraclavicular fossa. (B) Lateral view confirms lead misplacement with lead curving in a loop and then coursing anteriorly (black arrow) instead of descending and coursing anteriorly as would be seen in with a correctly placed right ventricular lead

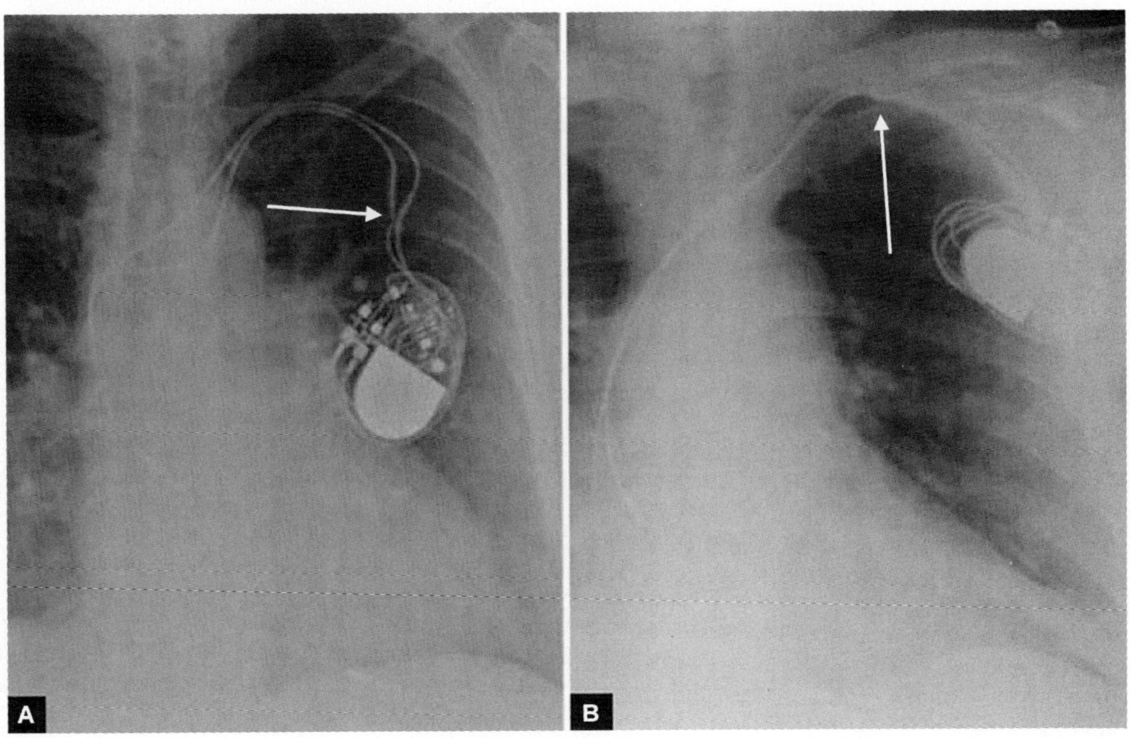


**Fig. 29.71:** Malfunctioning leads. (A) A 56-year-old female with a dual chamber malfunctioning pacemaker. Chest X-ray PA view shows the pacemaker malfunction is due to a kinked lead (white arrow). (B) An 86-year-old male with a malfunctioning dual chamber pacemaker. Chest X-ray AP view shows malfunction is due to pinching of the lead (white arrow) before entering the subclavian vein by the clavicle

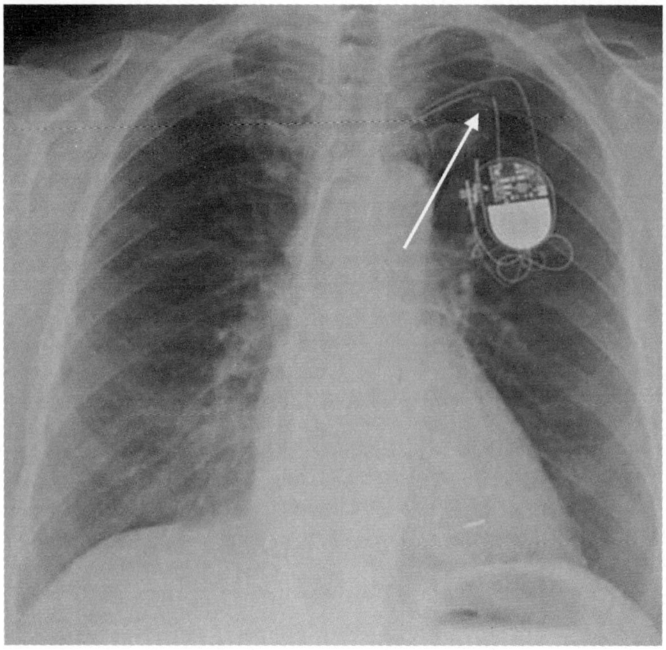

**Fig. 29.72:** Complete lead fracture. PA chest X-ray of a malfunctioning pacemaker due to lead complete fracture shows discontinuation of the lead wire (white arrow) proximal to the generator with wide gaps among the lead segments representing dislodgement and migration

surveillance but, more importantly, is also on the interface and interaction of the patient and pacemaker. A policy statement developed and published by the HRS notes that appropriate medical follow-up begins with patient and

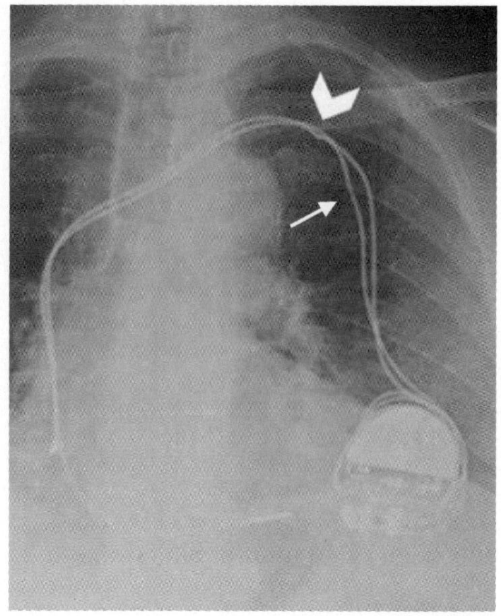

**Fig. 29.73:** Pinched lead and 'incomplete' lead fracture. An 84-year-old female with a malfunctioning dual chamber pacemaker. Chest X-ray PA view shows pacemaker malfunction is due to pinching of lead wire by the clavicle (white arrowhead). The relative thinning of caliber of the other lead (white arrow) simulates an incomplete fracture, but is in fact caused by the tie-down, which affixes the lead to the chest wall

family education before a pacemaker is implanted and continues throughout the patient's life (as opposed to the life of the device). Major goals of follow-up include optimization of pacemaker function, ongoing patient and family education, early identification of potential problems,

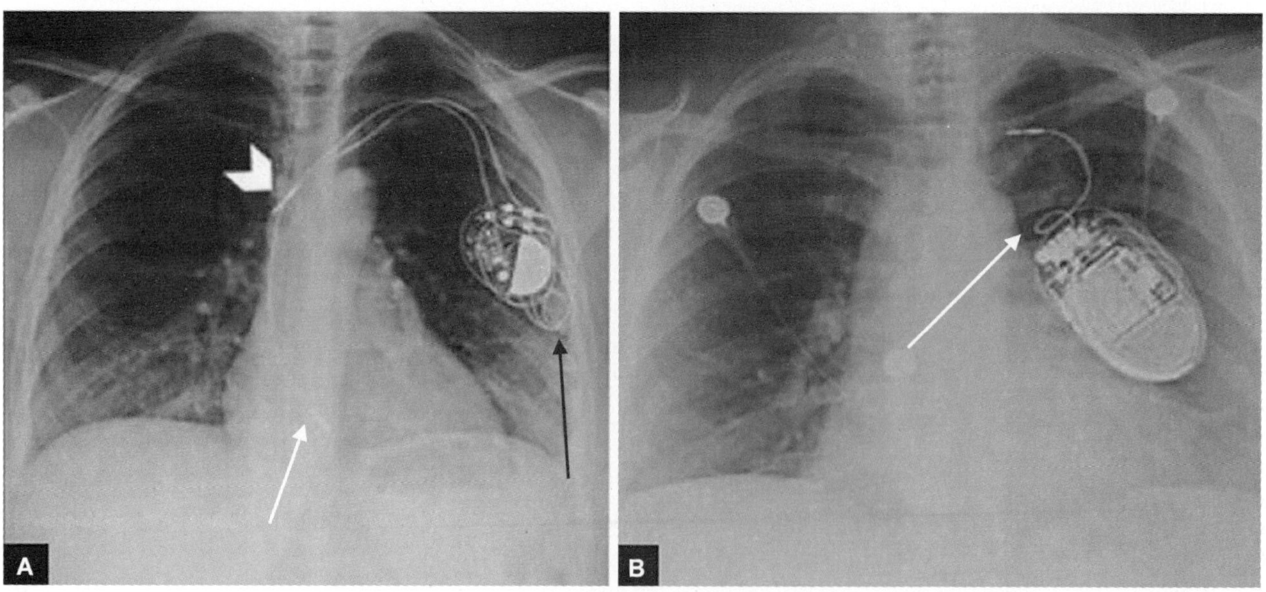


**Fig. 29.74:** Twiddler syndrome. (A) A 29-year-old female with a dual chamber pacemaker with twiddler syndrome. Chest X-ray PA view shows the generator has been rotated by the patient causing the lead wires to dislodge and wind around the generator (black arrow). The right atrial lead (white arrowhead) has been removed from the right atrial appendage and lies in the superior vena cava and the right ventricular lead (white arrow) now lies within the right atrium. (B) A 54-year-old female with single-chamber pacemaker and a severe case of twiddler syndrome. Chest X-ray PA view shows the lead wire, has been completely reeled around the generator (white arrow) causing the patient to receive no cardiac electrical therapy

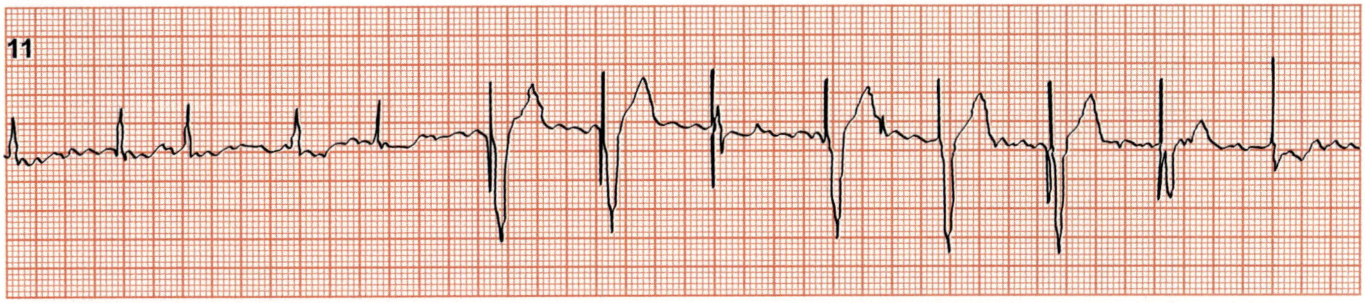


**Fig. 29.75:** VVI pacemaker with fusion beats (pseudomalfunction). This VVI pacemaker was implanted in a patient with atrial fibrillation and intermittent symptomatic complete heart block. In the lead II rhythm strip, the first five QRS complexes are normal in morphology and irregular, as would be expected in atrial fibrillation. The next two QRS complexes are wide and preceded by a pacemaker spike. This represents normal sensing and pacing. The eighth QRS complex is narrow but preceded by a pacemaker spike. The spikes occur at a fixed and regular interval. In this instance, spontaneous ventricular depolarization had begun at approximately the time the pacemaker discharged. The 12th QRS complex in the sequence represents a fusion beat. Within the QRS complex of the 13th beat, a pacemaker spike is visible. Again, this represents nearly simultaneous conduction of a supraventricular beat and pacemaker electrical discharge. At first glance, this may appear to be failure to sense; however, the pacemaker is functioning normally and competing with the underlying rhythm

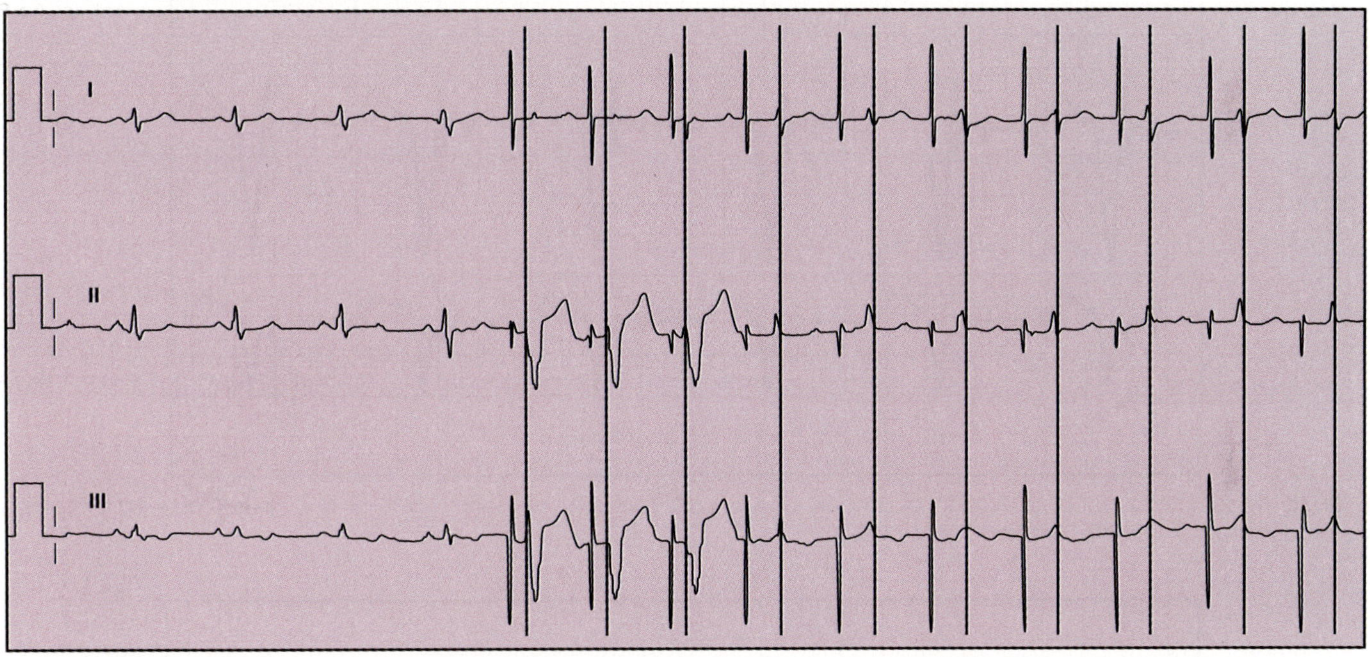


**Fig. 29.76:** This is a rhythm strip from a patient with a newly implanted ventricular lead. The patient also has an atrial lead. His pacemaker is a dual chamber DDD Medtronic pacemaker. A magnet was placed over the pacemaker in the middle of the recording

and timely identification of the need for battery and/or generator replacement. Although, some follow-up may be provided by the patient's primary physician, the HRS recommends that scheduled follow-up also be performed by physicians and support personnel trained in the management and evaluation of pacemaker therapy. Two major types of follow-up are generally used to evaluate and manage the patient with a permanent pacemaker: TTM and direct evaluation.

## TRANSTELEPHONE MONITORING

Transtelephone monitoring has been used for more than 30 years in the follow-up and management of persons with permanent pacemakers (Figs 29.83–29.87). TTM provides a relatively inexpensive, convenient method for monitoring battery function and screening pacemaker function. There are several advantages/benefits of TTM. It permits monitoring of pacemaker function in patients who live a considerable distance from an appropriate pacemaker follow-up center. Also, studies have shown that patients are more likely to use TTM than to make an appointment at a follow-up center, if they are concerned about a possible pacemaker malfunction. Another advantage is the cost of TTM; it is less costly than a direct evaluation. TTM has been found to be effective in detecting major pacemaker problems, such as failure to sense and failure to pace (i.e.

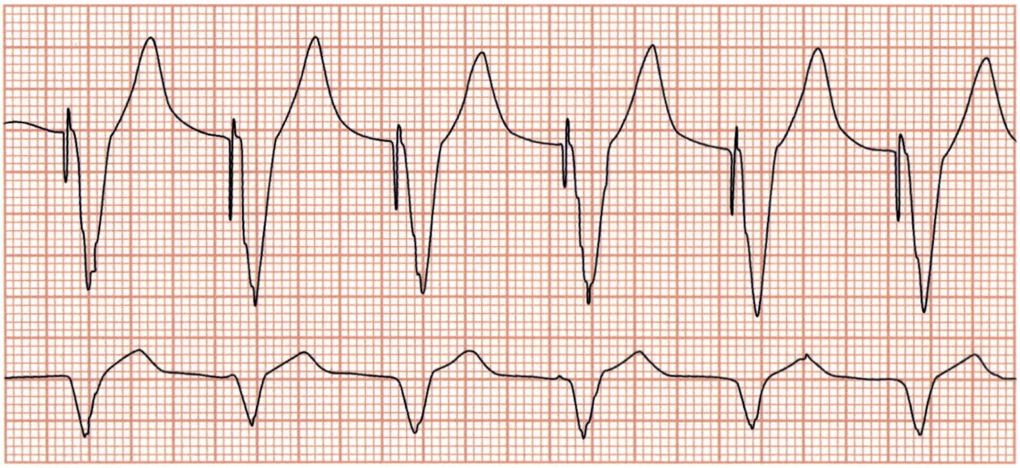

**Fig. 29.77:** Artificially induces electronic stimulus that paces the patient's rhythm causing a blip or spike on the ECG waveform

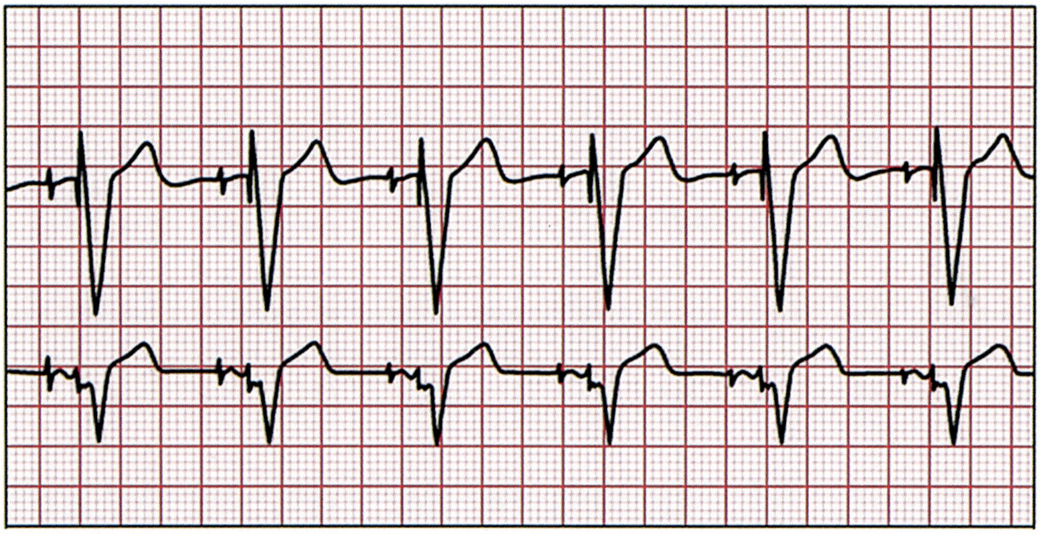

**Fig. 29.78:** AV sequential pacemaker (dual chamber). One spike followed by an abnormal P (atrial capture) followed by a second spike producting a wide QRS (ventricular capture)

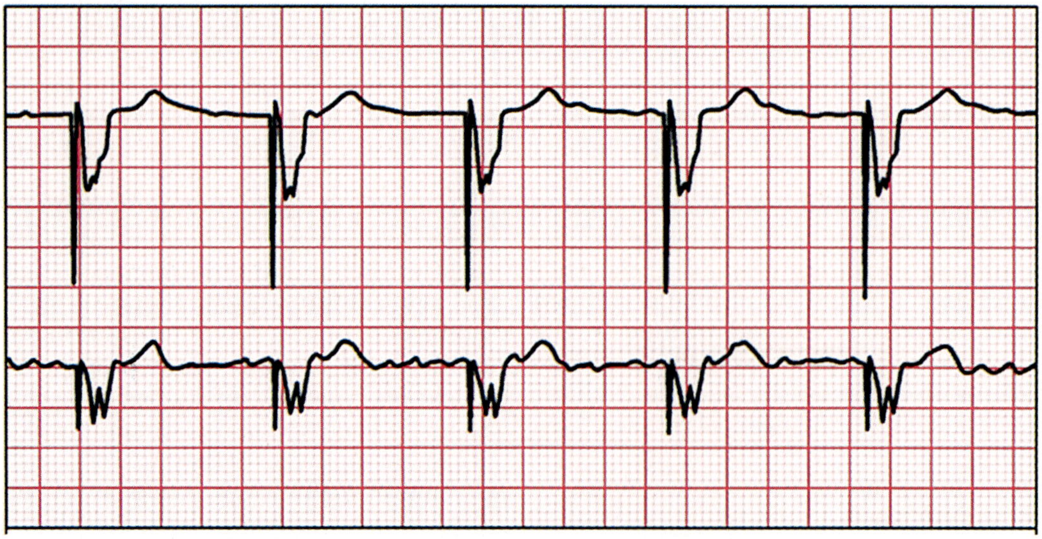

**Fig. 29.79:** Ventricular pacemaker (single chamber)—ventricular pacing in atrial fibrillation showing one spike producing a wide QRS (ventricular capture)

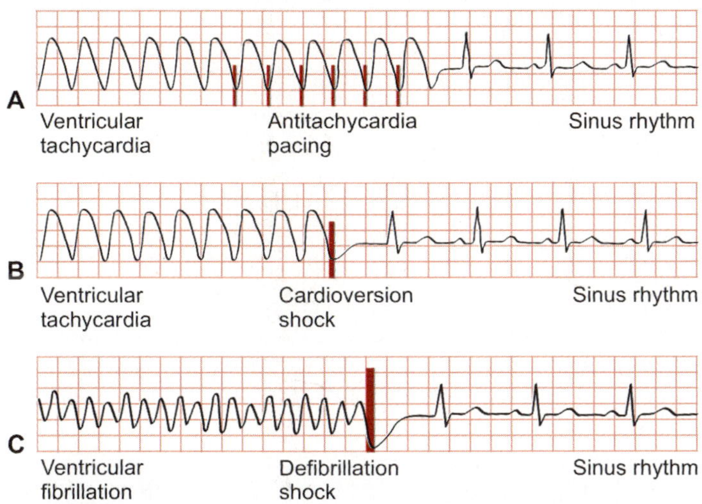


**Fig. 29.80:** Tiered arrhythmia therapy and implanted cardioverter-defibrillators (ICDs). These devices are capable of automatically delivering staged therapy in treating ventricular tachycardia (VT) or ventricular fibrillation (VF), including antitachycardia pacing (A) and cardioversion shocks (B) for VT, and defibrillation shocks (C) for VF

output failure). It can also monitor basic battery status and evaluate the battery function for indications that the battery is becoming depleted. Interrogation of the pacemaker generator cannot be done using TTM; data about the remaining voltage in the battery, programmed settings, and other specific information may only be obtained by telemetry interrogation using a programmer in a direct evaluation visit. Although, TTM is useful in screening for major problems, it has limited usefulness in correction of the problem. A person-to-person appointment in a pacemaker clinic or follow-up center is usually required to correct problems discovered during TTM.

## TROUBLESHOOTING ANTIBRADYCARDIA PACEMAKER FUNCTION

Pacemaker malfunctions may occur at any point during the life of a pacemaker. Malfunctions may be detected either through routine TTM or during extensive evaluation of pacemaker function during an annual or biannual direct evaluation visit. Indications of pacemaker malfunctions may also be detected initially during routine medical appointments or hospitalizations for the management of conditions not related to the pacemaker. The most common pacemaker problems include end of battery life, failure to capture, failure to pace and failure to sense.

## END OF BATTERY LIFE

With early pacemakers, the end of battery life often occurred abruptly and unpredictably, resulting in a dramatic, detrimental reduction in pacing rate and output voltage. Emergent replacement of the generator was required. With the advances in pacemaker technology, the end of battery life is a gradual and expected event. Through the use of TTM and pacemaker generator interrogation, the physician is able to watch progression of battery usage and measure specific indicators that point to the need to replace the generator and battery within a few weeks to months before problems develop. These indicators have been termed 'elective replacement indicators.' Elective replacement indicators are device specific; information about the indicators for a specific device should be obtained from the manufacturer. Various indicators may be used.

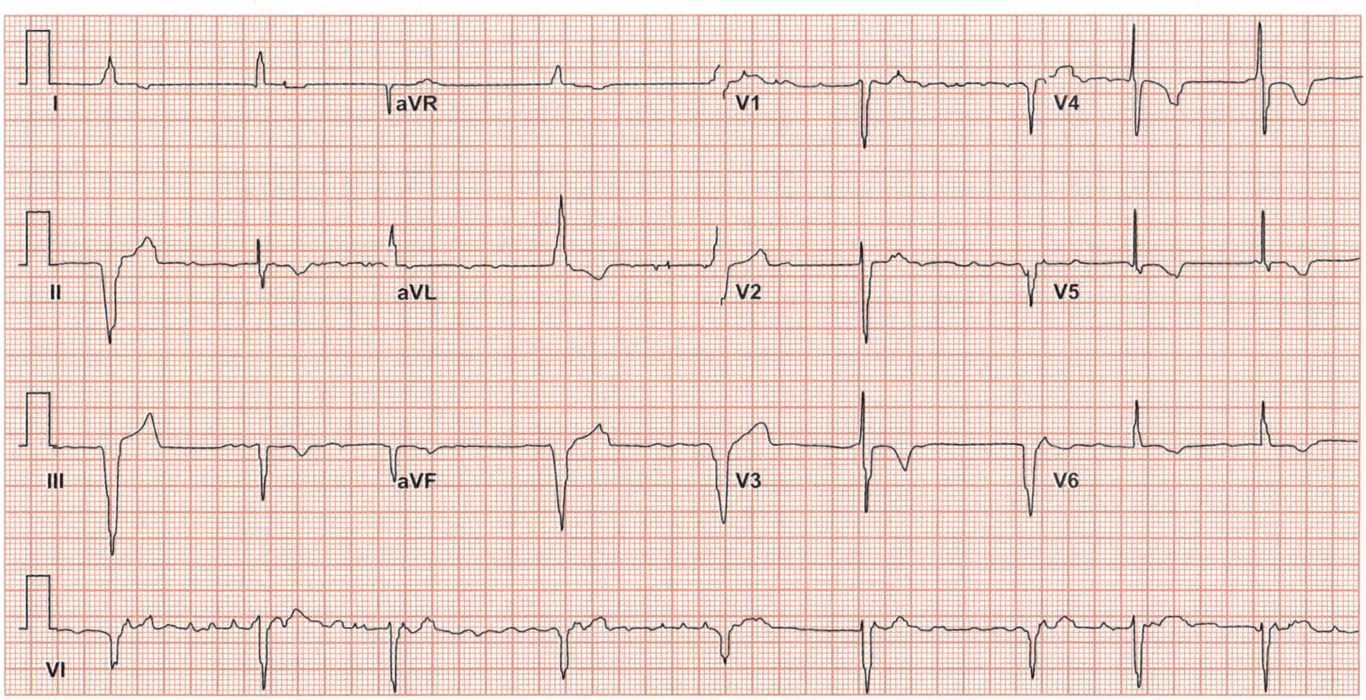


**Fig. 29.81:** DDD pacemaker is programmed to the VVI mode with no atrial sensing

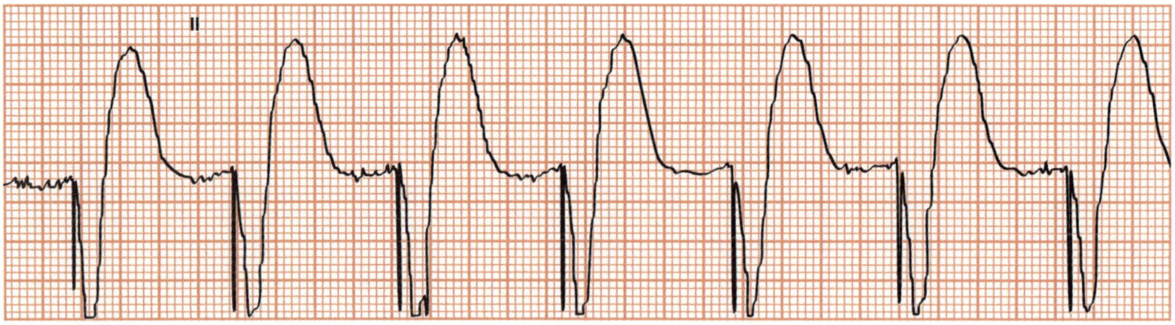


**Fig. 29.82:** Normal VVIR pacemaker function. The strip shows a heart rate of approximately 70 bpm; this falls within the lower and upper rate limits of patient BB's pacemaker. Ventricular pacer spikes are present in front of each QRS complex. The QRS complex shows the typical configuration for a paced QRS. Each pacer spike is followed by a paced QRS; there are no random pacemaker spikes or excessive pauses between beats

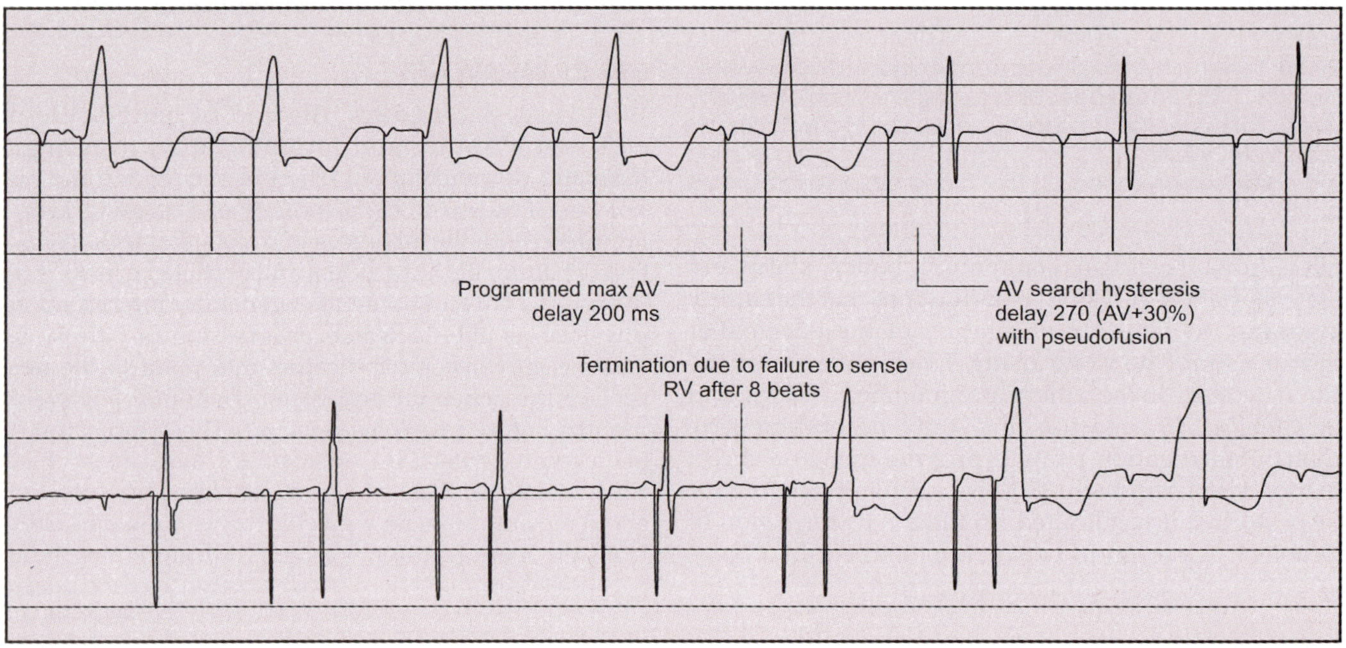


**Fig. 29.83:** An example of AV search hysteresis on telemetry is shown. The dual chamber pacemaker (Guidant Insignia I Plus; DDDR 70-130; base-rate AV delay 200 ms) is pacing at the lower rate limit at the longest of the dynamic AV delay. The AV delay increases to almost 270 ms, 30% longer than the programmed AV delay for 8 cycles. In this case, the algorithm failed to sense the intrinsic narrow QRS as it fell just beyond the extended AV delay, resulting in pseudofusion. Due to the lack of sensing during the 8 cycles, the AV delay then shortens to the programmed delay of 200 ms and re-attempts the algorithm in 32 cycles

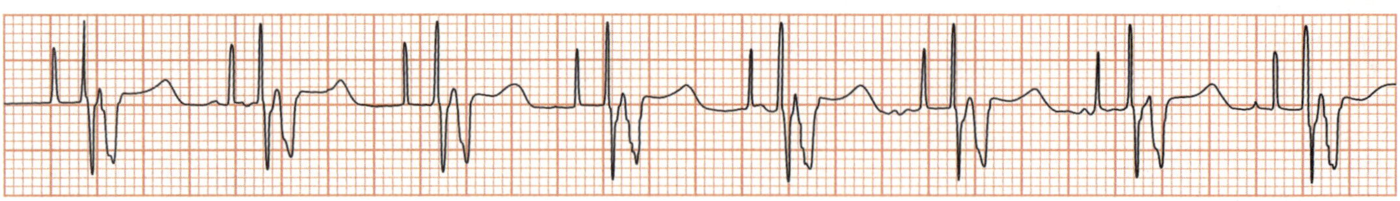

**Fig. 29.84:** Continuous telemetry monitoring is initiated and strip is obtained. It does not show any evidence of pacing problems; each beat is initiated by a P-wave, and each beat is followed by a paced QRS complex. Every QRS is paced, and the rate falls within the rate setting programmed for the pacemaker

The most common is a gradual decline in the rate of the pacemaker when a magnet is applied. Other indicators include a change in pacing mode. For example, a VVIR may change to VVI when the battery is nearing depletion. Even with the new technology and improved pacemaker batteries, unexpected catastrophic battery failure is possible. Catastrophic battery failure results in gross, complete malfunctioning of the pacemaker and severe patient compromise for those who are pacemaker dependent. Emergent treatment with an external or temporary pacemaker is usually required until the pacemaker generator can be replaced.

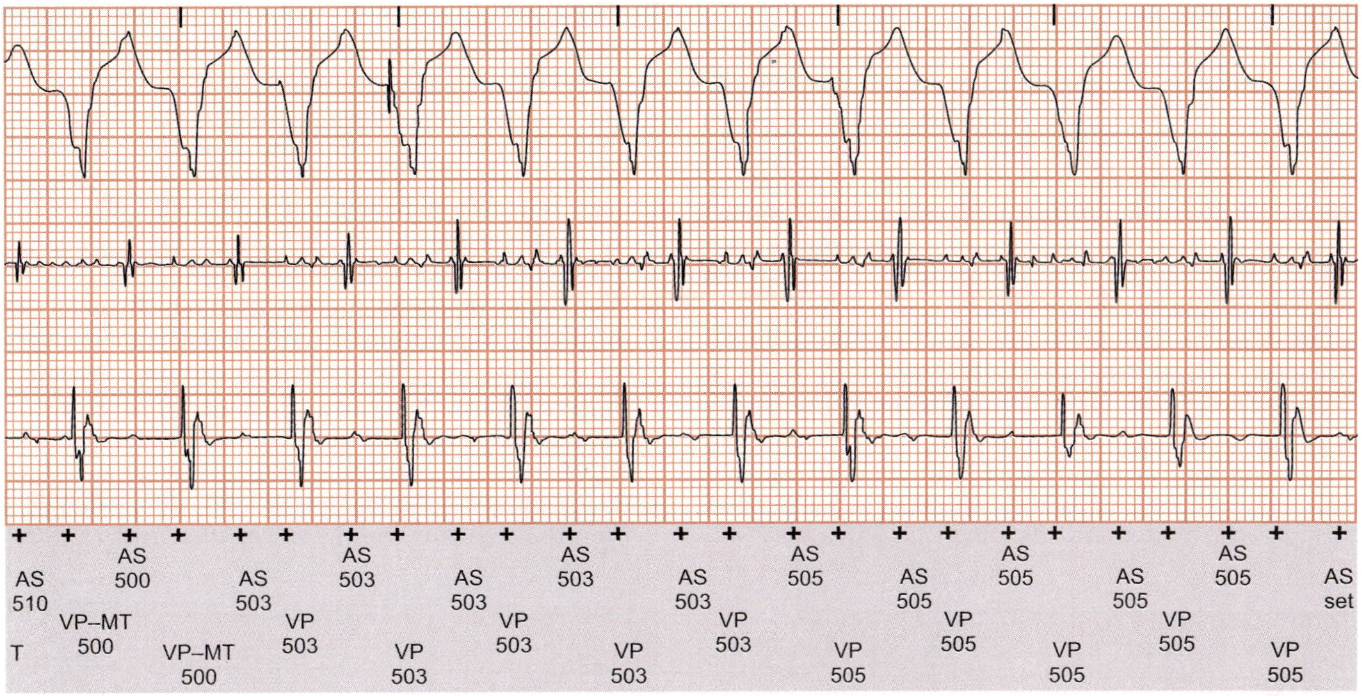


**Fig. 29.85:** Telemetered ECG tracing with surface lead II (top) and intracardiac electrograms [atrial electrogram (center) and ventricular electrogram (lower)] and marker channel (bottom) showing pacemaker-mediated tachycardia (PMT). The intracardiac markers indicate that the retrograde P-waves, labeled AS for atrial-sensed event, occur 280 milliseconds after the ventricular-paced beats, labeled VP

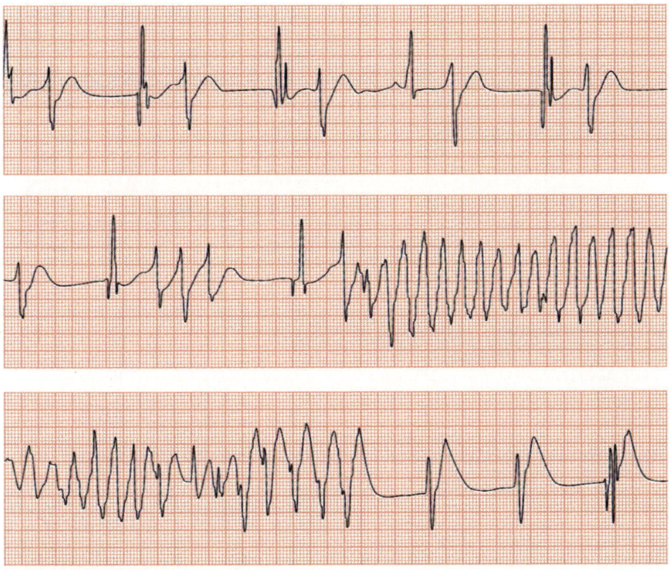

**Fig. 29.86:** Continuous telemetry strip showing episode of TdP in a patient with a dual-chamber pacemaker. This 75-year-old woman with sinus node dysfunction was started on quinidine and diltiazem in the hospital. The normally functioning pacemaker was programmed to the DDD mode with a lower rate of 50 beats per minute. She developed a junctional escape rhythm at around 50 bpm. Late-coupled ventricular bigeminy is followed by a three-beat run of ventricular tachycardia and then a 6-second run of TdP. The apparent ventricular undersensing is the result of 'safety pacing' after sensing the ventricular electrogram in the nonphysiologic AV delay period after the atrial artifact. Torsades de pointes was suppressed by increasing the pacing rate

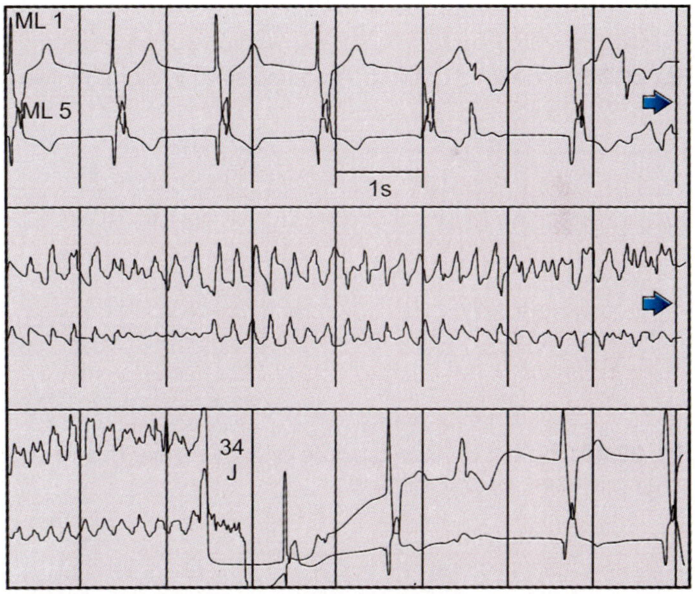


**Fig. 29.87:** Two-channel Holter monitor of an episode of sotalol-induced ventricular fibrillation in a patient with an implantable defibrillator with single chamber ventricular pacing. Sotalol had been started in the outpatient setting for the suppression of recurrent AF. The pacing rate had been left programmed at 44 bpm in an attempt to maintain AV synchrony. He developed bradycardia with continuous ventricular pacing. A late-coupled ventricular premature beat initiates an episode of TdP that rapidly degenerates into ventricular fibrillation. A 34-J shock from the defibrillator terminates the arrhythmia with re-emergence of the ventricular paced rhythm

## FAILURE TO CAPTURE

Failure to capture occurs when a correctly delivered pacing impulse fails to depolarize the heart (Figs 29.88–29.91). On ECG tracing, the pacemaker spike appears at the proper time, but it is not followed by the expected P-wave or QRS complex. In the initial period following pacemaker implantation, failure to capture may be caused by dislodgment of the pacemaker leads or poor positioning of the electrodes on the lead tip. Later in the life of the pacemaker, failure to capture may be caused by:

- An increase in fibrotic or scar tissue at the site of the lead implantation. Because scar tissue conducts electrical impulses poorly, an increase in voltage or output may be required for capture to occur.
- Fracture of the pacemaker lead. Although, pacemaker leads are designed to be extremely flexible and withstand considerable motion and twisting, the wires may still fracture. Fracture of a pacemaker lead prevents the impulse produced by the generator from being transmitted to the electrode at the lead tip.
- The connection between the pacemaker lead and the generator may have become loosened. The end of the pacemaker lead fits into the connector block on the outside of the generator. If this connection loosens, the electrical impulse will not effectively be transmitted to the electrode on the tip of the lead.
- Damage to the insulation on the lead. A break in the insulation also interferes with the effective delivery of the electrical impulse to the myocardium.
- Battery failure. This results in the generation of an impulse that is too low in voltage to depolarize the heart effectively.
- Effects of metabolic changes or medications that change the effective threshold for capture and require an

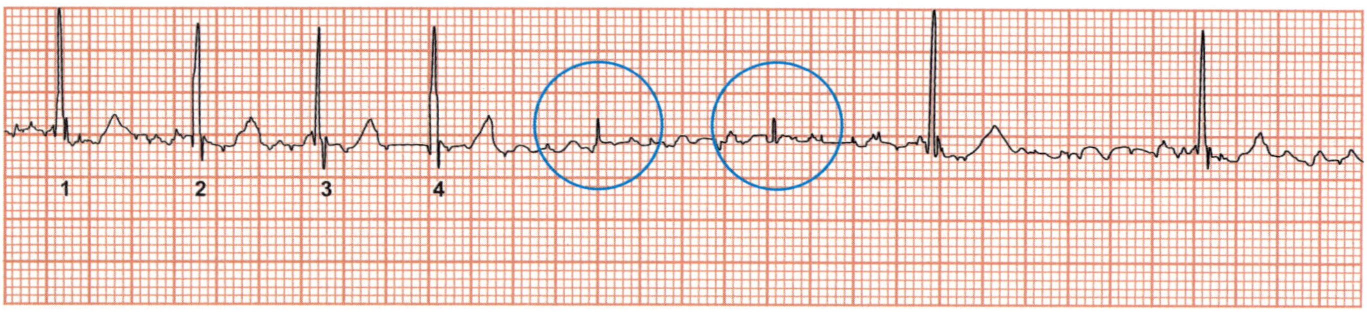


**Fig. 29.88:** A failure to capture. Following beat 4, there are two pacemaker spikes that are not followed by ventricular depolarization

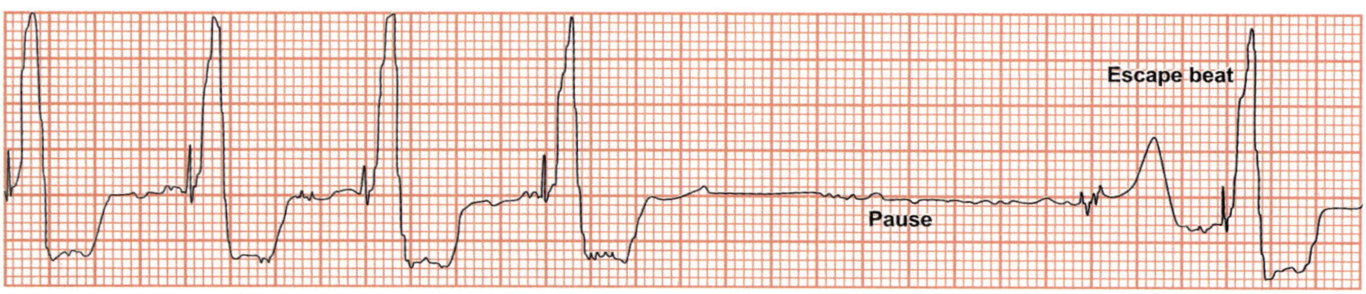


**Fig. 29.89:** The patient has a pause of a little more than 2 seconds followed by escape beat. The pacemaker has failed to fire a pacing impulse as programmed

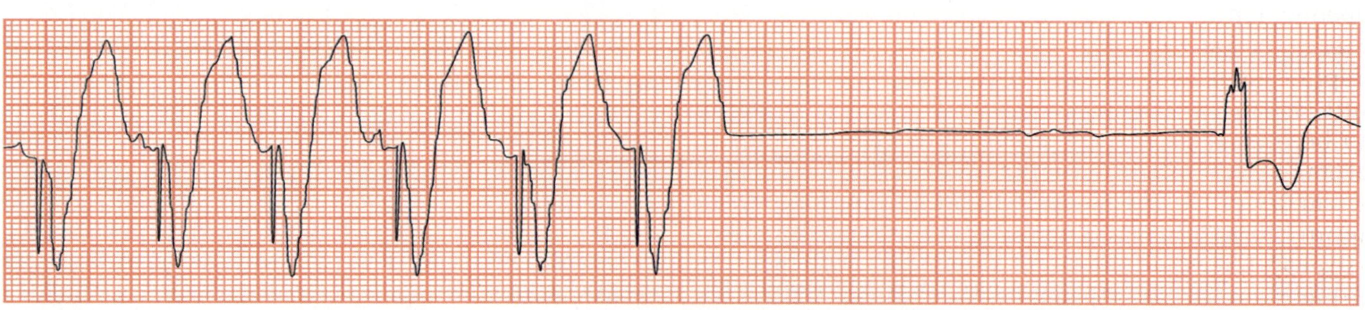

**Fig. 29.90:** A pause of approximately 3 seconds. The pause is followed by an escape beat. As there are no pacemaker spikes present during the pause, the pacemaker malfunction appears to be failure to fire. Patient should obtain immediate medical care

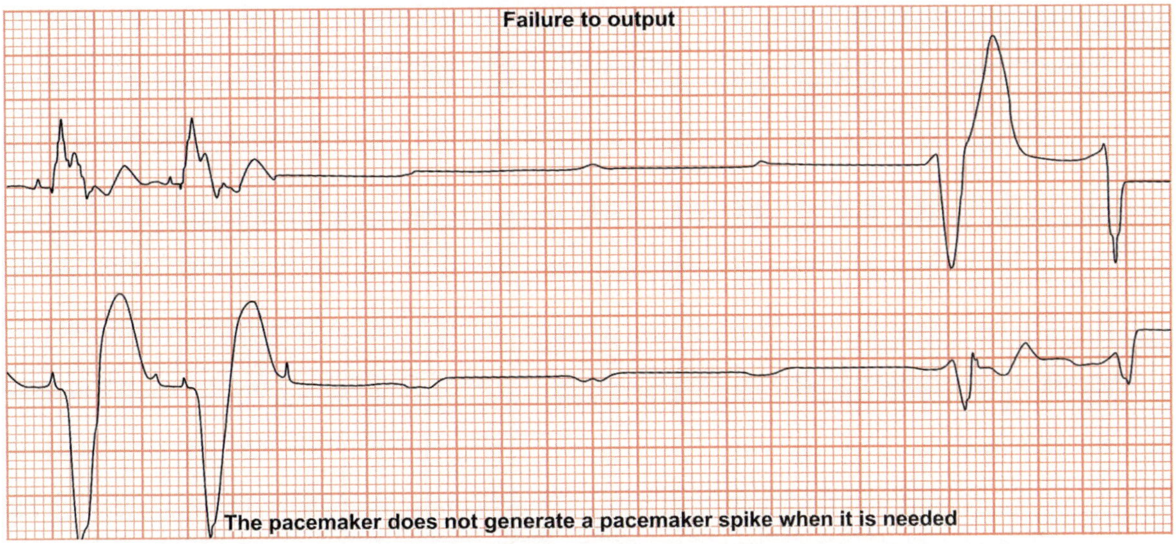


**Fig. 29.91:** Electrocardiogram showing failure to output in pacemaker malfunction

increase in voltage for depolarization to occur. Metabolic abnormalities that can affect capture threshold include hyperkalemia, hypercarbia, acidosis, alkalosis, severe hyperglycemia or hypoxemia. Drugs associated with the development of an increased capture threshold include beta-adrenergic blockers, flecainide, quinidine, amiodarone and procainamide. Reprogramming the capture threshold may correct the problem; however, in some cases, the metabolic abnormality should be corrected before the capture threshold can be effectively reprogrammed.

### Myocardial Ischemia and Myocardial Infarction

Depending on the cause, failure to capture may occur infrequently, intermittently, or continuously. The effects of the failure to capture depend on how frequently the pacemaker fails to capture, the extent to which the patient is pacemaker dependent and the effectiveness of the patient's underlying rhythm in maintaining cardiac output.

Persons who are not pacemaker dependent or who have only infrequent failure to capture may experience symptoms, such as bradycardia, shortness of breath, hypotension, dizziness, weakness, or reoccurrence of preimplantation symptoms. Persons who are pacemaker dependent may experience severe bradycardia or asystole. Emergency measures, such as external noninvasive or temporary transvenous pacing may need to be employed until the specific cause of the pacemaker malfunction can be identified and corrected. Often, revision of the pacemaker leads and/or generator is required to correct the causes of failure to capture. An apparent failure to capture may also be caused by inappropriate sensing or inappropriate timing intervals. If the pacemaker fires during the refractory period, the pacing impulse will not produce depolarization. Reprogramming the timing intervals or troubleshooting the sensing function is indicated (Fig. 29.92).

## FAILURE TO PACE

Failure to pace (also referred to as failure to output) occurs when the pacemaker should deliver a pacing impulse but does not (Fig. 29.93). On ECG tracing, failure to pace is characterized by a prolonged interval between two beats that exceeds the timing interval for the low rate limit. Clinically, that indicated the need for a pacemaker. Due to battery depletion failure to pace can result in pauses and a bradycardic rate that may precipitate symptoms of decreased cerebral perfusion, including syncope, near syncope, confusion and dizziness. Common causes of failure to pace include battery failure, fracture or dislodgment of the pacemaker lead, a loose connection between the pacemaker generator and the pacemaker lead, generator or circuitry failure and oversensing. Oversensing occurs when the sensing circuit inappropriately interprets some other stimulus as cardiac depolarization and inhibits delivery of a pacing impulse. A common cause of oversensing is electromagnetic interference. Failure to pace may occur intermittently, or it may occur 100% of the time. The effect on the patient depends on the frequency of the failure to pace and the patient's degree of dependence on the pacemaker to maintain an effective cardiac output. If the failure to pace is caused by oversensing, the problem may be temporarily corrected by putting the pacemaker into magnet mode. In an emergency, this may be performed through TTM. When the pacemaker is placed in magnet mode, the sensing function is turned off and the pacemaker fires asynchronously at a fixed rate. Permanent correction of failure to pace may require noninvasive reprogramming of the pacemaker's settings or the replacement of the pacemaker generator or leads.

## FAILURE TO SENSE

Failure to sense (i.e. undersensing) occurs when the pacemaker fires randomly at any point during the cardiac cycle instead of at the indicated or appropriate time

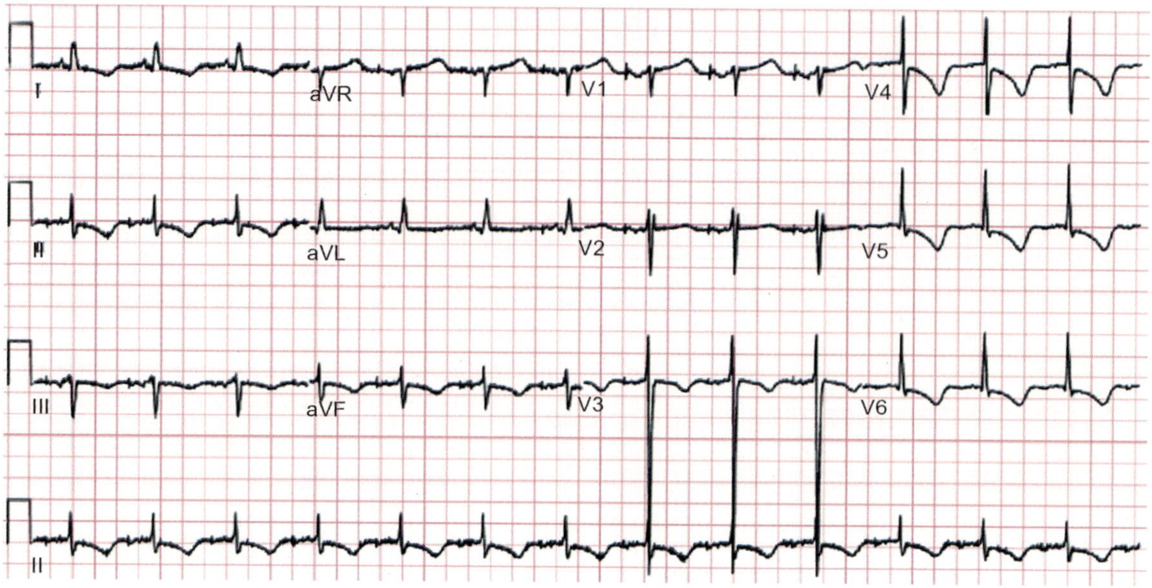


**Fig. 29.92:** Post-automatic implantable cardioverter defibrillator ECG shows pacemaker rhythm and prolonged QTc interval (600 msec)

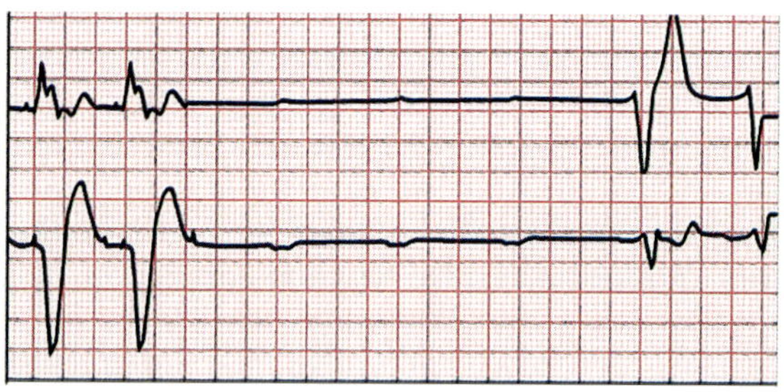

**Fig. 29.93:** Electrocardiographic tracing from a patient with a DDD pacemaker. Pacing artifact fail to result in ventricular depolarization, that is, failure to capture. In this patient, intermittent ventricular failure to capture was due to lead dislodgment

(Figs 29.94 and 29.95). In failure to sense, the pacemaker fails to detect previous electrical activity and the pacemaker fires inappropriately. The ECG tracing shows random pacemaker spikes appearing throughout the ECG tracing. Failure to sense causes the pacemaker to compete with the heart's intrinsic rhythm. The presence of random atrial spikes does not usually present a major problem; these spikes may interfere with the optimal functioning of the pacemaker, but because they are low in voltage, they do not usually precipitate the development of a chaotic electrical rhythm in the heart.

The presence of random ventricular spikes presents more of a problem. Under certain circumstances, such as in the presence of myocardial ischemia or acute MI, random pacemaker spikes falling at a vulnerable point in the cardiac cycle may trigger an erratic, ineffective rhythm. Failure to sense may be caused by multiple factors; some of these are not true malfunctions, but are the result of pacemaker programming. For example, a paced beat is normally followed by a period in which the pacemaker is refractory and does not sense any intrinsic electrical activity. If a premature beat occurs during the pacemaker's refractory period, the pacemaker may not sense it and may appear to fire 'early.' The presence of multiple or frequent pacemaker spikes that occur randomly throughout a tracing are an indication of a true malfunction. Causes of failure to sense include poor electrode position or dislodged electrode, break in the pacemaker lead's insulation, battery failure, inappropriate programming of sensitivity of the pulse generator, a nondocumented change in programming to asynchronous mode or MI. If failure to sense is caused by programming problems, noninvasive reprogramming of the pacemaker settings may correct the problem. A failure to sense caused by problems with the generator, circuitry or leads requires replacement of the broken component.

## BIVENTRICULAR PACING

Heart failure continues to be a major healthcare concern in the United States. Management of heart failure is a major consumer of healthcare resources; it is estimated that more Medicare dollars are spent on the management of heart failure than any other diagnosis. For the individual, heart failure results in a decreased quality of life, frequent hospital admissions, and poor overall prognosis. Heart failure worsens as the disease progresses and prescribed medications become less and less effective. Other treatment options, such as heart transplant and ventricular assist devices, are available to only a small percentage of people.

Advances in pacemaker technology have provided a new therapy option for patients in severe heart failure. Cardiac resynchronization therapy (CRT), also referred to as atrial-synchronized biventricular pacing or simply biventricular pacing, has been found to be effective in persons with New York Heart Association (NYHA) Class III or Class IV heart failure who meet certain criteria (Figs 29.96 and 29.97).

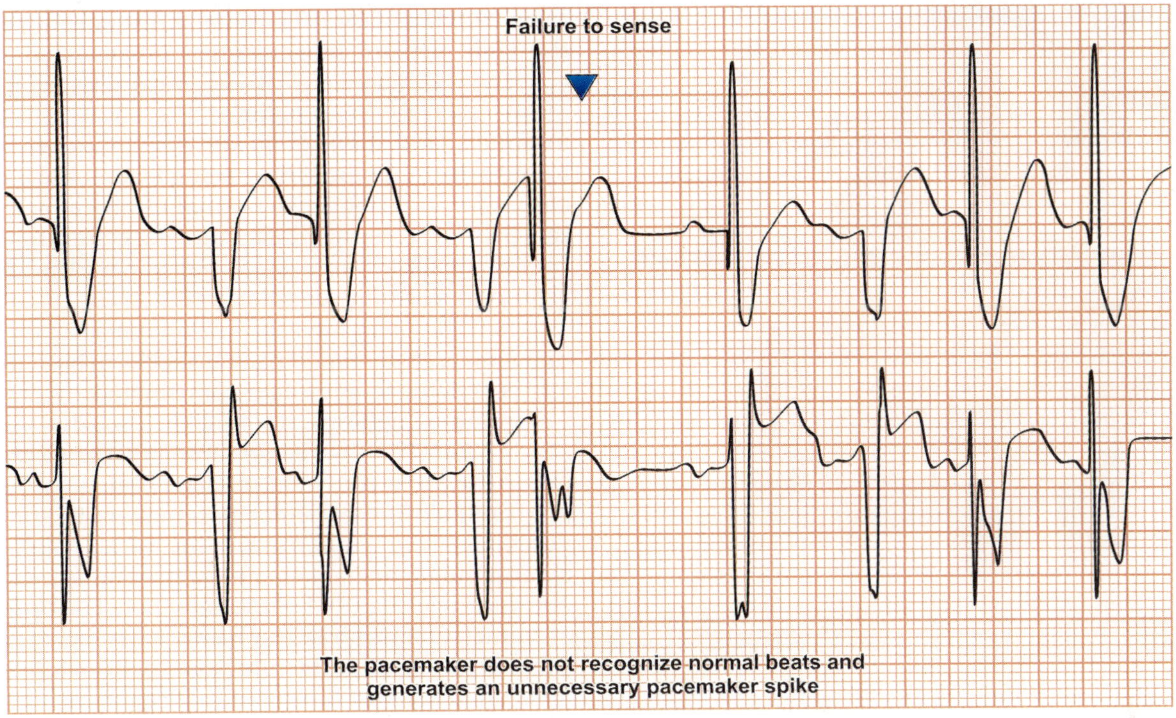


**Fig. 29.94:** Electrocardiogram showing failure of sensing in pacemaker malfunction

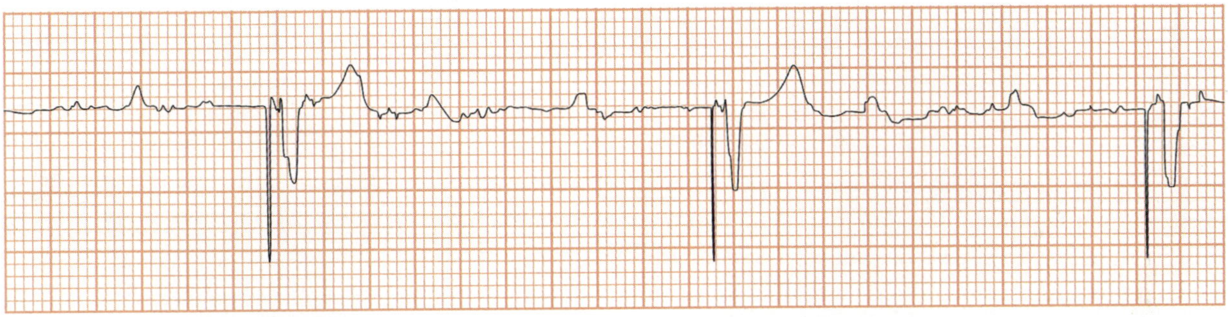

**Fig. 29.95:** Loss of atrial pacing because of oversensing preceding T-wave. Ventricular pacing set at a low rate

## BIVENTRICULAR PACING SYSTEMS

A biventricular pacing system (Figs 29.98 and 29.99) consists of two parts:

- A pulse generator that holds the power source (i.e. battery) and the electronic circuitry needed to generate and deliver pacing impulses to the heart.
- Pacemaker leads that can sense electrical activity and deliver pacing impulses to the heart as programmed. Unlike a traditional dual chamber pacemaker, which uses two pacemaker leads (one in the right atrium and one in the right ventricle), a biventricular system uses three leads—one for the right atrium, one for the right ventricle and one for the left ventricle. Placement of a biventricular pacemaker is, in many ways, similar to the placement of a standard antibradycardia pacemaker. The pacemaker generator is generally implanted in a pacemaker pocket created in the subcutaneous tissue located on top of the pectoralis muscle. The right atrial and right ventricular leads are inserted using a standard transvenous approach and attached to the endocardial surface of the right atrium and right ventricle respectively.

The major difference in implantation of a biventricular pacemaker is the placement of the left ventricular lead. Left ventricular leads are technically more difficult to place than leads in either the right atrium or right ventricle; proper positioning of the left ventricular lead is crucial to effective biventricular pacing. Left ventricular leads are not placed on the endocardium. Instead, they are inserted transvenously and passed to the coronary sinus, a structure that drains blood from the epicardial surface of the heart. The left ventricular lead is passed through the coronary sinus into one of the venous branches lying over the left ventricle. Because it lies in a venous vessel on the outside of the heart, the left ventricular lead cannot be held in place by tines or a screw, but rather is wedged into position. In some patients, transvenous placement of the left ventricular lead in the proper position cannot be achieved. The

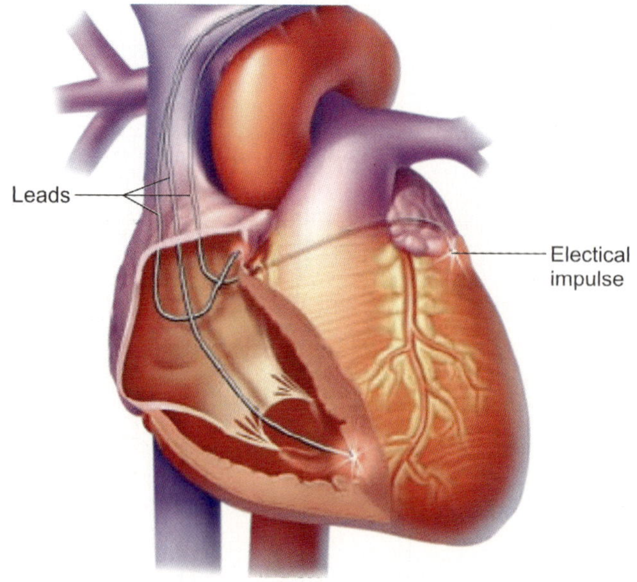


**Fig. 29.96:** Endocardial and epicardial leads in biventricular pacing along with their respective areas of connection for CRT

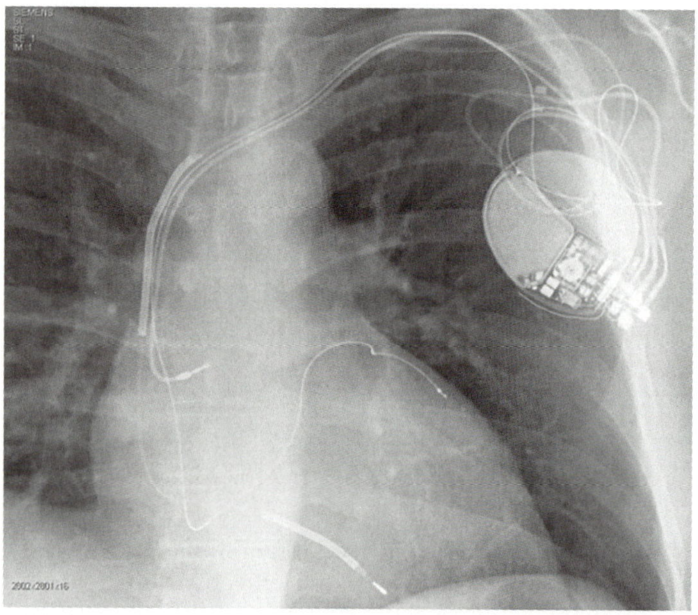

**Fig. 29.97:** Chest X-ray showing implantation of three leads including a left ventricular lead placed in a branch of the coronary sinus (cardiac resynchronisation therapy)

physician may offer these patients the option of undergoing a surgical procedure (i.e. minithoracotomy) for placement of the left ventricular lead.

## BIVENTRICULAR PACING FUNCTIONS

For biventricular pacing to be effective in producing coordinated contraction of both right and left ventricles, the pacemaker must achieve 100% capture in both ventricles (Figs 29.100 and 29.101). Initially, the sensing electrode in the right atrium monitors for normal atrial electrical activity. If it senses normal electrical activity, it relays that information to the generator. The atrial pacing circuit is inhibited, and the pacemaker does not deliver a pacing impulse through the atrial pacing lead. If the atrial sensing electrode does not sense normal electrical activity within the preprogrammed interval, the generator delivers a pacing shock through the atrial pacing lead to the right atrium to stimulate depolarization.

After the atria have been depolarized, the generator delivers carefully timed pacing shocks to both the right and left ventricles to stimulate coordinated contraction. Two programmed settings are crucial to produce coordinated contraction. The first is the timing of the electrical stimulation to each ventricle. Initially, electrophysiologists programmed biventricular pacemakers to stimulate both ventricles simultaneously. The newest generation of biventricular pacemakers can be programmed to stimulate one ventricle slightly before the other. The optimal timing of ventricular contraction has not yet been determined. Electrophysiologists may use echocardiography to determine the best timing sequence for each patient.

The second vital setting is the length of the atrioventricular delay. Atrioventricular delay is a programmable

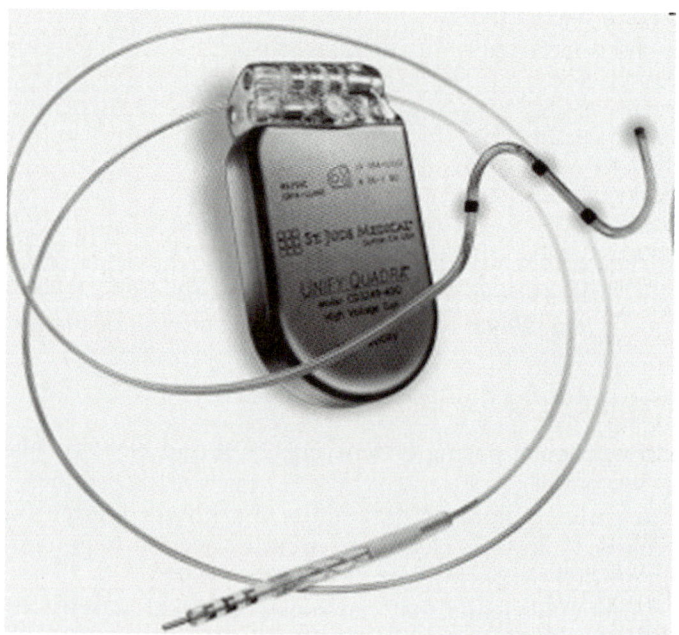


**Fig. 29.98:** The ENERGEN cardiac resynchronization therapy defibrillator (CRT-D) and implantable cardioverter defibrillator (ICD) is used to treat heart failure and sudden cardiac death. The system is designed to simplify and reduce the time needed for the implant procedure by combining three separate lead terminals into one integrated connector and reducing the number of connections and set screws needed in the device header. In addition, some patients will receive a remote monitoring system where an at-home communicator will allow physicians to monitor the patient's device, as well as vital signs, such as blood pressure and weight, in order to better manage this complex disease

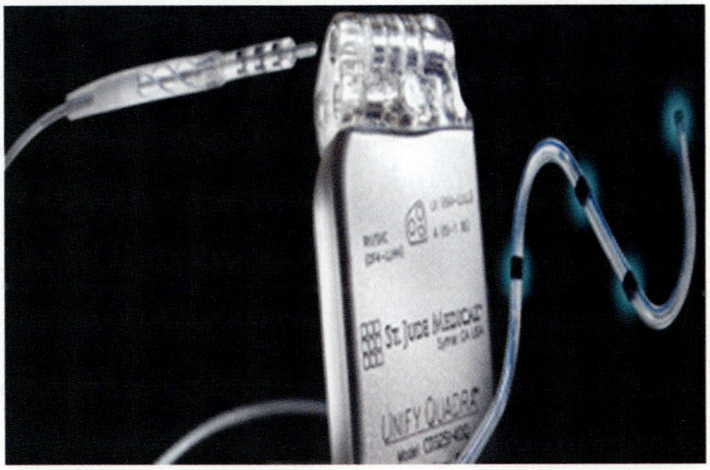

**Fig. 29.99:** A quadripolar pacing system quadripolar pacing system having received European approval in September, St. Jude Medical now announced FDA clearance of its Unify Quadra cardiac resynchronization therapy defibrillator (CRT-D) and the matching Quartet Left Ventricular Quadripolar Pacing Lead. The lead features four electrodes and the CRT-D is able to take advantage of them by providing up to ten different pacing configurations. Because the electrodes cover a greater area, precise placement of the lead is less critical as adjustments of the electrical signal can be made via software. Like many other implantable devices from St. Jude, the Unify Quadra can wirelessly interface with the Merlin. Net system for reporting both on the health of the patient and the status of the device. The Quartet lead, used as part of the Unify Quadra system—features four electrodes spaced over 4.7 centimeters, enabling up to 10 pacing configurations. Multiple pacing configurations allow the physician to implant the lead in the most stable position without making trade-offs in electrical performance. This includes pacing closer to the base of the left ventricle, which recent studies associate with better patient outcomes and which may be more difficult with traditional bipolar leads. The quadripolar pacing electrodes also provide physicians more options to optimize CRT performance, such as pacing around scar tissue in the heart and avoiding the most common pacing complications. The many benefits conferred from the Quartet lead's unconventional pacing have been demonstrated by implanters around the world and reported in a number of published studies

setting; it determines the interval of time that elapses between atrial and ventricular depolarization. To help ensure 100% capture of both right and left ventricular depolarization, the programmed atrioventricular interval should be shorter than the heart's intrinsic atrioventricular delay. Echocardiography can be used to guide the programming of the atrioventricular delay setting for each person.

## ATRIAL-SYNCHRONIZED BIVENTRICULAR PACING PATTERNS

Normal pacing patterns for biventricular pacemakers are different than the pacing patterns for traditional dual chamber antibradycardia pacemakers. In biventricular pacing, a P-wave should be present before each beat. This P-wave might be the patient's intrinsic P-wave, or it might be paced with a pacemaker spike present before the P-wave. Every P-wave (either paced or intrinsic) should be followed by a paced QRS complex. Depending on the model of biventricular pacemaker, there may be a single ventricular spike before the QRS complex, or there may be two spikes.

## CRITERIA FOR BIVENTRICULAR PACEMAKER IMPLANTATION

According to the American College of Cardiology and the American Heart Association, patients with left ventricular ejection fraction less than or equal to 35%, sinus rhythm, and New York Heart Association (NYHA) functional class III or ambulatory class IV symptoms despite recommended optimal medical therapy and who have cardiac dyssynchrony, which is currently defined as a QRS duration greater than or equal to 0.12 seconds, should receive cardiac resynchronization therapy, with or without an ICD, unless contraindicated.

*Level of evidence:* IA (sufficient evidence from multiple randomized trials or meta-analyses). Based on data from major clinical trials, a patient should meet the following criteria to be eligible for biventricular pacemaker implantation:

- A left ventricle ejection fraction of 35% or less
- New York Heart Association class III functional or class IV ambulatory heart failure
- Persistently symptomatic despite optimal drug therapy
- Presence of ventricular dyssynchrony, defined as a QRS duration that is greater than or equal to 0.12 seconds (or 120 ms)

The use of biventricular pacing for persons who meet these criteria has received a category I recommendation in the ACC/AHA heart failure guidelines as well as in the ACC/AHA/HRS pacemaker implantation guidelines.

Initially, biventricular pacemakers were only approved for use with persons who were in normal sinus rhythm and did not require antibradycardia pacing or device therapies for ventricular tachycardia or ventricular fibrillation. Devices are now approved for biventricular and antibradycardia pacing and may be combined with an implantable cardiodefibrillator (ICD).

In addition to the criteria established by the clinical trial data, some electrophysiologists also require that the patient show evidence of ventricular dyssynchrony on echocardiogram.

## CLINICAL CARE OF THE PERSON UNDERGOING BIVENTRICULAR PACEMAKER IMPLANTATION

### Preoperative Care

Preoperative preparation of the patient for transvenous insertion of a biventricular pacemaker is very similar to the preparation previously discussed for antibradycardia pacemakers. The same precautions and patient education are applicable in this case.

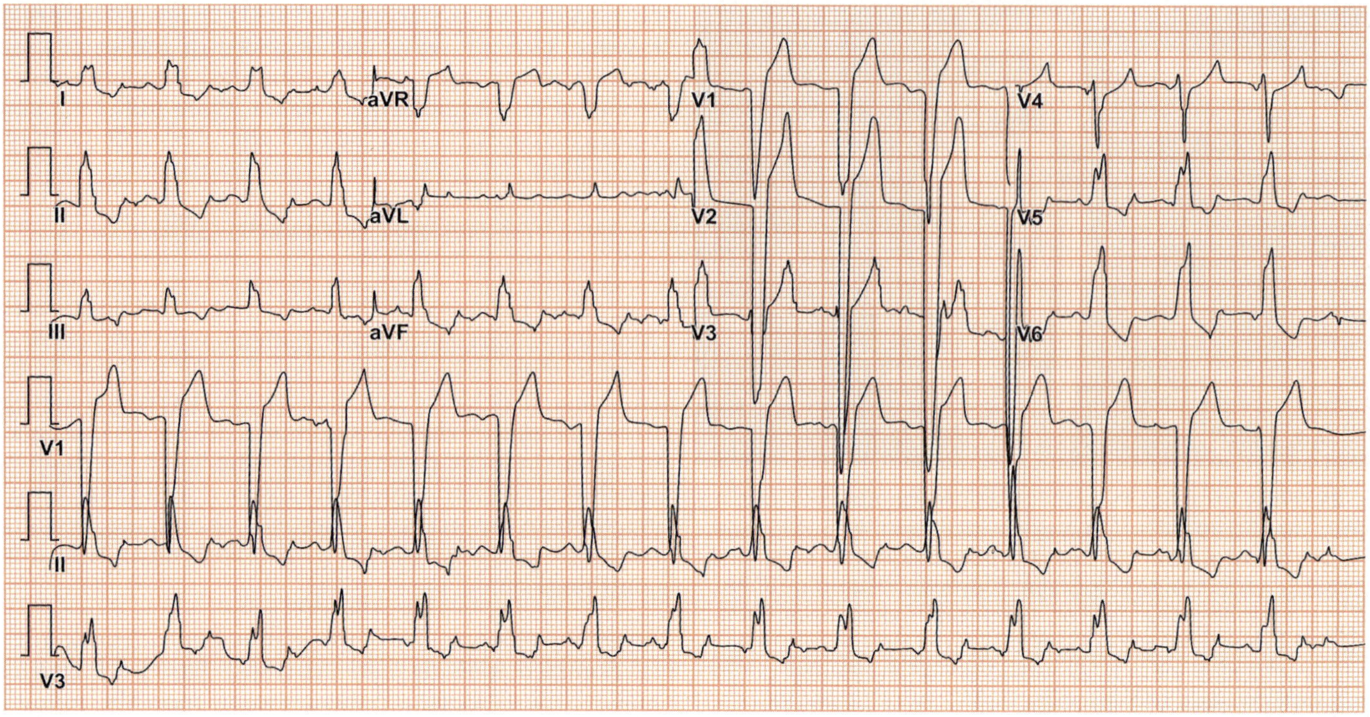


**Fig. 29.100:** Electrocardiogram showing normal sinus rhythm with left bundle branch block. Note that QRS duration is 152 ms

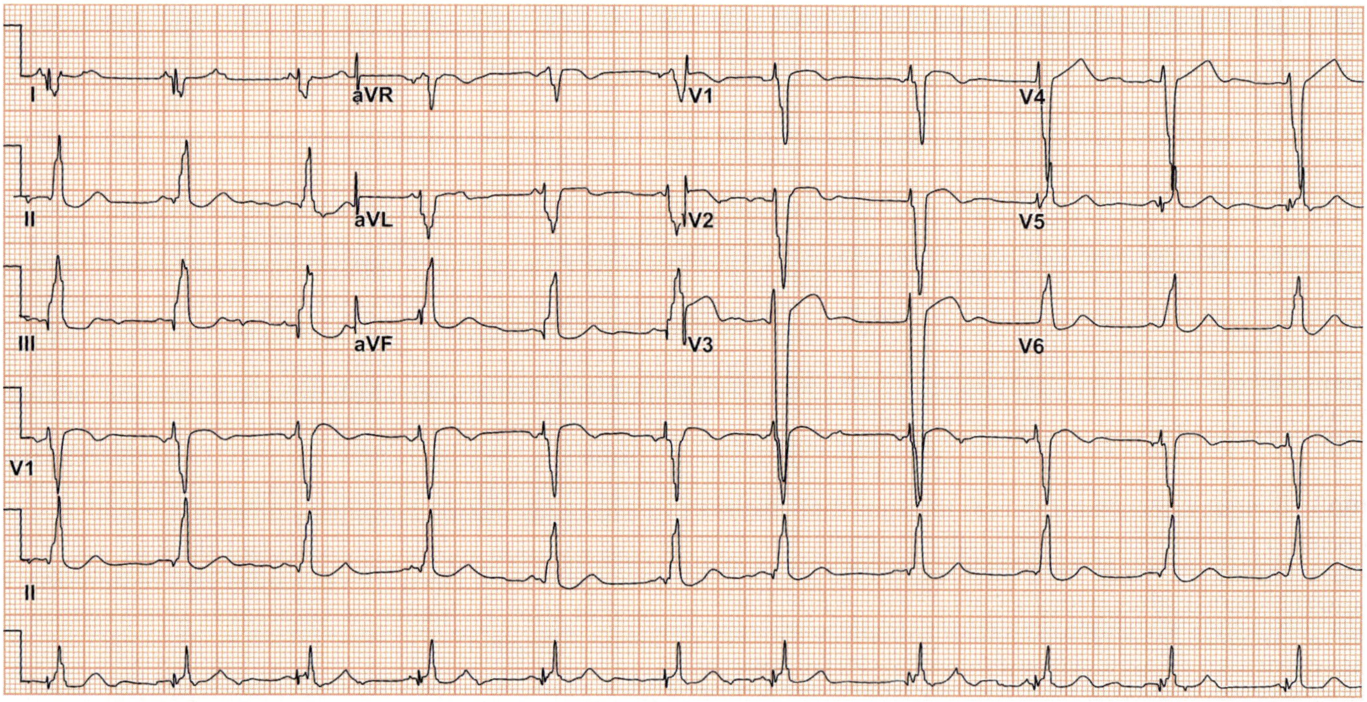


**Fig. 29.101:** Electrocardiogram (ECG) after cardiac resynchronization therapy defibrillator implantation. Note that QRS duration (130 ms) is narrowed compare with previous ECG

## Risks of Procedure

In addition to the usual risks associated with pacemaker implantation, implantation of a biventricular pacemaker carries additional risks specifically related to the left ventricular lead placement, including dissection or perforation of the coronary sinus. Although, these complications have been rare, their occurrence results in significant morbidity and mortality.

### Postimplantation Care

Care of the patient following successful biventricular pacemaker implantation is similar to that for patients who have undergone antibradycardia pacemaker implantation. Vital signs are monitored, and the pacemaker pocket is assessed for signs of bleeding or hematoma formation (Figs 29.102–29.105).

The patient's ECG is continuously monitored to evaluate the pacemaker's function. Due to the sophistication of today's pacemakers and the complexity of the programming involved, the assessment and evaluation of biventricular pacing is the responsibility of a specially trained physician. Nurses caring for the patient in the postoperative period should be alert to signs and symptoms that indicate a potential problem with the pacemaker, its leads, or its programming. Pertinent signs and symptoms include:

- Complete absence or intermittent absence of a ventricular pacing spike. To be effective in restoring ventricular synchrony, a biventricular pacemaker should achieve and maintain 100% ventricular capture. Loss of the ventricular pacing spike may indicate a problem with the pacemaker's programming and the atrioventricular delay interval.
- Intermittent or Complete loss of ventricular capture. As always, the loss of capture may indicate problems with one or more of the leads.
- Decrease in duration of QRS complex. Effective biventricular pacing should shorten the amount of time it takes for the ventricles to depolarize, resulting in a decrease in QRS duration.
- Sudden increase in QRS duration back to the patient's preimplantation baseline. A sudden increase in the duration of the QRS may indicate that synchronized ventricular contraction is no longer occurring. Loss of synchronization in the immediate postimplantation period is usually due to a loss of left ventricular pacing. Causes may include fracture or dislodgment of the left ventricular lead, a loose connection between the pacemaker generator and the pacemaker lead, or circuitry failure.

### When Left Ventricular Lead Placement Is Unsuccessful

On occasion, the physician will be unable to successfully position the left ventricular lead through a transvenous approach. Medical management options include:

- Re-attempting transvenous placement of the left ventricular lead at a later time
- Referring the patient to the appropriate surgical service for surgical placement of the left ventricular lead
- Recommending that no further attempts be made to implant the left ventricular lead.

### *Preparation for Discharge*

Prior to the patient's discharge, the physician will evaluate the effectiveness of the pacemaker's programmed settings. An echocardiogram may be performed to assist the physician in identifying and programming optimal settings for each patient

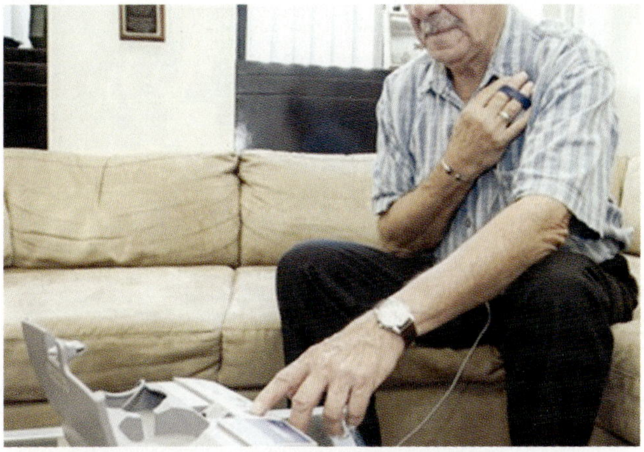

**Fig. 29.102:** Patients with implanted defibrillators and pacemakers are benefitting from technology that reduces the number of times they have to come to the hospital for treatment. A remote monitoring system called Medtronic CareLink

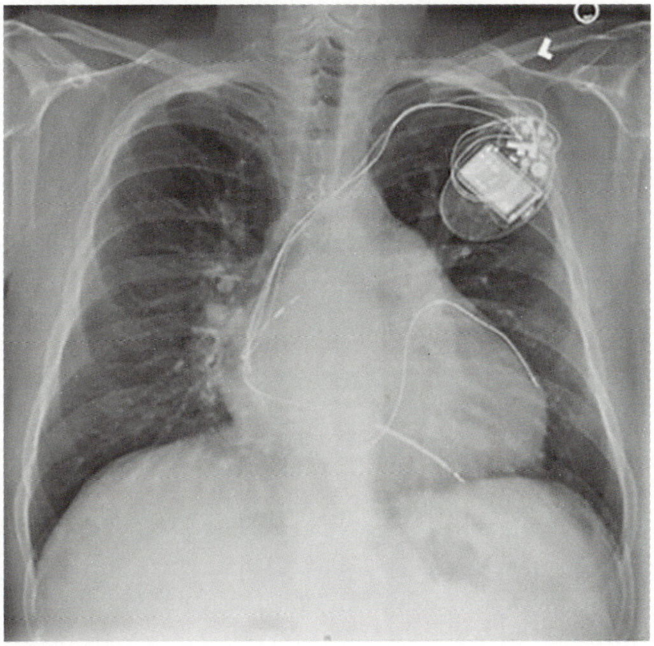

**Fig. 29.103:** An elderly patient with dilated cardiomyopathy was operated for CRT-LV D. This radiograph is showing leads in RV, coronary sinus and implantable cardioverter defibrillators (ICDs) (left infraclavicular region)

### *Discharge Education*

Key points in discharge education following biventricular pacemaker implantation include:

- Incision care and temporary restrictions
- Basic safety measures
- Adherence to medication therapy and diet restrictions. Stress to the patient that biventricular pacing does not replace other therapies for the management of heart

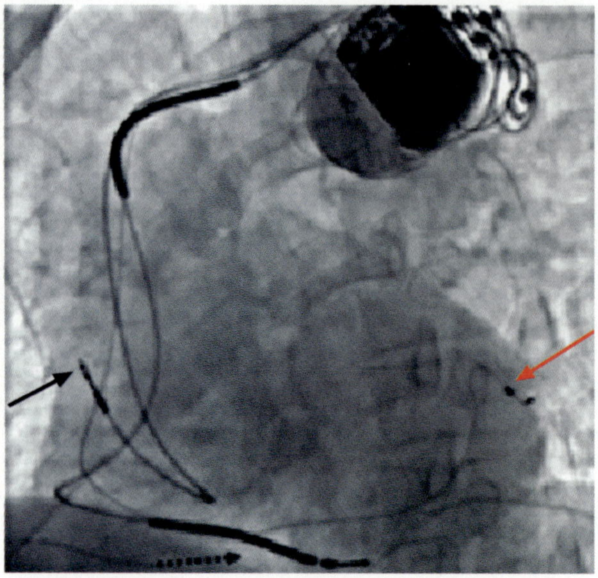

**Fig. 29.104:** Three leads can be seen in this photograph of a cardiac resynchronization device—a right atrial lead (solid black arrow), a right ventricular lead (dashed black arrow), and a coronary sinus lead (red arrow). The coronary sinus lead wraps around the outside of the left ventricle, enabling pacing of the left ventricle. Note that the right ventricular lead in this case has two thickened aspects that represent conduction coils and that the generator is larger than typical pacemaker generators, demonstrating that this device is both a pacemaker and a cardioverter-defibrillator, capable of delivering electrical shocks for dangerously fast abnormal ventricular rhythms

failure; adherence to prescribed medications and diet restrictions is still necessary.

- Self-monitoring of symptoms. Persons who respond to CRT will experience gradual improvement in activity tolerance, quality of life, and activities of daily living. Instruct the patient to note his or her current symptoms and current activity level. Encourage the patient to note even small improvements in his/her symptoms and exercise tolerance. Instruct the patient to notify his/her physician if symptoms either abruptly worsen or return to preimplantation levels. An abrupt increase in symptoms may indicate a loss of resynchronization. Loss of resynchronization can be caused by lead failure or lead displacement (most commonly the left ventricular lead), device malfunction, or problems with the programmed intervals.

## Complications in Paced Patients

Complications in paced patients are shown in Figures 29.106–29.110.

### *Pacemaker Syndrome*

First identified in the 1970s, pacemaker syndrome is a complex of signs and symptoms that occur when AV synchrony is lost during pacing and relieved when AV synchrony is restored. Once thought to occur solely with VVI pacing, pacemaker syndrome has also been shown to occur under certain circumstances with other types of pacemakers. Pacemaker syndrome should be suspected any

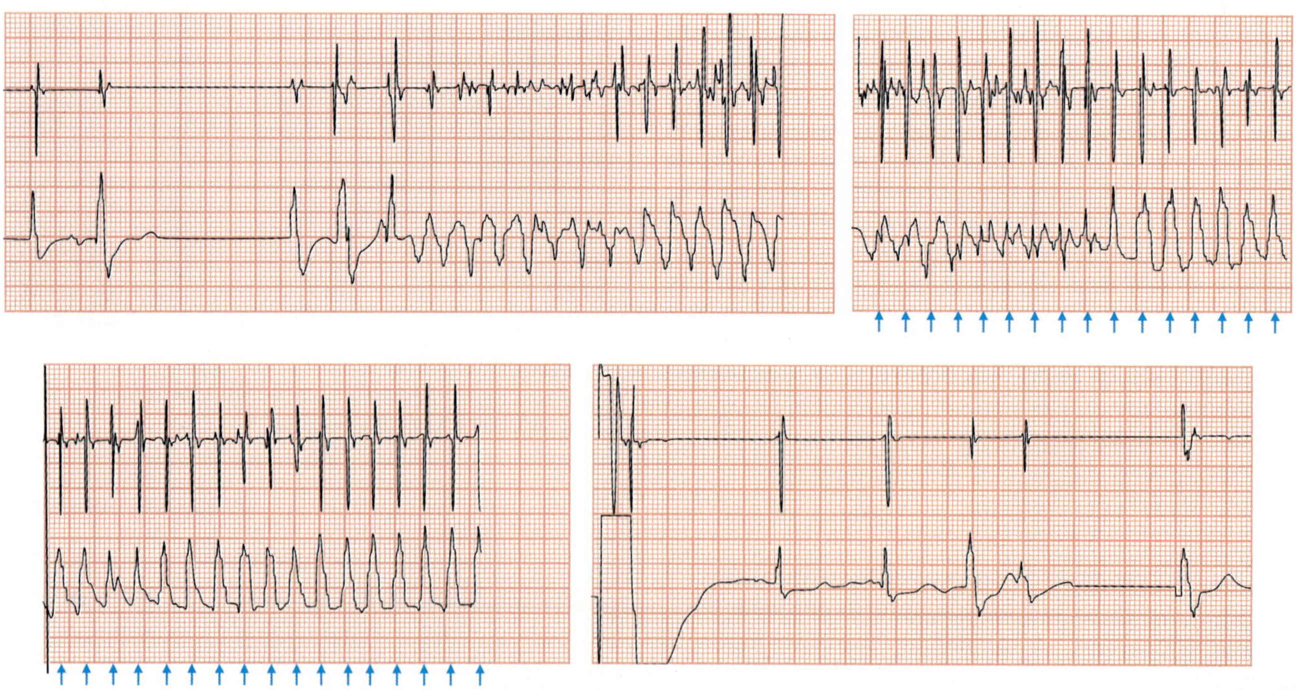

**Fig. 29.105:** Ventricular tachycardia. AICD firing recordings obtained from an automatic implantable cardiodefibrillator (AICD) in a 40-year-old patient with aortic stenosis, s/p left ventricular apical-descending aortic conduit and aortic valve replacement. The patient also had prolonged QT interval and documented episodes of ventricular tachycardia which prompted placement of the AICD. The intracardiac recording in the top left panel show initiation of a wide complex tachycardia that continues in the top right and lower left panels. A 21 joule shock is delivered in the beginning of the lower right panel resulting in resumption of sinus rhythm

time. The patient experiences a recurrence of preimplantation symptoms in the presence of a well-functioning pacemaker. The definition of pacemaker syndrome varies; some define it in terms of the presence of syncope, presyncope or malaise. Others suggest that pacemaker syndrome may be present in a patient who fails to achieve his or her optimal functional status following pacemaker implantation. Pacemaker syndrome may be defined as a constellation of specific symptoms that occur in the setting of a temporary or permanent pacemaker and result from loss of physiologic timing of atrial and ventricular contractions. The exact incidence of pacemaker syndrome is unclear; estimates range widely from 7% up to 85%, depending on which definition of pacemaker syndrome is applied.

### *Pathophysiology*

The primary cause of pacemaker syndrome appears to be the loss of AV synchrony that occurs with pacing. When AV synchrony is lost, atrial contraction and ventricular contraction are not coordinated. Active ventricular filling that normally occurs when the atria contract just before ventricular depolarization cannot occur; left ventricular filling is decreased and cardiac output drops. It is estimated that up to 20% of an individual's cardiac output comes from active ventricular filling. With the drop in cardiac output, the patient may experience signs and symptoms similar to those he/she experienced prior to implantation. These may include syncope, presyncope, confusion, dizziness or lightheadedness. In addition, when AV synchrony is lost, atrial contraction may occur during the time that the mitral and tricuspid valves are closed. Atrial contraction against closed valves results in an increase in volume and pressure in the atria, which in turn may trigger a vagal response resulting in syncope, presyncope, and hypotension. The elevation in atrial and pulmonic pressures also may result in symptoms of congestive heart failure.

### Crosstalk and Ventricular Safety Pacing

Crosstalk is the inappropriate sensing of far-field signals from the opposite cardiac chamber, causing pacing inhibition or oversensing. One of the most serious manifestations of crosstalk in a dual chamber pacing system is oversensing of far-field atrial stimuli, resulting in ventricular inhibition and asystole in the 'pacemaker-dependent' patient. The atrioventricular interval (AVI) thus encompasses multiple refractory and blanking intervals on each atrial/ventricular channel, as well as on the 'opposite' channel to prevent crosstalk (Figs 29.109–29.111).

## LONG-TERM FOLLOW-UP

Long-term follow-up focuses on device surveillance and monitoring of the patient's clinical status. The biventricular pacemaker should be interrogated on a regular basis to

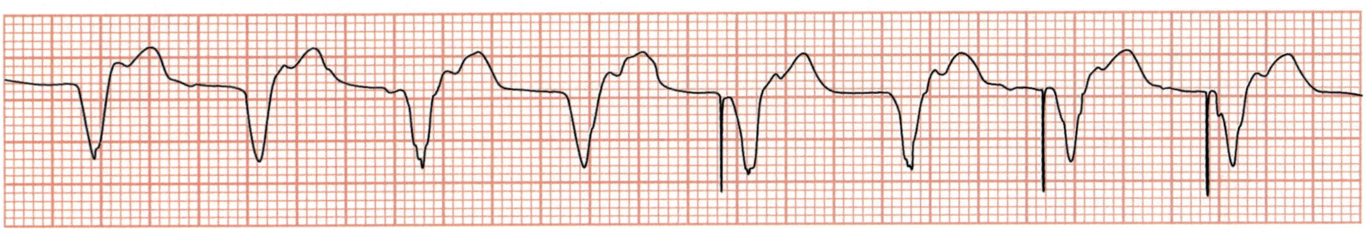

**Fig. 29.106:** Pacemaker syndrome—retrograde P-waves are evident

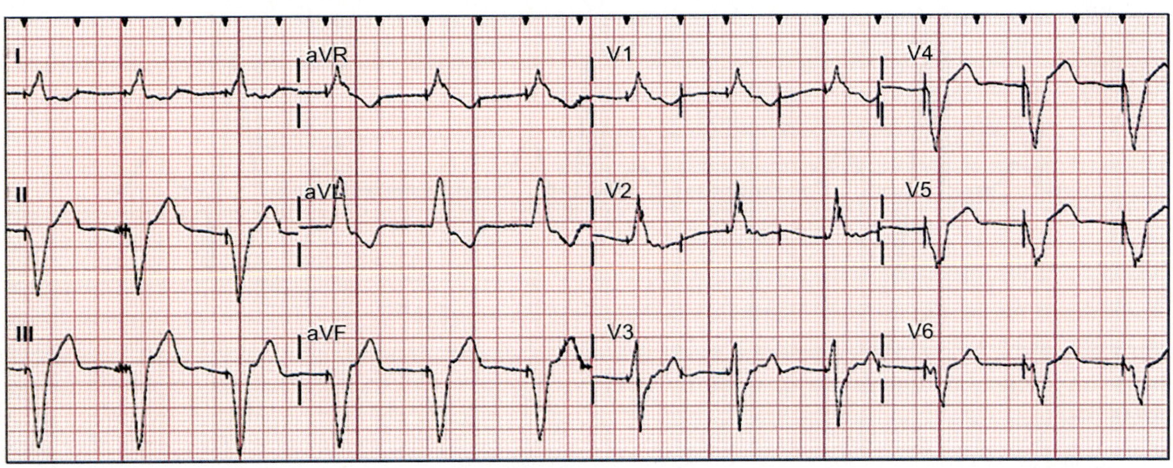


**Fig. 29.107:** High frequency pacing may occasionally be a sign of serious pacemaker malfunction (runaway pacemaker) or appropriate response to an arrhythmia (tracked sinus/atrial tachycardia). In dual chamber systems, proper identification of pacing spikes is necessary for troubleshooting. In this tracing, 150/minute pacing seems to be capturing 2:1. Note, however, that the pacing is regularly irregular (short-long) and the spike morphology is alternating in V1—every other one is an atrial spike. The patient is in atrial fibrillation, which is undersensed and the DDD pacemaker is delivering dual chamber stimulation at 70/minute with an AV delay of 400 ms

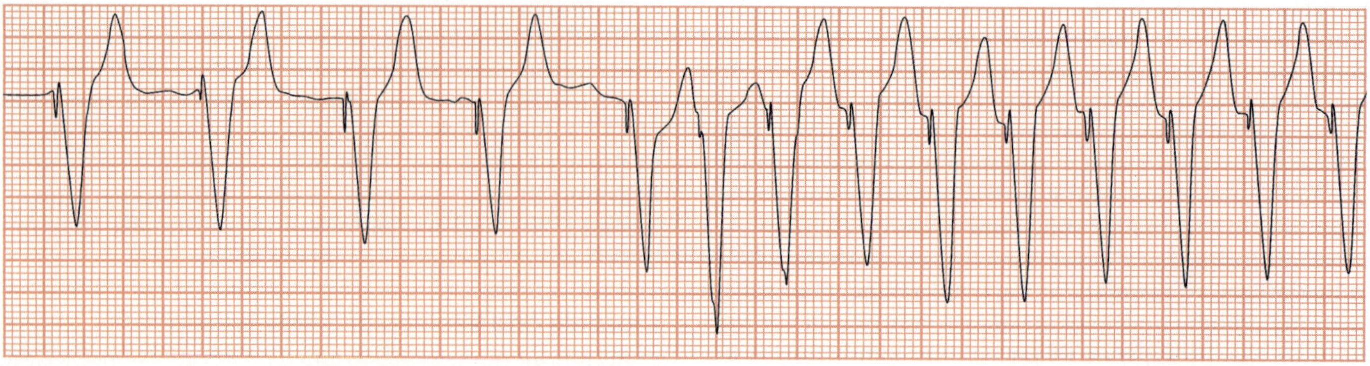

**Fig. 29.108:** The most commonly reported pacemaker mediated tachycardia is 'endless loop tachycardia' which occurs in patients with dual chamber pacemakers

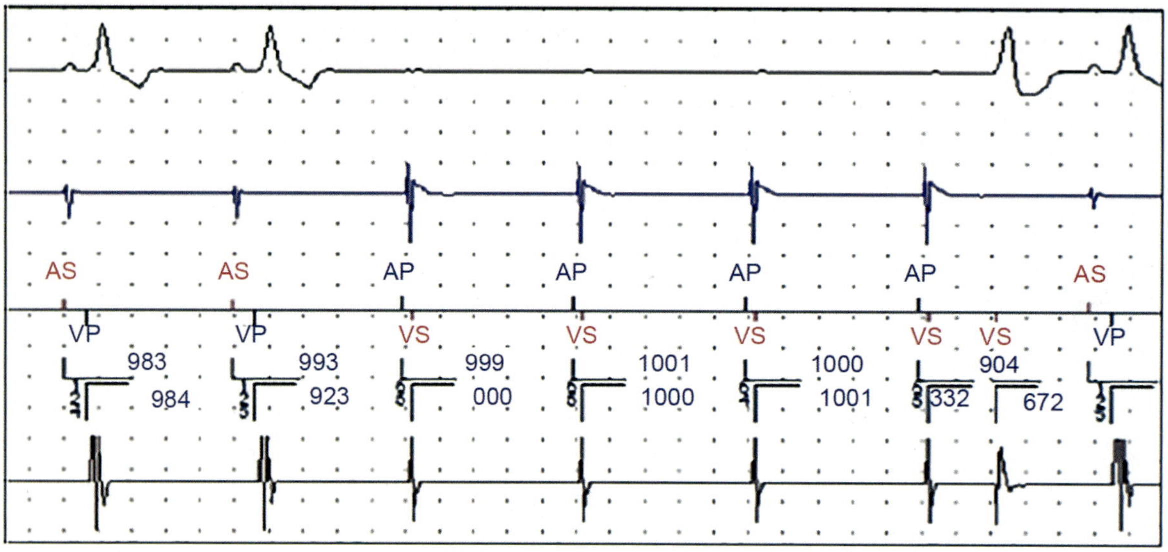


**Fig. 29.109:** AV crosstalk. Atrial pacing spike will be detected in the ventricle. Will inhibit ventricular pacing

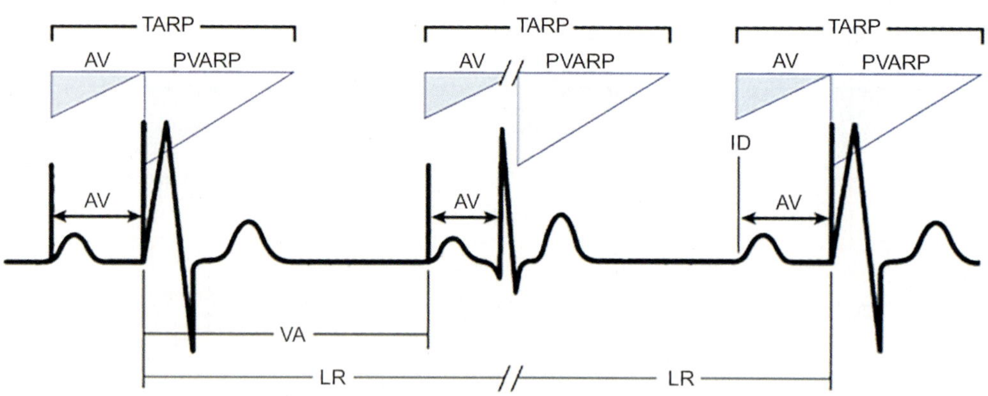


**Fig. 29.110:** The timing cycle in DDD consists of a lower rate (LR) limit, an atrioventricular interval (AVI), a postventricular atrial refractory period (PVARP) and an upper rate limit. The AVI and PVARP together comprise the total atrial refractory period (TARP). ID=intrinsic deflection

verify battery status, lead status, and appropriate device functioning. Sources differ in the recommended frequency of monitoring. Some recommend interrogation as often as every 3 months; others recommend a 6-month interval.

During follow-up visits, the patient's symptoms and overall disease progression should be assessed. Indications that the patient is responding favorably to the CRT include increased exercise tolerance, increased ability to participate in activities of daily living, improved quality of life, fewer unscheduled physician or urgent care visits, fewer hospitalizations or emergency room visits for symptom management and shortened length of stay when hospitalization is required. The patient's adherence to prescribed medical therapies, including medications, diet and lifestyle changes, should also be assessed.

For patients who do not respond to CRT as expected or who are responding very slowly, additional medical interventions may be employed. The physician may choose to increase the prescribed doses of beta blockers and/or ACE inhibitors. Patients with biventricular pacemakers may be able to tolerate increased doses of these medications; the increased doses will further block the neurohormonal processes that cause worsening symptoms. As a result, the patient may experience a gradual reduction in symptoms and an increase in activity tolerance. The physician may prescribe measures to increase physical reconditioning. Some patients, particularly those with NYHA class IV heart failure, are debilitated and require very slow, gradual increases in physical activity to reverse the deconditioning effects of their disease.

Patients should be assessed for any problems or symptoms that indicate a loss of ventricular resynchronization. These symptoms can be overt, such as an obvious worsening of heart failure symptoms and decrease in exercise tolerance, or they may be more subtle, consisting of vague complaints of increasing weakness and fatigue. If symptoms are present, assessment of pacemaker function, including the left ventricle pacing threshold and left ventricle capture, should be performed. The programmed AV interval should be evaluated to see if it is too long, thus allowing the patient's intrinsic conduction to trigger ventricular depolarization. The patient's ECG should be assessed for the presence of increasing premature ventricular contractions (PVCs). Frequent PVCs can inhibit the pacemaker from firing and will result in a loss of ventricular synchrony. If increasing PVCs are present, the patient's overall status should be assessed to determine the cause. The physician may consider prescribing anti-arrhythmic medications to limit or stop the PVCs. Increasing symptoms of heart failure can also be an indication that the patient's disease is continuing to progress toward its end stage.

Biventricular pacing remains a major focus in pacemaker research. Other areas that have been identified for further research include:

- Use of echocardiography to determine presence of ventricular dyssynchrony in patients with a narrow QRS complex
- Use of CRT in persons with NYHA class II heart failure to improve ejection fraction and reverse destructive left ventricular remodeling
- Better identification of persons who will respond to CRT
- Exploration of the effects of right ventricular pacing on left ventricular function and the development of left ventricular dyssynchrony
- Improvement of pacemaker design, function, lead systems and battery life

## EMERGING TRENDS IN PACEMAKER THERAPY

Emerging trends in pacemaker therapy are shown in Figures 29.114–29.120.

### The World's First Leadless Pacemaker

The world's first leadless pacemaker, developed by an Indian-origin scientist, Dr Vivek Reddy, has shown promising results after 1 year of human trials on 32 patients who received the pacemaker.

'This is the first time, we have seen one-year follow-up data for this innovative, wireless cardiac pacing technology.

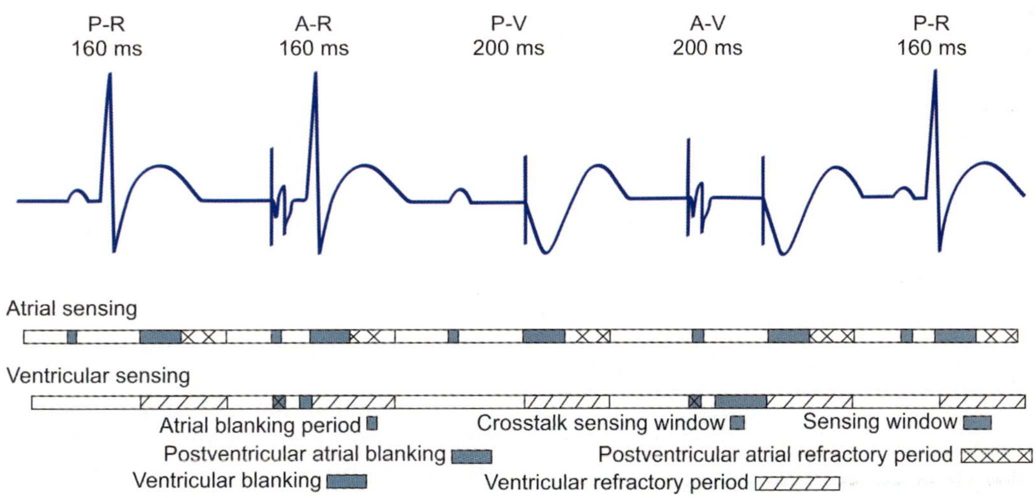


**Fig. 29.111:** DDD refractory periods. The lower rate is 60 beats per minute or 1000 ms in this example of ventricular-based timing. The atrial escape interval, the time from the R-A or V-A, is 800 msec, equal to 1000 msec minus the A-V interval of 200 msec. A=paced atrial event; P=sensed atrial event; R=sensed ventricular event; V=paced ventricular event. The refractory periods and sensing windows are given on the atrial and ventricular sensing channels. On the atrial channel, the atrial blanking period is after an atrial paced or sensed (usually) event. After a sensed or paced ventricular event, on the atrial channel, there may be a postventricular atrial blanking period followed by a postventricular atrial refractory period. On the ventricular channel, the ventricular sensed or paced event creates a ventricular refractory period. On the ventricular channel after an atrial paced event, there is a cross-channel ventricular blanking period, usually followed by a crosstalk safety pacing window and an alert period

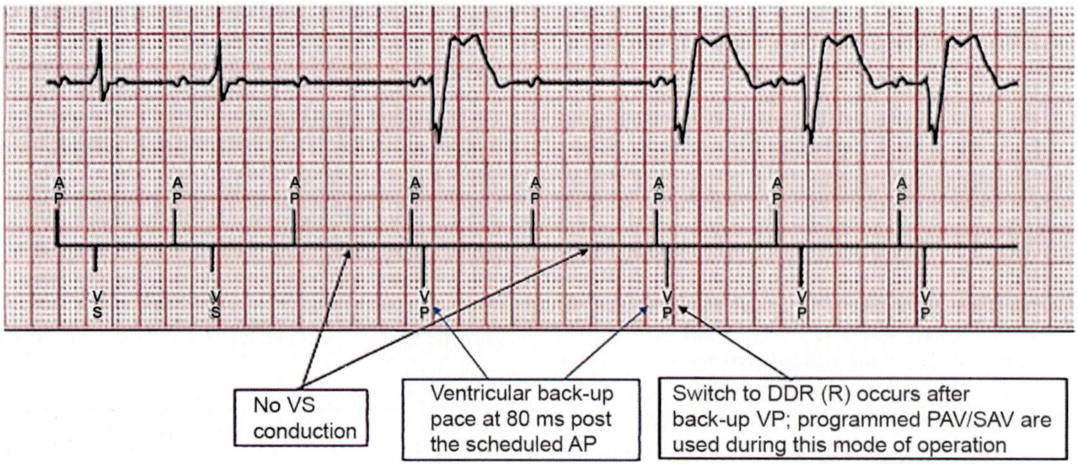


**Fig. 29.112:** MVP AAI(R) to DDD(R) pacing (MVP) managed ventricular operation switch from AAI(R) to temporary DDD(R) mode ventricular support if loss of A-V conduction is persistent. Two out of four most recent A-A intervals with no conducted VS event no VS conduction ventricular back-up pace at 80 ms post the scheduled AP switch to DDD(R) occurs after back-up VP; programmed PAV/SAV are used during this mode of operation

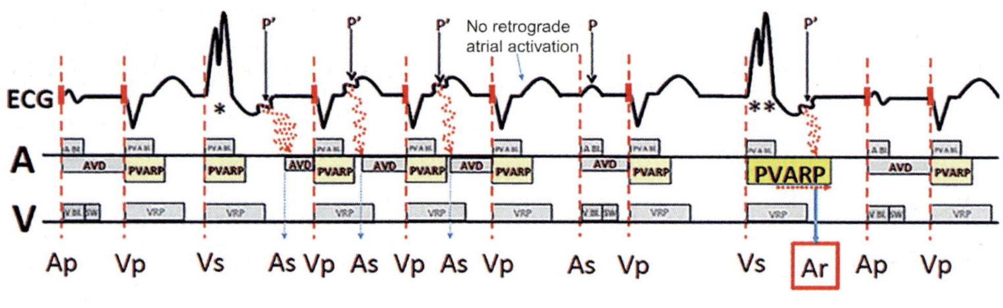


**Fig. 29.113:** Method of prevention of re-entrant tachycardia onset in pacemaker

Our results show the leadless pacemaker is comparable to traditional pacemakers,' said Reddy, director of arrhy thmia services at the Mount Sinai Hospital here.

The findings further support the promising performance and safety of this minimally-invasive, non-surgical pacing device.

The leads-free pacemaker is implanted by a cardiac electrophysiologist directly inside the heart during a catheter-guided procedure through the groin via the femoral artery. The device, resembling a small, metal silver tube, is only a few centimeters in length, making it less than ten percent the size of a traditional pacemaker. The follow-up study evaluated 32 patients with a slowed heartbeat (bradycardia) who successfully received St. Jude Medical's 'Nanostim' leadless pacemaker at two hospitals in Prague and one in Amsterdam. 'There was no experience of infections or failure to sense, pace or communicate with the pacemaker,' Reddy noted. The leadless cardiac pacemaker is placed directly inside a patient's heart without surgery during a catheter-guided procedure through the groin via the femoral vein.

The device, resembling a tiny, silver tube and smaller than a triple-A battery, is only a few centimetres in length, making it less than 10% the size of a traditional pacemaker.

It works by closely monitoring the heart's electrical rhythms and if the heart beat is too slow, it provides electrical stimulation therapy to regulate it.

"More long-term follow-up of these 'leadless' study patients will further our understanding of the potential advantages, benefits, and complication risks of leadless pacemaker technology, along with additional ongoing, larger trials," Reddy said.

More than four million patients globally have a pacemaker, and 700,000 new patients receive one each year. Reddy presented the one-year 'leadless' study data findings at 'Heart Rhythm 2014,' the Heart Rhythm Society's 35th annual scientific sessions in San Francisco city in the United States May 9, the hospital or access a computer connected to the hospital network. A remote cardiologist can now use AirStrip Cardiology to precisely measure ECG waveforms, helping on-site ED clinicians determine, e.g. if a patient requires cath lab intervention.

## SUMMARY

Due to research and advances in pacemaker technology, pacemaker therapy may be successfully used in the management of persons who have symptomatic bradycardia and in persons with heart failure who meet

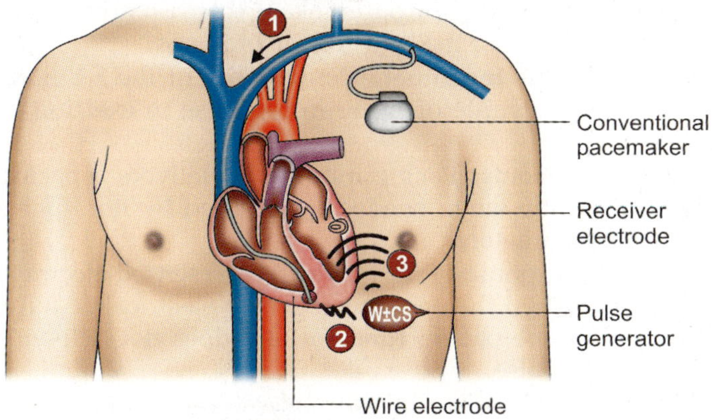


**Fig. 29.114:** Leadless pacemaker. EBR systems, a start-up out of Sunnyvale California, and Cambridge Consultants, the technology design and development firm, have developed a leadless pacemaker system for patients with advanced heart failure. The wireless cardiac stimulation system (WiCS) comprises two units, an implantable electrode and an external control unit. The electrode incorporates an ultrasonic, wireless receiver and delivers an electrical stimulus to the heart based on triggering signals from the external control unit. In its current iteration the WiCS system is designed to work with conventional pacemakers/ defibrillators pacing the right ventricle of patients requiring biventricular pacing. The WiCS external control unit senses the pacing stimulus delivered to the right ventricle and initiates a burst of stimulus from the electrode implanted in the left ventricle. According to the company, the wireless left ventricular pacing approach removes the need for complex surgery and the complications often associated with the coronary sinus leads used to pace the left ventricle

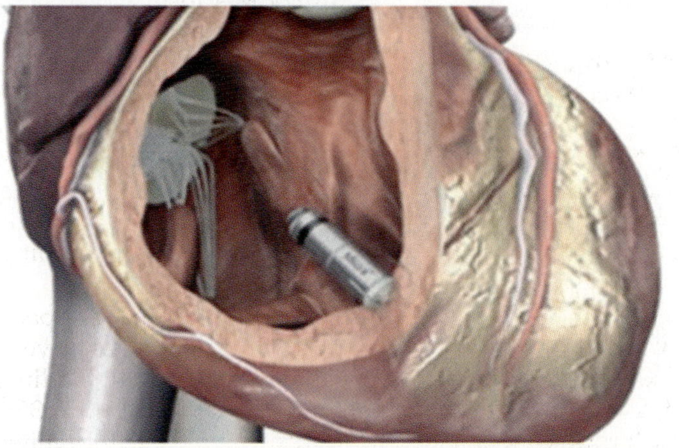

**Fig. 29.115:** Leadless pacemaker implanted by Dr Vivek Reddy MD, launches international LEADLESS II clinical research trial testing a miniature-sized, leadless pacemaker placed inside the heart without surgery

criteria for ventricular dyssynchrony. For antibradycardia pacing, definitive diagnosis requires the correlation of the bradyarrhythmia with the occurrence of symptoms of decreased cerebral blood flow, such as syncope, presyncope, dizziness and confusion. Ambulatory, ECG monitors provide valuable assistance in the documentation and correlation of symptoms with episodes of brady-

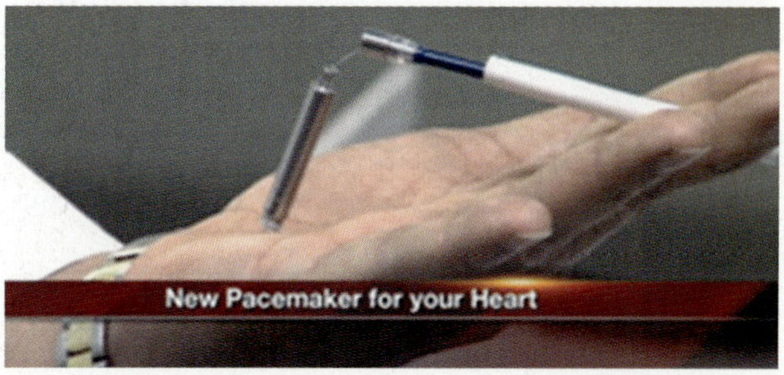


**Fig. 29.116:** Tiny leadless pacemaker less than 10% the size of a traditional pacemaker

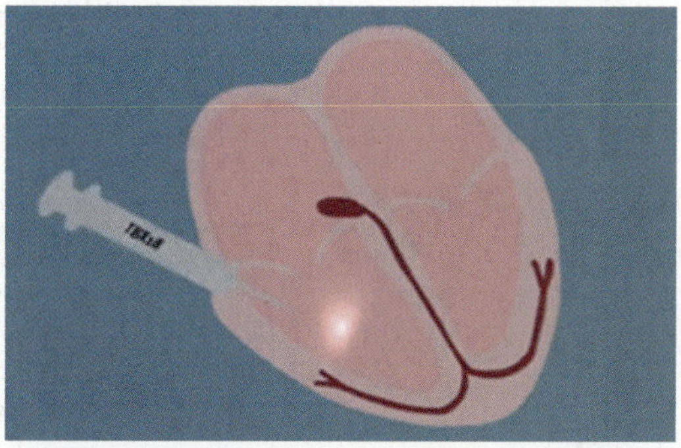

**Fig. 29.117:** Gene therapy is a procedure where genes (or segments of DNA) are inserted into a cell and the cell then takes up the gene and incorporates it into its own genome

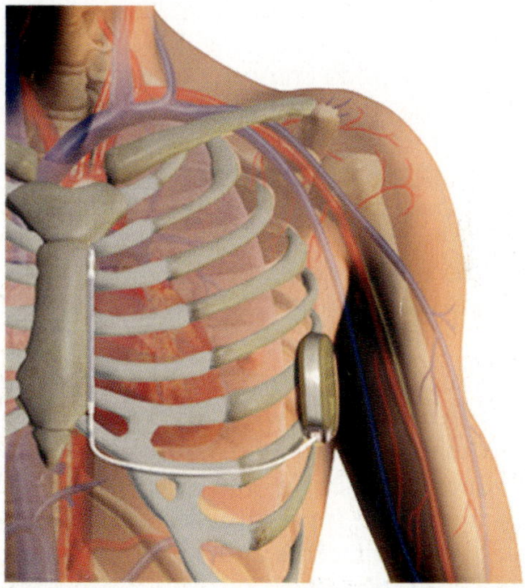

**Fig. 29.118:** Subcutaneous implantable cardiac defibrillator in position. The S-ICD System is designed to provide the same protection from sudden cardiac arrest as transvenous ICDs. The system has two main components—(1) the pulse generator, which powers the system, monitors heart activity, and delivers a shock if needed, and (2) the electrode, which enables the device to sense the cardiac rhythm and deliver shocks when necessary. Both components are implanted just under the skin, the generator at the side of the chest, and the electrode beside the breastbone. Unlike transvenous ICDs, the heart and blood vessels remain untouched. Implantation with the S-ICD system is straightforward using anatomical landmarks, without the need for fluoroscopy (an X-ray procedure that makes it possible to see internal organs in motion). Fluoroscopy is required for implanting the leads attached to transvenous ICD systems

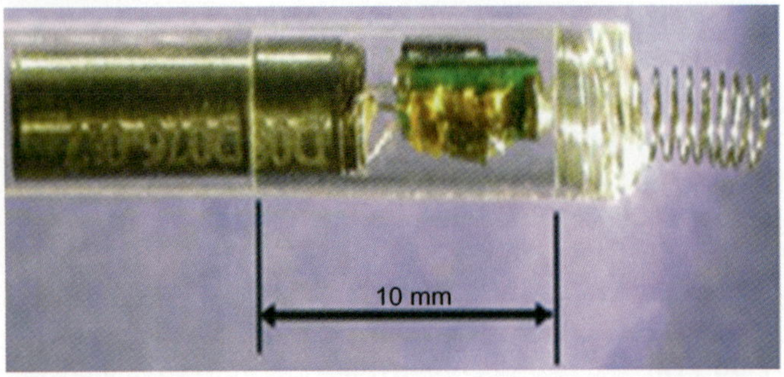


**Fig. 29.119:** Original mechanical concept for the fetal pacemaker and its deployment. University of Southern California's fetal pacemaker measures just 20 millimeters and is implanted directly onto the baby's heart using a cannula during noninvasive surgery. If successful, researchers hope that this type of pacemaker could someday be used to treat adults as well

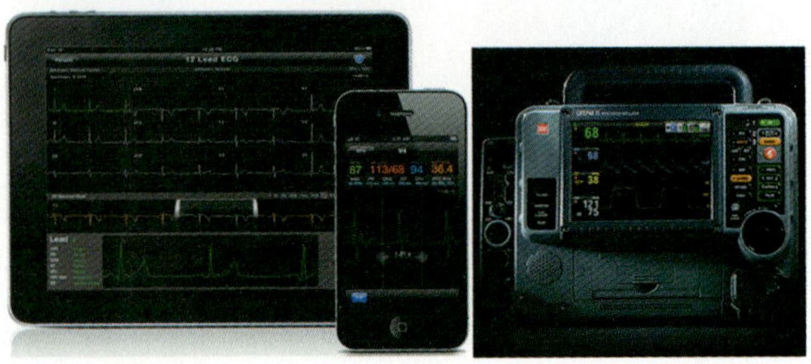

**Fig. 29.120:** Defibrillator/Monitors to transmit cardiac data to physician iPhones/iPads defibrillator/monitors to transmit cardiac data to physician iPhones/iPads AirStrip's CARDIOLOGY app, allowing doctors to provide immediate assistance to EMS crews handling complicated patients.The integrated solution empowers clinicians to communicate immediately with the EMS crew to provide the clinical assistance needed to properly care for the patient while EN route, direct them to the appropriate care facility and prepare for the arrival of the patient accordingly. With the integrated solution, these capabilities are available to clinicians anytime, anywhere on their smartphone or tablet device

arrhythmias. Pacing may also be used to provide CRT for persons with heart failure who have developed a loss of normal coordinated ventricular contraction as a result of the ventricular remodeling that occurs in heart failure. Selection of a specific type of pacemaker is based on an evaluation of patient factors and technical considerations. Follow-up care, including ongoing patient and family education, is vital in the effective management of the patient with a permanent pacemaker.

## GLOSSARY OF TERMS

- **Asynchronous mode:** Pacing mode in which the sensing function is turned off. The pacemaker delivers a pacing impulse at a set rate without regard for the heart's intrinsic electrical activity. It is the default setting for magnet mode in some pacemakers.
- **Atrioventricular interval:** Programmable setting on DDD and VDD pacemakers that defines the length of time that should occur between atrial depolarization and delivery of a ventricular pacing impulse. Roughly corresponds to the P-R interval in normal condition.
- **Capture:** Ability of the pacemaker to consistently trigger depolarization in the heart chamber paced.
- **Chronotropic incompetence:** Inability of the SA node to increase its rate of firing in response to exertion or stress.
- **Demand pacing:** Pacing mode that delivers a pacing impulse only when needed (as defined by its programmed parameters).
- **Inhibit:** Response of the pacemaker to sensed electrical activity. When the pacemaker senses electrical activity, it inhibits the pacing function and does not deliver a pacing impulse.
- **Pacing:** The ability of the pacemaker to deliver an electrical impulse through the pacemaker lead to the heart to stimulate depolarization.
- **Retrograde AV conduction:** Occurs when the electrical impulse spreads back from the ventricles across the AV node into the atria.
- **Sensing:** The ability of the pacemaker to recognize electrical activity in the heart.
- **Sensing threshold:** The largest electrical signal (ventricular or atrial) that can be consistently recognized by the sensing circuit.
- **Stimulation threshold:** The amount of electrical energy needed to depolarize the heart.
- **Triggered:** Pacemaker response to sensed electrical activity. When the pacemaker recognizes electrical activity, it triggers the pacemaker to deliver a pacing impulse at a preprogrammed interval.

### KEY POINTS

- The primary purpose of a pacemaker is to maintain an adequate heart rate, either because of the heart's native pacemaker is not fast enough, or there is a block in the heart's electrical conduction system.
- A pacemaker is composed to two parts, the pacing electrodes, or leads, which are wires that are inserted directly into the heart, and a pacemaker generator, which is surgically implanted in the chest wall.
- Rate responsive pacing allows the device to sense the physical activity of the patient and respond appropriately by increasing or decreasing the base pacing rate via rate response algorithms.
- A pacemaker monitors the heart's native electrical rhythm. When the pacemaker does not detect a heartbeat within a normal beat-to-beat time period, it will stimulate the ventricle of the heart with a short low voltage pulse. This sensing and stimulating activity continues on a beat by beat basis.
- Sometimes, devices resembling pacemakers, called implantable cardioverter defibrillators (ICDs), are implanted. An ICD has the ability to treat many types of heart rhythm disturbances by means of pacing, or defibrillation.
- Rate responsive pacing allows the device to sense the physical activity of the patient and respond appropriately by increasing or decreasing the base pacing rate via rate response algorithms.

- The outer casing of pacemakers is so designed that it will rarely be rejected by the body's immune system.
- Transcutaneous pacing (TCP) is an emergency procedure that acts as a bridge until transvenous pacing or other therapies can be applied.
- There are three basic types of permanent pacemakers, single-chamber pacemaker, dual chamber pacemaker, and rate-responsive pacemaker.
- Emergency clinicians must be familiar with the indications for pacemaker placement and aware of the complications associated with implantation. A systematic approach to evaluating the pacemaker is key to expeditious diagnosis of device malfunction. This includes careful history taking, a thorough physical examination of the patient, and accurate interpretation of the 12-lead ECG and chest radiographs. Device interrogation is a critical step in troubleshooting with regard to both pacemaker and antitachycardia functions.

## BIBLIOGRAPHY


1. Abraham WT, Fisher WG, Smith AL, et al. Cardiac resynchronization in chronic heart failure. N Engl J Med 2002; 346(24):1845–853. (Prospective randomized controlled; 453 patients).
2. Al-Bawardy R, Krishnaswamy A, Bhargava M, et al. Tricuspid regurgitation in patients with pacemakers and implantable cardiac defibrillators: a comprehensive review. Clin Cardiol 2013;36(5):249–54 (Review).
3. Altun A, Erdogan O. Pacemaker lead failure suggestive of crush injury. Cardiol Rev 2003;11(5):256. (Case report).
4. American College of Emergency Physicians, Society for Cardiovascular Angiography and Interventions, O'Gara PT, et al. 2013 ACCF/AHA guideline for the management of ST-elevation myocardial infarction: a report of the American College of Cardiology Foundation/American Heart Association Task Force on Practice Guidelines. J Am Coll Cardiol. 2013;61(4):e78–140 (Guideline).
5. Ammirati F, Colivicchi F, Santini M, et al. Permanent cardiac pacing versus medical treatment for the prevention of recurrent vasovagal syncope: a multicenter, randomized, controlled trial. Circulation 2001;104(1):52–7 (Prospective randomized; 93 patients).
6. Andersen HR, Nielsen JC, Thomsen PE, et al. Long-term follow-up of patients from a randomised trial of atrial versus ventricular pacing for sick-sinus syndrome 1997;350(9086): 1210–6 (Prospective observational; 225 patients).
7. Athan E, Chu VH, Tattevin P, et al. Clinical characteristics and outcome of infective endocarditis involving implantable cardiac devices. JAMA 2012;307(16):1727–35 (Prospective cohort; 2760 patients).
8. Barold SS, Herweg B, Giudici M. Electrocardiographic follow-up of biventricular pacemakers. Ann Noninvasive Electrocardiol 2005;10(2):231–55. (Review).
9. Barold SS, Herweg B. The effect of hyperkalaemia on cardiac rhythm devices. Europace 2014 (Review).
10. Becker R, Ruf-Richter J, Senges-Becker JC, et al. Patient alert in implantable cardioverter defibrillators: toy or tool? J Am Coll Cardiol 2004;44(1):95–98 (Prospective cohort; 240 patients).
11. Bernstein AD, Daubert JC, Fletcher RD, et al. The revised NASPE/BPEG generic code for antibradycardia, adaptive-rate, and multisite pacing. North American Society of Pacing and Electrophysiology/British Pacing and Electrophysiology Group. Pacing Clin Electrophysiol 2002;25(2):260–4 (Guideline).
12. Birnie DH, Tang AS. The problem of non-response to cardiac resynchronization therapy. Curr Opin Cardiol 2006;21(1):20–26 (Review).
13. Bracke F, Meijer A, Van Gelder B. Venous occlusion of the access vein in patients referred for lead extraction: influence of patient and lead characteristics. Pacing Clin Electrophysiol. 2003;26(8):1649–52. (Retrospective observational; 89 patients)
14. Brandt J, Anderson H, Fahraeus T, et al. Natural history of sinus node disease treated with atrial pacing in 213 patients: implications for selection of stimulation mode. J Am Coll Cardiol 1992;20(3):633–639 (Prospective observational; 213 patients).
15. Brignole M, Menozzi C, Lolli G, et al. Natural and unnatural history of patients with severe carotid sinus hypersensitivity: a preliminary study. Pacing Clin Electrophysiol 1988;11(11 Pt 2):175–180 (Retrospective observational; 5287 patients).
16. Brignole M, Menozzi C, Lolli G, et al. Validation of a method for choice of pacing mode in carotid sinus syndrome with or without sinus bradycardia. Pacing Clin Electrophysiol 1991;14(2 Pt 1):196–203 (Prospective observational; 60 patients).
17. Bristow MR, Saxon LA, Boehmer J, et al. Cardiac-resynchroni-zation therapy with or without an implantable defibril-lator in advanced chronic heart failure. N Engl J Med 2004; 350(21):2140–50 (Prospective randomized; 1520 patients).
18. Brown KR, Carter W, Jr. Lombardi GE. Blunt trauma-induced pacemaker failure. Ann Emerg Med. 1991;20(8):905–7 (Case report).
19. Chan TC, Cardall TY. Electronic pacemakers. Emerg Med Clin North Am 2006;24(1):179–94 (Review).
20. Cleland JG, Daubert JC, Erdmann E, et al. The effect of cardiac resynchronization on morbidity and mortality in heart failure. N Engl J Med 2005;352(15):1539–49 (Prospective randomized; 813 patients).
21. Connolly SJ, Sheldon R, Roberts RS, et al. The North American Vasovagal Pacemaker Study (VPS). A randomized trial of permanent cardiac pacing for the prevention of vasovagal syncope. J Am Coll Cardiol 1999;33(1):16–20 (Prospective randomized; 54 patients).
22. Connolly SJ, Sheldon R, Thorpe KE, et al. Pacemaker therapy for prevention of syncope in patients with recurrent severe vasovagal syncope: Second Vasovagal Pacemaker Study (VPS II): a randomized trial. JAMA 2003;289(17):2224–9 (Prospective randomized; 100 patients).
23. Cowie MR, Sarkar S, Koehler J, et al. Development and validation of an integrated diagnostic algorithm derived from parameters monitored in implantable devices for identifying patients at risk for heart failure hospitalization in an ambula-tory setting. Eur Heart J 2013;34(31):2472–80 (Retrospective observational; 2231 patients).

24. Credner SC, Klingenheben T, Mauss O, et al. Electrical storm in patients with transvenous implantable cardioverter-defibrillators: incidence, management and prognostic implications. J Am Coll Cardiol 1998;32(7):1909–15 (Prospective cohort; 136 patients).
25. Das G, Staffanson DB. Selective dysfunction of ventricular electrode-endocardial junction following DC cardioversion in a patient with a dual chamber pacemaker. Pacing Clin Electrophysiol 1997;20(2 Pt 1):364–5 (Case report).
26. Dretzke J, Toff WD, Lip GY, et al. Dual chamber versus single chamber ventricular pacemakers for sick sinus syndrome and atrioventricular block. Cochrane Database Syst Rev 2004(2):CD003710 (Systematic review).
27. Ellenbogen KA, Hellkamp AS, Wilkoff BL, et al. Complications arising after implantation of DDD pacemakers: the MOST experience. Am J Cardiol 2003;92(6):740–1 (Retro-spective observational; 2010 patients).
28. Emilsson K, Oddsson H, Allared M, et al. An unusual cause of high threshold values at pacemaker implantation. Pacing Clin Electrophysiol 1997;20(2 Pt 1):366–7 (Case report).
29. Epstein AE, DiMarco JP, Ellenbogen KA, et al. 2012 ACCF/AHA/HRS focused update incorporated into the ACCF/AHA/HRS 2008 guidelines for device-based therapy of cardiac rhythm abnormalities: a report of the American College of Cardiology Foundation/American Heart Association Task Force on Practice Guidelines and the Heart Rhythm Society. J Am Coll Cardiol 2013;61(3):e6–e75 (Guideline).
30. Epstein AE, DiMarco JP, Ellenbogen KA, et al. ACC/AHA/HRS 2008 guidelines for device-based therapy of cardiac rhythm abnormalities: a report of the American College of cardiology/American Heart Association Task Force on Practice Guidelines (Writing Committee to Revise the ACC/AHA/NASPE 2002 guideline update for implantation of cardiac pacemakers and antiarrhythmia devices) developed in collaboration with the American Association for Thoracic Surgery and Society of Thoracic Surgeons. J Am Coll Cardiol 2008;51(21):e1–e62 (Guideline).
31. European Heart Rhythm Association, European Society of Cardiology, Heart Rhythm Society, et al. 2012 EHRA/HRS expert consensus statement on cardiac resynchronization therapy in heart failure: implant and follow-up recommendations and management. Europace 2012;14(9):1236–86. (Guideline).
32. European Society of Cardiology, European Heart Rhythm Association, Brignole M, Auricchio A, Baron-Esquivias G, et al. 2013 ESC guidelines on cardiac pacing and cardiac resynchronization therapy: the Task Force on Cardiac Pacing and Resynchronization Therapy of the European Society of Cardiology (ESC). Developed in collaboration with the European Heart Rhythm Association (EHRA). Europace 2013;15(8):1070–118 (Guideline).
33. Farwell D, Patel NR, Hall A, et al. How many people with heart failure are appropriate for biventricular resynchronization? Eur Heart J 2000;21(15):1246–50 (Retrospective observational; 721 patients).
34. Fishberger SB, Mehta D, Rossi AF, et al. Variable effects of adenosine on retrograde conduction in patients with atrioventricular nodal reentry tachycardia. Pacing Clin Electrophysiol 1998;21(6):1254–7 (Prospective nonrandomized trial; 13 patients).
35. Friedman PA, McClelland RL, Bamlet WR, et al. Dual-chamber versus single-chamber detection enhancements for implantable defibrillator rhythm diagnosis: the detect supraventricular tachycardia study. Circulation 2006;113(25):2871–9 (Randomized controlled trial; 400 patients).
36. Furman S. Defibrillator twiddler's syndrome. Ann Thorac Surg 1995;59(2):544–6 (Comment).
37. Gang UJ, Hvelplund A, Pedersen S, et al. High-degree atrio-ventricular block complicating ST-segment elevation myocardial infarction in the era of primary percutaneous coronary intervention. Europace 2012;14(11):1639–45 (Retrospective observational; 2073 patients).
38. Gehi AK, Mehta D, Gomes JA. Evaluation and management of patients after implantable cardioverter-defibrillator shock. JAMA 2006;296(23):2839–47 (Review).
39. Gillis AM, Russo AM, Ellenbogen KA, et al. HRS/ACCF expert consensus statement on pacemaker device and mode selection. Developed in partnership between the Heart Rhythm Society (HRS) and the American College of Cardiology Foundation (ACCF) and in collaboration with the Society of Thoracic Surgeons. Heart Rhythm 2012;9(8):1344–65 (Guideline).
40. Gimbel JR, Cox JW Jr. Electronic article surveillance systems and interactions with implantable cardiac devices: risk of adverse interactions in public and commercial spaces. Mayo Clin Proc 2007;82(3):318–22 (Case series; 2 patients).
41. Glikson M, Friedman PA. The implantable cardioverter defibrillator. Lancet 2001;357(9262):1107–17 (Review).
42. Go AS, Mozaffarian D, Roger VL, et al. Heart disease and stroke statistics—2014 update: a report from the American Heart Association. Circulation 2014;129(3):e28–e292 (executive summary).
43. Greenspon AJ, Patel JD, Lau E, et al. Trends in permanent pace-maker implantation in the United States from 1993 to 2009: increasing complexity of patients and procedures. J Am Coll Cardiol 2012;60(16):1540–5 (Retrospective observational; 2.9 million patients).
44. Gross JN, Platt S, Ritacco R, et al. The clinical relevance of electromyopotential oversensing in current unipolar devices. Pacing Clin Electrophysiol 1992;15(11 Pt 2):2023–7 (Prospective observational; 34 patients).
45. Gurevitz O, Lipchenca I, Yaacoby E, et al. ST-segment deviation following implantable cardioverter defibrillator shocks: incidence, timing, and clinical significance. Pacing Clin Electro-physiol 2002;25(10):1429–32 (Prospective obser-vational; 28 patients).
46. Hauser RG, Hayes DL, Kallinen LM, et al. Clinical experience with pacemaker pulse generators and transvenous leads: an 8-year prospective multicenter study. Heart Rhythm 2007;4(2):154–60 (Prospective observational; 2652 pulse generators, 615 leads).
47. Hayes DL, Holmes DR Jr, Gray JE. Effect of 1.5 tesla nuclear magnetic resonance imaging scanner on implanted permanent pacemakers. J Am Coll Cardiol 1987;10(4):782–6 (Cross-sectional; 8 patients).
48. Higgins SL, Hummel JD, Niazi IK, et al. Cardiac resynchronization therapy for the treatment of heart failure in patients

with intraventricular conduction delay and malignant ventri-cular tachyarrhythmias. J Am Coll Cardiol 2003; 42(8): 1454–9 (Prospective randomized controlled; 490 patients).
49. Higgins SL, Suh BD, Stein JB, et al. Recurrent twiddler's syndrome in a nonthoracotomy ICD system despite a Dacron pouch. Pacing Clin Electrophysiol 1998;21(1 Pt 1):130–3 (Case report).
50. Huang SK, Ezri MD, Hauser RG, et al. Carotid sinus hyper-sensitivity in patients with unexplained syncope: clinical, electrophysiologic, and long-term follow-up observations. Am Heart J 1988;116(4):989–96 (Prospective observational; 76 patients).
51. Jacob S, Panaich SS, Maheshwari R, et al. Clinical applications of magnets on cardiac rhythm management devices. Europace 2011;13(9):1222–30 (Review).
52. Jilek C, Tzeis S, Vrazic H, et al. Safety of screening procedures with hand-held metal detectors among patients with implanted cardiac rhythm devices: a cross-sectional analysis. Ann Intern Med 2011;155(9):587–92 (Cross-sectional; 388 patients).
53. Kahloon MU, Aslam AK, Aslam AF, et al. Hyperkalemia induced failure of atrial and ventricular pacemaker capture. Int J Cardiol 2005;105(2):224–6. (Case report).
54. Kanal E, Borgstede JP, Barkovich AJ, et al. ACR Blue Ribbon Panel response to the AJR commentary by Shellock and Crues on the ACR white paper on MR safety. AJR Am J Roentgenol 2003;180(1):31–5 (Comment).
55. Karumbaiah K, Omar B. ST-elevation myocardial infarction in the presence of biventricular paced rhythm. J Emerg Med 2013;45(2):e35–e40. (Case report).
56. Kiviniemi MS, Pirnes MA, Eranen HJ, et al. Complications related to permanent pacemaker therapy. Pacing Clin Electrophysiol. 1999;22(5):711–20. (Retrospective observational; 446 patients).
57. Kutinsky IB, Jarandilla R, Jewett M, et al. Risk of hematoma complications after device implant in the clopidogrel era. Circ Arrhythm Electrophysiol 2010;3(4):312–8. (Prospective observational; 935 patients).
58. Lamas GA, Lee KL, Sweeney MO, et al. Ventricular pacing or dual-chamber pacing for sinus-node dysfunction. N Engl J Med 2002;346(24):1854–62 (Randomized controlled trial; 2010 patients).
59. Lampert R, Hayes DL, Annas GJ, et al. HRS expert consensus statement on the management of cardiovascular implantable electronic devices (CIEDs) in patients nearing end of life or requesting withdrawal of therapy. Heart Rhythm 2010; 7(7):1008–26 (Consensus statement).
60. Levine GN, Gomes AS, Arai AE, et al. Safety of magnetic resonance imaging in patients with cardiovascular devices: an American Heart Association scientific statement from the Committee on Diagnostic and Interventional Cardiac Catheterization, Council on Clinical Cardiology, and the Council on Cardiovascular Radiology and Intervention: endorsed by the American College of Cardiology Foundation, the North American Society for Cardiac Imaging, and the Society for Cardiovascular Magnetic Resonance. Circulation 2007;116(24):2878–91 (Scientific statement).
61. Lewalter T, Schimpf R, Kulik D, et al. Comparison of spontaneous atrial fibrillation electrogram potentials with the P-wave electrogram amplitude in dual chamber pacing with unipolar atrial sensing. Europace 2000;2(2):136–40 (Prospective observational; 42 patients).
62. Linde C, Abraham WT, Gold MR, et al. Randomized trial of cardiac resynchronization in mildly symptomatic heart failure patients and in asymptomatic patients with left ventri-cular dysfunction and previous heart failure symptoms. J Am Coll Cardiol 2008;52(23):1834–43 (Randomized controlled; 610 patients).
63. Link MS, Hellkamp AS, Estes NA 3rd et al. High incidence of pacemaker syndrome in patients with sinus node dys-function treated with ventricular-based pacing in the Mode Selection Trial (MOST). J Am Coll Cardiol 2004;43(11):2066–71 (Prospective cohort; 182 patients).
64. Madias JE. The nonspecificity of ST-segment elevation >5.0 mm in V1-V3 in the diagnosis of acute myocardial infarction in the presence of ventricular paced rhythm. J Electrocardiol 2004;37(2):135–9. (Case report).
65. Maisel WH, Moynahan M, Zuckerman BD, et al. Pacemaker and ICD generator malfunctions: analysis of Food and Drug Administration annual reports. JAMA 2006;295(16):1901– 6 (Retrospective observational).
66. Maisel WH. Pacemaker and ICD generator reliability: meta-analysis of device registries. JAMA 2006;295(16):1929–34 (Meta-analysis; 3365 patients).
67. Maloy KR, Bhat R, Davis J, et al. Sgarbossa Criteria are highly specific for acute myocardial infarction with pacemakers. West J Emerg Med 2010;11(4):354–7. (Retrospective cohort; 57 patients).
68. Mandal S, Pande A, Mandal D, et al. Permanent pacemaker-related upper extremity deep vein thrombosis: a series of 20 cases. Pacing Clin Electrophysiol 2012;35(10):1194–8 (Case series; 20 patients).
69. McMullan J, Valento M, Attari M, et al. Care of the pace-maker/implantable cardioverter defibrillator patient in the ED. Am J Emerg Med 2007;25(7):812–22 (Review).
70. McPherson CA, Manthous C. Permanent pacemakers and implantable defibrillators: considerations for intensivists. Am J Respir Crit Care Med 2004;170(9):933–40 (Review).
71. Misiri J, Kusumoto F, Goldschlager N. Electromagnetic inter-ference and implanted cardiac devices: the nonmedical environment (part I). Clin Cardiol 2012;35(5):276–80 (Review).
72. Misiri J, Kusumoto F, Goldschlager N. Electromagnetic interference and implanted cardiac devices: the medical environ-ment (part II). Clin Cardiol 2012;35(6):321–8 (Review).
73. Mollazadeh R, Mohimi L, Zeighami M, et al. Hemodynamic effect of atrioventricular and interventricular dyssynchrony in patients with biventricular pacing: implications for the pacemaker syndrome. J Cardiovasc Dis Res 2012;3(3):200–3 (Cross-sectional; 40 patients).
74. Mond HG, Proclemer A. The 11th world survey of cardiac pacing and implantable cardioverter-defibrillators: calendar year 2009—a World Society of Arrhythmia project. Pacing Clin Electrophysiol 2011;34(8):1013–27 (Survey; 1.02 mil-lion implantations).

75. Montefoschi N, Boccadamo R. Propafenone induced acute variation of chronic atrial pacing threshold: a case report. Pacing Clin Electrophysiol 1990;13(4):480–3 (Case report).
76. Morley CA, Perrins EJ, Grant P, et al. Carotid sinus syncope treated by pacing. Analysis of persistent s-symptom and role of atrioventricular sequential pacing. Br Heart J 1982; 47(5):411–8 (Case series; 70 patients).
77. Moss AJ, Hall WJ, Cannom DS, et al. Cardiac-resynchronization therapy for the prevention of heart-failure events. N Engl J Med 2009;361(14):1329–38 (Prospective randomized controlled; 1820 patients).
78. Mulpuru SK, Patel DV, Wilbur SL, et al. Electrical storm and termination with propofol therapy: a case report. Int J Cardiol 2008;128(1):e6–e8 (Case report).
79. Nademanee K, Taylor R, Bailey WE, et al. Treating electrical storm: sympathetic blockade versus advanced cardiac life support-guided therapy. Circulation 2000;102(7):742–7 (Prospective nonrandomized trial; 49 patients).
80. Nazarian S, Hansford R, Roguin A, et al. A prospective evalua-tion of a protocol for magnetic resonance imaging of patients with implanted cardiac devices. Ann Intern Med 2011;155(7):415–24. (Prospective nonrandomized trial; 438 patients, 555 MRI studies).
81. Nielsen JC, Thomsen PE, Hojberg S, et al. A comparison of single-lead atrial pacing with dual-chamber pacing in sick sinus syndrome. Eur Heart J 2011;32(6):686–96 (Prospective randomized; 1415 patients).
82. Ofman P, Rahilly-Tierney C, Djousse L, et al. Pacing system malfunction is a rare cause of hospital admission for syncope in patients with a permanent pacemaker. Pacing Clin Electrophysiol. 2013;36(1):109–12. (Retrospective observational; 162 patients)
83. Okmen E, Erdinler I, Oguz E, et al. An electrocardiographic algorithm for determining the location of pacemaker electrode in patients with right bundle branch block configuration during permanent ventricular pacing. Angiol-ogy 2006;57(5):623–30. (Retrospective observational; 25 patients).
84. Ortega-Carnicer J, Benezet J, Benezet-Mazuecos J. Hyperkalaemia causing loss of atrial capture and extremely wide QRS complex during DDD pacing. Resuscitation 2004;62(1):119–20. (Case report).
85. Osmonov D, Ozcan KS, Erdinler I, et al. Cardiac device-related endocarditis: 31-years' experience. J Cardiol 2013;61(2):175–80. (Retrospective observational; 5287 patients).
86. Parry SW, Steen N, Bexton RS, et al. Pacing in elderly recurrent fallers with carotid sinus hypersensitivity: a randomised, double-blind, placebo controlled crossover trial. Heart 2009;95(5):405–9. (Randomized controlled crossover trial; 34 patients).
87. Patton KK, Levy M, Viswanathan M. Atrial lead dysfunction: an unusual feature of hypothyroidism. Pacing Clin Electrophysiol 2008;31(12):1650–2 (Case report).
88. Pavia S, Wilkoff B. The management of surgical complications of pacemaker and implantable cardioverter-defibrillators. Curr Opin Cardiol 2001;16(1):66–71 (Review).
89. Pinski SL. Emergencies related to implantable cardioverter-defibrillators. Crit Care Med 2000;28(10 Suppl):N174–N180 (Review).
90. Platonov MA, Gillis AM, Kavanagh KM. Pacemakers, implantable cardioverter/defibrillators, and extracorporeal shockwave lithotripsy: evidence-based guidelines for the modern era. J Endourol 2008;22(2):243–7 (Guideline).
91. Raviele A, Giada F, Menozzi C, et al. A randomized, double-blind, placebo-controlled study of permanent cardiac pacing for the treatment of recurrent tilt-induced vasovagal syncope. The vasovagal syncope and pacing trial (SYNPACE). Eur Heart J 2004;25(19):1741–8 (Prospective randomized controlled; 29 patients).
92. Reddy VY, Knops RE, Sperzel J, et al. Permanent leadless cardiac pacing: results of the LEADLESS trial. Circulation 2014 (Prospective nonrandomized trial; 33 patients).
93. Rodriguez Y, Garisto J, Carrillo RG. Management of cardiac device-related infections: a review of protocol-driven care. Int J Cardiol 2013;166(1):55–60 (Retrospective observational; 350 patients).
94. Sack S, Wende CM, Nagele H, et al. Potential value of automated daily screening of cardiac resynchronization therapy defibrillator diagnostics for prediction of major cardiovascular events: results from Home-CARE (Home Monitoring in Cardiac Resynchronization Therapy) study. Eur J Heart Fail 2011;13(9):1019–27 (Prospective cohort; 377 patients).
95. Santos KR, Adragao P, Cavaco D, et al. Diaphragmatic myopotential oversensing in pacemaker-dependent patients with CRT-D devices. Europace 2008;10(12):1381–6 (Retrospective observational; 37 patients).
96. Sarko JA, Tiffany BR. Cardiac pacemakers: evaluation and management of malfunctions. Am J Emerg Med 2000;18(4): 435–40 (Review).
97. Schiraldi F, Guiotto G, Paladino F. Hyperkalemia induced failure of pacemaker capture and sensing. Resuscitation 2008;79(1):161–4. (Case report).
98. Sgarbossa EB, Pinski SL, Gates KB, et al. Early electrocardiographic diagnosis of acute myocardial infarction in the presence of ventricular paced rhythm. GUSTO-I investigators. Am J Cardiol 1996;77(5):423–4. (Retrospective observa-tional; 17 patients).
99. Sham'a RA, Nery P, Sadek M, et al. Myocardial injury seco-ndary to ICD shocks: insights from patients with lead fracture. Pacing Clin Electrophysiol 2014;37(2):237–41 (Prospective observational; 22 patients).
100. Shamim W, Francis DP, Yousufuddin M, et al. Intraventricular conduction delay: a prognostic marker in chronic heart failure. Int J Cardiol 1999;70(2):171–8 (Retrospective observational; 241 patients).
101. Sipahi I, Chou JC, Hyden M, et al. Effect of QRS morphology on clinical event reduction with cardiac resynchronization therapy: meta-analysis of randomized controlled trials. Am Heart J 2012;163(2):260–7 (Meta-analysis; 5356 patients).
102. Smith SW, Dodd KW, Henry TD, et al. Diagnosis of ST-elevation myocardial infarction in the presence of left bundle branch block with the ST-elevation to S-wave ratio in a modified Sgarbossa rule. Ann Emerg Med 2012;60(6):766–76. (Retrospective cohort; 162 patients).
103. Stavrakis S, Lazzara R, Thadani U. The benefit of cardiac resynchronization therapy and QRS duration: a meta-analysis. J Cardiovasc Electrophysiol 2012;23(2):163–8 (Meta-analysis; 6501 patients).

104. Stevenson WG, Chaitman BR, Ellenbogen KA, et al. Clinical assessment and management of patients with implanted cardioverter-defibrillators presenting to nonelectro-physiologists. Circulation 2004;110(25):3866–9.(Review).
105. Sugrue DD, Gersh BJ, Holmes DR Jr. et al. Symptomatic "isolated" carotid sinus hypersensitivity: natural history and results of treatment with anticholinergic drugs or pacemaker. J Am Coll Cardiol 1986;7(1):158–62 (Prospective observational; 56 patients).
106. Sutton R, Brignole M, Menozzi C, et al. Dual-chamber pacing in the treatment of neurally mediated tilt-positive cardio-inhibitory syncope: pacemaker versus no therapy: a multi-center randomized study. The Vasovagal Syncope International Study (VASIS) Investigators. Circulation 2000;102(3):294–9 (Prospective randomized; 42 patients).
107. Sweeney MO, Bank AJ, Nsah E, et al. Minimizing ventricular pacing to reduce atrial fibrillation in sinus-node disease. N Engl J Med 2007;357(10):1000–8 (Prospective randomized; 1065 patients).
108. Sweeney MO, Hellkamp AS, Ellenbogen KA, et al. Adverse effect of ventricular pacing on heart failure and atrial fibril-lation among patients with normal baseline QRS duration in a clinical trial of pacemaker therapy for sinus node dys-function. Circulation 2003;107(23):2932–7 (Retrospective observational trial; 1339 patients).
109. Takasugi N, Kubota T, Kawamura I, et al. Sudden reversible pacemaker failure in a patient with cardiac sarcoidosis: an unfortunate case of ventricular septal pacing. Europace 2012;14(7):1061–2 (Case report).
110. Tandogan I, Ozin B, Bozbas H, et al. Effects of mobile telephones on the function of implantable cardioverter defibrillators. Ann Noninvasive Electrocardiol 2005;10(4): 409–13 (Cross-sectional; 43 patients).
111. Tandogan I, Temizhan A, Yetkin E, et al. The effects of mobile phones on pacemaker function. Int J Cardiol 2005;103(1):51–8 (Cross-sectional; 679 patients).
112. Tang AS, Wells GA, Talajic M, et al. Cardiac-resynchroni-zation therapy for mild-to-moderate heart failure. N Engl J Med 2010;363(25):2385–95 (Prospective randomized; 1798 patients).
113. Thambo JB, Bordachar P, Garrigue S, et al. Detrimental ventri-cular remodeling in patients with congenital complete heart block and chronic right ventricular apical pacing. Circulation 2004;110(25):3766–72 (Prospective cohort; 53 patients).
114. Tracy CM, Epstein AE, Darbar D, et al. 2012 ACCF/AHA/HRS focused update of the 2008 guidelines for device-based therapy of cardiac rhythm abnormalities: a report of the American College of Cardiology Foundation/American Heart Association Task Force on Practice Guidelines and the Heart Rhythm Society. Circulation [corrected] 2012;126(14): 1784–800 (Guidelines).
115. Trohman RG, Kim MH, Pinski SL. Cardiac pacing: the state of the art. Lancet 2004;364(9446):1701–19 (Review).
116. Uslan DZ, Tleyjeh IM, Baddour LM, et al. Temporal trends in permanent pacemaker implantation: a population-based study. Am Heart J 2008;155(5):896–903 (Retrospective observational; 1291 patients).
117. van Veldhuisen DJ, Maass AH, Priori SG, et al. Implementa-tion of device therapy (cardiac resynchronization therapy and implantable cardioverter defibrillator) for patients with heart failure in Europe: changes from 2004 to 2008. Eur J Heart Fail 2009;11(12):1143–51 (Retrospective observational).
118. Waller C, Callies F, Langenfeld H. Adverse effects of direct current cardioversion on cardiac pacemakers and electrodes Is external cardioversion contraindicated in patients with permanent pacing systems? Europace 2004;6(2):165–8. (Case report; 3 cases).
119. Webster G, Jordao L, Martuscello M, et al. Digital music players cause interference with interrogation telemetry for pacemakers and implantable cardioverter-defibrillators without affecting device function. Heart Rhythm 2008;5(4): 545–50 (Cross-sectional; 51 patients).
120. Whellan DJ, Ousdigian KT, Al-Khatib SM, et al. Combined heart failure device diagnostics identify patients at higher risk of subsequent heart failure hospitalizations: results from PARTNERS HF (Program to Access and Review Trending Infor-mation and Evaluate Correlation to Symptoms in Patients With Heart Failure) study. J Am Coll Cardiol 2010; 55(17):1803–10 (Retrospective observational trial; 694 patients).
121. Wolber T, Ryf S, Binggeli C, et al. Potential interference of small neodymium magnets with cardiac pacemakers and implantable cardioverter-defibrillators. Heart Rhythm 2007;4(1):1–4 (Cross-sectional; 70 patients).
122. Young JB, Abraham WT, Smith AL, et al. Combined cardiac resynchronization and implantable cardioversion defibrillation in advanced chronic heart failure: the MIRACLE ICD Trial. JAMA 2003;289(20):2685–94 (Prospective randomized controlled; 369 patients).

# 30 Ventricular Assist Devices

A ventricular assist device or VAD, is a mechanical circulatory device that is used to partially or completely replace the function of a failing heart. Some VADs are intended for short term use, typically for patients recovering from heart attacks or heart surgery, while others are intended for long term use (months to years and in some cases for life), typically for patients suffering from congestive heart failure.

Ventricular assist devices need to be clearly distinguished from artificial hearts, which are designed to completely take over cardiac function and generally require the removal of the patient's heart.

Ventricular assist devices are designed to assist either the right (RVAD) or left (LVAD) ventricle, or both at once biventricular assist device (BiVAD). Which of these types is used, depends primarily on the underlying heart disease and the pulmonary arterial resistance that determines the load on the right ventricle.

Left ventricular assist devices (LVADs) are most commonly used, but when pulmonary arterial resistance is high, right ventricular assistance becomes necessary.

Long term VADs are normally used to keep patients alive with a good quality of life while they wait for a heart transplantation (known as a 'bridge to transplantation'). However, LVADs are sometimes used as destination therapy and sometimes as a bridge to recovery. In the last few years, VADs have improved significantly in terms of providing survival and quality of life among recipients.

Heart failure is the final common pathway for many chronic heart diseases. With the aging of the population and advances in the treatment of cardiac disease, the number of patients with heart failure continues to increase. Although, the majority of patients will remain stable for several years with standard medicines and surgery, a growing number will develop symptoms of advanced heart failure and may be referred for evaluation for heart transplant. For selected patients, who are too ill to wait for a heart donor or who are not eligible for a heart transplant because of age or other medical problems, VADs offer life-saving therapy. Initially designed as temporary support to bridge patients to heart transplant, these devices are now available and increasingly being used as lifetime support or destination therapy. Improvements in device design, along with advances in surgical and medical management, have allowed VAD patients to return home, to work, and to their communities, with excellent quality of life. At the same time, however, unique challenges have been encountered.

## CLINICAL ASSESSMENT OF ADVANCED HEART FAILURE

Heart failure is a common cardiac condition in which the heart is unable to pump blood at a sufficient rate to meet the demands of the body. There are two major types of heart failure—one is associated with abnormal heart filling (sometimes called diastolic heart failure or heart failure with preserved ejection fraction), and the other is associated with abnormal heart emptying (also called systolic heart failure or heart failure with reduced ejection fraction). Most patients, who develop heart failure have had a prior injury or stress on the heart that caused the heart to weaken. Examples include a heart attack, high blood pressure, heart valve problems, and irregular heart rhythms. Exposure to toxins such as alcohol and chemotherapy can also cause heart failure. A smaller number of patients are born with a heart defect or a genetic mutation that leads to heart failure in adulthood. Other common medical conditions, such as diabetes, obesity, and chronic lung or kidney disease, can worsen heart failure (Fig. 30.1).

The major symptoms of heart failure include fatigue, shortness of breath, and fluid retention. In most patients, these symptoms can be relieved or stabilized with medications such as angiotensin-converting enzyme inhibitors, β-blockers, and diuretics (or fluid pills), along with changes in lifestyle and diet. Implantable heart devices,

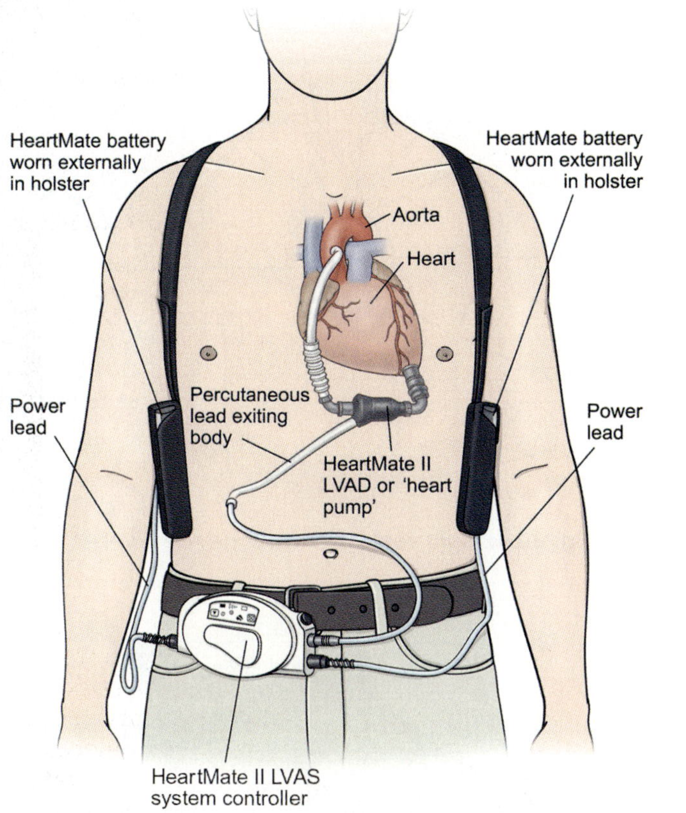


**Fig. 30.1:** Left ventricular assist device (LVAD) fitted over waist of the body alongwith its supporting connections

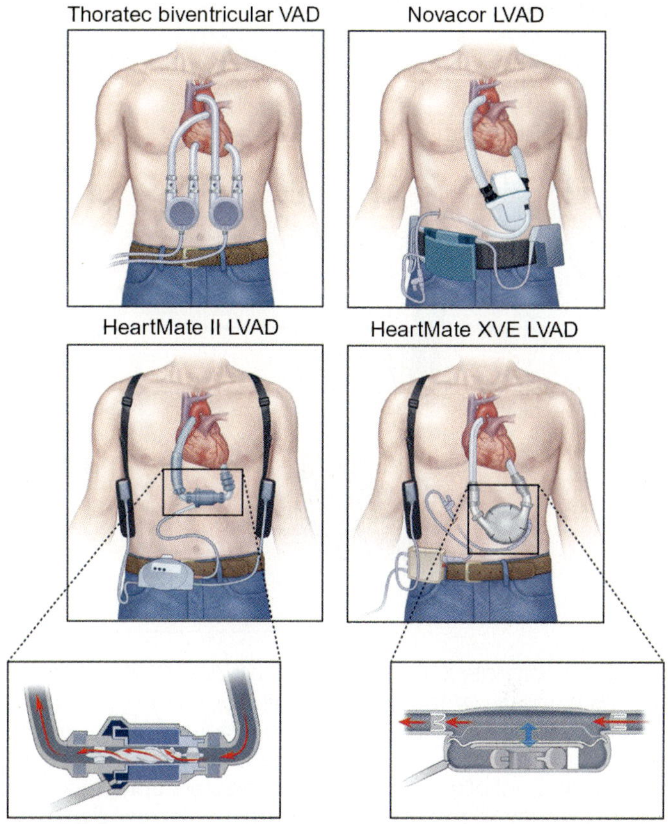


**Fig. 30.2:** Schematics of commonly used VADs mechanical support systems—thoratec VAD (top left), Novacor LVAD (top right), HeartMate II LVAD (bottom left) and HeartMate XVE LVAD (bottom right). Illustrations depicting the mechanisms of action of an axial flow and volume displacement pumps are shown for the HeartMate II and HeartMate XVE devices. The axial flow pump is a small device consisting of a continuously spinning impeller along a central shaft. Blood is drawn from the spinning blades of the impeller and propelled at 4–6 L/min with minimal hemolysis. The pulsatile pump of the HeartMate XVE uses an electromagnetic pusher plate to cyclically expand and decompress a chamber. The pusher plate can provide between 5 and 10 L/min of pulsatile blood flow *(Figure illustration by Rob Flewell)*

such as pacemakers and cardioverter-defibrillators, are also available to improve both the quality and duration of life. However, it is estimated that about 250,000 of the 7 million patients with heart failure living in the United States will develop symptoms of advanced heart failure. For carefully selected patients, heart transplantation offers a life-saving therapy. However, given the shortage of organ donors (there are approx. 2200 donor hearts available each year in the United States), the vast majority of patients with advanced heart failure will progress to end-stage disease. For some, mechanical circulatory support or VADs are available to take over the function of the failing heart.

## DIFFERENT TYPES OF VADS USED

Many different mechanical devices have been developed to support the failing heart, ranging from total artificial hearts to VADs (Figs 30.2–30.6). The main purpose of a VAD is to unload the failing heart and help maintain blood flow to vital organs. VADs were originally developed to serve as a temporary bridge to heart recovery, and then as a bridge to transplant. Over the past 10 years, however, VADs have been approved by the US Food and Drug Administration to provide permanent or lifetime support for patients with end-stage heart failure. Temporary VADs are also available and can be placed by cardiologists in the heart catheterization laboratory or by surgeons in the operating room. These devices provide short-term support while other medical problems (e.g. infection, kidney failure) can be treated, and the prognosis of the patient better defined.

## BRIDGE TO TRANSPLANT OR DESTINATION THERAPY

Ventricular assist devices are typically placed through a chest incision after the patient has been placed on a heart-lung bypass machine. There are three major components of the VAD—the inflow cannula, the outflow cannula and the pump itself. The inflow cannula is a large tube that drains blood from the heart into the pump; the outflow cannula returns blood to either the aorta (in a left ventricular assist device or LVAD) or pulmonary artery (in a right ventricular assist device). A minority of patients with failing left and right ventricles need biventricular assist devices or a total artificial heart to bridge them to transplant.

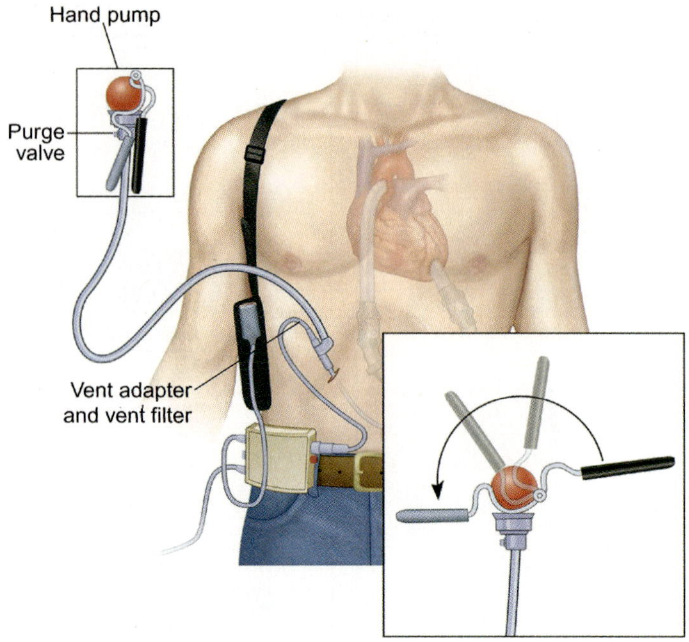


**Fig. 30.3:** HeartMate XVE hand pump. In cases of an emergency, such as a failure of the primary and backup drivers, a hand pump should be used immediately to restore flow to a pulsatile ventricular assist device (VAD). To use a hand pump properly, the system controller must be disconnected from the power source. Next, the hand pump bulb should be connected to the end of the driveline vent filter and the system primed by holding down the purge valve on the pump and collapsing the bulb. The hand pump delivers pulses of air to the pusher plate, generating a stroke volume. One hand pump is needed for each VAD. The pump should be squeezed approximately 60–90 times per minute to empty and fill the blood chambers (*Figure illustration by Rob Flewell*)

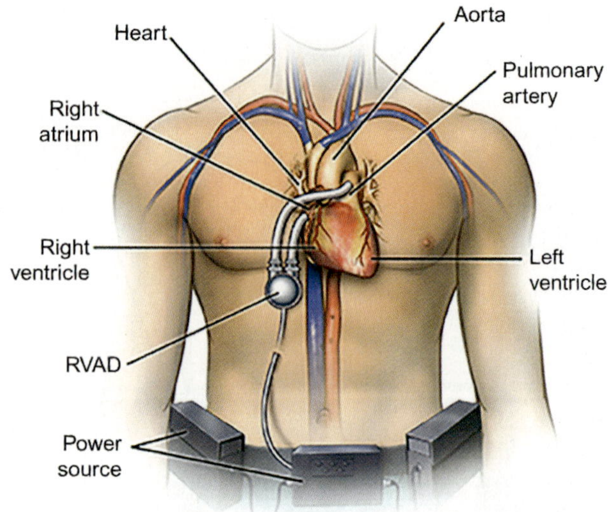


**Fig. 30.4:** Right ventricular assist device (RVAD)

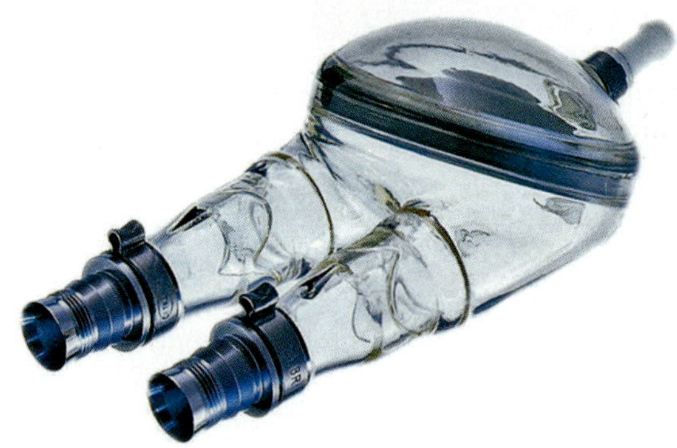

**Fig. 30.5:** EXCOR pediatric blood pump 30 ml for children up to 66 pounds device stablizes pediatric patients waiting for heart transplantation

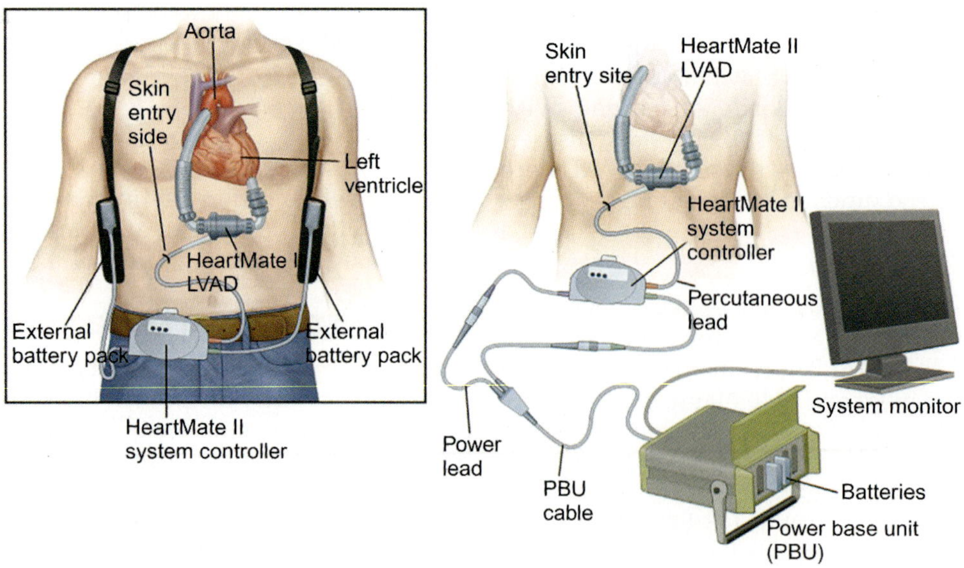


**Fig. 30.6:** Components of a continuous flow VAD. A continuous flow ventricular assist device (VAD) consists of a pump connected to the heart and aorta via an inflow cannula and an outflow cannula, respectively, an external driveline that powers the motor within the device, and a system controller. Power may be delivered through a power base unit (PBU) or battery packs, allowing increased mobility. (*Figure illustration by Rob Flewell.*) LVAD=left ventricular assist device

First-generation pumps were pulsatile, contained artificial heart valves, and ejected blood at rates typically between 80 times and 100 times per minute with the use of either forced air or electricity. Second-generation pumps circulate blood in a continuous fashion by use of an internal rotor that spins up to 15,000 times per minute (typical range, 8000–10,000 rpm). The major advantages of continuous-flow pumps are that they are smaller, quieter, easier to implant, and last longer than the older, pulsatile pumps. Currently approved VADs are implanted just below the diaphragm in the abdomen, or can sit outside of the body on top of the abdomen. Smaller pumps that can be implanted adjacent to the heart in the chest cavity or provide only partial heart support are under development. A driveline that contains the power wires exits the skin, usually on the right side of the abdomen, and connects to a controller that is worn on a belt. This controller is then connected to either a power-based unit that plugs into the wall or large batteries that can be worn in a holster or vest for portable use. The controller is the brain of the pump, and provides important information to the patient, caregivers, and medical team about VAD function and battery life. Less commonly used pumps that sit outside of the body connect directly to a portable driver on wheels that can be pulled like a small suitcase.

## CLINICAL INDICATIONS IN VADS IMPLANTATION

Ventricular assist devices are typically used for one of the three reasons—as a bridge to recovery, bridge to transplantation, or destination therapy (Table 30.1). Bridge to recovery is for patients who need only temporary support (e.g. days to weeks), during which time the heart recovers from an acute injury and the VAD is then removed. Examples include patients with a large heart attack or severe inflammation of the heart following a viral illness. In national databases, these patients make up <5% of the total VAD population. Bridge to transplant is the largest group to receive VADs. These patients are eligible for a heart transplant, but are too sick to wait for a donor heart to become available. Last, destination therapy patients are not eligible for heart transplant because of older age (e.g. >70 years) or other chronic medical problems, and receive a permanent VAD to treat end-stage heart failure. Another term that is sometimes used is bridge to candidacy for patients who might be eligible for transplant, but need a period of VAD support to see whether vital organ function, nutrition and strength can improve to allow successful heart transplant. In rare cases, patients with longstanding heart disease, VAD support may result in complete reversal of heart failure and allow the pump to be removed.

| **Table 30.1:** Components of VAD education and successful discharge home |
|---|
| Exercise and physical therapy |
| Nutrition |
| VAD self-care |
| Driveline site dressing changes |
| System controller checks |
| VAD log book |
| Activity restrictions |
| Responsibility of primary physicians, VAD coordinator and visiting nurses |
| Role of EMTs and local emergency rooms |
| Electric company and home power supply |

VAD=ventricular assist device; EMT=emergency medical technician

## PREOPERATIVE EVALUATION OF PATIENT

Candidates for implantation of a VAD undergo an extensive medical and psychosocial evaluation before a final decision about treatment. Typically, this evaluation occurs during a heart failure hospitalization, and includes cardiovascular testing, such as an echocardiogram (heart ultrasound), stress test and heart catheterization, and tests of other vital organ function, as well, including kidney, lung and liver function. A general medical evaluation, including an update of routine health maintenance screens (for example, mammogram, prostate examination and cholesterol blood test) and infectious disease screening (such as hepatitis, HIV and tuberculosis) are also performed. Appropriate vaccines are administered. In addition, patients are routinely evaluated by a VAD nutritionist, physical therapist, and pharmacist, and they undergo a dental examination.

A major focus of the evaluation is determining the potential for VAD therapy to improve quality of life while educating patients and families about the benefits and risks of VADs. Extensive teaching occurs during this process. Candidates must understand the VAD regimen before the implantation of the VAD, and they must show that they have adequate support and identify caregivers to be trained in the use of the device. These supports must be available to the VAD patient until they are able to independently care for the VAD. A VAD social worker and psychiatrist play key roles in this evaluation, and all patients must sign an informed consent form agreeing to the process. In addition, patients are asked to participate in a national database of VAD patients that is required for all Medicare-approved programs in the United States. Data are collected at the baseline evaluation, throughout the surgical admission, and on a regular basis during outpatient follow-up.

## RECOVERY FROM SURGERY, PREPARING FOR HOSPITAL DISCHARGE, AND RETURN HOME

The VAD operation takes between 6 and 10 hours. After surgery, patients spend on average 4–6 days in the cardiac surgery intensive care unit before being transferred to the step-down unit. This early period is focused on optimizing pump flow and monitoring for recovery of kidney, liver and lung function. Intravenous diuretics are often used to get rid of extra fluid that may have accumulated from heart failure or was given during the operation to support blood pressure. After the patient wakes up and is able to breathe on his/her own, ventilator support is removed. Surgical lines and drainage tubes are removed, and the patient is allowed to begin eating and taking oral medications. The keys to surgical success are early mobilization, good nutrition and physical therapy, and meticulous wound care, as well. For most patients with VADs, the blood must be carefully thinned with intravenous and then oral medications to avoid blood clot formation.

Preparing the patient and caregivers for discharge home is the primary responsibility of the VAD coordinator. The coordinator is typically a nurse practitioner or physician assistant who specializes in the care of patients with VADs. These individuals are extremely knowledgeable about all aspects of VAD care, including surgical and medical treatment and pump technology and support. They assist in obtaining the necessary equipment and supplies, and work closely with other VAD team members to ensure a successful outcome. Central to their role is proper training of the patient, family and community to allow a smooth transition home. If education and training are successful quality of life on the VAD will be maximized.

## POSTOPERATIVE PATIENT CARE AFTER VAD IMPLANTATION

The photograph depicting postoperative patient care is shown in Figure 30.7.

### Physical Exercise

Once patients have recovered from surgery, it is expected that they will work on regaining strength and increasing exercise tolerance. In the hospital, this process is coordinated by a physical therapist. Following discharge, some patients may feel comfortable initiating an exercise program at home. For others, enrollment in an outpatient cardiac rehabilitation program (often affiliated with a community hospital) provides support and helps to build confidence. The long-term goal is 30 minutes of submaximal aerobic exercise, such as walking or biking, daily.

### Dietary Management

Because of chronic illness and recurrent hospitalization, many patients with heart failure are malnourished at the time of VAD implantation. Poor nutrition can delay wound healing and increase the risk of infection; therefore, assessment by a nutritionist is critical to regaining strength and energy. During the hospitalization and sometimes after discharge, the nutritionist keeps a record of daily intake and makes recommendations for calorie and vitamin supplementation. Routine blood tests help track progress as well.

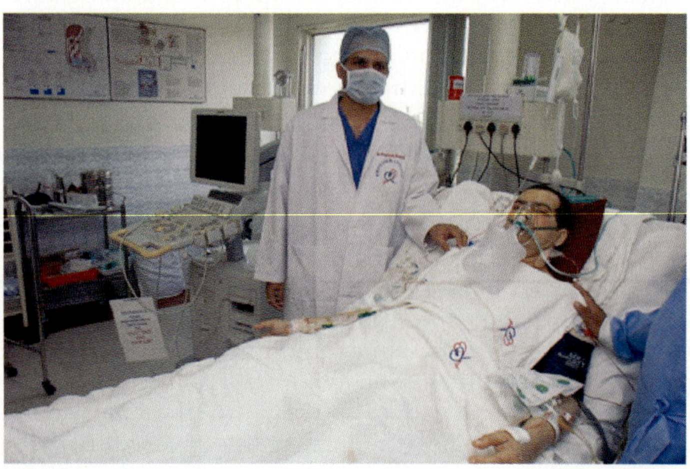

**Fig. 30.7:** Photograph of postoperative clinical assessment of VAD patient in ICU

### Ventricular Assist Device Self-care

In the hospital, nursing and medical staff are responsible for VAD care and proper function. Once at home, patients and caregivers must take over this job, which includes cleaning and checking equipment, changing the driveline dressing by the use of sterile technique, monitoring for infection, recording vital signs and VAD data, and making sure that batteries are working properly. Showers are allowed with proper equipment covering, but bathing and swimming are not possible with current VADs. Visiting nurses may assist in VAD care during the first 1 to 2 weeks after discharge, with a particular focus on dressing changes, medication adjustments, and laboratory draws.

### Restriction on Activities

Patients with ventricular assist device should avoid situations or environments that may increase the risk of infection, such as sick contacts or daycare centers, but they are not restricted from public gatherings. Good hygiene and regular handwashing are keys for anyone touching the VAD equipment or driveline dressing. Although, exercise is encouraged, strenuous activities or contact sports that could inadvertently lead to device damage or trauma to the driveline site are discouraged. Prolonged exposure to cold or heat should also be avoided. Restrictions on driving are specific to individual VAD programs and may be subject to state laws; patients are encouraged to speak with their VAD team about the safety and timing of resuming driving.

### Constant and Safe Power Source

Before discharge, the electric supply at home must be confirmed and undergo a safety check to ensure proper grounding for battery charging. In addition, the electric company is notified to place the VAD patient on a list for priority power restoration in the event of an electric outage. Planned power outages are avoided, and the company is requested not to turn off electricity in the event of a late or nonpayment. A VAD financial counselor is available to help resolve billing issues if they occur.

## RADIOGRAPHIC/MRI/CT IMAGING IN FOLLOW-UP OF VAD PATIENTS

Following uncomplicated surgery, patients will typically be discharged home to follow-up in the VAD clinic in 1–2 weeks, and monthly thereafter. The first several visits will involve a history and physical examination by the VAD physician, and review of medications and device function (e.g. alarms, battery life) by the VAD coordinator. The

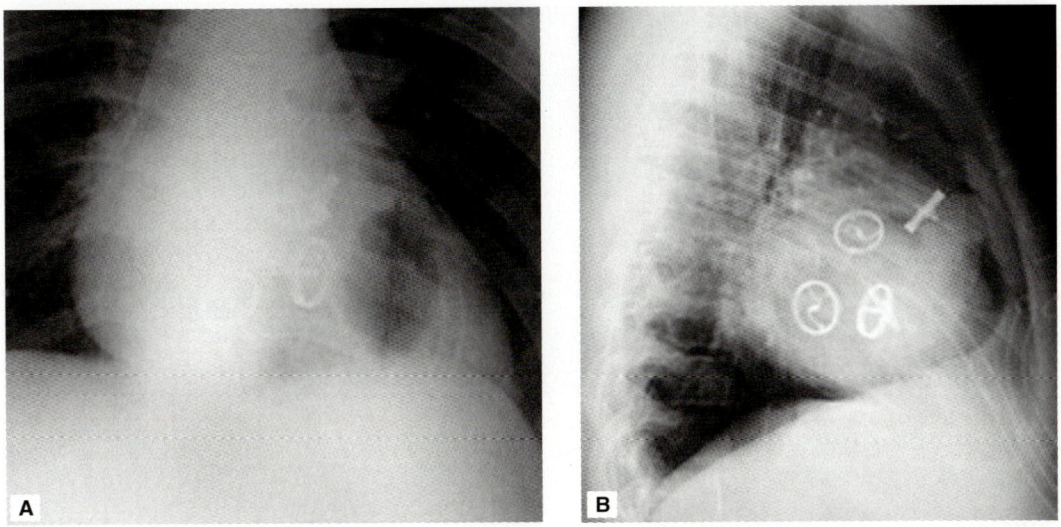


**Fig. 30.8:** Cropped frontal view (A) and full lateral view (B) of the chest show a CardioWest total artificial heart. Note the four prosthetic valves and the two coil, reinforced polyurethane tubes carrying pulses of compressed air to the two artificial ventricles

driveline dressing may be changed allowing for examination of the driveline site, especially if there is concern for infection (below). In some cases, the VAD surgeon may need to reevaluate the patient if there are unresolved surgical issues, such as instability of the chest wound, or remaining tubes to be pulled. Diet and exercise are reviewed with particular attention to heart-healthy foods and gradual increase in aerobic activities such as walking or biking. Emergency contact numbers and reasons to seek emergency care are reviewed.

Patients are asked to check their blood pressure (if possible), weight, and temperature daily, and to record values in a VAD log book. Specific device readings, such as pump speed and flow, are also recorded by hand. Diabetic patients are asked to keep a record of their blood sugars, because unusual fluctuations or high readings can be an early sign of infection. Outpatient consultation with a nutritionist or social worker is arranged as needed. Patients are encouraged to follow up with their primary care physicians and cardiologists within 1 month of discharge. In the event of an emergency department visit, patients and caregivers are taught to bring with them their VAD equipment, up-to-date medication list, VAD doctors' names and numbers, emergency contact and healthcare proxy information, and living will, if available (Figs 30.8–30.12).

## MEDICAL CARE ON A VAD

Medical care of VAD patients requires close attention to several issues, including treatment of high blood pressure, anticoagulation and heart rhythm disturbances. The majority of patients develop high blood pressure after VAD implantation, and this can have an impact on the durability of pump function and increase the risk of stroke. The first-generation pulsatile VADs were more likely to fail from bearing or internal valve wear if the blood pressure was not well controlled. With the second-generation continuous-flow pumps, blood pressure has a more direct impact on pump speed and flow. However, because of the nature of continuous blood flow, patients typically lack a pulse and the usual sounds heard with a stethoscope or picked up by an automatic blood pressure machine. Instead, average blood pressure must be measured by the use of a small ultrasound machine (or Doppler probe). When present, high blood pressure should be treated aggressively and may require more than 2 or 3 medications, such as angiotensin-converting enzyme (ACE) inhibitors, β-blockers and diuretics, to control. Reducing salt in the diet can also help.

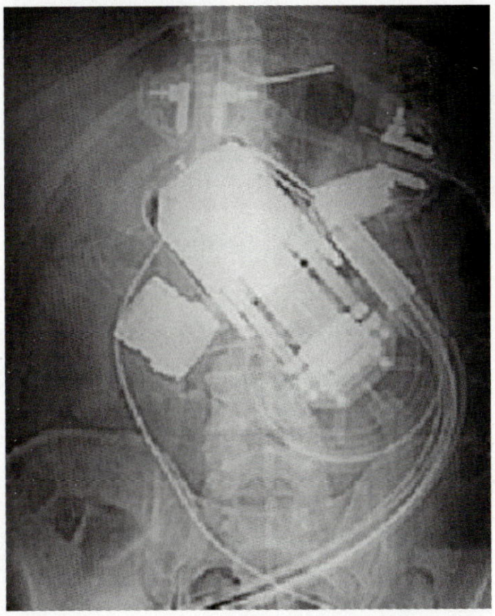

**Fig. 30.9:** Abdominal image shows a Novacor VAD

The current generation of mechanical pumps requires thinning of the blood (or anticoagulation) to prevent the formation of blood clots. These clots can cause dysfunction of the pump itself, or more typically, can embolize into the circulation and cause a transient ischemic attack, stroke or lack of blood flow to a limb or vital organ. The typical blood-

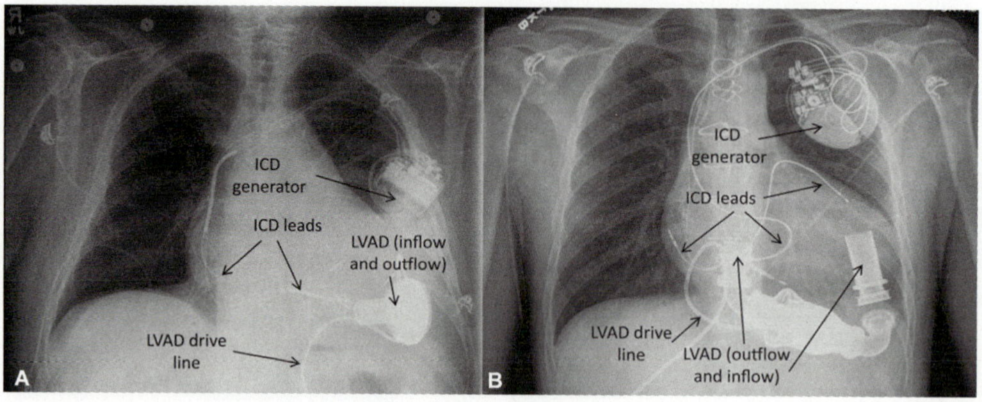


**Fig. 30.10:** Examples of implantable cardioverter-defibrillators (ICDs) with two different types of left ventricular assist devices (LVADs). Posterior-anterior chest X-ray projections of biventricular ICDs in the presence of HVAD (A) and HeartMate II, (B) models of LVAD

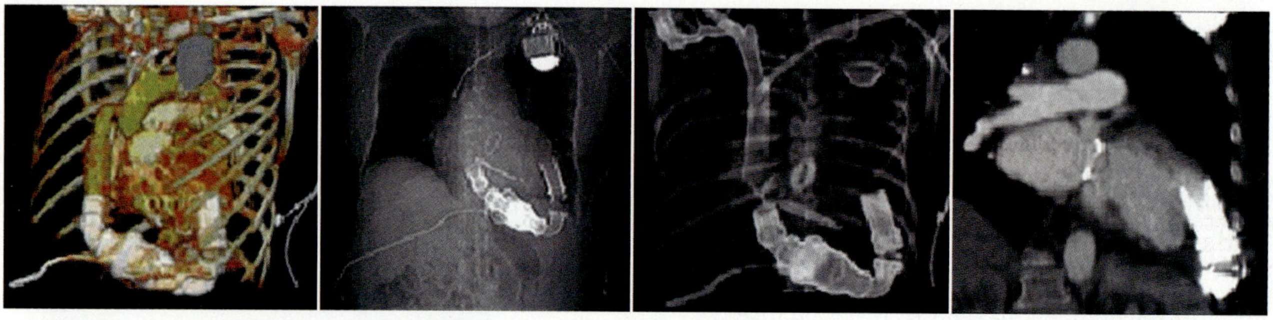

**Fig. 30.11:** From left to right showing total artificial heart with different noninvasive techniques including chest X-ray and MDCT

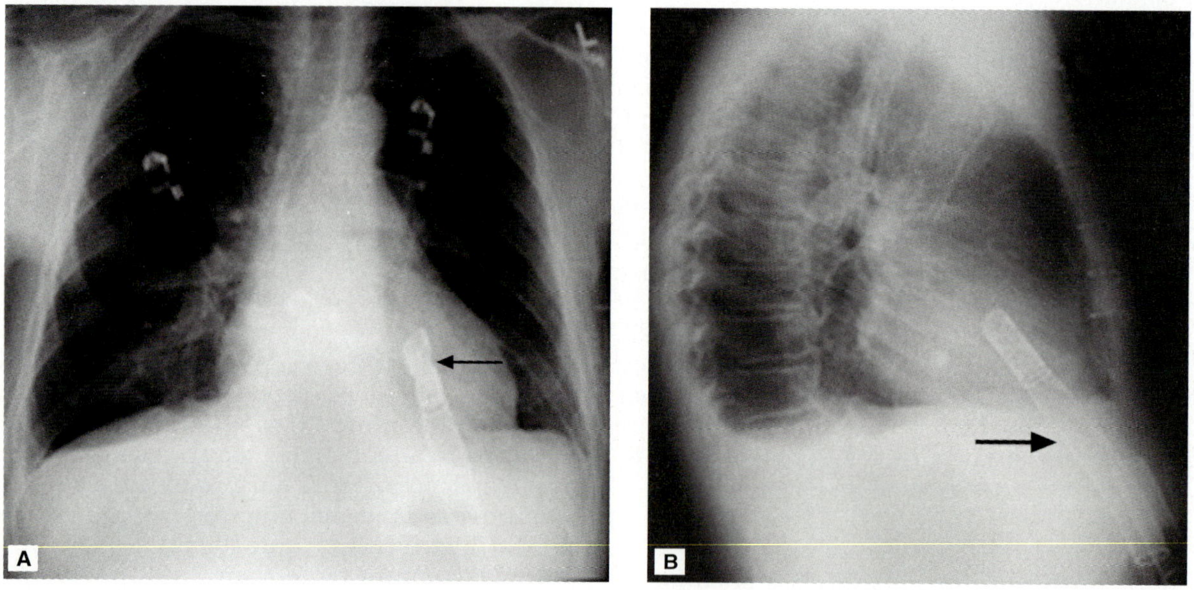


**Fig. 30.12:** Frontal (A) and lateral (B) views of the chest show a Thoratec left VAD (arrow)

thinning regimen for continuous-flow pumps includes the use of warfarin (which blocks the formation of clotting proteins by the liver) and a baby aspirin (which inactivates platelets). The level of anticoagulation is monitored regularly by checking a blood test called the international normalized ratio and adjusting the dose of warfarin. This is usually performed by a nurse specialist or pharmacist in a hospital- or office-based anticoagulation service. In the event of bleeding or clotting (below), the target international normalized ratio may need to be decreased or increased. Use of higher-dose aspirin or an additional antiplatelet agent, such as clopidogrel, is based on the patient's medical history (e.g. prior transient ischemic attack or coronary artery stent).

Patients with advanced heart failure often have a history of arrhythmias (heart rhythm disturbances) arising from the upper and/or lower chambers, and may have undergone placement of a pacemaker or cardioverter-defibrillator before VAD surgery. Some may also be receiving antiarrhythmic therapy. Therefore, it is critical for these patients to maintain follow-up with their device/heart rhythm specialists. Although, the majority of pacemakers/cardioverter-defibrillators are compatible with VADs, the internal settings may need to be adjusted after surgery to prevent unnecessary pacing or shocks. In some cases, a change in or addition of antiarrhythmic therapy may be necessary. Importantly, one sign of too much speed with a continuous-flow pump is the new occurrence of ventricular arrhythmias due to heart suction. In this situation, an echocardiogram can be used to optimize heart filling while adjusting pump speed.

## COMPLICATIONS OF VADS

Ventricular assist devices offer life-saving therapy and improve quality of life of patients with end-stage heart failure, but they are not free of complications. In the most recent studies, 80–90% of patients are alive at 1 year, and 60–70% are living at 2 years. Others have undergone successful heart transplant, been weaned off the VAD (bridge to recovery), or died while living on a VAD. Early problems after surgery include bleeding from the chest and right heart failure. Later problems include other sources of bleeding, infection, stroke or device malfunction.

### Bleeding

Most cardiac surgery, including VAD implantation, requires high levels of anticoagulation while the patient is on the heart-lung machine. This fact, along with the need for both chest and abdominal incisions and the poor nutritional status of many patients, increases the risk of early bleeding. Most patients can be managed with reversal of anticoagulation and transfusion of blood products, but some may need to return urgently to the operating room for bleeding control. After hospital discharge, patients are at increased risk of bleeding from the gastrointestinal tract and nose bleeds. There are several contributing factors, including anticoagulation and antiplatelet therapy (discussed above), nonpulsatile blood flow leading to blood vessel malformation in the gut, and pump-related changes in blood-clotting factors. Many patients take iron supplementation, whereas a minority requires weekly injections to stimulate red blood cell production from the bone marrow. For recurrent or life-threatening bleeding, anticoagulation may be discontinued completely.

### Right Heart Failure

Although, most patients with advanced heart failure have severe weakness of the left ventricle and undergo LVAD placement alone, a subgroup will also have weakness of the right ventricle that puts them at risk for developing right heart failure after LVAD surgery. Signs of right heart failure include swelling of the legs and abdomen, distention of neck veins and collection of fluid under the lungs. Inadequate filling of the LVAD and reduced blood flow can lead to weakness, poor appetite and organ dysfunction (e.g. kidney failure). Most cases of right heart failure can be managed with short-term support with intravenously administered medications and diuretics. More severe cases will require placement of a right ventricular assist device to bridge to transplant. Risk scores have been developed to help doctors predict which patients are likely to develop right heart failure and would benefit from initial placement of biventricular assist devices or a total artificial heart.

### Stroke

Patients with ventricular assist device are at risk of stroke, which can be caused by blood clots leaving the pump, high blood pressure or bleeding into the brain. The rates of stroke appear to have declined somewhat with the newer continuous-flow pumps, but the need for anticoagulation and ongoing risk of infection (which seems to increase the body's tendency to form clots) have not eliminated this complication. In older patients receiving VADs as destination therapy, underlying cerebrovascular disease may also increase the risk of stroke. Close monitoring of anticoagulation, optimal blood pressure control and meticulous wound care are important strategies for minimizing stroke risk. Lowering blood cholesterol with a healthy diet and cholesterol-lowering medications such as statins can also lower this risk.

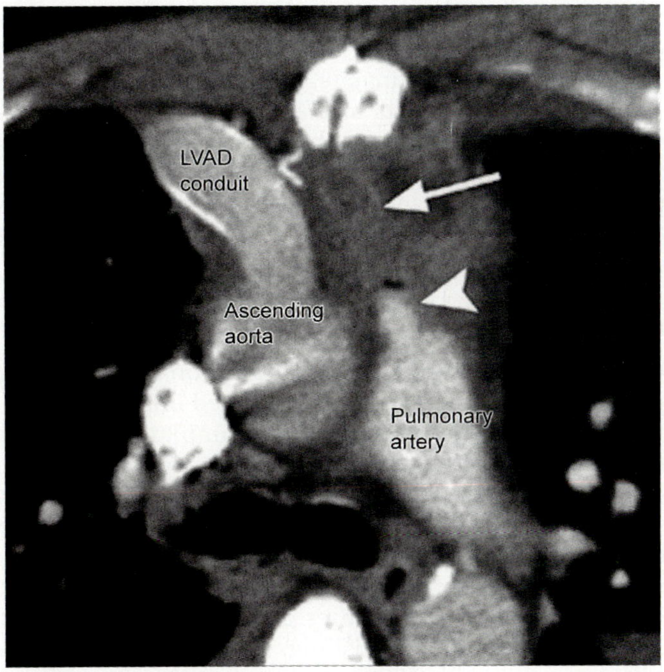


**Fig. 30.13:** A 57-year-old male with thrombosed right ventricular assist device (RVAD). Axial contrast-enhanced CT image shows thrombosis of the pulmonary artery RVAD conduit (arrow). However, the proximal portion is patent (arrowhead)

### Infection

Device infection (Fig. 30.13) can occur at any time during VAD support, but most frequently develops in the first few weeks or months after implant. Common bacteria that live on the skin, such as staphylococcus can gain access to the driveline and pump from the skin exit site. Alternatively, bacteria from the gut or urinary system can enter the bloodstream and secondarily infect the VAD. Patients who are immunosuppressed or have diabetes mellitus may be at increased risk for infections from uncommon organisms such as yeast. Depending on their severity and duration, driveline infections are treated with oral or intravenous antibiotics and daily wound care. Although, most driveline or cannula infections cannot be cured, they can usually be suppressed until the time of transplant and hardware removal. For a small number of patients, overwhelming infection and death may occur. As with most infections, the key is prevention. This includes meticulous care of the driveline exit site with the use of a mask and sterile gloves during dressing changes, stabilization of the driveline and avoiding activities that could lead to local trauma, and education of patients and caregivers about the early signs of infection, and the importance of prompt notification of the VAD team.

### Device Failure

With the first-generation pulsatile-flow pumps, device malfunction was a major cause of hospitalization and even death in VAD patients. These devices were designed for relatively short- or medium-term support to bridge patients to transplant. With the approval of pumps for destination therapy and increased waiting time for patients bridging to transplant, prolonged support (i.e. >1–2 years) was required. However, up to two-thirds or more of pumps failed during this period. Fortunately, the newer continuous-flow pumps with fewer parts and a simpler operation have demonstrated improved durability. Malfunction of wires, controllers and batteries still occurs, but these problems are relatively minor, indicated by alarms, and generally easy to repair. In rare instances, the entire VAD must be surgically replaced.

## QUALITY OF LIFE ON A VAD

Despite the possibility of complications with device therapy, most patients describe a marked improvement in their quality of life following VAD implantation. With normal blood flow to the body, symptoms of advanced heart failure resolve completely or are reduced to only a mild level. Patients are once again able to perform enjoyable activities such as exercise, travel and sex. For younger patients, return to work or school is possible, and older patients enjoy hobbies and outdoor activities, such as golf, hiking and fishing. In patient surveys, the ability to drive is mentioned as one of the biggest advantages to VAD treatment. Compared with medications or pacemakers, VADs improve quality of life to a far greater degree.

## FOCUS OF CURRENT RESEARCH

Until very recently, the heart was thought to be an organ that could not repair itself after suffering an injury, such as a heart attack or developing end-stage cardiomyopathy (primary heart muscle disease). Recent research, however, suggests that the heart can indeed repair itself with rest and new therapies. A group at the University of London showed that patients with long-standing cardiomyopathy, supported on an LVAD and treated with high-dose ACE inhibitors, β-blockers, and a medicine to stimulate new muscle growth, could recover heart function, allowing the LVAD to be safely removed. Others are working to harness the power of stem cell therapy to reverse heart failure on a VAD. While physicians and VAD coordinators wait for these and other major breakthroughs to occur, device companies continue to make progress in reducing pump size and improving battery life with the goal of designing a fully implantable pump.

## BIBLIOGRAPHY


1. A Study of Anginera In Patients Undergoing Coronary Artery Bypass Graft (CABG) Surgery". Clinicaltrials.gov (U.S. National Institutes of Health), 2009.
2. Assessment and management of heart failure after left ventricular assist device implantation circulation 2014; 129: 1161–6.
3. Benton, Susan. "HeartMate II Pivotal Clinical Trial Fact Sheet". Thoratec Corporation 2008.
4. Birks E, Tansley PD, Hardey J, George RS, Bowles CT, Burke M, Khaghani A, Banner NR, Yacoub MH. "Left Ventricular Assist Device and Drug Therapy for the Reversal of Heart Failure". New Eng J Med 2006;355(18):1873–84.
5. Dewey Todd. "The HeartMate II LVAS Pivotal Trial". Dallas: Cardiopulmonary Research Science and Technology Institute. Archived from the original on 2007.
6. Eisen Howard, Shelley Hankins. "Continuous Flow Rotary Left Ventricular Assist Device: Mechanical Circulatory Support 2.0". Journal of the American College of Cardiology (Elsevier) 2009;54(4):322–4.
7. Evaluation of the HeartWare LVAD System for the Treatment of Advanced Heart Failure". Baltimore: Johns Hopkins Medical 2009.
8. Fukamachi Kiyo; Smedira Nicholas. "Smaller, Safer, Totally Implantable LVADs: Fact or Fantasy?". American College of Cardiology Current Journal Review 2005;14(8):40–2.
9. Gavin Kara. "Exciting times for heart-assisting devices at U-M". Ann Arbor: University of Michigan 2008.
10. Heidelberg Cardiac Surgeons implant world's first new DeBakey Heart Assist Device". Insciences 2009.
11. Thoratec HeartMate II LVAS - P060040". Food and Drug Administration. Ann Arbor 2008.
12. HeartWare International Surpasses 50 Implants in the US. Biomedicine 2009.
13. Mager, Belinda . "FDA Approves HeartMate II Mechanical Heart Pump for Heart-Failure Patients Waiting for Organ Transplantation". New York: New York Presbytarian University Hospital 2008.

14. Maugh Thomas. "Transplant shows heart's reparative capabilities". Los Angeles Times, 2009.
15. Mechanical circulatory support for advanced heart failure: patients and technology in evolution. Circulation 2012; 125:1304–1315.
16. Miller Leslie, Pagani, Russell, John et al. "Use of a continu-ous flow device in patients awaiting heart transplan-tation". New England Journal of Medicine (Boston) 2007;357:885–96.
17. Osaki, Saturo; Edwards, Velez, Johnson, et al. "Improved surival in patients with ventricular assist device therapy: the University of Wisconsin experience". European Journal of Cardio-Thoracic Surgery (Elsevier) 2008;34(2):281–8.
18. Pagani Francis, Miller, Russell, Aaronson, et al. "Extended Mechanical Circulatory Support With a Continuous-Flow Rotary Left Ventricular Assist Device". Journal of American College of Cardiology 2007;54 (4).
19. Quinn, Dale. "VA study: heart-healing patch". Arizona Daily star 2009.
20. Shulman Allison, Martens, Christos, et al. "Comparisons of infection complications between continuous flow and pulsatile flow left ventricular assist devices". Journal of Thoracic Cardiovascular Surgery 2007;133:841–2.
21. Starling Randall, Naka, Boyle, Gonzalez-Stawinski, et al. "Initial FDA Post-Approval Study INTERMACS Registry Results with a Continuous Flow Left Ventricular Assist
22. Wilson SR, Givertz MM, Stewart GC, Mudge GH Jr, Ventri-cular assist devices: the challenges of outpatient manage-ment. J Am Coll Cardiol 2009;54:1647–59.

# 31 Noninvasive Cardiac Imaging

## CHEST RADIOGRAPHY

In medicine, a chest radiograph, colloquially called a chest X-ray (CXR), or chest film, is a projection radiograph of the chest used to diagnose conditions affecting the chest, its contents, and nearby structures (Fig. 31.1 A and B). Chest radiographs are among the most common films taken, being diagnostic of many conditions. Like all methods of radiography, chest radiography employs ionizing radiation in the form of X-rays to generate images of the chest. The mean radiation dose to an adult from a chest radiograph is around 0.02 mSv (2 mrem) for a front view (PA or posterior-anterior) and 0.08 mSv (8 mrem) for a side view (LL or latero-lateral).

The main regions where a chest X-ray may identify problems may be summarized as **ABCDEF** by their first letters:

- **A**irways, including hilar adenopathy or enlargement
- **B**reast shadows
- **B**ones, e.g. rib fractures and lytic bone lesions
- **C**ardiac silhoutte, detecting cardiac enlargement
- **C**ostophrenic angles, including pleural effusions
- **D**iaphragm, e.g. evidence of free air, indicative of perforation of an abdominal viscus
- **E**dges, e.g. apices for fibrosis, pneumothorax, pleural thickening or plaques
- **E**xtrathoracic tissues
- **F**ields (lung parenchyma), being evidence of alveolar flooding

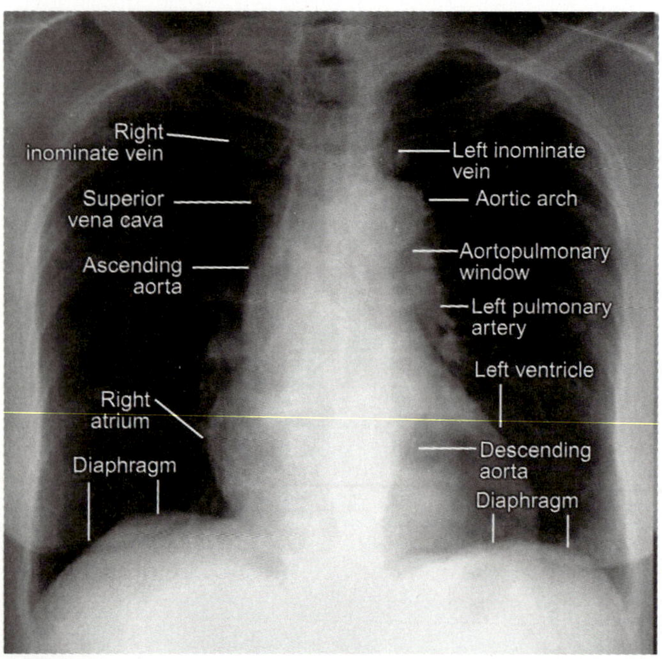


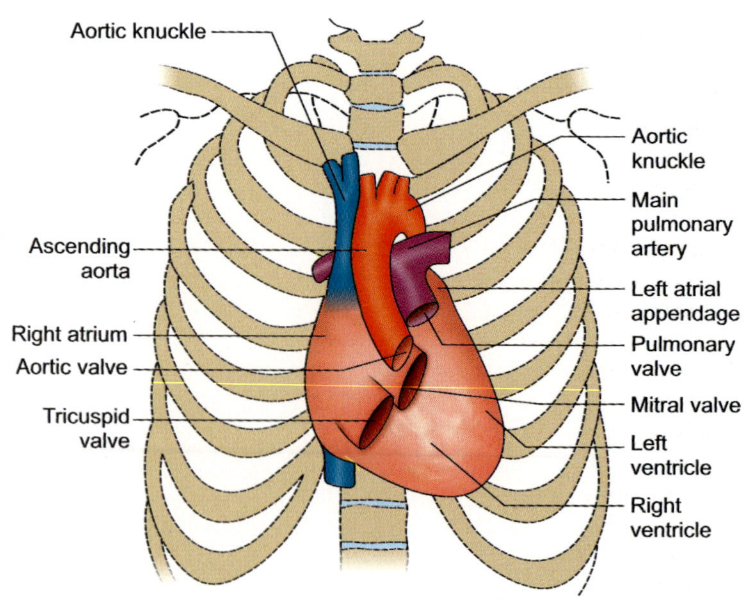


**Fig. 31.1 A:** (Left and right) Photograph of X-ray chest (PA view) and illustration showing various anatomical structures of heart and its great vessels (shown written with arrows on skiagram)

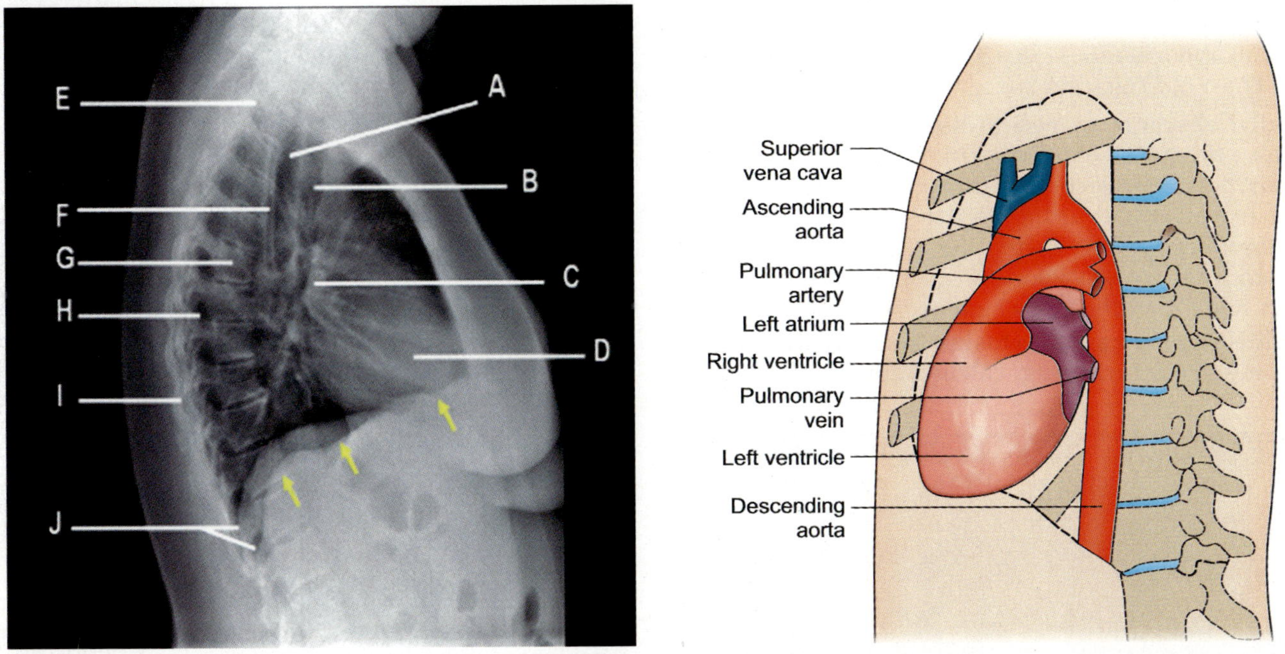


**Fig. 31.1B**: (Left and right) Photograph of X-ray chest (PA view) and illustration showing various anatomical structures of heart and its great vessels (shown written with arrows on skiagram). Structures that should be demonstrated on the left lateral chest radiograph include (A) esophagus, (B) trachea, (C) lung hill, (D) heart silhouette, (E) lung apices, (F) scapulae, (G) thoracic vertebra, (H) thoracic intervertebral foramen, (I) superimposed posterior ribs, (J) costophrenic angles and diaphragm (yellow arrows)

- Failure, e.g. alveolar air space disease with prominent vascularity with or without pleural effusions.

Good quality posteroanterior (PA) and lateral chest X-rays make an important contribution to the cardiac assessment.

## ASSESSMENT OF LOCATION OF CARDIAC SILHOUETTE AND STRUCTURAL ALTERATIONS IN CARDIOVASCULAR SYSTEM

### Cardiac Silhouette

Because the radiodensity of cardiac tissue is similar to that of blood intracardiac structures can rarely be identified unless they are calcified. However, the cardiac silhouette contrasts strongly with the adjacent radiolucent lung fields, permitting accurate appreciation of the heart size. The heart is long and thin in ectomorphic individuals, but is more bulky in endomorphic individuals. Nevertheless. the maximum transverse measurement should not exceed 50% that of the chest. Cardiac enlargement is caused either by pericardial effusion or by dilatation of the cardiac chambers and great vessels. Myocardial hypertrophy without chamber dilatation rarely causes radiographic cardiac enlargement.The ideal radiograph for assessing the heart and great vessels is the straight, erect, PA chest radiograph taken at full inspiration. PA radiographs image true heart size, as opposed to anteroposterior radiographs in which there is variable and indeterminate magnification. As a result of gravity, erect radiographs display small pulmonary vessels in the upper zone and larger ones in the lower; this sign of normality can not be assessed on a supine chest radiograph in which upper and lower zone vessels are equal in size. The high diaphragm and the commonly used short tube-to-film distance supine radiographs also lead to magnification of heart size. In addition, heart size affected by patient rotation. Because the long axis of the heart lies at about 45° to the sagittal plane patient rotation with the right shoulder forward (RAO) enlarges the cardiac image, whereas the reverse rotation (LAO) reduces it. Rotations such as these along the major axis of the body also affect the prominence of various great vessels (aorta and pulmonary arteries), making their evaluation unreliable.

### Heart size

Assessment of heart size is important because apparently enlarged hearts are usually abnormal, though there are exceptions. A small heart is generally not a useful finding.

*Transverse cardiac diameter:* It is the horizontal distance between the most rightward and leftward borders. A diameter of 15 cm is regarded as the upper limit of normal. If serial chest radiographs are available, a change in heart size can be assessed; a 1.5 cm difference in diameter is regarded as significant.

*Cardiothoracic ratio:* A cardiac diameter of 15 cm in a small individual is likely to be abnormal, and, to compensate for body size, the diameter is often expressed as a ratio (transverse cardiac diameter/transverse chest diameter). Conventionally, the transverse chest diameter is measured from the inside rib margin at the widest level of the chest. A CTR of 50% or less is generally considered normal and one of more than 55% is abnormal. The 50–55% range is a 'grey zone' that may or may not be abnormal.

### Pericardium

Two impotant abnormalities (Figs 31.2 and 31.3) which can be seen on chest radiography are:

1. **Congenital abscence of pericardium:** It include levo-position of the heart, confirmed by the absence of the right heart border projecting on the right of the vertebral column, as well as left cardiac border straightening and elongation ('Snoopy sign'), and the deep or very well-defined aortopulmonary window caused by the absence of pleura allowing lung to invaginate into this space.
2. **Pericarditis and pericardial effusion:** Pericardial disease may manifest as thickening, calcification or effusion.

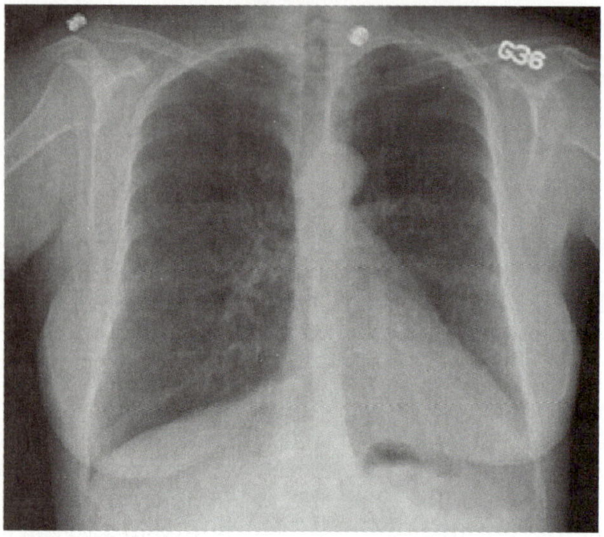

**Fig. 31.2:** Posteroanterior chest roentgenogram showing the leftward displacement of the heart and rectification of the left heart border, suggestive of left pericardial absence

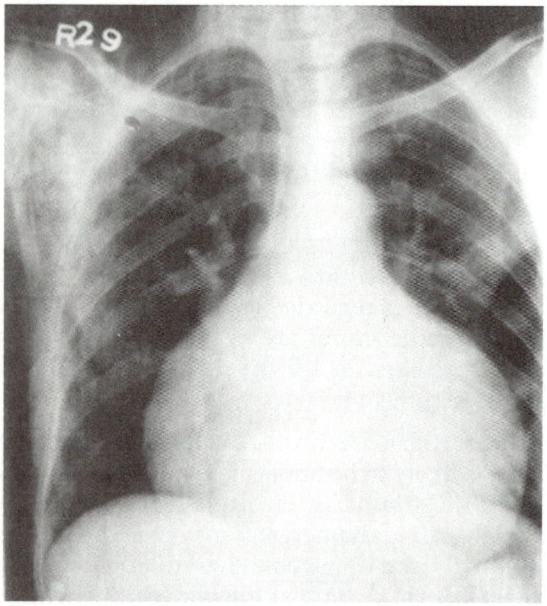

**Fig. 31.3:** X-ray chest (PA) view showing global cardiac enlargement with money bag configuration and olegaemic lung fields in patient with moderate pericardial effusion

Effusion is a cause of cardiomegaly. Cardiac enlargement caused by pericardial effusion is often nonspecific, but should be suggested by the following finding:
1. Featureless cardiac envelope
2. Rapid increase in heart size (over days)
3. Large heart with normal pulmonary vessels and lungs, particularly if cardiomegaly is a surprising finding in the clinical context.
4. Large heart with a small, isolated left pleural effusion
5. Occasionally, the pericardium is manifested as a line of soft tissue lying between darker mediastinal and epicardial fat, best seen on a lateral chest radiograph over the anterior aspect of the heart, low down behind the sternum; widening of this line beyond its normal 2 mm width is a specific sign of pericardial fluid or thickening. Rapid accumulation of sufficient pericardial fluid to cause tamponade may not enlarge the cardiac silhouette, because the fibrous pericardium takes time to stretch.

*Chamber size:* Assessment of chamber size and great vessel enlargement requires knowledge of the structures that form the border of the mediastinal silhouette. The chest radiograph is particularly accurate for assessing the left atrium (LA), is less so for the left ventricle (LV) and is poor for the right ventricle (RV) and right atrium (RA). It is fortunate that the chest radiograph allows accurate assessment of the LA because this chamber is commonly affected in adult heart disease and yet is inaccessible to clinical examination.

*Left atrium:* The signs of LA enlargement include:
1. Increased density in the region of the LA extending to the right of the spine, making the right heart denser than the left (Figs 31.4 and 31.5)
2. A visible right-hand margin to the LA, seen as a curvilinear border, convex inferolaterally through the right heart the 'distance from the midpoint of this curve to the nearest point of the left main stem bronchus is more than 7.0 cm.'
3. Elevation of the distal left main stem bronchus to a horizontal position on the PA chest radiograph, sometimes with widening of the carinal angle beyond the normal 80° on a lateral chest radiograph, the left main stem bronchus is elevated and angled backwards, out of alignment with the trachea.
4. A local convexity, where the LA appendage forms the mediastinal border just below the left main stem bronchus, appendage prominence with LA enlargement is unusual other than in chronic rheumatic heart disease.

#### *Causes of left atrial enlargement*
1. Mitral/Aortic valve disease
2. Reduced left ventricular compliance
3. Restrictive or hypertrophic cardiomyopathy
4. Systemic hypertension
5. Congestive cardiomyopathy
6. Ischaemic heart disease
7. Shunts (excluding atrial septal defect)
8. Left atrial myxoma

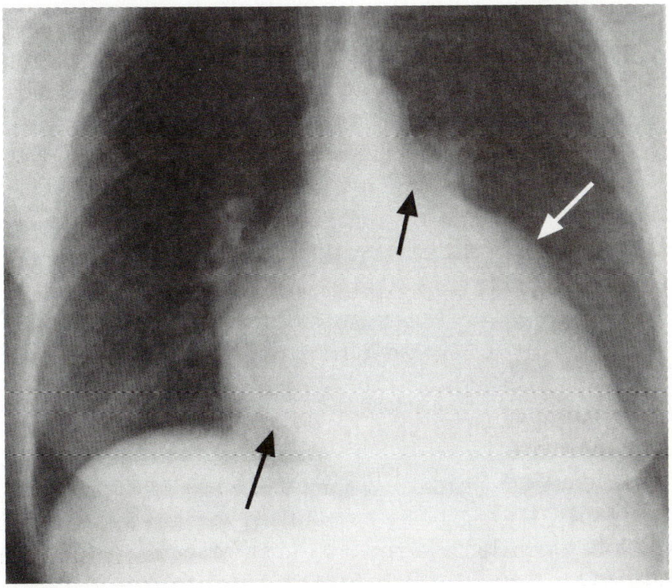

**Fig. 31.4:** Left atrial enlargement. There is an area of increased density overlying the right atrium with a curvilinear lower border (large black arrow). The distal left main stem bronchus is elevated (small black arrow) and the left atrial appendage bulges (white arrow)

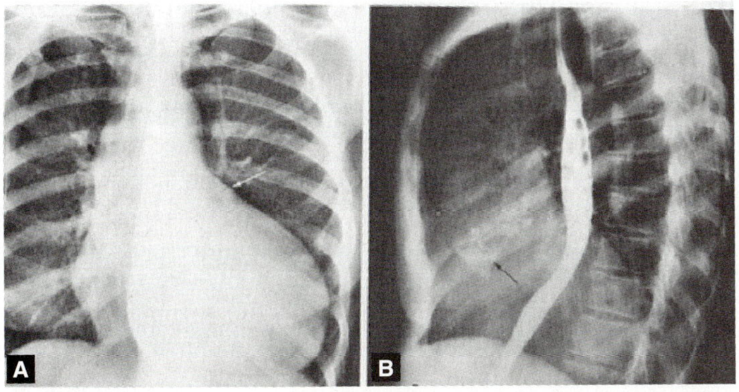


**Fig. 31.5:** Dilatation of the left ventricle in aortic valve disease. (A) Frontal view the cardiac silhouette is elongated downward and to the left, indicating left ventricular enlargement. There is slight prominence of the left atrial appendage (arrow). The esophagus is displaced medially. (B) Lateral view—the left ventricle is markedly enlarged and extends posterior to the esophagus. The aortic valve is densely calcified (arrow). The indentation on the anterior wall of the midesophagus is caused by the moderately dilated left atrium in patient with chronic aortic valvular stenosis

*Right atrium:* Assessment of RA size is too unreliable to be of use. But a buldge along the lower right cardiac border oblitrating cardiophrenic angle may be considered as a sign of right atrial enlargement.

*Left ventricle:* With LV enlargement, the LV contour elongates and the cardiac apex is displaced downwards and outwards. On the lateral radiograph, the inferoposterior aspect of the heart becomes lower and more posterior. LV left atrial enlargement may have an additional element of hypertrophy. In pure hypertrophy, however, the LV is commonly not enlarged and a contour change (a more rounded LV border) may or may not be present. Causes of LV enlargement are, with some exceptions, those of LA enlargement.

*Right ventricle:* Right ventricle enlargement in adult heart disease is often overshadowed and obscured by the enlargement of other chambers. It is seen most convincingly and commonly in congenital heart disease [Fallot's tetralogy and its variants, atrial septal defect (ASD)]. Principal findings are: a raised cardiac apex with a long, prominent upper contour and a shorter lower contour that turns medially; increased bulk of the anterior heart on lateral view, with the heart contacting the lower half, or more, of the sternum.

## Pulmonary Vessels

### Pulmonary Veins

The principal disorder affecting pulmonary veins is pulmonary venous hypertension (PVH). PVH is a common manifestation of adult heart disease (which is overwhelmingly left-sided). As pulmonary venous pressure rises, radiographic signs tend to occur in a sequence. Exceptions are not uncommon. It is related to the duration and rate of onset of PVH and the use of diuretic therapy. Indeed, modern therapy is so effective that there may be no evidence of PVH in LV disease sufficient to cause cardiac dyspnea.

*Redistribution of pulmonary vessel size:* It occurs at LA pressures of 16–22 cm $H_2O$. On an erect chest radiograph, upper zone vessels (arteries and veins) are normally smaller than lower zone vessels of the same generation; the discrepancy in diameter is about 1–3 mm. As pulmonary venous pressure rises, upper zone vessels (arteries and veins) increase in size and ultimately become wider than lower zone vessels. Distension of the upper venous trunk as it crosses the basal artery at the right hilum straightens the normal shallow V-shape of the lateral hilar contour.

*Interstitial edema:* It occurs at LA pressures of 22–30 cm $H_2O$. The lung interstitium is an interconnecting connective tissue framework that has central (perivascular, and peribronchial) and peripheral (interlobular and subpleural) components. As tissue fluids accumulate, these normally covert elements become visible (Figs 31.6 and 31.7).

*Causes of pulmonary venous hypertension:*

1. Aortic valve disease
2. Left ventricular disease
3. Myocardial ischemia
4. Cardiomyopathy
5. Reduced left ventricular compliance (e.g. hypertrophic cardiomyopathy)
6. Mitral valve disease
7. Left atrial myxoma
8. Pulmonary venous obstruction (veno-occlusive disease).

*Perihilar vessels:* These particularly in the perihilar and lower zones, become hazy and ill-defined and airway/ walls thicken.

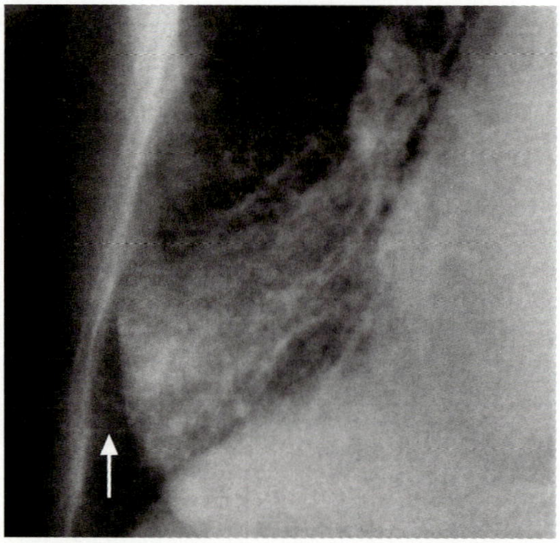

**Fig. 31.6:** Septal (Kerley) B lines—linear, non-branching horizontal lines about 2 mm wide and 1–2 cm long (arrow). When caused by raised pulmonary venous pressure, they are predominantly in the lower zone

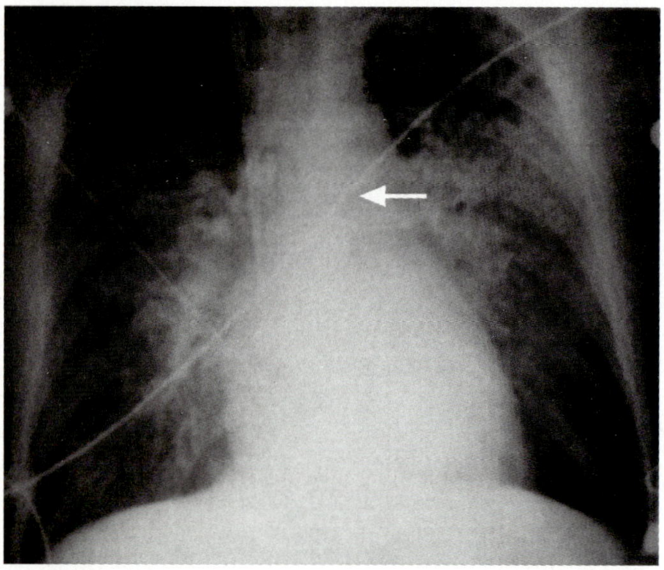

**Fig. 31.7:** Cardiogenic alveolar edema. Symmetrical airspace opacity with perihilar predominance is one characteristic pattern produced by cardiogenic edema

*Septal (Kerley) lines* appear. B lines are most commonly seen and are caused by edema of interlobular septa. They are straight, short (1–2 cm) horizontal lines that touch the parietal pleura and occur most commonly in the region of the costophrenic angles. Their width is usually 1–2 mm, but can be up to 5 mm. Septal B lines can be distinguished from small vessels because they do not branch, they touch the pleura and they are surprisingly dense for their width.

*Laminar effusions:* These are caused by fluid in pleural space, giving a vertical band of soft tissue density several millimetres wide against the lateral chest wall in, and just above, the costophrenic angle. Laminar effusions are often accompanied by septal lines, and their size provides a useful guideline for following the progress of heart failure.

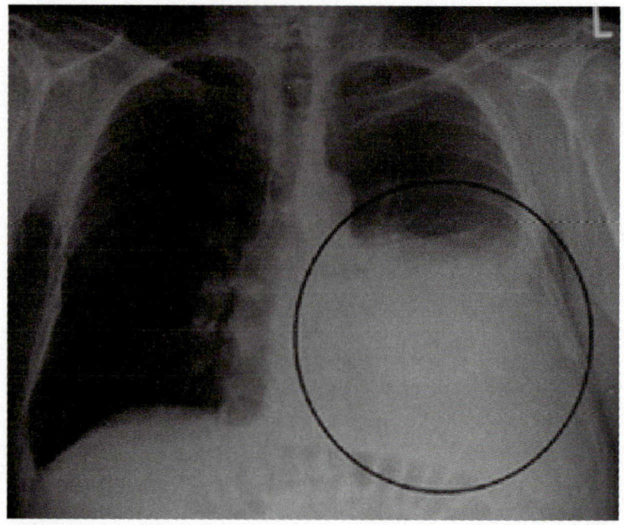

**Fig. 31.8:** A large left sided pleural effusion as seen on an upright chest X-ray

*Alveolar edema:* It occurs when the LA pressure exceeds 30 mmHg. Alveoli that have become filled with transudate become opaque (consolidation). The appearance is characterized by a pulmonary opacity of nondescript shape, with hazy margins. Characteristically, alveolar edema is bilateral with perihilar or lower zone predominance, but occasionally, it is unilateral or focal. Unlike infective consolidation, the appearance can change rapidly, particularly under the influence of diuretics.

**Pleural effusion** is a feature of PVH; it is commonly bilateral or right-sided and may vary in size from small to large. Pleural fluid is sometimes loculated and, when localized in the minor fissure, gives rise to a mass-like opacity that changes size with fluctuations in the degree of heart failure ('phantom tumour') (Fig. 31.8).

## Pulmonary Arteries and Veins

### *Main Pulmonary Artery*

The main pulmonary artery (MPA) forms a border between the aortic knuckle and the left main stem bronchus (Fig. 31.9). This segment is normally slightly concave, straight or slightly convex. Prominence of the MPA usually implies enlargement. Important causes of MPA prominence—pulmonary arterial hypertension is characterized by enlargement of both the MPA and the right and left hilar pulmonary arteries. The upper limit of normal diameter for the right pulmonary artery is 16 mm in men and 15 mm in women (measured 1 cm beyond the hilar point, the point at which the outer borders of the superior pulmonary vein and the basal pulmonary artery cross). Distal segmental and smaller vessels may be normal or reduced in size.

*Causes of a prominent main pulmonary artery*

1. Pulmonary arterial hypertension
2. Increased flow; L-R shunts
3. Mycotic aneurysm

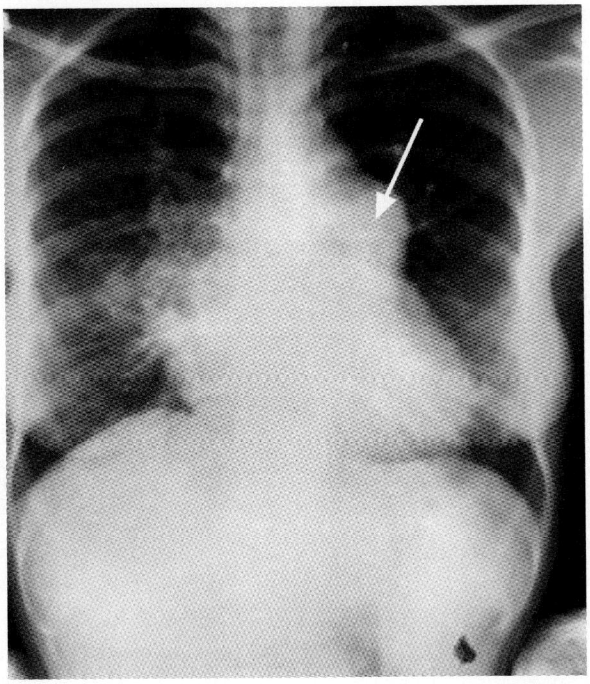

**Fig. 31.9:** Pulmonary arterial hypertension in a 16-year-old boy. The principal finding is prominence of the main pulmonary artery (arrow). In addition, the right and left pulmonary arteries are slightly widened

4. Pulmonary valve stenosis
5. Displaced by large aortic root
6. Mediastinal mass
7. Corrected transposition of great vessels

*Causes of pulmonary arterial hypertension*

1. Pulmonary venous hypertension
2. Shunts; left-to-right
3. Eisenmenger's syndrome
4. Pulmonary embolism
5. Thromboembolism
6. Parasites
7. Chronic hypoxia
8. Diffuse fibrotic lung disease
9. Uncommon
10. Arteritis
11. Drugs/toxins
12. Idiopathic

**Plethora** is the term used to describe the pulmonary vascular pattern in which there is a generalized increase in vessel size (arteries and veins). This is associated with loss of the normal size differential between upper and lower zone vessels. Plethora is characteristic of left-to-right shunts and is also seen in veno-arterial mixing lesions (e.g. total anomalous pulmonary venous drainage, truncus arteriosus). Mildly plethoric lungs may be seen in cor pulmonale in chronic obstructive pulmonary disease). Left-to-right shunts cause enlargement of proximal and distal pulmonary vessels, resulting in plethora. Plethora invariably occurs in shunts with a pulmonary flow; systemic flow ratio of more than 2:1, but is often absent in small shunts (<1.5;1).

*Pulmonary Oligaemia:* It is a general reduction in pulmonary resselsize. The change is opposite to that in plethora and is caused by low pulmonary blood flow. Oligaemia is difficult to assess reliably; it is more commonly associated with congenital heart disease (e.g. Fallot's tetralogy, Fallot variants and occasionally pulmonary valve stenosis) than with adult-acquired disease (e.g. pulmonary embolism and tricuspid valve disease).

In children and young adults, the ascending aorta is not border-forming on a PA chest radiograph and the lateral margin of the descending aorta is straight. The aorta elongates and 'unfolds' outwards with age, commonly producing a right-sided convexity to the mediastinum between the superior vena cava and the RA (after 40 years of age) and a lateral bowing of the descending aortic border.

### Congenital Heart Defects

*Secundum atrial septal defect:* The findings are—a large, left-shifted heart, commonly with features of RV dilatation plethoric lungs with large proximal vessels, including the MPA, a small aortic knuckle and a left atrium of normal size (Fig. 31.10).

*Ventricular septal defect:* Radiological changes generally differ from those of an atrial septal defect (ASD) (Fig. 31.11).

1. The heart and the MPA are less enlarged and may even be normal if the shunt is small.
2. Plethora is also usually less striking than in an ASD and, if the shunt is small, some upper/lower differential in vessel size remains.
3. The left atrium is commonly enlarged.

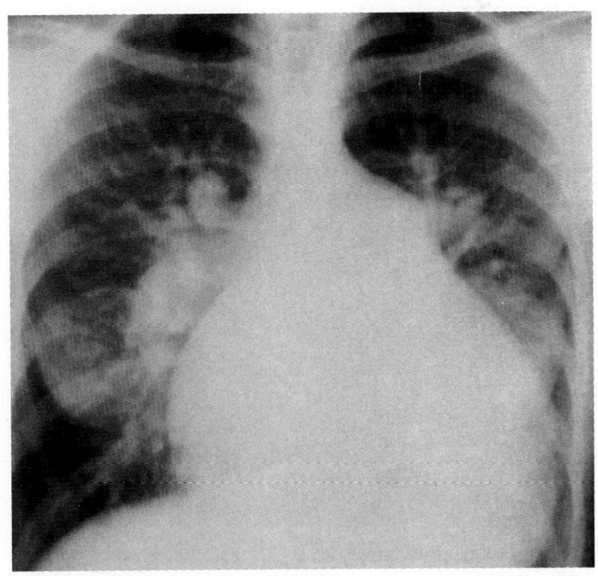

**Fig. 31.10:** Secundum atrial septal defect. The main and hilar pulmonary arteries (and veins) are large. The lungs are plethoric, with general enlargement of segmental and more distal vessels, and loss of the upper/lower zone size differential. Other characteristic features are the small (unidentifiable) aortic knuckle and the leftward shift of the heart

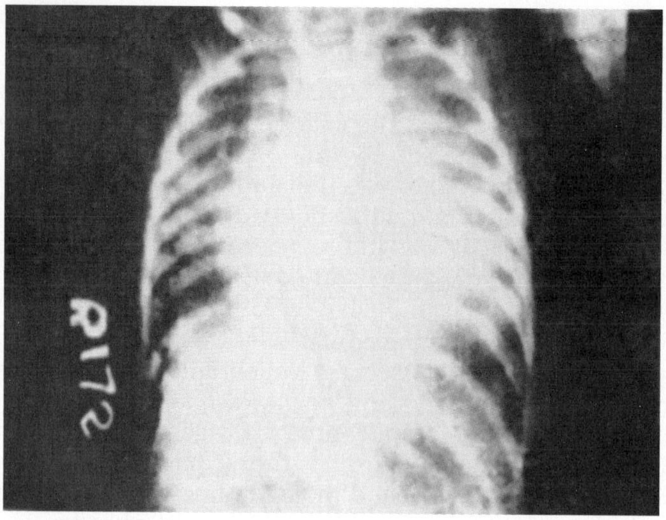



**Fig. 31.11:** Gross left ventricular enlargement with pulmonary plethora in a young child with L-R shunt with CCF

*Patent ductus arteriosus:* As in ventricular septal defect (VSD), heart enlargement and plethora may be slight or even absent in small shunts. The cardiac contour suggests LV enlargement, and mild LA enlargement is usually present. The most important features relate to the aortic arch and the MPA region. This is invariably abnormal, with a large knuckle or with flattening of the angle between the knuckle and the MPA. In adults, the ductus or the adjacent aorta may calcify (Fig. 31.12).

*Eisenmenger's syndrome:* In this syndrome there is raised pulmonary vascular resistance, shunt reversal and cyanosis produced by prolonged high flow through pulmonary vessels as the result of a left-to-right shunt. The important radiological difference from non-reversed shunts is that the lungs are no longer plethoric (Fig. 31.13).

*Coarctation of the aorta* (Fig. 31.14) is a localized congenital narrowing just beyond the left subclavian take-off. It is associated with other congenital anomalies (including bicuspid aortic valve) in about 70% of patients the ascending aorta and are characteristically most marked in the region of the aortic sinuses; because of this, they cause aortic regurgitation, and may be quite large without distorting the mediastinal envelope. Coarctation lead to inferior rib-notching (ribs three to eight) and an abnormal

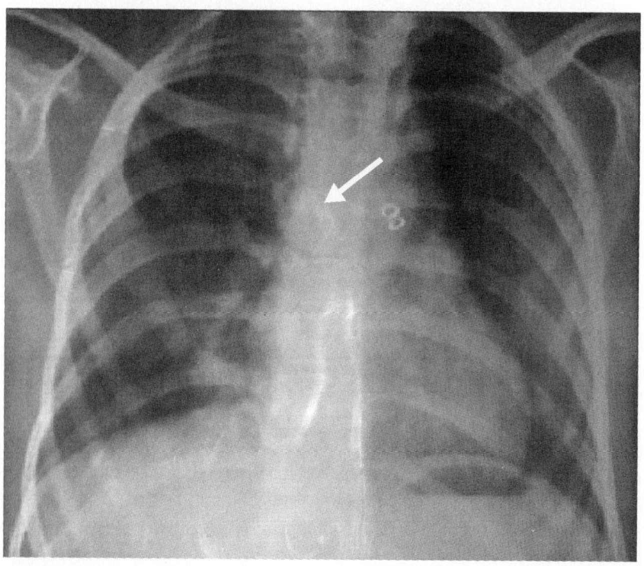

**Fig. 31.12:** Chest X-ray showing the old PDA clip in place

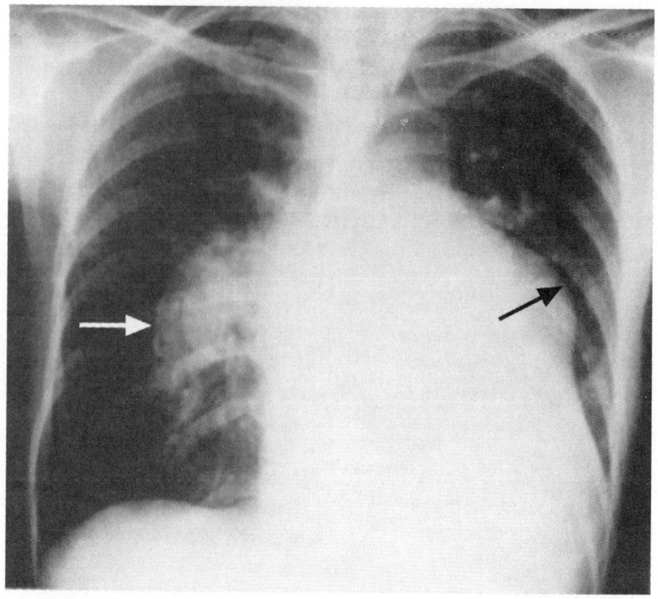

**Fig. 31.13:** Eisenmenger atrial septal defect. The left-sided bulge (black arrow) is caused by a massively enlarged main pulmonary artery

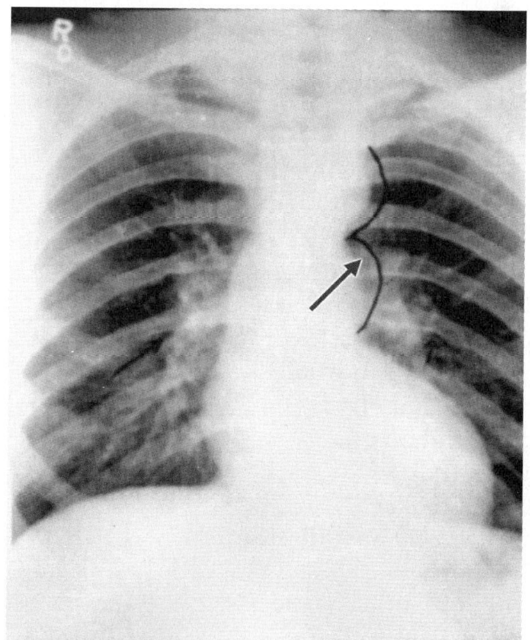

**Fig. 31.14:** Chest X-ray PA view showing prominence of left subclavian artery, abcent impression in the region of coarctation and distatal impression of descending aorta giving the configuration of number 3 as shown (arrow) in patient with coarctation of aorta

configuration of the aortic knuckle region, which may be high, low, flat or double. Heart size is usually normal, possibly with a contour suggesting LV hypertrophy, and occasionally there is mild LA enlargement. Slight prominence of the ascending aorta is common, and is caused by hypertension and/or a bicuspid aortic valve.

*Pulmonary stenosis* (Fig. 31.15)

*Dextrocardia* (Fig. 31.16)

*Transposion of great vessels (TGV)* (Fig. 31.17)

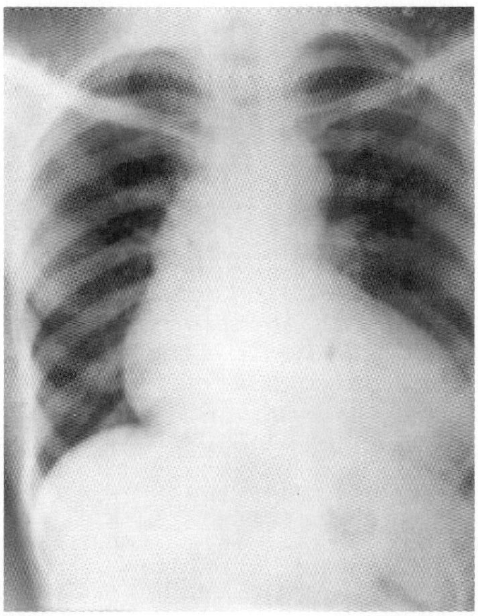

**Fig. 31.15:** Chest X-ray PA view showing, abscent pulmonary impression,olegaemic lung fields, upward lift of the cardiac apex and prominant bulge along the lower right border of the right atrium in an older child with congenital pulmonic stenosis with gross tricuspid regurgitation

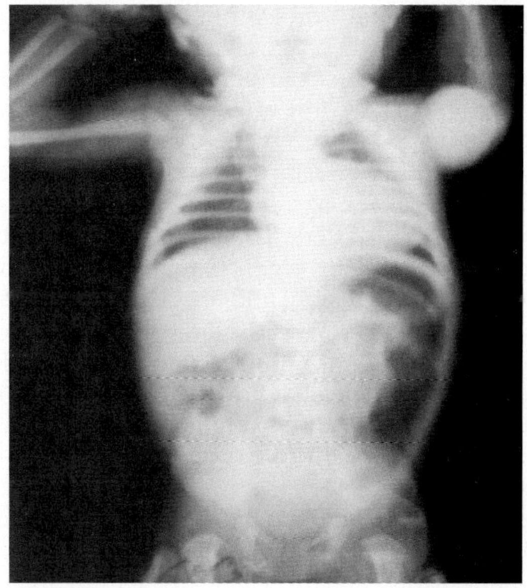

**Fig. 31.17:** Chest X-ray PA view showing wider base obliquily placed heart in the chest, abscent pulmonary impression and upward lift of the cardiac apex and egg shaped configuration of the heart in a child with dextro-transposion of great vessels

*Aortic aneurysm:* Aortic disease commonly manifests as an aneurysm, and it may be difficult to distinguish between aneurysm and unfolding aorta (Fig. 31.18). Observations suggesting that a prominent ascending aorta might be the result of aneurysm include:

1. Age >40 years
2. Absent or Disproportionately mild prominence of the descending aorta
3. Abnormally wide aortic arch (more than 40 mm). There may be radiographic clues to the cause of an aneurysm of the ascending aorta.

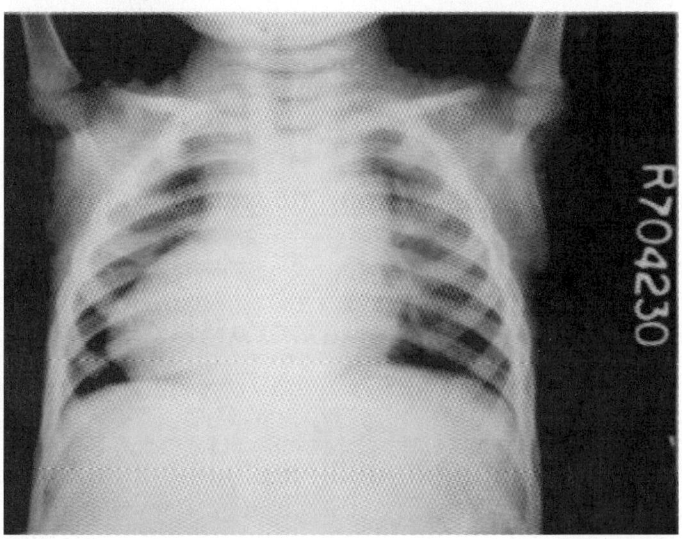


**Fig. 31.16:** Displacement of apex towards right. In the frontal view. The aortic arch is on the left and pulmonary impression is on the right side in a young hild patient with classical dextrocardia

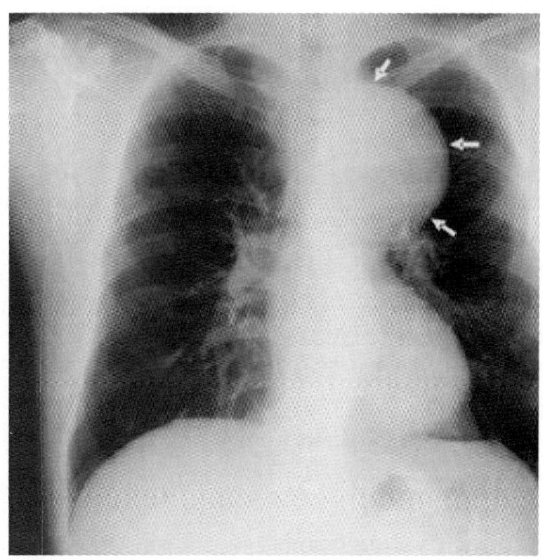

**Fig. 31.18:** Chest X-ray of a 31-year-old male patient, depicting a huge ballooning of the descending aorta (arrows) suggestive of aortic aneurysm

Although, the width of a prominent descending aorta cannot be assessed on a PA chest radiograph, it can be assessed on a lateral chest radiograph, on which its anterior and posterior borders are often outlined by lung, thus allowing distinction between aneurysm and unfolding.

- **Dissection of the aorta** appears as mediastinal widening. In addition, leakage of blood can cause haziness of the aortic outline, extrapleural opacity and pleural effusion.
- **Type A** dissections involve the ascending aorta with or without distal extension, and are treated surgically.
- **Type B** dissections start at the left subclavian artery and propagate distally into the descending aorta. They are usually treated medically. Previous radiographs may be useful because dissections often occur on the basis of a preexisting aneurysm (e.g. atherosclerosis, Marfan's cystic medial necrosis).

*The main radiographic clues to the cause of an aneurysm of the ascending aorta are:*

1. In hypertension, dilatation tends to be mild and generalized, and is often best appreciated in the arch
2. The ascending aorta and the arch are involved in aortic regurgitation, whereas aortic stenosis affects only the ascending aorta
3. Syphilis affects the ascending aorta and is characterized by thin, continuous and curvilinear marginal calcification that is bestseen on lateral radiographs
4. Calcification is qualitatively different in atheromatous aneurysms and comprises interrupted, irregular plaques; these aneurysms can affect any segment, but are most common in the descending aorta
5. Aneurysms in Marfan's syndrome typically affect the ascending aorta are characteristically most marked in the region of aortic sinuses; because of this they cause aortic regurgitation and may be quite large without distorting the mediastinal envelope

## Calcification

Both vascular and cardiac lesions may calcify and, if moderate, calcification may be seen on a chest radiograph (Figs 31.19 and 31.20). The optimal projection may be frontal or more commonly, lateral.

*Causes of cardiovascular calcification:*

- **Pericardium** *(Old infective, particularly tuberculous, and pericarditis)*
- **Myocardium**
  - *Old myocardial infarct*
- **Rheumatic heart disease (left atrium)**
  - *Mitral annular calcification*
- **Endocardium**
  - Jet lesions within chamber
  - Thrombus
  - Myxoma
  - Valvular dysfunctions
  - Rheumatic heart disease
  - Bicuspid/Senile aortic valve
  - Aortic homograft

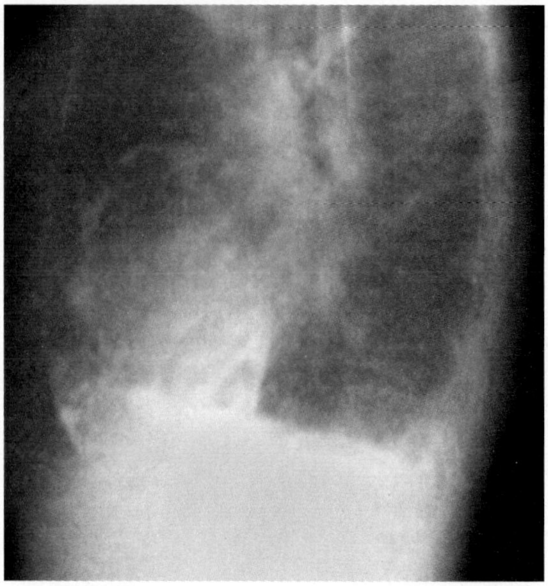

**Fig. 31.19:** Pericardial calcification. The calcification here is heavy and craggy with peripheral predominance. Sometimes, it has a more linear configuration. Almost invariably, it is easier to detect in lateral than in frontal views. Pericardial calcification usually follows pericarditis (particularly tuberculous, as in this case) and is commonly associated with constriction

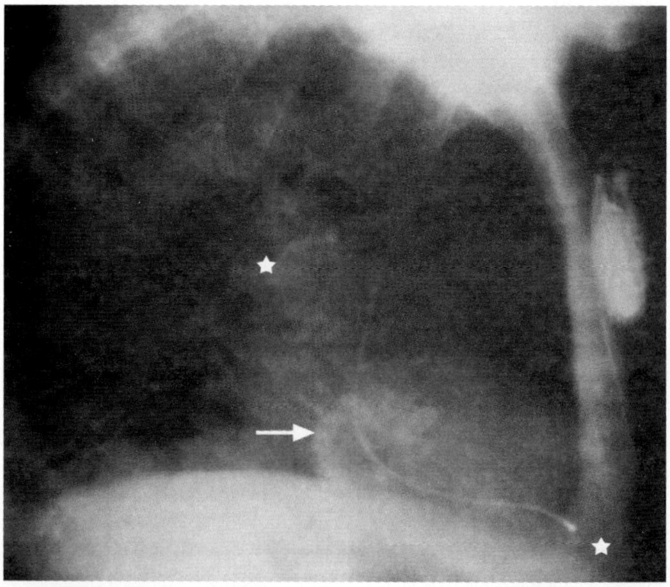

**Fig. 31.20:** Mitral annular calcification (arrow) commonly has a C-shaped configuration and lies in the region of the mitral valve (i.e. below a line joining the hilum and the anterior costophrenic angle, both marked with a star). It must not be confused with mitral valve calcification (often an easy distinction based on its configuration). Its presence is associated with systemic emboli and dysrhythmias (note the pacemaker in this patient)

- **Coronary artery**
  - *Atheroma*
- **Pulmonary artery**
  - *Pulmonary arterial hypertension*

- **Aorta**
  - *Atheroma*
  - *Aortitis*

### Ischemic Heart Disease

In acute myocardial infarction (MI), the chest radiograph enables assessment of haemodynamic disturbance, detects complications and excludes some other causes of chest pain. Haemodynamic disorder is manifested by pulmonary venous hypertension (PVH), which can occur despite a normal heart size (Figs 31.21 and 31.22) .

#### *Complications of Myocardial Infarction*

1. Mitral regurgitation is characterized by pulmonary venous hypertension, mild cardiomegaly and absent or mild LA enlargement.
2. The signs of VSD are similar to those of acute mitral regurgitation, and classic changes of plethora are not usually seen in the acute state.
3. Left ventricular aneurysm affects the anterolateral and apical parts of the LV in particular, producing either a large heart with a configuration of LV enlargement or a localized bulge to the LV border (apical or antero-laterally, that occasionally calcifies. Post-MI syndrome (Dressler's syndrome) is a delayed manifestation that gives rise to pericardial and pleural effusions, sometimes with basal lung consolidation.

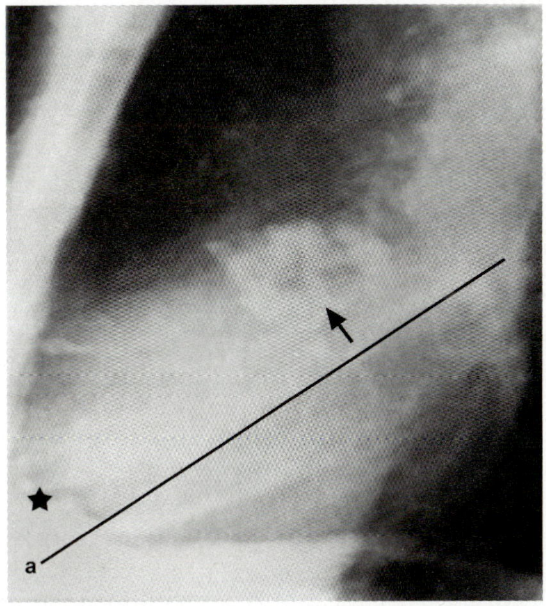


**Fig. 31.22:** Calcific, bicuspid aortic stenosis. A lateral view the aortic valve is heavily calcified (arrow), indicating severe stenosis, despite which the heart size is normal. The calcification is clear visible and typically lies above an imaginary line joining the costophrenic angle and the lung hilum (both marked with a star. The a-like configuration of the calcification is characteristic and clearly outlines the base and free margin of the two cusps

### Valvular Heart Disease

1. ***Mitral stenosis*** has characteristic radiological appearances. There is LA and LA appendage enlargement; the size of the LA correlates poorly with the degree of stenosis. Gross LA enlargement is not seen in pure mitral stenosis and indicates mitral regurgitation or a mixed lesion. *Mitral valve calcification* is present in longstanding, severe stenosis and is not a feature of mild disease. A normal heart size is common in uncomplicated disease. There is evidence of PVH. Pulmonary arterial hypertesion is evident in longstanding severe disease. At this stage, the heart usually becomes enlarged as the right-sided chambers dilate.

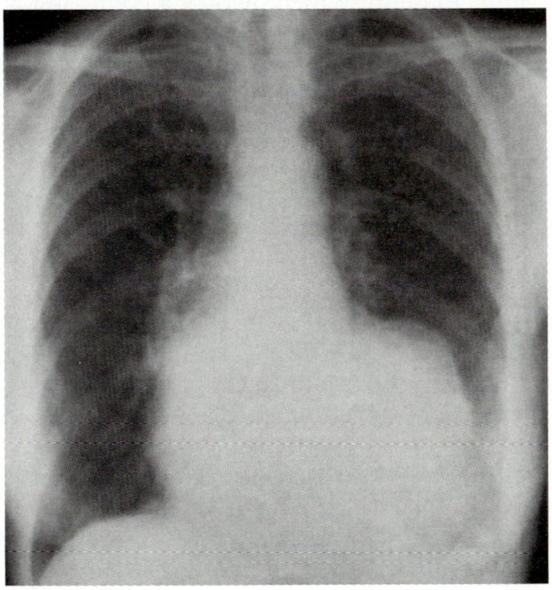

**Fig. 31.21:** Left ventricular aneurysm following old myocardial infarction. There is a pronounced bulge to the upper aspect of the left ventricular border. In this patient, the old infarct has also calcified in a thin, curvilinear manner

2. **Mitral regurgitation:** Radiological findings in mitral regurgitation differ in acute and chronic situations.
   a. ***Chronic mitral regurgitation:*** The heart is enlarged (with a contour of LV enlargement) and there is LA enlargement, which is often greater than in mitral stenosis. Signs of raised pulmonary venous pressure may be present but are often mild. In the absence of LV disease, heart size correlates with the severity of the mitral regurgitation.
   b. ***Acute mitral regurgitation:*** The main finding is gross pulmonary edema, often without overall enlargement of either the heart or the LA.
3. **Aortic stenosis:** It should be suspected if the radiograph shows:
   a. Aortic valve calcification with a normal heart size
   b. Cardiac contour that suggests left ventricular hypertrophy
   c. Prominence of the ascending aorta as a result of post-stenotic dilatation. With decompensation, the heart, including the LA, enlarges and signs of PVH develop.

4. **Aortic regurgitation:** The radiological signs of aortic regurgitation are:
   a. A large heart with a contour characteristic of LV dilatation.
   b. Mild LA enlargement (sometimes)
   c. A prominent ascending aorta caused by dilatation
   d. A calcified aortic valve (sometimes). PVH may be absent despite marked regurgitation and, when it develops, it is often late in the course of the disease.

### *Prosthetic Valves*

A large range of prosthetic valves is available (Fig. 31.23). Apart from homografts, all valves are radiopaque. Radiopaque components in prosthetic valves allow; identification of the type of valve, and usually indicate the direction of flow:

1. In hetrografts and caged valves, flow is from the base ring to the struit.
2. In the disc valves, the disc is often radiopaque, and the direction of flow is indicated if the disc is caught in an open position.
3. Because most replaced valves in adults are aortic or mitral knowledge of the direction of flow is usually sufficient to identify the valve site.
4. Occasionally, the tricuspid valve is replaced. This is oriented, from a flow point of view, like a mitral prosthesis, but it positioned more anteriorly and to the right. Some prosthetic valve abnormalities, including strut fracture and bioprosthesis calcification, can be detected on a chest radiograph.

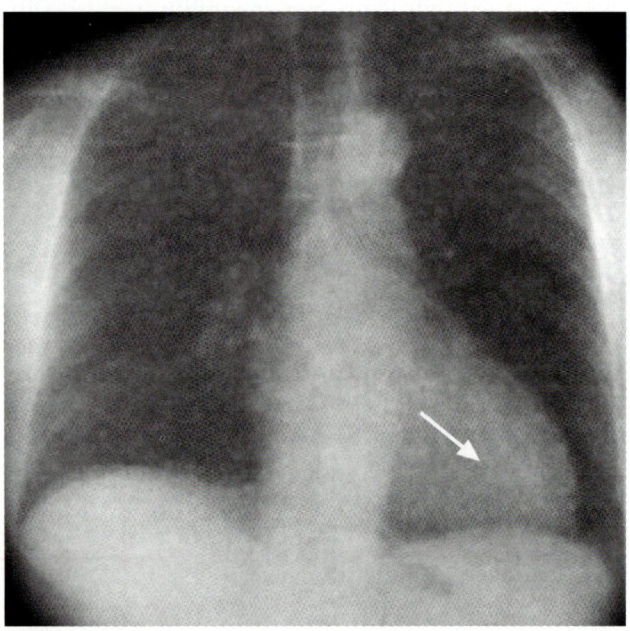

**Fig. 31.23:** Porcine (Carpentier-Edward) mitral valve replacement. Flow in such a prosthesis is from the 'base' to the tips of the stents and is indicated by the arrow. Flow in this direction could not be aortic but could be tricuspid or mitral. The position of the prosthesis to the left of the spine favours the latter

## ASSESSMENT OF EXTRATHORACIC, INTRATHORACIC AND INTRACARDIAC MEDICAL DEVICES

Chest devices are encountered on a daily basis by almost all radiologists. A multitude of extrathoracic materials, from intravenous catheters to oxygen tubing and electrocardiographic leads, frequently overlie the chest, neck and abdomen. Chest tubes, central venous catheters, endotracheal tubes and feeding tubes are very common. Cardiac surgery involves the use of many sophisticated devices and procedures, ranging from valve replacement to repair of complex congenital anomalies. Coronary artery bypass surgery is no longer considered unusual, and in many large medical centers, ventricular assist devices and total artificial hearts are frequently encountered. Breast implants are visible at standard chest radiography, and many ancillary devices not intended for treatment of cardiac or thoracic diseases are visible on chest radiographs. New devices are constantly being introduced, but most of them are variations on a previous theme. Knowing the specific name of a device is not important. It is important to recognize the presence of a device and to have an understanding of its function, as well as to recognize the complications associated with its use.

Chest radiography represents a significant percent of the workload of a diagnostic radiology department in a modern general hospital. The proliferation of intensive care units and the advances in the treatment of the very ill have greatly increased the numbers of examinations performed at the patient's bedside. Obtaining a daily chest radiograph is standard practice in most intensive care units, and any change in the patient's condition, or an intervention, can lead to several more studies in a given day. A medical center that has an active cardiothoracic surgery service and a busy trauma center generates large numbers of daily chest radiographs, many of which display a confusing array of medical apparatus used to treat and monitor patients. This article discusses the most common and important devices of the chest to help radiologists recognize their presence, have an understanding of their functions, and recognize the complications associated with their use.

### Extrathoracic Devices

Most life-support devices are within the patient's heart, blood vessels, lungs or pleura. Tubing, clamps, syringes and other apparatus often lie on or under the patient and are imaged with the chest during the radiographic examination.These objects are usually easy to recognize and of no great importance. Patients may also lie on trauma boards, foam mattresses, or other similar supports that may be visible on radiographs. Ventilator support tubing is almost always visible somewhere on a chest image, as are attachments such as temperature and humidity sensors. ECG electrodes are now so ubiquitous that even healthy newborns rarely escape having them applied. A versatile device commonly used in cardiac patients being transported by helicopter or ambulance is the external pacemaker-defibrillator.

Breast prostheses are usually recognizable on chest radiographs. Sometimes, breast reconstruction following mastectomy may require the gradual preparation of a pocket suitable for the prosthesis; in such cases, a tissue expander is used.

*Pleural devices:* Thoracostomy (chest) tubes are commonly used for evacuating fluid or air from the pleural space. They vary from 10–40 F in size, depending on the viscosity of the material to be evacuated, and the preferences of the individual physician involved in the treatment of the case.

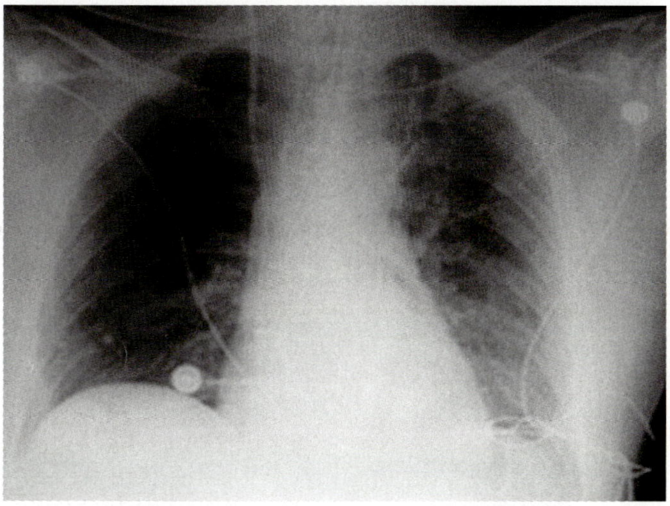

**Fig. 31.24:** Typical postoperative cardiac surgery chest radiograph. First postoperative study for a 58-year-old radiologist, who underwent coronary artery bypass graft (CABG) surgery. The image is underexposed and shows a confusing array of apparatus, including overlying oxygen tubing, a pulmonary artery catheter, a nasogastric tube, an endotracheal tube, a mediastinal drain, median sternotomy wires, mediastinal clips, electrocardiographic (ECG) leads, and incipient left lower lobe atelectasis and pleural fluid

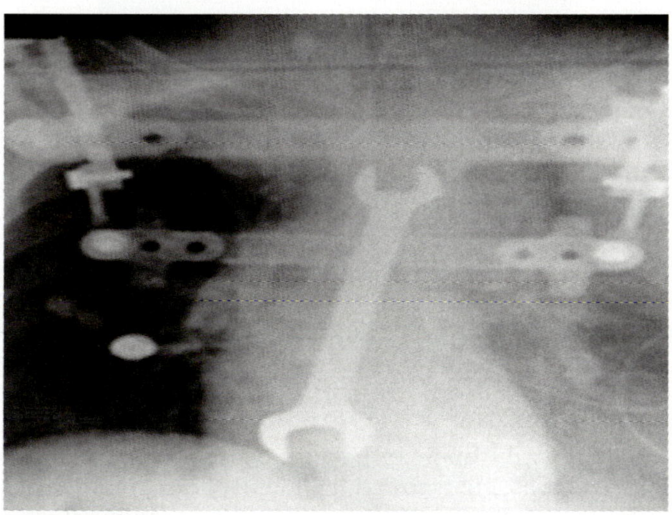

**Fig. 31.25:** Chest radiograph shows halo apparatus (with emergency wrench close at hand) for cervical spine stabilization

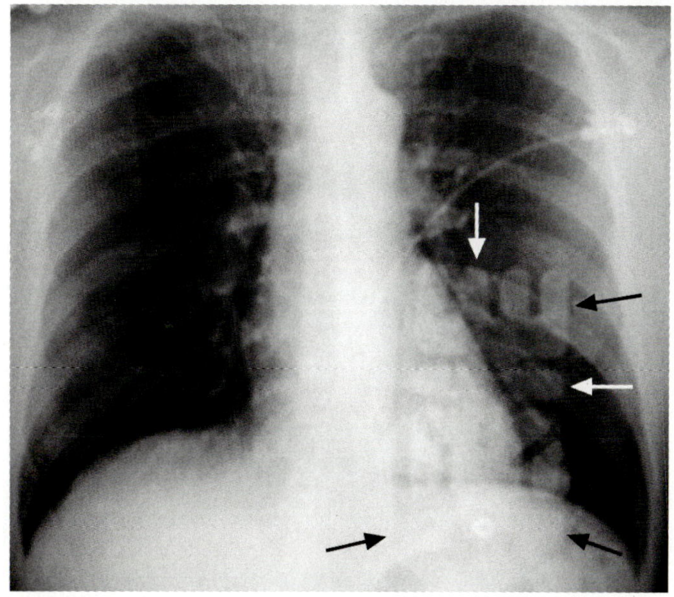

**Fig. 31.26:** Chest radiograph reveals an external pacemaker-defibrillator electrode plate overlying the left side of the chest. The rectangular Chinese character-like electrode (white arrows) goes on the patient's back, and the round electrode (black arrows) goes on the patient's front

The tube is usually placed anterosuperiorly to evacuate a pneumothorax and postero-inferiorly for fluid collections. The normally positioned tube lies on the surface of the expanded lung, between the visceral and parietal pleurae. Pigtail catheters may be used in place of standard thoracostomy tubes, and they are popular for empyema drainage and for installation of medication for treatment of an empyema. If the thoracostomy tube is not accomplishing, its task of adequate fluid drainage or reexpansion of a collapsed lung secondary to a pneumothorax, the tube is probably malpositioned. To accurately assess the position of a tube, both frontal and lateral views of the chest or even chest computed tomographic scans may be needed. A chest tube may enter an interlobar fissure, and with apposition of the visceral pleura of the two lobes, the end and side holes of the tube may become obstructed and the tube rendered ineffective. Malposition of chest tubes in lung parenchyma or subcutaneous soft tissues sometimes occurs. The proximal port of the chest tube may be in a superficial location outside the pleural cavity, or the tube may become kinked. The tube can also become occluded if its tip lies against the mediastinum.

In the era before antibiotics, a variety of pleural devices were used in the treatment of tuberculosis. These include 'ping-pong' ball plombage and wax plombage. Their appearance is quite dramatic, and they may occasionally be encountered in an older patient (Figs 31.24–31.26).

### Tracheal and Esophageal Devices

Endotracheal intubation is a life-saving procedure, but it can also be life-threatening if the tube is incorrectly positioned. In an adult, the tip of the tube should be situated

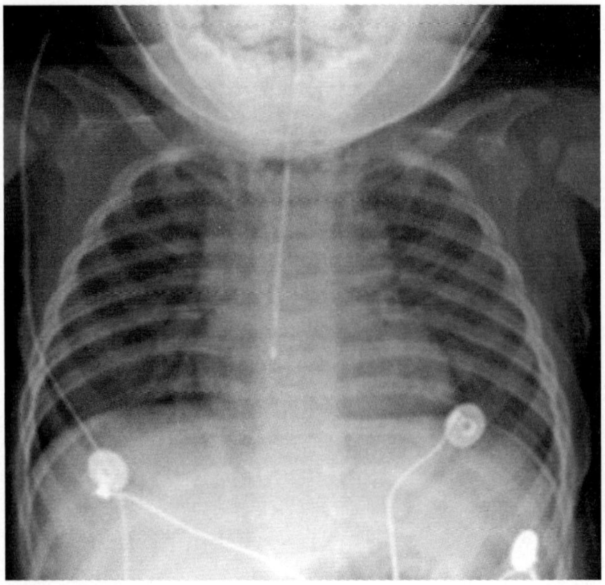

**Fig. 31.27:** Frontal chest radiograph of an infant shows a pH probe

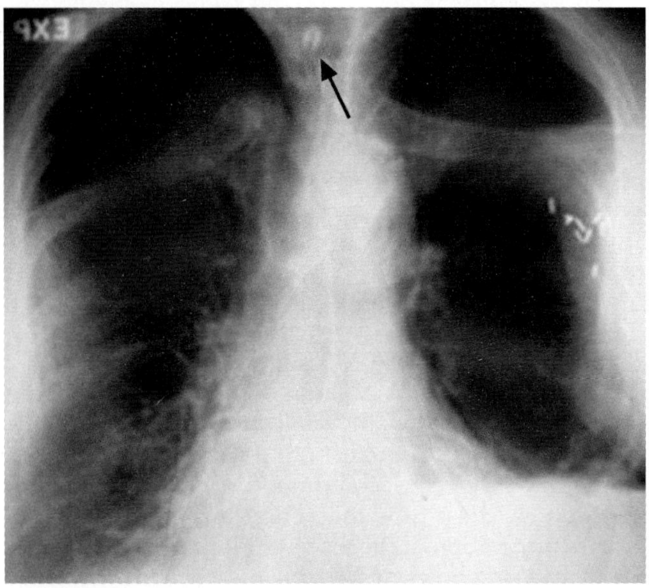

**Fig. 31.28:** Frontal chest radiograph demonstrates a tracheoesophageal voice prosthesis (arrow)

approximately 5 cm above the tracheal carina, so that excursions of 2 cm upward or downward (with neck extension or flexion) can be safely accommodated.

The carina may not be visible on every image, but the aortic 'knob' usually is. The carina is just caudad to the aortic arch, so that if the tip of the endotracheal tube is just above the aortic arch, it is in good position, midway between the vocal cords and the carina. When advanced too far, the endotracheal tube usually enters the right main bronchus, causing various combinations of hyperinflation and atelectasis of the two lungs, depending on the positions of the end and side holes. Besides being placed into the right bronchus, endotracheal tubes can also be

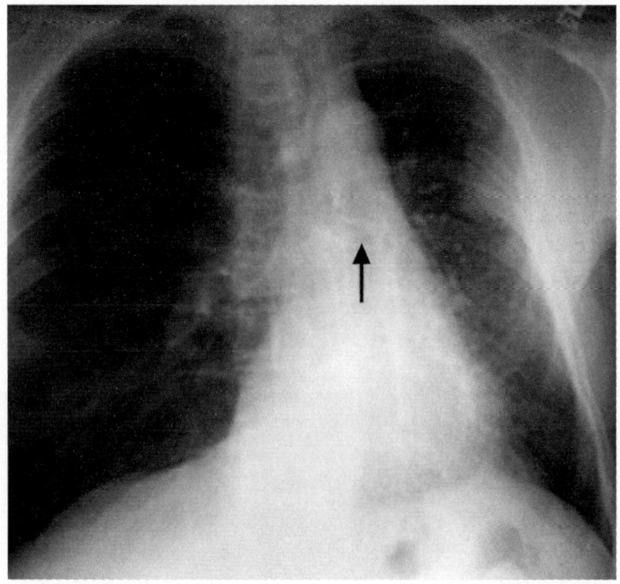

**Fig. 31.29:** Frontal view of the chest in a patient with a transplanted left lung reveals a left bronchial stent (arrow) and surgical clips

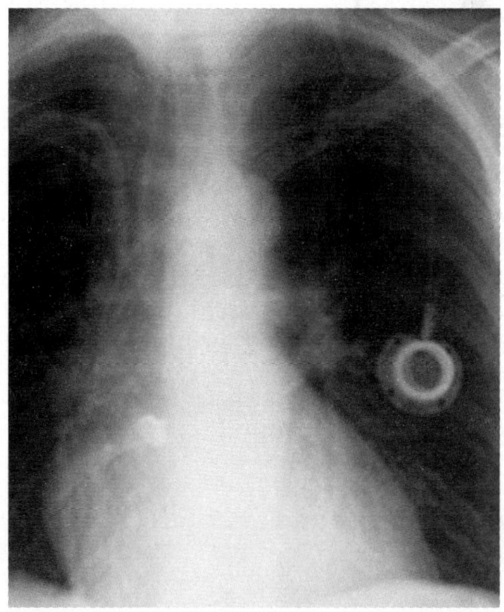

**Fig. 31.30:** Portable chest radiograph shows a right subclavian single-lumen central venous catheter and a left subcutaneous port catheter, which enters via the left subclavian vein. Both catheter tips are in the superior vena cava

inadvertently placed in the esophagus or in the soft tissues of the neck. Sometimes, a double-lumen endotracheal tube is deliberately used for differential ventilation of the two lungs to accommodate differences in compliance between them.

Nasogastric tubes and feeding tubes are frequently visualized passing through the mediastinum on their way to the stomach and intestines. Not infrequently, chest radiographs reveal medical devices in abnormal locations and unexpected foreign bodies.

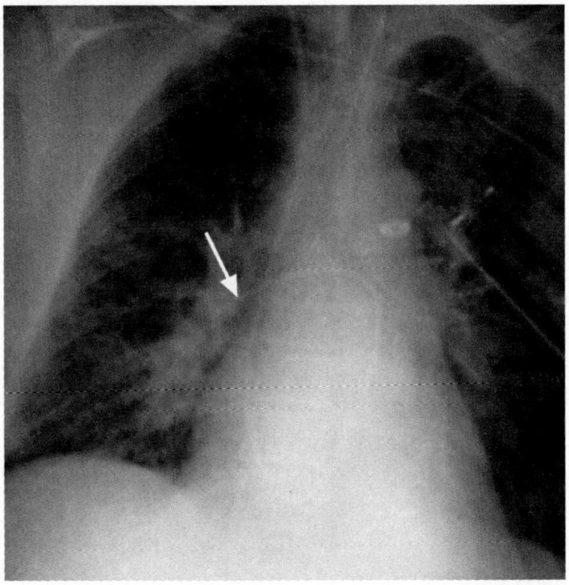

**Fig. 31.31:** Frontal chest radiograph shows a right jugular Swan-Ganz catheter with its tip (arrow) in the right lower pulmonary artery

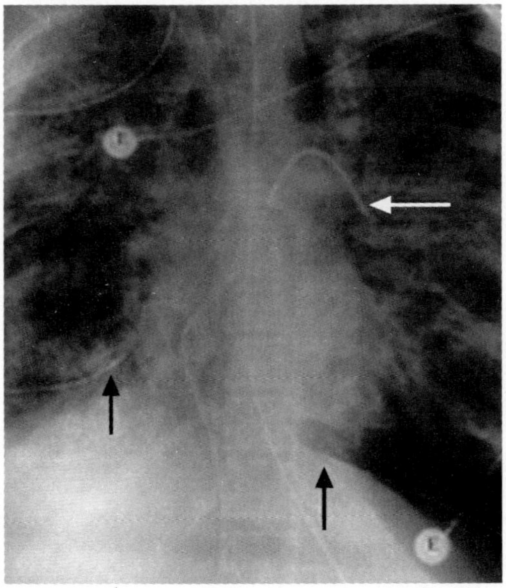

**Fig. 31.32:** Frontal chest radiograph shows a Swan-Ganz catheter (white arrow) in the left pulmonary artery via the inferior vena cava. Note also the bilateral chest tubes (black arrows) and ECG leads (E)

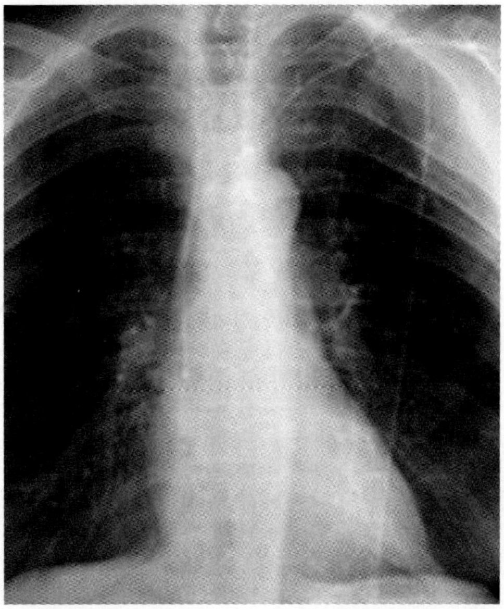

**Fig. 31.33:** Frontal view of the chest shows a left subclavian Groshong catheter with its tip in the proximal most portion of the superior vena cava

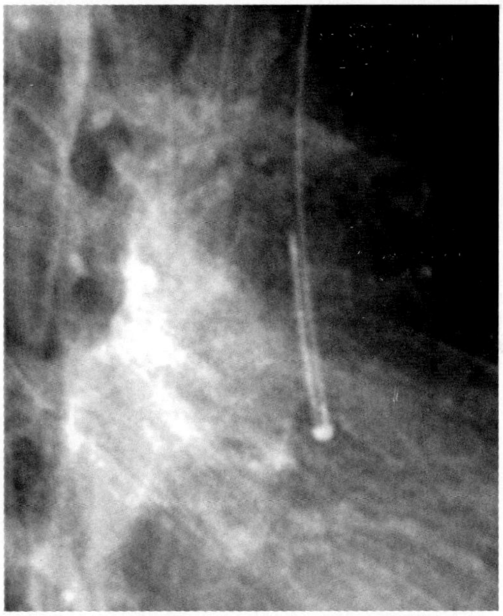

**Fig. 31.34:** Frontal view of the chest shows a left subclavian Groshong catheter with its tip in the proximal most portion of the superior vena cava

Esophageal balloons and esophageal stents used to treat benign and malignant esophageal disease may manifest themselves at chest radiography. Balloon dilatation and stent placement in the esophagus are safe, effective procedures for treating esophageal strictures and fistulas, and they provide reasonable palliative relief from malignant esophageal obstruction. Esophageal and gastric balloons are still occasionally used to treat bleeding varices. Probes to measure distal esophageal pH as part of a gastroesophageal reflux workup are sometimes seen and may be confused with a feeding tube, if one is not careful or if a proper patient history is not provided. The ideal location for the pH probe is the distal portion of the esophagus, just above the gastroesophageal junction.

Tracheostomy tubes and other tracheal and bronchial apparatus are not infrequently visible on chest radiographs. Tracheoesophageal voice prostheses are not common, but may occasionally be seen. Bronchial stents are occasionally seen in patients who have undergone lung transplantation and have developed a stricture at the anastomosis between the native tracheobronchial tree and the transplanted one. These stents may be metallic and easily recognized, or they may be composed of various plastic materials and be hard to recognize, especially if no history of stent placement or lung transplantation has been given.It is wise to look for these stents in all patients who have undergone lung transplantation (Figs 31.24–31.34).

## Vascular Devices

Vascular catheters of various types are now routinely used for monitoring hemodynamic function; for performing hemodialysis; and for administering fluids, medications,

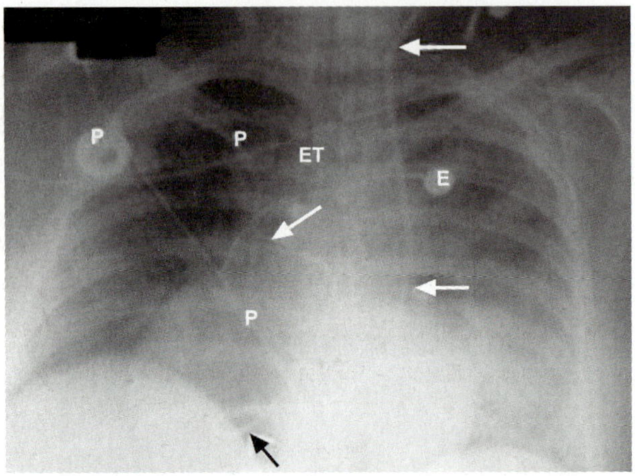


**Fig. 31.35:** Frontal view of the chest shows a left jugular Swan-Ganz catheter (arrows), which passes through a persistent left superior vena cava into the coronary sinus, through the right atrium and right ventricle, and into the right pulmonary artery. A subcutaneous port (P), an endotracheal tube (ET), an ECG lead (E) and a nasogastric tube (not labeled) are also seen

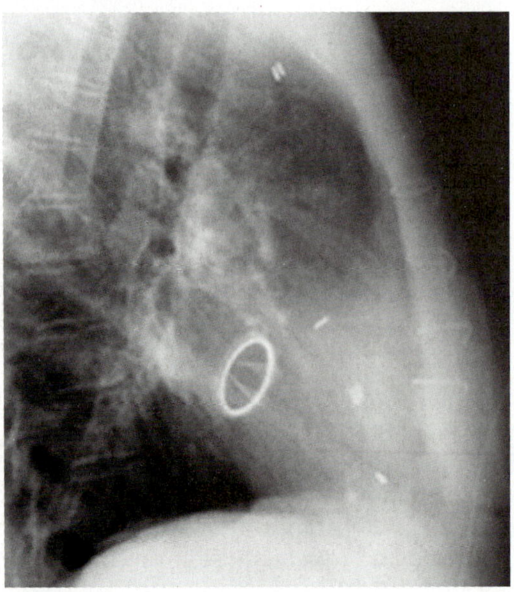

**Fig. 31.36:** Mechanical heart valve. Lateral view of the chest shows a Hemex tilting bileaflet mechanical mitral valve prosthesis. Median sternotomy wires and surgical clips are also evident

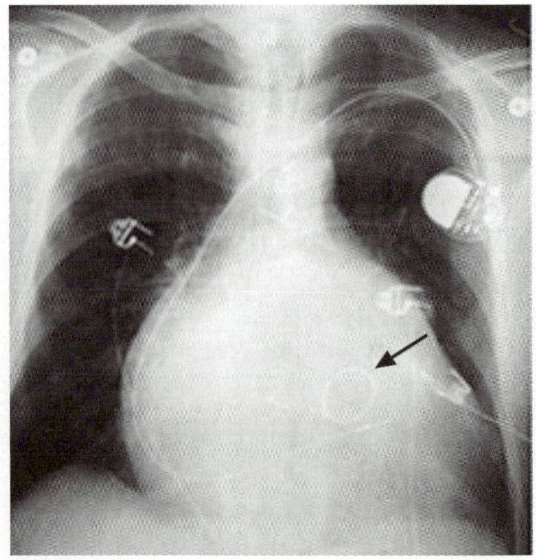

**Fig. 31.37:** Biologic heart valve. Frontal view of the chest shows a Hancock porcine mitral valve prosthesis (arrow). A single-lead pacemaker, ECG leads, and median sternotomy wires are also seen

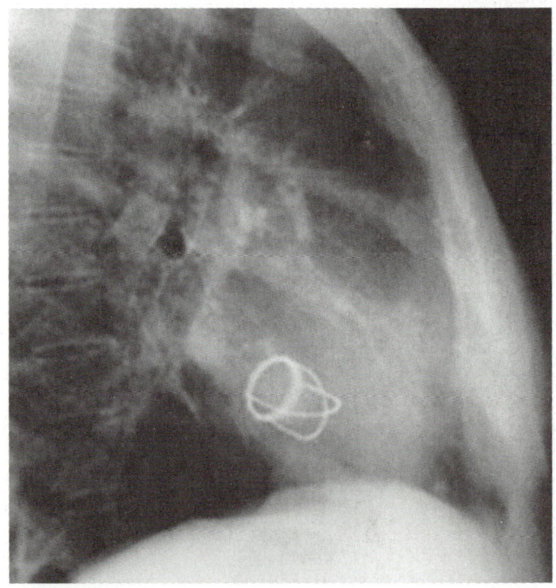

**Fig. 31.38:** Mechanical heart valve. Lateral view of the chest shows a Starr-Edwards caged ball mechanical mitral valve prosthesis

and nutrition (Figs 31.35–31.40). Some catheters are designed for short-term use in the postoperative or intensive care unit setting, whereas others are implanted for long-term use, such as those used in cancer patients. Venous devices are usually inserted, either percutaneously or surgically, via the subclavian, internal jugular, or femoral veins. Arterial devices usually are placed through the femoral artery, but sometimes the brachial or axillary route is employed.

Central venous catheters (also known as central venous pressure [CVP] catheters, central catheters, and central lines) typically have 1–3 lumens and are constructed out of

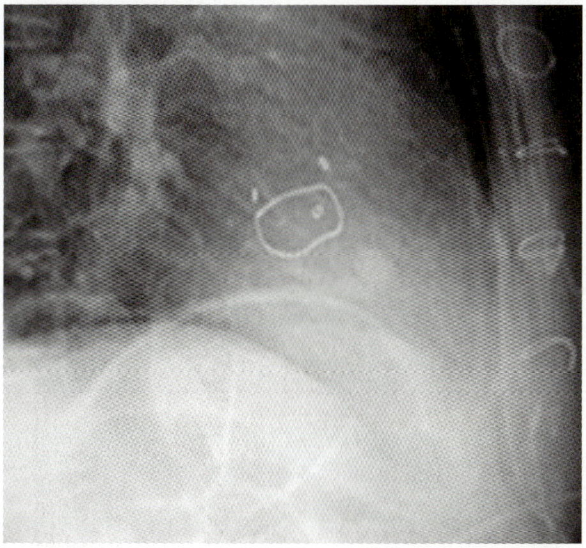

**Fig. 31.39:** Biologic heart valve. Collimated lateral view of the chest shows a Medtronic Hancock valve

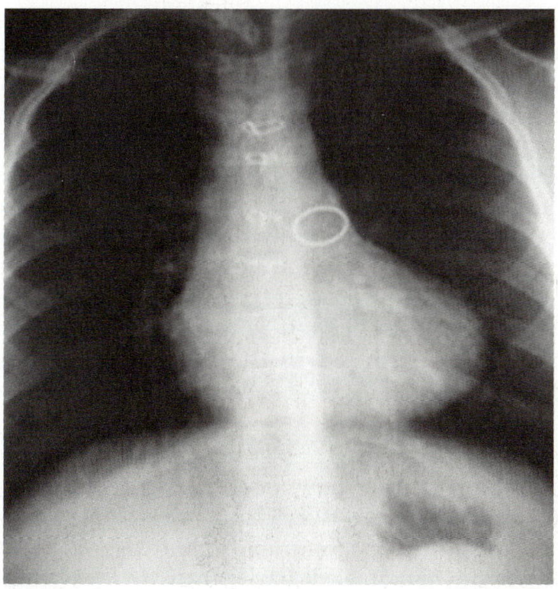

**Fig. 31.40:** Biologic heart valve. Frontal view of the chest shows a Hancock porcine valve prosthesis in a Rastelli conduit going from the right ventricle to the pulmonary artery

medical-grade silicone or polyurethane. The nomenclature for central catheters is confusing and inconsistent in daily use. For example, the terms *Hickman, Broviac, Leonard* and *Hohn* are trademarks of CR Bard, Inc. (Miami Lakes, Fla). Cordis sheath is a trademark of the Cordis Corporation (Covington, Ga). However, in many medical centers, these names are used generically to represent any central catheter, regardless of its actual construction, manufacturer or particular use.

Swan-Ganz is a registered trademark of Baxter International (Deerfield, Ill). This name has come to represent any type of multilumen catheter used for measuring hemodynamic pressures and cardiac output. A better term to use is *pulmonary artery catheter*. The Groshong (trademark of CR Bard) catheter is noted for its unusual closed, rounded. Near the tip in the side of the catheter is a three-position valve. The valve is designed to allow fluid to flow in and out through the valve, but it remains closed when it is not in use. This catheter does not require routine clamping or heparin solution to keep open. It does require periodic flushing with 0.9% normal saline.

There are also a variety of implantable access devices (subcutaneous ports), most commonly represented by the Port-A-Cath (trademark of CR Bard). Such devices are designed for easy, long-term access to the vascular system or peritoneal cavity. Port access is accomplished by percutaneous needle insertion. The port itself typically sits in the infraclavicular fossa, over the upper abdomen, or over the lower ribs. The port is usually connected to a central venous catheter or to an arterial catheter and can be used for instillation of fluids, medications, chemotherapeutic agents, parenteral nutritional solutions, and blood products. It can also be used for withdrawal of blood samples. There are almost as many types of access ports as there are types of standard central venous catheters.

A central venous catheter is ideally positioned in the superior vena cava for the monitoring of pressure or infusion of medication and nutrition. A catheter tip positioned in the right atrium increases the risk of perforation and cardiac arrhythmia. The same holds true for dialysis catheters. However, there is some controversy over the correct position for the tip of a central venous catheter. Some believe the usefulness and longevity of a catheter will be improved if its tip is positioned in the upper portion of the right atrium.

*Flow-directed, balloon-tipped catheters (pulmonary artery, Swan-Ganz catheters):* These are now widely used for monitoring circulatory hemodynamics. Accurate measurement of pulmonary arterial wedge pressure in a supine patient requires the catheter tip to be in the lower lobe (zone 3 of West) so that left atrial pressure, not alveolar pressure, is measured. Over a period of time, pulmonary artery catheters may migrate toward the periphery of the pulmonary bed and become lodged in a small pulmonary artery. Such migration can cause vessel injury by prolonged occlusion or by overdistention of the vessel when the catheter balloon is inflated. Also, pulmonary infarction can result from this situation. The period of time during which the balloon remains inflated and wedged should be limited, particularly in patients with pulmonary hypertension. A central location of the catheter tip near the lung hilum helps prevent pulmonary artery perforation and is a good 'parking' position for the catheter when it is not being used to measure pulmonary arterial wedge pressure.

The routine use of pulmonary artery catheters has been questioned by some authorities, but they are a common finding on intensive care unit portable chest radiographs. Even though these catheters are widely accepted and widely used, there are no definitive studies demonstrating their benefit.

Complications of catheter insertion vary with the catheters used and the sites employed. Catheter malposition usually involves the catheter passing into a tributary vessel rather than the one sought. The internal jugular vein, azygous arch and internal mammary vein are frequent sites of catheter malpositioning. Catheters may take an unusual course or position because of a congenital anomaly. Arterial puncture may lead to an abnormal catheter position with pulsatile flow in the catheter.

Pneumothorax is a common complication of unsuccessful attempts at subclavian or low jugular catheter insertion. Nerve injury is usually a complication of improper puncture technique. Vessel lacerations and perforations can produce hematomas, hemothorax and infusion of fluid into the mediastinum, thorax or other inappropriate space. Looping of catheters may lead to knotting. Pinching of catheters and catheter shearing usually occur at the site of entry and suture fixation.

Although, central venous catheters inserted into the subclavian vein or into the internal jugular vein represent the standard approach for establishing central venous access, a simpler, potentially less-injurious access to the central venous system is through the use of a peripherally inserted central catheter (PICC). PICC lines are smaller catheters that are peripherally inserted at or slightly proximal to the antecubital fossa, with the tip placed in the superior vena cava. They are often preferred over standard central lines in children.

## Cardiac Devices

Treatment of heart disease has probably fostered more development of sophisticated medical interventions than all the interventions designed for all other organs combined.

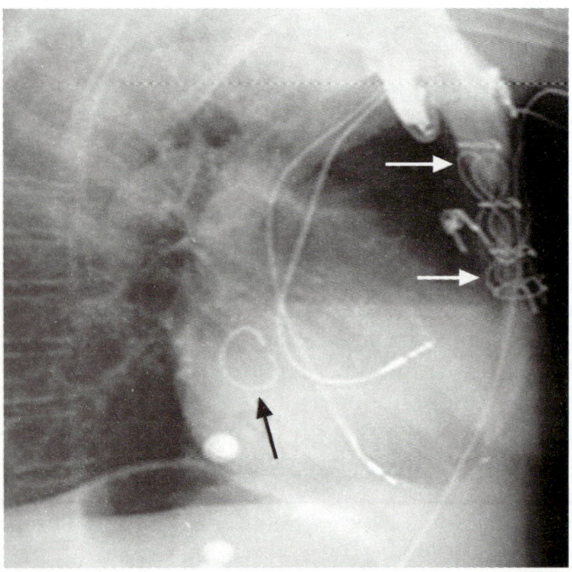

**Fig. 31.41:** Lateral view of the chest in an elderly patient shows a mitral annuloplasty ring (black arrow) and a dual-lead cardiac pacemaker. Sternal wires, surgical clips, and ECG leads are also present. The sternal wires are used to close a sternal dehiscence. The patient has both horizontal sternal wires and vertical intercostal wires (white arrows)

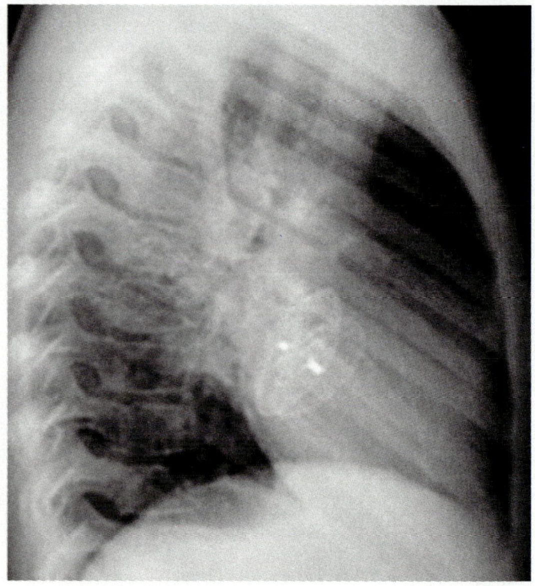

**Fig. 31.42:** Lateral view of the chest in a child shows an occlusion basket (umbrella) for treatment of an atrial septal defect

Coronary artery angioplasty, coronary artery stent placement, coronary artery bypass graft (CABG) surgery, the surgical correction of congenital cardiac defects, and even cardiac transplantation are no longer considered novel, experimental procedures. Cardiac pacemakers, valve prostheses and artificial hearts are sophisticated biomedical engineering products that have drastically altered the course of many cardiac disorders. Because chest radiography is commonly employed in the assessment of patients with heart disease, recognition of cardiac devices and the problems associated with them is important for all individuals involved in the care of these patients (Figs 31.41–31.42).

## Heart Valves

Heart valve prostheses have been used successfully since the 1960s, and there are two basic types—mechanical and biologic. The number, complexity, and use of prosthetic heart valves have increased dramatically to the point where most radiologists see them on a daily basis in their practices (Figs 31.43 and 31.44). Mechanical valves are composed of metals, polymers and ceramics. A mechanical valve functions basically as an occluder, moving passively with changes in pressure and flow within the heart. Most require life-long treatment with anticoagulants. Biologic valves contain tissue from human cadavers (homografts), porcine aortic cusps, or bovine pericardium (xenografts). Biologic valves are less durable than mechanical valves, with some deterioration developing, frequently 5–10 years after placement, but they do not usually require anticoagulant treatment.

There are many types of prosthetic cardiac valves, and it is not possible to discuss them in any detail in this article. Some mechanical valves include the Starr-Edwards (Edwards Lifesciences, Irvine, Calif), Bjork-Shiley (Pfizer, New York, NY), Medronic Hall (Medronic, Minneapolis,

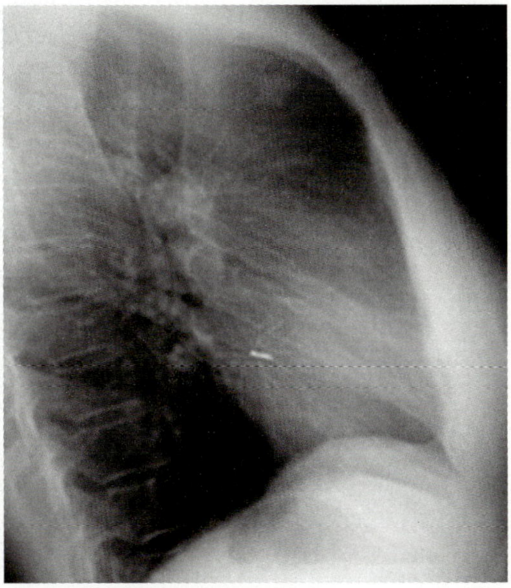

**Fig. 31.43:** Lateral view of the chest in an adult with an atrial septal defect shows an occlusion (filter) device

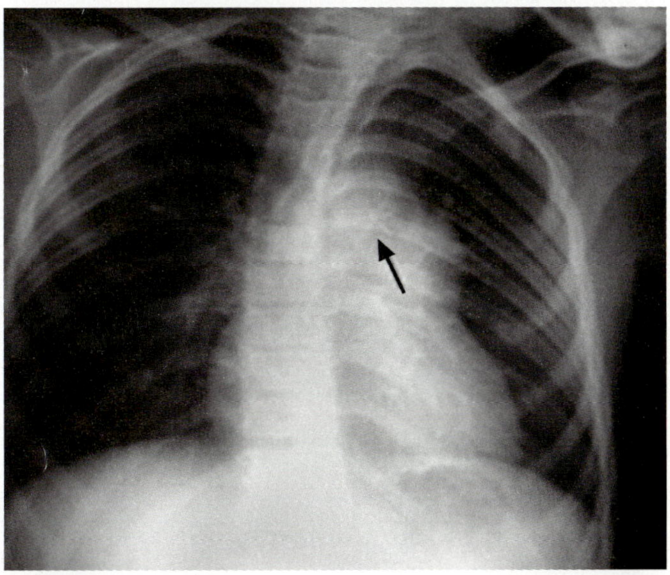

**Fig. 31.44:** Frontal view of the chest in a child shows an occlusion filter (arrow) used to close a patent ductus arteriosus

Minn), St Jude Medical (St Jude Medical, Inc, St Paul, Minn), Sorin Bicarbon (Sorin Biomedica, Italy), and the Carbomedics (Sorin Biomedica). Some bioprosthetic (biologic) heart valves include the Carpentier-Edwards (Edwards Lifesciences), Tissue Med (Aor Tech International PLC, United Kingdom) and the Hancock (Medtronic, Minneapolis, Minn). It is not important and often impossible to know the specific name of a particular prosthetic heart valve, but it is important to recognize its presence. Because prosthetic heart valves are used in a large variety of congenital and acquired conditions in both adults and children, it is frequently difficult to ascertain which native valve has been replaced by a prosthesis. The heart in such cases may be markedly enlarged, displaced, or altered by cardiac surgery. The mitral and aortic valves are those most commonly replaced, whereas prosthetic tricuspid valves are seen less often. Prosthetic pulmonary valves are rare. There are also various shunts or conduits used as part of a complex cardiac surgical procedure to correct congenital heart disease. These shunts may contain a prosthetic heart valve.

Sometimes, an annuloplasty ring may be used instead of a prosthetic cardiac valve to treat valvular regurgitation.The annuloplasty rings narrow and reshape the heart valve for proper functioning.

There are products designed to close nonphysiologic openings in the heart, such as a patent ductus arteriosus, atrial septal defect, or ventricular septal defect, without the need for open heart surgery. The first of these products was the Rashkind 'double umbrella' occlusion device (CR Bard) to close a patent ductus arteriosus. Other devices are the Bard Clamshell Septal Umbrella (CR Bard), the Amplatzer Septal Occluder (AGA Medical Corp, Golden Valley, Minn), and the Sideris device (AGA Medical) to close atrial septal defects, ventricular septal defects and other intracardiac communications. In general, these devices consist of a basket (umbrella) or filter placed in the defect to occlude it. They are often self-adjusting and lie flat against the atrial or ventricular septum. This flat design helps create a natural profile.

### Cardiac Pacemakers

Cardiac pacemakers are probably as common as prosthetic cardiac valves and are found in patients of all ages, although they are much more common in older adults being treated for abnormal cardiac rhythms caused by coronary artery disease (Figs 31.45–31.63). Cardiac pacemakers improve cardiac function, reduce the severity of clinical symptoms, and reduce mortality and morbidity.

A cardiac pacemaker is composed of two main elements—(a) a pulse generator and (b) lead wires with electrodes for

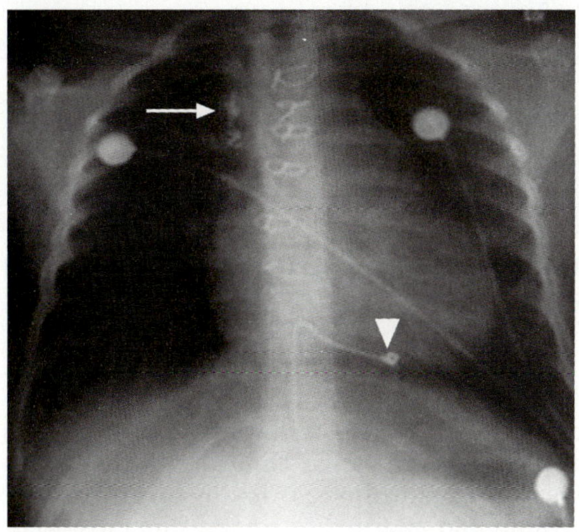

**Fig. 31.45:** Frontal view of the chest shows a single electrode epicardial 'corkscrew' subxiphoid pacemaker. There is also coils (white arrow) occluding a previous right Blalock-Taussig shunt. In addition, ECG leads and sternal wires are evident

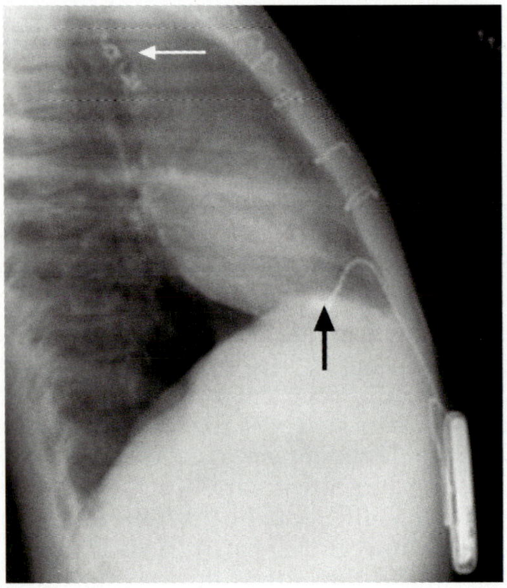

**Fig. 31.46:** Lateral view of the chest shows a single electrode epicardial 'corkscrew' subxiphoid pacemaker (arrowhead in a black arrow). There are also coils (white arrow) occluding a previous right Blalock-Taussig shunt. In addition, ECG leads and sternal wires are evident

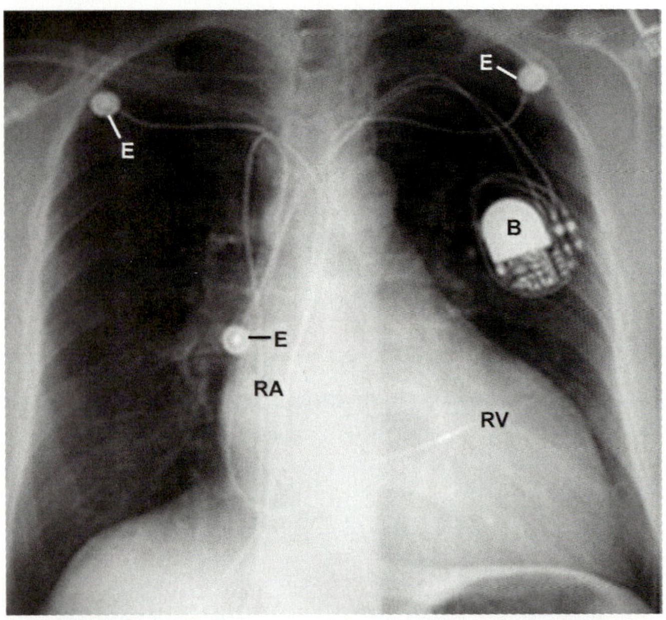


**Fig. 31.47:** Frontal view shows an atrioventricular sequential pacemaker with one electrode in the right atrial appendage (RA) and the other at the right ventricular apex (RV). Also shown are ECG leads (E) and the battery-control pack

contact with the endocardium or myocardium. Cardiac pacemakers were first used clinically in the 1960s, with stainless steel electrodes sewn directly onto the myocardium and attached to a fixed-rate pulse generator implanted in the subcutaneous tissues of the upper abdomen. Since then, there have been many advances, including small-caliber, fracture-resistant, transvenous leads and programmable multichamber atrioventricular

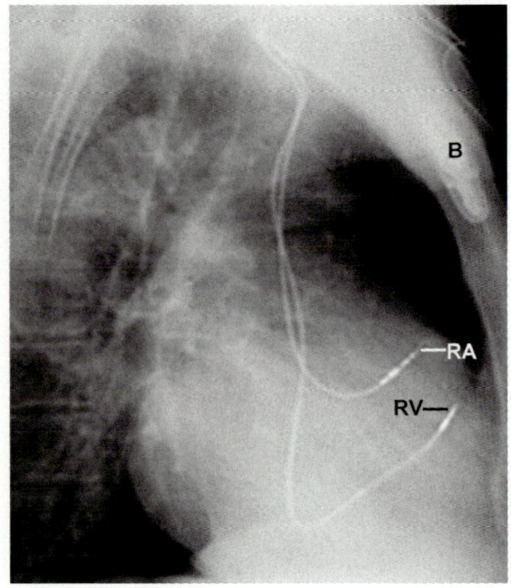


**Fig. 31.48:** Lateral view shows an atrioventricular sequential pacemaker with one electrode in the right atrial appendage (RA) and the other at the right ventricular apex (RV). Also shown are ECG leads (E) and the battery-control pack (B) for the pacemaker

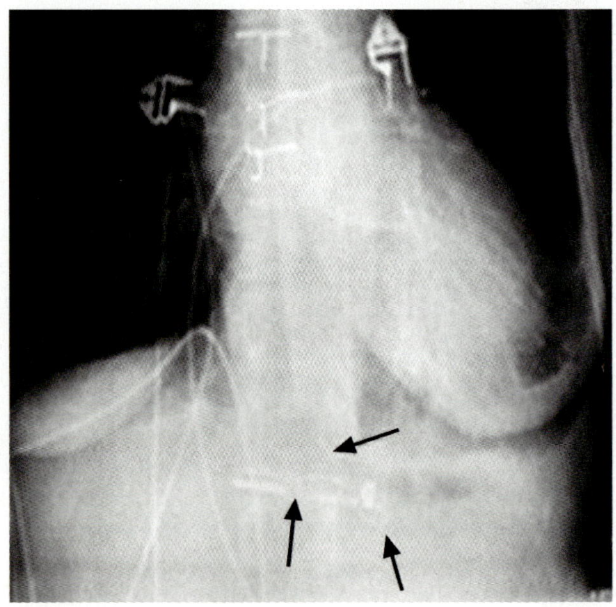

**Fig. 31.49:** Collimated frontal view of the chest shows typical epicardial pacing wires (arrows) coiled on the patient's anterior chest wall after heart surgery

pulse generators. The pacemaker generator (battery pack and control unit) is most commonly placed in the infraclavicular area.

There has been a steady improvement in pacemaker durability and utility. It is now possible for a patient traveling anywhere in the world to phone into his or her physician and have a scheduled periodic evaluation of pacemaker function over the phone. Pacemakers range from simple temporary epicardial electrodes to very

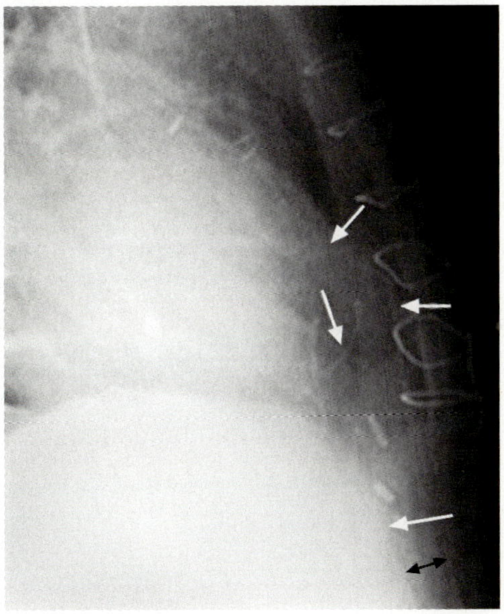

**Fig. 31.50:** Collimated lateral view of the chest shows the same epicardial pacing wires (arrows) as in a. Also shown but not labeled are sternal wires, surgical clips and a central venous catheter

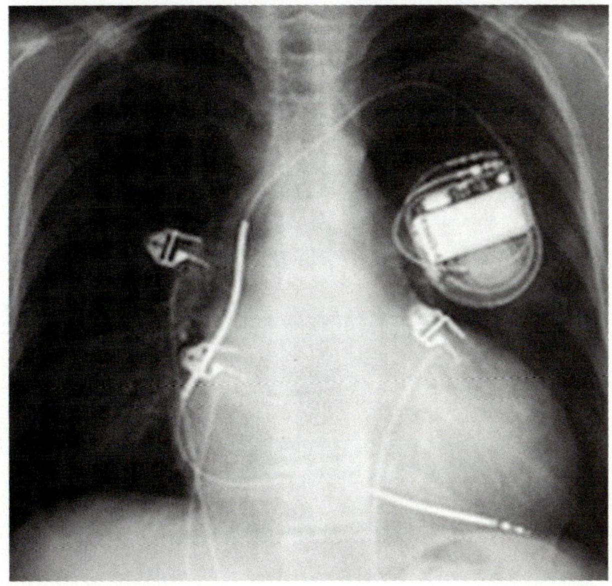

**Fig. 31.52:** Frontal view of the chest shows a typical automatic implantable cardioverter defibrillator

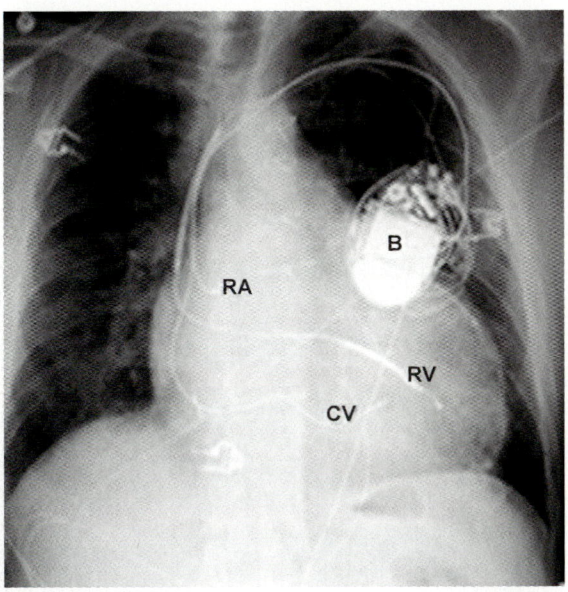


**Fig. 31.51:** Frontal view of the chest shows a combination biventricular pacemaker and an automatic implantable cardioverter defibrillator with a battery pack (B) and right atrial (RA), right ventricular (RV) and coronary venous (CV) leads. Note also the left ventricular calcification from a past myocardial infarction. The coronary venous lead is positioned in a vein draining the posterior inferior wall of the left ventricle, so that it can stimulate functional myocardial tissue rather than the nonfunctioning tissue represented by the ventricular wall calcification and probable myocardial aneurysm

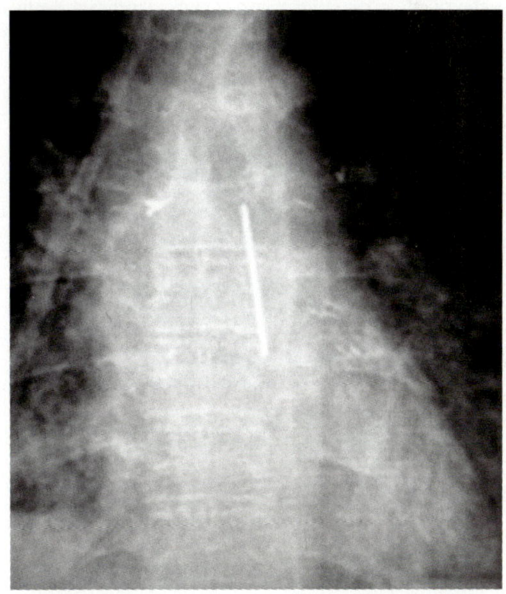

**Fig. 31.53:** Frontal view shows a sternal fixation pin or Kirschner wire. This sternal fixation was used for a patient who underwent lung transplantation in which a 'clamshell' chest incision was made, resulting in a transverse sectioning of the sternum. In this case, the sternum is best stabilized by a vertical fixation wire or pin. Note also the surgical clips overlying the heart and the root of the aorta

complex pacemakers with multiple atrial and ventricular leads. A single-lead intramyocardial pacer electrode may be appropriate in one patient, whereas a right atrial-biventricular synchronous pervenous device is indicated in another. Temporary, easily removable epicardial electrodes are now commonly placed at the time of cardiac surgery for immediate pacemaker access, should the need arise. The leads are simply pulled out through the incision when the patient is discharged from the hospital. Transvenous (pervenous) pacemaker leads are the most commonly used type today and are inserted through the subclavian or jugular vein with use of local anesthesia.

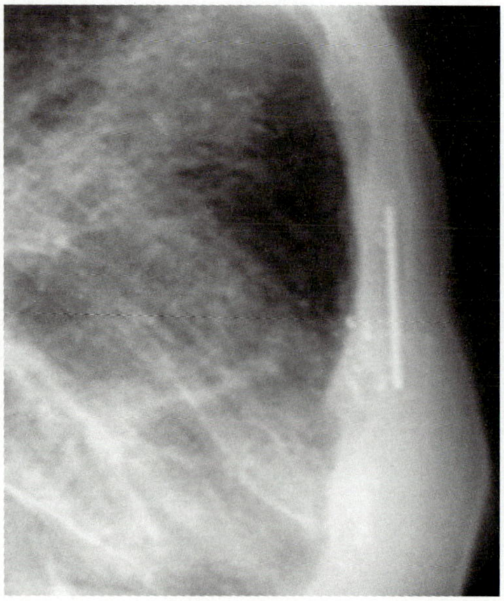

**Fig. 31.54:** Lateral view shows a sternal fixation pin or Kirschner wire. This sternal fixation was used for a patient who underwent lung transplantation in which a 'clamshell' chest incision was made, resulting in a transverse sectioning of the sternum. In this case, the sternum is best stabilized by a vertical fixation wire or pin. Note also the surgical clips overlying the heart and the root of the aorta

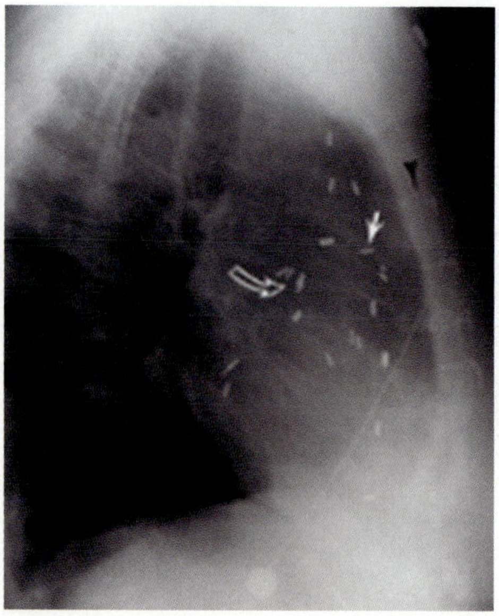

**Fig. 31.56:** Lateral view of the chest shows sternal wires (arrowhead), vascular clips of a saphenous vein bypass graft to the right coronary artery (curved arrow), and those of the left internal mammary graft to the left anterior descending coronary artery (straight arrow)

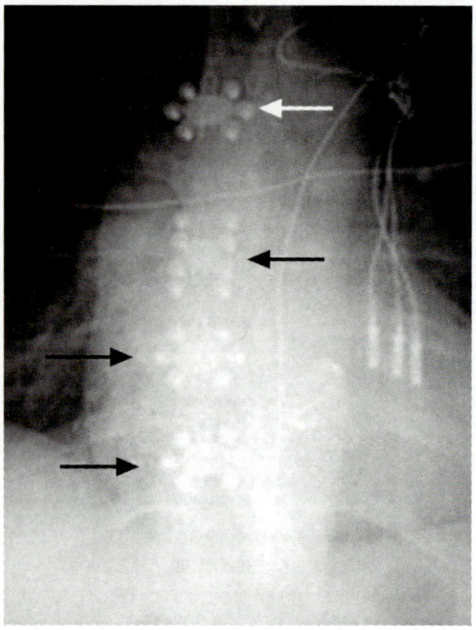

**Fig. 31.55:** Collimated view of a cardiac surgery patient shows a Synthes Maxillofacial Sternal Fixation System (Synthes, Paoli, Pa) (arrows)

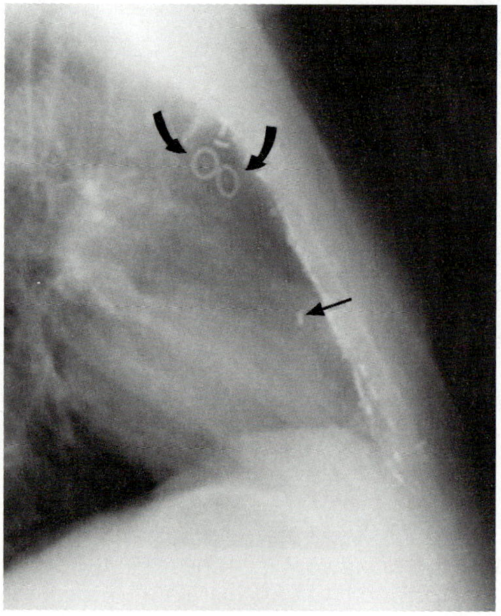

**Fig. 31.57:** Lateral view of the chest shows vascular clips of internal mammary artery bypass grafts (solid arrow) and marker rings on the ascending aorta around the ostia of two saphenous vein bypass grafts (open arrows)

Cardiac resynchronization therapy (CRT) or biventricular pacing is sometimes used to treat severe chronic congestive heart failure. Combined right and left ventricular pacing or left ventricular pacing alone may considerably improve heart function. CRT involves pre-excitation of the left ventricular wall by means of a lead placed in a tributary of the coronary sinus. There is often further benefit to the patient when CRT is combined with an implantable defibrillator, because there is a high risk of sudden death from ventricular tachycardia or ventricular fibrillation in all patients with heart failure. Current CRT usually involves atrial synchronized ventricular pacing to optimize atrioventricular timing with biventricular pacing to promote ventricular synchrony. CRT improves ejection fraction, left ventricular size and mitral regurgitation.

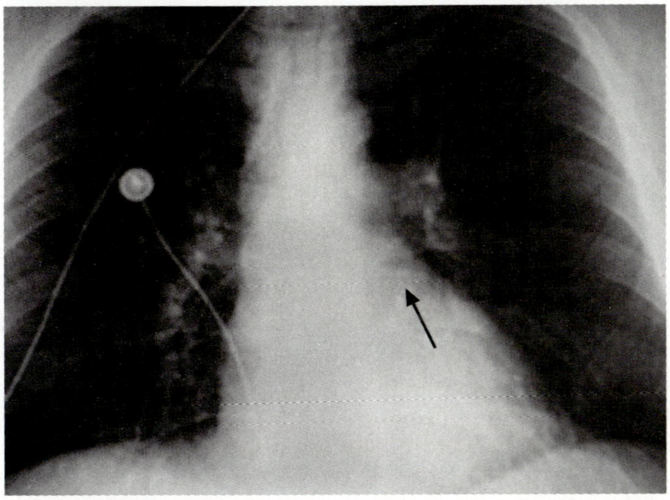

**Fig. 31.58:** Frontal view of the chest shows a left anterior descending coronary artery stent (arrow)

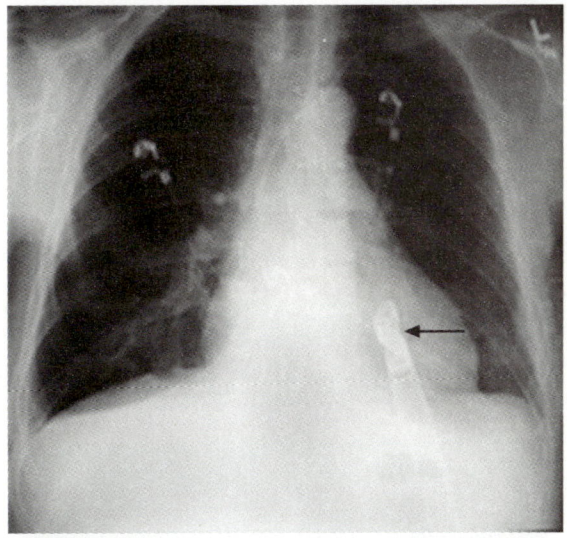

**Fig. 31.60:** Frontal view of the chest shows a thoratec left VAD (arrow)

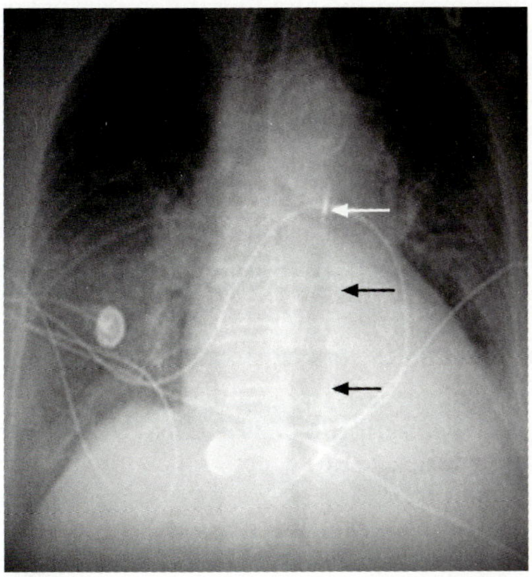

**Fig. 31.59:** Frontal view of the chest shows an intra-aortic counterpulsation balloon used in a patient with heart failure. The balloon (black arrows) is inflated. Usually, only the balloon tip (white arrow) is visible

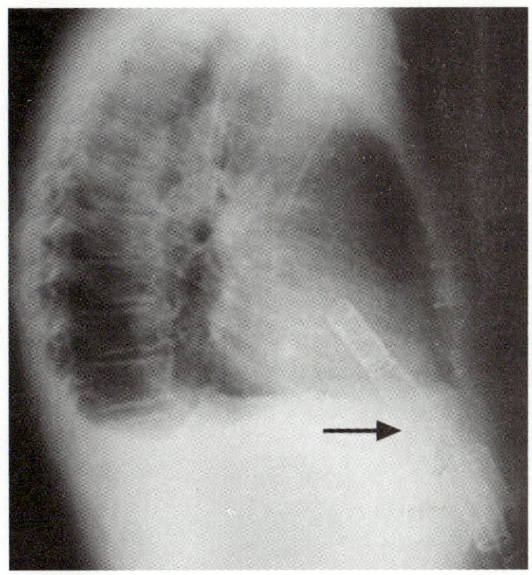

**Fig. 31.61:** Lateral view of the chest shows a thoratec left VAD (arrow)

There are several ways, pacemakers can be placed for left ventricular or biventricular pacing. In some cases, left ventricular epicardial leads are used. The leads go directly to the surface of the left ventricle, and they are usually associated with typical pacing electrodes in the right atrial appendage and right ventricular apex. In other cases, the left ventricular pacing electrodes are introduced through the coronary sinus and wedged into a left ventricular cardiac vein. In these instances, the position of the pacing leads may seem unusual, and detailed knowledge of the coronary venous anatomy is necessary for the radiologist and cardiologist to appreciate the location of the leads.

Because there can be such a wide variation in the proper positioning of pacemaker leads, it is often difficult for the average radiologist to know if a pacemaker is properly positioned. Frequent consultation with the cardiologists and cardiac surgeons in one's own medical center is important to gain familiarity with the pacemakers and therapeutic approaches used by the referring physicians. In this way, complications of pacemaker placement are more readily recognized and brought to the attention of the patient's physicians.

Pacemaker lead fracture is now rarely seen because of improvements in the flexibility of the metal alloys used in electrode construction. Even when they are broken, the ends frequently do not separate, so the radiograph does not show the fracture. Electronic testing has largely replaced radiography to investigate cases of suspected lead malfunction. After being in place for several weeks, pacemaker leads become 'epithelialized' and firmly

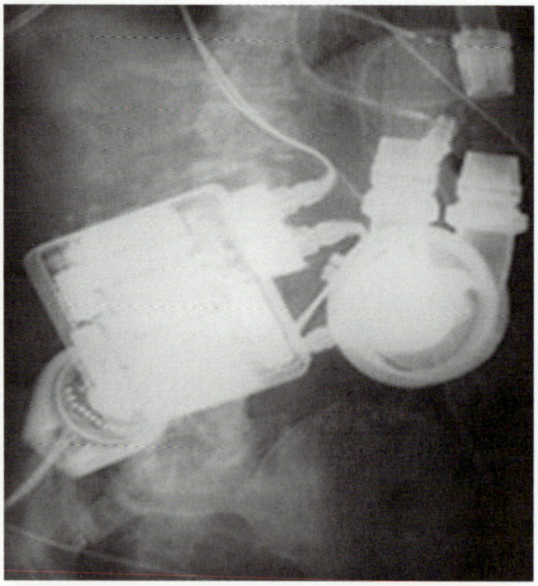

**Fig. 31.62:** Abdominal image shows a HeartMate VAD

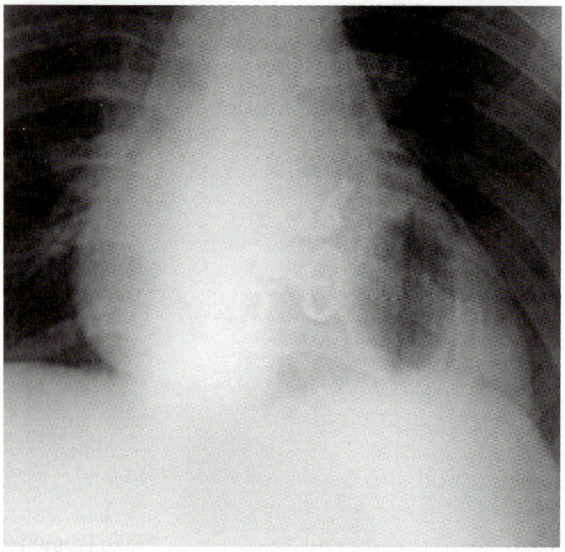

**Fig. 31.63:** Abdominal image shows a Novacor VAD

attached to the myocardial wall. When a pacemaker is changed, the leads are simply cut for removal of the control pack, and they are left in place because they are adherent to the heart. New leads are then placed with the new pacemaker. If a patient has had his or her pacemaker changed a number of times, there is often a bewildering array of wires about the heart. In this circumstance, it can be impossible to trace the currently functioning pacemaker leads back to the pacemaker battery pack. On rare occasion, a central venous catheter may interfere with a pacemaker lead.

The safety of magnetic resonance (MR) imaging studies for patients with cardiac pacemakers is an important matter and is subject to much discussion. Many radiologists and cardiologists consider MR imaging to be contraindicated for patients with a cardiac pacemaker. This approach is the safest, but it may not always be in the best interest of a patient with a cardiac pacemaker who needs an MR imaging study. There are circumstances in which a patient with a pacemaker may undergo MR imaging, especially if a 0.5 T unit is used. It may also be safe to perform MR imaging with an extremity system for patients with cardiac pacemakers and implantable cardioverter defibrillator systems. It must be emphasized that MR imaging should be performed on patients with a pacemaker or similar device only after the patient has been cleared for the study by his or her physicians. Such a study should be performed in a medical center with experienced staff who are able to monitor the patient before, during, and after the MR imaging study as well as treat any problems that arise from the study. MR imaging is generally safe for patients who have artificial heart valves, who have undergone coronary artery surgery, or who have retained epicardial pacemaker leads after cardiac surgery.

The automatic implantable cardioverter defibrillator (AICD or ICD) is a common cardiac device designed for both patient monitoring and therapy in case of ventricular tachycardia or fibrillation. The early AICD designs consisted of two shocking electrodes, two sensing electrodes, and a generator implanted in the abdominal wall. The new designs are completely different, consisting of various combinations of sensing and shocking electrodes. They are frequently combined with a pacemaker as a bundled system for the patient, treating both the patient's established arrhythmia and also acting as a fail-safe system should ventricular fibrillation or ventricular tachycardia occur.

### Coronary Artery Surgery and Stents

Since 1967, when the first aortocoronary saphenous vein bypass graft was performed, direct myocardial revascularization has gained wide acceptance. Revascularization techniques include CABG surgery, coronary artery angioplasty, and coronary artery stent placement. CABG surgery is probably the most common cardiac surgical procedure performed in adults. Until recently, CABG surgery was the primary surgical technique for treating coronary artery disease. Now, it is competing with coronary artery angioplasty and stent placement as well as improved noninterventional medical treatments for coronary artery disease. CABG surgery has been refined over the years and varies from center to center, which is reflected in the variety of devices seen in the postoperative chest radiographs of these patients. Median sternotomy is the usual surgical approach for CABG surgery, and sternal wires the common method of fixation of the two sternal segments. Vascular clips are used to occlude tributary branches of saphenous vein grafts and anterior intercostal branches of the internal mammary arteries. There may be a few clips or a great many, depending on the number and types of grafts used. Some surgeons place markers on the adventitia of the ascending aorta to indicate the proximal anastomoses of the bypass grafts. These markers, which facilitate subsequent graft angiography, vary considerably from center to center and even from surgeon to surgeon.

In many cases, CABG surgery has been supplanted by coronary artery angioplasty and stent placement. At present, almost 90% of coronary interventions include stent placement. Coronary artery stent placement was introduced in 1964 by Dotter and Judkins and has been in regular clinical use since the end of the 1980s. The objectives of coronary artery stent placement are to improve on the results of coronary artery balloon angioplasty, to reduce the occurrence of coronary artery restenosis, and to treat an acute or threatened closure of a coronary artery.

Before 1997, only two coronary artery stents were approved for clinical use in the United States—the Gianturco-Roubin I (Cook, Bloomington, Ind) and the Palmaz-Schatz (Johnson and Johnson, Warren, NJ). By 2002, over 40 stent designs were used in clinical practice. Many more are under investigation, including drug-coated stents.

Based on their method of expansion, coronary artery stents are divided into three groups—balloon expandable (most frequently used), self-expandable and thermally expandable. Most stents are composed of 316L stainless steel. Alternative stent designs have also incorporated nitinol, gold, tantalum and other metals. They must maintain elasticity, radial strength, biocompatibility and corrosion resistance. At present, the approved coronary artery stents range in size from 2.0–5.0 mm in diameter and 8.0–38.0 mm in length to accommodate the size of the target vessel. Stents of different designs have variable strut thickness. In addition to improvement in stent design and delivery technologies, further development includes covered stents, biodegradable stents and drug-delivery stents. Stent selection is determined by a variety of factors, including operator familiarity with the stent, lesion morphology and location and balloon delivery system characteristics. Complications associated with coronary artery stents are stent thrombosis and restenosis.

## Circulatory Assist Devices

The high mortality from cardiogenic shock continues to spur efforts to develop mechanical support for the circulatory system. It is estimated that 100,000 patients in the United States could benefit from heart transplantation. However, only 2,000 donor hearts are available each year. Most devices currently available provide temporary assistance until the damaged heart can recover or until a donor heart becomes available for transplantation. Most mechanical support for patients with heart failure consists of devices that assist the heart without replacing it (Figs 31.64–31.69).

Mechanical cardiac assist devices can be divided into three groups—(a) temporary cardiac assist devices, (b) permanent cardiac assist devices and (c) heart replacement devices. Examples of short-term cardiac assist devices are the intra-aortic balloon pump and newer left VADs, such as the TandemHeart (Cardiac Assist, Inc, Pittsburgh, Pa). The Biventricular System 5000 short-term VAD (ABIOMED, Danvers, Mass), e.g. is approved by the US Food and Drug Administration for treating postcardiotomy shock and as a bridge to either heart transplantation or implantation of a long-term device. It consists of two disposable, dual-chamber, extracorporeal blood pumps connected by transcutaneous cannulas to a console. This pump fills passively and ejects actively.

The intra-aortic counterpulsations balloon device (also known as IACB, IAB, IABP, IAC and IACD) is used to support the circulation after cardiac surgery or an acute myocardial infarction until the heart recovers adequate function of its own. The device consists of an inflatable balloon approximately 25 cm long mounted on a catheter, which is introduced via a femoral artery. The tip of the catheter is placed just distal to the left subclavian artery in the descending thoracic aorta.The balloon is inflated with

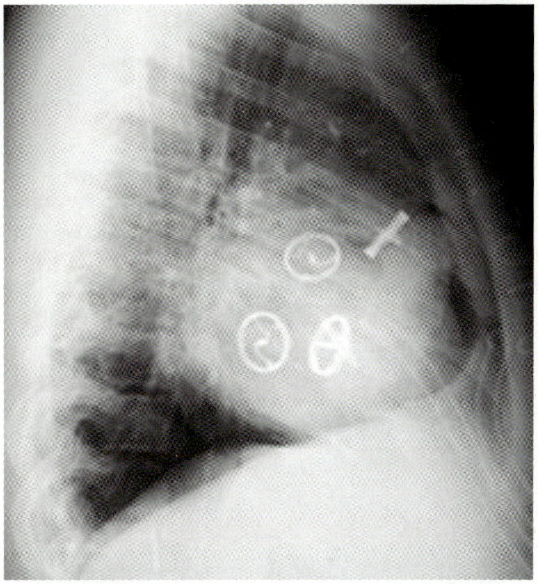

**Fig. 31.64:** Cropped frontal view of the chest shows a CardioWest total artificial heart. Note the four prosthetic valves and the two coil, reinforced polyurethane tubes carrying pulses of compressed air to the two artificial ventricles

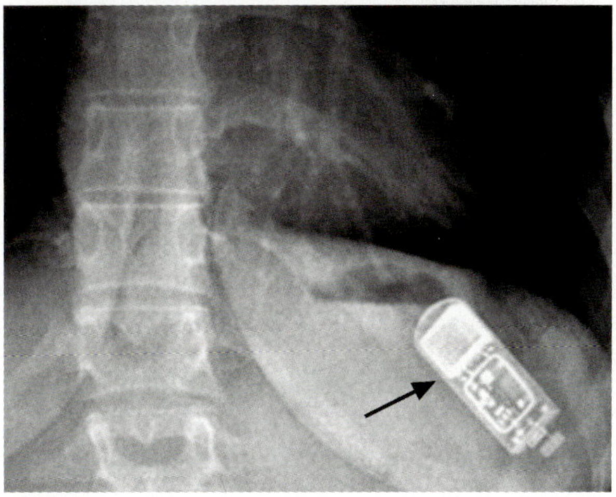

**Fig. 31.65:** Collimated frontal view of the chest shows an implantable loop recorder (arrow) in the left breast of a 25-year-old woman with a history of heart palpitations and surgical repair of a tetralogy of Fallot as a young child

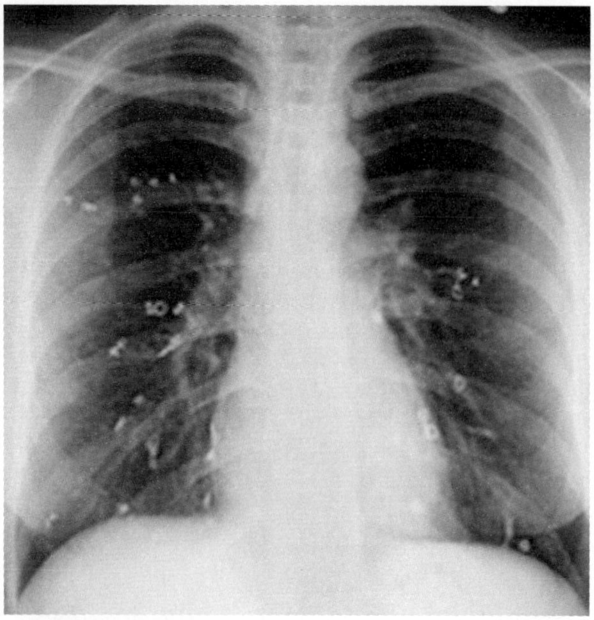

**Fig. 31.66:** Frontal view of the chest of a patient with hereditary hemorrhagic telangiectasia (Osler-Weber-Rendu disease) shows numerous coils, which had been used in multiple coil embolizations to treat repeated bouts of significant hemoptysis

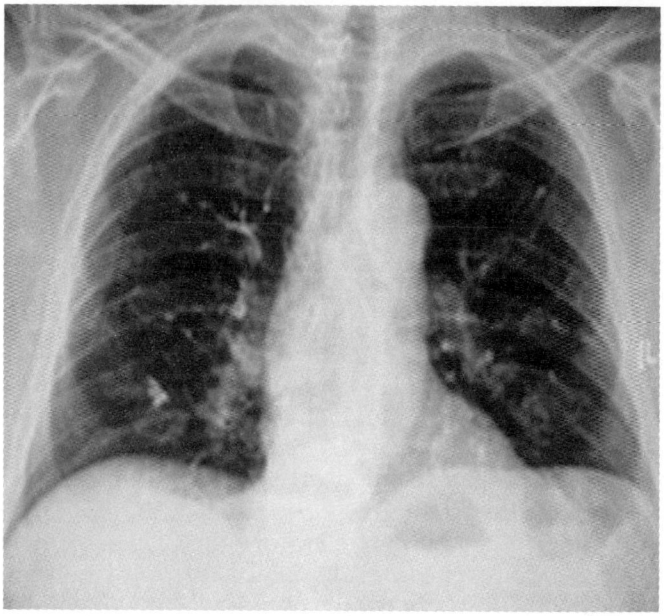

**Fig. 31.68:** Frontal views of the chest in a patient who had undergone vertebroplasty. The vertebroplasty material extruded from the vertebrae and entered the spinal venous system with ultimate embolization to the patient's lungs. The patient suffered no known sequelae

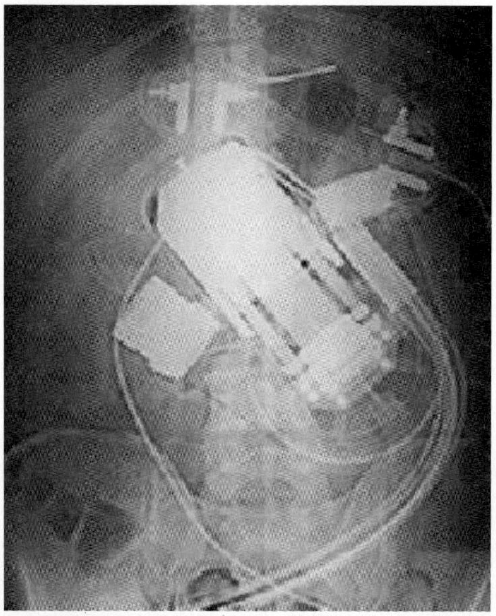

**Fig. 31.67:** Abdominal image shows a Novacor VAD

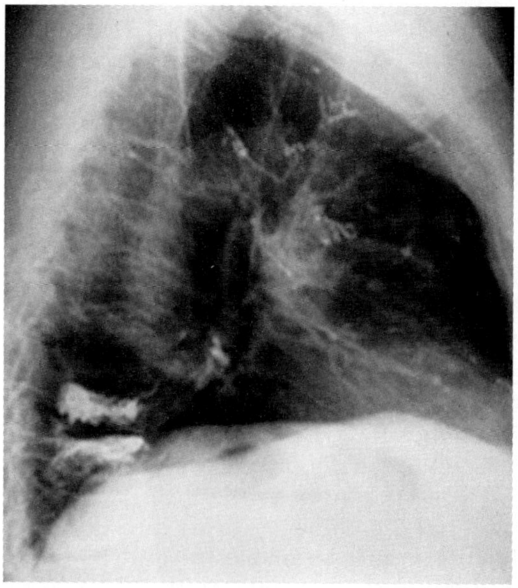

**Fig. 31.69:** Lateral views of the chest in a patient who had undergone vertebroplasty. The vertebroplasty material extruded from the vertebrae and entered the spinal venous system with ultimate embolization to the patient's lungs. The patient suffered no known sequelae

gas (carbon dioxide) during ventricular diastole to augment diastolic coronary artery perfusion and to reduce left ventricular afterload. This technique improves cardiac function by both increasing the oxygenation and decreasing the work requirements of the myocardium.

The mainstays of mechanical support for patients with severe congestive heart failure are VADs. These devices are mechanical pumps used for temporary or permanent blood circulation support. They can be used for a single right or left ventricle or for both ventricles. The left VADs are used in patients with end-stage heart failure, as a bridge to transplantation, but they may also be used as a destination therapy. These devices have been in clinical use since 1984. The HeartMate (Thoratec Corp, Pleasanton, Calif) became the first left VAD that was FDA-approved as a bridge to transplantation and for treating reversible cardiogenic shock. The newer, vented-electric HeartMate device is powered by an internal electric motor. This device has been in use since 1991. The HeartMate blood pump is a flexible polyurethane diaphragm within a titanium shell. The woven Dacron inflow and outflow cannulas each contain a 25-mm caged porcine xenograft valve.

Another left VAD is the Novacor pump (Novacor Corp, Oakland, Calif), which is implanted in the subcutaneous tissue of the left upper abdomen with power lines and sensors exiting *via* the right lower quadrant to connect with a control console. The pump takes blood through a Dacron conduit from the apex of the left ventricle and pumps it via another Dacron conduit to the aorta. Both the HeartMate and Novacor devices have a demonstrated durability for periods more than 2 years. Other similar or developing VADs include the Jarvik 2000 left VAD (Jarvik Heart, Inc. New York, NY), the MicroMed DeBackey VAD (MicroMed Technology, Inc, Houston, Tex), the HeartMate II and HeartMate III, the Incor (Berlin Heart, Hamburg, Germany), and the Terumo (Terumo Medical Corp, Somerset, NJ). The risks associated with implantation of a VAD include post-operative hemorrhage, sepsis, thromboembolism, renal failure, technical failure and neurologic sequelae. It is extremely important to note if any central venous catheter is near the tricuspid prosthetic valve of a VAD or total artificial heart. If a catheter becomes entangled in the valve, it can cause malfunction of the valve, which will in turn stop venous return to the heart, rapidly endangering the patient's life.

The total artificial heart requires removal of the native heart. It serves as a bridge to cardiac transplantation, but occasionally, it becomes the patient's permanent circulatory support for the rest of his or her life. The Jarvik 7 was the first attempt at an implantable artificial heart, but the recipient patients were completely hospital bound and suffered major complications. Other artificial hearts include the CardioWest (SynCardia Systems, Inc. Tucson, Ariz) and the AbioCor implantable replacement heart (ABIOMED. The AbioCor, for example, consists of two blood-pumping chambers; the right supplies blood to the lungs, and the left supplies the blood to the rest of the body. It is made of titanium and Angioflex (a proprietary polyether-based polyurethane plastic), and it is powered in part by an internal battery that can be recharged through the intact skin, obviating external power lines. Permanent implantable artificial hearts may be a reality in the not too distant future, but they still suffer the major hurdles of severe infections and thromboembolism, and their use remains very limited.

### Miscellaneous Devices

From time to time, other medical devices not commonly found at chest radiography may be seen. These devices include embolization coils, remote telemetry ECG monitoring devices, pericardial drainage catheters and left atrial catheters (Fig. 31.70). An interesting new device is the insertable (implantable) loop recorder, which is used for prolonged monitoring of the cardiac rhythm. It is a small electronic device implanted in the left pectoral region, and it can provide more than a year of continuous monitoring

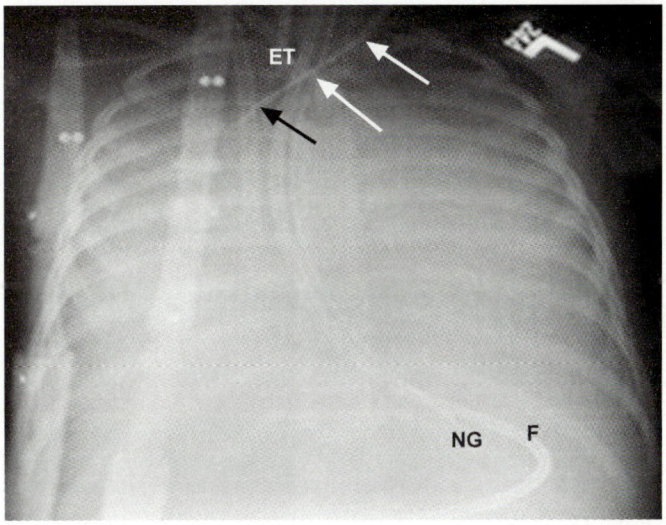


**Fig. 31.70:** Portable chest radiograph of a patient undergoing extracorporeal membrane oxygenation shows pulmonary edema in the lungs and the tubing going to the patient's right carotid artery and right jugular vein. Also seen are an endotracheal tube (ET), a right internal jugular vein catheter (black arrow), a left internal jugular vein catheter (white arrows), a nasogastric tube (NG), and a feeding tube (F)

that may be activated by the patient or automatically activated. It has a variety of uses including monitoring of patients with unexplained syncopal episodes and assessment of patients with atrial fibrillation, ventricular arrhythmias, or conduction disturbances.

Sometimes, unexpected neck, abdomen and spinal apparatus may be visible at chest radiography. Such objects include tracheostomy tubes; voice prostheses; neck drainage catheters; cervical, thoracic, or lumbar spine fixation apparatus; temperature monitoring catheters in the hypopharynx or esophagus; vagus nerve stimulators; abscess and biliary drainage catheters in the abdomen; umbilical arterial and venous catheters; and transjugular intrahepatic portosystemic shunts (TIPS) in the liver. Vertebroplasty is not uncommon, and in some medical centers extracorporeal membrane oxygenation apparatus may be seen in premature infants and other patients with severe heart and lung disease. Most of these devices have nothing to do with the cardiovascular or pulmonary structures in the chest, but they happen to overlie the chest or be visible on chest images, because they lie contiguous to the thorax in the neck, spine or upper abdomen. Recognizing and evaluating such apparatus is just as important as recognizing and evaluating apparatus primarily designed for the chest.

## EMERGENCY ECHOCARDIOGRAPHY (Transthoracic, Transesophageal, Doppler and Color-Doppler Echocardiography)

Point-of-care echocardiography using portable machines is an exciting development in emergency medicine (Figs 31.71–31.91 and Table 31.1). Recent improvements in

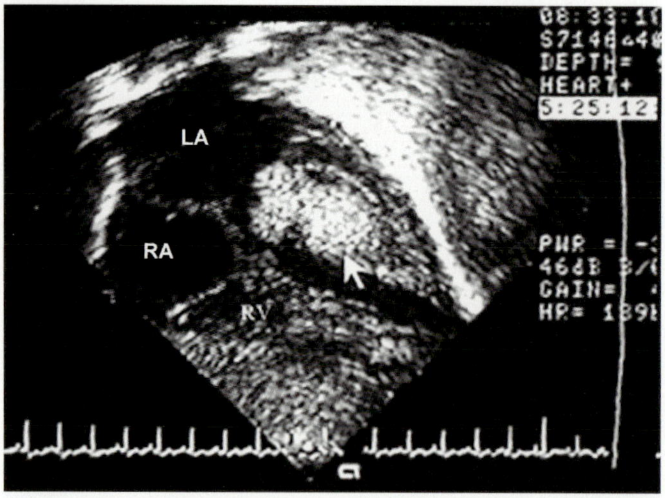


**Fig. 31.71:** Echocardiographic subcostal view of a patient with a large mass within the left ventricular cavity invading or connected to the anterior mitral valve leaflet. Mass within the left ventricle fills most of the ventricular cavity. LA=left atrium; RA=right atrium; RV=right ventricle; Arrow=left ventricular mass

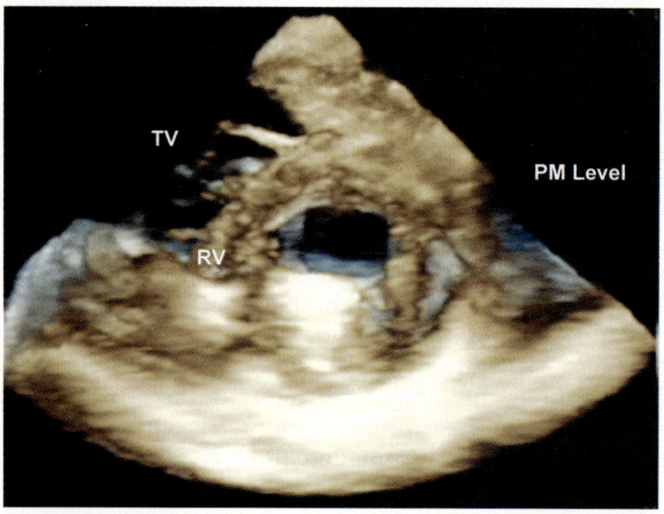


**Fig. 31.72:** 3D reconstruction of TEE view showing tumor mass occupying most of the right ventricle

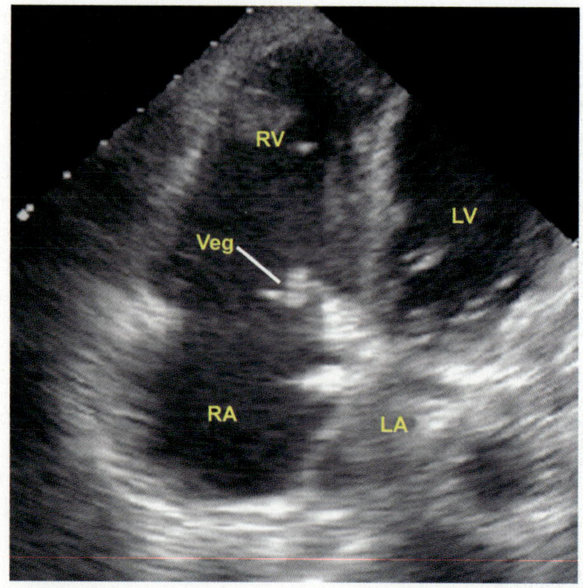


**Fig. 31.73:** Apical 4 C view showing vegetation on tricuspid valve

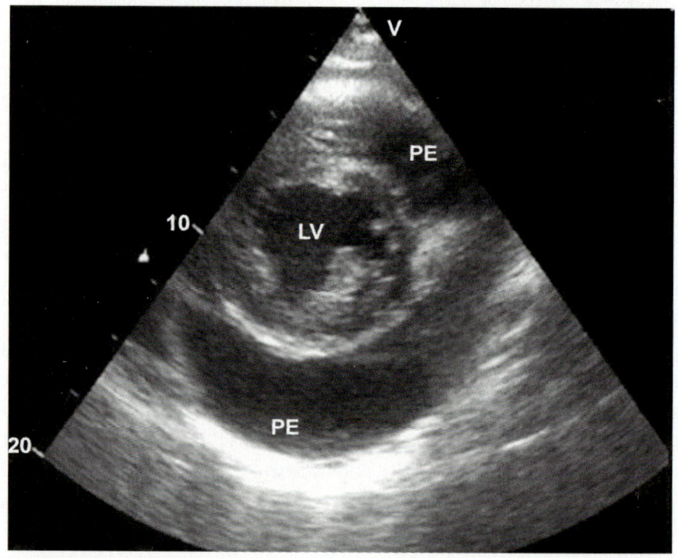


**Fig. 31.74:** Cardiac tamponade in a 50-year-old man with a 3-week history of malaise and dyspnea. Parasternal short-axis echocardiographic view shows a large circumferential pericardial effusion (PE) surrounding the left ventricle (LV)

ultrasound quality mean that emergency physicians are finding echocardiography useful in a variety of clinical settings. Evidence suggests that emergency physicians are able to master the skills of basic echocardiography sufficiently to improve patient care in the resuscitation scenario. Patients with clinical conditions, such as breathlessness, undifferentiated shock, chest pain and cardiac arrest may benefit. There is a steep learning curve involved in acquiring these skills and the specialty needs to take care in the way that its practitioners are accredited and perform echocardiography.

Ever since the birth of echocardiography, 50 years ago, this noninvasive diagnostic tool became a milestone in the clinical evaluation of cardiovascular patients, due to its diagnostic accuracy. Owing to advances in technology, the ultrasonic industry has recently produced hand-held devices (HHD) that are miniaturized, compact and battery-equipped echocardiographic systems. Basic versions of HHD, usually allow only bidimensional imaging and color flow Doppler analysis, but M-Mode visualization, continuous and pulsed wave Doppler imaging, ECG synchronization and other tools have recently been integrated in better-equipped HHD. These machines could offer some advantages compared with standard echocardiographic devices (SED), due to their simplicity of use, immediate availability at the patient's bedside, transportability and relatively low cost.

The potential usefulness of HHD has been successfully assessed in a wide range of clinical conditions. HHD has been reported to improve detection of relevant

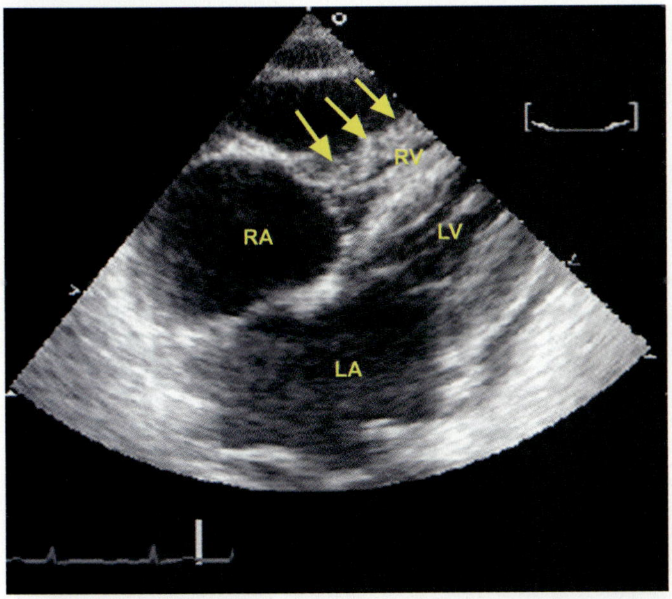


**Fig. 31.75:** Early diastolic collapse of right ventricular free wall (subcostal view) in cardiac tamponade

cardiovascular pathologies or unknown cardiac disorders, and to allow a good assessment of cardiac anatomy and function. Furthermore, they also have been shown to ensure a reliable assessment of left ventricular hypertrophy and abdominal aortic aneurysm. It has also been suggested that internists may use HHD without formal training in echocardiography and after a limited echo-training

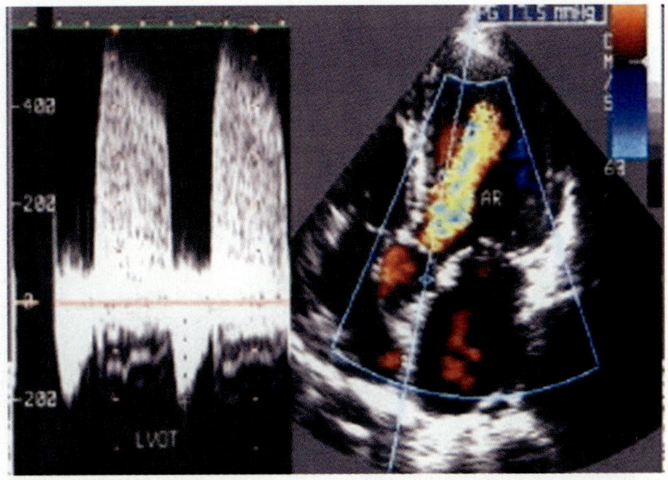


**Fig. 31.76:** Doppler echocardiogram showing aortic regurgitation (upward tracing in left panel) and color-Doppler echocardiogram showing aortic regurgitation (multicolored mosaic jet seen in left ventricle marked AR)

period. In addition, HHD has demonstrated acceptable accuracy during patient transport and in the context of ultrasound-guided pericardiocentesis and thoracentesis. However, HHD seems to have a narrower diagnostic field when compared with SED in the evaluation of critically ill patients.

Based on this evidence, HHD may be expected to become an important additional diagnostic tool during outpatients

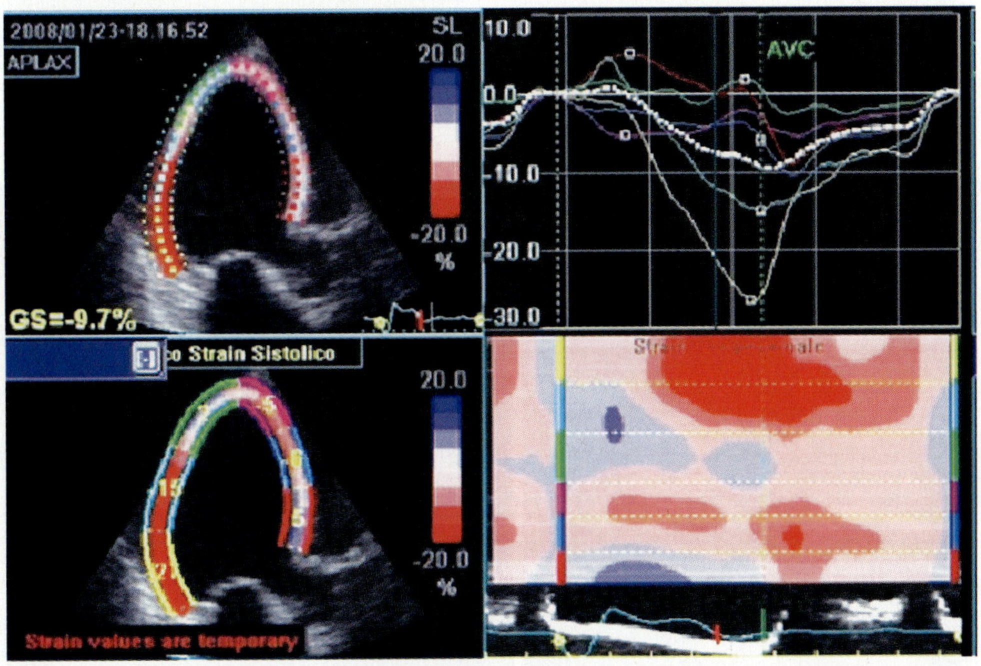


**Fig. 31.77:** Representation of 2D-strain (speckle tracking) of the left ventricle in the apical long axis view in a patient with systolic heart failure. The upper right panel depicts the strain curves sampled in each of the analyzed myocardial segments. It is also possible to calculate a global strain index (GS), which in this case is clearly diminished (GS = 9,7%; see upper left panel). The lower left panel shows peak systolic strain for each segment while the lower right panel shows longitudinal strain processed according to a color map of curvilinear anatomical M-mode. From top to bottom—the basal, mid and apical posterolateral wall, followed by the apical, mid, and basal interventricular anterior septum wall; in red the segments with higher contractility

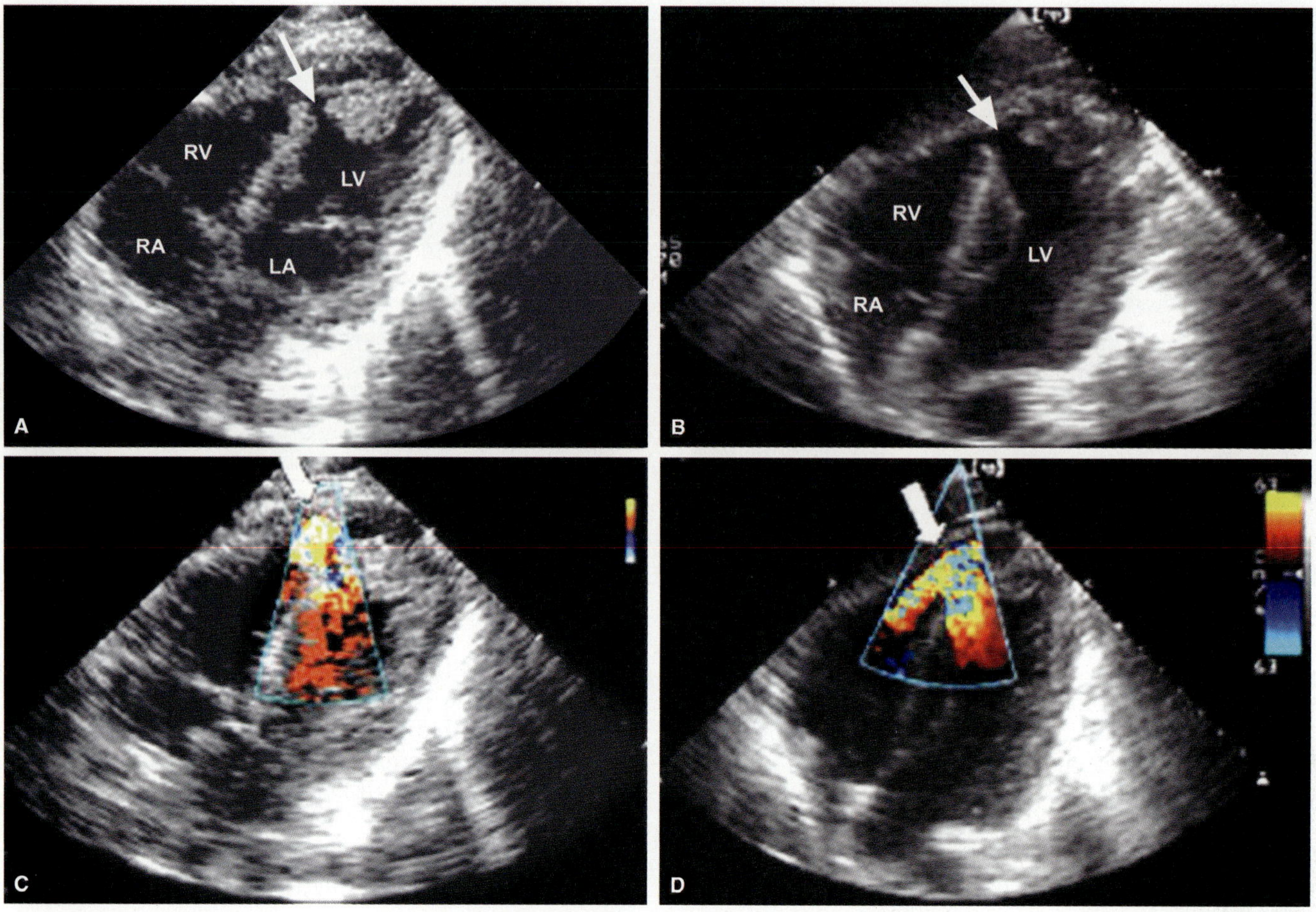


**Fig. 31.78:** Subcostal view in a ventilated patient sustaining severe multisystem trauma and a circulatory failure—(A), (C) using hand-held echocardiography, and (B), (D) using a full-featured echocardiographic platform. Two-dimensional echocardiography in both cases revealed a large ventricular septal defect (A and B, arrow). Color-Doppler mapping confirmed the presence of a large-left-to-right shunt (C and D, arrow). The patient underwent immediate surgical repair, which confirmed the diagnosis. LV=left ventricle; RV=right ventricle; LA=left atrium; RA=right atrium; AO=ascending aorta

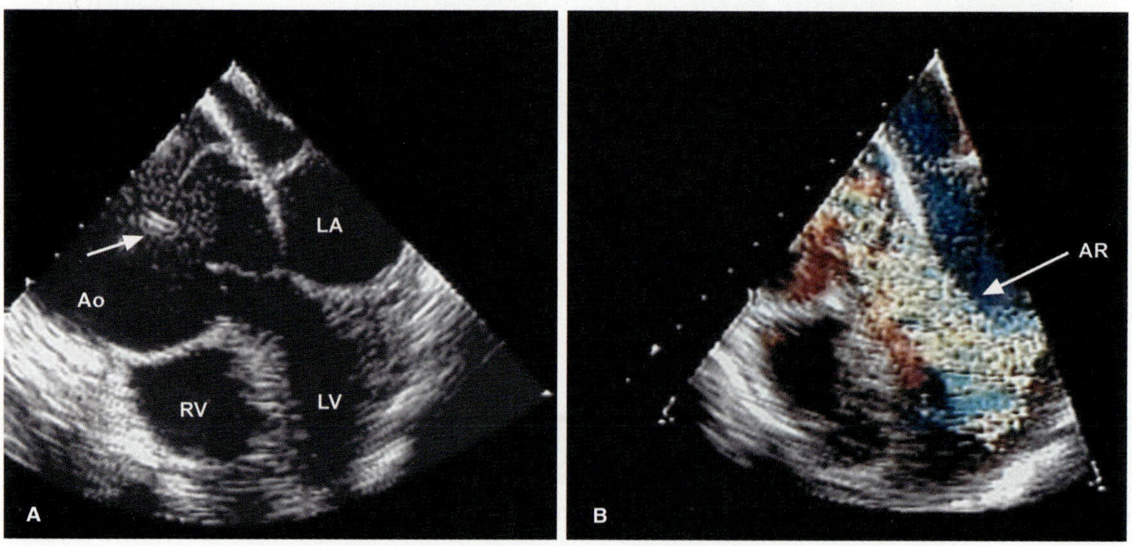


**Fig. 31.79:** Transesophageal still-frame echocardiographic view of a patient with a dilated aorta, aortic dissection, and severe aortic regurgitation. The arrow points to the intimal flap that is seen in the dilated ascending aorta. (A) The long-axis apex-down view of the black-and-white two-dimensional image in diastole. (B) Color-flow imaging that demonstrates a large mosaic jet of aortic regurgitation. AO=aorta; RV=right ventricle; AR=aortic regurgitation

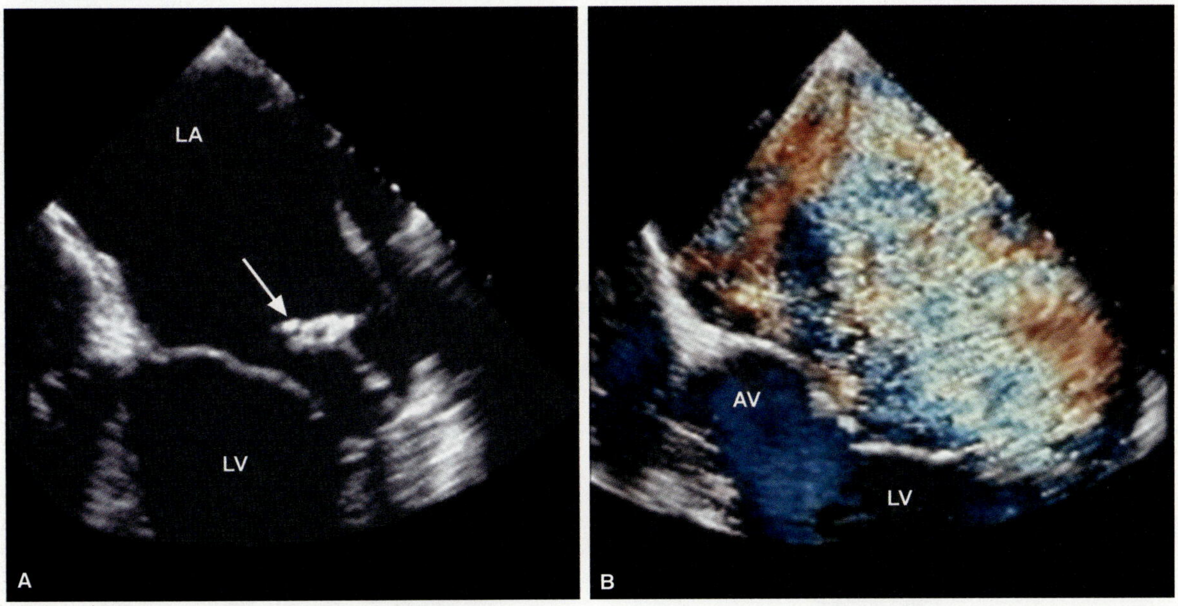


**Fig. 31.80:** (A) Transesophageal echocardiographic view of a patient with severe mitral regurgitation due to a flail posterior leaflet. The arrow points to the portion of the posterior leaflet that is unsupported and moves into the left atrium during systole; (B) color-flow imaging demonstrating a large mosaic jet of mitral regurgitation during systole. LA=left atrium; LV=left ventricle; AV=aortic valve

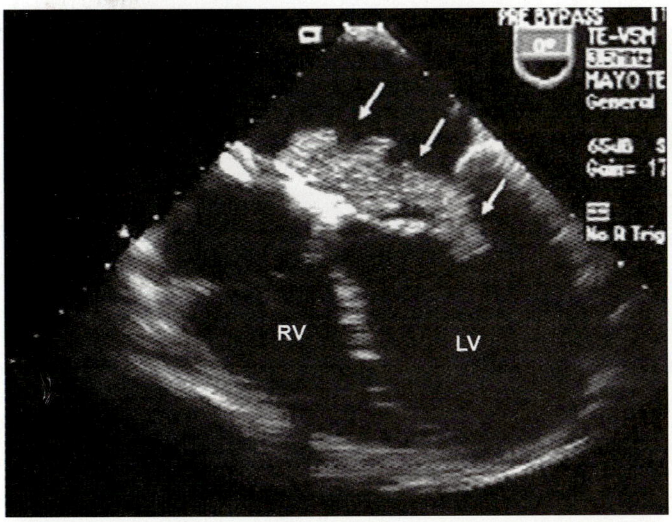


**Fig. 31.81:** Transesophageal still-frame echocardiographic images of a patient with a left atrial myxoma. There is a large echo-dense mass in the left atrium, attached to the atrial septum. The mass moves across the mitral valve in diastole. LV=left ventricle; RV=right ventricle

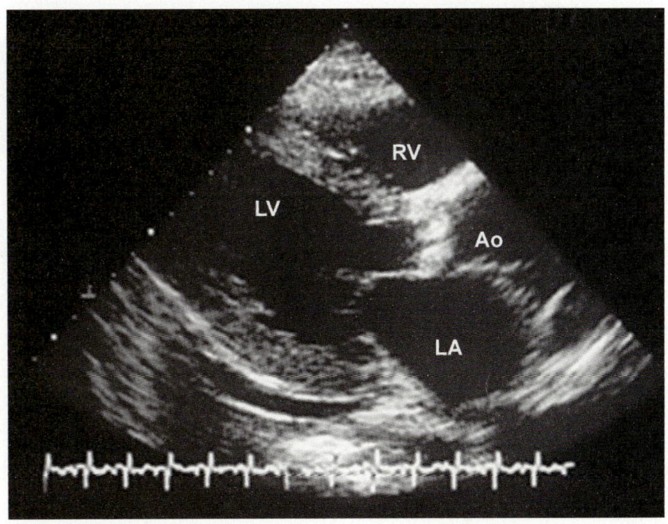


**Fig. 31.82:** Two-dimensional echocardiographic still-frame images from a patient with aortic stenosis. Parasternal long-axis view shows a heavily calcified aortic valve. RV=right ventricle; LV=left ventricle; Ao=aorta; LA=left atrium

cardiologic consulting or in non-cardiologic hospital sections. Nevertheless, the potential role of HHD in these settings has never been investigated.

Patients who present to the emergency department (ED) commonly report chest pain, shortness of breath or dyspnea on exertion. They are often tachycardic or even hypotensive. Unfortunately, history and physical examination alone often lack the sensitivity and specificity to accurately diagnose the underlying aetiology. Focused bedside echocardiography (FBE) is a valuable and increasingly available imaging modality that can be used to better manage these patients. Benefits of FBE include the following:

- Decreases time to diagnosis for pericardial effusions
- Helps diagnose pericardial effusions in cases of pulseless electrical activity
- Helps assess left ventricular function, even with limited views for in the setting of hypotension
- Helps assess volume status and CVP

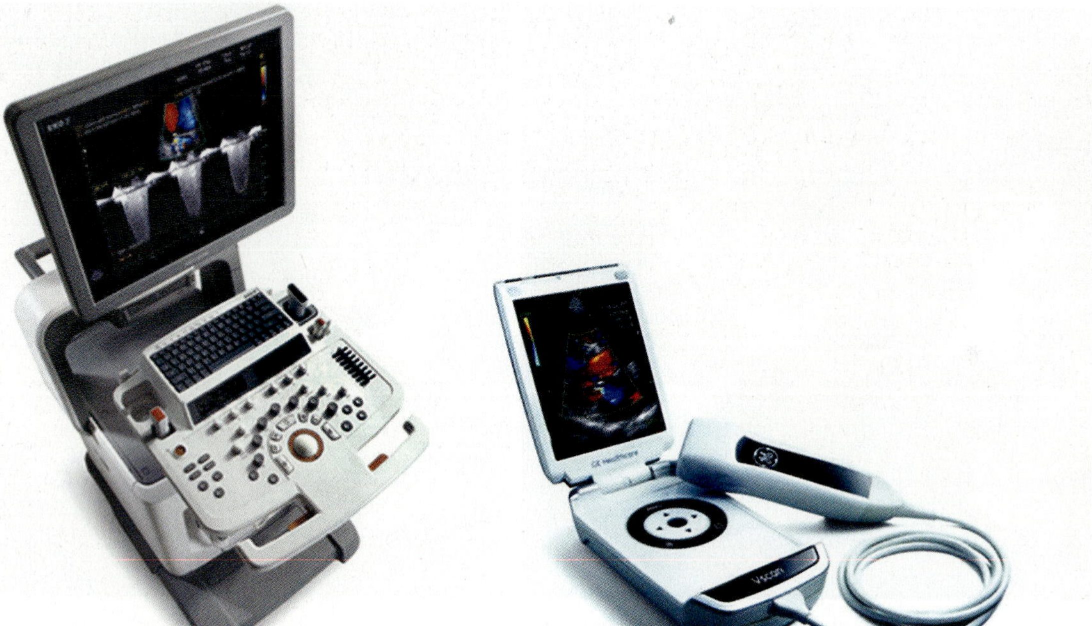

A B

**Fig. 31.83:** Echocardiographic machines which are commonly used in emergency department. (A) Portable, (B) V-Scan hand held echo machine

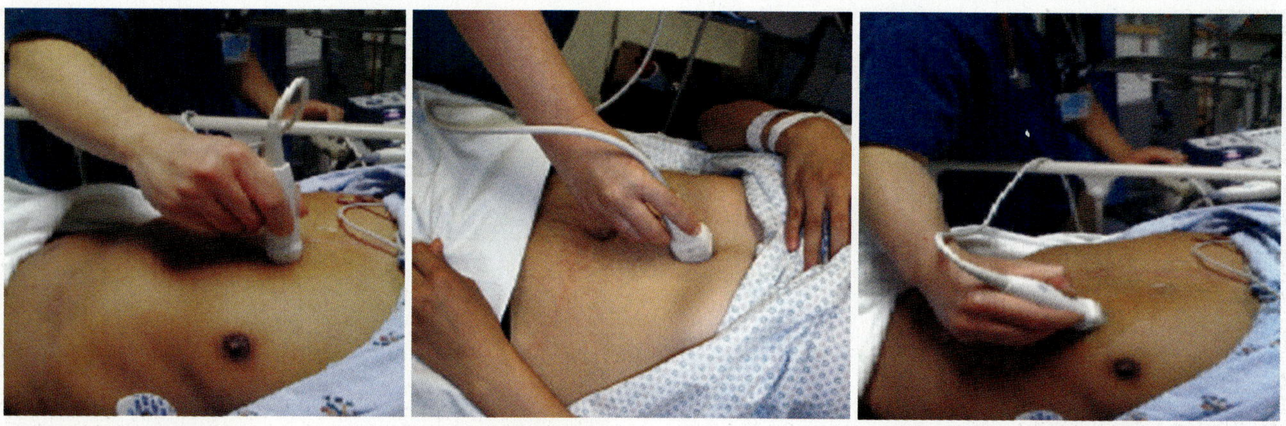

**Fig. 31.84:** Transthoracic approach showing different positions of transducer in obtaining echocardiographic information in emergent situation

- Helps diagnose decompensated congestive heart failure (FBE has been shown in some instances to even be more accurate than chest radiographs. It can be used alone or in conjunction with N-terminal pro-brain-type natriuretic peptide [NT-ProBNP] levels to help differentiate between congestive heart failure [CHF] and chronic obstructive pulmonary disease [COPD] in patients with shortness of breath)
- Helps diagnose deep vein thrombosis (DVT)
- While not sensitive for pulmonary embolism (PE), FBE findings can prompt pursuit of this diagnosis or risk stratify those patients who are found to have PE.
- Can be learned and integrated into clinical practice with limited training
- Can be performed at the bedside to avoid removing critically ill patients from the immediate clinical area.

The components of FBE include the following:

1. Subxiphoid four-chamber view
2. Parasternal long-axis and short-axis views
3. Apical four-chamber view
4. Subxiphoid long-axis view of the inferior vena cava (for assessment of CVP and volume status)
5. Assessment of the internal jugular vein (for assessment of CVP and volume status)
6. Examination of the femoral and popliteal veins (if DVT is suspected).

### Indications

Indications for FBE include the following:

- Any patient presenting with chest pain, shortness of breath or dyspnea on exertion

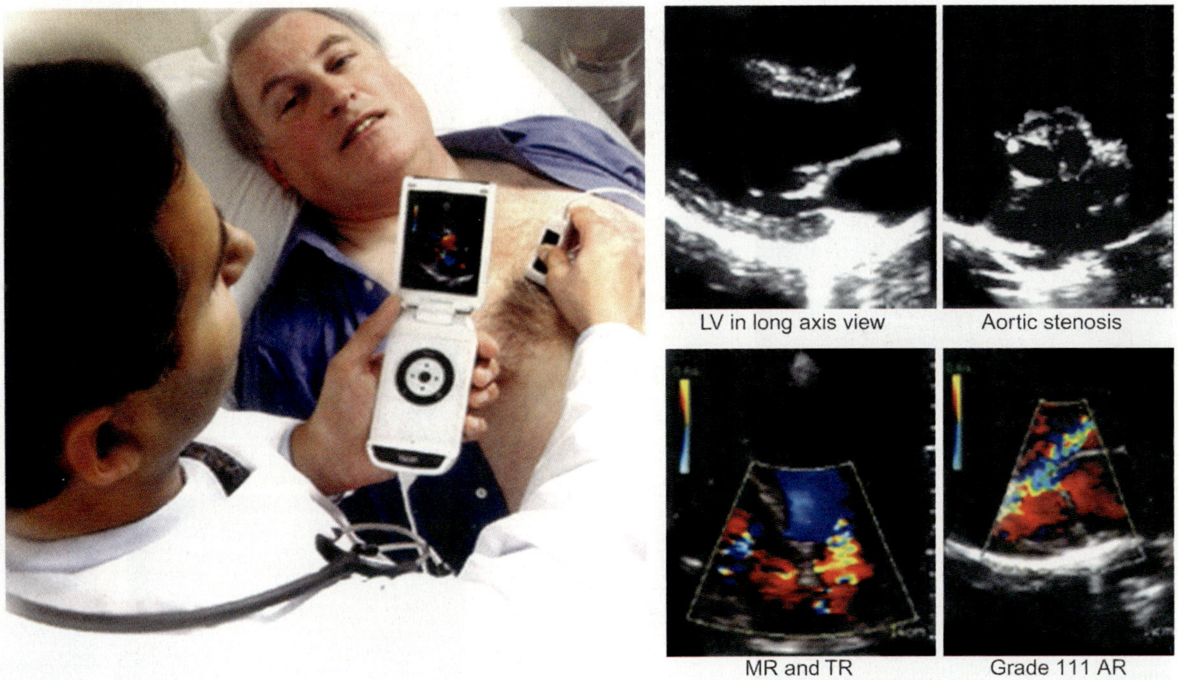


**Fig. 31.85:** Black and white and color flow scans obtained after application of hand held V-Scan technology

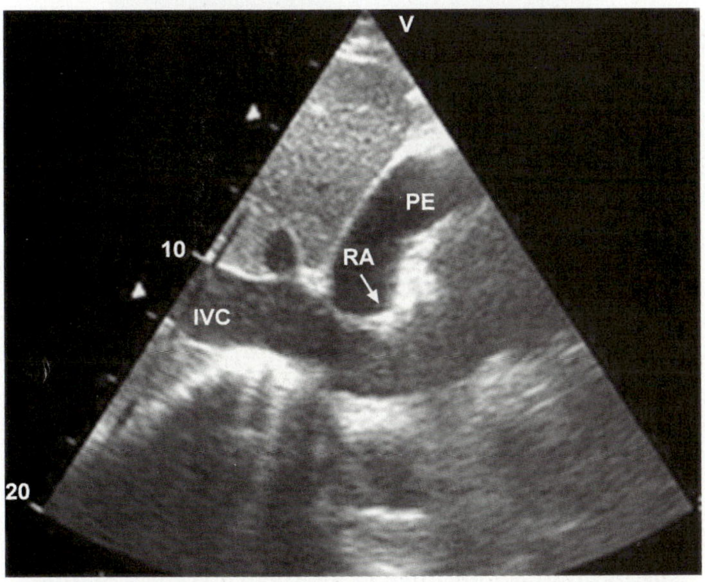


**Fig. 31.86:** Subcostal long-axis echocardiographic view shows diastolic collapse of the right atrium (RA) as well as a dilated and plethoric IVC. PE = pericardial effusion. Cardiac arrest later developed, and the patient required emergent pericardiocentesis

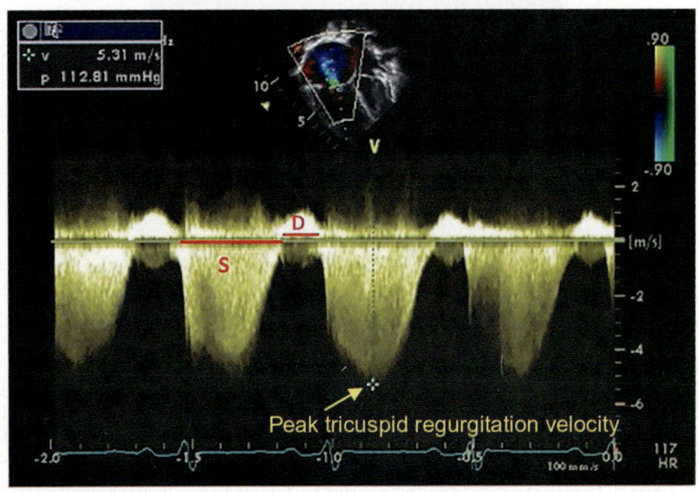


**Fig. 31.87:** Continuous Doppler echo scan shows gross tricuspid regurgitation with transvalvular pressure of 112.81 mmHg indicating severe pulmonary hypertension

- Code or Arrest situations, such as pulseless electrical activity (PEA)
- Suspected left- or right-sided heart failure
- Suspected pulmonary embolism
- Suspected cardiac tamponade
- Unexplained hypertension
- Unexplained hypotension
- Assessment of central venous pressure and volume status

### *Contraindications*

- When emergent interventions such as intubation, fluid resuscitation, or pressors are indicated, FBE should not delay the initiation of such treatment.
- While FBE can be difficult to perform in patients presenting in extremis or during ongoing resuscitations, the information obtained through FBE can be life-saving.

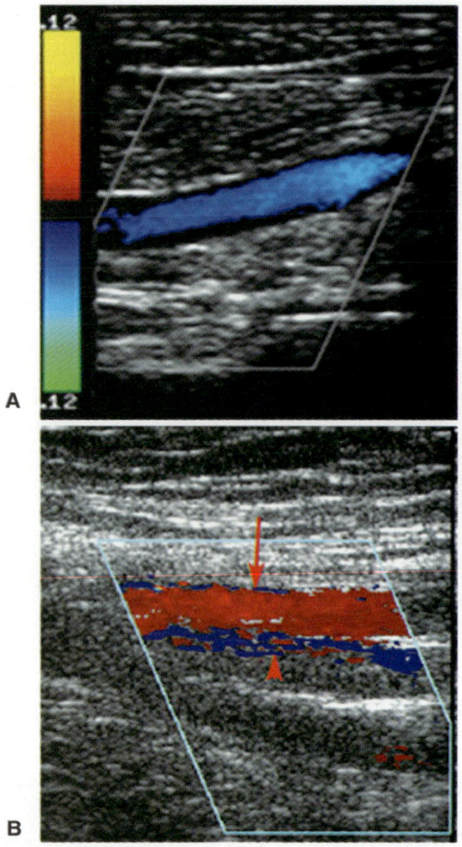

**Fig. 31.88:** (A) Longitudinal color-Doppler demonstrating normal blood flow in a peripheral vein. (B) Longitudinal color-Doppler image with transducer compression applied shows flow in the femoral artery (red arrow) and very minimal flow in the femoral vein (red arrowhead). The femoral vein does not compress with transducer pressure, indicating intraluminal thrombus

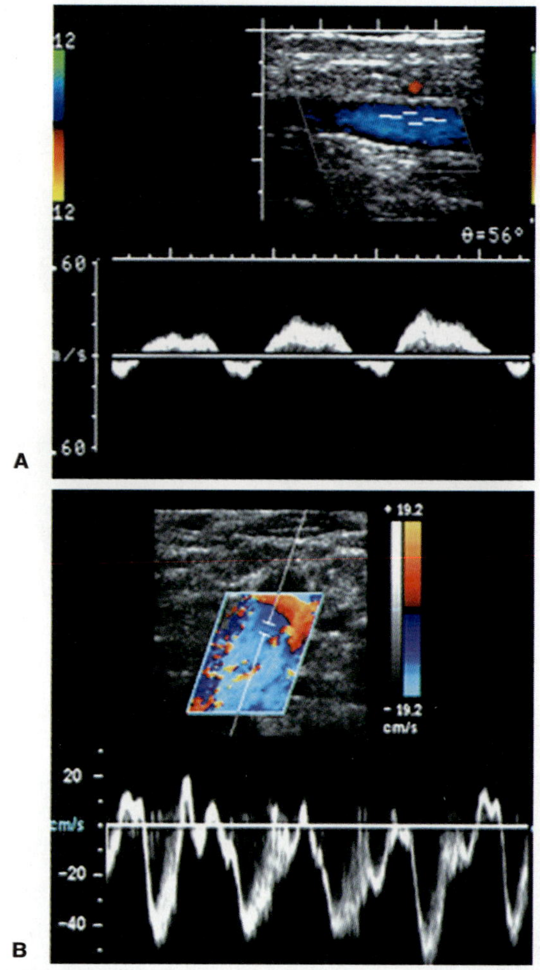


**Fig. 31.89:** (A) A Duplex Doppler demonstrating phasic flow in a normal peripheral vein. (B) Duplex Doppler demonstrating non-phasic flow in a peripheral vein with thrombosis

## Additional Cardiac Ultrasound Indications

*Cardiac ultrasonography for assessment of fluid status and intravascular volume:* The inferior vena cava (IVC) is important to evaluate because it can provide an assessment of the patient's fluid status and right atrial pressures.

- Measure the IVC diameter in both inspiration and expiration.
- The IVC should collapse with inspiration in the normal patient.
- The collapse index is obtained using the IVC diameter measurements in inspiration and expiration.

$$\text{Collapse index} = \frac{\text{Exp diameter} - \text{Insp diameter}}{\text{Exp diameter}} \times 100\%$$

  « A collapse index >50% suggests right atrial pressures < 10 mmHg, whereas a collapse index <50% suggests right atrial pressures >10 mmHg.

- A low collapse index (and, thus, elevated right atrial pressures) correlates with potentially life-threatening pathology, such as decompensated left heart failure, tamponade, tension pneumothorax, and massive pulmonary embolism (PE) causing right heart failure.
- Other possibilities include primary pulmonary hypertension, end-stage COPD and cor pulmonale and pulmonary fibrosis.
- Some clinicians consider the collapse index to be a bit cumbersome and prefer a more qualitative approach whereby the percent of collapse of the IVC with inspiration is indicative of a patient's volume status.
- A complete collapse of the IVC with inspiration is considered evidence of low CVP (<5 cm), a collapse of <50% is considered evidence of elevated CVP (>10 cm), and an increase in size of the IVC with inspiration is considered evidence of normal CVP (5–10 cm).
- Using this method, emergency physicians have over 80% correlation with formal echocardiography among patients with fluid overload, which is especially important among patients in whom the cause of dyspnea may not be obvious (e.g. patient with COPD and CHF).
- For those clinicians who prefer a more quantitative approach to fluid assessment with IVC measurements, the IVC diameter/aorta diameter (ICV/AO) index appears to be another option.

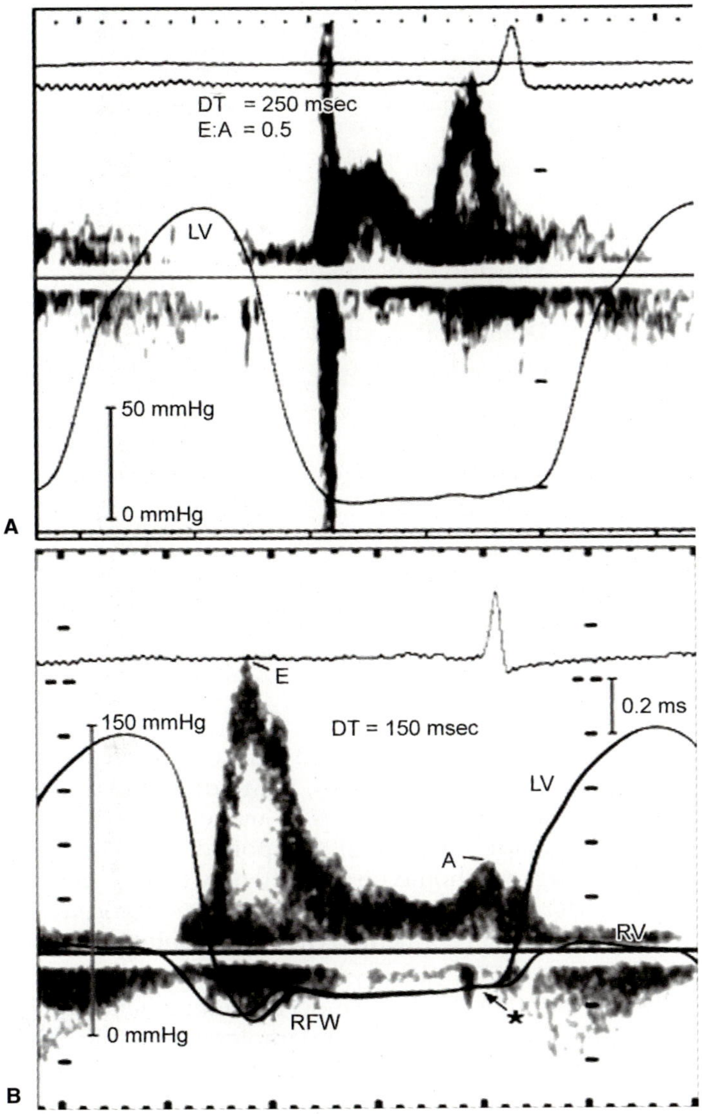


**Fig. 31.90:** High-fidelity left ventricular (LV) pressure curves superimposed on a mitral inflow velocity curve obtained by Doppler echocardiography. The ratio of early and late diastolic flows is termed the E:A ratio. The deceleration time (DT) measures the rate of decline of early velocity and reflects the effective operative compliance of the left ventricle. (A) In early stages of diastolic dysfunction, there is an abnormality of relaxation. There is a decrease in the early diastolic filling and an increase with filling at atrial contraction, resulting in a low E:A ratio of 0.5, with deceleration time (DT) of 250 ms. In this instance, the LV diastolic pressure is low at 6 mmHg. (B) As diastolic dysfunction progresses, there is a restriction to filling, in which there is a high early diastolic velocity and low velocity at atrial contraction resulting in a high E:A ratio of 3.0, with DT of 150 ms. In this instance, the LV diastolic pressure is markedly elevated to 34 mmHg

- The aorta diameter correlates with body surface area (BSA), age and sex, thus allowing for a more patient-specific assessment of fluid status.
- Furthermore, this allows providers to use the maximal IVC diameter without having to particularly time measurements relative to the respiratory cycle, which can be difficult in patients with severe dyspnea.

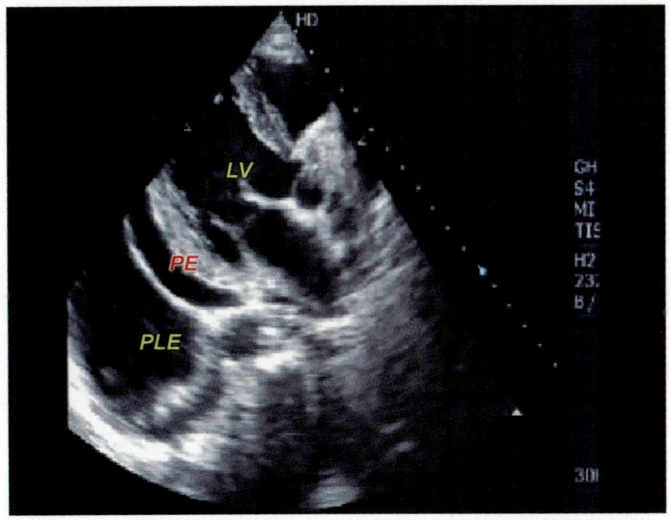


**Fig. 31.91:** Echo scan showing both pericardial and pleural effusions in patient with cardiac failure. PLE=pleural efusion and PE=pericardial effusion

- An IVC/AO index of 1.2 is normal. The index is lower in patients who are dehydrated and higher in patients with intravascular fluid overload.

*Cardiac ultrasonography for assessment of left ventricular function:* Left ventricular function can be assessed in several ways.

- The simplest and probably most effective method is to visualize the endocardial border and estimate the ejection fraction (EF) based on the change in left ventricle size between diastole and systole. Operators can then characterize the EF as 'normal' (>50% change) or 'diminished' (decreased movement of the left ventricular walls and only a small change in left ventricle size between diastole and systole).
- While this method may seem too simple, some emergency physicians find it to be easier to perform with limited training, and it has been shown to be as good as more quantitative methods in the evaluation of patients in the ED. In fact, several studies looking at emergency physicians' sonography of left ventricular function relied only on a gross visual assessment of left ventricular function without making any quantitative measurements.
- A more quantitative approach would be to obtain actual measurements of the left ventricle in both diastole and systole. Several methods for this approach have been suggested in the emergency medicine literature.

### The Moore-Tayal-Rose Protocol

- The diameter of the left ventricle can be measured at the level of the tips of the mitral leaflets in the parasternal long and short axes, while the area of the left ventricle can be determined by manually tracing the area of the left ventricle in the apical four-chamber or parasternal long views. The volume can then be estimated by multiplying the area by the length and comparing the volumes in diastole and systole.

**Table 31.1:** Selection of imaging tests

| | Echo | Nuclear | CT[a] | MRI[b] |
|---|---|---|---|---|
| LV size/function | Initial modality of choice | Available from gated SPECT or PET imaging | Best resolution | Best resolution |
| | Low cost, portable<br>Provides ancillary structural and hemodynamic information | | Highest cost | Highest cost |
| Valve disease | Initial modality of choice<br>Valve motion | | Visualize valve motion | |
| | Doppler hemodynamics | | Delineate abnormal flow | |
| Pericardial disease | Pericardial effusion<br>Doppler hemodynamics | | Pericardial thickening | Pericardial thickening |
| Aortic disease | TEE rapid diagnosis[c]<br>Acute dissection | | Image entire aorta<br>Acute aneurysm<br>Aortic dissection | Image entire aorta<br>Aortic aneurysm<br>Chronic dissection |
| Cardiac masses | TTE—large intracardiac masses<br>TEE—smaller intracardiac masses[c] | | Extracardiac masses<br>Myocardial masses | Extracardiac masses<br>Myocardiac masses |

[a]Contrast required; [b]Relative contraindication—pacemakers, metallic objects, claustrophobic; positron emission tomography; [c]When not seen on TTE. Echo=echocardiography; PET=positron emission tomography; SPECT=single-photon emission computed tomography;TEE=transesophageal echocardiography;TTE=transthoracic echocardiogram.

- In a study of 4 emergency physicians who completed 6 hours of videotape instruction on echocardiography, this method led to an 84% agreement rate with left ventricular function determined by cardiologists.
- This method was especially good at detecting severe left ventricular dysfunction in patients with decompensated congestive heart failure (CHF).

### The Randazzo-Snoey Protocol

- Left ventricular cross-sectional measurements are obtained in diastole and systole in 2 planes, using the subcostal, parasternal short axis, parasternal long axis or 4-chamber views. The EF is then calculated by dividing the systolic measurement by the diastolic measurement.
- In a study of 8 clinicians who underwent 3 hours of training, this method had an overall agreement of 86% with echocardiography read by cardiologists and was especially good at identifying patients with normal left ventricular function, which would help differentiate patients with COPD from those with CHF.

## Other Cardiac Pathologies

- ***Pericardial effusions***
  - Pericardial effusions are characterized by an anechoic stripe between the epicardium and pericardium. A small effusion can be physiologic, but must be differentiated from tamponade, which is a life-threatening cause of right heart failure that causes compression of the right heart. Sonographic signs of tamponade include diastolic collapse of the right heart (atrium or ventricle) and increased respiratory variation in mitral flow, which is known as 'sonographic pulsus paradoxus.' However, since many emergency physicians perform focused ultrasonography without Doppler flow capabilities, many do not even assess for a sonographic pulsus to make the diagnosis of tamponade. In general, tamponade is not a subtle finding and should be suspected by the presence of a moderate to large pericardial effusion and a wide pulse pressure or hemodynamic instability on clinical examination.
  - On the other hand, one must consider whether a small effusion is physiologic or pathologic, and that cannot be absolutely determined by a single echocardiogram. Therefore, the patient's clinical history, risk factors and particular differential diagnosis must also be considered. Be sure to arrange follow-up for repeat echocardiograms in all patients with an effusion identified by bedside echocardiography.
  - Physicians must also distinguish epicardial fat from a pericardial effusion, which is the most common cause of false positives among studies performed by emergency physicians. Differentiating between these conditions may be difficult, which is another reason that further evaluation is warranted in patients suspected of having a small effusion. Signs of epicardial fat include the presence of gray-scale echoes that move with the heart, anechoic stripes less than 1 cm thick, and the lack of an effect on myocardial function.
- ***Right ventricular abnormalities***
  - Many chronic conditions (e.g. pulmonary hypertension, cor pulmonale) may result in right ventricular dilatation and/or hypertrophy. However, sonographers need to be aware of the main signs of right ventricular strain, namely right ventricular dilation, right ventricular hypokinesis, abnormal septal motion

and tricuspid regurgitation. In particular, in the setting of an acute outflow obstruction (e.g. in massive PE, the size of the right ventricle closely approximates that of the left ventricle and, potentially, exceeds it.

- In the short-axis view, the right ventricle is normally crescent-shaped; if this is a rounded, dilated structure, it suggests elevated right-sided pressures, as seen.

## SINGLE-PHOTON EMISSION COMPUTED TOMOGRAPHY

(Figs 31.92 to 31.97)

Single-photon emission computed tomography is a well-validated method commonly used in daily practice in the diagnosis of coronary artery diseases (CAD). A radioactive tracer is injected, followed by imaging of its myocardial distribution using single photon emission computed tomography (SPECT). Exercise (e.g. treadmill) or pharmacologic (e.g. dobutamine or vasodilators) stress are commonly used. Unless contraindicated, vasodilators (e.g. adenosine, dipyridamole or, more recently, regadenason) are the first choice for pharmacologic stress, since they induce greater levels of hyperemia than β-adrenergic agonists. Adenosine is a direct-acting vasodilator, while dipyridamole inhibits cellular uptake and breakdown of adenosine. Regadenason is a recently introduced selective adenosine $A_{2A}$ receptor agonist that was US FDA approved in April 2008. It has been developed in an effort to minimize the complications and discomfort from the nonselective activation of $A_1$, $A_{2B}$ and $A_3$ receptors. Regadenason produces hyperemia with rapid onset (30s) and for a longer duration (~2–5 min) than adenosine. These drugs produce coronary vasodilation, resulting in limited hyperemia in regions supplied by arteries with obstructive CAD compared with regions supplied by arteries with no significant disease. Ischemia is induced infrequently with vasodilator administration because there is usually no major increase in myocardial oxygen demand. This heterogeneous perfusion is best detected with a blood flow tracer. Three perfusion tracers are commonly available—thallium (Tl)-201, technetium (Tc)-99m sestamibi and $^{99m}$Tc tetrofosmin. For tracer uptake and retention, all three agents require viable myocytes supplied by adequate perfusion.

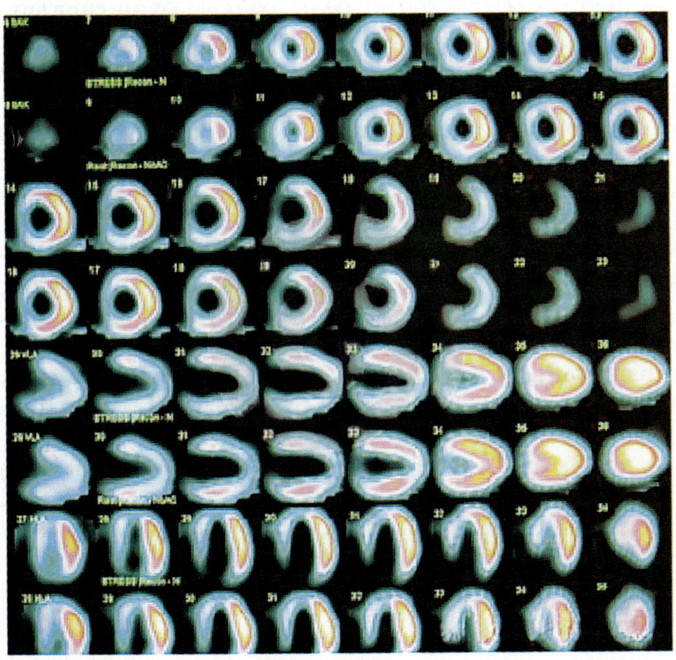

**Fig. 31.92:** Myocardial perfusion stress test—most popular test in the field of nuclear medicine imaging ,there are two parts ,which called rest and stress which can help cardiologist reveal real pathology in perfusion of myocardium

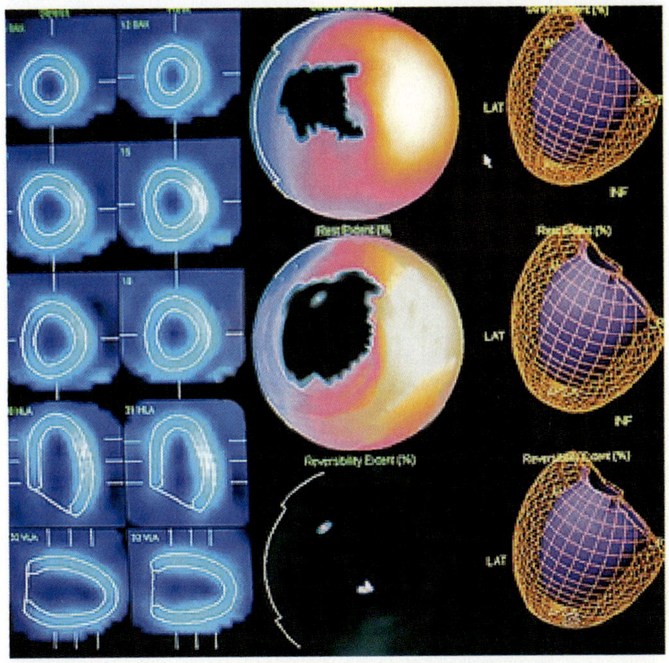

**Fig. 31.93:** Myocardial perfusion nuclear scan, rest and stress part presented myocardial scar as evidence of heart attack in past ,the black spots are on both parts of test in the same areas of upper and lower circles of image

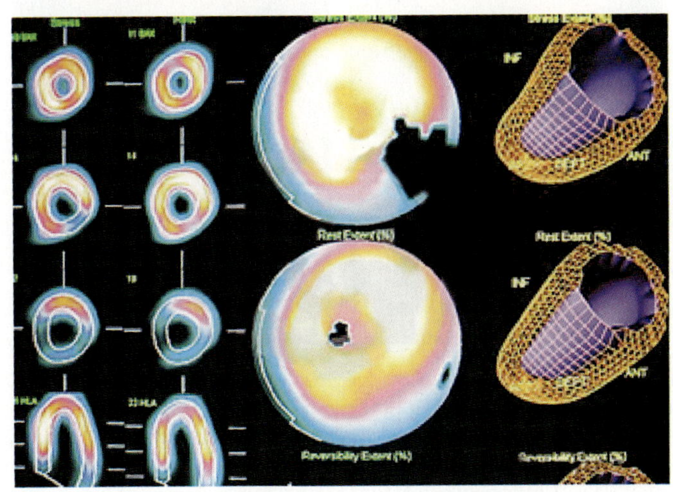

**Fig. 31.94:** Real cardiac ischemia revealed after stress myocardial perfusion nuclear test, there is area which is black on the stress part (upper circle), inferior, lateral part of wall of the heart

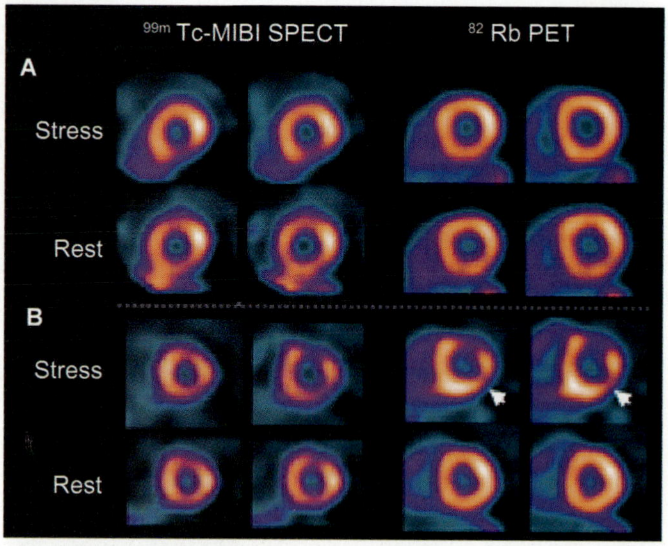


**Fig. 31.95:** Comparison of PET and SPECT perfusion imaging shown are matched, representative short-axis slices for single-photon emission computed tomography (SPECT) (left) and positron emission tomography (PET) (right) in 2 subjects with suspected coronary artery disease. Panel A illustrates improved specificity with PET. A fixed defect in the inferior wall on SPECT is absent on PET, suggesting the presence of a SPECT attenuation artefact. Panel B illustrates improved sensitivity with PET. Stress-induced perfusion defects in the anterior and inferolateral walls (arrows) are more clearly shown with PET versus SPECT

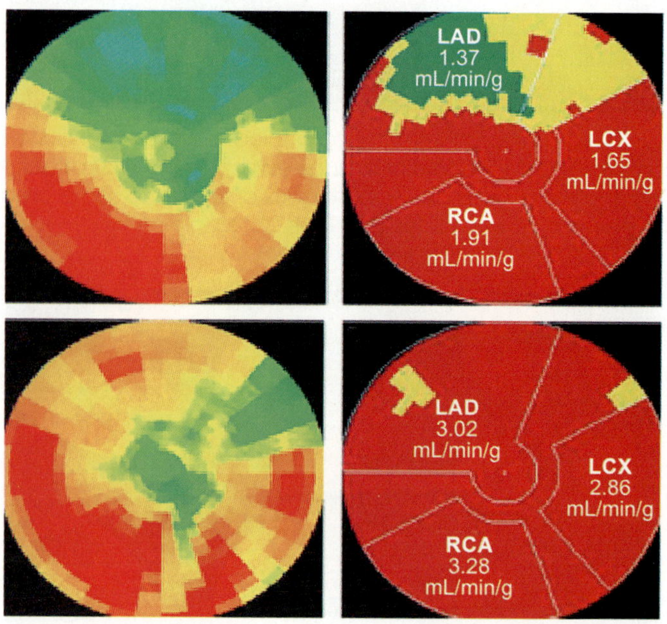


**Fig. 31.96:** Polar plots from MPS using technetium-99m SPECT (left) and nitrogen-13 ammonia PET (right) before (top) and 1 year after aggressive lipid-lowering therapy (bottom). The stress SPECT images show moderately reduced perfusion in the anterior and mid reduction infero-laterally and these areas improve after lipid lowering. However, the quantitative PET images show abnormal stress perfusion (<2 ml/g/min) in all three coronary territories and all areas improve after lipid lowering. The case illustrates the benefit of quantifying myocardial perfusion

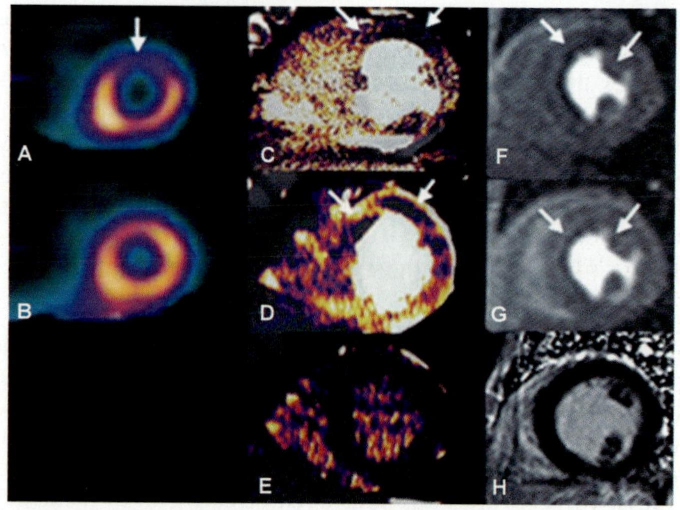


**Fig. 31.97:** Contrast-enhanced retrospectively ECG-gated DECT study in a 58-year-old man with abnormal SPECT. Short axis SPECT acquisitions during stress (A) and rest (B) show reversible perfusion defect in the left anterior descending (LAD) artery territory. Corresponding short axis DECT reconstructions reveal myocardial blood pool defects during both stress (C) and rest (D). DECT images show good agreement with perfusion cardiac MRI during stress (F) and rest (G) delineating a partially reversible sub-endocardial defect in the LAD territory. Late DECT image acquisition (6 minutes after iodine administration) shows no sign of delayed enhancement (i.e. myocardial infarct; (E). Similarly, there also is no evidence of hyperenhancement within the myocardium at delayed-enhancement cardiac MRI (15 minutes after gadolinium [Gd-DTPA] administration)

The agents are injected at peak exercise or during peak vasodilation. Two sets of images are obtained—once after stress and once at rest. Reconstructed images are displayed in the vertical long-, horizontal long- and short-axis projections. These can be viewed in grayscale or in various color-scale maps, which allow easier grading of severity of defects. Tracer uptake in myocardial segments is normalized to the region with maximal tracer uptake. Assessment is primarily visual and qualitative for routine scan interpretation. Reversible (stress-induced) defects identify viable regions supplied by obstructed vessels, while irreversible (fixed) defects reflect partial or transmurally infarcted myocardium. A standard method is to grade perfusion on a scale of 0–4, with 0 representing normal perfusion and 4 representing no visible tracer uptake. Display of rest and stress images in a single polar plot diagram representing all 17 segments of the LV with automated comparison of tracer uptake values with an established normal gender- and tracer-matched database also permits some degree of quantification of defect size and severity.

## Positron Emission Tomography

Positron emission tomography (PET) is another accurate method for assessing myocardial perfusion and metabolism in the evaluation of coronary disease. PET has been used as a research tool for many years, but has not seen extensive clinical application. Similar to SPECT, exercise (e.g. treadmill) or pharmacologic (e.g. dobutamine or vasodilators) stress is used. Pharmacologic stress imaging usually follows resting imaging after the initial activity has been allowed to decay. Three positron-emitting radiotracers are used clinically for cardiac PET imaging—$^{13}N$ and $^{82}Rb$ for assessing myocardial perfusion and $^{18}F$ deoxy-D-glucose (FDG) for evaluating myocardial glucose metabolism and viability assessment. Rb imaging is limited by the high cost of the Rb generator, which, together with the fixed high cost of PET cameras, necessitates two to three reimbursed studies per day to be economically feasible. $^{13}N$ requires an onsite cyclotron for its production and the current lack of reimbursement limits its clinical use. The short half lives of $^{82}Rb$ (75s) and $^{13}N$ (10 min) result in low radiation exposure for the patient, and allow other radionuclide imaging studies on the same day. The use of PET in myocardial perfusion imaging is expected to increase in the near future, with the regional distribution of positron-emitting radiotracers and the emergence of relatively low-cost PET systems.

Positron emission tomography imaging has been combined with computed tomography (CT) for attenuation correction. Hybrid scanners integrating PET and CT account for approximately 80% of new PET units installed. Attenuation-corrected images are displayed in cardiac short-axis, vertical long-axis and horizontal long-axis projections. An experienced reader will visually interpret the myocardial perfusion pattern. Similar to SPECT, a 5-point scoring system (0: normal uptake; 4: absent uptake) and a 17 LV segment model are used to compute a summed stress score, a summed rest score and a summed difference score.

From a large meta-analysis (n = 19 studies), the sensitivity and specificity of PET for the diagnosis of CAD were calculated as 92% (85–98%) and 85% (50–100%), respectively. The same study reported a positive likelihood ratio of 6.2 (CI: 3.3–11.8) and a negative likelihood ratio of 0.11 (CI: 0.08–0.14). On this basis, PET may be an excellent tool at confirming and excluding CAD. This diagnostic performance seems to be comparable to other functional stress-imaging modalities.

Contrary to SPECT, PET maintains its high diagnostic accuracy in women. Patterson et al. showed that sensitivity and specificity for the detection of CAD in women is equally high to that in men. Bateman and coworkers found that, of women who had undergone both stress SPECT and stress PET, both imaging tests had similar high sensitivity but the specificity of PET was significantly higher than for SPECT.

There are several advantages to PET. When compared with SPECT, image uniformity is probably the most important property of cardiac PET. This is because of its excellent spatial (2–4 mm) and temporal resolution. Bateman et al. found that the PET count exceeded that of SPECT by a factor of 2, despite the shorter imaging time of PET. Attenuation correction is also superior in eliminating attenuation artifacts. This may prove PET to be an attractive alternative to other imaging modalities in selected patients (e.g. obese patients) as an uncertain image finding of a noninvasive test is one of the factors prompting physicians to recommend further diagnostic procedures. In 2748 patients, Patterson et al. found a reduction in the number of uncertain ('probably' normal or abnormal) interpretations from 37% with $^{201}Tl$ SPECT to 21% with $^{82}Rb$ PET. PET with FDG has also shown promise in the assessment of atherosclerotic plaque inflammation, a feature that may be of significant clinical importance. Ogawa et al. have shown that macrophages are responsible for the FDG accumulation in vulnerable plaques. Since these plaques are rich with macrophages, FDG imaging was shown to be useful in the detection of vulnerable plaques.

A number of limitations, however, hamper the use of PET for myocardial perfusion assessment in daily practice. It is expensive and not widely available, especially outside of the United States of America. PET imaging is subject to a number of artifacts related to acquisition techniques, heart drift between rest and stress images, which leads to misregistration, and posterior artifacts due to highly attenuating structures (e.g. the spine). Similar to SPECT, PET has a limited ability in delineating the anatomical extent of disease in patients with multivessel stenosis. Radiation exposure also remains a concern. When combined with CT, a hybrid scan has an estimated radiation dose close to 13mSv.

## CARDIAC MAGNETIC RESONANCE IMAGING

Recently, MRI has emerged as a new noninvasive modality for detecting CAD (Figs 31.98–31.103). It uses high-intensity magnetic fields and radiofrequency to generate 3D/tomographic images with high resolution (~0.8 mm) and excellent tissue contrast. The two main imaging techniques employed in cardiovascular magnetic resonance (CMR) are spin echo imaging, which delineates the tissue structures of the heart as bright and the blood pool as dark (black-blood approach), and cine CMR, which produces

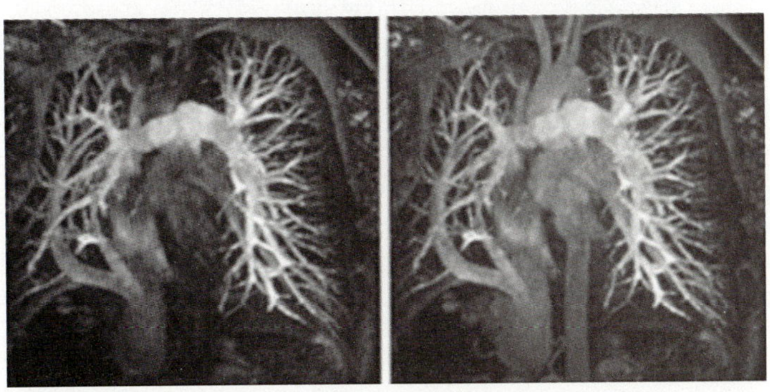

**Fig. 31.98:** Magnetic resonance angiography (MRA) scan of a patient with partial anomalous pulmonary venous drainage of the right lung into the inferior vena cava (scimitar syndrome). MRA is able to define the abnormal anatomic relationships of cardiac structures and great vessels in patients with congenital heart disease

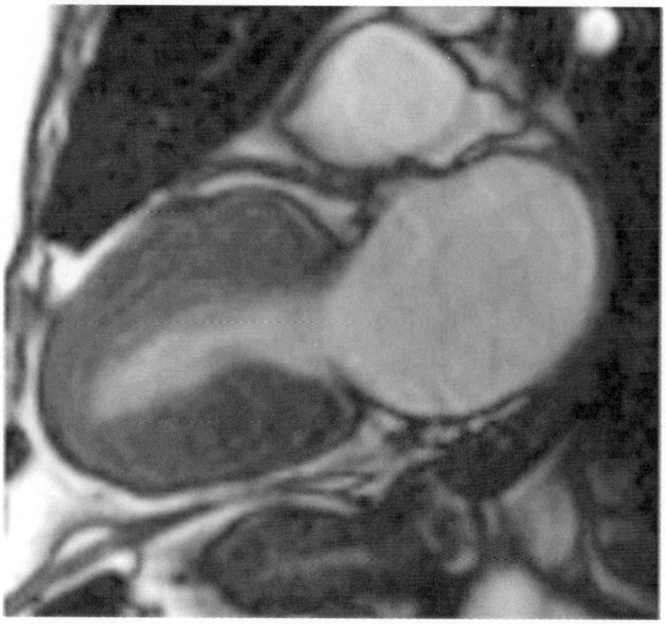

**Fig. 31.99:** MRI scan of a patient with hypertrophic cardiomyopathy, showing the severe increase in left ventricular wall thickness. Cardiac MRI is an ideal imaging modality for diagnosing cardiomyopathies

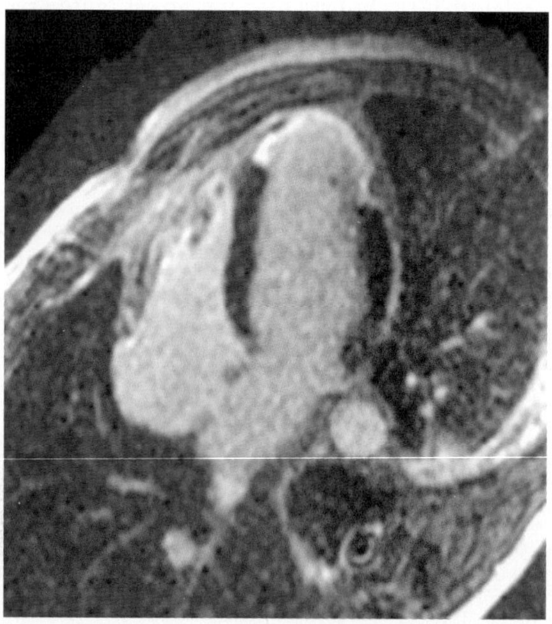

**Fig. 31.100:** MRI scan with delayed gadolinium enhancement in a patient with a large anteroapical infarction. The gadolinium (white area) accumulated in the extracellular space in the presence of cell death from myocardial infarction

images in which the blood pool appears as bright and cardiac tissue structure appears dark (bright-blood approach) using gradient echo-based rapid imaging sequences. Cines are typically obtained within single-breath holds using fast schemes. These schemes include fast low-angle shot (FLASH), steady-state with free precession

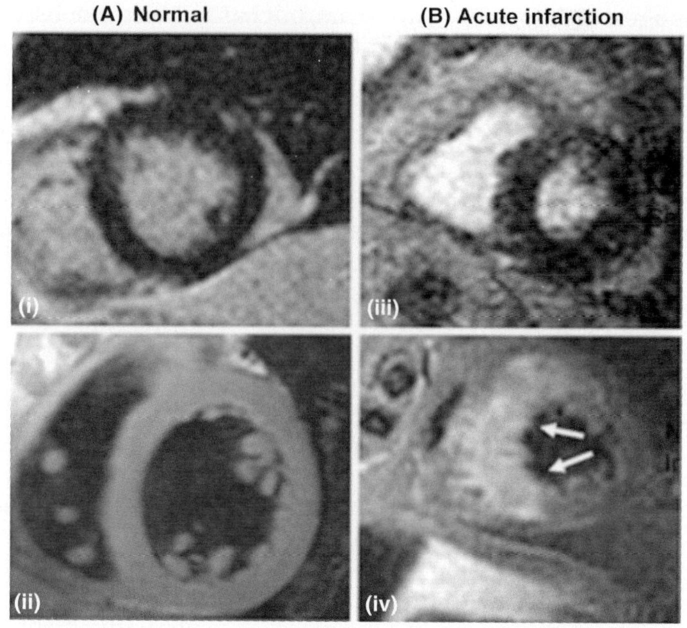


**Fig. 31.101:** (A) Normal delayed enhancement and 'edema'-sensitive images. (i) Delayed enhancement image illustrating normal black myocardium without infarction/fibrosis. (ii) A triple inversion recovery sequence that is T2-weighted demonstrating normal homogenous appearing gray myocardium. (B) A patient postmyocardial infarction and early revascularization without evidence of an infarction and an edematous myocardium in the septum. (iii) Delayed enhanced with normal black myocardium without infarction or fibrosis. (iv) A triple inversion recovery sequence illustrating edema in the septum without infarction. This is the area of 'salvaged' myocardium

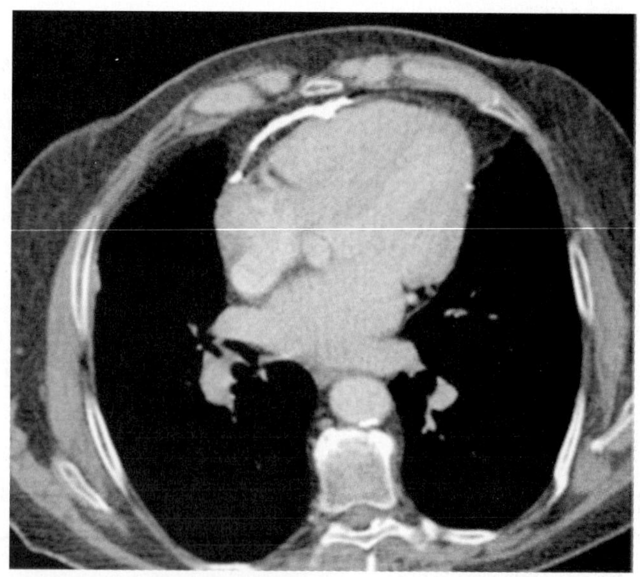

**Fig. 31.102:** CT scan showing pericardial calcification, seen as a white linear density anterior to the myocardium

(SSFP), spiral imaging and echo planar imaging (EPI). CMR evaluates the presence of CAD using three very different techniques; evaluation of wall motion and thickening

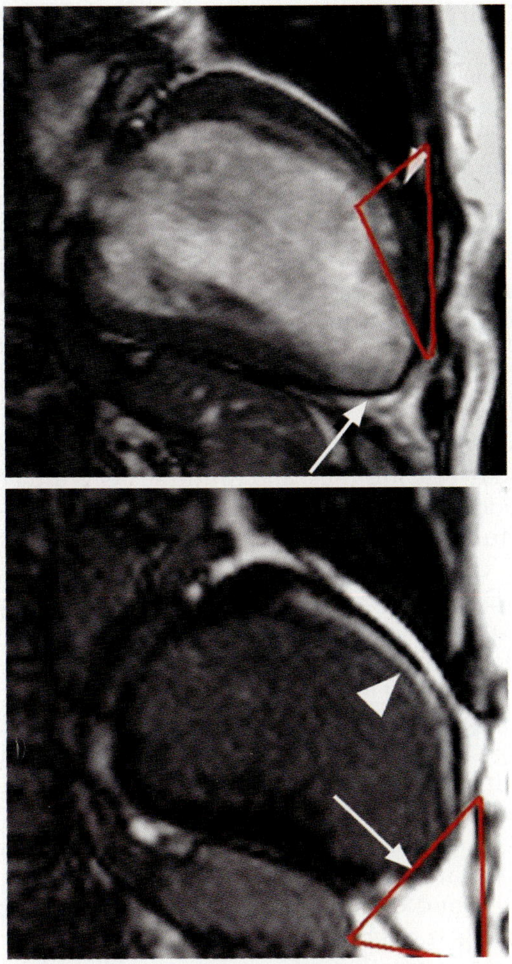

**Fig. 31.103:** Cardiac MRI to determine myocardium viability before revascularization. The whole concept of viability on cardiac MRI is based on the fact that all infarcts enhance vividly 10-15 minutes after intravenous contrast administration. Cardiac MRI shows the transmural extent of the infarct very reliably. It tells you that 'white is dead' (all infarcts irrespective of age enhance). In areas of hypokinesia, if there is a rim of 'black' or non-infarcted myocardium that is not contracting well, it indicates the presence of hibernating myocardium, which is likely to improve after revascularization of the artery supplying that particular territory. Viability imaging reliably allows identification of areas of hibernation and viable or non-viable myocardium. All infarcts irrespective of age enhance. The percentage involvement of the myocardial wall thickness by an infarct determines viability

during stress, dynamic first-pass perfusion imaging, which assesses for inducible perfusion defects, and anatomical assessment [coronary magnetic resonance angiography (MRA)], which provides noninvasive visualization of the coronary tree.

Assessment of wall motion with CMR utilizes dobutamine as the stress agent. Protocols similar to those implemented for dobutamine stress echo (SE) can be used for CMR. After rapid surveys to determine the exact heart axis, three short-axis planes (apical, mid and basal) and four- and two-chamber views are usually acquired. Images can be displayed as continuous cine loops using a quad-screen display for review of a 17-segment LV model. At each level of stress, LV segmental wall motion is assessed as normal, hypokinetic, akinetic or dyskinetic. Inducible ischemia is defined as deterioration of the segmental systolic wall motion within a myocardial segment observed in two orthogonal views.

When compared with invasive coronary angiography, the sensitivity and specificity of stress CMR detection of CAD by wall-motion analysis has been reported to be 83 and 86%, respectively, in a report pooling data from several investigations Stress MRI evaluation of wall motion has the advantage of providing high-quality images in most subjects, regardless of body habitus. The use of myocardial tagging, may also improve the sensitivity of wall-motion analysis. Tagging is a special radiofrequency modulation of the magnetized vector to obtain both line and grid representation of the myocardial segments to help assess regional heterogeneity of systolic segmental contraction.

An alternative approach to detect obstructive CAD by CMR is based on dynamic first-pass perfusion scanning. Adenosine is the preferred stressor agent. After acquisition of rest cine scans in the standard views (apical, mid and basal short-axis views; four- and two-chamber views), adenosine infusion is started. Within the last minute of the infusion, intravenous gadolinium (typical dose ranging from 0.05 to 0.15 mg/kg/min) is administered, and perfusion scanning is performed during breath holding. After a 10–15-min waiting period to allow for equilibration of the contrast agent with the myocardium, an identical rest perfusion scan is repeated. Interpretation of inducible perfusion defects is visually performed. The transmurality of a defect is determined from the single dynamic image showing the maximum extent of regional hypoenhancement. A regional hypoenhancement of at least 25% in any segment not visible on the rest perfusion scan is considered pathological. Alternatively, computer quantification of parameters, such as the signal-intensity upslope or regional contrast transit time, can be used to generate parametric relative perfusion maps or measures of relative perfusion index at rest and during stress. A myocardial perfusion reserve index (MPRI) of 1.1 (when the second smallest MPRI is used) has been suggested as a reasonable cut-off value.

The reported sensitivity of perfusion imaging averages 91%, with a specificity of 81% using coronary angiography as the gold standard Plein et al., showed that combined assessment of wall motion and perfusion yielded a sensitivity of 96% and a specificity of 83%, which was higher than the values for sensitivity and specificity of each method alone.

To date, few CMR studies have evaluated ischemia provocation in women. The study by Nagel et al., including 208 patients (61 women) revealed no significant differences in sensitivity, specificity and test accuracy of dobutamine CMR when compared with men. CMR maintains its high diagnostic accuracy in patients with single-vessel disease, which may be of particular value to female subsets of the population. CMR may also be well suited to women with chest pain due to microvascular disease and normal coronary arteries, a disease commonly known as syndrome

X. Owing to its high resolution, CMR can discriminate between subepicardial and subendocardial flow, which enables the detection of an abnormal subendocardial perfusion index in this syndrome.

The third approach for the detection of CAD by CMR uses anatomical assessment of the coronary tree by angiography. Using the natural T2-weighted signal difference between the blood in the coronary lumen and the surrounding myocardium, coronary artery contrast is generated without exogenous contrast administration. The reconstruction interval is usually performed during mid-diastole, when cardiac motion is the least and coronary flow is the greatest. The duration of data acquisition can vary from 50 to 150 ms per cardiac cycle, with the acquisition extending to several minutes. From pooled data, the sensitivity and specificity of coronary MRA on a patient level were 88 and 56%, respectively.

Cardiac MRI has the advantage of being a highly versatile modality because it provides multiple techniques in one imaging system. It does not involve exposure to radiation. CMR myocardial perfusion has the potential for significant clinical growth given greatly enhanced spatial resolution. The excellent resolution enables the assessment of subendocardial perfusion abnormalities. This may present a significant clinical advantage, since a subendocardial perfusion abnormality is a more sensitive sign of obstructive CAD compared with a transmural perfusion abnormality. The ability to detect subendocardial perfusion abnormalities may also reduce the possibility of false-negative studies owing to balanced multivessel CAD encountered with SPECT and PET imaging. In addition, CMR is well validated for quantifying the volumes, mass and function of the ventricles, and has become the gold standard against which other techniques are measured. Given its 3D nature, CMR does not rely on geometric assumptions, especially in the vertical heart, LV hypertrophy and with regional heterogeneity of CAD. This permits excellent interstudy reproducibility of volume and mass for both the LV and right ventricle. Other clinical applications of CMR include assessment of myocardial infarction and viability by combining delayed enhancement imaging, evaluation of infiltrative or inflammatory disease processes and study of pericardial and congenital diseases.

The disadvantages of CMR include that it is a relatively expensive technology with limited availability. Stress is still largely limited to pharmacologic agents. Exercise is avoided, owing to motion artifacts during imaging. Monitoring during testing can be suboptimal and ECG tracings and ST-segments can be altered by the strong magnetic field. The entire acquisition and image processing can be time consuming (30 minutes or more on average). Analysis times may be prolonged when quantitative assessment is performed. CMR cannot be used in patients with severe claustrophobia. It is also absolutely or relatively contraindicated in patients with pacemakers, defibrillators, certain aneurysm clips and other indwelling ferromagnetic materials. Gadolinium administration to patients with moderate-to-severe kidney disease (glomerular filtration rate <30 ml/min) has been associated with the syndrome of nephrogenic systemic fibrosis, although only rarely. CMR is feasible only in cooperative patients. The need for accurate gating with a stable heart rhythm and the ability to hold breath for long scan-acquisition time are other limitations. More recently, self-gating techniques have been described. These largely rely on cardiac tissue motion and blood flow, which eliminates the need for an external physiologic signal monitoring. Lack of established CMR sequences for first-pass perfusion imaging, standardized protocols for stress testing and analysis are other drawbacks that are being currently addressed.

Coronary MRA also suffers from a number of technical limitations, which continue to hinder its widespread clinical application. Visualization of the entire coronary tree requires several minutes, and multiple beats are needed to reconstruct the coronary arteries. Beat-to-beat variability in the duration of the cardiac cycle and the period of diastasis can produce image blurring. Only proximal and mid LAD and RCA segments can be assessed reliably. Visualization of the LCX is less successful, owing to the close relationship of the accompanying vein and adjacent blood pools of the left atrium and ventricle, in addition to a lower signal related to the greater distance from the receiving coil. The number of uninterpretable segments is still significant, and exclusion of up to 20% of all segments has been reported. In addition, coronary MRA can be affected by motion related to intrinsic cardiac contraction/relaxation and motion attributable to superimposed diaphragm and chest-wall movement during respiration. ECG gating is used to account for the intrinsic cardiac motion, while breath holding is required to reduce artifact from respiratory motion. To overcome some of these limitations, free-breathing navigator coronary MRA has been introduced. This system tracks the patient's diaphragmatic motion and pictures are only obtained when the diaphragm is 3–5 mm within its end expiratory position.

## MULTISLICE CARDIAC COMPUTED TOMOGRAPHY

The first experience with noninvasive coronary arteriography was described in 1995. Since its inception, substantial improvements in temporal and spatial resolution have been made (Figs 31.104–31.109). Mechanically, rotating gantries with a rotation time of less than 420 ms are now routinely used. The more recently introduced dual-source multislice computed tomographies (MSCTs) are able to attain a maximal temporal resolution as low as 83 ms in addition to superior spatial resolution to help improve coronary image quality at faster heart rates. The 64-slice MSCT systems have a spatial resolution of 0.4–0.7 mm. Systems capable of 256 or 320 slices with each gantry rotation are now available. MSCT scanners can be operated in a sequential (step and shoot) or spiral (helical) mode. Data acquisition is triggered by the patient's ECG in sequential mode or, in case of continuous acquisition imaging, the reconstruction is made through retrospective or prospective ECG gating. Imaging is performed within one single breath hold. Most patients undergoing MSCT

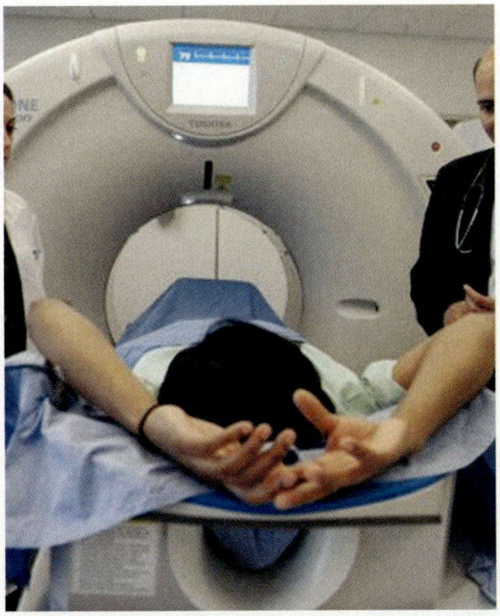

Fig. 31.104: Doctors talking with a patient before having a scan done with the new 320-multislice cardiac CT angiography machine in the emergency department

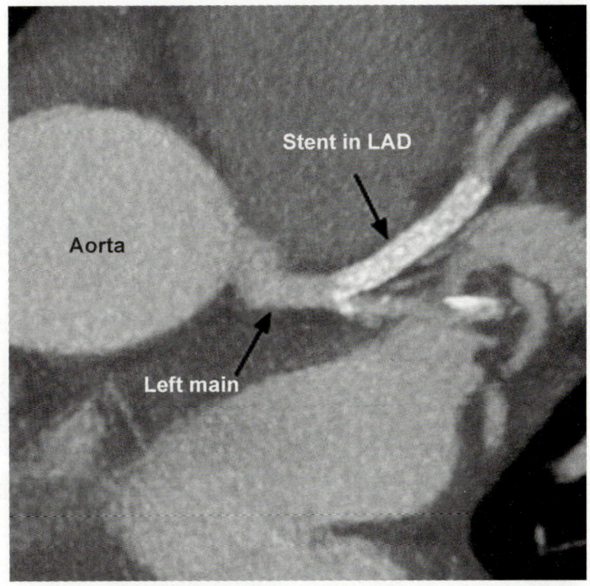


Fig. 31.106: A 320-multislice cardiac CT angiography in a patient before having stent in LAD artery (arrow)

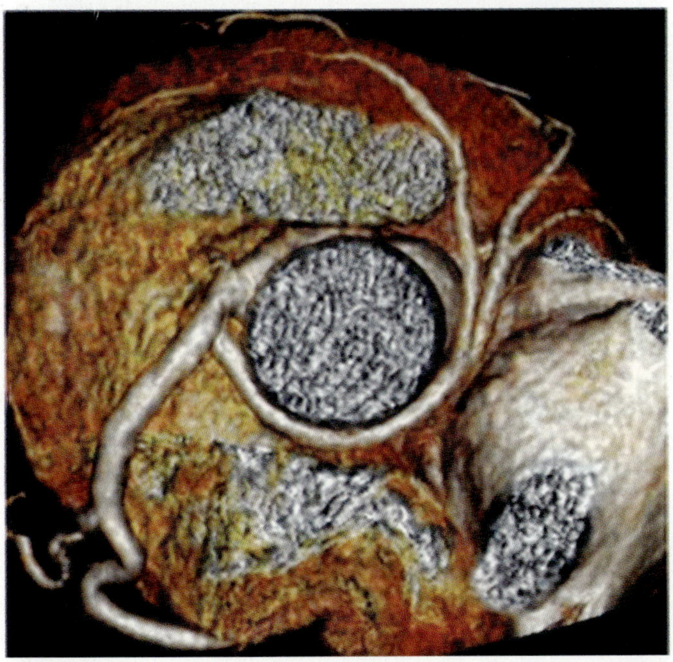

Fig. 31.105: Three-dimensional volume rendered image of a contrast enhanced CT angiogram illustrating an anomalous left coronary artery arising from the right coronary artery and traveling posterior to the aorta

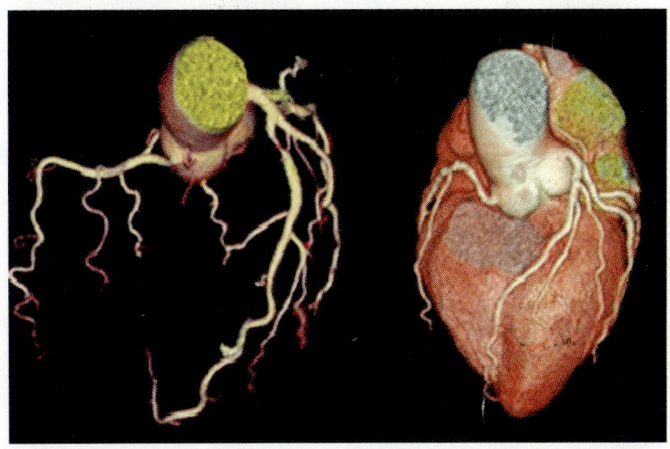

Fig. 31.107: Three-dimensional volume rendered image of a contrast enhanced CT angiogram demonstrating a normal left main coronary artery arising from the aorta and its two branches, the left anterior descending artery (left) and the circumflex artery (right) and right coronary artery (left panel)

receive oral or intravenous β-blockers to achieve a heart rate of less than 60–70 bpm to optimize acquisition of gated images during diastolic diastasis. For new dual-source MSCT, acceptable image quality has been obtained at heart rates up to 90 bpm. Sublingual nitroglycerin can also be administered before the scan to achieve adequate coronary vasodilation. The entire procedure can be performed in approximately 30 minutes with study acquisition requiring less than 10s.

When examining arteries, interpreters must review the images on workstations capable of 2D and 3D displays of the commonly available reconstruction formats. These include transaxial 2D image stacks, multiplanar reformation (MPR), maximum intensity projection (MIP), curved multiplanar reformation (cMPR) and volume-rendering technique (VRT) reconstructions. During segmental analysis, a combination of these reconstruction formats can be used, depending on the characteristics of the vessel being examined (e.g. presence of calcification and tortuosity). Each stenosis is interpreted in all three planes (sagittal, coronal and axial) using all postprocessed and axial raw

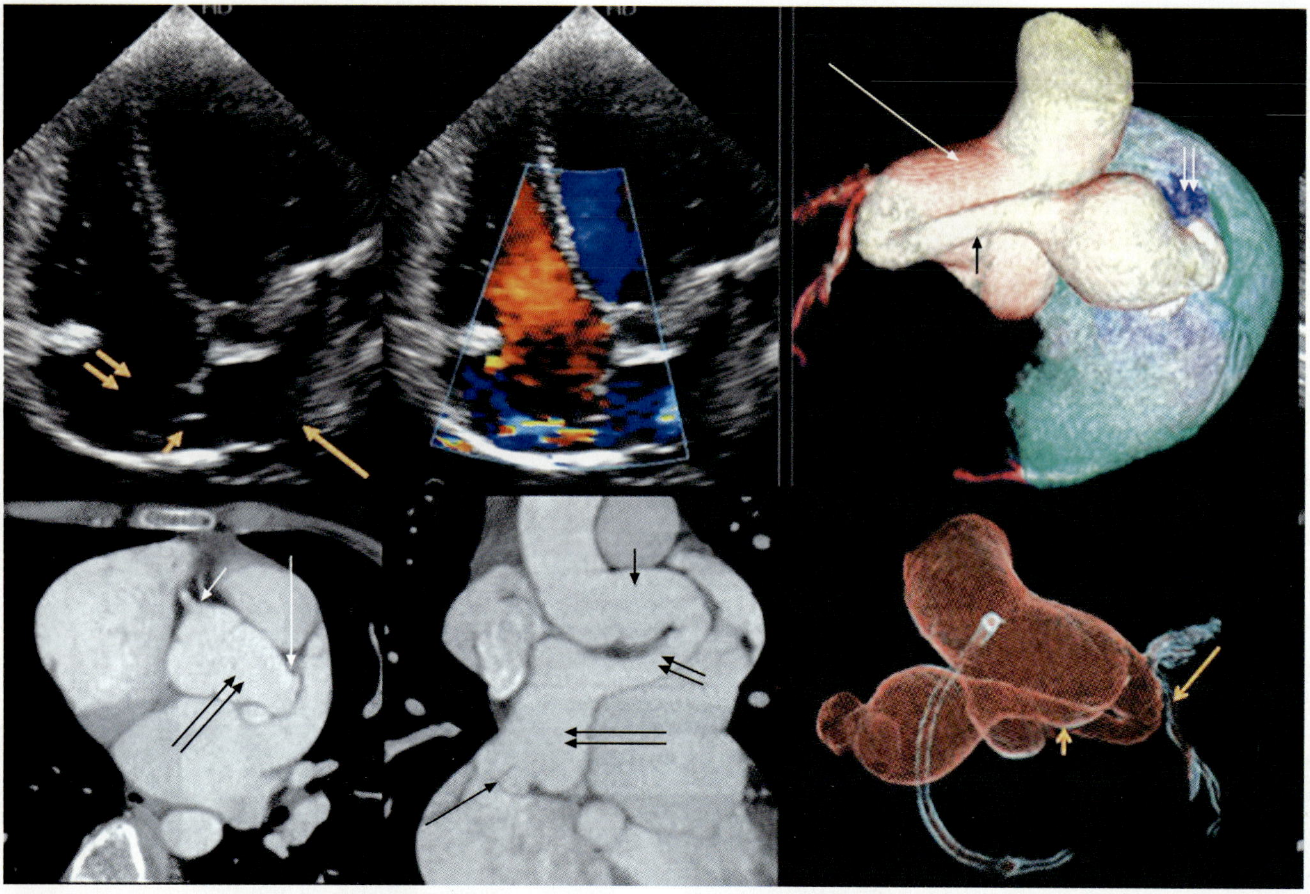

**Fig. 31.108:** Multislice CT imaging of ruptured left sinus of Valsalva aneurysm with fistulous track between left sinus and right atrium

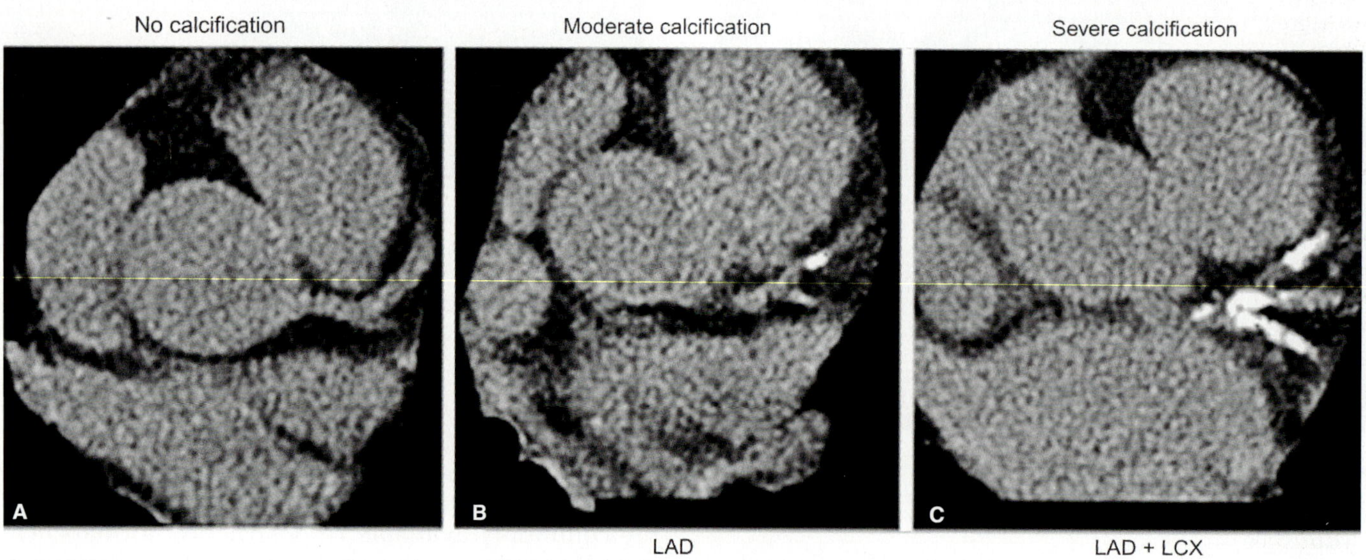


**Fig. 31.109:** CT scans of three patients showing the ability to detect coronary calcification. (A) Normal coronary arteries without calcification. (B) Calcification in the left anterior artery (LAD). (C) Severe calcification in the LAD and circumflex (CX) arteries

images. Coronary arteries are scored using the American Heart Association (AHA) coronary segmentation. The coronary tree should be examined initially for the course and branching of the main coronary vessels. Epicardial coronary arterial luminal stenosis is graded semiquantitatively as minimal (<30%), mild (30–49%), moderate (50–69%), severe (70–99%) or occluded.

Initial studies with four-slice technology showed encouraging results, with sensitivities and specificities ranging from 66–90% and from 71–99%, respectively.

However, the percentage of segments with nondiagnostic quality was very high (>25%). More recently, MSCT was reported to have high discriminative power to detect significant obstructive CAD with good sensitivity and specificity, which can reach the 90% range. As expected, considerably more segments are now available for evaluation (>90%). The reported specificity is considered to be on par with other noninvasive imaging modalities (mainly SE and SPECT), whereas the diagnostic sensitivity and negative predictive value (NPV) are higher with MSCT. For screening purposes, in properly selected patients, MSCT has excellent NPV reaching almost 100%, with a positive predictive value (PPV) of approximately 60%. As a result, a 'negative' MSCT excludes high-grade coronary stenosis with very high certainty, as long as image quality is diagnostic and all coronary segments are well seen. This may help identify patients who do not have to undergo an invasive angiography for CAD detection.

The limited available data suggest that MSCT maintains its diagnostic accuracy in women. In a study of 103 consecutive patients (51 men and 52 women) with known or suspected CAD, 64-slice MSCT had high diagnostic accuracy in all patients with no significant differences in accuracy on a segmental or vessel basis.

Multislice cardiac CT may have its greatest value in symptomatic patients with nondiagnostic functional tests or in those with suspected false-positive or -negative functional tests. The use of MSCT in these settings may help to avoid overutilization of invasive coronary angiography and exposure to unnecessary procedure-related risks. Another potential role of MSCT is in a specific subgroup of patients with a relative contraindication for physiologic testing. Patients with left bundle branch block (LBBB) may be better served by MSCT for evaluation of suspected CAD. Other imaging modalities may have lower specificity, PPV and higher false-positive results of CAD detection in those with LBBB. The diagnostic accuracy of MSCT for the detection of coronary stenosis was evaluated in 66 patients with LBBB without a history of CAD. The sensitivity and specificity values (97 and 95%, respectively) were similar to those in patients without LBBB. Another potential role of MSCT may include the workup of dilated cardiomyopathy in low- to intermediate-risk CAD patients. A single-center study reported that 64-slice MSCT correctly identified 60 out of 62 patients (97%) without and 28 out of 31 (90%) with ischemic cardiomyopathy. The reported accuracy of MSCT is higher than that reported for SPECT perfusion imaging and SE in distinguishing the cause of dilated cardiomyopathy.

Multislice cardiac CT can also been used for the detection of coronary artery calcification (CAC). Radiologic detection of CAC *in vivo* by fluoroscopy was first described in the late 1950s. The Agaston score is the most widely used and best-established measure of CAC for assessment of the diagnostic and prognostic value of CAC scanning. Use of age-, gender- and race-specific threshold values has improved diagnostic accuracy of CAC scanning. Other measures, such as the volume score and calcium mass, are often reported, and may prove superior to the Agaston score, but have been studied less well.

In both men and women presenting with chest pain, CAC detected by CT is highly sensitive for the presence of at least 50% of angiographic stenosis, but is only moderately specific, especially in individuals over 60 years of age. The absence of CAC is highly predictive of the absence of CAD. CAC scanning has also been shown to have incremental value in risk stratification above Framingham score and serum biomarkers. Currently, the screening of asymptomatic patients should be limited to clinically selected patients with an intermediate 10-year risk of coronary heart disease (between 10 and 20%), where the result can potentially lead to a change in management based upon reclassification to a lower or higher risk group. Other potential clinical applications of CAC scanning include workup of dilated cardiomyopathy in low-risk patients and emergency department evaluation of chest pain.

A primary disadvantage of MSCT in general is the radiation exposure, estimated to be between 7 and 21 mSv depending on the generation of the MSCT and the use of radiation-reducing algorithms. Supporters of the technique point out that there is little excess radiation exposure compared with diagnostic invasive coronary angiography (>5 mSv). The MSCT radiation dose imparts a small but non-negligible increase in the lifetime risk of cancer. This risk varies markedly and is much greater for women and younger patient Introduction of scanning algorithms using ECG-dependent dose modulation during spiral scan and a reduced tube voltage have been successful in reducing the radiation dose. More importantly, dose reduction does not influence diagnostic image quality The need for iodinated contrast (60–120 ml) makes MSCT relatively contraindicated in patients at risk for contrast-induced nephropathy or those with a history of allergy to contrast media.

The utility of MSCT is limited in certain patient populations in whom coronary segments cannot be visualized, or in whom the degree of stenosis cannot be assessed. These populations include older subjects or patients with chronic kidney disease with extensive coronary calcification, coronary stents or tortuous coronary arteries. As noted in the Assessment by Coronary Computed Tomographic Angiography of Individuals Undergoing Invasive Coronary Angiography (ACCURACY) trial, specificity was reduced in the presence of CAC (86 vs 53% for detection of ≥50% stenosis with calcium scores ≤400 vs >400 Agaston units). Dense coronary calcification tends to lead to an overestimation of diameter stenosis. Other patient-related factors that can interfere with the image quality include obesity, tachycardia, irregular heart rhythms or those unable to cooperate or hold their breath for 10–15s. These create 'stairstep artifacts' due to motion occurring between reconstruction of sequential heartbeats. MSCT also has lower sensitivity for exclusion of distal or branch vessel obstruction in segments less than 1.5 mm in size.

Multislice cardiac CT can be combined with PET and SPECT imaging. This combined approach would nonin-

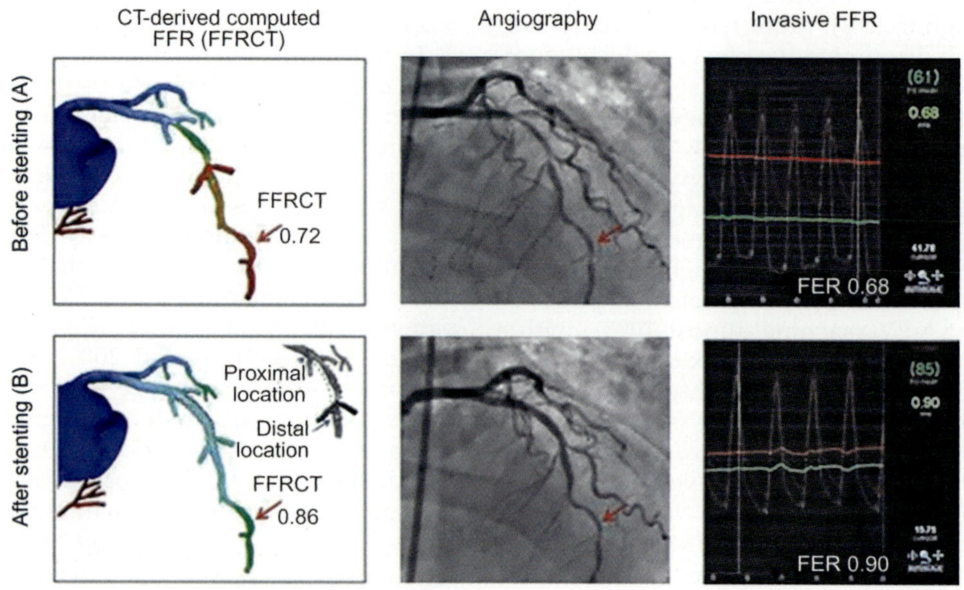


**Fig. 31.110:** Invasive and noninvasive functional assessment before and after revascularization. (A) Noninvasive fractional flow reserve (FFR) from coronary computed tomographic angiography data (FFRCT) of the left anterior descending (LAD) coronary artery was 0.72. Invasive coronary angiography and FFR confirmed the functionally significant LAD stenosis. (B) FFRCT demonstrated no ischemia in the LAD after virtual stenting, with a computed value of 0.86. Invasive FFR after stent implantation was 0.90

vasively provide comprehensive information (functional and anatomic) of the presence and physiological significance of the atherosclerotic coronary disease. It is conceivable that patients with known or suspected disease could be studied with sequential stress-rest perfusion imaging and CT angiography, allowing acquisition of superimposed images for the extent of abnormal coronary anatomy, perfusion and wall-motion abnormality. Early studies suggest that this hybrid modality has high sensitivity and specificity, and can add precision and confidence in deciding on the best therapeutic approach, reduce downstream unnecessary testing and be cost effective.

### Computed Fractional Flow Reserve Derived from Coronary CT Angiography

Recent advances in image-based modeling and computational fluid dynamics permit the calculation of coronary artery pressure and flow from typically acquired coronary CT scans. Computed fractional flow reserve (FFR) is the ratio of mean coronary artery pressure divided by mean aortic pressure under conditions of simulated maximal coronary hyperemia, thus providing a noninvasive estimate of fractional flow reserve computed tomography (FFRCT) at every point in the coronary tree. Prospective multicenter clinical trials have shown that computed FFRCT improves diagnostic accuracy and discrimination compared to CT stenosis alone for the diagnosis of hemodynamically significant coronary artery disease (CAD), when compared to invasive FFR as the reference gold standard. This promising new technology provides a combined anatomic and physiologic assessment of CAD in a single noninvasive test that can help select patients for invasive angiography and revascularization or best medical therapy (Fig. 31.110). Further evaluation of the clinical effectiveness and economic implications of noninvasive FFRCT are now being explored.

## BIBLIOGRAPHY

1. Bodner E, Frater R, eds. Replacement cardiac valves New York, NY: McGraw-Hill, 1992.
2. Dunbar RD, Mitchell R, Lavine M. Aberrant location of central venous catheters. Lancet 1981;1:711–5.
3. Fowler RA, Cook DJ. The arc of the pulmonary artery catheter. JAMA 2003;290:2732–34.
4. Funaki B. Central venous access: a primer for the diagnostic radiologist. AJR Am J Roentgenol 2002;179:309–18.
5. Gaur S, Achenbach S, Leipsic J, et al. Rationale and design of the HeartFlowNXT (HeartFlow analysis of coronary blood flow using CT angiography: NeXt sTeps) study. J Cardiovasc Comput Tomogr 2013;7:279–88.
6. Henry DA, Jolles H, Berberich JJ, Schmeizer V. The post-cardiac surgery chest radiograph: a clinically integrated approach. J Thorac Imaging 1989;4:20–41.
7. Henry DA, LeBolt S. Invasive hemodynamic monitoring: radiologist's perspective. RadioGraphics 1986;6:535–72.
8. Henschke CI, Yankelevitz DF, Wand A, Davis SD, Shiau M. Chest radiography in the ICU. Clin Imaging 1997;21: 90–103.
9. Hinke DH, Zandt-Stastny DA, Goodman LR, Quebbeman EJ, Krzywda EA, Andris DA. Pinch off syndrome: a complication of implantable subclavian venous access devices. Radiology 1990;177:353–6.
10. Hunt R, Hunter TB. Cardiac tamponade and death from perforation of the right atrium by a central venous catheter (letter). AJR Am J Roentgenol 1988;151:1250.

11. Katz JD, Cronau LH, Barash PG, Mandel SD. Pulmonary artery flow-guided catheters in the perioperative period: indications and complications. JAMA 1977;237: 2832–4.
12. Knutstad K, Hager B, Hauser M. Radiologic diagnosis and management of complications related to central venous access. Acta Radiol 2003;44:508–16.
13. Koo BK, Erglis A, Doh JH, et al. Diagnosis of ischemia-causing coronary stenoses by noninvasive fractional flow reserve computed from coronary computed tomographic angiograms. Results from the prospective multicenter DISCOVER-FLOW (Diagnosis of Ischemia-Causing Stenoses Obtained Via Noninvasive Fractional Flow Reserve) study. J Am Coll Cardiol 2011;58:1989–97.
14. Landay MJ, Estrera AS, Bordlee RP. Cardiac valve reconstruction and replacement: a brief review. RadioGraphics 1992; 12:659–71.
15. Landay MJ, Mootz AR, Estrera AS. Apparatus seen on chest radiographs after cardiac surgery in adults. Radiology 1990; 174:477–82.
16. Maffessanti M, Berlot G, Bortolotto P. Chest roentgenology in the intensive care unit: an overview. Eur Radiol 1998;8: 69–78.
17. McGee DC, Gould MK. Preventing complications of central venous catheterization. N Engl J Med 2003;348: 1123–33.
18. McLoud TC, Putman CE. Radiology of the Swan-Ganz catheter and associated pulmonary complications. Radiology 1975;116:19–22.
19. Min JK, Leipsic J, Pencina MJ, et al. Diagnostic accuracy of fractional flow reserve from anatomic CT angiography. JAMA 2012;308:1237–45.
20. Norgaard BL, Leipsic J, Sengupta S, et al. Quantitative assessment of image quality for determination of FFR by coronary computed tomography angiography (abstr). J Cardiovasc Comput Tomogr (Suppl) 2013;3:233.
21. Richard C, Warszawski J, Anguel N, et al. Early use of the pulmonary artery catheter and outcomes in patients with shock and acute respiratory distress syndrome: a randomized controlled trial. JAMA 2003;290:2713–20.
22. Swensen SJ, Peters SG, LeRoy AJ, Gay PC, Sykes MW, Tastek VF. Radiology in the intensive-care unit. Mayo Clin Proc 1991;66:396–410.
23. Therasse E, Oliva VL, Lafontaine E, Perreault P, Giroux M, Soulez G. Balloon dilatation and stent placement for esophageal lesions: indication, methods, and results. RadioGraphics 2003;23:89–105.
24. Trotman-Dickenson B. Radiology in the intensive care unit (part 2). J Intensive Care Med 2003;18:239–52.
25. Trotman-Dickenson B. Radiology in the intensive care unit (part I). J Intensive Care Med 2003;18:198–210.
26. Vesely TM. Central venous catheter tip position: a continuing controversy. J Vasc Interv Radiol 2003;14:527–34.
27. Wiener MD, Garay SM, Leitman BS, Wiener DN, Ravin CE. Imaging of the intensive care unit patient. Clin Chest Med 1991;12:169–98.
28. Zarshenas Z, Sparschu RA. Catheter placement and misplacement. Crit Care Clin 1994;10:417–36.

# 32 Recognition and Management of Pericardial Diseases

## Anatomy and Physiology

The pericardium is composed of the parietal pericardium (an outer fibrous layer) and the visceral pericardium (an inner serous membrane made of a single layer of mesothelial cells). The visceral pericardium is attached to the epicardial fat and reflects back on itself to form the parietal pericardium. The pericardium normally contains as much as 50 ml of an ultrafiltrate of plasma. Drainage occurs via the thoracic duct and the right lymphatic duct into the right pleural space (Fig. 32.1).

Pericardial physiology includes three main functions. First, through its mechanical function, the pericardium promotes cardiac efficiency by limiting acute dilation, maintaining ventricular compliance with preservation of the Starling curve, and distributing hydrostatic forces. The pericardium also creates a closed chamber with subatmospheric pressure that aids atrial filling and lowers transmural cardiac pressures. Second, through its membranous function, the pericardium shields the heart by reducing external friction and acting as a barrier against extension of infection and malignancy. Third, through its ligamentous function, the pericardium anatomically fixes the heart.

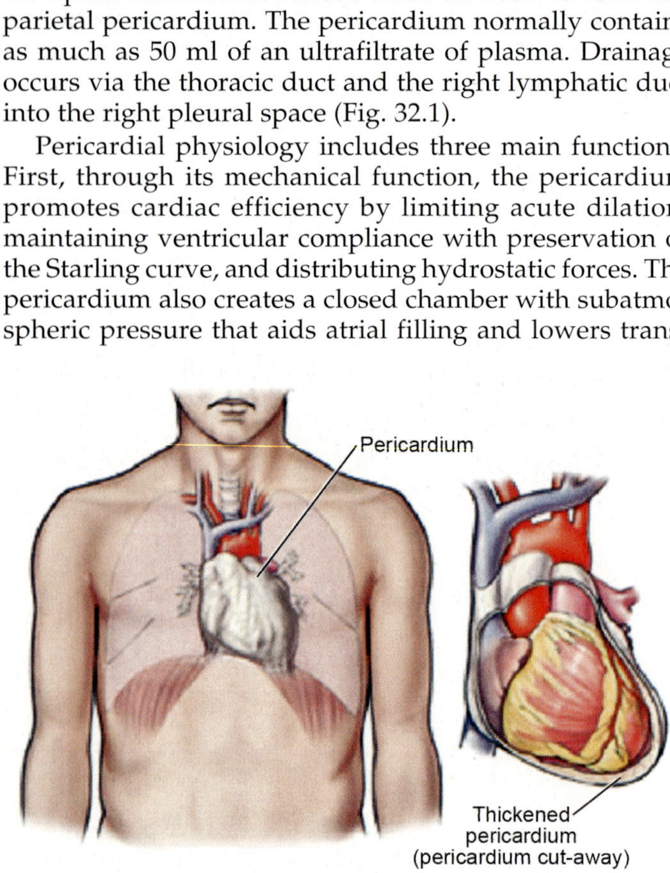


**Fig. 32.1:** Anatomy of pericardial sac in relation to surrounding vital structures of the heart, particularly myocardium and coronary vessels

*Absence of pericardium:* Partial absence of pericardium is much more common than complete absence. It may be associated with congenital anomalies, such as autism spectrum disorder (ASD), mitral stenosis, tetralogy of fallot (TOF) tricuspid regurgitation, patent ductus arteriosus and Eisenmenger physiology. Mitral valve prolapse may also be associated in this anomaly. In majority, it does not manifest with any symptom except chest pain due to torsion of the great vessels (Fig. 32.2).

Recurrent pulmonary infections may be a significant feature. Physical examination may reveal LV heave in the anterior or mid axillary line. A systolic murmur may be present and on occasion diastolic murmur has been reported. X-ray chest reveals shift of the heart to the left and its border elongated showing prominent seperation between the aorta and pulmonary artery. Lucencies caused by interposition of lung may be seen between the pulmonary artery segment and the aortic knob, and between the left hemidiaphragm and the base of the heart. Electrocardiogram in complete absence of the left side of the pericardium usually shows incomplete right bundle branch block (RBBB). In the presence of induced or spontaneous pneumothorax, air enters the pericardial space and outlines the percardium. Medium size defects may lead to herniation of the left atrium which may then strangulate and require surgical closure or enlargement of the defect to reduce the herniation and prevent recurrence.

The pericardium is a thin fibroelastic sac composed of two layers that separate the heart from the surrounding mediastinal structures. The outer layer of the pericardium is referred to as the fibrous pericardium and usually measures less than 2 mm in thickness. The inner portion of

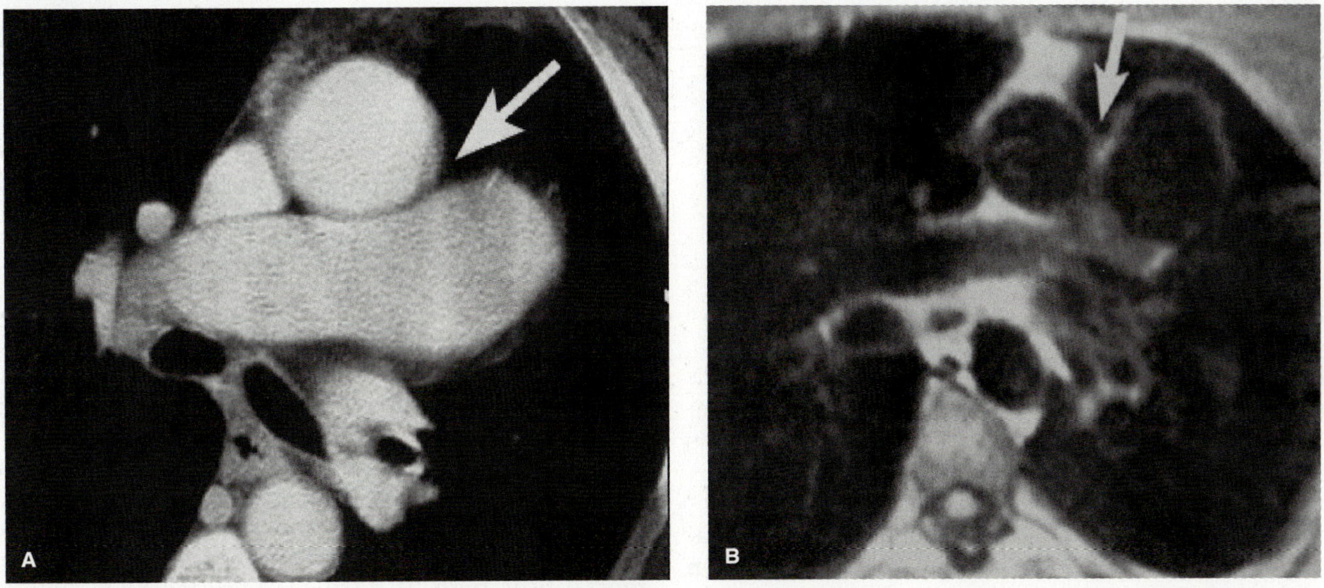


**Fig. 32.2:** Congenital absence of the pericardium. Axial contrast-enhanced CT scan (A) and ECG-gated T1-weighted SE image (B), show interposition of lung tissue between the aorta and the main segment of the pulmonary artery (arrow), indicating the absence of the pericardium in this area. Note the rotation of the heart toward the left

the pericardium is a two-layered sac called the serous pericardium. The visceral pericardium or epicardium is closely adherent to the underlying myocardium and is reflected upon itself to form the outer parietal pericardium which lines the fibrous sac. Between the two layers of the serous pericardium lies the pericardial cavity which normally contains up to 50 ml of pericardial fluid. While the pericardium is not critical for life, it serves important functions including maintenance of cardiac position within the chest and as a barrier to infection and inflammation.

## ACUTE PERICARDITIS

Acute pericarditis is an inflammatory process involving the pericardium that results in a clinical syndrome characterized by chest pain, pericardial friction rub, changes in the electrocardiogram (ECG) and occasionally, a pericardial effusion. Generally, the diagnosis requires 2 of these 3 features.

### Prevalence

Acute pericarditis is the admitting diagnosis in 0.1% of hospital admissions and 5% of admissions with chest pain. It occurs more commonly in men than in women.

### Aetiology

The most common form of acute pericarditis is idiopathic, which accounts for about 90% of cases (Box 32.1). Other common causes include infection, renal failure, myocardial infarction (MI), post-cardiac injury syndrome, malignancy, radiation and trauma. These are discussed in more detail later.

### Signs and Symptoms

Acute pericarditis typically presents with acute onset severe, sharp retrosternal chest pain, often radiating to the

**BOX 32.1:** Common causes of pericarditis and pericardial effusion

| | |
|---|---|
| **Idiopathic** | • Infectious<br>• Viral (including HIV)<br>• Bacterial<br>• Mycobacterial<br>• Fungal and protozoal |
| **Post-myocardial infarction (early and late)** | |
| **Postoperatively after open heart surgery** | |
| **Chest trauma** | • Blunt<br>• Sharp |
| **Radiation** | |
| **Malignancy** | • Primary: mesothelioma, angiosarcoma<br>• Metastatic: lung, breast, bone, lymphoma, melanoma |
| **Collagen vascular diseases** | • Rheumatoid arthritis<br>• Systemic lupus erythematosus |
| **Inflammatory/ infiltrative diseases** | • Sarcoidosis<br>• Amyloidosis |
| **Metabolic** | • Hypothyroidism<br>• Uremia |
| **Pharmacologic** | • Cromolyn sodium<br>• Doxorubicin<br>• Hydralazine<br>• Methysergide<br>• Minoxidil<br>• Penicillin<br>• Phenytoin<br>• Procainamide |

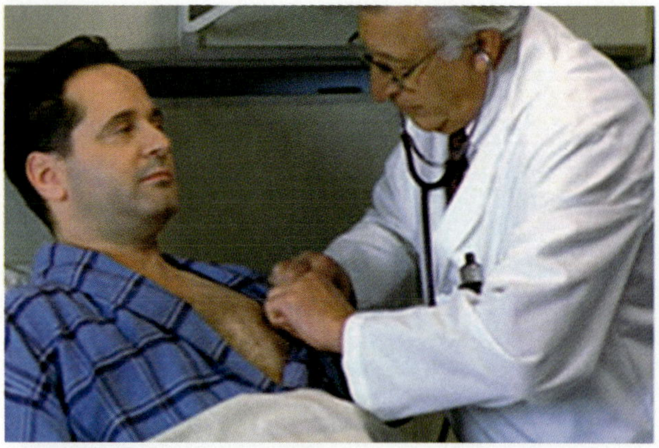

**Fig. 32.3:** Doctor assessing the cause of chest pain in a young person with past history of pulmonary tuberculosis

neck, shoulders or back. Positional changes are characteristic with worsening of the pain in the supine position and with inspiration; and improvement with sitting upright and leaning forward (Fig. 32.3 and Table 32.1).

Classically, a scratchy, grating, high-pitched friction rub (which has been likened to the squeak of leather of a new saddle) is heard. This is felt to be caused by fibrinous deposits in the inflamed pericardial space the timing of which can be mono-, bi-, or triphasic (corresponding to atrial systole, ventricular systole, and early ventricular diastole, respectively). It is best heard during inspiration at the left lower sternal border, with the patient leaning forward. The rub may disappear with the development of an effusion and impending cardiac tamponade.

## Specific Types

### *Idiopathic Pericarditis*

The cause of acute pericarditis is often difficult to establish, and idiopathic pericarditis remains the most common diagnosis. Most cases are presumed to have a viral aetiology.

### *Viral Pericarditis*

Coxsackievirus B and echovirus are the most common viruses, and a fourfold increase in antiviral titers is required for the diagnosis. Patients often experience a prodrome of an upper respiratory tract infection. The prognosis of viral pericarditis is generally good, with a self-limited course, and if uncomplicated, patients may be treated on an outpatient basis.

### *Purulent Pericarditis*

Before the antibiotic era, pneumonia was the prime cause of purulent pericarditis. Currently, causes include thoracic surgery, chemotherapy, immunosuppression, and hemodialysis, as well as extension from pneumonia and empyema. Presentation is usually acute with high fevers, chills, night sweats and dyspnea, but the classic findings of chest pain or friction rub are rare. Cardiac tamponade is common (42–77% of patients in selected series), and mortality is high. If purulent pericarditis is suspected, hospital admission, treatment with intravenous, broad-spectrum antibiotics and urgent drainage is recommended. Findings on pericardial fluid analysis include a high protein level (>6 g/dl), a low glucose level (<35 mg/dl), and a very high leukocyte count (6,000–240,000/mm$^3$).

### *Tuberculous Pericarditis*

Tuberculous pericarditis occurs in 1–2% of cases of pulmonary tuberculosis. It remains the leading cause of pericarditis in some developing countries. Immunocompromised or human immunodeficiency virus (HIV) positive patients are at increased risk. Nonspecific symptoms, such as dyspnea, fever, chills, and night sweats develop slowly, and a friction rub or chest pain is often absent. A patient with suspected or diagnosed pericardial tuberculosis should be hospitalized and antituberculous therapy started promptly. Analysis of the pericardial fluid shows high specific gravity, very high protein level (often >6 g/dl), and predominantly lymphocytic cells. A pericardial biopsy with

**Table 32.1:** Differential diagnosis of different clinical conditions with acute chest pain

| | Discription | Location | Radiation | Associations |
|---|---|---|---|---|
| Acute coronary syndromes | Crushing, tightening, squeezing or a pressure like | Retrosternal left anterior chest or epigastric | Rt. or Lt. shoulder, Rt. or Lt. arm/head, jaw | Dyspnea, diaphoresis and nausea |
| Pulmonary embolism | Heaviness, tightness | Whole chest (massive) or Focal chest (segmental) | None | Dyspnea, unstable vital signs, feling of impending doom if massive or just tachycardia, tachypnea if segmental |
| Aortic dissection | Ripping, tearing | Midline, substernal | Intrascapular area of back | Secondary arterial branch occlusion |
| Pneumothorax | Sudden, sharp, lancinating, and pleuritic | One side of chest | Shoulder, back | Dyspnea |
| Pericarditis/ temponade | Sharp, constant or pleuritic | Substernal | None | Fever, pericardial friction rub |
| Perforated esophagus | Sudden, sharp, and after forceful vomiting | Substernal | Back | Dyspnea, diaphoresis and signs of sepsis |

acid-fast bacilli polymerase chain reaction testing is recommended for all patients with suspected tuberculous pericarditis. However, a normal pericardial biopsy does not exclude the diagnosis.

### *Uremic and Dialysis-associated Pericarditis*

Uremic pericarditis occurs in 6–10% of patients with advanced renal failure before hemodialysis is initiated; blood urea nitrogen levels usually exceed 60 mg/dl. The typical ST-segment elevation on the ECG usually is absent. A large hemorrhagic effusion facilitated by impaired platelet function may occur, although tamponade is rare. Alternatively, a serous pericardial effusion related to fluid overload may occur. With both forms, initiation or intensification of hemodialysis is indicated, usually leading to improvement in 1–2 weeks.

### *Pericarditis Following Myocardial Infarction*

Post-MI pericarditis is a common complication (25–40% of patients with MI) and occurs early, within 3–10 days after the MI. Its development correlates with the extent of necrosis, is more common with anterior than inferior infarcts and is associated with a higher 1-year mortality rate as well as a higher incidence of congestive heart failure. The diagnosis of post-MI pericarditis requires symptoms or a new pericardial friction rub; a pericardial effusion alone is nonspecific. In addition to the typical ST-elevation seen with acute pericarditis that may be difficult to differentiate from the actual MI in this setting, findings on the ECG are persistently positive T-waves more than 2 days after MI or normalization of previously inverted T-waves.

### *Post-cardiac Injury Syndrome*

*Dressler's syndrome:* It typically occurs 2–3 weeks after MI or open heart surgery. An autoimmune component involving sensitization to myocardial self-antigens at the time of infarction is believed to be responsible. The fully expressed syndrome consists of pleuritic chest pain, fever, leukocytosis, and a pericardial friction rub. Pleural effusions or pulmonary infiltrates may be seen.

### *Malignancy*

Pericarditis associated with malignancy is caused mainly by metastatic disease. Pericarditis is common in metastasized bronchogenic or breast carcinoma, Hodgkin's disease, and lymphoma; it is rare in primary mesothelioma and angiosarcoma. Diagnosis is based on analysis of pericardial fluid cytology, which has a sensitivity ranging from 70–90% and a specificity of 95–100%.

### *Radiation Pericarditis*

Recent or remote mediastinal radiation can cause pericarditis at any time from weeks to months after the exposure.

### *Traumatic Pericarditis*

Sharp or blunt trauma and invasive cardiac procedures, such as electrophysiological ablation procedures, cardiac diagnostic, or interventional catheterization have been associated with pericardial irritation and inflammation.

## Diagnosis

The diagnosis of acute pericarditis remains a clinical one, based on history, physical examination, ECG and the echocardiogram. Other imaging studies, including computed tomography (CT) and magnetic resonance imaging (MRI) may be used in selected cases to investigate the pericardium.

### *Electrocardiography*

The ECG in acute pericarditis has four consecutive stages (Figs 32.4–32.7, Tables 32.2 and 32.3). Stage 1, characterized by diffuse concave-upwards ST-elevation and PR segment deviation in the direction opposite from the P polarity, is

**Table 32.2:** Stages of acute pericarditis by electrocardiography

| Stage | Time | ST-segment | T-wave | PR segment |
|---|---|---|---|---|
| 1 | Hours | Diffuse elevation | Upright | Leads $aV_R$, $V_1$: elevation; all others: depression |
| 2 | Days | Resolution | Flattening | Resolution |
| 3 | Days-weeks | — | Inversion | — |
| 4 | Days-weeks | — | Upright | |

**Table 32.3:** Electrocardiographic differentiation of acute pericarditis and myocardial infarction

| Parameter | Acute pericarditis | Acute myocardial infarction |
|---|---|---|
| ST-elevation | Diffuse in I, II and III<br>Originating from S wave<br>Concave upwards<br>Lead $V_6$: ST-T amplitude >0.24 mm | Focal—vascular territory<br>Originating from R wave<br>Convex upwards |
| ST-depression | Lead $aV_R$ only | Present; reciprocal changes to ST-elevation according to territory |
| PR segment | Leads $aV_R$, $V_1$: elevation frequent | Rare changes if atrial infarction is present |

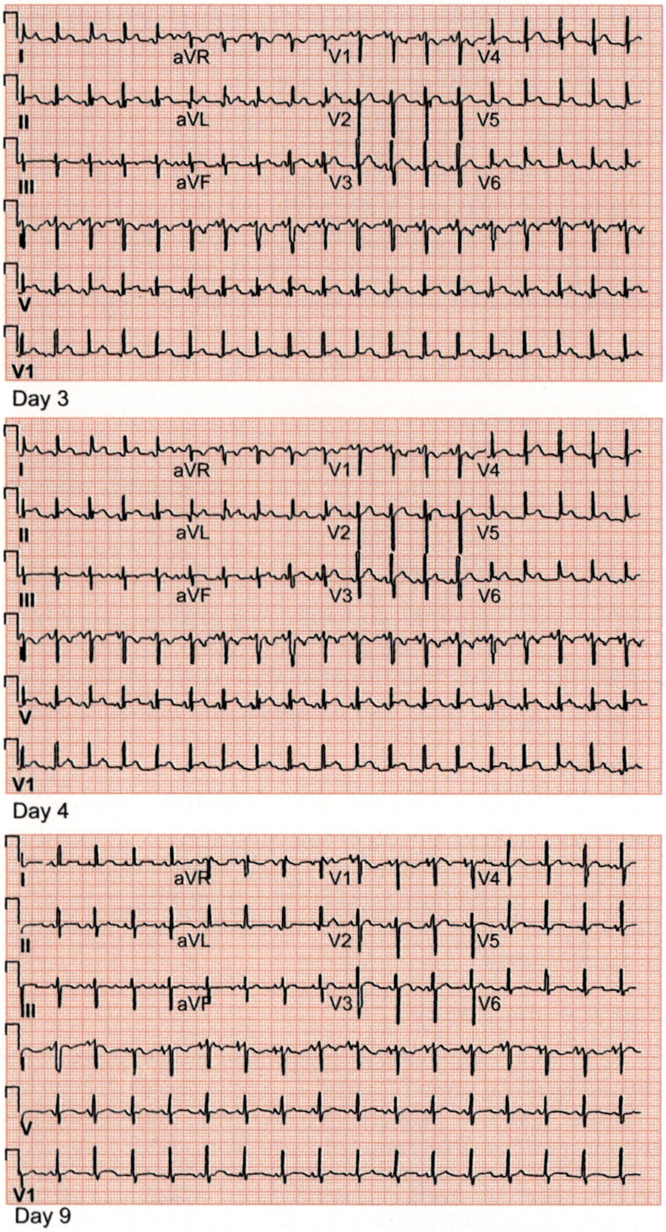


**Fig. 32.4:** Serial electrocardiograms obtained during recovery in the ICU that show resolution of the PR and ST-segment abnormalities noted previously

the most useful stage for the diagnosis of acute pericarditis. The distinction between pericarditis and acute MI is difficult at times, but there exist several helpful electrocardiographic clues. Troponin levels may be elevated in up to 50% of patients with pericarditis but in the absence of myocarditis, the prognosis remains unchanged.

### Blood Tests

Testing should include a complete blood count, markers of inflammation including erythrocyte sedimentation rate and/or C-reactive protein, markers of myocardial ischemia (troponins/CK-MB) to assess for myopericarditis, and assessment of renal function. Depending on presentation and clinical evaluation, additional blood testing may be necessary, such as viral titers, blood cultures, thyroid-stimulating hormone, antinuclear antibodies, HIV serology, or QuantiFERON-TB assay.

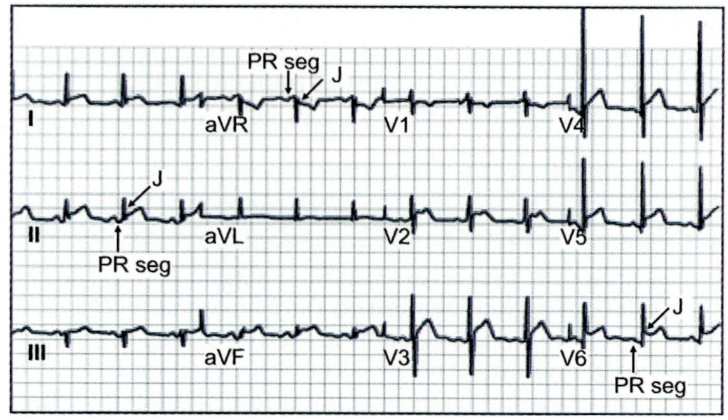


**Fig. 32.5:** Acute pericarditis , stage 1 ECG. J points, except aVR and V1, are elevated. T-waves are essentially normal. PR segments, except aVR and V1, are depressed. PR deviations are commonly absent in one limb lead (here, aVL)

### Chest Radiography

The chest radiograph may be entirely normal unless there is a pericardial effusion causing cardiomegaly or there are changes caused by an underlying disease (Fig. 32.8).

### Echocardiography

Trans-thoracic echocardiography (TTE) is used to detect and evaluate for pericardial effusion and any concomitant cardiac disease. Assessment of regional wall motion abnormalities can help differentiate acute pericarditis from myocardial ischemia. Echocardiography is essential in the presence of hemodynamic abnormalities, history of recent cardiac surgery, or if there is a clinical suspicion of a large or increasing pericardial effusion (Figs 32.9 and 32.10).

### Cardiac Computed Tomography and Cardiac Magnetic Resonance Imaging

Advanced imaging modalities are increasingly used in the diagnotic assessment of patients with acute pericarditis, and to help guide their management. Cardiac computed tomography (CCT) is useful to assess for loculated effusions and to evaluate for increased thickness of the pericardium, although these features are not diagnostic of acute pericarditis.

If there is clinical suspicion, CCT is useful in diagnosing the underlying aetiology of acute pericarditis, such as in the assessment of suspected malignancy-induced pericarditis. Inflammation of the pericardium produces characteristic changes that can be detected on cardiac magnetic resonance (CMR) imaging with very high sensitivity. Specifically, T2 weighted short-tau inversion recovery (STIR) imaging is useful for visualizing edema, while detection of a bright pericardium on late gadolinium enhancement (LGE) imaging is highly sensitive for pericardial inflammation.

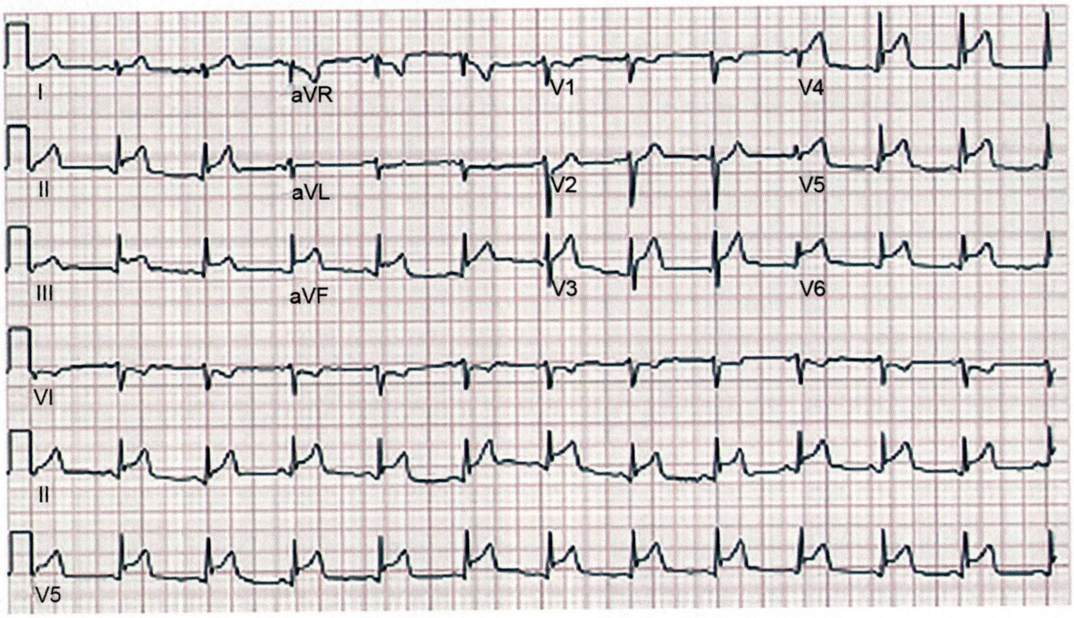


**Fig. 32.6:** ECG showing generalised ST-elevation in both limb and chest leads in patient with acute pericarditis without reciprocal changes

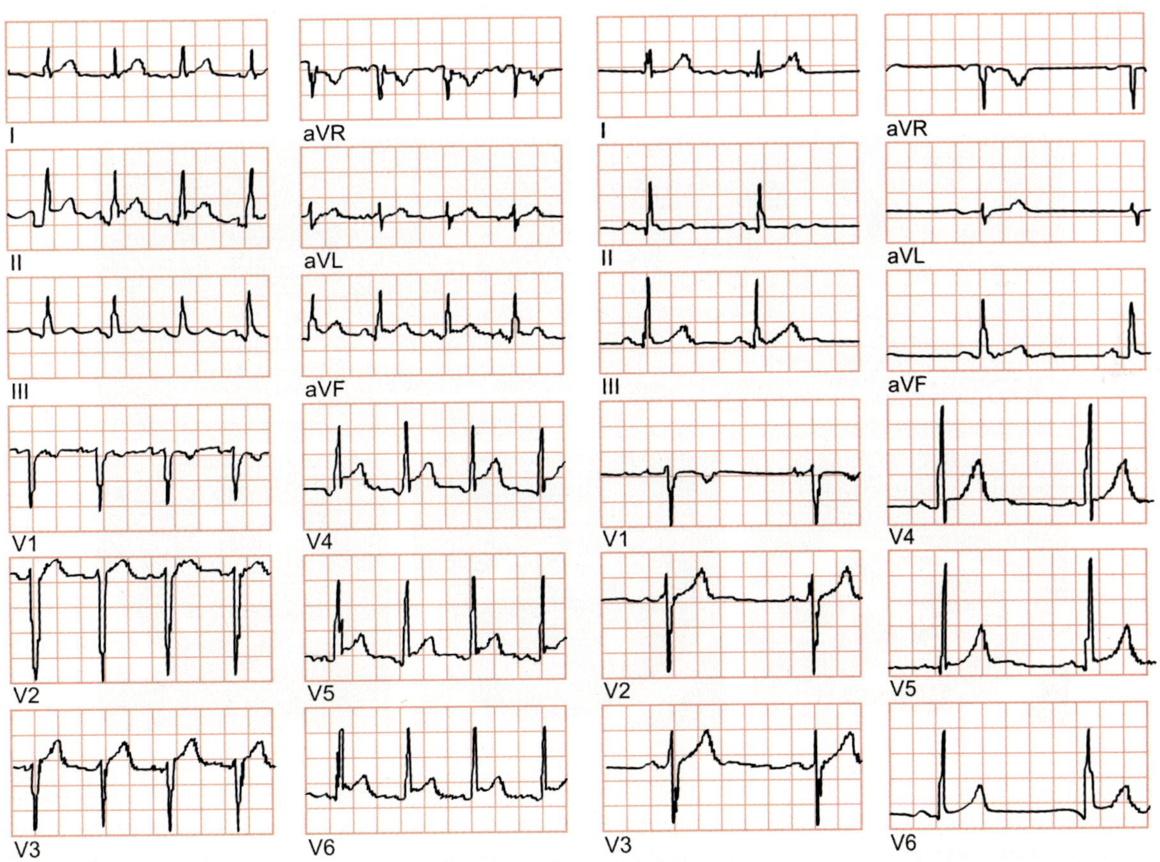


**Fig. 32.7:** Electrocardiograms contrast the pattern of ST-segment elevation characteristic of acute pericarditis (a) with the normal variant (early repolarization) pattern of ST-segment elevation (b). The normal variant pattern is associated with a normal or slow heart rate and has relatively tall R-waves and T-waves in V4, V5 and V6. The ST-segment elevation is less than 25% of the T-wave amplitude. In contrast, the acute pericarditis has PR depression and lower T-wave amplitude

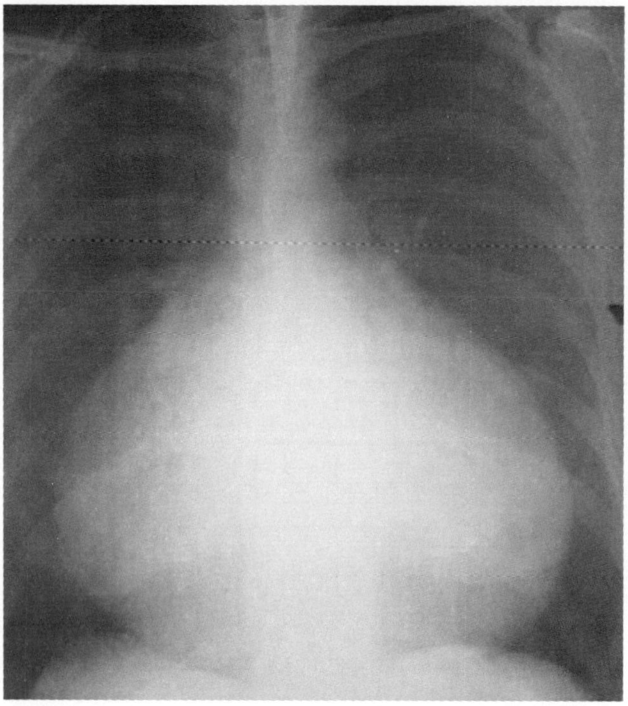

**Fig. 32.8:** Photograph of X-ray chest showing money bag or flask-shaped, enlarged cardiac silhouette in patient with moderate pericardial effusion

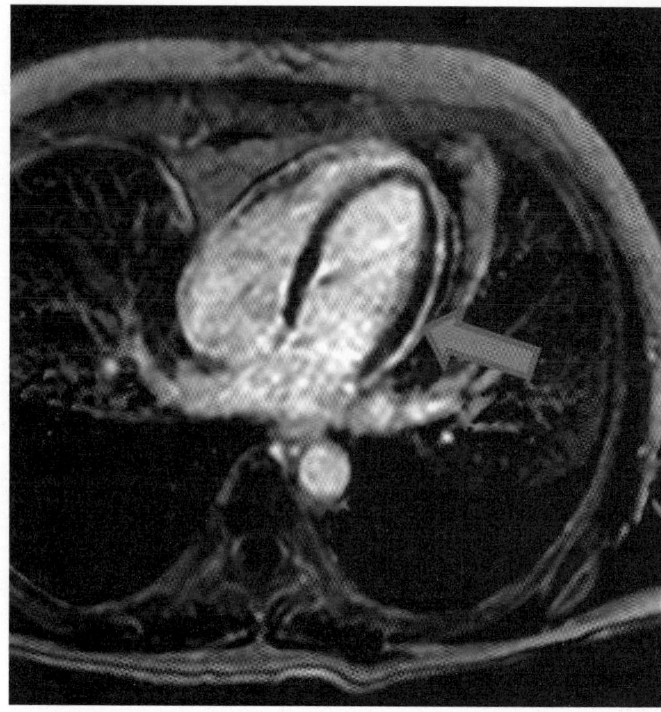

**Fig. 32.10:** Diffuse pericardial enhancement (arrow) on late Gadolinium enhancement in acute pericarditis. Repeat MRI performed after therapy shows near complete resolution of enhancement

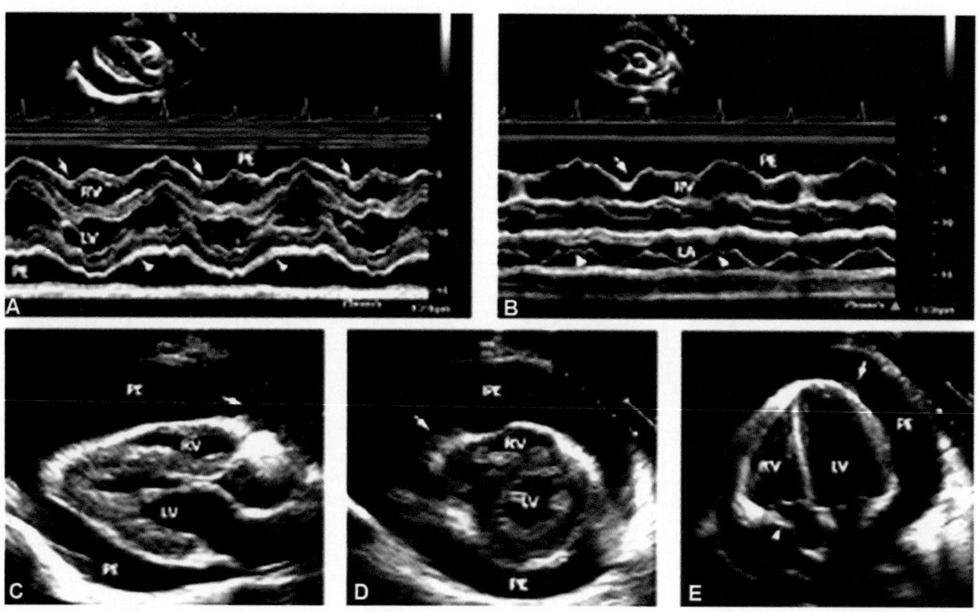


**Fig. 32.9:** Acute viral pericarditis complicated with a large pericardial effusion and cardiac tamponade in a 28-year-old man. (A) This 2D guided parasternal long-axis M-mode echo demonstrates a large pericardial effusion with significant diastolic compression of the RV anterior walls (arrows) and LV posterior walls (arrowheads). Also note the significant paradoxical interventricular septal motion, limited mitral valve opening, and electrical alternans on the electrocardiogram (ECG). (B) This 2D guided parasternal short-axis view M-mode echo demonstrates RV outflow tract (arrow) and LA (arrowheads) diastolic compression. (C, D) These 2D parasternal long-axis (C) and short-axis (D) views demonstrate a large circumferential pericardial effusion associated with severe visceral pericardial thickening with fronds and strands (arrows), RV and LV diastolic compression, and marked swinging of the heart with each heartbeat explaining the ECG electrical alternans. (E) This 2D apical four-chamber view demonstrates a large circumferential pericardial effusion associated with severe visceral pericardial thickening, including a mobile frond (arrow), marked swinging of the heart, and RV and especially significant (more than one-third of the cardiac cycle). RA=diastolic compression (arrowhead). LA=left atrium

### Treatment

Most cases of acute pericarditis are uncomplicated and self-limited, and may be treated on an outpatient basis. Indications for an advanced imaging modality, hospital admission, or both include clinical suspicion of a large effusion, hemodynamic instability, severe pain or other symptoms, suspicion of a serious underlying condition, or any other signs or symptoms of clinical instability or impending deterioration. Other features which suggest a more complex course include fever >38°C, subacute onset, lack of response to at least 1 week of anti-inflammatory therapy, myopericarditis, immunosuppression, trauma, or concurrent treatment with oral anticoagulant therapy.

#### *Medical Management*

In acute idiopathic and viral pericarditis, the aim of treatment is the resolution of pain and inflammation. For other etiologies of acute pericarditis treatment of the underlying disease is the mainstay of therapy. Combination therapy with colchicine and nonsteroidal anti-inflammatory drugs (NSAIDs) is recommended. Ibuprofen 600 mg or indomethacin 50 mg every 8 hours for 1–2 weeks followed by a gradual taper until resolution of symptoms and inflammatory markers, in combination with colchicine 0.6 mg twice daily (0.6 mg once daily if <70 kg) for 3 months is our standard recommendation.

Non-aspirin NSAIDs are contraindicated in the early period (<7–10 days) after MI (can predispose to cardiac rupture), and aspirin should be used instead (650–1,000 mg 3 times daily). Due to the risk of gastrointestinal toxicity, addition of gastrointestinal protection with a proton pump inhibitor is recommended in higher risk patient.

The randomized, open-label COPE (COlchicine for Acute PEricarditis) trial found that colchicine, in addition to aspirin, reduced the recurrence of pericarditis from 32.3% to 10.7% ($P = 0.003$). In the more recent randomized, double-blinded, placebo-controlled investigation on colchicine for acute pericarditis (ICAP) trial, a similar reduction in recurrent pericarditis was observed when colchicine was added to aspirin monotherapy (from 37.5% to 16.7%, $P < 0.001$). Unless their use is mandatory, anticoagulants should be avoided during the acute phase of pericarditis to reduce the risks of intrapericardial bleeding and tamponade.

Treatment with glucocorticoids should only be considered in recurrent pericarditis for patients with symptoms refractory to standard therapy, or in immune-mediated or uremic pericarditis. Use of steroids in acute pericarditis has been associated with recurrence. The correct dosing for steroid therapy remains controversial; however, our practice it to being with approximately 0.5 mg/kg/day with a prolonged and slow taper. As with non-aspirin NSAIDs, steroids should be avoided in post-MI pericarditis due to their impairment of scar formation and a consequently increased incidence of myocardial wall rupture.

#### *Pericardiectomy*

Pericardiectomy is not indicated in the management of acute pericarditis.

### Outcomes

Patients with uncomplicated acute pericarditis should have regular follow-up after the initial visit to ensure resolution of symptoms and rule out the development of constrictive symptoms.

## PERICARDIAL EFFUSION

Pericardial effusion is defined as an increased amount of pericardial fluid.

### Aetiology

The aetiology of a pericardial effusion can often be deduced from the clinical presentation, e.g. in patients who present with severe hypothyroidism, end-stage kidney failure, acute myocardial infarction, or who underwent a recent invasive cardiac procedure. The relative frequency of different etiologies of pericardial effusions depends on the geography and the patient population.

### Pathophysiology

The pericardial sac normally contains up to 50 ml of fluid; it can hold 80–200 ml of fluid acutely, and even up to 2 L if the fluid accumulates slowly.

### Signs and Symptoms

Pericardial effusions may be asymptomatic unless associated with inflammation or tamponade physiology. Other symptoms arise from the compression of surrounding structures (lung, stomach and phrenic nerve) or diastolic heart failure and include chest pressure or pain, dyspnea, nausea, abdominal fullness and dysphagia. Phrenic nerve irritation can cause hiccups.

With a small effusion, the physical examination is unremarkable. Larger effusions cause muffled heart sounds and, rarely, Ewart's sign (dullness to percussion, bronchial breath sounds and egophony below the angle of the left scapula).

### Diagnosis

#### *Electrocardiography*

Low voltage and electrical alternans may be seen if the effusion is large—the former due to increased distance from the chest leads, the latter caused by swinging of the heart within the effusion. These features in combination with sinus tachycardia should raise concern regarding the potential hemodynamic impact of the effusion and urgent assessment for tamponade physiology should be performed. Absence of hypotension should not dissuade the clinician from a possible diagnosis of pericardial effusion and tamponade, because hemodynamic instability usually does not occur until the patient nears circulatory collapse (Fig. 32.11).

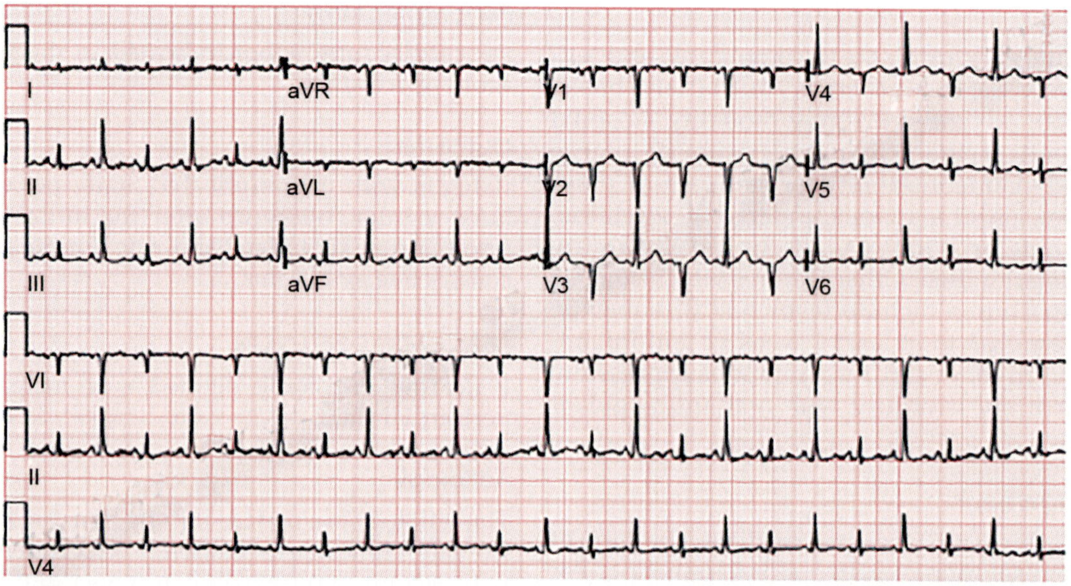


**Fig. 32.11:** ECG showing generalised low voltage graph with electrical alternans smaller QRS, flattening of ST-segment and T-wave inversion in patient with moderate pericardial effusion

### Chest Radiography

Cardiomegaly occurs if there is more than 250 ml of fluid in the pericardial sac. Displacement of the pericardial lining more than 2 mm away from the lower heart border is best seen on lateral film (Fig. 32.12).

### Echocardiography

Echocardiography is the main diagnostic tool used in the evaluation of pericardial effusion. A pericardial effusion causes an echo-free space between visceral and parietal pericardium; the extent of the space defines the size of the effusion. Large effusions can produce the picture of a swinging heart. Although, echocardiography is the imaging modality of choice for diagnosing a pericardial effusion, small loculated effusions pose a greater diagnostic challenge (Figs 32.13–32.15 and Table 32.4).

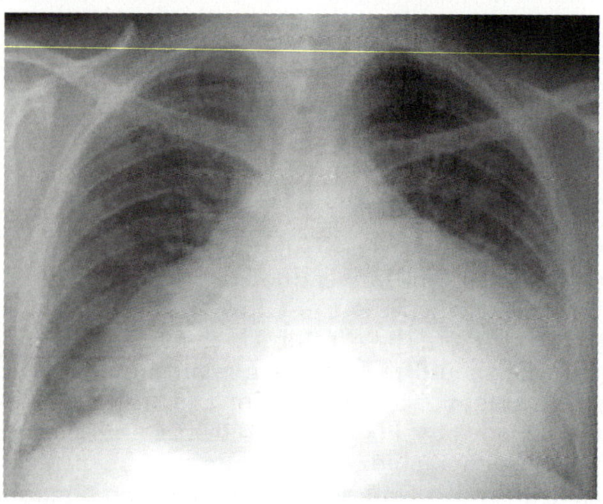

**Fig. 32.12:** X-ray chest (PA view). Massive cardiomegaly with normal lung field.

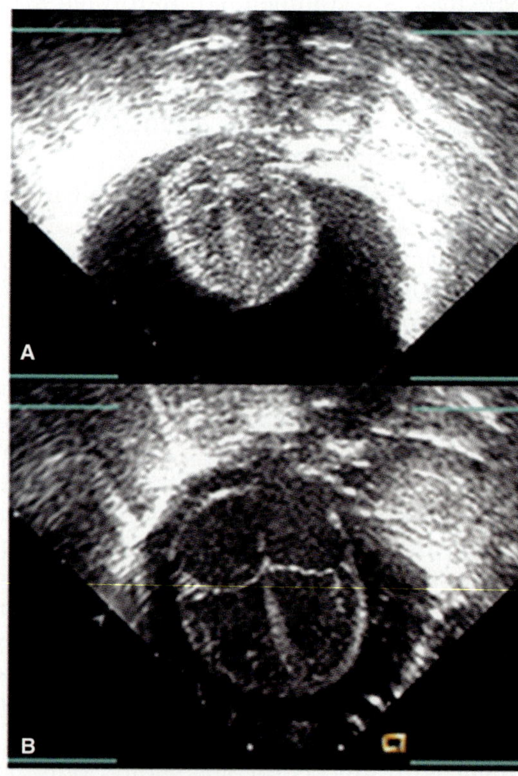


**Fig. 32.13:** (A) Initial echocardiogram shows a large pericardial effusion. (B) Followiing pericardiocentesis, the effusion is markedly decreased

**Table 32.4:** Sizing of pericardial effusion by echocardiography

| Parameter | Small | Medium | Large |
|---|---|---|---|
| Volume (ml) | <100 | 100–500 | >500 |
| Localization | Localized | Circumferential | Circumferential |
| Width (cm) | <1 | 1–2 | >2 |

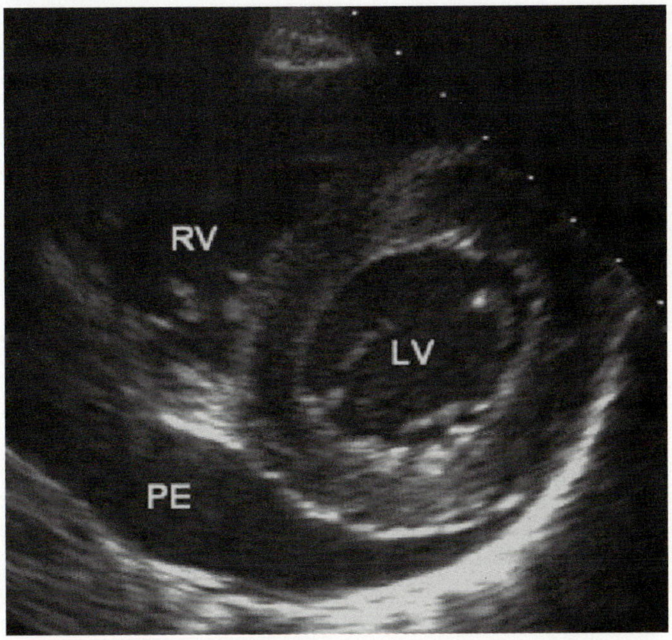


**Fig. 32.14:** Pericardial effusion from a parasternal short-axis echocardiographic view. RV=right ventricle; LV=left ventricle; PE=pericardial effusion

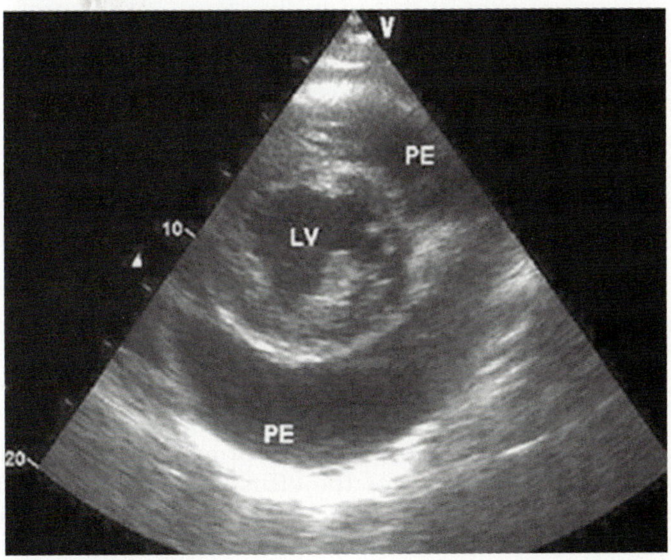


**Fig. 32.15:** Echocardiography. Moderate pericardial effusion with features of cardiac tamponade

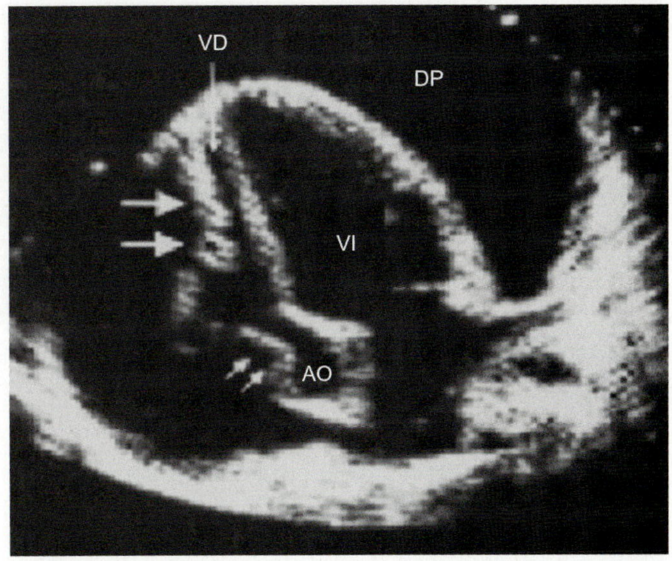


**Fig. 32.16:** Two-dimensional echocardiogram (4-chamber apical plane) showing a significant atrial (small arrows) and right ventricle (large arrows) collapse. The patient showed clinical signs of blockage. The collapse of both cavities is highly specific and has a high positive predictive value for tamponade. RA=right atrium; PE=pericardial effusion; RV=right ventricle; LV=left ventricle

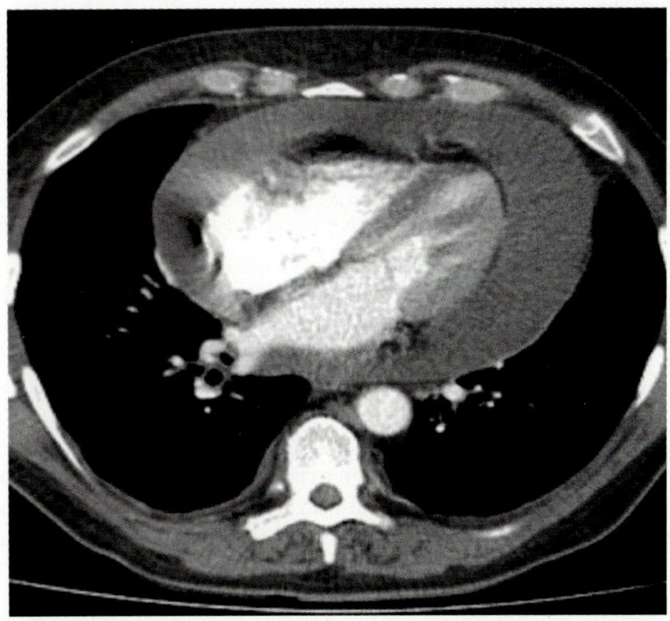

**Fig. 32.17:** Axial section from the CT chest showing the large circumferential pericardial effusion

### Magnetic Resonance Imaging and Computed Tomography

If there is a high level of clinical suspicion of a pericardial effusion and the TTE is nondiagnostic, alternative tomographic imaging should be considered. This is especially true for patients who have recently undergone open heart surgery, who frequently have echocardiographic studies with suboptimal imaging quality, and effusions which may be loculated and complex. Cardiac CT and MRI will also aid in differentiating an effusion from pericardial fat, pericardial cysts and pleural effusions, all of which can mimic a pericardial effusion (Figs 32.17–32.19).

### Laboratory Tests

Laboratory analysis in a patient with a pericardial effusion should include a complete blood count, chemistry panel, and erythrocyte sedimentation rate. Further testing should be done according to clinical suspicion.

### Analysis of Pericardial Fluid

The initial inspection should assess whether the fluid is hemorrhagic, purulent, or chylous. A red blood cell count

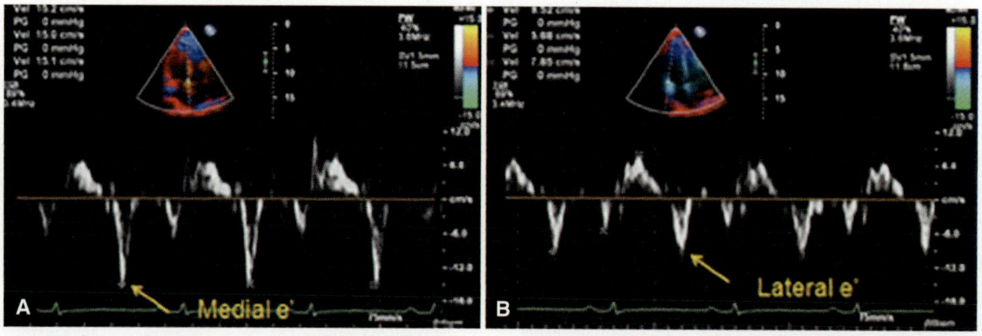


**Fig. 32.18:** Medial (A) and lateral (B) mitral annular tissue Doppler recording (apical window) in a patient with constrictive pericarditis. Note normal to increased early relaxation velocity (e'), with medial velocity greater than lateral (annulus reversus)

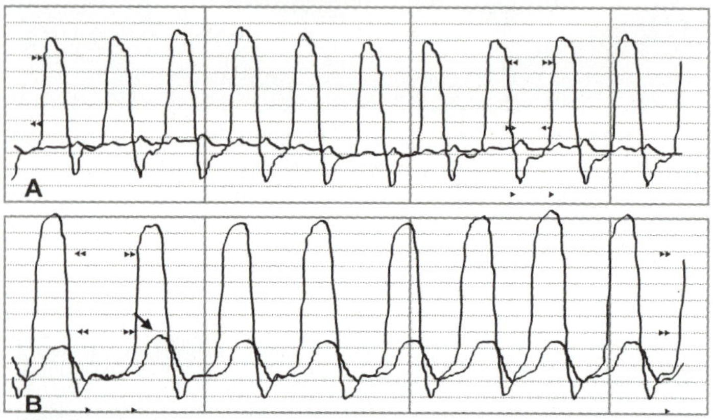


**Fig. 32.19:** Catheterization. (A) LV curve with diastolic dip-plateau and right atrial curve (equalized diastolic pressures). (B) Left ventricular (LV) and right ventricular (RV) pressure curve (equalized diastolic pressures). LV-RV pressure discordance during inspiration (arrow) in a patient with idiopathic effusive constrictive pericarditis

higher than 100,000/mm$^3$ is suggestive of trauma, malignancy, or pulmonary embolism (rare). Chylous fluid implies injury to the thoracic duct by trauma or infiltration. The fluid should be sent for a cell count; Gram stain; culture; cytology; acid-fast bacilli; determination of glucose, protein, and lactate dehydrogenase (LDH) levels; and specific gravity. The parameters have a high sensitivity for differentiating exudates versus transudates. An elevated protein level higher than 6.0 g/dl often indicates tuberculous, purulent, or parapneumonic effusion. An isolated increased fluid LDH level (>300 U/dl) with a normal serum LDH level is most likely caused by malignancy. A low pericardial fluid glucose level (<60–80 mg/dl) may be caused by parapneumonic, rheumatoid, tuberculous, or malignant effusion. However, no diagnostic test of pericardial fluid is specific for effusion associated with postpericardiotomy syndrome, radiation or uremic pericarditis, hypothyroidism, or trauma. The overall diagnostic yield of pericardial fluid analysis and biopsy is low (about 20%), emphasizing the importance of clinical history and examination.

## Treatment

The medical management of pericardial effusion is based on treating the underlying cause. Effusions causing pretamponade or tamponade require immediate drainage. Volume expansion and inotropic support may be used for hemodynamic stabilization pending drainage. In the immediate postoperative setting, surgical management and open drainage are preferred because of the high incidence of loculated effusions. Anti-coagulation should be avoided if possible.

### *Pericardiocentesis*

Pericardiocentesis should be performed for diagnostic purposes if the cause of the effusion is unclear, or if malignancy or a purulent effusion is suspected. Therapeutic pericardiocentesis should be performed for effusions

**Table 32.5:** Pericardial effusion–exudate versus transudate

| Parameter | Exudate | Transudate |
|---|---|---|
| Cause | Malignancy<br>Infectious, parainfectious<br>Postpericardiotomy syndrome<br>Collagen vascular disease | Radiation<br>Uremia<br>Hypothyroidism<br>Trauma |
| Specific gravity (g/ml) | >1.015 | <1.015 |
| Total protein (g/dl) | >3.0 | <3.0 |
| Fluid-to-serum protein ratio | >0.5 | <0.5 |
| Fluid-to-serum LDH ratio | >0.6 | <0.6 |
| Fluid-to-serum glucose ratio | <1.0 | >1.0 |

LDH = lactate dehydrogenase

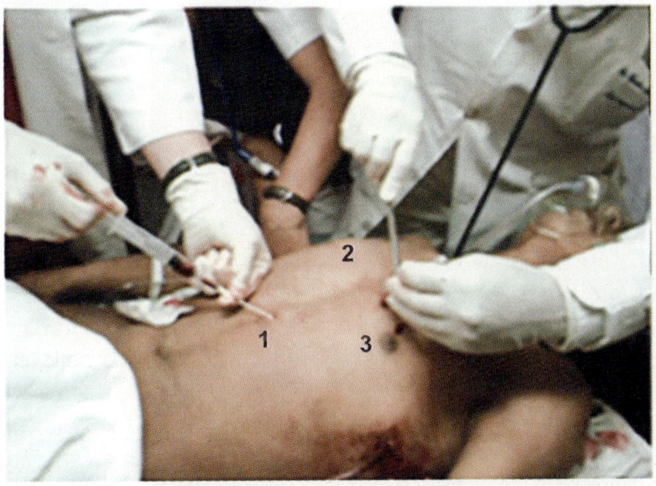


**Fig. 32.20A:** Different sites of pericardiocentesis in a patient with massive pericardial effusion (encircled arrow 1=epigastric, 2=parasternal, 3=apical regions over the chest)

amenable to percutaneous drainage that are causing pretamponade or tamponade physiology.

*Pericardiocentesis procedure:* It can be performed either using fluoroscopic (cardiac catheterisation laboratory) or echocardiographic guidance (Figs 32.20 and 32.21). ECG monitoring from the puncturing needle is not an adequate safeguard. Right heart catheterisation can be performed simultaneously with pericardiocentesis, allowing haemodynamic monitoring and exclusion of effusive-constrictive disease. The subxiphoid approach has been used most commonly, with a long needle with a mandrel (Johy or thin walled 18 gauge) directed towards the left shoulder at a 30° angle to the skin. This route is extrapleural and avoids the coronary, pericardial and internal mammary arteries. The operator intermittently attempts to aspirate fluid and injects small amounts of contrast medium. After aspiration of the fluid. The needle must be promptly replaced with a soft J tip guidewire which, after dilatation, is exchanged for a multi-holed pigtail catheter. It is prudent to drain the fluid in stepped amounts of <1 litre at a time to avoid acute right ventricular dilatation.

Echocardiographic guidance of pericardiocentesis is performed at the bedside. After identification of the shortest route to the effusion by echocardiography, the pericardium is entered intercostally (usually in the sixth or seventh rib space in the anterior axillary line). The feasibility of pericardiocentesis is high (93%) in patients with anterior effusion >10 mm, while the rate of success is only 58% with small, posteriorly located effusions. Fluoroscopic and haemodynamic monitoring contribute to a better outcome following the procedure (93.1% *vs* 73.3%), in comparison to emergency pericardial puncture with no imaging control. In addition, fluoroscopic guidance using the epicardial halo phenomenon significantly increased the feasibility of the procedure in patients with small effusions (200–300 ml; 92.6% *vs* 84.9%) and very small effusions <200 ml; 89.3% *vs* 76.7%).

Echocardiographic guidance improved efficacy to 96% for pericardiocentesis of loculated pericardial effusion after cardiac surgery and to 99% for rescue pericardiocentesis. The most serious, but rare, complications are lacerations/perforations of the myocardium and the coronary vessels. In addition, patients can experience air embolism, pneumothorax, arrhythmias (usually vasovagal bradycardia), and puncture of the peritoneal cavity or abdominal viscera. Internal mammary artery fistulas, acute pulmonary edema and purulent pericarditis have rarely been reported. The safety of pericardiocentesis was significantly improved with the introduction of echocardiographic or fluoroscopic guidance. Recent large echocardiographic series reported an incidence of major complications of 1.3–1.6%. In a large series of fluoroscopy, guided percutaneous pericardio-

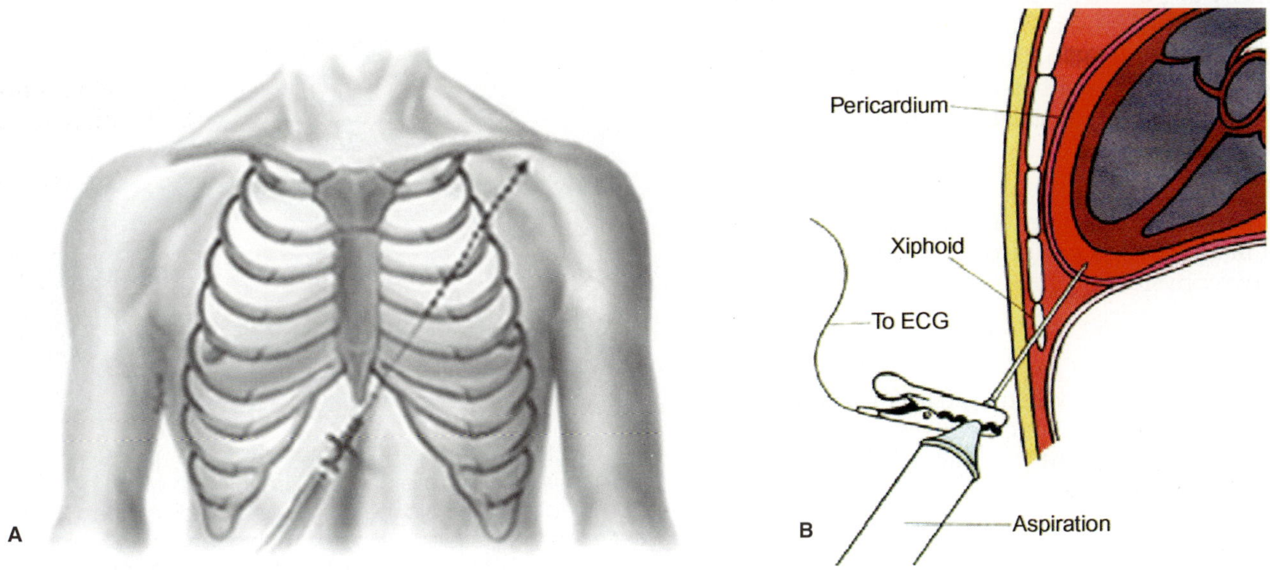


**Fig. 32.20B:** (A) Aspirating needle is positioned in epigastric region directing it towards the left shoulder. (B) Diagram showing technique of pericardiocentesis. Needle is inserted 2–4 cm below the junction of subxiphoid process and the left costal margin at an angle of 15–30°, so that it passes along the posterior aspect of the sternum until it enters the pericardial sac

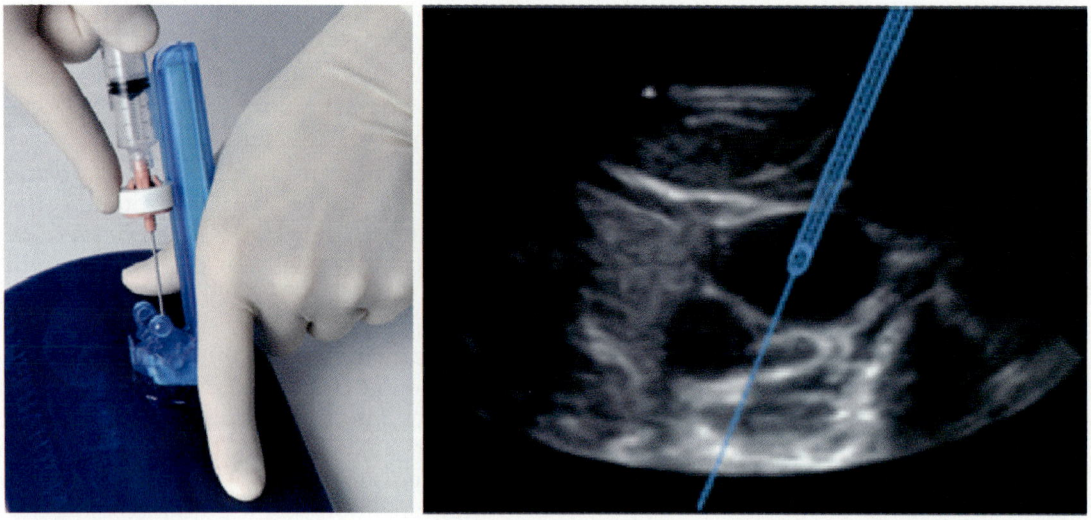

**Fig. 32.21:** AxoTrack needle guidance ultrasound probe for aspiration of pericardial effusion

centeses, cardiac perforations occurred in 0.9%, serious arrhythmias in 0.6%, arterial bleeding in 1.1 %, pneumothorax in 0.6%, infection in 0.3%, and a major vagal reaction in 0.3%. Incidence of major complications was also significantly reduced by utilising fluoroscopic guidance and the epicardial halo phenomenon. Pericardial constriction.

### *Surgical Treatment*

*Subxiphoid pericardiostomy*, also known as a pericardial window, may be done under local anesthesia. It has a high success rate, with few complications, and recurrence of fluid accumulation is rare.

*Percutaneous balloon pericardiotomy,* (Figs 32.22 and 32.23), is the least invasive of the surgical procedures. It is used primarily as palliative treatment for neoplastic effusions with a poor prognosis. The success rate for relieving reaccumulation of pericardial fluid is 85–92% at 30 days. It may be performed in the catheterization laboratory under fluoroscopy using a balloon-dilating catheter.

### Outcomes

After drainage, follow-up echocardiography should be performed in all patients to rule out reaccumulation and/ or constrictive physiology.

## CARDIAC TAMPONADE

Cardiac tamponade occurs when fluid accumulation in the finite serous pericardial space causes an increase in pressure, with subsequent cardiac compression and hemodynamic compromise.

### Prevalence

Of patients with large pericardial effusions, 25–30% develop tamponade.

### Pathophysiology

Elevated intrapericardial pressure leads to progressive limitation of diastolic ventricular filling, resulting in lowered cardiac output.

### Signs and Symptoms

#### *Symptoms*

Symptoms resulting from decreased cardiac output and congestion include dyspnea, chest discomfort, weakness, restlessness, agitation, drowsiness, oliguria and anorexia. If the tamponade develops acutely as a complication of an acute MI (free wall rupture) or trauma, the presentation is usually catastrophic, with shock or sudden death.

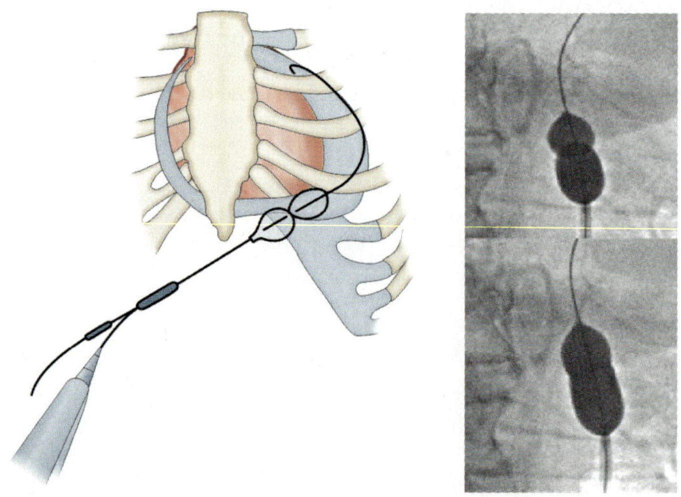

**Fig. 32.22:** Steps in single balloon pericardiotomy. **Step 1.** Introducer in the pericardium through which contrast has been injected to locate the parietal pericardium. **Step 2.** Balloon inserted in the parietal pericardium through a 0.035-inch guide. Before inflating, the introducer is removed slightly. **Step 3.** Progressive inflation of the balloon until the notch disappears, observing the typical hourglass image

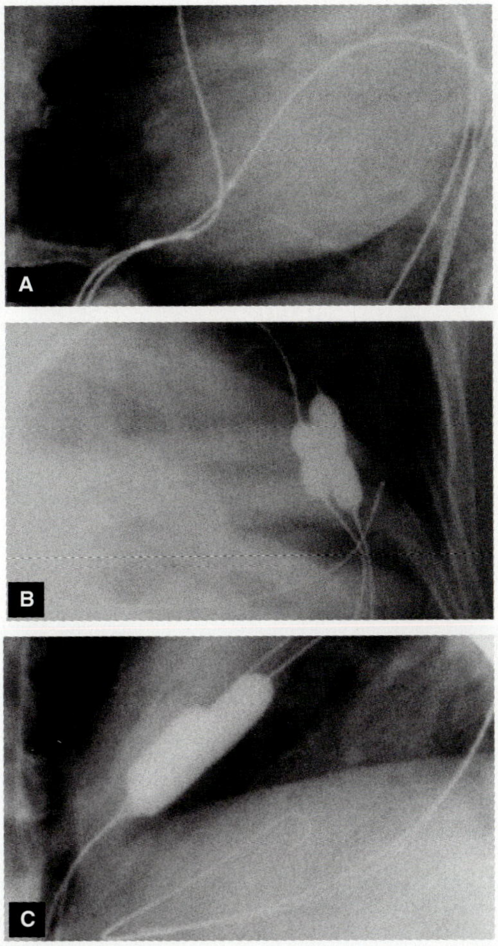


**Fig. 32.23:** (A) Two guidewires in the same tract separate from each other after their entrance into the pericardial cavity, so that the pericardial border can be defined clearly under fluoroscopy. (B) Double balloons were straddled over the pericardium. Both balloons were partially inflated and showed a central waist appearance. (C) Fully expanded double balloons creating a pericardial window

### *Physical Examination Findings*

The combination of the classic findings known as Beck's triad (hypotension, jugular venous distention, and muffled heart sounds) occurs in only 10–40% of patients. Tachycardia and tachypnea are common. Pulsus paradoxus is defined as an inspiratory decline in systolic blood pressure of more than 10 mmHg resulting from compression and poor filling of the left ventricle. Pulsus paradoxus is nonspecific and insensitive and can occur with extracardiac disease, such as severe chronic obstructive pulmonary disease or asthma.

## Diagnosis

The diagnosis of cardiac tamponade is a clinical diagnosis with echocardiagraphic comfirmation.

### *Electrocardiography*

The ECG may be unremarkable. Abnormal findings on ECG include tachycardia, electrical alternans), low voltage, and may include changes associated with acute pericarditis (Fig. 32.24).

### *Transthoracic Echocardiography*

Usually, a moderate-size or large pericardial effusion is present and leads to increasing compression and subsequent diastolic compression of the cardiac chambers, usually in the sequence right atrium, right ventricle, left atrium (with the lowest pressure chamber being affected first) (Figs 32.25–32.31). The most sensitive finding for tamponade physiology on the echocardiogram is inferior vena cava plethora, with absent inspiratory collapse; however this is not very specific. Right atrial inversion for greater than one thirds the cardiac cycle length is the most sensitive and specific sign. Right ventricular diastolic inversion may also been seen. Other, less-specific findings include excessive respiratory variations across the mitral

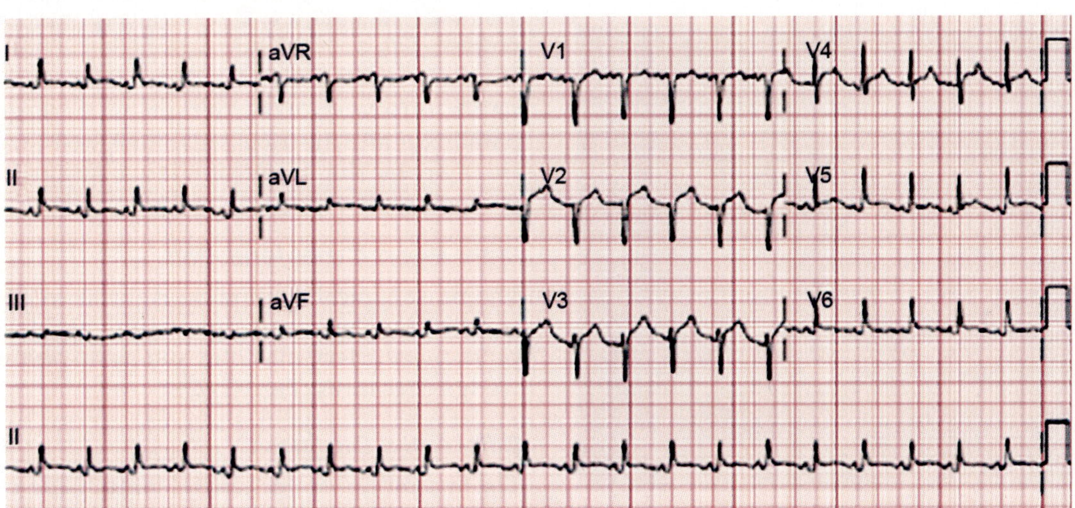


**Fig. 32.24:** Widespread ST-elevations PR depression as compared to ST-depression. Note: In aVR, there will be reciprocal changes and one will have PR elevation and ST-depression ('knuckle sign')

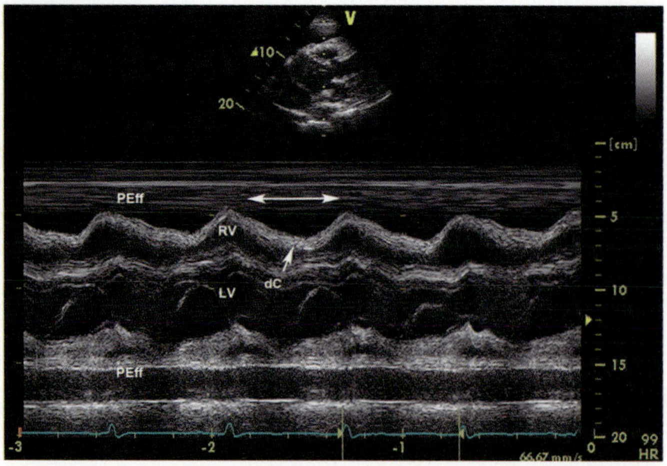


**Fig. 32.25:** M-Mode echoscan taken from the parasternal long-axis view in a patient with cardiac tamponade shows anterior and posterior pericardial effusion with diastolic collapse of RV

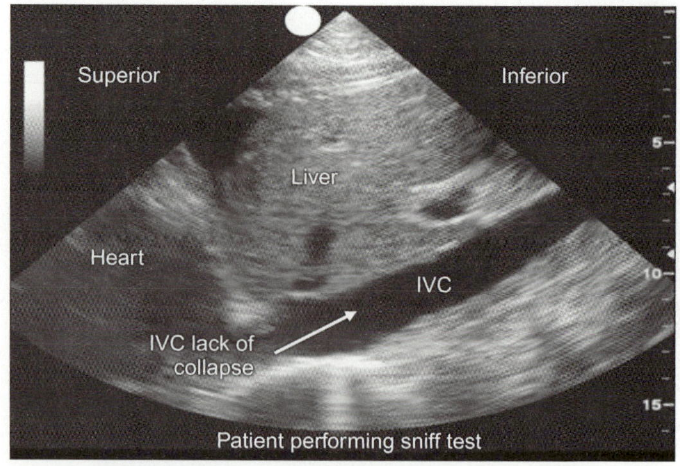


**Fig. 32.28:** Plethora of inferior vena cava. The presence of a dilated inferior vena cava with less than 50% collapse on forced inspiration, or sniff, correlates with an elevated central venous pressure and confirms tamponade physiology

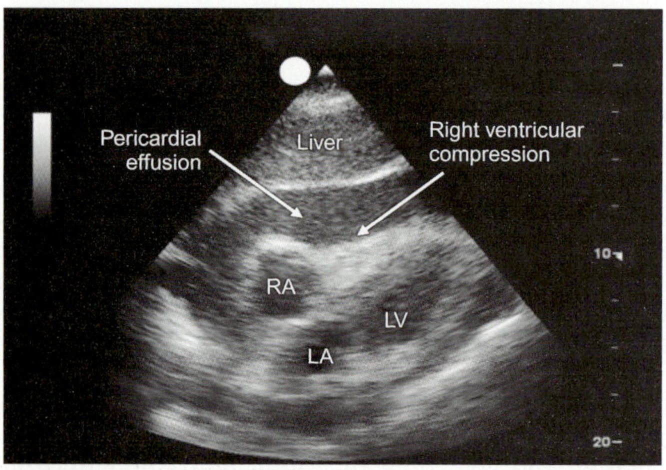


**Fig. 32.26:** Acute pericardial tamponade diastolic collapse of the right ventricle is noted on subxiphoid view. RA=right atrium; LV=left ventricle; LA=left atrium

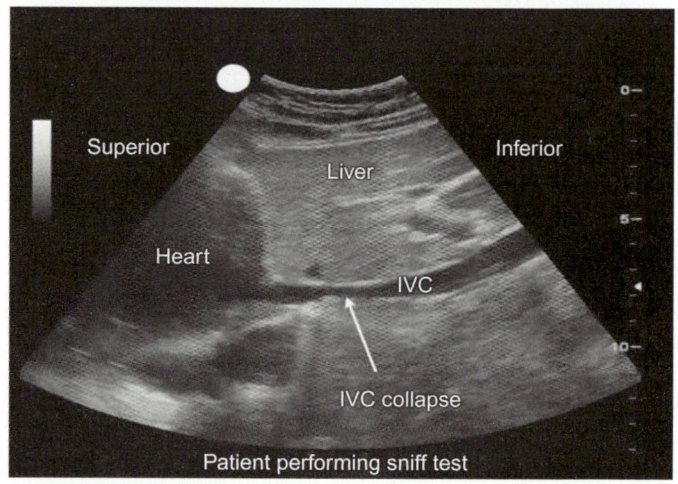


**Fig. 32.29:** Collapse of inferior vena cava. The presence of a small inferior vena cava with >50% collapse on forced inspiration, or sniff, correlates with a low central venous pressure and suggests the pericardial effusion is not causing obstructive tamponade physiology

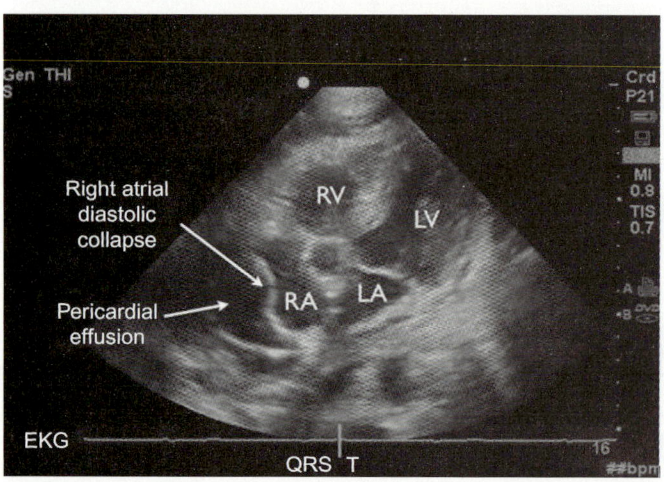


**Fig. 32.27:** Pericardial effusion with early tamponade. The right atrium is noted to have diastolic collapse, as timed with the T-wave on electrocardiogram monitoring at bottom. RV=right ventricle; RA=right atrium; LV=left ventricle; LA=left atrium

valve inflow (>30%), which is analogous to pulsus paradoxus and the tricuspid inflow (>60%). Absent diastolic flow from the hepatic views suggests tamponade physiology.

### Right Heart Catheterization

The most typical finding on right heart catheterization is equalization of mean right atrial, right ventricular and pulmonary artery diastolic, and mean pulmonary capillary wedge pressures (Fig. 32.32).

### Differential Diagnosis

The symptoms of pericardial tamponade can mimic those of right-sided heart failure, right ventricular infarction, constrictive pericarditis and pulmonary embolism. However, with the use of echocardiography and occasionally right heart catheterization, these may be distinguished.

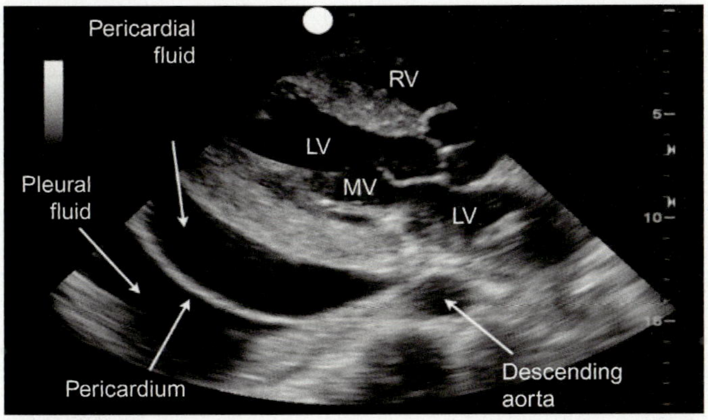


**Fig. 32.30:** Differentiation of a pericardial effusion from a pleural effusion. Note the descending aorta seen as a cylinder posterior to the left atrium. The posterior pericardial reflection is located anterior to the aorta. This allows determination of pericardial effusion, anterior to the pericardium, from a pleural effusion, posterior to the pericardium. RV=right ventricle; LV=left ventricle; LA=left atrium; MV=mitral valve

## Treatment

Patients with pretamponade and tamponade require immediate hospital admission and prompt pericardial drainage by pericardiocentesis. The drain catheter may be left in place for up to 48 hours, if drainage is slow or reaccumulation likely. If follow-up echocardiography documents fluid reaccumulation, a pericardial window should be considered, because the infection risk associated with a pericardial drain increases after 48 hours. Pending drainage, intravenous fluid expansion and inotropic support may be used for hemodynamically unstable patients.

# PERICARDIAL CONSTRICTION

Constrictive pericarditis refers to an abnormal scarring and loss of elasticity of the pericardium, resulting in impaired ventricular filling and decreased cardiac output.

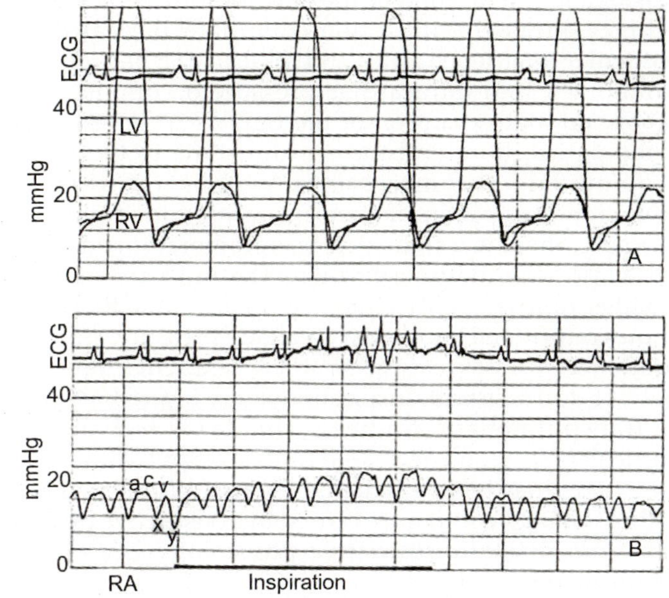


**Fig. 32.32:** Hemodynamic monitoring can confirm the diagnosis of pericardial tamponade. Equalization of diastolic pressures on the left and right sides of the heart, elevated right atrial pressure, and Kussmaul's sign (i.e. increase in right atrial pressure with inspiration) are noted

## Aetiology

The frequency of different causes of constrictive pericarditis depends on the population and geography in question. In developed countries, cardiac surgery and idiopathic constriction are the leading cause, while in certain developing countries tuberculous remains the number one aetiology.

## Pathophysiology

The initiating event results in a chronic inflammatory pericardial process, resulting in fibrinous scarring and

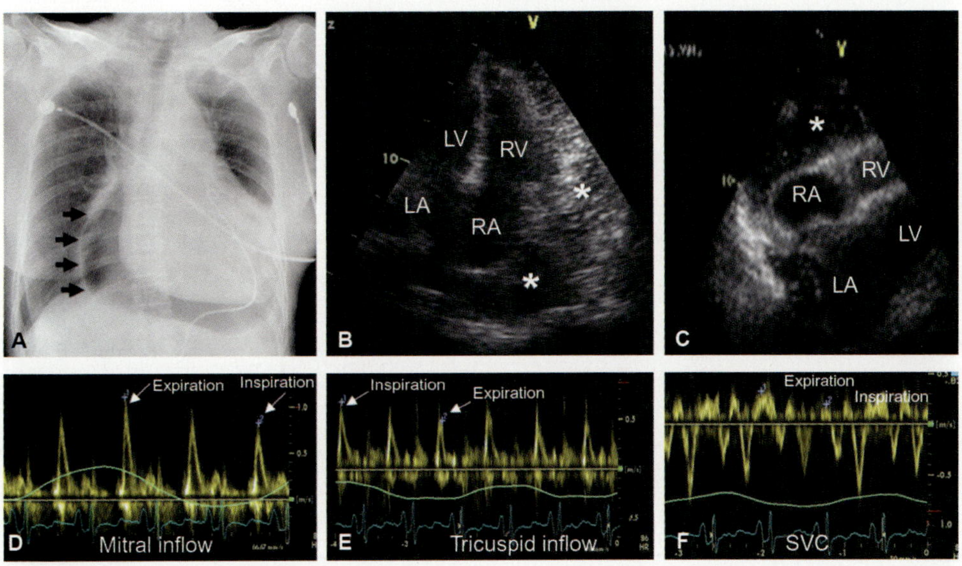


**Fig. 32.31:** (A) Chest radiograph shows air separating the pericardium from the heart indicating pneumopericardium (arrows). A transthoracic echocardiogram shows pericardial air microbubbles and effusion (B and C) with significant respiratory variation of tricuspid (D) and mitral (E) inflows and superior vena caval flow (F), confirming tamponade physiology

occasionally calcification of the pericardium. As the heart becomes encased with a non-compliant pericardium, ventricular interdependance and dissociation between the intrathoracic and intracardiac pressure occurs. In constriction, normal expansion of the right heart is restricted by the pericardium and the septum shifts to the left to accommodate the increase in venous return with inspiration; the opposite movement occurs with expiration. Normally, there is a reduction in intrathoracic and intracardiac pressure with inspiration. The rigid pericardium impedes normal ventricular expansion and therefore venous return and pulmonary venous pressure. Because intrathoracic pressure drops, but left ventricular pressure does not decrease with inspiration, there is a reduction in the transpulmonary gradient. This leads to impaired ventricular filling and decreased cardiac output. Ultimately, right and then left ventricular heart failure develop. Distinguishing heart failure caused by constrictive physiology from diastolic restrictive physiology is a classic diagnostic dilemma.

## Signs and Symptoms

### *Clinical Symptoms*

Symptoms are often vague and their onset is insidious; they include malaise, fatigue and decreased exercise tolerance. With progression of constrictive pericarditis, symptoms of right-sided heart failure (e.g. peripheral edema, nausea, abdominal discomfort and ascites) become apparent and usually precede signs of left-sided failure (e.g. exertional dyspnea, orthopnea and paroxysmal nocturnal dyspnea).

### *Physical Examination Findings*

Increased ventricular filling pressures cause jugular venous distention and Kussmaul's sign (paradoxical rise in jugular venous pressure on inspiration), which is sensitive but not specific for constrictive pericarditis. Auscultation may reveal muffled heart sounds and occasionally a characteristic pericardial knock (60–200 msec after the second heart sound), which is caused by sudden termination of ventricular inflow by the encasing pericardium .

Constrictive effusive pericarditis consists of a tense pericardial effusion in the presence of pericardial constriction, and both tamponade and constrictive signs and symptoms are present (Fig. 32.33).

## Diagnosis

### *Electrocardiography*

The ECG does not show specific findings, but low voltage may be seen (Fig. 32.34).

### *Laboratory Test Findings*

Brain natriuretic peptide (BNP) is a serum biomarker that can help distinguish constrictive pericarditis from

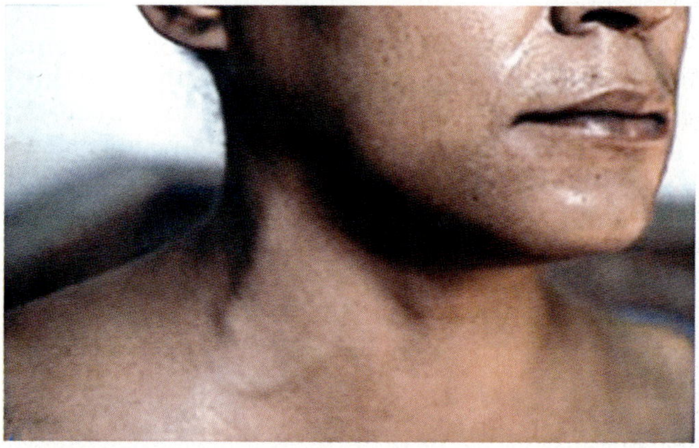

**Fig. 32.33:** Raised jugular venous pressure in constrictive pericarditis

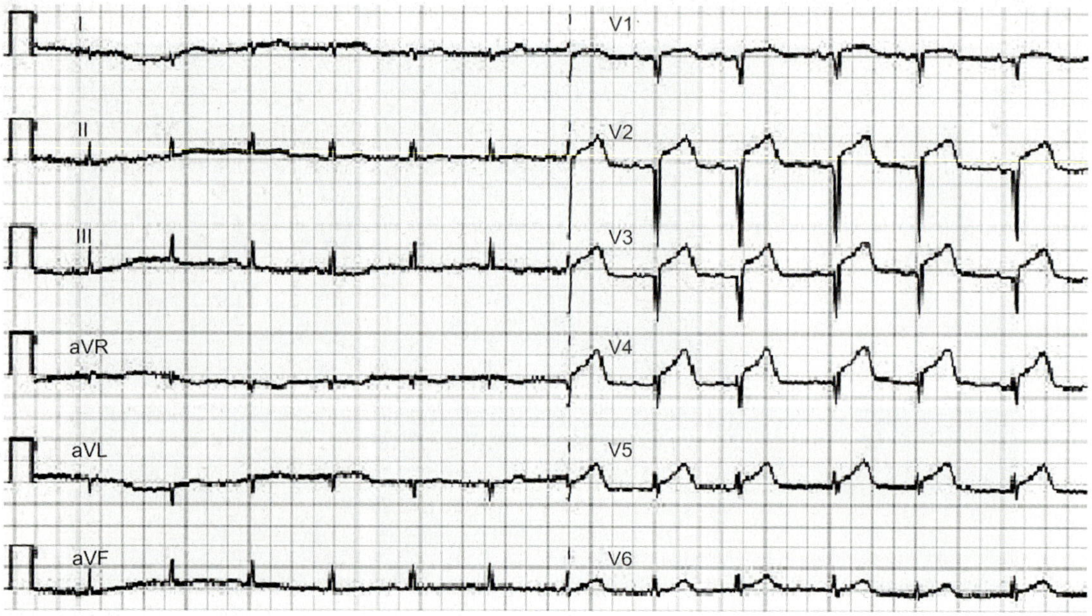


**Fig. 32.34:** Mixed constrictive-restrictive cardiomyopathy ECG—sinus rhythm (79/min) with absent progression of R-wave (V1-V4) along with ST-elevation

**Table 32.6:** Differentiation of pericardial constriction from restrictive cardiomyopathy

| | Pericardial constriction | Restrictive cardiomyopathy |
|---|---|---|
| **Physical examination** | | |
| Pulmonary congestion | Usually absent | Usually present |
| Jugular venous pulse | Prominent Y descent | |
| Early diastolic sound | Pericardial knock | S3 (low pitched) |
| Pericardial thickness | >2 mm (but <2 mm in 15%) | <2 mm |
| **Echo/Doppler findings** | | |
| LV myocardium | Normal | Sparkling myocardium in amyloid |
| Atrial size | +/– atrial enlargement | Atrial enlargement |
| Mitral annular diastolic velocity | Restricted | Restricted |
| Respiratory variation in E wave | >25% | <20% |
| Mitral annular diastolic velocity | >8 cm/s | <8 cm/s |
| **Biomarker** | | |
| B-type natriuretic peptide | <200 pg/ml | >600 pg/ml |
| **Hemodynamics** | | |
| Y descent | Prominent | Variable |
| PA systolic pressure | <50 mmHg | >60 mmHg |
| PCW-RA pressure | 0 | 5 mmHg |
| Reciprocal respiratory variation in right ventricular/left ventricular peak systolic pressure | Present | Absent |

PA=pulmonary arterial; PCW=pulmonary capillary wedge; RA=right atrial.

restrictive cardiomyopathy. Despite elevated filling pressures in both conditions, levels of BNP are significantly higher in restrictive cardiomyopathy (Table 32.6).

### *Chest Radiography*

Pericardial calcifications, pleural effusions and biatrial enlargement may be noted on the chest radiograph (Figs 32.35–32.37).

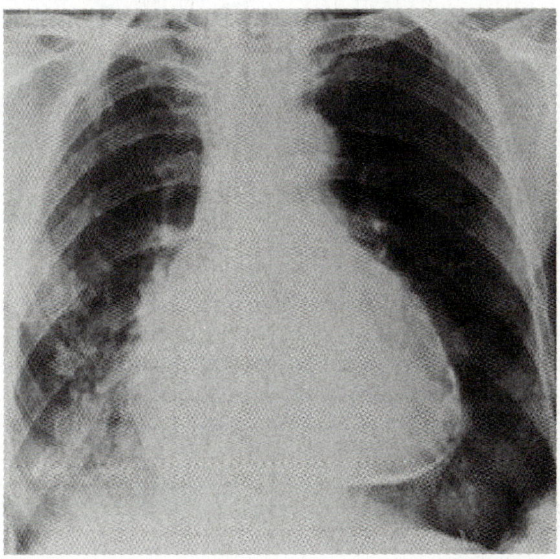

**Fig. 32.35:** Extensive pericardial calcifications on chest radiograph (posteroanterior projection). Extensive pulmonary infiltrates caused by tuberculosis can be noted

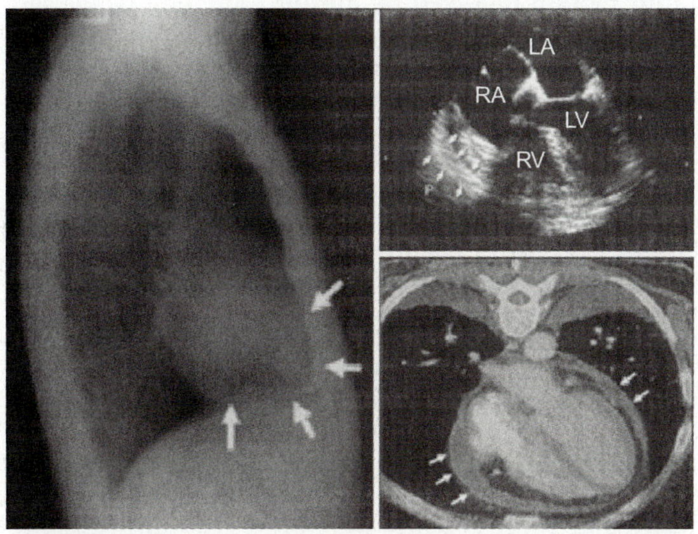


**Fig. 32.36:** Chest radiograph, transesophageal echocardiogram (TEE), and cardiac computed tomogram typical of constrictive pericarditis. (A) Pericardial calcification (arrows) on chest radiography is best seen from the lateral view over the right ventricle (RV) and across the diaphragmatic surface of the heart. Pericardial calcification reflects chronicity of constrictive pericarditis and is associated with a higher surgical mortality. (B) Thickness of the pericardium is often difficult to determine by transthoracic echocardiography, but TEE is usually reliable in measuring the pericardial thickness (arrows). (C) Increased pericardial thickness (arrows) can be visualized on computed tomogram of the same patient. LA=left atrium; LV=left ventricle; RA=right atrium

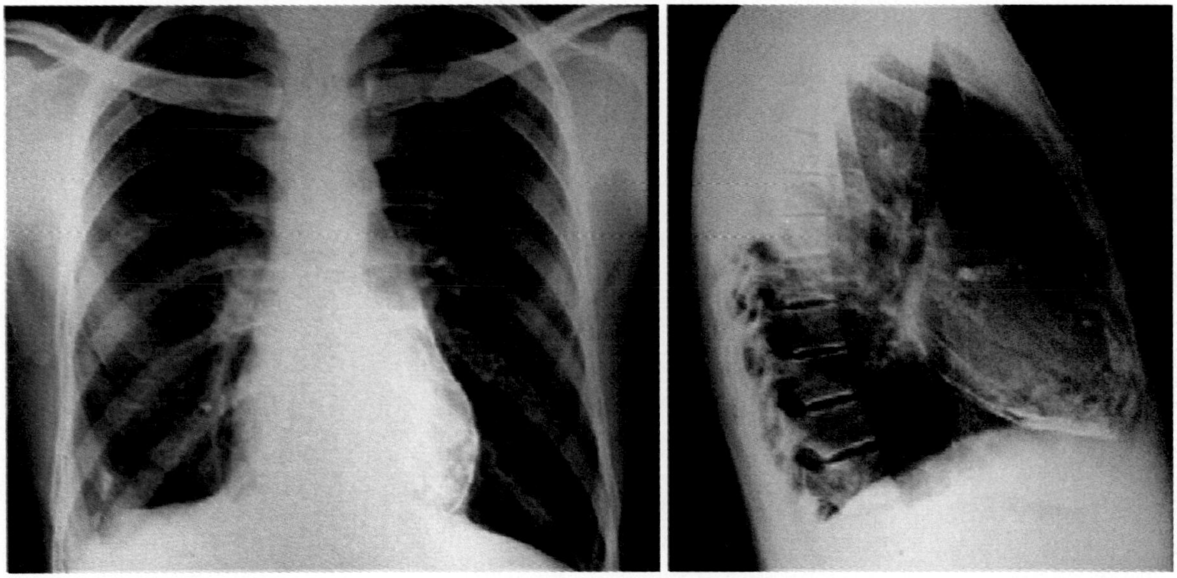

Fig. 32.37: (A) Chest X-ray, PA view, (B) lateral view, show pericardial calcification along anterior and interior borders.

### Echocardiography

Echocardiography is the best imaging modality for assessing hemodynamic parameters noninvasively (Figs 32.38–32.40). M-mode echocardiography is useful for looking for rapid motion followed by abrupt flattening of the left ventricular free wall in early and mid-diastole respectively.

Two-dimensional echocardiography may demonstrate a thickened pericardium (about one third of cases), myocardial tethering, abrupt cessation of left ventricular and right ventricular diastolic filling, biatrial enlargement, tubular deformity of the left ventricle, respirophasic septal shift, septal bounce and inferior vena cava plethora with absent inspiratory collapse. Doppler echocardiographic findings have the highest sensitivity and specificity for detecting constrictive physiology. Excessive respiratory variations in transmitral, transtricuspid, pulmonary venous, and hepatic vein flow are characteristic. Reduced lateral annular diastolic velocity (e′) compared to normal/increased velocity of the septal/medial annular velocity is termed annulus reversus and is a typical feature. Low tissue velocity at both medial and lateral annuli suggests restriction. More recently developed echocardiographic modalities, such as strain imaging have enhanced the ability to discriminate between restriction and constriction.

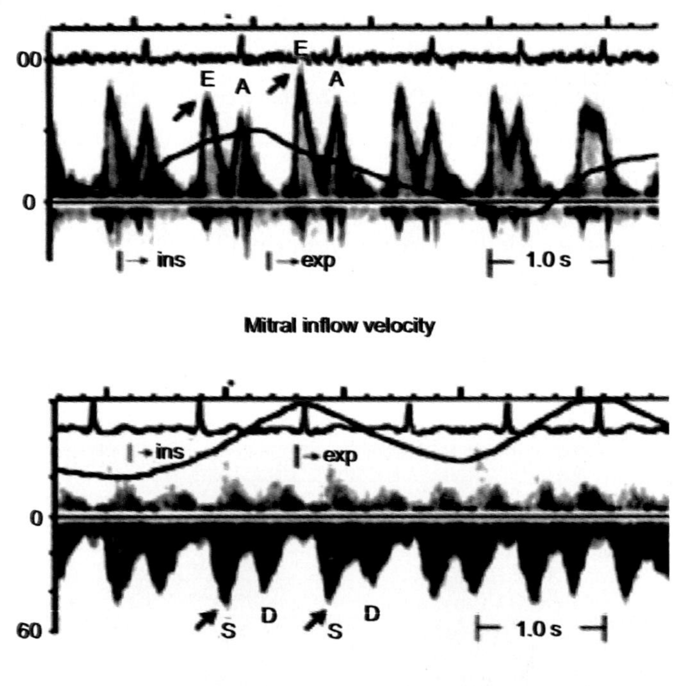


Fig. 32.38: Doppler mitral flow and superior vena caval velocity in a patient with pericardial constriction. There is marked (>25%) respiratory variation in the peak early diastolic initial flow velocity E (decreased during inspiration [ins] and increased during expiration [exp]). In contrast, there is less respiratory variation of the flow velocity in the vena cava. S=systole; D=diastole. *(Reproduced with permission from Boonyaratavej et al. 68 Copyright 1998, American College of Cardiology Foundation)*

### Right Heart Catheterization

Direct pressure measurements are performed, if there is doubt about the diagnosis. Characteristic features in the right atrium include elevated right atrial pressures, prominent x and y decents and Kussmaul sign. Square-root or dip-and-plateau right ventricular pressure waveforms reflect impaired ventricular filling. Because of the fixed and limited space within the stiff pericardium, end-diastolic pressure equalization (typically within 5 mmHg) occurs between these cardiac chambers. Pulmonary artery systolic pressures are usually normal in pericardial constriction; higher pulmonary pressures suggest a restrictive cardiomyopathy. The ratio of the right ventricular to left ventricular systolic pressure-time area during inspiration compared to expiration is a highly sensitive and specific means of differentiating constriction from restriction (Fig. 32.41).

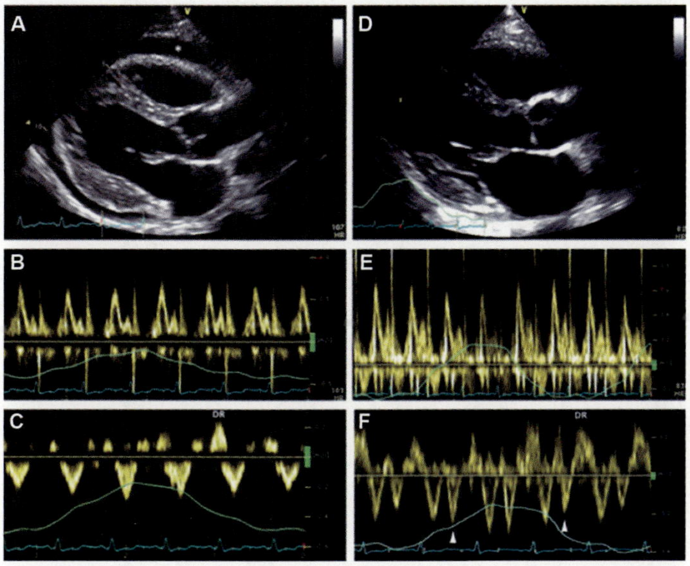


**Fig. 32.39:** Pre- and post-pericardiocentesis echo-Doppler features of effusive-constrictive pericarditis compared with cardiac tamponade and constrictive pericarditis. Prior to pericardiocentesis, medial and lateral é velocities were higher in ECP compared with tamponade; both ECP and tamponade patients had markedly decreased hepatic vein diastolic forward flow velocities. Inspiratory and expiratory mitral E/A ratios were higher in ECP compared with tamponade, but lower than those observed in CP. Post-pericardiocentesis, hepatic vein diastolic forward flow velocities increased in both ECP and tamponade. Hepatic vein diastolic reversal velocities decreased in tamponade but were unchanged in ECP

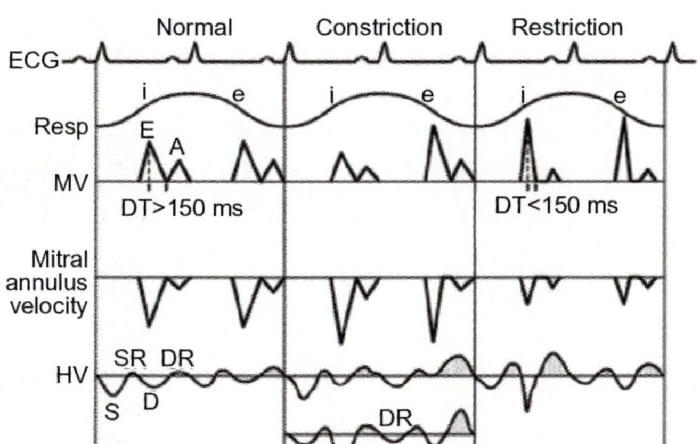


**Fig. 32.40:** Schematic diagram of Doppler echocardiographic features in constrictive pericarditis *vs* restrictive cardiomyopathy. Schematic illustration of Doppler velocities from mitral inflow (MV), mitral annulus velocity, and hepatic vein (HV). Electrocardiographic (ECG) and respirometer (Resp) recordings indicating inspiration (i) and expiration (e) are also shown. A=atrial filling; D=diastolic flow; DR=diastolic flow reversal; DT=deceleration time; E=early diastolic filling; S=systolic flow; SR=systolic flow reversal. Stippled areas under the curve represent flow reversal

### Magnetic Resonance Imaging and Computed Tomography

Computed tomography is the imaging modality of choice to evaluate the thickness of the pericardium and for pericardial calcification. Although, the finding of thickened pericardium on CT is specific for constriction, up to 18% of patients with constriction confirmed by other modalities do not have pericardial thickening. Computed tomography can also assist surgical planning (Figs 32.42–32.44).

While echocardiography is the first choice imaging modality for assesssment of constriction, for many patients CMR is becoming increasingly utilized in the initial evaluation, particularly, if any ambiguity remains regarding the diagnosis, if there is suggestion of active inflammation, or if the duration of symptoms has been brief. CMR is very useful to differentiate a small pericardial effusion from pericardial thickening. The superior signal-to-noise and contrast-to-noise ratio of CMR allows precise evaluation of the morphological and hemodynamic changes seen in pericardial constriction. Real-time cine sequences allow evaluation of the features described above in the 2D echocardiographic evaluation of pericardial constriction, which is useful, if echocardiographic images are suboptimal. Phase encoding velocity imaging potentially provides similar data to Doppler echocardiography but is not yet generally employed in routine practice. The main advantages of CMR over echo are the STIR and LGE sequences which permit evaluation of edema and inflammation that can impact management decisions.

### Treatment

The degree of constrictive physiology occurs along a spectrum of severity. Early forms may be difficult to diagnose without a high degree of clinical suspicion. It is increasingly recognized that some of these patients may respond to medical therapy, without surgical intervention; this is referred to as transient constrictive pericarditis. Inflammation seen on LGE, CMR images is a good predictor of those patients that may respond to anti-inflammatory therapy.

Medical treatment is limited in chronic constrictive pericarditis in the absence of active inflammation. Diuretics and a low-sodium diet may be tried for patients with mild to moderate (New York Heart Association Class I or II) heart failure symptoms or contraindications to surgery. For patients that do not respond to medical treatment, pericardiectomy is advised.

For effusive-constrictive pericarditis therapy includes pericardiocentesis initially, followed by treatment with anti-inflammatory agents. Frequently, pericardiectomy is necessary for long-term management.

### Outcomes

Recurrence following surgery is caused mainly by incomplete resection of the pericardium. Without surgical treatment, biventricular failure develops. Long-term survival after pericardiectomy is worse than matched controls but this is mainly related to the underlying aetiology.

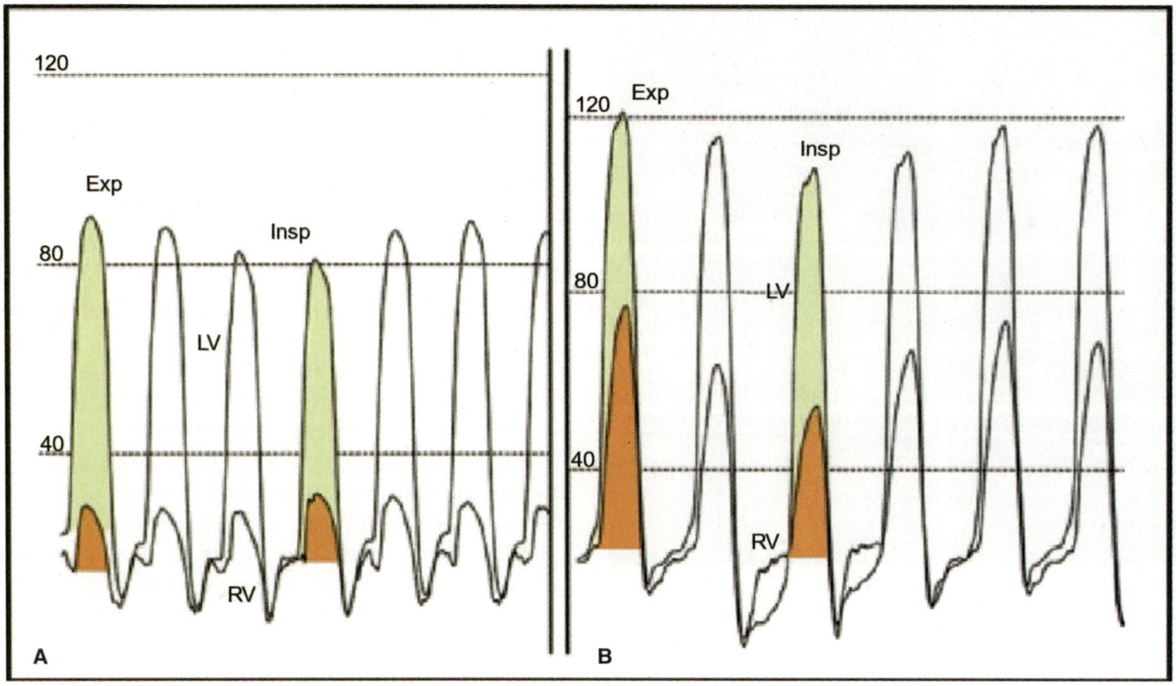


**Fig. 32.41:** Ventricular interdependence and respiratory variation in ventricular filling in constrictive pericarditis and restrictive cardiomyopathy. Ventricular interdependence is observed in simultaneous recordings of left ventricular (LV) and right ventricular (RV) pressures. (A) In constrictive pericarditis, inspiration (Insp) induces less filling of the LV, and the area of the LV pressure curve decreases (yellow shaded area) as compared with expiration (Exp). The opposite changes occur in the RV, so that area of the RV pressure curve increases with Insp (orange shaded area). Ejection time also varies with respiration in opposite directions in LV and RV. This discordant pressure change between the LV and RV occurs in constrictive pericarditis. (B) In restrictive cardiomyopathy, the changes in LV and RV systolic pressures with respiration are concordant. During Insp, the area of the RV pressure curve decreases (orange shaded area) as compared with Exp. The area of the LV pressure curve (yellow shaded area) is unchanged during Insp as compared with Exp. Note that both patients have early rapid filling and elevation and end-equalization of the LV and RV pressures at end Exp

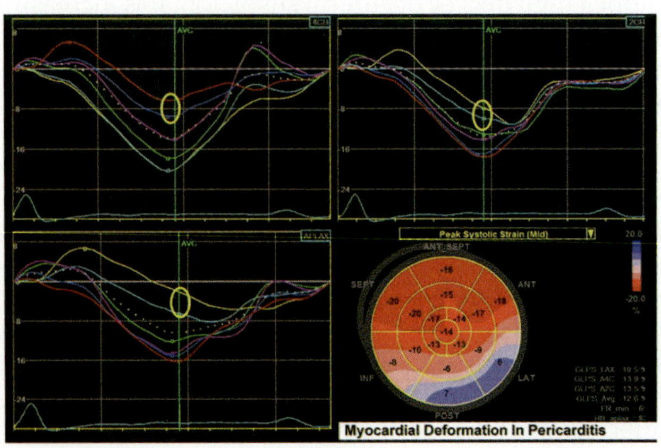


**Fig. 32.42:** Deformation analysis reveals a markedly reduced global longitudinal strain of only 12.6% despite the preserved LVEF. There are clear regional abnormalities seen which are highlighted with the yellow circles in the figure below. The basal and mid segment of the inferior, posterior and lateral wall show a reduced peak systolic strain. These segments are those directly adjacent to the pericardium ans reflects the adhesion of the pericardium to the myocardium, in turn restricting the longitudinal movement during systole. The segments that are not in contact to the pericardium (i.e. the septal wall) are unaffected since the myocardium is unaffected in this disease process

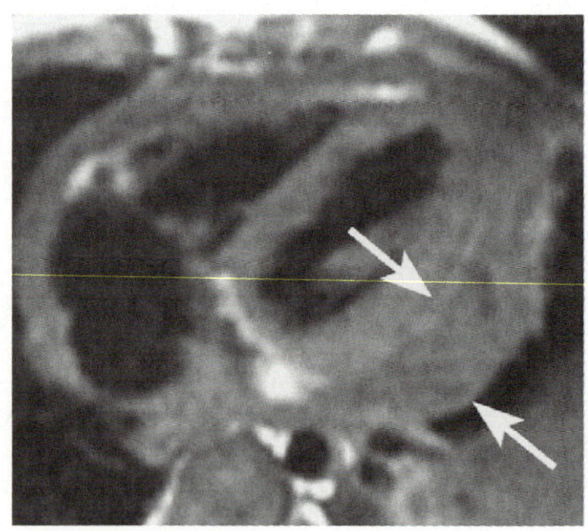

**Fig. 32.43:** Effusive constrictive pericarditis secondary to viral infection in a young adolescent with symptoms of heart failure. (A) Axial ECG-gated T1-weighted SE image shows a crescent-shaped area of intermediate signal intensity (arrows) surrounding the ventricles, which indicates either pericardial thickening or pericardial effusion. (B) Axial gadolinium-enhanced fat-saturated T1-weighted SE image shows marked thickening and enhancement in the pericardium (arrows), findings consistent with inflammation. A moderate-sized pericardial effusion is also depicted

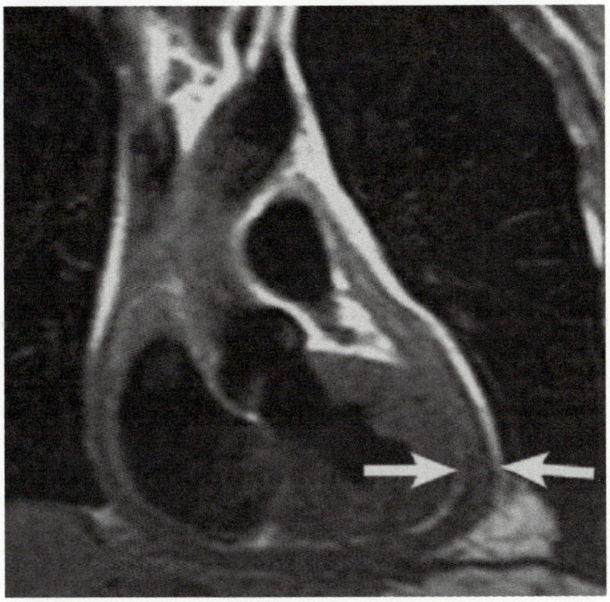

**Fig. 32.44:** Constrictive pericarditis in a young lady who presented with symptoms of constriction. Coronal ECG-gated T1-weighted SE image shows abnormally thickened pericardium (arrows) outlined by epicardial and anterior mediastinal fat

## KEY POINTS

### Acute Pericarditis

- Acute pericarditis manifests with acute positional and pleuritic chest pain, ECG changes, is sometimes accompanied by a pericardial rub, and is often associated with pericardial effusion.
- In the United States, 90% of cases of acute pericarditis are idiopathic.
- Non-aspirin NSAIDs and colchicine should be used for most patients, except for those with post-MI pericarditis (they should receive aspirin and colchicine).
- Colchicine reduces the recurrence of pericarditis.
- Steroids can increase the recurrence rate of pericarditis and the risk of acute myocardial rupture. They should be reserved for cases where steroids are indicated to treat the underlying cause of the effusion, or for recurrent/resistant pericarditis.

### Effusion and Cardiac Tamponade

- The pericardial sac normally contains up to 50 ml of fluid; it can hold 80–200 ml of fluid acutely, and even up to 2 L, if the fluid accumulates slowly. There are a wide range of medical conditions that can precipitate a pericardial effusion; the aetiology can often be deduced from the clinical presentation. In the absence of hemodynamic compromise, treatment of the underlying medical condition is indicated. Cardiac tamponade is a clinical diagnosis made by documenting one or more of the following in the presence of a pericardial effusion—tachycardia, pulsus paradoxus (>10 mmHg inspiratory decline in systolic BP), jugular venous distention, and muffled heart sounds.The signs depend on the volume of fluid in the pericardial sac and the rate at which the fluid accumulates.

*Contd...*

*Contd...*

- Echocardiography can confirm the diagnosis at an early stage and help with the drainage of the effusion.
- Pericardiocentesis should be performed for diagnostic purposes, if the cause is unclear or if purulent infection is suspected. Therapeutic pericardiocentesis should be performed, if there is evidence of hemodynamic compromise.

### Constrictive Pericarditis

- Constrictive pericarditis results from an abnormal scarring of the pericardium that causes impairment of diastolic filling.
- A diagnostic challenge often lies in differentiating constriction from restriction. The diagnosis can be made by noting hemodynamic derangements on echocardiography/CMR/right heart catheterization and a thickening of the pericardium on echo/CT/MRI.
- About 20% of patients do not demonstrate thickening of the pericardium by CT.
- For patients that do not respond to medical therapy, the treatment of choice is surgical excision of the pericardium.

## BIBLIOGRAPHY


1. Bilchick KC, Wise RA. Paradoxical physical findings described by Kussmaul: pulsus paradoxus and Kussmaul's sign. Lancet 2002;359:1940–2.
2. Bogaert J, Francone M. Pericardial disease: value of CT and MR imaging. Radiology 2013;267:340–56.
3. Corey GR, Campbell PT, Van Trigt P, et al. Etiology of large pericardial effusions. Am J Med 1993;95:209–13.
4. Curtiss EI, Reddy PS, Uretsky BF, Cecchetti AA. Pulsus paradoxus: definition and relation to the severity of cardiac tamponade. Am Heart J 1988;115:391–8.
5. Dunn PM, MacNichol J, Krekeler MM, Rotter SM, Brown K. Roentgenograms in pericardial effusion. JAMA 1987;258: 1890–91.
6. Feng D, Glockner J, Kim K, et al. Cardiac magnetic resonance imaging pericardial late gadolinium enhancement and elevated inflammatory markers can predict the reversibility of constrictive pericarditis after anti-inflammatory medical therapy: a pilot study. Circulation 2011;124:1830–37.
7. Fowler NO, Tuberculous pericarditis. JAMA 1991;266: 99–103.
8. Haley JH, Tajik AJ, Danielson GK, Schaff HV, Mulvagh SL, Oh JK. Transient constrictive pericarditis: causes and natural history. J Am Coll Cardiol 2004;271–5.
9. Imazio M, Adler Y. Management of pericardial effusion. Eur Heart J 2013;34:1186–97.
10. Imazio M, Bobbio M, Cecchi E, et al. Colchicine in addition to conventional therapy for acute pericarditis: results of the COlchicine for acute PEricarditis (COPE) trial. Circulation 2005;112:2012–6.
11. Imazio M, Brucato A, Mayosi BM, et al. Medical therapy of pericardial diseases: part I: idiopathic and infectious pericarditis. J Cardiovasc Med (Hagerstown) 2010;11:712–2.
12. Imazio M, Brucato A, Mayosi BM, et al. Medical therapy of pericardial diseases: part II: noninfectious pericarditis,

pericardial effusion and constrictive pericarditis. J Cardiovasc Med (Hagerstown) 2010;11:785–94.

13. Imazio M, Spodick DH, Brucato A, Trinchero R, Adler Y. Controversial issues in the management of pericardial diseases. Circulation 2010;121:916–28.
14. Khan AH. The postcardiac injury syndromes. Clin Cardiol 1992;15:67–72.
15. Klein AL, Abbara S, Agler DA, et al. American Society of Echocardiography clinical recommendations for multimodality cardiovascular imaging of patients with pericardial disease: endorsed by the Society for Cardiovascular Magnetic Resonance and Society of Cardiovascular Computed Tomography. J Am Soc Echocardiogr 2013;26: 965–1012.e15.
16. Kusunose K, Dahiya A, Popoviae ZB, et al. Biventricular mechanics in constrictive pericarditis comparison with restric-tive cardiomyopathy and impact of pericardiectomy. Circ Cardiovasc Imaging 2013;6:399–406.
17. LeWinter MM. Pericardial diseases. Libby P, Bonow RO, Mann DL, Zipes DP, eds. In: Braunwald's Heart Disease: A Textbook of Cardiovascular Medicine, Single Volume. 8th edition. Philadelphia, PA: Saunders. 2007;1829–53.
18. Leya FS, Arab D, Joyal D, et al. The efficacy of brain natri-uretic peptide levels in differentiating constrictive peri-carditis from restrictive cardiomyopathy. J Am Coll Cardiol 2005;45:1900–2.
19. Lotrionte M, Biondi-Zoccai G, Imazio M, et al. International collaborative systematic review of controlled clinical trials on pharmacologic treatments for acute pericarditis and its recurrences. Am Heart J 2010;160:662–70.
20. Maisch B, Seferoviae PM, Ristiae AD, et al. Guidelines on the diagnosis and management of pericardial diseases executive summary; the task force on the diagnosis and management of pericardial diseases of the European Society of Cardio-logy. Eur Heart J 2004;25:587–610.
21. Meyers DG, Meyers RE, Prendergast TW. The usefulness of diagnostic tests on pericardial fluid. Chest 1997;111:1213–21.
22. Oliva PB, Hammill SC, Edwards WD. Electrocardiographic diagnosis of postinfarction regional pericarditis. Ancillary observations regarding the effect of reperfusion on the rapi-dity and amplitude of T-wave inversion after acute myocar-dial infarction. Circulation 1993;88:896–904.
23. Rostand SG, Rutsky EA. Pericarditis in end-stage renal disease. Cardiol Clin 1990;8:701–7.
24. Sagristà-Sauleda J, Mercé AS, Soler-Soler J. Diagnosis and management of pericardial effusion. World J Cardiol 2011; 3:135–43.
25. Sagristà-Sauleda J, Permanyer-Miralda G, Candell-Riera J, Angel J, Soler-Soler J. Transient cardiac constriction: an unrecognized pattern of evolution in effusive acute idiopathic pericarditis. Am J Cardiol 1987;59:961–6.
26. Sugiura T, Iwasaka T, Takayama Y, et al. Factors associated with pericardial effusion in acute Q-wave myocardial infarc-tion. Circulation 1990;81:477–81.
27. Syed FF, Ntsekhe M, Mayosi BM, Oh JK. Effusive-constrictive pericarditis. Heart Fail Rev 2013;18:277–287.
28. Szabó G, Schmack B, Bulut C, et al. Constrictive pericarditis: risks, aetiologies and outcomes after total pericardiectomy: 24 years of experience. Eur J Cardiothorac Surg 2013;44:1023–1028; discussion 1028.
29. Talreja DR, Edwards WD, Danielson GK, et al. Constrictive pericarditis in 26 patients with histologically normal pericardial thickness. Circulation 2003;108:1852–57.
30. Taylor AM, Dymarkowski S, Verbeken EK, Bogaert J. Detection of pericardial inflammation with late-enhancement cardiac magnetic resonance imaging: initial results. Eur Radiol 2006;16:569–74.
31. Wood JE, Mahnensmith RL. Pericarditis associated with renal failure: evolution and management. Semin Dial 2001;14: 61–6.

# 33 Radiation and Chemotherapeutic Agents Related Heart Diseases

New anticancer therapies have led to a long life expectancy for many patients; however, treatment-related comorbidities have become an issue for long-term cancer survivors. Cardiac toxicity is one of most feared side-effects of anticancer agents, so that the gain in life expectancy due to anticancer therapy might be countered by increased mortality not only due to cardiac problems, above all heart failure (HF), but also myocardial ischaemia, arrhythmias, hypertension and thromboembolism (Fig. 33.1).

Detection of cardiac injury is crucial since it may facilitate early therapeutic measures.

The incidence of cardiotoxicity depends on different factors related to oncological therapies (type of drug, dose administered during each cycle, cumulative dose, schedule of administration, route of administration, combination of other cardiotoxic drugs or association with radiotherapy) and to patient [age, presence of cardiovascular (CV) risk factors, previous cardiovascular disease (CVD) and prior mediastinal radiation therapy].

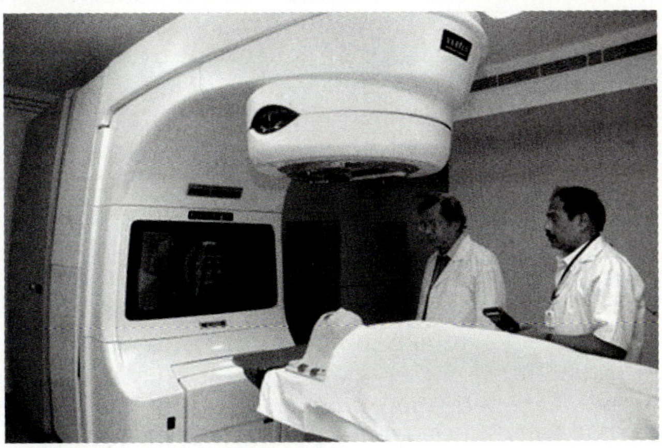

**Fig. 33.1:** Radiation unit with properly installed machine for the treatment of various types of cancers in one of the medical institutions of India

## CARDIOVASCULAR TOXICITY OF CHEMOTHERAPEUTIC AGENTS

### Drugs Associated with Heart Failure

#### *Anthracycline Cardiotoxicity*

The incidence of anthracycline-induced cardiotoxicity (AIC) varies depending on medication and cumulative dose—for doxorubicin from 4% to >36% in patient receiving 500–550 mg/m$^2$; epirubicin or idarubicin appears to have lower incidence of HF. However, it has been shown that the longer the follow-up, the higher the incidence of cardiac dysfunction.

AIC has been categorized as acute (transient decline in myocardial contractility immediately after infusion, incidence <1%), early onset chronic progressive (within first year after treatment, incidence 1.6–2.1%), late onset chronic progressive, presenting as dilated cardiomyopathy (CMP) from at least 1 year after completion of therapy, until 10–30 years from the first dose of treatment. There are several hypotheses to explain the mechanism of AIC, but free radical formation is generally accepted as the main mechanism; apoptosis also has a prominent role in the myocardial cell loss that has been demonstrated in such cases. Risk factors for AIC, besides cumulative dose, are intravenous high single dose, time of drug infusion <30 minutes, history of prior irradiation, use of other concomitant agents, such as cyclophosphamide, trastuzumab, paclitaxel, female gender, young or old age, underlying cardiovascular disease and increase in time elapsed since therapy administration. Among anthracyclines, liposomal doxorubicin showed reduced cardiotoxicity, albeit at the cost of hand–foot syndrome and sometimes other skin toxicity; thus it could be preferable in selected patients at high risk of HF.

Mitoxantrone, an antraquinone derivative, can cause cardiotoxicity that is similar to AIC; myocarditis and arrhythmias can be seen acutely with infusion, and after

1 year of monotherapy 3–4% of patients have reduction in left ventricular ejection fraction (LVEF).

### Targeted Drug Cardiotoxicity

Targeted drugs are compounds acting through inhibition of specific target molecules; in the context of anticancer therapy, protein kinases, because of their critical role in cell signal transduction, are the most attractive targets.

In clinical practice, there are two main classes of drug targeting tyrosine kinase receptors for growth factors; monoclonal antibodies (trastuzumab and bevacizumab) and small molecule tyrosine kinase inhibitors (TKIs—lapatinib, imatinib, sorafenib and sunitinib).

- Trastuzumab, a humanized monoclonal antibody that targets the extracellular portion of the human epidermal growth factor receptor 2 (HER2), is widely used in the treatment of HER2-positive breast cancer. The incidence of trastuzumab-related HF is 2–7%; it increases with age >50 years, border-line LVEF before treatment, history of CVD and prior treatment with anthracycline and it rises to 27% when trastuzumab is used concurrently with anthracycline plus cyclophosphamide. Unlike AIC, trastuzumab toxicity is not dose related, and it is frequently reversible.
- Bevacizumab, a recombinant humanized monoclonal antibody against vascular endothelial growth factor (VEGF) receptor, can be associated with HF or arterial thromboembolic events or venous thromboembolism, and it can induce severe hypertension.
- Lapatinib, a kinase inhibitor targeting internal HER2 and epidermal growth factor receptor, seems to have a low incidence of HF or other adverse cardiac effects.
- Imatinib, whose mechanism of cardiac injury is represented by mitochondrial dysfunction, has demonstrated deleterious effects on cardiomyocytes, in culture and *in vivo;* actually the precise rate of associated cardiotoxicity and its reversibility is still unknown and needs further investigation.
- Sunitinib and sorafenib, multitarget TKIs, have hypertension as the most common side-effect, but HF also is reported, especially in patients with a previous history of hypertension and coronary heart disease.

### Alkylating Agent-correlated Cardiotoxicity

The incidence of HF reported with cyclophosphamide therapy ranges from 7% to 28%; the risk of cardiotoxicity is dose related (>150 mg/kg and 1.5 g/m$^2$/day), occurs normally within 10 days after administration of the first dose, and it is also correlated to prior anthracycline or mitoxantrone therapy or mediastinal irradiation.

### Drugs Correlated with Myocardial Ischemia/ Thromboembolism

The most commonly described cardiotoxic effect of fluorouracil (5-FU) is angina-like chest pain, with incidence ranging from 1% to 68% in the literature; cardiac events occur generally within 5 days after first administration, and ischaemic changes on ECG have been reported in 68% of patients; risk factors are high dose (>800 mg/m$^2$), continuous infusion of medicament, history of CVD, prior mediastinal radiation, concurrent use of chemotherapy; possible mechanisms of cardiotoxicity are coronary artery thrombosis, interaction with coagulation system, vasospasm, direct toxicity on myocardium.

- Paclitaxel can induce a large spectrum of cardiac disturbances of multifactorial aetiology, including ventricular arrhythmias, bradycardia, several degrees of atrioventricular conduction block, bundle branch block (effects caused by the paclitaxel vehicle Cremophor EL) and cardiac ischaemia, although these disturbances do not seem to result in serious sequelae in most patients; however, the clinical use of doxorubicin–paclitaxel combinations is limited by a higher incidence of the cardiac toxicity known to be induced by doxorubicin alone.
- Cisplatin has been shown to increase the risk of thrombotic events, such as deep vein thrombosis or pulmonary embolism, but specific cardiotoxicity is rarely reported.

## MONITORING OF CARDIOTOXICITY

### Cardiovascular Evaluation of Patients before Treatment with Anticancer Agents

All patients undergoing chemotherapy should have prior careful clinic evaluation and assessment of CV risk factors or comorbidities. Frequent vital signs monitoring is recommended during chemotherapeutic agent infusion, particularly with 5-FU or paclitaxel [A].

Electrocardiography (ECG) and clinic cardiovascular evaluation are useful to screen signs of cardiomyopathy, conduction disturbances, QT interval, before beginning anticancer therapy with anthracycline or paclitaxel or small molecule TKIs. With respect to imaging techniques, baseline Doppler echocardiogram (DEcho) is requested to assess cardiac function in patients undergoing therapy with anthracycline, particularly in the presence of CV risk factors, age >60 years, previous CVD, prior mediastinal irradiation (A); baseline DEcho is needed to assess cardiac function in all patients undergoing therapy with trastuzumab, particularly in patients previously treated with anthracycline (A). Left ventricular (LV) fractional shortening and ejection fraction (LVEF) are the most common indexes for cardiac function assessment before starting oncological therapy, LVEF <54% is identified as a risk factor for development of HF in patients undergoing treatment with trastuzumab. Multiple gated acquisition myocardial scintigraphy allows a very reliable assessment of LVEF, but its use is limited because of radiation exposure.

Magnetic resonance imaging (MRI), used to assess myocardial function, to evaluate myocardial perfusion and for tissue characterization, is not an ideal first-line screening test at present, but may have potential in the future.

With cardiac computed tomography (CT) up to today image quality is better than MRI but, because of considerable radiation dose, it is not considered a useful method to assess cardiac function.

### Monitoring during and After Anticancer Therapy

Endomyocardial biopsy represents the most reliable method for evaluation of myocardial damage, but its very limited feasibility in daily clinical practice limits its use in cardiotoxicity monitoring.

Among the imaging techniques, echo offers several advantages; it can assess LV systolic and diastolic dysfunction, heart valve disease, pericarditis and pericardial effusion and carotid artery lesions. LV fractional shortening and LVEF are the most common indexes of LV systolic function for cardiac function assessment in oncology. LVEF is, however, not a very sensitive parameter in detecting early alterations in myocardial function. It is now recognized that the Doppler-derived diastolic indexes represent an early sign of LV dysfunction in cancer patients, so that evaluation of mitral diastolic flow pattern, early peak flow velocity to atrial peak flow velocity (E/A) ratio, deceleration time of E wave and isovolumic relaxation time can be useful to detect diastolic changes of LV function before systolic dysfunction occurs. Pulsed tissue Doppler may be easily performed during a standard Doppler echocardiographic examination; it has been successfully applied in several clinical setting and appears reliable in providing quantitative information on myocardial diastolic relaxation and systolic performance (E′ wave, A′ wave and S wave velocity). Tissue Doppler of LV lateral mitral annulus has a recognized prognostic role and, in combination with pulsed wave (PW) Doppler of mitral inflow, provides accurate information about the degree of LV filling pressure. Early changes in LV myocardial function of oncology patients were found by pulsed tissue Doppler of multiple LV sites.

B-type natriuretic peptide (BNP) is a cardiac hormone released by the myocardium in response to volume overload. An increase in BNP plasma level reflects an increased filling pressure of the LV as it occurs in LV dysfunction. Its value can rise when the HF is yet clinically unapparent and increases further according to HF severity. High levels of BNP correlate with LV dysfunction in cancer patients treated with oncological therapy. Nevertheless, further studies are requested to confirm the sensitivity and the specificity of this parameter.

Troponin is a specific and sensitive marker for detection of myocardial ischaemia, but elevation of troponin levels have been reported also after anthracycline therapy predicting subclinical and clinical cardiac morbidity and mortality; its use is limited because it needs numerous serial controls of serum levels at different time intervals.

## RECOMMENDATIONS FOR CARDIOTOXICITY MONITORING AND MANAGEMENT

Patients undergoing anticancer therapy should be encouraged to follow standard guidelines for reducing CV risk, such as blood pressure control, lipid level reduction, smoking cessation and lifestyle modifications.

- Periodic monitoring of cardiac function with DEcho is suggested especially for anthracyclines and their derivates or monoclonal antibodies.
- Baseline clinical and ECG evaluation are recommended in all patients undergoing anthracycline therapy (III, A).
- Assessment of baseline systolic and diastolic cardiac function with DEcho should be conducted before treatment with monoclonal antibodies (III, A) or anthracyclines and their derivates in patients aged >60 years, or with cardiovascular risk factors such as hypertension, hypercholesterolaemia, diabetes, obesity or previous treatment with 5-hydroxytryptamine-2B agonists (in Parkinson or obese patients) potentially inducing cardiac valvulopathy, or documented cardiopathy or previous thoracic radiotherapy (III, A).
- Further evaluations of LVEF are recommended, even in asymptomatic patients, according to the follow timing; after administration of half the planned dose of anthracycline, or after administration of cumulative dose of doxorubicin 300 mg/m$^2$, epirubicin 450 mg/m$^2$ or mitoxantrone 60 mg/m$^2$ (III, A) or after administration of a cumulative dose of doxorubicin of 240 mg/m$^2$ or epirubicin 360 mg/m$^2$ in patients aging <15 years or >60 years (III, B); before every next administration of anthracycline (III, A); after 3, 6 and 12 months from the end of therapy with anthracycline (III, B).
- During the echocardiographic assessments, patterns of PW Doppler of LV inflow tract and TDI-PW Doppler of mitral anulus should also be evaluated to detect initial signs of LV dysfunction that might occur before reduction of LVEF.
- Periodic monitoring (every 12 weeks) of cardiac function is also suggested for those patients receiving monoclonal antibodies, especially if previously treated with anthracycline (III, A).
- Assessment of cardiac function is recommended 4 and 10 years after anthracycline therapy in patients who were treated at <15 years of age (III, B), or even at age >15 years but with cumulative dose of doxorubicin of >240 mg/m$^2$ or epirubicin >360 mg/m$^2$ (III, B).
- LVEF reduction of ≥20% from baseline despite normal function or LVEF decline <50% necessitate reassessment or discontinuation of therapy and further frequent clinical and echocardiographic checks.
- Aggressive medical treatment of those patients, even asymptomatic, who show LV dysfunction at DEcho after anthracycline therapy is mandatory, especially if the neoplasia could have a long-term survival; it consists of angiotensin converting enzyme (ACE) inhibitors and β-blockers and the earlier HF therapy is begun (within 2 months from the end of anthracycline therapy), the better the therapeutic response.
- A predictive role for biomarkers of cardiotoxicity caused by cancer therapy is not well defined enough to include them as routine screening measurements. Nevertheless, as persistent increases in cardiac troponin I or BNP concentrations seem to identify patients at risk of cardiotoxicity [except in the presence of the syndrome of inappropriate antidicretic hormone (ADH) secretion for the latter], a useful approach, even if rather costly and still controversial, is performing baseline assessment

of biomarker concentrations and periodic measurements during therapy (at the end of chemotherapy administration, after 12, 24, 36, 72 hours and 1 month later for troponin I; at the end of medicament infusion and after 72 hours for BNP) to identify patients who need further cardiac assessment (III, C).

## RADIOTHERAPY-RELATED HEART DISEASE

A considerable amount of literature supports evidence of radiation-related heart injury after radiotherapy (RT) to the chest. The most appropriate groups of patients, where radiation-associated cardiac injuries are of clinical importance, are those with curable malignancies irradiated at a relatively younger age, so there is enough time to develop clinically significant late cardiac injury. Such malignancies are mainly Hodgkin's lymphoma and early-stage breast cancer, while there is an increasing number of lung and oesophageal cancer patients with long-term controlled disease who could develop post-RT cardiac sequelae.

Radiation-associated CV toxicity may be progressive. Complex, combined disease of heart coronary arteries, valves, myocardium and conduction system as well as diastolic dysfunction may be seen. Estimates of relative risk of fatal CV events after mediastinal irradiation for Hodgkin's disease ranges between 2 and 7 and after irradiation for left-sided breast cancer from 1.0 to 2.2.

Risk factors for radiation-associated heart damage include dose >30–35 Gy, dose per fraction >2 Gy, large volume of irradiated heart, younger age at exposure, longer time since exposure, use of cytotoxic chemotherapy, endocrine therapy or trastuzumab, presence of other risk factors, such as diabetes, hypertension, dyslipidaemias, obesity, smoking, etc.

### Evidence from Breast Cancer Patients

In the last update of the Early Breast Cancer Trialists' Collaborative Group (EBCTCG) meta-analysis on loco-regional RT, comparison of CV mortality between patients treated with and without RT has shown a statistically significant relative risk of 1.27. A similar latent time was estimated in an overview of trials started before 1975. In a Swedish study that included 55000 patients a mortality ratio of all CV disease for left versus right side in a period of >10 years after treatment was 1.10 [95% confidence interval (CI) 1.03–1.18] for all CV diseases and 1.13 (95% CI 1.03–1.25) for deaths from ischaemic disease. Other studies confirm those results.

### Evidence from Hodgkin's Lymphoma Patients

Mediastinal radiotherapy can cause a variety of CV complications, such as pericarditis, myocardial fibrosis, coronary artery disease, valvular abnormalities and conduction disturbances. Restrictive cardiomyopathy, valvular defects and conduction defects, persistent tachycardia and blunted haemodynamic responses to exercise are usually diagnosed. Nevertheless, myocardial infarction is the major cause of higher long-term mortality in survivors of Hodgkin's disease.

It is very important to note that death due to cardiac causes is estimated to be responsible for about one-quarter of the mortality from reasons other than Hodgkin's disease itself, which equals 2–5% of overall mortality in those with Hodgkin's disease.

### Cardiac Structures Affected by Radiation

Injury of the various structures and tissues in the heart can cause a spectrum of radiation-induced CV diseases (Figs 33.2–33.19 and Table 33.1).

- Arteritis of the endothelium of coronary arteries can cause premature coronary artery disease and atherosclerosis mainly in left anterior descending and right coronary artery. Time of appearance is 10–15 years after RT.
- Acute pericarditis and symptomatic (haemodynamic compromise with constriction or tamponade) or asymptomatic chronic pericardial effusion, appears usually 6–12 months following RT.
- Myocarditis and congestive heart failure due to non-specific diffuse interstitial fibrosis.
- Valvular stenosis and regurgitation mainly of mitral and aortic valves.
- Fibrosis of the conduction system and disturbed heart rate and complete or incomplete heart block.
- Some indirect implications on the heart may result from irradiation of adjacent structures. Lung and mediastinal fibrosis may result in respiratory insufficiency, pneumonic hypertension and may complicate any potential heart surgery. Hypothyroidism may affect the lipid profile and CV function. Mediastinal venous and lymph vessel obstruction may cause pericardial effusion or chylothorax.

Radiation tolerance doses for the above late-effects have been estimated to be between 30 and 40 Gy.

### Recommendations to Reduce Cardiac Toxicity in Patients Treated by Radiotherapy

There is some evidence that newer irradiation techniques seem to decrease the risk of RT-induced cardiac disease, but a longer follow-up time is needed to confirm it. Modern RT techniques include three-dimensional treatment planning with dose volume histogram (DVH) for accurate heart volume and dose calculation. Linear accelerator photons and multiple-field conformal or intensity-modulated radiotherapy (IMRT) are desirable for chest irradiation.

For (left) breast/chest wall RT, 6 MV or occasionally higher energy photons (for large breasts) from a linear accelerator should be used.

The introduction of cardiac-sparing lead block during standard simulator planning will result in cardiac irradiation being at least partially avoided in many patients.

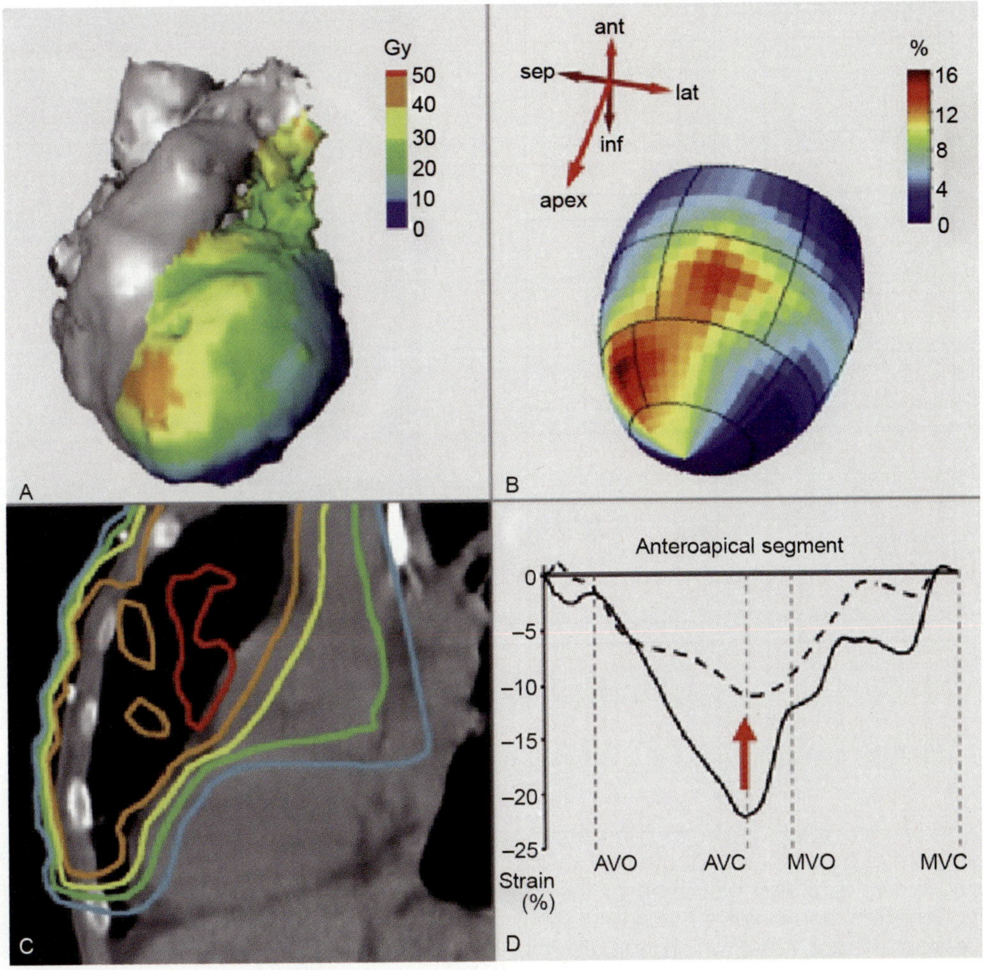


**Fig. 33.2:** Echocardiography. Acute radiation effects on regional myocardial function; comparison between radiation dose distribution (A and B) and regional myocardial function decrease measured by tissue Doppler-derived longitudinal myocardial strain (C and D) after radiotherapy in a patient with left-sided breast cancer. Note the regional concordance between irradiated area and regional dysfunction (modified from Jurcut et al.)

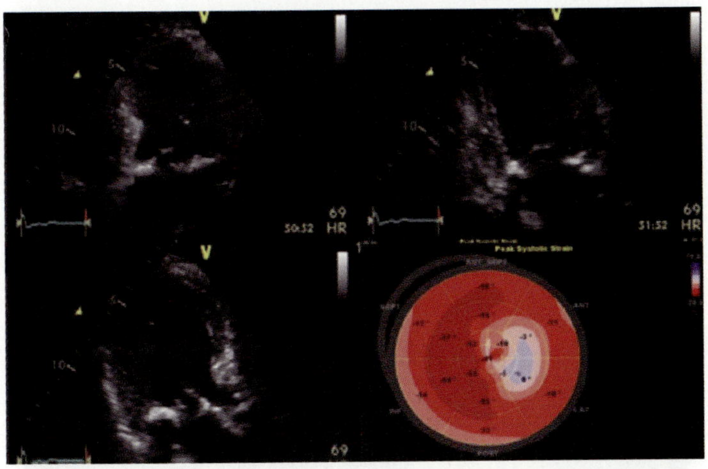

**Fig. 33.3:** Echocardiography. Longitudinal left ventricular (LV) function assessed by 2D speckle tracking imaging of a patient with radiation-induced valvular heart disease and LV dysfunction. LV ejection fraction was normal while a Bull's eye plot of LV longitudinal strain (lower right panel) demonstrates impaired regional longitudinal function (light colors)

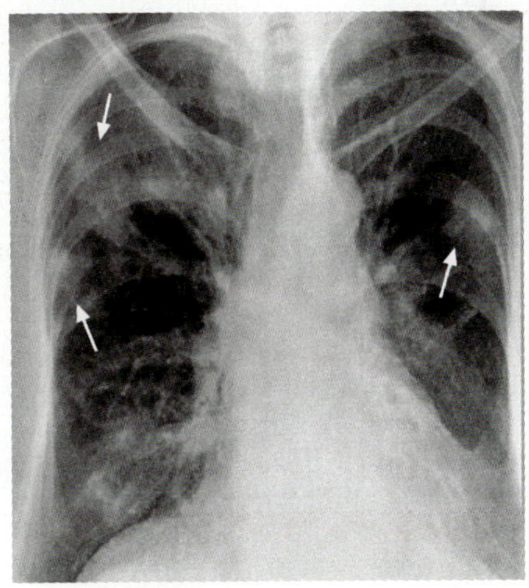

**Fig. 33.4:** Cyclophosphamide-induced BOOP in a 72-year-old woman with malignant thymoma, fever, nonproductive cough, and dyspnea. (a) Posteroanterior chest radiograph shows scattered, poorly defined peripheral opacities (arrows). (b) Follow-up posteroanterior chest radiograph obtained 2 weeks later shows progressive peripheral consolidation. Wedge resection biopsy of the middle lobe revealed findings of BOOP

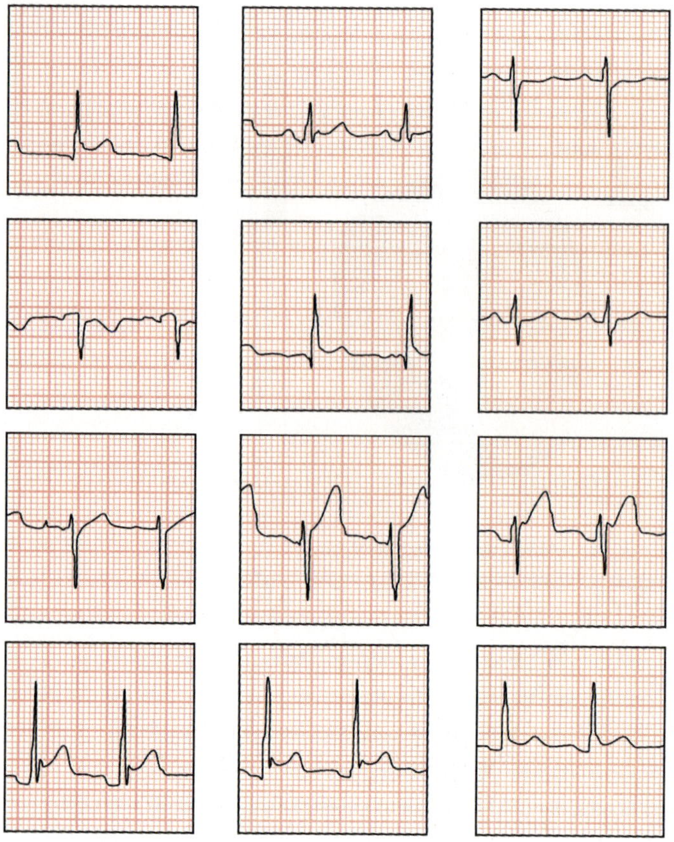

**Fig. 33.5:** Electrocardiogram of a patient with acute pericarditis following radiotherapy, showing diffuse elevation of the ST-segment with upwards concavity and positive T-waves (stage I) and PR-segment depression at leads V2-V4, which indicates the presence of a atrial injury curve

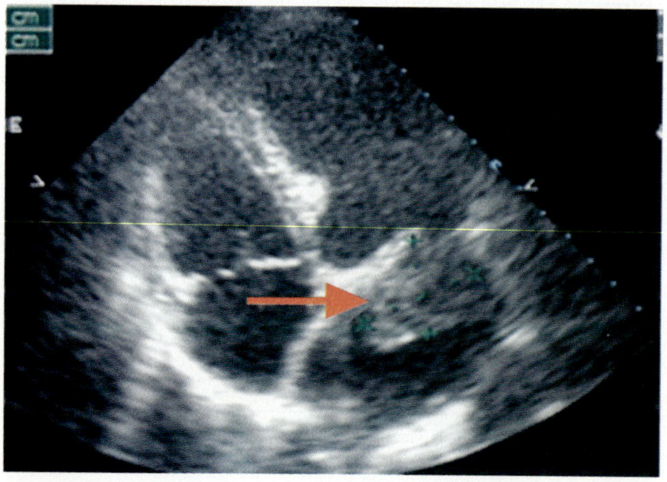

**Fig. 33.6:** Echocardiogram, four-chamber view. The patient was a 56-year-old female with a history of malignant pleural mesothelioma, who underwent pleurectomy and postoperative chemotherapy followed by 45 Gy radiation to the left chest. The patient developed post-radiation sarcoma on the mitral valve 14 years later. The echocardiogram shows a 2.8 × 3.6 cm echogenic mass attached to the posterior leaflet of the mitral valve that was prolapsing into the left ventricle on diastole. The arrow indicates the mass on the mitral valve

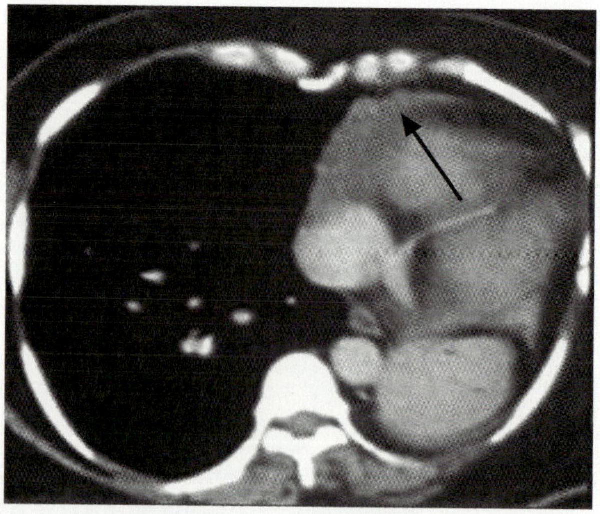

**Fig. 33.7:** Radiation-induced pericarditis after left pneumonectomy. Axial CT scans 6 months following the completion of radiation therapy shows mild pericardial effusion (arrow)

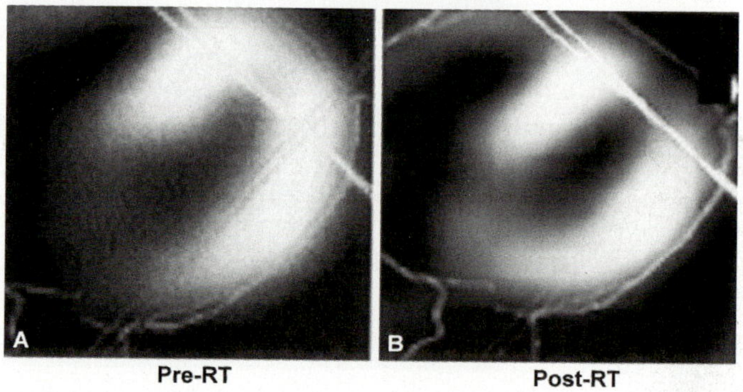


**Fig. 33.8:** Representative axial images pre-radiation therapy (RT) (A) and post-RT (B) cardiac single-photon emission computed tomography scans. The deep tangent border is shown as the solid line. A new perfusion defect in the anterior left ventricle after radiation is seen

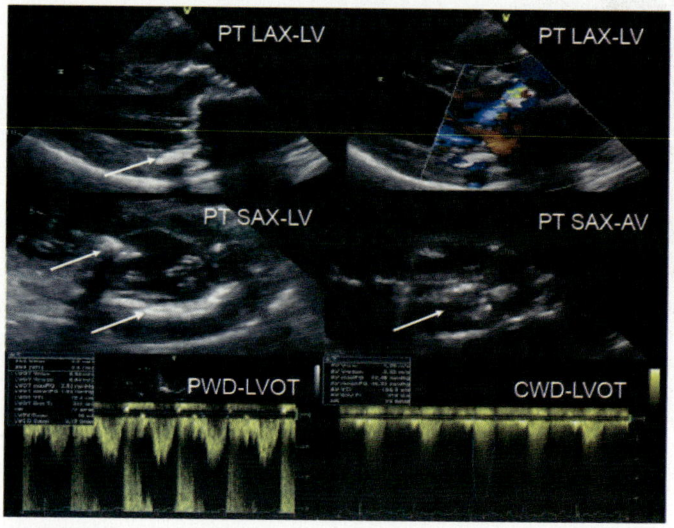


**Fig. 33.9:** Echocardiography. Example of a patient with radiation-induced valvular heart disease. Extensive calcifications of the aortic and mitral valve (arrows) and of the left ventricle. Significant aortic stenosis and regurgitation

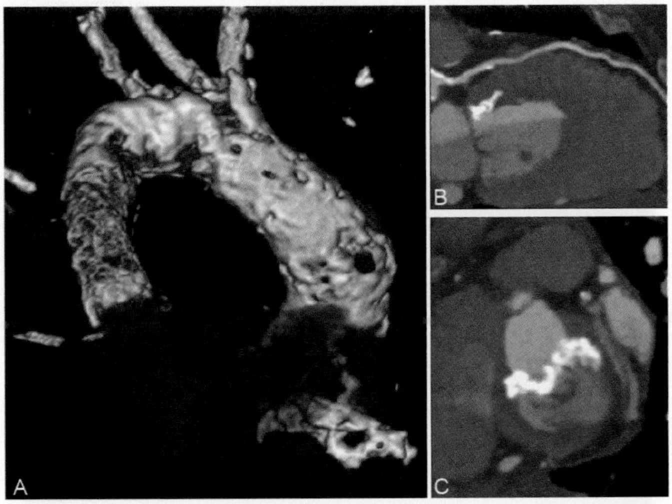


**Fig. 33.10:** Cardiac CT. Cardiovascular disease after radiation therapy; extensive vascular disease of the aorta and brachiocephalic branches, CAD that required bypass graft surgery and mitral valve disease in a 35-year-old woman who underwent extensive mediastinal radiation therapy because of Hodgkin's lymphoma at the age of 7

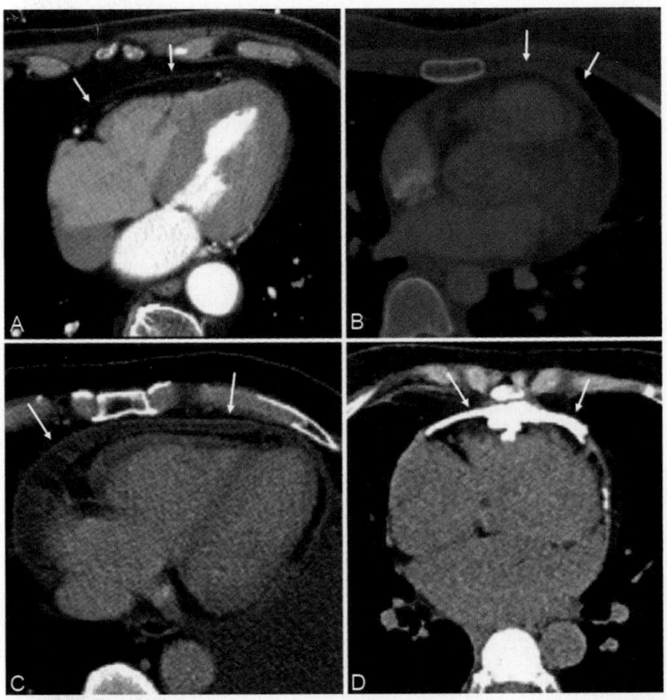


**Fig. 33.11:** Cardiac CT of the pericardium. (A) Normal pericardium, (B) thickened pericardium, (C) pericardial effusion and hyper-enhanced pericardial layers and (D) pericardial calcification

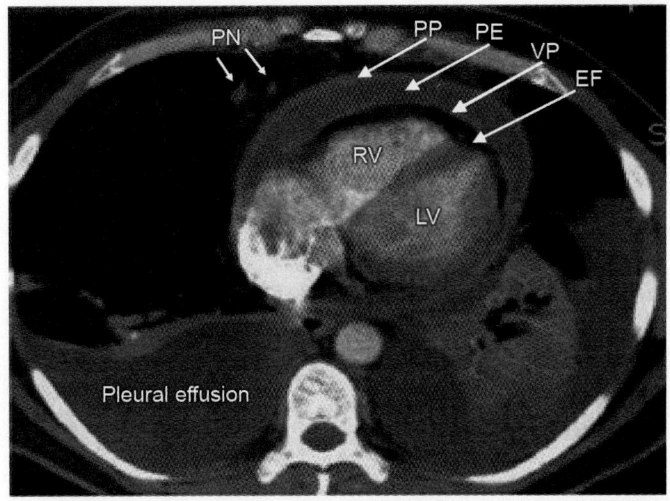


**Fig. 33.12:** Cardiac CT. Pericardial effusion; parietal pericardium (PP), pericardial effusion (PE), visceral pericardium (VP), epicardial at (EF), right ventricle (RV), left ventricle (LV) and pericardial lymph nodes (PN)

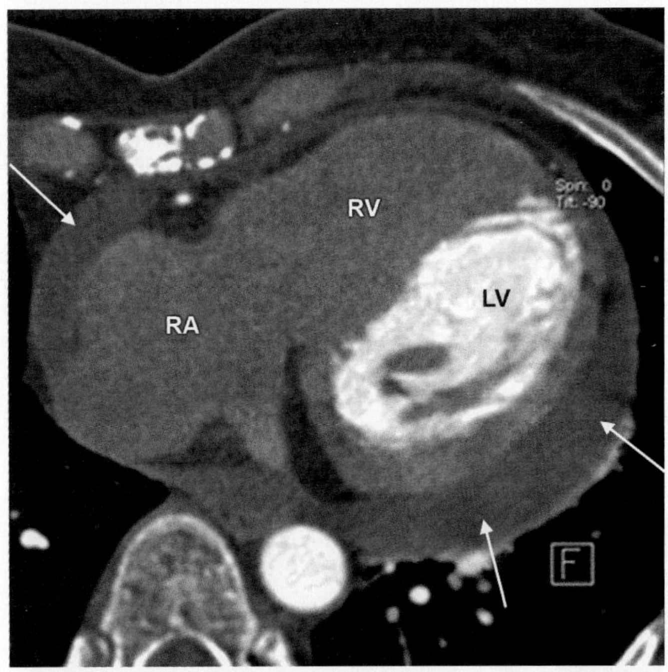


**Fig. 33.13:** Chronic pericardial effusion in a 54-year-old female patient with Hodgkin's disease seen in contrast-enhanced 64-slice CT. The arrows point at the pericardial effusion (LV=left ventricle; RV=right ventricle; RA=right atrium). Due to the timing of the scan relative to contrast injection, only the blood in the left ventricle is contrast-enhanced, hence, the low attenuation in the right-sided chambers

The use of a four-field IMRT technique can offer better sparing than the partial shielding technique as the maximum heart depth is increased. The IMRT plans also showed improved dose homogeneity within the planning target volume (PTV) but may be associated with increased irradiation of the contralateral breast. It has been proposed that maximum heart distance (MHD), i.e. the maximal distance between anterior cardiac contour and posterior tangential field edges as seen on beam's eye view is a reliable predictor of the mean heart dose in left-tangential breast or chest wall irradiation, and may be useful in centres

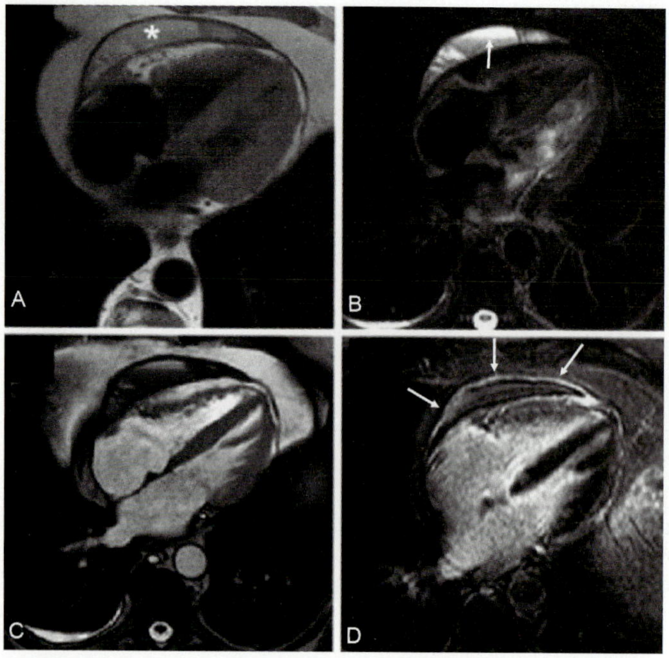


**Fig. 33.14:** Inflammatory-effusive constrictive pericarditis in 67-year-old man presesnting with increasing complaints of dyspnea. Transthoracic and transoesophageal echocardiography were inconclusive to rule out pericardial pathology. Dark-blood, T1-weighted (A) and T2-weighted STIR (B) fast spin-echo CMR, CMR (C) and LGE CMR (D). Located pericardial effusion (*asterisk*, A) with several fibrous layers, fluid–fluid level (arrow, B), several fibrous strands, and thickened appearance of the pericardial layers strongly enhancing the following administration of gadolinium contrast agent (arrow, D). The compression of the right ventricular free wall is well visible on CMR (C). Real-time CMR shows in spiratory septal inversion with an increased total respiratory septal shift confirming constrictive component. Pericardiectomy was performed showing chronically inflamed and fibrotically thickened pericardial layers with a collection of old blood

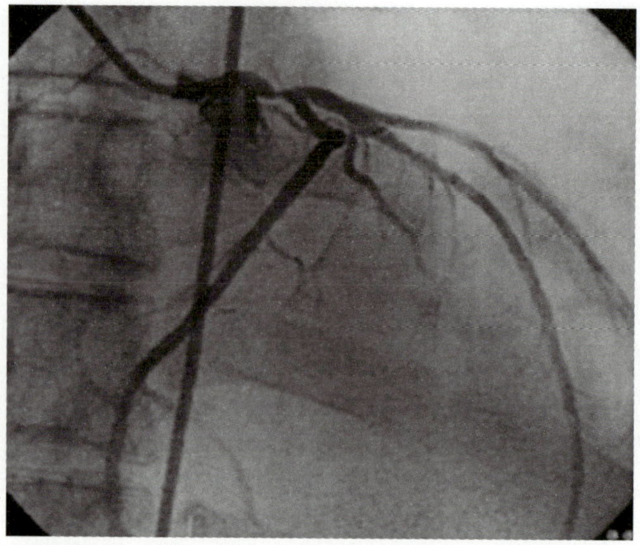

**Fig. 33.16:** A 45-year-old man presented with a 5 week history of worsening exertional dyspnea and orthopnea. He had also noted mild, bilateral ankle swelling. The patient had been diagnosed with stage III Hodgkin's lymphoma in 1968 at the age of 21. During the same year, he underwent total nodal irradiation followed by chemotherapy in 1971. He had remained entirely asymptomatic over the course of the next 24 years with no evidence of relapse. Cardiac catheterisation undertaken soon after admission revealed a tight left main stem stenosis with a left dominant system. Left ventriculogram showed severe, global hypokinesia, and raised left ventricular end diastolic pressure (22 mmHg). Urgent coronary artery bypass graft surgery was carried out. He made an uncomplicated recovery and his condition improved sufficiently to allow discharge 8 days following the procedure. His heart failure slowly resolved and repeat transthoracic echocardiogram performed 6 months after surgery showed an unequivocal improvement in left ventricular function. Left ventricular ejection fraction continued to improve and increased from 23% at 2 months to 42% at 2 years. He currently remains entirely asymptomatic off all medication

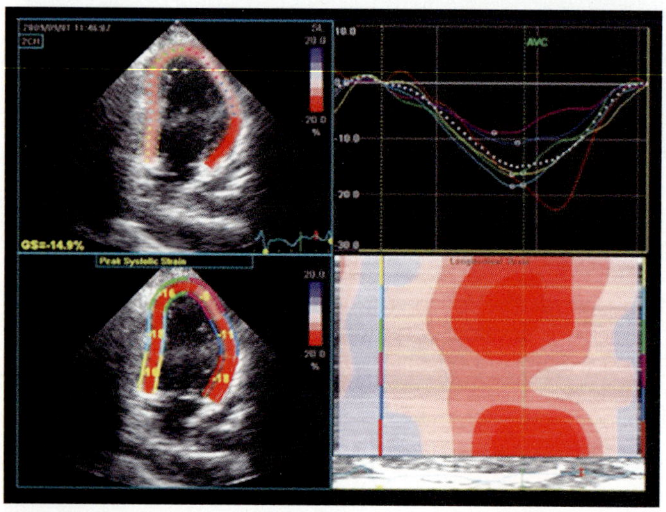


**Fig. 33.15:** Two-dimensional-based strain of a patient with anthracycline-induced cardiomyopathy. The mid and apical segments of the anterior wall exhibit abnormal regional strain

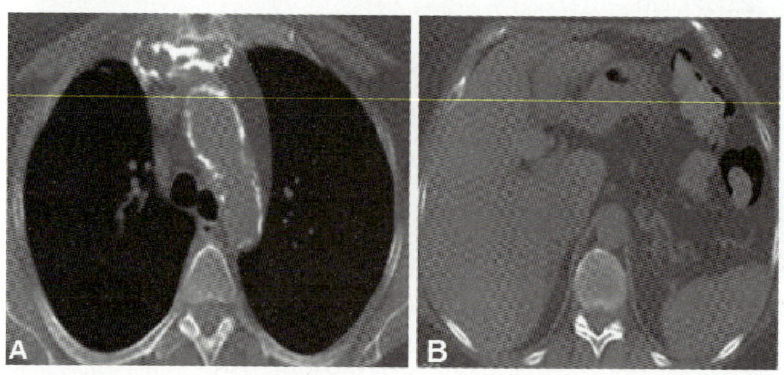


**Fig. 33.17:** (A) Radiation-induced aortitis in a 50-year-old woman with a remote history of radiation therapy for mediastinal lymphoma. (B) Shows a densely calcified residual mass in the anterior mediastinum, as well as significant calcification of the aortic wall within the radiation field

where three-dimensional cardiac dose assessment is not routinely available. A strong linear correlation was found between the MHD and the mean heart dose; for every 1 cm

**Table 33.1:** Radiation effects on the heart

| Acute | Long term |
|---|---|
| **Pericarditis** | |
| • Acute exudative pericarditis is rare and often occurs during radiotherapy as a reaction to necrosis/inflammation of a tumour located next to the heart.<br>• Delayed acute pericarditis occurs within weeks after radiotherapy and can be revealed by either an asymptomatic pericardial effusion or a symptomatic pericarditis. Cardiac tamponade is rare. Spontaneous clearance of this effusion may take up to 2 years. | • Delayed chronic pericarditis appears several weeks to years after radiotherapy. In this type, extensive fibrous thickening, adhesions, chronic constriction and chronic pericardial effusion can be observed. It is observed in up to 20% of patients within 2 years following irradiation.<br>• Constrictive pericarditis can be observed in 4–20% of patients and appears to be dose-dependent and related to the presence of pericardial effusion in the delayed acute phase. |
| **Cardiomyopathy** | |
| • Acute myocarditis related to radiation-induced inflammation with transient repolarization abnormalities and mild myocardial dysfunctions. | • Diffuse myocardial fibrosis (often after a >30-Gy radiation dose) with relevant systolic and diastolic dysfunction, conduction disturbance and autonomic dysfunction.<br>• Restrictive cardiomyopathy represents an advanced stage of myocardial damage due to fibrosis with severe diastolic dysfunction and signs and symptoms of heart failure. |
| **Valve disease** | |
| • No immediate apparent effects. | • Valve apparatus and leaflet thickening, fibrosis, shortening and calcification predominant on left-sided valves (related to pressure difference between the left and right side of the heart).<br>• Valve regurgitation more commonly encountered than stenosis.<br>• Stenotic lesions more commonly involving the aortic valve.<br>• Reported incidence of clinically significant valve disease: 1% at 10 years; 5% at 15 years, 6% at 20 years after radiation exposure.<br>• Valve disease incidence increases significantly after ≥20 years following irradiation; mild AR up to 45%, >moderate AR up to 15%, AS up to 16%, mild MR up to 48%, mild PR up to 12%. |
| **Coronary artery disease** | |
| • No immediate apparent effects (Perfusion defects can be seen in 47% of patients 6 months after radiotherapy and may be accompanied by wall-motion abnormalities and chest pain. Their long-term prognosis and significance are unknown). | • Accelerated CAD appearing in the young age.<br>• Concomitant atherosclerotic risk factors further enhance the development of CAD.<br>• Latent until at least 10 years after exposure (patients younger than 50 years tend to develop CAD in the first decade after treatment, while older patients have longer latency periods).<br>• Coronary ostia and proximal segments are typically involved.<br>• CAD doubles the risk of death; relative risk of death from fatal myocardial infarction varies from 2.2 to 8.8. |
| **Carotid artery disease** | |
| • No immediate apparent effects. | • Radiotherapy-induced lesions are more extensive, involving longer segments and atypical areas of carotid segments.<br>• Estimated incidence (including subclavian artery stenosis) about 7.4% in Hodgkin's lymphoma. |
| **Other vascular disease** | |
| • No immediate apparent effects. | • Calcification of the ascending aorta and aortic arch (porcelain aorta)<br>• Lesion of any other vascular segments present within the radiation field. |

AR=aortic regurgitation; AS=aortic stenosis; CAD=coronary artery disease; MR=mitral regurgitation; PR=pulmonary regurgitation.

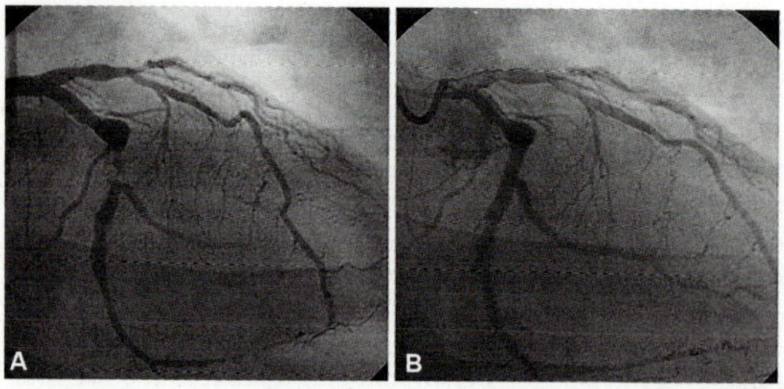


**Fig. 33.18:** (A) Angiogram demonstrating thrombotic subtotal occlusion of the left circumflex coronary artery in the setting of home 5-FU infusion highlighting the importance of careful pre-administration cardiac evaluation and close monitoring during drug administration. (B) Angiogram in the same projection following percutaneous coronary intervention with a bare metal stent relieving obstruction

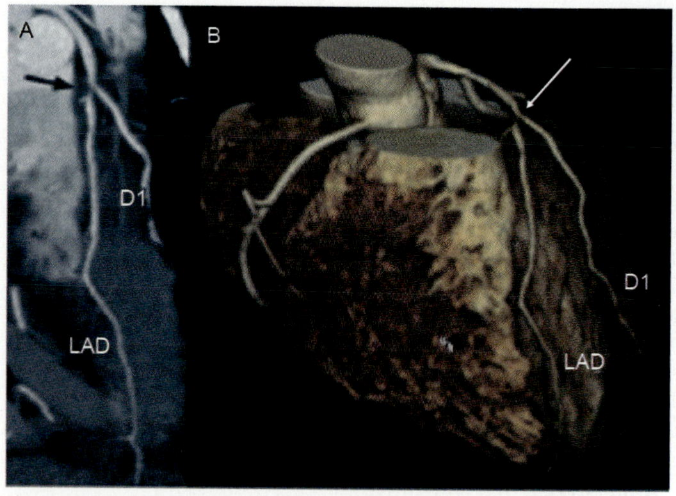


**Fig. 33.19:** Cardiac CT, CAD—a 41-year-old man with severe obstructive coronary disease of the left anterior-diagonal bifurcation (arrow), only a few years after mediastinal radiation therapy because of Hodgkin's lymphoma by angiographic (A) and CCT (B) imaging

increase in MHD, the mean heart dose increased by 2.9% on average (95% CI 2.5–3.3). Electron beams can be used for the treatment of superficial structures, such as in the internal mammary lymph nodes or the boost dose on the breast after tumorectomy, in the treatment of breast cancer.

For mediastinal RT, high-energy photons from a linear accelerator should be used to treat patients with equal weighting of anterior and posterior portals (instead of anterior weighting), all fields should be treated on each RT fraction, use of a subcarinal block after a dose of 30 Gy, and use of shrinking-field technique are the most important parameters to minimize heart exposure. As Adams et al., has stated, although permanent complications tend to occur less frequently under a total dose of 40 Gy, it is not a good idea to systematically limit treatment, which may be inadequate to control the neoplastic disease.

## TREATMENT OF RADIOTHERAPY-RELATED HEART COMPLICATIONS

Radiation-induced heart diseases are treated as non-radiation-related ones, but with special attention to the changes radiation causes to the heart and other structures of the chest.

### Monitoring of Cardiac Function after Chest Radiotherapy

Patients at high risk for radiotherapy-induced complications are those treated as children or young adults for Hodgkin's lymphomas with a mediastinal/heart dose of less than 30 Gy, mainly with what it, are called outdated RT techniques (see above). Those patients should be informed and followed up closely (III, A). Radiation-related heart toxicity is extremely rare during RT. Breast cancer patients treated by cytotoxic chemotherapy or monoclonal antibodies should be monitored. Patients treated by postoperative breast RT (with or without adjuvant endocrine treatment) are not regularly monitored for cardiac problems although RT should be considered as a risk factor when heart disease is diagnosed in those patients

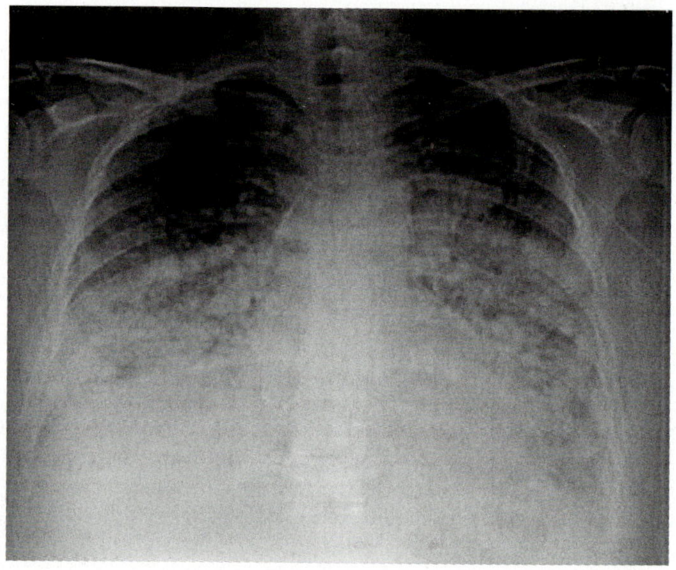

**Fig. 33.20:** The portable chest radiograph reveals bilateral airspace opacities and bilateral pleural effusions. These findings are nonspecific, but in the patient with acute promyelocytic leukemia on induction therapy with ATRA or ATO, differentiation syndrome should be considered. Patients have weight gain, fever, hypoxemia, respiratory distress, hypotension, renal and hepatic dysfunction, serositis (resulting in pleural and pericardial effusions), alevolar infiltrates (hemorrhage and myeloid cells), interstitial infiltrates (edema and myeloid cells) and peripheral edema. Patients are treated with dexamethasone until symptoms resolve. In severe cases (patients with respiratory distress or acute renal failure) ATRA and ATO are stopped until the patient recovers

(III, B). Data to support definitive recommendations on various tests and their frequency do not exist. However, RT-induced risk is lifelong and requires long-term follow-up. Screening and monitoring of heart function is identical to the standard tests and procedures cardiologists use for other patients, and consequently the follow-up protocols are based on departmental or personal experience and on each patient's needs and clinical picture. There is therefore a need for both oncologists and cardiologists to be aware of the risks and underlying pathophysiology of RT-related heart complications. Apart from clinical examination and medical history, tests usually requested depend on the studied abnormality (Fig. 33.20).

## BIBLIOGRAPHY


1. Adams JM, Lipsitz SR, Colan SD, et al. Cardiovascular status in long-term survivors of Hodgkin's disease treated with chest radiotherapy. J Clin Oncol 2004;22:3139–48.
2. Adams MJ, Hardenbergh PH, Constine LS, et al. Radiation-associated cardiovascular disease. Crit Rev Oncol Hematol 2003;45:55–75.
3. Adams MJ, Lipshultz SE, Schwartz C, et al. Radiation-associated cardiovascular disease: manifestations and management. Semin Radiat Oncol 2003;13:346–56.
4. Altena R, Perik PJ, van Veldhuisen DJ, et al. Cardiovascular toxicity caused by cancer treatment: strategies for early detection. Lancet Oncol 2009;10:391–9.
5. Batist G, Ramakrishnan G, Rao CS, et al. Reduced cardio-toxicity and preserved antitumor efficacy of liposome-encapsulated doxorubicin and cyclophosphamide compared with conventional doxorubicin and cyclophosphamide in randomized, multicenter trial of metastatic breast cancer. J Clin Oncol 2001;19:1444–54.
6. Benvenuto GM, Ometto R, Fontanelli A, et al. Chemotherapy-realted cardiotoxicity: new diagnostic and preventive strategies. Ital Heart J 2003;4:655–67.
7. Boivin JF, Hutchison G, Lubin J, et al. Coronary artery disease mortality in patients treated for Hodgkin's disease. Cancer 1992;69:1241–7.
8. Brosius FC, Waller BF, Roberts WC. Radiation heart disease: analysis of 16 young (aged 15–33 years) necropsy patients who received over 3,500 rads to the heart. Am J Med 1981; 70:519–30.
9. Carlson RG, Mayfield W, Normann S, et al. Radiation-associated valvular disease. Chest 1991;99:538–45.
10. Cheitlin MD, Armstrong WF, Aurigemma GP, et al. ACC/AHA/ASE 2003 Guideline update for the clinical application of echocardiography. Circulation 2003;108:1146–62.
11. Darby S, McGale P, Peto R,et al. Mortality from cardio-vascular disease more than 10 years after radiotherapy for breast cancer: nationwide cohort study of 90,000 Swedish women. BMJ 2003;326:256–7.
12. Darby SC, McGale P, Taylor CW, et al. Long-term mortality from heart disease and lung cancer after radiotherapy for early breast cancer: prospective cohort study of about 300,000 women in US SEER cancer registries. Lancet Oncol 2005;6: 557–65.
13. Demirci S, Nam J, Hubbs JL, et al. Radiation-induced cardiac toxicity after therapy for breast cancer: interaction between treatment era and follow-up duration. Int J Radiat Oncol Biol Phys 2009;73:980–7.
14. Di Lorenzo G, Autorino R, Bruni G, et al. Cardiovascular toxicity following sunitinib therapy in metastatic renal cell carcinoma: a multi center analysis. Ann Oncol 2009;20:1535–42.
15. Early Breast Cancer Trialists' Collaborative Group. Effects of radiotherapy and of differences in the extent of surgery for early breast cancer on local recurrence and 15-year survival: an overview of the randomised trials. Lancet 2005;366:2087–106.
16. Geyer CE, Forster J, Lindquist D, et al. Lapatinib plus capecitabine for HER2-positive advanced breast cancer. N Engl J Med 2006;355:2733–43.
17. Gharib MI, Burnett AK. Chemotherapy-induced cardio-toxicity: current practice and prospects of prophylaxis. Eur J Heart Fail 2002;4:235–42.
18. Giordano SH, Kuo YF, Freeman JL, et al. Risk of cardiac death after adjuvant radiotherapy for breast cancer. J Natl Cancer Inst 2005;97:419–24.
19. Glanzmann C, Kaufmann P, Jenni R, et al. Cardiac risk after mediastinal irradiation for Hodgkin's disease. Radiother Oncol 1998;46:51–62.
20. Grenier MA, Lipshultz SE. Epidemiology of anthracycline cardiotoxicity in children and adults. Semin Oncol 1998; 25(4 Suppl 10):72–85.
21. Gustavsson A, Eskilsson J, Landberg T, et al. Late cardiac effects after mantle radiation in patients with Hodgkin's disease. Ann Oncol 1990;1:355–63.
22. Hancock SL, Tucker MA, Hoppe RT. Factors affecting late mortality from heart disease after treatment for Hodgkin's disease. JAMA 1993;270:1949–55.
23. Hanrahan EO, Gonzalez-Angulo AM, Giordano SH, et al. Overall survival and cause-specific mortality of patients with stage T1a, bN0M0 breast carcinoma. J Clin Oncol 2007;25: 4952–60.
24. Heidenreich PA, Hancock SL, Lee BK, et al. Asymptomatic cardiac disease following mediastinal irradiation. J Am Coll Cardiol 2003;42:743–9.
25. Heidenreich PA, Hancock SL, Vagelos RH, et al. Diastolic dysfunction after mediastinal irradiation. Am Heart J 2005;150:977–82.
26. Hojris I, Overgaard M, Christensen JJ, Overgaard J. Morbidity and mortality of ischaemiac heart disease 3083 high-risk breast cancer patients given adjuvant systemic therapy treatment with or without postmastectomy irradiation: analysis of DBCG 82b and 82c randomised trials. Lancet 1999;354:1425–30.
27. Jurcut R, Wildiers H, Ganame J, et al. Detection and monitoring of cardiotoxicity-what does modern cardiology offer? Support Care Cancer 2008;16:437–45.
28. Keefe DL. Trastuzumab-associated cardiotoxicity. Cancer 2002;95:1592–600.
29. Kreuser ED, Voller H, Behles C, et al. Evaluation of late cardiotoxicity with pulsed Doppler echocardiography in patients treated for Hodgkin's disease. Br J Haematol 1993;84:615–22.
30. Lee CK, Aeppli D, Nierengarten ME. Int J Radiat Oncol Biol Phys. Vol. 48. 2000. The need for long-term surveillance for patients treated with curative radiotherapy for Hodgkin's disease: University of Minnesota experience; pp 169–79.

31. Lenihan DJ, Esteva FJ. Multidisciplinary strategy for managing cardiovascular risks when treating patients with early breast cancer. Oncologist 2008;13:1224–34.
32. Levine MN. Trastuzumab cardiac side effects: only time will tell. J Clin Oncol 2005;23:7775–6.
33. Lipshultz SE, Alvarez JA, Scully RE. Anthracycline associated cardiotoxicity in survivors of childhood cancer. Heart 2008;94:525–33.
34. Lipshultz SE, Sallan SE. Cardiovascular abnormalities in long-term survivors of childhood malignancy. J Clin Oncol 1993;11:1199–203.
35. Lund MB, Ihlen H, Voss BM, et al. Increased risk of heart valve regurgitation after mediastinal radiation for Hodgkin's disease: an echocardiographic study. Heart 1996;75:591–5.
36. Mackey JR, Clemons M, Côté MA, et al. Cardiac management during adjuvant trastuzumab therapy: recommendations of the Canadian Trastuzumab Working Group. Curr Oncol 2008;15:24–35.
37. Nagy AC, Cserép Z, Tolnay E, et al. Early diagnosis of chemotherapy-induced cardiomyopathy: a prospective tissue Doppler imaging study. Pathol Oncol Res 2008;14:69–77.
38. Nixon AJ, Manola J, Gelman R, et al. No long-term increase in cardiac-related mortality after breast-c.
39. Pai VB, Nahata MC. Cardiotoxicity of chemotherapeutic agents: incidence, treatment and prevention Drug Saf 2000; 22:263–302.
40. Paszat L, Mackillop WJ, Groome PA, et al. Mortality from myocardial infraction after adjuvant radiotherapy for breast cancer in the surveillance, epidemiology and end-results cancer registries. J Clin Oncol 1998;16:2625–31.
41. Piovaccari G, Ferretti RM, Prati F, et al. Cardiac disease after chest irradiation for Hodgkin's disease: incidence in 108 patients with long follow up. Int J Cardiol 1995;49:39–43.
42. Ramaekers D, Ector H, Aubert AE, et al. Heart rate variability and heart rate in healthy volunteers: Is the female autonomic system cardioprotective? Eur Heart J 1998;19:1334–41.
43. Raschi E, Vasina V, Ursino MG, et al. Anticancer drugs and cardiotoxicity: insights and perspectives in the era of targeted therapy. Pharmacol Ther 2010;125:196–218.
44. Rutqvist LE, Johanson H. Mortality by laterality of the primary tumor among 55,000 breast cancer patients from the Swedish Cancer Registry. Br J Cancer 1990;61:866–8.
45. Sandri MT, Salvatici M, Cardinale D, et al. N-terminal pro-B-type natriuretic peptide after high-dose chemotherapy: a marker predictive of cardiac dysfunction? Clin Chem 2005; 58:1405–10.
46. Schmidinger M, Zielinski CC, Vogl UM. Cardiac toxicity of sunitinib and sorafenib in patients with metastatic renal cell carcinoma. J Clin Oncol 2008;32:5204–11.
47. Seidman AD, Berry D, Cirrincione C, et al. Randomized phase III trial of weekly compared with every-3-weeks paclitaxel for metastatic breast cancer, with trastuzumab for all HER-2 overexpressors and random assignment to trastuzumab or not in HER-2 nonoverexpressors: final results of Cancer and Leukemia Group B protocol 9840. J Clin Oncol 2008;26:1642–9.
48. Silber JH, Cnaan A, Clark BJ, et al. Enalapril to prevent cardiac function decline in long-term survivors of pediatric cancer exposed to anthracyclines. J Clin Oncol 2004;22: 820–8.
49. Singal PK, Iliskovic N. Doxorubicin-induced cardiomyopathy. N Engl J Med 1998;339:900–5.
50. Stewart JR, Fajardo LF, Gillette SM, et al. Radiation injury to the heart. Int J Radiat Oncol Biol Phys 1995;31: 1205–11.
51. Swain SM, Whaley FS, Ewer MS. Congestive heart failure in patients treated with doxorubicin: a retrospective analysis of three trials. Cancer 2003;97:2869–79.
52. Swerdlow AJ, Higgins CD, Smith P, et al. Myocardial infarc-tion mortality risk after treatment for Hodgkin disease: a Colla-borative British Cohort Study. J Natl Cancer Inst 2007;99:206–14.
53. Tassan-Mangina S, Codorean D, Metivier M, et al. Tissue Doppler imaging and conventional echocardiography after anthracycline treatment in adults: early and late alterations of left ventricular function during a prospective study. Eur J Echocardiogr 2006;7:141–6.
54. Taylor CW, McGale P, Darby SC. Cardiac risks of breast-cancer radiotherapy: a contemporary review. Clin Oncol 2006;18:236–46.
55. Ye ET, Bickford CL. Cardiovascular complications of cancer therapy JACC 2009;53:2231–47.
56. Yeh ET, Tong AT, Lenihan DJ, et al. Cardiovascular complications of cancer therapy: diagnosis, pathogenesis and management. Circulation 2004;109:3122–31.

# 34 Cardiovascular Effects of Hypothermia

Hypothermia is usually readily apparent in the setting of severe environmental exposure. In elderly patients or 'indoor' patients, or for a patient—particularly a wet patient, with exposure to less extreme cold, the history may be subtle and less obvious. These patients may have a higher mortality rate secondary to a longer time to diagnosis and increased age and fragility. Mild or moderate hypothermia can present with misleading symptoms, such as confusion, dizziness, chills, or dyspnea.

A patient's companions often note initial symptoms in the field. Symptoms can include mood change, irritability, poor judgment, and lassitude. Companions may note the patient to demonstrate paradoxical undressing (a severely hypothermic person removes clothing in response to prolonged cold stress) or rhythmic or repeated motions such as rocking. Slurred speech and ataxia may mimic a stroke, alcohol intoxication, or high-altitude cerebral edema. Similarly, profound hypothermia may present as coma or cardiac arrest.

In an urban environment, the use of alcohol or illicit drugs, overdose, psychiatric emergency, and major trauma all are associated with an increased risk of hypothermia.

## PHYSICAL EXAMINATION

The key to establishing a diagnosis of hypothermia is rapid determination of true core temperature (Fig. 34.1 and Table 34.1). In the emergency department, core temperature is best measured using a low-reading temperature probe in the bladder or rectum or an esophageal probe. In the field, core temperature may be more difficult to establish reliably. A special low-reading thermometer can be used orally or rectally, but it may not reflect a true core temperature. Care should be taken not to rely on a temperature from a rectal thermometer lodged in stool because an inaccurately low core temperature can be recorded; the probe's reading will also lag behind the core temperature during rewarming. Additionally, a thermometer may become dislodged; be suspicious if a core temperature reading is identical to the room temperature (Tables 34.2 and 34.3).

- Obtaining a core temperature may help prevent erroneous diagnosis for patients with an altered mental status due to stroke, drug overdose, alcohol intoxication, or mental illness. Standard temperature measuring devices commonly used for triage may lack the capability to report unusually low temperature; obtain a core temperature reading for any patient suspected of being significantly hypothermic.
- At a given temperature, specific physical examination findings vary among patients. However, an examination does provide a frame of reference for dividing presenting symptoms into mild, moderate, and severe hypothermic signs.

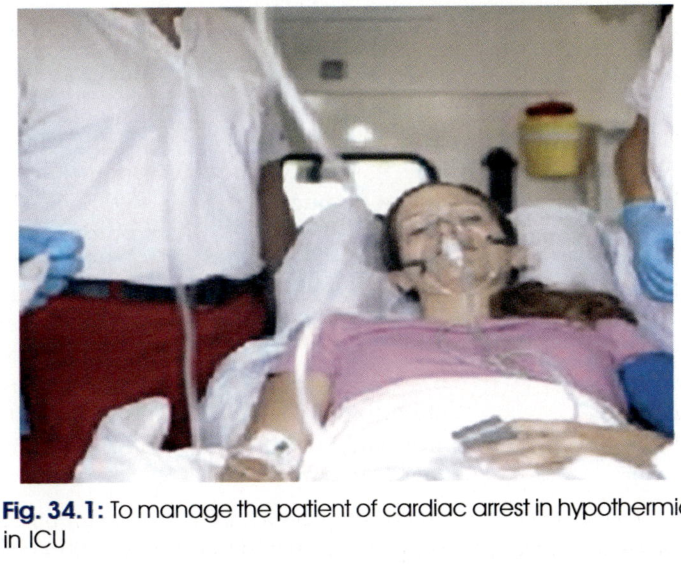

**Fig. 34.1:** To manage the patient of cardiac arrest in hypothermia in ICU

**Table 34.1:** Signs and symptoms of hypothermia by severity

| Mild | Neurologic | Severe |
|---|---|---|
| **Neurologic** | | |
| Amnesia, confusion progressing to dellrium, dysarthria, impaired judgment, hyperreflexia, clumsiness | Agitation, halluclnations, lethargy, dilated puplis with loos of reflex, hyporeflexia | Areflexia, loss of ocular reflexes, coma |
| **Cardiovascular** | | |
| Tachycardia, increased cardiac output, peripheral vasoconstriction | Progressive bradycardia unresponsive to atropine, decreased BP, decreased cardiac output, arrhythmias, increased QT interval, Osborn waves on ECG | Atrial fibrillation, second- and third-degree heart block, ventricular fibrillation (<28°C), asystole (<20°C), decreased systemic vascular resistance |
| **Respiratory** | | |
| Tachypnea, bronchorrhea, bronchospasm | Hypoventilation, decreased oxygen consumption, decreased $CO_2$ production respiratory addosis, loss of cough reflex | Pulmonary edema, adult respiratory distress syndrome, apnea |
| **Renal** | | |
| Bladder atony, cold diuresis | Cold diuresis, hyperkalemia, lactic acidosis, acute renal failure, decreased renal perfusion | Decreased renal perfusion, oliguria |
| **Musculoskeletal** | | |
| Increased shivering, hypertonia | Decreased shiver, muscular rigidity | Patient may appear dead, rhabdomyolysis |
| **Metabolic/endocrine** | | |
| Increased metabolic rate, hyperglycemia | Decreased metabolic rate, hyperglycemia or hypoglycemia | |
| **Hematologic** | | |
| Hemoconcentration, decreased platelet count, decreased WBC count, hypercoagulability, disseminated intercellular coagulopathy | | |
| **GI** | | |
| Ileus | Pancreatitis, gastric erosions, hepatic dysfunction | |

Data from Blem J et al. Mellet M, Hanania NA and Zimmerman JL, and Writers LE Jr

**Table 34.2:** Classification of hypothermia

| | |
|---|---|
| Mild | 32–35°C (90–95°F) |
| Moderate | 28–32°C (82–90°F) |
| Severe | Less than 28°C (82°F) |

## MILD HYPOTHERMIA (32–35°C)

- Between 34°C and 35°C, most people shiver vigorously, usually in all extremities.
- As the temperature drops below 34°C, a patient may develop altered judgment, amnesia, and dysarthria. Respiratory rate may increase.

**Table 34.3:** Physiologic effects of hypothermia by organ system and severity

| | Mild—32–35°C (89.6–95°F) | Moderate 32–35°C (82.4–89.6°F) | Severe <28°C (82.4°F) |
|---|---|---|---|
| Cardiovascular | • HR, • CO | • HR, • BP, • CO Prolonged cardiac conduction intervals, Osborn wave, afib | • Vfib, • Asystole hypertension |
| Respiratory | • RR, • Respiratory alkalosis | • $VO_2$, • RR, • Respiratory acidosis, • Brochorrhea, • Cough reflex, • Ciliary txn | • $VO_2$ • Pulmonary edema |
| Neurologic | • Ataxia, • Apathy, • Amnesia, dysarthria | • Pupils dilate • Pupillary reflex, paradoxical undressing, stupor, • LOC | • Areflexia, • EEG activity • Corneal, OC reflex, • CBF; no movement/pain response |
| Renal | Cold duresis | • Cold duresis, • GFR, metabolic acidosis | Oliguria |
| Metabolic | • Insulin release/uptake • Hyperglycemia | • Shivering | No shivering |

Afib=atrial fibrillation; BP=blood pressure; CO=cardiac output; CBF=central blood flow; GFR=glomerular filtration rate; HR=heart rate; OC=oculocephalic; RR=respiratory rate; Vfib=ventricular fibriltation; $VO_2$=oxygen consumption

- At approximately 33°C, ataxia and apathy may be seen. Patients generally are stable hemodynamically and able to compensate for the symptoms.
- In this temperature range, the following may also be observed: hyperventilation, tachypnea, tachycardia, and cold diuresis as renal concentrating ability is compromised.

### MODERATE HYPOTHERMIA (28–32°C)

- Oxygen consumption decreases, and the CNS depresses further; hypoventilation, hyporeflexia, decreased renal flow, and paradoxical undressing may be noted.
- Most patients with temperatures of 32°C or lower present in stupor.
- As the core reaches temperatures of 31°C or below, the body loses its ability to generate heat by shivering.
- At 30°C, patients develop a higher risk for arrhythmias. Atrial fibrillation and other atrial and ventricular rhythms become more likely. The pulse continues to slow progressively, and cardiac output is reduced. J wave may be seen on ECG in moderate hypothermia.
- Between 28°C and 30°C, pupils may become markedly dilated and minimally responsive to light, a condition that can mimic brain death.

### SEVERE HYPOTHERMIA (<28°C)

- At 28°C, the body becomes markedly susceptible to ventricular fibrillation and further depression of myocardial contractility.
- Below 27°C, 83% of patients are comatose.
- Pulmonary edema, oliguria, coma, hypotension, rigidity, apnea, pulselessness, areflexia, unresponsiveness, fixed pupils, and decreased or absent activity on EEG are all seen.

## Causes

- Decreased heat production
  - Several etiologies related to endocrine derangements may cause decreased heat production. These include hypopituitarism, hypoadrenalism, and hypothyroidism. Consider all these conditions in patients presenting with unexplained hypothermia who fail to rewarm with standard therapy.
  - Other causes include severe malnutrition or hypoglycemia and neuromuscular inefficiencies seen in the extremes of age.
- Increased heat loss
  - This category includes accidental hypothermia due to both immersion etiologies and nonimmersion etiologies and is the most common form of hypothermia encountered in the emergency department.
  - Patients may present with induced vasodilatation from pharmacologic or toxicologic agents.
  - Erythrodermas, such as burns or psoriasis, that decrease the body's ability to preserve heat, or iatrogenic etiologies, such as cold infusions, overenthusiastic treatment of heatstroke, or emergency deliveries, may cause hypothermia due to increased heat loss.

**Table 34.4:** Predisposing factors for hypothermia

| | | |
|---|---|---|
| **Decreased heart production** | | |
| Beta-blockers | Hypopituitarism | Malnutrition |
| Decreased ability to shiver or exercise | hypothyroidism | Neuroleptics |
| Endocrine failure | inadequate fuel | Neuromuscular disease |
| Hypoadernalism | Infancy | Old age |
| Hypoglycemia | | |
| **Impaired thermoregulation** | | |
| Diabetes mellitus | Peripheral neuropathy | Stroke |
| Nervous system dysfunction | Spinal cord injuries | Wernicke encephalopathy |
| Parkinson's disease | | |
| **Impeded circulation** | | |
| Dehydration | Mechanical obstruction | Tight-fitting clothes |
| Diabetes mellitus | Peripheral vascular disease | Tobacco use |
| **Increased heat loss** | | |
| Burns | Ethanol and durg use | Infancy |
| Disordes and diseases of the skin | Exfollative dermatitis | Psoriasis |
| Environmental exposure | Increased body-to-surface ratio | |
| **Medications** | | |
| Barbiturates | Ethanol use | Phenothiazines |
| Benzodiazepines | Neuroleptics | Tricyclic antidepressants |
| Beta-blockers | Opioids | |

Data from Biam J et al., Mellet M, Henaria NA and Zimmerman JL, Fetrone P et al., Dand DF et al., MMMR and Woodhouse P et al.

- Impaired thermoregulation
    - A variety of causes may be associated with impaired thermoregulation, but, generally, it is associated with failure of the hypothalamus to regulate core body temperature.
    - This may occur with CNS trauma, strokes, toxicologic and metabolic derangements, intracranial bleeding, Parkinson disease, CNS tumors, Wernicke disease, and multiple sclerosis.
- Miscellaneous causes include sepsis, multiple trauma, pancreatitis, prolonged cardiac arrest, and uremia.
- Hypothermia may be related to drug administration; such medications include beta-blockers, clonidine, meperidine, neuroleptics, and general anesthetic agents. Ethanol, phenothiazines, and sedative-hypnotics also reduce the body's ability to respond to low ambient temperatures.

Severe hypothermia can cause marked QTc prolongation, often in association with bradyarrhythmias (especially slow AF), Osborn waves and shivering artifact.

## MANAGEMENT

### Prehospital Care

Prehospital management focuses on preventing further heat loss, rewarming the body, core temperature, and avoiding precipitating ventricular fibrillation or another malignant cardiac rhythm. This should be the preeminent concern. Conscious patients can develop ventricular fibrillation suddenly; prehospital workers, particularly those operating in remote search- and -rescue operations, should avoid inadvertent jerky movement of severely hypothermic patients. Patients who develop hypothermia-induced dysrhythmia in the field may be beyond resuscitation. How the hypothermic heart deteriorates into the rhythm of ventricular fibrillation remains under debate (Flowchart 34.1).

### Arrhythmia in Hypothermic Patient (Figs 34.2–34.11)

- Patients developing hypothermia from cold-water immersion appear to be at high risk of fibrillation; rescuers probably are justified in instructing such

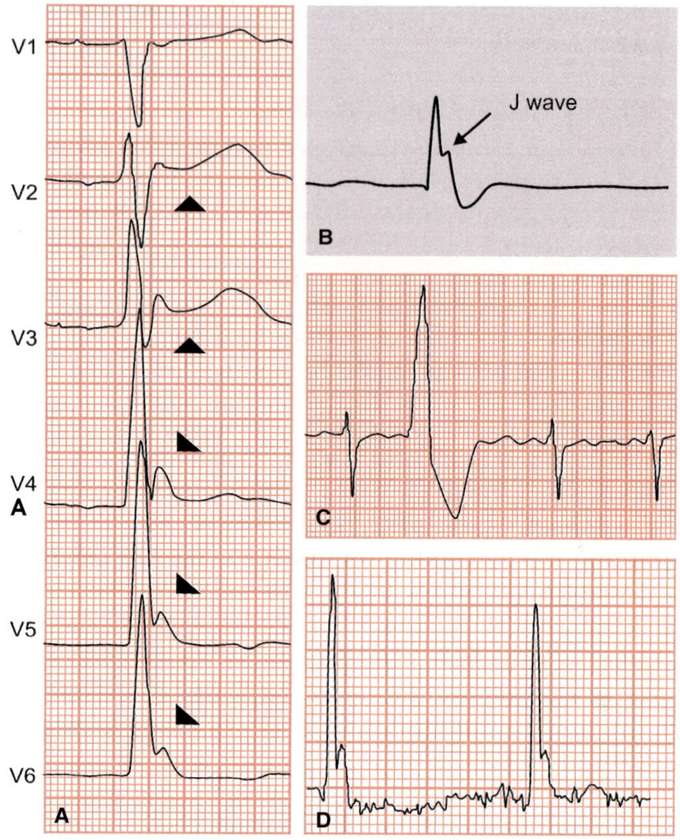


**Fig. 34.2:** (A) Detail of the admission ECG shows the Osborn waves and the Brugada-like ECG pattern with saddleback-type ST-segment elevation in V1 and V2. (B) Showing J wave as Osborn wave. (C) showing ventricular ectopic and (D) shows J-waves along with shivering pattern in different severity of hypothermia

**Flowchart 34.1:** Hypothermia prevention guidelines

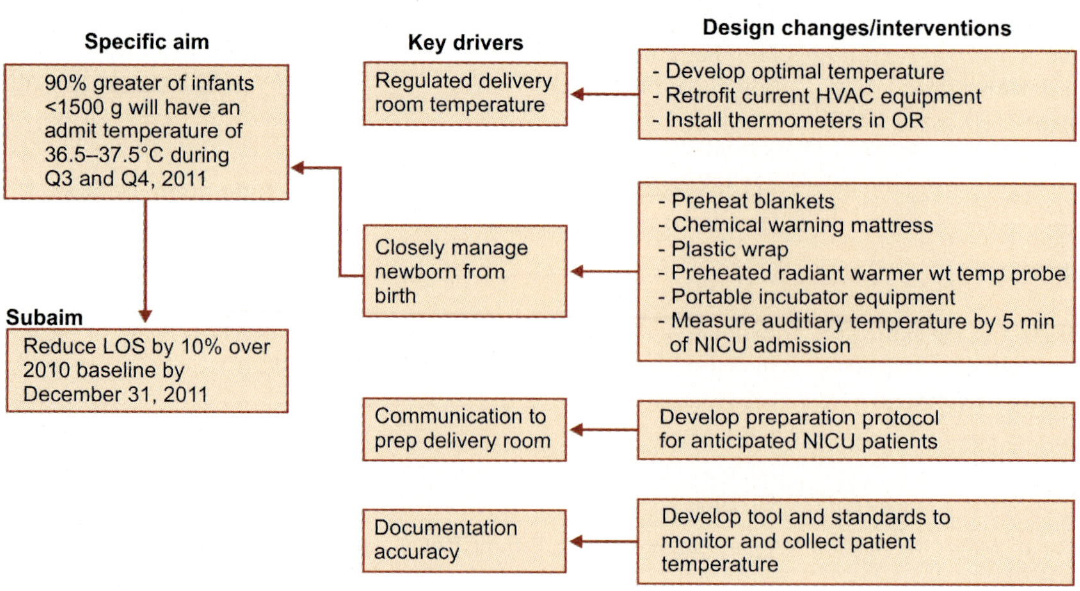

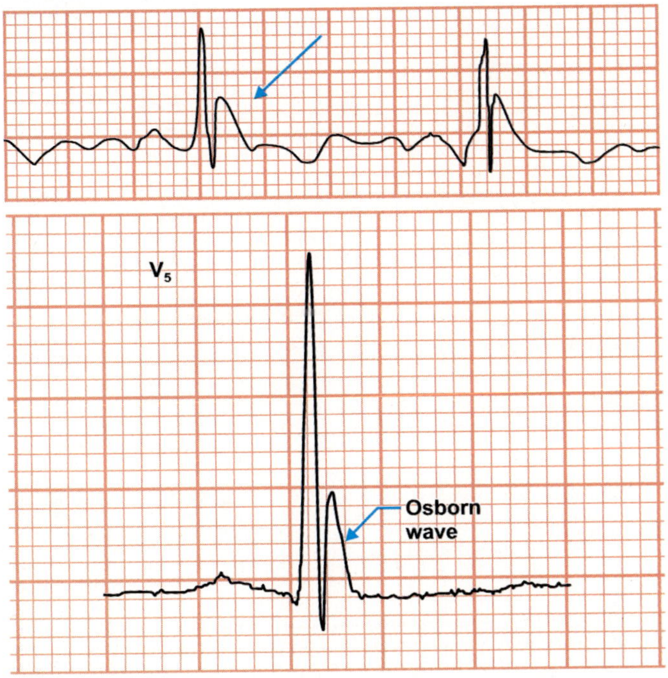


**Fig. 34.3:** Osborn wave. 81-year-old male with BP 80/62 and temperature 89.5°F (31.94°C). A 12 lead ECG of a patient with a body temperature of 32°C. Note the sinus bradycardia, the prolonged QT interval (QTc is not prolonged) and the Osborn J wave, most prominently in leads V2–V5. An ECG of a patient with a body temperature of 28°C. In hypothermia a number of specific changes can be seen—sinus bradycardia, prolonged QTc-interval, ST-segment elevation (inferior and left precordial leads), and Osborn waves (slow deflections at the end of the QRS-complex)

patients to minimize motion and to await careful extrication.

- Anecdotal reports of sudden cardiac death associated with tracheal intubation appear to be exaggerated, particularly if a patient is adequately preoxygenated.
- Both cardiac pacing and atropine are generally ineffective for bradyarrhythmia.
- Lidocaine is ineffective in preventing hypothermia-induced ventricular dysrhythmias.
- Many authors have advocated prophylactic bretylium in cases of severe hypothermia when spontaneous conversion to ventricular fibrillation is possible. This recommendation is due to the success of such therapy both in controlled animal studies and in anecdotal human reports.
- Cardiac dysrhythmias begin to develop at a core temperature of 30°C.
- Ventricular fibrillation susceptibility is greatest below the core temperature of 22°C.
- Bretylium (5 mg/kg initially) is recommended for any hypothermic patient manifesting significant new ventricular ectopy or frank dysrhythmia. However, bretylium has been discontinued by all manufacturers resulting in a worldwide shortage and has been unavailable to many centers since 1999.
- Although the optimal dosage and ideal infusion rate for bretylium are unknown, consider prophylactic bretylium for patients with core temperatures below 30°C.
- To prevent cardiac dysrhythmia with continued hypothermia, rescuers or paramedics should attempt rewarming in the field (a notable exception would be isolated frostbite injury in which limb rewarming would preclude self-rescue because of pain).
- Gently place patients in an environment most favorable to reducing further heat loss from evaporation, radiation, conduction, or convection.
- Remove wet clothing, and replace it with dry blankets or sleeping bags.
- Initiate active external rewarming with heat packs (e.g. hot water bottles, chemical packs) placed in the axillae, on the groin, and on the abdomen.
- Be aware of the risk of causing body surface burns from exuberant active external rewarming.
- In dire circumstances, when heat packs are unavailable, rescuers can provide skin-to-skin contact with patients.
- Ventricular fibrillation in a cold patient is a desperate event. Generally, defibrillation is ineffective at hypothermic core temperatures and when equipment for heroic attempts at resuscitation is unavailable. In such circumstances, attempt a round of chemical conversion with intravenous bretylium (if available), followed by extended cardiopulmonary resuscitation (CPR) until rescuers can begin active rewarming and perform successful defibrillation.

**Emergency Department Care** (Figs 34.12–34.14)

- Patients with respiratory failure should be endotracheally intubated and placed on a mechanical ventilator. Intubation and insertion of vascular catheters should not be delayed but performed gently while closely monitoring cardiac rhythm for ventricular fibrillation.
- Measure core temperatures using a low-reading esophageal, rectal, or bladder thermometer. Tympanic thermometers are unreliable in a setting of profound hypothermia and should not be used. If using a rectal probe, be careful not to insert it into stool.
- Determine whether a cold patient is profoundly or mildly hypothermic.
  - Profoundly hypothermic patients present with stupor or cardiac dysrhythmia (regardless of the recorded temperature) and a core temperature of 30°C or lower.
  - Mildly hypothermic patients may be rewarmed in any available manner (e.g. warm blankets, removal of cold, and wet clothing) since their risk for cardiac dysrhythmia is low. Surface rewarming is adequate in these cases, but it is ineffective in very low body temperatures and carries an additional risk of temperature after drops and shock secondary to peripheral vasodilation.
- Remove any wet clothing, and replace it with warm, dry materials.

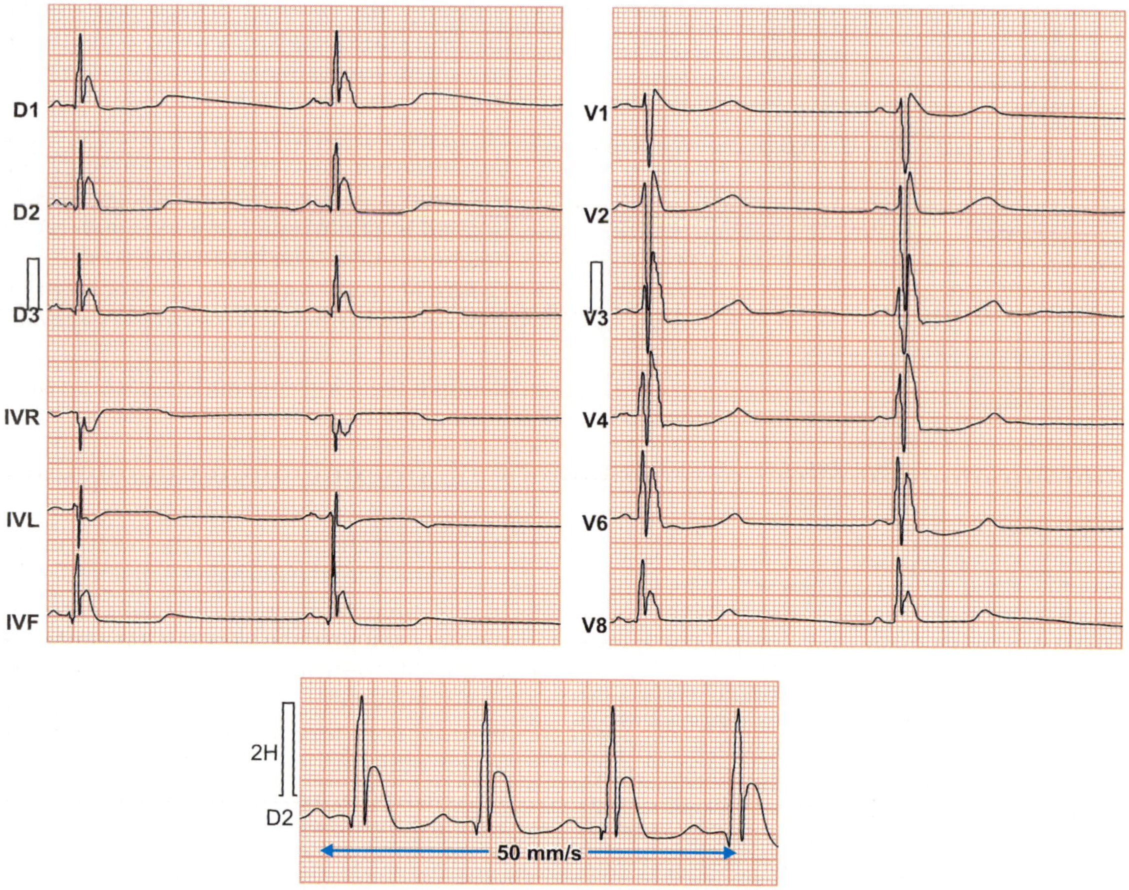


**Fig. 34.4:** Typical ECG of a patient with hypothermia showing extreme sinus bradycardia at 30 beats/min, and positive deflection (J wave) between the QRS complex and the ST-segment, especially visible in inferior and V5 through V6 leads

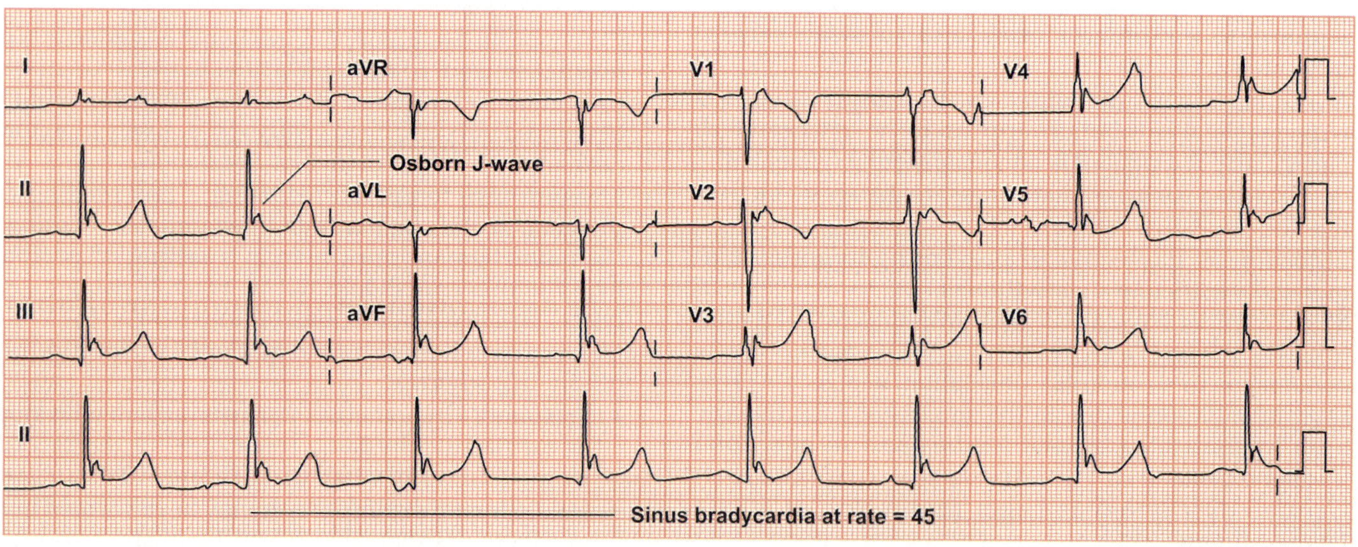


**Fig. 34.5:** ECG showing classical Osborn J-wave and sinus bradycardia in a patient with hypothermia

- Profound hypothermia is a true emergency, warranting the same resource-intensive resuscitation as myocardial infarction. Direct treatment at maintaining or restoring cardiac perfusion; maximizing oxygenation is indicated for a prolonged period of time until the core temperature is at least 32°C.
- Do not attempt resuscitation on the patient with a frozen chest where compressions are not possible.
- Gingerly handle patients identified with profound hypothermia, and take immediate measures to prevent degeneration of cardiac activity into malignant dysrhythmia.

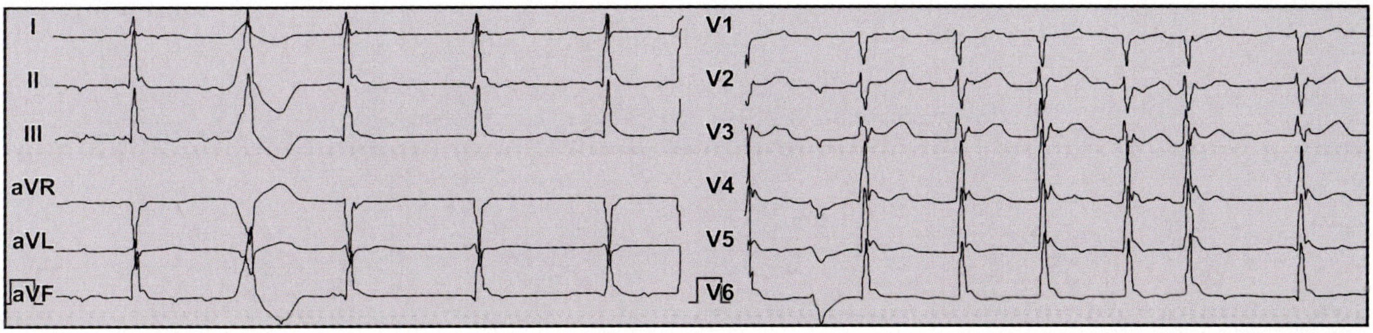


**Fig 34.6:** A 12-channel surface ECG obtained at the patient's admission shows sinus bradycardia, QT-interval prolongation, atrial and ventricular ectopy, prominent Osborn waves in all leads, a right bundle-branch block pattern, and a saddleback-type ST-segment elevation in $V_1$ and $V_2$

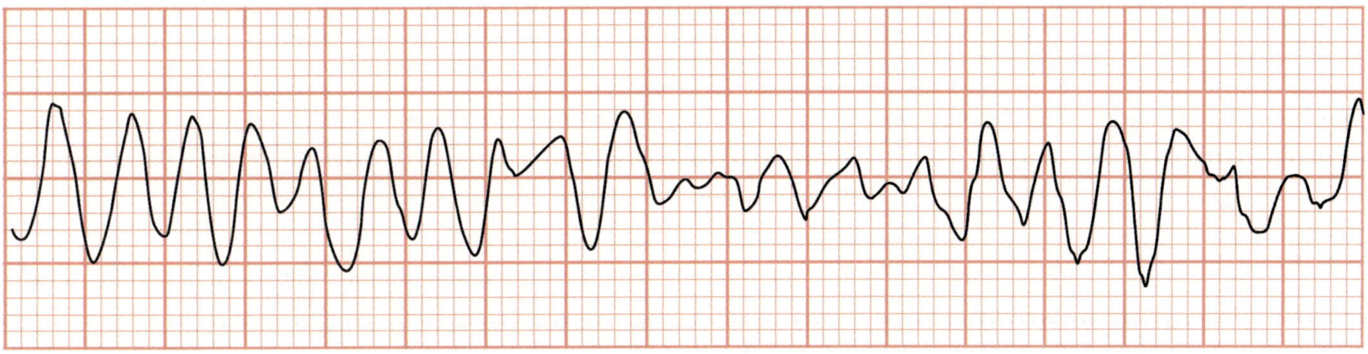

**Fig. 34.7:** ECG rhythm, rate, P-wave, PR-interval, T-wave, can not be determined and the duration of the QRS can not be determined. VF appears as fibrillatory waves with no recognisable pattern

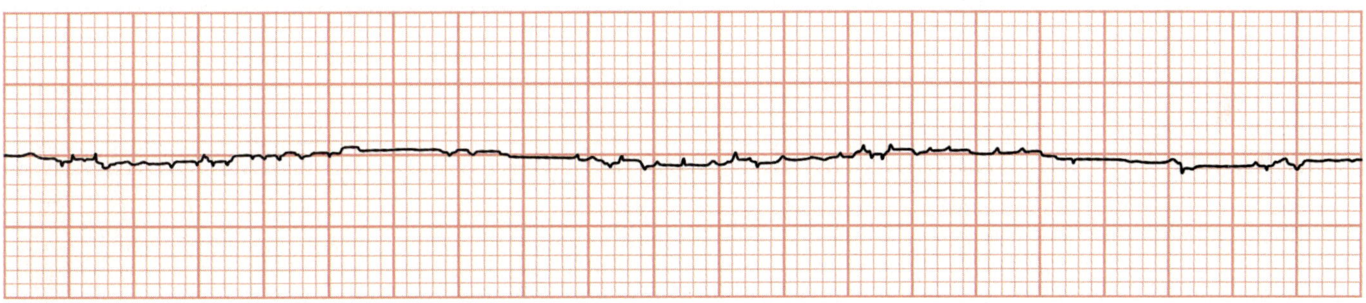

**Fig. 34.8:** ECG showing asystole as ventricular standstill. Patient unresponsive with no electrical activity in the heart and no $CO_2$. This is an arrest situation

- Profoundly hypothermic patients who demonstrate cardiac ectopy may be ideal candidates for bretylium, if available. Administer an initial dose of 5 mg/kg IV (repeated at 10 mg/kg, as needed) to prevent ventricular fibrillation.
  - Lidocaine is ineffective for treatment of hypothermia-induced dysrhythmias.
  - While no randomized human trials have been reported, at least 4 animal trials and two human case reports support using bretylium for any patient with profound hypothermia. Based on such evidence, the United States Wilderness Emergency Medical Services Institute recommends using empiric bretylium for profound hypothermia.
- Initiate warmed, humidified oxygen; provide heated intravenous saline; and place warmed blankets or heat lamps around a hypothermic patient.
- Lactated Ringer solution is not recommended because a hypothermic liver cannot metabolize lactate.
- Although many texts suggest that intravenous fluids be heated to 45°C, this temperature choice is based on convenience of previous study designs rather than any hard evidence. A trial using fluids heated to 65°C demonstrated more efficacy in treating severe hypothermia.

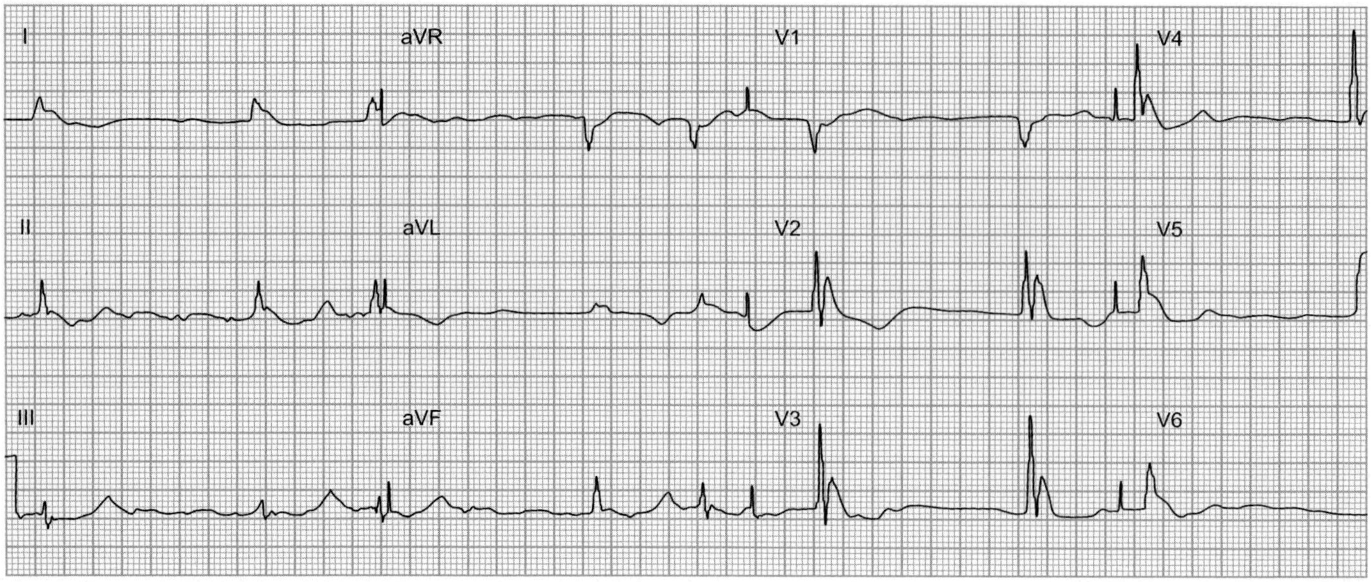


**Fig. 34.9:** Atrial fibrillation and Osborn J waves in a person with hypothermia. Note what could be mistaken for ST elevation

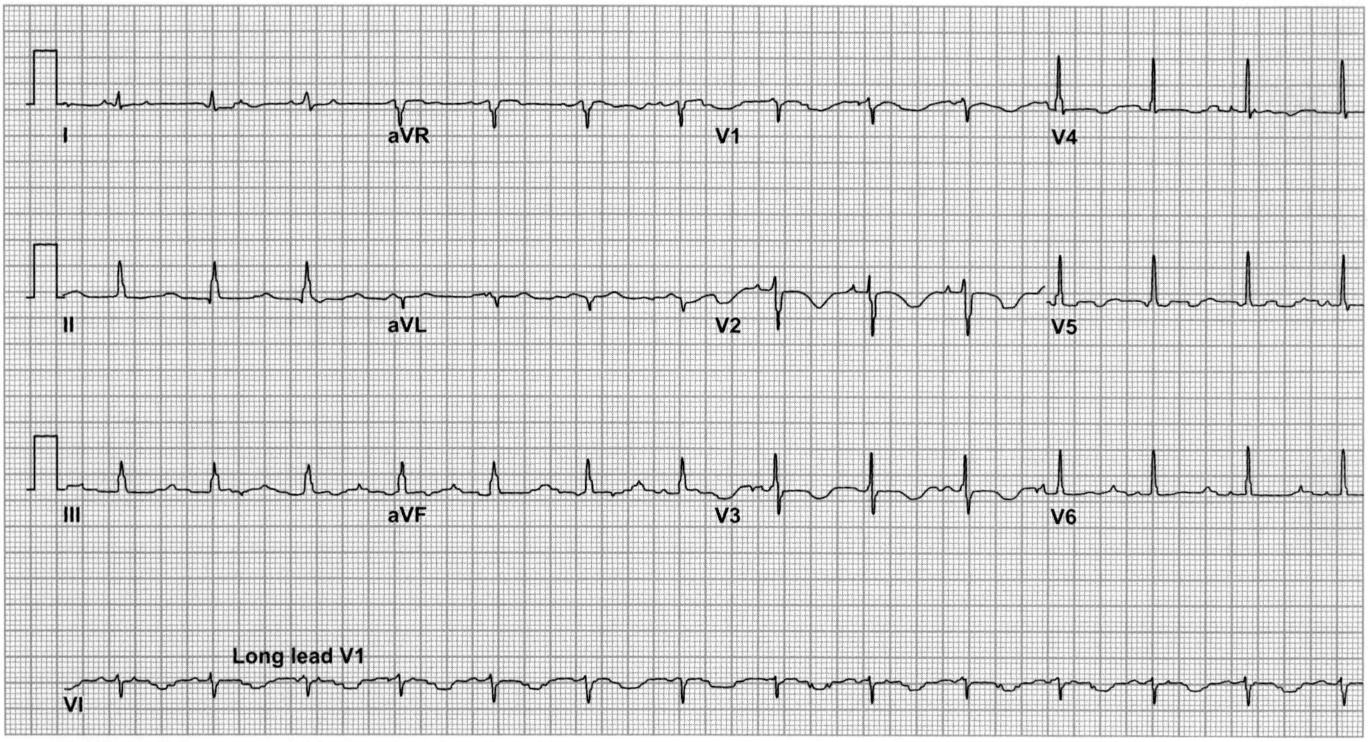


**Fig. 34.10:** ECG showing sinus rhythm, normalization of QRS waves (88 milliseconds), resolution of Osborn J-waves and improvement in $QT_C$ interval in patient with body temperature of 88.3°F (31.3°C)

- Emergency departments that routinely treat hypothermia can keep blankets and intravenous fluid bags in a shared heater.
- In urgent situations, intravenous fluids that contain no dextrose or blood can be heated in a microwave oven.
- Once these simple measures have been applied, consider more difficult rewarming therapies.
- Optimal rewarming techniques depend upon a patient's condition. Treatment is often limited by hospital availability and physician inexperience with rewarming approaches. If core body temperature does not respond to warming efforts, underlying infection or endocrine derangements must be considered.
- A patient who is not becoming progressively colder, is conscious, and has a perfusing cardiac rhythm may not

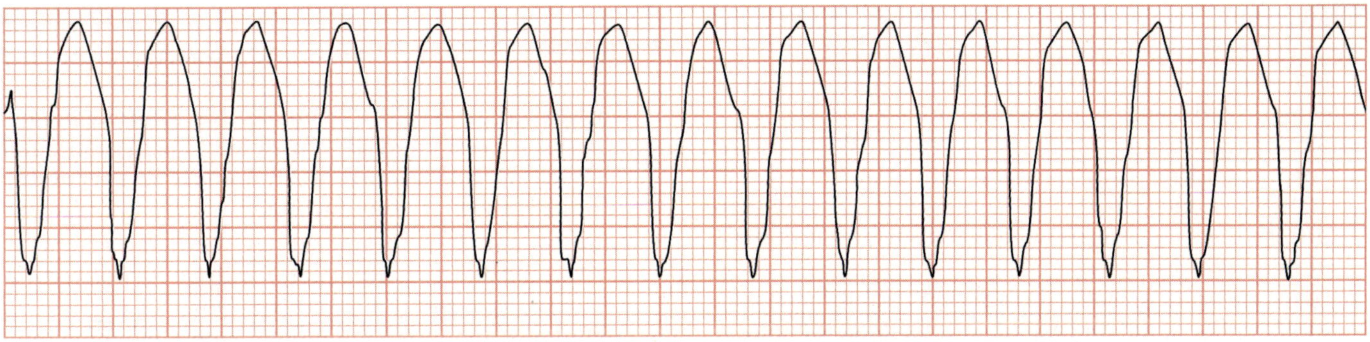

**Fig. 34.11:** ECG showing monomorphic ventricular tachycardia in severe hypothermia

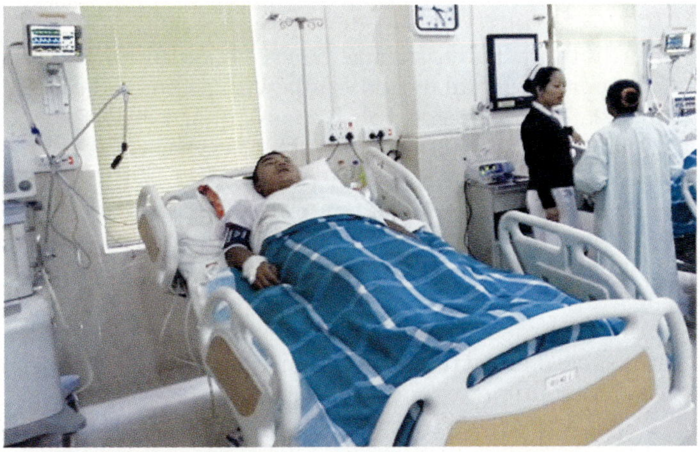

**Fig. 34.12:** Management of hypothermic injuries. The severity of frostbite injuries can now be assessed with triple phase bone scanning, allowing early prediction of likely subsequent tissue loss. Early hyperbaric oxygen therapy appears to improve outcome and the use of intravenous drugs such as synthetic prostaglandin analogues infusions and tissue plasminogen activator have been shown to reduce amputation rates. In non-freezing cold injuries the early administration of analgesia, the avoidance of secondary exposure, and the use of infrared thermography to assess the injuries are among newer approaches being introduced

require intensive intervention beyond the methods already discussed.

- Debate centers on interventions for patients who are worsening, are comatose, have nonperfusing rhythms, or appear dead. Most texts advocate aggressive therapy for severely hypothermic patients, basing the recommendation on anecdotal reports of success.
- Researchers recently confirmed justification for aggressive treatment in a 16-year longitudinal review of profound hypothermia. In this series of 32 Swiss patients presenting with hypothermia and cardiac arrest, 15 patients were resuscitated with aggressive techniques, and all 15 patients showed full neurologic recovery.
- In an older review, rewarming at rates faster than 2°C/h was noted to reduce mortality when compared with slower rates.

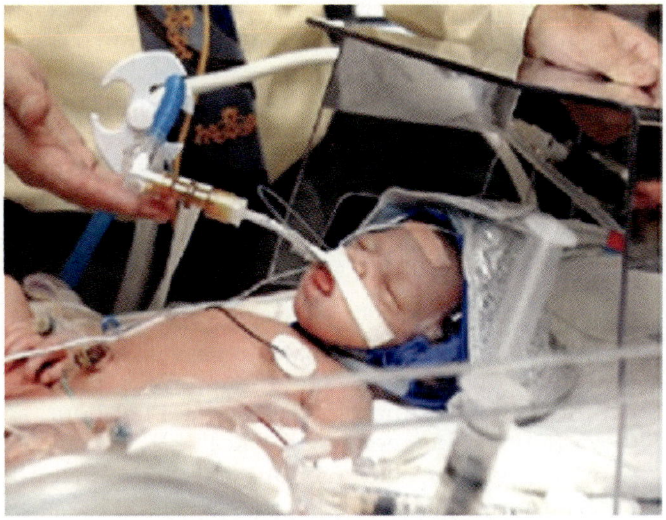

**Fig. 34.13:** Neonatal hypothermia treatment with cooling cap

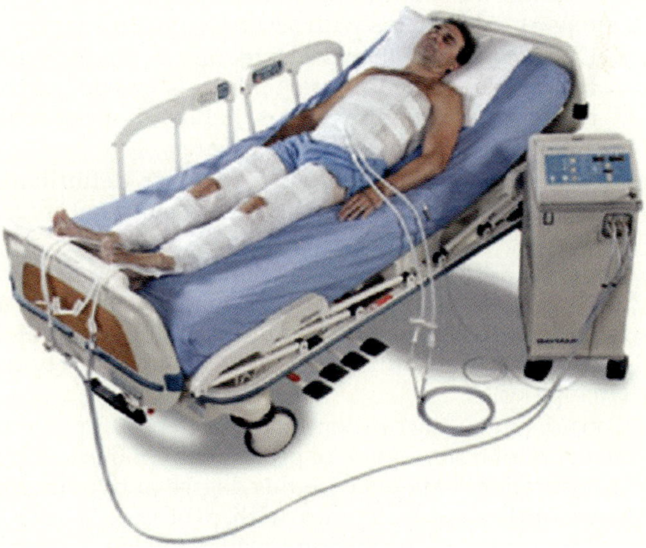

**Fig. 34.14:** Gaymar Medi-Therm III offers warming and cooling options

- An optimal warming strategy is elusive. Some have postulated that rapidly warming a patient to 33°C and maintaining him or her at that temperature, using hypothermia therapeutically as though he or she was a cardiac arrest patient might be beneficial.

- For simplicity, aggressive rewarming methods can be categorized as slow, moderate, or rapid.
- Slow rewarming provides heat from 17–30 kcal/h, corresponding to increasing temperature by 0.3–1.2°C/h (comparisons are somewhat difficult since different study groups used different measurements of heat gain.)
- Slow rewarming methods include IV solutions heated to 45°C (17 kcal/h); heated, humidified oxygen by mask (30 kcal/h or 0.7°C/h); warmed blankets (0.9°C/h); and heated, humidified oxygen via endotracheal tube (1.2°C/h).
- If intact, a patient's endogenous physiologic mechanisms (other than shivering) provide similar rates of rewarming (30 kcal/h).
- Moderate rewarming methods provide heat at approximately 3°C/h. Methods include warmed gastric lavage (2.8°C/h), intravenous solutions heated to 65°C (2.9°C/h), and peritoneal lavage with 45°C fluid at 4 L/h (70 kcal/h or 3 °C/h).

- Rapid rewarming methods provide heat at levels higher than 100 kcal/h.
  - Methods include thoracic lavage at 500 mL/min (6.1°C/h), cardiopulmonary bypass (400 kcal/h or 18°C/h), thoracic lavage at 2 L/min (19.7°C/h), ECMO, and AV dialysis [1–4 degrees per hour, and warm-water immersion (1500 kcal/h)].
  - In comparison, endogenous shivering provides rewarming at a rate of 300 kcal/h.
  - No noninvasive technique rewarms as rapidly as full-body immersion in warm water. Known as the Hubbard tank technique, immersion has successfully rewarmed humans with severe hypothermia.
  - Unfortunately, patients who require rapid rewarming in the emergency department also need cardiac monitoring and intravenous therapy, both of which are difficult to manage under water.
  - Defibrillation also is difficult; however, defibrillation is likely futile once a patient's core temperature falls below 30°C.
- Initiate CPR for hypothermic patients who deteriorate into ventricular fibrillation. These patients also warrant immediate weight-based defibrillation (2 J/kg), along with prompt administration of high-dose bretylium (10 mg/kg).
- Consider initiating cardiopulmonary bypass for any case of ventricular fibrillation or profound hypothermia with deterioration. Patients with this degree of hypothermia have optimized outcomes with procedures such as cardiopulmonary bypass and pleural lavage. However, these methods are invasive, often unavailable, and infrequently used and as such are subject to user-inexperience.
- Ventricular fibrillation should be treated immediately with defibrillation, despite the fact that most other dysrhythmias will correct with warming alone. If initial attempts at defibrillation are unsuccessful, further attempts at defibrillation and antiarrhythmic intravenous medications should be held until the patient is warmed to above 30°C. During this interval, basic life support is continued. If ventricular fibrillation persists despite rewarming, current AHA guidelines recommend administration of amiodarone.
- Although studies in emergency medicine are lacking, cardiothoracic surgeons who induce hypothermia to perform open-heart procedures rewarm patients on a daily basis using open cardiac massage with warmed saline solution. Therefore, a desperate case of severe hypothermia may warrant consideration of direct cardiac rewarming via open emergency department thoracotomy with open cardiac massage.
- Cardiothoracic bypass has been successful for treating cases of accidental hypothermia with prolonged cardiac arrest. To be successful, bypass must be performed rapidly. If a delay is expected, the physician can expedite bypass during an interim period by placing cordis catheters in the patient's femoral vein and artery. Groin cutdowns may be necessary to facilitate such placement; if cutdowns are needed, perform them without hesitation. If bypass is unavailable or delayed, 2 previously described methods of internal rewarming are available, heated thoracic lavage and arteriovenous (AV) heated countercurrent exchange.
  - The literature describes 2 methods of thoracic lavage; the simplest method uses available equipment and provides rewarming rates equivalent to cardiopulmonary bypass.
  - The technique involves placing 2 left-sided, 38 French chest tubes (third intercostal space midclavicular line and sixth intercostal space midaxillary line). Isotonic saline, in 3-liter bags heated to at least 41°C, is infused through the anterior tube at 2 L/min, then drained by gravity via the posterior tube. When warmed saline was not available, physicians successfully infused warmed tap water.
  - The AV heating method, developed at the University of Washington, uses a modified bypass technique for rapid blood rewarming using a level one fluid warmer that is familiar to physicians experienced in trauma resuscitation. The treatment is preferred for patients with profound hypothermia and markedly depressed hemodynamic status or cardiac arrest.
  - AV heating requires a spontaneous pulse, since the patient's intrinsic blood pressure drives flow through the countercurrent module (In true cardiothoracic bypass, an external pump is built into the machine).
  - Catheters are placed into the femoral artery and venous cordis.
  - Once catheters are placed, the arterial output is connected to the inflow port of a level one countercurrent warmer, where intravenous fluids are connected. The outflow port is connected to the femoral venous catheter.

- Water is circulated, at a temperature preset on the level one device, around the blood-containing tubing; the blood warms as it flows through the counter-current module.
- The AV method has rewarmed profoundly hypothermic patients 5 times more rapidly (39 min vs 199 min) than standard methods and was demonstrated to decrease the mortality rate.
- In an alternative endovascular warming technique, a catheter is advanced into the inferior vena cava and circulates warmed fluids. The catheter acts as indwelling radiator as it is connected to an esophageal temperature probe and uses a feedback loop to attain and maintain programmed patient temperature. By this method, the core body temperature may be elevated at a rate of 3 degrees an hour. Additionally, it is an invasive technique to raise core temperaturethat utilizes skills that emergency physicians are already well trained and comfortable with.

- Vasodilation increases the vascular space; consequently, patients that have been hypothermic for more than 45–60 minutes often require fluid administration. Hypotension should be addressed with volume resuscitation; inotropic agents, such as dopamine, should be avoided unless the hypotension is refractory to intravenous fluids due to the possible cardiac stimulation/ectopy that pressors may induce.
- Probes for pulse oximetry placed on the ears or the forehead appear to be less influenced by the peripheral vasoconstriction of the digits associated with decreased body temperature.
- Assessment should include a total body survey to exclude local cold-induced injuries.

## COLD INJURY (FREEZING AND NONFREEZING DAMAGE) OF LIMBS (Figs 34.15 and 34.16)

### *What is a cold injury?*

A cold injury is any disruption of internal processes, damage or death to tissue and associated complications that results from exposure to cold. This includes cold weather, cold water, snow, ice and liquid gas. Although the body has various means to tolerate and cope with cold, minimize damage and regulate the internal temperature, there comes a point where this is insufficient. Cold injury is dependent on the temperature of the environment or substance and the duration of exposure. The injury may also be determined by clothing and other other protective gear that can play a role in minimizing the severity of the injury.

### Cold Injury Types

There are two ways of classifying cold injury. Firstly it is based on whether a part of the body or the entire body is affected. Secondly it is determined by the degree of cold exposure and whether the tissue fluids freeze or not.

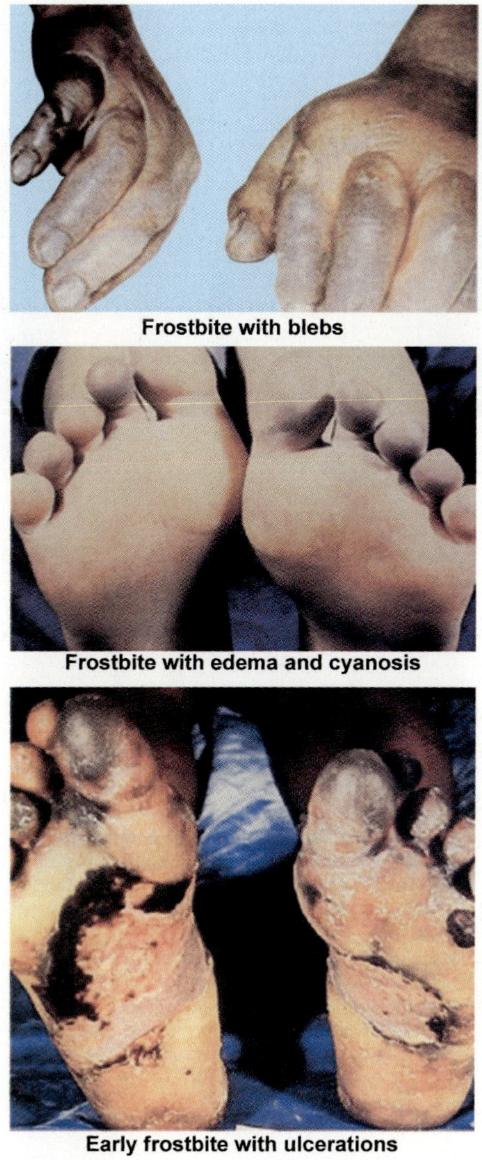


**Fig. 34.15:** Physical features of freezing cold Injury affecting limbs

### Localized or Systemic

- Localized cold injury means that only a part of the body is affected or sometimes several parts. The extremities are obviously the most likely to be affected as it is the farthest away from the trunk where most of the body heat is generated. Furthermore heat is lost in transit to the extremities and in most instances it is the extremities that are most exposed or in contact with cold. Therefore, it is also known as peripheral cold injuries.
- Systemic hypothermia is where the entire body is affected as the core temperature drops below 35 degrees Celsius or in severe cases it dips lower than 32 degrees Celsius. All organs and structures are affected and the most significant impact may be noted in the cardiovascular system (heart and blood vessels circulating blood) and the central nervous system (brain and spinal

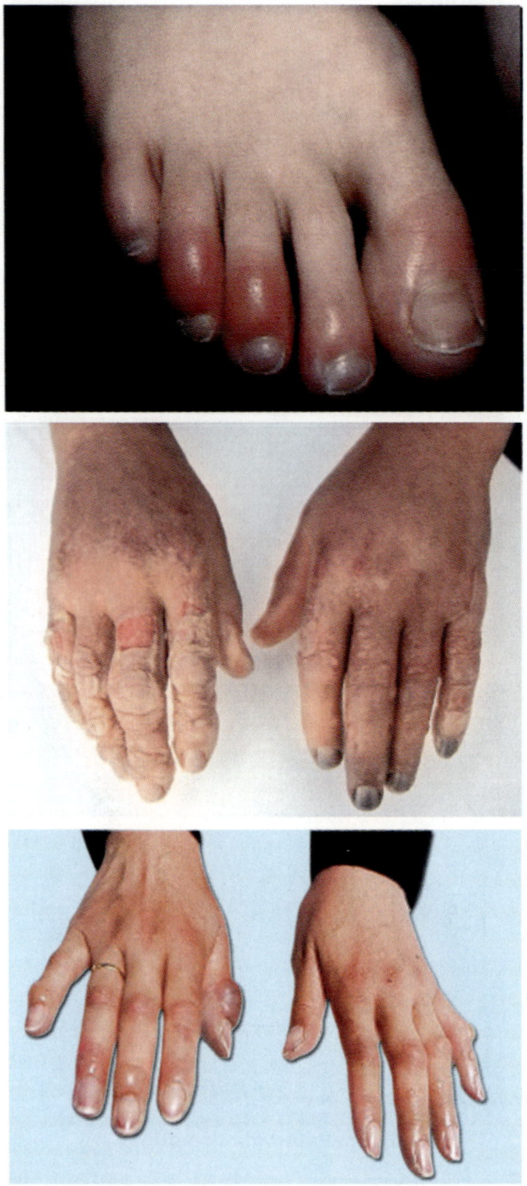

Fig. 34.16: Different types of frostbite injury of hands and feet

cord). Hypothermia is not discussed further in this article as it is separate and extensive syndrome.

### Freezing and Nonfreezing

Freezing and nonfreezing injuries depend on whether the tissue fluid freezes or not. Severe and serious damage occurs when there is freezing. Ice crystals form outside the cells in the surrounding tissue fluid thereby dehydrating the cell. Fluid is the main medium in the body for all processes and once it freezes, exchange of nutrients, gases and other biochemical processes will cease. Tissue death is inevitable.

### Nonfreezing Cold Injury

The two types of nonfreezing cold injuries are chillblain (pernio) and immersion foot (trench foot). Although frostnip is a milder form of cold injury than chillblains, it is discussed further under freezing cold injury as it is a form of mild frostbite.

### Chillblain

This type of cold injury arises with exposure to temperatures that do not cause freezing of the tissue fluids. It includes damp condition. The injury to the tissue is largely reversible. Blood vessels become inflamed and red raised lesions form on the skin. Sometimes blisters, erosions and ulcers may form on the skin surface.

### Immersion Foot

Immersion foot, also known as trench foot, occurs with prolonged exposure to wet conditions although it is not freezing temperatures. The feet are most commonly affected and this condition was widely seen in the trench battles of World War I. The heat loss may reduce the temperature to almost freezing point. Blood vessels and nerves are affected.

### Freezing Cold Injury

#### *Frostnip*

This type of cold injury is the mildest. It is seen as a prelude to frostbite. In frostnip the outer layers are affected and is also known as superficial frostbite. If there is intervention, then frostbite can be prevented.

#### *Frostbite*

This is the most severe type of cold injury. There are several effects that arise with this type of cold injury. The cold causes direct tissue damage, ice crystals also damages cells, dehydration of cells are seen with ice crystal formation, blood flow slows, blood clots form and there is ischemia (injury) with inadequate oxygen supply of the affected tissue. There are four stages of frostbite with the fourth being the most severe where tissue death occurs.

- First-degree frostbite—redness and swelling.
- Second-degree frostbite—large clear blisters along the length of the affected area.
- Third-degree frostbite—large blood-filled vesicles.
- Fourth-degree frostbite—tissue death (necrosis) and gangrene.

First and second degree frostbite are limited to the skin and subcutaneous tissue. Therefore it is also known as superficial frostbite. Third and fourth degree frostbite affects deeper tissue like the muscles, tendons, blood vessels and nerves. It is also referred to as deep frostbite.

### Cold Injury Causes

Although the causes are largely the same for all types of cold injury, there may be slight variations in that certain causative factors are more likely to cause one cold injury rather than another. The temperature exposure and duration are other factors that need to be considered in the type of injury. However, in broad terms cold injury is due to exposure to or contact with:

- Weather—cold, wet and windy
- Ice and snow
- Liquid gases like liquid nitrogen
- Immersion in running or standing water
- Freezer
- Frozen metal

### Risk Factors

There is a greater risk of cold injury with a lack of protective gear, inadequate thermal clothing and inappropriate shelter with insulation. There are also various physiological (non-disease changes in the body) and pathological (diseases) factors that also increase the risk of cold injury.

- Old age
- Alcohol misuse
- Anorexia nervosa
- Arthritis
- Diabetes mellitus
- Head trauma
- Illicit drug abuse
- Immobilization
- Infections
- Malnutrition
- Peripheral vascular disease
- Prescription medication
- Psychiatric illness
- Raynaud phenomenon
- Severe exhaustion
- Stroke
- Thyroid disease

### Cold Injury Symptoms

The different signs and symptoms seen with cold injury have been discussed under the freezing and nonfreezing types. Some of these symptoms develop in specific stages that arise over time. However, as a general overview, the signs and symptom of peripheral cold injury includes:

- Numbness and tingling
- Burning and severe pain
- White to blue discoloration of the skin
- Redness and swelling of the affected part
- Blisters, erosions and ulcers
- Necrosis and gangrene
- Loss of function of the affected part

### Cold Injury Diagnosis

Cold injuries are a clinical diagnosis meaning that it is made based on the presence of signs and symptoms indicative of a cold injury with a recent history of cold exposure. The severity of the tissue damage is indicative of the temperature and duration of exposure. Further tests may not be necessary but can be helpful in identifying the extent of the injury and biochemical changes in the body as a consequence of cold exposure.

*These investigations may include* (Table 34.5)

- Blood tests - CBC count, sedimentation rate, serum protein electrophoresis (SPEP) and quantitative immunoglobulins. These tests are mainly useful for chillblains. Overall blood tests have little value in diagnosing and assessing frostbite.
- X-ray
- CT scan
- Angiography
- Scintigraphy
- Bone scans

### Cold Injury Treatment

The goals of treatment for cold injuries include:

- Preventing further heat loss and exposure to cold by dressing the site, using appropriate clothing and providing insulation.
- Rewarming the area is done by the use of warm water and whirlpool baths (hydrotherapy).
- Restoring or improving blood flow by using warmth, anti-clotting and clot busting agents.
- Increasing oxygen perfusion through hyperbaric oxygen therapy.

**Table 34.5:** Laboratory studies in hypothermia

| Study | Utilization |
|---|---|
| CBC | Possible evidence of infection |
| Electrolytes | Hypokalemia or hyperkalemia |
| Glucose | Hypoglycemia may have precipitated hypothermia or may be the consequence of it |
| Renal function | Serum urea nitrogen and creatinine values may be elevated because of decreased glomerular flow rate |
| Arterial blood gases | Used to assess aacid-base status. Use uncorrected values in hypothermia. |
| Coagulation studies | Presence of bleeding diatheses. Use uncorrected values in hypothermia. |
| Blood alcohol level | Intoxication |
| Urinalysis | Toxicology screen |
| Thyroid function studies | Hypothyroidism |

Data from Hanenia NA and Zimmerman JL, Machem CC, Comeli HM, and Eddy VA et al.

**Table 34.6:** Rewarming techniques according to the degree of hypothermia

| Degree | Rewarming technique |
|---|---|
| Mild | Passive rewarming |
| Moderate | Active external rewarming |
| Severe | Active internal rewarming |

- Preventing infections and other injuries to the damaged area by administering antibiotics, dressing the wound and avoiding use of the affected area.
- Removing dead tissue through debridement although this is limited to superficial injuries. Removal of the affected area (amputation) where there is deep necrosis and gangrene.

### Cold Injury Rewarming

This is one of the single most important measures in treating and managing cold injury. Rewarming may require gentle heat and massage for nonfreezing injuries while conditions like frostbite needs more controlled techniques. Warm water may be used to bathe the area thereby thawing the tissue in frostbite. Direct heat should never be applied to the skin as it can cause burns. Although warm water baths are widely used, whirlpool baths where the water is constantly circulating are preferable. This ensures that the water is maintained at a constant temperature. Passive or active rewarming may also be necessary if there is systemic hypothermia. This involves the use of thermal blankets to help the body temperature increase on its own (passive), or addition of heat to assist in restoring the body temperature (active).

Superficial frostbite may require between 15 minutes to 30 minutes of rewarming whereas up to 1 hour of rewarming may be needed for deep frostbite. Insufficient rewarming is one of the main shortfalls in treating frostbite in the early stages. However, rewarming is not advised if there is a chance of re-exposure to cold and likelihood of frostbite recurring. Massage of the affected area should be avoided in frostbite. Rewarming will lead to pain as inflammation arises and the nerve activity gradually restores. Ibuprofen, acetaminophen and aspirin are milder drugs that may help with pain management but in severe cases, opioid analgesics like morphine may be required.

## BIBLIOGRAPHY


1. Abella BS, Rhee JW, Huang KN, Vanden Hoek TL, Becker LB. Induced hypothermia is underused after resuscitation from cardiac arrest: a current practice survey. Resuscitation. 2005;64(2):181–6.
2. Alam HB, Rhee P, Honma K, et al. Does the rate of rewarming from profound hypothermic arrest influence the outcome in a swine model of lethal hemorrhage? J Trauma 2006;60(1):134–46.
3. Bernard SA, Gray TW, Buist MD, et al. Treatment of comatose survivors of out-of-hospital cardiac arrest with induced hypothermia. N Engl J Med 2002;346(8):557–63 [Medline].
4. Biancolini CA, Del Bosco CG, Jorge MA, Poderoso JJ, Capdevila AA. Active core rewarming in neurologic, hypothermic patients: effects on oxygen-related variables. Crit Care Med 1993;21(8):1164–68.
5. Biem J, Koehncke N, Classen D, Dosman J. Out of the cold: management of hypothermia and frostbite. CMAJ 2003; 168(3):305–11.
6. Britt LD, Dascombe WH, Rodriguez A. New horizons in management of hypothermia and frostbite injury. Surg Clin North Am 1991;71(2):345–70.
7. Brunette DD, Sterner S, Robinson EP, Ruiz E. Comparison of gastric lavage and thoracic cavity lavage in the treatment of severe hypothermia in dogs. Ann Emerg Med 1987;16(11):1222–7.
8. Buckley JJ, Bosch OK, Bacaner MB. Prevention of ventricular fibrillation during hypothermia with bretylium tosylate. Anesth Analg 1971;50(4):587–93.
9. Casas F, Alam H, Reeves A, Chen Z, Smith WA. A portable cardiopulmonary bypass/extracorporeal membrane oxygenation system for the induction and reversal of profound hypothermia: feasibility study in a Swine model of lethal injuries. Artif Organs 2005;29(7):557–3.
10. Centers for Disease Control and Prevention (CDC). Hypo-thermia-related deaths—United States, 2003–2004. MMWR Morb Mortal Wkly Rep 25 2005;54(7):173–5.
11. Danzl DF, Pozos RS, Auerbach PS, et al. Multicenter hypo-thermia survey. Ann Emerg Med 1987;16(9):1042–55.
12. Danzl DF, Pozos RS, Hamlet MP. Accidental hypothermia. In: Wilderness Medicine pp. 51–103.
13. Danzl DF, Pozos RS. Accidental hypothermia. N Engl J Med 1994;331(26):1756–60.
14. ECC Committee, Subcommittees and Task Forces of the American Heart Association. American Heart Association Guidelines for Cardiopulmonary Resuscitation and Emergency Cardiovascular Care. Circulation 2005; 112(24 Suppl):IV1–203.
15. Elbaz G, Etzion O, Delgado J, Porath A, Talmor D, Novack V. Hypothermia in a desert climate: severity score and mortality prediction. Am J Emerg Med 2008;26(6):683–688.
16. Fildes J, Sheaff C, Barrett J. Very hot intravenous fluid in the treatment of hypothermia. J Trauma 1993;35(5):683–686; discussion 686–7.
17. Gentilello LM, Cobean RA, Offner PJ, Soderberg RW, Jurkovich GJ. Continuous arteriovenous rewarming: rapid reversal of hypothermia in critically ill patients. J Trauma 1992;32(3):316–25;
18. Headdon WG, Wilson PM, Dalton HR. The management of accidental hypothermia. BMJ 2009;338:b2085 [Medline].
19. Jurkovich GJ. Environmental cold-induced injury. Surg Clin North Am 2007;87(1):247-67, viii [Medline].
20. Kanzenbach TL, Dexter WW. Cold injuries. Protecting your patients from the dangers of hypothermia and frostbite. Postgrad Med 1999;105(1):72–8.
21. Keatinge WR. Hypothermia: dead or alive? BMJ 1991; 302(6767):3-4.
22. Ko CS, Alex J, Jeffries S, Parmar JM. Dead? Or just cold: profoundly hypothermic patient with no signs of life. Emerg Med J 2002;19(5):478–79.

23. Laniewicz M, Lyn-Kew K, Silbergleit R. Rapid endovascular warming for profound hypothermia. Ann Emerg Med 2008; 51(2):160–3.
24. Launay JC, Savourey G. Cold adaptations. Ind Health 2009; 47(3):221–7.
25. Long WB 3rd, Edlich RF, Winters KL, Britt LD. Cold injuries. J Long Term Eff Med Implants 2005;15(1):67–78.
26. McCullough L, Arora S. Diagnosis and treatment of hypothermia. Am Fam Physician 2004;70(12):2325–32.
27. Murphy K, Nowak RM, Tomlanovich MC. Use of bretylium tosylate as prophylaxis and treatment in hypothermic ventricular fibrillation in the canine model. Ann Emerg Med 1986;15(10):1160–6.
28. Plaisier BR. Thoracic lavage in accidental hypothermia with cardiac arrest—report of a case and review of the literature. Resuscitation 2005;66(1):99–104.
29. Polderman KH. Mechanisms of action, physiological effects, and complications of hypothermia. Crit Care Med 2009; 37(7 Suppl):S186–202.
30. Romet TT, Hoskin RW. Temperature and metabolic respo-nses to inhalation and bath rewarming protocols. Aviat Space Environ Med 1988;59(7):630–4.
31. Savard GK, Cooper KE, Veale WL, Malkinson TJ. Peripheral blood flow during rewarming from mild hypothermia in humans. J Appl Physiol 1985;58(1):4–13.
32. Schewe JC, Heister U, Fischer M, Hoeft A [Accidental urban hypothermia. Severe hypothermia of 20.7 degrees C]. Anaesthesist 2005;54(10):1005–11.
33. Sessler DI. Thermoregulatory defense mechanisms. Crit Care Med 2009;37(7 Suppl):S203-10 [Medline].
34. Spencer SM, Roeseler J, Verschuren F, Reynaert M, Thys F. Metabolism study in an 88-year-old woman with severe hypothermia during rewarming procedures. Am J Emerg Med 2007;25(8):986.e1–3.
35. Ulrich AS, Rathlev NK. Hypothermia and localized cold injuries. Emerg Med Clin North Am 2004;22(2): 281–98.
36. Vachiery JL, Reuse C, Blecic S, Contempre B, Vincent JL. Bretylium tosylate versus lidocaine in experimental cardiac arrest. Am J Emerg Med 1990;8(6):492–5.
37. Walpoth BH, Walpoth-Aslan BN, Mattle HP, et al. Outcome of survivors of accidental deep hypothermia and circulatory arrest treated with extracorporeal blood warming. N Engl J Med 1997;337(21):1500–5.

# 35 Neonatal Cardiac Emergencies

The approach to the infant with a cardiac emergency begins with identification of the unstable or critically ill child and proceeds rapidly into stabilization and provision of immediate therapies. Support of oxygenation, ventilation, and circulation will precede identification of specific cardiac lesions. The emergency clinician can use clinical findings, chest X-ray, and electrocardiographic information to plan emergent intervention. Infants in the first days of life who present with circulatory collapse secondary to obstruction of pulmonary or systemic blood flow (ductus dependent) conditions can be stabilized with prostaglandin E infusion. The more common presentation of cardiac disease in the first month of life is congestive heart failure. Infants with congestive heart failure require respiratory support, careful fluid management, and inotropic support. Many congenital heart diseases (CHDs) present in the neonatal period. Critical congenital heart defects has an incidence of 3–3.5/1,000 live births (almost half of all CHDs). These have been defined as lesions that are 'duct dependent' [i.e. dependent on a patent ductus arteriosus (PDA) for pulmonary or systemic bloodflow] or require intervention (surgical or catheter) within the first month in order to sustain life or prevent major morbidity. In addition, common neonatal arrhythmias can also present as emergencies. A clear appreciation of the pathophysiology of each particular CHD requires a sound understanding of the fetal, transitional and neonatal circulations, i.e. the normal physiological changes that occur after birth. As detailed antenatal anomaly scanning is not routinely available, the majority of neonates with critical CHD present clinically without a known diagnosis. Even when available, detection rates for CHD are modest, currently ranging from 57 to 67%. Despite the numerous different cardiac lesions, there is only a limited spectrum of clinical presentations that the practitioner is likely to encounter. A severely ill neonate with cyanosis and respiratory distress is a diagnostic challenge. The clinician must perform a rapid evaluation to determine whether congenital heart disease is a cause so that potentially life-saving measures can be instituted.

*Differential diagnosis:* The causes of cyanosis can be classified as respiratory, cardic, central nervous system (CNS) or other disorders.

*Evaluation:* During a physical examination if an infant appears blue, the following questions need immediate answer:

1. **Does the infant have respiratory distress?**
   If the infant has increased respiratory effort with increased rate, retractions and nasal flaring, respiratory disease should be high on the list of differential diagnosis. Cyanotic heart disease usually presents without respiratory symptoms but can have effotless tachypnea (rapid respiratory rate without retractions).
2. **Does the infant have murmor?**
   A murmor usually implies heart disease. Transposition of great vessels can present without a murmor.
3. **Is the cyanosis continous, intermittent, sudden in oncet or occurring only with feeding?**
   Intermittent cyanosis is more common with neurologic disorders, as these infants may have apneic spells alternating with periods of normal breathing. Continuous cyanosis is usually associated with intrinsic lung disease or heart disease. Cyanosis with feeding may occur with esophageal atresia and severe esophageal reflux. Cyanosis that disappears with crying may signify choanal atresia. The common causes of cyanosis could be discussed as follows.

   *Cardiac diseases*

   1. All cyanotic heart diseases includin transposition of great arteries, total anomalous pulmonary venous return, Ebstein's anomaly, tricuspid atresia, pulmonary atresia, pulmonary stenosis, tetralogy of Fallot, patent ductus arteriosus and ventricular septal defect.
   2. Persistent pulmonary hypertension
   3. Severe congestive heart failure.

*Respiratory diseases*

1. Lung diseases
   a. Hyaline membrane disease
   b. Transiet tachypnea of the newborn
   c. Pneumonia
   d. Meconium aspiration
2. Air leak syndrome
3. Congenital defects (e.g. diaphragmatic hernia, hypoplastic lungs, lobar emphysema, cystic adenomatoid malformation and diaphragmal abnormality)

*CNS diseases*

Periventricular-intraventricular hemorrhage, meningitis and primary seizure disorder can all cause cyanosis. Neuromuscular disorders such as Werdnong-Hoffmann disease and congenital myotonic dystrophy can cause cyanosis.

*Other disorders*

1. Methemoglobinemia
2. Polycythemia/hyperviscostiy syndrome
3. Hypothermia
4. Hypoglycemia
5. Sepsis
6. Pseudocyanosis caused by fluorescent lighting
7. Respiratory depression secondary to maternal medications (e.g. magnesium sulfate and narcotics)
8. Shock
9. Upper airway obstruction. Choanal atresia is nasal passage obstruction caused most commonly by a bony abnormality. Other causes are laryngeal web, tracheal stenosis, goiter and Pierre Robin syndrome.

4. **Is there differential cyanosis?**
   If there is cyanosis of upper or lower part of the body only, this usually signifies serious heart disease. The more common pattern is cyanosis restricted to the lower part of the body, which is seen in patients with patent ductus arteriosus with left-to-right shunt. Cyanosis restricted tothe upper half of the body is seen occasionally in patients with pulmonary hypertension, patent ductus arteriosus, coarctation of aorta and D-transposition of great arteries.
5. **What is the prenatal and delivery history?**
   An infant of a diabetic mother has increased risk of hypoglycemia, polycythemia, respiratory distress syndrome and heart disease. Infection, which can occur with premature rupture of membranes, may cause shock and hypotension with resultant cyanosis. Amniotic fluiod abnormalities, such as oligohydramnios (associated with hypoplastic lungs) or polyhydramnios (associated with esophageal atresia), may suggest a cause for cyanosis. Cesarean section is associated with increased respiratory distress.

## HEART DISEASE IN NEWBORN BABY

Congenital heart disease produces cyanosis when obstruction to right ventricular outflow causes intracardiac right-to-left shunting or when complex anatomic defects, unassociated with pulmonary stenosis, cause an admixture of pulmonary and systemic venous return in the heart. Cynosis from pulmonary edema may also develop in patients with heart failure caused by left-to-right shunts, although the degree is usually less severe. Cyanosis may becaused by persistence of fetal pathways, e.g. right-to-left shunting across theforamen ovale and ductus arterious in the presence of persistent pulmonary hypertension of the newborn (PPHN).

### Cardiac Evaluation of Newborn Infant

In the cardiac evaluation of the newborn infant, understanding the circulatory status at birth is very important. As the result of fetal circulation, newborn infants have right ventricular (RV) dominance associated with a thick RV wall, elevated pulmonary vascular resistance (PVR), and a thick medial layer of the pulmonary arterioles. The thick pulmonary artery smooth muscle gradually becomes thinner, and it resembles that of the adult by the time the baby is age 6–8 weeks. Most perinatal changes in hemodynamics are related to the thinning of the pulmonary vascular smooth muscle, resulting in a gradual fall in the PVR and a loss of RV dominance of the neonate. Premature infants in general have less RV dominance than full-term infants, and the PVR is not as high in the full-term neonate, which adds variability to the process. Because of these unique aspects of the perinatal circulatory system, the basic tools in the initial cardiac evaluation discussed are less reliable and the findings may be different in the newborn infant. Therefore, echo studies are commonly performed in the neonatal cardiac evaluation. Some important aspects of normal and abnormal findings in physical examination, electrocardiograpgy (ECG), and chest X-ray films of the neonate are briefly reviewed in this chapter.

### Physical Examination (Figs 35.1, 35.2 and Table 35.1)

1. Normal physical findings that are unique in normal newborn infants are:
   a. Heart rate is generally faster (usually over 100 beats/min, with normal ranges from 70 beats/min to 180 beats/min) than that of older children and adults.
   b. A varying degree of acrocyanosis is the rule rather than the exception.
   c. Mild arterial desaturation with arterial $PO_2$ as low as 60 mmHg is not unusual in an otherwise normal neonate. This may be caused by an intrapulmonary shunt through an as yet unexpanded portion of the lungs or by a right-to-left arterial shunt through the patent foramen ovale (PFO).
   d. There is relative hyperactivity of the RV, with the point of maximal impuls (PMI) at the lower left sternal border (LLSB) rather than at the apex.
   e. The second heart sound (S2) may be single in the first days of life, and occasionally an ejection click (reflecting pulmonary hypertension) is audible.
   f. An innocent heart murmur may be present. The most common one in this age group is the pulmonary flow murmur of the newborn infant.

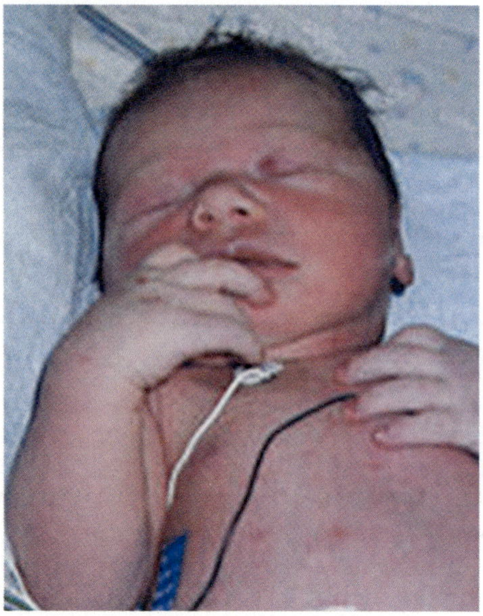

**Fig. 35.1:** A *cyanotic newborn*, or 'blue baby'. Note the blue coloration of the fingertips

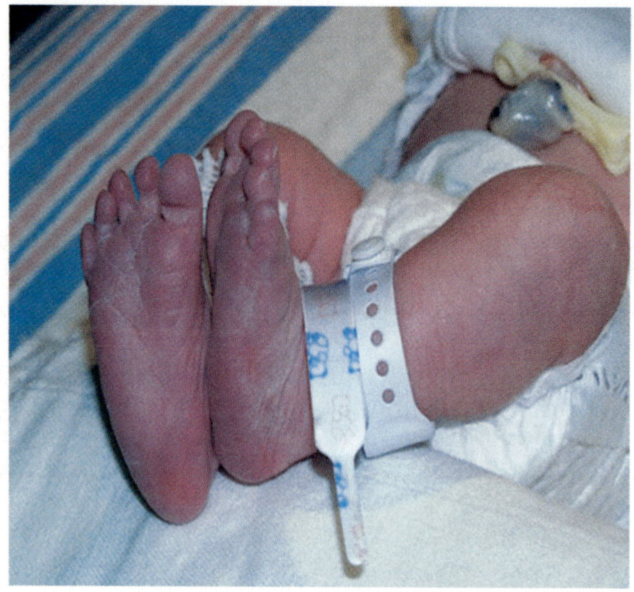

**Fig. 35.2:** Cyanosis of both the feet

**Table 35.1:** Distinction between respiratory and cardiac cyanosis in the neonate

| | Respiratory | Cardiac |
|---|---|---|
| History | Risk factors, e.g. meconium-stained liquor, prematurity, CNS depression | Suggestive antenatal scan, infant of diabetic mother, syndromes, previous children with CHD, etc. |
| Onset | At birth | Hours to days after birth |
| Examination | Respiratory distress tochypnoea, grunting, recession | Comfortable unless duct dependent pulmonary circulation with closing PDA |
| Auscultation | Lung crackles/wheezes, reduced air entry | Clear lungs, normal air entry, murmur not always prsent |
| Blood gas | High $pCO_2$, low $pO_2$ | Normal/low $pCO_2$, low $pO_2$ |
| Hyperoxia test* | Passed | Failed |
| Chest X-ray | Lung infiltrates, normal heart size | Clear lung fields, oligaernia or plethora, heart normal or enlarged, 'typical' cardiac silhouette† |
| ECG | Normal | May be abnormal and provide due to diagnosis |

*Hyperoxia testmeasure right radial or brachial arterial $pO_2$ in 100% $O_2$ (closed headbox or rebreather mask for 10–15 min): $pO_2$ <150 mmHg (20 kPa) → cardiac, $pO_2$ >150 mmHg → respiratory (note: there may be a few exceptions to this rule)

†'Typical' X-ray patterns are only occasionally seen—'egg on the side' (narrow mediastinum) for transposition, boot heart for tetralogy/pulmonary (and sometimes tricuspid) atresia, 'snowman' sign for supracardiac total anomalous pulmonary venous drainage (TAPVD), cardiomegaly with plethora for truncus arteriosus.

g. Peripheral pulses are easily palpable in all extremities, including the foot, in every normal infant.

2. Additional important features of premature infants are:
   a. The pulmonary flow murmur of the newborn infant is more frequent and louder in premature than in full-term infants.
   b. The likelihood of a patent ductus arteriosus (PDA) murmur is greater in premature infants.
   c. The peripheral pulses normally appear bounding because of the lack of a normal amount of subcutaneous tissue.
3. *Abnormal phycical findings:* The following abnormal physical findings cardiac pathology.
   a. Cyanosis, particularly when it does not improve with oxygen administration, requires further evaluation.
   b. Decreased or absent peripheral pulses in the lower extremities suggest coarctation of aorta (COA). Generalized weak peripheral pulses suggest hypoplastic left heart syndrome (HLHS) or circulatory shock. Bounding peripheral pulses suggest an aortic run-off lesion such as PDA or persistent truncus arterious.
   c. Tachypnea of greater than 60 breaths/min with or without retraction is abnormal.
   d. Hepatomegaly may suggest a heart defect manifesting with congestive heart failure (CHF). A midline liver suggests asplenia or polysplenia syndrome.
   e. A heart murmur may be a presenting sign of congenital heart disease (CHD). However, innocent murmurs are more common than pathologic murmurs.

f. An irregular rhythm or abnormal heart rate may suggest cardiac arrhythmias.

g. Blood pressure readings in the lower extremities 6–7 mmHg lower than those in the arm require further evaluation for COA.

### Blood Gases

Normal 1-day-old infant may have $PO_2$ as low as 60 mmHg, but transcutaneous oxygen saturation is higher than 90%.

### Electrocardiographraphy (Figs 35.3–35.8)

1. The normal ECG of a newborn infant is different from that of a child or an adult as follows:
    - Sinus tachycardia with a rate as high as 180 beats/min.
    - A rightward QRS axis with a mean of +125 degrees and a maximum of +180 degrees.
    - Relatively small voltages for the QRS complex and the T-wave.

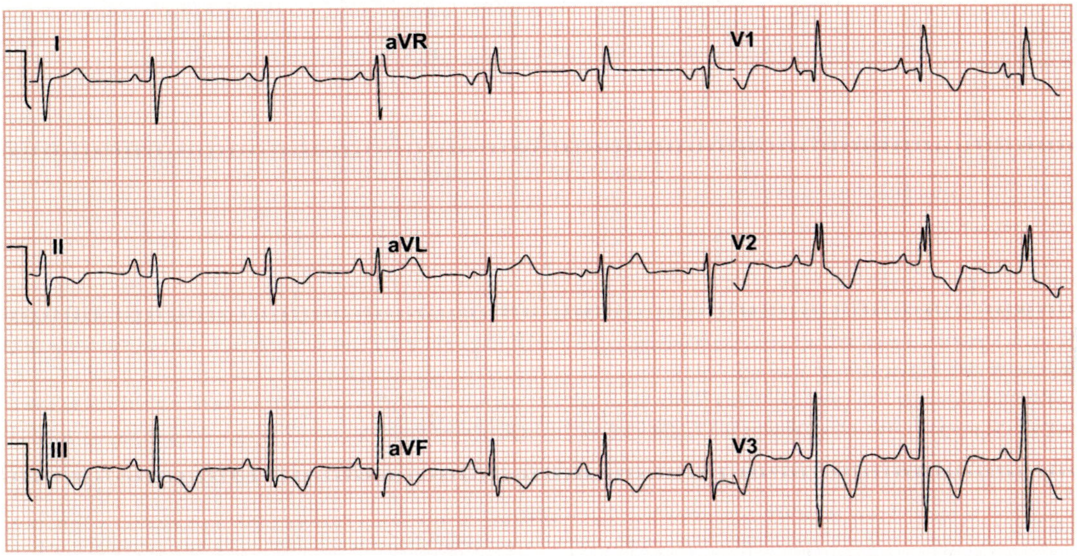


**Fig. 35.3:** ECG in TOF showing right axis deviation (+150 degrees). P pulmonale (P-wave in lead II >2.5 mm). Incomplete RBBB. Right ventricular strain pattern with T-wave inversion and ST-depression in the right precordial (V1–3) and inferior (II, III, aVF) leads

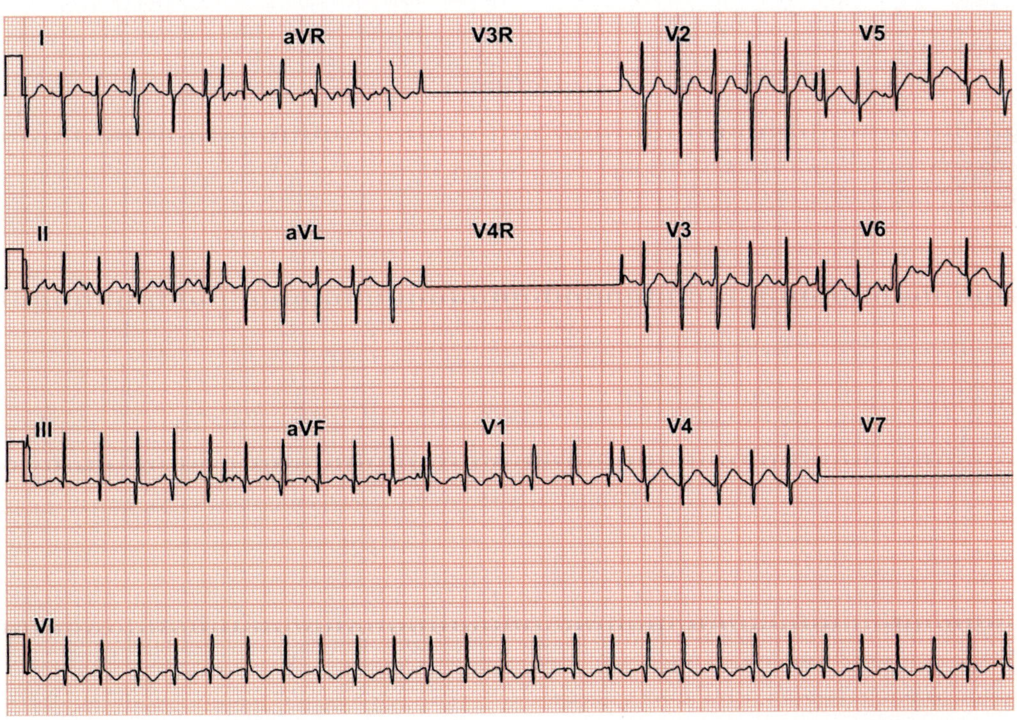


**Fig. 35.4:** d-TGA. Electrocardiogram obtained from a 3-day-old neonate. The tracing demonstrates right axis deviation and right ventricular predominance

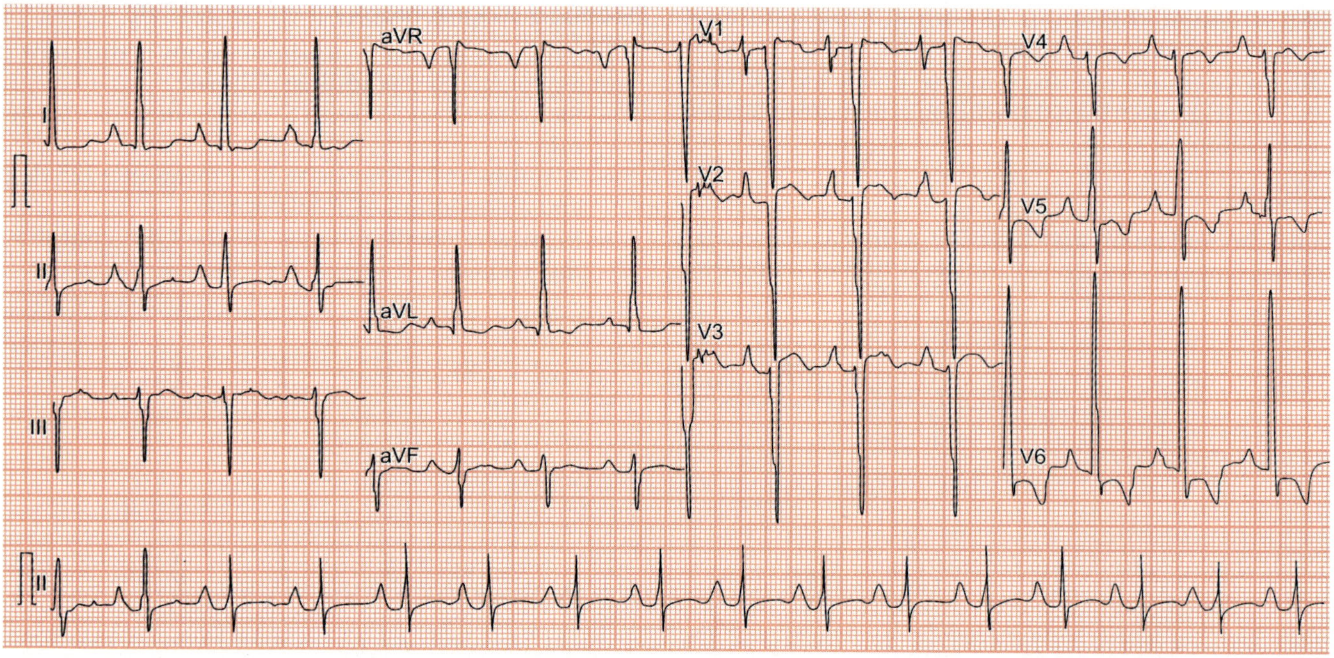


**Fig. 35.5:** Electrocardiography in tricuspid atresia reveals right atrial hypertrophy, an abnormal and superiorly oriented major QRS vector, the so-called left axis deviation in the frontal plane, left ventricular hypertrophy, and decreased right ventricular forces. Right atrial hypertrophy, manifested by tall and peaked P-waves (P-tricuspidale) in lead II and right chest leads may be present in 75% of patients with tricuspid atresia. In the so-called P-tricuspidale with a double peak, spike and dome configuration may be present

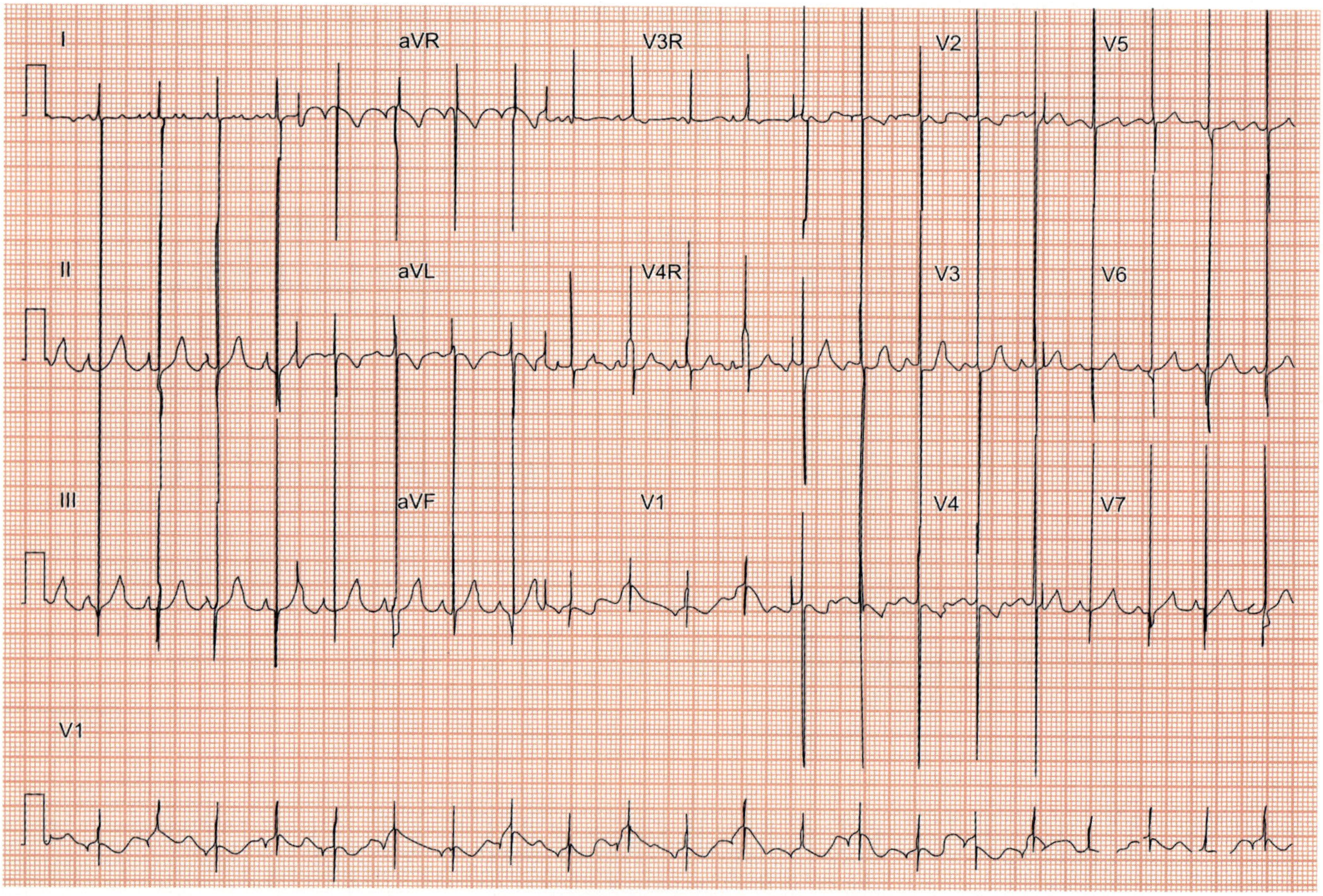


**Fig. 35.6:** Truncus arteriosus. Electrocardiogram obtained in a 4-month-old infant with type II truncus arteriosus. The tracing shows normal sinus rhythm, right atrial enlargement (peaked P-wave in lead II), right ventricular hypertrophy (tall R-wave V4R), right ventricular strain (flat or upright T-waves in anterior chest leads), and left ventricular hypertrophy (tall R-waves in lateral chest leads)

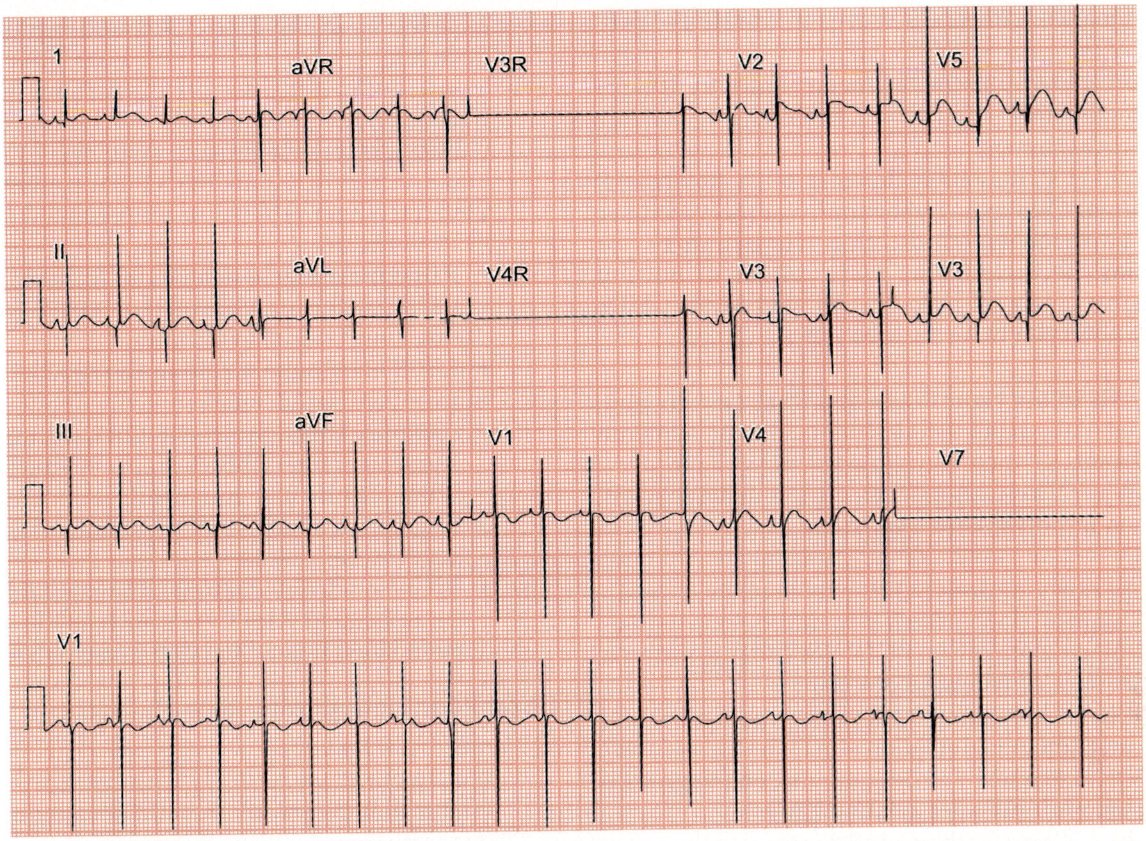


**Fig. 35.7:** Pulmonary atresia with intact IVS. Electrocardiogram 9-day-old infant with pulmonary atresia, intact ventricular septum with tracing showing left axis deviation for age (68 degrees), right atrial enlargement (peaked P-waves in lead II), and left ventricular hypertrophy

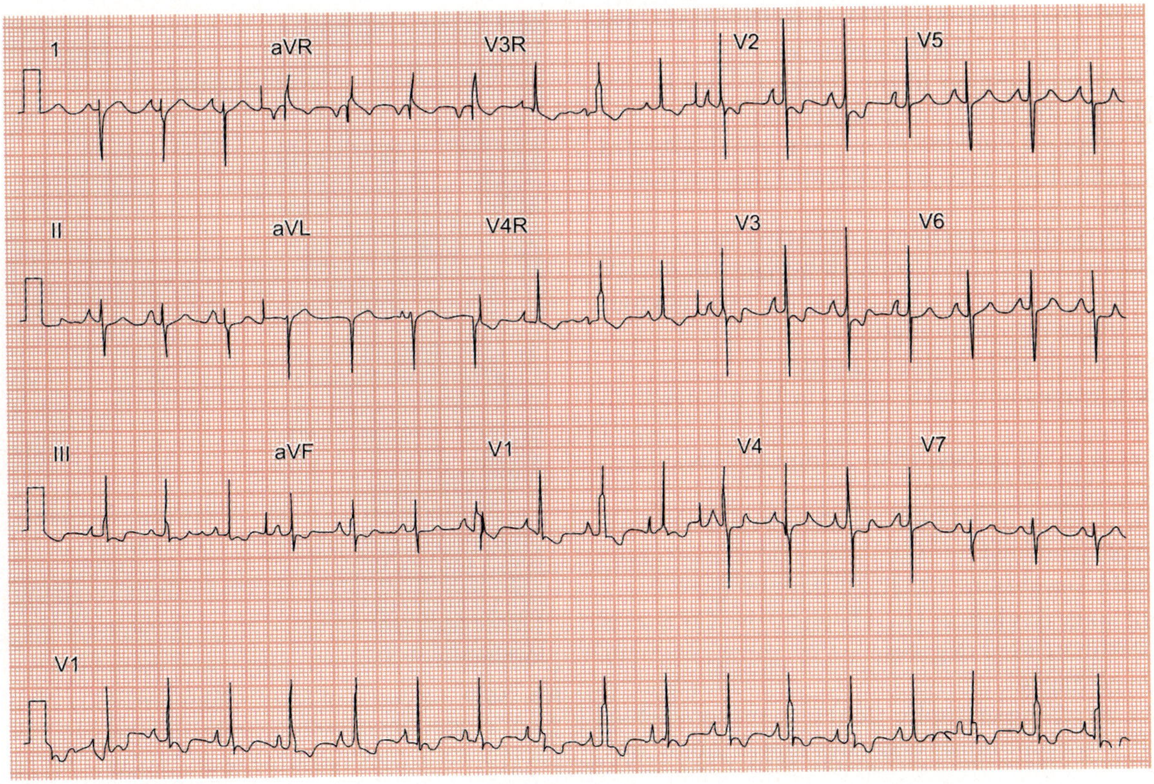


**Fig. 35.8:** The tracing shows right axis deviation, right atrial enlargement, right ventricular hypertrophy, and right ventricular strain (inverted T-waves in the anterior leads). In a patient with Eisenmenger syndrome

- RV dominance with tall R waves in the RPLs (V4R, V1 and V2).
- Occasional Q-waves in V1 (seen in about 10% of normal neonates)
- Benign arrhythmias

2. An abnormal ECG may be in the form of an abnormal P axis, abnormal QRS axis, hypertrophy of the ventricles or atria, vantricular conduction disturbances, or arrhythmias. Because of the wide ranges of normal values, many newborn infants with significant CHDs may show a normal ECG for their age.

A. *P axis*
- A P axis in the right lower quadrant (+90 to +180 degrees) suggests atrial situs inversus, asplenia syndrome, or incorrectly placed ECG electrodes.
- A superor P axis suggests an ectopic atrial rhythm, as seen in polysplenia syndrome.

B. *QRS axis*
- A superiorly oriented QRS axis between 0 and -150 degrees (left anterior hemiblock) suggests partial or complete ECD, including splenic syndromes, or tricuspid atresia.
- A QRS axis less than +30 degrees is abnormal and indicates left axis deviation (LAD) in the neonate. The QRS between +30 degrees and +60 degrees is unusual and indicates relative LAD.
- A QRS axis greater than +180 degrees (in the range of –150 to –180 degrees) may indicate RAD.

C. *Left ventricular hypertrophy* (LVH) is suggested in the newborn infant when the following are present:
- Left atrial hypertrophy (LAD) or relative LAD (less than +60 degrees) for the neonate.
- An R/S progression in the precordial leads that resembles the adult R/S progression.
- QRS voltages demonstrating abnormal leftward and posterior forces or abnormal inferior forces for age.

D. *Right ventricular hypertrophy* (RVH) is difficult to diagnose because of the normal dominance of the RV at this age. However, the following are helpful clues to RVH in the newborn infant.
- S waves in lead I 12 mm or greater
- Pure R waves with no S waves in V1 greater than 10 mm.
- R waves in V1 greater than 25 mm or R waves in aVR greater than 8 mm.
- A qR pattern in V1 (this is also seen in 10% of normal neonates).
- Upright T-waves in V1 after 3 days of age.
- Right axis deviation (RAD) with the QRS axis greater than +180 degrees.

E. *Atrial hypertrophy*
- Right atrial hypertrophy (RAH) is present when the P-wave amplitude is greater than 3 mm in any lead.
- Left atrial hypertrophy (LAH) is when the P-wave duration is 0.08 sec or greater (usually with notched P-waves in the limb leads and biphasic P-waves in V1).

F. Ventricular conduction disturbances (i.e. right bundle branch block (RBBB), left bundle branch block (LBBB), Wolff-Parkinson-Wite (WPW) syndrome, and intraventricular block) are present when the QRS duration is 0.07 sec or more (not 0.1 sec or greater as in the adult).
- RBBB may be associated with Ebstein anomaly and COA in the newborn. It is sometimes seen in otherwise normal neonates.
- LBBB is extremely rare in the newborn infant.
- Intraventricular block (with a widening of the QRS complex throughout the QRS duration) is more significant than RBBB because it is often associated with significant metabolic abnormalities (e.g. hypoxia, acidosis and hyperkalemia) and diffuse myocardial diseases.
- WPW syndrome may be an isolated finding or may be associated with CHDs such as Ebstein anomaly or L-TGA. It is a frequent cause of SVT.

**Chest Roentgenography** (Figs 35.9–35.16)

1. *Normal CXR findings*
- The cardiothoracic (CT) ratio of normal newborn infants may be greater than 0.5 because of inadequate inspiration and a large thymic shadow.
- The thymic shadow may have any of several shapes, including a classic sail sign, or may have undulant or

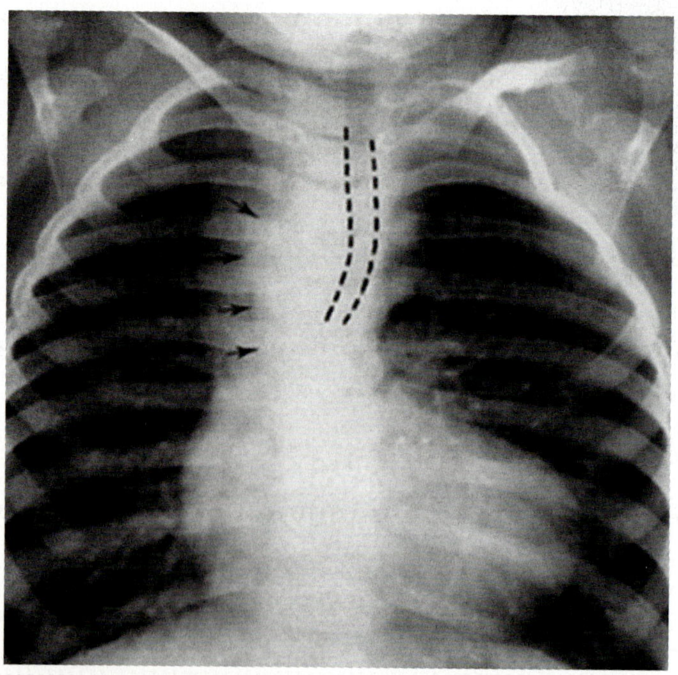

**Fig. 35.9:** Tetralogy of Fallot. Plain films may classically show a 'boot shaped' heart with an upturned cardiac apex due to right ventricular hypertrophy and concave pulmonary arterial segment. Most infants with TOF however may not show this finding. Pulmonary oligaemia due to decreased pulmonary arterial flow. Right sided aortic arch is seen in 25%

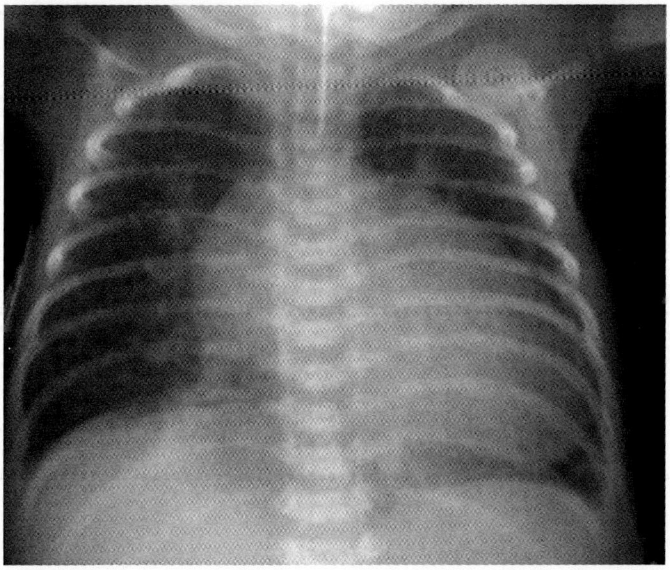

**Fig. 35.10:** Transposition of great arteries. A frontal chest radiograph classically shows cardiomegaly with a cardiac contours classically described as appearing like an egg on a string. There is often an apparent narrowing of the superior mediastinum as a result of the aortic and pulmonary arterial configuration, i.e. parallel in D-loop transposition, with main pulmonary artery posterior to the aorta

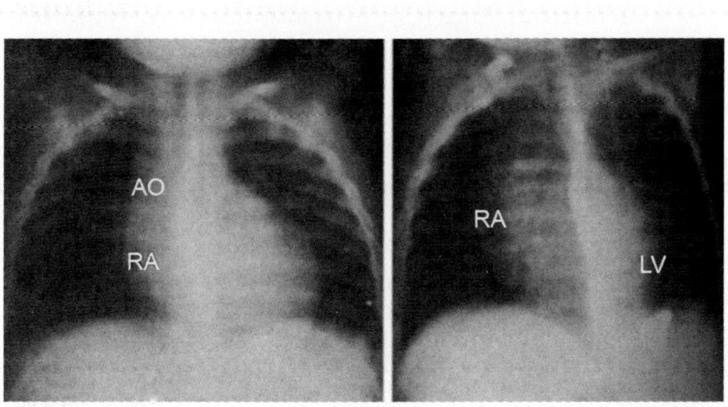


**Fig. 35.11:** Tricuspid atresia. Chest X-ray in a patient with tricuspid atresia demonstrating the following features—(a) reduced pulmonary blood flow, prominent aortic root (AO) and right atrium (RA); (b) the left anterior oblique projection on the right side shows distinctive humped appearance of the anterior cardiac silhouette due to right atrial (RA) enlargement in the absence of a right ventricle. The left ventricle (LV) is enlarged. (c) A right aortic arch may be observed in some cases

smooth borders, either unilateral or bilateral, on the upper mediastinum.

- Cardiac silhouette is not always as well defined in neonates as in older children.
- Evaluation of pulmonary vascular markings in the neonate poses a special problem. Although a reduced PBF is usually easier to detect (and indicates serious cyanotic CHD), increased vascularity is not always apparent even when the pulmonary blood flow is large. The distinction between increased PBF and pulmonary venous congestion is often difficult.

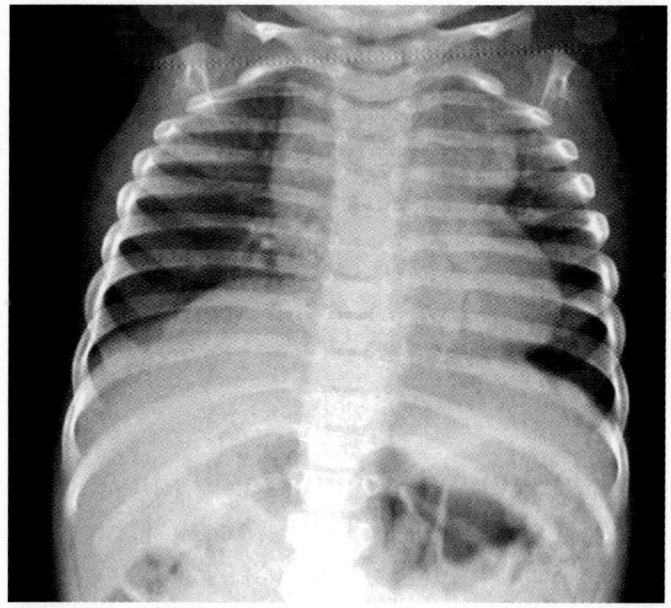

**Fig. 35.12:** TAPVC—plain film. The right heart is prominent in TAPVR because of the increased flow volume, but the left atrium remains normal in size. Types I and II result in cardiomegaly. The supracardiac variant (type I) can classically depict a snowman appearance on a frontal chest radiograph, also known as figure of 8 heart. The dilated vertical vein on the left, brachiocephalic vein on top, and the superior vena cava on the right form the head of the snowman; the body of the snowman is formed by the enlarged right atrium

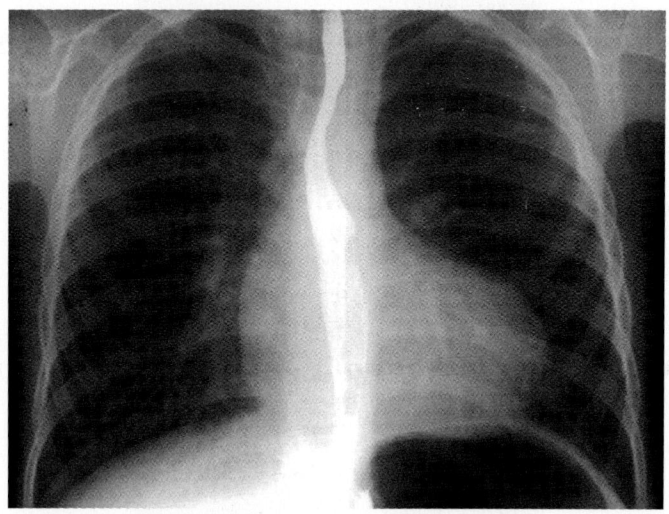

**Fig. 35.13:** Truncus arteriosus. Chest radiograph. Often shows moderate cardiomegaly with pulmonary plethora (mainly as a result of collateral formation) and widened mediastinum. However, the main pulmonary artery (arising from common trunk) may be small/unusual in position which may result in narrow mediastinum. This along with moderate cardiomegaly and pumonary plethora gives an appearance that is similar to D-loop transposition of great arteries. Right-sided aortic arch may be seen (see barium meal indentation)

2. *Abnormal chest X-ray findings:* A cardiac problem is suggested by an abnormal size, position, or silhouette

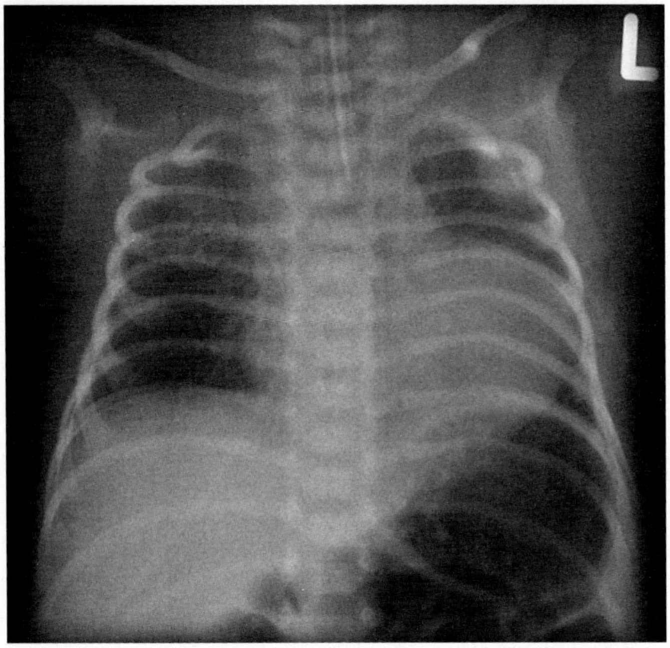

**Fig. 35.14:** Pulmonary atresia/stenosis. Chest radiograph PA-VSD—normal or mildly enlarged heart with poor/diminished pulmonary arterial vascular markings asymmetrical vascular suggest stenosis within pulmonary arterial tree, there can be plethora due to horizontal arteries forming aortopulmonary collaterals mottled appearance as the lung periphery may suggest pleuro-pulmonary collateral formation

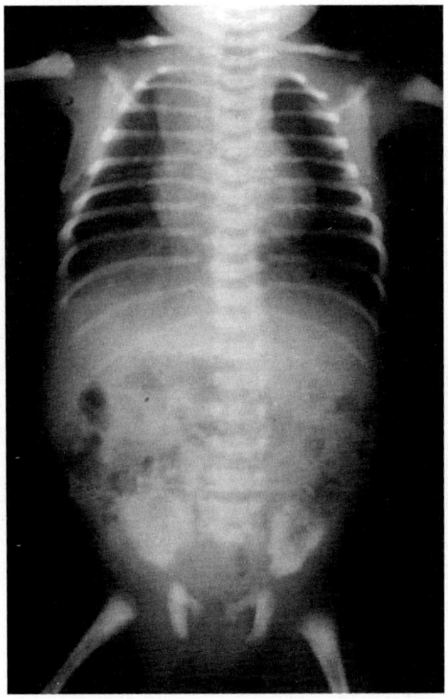

**Fig 35.15:** X-ray chest PA view. The radiograph shows a functioning heart with a single atrium and a single ventricle, as well as a degree of sacral dysgenesis

of the heart, by an abnormal shape or position of the liver, and by increased or decreased pulmonary vascularity on CXR films.

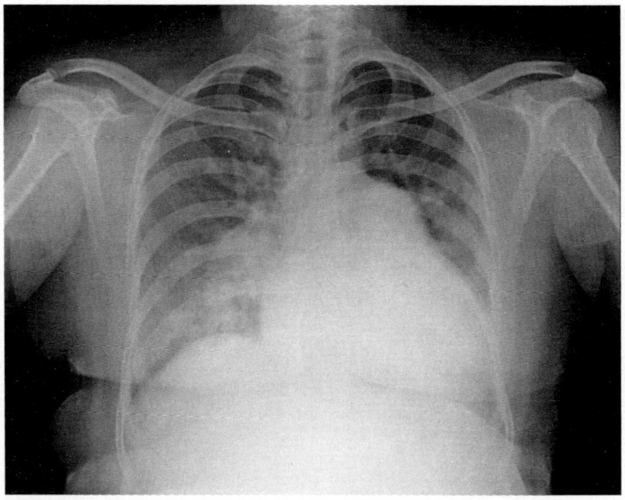

**Fig. 35.16:** X-ray chest PA view showing prominent MPA and its branches and generalized congestion of both central and peripheral arterioles in infant with primary pulmonary arterial hypertension

a. *Heart size*
   - The CT ratio is of limited value, since that of normal neonates is usually greater than 0.5. Many serious CHDs that eventually result in cardiomegaly show a normal heart size in neonates. Unequivocal cardiomegaly may be due to CHD [such as ventricular septal defect (VSD), PDA, transposition of the great arteries (TGA), Ebstein anomaly, hypoplastic left heart syndrome (HLHS), and other], myocarditis or cardiomyopathy, pericardial effusion, metabolic disturbance (e.g. hypoglycemia, severe hypoxemia, and acidosis), and overhydration or overtransfusion.
   - In the newborn infant who is intubated and on a ventilator, the heart size is greatly influenced by the ventilator setting. For example, a premature infant with a large-shunt
   - PDA may have a normal-sized heart on chest X-ray film if the ventilator settings are high, especially the positive end-expiratory pressure.

b. Abnormal cardiac silhouettes may be of considerable help in suggesting the correct diagnosis.
   - A boot-shaped heart (coeur en sabot) is seen in tetralogy of Fallot (TOF) and in tricuspid atresia.
   - An egg-shaped heart with narrow waist may be seen in TGA.
   - A large, globular heart is seen in Ebstein anomaly.

c. *Dextrocardia or mesocardia:* The presence of dextrocardia or mesocardia does not always indicate a serious heart defect. The segmental approach should be used for further evaluation. Four common situations seen in dextrocardia or mesocardia are situs inversus totalis with a normal heart, a rightward displacement of a normallyformed heart due to hypoplasia of the right lung, a complex cyanotic CHD, and asplenia or polysplenia syndrome.

d. *The situs of abdominal viscera:* A left-sided liver with the heart in the right side of the chest is seen in situs inversus totalis with normal heart. The liver and the cardiac apex on the same side suggest a complex cyanotic CHD. A midline liver suggests asplenia or polysplenia syndrome.
e. *Pulmonary vascular markings*
   - Increased pulmonary vascular marking (PVM) in a cyanotic infant suggest
   - TGA, persistent truncus arteriosus, or single ventricle. In an acyanotic infant, increased PVMs suggest VSD, PDA, or endocardial cushion defect (ECD).
   - Decreased PVMs suggest a critical cyanotic CHD with decreased pulmonary blood flow (PBF), such as pulmonary atresia, tricuspid atresia, TOF with severe pulmonary stenosis or atresia.
   - A ground-glass appearance or a reticulated pattern of the lung fields is characteristic of pulmonary venous obstruction.

## TT-two-dimensional and TEE-echocardiography in Congenital Heart Disease

Echocardiography is an important tool in providing the doctors with important information of the following (Figs 35.17–35.24):

- Size of the chambers, dimension, volume and the thickness of the walls.
- Pumping function: One can tell if the pumping power of the heart is normal or reduced to a mild or severe degree.
- Valve function: It identifies the structure, thickness and movement of each heart valve.
- Volume status: Low blood pressure can occur in the setting of poor heart function but may also be seen in reduced volume of circulating blood.
- Others: 'Pericardial effusion' or fluid in the pericardium (the sac that surrounds the heart), congenital heart disease, blood clots or tumors within the heart, active infection of the heart valves, abnormal elevation of pressure within the lungs.

The information obtained is essential in avoiding unnecessary cardiac catheterization and angiography in the absence of a cardiac defect, as well as in making a specific diagnosis.

## Umbilical Artery Line

A $PO_2$ value in a preductal artery (such as right radial artery) higher than that in a postductal artery (umbilical artery line) by 10–15 mmHg suggests an R–L shunt through a PDA. Such a differential $PO_2$ level may result from persistent pulmonary hypertension of the newborn (PPHN), critical AS, interrupted aortic arch, or coarctation of the aorta. An echo study will clarify the cause of the differential $PO_2$ levels.

Cardiology consultation is called for if a cardiac origin of cyanosis is suspected.

*Suggested approach to neonates with central cyanosis:* Although a significant heart murmur usually suggests a cardiac basis for the cyanosis, several of the more severe

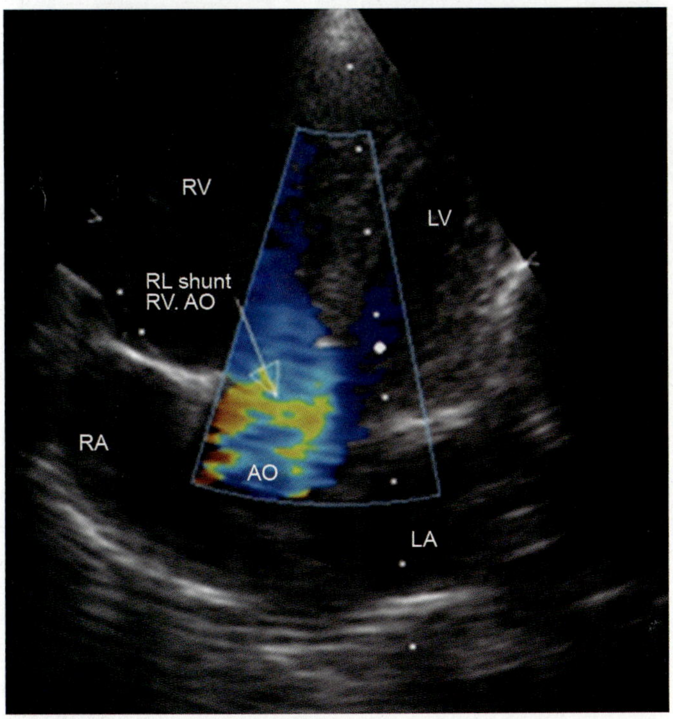


**Fig. 35.17:** Apical five chamber view in tetralogy of Fallot with color flow mapping (Color-Doppler imaging) in systole with right to left shunt across the VSD. Blue stream moving from right ventricle across the VSD to the aorta is clearly visualised in this frame. There is also a blue stream from the left ventricle to the aorta

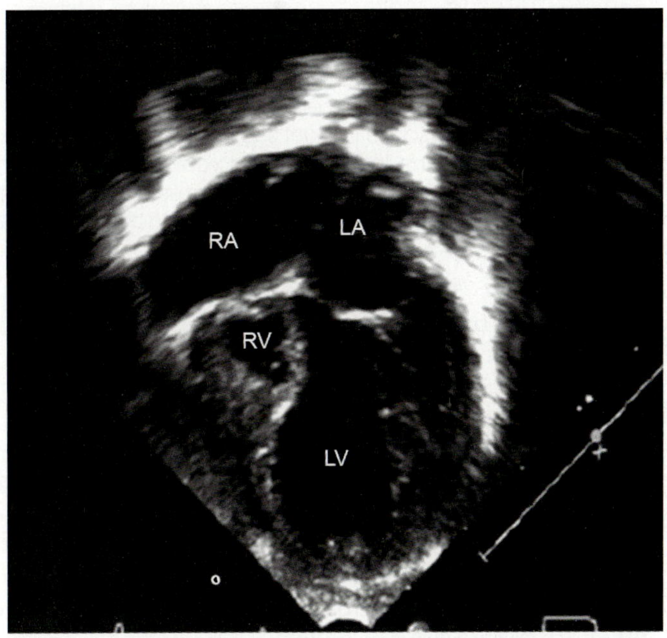


**Fig. 35.18:** Pulmonary atresia with intact ventricular septum. Apical four-chamber echocardiogram image in this newborn demonstrates the severely hypoplastic right ventricle (RV), too small to support any effective pulmonary blood flow, and requiring a single-ventricle palliative approach. A severely hypoplastic but patent tricuspid valve was present in this patient (LA=left atrium; LV=left ventricle; RA=right atrium)

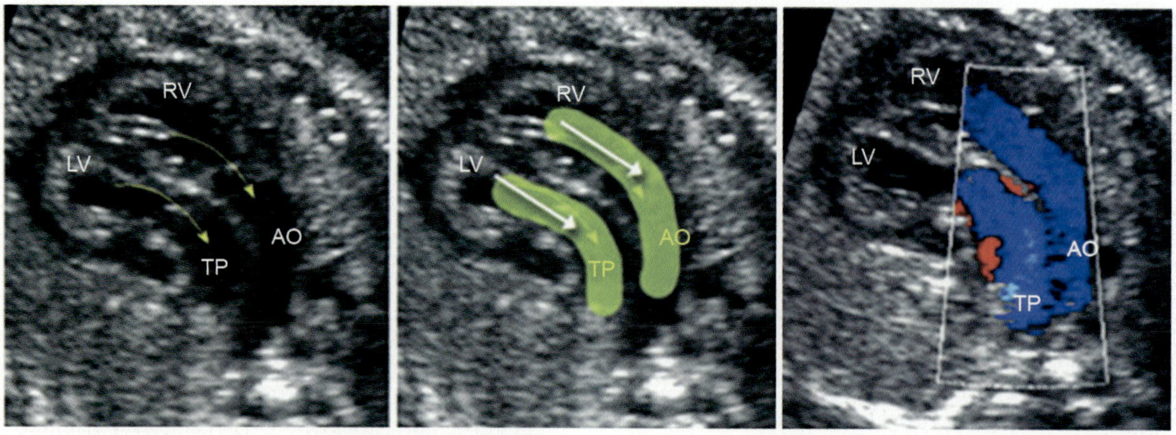


**Fig. 35.19:** Fetal ultrasonography demonstraes transposition of the great arteries with abnormal connection of the right ventricle (RV) with the aorta (AO) and the left ventricle (LV) with the pulmonary trunk (TP). Both great arteries show a parallel course

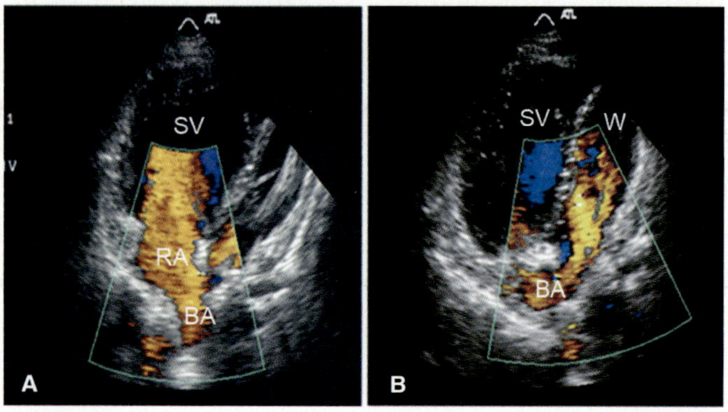


**Fig. 35.20:** (A) Modified apical image of D-transposition after baffle (Mustard) procedure. Pulmonary venous blood flows through a baffle (BA) to enter the right atrium (RA) and the systemic ventricle (SV), which is a morphologic right ventricle. The SV ejects into the aorta. There is no evidence of baffle stenosis. (B) Modified apical image from the same patient showing vena caval blood flow through a BA into the left atrium and venous ventricle (VV), which is a morphologic left ventricle. The venous ventricle ejects into the pulmonary artery. Again, there is no evidence of baffle stenosis

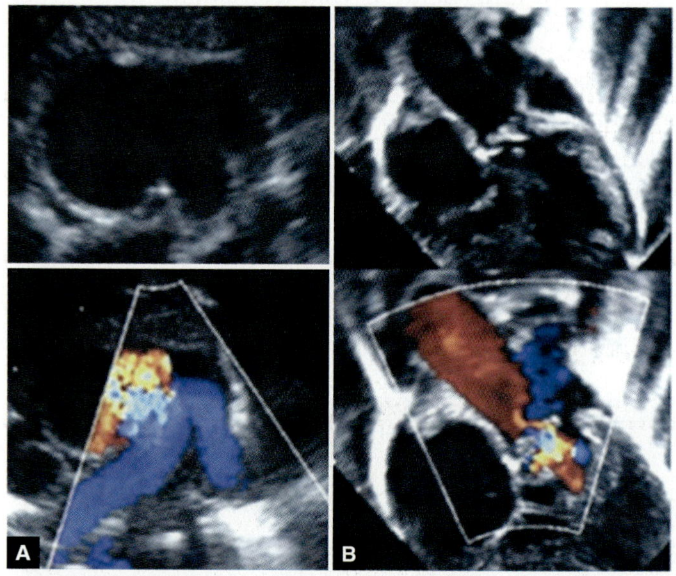


**Fig. 35.21:** (A) Suprasternal frontal view of truncus arteriosus. Notice that the branch pulmonary arteries come off the truncus without evidence of a clear main pulmonary artery; this is consistent with truncus type 2. (B) Subcostal left anterior oblique view of the truncus. 2D imaging is consistent with a thick truncal valve and the pulmonary arteries are seen coming off the trunk. Color-Doppler over the truncal valve shows flow acceleration

cardiac defects (transposition of the great vessels) may not initially be associated with a murmur.

## Heart Murmurs

1. **Innocent heart murmurs:** More than 50% of full-term newborn infants (and a higher percentage of premature infants) have an innocent systolic murmur at some time during the first week of life. Infants with innocent heart murmurs have normal ECG and chest X-ray findings.

   The four most common innocent murmurs in the newborn period are as follows:

   - Pulmonary flow murmur is most common. It is more often found in premature and small-for-gestational-age infants than in full-term infants. A soft systolic murmur (grade 1 to 2/6), heard best at the upper left sternal border (ULSB), transmits well to bozh sides of the chest, axillae, and the back.
   - Transient systolic murmur of PDA is soft (grade 1 to 2/6), audible at the ULSB and in the left infraclavicular area on the first day. It usually disappears shortly thereafter.
   - Transient systolic murmur of tricuspid regurgitation is indistinguishable from that of VSD and is most common in infants who had fetal distress or neonatal asphyxia.
   - Vibratory systolic innocent murmur is a counterpart of Still's murmur in older children. It is audible at the LLSB, apex, or midprecordium.

2. **Pathologic heart murmurs:** Most pathologic murmurs except atrial septal defect (ASD) are audible during the

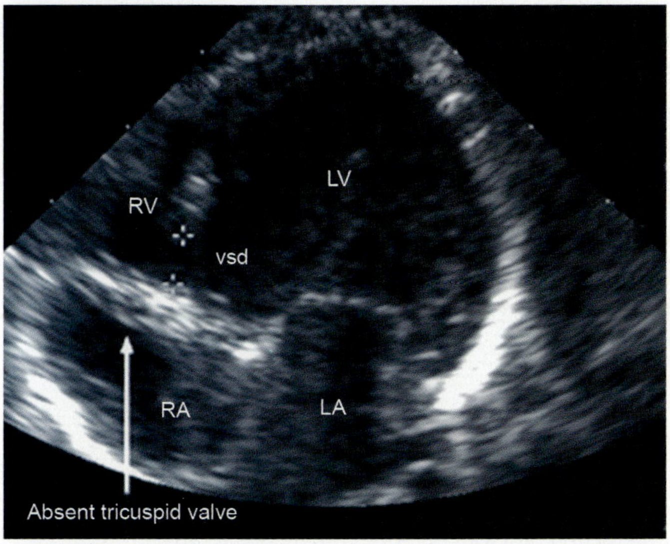


**Fig. 35.22:** TTE 4 chamber view shows abscence of tricuspid valve (arrow), a VSD (astrex) and a small RV. in a newborn with tricuspid atresia

first month of life. The time of appearance of a murmur depends on the nature of the defect.

- Heart murmurs of stenotic lesions [e.g. aortal stenosis (AS), pulmonary stenosis (PS)] are audible immediately after birth and persist, because they are independent of the level of the PVR.
- Heart murmurs of L–R shunt lesions, especially those of a large VSD, may appear later, when the PVR decreases. The murmur of ASD appears late in infancy or in childhood.
- The continuous murmur of a large PDA may not appear for 2–3 weeks.
- Instead, it is a crescendo systolic murmur with a slight or no diastolic component.

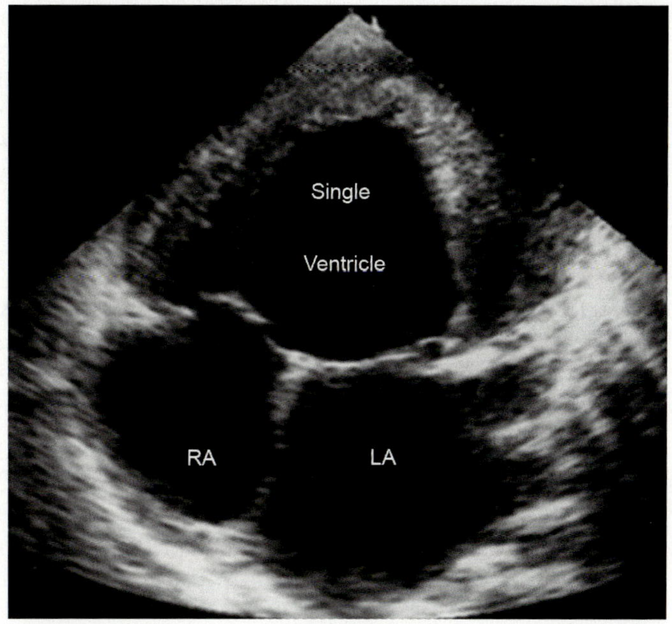


**Fig. 35.24:** 4C apical image showing single ventricle (LA=left atrium; LV,=left ventricle; RA=right atrium; RV=right ventricle)

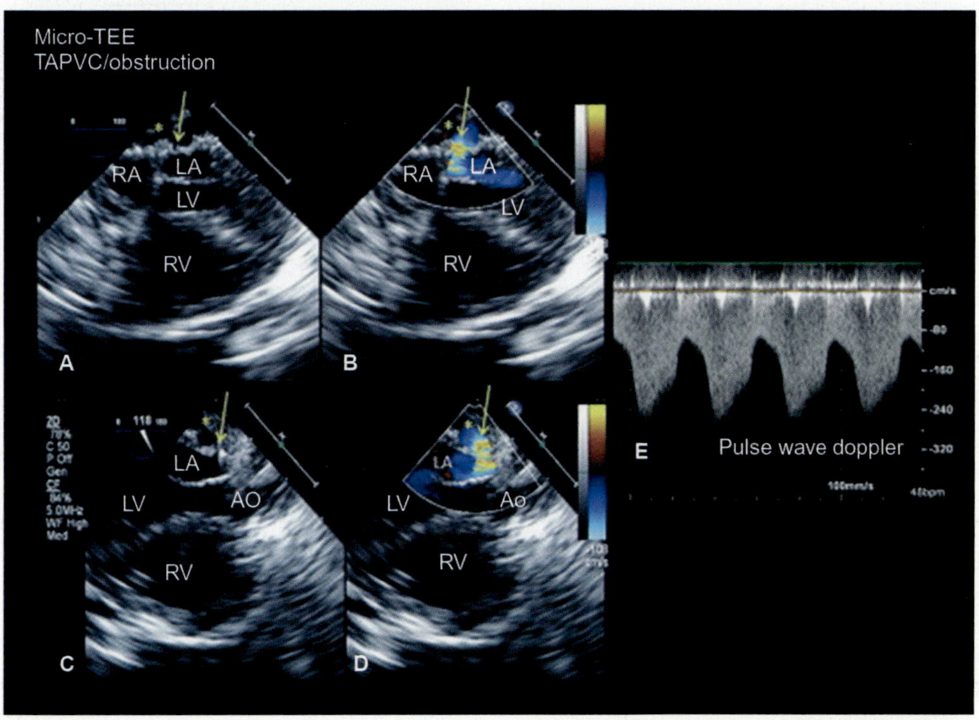


**Fig. 35.23:** Transesophageal echocardiograms using the microTEE transducer (Micro-TEE) in a patient with total anomalous pulmonary venous connection (TAPVC) with residual stenosis at the anastomosis of the pulmonary venous confluence (asterisk) to the left atrium (LA) (arrow). (A) Four-chamber two-dimensional echocardiographic view. (B) Four-chamber color-Doppler flow map. (C) Long-axis two-dimensional echocardiographic view. (D) Long-axis color-Doppler flow map. (E) Obstructive pattern pulsed-wave Doppler echocardiogram (Ao=Aorta; LV=left ventricle; RA=right atrium)

- Even in the absence of a murmur, a newborn infant may have a serious heart defect that requires immediate attention, e.g. severe cyanotic heart disease such as TGA or pulmonary atresia with a closing PDA. Infants who are in severe CHF may not have a loud murmur until the myocardial function is improved with anticongestive measures.

## LABORATORY INVESTIGATIONS

1. **Chest X-ray films may reveal pulmonary causes of cyanosis and urgency of the problem.** They will also hint at the presence and the type of any cardiac defects.
2. **Arterial blood gases on room air will confirm or rule out central cyanosis.** Elevated $PCO_2$ suggests pulmonary or central nervous system (CNS) problems. Low pH may be seen in sepsis, circulatory shock, or severe hypoxemia.
3. **Hyperoxia test is one method of distinguishing cyanotic congenital heart disease from pulmonary disease.** Neonates with cyanotic congenital heart disease usually do not have significantly raised arterial $PaO_2$ during administration of 100% oxygen. If the $PaO_2$ rises above 150 mmHg during 100% oxygen administration, an intracardiac shunt can usually be excluded, although the $PaO_2$ of some patients with cyanotic congenital heart lesions may be transiently increased to greater than 150 mmHg because of intracardiac streaming patterns. The $PaO_2$ in patiens with pulmonary disease generally increases significantly as ventilation-perfusion inequalities are overcome by oxygenadministration. In infants with a CNS disorder, the $PaO_2$ completely normalizes during artificial ventilation. Hypoxia in many heart lesions is profound and constant, whereas in respiratory disorders and in primary hypertension of the neonate (PPHN), arterial oxygen tension is not as low and often varies with time or changes in ventilator management. Hyperventilation may improve the hypoxia in neonates with PPHN and only occasionally in those with cyanotic heart disease.
4. **An ECG should be obtained if a cardiac origin of cyanosis is suspected.**

## HEART FAILURE IN THE NEWBORN INFANT

The clinical picture of CHF in the neonate may simulate another disorder such as meningitis, sepsis, pneumonia, or bronchiolitis. Tachypnea, tachycardia, pulmonary crackles or rhonchi, hepatomegaly, and weak peripheral pulses are common presenting signs. Heart murmur is either faint or absent. Cardiomegaly on chest X-ray film is always present, with or without increased PVMs or pulmonary edema (Table 35.2).

## HYPOPLASTIC LEFT HEART SYNDROME (Figs 35.25–35.28)

**Prevalence**: HLHS occurs in 1% of all CHDs and is the most common cause of death from CHD during the first month of life.

**Table 35.2:** Causes of congestive heart failure in the neonate

A. **Structural heart defects at birth**
- Hypoplastic left heart syndrome (HLHS)
- Severe tricuspid or pulmonary regurgitation
- Large systemic AV fistula

**Week 1**
- TGA
- Large PDA in premature infant
- Total anomalous pulmonary venous return (TAPVR) below diaphragm

**Week 1–4**
- Critical AS or PS
- Preductal COA

B. **Noncardiac causes**
- Birth asphyxia (resulting in transient myocardial ischemia)
- Metabolic: Hypoglycemia, hypocalcemia
- Severe anemia (as seen in hydrops fetalis)
- Neonatal sepsis
- Overtransfusion or overhydration

C. **Myocardial disease**
- Myocarditis
- Transient myocardial ischemia (with or without birth asphyxia)
- Catdiomyopathy (seen in infants of diabetic mothers)

D. **Disturbances in heart rate**
- Supravetricular tachycardia (supraventricular tachycardia (SVT) or
- Paroxysmal atrial tachycardia (PAT)
- Atrial flutter or fibrillation
- Congenital heart block (when associated with CHD). The time of onset of CHF varies rather predictably with the type of CHD. Two important CHDs that present with CHF in the newborn period are hypoplastic leftheart syndrome (HLHS) and large PDA in premature infants. Transient myocardial ischemia and infants of diabetic mothers are other causes of CHF in the neonate.

### Pathology and Pathophysiology

1. HLHS includes a group of closely related anomalies characterized by hypoplasia of the left ventricul (LV) (from atresia or severe stenosis of the aortic and/or mitral valves) and hypoplasia of the ascending aorta and aortic arch. The LA is small, and the atrial septum is frequently intact other than the PFO.
2. During fetal life the pulmonary vascular resistance (PVR) is higher than the systemic vascular resistance (SVR), and the dominant RV maintains normal perfusing pressure in the descending aorta through the ductal R-L shunt, even in the presence of the nonfunctioning hypoplastic LV. However, difficulties arise after birth, primarily from two factors:
   a. Reversal of the vascular resistance in the two circuits with the SVR higher than the PVR, and
   b. Closure of the PDA. The end result is a marked decrease in systemic cardiac output and aortic pressure, resulting in circulatory shock and metabolic

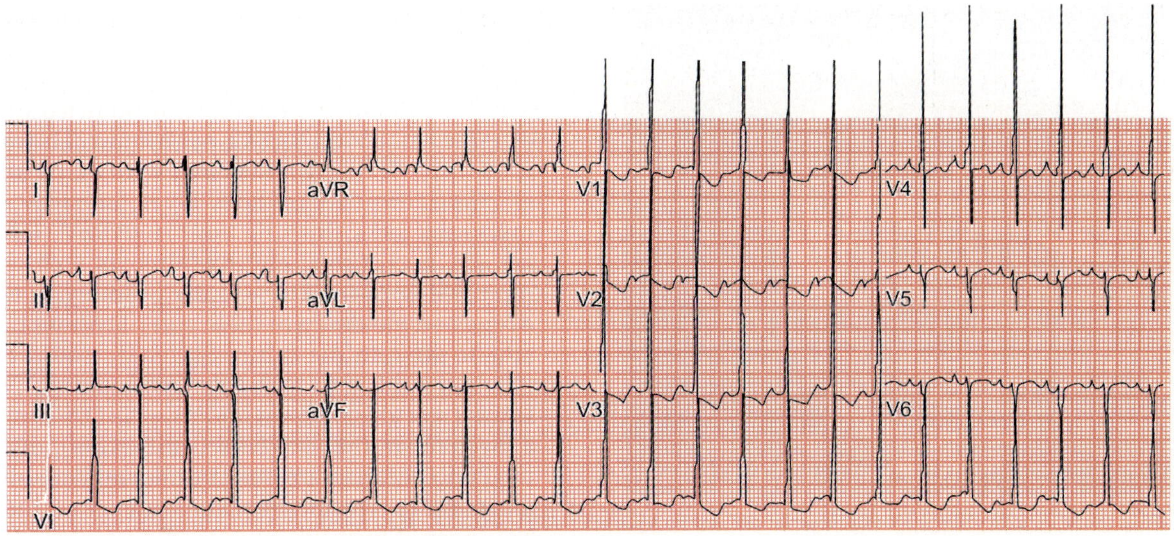


**Fig. 35.25:** 12-lead ECG from a 1-week-old infant with hypoplastic left heart syndrome. The ECG demonstrates marked right ventricular hypertrophy with strain

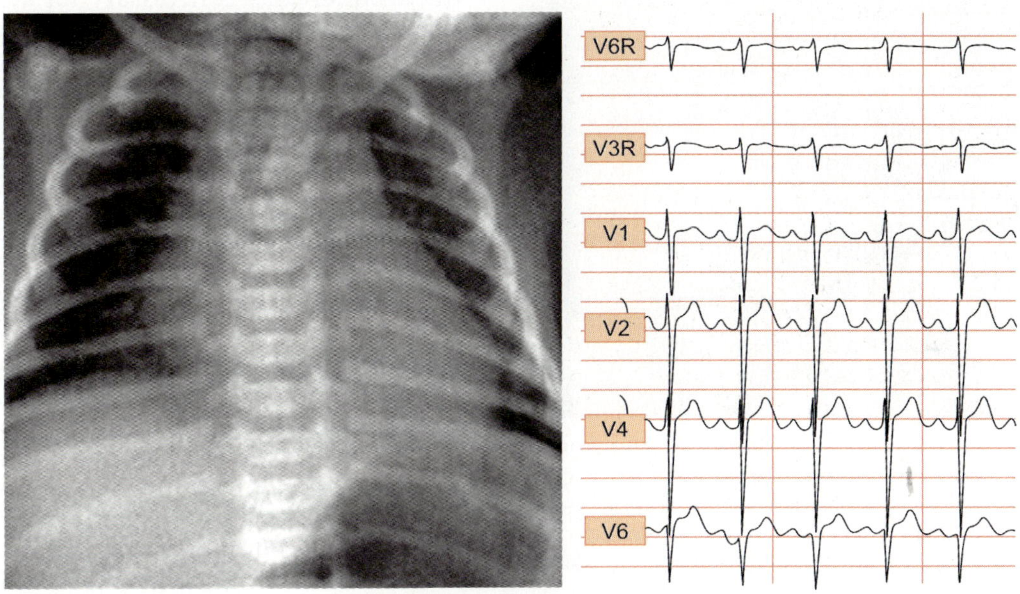


**Fig. 35 26:** Chest X-ray (A) and ECG (B) of our patient on the first day of life. Although the chest X-ray was normal, the ECG (V leads) showed tiny R and deep S waves with elevated ST- segments in left precordial leads (V2: +0.6 mV; V6: +0.42 mV), indicating myocardial damage

acidosis. An increase in PBF in the presence of the nonfunctioning LV results in an elevated LA pressure and pulmonary edema.

### Clinical Manifestations

1. The neonate is critically ill in the first few hourse to days of life, with mild cyanosis, tachycardia, tachypnea, and pulmonary crackles.
2. Poor peripheral pulses and vasoconstricted extremities are characteristic. The S2 is loud and single. Heart murmur is usually absent, but a grade 1 to 3/6 ejection systolic murmur may be present over the precordium.
3. The ECG shows RVH. Rarely, left ventricular hypertrophy (LVH) pattern is present because V5 and V6 electrodes are placed over the dilated RV.
4. Chest X-ray films show pulmonary venous congestion or pulmonary edema. The heart is only mildly enlarged.
5. The arterial blood gas determination reveals severe metabolic acidosis in the presence of a slightly decreased $PO_2$, a characteristic finding of this condition.
6. Echo findings are diagnosticand usually obviate cardiac catheterization. Severe hypoplasia of the aorta and aortic annulus and the absent or distorted mitral valve are usually imaged. The LV cavity is diminutive.

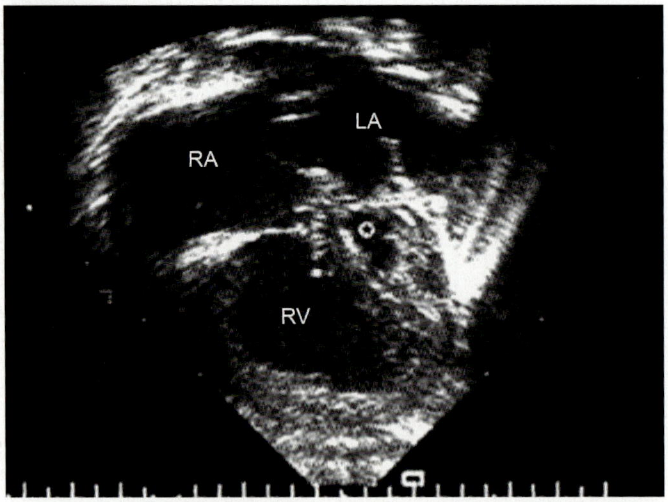


**Fig. 35.27:** This echocardiographic still frame shows a four-chamber view of the heart in a patient with hypoplastic left heart syndrome (HLHS). A large right ventricle (RV) and hypoplastic left ventricle (star) are seen (RA=right atrium, LA=left atrium)

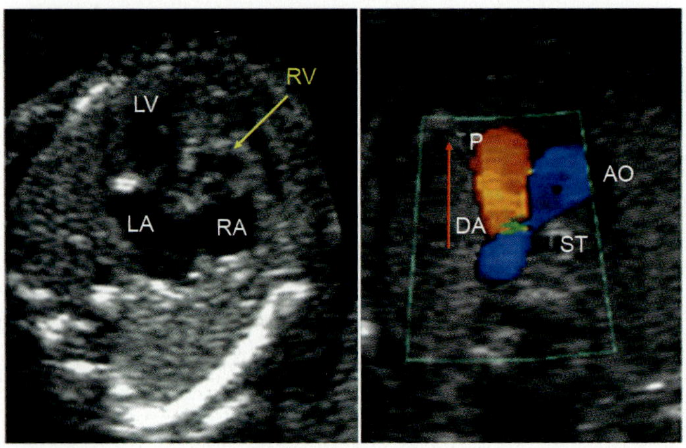


**Fig. 35.28:** Hypoplastic right ventricle (arrow) in a fetus with pulmonary atresia and intact ventricular septum (a). Color doppler of the four-chamber view with asymmetric flow between the left heart and right heart. Pulmonary valve atresia can be diagnosed using color-Doppler by visualizing the great vessels—aorta (AO) and pulmonary trunk (TP)—in the upper thorax and demonstrating the retrograde flow from the descending aorta across the ductus arteriosus toward the pulmonary valve

The RV cavity is markedly dilated, and the tricuspid valve is large. A partially constricted PDA may be imaged.

7. Progressive hypoxemia and acidosis result in death, usually in the first month of life.

## Management

1. Preoperatively the goal is to achieve adequate systemic oxygen delivery. Patency of the ductus arteriosus is critical for survival until surgery. Blood flow to the pulmonary and systemic circulations should be nearly balanced (goal p/s ratio of 1). The immediate therapy for all infants with HLHS is an intravenous infusion of prostaglandin E1 (PGE1) in order to pharmacologically manipulate the ductus arteriosus (DA) and maintain ductal patency. A continuous infusion of the prostaglandin is initiated, preferably through a central catheter, at a rate of 0.05–0.1 µg/kg per minute. However, numerous side effects are associated with PGE1 infusion such as respiratory depression, fever, lethargy, irritability, myoclonic jerks, flushing, edema, pyloric stenosis, hyperostosis, necrotizing enetrocolitis, as well as structural remodeling of the DA and the pulmonary vessels, with a reported incidence of these complications ranging from 10% to 40%. In the future Sildenafil could be a reasonable alternative to PGE1 for maintaining DA patency, since it can also prevent and reverse DA closure through a mechanism that is distinct, and eventually safer, from the PGE1 mechanism. An audible murmur and adequate peripheral perfusion provide evidence of ductal patency; however, Doppler echocardiography is needed to confirm flow. Once the ductus is open, the rate of infusion may be reduced to decrease the risk for potential adverse effects.Unrestricted blood flow through the ductus arteriosus is necessary for systemic perfusion. Sometimes even a temporary discontinuation of the prostaglandin infusion is possible, with careful monitoring of blood pressure and urine volume as well as frequent echocardiographic examinations, in order to enable maintenance of balance between systemic and pulmonary blood flow. The pulmonary/systemic (p/s) ratio preoperatively is dictated by the adequacy ofthe interatrial communication. An infant with a mildly restrictive interatrial communication may have balanced circulation and remain in a clinically stable condition as long as the ductus arteriosus remains open. Oxygen saturations of 75–85% by pulse oximetry suggest adequate balance between systemic and pulmonary blood flow. Ventilatory support may be needed for apneic episodes or tenacious secretions, both common adverse effects of treatment with prostaglandin E1. Judicious use of inotropic support is initiated if evidence of low cardiac output is detected. Infusion of dopamine at a rate of 3–5 µg/kg per minute usually results in improved ventricular function. High-dose inotropic support should be used with caution because it can result in increased SVR and cause a shift in the p/s ratio to greater than 1. In our institution we do not recommend the use of dopamine as a 'standard' since we consider it a 'dirty' drug with a lot of potential unexpected effects. Diuretics may be necessary to help alleviate the increased volume load on the right ventricle. Infants with an unrestrictive interatrial communication may be in a stablecondition initially, but signs of congestive heart failure may develop as the PVR (pulmonary vascular resistance) decreases. When oxygen saturations areapproximately 90%, systemic blood flow may be reduced, resulting in tissue hypoperfusion, metabolic acidosis, and a low cardiac output state. In infants with high oxygen saturation and evidence of tissue hypoperfusion, controlled mechanical ventilation is

often initiated to improve the p/s ratio and systemic cardiac output. Severe tricuspid regurgitation (TR) could be another issue that complicates the lifeof the intensivist dealing with a newborn with HLHS. Good preoperative management with mechanical ventilation in order to lower the degree of TR results in a better short-term prognosis of stage 1 Norwood operation The goal of respiratory management is to increase pulmonary vascular resistance and decrease systemic vascular resistance. The p/s ratio can be manipulated by increasing PVR by increasing the $PaCO_2$. $PaCO_2$ can be increased by adding supplemental inspired carbon dioxide, a potent pulmonary vasoconstrictor, to theventilator circuit. This approach for increasing $PaCO_2$ is preferred overhypoventilation, which may lead to atelectasis. PVR can also be increased by decreasing the concentration of inspired oxygen by adding supplemental nitrogen gas to attain a fraction of inspired oxygen of 0.17–0.19. PVR can also be increased by maintaining the hematocrit at greater than 0.40, a state that optimizes oxygen carrying capacity and increases the viscosity of the blood. Although these medical management strategies may provide temporary palliation, infants with marked pulmonary overcirculation and systemic hypoperfusion benefit from early surgical correction, because the methods to reverse this situation have limited effectiveness. Infants with HLHS who are born with a severely restricted or no interatrial communication, a rare occurrence, have profound hypoxemia. In fact, morbidityand mortality remain high in the subset of patients with an intact or very restrictive atrial septum. The severe restriction of blood flow across the atrial septum results in a life-threatening situation and these patients, which present with severe cyanosis and hemodynamic instability, require urgent postnatal cardiac catheterization to relieve the septal obstruction and improve oxygenation. Relief of the obstruction can be achieved by a balloon atrial septostomy or blade-septostomy at the time of cardiac catheterization or a surgical atrial septectomy. The tenuous condition of these infants makes each of these interventions high risk. The choice of intervention depends on the severity of the obstruction, the infant's cardiac anatomy and physiology, and the experience of the available medical and surgical team.

2. **Surgical:** Three options are available in the management of these infants; do nothing or choose one of two surgical options. The surgical options are the Norwood operation (followed by a Fontan operation) and cardiac transplantation.
   a. *Norwood operation*
      - The first-stage Norwood operation is performed on the neonate. This operation consists of (1) division of the MPA and closure of the distal stump, (2) a right-sided Gore-Tex shunt (usually a 4-mm tube) to provide PBF, (3) excision of the atrial septum (for adequate interatrial mixing), and (4) construction of a new aortic arch between the proximal mainpulmonary artery (MPA) and the hypoplastic ascending aorta and aortic archm using an aortic or pulmonary artery allograft. The surgical mortality rate is 35% or higher.
      - A cavopulmonary shunt (or bidirectional Glenn operation) is carried out at 6 months of age. Mortality is less than 5%.
      - A modified Fontan operation is carried out when the patient is a year and a half old. Overall survival after the Fontan operation is about 50% at 4 years.

   b. *Cardiac transplantation:* It is considered to be the procedure of choice in some centers. The transplantation is not a cure for the defect but creates a lifelong medical problem, the threat of infection and rejection.

### Premature Neonates with a Large PDA (Figs 35.29–35.32)

*Prevalence:* Significant PDA with CHF occurs in 15% of prematures with a birth weight of less than 1,750 g and in 40–50% of those with a birth weight of less than 1,500 g.

*Pathophysiology:* This is a special problem in premature infants who have been recovering from hyaline membrane disease. With improvement in oxygenation the PVR drops rapidly, but the ductus remains patent because its responsiveness to oxygen is immature in the premature newborn infant.

The resulting large L-R ductal shunt makes the lungs stiff, and weaning the infant from ventilator and oxygen therapy becomes difficult. Infants who remain on ventilators for a long time develop bronchopulmonary

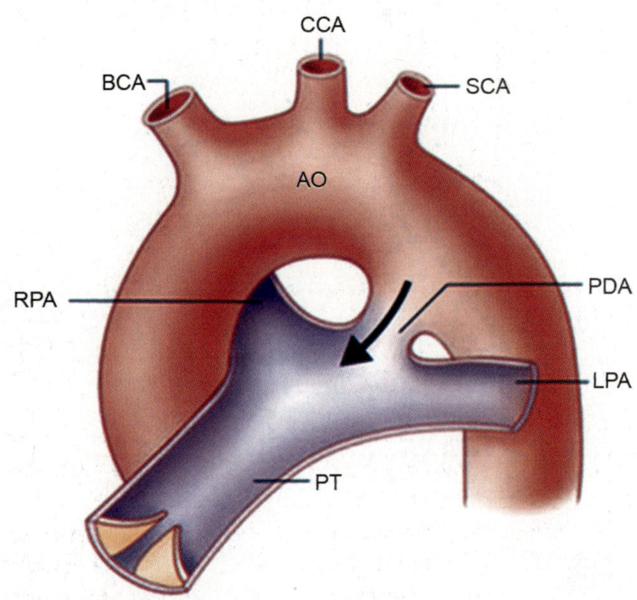


**Fig. 35.29:** The anatomy of a patent ductus arteriosus is shown. Note the relation between the position of the ductus, the left subclavian artery, and the pulmonary artery bifurcation (AO=aorta; BCA=brachiocephalic; CCA=common carotid artery; L=left; PDA=patent ductus arteriosus; PT=pulmonary trunk; RPA=right pulmonary artery; SCA=subclavian artery)

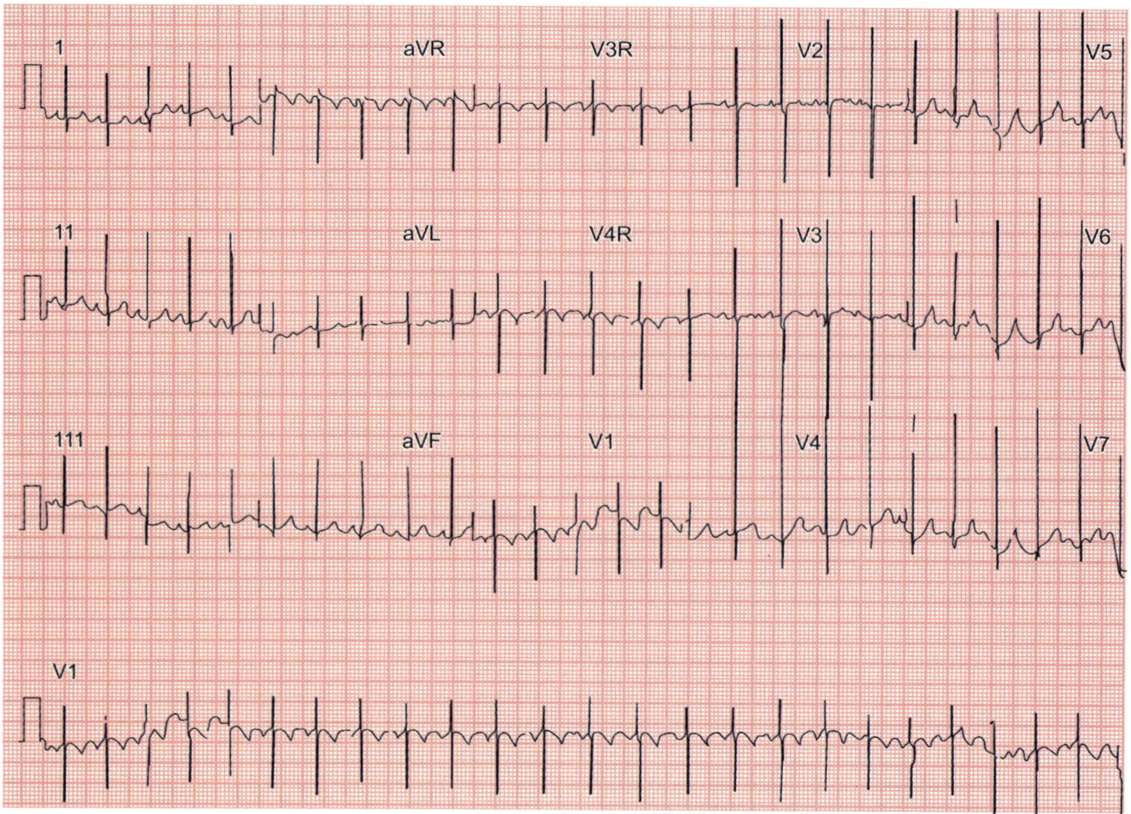


**Fig. 35.30:** ECG trace in a 3-month-old infant with large (5 mm) PDA associated with one-half systemic pulmonary artery pressure and left-sided volume overload. The tracing shows left atrial enlargement (biphasic P-wave V1) and left ventricular hypertrophy (27 mm R wave V6)

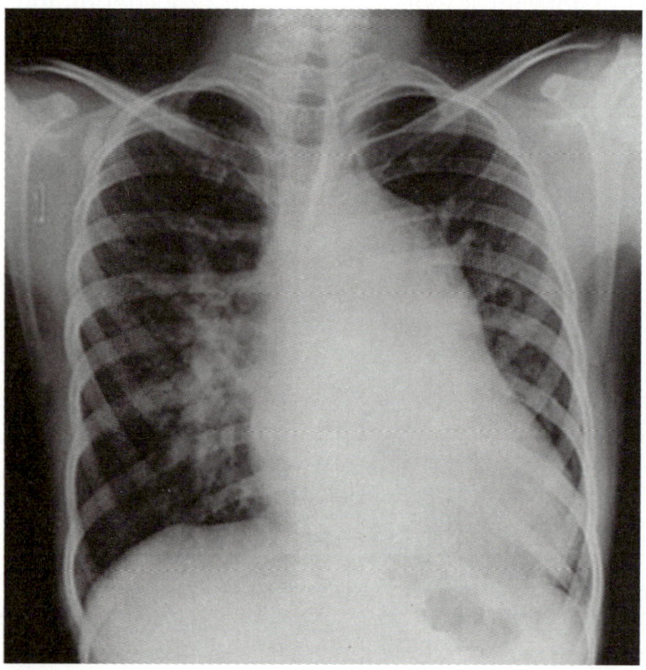

**Fig. 35.31:** Patent ductus arteriosus. PA view of the chest shows cardiomegaly with enlargement of the left ventricle and left atrium, dilatation of the main pulmonary artery segment, prominence of the central pulmonary arteries, and overall diffuse increase in pulmonary vascularity. The right ventricle may also show enlargement when pulmonary hypertension is present

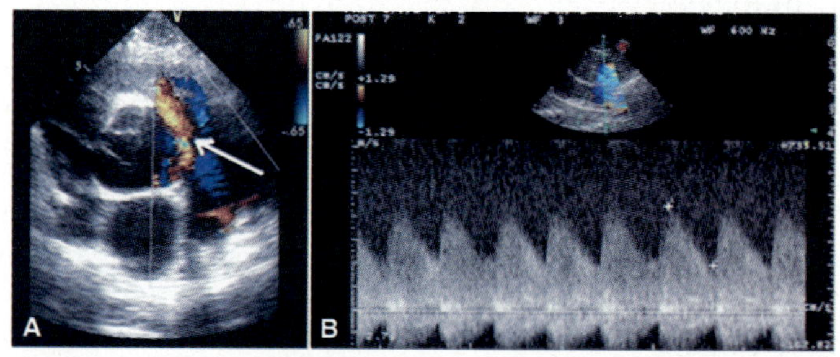


**Fig. 35.32:** (A) Transthoracic echocardiography image showing the patent ductus arteriosus (arrow). (B) Color-Doppler echo scan shows contineous blood flow through PDA both during systole and diastole

dysplasia with resulting pulmonary hypertension (cor pulmonale) and right-sided heart failure.

## Clinical Manifestations

1. The history usually reveals that a premature infant with hyaline membrane disease has made some improvement during the first few days after birth, but this is followed by inability to wean the infant from the ventilator or a need to increase ventilator settings or oxygen requirement in 4–7-day-old premature infants. Apneic spells or episodes of bradycardia may be initial signs in infants who are not on ventilators.

2. Bounding peripheral pulses and a hyperactive precordium are usually present. The classic continuous murmur of PDA at the ULSB is diagnostic, but the murmur is sometimes systolic only at the middle and upper LSB. Premature infants who are fluid overloaded or retaining fluid may also present with the hyperdynamic precordium, an ejection systolic murmur, bounding pulse, and wide pulse pressure.
3. Electrocardiogram may be normal or may show LVH with LA enlargement with larger sized shunt.
4. Chest X-ray films show cardiomegaly and evidence of pulmonary edema or pulmonary venous congestion in addition to varying degrees of the lung disease.
5. 2D echo study confirms the diagnosis. It provides anatomic information about the diameter, length, and shape of the ductus. The Doppler study of the ductus (with the sample volume placed at the pulmonary end of the ductus) provides important functional information such as ductal shunt patterns (pure L-R, bidirectional, or predominant R-L shunt), pressure in the PA, and magnitude of the ductal shunt or pulmonary perfusion status. An indirect estimate of the magnitude of the shunt can be made by the LA and LV dimensions.

*Management:* For symptomatic infants, either pharmacologic (indomethacin) or surgical closure of the ductus is indicates. A small PDA that is not causing CHF should be followed up medically for 6 months without surgical ligation because of the possibility of spontaneous closure.

1. Indomethacin (a prostaglandin synthetase inhibitor), 0.2 mg/kg IV every 12 hours for up to 3 doses, may be used on selected cases. A second course is occasionally necessary for adequate ductal closure. Contraindications to the use of indomethacin include (1) BUN over 25 mg/dl or creatinine levels over 1.8 mg/dl, (2) a platelet count below 80,000/mm$^3$, (3) a bleeding tendency (including intracranial hemorrhage), (4) necrotizing enterocolitis, and (5) hyperbilirubinemia.
2. A European study showed that ibuprofen given IV (10 mg/kg followed by 5 mg/kg every 24 hours, two times), starting on the third day of life, was as effective as indomethacin (0.2 mg/kg IV every 12 hours, three times), with a lower incidence of oliguria and a less deleterious effect on the cerebral blood flow than indomethacin. However, ibuprofen is not approved for use in premature PDA in this country.
3. If the medical treatment is unsuccessful or if the use of indomethacin is contraindicated, a surgical ligation of the ductus is indicated. The standard operative approach to the PDA has been through a posterolateral thoracotomy. The safety, effectiveness, and minimally invasive nature of video-assisted thoracoscopic surgery (VATS) have been reported for premature PDA. Advantages of the technique may include no need to cut the muscle and to spread ribs, thus a reduced compromise of respiratory mechanics and of chest wall deformity.

### Persistent Pulmonary Hypertension of the Newborn (Persistent Fetal Circulation)

Persistent pulmonary hypertension of the newborn (PPHN) occurs in term and post-term infants (Figs 35.33–35.36). Predisposing factors include birth asphyxia, meconium aspiration pneumonia, early-onset sepsis, hypoglycemia, polycythemia, maternal use of nonsteroidal anti-inflammatory drugs with in utero constriction of the ductus arterious, and pulmonary hypoplasia as a result of diaphragmatic hernia, amniotic fluid leak, oligohydramnions, or pleural effusions. PPHN is often idiopathic. Some patients with PPHN have low plasma arginine and nitric oxide metabolite concentrations and polymorphisms of the carbamoyl phosphate synthase gene, findings suggestive of a possible subtle defect in nitric oxide production. The incidence is 1/500–1,500 live births with a wide variation between different clinical centers.

*Pathophysiology:* Persistence of the fetal circulatory pattern of right-to-left shunting through the PDA and foramen ovale after birth is due to excessively high pulmonary vascular resistance. Fetal pulmonary vascular resistance is usually elevated relative to fetal systemic or postnatal pulmonary pressure. This fetal state permits shunting of oxygenated umbilical venous blood to the left atrium (and brain) through the foramen ovale and bypasses the lungs through the ductus arterious to the descending aorta. After birth, pulmonary vascular resistance normally declines rapidly as a consequence of vasodilation secondary to gas filling the lungs, a rise in postnatal $PaO_2$, a reduction in $PCO_2$, increased pH, and release of vasoactive substances. Increased neonatal pulmonary vascular resistance may (1) be maladaptive from an acute injury (e.g. not demonstrating normal vasodilation in response to increased oxygen and other changes after birth); (2) be the result of increased pulmonary artery medial muscle thickness and extension of smooth muscle layers into the usually nonmuscular, more peripheral pulmonary arterioles in response to chronic fetal hypoxia; (3) be due to pulmonary hypoplasia (diaphragmatic hernia, Potter syndrome); (4) be obstructive as a result of polycythemia or total anomalous pulmonary venous return; or be due to alveolarcapillary dysplasia, a lethal, possibly familial disorder characterized by a thickened alveolar septum and a reduced number of small pulmonary arteries and capillaries. Apart from the aetiology, profound hypoxia from right-to-left shunting and normal or elevated $PCO_2$ are present.

*Clinical manifestations:* Infants become ill in the delivery room or within the first 12 hours of life. PPHN related to polycythemia, idiopathic causes, hypoglycemia, or asphyxia may result in severe cyanosis with tachypnea, although initially, signs of respiratory distress may be minimal. Infants who have PPHN associated with meconium aspiration, group B streptococcal pneumonia, diagphragmatic hernia, or pulmonary hypoplasia usually exhibit cyanosis, grunting, flaring, retractions, tachycardia, and shock. Multiorgan involvement may be present.

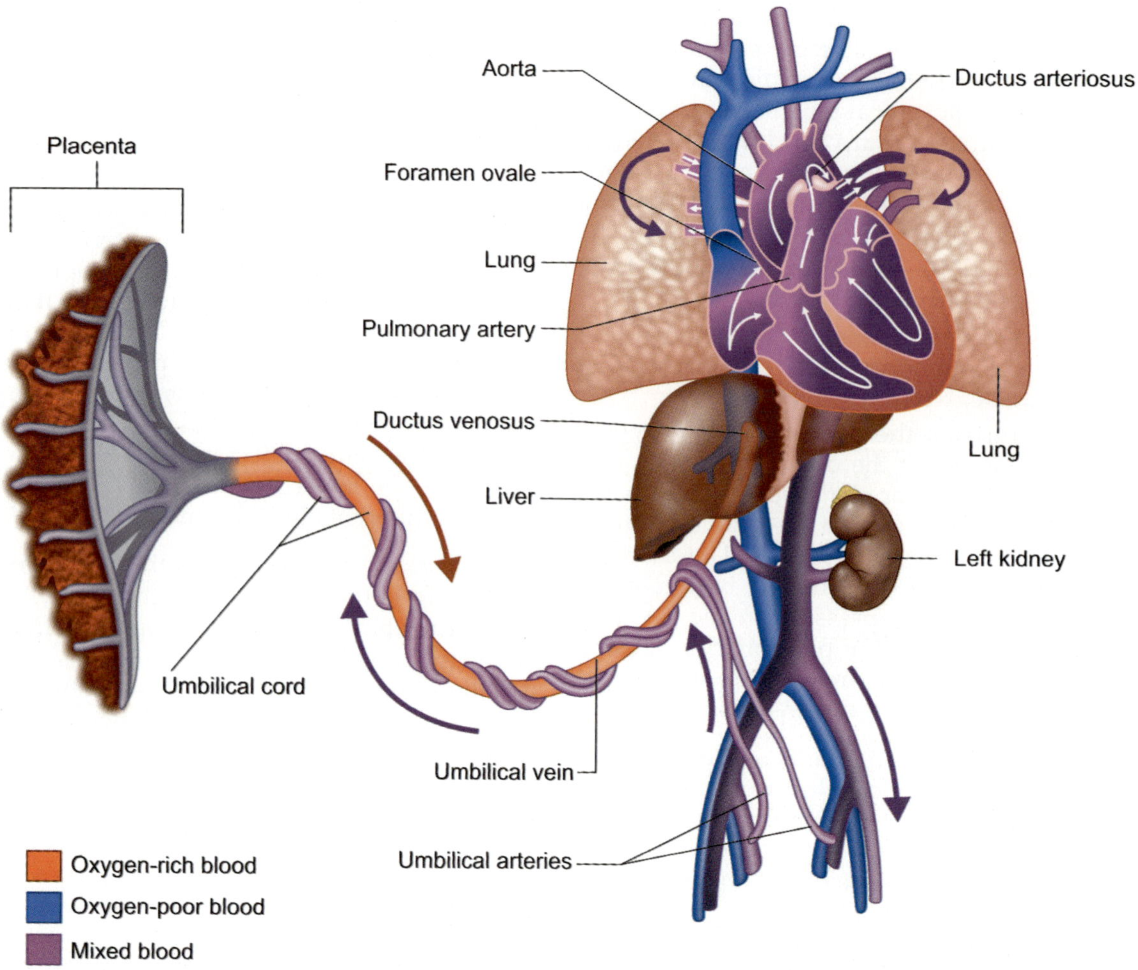


**Fig. 35.33:** Hemodynamics in persistent fetal circulation

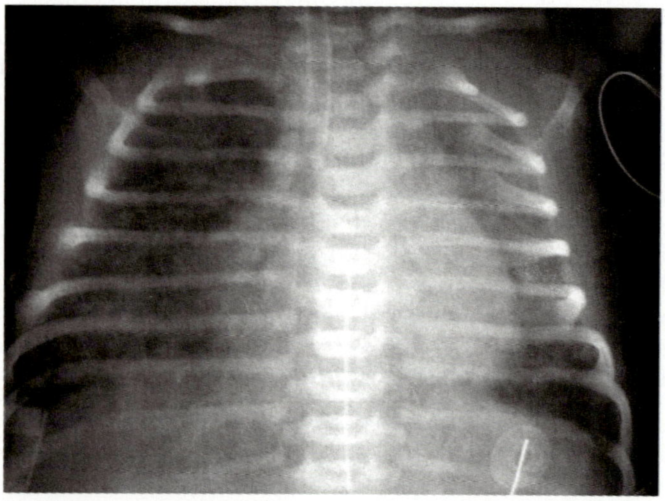

**Fig. 35.34:** Meconium aspiration. Radiograph obtained shortly after birth shows ill-defined, predominantly perihilar opacities in the lungs; these are more severe on the right than on the left. The lungs are hyperexpanded. The neonate's heart size is within normal limits

Myocardial ischemia, papillary muscle dysfunction with mitral and tricuspid regurgitation, and cardiac stunning produce cardiogenic shock with decreased pulmonary blood flow, tissue perfusion, and oxygen delivery. The hypoxia is quite labile and often out of proportion to the findings on chest roentgenograms.

*Diagnosis:* PPHN should be suspected in all term infants who have cyanosis with or without fetal distress, intrauterine growth restriction, meconium-stained amniotic fluid, hypoglycemia, polycythemia, diaphragmatic hernia, pleural effusions, and birth asphyxia. Hypoxia is universal and is unresponsive to 100% oxygen given by oxygen hood, but it may respond transiently to hyperoxic hyperventilation administered after endotracheal intubation or to the application of a bag and mask. A $PaO_2$ gradient between a preductal (right radial artery) and a postductal (umbilical artery) site of blood sampling greater than 20 mmHg suggest right-to-left shunting through the ductus arteriosus.

Real-time echocardiography combined with Doppler flow studies demonstrates right-to-left shunting across a patent foramen ovale and a ductus arteriosus. Deviation of the intra-atrial septum into the left atrium is seen in severe PPHN. Tricuspid or mitral insufficiency may be noted on auscultation as a holosystolic murmur and can be visualized echocardiographically together with poor contractility when PPHN is associated with myocardial

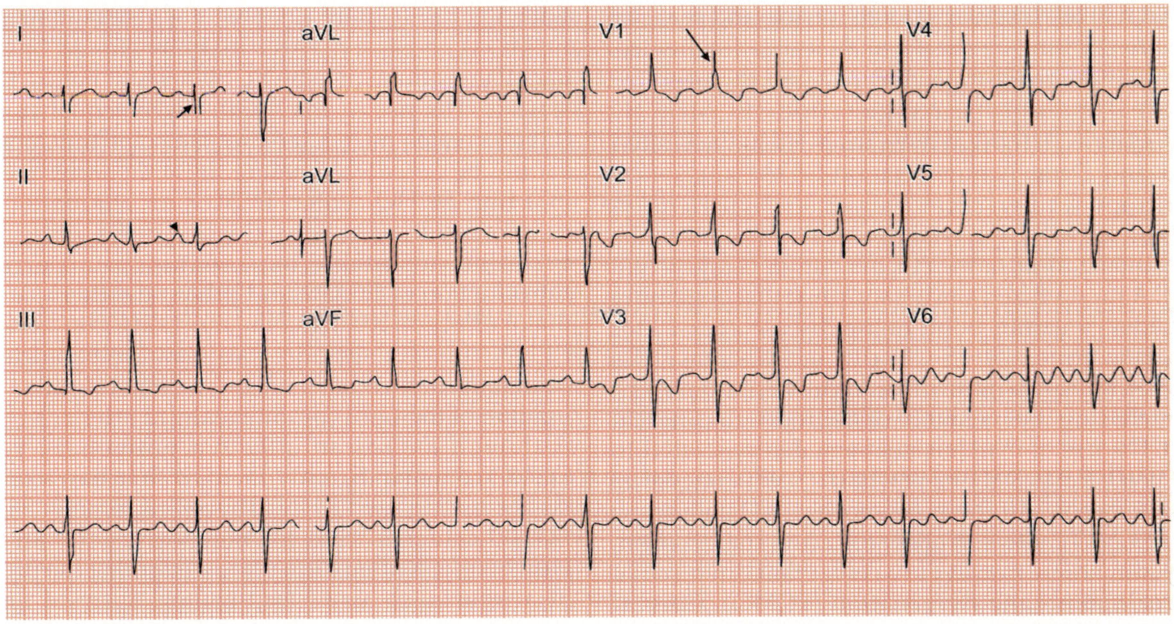


**Fig. 35.35:** Primary pulmonary hypertension. Electrocardiogram demonstrating the changes of right ventricular hypertrophy (long arrow) with strain in a patient with primary pulmonary hypertension. Right axis deviation (short arrow), increased P-wave amplitude in lead II (black arrowhead), and incomplete right bundle branch block (white arrowhead) are highly specific but lack sensitivity for the detection of right ventricular hypertrophy

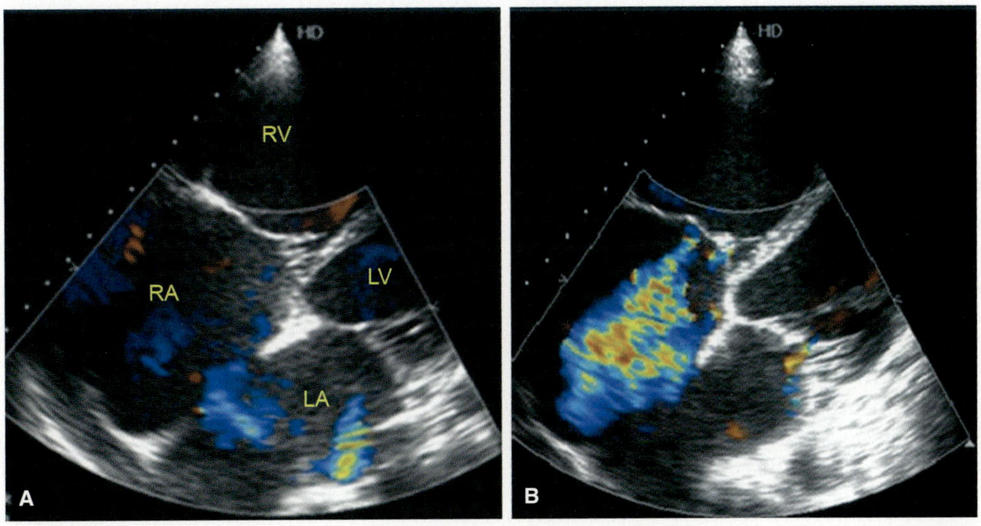


**Fig. 35.36:** (A) Color-Doppler echocardiography shows reversal of flow across ASD secundum. (B) Shows gross TR with raised pulmonary artery pressure in patient with Eisenmenger syndrome

ischemia. The degree of tricuspid regurgitation can be used to estime pulmonary artery pressure. The second heart sound is accentuated and not split. In asphyxia-associated and idiopathic PPHN, the chest roentgenogram is normal, whereas in PPHN associated with pneumonia and diaphragmatic hernia, it shows the specific lesions of parenchymal opacification and bowel in the chest, respectively. The differential diagnosis of PPHN includes cyanotic heart disease (especially obstructed total anomalous pulmonary venous return) and the associated etiologic entities that predispose to PPHN (e.g. hypoglycemia, polycythemia and sepsis).

*Treatment:* Therapy is directed toward correcting any predisposing disease (hypoglycemia, polycithemia) and improving poor tissue oxygenation. The response to therapy is often unpredictable, transient, and complicated by the adverse effects of drugs or mechanical ventilation. Initial management includes oxygen administration and correction of acidosis, hypotension, and hypercapnia. Persistent hypoxia should be managed with intubation and mechanical ventilation.

Treatment with inhaled nitric oxide (iNO) is indicated for newborns with an oxygen index (OI) of less than 25. Nitric oxide (NO) is an endothelially derived gas signaling molecule that relaxes vascular smooth muscle and that can be delivered to the lung by means of an inhalation device. In two large, randomized trials, NO reduced the need for extracorporeal membrane oxygenation (ECMO) by approximately 40%. Although these trials led to the United States Food and Drug Administration (FDA) approving iNO as a therapy for persistent pulmonary hypertension of the newborn (PPHN), iNO did not reduce mortality, the length of hospitalization, or the risk of neurodevelopmental impairment. A randomized study confirmed that beginning iNO at a milder or earlier point in the disease course (for an oxygenation index of 15–25) did not decrease the incidence of ECMO and/or death or improve other patient outcomes, including the incidence of neurodevelopmental impairment.The use of iNO has not been demonstrated to reduce the need for ECMO in newborns with congenital diaphragmatic hernia. In these newborns, iNO should be used in non-ECMO centers to allow for acute stabilization, followed by immediate transfer to a center that can provide extracorporeal membrane oxygenation (ECMO). Contra-indications to iNO include congenital heart disease characterized by left ventricular outflow tract obstruction (e.g. interrupted aortic arch, critical aortic stenosis, hypoplastic left heart syndrome) and severe left ventricular dysfunction.The appropriate starting dose is 20 ppm. Doses higher than this have not been shown to be more effective and have been associated with adverse effects, including methemoglobinemia and increased levels of nitrogen dioxide ($NO_2$). Appropriate lung recruitment and expansion are essential to achieve the best response. If a newborn has severe parenchymal lung disease and PPHN, strategies such as HFV may be required. Most newborns require iNO for less than 5 days. In general, the dose can be weaned to 5 ppm after 6–24 hours of therapy. The dose is then slowly weaned and discontinued when the $FiO_2$ is less than 0.4–0.6 and the iNO dose is 1 ppm. Abrupt discontinuation at higher doses should be avoided because it may cause abrupt rebound pulmonary hypertension. In centers that do not have immediate availability of ECMO support, use of iNO must be approached with caution. Because iNO cannot be abruptly discontinued, transport with iNO is usually needed if a subsequent referral for ECMO is necessary. This capability should be determined in collaboration with the ECMO center before treatment is started. The use of iNO with high frequency ventilation (HFV) creates particular problems for transport, and this should be considered before these therapies are combined in a non-ECMO center. ECMO, an adaptation of cardio-pulmonary bypass, is used when optimal support fails to maintain acceptable oxygenation and perfusion. The introduction of ECMO and other new therapies has had a major effect on reducing the mortality rate associated with PPHN. ECMO support can now be provided using a double-lumen catheter in the internal jugular vein; thus, ligation of the right common carotid artery can be avoided. Although iNO is an effective pulmonary vasodilator, ECMO remains the only therapy that has been proven to be life-saving for PPHN. Therefore, timely transfer to an ECMO center is vital for newborns with severe PPHN. However, it is often difficult to determine the proper timing of a referral to an ECMO center. Referral and transfer should occur before refractory hypoxemia develops. Early consultation and discussion with clinicians at the ECMO center is strongly recommended. Continuous delivery of NO is required during transport. Baseline criteria for newborns considered for ECMO are generally as follows:

- Gestation of more than 34 weeks
- Weight more than 2000 g
- No major intracranial hemorrhage on cranial sonograms (i.e. larger than a grade II hemorrhage)
- Reversible lung disease or mechanical ventilation for 7–14 days
- No evidence of lethal congenital anomalies or inoperable cardiac disease

### Transient Myocardial Ischemia (Figs 35.37–35.43)

*Prevalence:* Transient myocardial ischemia is a rarely recognized condition; the prevalence is unknown.

*Pathology and pathophysiology:*

1. Subendocardial ischemia or necrosis (possibly secondary to hypoxic pulmonary vasoconstriction) occurs in the

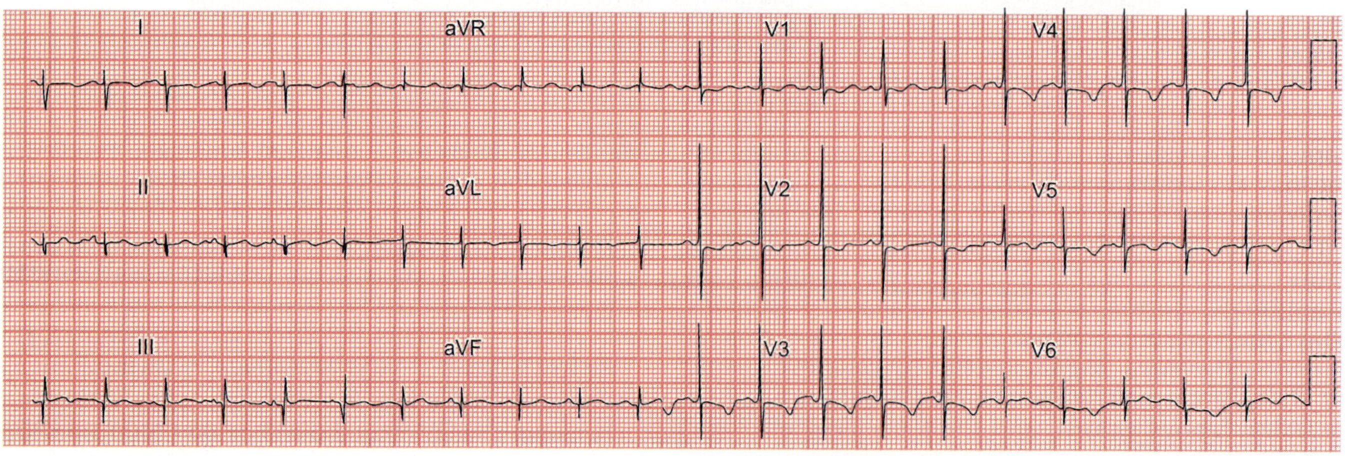


**Fig. 35.37:** This baby had birth asphyxia and myocardial damage with ECG changes (T-wave inversion in all the V leads with narrow waves in the inferior leads). There was myocardial dysfunction and an increased troponin T level

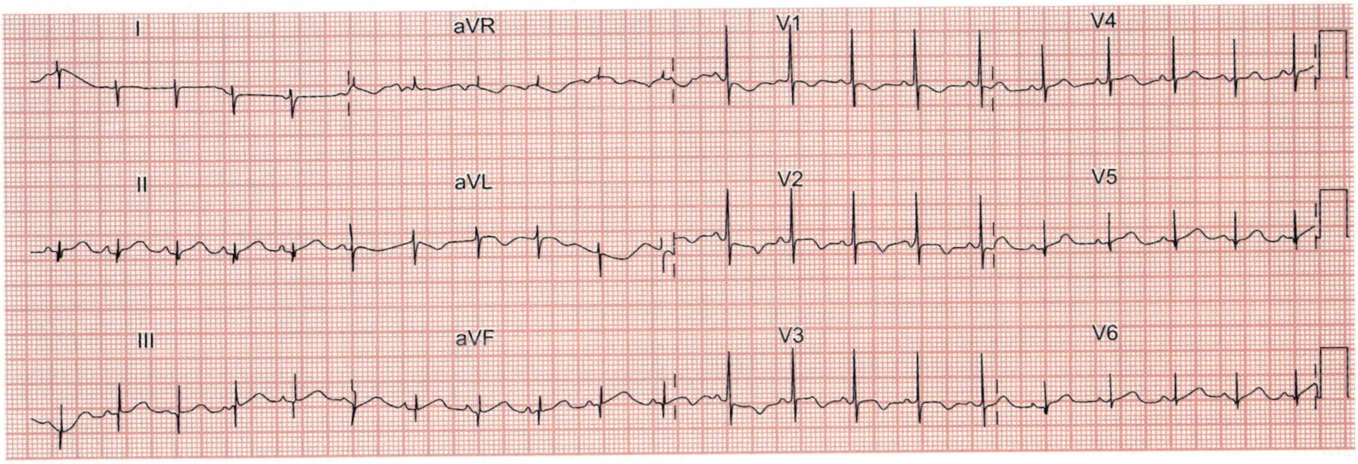


**Fig. 35.38:** The ECG changes started to resolve over the subsequent few days with improvement in myocardial function and there were no long-term sequelae

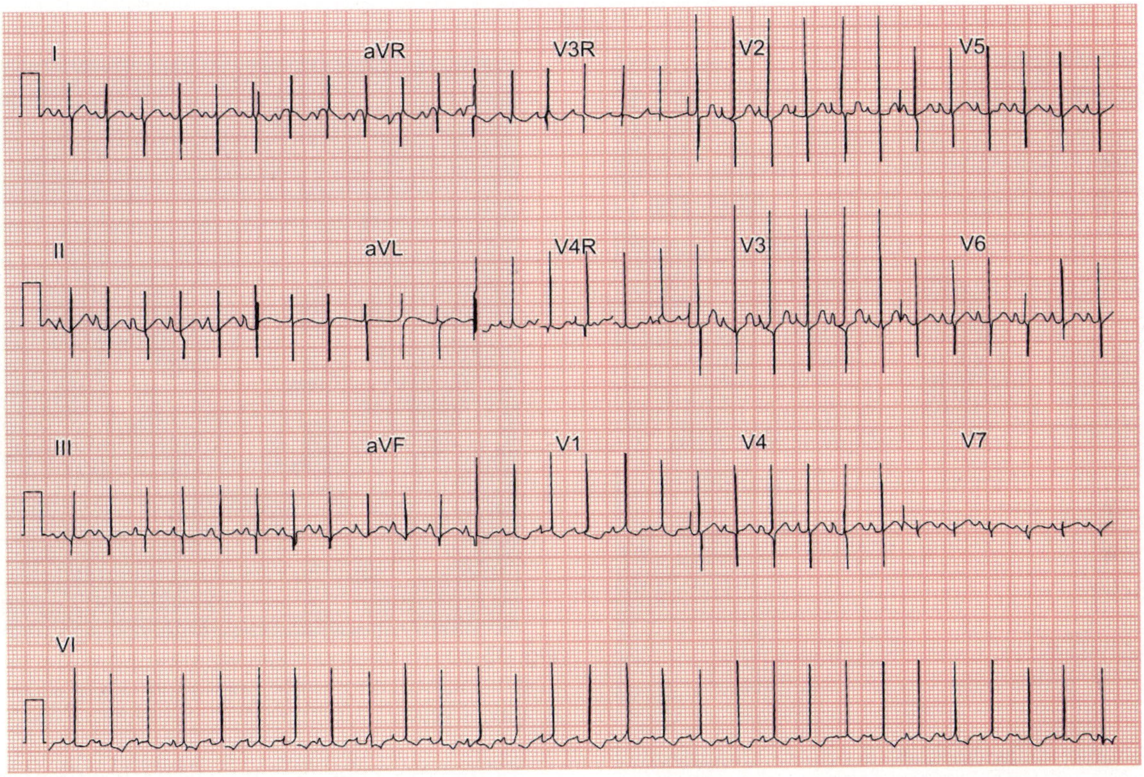


**Fig. 35.39:** TAPVR. Electrocardiogram obtained in a 10-days old infant with total anomalous pulmonary venous return to the coronary sinus. The tracing shows right atrial enlargement (peaked P-waves in lead II) and right ventricular hypertrophy

papillary muscles and other areas of the ventricles in the newborn infant who had prenatal or perinatal hypoxia and distress.

Evidence of pulmonary hypertension, bidirectional shunts at the atrial and/or ductal levels, and TR are usually present. Variable degrees of LV dysfunction are demonstrable by echocardiography.

2. Three levels of severity have been recognized.
   a. Transient tachypnea of the newborn is the mildest form of the condition. Mild LV dysfunction leads to fluid retention, pulmonary edema, and reduced lung compliance producing tachypnea.
   b. Transient tricuspid (or mitral) regurgitation results from papillary muscle infarction (evidenced by elevated serum levels of creatine phosphokinase MB fraction).
   c. Severe CHF with cardiogenic shock is the most severe form of myocardial dysfunction seen in the newborn infant.

### Clinical Manifestations

1. Tachypnea develops usually in full-term neonates with a low Apgar score. Mild cyanosis may also be present.
2. A systolic murmur of TR or MR is commonly present. Rarely, CHF with gallop rhythm, hypotension, and vascular collapse result.

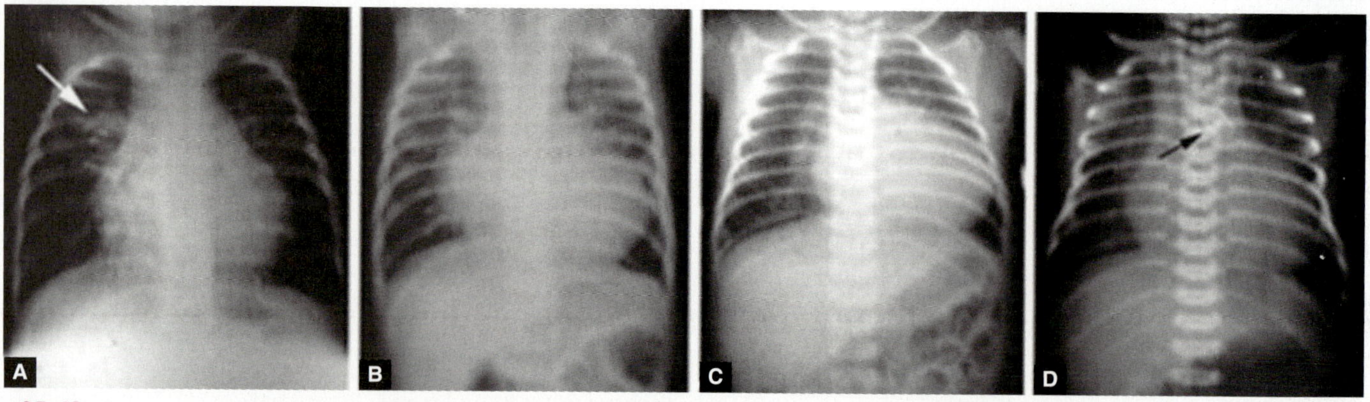


**Fig. 35.40:** Chest X-rays showing the different degrees of cardiomegaly and pulmonary congestion in neonates with heart failure syndrome. (A) Films of patients with aortic coarctation, with associated pneumonia (white arrow); (B) the film of a newborn with a double outflow tract of the right ventricle and severe pulmonary hypertension. (C) Film is typical of the 'lying egg' cardiomegaly of type I truncus arteriosus. (D) Film shows a hypoplastic left heart syndrome, in severe heart failure, with a stent placed at the level of the ductus arteriosus (black arrow) as palliative therapy

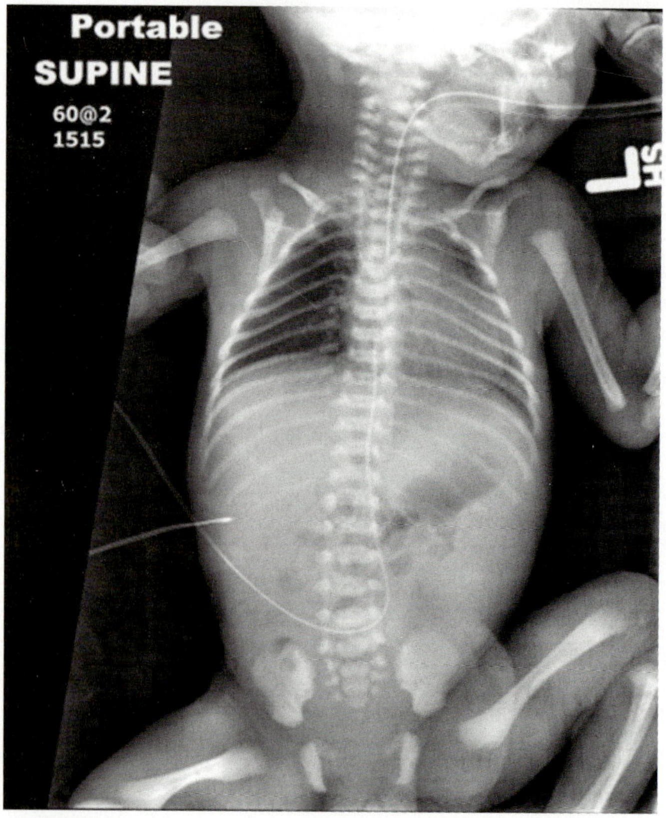


**Fig. 35.41:** The upper chest X-ray has an endotracheal tube near the carina (probably should be pulled back a bit). It also has cardiomegaly with vascular congestion. The line coming up from below is an umbilical venous catheter in the inferior vena cava

3. The ECG may show generalized flat T-waves and minor ST-segment depression.

   Abnormal Q-waves suggestive of anterior or inferior infarction may be seen.
4. **Chesy X-ray** shows varying degrees, sometimes marked, of cardiomegaly. PVMs may be increased due to

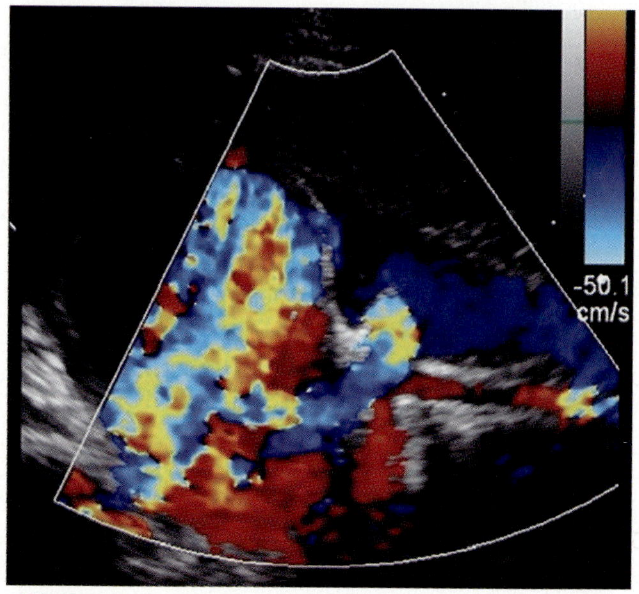


**Fig. 35.42:** Parasternal short axis view showing anomalous origin of left coronary artery from pulmonary artery, showing flow in the coronary artery

pulmonary venous congestion (described as wet lung) in severely affected neonates.

5. **Echo study** reveals varying degrees of myocardial dysfunction, including an enlarged LA and/or LV, decreased contractility of the LV, and mitral regurgitation (MR).
6. **Laboratory studies** may reveal mild reduction of $PO_2$ and pH (but usually without $CO_2$ retention), hypoglycemia, and elevated CPK MB fraction in patients with significant TR. A myocardial perfusion scan may show a diffuse impairment of thallium-201 uptake (different from myocarditis, in which myocardial perfusion is normal).
7. Infants with transient myocardial ischemia usually recover unless it is associated with severe acidosis, CNS damages, or advanced sepsis.

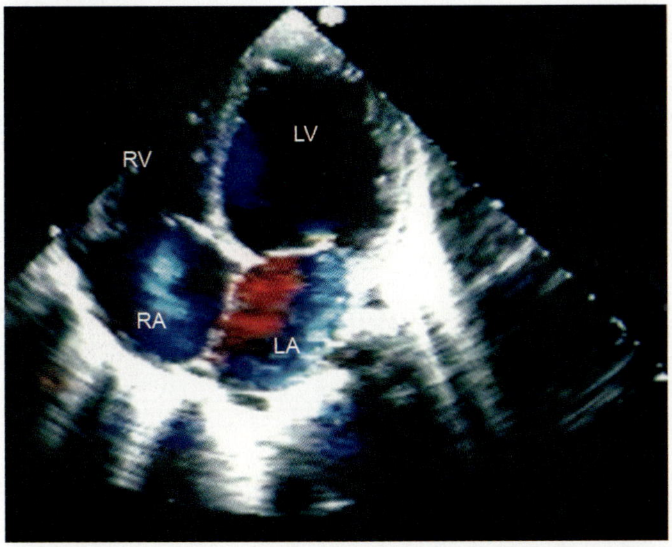


**Fig. 35.43:** This is a color-Doppler echocardiogram obtained from apical four-chamber view revealing a dilated left atrium and left ventricle with the blue jet of mitral regurgitation in a child myocardial ischemia. Mild tricuspid regurgitation is also shown

### *Management*

1. Supportive measures with administration of oxygen, correction of acidosis, and treatment of hypogycemia are all that are required for mild cases.
2. For severely affected infants, ventilatory assistance, short-acting inotropic agents (such as dopamine), a vasodilator agent, and fluid restriction and diuretic(s) may be indicated.

## Emergency Treatment if Cyanotic CHD is Suspected

If a cyanotic CHD is suspected, PGE1 should be started or made available (Figs 35.44–35.53). The starting dose is 0.05–0.1 µg/kg/min, administered in a continuous IV drip. When the desired effects (increased $PO_2$, increased systemic blood pressure, and improved pH) are achieved, the dose should be reduced step-by-step to 0.01µg/kg/min. When there is no effect with the initial starting dose, it may be increased to 0.4 µg/kg/min. If echocardiography is not immediately available, the clinician caring for a newborn with possible cyanotic heart disease should not hesitate to start a prostaglandin infusion (for a possible ductal-dependent lesion). Because of the risk of hypoventilation associated with prostaglandins, a practitioner skilled in neonatal endotracheal intubation must be available. Three common side effects of prostaglandin E1 IV infusion are apnea (12%), fever (14%), and flushing (10%).

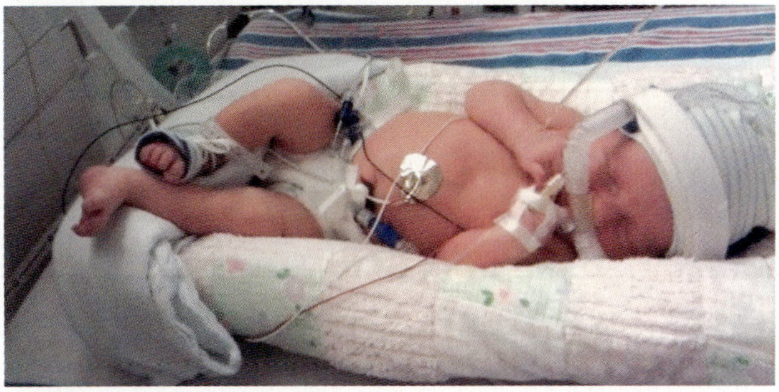

**Fig. 35.44:** Resuscitative measures including contineous positive pressure ventilation in a baby with cardiogenic shock

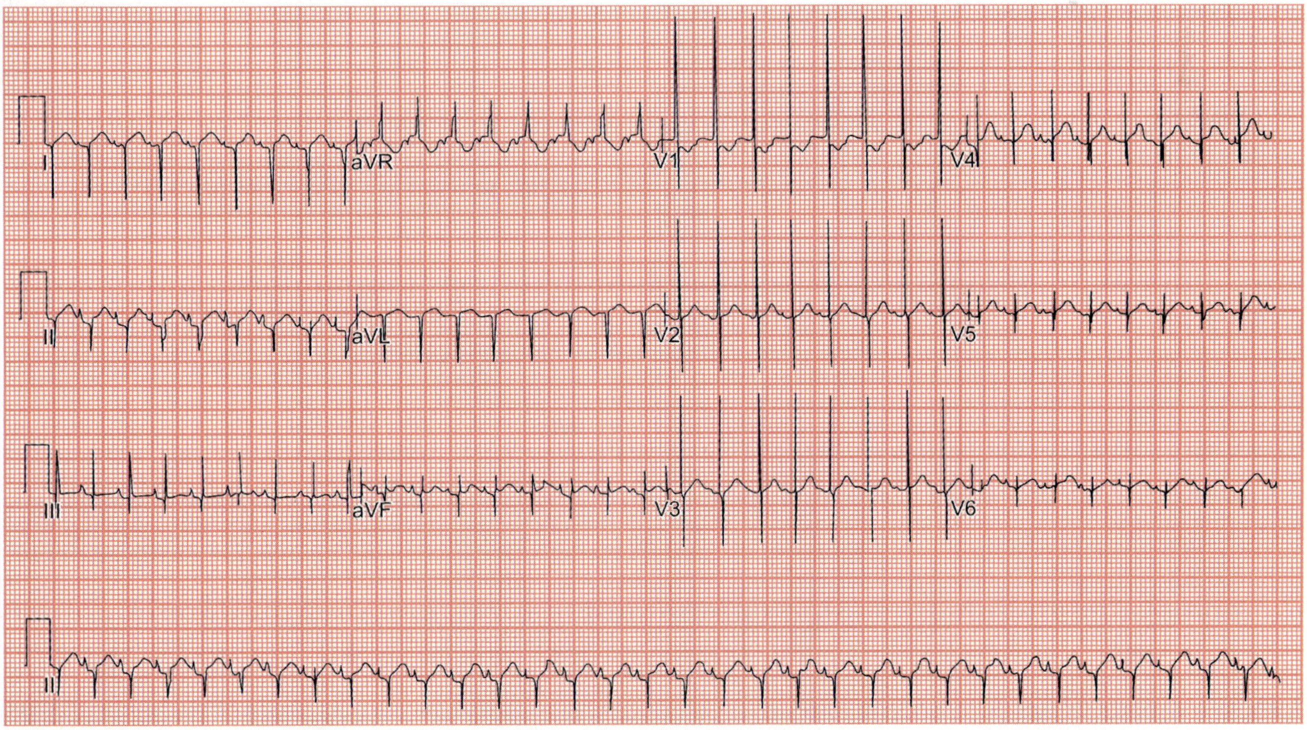


**Fig. 35.45:** Atrial flutter in a newborn with atrial rate of 375 and ventricular rate of 185 bpm. Note the typical 'sawtooth' appearance and mostly showing atrial flutter with 4 or 5:1 block

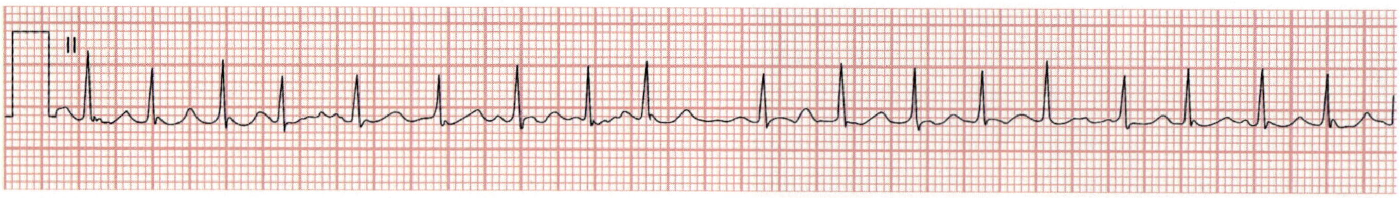


**Fig. 35.46:** Electrocardiogram (ECG) rhythm strip (about 7.6 s) showing atrial fibrillation. Note the irregular, rapid ventricular (QRS) response

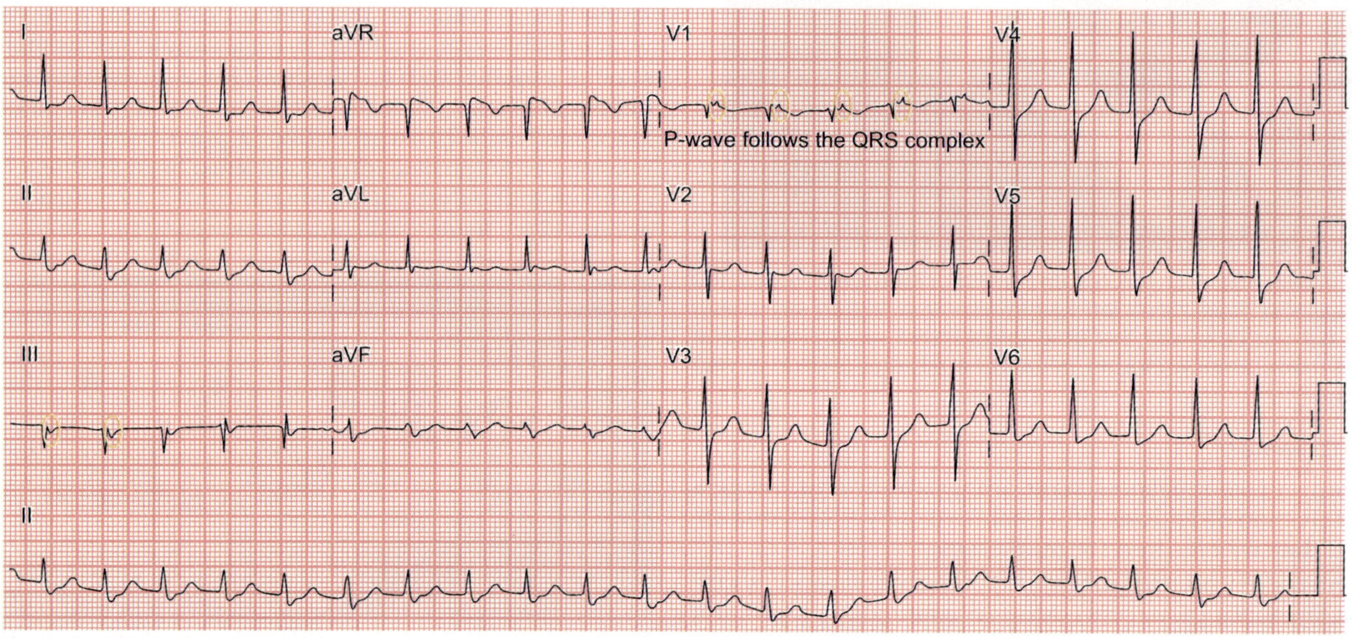


**Fig. 35.47:** Orthodromic atrioventricular re-entrant tachycardia. A re-entry circuit may also be established by a premature impulse traveling in an anterograde manner through a manifest accessory pathway and in a retrograde manner through the AV node; this is called antidromic AVRT. While the orthodromic AVRT is typically a narrow-complex tachycardia, antidromic AVRT inscribes a bizarre, wide-complex tachycardia

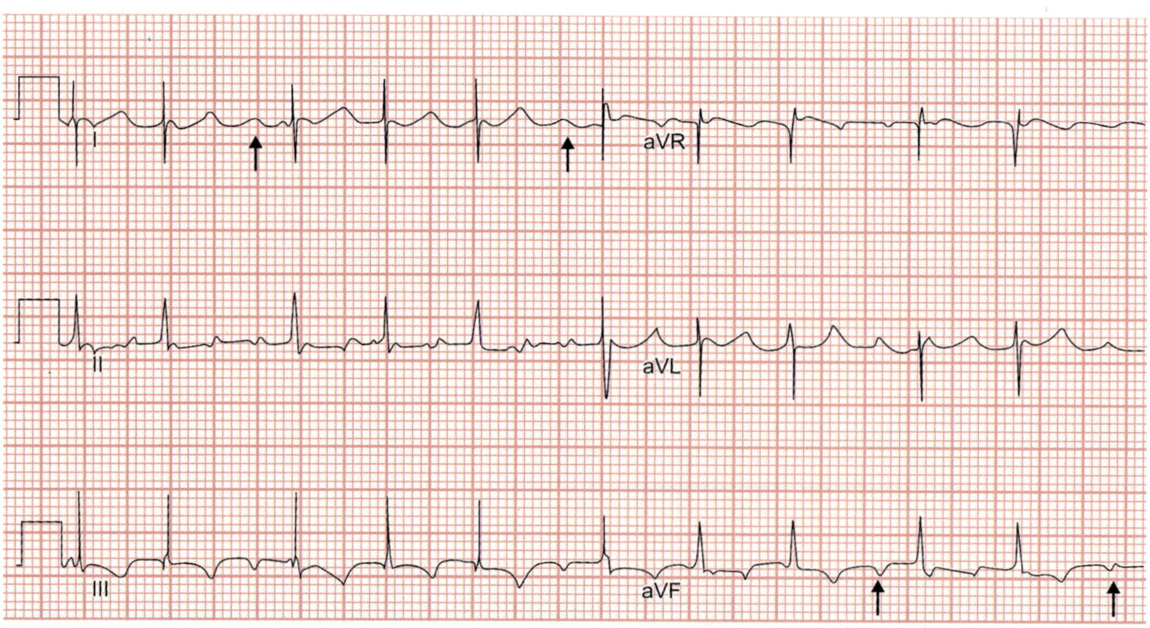


**Fig. 35.48:** A limb-lead ECG (at half standard; 5 mm/mV) demonstrating ectopic atrial tachycardia with an atrial cycle length of 220 ms and variable atrioventricular conduction. The P-wave morphology (arrows) suggests a lateral right atrial origin with a positive P-wave in lead I and a biphasic P-wave in lead AVF. A narrow-complex QRS is seen with 2:1 and 3:1 atrioventricular conduction

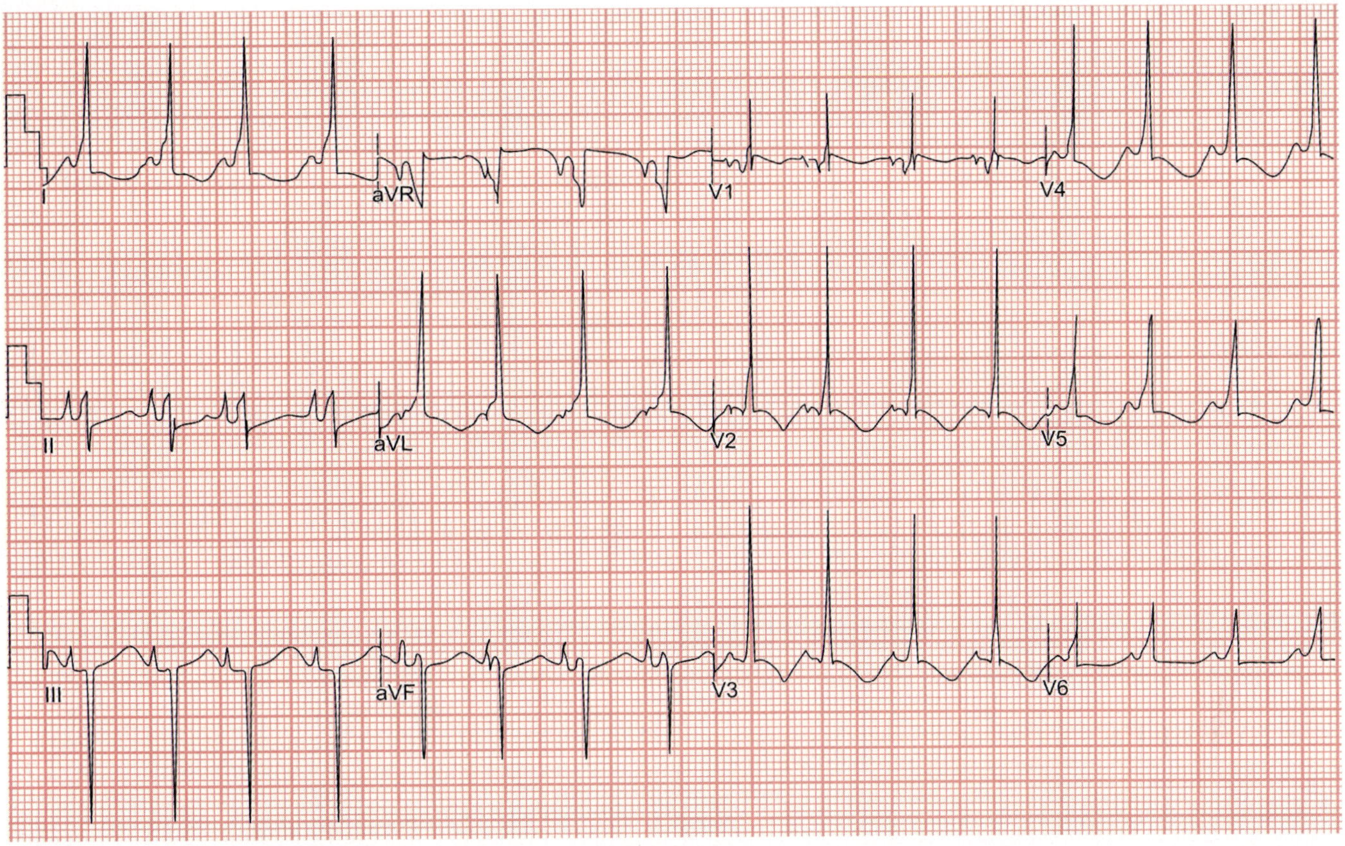


**Fig. 35.49:** A 12-lead ECG demonstrates pre-excitation (Wolff-Parkinson-White syndrome) during sinus rhythm. The precordial delta wave transitions from negative in V1 to positive between leads V2 and V3, consistent with a septal accessory pathway. Although a net positive QRS polarity in V1 suggests a left-sided accessory pathway in older patients, its significance is unclear in neonates who have predominant right-sided forces

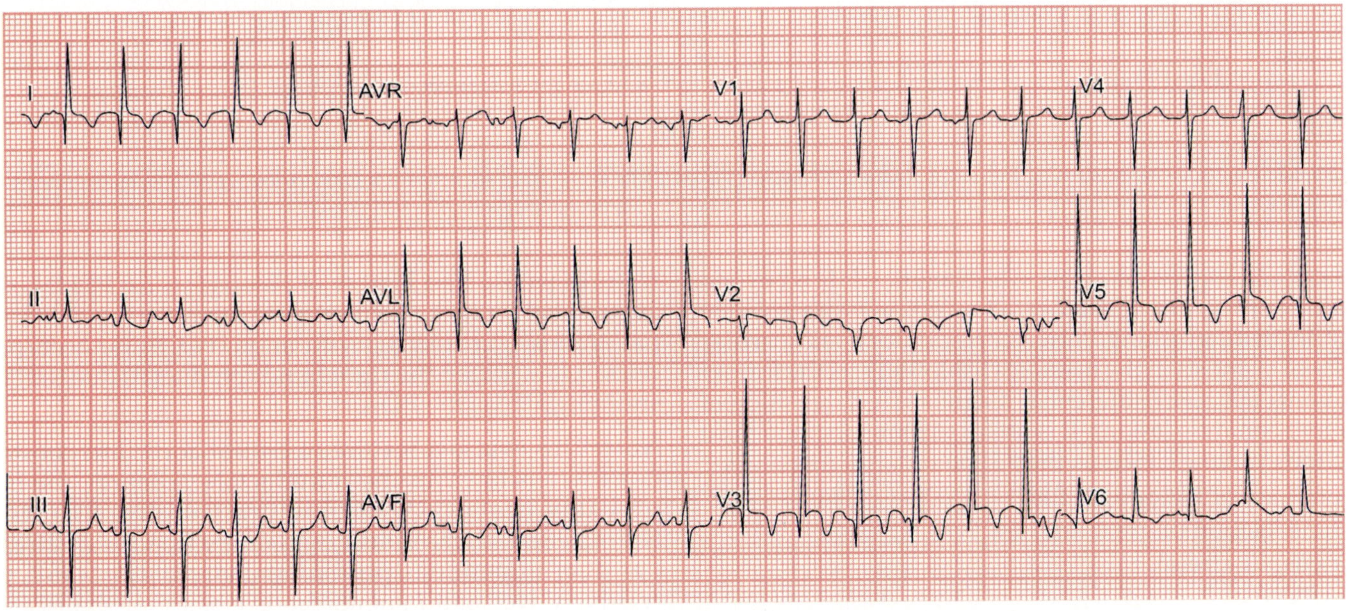


**Fig. 35.50:** ECG of an infant who presented in congestive cardiac failure, reveals deep Q-waves in leads I, aVL, V2 and V3, indicating an anterolateral myocardial infarct pattern. Deep Q-waves are also seen in V5 Q-waves represent the depolarisation of the interventricular septum. They are normally visible in lead I, II, III, aVF, V5, V6, but their duration should be less than 0.03 s, and they should be less than 5 mm deep. This patient, who had cardiogenic shock secondary to cardiomyopathy, had an anomalous left coronary artery from the pulmonary artery (ALCAPA). The condition, diagnosable by ECG, is surgically correctable

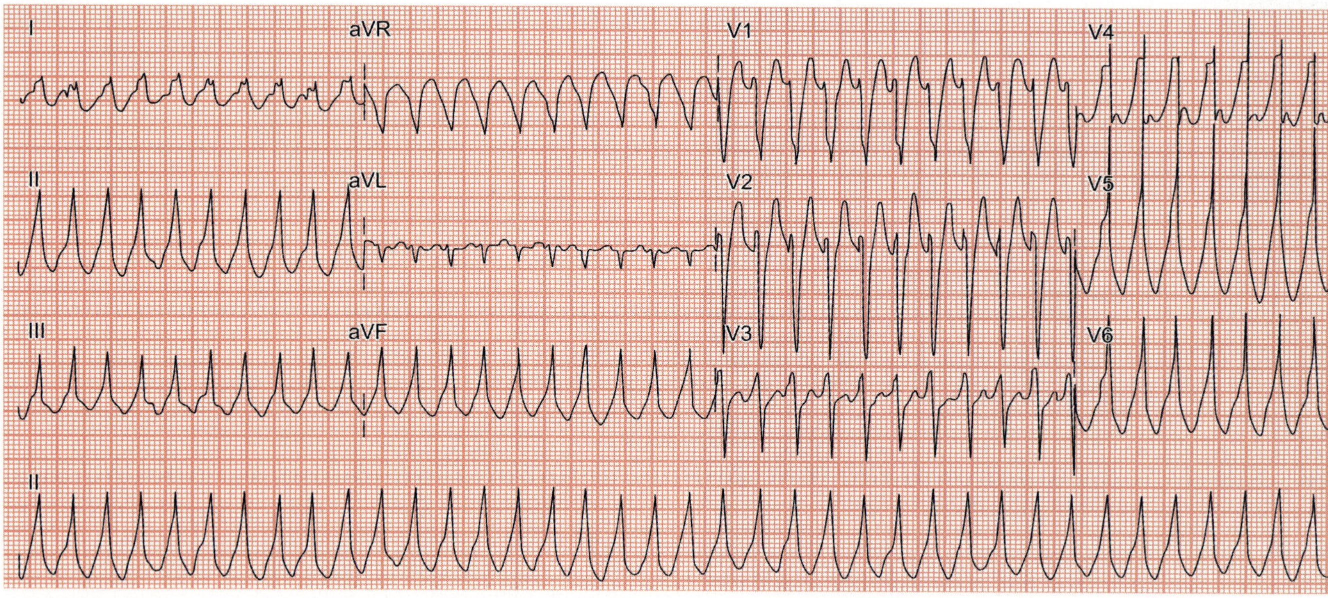

**Fig. 35.51:** EKG of ventricular tachycardia in a child with enteroviral encephalitis complicated with fulminant myocarditis

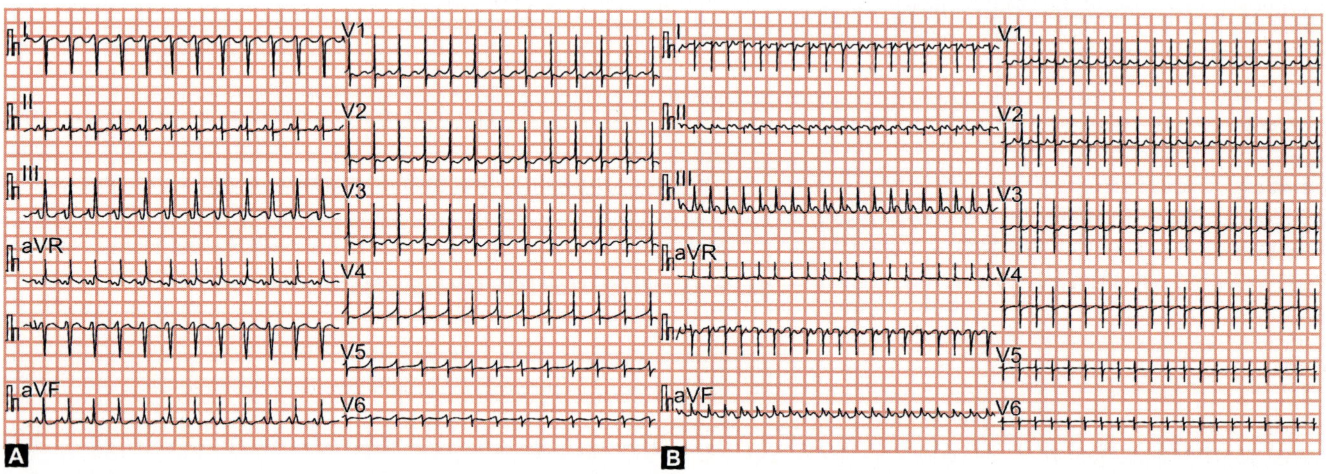

**Fig. 35.52:** Electrocardiogram of the sinus rhythm showed pre-excitation (A) and supraventricular tachycardia (B) in an infant with intracardiac tumor

*Cyanosis:* A detailed description of cyanotic CHD is beyond the scope of this article. Rather, a few pointers are given to assist in distinguishing between respiratory and cardiac causes of cyanosis in the neonate (Table 35.1), as the former represents the main differential diagnosis, with mention of the more common lesions. It is useful to remember the most common cyanotic CHDs as the 5 Ts in order of frequency:

- Tetralogy of Fallot with fits
- Transposition of great arteries,
- Tricuspid atresia,
- TAPVD,
- Truncus arteriosus,
- Pulmonary atresia/stenosis.

In addition, an important differential is persistent pulmonary hypertension of the newborn (PPHN)—suggestive features would be a history of risk factors for PPHN (such as perinatal asphyxia or meconium aspiration) and differential cyanosis, i.e. oxygen saturation/$PO_2$ in the feet (postductal) lower than the right hand (preductal) due to R to L shunting across the PDA.

***Note:*** This is also a feature of critical aortic arch obstructions (see below). In the introductory scenario, the baby probably has an RV outflow tract obstructive lesion (extreme tetralogy, critical pulmonary stenosis or atresia), i.e. duct-dependent pulmonary circulation, and was relatively well until spontaneous closure of the PDA on day 2 caused acute hypoxaemia and acidosis.

### Management

- Open the PDA ASAP. Mainstay therapy for reopening a PDA and keeping it open is prostaglandin E1

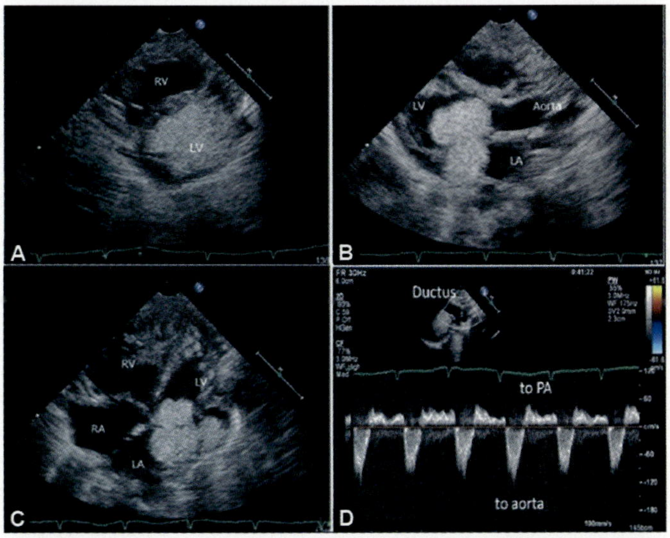


**Fig. 35.53:** Echocardiography shows a large tumor widely extended from the left atrium (LA) through mitral valve to the left ventricle (LV) in the short (A), parasternal (B), and four-chamber (C) views. Doppler ultrasound showed reversed ductus flow from pulmonary artery to aorta which dominant to ductus flow from aorta to pulmonary artery (D) (RA=Right atrium, RV=Right ventricle, LA=Left atrium, LV=Left ventricle, PA=Pulmonary artery)

(alprostadil) IV infusion (starting dose 50–100 ng/kg/min, if poor response (saturations and acidosis not improving) increase to maximum 300–400 ng/kg/min, maintenance dose 10–25 ng/kg/min) or prostaglandin E2 (dinoprostone) orally/via nasogastric tube [dose 25 μg/kg or quarter tablet (500 μg strength) every ½–1 hour] the latter should be available at all hospitals as an emergency drug, the former usually only at referral centres. Oral PGE2 is very safe (baby unlikely to come to any harm if diagnosis is not cyanotic CHD), but IV PGE1 can cause apnoea/hypoventilation and hypotension; hence used more in ICU or high-care settings. Prostaglandins may be used to attempt reopening of a PDA in a neonate up to 30 days of age.

- *Blood volume expansion*: 10 ml/kg 0.9% saline IV bolus, repeat as needed until liver edge palpable–to improve preload and hence encourage further opening of the PDA and pulmonary blood flow through the duct.
- Sodium bicarbonate empirically (as acidosis aggravates hypoxic pulmonary vasoconstriction)—1 mmol/kg IV as a 4.2% solution, repeat according to blood gas.
- Correct other derangements, e.g. hypoglycaemia, hypocalcemia, concomitant sepsis.
- Oxygen administration—aiming for saturations 75–85% (depending on exact diagnosis).
- Inotropes/vasopressors may be indicated to maintain adequate systemic perfusion and encourage pulmonary perfusion (by increasing systemic vascular resistance).
- If poor response to above, intubation/ventilation with sedation +/– paralysis to minimise metabolic demands and improve oxygenation.
- Consult with pediatric cardiologist and, once stabilised, transfer to tertiary centre for definitive diagnosis (usually with echocardiography) and management. This may entail cardiac catheterisation and often palliative surgery (e.g. modified Blalock-Taussig shunt).

### Shock

The practitioner faced with a shocked neonate needs to have a high index of suspicion for CHD as the presentation can often be mistaken for neonatal sepsis. The usual lesions implicated are the critical left-sided outflow tract obstructions such as critical aortic stenosis (AS), hypoplastic left heart syndrome (HLHS), critical coarctation and interrupted aortic arch, which all represent duct-dependent systemic circulations. These are also the most commonly missed critical CHD diagnoses. In critical AS and HLHS the R to L PDA flow provides all the systemic perfusion and in the arch obstructions provides flow to the lower body causing differential cyanosis (pink arms and blue feet). However, this sign is less prominent or absent if there is intracardiac mixing of systemic and pulmonary venous blood (e.g. coexistent large ASD or VSD). Important, and often missed (suggesting an arch obstruction), are discrepant pulses (as in the above scenario) and blood pressure (lower limb blood pressure less than that of upper limb, or even undetectable). Radiofemoral delay is impossible to detect at the fast heart rates of neonates—rather examine for diminished volume or absent pulses. The above neonate likely has a critical aortic arch obstruction with acute loss of lower body perfusion causing shock and metabolic acidosis after spontaneous ductal closure on day 5–6 (preserved brain perfusion, hence alert). He needs resuscitation as follows:

#### Management

- Arrange urgent admission to ICU and do not delay treatment.
- Again open the PDA ASAP. Prostaglandin therapy as above for duct-dependent pulmonary circulation. Note that oral PGE2 may be less reliable as gut absorption may be compromised in this setting. However, oral PGE2 must be started if IV PGE1 is not available.
- Blood volume expansion—0.9% saline in 5–10 ml/kg aliquots, monitoring liver size, to assist opening the PDA and improving systemic perfusion (baby also likely to be hypovolemic with poor feeding and vomiting).
- The rest of the resuscitation and stabilisation would be similar to the above approach for cyanosis, e.g. inotropes (especially if coexistent LV dysfunction), oxygen to achieve preductal saturations (>85% in this case), and often mechanical ventilation.
- It is important to check for and manage end-organ damage such as renal failure, liver dysfunction and gut ischemia/necrotising enterocolitis as per routine ICU protocols.
- Transfer to tertiary centre for definitive management—confirmation of diagnosis by echocardiography and, usually, primary surgical repair of the arch obstruction.

### Tachyarrhythmias

The most common neonatal tachyarrhythmias (excluding sinus tachycardia which usually does not exceed 220/min) are atrioventricular re-entry tachycardia (AVRT) (associated with an accessory AV pathway) followed by atrial flutter. Less likely causes include AV node re-entry tachycardia, ectopic and multifocal atrial tachycardia and junctional tachycardias. Note that these are all narrow QRS complex tachycardias. Wide complex tachycardias are less commonly seen and, as for older children, merit urgent consultation with a pediatric cardiologist. They are best regarded and treated as ventricular tachycardia rather than SVTs with aberrant conduction. You decide to administer adenosine. This has only a very transient effect slowing the rate to about 130/min—after a few seconds the rate is again 280/min.

### Management

- *Atrial flutter:* Adenosine is not effective. The treatment of choice is synchronised DC cardioversion—as little as 0.5 J/kg is often enough to cardiovert to sinus rhythm. Ensure that pediatric paddles are used with adequate electrode jelly and the correct application front and back of the chest for a neonate. Remember to sedate the baby for comfort.
- *AVRT:* Similar approach as for older children—if shocked, initial attempt at vagal manoeuvre and, if unsuccessful, progress immediately to synchronised DC cardioversion 1 J/kg, then 2 J/kg if no response or adenosine, whichever is quicker to administer. The starting dose of adenosine for neonates is 150 μg/kg rapid IV bolus; if no response, increase by 50 μg/kg every 2 minutes to a maximum single dose of 300 μg/kg. 'Wide complex tachycardia (probable VT); synchronised DC cardioversion 1 J/kg, then 2 J/kg if no response (sedate if conscious without delaying cardioversion).' Treat any aggravating and reversible factors, e.g. hypoglycemia, electrolyte imbalance, acidosis.
- It is good practice to record the tachyarrythmia on a 12-lead ECG as well as a rhythm strip before and during any therapy (cardioversion or adenosine as in the above case) so that the rhythm can be analysed by a cardiologist.
- If still no response, consult a pediatric cardiologist and refer to a tertiary centre (options include amiodarone, digoxin or propranolol, depending on the diagnosis) (Tables 35.3 and 35.4).

### Bradyarrhythmias

The commonest cause of bradycardia in the neonate (defined as a heart rate <75b/min) is congenital complete heart block. It is often associated with maternal lupus erythematosus or other connective tissue diseases (which are often asymptomatic in the mother). Less commonly, cases may be isolated or associated with CHD.

**Table 35.3:** Dosage, advantages, and side effects of drugs used for treatment of AF

| Drug | Adult dosage | Advantages | Side effects |
|---|---|---|---|
| Esmolol | 500 μg/kg over 1 min then 0.05–0.2 mg/kg/min | Short-acting effect and short duration | Might worsen congestive heart failure; can cause bronchospasm, hypotension; AVB |
| Atenolol | 1–5 mg IV over 5 min repeat after 10 min then 50–100 mg b.i.d. PO | Rapid onset of rate control (IV) | |
| Metoprolol | 1–5 mg IV over 2 min then 50–100 mg b.i.d. PO | Rapid onset of rate control (IV) | |
| Digoxin | 0.25–10 mg IV then 0.125–0.5 mg/day IV/PO | Can be used in heart failure | Nausea, AVB moderate effect in POAF |
| Verapamil | 2.5–10 mg IV over 2 min then 80–12 mg/day b.i.d. PO | Short-acting effect | Might worsen congestive heart failure, AVB |
| Amiodarone | 2.5–5 mg/kg IV over 20 min then 15 mg/kg or 1.2 g over 24 h | Can be used in patients with severe LV dysfunction | Thyroid and hepatic dysfunction, torsades de pointers, pulmonary fibrosis, photosensitivity and bradycardia |
| Procainamide | 10–15 mg/kg IV up to 50 mg/min | Therapeutic levels quickly achieved | Hypotension, fever, accumulates in renal failure, can worsen heart failure, requires drug level monitoring |
| Ibutilide | 1 mg IV over 10 min, can repeat after 10 min if no effect | Easy to use | Torsades de pointes more frequent than amiodarone and procainamide |

IV=intravenous; LV=left ventricular; AVB=atrioventricular block; b.i.d.=twice daily; PO=by mouth

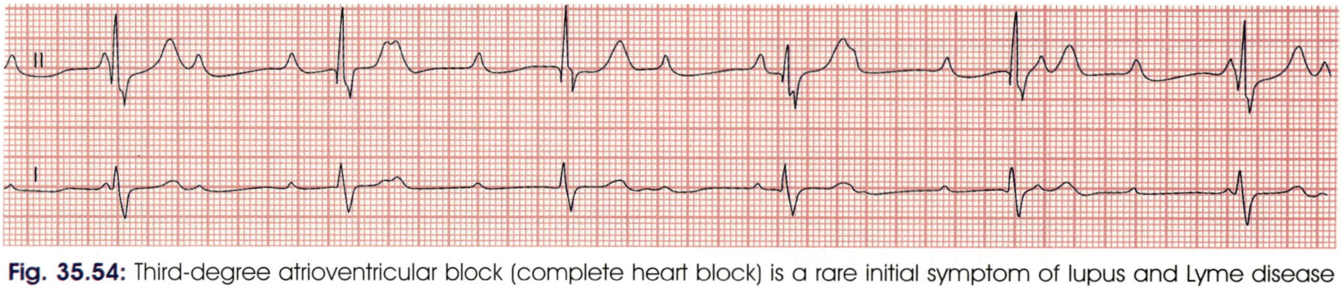


**Fig. 35.54:** Third-degree atrioventricular block (complete heart block) is a rare initial symptom of lupus and Lyme disease

**Table 35.4:** Dosage, therapeutic level and effect, and adverse effect of drugs used for treatment of cardiac arrhythmias

| Condition and drug | Dose range | Therapeutic level and effect | Adverse effects |
|---|---|---|---|
| **Atrial flutter** | | | |
| Digoxin | LD 1,200 µg per 24 h IV in 3 divided doses; MD 375–750 µg daily PO in two equal daily doses | 0.7–2.0 µg/ml<br>Mild nausea, fatigue and sinus bradycardia, first-degree atrioventricular block, rare noctural | Severe nausea and/or vomiting, severe sinus bradycardia or atrioventricular block, maternal and fetal proarrhythmia |
| Sotalol | 160–480 mg daily in two equal daily doses or every 8 h PO | Wenchebach atrioventricular block | Nausea and/or vomiting, dizziness, fatigue, bundle branch block and maternal and/or fetal proarrhythmia |
| **Supraventicular tachycardia*** | | | |
| Recalinide† | 100–300 mg daily in equal doses given every 8 h PO | 0.7–2.8 µg/ml<br>Maternal and/or fetal sinus bradycardia, first-degree atrioventricular block, P and QRS widening, QT prolongation | Nausea and/or vomiting maternal and/or fetal thyroid dysfunction, photosensitivity rash, thrombocytopenia, bundle branch block, proarrhythmia, torsades de pointes in fetuses with long QT syndrome |
| Amiodarone† | LD 1,800–2,400 mg daily in equal doses given every 6 h for 48 h; MD 200–600 mg daily PO | | |
| Procalnomide† | LD 500–600 mg over 20 min IV; MD 2–6 mg/min IV Initially 1,250 mg, followed in 1 h by 750 mg, then 250–1,000 mg every 3–6 h PO | 4–10 µg/ml<br>Uterine irritability, QT prolongation | Nausea and/or vomiting, hypotension proarrhythmia, blood dyscrasias |
| **Ventricular tachycardia†** | | | |
| Magnesium sulfate | LD 2–4 g IV followed by 1–2 g/h IV | 1.5–3.0 mmol/L | Fatigue, central nervous system symptoms, stop for loss of patellar reflex at levels of 3.5–5.0 mmol/L, cardiac arrhymias at high levels |
| Lidocaine | LD 1.0–1.5 mg/kg IV followed by 1–2 g/h IV | 1.5–5.0 µg/ml | Central nervous system symptoms |
| Proprandol | 40–80 mg every 8 h PO | NA<br>Increased uterine tone, bronchoconstriction | Fetigue, bradycardia and hypotension |
| Deamethasone | LD 4–8 mg PO; MD 4 mg daily | NA<br>Fluid retention | Similar to other corticosteroids. Short-term use preferred, fetal growth restriction |
| Sotalol | 160–480 mg daily in two equal daily doses or every 8 h PO | NA<br>Bradycardia, first-degree atrioventricular block, P and QRS widening QT prolongation | Nausea and/or vomiting, dizziness, fatigue, bundle branch block, maternal and/or fetal proarrhythmia |

*Sotalol or digoxin dose as for atrial flutter are also commonly used to treat supraventricular tachycardia.
†These doses of amiodarone, flocatrindo and procalnamide can be used to treat either ventricular or supraventricular tachycardias (IV=Intravenous; IVCD=Intraventricular conduction delay; LD=Loading dose; MD=Maintenance dose; PO=Oral.

### *Acute management*

- The majority of neonates (with heart rates above 50–55 bpm) will be asymptomatic with good cardiac output and hence will not require immediate treatment—they may be referred, on the same admission, to a pediatric cardiologist for exclusion of structural heart disease and ongoing observation.
- If the neonate is symptomatic (signs of heart failure or cardiogenic shock), treat as for the older child—positive chronotropes (atropine, adrenaline or isoprenaline), blood volume expansion and temporary pacing under sedation (transcutaneous or trans-oesophageal).
- Eventually all patients will require permanent cardiac pacing but this can often be delayed for years in the stable patient.

## Acute Congestive Heart Failure

Many of the critical CHDs as well as the arrhythmias can present with acute heart failure (HF). The important point is to differentiate HF from respiratory distress due to lung disease or neonatal sepsis –as in older children, useful clues for HF are cardiomegaly and hepatomegaly.

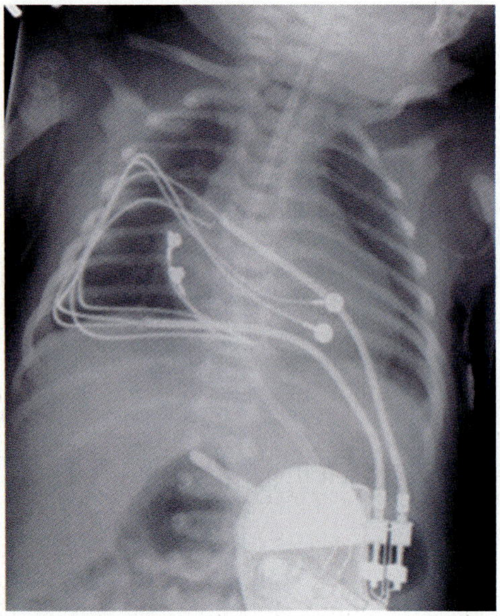

**Fig. 35.55:** A baby girl was born prematurely at 34 weeks, weighing 1.5 kg. The baby was diagnosed with a complete heart block in the 28th week of mothers pregnancy. The baby had a permanent pacemaker during 20th minute of her life. This is considered as the worlds smallest baby to receive a permanent cardiac pacemaker on 5th, march 2015 in Mumbai

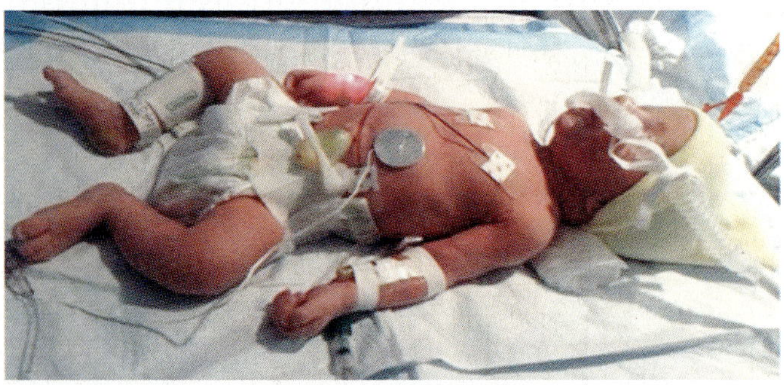

**Fig. 35.56:** A newborn lying on the cot fitted with monitoring and resuscitative equipments for the management of heart failure

*Management*

- Nonpharmacological measures, e.g. fluid restriction, nutritional support, oxygen and ventilatory support as indicated, correct aggravating factors such as anemia or sepsis.
- Diuretics, usually furosemide 0.5–1 mg/kg 8–12-hourly IV or orally with spironolactone 1 mg/kg 12-hourly per mouth.
- ACE inhibitors are generally contraindicated in neonates (high risk of severe hypotension and renal failure).
- Inotropes/vasodilators such as dobutamine may be indicated in severe HF.
- Refer to tertiary pediatric cardiac centre (on the same admission) for definitive management. The above-described neonate is found to have truncus arteriosus and proceeds to full surgical repair after 5 days of stabilisation on antifailure treatment as above.

### Treatment of Hydrops Fetalis

Treatment depends on the cause. During pregnancy, treatment may include:

- Medicine to cause early labor and delivery of the baby
- Early cesarean delivery if condition gets worse
- Intrauterine fetal blood transfusion
- Treatment for a newborn may include:
  - Direct transfusion of packed red blood cells (compatible with the infant's blood type) and an exchange transfusion to rid the baby's body of the substances that are destroying the red blood cells.
  - Needle aspiration to remove extra fluid from around the lungs and belly area
  - Medicines to control congestive heart failure and help the kidneys remove extra fluids
  - Methods to help the baby breathe, such as a breathing machine (Prognosis)
  - Hydrops fetalis often results in death of the infant shortly before or after delivery. The risk is highest among the most premature babies and those who are severely ill at birth.
- Possible complications
  - A form of central nervous system damage called kernicterus may occur.
- Prevention
  - Rh incompatibility, which can lead to this condition, can be prevented if the mother takes a medicine called RhoGAM at certain times during and after pregnancy.

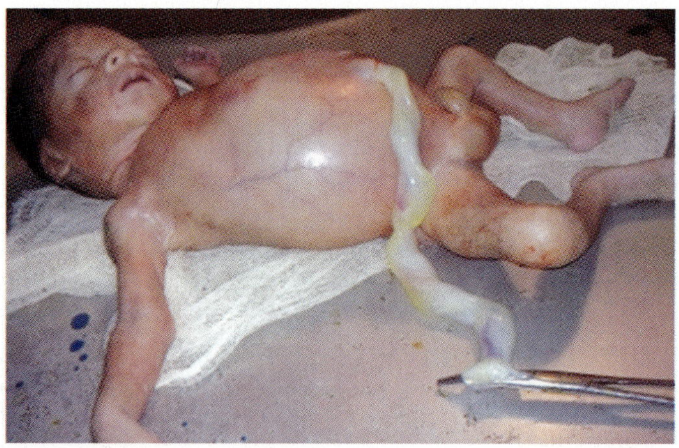

**Fig. 35.57:** Generalized edema of the body, ascites, hepatomegaly, jaundice, severe anemia and heart failure

## SUMMARY

The practitioner faced with an acutely ill neonate needs to have a high index of suspicion for a cardiac aetiology. Obvious clues would include all of the above presentations. A thorough cardiovascular examination should always be undertaken—without delaying emergency care—including a hyperoxia test in the cyanosed neonate, a check for discrepant pulses and blood pressures, and differential cyanosis. A chest X-ray and 12-lead ECG are essential firstline investigations to narrow the differential diagnosis. Immediate stabilisation as outlined above, followed by prompt referral to a tertiary centre, provides the best opportunity to minimise morbidity and mortality.

## BIBLIOGRAPHY


1. Atz AM, Feinstein JA, Jonas RA. Preoperative management of pulmonary venous hypertension in hypoplastic left heart syndrome with restrictive atrial septal defect. Am J Cardiol 1999;83:1224–8.
2. Baba K, Ohtsuki S, Kamada M, Kataoka K, Ohno N, Okamoto Y, et al. Preoperative management for tricuspid regurgitation in hypoplastic left heart syndrome. Ped Internat 2009;51:399–404.
3. Bahrami KR, Van Meurs KP. ECMO for neonatal respiratory failure. Semin Perinatol 2005;29(1):15–23.
4. Behrman RE, Kliegman RM, Jenson HB. Nelson Textbook of Pediatrics 17th ed. Philadelphia: WB Sauders, 2004.
5. Chambers CD, Hernandez-Diaz S, Van Marter LJ, Werler MM, Louik C, Jones KL, et al. Selective serotonin-reuptake inhibitors and risk of persistent pulmonary hypertension of the newborn. N Engl J Med 2006;354(6):579–87.
6. Dorfman AT, Marino BS, Wernovsky G, Tabbutt S, Ravishankar C, Godinez RI, et al. Critical heart disease in the neonate: Presentation and outcome at a tertiary care center. Pediatr Crit Care Med 2008;9:193–202.
7. Farrow KN, Fliman P, Steinhorn RH. The diseases treated with ECMO: focus on PPHN. Semin Perinatol 2005;29(1):8–14.
8. Fricker FJ. Hypoplastic Left Heart Syndrome – Diagnosis and early management. Neo Reviews 2008;9:253.
9. Gomella TL. Neonatology: Management, Procedures, On-Call Problems. Diseases, and Drugs 4th ed. Appleton & Lange; 1999.
10. Hoffmann GM, Ghanayem NS, Kampine JM, Berger S, Mussatto KA, Litwin SB, et al. Venous saturation and the anaerobic threshold in neonates after the Norwood procedure for hypoplastic left heart syndrome. Ann Thorac Surg 2000;70:1515–21.
11. Konduri GG, Solimano A, Sokol GM, Singer J, Ehrenkranz RA, Singhal N, et al. A randomized trial of early versus standard inhaled nitric oxide therapy in term and near-term newborn infants with hypoxic respiratory failure. Pediatrics 2004;113(3 Pt 1):559–64.
12. Lewis AB, Freed MD, Heymann MA, Roehl SL, Kensey RC. Side effects of therapy with prostaglandin E1 in infants with critical congenital heart disease. Circulation 1981;64:893–898.
13. Metra M, Giubbini R, Nodari S, et al. Differential effects of beta-blockers in patients with heart failure: A prospective, randomized, double-blind comparison of the long-term effects of metoprolol versus carvedilol. Circulation 2000; 102(5):546–51.
14. Miller SP, McQuillen PS, Hamrick S, Xu D, Glidden DV, Charlton N. Abnormal brain development in newborns with congenital heart disease. N Engl J Med 2007;357:1928–38.
15. Newburger JW, Jonas RA, Wernovsky G. A comparison of the preoperative neurologic effects of hypothermic circulatory arrest versus low-flow cardiopulmonary bypass in infant heart surgery. N Engl J Med 1993;329:1057–64.
16. Pawlik TD, Porta NF, Steinhorn RH, Ogata E, deRegnier RA. Medical and financial impact of a neonatal extracorporeal membrane oxygenation referral center in the nitric oxide era. Pediatrics 2009;123(1):e17–24.
17. Rosenthal D, Chrisant MR, Edens E, et al. International Society for Heart and Lung Transplantation: Practice guide-lines for management of heart failure in children. J Heart Lung Transplant 2004;23(12):1313–33.
18. Rychik J, Rome JJ, Collins MH, DeCampli WM, Spray TL. The hypoplastic left heart syndrome with intact atrial septum: atrial morphology, pulmonary vascular histopathology and outcome. J Am Coll Cardiol 1999;34: 554–60.
19. Senka Mesihoviæ- Dinareviæ. Djeèija kardiologija: od fetusa do adolescenta. Medicinski fakultet, Sarajevo; 2000.
20. Shaddy RE, Tani LY, Gidding SS, et al. Beta-blocker treatment of dilated cardiomyopathy with congestive heart failure in children: a multi-institutional experience. J Heart Lung Transplant 1999;18:269–74.
21. Shaddy RE. Optimizing treatment for chronic congestive heart failure in children. Crit Care Med 2001;29(10 Suppl): S237–40.
22. Shah PS, Ohlsson A. Sildenafil for pulmonary hypertension in neonates. Cochrane Database Syst Rev 2011; CD005494.
23. Singh GH, Fong LV, Salmon AP, Keeton BR. Study of low dosage prostaglandin–usages and complication. Eur Heart J 1994;15:377–81.
24. Steinhorn RH, Kinsella JP, Pierce C, Butrous G, Dilleen M, Oakes M, et al. Intravenous sildenafil in the treatment of neonates with persistent pulmonary hypertension. J Pediatr 2009;155(6):841–7.
25. Steinhorn RH. Nitric oxide and beyond: new insights and therapies for pulmonary hypertension. J Perinatol 2008;28 Suppl 3:S67–71.
26. Tabbutt S, Nord AS, Jarvik GP. Neurodevelopmental outcomes after staged palliation for hypoplastic left heart syndrome. Pediatrics 2008;121:476–83.
27. Taketomo CK, Hurlburt-Hodding J, Kraus DM. Pediatric drug handbook, 1997–1998.
28. Thiebaud B, Michelakis E, Wu XC, Harry G, Hashimoto K, Archer SL. Sildenafil Reverses $O_2$ constriction of the rabbit Ductus Arteriosus by inhibiting Type 5 phosphodisesterase and activating BK Ca Channels. Ped Res 2002;52:19–24.
29. UK collaborative randomised trial of neonatal extracorporeal membrane oxygenation. UK Collaborative ECMO Trail Group. Lancet 1996;348(9020):75–82.
30. Walsh-Sukys MC, Tyson JE, Wright LL, Bauer CR, Korones SB, Stevenson DK, et al. Persistent pulmonary hypertension of the newborn in the era before nitric oxide: practice varia-tion and outcomes. Pediatrics 2000;105(1 Pt 1):14–20.
31. Wung JT, James LS, Kilchevsky E, James E. Management of infants with severe respiratory failure and persistence of the fetal circulation, without hyperventilation. Pediatrics 1985; 76(4):488–94.

# 36 Fetal Cardiac Emergent Interventions (An Overview)

The potential benefits of fetal cardiac intervention (FCI) have been realized for many years. In 1975, Eibschitz et al. reported intrapartum treatment of fetal ventricular tachycardia by administering propranolol to the mother, and as early as 1986, in-utero pacing was attempted for complete heart block in a human fetus. Recently, however, interest in FCI has accelerated. As with other fetal interventions, FCI can only become a highly useful clinical tool if it is applied to conditions in which a feasible mode of therapy is available and either the fetus is at risk for demise as a result of the condition or intervention may alter the evolution of the condition such that the severity of the postnatal disease is substantially reduced. For conditions in which the fetus is at high risk for prenatal or neonatal death, the rationale for FCI is obvious, to improve survival. If death is not imminent but the disease is likely to have major life-long morbidity, the rationale is that FCI will modify the course of cardiac growth, function, and/or development in-utero sufficiently to alter postnatal outcome and justify the potential risks of the procedure. Prenatal intervention may also allow the fetus to recover in the supportive in-utero environment, during a developmental period when there is enhanced wound healing and the capacity for myocyte proliferation (Figs 36.1–36.3).

This construct rightfully emphasizes death or significant morbidity as therapeutic targets. FCI can entail substantial short-term risk to the fetus, uncertain long-term risk to the fetus and child, and at least some risk to the mother. There are no known medical benefits to the mother. With that risk profile, FCI will not be embraced by the maternal-fetal medicine and cardiology communities unless it is used to treat serious conditions in which the potential benefits to the fetus are high and can be achieved in a reasonable percentage of cases.

Although many recent publications have dealt with closed, 'minimally invasive' FCI, there is a considerable body of evidence regarding pharmacological and surgical FCI as well. This review will touch on all of these topics, with a focus on the most recent literature.

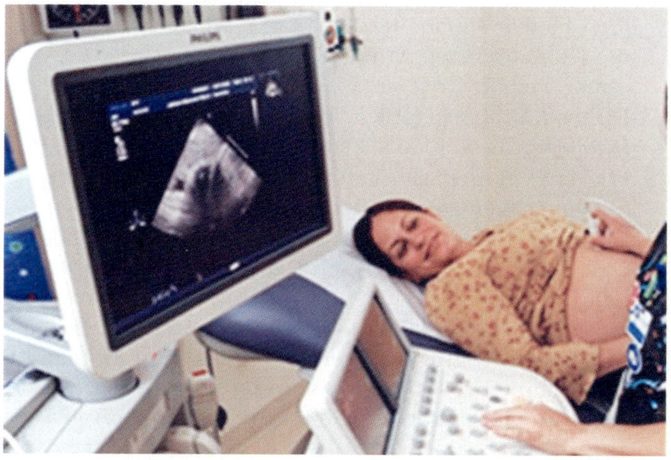

**Fig. 36.1:** Doctor performing foetal echocardiography

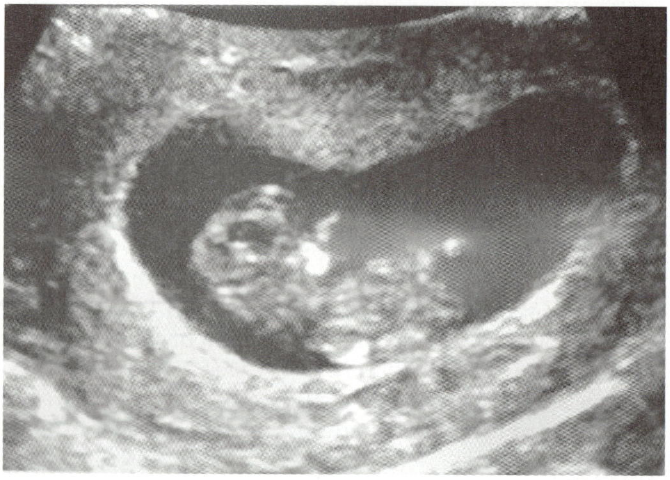

**Fig. 36.2:** Abdominal ultrasound showing viable intrauterine 10 weeks old foetus

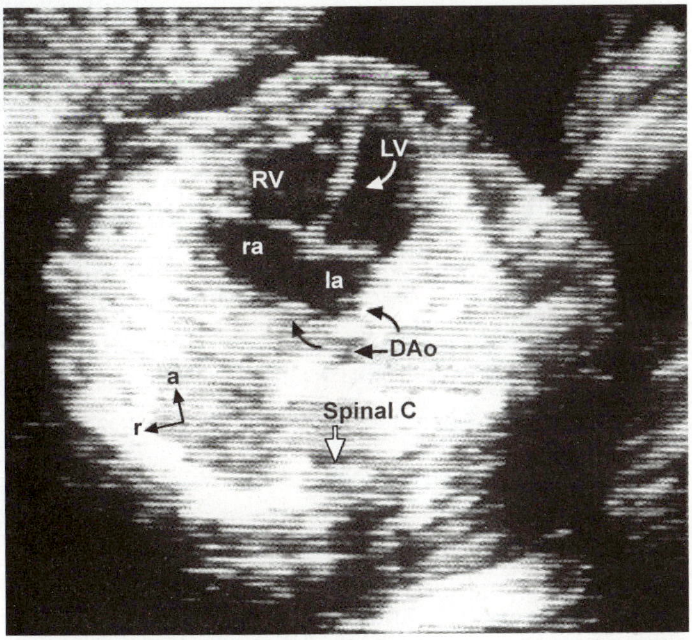


**Fig. 36.3:** Fetal echocardiography showing well formed four chambers of the heart with concordant A–V valves communicating through their respective chambers

## FETOSCOPIC AND ULTRASONOGRAPHIC TECHNIQUES IN FCI

These are useful not only in diagnosis of congenital heart defects in-utero but also helps in the management of critical cardiovascular disorders (Figs 36.4–36.13).

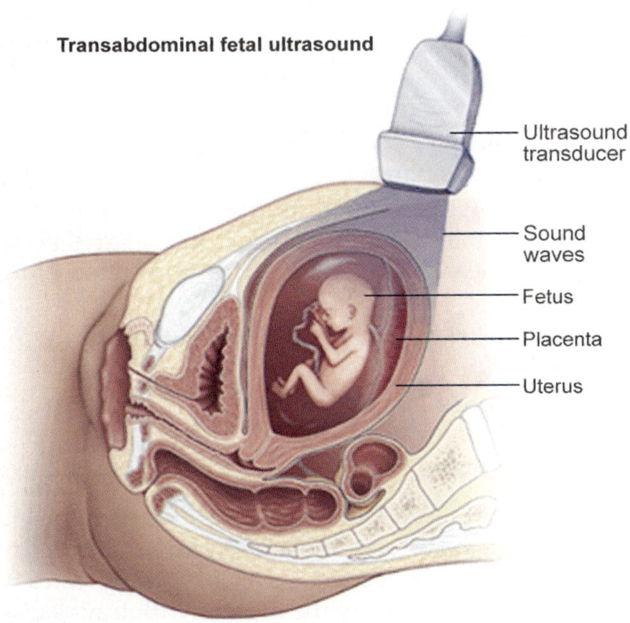


**Fig. 36.4:** Ultrasound beam striking at different parts of fetus for their identification and perfomance of selected percutaneous intervention

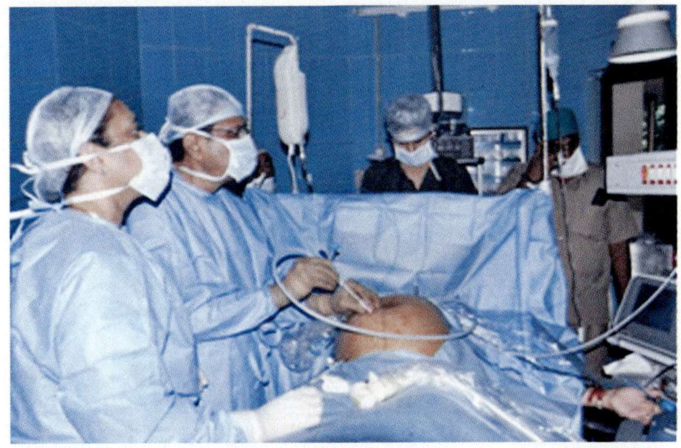

**Fig. 36.5:** A team of doctors performing fetoscopy procedure on a pregnant woman for assessment of fetal health

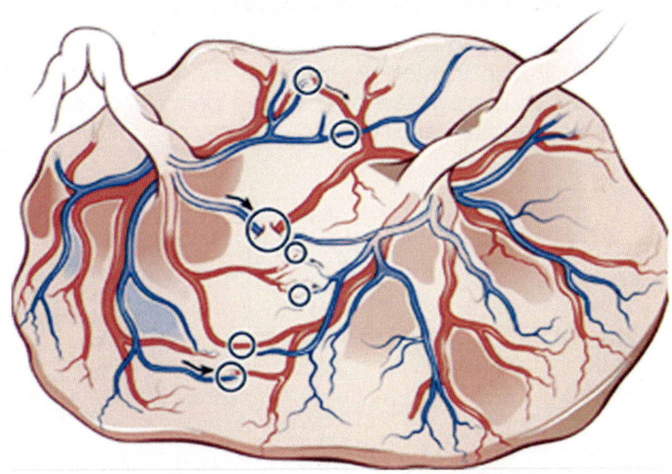

**Fig. 36.6:** Drawing of the shared placenta in twin-to-twin transfusion syndrome. Multiple vessels connect both fetuses over what is called 'anastomoses' (open circles). These anastomoses are the subject of laser coagulation

## FETAL ULTRASONOGRAPHY IN DIAGNOSIS AND MANAGEMENT OF CONGENITAL DISORDERS

(Figs 36.14–36.28)

### Fetal Visualization—Ultrasound

Ultrasound is a noninvasive procedure for imaging fetal anatomy. It is harmless to both the fetus and the mother. Ultrasound can evaluate gestational age, as well as identify twins; fetal position; placental location; fetal growth, development, and movement; and any structural birth defects. It also can assess amniotic fluid volume.

Many fetal organ systems and anatomical lesions, including some genitourinary, gastrointestinal, skeletal, and central nervous system abnormalities and congenital cardiopathies, can be visualized by ultrasound between 16–20 weeks' gestation. Using ultrasound, Romain et al. carried out prenatal detection of congenital cataract in an unborn fetus with trisomy. Aslan et al. carried out prenatal diagnosis of Neu-Laxova syndrome at 38 weeks' gestation.

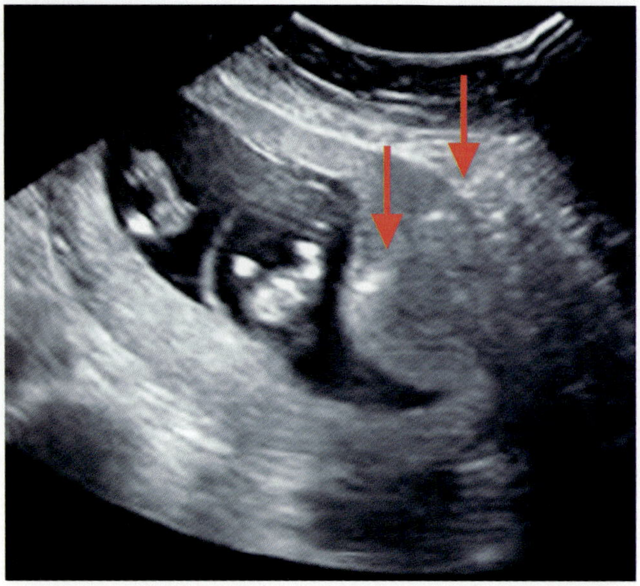

**Fig. 36.7:** Fetal skin biopsy is the optimal way to evaluate ambiguity that occasionally arises in the interpretation of amniocentesis data. These biopsies are performed without a hospital stay, and under ultrasound guidance

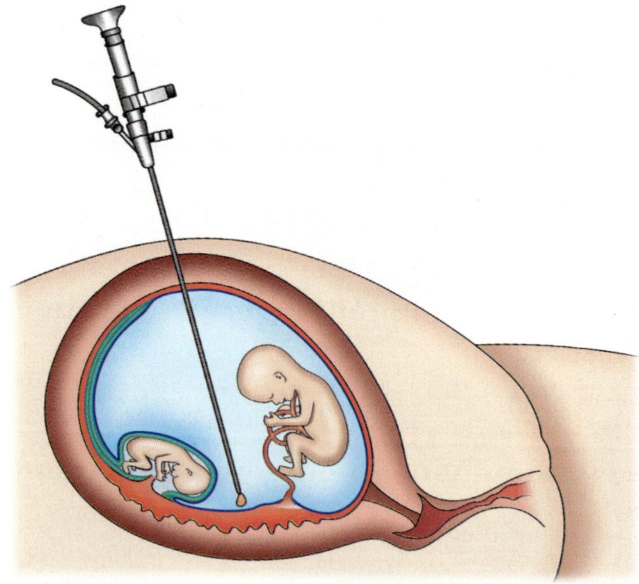

**Fig. 36.9:** A fetoscopic laser treatment. A cannula has been placed through the abdominal wall, through which a scope and laser beam has been passed. The connecting vessels are identified and subsequently destroyed

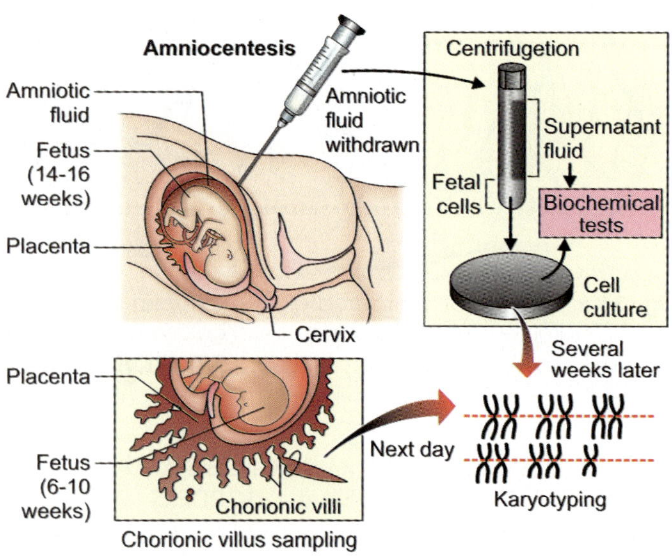


**Fig. 36.8:** The technique of amniocentesis for identification of fetal genetic disorders

Ultrasound also is used to guide invasive sampling, such as amniocentesis, CVS, cordocentesis, and various fetal biopsies.

Bernard et al. found that spina bifida may be detected early in pregnancy with biparietal diameter (BPD) on ultrasound. BPD is lower in spina bifida babies. Half of the deformities could be detected by this modality.

### Fetal Visualization—Fetal echocardiography

Fetal echocardiography can be performed at 15 weeks' gestation and beyond. When this technique is used with duplex or color flow Doppler, it can identify a number of major structural cardiac defects and rhythm disturbances. By fetal echocardiography, Saygili et al. diagnosed absent pulmonary valve syndrome in a male infant prenatally at 22 weeks' gestation. Fetal echocardiography is recommended in cases where cardiac defects are suspected, including the following:

- Identification of an extracardiac malformation on routine ultrasound
- Abnormality of another major organ system
- Suspected genetic disease or fetal chromosome abnormality associated with heart defects
- Exposure to potentially teratogenic agents
- Family history of congenital heart defects, particularly in a parent or sibling
- Maternal diseases, such as diabetes or phenylketonuria associated with fetal structural heart defects, in particular heart blocks, such as lupus or other immune disorders
- Alcohol or drug consumption by mother during pregnancy
- Maternal rubella infection during pregnancy

## PHARMACOLOGICAL FCI

The first reported and most entrenched mode of FCI is pharmacological therapy, most often for fetal arrhythmia or heart block. Pharmacological FCI typically consists of medication taken orally by the mother with transplacental passage to the fetus, but it may be provided directly through the umbilical vein or by fetal intramuscular or intravascular injection (Table 36.1).

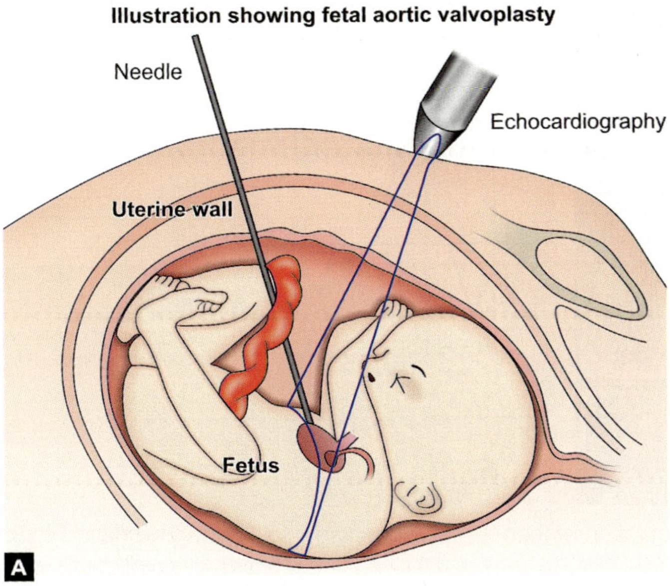


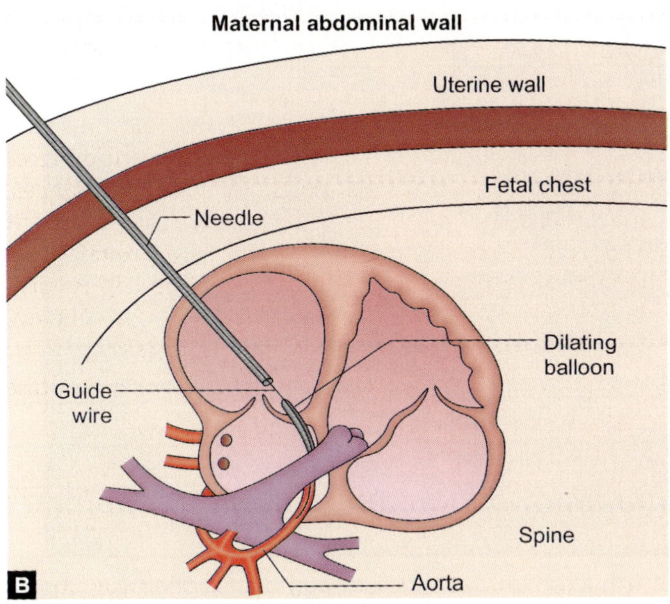


**Fig. 36.10:** (A and B) Deal fetal position and cannula course. Fetal left chest is anterior, and pathway from maternal abdomen to LV apex is unobstructed. This pathway, which corresponds to cannula course, continues from LV apex to aortic valve

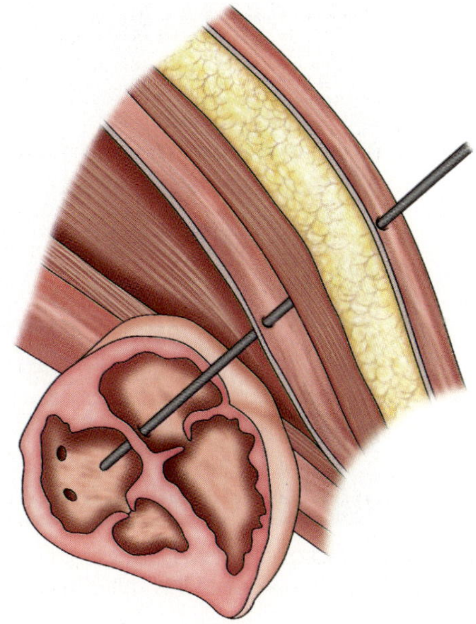

**Fig. 36.11:** Optimal fetal position and needle trajectory for atrial septoplasty. The right atrium is punctured through the fetal chest and the needle advanced through the atrial septum, which is thickened and bows tensely into the right atrium

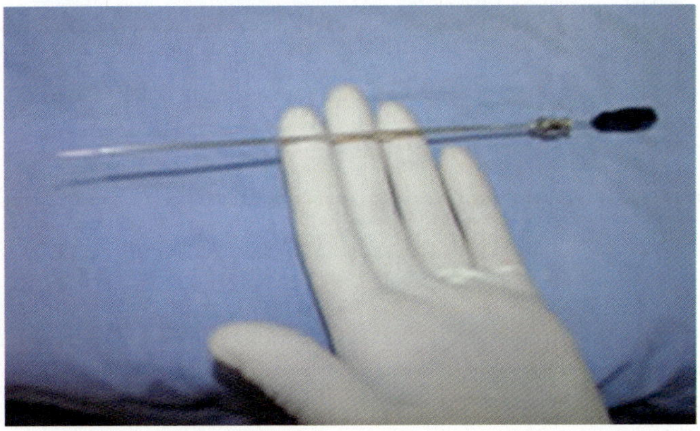

**Fig. 36.12:** Chiba needle used for fetal invasive procedures

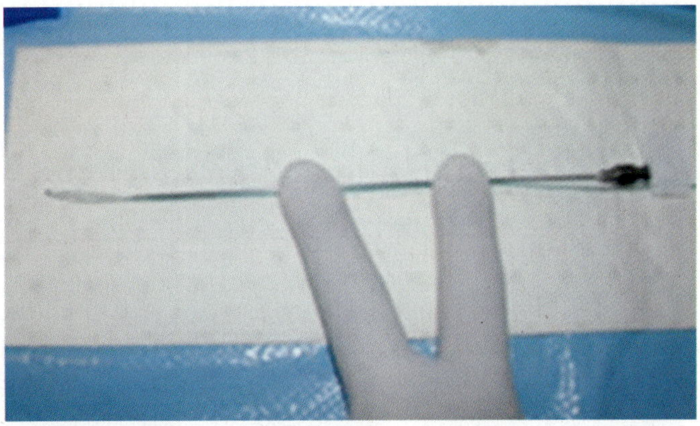

**Fig. 36.13:** Balloon angioplasty preassembled on guide that will be introduced through the needle Chiba to dilate the aortic valve

## FETAL TACHYARRHYTHMIAS

Pharmacological FCI was first described by Eibschitz et al. who treated fetal tachycardia with propranolol in 1975 (Figs 36.29–36.32). Maternal digoxin was first used to treat fetal supraventricular tachycardia several years later. Fetal supraventricular tachycardia, most often atrioventricular (AV) re-entry or atrial flutter, probably remains the most common indication for pharmacological FCI. Over the years, most antiarrhythmic agents have been used to treat fetal supraventricular tachycardia. Digoxin has been a mainstay of therapy; other agents have come io more common use recently, including sotalol, darone, and

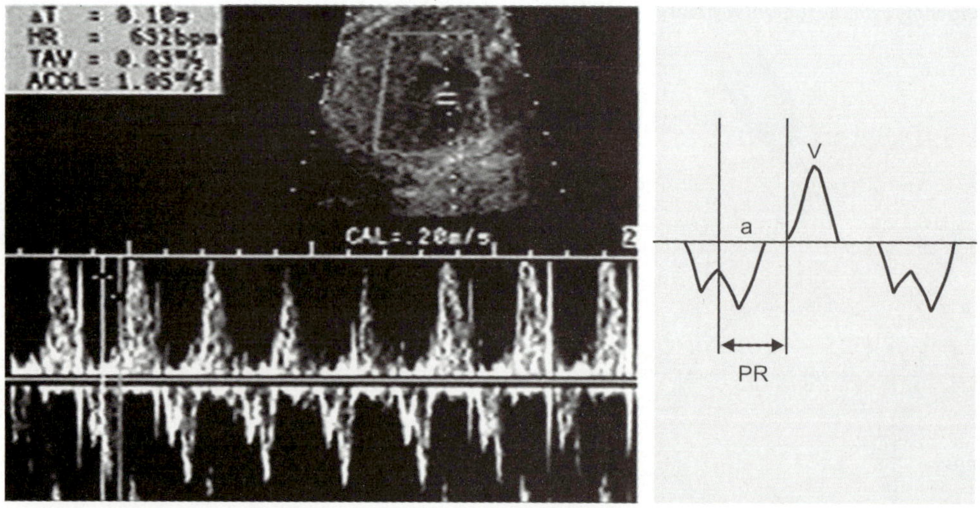


**Fig. 36.14:** Mitral valve and aortic valve Doppler in a 20-week fetus. Calculation of the PR interval to assess for first degree heart block is made measuring from the onset of the mitral a wave to the onset of the aortic outflow wave (a=mitral a wave, V=aortic outflow)

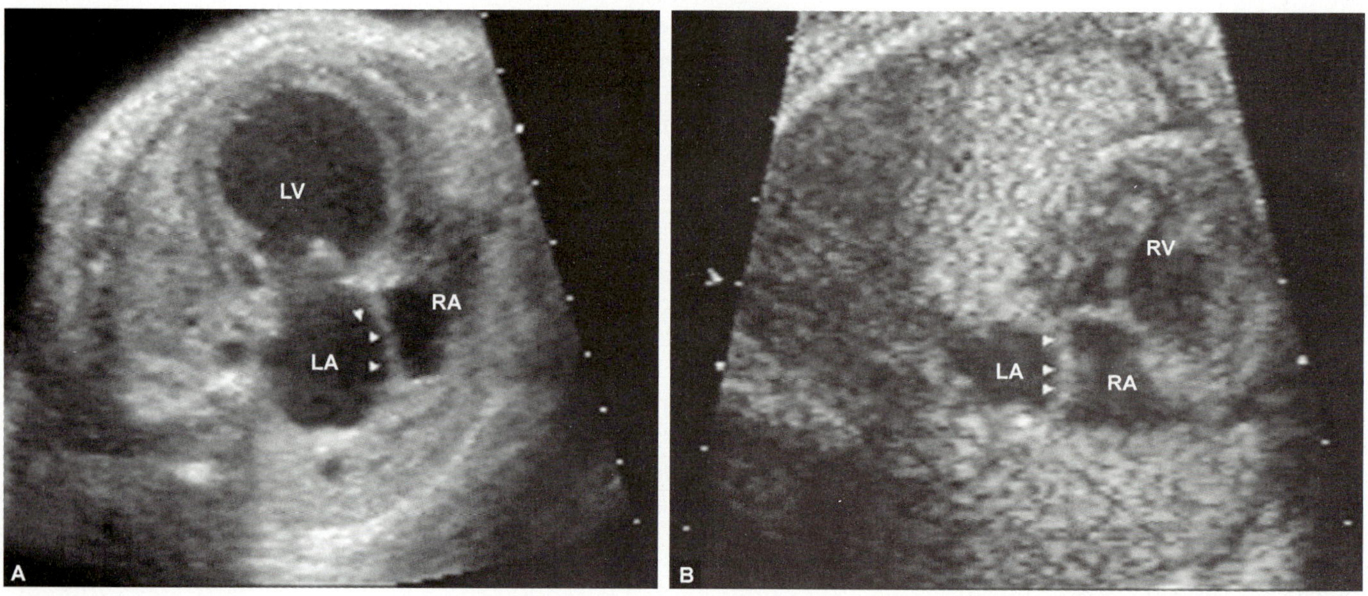


**Fig. 36.15:** Fetal echocardiographic apical view of the heart in a fetus with foramen ovale closure and ductus arteriosus closure and transposition of the great arteries (A) and in a fetus with foramen ovale closure and hypoplastic left heart syndrome (B) (RA=right atrium, RV=right ventricle, LA=left atrium, LV=left ventricle, arrows demarcate the atrial septum)

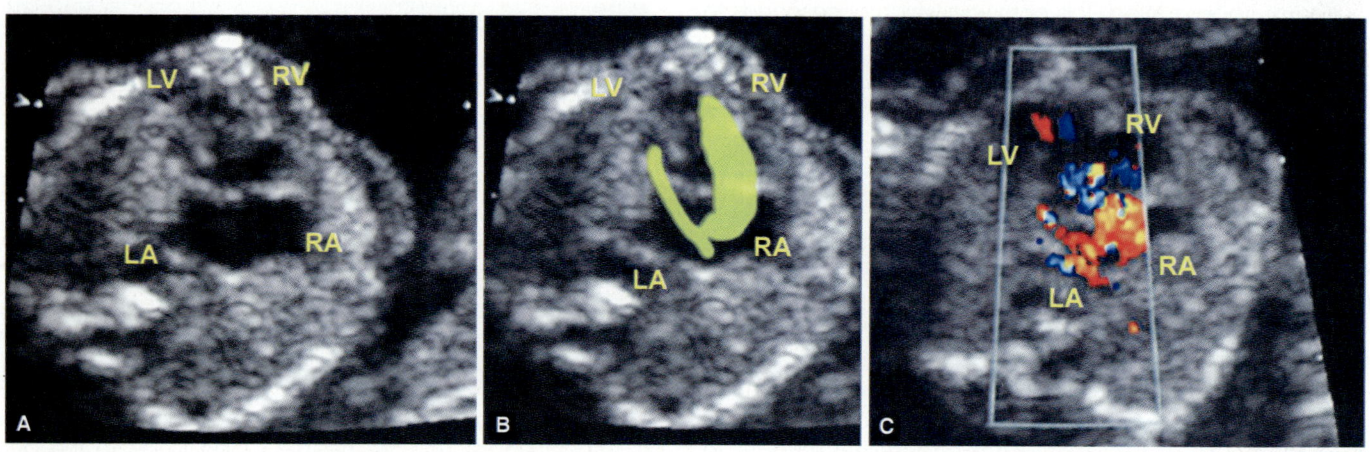


**Fig. 36.16:** (A and B) Hypoplastic left heart syndrome—the left ventricle diminutive, with color-Doppler, (C) there is an asymmetric color perfusion of the chambers

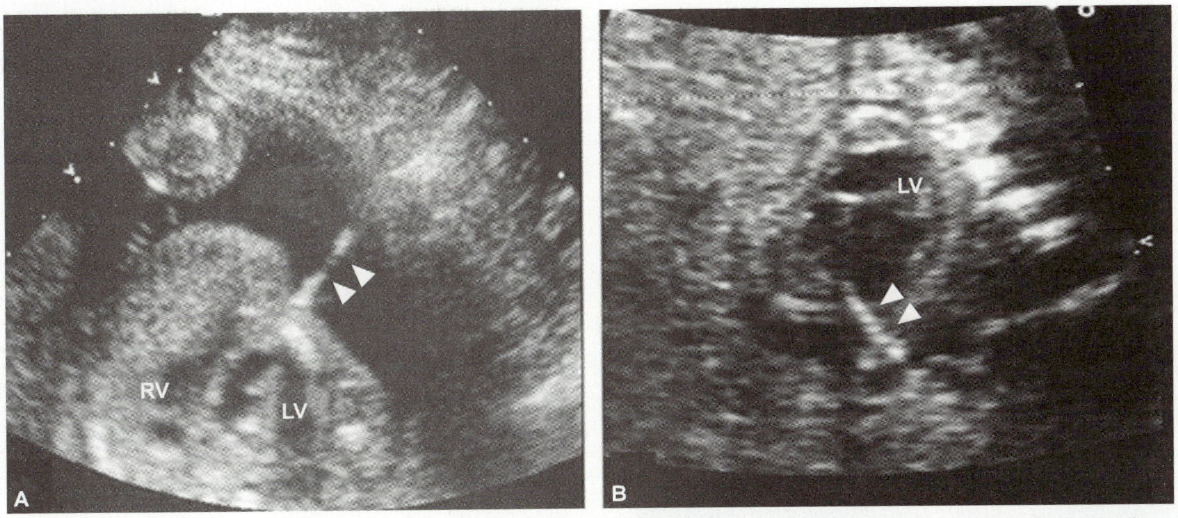


**Fig. 36.17:** Fetal echocardiographic views of aortic balloon dilation in fetuses with aortic stenosis. (A) Note the needle approaching the left ventricular apex. (B) Note the wire crossing the left ventricular outflow tract. Note the balloon being inflated at the level of the aortic valve (RV=right ventricle, LV=left ventricle, arrows demarcate needle, wire, or balloon during the procedure. Images courtesy of Dr Wayne Tworetsky from Boston Children's Hospital)

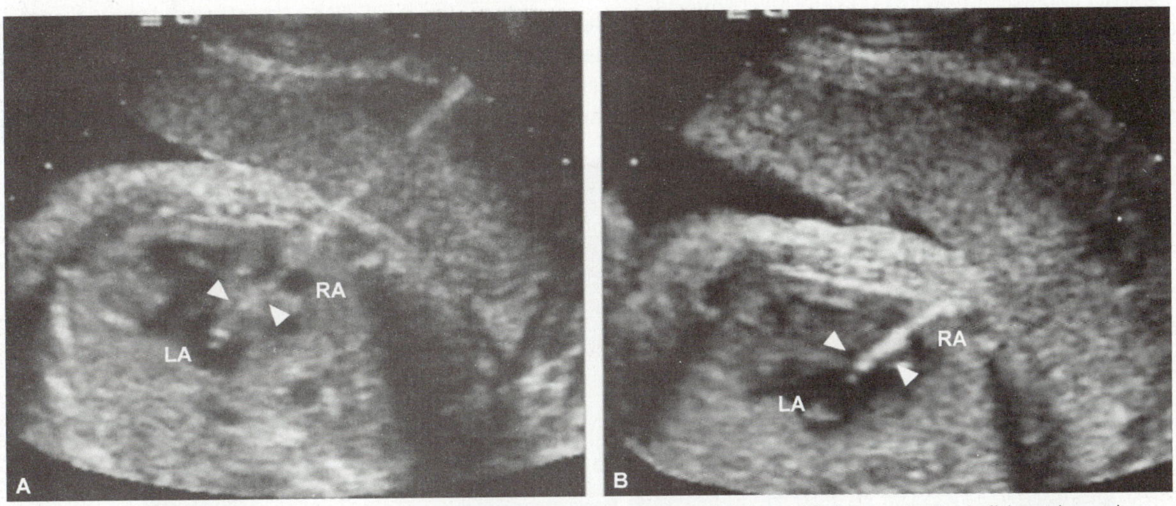


**Fig. 36.18:** Fetal echocardiographic views of an atrial septal dilation in a fetus with hypoplastic left heart syndrome and an intact atrial septum. (A) Note the needle crossing the atrial septum. (B) Note the balloon crossing the atrial septum (RA=right atrium, LA=left atrium, arrows demarcate the needle or balloon for the procedure)

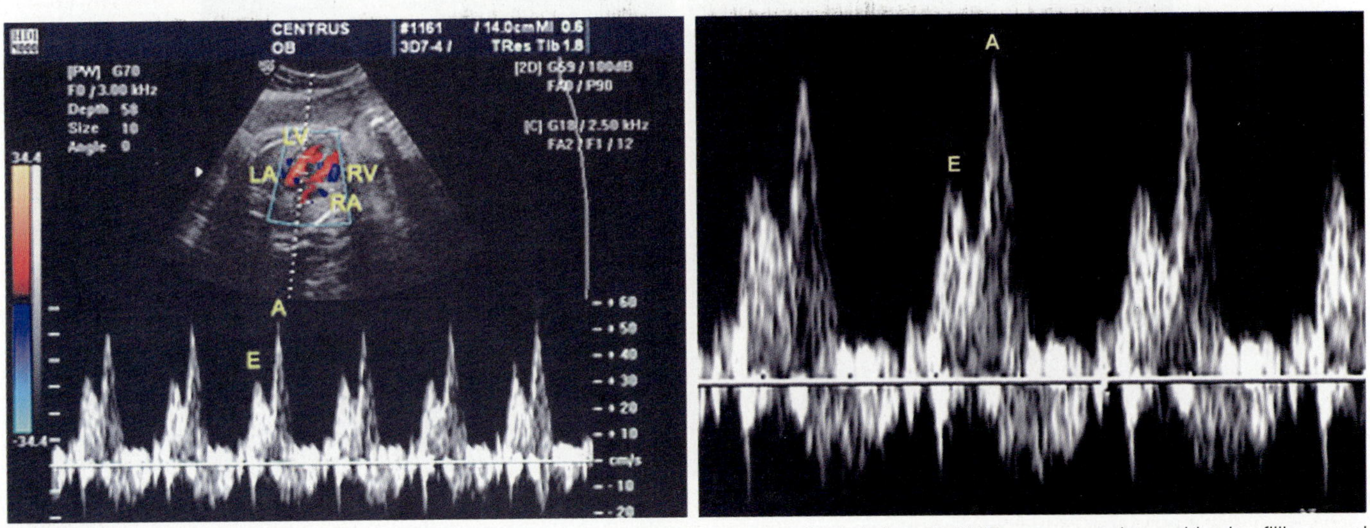


**Fig. 36.19:** Low velocity waveform across the tricuspid valve at 28 weeks of gestation (left) (E-wave=early ventricular filling and A-wave=atrial ventricular filling)

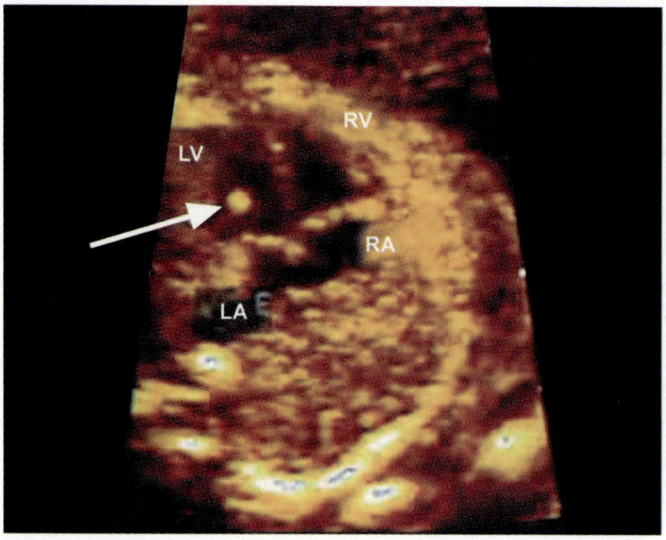


**Fig. 36.20:** Four-chamber view. Note the white arrow pointing the echogenic foci in the left ventricle. Echogenic foci are usually of no pathological significance and in more than 90% of cases the resolve by the third trimester or during pregnancy. However, they are sometimes associated with cardiac defects and chromosomal abnormalities. For isolated hyperechogenic foci the risk for trisomy 21 may be 3 times the background maternal age and gestation related risk

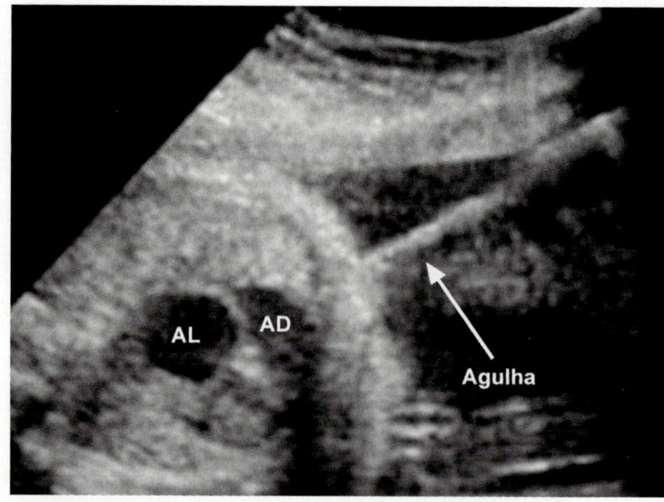


**Fig. 36.22:** Ultrasound image of fetal atrioseptostomy. The balloon is being inflated at the atrial level. Note the interatrial septum tense and bulging into the right atrium due to left atrial hypertension. AD=right atrium; AE=left atrium

flecainide. Transplacental therapy with first-line agents is usually effective in nonhydropic fetuses, but outcomes remain suboptimal, with fetal death in 10% of cases overall and a higher percentage of fetuses with hydrops.

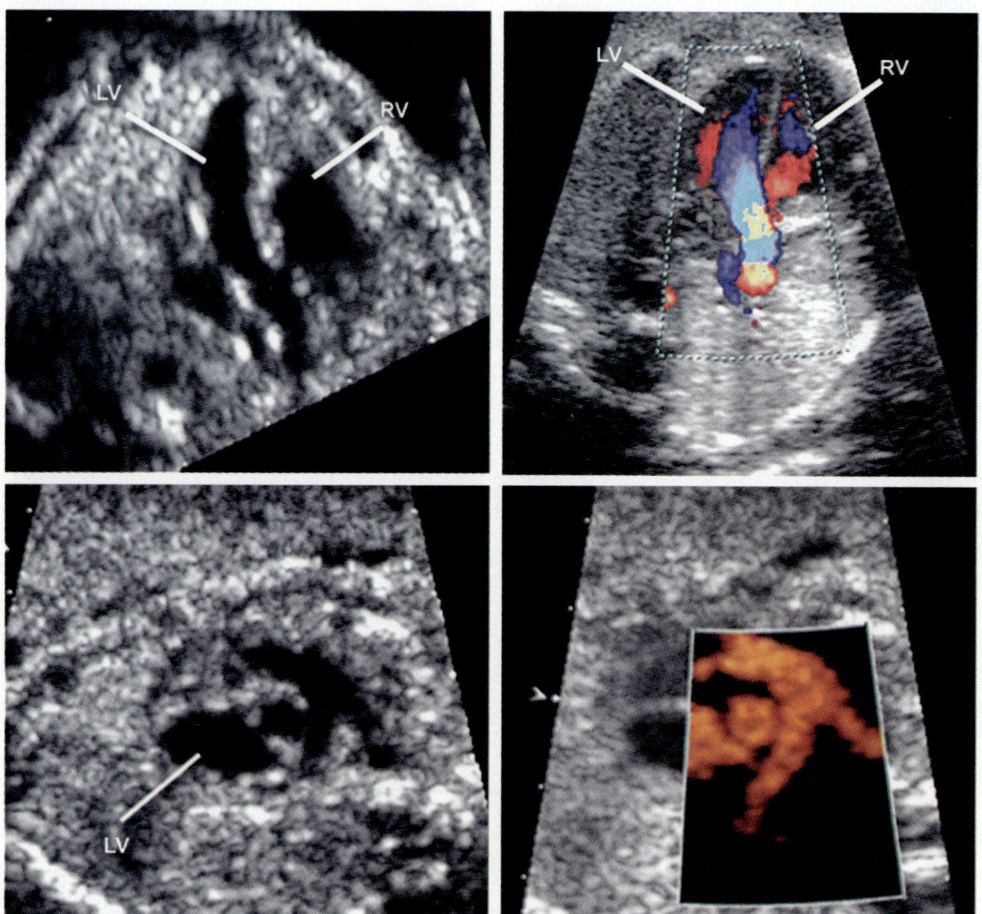


**Fig. 36.21:** Five-chamber view of the fetal heart with superimposed color-Doppler showing the aorta (blue) originating from the left ventricle (top). Short-axis view of the fetal heart with superimposed color-Doppler showing the pulmonary artery originating from the right ventricle (bottom)

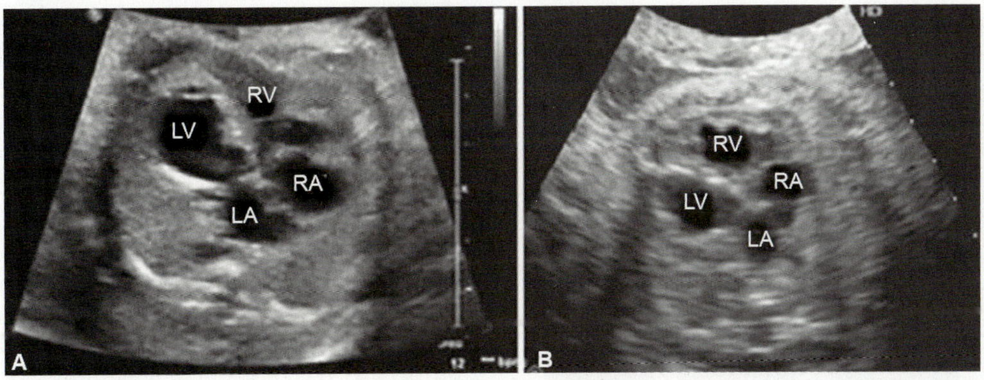


**Fig. 36.23:** Fetal echocardiogram. Fetus with critical aortic valve stenosis. (A) The left ventricle is dilated with signs of diffuse endocardial fibroelastosis, and we note a mild pericardial effusion. (B) After the valvuloplasty note a significant improvement in left ventricular dilatation has observed 3 days after the procedure. RA=right atrium; LA=left atrium; RV=right ventricle

The optimal therapeutic strategy for fetal supraventricular tachycardia has not been determined in a standardized trial, and practice varies. The indications for therapy may depend on fetal age and disease severity. When hydrops is present, pharmacological FCI may help as a bridge to delivery and postnatal treatment. In preterm fetuses, sustained tachycardia should probably be treated regardless of cardiac dysfunction or hydrops, because these sequelae can develop rapidly. For intermittent tachycardia, treatment is generally unnecessary, unless hydrops or

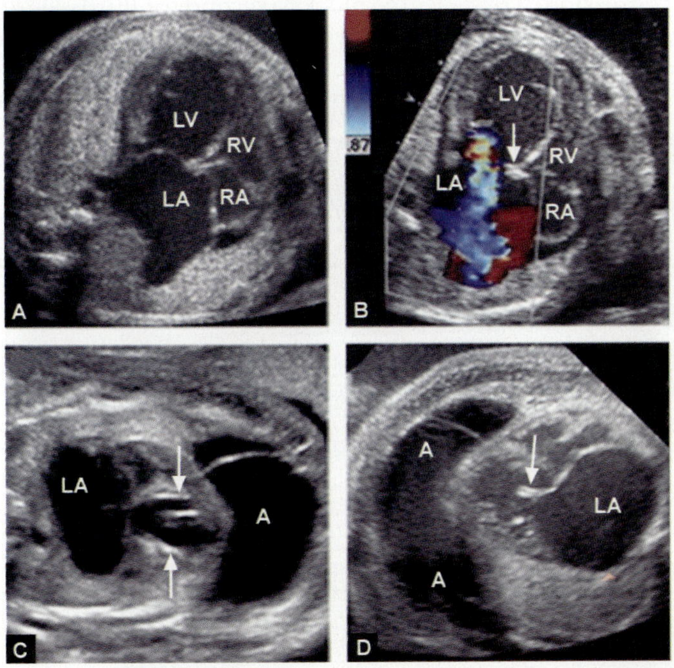


**Fig. 36.24:** Fetal echocardiogram images. (A) Fetal echocardiogram in a four-chamber view, demonstrating severe left atrial (LA) enlargement, with bowing of the atrial septum (*) into the right atrium (RA) and partial obstruction of the tricuspid valve. The right ventricle (RV) is compressed by a dilated left ventricle (LV). (B) Doppler color flow image in a four-chamber view from the same fetus demonstrating severe LA and LV enlargement, severe mitral regurgitation, and an anatomically abnormal mitral valve with an echogenic anterior leaflet (arrow). There is significant compression of the RA and RV (C and D). These oblique transverse images from a different fetus demonstrate severe LA enlargement, ascites (A), and moderate to severe LV endocardial fibroelastosis (arrows). In D, the anterior leaflet of the mitral valve (arrow) is bright and immobile

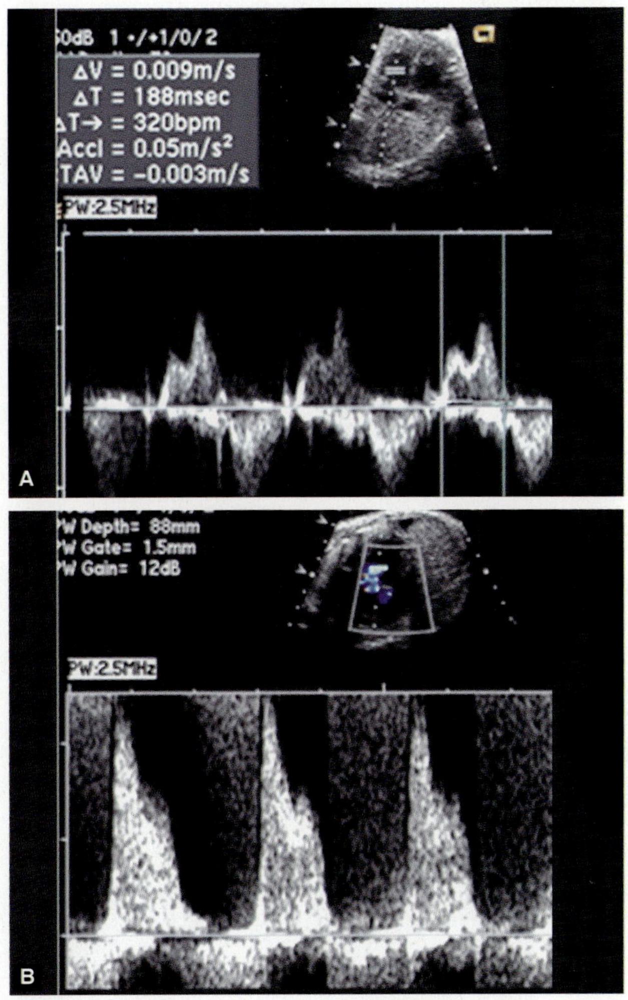


**Fig. 36.25A and B:** Mitral and tricuspid valve Doppler inflow patterns. (A) Normal mitral valve Doppler. (B) Abnormal Doppler with a partially fused mitral valve inflow pattern

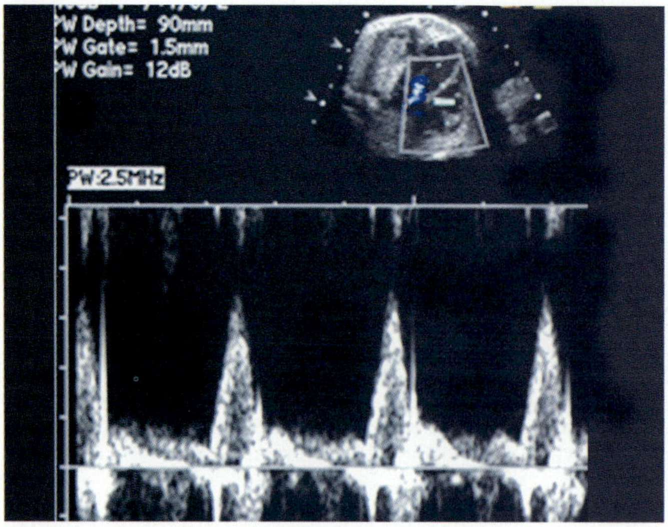


**Fig. 36.25C:** Mitral and tricuspid valve. Doppler inflow patterns—tricuspid valve monophasic Doppler pattern

cardiac dysfunction is evident. Transplacental delivery of some drugs is impaired in the setting of hydrops, and supraventricular tachycardia may be refractory for other reasons as well. In such circumstances, intravascular administration and/or oral agents with better placental uptake kinetics may be indicated. Direct administration, usually by percutaneous umbilical venous injection, introduces the risks of cordocentesis and is reserved for high-acuity refractory cases.

## FETAL BRADYCARDIA

Sustained fetal bradycardia may be caused by sinus node dysfunction, long-QT syndrome, AV block, or fetal distress with acidosis (Figs 36.33–36.38). The most common fetal bradyarrhythmia and the primary indication for FCI is high-grade AV block. The potential consequences of fetal AV block are cardiomyopathy and hydrops. AV block in the fetus generally occurs in association with either maternal autoimmune disease, malformation syndromes such as heterotaxy, or L-loop transposition of the great arteries.

Autoimmune fetal AV block can be treated with maternal administration of dexamethasone and/or sympathomimetic agents. Several recent multicenter studies found that transplacental dexamethasone did not reverse high-grade block, although it may have prevented the progression of first-degree block to second- or third-degree block, and it was associated with a higher risk of premature

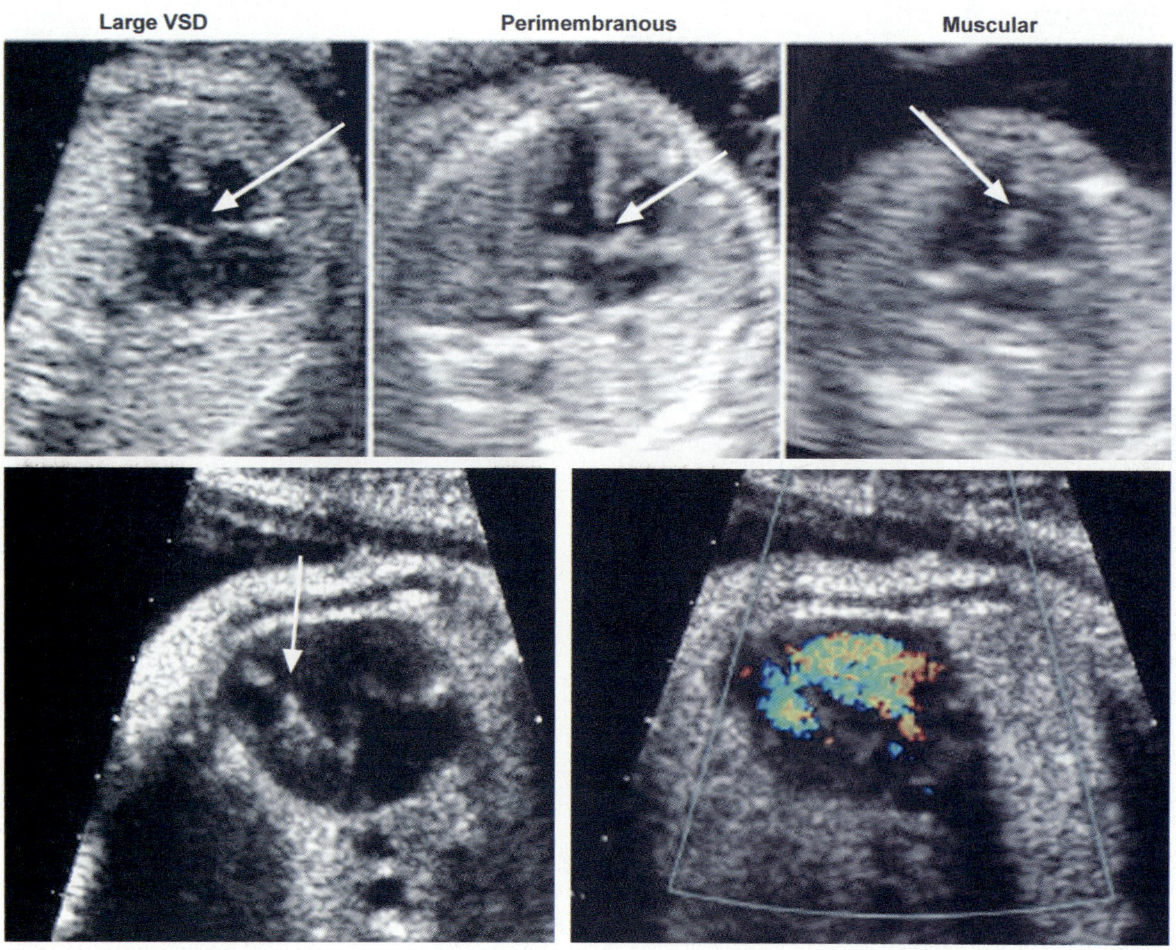


**Fig. 36.26:** Foetal echocardiogram showing different types of VSD

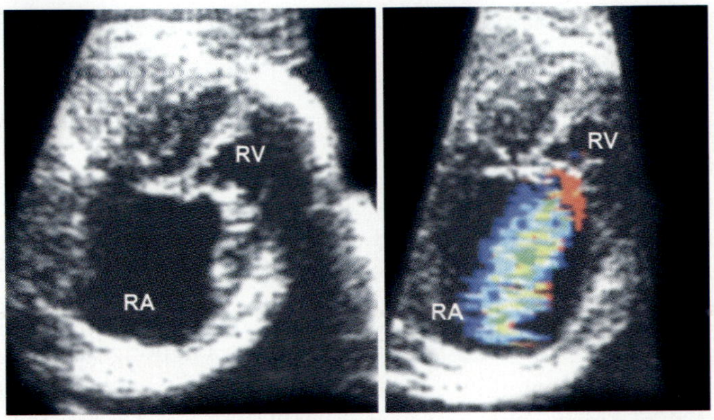


**Fig. 36.27:** Foetal echocardiogram showing tricuspid valve dysplasia with severe tricuspid insufficiency and cardiomegaly. Retrograde flow from the right ventricle (RV) to the right atrium (RA) is seen in blue and turbulence is coded by green pixels

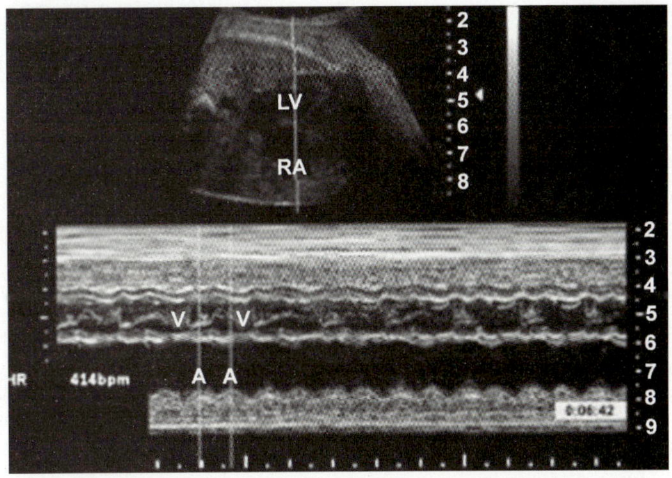


**Fig. 36.29:** M-mode tracing using a four-chamber view to demonstrate atrial (A) and ventricular (V) wall motions. The M-mode is directed simultaneously through the left ventricle (LV) and right atrium (RA). There is atrial flutter with an atrial rate of 414 beats/min (bpm), functional 2:1 atrioventricular block, and a regular ventricular rate of 207 bpm

birth and growth restriction. Other studies reported that dexamethasone, typically in association with β-adrenergic agonists when significant bradycardia was present, improved the overall prognosis in fetuses with autoimmune AV block. Sympathomimetic agents may increase the heart rate in fetuses with bradycardia due to AV block or sinus node dysfunction, but they do not restore AV synchrony. It is unclear whether in utero β-adrenergic stimulation improves outcome, because the postnatal management of AV block associated with complex congenital heart disease is challenging under any circumstances.

## FETAL HYDROPS DUE TO OTHER CARDIAC CAUSES

Transplacental treatment with digoxin has also been described for fetal hydrops resulting from other conditions, including structural anomalies (e.g. Ebstein's anomaly, absent pulmonary valve syndrome), right heart dysfunction from left heart disease, premature closure of the ductus arteriosus, intrauterine myocardial infarction, cardiac tumor, cardiomyopathy, and others (Figs 36.39–36.57). These are uncommon conditions, with published reports limited to individual cases, so the efficacy of digoxin in their management is unknown.

### Maternal Hyperoxia

Maternal hyperoxia, which affects fetal vascular function and hemodynamics, has been used to assess placental function and treat intrauterine growth retardation, but its benefits have not been established. Recently, Szwast et al. reported using maternal hyperoxia to assess pulmonary vasoreactivity in fetuses with hypoplastic left heart

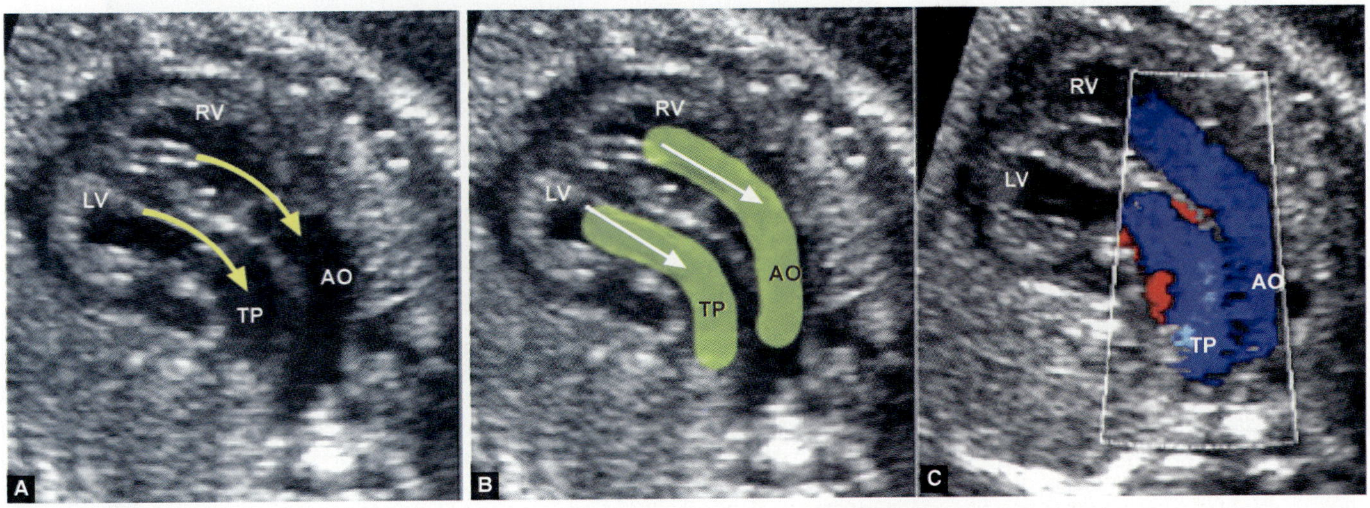


**Fig. 36.28:** (A to C) Fetal echocardiogram showing transposition of the great arteries demonstrating the abnormal connection of the right ventricle (RV) with the aorta (AO) and the left ventricle (LV) with the pulmonary trunk (TP). Both great arteries show a parallel course associated with tricuspid atresia

**Table 36.1:** Pharmacological interventions in fetal arrhythmias

| Condition and drug | Dose range | Therapeutic level and effect | Adverse effects |
|---|---|---|---|
| ***Atrial flutter*** | | | |
| Digoxin | LD 1,200 µg per 24 h IV in 3 divided doses;<br>MD 375–750 µg daily PO in two equal daily doses | 0.7–2.0 ng/ml<br>Mild nausea, fatigue and sinus bradycardia, first-degree atrioventricular block, rare noctumal Wenchebach atrioventricular block | Severe nausea and/or vomiting, severe sinus bradycardia or atrioventricular block, maternal and fetal proarrhythmia |
| Sotalol | 160–480 mg daily in two equal daily doses or every 8 h PO | NA<br>Improved survival, bradycardia, first-degree atrioventricular block, P and QRS widening, QT prolongation | Nausea and/or vomiting, dizziness, fatigue, bundle branch block, maternal and/or fetal proarrhythmia |
| ***Supraventricular tachycardia**** | | | |
| Flecainide‡ | 100–300 mg daily in equal doses given every 8 h PO | 0.2–1.0 µg/ml<br>Mild IVCD, headache, QT prolongation | Visual and central nervous system symptoms, bundle branch block, QT prolongation, fetal or neonatal proarrhythmia |
| Amiodarone‡ | LD 1,800–2,400 mg daily in equal doses given every 6 h for 48 h;<br>MD 200–600 mg daily PO | 0.7–2.8 µg/ml<br>Maternal and/or fetal sinus bradycardia, cardia, first-degree atrioventricular block, P and QRS widening, QT prolongation | Nausea and/or vomiting, maternal and/or fetal thyroid dysfunction, photosensitivity rash, thrombocytopenia, bundle branch block, proarrhythmia, torsades de pointes in fetuses with long QT syndrome |
| Procainamide‡ | LD 500–600 mg over 20 min IV;<br>MD 2–6 mg/min IV initially 1,250 mg, followed in 1 h by 750 mg, then 250–1,000 mg every 3–6 h PO | 4–10 µg/ml<br>Uterine irritability, QT prolongation | Nausea and/or vomiting, hypotension, proarrhythmia, blood dyscrasias |

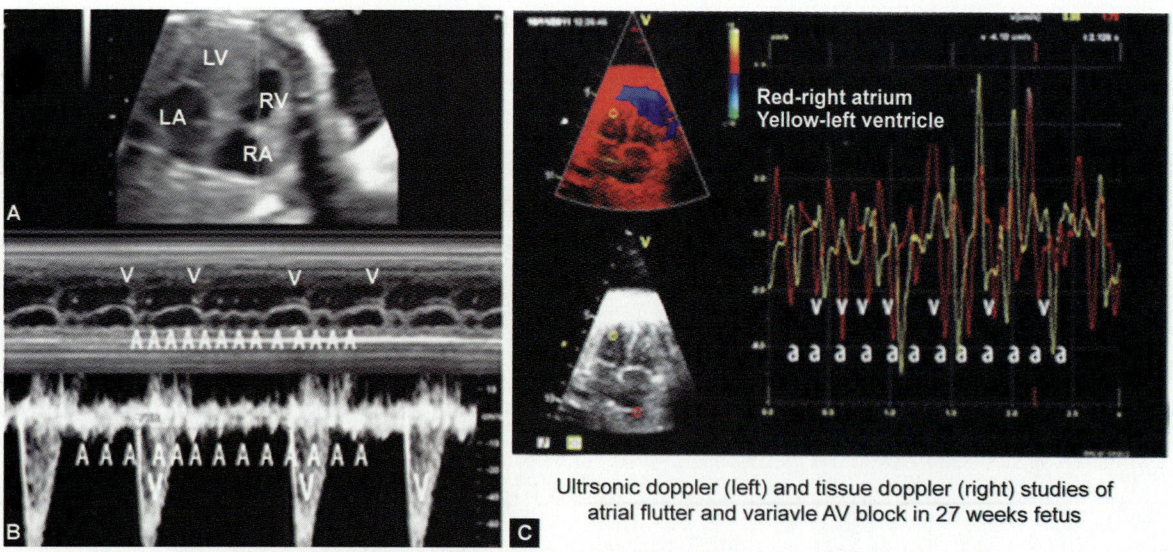


Ultrsonic doppler (left) and tissue doppler (right) studies of atrial flutter and variavle AV block in 27 weeks fetus

**Fig. 36.30:** Assessment of a 27-week fetus with atrial flutter and variable A-V conduction. (A) M-mode tracings demonstrate the timing of atrial A and ventricular V contractions. (B) Simultaneous superior vena cava and ascending aortic pulsed Doppler spectra show timing of a wave reversal in atrial systole in the superior vena cava A and forward flow in the aorta during ventricular systole V. (C) Tissue color-Doppler tracings also demonstrate the temporal relationship between atrial A and ventricular V contractions by changes in myocardial velocities. The atrial rate (A-atrial contraction or systolic flow) is roughly 300 bpm whereas the ventricular rates (V-ventricular contraction or systolic flow) range from 100–200 bpm. A=atrial

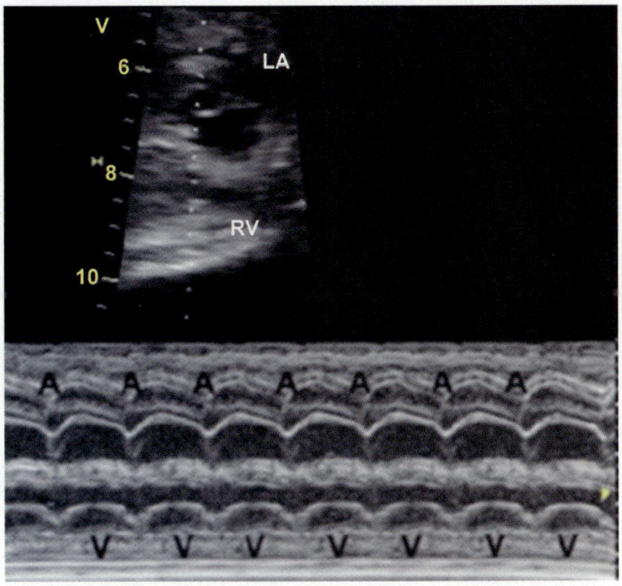


**Fig. 36.31:** SVT with a heart rate of 240 bpm. M-mode tracing through the right atrium (bottom) and the right ventricle (top). There is 1:1 AV-conduction with a short AV-interval

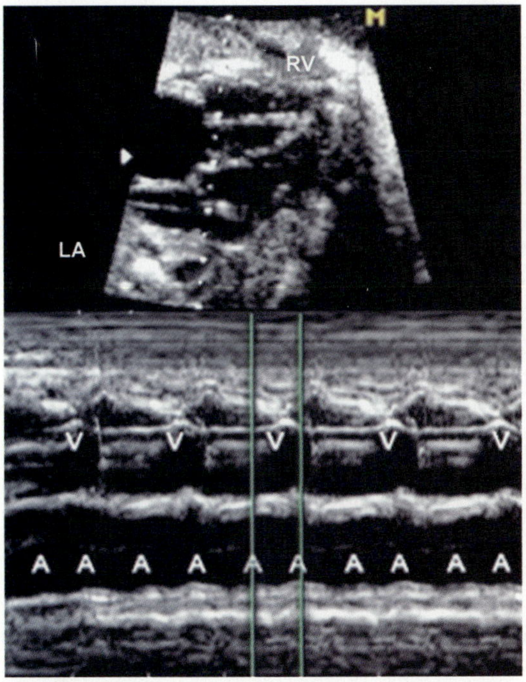


**Fig. 36.32:** Atrial flutter. Simultaneous M-mode tracing to record the RV and LA freewall movements during the cardiac cycles. The atrial rate is very fast and regular at 462 bpm while the ventricular rate is 231 bpm suggesting 2:1 AV conduction

syndrome (HLHS) and found diminution of the normal pulmonary arterial flow response to predict fetuses at high risk for critical atrial septal restriction after birth. Although not therapeutic, maternal hyperoxia in this application is a form of pharmacological transplacental FCI that may have implications for postnatal intervention and other methods of prenatal intervention.

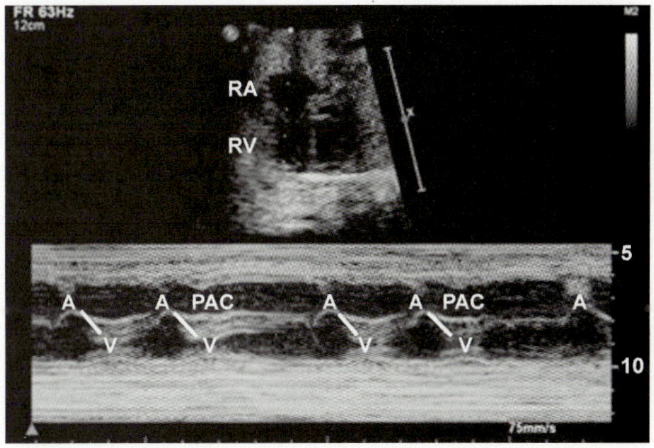


**Fig. 36.33:** Blocked PAC. M-mode tracing from a four-chamber view with the transducer beam through the RA and the RV. There are blocked PACs in a trigeminy pattern. Only the normal atrial contractions (A) are followed by a ventricular contraction (V)

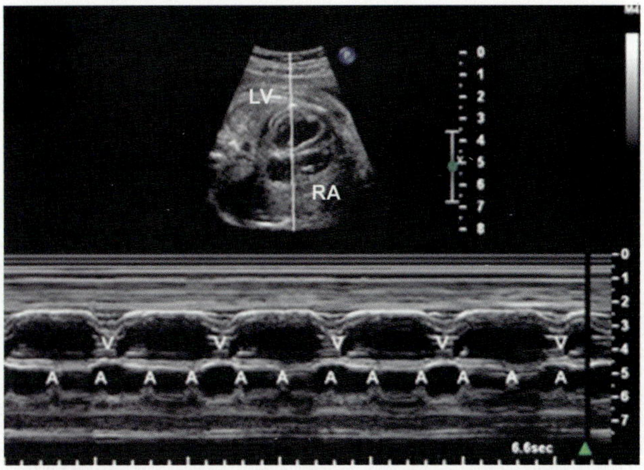


**Fig. 36.34:** Complete heart block. M-mode tracing from a four chamber view with the transducer beam through the RA and the LV. There are regular atrial contractions (A) with a normal heart rate of 125 bpm and independent ventricular contractions (V) with a heart rate of 50 bpm

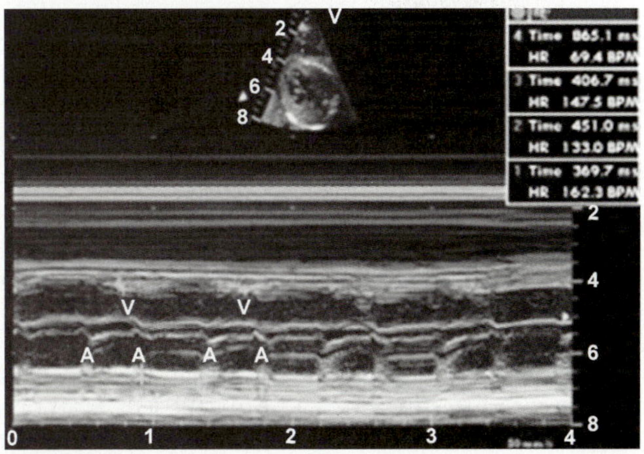


**Fig. 36.35:** M-mode echocardiography at 20 weeks showing significant fetal bradycardia (V–V: 67 beats/min) related to atrial bigeminy. There is atrial beat-to-beat variation with the premature atrial beats (A–A interval: 370 ms) being blocked and the normal atrial impulses (450 ms) being conducted. A repeat echocardiogram showed normal cardiac rhythm 1 week later

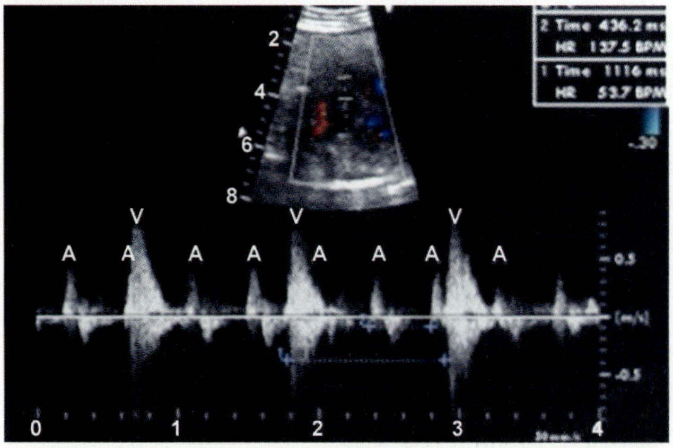


**Fig. 36.36:** Simultaneous Doppler of the aorta and superior vena cava showing complete atrioventricular block. The atrial (A-A) rate was 138 beats/min (bpm) and the ventricular (V-V) rate was 54 bpm, with complete atrioventricular dissociation

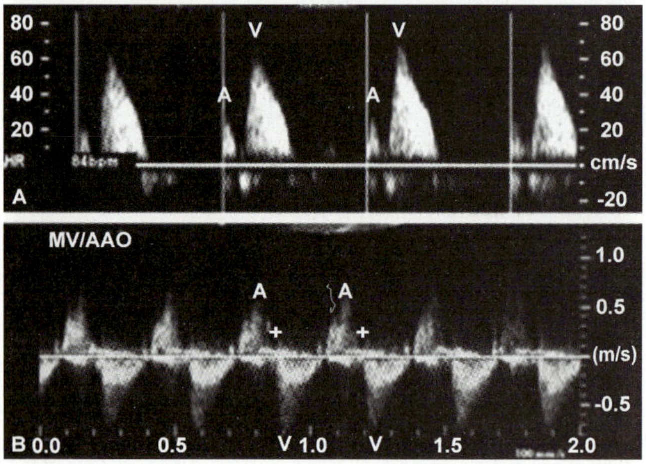


**Fig. 36.37:** Pulsed Doppler flow modalities. (A) Simultaneous ascending aorta (V) and superior vena cava (A). Doppler flow recording at 20 weeks of gestation showing sinus bradycardia with normal 1:1 atrioventricular conduction. (B) Simultaneous inflow/outflow Doppler of a 19-week fetus with long ventriculo-atrial tachycardia of 190 beats/min due to fetal thyrotoxicosis. The mother had a medical history of Graves' disease for which she had been treated with propylthiouracil and radioactive iodine

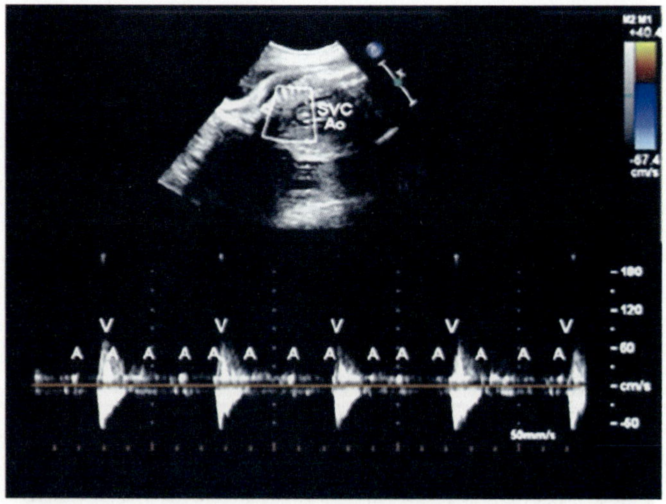


**Fig. 36.38:** Simultaneous pulse wave Doppler of the aorta and vena cava superior of a fetus with complete heart block showing backflow following atrial contractions (A) in the superior vena cava with an atrial rate of 140/min (A) and in the same direction aortic outflow following ventricular contractions (V) which are independent with a regular rate of 60/min

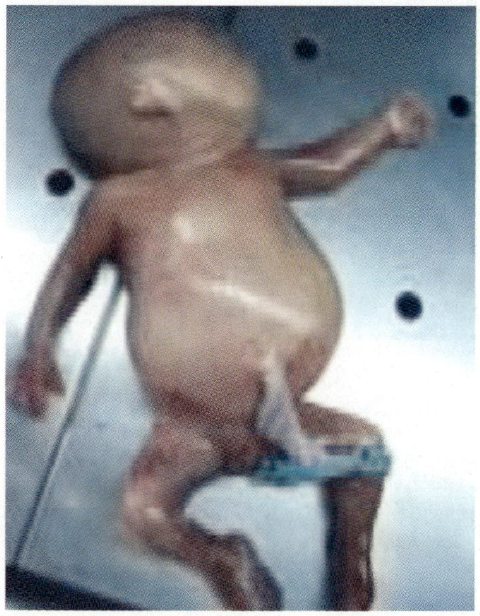

**Fig. 36.39:** A 22 weeks of gestation fetus with generalized hydropic aspect. Subcutaneous edema and abdominal distention secondary to ascites

## Open Fetal Cardiac Intervention

For the present review, 'open FCI' denotes any intervention in which the uterus is opened surgically or accessed through a surgical trochar $\geq$3 mm in diameter, which includes most fetoscopic techniques. This delineation is based on reports that preterm labor occurs in 80% of fetal surgical procedures in which a single 10F (3.3 mm) port is used and almost universally with larger ports or incisions (Table 36.2) (Fig 36.58).

### *Experimental Fetal Cardiac Surgery*

Research on fetal cardiac surgery has been performed for more than 25 years. The major focus of investigation has been the pathophysiology of extracorporeal circulatory bypass, which is likely to be necessary for fetal cardiac surgery. In early studies, it was shown that a 1–1.5 kg lamb fetus could be placed on and separated from cardiac bypass reproducibly, but that post-bypass fetal demise was imminent. Further work in sheep, goats, and primates has furthered our knowledge of the pathophysiology of fetal cardiac bypass and the feasibility of fetal cardiac surgery. Survival to term can now be achieved in a high percentage of cases.

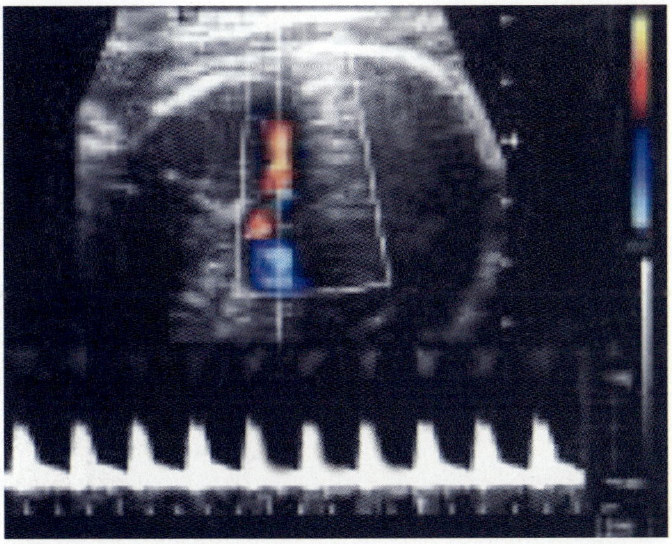

**Fig. 36.40:** Hydrops. During diagnostic evaluation a meticulous ultrasound must be performed in order to detect fetal or placental malformations and to exclude fetal anemia by Doppler study of the peak systolic velocity of the middle cerebral artery

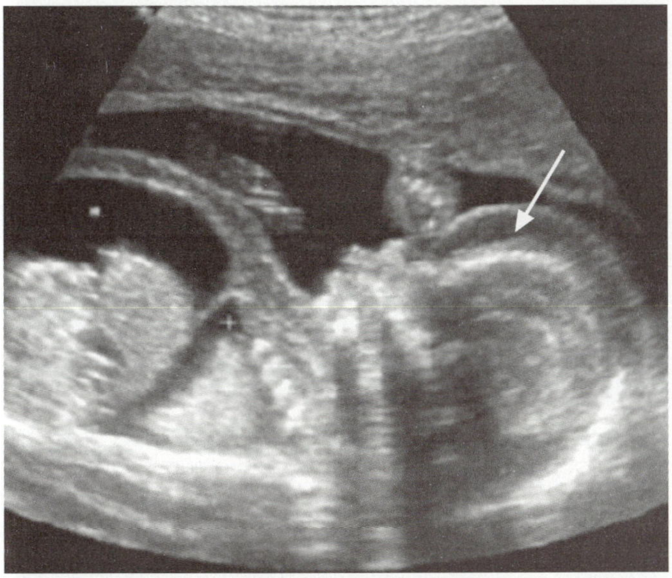

**Fig. 36.41:** Hydrops. Severe ascites (*), pleural effusion (+) subcutaneous edema (white arrow)

### *Cardiovascular and Placental Response to Extracorporeal Circulation*

The most significant response to fetal bypass when the placenta is incorporated as the oxygenator is severe placental dysfunction characterized by increased vascular resistance, reduced blood flow, and consequent impairment in fetal gas exchange, with fetal acidosis rapidly ensuing during and after bypass. The pathophysiology of post-bypass placental dysfunction is multifactorial and includes bypass-induced production of prostanoids, endothelial dysfunction, leukocyte and complement activation, and other endogenous vasoactive and inflammatory pathways. Fetal cardiac bypass and surgery may also lead to changes

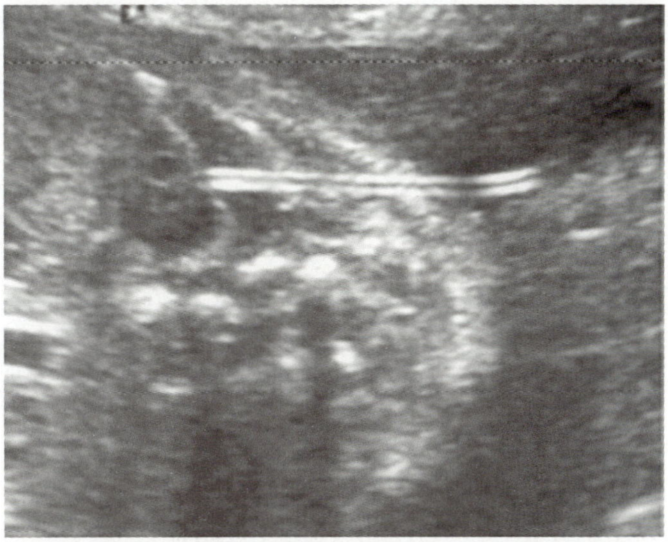

**Fig. 36.42:** Placement of a catheter in one of the cysts connecting with the amniotic cavity

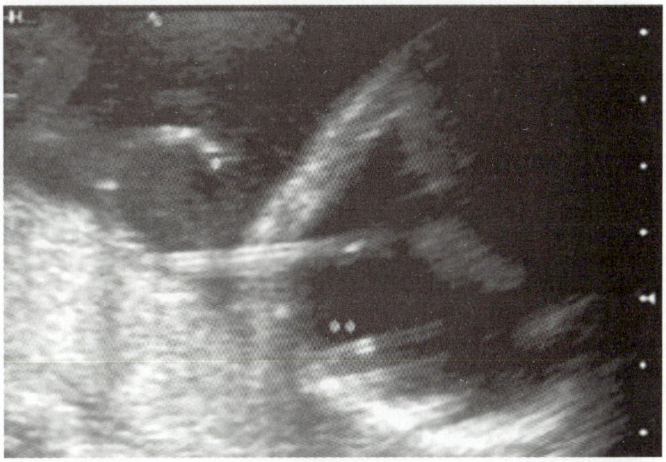

**Fig. 36.43:** Left pleural effusion. Pleuroamniotic shunting (pig tail). One of the ends is within the amniotic cavity (*) the other (**) in the pleural cavity. It allows to drain the effusion, decompress the lung and prevent pulmonary hypoplasia

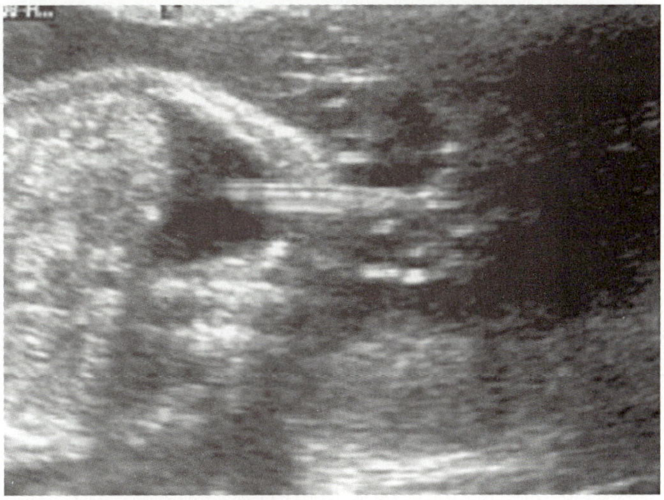

**Fig. 36.44A:** Thoracoamniotic shunt

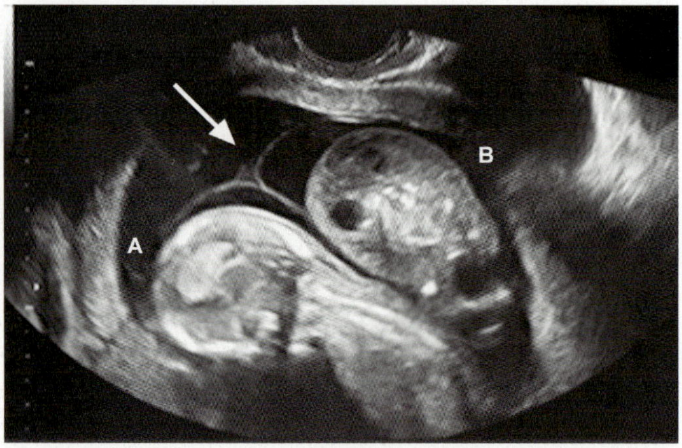


**Fig. 36.44B:** Two-dimensional cross section at 12 postmenstrual weeks showing monochorionic-diamniotic twins. The arrow points to the dividing membranes. Note the pump twin A, on the left and the grossly abnormal acardiac twin B, on the right with absence of the head and heart

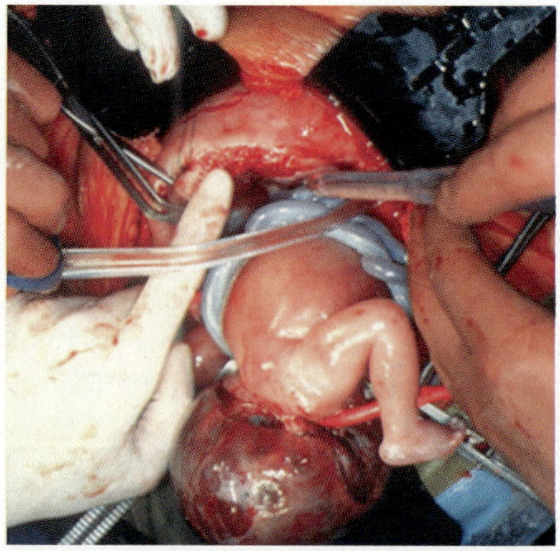

**Fig. 36.44C:** The first prenatal resection of SCT for fetal hydrops was performed, and despite successful resection of the mass and resolution of fetal hydrops, fetus could not survive

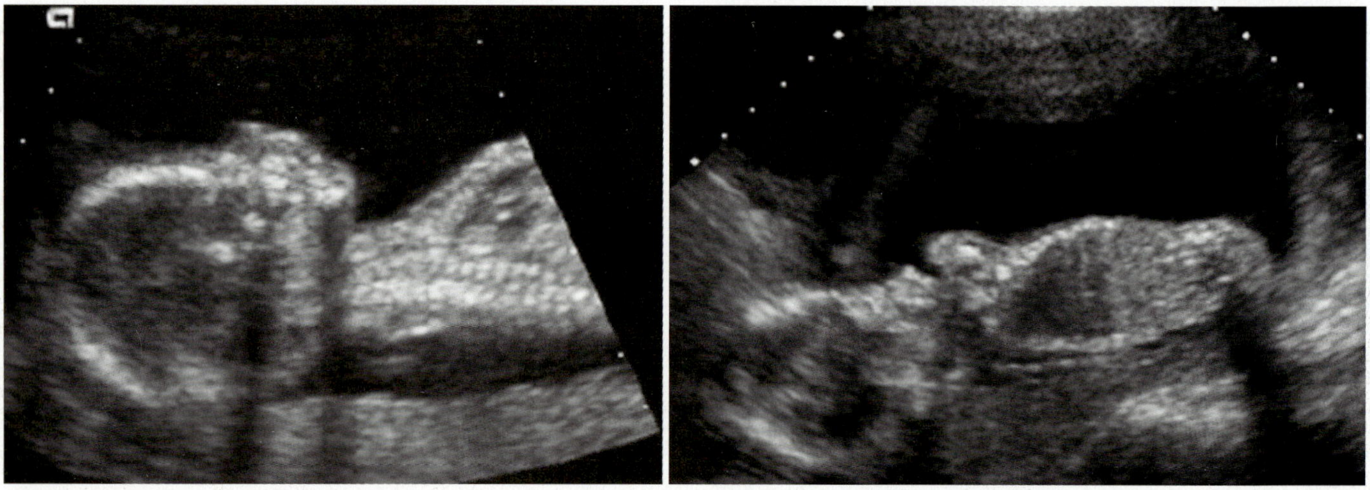

**Fig. 36.45:** Amniotic fluid volume alters imaging. The large baby on the left (recipient) has increased amniotic fluid, so a clear profile and clear imaging are obtained. The donor, on the right, is tightly wrapped in his membrane and imaging is very indistinct

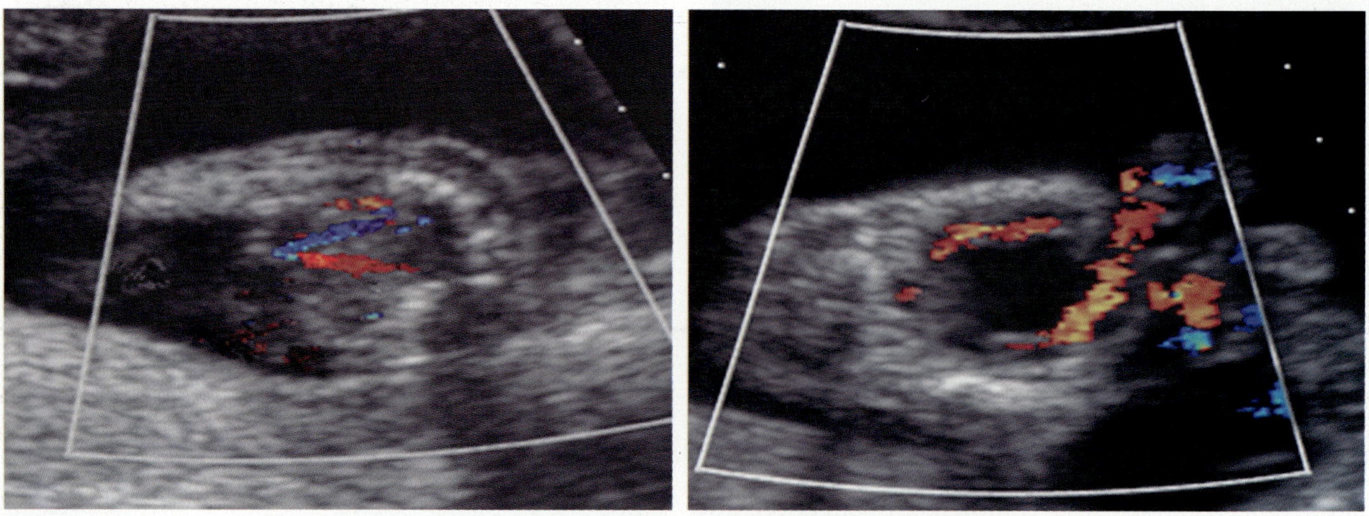

**Fig. 36.46:** The donor on the left has no visible bladder (the colored lines represent umbilical arteries, one on each side of the bladder, which is empty). The recipient on the right has a continuously over-filled bladder (the black circle in between the two arteries)

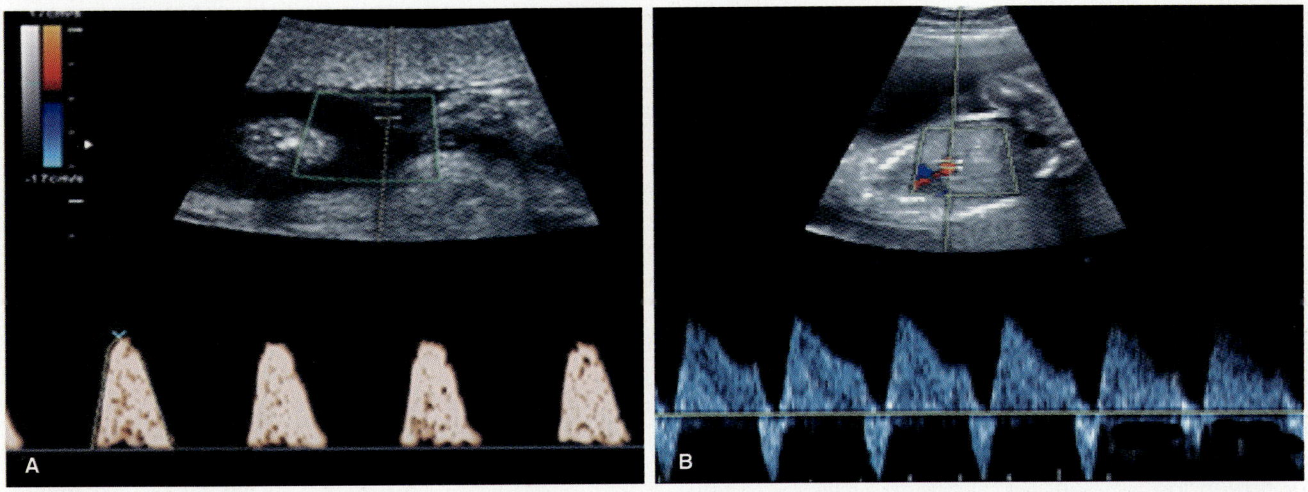


**Fig. 36.47:** Each baby has circulatory problems as TTTS progresses. (A) The donor has severe placental resistance and very low blood flow to the placenta. (B) The recipient is struggling with heart failure, with blood running backward during the cardiac cycle

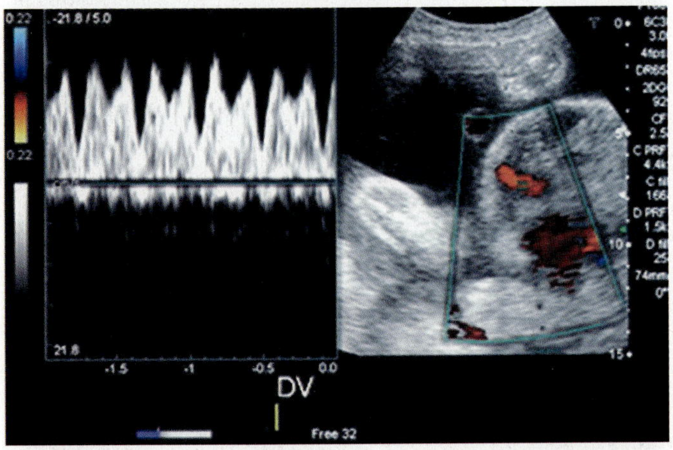


**Fig. 36.48:** Twin-twin transfusion syndrome. The ductus venosus flow in the recipient twin is still within acceptable limits, though the atrial contraction 'a' wave is almost reaching the baseline. Such a flow pattern needs to be monitored closely

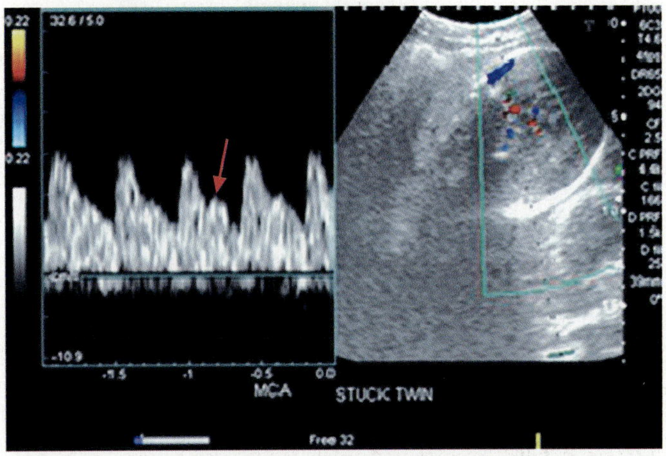


**Fig. 36.50:** Twin-twin transfusion syndrome. Middle cerebral artery Doppler of the donor (stuck) twin shows high diastolic flow (arrow), suggesting a brain-favoring effect and fetal adaptation to hypoxemia

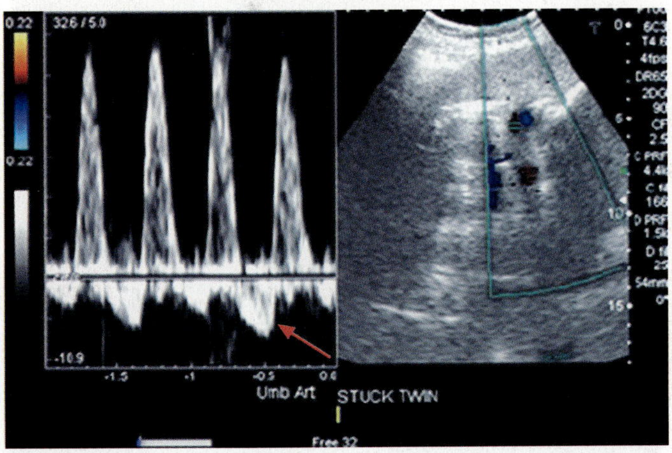


**Fig. 36.49:** Twin-twin transfusion syndrome. Umbilical artery Doppler of the donor (stuck) twin shows diastolic reversal (arrow). This is a predictor of poor outcome

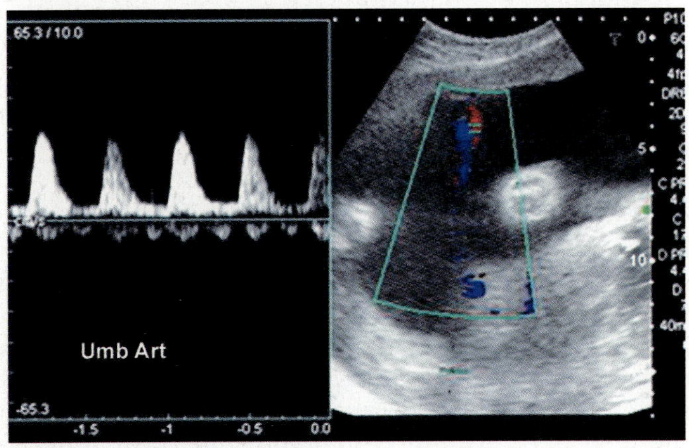


**Fig. 36.51:** Twin-twin transfusion syndrome. Umbilical artery Doppler in the recipient twin. The flow pattern is unidirectional, but the diastolic flow is very low. This is an indicator of a poor prognosis

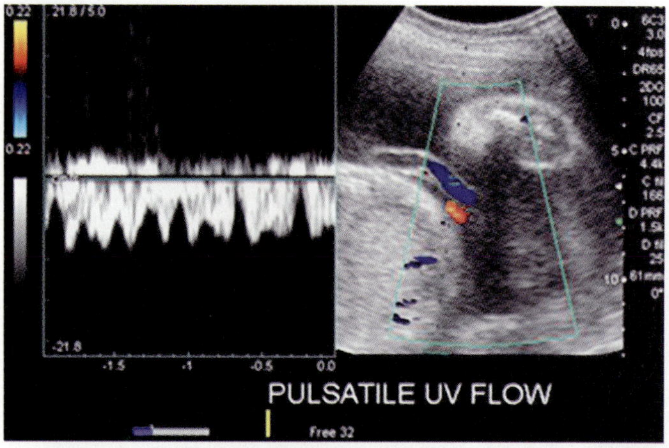


**Fig. 36.52:** Twin-twin transfusion syndrome. Pulsatile umbilical venous flow in the recipient twin suggests a critically ill fetus. Normal umbilical venous flow is continuous and nonpulsatile, with phasic/respiratory variations at times

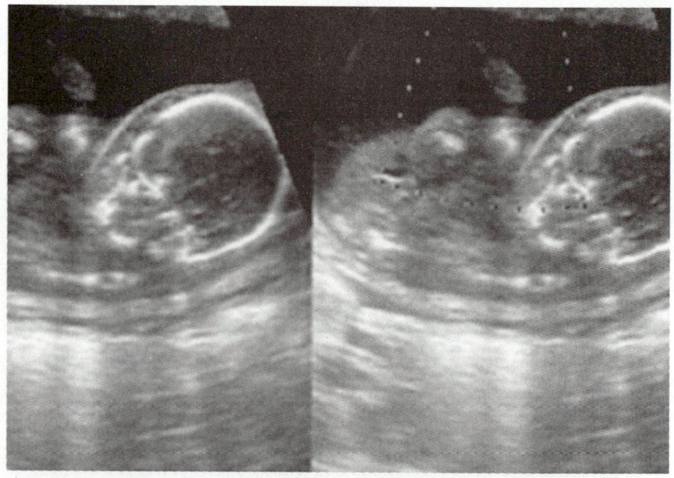

**Fig. 36.54:** Absent blood flow in the umbilical cord of the second twin after radiofrequency cord ablation

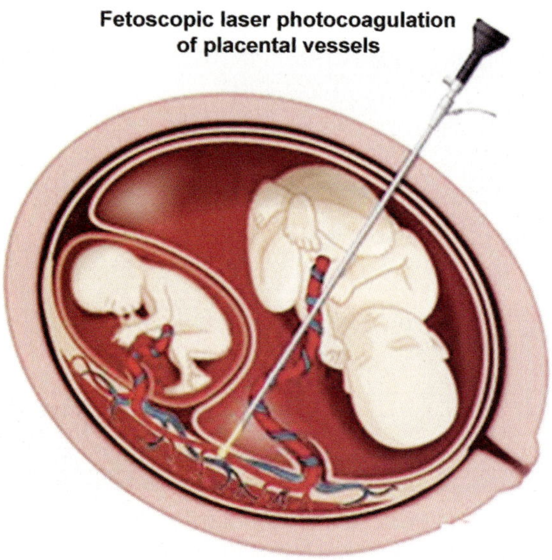


**Fig. 36.53:** Placental vessels supply in twin-to-twin transfusion syndrome and applicability of radiofrequency ablation in coagulation of blood supply to the weeker fetus in order to save the other fetus

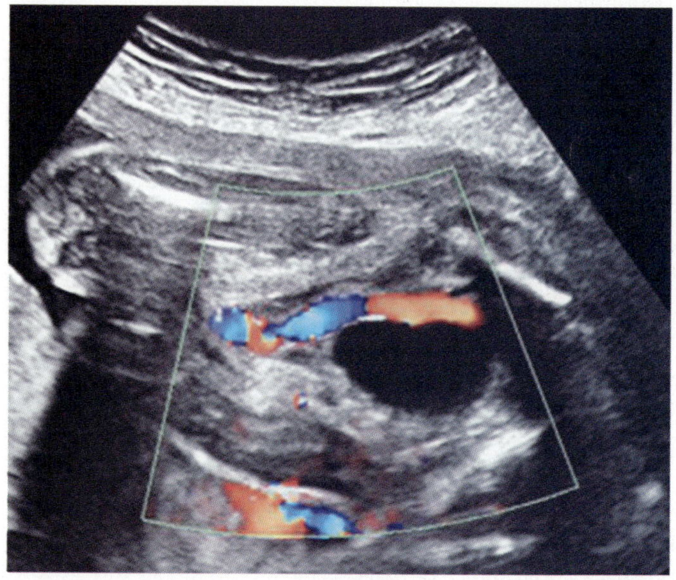

**Fig. 36.55:** Color-Doppler image of single umbilical artery around the fetal bladder

on the maternal side of the placenta, with reduction in uterine arterial flow and consequent impairment of fetoplacental gas exchange.

### *Fetal Cardiac Function and the Fetal Stress Response*

Fetal cardiac bypass and surgery induce a significant stress response that has important effects on fetal hemodynamics independent of the placental dysfunction discussed above. The stress response stimulates a rise in endogenous fetal catecholamines, which increases total vascular resistance and cardiac afterload. Because the contractile apparatus of the fetal myocardium is immature, the heart tolerates increased afterload poorly. In ovine fetal bypass studies, survival to term was first achieved with spinal anesthesia to blunt the stress response and indomethacin to block prostaglandin synthesis. More recently, it was shown that

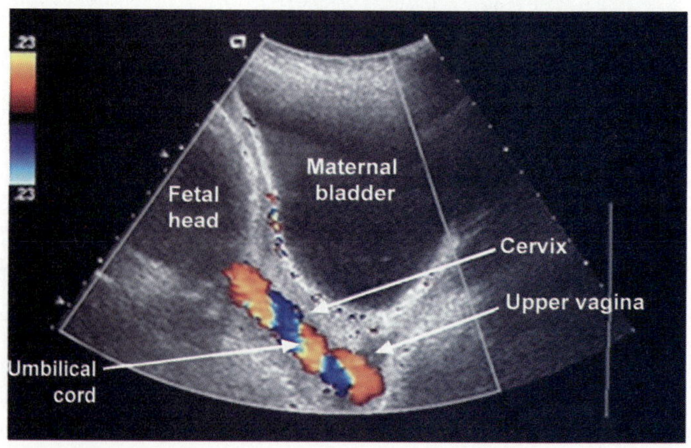


**Fig. 36.56:** Fetal color-Doppler echocardiography shows umbilical cord prolapse at 29 weeks' gestation

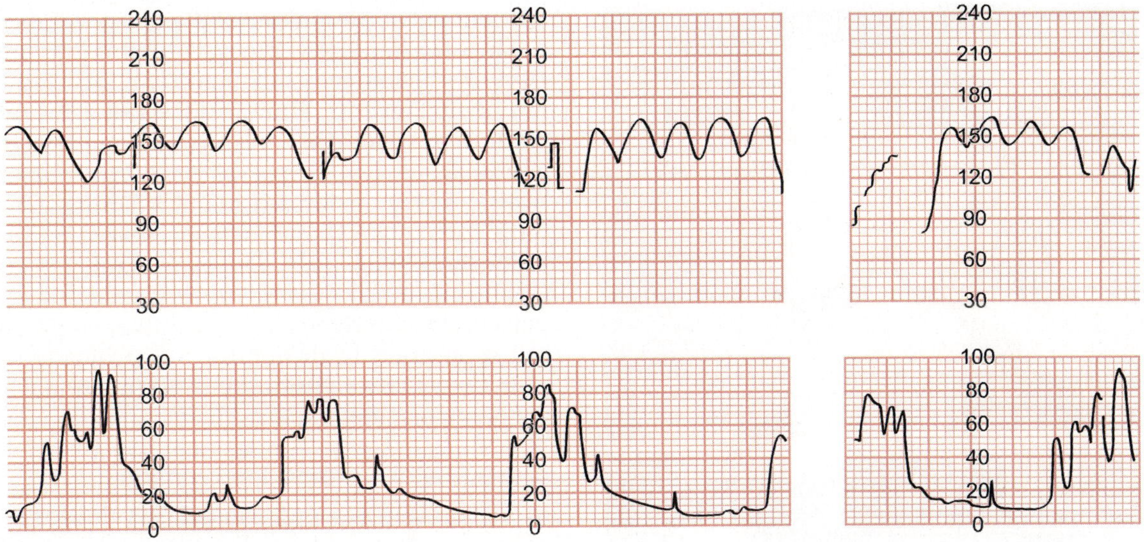


**Fig. 36.57:** Intrapartum cardiotocograph tracing (term gestation) in a patient with placental abruption revealing a sinusoidal fetal heart rate pattern just before delivery

**Table 36.2:** Congenital cardiovascular anomalies potentially amenable to FCI

| Indication for intervention and condition | Actual or possible FCI |
|---|---|
| MR indicates mitral regurgitation | |
| Risk of fetal or early neonatal death | |
| Fetal tachycardia with hydrops | Maternal antiarrhythmic pharmacotherapy |
| Structural anomalies causing hydrops | Maternal digoxin |
| Congenital heart block | Pacemaker; maternal antiarrhythmic and/or b-adrenergic pharmacotherapy |
| Severe Ebstein malformation | Tricuspid valve repair; tricuspid valve occlusion |
| Severe congenital MR with AS and intact atrial septum | Balloon or surgical aortic valvuloplasty; creation of atrial septal defect |
| HLHS with intact atrial septum | Creation of atrial septal defect |
| Obstructed, totally anomalous pulmonary venous return | Stenting of obstructed vertical vein/ductus venosus; surgical repair |
| Risk of primary anomaly evolving into more severe condition | |
| Fetal AS with evolving HLHS | Balloon or surgical aortic valvuloplasty; resection of endocardial fibroelastosis |
| PA/IVS with evolving hypoplastic right heart | Percutaneous or open pulmonary valve perforation and dilation |
| Premature closure of ductus arteriosus with evolving pulmonary hypertension | Ductal stenting |
| Absent pulmonary valve syndrome with evolving bronchomalacia | Pulmonary arterioplasty and/or valvuloplasty |

fetal bypass leads to cardiac injury, reflected in troponin elevation and increased plasma natriuretic peptides. Calcium-handling properties of the fetal myocardium differ from the more mature state, and recent studies have started to define strategies for myocardial protection during fetal open heart surgery.

### Technical Considerations for Fetal Cardiac Surgery

In experimental fetal cardiac bypass, surgical exposure, intervention, and cardiac bypass have proven technically feasible. Nevertheless, successful fetal bypass requires consideration of several technical adaptations.

Placental function during fetal bypass is altered by inclusion or exclusion of the placenta in the bypass circuit. Placental inclusion obviates the need for an extracorporeal oxygenator, which decreases contact activation of inflammatory and vasoactive mediators. On the other hand, inclusion of the high-capacitance, low-resistance placenta in the circuit requires high flow rates, which can be limited by cannula size. Placental perfusion during bypass also

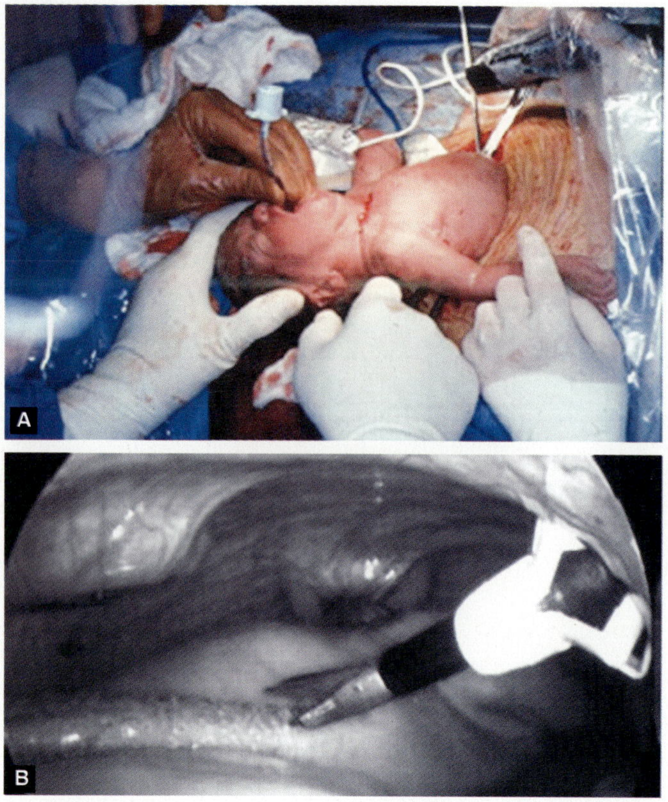

Fig. 36.58: (A and B) Fetus undergoing ex-utero intrapartum treatment

causes placental endothelial damage and dysfunction, although these effects may be mitigated when bypass is performed with pulsatile rather than continuous flow, possibly owing to preserved nitric oxide production during the former.

The systemic effects of postnatal cardiopulmonary bypass are known to result in part from blood contact with artificial surfaces in the bypass circuit. Thus, miniaturization of the fetal bypass circuit has been a technical priority. For example, in fetuses undergoing cardiac bypass with a modified bypass circuit that uses an in-line axial flow pump and no maternal blood prime, placental function was preserved relative to control fetuses in which a conventional circuit was used. Despite these difficulties, models of congenital heart disease created in-utero confirm the feasibility of operating on the heart of the lamb fetus with survival to full term.

### Fetoscopic and Adjunctive Forms of Closed FCI

Fetoscopic access has been investigated as an approach to FCI and fetal monitoring during cardiac and noncardiac interventions. Although the relative risks of percutaneous and fetoscopic access have not been assessed, port-access uterine entry for fetoscopic FCI may carry a higher risk of premature labor than percutaneous access.

### Open FCI in Humans

The first reported open FCI procedure in a human fetus was pacemaker placement for complete AV block. Subsequently, animal models were developed to evaluate pacing for fetal AV block, but this has not become a clinically viable treatment strategy, isolated human cases not withstanding. Human FCI aided by fetoscopy and cardioscopy has also been reported, with technical success and fetal survival in several cases. We are aware of 1 open heart surgery performed in a third-trimester human fetus with tricuspid valve dysplasia, severe tricuspid regurgitation, and hydrops by Dr Frank Hanley in 2003 (personal communication, June 6, 2009). Cardiopulmonary bypass was initiated and the tricuspid valve repaired successfully, but separation from bypass was prevented by anatomic pulmonary atresia (thought to be functional atresia before surgery), and the fetus died.

## Closed Fetal Cardiac Intervention

In the present review, 'closed FCI' indicates mechanical interventions in which the uterus is not opened or accessed with a port ≥3 mm in diameter (Figs 36.59–36.61). In practice, closed FCI consists primarily of percutaneous interventions in which an 18- to 19-gauge needle is used to gain uterine and fetal access. The first reported case of closed FCI was a balloon aortic valvuloplasty performed in 1989. Since then, FCI has been reported in human fetuses with aortic stenosis (AS), HLHS with atrial septal restriction, pulmonary atresia or stenosis, and AV block. In 2000, a program for FCI,was started, initially to treat fetal AS with evolving HLHS, then expanding to include HLHS with an intact or highly restrictive atrial septum, pulmonary atresia with an intact ventricular septum (PA/IVS) and evolving hypoplastic right heart syndrome, and structural anomalies causing hydrops.

Typically, FCI is performed,using a percutaneous ultrasound-guided approach with maternal and fetal anesthesia; in a minority of cases, laparotomy without hysterotomy is used to facilitate fetal imaging or access. All of the procedures we perform consist of opening an atretic or restrictive valve or septum, and instrumentation is limited and simple, with an access cannula, a guidewire,

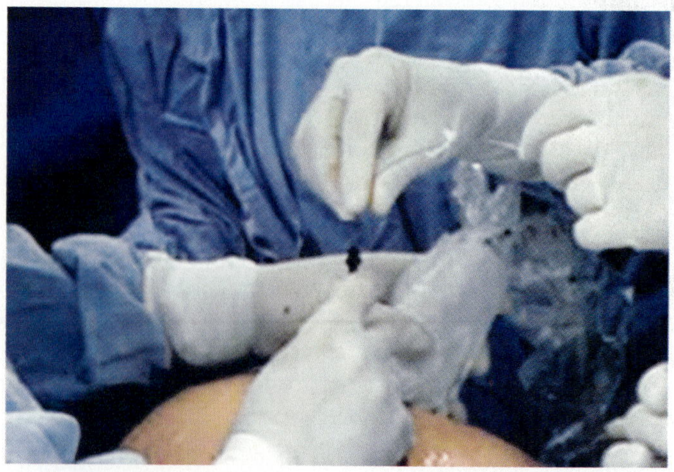

Fig. 36.59: Experts performing aortic valvoplasty with premounted balloon in the needle that is positioned below the aortic valve with the help of maternal transabdominal ultrasound monitoring

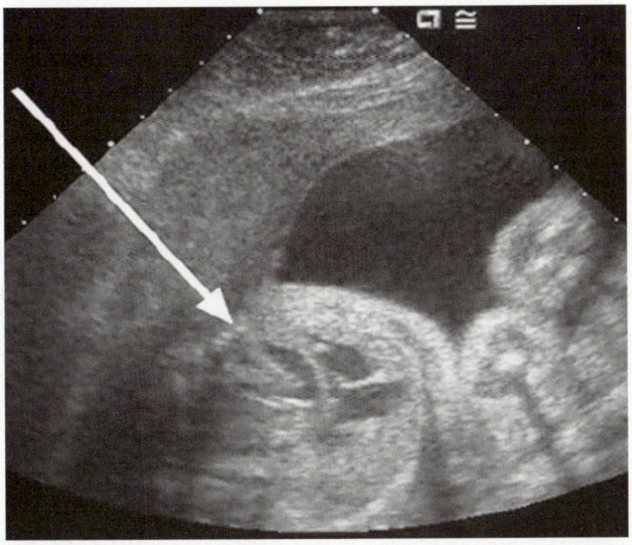

**Fig. 36.60:** Fetal aortic stenosis, intraoperative image illustrating the needle trajectory that will afford access to the left ventricle and aortic valve. The initial needle course must be precise, as very little manipulation is possible once the device has punctured the left ventricle

an angioplasty balloon and/or stent, and sometimes an additional needle to enter the heart or perforate an atretic valve or septum. With the exception of an 18-gauge curved-tip cannula that was developed specifically for FCI.

## FETAL AORTIC VALVULOPLASTY

The most common closed FCI procedure is aortic valvuloplasty, and the primary indication for fetal aortic valvuloplasty is to alter the in utero natural history of midgestation fetal AS with evolving HLHS (Figs 36.62–36.67). Some patients with HLHS are diagnosed during the second trimester with valvar AS and a normal-sized or dilated left ventricle (LV) and evolve to HLHS over the course of gestation. In other fetuses diagnosed with AS in midgestation, left heart growth and function will remain sufficient for a biventricular outcome. Several abnormal physiological features are associated with progression to HLHS. Retrograde flow in the transverse aortic arch, severe LV dysfunction, monophasic and short mitral valve inflow, and left-to-right flow across the foramen ovale. Thus, one can reliably predict which midgestation fetuses with AS will evolve to HLHS. The potential benefit of FCI for

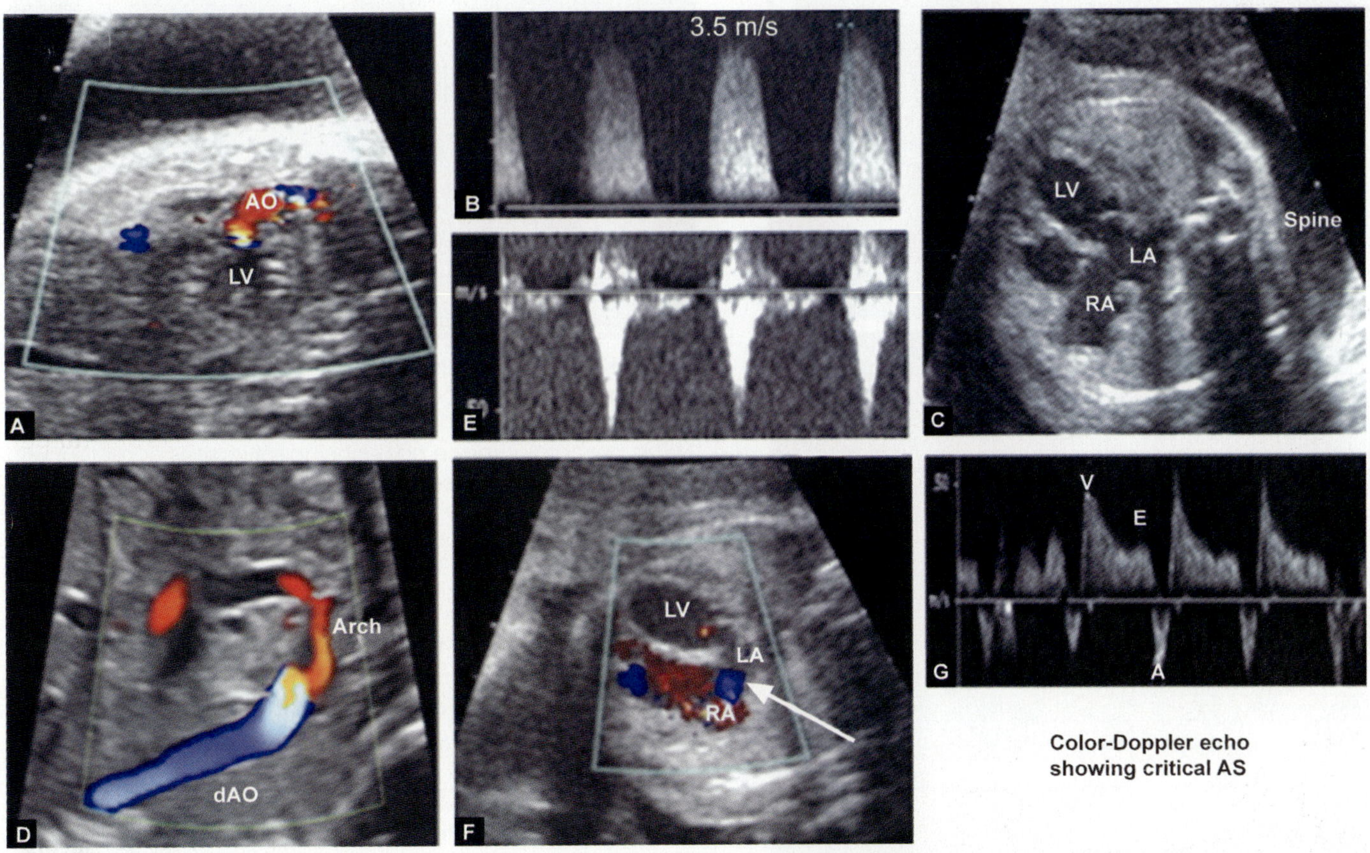


**Fig. 36.61:** Critical AS encountered in a mid-trimester fetus. (A) Early in gestation the left ventricle was hypertrophied and there was turbulent forward flow by color-Doppler through the aortic valve. (B) CW Doppler interrogation suggested the peak aortic valve gradient was 30–35 mmHg. As the obstruction worsened. (C) The LV became dilated with reduced systolic function and (D) eventually retrograde flow was observed through the distal arch. (E) In addition to systolic dysfunction, a uniphasic rather than biphasic Doppler inflow pattern was observed suggesting reduced LV diastolic function, a feature associated with progressive LV hypoplasia. (F) Increased LV filling pressure resulted in left to right atrial level shunting (arrow). (G) As a consequence of increased left atrial pressure, there was reversal of flow during atrial systole in the pulmonary veins (A=flow in atrial systole; V=flow in ventricular systole; E=flow through the pulmonary veins in early ventricular diastole; LV=left ventricle; RA=right atrium; LA=left atrium; Ao=aorta; dAo=descending aorta)

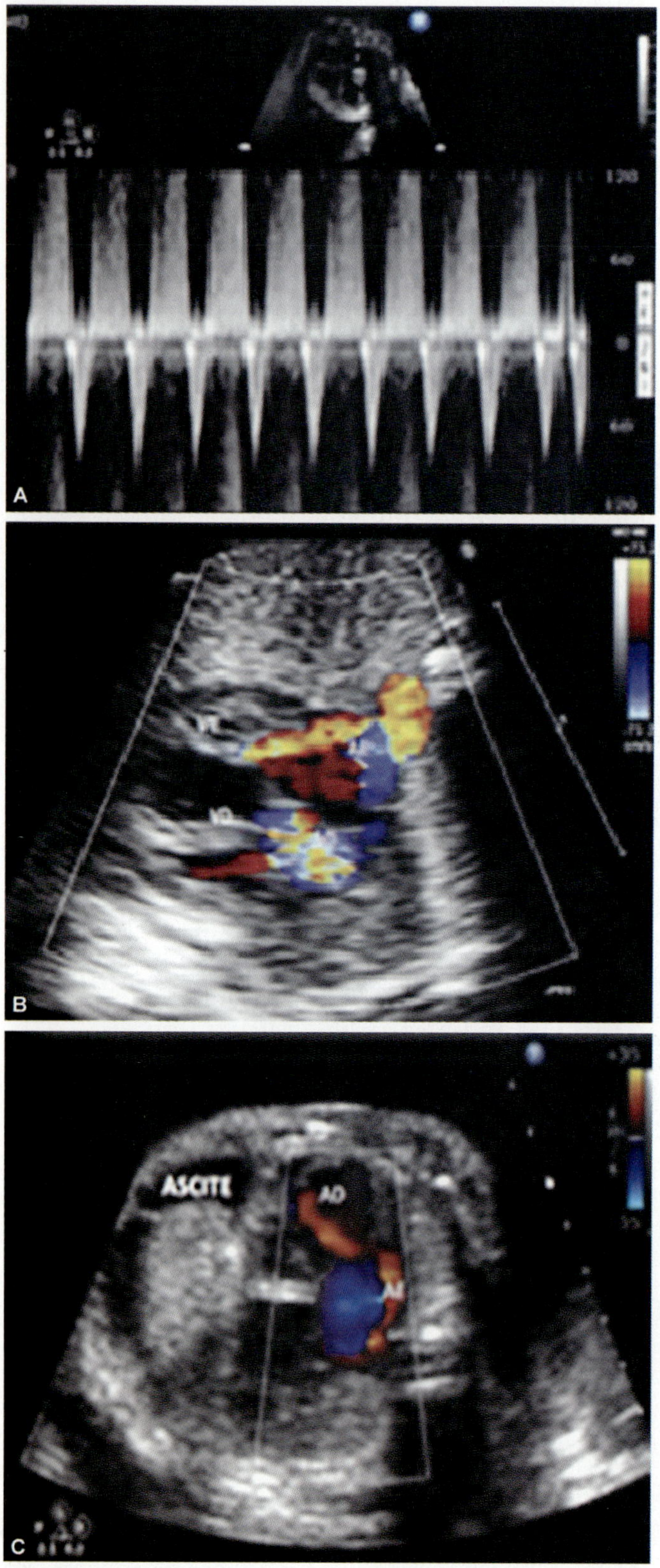


**Fig. 36.62:** Echocardiographic images of fetus with aortic stenosis with parameters indicative of progression to left ventricular hypoplasia. (A) Color-Doppler of the mitral valve demonstrating single-phase left ventricular filling and mitral insufficiency importance. (B) Reverse flow in the ascending aorta. (C) Left-right flow through the atrial septum

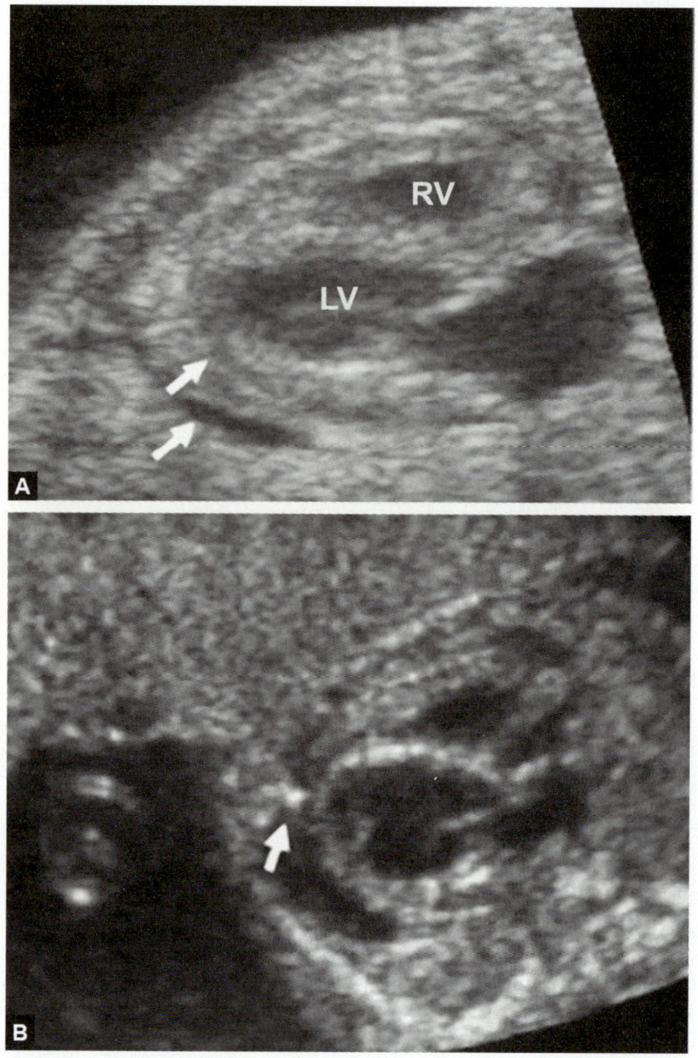


**Fig. 36.63:** Long-axis echocardiograms demonstrating a partially coagulated hemopericardium after transventricular fetal aortic valvuloplasty (A) and drainage of a hemopericardium (B). (A) The pericardial space has echolucent regions consistent with liquid blood and echogenic areas consistent with thrombus; arrows demarcate the epicardial surface of the LV and the pericardium. (B) The arrow is positioned over the hemopericardium and indicates the tip of the pericardiocentesis needle

evolving HLHS is that decreasing LV afterload or promoting flow through the left heart may help prevent progressive left heart dysfunction and hypoplasia over the subsequent course of gestation and, in the process, prevent evolution to HLHS.

The first known fetal aortic valvuloplasty was performed in 1989. Kohl et al. reviewed the published experience with this procedure in 2000. From 1989 to 1997, 12 cases were performed in third-trimester fetuses with AS or atresia (not midgestation AS with evolving HLHS) at 6 centers. A balloon was passed across the valve and expanded in 7 of the 12 fetuses, but only 1 of these 7 survived beyond the newborn period. This early experience highlighted several important issues, including the technical feasibility of third-

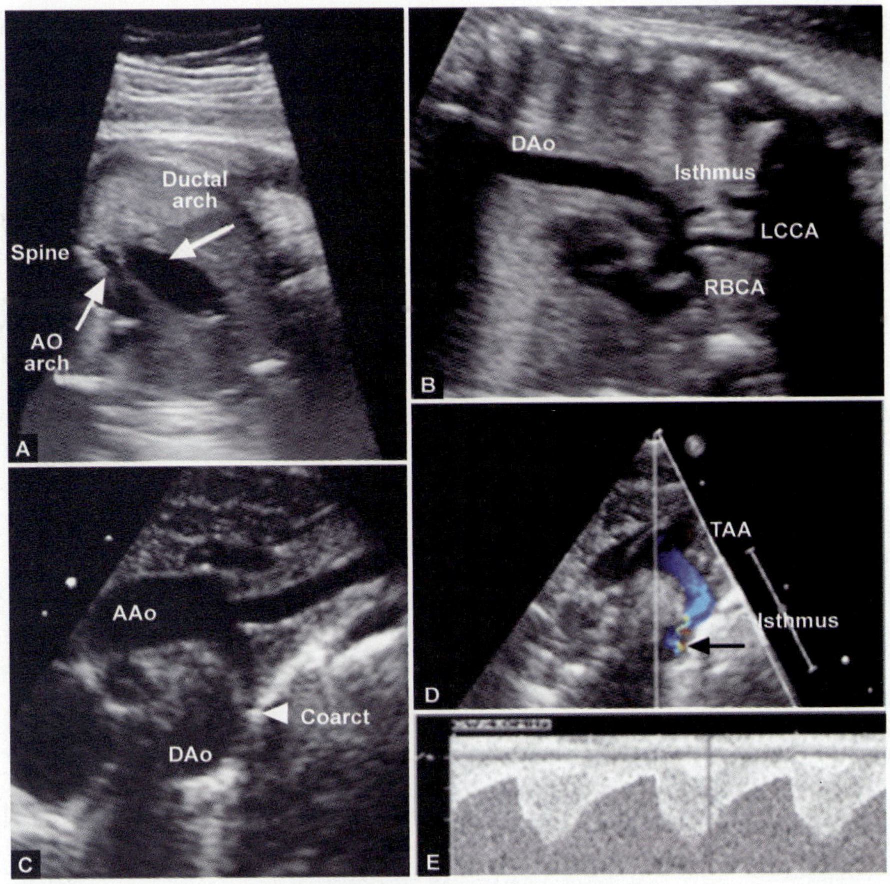


**Fig. 36.64:** Images obtained from a 35-week fetus with gastroschisis and postnatal coarctation. The only cardiac finding before birth was (A) a discrepancy in the aortic and ductal arches shown in a cross-sectional view through the fetal chest and (B) mild transverse and distal arch hypoplasia. With ductus arteriosus constriction after birth there was progressive severe discrete distal arch obstruction with (C) a very small lumen (arrow) and high velocity continuous flow by (D) color and (E) CW Doppler (systolic gradient 64 mmHg) prompting surgical intervention (AO=aortic; DAo=descending aorta; RBCA=right brachiocephalic artery; LCCA=left common carotid artery; TAA=transverse aortic arch; AAo=ascending aorta; DAo=descending aorta)

trimester closed FCI, the importance of delivering the valvuloplasty balloon through an access cannula without a sharp edge, and the risk and potential consequences of fetal bradycardia.

After an initial learning curve, technical success has been achieved consistently in 75–80% of procedures. When the valve is dilated, there is immediate improvement in flow across the aortic valve, and there may be an obvious decrease in LV size. Moderate or severe postdilation aortic regurgitation (AR) occurs in nearly 40% of technically successful procedures. As with postnatal aortic valvuloplasty, the larger the balloon–annulus diameter ratio, the higher the likelihood of significant AR, but in contrast to neonatal aortic valvuloplasty, the target ratio is 1.1 to 1.2 instead of 0.9.

After successful fetal aortic valvuloplasty, in-utero aortic and mitral valve growth are improved relative to control fetuses, but there is no difference in LV short- or long-axis growth velocity. In contrast to the modest changes in left heart growth, there are clear beneficial changes in left heart physiology after fetal aortic valvuloplasty, as reported previously. Namely, after successful FCI, the left heart physiological parameters reported by Makikallio et al. to predict progression to HLHS were improved in a large majority of successfully treated fetuses but not in controls that were similar before intervention. In summary, there is solid evidence that balloon dilation of the aortic valve in fetuses with AS and evolving HLHS improves left heart physiology and leads to improved growth of the aortic and mitral valves but has no apparent effect on LV growth per se.

Ultimately, the goal of FCI for AS with evolving HLHS is to alter left heart physiology and growth sufficiently to allow postnatal survival with a healthy biventricular circulation. In recently published experience, just over 30% of patients who underwent technically successful FCI for this indication had a biventricular circulation from birth, and another 8% were converted to a biventricular circulation after initial univentricular palliation. Patients with larger LV size and higher LV pressure at the time of intervention are more likely to have a biventricular outcome. Using multivariable analysis, identification of a cohort of patients with essentially no chance of biventricular outcome was done and modified the selection criteria to exclude patients who fall below a defined threshold score. It has become

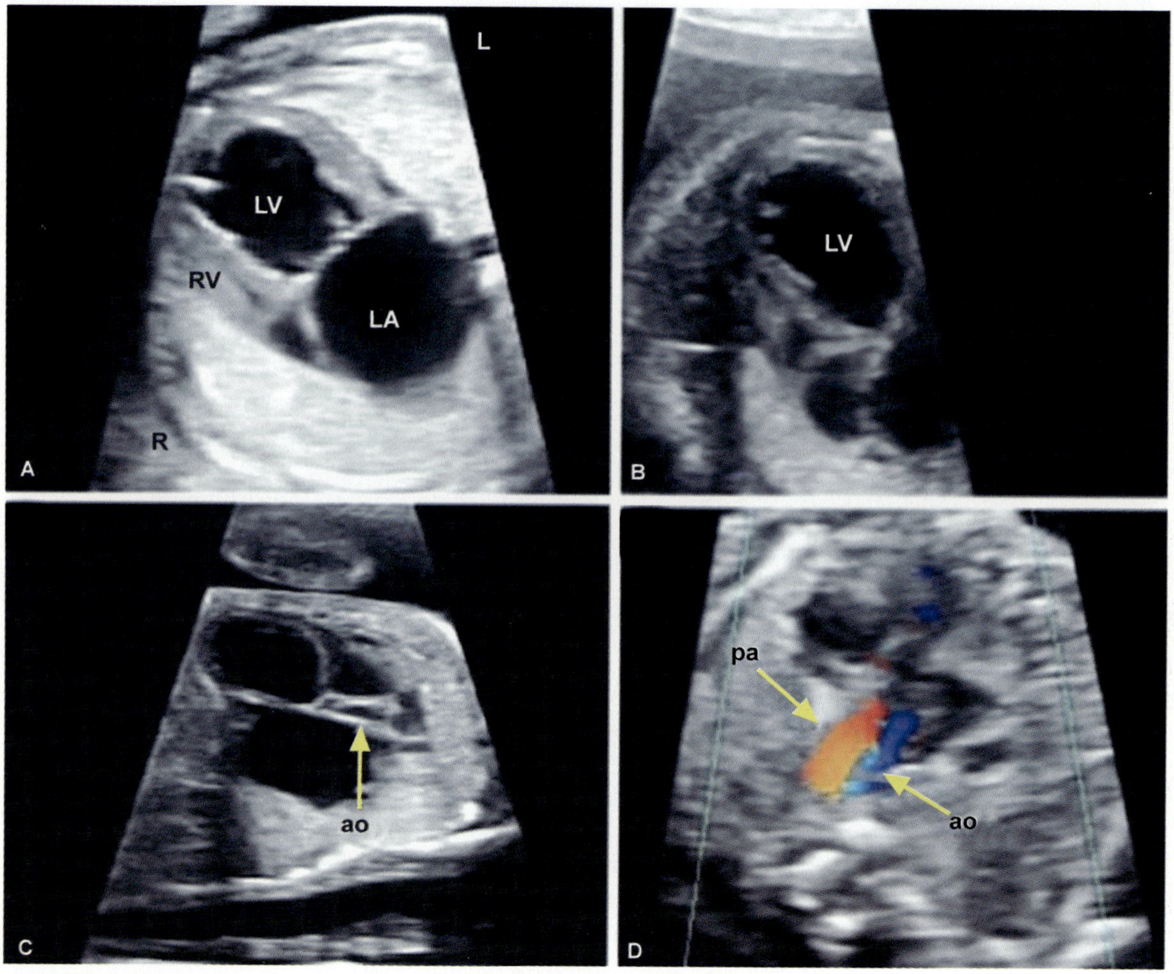


**Fig. 36.65:** Echocardiographic images. (A and B) Dilated left ventricle, left atrium and compressed right ventricle, (C) critical aortic stenosis, (D) in the three-vessel and tracheal view, the aortic diameter is much smaller than the pulmonary artery with reversed flow in the aortic arch

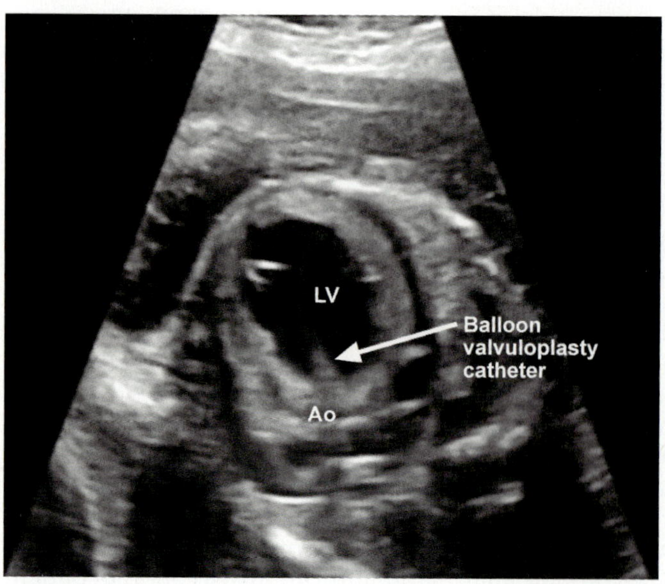


**Fig. 36.66:** Echocardiographic image showing introducer cannula and balloon catheter inflation in the aortic valve

clear that prenatal intervention is not a standalone intervention. In all cases that have gone on to biventricular outcome postnatally, postnatal interventions have been required, including repeat aortic valvuloplasty in most cases, temporary left atrial decompression, and frequently surgical intervention such as coarctation repair, resection of endocardial fibroelastosis, and mitral valvuloplasty.

Almost half of fetuses undergoing prenatal aortic valvuloplasty experience a combination of bradycardia and right ventricular dysfunction of variable severity. Fetal hemodynamic instability occurs almost exclusively in fetuses undergoing ventricular puncture (as opposed to atrial access) and may become evident either before the balloon is introduced into the ventricle, during dilation, or even after removal of equipment from the fetal heart. In early experience, these were treated with intramuscular or intracardiac epinephrine, but currently use a prophylactic approach, introducing epinephrine and bicarbonate through the balloon catheter at the time of intervention, regardless of whether bradycardia and right ventricular dysfunction have been identified. If subsequent treatment

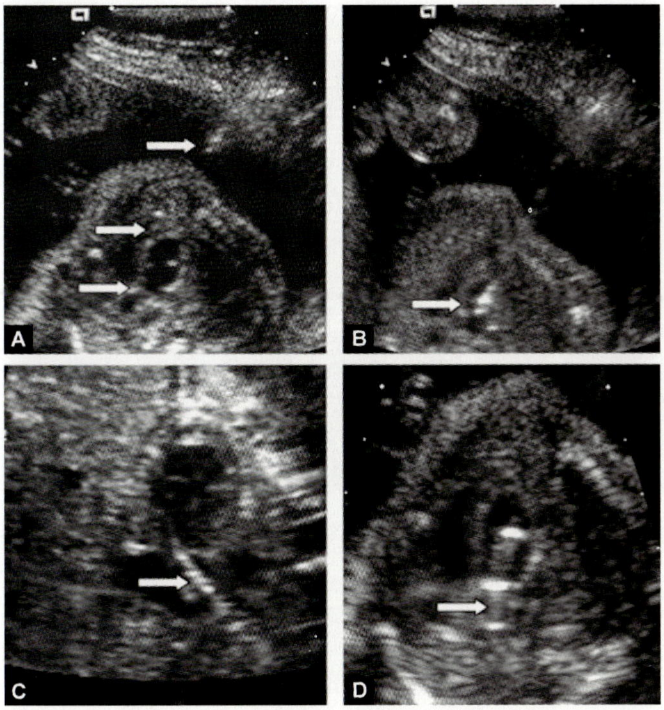


**Fig. 36.67:** Ultrasound images of technically successful percutaneous in-utero aortic valvuloplasty. (A) LV before intervention. Four-chamber view demonstrating echogenic LV, apex-forming RV, and alignment of needle (arrow), LV apex (arrow), aortic valve, and ascending aorta (arrow). (B) Cannula in LV. After LV puncture with cannula, LV appears smaller. Cannula can be seen as echo-bright line in LV, with its tip directed at aortic valve (arrow). (C) Guidewire across aortic valve in ascending aorta (arrow). (D) Balloon across valve. Correct position of balloon across aortic valve is confirmed by external measurements of catheter and by ultrasound imaging. Balloon inflation appears as movement of bright reflection along line of LV outflow track and across level of valve (arrow)

is necessary, intracardiac or intramuscular medication is given as well. In addition to fetal hemodynamic instability, hemopericardium is also common and may be accompanied by bradycardia. The hemopericardium is frequently small (less than 1—2 mm) but may be substantially larger, in which case percutaneous drainage is attempted, usually with successful removal of fluid. In fetuses that develop hemodynamic instability or hemopericardium, treatment generally results in restoration of an adequate circulation. The pathophysiology and inciting factors for hemodynamic instability are not entirely clear but are likely the result of some combination of fetal hypoxemia and autonomic or direct response to ventricular compression and puncture. The foundation for FCI in fetuses with AS and evolving HLHS is the belief that a biventricular circulation is superior to a univentricular circulation. Of course, this is not a simple dichotomous calculus, because all univentricular or biventricular circulations are not of equal functional quality. Although this determination is central to the debate about the practice of FCI, the details are beyond the scope of this review. Another potential benefit of FCI for AS, in the event that a biventricular circulation is not achieved, is a greater contribution of the left side of the heart to the functionally univentricular circulation, which may improve its efficiency and/or durability.

The risks of fetal aortic valvuloplasty for AS with evolving HLHS have not been defined completely.

In the final analysis, the risk-benefit analysis of FCI for evolving HLHS depends to a large extent on individual opinions about the importance of biventricular versus univentricular physiology, and it must take into account both the chronic morbidity and mortality risks of a functionally univentricular circulation and the unknown longer-term risks of a biventricular circulation after FCI. The robustness and health of a biventricular circulation can vary, and the presence of multilevel left heart disease may significantly impact the health of a biventricular circulation. Thus, any risk-benefit analysis before FCI is necessarily speculative and based on the limited available data, as well as being situated in the context of evolving management options and outcomes in patients with both univentricular and biventricular heart disease.

## FETAL HLHS WITH INTACT OR HIGHLY RESTRICTIVE ATRIAL SEPTUM

Although neonatal survival in infants with HLHS continues to improve, outcomes among certain subsets of patients remain poor; one of the strongest risk factors for early mortality is an intact or highly restrictive atrial septum (Figs 36.68–36.72). Although limited pulmonary venous egress may be well tolerated in utero, neonates with major septal restriction are at substantially higher risk of death than those without. There are two primary problems associated with this condition—(1) profound hypoxemia after birth due to restricted outflow from the pulmonary veins, which results in little effective pulmonary blood flow, and (2) chronic pulmonary venous hypertension in-utero due to restriction to left atrial outflow, which results in

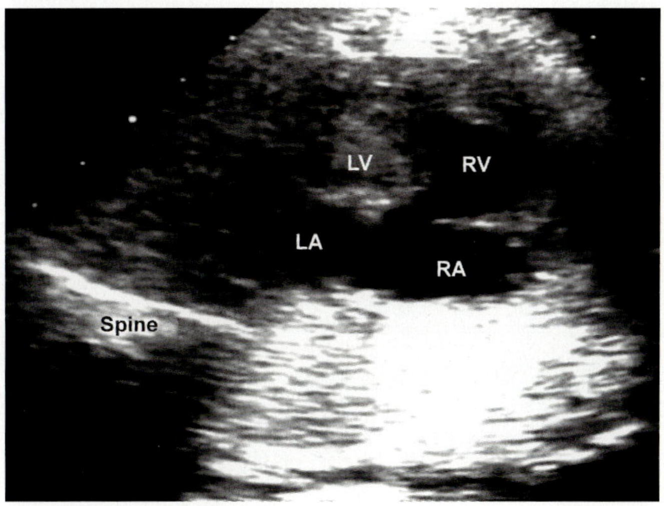


**Fig. 36.68:** Ultrasonography showing small sized left atrium, hypoplastic heart forming the apex and atresic mitral valve in an unborn baby with hypoplastic left heart syndrome

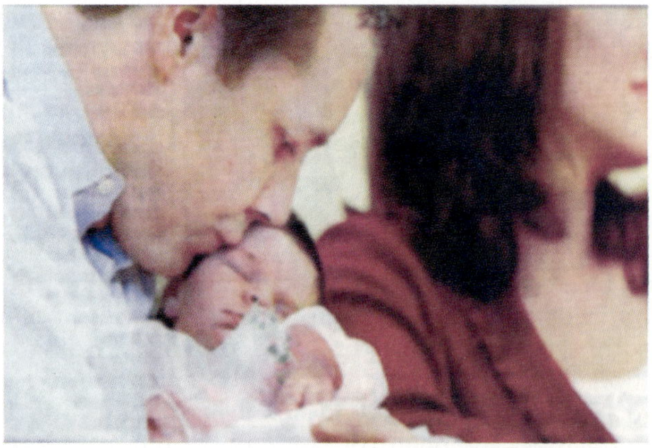

**Fig. 36.69:** Photograph of a newborn baby. Grace out of US National couple with mother Angela VanDer-werken of Virginia who became worlds first baby to receive intrauterine stent for the treatment of hypoplastic left heart syndrome when this baby was 7 months old in the womb of the mother. This surgery was performed by the team of experts under chief surgeon Dr James Lock, at children hospital Boston and Brigham and women hospital, Boston

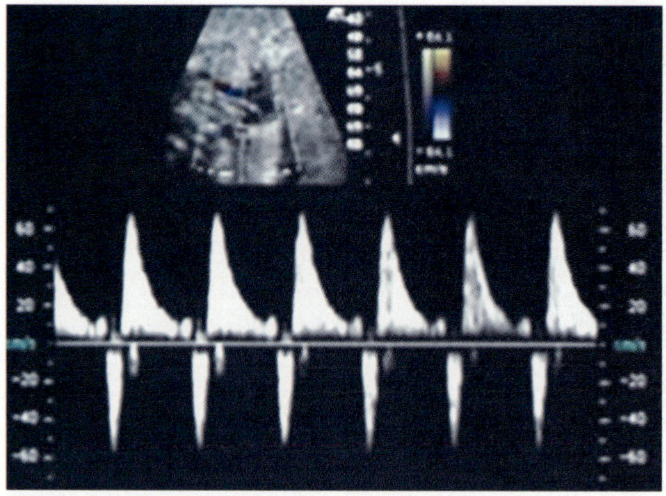

**Fig. 36.71:** Pulmonary vein Doppler of fetal carrier syndrome showing hypoplasia of the left heart with critically restrictive foramen ovale. Note that the flow is bidirectional wave at the expense of the reverse flow

pulmonary venous thickening and perioperative morbidity and mortality. Thus, even if postnatal opening of the atrial septum is rapid and effective, damage to the pulmonary vasculature may contribute to further mortality in the first few weeks or months of life.

In fetuses with HLHS and an intact atrial septum, FCI may improve both of the major problems posed by the restriction of pulmonary venous outflow. If the left atrium can be decompressed before birth, the profound perinatal hypoxemia and acidosis and their associated morbidities may be prevented. If left atrial decompression can be achieved sufficiently early in gestation, adverse pulmonary venous remodeling may also be prevented. Physiologically, the earliest possible treatment of left atrial hypertension on diagnosis of atrial septal restriction should maximize the benefit of normalizing the developmental conditions for the pulmonary vasculature.

Recently some workers have reported their experience with FCI in 21 fetuses with HLHS and an intact or highly restrictive atrial septum. Prenatal atrial septoplasty for this condition has also been reported by others with various monitoring and interventional approaches. The atrial septum is crossed and an interatrial communication created in all cases, either with balloon dilation or placement of a stent. Among neonates delivered after FCI for HLHS with significant atrial septal restriction, surgical survival remains quite poor (58%); however, in-utero creation of an atrial septal defect does appear to have some benefit in terms of preoperative management, because neonates with an interatrial defect <3 mm after FCI had higher oxygen saturation at birth and are less likely to need urgent postnatal

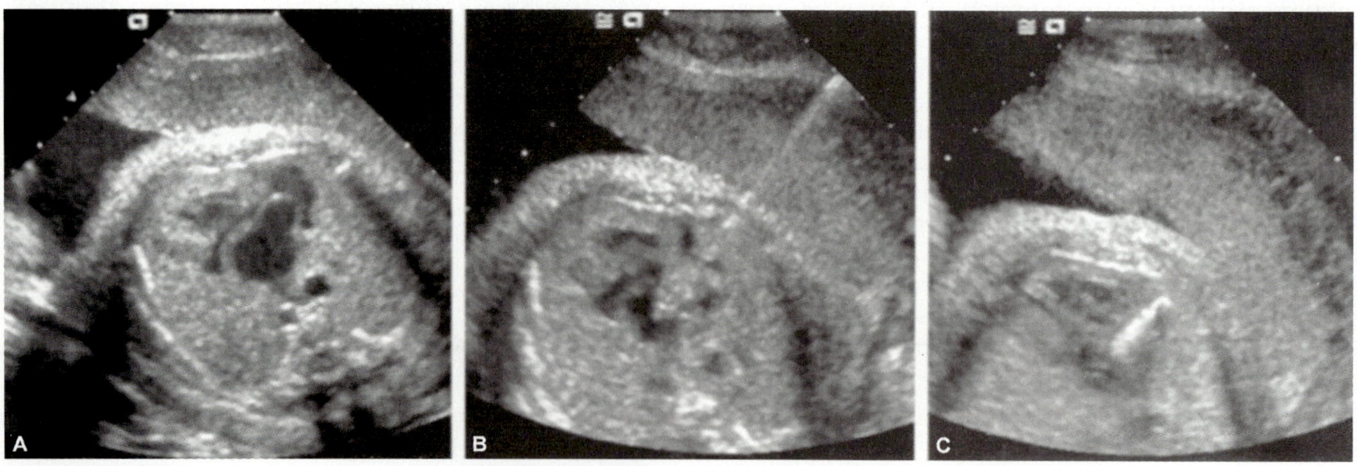


**Fig. 36.70:** Creation of an atrial septal defect in-utero for fetuses with hypoplastic left heart syndrome and intact or highly restrictive atrial septum. Transabdominal ultrasound image of heart in 1 fetus with dilated left atrium and thin, bulging atrial septum before atrial septal puncture (A), during septal puncture with Chiba needle (B), and during dilation with 3 mm coronary angioplasty balloon (C)

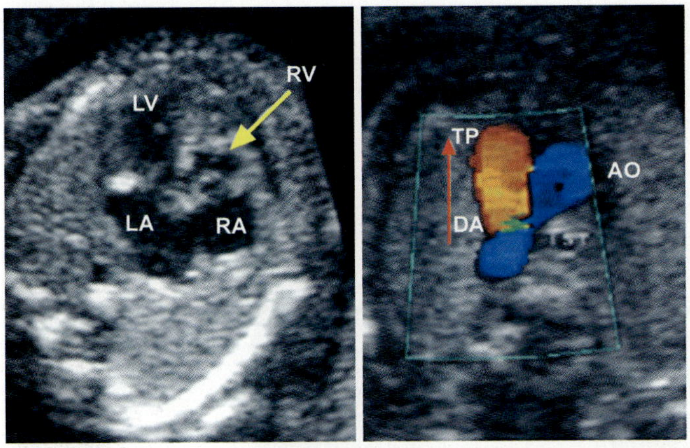


**Fig. 36.72:** Hypoplastic right ventricle (arrow) in a fetus with pulmonary atresia and intact ventricular septum (A). Color-Doppler of the four chamber view with asymmetric flow between the left heart and right heart. Pulmonary valve atresia can be diagnosed using color-Doppler by visualizing the great vessels—aorta (Ao) and pulmonary trunk (TP)—in the upper thorax and demonstrating the retrograde flow from the descending aorta across the ductus arteriosus toward the pulmonary valve

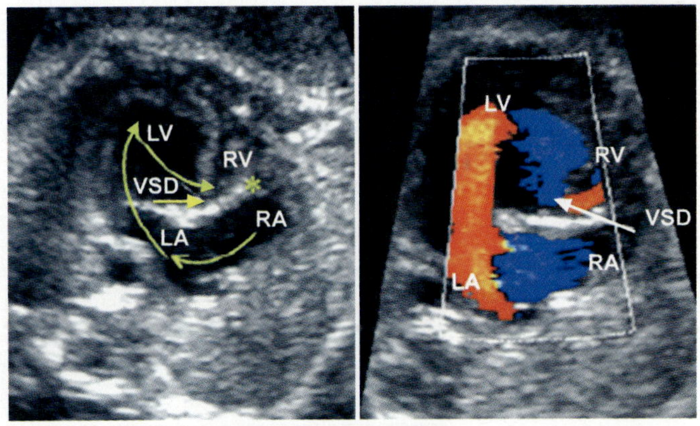


**Fig. 36.73:** Tricuspid atresia (*) and ventricular septal defect (VSD). Arrows show the direction of flow; due to the atresia of the tricuspid valve, blood entering the right atrium cannot enter directly into the right ventricle and it flows to the left atrium, left ventricle and across the VSD to the hypoplastic right ventricle (right)

left atrial decompression. Although assessment of any postnatal survival benefit of FCI in patients with HLHS and an intact atrial septum will require more extensive experience, the potential to avert immediate postnatal deterioration has been demonstrated, and FCI indicated for the comprehensive management of these high-risk fetuses.

## RIGHT SIDED FETAL CARDIAC LESIONS

### *Fetal Pulmonary Atresia with Evolving Hypoplastic Right Heart*

Fetal intervention for severe right ventricular outflow obstruction via transthoracic per-ventricular balloon pulmonary valvuloplasty has also been attempted. The role of intervention is to promote right heart functional development and to improve the possibility of postnatal biventricular circulation (Figs 36.73–36.75).

Fetal pulmonary atresia with intact ventricular septum. Right ventricle is small and hypertrophied at 27 weeks, with tricuspid valve size 3 standard deviations below normal for gestational age. This would represent borderline candidate for fetal procedure, as success with postnatal therapy alone is likely.

Isolated case reports and one series have described this procedure. In a series of 10 affected fetuses, a group from Boston reported technical success in 60% of fetuses along with subsequent in-utero growth of right heart structures, 40% of whom were able to achieve biventricular circulation after birth.

Identification of potential candidates is generally based on the risk of progression to univentricular circulation if left untreated, though this risk is less well defined for fetuses with right heart obstruction than for those with aortic valve obstruction.

Reviews of the evolution of severe pulmonary outflow tract obstruction have shown that a preprocedure tricuspid valve annulus dimension of more than 3 standard deviations below gestational age-based normal values and diminutive size of the pulmonary valve and the outflow are more likely to be associated with evolution of right heart hypoplasia sufficient to preclude biventricular circulation at birth despite aggressive postnatal intervention. This should guide future attempts at fetal pulmonary valvuloplasty.

Therefore, although technical success is possible for fetal aortic and pulmonary valvuloplasty and atrial septoplasty, further work is needed before these techniques are widely adopted, in part because of the rarity of the lesions for which intervention would be warranted.

For instance, of all cases of HLHS encountered in one large referral center over several years, only 1.6% involved a dilated left heart and suspected critical aortic stenosis at initial prenatal diagnosis. Fewer than one-quarter of infants with left-side hypoplasia have been observed to have some degree of clinically important atrial septal restriction, and many of these infants may have sufficient decompression in the preoperative period.

Ideally, randomized multicenter trials that include long-term follow-up of patients who have undergone these procedures will provide the most definitive conclusions as to efficacy, safety, and superiority over current palliative pathways that include only postnatal interventions.

## FETAL COMPLETE HEART BLOCK

Complete heart block in the fetus can be a life-threatening emergency that may present without warning. Diagnosis relies on fetal M-mode and Doppler ultrasonography to relate atrial and ventricular mechanical events. Heart block in the fetus may be associated with structural heart disease, may result from maternal autoimmune disease, or may be idiopathic (Figs 36.76–36.78).

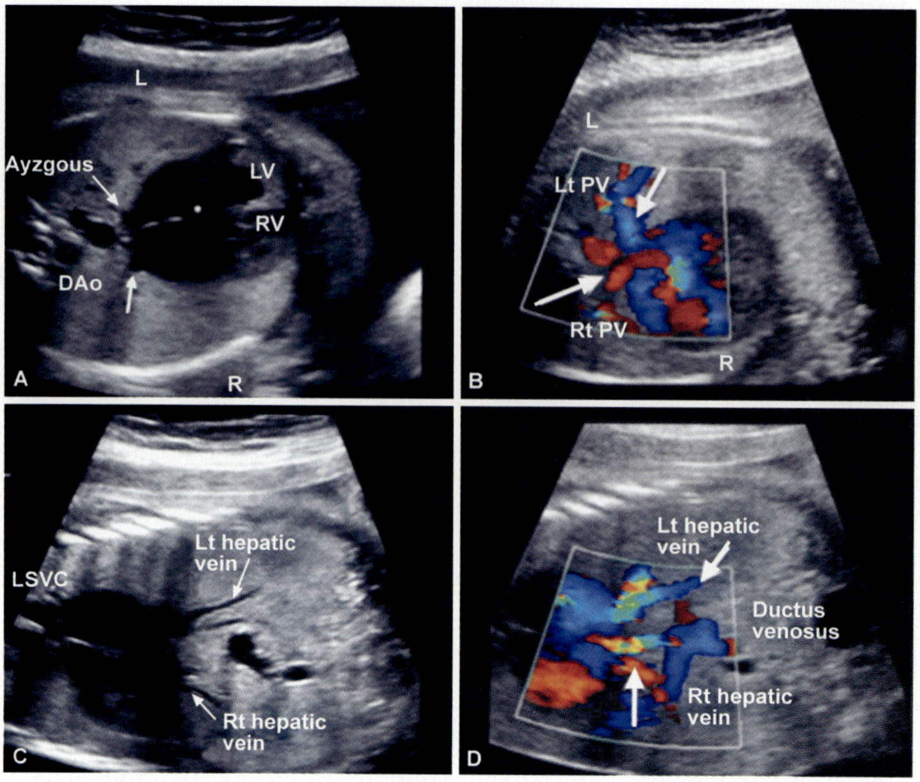


**Fig. 36.74:** Images from a 30-week fetus with left atrial isomerism, mesocardia and anomalous systemic and pulmonary venous connections. Left and right pulmonary veins (A and B, arrows) and left and right hepatic veins (C and D, arrows) can be seen connecting on either side of the atrial septum by 2D and color flow map imaging. A coronary sinoseptal defect was identified (*). The dilated azygous vein connected with a left superior vena cava that drained into the left sided atrium. Surgical repair with intra-atrial baffling of systemic and pulmonary veins was used to correct this lesion at 9 months. L=left; R=right; Lt=left; Rt=right; DAo=descending aorta; RV=right ventricle; LV=left ventricle; PV=pulmonary vein; LSVC=left superior vena cava

In most cases associated with a structurally normal heart, maternal autoantibodies are present in the maternal serum. The mothers may not show clinically apparent symptoms of lupus or Sjögren syndrome; however, in both, transplacental passage of the antibodies can potentially cause inflammation and fibrosis at the atrioventricular (AV) node in particular.

Although some success has been reported with administration of corticosteroids to the mother of a fetus with first- or second-degree AV block, pharmacologically effective options are available for treatment of third-degree or complete heart block, and fetuses with low intrinsic ventricular rates are at risk for significant morbidity and mortality. Administration of beta-mimetics to increase fetal heart rate have somewhat improved fetal survival.

A few isolated investigators over the past two decades have attempted treatment to increase ventricular rates in the face of hydrops and imminent demise of the fetus in the form of implantation of fetal pacemakers. The results appeared mixed, with some reporting initial good results, with complete resolution of hydrops and achievement of normal heart rates.

Theoretically, this approach should provide relief in the gestational period wherein the insult is the most severe, prolonging pregnancy and promoting feasibility of early postnatal permanent pacemaker implantation. However, to date, no survivors following institution of fetal pacing have been reported.

Previous approaches have relied on the placement of an epicardial pacing lead on the fetal heart with an extrauterine pulse generator implanted in the maternal abdomen, with failure attributed to lead dislodgment due to fetal movement. Owing to a lack of information regarding successful performance of this procedure, this approach is not discussed further in this article.

## FETAL PULMONARY ATRESIA WITH INTACT VENTRICULAR SEPTUM (PA/IVS)

It occurs as a spectrum of hypoplastic right heart disease, with cases at the mild end of the spectrum amenable to biventricular repair and those with more severe right heart hypoplasia managed with univentricular palliation or transplantation (Fig 36.79). In newborns with PA/IVS, the likelihood of a biventricular outcome can be estimated from the Z-score of the tricuspid valve annulus, with a Z-score above 3 associated with biventricular outcome and below 3 with univentricular palliation.

The potential role of FCI in fetuses with PA/IVS is to promote right heart growth and functional development and increase the chance of a biventricular circulation

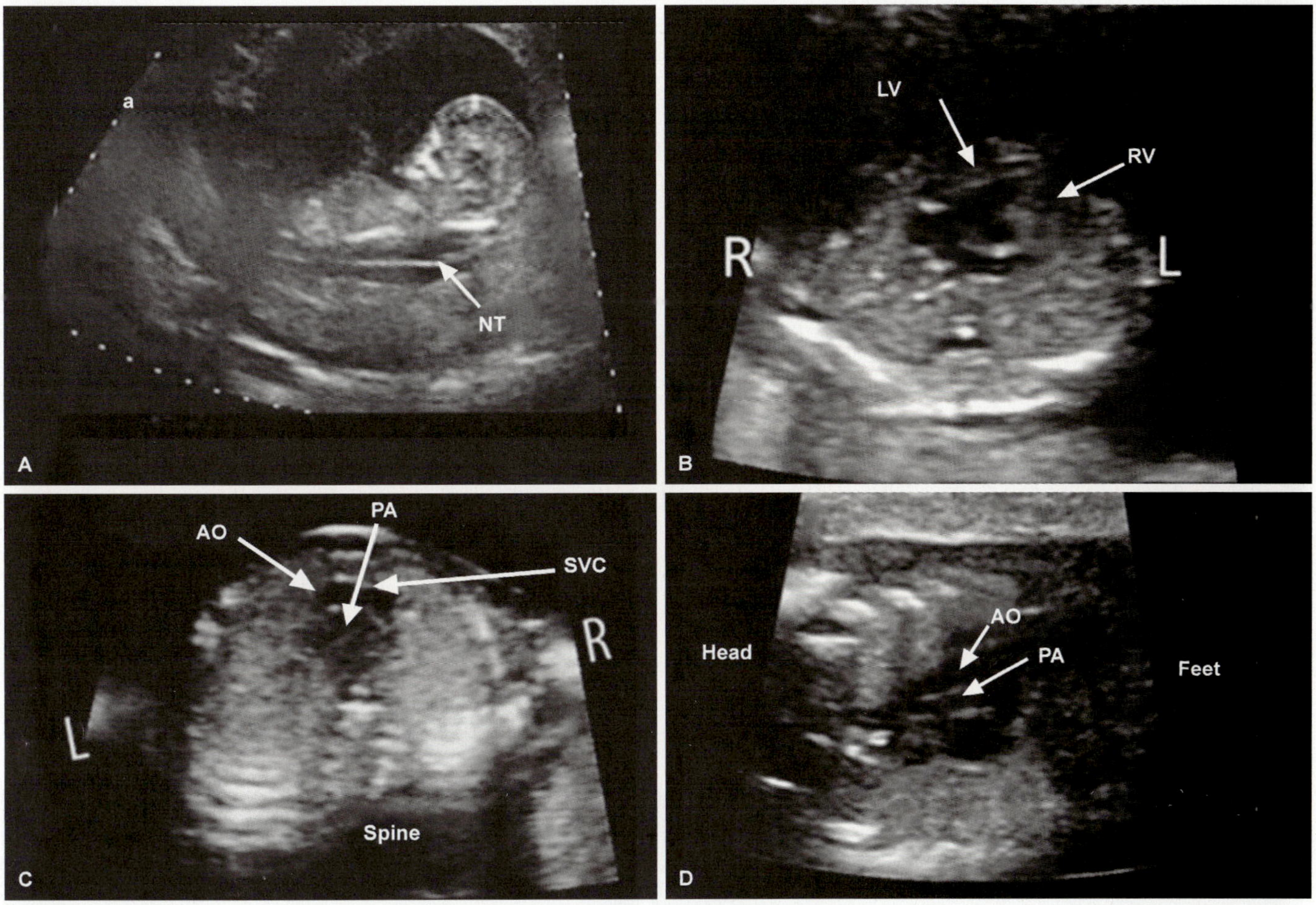


**Fig. 36.75:** 12 and 37 weeks gestational age fetus with (A) a 7 mm nuchal translucency (NT). (B) On further assessment, the four-chamber revealed levocardia inverted ventricles and a mildly foreshortened left sided right ventricle. At 14 weeks, the presence of L-transposition ('corrected transposition') of the great arteries demonstrated by (C) an abnormal 3 vessel view with an anterior and leftward aorta arising from the right ventricle and posterior pulmonary artery from the left ventricle and (D) parallel arrangement of the great arteries (L=left; R=right; AO=ascending aorta; PA=pulmonary artery; LV=left ventricle; RV=right ventricle; SVC=superior vena cava

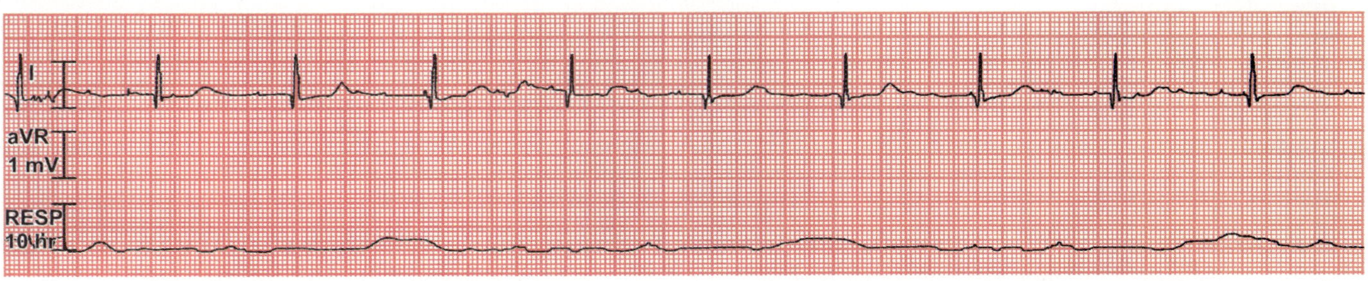


**Fig. 36.76:** Electrocardiography—complete atrioventricular block before pacemaker implantation

after birth. Identification of potential candidates for FCI for PA/IVS should be based on the risk of progression to a functionally univentricular circulation postnatally without FCI and the possibility of altering that progression prenatally. There is limited information about predictors of postnatal outcomes in fetuses with PA/IVS. Both anatomic and physiological characteristics are likely to be important, but many patients are in the middle of the severity spectrum, and postnatal management strategy plays an important role in the ultimate outcome.

On the basis of this limited experience, it appears that prenatal pulmonary valve perforation and dilation may be performed successfully in midgestation fetuses, with maintenance of valvar patency throughout gestation and apparently improved growth of right heart structures. The effects of this strategy on right heart functional development and postnatal outcome remain to be determined. Because postnatal outcomes for the majority of patients with PA/IVS are usually favorable, it may be more of a challenge to appropriately select patients and

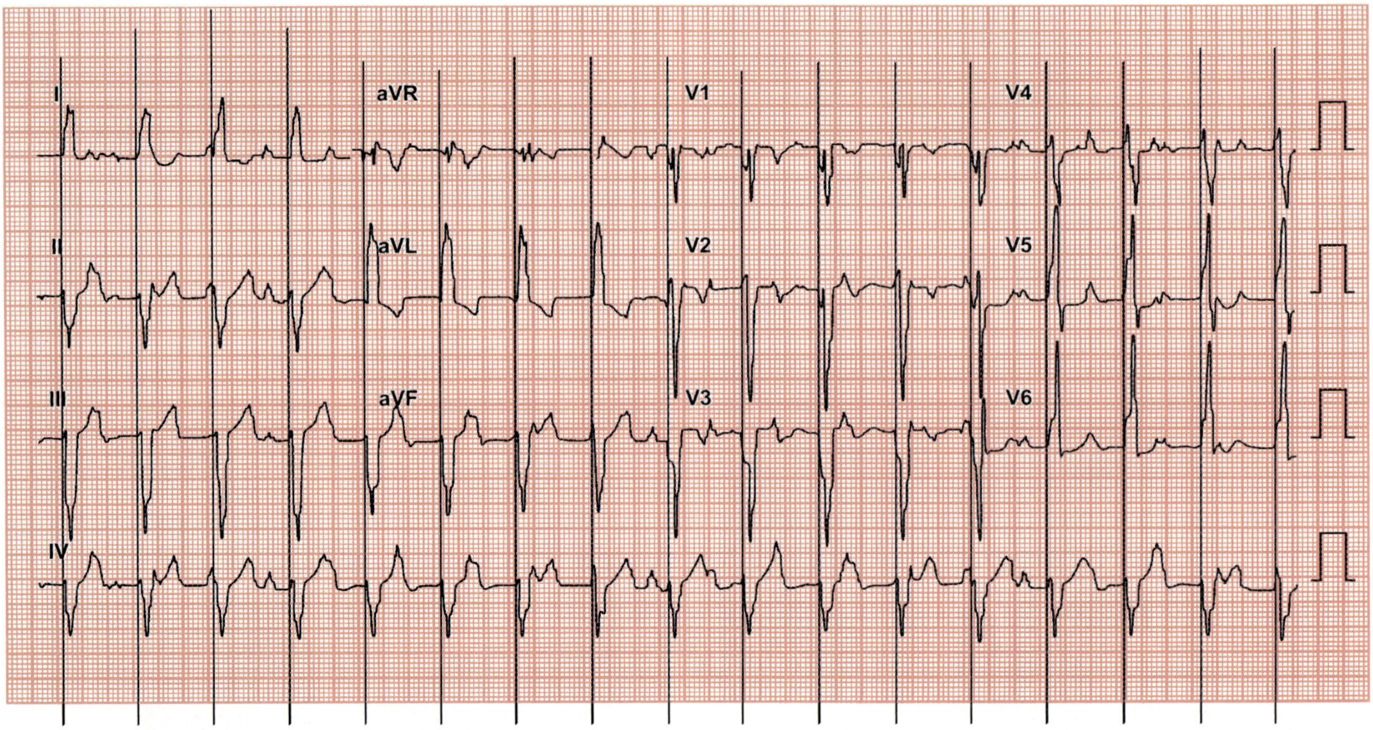


**Fig. 36.77:** Electrocardiography—regular ventricular pacing rhythm after pacemaker implantation

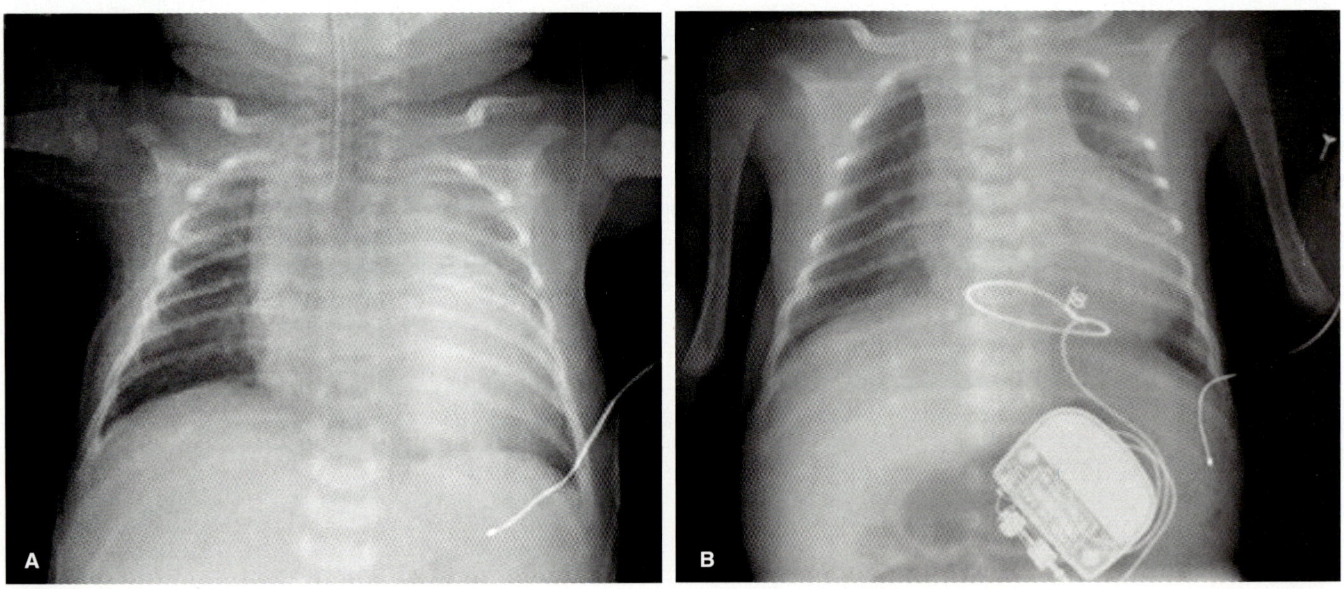


**Fig. 36.78:** (A) Chest X-ray—cardiomegaly and impending congestive heart failure before pacemaker implantation. (B) Chest X-ray—normal heart size after pacemaker implantation

demonstrate effectiveness than for the previously discussed anomalies.

### Twin-to-twin Transfusion Syndrome

*Most pregnancies result in one baby. In about one in 80 pregnancies, twins are conceived. This can occur in one of two ways* (Figs 36.80–36.82).

The more common way (which accounts for two-thirds of cases) is for the two different sperm to fertilize two different eggs, resulting in what is called a dizygotic (DZ) twin gestation. These twins are often called fraternal twins. In this type of twinning each twin has its own sac of amniotic fluid and its own placenta (afterbirth). Dizygotic twins have two sets of membranes surrounding their amniotic fluid sacs (one inner amnion layer and one outer chorion layer), and therefore they are known as diamniotic, dichorionic.

In about one-third of twin pregnancies, one sperm fertilizes one egg, but this splits into two embryos resulting

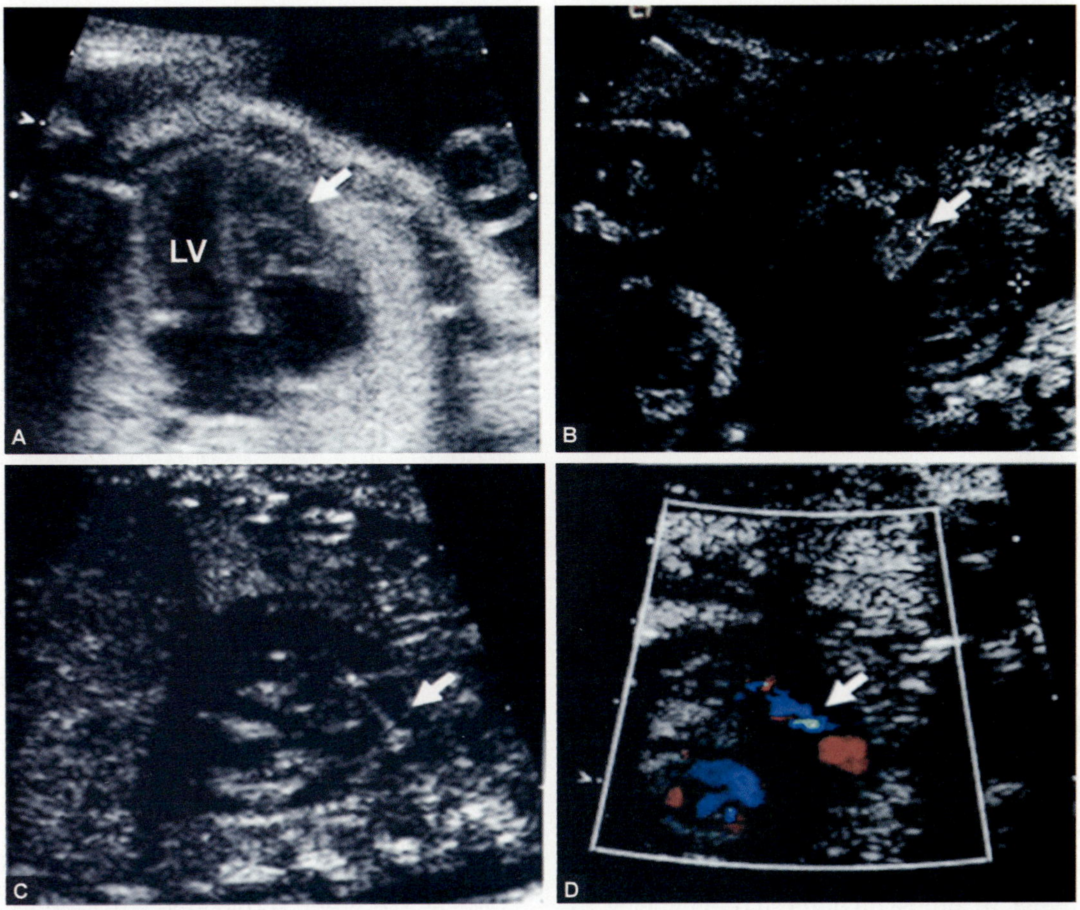


**Fig. 36.79:** Echocardiographic images obtained during the intervention for patient. (A) This four-chamber view demonstrates a hypoplastic RV (arrow). (B) In this oblique projection, the 19-gauge cannula can be seen passing through the uterus, amniotic cavity, and chest wall of the fetus and approaching the RV outflow tract (arrow). (C) This short-axis image demonstrates the tip of the Chiba needle in the pulmonary artery (arrow). (D) After successful valvuloplasty, color-Doppler ultrasound flow imaging demonstrates an antegrade jet of flow across the patent PV (arrow)

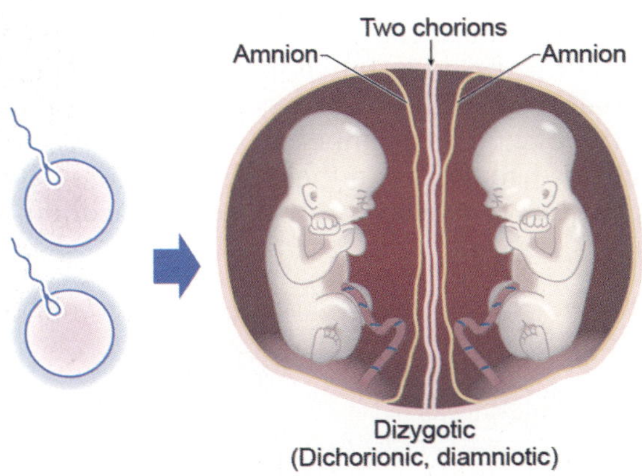


**Fig. 36.80:** Dizygotic (dichorionic and diamniotic) fetuses

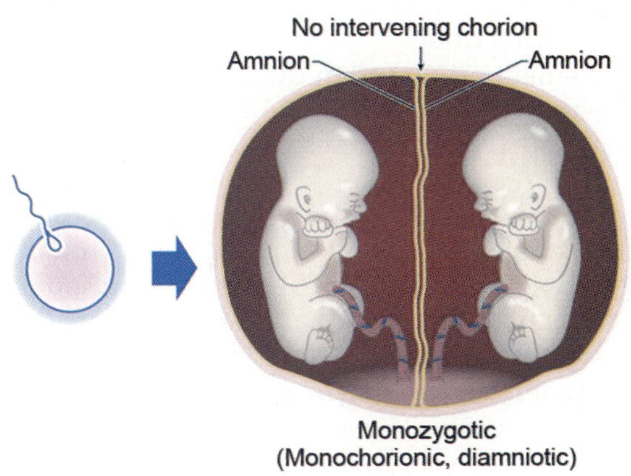


**Fig. 36.81:** Monozygotic (monochorionic and diamniotic) fetuses

in what is known as monozygotic (MZ) twins. These twins are often referred to as identical twins since they have the same genetic material. Approximately one-third of MZ twins look just like fraternal twins on prenatal ultrasound since there are two separate amniotic sacs and two separate placentas. However, in two-thirds of identical twins, each twin has its own amniotic sac but shares a common placenta. This type of MZ twinning is called monochorionic, diamniotic since there is an inner layer surrounding the amniotic sac of each twin, but there is only one common

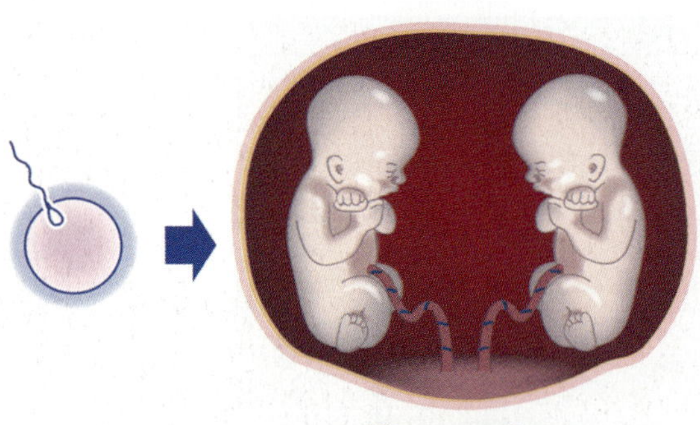


**Fig. 36.82:** Monozygotic (monochorionic and monoamniotic) fetuses

outer layer (chorion) surrounding both of the sacs. This type of twinning occurs in approximately one in 360 pregnancies. Monochorionic twins are at higher risk for complications since they share a common placenta. Less than 1% of identical twins (about one in 2,400 pregnancies) will have one amniotic sac and one placenta for both twins. This type of twinning is referred to as monchorionic, monoamniotic twinning. These twins are at very high risk for loss of the pregnancy due to entangled umbilical cords.

### What is Twin-twin Transfusion Syndrome and How Does One Get it?

This condition occurs only in those identical twins that are monochorionic, diamniotic (one-third of all identical or monozygotic twins). In almost all of these pregnancies, the single placenta contains blood vessel connections between the twins. For reasons that are not clear, in 15–20% of monochorionic, diamniotic twins, the blood flow through these blood vessel connections becomes unbalanced, resulting in a condition known as twin-twin transfusion syndrome (TTTS). This is not an inherited or genetic condition. It is not caused by something that a mother or father has done or not done.

In TTTS, the smaller twin (often called the donor twin) does not get enough blood while the larger twin (often called the recipient twin) becomes overloaded with too much blood.

In an attempt to reduce its blood volume, the recipient twin will increase the urine it makes. This will eventually result in the twin having a very large bladder on ultrasound, as well as too much amniotic fluid around this twin. This is known as polyhydramnios.

At the same time, the donor twin will produce less than the usual amount of urine. The amniotic fluid around the donor twin will become very low or absent. This is known as oligohydramnios.

As the disease progresses, the donor will produce so little urine that its bladder may not be seen on ultrasound. The twin will become wrapped by its amniotic membrane (known as a 'stuck' twin). Often the polyhydramnios of the recipient twin is the first thing noticed by the patient due a sudden increase in the size of the uterus. Clothes may become tight fitting over a short period of time. At other times the differences in the amniotic fluid volumes between the twins is only noted at the time of a routine ultrasound.

### How is Twin-twin Transfusion Syndrome Diagnosed?

The diagnosis of TTTS is made with an ultrasound evaluation that shows a twin pregnancy with one placenta, twins of the same sex in separate amniotic sacs, and polyhydramnios in the recipient's sac and oligohydramnios in the donor's sac. Amniotic fluid volume is measured with ultrasound by determining the deepest pocket measurement from the patient's skin to her back. This measurement is known as the maximum vertical pocket (MVP) (Fig. 36.83).

### What are the Twin-twin Transfusion Syndrome Five Stages of Classification?

Quintero1 has proposed five stages of TTTS based on ultrasound findings (Fig 36.84):

- **Stage I:** This is the initial way that TTTS is seen on ultrasound. In stage I, there is oligohydramnios in the donor's sac with an MVP of two centimeters or less (three-quarters of an inch) and polyhydramnios in the recipient's sac with a maximum vertical pocket of fluid of 8 cm or more (just over 3 inches). The bladder of the donor baby is still seen.
- **Stage II:** As defined above, there is polyhydramnios and oligohydramnios, but the bladder is no longer seen in the donor twin during the ultrasound evaluation.
- **Stage III:** Blood flow in the fetus can be measured with a special type of ultrasound called Doppler. In addition to the findings of stages I and II, careful study of the blood flow in the umbilical cord and fetal ductus venosus (the large blood vessel in the fetus that returns blood to the heart from the placenta) reveals abnormal patterns in stage III. These patterns can occur in either or both fetuses.

In the umbilical cord, the diastolic flow can be either absent or reversed in the umbilical artery. This pattern is usually seen in the donor twin. In the ductus venosus, the diastolic flow can either be absent or reversed. This pattern is usually see in the recipient twin due to early heart failure. The recipient twin can also exhibit leakage

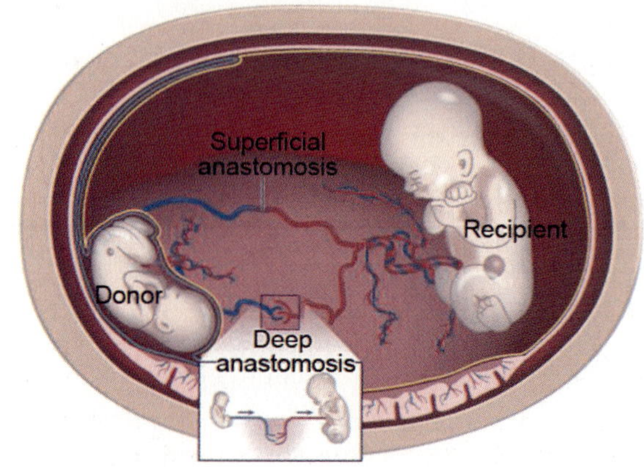


**Fig. 36.83:** Anastomosis in twin-twin transfusion syndrome

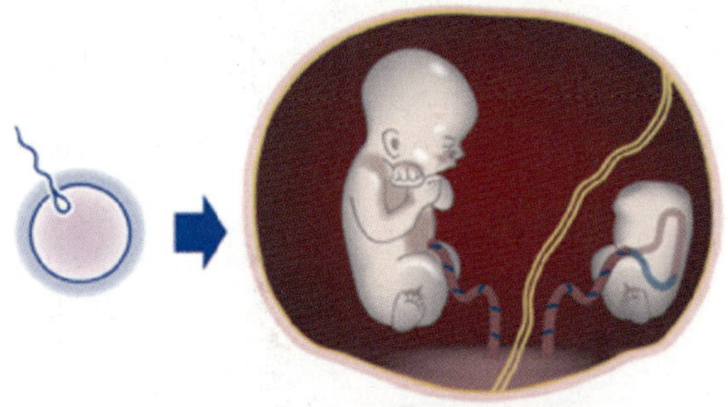


**Fig. 36.84:** Trap sequence (twin-reversed arterial perfusion sequence) in twin-twin transfusion syndrome

across the main valve on the right side of the heart, this is known as tricuspid regurgitation.

- **Stage IV:** One or both babies shows signs of hydrops. This means there is excess fluid in parts of the baby such as swelling of the skin around the head (scalp edema), fluid in the abdomen (ascites), fluid around the lungs (pleural effusions) or fluid around the heart (pericardial effusion). These findings are evidence of heart failure and are typically seen in the recipient twin.
- **Stage V:** One or both babies have died. The survival of the twins is poorer when there is progression to a higher stage over time. It has been estimated that half of patients will progress to a higher stage, 30% will remain at the same stage and 20% will improve to a lower stage.

### *What is an Acardiac Twin or Twin Reversed Arterial Perfusion (TRAP) Syndrome?*

An usual form of TTTS occurs in about one in 15,000 pregnancies. In these monochorionic twins, one twin develops normally while the other twin fails to develop a heart as well as other body structures. The abnormal twin is called an acardiac twin. In these pregnancies, the umbilical cord from the acardiac twin branches directly from the umbilical cord of the normal twin. Blood flow to the acardiac twin comes from the normal twin, which is also known as a pump twin. This blood flow is reversed from the normal direction leading to the name for this condition—twin reversed arterial perfusion syndrome or TRAP. In some cases the blood flow from the pump twin to the acardiac twin stops on its own and the acardiac twin stops growing. In other cases, the flow continues and the acardiac twin continues to increase in size. This eventually leads to heart failure and polyhydramnios in the pump twin. Without treatment, more than 50% of cases of TRAP will result in the death of the pump twin.

### *What is the Outcome for Twin-twin Transfusion Syndrome (TTTS)?*

There are a number of ways to treat TTTS, any of which many be the correct method depending on ultrasound findings, the gestational age of the pregnancy and a couple's specific needs.

Left untreated, TTTS prior to 24 weeks' gestation (6 months of pregnancy), 80–90% of cases are associated with the loss of one or both twins. If one of the twins should die, the blood vessel connections in the placenta can place the surviving twin at risk for long-term brain damage in as many as one-third of cases. In general, more advanced stages of TTTS have a worse prognosis than the earlier stages. When severe TTTS occurs at a very early gestational age (prior to 16 weeks or the fourth month of pregnancy), the option of termination of the pregnancy can be considered due to the grim prognosis.

The various therapies that are available target either the unequal fluid between the twins' sacs or interrupt the blood vessel communications between the twins on the single placenta. The successful outcome of these treatments has been based on the number of babies that survive, as well as the number of babies who do not have brain damage. The treatments that are currently available are described below.

## Treatments

### *Reduction Amniocentesis*

Serial amniocentesis involves the removal of the excessive amniotic fluid from the sac of the recipient twin using a needle that is passed through the maternal abdomen.

The amount of amniotic fluid removed will vary based on the initial volume in the recipient sac, the gestational age and the development of uterine contractions during the procedure. As a general rule no more than three liters (approximately two and one-half quarts) of amniotic fluid is removed at any one time. The procedure is usually completed within 30 minutes or less. The procedure may temporarily restore the balance in the amniotic fluid in both twins' sacs. This technique may be useful for milder cases of TTTS that occur later in pregnancy.

However, reduction amniocentesis usually requires repeat procedures to be undertaken every few days to weekly when the fluid returns to high levels. The procedure is generally not thought to be effective for more advanced stages of TTTS (stages III and IV).

Complications of repeated amniocenteses for the treatment of TTTS include premature labor with early delivery in 3% of cases, premature rupture of the membranes in 6% of cases, infection in about 1% of cases, and premature separation of the placenta from the wall of the womb (called an abruption) in 1% of cases.

Pregnancies managed with serial reduction amniocentesis on average deliver by 29–30 weeks of gestation (approximately ten weeks prior to the 'due date'). If there is progression of TTTS to a more advanced stage, serial amniocenteses will reduce the success rate for such procedures such as laser (see below). Reported survival rates have varied from 18– 83%, with a recent study noting that just over half (56%) of severe TTTS cases managed with reduction amniocentesis will end with at least one infant without brain damage. Approximately, 20–25% of the TTTS survivors from pregnancies treated with reduction amniocentesis have been found to have long-term developmental delay.

### Septostomy

Septostomy (Fig. 36.85) (also known as microseptostomy) is the creation of a hole in the membrane between the babies' sacs using a needle. This causes fluid to move from the amniotic sac with excessive fluid (the recipient's sac) into the sac with absent or low fluid (donor's sac). Since septostomy is performed with a needle that is used to perform amniocentesis, complications of infection, premature labor and premature rupture of the membranes are rare. Septostomy carries the additional potential risk for the hole to become larger between the two sacs and could even allow the babies to share the same amniotic space if the entire separating membrane becomes disrupted. This has been reported to occur in 3% of septostomies. In the worst case scenario, the umbilical cords of the twins could become entangled, leading to the death of one or both fetuses. In one large series, survival to birth was 80% for at least one twin and was 60% for both twins. Patients undergoing septostomy typically require fewer procedures than those treated with amnioreduction. There is no data currently available regarding neurologic outcome in survivors of septostomy.

### Selective Laser Ablation of the Placental Anastomotic Vessels

In more advanced stages of TTTS (stage II and higher) laser ablation of the communicating vessels on the placenta between the twin fetuses can be a curative procedure (Fig. 36.86).

The procedure is performed in an operating room. After the patient's abdomen has been washed with an antiseptic and covered with sterile paper drapes, an ultrasound is performed to determine the appropriate spot to enter the uterus. The skin is then injected with an anesthetic medication to 'numb' the area and deep tissues directly under the selected site. An anesthesiologist will also administer medications through an intravenous line to produce sedation. A small skin cut is made to allow the introduction of a thin hollow tube and needle. The instruments are inserted under ultrasound guidance into the amniotic sac of the recipient twin. The needle is removed and a telescope (fetoscope) with a thin fiber to carry the laser energy is then inserted through the hollow tube. The fetoscope is used to look directly at the blood vessels on the surface of the placenta. Vessels that are found to communicate between the twins are then closed using laser light energy. At the completion of the surgery, the extra-amniotic fluid in the recipient twin's sac is removed to achieve a normal volume. The procedure may take 45 minutes to 2 hours depending on the difficulty of the case.

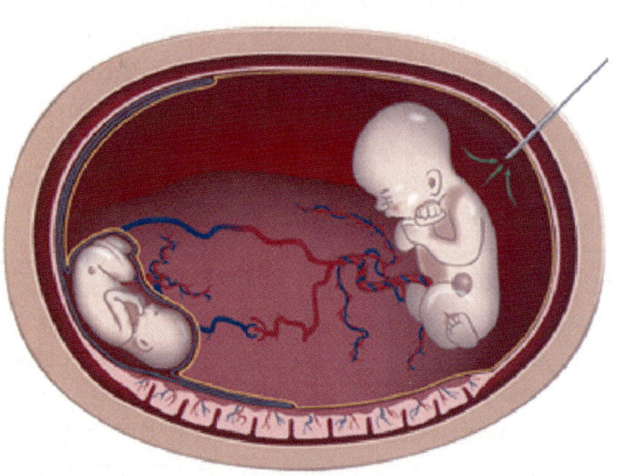

**Fig. 36.85:** Reduction amniocentesis septostomy (also known as microseptostomy)

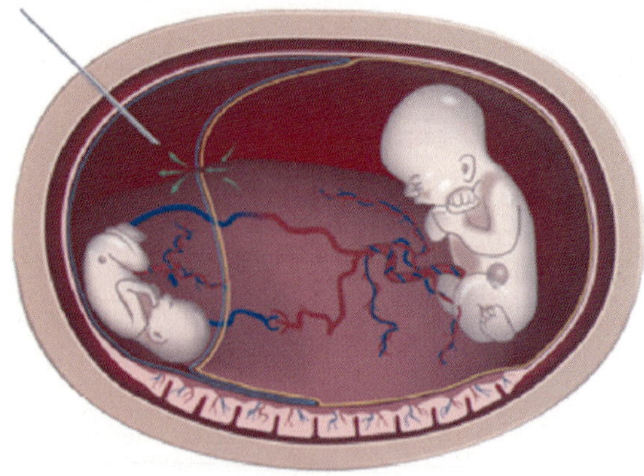

**Fig. 36.86:** Selective laser ablation of the placental anastomotic vessels

Because the fetoscope requires a larger hole to be made into the amniotic cavity than would be the case with an amnioreduction or septostomy procedure, laser ablation is associated with a higher risk of complications such as premature contractions, premature rupture of the membranes (15–20% of cases), placental separation (2%) and infection. For this reason, special medications to prevent contractions and antibiotics to prevent infection will be given before and after the procedure. In addition, laser therapy may be associated with unique risks since the laser energy may cause certain areas of the placenta or blood vessels on the surface of the placenta to bleed.

Laser ablation has been shown to result in the survival of at least one twin in 70–80% of cases and both twins in one-third of cases. Should one fetus die after the procedure, the likelihood that the surviving fetus will develop complications is reduced from 35% to approximately 7%. This is because the babies are no longer sharing blood vessels between them. In one-third of cases, neither twin will survive. Studies to date have indicated that approximately 8% of survivors following laser ablation will have a long-term mental handicap. This is approximately half of the rate of problems seen in survivors treated with amnioreduction.

### Selective Cord Coagulation

In some cases, a couple may make the difficult decision to proceed with the purposeful loss of one twin to save the

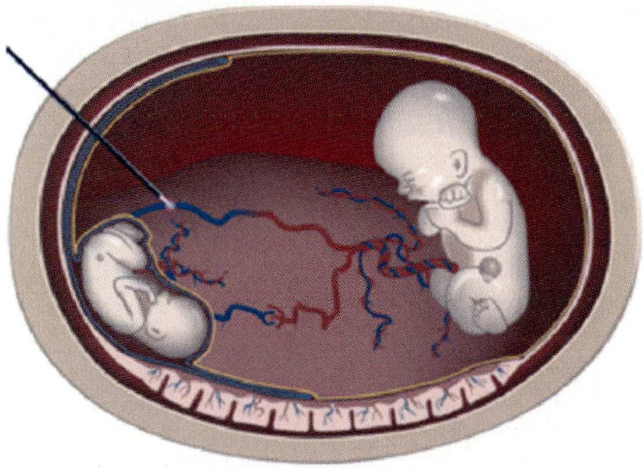

**Fig. 36.87:** Laser ablation of the placental anastomotic vessels selective cord coagulation

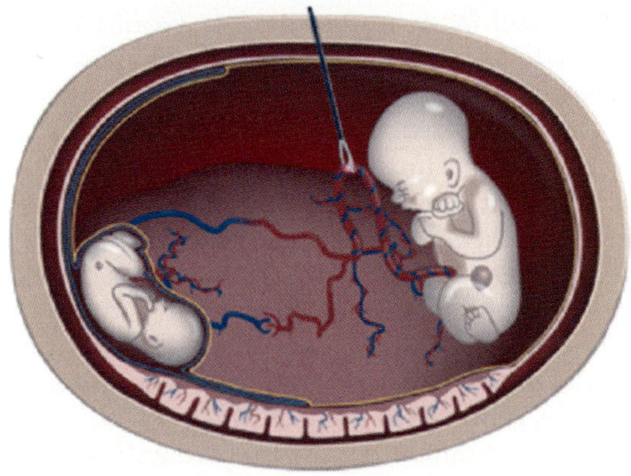

**Fig. 36.88:** Selective cord coagulation radiofrequency ablation

other twin. This procedure is used when laser ablation of the connecting vessels is not possible or if one of the twins is so close to death that laser ablation would likely not be successful. By stopping the flow in the cord of the dying twin, the other twin can be protected from the consequences of its sibling's death. The procedure is performed through the use of a special forceps that is placed into the amniotic sac of the recipient twin while watching with ultrasound. The umbilical cord is then grasped and electrical current is applied to burn (coagulate) the blood vessels in the cord so that the blood flow will stop to this fetus. The communication between the fetuses is definitively ended; however, this eliminates the chance of survival for one of the twins. Complications of this procedure include premature delivery and premature rupture of the membranes. Rupture of the membranes has been reported to occur in about 20% of cases. Survival of the one remaining fetus can be expected in 85% of cases (Fig. 36.87).

### Radiofrequency Ablation

This procedure is usually reserved for TRAP sequence. The umbilical cord of the acardiac fetus is usually very short and difficult to see on ultrasound (Fig. 36.88). As a result, it is often difficult to stop the blood flow into the acardiac fetus by coagulation of the umbilical cord. For this reason, a major blood vessel in the acardiac fetus is often targeted as the site for occlusion of blood flow. This can be accomplished through the use of a radiofrequency ablation catheter. In this procedure, a specialized needle is passed into the amniotic fluid and then into the body of the acardiac fetus. A special current is then applied to the needle to burn the area around the major blood vessel in the abnormal fetus. This will stop the blood flow and allow the pump twin (normal twin) to no longer have to send blood to the acardiac twin. Complications of infection, premature contractions and premature rupture of the membranes can occur as in any needle procedure. In one series, the risk for premature rupture of the membranes was 8%. In this same series, the chance for a successful live birth for the pump twin was 90%.

### What can I Expect After Surgery?

Following surgery, you will be taken to the recovery room in labor and delivery or a labor room where you and your fetus or fetuses will be closely monitored. Your abdomen will be a little tender or sore once the local anesthetic wears off. You may be given medications after surgery to relax the uterus and stop any contractions. The pain and discomfort after surgery is usually minimal. If needed, pain relief medicine is available. Your spouse or other support person may remain with you in your room. Following surgery, you may have food as tolerated. You will be admitted to the hospital for an overnight stay. That night, activity is restricted to bathroom privileges only, but this depends upon your specific condition. You will undergo an ultrasound the day after surgery to determine how the babies are doing.

### What can I Expect After I am Discharged Home?

You will then be discharged home to the care of your primary obstetrician and/or your referring maternal-fetal medicine specialist. Your instructions will include bed rest with bathroom privileges for 7 days after the surgery, with a gradual increase in activity. We will also ask that you get a thermometer and take your temperature 3 times per day. You should notify your primary obstetrician for any increase above 100.4°F of an oral temperature. The site of the surgery can get wet in a shower within 24 hours of the procedure. You can remove the steri-strips over the incision yourself 1 week after the surgery.

After 4 weeks you can resume normal activity based on your pregnancy condition and the comfort level of your primary obstetrician. Weekly ultrasounds are recommended for the next month. After that time, if all is going well, ultrasounds are performed as directed by your doctor.

Although you are returning home, we will continue to follow your pregnancy closely through our care coordinator. Please make arrangements with your doctor to forward your ultrasound reports and any other pertinent information to us. We also ask that you inform your obstetrician and labor nurse that we would like to have your placenta sent back to us after you delivery. This information is useful to further our knowledge and will assist in the future treatment of patients with TTTS.

Social services and pastoral care are available for all our patients and their families. If you would like to see them at any time, you need only to request it and they can be contacted. We are sensitive to the psychological, social and spiritual needs of our families. We will provide any support that is necessary. Please contact us if you have any questions, concerns or special requests. For our out of town patients, we realize that traveling may be difficult or stressful and want you to know that we will do everything we can to accommodate your special needs and schedule.

## FUTURE DIRECTIONS

There is much that remains to be learned about the benefits and potential adverse effects of FCI. Although pharmacological FCI is well established in the management of fetal arrhythmias and heart block, there is room for improvement nonetheless. In addition, novel pharmacological strategies, such as maternal hyperoxia, and the prospect of other agents for other conditions will inevitably emerge. On the basis of the experimental evidence, open FCI appears feasible, although the indications for and establishment of open FCI in humans must be explored critically. There are severe congenital cardiac anomalies for which more complex interventions may be beneficial, such as severe Ebstein's malformation with fetal hydrops.

Ultimately, the utility of FCI will depend on a variety of clinical and technological factors, including more frequent, earlier diagnosis of congenital heart disease in-utero, characterization of prognostic features in fetuses with congenital heart disease, better understanding of the capacity and optimal gestational windows for cardiovascular remodeling after FCI, and improved and focused technology. Advances in imaging and instrumentation should facilitate greater precision and effectiveness of intervention and may open the door to procedures for more complex indications. More sophisticated image-guided or robotic interventional approaches to closed FCI are being explored and may help improve precision and success, potentially shifting the gestational horizon to allow safe intervention in younger fetuses. At the same time, as experience with FCI accumulates, risk profiles can be expected to improve, which may facilitate FCI for less severe conditions if such procedures can be expected to improve outcomes.

## BIBLIOGRAPHY


1. Ahuja P, Sdek P, MacLellan WR. Cardiac myocyte cell cycle control in development, disease, and regeneration. Physiol Rev 2007;87:521–44.
2. Arzt W, Tulzer G, Aigner M, Mair R, Hafner E. Invasive intrauterine treatment of pulmonary atresia/intact ventricular septum with heart failure. Ultrasound Obstet Gynecol 2003; 21:186–8.
3. Battaglia C, Artini PG, D'Ambrogio G, Bencini S, Galli PA, Genazzani AR. Maternal hyperoxygenation in the treatment of mild intrauterine growth retardation: a pilot study. Ultrasound Obstet Gynecol 1994;4:472–5.
4. Carpenter R, Strasburger JF, Garson A, Smith RT, Deter RL, Englehardt H. Fetal ventricular pacing for hydrops secondary to complete atrioventricular block. J Am Coll Cardiol 1986;8:1434–6.
5. Cortes RA, Farmer DL. Recent advances in fetal surgery. Semin Perinatol 2004;28:199–211.
6. Dickinson JE, Evans SF. The progression of disease stage in twin-twin transfusion syndrome. J Matern Fetal Neonatal Med 2004;16:95–101.
7. Eibschitz I, Abinader EG, Klein A, Sharf M. Intrauterine diagnosis and control of fetal ventricular arrhythmia during labor. Am J Obstet Gynecol 1975;122:597–600.
8. Fenton KM, Heinemann MK, Hanley FL. Exclusion of the placenta during fetal cardiac bypass allows improved systemic perfusion and provides important information about the mechanism of placental injury. J Thorac Cardiovasc Surg 1993;105:502–12.
9. Fenton KN, Heinemann MK, Klautz RJM, Liddicoat JR, Hanley FL. Inhibition of fetal stress response improves cardiac output and gas exchange after fetal cardiac bypass. J Thorac Cardiovasc Surg 1994;107:1416–22.
10. Fenton KN, Zinn HE, Heinemann MK, Liddicoat JR, Hanley FL. Long-term survivors of fetal cardiac bypass in lambs. J Thorac Cardiovasc Surg 1994;107:1423–7.
11. Fesslova V, Vignati G, Brucato A, De Sanctis M, Butera G, Pisoni MP, Chiappa E, Acaia B, Meroni PL. The impact of treatment of the fetus by maternal therapy on the fetal and postnatal outcomes for fetuses diagnosed with isolated complete atrioventricular block. Cardiol Young 2009;19:282–90.
12. Friedman DM, Kim MY, Copel JA, Llanos C, Davis C, Buyon JP. Prospective evaluation of fetuses with autoimmune-associated congenital heart block followed in the PR Interval and Dexamethasone Evaluation (PRIDE) Study. Am J Cardiol 2009;103:1102–6.
13. Galindo A, Gutierrez-Larraya F, Velasco JM, de la Fuente P. Pulmonary balloon valvuloplasty in a fetus with critical pulmonary stenosis/atresia with intact ventricular septum and heart failure. Fetal Diagn Ther 2006;21:100–4.
14. Gurtner GC, Werner S, Barrandon Y, Longaker MT. Wound repair and regeneration. Nature 2008;453:314–21.
15. Hecher K, Plath H, Bregenzer T, Hansmann M, Hackeloer BJ. Endoscopic laser surgery versus serial amniocenteses in the treatment of severe twin-twin transfusion syndrome. Am J Obstet Gynecol 1999;180:717–24.
16. Jaeggi ET, Fouron JC, Silverman ED, Ryan G, Smallhorn J, Hornberger LK. Transplacental fetal treatment improves the outcome of prenatally diagnosed complete atrioventricular block without structural heart disease. Circulation 2004;110: 1542–8.
17. Kleinman CS, Donnerstein RL, DeVore GR, Jaffe CC, Lynch DC, Berkowitz RL, Talner NS, Hobbins JC. Fetal echocardiography for evaluation of in utero congestive heart failure. N Engl J Med 1982;306:568–75.
18. Kohl T, Breuer J, Heep A, Wenningmann I, Weinbach J, Gembruch U. Fetal transesophageal echocardiography

during balloon valvuloplasty for severe aortic valve stenosis at 28+6 weeks of gestation. J Thorac Cardiovasc Surg 2007; 134:256–7.
19. Kohl T, Müller A, Tchatcheva K, Achenbach S, Gembruch U. Fetal transesophageal echocardiography: clinical introduction as a monitoring tool during cardiac intervention in a human fetus. Ultrasound Obstet Gynecol 2005;26:780–5.
20. Kohl T, Sharland G, Allan LD, Gembruch U, Chaoui R, Lopes LM, Zielinsky P, Huhta J, Silverman NH. World experience of percutaneous ultrasound-guided balloon valvuloplasty in human fetuses with severe aortic valve obstruction. Am J Cardiol 2000;85:1230–3.
21. Kunisaki SM, Jennings RW. Fetal surgery. J Intensive Care Med 2008;23:33–51.
22. Lee H, Wagner A, Bobert B, et al. Radiofrequency ablation for TRAP sequence. Am J Obstet Gynecol 2005;191:S18.
23. Maeno Y, Himeno W, Saito A, Hiraishi S, Hirose O, Ikuma M, Inamura N, Kawataki M, Mizukami A, Ota M, Shiraishi H, Satomi G, Kato H. Clinical course of fetal congenital atrioventricular block in the Japanese population: a multi-centre experience. Heart 2005;91:1075–9.
24. Mari G, Roberts A, Detti L, et al. Perinatal morbidity and mortality rates in severe twin-twin transfusion syndrome: results of the International Amnioreduction Registry. Am J Obstet Gynecol 2001;185:708–15.
25. Marshall AC, Levine J, Morash D, Silva V, Lock JE, Benson CB, Wilkins-Haug LE, McElhinney DB, Tworetzky W. Results of in utero atrial septoplasty in fetuses with hypoplastic left heart syndrome. Prenat Diagn 2008;28:1023–8.
26. Marshall AC, van der Velde ME, Tworetzky W, Gomez CA, Wilkins-Haug L, Benson CB, Jennings RW, Lock JE. Creation of an atrial septal defect in utero for fetuses with hypoplastic left heart syndrome and intact or highly restrictive atrial septum. Circulation 2004;110:253–8.
27. McElhinney DB, Marshall AC, Wilkins-Haug LE, Brown DW, Benson CB, Silva V, Marx GR, Mizrahi-Arnaud A, Lock JE, Tworetzky W. Predictors of technical success and postnatal biventricular outcome after in utero aortic valvuloplasty for aortic stenosis with evolving hypoplastic left heart syndrome. Circulation 2009;120:1482–90.
28. Mizrahi-Arnaud A, Tworetzky W, Bulich LA, Wilkins-Haug LE, Marshall AC, Benson CB, Lock JE, McElhinney DB. Pathophysiology, management, and outcomes of fetal hemodynamic instability during prenatal cardiac intervention. Pediatr Res 2007;62:325–30.
29. Moise KJ, Jr., Dorman K, Lamvu G, et al. A randomized trial of amnioreduction versus septostomy in the treatment of twin-twin transfusion syndrome. Am J Obstet Gynecol 2005; 193:701–7.
30. Newburger JW, Keane JF. Intrauterine supraventricular tachycardia. J Pediatr 1979;95:780–6.
31. Oudijk MA, Michon MM, Kleinman CS, Kapusta L, Stoutenbeek P, Visser GH, Meijboom EJ. Sotalol in the treatment of fetal dysrhythmias. Circulation 2000;101: 2721–6.
32. Parry AJ, Petrossian E, McElhinney DB, Reddy VM, Hanley FL. Neutrophil degranulation and complement activation during fetal cardiac bypass. Ann Thorac Surg 2000;70: 582–9.
33. Patel D, Cuneo B, Viesca R, Rassanan J, Leshko J, Huhta J. Digoxin for the treatment of fetal congestive heart failure with sinus rhythm assessed by cardiovascular profile score. J Matern Fetal Neonatal Med 2008;21:477–82.
34. Pomini F, Noia G, Mancuso S. Hypothetical role of prosta-glandins in the onset of preterm labor after fetal surgery. Fetal Diagn Ther 2007;22:94–9.
35. Quintero RA, Dickinson JE, Morales WJ, et al. Stage-based treatment of twin-twin transfusion syndrome. Am J Obstet Gynecol 2003;188:1333–40.
36. Quintero RA, Huhta J, Suh E, Chmait R, Romero R, Angel J. In utero cardiac fetal surgery: laser atrial septotomy in the treatment of hypoplastic left heart syndrome with intact atrial septum. Am J Obstet Gynecol 2005;193:1424–8.
37. Quintero RA, Morales WJ, Allen MH, Bornick PW, Johnson PK, Kruger M. Staging of twin-twin transfusion syndrome. J Perinatol 1999;19:550–5.
38. Reddy VM, Liddicoat JR, Klein JR, McElhinney DB, Wampler RK, Hanley FL. Fetal cardiac bypass using an in-line axial flow pump to minimize extracorporeal surface and avoid priming volume. Ann Thorac Surg 1996;62:393–400.
39. Reddy VM, Liddicoat JR, Klein JR, Wampler RK, Hanley FL. Long-term fetal outcome after fetal cardiac bypass: fetal survival to full term and organ abnormalities. J Thorac Cardiovasc Surg 1996;111:536–44.
40. Reddy VM, McElhinney DB, Rajasinghe HA, Liddicoat JR, Hendricks-Munoz K, Fineman JR, Hanley FL. Role of the endothelium in placental dysfunction after fetal cardiac bypass. J Thorac Cardiovasc Surg 1999;117:343–51.
41. Reddy VM, McElhinney DB, Rajasinghe HA, Rodriguez JL, Hanley FL. Cytokine response to fetal cardiac bypass. J Matern Fetal Invest 1998;8:46–9.
42. Richter RC, Slate RK, Rudolph AM, Turley K. Fetal blood flow during hypothermic cardiopulmonary bypass in utero. J Cardiovasc Surg 1985;26:86.
43. Sabik JF, Assad RS, Hanley FL. Prostaglandin synthesis inhibition prevents placental dysfunction after fetal cardiac bypass. J Thorac Cardiovasc Surg 1992;103:733–42.
44. Sabik JF, Heinemann MK, Assad RS, Hanley FL. High dose steroids prevent placental dysfunction after fetal cardiac bypass. J Thorac Cardiovasc Surg 1994;107:116–25.
45. Schmolling J, Renke K, Richter O, Pfeiffer K, Schlebusch H, Höller T. Digoxin, flecainide, and amiodarone transfer across the placenta and the effects of an elevated umbilical venous pressure on the transfer rate. Ther Drug Monit 2000;22: 582–8.
46. Selamet Tierney ES, Wald RM, McElhinney DB, Marshall AC, Benson CB, Marcus EN, Marx GR, Levine JC, Wilkins-Haug L, Lock JE, Tworetzky W. Changes in left heart hemodynamics after technically successful in utero aortic valvuloplasty. Ultrasound Obstet Gynecol 2007;30:715–20.
47. Senat MV, Deprest J, Boulvain M, Paupe A, Winer N, Ville Y. Endoscopic laser surgery versus serial amnioreduction for severe twin-to-twin transfusion syndrome. N Engl J Med 2004;351:136–44.
48. Strasburger JF, Cuneo BF, Michon MM, Gotteiner NL, Deal BJ, McGregor SN, Oudijk MA, Meijboom EJ, Feinkind L, Hussey M, Parilla BV. Amiodarone therapy for drug-refractory fetal tachycardia. Circulation 2004;109:375–9.

49. Suh E, Quintessenza J, Huhta J, Quintero R. How to grow a heart: fibreoptic guided fetal aortic valvotomy. Cardiol Young 2006;16(Suppl 1):43–6.
50. Szwast A, Tian Z, McCann M, Donaghue D, Rychik J. Vaso-reactive response to maternal hyperoxygenation (MH) in the fetus with hypoplastic left heart syndrome (HLHS). Circ Cardiovasc Imaging. 2009 Dec 31. [Epub ahead of print.]
51. Taylor MJ, Govender L, Jolly M, Wee L, Fisk NM. Validation of the Quintero staging system for twin-twin transfusion syndrome. Obstet Gynecol 2002;100:1257–65.
52. Tulzer G, Arzt W, Franklin RC, Loughna PV, Mair R, Gardiner HM. Fetal pulmonary valvuloplasty for critical pulmonary stenosis or atresia with intact septum. Lancet 2002;360:1567–8.
53. Turley K, Vlahakes GJ, Harrison MR, Messina L, Hanley F, Uhlig PN, Ebert P. Intrauterine cardiothoracic surgery: the fetal lamb model. Ann Thorac Surg 1982;34:422–6.
54. Tworetzky W, McElhinney DB, Marx GR, Benson CB, Brusseau R, Morash D, Louise E, Wilkins-Haug LE, Lock JE, Marshall AC. In utero valvuloplasty for pulmonary valve atresia with hypoplastic right ventricle: techniques and outcomes. Pediatrics 2009 Aug 24. [Epub ahead of print.]
55. Tworetzky W, Wilkins-Haug L, Jennings RW, van der Velde ME, Marshall AC, Marx GR, Colan SD, Benson CB, Lock JE, Perry SB. Balloon dilation of severe aortic stenosis in the fetus: potential for prevention of hypoplastic left heart syndrome: candidate selection, technique, and results of successful intervention. Circulation 2004;12:2125–31.
56. van den Heuvel F, Bink-Boelkens MT, du Marchie Sarvaas GJ, Berger RM. Drug management of fetal tachyarrhytmias: are we ready for a systematic and evidence-based approach? Pacing Clin Electrophysiol 2008;31(Suppl 1): S54–S57.
57. Wilkins-Haug LE, Tworetzky W, Benson CB, Marshall AC, Jennings RW, Lock JE. Factors affecting technical success of fetal aortic valve dilation. Ultrasound Obstet Gynecol 2006; 28:47–52.

# 37 Heart Transplantation in Adults

A heart transplant, or a cardiac transplant, is a surgical transplant procedure performed on patients with end-stage heart failure or severe coronary artery disease. As of 2008 the most common procedure is to take a working heart from a recently deceased organ donor (cadaveric allograft) and implant it into the patient. The patient's own heart is either removed (orthotopic procedure) or, less commonly, left in place to support the donor heart (heterotopic procedure). Postoperation survival periods average 15 years. Heart transplantation is not considered to be a cure for heart disease, but a life-saving treatment intended to improve the quality of life for recipients.

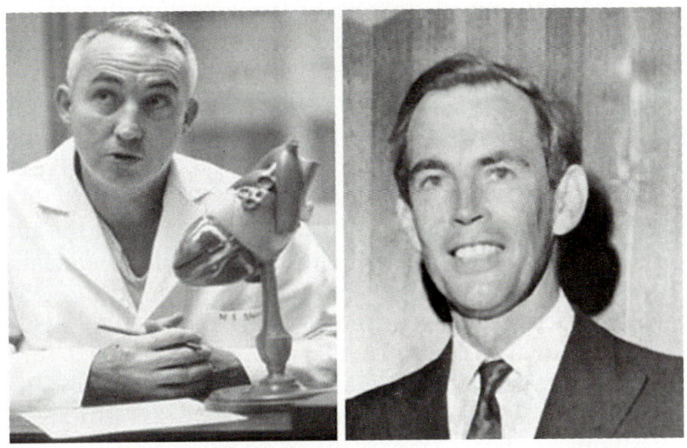

**Fig. 37.1: Norman Shumway (Left)** who is widely regarded as the father of heart transplantation and the world's first adult human heart transplant was performed by a South African cardiac surgeon, **Christiaan Barnard (Right)**, utilizing the techniques developed and perfected by Shumway and Richard Lower

## History

In 1945 the Soviet Pathologist Nikolai Sinitsyn successfully transplanted a heart from one frog to another frog and from one dog to another without killing any. **Norman Shumway** is widely regarded as the father of heart transplantation although the world's first adult human heart transplant was performed by a South African cardiac surgeon, **Christiaan Barnard**, utilizing the techniques developed and perfected by Shumway and Richard Lower. Barnard performed the first transplant on Louis Washkansky on December 3, 1967 at the Groote Schuur Hospital in Cape Town, South Africa. Adrian Kantrowitz performed the world's first pediatric heart transplant on December 6, 1967, at Maimonides Hospital in Brooklyn, New York, barely three days after Christiaan Barnard's pioneering procedure. Norman Shumway performed the first adult heart transplant in the United States on January 6, 1968, at the Stanford University Hospital (Fig. 37.1).

Worldwide, about 3,500 heart transplants are performed annually. The vast majority of these are performed in the United States (2,000–2,300 annually). Cedars-Sinai Medical Center in Los Angeles, California, currently is the largest heart transplant center in the world, having performed 119 adult transplants in 2013 alone. About 800,000 people have NYHA Class IV heart failure symptoms indicating advanced heart failure. The great disparity between the number of patients needing transplants and the number of procedures being performed spurred research into the transplantation of nonhuman hearts into humans after 1993. Xenografts from other species and man-made artificial hearts are two less successful alternatives to allografts.

## FIRST HEART TRANSPLANT IN INDIA

AIIMS is the first Indian center to perform a successful cardiac transplant. The surgery was performed by **Dr Panangipalli Venugopal**, the exdirector of AIIMS in 1994. The Organ Transplant Bill 1994 was passed in the Indian Parliament in May 1994 which legalized the organ transplants in India. The Bill was on the Table of the President of India for final approval when Dr Venugopal led a team of doctors to perform the first successful heart transplant in India on 3 August 1994. This was the first of the 26 heart transplant procedures performed by Dr Venugopal.

Another heart surgeon from India, i.e. Dr KM Cherian performed the first coronary artery bypass surgery in India in 1975. He also performed the country's first heart transplant, first infant cardiac surgery and the first heart and lung transplant (1999). Pioneering pediatric cardiac surgery in India, Cherian has pioneered the first coronary artery bypass surgery in India [as well as the first heart transplant after the legislation of brain death in India; the first bilateral lung transplant; the first pediatric heart transplant; the first auto transplant; and the first heart and lung transplant (1999).

The University of Michigan Cardiac Transplant Program is the leading cardiac transplant center in Michigan, performing over 30 cardiac transplants a year. The cardiovascular center has three adult cardiac transplant surgeons and seven heart failure and transplant cardiologists with advanced training in managing the complexities of this patient population. Because the University of Michigan is a high volume transplant center, we provide the multidisciplinary care required for the complex transplant patient, encompassing specialists in advanced circulatory support, cardiac critical care, nutrition, social work, congenital heart disease, inherited cardiomyopathies, and transplant infectious disease. We also enroll all patients under the care of a University of Michigan cardiac transplant specialist into our post-transplant telemanagement program. As a result of this multidisciplinary approach, University of Michigan Cardiac Transplant Program boasts a 91% three year post-transplant survival, compared to an expected survival of 79%. We have performed nearly 800 adult heart transplants. A heart transplant is an operation in which the diseased heart in a person is replaced with a healthy heart from a deceased donor. Ninety percent of heart transplants are performed on patients with end-stage heart failure. Heart failure is a condition in which the heart is damaged or weakened and can't pump enough blood to meet the body's needs. 'End-stage' means the condition has become so severe that all treatments, other than heart transplant, have failed.

### Overview

Heart transplants are done as a life-saving measure for end-stage heart failure when medical treatment and less drastic surgery have failed. Because donor hearts are in short supply, patients who need a heart transplant go through a careful selection process. They need to be sick enough to need a new heart, yet healthy enough to receive it. Survival rates for people receiving a heart transplant have improved over the past 5–10 years-especially in the first year after the transplant. About 88% of patients survive the first year after transplant surgery, and 72% survive for 5 years. The 10-year survival rate is close to 50%, and 16% of heart transplant patients survive 20 years. After the surgery, most heart transplant recipients (about 90%) can come close to resuming their normal daily activities. However, fewer than 40% return to work for many different reasons.

## THE HEART TRANSPLANT PROCESS

The heart transplant process starts when doctors refer patients with end-stage heart failure to a heart transplant center for evaluation. Patients found to be eligible for a heart transplant are placed on a waiting list for a donor heart. Heart transplant surgery is done in a hospital when a suitable donor heart is found. After the transplant, patients are started on a lifelong health care plan involving multiple medicines and frequent medical monitoring.

### Indications of a Heart Transplant

- Most patients referred to a heart transplant center have end-stage heart failure.
- Of these patients, close to half have heart failure as a result of coronary artery disease.
- Others have heart failure caused by hereditary conditions, viral infections of the heart, or damaged heart valves and muscles due to factors such as the use of certain medicines and alcohol, and pregnancy.
- Most patients considered for a heart transplant have exhausted attempts at less invasive treatments and have been hospitalized a number of times for heart failure.

### Preoperative Assessment of a patient before Heart Transplant

The heart transplant specialists at the heart transplant center will determine whether a patient is eligible for a transplant. Specialists often include a (Fig. 37.2):

- Cardiologist (a doctor who specializes in treating heart problems)
- Cardiac surgeon (a doctor who performs the surgery)
- Transplant coordinator (a person who makes arrangements for the surgery, such as transportation of the donor heart)
- Social worker

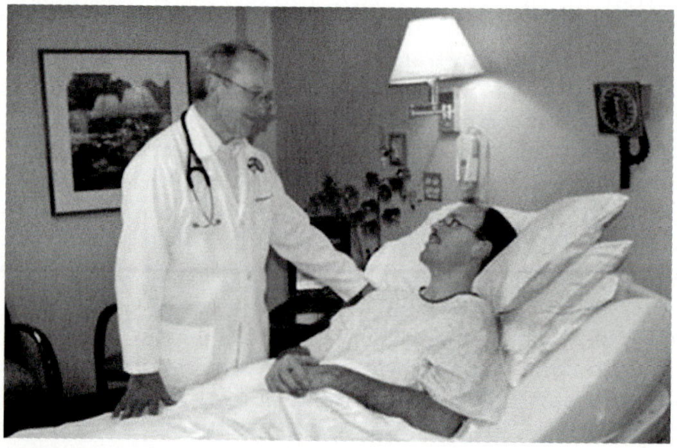

**Fig. 37.2:** Preoperative clinical assessment of a patient waiting a heart transplant

- Dietitian
- Psychiatrist

### Contraindications

Some patients are less suitable for a heart transplant, especially if they suffer from other circulatory conditions related to the heart. The following conditions in a patient increase the chances of complications:

- Kidney, lung, or liver disease
- Insulin-dependent diabetes with other organ dysfunction
- Life-threatening diseases unrelated to heart failure
- Vascular disease of the neck and leg arteries
- High pulmonary vascular resistance
- Recent thromboembolism
- Age over 60 years (some variation between centers)
- Substance abuse, notably tobacco smoking (which increases the chance of lung disease)

## WHAT TO EXPECT BEFORE A HEART TRANSPLANT?

### The Heart Transplant Waiting List

Patients who are eligible for a heart transplant are placed on a waiting list for a donor heart. This waiting list is part of a national allocation system for donor organs run by the organ procurement and transplantation network (OPTN).

To make sure that organs are distributed fairly, OPTN has policies on how donor hearts are allocated. These policies are based on the urgency of need, the organs that are available for transplant, and the location of the patient who is receiving the heart (the recipient). Organs are matched for blood type and size of donor and recipient.

### The Donor Heart

Guidelines on how a donor heart is selected require that the donor meet the legal requirement for brain death and that the appropriate consent forms are signed. Guidelines suggest that the donor be younger than 65 years of age, have little or no history of heart disease or trauma to the chest, and not be exposed to hepatitis or HIV. It's also recommended that the donor heart not be without blood circulation for more than 4 hours.

### Waiting Times

Approximately 3,000 people in the United States are on the waiting list for a heart transplant on any given day. About 2,000 donor hearts are available each year. Wait times vary from days to several months and will depend on a recipient's blood type and condition.

A person may be taken off the list for some time if he or she has a serious medical event such as a stroke, infection, or kidney failure. Time spent on the waiting list plays a part in who receives a donor heart. For example, if a donor heart becomes available and there are two recipients with equal need, the recipient who has been waiting longer will usually get the heart.

### Ongoing Medical Treatment

Patients on the waiting list for a donor heart receive ongoing treatment for heart failure and other medical conditions.

- Treating arrhythmias (irregular heartbeats), for example, is very important because they can cause sudden cardiac arrest in people who have heart failure. As a result, many transplant centers will place implantable cardioverter defibrillators (ICDs) in patients before surgery. An ICD is a small device that's placed in the chest or abdomen to help control life-threatening arrhythmias.
- Another treatment that may be recommended to waiting list patients is an implanted mechanical pump called a ventricular assist device (VAD), which helps the heart pump blood.
- Regular outpatient care for waiting list patients may include frequent exercise testing, assessing the strength of the heartbeat, and right cardiac catheterization (a test to measure blood pressure in the right side of the heart).

## CONTACT WITH THE TRANSPLANT CENTER DURING THE WAIT

People on the waiting list are often kept in close contact with the transplant center because most donor hearts must be transplanted within 4 hours after removal from the donor.

At some heart transplant centers, recipients receive a pager so the center can contact them at any time. They are asked to notify the transplant center if they're going out of town. Recipients often need to be prepared to arrive at the hospital within 2 hours of being notified about a donor heart.

Not all patients who are called to come to the hospital will get a heart transplant. Sometimes, at the last minute, the donor heart is found to be unsuitable for certain patients. Other times, patients from the waiting list are called to come in as possible substitutes in case something happens with the selected recipient.

## DURING A HEART TRANSPLANT

Just before the heart transplant surgery, patients will receive general anesthesia (that is, they are temporarily put to sleep) (Fig. 37.3).

- A bypass machine is hooked up to the arteries and veins of the heart. The machine pumps blood through the patient's lungs and body while the diseased heart is removed and the donor heart is sewn into place.
- Heart transplant surgery usually takes about 4 hours. Patients often spend the first days after surgery in the intensive care unit of the hospital.

## AFTER A HEART TRANSPLANT

### In the Hospital

- The amount of time a heart transplant recipient spends in the hospital will vary with each person. It often involves 1–2 weeks in the hospital and 3 months of moni-

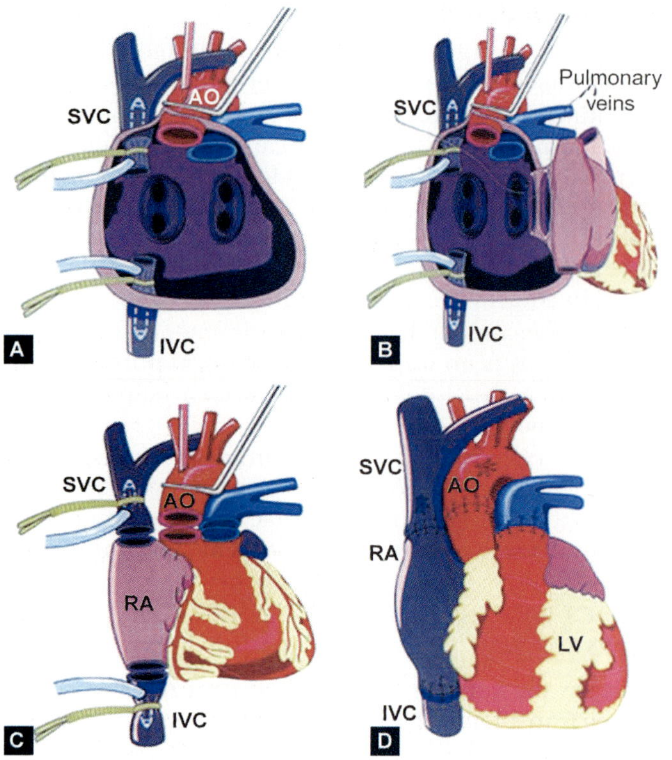


**Fig. 37.3:** (A) Recipient anatomy after native heart removed, (B) First anastomosis. Donor left pulmonary veins to recipient left pulmonary veins, (C) donor heart after completion of pulmonary venous anastomosis, (D) completed transplant

toring by the transplant team at the heart transplant center.
- Monitoring may include frequent blood tests, pulmonary (lung) function tests, EKGs (electrocardiograms), echocardiograms, and biopsies of the heart tissue.
- A heart biopsy is a standard test used to see whether your body is rejecting the new heart. It might be done frequently in the weeks after a transplant. During a heart biopsy, a tiny grabbing device is inserted into a vein of the neck or groin (upper thigh).
- The device is threaded through the vein to the right atrium of the new heart to take a small tissue sample. The tissue sample is checked for signs of rejection.

### Watching for Signs of Rejection

The new heart is a 'foreign body,' which your immune system may attack if you're not receiving enough medicine to suppress your immune system after the surgery. Therefore, you and the transplant team will work together to protect the new heart by watching for signs of rejection. These signs include:
- Shortness of breath
- Fever
- Fatigue (tiredness)
- Weight gain (retaining fluid in the body)
- Reduced amounts of urine (problems in the kidneys can cause this)
- You and the team also will work together to manage the transplant medicines and their side effects, prevent infections, and continue treatment of ongoing medical conditions.
- You may be asked to monitor your temperature, blood pressure, and pulse when you go home.

### Preventing Rejection

- You will need to take medicine to suppress your immune system so that the new heart will not be rejected. These transplant medicines are called immunosuppressants.
- They're a combination of medicines that are tailored to your situation. Often, they include cyclosporine, tacrolimus, MMF (mycophenolate mofetil), and steroids such as prednisone.
- Transplant medicines may need to be switched or adjusted if they are not effective or have too many side effects.

## MANAGING TRANSPLANT MEDICINES AND THEIR SIDE EFFECTS

You will have to manage multiple medicines. Setting up a routine for taking medicine at the same time each day and for refilling prescriptions is helpful. It's crucial to never run out of medicine. It may help to always use the same pharmacy. Keep a list of all medicines with you at all times in case of an accident. When traveling, keep extra doses of medicine with you, not packed in the luggage. Bring your medicine with you to all doctor visits. Side effects from medicines can be serious. These include:
- Risk of infection,
- Diabetes,
- Osteoporosis (thinning of the bones),
- High blood pressure,
- Kidney disease,
- Cancer—especially lymphoma and skin cancer.

Discuss any side effects of the medicines with your transplant team, because the dose of a given medicine or the medicine itself can be changed. Report all new medicines to your transplant coordinator.

### Preventing Infection

Some transplant medicines can increase your chances of developing infections. You may be asked to watch for signs of infection, including:
- Fever, sore throat, cold sores, and flu-like symptoms.
- Signs of possible chest or lung infections could include shortness of breath, cough, and a change in the color of sputum (spit).
- The incision must be checked for redness, swelling, or drainage. It's especially important to look for signs of infection, because transplant medicines can often mask these signs.
- Discuss with your doctor measures you should take to reduce your chances of developing infections. For example, your doctor may recommend that you avoid

contact with animals or crowds of people in the first few months after your transplant.

- Regular dental care also is important. Your doctor may prescribe you antibiotics before any dental work to prevent infections.

### Pregnancy

Many successful pregnancies have occurred after heart transplant surgeries; however, special care is important. If you've had a heart transplant, talk with your doctor before planning a pregnancy.

## RISKS OF A HEART TRANSPLANT SURGERY

Although heart transplant surgery is a life-saving measure, it has many risks. Careful monitoring, treatment, and regular medical care can prevent or help manage some of these risks.

Risks of heart transplant include:

- Failure of the donor heart
- Complications from medicines
- Infection
- Cancer
- Problems that arise from not following lifelong health care plans
- Failure of the donor heart
- Over time the new heart may fail due to the same reasons that caused the original heart to fail. Failure of the donor heart also can occur if the body rejects the donor heart or if blood vessel disease develops in the new heart and causes it to fail. This blood vessel disease is called cardiac allograft vasculopathy (CAV).
- Patients who receive a heart transplant that fails can be considered for another transplant (called a retransplant).

### Primary Graft Dysfunction

The most frequent cause of death in the first 30 days after transplant is when the new donor heart fails and isn't able to function. This is called primary graft dysfunction. Factors such as shock or trauma to the donor heart or narrowed blood vessels in the recipient's lungs can cause primary graft dysfunction. Medicines (for example, inhaled nitric oxide and intravenous nitrates) may be used to treat this condition.

### Rejection of the Donor Heart

Rejection is one of the leading causes of death in the first year after transplant. The recipient's immune system sees the new heart as a 'foreign body' and attempts to destroy or reject it. During the first year, 25% of patients have signs of a possible rejection at least once. Half of all possible rejections happen in the first 6 weeks after surgery, and most happen within 6 months of surgery.

### Cardiac Allograft Vasculopathy

CAV is a chronic (ongoing) disease in which the walls of the new heart's coronary arteries become thick, hard, and lose their elasticity. CAV can destroy the circulation of blood in the donor heart and cause serious damage.

CAV is a leading cause of donor heart failure and death in the years following transplant surgery. It can cause heart attack, heart failure, dangerous arrhythmias, and sudden cardiac arrest.

### Complications from Medicines

Taking daily medicines that stop the immune system from attacking the new heart is absolutely critical, even though the medicine combinations have serious side effects.

Cyclosporine and other medicines can cause kidney damage. Kidney damage affects more than 25% of patients in the first year after transplant. Five percent of transplant patients will develop end-stage kidney disease in 7 years.

### Infection

When the immune system—the body's defense system—is suppressed, the patient is at increased risk for infection. Infection is a major cause of hospital admission for heart transplant patients and a leading cause of death in the first year after transplant.

### Cancer

Suppressing the immune system leaves patients at risk for cancers and malignancies. Malignancies are a major cause of late death in heart transplant patients—nearly 25% of heart transplant deaths occur within 3 years after transplant.

The most common malignancies are tumors of the skin and lips (patients at highest risk are older, male, and fair-skinned) and malignancies in the lymph system such as non-Hodgkins lymphoma.

### Other Complications

- High blood pressure develops in more than 70% of heart transplant patients in the first year after transplant and in nearly 95% of patients in 5 years.
- High levels of cholesterol and triglycerides in the blood develop in more than 50% of heart transplant patients in the first year after transplant and in 84% of patients in 5 years.
- Osteoporosis can develop or worsen in heart transplant patients. This is a condition in which bones gradually become thinner and weaker.

### Complications from Not Following Lifelong Health Care Plans

Not following a lifelong treatment plan increases the risk of all heart transplant complications. Heart transplant recipients are asked to closely follow their doctors' instructions and monitor their own health status throughout their lives.

Lifelong health care includes taking multiple medicines on a strict schedule, watching for signs and symptoms of complications, keeping all medical appointments, and stopping unhealthy behaviors such as smoking.

## HEART TRANSPLANT SURGICAL PROCEDURES

### Preoperative

A typical heart transplantation begins when a suitable donor heart is identified. The heart comes from a recently deceased or brain dead donor, also called a beating heart cadaver. The patient is contacted by a nurse coordinator and instructed to come to the hospital for evaluation and presurgical medication. At the same time, the heart is removed from the donor and inspected by a team of surgeons to see if it is in suitable condition. Learning that a potential organ is unsuitable can induce distress in an already fragile patient, who usually requires emotional support before returning home. The patient must also undergo emotional, psychological, and physical tests to verify mental health and ability to make good use of a new heart. The patient is also given immunosuppressant medication so that the patient's immune system does not reject the new heart.

### Operative

Once the donor heart passes inspection, the patient is taken into the operating room and given a general anesthetic. Either an orthotopic or a heterotopic procedure follows, depending on the conditions of the patient and the donor heart (Fig. 37.4).

### Orthotopic Procedure

The orthotopic procedure begins with a *median sternotomy*, opening the chest and exposing the *mediastinum*. The *pericardium* is opened, the *great vessels* are *dissected* and the patient is attached to *cardiopulmonary bypass*. The donor's heart is injected with *potassium chloride* (KCl). Potassium chloride stops the heart beating before the heart is removed from the donor's body and packed in ice. Ice can usually keep the heart usable for 4–6 hours depending on preservation and starting condition. The failing heart is removed by transecting the great vessels and a portion of the left atrium. The patient's pulmonary veins are not transected; rather a circular portion of the *left atrium* containing the *pulmonary veins* is left in place. The donor heart is trimmed to fit onto the patient's remaining left atrium and the great vessels are *sutured* in place. The new heart is restarted, the patient is weaned from cardiopulmonary bypass and the chest cavity is closed. The orthotopic procedure was developed by Shumway and Lower at Stanford-Lane Hospital *in San Francisco in 1958*.

In the heterotopic procedure, the patient's own heart is not removed. The new heart is positioned so that the chambers and blood vessels of both hearts can be connected to form what is effectively a 'double heart'. The procedure can give the patient's original heart a chance to recover, and if the donor's heart fails (e.g. through rejection), it can later be removed, leaving the patient's original heart. Heterotopic procedures are used only in cases where the donor heart is not strong enough to function by itself (because either the patient's body is considerably larger

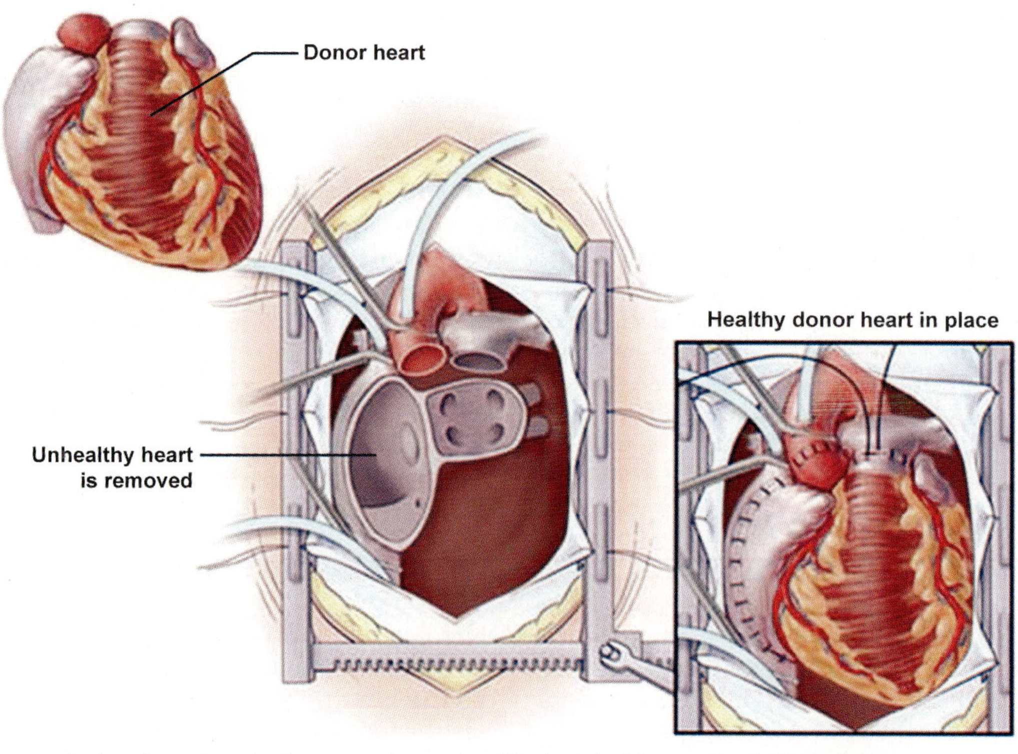


**Fig. 37.4:** The placement of a donor heart after removing unhealthy heart of the patient. While the back of the patient's left atrium and great vessels are *left in place*

than the donor's, the donor's heart is itself weak, or the patient suffers from pulmonary hypertension).

### *'Living Organ' Transplant*

In February 2006, at the Bad Oeynhausen Clinic for Thorax and Cardiovascular Surgery, Germany, surgeons successfully transplanted a 'beating heart' into a patient. Rather than cooling the heart, the living organ procedure keeps it at body temperature and connects it to a special machine called an Organ Care System that allows it to continue pumping warm, oxygenated blood. This technique can maintain the heart in a suitable condition for much longer than the traditional method.

### *Nonbeating Heart Transplant*

The first successful nonbeating heart transplant was achieved in Australia in 2014, performed by cardiothoracic surgeon Kumud Dhital. The transplant was made possible by the development of preservation technology able to preserve a heart, resuscitate it and to assess the function of the heart. The first patient to have this surgery was 57-year-old Michelle Gribilas. Papworth Hospital in England (where the first nonbeating heart transplant in Europe was carried out) stated that the technique could increase the number of hearts available for transplant by at least 25%.

### *Postoperative Transplanted Heart in the Thorax of Recipient*

The patient is taken to the ICU to recover. When they wake up, they move to a special recovery unit for rehabilitation (Fig. 37.5). The duration of in-hospital, post-transplant care depends on the patient's general health, how well the heart is working, and the patient's ability to look after the new heart. Doctors typically prefer that patients leave the hospital 1–2 weeks after surgery, because of the risk of infection and presuming no complications. After release, the patient returns for regular check-ups and rehabilitation. They may also require emotional support. The frequency of hospital visits decreases as the patient adjusts to the transplant. The patient remains on immunosuppressant medication to avoid the possibility of rejection. Since the vagus nerve is severed during the operation, the new heart beats at around 100 beats per minute unless nerve regrowth occurs.

Immunosuppressive agents are continued in the intensive care unit. The patient is regularly monitored to detect rejection. This surveillance can be performed via frequent biopsy or a gene expression blood test known as AlloMap Molecular Expression Testing. Typically, biopsy is performed immediately post-transplant and then AlloMap replaces it once the patient is stable. The transition from biopsy to AlloMap can occur as soon as 55 days after the transplant.

## Postoperative Laboratory Investigations

**ECG:** Shows recipient P-waves in patient with orthotopic heart transplant (Fig. 37.6).

**Echocardiography:** It has become vitally important for cardiac assessment of patients following heart transplant (HTx) (Figs 37.7–37.9).

## Cineangiogaphy (Figs 37.10 and 37.11)

### *Intravascular Ultrasound*

Although annual angiography is the recommended screening method, its sensitivity for detecting coronary disease in transplanted hearts is low (positive predictive value of only 44% compared to IVUS) (Fig. 37.12).

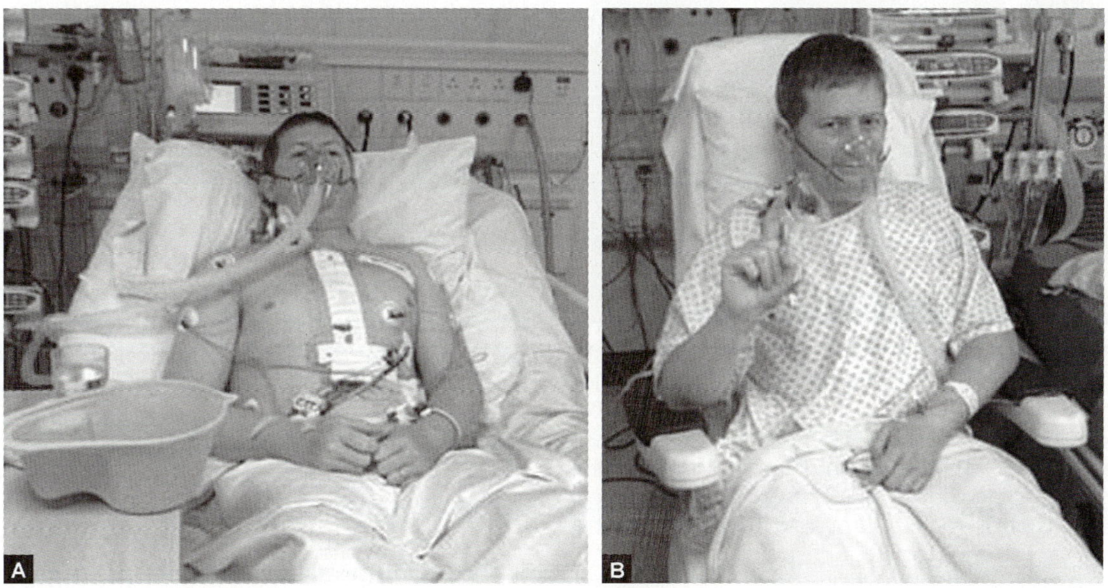

**Fig. 37.5:** (A) Immediate after surgery in ICU with all necessary gadgets on (B) (postoperative ) An adult patient who had chronic heart failure was operated for heart transplantation. He has improved from his heart failure and felt relaxed during his postoperative period in ICU

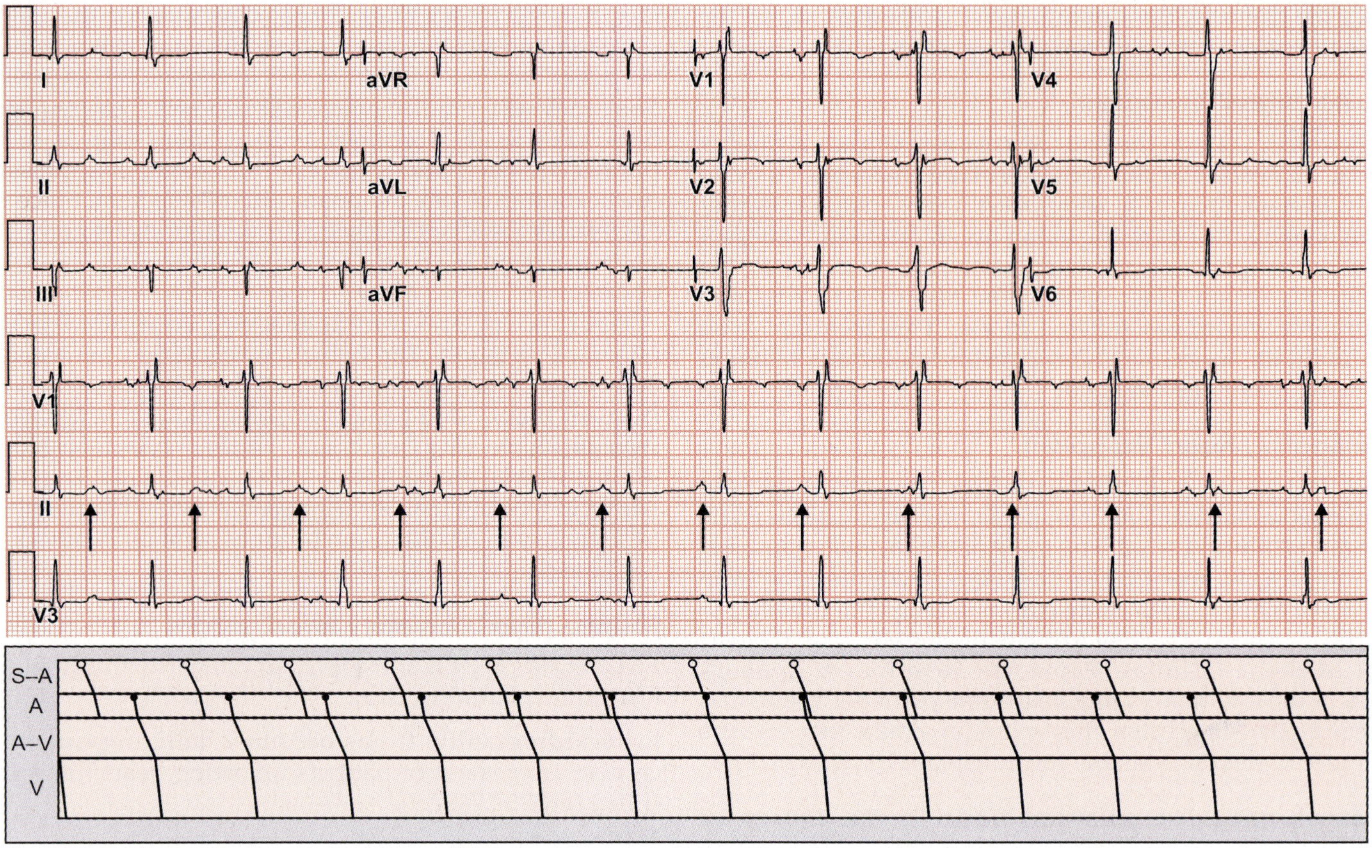


**Fig. 37.6:** ECG shows orthotopic heart transplant. Recipient P-waves (arrows)

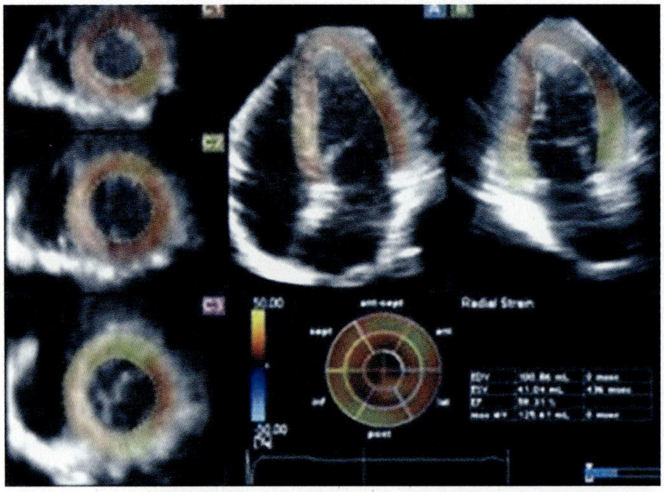


**Fig. 37.7:** Analysis of myocardial deformation in heart transplant patients. Echocardiography has become vitally important for cardiac assessment of patients following heart transplant (HTx). The present work will investigate whether the contractile behaviour of the transplanted heart differs in general from that of healthy subjects. Myocardial deformation will therefore be evaluated using three-dimensional speckle tracking technology. The transplant patients will undergo regular echocardiographic examinations as a part of outpatient follow-up examinations. The purpose of the study is to develop prognostic echocardiographic parameters in order to detect threatened rejection of the transplant earlier on

Conventional angiography does not assess the arterial wall and the vascular remodeling that results from CAV may hinder its diagnosis. IVUS overcomes these limitations and is considered the gold standard exam and the most sensitive for early detection of CAV. Maximal intimal thickening evaluation should be based on automated pullback in one or more epicardial vessels over a 40–50 mm segment. Intimal thickening of >0.5 mm in the first year post-transplant is a risk marker for mortality and nonfatal major cardiovascular events and predicts the development of CAV within five years. IVUS can thus be used to assess the risk of developing the disease, determine prognosis and guide therapy, but this indication is not fully consensual.

The current ISHLT guidelines state that conventional coronary angiography should be performed annually or biannually to assess the development of CAV. Patients free of CAV at 3–5 years after transplantation, especially those with renal insufficiency, may undergo less frequent invasive evaluation. IVUS in conjunction with coronary angiography at 4–6 weeks after transplantation is an option if there is suspicion of donor coronary disease (donor age >35 years), but is not performed in most centers, while at one year it can detect rapidly progressive CAV and provide prognostic information. Follow-up coronary angiography is recommended 6 months after percutaneous coronary intervention because of high restenosis rates in cardiac transplant recipients.

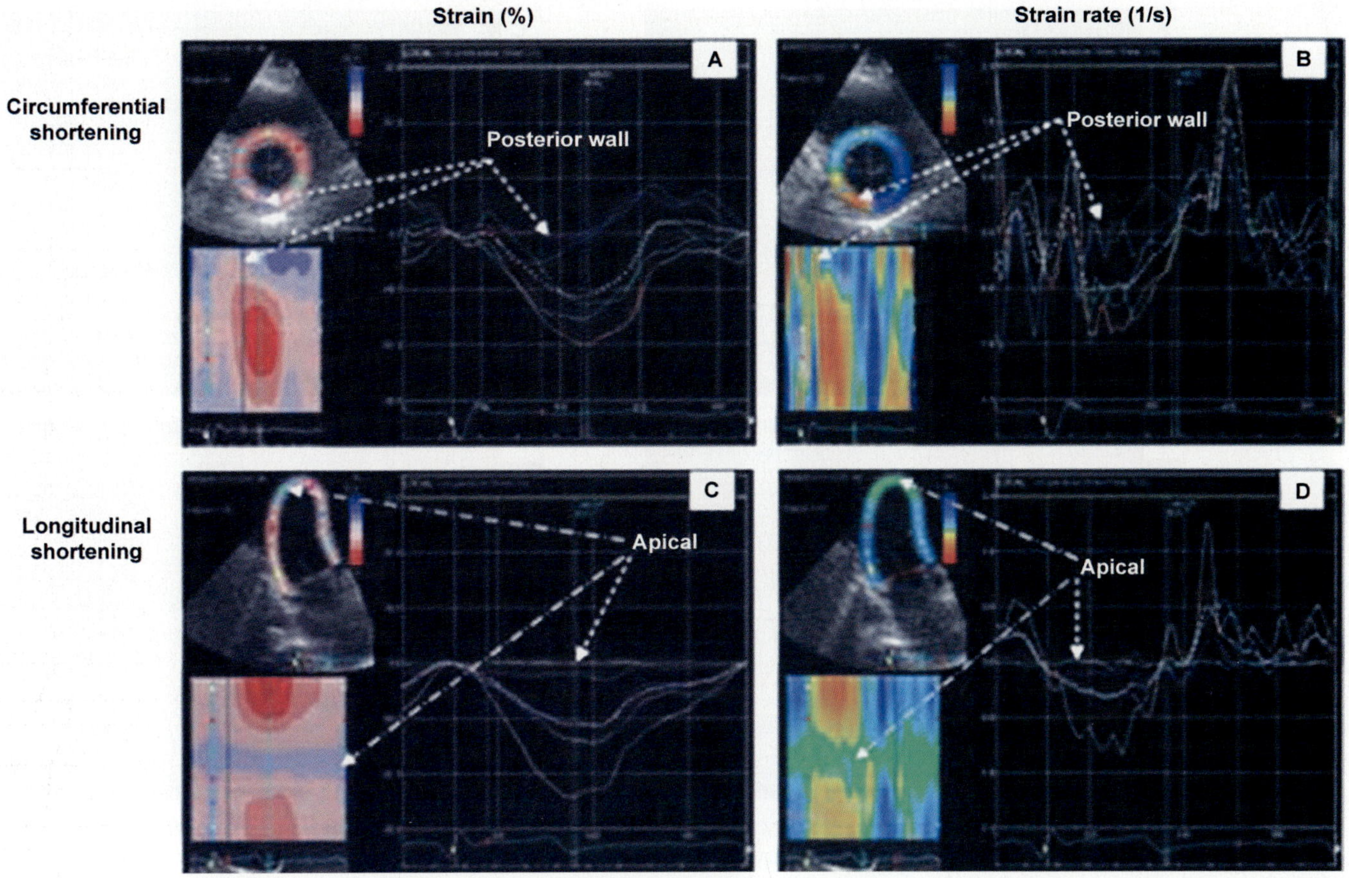


**Fig. 37.8:** Strain and strain rate images in heart transplant recipients with focal stenoses of coronary arteries. (A and B) Circumferential strain and strain rate in a patient with stenosis of the right coronary artery. (C and D) Longitudinal strain and strain rate in a patient with stenosis of the left anterior descending coronary artery [Dandel et al. JHLT 2008;27(2):S95–96]

## THE HEART BIOPSY REGIMEN

Heart biopsies are a necessary part of careful, comprehensive monitoring to evaluate whether the body is accepting the new organ. Biopsies are performed by placing an IV line, usually from the right neck, and passing a delicate scissor device through the veins and into the right ventricle.

There, under X-ray or echocardiogram guidance, several small pieces of the right ventricle are removed for microscopic examination. If we see evidence of immune injury to the heart (either infiltration of cells called lymphocytes, or evidence that protein antibodies may be building up against the heart), then additional therapy may be prescribed to reverse this acute rejection process. In almost every instance this therapy is successful at reversing the rejection.

### Immunosuppressive Medication

Transplantation has become so successful in recent years in large part through the development of new, more effective drugs which prevent donated organs. These drugs inhibit the body's immune system from identifying the new organ as foreign, or 'non-self', and then from trying to destroy it. It is necessary for all patients to take immunosuppressive medication for the rest of their lives following transplant. A successful transplant can be undermined very quickly by the failure of patients to take their medications appropriately and responsibly (Table 37.1).

### Postoperative Exercise Programme

Organ transplantation is one of the medical miracles or the 20th century. It has the capacity to substantially improve exercise performance and quality of life in patients who are severely limited with chronic organ failure (Fig. 37.13). We focus on the most commonly performed solid-organ transplants and describe peak exercise performance following recovery from transplantation. Across all of the common transplants, evaluated significant reduction in VO2peak is seen (typically renal and liver 65–80% with heart and/or lung 50–60% of predicted). Those with the lowest VO2peak pretransplant have the lowest VO2peak post-transplant. Overall very few patients have a VO2peak in the normal range. Investigation of the cause of the reduction of VO2peak has identified many factors pre- and post-transplant that may contribute. These include organ-specific factors in the otherwise well-functioning allograft (e.g. chronotropic incompetence in heart transplantation) as well as allograft dysfunction itself (e.g. chronic lung

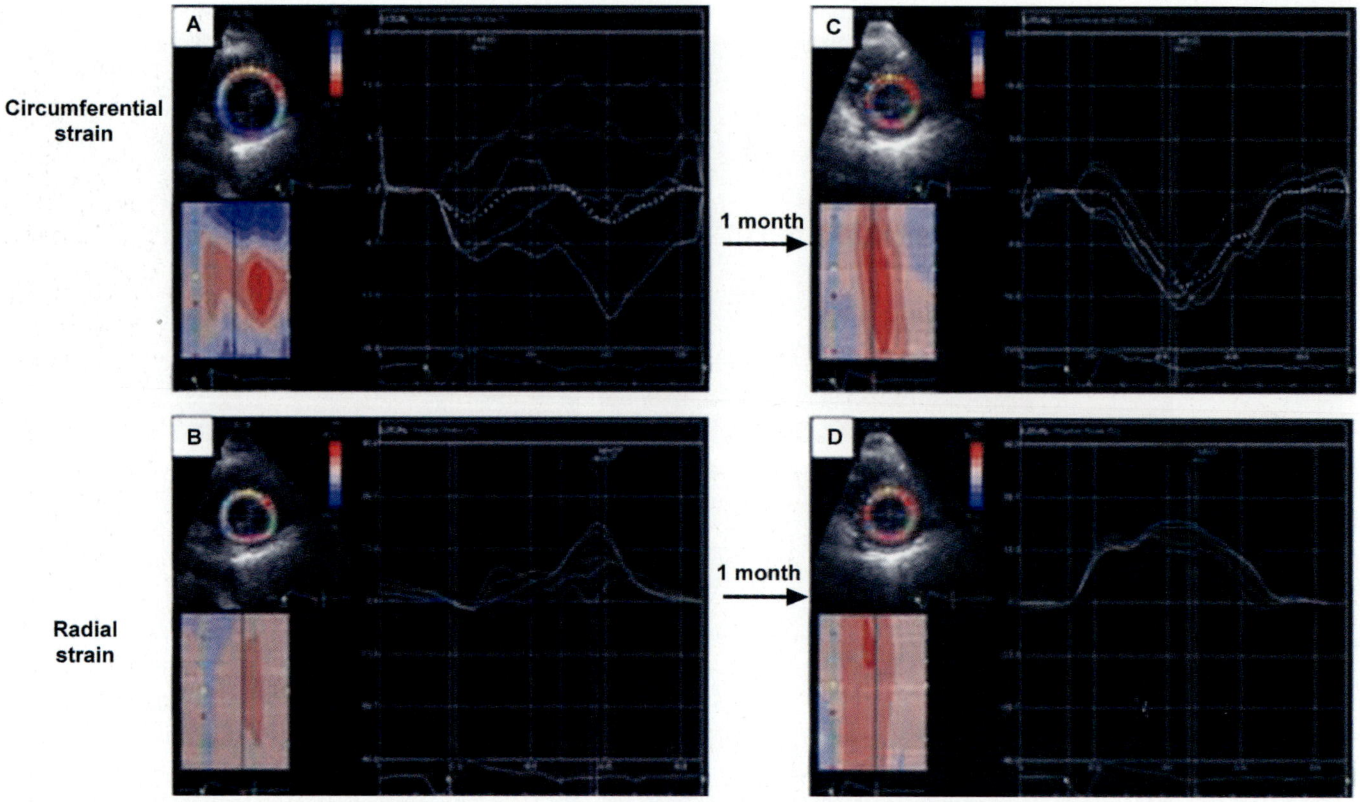


**Fig. 37.9:** Time course of 2D-strain images recorded during reduction of the LVAD (type incor) rate in a patient with idiopathic dilated cardiomyopathy who showed relevant myocardial recovery during mechanical unloading. After LVAD implantation, the global strain values were low and regional strain curves showed important dyssynchrony (A and B). One month later global strain values were several times higher and regional strain curves indicated uniform circumferential shortening and radial thickening (C and D), (Dandel et al. 2007, oral abstract, AHA Scientific Sessions)

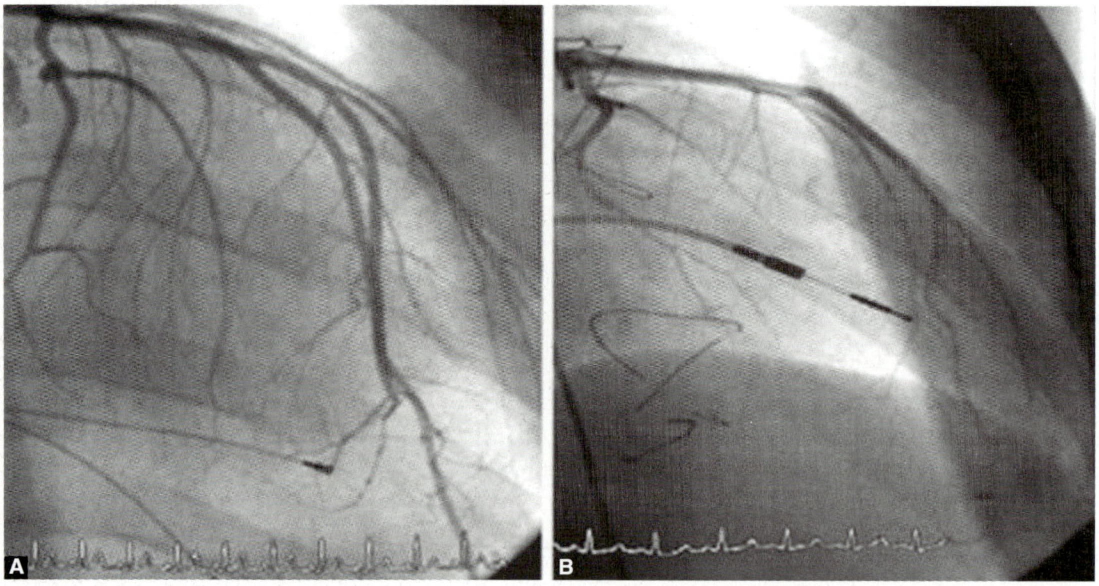


**Fig. 37.10:** Angiographic studies from 2 patients. (A) A patient without signs of CAD. (B) Signs of CAD with peripheral obliterations and B2 lesions with an intramyocardial pacemaker electrode (IMEG) in place

allograft dysfunction). However, looking across all transplants, a pattern emerges. A low muscle mass with qualitative change in large exercising skeletal muscle groups is seen pretransplant. Many factor post-transplant

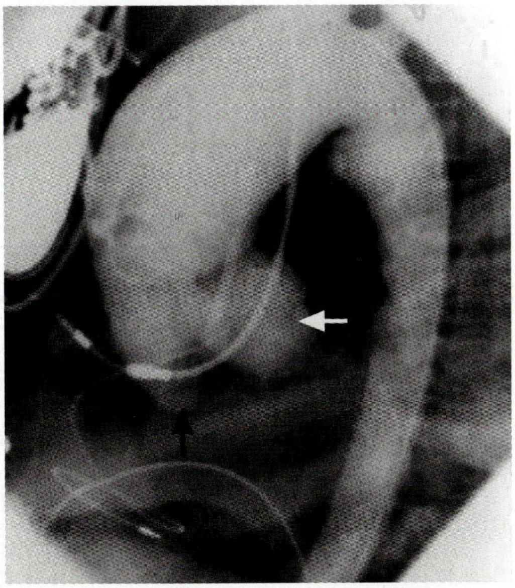

Fig. 37.11: Lateral aortogram confirming false aneurysm posteriorly (open arrow). Note large ascending aorta and absence of distal aortic rupture after heart transplantation (closed arrow=native aortic root)

aggravate these changes or prevent them recovering, especially calcineurin antagonist drugs which are key immunosuppressing agents. This results in the reduction of VO2peak despite restoration of near normal function of the initially failing organ system. As such organ transplantation has provided an experiment of nature that has focused our attention on an important confounder of chronic organ failure-skeletal muscle dysfunction.

According to some workers partial normalization of HR was achieved by 71% of heart transplantation patients at 12 months, with significant changes occurring within 6 months in most subjects. These findings should contribute to reducing the exercise restrictions that apply to the denervated heart.

## Prognosis

The prognosis for heart transplant patients following the orthotopic procedure has increased over the past 20 years, and as of June 5, 2009, the survival rates were:

- 1 year: 88.0% (males), 86.2% (females)
- 3 years: 79.3% (males), 77.2% (females)
- 5 years: 73.2% (males), 69.0% (females)

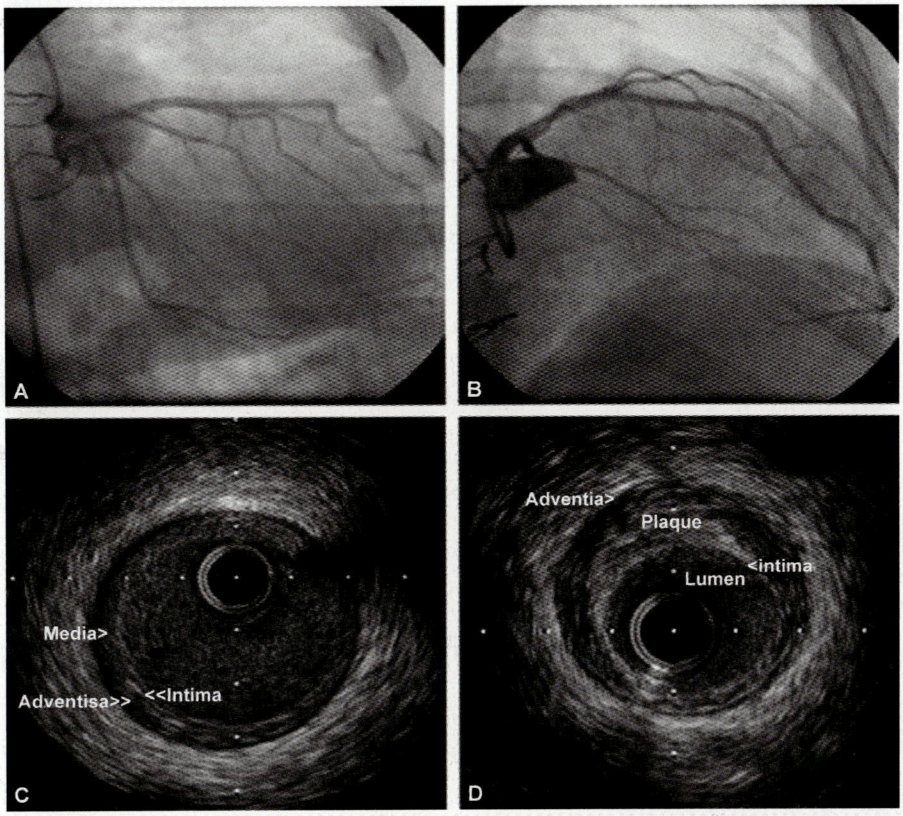


Fig. 37.12: Intravascular ultrasound images of the anterior descending artery in a patient transplanted 5 years previously, showing both the concentric intimal thickening typical of cardiac allograft vasculopathy (C) and an eccentric plaque typical of atherosclerotic coronary disease (D). Coronary angiography did not suggest disease in this artery (A and B)

**Table 37.1:** Immunosuppressive medication, action and side effects

| Type | Drug | Action | Side Effects |
|---|---|---|---|
| Calcineurin inhibitor | Prograf or cyclosporine | Prevents rejection | • Increased risk of infection<br>• Numbness or tingling in hands, feet and mouth<br>• Tremors<br>• Hair growth<br>• Hot flashes<br>• Overgrowth and swelling of gums<br>• High blood pressure<br>• Kidney dysfunction<br>• Increased blood sugar |
| Calcineurin inhibitor | Rapamune | Prevents rejection | • Low white count and platelets<br>• Increases cholesterol<br>• Delayed healing<br>• Fluid retention |
| Antiproliferative agent | Cellcept or Imuran | Prevents rejection | • Nausea<br>• Stomach cramps<br>• Diarrhea<br>• Increased blood sugar<br>• Low white blood counts |
| Antibody therapy | OKT3<br>ATGAM<br>Thymoglobulin<br>Dicluzimab<br>Basiliximab | Prevents or reverses acute rejection | • Fever<br>• Chills<br>• Flu-like symptoms<br>• Rash |
| Steroids | Prednisone | Prevents rejection | • Increased risk of infection<br>• Stomach irritation<br>• Swelling of face (chipmunk cheeks), hands or ankles<br>• Weight gain<br>• High blood sugar<br>• Skin changes<br>• Muscle weakness<br>• Mood changes<br>• Brittle bones |

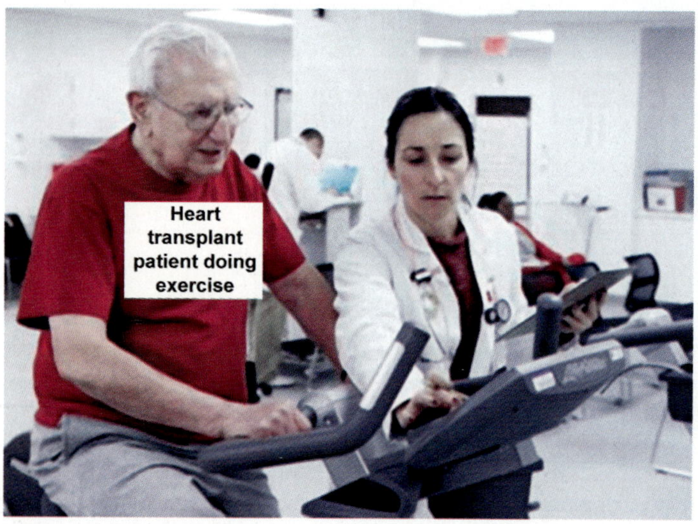


**Fig. 37.13:** Heart transplant recipient is subjected to cycle exercise in order to know the capacity and effect of exercise on his vital parameters

## BIBLIOGRAPHY


1. Arnaoutakis GJ, George TJ, Allen JG, Russell SD, Shah AS, Conte JV, et al. Institutional volume and the effect of recipient risk on short-term mortality after orthotopic heart transplant. J Thorac Cardiovasc Surg 2012;143(1):157–67.
2. Caves PK, Stinson EB, Billingham M, Shumway NE. Percutaneous transvenous endomyocardial biopsy in human heart recipients. Experience with a new technique. Ann Thorac Surg 1973;16(4):325–36.
3. Chan MC, Giannetti N, Kato T, et al. Severe tricuspid regurgitation after heart transplantation. J Heart Lung Transplant 2001;20(7):709–17.
4. Copeland JG, Emery RW, Levinson MM, et al. Selection of patients for cardiac transplantation. Circulation 1987;75(1): 2–9.
5. Davies RR, Russo MJ, Yang J, et al. Listing and transplanting adults with congenital heart disease. Circulation 2011;123(7): 759–67.
6. Ford MA, Almond CS, Gauvreau K, Piercey G, Blume ED, Smoot LB, et al. Association of graft ischemic time with

survival after heart transplant among children in the United States. J Heart Lung Transplant 2011;30(11):1244–9.
7. Griepp RB, Ergin MA. The history of experimental heart transplantation. J Heart Transplant 1984;3:145.
8. Griffith BP, Hardesty RL, Deeb GM, et al. Cardiac transplantation with cyclosporin A and prednisone. Ann Surg 1982;196(3):324–9.
9. Heart Failure Society of America. The Stages of Heart Failure New York Heart Association (NYHA) Classification. Heart, Failure Society of America Accessed, 2009.
10. Hill JD. Bridging to cardiac transplantation. Ann Thorac Surg 1989;47(1):167-71.
11. Hofflin JM, Potasman I, Baldwin JC, et al. Infectious complications in heart transplant recipients receiving cyclosporine and corticosteroids. Ann Intern Med 1987;106(2):209–16.
12. Holman WL, Kormos RL, Naftel DC, Miller MA, Pagani FD, Blume E, et al. Predictors of death and transplant in patients with a mechanical circulatory support device: a multi-institutional study. J Heart Lung Transplant 2009;28(1): 44–50.
13. Hunt J, Lerman M, Magee MJ, et al. Improvement of renal dysfunction by conversion from calcineurin inhibitors to sirolimus after heart transplantation. J Heart Lung Transplant 2005;24(11):1863–7.
14. Kaczmarek I, Sadoni S, Schmoeckel M, et al. The need for a tailored immunosuppression in older heart transplant recipients. J Heart Lung Transplant 2005;24(11):1965–8.
15. Kfoury AG, Renlund DG, Snow GL, Stehlik J, Folsom JW, Fisher PW, et al. A clinical correlation study of severity of antibody-mediated rejection and cardiovascular mortality in heart transplantation. J Heart Lung Transplant 2009;28(1): 51–7.
16. Khan MS, Mery CM, Zafar F, Adachi I, Heinle JS, Cabrera AG, et al. Is mechanically bridging patients with a failing cardiac graft to retransplantation an effective therapy? Analysis of the United Network of Organ Sharing database. J Heart Lung Transplant 2012.
17. Kilic A, Conte JV, Shah AS, Yuh DD. Orthotopic Heart Transplantation in Patients With Metabolic Risk Factors. Ann Thorac Surg 2012.
18. Kramer BL, Massie BM, Topic N. Controlled trial of captopril in chronic heart failure: a rest and exercise hemodynamic study. Circulation 1983;67(4):807–16.
19. Lee I, Localio R, Brensinger CM, Blumberg EA, Lautenbach E, Gasink L, et al. Decreased post-transplant survival among heart transplant recipients with pre-transplant hepatitis C virus positivity. J Heart Lung Transplant 2011;30(11): 1266–74.
20. McGee E, McCarthy PM, Hoercher KJ, et al. Donor Tricuspid Annuloplasty Reduces Post-Transplant Tricuspid Regurgitation (Abstract 22). The Kaufman Center for Heart Failure, The Cleveland Clinic. International Society for Heart and Lung Transplantation Meeting, San Francisco, 2004.
21. Miller CA, Sarma J, Naish J, Yonan N, Williams SG, Shaw SM, et al. Multiparametric Cardiovascular Magnetic Resonance Assessment of Cardiac Allograft Vasculopathy. J Am Coll Cardiol 2013.
22. Moriguchi J, Davis S, Jocson R, Esmailian F, Ardehali A, Laks H, et al. Successful use of a pneumatic biventricular assist device as a bridge to transplantation in cardiogenic shock. J Heart Lung Transplant 2011;30(10):1143–7.
23. Overcast TD, Evans RW, Bowen LE, et al. Problems in the identification of potential organ donors. Misconceptions and fallacies associated with donor cards. JAMA 1984;251(12): 1559–62.
24. Pedotti P, Mattucci DA, Gabbrielli F, Venettoni S, Costa AN, Taioli E. Analysis of the complex effect of donor's age on survival of subjects who underwent heart transplantation. Transplantation 2005;80(8):1026–32.
25. Portner PM, Oyer PE, Pennington DG, et al. Implantable electrical left ventricular assist system: bridge to transplantation and the future. Ann Thorac Surg 1989;47(1): 142–50.
26. Ramakrishna H, Jaroszewski DE, Arabia FA. Adult cardiac transplantation: A review of perioperative management Part- I. Ann Card Anaesth 2009;12(1):71–8.
27. Reichart B, Brandl U. 40 years of heart transplantation and the DFG-Transregio Research Group Xenotransplantation. Xenotransplantation 2008;15(5):293–4.
28. Sauer H. Recent advances using stem cell-derived cardiac and vascular cells for cardiomyoplasty. Xenotransplantation 2008;15(5):306.
29. Schuh A, Liehn EA, Sasse A, Schneider R, Neuss S, Weber C, et al. Improved left ventricular function after transplantation of microspheres and fibroblasts in a rat model of myocardial infarction. Basic Res Cardiol. Jan 12 2009;
30. Sweeney MS, Macris MP, Frazier OH, et al. The treatment of advanced cardiac allograft rejection. Ann Thorac Surg 1988; 46(4):378–81.
31. Tambur AR, Pamboukian SV, Costanzo MR, et al. The presence of HLA-directed antibodies after heart transplantation is associated with poor allograft outcome. Transplantation 2005;80(8):1019–25.
32. Tremmel JA, Ng MK, Ikeno F, Hunt SA, Lee DP, Yeung AC, et al. Comparison of drug-eluting versus bare metal stents in cardiac allograft vasculopathy. Am J Cardiol 2011;108(5): 665–8.
33. Ye F, Ying-Bin X, Yu-Guo W, Hetzer R. Tacrolimus versus cyclosporine microemulsion for heart transplant recipients: a meta-analysis. J Heart Lung Transplant 2009;28(1):58–66.

# 38 Toxicologic Cardiovascular Emergencies

## DIGITALIS TOXICITY

The therapeutic properties of cardiac glycosides (e.g. digoxin, a product of the foxglove plant) have been known since the days of the Roman Empire. The ancient Romans used red squill, a cardiac glycoside derived from the sea onion, as a diuretic and heart medicine. Cardiac glycosides are found in certain flowering plants such as oleander and lily-of-the-valley. Certain herbal dietary supplements also contain cardiac glycosides (Figs 38.1 and 38.2).

Physicians first studied digoxin in the 18th century. William Withering published his classic account of foxglove and some of its medical uses in 1785, remarking upon his experience with digitalis. Indians in South America had used cardiac glycosides in their dart poisons. Digitalis toxicity was well known in previous centuries, and some have suggested that the toxic visual symptoms of digitalis may have played a role in Van Gogh's use of swirling greens and yellows. During the early 20th century, the drug was introduced as treatment of atrial fibrillation. Only subsequently was the value of digitalis for the treatment of congestive heart failure (CHF) established. The syndrome of digoxin toxicity was originally described in 1785 by Withering. It is a disorder that is characterized by poisoning due to consumption of excessive amounts of digoxin, a chemical found in plants of the genus Digitalis. Poisoning may also occur due to intake of small amounts of digoxin over an extended period of time.

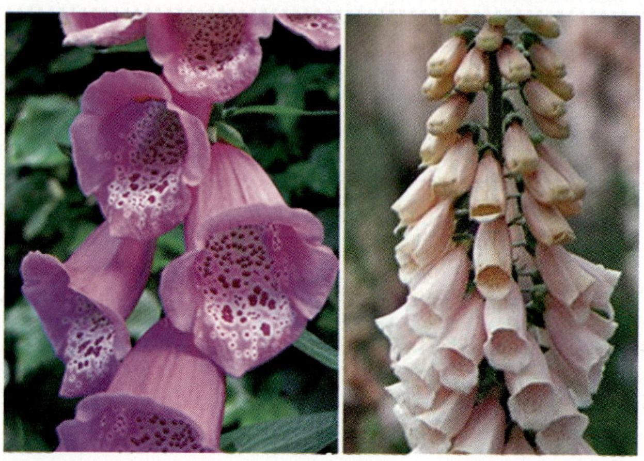

Fig. 38.1: The plant of Foxglove. Foxglove's drooping pink or white flowers may be pretty, but they can be highly toxic

### Frequency

Approximately 0.4% of all hospital admissions, 1.1% of outpatients on digoxin, and 10–18% of nursing home

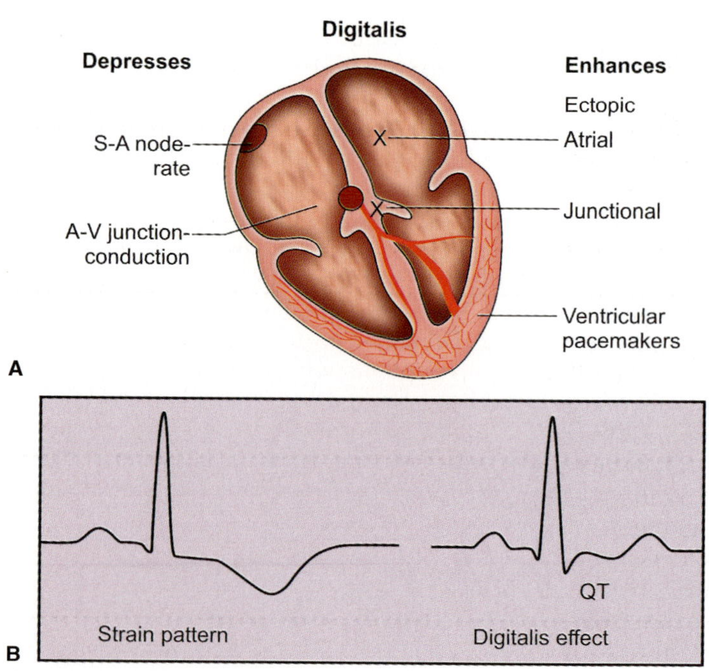


Fig. 38.2: (A) Diagram depicting the effect of digitalis on the conduction system of the heart. (B) Showing ST-segment morphology in strain pattern and digitalis effect which is commonly misken with myocardial strain pattern

patients develop toxicity. In 2006, the American Association of Poison Control Centers reported an incidence of 2610 toxic digitalis exposures. The overall incidence of digoxin toxicity has decreased because of a number of factors including increased awareness of drug interactions, decreased use of digoxin to treat heart failure and arrhythmias, and the availability of accurate rapid radioimmunoassays to monitor drug levels. Although the number of digitalis exposures is far less than the incidence of calcium channel blocker toxicity (10,031 cases) or beta-blocker toxicity (18,253 cases), the mortality rate from digitalis toxicity is far higher with 22 deaths reported versus 13 deaths from calcium channel antagonists and only 4 deaths attributed to beta-blocker toxicity.

Cardiovascular drug poisoning including digitalis toxicity ranks as the third leading cause of death from all poisonings in 2006. Data from the 2007 Annual Report of the American Association of Poison Control Centers is similar to previous data, with 2565 digitalis exposures reported. However, fatalities were lower, with 10 deaths reported.

### Global Incidence

Approximately 2.1% of inpatients on digoxin and 0.3% of all admissions develop toxicity.

### Mortality/Morbidity

- Morbidity is usually 4.6–10%; however, morbidity is 50% if the digoxin level is greater than 6 ng/ml.
- Mortality due to digoxin exposure varies with the population studied. Adult mortality depends on underlying comorbidity. In general, older people have a worse outcome than adults who, in turn, have a worse outcome than children.

### Age

Advanced age (>80 year) is an independent risk factor and is associated with increased morbidity and mortality.

### Signs and Symptoms of Digoxin Toxicity

The symptoms of digoxin toxicity range from obvious to nonspecific. Obvious signs of digoxin poisoning may include vomiting, nausea, hypotension, or hypothyroidism. It can be difficult to recognize digoxin toxicity in patients, however, since the symptoms may be attributed to the underlying condition for which digoxin is prescribed. Signs and symptoms of life-threatening or potentially life-threatening digoxin toxicity include but are not limited to severe ventricular arrhythmia including sinus ventricular tachycardia or fibrillation; progressive bradycardia second- or third-degree heart block not responsive to atropine serum potassium levels exceeding 5.5 mEq/L in adults or 6 mEq/L in children with rapidly progressive signs and symptoms of digoxin toxicity; neurologic symptoms (e.g. visual disturbances, disorientation, and confusion). Diagnosing digoxin toxicity can also be difficult because about 30% of patients with digoxin toxicity have no symptoms. It may be helpful to know who's at risk for digoxin toxicity and the side effects of digitalis treatment to facilitate proper diagnosis.

### Physical Examination

Hemodynamic instability is related directly to the presence of a dysrhythmia or acute congestive heart failure (CHF).

- Cardiovascular findings on physical examination relate to the severity of CHF, dysrhythmias, or hemodynamic instability.
  - Digoxin toxicity may cause any dysrhythmia. Classically, dysrhythmias that are associated with increased automaticity and decreased AV conduction occur (i.e. paroxysmal atrial tachycardia with 2:1 block, accelerated junctional rhythm, or bidirectional ventricular tachycardia [torsade de pointes]
  - Premature ventricular contractions (PVCs) are the most common dysrhythmia. Bigeminy or trigeminy occurs frequently.
  - Sinus bradycardia and other bradyarrhythmias are very common. Slow atrial fibrillation with very little variation in the ventricular rate (regularization of the R-R interval) may occur.
  - First-degree heart block, second-degree AV block, complete AV dissociation, and third-degree heart block are also very common.
  - Rapid atrial fibrillation or atrial flutter is rare.
  - Ventricular tachycardia is an especially serious finding.
  - Cardiac arrest from asystole or ventricular fibrillation is usually fatal.
    - Gastrointestinal symptoms are common, but the abdominal examination is usually nonspecific.
    - Neurological findings are related to changes in sensorium or mental status. Lateralizing findings usually indicate another disease process.
    - Visual changes occur, but the pupils are spared, and objective findings are few.
    - Drug-induced fever does not occur.

### Aetiological Factors

- Deteriorating renal function, dehydration, electrolyte disturbances, or drug interactions usually precipitates chronic toxicity. Acute overdose or accidental exposure to plants containing cardiac glycosides may cause acute toxicity.
- Hypokalemia, hypernatremia, or hypomagnesemia increases the toxic cardiovascular effects of digoxin because of their depressive effects on the $Na^+/K^+$ ATPase pump. Digoxin toxicity does not cause hypokalemia, but hypokalemia can worsen digoxin toxicity. Hyperkalemia is the usual electrolyte abnormality precipitated by digoxin toxicity, primarily in the acute setting. Hyperkalemia may be associated with acute renal failure that subsequently precipitates digoxin toxicity. Chronic digoxin toxicity does not usually cause hyperkalemia.
- Acidosis depresses the $Na^+/K^+$ ATPase pump and may cause digoxin toxicity.

- Myocardial ischemia suppresses the $Na^+/K^+$ ATPase pump and independently alters myocardial automaticity. Digoxin toxicity is more likely in this setting.
- Erroneous dosing, especially in infants receiving parenteral digoxin, unfortunately, is a frequent cause of digoxin toxicity and is usually associated with high mortality. Hypothyroid patients are prone to digoxin toxicity secondary to decreased renal excretion and a smaller volume of distribution.

### Risk Factors in Digoxin Toxicity

Which patients may be at higher risk for digoxin toxicity? Recognizing digoxin toxicity may be difficult, but it may help to know what to look for. Patients at risk of digoxin toxicity are typically older and have comorbidities.

Risk factors for digoxin toxicity include:

- Advanced age (>80 years)
- Decrease in renal clearance or loss of renal function due to chronic disease
- Hypokalemia
- Hypomagnesemia
- Hypothyroidism
- Multiple concomitant prescription drugs
- Macrolide antibiotics
- Drugs that impair renal function
- Drugs that cause hypokalemia

When diagnosing digoxin toxicity, pay attention to these risk factors. Patients undergoing digoxin therapy who exhibit these risk factors should be closely monitored so that any signs of digoxin poisoning are identified early to ensure timely treatment.

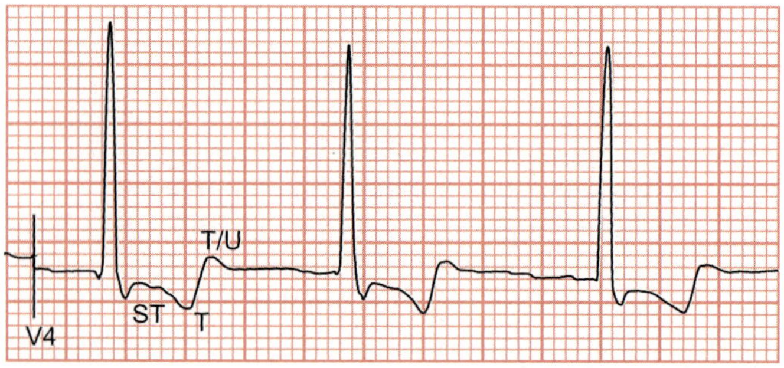


**Fig. 38.3:** ECG. Downslowping ST-depression with abnormal T-waves and shortened QT intervals on EKG in the digitalis effect

### Diagnosis in Digoxin Toxicity

Patients suspected of having this condition should undergo an ECG examination. A measurement of serum digoxin concentrations should be carried out. Measurement is, however, only truly reflective after completion of distribution (4–6 hours after last dosage). It usually requires two levels to make sure of the distributed levels.

### ECG Changes in Digoxin Toxicity

In case of digitalis use and digitalis toxicity, some characteristic Electrocardiographic (ECG) changes can be seen (Figs 38.2–38.11). At therapeutic levels, digoxin gives rise to characteristic changes in ECG readings such as scooping of the ST-segments or prolongation of the PR segment. On

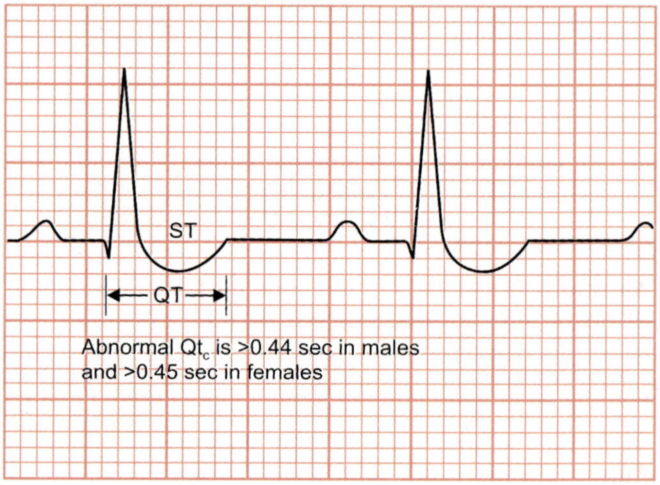


**Fig. 38.4:** Digoxin effect refers to the presence on the ECG such as downsloping ST-depression with a characteristic 'sagging' appearance, flattened, inverted, or biphasic T-waves. and shortened QT interval. Classic scooped out ST-segment. Other features of digoxin effect are mild PR interval prolongation of up to 240 ms (due to increased vagal tone), prominent U-waves, peaking of the terminal portion of the T-waves and J point depression (usually in leads with tall R-waves)

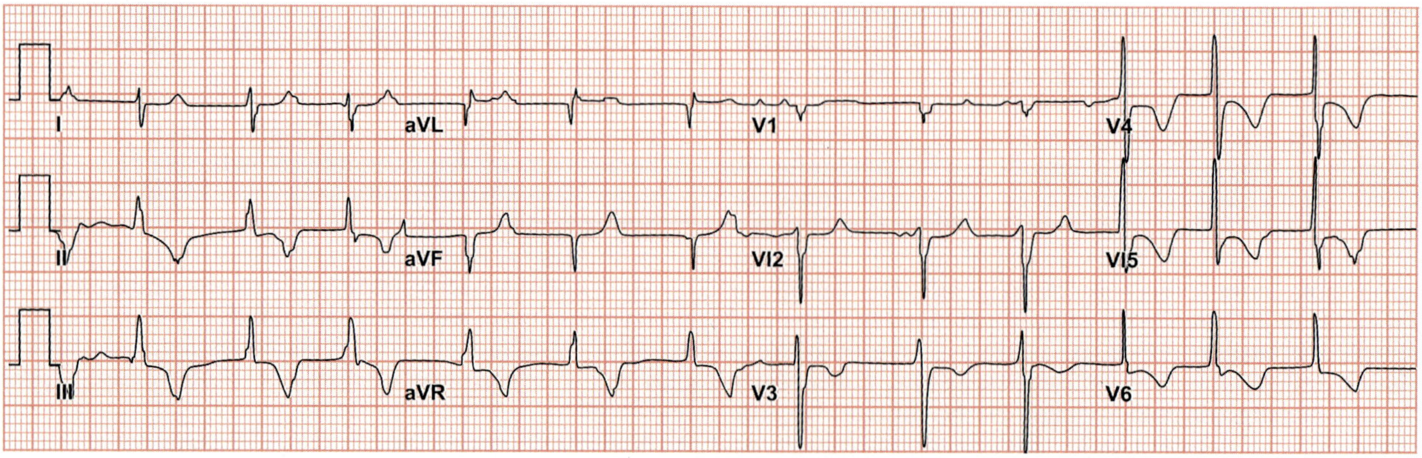


**Fig. 38.5:** ECG showing generalised ST-depression and T-wave inversion as seen in digitalis toxicity

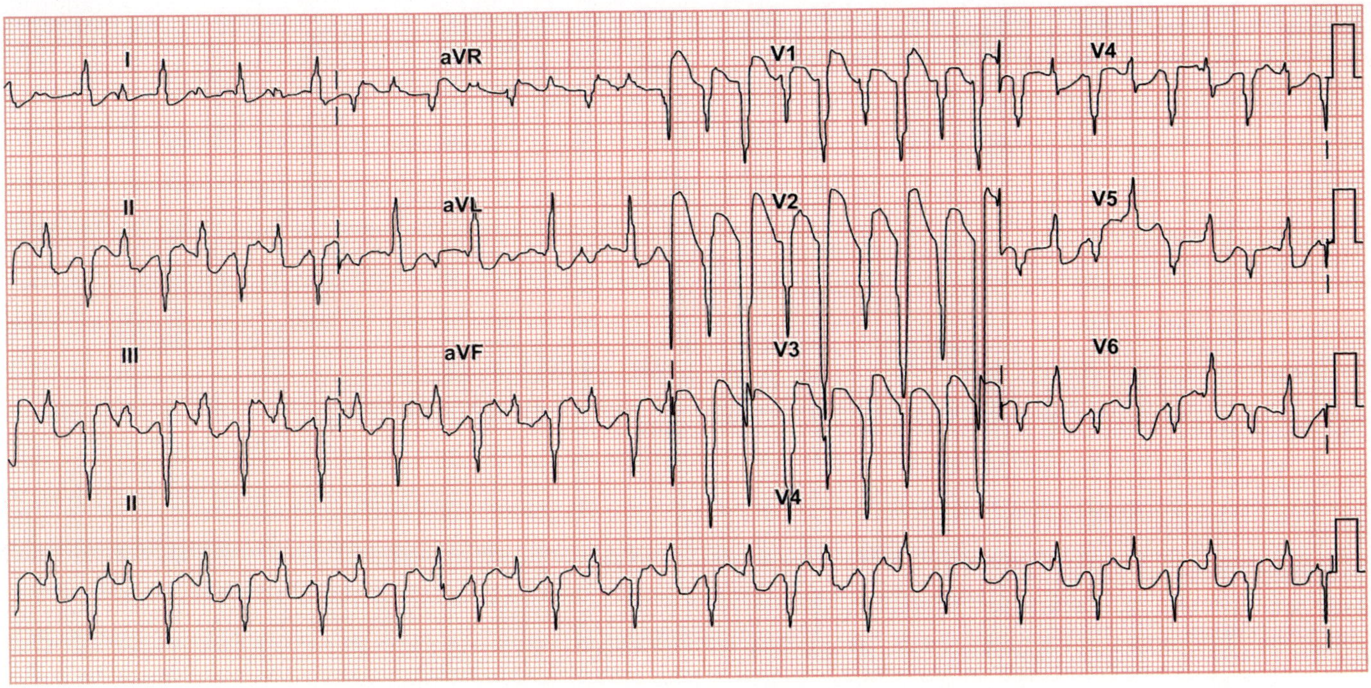


Fig. 38.6: Bidirectional tachycardia in patient with digoxin toxicity

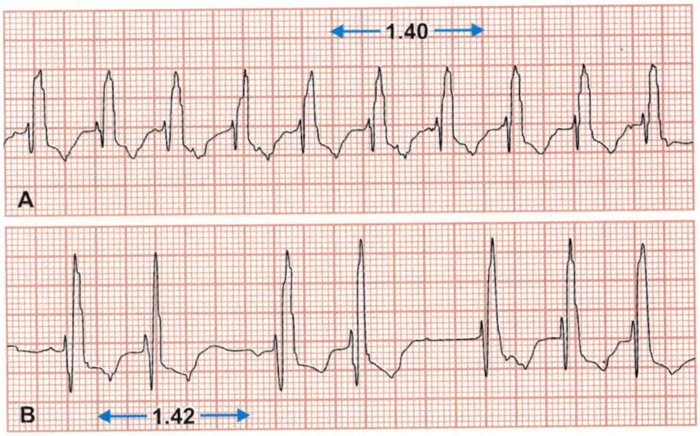


Fig. 38.7: Junctional tachycardia (A) and junctional tachycardia with exit block (B) due to digitalis intoxication

the other hand, digitalis toxicity may give rise to myriad changes in ECG readings.

- Bioavailability varies depending on the drug formulation.
    - Lanoxin has 25% less bioavailability than lanoxicaps.
    - Toxicity may occur by increasing bioavailability.
    - Certain antibiotics that suppress intestinal flora may increase absorption of digoxin.
- Drug interactions are one of the most common causes of digoxin toxicity.
    - Some medications directly increase digoxin plasma levels; other medications alter renal excretion or induce electrolyte abnormalities.
    - Drugs that have been reported to cause digoxin toxicity include the following:
        - Amiloride—may reduce the inotropic response to digoxin

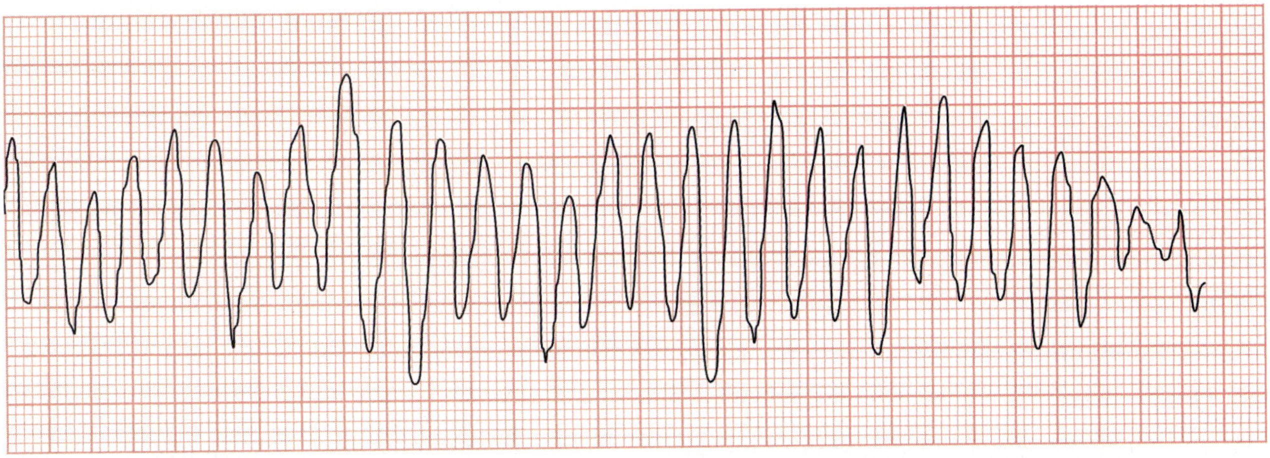

Fig. 38.8: ECG showing undulating graph as seen in torsades de pointes in digitalis toxicity

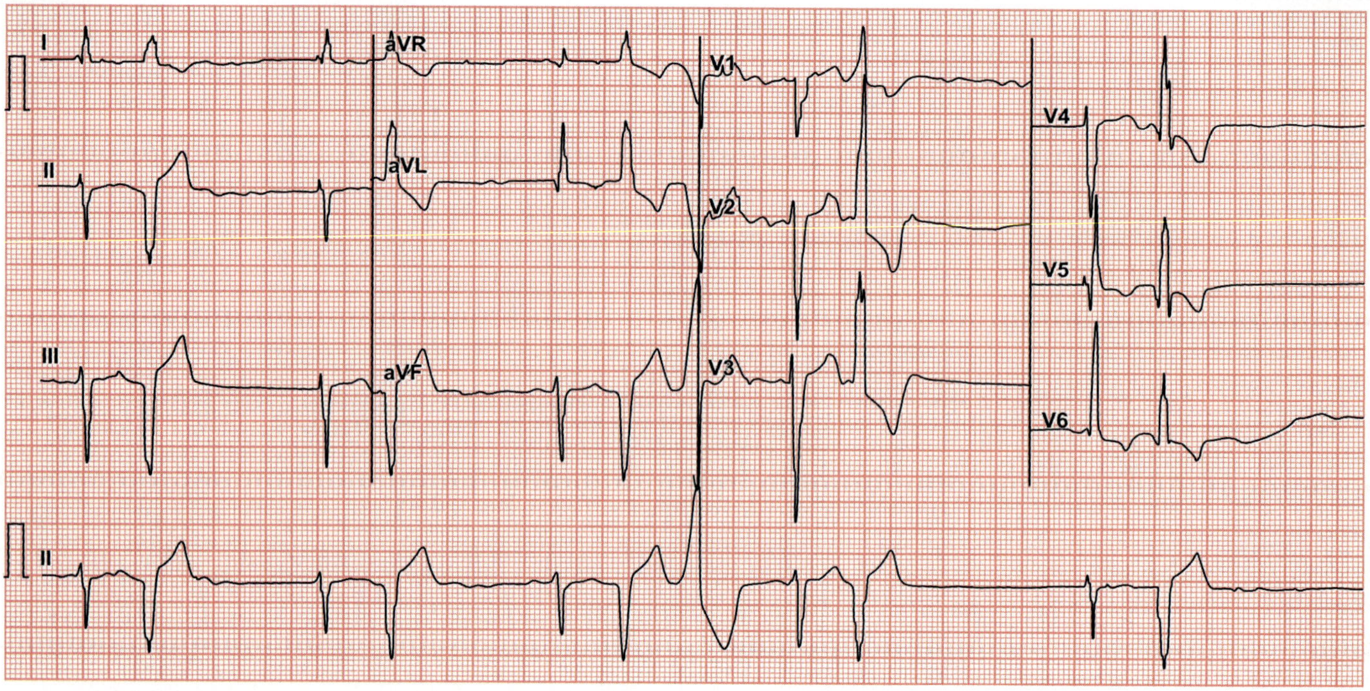


**Fig. 38.9:** Atrial fibrillation with slow ventricular rate, ventricular bigeminy, bidirectional ventricular ectopy as seen in digitalis toxic

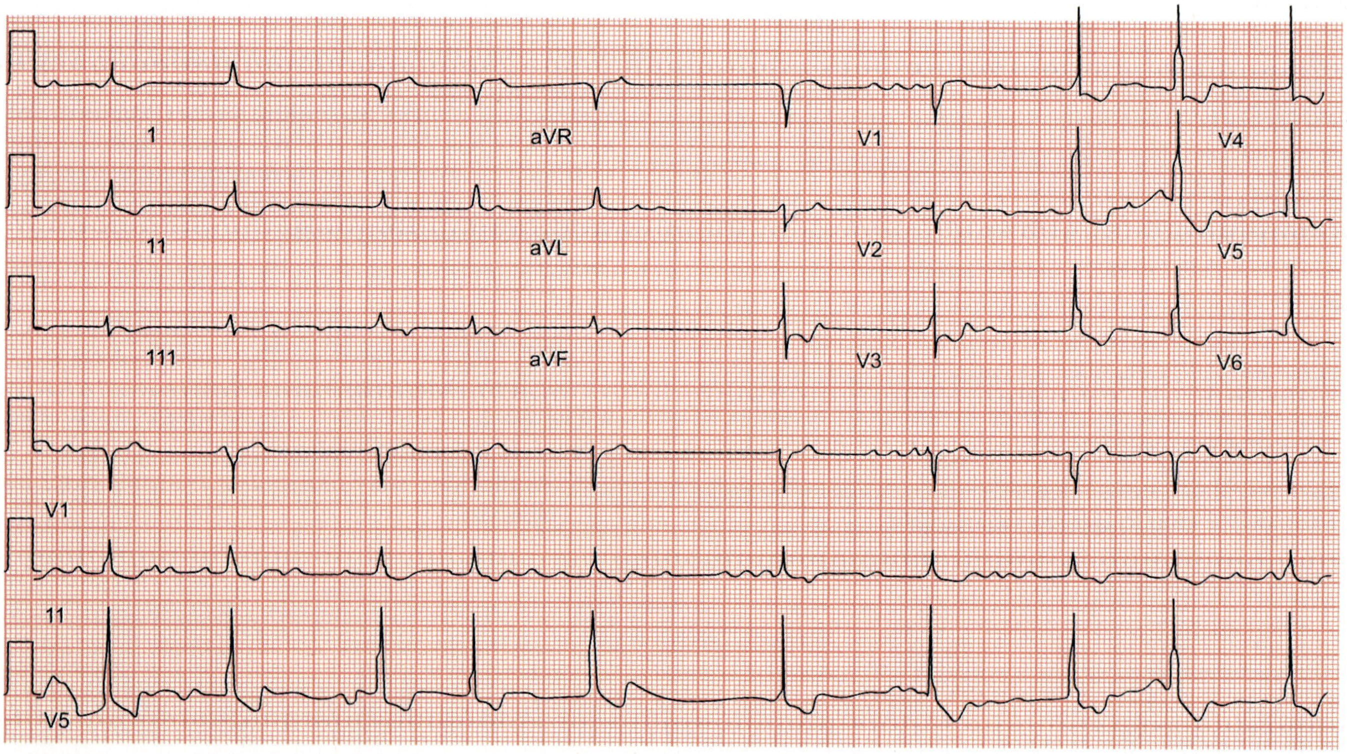


**Fig. 38.10:** ECG showing (1) atrial fibrillation with bradycardia, (2) ST-segment depression consistent with digoxin effect. The ECG shows a downsloaping ST-segment depression in multiple leads that are shaped like the 'reverse check mark sign' or a 'scooped out' appearance. This pattern is typical of digoxin. This may occur at normal digoxin levels in some people, but becomes more common as the digoxin level increases

* Amiodarone reduces renal and nonrenal clearance of digoxin and may have additive effects on the heart rate
* Benzodiazepines (alprazolam, diazepam) have been associated with isolated reports of digoxin toxicity
* Beta-blockers (propranolol, metoprolol, and atenolol) may have additive effects on the heart rate; carvedilol may increase digoxin blood levels in addition to potentiating its effects on the heart rate

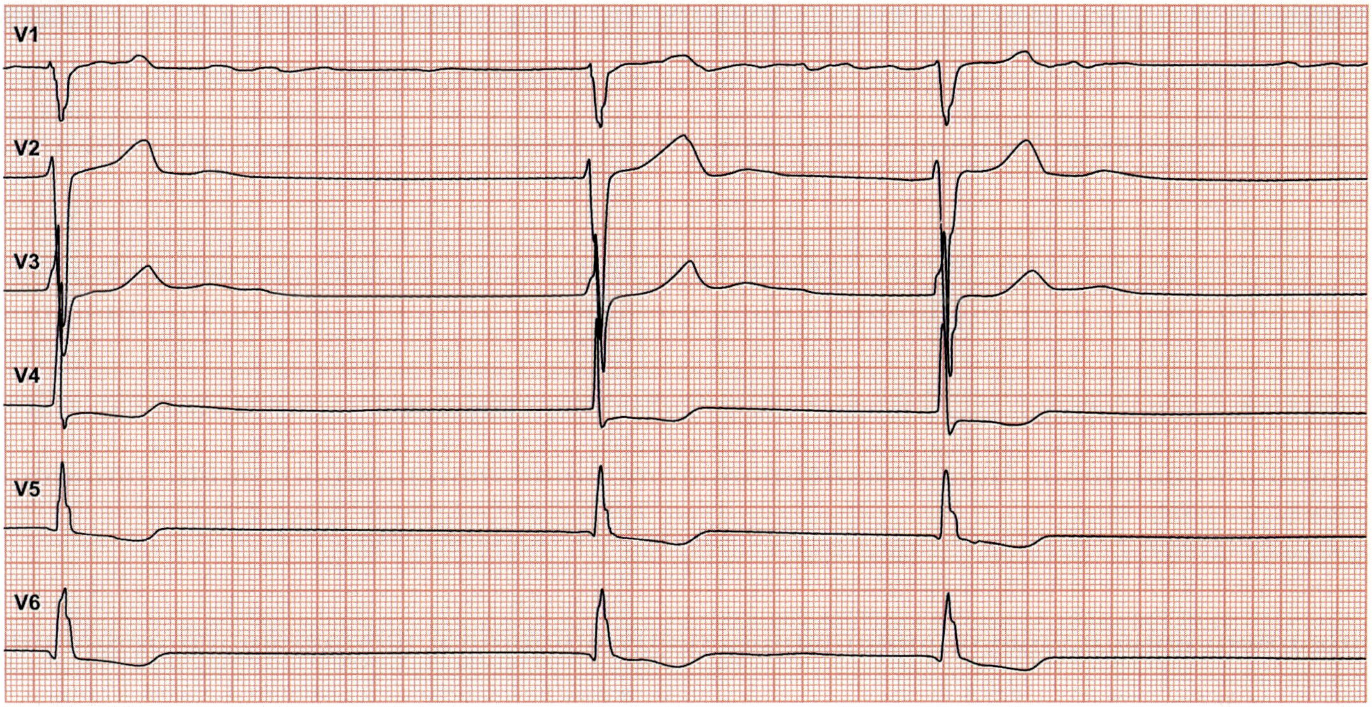


**Fig. 38.11:** ECG displays atrial fibrillation with slow ventricular response. There is a high degree of AV block, resulting in a bradycardic rate at 35 bpm (50 mm/s). The axis is in the normal quadrant and at 60 degrees. Limb leads show T-wave flattening, and there is perhaps a slight ST-segment depression visible in leads II and AVF. There is a quite prominent U-wave. Normally, the U-wave is best appreciated in the lateral precordial leads (V5–V6). Here however, it is seen in leads V2 and V3. The classic ST-segment morphology induced by digitalis both at therapeutic and toxic serum levels, is the 'coved' or 'scooped', or sometimes referred to as 'bowl shaped' ST-segment depression. It is sometimes described as if the ST-segment has been dragged downwards from a point at the middle of the segment. Digitalis intoxications may however, manifest with or without the classic morphology even at high serum levels. The classic digitalis effect on the ST-segment is sometimes called the Cohn effect, named after Alfred E Cohn, the American cardiologist

* Calcium channel blockers—diltiazem and verapamil increase serum digoxin levels; not all calcium channel blockers share this effect.
  - Cyclosporine may increase digoxin levels, possibly due to reduced renal excretion.
  - Erythromycin, clarithromycin, and tetracyclines may increase digoxin levels.
  - Propafenone increases digoxin level; effects are variable.
  - Quinidine increases digoxin level substantially but clinical effect is variable; related drugs such as hydroxychloroquine or quinine may also affect levels.
  - Propylthiouracil may increase digoxin levels by reducing thyroid hormone levels.
  - Indomethacin.
* Spironolactone may interfere with digoxin assays; may directly increase digoxin levels; may alter renal excretion.
* Hydrochlorothiazide.
* Furosemide and other loop diuretics.
* Triamterene.
* Amphotericin B may precipitate hypokalemia and subsequent digoxin toxicity.
* Succinylcholine increased risk of dysrhythmias has been reported.
* Herb/nutraceutical avoid ephedra (risk of cardiac stimulation); avoid natural licorice (causes sodium and water retention and increases potassium loss).

Clinical digoxin toxicity represents a complex interaction between digoxin and various electrolyte and renal abnormalities. A patient with normal digoxin levels (0.5–2 ng/ml) but renal insufficiency or severe hypokalemia may have more serious cardiotoxicity than a patient with high digoxin levels and no renal or electrolyte disturbances.

## Management

- It can be difficult to conduct treatment of digitalis toxicity. This is due to the fact that the condition of the heart of a diseased individual is highly fragile due to toxic effects of digoxin. Cure may include nonserious treatment such as,
  - Monitoring cardiac condition
  - Use of intravenous fluids
  - Use of potassium supplements

Medications may also be used to bind digoxin in the intestine. This will help prevent absorption of the chemical into the bloodstream. Digibind is a popular drug of this type. It is used as an antidote for dgoxin toxicity. It is not advisable to induce vomiting in DT sufferers as it can put further stress on hearts with reduced cardiac rate. It is also unwise to stimulate vomiting in patients suffering from other damaging conditions. In emergency cases, afflicted individual should necessarily be assisted in breathing to keep them alive for long enough to receive treatment. Cure, in such cases, can involve removing the contents of the stomach with the aid of tubes. In cases where toxic effects have developed occurred over an extended time period, drugs may be required to reverse the harmful effects. Effective management of this condition depends on early recognition of its association with dysrhythmia and/or any noncardiac manifestation.

Management involves:

1. Assessment of the severity of the problem
2. Assessment of the cause of toxicity, such as reduced renal clearance, the prescribed dosage, and concurrent medications
3. Assessing whether overdosage is intentional or accidental
4. Considering factors that influence treatment, such as age, chronicity of digoxin intoxication, medical history, existing renal insufficiency and/or heart disease
5. Taking ECG changes into account
6. Constant hemodynamic assessment, involving cardiac monitoring and 12-lead ECG
7. Immediate electrolyte level measurement

Treatment of digitalis toxicity should include the withdrawal of the cardiac glycoside and the elimination of all factors enhancing the toxic effects of digitalis. When the arrhythmia is causing hemodynamic instability or when there is ventricular irritability, treatment with antiarrhythmic agents is indicated. Potassium chloride, lidocaine and diphenylhydantoin are the drugs of choice in the treatment of tachyarrhythmias and ventricular premature beats. Atropine can be used to counteract the vagal effect of digitalis in bradycardia and heart block. If atropine is ineffective, the placement of a temporary artificial pacemaker may be necessary. When congestive heart failure is a complication, the use of a vasodilator to decrease ventricular preload and afterload will improve the mechanical efficiency of the heart, increase cardiac output and relieve pulmonary congestion.

### DigiFab®

DigiFab® Digoxin Immune Fab (Ovine) is a sterile, purified, lyophilized preparation of digoxin-immune ovine Fab (monovalent) immunoglobulin fragments.

Each vial of DigiFab® Digoxin Immune Fab (Ovine), which will bind approximately 0.5 mg digoxin, contains 40 mg of digoxin immune Fab, 75 mg (approx.) of mannitol USP, and 2 mg (approx.) sodium acetate USP as a buffering agent.

The product contains no preservatives and is intended for intravenous administration after reconstitution with 4 ml of sterile water for injection USP. DigiFab® Digoxin Immune Fab (Ovine has the following benefits such as it:

- Rapidly binds to and neutralizes digoxin with measurable results
- Rapidly reduces levels of free digoxin to undetectable
- More than 40% of digoxin excreted by 24 hours
- 93% of patients resolved their digoxin poisoning by 20 hours.

## CALCIUM CHANNEL BLOCKER

Calcium channel blockers (CCBs) were initially introduced for use in the United States in 1981, and extended-release formulations were available 10 years later. Indications for use of these drugs are angina, hypertension, arrhythmias, and migraine prophylaxis.

Calcium channel blocker overdose is rapidly emerging as one of the most lethal prescription drug ingestions. Overdose by immediate-release agents is characterized by rapid progression to hypotension, bradyarrhythmias, and cardiac arrest. Overdose by extended-release formulations can result in delayed onset of arrhythmias, shock, sudden cardiac collapse, and bowel ischemia.

### Pathophysiology

Calcium channel blockers have the following four cardiovascular effects:

1. Peripheral vasodilatation
2. Negative chronotropy (decreased heart rate)
3. Negative inotropy (decreased cardiac contractility)
4. Negative dromotropy (decreased cardiac conduction)

Other physiologic responses to calcium channel blocker overdose include suppression of insulin release from the pancreas and decreased free fatty acid utilization by the myocardium. These factors produce hyperglycemia, lactic acidosis, and depressed cardiac contractility.

## BETA-BLOCKER

Beta-adrenergic antagonists (i.e. beta-blockers) have been in use for nearly 50 years. In addition to their traditional role in treating hypertension and other cardiovascular disorders, beta-blockers are also used for additional purposes such as migraine headaches, hyperthyroidism, glaucoma, anxiety, and various other disorders. As a result of their expanded use, the incidence of overdose with these agents has also increased (Figs 38.12 and 38.13).

### Pathophysiology

Understanding the direct and indirect effects of beta-receptor blockade is crucial to rapid identification and appropriate treatment of beta-blocker toxicity. Beta-blockers act as competitive inhibitors of catecholamines, exerting their effects at both central and peripheral receptors. Blockade of beta-receptors results in decreased production of intracellular cyclic adenosine monophos-

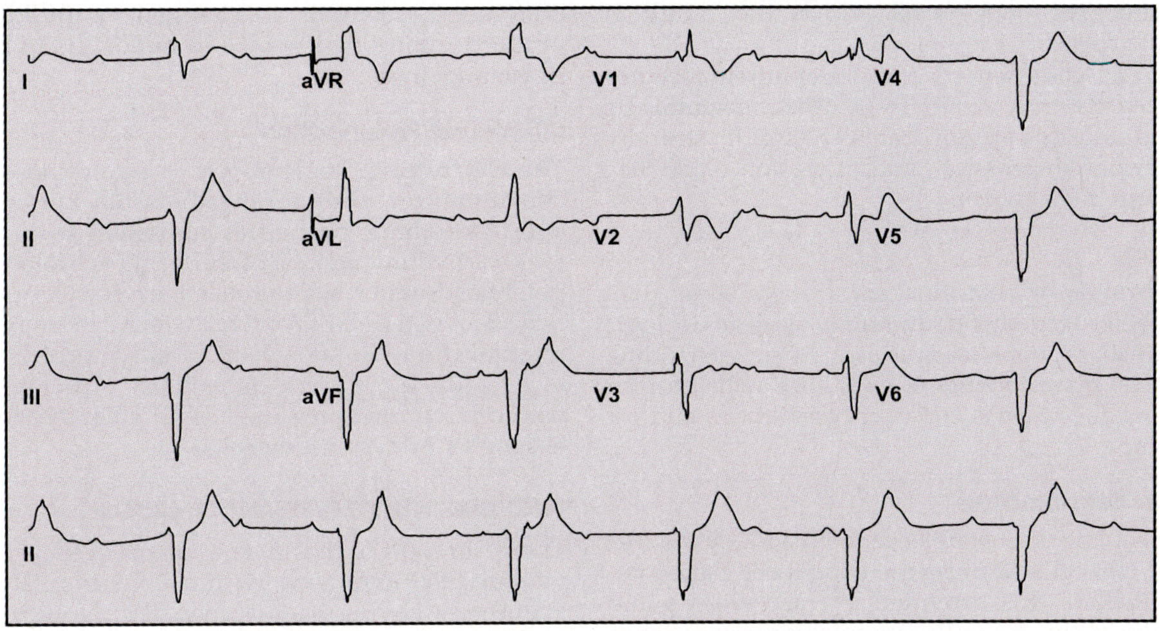


**Fig. 38.12:** Propranolol therapy showing bradycardia—complete heart block with marked Na channel blockade

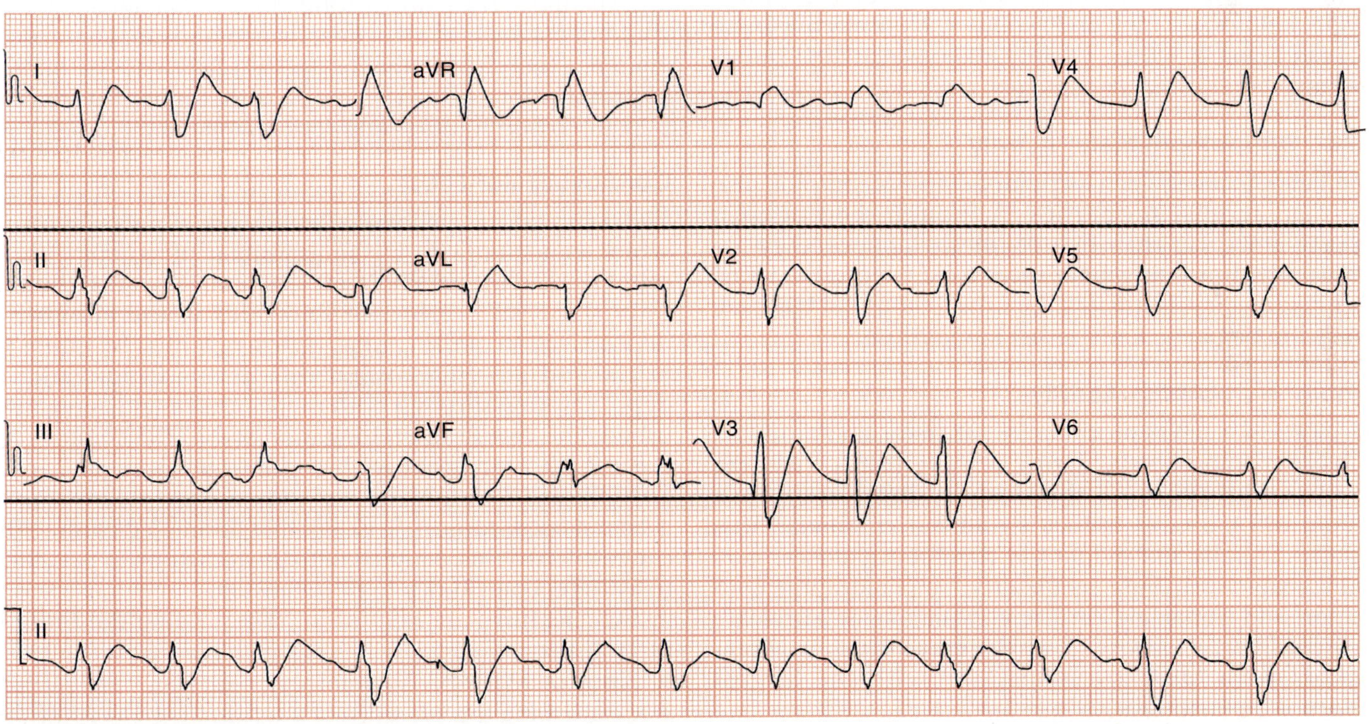


**Fig. 38.13:** Propranolol is a lipid soluble, noncardioselective beta-blocker with sodium-channel blocking effects. Propranolol is a lipid soluble, noncardioselective betablocker with sodium-channel blocking effects. A 27-year-old female weighing 60 kg presents to ED approximately one hour after swallowing 70 × 40 mg propranolol tablets (=2.8 grams) with suicidal intent. At the time of assessment she is drowsy (GCS 13) with a heart rate of 46 bpm and BP 100/60. Fifteen minutes earlier she had been awake and able to give a history to paramedics. ECG shows sinus bradycardia of 45 bpm with PR interval 210 ms, QRS duration 115 ms, QT-interval 380 ms and a small R wave in aVR of approximately 2 mm in height

phate (cAMP) with a resultant blunting of multiple metabolic and cardiovascular effects of circulating catecholamines. Beta1-blockers reduce heart rate, blood pressure, myocardial contractility, and myocardial oxygen consumption. Beta2-receptor blockade inhibits relaxation of smooth muscle in blood vessels, bronchi, the gastrointestinal system, and the genitourinary tract. In addition, beta-adrenergic receptor antagonism inhibits both glycogenolysis and gluconeogenesis, which may result in hypoglycemia.

Other than the direct effects of the beta-adrenoreceptor blockade, toxicity may result from other mechanisms including sodium and calcium channel blockade, centrally mediated cardiac depression, and alteration of cardiac myocyte energy metabolism.

### Pharmacology

Numerous brands of beta-blockers are available; they comprise a heterogeneous drug family with toxicologic characteristics that vary between classes. An understanding of the different characteristics of each class is helpful for understanding the various clinical presentations and for guiding therapy.

### Nonselective Beta-blockers

Propranolol was the first beta-blocker with widespread use; much of the clinical and overdose experience that exists with beta-blockers was provided by case reports and clinical studies of this drug. Propranolol is a nonselective beta-blocker, demonstrating equal affinity for both beta1- and beta2-receptors. Other nonselective beta-blockers include nadolol, timolol, and pindolol. Nonselective beta-blockers exert a wider variety of extracardiac manifestations.

### Intrinsic Sympathomimetic Activity

Some beta-blockers, such as pindolol and acebutolol, also have beta-agonist properties. Although their agonist property is weaker than that of catecholamines, they are capable of stimulating beta-receptors, especially when catecholamine levels are low. Of note, acebutolol has been reported to be particularly lethal in overdose.

### Membrane-stabilizing Activity

Beta-blockers, such as propranolol, labetalol, and pindolol, can have membrane-stabilizing activity (MSA) (e.g. the quinidine-like effects of the class IA antidysrhythmic effects). MSA blocks myocyte sodium channels. This property, usually not evident at therapeutic doses, may significantly contribute to toxicity by prolonging QRS duration and impairing cardiac conduction. Seizures are more commonly observed in drugs with MSA. Beta-blockers with MSA are associated with the largest proportion of fatalities.

### Lipid Solubility

Lipid solubility is higher in agents such as propranolol and carvedilol but lower in agents such as atenolol and nadolol. It may influence the degree of central nervous system (CNS) effects and utility of hemodialysis or hemoperfusion. High lipid solubility leads to a larger volume of distribution and better CNS penetration. Lipophilic beta-blockers are primarily metabolized by the liver. Propanolol is among these, and its active metabolite (4-OH propranolol) prolongs its biological activity. Conversely, hydrophilic beta-blockers have a small volume of distribution and are eliminated essentially unchanged by the kidneys; this property allows hydrophilic beta-blockers to be removed by hemodialysis.

### QT-interval Prolongation

The electrophysiologic effects of sotalol deserve special consideration. Unlike other beta-blockers, sotalol has antidysrhythmic properties consistent with the type III antidysrhythmic agents. Class III agents prolong the action potential duration and the effective refractory period of AV and atrioventricular myocytes, which can lengthen the QT-interval duration and result in polymorphic ventricular tachycardia (i.e. torsade de pointes). Toxicity with sotalol has been reported to result in ventricular dysrhythmias for as long as 2 days postingestion.

## TRICYCLIC ANTIDEPRESSANT OVERDOSE

The first report of the adverse effects of tricyclic overdose was in 1959 and came within 2 years of their clinical usefulness having been recognised. Now tricyclics are identified as one of the most frequently ingested substances in self-poisoning along with paracetamol, benzodiazepines and alcohol. They are second only to analgesics as the commonest drug taken in fatal drug overdose. There is also evidence that the number of deaths relative to the number of prescriptions issued is significantly higher for tricyclics in comparison to other antidepressants.

### Cardiovascular Effects

The commonest cardiovascular effect is sinus tachycardia, which is attributable to the inhibition of norepinephrine reuptake and the anticholinergic action. However, the most important toxic effect of tricyclics is the slowing of depolarisation of the cardiac action potential by inhibition of the sodium current and this delays propagation of depolarisation through both myocardium and conducting tissue. This results in prolongation of the QRS complex and the PR/QT intervals with a predisposition to cardiac arrhythmias. This inhibition of sodium flux into myocardial cells can occur to such an extent that depressed contractility can result and this, coupled with the reduction in peripheral resistance, contributes to hypotension.

ECG features are helpful for determining the presence of TCA toxicity:

- Sinus tachycardia is commonly seen
- Confirming the presence of a terminal 40 ms rightward axis shift, seen as an R wave deflection in aVR or an S wave in I or aVL, is the standard test for diagnosing TCA overdose
- QRS duration >100 ms is seen in TCA toxicity, but its absence does not exclude the diagnosis. Classic **ECG changes** (Figs 38.14–38.17).

Other ECG changes which can occur in TCA poisoning include:

- Prolonged QTc duration
- Prolonged PR interval
- AV block

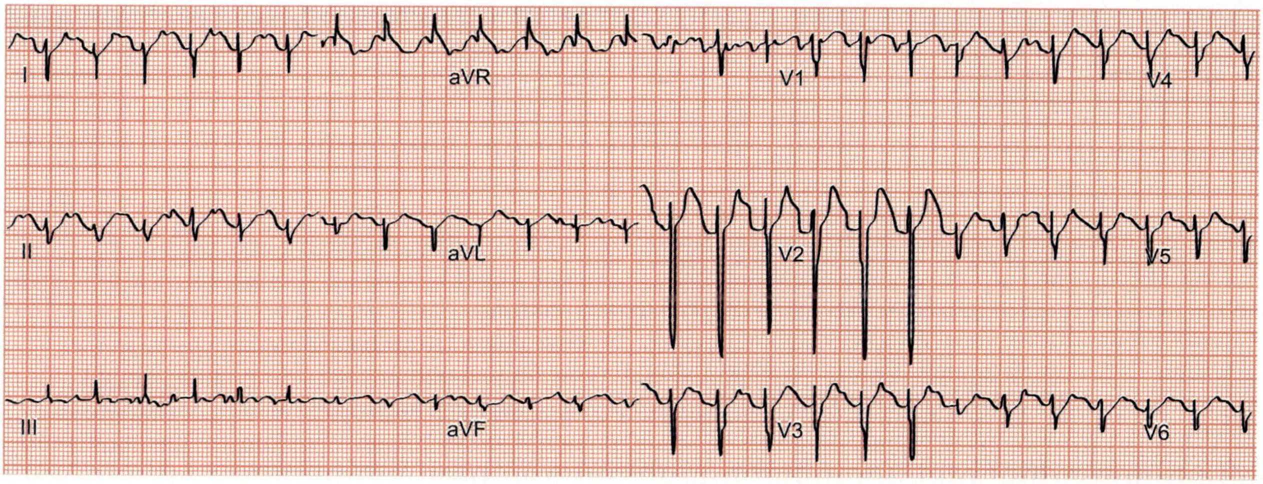


**Fig. 38.14:** (TCA ingestion) 12-lead ECG with a sinus tachycardia characterized by a widened QRS complex, deep S-wave in lead I, and prominent R-wave in lead aVR. These findings are consistent with cardiotoxicity resulting from TCA ingestion. Reprinted with permission from Mattu A, Brady WJ: ECGs for the Emergency Physician. BMJ Publishing, London, 2004, pg 110

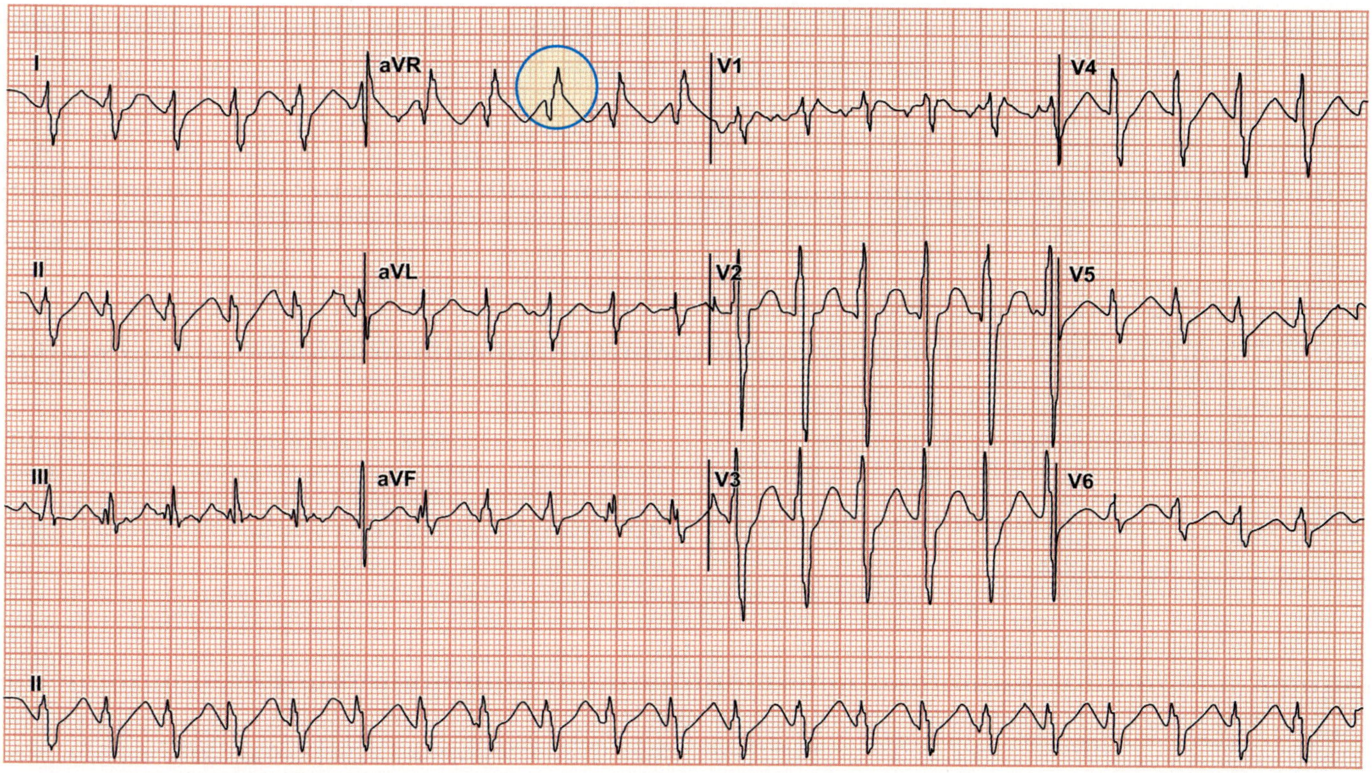


**Fig. 38.15:** Cyclic antidepressants block fast sodium channels leading to intraventricular conduction delay, widening of the QRS (with subsequent prolongation of QTc), and rightward axis deviation. The characteristic QRS >100 msec with a prominent terminal R in aVR (shown) is concerning and predictive of both ventricular arrhythmia onset and seizure activity. Tricyclic antidepressants (e.g. imipramine, desipramine, and amitriptyline) are regularly prescribed for treating chronic neuropathic pain, enuresis, and refractory depression. A child who ingested a cyclic antidepressant should be admitted for cardiac monitoring and serial ECGs. Any widening of the QRS >100 msec should be treated with a bicarbonate drip (1–2 mEq/kg/hr) to overcome sodium-channel blockade

- Nonspecific ST- and T-wave changes
- Downward sloping ST- elevation in leads V1 to V3 with right bundle branch block (Brugada's wave).

Once QRS prolongation is confirmed, rapid administration of 1—2 mEq/kg of sodium bicarbonate will provide enough sodium substrate to narrow the QRS duration in the setting of a sodium channel blocker. Importantly, narrowing of the QRS confirms only the presence of a sodium channel blocker (i.e. cocaine or diphenhydramine) and not specifically a TCA.

Serum TCA levels can be obtained but are not as valuable as the ECG. Also, serum TCA levels are not rapidly

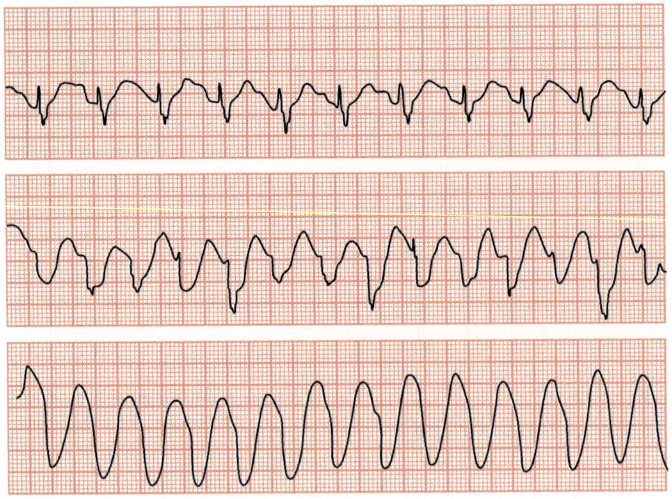

**Fig. 38.16:** ECG shows widened QRS ventrcular tachycardia in patient with tricyclic antidepressant drug

available and should never be used to guide management in the setting of an acute TCA overdose.

The overall incidence of serious cardiovascular arrhythmias is low. In one series four patients from 153 admitted to an intensive care unit had either a nodal or ventricular arrhythmia and only 3 of 225 patients admitted to another intensive care unit developed arrhythmias. Hypotension is more common with an incidence of 14–51% having been reported.

Management plan for treatment of tricyclic overdose:

- Assess and treat ABCs as appropriate.
- Examine for clinical features
- Check urea and electrolytes—look for low potassium
- Check arterial blood gases—look for acidosis
- Perform electrocardiograph—look for QRS >0.16 seconds
- Consider gastric lavage only if within one hour of a potentially fatal overdose.
- Give 50 grams of charcoal within one hour of ingestion.
- Give sodium bicarbonate (50 ml of 8.4%) if:
  a. pH <7.1
  b. RS >0.16 seconds
  c. Arrhythmias
  d. Hypotension
- Arrhythmias: Avoid antiarrhythmics
- Correct hypoxia, hypotension, acidosis, and hypokalemia
- Give sodium bicarbonate.
- Hypotension: Give intravenous fluids
- Consider inotropes
- Cardiac arrest: Prolonged resuscitation may be successful
- Monitoring: Patients who display signs of toxicity should be monitored for a minimum of 12 hours.

## COCAINE TOXICITY

The ancient Incas of Peru believed cocaine to be a gift from the gods. However, it is a modern-day curse to the emergency physician. Aside from alcohol and tobacco, cocaine is the most common cause of drug-related ED visits in the United States, accounting for 548,608 ED visits in 2006 (CI, 374,579–722,636), nearly twice the number according to the drug abuse warning network (DAWN) as marijuana or hashish, the second leading cause at 290,000 visits. Heroin-related visits are estimated at 190,000.

Patients who present to the ED with cocaine toxicity often also have other drugs present; in fact, the combined use of alcohol and cocaine may be the major cause of drug-related deaths.

Across the spectrum of acute and chronic effects, nearly every organ system can be effected. Trauma is often associated with cocaine use. Even the absence of cocaine may precipitate an ED visit due to withdrawal symptoms (Fig. 38.18).

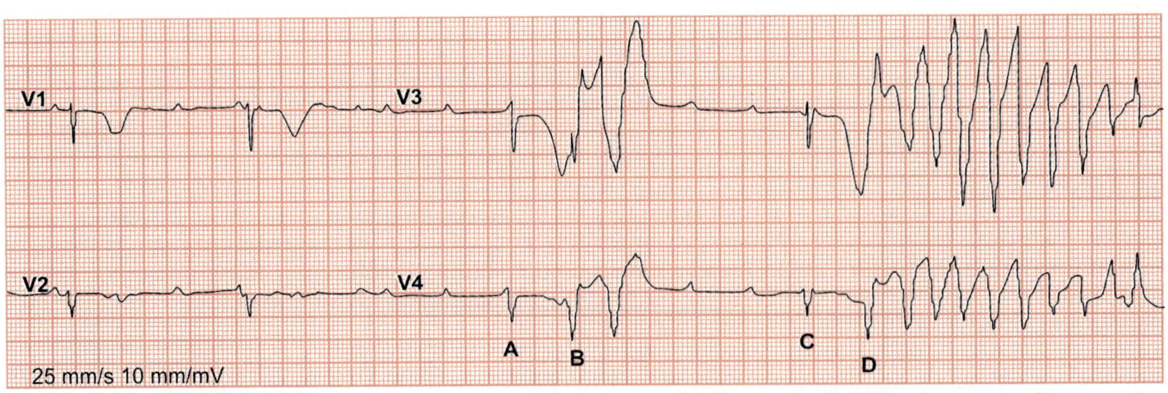


**Fig. 38.17:** Bradycardia-associated TdP in a patient who presented initially with complete atrioventricular block. Note the typical short-long-short QRS complex interval initiation sequence—a supraventricular escape beat (A) is followed by two premature ventricular extrasystoles (B) after a short coupling interval, which is followed, after a long AV block-induced pause after the ventricular extrasystoles, by a supraventricular beat (C) and another short-coupled premature ventricular depolarization (D), which is the first beat of the TdP. The QTc in the preceding supraventricular beats is 480 ms

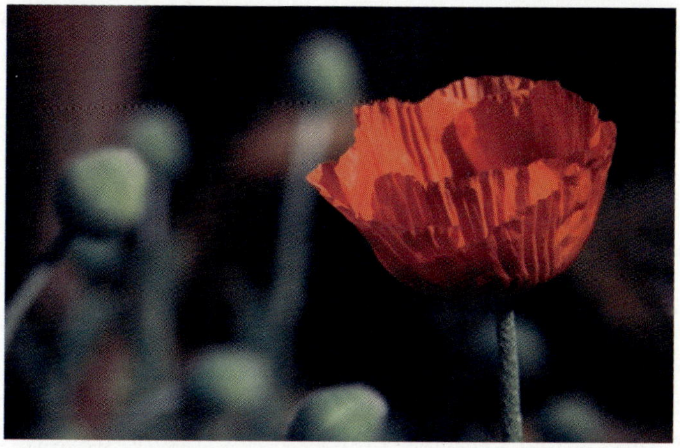

**Fig. 38.18:** The plant of opium poppy. Perhaps no plant has a more intricate global history than the opium poppy. The plant was used for medicinal purposes in China for centuries. In the early 19th century, the delicate herb gave rise to the powerful analgesic morphine that is still used to kill pain today. But opium has a dark side. It is also the source of the body-wrecking drug heroin

## Pathophysiology

Tachydysrhythmias cause most acute cocaine-related nontraumatic deaths. Other causes of sudden death include stroke, subarachnoid hemorrhage, hyperthermia, and the consequences of agitated delirium. Myocardial infarction (MI) can result from acute vasospasm, dysrhythmia, or chronic accelerated atherogenic disease.

## Dysrhythmia

Cardiovascular effects result primarily from direct actions on the heart and secondarily from effects on the CNS. Central and peripheral adrenergic stimulation results from inhibition of norepinephrine and dopamine reuptake at preganglionic sympathetic nerve endings. By preventing catecholamine reuptake at presynaptic terminals, cocaine causes catecholamine to accumulate at the postsynaptic membranes.

Without presynaptic reuptake, the action of a neurotransmitter on its receptors becomes sustained. Effects of endogenous catecholamines are thereby potentiated, resulting in tachycardia, hypertension, vasoconstriction, and increased myocardial oxygen consumption. Although cocaine-related tachydysrhythmias result primarily from increases in catecholamine levels, the local anesthetic properties of cocaine can impair impulse conduction in the ventricle, providing a substrate for re-entrant ventricular dysrhythmias.

- People who abuse cocaine may be exposed to toxic levels of circulating catecholamines. In one study, 48 mg of cocaine more than doubled circulating levels of norepinephrine (420 pg/ml increased to 900 pg/ml). However, most cocaine-related dysrhythmic fatalities occur in patients with low or modest levels of cocaine use. This finding suggests that the mechanism of death may be different in long-term cocaine users, in whom sudden death is most likely the consequence of adrenergic effects and long-term catecholamine toxicity.
- In rat studies, long-term use markedly increased norepinephrine content of the left ventricle. This theoretically suggests that long-term cocaine users could be at increased risk of malignant arrhythmia if excess norepinephrine also accumulates in the human left ventricle. Of note, coincident with the increase in ventricular catecholamine concentration, the rate of catecholamine synthesis was reduced, reflecting physiologic attempts to decrease sympathetic tone secondary to chronic cocaine stimulation. Alterations in cardiac histology may produce an arrhythmogenic anatomic substrate. Independent of coronary artery disease or clinically documented MI, cocaine use may induce scattered foci of myocarditis, microfocal fibrosis, and contraction band necrosis, the severity of which is correlated with serum and urine concentrations of cocaine. Although common in the hearts of cocaine and other stimulant abusers, such findings are found in only a minority of hearts examined.
- Other conditions providing an anatomic arrhythmogenic substrate include the accessory pathways resulting in Wolff-Parkinson-White (WPW) syndrome, and left ventricular enlargement.
- In patients with an arrhythmogenic anatomic substrate, even low levels of cocaine can cause tachydysrhythmias. In a study of 19 people who had survived cocaine-related cardiac arrest, had asystolic arrest because of massive overdose) and the remaining 11 had arrest resulting from ventricular fibrillation (VF). Of the latter group, all had an anatomic substrate for the dysrhythmia; patients had an MI, had WPW, and 6 had left ventricular hypertrophy or cardiomyopathy. On subsequent electrophysiologic testing, several patients had dysrhythmias, which were induced only after they had been given cocaine.
- Normal electrical conduction may become disrupted in cardiomegaly, which can be observed with chronic cocaine use. Rat studies have demonstrated that cocaine causes genetic changes in cardiac myocytes. Hemodynamic overload results in the production of high levels of atrial natriuretic factor (ANF). Increased levels of mRNA coding for ANF were measurable within 4 hours after rats were injected with 40 mg/kg of cocaine. When that same dose was administered to rats over 28 days, levels of mRNA coding for collagen and heavy-chain myosin increased, and left ventricular mass increased by 20%. Increased collagen production and increased left ventricular mass are independent risk factors for sudden death. Similar findings also are observed in humans. The hearts of cocaine users are 10% heavier than those of nonusers. In a study of 200 asymptomatic patients in a rehabilitation program who had used cocaine long term, one-third had increased QRS voltage, indicative of left ventricular enlargement. Another study of asymptomatic patients in rehabilitation revealed that more than 40% had an echocardiographically demonstrable increased left ventricular mass.

- An autopsy study conducted by Darke, Kay, and Duflou (2006) compared cardiovascular and cerebrovascular pathology in decedents dying of cocaine toxicity, opioid toxicity, and those dying of hanging who were toxicologically negative for cocaine or opioids. With gender, effects of age, and body mass index (BMI) having been controlled for, 1 in 7 cocaine users were found to have left ventricular hypertrophy, two and one-half times the odds of such a pathologic diagnosis being made in either comparison group. In patients with enlarged hearts due to long-term exposure to high levels of cocaine, even low cocaine levels can be lethal.
- Cocaine also has quinidine-like direct cardiotoxic effects, causing intraventricular conduction delay, as reflected by widening of the QRS and prolongation of the QT segment. In large doses, blockade of the fast sodium channels prolongs the slope of phase 0 of the cardiac action potential, which may result in a negative inotropic response, bradycardia, and, often as a precursor to death, hypotension from decreased contractility and dysrhythmia.
- With high blood levels of cocaine, such as those observed in a body packer or body stuffer when a cocaine packet ruptures, or in a binge user with large cocaine supply, the membrane-stabilizing effects of cocaine may cause cardiac arrest from asystole. In such cases, blood levels may exceed 50,000 ng/ml. Cardiac arrest is even more likely if the patient also has been consuming alcohol, with resultant production of cocaethylene. Tolerance rapidly develops to the euphoriant effects of cocaine but not to its local anesthetic effects of membrane stabilization.

### MI and Acute Coronary Syndromes (Figs 38.19–38.22)

- A 2001 nationally representative study of 10,085 American adults aged 18–45 years found that regular use of cocaine was associated with an increased likelihood of MI. Approximately 1 of every 4 nonfatal MIs was attributable to frequent use of cocaine (defined in this study as >10 uses in a lifetime).
- Patients with cocaine-related MI often have fixed atherosclerotic lesions. Cocaine can induce increased heart rate and BP, resulting in increased myocardial oxygen demand. The additional metabolic requirements may convert an asymptomatic obstruction into one of clinical significance.
- Substantial evidence indicates that cocaine use causes accelerated coronary atherosclerosis. According to a 1995 study of trauma fatalities among men with a mean age of 34 years and an incidental finding of cocaine metabolites, 25% had lesions in 2 or more vessels, and 19% had disease in 3–4 vessels. Of the control subjects, only 6% had 2-vessel disease, and none had 3- or 4-vessel disease. In another study of 22 long-term cocaine users with a mean age of 32 years, all of whom died suddenly with detectable serum cocaine levels, severe narrowing of more than 75% cross-sectional area was found in 1 or more coronary arteries in 36% of patients.
- Hollander and Hoffman reviewed and analyzed the literature of 91 patients with cocaine-induced MI. Cardiac catheterization in 54 patients demonstrated that 31% had significant coronary atherosclerosis. Autopsy studies of patients with cocaine-related MI revealed atherosclerotic lesions in more than one half of patients. In another review of medical examiners' records, 495

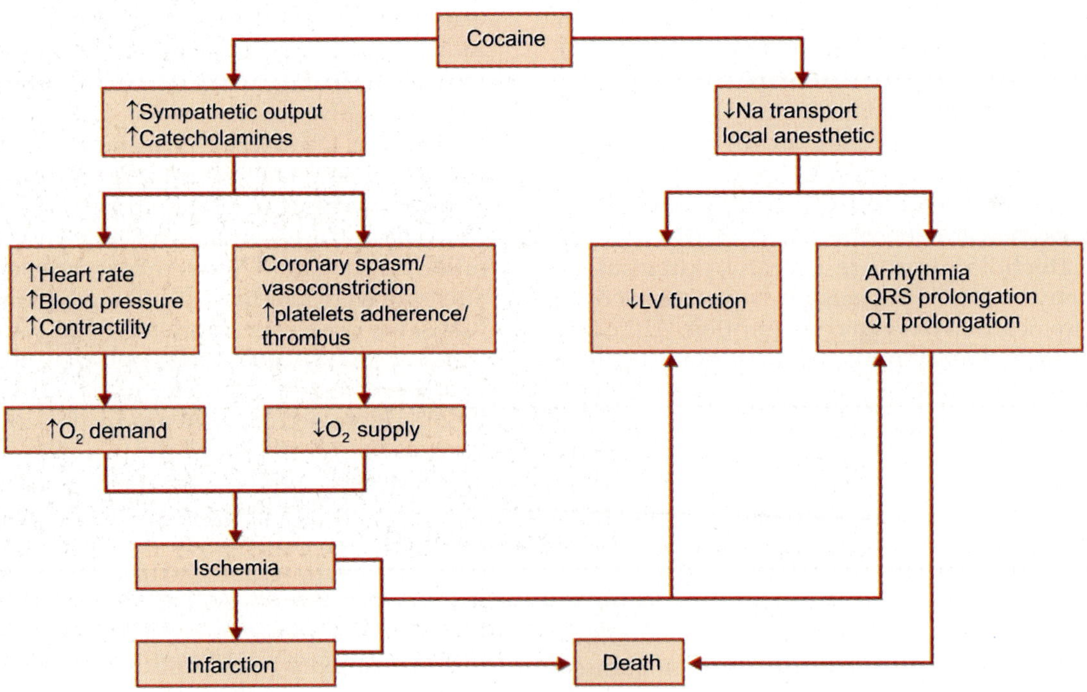


**Fig. 38.19:** Acute effects of cocaine on the cardiovascular system

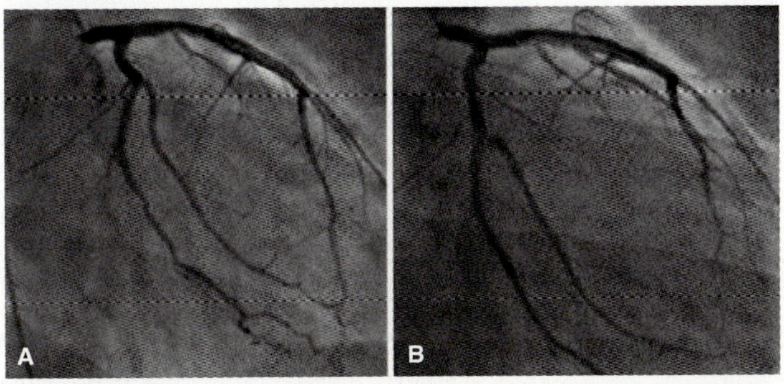


**Fig. 38.20:** Coronary artery dissection secondary to cocaine abuse. Coronary angiography, on the second day, revealed a dissection extending from the proximal to midsegment of left anterior descending (LAD) coronary artery with normal left circumflex and right coronary arteries (A and B). Left ventriculogram showed moderate left ventricular systolic dysfunction. Primary percutaneous intervention was not considered due to late presentation and ECG evidence of completed infarct, as well as insignificant symptoms. In view of possible cocaine-induced vasospasm related anterolateral STEMI, it was decided to manage the patient conservatively with nitrate infusion, diltiazem, dual antiplatelet and low molecular weight heparin (LMWH) after consultation with a specialist. Subsequently, he had two more admissions with chest pain and a small rise in troponin levels. His case was, therefore, rediscussed at our cardiology MDT meeting, where a decision to perform a repeat diagnostic coronary angiogram was suggested before any further intervention. Fortunately, his repeat coronary angiogram revealed spontaneously healed dissection (A)

deceased patients had positive toxicologic findings of cocaine; 6 of them, whose mean age was 29 years, had MI with total thrombotic occlusion primarily involving the left anterior descending coronary artery. All of the patients had significant coronary atherosclerosis, with 83% having lesions that caused luminal stenosis of more than 75% cross-sectional area in 1 or more vessels.

- Of the patients reviewed by Hollander and Hoffman, 24% had a thrombotic occlusion in the absence of clinically significant coronary disease. Cocaine's effect of increasing levels of plasma plasminogen activator enhances clot formation. In addition, cocaine activates platelets both directly and indirectly by means of an alpha-adrenergic–mediated increase in platelet aggregation.
- Cocaine increases production of the potent vasoconstrictor endothelin, and simultaneously decreases production of nitrous oxide, a powerful vasodilator. As a result of alpha-adrenergic stimulation, cocaine may exert a direct vasoconstrictive effect by increasing the influx of calcium across endothelial cell membranes. These factors may produce coronary artery spasm. Although this may occur even in patients who do not have significant coronary artery disease, spasm is most pronounced in portions of the coronary artery that are already narrowed. Therefore, in patients who do have high-grade obstruction, including patients whose stenoses were previously asymptomatic, coronary artery spasm of even modest degree can have devastating consequences.
- In healthy coronary arteries, endothelial cells release endothelium-derived relaxing factor (EDRF) and prostacyclin, which interact synergistically to relax vascular smooth muscle and inhibit platelet adhesion and aggregation. Mild atherosclerosis and hypercholesterolemia impair endothelium-mediated vasodilation in coronary arteries, and animal studies suggest that endothelial dysfunction predisposes a person to vasoconstriction and arterial spasm. Hypersensitivity to the vasoconstrictor effects of catecholamines has also been demonstrated in humans with endothelial dysfunction. Therefore, individuals with mild coronary disease who use cocaine may be predisposed to occlusive vascular spasm at the site of early atherosclerotic lesions.

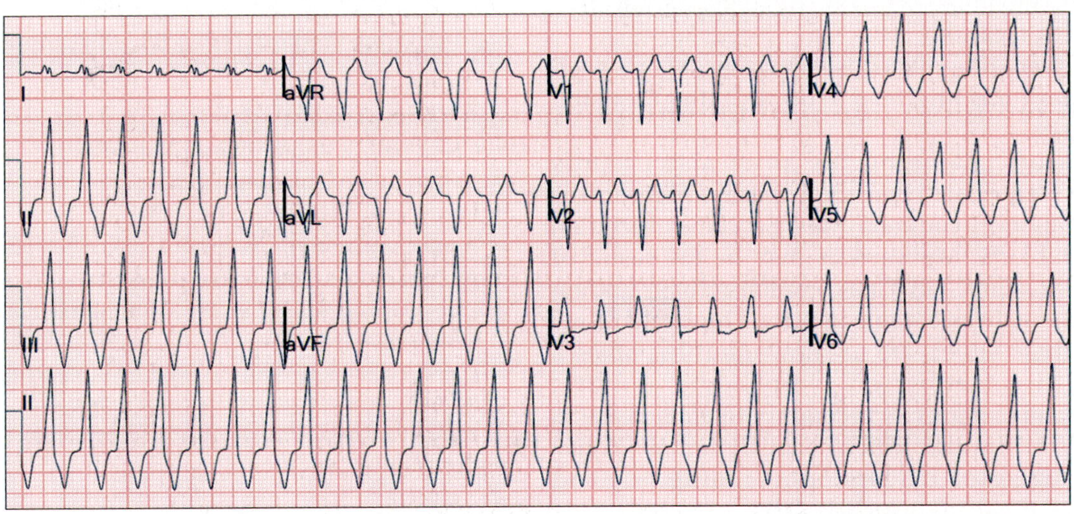


**Fig. 38.21:** Cocaine induced wide complex tachycardia at the rate of 170 bpm, with QRS duration of 124 ms

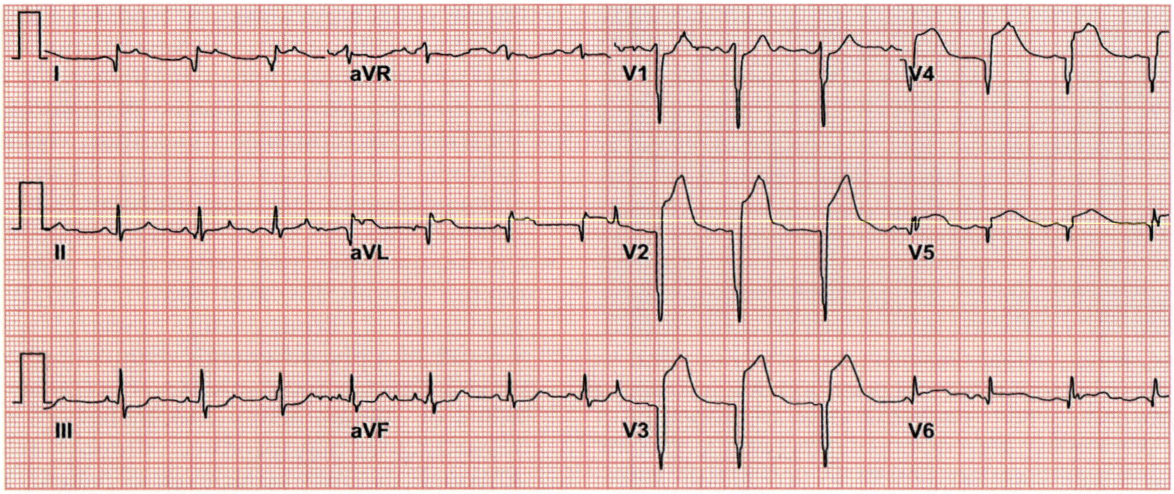


**Fig. 38.22:** Significant pathologic Q-waves (V2–6, I, aVL) plus marked ST-segment elevation are evidence for this large anterior/anterolateral MI. The exact age of the infarction cannot be determined without clinical correlation and previous ECGs, but this is likely a recent MI due to cocaine toxicity

- The combination of intimal hyperplasia, accelerated atherosclerosis, and endothelial dysfunction create a prothrombotic milieu.
- Cocaine also potentiates platelet thromboxane production and decreases protein C and antithrombin III production, as well as the production and release of prostacyclin. Aggregating platelets are an important source of serotonin. In patients with dysfunctional endothelium, serotonin causes intense vasoconstriction because of its unopposed effects on vascular smooth muscle.
- Chronic use appears to deplete stores of dopamine in peripheral nerve terminals. In patients undergoing cocaine withdrawal, more than one-third have frequent episodes of ST-segment elevation (similar to variant angina), as documented on Holter monitoring. Inhibition of dopamine-mediated coronary vasodilatation secondary to dopamine depletion has been advanced as the hypothetical cause.
- Patients with cocaine-related ischemic chest pain, even those who have had MIs, tend to do well after they stop using cocaine.
- The effects of cocaine on the heart also include myocarditis and dilated cardiomyopathy. Myocarditis may be 5 times more common among cocaine users than in control subjects. Myocarditis may be the result of microvascular injury, and it is a common autopsy finding in patients dying from cocaine toxicity. The mechanisms producing these effects are unknown, but hypotheses include a direct effect on lymphocyte activity, myocardial cell cytotoxicity secondary to an increase in the activity of natural killer cells, hypersensitivity reactions (suggested by eosinophilic infiltrate), and induction of focal myocarditis from catecholamine administration.
- Cocaine causes a direct negative inotropic effect on cardiac muscle, resulting in transient toxic cardiomyopathy. In one small series, 8 of 10 subjects who used cocaine long term had chest pain without MI but left ventricular ejection fractions less than 50%. In a case report, Jouriles describes a 35-year-old woman with hypotension, seizures, and hypoxemia who had an ejection fraction of 10% after smoking crack cocaine.

### Cardiovascular Findings (Table 38.1)

- Cardiopulmonary complaints are the most common presenting manifestations of cocaine abuse and include chest pain (frequently observed in long-term use or overdose), MI, arrhythmia, and cardiomyopathy. In individuals with cocaine-associated MI, median times to the onset of chest pain vary with the route or form of cocaine use—30 minutes for intravenous use, 90 minutes for crack, and 135 minutes for intranasal use.
- Chest pain may be observed in as many as 40% of patients presenting to the ED after admitting to cocaine

**Table 38.1:** Cardiovascular complications of cocaine

- Sudden death
- Acute myocardial infarction
- Chest pain without myocardial infarct
- Acute, reversible myocarditis
- Irreversible heart muscle disease
- Acute, severe hypertension
- Acute aortic dissection, rupture
- Electrocardiographic changes—sinus tachycardia, premature ventricular complexes
- Wolff-Parkinson-White arrhythmias, ventricular tachycardia, torsade de pointes, ventricular fibrillation prolongation of QTc, and early repolarization (ST-segment) changes
- Pneumopericardium
- Stroke
- Subarachnoid hemorrhage
- Accelerated coronary atherosclerosis
- Intimal hyperplasia of coronary vessels

use. In a study of urban and suburban EDs, cocaine or its metabolites were found in 17% of patients presenting with chest pain. This starkly contrasts with the pretest estimated prevalences of 2–4% for the suburban study site and 10% for the urban sites. The mean age of patients with chest discomfort and positive assays for cocaine was 36 years.

- Include cocaine use in the differential diagnosis of any acute vascular problem.
- Vascular spasm may cause blindness, renal infarction, limb ischemia, and intestinal ischemia. Limb ischemia may occur after intra-arterial injection. This may be accidental, or intentional due to the unavailability of veins because of sclerosis secondary to repetitive puncture, or due to the desired effects from arterial injection.

**Aortic dissection** may also be associated with cocaine use.

- Hypertension occurs frequently.
- Cocaine-associated VF
- Prolonged resuscitative efforts are recommended in AHA Guidelines 2005 for patients with cardiopulmonary arrest in a setting of drug intoxication.
- Hypotheses about the causes of cocaine-associated VF, if confirmed, have treatment implications. In one study, when the heart rate is held constant, alpha-adrenergic but not beta-adrenergic receptor antagonists prevented cocaine-induced VF. Cocaine activation of myocardial alpha-adrenergic receptors, specifically alpha1A-adrenergic receptors, may substantially contribute to VF during myocardial ischemia. Activation of these receptors elevates cytosolic calcium levels and provokes delayed after-depolarizations. Therefore, calcium overload may be the final common pathway linking enhanced adrenergic activity to cocaine-induced VF.
- This observation raises a question as to the role, if any, of calcium antagonists in cocaine toxicity. Studies supporting the use of calcium channel blockers have been performed only in animal models. Consistent with a local anesthetic mechanism of its toxic effects, calcium channel blockers have not been shown to reduce cocaine toxicity in humans. Furthermore, they increase the lethality of cocaine. This additive lethality may result from the negative inotropic effects shared by these agents.

### Cocaine-associated Cardiac Dysrhythmias

- Ventricular ectopy is usually transient and is managed with careful observation and escalating doses of benzodiazepine to blunt the hypersympathetic state by modulating cocaine-induced CNS stimulation. Treat malignant ventricular ectopy and perfusing VT by ensuring good oxygenation, by treating the hyperadrenergic state with escalating doses of benzodiazepine, and by administering appropriate antidysrhythmic medications if ventricular arrhythmias persist. Ensure that a defibrillator is readily available.
- Malbrain et al. recommend the use of an antidysrhythmic agent, such as bretylium (though now rarely found on code carts). Another pharmacologic option is magnesium sulfate, though caution is necessary because it may cause hypotension.
- Consider sodium bicarbonate for treating dysrhythmias resulting from the direct toxic effects of cocaine, such as when sodium channel blockade causes a QRS >100 milliseconds. Dual mechanisms of action have been proposed for its therapeutic effects—(1) Alterations in pH may change the conformation of the sodium channel, and (2) increased extracellular sodium concentrations may override sodium channel blockade. Hourly measurements of blood pH are indicated, with appropriate adjustments until the blood pH is properly controlled. End points of bicarbonate therapy are a serum pH of 7.50–7.55.
- Paroxysmal SVT (PSVT), atrial flutter, and rapid atrial fibrillation are generally short-lived and do not require immediate treatment. Use escalating doses of benzodiazepine to treat hemodynamically stable patients with persistent supraventricular arrhythmias to blunt the hypersympathetic state by modulating cocaine-induced stimulation of the CNS, taking caution not to depress consciousness and create a need for respiratory assistance. In drug-induced hemodynamically significant tachycardia, the pathophysiologic mechanism responsible may be increased automaticity, triggered activity, or re-entry phenomenon. Tachycardia caused by increased automaticity will not be responsive to interventions such as adenosine and synchronized cardioversion. Benzodiazepines are generally safe and effective in drug-induced hemodynamically significant tachycardia (HST).

### Cocaine-associated Chest Pain

- Chest pain may result from musculoskeletal, cardiovascular, pulmonary, or other causes. In patients with cocaine-related chest pain, assume that cardiac ischemia is present until this is proven otherwise. Accordingly, the ED approach to such patients, in addition to oxygen, intravenous access, and monitoring, includes the steps outlined below.
- The hypertonic content of the drug packet attracts water, making the ingested packages especially prone to rupture or leakage resulting in toxicity.
- Potent polypharmaceutic overdose is also common, resulting from an attempt to swallow all of the illegal drugs on site.
- The administration of activated charcoal has been recommended to adsorb any toxins from leaking bags, from ruptured bags, or that were liberated during enhancement of bowel transit (e.g. whole-bowel irrigation). Treatment of asymptomatic patients should include laxatives (e.g. sodium sulfate, magnesium sulfate, magnesium citrate, psyllium hydrophilic mucilage) or whole-bowel irrigation, several doses of activated charcoal, and close observation.

- If a polyethylene glycol electrolyte lavage solution (e.g. GoLYTELY, Colyte) is to be used for whole-bowel irrigation, Malbrain cautions that it must follow the administration of activated charcoal because the maximal adsorptive capacity of activated charcoal is at pH 7 and the polyethylene glycol electrolyte lavage solution has a pH of 8.38. Do not use paraffin-containing laxatives (e.g. lansoyl) because they degrade latex. Avoid endoscopic manipulation and enemas because the drug packet may be ruptured. Contraindications to whole-bowel irrigation include ileus, GI hemorrhage, or bowel perforation.
- Monitor body stuffers for several hours. Body packers may require hours to days of hospitalization until all the packets have been passed. Surgical intervention is needed if patients present with serious signs or symptoms or intestinal obstruction.
- Intoxicated with (but not directly due to) the drug, pathology associated with drug administration and pathology resulting from pharmacological action of the drug.
- Cardiac complications are the commonest cause of death amongst cocaine users, and can occur after acute or chronic abuse.
- Chest pain, myocardial ischemia and infarction, cardiac dysrhythmias and sudden death have been reported. Myocarditis and aortic rupture may also occur, but rarely.
- Ischemia and infarction usually occur in chronic abusers, but infarction can occur after initial use of cocaine. Cocaine (usually) has a positive inochronotropic action on the heart, through peripheral and central stimulation of the sympathetic nervous system, and increased adrenal medullary epinephrine production.
- Heart rate, blood pressure, systemic vascular resistance, and left ventricular rate-pressure product are acutely increased, and myocardial oxygen demand is increased in parallel.
- However, myocardial oxygen delivery is reduced, due to raised left ventricular end diastolic pressure, myocardial arteriolar vasoconstriction, reduced coronary diastolic filling time during tachycardia and cocaine-induced coronary artery vasospasm. Myocardial ischemia results from the imbalance between oxygen supply and demand. Q or non-Q-wave infarcts may ensue. Coronary artery dissection has been reported. Spasm may be worsened by the coadministration of cigarette smoke (which elevate carboxyhemoglobin levels and increase blood viscosity, which further reduces myocardial oxygen supply). Infarction is made more likely by the prothrombotic effects of cocaine. Platelet aggregation and activation are enhanced, and fibrinolysis is decreased (by an increase in levels of endogenous tissue plasminogen activator inhibitor). Underlying heart disease is not a prerequisite for the development of cocaine-related ischemia and infarction, but its presence significantly increases the likelihood of infarction and worsens the prognosis after infarction. Coronary atherosclerosis reduces the arterial endothelial release of coronary vasodilators (nitric oxide and prostacycline), enhancing coronary vasospasm at the site of atherosclerotic plaque. In addition, endothelial damage may occur after coronary vasospasm, promoting further atherosclerotic change, and thrombosis. Moreover, platelet activation releases smooth muscle growth factors, which promote vascular hyperplasia and coronary luminal occlusion. Indeed, cocaine appears to be an independent accelerant of coronary atherosclerosis.
- Cocaine-related chest pain annually accounts for 37,000 admissions to hospital in the United States. The pain is commonly described as sharp, stabbing or pleuritic, and may represent ischemia secondary to coronary vasospasm. Chest pain is invariably present prior to cocaine-related infarction. 6% with chest pain proceed to infarction. 4% die after infarction, 4–12% develop life-threatening arrhythmias, and congestive cardiac failure occurs in 5–7%. Electrocardiography is only sensitive for infarction in one-third of cases of cocaine-related chest pain (compared to 61% of noncocaine-related chest pain, though abnormalities are seen in two-thirds. CK and CK-MB levels may be raised in cocaine users who have not had an infarct (due to increased motor activity, seizures, hyperthermia, and rhabdomyolysis). Troponin I levels may be more beneficial in diagnosing cocaine-related myocardial infarction.
- Cocaine ingestion may result in cardiac dysrhythmia. Initial ingestion may be associated with bradycardia, although tachycardia is most common. Multifocal ventricular ectopics, ventricular tachycardia, ventricular fibrillation and asystole occur with increasing dose. Sudden death, accounting for the majority of cocaine-related deaths, is most likely attributable to a combination of dysrhythmia and cardiomyopathy. Several mechanisms contribute to cocaine induced dysrhythmia —myocardial ischemia, raised plasma catecholamine concentrations, centrally upregulated sympathetic nervous system outflow, hyperpyrexia, metabolic acidosis and cardiac myocyte membrane stabilisation by cocaine (by interference with transmembranal $Na^+$ and $Ca^{2+}$ flux). Intracardiac nerve impulses undergo slowed, heterogeneous depolarisations, with prolonged repolarisations.More recently, cocaine and cocaethylene have been shown to effectively block HERG-related (human ether-a-go-go-related gene) potassium channels, thereby suppressing the delayed-rectifier potassium current [I(K)] resulting in prolongation of cardiac repolarisation. Re-entrant dysrhythmias occur, and may be promoted by the formation of myocardial contraction bands, which are noncontracting, disorganised, amorphous masses of cardiac myofibrils that are associated with prolonged, high intake of cocaine (amongst other causes). Massive doses of cocaine can result in ventricular standstill. Left ventricular hypertrophy occurs in 54% of cocaine abusers and regional wall motion abnormalities in 21%. Contractile dysfunction may occur with prolonged, high

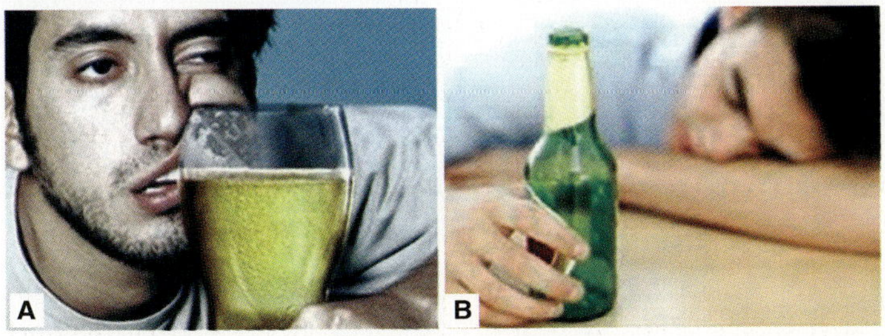


**Fig. 38.23:** (A) A person showing drinking alcohol and his bodily attitude depicts its intoxicating effect. (B) An adolescent is consuming over dose of alcohol with drowsiness

dose abuse, secondary to the effects of catecholamines, progressive myocytolysis, and focal fibrosis (in response to recurrent episodes of myocardial ischemia and infarction) and myocardial contraction band formation. In addition, cocaine directly causes myocyte apoptosis (particularly during episodes of oxidative stress). Poor contractile function may be reversible by reducing (and maintaining) circulating catecholamine levels to the normal range. Cocaine-related myocarditis may occur in a to toxic, dose-dependent manner, secondary to a hypersensitivity (dose-independent) reaction. Toxic myocarditis was found in 20% of cocaine abusers at autopsy, and is manifest by small areas of myocardial necrosis and loss of cardiac myofibrils. Cocaine-related chest pain may be a symptom of myocarditis.

- Cocaine-related episodes of hypertension, in the presence of atherosclerotic blood vessels, can result in potentially fatal aortic dissection or rupture.This usually involves the ascending aorta. Aortic root dissection may impinge coronary artery blood flow, leading to further myocardial infarction.

## ALCOHOL ABUSE

All patients with dilated cardiomyopathy should be asked about alcohol consumption. In addition, macrocytosis is a good indicator of chronic alcohol abuse, even when liver function tests are normal. Susceptibility to the adverse effects of alcohol on the heart is apparently individual. Susceptibility is demonstrated by the presence of immunoglobin A on the sarcolemma and muscle of small blood vessels at biopsy of patients with alcoholic cardiomyopathy (Fig. 38.23).

Alcohol abuse causes the diffuse myocardial damage seen in other primary myocardial diseases. However, fewer than one-half of patients present with symptoms of congestive heart failure (CHF), whereas in other primary myocardial diseases CHF.is the predominant feature. A significant number of patients with alcoholic cardiomyopathy present with arrhythmias and chest pain.

The EKG of patients with alcoholic cardiomyopathy may be normal or display nonspecific changes. As disease of the ventricle progresses, poor R-wave progression is

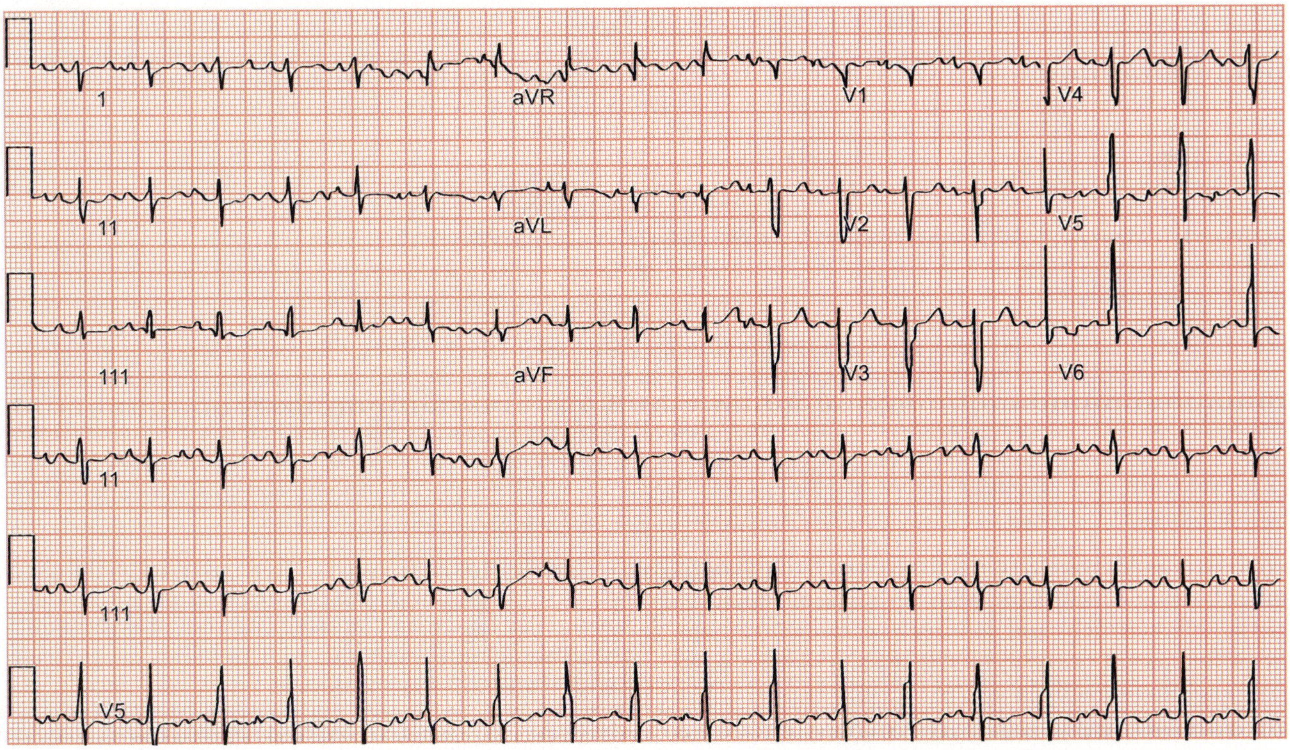


**Fig. 38.24:** A 58-year-old woman has abused cocaine and alcohol for 4 years. She has been followed for 2 years for a dilated cardiomyopathy, presumably precipitated by substance abuse, but she frequently fails to keep her appointments. She has no structural abnormalities of the heart. The ECG shows sinus tachycardia, right atrial enlargement, and right axis deviation. Sinus tachycardia is defined as a sinus rhythm (consistent, single P-wave for each QRS complex) at a rate exceeding 100 beats/min. Right atrial enlargement criteria include a P-wave amplitude exceeding 2.5 mm in lead II and/or exceeding 1.5 mm in V1

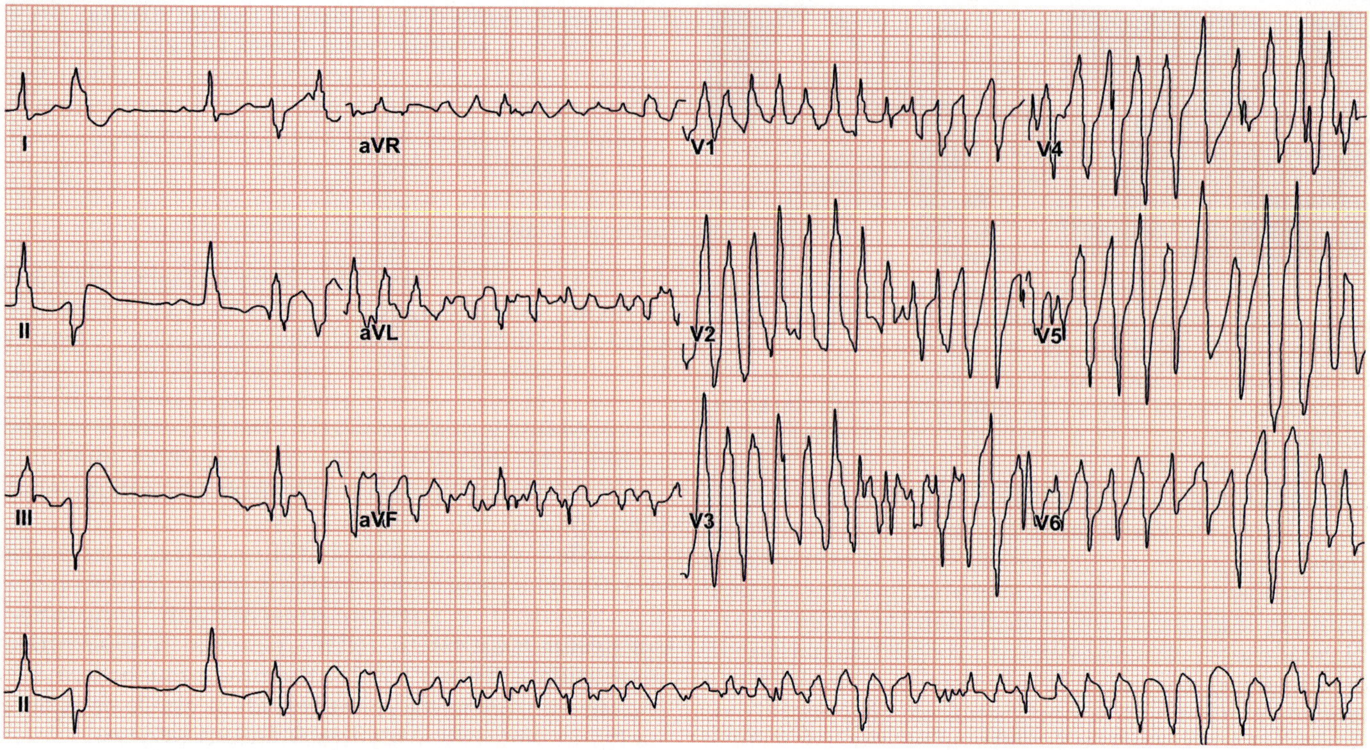


**Fig. 38.25:** Ventricular tachycardia in patient with chronic alcohol ingestion

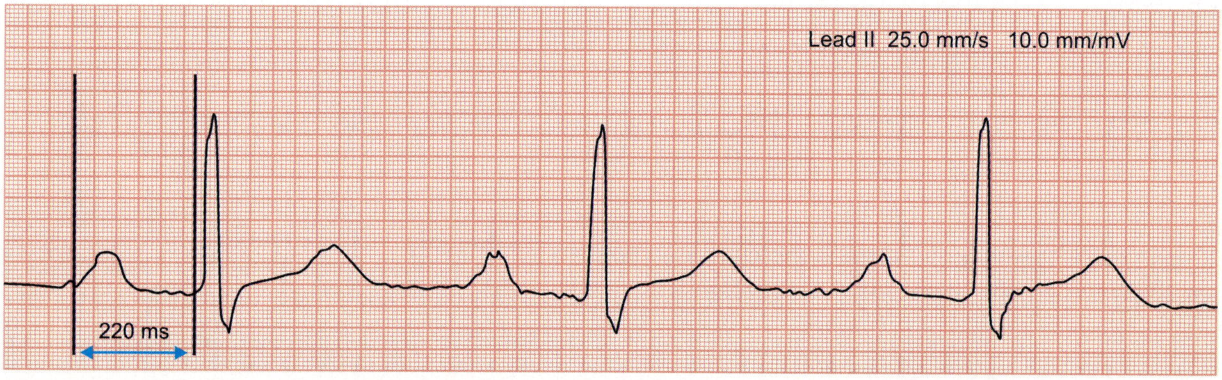


**Fig. 38.26:** ECG of an adolescent who was in a subcomatose condition after binge drinking. His serum alcohol concentration was 3.7 g/L. The next morning, before transfer to the pediatric ward, he developed a third-degree atrioventricular (AV) block. This recovered spontaneously after a precordial thump. Retrospectively, electrocardiography showed an increasing PR prolongation (200–300 ms) before the removal of the infusion needle. ECG recordings several hours later showed a first-degree AV block, which was no longer seen during follow-up, 1 month later. The authors conclude that acute alcohol poisoning has the potential to prolong the PR interval in young, healthy adolescents without pre-existing first-degree AV block and provoke a third-degree AV block after vagal stimulation. It is yet another potential danger of acute alcohol intoxication in this age group

common, reflecting conduction delay. In addition, enlargement of the left ventricle and left and/or right atrium is common, whereas left or right bundle branch block is seen in 10% of patients (Figs 38.24–38.26).

Supraventricular arrhythmias predominate in patients without overt cardiomyopathy and in patients with acute intoxication; atrial fibrillation is the most prominent. The aetiology appears to be moderate delays in conduction, which cause acute arrhythmias or 'holiday heart.' Acute arrhythmias are seen in heavy, binge drinking, in chronic abuse, or in special circumstances (e.g. prolonged sleeplessness) without chronic abuse. The risk of supraventricular arrhythmias with 6 or more drinks/day is increased by . Atrial flutter also is common.

Alcohol induces a number of pathologic changes to the heart. The classic manifestation include:

- Heart failure from dilated cardiomyopathy
- Dilated cardiomyopathy is an irreversible process in which the ventricular wall thickness is normal but the ventricular chambers are enlarged, giving the appearance of thinned walls

- Patients have subsequent systolic dysfunction and are at risk for arrhythmias
- Thromboembolism
- Sudden death
- Holiday heart syndrome refers to the development of rhythm disturbances after alcohol use in patients without structural heart disease
- Atrial fibrillation is the most common disturbance, and most cases are self-limiting

## TOBACCO ABUSE

The link between smoking and cardiovascular disease was initially proposed to explain the marked rise in the incidence of coronary heart disease in smokers after World War I.

Since then a wealth of data has shown that smoking predisposes to virtually every clinical manifestation of cardiovascular disease including myocardial infarction (MI) and other acute coronary syndromes, stable angina, sudden death, ischemic and hemorrhagic stroke, aortic aneurysm and peripheral vascular disease. The Framingham Heart Study demonstrated that men and women who had never smoked lived 6.2 and 4.9 years longer, respectively, free of cardiovascular disease than cigarette smokers.' Among smokers with a history of cardiovascular disease, men and women who had never smoked lived 2.4 and 2.7 years longer, respectively, than smokers (Fig. 38.27).

- These differences are the result of the increased rate of cardiovascular disease, the increased rate of mortality when cardiovascular disease is estabished and the higher rate of mortality from noncardiovascular diseases associated with smoking. Smoking interacts synergistically with blood lipid levels resulting in markedly increased rates of cardiovascular disease in populations with high cholesterol levels.
- The recent INTERHEART study demonstrated that the risk of acute MI associated with smoking is consistent across a wide range of populations with diverse lifestyles and socioeconomic development.
- This risk is closely related to the number of cigarettes smoked even at low smoking levels. Previous studies have shown that the risk of fatal and nonfatal coronary artery disease is doubled among very light smokers of 1–4 cigarettes a day, especially in women.
- Smoking may be relatively more damaging for women than for mens. Smoking cigarettes with filters or low-tar cigarettes does not ameliorate the harm because smokers obtain their preferred amount of nicotine (and accompanying carbon monoxide and pro-oxidant gases) by taking more frequent and deeper puffs or by blocking the ventilation holes in the filter. In terms of attributable risk, the impact of smoking on coronary artery disease is most marked in young and middle-aged individuals. In smokers younger than 50 years about one-half of nonfatal MI is due to smoking.

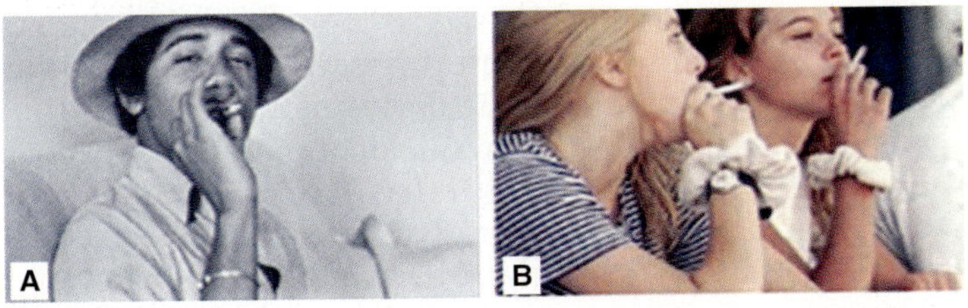

**Fig. 38.27:** (A) Adolescent is busy in smoking cigarette. (B) Two young girls smoking cigarettes on road side

- Attributable risk decreases in older age groups and about one-fifth of nonfatal Mis are attributable to smoking in men and women aged 60–64 years. Smoking cessation, even at the age of 60 years or later, reduces cardiovascular risk substantially. Cohort studies have generally shown that most of the drop in the excess risk of coronary artery disease mortality among former smokers occurs in the first 2–3 years of cessation. Thereafter, the rate of decline slows and it may take up to 10–15 years for former smokers to reach the same risk level as that of lifelong nonsmokers. In patients with coronary artery disease, stopping smoking is associated with an estimated 36% reduction in mortality compared with continuing smokers'. Such a large decrease in risk is similar to that observed with statin therapy. It occurs on top of such therapy and is extremely cost-effective.

1. **Smoking causes death**
   - The adverse health effects from cigarette smoking account for an estimated 443,000 deaths, or nearly one of every five deaths, each year in the United States.
   - More deaths are caused each year by tobacco use than by all deaths from human immunodeficiency virus (HIV), illegal drug use, alcohol use, motor vehicle injuries, suicides, and murders combined.
   - Smoking causes an estimated 90% of all lung cancer deaths in men and 80% of all lung cancer deaths in women.
   - An estimated 90% of all deaths from chronic obstructive lung disease are caused by smoking.
2. **Smoking and increased health risks:** Compared with nonsmokers, smoking is estimated to increase the risk of:
   - Coronary heart disease by 2–4 times,
   - Stroke by 2–4 times,
   - Men developing lung cancer by 23 times,
   - Women developing lung cancer by 13 times, and dying from chronic obstructive lung diseases (such as chronic bronchitis and emphysema) by 12–13 times.
3. **Smoking and cardiovascular disease** (Figs 38.28–38.30)
   - Smoking causes coronary heart disease, the leading cause of death in the United States.
   - Cigarette smoking causes reduced circulation by narrowing the blood vessels (arteries) and puts smokers at risk of developing peripheral vascular

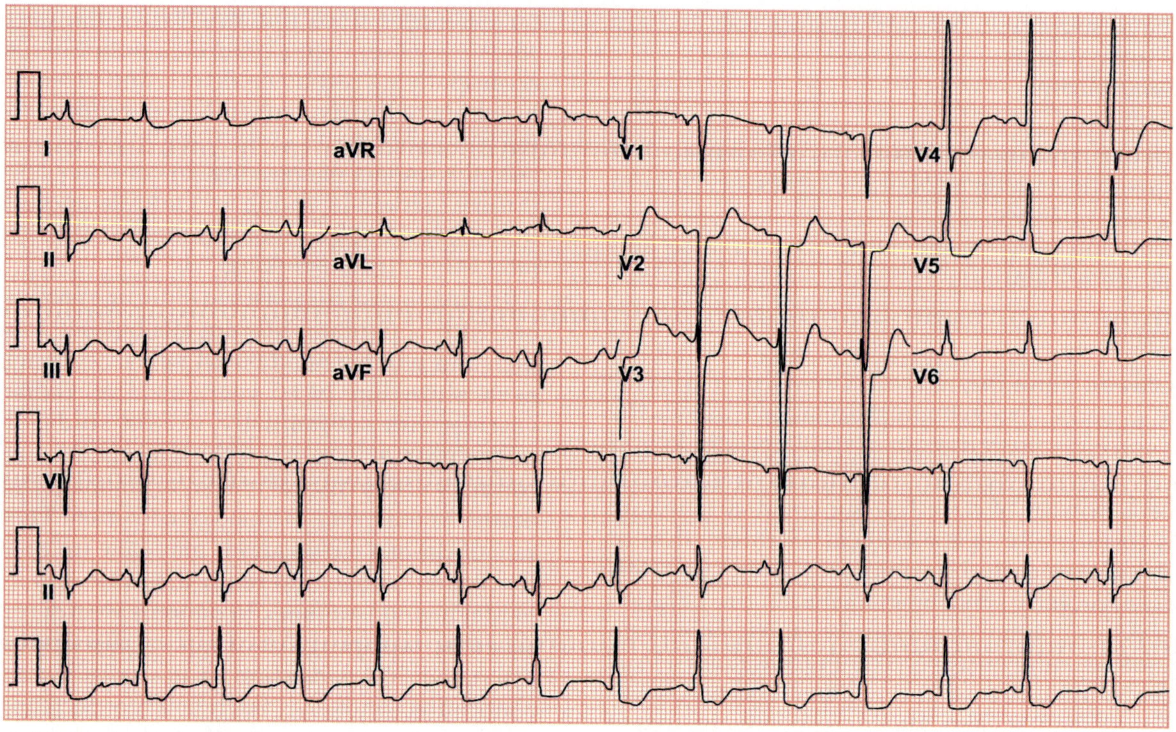


**Fig. 38.28:** A 12-lead electrocardiogram example of ischemic anterolateral ST-segment depression in a patient with habit of chronic smoking

disease (i.e. obstruction of the large arteries in the arms and legs that can cause a range of problems from pain to tissue loss or gangrene)

- Smoking causes abdominal aortic aneurysm (i.e. a swelling or weakening of the main artery of the body the aorta, where it runs through the abdomen).

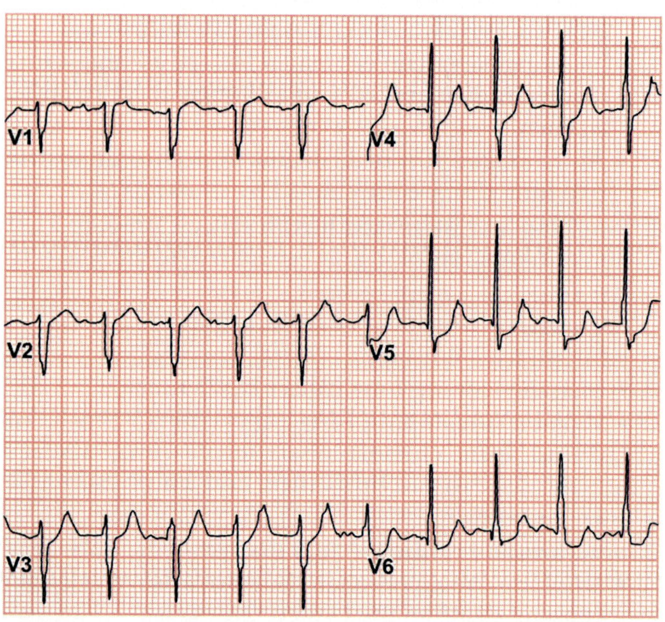


**Fig. 38.29:** 50-year-old businessman sedentary, obese (BMI=32), cigar-smoking began to notice a choking sensation in his chest with exertion which was relieved by rest ECG showed ST-depression in V4–V6 as a part of ischemic heart disease

## YELLOW OLEANDER POISONING

In nature, a wide variety of cardiotonic steroids is found in plants, the insects that feed on them and in the parotid glands and skin of some toads. All these natural drugs contain a steroid nucleus with a lactone ring, five-membered in the case of cardenolides, six-membered in bufadienolides. The cardiac glycosides have a carbohydrate or sugar moiety attached through an oxygen bridge to carbon 3 of the 'A' ring of the steroid. The myocardial effects of these compounds are attributable to increased intracellular concentrations of $Ca^{2+}$ and $Na^{+}$ resulting from inhibition of the trans-membrane $Na^{+}/K^{+}$ ATPase pump (Fig. 38.31).

- The digitalis glycosides are by far the best known of the cardiac glycosides but many hundreds of others have been identified in different species of plants from at least 12 different families. The apo-cyanaceae is source of African arrow poisons and also contains many of the most beautiful but deadly tropical flowers such as yellow oleander. The yellow oleander contains at least eight different cardiac glycosides. All parts of the plant are dangerous, especially the seeds. Ingestion of oleander seeds or leaves is a common cause of accidental poisoning worldwide, particularly among children. The oleander has been used for suicide, homicide, abortion and as herbal remedies in India, Thailand, Brazil and elsewhere. Yellow oleander glycosides proved effective in patients with heart failure and atrial fibrillation. However, digitoxin or ouabains have been preferred because of less frequent gastrointestinal side-effects. Most of our patients were healthy before their poisoning.

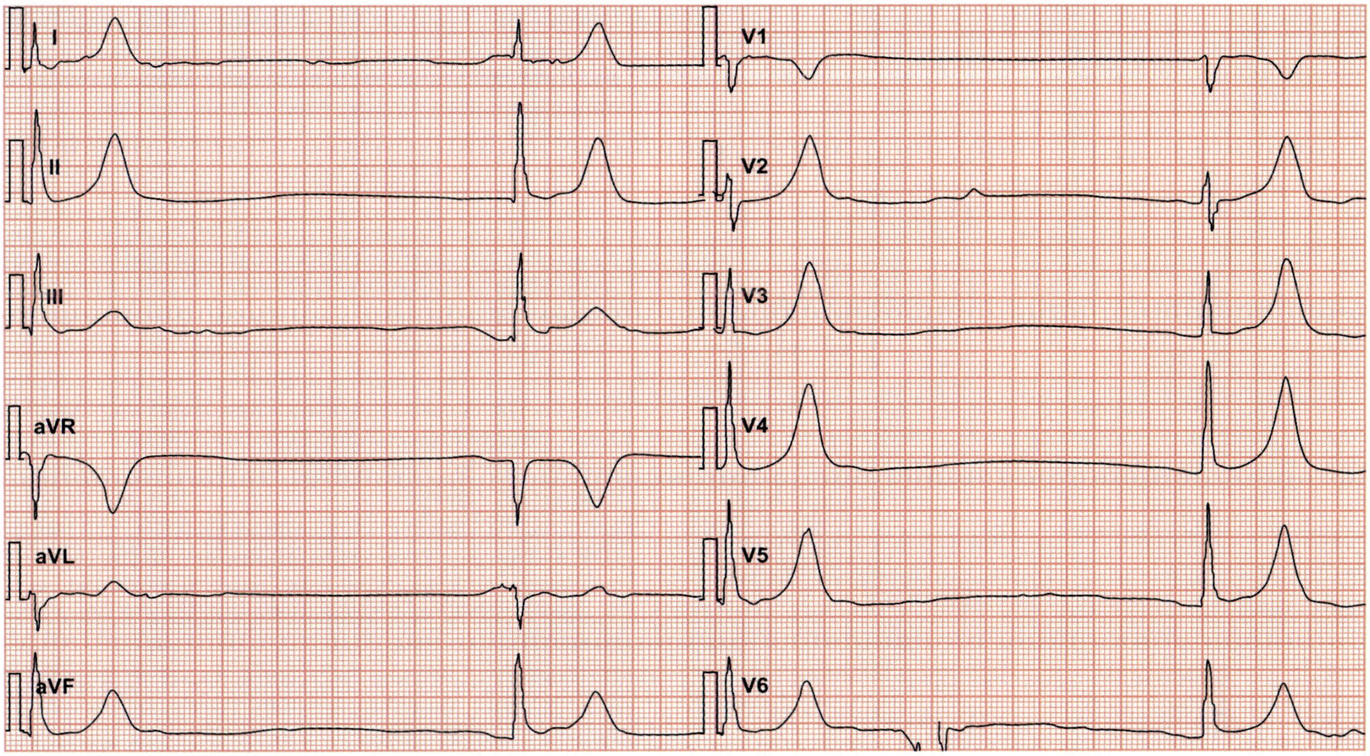


**Fig. 38.30:** ECG showed extreme sinus bradycardia in 60-year-old man after alcohal intoxication

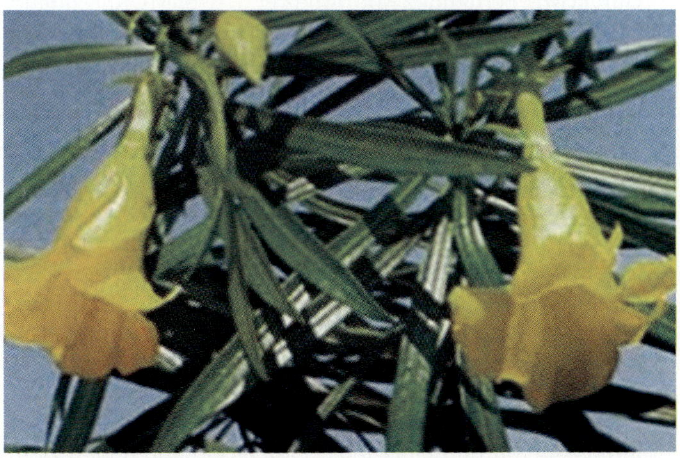

**Fig. 38.31:** Plant yellow oleander with leaves and flower

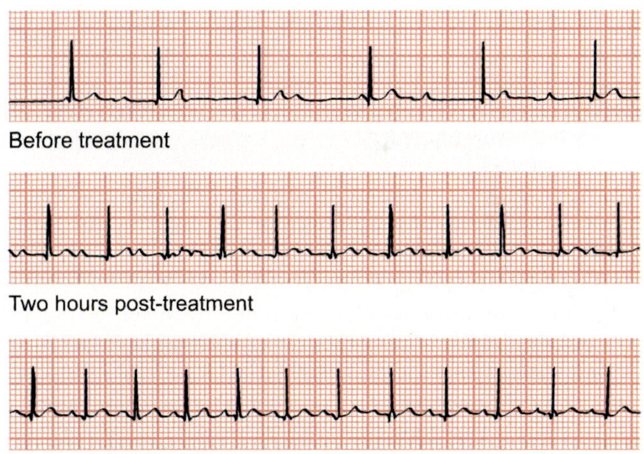


**Fig. 38.32:** Electrocardiogram in yellow oleander poisoning showing 2.1 AV block (upper strip) and complete resolution of cardiac arrhythmia after treatment with antidigitoxin antibodies

This differs markedly from patients with digoxin poisoning and majority of patients with digoxin overdose are on multiple drug treatment. As a result of the patients' young age and previously healthy state, the cardiac arrhythmias induced by oleander poisoning are unlikely to result from pre-existing conditions. Most symptomatic patients had conduction defects affecting the sinus or AV node and in 27% of the severe cases, both nodes were significantly affected.

- Rhythms characteristic of Mobitz type II AV conduction block, although reported to be rare in isolated digoxin poisoning, occurred in several cases of the oleander poisoning (Fig. 38.32).

**Carbon monoxide effects poisoning:** CO can cause harmful health effects by reducing oxygen delivery to the body's organs (like the heart and brain) and tissues. At extremely high levels, CO can cause death. Exposure to CO can reduce the oxygen-carrying capacity of the blood (Fig. 38.33).

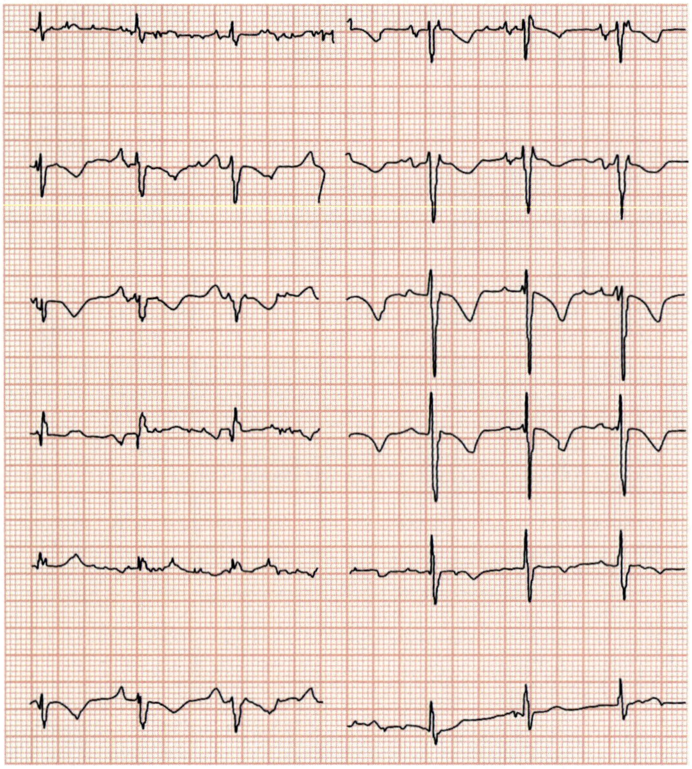

**Fig. 38.33:** 12-lead ECG from a patient with severe CO poisoning (CO hemoglobin of 39.1%) showing signs of myocardial ischemia as suggested by T-wave inversion in the precordial and inferior limb leads. An elevated troponin level (troponin I level of 11.8 g/L) confirmed the presence of myocardial injury

## BIBLIOGRAPHY


1. Aarnoudse AL, Dieleman JP, Stricker BH. Age- and gender-specific incidence of hospitalisation for digoxin intoxication. Drug Saf 2007;30(5):431–6.
2. Ahmed A, Waagstein F, Pitt B, White M, Zannad F, Young JB, et al. Effectiveness of digoxin in reducing one-year mortality in chronic heart failure in the Digitalis Investigation Group trial. Am J Cardiol 2009;103(1):82–87 [Medline].
3. Ali KM. Collateral effects of antiarrhythmics in pediatric age. Curr Pharm Des 2008;14(8):782–7.
4. Alonso A, Garcia Rodriguez LA, Logroscino G, et al. Use of antidepressants and the risk of Parkinson's disease: a prospective study. J Neurol Neurosurg Psychiatry. 2009; 80:671–5.
5. Anthenelli R, Dale L. Rimonabant helps cigarette smokers stop smoking and prevents post-cessation weight gain: results from the STRATUS-US trial. In: Final Program and Abstracts of 6th Annual Conference of the SRNT Europe; Tubingen, Germany, 2004, p. 35.
6. Bailey B, Buckley NA, Amre DK. A meta-analysis of prog-nostic indicators to predict seizures, arrhythmias or death after tricyclic antidepressant overdose. J Toxicol Clin Toxicol 2004;42(6):877–88.
7. Belson MG, Gorman SE, Sullivan K, Geller RJ. Calcium channel blocker ingestions in children. Am J Emerg Med 2000;18(5):581–6.
8. Benson BE, Spyker DA, Troutman WG, Watson WA, Bakhireva LN. Amlodipine toxicity in children less than 6 years of age: a dose-response analysis using national poison data system data. J Emerg Med 2009;1.
9. Brayer AF, Wax P. Accidental ingestion of sustained release calcium channel blockers in children. Vet Hum Toxicol 1998; 40(2):104–6.
10. Bronstein AC, Spyker DA, Cantilena LR Jr, Green JL, Rumack BH, heard SE. 2007 Annual Report of the American Association of Poison Control Centers' National Poison Data System (NPDS): 25th Annual Report. Clin Toxicol (Phila) 2008;46(10):927–1057.
11. Bronstein AC, Spyker DA, Cantilena LR Jr, Green JL, Rumack BH, Giffin SL. 2008 Annual Report of the American Association of Poison Control Centers' National Poison Data System (NPDS): 26th Annual Report. Clin Toxicol (Phila) 2009;47(10):911–1084.
12. Bronstein AC, Spyker DA, Cantilena LR Jr, Green JL, Rumack BH, Giffin SL. 2008 Annual Report of the American Association of Poison Control Centers' National Poison Data System (NPDS): 26th Annual Report. Clin Toxicol (Phila) 2009;47(10):911–1084.
13. Bronstein AC, Spyker DA, Cantilena LR Jr, Rumack BH, Dart RC. 2011 Annual report of the American Association of Poison Control Centers' National Poison Data System (NPDS): 29th Annual Report. Clin Toxicol (Phila) 2012; 50(10):911–1164.
14. Cepeda Piorno J, Pobes Martínez de Salinas A, González García ME, Fernández Rodríguez E. [Use of MDRD equation to detect occult renal failure and reduce the risk of digitalis overdose]. Nefrologia 2009;29(2):150–5.
15. Chan AL, Wang MT, Su CY, Tsai FH. Risk of digoxin intoxication caused by clarithromycin-digoxin interactions in heart failure patients: a population-based study. Eur J Clin Pharmacol 2009;65(12):1237–43.
16. Coe JW, Brooks PR, Vetelino MG et al. Varenicline: an a4j32 nicotinic receptor partial agonist for smoking cessation. J Med Chem 2005;48: 3474–7.
17. Cohen C, Perrault G, Voltz C et al. SR141716, a central cannabinoid (CB1) receptor antagonist, blocks the motivational and dopamine-releasing effects of nicotine in rats. Behav Pharmaco 2002;13:451–63.
18. D'Agostino ML, Risser J, Robinson-Bostom L. Imipramine-induced hyperpigmentation: a case report and review of the literature. Journal of Cutaneous Pathology 2008;36:799–803.
19. Derlet RW, Horowitz BZ. Cardiotoxic drugs. Emerg Med Clin North Am 1995;13(4):771–91.
20. DeWitt CR, Waksman JC. Pharmacology, pathophysiology and management of calcium channel blocker and beta-blocker toxicity. Toxicol Rev 2004;23(4):223–38.
21. Eisner DA, Kashimura T, Venetucci LA, Trafford AW. From the ryanodine receptor to cardiac arrhythmias. Circ J 2009;73(9):1561–7.
22. Fagerstrom K, Balfour DJK. Neuropharmacology and potential efficacy of new treatments for tobacco dependence. Expert Opin Investig Drugs 2006;15:107–16.
23. Gheorghiade M, van Veldhuisen DJ, Colucci WS. Contemporary use of digoxin in the management of cardiovascular disorders. Circulation 2006;113(21):2556–64.

24. Gonzalez S, Cascio MG, Fernandex-Ruiz J et al. Changes in endo-cannabinoid content in the brain of rats chronically exposed to nicotine, ethanol or cocaine. Brain Res 2002;954: 73–81.
25. Haynes K, Heitjan D, Kanetsky P, Hennessy S. Declining public health burden of digoxin toxicity from 1991 to 2004. Clin Pharmacol Ther 2008;84(1):90–94. [Medline].
26. Horowitz BZ, Rhee KJ. Massive verapamil ingestion: a report of two cases and a review of the literature. Am J Emerg Med 1989;7(6):624–31.
27. Koren G, Parker R. Interpretation of excessive serum concentrations of digoxin in children. Am J Cardiol 1985; 55(9):1210–4.
28. Kulig K, Bar-Or D, Cantrill SV, Rosen P, Rumack BH. Management of acutely poisoned patients without gastric emptying. Ann Emerg Med 1985;14(6):562–7.
29. Kwadijk-de Gijsel S, Bijl MJ, Visser LE, et al. Variation in the CYP2D6 gene is associated with a lower serum sodium concen-tration in patients on antidepressants. British Journal of Clinical Pharmacology 2009;68:221–5.
30. Lester L, McLaughlin S. SALT: a case for the sodium channel blockade toxidrome and the mnemonic SALT. Ann Emerg Med 2008;51(2):214.
31. Liebelt EL, Francis PD, Woolf AD. ECG lead aVR versus QRS interval in predicting seizures and arrhythmias in acute tricyclic antidepressant toxicity. Ann Emerg Med 1995; 26(2):195–201.
32. Liebelt EL, Ulrich A, Francis PD, Woolf A. Serial electrocardiogram changes in acute tricyclic antidepressant overdoses. Crit Care Med 1997;25(10):1721–6.
33. Litovitz TL, Klein-Schwartz W, White S, Cobaugh DJ, Youniss J, Drab A, et al. 1999 annual report of the American Association of Poison Control Centers Toxic Exposure Surveillance System. Am J Emerg Med 2000;18(5): 517–74.
34. Mahdyoon H, Battilana G, Rosman H, Goldstein S, Gheorghiade M. The evolving pattern of digoxin intoxication: observations at a large urban hospital from 1980 to 1988. Am Heart J 1990;120(5):1189–94.
35. Marubio LM, Gardier AM, Durier S et al. Effects of nicotine in the dopaminergic system of mice lacking the alpha4 subunit of neuronal nicotinic acetylcholine receptors. Eur J Neurosci 2003;17:1329.
36. Nides M, Oncken C, Gonzales D et al. for the varenicline study group. Smoking cessation with varenicline, a selective a4f\2 nicotinic receptor partial agonist. Arch Intern Med 2006; 166:1561–8.
37. Oncken C, Gonzales D, Nides M et al. for the varenicline study group. Efficacy and safety of the novel selective nicotinic acetylcholine receptor partial agonist, varenicline, for smoking cessation. Arch Intern Med 2006;166: 1571–1577.
38. Ranniger C, Roche C. Are one or two dangerous? Calcium channel blocker exposure in toddlers. J Emerg Med 2007; 33(2):145–54.
39. Rollema H, Coe Jw. Discovery and pharmacology of vareni-cline: an a4f\2 partial agonist for smoking cessation. Int J Neuropsychopharmacology 2006;9(suppl 1):S55.
40. Rosenberg LB, Whang W, Shimbo D, et al. Exposure to tricyclic antidepressants is associated with an increased risk of incident CHD events in a population-based study. International Journal of Cardiology 2009;epub ahead of print.
41. Tapper AR, McKinney SL, Nashmi R et al. Nicotine activation of a4 receptors: sufficient for reward, tolerance, and sensitization. Science 2004;306:1029–32.
42. Thacker D, Sharma J. Digoxin toxicity. Clin Pediatr (Phila) 2007;46(3):276–9.
43. The Internet Drug Reference Top 300 Prescriptions for 2005. RxList. Available athttp://www.rxlist.com/script/main/art.asp?articlekey=79509. Accessed: March 4, 2010.

# 39 Sudden Cardiac Death

Sudden cardiac death (SCD) is an unexpected death due to cardiac causes occurring in a short time period (generally within 1 h of symptom onset) in a person with known or unknown cardiac disease. Most cases of SCD are related to cardiac arrhythmias. Approximately half of all cardiac deaths can be classified as SCDs. SCD represents the first expression of cardiac disease in many individuals who experience out-of-hospital cardiac arrest. It is estimated that more than 7 million lives per year are lost to SCD worldwide, including over 300,000 in the United States (Fig. 39.1).

## PATHOPHYSIOLOGY

The most common electrophysiologic mechanisms leading to SCD are tachyarrhythmias such as ventricular fibrillation (VF) or ventricular tachycardia (VT). Interruption of tachyarrhythmias, using either an automatic external defibrillator (AED) or an implantable cardioverter defibrillator (ICD), has been shown to be an effective treatment for VF and VT. The implantable defibrillator has become the central therapeutic factor in the prevention and treatment of sudden cardiac death. Patients with tachyarrhythmias, especially VT, carry the best overall prognosis among patients with sudden cardiac arrest (SCA).

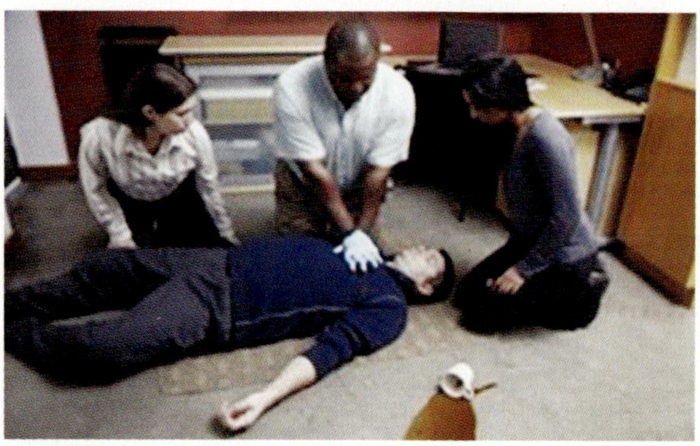

**Fig. 39.1:** Young person lying flat on the ground with sudden cardiac arrest

There are multiple factors at the organ (e.g. imbalance of autonomic tone), tissue (e.g. re-entry, wave break, and action potential duration alternans), cellular (e.g. triggered activity, and automaticity) and subcellular (abnormal activation or deactivation of ion channels) level involved in generation of VT or VF in different conditions. An anatomical or a functional block in the course of impulse propagation may create a circuit with the wave front circling around it and resulting in VT. Other mechanisms such as wave break and collisions are involved in generating VF from VT. While at the tissue level the above-mentioned re-entry and wave break mechanisms are the most important known mechanisms of VT and VF, at the cellular level increased excitation or decreased repolarization reserve of cardiomyocytes may result in ectopic activity (e.g. automaticity, triggered activity), contributing to VT and VF initiation.

At the subcellular level, altered intracellular $Ca^{2+}$ currents, altered intracellular $K^+$ currents (especially in ischemia), or mutations resulting in dysfunction of a sodium channel ($Na^+$ channelopathy) can increase the likelihood of VT and VF.

Approximately, 20–30% of patients with documented sudden death have bradyarrhythmia or asystole at the time of initial contact. Oftentimes, it is difficult to determine with certainty the initiating event in a patient presenting with a bradyarrhythmia because asystole and pulseless electrical activity (PEA) may result from a sustained VT. Less commonly, an initial bradyarrhythmia producing myocardial ischemia may then provoke VT or VF.

Most cases of SCD occur in patients with structural abnormalities of the heart. Myocardial infarction (MI) and post-MI remodeling of the heart is the most common structural abnormality in patients with SCD. In patients who survive a myocardial infarction, the presence of premature ventricular contractions (PVCs), particularly complex forms such as multiform PVCs, short coupling intervals (R-on-T phenomenon), or VT (salvos of 3 or more ectopic beats), reflect an increased risk of sudden death. However suppression of the PVCs with antiarrhythmic drugs increases mortality, owing to the proarrhythmic risk of currently available medications.

Hypertrophic cardiomyopathy and dilated cardiomyopathy are associated with an increased risk of SCD. Various valvular diseases such as aortic stenosis are associated with increased risk of SCD. Acute illnesses, such as myocarditis, may provide both an initial and sustained risk of SCD due to inflammation and fibrosis of the myocardium.

Less commonly, SCD happens in patients who may not have apparent structural heart disease. These conditions are usually inherited arrhythmia syndromes.

Even though many patients have anatomic and functional cardiac substrates that predispose them to develop ventricular arrhythmias, only a small percentage develop SCD. Identifying the patients at risk for SCD remains a challenge. **The strongest known predictor of SCD is significant left ventricular dysfunction of any cause.** The interplay between the regional ischemia, LV dysfunction, and transient inciting events (e.g. worsened ischemia, acidosis, hypoxemia, wall tension, drugs and metabolic disturbances) has been proposed as being the precipitator of sudden death.

## RISK FACTORS OF SCD

Because sudden cardiac arrest is so often linked with coronary artery disease, the same factors that put you at risk of coronary artery disease and of sudden cardiac arrest (Fig. 39.2). These include:

- A family history of coronary artery disease
- Smoking
- High blood pressure
- High blood cholesterol
- Obesity
- Diabetes
- A sedentary lifestyle
- Drinking too much alcohol (more than 1–2 drinks a day)
- Other factors that may increase your risk of sudden cardiac arrest include:
  - A previous episode of cardiac arrest or a family history of cardiac arrest
  - A previous heart attack
  - A personal or family history of other forms of heart disease, such as heart rhythm disorders, congenital heart defects, heart failure and cardiomyopathy
  - Age—the incidence of sudden cardiac arrest increases with age, especially after age 45 for men and age 55 for women
  - Being male—men are 2–3 times more likely to experience sudden cardiac arrest
  - Using illegal drugs, such as cocaine or amphetamines
  - Nutritional imbalance, such as low potassium or magnesium levels.

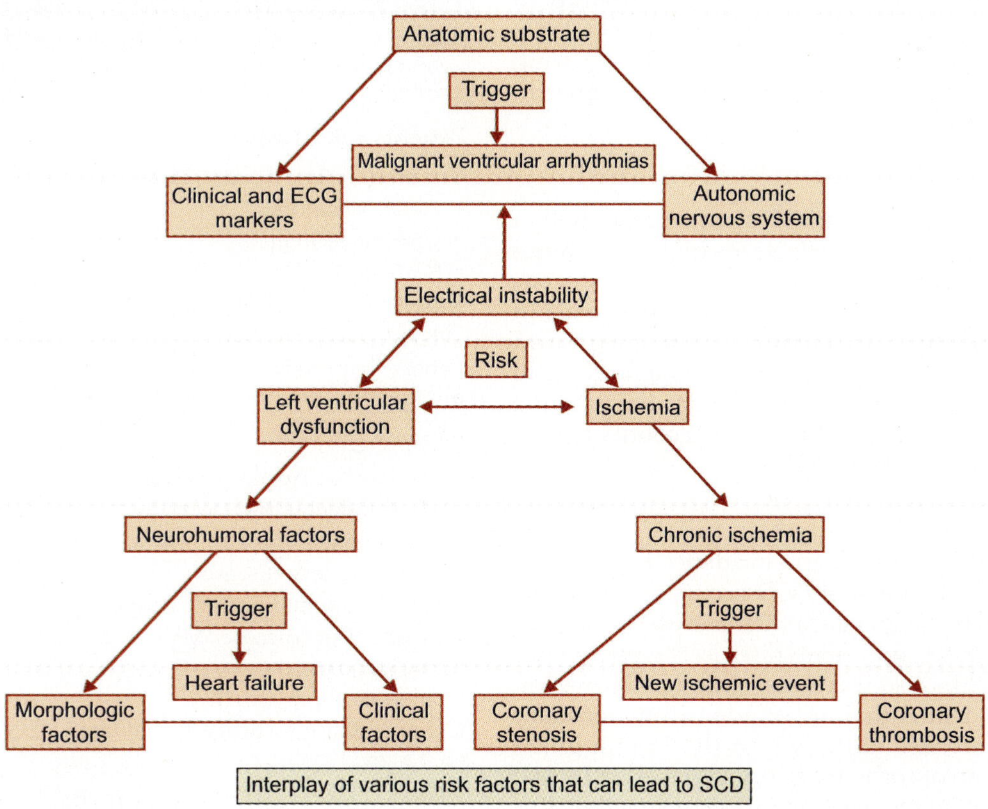


**Fig. 39.2:** Interplay of various risk factors that can lead to sudden cardiac death

## MORTALITY/MORBIDITY

Of more than 300,000 deaths attributed to SCD in the United States each year, a large portion (as many as 40%) are unwitnessed. For most people who experience SCD, their survival depends on the presence of individuals who are competent in performing basic life support, the rapid arrival of personnel and apparatus for defibrillation and advanced life support, and transfer to a hospital. Even under ideal circumstances, only an estimated 20% of patients who have out-of-hospital cardiac arrest survive to hospital discharge. In a study of out-of-hospital cardiac arrest survival in New York City, only 1.4% of patients survived to hospital discharge. Other studies in suburban and rural areas have indicated higher rates of survival (as high as 35%). Placement of automatic external defibrillators throughout communities and training people to use them has the potential to markedly improve outcomes from SCD. Upon emergency department (ED) presentation, the most important determinants of survival include (1) an unsupported systolic blood pressure (SBP) greater than 90 mmHg, (2) a time from loss of consciousness to return of spontaneous circulation (ROSC) of less than 25 minutes, and (3) some degree of neurological responsiveness. A major adverse outcome from a SCD event is anoxic encephalopathy, which occurs in 30–80% of cases.

### Race

Most studies demonstrate inconclusive data with regard to racial differences as they relate to the incidence of sudden death. Some studies suggest that a greater proportion of coronary deaths were 'sudden' in blacks compared to whites. In a report by Gillum et al. on SCD from 1980–1985, the percentage of coronary artery disease deaths occurring out of the hospital and in EDs was found to be higher in blacks than in whites.

### Sex

Men have a higher incidence of SCD than women, with a ratio of 3:1. This ratio generally reflects the higher incidence of obstructive coronary artery disease in men. Recent evidence suggests that a major sex difference may exist in the mechanism of myocardial infarction. Basic and observational data point to the fact that men tend to have coronary plaque rupture, while women tend to have plaque erosion. Whether this biologic difference accounts for the male predominance of SCD is unclear.

### Age

The incidence of SCD parallels the incidence of coronary artery disease, with the peak of SCD occurring in people aged 45–75 years. The incidence of SCD increases with age in men, women, whites, and nonwhites as the prevalence of coronary artery disease increases with age. However, the proportion of deaths that are sudden from coronary artery disease decreases with age. In the Framingham study, the proportion of coronary artery disease deaths that were sudden was 62% in men aged 45–54 years, but this percentage fell to 58% in men aged 55–64 years and to 42% in men aged 65–74 years. According to Kuller et al. 31% of deaths are sudden in people aged 20–29 years.

### History

Obtaining a thorough history from the patient, family members, or other witnesses is necessary to obtain insight into the events surrounding the sudden death. Patients at risk for SCD may have prodromes of chest pain, fatigue, palpitations, and other nonspecific complaints. History and associated symptoms, to some degree depend on the underlying aetiology of SCD. For example, SCD in an elderly patient with significant coronary artery disease may be associated with preceding chest pain due to a myocardial infarction, while SCD in a young patient may be associated with history of prior syncopal episodes and/or a family history of syncope and SCD and due to inherited arrhythmia syndromes. As many as 45% of persons who have SCD were seen by a physician within 4 weeks before death, although as many as 75% of these complaints were not related to the cardiovascular system. A prior history of LV impairment (ejection fraction < 30–35%) is the most potent common risk factor for sudden death. Risk factors that relate to coronary artery disease and subsequent myocardial infarction and ischemic cardiomyopathy also are important and include a family history of premature coronary artery disease, smoking, dyslipidemia, hypertension, diabetes, obesity, and a sedentary lifestyle. Specific considerations include the following (Table 39.1).

**Table 39.1:** Causes of SCD in patients above and below 50 years of age. Approximations with potential bias (data from young patients mainly from US and European registries on SCD in athletes.

| | |
|---|---|
| **Patients = 50 years** | |
| Coronary artery disease, ischemic cardiomyopathy | |
| • Acute ischemia | 75–80% |
| • Chronic ischemia | |
| • Scar-related VT | |
| • Ventricular remodeling | |
| Dilated cardiomyopathy | 15–20% |
| Others (hypertensive heart disease, aortic stenosis, myocarditis, etc. | 5–10% |
| **Patients <50 years** | |
| Hypertrophic cardiomyopathy | 5–30% |
| Arrhythmogenic right ventricular cardiomyopathy | 5–25% |
| Myocarditis | 6–10% |
| Coronary artery disease | 5–20% |
| Coronary anomalies (incl. tunneled LAD) | 2–20% |
| Valvular heart disease (MVP, congenital HD, aortic stenosis, etc.) | 5–10% |
| Dilated cardiomyopathy | 2–4% |
| Channelopathies (Brugada syndrome, LQTS, SQTS, CPVT, etc.) | 3–5% |
| Others | 3–20% |

*Coronary artery disease*
- Previous cardiac arrest
- Syncope
- Prior myocardial infarction, especially within 6 months
- Ejection fraction less than 30–35%
- History of frequent ventricular ectopy (more than 10 PVCs per hour or nonsustained VT).

*Dilated cardiomyopathy*
- Previous cardiac arrest
- Syncope
- Ejection fraction less than 30–35%
- Use of inotropic medications

*Hypertrophic cardiomyopathy*
- Previous cardiac arrest
- Syncope
- Family history of SCD
- Symptoms of heart failure
- Drop in SBP or ventricular ectopy upon stress testing
- Palpitations
- Most are asymptomatic

*Valvular disease*
- Valve replacement within 6 months
- Syncope
- History of frequent ventricular ectopy
- Symptoms associated with severe uncorrected aortic stenosis or mitral stenosis

*Long QT syndrome*
- Family history of long QT and SCD
- Medications that prolong the QT interval
- Bilateral deafness

### Wolff-Parkinson-White (WPW) Syndrome (with Atrial Fibrillation or Atrial Flutter with Extremely Rapid Ventricular Rates)

With extremely rapid conduction over an accessory pathway, degeneration to VF can occur (Fig. 39.3).

*Other*

Brugada syndrome, arrhythmogenic right ventricular (RV) cardiomyopathy/dysplasia, and others.

## PHYSICAL EXAMINATION

The physical examination may reveal evidence of underlying myocardial disease or may be entirely normal, depending on the underlying cause. Initial evaluation studies show that patients who survive to ED presentation can be stratified by a cardiac arrest score, which has excellent diagnostic value. The cardiac arrest score, developed by Thompson and McCullough, can be used for patients with witnessed out-of-hospital cardiac arrest and is defined by the following criteria.

*Clinical characteristic points*
- ED SBP greater than 90 mmHg = 1 point
- ED SBP less than 90 mmHg = 0 points

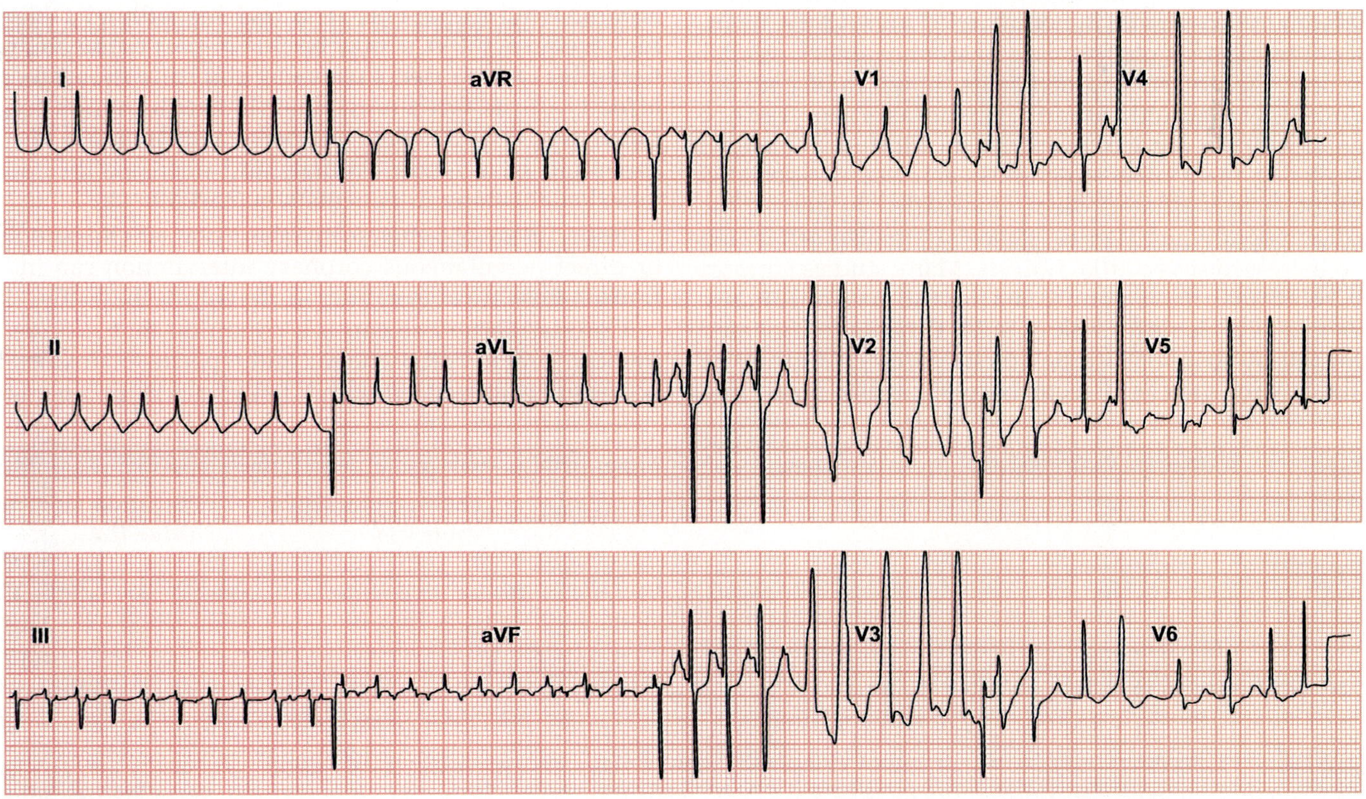


**Fig. 39.3:** Atrial fibrillation with a rapid ventricular response rate during Wolff-Parkinson-White syndrome. Initial atrioventricular reentrant tachycardia

- Time to ROSC less than 25 minutes = 1 point
- Time to ROSC more than 25 minutes = 0 points
- Neurologically responsive = 1 point
- Comatose = 0 point
- Maximum score = 3 points

Patients with a score of 3 points can be expected to have an 89% chance of neurologic recovery and an 82% chance of survival to discharge.

McCullough indicates that even in the setting of ST-elevation and early invasive management with primary angioplasty and intraaortic balloon pump insertion, patients with low cardiac scores are unlikely to survive.

Severe anoxic encephalopathy in patients with scores of 0, 1, or 2 mitigates conservative management with empiric supportive and medical therapy. Given the very poor actuarial survival rates for these patients, invasive management with catheterization and electrophysiology studies (EPS) is rarely justified.

## ETIOLOGICAL FACTORS

### Ischemic Heart Disease

Cardiac arrest due to ventricular arrhythmias may be due to post-MI remodeling of the heart with scar formation and interstitial fibrosis (intramyocardial collagen deposition) or to acute MI/ischemia (Table 39.2). A chronic infarct scar can serve as the focus for re-entrant ventricular tachyarrhythmias. This can occur shortly after the infarct or years later. Interestingly, post-MI remodeling and ischemic cardiomyopathy may be associated with increased interstitial fibrosis even in noninfarcted areas of the heart. Interstitial fibrosis can provide anatomical block similar to a scar. Fibroblasts and myocytes shown to be coupled through gap junctions and fibroblasts can reduce repolarization reserve of myocytes. In addition to post-MI remodeling, many other structural heart diseases associated with SCD (e.g. dilated cardiomyopathy, hypertrophic cardiomyopathy, and aortic stenosis) are also associated with increased myocardial fibrosis. Many studies support the relationship of symptomatic and asymptomatic ischemia as a factor for risk of SCD. Patients resuscitated from out-of-hospital cardiac arrest represent a group of patients with increased recurrence of cardiac arrest and have been shown to express an increased incidence of silent ST-segment depression. Experiments inducing myocardial ischemia in animal models have a strong relationship with the development of VF. However, in patients with prior myocardial infarction and scarring, ventricular arrhythmias, especially VT, do not require an acute ischemic trigger.

In postmortem studies of people who have died from SCD, extensive atherosclerosis is a common pathologic finding. In survivors of cardiac arrest, coronary heart disease with vessels showing greater than 75% stenosis is observed in 40–86% of patients, depending on the age and sex of the population studied. Autopsy studies show similar results; in one study of 169 hearts, approximately 61% of patients died of SCD, and more than 75% stenosis in 3 or 4 vessels and similar severe lesions were present in at least 2 vessels in another 15% of cases. No single coronary artery lesion is associated with an increased risk for SCD. Despite these findings, only approximately 20% of SCD-related autopsies have shown evidence of a recent MI. A greater proportion of autopsies (40–70%) show evidence of a healed MI. Many of these hearts also reveal evidence of plaque fissuring, hemorrhage, and thrombosis.

The Cardiac Surgery Study (CASS) showed that improving or restoring blood flow to an ischemic myocardium decreased the risk of SCD, especially in patients with 3-vessel disease and heart failure, when compared with medical treatment over a 5-year period.

The efficacy of beta-blocking agents, such as propranolol, in decreasing sudden death mortality, especially when administered to patients who had MI with VF, VT, and high-frequency PVCs, may be due in part to the ability of beta-blockers to decrease ischemia, but they are also effective in,ts with nonischemic cardiomyopathy for reduction of SCD. Beta-blockers also increase the VF threshold in ischemic animals and decrease the rate of ventricular ectopy in patients who had MI.

Reperfusion of ischemic myocardium with thrombolysis or direct percutaneous coronary intervention can induce transient electrical instability different mechanisms.

Coronary artery spasm is a condition that exposes the myocardium to both ischemia and reperfusion insults. It is occasionally associated with VT, VF, and SCD. Since some

**Table 39.2:** Combining noninvasive tests for predicting arrhythmic events after myocardial infarction

| | Positive predictive value (%) | Negative predictive value (%) |
|---|---|---|
| VPB on Holter | 5–15 | >90 |
| NSVT on Holter | 20–50 | 72–93 |
| LVEF ≤40% + frequent or complex VPB on Holter | 15–40 | 94–95 |
| LVEF ≤40% + frequent VPB or NSVT on Holter | 15 | 98 |
| QRS duration ≥120 ms + frequent VPB or NSVT on Holter | 24 | 97 |
| LVEF ≤40% + QRS duration ≥120 ms + frequent VPB or NSVT on Holter | 32 | 97 |
| Reduced HRV + frequent or complex VPB on Holter | 34–53 | 77–96 |
| LVEF ≤40% + reduced HRV + frequent VPB on Holter | 50 | |

of the episodes of coronary vasospasm may be silent, this disease should be considered in a patient with unexplained SCA. The exact mechanism of ventricular arrhythmia in coronary vasospasm is not known, but factors associated with both ischemia and reperfusion may contribute in induction of arrhythmia.

Nonatherosclerotic coronary artery abnormalities, including congenital lesions, coronary artery embolism, coronary arteritis, and mechanical abnormalities of the coronary artery, have been associated with an increased incidence of sudden death.

### Nonischemic Cardiomyopathies

Patients with nonischemic cardiomyopathies represent the second largest group of patients who experience SCD in the United States. Nonischemic myopathies, for the purpose of this article, can be divided into the categories dilated and hypertrophic (Table 39.3).

### Dilated Cardiomyopathy

Dilated cardiomyopathy can result from prior ischemia and myocardial infarction or from nonischemic causes (Fig. 39.4). Nonischemic dilated cardiomyopathy (DCM) is becoming increasingly more common, with an incidence of approximately 7.5 cases per 100,000 persons each year. Of cases of SCD, 10% are estimated to be attributable to DCM. The prognosis is very poor for these patients, with a 1-year mortality rate of 10–50%, depending on the New York Heart Association functional class; approximately 30–50% of these deaths are SCD.

The causes of DCM are uncertain; viral, autoimmune, genetic, and environmental (alcohol) origins are implicated. The predominant mechanism of death appears to be ventricular tachyarrhythmia, although bradyarrhythmia and electromechanical dissociation also have been observed, especially in patients with advanced LV dysfunction. Extensive fibrosis of the subendocardium, leading to dilated ventricles and subsequent generation of re-entrant tachyarrhythmias, is a proposed factor in mechanism of sudden death. Multiple factors have been shown to contribute to increased risk for SCD in this population. The most important hemodynamic predictor is an increase in end-diastolic pressure and subsequent wall tension. Other important factors are increased sympathetic tone, neurohumoral activation, and electrolyte abnormalities.

Many drugs used in the treatment of heart failure, such as antiarrhythmics, inotropic agents, and diuretics, have direct or indirect (e.g. through electrolyte abnormalities) proarrhythmic properties, which may provoke arrhythmias in some cases. Potassium-sparing diuretics may be helpful in decreasing SCD.

Nonsustained ventricular tachycardia (NSVT) is common in patients with dilated cardiomyopathy and approximately 80% of persons with DCM have abnor-

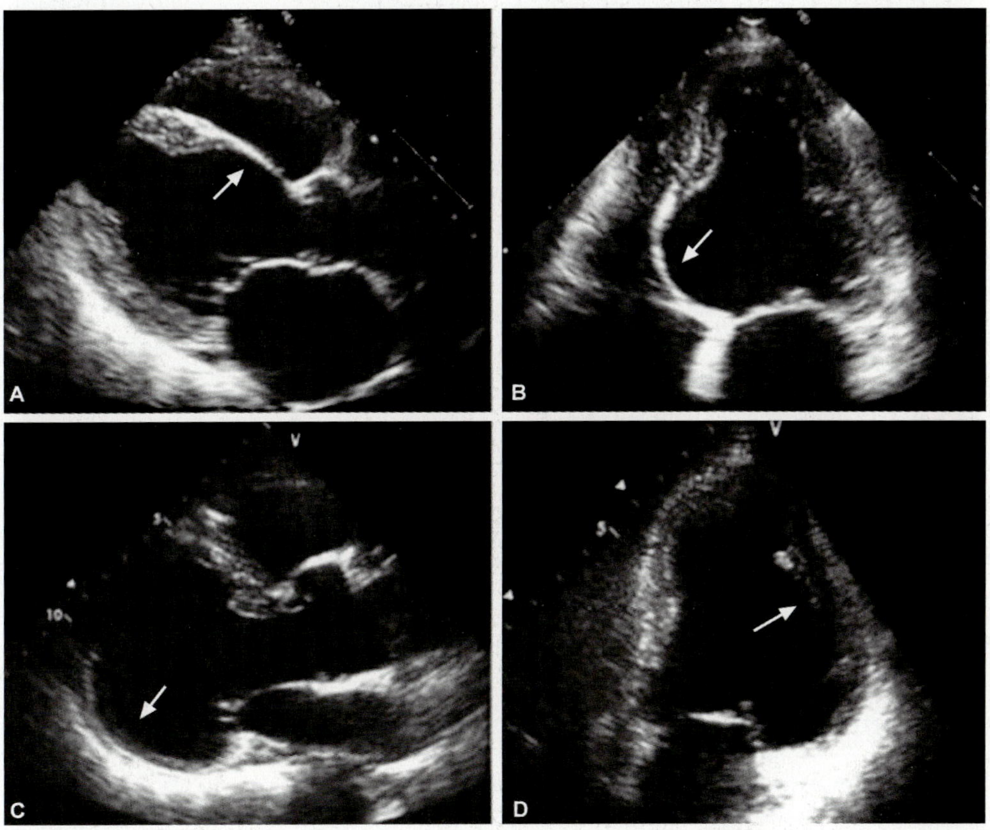

**Fig. 39.4:** 2-D echocardiographic images suggestive of dilated cardiomyopathy characterized by thinning and akinesia of the basal septum (A and B). Aneurysmal dilatation involving inferior or posterolateral wall (C and D)

**Table 39.3:** Risk stratification techniques, clinical considerations and markers for SCD in patients with idiopathic dilated, hypertrophic and arrhythmogenic right ventricular cardiomyopathies

| Disease entity | Features |
|---|---|
| Idiopathic dilated cardiomyopathy | 1. Clinical characteristics<br>a. Prior cardiac arrest<br>b. Family history of SCD<br>c. Unexplained syncope<br>d. Holter/event monitor: Spontaneous NSVT/VT<br>e. Stress testing/6 min walk: Poor functional capacity, abnormal heart rate recovery<br>f. Comorbid conditions<br>2. Myocardial substrate abnormalities/Noninvasive imaging<br>a. Sinus rhythm ECG: Prolonged QRS duration, QRS notching/fragmentation, epsilon-equivalents<br>b. Abnormal SAECG<br>c. TTE: Reduced LVEF, increased LV end-diastolic diameter, ventricular dyssynchrony<br>d. CMRI—delayed gadolinium enhancement<br>e. EP study—inducible ventricular arrhythmias; extensive low voltage/abnormal signals on electroanatomic mapping (apical extension); large midepicardial scar burden, multiple VT morphologies, hemodynamically intolerable VT, recurrent VT at post-ablation noninvasive programmed stimulation<br>3. Repolarization abnormalities<br>a. Abnormal QT interval/QT dispersion<br>b. T-wave alternans<br>c. Early repolarization<br>4. Autonomic dysfunction<br>a. Reduced short and long-term heart rate variability<br>b. Increased HR 'turbulence'<br>c. Barorecepor hypersensitivity |
| Hypertrophic cardiomyopathy | 1. Clinical characteristics<br>a. Prior cardiac arrest<br>b. Family history of SCD<br>c. Holter/event monitor: Spontaneous VT, high NSVT burden<br>d. Unexplained syncope<br>e. Stress testing: Hyotensive blood pressure response<br>2. Myocardial substrate abnormalities/Noninvasive imaging<br>a. TTE: severe LVH (septal wall thickness >3 mm); large LV outflow tract dynamic gradient; apical variant<br>b. CMRI: Delayed gadolinium enhancement<br>c. EP Study: High DFTs, inducible ventricular arrhythmias; extensive low voltage/abnormal signals on electroanatomic mapping; large midepicardial scar burden, maltiple VT morphologies, hemodynamically intolerable VT<br>3. Genotype: Unfavorable genotype/multiple concomitant mutations |
| Arrhythmogenic right ventricular cardiomyopathy | 1. Clinical characteristic<br>a. Unexplained syncope<br>b. ≥1 family member with SCD<br>c. Spontaneous NSVT/VT (typically LBBB morphology and superior axis<br>d. RBBB morphology VT suggestive of LV involvement<br>2. Myocardial substrate abnormalities/Noninvasive imaging<br>a. ECG: Precordial T-wave inversions, epsilon waves, delayed terminal QRS activation (parietal block)<br>b. TTE: Extensive regional RV akinesia, dyskinesia or aneurysms; dilated right ventricular outflow tract<br>c. CMRI: Reduced RVEF, extensive regional RV akinesia, dyskinesia; microaneurysms, dyssynchronous RV contraction, incareased RVEDV/BSA ratio<br>d. EP study: Extensive areas of low voltage, biventricular involvement, inducible ventricular arrhythmias; extensive low voltage/abnormal signals on electroanatomic mapping; large mid-epicardial scar burden, multiple VT morphologies, hemodynamically intolerable VT<br>3. Genotype: Pathogenic desmosomal mutations |

SCD=sudden cardiac death; NSVT=nonsustained ventricular tachycardia; VT=ventricular tachycardia; ECG=electrocardiogram; SAECG=signal-averaged electrocardiogram; TTE=transthoracic echocardiogram; LV=left ventricle; LVEF=left ventricular ejection fraction; CMRI=cardiac magnetic resonance imaging; EP=electrophysiologic; LVH=left ventricular hypertrophy; DFT=defibrillation threshold; RV=right ventricle; RVEF=right ventricular ejection fraction; RVEDV/BSA=right ventricular end-diastolic volume to body surface area ratio; L/RBBB=left or right bundle branch block.

malities on Holter monitoring. Although NSVT may be a marker, it has not been shown to be a reliable predictor of SCD in these patients. Recent studies have shown possibility of increased mortality following suppression of NSVT by antiarrhythmic medications due to proarrhythmic properties of these medications and involvement of several other factors in generation of VT and VF. Given the possibility of sustained VT being the underlying cause, a history of syncope should be aggressively pursued. Unexplained syncope, especially in patients with class 3 or 4 heart failure, has been shown to be a predictor of SCD in most patients with cardiomyopathy.

### Hypertrophic Cardiomyopathy

Hypertrophic cardiomyopathy (HCM) is an autosomal-dominant, incompletely penetrant genetic disorder resulting from a mutation in one of the many (>45) genes encoding proteins of the cardiac muscle sarcomere (Fig. 39.5). Among the genetic abnormalities described, mutations in the genes coding for the beta-myosin heavy chains, and cardiac troponin T make up most cases. Other mutations may include alpha-myosin heavy chain *MYH6*), cardiac troponin C (*TNNC1*), alpha-tropomyosin (*TPM1*), myosin binding protein-C (*MYBPC3*), cardiac troponin (*TNNI3*), essential and regulatory light-chain genes (*MYL3* and *MYL2*, respectively), cardiac alpha-actin gene (*ACTC*), and titin (*TTN*). The incidence of SCD in this population is 2–4% per year in adults and 4–6% per year in children and adolescents. HCM is the most common cause of SCD in people younger than 30 years.

The vast majority of young people who die of HCM are previously asymptomatic. The patients may experience SCD while at rest or with mild exertional activity; however, in a significant portion of these patients, the SCD event occurs after vigorous exertion. HCM is the single greatest cause of SCD in young athletes and, hence, is the major entity for which to screen during the physical examination of an athlete.

The mechanism of SCD in HCM is not entirely understood. Initially, it was thought to be due to obstruction of the outflow tract because of catecholamine stimulation. However, later studies suggested that individuals with nonobstructive HCM are at high risk for SCD as well, primarily related to VT or VF. The mechanism of arrhythmia in this setting is not clear, and hypertrophy may be a part of cardiac remodeling in these patients that provides the substrate for lethal arrhythmia.

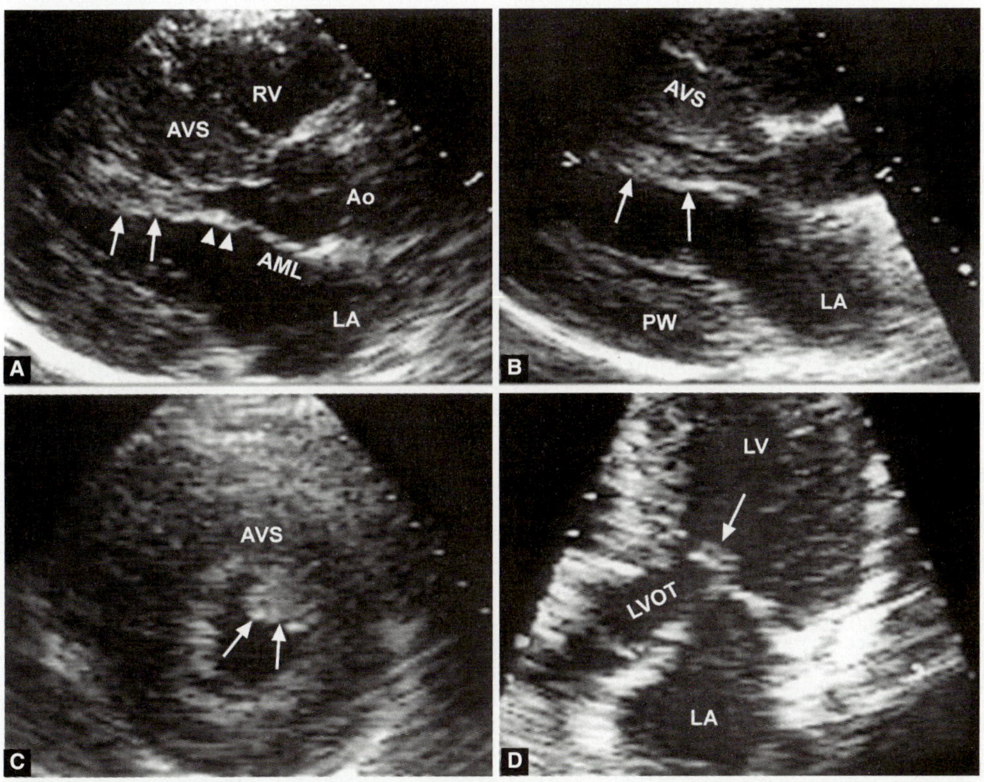


**Fig. 39.5:** Two-dimensional echocardiographic stop-frame images from patient demonstrating spectrum of morphological and functional abnormalities. (A) Rotated parasternal long-axis view in systole showing direct anatomic continuity between hypertrophied anterolateral papillary muscle (arrows) and anterior mitral leaflet (AML; arrowheads), and midcavitary muscular apposition between papillary muscle and anterior ventricular septum (AVS). (B) Long axis with further rotation showing length of midcavity apposition between papillary muscle (arrows) and AVS. (C) Parasternal short-axis view showing exaggerated anterior position of anterolateral papillary muscle (arrows). (D) Apical view showing SAM and sharp angulated bend of both mitral leaflets (arrow) (without septal contact) created by a portion of mitral valve unencumbered by direct papillary muscle insertion. (Ao=aorta; LA=left atrium; LVOT=left ventricular outflow tract; LV=left ventricle; PW=posterior wall; RV=right ventricle)

Rapid or polymorphic symptomatic NSVT may have better predictive value compared with asymptomatic and monomorphic NSVT. Other clinical markers that may have predictive value for SCD in patients with HCM are young age at onset, thickness of the septum, and family history of SCD.

### Arrhythmogenic Right Ventricular Cardiomyopathy

Arrhythmogenic RV cardiomyopathy is characterized by replacement of the RV wall with fibrofatty tissue. Involvement of the interventricular septum and left ventricle is associated with poorer outcomes.

About 30–50 of cases occur as a phenotypically apparent familial disorder. Several genetic defects, including mutations in the desmoplakin domain locus on chromosome 6 and the ryanodine receptor locus on chromosome 1 (although this has been debated), have been correlated with SCD. Again, interstitial fibrosis plays an important role in ventricular arrhythmia in this condition. Autosomal dominant inheritance is common, but autosomal recessive transmission has been reported for select mutations. The autosomal recessive form, Naxos disease (named after the Greek Island), has been reported in a geographically isolated area mainly in Mediterranean countries and is usually associated with wooly hair and palmoplantar keratoderma or similar skin disorder. This disorder is associated with mutation in the gene for plakoglobin, a protein involved in cellular adhesion, found on chromosome 17p.

Arrhythmogenic RV dysplasia affects men more often than women. The annual incidence rate of SCD in this population is approximately 2%. Patients may present with signs and symptoms of RV hypertrophy and dilation, often with sustained monomorphic or polymorphic VT of a left bundle-branch block morphology with an axis usually between negative 90–100°.

Atrial arrhythmias may be present in as many as 25% of patients. Syncope and sudden death often are associated with exercise. In many patients, sudden death is the first manifestation of the disease. Clinicians should be alerted to the epsilon wave finding on ECG studies (see the image below). The epsilon wave can be present in as many as 23% of patients after the first VT event. The percentage of patients with the epsilon wave finding on ECG increases to 27% and 34% at 5 and 10 years, respectively, after the first VT event.

Uhl anomaly is a condition in which the RV wall is extremely thin secondary to apposition of endocardial and epicardial layers.

### Valvular Disease

Prior to the advent of surgical therapy for valvular heart disease, SCD was fairly common in patients with progressive aortic stenosis (Figs 39.6 and 39.7). Most aortic stenosis deaths were sudden. In a study by Chizner et al. of 42 patients who had isolated aortic stenosis and did not undergo valve replacement, as many as 56% of deaths were sudden at 5 years of follow-up. Of these 42 patients, 32 were symptomatic and 10 were asymptomatic. The mechanism of sudden death is unclear, and both malignant ventricular arrhythmia and bradyarrhythmia have been documented.

The incidence of SCD has decreased significantly with advent of aortic valve replacement. However, it still accounts for the second most common cause of death postoperatively in this population and especially in those with prosthetic and heterograft aortic valve replacement. The incidence of SCD after aortic valve surgery is highest in the first 3 weeks after the procedure and then plateaus at 6 months of follow-up.

### Other Valvular Lesions

The risk of SCD is much lower in other valvular diseases compared with aortic stenosis.

Aortic insufficiency usually presents with signs of heart failure and progressive LV dilatation. As part of this

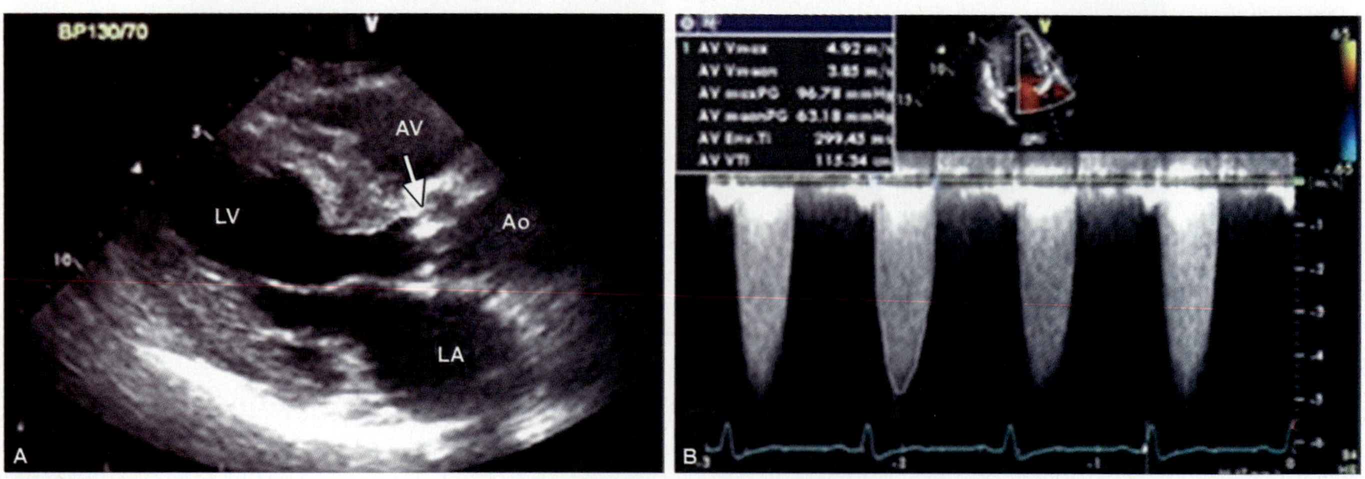


**Fig. 39.6:** Transthoracic echocardiography before the transcatheter aortic valve implantation. (A) Parasternal long axis view shows heavily calcified stenotic aortic valve. (B) Pressure gradient over aortic valve by Doppler (maximal pressure gradient 97 mmHg, mean pressure gradient 63 mmHg). (AV=aortic valve, Ao=aorta, LV=left ventricle, LA=left atrium)

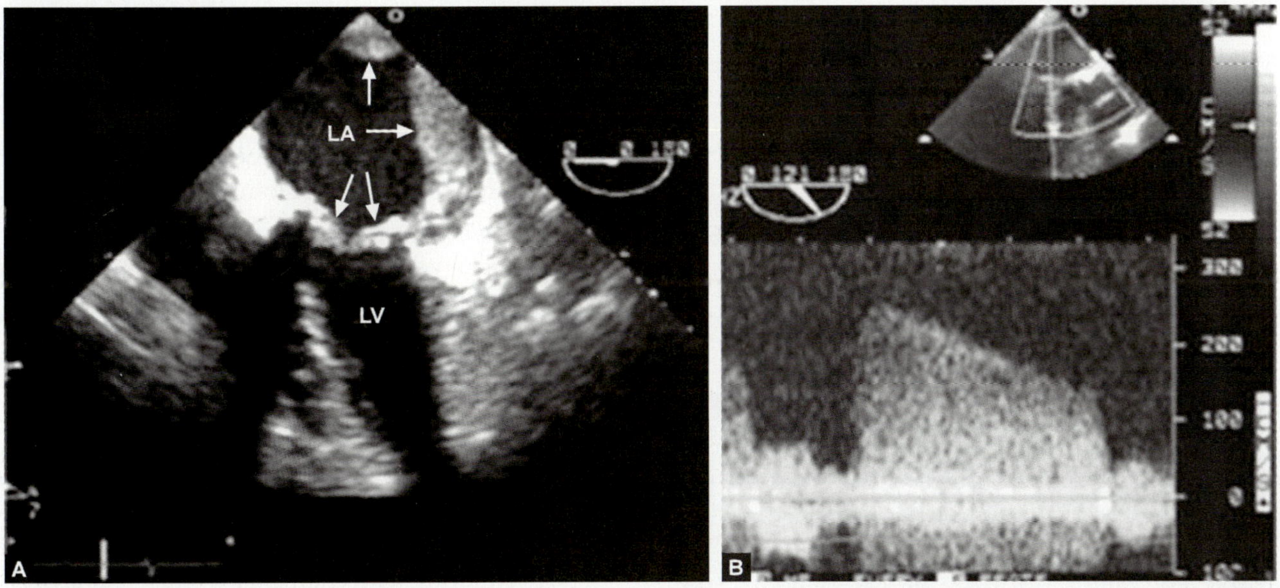


**Fig. 39.7:** TEE performed on the 15th postoperative day. (A) Midesophageal transverse view in diastole showing diffuse thrombosis of the bioprosthetic mitral valve leaflets (arrows) causing severe leaflet restriction and stenosis. Large immobile thrombi are adherent to the left atrial (LA) wall (double arrows). (B) Transmitral continuous-wave Doppler showing severe mitral stenosis. Estimated mitral valve area using the pressure half time formula is 0.6 $cm^2$, and the mean transvalvular gradient is 14 mmHg. LV indicates left ventricle

process, re-entrant or automatic ventricular foci may develop and ultimately lead to a symptomatic ventricular arrhythmia. After valve replacement, LV wall tension can be expected to reduce and the risk of arrhythmia can be expected to decrease.

**Mitral stenosis** is becoming increasingly uncommon in the United States because of widespread use of antibiotics in primary streptococcal infections. SCD due to mitral stenosis is very rare.

The incidence of SCD is low in patients with mitral valve prolapse (MVP). MVP has a 5–7% incidence in the general population. In clinically significant MVP, the risk of SCD seems to rise along with total mortality. Kligfield et al. estimated that the incidence of sudden death varies with the presence of symptoms and the severity of mitral regurgitation. Ventricular tachyarrhythmias are the most frequent arrhythmia in patients with SCD. Risk factors for SCD to consider in these patients include a family history of SCD, echocardiographic evidence of a redundant mitral valve, repolarization abnormalities, and lengthening of the corrected QT interval (>420 ms in women and >450 ms in men).

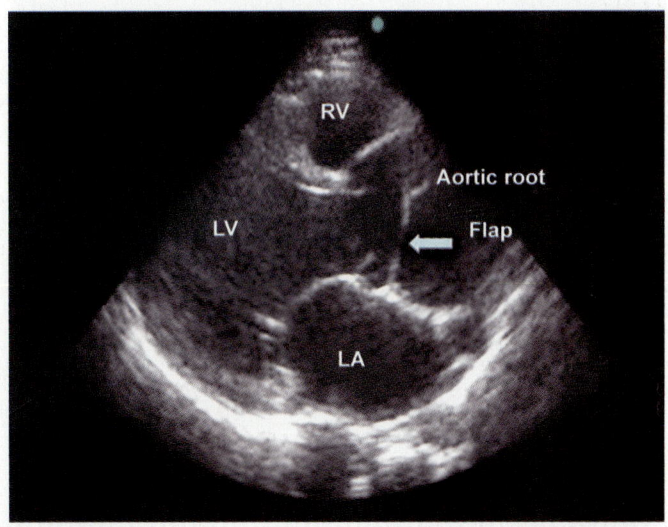


**Fig. 39.8:** Two-dimensional echocardiogram from a patient. Left parasternal long axis in systole shows the intimal dissection flap and severe aortic regurgitation. LV=left ventricle; LA=left atrium; RV=right ventricle

## Congenital Heart Disease

In the pediatric and adolescent age groups, SCD occurs with an incidence of 1.3–8.5 cases per 100,000 patients annually, accounting for approximately 5% of all deaths in this group (Fig. 39.8). The causes of SCD are much more diverse in children than adults. In reviewing 13 studies involving 61 children and adolescents with SCD, Driscoll found 50% of cases were due to HCM; 25% were due to anomalous origin of the left coronary artery; and the remaining patients had aortic stenosis, cystic medial necrosis, and sinus node artery obstruction. The following is a classification of SCD in the pediatric population.

In patients with known, previously recognized (including repaired) congenital heart disease, abnormalities associated with SCD include the following:

- Tetralogy of Fallot
- Transposition of the great arteries
- Fontan operation
- Aortic stenosis
- Marfan syndrome

**Mitral Valve Prolapse** (Figs 39.9–39.12)

- Hypoplastic left heart syndrome
- Eisenmenger syndrome
- Congenital heart block
- Ebstein anomaly

In patients with known, previously recognized (including repaired) heart disease, acquired causes of SCD include the following:

- Kawasaki syndrome
- DCM or myocarditis

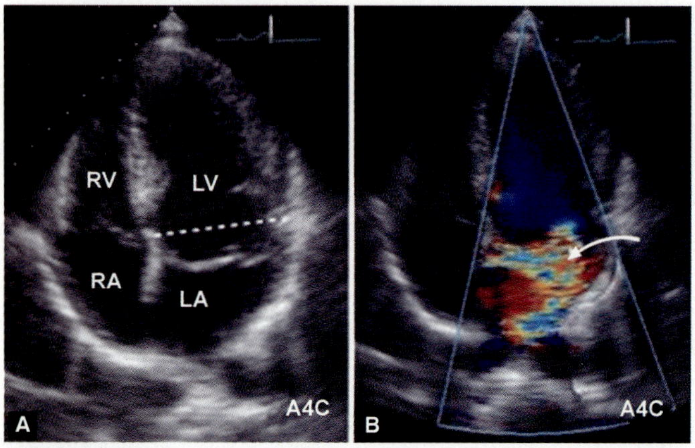


**Fig. 39.9:** Bileaflet prolapse is easily visualized in the apical four-chamber (A4C) view (A). Severe mitral regurgitation was present (B)

In patients with previously unrecognized heart disease who have structural heart disease, causes of SCD include the following:

- HCM
- Congenital coronary artery abnormalities
- Arrhythmogenic RV cardiomyopathy.

In patients with previously unrecognized heart disease who do not have structural heart disease, causes of SCD include the following:

- Long QT syndrome
- Primary ventricular tachycardia and ventricular fibrillation
- Primary pulmonary hypertension
- Commotio cordis—traumatic blow to the chest wall (e.g. from a hockey puck or baseball) causing VT/VF and SCD in the absence of significant identifiable trauma.

The predominant mechanism is ventricular arrhythmias. In tetralogy of Fallot after postoperative correction of the anomaly, as many as 10% of these patients have VT and the incidence of sudden death is 2–3%. In the Fontan procedure, i.e. to correct a physiologic single ventricle, even atrial arrhythmias can cause severe hemodynamic compromise and arrhythmic death. Patients who develop secondary pulmonary hypertension (Eisenmenger syndrome), despite attempted correction of the anatomic defects, have a very poor prognosis. The terminal event may be bradycardia or VT progressing to VF.

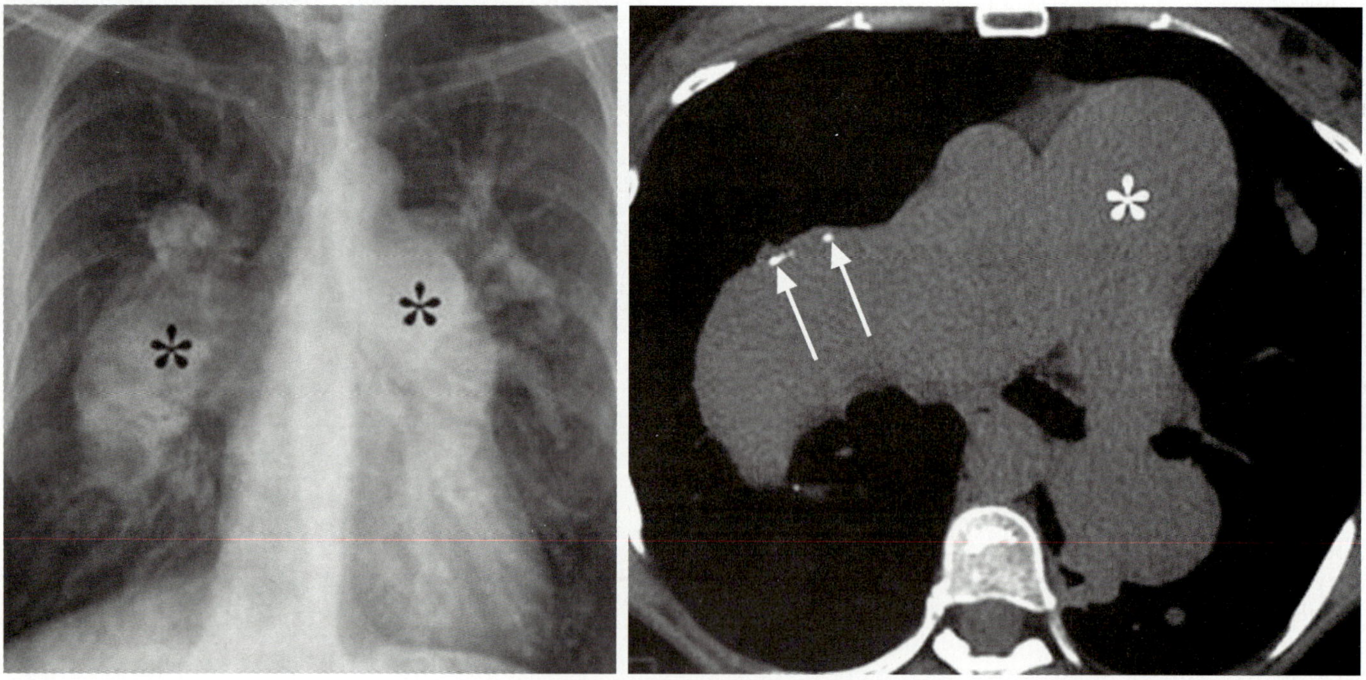

**Fig. 39.10:** A woman with pulmonary hypertension secondary to an uncorrected ostium secundum atrial septal defect (Eisenmenger syndrome) of several years evolution. The chest radiograph shows marked dilatation of the pulmonary arteries (black asterisks). Unenhanced MSCT depicts marked dilatation of the pulmonary arteries (white asterisk), and calcifications in the pulmonary artery trunk and right main pulmonary artery (black arrows) due to chronic pulmonary artery hypertension. The patient was treated with bilateral lung transplantation and surgical closure of the atrial septal defect in the same procedure

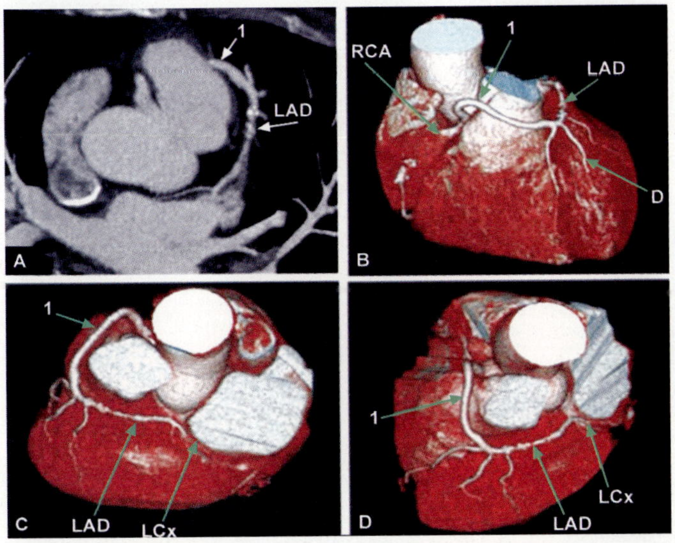


**Fig. 39.11:** (A to D) Maximum intensity projection and volume rendering reconstructions of a case of absent left main coronary artery, a large anomalous arterial structure (1) with preinfundibular course supplies both LADs, LCx and their branches. RCA is occluded. (D) Diagonal artery (LAD=left anterior descending; LCx=left circumflex; RCA=right coronary artery

## Primary Electrophysiologic Abnormalities

This generally represents a group of abnormalities in which patients have no apparent structural heart disease but have a primary electrophysiologic abnormality that predisposes them to VT or VF. Some imaging techniques have detected abnormal sympathetic neural function in these patients. An ECG study can provide clues to the diagnosis; consider a familial component to these conditions. Normal early repolarization may be associated with increased SCD, though this often represents a benign finding. Results from the cardiac arrest survivors with preserved ejection fraction registry (CASPER) suggest early repolarization is present in a significant proportion of causally diagnosed and idiopathic VF.

## Long QT Syndrome

Idiopathic long QT syndrome, in which patients have a prolonged QT with a propensity to develop malignant ventricular arrhythmias, is a rare familial disorder (Figs 39.13 and 39.14).

Two inheritance patterns of congenital long QT syndrome have been described. The Jervell-Lange-Nielsen syndrome, associated with congenital deafness, has an autosomal-recessive pattern of inheritance. The Romano-Ward syndrome is not associated with deafness and has an autosomal dominant pattern of inheritance with variable penetration. This syndrome accounts for 90% of long QT syndrome cases. More than 200 mutations in the 10 or more genes related to long QT syndrome have been found. Among the most common are mutations of *SCN5A* on chromosome 3, the *HERG* gene on chromosome 7, and the *KVLTQT1* gene on chromosome 11.

Alteration in the function of a myocellular channel protein that regulates the potassium flux during electrical repolarization is thought to be causative, though in some subsets of long QT syndrome, such as those with mutations in *SCN5A* (long QT3), Na channels are primarily impaired. A relationship with sympathetic nervous system imbalance also appears to exist. The prolongation that occurs makes these patients susceptible to develop a specific form of VT called torsade de pointes.

The clinical course of patients with long QT syndrome is quite variable, with some patients remaining asymptomatic while others develop torsade de pointes with syncope and sudden death. Symptoms and SCD are more common among homozygous individuals (those with two copies of the mutant allele), compared with heterozygous individuals (who have a single mutant allele). The risk of SCD is impacted by environmental factors such as hypokalemia, medications and the presence of sinus pauses. SCD in these patients also has been associated with emotional extremes, auditory auras or stimulation, and vigorous physical activity. Symptoms usually begin in childhood or adolescence.

The probability that a specific patient has congenital long QT syndrome is divided to low, intermediate, and high probability based on the following criteria—(1) ECG criteria including long QT, torsade de pointes, notched T-wave, T-wave alternans, bradycardia for age; (2) clinical criteria including syncope with or without stress, deafness; and (3) family history of long QT syndrome or SCD.

When measuring QTc, selecting rhythm strips that have minimal variability of RR intervals and a stable heart rate is important.

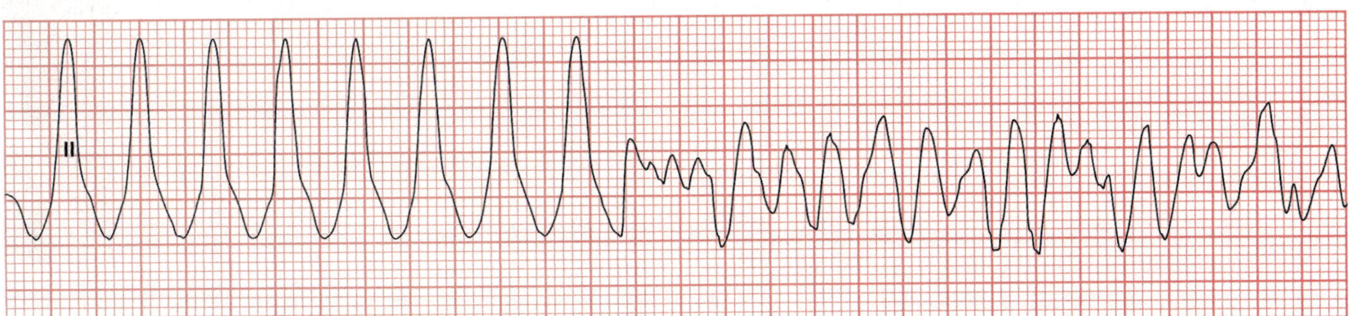


**Fig. 39.12:** Monomorphic ventricular tachycardia changing to ventricular fibrillation. The rhythm is irregular because of the transition from ventricular tachycardia to ventricular fibrillation. The monomorphic ventricular tachycardia has a rate of 187/min. This degenerates into a coarse ventricular fibrillation

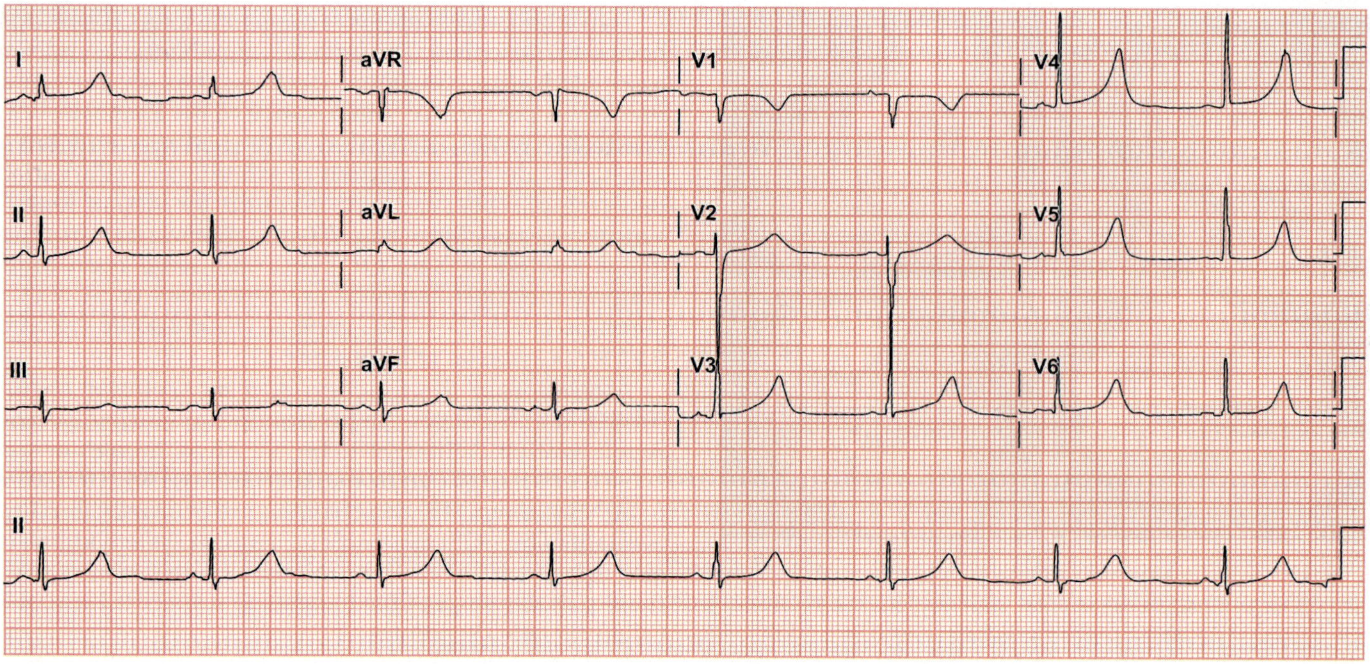


**Fig. 39.13:** ECG findings in type 1 long QT syndrome

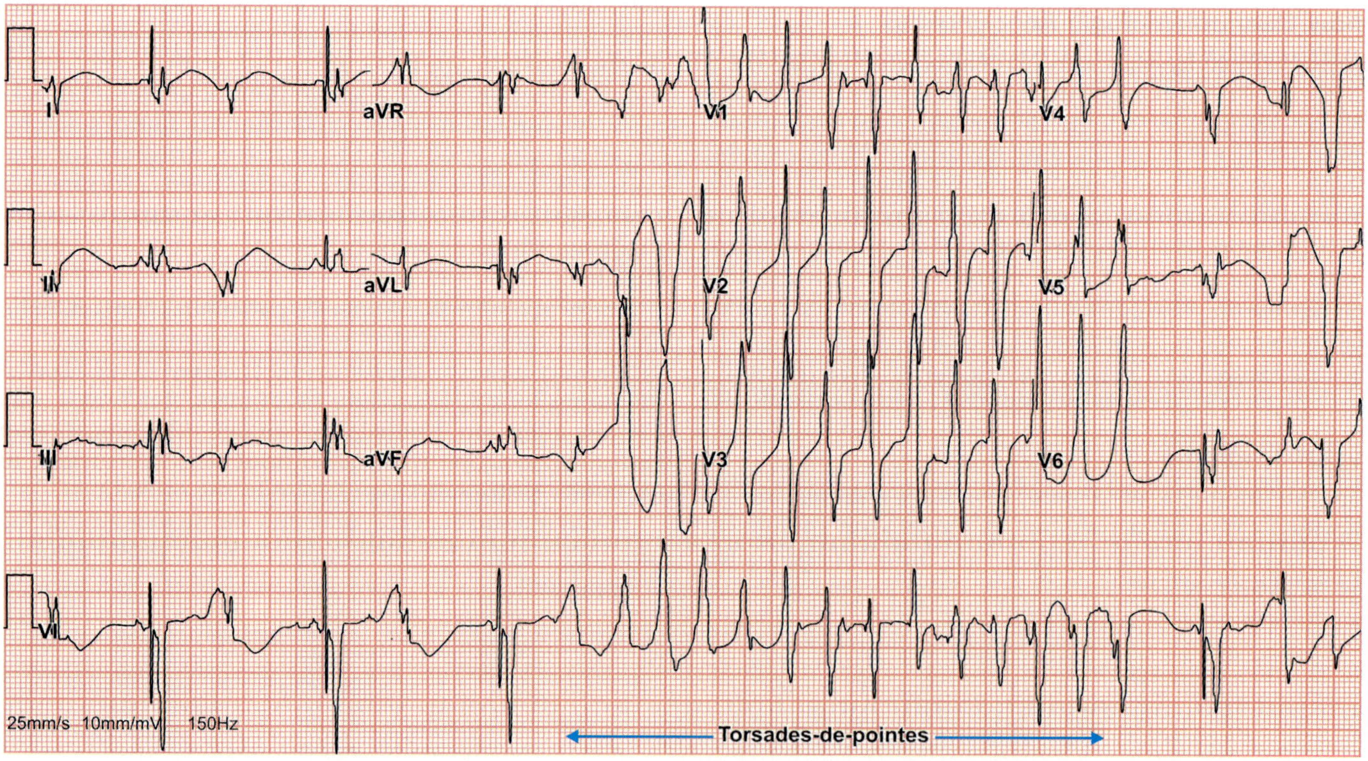


**Fig. 39.14:** ECG showing long QT syndrome with torsades de pointes

Treatment for long QT syndrome includes beta-blockers and often pacemaker or ICD implantation. Beta-blockers decrease the overall mortality in patients with long QT syndrome. However, they do not eliminate the risk of syncope, cardiac arrest, and SCD completely. They are not effective in patients with mutation in Na channel genes (long QT3). Torsade de pointes in patients with long QT syndrome is associated with bradycardia and pauses. Therefore, a pacemaker can prevent torsade de pointes in these patients by preventing bradycardia. ICD therapy may be indicated in patients with recurrent symptoms despite treatment with beta-blockers.

### Acquired Long QT Syndrome

A number of antiarrhythmics (especially class Ia and class III) and other medications, electrolyte abnormalities, cerebrovascular diseases, and altered nutritional states are known to cause QT prolongation and put patients at risk for torsade de pointes. This usually occurs when QT prolongation is associated with a slow heart rate and hypokalemia.

The QT interval is prolonged in as many as 32% of patients with intracranial hemorrhage (especially in subarachnoid hemorrhages). Lesions in the hypothalamus are thought to lead to this phenomenon.

Reports of sudden death due to ventricular arrhythmia in patients with hypocalcemia, hypothyroidism, nutritional deficiencies associated with modified starvation diets, and in patients who are obese and on severe weight-loss programs have been reported.

Class Ia antiarrhythmic drugs that cause acquired long QT syndrome include quinidine, disopyramide, and procainamide. Class III antiarrhythmic drugs that cause acquired long QT syndrome include sotalol, *N*-acetyl procainamide, bretylium, amiodarone, and ibutilide.

Other drugs that cause acquired long QT syndrome include bepridil, probucol, tricyclic and tetracyclic antidepressants, phenothiazines, Haldol, antihistamines (e.g. terfenadine, astemizole), antibiotics (e.g. erythromycin, sulfamethoxazole/trimethoprim), chemotherapeutics (e.g. pentamidine, anthracycline), serotonin antagonists (e.g. ketanserin, zimeldine), and organophosphorus insecticides. Electrolyte abnormalities that cause acquired long QT syndrome include hypokalemia, hypomagnesemia, and hypocalcemia.

Altered nutritional states and cerebrovascular disease that cause acquired long QT syndrome include intracranial and subarachnoid hemorrhages, stroke, and intracranial trauma.

Hypothyroidism and altered autonomic status (e.g. diabetic neuropathy) can cause acquired long QT syndrome.

Hypothermia can cause acquired QT prolongation. The ECG will typically also demonstrate an Osborn wave, a distinct bulging of the J point at the beginning of the ST-segment. This ECG finding resolves upon warming.

### Short QT Syndrome

The short QT syndrome is a newly recognized syndrome, first time described in 2000, which can lead to lethal arrhythmias and SCD (Figs 39.15 and 39.16). Three mutations in potassium channels have been described that lead to gain of function in potassium channels and shortening of action potential and decreased QT interval.

To diagnose short QT syndrome, the QTc should be less than 330 msec and tall and peaked T-waves should be present. Clinical manifestations are variable from no symptoms, to palpitations due to atrial fibrillation, syncope due to VT, and SCD. VF is easily inducible at electrophysiology study in these patients, and SCD can happen at any age.

A study by Gollob et al. proposes diagnostic criteria that include QTc interval, J point-to-T peak interval, clinical history [e.g. SCA, atrial fibrillation (AF), syncope], family history and genotyping.

Although antiarrhythmic medications, such as sotalol, ibutilide, and procainamide, have been proposed as a therapy (to prolong the QT), data to support this approach

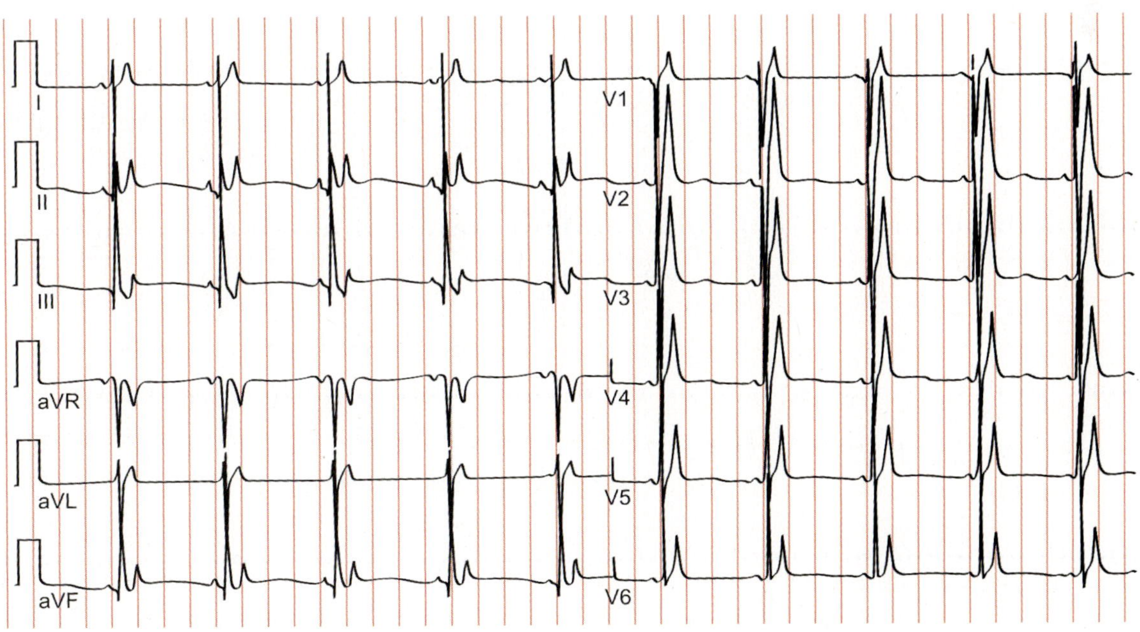


**Fig. 39.15:** ECG showing short QT interval. Lack of the normal changes in QT interval with heart rate. Peaked T-waves, particularly in the precordial leads. QT <320 ms and a QTc <340 ms with no evidence of structural heart disease

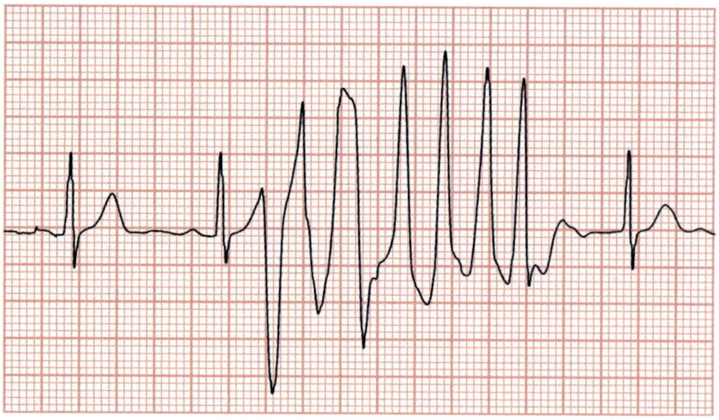

**Fig. 39.16:** Self-terminating episode of polymorphic VT in a patient with SQTS–lead $V_3$. The episode is precipitated by an extrasystole with a very short coupling interval

are insufficient at present. ICD placement may be considered to prevent VT and SCD, although T-wave oversensing, resulting in inappropriate ICD discharges, has been problematic.

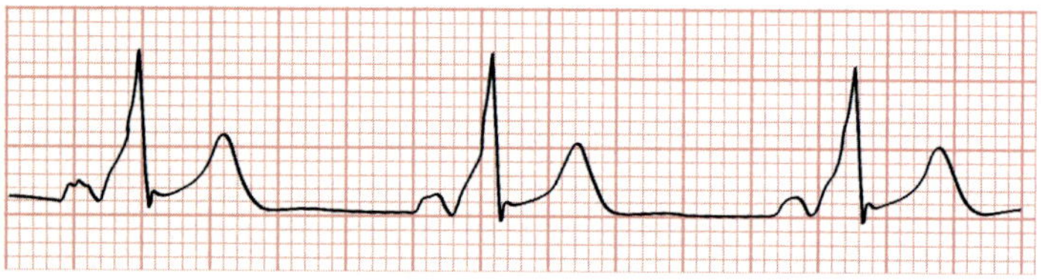

**Fig. 39.17:** ECG findings in the Wolff-Parkinson-White syndrome are short PR interval (<120 ms), broad QRS (>100 ms), and a slurred upstroke to the QRS complex (the delta wave)

Because no long-term outcome data are available, Giustetto et al. investigated the clinical characteristics and the long-term course of a large cohort of patients with short QT syndrome (defined as QT of ≤ 360 ms). Their findings suggest short QT syndrome carries a high risk of sudden death in all age groups, with the highest risk in symptomatic patients. Hydroquinidine therapy appeared to reduce the antiarrhythmic event rate from 4.9% to 0%. However, this was a small registry studying a rare disease; thus, the true benefit is unclear.

### Wolff-Parkinson-White Syndrome

WPW syndrome is a recognized but rare cause of sudden death (Figs 39.17 and 39.18). The existence of an atrioventricular accessory pathway in this syndrome results in ventricular preexcitation, which appears with short PR interval, wide QRS complex, and delta wave on ECG. The refractory period in the anterograde direction of accessory pathway determines the ventricular rate in the setting of atrial fibrillation and WPW. Most patients with WPW syndrome and SCD develop atrial fibrillation with a rapid ventricular response over the accessory pathway, which induces VF. In a study by Klein et al of 31 patients with VF and WPW syndrome, a history of atrial fibrillation or reciprocating tachycardia was an important predisposing factor. The presence of multiple accessory pathways, posteroseptal accessory pathways, and a pre-excited R–R interval of less than 220 ms during atrial fibrillation are associated with higher risk for SCD.

Symptomatic patients should be treated by antiarrhythmic medications (e.g. procainamide), catheter ablation of the accessory pathway, or electrical cardio-

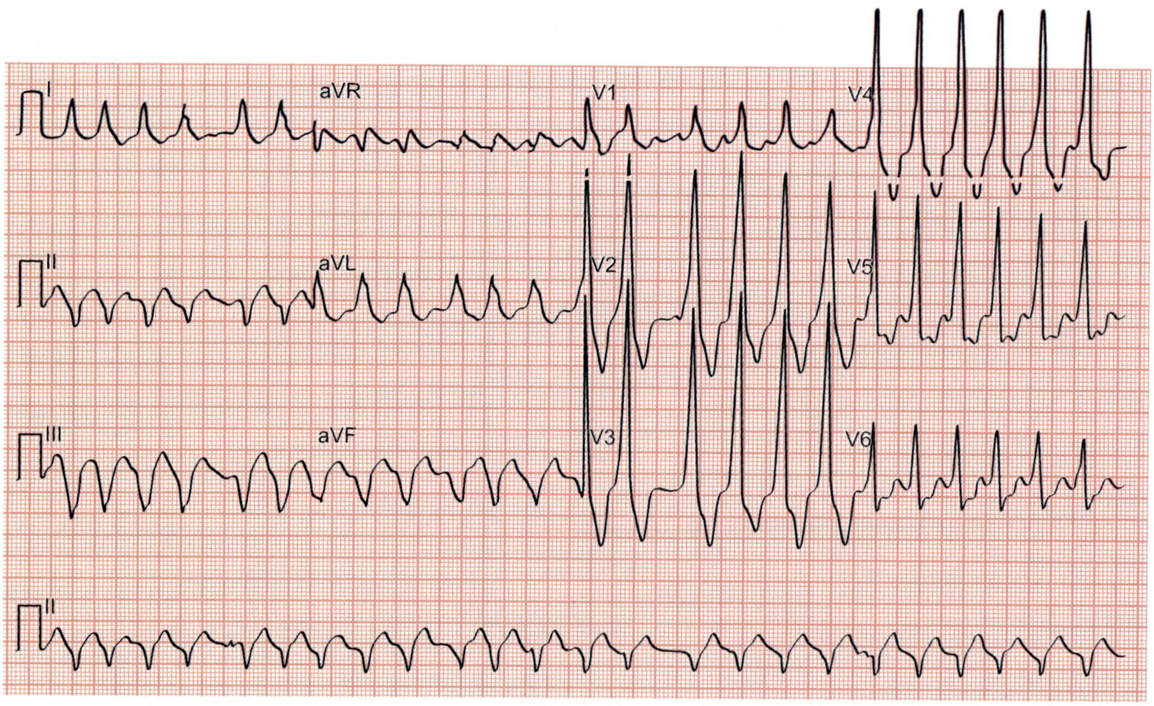


**Fig. 39.18:** Electrocardiogram of a patient showing atrial fibrillation with W-P-W syndrome

version depending on the severity and frequency of symptoms. Asymptomatic patients may be observed without treatment.

Medications such as digoxin, adenosine, and verapamil that block the AV node are contraindicated in patients with WPW and atrial fibrillation because they may accelerate conduction through the accessory pathway, potentially causing VF and SCD.

## Brugada Syndrome

In 1992, Brugada and Brugada described a syndrome of a specific ECG pattern of right bundle-branch block and ST-segment elevation in leads $V_1$ through $V_3$ without any structural abnormality of the heart, that was associated with sudden death (Figs 39.19 and 39.20).

In 25–30% of these patients, a mutation in *SCN5A* on chromosome 3 is detected. This mutation results in a sodium channelopathy. The most common clinical presentation is syncope, and this mutation is most common in young males and in Asians. It is associated with VT, VF, and SCD.

Three ECG types of Brugada pattern are described. Only type 1, which consists of a coving ST-elevation in $V_1$ to $V_3$ with downsloping ST-segment and inverted T-waves, pseudo RBBB pattern with no reciprocal ST changes and normal QTc, is specific enough to be diagnostic for Brugada syndrome when it is associated with symptoms. The other two ECG patterns of Brugada are not diagnostic, but they merit further evaluation.

The Brugada ECG pattern can be dynamic and not found on an index ECG. When clinical suspicion is high, a

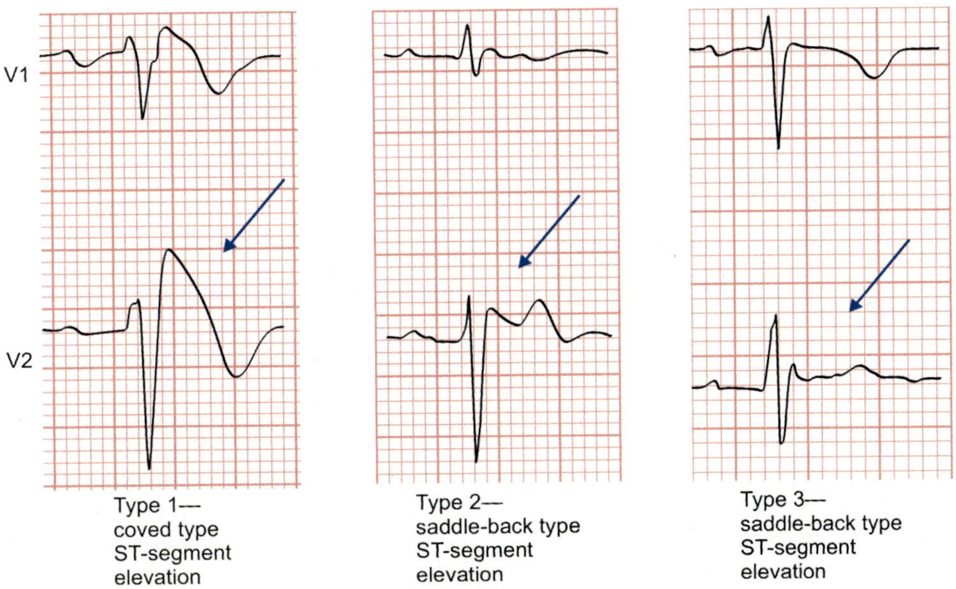


**Fig. 39.19:** Showing ECG criteria of different types of Brugada syndrome as seen in lead V1 and V2

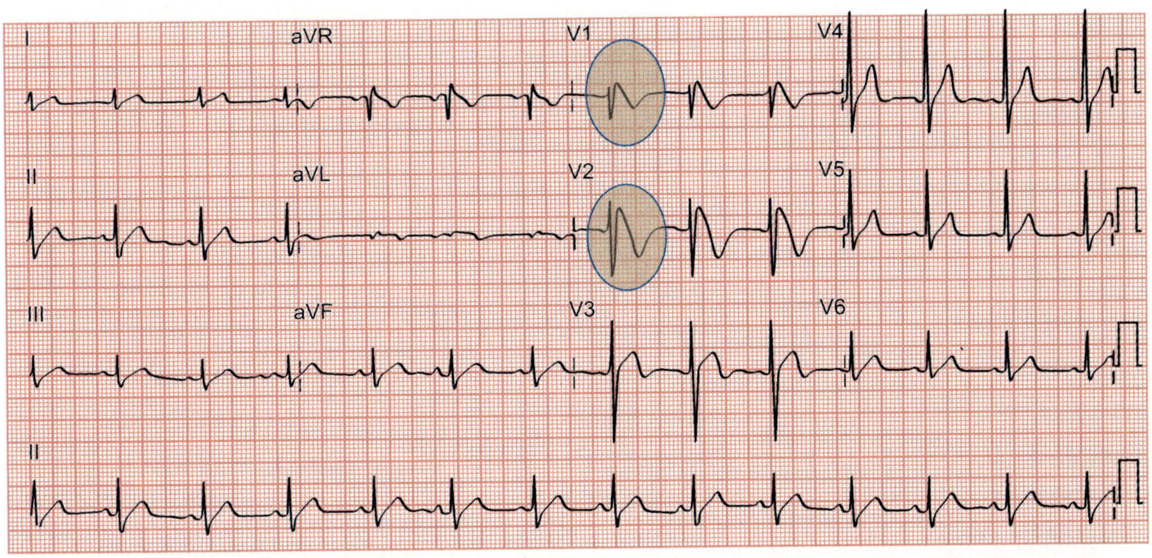


**Fig. 39.20:** Brugada syndrome–rSr′ pattern with a saddle-shaped elevated ST-segment and a negative T-wave is seen in lead V1 and V2

challenge test with procainamide or some other Na channel blocker may be diagnostic by reproducing the type 1 ECG pattern.

Although antiarrhythmic medications, catheter ablation and pacemaker therapies all have potential, in young and symptomatic patients, an ICD should be implanted to prevent VF and SCD. ICD therapy is the only proven treatment to date. Whether ICD placement is indicated in older or asymptomatic patients is controversial at present.

A prospective study by Delise, et al. suggests using a combination of clinical risk factors (syncope and family history of SCD) with VT inducibility in EP study to risk stratify patients with the type 1 ECG pattern of Brugada syndrome (Fig. 39.21).

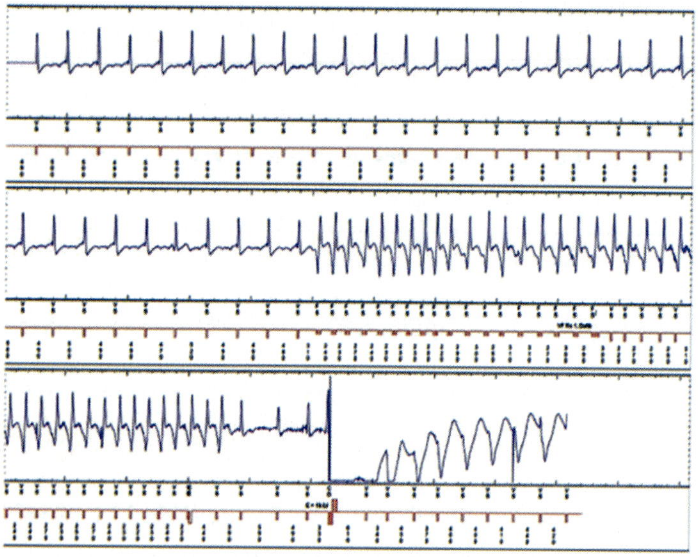

**Fig. 39.21:** Self-terminated nonsustained ventricular tachycardia leading to an inappropriate shock. An implantable cardioverter-defibrillator (ICD) electrogram demonstrating nonsustained ventricular tachycardia that self-terminates and is followed by an inappropriate ICD shock

**Catecholaminergic polymorphic ventricular tachycardia (CPVT)** is a syndrome that presents with polymorphic VT, syncope, or SCD, and in about half of these patients, a mutation in one of two different genes have been detected (Fig. 39.22).

The polymorphic VT is characteristically induced by emotional or physical stress (e.g. exercise stress test). The medical therapy of choice is administration of beta-blockers, and ICD may be indicated. New data may support the use of flecainide in the treatment of this disease. Primary ventricular fibrillation occurs in a structurally normal heart due to idiopathic aetiology. An estimated 3–9% of cases of VT and VF occur in the absence of myocardial ischemia. As many as 1% of patients with out-of-hospital cardiac arrest have idiopathic VF with no structural heart disease. As many as 15% of patients younger than 40 years who experience VF have no underlying structural heart disease. Viskin and Behassan noted that of 54 patients with idiopathic VF, 11 patients had histologic abnormalities on endomyocardial biopsy.

SCD is often the first presentation of VF in patients at risk but who have had no preceding symptoms. In those patients who survive, VF may recur in as many as one-third of patients. The options for medical therapy include beta-blockers and class 1A antiarrhythmic drugs, but limited data are available regarding their efficacy. The mainstay of treatment is preventing VF by ICD placement. Mapping and radiofrequency ablation of the triggering foci is an option for those patients who experience frequent episodes of VF following ICD placement. Right ventricular outflow tract (RVOT) tachycardia is the most common form of idiopathic VT, comprising 70–80% of all idiopathic VTs. RVOT tachycardia is a very rare cause of SCD. It also has been referred to as exercise-induced VT,

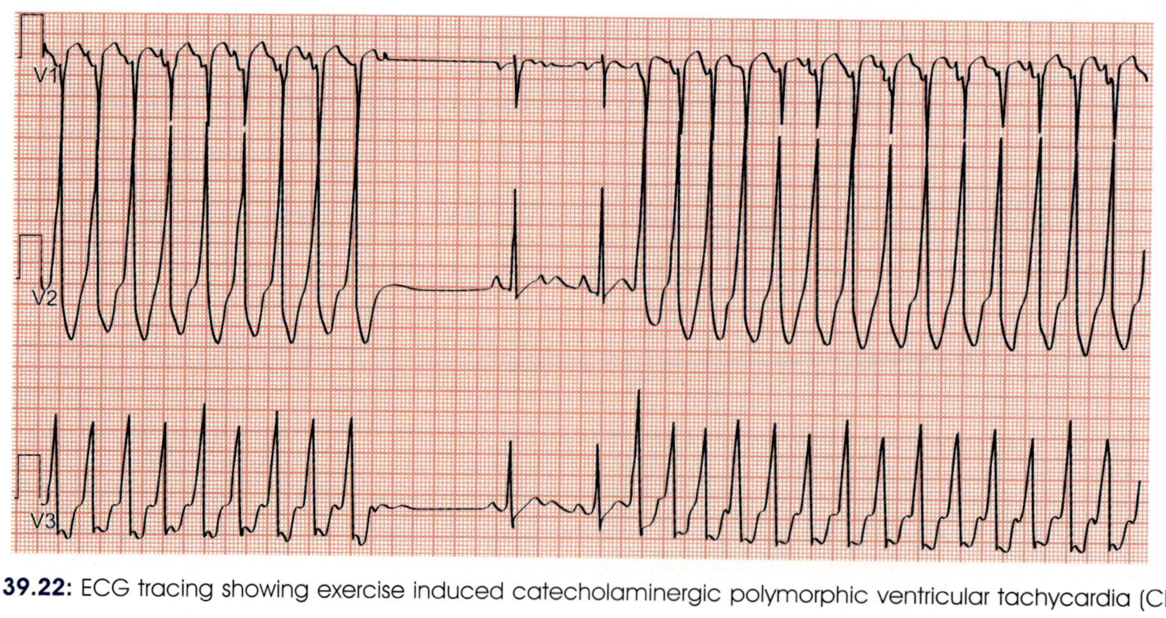


**Fig. 39.22:** ECG tracing showing exercise induced catecholaminergic polymorphic ventricular tachycardia (CPVT)

adenosine-sensitive VT, and repetitive monomorphic VT (Fig. 39.23).

RVOT tachycardia occurs in patients without structural heart disease and arises from the RV outflow region. Current data suggest that triggered activity is the underlying mechanism of RVOT tachycardia. RVOT tachycardia is believed to be receptor-mediated because exogenous and endogenous adenosine can terminate this process. Manoeuvres that increase endogenous acetylcholine also have been demonstrated to antagonize this process.

**Symptoms** typical of RVOT tachycardia include palpitations and presyncope or syncope, often occurring during or after exercise or emotional stress. VT also can occur at rest. The ECG during VT displays a left bundle-branch block/inferior axis morphology.

**Treatment** is based on frequency and severity of symptoms. The first line of therapy is a beta-blocker or calcium channel blocker. Patients with symptoms not relieved by medical therapy are best treated with radiofrequency catheter ablation. Successful ablation is reported in 83–100% of cases.

### Other Causes of Sudden Death

Two major causes of sudden cardiopulmonary death deserve mention.

**Pulmonary embolism** is a frequent cause of sudden death in people at risk. Risk factors include previous personal or family history of deep venous thromboembolism, malignancy, hypercoagulable states, and recent mechanical trauma such as hip or knee surgery (Figs 39.24–39.26).

**Aortic dissection or aneurysmal rupture** is the other major cause of out-of-hospital nonarrhythmic cardiovascular death. Predisposing factors for aortic dissection include genetic deficiencies of collagen such as Marfan syndrome, Ehlers-Danlos syndrome, and aortic cystic medial necrosis.

## DIAGNOSTIC CONSIDERATIONS

Other conditions to be considered in patients with suspected sudden cardiac death include arrhythmogenic RV dysplasia and Brugada syndrome.

Important considerations include the following:

- Recognize and initiate early management of patients with ischemic heart disease. The importance of this cannot be overestimated, because approximately 80% of SCD cases can be attributed to ischemic heart disease.
- Use appropriate medical therapy for ischemic heart disease (e.g. beta-blockers).
- It is very important to involve a specialist in cardiovascular disease in the care of patients who have had a cardiac arrest or have symptoms of ischemic heart disease, valvular disorders, or presentations with complex arrhythmias.

It is very important to educate patients about the consequences of noncompliance with medical therapy.

For patient education information, see the heart health center and healthy living center, as well as chest pain, heart rhythm disorders, coronary heart disease, heart attack, and cardiopulmonary resuscitation (CPR).

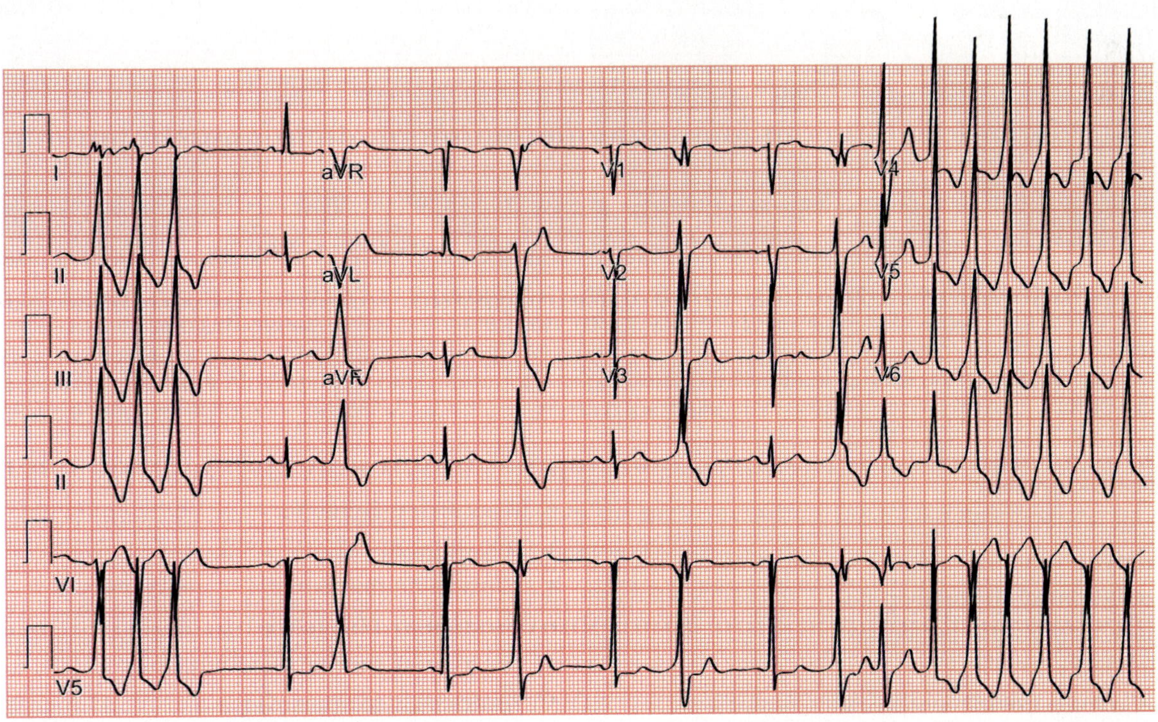


**Fig. 39.23:** Electrocardiogram illustrating repetitive monomorphic right ventricular outflow tract ventricular tachycardia, left bundle branch block morphology, and an inferior axis

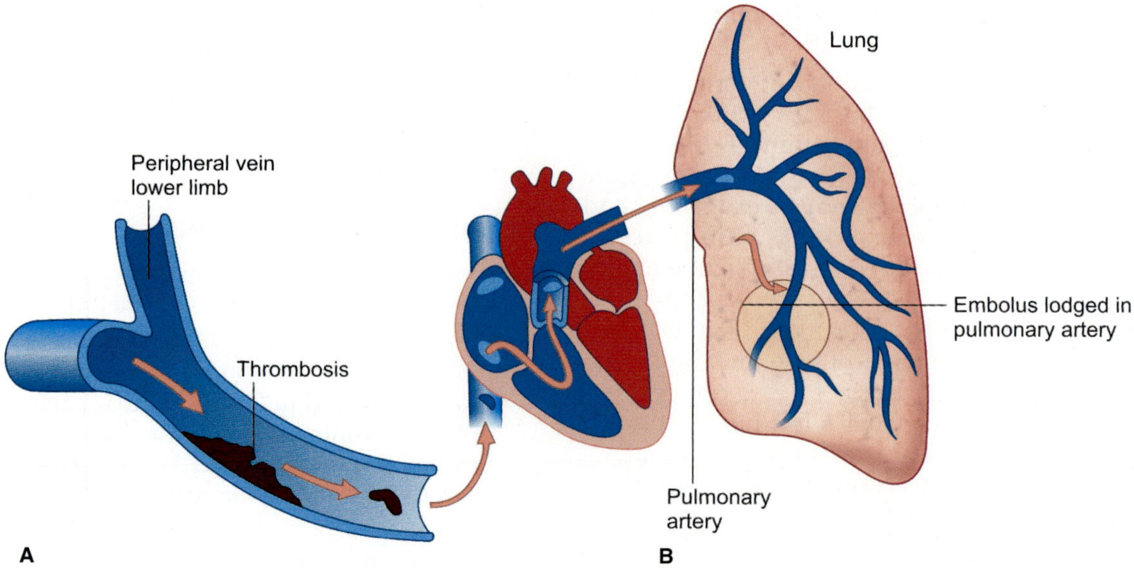


**Fig. 39.24:** Diagram showing route of thrombosis from peripheral lower limb (A) to one of the major or minor pulmonary arteries (B)

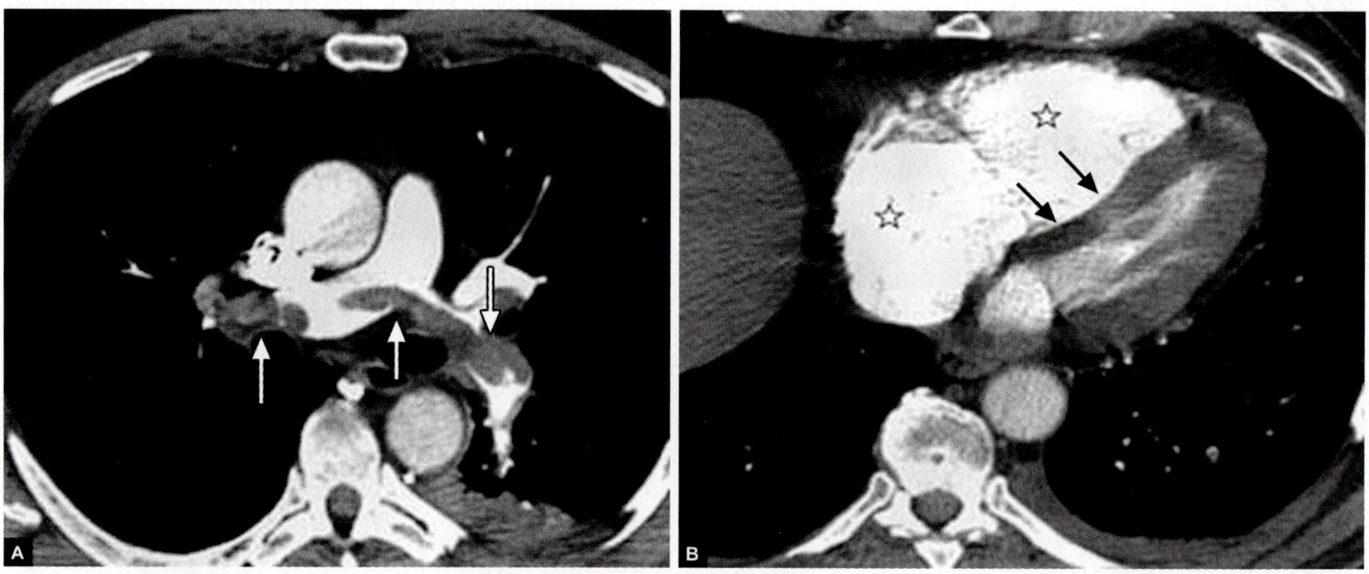


**Fig. 39.25:** CT pulmonary angiogram demonstrates a saddle embolus and signs of right heart strain in a 54-year-old man. (A) Axial contrast-enhanced image obtained at the level of the main pulmonary artery shows low density material (arrows) within the left and right main pulmonary arteries, crossing the bifurcation of the main PA. This is consistent with a saddle embolus. (B) Axial contrast-enhanced image obtained at the level of the heart shows enlarged right atrium and right ventricle (stars) with leftward bowing of the interventricular septum (arrows) and narrowing of the luminal diameter of the left ventricle, indicative of right heart strain.

## Differential Diagnoses

- Aortic stenosis
- Cardiomyopathy, dilated
- Cardiomyopathy, hypertrophic
- Coronary artery atherosclerosis
- Ebstein anomaly
- Lown-Ganong-Levine syndrome
- Myocardial infarction
- Myocardial ischemia
- Tetralogy of Fallot
- Torsade de pointes
- Ventricular fibrillation
- Ventricular premature complexes
- Ventricular tachycardia
- Wolff-Parkinson-White syndrome

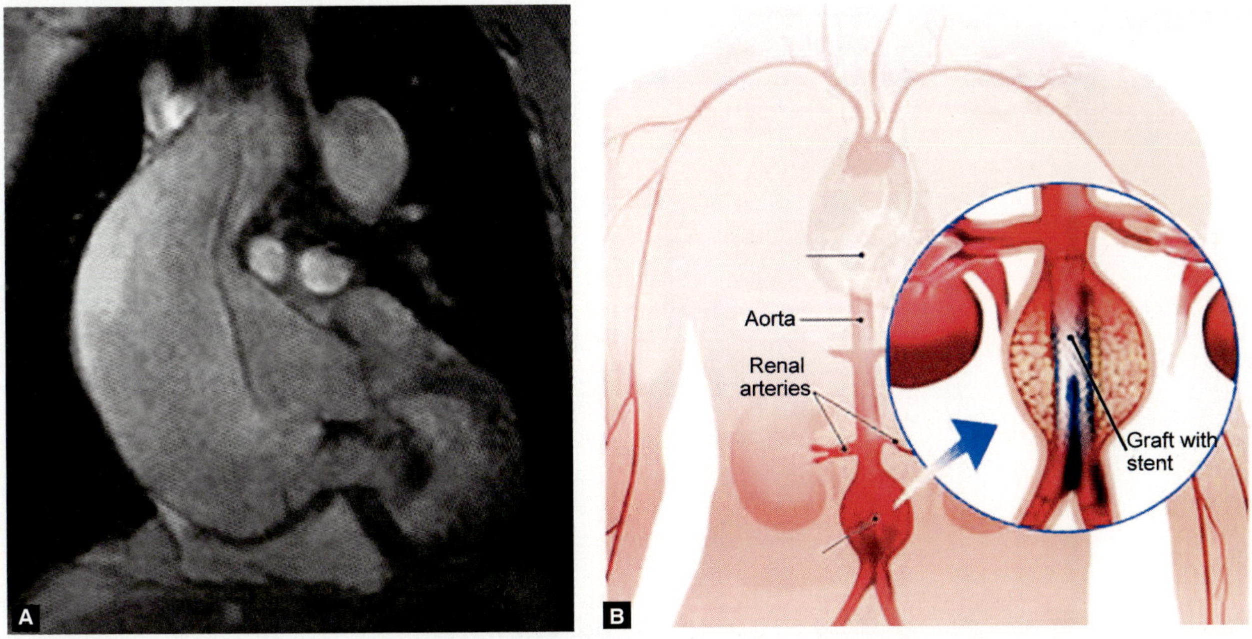


**Fig. 39.26:** (A) Magnetic resonance angiography of a large ascending aortic aneurysm with a proximal (type A) dissection. There is a dissection flap extending from the aortic sinuses to the arch, (B) shows aneurysm of the abdominal aorta

## LABORATORY STUDIES

Laboratory studies in the workup of sudden cardiac death include the following:

- *Cardiac enzymes (creatine kinase, myoglobin and troponin)*: Elevations in these enzyme levels may indicate ischemia and MI. The extent of myocardial damage usually can be correlated to the extent of elevation in the enzyme levels. Patients are at increased risk for arrhythmia in the peri-infarct period.
- *Electrolytes, calcium, and magnesium*: Severe metabolic acidosis, hypokalemia, hyperkalemia, hypocalcemia, and hypomagnesemia are some of the conditions that can increase the risk for arrhythmia and sudden death.
- *Quantitative drug levels (quinidine, procainamide, tricyclic antidepressants and digoxin)*: Drug levels higher than the levels indicated in the therapeutic index may have a proarrhythmic effect. Subtherapeutic levels of these drugs in patients being treated for specific cardiac conditions also can lead to an increased risk for arrhythmia. Most of the antiarrhythmic medications also have a proarrhythmic effect.
- *Toxicology screen*: Looking for drugs, such as cocaine, that can lead to vasospasm-induced ischemia is warranted if suspicion exists. Obtaining levels of drugs (antiarrhythmics) also may be warranted.
- *Thyroid-stimulating hormone*: Hyperthyroidism can lead to tachycardia and tachyarrhythmias. Over a period of time, it also can lead to heart failure. Hypothyroidism can lead to QT prolongation.
- *Brain natriuretic peptide (BNP)*: BNP has predictive value especially in post MI patients and in patients with heart failure. Although preliminary and not conclusive, emerging data support the notion that an elevated BNP level may provide prognostic information on the risk of SCD, independent of clinical information and LVEF.

### Chest Radiography

This may reveal whether someone is in congestive heart failure. It also can show signs suggesting LV enlargement or RV enlargement. Signs of pulmonary hypertension also may be evident on the chest radiograph (Figs 39.27–39.29).

### Echocardiography

Two-dimensional echocardiography with Doppler is essential in the evaluation of SCD (Fig. 39.30). A number

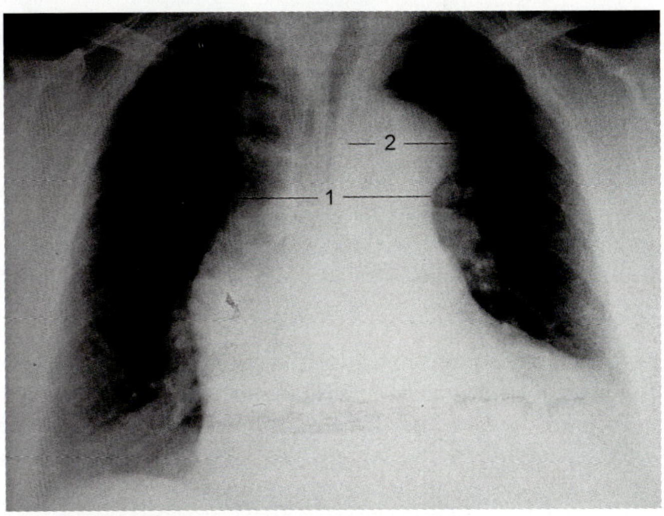


**Fig. 39.27:** X-ray chest PA view showing wide aortic knob in aortic dissection in patient who presented in ED department with severe chest pain and died suddenly

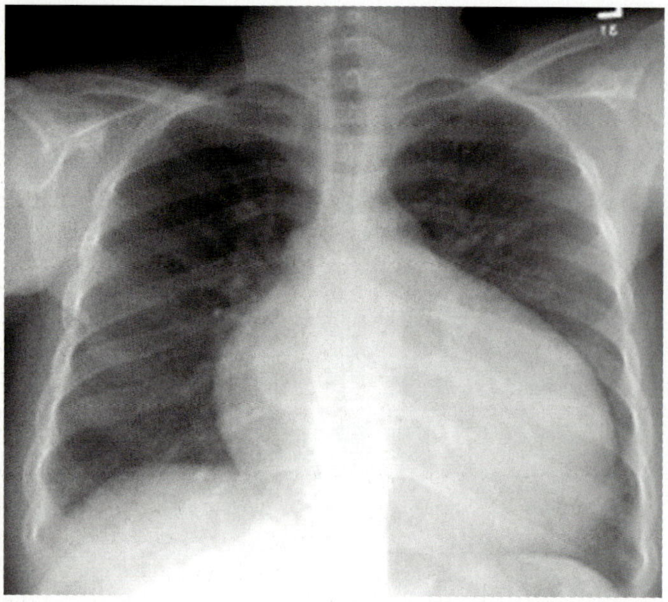

**Fig. 39.28:** X-ray chest PA view showing diffuse cardiomegaly with dominant LV and LA in dilated cardiomyopathy

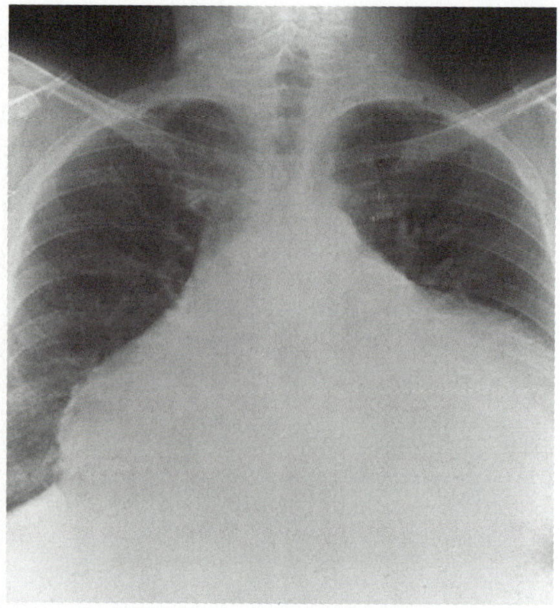

**Fig. 39.29:** X-ray chest PA view. Chest radiograph of cardiomegaly. This patient had a very large pericardial effusion

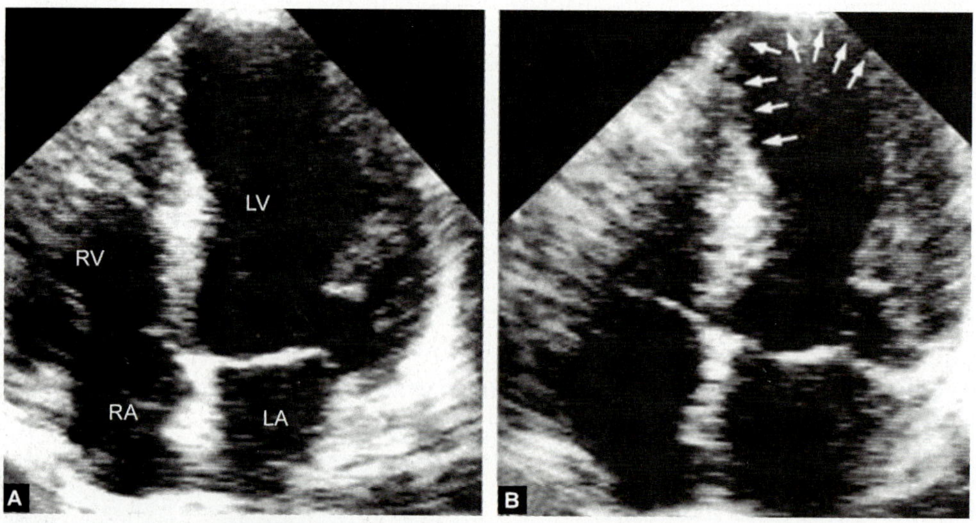


**Fig. 39.30:** Echocardiographic wall motion abnormality coronary artery disease. (A) Two-dimensional echocardiographic apical four-chamber view at end-diastole. (B) Two-dimensional echocardiographic apical four-chamber view at end-systole. The right ventricle (RV) and the septal and lateral walls at the base of the left ventricle (LV) demonstrate normal inward motion from diastole through systole; however, the distal septum and apex demonstrate akinesis (arrows in B). The wall motion abnormality demonstrated in this frame was caused by ischemia from a lesion in the mid-left anterior descending artery. LA=left atrium; RA=right atrium. [From MH Picard, AE Weyman. Echocardiography in chronic ischemic heart disease, in GA Beller (ed): Chronic Ischemic Heart Disease, vol 5, in E Braunwald (series ed): Atlas of Heart Diseases, Philadelphia: Current Medicine, 1996, pp. 4.2]

of studies have demonstrated that the use of two-dimensional echocardiogram to evaluate left wall motion abnormalities after an acute MI (using the LV wall-motion score index) is useful in predicting the risk for major cardiac events, including sudden death. A decrease in the ejection fraction and worsening wall motion abnormalities upon exercise echocardiography in patients who have had an MI has been suggested to confer increased risk of cardiac death.

## Nuclear Imaging

Resting thallium or technetium-99m scintigraphy is helpful in assessing myocardial damage after MI (Figs 39.31–39.35). A larger defect has been associated with greater risk for future cardiac events. Exercise nuclear scintigraphy is very sensitive for detecting the presence, extent, and location of myocardial ischemia. Gibson et al. found that pharmacologic-stress nuclear (dipyridamole or adenosine)

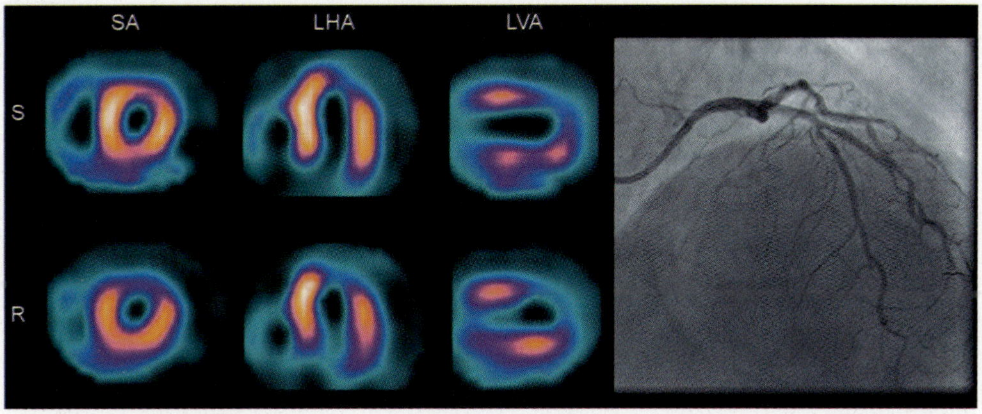


**Fig. 39.31:** Single-photon emission computed tomography myocardial perfusion with 99mTc-tetrofosmin of a patient with chronic anterior infarction and paradoxical scintigraphic pattern, criteria of viability, and permeable anterior descending artery. LHA=long horizontal axis; LVA= long vertical axis; R=rest; S=stress; SA=short axis. (Images courtesy of Dr. M. Nazarena Pizzi, Hospital Universitari Vall d'Hebron, Barcelona)

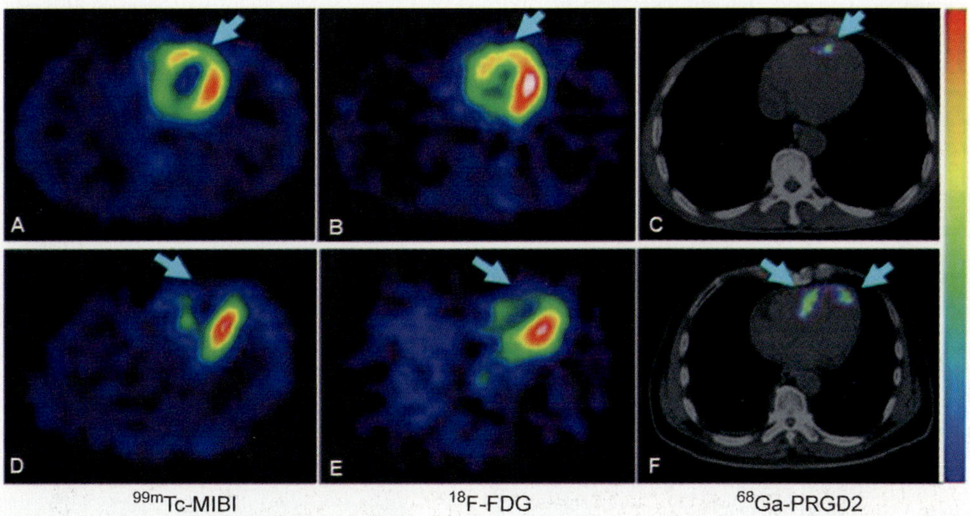


**Fig. 39.32:** Comparison of a patient with slight myocardial infarction (MI) and a patient with severe MI. Upper row: In a 58-year-old man at the 5th day after the event, a small apical region with decreased 99mTc-MIBI perfusion (A, arrow) and 18F-FDG metabolism (B, arrow) showed mild 68Ga-PRGD2 accumulation (C, arrow), with a pSUV of 0.62. Lower row: In a 45-year-old woman on the 7th day after the event, an apical defect on 99mTc-MIBI perfusion images (D, arrow) and 18F-FDG metabolism images (E, arrow) corresponded with moderate 68Ga PRGD2 uptake (F, arrows), with a pSUV of 2.02

scintigraphy was better than submaximal exercise ECG and coronary angiography in predicting cardiac death and other cardiac events. These tests can be very helpful in patients with low functional capacity such as chronic obstructive pulmonary disease, peripheral vascular disease, or orthopedic problems. The multi-center post-infarction research group provided evidence that resting ejection fraction was the most important noninvasive predictor of SCD and other cardiac events in patients with MI.

## Magnetic Resonance Imaging

- **Electrocardiogram** (Figs 39.39–39.41): This study is indicated in all patients. Evidence of MI, prolonged QT interval, short QT interval, epsilon wave, Brugada sign, short PR, a WPW pattern, or other conditions should be sought.
- **Signal-averaged ECG** [SAECG (Figs 39.42–39.45)] has been variably reported to be useful in analysis of patients with SCD. What may be more useful is analysis of T-wave alternans in patients with VT, VF, and/or SCD. Small changes in T-amplitude are not detected in 12-lead ECG. Microvolt T-wave alternans (MTWA) amplifies the alternans and may be used in the workup to predict the risk of SCD. MTWA appears to have high negative predictive value for the risk of SCD in patient with low LVEF (<35%). In addition, a pooled-analysis from 5 prospective studies showed that SCA happens in approximately 3% of patients with an abnormal MWTA

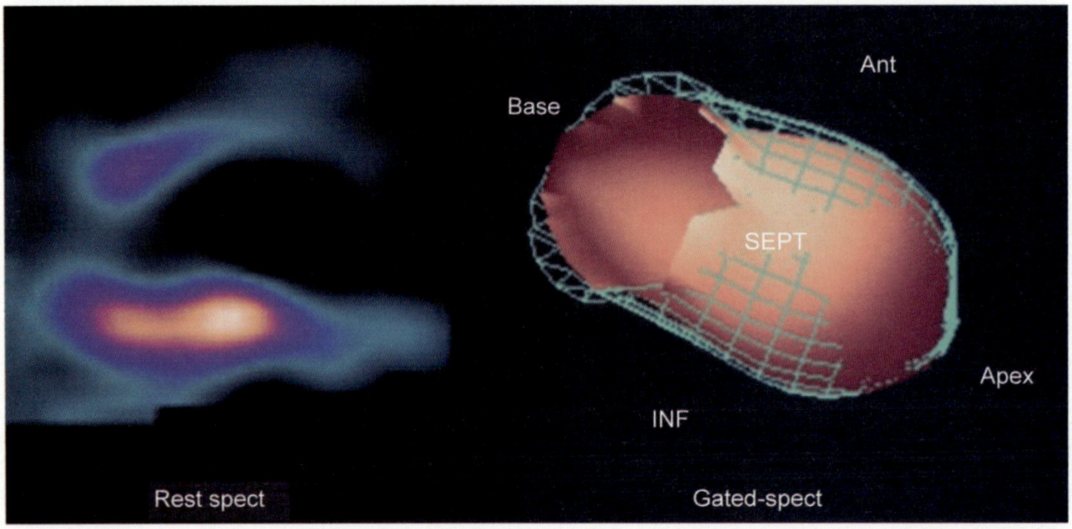


**Fig. 39.33:** SPECT images of myocardial perfusion at rest (vertical long-axis view) of a patient with anterior infarction and criteria of myocardial viability. The apical akinesia region (right) indicates to moderate (grade 2) perfusion uptake defect (left). End-diastolic volume, 123 ml; end-systolic volume, 81 ml; ejection fraction, 34%. Ant=anterior; Inf=inferior; SPECT=single-photon emission computed tomography

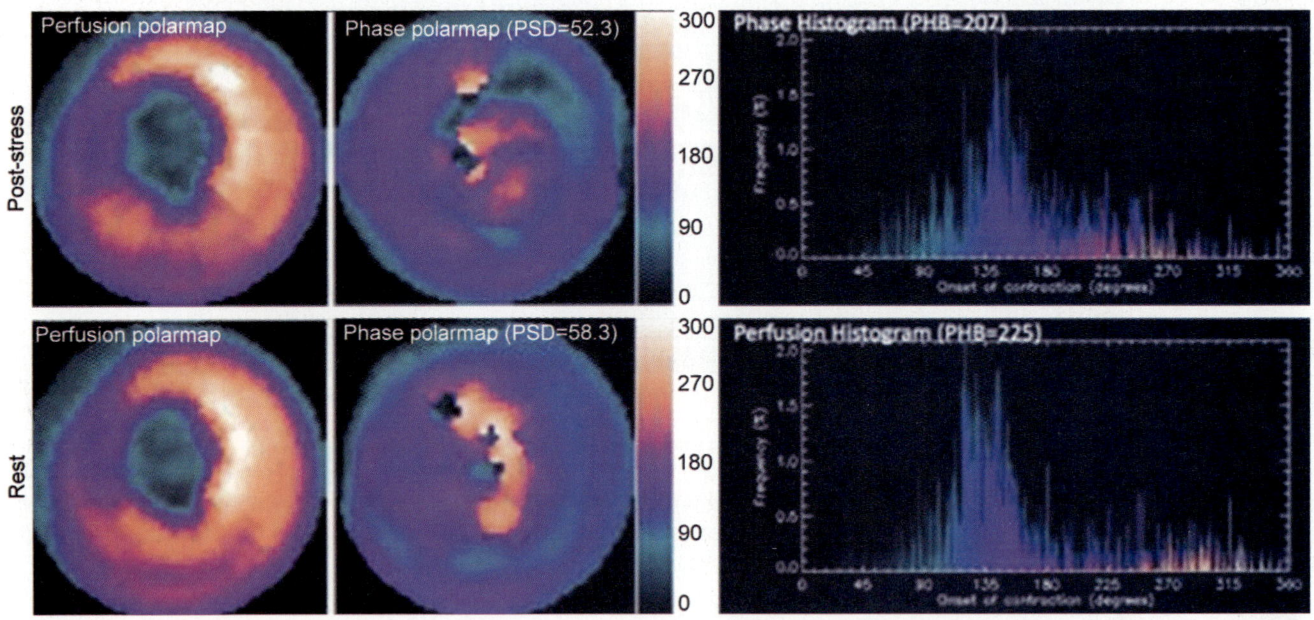


**Fig. 39.34:** An example patient with severe LV dysfunction (LVEF=24%) and myocardial infarction (summed stress score=33). Even though severe reduction in perfusion uptake in the infarct region might impact the phase measurement, the global LV dyssynchrony parameters were not significantly different between the post-stress and resting scans

test and LVEF >35%, suggesting that MTWA may be considered as a tool to identify patients at risk for SCA However, further studies are required to determine how MTWA alone or perhaps in combination with other electrophysiologic tools can be used to risk stratify the patients at risk for SCA.

- **Genetic testing:** The value of genetic testing in conditions such as congenital long QT and HCM is still being evaluated. Some studies have recommended the testing of siblings and close relatives of people with SCD due to these conditions (Fig 39.46).

## Procedures

### Coronary Angiography

Perform cardiac catheterization in patients who survive SCD to assess the state of ventricular function and the

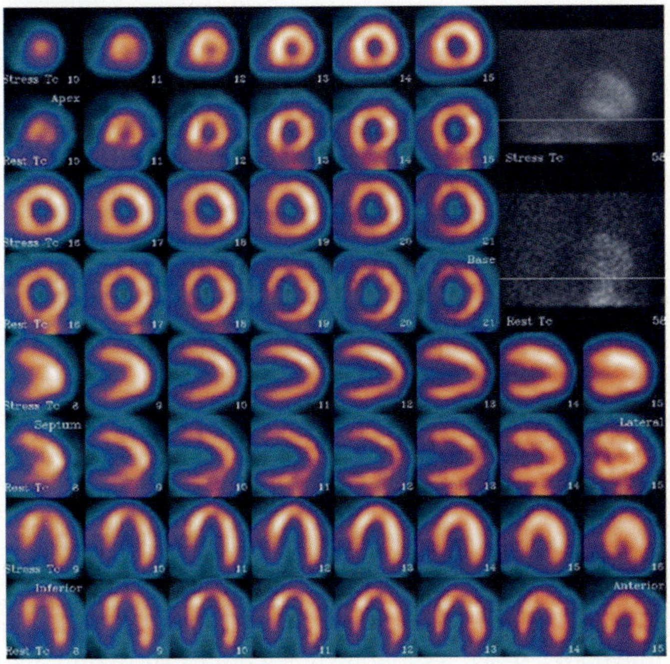


**Fig. 39.35:** Myocardial perfusion imaging was performed with dipyridamole stress test using one day Tc-99m-tetrofosmin rest-stress protocol. There were no symptoms or ECG changes to suggest dipyridamole induced myocardial ischemia. The images do not show any reversible perfusion defects to suggest presence of dipyridamole induced myocardial ischemia. Left ventricle is dilated (EDV 176 ccs) and hypertrophied. Gated images show global hypokinesis with an ejection fraction of 34%. These findings suggest nonischemic cardiomyopathy. Echocardiography showed left ventricular hypertrophy and dilatation with a globally reduced ejection fraction of 30–40%

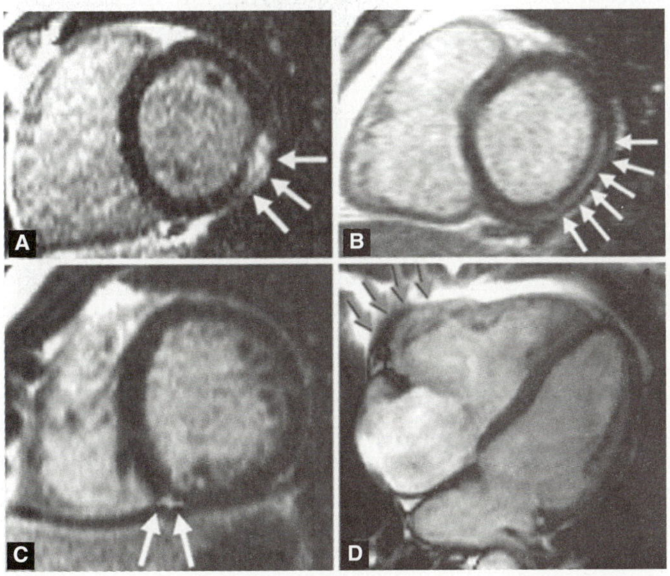


**Fig. 39.36:** CMR imaging. (A) through (C)—short-axis cuts demonstrating LV in a subepicardial distribution at the inferolateral wall (A), at the inferior wall-septal junction (B), and in a midmyocardial distribution at the inferolateral wall (C). (D) Steady-state free-precession image in 4-chamber view showing localized dilation at the subtricuspid region of the RV (gray arrows)

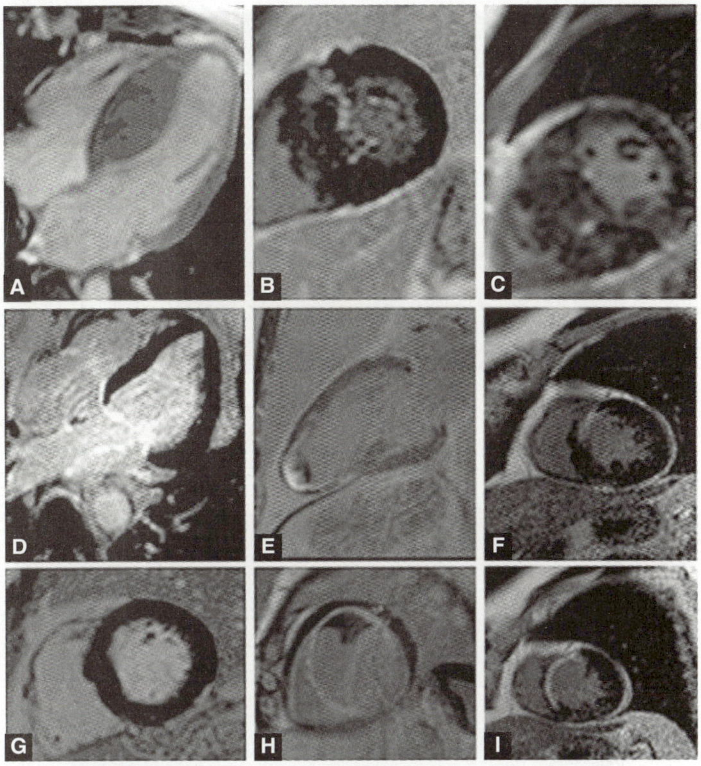


**Fig. 39.37:** CMR and risk stratification for SCD. The top panel shows patients with HCM with severe asymmetric septal hypertrophy (A) and LGE in the septum, especially near RV insertion (B). No LGE is seen in the other walls. Another HCM with severe LVH but a lesser degree of LGE (C). Both severe LVH (>30 mm) and extent of LGE predict SCD risk. Middle and lower panels—show normal heart with no LGE (D, G) and varieties of scar (E, F, H, I). Apical scar (E) and anterioseptal scar (F) with mild heterogeneity, while H and I shows varying extent and thickness —H is a full thickness scar in most of the septum and this is non-viable myocardium. I shows a partial thickness scar with islands of tissue that is not scar—these might be substrates for arrythmia. Presence of scar and scar heterogeneity predict arrhythmic events better than current parameters like EF etc. There is a good-sized LV apical clot (E and H). LGE=late gadolinium enhancement.

severity and extent of CAD. The number of vessels with severe obstruction and the degree of LV dysfunction are important variables in predicting cardiac events. Ejection fraction is the best predictor of significant cardiac events and survival. Coronary angiography also can help identify coronary anomalies and other forms of congenital heart disease. Angiography is performed with the aim of identifying patients who may benefit from revascularization. Revascularization is indicated when ischemic myocardium is present as the underlying substrate of VT/VF (Figs 39.47 and 39.48).

### Electrophysiology Studies and Deformation Imaging

In targeted patients, EPS play diagnostic, prognostic, and therapeutic roles (Figs 39.49 and 39.60). EPS usually are performed after ischemic and structural heart disease has been diagnosed and addressed. These studies have been

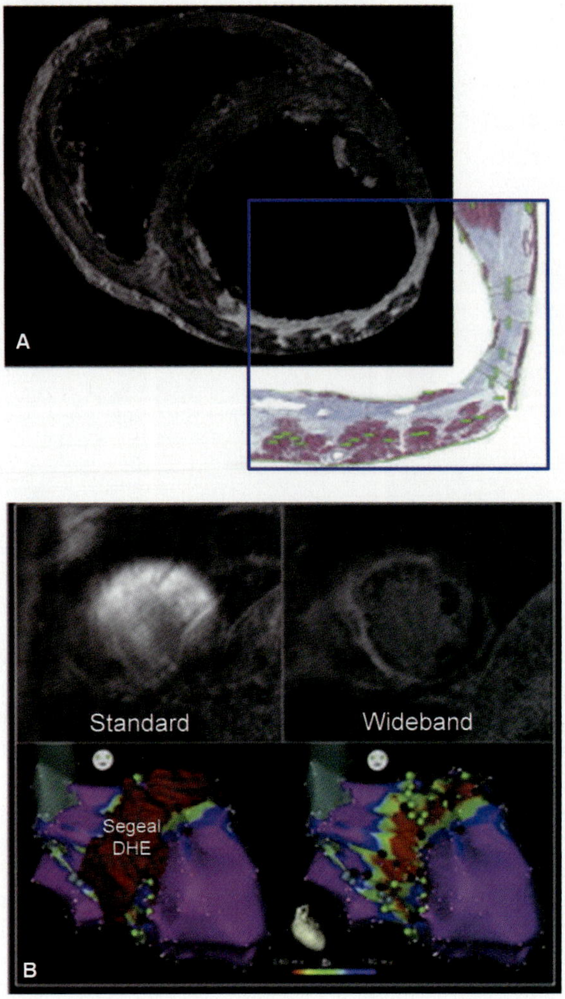


**Fig. 39.38:** Characterization of ischemic heart disease substrates—magnetic resonance imaging. (A) An ex-vivo magnetic resonance image (MRI) of an infarcted porcine heart is shown (top image), with the corresponding Masson's trichrome stain of the same region shown in the inset. The high resolution of this MRI image relative to the histologic image can be readily recognized. It should be noted that artifacts created by cardiac motion and presence of thoracic structures are not present in ex-vivo MR images. (B) The top left and right images depict an MR image before and after application of the WIDEBAND method of device artifact attenuation. The bottom left and right images depict the corresponding voltage map (right anterior oblique projection of left ventricular endocardium) showing consistency between the WIDEBAND (left) and electroanatomic (right) location of scar. Adapted from Stevens SM, Tung R, Rashid S et al. Heart Rhythm 2013

used to identify patients who have inducible versus noninducible sustained monomorphic VT. The presence of inducible sustained VT, at baseline or when the patient is on antiarrhythmic medications, confers a higher risk for sudden death. Significantly lower ventricular function also has been observed in patients with inducible sustained VT. Inducible bundle-branch re-entrant VT can be seen in patients with DCM and in the postoperative period after valvular replacement. As many as 20% of patients with HCM have inducible sustained monomorphic VT.

The identification of accessory pathways also is possible with these studies. EPS are performed with an eye toward the following:

- Ablation of VT foci, e.g. bundle branch VT, RVOT VT, and some cases of idiopathic LV tachycardia
- ICD implantation, which is generally the case in survivors of SCD

## MEDICAL CARE

Advanced cardiac life support (ACLS): In the event of cardiac arrest, the immediate implementation of ACLS guidelines is indicated. Widespread interest in improving rates of public ACLS training with a special emphasis on use of early defibrillation by public service personnel (e.g. police, fire, and airline attendants) exists. Through these measures, the greatest public health benefits can be achieved in the fight against sudden death. In 2010, the American Heart Association (AHA) published new guidelines for cardiopulmonary resuscitation and emergency cardiovascular care science.

The 2009 American Heart Association Cardiac Arrest Survival Summit released consensus recommendations for implementation strategies to optimize the care of patients with out-of-hospital sudden cardiac arrest (OHCA). These recommendations included collection of national data on OHCA and local culture changes because incomplete implementation of existing standards was seen as the limiting problem.

In general, ACLS guidelines should be followed in all cases of SCA; however, depending on the presented rhythm, the following should be considered in acute therapy of SCA:

### Bystander CPR

The best techniques for bystander CPR continue to evolve based on rigorous scientific evaluation and considerations of practical applicability. Recent data suggest, for example, that compression-only CPR may be of equal or greater effectiveness than traditional compression plus ventilation techniques. Adielsson et al. suggest that the long-term perspective data among patients in VF or pulseless VT who were given bystander CPR revealed that survival to 1 month after VF almost doubled. Berdowski and colleagues in a recent cohort study demonstrated that the bystander use of automated external defibrillators can reduce the time to defibrillation from 11 minutes to 4.1 minutes and improves neurologically intact survival to discharge from 14.3% to 49.6%. That observation is consistent with already known facts that the main initiating mechanisms of sudden cardiac death are ventricular tachycardia and ventricular fibrillation, and that time to defibrillation is a critical factor in restoring the rhythm. The conclusion that may be drawn from the above studies is that immediate chest compression

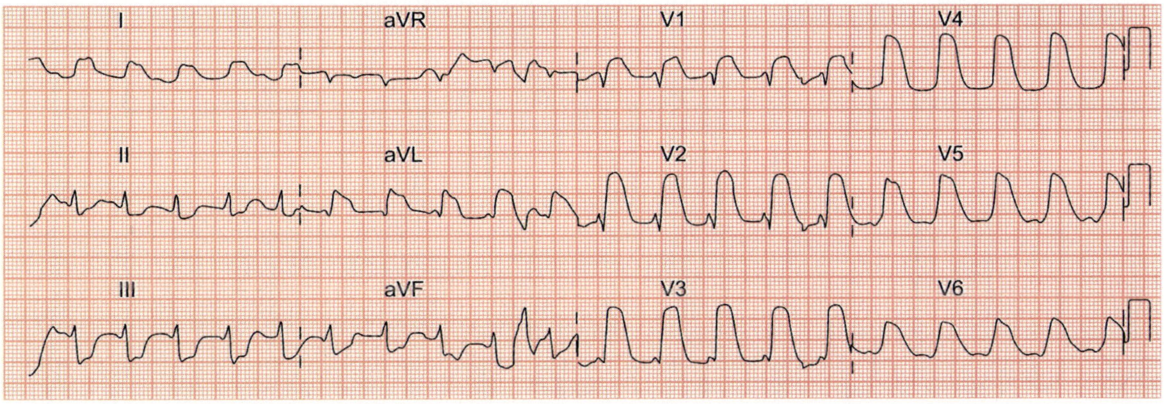


**Fig. 39.39:** Extensive anterior MI ('tombstoning' pattern). Massive ST-elevation with 'tombstone' morphology is present throughout the precordial (V1–6) and high lateral leads (I, aVL). This pattern is seen in proximal LAD occlusion and indicates a large territory infarction with a poor LV ejection fraction and high likelihood of cardiogenic shock and death

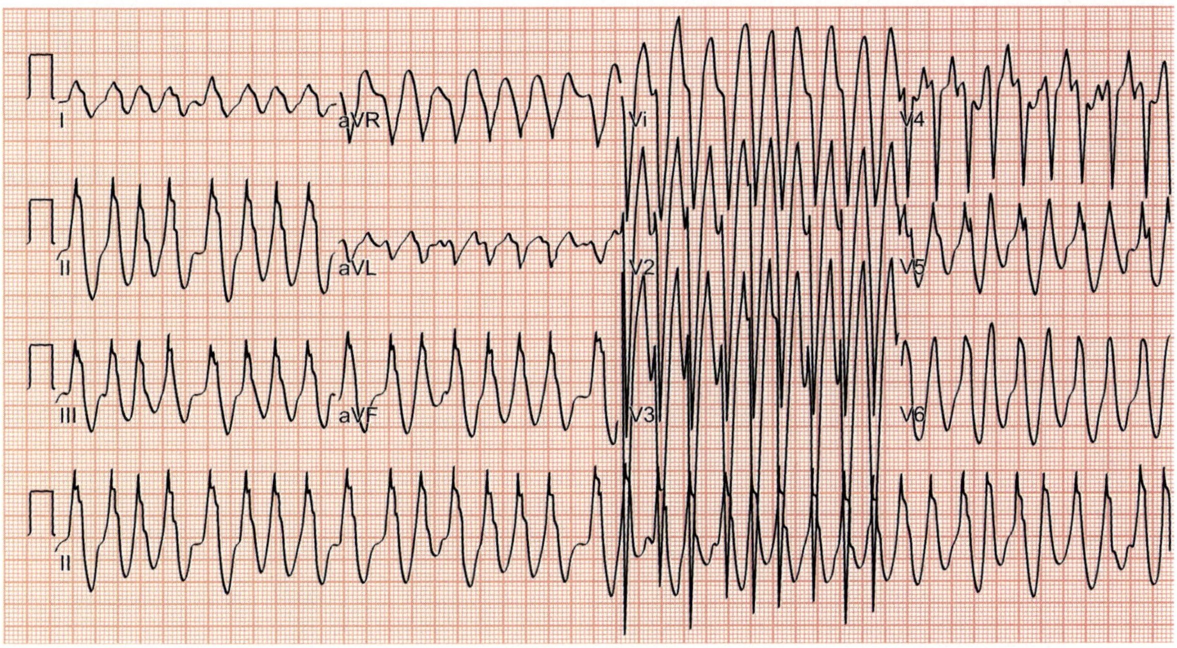


**Fig. 39.40:** ECG trace showing features of W-P-W syndrome with atrial fibrillation

and defibrillation are the most important interventions to improve the outcome in sudden cardiac arrest, whereas ventilation does not play as important a role.

## Ventricular Arrhythmia (VF and VT)

Defibrillation is the mainstay of the acute therapy of SCA due to VF or VT. Epinephrine (1 mg q3–5 min) or vasopressin (40 U single dose) are given. Amiodarone (300 mg IV push and 150 mg repeat IV push if needed) and lidocaine (1 mg/kg IV push q3–5 min up to 3 doses) can be used as antiarrhythmic drugs if defibrillation does not control the VF/VT. In case of polymorphic VT or suspected hypomagnesemia, 1–2 g IV push of magnesium is recommended.

## Pulseless Electrical Activity

Epinephrine (1 mg q3–5 min) can be used as there is no evidence supporting the use of vasopressin in pulseless electrical activity (PEA). Atropine (1 mg q3–5 min) should be used in case of bradycardia. Sodium bicarbonate (1 meq/kg) should be given if there is associated hyperkalemia and its use may be considered in long arrest intervals and suspected metabolic acidosis.

## Asystole

One study suggested that vasopressin is more effective in acute therapy of asystole than epinephrine. Atropine and sodium bicarbonate are used with similar indications in PEA.

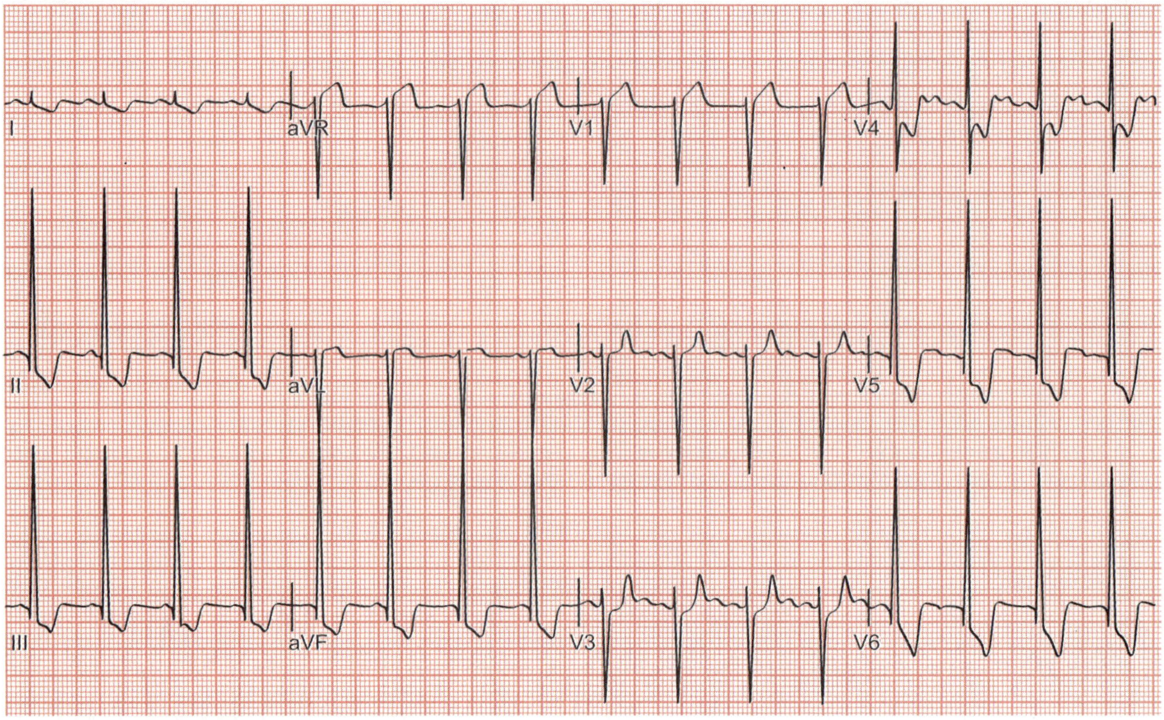


**Fig. 39.41:** ECG trace shows abnormal ST-segments, deeply flipped T-waves, tall R apical waves in leads II, III, aVF and V4–V6 with deep Q-waves in patient with hypertrophic cardiomyopathy

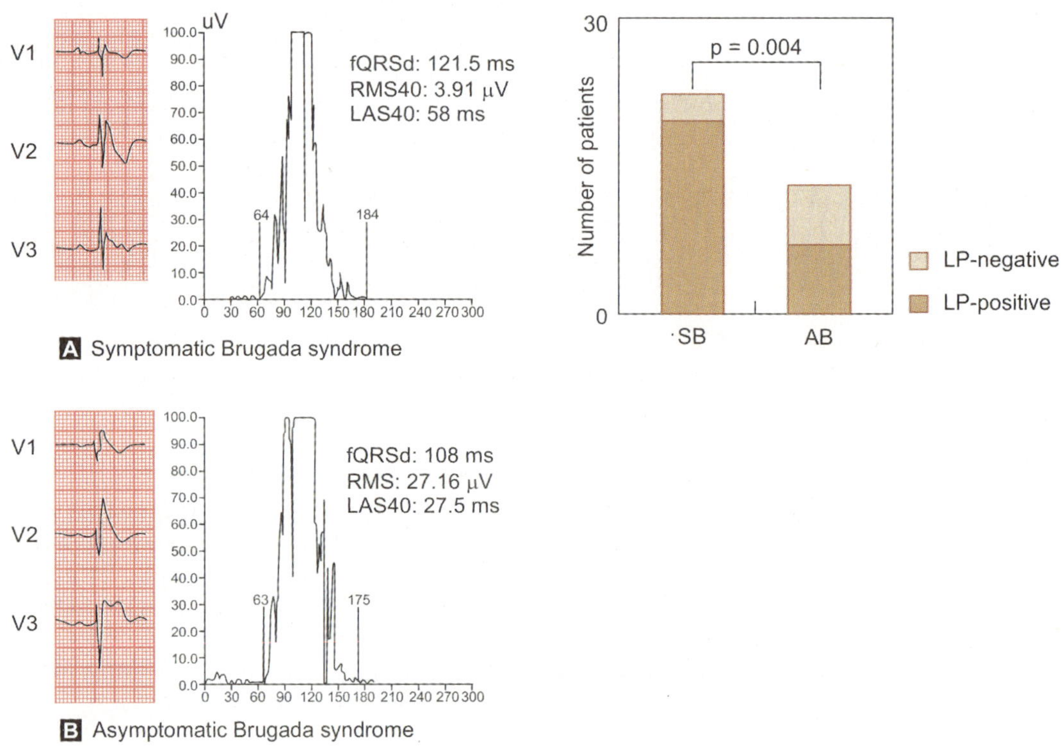


**Fig. 39.42:** Signal-averaged ECGs in Brugada syndrome. (A) Typical ECGs (V1–V3) in a patient with symptomatic Brugada syndrome (a) and with asymptomatic Brugada syndrome (b), and typical signal-averaged ECGs. Respective parameter values as calculated from signal-averaged ECGs are shown in the upper right. (B) Positivity rates of late potential (LP) in symptomatic Brugada syndrome (SB) and asymptomatic Brugada syndrome (AB). LP was positive in 25 (92.6%) of 27 patients with SB and in 8 (47.1%) of 17 patients with AB. Therefore, the LP positivity rate was significantly higher in the SB group (P = 0.0004)

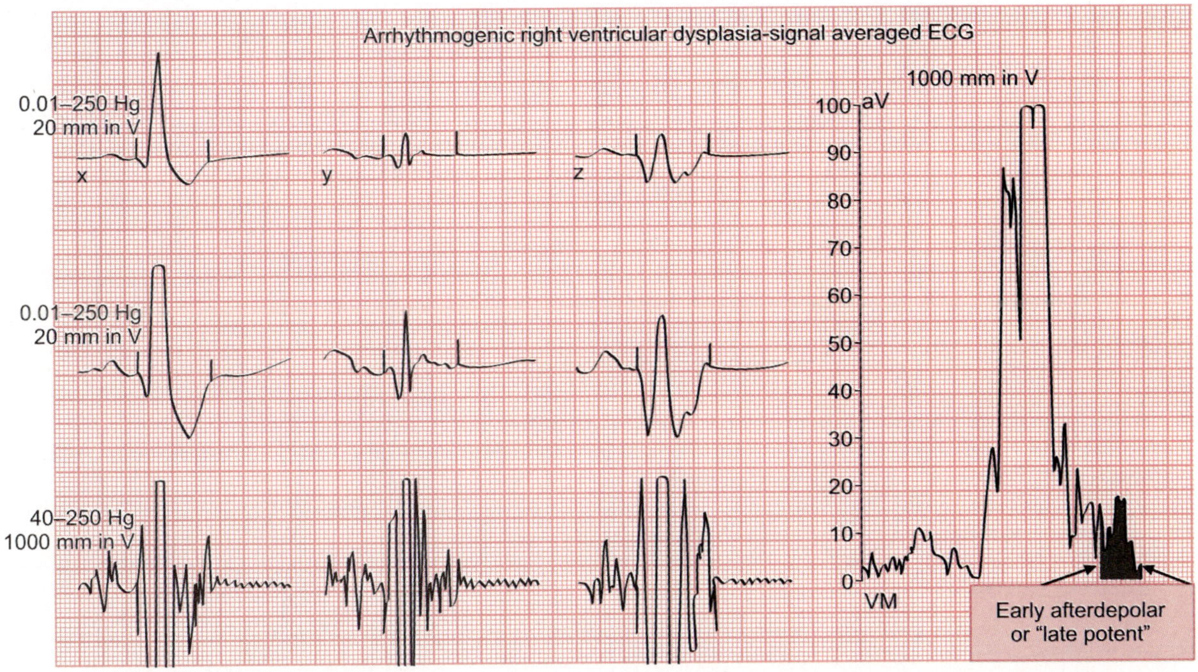


**Fig. 39.43:** A signal averaged ECG is a diagnostic test that averages multiple QRS complexes over a 10-minute time period or at least 250 QRS complexes in order to see minute changes in the electrical activity that is not apparent on the standard 12-lead ECG. 'Early afterdepolarizations' or 'late potentials' may be seen after the QRS complex and is thought to increase the risk of ventricular arrhythmias, although this is controversial. These are also prominent in patients with arrhythmogenic right ventricular dysplasia (ARVD)

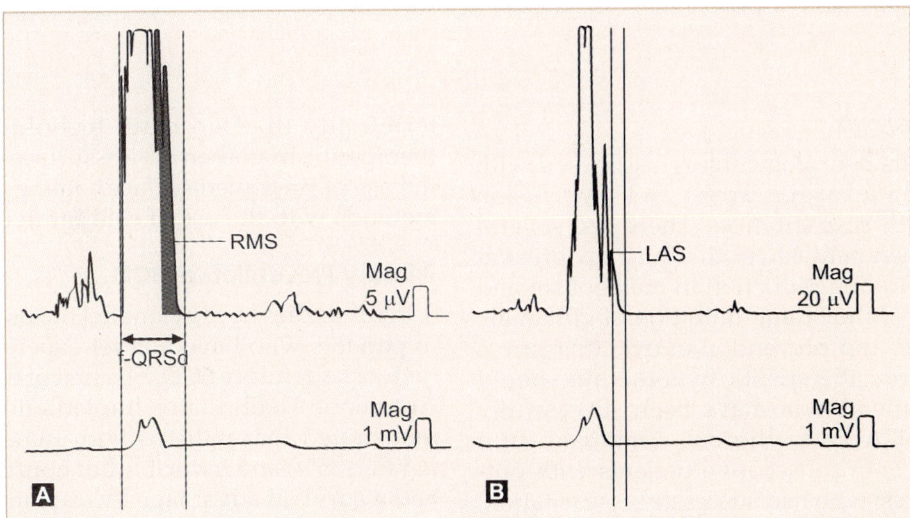


**Fig. 39.44:** Evaluation of myocardial ischemia in Kawasaki disease by dobutamine stress signal-averaged ventricular late potentials. Measurement (A) f-QRSd=filtered QRS duration, RMS= root mean square voltage during 40 ms in the filtered QRS terminal part. (B) LAS–duration of signal under 40 μV

## Medical Stabilization

Careful postresuscitative care is essential to survival because studies have shown a 50% repeat in hospital arrest rate for people admitted after an SCD event. Treatment of myocardial ischemia, heart failure, and electrolyte disturbances are all justified by the results of multiple acute MI and congestive heart failure randomized trials. Empiric beta-blockers are reasonable in many circumstances because of favorable properties.

**Causes.** Empiric antiarrhythmics, including amiodarone, should not supersede ICD implantation unless control of recurrent VT is needed while the patient is in the hospital.

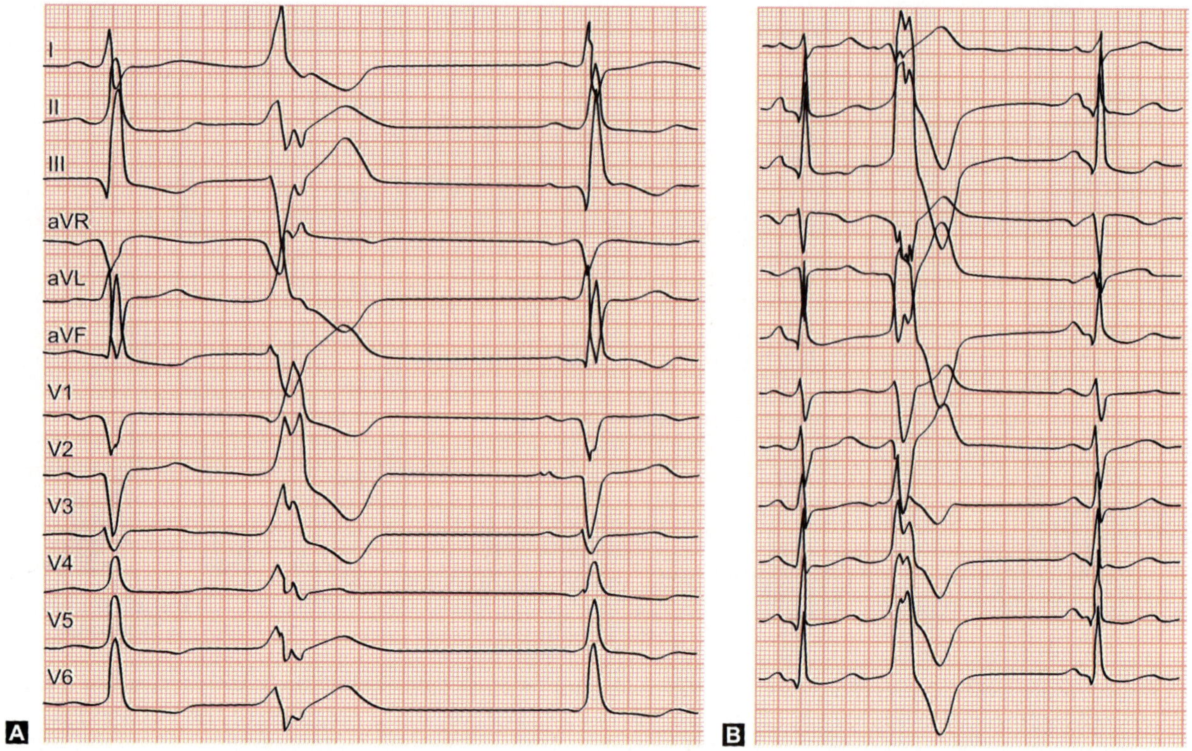


**Fig. 39.45:** The duration of the ventricular ectopic beat (>170 ms) has been shown to correlate with the presence and severity of structural heart disease. (A) Demonstrates a broad fractionated ventricular premature beat from a patient with ischemic heart disease (ventricular ectopic QS interval 208 ms). (B) Demonstrates a narrow ventricular premature beat originating in the right ventricular outflow tract from a patient with a structurally normal heart (ventricular ectopic QS interval 147 ms). Paper speed 50 mm/s

### *Therapeutic Hypothermia*

This intervention limits neurologic injury associated with brain ischemia during a cardiac arrest and reperfusion injury associated with resuscitation. There are several plausible ways that therapeutic hypothermia may prevent neurologic injury, including reduction in metabolism and oxygen consumption of the brain, inhibition of glutamate and dopamine release, and prevention of oxidative stress and apoptosis. Therefore, therapeutic hypothermia should be considered for patients who have been successfully resuscitated from SCA and who are comatose. In a prospective study of 1145 consecutive patients with out-of-hospital cardiac arrest who had successful resuscitation, therapeutic hypothermia was associated with increased odds of good neurological outcome (odds ratio, 1.9; 95% confidence interval, 1.18–3.06) in patients with VT or VF. Therapeutic hypothermia is more effective in patients with initial rhythm of VF/VT but is also recommended for patients presenting with asystole and PEA.

Patients who should not receive this therapy include: (1) those with tympanic membrane temperature below 30°C at the time of presentation, (2) those who were comatose before SCA, (3) those who are pregnant, (4) those who have inherited coagulation disorders, and (5) those who are terminally ill. Two main techniques for induction of therapeutic hypothermia are surface cooling methods with the use of precooled surface cooling pads and core cooling methods with the use of cold intravenous fluids.

## Primary Prevention of SCD

Several studies have evaluated the use of prophylactic ICDs in patients who have not yet experienced SCD but are at high risk for future SCD. The first of these trials, Multicenter Automatic Defibrillator Implantation Trial (MADIT) demonstrated that patients with ischemic cardiomyopathy (LVEF ≤35%) and inducible but nonsuppressible VT on EPS had a survival advantage by implanting an ICD.

This study was followed by MADIT-2, demonstrating that post-MI patients with an LVEF ≤30% have a survival benefit with ICD implantation. The defibrillators in nonischemic cardiomyopathy treatment evaluation (DEFINITE) study showed that implantation of an ICD reduced the risk of sudden cardiac death in a patient population of nonischemic cardiomyopathy (LVEF <36%) who also had PVCs or nonsustained VT.

Finally, the Sudden Cardiac Death in Heart Failure Trial (SCD-Heft) demonstrated that patients with either ischemic or nonischemic cardiomyopathy on optimal medical

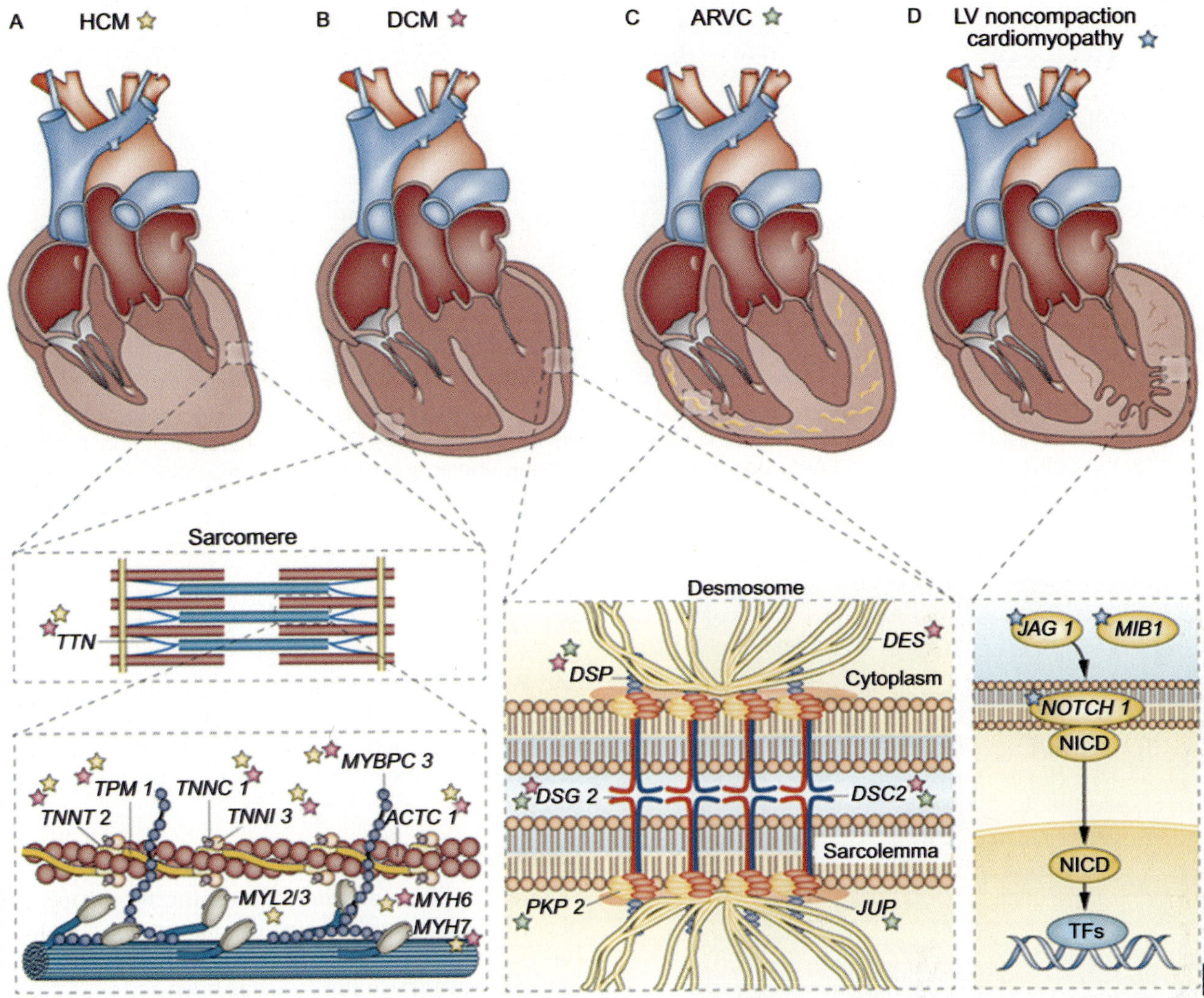


**Fig. 39.46:** Genetic mechanisms of cardiomyopathies. (A) Mutations in TTN and other genes encoding sarcomeric proteins have been shown to cause HCM (yellow stars). (B) Similarly, mutations in genes encoding either sarcomeric or desmosomal proteins have been linked with DCM (pink stars). (C) Mutations in genes encoding desmosomal proteins have also been implicated in the pathogenesis of ARVC (green stars). (D) Mutations involved in the NOTCH1 signalling pathway are thought to underlie LV noncompaction cardiomyopathy (blue stars). ARVC=arrhythmogenic right ventricular cardiomyopathy; DCM=dilated cardiomyopathy; HCM= hypertrophic cardiomyopathy; LV=left ventricular; NICD1= NOTCH1 intracellular domain; TF=transcription factor. Permission for inset panels from parts a–c obtained from NPG© Hershberger, R. E. et al. Nat Rev Cardiol 2013;10:531–547

therapy, LVEF ≤35%, and NYHA II or III treated with an ICD demonstrate greater survival as compared with either amiodarone or placebo.

The recent Home Automated Defibrillator Trial (HAT) demonstrated no survival benefit for the use of a home AED in patients surviving a recent anterior MI who were not candidates for an ICD. However, the overall mortality and incidence of SCD was much lower than predicted from previous data and the noncardiac mortality was as high as cardiac mortality in the population of this study. These factors led to much less power than initially projected in this trial to detect a significant difference in the mortality rate between the arms.

The use of microvolt T-wave alternans (MTWA) to determine which patients with depressed LV systolic function would best benefit from prophylactic ICD placement has been the subject of several recent clinical trials. To date, the results of these clinical trials has not been conclusive.

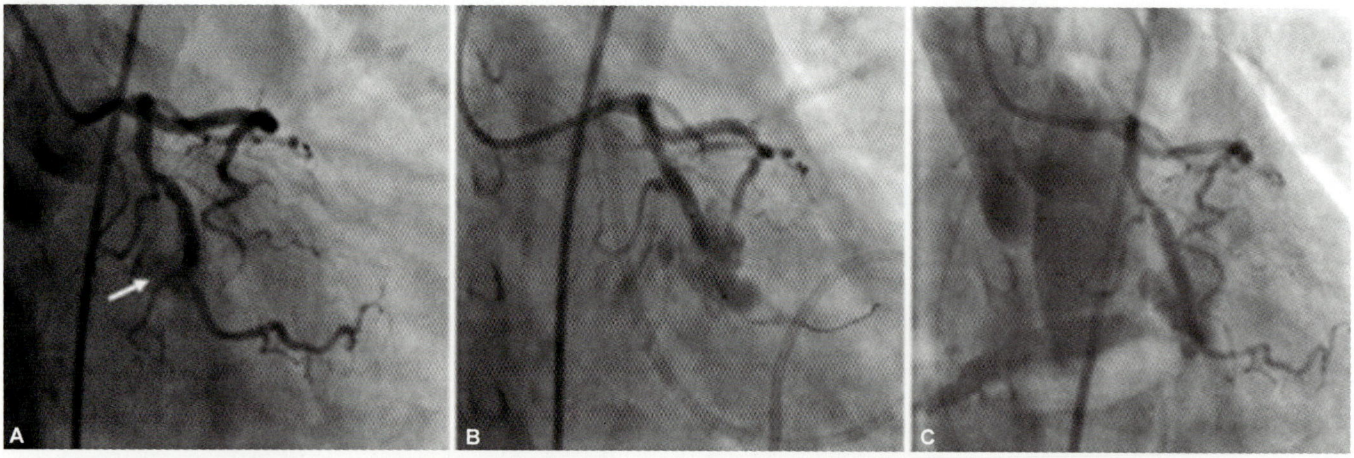


**Fig. 39.47:** Coronary angiogram after cardiovascular resuscitation due to sudden cardiac arrest in general ward. (A) Angiogram showed type III coronary perforation with bleeding at the previous stent implantation site (arrow). (B) Before inflation, first Jo graft stent was placed for the active bleeding site. (C) After stenting of two graft stents, the final angiogram during cardiovascular resuscitation showed no additional bleeding

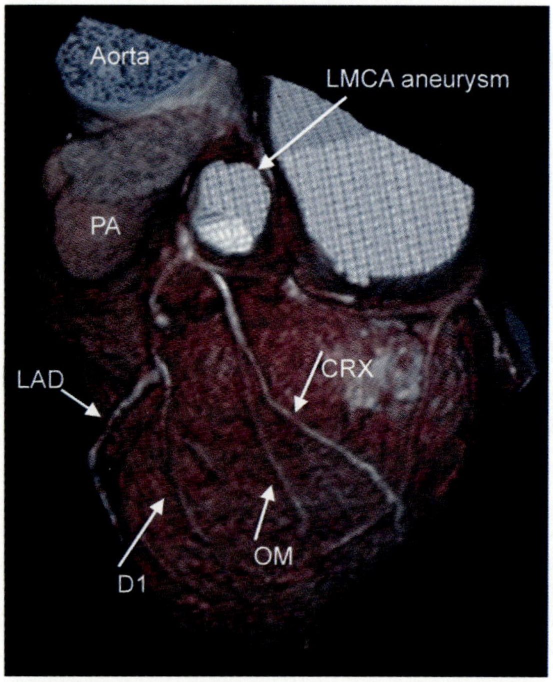


**Fig. 39.48:** MDCT showing giant aneurysm of left main coronary artery

## SURGICAL CARE

### Temporary Cardiac Pacing

Transcutaneous or transvenous cardiac pacing may be considered in the patients with bradycardia and asystole.

### Radiofrequency Ablation

Radiofrequency ablation, now routinely available, may be indicated for patients with accessory pathways, bundle-branch block VT, RVOT VT, idiopathic LV tachycardia, and more rare forms of automatic focus VT. Unfortunately, most cases of SCD are not amenable to radiofrequency ablation and require ICD implantation. Radiofrequency ablation may be useful in the treatment of patients with SCD who experience frequent recurrent VT/VF after ICD placement, especially those who require frequent defibrillation (Fig 39.61).

### Cardioverter Defibrillator Therapy

Several multicenter trials examining the prophylactic use of cardioverter defibrillator therapy in patients at high risk for SCD have been performed. The annual SCD rate in patients with these devices has been reduced from 25% to 1–2%. Studies have shown that in patients at high risk in whom electrophysiologic-guided therapy with antiarrhythmics has failed, ICD placement is beneficial. In several studies comparing ICD placement to antiarrhythmic therapy in patients with VT and/or prior cardiac arrest, ICD placement has been shown to be associated with decreased mortality. The use of ICDs for primary prevention of SCD is now standard care for most patients with LVEF ≤35%. Newer ICDs with pacing capabilities have addressed bradyarrhythmias either causing or complicating VT or VF (Fig. 39.62).

### Cardiac Surgery

Cardiac surgery can be a primary treatment for SCD via a variety of strategies. Surgical treatment in patients with ventricular arrhythmias and ischemic heart disease includes coronary artery bypass grafting (CABG) (Figs 39.63–39.66).

The CASS study illustrated that patients with significant CAD and operable vessels who underwent CABG had a decrease in the incidence of sudden death when compared to patients on conventional medical treatment. The reduc-

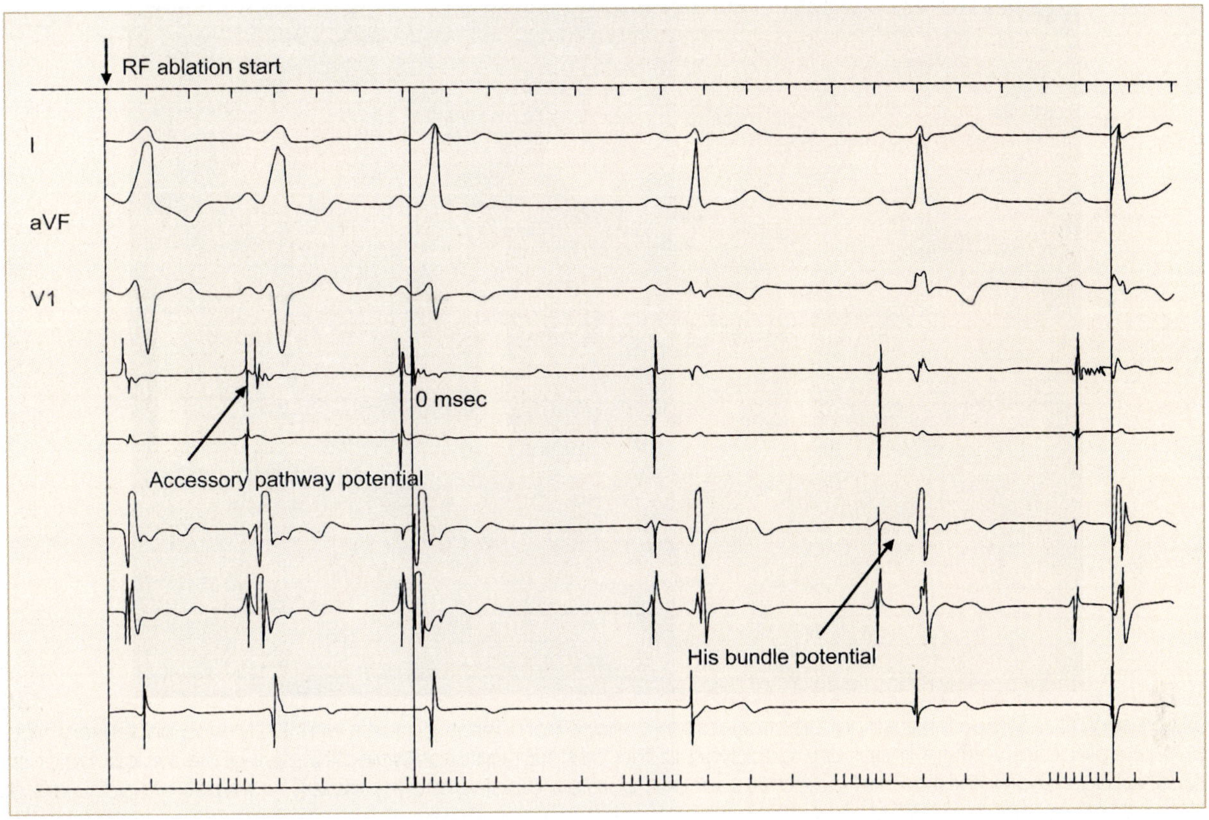


**Fig. 39.49:** Accessory pathway potential and local AV fusion at successful RF ablation site with loss of pre-excitation and return of normal HV interval

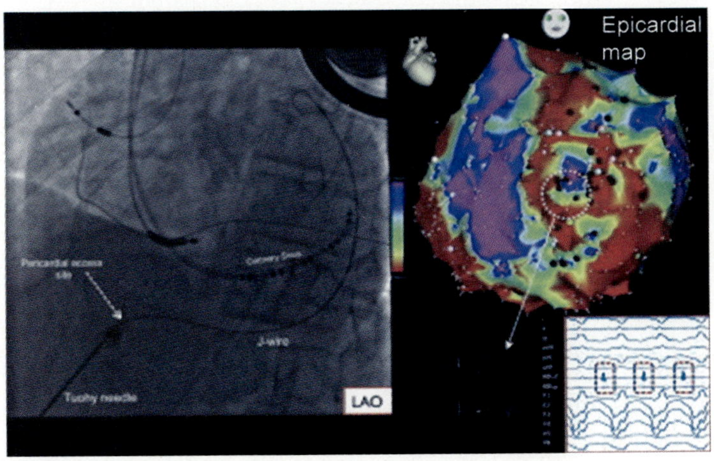


**Fig. 39.50:** Epicardial access and mapping for ventricular tachycardia (VT). The left panel depicts an image of epicardial access in the left anterior oblique (LAO) projection. The Tuohy needle is seen entering the pericardium as indicated, small amounts of contrast are injected during the course of the needle to identify structures passed in its trajectory. A J-tipped wire passed through the needle into pericardial space outlines the lateral heart border in LAO. The right panel image depicts an epicardial voltage map in the LAO projection. A site with late potentials during baseline paced rhythm is shown (broken white circle and inset), as well as the diastolic potentials recorded during VT

tion was most evident in patients who had three-vessel disease and CHF.

Surgical treatment of ventricular arrhythmias in patients with nonischemic heart disease includes excision of VT foci after endocardial mapping and excision of LV aneurysms. This is performed with decreasing frequency, because of perioperative mortality and the alternative, transvenous ICD implantation.

**Aortic valve replacement** is associated with improved outcome in patients with hemodynamically significant valvular stenosis and well-preserved ventricular function. In patients with MVP associated with significant valvular regurgitation and LV dysfunction, malignant tachyarrhythmias and SCD have been reported. These patients are candidates for mitral valve repair or replacement. Orthotopic heart transplantation is indicated in cases of SCD and refractory heart failure in which significant improvement in actuarial survival is expected. Given a limited donor service, this form of treatment is expected to be beneficial for very few people who survive SCD.

Patients with long QT syndrome who do not respond to beta-blockers are candidates for ICD implantation or high thoracic left sympathectomy.

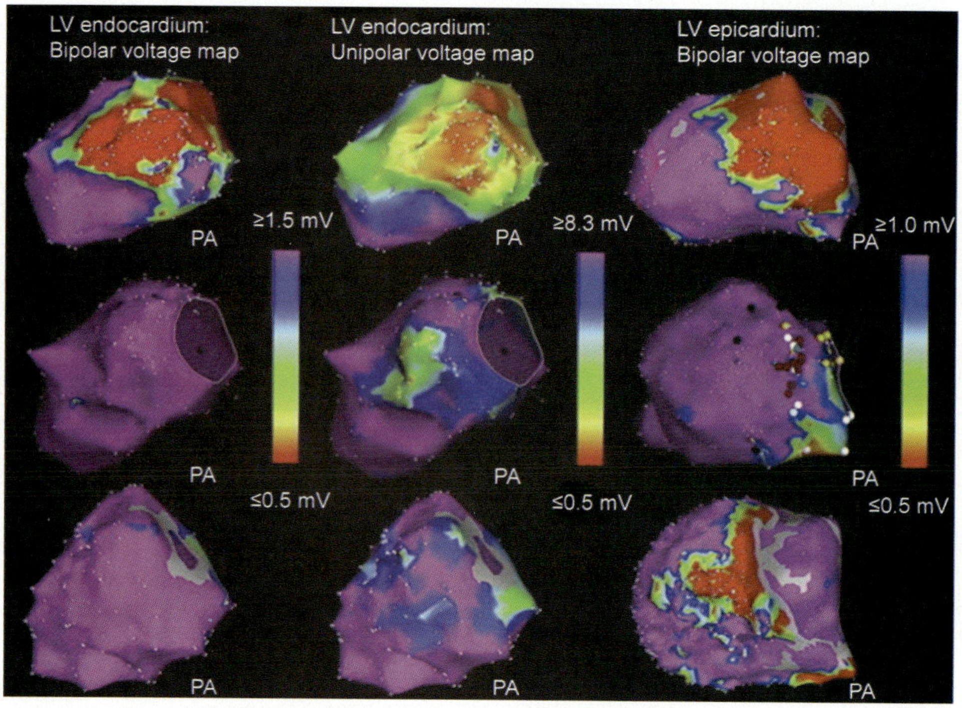


**Fig. 39.51:** Representative three-dimensional electroanatomic maps from three patients with IDCM who underwent VT ablation. LV endocardial and epicardial voltage maps are displayed in the posterior-anterior projection, using the typical color spectrum to represent tissue voltage characteristics (red indicates scar and purple indicates healthy tissue). Two types of signals are displayed in which 'bipolar' reflects a narrower field of view and 'unipolar', which encompasses tissue characteristics further from the catheter tip. (Patient A) low endocardial and epicardial voltage is present in the perivalvular region consistent with transmural scar. (Patient B) normal endocardial and epicardial bipolar voltage but abnormal unipolar voltage, suggestive of isolated mid-myocardial scar. (Patient C) normal endocardial voltage but patchy scar in the basal-lateral epicardium extending to the midwall. LV=left ventricle; PA=posterior-anterior projection; mV=millivolt

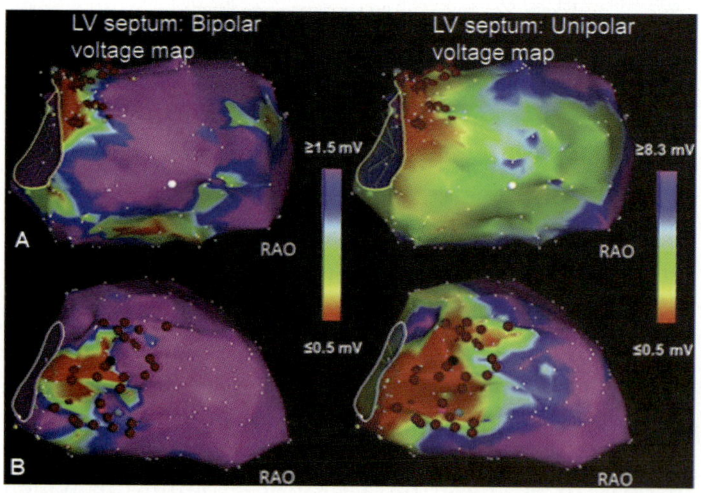


**Fig. 39.52:** Representative three-dimensional electroanatomic maps of two patients with IDCM and VT arising from the interventricular septum. LV bipolar and unipolar voltage is displayed in the right anterior oblique projection. Note that patients A and B possess septal VT substrate with a large intramural component, as indicated by limited bipolar low voltage and more extensive areas of unipolar low voltage. Sites of radiofrequency lesions are shown (red markers). LV=left ventricle; RAO=righanterior oblique projection; mV=millivolt

## Consultations

A cardiologist always should be participating in the care of these patients. Cardiac electrophysiologists should be involved in the care of these patients, which generally involves ICD implantation.

Other consultations for expertise include an interventional cardiologist and cardiac surgeon, and are made on an individual basis.

## Diet

Patients with coronary artery disease are advised to follow a diet low in fat and cholesterol. Patients with severe heart failure should monitor their fluid and sodium intake.

# MEDICATION SUMMARY

Medications are prescribed on an individual basis, depending on the underlying cause of SCD.

## Transfer

Patients should be at centers where intensive cardiac monitoring and appropriate invasive and noninvasive studies can be performed. In general, a cardiovascular service, including interventional cardiology, electrophysiology, and cardiac surgery, is needed.

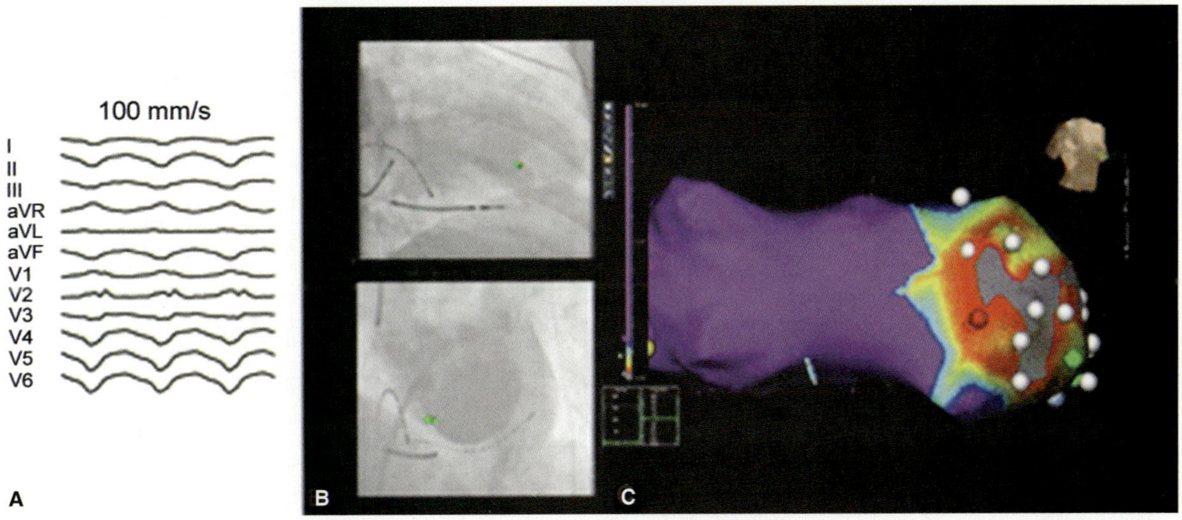


**Fig. 39.53:** Substrate analysis in a patient with a remote anterior myocardial infarction, a large aneurysm of the left ventricle, and ventricular tachycardia. (A) The 12-lead ECG of the tachycardia with a speed of 100 mm/s. (B) The left ventricular aneurysm as depicted with left ventriculography. In this case, the novel MediGuide™ Technology (St Jude Medical Inc., St Paul, MN, USA) for catheter navigation on pre-recorded cine loops was applied. (C) Voltage mapping of the left ventricle in the electrophysiology laboratory with the use of the Ensite NavX™ system (St Jude Medical Inc.). In the reconstructed three-dimensional model of the left ventricle, the grey color depicts scar, the purple depicts healthy myocardium, and the colors in-between depict diseased myocardium based on the voltage of the local electrograms at the different points of the left ventricle

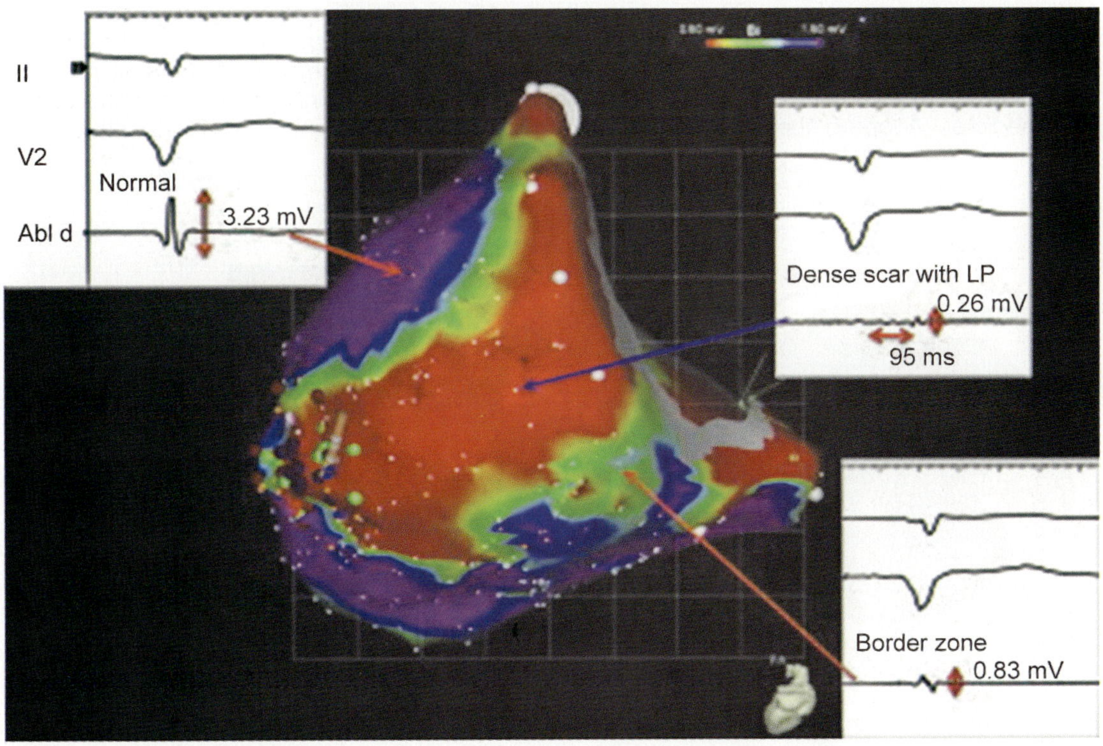


**Fig. 39.54:** Bipolar electrogram morphology in ischemic heart disease substrates. Representative examples of bipolar electrograms (and amplitudes) recorded from regions of 'normal', dense scar, and border zone myocardium are shown superimposed onto a voltage map (0.5–1.5 mV). A significant portion of the electrograms recorded in the dense car region are 'late' (i.e. occur well after the surface QRS) and are very low in amplitude (<0.5 mV)

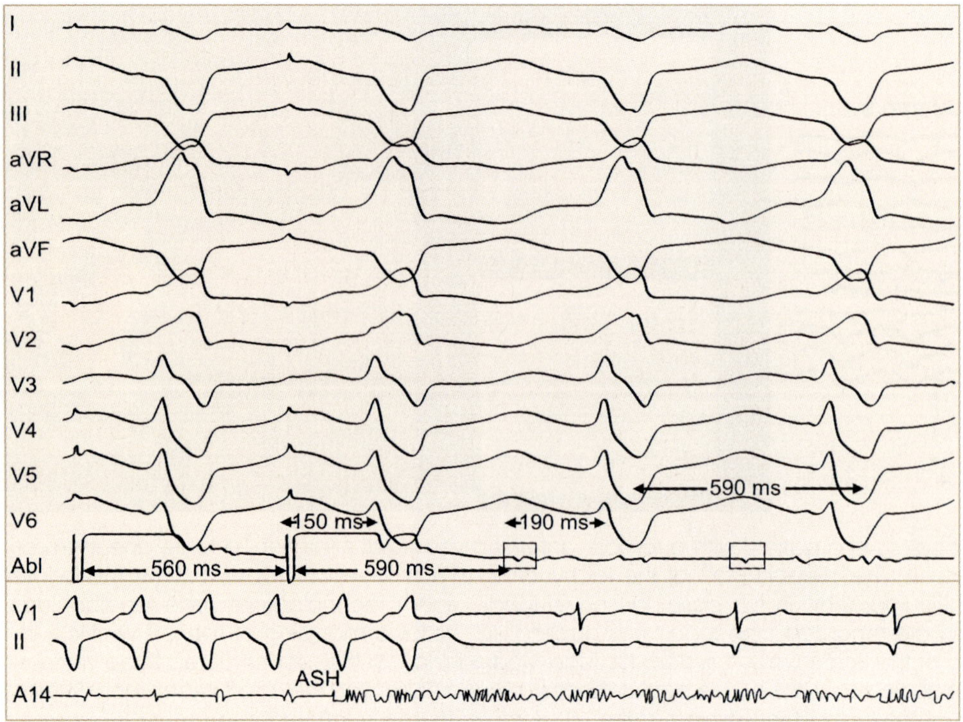


**Fig. 39.55:** Entrainment and ablation of monomorphic ventricular tachycardia (MMVT). Top panel—an MMVT with a cycle length of 590 ms is entrained at 560 ms. The post-pacing interval (PPI) is 590 ms, and exactly matches the TCL. The stimulus to QRS (Stim-QRS) interval shown on the last paced complex is 190 ms, which also exactly matches the electrogram to QRS (EGM-QRS) interval at 190 ms. The entrainment demonstrated here is also concealed (paced QRS morphology is identical to MMVT QRS morphology, i.e. no evidence of QRS fusion). These conditions (PPI=TCL, Stim-QRS=EGM-QRS, and concealed entrainment) confirm that the site is a protected and critical isthmus for this MMVT. Lower panel—ablation at the site with entrainment characteristics demonstrated above terminates MMVT immediately. Adapted from Tung R, Boyle NG, Shivkumar K. Circulation. 2011;123(20):2284–2288

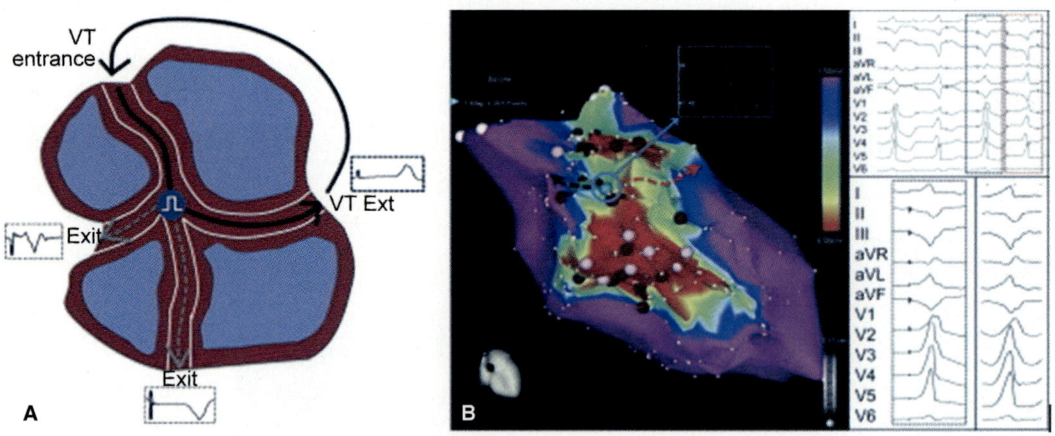


**Fig. 39.56:** Multiple exit sites and channels. (A) Schematic representation of interconnected channels with a common isthmus, and three spatially separate exits, each producing a distinct QRS morphology. (B) The image on the left depicts the electroanatomic map from a patient with inferior wall low voltage areas (0.5–1.5 mV). The electrogram recorded at an isthmus site (inset, indicated by blue circle and arrow) with two exits is shown. Pacing at this site produced two distinct QRS morphologies and two stimulus to QRS intervals (black and red box in top right tracing). One of the paced QRS morphologies (black box) matches the clinical VT (shown in right lower tracing). Adapted from Tung R, Mathuria N, Michowitz Y et al. Circ Arrhythmia Electrophysiol 2012;5:264–272

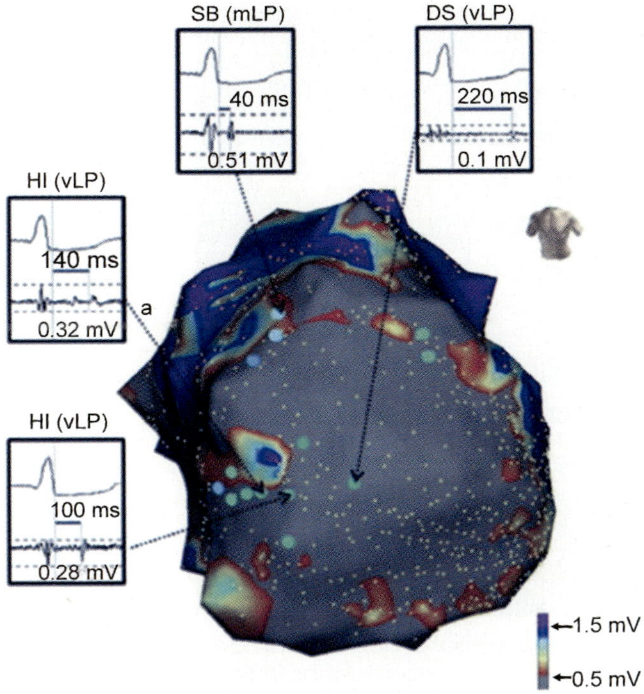


**Fig. 39.57:** Distribution of late potentials in ischemic heart disease substrates. An electroanatomic map is shown in anteroposterior view depicting an anterior myocardial infarction, with heterogeneous islets (HIs, regions of preserved voltage within dense scar) shown. Very late potentials (VLPs, green tags) were recorded around HIs or dense scar (DS) areas. Mid-late potentials (MLPs, blue tags) were recorded at scar border SB between DS and normal tissue. Yellow dots reflect electrogram sampling points. Adapted from Nakahara S, Tung R, Ramirez RJ et al. Heart Rhythm 2010;7:1817–1824

## Prognosis

Prognosis of morbidity and mortality for people who have had SCA can be made using the cardiac arrest score developed by McCullough and Thompson (*see* Physical). The detection of the underlying cause of SCD and available treatment options play an important role in the natural history and prognosis of SCD. SCD/SCA is a frequently encountered problem for emergency physicians, internists, and cardiologists. Ischemic cardiomyopathy in all adult cases and HCM in pediatric and adolescent cases are at the top of the list of causes of SCA. The clinical course, once the patient is resuscitated, largely is predicted by the ED presentation of hemodynamic stability, early neurologic recovery, and the duration of the resuscitation. Patients who survive the initial phases require a systematic evaluation of LV performance, myocardial perfusion, and electrophysiologic instability. Survivors of SCA have a recurrence rate on the order of 20–25% per year, making ICD implantation important in the majority of these patients. ICD implantation saves lives. Risk stratification will continue to be an area of active research. Preventive measures, at their roots, are measures of coronary artery disease prevention. Efforts to inform and train the public about external defibrillator use likely will have a great public health impact on improving survival rates of SCA. However, more basic and clinical research is required to understand the mechanism of VF/VT and to be able to identify the patients at risk who benefit from ICD therapy.

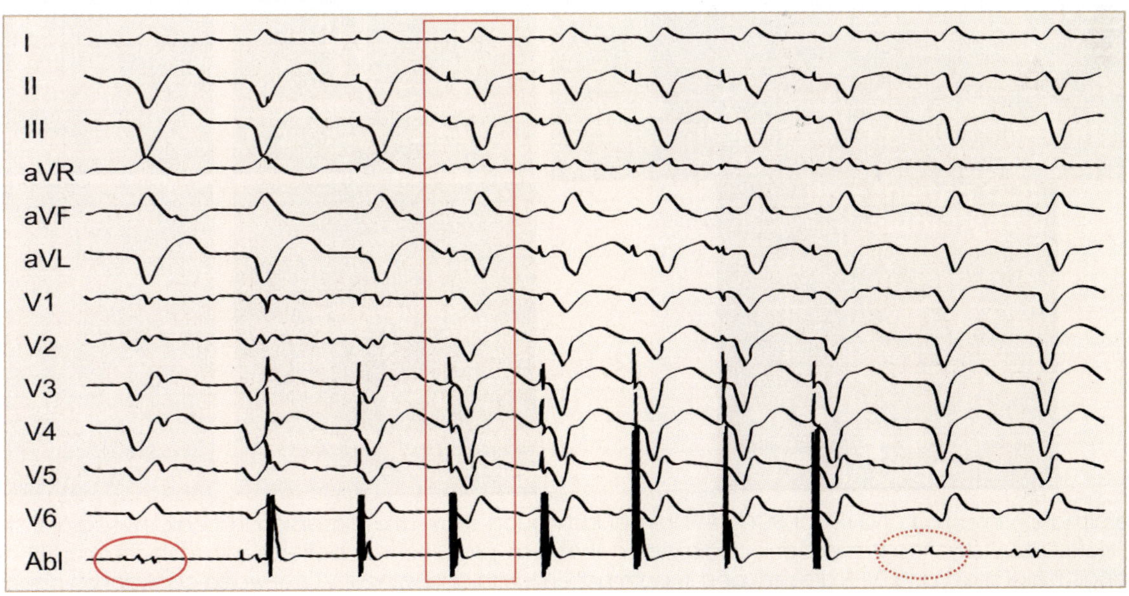


**Fig. 39.58:** Pace map induction (PMI). A representative tracing showing PMI. Low amplitude electrograms with split potentials (solid red circle on ablation catheter, Abl) recorded at a site from which pacing induced a monomorphic ventricular tachycardia (MMVT). The red box indicates the first beat of MMVT. The split potentials become diastolic potentials during MMVT (broken red circle)

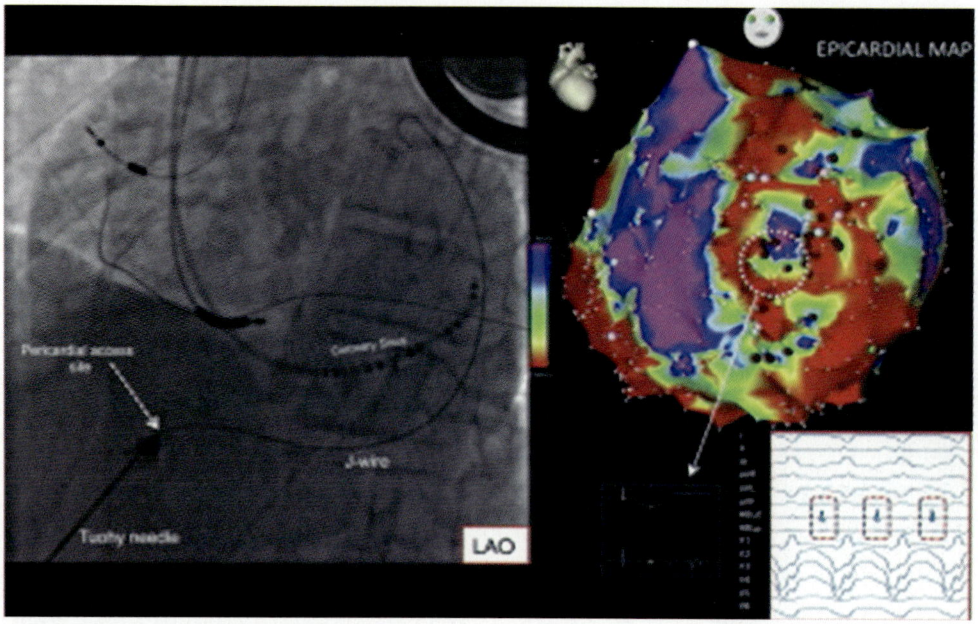


**Fig. 39.59:** Epicardial access and mapping for ventricular tachycardia (VT). The left panel depicts an image of epicardial access in the left anterior oblique (LAO) projection. The Tuohy needle is seen entering the pericardium as indicated, small amounts of contrast are injected during the course of the needle to identify structures passed in its trajectory. A J-tipped wire passed through the needle into pericardial space outlines the lateral heart border in LAO. The right panel image depicts an epicardial voltage map in the LAO projection. A site with late potentials during baseline paced rhythm is shown (broken white circle and inset), as well as the diastolic potentials recorded during VT

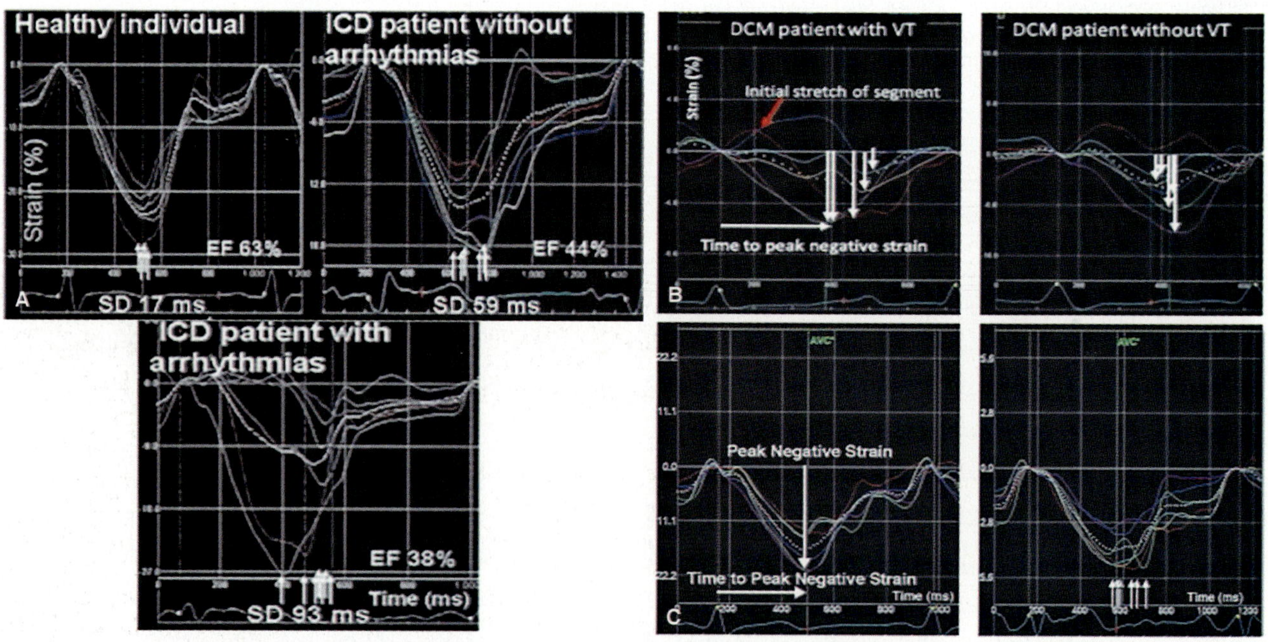


**Fig. 39.60:** Deformation imaging and risk of SCD. (A) Normal individuals show little dispersion in peak myocardial strain timing but abnormal ventricles show significant mechanical dispersion that was prominent in patients with arrhythmias. (B) In patients with DCM, global longitudinal strain and LVEF are reduced in both patients with and without VT but worse contraction dispersion was seen in a patient with VT. (C) Similarly, dispersion is worse in post-MI patients who have arrhythmic events. Modified from Haugaa et al. J Am Coll Cardiol Img 2010;3:247–256; JASE 2012;25,667–673; J Am Coll Cardiol Img 2013;6:2013;841–850

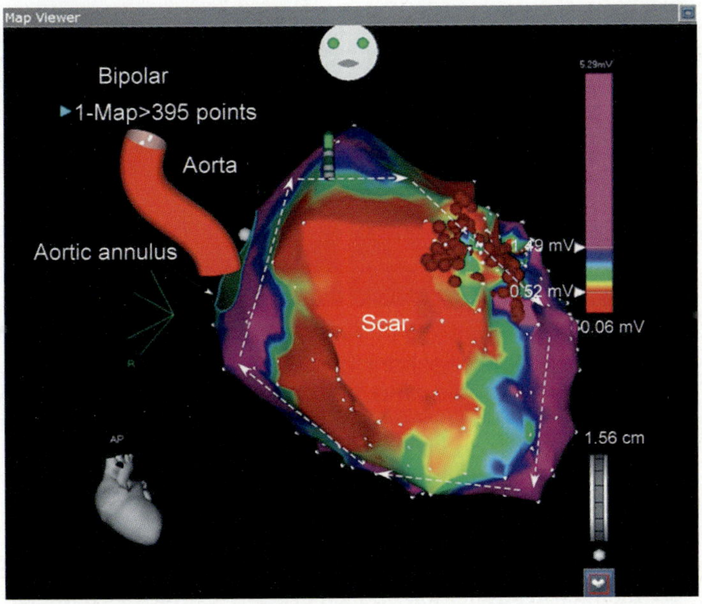


**Fig. 39.61:** The picture shows the anteroposterior projection of the enlarged left ventricle with a large scar on almost all the anterior wall. Any voltage bellow 0.5 mV (red color) was considered scar and any voltage above 1.5 mV were considered normal myocardium (purple color). In between them three transitional tissues are collared in yellow, green and blue. No tissue penetrated the scar and no central pathways could be mapped. The arrows show the large re-entry cycle around the scar. Normal myocardium is around the scar and constitutes the re-entry circle. The ablation points (red dots) block the isthmus between two scars

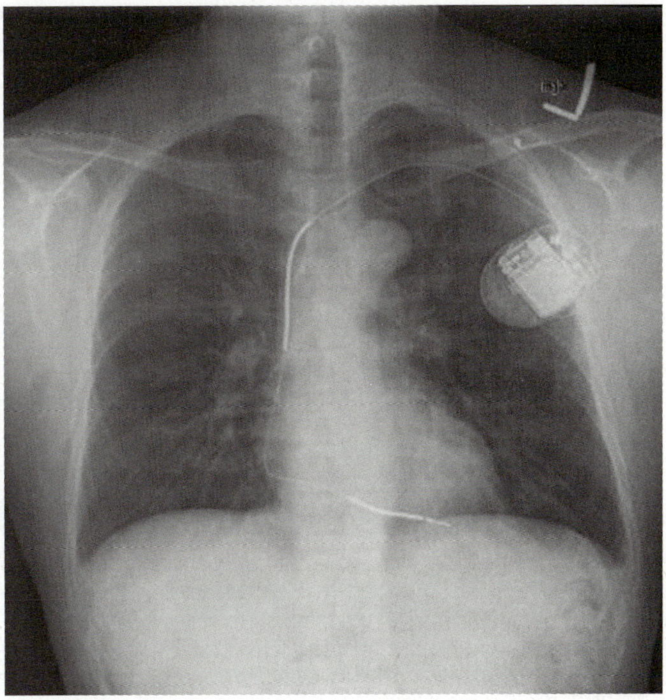

**Fig. 39.62:** A normal chest X-ray after placement of an ICD, showing the ICD generator in the upper left chest and the ICD lead in the right ventricle of the heart. Note the two opaque coils along the ICD lead

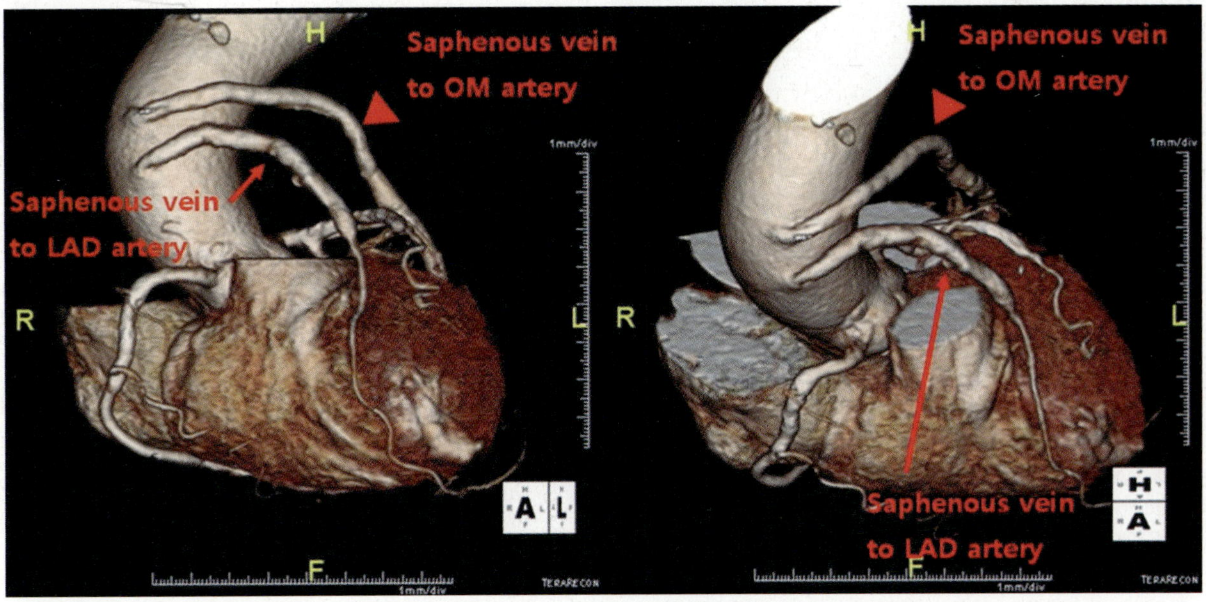


**Fig. 39.63:** Saphenous vein grafts. Three-dimensional volume-rendered images show the typical appearance of right (arrow) and left (arrowhead) saphenous vein grafts (SVGs) sutured to the anterior aorta. The right SVG is attached to the mid-portion of left anterior descending (LAD) artery and the left SVG is attached to the obtuse marginal (OM) artery

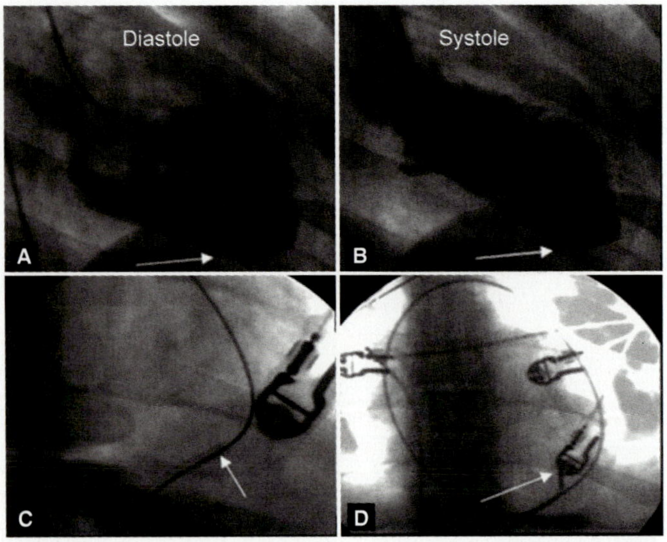


**Fig. 39.64:** (A) Inferolateral left ventricular aneurysm in diastole (arrow). A black line is drawn to indicate its border. (B) Inferolateral left ventricular aneurysm in systole (arrow). A black line is again drawn to indicate its border. (C) Access to the epicardial space with the ablation catheter. (D) Tip (8 mm) of the ablation catheter at the successful radiofrequency ablation lesion

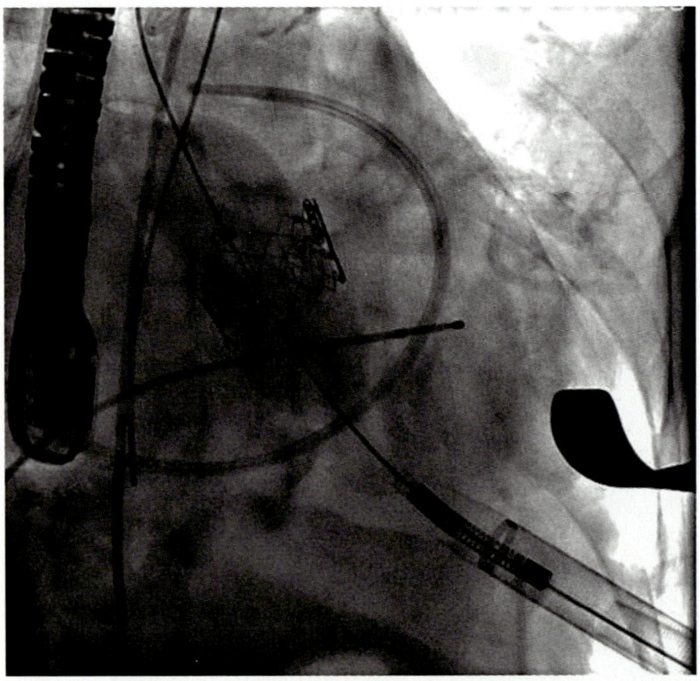

**Fig. 39.65:** The valve is deployed in position during direct fluoroscopic visualization with a brief period of rapid ventricular pacing to reduce ejection in an elderly person with severe aortic stenosis

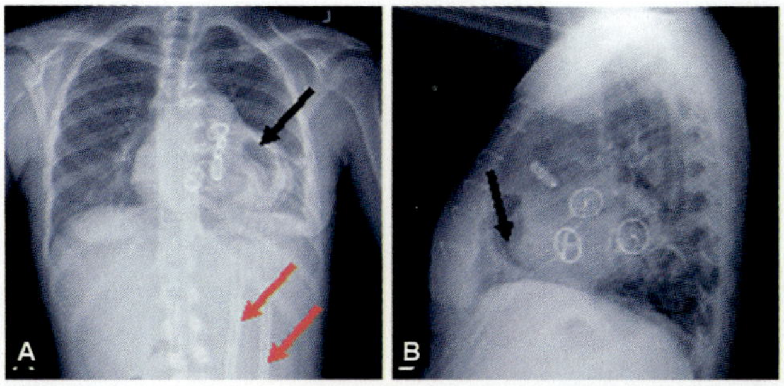


**Fig. 39.66:** Posteroanterior (A) and lateral (B) chest X-ray views of a patient with a total mechanical heart. The black arrows indicate pneumatic chambers, and the red arrows show the airflow cables. The native cardiac valves have been removed; all valves are part of the mechanical heart

## BIBLIOGRAPHY


1. Adielsson A, Hollenberg J, Karlsson T, et al. Increase in survival and bystander CPR in out-of-hospital shockable arrhythmia: bystander CPR and female gender are predictors of improved outcome. Experiences from Sweden in an 18-year perspective. Heart 2011;97(17):1391–6.
2. Altemose GT, Buxton AE. Idiopathic ventricular tachycardia. Annu Rev Med 1999;50:159–77.
3. American Heart Association Guidelines for Cardiopulmonary Resuscitation and Emergency Cardiovascular Care Science Circ 2010;
4. Anderson KP, Freedman RA, Mason JW. Sudden death in idiopathic dilated cardiomyopathy. Ann Intern Med 1987; 107(1):104–6.
5. Antiarrhythmics Versus Implantable Defibrillators Investigators. A comparison of antiarrhythmic-drug therapy with implantable defibrillators in patients resuscitated from near-fatal ventricular arrhythmias. The Antiarrhythmics versus Implantable Defibrillators (AVID) Investigators. N Engl J Med 1997;337(22):1576–83.
6. Bardy GH, Lee KL, Mark DB, et al. Amiodarone or an implant-able cardioverter-defibrillator for congestive heart failure. N Engl J Med 2005;20;352(3):225–37.
7. Bardy GH, Lee KL, Mark DB, et al. Home Use of Automated ExternalDefibrillators for Sudden Cardiac Arrest. N Engl J Med 2008;24;358(17):1793–804.
8. Bayes de Luna A, Coumel P, Leclercq JF. Ambulatory sudden cardiac death: mechanisms of production of fatal arrhythmia on the basis of data from 157 cases. Am Heart J 1989;117(1): 151–9.
9. Belhassen B, Viskin S. Idiopathic ventricular tachycardia and fibrillation. J Cardiovasc Electrophysiol 1993;4(3):356–68.
10. Benditt DG, Pritchett LC, Smith WM, et al. Characteristics of atrioventricular conduction and the spectrum of arrhythmias in Lown-Ganong-Levine syndrome. Circulation 1978; 57(3): 454–65.
11. Berdowski J, Blom MT, Bardai A, Tan HL, Tijssen JG, Koster RW. Impact of Onsite or Dispatched Automated External Defibrillator Use on Survival After Out-of-Hospital Cardiac Arrest. Circulation 2011;124(20):2225–32.
12. Berger S, Dhala A, Friedberg DZ. Sudden cardiac death in infants, children, and adolescents. Pediatr Clin North Am 1999;46(2):221–34.
13. Beta-blocker Heart Attack Research Group. A randomized trial of propranolol in patients with acute myocardial infarction. I. Mortality results. JAMA 1982;247(12):1707–14.
14. Bigger JT, Fleiss JL, Kleiger R. The relationships among ventricular arrhythmias, left ventricular dysfunction, and mortality in the 2 years after myocardial infarction. Circulation 1984;69(2):250–8.

15. Bigger JT. Prophylactic use of implanted cardiac defibrillators in patients at high risk for ventricular arrhythmias after coronary-artery bypass graft surgery. Coronary Artery Bypass Graft (CABG) Patch Trial Investigators. N Engl J Med 1997;337(22):1569–75.
16. Blackstone EH, Kirklin JW. Death and other time-related events after valve a replacement. Circulation 1985;72(4): 753–67.
17. Bobrow BJ, Spaite DW, Berg RA, Stolz U, Sanders AB, Kern KB. Chest compression-only CPR by lay rescuers and survival from out-of-hospital cardiac arrest. JAMA 2010; 304(13):1447–54.
18. Bromberg BI, Lindsay BD, Cain ME. Impact of clinical history and electrophysiologic characterization of accessory pathways on management strategies to reduce sudden death among children with Wolff-Parkinson-White syndrome. J Am Coll Cardiol 1996;27(3):690–5.
19. Brooks A, Schinde V, Bateman AC, Gallagher PJ. Interstitial fibrosis in the dilated non-ischaemic myocardium. Heart 2003;89(10):1255–6.
20. Brugada J, Brugada R, Brugada P. Right bundle-branch block and ST-segment elevation in leads V1 through V3: a marker for sudden death in patients without demonstrable structural heart disease. Circulation 1998;97(5):457–60.
21. Brugada P, Brugada J. A distinct clinical and echocardiographic syndrome: right bundle branch block, persistent ST-segment elevation with normal QT interval and sudden cardiac death. PACE 1991;14:746–51.
22. Brugada R, Hong K, Cordeiro JM. Short QT syndrome. CMAJ 2005;173(11):1349–54.
23. Burkart F, Pfisterer M, Kiowski W. Effect of antiarrhythmic therapy on mortality in survivors of myocardial infarction with asymptomatic complex ventricular arrhythmias: Basel Antiarrhythmic Study of Infarct Survival (BASIS). J Am Coll Cardiol 1990;16(7):1711–8.
24. Burke AP, Farb A, Malcom GT. Coronary risk factors and plaque morphology in men with coronary disease who died suddenly. N Engl J Med 1997;336(18):1276–82.
25. Cairns JA, Connolly SJ, Roberts R. Randomised trial of outcome after myocardial infarction in patients with frequent or repetitive ventricular premature depolarisations: CAMIAT. Canadian Amiodarone Myocardial Infarction Arrhythmia Trial Investigators. Lancet 1997;349(9053): 675–682.
26. Cardiac Arrhythmia Suppression Trial Investigators. Preliminary report: effect of encainide and flecainide on mortality in a randomized trial of arrhythmia suppression after myocardial infarction. The Cardiac Arrhythmia Suppression Trial (CAST) Investigators. N Engl J Med 1989; 321(6):406–12.
27. Chang D, Goldstein S. Sudden cardiac death in ischemic heart disease. Compr Ther 1997;23(2):95–103.
28. Chizner MA, Pearle DL, deLeon AC. The natural history of aortic stenosis in adults. Am Heart J 1980;99(4):419–24.
29. Corrado D, Basso C, Thiene G. Spectrum of clinicopathologic manifestations of arrhythmogenic right ventricular cardio-myo-pathy/dysplasia: a multicenter study. J Am Coll Cardiol. 1997;30(6):1512–20.
30. Davies MJ, Thomas A. Thrombosis and acute coronary-artery lesions in sudden cardiac ischemic death. N Engl J Med 1984; 310(18):1137–40.
31. Davies MJ. The investigation of sudden cardiac death. Histopathology 1999;34(2):93–8.
32. de Vreede-Swagemakers JJ, Gorgels AP, Dubois-Arbouw WI, van Ree JW, Daemen MJ, Houben LG, et al. Out-of-hospital cardiac arrest in the 1990's: a population-based study in the Maastricht area on incidence, characteristics and survival. J Am Coll Cardiol 1997;30(6):1500–5.
33. Delise P, Allocca G, Marras E, et al. Risk stratification in individuals with the Brugada type 1 ECG pattern without previous cardiac arrest: usefulness of a combined clinical and electrophysiologic approach. Eur Heart J 2011;32(2):169–76.
34. DeRose JJ, Banas JS, Winters SL. Current perspectives on sudden cardiac death in hypertrophic cardiomyopathy. Prog Cardiovasc Dis 1994;36(6):475–84.
35. Derval N, Simpson CS, Birnie DH, et al. Prevalence and Characteristics of Early Repolarization in the CASPER Registry Cardiac Arrest Survivors With Preserved Ejection Fraction Registry. J Am Coll Cardiol 2011;58(7):722–8.
36. Domanski MJ, Zipes DP, Schron E. Treatment of sudden cardiac death. Current understandings from randomized trials and future research directions. Circulation 1997;95(12): 2694–9.
37. Doval HC, Nul DR, Grancelli HO. Nonsustained ventricular tachycardia in severe heart failure. Independent marker of increased mortality due to sudden death. GESICA-GEMA Investigators. Circulation 1996;94(12):3198–203.
38. Doyle JT, Kannel WB, McNamara PM. Factors related to suddenness of death from coronary disease: combined Albany-Framingham studies. Am J Cardiol 1976;37(7): 1073–8.
39. Driscoll DJ, Edwards WD. Sudden unexpected death in children and adolescents. J Am Coll Cardiol 1985;5(6 Suppl): 118B–21B.
40. Dumas F, Grimaldi D, Zuber B, et al. Is hypothermia after cardiac arrest effective in both shockable and nonshockable patients?: insights from a large registry. Circulation 2011; 123(8):877–86.
41. Echt DS, Liebson PR, Mitchell LB. Mortality and morbidity in patients receiving encainide, flecainide, or placebo. The Cardiac Arrhythmia Suppression Trial. N Engl J Med 1991; 324(12):781–8.
42. Ehtisham J, Watkins H. Is Wolff-Parkinson-White syndrome a genetic disease?. J Cardiovasc Electrophysiol 2005;16(11): 1258–62.
43. Ezekowitz JA, Rowe BH, Dryden DM, et al. Systematic review: implantable cardioverter defibrillators for adults with left ventricular systolic dysfunction. Ann Intern Med 2007;21;147(4):251–62.
44. Fielitz J, Hein S, Mitrovic V, et al. Activation of the cardiac renin-angiotensin system and increased myocardial collagen expression in human aortic valve disease. J Am Coll Cardiol 2001;37(5):1443–9.
45. Garson A, McNamara DG. Sudden death in a pediatric cardiology population, 1958 to 1983: relation to prior arrhythmias. J Am Coll Cardiol 1985;5(6 Suppl):134B–137B.

46. Gillum RF. Coronary heart disease in black populations. I. Mortality and morbidity. Am Heart J 1982;104(4 Pt 1): 839–851.
47. Gillum RF. Sudden coronary death in the United States: 1980-1985. Circulation 1989;79(4):756–65.
48. Gilman JK, Jalal S, Naccarelli GV. Predicting and preventing sudden death from cardiac causes. Circulation 1994;90(2): 1083–92.
49. Giustetto C, Schimpf R, Mazzanti A, et al. Long-Term Follow-Up of Patients With Short QT Syndrome. J Am Coll Cardiol 2011;58(6):587–95.
50. Goldberger JJ. Treatment and prevention of sudden cardiac death: effect of recent clinical trials. Arch Intern Med 1999; 159(12):1281–7.
51. Goldstein S, Landis JR, Leighton R. Characteristics of the resuscitated out-of-hospital cardiac arrest victim with coro-nary heart disease. Circulation 1981;64(5):977–84.
52. Goldstein S. The necessity of a uniform definition of sudden coronary death: witnessed death within 1 hour of the onset of acute symptoms. Am Heart J 1982;103(1):156–9.
53. Gollob MH, Redpath CJ, Roberts JD. The Short QT Syndrome Proposed Diagnostic Criteria. J Am Coll Cardiol 2011;57(7): 802–12.
54. Gottlieb SS. The use of antiarrhythmic agents in heart failure: implications of CAST. Am Heart J 1989;118(5 Pt 1):1074–7.
55. Gulati A, Jabbour A, Ismail TF, Guha K, Khwaja J, Raza S, et al. Association of fibrosis with mortality and sudden cardiac death in patients with nonischemic dilated cardiomyopathy. JAMA 2013;309(9):896–908.
56. Haïssaguerre M, Derval N, Sacher F, Jesel L, Deisenhofer I, de Roy L, et al. Sudden cardiac arrest associated with early repolarization. N Engl J Med 2008;358(19):2016–23.
57. Holmes DR, Davis KB, Mock MB. The effect of medical and surgical treatment on subsequent sudden cardiac death in patients with coronary artery disease: a report from the Coronary Artery Surgery Study.Circulation 1986;73(6): 1254–63.
58. Holzer M. Targeted temperature management for comatose survivors of cardiac arrest. N Engl J Med 2010;363(13): 1256–64.
59. Ikeda Y, Yutani C, Huang Y, et al. Histological remodeling in an ovine heart failure model resembles human ischemic cardiomyopathy. Cardiovasc Pathol 2001;10(1):19–27.
60. Iseri LT, Humphrey SB, Siner EJ. Prehospital brady-asystolic cardiac arrest. Ann Intern Med 1978;88(6):741–5.
61. Itoh H, Horie M, Ito M. Arrhythmogenesis in the short-QT syndrome associated with combined HERG channel gating defects: a simulation study. Circ J 2006;70(4):502–8.
62. Jaoude SA, Leclercq JF, Coumel P. Progressive ECG changes in arrhythmogenic right ventricular disease. Evidence for an evolving disease. Eur Heart J 1996;17(11):1717–22.
63. Kadish A, Dyer A, Daubert JP, et al. Prophylactic defibrillator implantation in patients with nonischemic dilated cardio-myo-pathy. N Engl J Med 2004;20;350(21):2151–8.
64. Kannel WB, Cupples LA, D'Agostino RB. Sudden death risk in overt coronary heart disease: the Framingham Study. Am Heart J 1987;113(3):799–804.
65. Kuller LH. Sudden death—definition and epidemiologic considerations. Prog Cardiovasc Dis 1980;23(1):1–12.
66. Kunavarapu C, Bloomfield DM. Role of noninvasive studies in risk stratification for sudden cardiac death.Clin Cardiol 2004;27(4):192–7.
67. Ladich E, Virmani R, Burke A. Sudden cardiac death not related to coronary atherosclerosis. Toxicol Pathol 2006; 34(1):52–7.
68. Latini R, Maggioni AP, Flather M. ACE inhibitor use in patients with myocardial infarction. Summary of evidence from clinical trials. Circulation 1995;92(10):3132–7.
69. Lerman BB, Stein KM, Markowitz SM. Idiopathic right ventricular outflow tract tachycardia: a clinical approach. Pacing Clin Electrophysiol 1996;19(12 Pt 1):2120–37.
70. Lombardi G, Gallagher J, Gennis P. Outcome of out-of-hospital cardiac arrest in New York City. The Pre-Hospital Arrest Survival Evaluation (PHASE) Study. JAMA 1994; 271(9):678–83.
71. Makikallio TH, Barthel P, Schneider R. Frequency of sudden cardiac death among acute myocardial infarction survivors with optimized medical and revascularization therapy. Am J Cardiol 2006;15;97(4):480–4.
72. Marcus FI, Fontaine GH, Guiraudon G. Right ventricular dysplasia: a report of 24 adult cases. Circulation 1982; 65(2): 384–98.
73. Maron BJ, Bonow RO, Cannon RO. Hypertrophic cardiomyopathy. Interrelations of clinical manifestations, pathophysiology, and therapy (2). N Engl J Med 1987; 316(14): 844–52.
74. Maron BJ, Epstein SE, Roberts WC. Causes of sudden death in competitive athletes. J Am Coll Cardiol 1986;7(1):204–14.
75. Maron BJ, Shirani J, Poliac LC. Sudden death in young competitive athletes. Clinical, demographic, and pathological profiles. JAMA 1996;276(3):199–204.
76. Maseri A, Severi S, Marzullo P. Role of coronary arterial spasm in sudden coronary ischemic death. Ann N Y Acad Sci 1982;382:204–17.
77. McCullough PA, Thompson RJ, Tobin KJ. Validation of a decision support tool for the evaluation of cardiac arrest victims. Clin Cardiol 1998;21(3):195–200.
78. Mehra R. Global public health problem of sudden cardiac death. Journal of Electrocardiology 2007;40(6 Suppl): S118–122.
79. Merchant FM, Ikeda T, Pedretti RF, Salerno-Uriarte JA, Chow T, Chan PS, et al. Clinical utility of microvolt T-wave alternans testing in identifying patients at high or low risk of sudden cardiac death. Heart Rhythm 2012;9(8):1256–1264.e2.
80. Metoprolol in Acute Myocardial Infarction Trial Research Group. Metoprolol in acute myocardial infarction (MIAMI). A randomised placebo-controlled international trial. The MIAMI Trial Research Group. Eur Heart J 1985;6(3):199–226.
81. Moss AJ, Hall WJ, Cannom DS, et al. Improved survival with an implanted defibrillator in patients with coronary disease at high risk for ventricular arrhythmia. N Engl J Med 1996; 26;335(26):1933–40.
82. Moss AJ, Schwartz PJ, Crampton RS. The long QT syndrome. Prospective longitudinal study of 328 families. Circulation 1991;84(3):1136–44.
83. Moss AJ, Zareba W, Hall WJ, et al. Prophylactic implantation of a defibrillator in patients with myocardial infarction and

reduced ejection fraction. N Engl J Med 2002;21;346(12): 877–83.

84. Moss AJ. Prognosis after myocardial infarction. Am J Cardiol 1983;52(7):667–9 [Medline].
85. Myerburg RJ, Castellanos A. Cardiac arrest and sudden cardiac death. In: Brunwald E, ed. Heart Disease: A Textbook of Cardiovascular Medicine. 4th ed. Philadelphia, Pa: WB Saunders, 1992:756–89.
86. Myerburg RJ, Estes D, Zaman L. Outcome of resuscitation from bradyarrhythmic or asystolic prehospital cardiac arrest. J Am Coll Cardiol 1984;4(6):1118–22.
87. Myerburg RJ, Kessler KM, Castellanos A. Sudden cardiac death. Structure, function, and time-dependence of risk. Circulation 1992;85(1 Suppl):I2–10.
88. Nademanee K, Singh BN, Stevenson WG. Amiodarone and post-MI patients. Circulation 1993;88(2):764–74.
89. Napolitano C, Bloise R, Priori SG. Long QT syndrome and short QT syndrome: how to make correct diagnosis and what about eligibility for sports activity. J Cardiovasc Med (Hager-stown) 2006;7(4):250–6.
90. Narasimhan C, Jazayeri MR, Sra J. Ventricular tachycardia in valvular heart disease: facilitation of sustained bundle-branch re-entry by valve surgery. Circulation 1997;96(12): 4307–713.
91. Neumar RW, Barnhart JM, Berg RA, et al. Implementation Strategies for Improving Survival After Out-of-Hospital Cardiac Arrest in the United States: Consensus Recommendations From the 2009 American Heart Association Cardiac Arrest Survival Summit. Circulation 2011;123(24):2898–910.
92. Neuspiel DR, Kuller LH. Sudden and unexpected natural death in childhood and adolescence. JAMA 1985;254(10): 1321–5.
93. Prystowsky EN. Prevention of sudden cardiac death. Clin Cardiol 2005;28(11 Suppl 1):I12–18.
94. Rosen MR, Jause MJ, Myerburg RJ. Arrhythmias induced by coronary artery occlusion: what are the electrophysiologic mechanisms? In: Hearse DJ, Mannings AS, Janse M, (Eds.) Life-Threatening Arrhythmias During Ischemia and Infarction. New York, NY: Raven 1987;11–47.
95. Sarkozy A, Brugada P. Sudden cardiac death and inherited arrhythmia syndromes. J Cardiovasc Electrophysiol 2005;16 (Suppl 1):S8–20.
96. Schoenfeld MH, McGovern B, Garan H. Determinants of the outcome of electrophysiologic study in patients with ventricular tachyarrhythmias. J Am Coll Cardiol 1985;6(2): 298–306.
97. Shirani J, Pick R, Roberts WC, Maron BJ. Morphology and significance of the left ventricular collagen network in young patients with hypertrophic cardiomyopathy and sudden cardiac death. J Am Coll Cardiol 2000;35(1):36–44.
98. Sovari AA, Cesario D, Kocheril AG, Brugada R. Multiple episodes of ventricular tachycardia induced by silent coronary vasospasm. J Interv Card Electrophysiol 2008; 21(3):223–6.
99. Spirito P, Seidman CE, McKenna WJ. The management of hypertrophic cardiomyopathy. N Engl J Med 1997;336(11): 775–85.
100. Sra J, Akhtar M. Recent advances in understanding the mechanisms, diagnosis and treatment of congenital and acquired long QT syndrome. Indian Heart J 1996;48(6):639–51.
101. Stern S, Tzivoni D. Ventricular arrhythmias, sudden death, and silent myocardial ischemia. Prog Cardiovasc Dis 1992; 35(1):19–26.
102. Stevenson WG, Stevenson LW, Middlekauff HR. Sudden death prevention in patients with advanced ventricular dysfunction. Circulation 1993;88(6):2953–61.
103. Stiles S. Gd-Enhanced CMR Risk-Stratifies in Ischemics, Nonischemics; Clinical Value Uncertain. Medscape News 2013. Available at http://www.medscape.com/viewarticle/780491. Accessed 2013.
104. Tamburro P, Wilber D. Sudden death in idiopathic dilated cardiomyopathy. Am Heart J 1992;124(4):1035–45.
105. Tapanainen JM, Lindgren KS, Makikallio TH. Natriuretic peptides as predictors of non-sudden and sudden cardiac death after acute myocardial infarction in the beta-blocking era. J Am Coll Cardiol 2004;43(5):757–63.
106. Thompson RJ, McCullough PA, Kahn JK. Early prediction of death and neurologic outcome in out-of-hospital sudden death survivors in the emergency department. Circulation 1996;94:I–356.
107. Thompson RJ, McCullough PA, Kahn JK. Prediction of death and neurologic outcome in the emergency department in out-of-hospital cardiac arrest survivors. Am J Cardiol 1998;81(1): 17–21.
108. Viskin S, Lesh MD, Eldar M. Mode of onset of malignant ventricular arrhythmias in idiopathic ventricular fibrillation. J Cardiovasc Electrophysiol 1997;8(10):1115–20. [Medline].
109. Watanabe H, Chopra N, Laver D, Hwang HS, Davies SS, Roach DE. Flecainide prevents catecholaminergic poly-morphic ventricular tachycardia in mice and humans. Nat Med 2009;15(4):380–3.
110. Watkins H, McKenna WJ, Thierfelder L. Mutations in the genes for cardiac troponin T and alpha-tropomyosin in hypertrophic cardiomyopathy. N Engl J Med 1995;3 32(16): 1058–64.
111. Wellens HJ, Durrer D. Wolff-Parkinson-White syndrome and atrial fibrillation. Relation between refractory period of accessory pathway and ventricular rate during atrial fibril-lation. Am J Cardiol 1974;34(7):777–82.
112. Wenzel V, Krismer AC, Arntz HR, et al. A comparison of vasopressin and epinephrine for out-of-hospital cardiopulmonary resuscitation. N Engl J Med 2004;8;350(2): 105–13.
113. Westenskow P, Splawski I, Timothy KW. Compound muta-tions: a common cause of severe long-QT syndrome. Circulation 2004;109(15):1834–41.
114. Winslow RD, Mehta D, Fuster V. Sudden cardiac death: mechanisms, therapies and challenges. Nat Clin Pract Cardiovasc Med 2005;2(7):352–60.
115. Yusuf S, Peto R, Lewis J. Beta blockade during and after myocardial infarction: an overview of the randomized trials. Prog Cardiovasc Dis 1985;27(5):335–71.
116. Zipes DP, Wellens HJ. Sudden cardiac death. Circulation 1998;98(21):2334–51.

# 40 Hematological Disorders Affecting Cardiovascular System in Emergency Department

## ANEMIA AS A RISK FACTOR FOR CARDIOVASCULAR DISEASE

Anemia as a risk factor for cardiovascular disease. In the present review we examine the physiologic response to chronic anemia and describe potential adverse effects of anemia on myocardial and large arterial remodeling. The present observational data demonstrating that anemia is a risk factor for cardiovascular disease (CVD) outcomes in patients with chronic kidney disease and patients with heart failure. This also presents data that have evaluated the relationship of level of hematocrit to CVD outcomes in patients with ischemic heart disease and in patients in the general population. The results from the latter studies have been inconclusive and have been limited by lack of knowledge of the cause of anemia. This is potentially important because iron deficiency anemia may, in fact, improve endothelial function (Fig. 40.1).

Chronic anemia may have adverse effects on myocardial and large arterial remodeling. Decreased iron stores and, therefore, potentially, iron-deficiency anemia may, however, improve endothelial function and thereby decrease cardiovascular disease (CVD) outcomes. In this review we discuss observational and controlled trials that have evaluated the effect and treatment of chronic anemia on CVD outcomes in three populations—patients with chronic kidney disease (CKD); patients with CVD; and subjects in the general population.

## PATHOPHYSIOLOGY

### Effects of Anemia on the Myocardium

Although the exact role of anemia in promoting CVD is currently not well understood, maintenance of adequate tissue oxygenation in the anemic state is achieved by both nonhemodynamic and hemodynamic adaptations. Nonhemodynamic adaptations include increases in erythropoietin production and increases in intraerythrocytic concentrations of diphosphoglycerate. Hemodynamic changes include systemic arterial dilatation, which leads to a decreased systemic vascular resistance, and reduced afterload, which in turn may increase stroke volume.

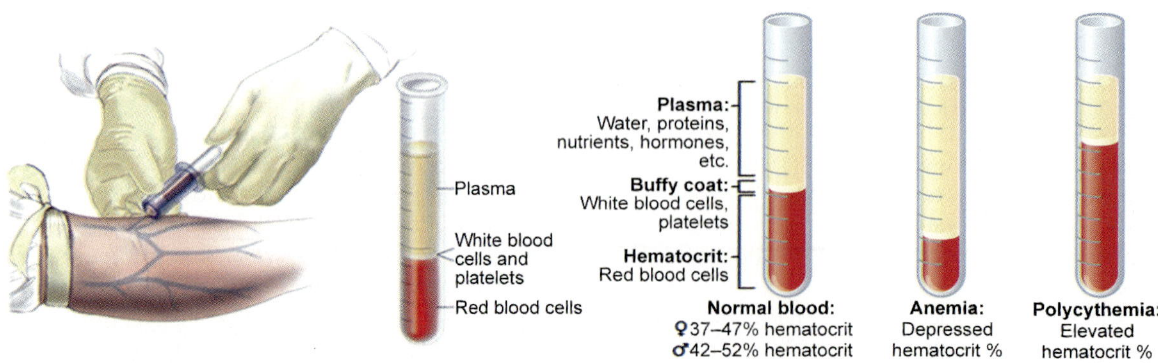


**Fig. 40.1:** Complete blood count (CBC). Blood is collected by inserting a needle into a vein and allowing the blood to flow into a tube. The blood sample is sent to the laboratory and the red blood cells, white blood cells, and platelets are counted. The CBC is used to test for, diagnose, and monitor many different conditions

Anemia also results in decreased blood viscosity, which increases venous return and thus, augments preload. Finally, the presence of anemia activates the sympathetic nervous system, which results in an increase in heart rate. Increased preload, heart rate, and stroke volume, as well as reduced afterload all act to raise cardiac output.

Over the long term, adaptations that initially increase cardiac output may lead to left ventricular enlargement and eccentric left ventricular hypertrophy (LVH), characterized by increased LV internal dimensions and a normal ratio of wall thickness to cavity diameter. The latter is well appreciated in patients with sickle cell disease, as well as in patients who are anemic secondary to their CKD. Patients with CKD also have a high prevalence of comorbid conditions such as hyperparathyroidism and a high calcium/phosphorus product, which may contribute to myocardial fibrosis and calcium deposition. In this setting, the effects of anemia on myocardial remodeling may be aggravated, resulting in more severe LVH and less reversible pathology. Left ventricular hypertrophy, in turn, may predispose to heart failure or aggravate ischemic heart disease (IHD). It remains unknown whether more subtle changes in cardiac remodeling may occur in patients with less severe degrees of anemia and in patients with other causes of anemia (Fig. 40.2).

### Effects of Anemia on the Blood Vessel Wall

Chronic anemia may also adversely affect large blood vessels, resulting in arterial hypertrophy and remodeling, occurring as a result of sustained increases in cardiac output. In theory, this may reverse the early vasodilatation characteristic of anemia and lead to increased systemic vascular resistance, which further contributes to the development of LVH. Early on, these changes may be reversible; however, in conditions such as CKD, they may become permanent.

### Effects of Anemia on Precipitating Ischemia in Subjects with Prevalent CVD

It has been shown that the resting human heart can withstand acute severe isovolemic anemia as low as 5.0 g/dl, without evidence of inadequate systemic oxygenation. Acute isovolemic hemoglobin reduction to 5.0 g/dl in 33 healthy resting subjects produced no evidence of hypoxia, assessed by change in oxygen consumption or an increase in plasma lactate concentration. Analysis of Holter readings suggests that at this level of hemoglobin concentration in the resting healthy population, myocardial ischemia would occur only infrequently. However, animal experiments and studies in postoperative patients with CVD suggest that the presence of IHD may significantly impair the heart's ability to tolerate low levels of hemoglobin.

## OTHER REASONS WHY ANEMIA MAY BE ASSOCIATED WITH CVD OUTCOMES

It is important to recognize that, although studies may demonstrate an association between anemia and CVD outcomes, this does not necessarily imply that anemia is the cause and, therefore, a treatable cause of CVD. That is, confounding from unmeasured factors, or residual confounding from measured factors may be playing a role. Two examples include the following: (1) anemia may be associated with an unmeasured risk factor, such as inflammatory status, which in turn is the cause of both the anemia and the causal risk factor associated with CVD; and (2) anemia may be a marker of the severity of underlying

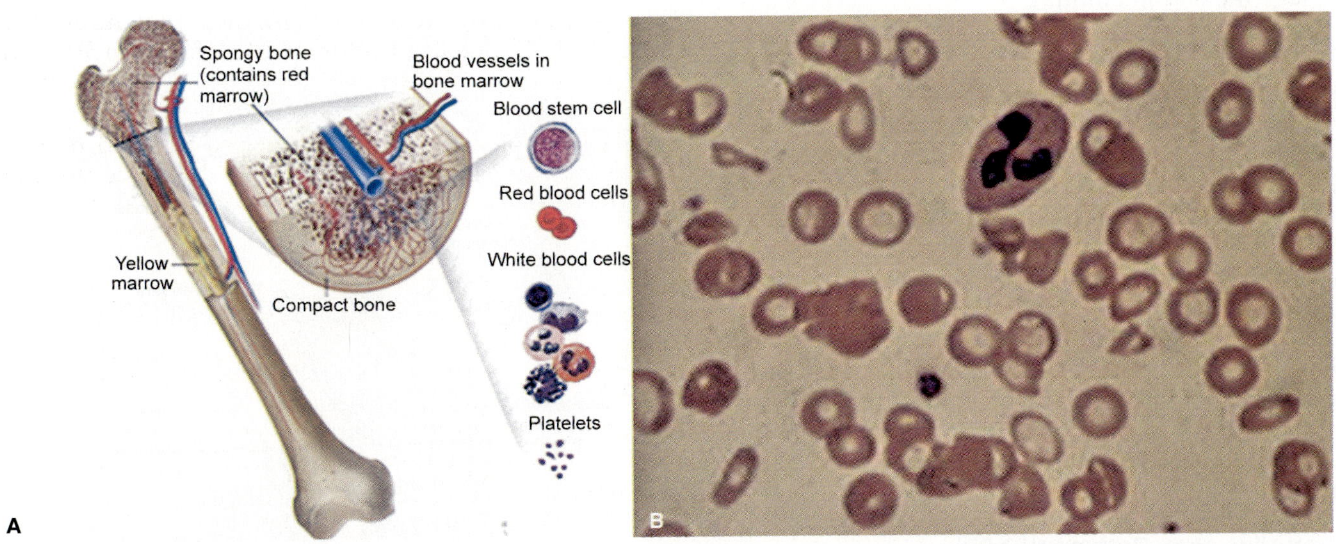


**Fig. 40.2:** (A) Anatomy of the bone. The bone is made up of compact bone, spongy bone, and bone marrow. Compact bone makes up the outer layer of the bone. Spongy bone is found mostly at the ends of bones and contains red marrow. Bone marrow is found in the center of most bones and has many blood vessels. There are two types of bone marrow—red and yellow. Red marrow contains blood stem cells that can become red blood cells, white blood cells, or platelets. Yellow marrow is made mostly of fat (B). Blood smear of a person with iron-deficiency anemia at 40X enhancement

heart disease. For example, in patients with heart failure, anemia may be due to hemodilution associated with the severity of heart failure.

## DOES THE CAUSE OF ANEMIA AFFECT CVD RISK? A POTENTIAL PROTECTIVE EFFECT OF IRON DEFICIENCY

In 1981, Sullivan proposed that iron depletion and, by inference, potentially iron-deficiency anemia may protect against IHD. Although controversial, there have been several lines of support for this hypothesis.

### Different Rates of IHD incidence in Men and Women

The crude IHD death rate in United States men and women aged 35–74 is 219 and 91 per 100,000 population, respectively. The incidence of IHD is consistently higher in men of all age groups compared to women in the same age groups, with the maximal difference of 300% in the 45–54 age group. The difference in the incidence of IHD appears to parallel the changes in iron stores seen with increasing age. In men, iron stores, assessed by serum ferritin concentration, rise after adolescence. In women, iron stores remain low and only begin to rise after the age of 45 years. The maximal sex difference in serum ferritin level is reached at approximately 45 years of age.

### Why Iron Deficiency may be Protective

Redox-active iron may contribute to lipid peroxidation, endothelial cell activation, and generation of reactive oxygen species. Increased oxidative stress, in turn, may be associated with impaired action of endothelium-derived nitric oxide in patients with atherosclerosis, thus contributing to endothelial dysfunction. Iron chelation has been shown to improve endothelial function in patients with coronary artery disease, supporting the theory that iron may damage the endothelium.

### Observational Studies Linking Iron Stores to IHD

Some, but not all, studies have noted an association between increased iron stores and risk of IHD. For example, a study of 9920 Canadian men and women demonstrated an association between levels of serum iron and risk of fatal acute myocardial infarction. The rate ratio in the highest category of serum iron levels compared to the lowest category was 2.18 for men and 5.53 for women, respectively. Studies from the Framingham population have also been consistent with the iron hypothesis. That is, the risk of IHD in women increased equally by natural menopause or by surgical menopause (independent of oophorectomy). Thus, uterine factors, rather than hormonal factors, might be responsible for the protection of premenopausal women against IHD.

### Blood Donation may Reduce IHD Risk

If iron deficiency was protective, one could hypothesize that frequent donation of blood may reduce IHD. In fact, in a prospective cohort of 2682 Finnish men followed for up to 5.5 years, blood donation was shown to decrease the risk of myocardial infarction by 86%. This finding, however, has not been consistent. For example, although 655 blood donors had half the risk of CVD events compared to 3200 nondonors in an unadjusted analysis, this difference was no longer significant after adjustment for potential confounders.

## OBSERVATIONAL STUDIES AND INTERVENTIONAL TRIALS RELATING ANEMIA TO CVD OUTCOMES

### Patients with CKD

#### *Relationship between Anemia and LVH in Patients with Reduced Glomerular Filtration Rate*

In a cross-sectional study of 175 patients attending a kidney disease clinic, Levin et al. evaluated the relationship of hemoglobin level to echocardiographic findings. The population consisted of 115 men and 60 women with mean age of 51 (range, 20–82). Mean creatinine clearance (Ccr) was 25.5 ml/min, and LVH was present in 38.9% of the population. The authors demonstrated that anemia and systolic blood pressure were the most important modifiable risk factors associated with the presence of LVH. In multiple logistic regression analysis each 1 g/dl decrease in hemoglobin was associated with a 6% increase risk of LVH (P = 0.0062). Similar results have been noted in other studies (Fig. 40.3).

Results of longitudinal studies have also demonstrated an association between hemoglobin and left ventricular parameters. For example, Levin et al. evaluated factors associated with LV growth (LVG) in a prospective study of 246 patients with echocardiograms at baseline and 12 month follow-up. The overall prevalence of LVH at baseline was 36%. Left ventricular growth, defined by an increase in left ventricular mass index (LVMI) openface>20% or >20 g/m$^2$ from baseline to 12 months, occurred in 25% of the population. Multivariable regression analysis demonstrated a 1.32 increased odds of LVG for each 0.5 g/dl

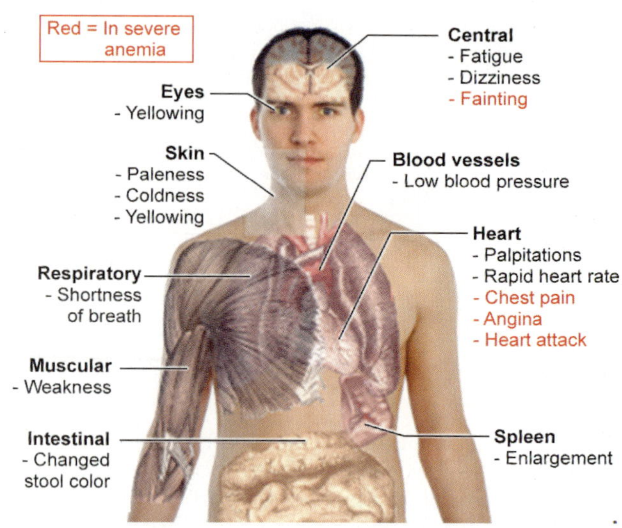


**Fig. 40.3:** Features of anemia

decrease in hemoglobin (P = 0.004). Combined, the results of both of these studies suggest that the presence of anemia may be a risk factor for LVG and development of LVH early in the course of CKD.

### *Treatment of Anemia in Patients with reduced Glomerular Filtration Rate*

There have been a number of small nonrandomized studies that have demonstrated improvement of cardiac parameters with correction of anemia in patients in the earlier stages of CKD. Portoles et al. studied 11 patients with reduced GFR who received recombinant human erythropoietin for a 6-month period. The hemoglobin increased from 9.0 to 11.7 g/dl, and there was a trend toward decreased LV thickness and a significant decrease in LVMI (178–147 $g/m^2$) following treatment. Similarly, Hayashi et al. studied 9 patients with reduced glomerular filtration rate (GFR), with a mean hematocrit (Hct) of 23.6% and mean LVMI of 140.6 $g/m^2$ at baseline. These patients were initially partially treated to a goal Hct of 30% and subsequently to a goal Hct of 40%. Left ventricular mass index decreased to 126.9 $g/m^2$ after partial correction of the anemia (Hct, 32%), and to 111.2 $g/m^2$ after full correction of the anemia (Hct, 39%) (P < 0.0001). Finally, randomized trials have demonstrated significant beneficial cardiovascular effects in terms of exercise capacity after treatment of anemia.

Of interest are two ongoing studies. The first is the correction of hemoglobin and outcomes in renal insufficiency (CHOIR) study, which randomized 2000 patients with a baseline hemoglobin of 10.5–11 g/dl to a target hemoglobin of 13–13.5 g/dl with the use of recombinant human erythropoietin versus placebo. The primary outcome is a composite of all-cause mortality, myocardial infarction, stroke, and hospitalization for congestive heart failure. The second is the cardiovascular reduction by early anemia treatment with epoetin beta (CREATE) Study, which randomized patients to immediate treatment with epoetin beta to a target hemoglobin of 13–15 g/dl, or to late treatment with a target hemoglobin of 10.5–11.5 g/dl, once their hemoglobin levels have fallen below 10.5 g/dl. The primary outcome is time to first cardiovascular event.

### *Relationship between Anemia and CVD Outcomes in Dialysis Patients*

Decreased hemoglobin levels have been associated with a higher risk for CVD events in dialysis patients. For example, in a cohort of 432 dialysis patients followed for an average of 41 months, each g/dl lower hemoglobin was associated with a 1.28 (P = 0.018), 1.20 (P = 0.046), and 1.14 (P = 0.024) adjusted risk of de novo and recurrent congestive failure, as well as all-cause mortality, respectively. More recently, Collins et al. studied a cohort of >~67,000 United States Renal Data System hemodialysis patients and assessed the effect of baseline Hct on the risks of cardiac mortality at 1 year. In multivariable analysis, they demonstrated that for patients with Hct values of ≥36%, cardiac mortality rates were not different when compared with patients with hematocrit values of 33–36%. Patients with Hct <30% or 30–33% were found to have a higher risk of cardiac death than patients with Hct 33–36% [relative risk (RR) of 1.57 and 1.25, respectively; (P <0.001 for both)].

### Treatment of Anemia in Dialysis Patients

Uncontrolled studies have suggested that treatment of anemia is associated with reduction in left ventricular mass and favorable outcomes, such as decreased all-cause and CVD mortality in dialysis patients. Similarly, treatment of anemia from a Hct of 25–34% has been shown to decrease exercise-induced myocardial ischemia, diagnosed by EKG monitoring. The results from randomized controlled trials have, however, been less conclusive. The Normal Hematocrit Trial enrolled >1200 patients with IHD or congestive heart failure who were randomized to a Hct goal of either 30 or 42%. The primary end-points were time to first myocardial infarction or death. Patients randomized to the higher Hct group showed a trend toward increased mortality (though not significant) compared to patients in the lower Hct group. The exact explanation for these results remains unknown although potential reasons included increased access thrombosis in the higher Hct target, as well as increased iron use in the higher Hct group. The Canadian Normalization of Hemoglobin Trial randomized a total of 146 patients with either asymptomatic concentric LVH or LV dilatation to receive doses of recombinant human erythropoietin designed to achieve a target hemoglobin (Hb) level of either 10 or 13 g/dl. Results showed that in the concentric LVH group and in the LV dilatation group, the changes in LVMI and LV volume index, respectively, were similar at both target Hb concentrations. However, patients with concentric LVH were less likely to develop progressive LV dilatation if they were randomized to the high Hb target. Results are now being awaited from a larger ongoing controlled trial in 544 asymptomatic patients with concentric LVH and normal LV cavity volume who are being randomized to a target Hb of 14 g/dl versus 10– 11 g/dl. The primary study outcome is percent change in LV cavity volume and secondary outcomes, is percent change in LV mass. These trials suggest that, although there may be some benefit to treatment of anemia in hemodialysis patients prior to development of clinical CVD, additional trials should be conducted in the earlier stages of CKD to evaluate whether many of the cardiac changes that occur as GFR declines can be prevented.

## Patients with Heart Failure

### *Prevalence of Anemia in Heart Failure*

The prevalence of anemia is high in patients with heart failure, increasing as the severity of the heart failure worsens. For example, Silverberg demonstrated that the prevalence of anemia (Hb <12 g/dl) was 9.1% and 19.2% in patients with New York Heart Association (NYHA) functional class I or II, respectively, while it was as high as 79.1% in patients with NYHA functional class IV.

### Relationship between Anemia and Outcomes

Several studies have now demonstrated that the presence of anemia is an independent risk factor for outcomes in patients with heart failure. For example, in the Studies of Left Ventricular Dysfunction (SOLVD), each 1% lower Hct at baseline was associated with a 3% increase risk in all-cause mortality in multivariable analysis. Similar findings were noted in a study by Horwich et al. who demonstrated an inverse association between Hb level and mortality in a study of 1061 patients with advanced heart failure (NYHA functional class III or IV and LVEF <40%). In multivariable analysis, each 1 g/dl lower Hb was associated with a relative risk of 1.13 (CI, 1.045–1.22) for all-cause mortality.

### Treatment of Anemia in Heart Failure

In an uncontrolled study, Silverberg et al. used a combination of subcutaneous erythropoietin and intravenous iron to correct anemia in 26 patients with persistent, severe heart failure. Treatment resulted in improvements in mean Hb from 10.2 to 12.1 g/dl (P = 0.001), and a decrease in mean NYHA functional class from 3.7 to 2.7. In addition, the dose of diuretics and the number of hospitalizations decreased. In a controlled trial, Silverberg et al. randomized 32 patients with moderate to severe heart failure and Hb levels of 10.0–11.5 g/dl, to a target Hb of 12.5 g/dl versus placebo. Intravenous iron and erythropoietin were used in the treatment group to achieve the Hb goal. The treatment group showed an improvement in NYHA functional class by 42%, in contrast to patients with untreated anemia, who showed a decline in NYHA class. There was also a reduction in the need for oral and intravenous diuretics, as well as hospitalizations in the treatment compared with the placebo group. Finally, Mancini et al. have studied the effect of treatment of anemia on exercise performance in patients with heart failure. Twenty-six patients with anemia and heart failure were randomized to receive erythropoietin or placebo for 3 months. Results revealed that patients in the treatment group had increased peak oxygen consumption and exercise capacity in comparison with the placebo group.

### Patients with Coronary Artery Disease

The frequency and impact of reduced Hct was investigated in a retrospective analysis of medicare beneficiaries 65 years or older who were hospitalized with acute myocardial infarction·The authors noted that patients with lower Hct values on admission had higher 30-day mortality rates. Furthermore, blood transfusion was associated with a reduction in 30-day mortality among patients whose Hct on admission ranged from 5.0 to 24.0% (adjusted odds ratio, 0.22; 95% CI, 0.11–0.45) to 30.1–33.0% (adjusted odds ratio, 0.69; 95% CI, 0.53–0.89). The authors concluded that transfusion might improve outcomes in elderly patients who are anemic and who have suffered an acute myocardial infarction. However, not all studies are consistent with this finding. A recent study examined the association of anemia with 1-year mortality among 30,341 patients hospitalized with acute myocardial infarction in 1986 (prethrombolytic era, $N = 15{,}584$) and 1996 (thrombolytic era, $N = 14{,}757$). In unadjusted analyses, a higher mortality was observed among patients with acute myocardial infarction and anemia. However, after adjustment for demographics, severity of CVD, and other comorbid conditions there was no difference in the anemic group compared with the non-anemic group.

## CONCLUSION

Anemia appears to be an independent risk factor for surrogates of CVD, such as LVH, and with clinical CVD outcomes in patients with CKD or heart failure. In these two populations, randomized controlled trials are needed to assess if this is due to a cause-and-effect relationship and whether treatment of anemia can reduce CVD outcomes. In patients with IHD and in subjects in the general population the relationship between anemia with CVD is inconclusive. Future observational studies that evaluate this relationship should attempt to identify both the cause of the anemia as well as surrogates of CVD. The reason for the latter is that anemia itself may result in ventricular remodeling and LVH, while iron-deficiency anemia could theoretically improve endothelial function. Therefore, the possibility of competing risks may be at play.

## THE ROLE OF ANEMIA IN THE PROGRESSION OF CONGESTIVE HEART FAILURE

Heart failure (HF) is a common disease associated with poor prognosis. Anemia is commonly associated with HF due to bone marrow depression, reduced availability of iron and hemodilution, and is sometimes aggravated by too frequent blood testing. Low hemoglobin is very detrimental to the hemodynamic state of the patient with decreased cardiac output as it further diminishes the oxygen supply to the tissues. When anemia is associated with HF. and renal failure, the patient enters a vicious cycle called cardio renal anemia syndrome. The prognosis of patients with HF is worse as the hemoglobin is lower and even mild anemia is associated with <1 year survival. Aggressive correction of the anemia by subcutaneous injections of erythropoietin and intravenous iron has been shown to improve the functional capacity and quality of life of patients with cardiorenal anemia syndrome and to reduce the need for hospitalization. However, intravenous iron can be detrimental because of increased formation of free radicals, oxidative stress and risk of infection. The level of hemoglobin needed to be achieved is not clear, but it seems indicated to maintain it above 12 g%.

### Anemia in Chronic Heart Failure

Anemia occurs commonly in patients with chronic heart failure (CHF) and has been proposed as a novel therapeutic target in this patient population. The present review will summarize the current knowledge of the prevalence, causative factors, and pathophysiological correlates of anemia in CHF. Potential risks and benefits of therapy with erythropoietic agents for the treatment of anemia in CHF will also be discussed.

### Prevalence of Anemia in CHF

Estimates of the prevalence of anemia in patients with CHF and low ejection fraction range widely from 4–61% (median 18%).Variability in estimated prevalence is partly attributable to use of inconsistent definitions of anemia in individual reports. The World Health Organization definition of anemia (hemoglobin concentration <13.0 g/dl in men and <12.0 g/dl in women) takes into account known gender differences in distribution of hemoglobin values, whereas the National Kidney Foundation defines anemia as hemoglobin ≤12 g/dl in men and postmenopausal women. These standard definitions of anemia are not based on well-established physiological or population norms. Published reports in CHF populations have used these and other study-specific definitions of anemia (including other arbitrary or statistically defined hemoglobin and hematocrit categories and administrative diagnostic codes from hospital records). Despite these inconsistencies in the definition of anemia cases, most studies indicate that the prevalence of anemia is increased in CHF populations with comorbid kidney disease, advanced age, and more severe symptoms (range, 30–61%) when compared with less symptomatic ambulatory populations (range, 4–23%). In patients with CHF and preserved ejection fraction, the few published reports indicate that anemia is also highly prevalent in this group.

## UNDERLYING CAUSE OF ANEMIA IN CHF

Anemia occurs when there is a deficiency in new erythrocyte production relative to the rate of removal of aged erythrocytes (Fig. 40.4). Erythropoietin, a 30.4 kDa glycoprotein growth factor produced primarily by kidney, is the key component of the homeostatic system for regulation of red blood cell mass and tissue oxygen delivery. Erythropoietin prevents the programmed cell death of erythrocyte progenitor cells and thereby stimulates their proliferation, maturation, and terminal differentiation. Any abnormality that reduces renal secretion of or bone marrow response to erythropoietin may result in anemia. Iron deficiency is present in <30% of anemic patients with CHF, so the majority of observed anemia is normocytic, often classified as anemia of chronic disease. Although risk factors for anemia identified in cross-sectional studies do not provide evidence of a causal link, these observations suggest that several distinct mechanisms may commonly contribute to anemia in patients with CHF. Chronic kidney disease is a common comorbidity in patients with CHF and is a strong independent predictor of increased risk of anemia in several studies. In chronic kidney disease populations without heart failure, moderate to severe kidney disease [defined as glomerular filtration rate (GFR) <60 ml/min] is associated with diminished erythropoietin production and a progressive decrease in hemoglobin values that is linearly related to reduction in GFR. The estimated prevalence of at least moderate chronic kidney disease (defined as GFR <60 ml/min) in CHF populations is 20–40%.

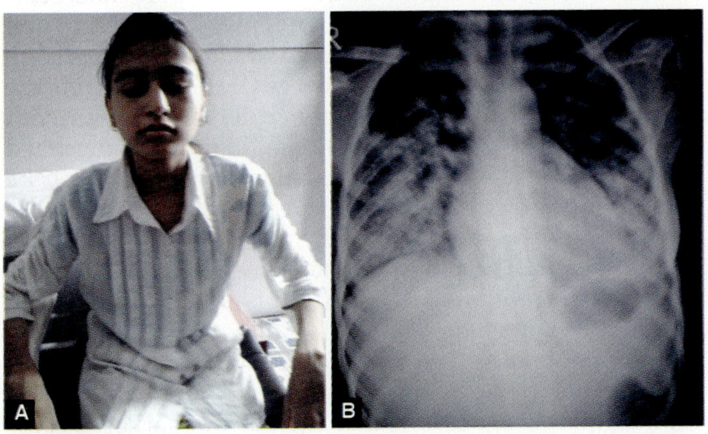


**Fig. 40.4:** (A) Photograph of a 16-year-old girl who presented with severe anemia (Hb <6.0 g/dl) exertional dyspnea, pallor, poor appetite, lethargy and reduced sleep. (B) Chest X-ray showed bilateral fluffy shadows due to congestive heart failure which got reduced with decongestive therapy within 2 weeks of follow up

Anemia is frequently associated with decreased body mass index in published reports, a finding that suggests that patients with cachexia are at greater risk for anemia. Serum levels of proinflammatory cytokines are increased in cachectic patients with CHF and may contribute to development of anemia by several mechanisms. Proinflammatory cytokines including tumor necrosis factor-α (TNF-α), interleukin-1, and interleukin-6 have been shown to disrupt multiple aspects of erythropoiesis, including reduction of renal erythropoietin secretion, suppression of erythropoietin activity in red blood cell precursors in the bone marrow level, and reduction of bioavailability of iron stores for hemoglobin synthesis. Proinflammatory cytokines also increase levels of the liver-derived peptide hormone, hepcidin. Hepcidin interacts with ferroportin and other iron transport proteins in the enterocyte to inhibit gut iron absorption and thereby reduces iron bioavailability for hemoglobin synthesis. In a mouse model of heart failure induced by myocardial infarction, anemia was linked to activation of the TNF-α/Fas signaling pathway. The number of bone marrow progenitor cells and the proliferative capacity of these cells were reduced by 40% to 50% in heart failure mice when compared with control animals. A 3-fold increase in apoptosis among progenitor cells in heart failure mice was significantly correlated with the increase of TNF-α/Fas expression in bone marrow natural killer and T cells. In patients with CHF, increased levels of proinflammatory cytokines (TNF-α and soluble TNF receptors) or other blood markers of inflammation (C-reactive protein) are inversely related to the hemoglobin level. The renin-angiotensin system plays an integral role in the normal regulation of plasma volume and red blood cell volume. Increased angiotensin II signaling in the kidney alters peritubular oxygen tension, a key regulatory factor for erythropoietin secretion. Reduced oxygen tension in the peritubular fibroblasts of the renal cortex is associated with increased intracellular concentrations of reactive oxygen species, which, in turn, increases activation of hypoxia inducible factor-1 (HIF-1) and erythropoietin gene expression. Angiotensin II increases erythropoietin secretion by reducing renal blood flow and increasing proximal tubular reabsorption. Angiotensin II may also have direct stimulatory effects on bone marrow erythrocyte precursors. Erythropoietin levels are modestly increased in patients with CHF in proportion to measures of activation of the renin-angiotensin system. Inhibition of the renin-angiotensin system with either ACE inhibitors or angiotensin receptor blockers is associated with decreased erythropoietin production and reduced hemoglobin levels. ACE also catalyzes the breakdown of Ac-SDKP, a tetrapeptide inhibitor of erythropoiesis. In ACE inhibitor-treated anemic CHF subjects with low serum ACE activity, Ac-SDKP levels are increased when compared with nonanemic CHF subjects. Serum taken from anemic patients with CHF with high levels of Ac-SDKP inhibited formation of erythroid precursors in culture when compared with serum from nonanemic CHF or healthy control subjects. The effects of ACE inhibition on hematocrit are complex as ACE inhibition may decrease red cell production and also reduce plasma volume (see discussion on hemodilution below). In clinical trials, pharmacological inhibition of the renin-angiotensin system is associated with small but statistically significant reduction in hemoglobin levels.

Anemia is frequently associated with clinical signs and symptoms of congestion, a finding that suggests that plasma volume expansion may contribute to anemia in CHF by a process of hemodilution. In 37 ambulatory nonedematous anemic patients with CHF, a radiolabeled albumin technique for direct measurement of plasma volume demonstrated 46% of the patients with low hematocrit values had normal red blood cell volume such that the anemia was entirely attributable to expanded plasma volume and consequent hemodilution. Patients with hemodilution were clinically similar to patients with reduced red blood cell volume but were at greater risk for mortality during follow-up. The impact of hemodilution on treatment approaches in anemic patients with CHF is uncertain. Administration of erythropoietic agents to increase red blood mass in hemodilution patients could further increase total blood volume with possible adverse clinical consequences. Alternatively, it is possible that more aggressive treatment with diuretics could reduce plasma volume and effectively correct anemia in hemodilution patients.

### Pathophysiology in Anemia

Severe reduction in hemoglobin (4–5 g/dl) is associated with sodium and water retention, reduction of renal blood flow and glomerular filtration rate, and evidence of neurohormonal activation in the absence of organic heart disease. These cardiorenal responses may be attributable to the effects of severe anemia on blood viscosity, oxygen tension in the microvasculature, and nitric oxide availability. Lesser degrees of anemia may contribute to neurohormonal activation and disease progression in patients with CHF. In patients with β-thalassemia syndromes, heart failure is a common complication that is likely mediated by the hemodynamic and neurohormonal effects of severe chronic anemia and iron overload secondary to chronic transfusion requirements. Aggressive iron chelation therapy greatly reduces but does not eliminate the risk of heart failure in these patients.

Hemoglobin content in blood is an important determinant of oxygen delivery to skeletal muscle during exercise. Patients with CHF lack normal physiological reserve to compensate for decreased hemoglobin and may manifest decreased aerobic capacity in response to mild degrees of anemia. Several investigators have reported association between reduced hemoglobin and greater functional impairment as defined by New York Heart Association classification. Kalra and colleagues reported a linear relation between reduced hemoglobin values and peak oxygen consumption in anemic patients with CHF with hemoglobin <13.0 g/dl.

Cardiac mass increased by 25% in a rat model of chronic anemia. An inverse relation between hemoglobin value or hematocrit value and left ventricular hypertrophy has also described in clinical studies of patients with dialysis-dependent and predialysis chronic kidney disease. In a subgroup of patients with CHF enrolled in the Randomized Etanercept North American Strategy to Study Antagonism of Cytokines (RENAISSANCE) trial with available cardiac MRI data, a 1 g/dl increase in hemoglobin was associated with a 4.1-g/m$^2$ decrease in left ventricular mass over 24 weeks. This observation was independent of study drug treatment and does not provide evidence of a causal relation between changes in hemoglobin levels and changes in left ventricular mass. In two randomized trials of patients with chronic kidney disease, increased hemoglobin in response to erythropoietic agents was not associated with reduction in left ventricular hypertrophy.

### Anemia and Clinical Outcomes

Reduced hemoglobin in patients with CHF has been repeatedly shown to be independently associated with increased risk of hospitalization and all-cause mortality These findings in a diverse array of CHF populations are remarkably concordant and generally suggest a linear association between reduced hemoglobin and increased mortality risk. In studies that analyzed hemoglobin as a continuous variable, a 1-g/dl decrease in hemoglobin was independently associated with significantly increased mortality risk. The potential mechanisms linking anemia to increased mortality risk in CHF have not been characterized but may be related to changes in ventricular loading conditions and cardiac structure, altered neurohormonal activation, or reduced free radical scavenging capacity. It is also possible that anemia is a marker of more severe underlying myocardial disease.

### Treatment Approaches

The clinical utility of blood transfusion in anemic cardiovascular disease populations is controversial. According to the guidelines from the American College of Physicians and the American Society of Anesthesiology, the 'transfusion threshold' for patients without known risk factors for cardiac disease is a hemoglobin level in the range of 6–8 g/dl. In 78,974 elderly patients hospitalized with acute myocardial infarction, blood transfusion was associated with a significantly lower 30-day mortality rate among patients with a hematocrit ≤30% on admission. In 838 critically ill patients (26% with cardiovascular disease), maintaining hemoglobin at 10–12 g/dl did not provide additional benefits on 30-day mortality compared with maintaining hemoglobin at 7–9 g/dl. Blood transfusion may be associated with other adverse effects including immunosuppression with increased risk of infection, sensitization to HLA antigens, and iron overload. Given this profile of risks and benefits, transfusion may be considered as an acute treatment for severe anemia on an individualized basis but does not appear to be a viable therapeutic strategy for the long-term management of chronic anemia in CHF.

Although erythropoietin levels are modestly elevated in patients with CHF, the increase is less than that observed in other anemic populations. Accordingly, anemia in CHF may be responsive to exogenous erythropoietin supplementation. The primary mechanism by which erythropoietin stimulates red blood cell production is inhibition of apoptosis of bone marrow erythrocyte progenitors. The erythropoietin receptor is a member of the cytokine class I receptor superfamily. Ligand binding of erythropoietin to the homodimeric erythropoietin receptor activates antiapoptotic signal transduction pathways. Bone marrow erythroid progenitor cells escape from apoptosis and proliferate to result in the growth and maturation of proerythroblasts and normoblasts. Subsequently, reticulocytosis occurs and hemoglobin concentration rises.

### Erythropoietic Agents

There are three currently available erythropoietic agents for treatment of anemia: ***epoetin-α, epoetin-β*** (both of which are recombinant human erythropoietin [rHuEpo]), and ***darbepoetin-α***. rHuEpo was first synthesized in 1985, 2 years after the erythropoietin gene was cloned, and was approved by the United States Food and Drug Administration for clinical use for treatment of anemia in end-stage chronic kidney disease in 1988. Early studies in dialysis-dependent patients with chronic kidney disease showed that intravenous or subcutaneous administration of 150–200 IU/kg per week (in 1–3 divided doses) increased hemoglobin concentrations to 10–12 g/dl in 83–90% of anemic patients with chronic kidney disease. Plasma half-life of rHuEpo after intravenous dosing is 6–8 hours. Approximately 25% of the administered dose is absorbed after subcutaneous dosing, but the plasma half-life is increased to >24 hours. The amount of subcutaneous rHuEpo needed to achieve hemoglobin targets in patients with chronic kidney disease is approximately 25% less than that needed for intravenous dosing. Darbepoetin-α is a long-acting, N-linked supersialylated analog of human erythropoietin approved by the US Food and Drug Administration for the treatment of anemia in patients with chronic kidney disease in 2001. Compared with both native and recombinant erythropoietin, it has stronger affinity for erythropoietin receptor and longer plasma half-life of approximately 48 hours, with consequent longer dosing intervals of 1–2 weeks during maintenance therapy.

The effect of rHuEpo treatment on anemic patients with CHF was first reported by Silverberg and his colleagues. In an open-label study design, 26 anemic chronic HF patients (NYHA class III–IV and hemoglobin <12 g/dl) were treated with subcutaneous rHuEpo (mean dose, 5277 IU/wk) and intravenous iron sucrose (mean dose, 185 mg/mo) with 4–15 months of follow-up duration (mean, 7 months). rHuEpo therapy increased mean hemoglobin from 10.2–12.1 g/dl and was associated with improved NYHA function class (3.7 ± 0.5 at baseline to 2.7 ± 0.7, $P$ <0.05), increased left ventricular ejection fraction (28 ± 5% at baseline to 35 ± 8%, $P$ <0.001), and reduced need for oral and intravenous furosemide. The same investigators subsequently reported a randomized open-label trial with a mean follow-up duration of 8 months to compare the effects of partial correction of anemia with subcutaneous rHuEpo and intravenous iron sucrose therapy versus usual care in 32 patients with severe CHF and anemia (NYHA class III–IV and hemoglobin <11.5 g/dl). When compared with usual care, the rHuEpo therapy (4000 IU 1–3 times weekly subcutaneously plus intravenous iron sucrose 200 mg every 2 weeks) significantly increased the hemoglobin level (10.3–12.9 g/dl versus 10.9–10.8 g/dl, $P$<0.0001), improved NYHA functional class (rHuEpo 3.8 ± 0.4 to 2.2±0.7 versus usual care 3.5 ± 0.7 to 3.9 ± 0.3, $P$ <0.0001), and decreased hospitalization days (rHuEpo 13.8 ± 7.2 to 2.9 ± 6.6 days versus usual care 9.9±4.8 versus 15.5 ± 9.8 days, $P$ <0.0001). An uncontrolled clinical series from the same investigators demonstrated comparable clinical benefits of rHuEpo in 179 patients with CHF and concomitant predialysis chronic kidney disease. Mancini and colleagues conducted a single-blinded, randomized, placebo-controlled trial of rHuEpo therapy in 26 patients with advanced CHF and anemia (hematocrit <35%). Patients received subcutaneous rHuEpo 5000 IU 3 times per week adjusted to raise hematocrit to >45% for up to 3 months or a single subcutaneous injection of saline. Supplemental oral iron and folate were also given to the patients who received rHuEpo therapy. Compared with the placebo group, rHuEpo therapy was associated with significant increases in hemoglobin (11.0 ± 0.5 to 14.3 ± 1.0 g/dl, $P$ <0.05), peak oxygen uptake (11.0 ± 1.8 to 12.7 ± 2.8 ml/min per kilogram, $P$ <0.05), and treadmill exercise duration (590±107 to 657 ± 119 seconds,$P$<0.004). The increases in hemoglobin levels were linearly associated with the increase in peak oxygen uptake ($r$=0.53, $P$ <0.02). Subjects with both hemodilution anemia and true anemia with reduced red blood cell volume appeared to derive comparable improvement in exercise capacity in response to rHuEpo therapy. In the hemodilution subgroup with expanded plasma volume, the rise in measured hematocrit in response to rHuEPO treatment was primarily due to a decrease in plasma volume. As diuretic dosing did not change during the study, this finding suggests that erythropoietin has direct or indirect effects on renal regulation of plasma volume.

The pharmacokinetic and pharmacodynamic profile of ***darbepoetin-α*** was compared in 33 anemic CHF patients (hemoglobin ≤12.5 g/dl) versus 30 healthy subjects. Darbepoetin-α administered once monthly at doses of 2.0 μg/kg or higher produced a sustained increase in hemoglobin concentration in anemic patients with CHF without severe drug-related adverse events. The effect of treatment with darbepoetin-α (0.7 μg/kg subcutaneously every 2 weeks for 26 weeks) on exercise tolerance in 41 anemic patients with CHF (hemoglobin 9–12 g/dl) was evaluated in a randomized placebocontrolled trial. An abstract report of the study findings indicates favorable effects of darbepoetin-α on exercise duration and quality of life when compared with placebo. A larger double-blinded, placebo-controlled, randomized trial, Studies of Anemia in Heart Failure Trial (STAMINA HeFT), was undertaken to determine whether increased hemoglobin in response to darbepoetin-α can improve exercise capacity and quality of life in 300 anemic patients with CHF. The study has completed enrollment, but results have not yet been published.

### Potential Risks of Erythropoietic Therapy

Erythropoietic agents are associated with increased risk of thrombosis. Increased thrombotic risk may be partly attributable to effects of increased hemoglobin levels on blood viscosity or platelet–erythrocyte interactions or to direct effects of erythropoietin in platelets or vascular endothelial cells. Clinical studies on the incidence of thrombotic events associated with chronic rHuEpo therapy in anemic patients with end-stage renal disease on dialysis have reported mixed findings. In the largest randomized clinical trial to date, Besarab and colleagues compared the effects of treatment with rHuEpo to a low target hematocrit of 30% versus a normal range target hemoglobin of 42% in 1233 patients with hemodialysis-dependent end-stage chronic kidney disease and comorbid heart disease. This study was terminated prematurely because of a trend toward increased relative risk of death or nonfatal myocardial infarction in the group assigned to the normal hemoglobin target when compared with group assigned to the target hematocrit of 30% (relative risk, 1.3, 95% CI, 0.9–1.9). The mechanisms underlying this observation are uncertain, as within each treatment group, higher hemoglobin values were associated with reduced risk. In a retrospective study of anemic patients with cervical cancer, chronic rHuEpo therapy was associated with increased risk of deep vein thrombosis that was independent of hematocrit. rHuEPO therapy has also been associated with increased risk of all-cause mortality in two randomized, placebo-controlled trials of patients with breast cancer and head and neck cancer. Thrombotic events were not common causes of death in these studies. Although the findings in chronic kidney disease and cancer populations may not be directly pertinent to patients with CHF, these findings raise concerns and emphasize the need for additional trials to determine the long-term safety and efficacy of erythropoietic agents in the CHF population. In the small clinical trials of anemic patients with CHF summarized above, no thrombotic events or other adverse effects of erythropoietic agents have been reported in approximately 300 patients. Antiplatelet and anticoagulant medications commonly prescribed in patients with CHF may mitigate prothrombotic effects of erythropoietic agents.

Chronic rHuEPO therapy is frequently associated with increased blood pressure. Increased blood pressure during chronic erythropoietic therapy may be attributable to increased blood viscosity due to increased red cell mass, altered neurohormonal milieu, and direct effects on microvascular structure and function. In patients with chronic kidney disease, risk factors for hypertension include rapid increase in hematocrit during therapy, a low baseline hematocrit before rHuEpo administration, high doses and intravenous route of rHuEPO administration, the presence of native kidneys, and a genetic predisposition to hypertension. In the study of anemic subjects with CHF by Mancini and colleagues, treatment with rHuEPO did not change blood pressure at rest or during exercise and did not change forearm vascular resistance as measured with venous occlusion plethysmography. Other rare serious side effects reported with rHuEPO therapy include seizures and pure red cell aplasia caused by antibody formation against erythropoietin.

### Role of Iron Supplementation

Although frank iron deficiency is apparent in only a minority of anemic patients with CHF, functional iron deficiency, which is characterized by reduced availability of tissue iron stores for erythropoiesis, may be a common problem in the CHF population. Available small studies in anemic patients with CHF demonstrated significant increases in hemoglobin values in response to rHuEpo with intravenous or oral iron supplementation. Current guidelines from the National Kidney Foundation recommend use of intravenous iron to maintain serum ferritin level of 100 to 800 ng/ml and a transferrin saturation 20–50% to optimize the clinical response to erythropoietic agents. Although intravenous iron sucrose and iron gluconate preparations are not associated with anaphylaxis and are generally well tolerated in chronic kidney disease populations, there are concerns that excess iron stores may be associated with increased risk of infection and cardiovascular events. Additional work is needed to determine the safety and efficacy of intravenous iron supplementation in anemic patients with CHF with functional iron deficiency.

### Recommendations for Current Practice

There is little discussion of assessment and treatment options for anemia in recent CHF clinical guidelines. On the basis of available data, we recommend serial measurement of hemoglobin in patients with CHF at

6-month intervals in order to identify the subset of patients with anemia who may benefit from further assessment and treatment. In patients with anemia (defined by World Health Organization criteria), further assessment including evaluation for iron or other nutritional deficiencies and estimation of glomerular filtration rate should be performed. For the subpopulation of patients with CHF with moderate-to-severe anemia (hemoglobin <11 g/dl) and concomitant moderate to severe chronic kidney disease (estimated glomerular filtration rate ≤60 ml/min), current guidelines of the National Kidney Foundation recommend treatment with erythropoietic agents and supplemental iron to a target hemoglobin of 12 g/dl. The primary goal of treatment is to improve quality of life; there are no clinical outcome trials in predialysis patients with chronic kidney disease that support use of erythropoietic agents. Given the absence of data on long-term clinical outcomes in patients with CHF and the concerns raised by the finding of increased mortality rates in other anemic populations, treatment with erythropoietic agents in patients with CHF with less severe degrees of anemia and preserved renal function is not recommended until more data on safety and efficacy is available.

### Future Directions

The erythropoietin receptor is present in a variety of cells not directly involved in erythropoiesis, including endothelial cells, vascular smooth muscle cells, neuronal cells, and myocardium. Cytoprotective antiapoptotic effects of erythropoietin have been reported in animal models of central nervous system injury and in experimental models of myocardial hypoxia or ischemia-reperfusion injury. Because ongoing apoptosis has been postulated to be an important mechanism of myocyte loss in CHF, the antiapoptotic effects of rHuEpo in cardiovascular tissues suggest a potential therapeutic role beyond the treatment of anemia. Certain derivatives of naturally occurring erythropoietin (carbamylated erythropoietin and erythropoietin mutants) do not bind to the classical erythropoietin receptor nor promote erythropoiesis and yet have been shown to confer neuroprotection in experimental models of stroke, spinal cord compression, and diabetic neuropathy. These derivatives appear to mediate cytoprotective effects via specific binding to a heterodimeric receptor complex consisting of the erythropoietin receptor and common β-receptor. Derivatives designed to target this heteroreceptor could potentially provide therapeutic cytoprotection without stimulating erythropoiesis in nonanemic CHF or other cardiovascular disease populations.

## GUIDANCE FOR ANEMIA IN HEART DISEASE

- Blood transfusions should be used restrictively and erythropoiesis-stimulating agents (ESAs) should not be used at all for treating anemia in patients with heart disease, according to recommendations from the American College of Physicians.
- In hospitalized patients with coronary heart disease, red blood cell transfusions should be used only for more severe anemia, with a hemoglobin level of 7–8 g/dl—versus higher levels—used as a threshold to determine treatment, recommended Amir Qaseem, MD, PhD, and colleagues on behalf of the college's clinical guidelines committee.
- And patients with congestive heart failure or coronary heart disease should not receive ESAs for mild-to-moderate anemia because of a lack of proven benefit and the potential for increased risks of death and venous thromboembolism, they advised.
- The guideline was published in the Dec. 3 issue of Annals of Internal Medicine.
- Although anemia occurs frequently in patients with heart disease — in up to one-third of patients with heart failure and 10–20% of those with coronary disease — and has been associated with poorer outcomes, the benefits of treating milder forms of the condition in these patients has not been well established.
- The ACP based their recommendations on evidence of the utility of using red blood cell transfusions, ESAs, or iron replacement to treat anemia in adult patients with heart disease that was reviewed by Devan Kansagara, MD, of the Portland VA Medical Center and Oregon Health and Science University, and colleagues.
- Although the quality of evidence was generally low, studies of both medical and surgical patients suggested that treating milder anemia (hemoglobin levels above 10 g/dl) with red blood cell transfusions versus restricting their use to patients with hemoglobin levels below 10 g/dl did not reduce the risk of mortality.
- The risk of cardiovascular events—including myocardial infarction, congestive heart failure exacerbation, arrhythmia, or cardiac death—tended to be lower with more liberal use of transfusions, although the reduction did not reach statistical significance in combined medical and surgical populations (RR 0.64, 95% CI 0.38–1.09). The findings were similar in patients undergoing surgery.
- The data were insufficient to determine whether transfusions improved quality of life or exercise capacity, and there was little information about potential harms. None of the trials reported an increase in adverse events with liberal versus restrictive use of transfusions, however.
- 'Current evidence does not support the benefit of liberal blood transfusions in patients with asymptomatic anemia and heart disease,' Qaseem and colleagues wrote. The recommendation for restrictive use of transfusions was considered a weak recommendation based on low-quality evidence.
- They added, 'the probability that transfusion may be beneficial is higher in patients with lower hemoglobin levels (less than 7 g/dl) and lower in less anemic patients (hemoglobin greater than 10 g/dl).'
- The evidence was stronger regarding the use of ESAs in patients with heart disease; use of the drugs did not consistently affect mortality, cardiovascular events,

exercise capacity, quality of life, or the rate of hospitalization, but did increase the risk of venous thrombosis in patients with heart failure.

- 'The ACP does not support the use of ESAs for treating patients with mild-to-moderate anemia and heart disease because the harms outweigh the benefits for these patients,' the authors wrote. The recommendation for avoiding ESAs was considered a strong one based on moderate-quality evidence.
- In general, there was inadequate evidence to determine the long-term benefits of giving intravenous iron to patients with heart disease and anemia caused by an iron deficiency, although some evidence pointed toward short-term improvements in exercise tolerance and duration and quality of life and reductions in cardiovascular events and mortality in patients with stable systolic heart failure.

## RELATIONSHIP BETWEEN BLOOD DISORDERS AND THE CARDIOVASCULAR SYSTEM

The fundamental relationship between blood disorders and the cardiovascular system originates within multiple points of interface, ranging from the heart and its structural constituents to include heart chambers, valves, coronary arteries, coronary veins, and the cerebrovascular and peripheral vasculature. While the cellular components of circulating blood derive their primary origin from multipotent progenitor cells, plasma-based components, which include coagulation proteins, are mostly born of hepatic synthesis and endothelial cells. Here we provide a focused overview of nononcological blood disorders and their potential impact on the arterial circulatory system as common phenotypes, including myocardial infarction, ischemic stroke and peripheral arterial occlusive events. Venous thromboembolism is employed in our discussion as a clinical template. We also provide practical steps and guidance for diagnostic testing and management in routine clinical practice (Fig. 40.5).

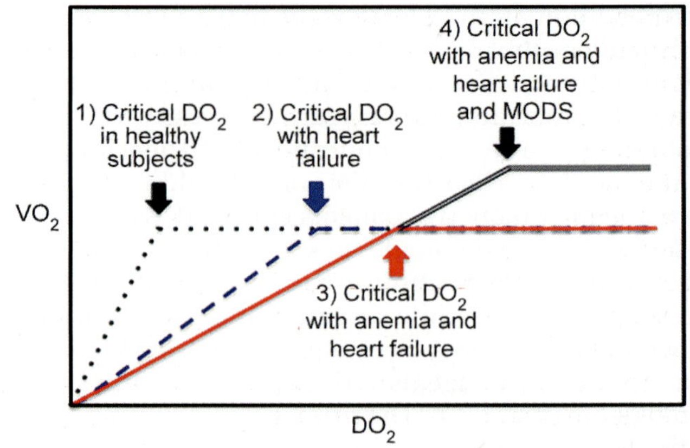


**Fig. 40.5:** Critical oxygen delivery ($DO_2$), cardiac failure, anemia and multiple organ dysfunction syndrome (MODS). X axis: systemic $DO_2$; Y axis: global oxygen consumption ($VO_2$). Critical $DO_2$: level below which $DO_2$ does not meet oxygen demand ($O_2$ supply dependency). (1) In healthy subjects (dotted black and white line), as $DO_2$ decreases, $VO_2$ remains constant by compensatory mechanisms (increased cardiac output and cellular $O_2$ extraction). (2) Cardiac failure limits compensatory increase in cardiac output (hatched blue line). (3) This limitation is worst in patients with anemia and heart failure (plain red line) because low hemoglobin decreases arterial oxygen content ($CaO_2$). (4) Severe cardiac dysfunction may be associated with systemic inflammatory response syndrome (SIRS) and multiple organ dysfunction syndrome (MODS), both of which increase systemic $VO_2$ and therefore critical $DO_2$ (double black line)

Blood is the medium for exchanging oxygen, nutrients, and waste products throughout the body, and consists of plasma, blood cells (red blood cells, white blood cells), and platelets. Platelets play an important role in clotting, white blood cells are responsible for inflammation, and red blood cells carry oxygen and nutrients to all tissues of the body and carry waste products away from the organs. Any abnormality of these blood components can result in hematologic disorders. While disorders involving platelets and coagulation that can lead to thrombosis and/or bleeding are of primary concern for most cardiologists, disorders involving red blood cells and platelets can also affect the mechanics of blood flow and blood viscosity. Our understanding of hematologic disorders has advanced steadily in recent years, particularly with the development of genetics and molecular biologic techniques. Here we provide a focused overview of nononcologic blood disorders and their potential impact on the arterial circulatory system, including the common phenotypes of myocardial infarction, ischemic stroke, and peripheral arterial occlusive events. Venous thromboembolism (VTE) is employed as a clinical template to heighten awareness of a common problem faced by all clinicians and to distinguish blood disorders which are unique to the venous and to the arterial circulatory systems. Anemia and red blood cell transfusion in critically ill cardiac patients. Anemia and red blood cell (RBC) transfusion occur frequently in hospitalized patients with cardiac disease. In this narrative review, we report the epidemiology of anemia and RBC transfusion in hospitalized adults and children (excluding premature neonates) with cardiac disease, and on the outcome of anemic and transfused cardiac patients. Both anemia and RBC transfusion are common in cardiac patients, and both are associated with mortality. RBC transfusion is the only way to rapidly treat severe anemia, but is not completely safe. In addition to hemoglobin (Hb) concentration, the determinant(s) that should drive a practitioner to prescribe a RBC transfusion to cardiac patients are currently unclear. In stable acyanotic cardiac patients, Hb level above 70 g/L in children and above 70–80 g/L in adults appears safe. In cyanotic children, Hb level above 90 g/L appears safe. The appropriate threshold Hb level for unstable cardiac patients and for children younger than 28 days is unknown. The optimal transfusion strategy in cardiac patients is not well characterized. The threshold at which the risk of anemia outweighs the risk of transfusion is not known. More studies are needed to determine when RBC transfusion is indicated in hospitalized patients with cardiac disease.

Anemia and red blood cell (RBC) transfusion occur frequently in hospitalized patients with cardiac disease. In this narrative review, we report the epidemiology of anemia and RBC transfusion in hospitalized adults and children (excluding premature neonates) with cardiac disease, and on the outcome of anemic and transfused cardiac patients. Both anemia and RBC transfusion are common in cardiac patients, and both are associated with mortality. RBC transfusion is the only way to rapidly treat severe anemia, but is not completely safe. In addition to hemoglobin (Hb) concentration, the determinant(s) that should drive a practitioner to prescribe a RBC transfusion to cardiac patients are currently unclear. In stable acyanotic cardiac patients, Hb level above 70 g/L in children and above 70–80 g/L in adults appears safe. In cyanotic children, Hb level above 90 g/L appears safe. The appropriate threshold Hb level for unstable cardiac patients and for children younger than 28 days is unknown. The optimal transfusion strategy in cardiac patients is not well characterized. The threshold at which the risk of anemia outweighs the risk of transfusion is not known. More studies are needed to determine when RBC transfusion is indicated in hospitalized patients with cardiac disease.

## CARDIOVASCULAR EFFECT OF SICKLE CELL DISEASE WITH CHRONIC HEMOLYTIC ANEMIA

Sickle cell disease is characterized by recurrent episodes of ischemia-reperfusion injury to multiple vital organ systems and a chronic hemolytic anemia, both contributing to progressive organ dysfunction. The introduction of treatments that induce protective fetal hemoglobin and reduce infectious complications has greatly prolonged survival. However, with increased longevity, cardiovascular complications are increasingly evident, with the notable development of a progressive proliferative systemic vasculopathy, pulmonary hypertension (PH), and left ventricular diastolic dysfunction.

Pulmonary hypertension is reported in autopsy studies, and numerous clinical studies have shown that increased pulmonary pressures are an important risk marker for mortality in these patients. In epidemiological studies, the development of PH is associated with intravascular hemolysis, cutaneous leg ulceration, renal insufficiency, iron overload, and liver dysfunction. Chronic anemia in sickle cell disease results in cardiac chamber dilation and a compensatory increase in left ventricular mass. This is often accompanied by left ventricular diastolic dysfunction that has also been a strong independent predictor of mortality in patients with sickle cell disease. Both PH and diastolic dysfunction are associated with marked abnormalities in exercise capacity in these patients. Sudden death is an increasingly recognized problem, and further cardiac investigations are necessary to recognize and treat high-risk patients (Fig. 40.6).

### Pulmonary Hypertension

#### *Mechanisms of Disease and Clinical Risk Factors*

Pulmonary hypertension (PH) represents one of the major emerging vasculopathic complications of SCD as this patient population ages (Fig. 40.7). Hemolytic anemia has been proposed as an important mechanism leading to pulmonary vasculopathy, hemoglobin, when decompartmentalized from the red cell, will react with nitric oxide (NO) at the near diffusion limit, to oxidize the NO to nitrate. This reaction is so fast and irreversible that even levels of cell-free plasma hemoglobin of only 6–10 μm are sufficient to inhibit all NO signaling and produce vasoconstriction. In addition to cell-free hemoglobin, hemolysis releases other red cell enzymes that have the potential to inhibit

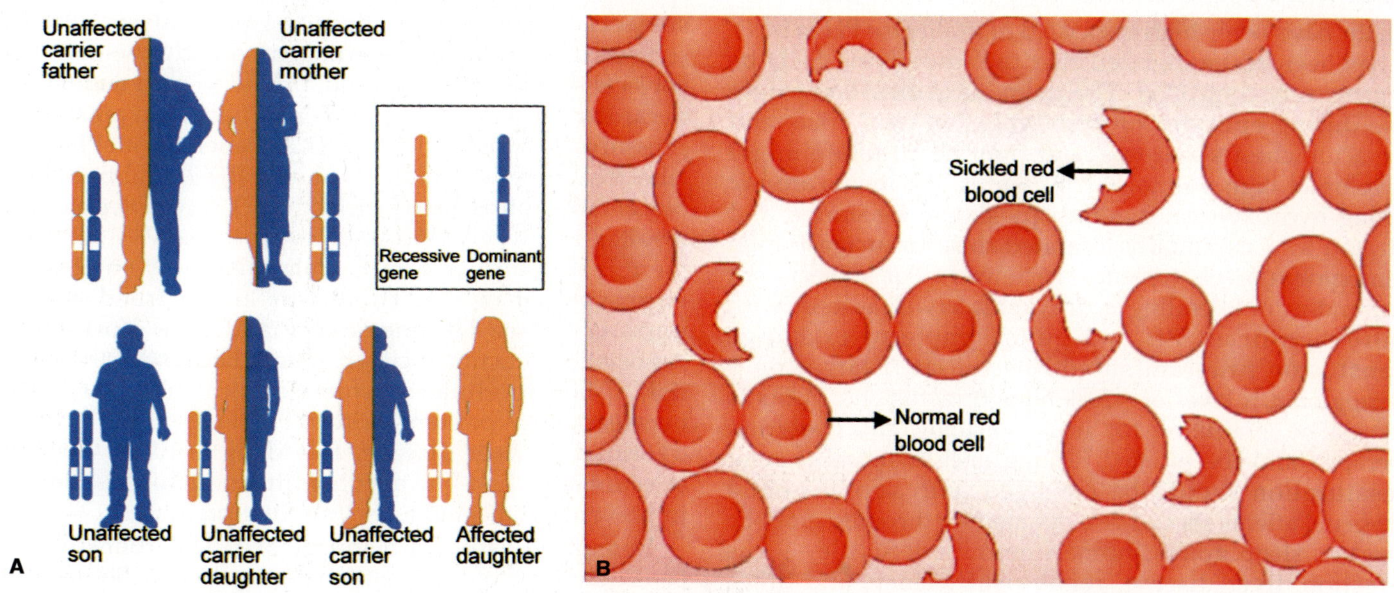


**Fig. 40.6:** (A) Genetic transmission of beta-thalassemia. (B) A simple blood test can diagnose sickle cell anemia. The blood cells will show up in the shape of sickles or crescents under a microscope

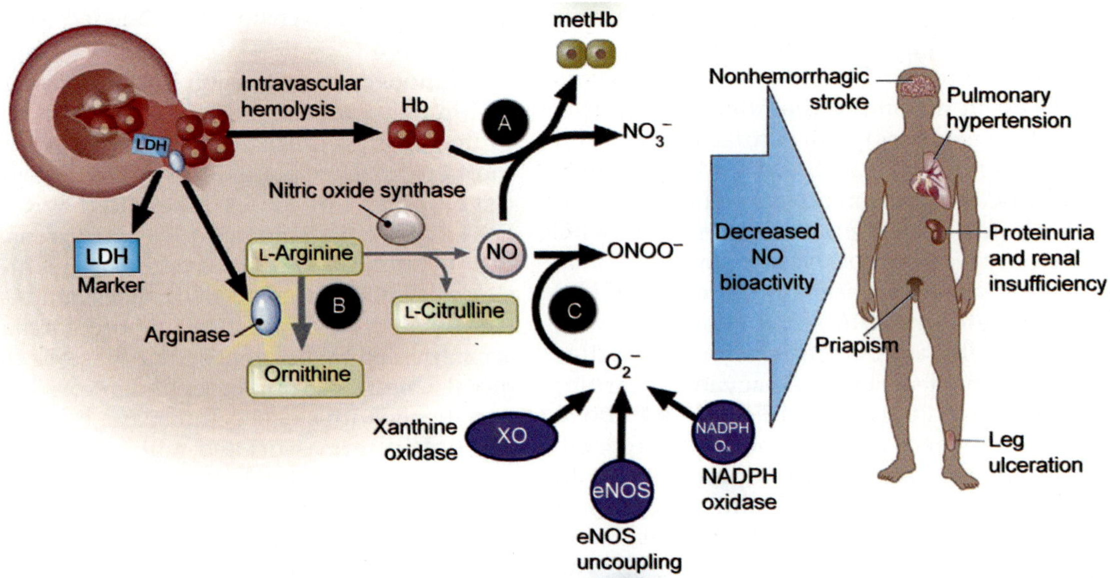


**Fig. 40.7:** Mechanisms of PH in SCD patients. A pulmonary vessel with severe intimal and smooth muscle proliferation is shown from a 35-year-old patient with sickle cell disease (SCD) who died suddenly with known pulmonary arterial hypertension. Mechanisms that contribute to the development of pulmonary hypertension (PH) identified in animal and human studies are summarized. ADMA=asymmetric dimethylarginine; ET=endothelin; NADPH=nicotinamide adenine dinucleotide phosphate; NOS=nitric oxide synthase; ROS=reactive oxygen species; TGF=transforming growth factor

NO signaling. Arginase 1 is present in abundance in red cells and metabolizes arginine to ornithine, reducing arginine availability for NO synthesis. In addition, other independent factors that contribute to the development of PH in this population include surgical splenectomy and functional asplenia, thromboembolism, lung fibrosis and hypoxemia, increases in other vasoactive mediators such as placental growth factor and endothelin (ET)-1, renal insufficiency, and genetic factors.

### Treatment Options for PH in SCD

On the basis of the high associated mortality for PH in SCD, it has been recommended that the underlying SCD be aggressively controlled. The pulmonary pressures might rise during episodes of vaso-occlusive pain crisis and the acute chest syndrome, and right heart failure might develop at high pulmonary pressures. If patients are not taking hydroxyurea, this therapy should be started and titrated to a maximally tolerated dose to increase fetal hemoglobin levels (recently reviewed). For subjects not responding or tolerating hydroxyurea as well as those with more significant PH, a regular simple or exchange transfusion program should be initiated targeting a hemoglobin S level of <20% after transfusions. Patients should be evaluated for iron overload, and chelation therapy should be initiated. Resting, nocturnal, and exercise desaturation should be managed with supplemental oxygen. Patients should be evaluated for thrombo-embolic disease, sleep apnea, human immunodeficiency virus infection, liver disease, renal insufficiency, and other conditions that could contribute to the development or evolution of PH.

In patients with PAH defined by right heart catheterization (mPAP ≥25 mmHg, pulmonary capillary wedge pressure <15 mmHg, and an elevated transpulmonary gradient ≥10 to 12 mmHg), therapy with PAH-specific therapies can be considered. Although PAH represents a common complication in patients with SCD, with a high associated morbidity and mortality, there exist no large randomized placebo-controlled trials to guide therapy decisions. A trial of bosentan, an ET A and B receptor blocker, was stopped early on the basis of a decision by the sponsor, with only approximately 15 sites activated and 27 subjects enrolled. An underpowered analysis of these subjects showed no evident increase in adverse events in subjects receiving therapy and a trend toward an increase in cardiac output but no significant changes in pulmonary pressures. In a case series of 17 SCD patients with PH, open label treatment with either bosentan (ET A and B receptor blocker) or ambrisentan (a selective ET A receptor blocker) resulted in lower NT-proBNP levels, lower TRV measurements, and higher 6-min walk distance, suggesting improvement in PH. There was also a trend toward improved Borg Dyspnea Score and New York Heart Association functional classification. Because of the lower risk of hepatocellular dysfunction on ambrisentan and because many patients with SCD have comorbid iron overload or liver disease, this drug is likely the best selection as a first-line agent, with simultaneous diuresis to prevent edema and a rise in filling pressures.

Phosphodiesterase 5 inhibitor (PD5) therapy was considered one of the most promising approaches to SCD-associated PH, because these agents seem to be effective in both PAH and pulmonary venous hypertension related to diastolic dysfunction. A small open label study of sildenafil in patients with SCD who were taking maximal hydroxyurea therapy or transfusions revealed significant reductions in TRV and NT-proBNP and increases in 6-min walk distance. However, a large multi center trial of sildenafil was discontinued early on the basis of an unexpected increase in hospital stay for pain (45% of sildenafil, 22% placebo, $p=0.022$). Consistent with these observations, the use of PD5s in other PAH patient populations and in large clinical trials of patients with erectile dysfunction has been associated with an increase in the incidence of myalgias and back pain that could have contributed to the increase in the pain reported in the current study. It is increasingly evident that back pain and myalgias represent a class effect of PD5 inhibitors. Therapy with PD5 inhibitors should only be used, on the basis of the results of the Walk-PHASST sildenafil treatment study, in SCD patients that are extremely well-controlled on hydroxyurea and transfusion therapy and should not be considered a first-line therapy.

## LV Dysfunction

### LV Dilation

Cardiac complications are a common feature of SCD and are felt to be an important cause of the morbidity and mortality associated with this disease. The chronic anemia of SCD results in an increase in cardiac output with only a minimal increase in heart rate. Left ventricular stroke volume increases with significant dilation of the LV, and the degree of LV dilation is closely linked to the degree of anemia. The dilated LV adapts to the increased wall stress by developing eccentric hypertrophy in which wall thickening is increased and myofibers are elongated. Eccentric hypertrophy allows the LV to adapt to chronic volume overload by initially preserving diastolic compliance and maintaining normal filling pressures.

### Increased LV Mass and Diastolic Dysfunction

Over time, progressive dilation leads to increased wall stress and an increase in LV mass (Fig. 40.8). Early studies of SCD found evidence of increasing LV mass with increasing age as well as impaired LV filling. The presence of increased mass in both children and adults has been confirmed in the majority of imaging studies. Invasive right heart catheterization measurements of patients with PH (mean PAP $\geq$25 mmHg) show evidence of diastolic dysfunction in approximately one-half of the patients. Screening echocardiography studies show a significant variation in the prevalence of diastolic dysfunction, due to the well-known difficulty in the noninvasive diagnosis of diastolic dysfunction.

Although a tissue Doppler-derived E/e′ ratio >15 is accepted as a predictor of high LV filling pressure in the setting of LV dysfunction, the application of this in patients with preserved systolic function has been difficult. Kasner et al. studied patients with heart failure and normal ejection fraction and found that an increased E/e′ ratio above 8 was a useful noninvasive predictor of diastolic dysfunction. This ratio has not been prospectively validated in the different hemodynamic circumstances of SCD. Nonetheless, a retrospective review of the NIH cohort patients undergoing echocardiography and cardiac catheterization within 72 h suggested that the E/e′ ratio is useful to predict a pulmonary capillary wedge pressure >15 mmHg.

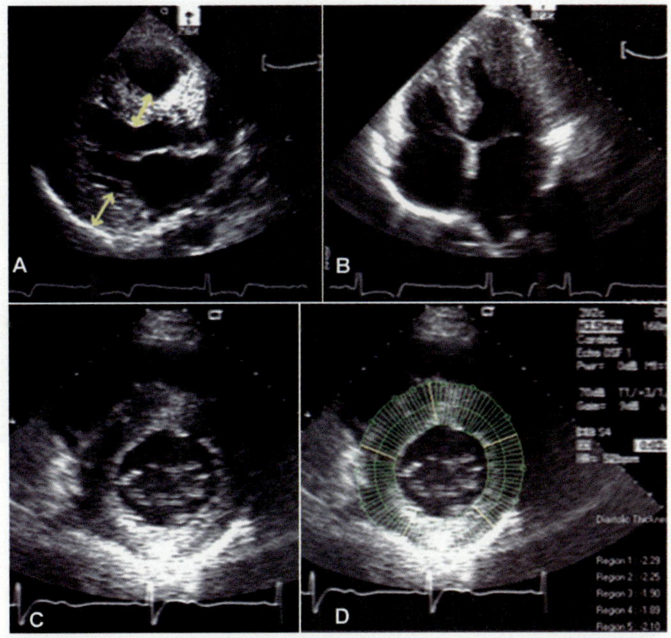


**Fig. 40.8:** Representative 2D echocardiogram of a 49-year-old male Fabry patient. (A) Parasternal long-axis window at end-diastole. Yellow arrows indicate standard ASE measurements of the interventricular septum and posterior wall at the base. (B) Apical four-chamber window at end-systole. Severe concentric left ventricular hypertrophy (LVH) and preserved ejection fraction is shown. (C) Parasternal short-axis window at end-diastole. (D) Radial chord method utilized to measure regional left ventricular wall thickness

### LV systolic Dysfunction

Although 'heart disease' and 'heart failure' have traditionally been considered common in adult SCD patients, recent large screening echocardiographic studies indicate that LV systolic function is preserved in the majority of SCD patients studied in a resting state, and the presence of segmental wall motion abnormalities is rare. When LV dysfunction is present, it has been seen particularly in older patients and those with associated conditions such as hypertension and renal (Figs 40.9 and 40.11).

### Right Ventricular Dysfunction

Imaging studies of SCD patients at steady state without PH have shown dilated right heart chambers without significant right ventricular dysfunction in most cases. During acute chest syndrome, pulmonary pressures increase, and in a series of 84 consecutive hospital admissions, cor pulmonale was seen in 13% of patients. All of

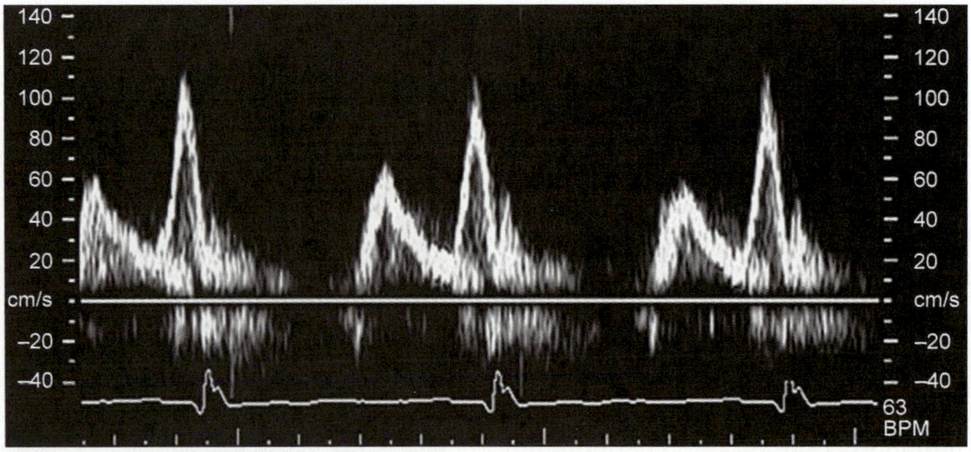


**Fig. 40.9:** Trans-mitral-valve Doppler flow tracing in a patient with mild diastolic dysfunction (abnormal relaxation). The E-to-A-wave ratio is less than 1.0

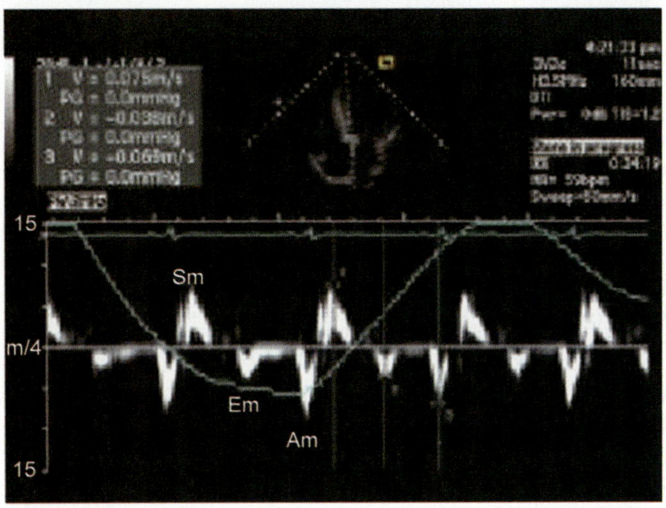


**Fig. 40.10:** Tissue Doppler showing systolic myocardial velocity (Sm) and diastolic myocardial velocity during early filling (Em) and atrial contraction (Am)

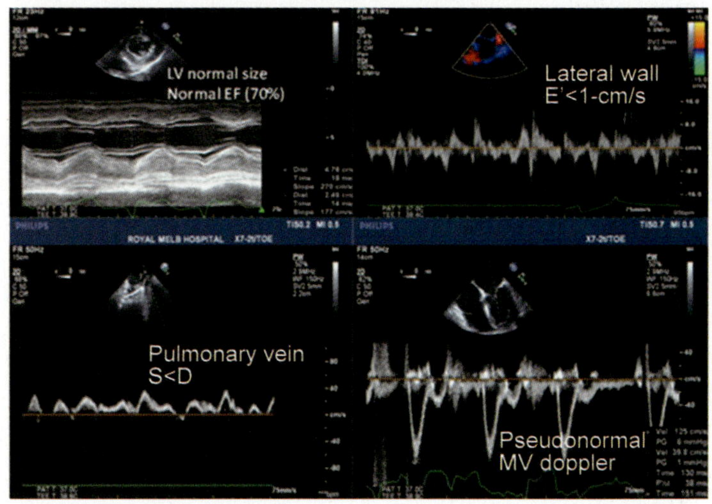


**Fig. 40.11:** Typical diastolic failure (small stiff heart) typically Grade 2 American Society of Echocardiography (ASE). This is a common pattern in the periopertive setting. Typically cardiac index (CI) 1.8–2.2 l/min/m$^2$. Pulmonary artery wedge pressur (PCWP) >15 mmHg

these patients had a TRV ≥3 m/s during the acute event, and they were at particularly high risk for multiorgan failure and sudden death.

Acute pressure overload on top of a chronic pulmonary vasculopathy is felt to be the reason for acute right ventricular decompensation.

### *Myocardial Infarction*

Myocardial ischemia and infarction have been reported to occur in SCD, but in almost all cases evaluated in the published data and in our practice at the National Institutes of Health, coronary angiography reveals normal coronary arteries. Case reports of patients presenting with acute crisis have shown ECG abnormalities, nuclear perfusion defects, magnetic resonance imaging abnormalities, and troponin elevations suggestive of acute myocardial infarction. These findings have been attributed to acute and chronic microvascular occlusion in the setting of chronic endothelial damage, a procoagulant state, and the systemic vasculopathy previously described. Reversal of the cardiac abnormalities has been seen after exchange transfusion and aggressive supportive care for the ischemia; however, evidence-based guidelines for treatment with antiplatelet agents, anticoagulation, and thrombolytics are lacking.

### *Functional Capacity*

Marked abnormalities in exercise capacity have consistently been seen in SCD patients. In addition to possible cardiac filling abnormalities, suggested mechanisms for this limitation in patients studied with cardiopulmonary testing include the anemia itself, pulmonary vascular disease, peripheral vascular disease, and/or a myopathy. The 6-min walk test is a useful measure of functional capacity in this population, and the walk distance correlates directly with peak oxygen consumption and indirectly with the severity of the PH. Despite mild increases in pulmonary pressures and pulmonary vascular resistance, studies of SCD patients have shown more severely reduced 6-min walk distances compared with patients with primary PAH.

### Cardiac Iron Overload

Myocardial iron deposition has been considered as one aetiology for the cardiac abnormalities seen in SCD. Although autopsy studies have documented myocardial iron deposition, magnetic resonance imaging studies using T2* measurements suggest that this finding is rare even in the presence of a significant transfusion history, systemic iron overload, and/or hepatic iron overload. The rate of transfusional iron overload in the liver is lower for sickle cell patients than for myelodysplastic syndromes or thalassemia major, perhaps due to the intermittent nature of the transfusions or the systemic inflammatory state that limits cellular iron accumulation. In SCD patients, ferritin levels have been found to be a univariate predictor of mortality. Myocardial T2* measurements are associated with LV dysfunction and cardiac arrhythmias in thalassemia, but this relationship has not been established in SCD, suggesting that other etiologies for myocardial dysfunction might be more prevalent.

### Dysrhythmia

Electrocardiographic abnormalities, including QT prolongation, are not uncommon in SCD patients at rest. Liem et al. reported a 38% prevalence of QT prolongation in children and young adults, but they did not find a correlation between the QT measurement and LV hypertrophy in their series. Maisel et al. studied 30 SCD patients with 24-h electrocardiographic monitoring during acute crisis and found significant arrhythmias in 80% of the patients, with over one-half the patients having ventricular arrhythmias.

### Sudden Death

Sudden death is an increasingly recognized and reported mechanism of death in the aging SCD population. This occurs in the setting of hospital stay with sepsis or multi-organ failure, during recovery from a routine vaso-occlusive event, or at home. Although this was historically ascribed to narcotic 'overdose,' it is now clear that this is a direct complication of pulmonary vascular and cardiac disease. In a large autopsy series of 306 SCD patients, Manci et al. found that death was sudden and unexpected in 40% of patients and was usually associated with acute events. Although clinical examination of these patients had reported underlying chronic organ injury in 25% of patients, they found pathologic evidence of chronic organ injury in 75% of patients, suggesting that the severity of the underlying disease was often underestimated by clinicians. More recent autopsy series have shown that cardiopulmonary causes account for the majority of deaths, with sudden death/pulseless electrical activity, heart failure/ myocardial infarction, and pulmonary thromboembolism/ PH being the most common findings at the time of death.

## CARDIOVASCULAR EFFECTS IN THALASSEMIAS

(Figs 40.12–40.14)

### Chronic Anemia

Patients with chronic anemia increase their cardiac output to maintain oxygen delivery, resulting in increased cardiac dimensions and heart rate. Anemic patients have larger hearts on CXR, echo, and MRI measurements than patients with normal hemoglobin levels, even without any other pathology. Thus, normative data generated from non-anemic patients is inappropriate for patients with hemoglobinopathies. The larger cardiac dimensions, stroke volumes, and heart rates carry metabolic cost; chronically anemic patients have higher resting oxygen consumption and decreased reserves. Increased resting metabolism is also a source of increased oxidative stress, independent of the free-radical effects of iron. Patients with thalassemia have low or normal blood pressures, despite their increased cardiac output, because they have lower vascular resistance. Lower tonic vascular tone partially compensates for the increased chamber dimensions, but it leaves patients

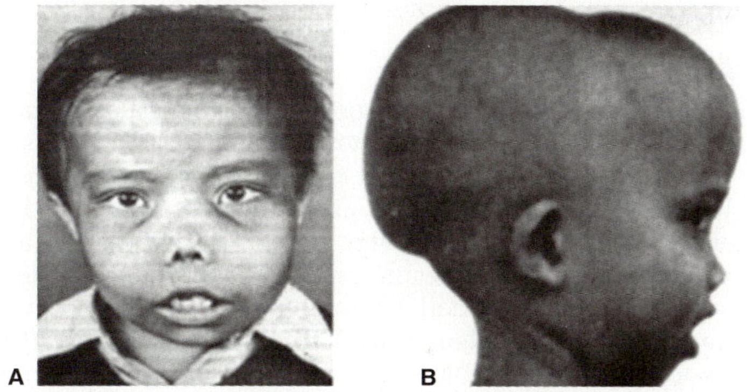


**Fig. 46.12:** (A) Photograph showing prominence of frontal, parietal, and maxillary bones due to bone marrow hypertrophy, depressed bridge of nose and typical pallor giving an impression of 'mongoloid facies' in a young patient with thalassemia major. (B) Showing enlargement of skull bones in a child with longstanding beta-thalassemia.

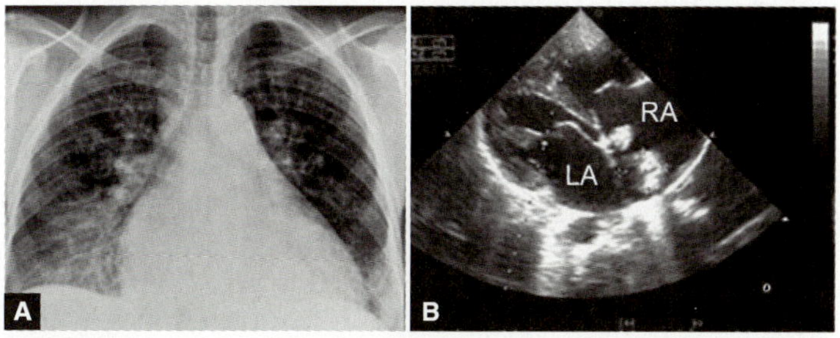


**Fig. 40.13:** (A) Cardiomegaly and pulmonary congestion due to heart failure in patient with longstanding beta-thalassemia. (B) Transthoracic echocardiographic examination revealed two mobile, homogenous masses suggesting thrombus or myxoma at two separate locations in the right atria. Both atrial and ventricular dimensions and functions were normal. A transesophageal echocardiogram confirmed the presence of the two masses

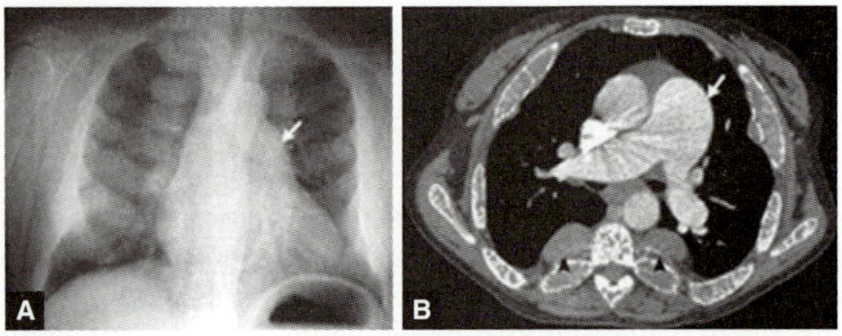

**Fig. 40.14:** Chest radiography (A, arrow) and computed tomography (B, arrow) show enlarged central pulmonary arteries owing to pulmonary arterial hypertension. In patients with thalassemia, such enlargement is thought to arise from chronic anemia, hemolysis, and an increased tendency for microscopic thrombi to form within the pulmonary vasculature. Bilateral paravertebral soft-tissue masses (B, arrowheads), as well as marked medullary expansion of the bony structures (with the ribs showing the most pronounced involvement), were also present, findings that are associated with compensatory extramedullary hematopoiesis

vulnerable to the endothelial toxicity of iron overload as well as making them less tolerant and responsive to the effects of afterload-reducing agents.

### Splenectomy

Hypersplenism is relatively common in the thalassemias and may necessitate spleen removal. Splenectomy may also be performed to lower blood transfusion requirements. However, the spleen plays a critically important role in removing hematologic debris from the cardiovascular system. Phosphatidylserine positive platelets, platelet fragments, and red cell fragments are powerful pro-coagulants. They also inhibit nitric oxide, stimulate vasoconstricting substances such as endothelin and vasoconstricting prostaglandins, and produce endothelial proliferation. The spleen also removes brittle senescent red cells from the circulation, suppressing intravascular hemolysis. Cell-free hemoglobin is a powerful oxidant and scavenger of nitric oxide. As a result, splenectomy is a strong risk factor for intravascular thrombosis and pulmonary hypertension.

### Iron Overload

Patients with thalassemia develop iron overload through increased iron absorption and transfusional therapy. Iron is toxic to all the endocrine glands that support the heart. Insulin-resistance and frank diabetes are relatively common. Hyperglycemia and insulin resistance are powerful oxidative stressors to the heart, worsening the effects of iron overload. Proper insulin sensitivity is also vital for efficient cardiac energy utilization. Iron may also poison the thyroid and parathyroid gland, impairing metabolism and calcium regulation respectively. Iron-mediated adrenal insufficiency may also manifest itself during metabolic stress. Deficiencies of growth hormone and the sex steroids impair cardiac function. Iron-mediated endocrine toxicity must be excluded in TM patients with cardiac failure.

### Nutritional Deficiencies

The hemoglobinopathies are a hypermetabolic state and inherently produce chronic oxidative stress. Broad-spectrum nutritional deficiencies are prevalent and may reinforce disease toxicity. Fat-soluble vitamin depletion is common, including vitamin A, D, E, and K, suggesting fat malabsorption. The mechanisms and consequences are unknown. Vitamin D deficiency is associated with increased cardiac iron and decreased function, but causation has not been proven. Many trace metals are decreased, including selenium, zinc, and copper. B-vitamin levels are also low, particularly thiamine, riboflavin, and folate, most likely from consumption during ineffective erythropoiesis. Severe thiamine deficiency can have neurological and cardiac toxicity, whereas deficient riboflavin and folate may result in elevated homocysteine and endothelial toxicity. Carnitine deficiency is also relatively common in thalassemia and can impair cardiac function.

### Lung Disease

The heart and lungs are intimately coupled. Patients with thalassemia major develop mild, nonprogressive restrictive lung disease. In homogeneous ventilation and small airways disease is common but diffusion capacity (when corrected for hemoglobin) is normal suggesting that vascular networks are normal at the alveolar level. Both the aetiology and the consequences of these changes are unknown.

## IRON CARDIOMYOPATHY

### Mechanisms

Figure 40.15 represents the pathophysiology of iron cardiomyopathy, artificially divided into iron uptake, iron storage, and iron toxicity. The heart takes up physiologic amounts of iron through transferrin receptors, but this process is tightly regulated and does not lead to iron overload. When transferrin-binding capacity is exceeded, circulating low molecular weight non-transferrin-bound iron (NTBI) species appear. NTBI is oxidatively active and can enter through nonspecific, poor-regulated cation channels in the heart, leading to cardiac iron overload. Several channel mechanisms have been proposed, including L-type voltage-dependent calcium channels, but much more work is necessary to characterize cardiac iron-uptake processes.

## PROSTHETIC HEART VALVES (Fig 40.16)

### Hemolysis

Blood tests for hemolysis (lactate dehydrogenase) should be part of routine follow-up. A large proportion (50–95%) of patients with mechanical valves have some degree of intravascular hemolysis. However, anemia caused by hemolysis is rare unless prosthetic regurgitation has occurred. Patients with mild-to-moderate anemia can generally be treated conservatively with iron and folate,

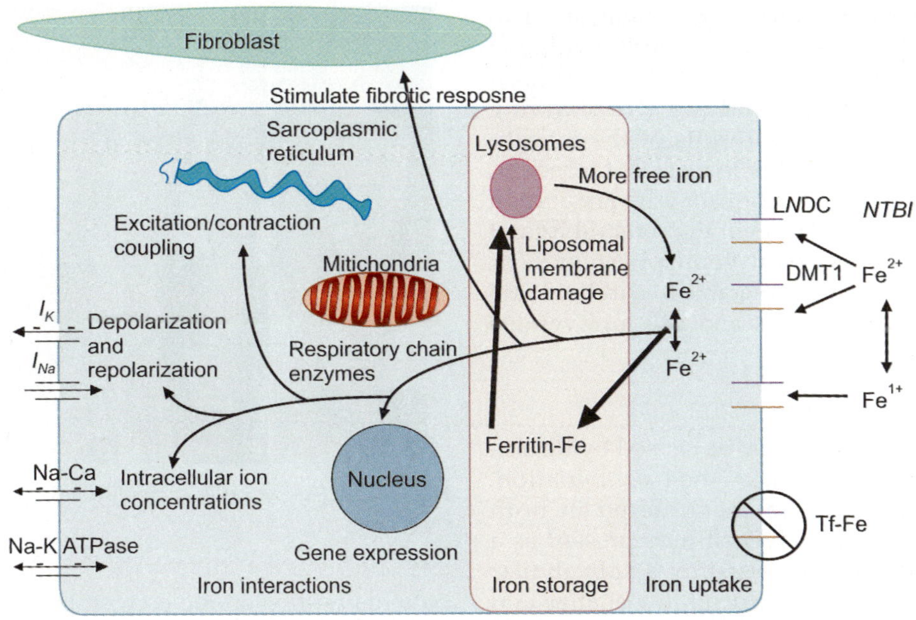


**Fig. 40.15:** Pathophysiology of iron cardiomyopathy, artificially divided into iron uptake, iron storage, and iron toxicity

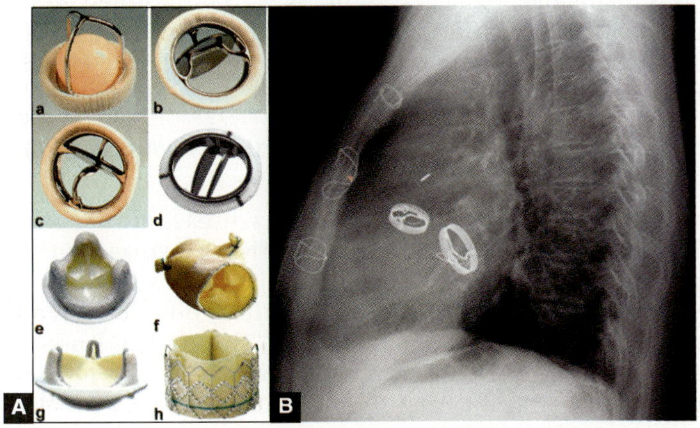


**Fig. 40.16:** (A) Various types of prosthetic heart valves. (B) X-ray chest lateral view shows mitral and aortic prosthetic valves

beta-blockers, and erythropoietin. However, repeat valve surgery or surgical repair of a paravalvular leak may be needed when prosthetic valve hemolysis is associated with severe refractory anemia.

## Anticoagulant-related Hemorrhage

In patients on long-term anticoagulation, the annual risk of a hemorrhagic event is ≈1% per patient-year. Randomized comparative studies of bioprosthetic versus mechanical prostheses reported that thromboembolism rates are similar with the two types of valves but bleeding is more common with a mechanical valve. In patients with mechanical valves, the bleeding events are most often due to excessive anticoagulation, which can be managed by withholding warfarin and monitoring the level of anticoagulation with serial INR determinations.

## Long-term Complications: Identification and Management

Mechanical valves have a substantial risk of thromboemboli and thrombotic obstruction and therefore require long-term anticoagulation therapy, which in turn is associated with an increased risk of hemorrhagic complications. Nonetheless, contemporary mechanical valves have excellent durability. In contrast, bioprosthetic valves have a low risk of thromboembolism without anticoagulation, but their durability is limited by calcific or noncalcific tissue deterioration.

## Thromboembolic and Bleeding Complications

Thromboembolic complications are an important cause of morbidity and mortality in patients with a prosthetic heart valve, with an estimated incidence of clinical events ranging from 0.6 to 2.3% per patient-year. The risk of thromboembolic complications is similar for patients with mechanical valves on warfarin therapy and bioprosthetic valves without warfarin therapy. The risk of thromboembolism depends not only on prosthesis type but also on valve position and thrombogenicity, patient risk factors, and antithrombotic treatment.

## Systemic Emboli

In patients with a prosthetic valve, thromboembolic events are presumed to be related to the valve unless proven otherwise. The presence of a thrombus on the prosthesis may not be confirmed by echocardiography because the thrombus is no longer present, is too small to be detected, or is occulted by the shadowing caused by the valve components. The first step in the management of a patient with a prosthetic valve and a systemic embolic event is to carefully assess the adequacy of anticoagulation control. If it is inadequate, therapy is adjusted or reinstituted to achieve and maintain a therapeutic effect. If anticoagulation has been adequate, warfarin therapy should be increased to achieve a higher INR target, and not withstanding bleeding risk assessment and the results of the investigation, aspirin may also be added or increased. Moreover, in patients with recent cerebral embolism who are at high risk for hemorrhagic transformation of the cerebral infarct (infarct size >35% of the cerebral hemisphere and/or uncontrolled hypertension), it is preferable to withhold oral anticoagulation for at least 5 days and use intravenous heparin in the meantime.

### Prosthesis Thrombosis

Obstruction of prosthetic valves may be caused by thrombus formation, pannus ingrowth, or their combination. Pannus ingrowth alone may be encountered in both bioprosthesis and mechanical valves. It may present as a slowly progressive obstruction caused by a subvalvular annulus, in which case it may be difficult to visualize and thus distinguish from progressive structural valve deterioration (SVD). Valve thrombosis is most often encountered in patients with mechanical valves and inadequate antithrombotic therapy. Thrombosis also may be seen in bioprosthetic valves where it most often occurs in the early postoperative period. Pannus and thrombosis may be present alone or in combination and cause acute or subacute valve obstruction. The incidence of obstructive valve thrombosis varies between 0.3% and 1.3% per patient-year in patients with mechanical valves.

## HEMATOLOGIC DISORDERS IN PATIENTS WITH CYANOTIC CONGENITAL HEART DISEASE

Hematologic management of adults with cyanotic congenital heart disease has received little recent attention.

The lack of practical therapeutic guidelines prompted us to consolidate our observations on 124 cyanotic adults for general physicians, cardiologists, and hematologists who care for these patients. Specific attention focused on regulation of erythrocyte mass and concepts of compensated and decompensated erythrocytosis, symptoms of deficient tissue oxygen transport, hyperviscosity and iron deficiency, the potential relation between elevated hematocrit levels and brain injury, hemostasis, urate metabolism, and renal function. Cerebral infarction was not seen in any patient. Phlebotomy is best reserved for treatment of symptomatic hyperviscosity. Iron therapy is indicated for symptomatic iron deficient erythropoiesis. Abnormal hemostatic mechanisms are the rule. Antithrombotic medications have little or no role in treatment (Fig. 40.17).

Hyperuricemia is the result of abnormal renal uric acid excretion not urate overproduction, and serves as a marker of abnormal renal function. Drugs that promote urate excretion are the preferred maintenance treatment in symptomatic hyperuricemic patients. Erythrocytosis, thrombocytopenia, platelets function defects, coagulation factors deficiencies are the main hematologic disorders in

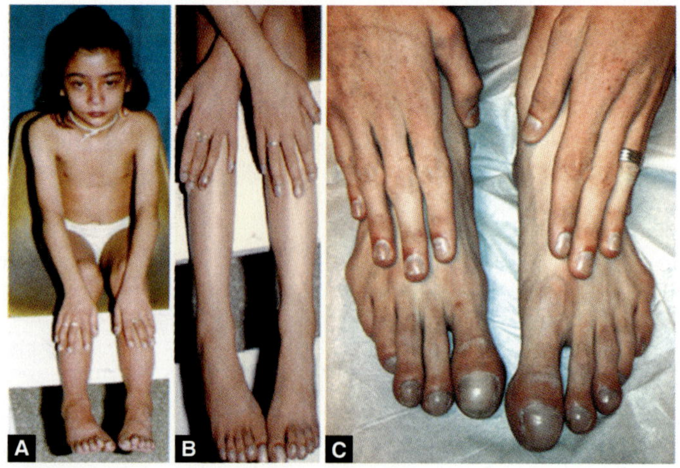

**Fig. 40.17:** (A) Cyanotic child. (B) Digital clubbing. (C) Differential cyanosis

patients with cyanotic congenital heart disease. They are responsible for increased bleeding tendency and contraindication of anticoagulation. Phlebotomy in this group of patients should be recommended when erythrocytosis is accompanied by clinical symptoms. Excessive phlebotomy can lead to iron deficiency and cause hyperviscosity symptoms. The iron supplementation should be closely monitored.

### *Cerebrovascular Events in Adult Patients with Cyanotic Congenital Heart Disease*

Adults with cyanotic congenital heart disease are at risk of having cerebrovascular events. This risk is increased in the presence of hypertension, atrial fibrillation, history of phlebotomy and microcytosis, the latter condition having the strongest significance ($p < 0.005$). This finding leads us to endorse a more conservative approach toward phlebotomy and a more aggressive approach toward treating microcytosis in adults with cyanotic congenital heart disease.

## COAGULATION ABNORMALITIES AND CARDIOVASCULAR DISEASE

In patients with excessive venous thrombosis, genetic defects predisposing to thrombosis can be found in 60–80%. Increased plasma levels of coagulation proteins such as fibrinogen and plasminogen activator inhibitor-1 (PAI-1) are associated with an increased risk of myocardial infarction. However, despite the presence of polymorphisms that regulate plasma levels of factor VIII, PAI-1, and fibrinogen the association between common polymorphisms of these coagulation protein and ischemic cardiac disease remains ambiguous. Up to 10% of the population have defects that predispose them to excessive venous thrombosis. In spite of the essential role of thrombosis in coronary ischemic syndrome, no convincing evidence has implicated the two most common venous hypercoagulable states in ischemic heart disease. Pathogenic polymorphisms in the platelet fibrinogen and collagen receptors remains an area of intense research interest. Finally, it has been shown that lipoproteins can act as mediators of coagulation processes. There are several systemic changes in hemostasis and fibrinolysis in atherosclerosis. In this study, the association between the degree of coronary atheromatosis and two key components of the coagulation system were evaluated. Once a thrombus resulting from a hypercoagulability condition is formed it is dissolved by the fibrinolytic system. So, researchers have hypothesized that a decrease in fibrinolytic activity could be a risk factor for ischemic events. It is still unclear in the literature whether the quantity of plasminogen that is transformed into plasmin is linearly correlated to plasminogen levels. Plasminogen plasma concentration does not vary significantly in normal blood coagulation. In the present study, the average values obtained for plasminogen did not show statistically significant differences between the three groups and remained within the normal range indicated for the method. An independent and unexpected association between high plasminogen levels and CAD risk has been reported previously, since decreased plasminogen levels suggest the generation of less plasmin and signal impaired fibrinolytic activity, which favors the deposit of fibrin and contributes to atherothrombosis. However, plasminogen has several nonfibrinolytic roles the most important of which is related to the inflammatory process. Plasminogen is directly linked to monocyte recruitment during inflammatory response and there is evidence that interleukin-6 may increase the plasminogen gene expression. So, it is likely that the increase in plasminogen plasma concentration is secondary to the inflammatory process present in subclinical atherosclerotic lesions. This may, at least in part, justify the presence of the positive correlation found in this study between plasminogen and fibrinogen levels ($r = 0.46$; p-value $<0.0001$).

Few studies have shown the participation of plasminogen in the local process of atherothrombosis. Likewise, in the present study, plasminogen levels were not correlated to the presence or severity of CAD and did not bring additional benefits, at least for subjects with the diagnosis of CAD. Similar observations were made by Hoffmeister et al. in a case-control study; the authors failed to find any association between elevated levels of plasminogen and stable CAD in German patients. Some systemic inflammation markers may indicate the severity of the inflammatory process and their levels were recently associated to CAD. Similar results were reported by Giannitsis et al. who found that the mean values for the plasma levels of fibrinogen increased progressively as the CAD became more severe, although these values remained within the normal range. This current study also showed that, despite being within the normal range, plasma fibrinogen levels are significantly higher in patients with mild/moderate and severe atheromatosis than in angiographically normal subjects. The association between hyperfibrinogenemia and the progression of CAD has been widely reported. It is well-known that hyperfibrinogenemia is associated to acute coronary events and may be partly a cause and not just a consequence of the lesion as fibrinogen is a protein that appears in the acute phase and as the atherosclerotic process presents inflammatory components.

As this is a cross-sectional study, we evaluated associations, not predictions nor causation. Another important limitation is the fact that our observations are based on a small group of patients; further studies involving larger numbers of patients may elucidate the association between plasma levels of plasminogen and the severity of coronary stenosis. Our findings relate to a group of patients that, according to cardiologists, require coronary angiography and thus our subjects with no coronary stenosis may not be representative of the general population. Platelets have been implicated in the pathogenesis of coronary artery disease, and a number of studies have examined platelet function and coagulation parameters in such patients.

Different studies demonstrated significant elevations in platelet coagulant activities concerned with the initiation and early stages of intrinsic coagulation in patients with chest pain and angiographically demonstrated coronary artery disease as compared with those with chest pain but normal coronary angiograms. In addition, compared with in patients with normal coronary angiograms, significant decreases in antithrombin III functional activity were observed in patients with documented coronary artery disease without concomitant decreases in antithrombin III antigen levels. The results of various assays of the platelet coagulant activities reflect the role of platelets at different stages of intrinsic coagulation.

## COMPLICATIONS OF ORAL ANTICOAGULANTS IN CARDIOVASCULAR DISEASE

Thromboembolism is a common complication of heart disease. The decision to prescribe an anticoagulant to prevent thromboemboli should be based on a particular patient's risk without treatment and the likely benefit and side effects of the proposed treatment.

This meta-analysis of randomized trials includes data from more than 20,000 patients with established CAD. Clear reductions in total mortality, MI, and stroke occurred among patients treated with oral anticoagulants (OA) at high intensity (INR 2.8 to 4.8), although this therapy was also associated with a significant increase in major bleeding. Conversely, low-intensity OA (INR <2.0) in the presence of aspirin does not confer any benefit over aspirin alone but still increases major bleeding episodes. Moderate-intensity OA reduced recurrent ischemic events by 16% compared with controls. For moderate- or high-intensity OA, the reduction in CV events was 21% compared with aspirin, and when used together with aspirin, moderate-to-high-intensity OA reduced recurrent ischemic events by 12% compared with aspirin alone. A comparison of moderate- or high-intensity OA alone versus the combination of moderate-intensity OA plus aspirin may be more effective than moderate-to-high-intensity OA alone, although with the paucity of current data, this cannot be confirmed. Certainly there is no apparent significant increase in bleeding with the combination of moderate-intensity OA and aspirin compared with OA alone. This supports other evidence that it is the INR intensity rather than the simultaneous use of antiplatelet agents with OA that leads to bleeding episodes and justifies careful monitoring of the INR for patients who are receiving OA.

The data presented in this overview represent the *observed* treatment effects because the summary estimates included all patients whether they were actually compliant with the intended therapy or not. Therefore, these estimates are conservative, represent an intention-to-treat analysis, and are likely to be an underestimate of the *true* risk reduction achievable with OA when compliance is maximized and the target INR is achieved. An example of the effect of noncompliance on the overall estimate of treatment effect comes from the OASIS-2 trial. In this trial, OA and aspirin versus aspirin alone was associated with a small nonsignificant reduction in CV death, MI, and stroke (7.6% vs 8.3%; risk reduction, 0.90; 95% CI, 0.72–1.14; p = 0.40). However, at the end of the follow-up period, only 63.7% of patients who had been randomized to receive OA and aspirin were actually receiving their OA. Compliance with OA varied significantly between the 14 countries participating in the trial. The 'good compliance' countries were those in which compliance with OA was at least 70% at 35 days; 'poor compliance' countries had <70% at 35 days. In the 'good compliance' countries, the combination of OA and aspirin was associated with a significant 32% reduction in CV death, MI, and stroke (6.1% vs 8.9%; risk reduction, 0.68; 95% CI, 0.48–0.95; p = 0.02) compared with aspirin alone. Conversely, in 'poor compliance' countries, no reduction in the composite outcome of CV death, MI or stroke was observed. As expected, there was a larger relative increase in major bleeding among the 'good compliance' countries compared with the 'poor compliance' countries (2.71 vs 1.58). Therefore, in the high compliance subgroup, OA and aspirin use was associated with a relative risk reduction three times that observed with OA and aspirin using the intent-to-treat approach. This review provides evidence that among CAD patients the combination of moderate-intensity OA plus aspirin is more effective than aspirin alone and is relatively safe. This combination should be considered for high-risk patients with CAD, including those who suffer a CV event while receiving aspirin monotherapy (e.g. an aspirin failure). The potential benefits of OA therapy in reducing serious clinical events such as MI, stroke, and death should be weighed against the risk that OA might cause life-threatening bleeding. Clinical algorithms can assist clinicians in making such judgments. Recently, dual antiplatelet therapy has been shown to be superior to aspirin alone in preventing recurrent MI, stroke, and CV death among patients with ACS. The efficacy and safety profiles comparing dual antiplatelet therapy with moderate-intensity OA and aspirin have not been adequately evaluated, and future studies should address this question.

## KEY POINTS

- Whether anticoagulant treatment should be started depends on the balance between the risk of thrombomboli without treatment and the likely benefits of treatment in each patient
- Factors increasing the risk of bleeding include serious concomitant disease, previous gastrointestinal bleeding, uncontrolled hypertension, and immobility
- Factors that cumulatively increase the risk of thromboembolism in nonrheumatic atrial fibrillation include age over 60, recent congestive heart failure, hypertension (treated or untreated), previous thromboembolism, and the presence of a large atrium or of global left ventricular dysfunction
- Cardioversion of nonrheumatic atrial fibrillation (including fibrillation of new onset) is associated with an increased thromboembolic risk, which is reduced by anticoagulant treatment
- Heparin and aspirin are both beneficial in unstable angina
- Anticoagulants should be considered after myocardial infarction in patients with an increased risk of thromboemboli: patients in atrial fibrillation and those with persistent heart failure.

## BIBLIOGRAPHY


1. Al-Ahmad A, Rand WM, Manjunath G, Konstam MA, Salem DN, Levey AS, Sarnak MJ. Reduced kidney function and anemia as risk factors for mortality in patients with left ventricular dysfunction. J Am Coll Cardiol 2001;38:955–62.
2. Alhenc-Gelas M, Gandrille S, Aubry ML, Aiach M. Thirty-three novel mutations in the protein C gene. French INSERM network on molecular abnormalities responsible for protein C and protein S. Thromb Haemost 2000;83:86–92.
3. Ali Ghasemi, Mohsen Horri, Yaser Salahshour. Coagulation Abnormalities in Pediatric Patients with Congenital Heart Disease: A Literature Review 2014;2:141–3.
4. Allaart CF, Poort SR, Rosendaal FR, Reitsma PH, Bertina RM, Briet E. Increased risk of venous thrombosis in carriers of hereditary protein C deficiency defect. Lancet 1993;341:134–8.
5. Anand IS, Chandrashekhar Y, Ferrari R, et al. Pathogenesis of edema in chronic severe anaemia: Studies of body water and sodium, renal function, haemodynamic variables, and plasma hormones. Br Heart J 1993;70:357–62.
6. Anand IS, Chandrashekhar Y, Ferrari R, Poole-Wilson PA, Harris PC. Pathogenesis of edema in chronic severe anaemia: studies of body water and sodium, renal function, haemodynamic variables, and plasma hormones. Br Heart J 1993;70:357–62.
7. Anand IS, Chandrashekhar Y, Wander GS, Chawla LS. Endothelium-derived relaxing factor is important in mediat-ing the high output state in chronic severe anemia. J Am Coll Cardiol 1995;25:1402–7.
8. Anand IS, Kuskowski MA, Rector TS, Florea VG, Glazer RD, Hester A, Chiang YT, Aknay N, Maggioni AP, Opasich C, Latini R, Cohn JN. Anemia and change in hemoglobin over time related to mortality and morbidity in patients with chronic heart failure: results from Val-HeFT. Circulation 2005;112:1121–7.

9. Anand IS. Anemia and chronic heart failure implications and treatment options. J Am Coll Cardiol 2008;52:501–11.
10. Anand S, Yusuf S. Oral anticoagulant therapy in patients with coronary artery disease: a meta-analysis JAMA 1999; 282:2058–67.
11. Androne AS, Katz SD, Lund L, et al. Hemodilution is common in patients with advanced heart failure. Circulation 2003;107:226–9.
12. Androne AS, Katz SD, Lund L, LaManca J, Hudaihed A, Hryniewicz K, Mancini DM. Hemodilution is common in patients with advanced heart failure.Circulation 2003;107: 226–9.
13. Antithrombotics Trialists' Collaboration Collaborative meta-analysis of randomised trials of antiplatelet therapy for prevention of death, myocardial infarction, and stroke in high risk patients BMJ 2002;324:71–86.
14. Arnold DM, Nazi I, Kelton JG. New treatments for idiopathic thrombocytopenic purpura: rethinking old hypotheses. Expert Opin Investig Drugs 2009;18:805–19.
15. Aubrun C, Nichol A, Cooper DJ, Bellomo R. Age of red blood cells and transfusion in critically ill patients. Ann Intensive Care 2013;4:2.
16. Bateman ST, Lacroix J, Boven K, Forbes P, Barton R, Thomas N, Jacobs B, Markovitz B, Goldstein B, Hanson J, Randolph AG. for the Pediatric Acute Lung Injury and Sepsis Investigator's (PALISI) Network. Anemia, blood loss and blood transfusion in North American children in the intensive care unit. Am J Respir Crit Care Med 2008;4:26–33.
17. Bates SM, Greer IA, Pabinger I, Sofaer S, Hirsh J. Venous thromboembolism, thrombophilia, antithrombotic therapy, and pregnancy: American College of Chest Physicians Evidence-Based Clinical Practice Guidelines. 8th ed. Chest 2008;133:S844–86.
18. Belcher JD, Marker PH, Weber JP, Hebbel RP, Vercellotti GM. Activated monocytes in sickle cell disease: potential role in the activation of vascular endothelium and vaso-occlusion. Blood 2000;96:2451–9.
19. Berry C, Hogg K, Norrie J, Stevenson K, Brett M, McMurray J. Heart failure with preserved left ventricular systolic function: a hospital cohort study. Heart 2005;91:907–13.
20. Bertina RM, Koeleman BP, Koster T, Rosendaal FR, Dirven RJ, De Ronde H, et al. Mutation in blood coagulation factor V associated with resistance to activated protein C. Nature 1994;369:64–7.
21. Besarab A, Bolton WK, Browne JK, Egrie JC, Nissenson AR, Okamoto DM, Schwab SJ, Goodkin DA. The effects of normal as compared with low hematocrit values in patients with cardiac disease who are receiving hemodialysis and epoetin. N Engl J Med 1998;339:584–90.
22. Brines M, Grasso G, Fiordaliso F, Sfacteria A, Ghezzi P, Fratelli M, Latini R, Xie QW, Smart J, Su-Rick CJ, Pobre E, Diaz D, Gomez D, Hand C, Coleman T, Cerami A. Erythropoietin mediates tissue protection through an erythropoietin and common beta-subunit heteroreceptor. Proc Natl Acad Sci USA 2004;101:14907–12.
23. Brouwer JL, Lijfering WM, Ten Kate MK, Kluin-Nelemans HC, Veeger NJ, Van der Meer J.High long-term absolute risk of recurrent venous thromboembolism in patients with hereditary deficiencies of protein S, protein C or anti-thrombin. Thromb Haemost 2009;101:93–9.
24. Brucks S, Little WC, Chao T, Rideman RL, Upadhya B, Wesley-Farrington D, Sane DC. Relation of anemia to diastolic heart failure and the effect on outcome. Am J Cardiol 2004;93:1055–7.
25. Bunn HF. Pathogenesis and treatment of sickle cell disease. N Engl J Med 1997;337:762–9.
26. Burt MJ, Halliday JW, Powell LW. Iron and coronary heart disease. BMJ 1993;307:575–6.
27. Calvillo L, Latini R, Kajstura J, Leri A, Anversa P, Ghezzi P, Salio M, Cerami A, Brines M. Recombinant human erythropoietin protects the myocardium from ischemia-reperfusion injury and promotes beneficial remodeling. Proc Natl Acad Sci USA 2003;100:4802–6.
28. Cantin B, Després JP, Lamarche B, Moorjani S, Lupien PJ, Bogaty P, Bergeron J, Dagenais GR. Association of fibrinogen and lipoprotein(a) as a coronary Heart disease risk factor in men (The Quebec Cardiovascular Study). Am J Cardiol 2002;89(6):662-6.
29. Carson JL, Duff A, Poses RM, et al. Effect of anaemia and cardiovascular disease on surgical mortality and morbidity. Lancet 1996;348:1055–60.
30. Castoldi E, Brugge JM, Nicolaes GA, Girelli D, Tans G, Rosing J. Impaired APC cofactor activity of factor V plays a major role in the APC resistance associated with the factor V Leiden (R506Q) and R2 (H1299R) mutations. Blood 2004; 103: 4173–9.
31. Cerami A, Brines M, Ghezzi P, Cerami C, Itri LM. Neuroprotective properties of epoetin alfa. Nephrol Dial Transplant 2002;17(Suppl 1):8–12.
32. Chalmers TC, Matta RJ, Smith H, Kunzler AM. Evidence favouring the use of anticoagulants in the hospital phase of acute myocardial infarction. N Engl J Med 1977;297: 1091–6.
33. Chang JJ, Parikh CR. When heparin causes thrombosis: significance, recognition, and management of heparin-induced thrombocytopenia in dialysis patients. Semin Dial 2006;19:297–304.
34. Cheung JY, Miller BA. Molecular mechanisms of erythropoietin signaling. Nephron 2001;87:215–22.
35. Churchill DN, Muirhead N, Goldstein M, Posen G, Fay W, Beecroft ML, Gorman J, Taylor DW. Probability of thrombosis of vascular access among hemodialysis patients treated with recombinant human erythropoietin. J Am Soc Nephrol 1994; 4:1809–13.
36. Cleland JG, Coletta AP, Clark AL, Velavan P, Ingle L. Clinical trials update from the European Society of Cardiology Heart Failure meeting and the Am College of Cardiology: darbe-poetin alfa study, ECHOS, and ASCOT-BPLA. Eur J Heart Fail 2005;7:937–9.
37. Cleland JG, Sullivan JT, Ball S, Horowitz JD, Agoram B, Rosser D, Yates W, Tin L, Fuentealba P, Burton PB. Once-monthly administration of darbepoetin alfa for the treatment of patients with chronic heart failure and anemia: a pharma-co-kinetic and pharmacodynamic investigation. J Cardiovasc Pharmacol 2005;46:155–61.
38. Cook JD, Lipschitz DA, Miles LE, et al. Serum ferritin as a measure of iron stores in normal subjects. Am J Clin Nutr 1974;27:681–7.
39. Cooper CE. Nitric oxide and iron proteins. Biochim Biophys Acta 1999;1411:290–309.

40. Corwin HL, Gettinger A, Pearl RG, Fink MP, Levy MM, Abraham E, MacIntyre NR, Shabot MM, Duh MS, Shapiro MJ. The CRIT Study: anemia and blood transfusion in the critically ill-current clinical practice in the United States. Crit Care Med 2004;4:39–52.
41. Cromie N, Lee C, Struthers AD. Anaemia in chronic heart failure: what is its frequency in the UK and its underlying causes? Heart 2002;87:377–8.
42. Dahlback B. The protein C anticoagulant system: inherited defects as basis for venous thrombosis. Thromb Res 1995; 77:1–43.
43. Day SM, Duquaine D, Mundada LV, Menon RG, Khan BV, Rajagopalan S, Fay WP. Chronic iron administration increases vascular oxidative stress and accelerates arterial thrombosis. Circulation 2003; 107: 2601–6.
44. De Luca G, Verdoia M, Cassetti E, Schaffer A, Cavallino C, Bolzani V, Marino P; Novara Atherosclerosis Study Group (NAS). High fibrinogen level is an independent predictor of presence and extent of coronary artery disease among Italian population. J Thromb Thrombolysis 2011;31(4):458–63.
45. De Mattia D, Del Vecchio GC, Russo G, De Santis A, Ramenghi U, Notarangelo L, et al. Management of chronic childhood immune thrombocytopenic purpura: AIEOP consensus guidelines. Acta Haematol 2010;123:96–109.
46. Denman Hammond, Robert Stantona, Gerald S Gilchrist, Henry Ekert. Hemostasis in cyanotic congenital heart disease. The Journal of Pediatrics 1970:769;221–30.
47. Dentali F, Crowther M, Ageno W. Thrombophilic abnor-malities, oral contraceptives, and risk of cerebral vein thrombosis: a meta-analysis. Blood 2006;107:2766–73.
48. Devendra GP, Hart SA, Whitney EJ, Krasuski RA. Impact of fibrinogen levels on angiographic progression and 12-year survival in the armed forces regression study. Angiology 2010;61(4):333–7.
49. Diaz-Ricart M, Etebanell E, Cases A, Lopez-Pedret J, Castillo R, Ordinas A, Escolar G. Erythropoietin improves signaling through tyrosine phosphorylation in platelets from uremic patients. Thromb Haemost 1999;82:1312–7.
50. Duffy S, Biegelson E, Holbrook M, et al. Iron chelation improves endothelial function in patients with coronary disease. Circulation 2001;103:2799–804.
51. Duke M, Abelmann WH. The hemodynamic response to chronic anemia. Circulation 1969;39:503–15.
52. Ebert BL, Bunn HF. Regulation of the erythropoietin gene. Blood 1999;94:1864–77.
53. Eschbach JW, Abdulhadi MH, Browne JK, Delano BG, Downing MR, Egrie JC, Evans RW, Friedman EA, Graber SE, Haley NR, Korbet S, Krantz SB, Lundin AP, Nissenson AR, Ogden DA, Paganini ED, Rader B, Rutsky EA, Stivelman J, Stone WJ, Teschan P, van Stone JC, van Wyck DB, Zuckerman K, Adamson JW. Recombinant human erythro-poietin in anemic patients with end-stage renal disease: results of a phase III multicenter clinical trial. Ann Intern Med 1989;111:992–1000.
54. Ezekowitz JA, McAlister FA, Armstrong PW. Anemia is common in heart failure and is associated with poor outcomes: insights from a cohort of 12 065 patients with new-onset heart failure. Circulation 2003;107:223–225.
55. Felker GM, Gattis WA, Leimberger JD, Adams KF, Cuffe MS, Gheorghiade M, O'Connor CM. Usefulness of anemia as a predictor of death and rehospitalization in patients with decompensated heart failure. Am J Cardiol 2003;92:625–8.
56. Feudjo-Tepie MA, Robinson NJ, Bennett D. Prevalence of diagnosed chronic immune thrombocytopenic purpura in the US: analysis of a large US claim database: a rebuttal. J Thromb Haemost 2008;6:711–712.
57. Fiordaliso F, Chimenti S, Staszewsky L, Bai A, Carlo E, Cuccovillo I, Doni M, Mengozzi M, Tonelli R, Ghezzi P, Coleman T, Brines M, Cerami A, Latini R. A nonerythropoietic derivative of erythropoietin protects the myocardium from ischemia-reperfusion injury. Proc Natl Acad Sci USA. 2005; 102: 2046–51.
58. Fiore LD, Ezekowitz MD, Brophy MT, et al. Department of Veterans Affairs Cooperative Studies Program Clinical Trial comparing combined warfarin and aspirin with aspirin alone in survivors of acute myocardial infarction: primary results of the CHAMP study Circulation 2002;105:557–63.
59. Fitzhugh CD, Lauder N, Jonassaint JC, Telen MJ, Zhao X, Wright EC, et al. Cardiopulmonary complications leading to premature deaths in adult patients with sickle cell disease. Am J Hematol 2010;85:36–40.
60. Foley RN, Parfrey PS, Morgan J, Barre PE, Campbell P, Cartier P, Coyle D, Fine A, Handa P, Kingma I, Lau CY, Levin A, Mendelssohn D, Muirhead N, Murphy B, Plante RK, Posen G, Wells GA. Effect of hemoglobin levels in hemodialysis patients with asymptomatic cardiomyopathy. Kidney Int 2000;58:1325–35.
61. Folsom AR, Aleksic N, Park E, Salomaa V, Juneja H, Wu KK. Prospective study of fibrinolytic factors and incident coronary artery disease. The Atherosclerosis Risk in Communities (ARIC) Study. Arterioscler Thromb Vasc Biol 2001;21(4):611–617.
62. Fuste B, Serradell M, Escolar G, Cases A, Mazzara R, Castillo R, Ordinas A, Diaz-Ricart M. Erythropoietin triggers a signal-ing pathway in endothelial cells and increases the thrombo-genicity of their extracellular matrices in vitro. Thromb Haemost 2002;88:678–85.
63. Fyhrquist F, Karppinen K, Honkanen T, Saijonmaa O, Rosenlof K. High serum erythropoietin levels are normalized during treatment of congestive heart failure with enalapril. J Intern Med 1989;226:257–60.
64. Galli M, Luciani D, Bertolini G, Barbui T. Lupus anticoagulants are stronger risk factors for thrombosis than anti-cardiolipin antibodies in the antiphospholipid syndrome: a systematic review of the literature. Blood 2003;101:1827–32.
65. Gandhi K, Aronow WS, Desai H, Amin H, Sharma M, Lai HM, et al. Cardiovascular manifestations in patients with thrombotic thrombocytopenic purpura: a single-center experience. Clin Cardiol 2010;33:213–6.
66. Gandrille S, Borgel D, Sala N, Espinosa-Parrilla Y, Simmonds R, Rezende S, et al. Scientific and Standardization Committee Communication: Protein S Deficiency: A Database of Mutations.
67. Ghali JK, Anand IS, Abraham WT, Fonarow GC, Greenberg B, Krum H, et al. Randomized double-blind trial of darbe-poetin alfa in patients with symptomatic heart failure and anemia. Circulation 2008;117:526–35.
68. Gibbons GH, Dzau VJ. The emerging concept of vascular remodeling. N Engl J Med 1994;330:1431–8.

69. Gladwin MT, Vichinsky E. Pulmonary complications of sickle cell disease. N Engl J Med 2008;359:2254–65.
70. Gladwin MT, Vichinsky E. Pulmonary complications of sickle cell disease. N Engl J Med 2008;359:2254–65.
71. Goodnough LT, Brecher ME, Kanter MH, AuBuchon JP. Transfusion medicine: first of two parts–blood transfusion. N Engl J Med 1999;340:438–47.
72. Greaves SC, Gamble GD, Collins JF, et al. Determinants of left ventricular hypertrophy and systolic dysfunction in chronic renal failure. Am J Kidney Dis 1994;24:768–76.
73. Hassell KL. Population estimates of sickle cell disease in the U.S. Am J Prev Med 2010;38:S512–21.
74. Hayabuchi Y, Matsuoka S, Akita H, Kuroda Y. Hyperuricaemia in cyanotic congenital heart disease. Eur J Pediatr 1993;152:873–689.
75. Haywood LJ. Cardiovascular function and dysfunction in sickle cell anemia. J Natl Med Assoc 2009;101:24–30.
76. Haywood S, Liesner R, Pindora S, Ganesan V. Thrombophilia and first arterial ischaemic stroke: a systematic review. Arch Dis Child 2005;90:402–5.
77. Head CA, Swerdlow P, McDade WA, Joshi RM, Ikuta T, Cooper ML, et al. Beneficial effects of nitric oxide breathing in adult patients with sickle cell crisis. Am J Hematol 2010; 85:800–2.
78. Henke M, Laszig R, Rube C, Schafer U, Haase KD, Schilcher B, Mose S, Beer KT, Burger U, Dougherty C, Frommhold H. Erythropoietin to treat head and neck cancer patients with anaemia undergoing radiotherapy: rando-mised, double-blind, placebo-controlled trial. Lancet 2003; 362:1255–60.
79. Hitoshi Horigome, Yuji Hiramatsu, Osamu Shigeta, Toshiro Nagasawa, Akira Matsui, Overproduction of platelet micro-particles in cyanotic congenital heart disease with poly-cythemia. J Am Coll Cardiol 2002;39:1072–1077.
80. Ho WK, Hankey GJ, Quinlan DJ, Eikelboom JW. Risk of recurrent venous thromboembolism in patients with common thrombophilia: a systematic review. Arch Intern Med 2006;166:729–36.
81. Hoffmeister HM, Heller W, Seipel L. Blood coagulation and fibrinolysis in atherosclerosis. Z Kardiol 1999;88(5):315–23 [German].
82. Horina JH, Schwaberger G, Brussee H. et al. Increased red cell 2,3-diphosphoglycerate levels in haemodialysis patients treated with erythropoietin. Nephrol Dial Transplant 1993;8: 1219–22.
83. Horwich TB, Fonarow GC, Hamilton MA, MacLellan WR, Borenstein J. Anemia is associated with worse symptoms, greater impairment in functional capacity and a significant increase in mortality in patients with advanced heart failure. J Am Coll Cardiol 2002;39:1780–6.
84. Hurlen M, Smith P, Arnesen H. Effects of warfarin, aspirin and the two combined, on mortality and thrombo-embolic morbidity after myocardial infarction. The WARIS-II (Warfarin-Aspirin Reinfarction Study) design Scand Cardiovasc J 2000;34:168–71.
85. Huynh T, Theroux P, Bogaty P, Nasmith J, Solymoss S. Aspirin, warfarin, or the combination for secondary prevention of coronary events in patients with acute coronary syndromes and prior coronary artery bypass surgery Circulation 2001;103:3069–74.
86. Institute of Medical Genetics, Cardiff. Human Gene Mutation Database. Seligsohn U, Lubetsky A. Genetic susceptibility to venous thrombosis. N Engl J Med 2001;344:1222–31.
87. International Anticoagulation Review GroupCollaborative analysis of long-term anticoagulant administration after acute myocardial infarction. Lancet 1970;7640;203–9.
88. Ishani A, Weinhandl E, Zhao Z, Gilbertson DT, Collins AJ, Yusuf S, Herzog CA. Angiotensin-converting enzyme inhibitor as a risk factor for the development of anemia, and the impact of incident anemia on mortality in patients with left ventricular dysfunction. J Am Coll Cardiol 2005;45: 391–9.
89. IV. NKF-K/DOQI Clinical Practice Guidelines for Anemia of Chronic Kidney Disease: update 2000. Am J Kidney Dis 2001;37:S182–S238.
90. Jensen JD, Eiskjaer H, Bagger JP, Pedersen EB. Elevated level of erythropoietin in congestive heart failure relationship to renal perfusion and plasma renin. J Intern Med 1993;233: 125–30.
91. Jovin IS, Muller-Berghaus G. Interrelationships between the fibrinolytic system and lipoproteins in the pathogenesis of coronary atherosclerosis. Atherosclerosis 2004;174(2): 225–33.
92. Kannel WB, Hjortland MC, McNamara PM, et al. Menopause and risk of cardiovascular disease: The Framingham study. Ann Intern Med 1976;85:447–52.
93. Kato GJ, Hebbel RP, Steinberg MH, Gladwin MT. Vasculopathy in sickle cell disease: Biology, pathophysiology, genetics, translational medicine, and new research directions. Am J Hematol 2009;84:618–25.
94. Kaul DK, Finnegan E, Barabino GA. Sickle red cell-endo-thelium interactions. Microcirculation 2009;16:97–111.
95. Kaul DK, Hebbel RP. Hypoxia/reoxygenation causes inflammatory response in transgenic sickle mice but not in normal mice. J Clin Invest 2000;106:411–20.
96. Khor B, Van Cott EM. Laboratory evaluation of hypercoagulability. Clin Lab Med 2009;29:339–66.
97. Kiss JE. Thrombotic thrombocytopenic purpura: recognition management. Int J Hematol 2010;91:36–45.
98. Konstantinos Dimopoulos, Gerhard-Paul Diller, Georgios Giannakoulas, et al. Anemia in Adults With Congenital Heart Disease Relates to Adverse Outcome. J Am Coll Cardiol 2009;54:2093–100.
99. Kosiborod M, Smith GL, Radford MJ, Foody JM, Krumholz HM. The prognostic importance of anemia in patients with heart failure. Am J Med 2003;14:112–9.
100. Kumor-Kurek M, Siudalska H. Hematologic disorders in patients with cyanotic congenital heart disease. Pol Merkur Lekarski 1999:7;82–4.
101. Lacroix J, Hébert PC, Fergusson D, Tinmouth A, Blajchman MA, Callum J, Cook D, Marshall J, McIntyre L, Turgeon A. for the ABLE study group, and the Canadian Critical Care Trials Group. The age of blood evaluation (ABLE) randomized controlled trial: study design. Transfus Med Rev 2011; 4:197–205.
102. Lacroix J, Tucci M. Impact clinique de la durée d'entreposage des globules rouges avant transfusion. Transfus Clin Biol 2011;4:97–105.
103. Lawler PR, Filion KB, Dourian T, Atallah R, Garfinkle M, Eisenberg MJ. Anemia and mortality in acute coronary

syndromes: a systematic review and meta-analysis. Am Heart J 2013;4:143–53.

104. Leist M, Ghezzi P, Grasso G, Bianchi R, Villa P, Fratelli M, Savino C, Bianchi M, Nielsen J, Gerwien J, Kallunki P, Larsen AK, Helboe L, Christensen S, Pedersen LO, Nielsen M, Torup L, Sager T, Sfacteria A, Erbayraktar S, Erbayraktar Z, Gokmen N, Yilmaz O, Cerami-Hand C, Xie QW, Coleman T, Cerami A, Brines M. Derivatives of erythropoietin that are tissue protective but not erythropoietic. Science 2004;305:239–42.
105. Levin A, Singer J, Thompson CR, et al. Prevalent left ventricular hypertrophy in the predialysis population: Identifying opportunities for intervention. Am J Kidney Dis 1996;27:347–54.
106. Levin A, Thompson CR, Ethier J, et al. Left ventricular mass index increase in early renal disease: Impact of decline in hemoglobin. Am J Kidney Dis 1999;34:125–34.
107. Levine RL, McCollum D, Hursting M. How frequently is venous thromboembolism in heparin-treated patients associated with heparin-induced thrombocytopenia? Chest 2006;130:681–7.
108. Levy PS, Kim SJ, Eckel PK, et al. Limit to cardiac compensation during acute isovolemic hemodilution: Influence of coronary stenosis. Am J Physiol 1993;265:H340–9.
109. Lewis AB, Freed MD, Heymann MA, Roehl SL, Kensey RC. Side effects of therapy with prostaglandin E1 in infants with critical congenital heart disease. Circulation 1981;64: 893–8.
110. Leyland-Jones B, Semiglazov V, Pawlicki M, Pienkowski T, Tjulandin S, Manikhas G, Makhson A, Roth A, Dodwell D, Baselga J, Biakhov M, Valuckas K, Voznyi E, Liu X, Vercammen E. Maintaining normal hemoglobin levels with epoetin alfa in mainly nonanemic patients with metastatic breast cancer receiving first-line chemotherapy: a survival study. J Clin Oncol 2005;23:5960–72.
111. Lijnen HR, Collen D. Mechanisms of physiological fibrinolysis. Baillieres Clin Haematol 1995;8(2):277–90.
112. Lill MC, Perloff JK, Child JS. Pathogenesis of thrombocytopenia in cyanotic congenital heart disease. Am J Cardiol 2006;98:254–8.
113. Lim W, Crowther MA, Eikelboom JW. Management of antiphospholipid antibody syndrome: a systematic review. JAMA 2006;295:1050–7.
114. London GM, Parfrey PS. Cardiac disease in chronic uremia: pathogenesis. Adv Ren Replace Ther 1997;4:194–211.
115. Long BR, Leya F. The role of antiphospholipid syndrome in cardiovascular disease. Hematol Oncol Clin North Am 2008; 22:79–94.vi-vii.
116. Luc G, Bard JM, Juhan-Vague I, Ferrieres J, Evans A, Amouyel P, Arveiler D, Fruchart JC, Ducimetiere P; PRIME Study Group. C-reactive protein, interleukin-6 and fibrinogen as predictors of coronary heart disease. Arterioscler Thromb Vasc Biol 2003;23(7):1255–61.
117. Machado RF, Martyr S, Kato GJ, Barst RJ, Anthi A, Robinson MR, et al. Sildenafil therapy in patients with sickle cell disease and pulmonary hypertension. Br J Haematol 2005; 130:445–53.
118. Maggioni AP, Opasich C, Anand I, Barlera S, Carbonieri E, Gonzini L, Tavazzi L, Latini R, Cohn J. Anemia in patients with heart failure: prevalence and prognostic role in a controlled trial and in clinical practice. J Card Fail 2005;11: 91–8.
119. Mahmoodi BK, Brouwer JL, Veeger NJ, Van der Meer J. Hereditary deficiency of protein C or protein S confers increased risk of arterial thromboembolic events at a young age: results from a large family cohort study. Circulation 2008;118:1659–67.
120. Maksimowicz-McKinnon K, Selzer F, Manzi S, Kip KE, Mulukutla SR, Marroquin OC, et al. Poor 1-year outcomes after percutaneous coronary interventions in systemic lupus erythematosus: report from the National Heart, Lung, and Blood Institute Dynamic Registry. Circ Cardiovasc Interv 2008;1:201–8.
121. Mann JF. Hypertension and cardiovascular effects–long-term safety and potential long-term benefits of r-HuEPO. Nephrol Dial Transplant 1995;10(Suppl 2):80–4.
122. Manttari M, Manninen V, Huttunen JK, et al. Serum ferritin and ceruloplasmin as coronary risk factors. Eur Heart J 1994; 15:1599–603.
123. Marchiori A, Mosena L, Prins MH, Prandoni P. The risk of recurrent venous thromboembolism among heterozygous carriers of factor V Leiden or prothrombin G20210A mutation. A systematic review of prospective studies. Haema-tologica 2007;92:1107–14.
124. Marques MB. Thrombotic thrombocytopenic purpura and heparin-induced thrombocytopenia: two unique causes of life-threatening thrombocytopenia. Clin Lab Med 2009; 29:321–38.
125. Maschio G. Erythropoietin and systemic hypertension. Nephrol Dial Transplant 1995;10(Suppl 2):74–9.
126. McClellan WM, Flanders WD, Langston RD, Jurkovitz C, Presley R. Anemia and renal insufficiency are independent risk factors for death among patients with congestive heart failure admitted to community hospitals: a population-based study. J Am Soc Nephrol 2002;13:1928–36.
127. McCullough PA, Lepor NE. Anemia: a modifiable risk factor for heart disease. Introduction. Rev Cardiovasc Med 2005;6 (Suppl 3):S1–S3.
128. McMurray JJ, Anand IS, Diaz R, Maggioni AP, O'Connor C, Pfeffer MA, et al. Design of the Reduction of Events with Darbepoetin alfa in Heart Failure (RED-HF): a Phase III, anaemia correction, morbidity-mortality trial. Eur J Heart Fail 2009;11:795–801.
129. Metivier F, Marchais SJ, Guerin AP, et al. Pathophysiology of anaemia: Focus on the heart and blood vessels. Nephrol Dial Transplant 2000;15(Suppl 3):S14–S18.
130. Meyers DG, Strickland D, Maloley PA, et al. Possible association of a reduction in cardiovascular events with blood donation. Heart 1997;78:188–93.
131. Mitka M. Researchers probe anemia-heart failure link. JAMA 2003;290:1835–8.
132. Moon C, Krawczyk M, Ahn D, Ahmet I, Paik D, Lakatta EG, Talan MI. Erythropoietin reduces myocardial infarction and left ventricular functional decline after coronary artery ligation in rats. Proc Natl Acad Sci USA 2003;100: 11612–17.
133. Morrison HI, Semenciw RM, Mao Y, et al. Serum iron and risk of fatal acute myocardial infarction. Epidemiology 1994; 5:243–6.

134. Mozaffarian D, Nye R, Levy WC. Anemia predicts mortality in severe heart failure: the prospective randomized amlodipine survival evaluation (PRAISE). J Am Coll Cardiol 2003; 41:1933–9.
135. Mrug M, Stopka T, Julian BA, Prchal JF, Prchal JT. Angio-tensin II stimulates proliferation of normal early erythroid progenitors. J Clin Invest 1997;100:2310–4.
136. Nand S, Wong W, Yuen B, Yetter A, Schmulbach E, Gross Fisher S. Heparin-induced thrombocytopenia with thrombosis: incidence, analysis of risk factors, and clinical outcomes in 108 consecutive patients treated at a single institution. Am J Hematol 1997;56:12–6.
137. Neskovic AN, Stankovic I, Milicevic P, Aleksic A, Vlahovic-Stipac A, Calija B, et al. Primary PCI for acute myocardial infarction in a patient with idiopathic thrombocytopenic purpura. A case report and review of the literature. Herz 2010;35:43–9.
138. Norstrom E, Thorelli E, Dahlback B. Functional characterization of recombinant FV Hong Kong and FV Cambridge. Blood 2002;100:524–30.
139. Osarogiagbon UR, Choong S, Belcher JD, Vercellotti GM, Paller MS, Hebbel RP. Reperfusion injury pathophysiology in sickle transgenic mice. Blood 2000;96:314–20.
140. Palareti G, Valdre L, Favaretto E, Bovina V, Cini M, Legnani C. No early signs of atherosclerotic alterations in carriers of inherited thrombophilia. Eur J Intern Med 2010;21:273–7.
141. Papageorgiou N, Tousoulis D, Siasos G, Stefanadis C. Is fibrino-gen a marker of inflammation in coronary artery disease? Hellenic J Cardiol 2010;51(1):1-9. Comment in: Kostis JB. Hellenic J Cardiol 2010;51(5):475; author reply 475.
142. Park YA, Waldrum MR, Marques MB. Platelet count and prothrombin time help distinguish thrombotic thrombocytopenic purpurahemolytic uremic syndrome from disseminated intravascular coagulation in adults. Am J Clin Pathol 2010;133:460–5.
143. Parsa CJ, Matsumoto A, Kim J, Riel RU, Pascal LS, Walton GB, Thompson RB, Petrofski JA, Annex BH, Stamler JS, Koch WJ. A novel protective effect of erythropoietin in the infarcted heart. J Clin Invest 2003;112:999–1007.
144. Perloff JK, Marelli AJ, Miner PD. Risk of stroke in adults with cyanotic congenital heart disease. Circulation 1993; 87:1954–1959.
145. Pfeffer MA, Burdmann EA, Chen CY, Cooper ME, De Zeeuw D, Eckardt KU, et al. A trial of darbepoetin alfa in type 2 diabetes and chronic kidney disease. N Engl J Med 2009; 361:2019–32.
146. Platt OS, Brambilla DJ, Rosse WF. Mortality in sickle cell disease. Life expectancy and risk factors for early death [see comments]. N Engl J Med 1994;330:1639–44.
147. Platt OS. Sickle cell anemia as an inflammatory disease [comment]. J Clin Invest 2000;106:337–8.
148. Portoles J, Torralbo A, Martin P, et al. Cardiovascular effects of recombinant human erythropoietin in predialyis patients. Am J Kidney Dis 1997;29:541–8.
149. Pratico D, Pasin M, Barry OP, et al. Iron-dependent human platelet activation and hydroxyl radical formation: Involvement of protein kinase C. Circulation 1999;99:3118–24.
150. Rao SV, Jollis JG, Harrington RA, Granger CB, Newby LK, Armstrong PW, et al. Relationship of blood transfusion and clinical outcomes in patients with acute coronary syndromes. JAMA 2004;292:1555–62.
151. Raskob GE, Silverstein R, Bratzler DW, Heit JA, White RH. Surveillance for deep vein thrombosis and pulmonary embolism: recommendations from a national workshop. Am J Prev Med 2010;38:S502–509.
152. Rauchhaus M, Doehner W, Francis DP, Davos C, Kemp M, Liebenthal C, Niebauer J, Hooper J, Volk HD, Coats AJ, Anker SD. Plasma cytokine parameters and mortality in patients with chronic heart failure. Circulation 2000;102: 3060–7.
153. Reed SD, Li Y, Ellis SJ, Isitt JJ, Cheng S, Schulman KA, Whellan DJ. Associations between hemoglobin level, resource use, and medical costs in patients with heart failure: findings from HF-ACTION. J Card Fail 2012;4:784–91.
154. Rees DC, Cox M, Clegg JB. World distribution of factor V Leiden. Lancet 1995;346:1133–4.
155. Rees DC, Williams TN, Gladwin MT. Sickle-cell disease. Lancet 2010;376:2018–31.
156. Revicki DA, Brown RE, Feeny DH, et al. Health-related quality of life associated with recombinant human erythro-poietin therapy for predialysis chronic renal disease patients. Am J Kidney Dis 1995;25:548–54.
157. Ridker PM, Hennekens CH, Lindpaintner K, Stampfer MJ, Eisenberg PR, Miletich JP. Mutation in the gene coding for coagulation factor V and the risk of myocardial infarction, stroke, and venous thrombosis in apparently healthy men. N Engl J Med 1995;332:912–7.
158. Rosendaal FR, Doggen CJ, Zivelin A, Arruda VR, Aiach M, Siscovick DS, et al. Geographic distribution of the 20210 G to A prothrombin variant. Thromb Haemost 1998;79:706–8.
159. Saigo M, Hsue PY, Waters DD. Role of thrombotic and fibrinolytic factors in acute coronary syndromes. Prog Cardiovasc Dis 2004;46(6):524–538.
160. Salisbury AC, Alexander KP, Reid KJ, Masoudi FA, Rathore SS, Wang TY, et al. Incidence, correlates, and outcomes of acute, hospital-acquired anemia in patients with acute myocardial infarction. Circ Cardiovasc Qual Outcomes 2010; 3:337–46.
161. Salomaa V, Rasi V, Kulathinal S, Vahtera E, Jauhiainen M, Ehnholm C, et al. Hemostatic factors as predictors of coronary events and total mortality: the FINRISK 92 hemostasis study. Arterioscler Thromb Vasc Biol 2002;22(2): 353–8.
162. Scazziota A, Altman R. El mecanismo de la hemostasia normal. Rev Iberoamer Thromb Hemostasia 1996;1:9–26.
163. Scully M, Yarranton H, Liesner R, Cavenagh J, Hunt B, Benjamin S, et al. Regional UK TTP registry: correlation with laboratory ADAMTS 13 analysis and clinical features. Br J Haematol 2008;142:819–26.
164. Selwyn AP. Prothrombotic and antithrombotic pathways in acute coronary syndromes. Am J Cardiol 2003;91(12A): 3H-11H.
165. Sharma R, Francis DP, Pitt B, Poole-Wilson PA, Coats AJ, Anker SD. Haemoglobin predicts survival in patients with chronic heart failure: a substudy of the ELITE II trial. Eur Heart J 2004;25:1021–8.
166. Shelonitda S. Rose, Ashish A. Shah, Donald R. Hoover, and Parvin Saidi, Cyanotic Congenital Heart Disease (CCHD)

with Symptomatic Erythrocytosis.J Gen Intern Med 2007;22: 1775–7.

167. Silverberg DS, Wexler D, Blum M, Keren G, Sheps D, Leibovitch E, Brosh D, Laniado S, Schwartz D, Yachnin T, Shapira I, Gavish D, Baruch R, Koifman B, Kaplan C, Steinbruch S, Iaina A. The use of subcutaneous erythropoietin and intravenous iron for the treatment of the anemia of severe, resistant congestive heart failure improves cardiac and renal function and functional cardiac class, and markedly reduces hospitalizations. J Am Coll Cardiol 2000; 35:1737–44.
168. Smith WR, Penberthy LT, Bovbjerg VE. Daily assessment of pain in adults with sickle cell disease. Ann Intern Med 2008; 148:94–101.
169. Steinberg MH, McCarthy WF, Castro O, Ballas SK, Armstrong FD, Smith W, et al. The risks and benefits of long-term use of hydroxyurea in sickle cell anemia: A 17.5 year follow-up. Am J Hematol 2010;85:403–8.
170. Steinberg MH. Management of sickle cell disease. N Engl J Med 1999;340:1021–30.
171. Stenson PD, Ball EV, Howells K, Phillips AD, Mort M, Cooper DN. The Human Gene Mutation Database: providing a comprehensive central mutation database for molecular diagnostics and personalized genomics. Hum Genomics 2009;4:69–72.
172. Sullivan JL. Iron and the sex difference in heart disease risk. Lancet 1981;1:1293–4.
173. Sullivan JL. Iron therapy and cardiovascular disease. Kidney Int Suppl 1999;69: S135–S137.
174. Sullivan JL. Iron, hematocrit, and the sex difference in heart disease. Arch Pathol Lab Med 1993;117:966–7.
175. Swedberg K, Cleland J, Dargie H, Drexler H, Follath F, Komajda M, Tavazzi L, Smiseth OA, Gavazzi A, Haverich A, Hoes A, Jaarsma T, Korewicki J, Levy S, Linde C, Lopez-Sendon JL, Nieminen MS, Pierard L, Remme WJ. Guidelines for the diagnosis and treatment of chronic heart failure: executive summary (update 2005): The Task Force for the Diagnosis and Treatment of Chronic Heart Failure of the European Society of Cardiology. Eur Heart J 2005;26: 1115–40.
176. Swisher KK, Terrell DR, Vesely SK, Kremer Hovinga JA, Lammle B, George JN. Clinical outcomes after platelet transfusions in patients with thrombotic thrombocytopenic purpura. Transfusion 2009;49:873–87.
177. Syrovets T, Simmet T. Novel aspects and new roles for the serine protease plasmin. Cell Mol Life Sci 2004;61(7–8): 873–85.
178. Szachniewicz J, Petruk-Kowalczyk J, Majda J, Kaczmarek A, Reczuch K, Kalra PR, Piepoli MF, Anker SD, Banasiak W, Ponikowski P. Anaemia is an independent predictor of poor outcome in patients with chronic heart failure. Int J Cardiol 2003;90:303–8.
179. Tang YD, Katz SD. The prevalence of anemia in chronic heart failure and its impact on the clinical outcomes. Heart Fail Rev 2008;13:387–92.
180. Tanner H, Moschovitis G, Kuster GM, Hullin R, Pfiiffner D, Hess OM, Mohacsi P. The prevalence of anemia in chronic heart failure. Int J Cardiol 2002;86:115–21.
181. Teehan BP, Krantz S, Stone WA, et al. Double-blind, placebo-controlled study of the therapeutic use of recombinant human erythropoietin for anemia associated with chronic renal failure in pre-dialysis patients. Am J Kidney Dis 1991; 18:50–9.
182. Ten Berg JM, Kelder JC, Suttorp MJ, et al. Effect of coumarins started before coronary angioplasty on acute complications and long-term follow-up: a randomized trial. Circulation 2000;102:386–91.
183. Terrell DR, Beebe LA, Vesely SK, Neas BR, Segal JB, George JN. The incidence of immune thrombocytopenic purpura in children and adults: A critical review of published reports. Am J Hematol 2010;85:174–80.
184. Terrell DR, Vesely SK, Hovinga JA, Lammle B, George JN. Different disparities of gender and race among the thrombotic thrombocytopenic purpura and hemolytic-uremic syndromes. Am J Hematol 2010;85:844–7.
185. Terrovitis JV, Anastasiou-Nana M, Kaldara E, Drakos SG, Nanas SN, Nanas JN. Anemia in heart failure: pathophysiologic insights and treatment options. Future Cardiol 2009; 5:71–81.
186. Thachil J. Nitric oxide in immune thrombocytopenic purpura. Hematology 2009;14:59–62.
187. The OASIS investigators effects of long-term, moderate-intensity oral anticoagulation in addition to aspirin in unstable angina. J Am Coll Cardiol 2001;37:475–85
188. Tinmouth A, Fergusson D, Chin-Yee I, Hebert PC. Clinical consequences of red cell storage in the critically ill. Transfusion 2006;4:2014–27.
189. Tsai HM. Pathophysiology of thrombotic thrombocytopenic purpura. Int J Hematol 2010;91:1–19.
190. Tsujita K, Nikolsky E, Lansky AJ, Dangas G, Fahy M, Brodie BR, et al. Impact of anemia on clinical outcomes of patients with ST-segment elevation myocardial infarction in relation to gender and adjunctive antithrombotic therapy (from the HORIZONS-AMI trial). Am J Cardiol 2010;105: 1385–94.
191. Tuomainen TP, Salonen R, Nyyssonen K, et al. Cohort study of relation between donating blood and risk of myocardial infarction in 2682 men in eastern Finland. BMJ 1997;314: 793–4.
192. Valles J, Santos MT, Aznar J, Martinez M, Moscardo A, Pinon M, Broekman MJ, Marcus AJ. Platelet-erythrocyte interactions enhance alpha(IIb) beta(3) integrin receptor activation and P-selectin expression during platelet recruitment: down-regulation by aspirin ex-vivo. Blood 2002; 99:3978–84.
193. Vallet B, Robin E, Lebuffe G. Venous oxygen saturation as a physiologic transfusion trigger. Crit Care 2010;4:213.
194. van Der Bom JG, de Maat MP, Bots ML, Haverkate F, de Jong PT, Hofman A, et al. Elevated plasma fibrinogen: cause or consequence of cardiovascular disease? Arterioscler Thromb Vasc Biol 1998;18(4):621–5.
195. van der Meer P, Lipsic E, Westenbrink BD, van de Wal RM, Schoemaker RG, Vellenga E, van Veldhuisen DJ, Voors AA, van Gilst WH. Levels of hematopoiesis inhibitor N-acetyl-seryl-aspartyl-lysyl-proline partially explain the occurrence of anemia in heart failure. Circulation 2005;112:1743–7.
196. van der Meer P, Voors AA, Lipsic E, Smilde TD, van Gilst WH, van Veldhuisen DJ. Prognostic value of plasma erythropoietin on mortality in patients with chronic heart failure. J Am Coll Cardiol 2004;44:63–7.

197. Vaziri ND. Mechanism of erythropoietin-induced hypertension. Am J Kidney Dis 1999;33:821–8.
198. Vincent JL, Baron JF, Reinhart K, Gattinoni L, Thijs L, Webb A, Meier-Hellmann A, Nollet G. For the ABC Investigators. Anemia and blood transfusion in critically ill patients. JAMA 2002;4:1499–507.
199. Warkentin TE, Greinacher A, Koster A, Lincoff AM. Treatment and prevention of heparin-induced thrombocytopenia: American College of Chest Physicians Evidence-Based Clinical Practice Guidelines. 8th ed. Chest 2008;133:S340–80.
200. Warkentin TE, Sheppard JA, Moore JC, Cook RJ, Kelton JG. Studies of the immune response in heparin-induced thrombocytopenia. Blood 2009;113:4963–9.
201. Weiskopf RB, Viele MK, Feiner J, et al. Human cardiovascular and metabolic response to acute, severe isovolemic anemia. JAMA 1998;279:217–21.
202. Wells PS, Blajchman MA, Henderson P, Wells MJ, Demers C, Bourque R, et al. Prevalence of antithrombin deficiency in healthy blood donors: a cross-sectional study. Am J Hematol 1994;45:321–4.
203. Werdehoff SG, Moore RB, Hoff CJ, et al. Elevated plasma endothelin-1 levels in sickle cell anemia: Relationships to oxygen saturation and left ventricular hypertrophy. Am J Hematol 1998;58:195–9.
204. Wexler D, Silverberg D, Sheps D, Blum M, Keren G, Iaina A, Schwartz D. Prevalence of anemia in patients admitted to hospital with a primary diagnosis of congestive heart failure. Int J Cardiol 2004;96:79–87.
205. Winearls CG. Recombinant human erythropoietin: 10 years of clinical experience. Nephrol Dial Transplant 1998;13 (Suppl 2):3–8.
206. Witte K, Thackray S, Clark AL, Cooklin M, Cleland JG. Clinical trials update: improvement-hf, copernicus, mustic, aspect-ii, apricot and heart. Eur j heart fail 2000;2: 455–60.
207. Wu H, Lee SH, Gao J, Liu X, Iruela-Arispe ML. Inactivation of erythropoietin leads to defects in cardiac morphogenesis. Development 1999;126:3597–605.
208. Wun T, Law L, Harvey D, Sieracki B, Scudder SA, Ryu JK. Increased incidence of symptomatic venous thrombosis in patients with cervical carcinoma treated with concurrent chemotherapy, radiation, and erythropoietin. Cancer 2003; 98:1514–20.
209. Young G, Albisetti M, Bonduel M, Brandao L, Chan A, Friedrichs F, et al. Impact of inherited thrombophilia on venous thromboembolism in children: a systematic review and meta-analysis of observational studies. Circulation 2008; 118:1373–82.
210. Youssoufian H, Longmore G, Neumann D, Yoshimura A, Lodish HF. Structure, function, and activation of the erythropoietin receptor. Blood 1993;81:2223–36.
211. Zakarija A, Bandarenko N, Pandey DK, Auerbach A, Raisch DW, Kim B, et al, Clopidogrel-associated TTP. An update of pharmacovigilance efforts conducted by independent resear-chers, pharmaceutical suppliers, and the Food and Drug Administration. Stroke 2004;35:533–7.

# 41 Cardiovascular Emergencies in Young Athletes

The majority of sudden deaths in young athletes occur in the context of underlying inherited or genetic cardiac disorders. The evaluation of every athlete regarding underlying cardiac disease is impractical and therefore needs to be targeted at those who are at a higher risk. A practical approach would be to channel efforts towards athletes with cardiac symptoms, those with a family history of inherited cardiac disease, and those with a family history of premature sudden death. There are potential pitfalls in the evaluation of young athletes using noninvasive tests when making the distinction between physiological adaptations to exercise and cardiac pathology. Physicians evaluating young athletes need to be aware of the spectrum of physiological adaptations and to be familiar with conditions responsible for sudden death in this population.

Athlete's heart is a constellation of structural and functional changes that occur in the heart of people who train for >1 hour most days.

The changes are asymptomatic; signs include bradycardia, a systolic murmur, and extra heart sounds. ECG abnormalities are common. Diagnosis is clinical or by echocardiography. No treatment is necessary. Athlete's heart is significant because it must be distinguished from serious cardiac disorders. Intensive, prolonged endurance and strength training produces many physiologic adaptations. Volume and pressure loads in the left ventricle (LV) increase, which, over time, increase LV muscle mass, wall thickness, and chamber size. Maximal stroke volume and cardiac output increase, contributing to a lower resting heart rate and longer diastolic filling time. Lower heart rate results primarily from increased vagal tone, but decreased sympathetic activation and other nonautonomic factors that decrease intrinsic sinus node activity may play a role. Bradycardia decreases myocardial $O_2$ demand; at the same time, increases in total Hb and blood volume enhance $O_2$ transport. Despite these changes, systolic function and diastolic function remain normal. Structural changes in women are typically less than those in men of the same age, body size, and training. While the entity of athlete's heart has been recognized for over 100 years, only in the past two decades has the application of echocardiography and other noninvasive imaging techniques permitted definition with some precision of the alterations in cardiac dimensions associated with athletic (Figs 41.1–41.5) conditioning. Echocardiography has demonstrated that long-term athletic training leads to an increase in left ventricular mass due to increases in left ventricular diastolic cavity dimension, wall thickness, or both. These changes in cardiac morphology are relatively mild in absolute terms, and the differences between athlete and nonathlete populations are statistically significant but generally small. Furthermore, cardiac alterations associated with training differ somewhat depending on the particular sport in which

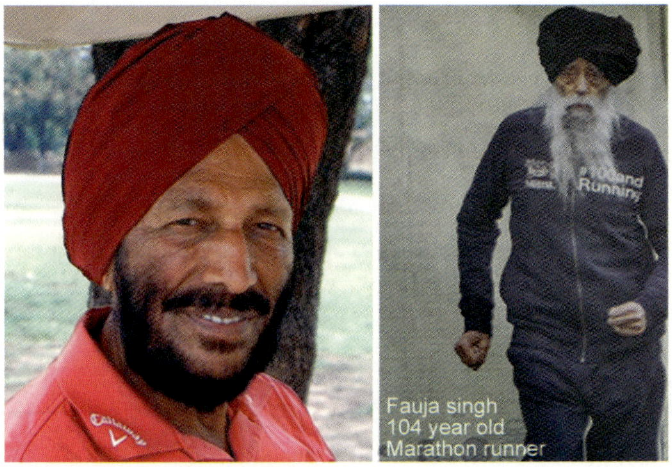


**Fig. 41.1:** Two India's athletics icons Milkha Singh (80 years), and S. Fauja Singh (104 years) who are encouraging many Indian young athletes to take part in diffrent games. Playing games tones up your cardiovascular system and prolongs your life and one may remain drug and disease free even more than 100 years like these two living legendaries

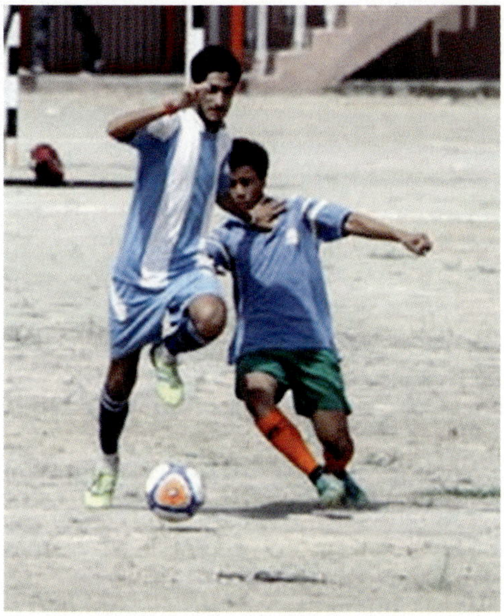

**Fig. 41.2:** Young footballers in dribbling and weaving tussle during inter-school football match

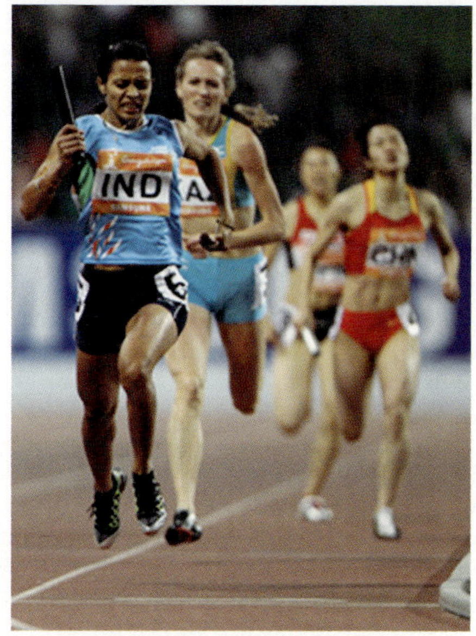


**Fig. 41.3:** Young international athletes including Indian taking part in running competition

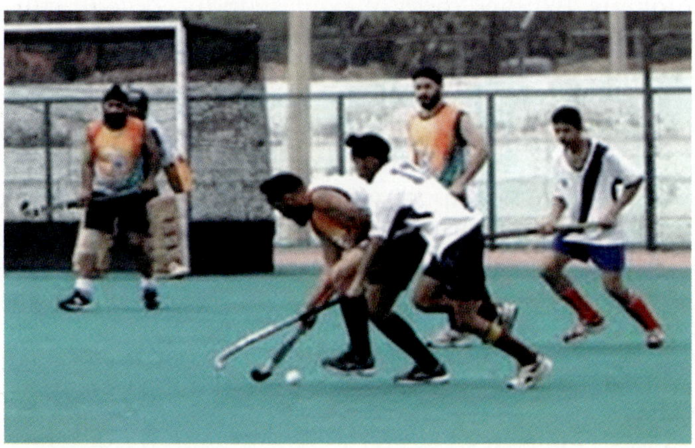

**Fig. 41.4:** Players in action during hockey match at KK Hakku Stadium, Jammu

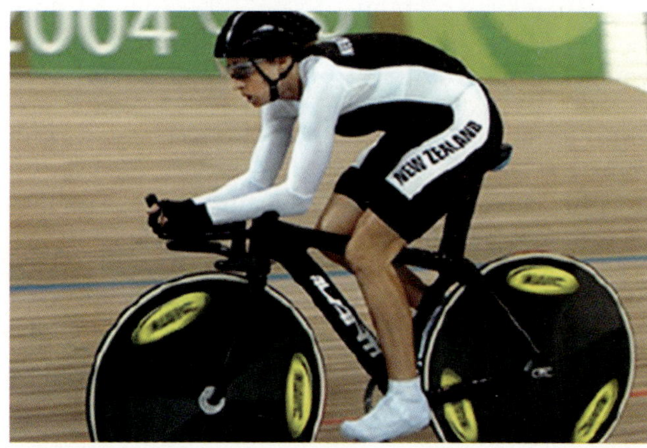


**Fig. 41.5:** A young athlete taking part in cycle race

the individual athlete participates. In particular, the changes in left ventricular wall thickness, cavity dimension, or both associated with long-term athletic training may be more striking in certain sports such as distance running, swimming, cycling, and rowing/canoeing. The differential diagnosis with cardiac disease is more likely to be raised in athletes training in such sports.

## WHAT IS ATHLETES HEART?

### DEFINITION OF ATHLETIC HEART SYNDROME

Athletic heart syndrome, (AHS) also known as athlete's heart, athletic bradycardia or exercise-induced cardiomegaly is a nonpathological condition commonly seen in sports medicine, in which the human heart is enlarged, and the resting heart rate is lower than normal.

### ATHLETIC HEART HISTORICAL PERSPECTIVES

The concept that the cardiovascular system of trained athletes differs structurally and functionally from others in the normal general population remarkably extends over a century. During that time, there has also been periodic controversy about the true nature of athlete's heart, i.e. whether the findings are physiologically adapted, benign, and related only to training, or alternatively are potentially pathological and the harbinger of disease and disability.

The clinical entity of athlete's heart has been defined with increasing precision using a variety of techniques. Henschen is credited with the first description in 1899, using only a basic physical examination with careful percussion to recognize enlargement of the heart caused by athletic activity in cross-country skiers. Henschen concluded that both dilatation and hypertrophy were present, involving both the left and right sides of the heart, and these changes were normal and favorable – 'Skiing causes an enlargement of the heart which can perform more work than a normal heart.'

Subsequent investigators used quantitative chest radiography to show that heart size was increased in athletes, particularly those engaged in endurance sports with large aerobic requirements. Some early observers even regarded the heart of the trained athlete to be weakened owing to the 'strain' created by continuous and excessively strenuous training and believed that athletes were subject to deteriorating cardiac function and heart failure.

## WHAT IS ATHLETIC HEART SYNDROME?

Athletic heart syndrome is a heart condition that may occur in people who exercise or train for more than an hour a day, most days of the week. Athletic heart syndrome isn't necessarily bad for you—if you're an athlete. And it's not what makes young athletes expire in mid-court. While it does lead to structural changes in the heart, a person with the condition usually doesn't notice any symptoms. Athletic heart syndrome doesn't require treatment and is important to diagnose only to rule out heart problems that are serious.

Like any other muscle, the heart gets stronger with exercise. Endurance exercises such as jogging, swimming, and cycling can make the organ bigger, allowing it to pump more blood with every beat. Short, intense workouts such as weight lifting further increase the pumping power by thickening the walls of the heart.

Just as body builders sculpt their abs and biceps into highly unusual shapes, many hardcore competitive athletes develop extraordinary hearts. Not only is the heart extra large and thick, it also may produce some irregular rhythms (arrhythmia). A person with athletic heart syndrome may also have a markedly slow resting heart rate, in the range of 35–50 beats a minute. In addition, electrical impulses can take strange routes across the heart, causing abnormal readings on an electrocardiogram (ECG or EKG). Together, these changes produced by exercise are called athletic heart syndrome.

## PHYSIOLOGY OF ATHLETIC HEART SYNDROME

Cardiovascular adaptations to exercise have been systematically defined and differ with respect to the type of conditioning; endurance training (sometimes also described as dynamic, isotonic, or aerobic) such as long-distance running and swimming; and strength training (also referred to as static, isometric, power, or anaerobic) such as wrestling, weightlifting, or throwing heavy objects. Sports such as cycling and rowing are examples of combined endurance and strength exercise. Most athletic disciplines to some extent combine endurance and strength modes of physical conditioning, and training-related physiological alterations represent a complex set of central and peripheral mechanisms operating at structural, metabolic, and regulatory levels.

Acute responses to endurance exercise training include substantial increases in maximum oxygen consumption, cardiac output, stroke volume, and systolic blood pressure, associated with decreased peripheral vascular resistance. The immediate results of strength conditioning include only mildly increased oxygen consumption and cardiac output but substantial increases in blood pressure, peripheral vascular resistance, and heart rate.

Long-term cardiovascular adaptation to dynamic training produces increased maximal oxygen uptake due to increased cardiac output and arteriovenous oxygen difference. Strength exercise results in little or no increase in oxygen uptake. Thus, endurance exercise predominantly produces volume load on the left ventricle (LV), and strength exercise causes largely a pressure load.

## CARDIAC ENLARGEMENT: PATHOLOGY VERSUS PHYSIOLOGICAL ADAPTATION

The phenotypic overlap between exercise-induced cardiac remodeling and pathological structural heart disease is widely appreciated. Cardiac structural abnormality of unclear origin and significance may be detected during preparticipation cardiovascular disease screening, routine health examinations, or evaluation of the athlete with symptoms. Extreme cases of exercise-induced ventricular remodeling may be difficult to differentiate from mild forms of hypertrophic cardiomyopathy, familial or acquired dilated cardiomyopathy, and arrhythmogenic RV cardiomyopathy. The clinical task of differentiating marked exercise-induced remodeling from these important forms of disease remains important, with implications including sport restriction, pharmacological therapy, and placement of an implantable cardiac defibrillator. The overlap between features of the athlete's heart and characteristics of cardiomyopathy, specifically hypertrophic cardiomyopathy, that may affect young athletes has been coined the Maron gray zone. A valuable schema for approaching the athletic patient with LV hypertrophy of unclear origin has been presented, and remains useful in clinical practice. It is noteworthy that this diagnostic approach was developed at a time when noninvasive cardiovascular imaging was in its infancy and, for the most part, restricted to basic two-dimensional echocardiography. Recent advances in cardiovascular diagnostics have proven to be useful additions to these original criteria. Functional myocardial echocardiography, including tissue Doppler and speckle-tracking imaging, permits detailed and accurate assessment of myocardial function. Tissue Doppler imaging permits assessment of myocardial relaxation and contraction velocity. Across numerous studies, early diastolic relaxation velocity has been shown to be normal or increased in athletes with LV hypertrophy resulting from exercise-induced remodeling. In contrast, pathological forms of LV hypertrophy are typically associated with reduced early diastolic relaxation velocity and peak systolic tissue velocity. Tissue strain and strain rate may also provide useful insight into the origin of LV hypertrophy in athletes.

Cardiac magnetic resonance imaging has similarly emerged as an invaluable tool for the evaluation of the athlete with indeterminate cardiac enlargement. Cardiac magnetic resonance allows highly accurate assessment of myocardial thickness, chamber volumes, tissue composition, extracardiac anatomy, and cardiac magnetic resonance-derived reference values in athletes have been published. Importantly, the use of gadolinium contrast with delayed imaging provides information about the presence and location of myocardial fibrosis. Recent data document myocardial fibrosis patterns that are relatively specific to certain cardiomyopathies and highlight the utility of cardiac magnetic resonance for the assessment of indeterminate cardiac enlargement in the athlete. At the present time, we use cardiac magnetic resonance in athletes with either indeterminate echocardiographic imaging or clinical features that suggest a diagnosis that may not be definitively assessed by echocardiography (i.e. myocarditis). The interested reader is referred to a recently published comprehensive review on this topic. At the present time, there is no single diagnostic test with adequate accuracy for differentiating adaptive from pathological cardiomyopathy. Consequently, we encourage clinicians faced with this diagnostic dilemma to begin the assessment with an integrated consideration of personal and family medical history, 12-lead ECG, and echocardiography. In many cases, this relatively basic but informative triad will provide sufficient information for informed diagnostic decision making. In cases that remain unclear after this initial evaluation, further measures, including tissue Doppler echocardiography, speckle-tracking echocardiography, magnetic resonance imaging, cardiopulmonary exercise testing, prescribed detraining, and disease-specific genetic testing, may be considered.

## THE 'ATHLETIC HEART SYNDROME' A CRITICAL REVIEW

Cardiological findings in athletes are often similar to those observed in clinical cases. Electrocardiographic and cardiac imaging abnormalities as well as physical findings may be the same in both of these groups. Bradycardia and rhythm disturbances are the most common abnormalities in athletes. Most athletes with abnormal electrocardiograms are asymptomatic and numerous investigators have failed to detect heart disease in association with such electrocardiograms.

In contrast to cardiac dysfunction observed in clinical cases, enhanced or normal ventricular systolic and diastolic function have been reported in athletes. In endurance athletes, this is associated with very high values for maximal aerobic power ($VO_{2max}$). Absolute and body size-normalised cardiac dimensions in most athletes do not approach values from chronic disease states, and may not exceed echocardiographic normal limits. In addition, pathological and physiological enlargement appear to be biochemically and functionally different. Myosin ATPase enzyme expression and calcium metabolism are different in rats with pathologically or physiologically induced enlargement. The reported biochemical differences underlie systolic and diastolic dysfunction in pathological enlargement. Conversely, trained rodents and humans have demonstrated enhanced systolic and diastolic function. It is important to note that cardiac enlargement observed in athletes is the result of normal adaptation to physical conditioning and/or hereditary influences. Conversely, pathological changes result from disease processes which can lead in turn to reduced function, morbidity and mortality. Since the mid-1970s echocardiography has been used to compare cardiac dimensions in male endurance- and resistance-trained athletes. A sport-specific profile of eccentric and concentric enlargement has been documented in endurance and resistance athletes, respectively. Subsequent studies of athletes have examined factors such as age, sex and degree of competitive success to determine their contribution to these sport-specific cardiac profiles. Unique athletic subgroups have also been analysed and have included ballet dancers, rowers, basketball players and triathletes. However, there is a paucity of data on cardiac dimensions in female athletes. Finally, physical conditioning studies have also examined echocardiographic dimensions before and after endurance and resistance training. Significant enlargement of internal dimensions, wall thickness or left ventricular mass have been reported but such increases are relatively small and by no means universal. Several conflicting explanations for enlarged cardiac dimensions appear in the literature. Chronic volume and pressure hemodynamic overloading during physical conditioning has been proposed to explain eccentric and concentric cardiac enlargement in endurance- and resistance-trained athletes respectively. However, twin studies suggest that hereditary factors may be important determinants of cardiac dimensions and/or the degree of cardiac adaptability to physical conditioning.

## DIAGNOSIS OF ATHLETIC HEART SYNDROME

Athlete's heart is usually an incidental finding during a routine screening or during tests for other medical issues. An enlarged heart can be seen at echocardiography or sometimes on a chest X-ray. Similarities at presentation between athlete's heart and clinically relevant cardiac problems may prompt electrocardiography (ECG) and exercise cardiac stress tests.

The ECG can detect sinus bradycardia, a resting heart rate of fewer than 60 beats per minute. This is often accompanied by sinus arrhythmia. The pulse of a person with athlete's heart can sometimes be irregular while at rest, but usually returns to normal after exercise begins (Fig. 41.6, Tables 41.1 and 41.2).

Regarding differential diagnosis, left ventricular hypertrophy is usually indistinguishable from athlete's heart and at ECG, but can usually be discounted in the young and fit.

It is important to distinguish between athlete's heart and hypertrophic cardiomyopathy, a serious cardiovascular disease characterised by thickening of the heart's walls, which produces a similar ECG pattern at rest. This genetic disorder is found in 1 out of 500 Americans and is a leading cause of sudden cardiac death in young athletes (although only about 8% of all cases of sudden death are actually exercise-related).

**Table 41.1:** Specific athlete characteristics needed for cardiovascular testing according to American Heart Association recommendations

| Type of examination | Characteristics |
|---|---|
| Personal history | • Exertional chest pain or discomfort<br>• Unexplained syncope or near-syncope, assumed not vasovagal<br>• History of hypertension<br>• Excessive exertional and unexplained dyspnea/fatigue<br>• History of previously recognized heart murmur |
| Family history | • Sudden and unexpected premature death in at least one relative before age 50 years<br>• Disability from heart disease in a close relative <50 years old<br>• Previously diagnosed inheritable heart disease in family members including, but not limited to, hypertrophic cardiomyopathy, dilated cardiomyopathy, congenital long QT syndrome or other ion channelopathies, Marfan syndrome, or clinically important arrhythmias |
| Physical examination | • Heart murmur<br>• Abnormal femoral pulses, suggestive of aortic coarctation<br>• Physical stigmata of Marfan syndrome<br>• Abnormal brachial artery blood pressure for age (taken in both arms in a sitting position) |

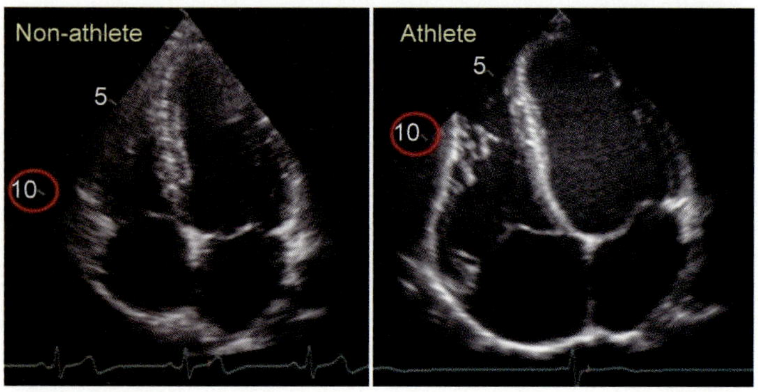


**Fig. 41.6:** Echo scans in 4C apical views showing dilatation of athlete heart in comparison to normal heart

## IS ATHLETIC HEART SYNDROME DANGEROUS?

An enlarged heart, arrhythmia, and unusual ECG readings would all be signs of serious trouble for the average person. In fact, the rhythms and ECG readings associated with athletic heart syndrome often mimic life-threatening disorders. But athletic heart syndrome itself is harmless. The 'abnormal' changes in the athlete's heart are actually a testament to the body's ability to adapt.

If an athlete has symptoms of chest pain, reports irregular beats, or has passed out, he or she should get a medical exam to pinpoint the problem. Your doctor may want to run extra tests to determine whether the symptoms are a normal sign of your body's ability to adapt to training, or whether there's some abnormality in your heart. These tests may include an electrocardiogram, sonogram (a picture of the heart using sound waves), or another type of test.

Of course, some athletes really do have heart trouble. Occasionally, seemingly healthy young basketball or football players drop dead in the middle of a game or a practice. In almost every case, doctors trace the death to an unsuspected condition, such as congenital heart disease, but one that has nothing to do with athletic heart syndrome.

**Table 41.2:** Common ECG findings in athletes. Training-related ECG alterations are common, physiological adaptations to regular exercise and are considered normal variants in athletes

| Normal ECG |
|---|
| Sinus bradycardia |
| Sinus arrhythmia |
| First-degree AV block |
| Incomplete RBBB |
| Early repolarisation |
| Isolated QRS voltage criteria for LVH |

- Isolated increases in QRS amplitude are common in trained athletes. However, QRS voltage criteria for LVH+ any nonvoltage criteria for LVH (such as atrial enlargement, left axis deviation, a strain pattern of repolarisation, ST-segment depression, T-wave inversion or pathological Q-waves) are abnormal and require further evaluation
- AV, atrioventricular; LVH, left ventricular hypertrophy; RBBB, right bundle-branch block

## HOW IS ATHLETIC HEART SYNDROME TREATED?

Since athletic heart syndrome is harmless, there's no reason to treat it unless you experience regular light-headedness, chest pains, or you lose consciousness. If you really want a 'normal' heart again, all you have to do is stop exercising. Soon, your heart, along with the rest of your body, will sag back into its former shape. But why not keep everything extra strong and healthy for a while? You should be proud of your athletic body, heart included.

### Emergency Planning

Cardiac emergencies are frightening events and can lead to chaos and confusion on the playing field. Proper emergency planning increases the likelihood of a coordinated, efficient response and a good outcome. Potential first responders to a cardiovascular emergency during training and competition should be identified. In United States high schools, certified athletic trainers and coaches were the most likely first responders (47% and 33%, respectively). Additional personnel may include physiotherapists, strength and conditioning coaches, team physicians, officials and other staff or administrators. All personnel responsible for the care or training or athletes should be educated in the recognition of cardiac emergencies, CPR, AED use and have specific knowledge of the location of the nearest AED.

A communication system should be available at all venues to activate the local emergency medical system and any on-site response team. Transportation routes for emergency vehicles to access the specific location, as well as appropriate hospital facilities, should be predetermined.

Access to early defibrillation must be ensured through the strategic placement of AEDs. The chance of survival decreases approximately 10% with every minute defibrillation is delayed. The recommended time from collapse to first shock is less than 3 min.The number of AEDs and location, whether mounted or portable, is unique for every venue. AEDs should be registered with the local emergency medical system and checked regularly (per manufacturer recommendations) for maintenance or replacement of the device battery and leads. An extra set of pads should be available with every device in case the primary set is damaged or does not adequately adhere to the victim's chest. Supplies to remove clothing and improve adhesiveness of the pads should also be available and include a scissors, razor, towel and antiperspirant spray. Other emergency equipment is dependent on the level of training of the first responders and may include bag-valve masks, advanced airways, pulse oximetry, supplemental oxygen, sphygmomanometer, intravenous fluids and medications such as aspirin and nitroglycerin. A written emergency action plan should be developed for every sporting venue and organisation. The plan should be coordinated with the local emergency medical services system and any on-site safety or security officials. It should also include information on documenting and reporting a cardiac event after the initial resuscitation. Regular review and rehearsal of the plan (at least once annually) should be done with all potential responders.

## Evaluation of Athletes Health Status Prior to Participation in Competitive Games

### *Symptoms and Signs*

There are no symptoms. Signs vary but may include bradycardia; an LV impulse that is laterally displaced, enlarged, and increased in amplitude; a systolic ejection (flow) murmur at the left lower sternal border; a third heart sound (S3) due to early, rapid diastolic ventricular filling; a fourth heart sound (S4), heard best during resting bradycardia because diastolic filling time is increased; and hyperdynamic carotid pulses. These signs reflect structural cardiac changes that are adaptive for intense exercise.

### *Clinical Evaluation*

Findings are typically detected during routine screening or during evaluation of unrelated symptoms. Most athletes do not require extensive testing, although ECG is often warranted. If symptoms suggest a cardiac disorder (e.g. palpitations, chest pain), ECG, echocardiography, and exercise stress testing are done. Athlete's heart is a diagnosis of exclusion; it must be distinguished from disorders that cause similar findings but are life-threatening (e.g. hypertrophic or dilated cardiomyopathies, ischemic heart disease, arrhythmogenic right ventricular dysplasia).

### *Electrocardiography*

Numerous changes in rhythm and ECG morphology can occur; they correlate poorly with level of training and cardiovascular performance. The most common ECG findings are shown in Figs 41.7–41.23 and Tables 41.3– 41.5.

Rarely, heart rate is <40 beats/min. Sinus arrhythmia often accompanies the slow heart rate. Resting bradycardia may also predispose to atrial or ventricular ectopy

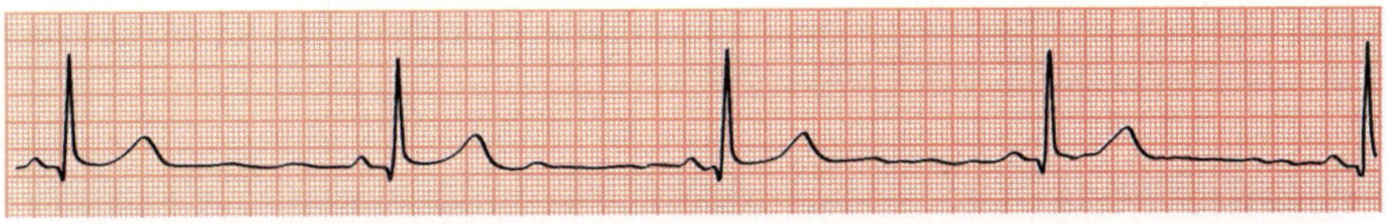

**Fig. 41.7:** ECG trace taken in one of the athletes showing sinus bradycardia

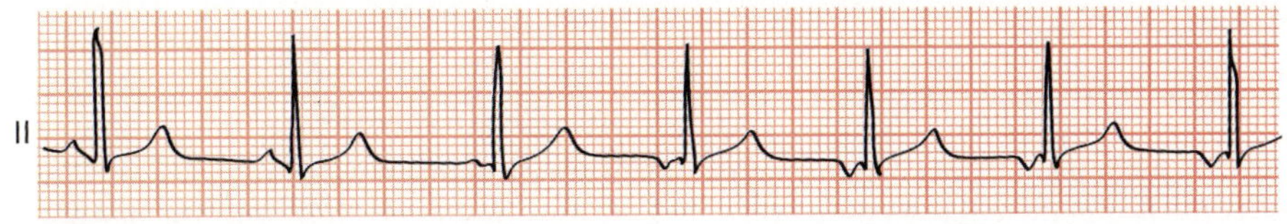


**Fig. 41.8:** Wandering atrial pacemaker is a benign rhythm change where the pacemaker site shifts from the sinus node into the atrial tissues. P-wave morphology varies with the pacemaker site

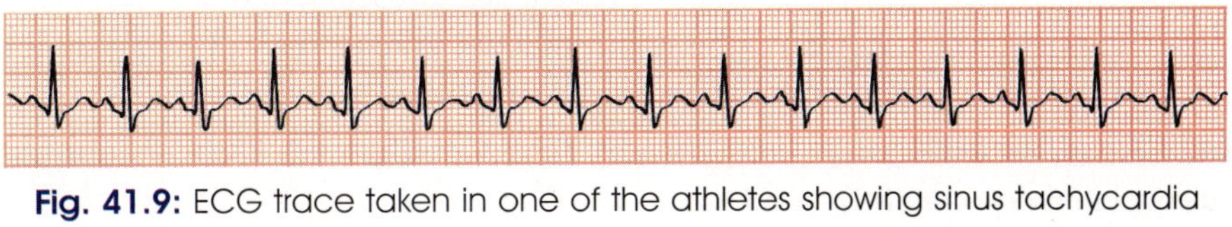

**Fig. 41.9:** ECG trace taken in one of the athletes showing sinus tachycardia

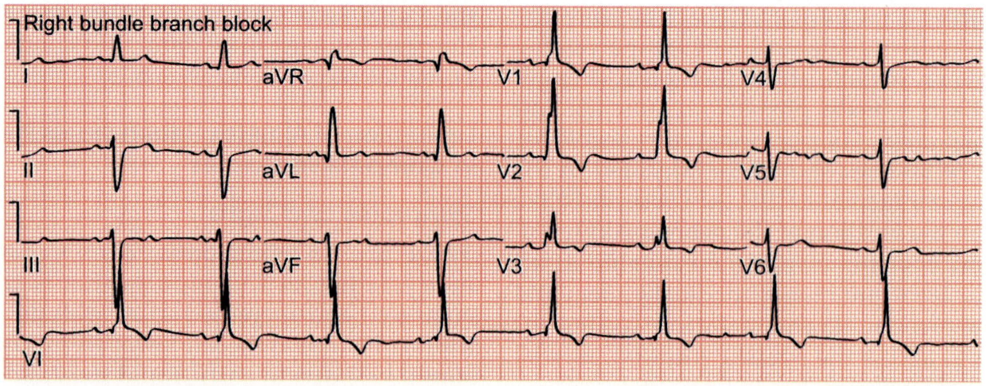


**Fig. 41.10:** ECG showing complete RBBB, the duration of the QRS complex is >0.10 seconds. With incomplete RBBB an rSR′ pattern will be seen in lead V1 but the QRS duration will be within the limits of normal. An rSR′ or rR′ pattern, with the initial r-wave less than the R′ or r′, in leads V1 through V3 may be present. In leads I and V6 the S-wave is wide. The QRS axis may be normal or there may be right or left axis deviation. The T-wave is almost always inverted in lead V1 and may be inverted in V2. In the other precordial leads, and in the limb leads, the T-wave is directed opposite to the terminal portion of the QRS complex

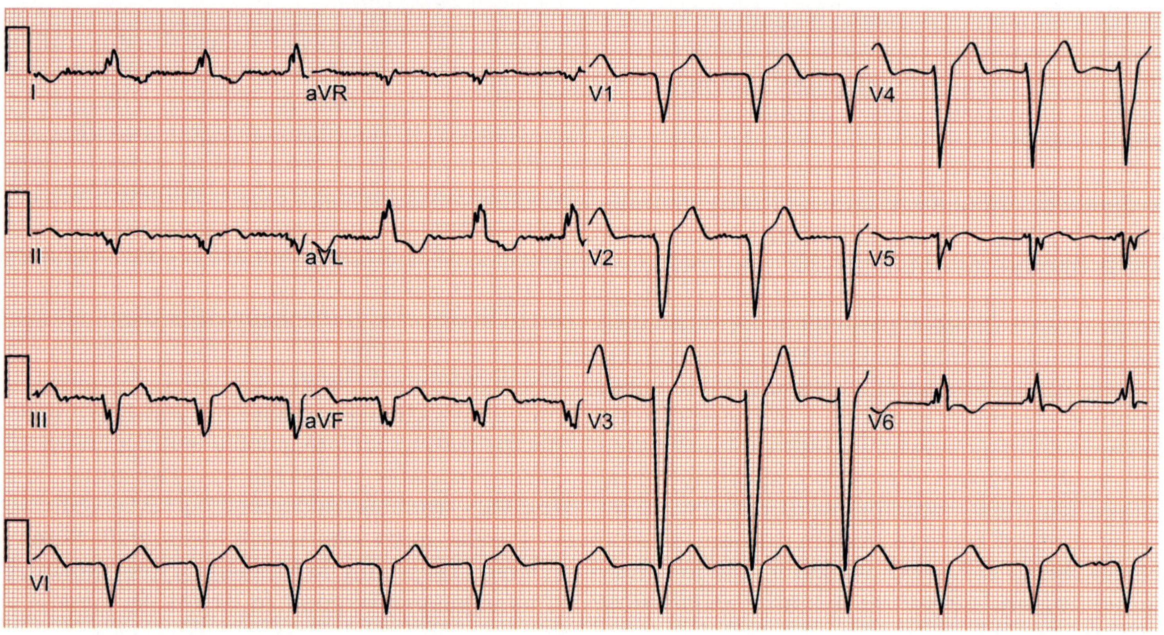


**Fig. 41.11:** ECG trace showing LBBB with notched, widened QRS complexs in leads 1, AVL V5, V6 and deep S-waves in precordial leads V1–V4 in one of the athletes taking part in competitive games

**Table 41.3:** Classification of abnormalities of the athlete's electrocardiogram

| Group 1: Common and training-related ECG changes | Group 2: Uncommon and training-unrelated ECG changes |
|---|---|
| Sinus bradycardia | T-wave inversion |
| First-degree AV block | ST-segement depression |
| Incomplete RBBB | Pathological Q-waves |
| Early repolarization | Left atrial enlargement |
| Isolated QRS voltage criteria for left ventricular hypertrophy | Left-axis deviation/left anterior hemiblock |
| | Right-axis deviation/left posterior hemiblock |
| | Right ventricular hypertrophy |
| | Ventricular pre-excitation |
| | Complete LBBB or RBBB |
| | Long or short-QT interval |
| | Brugada-like early repolarization |

RBBB=right bundle-branch block; LBBB=left bundle-branch block.

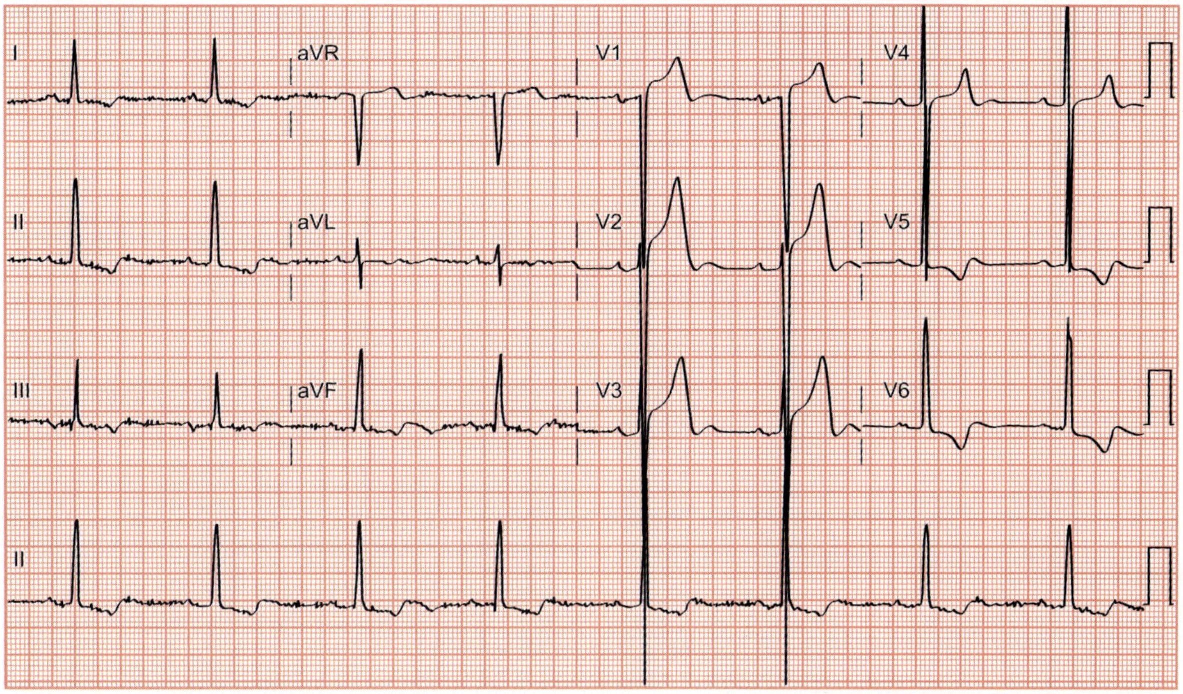


**Fig. 41.12:** ECG trace showing massively increased QRS voltages—the S-waves in V3 are so deep they are literally falling off the page. The ST-elevation in V1–3 is simply in proportion to the very deep S waves ('appropriate discordance'). The LV strain pattern is seen in all leads with a positive R-wave (V5–6, I, II, III, aVF)

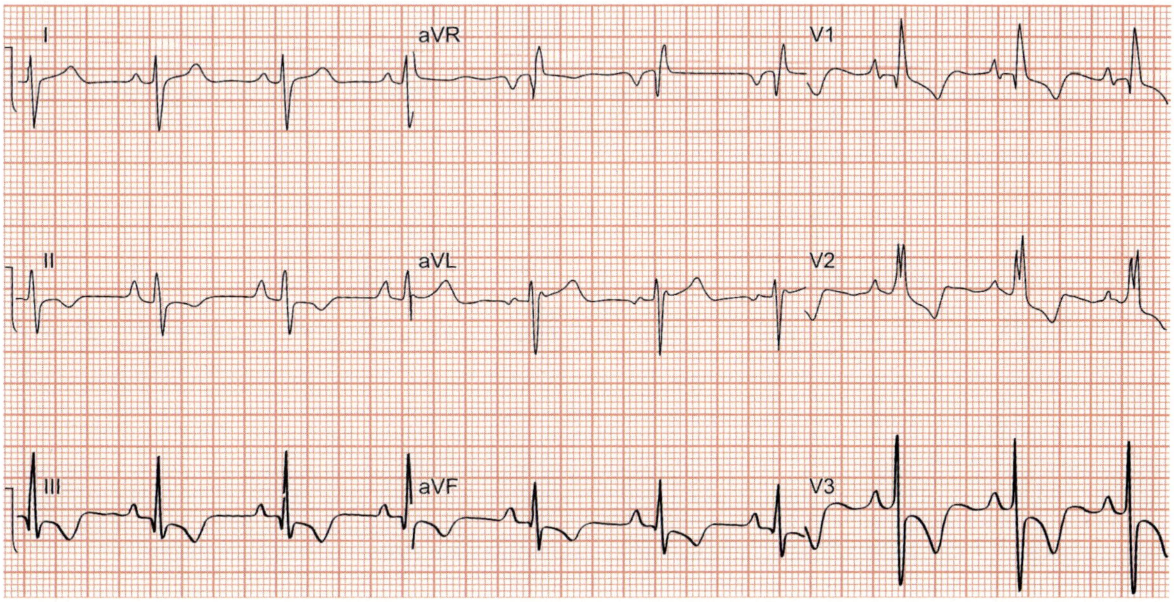


**Fig. 41.13:** ECG trace showing right axis deviation (+150 degrees). P pulmonale (P-wave in lead II >2.5 mm). Incomplete RBBB. Right ventricular strain pattern with T-wave inversion and ST-depression in the right precordial (V1-3) and inferior (II, III, aVF) leads

(including couplets and bursts of nonsustained ventricular tachycardia); pauses after ectopic beats do not exceed 4 sec.

There is an association between HCM and Wolff-Parkinson-White (WPW) syndrome; ECG features of WPW were seen in 33% of patients with HCM in one study. At least one genetic mutation has been identified that is associated with both conditions. Atrial fibrillation and supraventricular tachycardias are common. Ventricular dysrhythmias (e.g. VT) also occur and may be a cause of sudden death.

## Imaging Studies (Figs 41.24–41.30 and Table 41.6)

### *Echocardiography*

Echocardiography can usually distinguish athlete's heart from cardiomyopathies but the distinction is not always

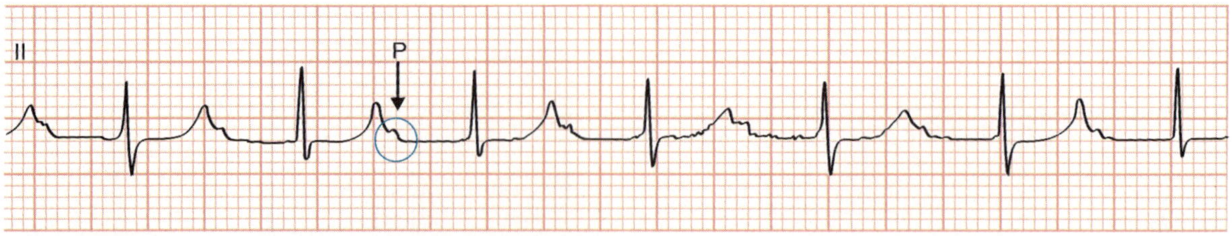


**Fig. 41.14:** ECG trace showing marked first degree heart block (PR interval >300 ms, P-waves are buried in the preceding T-wave)

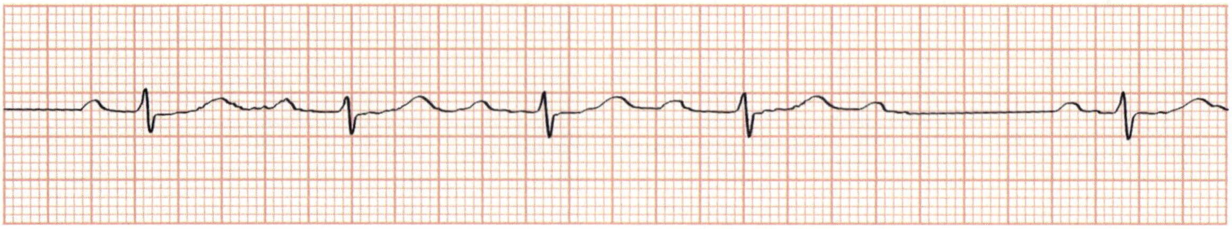

**Fig. 41.15:** ECG trace showing type I (Mobitz) AV block. There is progressive prolongation of the PR interval culminating in a nonconducted P-wave. The PR interval is the longest immediately before the dropped beat. The PR interval is shortest immediately after the dropped beat

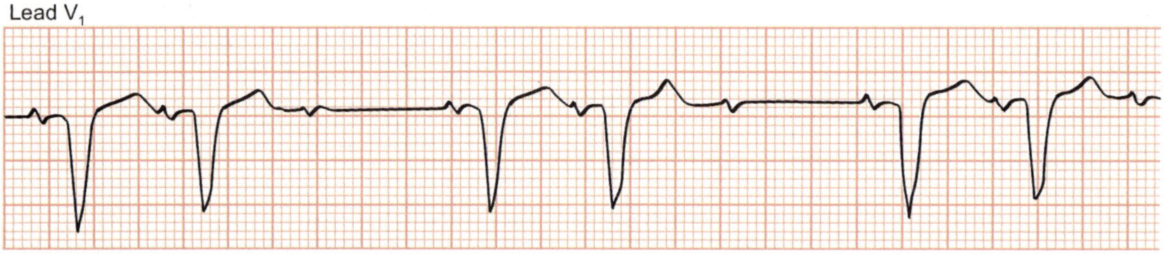


**Fig. 41.16:** ECG trace showing type II (Mobitz) AV block. The PR intervals are constant until a nonconducted P-wave occurs. There must be *two consecutive constant* PR intervals to diagnose type II AV block (i.e. if there is 2:1 AV block we can't be sure if its type I or II). The RR interval of the pause is *equal to* the two preceding RR intervals

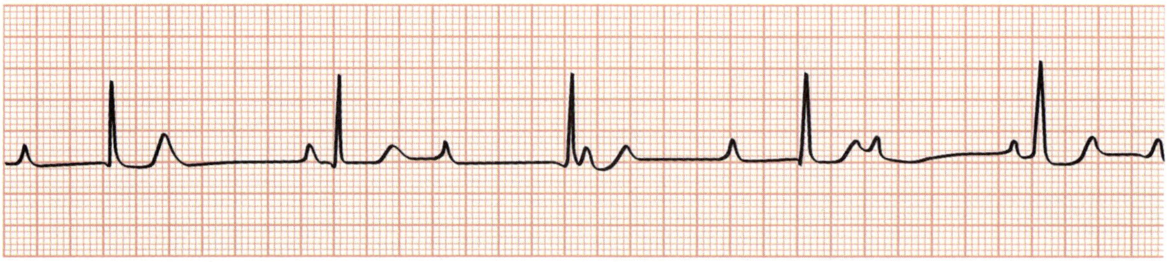

**Fig. 41.17:** ECG trace showing complete heart block, there is complete absence of AV conduction—*none* of the supraventricular impulses are conducted to the ventricles. Perfusing rhythm is maintained by a junctional or ventricular escape rhythm. Alternatively, the patient may suffer ventricular standstill leading to syncope (if self-terminating) or sudden cardiac death (if prolonged). Typically the patient will have severe bradycardia with independent atrial and ventricular rates, i.e. AV dissociation

clear because there is a continuum from physiologic to pathologic cardiac enlargement. The zone of overlap between the athlete's heart and cardiomyopathy is left ventricular septal thickness between 13 mm to 15 mm in men and 11 mm to 13 mm in women. In this overlap area, the presence of mitral valve systolic anterior motion strongly suggests hypertrophic cardiomyopathy. In general, echocardiographic changes correlate poorly with level of training and cardiovascular performance. Trace mitral regurgitation and tricuspid regurgitation are commonly detected.

### Stress Testing

During exercise stress testing, heart rate remains lower than normal at submaximal stress and increases appropriately and comparably to nonathletes at maximal stress; it rapidly recovers after exercise (Figs 41.31–41.36). BP response is normal. Systolic BP increases, diastolic BP falls, and mean BP stays relatively constant. Many resting ECG changes decrease or disappear during exercise; this finding is unique to athlete's heart, distinguishing it from pathologic conditions. However, pseudonormalization of T-wave inversions could reflect myo-

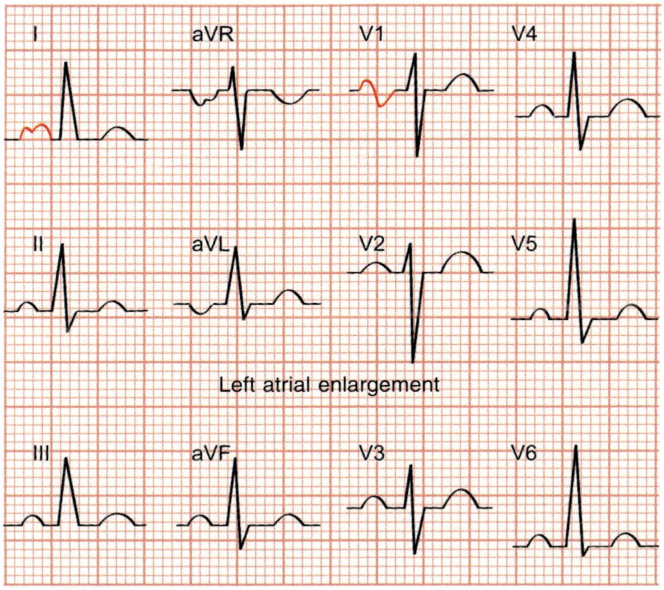


**Fig. 41.18:** Left atrial enlargement. ECG trace showing P-wave with a broad (>0.04 sec or 1 small square) and deeply negative (>1 mm) terminal part in V1 P-wave duration >0.12 sec in leads I and/or II

cardial ischemia and thus warrants further investigation in older athletes.

## Differential Diagnosis between Athlete's Heart and Cardiovascular Disease

- **Dilated cardiomyopathy:** In an important minority of athlets, the increase in left ventricular diastolic cavity dimension that occurs with training overlaps with that characteristic of certain known pathological entities. For example, while left ventricular end-diastolic cavity dimension in athletes is usually in the range of 53–58 mm, in some individuals it may extend into what may be regarded as the pathological range of >58 mm and

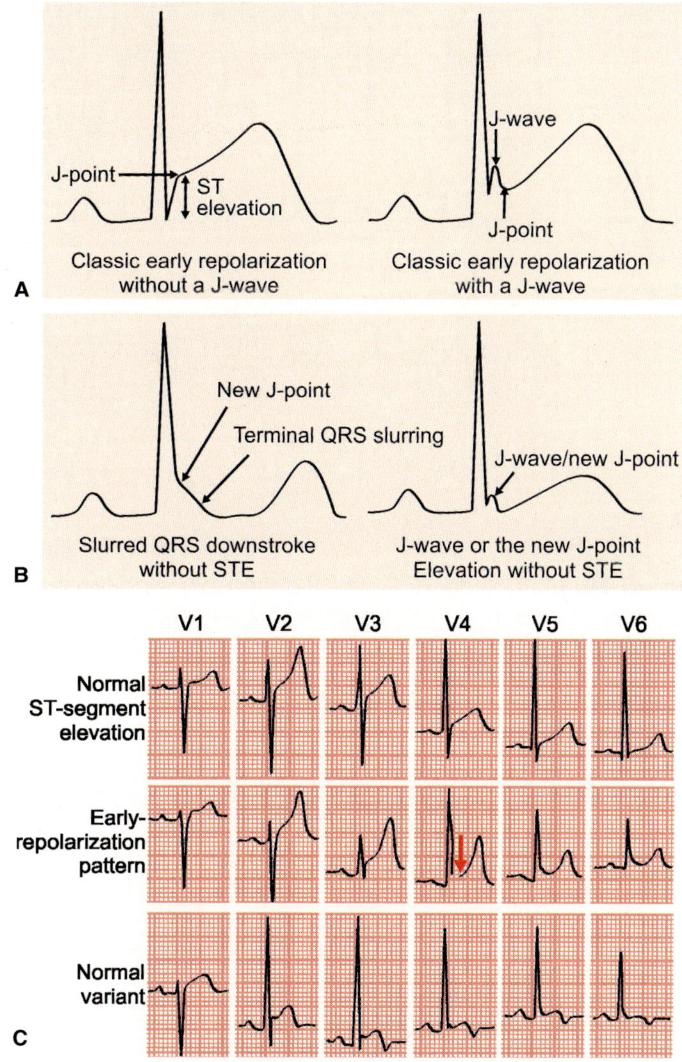


**Fig. 41.19:** (A and B) Illustrations and (C) a 12-lead electrocardiogram showing type I (inferolateral) early repolarization pattern (ERP) (red arrow indicates J-wave elevation)

**Table 41.4:** Criteria for positive 12-lead ECG in athletes

**P-wave**

Left atrial enlargement: Negative portion of the P-wave in lead V1 = 0.1 mV in depth and 0.04 s in duration

Right atrial enlargement: Peaked P-wave in leads II and III or V1 = 0.25 mV in amplitude

**QRS complex**

Frontal plane axis deviation: right = +120° or left –30° to –90°

increased voltage amplitude of R- or S-wave in a standard lead = 2 mV, S wave

in lead V1 or V2 = 3 mV, or R wave in lead V5 or V6 = 3 mV; abnormal Q-waves = 0.04 s in duration or = 25% of the height of the ensuring R-wave or QS pattern in two or more leads; right or left bundle-branch block with QRS duration = 0.12 s; R- or R′-wave in lead V1 = 0.5 mV in amplitude and R/S ratio = 1.

**ST-segment, T-waves and QT interval**

ST-segment depression or T-wave flattening or inversion in two or more leads

Prolongation of heart rate corrected QT interval > 0.44 s in males and > 0.46 s in females

**Rhythm and conduction abnormalities**

Premature ventricular beats or more severe ventricular arrhythmias

Supraventricular tachycardias, atrial flutter, or atrial fibrillation; short PR interval (< 0.12 s) with or without delta wave; sinus bradycardia with resting heart rate = 40 beats/min first (PR = 0.21 s)[a], second or third degree atrioventricular block.

[a]Not shortening with hyperventillation or limited exercise test. Modified from Corrado et al.

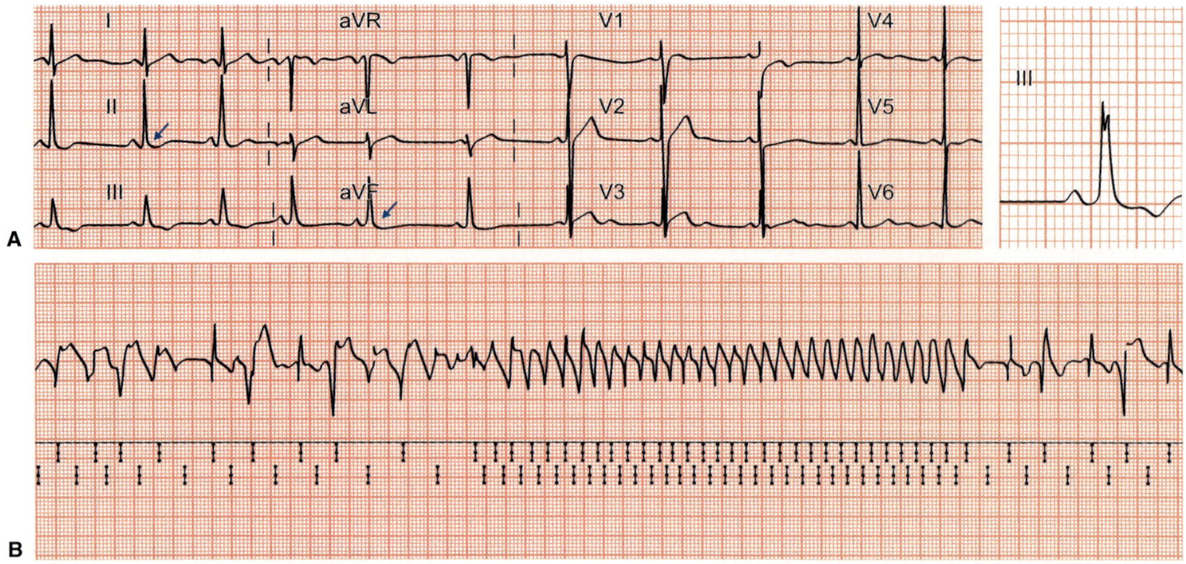


**Fig. 41.20:** (A) 12-lead ECG showing the early repolarization pattern in the inferior leads (arrows) and the fractionated QRS with negative T-wave in lead III (magnified view on the right side; the fractionation of the QRS was interpreted as a giant J-wave). (B) Nonsustained ventricular fibrillation as recorded by the loop recorder (VS, ventricular sensed event by the device; FS, ventricular fibrillation sensing by the device, vertical values representing the instantaneous cycle length durations between successive ventricular events)

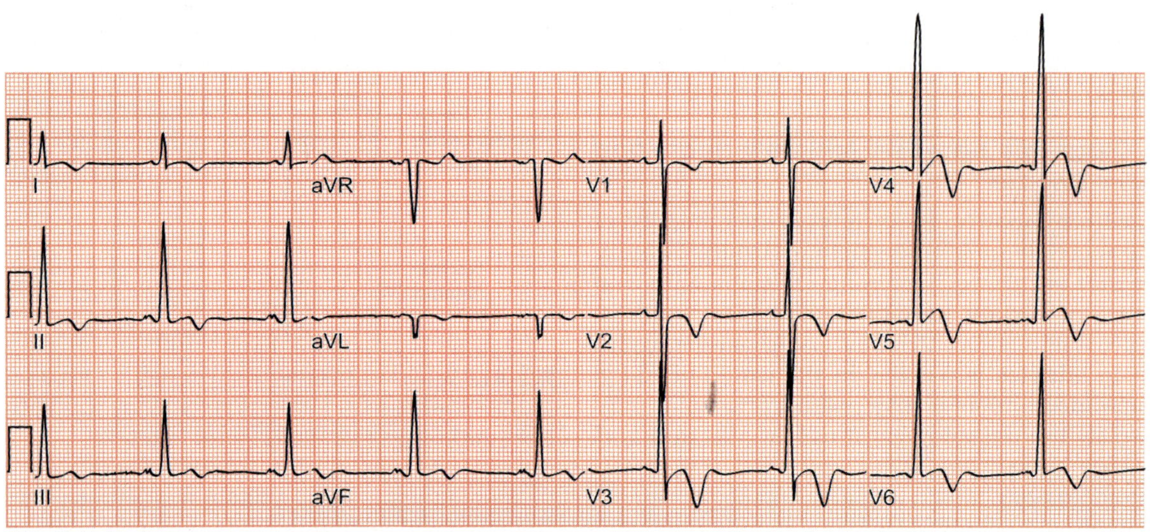


**Fig. 41.21:** ECG shows the typical pattern of apical HCM. Large precordial voltages. Giant T-wave inversions in the precordial leads. Inverted T-waves are also seen in the inferior and lateral leads

thereby resemble dilated cardiomyopathy. However, the absence of left ventricular systolic dysfunction is usually sufficient to distinguish this physiological ventricular enlargement induced by training from that due to dilated cardiomyopathy.

- **Myocarditis:** Myocarditis, a disorder associated with a heterogeneous clinical profile, has recently been incriminated as the possible cause of some highly publicized deaths in athletes. While myocarditis usually has an infectious origin, it can also be a consequence of drug abuse. Sudden cardiac death may occur in its active or healed phases as a consequence of complex arrhythmias that develop in the setting of an unstable myocardial electrical substrate. In an athlete with myocarditis, left ventricular cavity enlargement may be due to the disease, to athletic training, or to a combination of these, but the differential diagnosis with athlete's heart is usually resolved by the presence of clinically relevant and overt arrhythmias, cardiac symptoms such as syncope, presyncope and palpitations, or heart failure with systolic dysfunction. In some instances, the diagnosis may also be clarified by histological examination of myocardium obtained by endomyocardial biopsy.
- **Right ventricular dysplasia:** Arrhythmogenic right ventricular dysplasia (or cardiomyopathy) is a heart muscle disorder of unknown cause that is characterized pathologically by fibrofatty replacement of the right ventricular myocardium. The clinical and phenotypic profile is variable but includes structural and functional abnormalities of the right ventricle, ventricular and

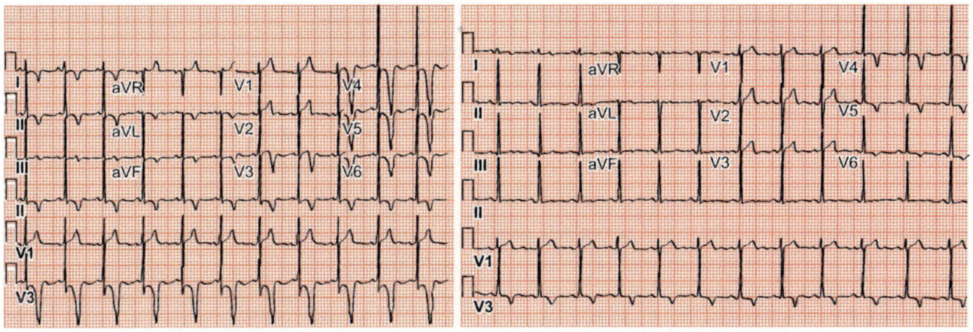

**Fig. 41.22:** 12-lead ECG of an asymptomatic athlete with HCM. The disease was suspected at preparticipation evaluation. Thanks to ECG abnormalities consisting of increased QRS voltages and inverted T-waves in lateral leads. HCM was diagnosed by echocardiography afterwards

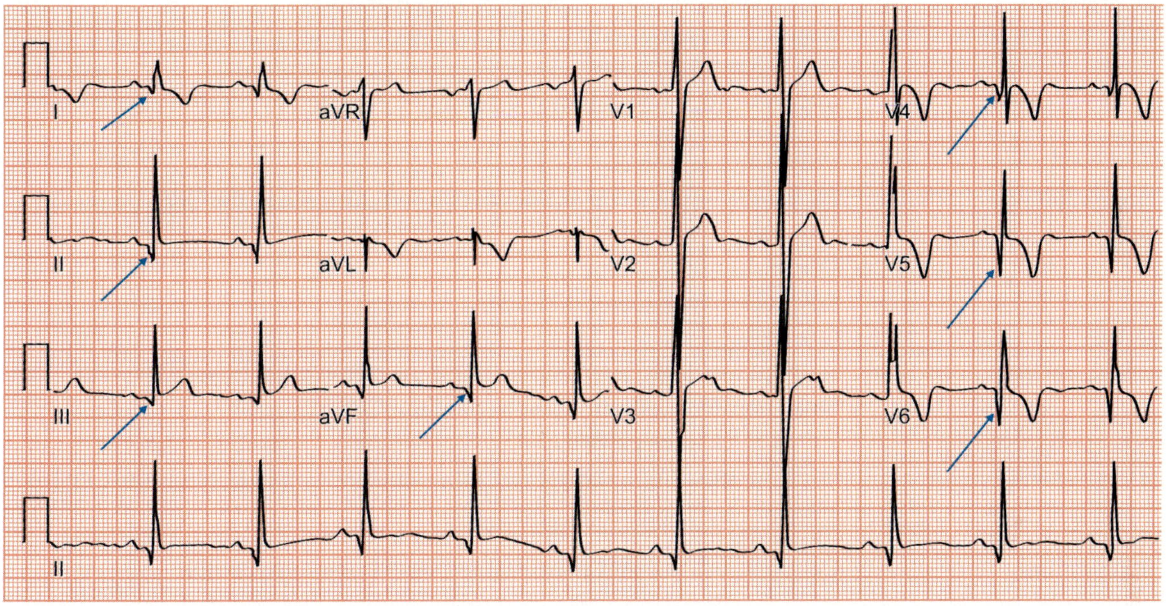

**Fig. 41.23:** ECG shows left ventricular hypertrophy results in increased precordial voltages and nonspecific ST-segment and T-wave abnormalities. Asymmetrical septal hypertrophy produces deep, narrow ('dagger-like') Q-waves in the lateral (V5-6, I, aVL) and inferior (II, III, aVF) leads. These may mimic prior myocardial infarction, although the Q-wave morphology is different; infarction Q-waves are typically >40 ms duration while septal Q-waves in HCM are <40 ms. Lateral Q-waves are more common than inferior Q-waves in HCM. Left ventricular diastolic dysfunction may lead to compensatory left atrial hypertrophy, with signs of left atrial enlargement ('P mitrale') on the ECG

supraventricular arrhythmias, familial occurrence, and the risk for sudden cardiac death. Indeed, it has been suggested that right ventricular dysplasia is an important cause of sudden death in the young, including competitive athletes, largely on the basis of reports from the north-eastern (Veneto) region of Italy.

Because highly trained athletes may demonstrate right ventricular enlargement and a variety of depolarization, repolarization, and conduction abnormalities on the ECG, the differential diagnosis between athlete's heart and right ventricular dysplasia may arise. Noninvasive identification of right ventricular dysplasia by echocardiography may be difficult because of technical limitations in imaging right ventricular structure and assessing function in these patients and because the spectrum of the disease is broad and includes mild morphological forms with subtle manifestations. Magnetic resonance imaging, however, promises enhanced noninvasive diagnosis of this condition. The demonstration of right ventricular segmental or global dysfunction or substantial right ventricular cavity enlargement would support the diagnosis of right ventricular dysplasia; alternatively, thickening or enlargement of the left ventricle would be most consistent with athlete's heart.

- **Hypertrophic cardiomyopathy:** The greatest difficulty in distinguishing clinically between athlete's heart and structural heart disease most frequently arises with respect to HCM, since many of the other cardiac disorders that cause sudden death in a young athletic population can be identified independently of any changes in cardiac morphology typically associated with

**Table 41.5:** Abnormal ECG criteria in athletes. Any abnormal finding is considered training-unrelated and suggests the possibility of underlying pathological disease, required further diagnostic investigation

| Abnormal ECG finding | Definition |
|---|---|
| T-wave inversion | >1 mm in depth from baseline in two or more adjacent leads not including aVR or V1 |
| ST-segment depression | ≥1 mm in depth in two or more adjacent leads |
| Pathological Q-waves | >3 mm in depth or >0.04 s in duration in two or more leads |
| Complete left bundle-branch block | QRS >0.12s, predominantly negative QRS complex in lead $V_1$ (QS or rS and upright monophasic R-wave in leads I and $V_6$ |
| Complete right bundle-branch block | QRS >0.12 s, terminal R wave in lead $V_1$ (rsR′) and wide terminal S-wave in leads I and $V_6$. |
| Intraventricular conduction delay | Nonspecific, QRS > 0.12 s |
| Left atrial enlargement | Prolonged P-wave duration of >0.12 s in lead I or II with negative portion of the P-wave ≥1 m in depth and ≥0.04 s in duration in lead $V_1$ |
| Left axis deviation | –30° to 90° |
| Right atrial enlargement | High/pointed P-wave ≥2.5 mm in lead II and III or $V_1$ |
| Right ventricular hypertrophy | Right axis deviation ≥120°, tall R-wave in V1 + persistent precordial S wave (R – $V_1$ + S – $V_5$ >10.5 mm) |
| Mobitz type II 2° AV block | Intermittently nonconducted P-wave not preceded by PR prolongation and not followed by PR shortening |
| 3° AV block | Complete heart block |
| Ventricular pre-excitation | PR interval <0.12 s with a S-wave (slurred upstroke in the QRS complex) |
| Long QT interval | QTc ≥0.47 s (99% men) |
| | QTc ≥0.18 s (99% women) |
| | QTc ≥0.50 s (unequivocal LQTS) |
| Short QT interval | QTc ≤0.34 s |
| Brugada-like ECG pattern | High take-off and downsloping ST-segment elevation in $V_1$-$V_3$ |
| Epsilon wave | Small negative deflection just beyond the QRS in $V_1$ or $V_2$ |
| Profound sinus bradycardia | <30 BPM or sinus pauses ≥3 s |
| Atrial tachyarrhythmias | Supraventricular tachycardia, atrioventricular nodal re-entrant tachycardia, atrial fibrillation, atrial flutter |
| Premature ventricular contractions | ≥2 per tracing |
| Ventricular arrhythmias | Couplets, triplets, and nonsustained ventricular tachycardia |

AV=atrioventricular; BPM=beats per minute; LQTS=long QT syndrome.

training. The basic definition of HCM used here is that of a patient (or athlete) with evidence of a hypertrophied and nondilated left ventricle in the absence of another cardiac or systemic disease that could itself cause hypertrophy of the magnitude present in that individual.

**Wall thickness:** In the vast majority of competitive athletes, absolute left ventricular wall thickness is normal or only mildly increased (12 mm). In some athletes, however, the increase in left ventricular wall thickness may be more substantial, up to 16 mm, unavoidably raising the possibility of HCM. In patients with HCM, the increase in left ventricular wall thickness is usually marked; the average wall thickness reported in most echocardiographic studies of this disease is 20 mm, ranging to >50 mm. However, an important minority of patients with HCM show relatively mild left ventricular hypertrophy with wall thickness values in the range of 13–15 mm, and many of these patients are asymptomatic. Therefore, a diagnostic dilemma arises in those athletes who fall into this morphological 'gray zone' between physiological hypertrophy and HCM. While this distinction cannot be resolved with certainty in some of these athletes, careful analysis of several echocardiographic and clinical features permits this diagnostic differentiation in most.

## Cardiac Arrhythmia in Young Athletes (Figs 41.46–41.53)

### Atrial Fibrillation

Treatment of atrial fibrillation in young athletes is similar to other young patient populations. There is little evidence that calcium channel blockers and beta-blockers reduce episodes of atrial fibrillation, but rather make them less symptomatic when they occur. Antiarrhythmic drugs are typically quite effective in individuals without heart disease.

Type 1C agents such as flecainide or propafenone are generally preferred as initial agents because of the safety profile and efficacy of these drugs. Rapid atrial flutter can be especially troubling with flecainide and for this reason a rate controlling agent such as a beta-blocker or calcium channel blocker is generally recommended. The use of

| | Athlete heart | Nonathlete heart |
|---|---|---|
| **Left ventricular function** | | |
| Morphology | IVSd 8–16* mm **<13 mm** LVIDd 49–73 mm **<65 mm** LVM 113–618* g **<400 g** | IVSd 6–10 mm LVIDd 42–59 mm LVM 88–224 g |
| Volumes/ EF(%) | LVEDV 130–260 ml EF **<240 ml** 41–77% **>48%** | LVEDV 67–155 ml EF >55% |
| Tissue Doppler | $S_m$ 6.5–14 cm/s $E_m$ 7.5–16 cm/s | $S_m$ >6 cm/st $E_m$ >8 cm/s |
| Strain Strain rate | Not clearly different from nonathletes | Normal values not established |
| LA size | 22–55 mm (diameter) | 30–40 mm (diameter) |
| **Right ventricular function** | | |
| RVFAC | 26–60% | 32–60% |
| Volumes/ EF (%) | RVEDV 130–260 ml RVEF >45% | RVEDV 60–150 ml RVEF >50% t |

**Fig. 41.24:** Changes in morphology and function in an athlete's heart. Ranges of values for athletes' hearts are obtained from published studies. Proposed cutoff values for athletes (bold) beyond which pathology may be considered. *IVSd and LVM ranges include black athletes; †Normal ranges not validated. EF=ejection fraction; IVSd=interventricular septal defect; LA=left atrial; LVEDV=left ventricular end-diastolic volume; LVIDm=left ventricular internal diameter at midventricle; LVM=left ventricular mass; RVEDV=right ventricular end-diastolic volume; RVEF=right ventricular ejection fraction; RVFAC=right ventricular function area change

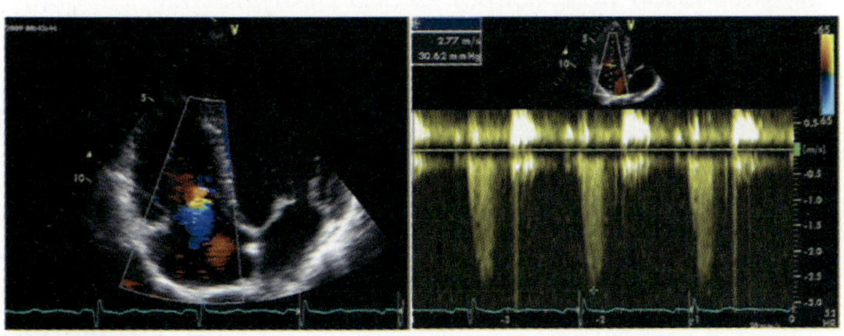

**Fig. 41.25:** Maximal tricuspid regurgitation peak velocity in an athlete, measured from the spectral profile of the tricuspid regurgitation jet in the apical four-chamber view

amiodarone is not advised because of the young age of the athletes and the long-term toxicity of amiodarone. Whether dronedarone will play a role in the management of atrial fibrillation in young athletes is not yet clear. Ablation of atrial fibrillation is a particularly attractive option for

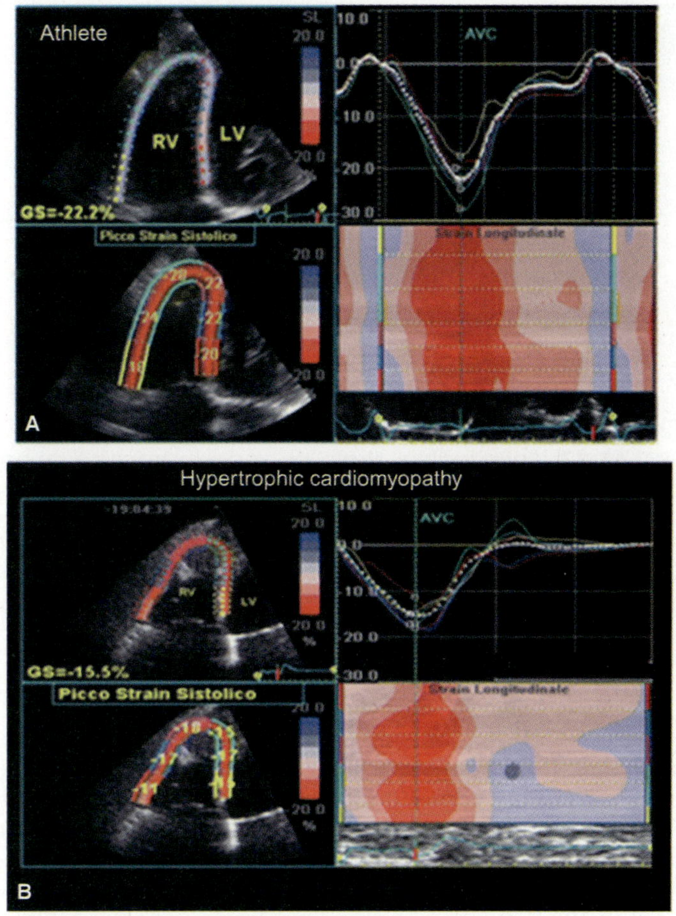


**Fig. 41.26:** Right ventricular two-dimensional speckle-tracking strain echocardiography pattern in an athlete and in a patient with hypertrophic cardiomyopathy (A and B, respectively)

athletes as they generally are young, have normal hearts and face a lifetime of atrial fibrillation risk.Pulmonary vein isolation would be a reasonable first step in the ablation of atrial fibrillation in athletes with more aggressive ablation options reserved for those who fail pulmonary vein isolation.

**Atrial flutter** is unusual in the individual without heart disease; when present, a stress test and echocardiogram are necessary to rule out the presence of structural heart disease.

Radiofrequency ablation is preferable to antiarrhythmic agents in individuals with atrial flutter because of the high likelihood of cure and the low risk of the procedure. Anticoagulation in atrial fibrillation and atrial flutter is not different than in nonathletes.

**Wolff-Parkinson White (WPW)** is not more common in the athlete, but athletes with WPW may be at higher risk for sudden death due to the high sympathetic drive seen with competition and with training.

For this reason most authorities recommended risk stratification of individuals with WPW. Risk stratification may be performed by rapid atrial pacing, by induction of atrial fibrillation in the electrophysiological laboratory

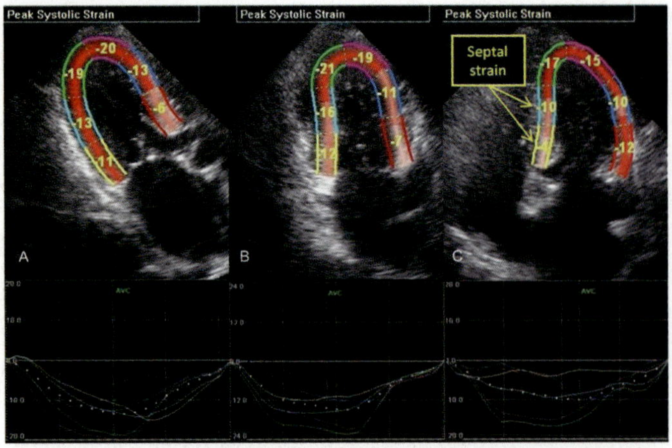


**Fig. 41.27:** Longitudinal strain by speckle tracking echocardiography from a patient with obstructive HCM. (A) Apical short axis; (B) apical two-chamber; (C) apical four-chamber. Global longitudinal strain was obtained by averaging the maximum systolic shortening in a 16-segment model (6 basal, 6 mid, and 4 apical segments). Septal longitudinal strain was defined as mean of two septal segments (basal and mid-segments from apical four-chamber view)

and sometimes by stress testing. The 36th Bethesda guidelines recommend ablation for multiple bypass tracts or if the bypass tract can conduct rapidly enough to sustain a tachycardia of greater than 240 bpm. ESC guidelines are more aggressive and recommend ablation for all asymptomatic WPW athletes age 12 years because of the relative ease of ablation and the life-long risk of SCD. In individuals who refuse ablation, competitive sports are allowed provided that short pre-excited cycle lengths of <240 ms at rest and <220 on isoproterenol or exercise during atrial fibrillation are not present. Both European and Bethesda Guidelines recommend radiofrequency ablation for the symptomatic athlete with WPW.

**Supraventricular tachycardias** such as AV nodal reentrant tachycardia, AV reciprocating tachycardia, and atrial tachycardia are not more common in athletes. Similar to nonathletes, when these arrhythmias occur initial treatment may be with beta-blockers and calcium channel blockers. However, in both the 36th Bethesda Guidelines

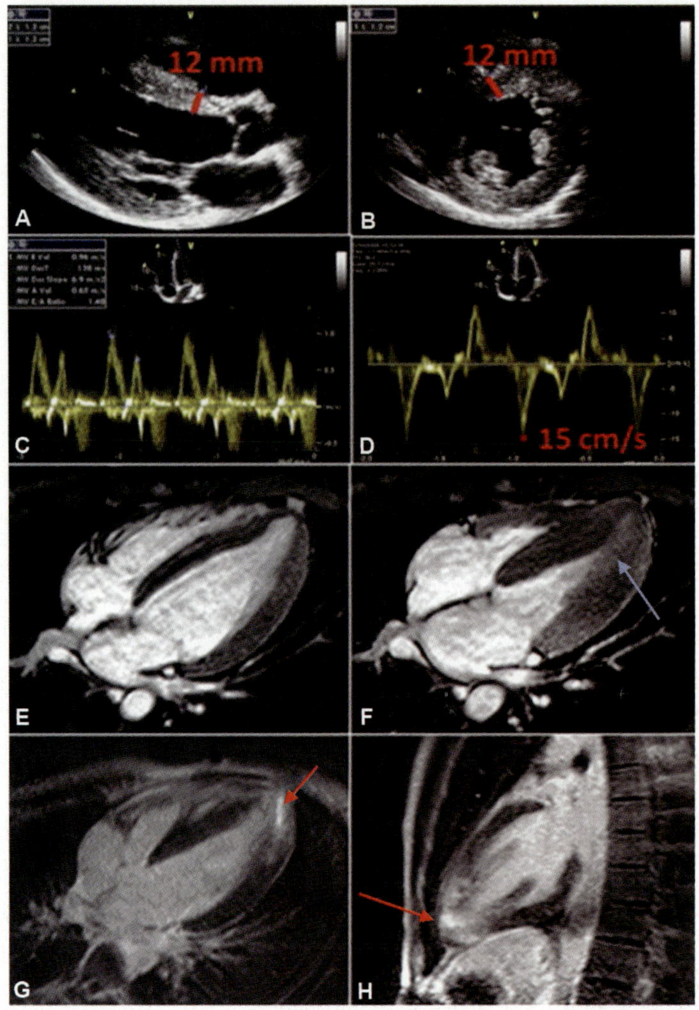


**Fig. 41.28:** A young athlete with hypertrophic cardiomyopathy example of the importance of CMR in diagnosing HCM in a young athlete who presented with aborted sudden cardiac death and in whom echocardiography was not diagnostic. Left ventricular wall thickness of 12 mm was within ranges accepted for his athletic training (A and B). Mitral inflow and early diastolic annular motion were normal (C and D). The concentric nature of the hypertrophy was atypical for an athlete (E=diastole, F=systole) resulting in intracavity obstruction (blue arrow). T1-weighted images after the administration of gadolinium contrast (G and H) demonstrate apical scarring (red arrows)

**Table 41.6:** Differences between atheletic heart syndrome and cardiomyopathy

| Feature | Athletic heart syndrome | Cardiomyopathy |
|---|---|---|
| Left ventricular hypertrophy | <13 mm | > 15 mm |
| Left ventricular end-diastolic diameter | <60 mm | > 70 mm |
| Diastolic function | Normal (E: A ratio >1) | Abnormal (E:A ratio <1) |
| Septal hypertrophy | Symmetric | Asymmetric (in hypertrophic cardiomyopathy) |
| Family history | None | May be present |
| BP response to exercise | Normal | Normal or reduced systolic BP response |
| Deconditioning | Left ventricular hypertrophy regression | No left ventricular hypertrophy regression |

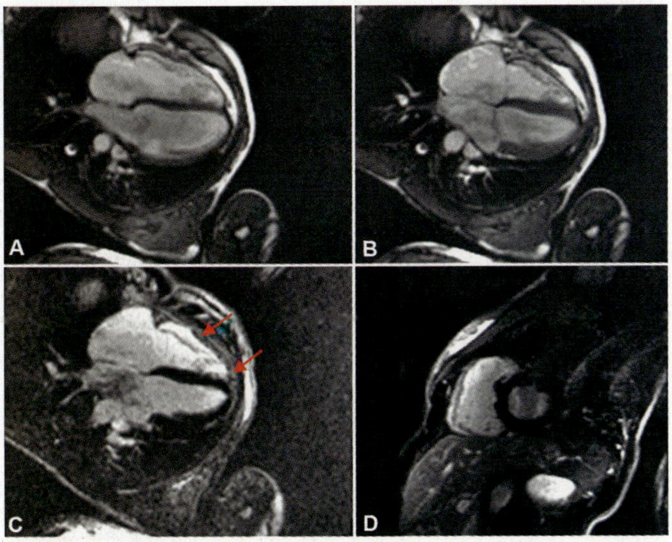

**Fig. 41.29:** An athlete with ventricular tachycardia and an abnormal right ventricle cardiovascular magnetic resonance study of an elite triathlete after sustained ventricular tachycardia. Cine images in diastole (A) and systole (B) demonstrate an enlarged right ventricle (RV) with reduced systolic function. Note also the septal shift in diastole suggesting significant volume loading. T1-weighted (late gadolinium enhancement) images (C and D) demonstrate increased signal (arrows) of uncertain significance given the spatial resolution constraints within the thin walled RV. A RV focus was identified on electrophysiology studies, which correlated with fibrosis on biopsy

and the European Guidelines, definitive treatment such as ablation is generally preferred because of the young age and lifetime risk of these arrhythmias.Atrial premature contractions are common in many individuals and may be symptomatic or asymptomatic.

If symptomatic, atrial premature beats can be treated with beta-blockers; however, reassurance is usually reasonable enough treatment.

### *Idiopathic Ventricular Tachycardia*

The two most common cardiac regions for idiopathic ventricular tachycardias are the right ventricular outflow tract and the left posterior fascicle. Both of these ventricular tachycardias can be triggered by exercise and both these ventricular tachycardias are readily curable with ablation. They are also adenosine and verapamil sensitive. In individuals with these idiopathic ventricular tachycardias strong consideration should be given to ablation as the ablation is curative and of relatively low risk.

## Deep Vein Thrombosis (DVT) or Pulmonary Embolism (PE) in Athletes (Figs 41.54–41.59)

The diagnosis of deep vein thrombosis (DVT) or pulmonary embolism (PE) in athletes, who exhibit classic symptoms, may be delayed or even missed because such medical problems are often not considered by healthcare providers or by the affected athlete. No studies have been done to determine whether athletes are at a higher, the same, or

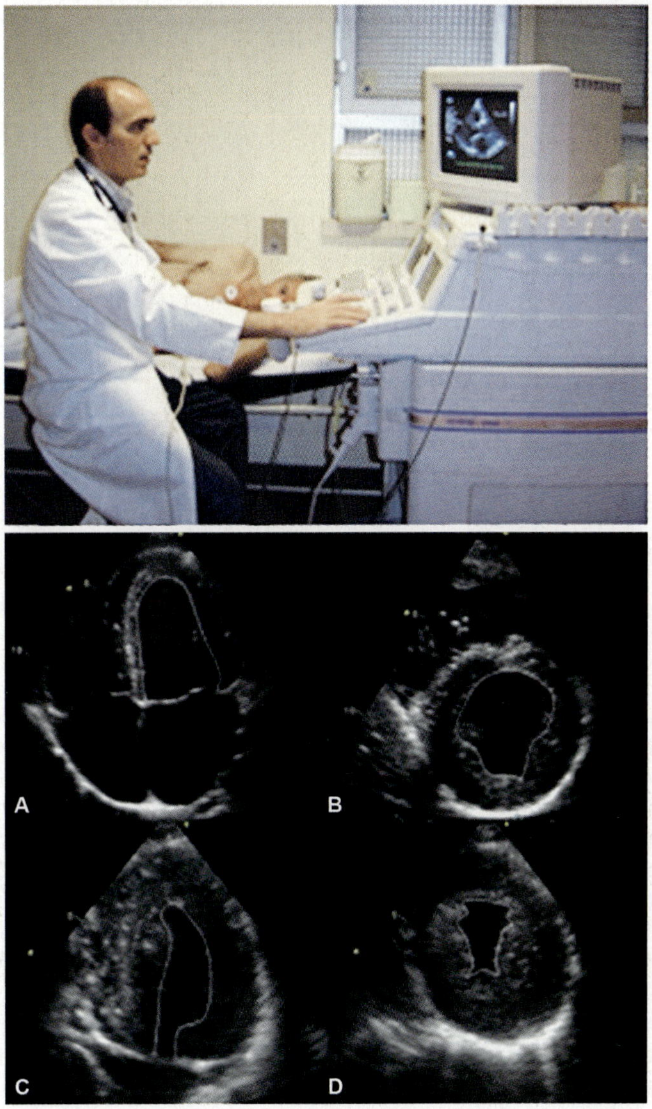

**Fig. 41.30:** Stress echocardiography to exclude a cardiomyopathy exercise can be used to differentiate low systolic function from a myopathic process. Imaging during exercise is critical in athletes and can be achieved using a recumbent ergometer (top panel). End systolic frames at rest (A and B) and peak exercise (C and D) demonstrate excellent augmentation of low-normal resting function

lower risk for developing blood clots than non-athletes. Blood clots are uncommon in young, healthy individuals—and most athletes are young and healthy. So, for that reason, DVT, PE, and arterial clots in athletes are not the norm.

To understand the problematic issues facing an athlete and the attending caregiver it is important to first understand the condition terminology. Our body is composed of an endless tunnel of arteries and veins through which blood flows throughout the body. Arteries are the blood vessels through which the blood flows from the heart into the periphery—the brain, the internal organs, the legs, and the arms. A clot in an artery leads to stroke, heart attack, or limb threatening peripheral arterial clot causing a

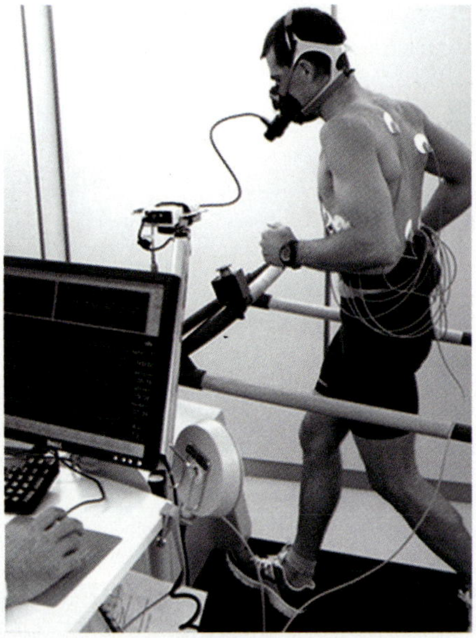

**Fig. 41.31:** Exercise stress testing being conducted for participation in atheletic events

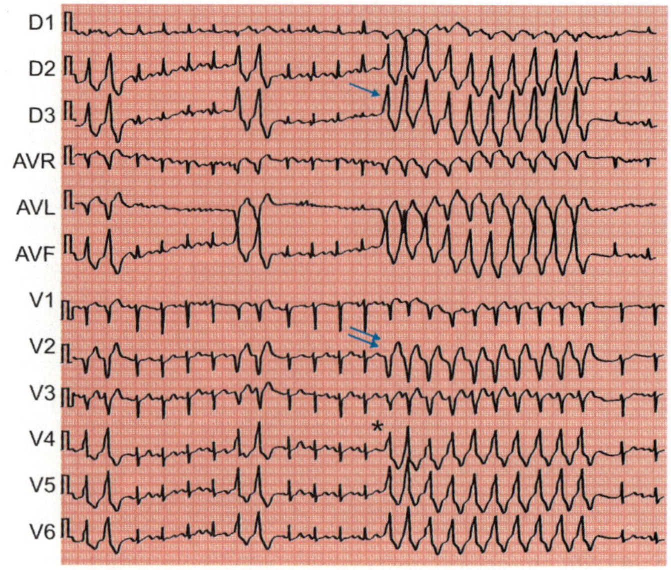


**Fig. 41.32:** Exercise-induced right ventricular outflow tract ventricular tachycardia in a 16-year-old female volleyball player. The figure shows the 12-lead electrocardiographic tracing during exercise stress testing (workload of 150 W; sinus heart rate 130 beats/min). From the left, two ventricular couplets and a nonsustained episode of right ventricular outflow tract ventricular tachycardia (arrow) are induced by exercise. The episode of ventricular tachycardia lasts 10 beats, with a minimum R2R2 interval of >400 ms, which is slightly symptomatic for palpitations. The premature ventricular beat morphology is like left bundle branch block in precordial leads (double arrow), with inferior axis in peripheral leads (one arrow) and with R/S transition in lead V4 (asterisk). At 15-year follow-up, the athlete showed complete reversibility of the arrhythmia during exercise testing and the absence of cardiovascular events with continuation in competitive sports

painful, cold, and pale extremity. Many people think of blood clots as a problem occurring in elderly people, but not in young and apparently healthy individuals. Symptoms may, therefore, be misinterpreted as something less serious. The leg symptoms from DVT are often interpreted as 'muscle tear,' a 'Charlie horse,' a 'twisted ankle,' or shin splints, while the chest symptoms from PE are attributed to a pulled muscle, costochondritis (inflammation of the joint between ribs and breast bone), bronchitis, or a 'touch of pneumonia.' Veins are the vessels through which blood is carried back to the heart. A clot in the deep veins of legs, arms, pelvis, abdomen, or around the brain is called a deep vein thrombosis (DVT). If a piece of clot breaks off from a leg or arm DVT it can travel into the lung causing a life-threatening condition known as a pulmonary embolism (PE).

### Athlete-specific Risk Factors for Clots

Being apparently healthy and being an athlete does not prevent a person from developing blood clots. Several circumstances put the athlete, as well as the nonathlete, at increased risk for DVT and PE. Athletes, coaches and trainers should be particularly aware of these risk factors (Figs 41.60–41.64).

*Blood clots can occur when:*

- There is a disparity between the two systems that balance the clotting process in our blood; either
  A. Too much activity of the proteins and blood platelets that form clots (the procoagulant system), or
  B. Too little activity of the system that dissolves blood clots as they form the fibrinolytic system
- There is trauma to the blood vessel wall, as may occur after a bone fracture or in thoracic outlet obstruction
- Blood return from the extremities to the heart is impaired, such as when sitting with bent legs in cramped positions for a prolonged period of time
- The blood is 'thicker' than usual, as occurs when an athlete is dehydrated, using the drug erythropoietin (EPO), or has received excessive blood transfusions (blood doping).
- Unfortunately, there are few studies investigating the influence that physical training has on blood clot formation and dissolution. So, the exact net effect of training on this equilibrium is unknown. It is known, for example, that blood levels of the clotting protein 'factor VIII' increase with exercise and that the elevation persists during recovery. Theoretically, this could lead to an increased risk of blood clots in athletes. However, data also indicate that the fibrinolytic system that dissolves blood clots is overactive in people who exercise. With this over activity present, the athlete would be protected from having a blood clot. Yet, the net effect of these changes in the athlete is not known.

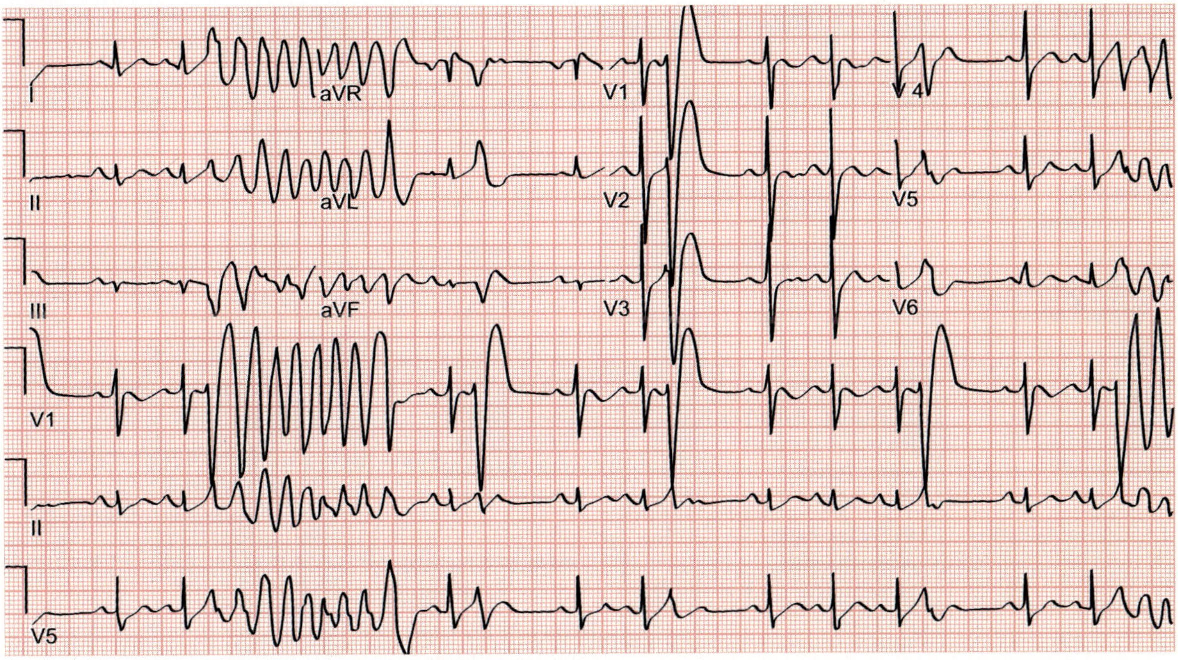


**Fig. 41.33:** Exercise-induced polymorphic ventricular tachycardia in a 20-year-old elite male swimmer

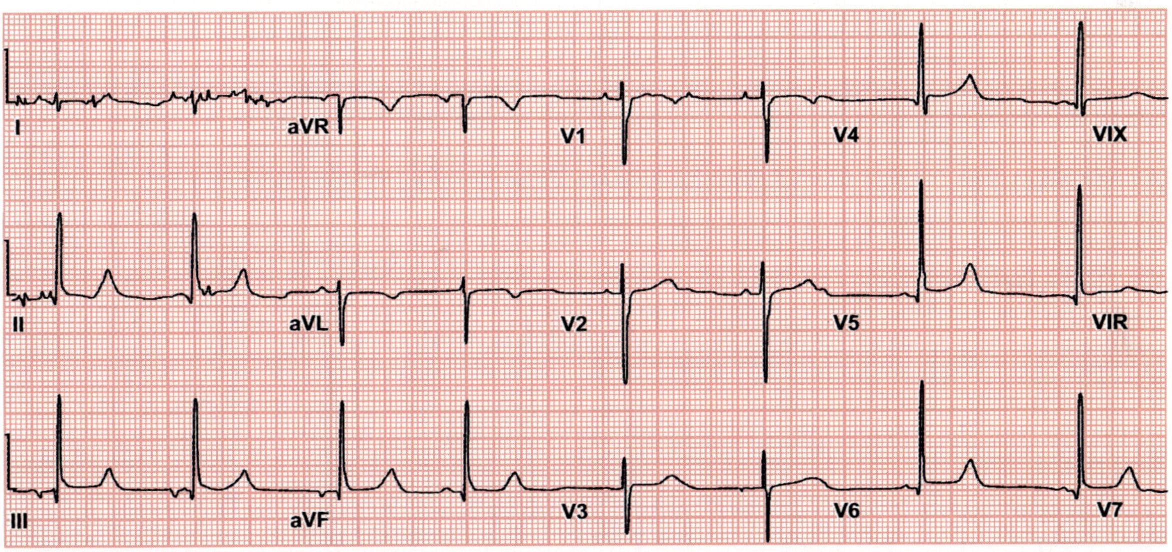


**Fig. 41.34:** Post-exercise ECG showing a prolonged corrected QT interval (QTc) of 490 milliseconds, with abnormal T-wave morphology. The QTc prolonged with exercise stress testing in the recovery period to 520 milliseconds, confirming the impression of long QT syndrome (LQTS). He was started on 10 mg of nadolol twice daily and was asked to stop competitive swimming. She was advised to avoid caffeine and stimulants, and not to take medications known to further prolong the QT interval

- A detailed scientific discussion of the coagulation issues relevant to exercise and training can be found in a recently published review. However, the conclusions are sparse and vague, because of a lack of data and conflicting results from different studies.

### *Risk Factors for DVT and PE in Athletes*

The most common clots occurring in athletes are DVT of the leg and PE. Factors that increase the risk for an athlete, as well as the nonathlete. A few unique risk factors predisposing the young and the athlete to DVT and PE are:

- **Thoracic outlet obstruction:** In some individuals an extra (cervical) rib or excess muscle or tendon tissue compress the big vein in the upper chest (subclavian vein) that drains the blood from the arm. This compression typically gets worse when the arm is lifted up. This obstruction, often combined with repeated trauma to the vein (due to throwing activities or gymnastics maneuvers), may cause a DVT to form

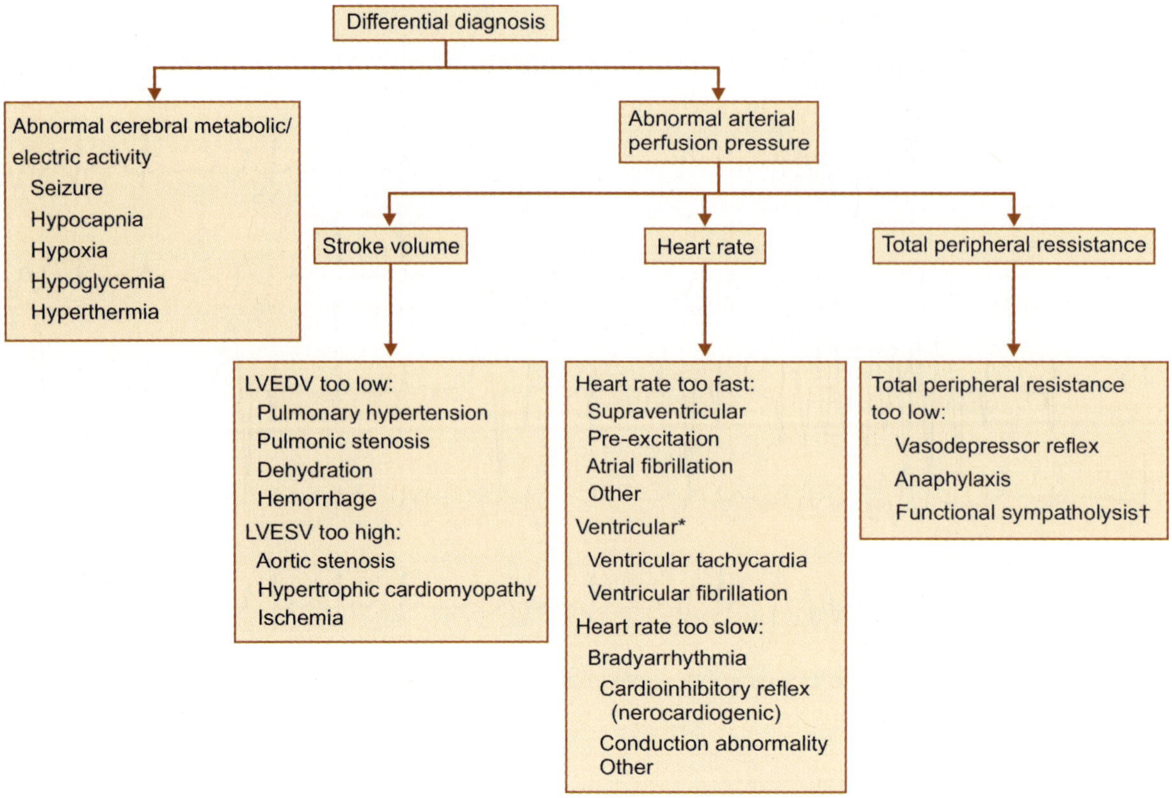


**Fig. 41.35:** Differential diagnosis of exercise-related syncope in young athletes. Arterial perfusion pressure is a function of the 'triple product' of heart rate 3 stroke volume 3 total peripheral resistance. (LVEDV=left ventricular end-diastolic volume; LVESV=left ventricular end-systolic volume). Information from Levine BD, Buckey JC, Fritsch JM, Yancy CW Jr, Watenpaugh DE, Snell PG. Physical fitness and cardiovascular regulation: mechanisms of orthostatic intolerance. J Appl Physiol 1991;70:112–22

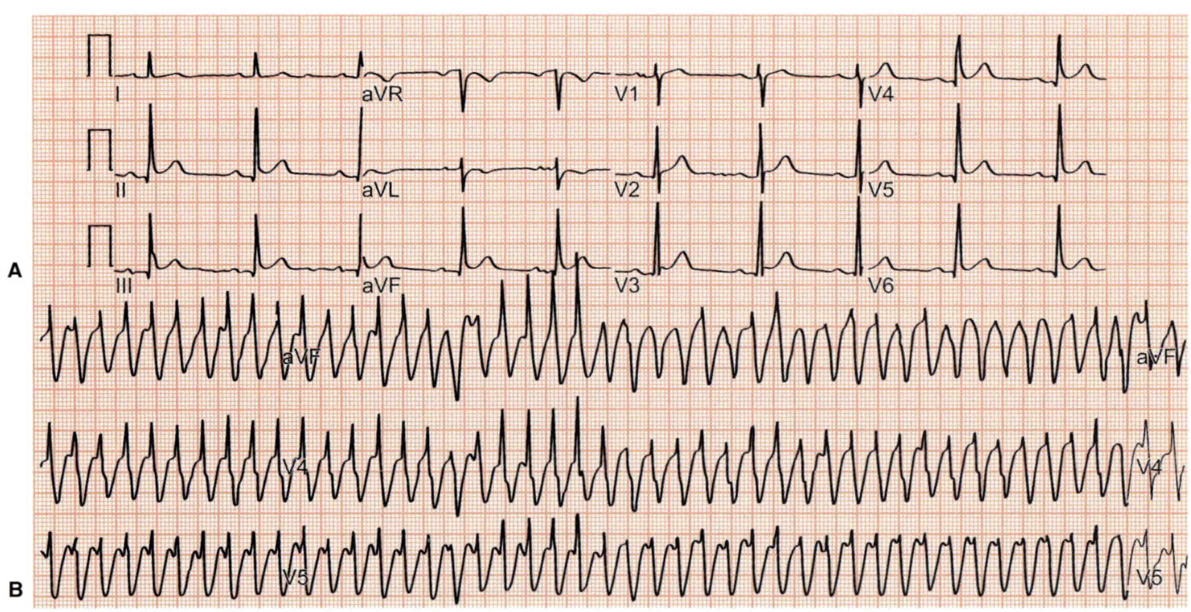


**Fig. 41.36:** Note the features of ERPV in the baseline ECG (A) recorded immediately before an exercise stress test (B) that resulted in torsade de pointe

in this area, extending into the arm veins. This is termed 'effort thrombosis' or 'thoracic outlet obstruction/ syndrome.' If the DVT resolves, such as after clot buster treatment, resection of the extra rib or the excess tissue may be indicated to increase space in the thoracic outlet.

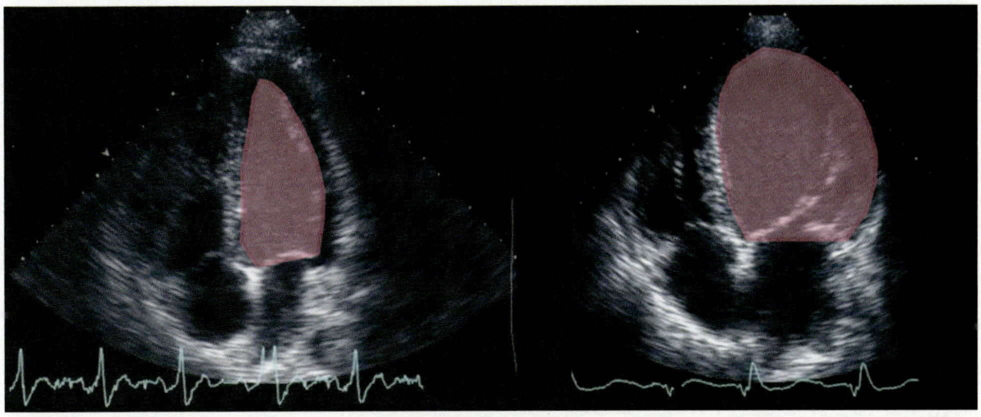

**Fig. 41.37:** Apical 4C views show dilated thin LV and LA with low LVEF

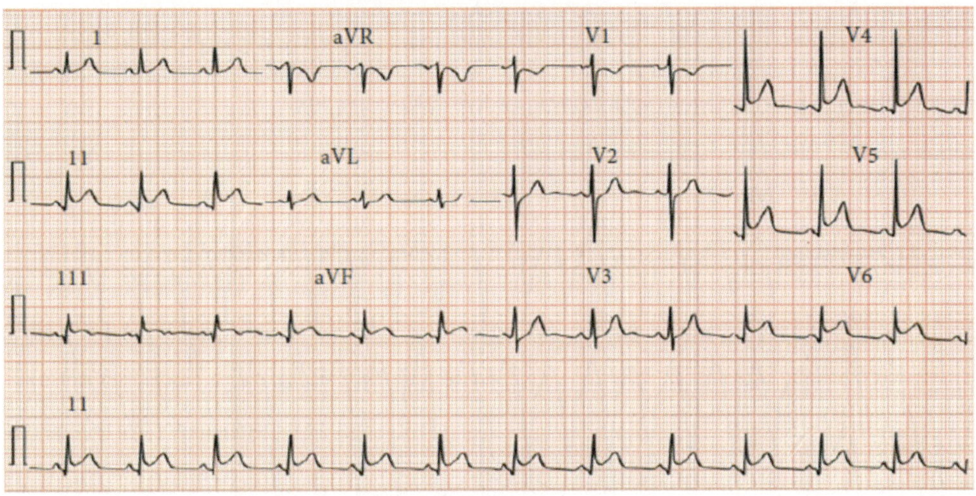


**Fig. 41.38:** 12-lead electrocardiogram showing ST-segment elevation of 2 mm in leads II, III, aVF, V4, V5, and V6

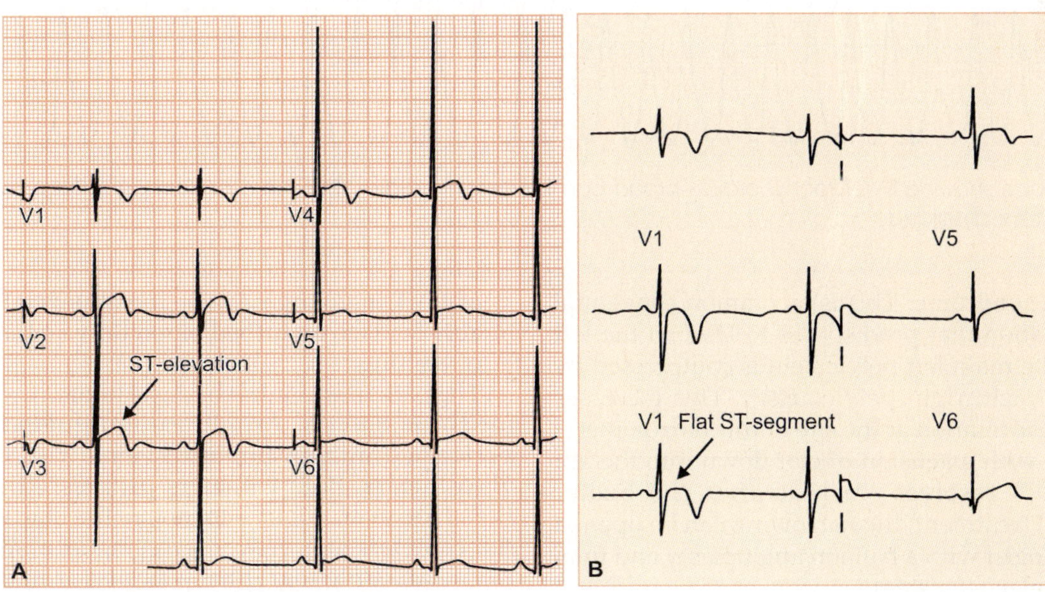


**Fig 41.39:** (A) Normal variant repolarisation changes in a black/African athlete characterised by domed ST-segment elevation and T-wave inversion in V1–V4. (B) Pathological T-wave inversion in V1–V3. Note the isoelectric ST-segment. The absence of ST-segment elevation prior to T-wave inversion makes this ECG abnormal. Additional testing is required to rule out arrhythmogenic right ventricular cardiomyopathy

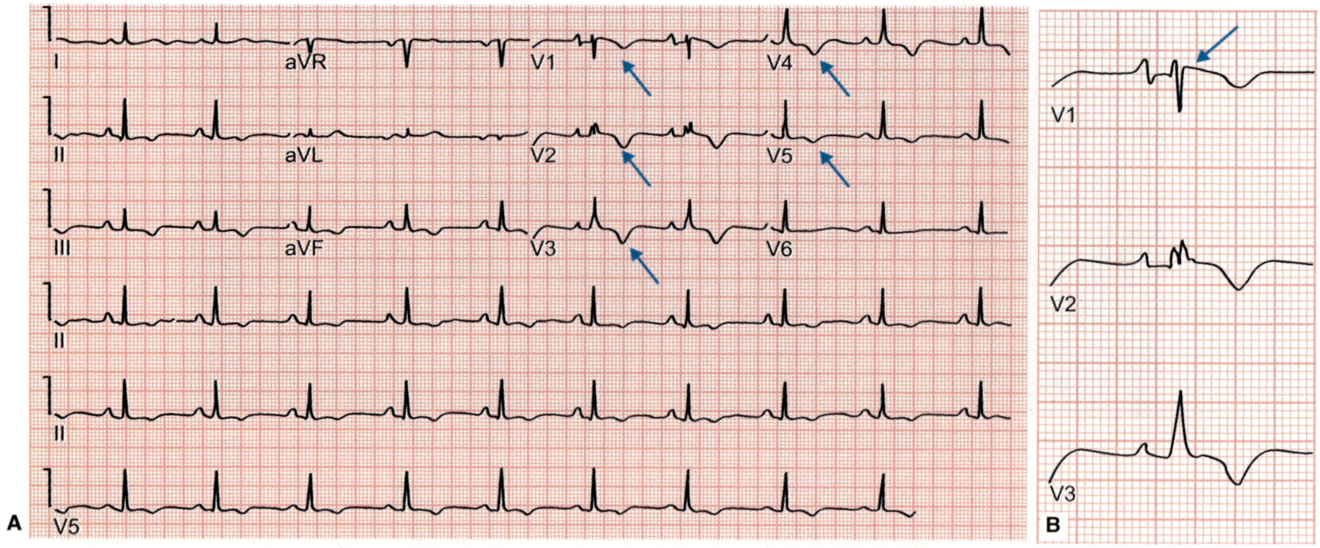


**Fig. 41.40:** ECG from a patient with arrhythmogenic right ventricular cardiomyopathy. (A) Inverted T-waves in leads V1–V5. (B) A subtle epsilon wave with notching in V1 at the terminal portion of the QRS complex

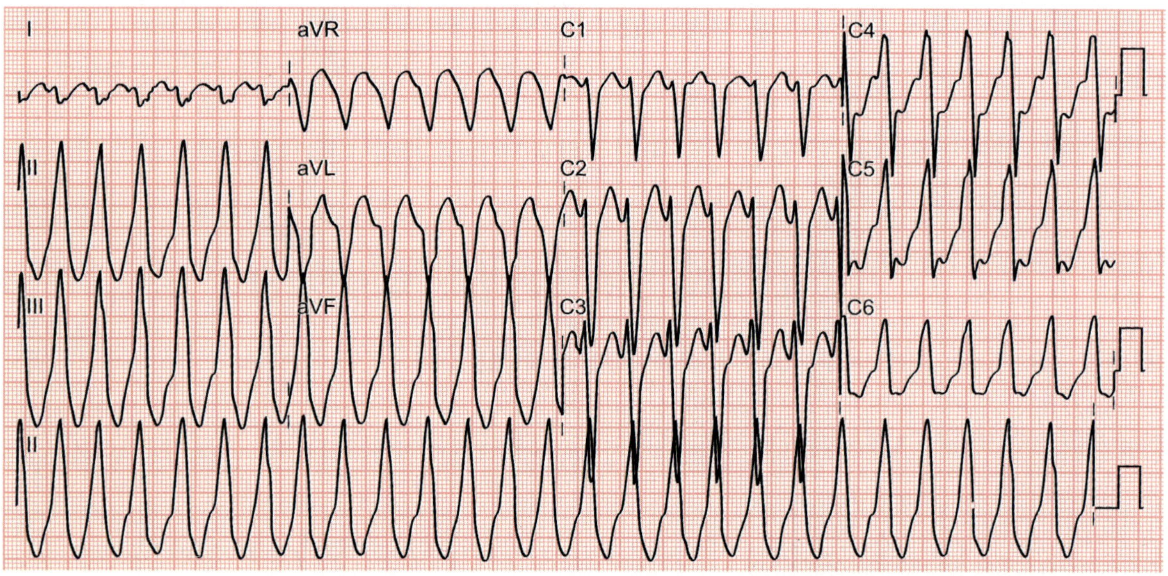


**Fig. 41.41:** ECG trace showing RVOT tachycardia—broad complex tachycardia. LBBB-like morphology. Inferior axis (+90 degrees) due to right ventricular dysplasia

- **May-Thurner syndrome:** This is a common congenital anatomic variation that predisposes to DVT in the left leg, because the main left pelvic vein is compressed by the overlying main right pelvic artery. This increases the risk of clot formation at the site of this narrowing in the left pelvis with extension of clot down into the left leg. If the DVT resolves, such as after clot buster (thrombolytic) treatment, the narrowing can be opened up by a radiologist with a balloon angioplasty and then kept open by placing a stent.
- **Congenital absence or malformation of the vena cava:** Congenital abnormalities of the anatomy of the big vein in the abdomen (vena cava) or pelvic veins can be a cause of DVT in young people. The abnormal anatomy probably leads to disturbed blood flow and an increased risk of clotting.

The patient was intravenously heparinized and prepared for thrombolysis. An ultrasound-guided puncture was performed in both popliteal veins with multiperforated 5F catheters. Both catheters progressed easily until the IVC. However, about 5 cm above the iliac vein confluence, the catheters stopped progressing at a site lateral to the IVC wall. Phlebography was performed, confirming a voluminous thrombosis with increased iliac arteries and extensive collateral circulation above those veins, with no contrast in the IVC. Due to the hypothesis of extrinsic IVC compression, thrombolysis was not performed.

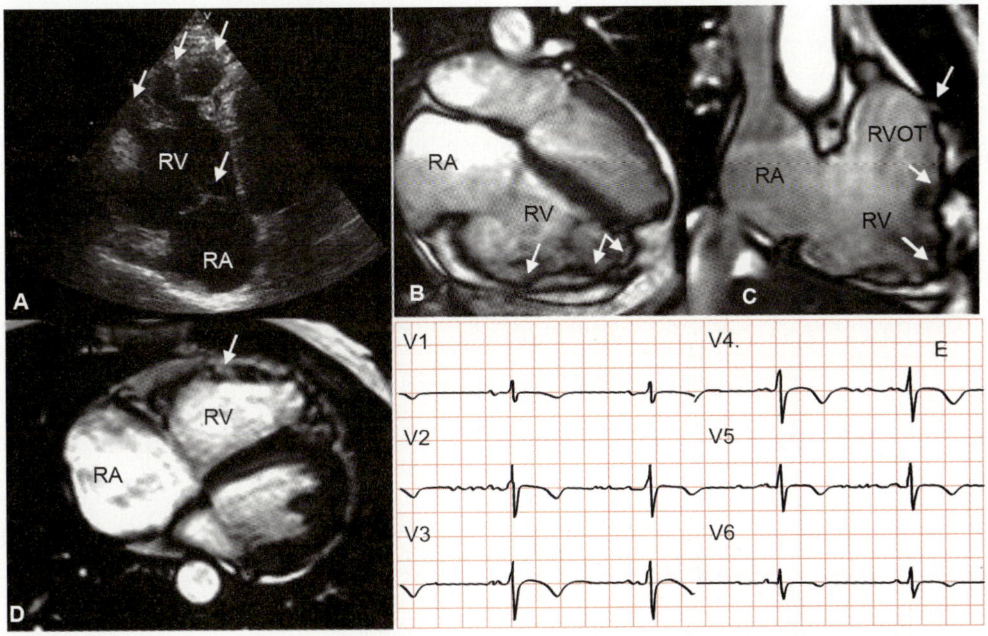


**Fig. 41.42:** (A) Echo, (B, C and D) CT/MRI, and (E) features of arrythmogenic cardiomyopathy

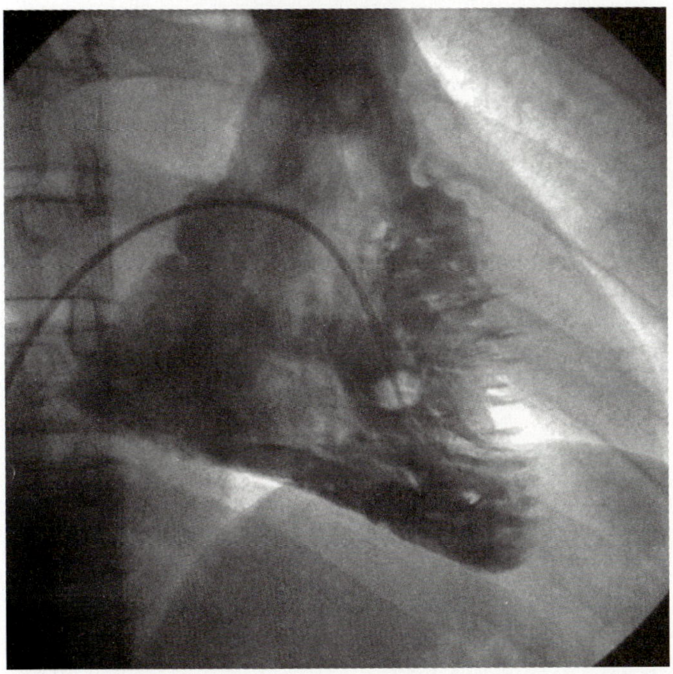

**Fig. 41.43:** Right ventriculogram showing akinetic/dyskinetic areas with diastolic septal bulge ('stack of coins') compatible with arrhythmogenic right ventricular dysplasia

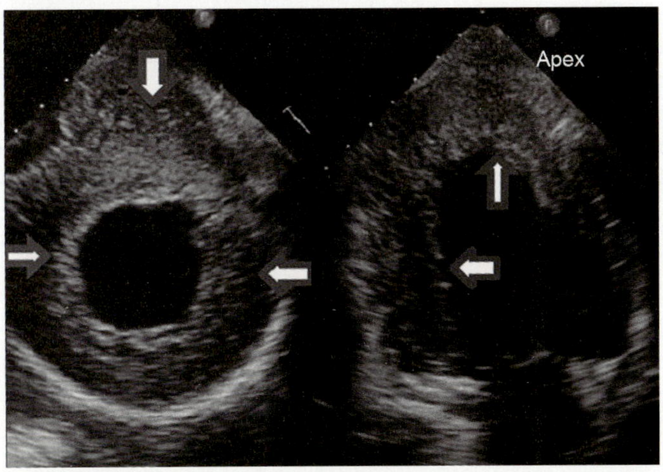


**Fig. 41.44:** Echocardiogram showing short axis (left) and two chamber view (right) in patient with HOCM affecting more than one segment including the apex (arrows)

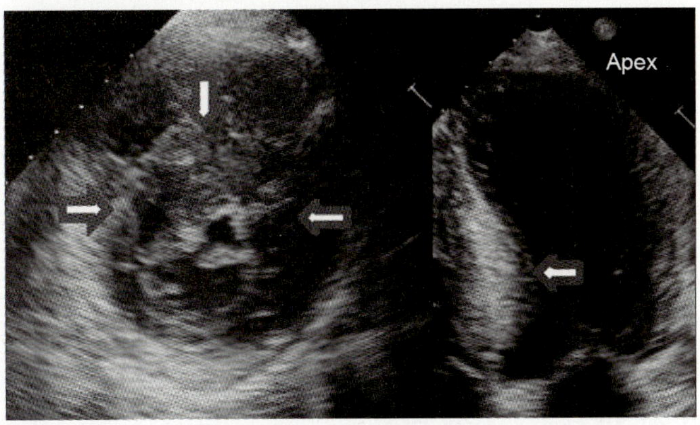


**Fig. 41.45:** Echocardiogram showing hypertrophy of more than one segment (arrows) in short axis and long axis but sparing the apex in patient with HOCM

Treatment decisions for people affected with blood clots must be individualized. This is particularly true for young, apparently healthy individuals, such as athletes. In the case of unexplained DVT, testing for an inherited or acquired clotting disorder may be appropriate. When first diagnosed with the DVT, clot buster medication (fibrinolytic or thrombolytic therapy) should be considered to quickly dissolve the clot. However, clot buster treatment has not been systematically studied to determine whether it really

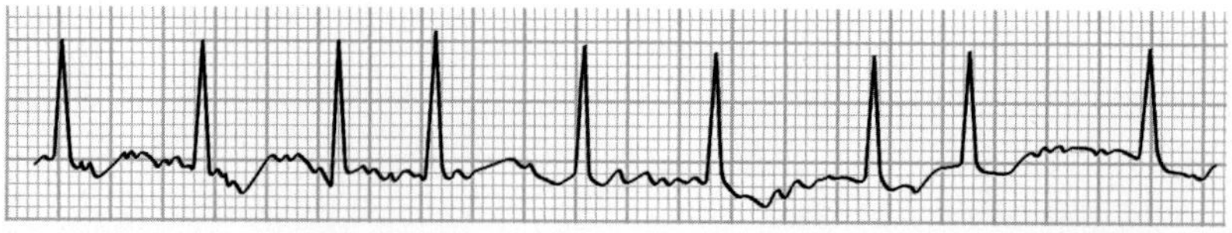

**Fig. 41.46:** ECG trace showing atrial fibrillation in a young athlete

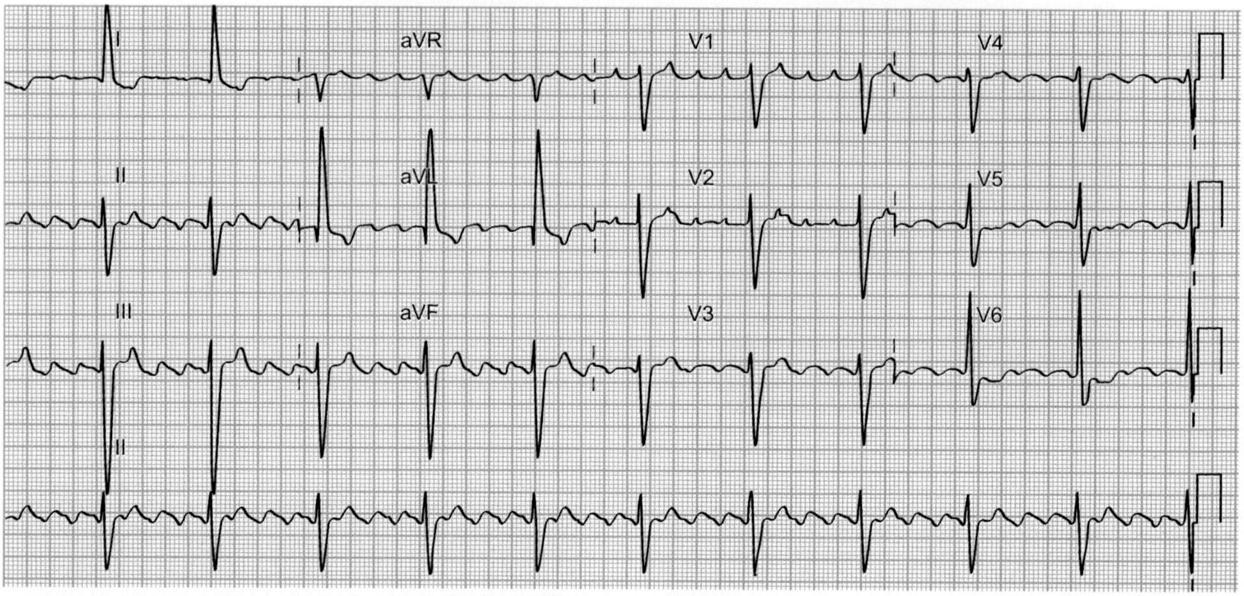


**Fig. 41.47:** ECG trace showing atrial flutter with 4:1 block. There are inverted flutter waves in II, III + aVF at a rate of 260 bpm. There are upright flutter waves in V1–2 (= anticlockwise circuit). There is 4:1 block, resulting in a ventricular rate of 65 bpm. The relatively slow ventricular response suggests treatment with an AV nodal blocking agent

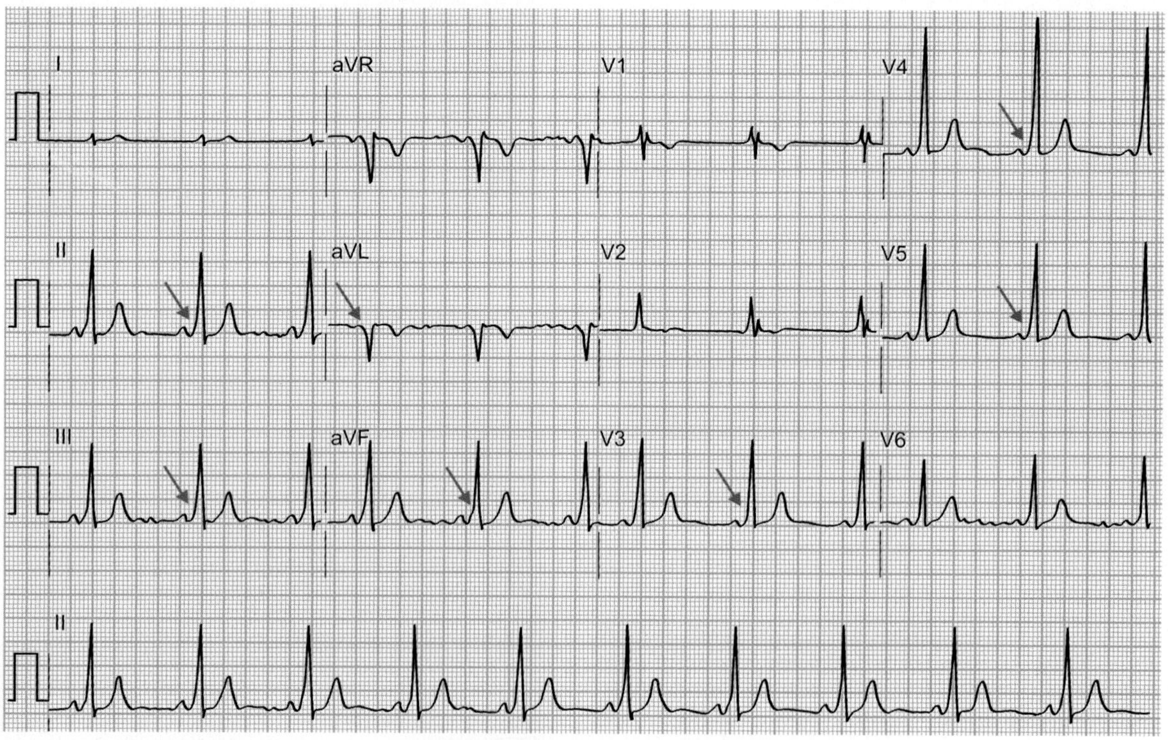


**Fig. 41.48:** ECG in WPW. PR interval <0.12 seconds, P-waves of normal appearance; QRS complex is wide, with a longer duration than 0.12 seconds. The presence of delta waves. Slow enrollment or thickening of the initial portion of the QRS complex (delta wave) is the most important criterion for diagnosis of Wolff-Parkinson-White syndrome. Delta wave length ranges between 0.02–0.07 seconds. Secondary changes of ST-segment and T-wave, which are showing a opposite direction from the QRS complex and delta wave

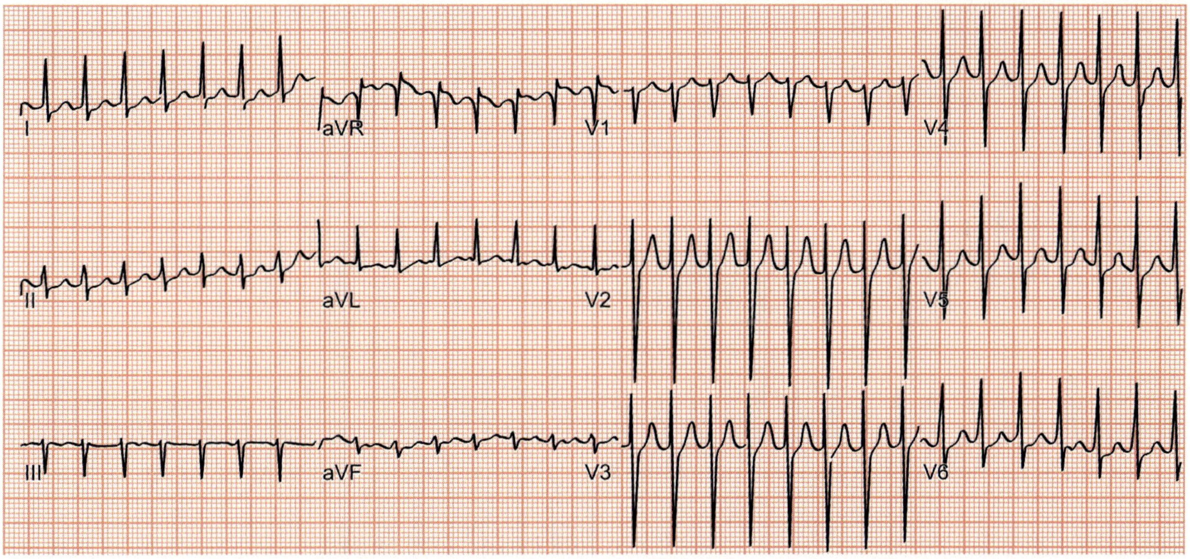


**Fig. 41.49:** ECG showing supraventricular tachycardia-AV nodal re-entry. AV nodal re-entry is a form of SVT that establishes its atrioventricular circuit entirely within the AV node. The heart rate is usually regular, between 150 bpm to 250 bpm (below=186 bpm). The QRS complex is narrow with a duration less than 0.2 seconds and a conduction ratio of 1:1. P-waves are buried within the QRS complex although they may be visible at the end of the complex as a distortion of the terminal forces. Due to the fact that atrial activation originates from the inferior aspect of the right atrium. P-wave polarity is negative in leads II, III and aVF. This form of SVT is usually benign and is easily converted to sinus rhythm by vagal manoeuvres

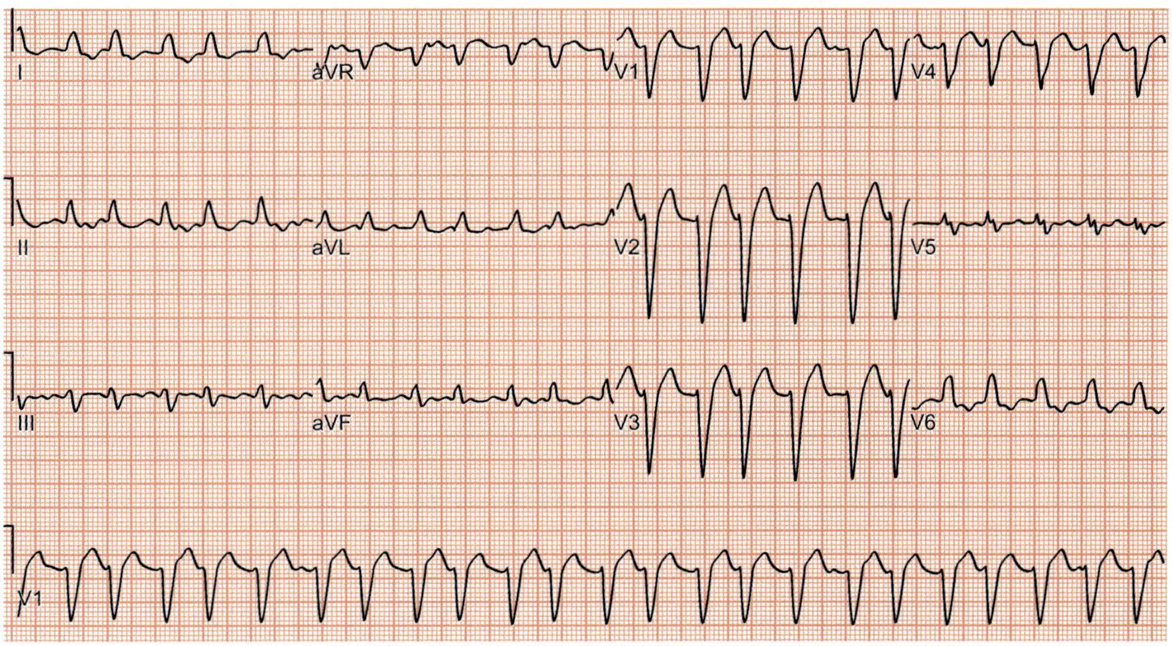


**Fig. 41.50:** ECG findings—supraventricular tachycardia with aberrancy

decreases the risk for long-term damage to the veins of the leg and arm, i.e. the post-thrombotic syndrome.

## Sudden Cardiac Arrest in Young Athletes

Each year between 10–12 million kids in the United States. participate in sports. The tragedy of a sudden death in an otherwise 'presumably healthy' child causes not only sadness, but concern as to how the death might have been prevented. Doctors are often asked, 'is not there a test or something to prevent this'? Depending on the studies I have read, the sudden cardiac death of a child or adolescent accounts for about 100 deaths a year in the United States. The prevalence rate for sudden cardiac death is 1:100,000–200,000 and is higher among males than females. Statistics show that 90% of these sudden deaths occur immediately post-training or competition with football and basketball

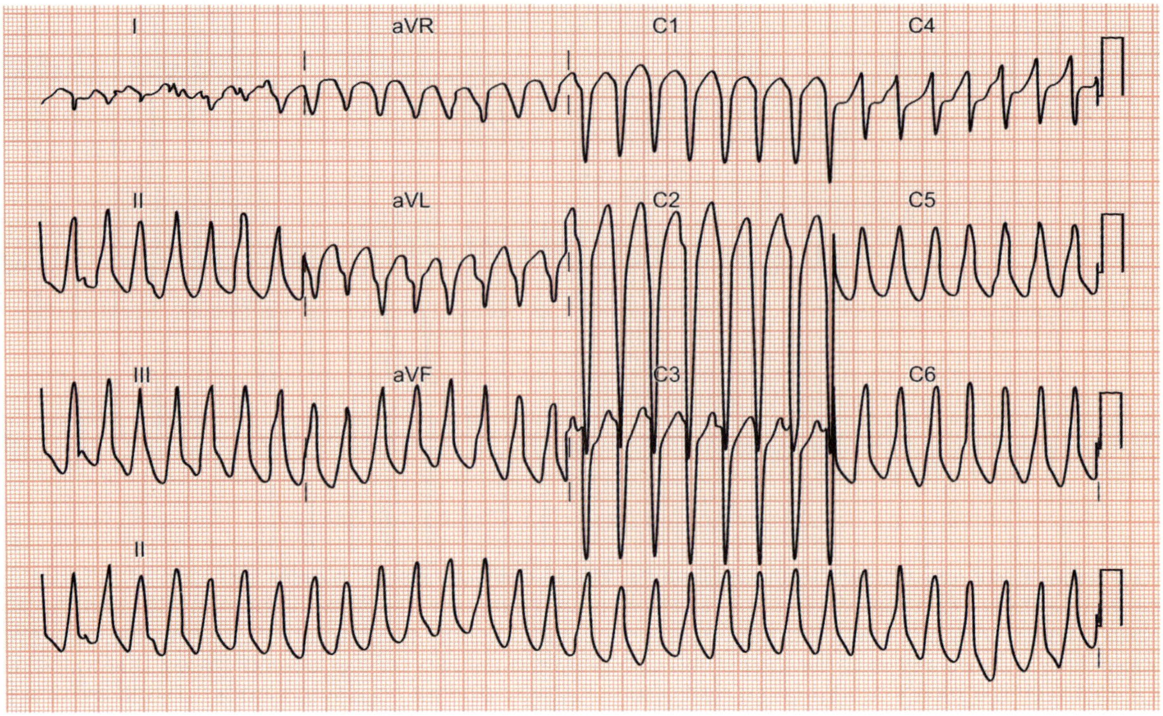


**Fig. 41.51:** Left-bundle branch block ventricular tachycardia with inferior axis (right ventricular outflow tract origin)

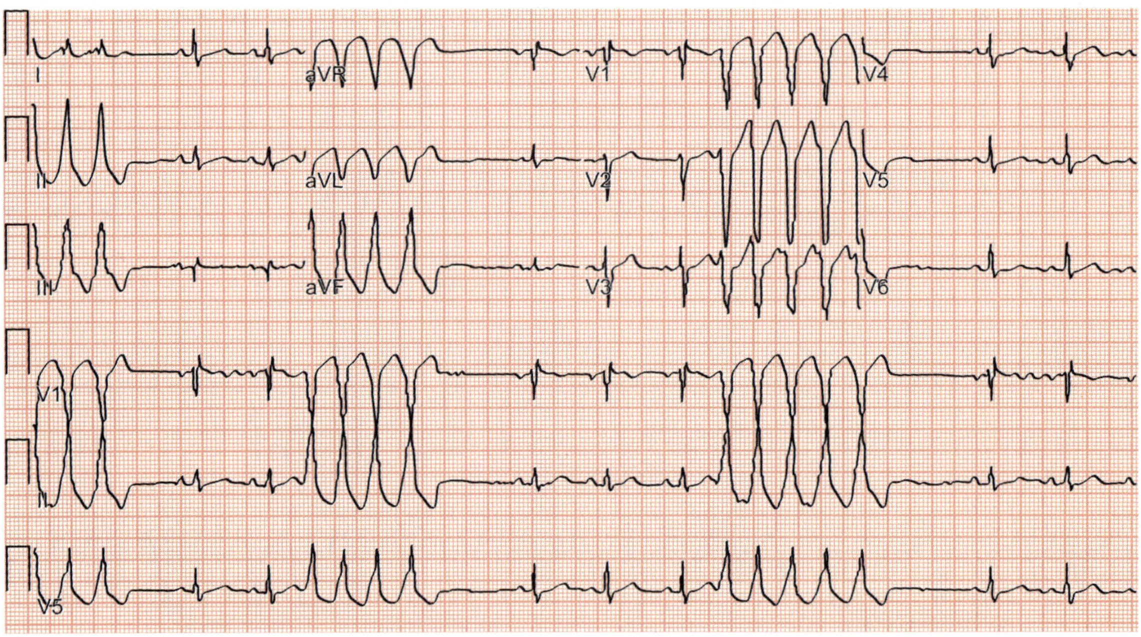


**Fig. 41.52:** ECG showing nonsustained monomorphic ventricular tachycardia

having the highest incidence. In 2007 the American Heart Association came out with guidelines to evaluate athletes who may be at risk for sudden cardiac death. The most important screening mechanism has been found to be the 'gold standard' in medicine, a thorough history and physical exam. The history that should be taken on any athlete who is being screened for sports participation should include a history of any unexplained or sudden death in a family member. Are there any family members with unexplained fainting episodes or seizures? Are there family members who had unexplained deaths (drowning or single car accidents)? Are there any family members with a known genetic disorder that predisposes to sudden cardiac death? The history should also ask about any fainting (syncope) in the athlete. After a good history is taken (which should be updated yearly), the child/

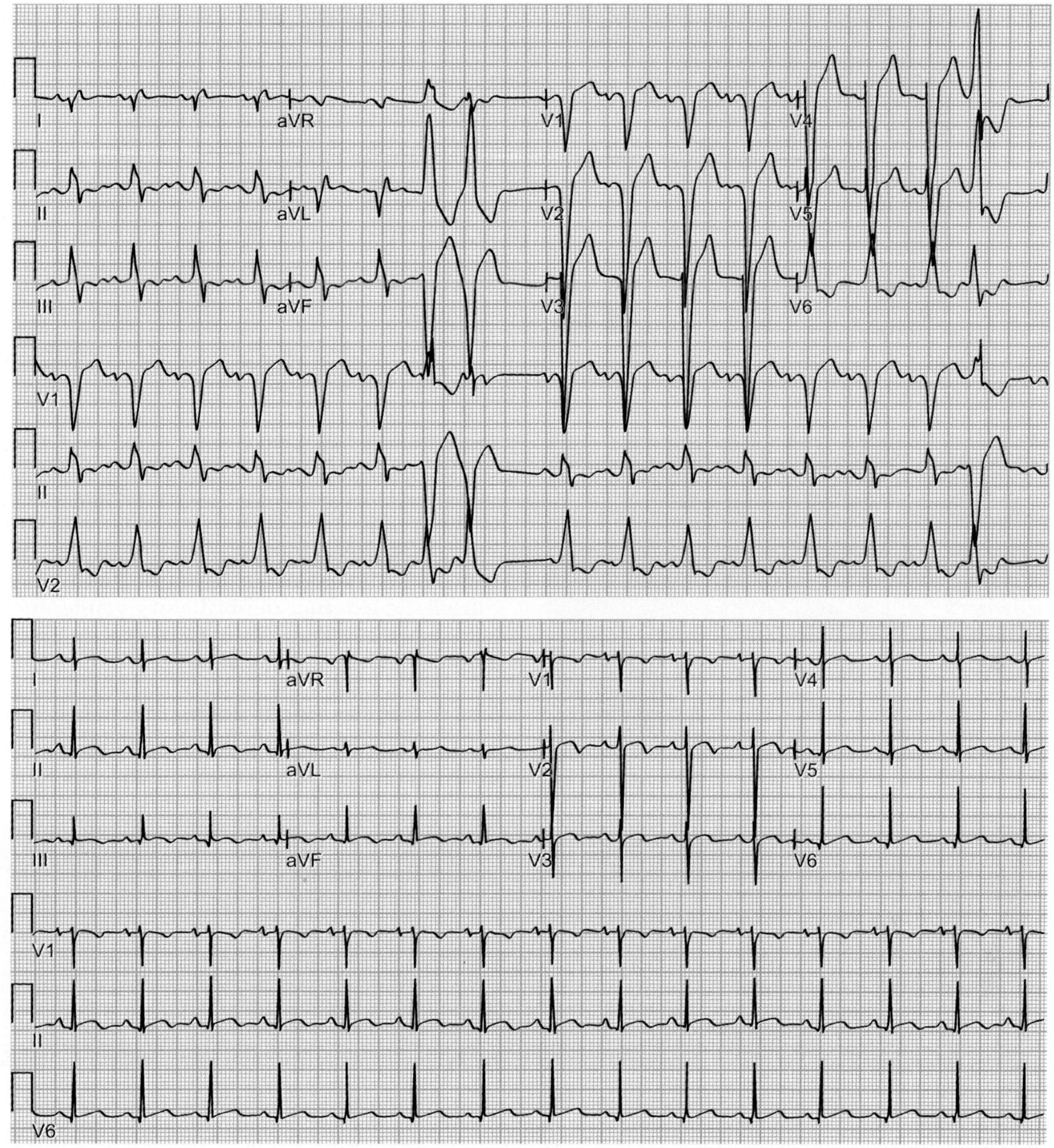


**Fig. 41.53:** 12-lead ECGs from a young black athlete with arrythmogenic cardiomyopathy. (A) Sinus tachycardia (rate about 101/min) with LBBB accompanied by RAD (here about 108°). Frequent multifocal PVCs (both singly and in pairs) and left atrial enlargement. (B) Same patient about 5 months later status—postorthotopic heart transplant

adolescent needs a complete and thorough physical exam. This exam should include blood pressure measurements, and a careful cardiac exam looking for new murmurs. Symptoms such as palpitations during exercise, visual changes, fainting while exercising or immediately after exercise, and chest pain should all warrant further evaluation. Studies show that about half of pediatric patients who succumb to sudden cardiac death had experienced a warning sign. There are about 20 causes for SCD, with the most common causes being hypertrophic cardiomyopathy, anomalous coronary artery, and myocarditis. While some may advocate routine EKG screening and echocardiograms on athletes (this is done in Italy), many studies have been done which show that it would take the screening of 200,000 student athletes to prevent 1 death. At the same time you will certainly identify some children with clear risk factors for SCD, but for every positive finding there may be 10–20 athletes who have 'borderline' or questionable findings that would require even more expensive follow up. These pediatric patients might also be told they cannot participate in sports during the evaluation time and some might be told that they cannot

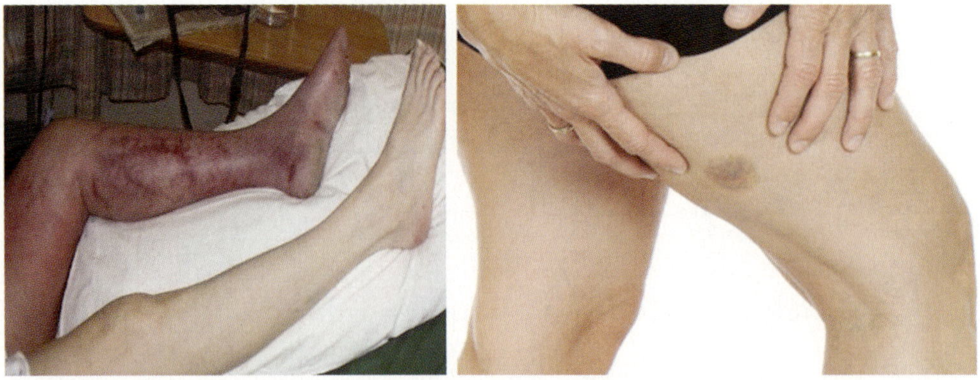

**Fig. 41.54:** Two athletes who developed venous thromboses after exhaustive competitive games

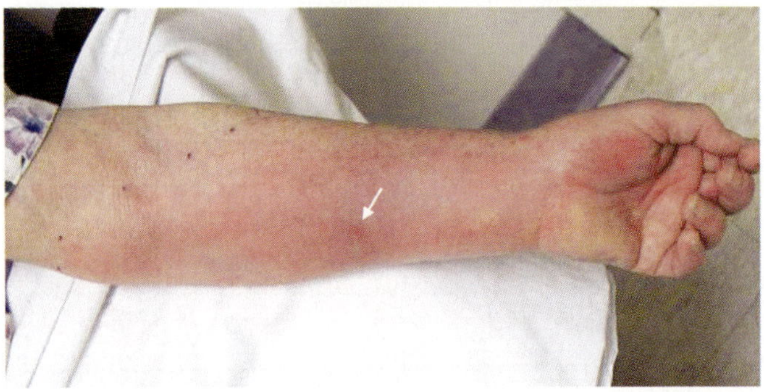

**Fig. 41.55:** An athlete who developed venous thromboses after extensive exercise

participate even if they were not found to have disease, but were excluded just due to liability concerns. There does not seem to be one right answer to this issue. If your child is going to begin competitive sports make sure to see your pediatrician for a complete physical exam including a good family history. Also advocate that your school have automatic external defibrillators viable at all times and personnel that know how to use them. That's your daily dose for today. We'll chat again tomorrow.

### Risk of Sudden Death during Sports Performance

Little is known about the risk of sudden death associated with exercise in young competitive athletes, and whether

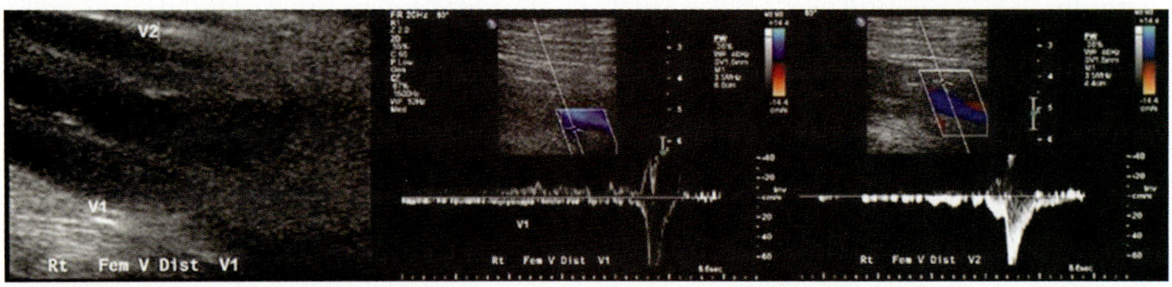


**Fig. 41.56:** The ultrasound image (left) shows the distal femoral vein, which is duplicated. The wave form in both branches is also shown

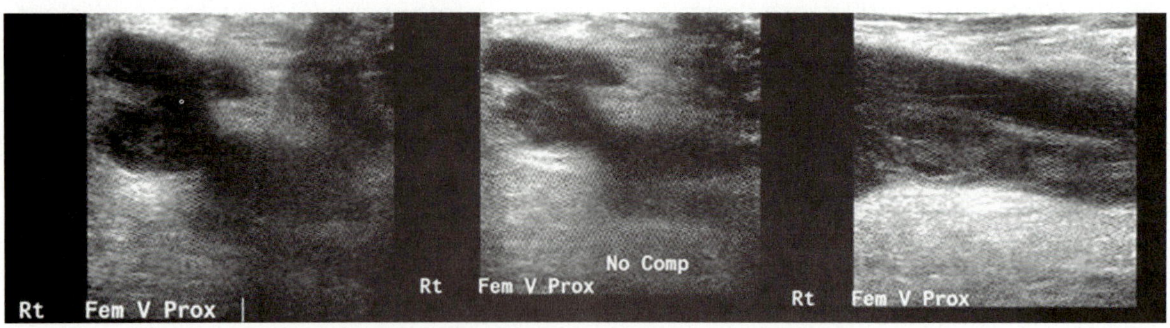


**Fig. 41.57:** These three views of the proximal femoral vein show the diameter of an occluding thrombus within the vessel. The middle image shows no compression of the vessel; the longitudinal image on the right shows the length of the thrombus. This clot extends into the profunda femoris and greater saphenous veins, as we shall see shortly. A clot this large can break away from the vessel wall becoming an embolus that may lodge in the pulmonary veins or go upward to occlude blood supply to the brain

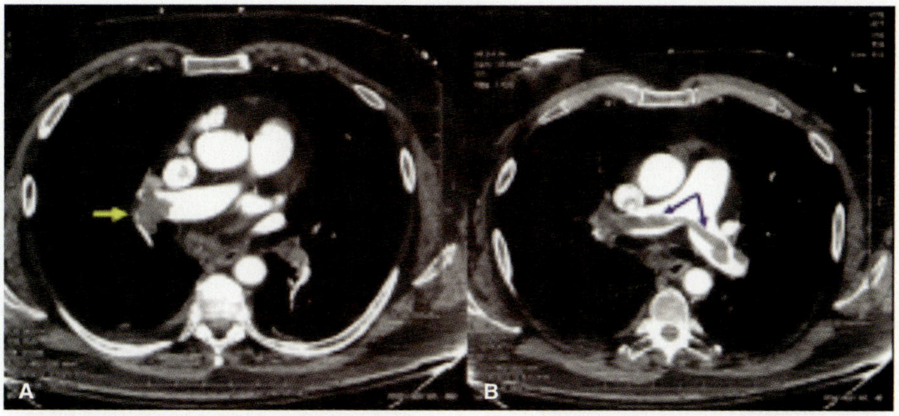


**Fig. 41.58:** These two axial CT images show profound pulmonary emboli. (A) The embolus almost completely blocks the right pulmonary artery (yellow arrow). (B) An extensive saddle embolus forming in both pulmonary arteries and becoming extensive. Both of these types of pulmonary emboli are life-threatening and require immediate medical attention

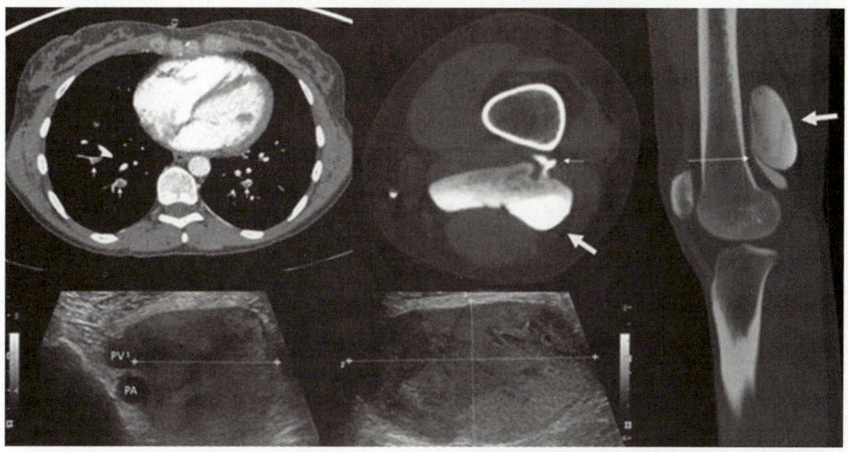

**Fig. 41.59:** Popliteal vein aneurysm presenting as recurrent pulmonary embolism

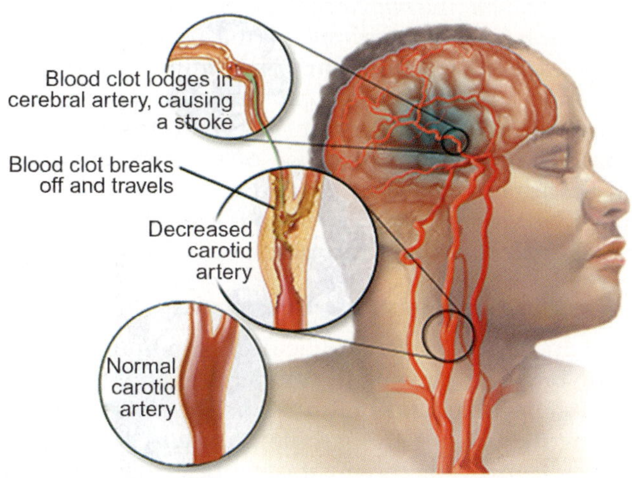


**Fig. 41.60:** The pathogenesis of development of cerebral stroke in an athlete

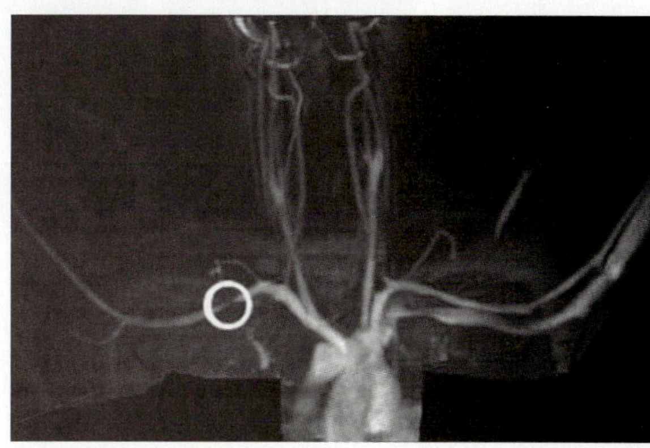

**Fig. 41.61:** MRI scan of the thoracic outlet showing compression of the subclavian artery

the benefits of sports activity outweigh the hazards of exercise-related fatal events is a clinical dilemma. For the purpose of this consensus document, we consider young competitive athletic individuals who are aged 35 years or less and are engaged in a regular fashion in exercise training as well as participating in official athletic competitions. Competition is intended as an organized team or individual sport event, placing high premium on athletic excellence and achievement (Figs 41.65–41.76).

Characteristics of competitive athletes are their strong inclination to extend themselves physically to their limits and to improve performance. Recently, Corrado et al. assessed the incidence of sudden death in the athletic and

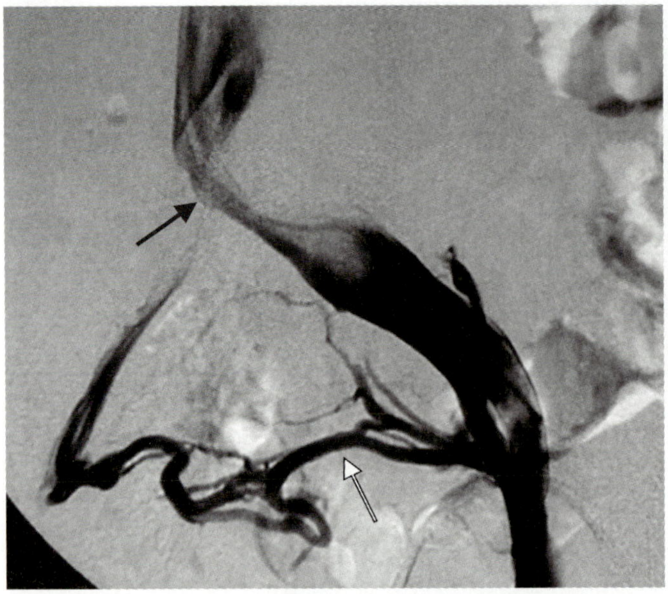

**Fig. 41.62:** Subtracted frontal venogram shows left iliac vein in May-Thurner syndrome. Note the compressed left common iliac vein (black arrow) and contralateral venous drainage via pelvic venous collaterals (white arrow)

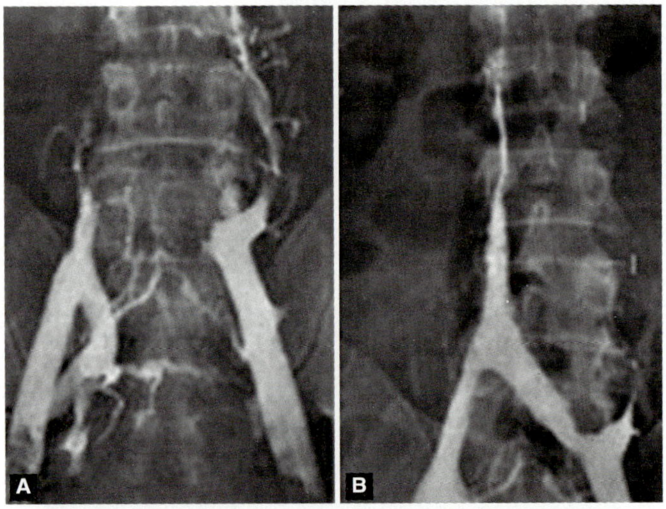


**Fig. 41.63:** (A) Occluded IVC and common iliac, (B) after urokinase infusion

nonathletic young population (12–35 years old) of the Veneto Region of Italy and showed that competitive sports activity enhances by 2.5-fold the risk of sudden death in adolescents and young adults. In this study, young competitive athletes who died suddenly were affected by silent cardiovascular diseases, predominantly consisting of cardiomyopathies, premature coronary artery disease, and congenital coronary anomalies. Therefore, sports activity was not per se a cause of the increased mortality; rather, it acted as a trigger of cardiac arrest upon those underlying cardiovascular diseases predisposing to life-threatening ventricular arrhythmias. Thus, it seems ethically and clinically justifiable that every effort should

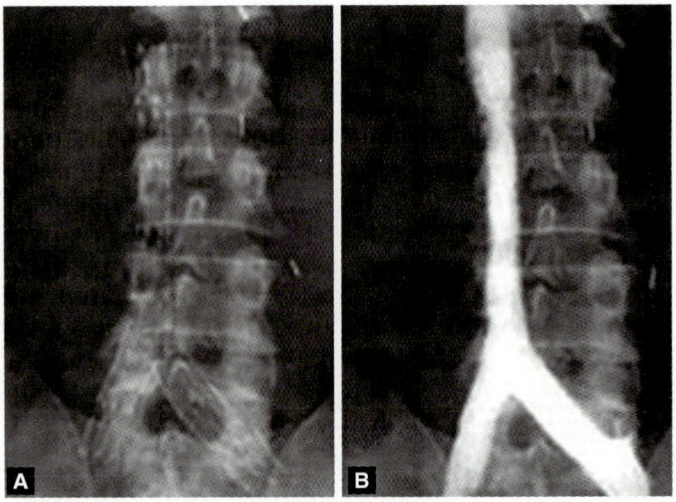


**Fig. 41.64:** (A) After stent placement, (B) 5-month follow up venogram

be made to recognize in good time such diseases that the athlete is at risk, with the perspective that disqualification of affected individuals makes the prevention of athletic field death possible.

A variety of cardiovascular diseases have been identified as potential causes of sudden death in young competitive athletes (<35 years old). The vast majority of these deaths occur on the athletic field during severe exertion in the context of training or competition. Each of the responsible diseases is also known to cause sudden death in nonathletes.

### Hypertrophic Obstructive Cardiomyopathy

Hypertrophic cardiomyopathy (HCM) is a primary disease of the *myocardium* (the *muscle* of the *heart*) in which a portion of the myocardium is *hypertrophied* (thickened) without any obvious cause, creating functional impairment of the cardiac muscle. It is a leading cause of *sudden cardiac death* in young athletes. The occurrence of hypertrophic cardiomyopathy is a significant cause of sudden unexpected cardiac death in any age group and as a cause of disabling cardiac symptoms. Younger people are likely to have a more severe form of hypertrophic cardiomyopathy.

### Congenital Coronary Artery Anomalies

Sudden and unexpected cardiac deaths in young subjects are rare, but tragic events in competitive athletes assume high public profile, and that unavoidably raise questions regarding the underlying pathological causes and clinical strategies to prevent these catastrophes. Various pathological investigations have reported that several structural cardiovascular abnormalities are responsible for sudden death in young athletes, but hypertrophic cardiomyopathy is the most common disease in US autopsy-based series, and right ventricular cardiomyopathy predominates in young Italian athletes. Nevertheless, congenital coronary artery anomalies (CCAA) are frequently found (in about 20% of cases), and they represent the second most frequent

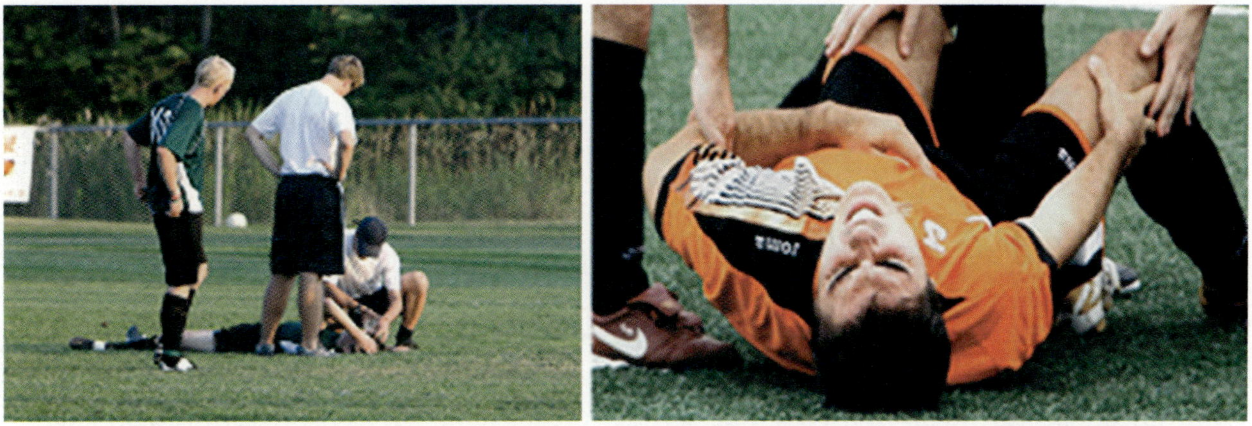

**Fig. 41.65:** Photographs showing unconscious athletes in the ground with resuscitative ground staff

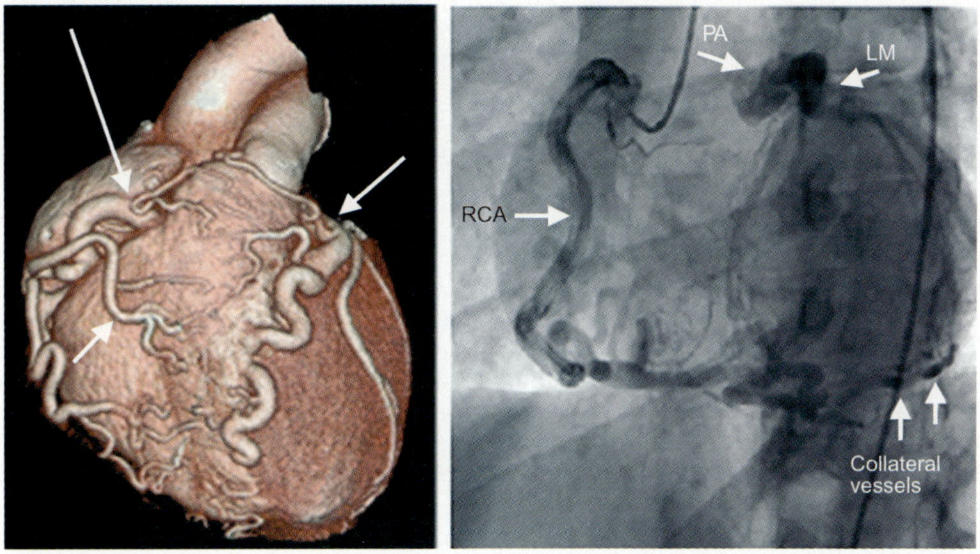


**Fig. 41.66:** Cronary artery anomalies. (A) Three-dimensional volume-rendered multidetector CT angiogram shows dilated intercoronary collateral arteries (arrowheads), which connect the tortuous RCA (long arrow) to the LCA (short arrow). (B) Cine-coronary angiography of the right coronary artery with collateral filling of the left coronary vascular territory, which connects directly to the pulmonary trunk

disease responsible for athletic field deaths. Specifically, the wrong sinus coronary artery origin, that is, the left main artery arising from the right anterior sinus (ALMCA), and the right coronary artery originating from the left sinus (ARCA), with a proximal course between aorta and pulmonary trunk, are the most frequent occurrences of CCAA.

### Myocarditis

Myocarditis is the reason for sudden cardiac death in 5–22% of athletes <35 years of age. Actually, parvovirus B19 and human herpes virus 6 are the most important pathogens. Clinical presentation of myocarditis is heterogeneous, with all courses between asymptomatic and fulminant reported. Especially in athletes it is important to take subtle discomforts seriously and initiate further evaluation. Electrocardiogram, laboratory parameters, serologic markers, and echocardiography are helpful in diagnosis of myocarditis, but are not specific. Magnetic resonance imaging (MRI) of the heart has become an important tool in the evaluation of patients with myocarditis and allows noninvasive appraisal of myocardial inflammation using late enhancement. However, MRI is not able to assess viral persistence. Therefore, endomyocardial biopsy (EMB) remains the gold standard in diagnosis of myocarditis. When considering EMB in these athletes one should not ignore spontaneous healing in 50% of patients with myocarditis. Contrariwise, specific therapy (e.g. immunosuppression, interferon and immunoglobulins) for myocarditis is only feasible after getting results of EMB. When myocarditis is verified, athletes have to withdraw from sport for at least 6 months. Before restarting physical activity, a detailed examination is necessary and most of the patients will undergo another EMB. For prevention of myocarditis and sudden cardiac death it is recommended to stop elite sport for 4 weeks

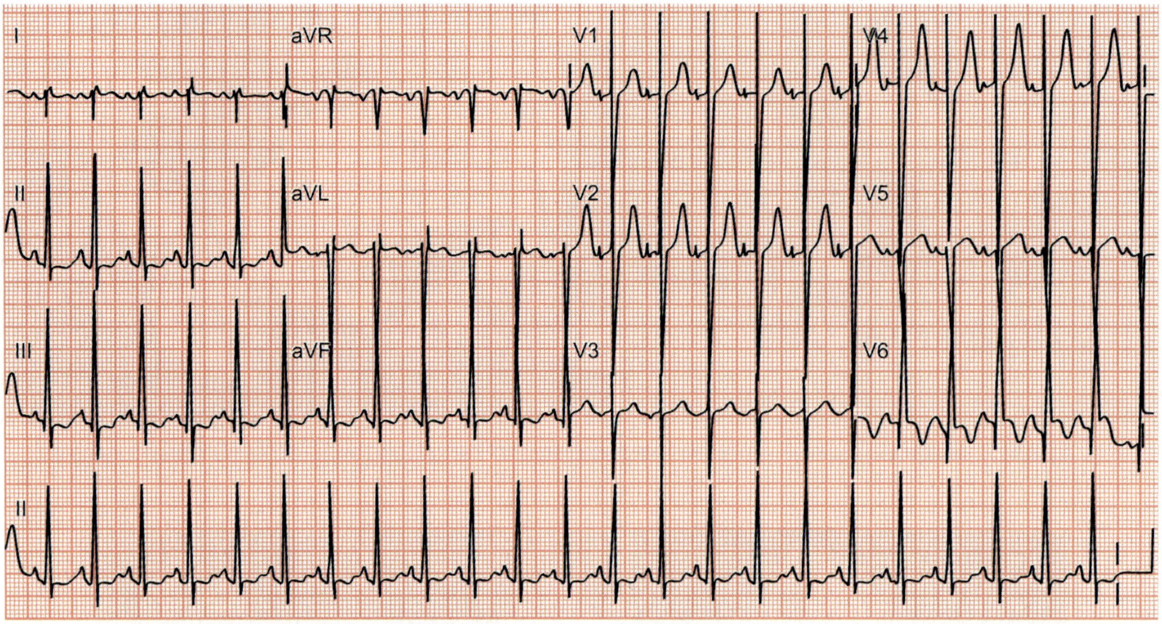


**Fig. 41.67:** ECG presentation in patient with ALCAPA. Typical prominent Q-waves are present in lead V6. Conversely, typical abrupt loss of R-waves in midprecordial leads and prominent Q-waves in leads I and aVL associated with ALCAPA are not present

after an unspecific infection. Whether moderate sport can be started earlier is unclear.

### Dilated Cardiomyopathy

In an important minority of athletes, the increase in left ventricular diastolic cavity dimension that occurs with training overlaps with that characteristic of certain known pathological entities. For example, while left ventricular end-diastolic cavity dimension in athletes is usually in the range of 53–58 mm, in some individuals it may extend into what may be regarded as the pathological range of >58 mm and thereby resemble dilated cardiomyopathy. However, the absence of left ventricular systolic dysfunction is usually sufficient to distinguish this physiological ventricular enlargement induced by training from that due to dilated cardiomyopathy.

### Marfan Syndrome

Marfan syndrome is an autosomal dominant genetic disease with variable penetrance, mostly caused by a mutation in the fibrillin-1 gene on chromosome 15. It has an increased risk for sudden death due to aortic dissection. It is characterized clinically by a diverse constellation of abnormalities variable in severity and involving primarily the ocular, skeletal, and cardiovascular organ systems.

The disease has an estimated incidence of 1 in 5000–7000 and has been shown to be more common in taller athletes such as basketball and volleyball players because tallness is one of the phenotypic expressions of the syndrome. Diagnosis is made according to the Ghent nosology if major criteria are present in two organ systems and a third is involved, or when there is a family history of Marfan syndrome. Skeletal abnormalities include arm span to

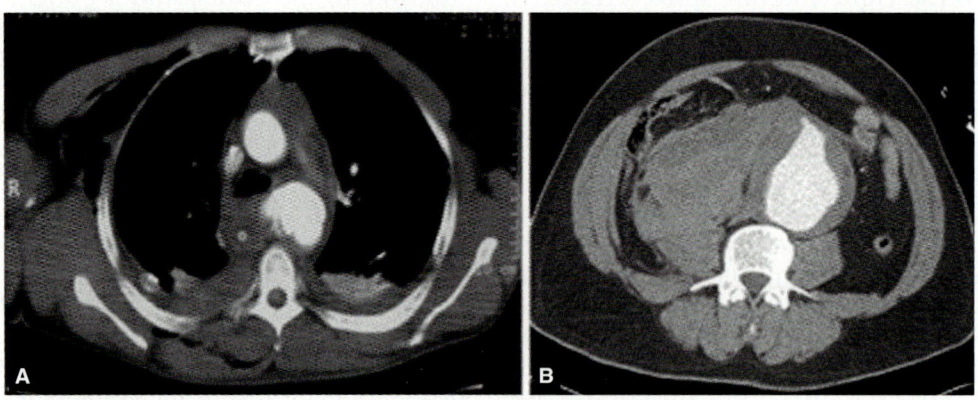


**Fig. 41.68:** (A) Axial source image of CT angiography showing traumatic aortic dissection. (B) Axial source image of CT angiography showing ruptured ascending aorta

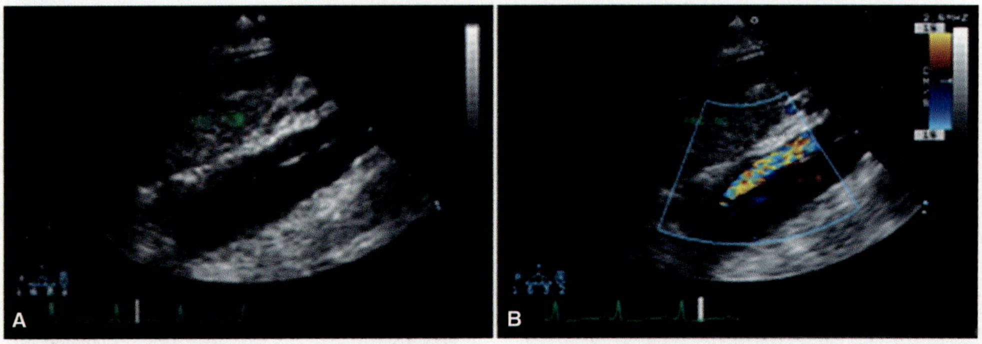


**Fig. 41.69:** Marfan syndrome in an athlete. An echocardiogram displaying the true lumen and false lumen of an aortic dissection. In the image (A), the intimal flap can be seen separating the two lumens. In the image (B) color flow during ventricular systole suggests that the upper lumen is the true lumen

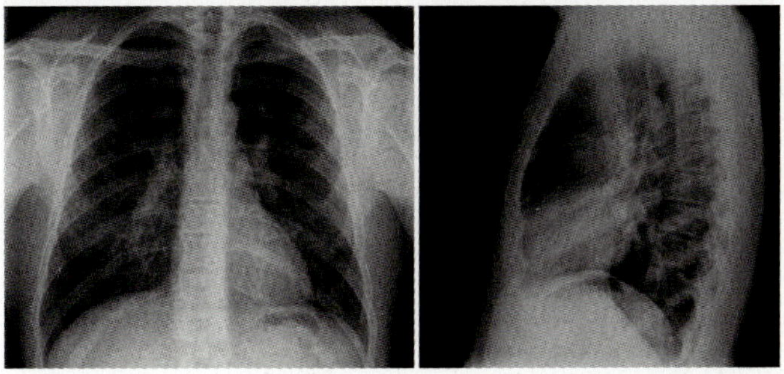

**Fig. 41.70:** The pictures of the chest by X-ray exam in two different visualizations show the pulmonary involvement showing Hilar lymphadenopathy in sarcoidosis in one of the competitive athletes

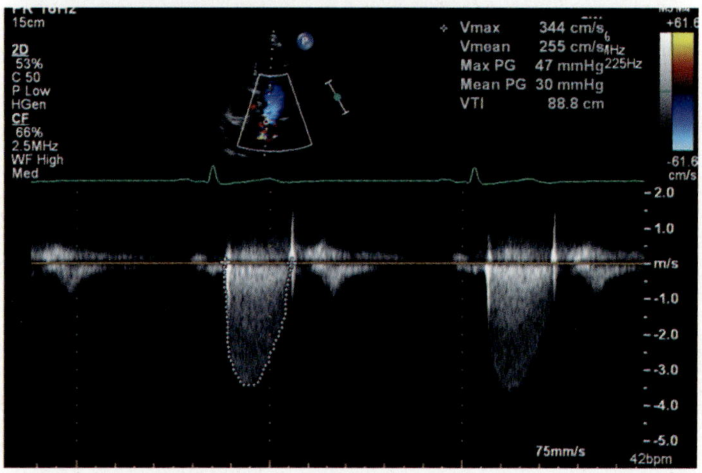


**Fig. 41.71:** Echo-Doppler study showing increase in gradient of the athletes in aortic valvular stenosis

height ratio greater than 1.05, tall stature, arachnodactyly, hyperextensibility and ligamentous laxity, scoliosis, and chest wall deformity (pectus excavatum or carinatum), in addition to ectopia lentis (lens dislocation).

Cardiovascular manifestations that impact on prognosis consist of progressive dilatation of the aortic root or descending aorta which are predisposed to dissection and rupture; and mitral valve prolapse with associated mitral regurgitation or LV systolic dysfunction, which may occasionally be predisposed to ventricular tachyarrhythmias and sudden death.

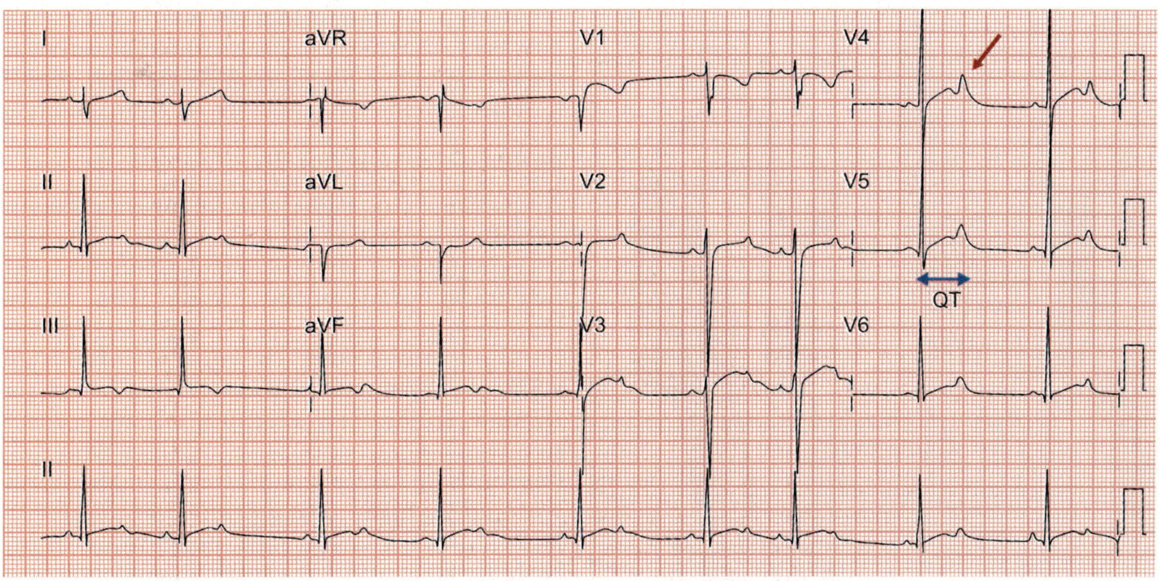


**Fig. 41.72:** ECG of an 18-year-old tennis player demonstrating a prolonged QT interval (>500 msec) with T-wave notching (arrow)

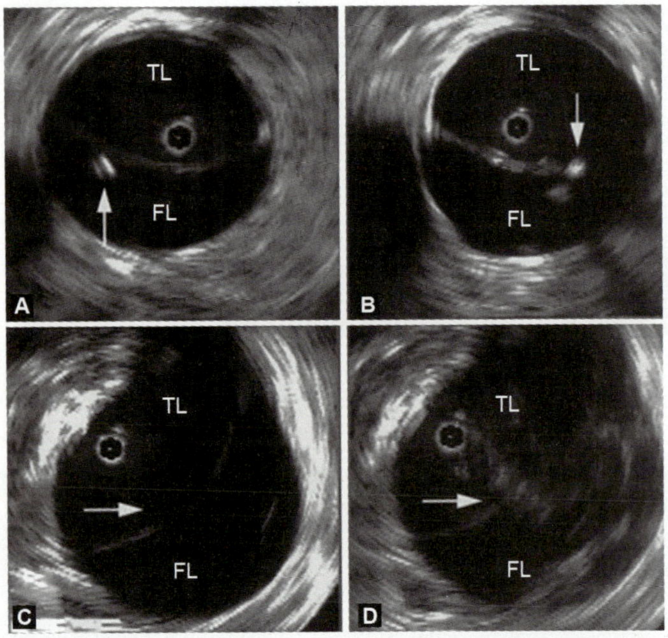


**Fig. 41.73:** IVUS imaging during procedure in aortic dissection. (A) Tip of needle positioned against membrane before membrane was punctured (arrow). (B) Needle lying across membrane after puncture (arrow). (C) After fenestration, opening created in membrane is well visualized (arrow), (D) Satisfactory flow of contrast from one lumen into other (arrow). TL=true lumen; FL=false lumen

Echocardiography can be used to measure and monitor the degree of aortic root dilation. The risk for aortic rupture is usually linked to marked enlargement of the aorta (transverse dimension greater than 50 mm). However, dissection can also occur with a normal (or near-normal) aortic root dimension. Weightlifting has been specifically associated with aortic dissection in athletes. The incidence of aortic dissection appears to decrease with earlier prophylactic surgical aortic root reconstruction and beta-blocker therapy.

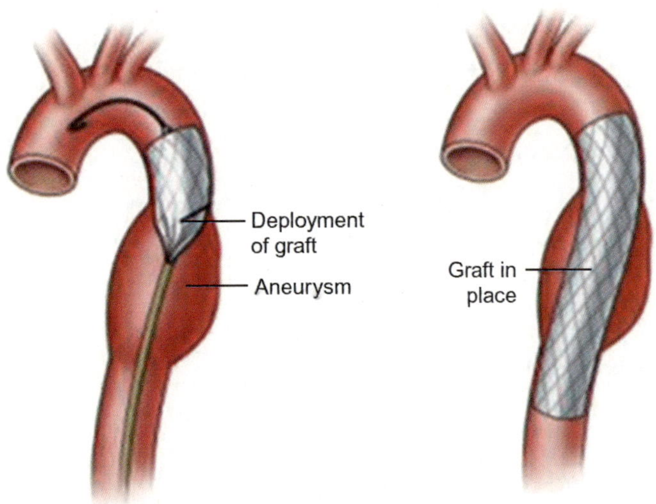


**Fig. 41.74:** Surgical repair in an athlete with Marfan syndrome

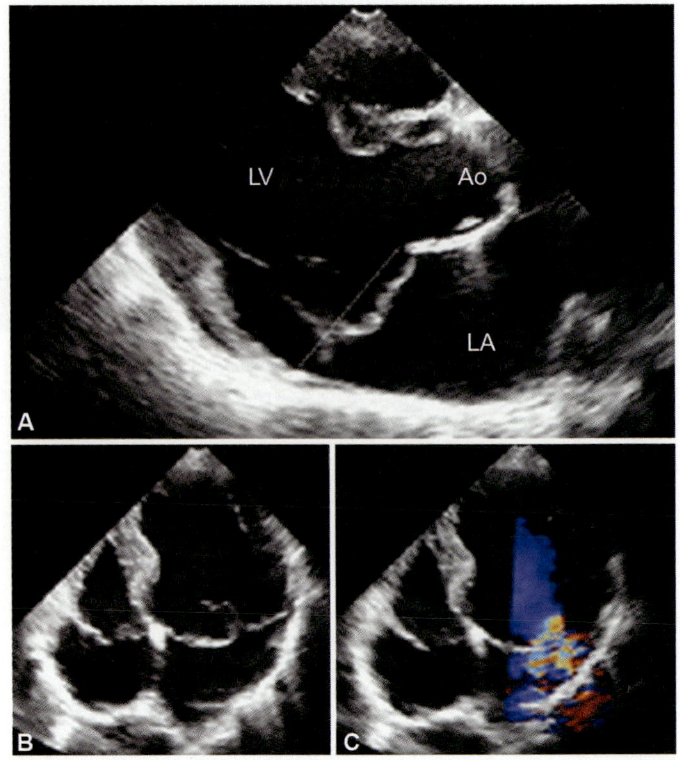


**Fig. 41.75:** Mitral valve prolapse. (A) Echocardiographic parasternal long-axis view showing the mitral leaflets prolapsing more than 2 mm above the plane of the mitral annulus (dotted line) during systole in a child with Marfan syndrome. (B) Echocardiographic apical four-chamber view showing bileaflet prolapse in the same patient. (C) Color-Doppler view showing moderate mitral regurgitation (Ao=aorta; LA=left atrium; LV=left ventricle)

Athletes with Marfan syndrome can participate in low and moderate static/low dynamic competitive sports if they do not have any of the aortic root dilatation or moderate-to-severe mitral regurgitation or family history of dissection or sudden death in a Marfan relative. It is recommended, however, that these athletes have an echocardiographic measurement of aortic root dimension repeated every 6 months for close surveillance of aortic enlargement.

### *Right Ventricular Dysplasia (in One Series)*

Arrhythmogenic right ventricular dysplasia (ARVD) is a cardiomyopathy with several time-dependent clinical presentations. The clinical characteristics depend on the penetration grade of the disease. There are two different histological patterns consisting of a lipomatous and a fibrolipomatous form. The presence of arrhythmias in the ARVD syndrome constitutes an important risk factor for sudden cardiac death in athletes. In this article, we describe two professional endurance athletes who died suddenly. One of these athletes had asymptomatic ARVD, the other had symptomatic polymorphic ventricular tachycardias. Both athletes showed fatty penetration of the disease in both the right and left ventricle; one of them also showed fatty involvement at the atrial level and in the other there

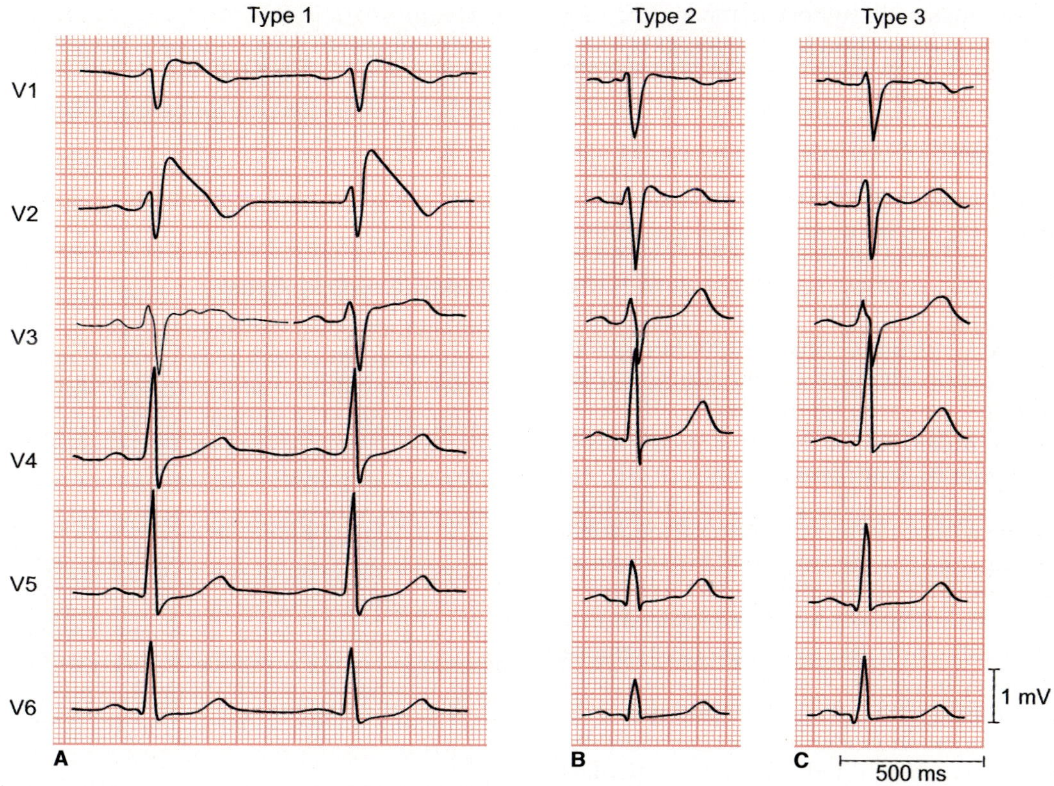


**Fig. 41.76:** Three types of ST-segment elevation in Brugada syndrome, as shown in the precordial leads on ECG in the same patient at different times. (A) Shows a type 1 ECG pattern with pronounced elevation of the J point (arrow), a coved-type ST-segment, and an inverted T-wave in V1 and V2. (B) Illustrates a type 2 pattern with a saddleback ST-segment elevated by >1 mm. (C) Shows a type 3 pattern in which the ST-segment is elevated and It; 1 mm. According to a consensus report (Antzelevitch, 2005), the type 1 ECG pattern is diagnostic of Brugada syndrome. Modified from Wilde, 2002

were signs of myocarditis consistent with ARVD. In the last few years magnetic resonance imaging has become an important diagnostic tool in patients with ARVD.

### Cardiac Sarcoidosis

Sarcoidosis is a multisystem granulomatous disorder of unknown aetiology, characterized by 'noncaseating granulomas' in different organs. Clinical signs are variable and dependent on the organ involved. Although it is often asymptomatic in athletes, considering the high level of athletic performance and the related risks due to the potential heart involvement, a particular diagnostic flow-chart to consider some other diagnoses is required.

### Aortic Valve Stenosis

In patients with aortic stenosis (AS), sudden death remains a particular concern. The following hypothesis have been proposed to explain the mechanism of sudden death in aortic stenosis. (1) An abnormal Betzold-Jarisch reflex (stimulation of left ventricular baroreceptors may lead to arterial hypotension, a fall in venous return and consequent bradycardia). (2) Ventricular tachyarrhythmias (inappropriate hypotension and a low cardiac output provoke coronary hypoperfusion, in patients who already have a predisposition through left ventricular hypertrophy). (3) Atrioventricular conduction disturbances [there is a contiguity between valvular-perivalvular calcification and the His-Purkinje system (there is also a high prevalence of conduction abnormalities in patients with AS)].

### QT-interval Prolongation Syndromes

Numerous conditions are associated with SCD; the focus for this article is the long QT syndrome (LQTS)—a disorder of the heart's electrical system. The prolonged Q-T interval that can be detected via an electrocardiograph (ECG). This prolonged Q-T interval represents the slower than normal passing of the electrical signal through the ventricles of the heart. This congenital syndrome is often asymptomatic. In some cases people with LQTS experience unexplained faints, seizures, or arrhythmias. Sudden death can be the first clinical manifestation. According to Pugh et al. (2011), genetic testing is available for people with prolonged QT on ECG and those with a family history of SCD. This test is particularly useful for patients who do not exhibit any of the symptoms that are typically associated with the condition. The diagnosis of LQTS should be considered for any athlete with a history of losing consciousness.

### Acute Aortic Dissection

Acute aortic dissection can occur at the time of intense physical exertion in strength-trained athletes like weight-lifters, bodybuilders, throwers, and wrestlers. Rapid rise in blood pressure and history of hypertension are the most common causes of aortic dissection in athletes. It is a very tragic event because of its high mortality rate of about 32% in young patients.

### Mitral Valve Prolapse

Mitral valve prolapse is probably the most common cardiac valve disorder, affecting approximately 5% of the population. Although it is genetically determined, its clinical manifestations do not usually become evident before adulthood. In the setting of a cardiology referral center, a mitral valve prolapse syndrome, consisting of nonspecific symptoms, repolarization changes on the electrocardiogram and arrhythmias, has been identified.

The prognosis of mitral valve prolapse is generally favorable but infrequent complications do occur and include transient ischemic attacks, progression of mitral regurgitation with or without ruptured chordae tendineae, infective endocarditis and sudden death. The symptoms and the complications are not usually related to physical activity. A permissive attitude toward participation of patients with mitral valve prolapse in competitive athletics is probably warranted; however, it would appear reasonable to disqualify athletes with mitral valve prolapse in the following circumstances—history of syncope; disabling chest pain; complex ventricular arrhythmias, particularly if induced or worsened by exercise; significant mitral regurgitation; prolonged QT interval; Marfan syndrome; and family history of sudden death.

### Brugada Syndrome

Brugada syndrome is a genetic disease resulting in a characteristic abnormal EKG pattern and increased risk of SCD. Arrhythmic events generally occur in early to mid-adulthood (22–45 years of age), are more likely at night, and men are more likely to be affected. Current treatment relies upon the implantable cardioverter-defibrillator (ICD), which can detect and correct an abnormal and potentially lethal heart rhythm. There has been a great deal of progress in recent years identifying the genetic causes of Brugada syndrome, with as many as 8 specific genes identified. Genetic screening is available for families with a history of Brugada syndrome, and can help identify individuals who are at risk for SCD, and those who are not at risk

## MANAGEMENT OF CARDIOVASCULAR EMERGENCIES (Fig. 41.77)

### Sudden Cardiac Arrest

Management of a cardiac emergency begins with prompt recognition, an accurate assessment and in uncertain cases the implementation of response protocols based on proper assumptions. SCA should be suspected in all cases of non-traumatic collapse, and in all cases in which an athlete is collapsed and unresponsive. There are a number of potential pitfalls when evaluating a collapsed athlete that may result in delayed recognition of SCA and resultant critical delays in resuscitation. Agonal breathing and occasional gasping often occur within the first minutes after SCA and can be misinterpreted as normal respirations. Accurate assessment of the presence or absence of a pulse in the emergency setting is also challenging and studies demonstrate that healthcare providers correctly diagnose pulselessness as little as 50% of the time. As a result, the 2010 American Heart Association and international guidelines for CPR recommend that healthcare providers spend no more than 10s assessing for a definitive pulse, and that lay responders not check for a pulse at all. In addition, brief myoclonic or seizure-like activity occurs in approximately half of young athletes with SCA. Thus, SCA must be assumed in any athlete with seizure-like activity until cardiac arrest is effectively ruled out.

In cases of presumed or confirmed SCA, key steps in management must occur rapidly, and often simultaneously. These include:

1. **Calling for help** and activating the local emergency medical response system

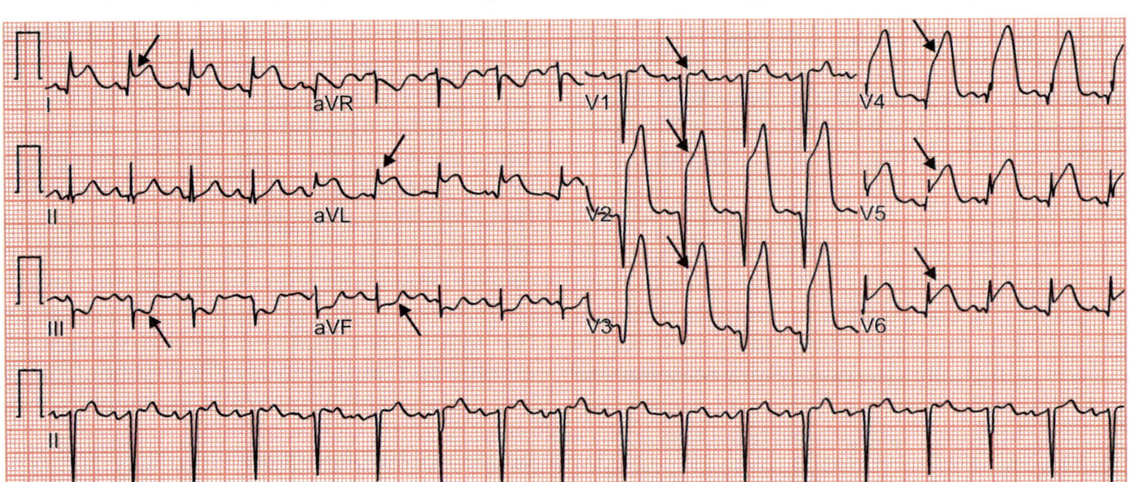


**Fig. 41.77:** ECG trace showing ST-segment elevation leads 1, AVL, V1–V6 and reciprocal changes in leads II, II and AVF in acute coronary syndrome (arrows)

2. **Beginning CPR with chest compressions**
3. **Retrieving and applying a defibrillator (if available)** for rhythm analysis and shock deployment (if indicated) as soon as possible. Most cases of SCA in the athletic setting are witnessed and involve more than one rescuer. Thus, one rescuer can perform CPR while another retrieves the AED if not already present.

**Recent CPR guidelines changed the basic life support sequence from 'A-B-C'** (airway, breathing and chest compressions) to 'C-A-B' (chest compressions, airway and breathing). In the A-B-C sequence, chest compressions are often delayed while the responder opens the airway to give mouth-to-mouth breaths or retrieves a barrier device or other ventilation equipment. By changing the sequence to C-A-B, chest compressions will be initiated sooner and may ensure that more victims receive chest compressions by rescuers unable or unwilling to provide ventilations. Hands-only (compression only) CPR is encouraged for the untrained lay rescuer and appears to achieve outcomes similar to those of conventional CPR (compressions with rescue breathing). Adequate chest compressions include a rate of 100/min with a depth of at least 2 inches, complete recoil of the chest in between compressions and minimisation of any pauses in compressions.

**Chest compressions** should be resumed immediately after shock delivery. Many victims will have pulseless electric activity or asystole after defibrillation. Thus, CPR is needed to provide perfusion to the myocardium during this critical period to decrease recurrent ventricular arrhythmias. Minimising the interval between stopping chest compressions and delivering a shock (i.e. the preshock pause) also improves the chance of shock success and patient survival. Resuscitative measures should be continued until the victim becomes responsive or a noncardiac cause of collapse is clearly identified.

### Acute Coronary Syndromes

Acute coronary syndrome (ACS) should be suspected in any athlete presenting with chest pain. Knowledge of an athlete's medical history and risk factors for coronary artery disease is helpful to guide management. Some symptoms attributed to ACS, such as diaphoresis, dyspnea, lightheadedness and nausea, may be more difficult to differentiate in the athletic setting. A focused assessment should include vital signs, heart and lung auscultation, and chest wall palpation as reproducible pain with palpation decreases the likelihood of ACS. When there is clinical suspicion for ACS, the athlete should be immediately removed from play, seated or laid supine and the local emergency medical system activated.

**Treatment** in hemodynamically stable patients includes aspirin 162–325 mg chewed and nitroglycerin 0.4 mg sublingual every 5 min up to three doses as needed for chest pain. If an AED is available, it should be retrieved as acute ischemia increases the risk of ventricular arrhythmias and SCA. New guidelines do not recommend routine use of oral beta-blockers and supplemental oxygen in the absence of hypoxia due to lack of evidence that shows a survival benefit. Patients with ACS or SCA are ideally transferred to hospital facilities capable of advanced cardiac care and immediate percutaneous coronary intervention with angiography or bypass surgery if indicated.

### Prognosis

Although gross structural changes resemble those in some cardiac disorders, no adverse effects are apparent. In most cases, structural changes and bradycardia regress with detraining, although up to 20% of elite athletes have residual chamber enlargement, raising questions, in the absence of long-term data, about whether athlete's heart is truly benign.

### Athlete-specific Challenges and Questions

Most often, an active individual—be it an athlete or one who remains physically fit through routine training and exercise—is suddenly stymied by the affects of his/her clotting incident. Questions, lots of questions, are poised to the caregiver. Of paramount importance for the athlete are particularly the two following issues:

#### *Can I Continue My Sport While on Warfarin?*

A solid medical assessment should be made whether the person who has had a blood clot can come off warfarin or should remain on it. Being on warfarin increases the risk for bleeding. Therefore, contact sports and sports with a risk for serious injury, such as football, hockey, basketball, soccer, gymnastics, alpine skiing, or boxing should not be pursued by a person on warfarin. However, athletes such as runners, bicyclists or triathletes may be able to continue their sport, but they should adapt their activities to avoid trauma that might put them at risk for bleeding (avoid situations leading to bicycle crashes, etc.). Individual blood thinning treatment plans can also be designed, such as (a) a decrease in warfarin dosage a few days prior to athletic events that would otherwise put the person at increased risk for bleeding, (b) switching the athlete who should be on long-term blood thinners to low molecular weight heparin shots during the athletic season and interrupting the shots for competitions that pose a risk for bleeding, (c) stopping blood thinners during the season and accepting a higher risk for blood clots during that time, but restarting warfarin during the off season. Finally, an athlete may decide to switch from a high risk bleeding competitive sport to one with a lower risk. Obviously, these are all very individual treatment decisions that should be thoroughly discussed between the patient's personal physician, the patient, and the team physician (if the patient is participating in a team sport).

#### *How Soon After a DVT or PE Can I Go Back to Training?*

Patients with a DVT may have significant extremity swelling and pain which may improve only slowly over weeks and months. Some residual symptoms may persist long-term, this is termed 'postthrombotic syndrome.' It appears that being highly active one month after a DVT is not detrimental; it may, actually be beneficial and lead to less symptoms of post-thrombotic syndrome. This can be used as an argument to encourage individuals to return to physical activity relatively soon after a DVT. Also, wearing individually fitted compression stockings decreases the long-term risk for post-thrombotic syndrome.

No official guidelines exist as to when and how quickly an athlete might return to exercising. Each patient will need an individualized exercise plan. It seems appropriate to refrain from any athletic activities for the first 10–14 days after an acute DVT or PE until the clot is more adherent to the blood vessel wall and the risk of having the clot break loose (causing a PE) has decreased. To lessen deconditioning during this period of relative inactivity, the athlete may do some strength training—arm and trunk exercises in the case of a leg DVT, leg and trunk exercises in the case of an arm DVT. The athlete may then increase activity between week 2 and 4 and return to pre-clot activity levels by week 4.

### How to Minimize the Risk for Clots?

Measures that the athlete and, for that matter, the non-athlete should take to minimize the risk for DVT or PE are listed in Table 41.3. For the athlete the most important ones are probably to (a) avoid dehydration, and (b) take breaks when traveling long distances.

### Psychosocial Implications

Athletes need to appreciate that significant deconditioning can occur after a DVT or PE. Depression can also set in after such a life-changing event. This is not surprising, given that athletes often view themselves as healthy and, from a health point of view, invincible, and now suddenly realize that they are vulnerable, sick, and sometimes even disabled. Patient support groups may be helpful in this situation, as may antidepressants.

### Hypercoagulability in Athletes

Risk factors for thromboembolism are well known, and athletes are placed under conditions that can result in exposure to several of these risk factors, which include travel, trauma, immobilization, hemoconcentration, and polycythemia. Presence of a genetic hypercoagulable disorder adds additional risk. Overall management is no different than in nonathletes. Thrombolysis is strongly recommended for upper extremity deep venous thrombosis (DVT) coupled with surgical decompression of obstructive structures if indicated. Thrombolytic therapy does not appear to be necessary for treatment of lower extremity DVT. Prevention of DVT with travel can be achieved through general techniques such as leg exercises, hydration, and loose fitting clothes. Aspirin before travel shows some benefits of protection, but individuals at higher risk may need low molecular weight heparin. Athletes should be screened during preparticipation physicals for thromboembolic risk. Individuals on anticoagulation therapy should not participate in collision or contact sports. Return to play with gradual increase in intensity is recommended with careful monitoring for recurrent venous thromboembolism and management of post-thrombotic symptoms.

## KEY RECOMMENDATIONS IN ATHLETES

**Planning for cardiac emergencies in the athletic setting**

- Establish an emergency action plan for each venue.
- Identify anticipated first responders (coaches, officials, administrators and the medical team) and provide training in Sudden cardiac arrest (SCA) recognition, cardiopulmonary resuscitation (CPR) and automated external defibrillators (AED) use.
- Develop an internal communication system and a means to activate the local emergency response system.
- Install AEDs in strategic locations and equip key medical staff with portable AEDs as needed to ensure early access to defibrillation (within 3 min of collapse)
- Register AEDs with the local emergency medical system.
- Identify the person responsible for AED maintenance.
- Determine routes for emergency vehicles to easily access each athletic venue in case of a cardiac emergency.
- Practice and review the emergency action plan at least annually with all potential first responders.
- Consider acquiring additional emergency equipment and medications depending on the population at risk and the experience of the medical providers.
- Coordinate onsite ambulances and other mobile responders for certain high-risk events.

**Management of cardiac emergencies in the athletic setting**

- Promptly recognise a cardiac emergency by maintaining a high level of suspicion.
- Assume SCA in any collapsed and unresponsive athlete.
- Avoid misdiagnosis as a result of agonal breathing and/or seizure-like activity.
- Elicit help from people nearby.
- Activate the local emergency response system.
- Begin chest compressions, retrieve an AED and apply it as soon as possible for defibrillation (if indicated).
- Continue CPR, AED use and resuscitative efforts until the victim becomes responsive or care is transferred to an emergency facility capable of advanced cardiac life support.
- In a conscious athlete suspected of having an acute coronary syndrome, provide aspirin and nitroglycerin, activate the emergency response system and monitor closely.

## BIBLIOGRAPHY


1. Berg RA, Hemphill R, Abella BS, et al. Part 5: adult basic life support: 2010 American Heart Association Guidelines for Cardiopulmonary Resuscitation and Emergency Cardiovascular Care. Circulation 2010;122:S685–705.
2. Borjesson M, Dugmore D, Mellwig KP, et al. Time for action regarding cardiovascular emergency care at sports

arenas: a lesson from the Arena study. Eur Heart J 2010;31: 1438–41.

3. Borjesson M, Serratosa L, Carre F, et al. Consensus document regarding cardiovascular safety at sports arenas: position stand from the European Association of Cardiovascular Prevention and Rehabilitation (EACPR), section of Sports Cardiology. Eur Heart J 2011;32:2119–24.
4. Corrado D, Basso C, Rizzoli G, et al. Does sports activity enhance the risk of sudden death in adolescents and young adults? J Am Coll Cardiol 2003;42:1959–63.
5. Crocco TJ, Sayre MR, Liu T, et al. Mathematical determination of external defibrillators needed at mass gatherings. Prehosp Emerg Care 2004;8:292–7.
6. Dahabreh IJ, Paulus JK. Association of episodic physical and sexual activity with triggering of acute cardiac events: systematic review and meta-analysis. JAMA 2011;305:1225–33.
7. Drezner JA, Courson RW, Roberts WO, et al. Inter-association task force recommendations on emergency preparedness and management of sudden cardiac arrest in high school and college athletic programs: a consensus statement. J Athl Train 2007;42:143–58.
8. Drezner JA, Rao AL, Heistand J, et al. Effectiveness of emergency response planning for sudden cardiac arrest in United States high schools with automated external defibrillators. Circulation 2009;120:518–25.
9. Drezner JA, Rogers KJ. Sudden cardiac arrest in intercollegiate athletes: detailed analysis and outcomes of resuscitation in nine cases. Heart Rhythm 2006;3:755–9.
10. Drezner JA. Preparing for sudden cardiac arrest—the essential role of automated external defibrillators in athletic medicine: a critical review. Br J Sports Med 2009;43:702–7.
11. Eberle B, Dick WF, Schneider T, et al. Checking the carotid pulse check: diagnostic accuracy of first responders in patients with and without a pulse. Resuscitation 1996;33: 107–16.
12. Eckart RE, Scoville SL, Campbell CL, et al. Sudden death in young adults: a 25-year review of autopsies in military recruits. Ann Intern Med 2004;141:829–34.
13. Field JM, Hazinski MF, Sayre MR, et al. Part 1: executive summary: 2010 American Heart Association Guidelines for Cardiopulmonary Resuscitation and Emergency Cardiovascular Care. Circulation 2010;122:S640–656.
14. Harmon KG, Asif IM, Klossner D, et al. Incidence of sudden cardiac death in national collegiate athletic association athletes. Circulation 2011;123:1594–1600.
15. Hazinski MF, Markenson D, Neish S, et al. Response to cardiac arrest and selected life-threatening medical emergencies: the medical emergency response plan for schools—a statement for healthcare providers, policymakers, school administrators, and community leaders. Ann Emerg Med 2004;43:83–99.
16. Hazinski MF, Nolan JP, Billi JE, et al. Part 1: executive summary: 2010 International Consensus on Cardiopulmonary Resuscitation and Emergency Cardiovascular Care Science with Treatment Recommendations. Circulation 2010; 122:S250–275.
17. Henkel DM, Witt BJ, Gersh BJ, et al. Ventricular arrhythmias after acute myocardial infarction: a 20-year community study. Am Heart J 2006;151:806–12.
18. Katz E, Metzger JT, Marazzi A, et al. Increase of sudden cardiac deaths in Switzerland during the 2002 FIFA World Cup. Int J Cardiol 2006;107:132–3.
19. Kim JH, Malhotra R, Chiampas G, et al. Cardiac arrest during long-distance running races. N Engl J Med 2012;366: 130–40.
20. Lapostolle F, Le Toumelin P, Agostinucci JM, et al. Basic cardiac life support providers checking the carotid pulse: performance, degree of conviction, and influencing factors. Acad Emerg Med 2004;11:878–80.
21. Larsen MP, Eisenberg MS, Cummins RO, et al. Predicting survival from out-of-hospital cardiac arrest: a graphic model. Ann Emerg Med 1993;22:1652–8.
22. Leusveld E, Kleijn S, Umans VA. Usefulness of emergency medical teams in sport stadiums. Am J Cardiol 2008;101: 712–4.
23. Luiz T, Kumpch M, Metzger M, et al. Management of cardiac arrest in a German soccer stadium. Structural, process and outcome quality. Anaesthesist 2005;54:914–22.
24. Maron BJ Sudden death in young athletes. N Engl J Med 2003;349:1064–75.
25. Maron BJ, Doerer JJ, Haas TS, et al Sudden deaths in young competitive athletes: analysis of 1866 deaths in the United States, 1980–2006. Circulation 2009;119:1085–92.
26. Maron BJ, Estes NA. Commotio cordis. N Engl J Med 2010; 362:917–27.
27. Maron BJ, Poliac LC, Roberts WO. Risk for sudden cardiac death associated with marathon running. J Am Coll Cardiol 1996;28:428–31.
28. Motyka TM, Winslow JE, Newton K, et al. Method for determining automatic external defibrillator need at mass gatherings. Resuscitation 2005;65:309–14.
29. O'Connor RE, Brady W, Brooks SC, et al. Part 10: acute coronary syndromes: 2010 American Heart Association Guide-lines for Cardiopulmonary Resuscitation and Emer-gency Cardiovascular Care. Circulation 2010;122: S787–817.
30. O'Doherty M, Tayler DI, Quinn E, et al. Five hundred patients with myocardial infarction monitored within one hour of symptoms. Br Med J (Clin Res Ed) 1983;286:1405–8.
31. Rea TD, Fahrenbruch C, Culley L, et al. CPR with chest compression alone or with rescue breathing. N Engl J Med 2010;363:423–33.
32. Ruppert M, Reith MW, Widmann JH, et al. Checking for breathing: evaluation of the diagnostic capability of emergency medical services personnel, physicians, medical students, and medical laypersons. Ann Emerg Med 1999; 34:720–9.
33. Strike PC, Perkins-Porras L, Whitehead DL, et al. Triggering of acute coronary syndromes by physical exertion and anger: clinical and sociodemographic characteristics. Heart 2006; 92:1035–40.
34. Swap CJ, Nagurney JT. Value and limitations of chest pain history in the evaluation of patients with suspected acute coronary syndromes. JAMA 2005;294:2623–9.
35. Thompson PD, Stern MP, Williams P, et al. Death during jogging or running. A study of 18 cases. JAMA 1979;242: 1265–7.
36. Toresdahl BG, Drezner JD, Rao AL, et al. Outcomes of sudden cardiac arrest in US high schools: a prospective study

from the national registry for AED use in sports. Clin J Sport Med 2011;20:137.

37. Tunstall Pedoe DS. Marathon cardiac deaths: the london experience. Sports Med 2007;37:448–50.
38. Virmani R, Robinowitz M, McAllister HA. Nontraumatic death in joggers. A series of 30 patients at autopsy. Am J Med 1982;72:874–82.
39. Waller BF, Roberts WC. Sudden death while running in conditioned runners aged 40 years or over. Am J Cardiol 1980;45:1292–300.
40. Wassertheil J, Keane G, Fisher N, et al. Cardiac arrest outcomes at the Melbourne Cricket Ground and shrine of remembrance using a tiered response strategy-a fore-runner to public access defibrillation. Resuscitation 2000;44:97–104.
41. Webner D, Duprey KM, Drezner JA, et al. Sudden cardiac arrest and death in United States marathons. Med Sci Sports Exerc 2012.
42. Wilbert-Lampen U, Leistner D, Greven S, et al. Cardiovascular events during World Cup soccer. N Engl J Med 2008; 358:475–483.
43. Willich SN, Lewis M, Löwel H, et al. Physical exertion as a trigger of acute myocardial infarction. Triggers and mechanisms of Myocardial Infarction Study Group. N Engl J Med 1993;329:1684–90.

# 42 Acute Cardiac Abnormalities in Electrolyte Imbalance

Electrolytes, or ions, are the charged particles in body fluids that help transmit electrical impulses for proper nerve, heart, and muscle function. The number of positive ions, called cations, and negative ions, called anions, is supposed to be equal. Anything that upsets this balance can have life-threatening consequences. There's a long list of conditions that lead to electrolyte imbalances, including dehydration, diabetic ketoacidosis, cancer, and even head injury. But renal disease is at the top of the list. It's the kidneys' job to control fluid, electrolyte, and acid-base balance. Because too much or too little of any one of the electrolytes quickly becomes a major problem of its own, doing everything possible to maintain the proper balance is a vital component of patient care. Therefore, monitoring electrolytes and checking for signs of an imbalance should be an integral part of your nursing assessment. Here, then, is a review of the role each electrolyte plays, the causes of imbalances, and the corrective measures required.

## Potassium (K), Magnesium (Mg), Calcium (Ca), and Phosphorus ($PO_4$) Imbalances

These can also alter the electrical equilibrium of the cells. The end result? Serious changes in cardiac conduction that can quickly turn lethal. Let's look at each of these electrolytes and the implications that an imbalance will have on your care (Table 42.1).

**Table 42.1:** Causes and altered levels of serum electrolytes

| Normal range | Causes of elevation | Cause of decline |
|---|---|---|
| Sodium (Na) 135–145 mEq/L | Hypernatremia: Excessive loss of water through GI system, lungs or skin; fluid restriction, certain diuretics, hypertonic IV solution, tube feeding; hypothalamic lesion, hyperaldosteronism, corticosteroid use, cushing's syndrome, diabetes insipidus | Hyponatremia: Congestive heart failure, cirrhosis, nephrosis, excess fluid intake, syndrome of inappropriate antidiuretic hormone secretion (dilutional hyponatremia) sodium depletion, loss of body fluids without replacement, diuretic therapy laxatives, nasogastric suctioning. Hypoaldosteronism, cerebral salf-wasting disease |
| Potassium (K) 3.5–5.0 mEq/L | Hyperkalemia: Aldosterone deficiency, sodium depletion, acidosis, trauma, hemolysis of red blood cells, and potassium-sparing diuretics | Hypokalemia: Lack of dietary intake of potassium, vomiting, nosogastric suctioning, potassium-depleting diurectics, aldosteronism, salt-wasting kidney disease, major GI surgery, diuretic therapy with inadequate potassium replacement |
| Calcum (Ca) 8.5-10.5 mEq/L | Hypercalcemia: Excessive vitamin D, immobility, hyperparathyroidism, potassium sparing diuretics, ACE inhibitors, malignancy of bone or blood | Hypocalcemia: Hypoparathyroidism, malabsorption, insufficient or inactivated vitamin D or inadequate intake of calcium, hypoalbuminemia, diuretic therapy diarrhea, acute pancreatitis, bone cancer, gastric surgery |
| Magnesium (Mg) 1.5–2.5 mg/dl | Hypermagnesemia: Excessive use of magnesium-containing antacids and laxatives, untreated diabetic ketoacidosis, excessive magnesium infusions. | Hypomagnesemia: Malabsorption related to GI disease, excessive loss of GI fluids, acute alcoholism/cirrhosis, diuretic therapy, hyper or hypothyroidism, pancreatitis, preeclampsia, and nasogastric suctioning fistula drainage |

But when the kidneys are not functioning properly, that correction does not take place. Not surprisingly, renal disease is the most common cause of hyperkalemia, but acidosis, aldosterone deficiency, sodium depletion, and excess oral intake of potassium supplements are among a number of other possible causes. Signs and symptoms of hyperkalemia include abdominal cramping, fatigue, lethargy, and muscle weakness or paralysis. Severe hyperkalemia will slow cardiac impulse conduction, producing classic changes on EKG. Tall, peaked T-waves are often seen first, followed by a prolonged PR interval and widened QRS complex, signifying delayed conduction, and a shortened QT interval. Left untreated, the excess potassium will continue to suppress conduction until cardiac arrest occurs. Severe hyperkalemia requires rapid action. Stop any potassium administration, and give IV calcium chloride or calcium gluconate, as ordered, to stimulate conduction. The doctor may also order IV sodium bicarbonate, insulin and 50% dextrose, or albuterol to try to shift potassium out of the bloodstream and back into the cells. Depending upon their kidney function, patients with hyperkalemia that is not severe may be given IV diuretics to promote potassium excretion by the kidneys or a resin such as sodium polystyrene sulfonate (kayexalate) that will bind potassium in the gut. But if these efforts fail, hemodialysis may be required in addition to treating the underlying cause. When it comes to hypokalemia, diuretic therapy with inadequate potassium replacement is the most common cause, but patients who lose large amounts of potassium through nasogastric suctioning and diarrhea, for instance, are also at risk. Interestingly, so, too, are patients who were recently hyperkalemic—especially when acidosis is the cause or they're given too much of a drug that brings the potassium down. In acidosis, as pH returns to normal, potassium returns to the cells, lowering serum potassium and increasing the risk of hypokalemia.

## POTASSIUM (Fig. 42.1)

### The Normal Range of $K^+$

It is 3.5–5.0 mEq/liter. Common causes for deviation, above and below this range, are discussed ahead.

## HYPOKALEMIA

### Symptoms

These include muscle weakness or tenderness, leg cramps, drowsiness, confusion, loss of appetite, abdominal distention, and abnormal cardiac conduction. Given too rapidly, IV potassium can cause cardiac arrest, so never administer it by IV push. Follow your institution's protocol, using a pump, if possible, to regulate the infusion so that it runs in over at least an hour when 15–20 mEqs are mixed in 100 ml of solution. Because potassium is very irritating to tissues, administration through a central line is recommended. For the same reason, you should give oral preparations with food to reduce gastric irritation and abdominal discomfort. Report continued complaints of abdominal pain or distention to the physician. This could be a sign of upper GI ulcers caused by potassium.

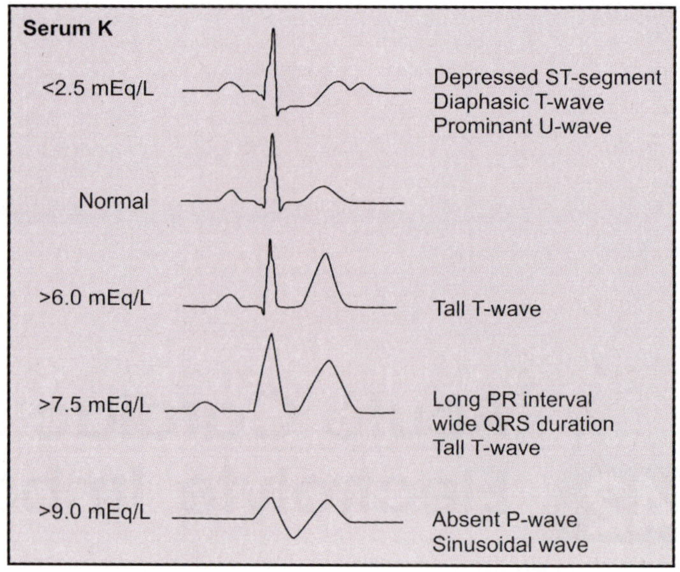


**Fig. 42.1:** Relationship between the representation of ECG and serial levels of serum potassium including hypo and hyperkalemia

### Etiological Factors

1. Underingestion
2. Underadministration
3. Diuretics
4. Nasogastric suction
5. Diuretic phase of acute tubular necrosis
6. After-relief of urinary tract obstruction
7. Renal tubular acidosis
8. Steroid treatment
9. Oral contraceptives
10. Hyperaldosteronism

### Electrocardiographic Findings Including Arrhythmias

*Look for flattened or inverted T-waves and a depressed ST-segment*. There are also decreased T-wave amplitude and increase in U-wave amplitude (Fig. 42.2). The lack of potassium makes cardiac muscle irritable, increasing the risk of premature atrial and/or ventricular contractions that can trigger ventricular tachycardia, which can progress to fibrillation and death. Initial treatment of hypokalemia, especially when it is accompanied by cardiac symptoms, focuses on replacing potassium. But this requires great care. The effects of high and low L+ levels on the electrocardiogram are given below. This electrolyte is the major intracellular cation. The 2% that is found in extracellular fluid is crucial to neuromuscular and cardiac function. Normally, elevated serum potassium stimulates the release of aldosterone, a hormone produced by the adrenal gland. In the kidneys, aldosterone triggers the excretion of potassium and the retention of sodium until serum potassium levels return to normal. Atrial, junctional, and ventricular ectopic rhythms all are common.

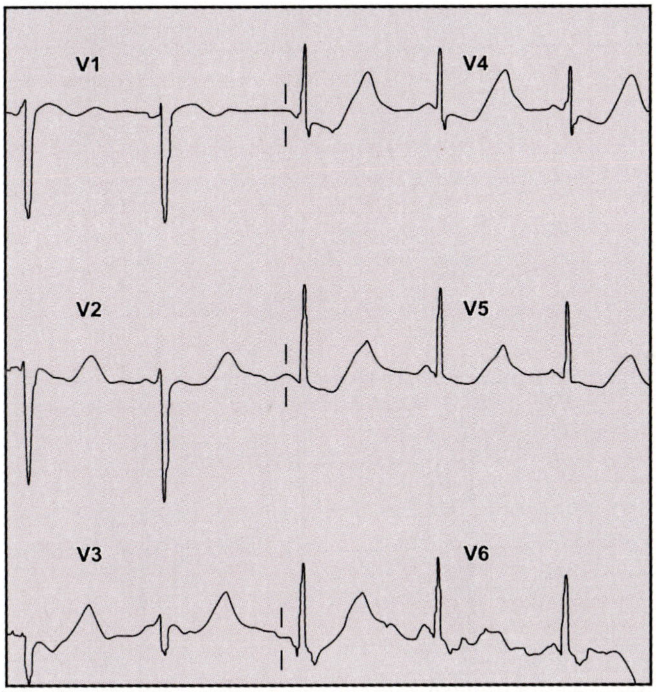


**Fig. 42.2:** Hypokalemia in a girl with anorexia nervosa and purgative abuse. Sinus rhythm. Normal axis. Narrow QRS complex. ST-depression V3–V5. 'Apparent' prolonged QT interval. T-waves unseparable from giant U-waves seen V2–6

### *Treatment*

1. Oral: KCl elixir or capsules; 10–30 mEq every 1–2 hours.
2. IV: Do not exceed 20 mEq/hour, and do not use a concentration greater than 50 mEq/liter.
3. Concurrent $Mg^{2+}$ replacement such as $MgSO_4$ 1g IV over 1 hour may be necessary.

### *Hypokalemia and Digitalis*

Digitalis has numerous effects on the heart. Some of the more clinically important ones are increased contractility, decreased AV conduction, and increased ventricular automaticity. Low $K^+$ enhances increased ventricular automaticity from digitalis.

## HYPERKALEMIA (Figs 42.3–42.6)

*Etiological factors:*

1. Overingestion
2. Overadministration
3. Acute renal failure
4. Chronic renal failure
5. Interstitial nephritis
6. Hypoaldosteronism
7. Rhabdomyolysis

*Electrocardiographic findings:*

1. Increased T-wave amplitude
2. Decreased P-wave amplitude
3. Increased PR interval
4. Increased QRS duration

### Hyperkalemia and Arrhythmias

Hyperkalemia causes a generalized suppression of conduction. AV nodal cells are the least sensitive to this suppression, and nodal or junctional rhythm is most

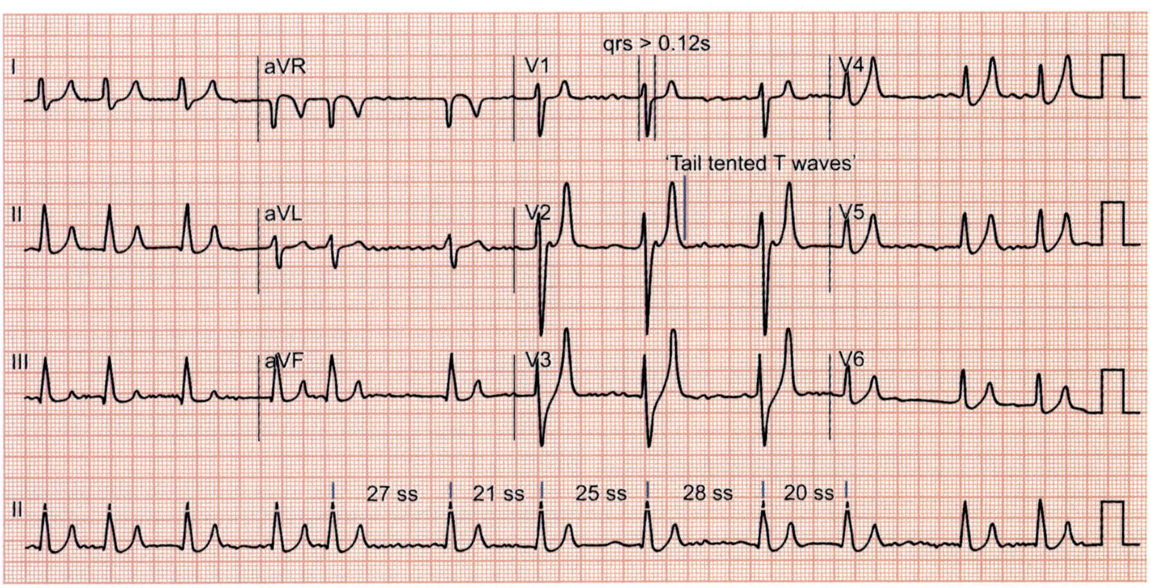


**Fig. 42.3:** ECG is taken from a man with severe hyperkalemia and illustrates many of the ECG changes associated with this metabolic abnormality. The T-waves are tall and rise rapidly to a narrow peak ('tall tented T-waves'). Also note, that the QRS complexes are wide (>/= 0.12s). These are classic and predictable ECG manifestations of significant hyperkalemia. Loss of P-waves is a feature of hyperkalemia. However, in this particular case the patient was in atrial fibrillation (hence, his irregular rhythm), a finding unrelated to his serum potassium

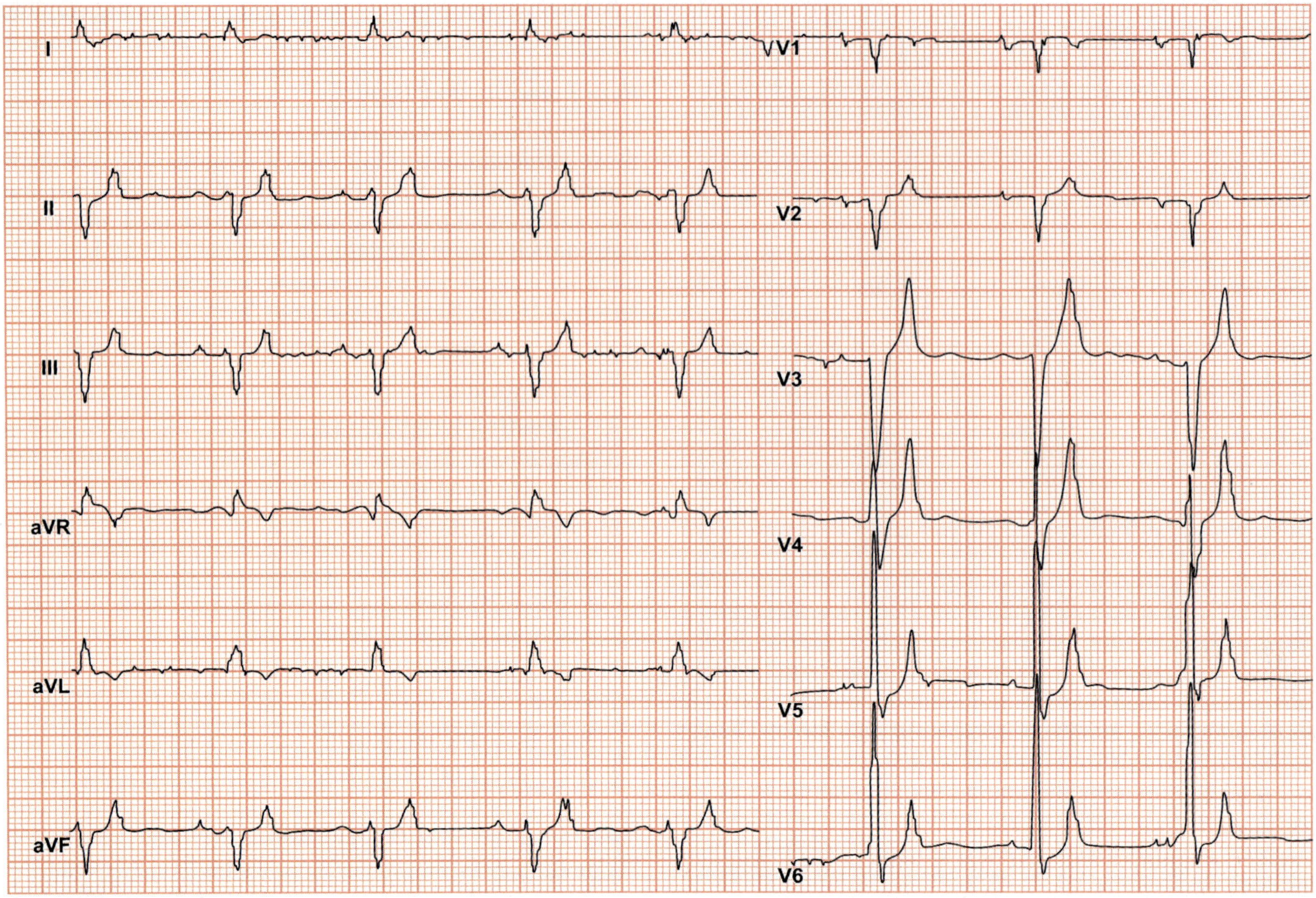


**Fig. 42.4:** 12-lead ECG from a patient with hyperkalemia ($K^+$ concentration of 7.1 mEq/L). Note the classic peaked T-waves in the precordial leads. The QTc interval (341 ms) is shortened

common. At $K^+$ serum concentrations> 12 meq/liter, ventricular fibrillation is very likely to occur.

### Treatment of Hyperkalemia

It includes one or more of the following:

1. Calcium gluconate: 5–10 ml of 10% solution IV, which can be repeated every 5 minutes three times; it is used only for $K^+$ level greater than 6.5 mEq/liter with ECG changes.
2. $NaHCO_3$, a 50 mEq ampule IV over 5 minutes can be used, but one should beware of $Na^+$ load.
3. D5W, a 50 ml ampule, plus 10 units regular insulin. IV over 5 minutes.
4. Sodium polystyrene sulfonate (kayexalate), 20–50 g in 100–200 ml sorbitol PO, which can be repeated every 3–4 hours up to 5 doses per day.

## CALCIUM AND PHOSPHORUS

These two electrolytes are inversely related in the blood, when calcium levels are high, phosphorus levels are low, and vice versa. Calcium is a cation with multiple functions, including transmitting nerve impulses, maintaining cell wall permeability, and activating the body's clotting mechanism. It's also involved in contracting cardiac and smooth muscle, generating cardiac impulses, mediating cardiac pacemaker function, and forming bones and teeth. Phosphorus, the major intracellular anion, also plays a major role in bone formation.It's necessary for energy production in the cells and for carbohydrate, protein, and fat metabolism, as well. Phosphorous also helps maintain acid-base balance by buffering hydrogen ions. Parathyroid hormone (PTH) is responsible for regulating calcium and phosphorus. When calcium levels are low, PTH increases calcium reabsorption, and blocks phosphorus from being reabsorbed. Hypocalcemia can result from diarrhea, diuretics, or acute pancreatitis. It can also be caused by malignancies that steal calcium for abnormal bone formation, conditions that affect the parathyroid gland and thus interfere with PTH production, and disorders that interfere with the availability of calcitrol, such as vitamin D deficiency and malabsorption syndromes. The drop in calcium that occurs in the presence of these disorders triggers a concomitant rise in phosphorus. But there are primary triggers for hyperphosphatemia to watch for, as well (Figs 42.7–42.13).

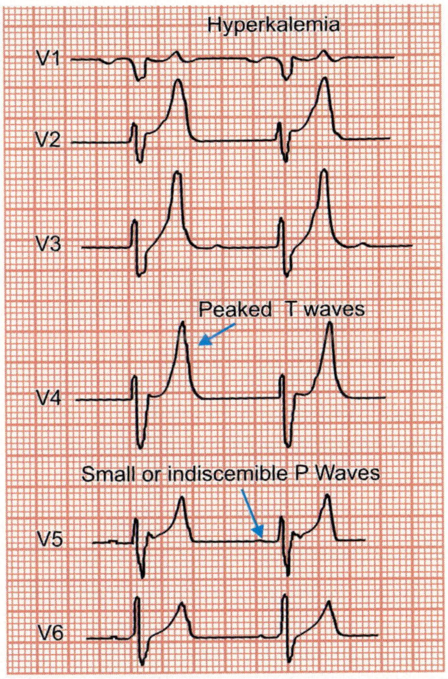


**Fig. 42.5:** Electrocardiography showing precordial leads in hyperkalemia

*Symptoms of hypercalcemia and hypophosphatemia*

- Lethargy, fatigue, changes in mental status, anorexia, nausea, diminished bowel sounds, and constipation.
- Patients may also complain of bone pain; flank and thigh pain is associated with stones formed by excess calcium in the kidneys.
- Neurologic abnormalities, including weakness, lethargy, coma, and tetany, can occur with deviations in serum $Ca^{2+}$ levels. Sinus arrest has been noted with hypercalcemia. Treatment may be needed for these and not specifically for cardiac status.

*Causes of hypercalcemia:* Excessive use of dietary supplements containing calcium and vitamin D, which increase calcium reabsorption, and hyperparathyroidism.

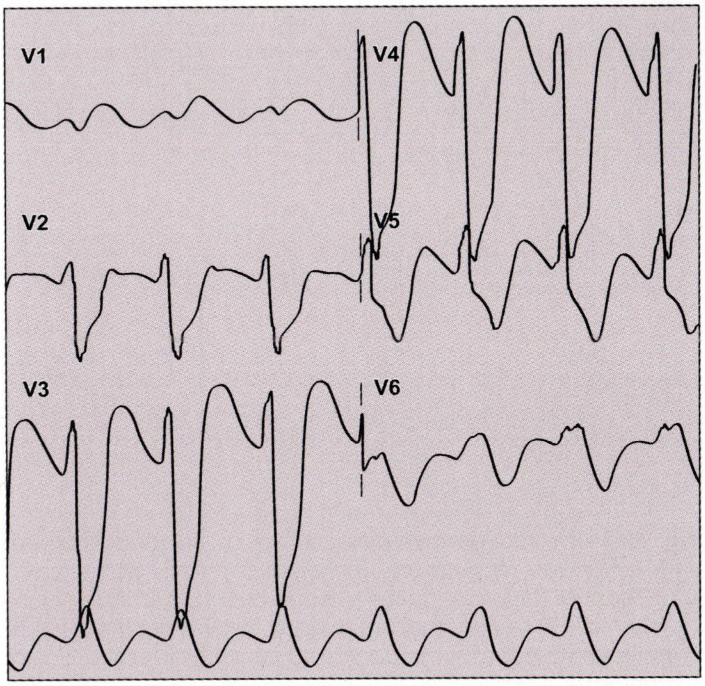


**Fig. 42.6:** Severe hyperkalemia in a patient with iatrogenic renal failure. The ECG abnormalities noted are absence of the P-wave. Extremely bizarre widened QRS complexes. Sine wave in appearance

A primary cause of low serum phosphorus is chronic alcoholism. The normal range of $Ca^{2+}$ is 8.5–10.5 mg/dl. Common causes for deviation, above and below this range, are as follows:

1. Hyperparathyroidism
2. Malignancy
3. Thiazides
4. Familial
5. Sarcoid
6. Vitamin D toxicity
7. Multiple endocrine neoplasia

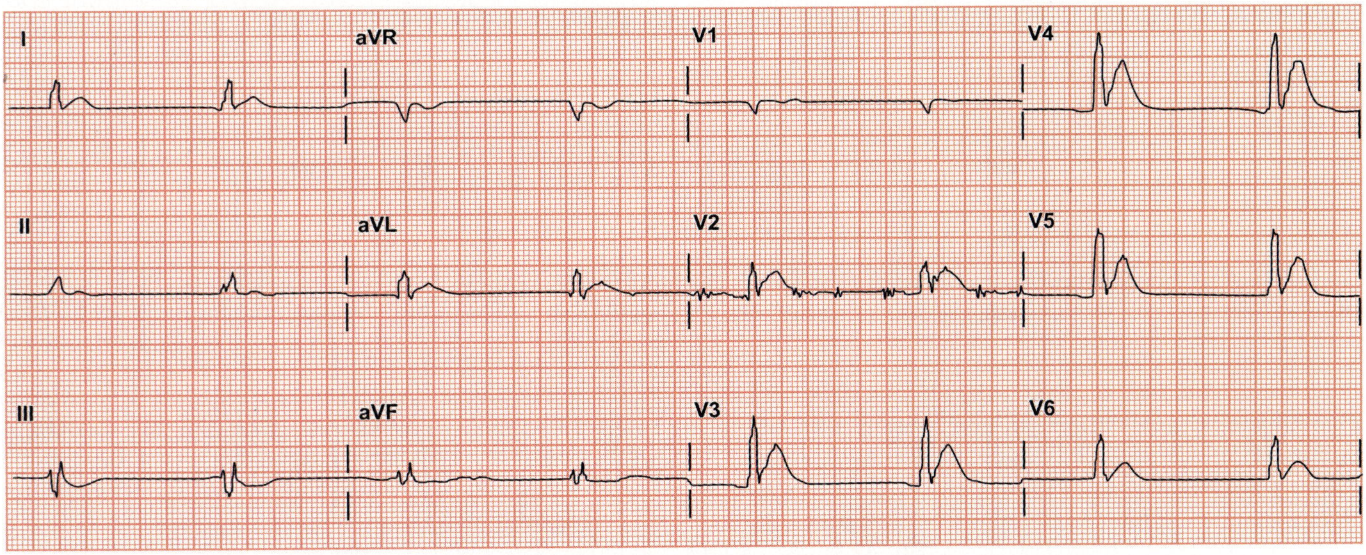


**Fig. 42.7:** Marked shortening of the QTc (260 ms) due to hypercalcemia

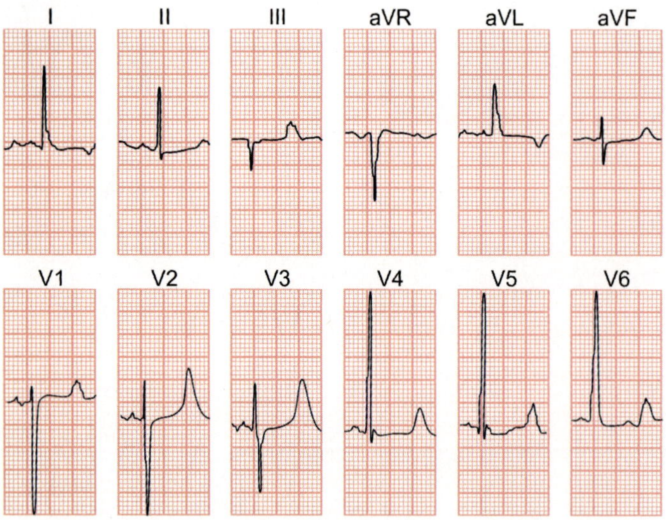


**Fig. 42.8:** This tracing was recorded from a 18-year-adolescent with advanced renal failure. The duration of the QT-interval is 0.56 second. This prolongation is due to hypocalcemia (a serum calcium of 1.8 mg %). The tent-shaped T-waves are the result of hyperkalemia (6.7 mEq/L). The tracing also shows left ventricular hypertrophy

*Electrocardiographic findings:* Shortened ST-segment and widened T-wave are commonly found.

### *Treatment of Hypercalcemia*

- Normal saline 1–2 liters IV every 4 hours
- Furosemide 80–120 mg IV every 4 hours
- Mithramycin 25 microgram/kg IV every 3–4 days.
- Calcitonin 4 units/kg SC every 12 hour

*Causes of hypocalcemia*

1. Hypoparathyroidism
2. Acute tubular necrosis
3. Chronic renal failure
4. Pancreatitis
5. Malabsorption
6. Malnutrition
7. Hyperphosphatemia

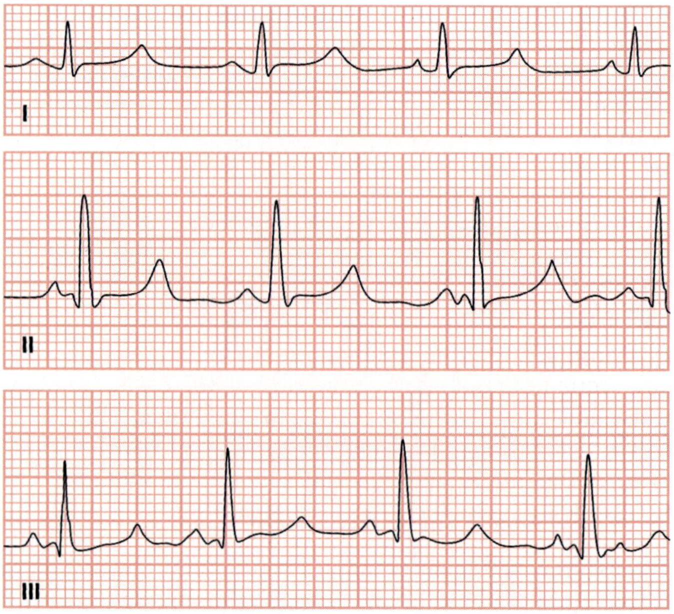


**Fig. 42.10:** Hypocalcemia of obscure endocrine origin in a 9-year-old school girl who was hospitalized at the age of 7 with classical symptoms and findings of Addison's disease. She responded well to treatment with deoxycorticosterone acetate (DOCA) and cortical extract. This tracing shows sinus arrhythmia at a rate averaging 70 complexes per minute, a PR-interval of 0.15 second, normal QRS complexes, upright T-waves, and long ST-segments. The QT duration is prolonged, and measures 0.42 second (the upper limit of normal is 0.39 second for this heart rate)

### *Treatment of Hypocalcemia*

*Oral*

- Calcium carbonate 500 mg 4 times a day.
- Vitamin D3, 0.25–1.0 microgram.
- Phosphate binders 30 ml PO 3 times a day if hypophosphatemia is present. IV route
- 10 ml 10% calcium gluconate over 5 minutes, then 50 ml in 500 ml D5W over 12 hours.

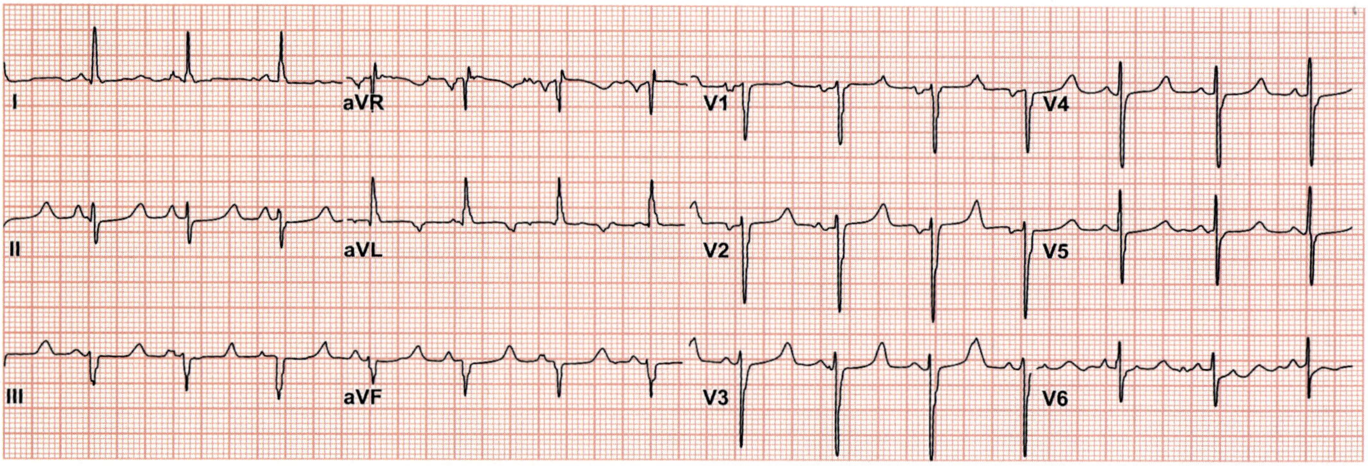


**Fig. 42.9:** QTc 510 ms due to hypocalcemia

*Electrocardiographic features including cardiac arrhythmias in hypercalcemia and hypocalcemia:* The effect of high and low $Ca^{2+}$ levels has been noted on the QT interval. It is shortened by hypercalcemia but is prolonged by hypocalcemia. Within the range of clinically encountered $Ca^{2+}$ levels (2–20 mg/dl), there are little or no arrhythmic effects. Hypertension and conduction abnormalities, such as AV blocks, that can progress to cardiac arrest.

### Hypercalcemia and Hypophosphatemia

(Figs 42.11–42.13)

**Symptoms of hypercalcemia and hypophosphatemia.** It can occur in patients with normal renal function if they abuse laxatives that are high in phosphorus or have too much of the mineral in their diet. Both hypocalcemia and hyperphosphatemia can cause:

- Lethargy, fatigue, bone or joint pain, and sudden seizures. Low calcium levels also produce neuromuscular symptoms, including tremors, cramps, and numbness or tingling in the extremities and around the mouth. Patients may also complain of nausea, abdominal distention, vomiting, or constipation and develop cardiac symptoms, including life-threatening ventricular dysrhythmias.
- EKG tracings will show prolonged ST-segments and QT intervals. Decreased cardiac output and vascular smooth muscle relaxation produce decreases in BP that can progress to circulatory collapse.

#### *Treatment*

- It focuses on increasing calcium and lowering phosphorus.
- Give IV calcium gluconate or calcium chloride or oral preparations, as ordered.
- Aluminum hydroxide gels that bind to phosphorus are given to increase elimination through the bowel.
- Patients with normal renal function may also receive the diuretic acetazolamide (diamox) to promote renal excretion of phosphorus.
- When necessary, hemodialysis is used to quickly correct hyperphosphatemia.

### MAGNESIUM (Figs 42.14–42.16)

- A prolonged PR interval, widened QRS complex, and lengthened QT interval. If a patient's renal function is normal.
- EKG changes associated with low serum magnesium are similar to those seen in hypokalemia—a flat or inverted T-wave and ST-segment depression. There is also a shortened QT interval. Treatment focuses on giving the patient magnesium—either in IV or oral form—as ordered to return levels to normal. This is especially important in patients recovering from an acute MI. Research has shown that maintaining adequate serum magnesium levels in these patients can significantly improve ventricular function and reduce mortality rates.

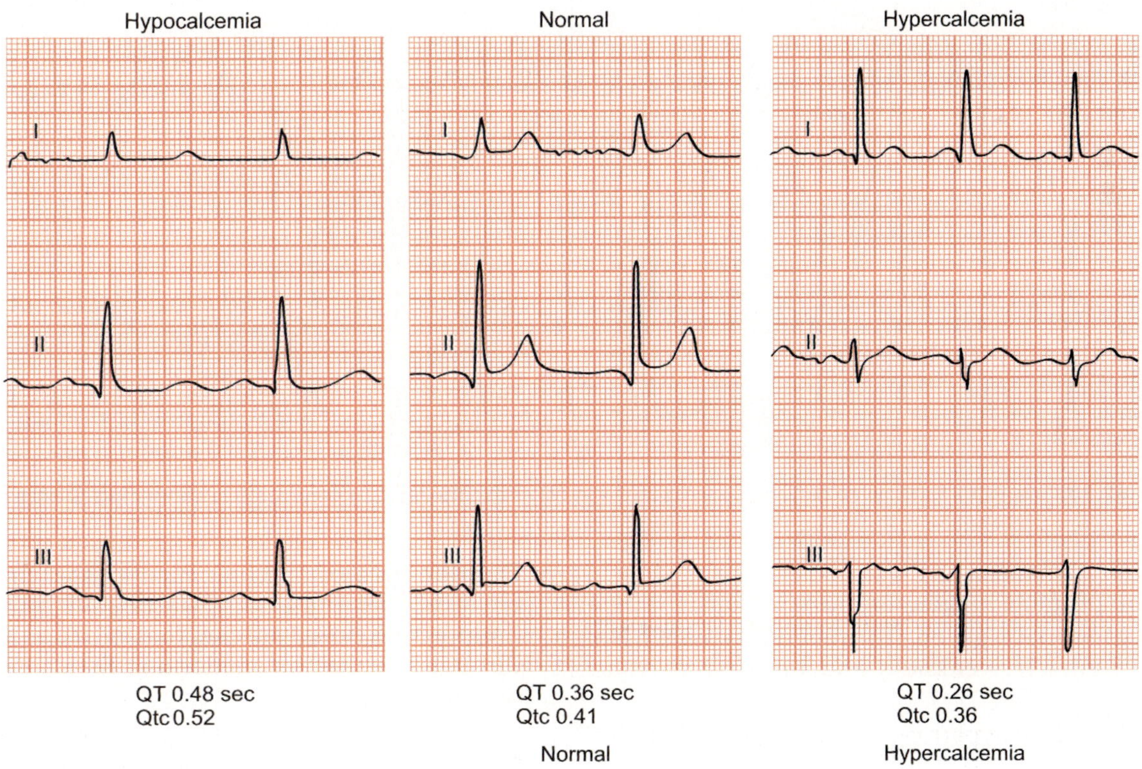


**Fig. 42.11:** ECG shows prolongation of QT interval is a patient with hypocalcemia

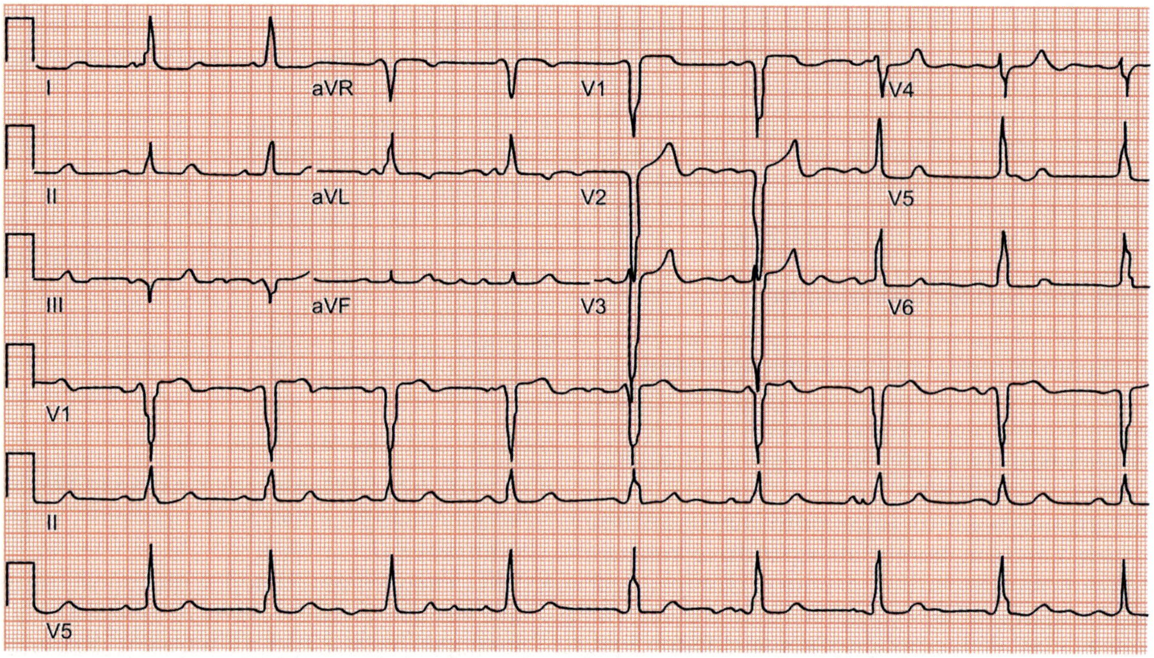


**Fig. 42.12:** The ECG findings of hypocalcemia include (1) a prolonged QT-interval, (2) a lengthened ST-segment

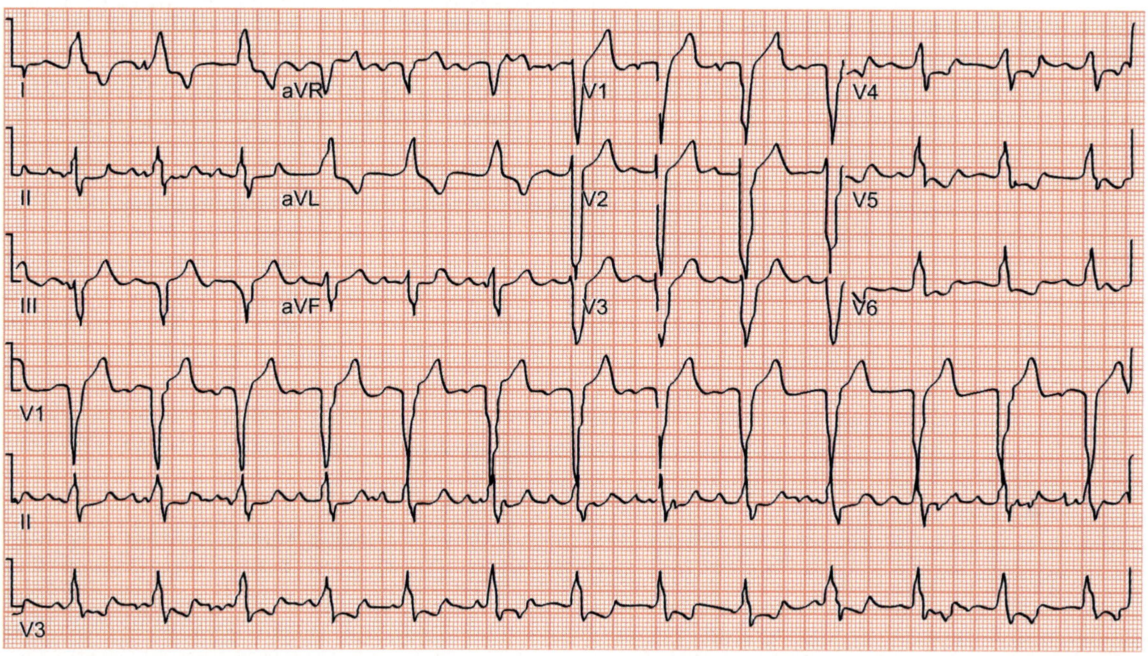


**Fig. 42.13:** The ECG findings of hypercalcemia include (1) a shortened QT-interval, (2) a shortened ST-segment

*Treatment may include:*

- Diuretics to promote magnesium loss.
- Calcium gluconate given intravenously can help counteract muscle weakness and improve cardiac function.
- Patients with severe hypermagnesemia and renal failure may need hemodialysis. The other side of the magnesium equation is hypomagnesemia. It's common in critically ill patients and is associated with high mortality rates.
- Diuretic therapy, chronic alcoholism, cirrhosis, pancreatitis, and pre-eclampsia can all cause excessive magnesium loss, as can losses from the GI tract through nasogastric suctioning, fistula drainage, and diarrhea.

This cation is found primarily in the cells and is responsible for reactions that involve muscle function, energy production, and carbohydrate and protein metabolism. Renal failure is the major cause of hypermagnesemia. Other causes include excessive intake of

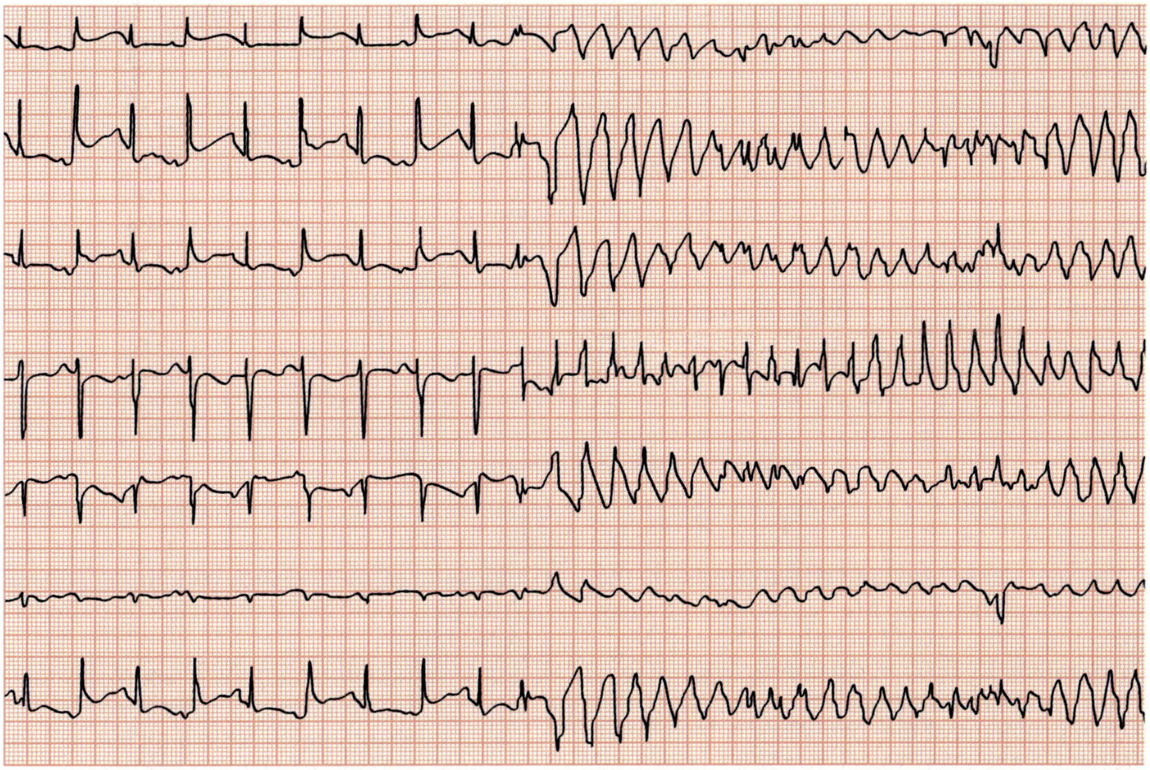

**Fig. 42.14:** Patients with hypokalemia or hypomagnesemia should have the condition corrected as these disorders can exaggerate the degree of QTc prolongation and increase the potential for TdP. Special attention should be given to electrolyte and acid-base balance in patients experiencing severe or prolonged diarrhea or in patients receiving concomitant diuretics

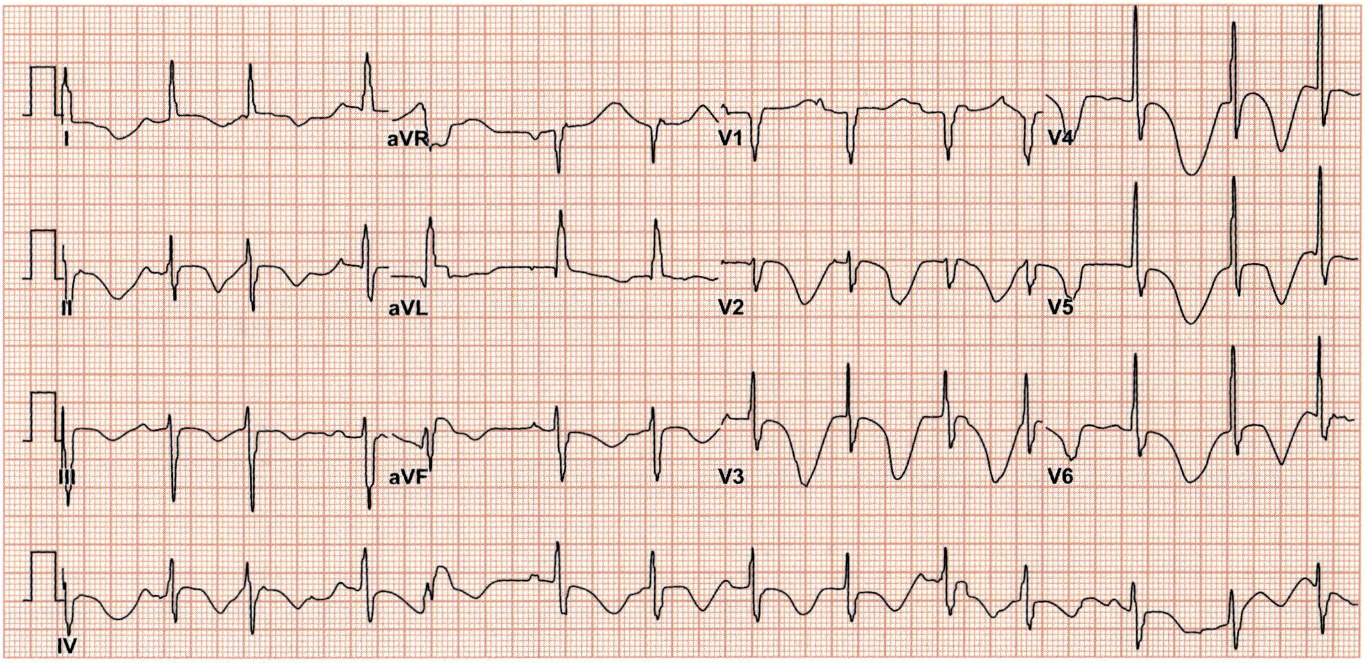


**Fig. 42.15:** Marked QT prolongation in an asymptomatic patient on erythromycin. Patient was also found to be profoundly hypomagnesemic and hypokalemic

magnesium-containing antacids and laxatives and conditions that produce acidosis such as diabetic ketoacidosis.

### Etiological Factors

The normal range of $Mg^{2+}$ is 1.4–2.0 mEq/liter. Renal insufficiency is the major cause of hypermagnesemia.

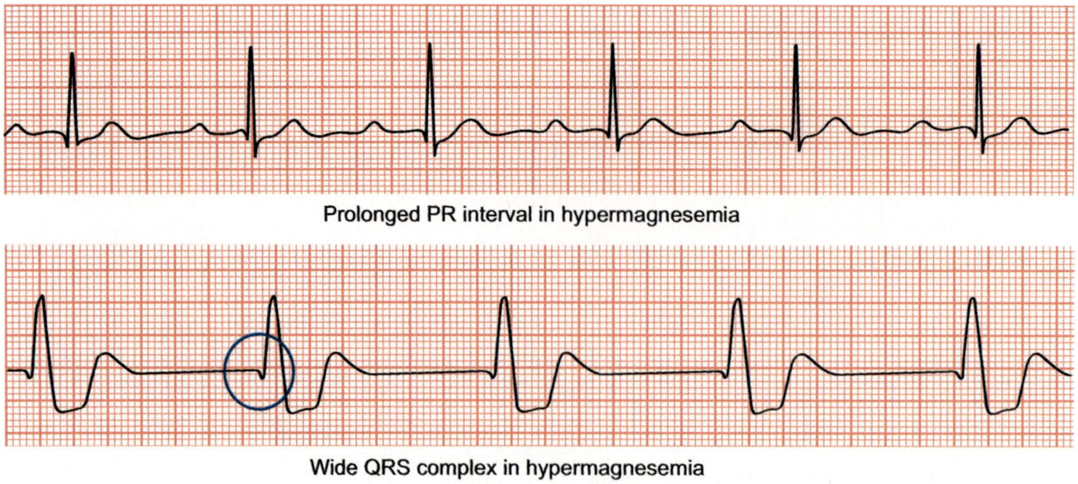


**Fig. 42.16:** ECG traces showing prolonged P-R interval and wide QRS complex in hypermagnesemia

Malnutrition, chronic alcoholism, and overdiuresis are the main causes of hypomagnesemia. $Mg^{2+}$ is the second most abundant intracellular ion, exceeded only by $K^+$ and $Mg^{2+}$ flux generally parallels $K^+$ flux. In dual deficiency states, repletion of one is difficult without the repletion of the other. The known problems of the correlating intracellular and extracellular $K^+$ are even worse for $Mg^{2+}$, since all factors influencing the $Mg^{2+}$ flux are not known.

### Signs and Symptoms of Hypomagnesemia

- Lethargy, altered mental status that can progress to coma, respiratory depression, and muscle weakness.
- Impaired cardiac conduction and contractility produce bradycardia and hypotension and can progress to a full cardiac arrest.
- Muscle weakness or tremors, anorexia, nausea, and dizziness, as well as neurologic changes including lethargy, confusion, and coma. Like hypokalemia, hypomagnesemia increases cardiac muscle irritability and the potential for ventricular dysrhythmias, especially in patients with a recent MI.

### Hypomagnesemia and Arrhythmias

$Mg^{2+}$ abnormalities are not clearly detectable on the surface ECG. In general, $Mg^{2+}$ is useful in conjunction with $K^+$ to abolish either automatic or re-entrant arrhythmias that may be due to low-to-normal $K^+$; these include atrial flutter and fibrillation, and ventricular ectopic beats.

### Treatment of Hypomagnesemia

Administer $MgSO_4$ 1 g, over 1 hour, this may be repeated every 2–4 hour, if required.

## Hypermagnesemia

### Causes

Most cases of hypermagnesemia are due to iatrogenic interventions and administration, especially errors in calculating appropriate infusions. Additional causes include the following:

- Ingestion of magnesium-containing substances such as vitamins, antacids, or cathartics by patients with chronic renal failure
- Acute renal failure (in the absence of dialysis)
- Excessive intravenous infusions of magnesium in patients being treated for eclampsia, asthma, torsade de pointes, or other cardiac arrhythmias
- In neonates, treatment of maternal eclampsia with magnesium, which passes through the placental circulation
- Decreased GI elimination and increased GI absorption of magnesium due to intestinal hypomotility from any cause
- GI medications that decrease motility, including narcotics and anticholinergics
- Hypomotility disorders such as bowel obstruction and chronic constipation
- Tumor lysis syndrome, by releasing massive amounts of intracellular magnesium
- Adrenal insufficiency (secondary hypermagnesemia)
- Rhabdomyolysis, like tumor lysis syndrome, by releasing significant amounts of intracellular magnesium
- Milk-alkali syndrome
- Hypothyroidism
- Hypoparathyroidism
- Neoplasm with skeletal muscle involvement
- Lithium intoxication
- Extracellular volume contraction, as in diabetic ketoacidosis (DKA)

### Electrocardiographic Findings in Hypermagnesemia

In summary, severe symptomatic hypermagnesemia may result from magnesium containing medications, which are generally considered benign. It should not be used in patients with renal failure even with CCPD. Our findings indicate that the ECG manifestations of hypermagnesemia are very similar to those of hyperkalemia, increasing the potential for misdiagnosis of hypermagnesemia. Serum magnesium concentrations should be measured in patients with renal insufficiency who present with these symptoms, thus preventing significant complications and possible fatal events. Prolonged PR interval and widened QRS complexare frequently found.

### Emergency Department Care

Although the effectiveness of dialysis in removing divalent cations is debated, some studies have demonstrated removal of a large amount of magnesium using this modality. Dialysis is best used when levels exceed 8 mEq/L, when life-threatening symptoms are present, or in patients with poor renal function.

- Assess the patient's ABCs and stabilize.
- Intubate if necessary.
- Treat hypotension with fluids.
- Treat arrhythmia as per advanced cardiac life support (ACLS) protocol or with treatment
- Obtain appropriate studies as discussed in workup.

## SODIUM

Sodium (Na), the most abundant cation in extracellular fluid, plays a key role in transmitting nerve impulses. It also helps maintain serum concentration, or osmolality. Water follows salt in the body, so a gain or loss in sodium results in a gain or loss in water. For instance, when you eat too much salt, the rise in serum osmolality triggers thirst and the release of antidiuretic hormone (ADH) from the pituitary gland. Thirst leads you to drink, while ADH signals the kidneys to hang onto water.The opposite is also true: Low serum osmolality from too little salt stops thirst and inhibits ADH release, allowing more water to be excreted by the kidneys (Figs 42.17–42.20).

Hypernatremia occurs when either too much water is lost or too much salt is taken in (you'll find a list of normal values and causes of electrolyte imbalances. The elderly are particularly at risk for hypernatremia following surgery or a fever because of volume depletion, and because of a

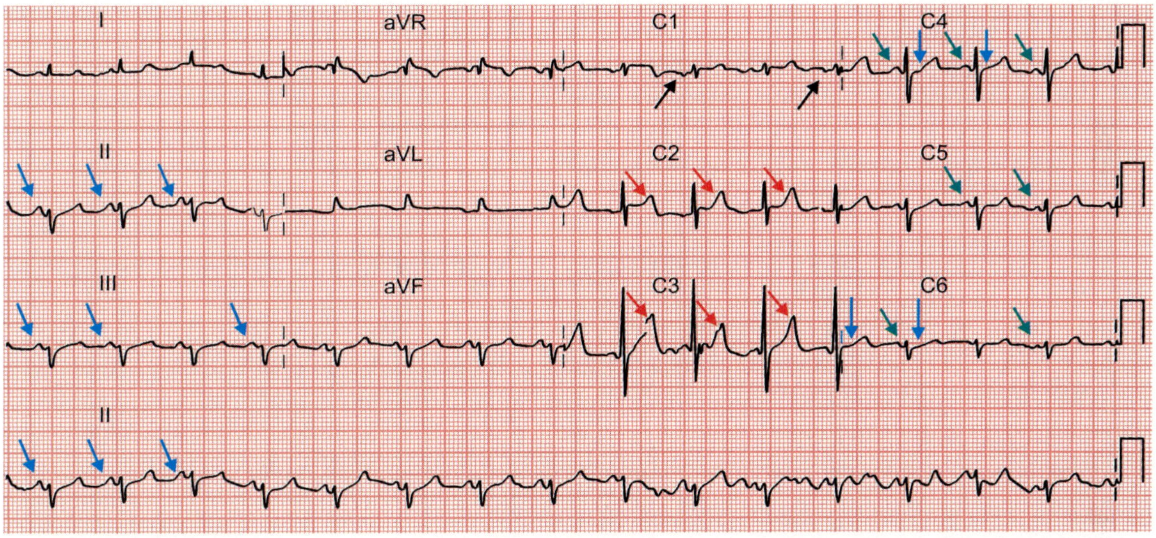


**Fig. 42.17:** ST-segment elevation in leads II, III, avF as well as in lateral leads V4–6 mimicking it, of acute inferolateral infarction in patient with severe hyponatremia

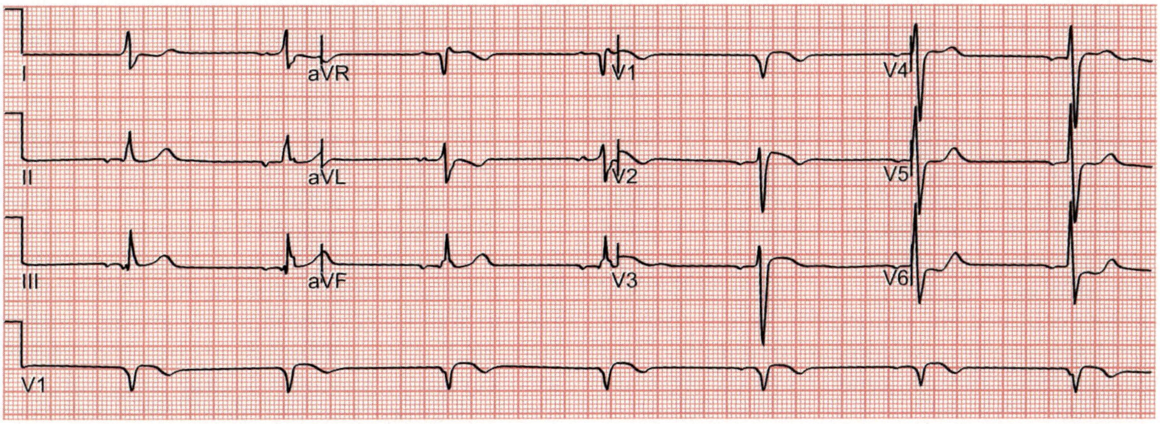


**Fig. 42.18:** 12-lead electrocardiogram obtained upon admission (serum sodium concentration of 101 mmol/L) showing ST-segment changes that resemble a Brugada ECG pattern. A downward coving of the ST-segment with T-wave inversion is present in the anterior precordial leads. The QRS exhibits late rightward forces

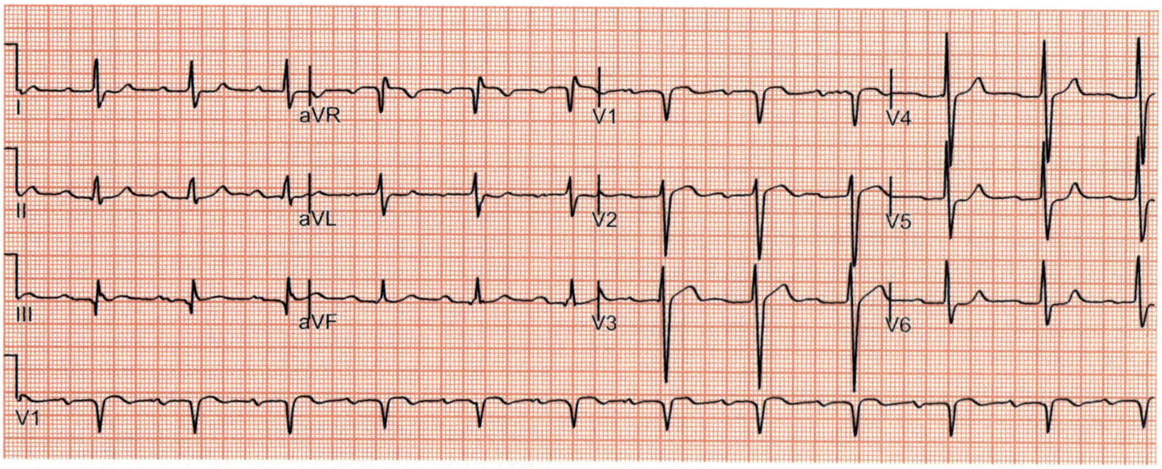


**Fig. 42.19:** 12-lead electrocardiogram showing normalization of ST-segment elevations at serum sodium concentration of 119 mmol/L. When compared with the admission ECG as shown in Fig. 42.18, the anterior precordial leads now exhibit a more normal ST-segment and T-wave pattern. A prolonged PR interval is also noted

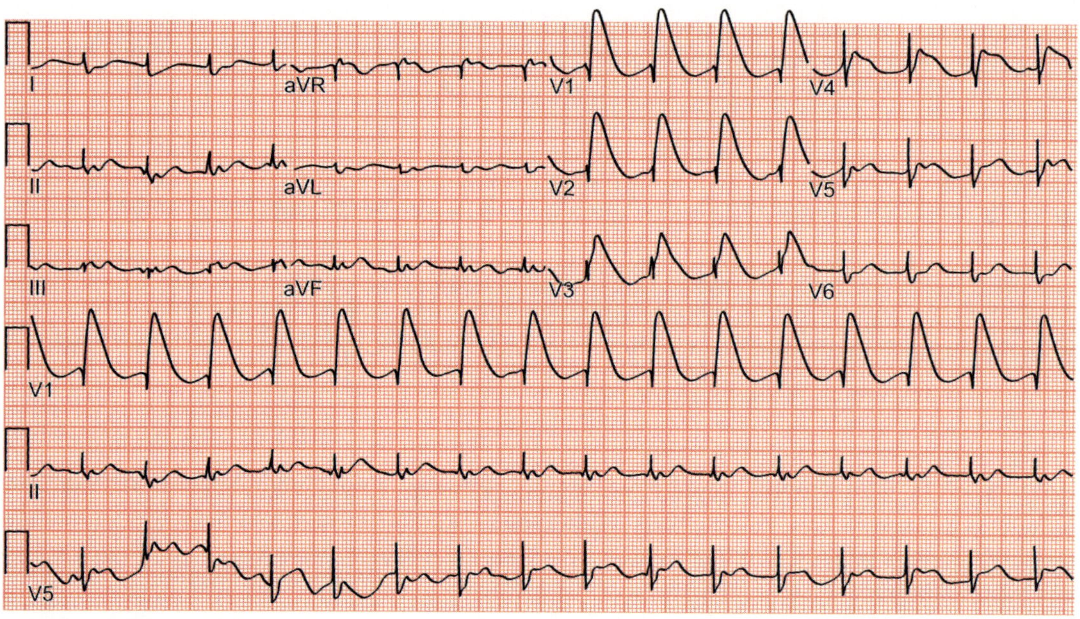


**Fig. 42.20:** The patient had a cardiac arrest most likely from sustained ventricular tachycardia secondary to a Brugada pattern. Hence, hyponatremia should be recognized as an important aetiology in the list of causes that unmask a Brugada pattern in patients with this channelopathy

diminished thirst mechanism. All patients on fluid restrictions and those receiving diuretic therapy, hypertonic IV solutions, or tube feedings are at risk, as well. So, too, are patients with diabetes, because of dehydration related to their hyperglycemia. Regardless of the cause, patients with hypernatremia may appear thirsty, tachycardic, and lethargic. As their cells become more dehydrated, patients may develop disorientation, weakness, irritability, and muscle twitching. Urine output is generally low as the body tries to compensate by hanging onto water. The exception is untreated diabetes insipidus, where a lack of ADH results in a high urine output—possibly as much as 20 liters in 24 hours. Regardless, though, of whether urine output is high or low, seizures, coma, or death may result if hypernatremia is left untreated. Correcting the situation requires that you focus on the underlying cause. That may be as simple as replacing volume orally or by the IV administration of isotonic solutions such as normal saline. Or it may be as complex as putting the patient on dialysis. Part of your routine nursing care for the hypernatremic patient will involve monitoring serum sodium and osmolality and administering fluids based on the results. You'll also carefully monitor intake and output, and avoid overhydration. The flip side of the sodium equation is hyponatremia, which usually occurs when the body loses more sodium than water or when excess water dilutes the normal sodium concentration. Dilutional hyponatremia can be caused by excess fluid intake, and conditions such as congestive heart failure or syndrome of inappropriate antidiuretic hormone secretion (SIADH). The neurological symptoms of hyponatremia are similar to those of hypernatremia—lethargy and confusion—with the possible addition of nausea and vomiting resulting from cerebral edema. Other signs and symptoms depend upon the cause. Patients who have lost sodium through diarrhea, certain diuretics, suctioning, or laxatives, for example, may show signs of dehydration, including tachycardia and hypotension. Those with dilutional hyponatremia may show signs of fluid overload, such as hypertension and difficulty breathing.

Treatment depends upon both the degree of sodium deficiency and the cause. In cases of mild hyponatremia, an increased intake of dietary sodium may be ordered, while patients who are both hyponatremic and hypovolemic may receive IV fluid replacement using solutions containing normal saline. Those with mild dilutional hyponatremia from overadministration of free water may need nothing more than the restriction of fluid intake. This approach is also appropriate for patients with hyponatremia caused by SIADH. Severe hyponatremia, however, is a medical emergency, permanent neurological damage can occur when serum sodium falls below 110 mEq/L. Giving hypertonic saline (3% NaCl) solution is the treatment of choice, but must be done with caution. A rapid increase in serum sodium can cause fluid overload and cardiac failure, as well as cerebral osmotic demyelination syndrome—a condition caused by osmotic injury to myelinated nerve fibers that leads to paralysis and death.

Consistent serum osmolality maintained through a balance of sodium and water intake and excretion. Normal serum range—136–144 mmol/L. Sodium-related disorders.

#### *Hyponatremia*

It is defined as <136 mmol/L.

#### *Symptoms*

- Nausea
- Headache
- Lethargy
- Emesis
- Severe hyponatremia can cause seizures, coma, and death.

### Causes

#### *Hyperosmolar Hyponatremia*

- Hyperglycemia—for every 100 mg/dl increase of glucose, serum Na is lowered by 1.7 mmol/L
- Iso-osmolarhyponatremia (pseudohyponatremia)
- Excess lipids or proteins in serum
- May or may not be an issue—results dependent on assay method used by laboratory
- Hypo-osmolar hyponatremia—three categories
- Hypovolemic—thiazide diuretics, osmotic diuresis, adrenal insufficiency, and ketonuria
- Isovolemic—syndrome of inappropriate antidiuretic hormone, hypothyroidism, HIV, and certain cancers
- Hypervolemic—psychogenic polydipsia, multiple tap-water enemas, and congestive heart failure

#### *Electrocardiographic Changes in Hyponatremia*

Severe hyponatremia may present with EKG changes of ST-segment elevation mimicking acute myocardial infarction. Severe hyponatremia has been associated rarely with EKG findings of Brugada syndrome of acute myocardial infarction.

#### *Treatment*

- Na deficit = (desired Na-measured serum Na) × 0.6 (males) or 0.5 (females) × body weight (in kg)
- Hypovolemic-saline replacement
- Severe symptoms—use 3% saline solution (513 mmol/L)
- Less severe symptoms—use normal saline solution
- Isovolemic or hypervolemic—fluid restriction.

#### *Hypernatremia*

It is defined as serum Na >144 mmol/L.

**Symptoms:** Mimics symptoms of hyponatremia.

#### *Causes*

- Water depletion
- Extrarenal losses
- Insensible losses (e.g. fever)
- Gastrointestinal losses (e.g. diarrhea)
- Renal losses
- Diabetes insipidus (central, nephrogenic)
- Hyperaldosteronism
- Cushing disease
- Salt gain–hypertonic solution or sodium bicarbonate

#### *Treatment*

- Fluid replacement. Free water deficit = [(measured plasma Na–140)/140] × body weight (in kg) × 0.6 (males) or 0.5 (females)
- Mild—oral fluids
- Severe—IV fluids; replace deficit with 5% dextrose in water.

### Acid-base Balance Imbalance

Chloride (Cl) and bicarbonate ($HCO_3$) are the major extracellular anions. While both play an important role in maintaining acid-base balance, bicarbonate is by far the star of the show. Bicarbonate is the body's major buffer system. It helps keep the ratio between acids and bases in a tight range that's numerically expressed as the pH (normal pH is 7.35 –7.45). A rise in pH above normal (alkalosis) or below normal (acidosis) causes cellular damage and can eventually lead to a patient's death. For its part, chloride exists in an inverse relationship with bicarbonate. When there's too little chloride, bicarbonate builds up, and metabolic alkalosis results. The flip side of this—too much chloride—is a bit more complicated. If chloride is high and sodium is normal, the patient may be acidotic. If chloride is high and the sodium is also high, the patient is likely to be dehydrated. One way to determine the cause of an acid-base imbalance is by calculating the anion gap. To calculate this gap, you need to take your patient's lab results and add the chloride and bicarbonate values. Then, subtract the sum of the two from the value for sodium. The normal anion gap range is 8–12.5. A high anion gap (>12) is indicative of conditions such as diabetic- or alcohol-induced keto-acidosis. A high anion gap may also be your first indication of lactic acidosis in patients with shock or sepsis. A normal anion gap with elevated chloride levels should also raise a flag for acidosis. That's because in cases of diarrhea and renal tubular acidosis, bicarbonate is lost, and chloride is retained to maintain electrical neutrality. Either way, interventions focus on treating the underlying cause of the acidosis. A low anion gap indicates alkalosis and hypo-chloremia from vomiting, nasogastric suctioning, or diuretic therapy. But other causes of alkalosis include Cushing's syndrome, excessive aldosterone secretion, and hypokalemia. Massive blood transfusions, over-administration of IV fluids containing bicarbonate, and excessive intake of antacids containing sodium bicarbonate can also cause bicarbonate levels to rise. Again, treatment focuses on resolving the underlying cause. Patients with alkalosis may receive acetazolamide. The drug lowers bicarbonate levels by increasing its excretion in the urine and prevents the formation of new bicarbonate. Prolonged use can lead to acidosis, however, so watch bicarbonate levels closely. Your careful attention to bicarbonate, chloride, and the other electrolytes mentioned here, can have a tremendous impact on your patient's well-being. Understanding what the lab values mean in relation to changes in a patient's condition can be a challenge. But getting a firm handle on things will ensure that you take the necessary steps to correct imbalances before the situation becomes dire.

The electocardiographic changes are, presumably, due to alterations in the concentration of electrolytes in the myocardium. But it is, usually, presumed that serum concentrations of electrolytes represent the myocardial levels. Hence, for any doubtful clinical and electrocardiographic findings, the serum concentrations of the concerned electrolyte is analyzed in the laboratory. Ninety-eight percent of the total body potassium is intracellular.

The determination of the serum potassium concentration is, therefore, poorly correlated with that of myocardial levels. It is also true that the serum potassium may be abnormally high or low with least electrocardiographic alterations. Yet there may be a situation in which one may find classical ECG changes. Attributed both to hyper and hypokalemia with normal serum potassium values.

Before one may comment upon the ECG changes in relation to various serum concentrations of the electrolytes, the following points of caution to be considered:

1. Digitalis may alter the ECG and the changes found in hypokalemmia closely resemble those due to excessive digitalis. Hypokalemia may potentiate digitalis dysrhythmia.
2. Associated coronary artery disease or hypertensive heart disease may modify the ECG changes, and obscure the changes due to electrolyte alterations.
3. ECG effects of hyperkalemia may be exaggerated by low sodium concentration, and higher sodium levels may obscure them.
4. Electrocardiographic abnormality is always individualized as abnormal serum postassium levels may not produce the same degree of alteration on ECG in all the patients screened.
5. Many systemic diseases, when coexisting. May produce alterations in the levels of both potassium and calcium at the same time. Hence, the electrocardiographic changes are, usually, not pertaining to one electrolyte only but to a composite graph of both the electrolytes. Clinically important electrolytes include potassium ($K^+$), calcium ($Ca^{2+}$) and magnesium ($Mg^{2+}$). They are responsible for the resting action potentials of cardiac cells, diastolic depolarization of pacemaker cells and excitation- contraction. $Mg^{2+}$ is a cofactor in the Na-K-ATPase pump that serves to generate high intracellular concentrations of $K^+$ and low intracellular concentrations of $Na^+$.

## BIBLIOGRAPHY


1. Acker CG, Johnson JP, Palevsky PM, Greenberg A. Hyperkalemia in hospitalized patients: causes, adequacy of treatment, and results of an attempt to improve physician compliance with published therapy guidelines. Arch Intern Med 1998;158:917–24.
2. Adhiyaman V, Asghar M, Oke A, White AD, Shah IU. Nephrotoxicity in the elderly due to co-prescription of angiotensin converting enzyme inhibitors and nonsteroidal anti-inflammatory drugs. JR Soc Med 2001;94:512–4.
3. Agus ZS, Wasserstein A, Goldfarb S. Disorders of calcium and magnesium homeostasis. Am J Med 1982;72(3):473–88.
4. Aslam S, Friedman EA, Ifudu O. "Electrocardiography is unreliable in detecting potentially lethal hyperkalaemia in haemodialysis patients." Nephrology, dialysis, transplantation: official publication of the European Dialysis and Transplant Association-European Renal Association 2002; 17(9):1639–42.
5. Balci AK, Koksal O, Kose A, Armagan E, Ozdemir F, Inal T, et al. General characteristics of patients with electrolyte imbalance admitted to emergency department. World J Emerg Med 2013;4(2):113–6.
6. Birrer RB, Shallash AJ, Totten V. Hypermagnesemia-induced fatality following epsom salt gargles(1). J Emerg Med 2002; 22(2):185–8.
7. Chang WT, Radin B, McCurdy MT. Calcium, magnesium, and phosphate abnormalities in the emergency department. Emerg Med Clin North Am 2014;32(2):349–66.
8. DeFronzo RA. Hyperkalemia and hyporeninemic hypo-aldosteronism. Kidney Int 1980;17:118–34.
9. Don BR, Sebastian A, Cheitlin M, Christiansen M, Schambelan M. "Pseudohyperkalemia caused by fist

clenching during phlebotomy". N Engl J Med 1990;322(18): 1290–2.

10. Elliott MJ, Ronksley PE, Clase CM, Ahmed SB, Hemmelgarn BR. "Management of patients with acute hyperkalemia". CMAJ 2010;182(15):1631–5. doi:10.1503/cmaj.100461. PMC 2952010.
11. Gennari FJ. Disorders of potassium homeostasis. Hypokalemia and hyperkalemia. Crit Care Clin 2002;18:273–88.
12. Grande Villoria J, Macias Nunez JF, Miralles JM, De Castro del Pozo S, Tabernero Romo JM. Hyporeninemic hypoaldosteronism in diabetic patients with chronic renal failure. Am J Nephrol 1988;8:127–37.
13. Guillaume T, Krzesinski JM. [Management of serum magnesium abnormalities]. Rev Med Liege 2003;58(7–8): 465–7.
14. Huggins RM, Kennedy WK, Melroy MJ, Tollerton DG. Cardiac arrest from succinylcholine-induced hyperkalemia. Am J Health Syst Pharm 2003;60:694–7.
15. Iolascon, A; Stewart, GW; Ajetunmobi, JF; et al. "Familial pseudohyperkalemia maps to the same locus as dehydrated hereditary stomatocytosis (hereditary xerocytosis)". Blood 1999;93(9):3120–3.
16. Juurlink DN, Mamdani MM, Lee DS, Kopp A, Austin PC, Laupacis A, et al. Rates of hyperkalemia after publication of the Randomized Aldactone Evaluation Study. N Engl J Med 2004;351:543–51.
17. Kaze Folefack F, Stoermann Chopard C. [Magnesium metabolism disturbances]. Rev Med Suisse 2007;3(101):605–606, 608, 610–1.
18. Kim HJ, Han SW. Therapeutic approach to hyperkalemia. Nephron 2002;92(Suppl 1):33–40.
19. Kratz A, Ferraro M, Sluss PM, Lewandrowski KB, Ellender Stacey, M Peters, Christine C, Kratz Alexander, Ferraro Maryjane, et al. "Case records of the Massachusetts General Hospital. Weekly clinicopathological exercises. Laboratory reference values". The New England Journal of Medicine 2004;351(15):1548–63.
20. Leitch SP, Patterson DJ. "Interactive effects of K+, acidosis, and catecholamines on isolated rabbit heart: implications for exercise.". Journal of Applied Physiology (Bethesda Md. 1985) 1994;77(3):1164–71.
21. Lin CH, Tu YF, Chiang WC, Wu SY, Chang YH, Chi CH. Electrolyte abnormalities and laboratory findings in patients with out-of-hospital cardiac arrest who have kidney disease. Am J Emerg Med 2013;31(3):487–93.
22. Lindinger, MI. "Potassium regulation during exercise and recovery in humans: implications for skeletal and cardiac muscle". J Mol Cell Cardiol 1995;27(4):1011–22. 70–5.
23. McFarlane SI, Sowers JR. Cardiovascular endocrinology 1: aldosterone function in diabetes mellitus: effects on cardiovascular and renal disease. J Clin Endocrinol Metab 2003;88: 516–23.
24. Musso CG. Magnesium metabolism in health and disease. Int Urol Nephrol 2009;41(2):357–62.
25. Pantanowitz L. Drug-induced hyperkalemia [Letter]. Am J Med 2002;112:334.
26. Perazella MA, Tray K. Selective cyclooxygenase-2 inhibitors: a pattern of nephrotoxicity similar to traditional nonsteroidal anti-inflammatory drugs. Am J Med 2001;111:64–7.
27. Perazella MA. Drug-induced hyperkalemia [Letter Reply]. Am J Med 2002;112:334–5.
28. Perazella MA. Drug-induced hyperkalemia: old culprits and new offenders. Am J Med 2000;109:307–14.
29. Pitt B, Zannad F, Remme WJ, Cody R, Castaigne A, Perez A, et al. The effect of spironolactone on morbidity and mortality in patients with severe heart failure. Randomized Aldactone Evaluation Study investigators. N Engl J Med 1999;341: 709–17.
30. Sevastos N, Theodossiades G, Efstathiou S, Papatheodoridis GV, Manesis E, Archimandritis AJ. "Pseudohyperkalemia in serum: the phenomenon and its clinical magnitude". J Lab Clin Med 2006;147(3):139–44.
31. Smith JC, Siddique H, Corrall RJ. Misinterpretation of serum cortisol in a patient with hyponatremia. BMJ 2004;328: 215–6.
32. Soave PM, Conti G, Costa R, Arcangeli A. Magnesium and anaesthesia. Curr Drug Targets 2009;10(8):734–43.
33. Su M, Stork C, Ravuri S, et al. "Sustained-release potassium chloride overdose". J Toxicol Clin Toxicol 2001;39(6): 641–8.
34. Surawicz B. "Relationship between electrocardiogram and electrolytes." American heart journal 1967;73(6):814–34.
35. Vanden Hoek TL. Morrison LJ, Shuster M, Donnino M, Sinz E, Lavonas EJ, Jeejeebhoy FM, Gabrielli A. "Part 12: cardiac arrest in special situations: 2010 American Heart Association Guidelines for Cardiopulmonary Resuscitation and Emergency Cardiovascular Care." Circulation 2010;122 (18 Suppl 3).
36. Witham MD, Gillespie ND, Struthers AD. Hyperkalemia after the publication of RALES. N Engl J Med 2004;351: 2448–50.
37. Wrenn KD, Slovis CM, Slovis BS. "The ability of physicians to predict hyperkalemia from the ECG." Annals of emergency medicine 1991;20(11):1229–32.
38. Yusuf S, Sleight P, Pogue J, Bosch J, Davies R, Dagenais G. Effects of an angiotensin-converting enzyme inhibitor, Ramipril, on cardiovascular events in high-risk patients. The Heart Outcomes Prevention Evaluation Study Investigators [published corrections appear in N Engl J Med 2000;342:1376; N Engl J Med 2000;342:748]. N Engl J Med 2000;342:145–53.

# 43 Scope of Telemedicine in Emergency Cardiology

An increasing number of medical specialties such as dermatology, oncology, radiology, surgery, cardiology, and psychiatry use telemedicine routinely. In a country like Greece, which consists of several small islands dispersed around a mountainous mainland with many remote parts, telemedicine is not only beneficial but rather necessary for high-quality healthcare provision to its population. The services of telemedicine in their modern form appeared in Greece in 1991. Due to the low reliability of the plain old telephone service (POTS) at the beginning of these efforts, the implementations became wireless, via satellite links. However, the digitization of the POTS and the general improvement of the telecommunication infrastructure, especially the deployment of GSM (global system for mobile communications) networks, which took place since then, have favoured further developments in the field.

Telecardiology and specifically transtelephonic electrocardiographic transmission (TET) remains the most widespread form of telemedicine since it can ensure a valid, reliable, and objective assessment of cardiac rhythm and function. However, its use in sports medicine is not so widely mentioned, and relevant studies are very scarce in the international literature. Perhaps the only known application in this area is the follow-up of patients with cardiovascular disease during their rehabilitation exercise (Figs 43.1–43.3).

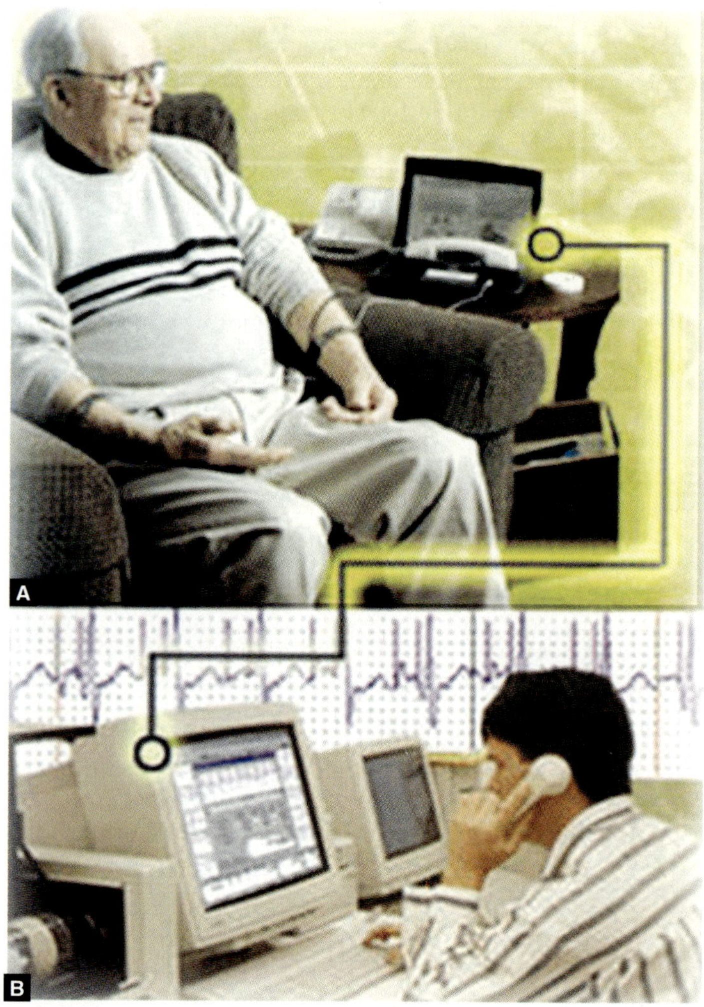

**Fig. 43.1:** (A) The patient is sitting comfortably in a room connected to pacemaker monitoring equipment. (B) The ECG record of the same patient is being monitored and information gathered is being transmitted by the trained worker to a specialist for necessary management

With the increasing number of individuals having physically active lifestyles, transient risk of cardiovascular events during exercise is not rare, especially among athletes with unrecognized cardiovascular diseases. Therefore, at least annual preparticipation screening is generally recommended prior to participation in sports. In order to increase the number of athletes properly tested, the screening program should be accurate, practical to apply under field conditions to large numbers of subjects, and have relatively low cost.

With advances in information communication technology, monitoring can go beyond just telephone calls

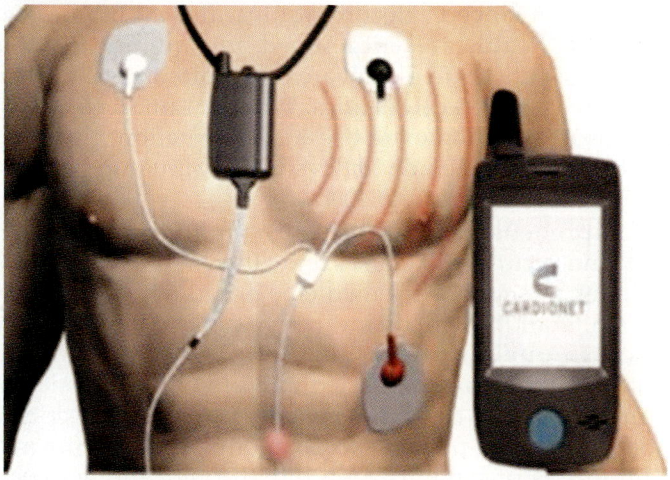


**Fig. 43.2:** The sensor sends ECG information about every heart beat to a small portable monitor

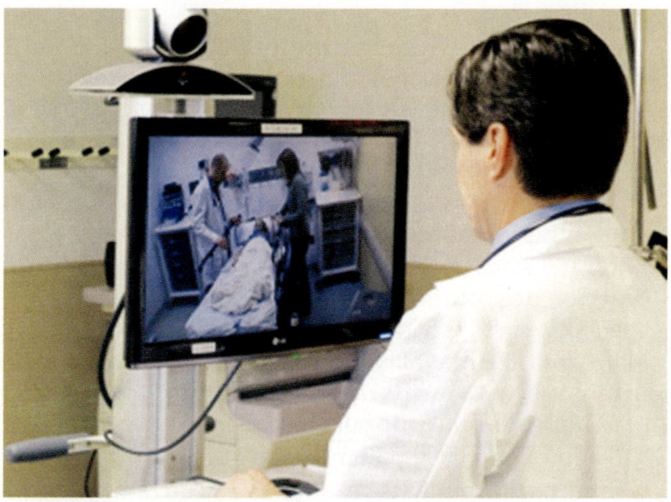

**Fig. 43.3:** The patient is being monitored in ICCU in a remote center through telesystem

requesting patient information. Telemonitoring involves the transfer of physiological data such as blood pressure, weight, electrocardiographic signals, or oxygen saturation through technology such as telephone lines, broadband, satellite, or wireless networks. Similar to structured telephone support, this strategy may lift some of the burden of geographic or funding barriers limiting in-home visits. By incorporating more data, telemonitoring also promises to detect HF deterioration earlier, allowing for more prompt and effective intervention. Two recent meta-analyses have suggested that telemonitoring in ambulatory HF patients can improve mortality by 17–47% during 6–12 months of follow-up and reduce hospitalizations by 7–48%. However, 2 large subsequent randomized controlled trials suggest caution before widely using telemonitoring. In the TELE-HF (Telemonitoring to Improve Heart Failure Outcomes) study, a telephone-based interactive voice-response system that obtained symptom and weight information provided no significant benefit over usual care in terms of all-cause rehospitalization rates or death. Similarly, the TIM-HF (Telemedical Interventional Monitoring in Heart Failure) study was not able to demonstrate a significant impact of telemonitoring on HF-related rehospitalization rates or mortality.

The negative findings of TELE-HF and TIM-HF highlight the complexity of home monitoring interventions. In contrast to more successful implementations of telemonitoring TELE-HF relied on patient-initiated communication; patients had to use a toll-free telephone system in which an automated voice asked a series of questions to which they had to respond by using a keypad. Fourteen percent of patients assigned to the telemonitoring arm never used the automated call-in system, and only 55% were still regularly using the system by the end of the study period. Also, nurses in TELE-HF were not empowered to change the medication regimen without physician consultation, thus adding a layer of communication and delay. Described by Desai and Stevenson as the 'circle of home management of HF', HF home management involves multiple components of which monitoring is only one factor. There also needs to be timely transmission of data, receipt of the information by the appropriate staff who can analyze and act on it, a feedback loop to the patient with directions, and sufficient patient empowerment to understand and implement the instructions. Also, although telemonitoring promises to reduce the need for in-person follow-up, it may actually increase the workload involved. In the TELE-HF study, although there were only 25 patients per site on average, there were 884 incidents per site requiring responses.

Mobile phone-based remote monitoring systems along with application-based support of HF patient education and disease management could be relatively inexpensive and convenient tools to improve HF home management. Mobile phones are now widely available and have considerable computational power, while being relatively inexpensive compared with dedicated remote monitoring hardware. These systems are also portable, enabling patients to be monitored anywhere with mobile phone reception. Initial studies have shown the potential of this approach in HF home management, but further studies are needed. The US Agency for Healthcare Research and Quality has recently provided substantial funding to support research into the use of wireless and telephone care management to reduce HF readmissions.

Patients with ST-elevation myocardial infarction (STEMI) should receive reperfusion therapy as soon as possible to reduce mortality and morbidity. Guidelines recommend primary percutaneous coronary intervention (PCI) as the preferable strategy, if this can be performed in a timely manner. One of the main obstacles to a more widespread use of primary PCI is the limited accessibility to PCI centers operating on a 24-h basis. Thus, to treat STEMI patients within the recommended time limits, early diagnosis is essential in order for patients to be transported to a PCI center in due time. This has led to an increased interest in prehospital diagnosis. The diagnostic modality of choice has been the electrocardiogram (ECG). The ECG is recorded in the field and interpreted by emergency physicians, paramedics or cardiologists receiving the ECG in the hospital by wireless transmission. This method is very robust and has been successfully implemented in several countries worldwide. Prehospital ECG diagnosis and field triage directly to primary PCI has been shown to decrease treatment delay significantly and is associated with a lower mortality. The electrocardiogram is recorded in the ambulance and sent wirelessly to a primary percutaneous coronary intervention center. The electrocardiogram is interpreted by the on-call cardiologist and after talking to the patient and/or paramedic a decision is made to either redirect the patient for primary percutaneous coronary intervention, in case of ST-elevation myocardial infarction, or send the patient to the nearest local hospital for further diagnosis and initial pharmacological therapy. PCI, percutaneous coronary intervention; STEMI, ST-elevation myocardial infarction.

The prehospital use of continuous ECG surveillance in the form of ST monitoring has been shown to provide important prognostic information and might further improve triage for tailored treatment regimens. Both ST monitoring and ECG diagnosis rely on optimal equipment for ECG recording. Through the years new hardware and analysis algorithms along with more practical lead positioning systems have been introduced and might help to further expand the indications and use of prehospital ECG recording and diagnosis.

## INDIAN SCENARIO OF TELEMEDICINE

Telemedicine is an innovative concept that circumvents geography and the nonavailability of trained medical personnel to offer immediate medical treatment and knowledge long distance. Narayana Hrudayalaya Health-city uses advanced telecommunications to administer affordable healthcare with speed and quality to large volumes of patients in distant areas in India, areas that often lack even basic medical facilities. With the same technology, it also shares medical expertise and information with other countries, which include Malaysia, Mauritius, and several sub-Saharan nations (Fig. 43.4).

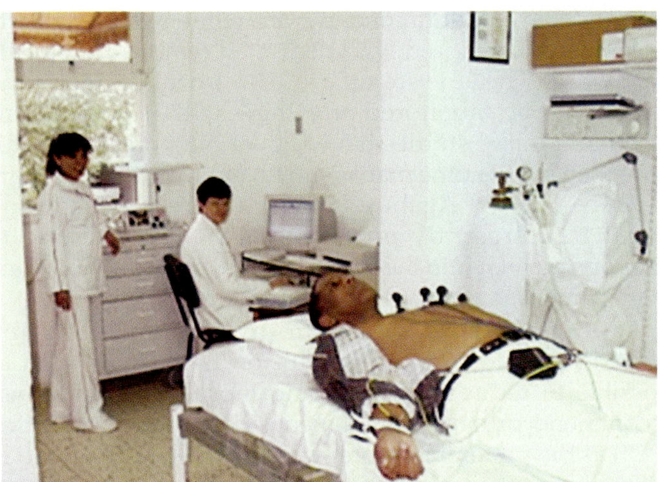

**Fig. 43.4:** An example of a 12-lead-ECG being transmitted via DES cardiovascular emergency situations follow the online tele-ECG transmission. In a nonemergency case, such as a routine clinical evaluation, ECG will be transmitted via internet. As a first step, ECG online transmission requires a phone call from a medical doctor or a nurse to the remote cardiologist advising that an ECG is being transmitted for analysis

Comprehensive medical solutions for emergencies, quick and accurate diagnoses and efficient patient care are the hallmarks of our telemedicine programme. Coronary care units and telemedicine centres in rural sectors are linked to our hospitals. Senior specialists sitting in tertiary centres guide paramedics and general physicians in remote areas to conduct screenings and stabilise critical patients. Free out-patient consultation is offered from afar to hundreds of patients each day through the network. Satellite connectivity is provided free of cost by the Indian Space Research Organisation (ISRO), and high speed telephone or integrated services digital network connectivity is also used.

Telemedicine diagnoses are often the first point of contact with overseas patients entering our international outreach programme, and the technology is subsequently useful for follow-up consultations once they are back in their home countries post-treatment.

Over the years, the telemedicine facility has grown to the following numbers:

- ISRO network covers 332 hospitals–299 remote/rural/district hospitals/health centers connected to 33 specialty hospitals located in major cities
- Narayana Hrudayalaya has created a network of 4–5 intensive care units and 20 telemedicine centers providing 24-hour support to patients
- Treated over 53,000 patients over the past 10 years
- Connected to patients in Malaysia, Tanzania, Nigeria, Burundi, Zambia, and Bangladesh
- Over 550 CME programmes conducted in the past 5 years

### Services Offered by Our Telemedicine Department

#### *Hrudaya Post*

All the district head post offices in Karnataka (25 in number) have been connected to Narayana Hrudayalaya through internet and software applications. A patient with medical reports could always walk in any district head PO with his medical reports hand it over to the postal staff for uploading the documents may it be paper documents, ECG or an angiogram. They would receive the analyzed reports within 24 hrs which would be handed over the counter or delivered to the doorstep of the patient by post. The services charges of the postal department vary from ₹100 to 125 depending on the number of documents and the post charges would be charged extra.

### Specifications for Setting up a Telemedicine Unit

The World Health Organisation defines telemedicine as 'The delivery of health care services, where distance is a

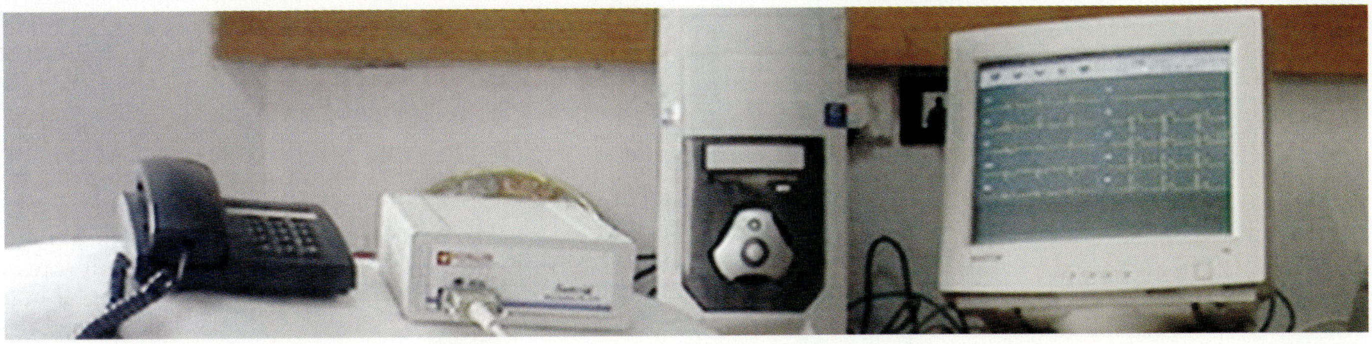

**Fig. 43.5:** Laboratory equipment in telemedicine. From left—telephone, ambulatory BP monitor and computer monitor has been connected to internet for transmission of data to a remotely placed specialist

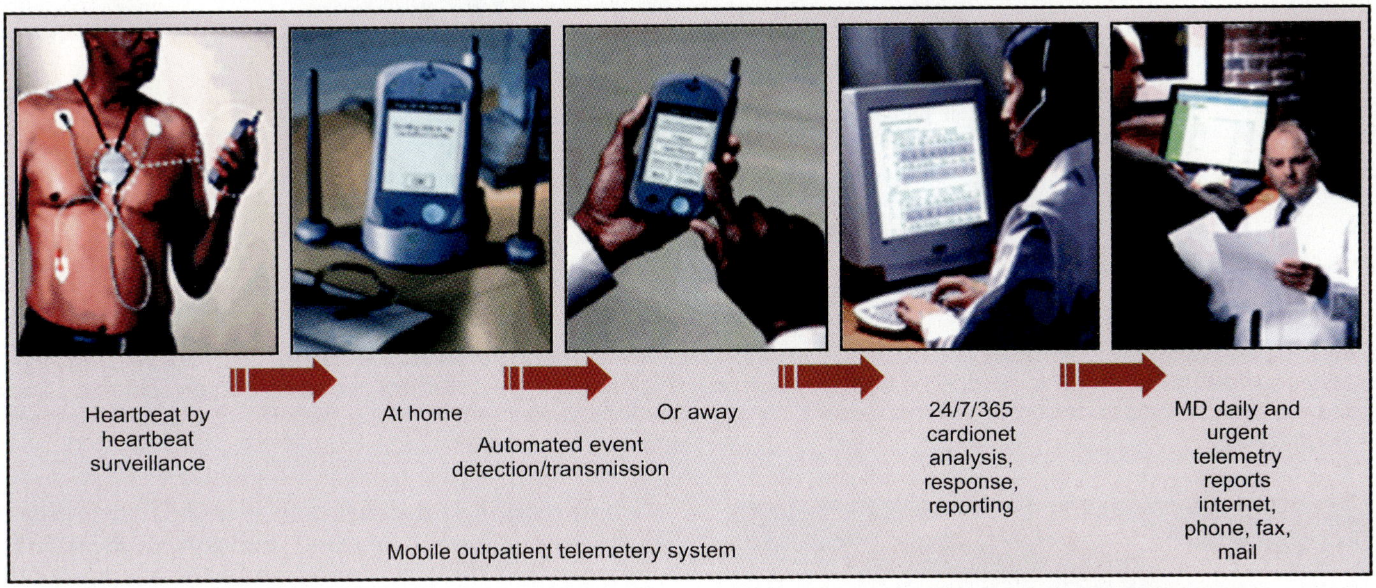


**Fig. 43.6:** Mobile cardiac outpatient telemetry (MCOT) system which reports patients cardiac records daily to the registered specialist through either fax or internet services

critical factor, by all healthcare professionals using information and communication technologies for the exchange of valid information for diagnosis, treatment and prevention of disease and injuries, research and evaluation, and for the continuing education of healthcare providers, all in the interests of advancing the health of individuals and their communities' (Figs 43.5–43.8).

### Required Infrastructure

An **airconditioned, soundproof room** with electrical outlets for connecting various equipments and a very good earthing pit.

### Recommendation

Five 15 amps sockets for UPS, five 5 amps socket for other diagnostic equipments, UPS of at least 3 kVA capacity. Curtains/Walls preferably light blue or Gray in color to give good contrast for video conferencing.

### Video Conferencing Hardware

A **television** preferably with 29 inches screen. Alternatively, if tele continuing medical education (CMEs) are planned a LCD projection on to a big screen.

*A Video conferencing system:* These can be:

1. Standalone codec based system (recommended)
2. PC based using PC add-on card codec
3. PC based with in-camera codec
4. PC based Web camera and software only codec.

### IT Hardware

A computer with printer and a scanner (capable of scanning X-ray films also or alternatively a X-ray digitiser).

Data such as images and video pictures that are not in digital format require to be converted to digital format for transmission. This is done using 'Codec' units (short for coder/decoder).

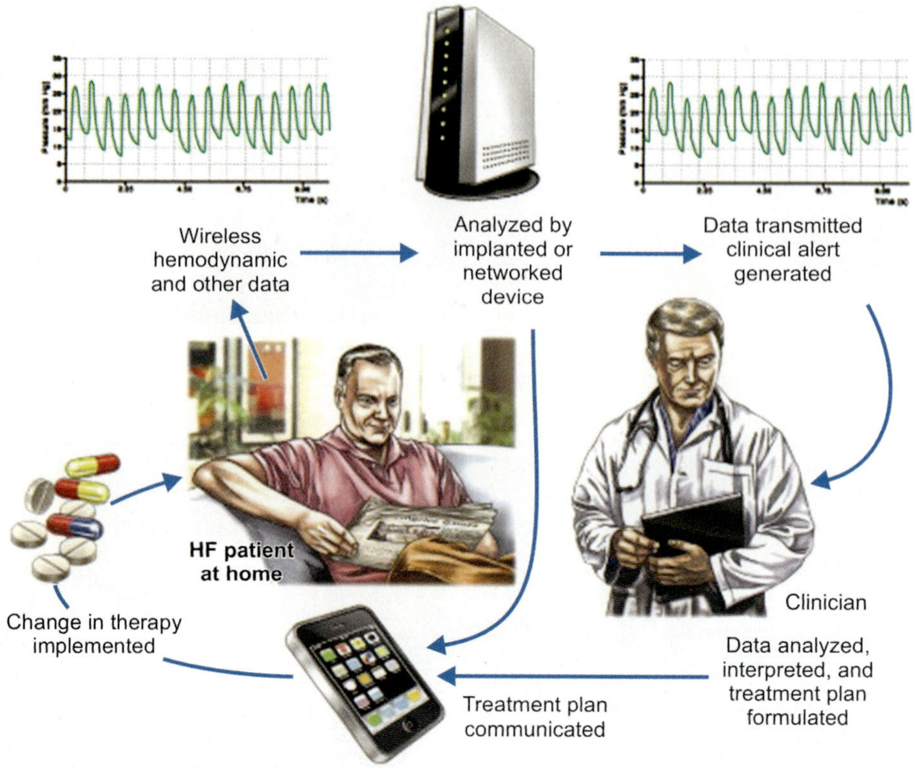


**Fig. 43.7:** Home hemodynamic monitoring of chronic HF changes in therapy can potentially be made more rapidly in response to wirelessly collected hemodynamic data. Even before symptoms develop, data are collected and alerts can be sent to a clinician for review or personalized treatment recommendations can be automatically generated on the basis of a prespecified algorithm (HF=heart failure)

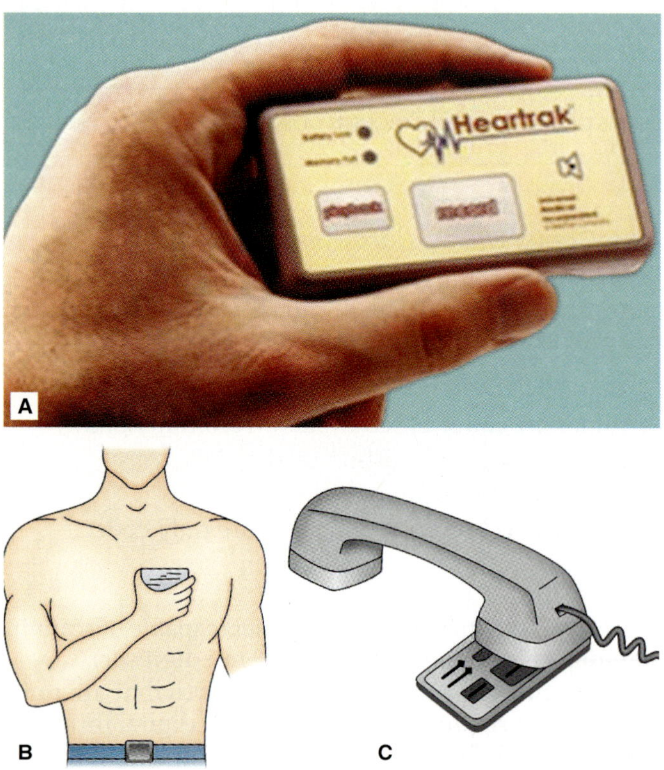


**Fig. 43.8:** (A) Heart tak monitor. (B) A patient placing the same over the heart area for record of ECG. (C) A telephone through which the recorded information is transmitted

Compression softwares help transmit large files in shorter time. Digital imaging and communications in medicine (DICOM) compression is the recommended standard for transmitting medical images.

### Connectivity Hardware

- Can be either terrestrial or satellite based.
- Terrestrial communication can be through analog modems, DSL modems, ISDN and broadband.
- Satellite communication is usually through VSATs (very small aperture terminals). Provides much better image transfer quality than terrestrial mode of communication as well as instantaneous global coverage.

### Medical Hardware

Various instrumentation that can be connected to the video-conferencing unit to directly relay data from the patient are:

- Digital 12-lead ECG, electronic stethescope, digital microscope, digital blood pressure monitor, skin camera, Doppler ultrasound and echocardiography equipment, etc.
- Stored images such as X-rays, ultrasound images, CT/MRI images or pathology slide images can be scanned in to a computer and transmitted. Moving video images of echocardiography can be transmitted by connecting the video player/DVD player to the video-conferencing system.

### Telecardiology Procedure

A transtelephonic monitor is a small electronic device used to record a patient's heart rhythm. Unlike other ambulatory monitors, the transtelephonic monitor (TTM) does not continuously record the heart rhythm over a short period of time. Instead, it is given to the patient for an extended period of time (weeks to months) and activated by the patient at the push of a button. The data from the TTM is then transmitted to our office (Figs 43.9 and 43.10).

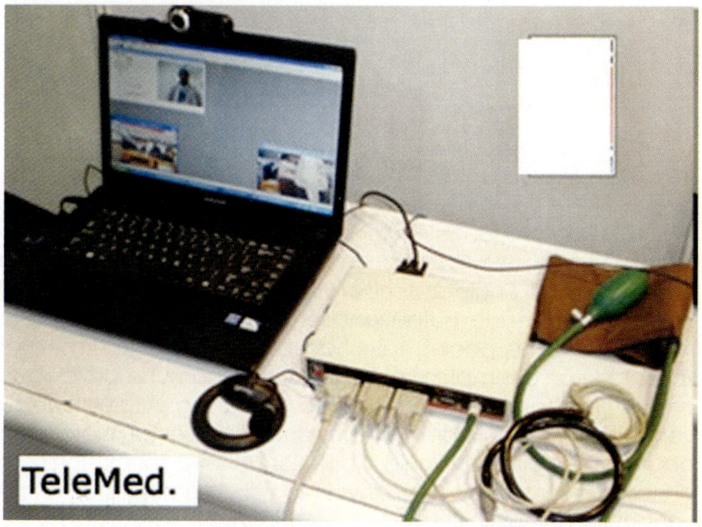


**Fig. 43.9:** Laboratory equipment in telemedicine

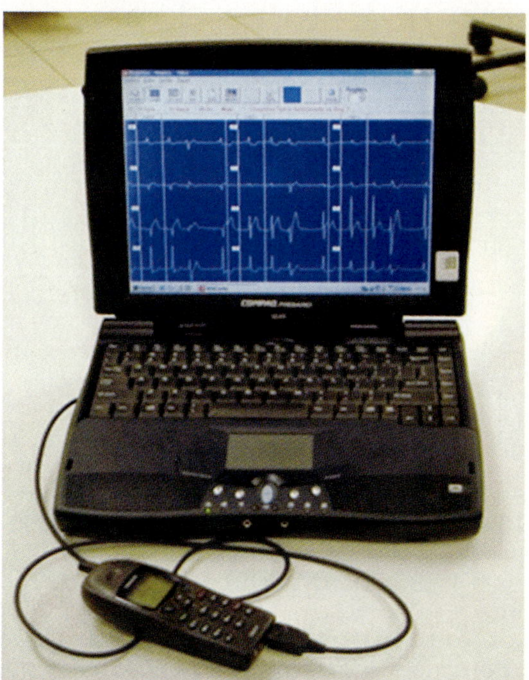

**Fig. 43.10:** Remote computer connected to a mobile phone of the digital tele-ECG system. The PC Anywhere 32 is the telecommunication software, which is installed in the host and the remote computers, a system that allows data transmission via phone for remote analysis

The device used for storing and transmitting the ECG was a portable electrocardiograph (Cardiette Excel 106 scp) with an internal modem and a capability of connecting to an external one with a transmission speed of up to 19.2 kbps. An important feature of the electrocardiograph was the compression of data before transmission, which allowed high quality 12-lead recordings to be sent in small files. In the absence of a fixed telephone line (POTS), a dual-band GSM (900/1800 MHz) modem was used (Siemens TC35 terminal) working with the circuit switched data (CSD) bearer service of a national operator with more than 99% geographical coverage and a nontransparent data rate of 9.6 kbps. The data calls from the electrocardiograph were terminated at a workstation running the software package Medibox Cardiobox of H&C Medical Devices SpA and connected with a modem to the POTS. The communication between the cardiologist sitting in front of this workstation and the medical team in the field for reporting was always carried out with a mobile phone. Following the initial assessment, 58 athletes were given further appointments for echocardiography, stress test, and 24-hour Holter monitoring of ECG or blood pressure.

Descriptive statistics were used to describe categorical variables. For statistical analysis, the statistics toolbox of MATLAB was used (The Mathworks Inc., MA, USA). The correlation coefficient was derived to assess the association between the reception level of GSM and the number of failed transmissions. A $P < .05$ was accepted as statistically significant.

### Telephonic ECG

T-ECG (telephonic ECG) is a mobile application for mobile devices. It replaces the remote central program for demodulate the audio signal produced by transtelephonic ECG devices and, displays, analyzes and archives the resulting chart (Fig. 43.11).

Mobile transtelephonic devices usually record 12-lead ECGs and transform the original electrical signals of the heart in a FM audio signal that can be transmitted over normal phone lines.

T-ECG converts the acoustic analog signal produced by the transtelephonic ECG devices in a digital representation and stores it in your mobile.

#### *Functions*

1. Demodulates the audio FM signal produced by the ECG device and stores digitally the signal;
2. Reconstructs the original analog signal and play it if necessary;
3. Displays the complete ECG chart on the screen;
4. Displays a detailed view of any single lead;
5. Produces a PDF document with the ECG;
6. Creates a patient record with basic information (name, age, sex, etc.);
7. Sends by mail the digital version in XML format to other device running T-ECG;
8. Sends by mail the PDF document with cardiologist diagnostic.

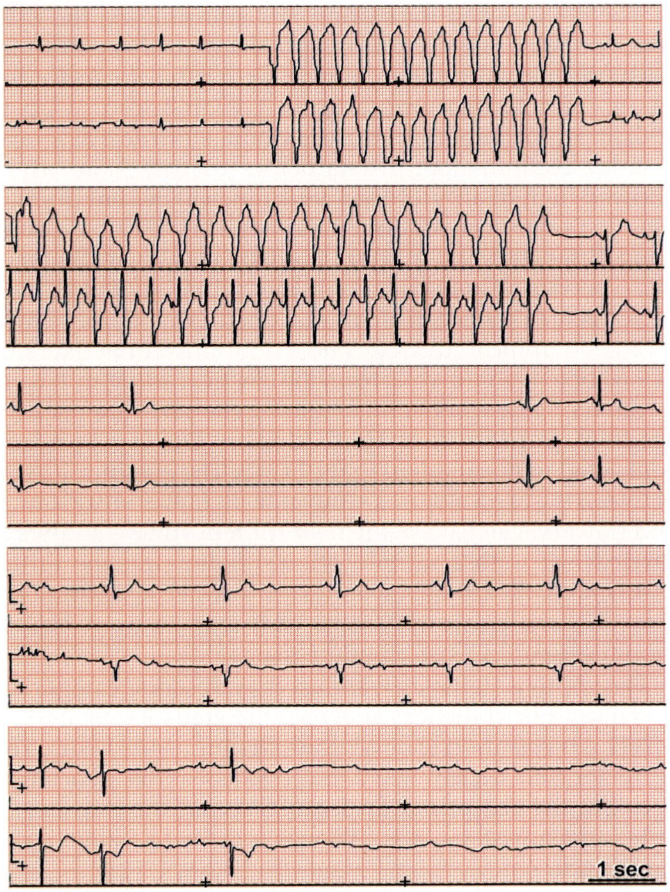


**Fig. 43.11:** Examples for cardiac arrhythmias in patients with acute cerebrovascular diseases detected by continuous telemetric ECG monitoring. The corresponding 2-trace ECG strips are shown. From top to bottom—nonsustained ventricular tachycardia HR=180 beats/min; spontaneous termination of a supraventricular tachycardia with pre-existing left bundle branch block; sinus arrest >5 seconds; AV block second degree; a systole in the context of atrial fibrillation (ECG=electrocardiogram; HR=heart rate; AV=atrioventricular)

## Electrocardiogram Recording before Reaching Referral Hospital

In the 1970s, Uhley reported their experiences in transmitting single-lead telemetry from the ambulance to the hospital for arrhythmia monitoring in patients with suspected cardiovascular disease. For several years, however, it was not possible to transmit a diagnostic-quality 12-lead ECG due to technical difficulties and unstable data networks. In 1987, Grim et al. published a paper on successful implementation of diagnostic-quality, 12-lead ECG transmission using new error-correcting digital transmission via cellular phone links. The new transmission technology was validated in other studies, showing the possible benefit of early and reliable diagnosis of acute myocardial infarction (Figs 43.12–43.17).

In the late 1990s the terms STEMI and non-ST-elevation acute myocardial infarction were introduced to ensure a more clinically and therapeutically relevant triage of acute myocardial infarction patients. This primarily relied on the

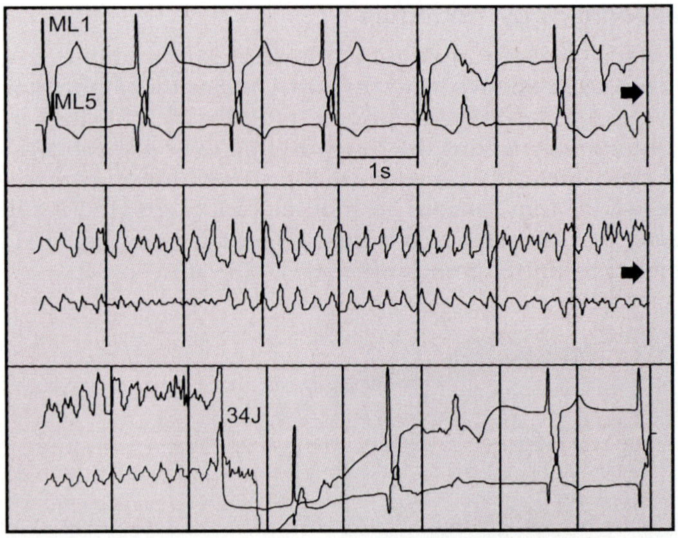


**Fig. 43.12:** Two-channel Holter monitor of an episode of sotalol-induced ventricular fibrillation in a patient with an implantable defibrillator with single-chamber ventricular pacing. Sotalol had been started in the outpatient setting for the suppression of recurrent AF. The pacing rate had been left programmed at 44 bpm in an attempt to maintain AV synchrony. He developed bradycardia with continuous ventricular pacing. A late-coupled ventricular premature beat initiates an episode of TdP that rapidly degenerates into ventricular fibrillation. A 34-J shock from the defibrillator terminates the arrhythmia with re-emergence of the ventricular paced rhythm

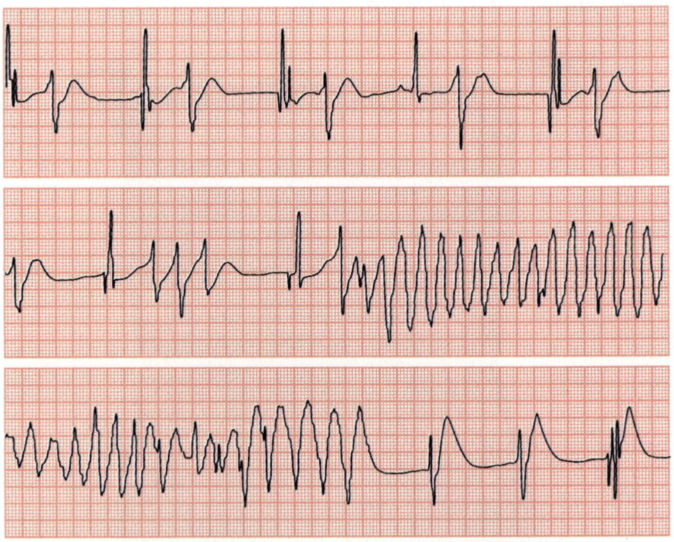

**Fig. 43.13:** Continuous telemetry strip showing episode of TdP in a patient with a dual-chamber pacemaker. This 75-year-old woman with sinus node dysfunction was started on quinidine and diltiazem in the hospital. The normally functioning pacemaker was programmed to the DDD mode with a lower rate of 50 beats per minute. She developed a junctional escape rhythm at around 50 bpm. Late-coupled ventricular bigeminy is followed by a three-beat run of ventricular tachycardia and then a 6-second run of TdP. The apparent ventricular undersensing is the result of 'safety pacing' after sensing the ventricular electrogram in the nonphysiologic AV delay period after the atrial artifact. Torsades de pointes was suppressed by increasing the pacing rate

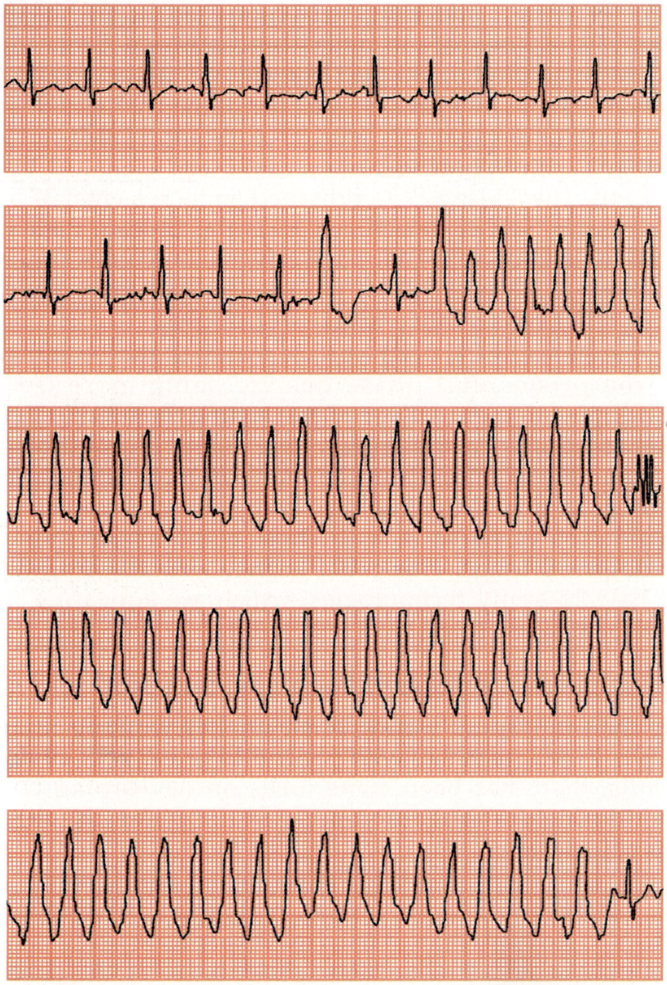

**Fig. 43.14:** Heart tak recorded ECG trace in which patient had SVT (top), VPC (middle) and finally ended up with ventricular tachycardia (bottom)

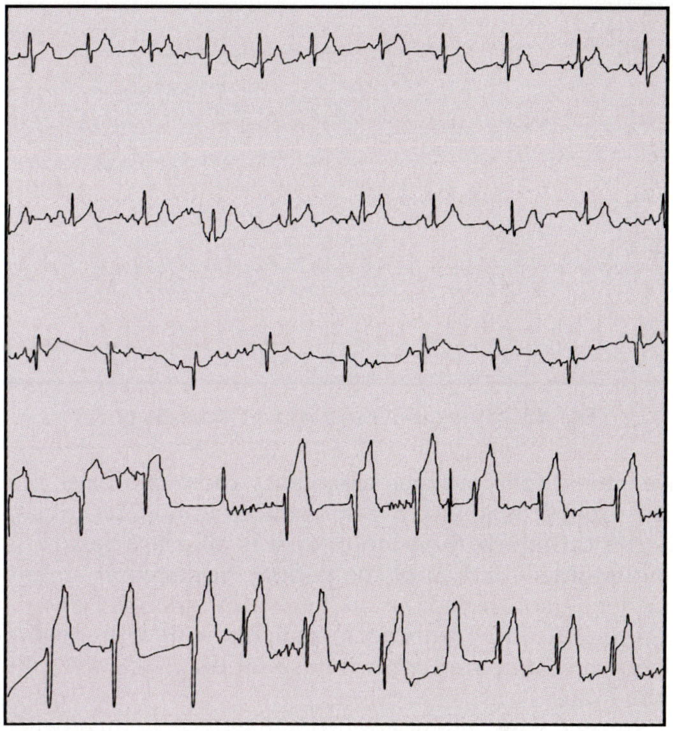

**Fig. 43.15:** Tele-ECG showing S-T elevation in V1–V6 as seen in acute anterior wall MI

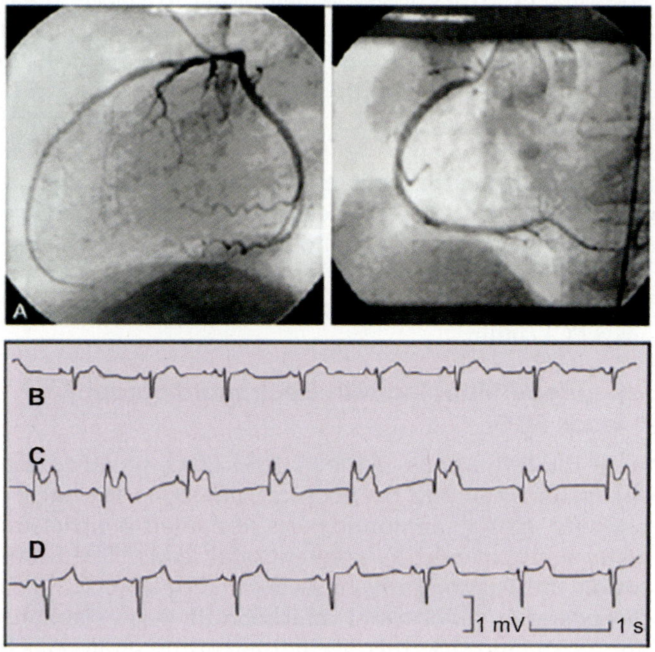


**Fig. 43.16:** (A) Angiograms showing only mild coronary disease, (B) Reference ECG. (C) ECG recorded during episode of palpitations, angina, and shortness of breath showing marked ST-segment elevation. (D) ECG recorded 5 minutes after episode; note that ST-segment is almost back to normal

large thrombolysis trials showing an improved outcome with the immediate use of lytic therapy for patients with STEMI. Early reperfusion therapy thereby became an important objective in the optimal treatment of STEMI and this led to a further interest in early diagnosis and optimal triage. In 2000, Wall et al. reported that prehospital diagnosis of acute myocardial infarction was associated with more rapid reperfusion therapy by thrombolysis, but the focus was still mainly on the in-hospital, emergency department delays in diagnosis.

However, this changed as several randomized trials and meta-analyses proved primary PCI to be a superior reperfusion strategy in STEMI patients, if performed in a timely manner.The limited access to PCI centers increased the focus on early diagnosis, allowing the patient direct admission or transfer to a PCI center as soon as possible.

In 2005, Terkelsen et al. demonstrated the benefit of prehospital ECG diagnosis and field triage to a primary PCI center in patients with STEMI. The study comprised 161 patients. A prehospital ECG was recorded in 106 patients, of them admitted directly to a primary PCI center. The time from first medical contact to balloon was a median 81 min shorter in patients with prehospital diagnosis and field triage compared to patients diagnosed in the hospital. Prehospital ECG diagnosis and field triage not only allows

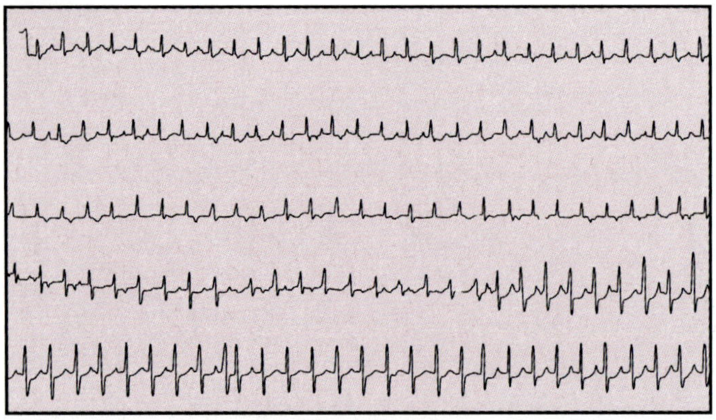

**Fig. 43.17:** Tele-ECG showing an episode of SVT

the patient to bypass the emergency room of a local, non-PCI-capable hospital, it also reduces in-hospital delays, as the catheterization laboratory is able to prepare for the imminent arrival of the patient. Sejersten et al. have further demonstrated this. In their study, door-to-PCI delay was significantly reduced in patients with a prehospital diagnosis compared with inhospital diagnosis (34 vs 97 min, P<.001).

Studies from many countries have reproduced these results despite varying geographic settings, health-care organizations and prehospital logistic set-ups.

Recently Sorensen et al. evaluated the routine use of prehospital ECG diagnosis and field triage in a larger region comprising both urban and rural surroundings. The authors found that prehospital diagnosis and triage reduces the importance of distance to primary PCI center, in as much as time from first medical contact to balloon inflation only varied 9 min between patients belonging to urban versus rural hospitals, with a median 10 km versus 40 km distance to the PCI center (further the study showed a decreased mortality in patients with prehospital diagnosis and triage. A recent Dutch study further emphasized the importance and value of prehospital diagnosis for patients living far from a PCI center.

## Body-surface Mapping with Electrocardiography (80-leads ECG)

One of the limitations of the 12-lead ECG, whether used in-hospital or in the prehospital phase, is the lack of sensitivity. Not all anatomic parts of the left ventricle are equally well covered by conventional leads. The infarct location most commonly missed on 12-lead ECG is the inferoposterior myocardial infarction. It was established many years ago that this limitation can be overcome by using additional leads, like V7–V9. Actual body-surface mapping often uses an 80-lead ECG, which improves the ability to detect acute myocardial infarction and thus improve the sensitivity of electrocardiography in large clinical series. The sensitivity for detection of troponin-confirmed acute myocardial infarction approaches 80% and c-statistics improve with a factor of almost 0.10.Right ventricular involvement complicating inferior STEMI can also be better detected by 80-lead body-surface mapping ECG. Recently a randomized trial compared the prevalence, clinical care patterns, and clinical outcomes of patients with STEMI identified on 80-lead but not on 12-lead (80-lead-only STEMI). The primary outcome of the trial was door-to-sheath time in patients with 80-lead-only STEMI versus patients with STEMI identified by 12-lead alone (12-lead STEMI). The 80-lead ECG provided an incremental 27.5% increase in STEMI detection versus the 12-lead. Patients with 80-lead-only STEMI have adverse outcomes similar to those of 12-lead STEMI patients but are treated with delayed or conservative invasive strategies.

The 80-lead ECG body-surface map has also been used in the prehospital phase despite being more time-consuming to mount. Even in this setting the sensitivity of the acute myocardial infarction detection method is comparable to findings in the more protected in-hospital setting. Despite these findings, body-surface mapping for evaluation of patients with chest pain has not gained widespread usage. This could change with the invention of easy to apply technologies, which are appearing for commercial use (Figs 43.18 and 43.19).

## Novel Electrocardiogram Recording and Lead System

As the prehospital setting often implies working under difficult circumstances with patients in a very poor clinical status, there has been some focus on developing ECG monitoring systems for simple, fast application with a durable design.

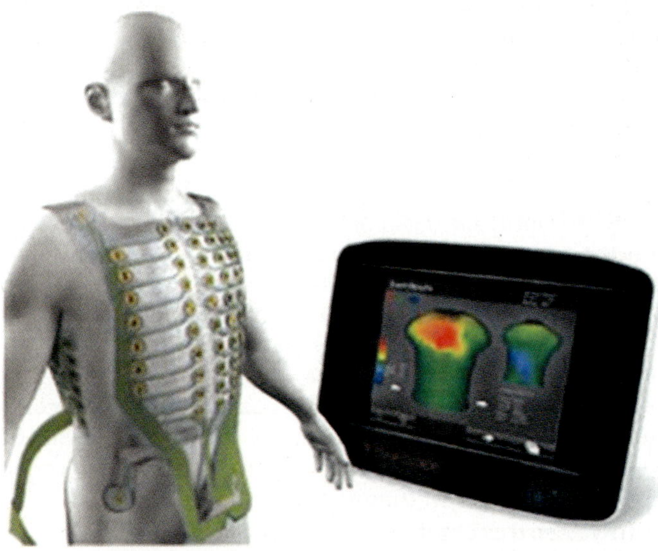

**Fig. 43.18:** Heartscape 80-lead 3D ECG system—Heartscape 80-lead 3D ECG system. The concept is not entirely new, as it is the successor to the PRIME ECG system which has the same amount of leads, and has been available since 2003. The Heartscape 3D ECG system aims to give a 360 degree electrocardiographic view of the heart, to helping in identifying myocardial infarcts without ST-segment elevation on traditional 12-lead ECGs, and in patients with left bundle branch block.Compared to traditional 12-lead ECG's, the system has shown to be more sensitive while retaining comparable specificity in detecting acute infarcts

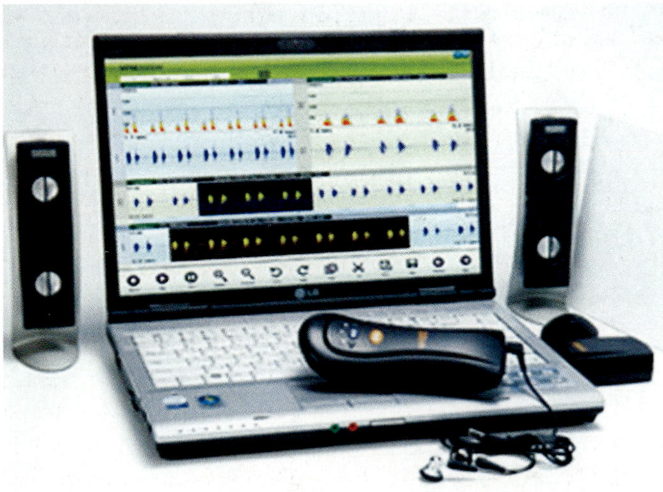

**Fig. 43.19:** AMD-3130 E-Scope stethoscope. The AMD-3130 E-Scope stethoscope utilizes state of the art electronic technology to amplify heart, breath and Korotkoff sounds so they become much easier to hear. The sound is pure and clean. Compared to acoustic stethoscopes, murmurs and faint lows are much more distinguishable

One such system (the EASI lead system), using only 4 leads to extract a full, diagnostic '12-lead' ECG, has been compared with a conventional 12-lead ECG by Sejersten et al. The authors report that the 4-lead EASI system was just as good for detecting acute, myocardial ischemia as the standard 12-lead ECG. Drew et al. also investigated the use of a more simple lead system in the synthesized 12-lead ST monitoring and real-time tele-electrocardiography initiative. The 5-lead ECG system used in this series of studies has proven effective in diagnosing ischemia and has reduced treatment delay in the study region (Northern California, United States).

## Telemeteric Healthcare and Device Monitoring

The combination of an aging population and continued developments of modern therapy within cardiology and internal medicine in general have led to an increasing prevalence of chronic diseases, including heart failure, and the need for implantable devices. This development has increased the need for continued and close contact between the patient and the healthcare system to ensure the optimal treatment for the individual. Consequently, the healthcare system is challenged by the still-increasing need for qualified healthcare professionals, and resources in general, as well as increasing costs. One way to approach this challenge is the use of telehealthcare, allowing the patient to be in close contact with the appropriate healthcare provider and exchanging valuable information needed for managing the patient's disease (Fig. 43.20).

Telehealthcare is defined as personal healthcare over a distance and consists of the following components—(a) data provided by the patient (e.g. blood pressure, pulse, weight, subjective information about health); (b) electronic transmission of data from the patient to a healthcare professional, and (c) personalized feedback tailored to the individual patient. Telehealthcare can be based on either real-time (synchronous), store-and-forward (asynchronous), or hybrid systems. Synchronous telehealthcare requires the availability of patient and healthcare provider at the same time and real-time processing of the patient's data, while asynchronous telehealthcare provides more flexibility for both the patient and healthcare provider.

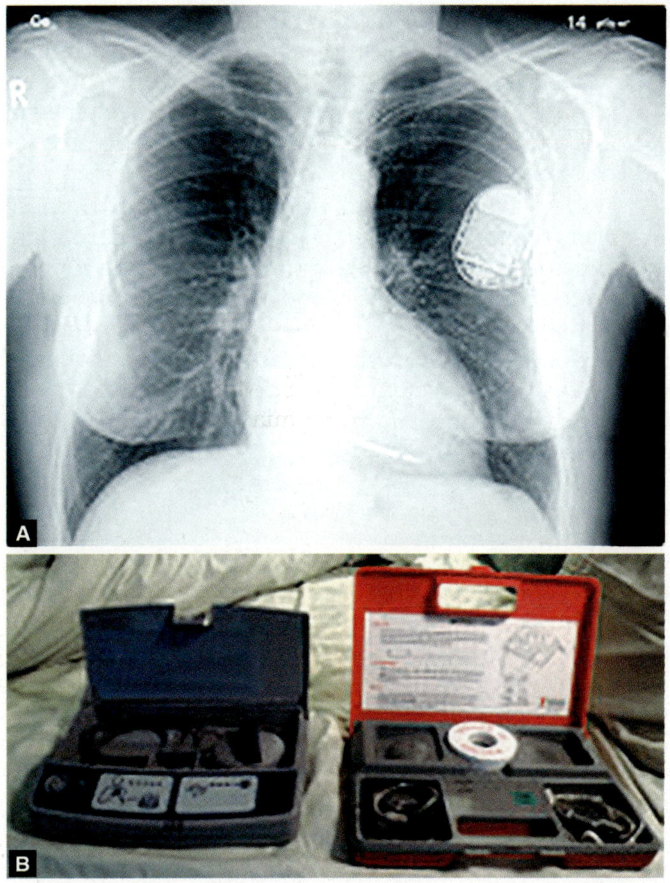


**Fig. 43.20:** (A) X-ray image of installed pacemaker showing wire routing. (B) Two types of remote monitoring devices used by pacemaker patients

The technology used in telehealthcare is a composite of portable medical imaging devices (e.g. blood pressure device), computer/smart phone, and the wireless communication infrastructure, requiring a stable network for data transmission. The transmitted data may then be stored at a receiving station for momentary or later processing and review.

Four generations of telehealthcare for remote management of patients have been proposed, a system of nonreactive data collection and analysis, with asynchronous transmission of data to a healthcare provider, e.g. from an event recorder, a system with a nonimmediate analytical or decision-making structure, with synchronous data transfer, allowing the healthcare provider to view data and recognize important changes, but delays may occur if the system is only active during the day, a remote patient management system with consistent analytical and decision-making support by a healthcare personal, even outside of office hours, and a fully integrated remote management system, where data from both invasive and noninvasive telemedical devices are linked in a telemedical platform and available for both the primary care provider and the telemedical center.

A wide variety of both noninvasive and invasive variables are available for telehealthcare within cardiology. Most are recorded manually by the patients via a device (e.g. systolic and diastolic blood pressure, pulse, 3-lead ECG, heart rate variability, bodyweight, oxygen saturation, blood glucose, natriuretic peptides). Others obtained from invasive devices are recorded automatically (e.g. impedance, incidence of arrhythmias, pulmonary and left atrial pressure.

## TELEMEDICINE AND HEART FAILURE

Heart failure is associated with substantial morbidity, mortality, and healthcare costs. Patients are often followed closely in heart failure clinics but admittance to a cardiology department is frequently required, and the 30-day readmission rate is high. Telehealthcare may be a solution, providing a way to identify and monitor subclinical congestion. The earlier identification and treatment of congestion together with improved coordination of care may prevent hospitalization (Figs 43.21–43.23).

Ideally, contact between a patient and a healthcare provider is established with technology enabling the two parties to see and hear each other via a microphone and a computer screen over large distances using a telephone or

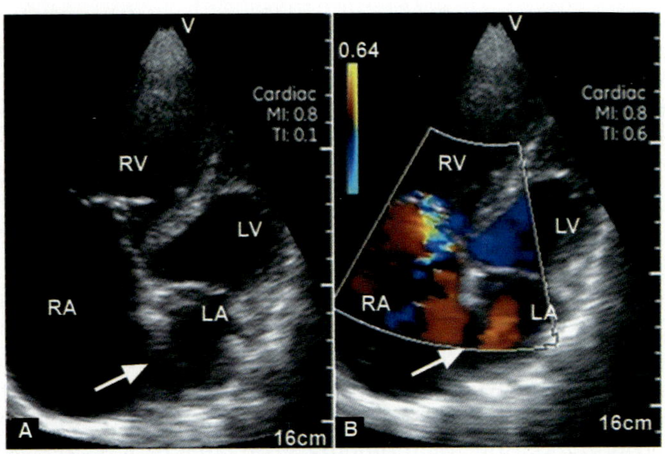


**Fig. 43.21:** Representative images taken from a 43-year-old man without a medical history presenting for evaluation of dyspnea from a remote place. The point-of-care diagnosis by the cardiology fellow properly identified the marked right ventricular dysfunction (parasternal long-axis view and abnormal motion typical of right ventricular overload. The fellow suspected an atrial septal defect on the basis of the suggestive echo dropout on apical four-chamber view (white arrowhead in A) but color flow Doppler, (B) did not demonstrate shunting across the atrial septum. Expert overread did not affirm the diagnosis of atrial septal defect

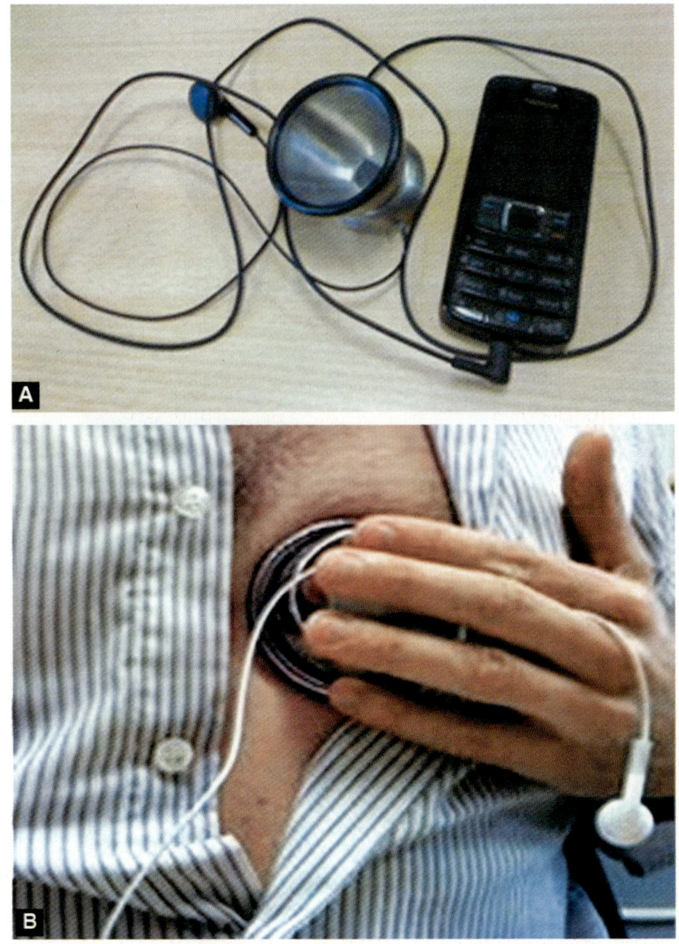

**Fig. 43.22:** (A) Mobile phone stethoscope and (B) its applicability over the chest of the patient

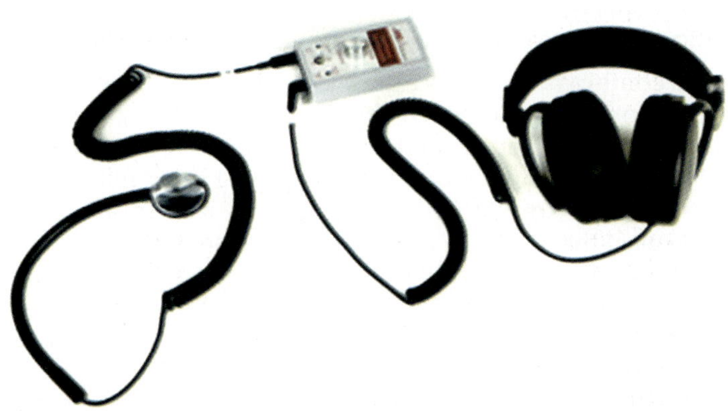

**Fig. 43.23:** AMD-3700 telephonic. It features low data bandwidth and high performance. Each module can operate on either transmit or receive mode auscultation bandwidth—20–1,400 Hz at low data communications bandwidth (19.2 kbps). Plugging chest piece automatically switches unit from send to receive mode bell/diaphragm (B/D) switch to enhance auscultation exam for both cardiac and pulmonary systems. Detachable chest piece assembly and detachable headset

satellite connection. One device is installed in the patient's home and one at the heart failure clinic. Preferably the patient's device is portable and capable of both videoconference and data transmission, and can be managed by the healthcare professional using a remote control.

According to individual arrangements patients could be instructed to record blood pressure, heart rhythm and weight, and give a subjective description of symptoms every morning, and then transmit data daily, just prior to or during a scheduled remote follow-up. Data can then be reviewed just before the videoconference with the patient, so treatment can be altered if needed. It is important that the healthcare professional be empowered to change medication regimens so delay is diminished and the correct treatment established in a timely manner.

Several advantages of the use of telehealthcare in heart failure have been reported. Patients get a better understanding of their disease by being responsible for monitoring and being involved in some self-managing, which enhances patient education and empowerment. This supports adherence to the planned treatment, but also ensures preventive care with early detection of disease exacerbations and timely management. Travel and waiting time is reduced or even abolished for the patient, and quality of life improves. Additionally, patients are at home in comfortable and safe surroundings and still in close contact with the hospital. An advantage for the hospital is that the technology leaves room for new and unstable patients, and long admittances to hospital may be prevented.

However, the effectiveness of telehealthcare by reducing morbidity and mortality in heart failure patients has not been established because results have been conflicting. Accordingly, meta-analyses have suggested that telehealthcare reduced morbidity and mortality but 2 prospective randomized clinical trials not including the metaanalyses did not support those findings. A possible explanation for this difference may be that the meta-analyses combined many small dissimilar studies of patients with varying risk profiles followed for different durations of time and with differences between studies in the intervention used. A newly published prospective randomized trial of 3230 patients with either obstructive pulmonary disease or heart failure showed that telehealthcare was associated with lower mortality, emergency admission rates, and shorter length of admission. An ongoing Danish study randomizes chronic heart failure patients to either traditional treatment in outpatient clinics or monitoring by telehealthcare. Another part of the study randomizes patients admitted with acute heart failure to traditional treatment in hospital versus early discharge and daily contact with the hospital via telehealthcare. The hypothesis is that at-home treatment of heart failure patients is feasible, effective, and safe, and thereby releases resources to other patient groups (personal communication).

In the studies mentioned above telehealthcare was based on noninvasive data, but other studies have investigated the management of heart failure patients using data from implantable devices. An increase in pulmonary vascular congestion is reflected by increased impedance, and thus intrathoracic impedance monitoring may be a valuable tool in the management of heart failure in patients, such as those with an implantable cardioverter-defibrillator (ICD). This is supported by a study that found significantly greater sensitivity to predict worsening heart failure events for intrathoracic impedance monitoring compared to acute weight increase. Likewise, left ventricular filling pressures and pulmonary artery pressures are correlated with clinical congestion, functional limitation, and poor prognosis in heart failure patients. Since the intracardiac and pulmonary artery pressures increase several days to weeks before the onset of clinical symptoms of congestion, close monitoring may provide early warning and assist appropriate management, including changes in medication. Abraham et al. used a wireless implantable hemodynamic monitoring system to measure pulmonary artery pressure, and reported that the use of the system significantly reduced the duration of hospital stays and the rate of hospital admissions related to heart failure, the latter by 30%.

In a study that monitored left atrial pressure, this monitoring was associated with reduced risk of acute decompensation and death. Additional randomized clinical trials using third- or fourth-generation telemedical systems that combine noninvasive and invasive variables with daily monitoring and management are needed to fully clarity the value of telehealthcare in cardiology.

## IMPLANTABLE DEVICES MONITORING WITH TELEMEDICINE

The number of patients with pacemakers and ICDs has increased tremendously over the years as indications have broadened to include more patient groups. According to guidelines, patients with a pacemaker or an ICD need a follow-up at 3–12 months and 3–6 months, respectively. Usually the follow-up visits include both an evaluation of the device function (including battery status and capture thresholds) and a clinical examination, which may result in reprogramming of the device or changes in medical treatment. These time-consuming visits can be a burden to the patient, as they often require long transportation, waiting time, and time off work. For the outpatient clinic, the many visits require both space and a large staff because of the workload associated with every visit.

Remote monitoring and remote follow-up by the use of telehealthcare offers an alternative management strategy. Preferably, the system should be able to automatically transmit data stored in the device to the outpatient clinic using the wireless global system for mobile communication network or a landline. Automatic wireless data transmission requires a pacemaker or ICD equipped with a micro-antenna for communication with a transmitter located close to the patient. This setup diminishes the need for patient compliance and increases the frequency of transmissions.

Several companies provide systems for automatic wireless data transmission. Data stored in the device's memory (e.g. battery voltage, lead characteristics, arrhythmias, and alerts) can be transmitted. The alerts may be based on a change in device performance (battery status, lead impedance), programming (disabling of ventricular fibrillation therapy, insufficient safety margins for sensing or capture), or medical data (arrhythmias, indication of lung fluid accumulation). Events that trigger an alert can be defined according to the individual patient. Data is usually transmitted to a central database, where it is processed and made available to the physician on a secure webpage. Additional notification by e-mail, SMS, fax, or phone messages may be valuable when critical data are available for consultation.

Many pacemakers and ICDs can automatically run tests like battery status, lead impedances, sensing and capture thresholds that used to be manually performed at the outpatient clinic. Both scheduled follow-up, with transmission of predefined data, and unscheduled monitoring can then be performed. Daily monitoring allows transmission of data with any predefined alerts to a physician. Consequently, remote monitoring may improve patient safety and quality of care. Depending on the need for reprogramming, clinic follow-ups are still needed because due to safety issues no system yet allows remote device programming.

The safety and clinical benefits conferred by telehealthcare in patients with implantable devices have been validated in several studies. In the COMPAS trial, long-term remote monitoring of pacemaker recipients was a safe substitute for conventional follow-ups, decreased the number of ambulatory visits, and enabled early detection of important clinical and device-related adverse events. Another study showed that half of the regularly scheduled visits could be omitted by the use of remote monitoring, without impairing patient safety. Additionally, only 6% of patients undergo device reprogramming or admittance to hospital during clinic visits, and thus 94% of these visits might as well be executed by remote monitoring. Remote monitoring could diagnose 99% of arrhythmia- or device-related problems in patients with an ICD, when combined with a clinical follow-up. In addition to fewer scheduled clinic visits, unscheduled visits following an ICD shock might be prevented by remote follow-up; after such an event the patient may perform manual upload of data, transmitted to the healthcare provider for immediate determination of whether the shock was appropriate or not, and whether device reprogramming or medical modifications are needed. Finally, several studies have demonstrated that remote monitoring reduces the time to event recognition and diagnosis and the time from the event to a clinical decision for the individual patient.

Remote monitoring is also advantageous in patients with paroxystic atrial fibrillation because alerts could identify the start-point of atrial fibrillation, resulting in an unscheduled follow-up either in office or by phone, and appropriate interventions (e.g. antiarrhythmic medication, anticoagulation or antiplatelet medication, external cardioversion, device reprogramming). In general, satisfaction is high and both patient and healthcare personals prefer remote follow-up over in-clinic visits (Figs 43.24–43.29).

## FUTURE CHALLENGES AND OPPORTUNITIES

The field of HF home monitoring has many additional avenues to investigate. Further studies to identify which patient population will derive the greatest benefit from home monitoring are needed. Also, identifying which variables are best to monitor requires further study, whether it be patient symptoms, directly recorded data such as heart rate, blood pressure, or pulmonary artery pressures, or calculated measurements such as intrathoracic impedance. Alternately, monitoring patient behaviors such as medication adherence may be more important. There are automated pill boxes that record whether pills have been taken and even pills with an edible sensor that trigger a signal when digested. Home testing and monitoring of biomarkers may also be of value. Use of serial natriuretic peptides has been found to be potentially useful in guiding care of HF patients in some but not all studies in the outpatient setting, with a meta-analysis of these trials suggesting that all-cause mortality may be reduced, particularly in patients younger than 75 years, without clear reduction in all-cause hospitalization. Home testing of these or other biomarkers should be further explored. As an increasing amount of information is gathered, however, one runs the risk of obtaining too much data to manage. Important alerts may get lost if an appropriate triage system is not in place.

Any successful approach will likely need to be multipronged. Monitoring alone, without adequate follow-up and feedback to the patient, is unlikely to be the solution that prevents HF readmissions or decompensation. Importantly, as many of the interventions, particularly the implanted hemodynamic monitoring devices, were tested in a select cohort of patients being followed up by

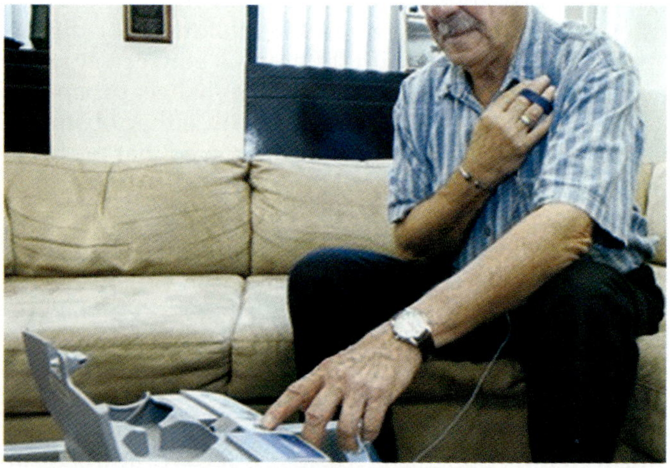

**Fig. 43.24:** Patients with implanted defibrillators and pacemakers are benefitting from technology that reduces the number of times they have to come to the hospital for treatment. A remote monitoring system called Medtronic CareLink

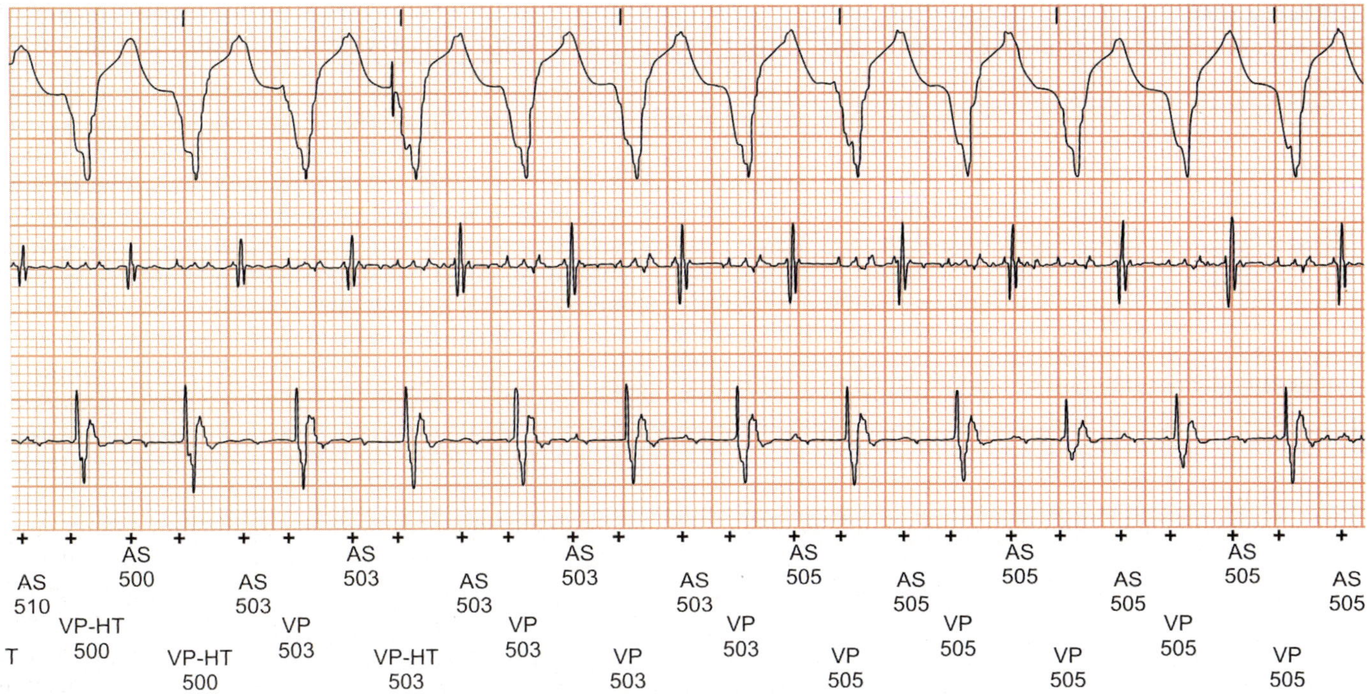


**Fig. 43.25:** Telemetered ECG tracing with surface lead II (top) and intracardiac electrograms [atrial electrogram (center) and ventricular electrogram (lower)] and marker channel (bottom) showing pacemaker-mediated tachycardia (PMT). The intracardiac markers indicate that the retrograde P-waves, labeled AS for atrial-sensed event, occur 280 milliseconds after the ventricular-paced beats, labeled VP

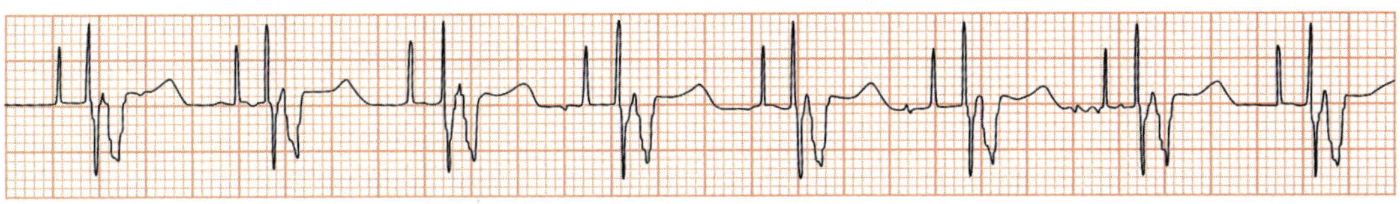

**Fig. 43.26:** Continuous telemetry monitoring is initiated and strip is obtained. it does not show any evidence of pacing problems; each beat is initiated by a P-wave, and each beat is followed by a paced QRS complex. Every QRS is paced, and the rate falls within the rate setting programmed for the pacemaker

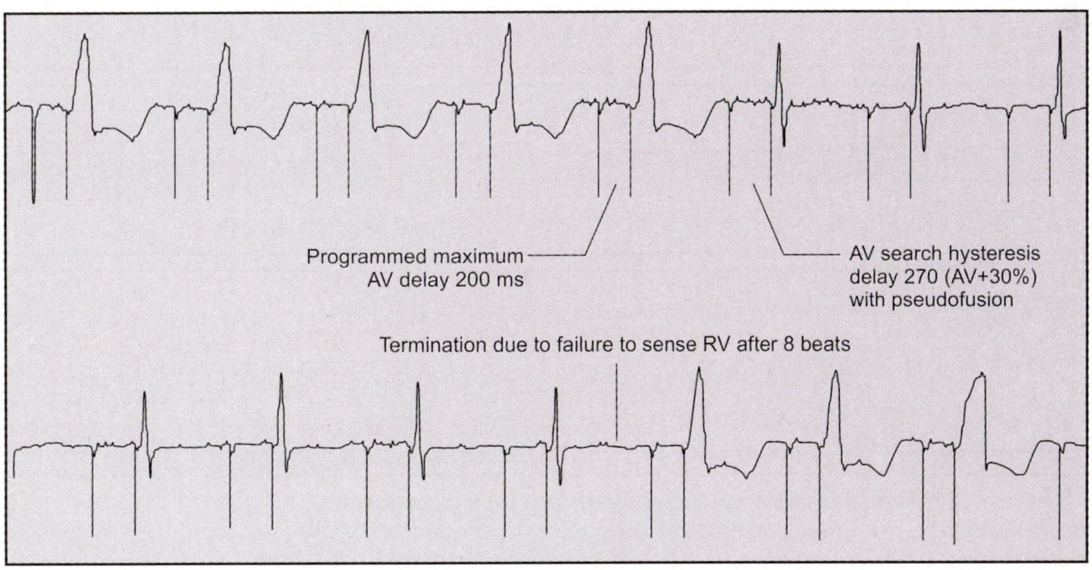


**Fig. 43.27:** An example of AV search hysteresis on telemetry is shown. The dual chamber pacemaker (Guidant Insignia I Plus; DDDR 70–130; base-rate AV delay 200 ms) is pacing at the lower rate limit at the longest of the dynamic AV delay. The AV delay increases to almost 270 ms, 30% longer than the programmed AV delay for 8 cycles. In this case, the algorithm failed to sense the intrinsic narrow QRS as it fell just beyond the extended AV delay, resulting in pseudofusion. Due to the lack of sensing during the 8 cycles, the AV delay then shortens to the programmed delay of 200 ms and reattempts the algorithm in 32 cycles

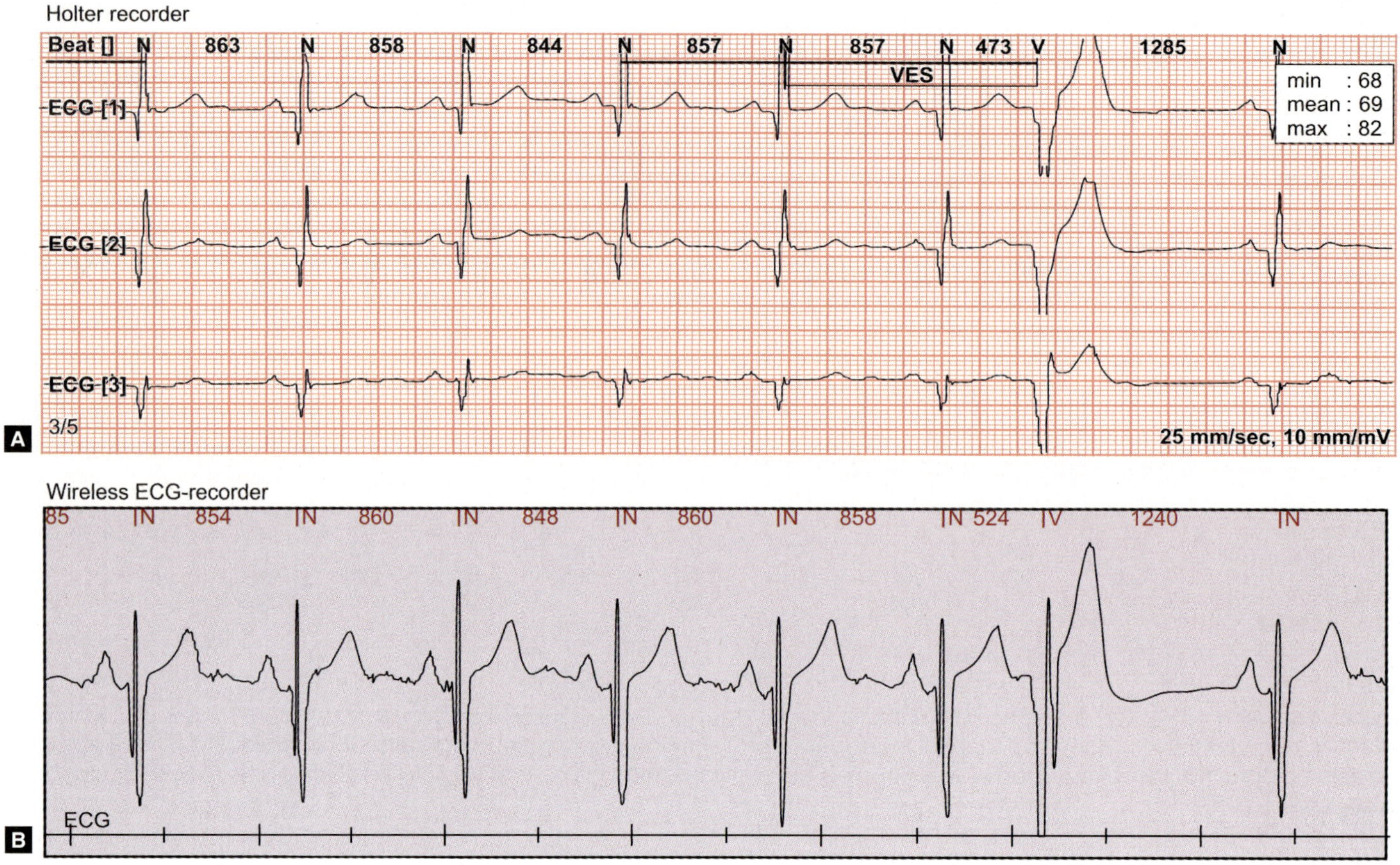


**Fig. 43.28:** Two snapshots of 7-s time-series of concurrent ECG recordings from the Holter recorder (A), and from the wireless ECG recorder (B)

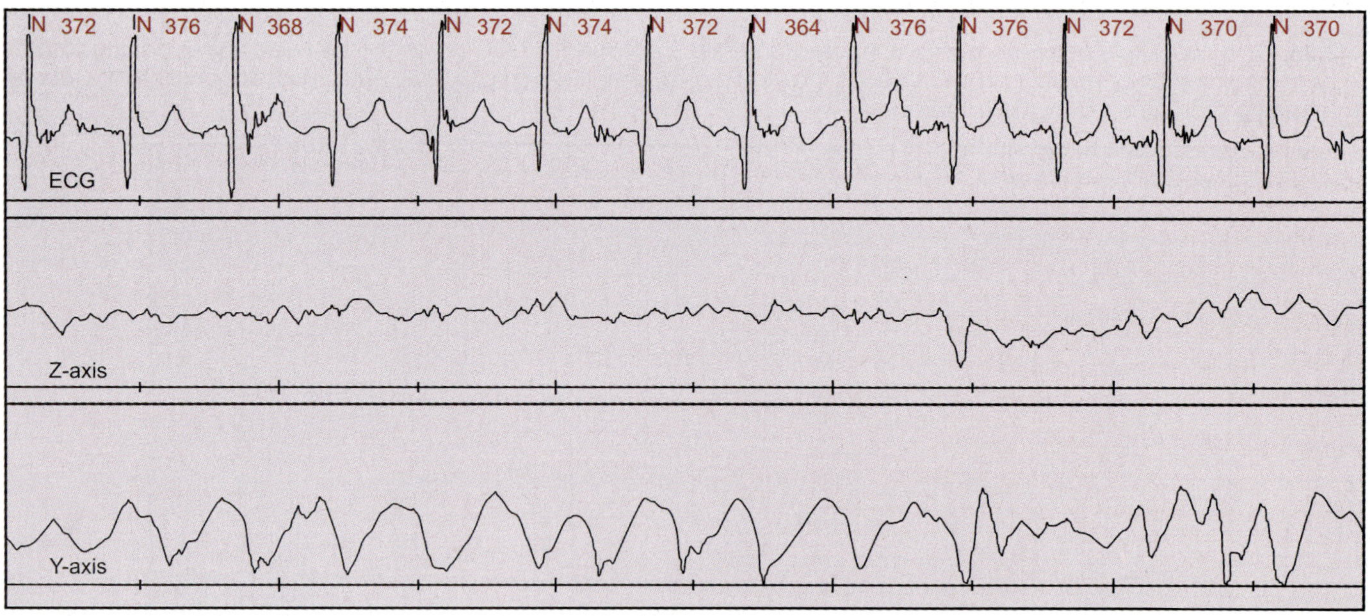


**Fig. 43.29:** Recordings obtained with the wireless ECG sensor system during outdoor football game training, where the upper curve shows the ECG signal, while the two lower curves show a signal from an accelerometer in Z-axis (sideways) and Y-axis (upwards) directions indicating the level of physical activity. The actual heart rate is approx. 160 b/min

experienced centers, additional study will be needed to determine whether the benefits can be generalized to a broader cohort of patients and more diverse group of clinicians and clinical practice settings. Although these strategies are developed to reduce the HF burden for the patient and society, these interventions themselves may also be costly. The ability to reimburse not only for the devices, but also for the training and education of patients and staff, will dictate how these interventions develop. Although chronic care management programs are potentially cost saving, the benefits from improved disease control and reduced hospitalization rates often accrue to the insurers rather than the ambulatory care practices responsible for providing that care. How these home monitoring programs are incorporated into the patient-provider relationship is also a work in progress. This prospect will require methods to ensure more effective and efficient collection of data, reliable transmission of information, and integration into an already busy workflow.

Telemedicine has revolutionized modern cardiology and provided the opportunity for consultations between doctors separated by long distances, even between continents. In the acute phase of heart disease, telemedicine has helped to deliver optimal care faster and in chronic disease consultation between doctor and patient decreases the need for outpatient visits. As these systems are further improved, so are patient outcomes. In the future, it is likely that smaller implantable devices will become available to provide wireless feedback to patients and doctors alike via telemedicine.

## BIBLIOGRAPHY


1. Abraham WT, Adamson PB, Bourge RC, Aaron MF, Costanzo MR, Stevenson LW, et al. Wireless pulmonary artery haemodynamic monitoring in chronic heart failure: a randomised controlled trial. Lancet 2011;377:658–6.
2. Abraham WT, Compton S, Haas G, Foreman B, Canby RC, Fishel R, et al. Intrathoracic impedance vs daily weight monitoring for predicting worsening heart failure events: results of the Fluid Accumulation Status Trial (FAST). Congest Heart Fail 2011;17:51–55.
3. Adams GL, Campbell PT, Adams JM, Strauss DG, Wall K, Patterson J, et al. Effectiveness of prehospital wireless transmission of electrocardiograms to a cardiologist via hand-held device for patients with acute myocardial infarction (from the Timely Intervention in Myocardial Emergency. NorthEast Experience [TIME-NE]). Am J Cardiol 2006;98:1160–4.
4. Adamson PB, Magalski A, Braunschweig F, Böhm M, Reynolds D, Steinhaus D, et al. Ongoing right ventricular hemodynamics in heart failure: clinical value of measurements derived from an implantable monitoring system. J Am Coll Cardiol 2003;41:565–71.
5. Allely EB. Synchronous and asynchronous telemedicine. J Med Syst 1995;19:207–12.
6. Andersen HR, Nielsen TT, Rasmussen K, Thuesen L, Kelbaek H, Thayssen P, et al. A comparison of coronary angioplasty with fibrinolytic therapy in acute myocardial infarction. N Engl J Med 2003;349:733–42.
7. Anker SD, Koehler F, Abraham WT. Telemedicine and remote management of patients with heart failure. Lancet 2011;378:731–9.
8. Atary JZ, De Visser M, Van den Dijk R, Bosch J, Liem SS, Antoni ML, et al. Standardised pre-hospital care of acute myocardial infarction patients: MISSION! guidelines applied in practice. Neth Heart J 2010;18:408–15.
9. Brugada P. What evidence do we have to replace in-hospital implantable cardioverter defibrillator follow-up?. Clin Res Cardiol 2006;95(Suppl 3):3–9.
10. Bui AL, Fonarow GC. Home monitoring for heart failure management. J Am Coll Cardiol 2012;59:97–104.
11. Burri H, Senouf D. Remote monitoring and follow-up of pacemakers and implantable cardioverter defibrillators. Europace 2009;11:701–9.
12. Chaudhry SI, Mattera JA, Curtis JP, Spertus JA, Herrin J, Lin Z, et al. Telemonitoring in patients with heart failure. N Engl J Med 2010;363:2301–9.
13. Clemmensen P, Sejersten M, Sillesen M, Hampton D, Wagner GS, Loumann-Nielsen S. Diversion of ST-elevation myocardial infarction patients for primary angioplasty based on wireless prehospital 12-lead electrocardiographic transmission directly to the cardiologist's handheld computer: a progress report. J Electrocardiol 2005;38(Suppl 4):194–8.
14. Crossley GH, Boyle A, Vitense H, Chang Y, Mead RH, CONNECT Investigators. The CONNECT (Clinical Evaluation of Remote Notification to Reduce Time to Clinical Decision) trial: the value of wireless remote monitoring with automatic clinician alerts. J Am Coll Cardiol 2011;57:1181–9.
15. Dieker HJ, Liem SS, El Aidi H, Van Grunsven P, Aengevaeren WR, Brouwer MA, et al. Pre-hospital triage for primary angioplasty: direct referral to the intervention center versus interhospital transport. JACC Cardiovasc Interv 2010;3: 705–11.
16. Drew B. Pre-hospital synthesized 12-lead ECG ischemia monitoring with trans-telephonic transmission in acute coronary syndromes. Pilot study results of the ST SMART trial. J Electrocardiol 2004;37(Suppl):214–21.
17. Drew BJ, Sommargren CE, Schindler DM, Benedict K, Zegre-Hemsey J, Glancy JP. A simple strategy improves prehospital electrocardiogram utilization and hospital treatment for patients with acute coronary syndrome (from the ST SMART Study). Am J Cardiol 2011;107:347–52.
18. Effectiveness of intravenous thrombolytic treatment in acute myocardial infarction. Gruppo Italiano per lo Studio della Streptochinasi nell'Infarto Miocardico (GISSI). Lancet 1986;1:397–402.
19. Epstein AE, Dimarco JP, Ellenbogen KA, Estes NA, Freedman RA, Gettes LS, et al. ACC/AHA/HRS 2008 Guide-lines for device-based therapy of cardiac rhythm abnormalities. Heart Rhythm 2008;5:e1–e62.
20. Giovas P, Papadoyannis D, Thomakos D, Papazachos G, Rallidis M, Soulis D, et al. Transmission of electrocardiograms from a moving ambulance. J Telemed Telecare 1998; 4(Suppl 1):5–7.
21. Grim P, Feldman T, Martin M, Donovan R, Nevins V, Childers RW. Cellular telephone transmission of 12-lead electrocardiograms from ambulance to hospital. Am J Cardiol. 1987;60:715–20.
22. Grines CL, Westerhausen DR, Grines LL, Hanlon JT, Logemann TL, Niemela M, et al. A randomized trial of

transfer for primary angioplasty versus on-site thrombolysis in patients with high-risk myocardial infarction: the Air Primary Angioplasty in Myocardial Infarction study. J Am Coll Cardiol 2002;39:1713–9.

23. Heidbüchel H, Lioen P, Foulon S, Huybrechts W, Ector J, Willems R, et al. Potential role of remote monitoring for scheduled and unscheduled evaluations of patients with an implantable defibrillator. Europace 2008;10:351–7.
24. Ho KK, Pinsky JL, Kannel WB, Levy D. The epidemiology of heart failure: the Framingham Study. J Am Coll Cardiol 1993; 22(Suppl 4):A6–A13.
25. Hoekstra JW, O'Neill BJ, Pride YB, Lefebvre C, Diercks DB, Peacock WF, et al. Acute detection of ST-elevation myocardial infarction missed on standard 12-Lead ECG with a novel 80-lead real-time digital body surface map: primary results from the multicenter OCCULT MI trial. Ann Emerg Med 2009;54:779–88.
26. Inglis SC, Clark RA, McAlister FA, Ball J, Lewinter C, Cullington D, et al. Structured telephone support or telemonitoring programmes for patients with chronic heart failure. Cochrane Database Syst Rev 2010;8:CD007228.
27. Jencks SF, Williams MV, Coleman EA. Rehospitalizations among patients in the Medicare fee-for-service program. N Engl J Med 2009;360:1418–28.
28. Keeley EC, Boura JA, Grines CL. Primary angioplasty versus intravenous thrombolytic therapy for acute myocardial infarction: a quantitative review of 23 randomised trials. Lancet 2003;361:13–20.
29. Klersy C, De Silvestri A, Gabutti G, Regoli F, Auricchio A. A meta-analysis of remote monitoring of heart failure patients. J Am Coll Cardiol 2009;54:1683–94.
30. Koehler F, Winkler S, Schieber M, Sechtem U, Stangl K, Böhm M, et al. Impact of remote telemedical management on mortality and hospitalizations in ambulatory patients with chronic heart failure: the telemedical interventional moni-toring in heart failure study. Circulation 2011;123: 1873–80.
31. Kudenchuk PJ, Maynard C, Cobb LA, Wirkus M, Martin JS, Kennedy JW, et al. Utility of the prehospital electrocardiogram in diagnosing acute coronary syndromes: the Myocardial Infarction Triage and Intervention (MITI) Project. J Am Coll Cardiol 1998;32:17–27.
32. Kushner FG, Hand M, Smith SC, King SB, Anderson JL, Antman EM, et al. 2009 focused updates: ACC/AHA guidelines for the management of patients with ST-elevation myocardial infarction (updating the 2004 guideline and 2007 focused update) and ACC/AHA/SCAI guidelines on percutaneous coronary intervention (updating the 2005 guideline and 2007 focused update) a report of the American College of Cardiology Foundation/American Heart Association Task Force on Practice Guidelines. J Am Coll Cardiol 2009;54:2205–41.
33. Le May MR, So DY, Dionne R, Glover CA, Froeschl MP, Wells GA, et al. A citywide protocol for primary PCI in ST-segment elevation myocardial infarction. N Engl J Med 2008;358: 231–40.
34. Mabo P, Victor F, Bazin P, Ahres S, Babuty D, Da Costa A, et al. A randomized trial of long-term remote monitoring of pacemaker recipients (the COMPAS trial). Eur Heart J 2012; 33:1105–11.
35. Martinoni A, Politi A, De Servi S. [Role of prehospital electrocardiogram in the early diagnosis of ST-elevation myocardial infarction]. G Ital Cardiol (Rome) 2010;11(10 Suppl 1): S53–S56.
36. Marzegalli M, Lunati M, Landolina M, Perego GB, Ricci RP, Guenzati G, et al. Remote monitoring of CRT-ICD: the multicenter Italian CareLink evaluation-ease of use, acceptance, and organizational implications. Pacing Clin Electrophysiol 2008;31:1259–64.
37. McLean S, Protti D, Sheikh A. Telehealthcare for long term conditions. BMJ 2011;342:d120.
38. Ornato JP, Menown IB, Peberdy MA, Kontos MC, Riddell JW, Higgins GL, et al. Body surface mapping vs 12-lead electrocardiography to detect ST-elevation myocardial infarction. Am J Emerg Med 2009;27:779–84.
39. Owens C, McClelland A, Walsh S, Smith B, Adgey J. Comparison of value of leads from body surface maps to 12-lead electrocardiogram for diagnosis of acute myocardial infarction. Am J Cardiol 2008;102:257–65.
40. Owens CG, McClelland AJ, Walsh SJ, Smith BA, Tomlin A, Riddell JW, et al. Prehospital 80-LAD mapping: does it add significantly to the diagnosis of acute coronary syndromes?. J Electrocardiol 2004;37(Suppl):223–32.
41. Pedersen SH, Galatius S, Hansen PR, Mogelvang R, Abildstrom SZ, Sorensen R, et al. Field triage reduces treatment delay and improves long-term clinical outcome in patients with acute ST-segment elevation myocardial infarction treated with primary percutaneous coronary intervention. J Am Coll Cardiol 2009;54:2296–302.
42. Raatikainen MJ, Uusimaa P, Van Ginneken MM, Janssen JP, Linnaluoto M. Remote monitoring of implantable cardioverter defibrillator patients: a safe, time-saving, and cost-effective means for follow-up. Europace 2008;10: 1145–51.
43. Randomised trial of intravenous streptokinase, oral aspirin, both, or neither among 17,187 cases of suspected acute myocardial infarction: ISIS-2. ISIS-2 (Second International Study of Infarct Survival) Collaborative Group. Lancet 1988; 2:349–60.
44. Ricci RP, Morichelli L, Santini M. Remote control of implanted devices through Home Monitoring technology improves detection and clinical management of atrial fibrillation. Europace 2009;11:54–61.
45. Santini M, Ricci RP, Lunati M, Landolina M, Perego GB, Marzegalli M, et al. Remote monitoring of patients with biventricular defibrillators through the CareLink system improves clinical management of arrhythmias and heart failure episodes. J Interv Card Electrophysiol 2009;24:53–61.
46. Sejersten M, Sillesen M, Hansen PR, Nielsen SL, Nielsen H, Trautner S, et al. Effect on treatment delay of prehospital teletransmission of 12-lead electrocardiogram to a cardiologist for immediate triage and direct referral of patients with ST-segment elevation acute myocardial infarction to primary percutaneous coronary intervention. Am J Cardiol. 2008; 101: 941–6.
47. Sejersten M, Wagner GS, Pahlm O, Warren JW, Feldman CL, Horácek BM. Detection of acute ischemia from the EASI-derived 12-lead electrocardiogram and from the 12-lead electrocardiogram acquired in clinical practice. J Electrocardiol 2007;40:120–6.

48. Sood S, Mbarika V, Jugoo S, Dookhy R, Doarn CR, Prakash N, et al. What is telemedicine? A collection of 104 peer-reviewed perspectives and theoretical underpinnings. Telemed J E Health 2007;13:573–90.
49. Sorensen JT, Terkelsen CJ, Norgaard BL, Trautner S, Hansen TM, Botker HE, et al. Urban and rural implementation of prehospital diagnosis and direct referral for primary percutaneous coronary intervention in patients with acute ST-elevation myocardial infarction. Eur Heart J 2011;32:430–6.
50. Steg PG, James SK, Atar D, Badano LP, Blömstrom-Lundqvist C, Borger MA, et al. ESC Guidelines for the management of acute myocardial infarction in patients presenting with ST-segment elevation: The Task Force on the management of ST-segment elevation acute myocardial infarction of the European Society of Cardiology (ESC). Eur Heart J 2012;33: 2569–619.
51. Steventon A, Bardsley M, Billings J, Dixon J, Doll H, Hirani S, et al. Effect of telehealth on use of secondary care and mortality: findings from the Whole System Demonstrator cluster randomised trial. BMJ 2012;344:e3874.
52. Terkelsen CJ, Kaltoft AK, Norgaard BL, Bottcher M, Lassen JF, Clausen K, et al. ST changes before and during primary percutaneous coronary intervention predict final infarct size in patients with ST elevation myocardial infarction. J Electrocardiol 2009;42:64–72.
53. Terkelsen CJ, Lassen JF, Nørgaard BL, Gerdes JC, Poulsen SH, Bendix K, et al. Reduction of treatment delay in patients with ST-elevation myocardial infarction: impact of prehospital diagnosis and direct referral to primary percutanous coronary intervention. Eur Heart J 2005;26:770–7.
54. Terkelsen CJ, Nørgaard BL, Lassen JF, Gerdes JC, Ankersen JP, Rømer F, et al. Telemedicine used for remote prehospital diagnosing in patients suspected of acute myocardial infarction. J Intern Med 2002;252:412–20.
55. Thygesen K, Alpert JS, Jaffe AS, Simoons ML, Chaitman BR, White HD, et al. Third universal definition of myocardial infarction. Eur Heart J 2012;33:2551–67.
56. Uhley HN. Electrocardiographic telemetry from ambulances. A practical approach to mobile coronary care units. Am Heart J 1970;80:838–42.
57. Varma N, Epstein AE, Irimpen A, Schweikert R, Love C, TRUST Investigators. Efficacy and safety of automatic remote monitoring for implantable cardioverter-defibrillator follow-up: the Lumos-T Safely Reduces Routine Office Device Follow-up (TRUST) trial. Circulation 2010;122: 325–32.
58. Wall T, Albright J, Livingston B, Isley L, Young D, Nanny M, et al. Prehospital ECG transmission speeds reperfusion for patients with acute myocardial infarction. N C Med J 2000;61:104–8.
59. Widimský P, Budesínský T, Vorác D, Groch L, Zelízko M, Aschermann M, et al. Long distance transport for primary angioplasty vs immediate thrombolysis in acute myocardial infarction. Final results of the randomized national multicentre trial-PRAGUE-2. Eur Heart J 2003;24:94–104.
60. Wilkoff BL, Auricchio A, Brugada J, Cowie M, Ellenbogen KA, Gillis AM, et al. HRS/EHRA Expert Consensus on the Monitoring of Cardiovascular Implantable Electronic Devices (CIEDs): description of techniques, indications, personnel, frequency and ethical considerations: developed in partnership with the Heart Rhythm Society (HRS) and the European Heart Rhythm Association (EHRA); and in collaboration with the American College of Cardiology (ACC), the American Heart Association (AHA), the European Society of Cardiology (ESC), the Heart Failure Association of ESC (HFA), and the Heart Failure Society of America (HFSA). Endorsed by the Heart Rhythm Society, the European Heart Rhythm Association (a registered branch of the ESC), the American College of Cardiology, the American Heart Association. Europace 2008;10:707–25.
61. Yu CM, Wang L, Chau E, Chan RH, Kong SL, Tang MO, et al. Intrathoracic impedance monitoring in patients with heart failure: correlation with fluid status and feasibility of early warning preceding hospitalization. Circulation 2005; 112: 841–8.
62. Zile MR, Bennett TD, St John Sutton M, Cho YK, Adamson PB, Aaron MF, et al. Transition from chronic compensated to acute decompensated heart failure: pathophysiological insights obtained from continuous monitoring of intracardiac pressures. Circulation 2008;118:1433–41.

# 44 Cardiovascular Emergencies in Air Traveling

To save the time and avoid physical discomforts lacs of people travel by aerial route annually all over the world both in domestic and international flights. These people include pregnant ladies, newly born infants, corporate business managers, sick and fragile elderly individual and patients for getting treatment ouside their residing countries. Currently, aerocrafts are fitted with latest medical equipment to face any emergent health problem and crew staff is well trained to administer first aid treatment. From time to time,trained crew personel always pass on medical tips for leg exercises in the prevention of pulmonary embolism. The patients with pacemakers and ICD need special care during longer duration international flights and are advised to make contact with their respective specialists through telemeteric equipments if possible (Fig 44.1).

Recent data drawn from several major US carriers between 1996 and 1997 show 15 deaths among approximately 1.4 million passengers. Cardiac events account for the greatest percentage of flight diversions and appear to represent the major cause of in-flight death. As more patients with severe cardiovascular disease travel, on-board cardiac events might be expected to increase.

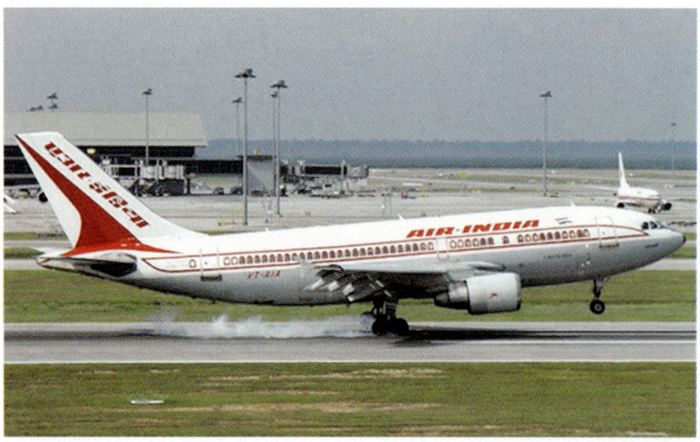

**Fig. 44.1:** An air-India aeroplane ready for an international flight

This chapter reviews the pathophysiology and delineate the risk for patients with cardiovascular disease of sudden death, DVT, and ischemia/infarction when they travel by air.

On 12 June 2001, the federal aviation administration (FAA) issued a final ruling mandating that passenger-carrying aircraft of more than 7,500-lb maximum payload capacity with at least one flight attendant carry at least one automated external defibrillator (AED) and an enhanced emergency medical kit.

All flight attendants will be required to receive initial and recurrent training on AED usage and in cardiopulmonary resuscitation (CPR). The rule becomes effective on 12 April 2004. Page et al. extrapolated from the data accumulated regarding AED use by one major US airline, and suggested that the widespread availability of AEDs on commercial airlines might prevent up to 93 in-flight deaths from ventricular fibrillation each year worldwide. Long-term survival rates in such patients range from 26 to 40%, which compares favorably with the 2–5% long-term survival rates often quoted for out-of-hospital arrests Air travel impacts on patients with cardiovascular disease in several ways. Patients with cardiovascular disease can be more sensitive to changes in arterial oxygen saturation. Airline cabins are not pressurized to provide an altitude that mimics sea level. Cabin altitude may vary during an individual flight, although the FAA mandates an effective cabin altitude of 8,000 ft at maximum flying altitude. The effective cabin altitude of a plane flying at 40,000 ft approaches 7,500 ft if the cabin pressure is maintained at 585 mmHg. The net effect of such pressure changes is to decrease arterial oxygen tension, which could provoke ischemia and arrhythmia in those most susceptible. The arterial oxygen tension in a healthy individual, with a resting $PaO_2$ of 98 at sea level, may fall to less than 60 mmHg at such pressures during a routine commercial air flight. One can estimate that inspired $PO_2$ will fall by 4 mmHg per 1000 ft above sea level.

## PRECAUTIONS TO BE OBSERVED BY TRAVELERS IN CASE OF CARDIOVASCULAR DISEASES (Tables 44.1–44.3)

- **Patients with chronic obstructive pulmonary disease:** Patients with concomitant pulmonary disease and even those without pulmonary compromise may require supplemental oxygen during air travel. It is recommended that any passenger with a partial pressure of arterial oxygen of less than 70 mm at sea level at rest should receive supplemental oxygen during air travel. Oxygen should be requested well in advance, and is typically only available at 2-L or 4-L flow rates. Most airlines will also require a letter of medical clearance from the patient's physician at least 48 hours prior to the flight. US air carriers will require a prescription for oxygen. Charges for in-flight oxygen vary widely. There are no specific data to support the routine use of in-flight oxygen in travelers who have suffered a recent myocardial infarction (MI) or have cardiac disease.
- **Patients with angina pectoris and myocardial ischemia:** Several studies have either demonstrated or suggested increased sympathetic activity at altitudes of 1,500–3,000 m. This is believed to be secondary to hypoxia at higher altitudes. Angina and ST-segment depression have been documented to occur at lower workloads in subjects at high altitude. Whereas one might expect an increase in anginal symptoms during air travel, studies of this patient population during air travel have not been performed. The relative inactivity during air travel may mitigate the decreased work capacity seen at altitude. Similarly, although arrhythmia might be expected to occur more commonly at altitude, given the increased sympathetic activity and increased hypoxia noted above, this has not been borne out in one very small study evaluating the response of elderly subjects to an altitude of 2,500 m. Levine et al. examined the response of 20 subjects with a mean age of 68 years to an altitude of 2,500 m. Two of the 20 had a history of significant arrhythmias. Estimated mean pulmonary artery pressure increased by 43% with acute exposure to altitude, probably secondary to hypoxia and sympathetic activation. No significant arrhythmias were noted in the study group at altitude, although the investigators did find an increase in ventricular premature beats. The very small study size limits the broad application of these results to the air traveler with cardiovascular disease.
- **Right- or left-sided heart failure:** The increase in pulmonary artery pressure noted by Levine et al. suggests that travelers with depressed ejection fractions might suffer from increased symptoms of right- or left-sided heart failure during air travel. No study has addressed this issue. Whereas measurement of pulmonary artery pressure during flight might be impractical, a retrospective survey of such patients addressing in-flight symptoms would be relatively easy to undertake.
- **Cardiac arrhythmias due to hypoxemia:** Air travel impacts on patients with cardiovascular disease in

| **Table 44.1:** In-flight medical kit content requirements on airlines |
|---|
| Sphygmomanometer |
| Stethoscope |
| Oropharyngeal airway—three sizes |
| Self-inflating manual resuscitation device with three masks |
| CPR mask—three sizes |
| Intravenous administration set |
| Adhesive tape |
| Saline solution—50 ml |
| Non-narcotic analgesic—325 mg, four tablets |
| Antihistamine tablets—25 mg, four tablets |
| Antihistamin injectable—50 mg, two doses |
| Atropine 0.5 mg–5 ml, four doses |
| Aspirin tablets—325 mg, four tablets |
| Bronchodilator, inhaled (metered dose inhaler or equivalent) |
| Dextrose—50% in 50 ml, two doses |
| Epinephrine 1:1,000–1 ml injectable, two doses |
| Epinephrine 1:10,000–2 ml injectable, two doses |
| Lidocaine—5 ml, 20 mg/ml, injectable, two doses |
| Nitroglycerin tablets—0.4 mg, 10 tablets |
| Automated external defibrillator |

CPR=cardiopulmonary resuscitation

| **Table 44.2:** Contraindications to air travel for patients with cardiac disease |
|---|
| Myocardial infarction within previous 2 weeks |
| Unstable angina |
| Coronary artery bypass graft within previous 2 weeks |
| Poorly compensated heart failure |
| Uncontrolled ventricular or supraventricular arrythmias |

| **Table 44.3:** General recommendations for air travelers with cardiac disease |
|---|
| Medication sufficient for the length of travel should be placed in carry-on luggage |
| Avoid in-flight meals high in sodium, alcohol, and caffeinated beverages. Drink generous amounts of water |
| Patients should carry a copy of their latest ECG, with and without pacing if applicable |
| Patient should carry cards containing information about implantable devices such as pacemakers and ICDs as well as intracoronary stents. These are available from the manufactures as well as individual physicians |
| Patients should carry an updated medication list with allergies |
| Airlines should be contracted >48 h in advance if supplemental oxygen is needed during the flight |
| Graduated below-wht-knee compression stocking (20–30 mmHg) should be considered for flights >5,000 km or 8 h |

ICD=implantable cardioverter defibrillator

several ways. Patients with cardiovascular disease can be more sensitive to changes in arterial oxygen saturation. Airline cabins are not pressurized to provide an altitude that mimics sea level. Cabin altitude may vary during an individual flight, although the FAA mandates an effective cabin altitude of 8,000 ft at maximum flying altitude. The effective cabin altitude of a plane flying at 40,000 ft approaches 7,500 ft if the cabin pressure is maintained at 585 mmHg. The net effect of such pressure changes is to decrease arterial oxygen tension, which could provoke ischemia and arrhythmia in those most susceptible. The arterial oxygen tension in a healthy individual, with a resting $PaO_2$ of 98 at sea level, may fall to less than 60 mmHg at such pressures during a routine commercial air flight. One can estimate that inspired $PO_2$ will fall by 4 mmHg per 1000 ft above sea level.

- **Dehydration during longer travel tour:** Dehydration has been a major concern with long-haul air travel, due to the 10% humidity of circulating air on commercial aircraft. Theoretically, dehydration could be expected to contribute to the deleterious effect of air travel on cardiac patients by effectively decreasing preload and therefore cardiac output. Whereas low humidity may lead to dry skin and eye irritation, it has not been proven to result in significant intravascular dehydration. Skjenna et al. cite data demonstrating that most patients actually gain weight secondary to increased fluid intake during air travel. Landgraf et al. simulated flight conditions in 12 healthy volunteers and found an average surplus in fluid balance of 1,100–1,200 ml. This corresponded to an average weight gain of approximately 1 kg. Nevertheless, dehydrating alcohol and caffeinated beverages should be avoided, and care should be taken to consume adequate fluids. Airline food is often quite high in sodium. The increased sodium load can present problems for travelers with congestive heart failure, who may be more sensitive to volume shifts than other cardiac patients. Mental stress may lead to cardiac ischemia in those with known coronary artery disease. Flying can be a significant stressor in many travelers, and represents a potential risk factor for in-flight ischemia as well. General recommendations for air travelers with cardiac disease are presented in. In addition to concern over the risks of ischemia in flight, a number of travelers experience MI while abroad or in close proximity to planned travel. The American Medical Association (AMA) commission on emergency medical services recommended in 1982 that travelers abstain from flying within 3 weeks of an MI. Major advances in angioplasty and coronary revascularization have occurred since the publication of these guidelines and should prompt a re-examination of prior recommendations. The American College of Cardiology recommends a 2-week waiting period prior to travel after an uncomplicated MI.
- **Air travel for patients with myocardial infarction:** Very few studies have evaluated the safety of air travel following MI. Cox et al. undertook the most extensive examination of the topic in their study of 196 patients with recent MI transported by two medical assistance companies on commercial airliners from December 1986 to October 1989. The majority of patients were men, with a mean age of 63 years. Electrocardiographic localization of the infarction was available for 93% of patients, although peak creatinine kinase values were not provided. Forty-five percent of patients suffered anterior circulation infarctions, whereas 34% of infarcts were localized to the inferior circulation by ECG. Only 4.1% of the patients underwent angioplasty or coronary bypass surgery. Medication data were available for 147 of the 196 study patients. Fifty-six patients were taking aspirin and 32 were taking beta-blockers at the time of transport. Nine patients required physician intervention during the flight. Of these nine, six undertook travel less than 14 days after MI. Cox et al. concluded that air travel may be safely undertaken within 2–3 weeks of MI when an accompanying physician is present. Zahger et al. came to a similar conclusion in their small study of 17 patients who suffered acute MI in Israel between May 1996 and May 1999. All patients were risk stratified and offered intervention when appropriate. Seven patients underwent angiography and five were revascularized. Patients flew home 18 ± 11 days after admission. Only five flew with medical escorts, and none of the original 17 patients

| **Table 44.4:** Recommendations for travelers with implant devices (ICD or Pacemaker) |
|---|
| Identification cards with the device type are available from the manufacturer in several languages |
| Patients should be advised not to lean on or linger around metal detector archways |
| Hand-held magnetic security devices should not be placed over an ICD. Patients should request a hand search. If this is not possible, security personnel should be cautioned not to hold a hand-held metal detector over an ICD for more than 1–2 s and to allow at least 30s to elapse before any second pass over the area of the ICD |
| Hand-held magnetic security devices may be used for travelers with pacemakers, but security personnel should be cautioned not to hold the magnet over the device for a prolonged period |
| Carry information card with device type, implantation information, physician contact information and manufacturer contact information |
| Patients should carry a copy of a recent ECG with and without pacing |
| Patients with ICDs who are subjected to frequent device firing should obtain physician contact information for their travel desination in the event that their device requires interrogation. Most major manufacturers maintain websites and toll-free helplines |
| Telephone line quality may limit the use of telephone pacemaker monitors outside of the US |

ICD=implantable cardioverter defibrillator

experienced significant in-flight events.The data by various workers suggest that air travel 2–3 weeks after an acute MI is reasonably safe when appropriate revascularization or angiography has been undertaken in high-risk patients. Medical escort may not be necessary. Placement of intracoronary stents should not result in activation of airport security systems. The increasing availability of AEDs on commercial flights may provide an increased measure of security for those who suffer from ventricular fibrillation during air travel. Evaluations of the use of AEDs on board US aircraft show survival rates for resuscitation ranging from 27 to 40%.

## PATIENTS WITH IMPLANTABLE PACEMAKER AND IMPLANTABLE CARDIOVERTER/DEFIBRILLATOR

As implantable pacemaker and implantable cardioverter/defibrillator (ICD) technology has advanced, a substantial percentage of patients with cardiac disease have undergone the implantation of such devices (Figs 44.2–44.5). Many pacemakers and ICDs can be interrogated and adjusted externally via a wireless communications link. Magnets producing a strong enough field will inhibit tachycardia therapy when placed on top of almost all ICD models while the magnet is in place. These features present several potential problems for those wishing to travel by air. The major manufacturers of pacemaker and ICD technology assert that their devices will not be harmed by airport security systems, although they caution that either device may be temporarily affected. Both ICDs and pacemakers may, in rare cases, set off airport metal detectors. All patients should carry a card from a physician or the manufacturer of the device. Pacemakers and ICDs may, theoretically, undergo temporary malfunction when exposed to airport metal detection equipment, but the few published studies have not shown significant interference with device function. All devices were interrogated before and after exposure. An external six-lead electrocardiogram was recorded during exposure. No change in parameters, inappropriate detection of nonsustained ventricular arrhythmias or suspension of therapies was observed.

Although the major manufacturers of ICD technology have not received any reports of delivery of ICD therapy due to exposure to hand-held metal detectors, there is a theoretical risk that the alternating magnetic field created by the hand-held wand might be detected by the device and lead to delivery of inadvertent shock therapy and/or temporarily inhibit an ICD's pacemaker output. It is is advised that patients with ICDs do not allow a search with a hand-held device and instead request a hand search. If a hand-held device is used, the examiner should be cautioned not to hold the magnet over the device for more than a few

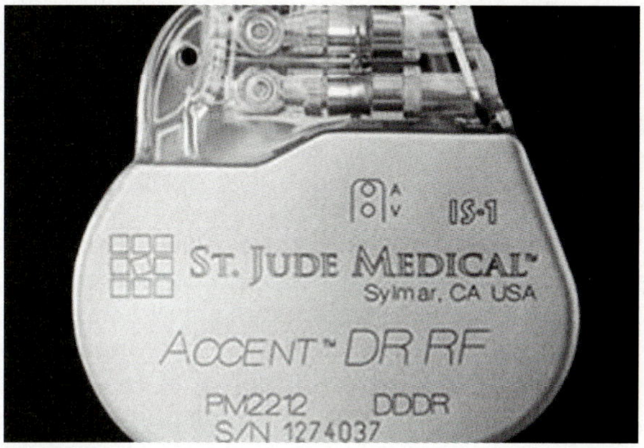


**Fig. 44.3:** The Accent™ RF pacemaker is the first to simplify patient management—from implant through follow-up—with wireless monitoring. With the intelligence to sense and automatically adjust device parameters, the Accent™ RF device, a wireless monitoring pacemaker, is designed to maintain effective therapy and enhance patient safety. The Accent™ RF pacemaker provides intelligent sensing and adjustment of selected device parameters and remote monitoring to help streamline follow-ups, simplify therapy optimization and enhance clinic efficiency

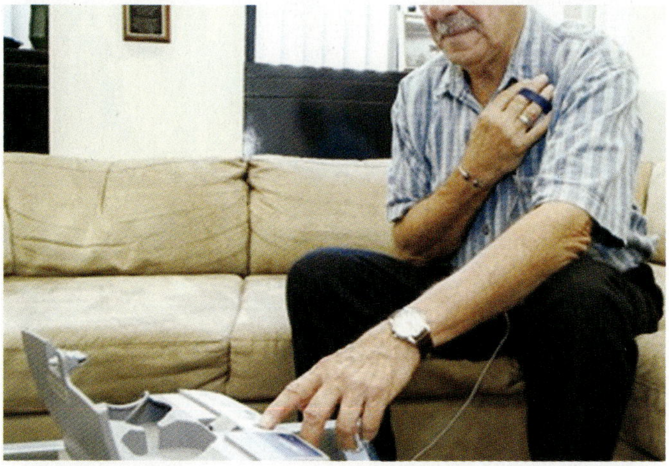

**Fig. 44.2:** Patients with implanted defibrillators and pacemakers are benefitting from technology that reduces the number of times they have to come to the hospital for treatment. A remote monitoring system called Medtronic CareLink

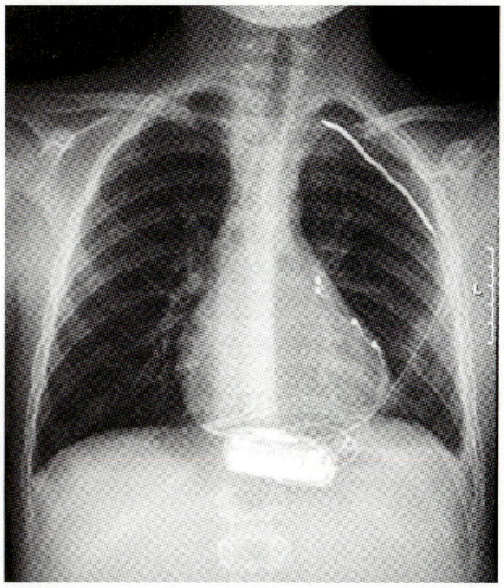

**Fig. 44.4:** Technique of ICD implantation as a prophylaxis to ventricular tachyarrhythmia induced sudden cardiac death

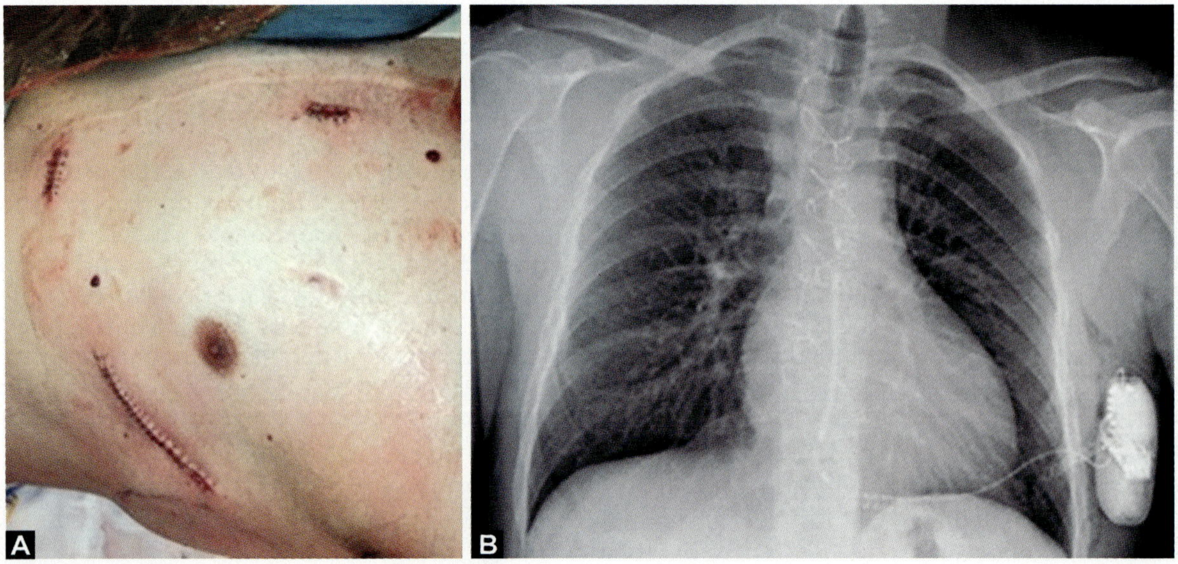


Fig. 44.5: View of the patient's chest after implantation of the automatic subcutaneous implantable device (A) and anteroposterior X-ray at 24 h postimplantation (B)

seconds. If a hand-held wand is passed over the device more than once, at least 30 s should elapse between each pass. Neither ICDs nor pacemakers should be affected by the in-flight environment (Tisch D, personal communication, 5 June 2002; Dostalek J, personal communication, 22 June 2002). Many manufacturers maintain websites and helplines to advise patients and physicians regarding their devices during travel.

Patients with ICDs may be shocked with an AED if their device fails while in flight, although device failure is no more common during air travel than at other times. All patients with implantable devices should carry an ID card detailing the type of device, their physician's contact information and the date of implantation. It is also advised that patients carry a copy of an ECG taken with and without pacing.

## DVT AND THROMBOEMBOLISM DURING AIR TRAVEL

These have long been proposed as possible complications of air travel. Pulmonary embolism (PE) has been suggested as a culprit in deaths related to air travel, although evidence linking air travel to DVT has been somewhat elusive (Figs 44.6, 44.7 and Table 44.5).

The Lonflit 1 study was planned to evaluate the incidence of DVT as a consequence of long fights in economy class. DVT diagnosis was made by comparing ultrasound scans 48h before flying and 24h after flying. The study evaluated 355 subjects at low risk for DVT and 389 at high risk, defined as prior DVT, malignancy within 2 years, limited mobility, coagulation disorders or large varicose veins. Subjects with artificial cardiac valves, diabetes, hypertension, renal or hepatic insufficiency and pacemakers were excluded. No DVTs were found in the low-risk group, whereas 2.8% of the high-risk group were found to have evidence of new thrombosis after an average of 12.4 hours of flying; almost all cases (94.7%) were observed in subjects sitting in

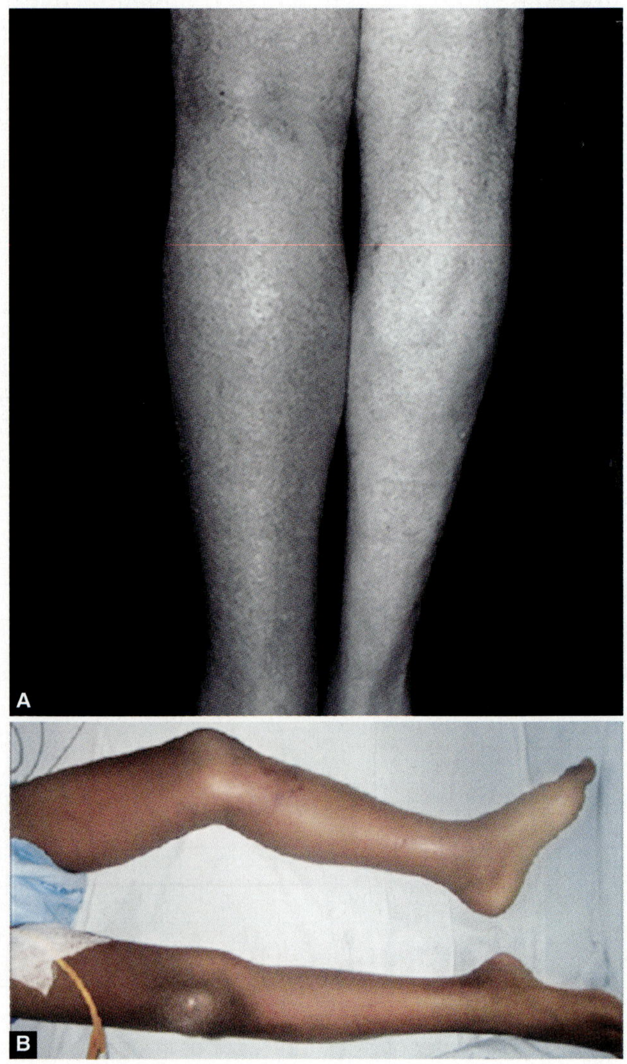


Fig. 44.6: (A and B) Deep vein thrombosis in the left leg of two patients

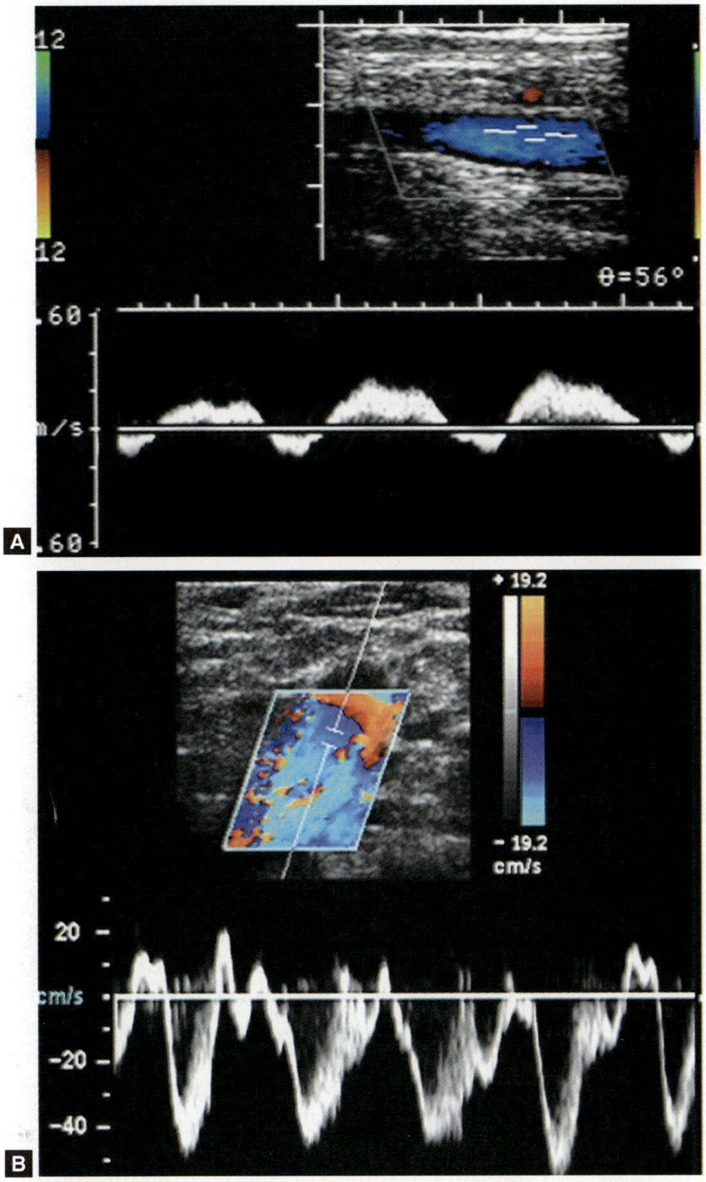

**Fig. 44.7:** (A) Normal peripheral vein. (B) Duplex Doppler demonstrating nonphasic flow in a peripheral vein with thrombosis

window or central seats. The putative mechanisms of increased risk during air travel include venous stasis, fluid retention, hemoconcentration secondary to dehydration, and increased erythropoietin levels. Decreased $PaO_2$ may also play a role by interfering with fibrinolysis and activating the coagulation cascade. Congestive heart failure has long been proposed as a risk factor for venous thromboembolism (VTE). Chronic hypercoagulability and venous stasis have both been proposed as possible mechanisms. Howell et al. found that a left ventricular ejection fraction (LVEF) between 20% and 44% was associated with an increased risk of VTE, with an odds ratio of 2.8 (95% CI 1.4–5.7%) in a population of Veteran's administration patients.LVEF <20% was associated with an odds ratio of 38.3 (95% CI 9.6–152.5%) for VTE.

Although it has been difficult to draw significant conclusions regarding the prevalence of DVT and PE secondary to air travel, compression stockings have been proven to decrease the incidence of calf DVT and may decrease the overall risk of more proximal DVT and PE. Scurr et al. presented compelling evidence that superficial calf DVT may be prevented by the use of graduated elastic compression stockings.The selection criteria excluded patients with cardiorespiratory disease, malignancy, and prior venous thrombosis. All subjects were over 50 years of age. None of the 115 patients who wore compression stockings were found to have calf DVTs after flights of more than 8 hours. The Lonflit-4 trial provided further evidence of the efficacy of compression stockings in the prevention of lower extremity venous thrombosis in low-to-medium-risk patients. No lower extremity venous thromboses were detected among 184 subjects in the group randomized to compression stockings, whereas four deep venous thromboses and two superficial thromboses were discovered in the control group of 188 patients. All subjects traveled for 7–8 hours by air in economy class. The Lonflit-2 trial supports the use of compression stockings in populations at high risk for DVT. In Lonflit-2, 833 subjects believed to be at high risk for DVT based on prior DVT, coagulation disorders, neoplastic disease, large varicose veins or limited mobility were prospectively randomized to below-the-knee compression stockings or no intervention during air travel lasting for an average of 12.4 h. Twenty-two DVTs were identified in 19 of the 422 subjects in the control group, whereas only one DVT was found in the 411 subjects who wore below-the-knee elastic compression

**Table 44.5:** Recommendations to prevent venous thromboembolism (VTE) in travelers with cardiac disease

1. **Low risk**—Travel <5,000 km or <8 h

   **Recommendations:** Mobilization and hydration ± compression stockings

2. **Moderate risk**—Travel >5,000 km ot >8 h, age >50 years, and a modifying factor such as large varicose veins; congestive heart failure with LVEF 20–44%; recent myocardial infarction; hormone replacement therapy oral contraceptive pills; pregnancy

   **Recommendations:** Compression stockings, mobilization, hydration, and aisle seating. While many consultants recommend aspirin for DVT prophylaxis in this population, there are no specific randomized trials to support this practice at present

3. **High risk**—Travel >5,000 km or >8 h in patients with prior VTE; known thrombophilia; recent major surgery within 6 weeks; malignancy within 2 years of travel; congestive heart failure with LVEF <20%

   **Recommendations:** Compression stockings, ailse seating, mobilization and hydration. One injection of low-molecular-weight heparin prior to flight should be considered in those not currently treated with warfarin. NB: It should be noted that these recommendations are based on the best available evidence. To date, only one randomized trial has evaluated the use of aspirin and low-molecular-weight heparin in high-risk populations.

stockings. In both groups, all subjects were seated in window or central seats.

## ASPIRIN THERAPY IN THE PREVENTION OF THROMBOEMBILISM AND PULMONARY EMBOLISM

The role of aspirin therapy in the prevention of VTE has been a subject of considerable debate. The most recent guidelines from the American College of Chest Physicians do not recommend the use of aspirin as prophylaxis for venous thrombosis, although the guidelines do not specifically address the issue of air travel and venous thrombosis.The authors cite the superior efficacy of other agents, notably low-molecular-weight heparin (LMWH), unfractionated heparin and warfarin, in making their recommendations. The prevention of pulmonary embolism and deep vein thrombosis with low dose aspirin. Pulmonary embolism prevention (PEP) trial randomized 13,356 patients undergoing surgery for hip fracture and 4,088 patients undergoing elective arthroplasty to 160 mg daily aspirin therapy or placebo started preoperatively and continued for 35 days. The use of other thromboprophylactic measures was permitted. Eighteen percent of patients were treated with unfractionated heparin, 26% with LMWH, and 30% with thromboembolic-deterrent stockings. Aspirin therapy reduced the risk of PE and DVT by 34% in the combined groups, with a similar proportional risk reduction in those treated with heparin. In those patients taking aspirin alone versus placebo, the risk of bleeding was 2.6 versus 2.5%. The concomitant use of other thromboprophylaxis and the high-risk nature of the patient population make any extrapolation to other populations quite difficult.

Lonflit-3 evaluated the efficacy of aspirin and LMWH in the prevention of DVT in 300 high-risk subjects traveling for more than 10 h by air. Patients were defined as high risk if they had had prior DVT, a coagulation disorder, obesity or severely limited mobility, malignancy within the preceding 2 years, or large varicose veins. Patients with cardiovascular disease, diabetes and hypertension were excluded. The control group received no intervention. The aspirin group received 400mg of aspirin daily for 3 days, beginning 12h before the start of air travel.

The LMWH group received one dose of enoxaparin 2–4 hours prior to the flight, based on a weight-adjusted protocol. Six DVTs were discovered in the control group involving four patients, whereas three DVTs involving three patients were found in the aspirin arm. The p-value for number of limbs involved was <.05, but was not statistically significant when the number of patients with DVT was analyzed. No DVTs were identified in the enoxaparin arm. The p-value was <.002 for limbs affected when compared to controls. The statistical significance of enoxaparin compared to aspirin was not given. It is difficult to make inferences for either the population in question or air travelers as a whole based on this study. The small size of the study, the small number of patients with DVT and the lack of statistical significance when numbers of patients with DVT are compared in the aspirin and placebo groups

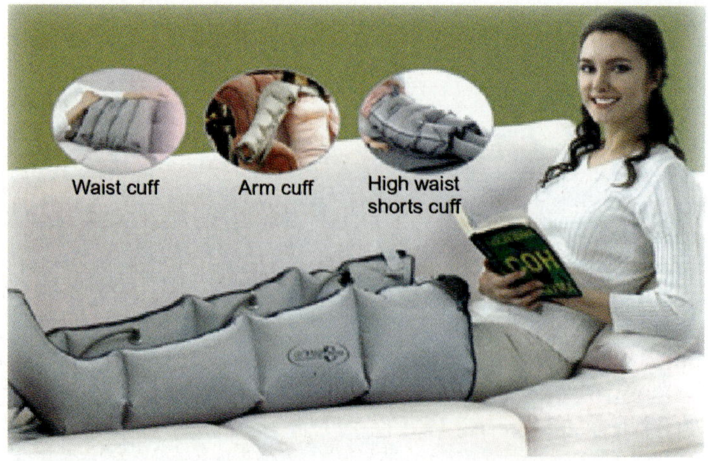


**Fig. 44.8:** Intermittent pneumatic compression in the prevention of venous thrombolism in the legs

do not allow justification of aspirin therapy in this group. The PEP trial would support the use of a 160 mg dose rather than 400 mg in any subsequent study. The use of LMWH has been shown to be efficacious in the prevention of DVT in high-risk populations and is recommended for DVT prophylaxis in high-risk postoperative patients. Lonflit-3 supports the utility of LMWH in high-risk populations during air travel. Role of compression stockings in the prevention of venous thrombolism in the legs (Fig. 44.8).

Compression stockings appear to represent a reasonable measure in all travelers over the age of 50 years who fly for more than 8 h or further than 5,000 km in a single journey. Whereas Lonflit-3 excluded patients with cardiovascular disease, many travelers with cardiac disease will be on chronic aspirin therapy prior to embarking on air travel. The appropriate dose of aspirin and its specific role in this population remain unclear. Lonflit-3 suggests that aspirin would not be of great utility in a moderate-risk population, as it did not significantly alter the incidence of DVT in a high-risk population. A retrospective trial analyzing the incidence of symptomatic DVT and PE in patients on chronic aspirin therapy would require a large number of patients, but is quite feasible. LMWH may prove useful in patients at particularly high risk for DVT who are not maintained on chronic anticoagulation. Avoidance of constrictive clothing, avoidance of leg crossing and participation in minor physical activity during flights are likely to have some efficacy as well, although this has not been proven. Aisle seating, avoidance of tobacco and alcohol-containing beverages, and increased consumption of fluids may also be of benefit.

## SUMMARY

The number of air travelers with cardiac disease will continue to increase. Advances in pacemaker, AICD and revascularization will allow many who could not travel only a few decades ago to do so with relative ease. This growing population will face a variety of hazards related to air travel, including in-flight ischemia, arrythmia, and venous thromboembolic events. Although there is a dearth of research specifically examining the air traveler with cardiac disease.

Future research is needed to further assess the risk of air travel after MI in the age of more complete revascularization and more aggressive antiplatelet therapy. None of the trials conduced so far recommend the use of glycoprotein IIb/IIIa inhibitors, clopidogrel, or drug-coated stents. AMA guidelines on this topic may require revision based on these advances. The current generation of pacemakers and ICDs would allow easy access to data regarding in-flight arrhythmia and might help to further elucidate the impact of altitude on the occurrence of ventricular and atrial arrhythmias. The increasing availability of AEDs will provide further data regarding the incidence of cardiac arrest as a cause of in-flight medical events and in-flight death.

## BIBLIOGRAPHY

1. Alexander JK. Coronary problems associated with altitude and air travel. Cardiol Clin 1995;13:271–8.
2. AMA Commission on Emergency Medical Services. Medical aspects of transportation aboard commercial aircraft. JAMA 1982;247(7):1007–11.
3. Ansell J. Air travel and venous thromboembolism—is the evidence in? N Engl J Med 2001;345(11):828–9.
4. Belcaro G, Cesarone MR, Shah SSG, et al. Prevention of edema, flight microangiopathy and venous thrombosis in long flights with elastic stockings. A randomized trial. Angiology 2002;53:635–45.
5. Belcaro G, Geroulakos G, Nicolaides MS, et al. Venous thromboembolism from air travel: the LONFLIT study. Angiology 2000;52:369–74.
6. Bendz B, Rostrop M, Sevre K, et al. Association between acute hypobaric hypoxia and activation of coagulation in human beings. Lancet 2000;356:1657–8.
7. Cesarone MR, Belcaro G, Nicolaides AN, et al. Venous thrombosis from air travel: the Lonflit 3 study. Angiology 2002;53:1–6.
8. Code of Federal Regulations, Title 14 CFR. Part 25.841. Washington, DC: US Government Printing Office, 1986. Cited in H Gong. Air travel and oxygen therapy in cardiopulmonary patients. Chest 1992;101:1104–13.
9. Cooperman Y, Zarfati Z, Laniado S. The effect of metal detector gates on implanted permanent pacemakers. PACE 1988;11:1386–7.
10. Cox GR, Peterson J, Bouchel L, et al. Safety of commercial air travel following myocardial infarction. Aviat Space Environ Med 1996;67(10):976–82.
11. Cummins RO, Chapman PJC, Chamberlin DA, et al. In flight deaths during commercial air travel: how big is the problem? JAMA 1988;259:1983–8.
12. DeJohn CA, Veronneau SJ, Wolbrink AM, et al. The evaluation of in-flight medical care aboard selected US air carriers: 1996 to 1997. Technical report no. DOT/FAA/AM-0013. Washington, DC: US Department of Transportation, Federal Aviation Administration, Office of Aviation Medicine, 2000.
13. Department of Transportation, Federal Aviation Administration, 14 CFR Part 135, 177. Fed Reg 2001;66(71);19045.
14. Ferrari E, Chevallier T, Chapelier A, et al. Travel as a risk factor for venous thromboembolic disease: a case-control study. Thorax 2000;55:s32–s36.
15. Geerts WH, Heit JA, Clagett GP, et al. Prevention of venous thromboembolism. Chest 2001;119:132s–175s.
16. Gendreau M, DeJohn C. Responding to medical events during commercial airline flights. N Engl J Med 2002;346(14):1067–73.
17. Gertler JP, Perry L, L'Italien G, et al. Ambient oxygen tension modulates endothelial fibrinolysis. J Vasc Surg 1993;18:939–46.
18. Gong H. Advising patients with pulmonary disease on air travel. Ann Intern Med 1989;111:349–51.
19. Gong H. Air travel and oxygen therapy in cardiopulmonary patients. Chest 1992;101:1104–13.
20. House of Lords Select Committee on Science and Technology. Fifth report. Chapter 6: Deep vein thrombosis, seating and stress. London: House of Lords, 2000.
21. Howell MD, Geraci JM, Knowlton AA. Congestive heart failure and outpatient risk of venous thromboembolism: a retrospective case-control study. J Clin Epidemiol 2001;54:810–6.
22. Kattenbeck K, Achtelik M, Weissmueller P, Trappe HJ. Interactions between implantable cardioverter defibrillators and metal detectors at airports: present or not? Europace Suppl 2000;1:D101.
23. Kazmers A, Groehn H, Meeker C. Acute calf vein thrombosis: outcomes and implications. Am Surg 1999; 65:1124–7.
24. Kolb C, Schmeider S, Lehmann G, et al. Do airport metal detectors interfere with implantable pacemakers or cardioverter-defibrillators? JACC 2003;41:2054–9.
25. Krantz DS, Sheps DS, Carney RM, Natelson BH. Effects of mental stress in patients with coronary artery disease: evi-dence and clinical implications. JAMA 2000;283:1800–2.
26. Landgraf ET, Vanslew B, Schulte-Huermann D, et al. Economy class syndrome: rheology, fluid balance, and lower leg edema during a simulated 12-hour long distance flight. Aviat Space Environ Med 1994;10:930–5.
27. Lapostolle F, Surget V, Borron S, et al. Severe pulmonary embolism associated with air travel. N Engl J Med 2001; 345(11):779–83.
28. Levine BD, Zuckerman JH, deFilippi CR. Effect of high-altitude exposure in the elderly: the tenth mountain division study. Circulation 1997;96(4):1224–32.
29. Medtronic Corporation. Guidelines: traveling and security systems. Available at: http://www.medtronic.com (accessed 1 Nov. 2003).
30. Morgan PJ, Alexander JK, Nicoli SA, et al. The patient with coronary disease at altitude: observations during acute exposure to 3100 meters. J Wilderness Med 1990;1:147.
31. O'Rourke MF, Donaldson E, Geddes JS. An Airline Cardiac Arrest Program. Circulation 1997;96:2849–53.
32. Page RL, Joglar JA, Kowal RC, et al. Use of automated external defibrillators by a US airline. N Engl J Med 2000; 343:17.
33. Paulter NG. Hand-held metal detectors for use in concealed weapon and contraband detection. NIJ Standard-0602.01.

Washington DC: US Department of Justice, National Institute of Justice, 2000:8–9.

34. Perez-Rodriguez E, Jimenez D, Diaz G, et al. Incidence of air travel-related pulmonary embolism at the Madrid-Barajas airport. Arch Intern Med 2003;163(22):2766–70.
35. Pinski SL. Emergencies related to implantable cardioverter-defibrillators. Crit Care Med 2000;28:N174–N180.
36. Pulmonary Embolism Prevention (PEP) Trial Collaborative Group. Prevention of pulmonary embolism and deep vein thrombosis with low dose aspirin: Pulmonary Embolism Prevention (PEP) trial. Lancet 2000;355:1295–302.
37. Robertson RM. Sudden death from cardiac arrest—improving the odds. N Engl J Med 2000;343:1259–60.
38. Roby H, Lee A, Hopkins A. Safety of air travel following acute myocardial infarction. Aviat Space Environ Med 2002; 73:91–6.
39. Rodenberg H. Prevention of medical emergencies during air travel. Am Fam Phys 1988;37:263.
40. Ryan ET, Kain KC. Primary care: health advice and immunization for travelers. N Engl J Med 2000;342(23):1716–25.
41. Ryan TJ, Anderson JL, Antman EM, el al. ACC/AHA guide-lines for the management of patients with acute myocardial infarction: executive summary. A report of the American College of Cardiology/American Heart Association Task Force on Practice Guidelines (Committee on Management of Acute Myocardial Infarction). Circulation 1996;94(9):2341–50.
42. Sarvesvaran R. Sudden natural deaths associated with commercial air travel. Med Sci Law 1986;26:35–8.
43. Schwarz T, Siegert G, Oettler W, et al. Venous thrombosis after long-haul flights. Arch Intern Med 2003;163(22): 2759–64.
44. Scurr JH, Machin SJ, Bailey-King S, et al. Frequency and prevention of symptomless deep-vein thrombosis in long-haul flights: a randomized trial. Lancet 2001;357:1485–9.
45. Skjenna OW, Evans JF, Moore M, et al. Helping patients travel by air. Can Med Assoc J 1992;144(3):287–93.
46. Stoller JK, Hoisington E, Auger G. A comparative analysis of arranging in-flight oxygen aboard commercial airline carriers. Chest 1999;115(4):991–5.
47. Zahger D, Leibowitz D, Tabb IK, et al. Long-distance air travel soon after an acute coronary syndrome: a prospective evaluation of a triage protocol. Am Heart J 2000;140: 241–2.

# Appendix

# Newer Innovations in the Field of Cardiology

## ANTI-AGING DRUG MAY BE JUST FIVE YEARS AWAY

LONDON : A new anti-aging drug may be just five years away, say scientists who have identified the role of an enzyme in muscle wasting and associated age-related problems. Researchers at the University of Birmingham believe that inhibiting the enzyme could hold the key to developing ways of preventing, or reversing, the adverse effects of aging. The research is a significant step in understanding the role played by the enzyme '11beta-HSD1' in the degenerative effects of ageing—including sarcopenia (age related muscle wasting). Researchers claim the anti-aging drug could be available to the general public within the next five years, according to the Mirror. The expression of 11beta-HSD1, responsible for activating the steroid hormone cortisol, was increased in the muscles of older females. About 134 healthy volunteers, aged between 20–80, underwent physical and biochemical tests at a clinical research facility. The findings show that expression of 11beta-HSD1 in skeletal muscles is increased 2.72-fold in women aged over 60 years of age, compared to those aged between 20 and 40. In male participants, no difference was seen. High levels of the enzyme aligned with increased levels of cortisol, reduced grip strength, insulin resistance and a poorer body composition profile. 'As yet, we do not know why it appears to only occur in women, it is obviously an interesting area for further research. We are planning to look at whether hormones such as estrogens could be involved,' Dr Zaki Hassan-Smith, from the University of Birmingham, said. The research team wanted to investigate novel ways of increasing the healthy life span—the years in which people can maintain active lifestyles without the debilitating impact of muscle wasting. 'Looking at this particular enzyme seemed like an intriguing way forward. We knew how it works in relation to Cushing's Syndrome, which is characterised by similar symptoms, and thought it would be worthwhile applying what we knew to the aging population,' said Hassan-Smith. Cushing's syndrome is a rare disease caused by high cortisol levels, and those who suffer from the syndrome see marked changes in their body composition. The effects can be devastating for patients who can develop features such as muscle wasting and weakness, weight gain, thinning of the bones, diabetes, high blood pressure and heart disease. At present there is no accepted pharmacological treatment for sarcopenia but pharmaceutical companies are developing and testing inhibitors of 11beta-HSD1 with a focus on treatments for such conditions as diabetes. The team is excited about taking the results of their study forward into future research, with one eye on adapting the inhibitors already in development to combat muscle aging. The study was published in the Journal of Clinical Endocrinology and Metabolism.

## HYPERTENSION GUIDELINES

The recommendations made by the individual members of JNC 8 are very narrow in scope and of possible interest to 'academicians' who seek evidence-based strategies but not of much practical value to the healthcare providers who actually treat hypertension. One example—the guidelines from the past members of JNC 8 suggest a threshold of >150/90 mmHg for patients 60 years or older whereas the ASH/ISH guidelines apply that level of BP threshold for patients >80 years. The suggestion for age dependent criteria for hypertension management made by the erstwhile JNC 8 were made on the basis of hand-picked studies in the elderly. The recommendation was based on the observation that a systolic BP of <140 mmHg was not superior to <150 mmHg. However, in the studies they cited, no harm was induced at a systolic BP <140 mmHg. In contrast, the ASH/ISH guidelines suggest a threshold of <140/90 mmHg for patients between ages 60 and 80 on the basis of data from 3 large studies—ALLHAT, VALUE, and ACCOMPLISH. The threshold for <150 mmHg (as opposed to <140 mmHg) applies only if you are 80 years of age or

**Table A-1:** Classification of blood pressure (age 18 and above) Indian guidelines 2013

| Category | SBP (mmHg) | DBP (mmHg) |
|---|---|---|
| Optimal | <120 | <80 |
| Normal | <130 | <85 |
| High normal | 130–139 | 85–89 |
| **Hypertension** | | |
| Stage 1 | 140–159 | 90–99 |
| Stage 2 | 160–179 | 100–109 |
| Stage 3 | >180 | >110 |
| **ISH** | | |
| Grade I | 140–159 | <90 |
| Grade II | >160 | <90 |

older. This has been a contentious point. Who can really argue that for a 60-year-old, a systolic BP level <140 mmHg is embarrassing! The proposal made by the JNC 8 panel members that the target BP for patients over 60 should be >150/90 mmHg has the potential of misinterpretation and laxity at a time when there is a hue and cry to improve the hypertension control rates in all ages. The elderly group is of paramount importance because of high risk, disease vulnerability, and high rates of 'resistant' hypertension. The burden of proof provided by the JNC 8 members was insufficient to reduce the burden of CVD.

### Take Home Practical Points

- The threshold to treat hypertension should be 140/90 mmHg in all patients <80 years.
- For individuals >80 years, the threshold to treat hypertension should be 150/90 mmHg.
- For patients with chronic kidney disease CVD, diabetes, and proteinuria, the blood pressure target should be between 130/80 mmHg and 140/90 mmHg.
- Keep in mind what I stated elsewhere – the issue in patients with hypertension is 'high' blood pressure and not 'low' blood pressure. No one is asking you to lower the BP levels deliberately to 110/60 mmHg or 90/50 mmHg. Common sense is still valid.
- Do not loosen the goal blood pressure levels but focus on achieving a blood pressure of <140/90 mmHg in persons under the age of 80 years; for individuals older than 80 years, achieve (if possible) the blood pressure level of 150/90 mmHg.
- Simple, no confusion, straight forward, and go for it.

## VALUE OF FFR IN CLINICAL PRACTICE

### *Key points*

- Fractional flow reserve (FFR) is a single highly reliable and reproducible invasive method to assess the ischemia producing potential of a lesion with accuracy of more than 90%
- Currently a cutoff value of less than 0.8 is recommended for revascularization
- Useful in assessment of intermediate coronary lesions in stable ischemic heart disease (left main disease, bifurcation disease, ostial disease, serial lesions, diffuse disease, old MI and collateralized vessels)
- In ACS patients it can be used for non-culprit lesions and after 7 days in the culprit lesions (not reliable in the culprit vessels in acute stage)
- While performing FFR important to equalize pressure sensor at the tip of the guide catheter after removing the introduced needle
- Pressure sensor should be placed at least 3 cm distal to the lesion
- Although a number of resting indices (resting Pd/Pa, IFR etc.) have been proposed, their diagnostic accuracy is around 80%. However, if resting Pd/Pa is <0.8 on maximal hyperemia, the FFR will be <0.8. If one is evaluating a single focal stenosis one can use the baseline criteria for revascularization.
- Hyperemia is essential to achieve a steady state of minimal microvascular resistance to correctly interpret lesion physiology in all lesions (single or serial or diffuse disease).
- For hyperemia IV adenosine or regadenoson is better than IC bolus for steady state and continuous pullback to assess serial lesions.
- Sometimes IV adenosine may not have adequate vasodilatory effect due to rapid peripheral metabolism. In such scenarios perform the response using incremental doses of IC adenosine bolus. For multivessel evaluation, IV adenosine is preferred over regadenoson because it has a longer lasting hemodynamic effect.
- Regadenoson has significantly larger blood pressure lowering effect than IV adenosine (caution in patients with borderline blood pressures).
- Slight variations in FFR values seen with respirations but use the lowest value in steady state.
- Pullback slowly along the entire length of the artery.
- Pullback to guide catheter to identify if there is any significant electronic drift.

**Table A-2:** Vasodilators for testing fractional flow reserve

| |
|---|
| **Epicardial vasodilators** |
| Nitroglycerin: 200–400 μg IC, administer 30s before first measurement |
| **Microvascular vasodilators** |
| Adenosine or ATP: ≥40 μg IC bolus in RCA, ≥80 μg IC bolus in LCA |
| Adenosine or ATP: 140 μg/kg/min IV (preferably through a central venous line) |
| Regadeonson (Rapiscan): 400 μg single bolus IC or peripheral IV |
| Papaverine: 10–12 mg in the RCA, 15–20 mg in the LCA |

IC=intracoronary; IV=intravenously; RCA=right coronary artery; LCA=left coronary artery; ATP=adenosine triphosphate.

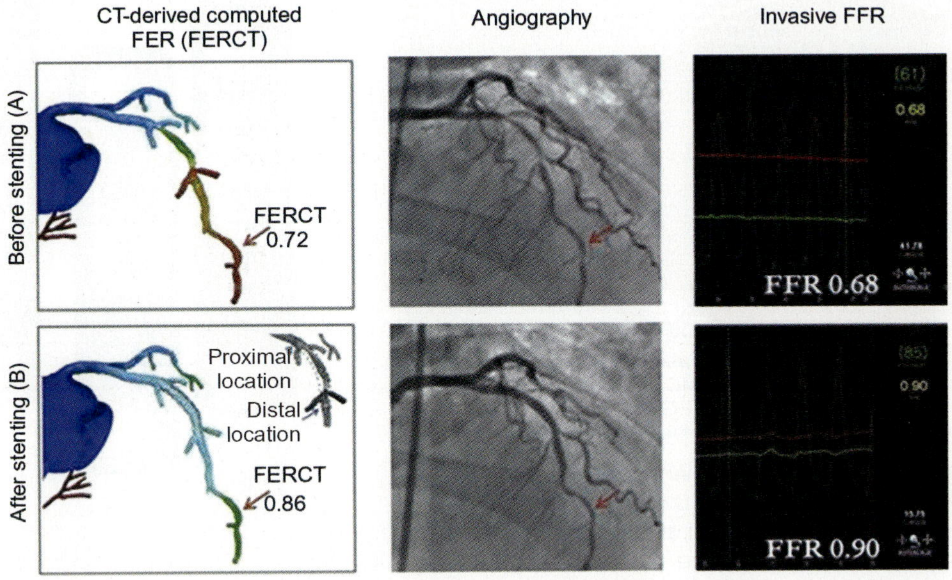


**Fig. A-1:** Invasive and noninvasive functional assessment before and after revascularization. (A) Noninvasive fractional flow reserve (FFR) from coronary computed tomographic angiography data (FFRCT) of the left anterior descending (LAD) coronary artery was 0.72. Invasive coronary angiography and FFR confirmed the functionally significant LAD stenosis. (B) FFRCT demonstrated no ischemia in the LAD after virtual stenting, with a computed value of 0.86. Invasive FFR after stent implantation was 0.90

## COMPUTED FRACTIONAL FLOW RESERVE DERIVED FROM CORONARY CT ANGIOGRAPHY

Recent advances in image-based modeling and computational fluid dynamics permit the calculation of coronary artery pressure and flow from typically acquired coronary computed tomography (CT) scans. Computed fractional flow reserve (FFRCT) is the ratio of mean coronary artery pressure divided by mean aortic pressure under conditions of simulated maximal coronary hyperemia, thus providing a noninvasive estimate of fractional flow reserve at every point in the coronary tree. Prospective multicenter clinical trials have shown that computed FFRCT improves diagnostic accuracy and discrimination compared to CT stenosis alone for the diagnosis of hemodynamically significant coronary artery disease (CAD), when compared to invasive FFR as the reference gold standard. This promising new technology provides a combined anatomic and physiologic assessment of CAD in a single noninvasive test that can help select patients for invasive angiography and revascularization or best medical therapy. Further evaluation of the clinical effectiveness and economic implications of noninvasive FFRCT are now being explored.

## VITAMIN D AND CARDIOVASCULAR DISEASE

Vitamin D is a fat soluble vitamin which also functions as a hormone. Now there is ample evidence that low levels of vitamin D has been found to be associated with diabetes, systemic hypertension, metabolic syndrome, coronary heart disease (CHD), heart failure and vascular inflammation.

The mechanism of vitamin D deficiency leading to atherosclerotic vascular disease is complex. It involves raised parathormone levels leading to heightened RAAS (renin-angiotensin-aldosterone system) activity, insulin resistance and inflammation. At the cellular level, vitamin D acts through the vitamin D receptor (VDR), which is found in virtually all tissues of the body including cardiovascular tissues like cardiomyocytes, endothelial, and vascular smooth muscle cells. Cardiovascular effects of vitamin D share the common initial steps of nuclear and plasma membrane VDR activation in the above cells.

There are few reports of association of CHD and vitamin D levels from India. An observational study of hospitalized patients with AMI from Bengaluru reported 83.5% prevalence of vitamin D deficiency. The association between low vitamin D levels and cardiovascular risk factors have also been noted in previous studies from India.

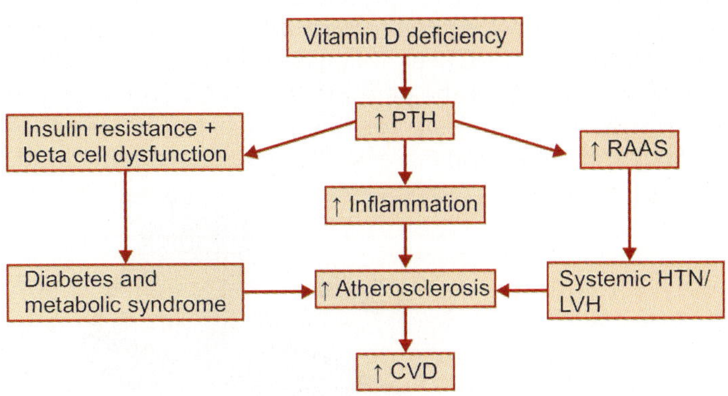


**Fig. A-2:** The mechanisms of vitamin D deficiency leading to atherosclerotic vascular disease. (PTH=parathyroid hormone, RAAS=renin angiotensin aldosterone system, HTN=hypertension, CVD=cardiovascular disease, LVH=left ventricular hypertrophy)

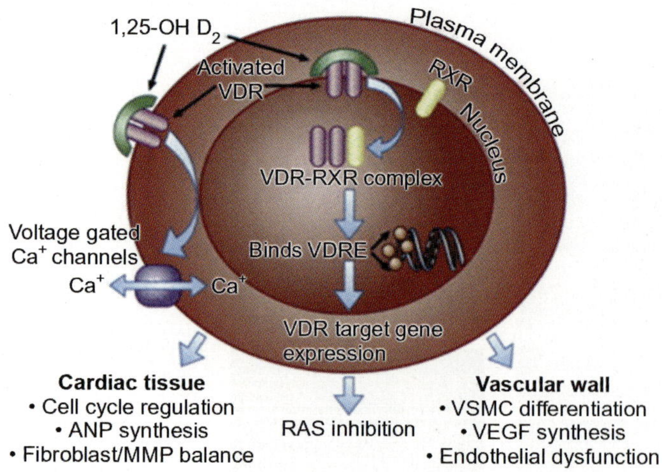


**Fig. A-3:** Mechanisms by which vitamin D deficiency may confer cardiovascular risk. Potential effects of vitamin D metabolism on the cardiovascular system are divergent, but share common initial steps of nuclear and plasma membrane VDR activation. VDR, vitamin D receptor; 1,25-OH $D_2$, 1,25-dihydroxyvitamin D; RXR, retinoid-X receptor; $Ca^+$, calcium cation; ANP, atrial natriuretic peptide; MMP, matrix metalloproteinases; VDRE, vitamin D response elements (promoter region of target genes); RAS, renin-angiotensin system; VEGF, vascular endothelial growth factor; VSMC, vascular smooth muscle cells. (Published with permission from EHJ, Ibhar Al Mheid et al. Vitamin D and cardiovascular disease: is the evidence solid? Eur Heart J. 2013 Dec;34(48):3691–8)

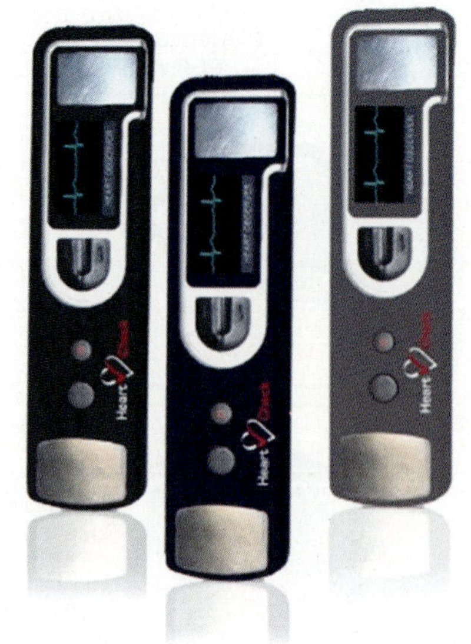

**Fig. A-4:** The HeartCheck Pen which would benefit persons interested in monitoring their health

## THE ECG OF THE FUTURE

What is electrocardiography (ECG), and why is it useful? ECG is the interpretation of the electrical activity of the heart over a period of time. It is used to measure the rate and regularity of heartbeats as well as the size and position of the chambers, the presence of any damage to the heart, and the effects of drugs or devices used to regulate the heart.

It sounds like having an ECG could be quite handy, right? Well yes, it would be, but who would want to spend thousands and have a large brick of a device lying around? *Look at the size of that thing below, not me!* How about something you can trust to deliver accurate results and slip into your shirt pocket? *Now we are talking.* CardioComm's new handheld HeartCheck™ Pen does just that, it puts the benefits of an ECG in the palm of your hand. You may see hypochondriacs lining up for this device, but its use goes well beyond those who have health obsession on the mind.

The HeartCheck Pen would benefit any person interested in monitoring his/her health due to heart disease. It could also be used to determine potential heart disease by assessing abnormal heart rhythms and muscle defects. From athletes to seniors, a wide range of consumers could benefit from this device.

'We feel the HeartCheck Pen is a true remote monitoring device because it is compact, easy to use, and takes accurate heart readings in only 30 seconds. The pen may be used from anywhere, including at home, the office, the gym or in remote areas which are often inaccessible to common ECG machines,' said Etienne Grima, CardioComm Solutions' CEO.

The device makes sending and storing ECGs easy. Up to 20 ECGs can be stored on the device, and once you hit that mark you can download the ECGs to your computer and print them off, or save some trees and send them electronically to your doc or clinic. The data can also be downloaded to GEMS™ Home, where repeated recordings can be managed in a personal health data record.

'What makes this product unique,' explained Grima, 'is that after a consumer sends a selected heart rate recording to the C4 medical call-center over the internet using GEMS™ Home, the actual ECG recording will be reviewed and interpreted by an attending C4 physician. The ECG

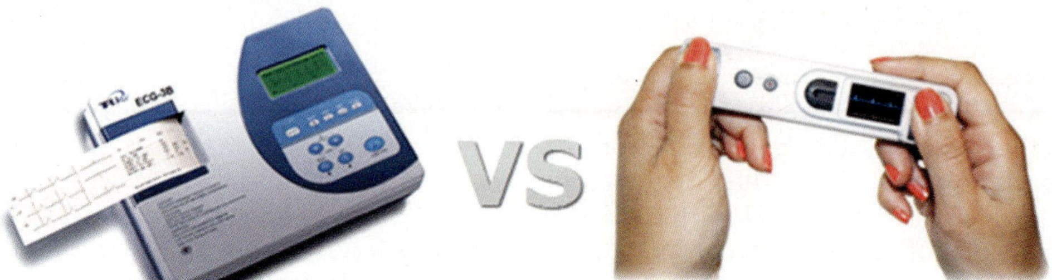


**Fig. A-5:** Comparing conventional (A) and pen type ECGs (B)

report will then be made available to the customer, again through GEM Home, where they may retrieve the ECG interpretation and use it in communicating with their own health care providers.'

The HeartCheck Pen definitely has some interesting advantages over its big brother, but is it something you would use?

## NEW ANDROID ECG SYSTEM TO PATIENTS, ATHLETES KEEP A CLOSE EYE ON HEART

A new smartphone-based device that may replace Holter monitors and help athletes achieve endurance goals is under development at VTT technical research centre of Finland. Some dangerous heart arrhythmias can be hard to detect since they often comes and go, and so can be missed at the doctor's office. Holter monitors have been used for decades to monitor the heart over extended periods of time, but they are bulky and inconvenient.

The new system straps on the chest of the user and sends ECG data over to an android smartphone wirelessly over bluetooth. A live chart can be examined and historical data can be passed to a cardiologist for review. Moreover, unlike the AliveCor and ECGCheck that are ECGs within an iPhone case, the form factor of the VTT device allows athletes to closely monitor their heartbeat during exercise, helping achieve goals while detecting **arrhythmia.**

### From VTT

The device measures ECG signals at a sufficiently high sampling rate, identifies individual heart beats and counts the interval between consecutive beats. The device is also equipped with an accelerometer. The signals are sent to a smartphone via bluetooth. The application displays ECG, heart rate and its variability. The signal from the accelerometer can also be used as a step counter.

Beat2Phone is the first device and software application developed for android phones that can be used to measure and save an ECG and to perform an extensive analysis of the data. The device also enables an advanced heart rate analysis, and GPS-based speed and distance measurements. Compared to wristband devices, smart phones represent the best available user interface technology.

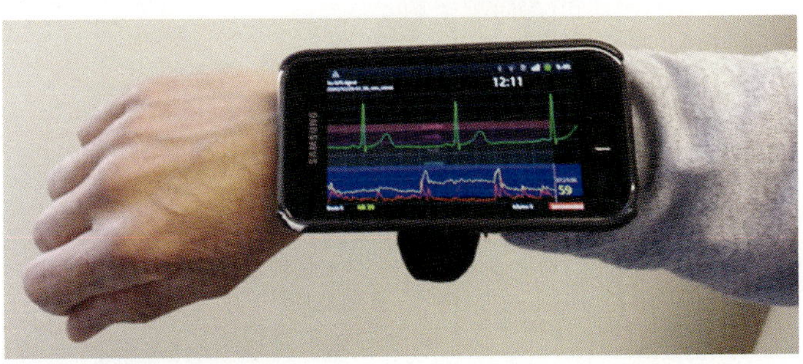

**Fig. A-6:** A new android ECG system for monitoring heart rhythm on the wrist of a person

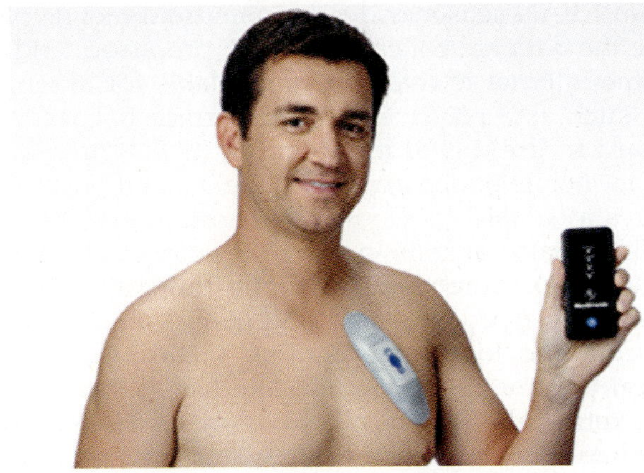

**Fig. A-7:** The SEEQ™ mobile cardiac telemetry system

## SEEQ MOBILE CARDIAC TELEMETRY SYSTEM

Short-term heart monitoring up to 30 days.

It may help your doctor diagnose and treat irregular heartbeats related to:

- Unexplained fainting
- Heart palpitations
- Atrial fibrillation
- Unexplained stroke

### The Simplest Solution

Unlike most external heart monitoring systems, SEEQ MCT features a discreet, patient-friendly design. You can easily apply the peel-and-stick wearable sensor yourself. It is like an adhesive bandage you wear on your chest. Once applied, the wearable sensor monitors your heart, records any irregular heart rhythms, and communicates through a cellular network to the Medtronic Monitoring Center via the transmitter you carry with you.

## MONITORING YOUR HEALTH WITH YOUR MOBILE PHONE ECG

The newly-developed low-power interface wirelessly transmits bio-signals retrieved by imec and Holst Centre's

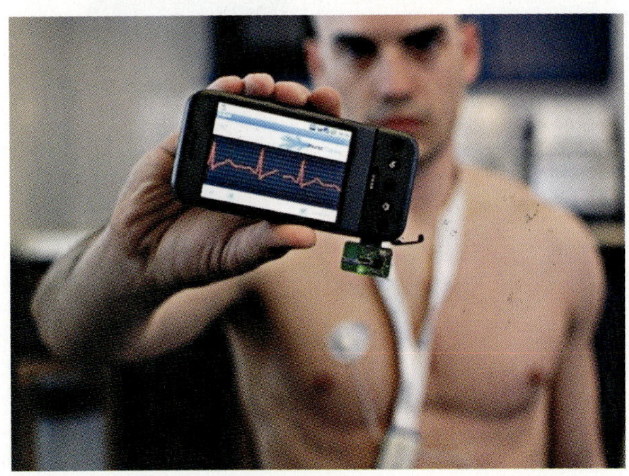

**Fig. A-8:** ECG signals wirelessly transmitted to an android mobile phone via a low-power interface

Human++ BAN sensor nodes to an android mobile phone where the data are collected, stored, processed, and sent over the internet to make them available for authorized users such as a physician. The interface is based on a standard secure digital input output (SDIO) interface on android mobile phones, enabling the integration of all the features available on Google's operating system (SMS, e-mail and data transmission over the internet, GPS to track user location). Moreover, the mobile phone's hardware is extended to operate with low-power communication protocols and low-power radios, enabling long-term medical telemonitoring. As the interface is based on the Linux kernel, the system is also easily portable on other Linux-based devices, such as PDA's or laptops. And, the system allows configuration of thresholds on the measured parameters and automatic sending of alerts such as SMS messages and e-mails based on these values.

## CARDIODEFENDER SMARTPHONE-BASED ECG, A 21ST CENTURY HOLTER MONITOR

**Everist Genomics**, an Ann Arbor, Michigan company, is set to release its CardioDefender diagnostic system, a smartphone ECG that can provide continuous readings throughout the day that can help detect arrhythmias that may be hard to spot in an office visit. The system uses a wrist watch-like device to collect data from electrodes and transmit it wirelessly via bluetooth to a smartphone that can then share it with clinicians monitoring the patient. CardioDefender, that recently won both FDA approval and EU's CE Mark, can activate an alarm to rapidly notify a physician of any particularly unwelcome graph via an email, page, or other electronic means.

- Fully mobile system; CardioDefender is the world's first ECG system which delivers hospital based quality ECG and arrhythmia analysis by integrating unique software, algorithms and data compression capabilities which enable a smartphone to perform as a mobile ECG.
- Real-time, heart-rhythm monitoring
- Beat-by-beat analysis of heart rhythm (as opposed to sampling some heart beats or part of a heart beat)
- Long-term monitoring capability; CardioDefender can perform up to 3 months of real-time, beat-by-beat quantitative patient monitoring and analysis
- Quantitative analysis and reporting; CardioDefender is a fully automated, quantitative ECG monitoring and arrhythmia event reporting system
- Comprehensive range of heart rhythm monitoring algorithms to enable automated detection and reporting of medically important arrhythmias to physicians and monitoring centers
- Abnormal heart rhythms reported directly to physicians mobile phone or computer; innovative and patent protected software and data compression technology means CardioDefender can report real-time results to a physician's smartphone, tablets, laptop and desk top computer (in addition to a cardiac monitoring center)
- Access to full, detailed ECG data captured during the monitoring period, including post-heart monitoring data processing for additional measurements
- Real-time reporting of symptomatic and asymptomatic arrhythmias; CardioDefender has the ability to capture and report both symptomatic and asymptomatic arrhythmias

## PEN ON THE PULSE: A BETTER WAY TO MEASURE BLOOD PRESSURE

Innovative pulse-reading technology is at the centre of the University of Queensland (UQ) blood pressure study to reduce cardiovascular disease.

In a world-first study, researchers from UQ are using innovative pulse-reading technology to measure blood pressure to reduce cardiovascular disease. Principal investigator, Associate Professor Jim Sharman and Professor Michael Stowasser from the UQ *School of Medicine* said the findings would provide a new and refined target

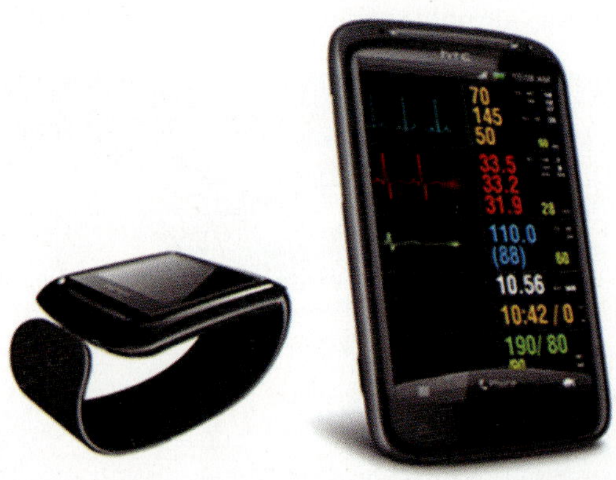


**Fig. A-9:** CardioDefender smartphone-based ECG, a 21st Century Holter Monitor. Real-time reporting of symptomatic and asymptomatic arrhythmias; CardioDefender has the ability to capture and report both symptomatic and asymptomatic arrhythmias

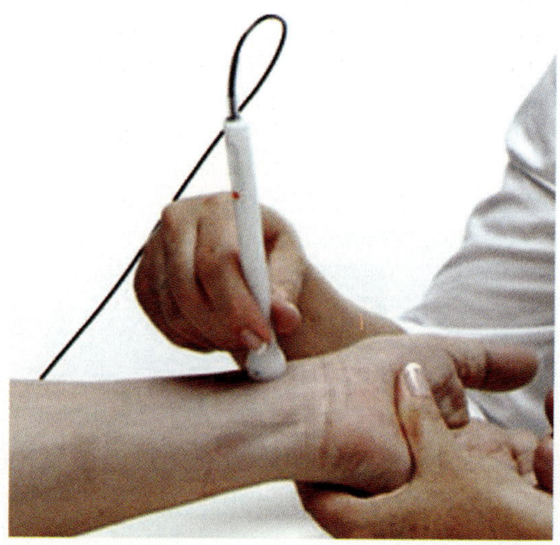

**Fig. A-10:** A newer pen on radial artery technique in the measurement of blood pressure

for blood pressure control to lower cardiovascular disease risk.

Associate Professor Sharman said hypertension was one of the major risk factors for cardiovascular disease, which was the cause of more deaths every year than any other disease.

'Maintaining good blood pressure control is seen as a key process in appropriate management of cardiovascular disease risk,' associate professor sharman said.

'Preliminary studies have indicated that the standard inflated arm cuff, a crude method that is over 100-years-old, may not necessarily be the best way to measure blood pressure on those who have hypertension.'

'In recent years, noninvasive techniques have been developed to give a more accurate estimate of blood pressure that the organs are exposed to, and central blood pressure.'

'The new method measures central blood pressure from the arterial pulse at the wrist using a pen-like device that has a pressure transducer at the tip, this is placed lightly on the pulse at the wrist and a mathematical formula is then used to synthesise central blood pressure.'

'The method is quick, reliable and provides important information on blood pressure that is above and beyond that using the old upper arm cuff method.'

In February this year the researchers made a major breakthrough by proving for the first time that targeted central blood pressure lowering is possible using a routine low-dose of a medication that is cheap, readily available and has a well-documented safety profile.

'This is a big reason why we got funding from the National Health and Medical Research Council to do this study,' Associate Professor Sharman said.

'We expect that evidence from this new trial will ultimately lead to a paradigm shift in the approach to treating patients with hypertension.'

'That is, central blood pressure will be considered a more important therapeutic target than conventional blood pressure measured at the upper arm.'

This new and refined method may be used in general medicine to help lower cardiovascular disease risk among a very broad group of people who have hypertension.

Male and females aged between 18 years and 70 years who have been diagnosed with hypertension and are taking at least one but no more than three medications for hypertension are invited to participate.

The study is over 24 months where participants will be asked to visit the Princess Alexandra Hospital every 3 months for the first 6 months then every 6 months for the next 18 months.

## WRIST REDUCING HIGH BLOOD PRESSURE VESSEL CLEANING MACHINE

### Product Description

Wrist reducing high blood pressure vessel cleaning machine.

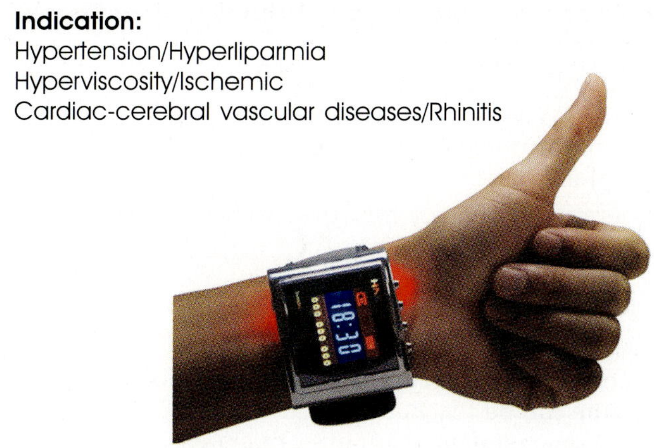


**Fig. A-11:** Wrist reducing high blood pressure vessel cleaning machine

### Indications

High blood pressure, hyperviscosity, hyperlipidemia, hypertension, diabetes, cardiovascular and cerebrovascular diseases

### Advantage

1. Low level laser irradiation, noninvasive, no side effect, no cross infection, pure green physiotherapy.
2. Above 90% therapeutic effect with positive clinical trial report provided.
3. As household physiotherapy devices, small size, intelligent design, easy operation and convenient carrying.
4. Great marketing margin exists.
5. Certification and patents protection provided with the passing of CE, RoHs, ISO9001 and ISO13485.

### Therapeutic Principle

HY30-D hypertention laser therapy watch is based on modern laser medicine and proven clinical practice. The device applies a low-level 650 nm wavelength laser. Our instrument utilizes explicit irradiation to change biological characteristics and remove fat layer/cholesterol from red blood cells, thereby improving the activity, deformability, and oxygen carrying capacity of cells to reduce the concentration of middle molecules in the bloodstream. This process improves hem rheological properties while lowering triglycerides and cholesterol for the effective treatment and prevention of heart and brain diseases.

### Function and Performance

1. Improving blood viscosity through laser blood irradiation.
2. Improving blood oxygen carrying capacity through laser blood irradiation.
3. Reducing blood-fat and total cholesterol through laser blood irradiation.
4. Quickly and effectively correct the abnormity of lipid metabolism and maintain the equilibrium level of the

lipid metabolism in the human body through laser blood irradiation.

5. Improving the partial blood circulation around the nasal cavities and the immunological competence of the nasal mucosa membranes through irradiation the nasal mucosa.
6. Therapeutic efficacy control on ischemic cardiac-cerebral vascular diseases.

### Features

1. Good clinical therapeutic effect, laser irradiation to three parts or acupoints of human body at the same time can be reached.
2. A laser stabilizer specially added to perform with more stability.
3. Our semiconductor laser devices are used by high quality imported laser head which has the long life-span.
4. Products owned five patents protection.
5. Humanistic and scientific design to fit human physiological curve and ergonomics.
6. Medical use of high capacity lithium battery for the energy-saving.
7. Using high-class and durable metal enclosure which is conducive to heat diffusion for the power stable.
8. Time and power are adjustable, very smart memory system.
9. Two output modes—pulse and continues, which have manual and automatic switch available.
10. Pluggable laser wire, more convenience in use and easier maintenance.

### Caution

1. Not suitable for the following groups: Cancer patient, pregnancy, patient with hemorrhagic diseases.
2. Children shall only use the instrument under the direction of their parents.
3. The elder patients and sensitive patients must accept the low-power and short-time treatment at the beginning, the rate of work could be increased as the body adjusts.

## NEXT GENERATION OF VITAL AND BLOOD PRESSURE MEASUREMENT

- Wear your CARUNDA24 on your wrist, just like a watch and monitor your blood pressure around the clock.
- Measure your blood pressure easily and comfortably, without a cuff.
- Your blood pressure will be displayed (and stored) immediately.
- Your personal data can be transferred to external devices for further analysis.
- Continuous measurements – without a cuff – overcome a 100 year limitation of traditional methods of measuring blood pressure.
- Follow the exciting process of developing a brand new system on these pages.

### Background

Today more than one billion people are suffering from high blood pressure (hypertension) and continuous surveillance should be available for these people. Over half of the population affected are not even aware of their disease according to the World Health Organisation. Monitoring vital functions is a must for these and other people suffering from other kind of serious diseases.

Vital functions include breathing, body (core) temperature and the cardiovascular system, in particular arterial pulse (wave) and arterial blood pressure. Today there are a several systems which deliver a variety of data, but only very few in the field of blood pressure. The well-known and widely used heart-rate-monitors show only one aspect of the pulse and not the whole pulse-wave.

CARUNDA24 solves this problem. The continuous, noninvasive measurement of the pulse wave provides you and your physician or health-care professional not only with blood pressure (diastolic and systolic) but also critical information about the quality of your pulse including the number and regularity of your heartbeat and the rate of increase in blood pressure.

Whether you are affected by high blood pressure, or simply want to take preventive action, CARUNDA24 will help increase awareness and early recognition of potential

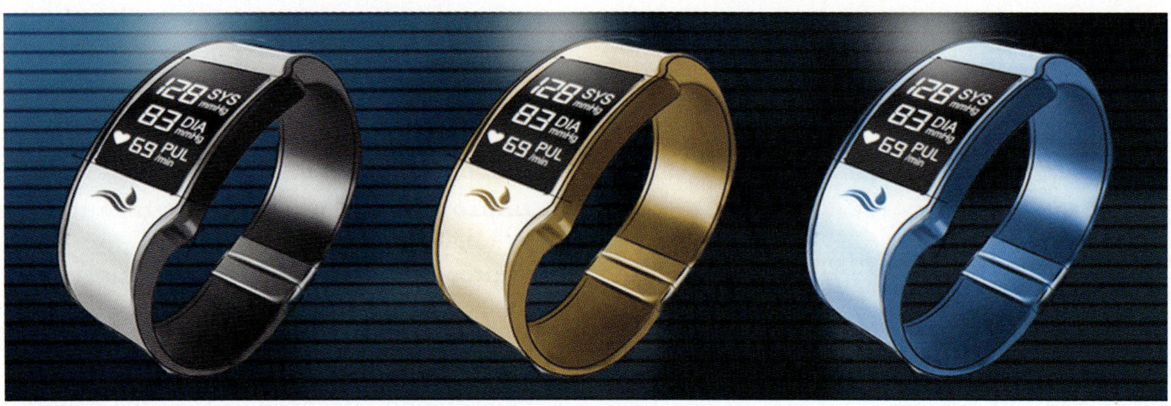


**Fig. A-12:** Next generation wristwatch type of vital and blood pressure measurement instrument

adverse events, enabling you reduce their risk of related health problems.

### What You Can Expect

With CARUNDA24 we aim to offer a medically certified system that meets the highest technical and medical requirements and is suitable for use in hospitals, medical practices as well as at home. CARUNDA24 looks—and can be worn—just like an ordinary watch, measuring the pulse wave and therefore the blood pressure (continuously) on the surface of the wrist. Data is displayed and stored instantly and can be transferred wirelessly to external equipment for detailed analysis.

Measuring blood pressure with CARUNDA24 is extremely simple – it can be measured for several hours; in fact all day long, if necessary, around the clock!

STBL aims to provide state of the art medical approved systems, that fullfil highest technological and medical standards. These systems should be able to be used in clinics, medical offices but also at home.

### Risks and Challenges

Even after a successful 'proof of concept', the road from clinical prototype to a commercially deliverable system is still full of challenges; which may be of a technical nature (as CARUNDA24 uses a new method which still has to be subjected to extensive testing) or in the validation process where unknown questions may arise.

At the start of 2014 the preperation of an extensive clinical proof of concept milestone was started which will lasted around 9 months. With the preparation of a new generation of prototypes can be begun in the first quarter of 2015 the earliest. In this and all further steps unknown questions may arise whicht could lead to further delays.

### Additional Applications

Due to the newly developed continuous measurement method and modern communication technologies CARUNDA24 systems could be used in the field of telemedicine, remote surveillance such as in nursing homes or intensive care units.

## NONINVASIVE GLUCOMETER FROM ORSENSE APPROVED IN EUROPE

The bulky device is illustrated in Fig. A-13, and the Fig. A-12 expected appearance of the next generation device based on the company's proprietary technology. The NBM-200G is based on OrSense's proprietary breakthrough technology that allows noninvasive measurement of analytes including glucose, hemoglobin, and oxygen saturation with very high sensitivity. The NBM-200G is operated by placing a ring-shaped probe around the patient's finger, which applies a gentle pressure to the finger, similar to that applied during noninvasive blood-pressure measurement and temporarily occludes the blood flow. During the occlusion, optical elements in the sensor perform a sensitive measurement of the light transmitted through the finger. This method, called occlusion spectroscopy, provides a quick, accurate and painless measurement of the patient's blood glucose. The method was tested on over 400 subjects, exhibiting comparable accuracy to invasive solutions, while providing superior ease of use and safety. In addition, the NBM-200G enables the identification of glucose trends and the detection of hypo- and hyperglycemia events and may also optimally answer the growing need for tight glycemic control in acute care settings, thereby reducing morbidity and mortality.

## 24 HOURS $SpO_2$ AMBULATORY BLOOD PRESSURE MONITORING COLOR LCD $SpO_2$ ABPM BP MONITOR

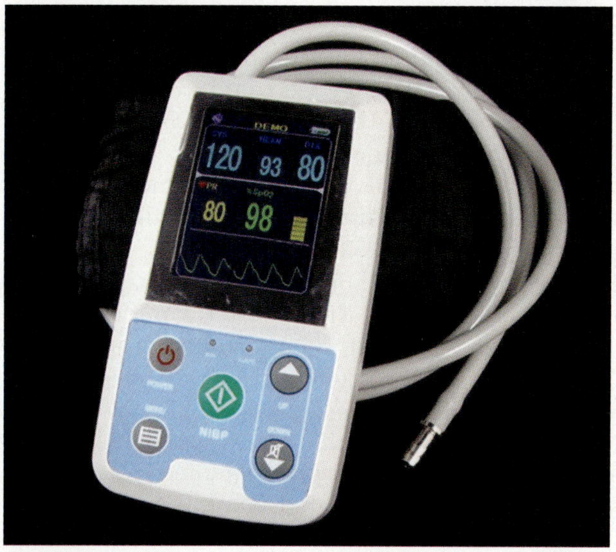


**Fig. A-14:** 24 hours $SpO_2$ ambulatory blood pressure monitoring Color LCD $SpO_2$ ABPM BP monitor

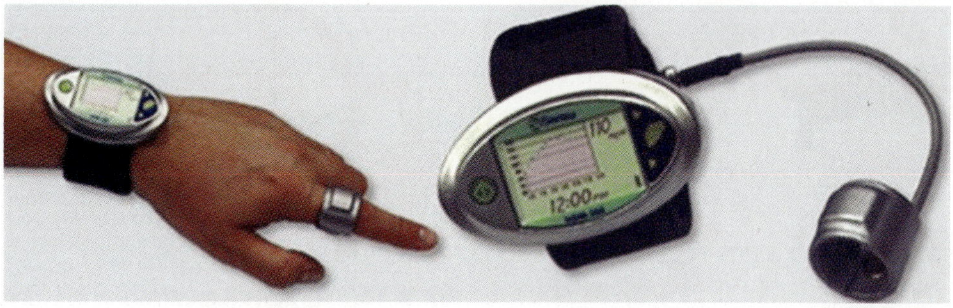


**Fig. A-13:** OrSense Ltd., a Nes Ziona, Israel company, is reporting that its NBM-200G noninvasive continuous monitor of blood glucose for diabetics has been granted the CE Mark of approval in the EU

## 2014 NEW WIRELESS/WIFI TREADMILL STRESS TEST SYSTEM FOR CARDIAC STRESS EXERCISE IN GYM/ HOME WITH CE AND ISO

- Wireless solution for cardiac stress exercise.
- Windows XP/VISTA operating system
- CardioScape provides an intuitive user interface with flexible configurations to facilitate ease-of-use
- Complete ST presentation
- In addition to continuous ST trends, CardioScape presents ST level and slope for all 12 average complexes and auto-comparison with reference complexes which can be edited both during and after the procedure.

### Wireless ECG Acquisition Option

- Wireless ECG module digitally transmits and receives diagnostic quality 12-lead ECG data without the need for a conventional tethered patient cable
- Source consistency filter
- CardioScape super anti-drift technology reduces noise and baseline artifact while preserving a diagnostic quality ECG signal
- Beat by beat review mode
- Post-test playback allows for full disclosure review of the entire test
- Comprehensive trends
- Display and print all kinds of trend graph such as HR, BP, METS, HR*BP, exercise trend, ST-segment level/ Influence/Slope/ST/HR, etc.
- Powerful case management
- CardioScape provides powerful case management and perfect case history input/output function
- Compatible with RS232 Treadmills
- CardioScape is compatible with Trackmaster, Cosmos, RAM, Schiller, Taeha, Trackmaster, Parker, Valiant
- CardioScape wireless ECG transmitter and receiver
- CardioScape advanced wireless telemetry revolutionizes traditional stress exercise and enables new levels of freedom in multi-modality stress testing. CardioScape stress exercise systems applies patented ECG algorithms and are designed to meet a complete range of stress exercise testing needs.

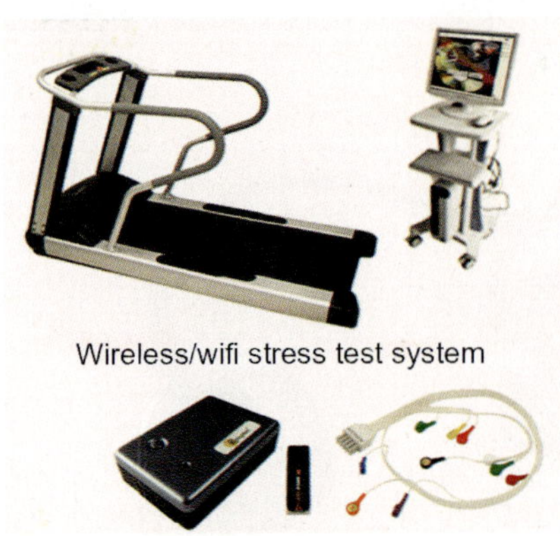


**Fig. A-15:** PC-based wireless treadmill ECG stress test system

### Freedom of Movement

CardioScape provides wireless freedom of movement for the patient and clinician.

### Diagnostic Quality

CardioScape wireless technology features full diagnostic ECG quality.

### Significant Artifact Reduction

The wireless soltuion eliminates artifact due to traditional cable movement, resulting in cleaner, higher quality tracing.

### Comfortable ECG Acquisition for Patient

CardioScape eliminate the need for traditional ECG patient cable.

## CLINICAL APPLICATION OF CENTRAL BLOOD PRESSURE

### What is Central Blood Pressure?

Central blood pressure is the pressure in the aorta, which is the large artery into which the heart pumps. The term *'central blood pressure'* usually refers to the pressure in the aorta near the heart.

### How is Central Blood Pressure Different from Normal Blood Pressure?

Normally, blood pressure is measured in the upper arm, which is a *'peripheral'* artery. Peripheral blood pressure is usually higher than central blood pressure due to the peripheral site being closer to locations from which echoes reverberate.

The degree to which the peripheral blood pressure is higher than central blood pressure depends partly on the stiffness of the arteries.

### Why is Central Blood Pressure Important?

Central pressure has been shown to more strongly relate to vascular disease and outcome than traditional upper arm blood pressure. It also can distinguish between the effects

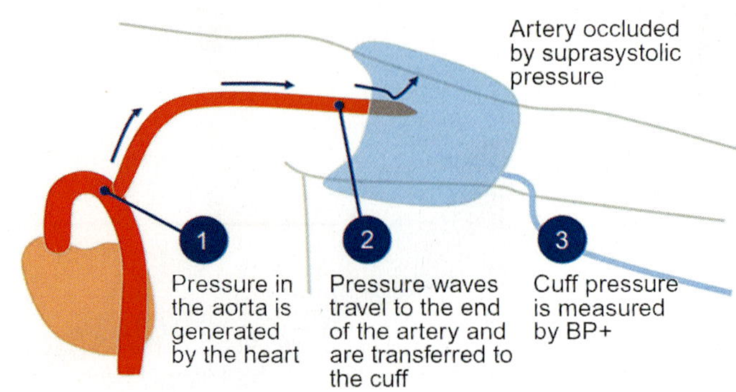


**Fig. A-16:** Diagram explaining basic understanding of central blood pressure mechanism

of different hypertension medications when upper arm blood pressure and pulse wave velocity do not.

Central blood pressure is the pressure that the heart has to pump against to get blood to flow to the rest of the body. Higher central blood pressures mean that the heart must work harder to do its job. This can eventually lead to heart failure. Central blood pressure also determines the pressure in the blood vessels feeding the brain. If central pressure is too high, it may cause aneurysms and strokes.

### How is Central Blood Pressure Measured?

Central blood pressure can be directly measured only using a pressure sensor or catheter inserted into the aorta (usually through an artery in the groin or wrist). This procedure is invasive and can lead to complications.

### How Does BP+ Measure Central Blood Pressure Noninvasively?

BP+ calculates central blood pressure using a physics-based model of the arteries between the aorta and the cuff. This model relate how pressure waves travel between the aorta and the occluded artery under the suprasystolic cuff, as shown in the diagram that follows.

### Central Aortic Systolic Pressure Monitoring Device

A-PULSE CASPal® is a simple device for the measurement of central aortic systolic pressure (CASP) in a simple clinic or home setting. It is a world-first portable CASP measurement device developed by HealthSTATS International. It is empowered by EVBP technology; a FDA listed and patented technology using modified applanation tonometry on the radial artery at the position of the wrist. It is completely noninvasive, painless and easy-to-operate.

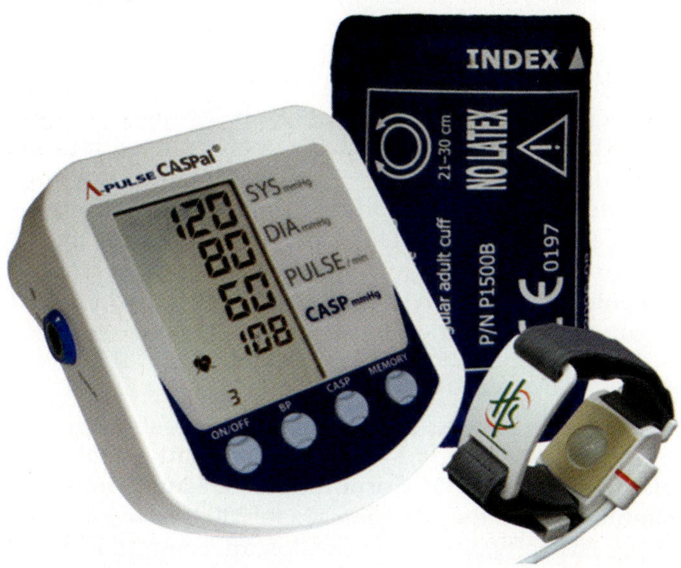


**Fig. A-17:** A-PULSE CASPal® is a simple device for the measurement of central aortic systolic pressure (CASP) in a simple clinic or home setting, using modified applanation tonometry on the radial artery at the position of the wrist

It is specially designed for home user for ease of use to obtain CASP.

*A-PULSE CASPal®* is a noninvasive blood pressure monitoring system which is designed to measure the central aortic systolic pressure (CASP) and additional arterial pulse waveform related indices based on arterial tonometry at the radial artery of the wrist. The system consists of four main elements:

- A-PULSE CASPal® monitor
- Wrist sensor module based on the technology of the BPro® monitor device
- Built-in software algorithm for blood pressure measurement and calculation based on the A-PULSE CASP® software
- Integrated oscillometric blood pressure module for calibration.

### What are the Advantages of the BP+ Approach to Central Pressure?

Central pressure is estimated noninvasively by using a mathematical relationship to a peripheral pressure. The degree to which this mathematical relationship matches any individual determines the accuracy of the central pressure estimate in that subject.

The BP+ technique has a number of advantages over empirical transfer function and statistical attempts at estimating central blood pressure.

Upper arm measurement means the distance between the sensor and the heart is much shorter than wrist or finger measurements, meaning less variability between the arterial geometry of individuals.

Cuff inflated to occlude the brachial artery means individual variations in downstream arteries can be ignored.

Physics-based model is applicable where statistical and empirical relationships are invalid. This is particularly true for stiff arteries.

### Does BP+ Require Calibration to Estimate Central Blood Pressure?

No external calibration is necessary to estimate central blood pressure using BP+ . Instead information already collected from the upper-arm blood pressure measurement is used.

### Does BP+ Assume Central Mean and Diastolic Pressures?

BP+ calculates central systolic, diastolic and mean pressures. Other technologies assume central diastolic and/or mean pressures are equal to peripheral blood pressures.

### How Accurate are BP+ Central Blood Pressure Estimates?

Central blood pressure estimates have been independently tested against an accepted noninvasive technique for central blood pressure estimation and indicates well within the requirements of American Association for the Advancement of Medical Instrumentation (AAMI) standard SP10. Details will be available in the proceedings of artery 2010.

### Does the Central Pressure Estimate Require Patient Height, Age, Sex, etc.?

The BP+ central pressure estimate is model-based, not statistics-based and does not require the use of any other patient measurements.

### Does Brachial Artery, Arm or Cuff Variation Affect Accuracy?

The suprasystolic waveform is calibrated from the peripheral blood pressure. Variations in the arm and cuff are therefore not significant.

The brachial artery is not nearly as affected by cardiovascular disease as other major blood vessels and so does not influence the accuracy of the artery model in this way.

### Is Augmentation Index Related to Central Blood Pressure?

Both augmentation index and central blood pressure are known to increase with the age of the subject and be related to cardiovascular outcome. However, they are thought to measure different aspects of arterial stiffness.

Blood pressure plays a significant role in determining the arterial wall structure. Elevated blood pressure can lead to remodelling of the arterial structure, to compensate for changes in wall stress which would affect the augmentation index.

### Are Cholesterol and Central Blood Pressure Related?

Cholesterol is a blood chemical indicator, which may or may not relate to functional measures of cardiovascular health such as central blood pressure. Nevertheless, some research suggests that patients with hypercholesterolemia exhibit increased central pulse pressure compared with normocholesterolemic controls.

## A POCKET-SIZED ECHOCARDIOGRAPHY MACHINE

### Will Vscan Ultrasound Technology Replace the Stethoscope?

Sometimes a never before seen idea is not necessary for frugal innovation. If a currently used product can be remade in such a way that it becomes more effective and valuable to society this is also an example of frugal innovation. GE has a great example of this type of innovation with their Vscan pocket sized ultrasound device.

The Vscan ultrasound device greatly increased the usability of ultrasound technology by making the device small enough that if can fit in a pocket. Traditional ultrasound equipment is much larger and often must be wheeled around on a large cart.

However the cost of Vscan is more impressive than its size. Traditional ultrasound equipment can cost up to $150,000 but Vscan costs only $7,700. This makes the device not only portable but effective for use in many situations.

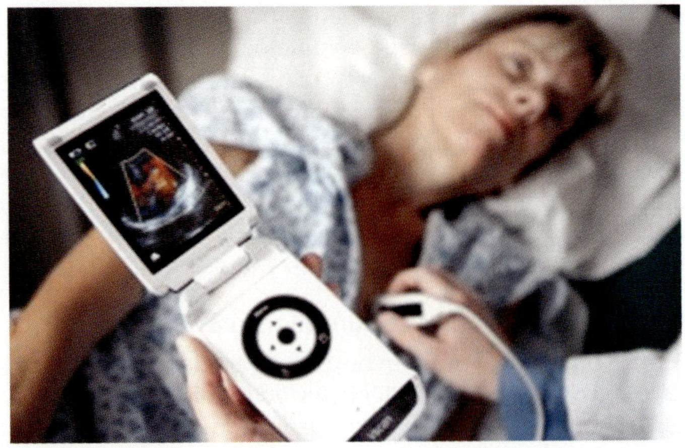

**Fig. A-18:** A patient being examined for his heart problem by a portable Vscan echocardiography

MIT Technology Review compares Vscan with the traditional stethoscope. The stethoscope has become iconic in the medical world but it's primary use is only to listen to the heart. Now doctors have access to technology that lets them look at a patients heart in real time.

## ELECTRONIC STETHOSCOPES: WHAT IS NEW FOR AUSCULTATION?

Although there is nothing wrong with traditional stethoscopes, taking the time to learn the nuances of digital auscultation will improve your diagnostic capabilities.

The stethoscope is perhaps the most iconic device associated with medical practice, and the most important part of the stethoscope will always be the part 'between the ear tips.' Because I last reviewed high-tech stethoscopes 5 years ago, I thought it appropriate to discuss the new technologies that can improve our ability to auscultate.

### *Murmurs are Common*

The incidence of *heart murmurs* can be as high as 80–90% in children, yet the vast majority of auscultated murmurs in children are not associated with structural *heart disease* and therefore are considered merely 'functional' or 'innocent' murmurs. This creates a dilemma for the pediatrician who, upon hearing a previously undocumented murmur in a child, must decide whether the murmur merits further investigation.

### *Murmur Interpretation Software*

Five years ago, murmur interpretation software was available from Zargis Medical, which had established a relationship with 3M Corporation (St Paul, Minnesota), manufacturer of the Littmann Model 3200 electronic stethoscope. The software, called cardioscan, communicated via bluetooth wireless connectivity to the stethoscope and prompted the user to record heart sounds from 4 positions on the patient's chest. The *software* would then analyze the recordings, report whether a murmur was present, and specify whether an echocardiogram was indicated.

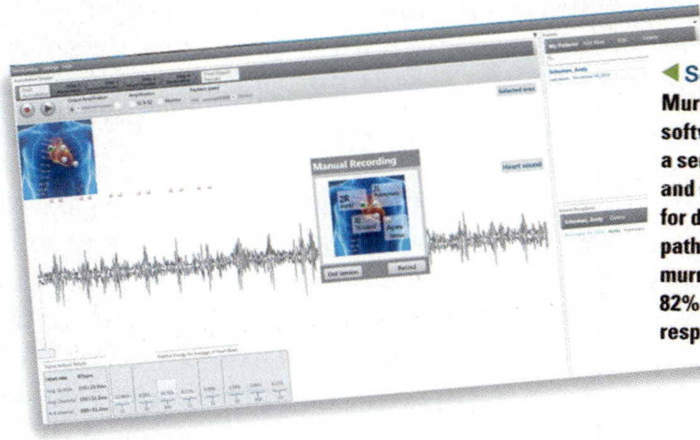


**Fig. A-19:** Features of SensiCardiac stethoscope

### An Update and Review of Instrument-based Vision Screening

Unfortunately, Zargis Medical went out of business, and its excellent murmur analysis software became unavailable. However, a South African company, Diacoustic Medical Devices (Stellenbosch, South Africa) recently introduced its own **SensiCardiac** software to analyze murmurs. One study performed in Australia on a limited number of patients indicated that the SensiCardiac software has a sensitivity and specificity for detecting pathologic murmurs of 82% and 88%, respectively. This is much better than the performance of PCPs in identifying pathologic murmurs, but less than that of cardiologists.

The SensiCardiac software is used in conjunction with the Littmann Model 3200 stethoscope and is accessed via a subscription service that costs $25 per month for up to 20 tests; $49 per month for up to 100 tests; and $99 per month for unlimited testing. The software is growing in popularity in areas of the world where access to cardiologists is limited. Keep in mind that the majority of heart sounds and murmurs occur in the frequency range of 5–800 Hz. Because human ears are most sensitive to sounds in the 500–4000 Hz frequency range, many murmurs ideally need to be amplified for them to be appreciated by examiners. Computers have no frequency limitations, and computer-assisted auscultation software such as SensiCardiac can improve the ability of physicians to diagnose pathologic murmurs.

### Advantages of Digital Stethoscopes

As a reviewer of *medical devices*, over the years I have had the opportunity to use a variety of electronic stethoscopes. These stethoscopes convert the acoustic signal of auscultated sounds into digital signals that can be processed for optimal listening. While we refer to these devices as electronic stethoscopes, it is more appropriate to refer to them as digital stethoscopes.

I have been an avid user of the Littmann 3200 stethoscope for many years and I will never go back to using a traditional stethoscope. Chief advantages of going electronic are the reduction or elimination of external sounds that interfere with optimal *auscultation*, as well as amplification of sounds across selected frequency ranges.

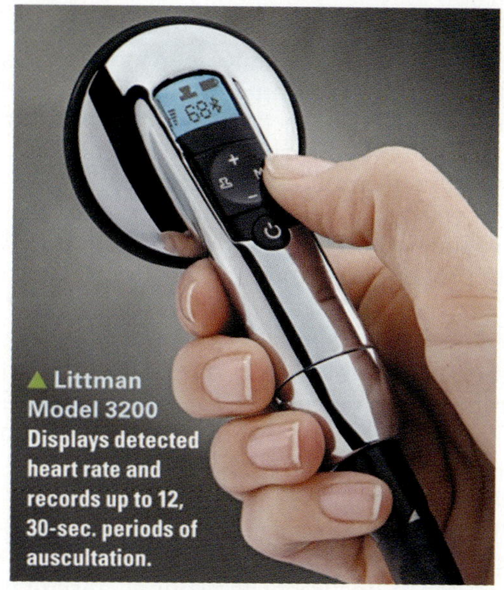


**Fig. A-20:** Features of Littmann 3200 stethoscope

Despite poor hearing, I can detect murmurs and lung sounds with my Littmann Model 3200 that colleagues using standard stethoscopes sometimes miss. The Littmann Model 3200 displays the detected heart rate and also enables me to record up to 12, 30-second periods of auscultation. Later, I can replay the recording for the parent merely by pushing a few buttons on the headpiece and placing the earpieces in the parent's ears. I find this extremely helpful in explaining a murmur or lung findings with parents and, as a consequence, they are more likely to understand and follow my recommendations.

While I have found the Littmann Model 3200 useful in detecting murmurs, its true utility, I think, lies in auscultation of lung sounds. Because it facilitates the auscultation of rales and rhonchi, I find I have substantially reduced the number of chest X-rays that I order. It does take time to learn the subtleties associated with auscultation with a digital stethoscope (distinguishing pathologic sounds from normal sounds), but given time and patience I am confident that most providers can become expert users of these devices.

#### *Littmann Models 3200 and 3100*

In addition to the features discussed above, the Model 3200 is powered by a single AA battery and has a bell, diaphragm, and combined frequency mode. You can download the free *StethAssist Heart and Lung Sound Visualization Software* from the 3M website (*bit.ly/StethAssist-software*) to either a Mac or PC for storage and display. The recordings also can be sent to cardiologists for analysis via the internet. The Littmann Model 3200 is quite affordable at about $400. If you want the acoustics of the 3200 but are not interested in its recording capability, combined frequency mode, and its ability to wirelessly connect to diagnostic software, you can purchase the *Littman Model 3100* for about $60 less.

### An Iconoclastic Electronic Stethoscope

Thinklabs (Centennial, Colorado) is an interesting company headed by a very interesting entrepreneur. Clive Smith is both a musician and an electrical engineer with a graduate degree from the California Institute of Technology, Pasadena. After years of research and development, Thinklabs has developed a new digital stethoscope that utilizes an electromagnetic diaphragm with a conductive inner surface to provide outstanding acoustics for auscultation.

### ViScope MD and CardioSleeve

Two other electronic stethoscopes are worth your consideration. The ***ViScope MD*** from HD Medical Group (Santa Clara, California) is the first 'visual' stethoscope that displays a simultaneous phonocardiogram on a high-resolution color screen.

With this device, you can essentially 'see' what you hear. It can capture 4, 10-second recordings and transfer this data to a computer to document the sounds auscultated. Like the Littmann Model 3200, it features noise cancellation as well as sound amplification, and it has a bell, diaphragm, and combined frequency mode. The ViScope MD integrates an internal algorithm that indicates whether a murmur is present. It has a rechargeable battery and sells for $600.

Finally, in the next quarter of this year, physicians can look forward to a unique stethoscope accessory that not only provides improved auscultation and bluetooth connectivity to mobile devices, but also adds 3-lead electrocardiogram capabilities as well. The device is called the **CardioSleeve** from Rijuven Corporation (Wexford, Pennsylvania) and it connects to most standard stethoscopes. The CardioSleeve communicates with a smartphone to display its results that can be uploaded to Rijuven servers for review and analysis. It is being promoted as a device that will improve our ability to detect pathologic murmurs as well as dysrhythmias, and it may be helpful in diagnosing long QT syndrome that is associated with sudden death in pediatric patients. The stethoscope accessory will be priced at $400, and a subscription to its online services will be reasonably priced. I look forward to trialing the device when it becomes available.

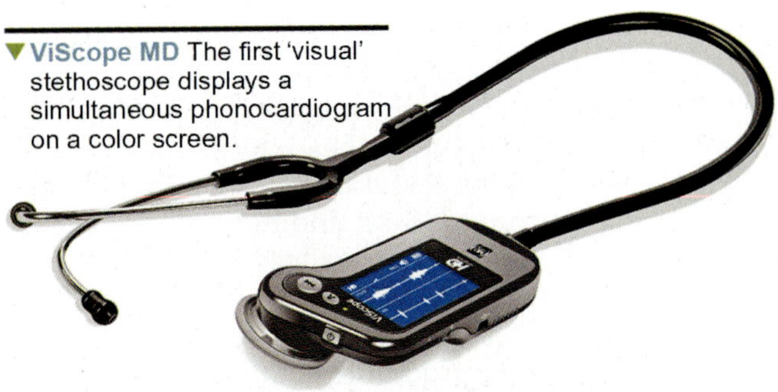


**Fig. A-21:** Features of ViScope MD stethoscope

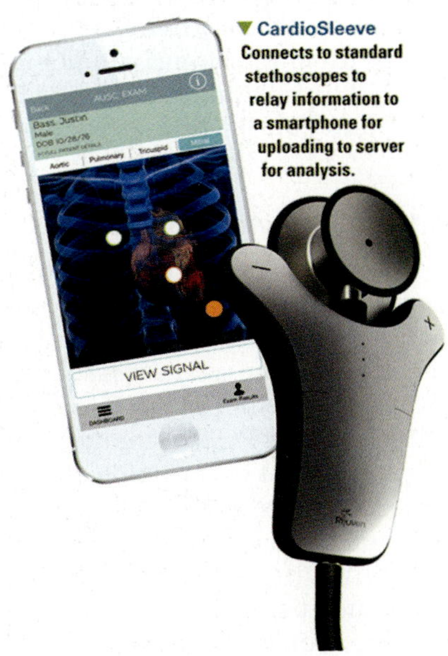


**Fig. A-22:** Features of CardioSleeve stethoscope

## CARDIONICS AMPLIFIED FOR THE HARD OF HEARING AND HEARING IMPAIRED ELECTRONIC STETHOSCOPE FOR PHYSICIAN

*Reviews*

The Cardionics Electronic Stethoscope for the hard of hearing and hearing impaired is designed to be worn on the belt or lab coat. Delivers improved sound quality, making physical diagnosis faster and easier. Amplifies heart, breath and bowel sounds or Korotkoff sounds without amplifying outside noise. Can also be used in a stress test situation on a treadmill.

- This product is compatible with cardionics extra headphones.
- Includes single adult diaphragm.
- Output allows attachment to PDA, computer, tape recorder or external earphones
- Sound selector switch allows listening in proper frequency for heart or breath sounds

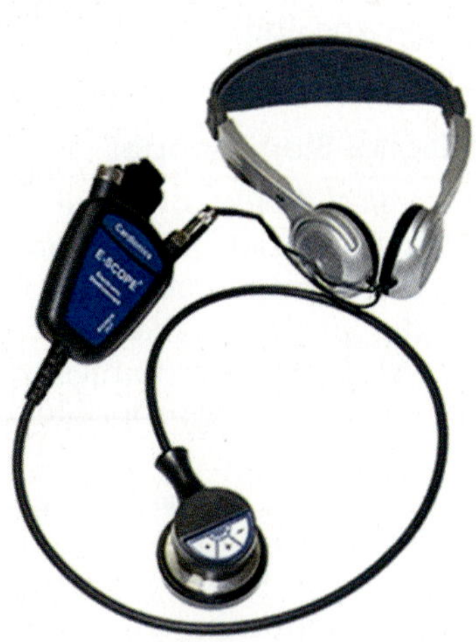

**Fig. A-23:** Features of cardionics amplified for the hard of hearing and hearing impaired electronic stethoscope for physician

- Exceptional sound quality with 64 gain positions
- One-year warranty against manufacturer's defects.

## CONTEMPORARY REVIEWS IN INTERVENTIONAL CARDIOLOGY

### Bioabsorbable Coronary Stents

Percutaneous coronary intervention (PCI) with bioabsorbable stents has created interest because the need for mechanical support for the healing artery is temporary, and beyond the first few months there are potential disadvantages of a permanent metallic prosthesis. Stents improve immediate outcomes, including profoundly reducing acute vessel occlusion after PCI by scaffolding intimal tissue flaps that have separated from deeper layers and by optimizing vessel caliber. They limit restenosis by preventing negative remodeling. The intimal hyperplastic healing response to PCI that contributes to restenosis, especially after bare metal stenting, can be limited by coating stents with antiproliferative medications.

Potential advantages of having the stent disappear from the treated site include reduced or abolished late stent thrombosis, improved lesion imaging with computed tomography or magnetic resonance, facilitation of repeat treatments (surgical or percutaneous) to the same site, restoration of vasomotion, and freedom from side-branch obstruction by struts and from strut fracture-induced restenosis. Bioabsorbable stents have a potential pediatric role because they allow vessel growth and do not need eventual surgical removal. The progression of stenosis seen within stents 7–10 years after stenting has been attributed, at least in part, to inflammation around metallic struts, which might argue for an absorbable stent. Progression is also observed late after balloon angioplasty. Some patients say they prefer an effective temporary implant rather than a permanent prosthesis.

Although the concept of bioabsorbable stents has created interest for >20 years, there are challenges in making a stent that has sufficient radial strength for an appropriate duration, that does not have unduly thick struts, that can be a drug delivery vehicle, and where degradation does not generate an unacceptable inflammatory response. We will review the different bioabsorbable stents that have been studied clinically and discuss the duration of the need for mechanical support and the potential amelioration of late stent thrombosis risk

### Bioabsorbable Therapeutics Stent

The bioabsorbable therapeutics stent (Bioabsorbable Therapeutics Inc, Menlo Park, Calif), a fully bioabsorbable sirolimus-eluting stent that also releases salicylic acid, has a polymer backbone that gives the stent the physical structure and a polymer coating that contains and controls the release of the antiproliferative.

The structure of the coating polymer is repeating salicylate molecules linked by adipic acid molecules. The stent backbone polymer structure is also repeating salicylate molecules but joined by different linker molecules. During absorption, the bonds between salicylic acid and linker molecules are hydrolyzed releasing the anti-inflammatory drug, salicylic acid. This anti-inflammatory agent is expected to counter the inflammation associated with PCI and with polymer degradation. Sirolimus is dissolved in the coating polymer that is applied to the abluminal surface of the stent backbone releasing the antiproliferative drug at a rate and dose similar to that of Cypher stents. Absorption of the stent, expected to be complete within 6–12 months, is by surface erosion. In the first-in-man Whisper trial, a stent with strut thickness of 200 μm and a crossing profile of 2.0 μm with a stent-to-artery coverage of 65% was implanted in 8 patients. Because of higher-than-expected intimal hyperplasia, a subsequent design iteration will have thinner struts, a higher dose of sirolimus, and a lower percent wall coverage.

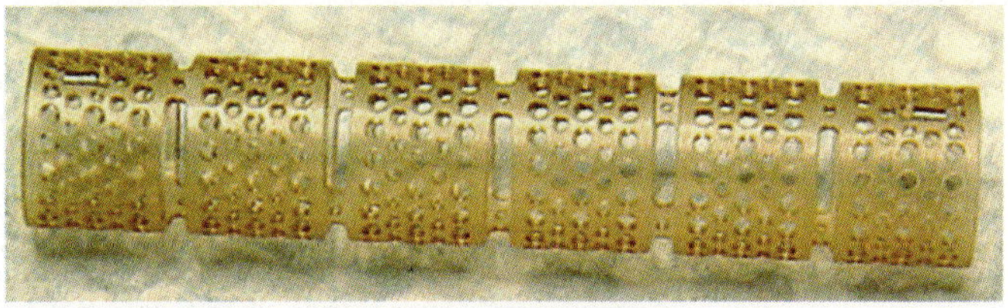

**Fig. A-24:** The bioabsorbable therapeutics stent has absorbable backbone and coating polymers constructed from repeating salicylate molecules joined by linker molecules. The coating contains and controls the release of sirolimus. The stent has a high stent-to-artery ratio of 65%. It has a strut thickness of 200 μm and crossing profile of 2.0 mm. It is balloon expandable and radiolucent

### How Long Do Coronary Arteries Need the Mechanical Support of a Stent?

Stents, essential components of contemporary PCI, scaffold intimal flaps that have separated from deeper layers, prevent early constrictive remodeling, and deliver antiproliferative drug to limit excessive healing. After this, a permanent implant is unnecessary and has potential disadvantages. After balloon angioplasty, preclinical and human studies have shown that restenosis is caused mainly by early constrictive remodeling (vessel shrinkage) and to a lesser extent by an hyperplastic healing response. Not all patients experience constrictive remodeling and some indeed have positive remodeling. Prevention of constrictive remodeling is the major reason stents limit restenosis. Over time, during the absorption process, an absorbable stent gradually loses its radial strength and ability to resist constrictive remodeling forces long before it is fully absorbed. What is not clear is how long the artery needs the support of a stent.

In a clinical study using serial angiography and IVUS after angioplasty and directional coronary atherectomy, there was some early positive remodeling up to 1 month and then between 1 month and 6 months there was luminal reduction due mainly to negative remodeling (reduction in external elastic lamina). Most angiographic restenosis after balloon angioplasty occurs between 1 month and

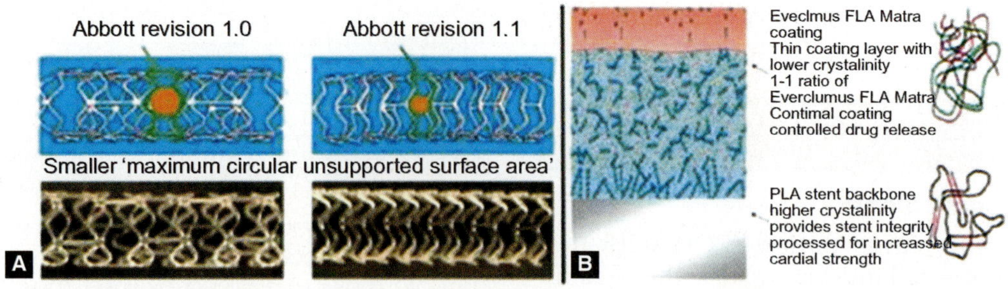


**Fig. A-25:** (A) The changes in scaffold design between revision 1.0 and revision 1.1, the Abbott Absorb biovascular scaffolds (BVS). Revision 1.1 has a higher radial strength as a consequence of reduced 'maximum circular unsupported surface area'. (B) Shows the material structure of the scaffolds, which is unchanged between the two revisions. (Images adapted and reprinted from Onuma Y et al. with permission from Europa Digital and Publishing 15; BVS 1.0 and BVS 1.1 images reprinted with permission from data on file at Abbott Vascular). Access the article online to view this figure in color

3 months and is rare thereafter. Absorption of a magnesium alloy stent in humans was rapid and mechanical support lasting days or weeks was too short to prevent constrictive remodeling and restenosis. These data taken together suggest that a mechanically intact stent is needed to counter negative remodeling and limit restenosis for somewhere between 1 month and 3 months. Stents are required to limit the constrictive remodeling in the first 6 months after balloon angioplasty. Because most patients have luminal enlargement between 6 months and 5 years after balloon angioplasty, a stent is not needed beyond 6 months. If, as has been postulated but not proven, the late luminal enlargement after balloon angioplasty is due to adaptive positive arterial remodeling, a circumferentially rigid stent may be disadvantageous in that it may obstruct this normal component of vessel healing.

In the Absorb trial, the polylactide BVS stent struts resisted the constrictive remodeling forces sufficiently, such that by 6 months on IVUS there was no vessel shrinkage (no change in external elastic lamina) although the stent itself had reduced in cross-sectional area by 11–12%. Between 6 months and 2 years, IVUS showed no change in vessel area (external elastic lamina), but the lumen increased in size and the stent was no longer identifiable by 2 years.The BVS stent clearly did its job of preventing negative remodeling; however, the duration for which radial support was provided is unclear.

## Will Bioabsorbable Stents Eliminate the Risk of Late Thrombosis at the PCI Site?

DES are a major breakthrough in interventional cardiology because they more than halve the need for repeat intervention compared with BMS.Although a small increase in thrombosis is offset by a reduced risk of complications associated with repeat revascularization. Late (6 month to 1 year) or very late (beyond 1 year) thrombosis is the feared complication of stenting that may result in myocardial infarction and death. Although late-stent thrombosis occurs with both BMS and DES, that after DES occurs later and as primary thrombosis, whereas that after BMS can be secondary to repeat intervention for restenosis. A worst case scenario is that the problem of late-stent thrombosis after first-generation DES implantation may be ongoing indefinitely as a registry of >8000 patients reported that it occurred at a constant rate of 0.6% per annum without diminution by 4 years. Indefinite continuation of dual antiplatelet therapy is not a practical solution because of expense and because a quarter of late-stent thromboses occurred in patients receiving dual antiplatelet therapy. In addition, dual antiplatelet therapy may be discontinued because of troublesome minor bleeding or to reduce the risk of bleeding during surgery.

An ideal DES would have no risk of late thrombosis and a fully bioabsorbable drug-eluting stent may fulfill this hope. Primary thrombosis at the treated site almost never occurred late after balloon angioplasty and has been described as the bane of stenting from the very beginning. Although multiple factors predispose to late thrombosis, it is reasonable to hope that it will be rare if a stent is completely absorbed because there would be no permanent metallic or polymeric foreign body exposed to blood even if endothelialization were functionally abnormal, delayed, or incomplete. If stent struts disappear, there can be no late stent malapposition. If the stent struts and coating are completely absorbed and the drug gone, there may be none of the ongoing chronic inflammation known to predispose to thrombosis. The endothelial regrowth after first-generation Taxus or Cypher stenting may be delayed but, in addition, may be functionally abnormal. Preliminary reports from some patients 2 years after BVS stent implantation raise the possibility of return of a functionally normal endothelium at the stented site because there was vasodilatation or absence of vasoconstriction downstream after acetylcholine administration. These observations will need to be confirmed in a larger trial. When the bioabsorbable coating of a metallic DES has been absorbed, all that remains is a BMS, and so the risk of late thrombosis may be limited to that of a BMS. However, even BMS have an ongoing risk of thrombosis that may be improved if there were no permanent foreign body in the vessel wall. An additional reason that a fully bioabsorbable DES may have a low risk of late thrombosis, perhaps lower than even late after balloon angioplasty.

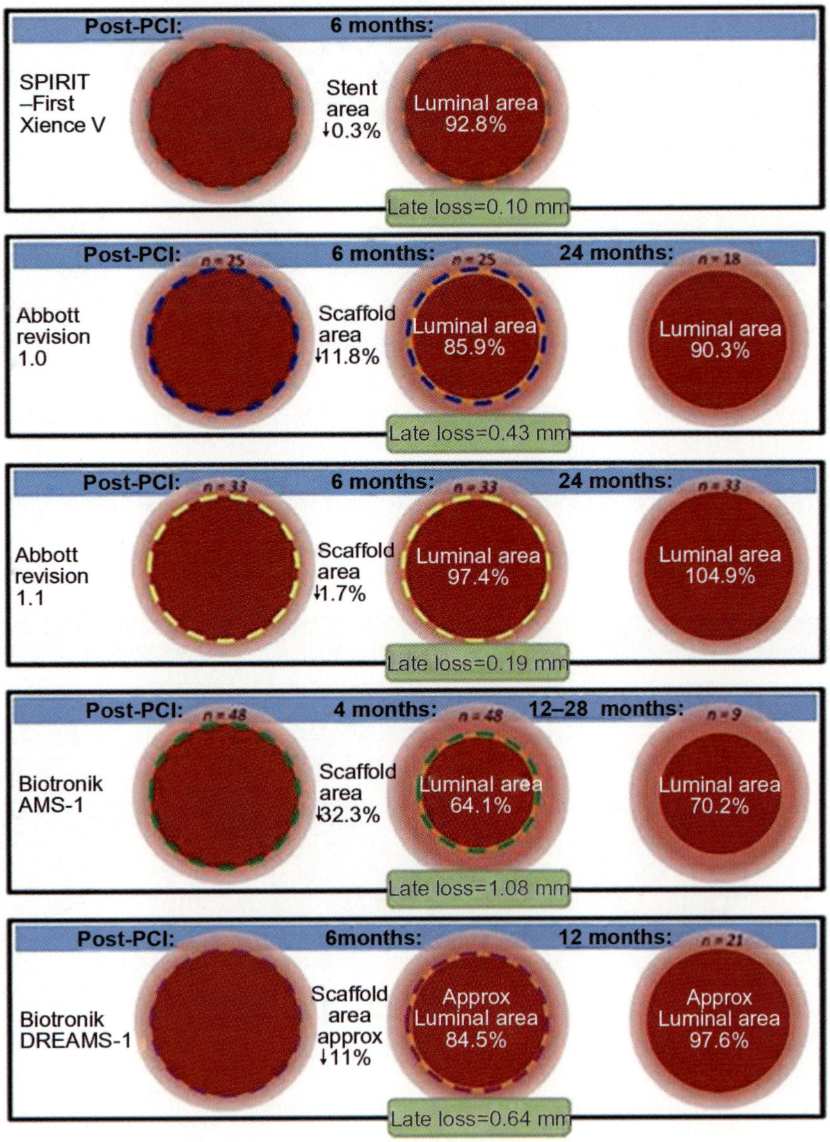


**Fig. A-26:** Comparison of bioabsorbable stent/scaffold and Xience V DES luminal area at follow-up (adapted from Garg and Serruys, Serruys Pres. TCT 2008 and 2011)

## SUMMARY OF STENT TECHNOLOGY

An ideal stent should furnish best acute outcomes after PCI by sealing intimal flaps and optimizing lumen size. It should control restenosis by limiting negative remodeling and by controlling excessive healing by delivery of an antiproliferative drug. Beyond 6 months, a permanent implant has no useful function and has possible disadvantages including the potential for late thrombosis. The concept of a stent that does its job and disappears has appeal. A number of different materials ranging from magnesium to a variety of polymers have been used to construct stents of different designs. Some of these are being tested in clinical trials. The best outcomes to date have been with the BVS everolimus-eluting PLLA stent where in the Absorb trial, cohort A at 2 years, the stent was safe in the small number of patients with simple lesions. Indeed, there is a suggestion of luminal enlargement between 6 months and 2 years, return of vasomotion, and endothelial function. These findings need to be confirmed in larger trials in more complex lesions. A hope is that a healed, normally functioning vessel free of foreign body and restenosis will be free of the risk of late thrombosis. Time will tell if this dream will come true.

## TRANSCATHETER AORTIC VALVE REPLACEMENT OR TVI

Transcatheter aortic valve replacement (TAVR) is a procedure for select patients with severe symptomatic aortic stenosis (narrowing of the aortic valve opening) who are not candidates for traditional open chest surgery or are high-risk operable candidates. TAVR is performed on a beating heart and does not require cardiopulmonary bypass. The TAVR valve is made of bovine (cow) pericardium and is supported with a metal stent. There are currently three approaches.

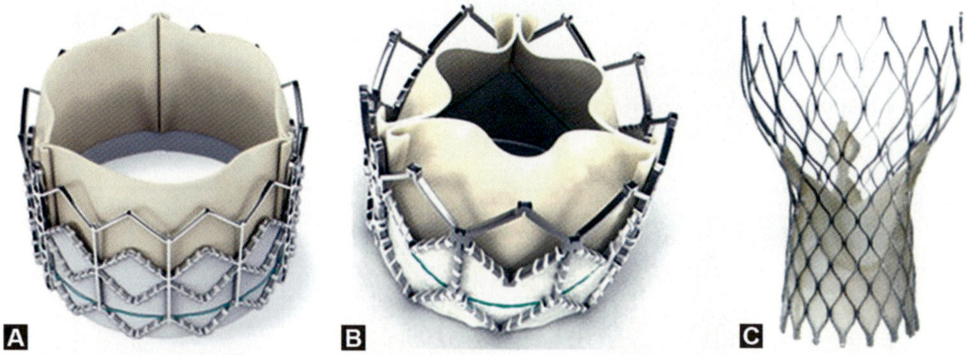


**Fig A-27:** Current widely available transcatheter valves. (A) The Edwards SAPIEN THV balloon-expandable valve (Edwards Lifesciences, Irvine, California) incorporates a stainless steel frame, bovine pericardial leaflets, x and a fabric sealing cuff. (B) The SAPIEN XT THV (Edwards Lifesciences) utilizes a cobalt chromium alloy frame and is compatible with lower profile delivery catheters. (C) The Medtronic CoreValve (Medtronic, Minneapolis, Minnesota) incorporates a self-expandable frame, porcine pericardial leaflets, and a pericardial seal

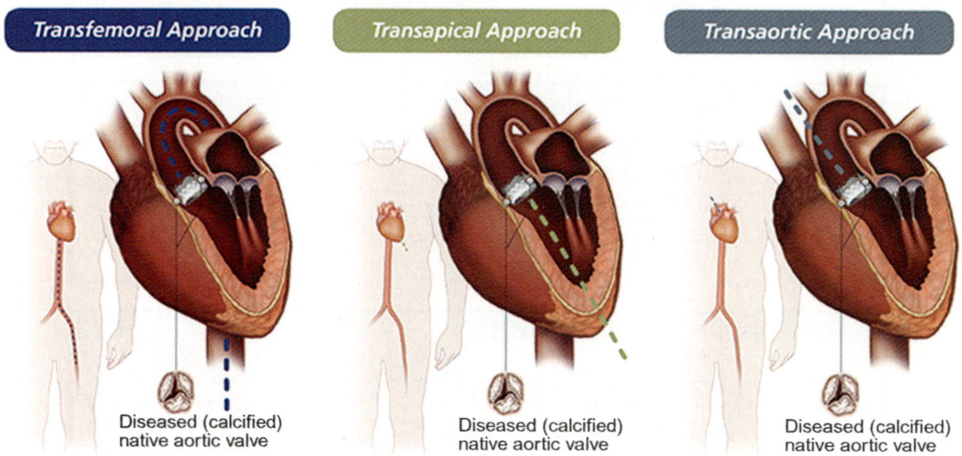


**Fig. A-28:** Different routes of aortic valve implantation

### Transfemoral Approach

A catheter is placed in the femoral artery (in the groin) similar to angioplasty, and guided into the chambers of the heart. A compressed tissue heart valve is placed on the balloon catheter and is positioned directly inside the diseased aortic valve. Once in position, the balloon is inflated to secure the valve in place. This procedure is performed with general anesthesia in a hybrid suite (which has both catheterization and surgical capabilities). A team of interventional cardiologists and imaging specialists,

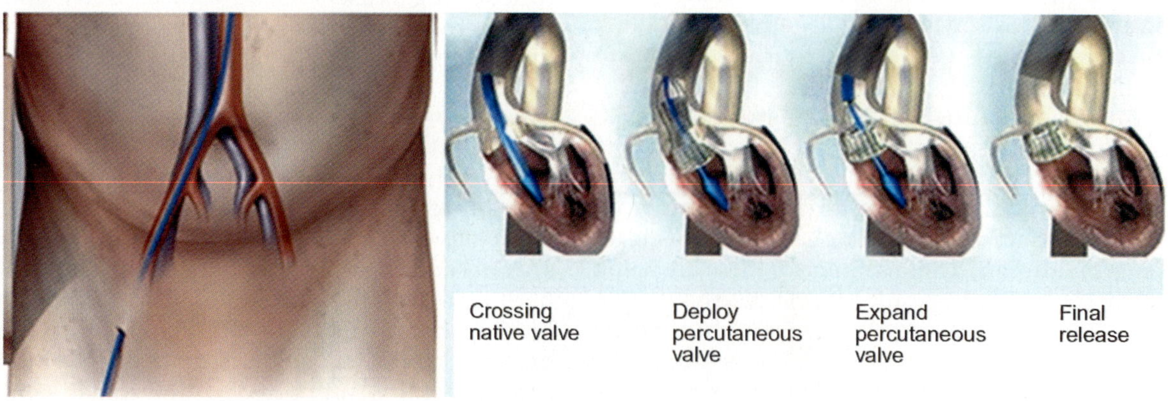


**Fig. A-29:** Different steps in transfemoral implantation of aortic valve

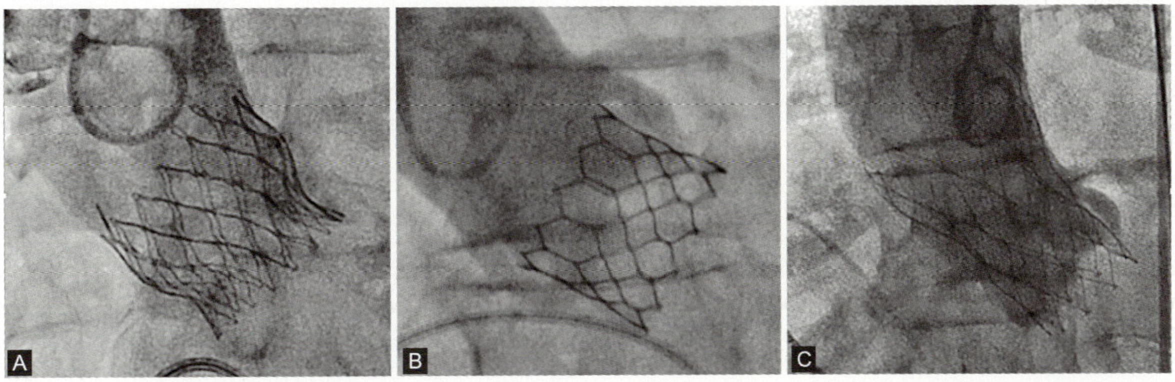

Fig. A-30: Fluoroscopic images of some newer valves undergoing early evaluation in patients. The CENTERA valve (A) is self-expandable and utilizes an electronic motorized release and retrieval system, while the S3 valve (B) incorporates an improved sealing system and utilizes a 14-F expandable sheath (Edwards Lifesciences, Irvine, California). (C) The Portico valve (St. Jude Medical Inc., St. Paul, Minnesota) is self-expandable, retrievable, and repositionable

heart surgeons and cardiac anesthesiologists work together, utilizing fluoroscopy and echocardiography to guide the valve to the site of the patient's diseased heart valve. Cleveland Clinic was one of three early pioneering centers in the USA and one of more than 20 centers involved in the randomized PARTNER trials (placement of aortic transcatheter valve) of TAVR. The one-year results of the PARTNER-B trial were released in September 2010. The inoperable patients involved in the PARTNER-B trial had severe symptomatic aortic stenosis and were not candidates for surgery. The patients were randomly selected to receive either TAVR or standard medical care. Among the inoperable patients who had TAVR, the procedure reduced their absolute risk of dying within a year by 20% (the risk of mortality at one year went from 50 to 30%).

The transfemoral approach is now approved by the FDA for patients who have severe, symptomatic aortic stenosis who are ineligible for open surgical replacement, based on the PARTNER-B trial results. It is not approved for patients who are eligible for traditional aortic valve surgery, patients with bicuspid aortic valves, endocarditis, or cannot tolerate anticoagulation/antiplatelet therapy.

### Investigational Transfemoral Approach

TAVR via femoral artery is now being tested for moderately high risk and high risk operable patients as well as inoperable patients in a new research trial PARTNER-II.

### Transapical Approach

The transfemoral approach requires the use of catheters large enough to place the transcatheter aortic valve replacement through. Patients with peripheral artery disease may not have arteries large enough to support the transfemoral approach. In this case, patients can be evaluated to participate in a research study (PARTNER-II) which uses the alternative transapical approach.

During the transapical procedure, the surgeon makes a 4-inch incision between the ribs. A compressed tissue heart valve is placed on the balloon catheter, inserted through the ribs into the apex of the left ventricle and positioned directly inside the diseased aortic valve. Once in position, the balloon is inflated to secure the valve in place. This procedure is performed under general anesthesia, in a hybrid operating room. A team of imaging and interventional cardiologists and heart surgeons work together, utilizing fluoroscopy and echocardiography to guide the valve to the site of the patient's diseased heart valve.

### Investigational Transaortic Approach

During the transaortic procedure, the surgeon makes a J shaped incision at the top of the sternum in between the

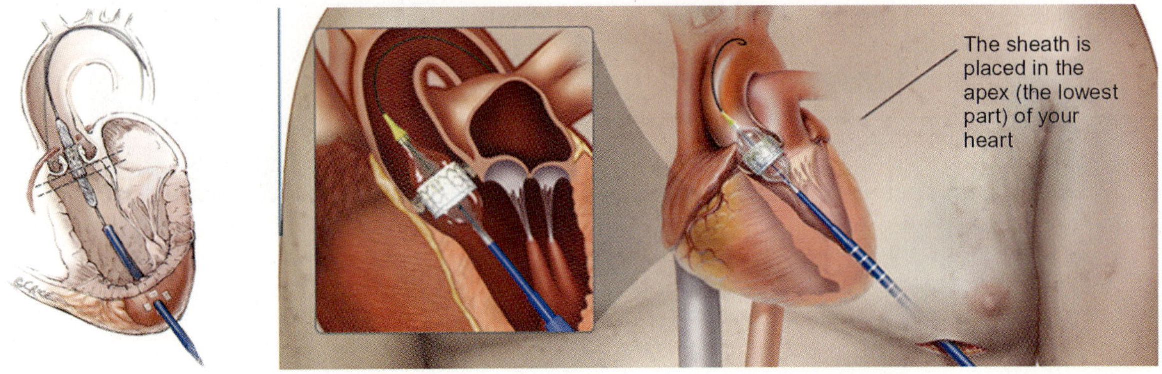


Fig. A-31: Transapical approach in implantation of aortic valve

manubrium and the sternum. A compressed tissue heart valve is placed on the balloon catheter, inserted into the aorta and positioned directly inside the diseased aortic valve. Once in position, the balloon is inflated to secure the valve in place.

### What You Should Know About TAVR?

TAVR is performed in high-risk and inoperable patients with aortic stenosis. All patients are careful evaluate to see if they are candidates for traditional surgical aortic valve replacement and then TAVR can be considered for treatment. The goal is to provide the best treatment for each individual patient.

Cleveland Clinic was involved in TAVR research since 2006 and has evaluated around 2000 patients and performed more than 220 procedures.

Transfemoral TAVR was recently approved by the FDA for inoperable patients.

There are ongoing research trials for TAVR for high-risk operable, moderate risk operable and inoperable patients. The positive results seen in the PARTNER trial were related to procedures performed at valve centers where there is a team approach between interventional cardiologists and surgeons.

The one year survival results for PARTNER-A, the high-risk patient population were similar in those who received surgery vs those who received TAVR.

There are still risks associated with TAVR as there is with surgical AVR. These should be taken into consideration in decision making.

### Total Endoscopic Aortic Valve Replacement

Surgical aortic valve replacement (SAVR) is continually evolving with minimal access procedures becoming more widespread thanks to the latest turning point, sutureless technology. Beyond the advantages linked to the elimination of sutures and knots (some of those devices carrying a Nitinol frame offer the possibility of being compressed, enabling their passage through a thoracoscopic trocar.

Total endoscopic aortic valve replacement (TEAVR) aims to further reduce surgical wall chest trauma by avoiding sternal fractures or costal spreading. Clinical advantages have already been shown during atrial septal defect (ASD) closure surgery, thus favoring total endoscopic approach over ministernotomy and minithoracotomy.

## WATCHMAN AND LARIAT PROCEDURES IN PREVENTION OF ATRIAL FIBRILLATION STROKE

The Watchman and Lariet procedures are among the newest procedures available to prevent afib related stroke.The most serious risk from atrial fibrillation is thromboembolic stroke. The left atrial appendage (LAA) is a pouch-like extension of the left atrium about the size of your thumb with a narrow opening into the left atrium. With atrial fibrillation, blood can pool and form clots in this appendage. If a blood clot breaks loose it may travel through the blood vessels and eventually plug a smaller vessel in the brain or heart. Doctors often prescribe the blood thinning medications such as coumadin to prevent blood clots, however, it can often cause serious side effects.

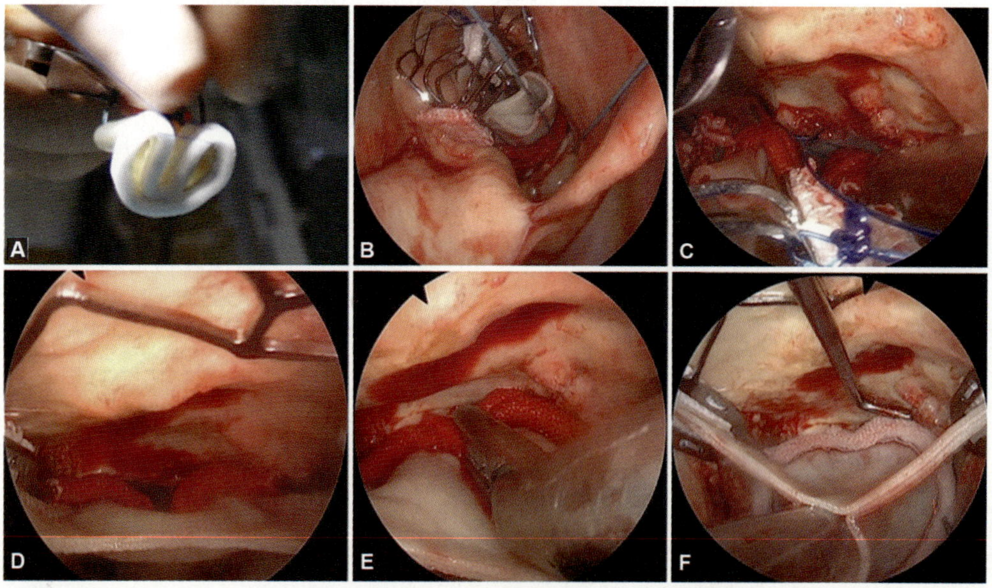

**Fig. A-32:** Deployment of the 3f enable valve through endoscopic technique. (A) The 3f enable valve is kept compressed by a prolene stitch before introduction in the trocar; (B) positioning of the noncoronary portion of the bioprosthesis; (C) positioning of the right portion of the bioprosthesis; (D) initial deployment of the folded leaflet after cutting the prolene stitch; (E) final deployment of the right portion of the bioprosthesis cuff; (F) final control of the sitting of the 3f enable valve (including hook control around the valve)

Today, the doctors at PHCVI can offer many patients an alternative such as the Watchman Device and Lariat procedure to prevent blood clots associated with atrial fibrillation.

### What is the Watchman Device?

The Watchman Device is a small, fabric-covered device permanently placed in the opening of the left atrial appendage to prevent harmful-sized blood clots from exiting and entering the bloodstream. It is made of materials that are well-tolerated by most patients, and intended for those with nonvalvular atrial fib, who require treatment for potential blood clotting and can tolerate coumadin.

*The procedure:* Watchman LAA closure is performed under local or general anesthesia in the cathaterization lab. The heart is reached through a hole made in the femoral vein in the upper thigh and the device is delivered to the LAA through a catheter under X-ray and ultrasound guidance. The procedure takes about an hour and requires an overnight hospital stay. It takes at least 45 days for the heart tissue to heal. It will be important to continue taking coumadin (your doctor will prescribe a lower dosage) and a daily aspirin. Your physician may also prescribe an antibiotic to prevent infection after surgery.

*What is the lariat procedure?* This permanent, one-time procedure has been found to be highly successful and poses fewer risks and less discomfort to patients than surgery. Performed under general anesthesia, the Lariat procedure uses two catheters carrying the Lariat suture delivery device. One of these catheters is inserted under the patient's rib cage; the other is sent to the heart's left atrial appendage (LAA). Once the catheters are in place, the device places and then tightens a loop stitch around the base of the left atrial appendage, sealing it off from the rest of the heart, blocking stroke-causing blood clots from traveling to the brain.

### Benefits of the Lariat Procedure

The Lariat procedure is a minimally invasive procedure that:

- Can reduce the risk of stroke by 85–90%
- Is suitable for patients who cannot undergo surgery
- Minimizes discomfort and promotes faster healing and quicker recovery.

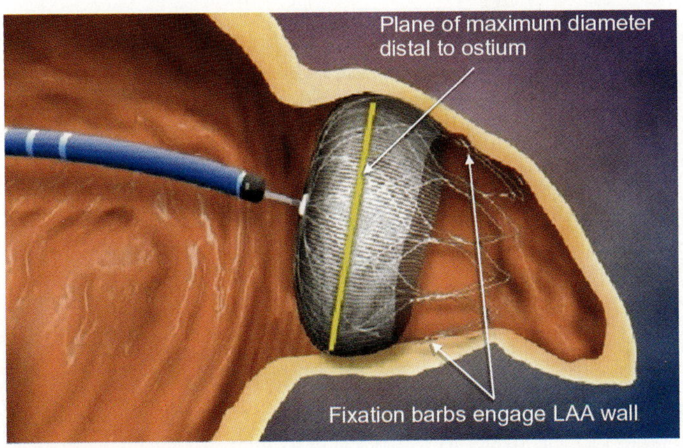


**Fig. A-33:** Watchman device for occlusion of left atrial appendage in the prevention stroke in atrial fibrillation

## CHEAP BLOOD PRESSURE—VERAPAMIL MAY REVERSE DIABETES-RELATED DEATH OF PANCREATIC BETA CELLS, CURES DIABETES IN MICE, HUMAN TRIALS ANNOUNCED

A common high-blood-pressure medication appears to reverse the diabetes-related death of pancreatic beta cells, according to a University of Alabama at Birmingham study published today in the journal *diabetes*.

The authors argue that the findings—while in human pancreatic islets and diabetic mice–could have clinical implications as physicians consider that calcium channel blockers may address two major, related diseases. They also found evidence in past clinical trials that the study drug verapamil may slow diabetes.

Beta cells secrete insulin to control blood sugar levels, but begin to die as patients develop type 1 or type 2 diabetes. No one suspected that calcium channel blockers might reverse beta cell death because the studies that led to their FDA approval measured their effect on heart attacks, not blood sugar. UAB researchers were surprised when hints of verapamil's effect were discovered amid their effort to design a drug to shut down a protein called TXNIP.

The team had published several papers over 10 years that describe the way high blood sugar uniquely turns on the gene for TXNIP, and how excessive TXNIP-signaling in diabetes signals cells to self-destruct. Recent studies also have suggested that lowering TXNIP levels in the heart lessens the damage caused by a heart attack.

'We long have felt that finding an oral medication that inhibits beta cell TXNIP expression would represent a major breakthrough, and now we have the first study showing that a drug already proven safe in years of clinical practice may halt the *development of diabetes*,' said Anath Shalev, MD, Director of the UAB comprehensive diabetes center and senior author of the paper. 'Our results are encouraging because patients with diabetes suffer from beta cell death as part of their disease, there has been no treatment targeting this problem and TXNIP-inhibition promises to reverse it.'

Of the nearly 26 million adult patients with diabetes, 67 percent also have high blood pressure.

Based on its findings, the UAB team has redoubled its original effort to design a new class of TXNIP-inhibitors. In partnership with the Southern Research Institute and the Alabama Drug Discovery Alliance, they are now screening a library of 300,000 molecules, a search they hope will yield drug candidates that reverse beta cell death without affecting blood pressure.

In cell studies, the team found that verapamil reduced TXNIP gene expression by 50%. In diabetic mice, verapamil treatment maintained normal glucose level, while glucose spiked in control mice. This was accompanied by an 80%

reduction in TXNIP levels in isolated islets of verapamil-treated animals.

Using molecular biology techniques, researchers were able to watch as expression of TXNIP, or thioredoxin-interacting protein, rose in beta cells to abnormal levels as mice became diabetic and then fell again as they received verapamil.

The team also found that treatment only reduced TXNIP gene expression when high blood sugar had driven it to abnormal levels, making the pathway 'extremely attractive' as a target for drugs, Shalev said. Future treatments conceivably could return TXNIP levels to normal in diabetic patients, but leave in place the basic level of TXNIP-signaling that cells rely on to regulate life processes. The results also suggest the drug is able to slow diabetes in mice with longstanding disease and is more effective when given early.

'The debate now should begin as to whether physicians should consider verapamil an additional treatment to protect beta cells in patients with both hypertension and diabetes, similar to the use of ACE inhibitors for kidney protection,' said Shalev, who also is a clinician. 'As it stands, it can take years before patients with diabetes receive verapamil, possibly missing a window of opportunity. Future clinical studies need to test whether or not earlier treatment could have a profound effect on diabetes progression by saving more beta cells.'

Though no one had previously established the link between calcium channel-blockers, TXNIP and beta cell death, past studies had hinted at a connection. Analysis of the INVEST trial revealed that newly diagnosed diabetes was less common in patients treated with verapamil, especially in the Hispanic population.

In addition to protecting insulin-producing cells, experiments also showed that verapamil countered insulin-resistance that makes the hormone less able to lower blood-sugar levels in diabetic patients. Theory has it that lowering TXNIP levels counters this by increasing glucose uptake in the tissues targeted by insulin (e.g. muscle and fat), a phenomenon observed in mice lacking the TXNIP gene.

Shalev's team spent years establishing TXNIP as the mandatory link between high blood sugar and beta cell death. The effort reached its first milestone in 2002 in a study that demonstrated the gene for TXNIP had the greatest increase in expression —11-fold greater than any of the 6,000 genes expressed in pancreatic islets — in the face of rising glucose levels. In 2005, the team identified the DNA region that turns on the TXNIP gene in response to high sugar in beta cells and later showed that the carbohydrate response element-binding protein (ChREBP) attaches to DNA there.

Their next paper in 2008 revealed that genetic deletion of TXNIP protects against type 1 and type 2 diabetes and too much TXNIP-signaling shuts down the Akt/Bcl-xL pathway that keeps beta cells alive.

TXNIP stands for thioredoxin-interacting protein, and the overactive TXNIP signaling seen in diabetes sharply reduces the antioxidant activity of the protein thioredoxin. The team had found previously that that higher TXNIP levels in the mitochondria of beta cells increase the chances it will pull thioredoxin off of the protein it would otherwise shut down, apoptosis-signaling kinase 1. Once free, this enzyme initiates a chain reaction that ends in beta cell death.

Shalev's team also has now shown that calcium channel-blockers inhibit signaling through the enzyme calcineurine, which increases ChREBP phosphorylation and keeps it from getting into the beta cell nucleus. With less ChREBP, extra TXNIP gene expression is shut down.

## DELHI BASED DUO BUILD WORLD'S CHEAPEST AND SMALLEST VENTILATOR THAT FITS IN POCKET

Good news for patients who are advised to stay on a ventilator. They can now breathe comfortably by using this *mini* ventilator. The world's cheapest and smallest ventilator, developed by AIIMS in collaboration with a private company, can easily fit into your pocket, according to PTI. This invention is the is the brainchild of Dr Deepak Agrawal, professor in the department of neurosurgery at AIIMS, who joined with Diwakar Vaish, a robotics researcher at A-SET Robotics to make the device.

Diwakar Vaish (25) said, 'It is almost 450 times smaller than the conventional ventilators and can be moved around easily,' as per Hindustan Times.

There are lot of patients in AIIMS and in hospitals across India who are required to be on ventilator for a prolonged period and are unable to arrange them because of the exorbitant costs and the technical expertise required to operate them. 'We have 10–15 such patients in the neuro-surgery department itself who are on ventilator for the last two years or more,' said Dr Agrawal. This ventilator is easy to use and soon will be available in the market for a price at less than ₹ 15,000. 'We are using the ventilator on some patients as pilot,' he added. Currently, a basic ventilators is priced above 2.5 lakhs in the market, as per PTI.

The ventilator can be controlled with an android app and it uses an artificial intelligence algorithm to adjust air supply for normal breathing of the patient, as per HT. Vaish

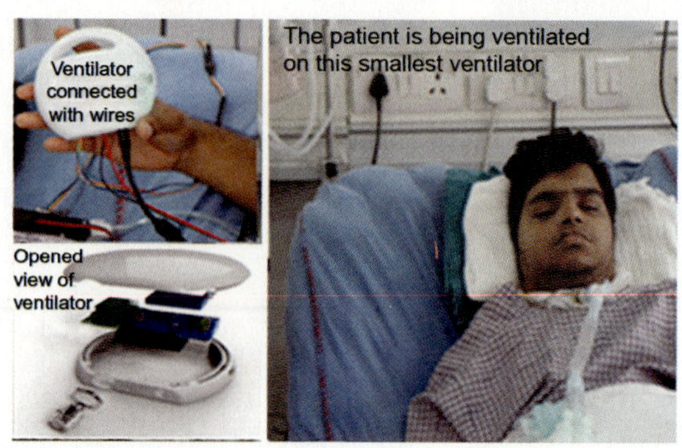


**Fig. A-34:** The world's cheapest and smallest ventilator, developed by AIIMS in collaboration with a private company, can easily fit into your pocket

said, 'There is no requirement for oxygen cylinders, which cost between ₹ 3,000 and ₹ 4,000 a day.' 'It works by pushing the atmospheric air into the lungs of the patients who cannot breathe on their own. The disposable ventilators currently in use also push in air, but they do it at a fixed frequency that does not necessarily match the patient's breathing pattern, which may cause low oxygen saturation. This device synchronises ventilator air support with the normal breathing pattern,' Dr Agrawal was quoted as saying by HT.

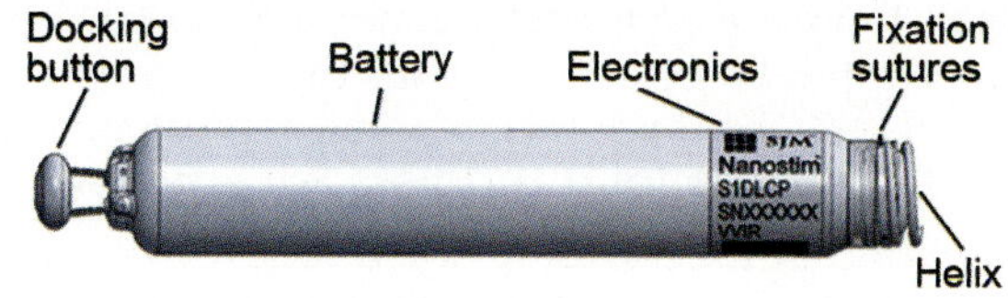


**Fig. A-36:** The St. Jude Medical Nanostim™ leadless pacemaker (reproduced with permission from St. Jude Medical Inc.). The various components of the pacemaker have been shown in this figure

## CURRENT INNOVATIONS IN PACEMAKER THERAPY

In recent years, more and more pacemakers have been implanted, with the result that not only cardiological specialists are increasingly being confronted by such patients. In view of the multiplicity of the implanted systems, every general practitioner should have a basic knowledge of their various functions. Functional pacemaker disorders may result in an acute emergency that requires immediate attention. Current innovations in pacemaker therapy would be discussed under the following headings such as:

1. Leadless pacemaker therapy
2. Left ventricular resynchronization therapy with leadless pacemaker
3. Leadless pacing—current status and future perspectives
4. Advances in implantable cardioverter defibrillator (ICD) technology
5. Battery life, MRI-safe ICDs, reducing shocks and reducing implanted hardware.

A *pacemaker* is a device that sends small electrical impulses to the heart muscle to maintain a suitable heart rate or to stimulate the lower chambers of the heart (ventricles).

### What is Leadless Pacemaker?

Pacemakers are used to treat patients with brady-arrythmias, slow heart rhythms that may occur as a result of disease in the heart's conduction system (such as the SA node, AV node or His-Purkinje network). A leadless pacemaker is small self-contained device that is inserted in the right ventricle of the heart.

### What are the Benefits of a Leadless Pacemaker?

- It does not require connecting leads (wires) or a generator, or a creation of a surgical pocket on the chest. These are the most common causes of traditional pacemaker complications over the long-term, and may affect up to 1 in 10 patients.
- When the leadless device is in place, there is no lump under the skin on the chest or leads anchored to the muscle bed. Sometimes these cause minor discomfort for patients who live with traditional pacemakers. The incisional access for a traditional pacemaker and each generator replacement leaves a scar that is a cosmetic concern for some patients.
- The procedure uses a catheter to place the device. The procedure typically takes less time than a traditional pacemaker implant procedure.

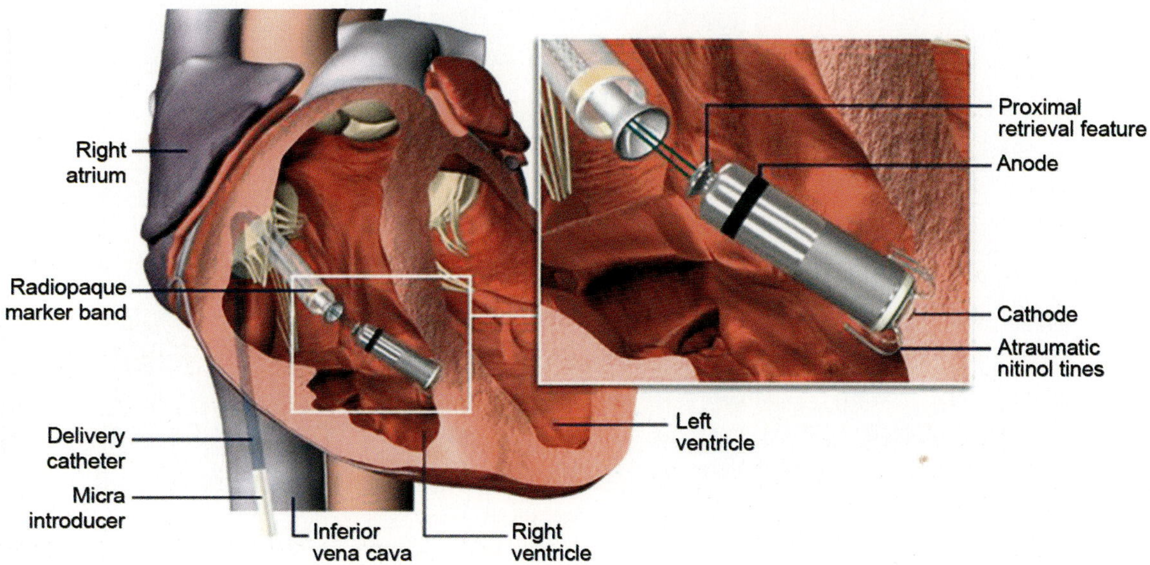


**Fig. A-35:** The route, site and morphological features of leadless pacemaker

- Because there are no wires or generator, you do not need to limit upper body activity after the implant.

### Who is a Candidate for a Leadless Pacemaker?

Not everyone is a candidate for a leadless pacemaker. Currently, the device is available only for patients with certain medical conditions and a slow heart rate (bradycardia) who need single-chamber pacing only. Like all pacemakers, leadless pacemakers require approval by the Food and Drug Administration (FDA) and sometimes there are additional restrictions upon availability for an individual patient. Your doctor can tell you if you are a candidate for a leadless pacemaker after a review of your medical history, heart rhythm, and the results of medical tests. You may need an echocardiogram (ultrasound of the heart) or other noninvasive tests.

### Contraindications in Leadless Pacemakers

These devices are contraindicated in individuals who require:

- Dual-chamber pacing or who have demonstrable pacemaker syndrome.
- Current devices are not MRI compatible.
- Leadless pacemakers are contraindicated in patients with implantable cardioverter-defibrillators, as high-voltage shocks could damage the pacemaker, and the effect of the pacemaker on shock effectiveness is unknown.
- Leadless devices should be avoided in individuals with elevated right ventricular pressures because of higher theoretical risk of embolization.
- The presence of mechanical tricuspid valves or inferior vena cava filters also precludes the use of leadless pacemakers.

### How is the Leadless Pacemaker Implanted?

After puncture of the right femoral artery, a 12F vascular introducer was inserted in conjunction with an arterial closure device (ProStar XL or Perclose Proglide 6F, Abbot Vascular Inc.). A 12F deflectable sheath (WiCS-LV) was introduced into the LV via a transaortic approach using a 180 cm soft-tip guide wire (0.032 or 0.035) and a dilator. Intravenous heparin was administered to attain and maintain an activation clotting time level in the range of 200–250. The dilator/wire was exchanged for a catheter with the electrode at the distal tip and equipped with a detachable connection to the electrode. This connection retains the electrode on the catheter prior to deployment and also provides a direct electrical contact to the cathode of the electrode for electrogram monitoring and pacing. With the electrode retained within the tip of the sheath, the sheath was steered under fluoroscopic guidance to a targeted LV implant site. Radiopaque contrast was administered through the catheter and used to discern sheath contact with the LV. Tissue viability was confirmed using the electrogram and by pacing threshold. The procedure takes about 30 minutes to complete, although this can vary patient-to-patient based on individual anatomical consideration.

### What Happens After the Procedure?

You will need to lie flat and keep the leg straight for 2–6 hours after the procedure. This prevents bleeding from the access site. Do not try to sit or stand. A sterile dressing will be placed on your groin area to protect it from infection. You will spend the night in the hospital and will be able to go home after your device check and a chest X-ray.

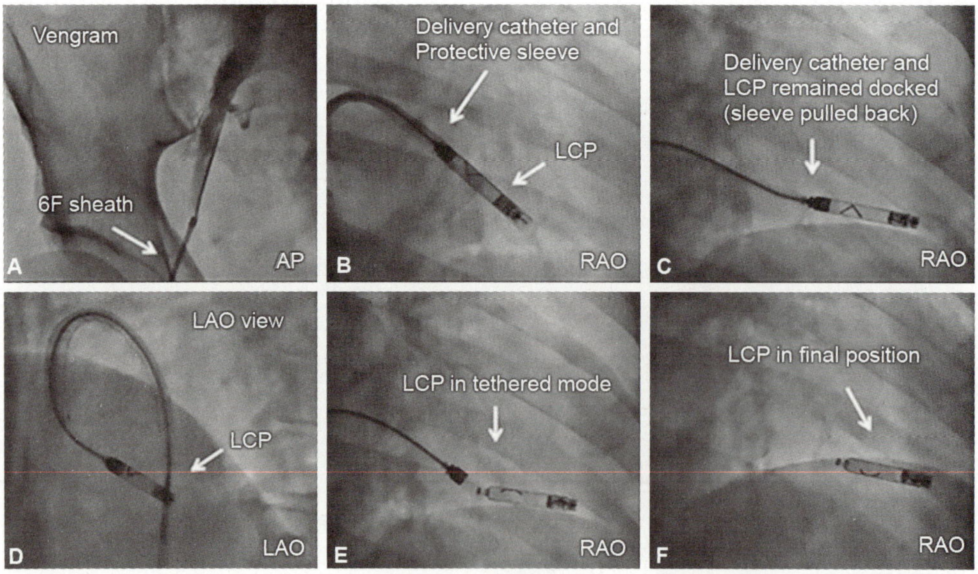


**Fig. A-37:** Leadless cardiac pacemaker implantation steps. (A) A venogram may optionally be performed. (B) The LCP is positioned into the RV by deflecting the catheter and placed 0.5–1 cm from the RV apex. (C and D) Protective cover is pulled back to expose the flexible part of the catheter. (E) The pacemaker is undocked from the delivery catheter while a tethered connection is maintained. In case the position is suboptimal, the LCP can be re-engaged, unscrewed, and repositioned. (F) The LCP is released by rotating the release knob of the catheter

### What are the Risks of a Leadless Pacemaker Implant?

Every procedure has complications associated with it. The most common possible problems after a leadless pacemaker implant involve the incision site, such as swelling and bleeding. These are not typically life-threatening but may lead to a longer hospital stay or slower recovery.

More serious but rare complications include the device moving out of place (dislodgement) or internal bleeding, such as pericardial effusion or tamponade.

*Follow-up:* Follow up after a leadless pacemaker is similar to a traditional schedule with noninvasive checks.

First-in-man implantation of leadless ultrasound-based cardiac stimulation pacing system; novel endocardial left ventricular resynchronization therapy in heart failure patients.

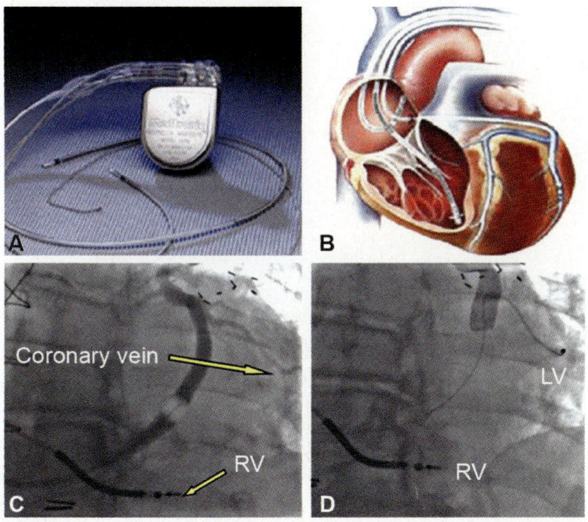


**Fig. A-38:** (A) Morphological features and attachment in of biventricular pacemaker. (B) Transvenous RV and transcoronary sinus epicardial vessel routes in biventricular pacing. (C) Cine angiography radiological depiction of catheter in coronary venous and RV locations (arrows). (D) Cine angio demonstrates final positions of pacemaker leads in LV and RV as normally seen in biventricular pacing

*Transthoracic echocardiography imaging* was performed to view the distal end of the sheath and to insure proper alignment. By advancing the catheter the electrode's anchor barbs were attached to the LVendo wall. Contrast injections through the catheter in two fluoroscopic views confirmed insertion of the anchor barbs, the electrode was released, and detachment was confirmed by changes in the electrogram signal. The sheath was withdrawn, the artery was secured with the closure device, and heparin was stopped to reduce the ACT level to below 180 s prior to the implantation of the transmitter.

A 3 cm incision in a left lateral or in an abdominal position and a 6 cm incision over the previously identified ICS were made to create the subcutaneous pockets for the battery and transmitter. Tunnelling between the two incisions passed the interconnect cable from the transmitter to connect the battery, then both were inserted in their pockets.

Programming the transmitter was performed to enable sensing the RV pacing signal and to trigger acoustic transmissions to the electrode in the LV. After observation of biventricular pacing on 12-lead ECG, the transmitter and battery were sutured in place.

The importance of specific-site pacing is increasingly recognized in cardiac resynchronization therapy (CRT). Using current pacing technology, site selection is still largely limited by coronary vein anatomy, whereas left ventricular (LV) endocardial pacing using current lead technology is risky and challenging. To overcome limitations and complications with current LV pacing, the feasibility of a new technology enabling LV endocardial stimulation without the use of a lead is being evaluated in patients.

### Methods and Results

Patients presented in this report are part of the wireless stimulation endocardially for CRT trial (WiSE-CRT) study investigating the safety and performance of the WiCS®-LV

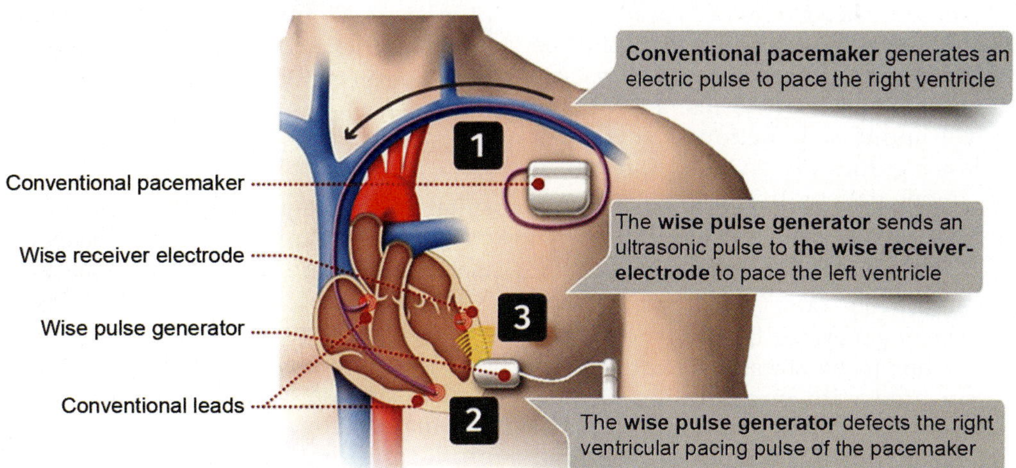


**Fig. A-39:** Different components of a novel endocardial left ventricular resynchronization therapy

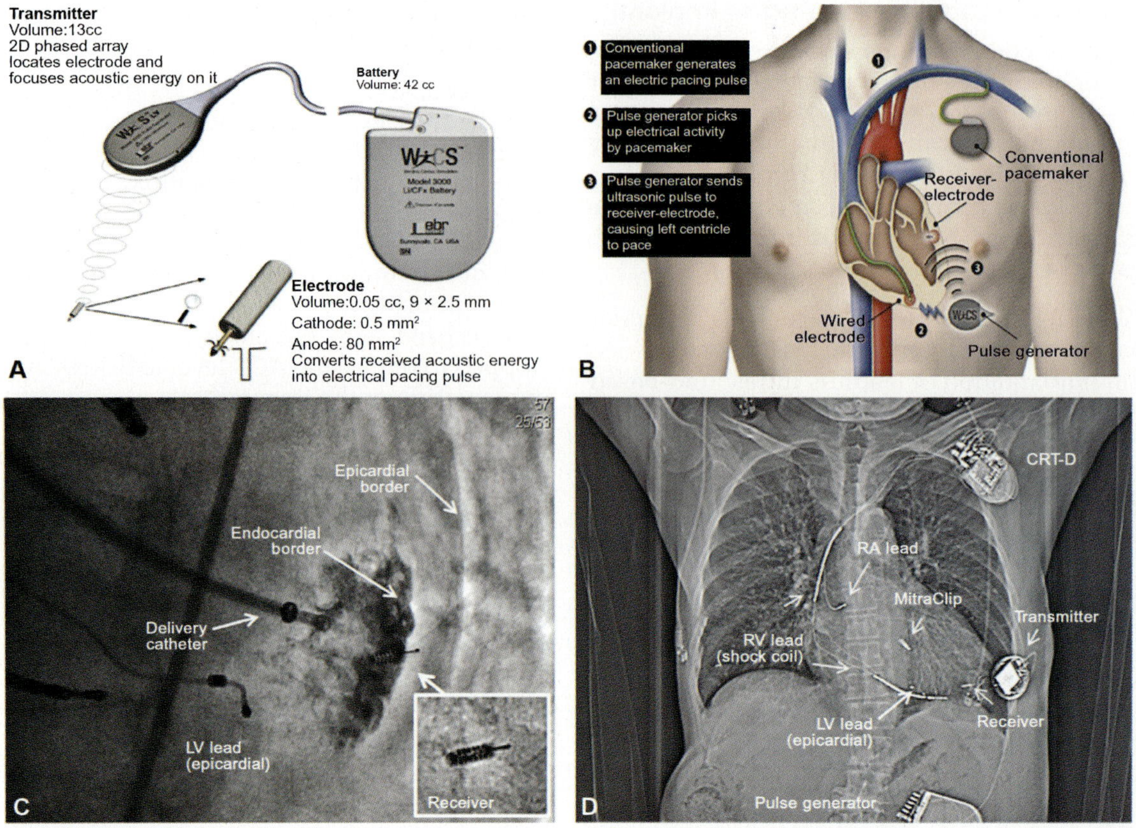


**Fig. A-40:** (A) The WiCS-LV technology. Piezoelectric transducers transmit ultrasound, then the mechanical energy is harvested and converted to an electrical output. The electrode is attached to the LV endocardium by anchor barbs. A woven polyester casing aids endothelialization. (B) WiCS-LV is coimplanted with a pacemaker, ICD, or CRT device. It provides biventricular pacing by sensing the RV pacing output of the coimplant and generating ultrasound targeted at the electrode that is converted to an electrical output to pace the LV. (C) Under fluoroscopic guidance using radiopaque contrast the sheath is positioned to the LV wall and the electrode anchored to the tissue. Contrast injection in this view illustrates the electrode attachment is clearly past the endocardial border. (D) Chest and abdomen X-ray showing the CRT-D in the left subclavicular region; RA lead; RV lead; and LV lead in the CS. Also shown are MitraClip; WiCS transmitter, receiver, and pulse generator battery

system, an implantable cardiac pacing system capable of leadless pacing based on converting ultrasound energy to electrical energy. Three patients are presented—(i) a patient with an existing implantable defibrillator, (ii) a patient with a CRT system whose LV lead does not capture, and (iii) a CRT patient classified as a nonresponder. All three patients were successfully treated. Acute electrical pacing thresholds ranged from 0.7–1.0 V at 0.5 ms; all patients retained captured at 6 months. Functional New York Heart Association class significantly changed (pre: III in two patients, and IV in one patient; post: I in one patient, II in one patient, and II–III in one patient), and LV ejection fraction increased from 23.7 ± 3.4% to 39 ± 6.2% ($P < 0.017$).

*Leadless pacing: current status and future perspectives:* Despite all the enthusiasm generated by these novel and remarkable devices, it has to be stressed that the periprocedural risks associated with implantation require attention. For two out of the three systems, clinical trials have either been terminated or put temporarily on hold because of severe complications, including death. Cardiac perforation and tamponade seem to be issues that need to be addressed. Device design, especially as regards the fixation mechanism, should be carefully evaluated and if necessary adapted. A safe implantation technique that is applicable to a broad clinical setting is desirable. This will also require proper education and training of implanting physicians. Evaluation of these devices in clinical studies and registries will be necessary to judge the benefit-to-risk profile, especially in the long-term.

Future steps that may be taken are the development of leadless multichamber devices that communicate with each other. Such new devices would make leadless pacing suitable for a much larger population. Boston Scientific is currently developing a leadless pacemaker system, which may in the future be complementary to their subcutaneous ICD (e.g. for delivering antitachycardia or antibradycardia pacing, or for enhancing arrhythmia diagnosis). Research is currently underway for harvesting kinetic energy from cardiac motion to fuel pacemaker function (similarly to automatic watches). Intracardiac pacemakers may one day profit from such technology, thereby dispensing with the need for device replacement. Intravascular defibrillators are another next step, and initial results of an investigational device have recently been published.

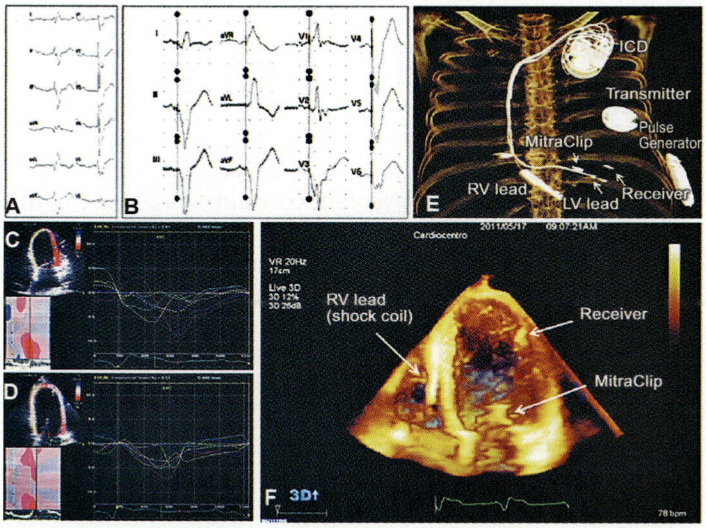


Fig. A-41: (A) A surface 12-lead ECG demonstrates sinus rhythm. (B) Simultaneous right ventricle and LVendo pacing. (C) Related longitudinal strain echocardiographic evaluation. (D) Dyssynchrony with intrinsic rhythm with delays in septal and lateral LV wall segments, but significant reduction of mechanical dyssynchrony during simultaneous right ventricle and LVendo pacing. (E) Cardiac tomography scan showing an ICD, a MitraClip device, the ultrasound generator, and the endo-cardial electrode (receiver). (F) A three-dimensional echocardiographic view demonstrating the electrode in the LV wall post-implant

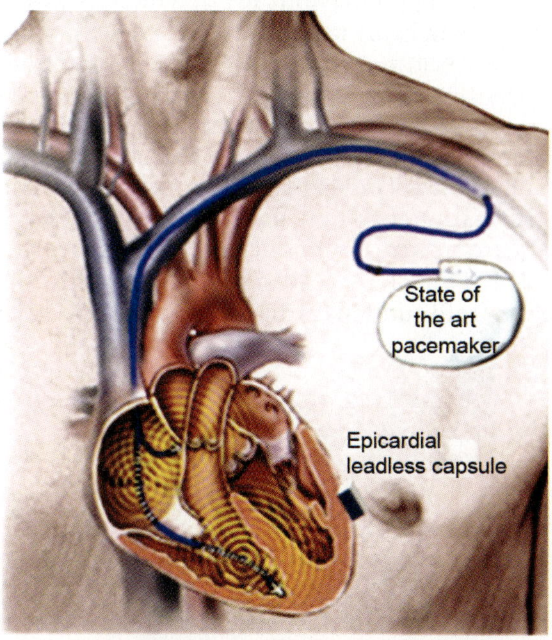


Fig. A-42: Epicardial leadless capsule unit 3D module with electronic chips and battery. Capacitors to be integrated in PICS technology. Mechanical design of capsule with 3D accelerometer without energy scavenger

## ADVANCES IN IMPLANTABLE CARDIOVERTER DEFIBRILLATOR TECHNOLOGY

There have been several recent advancements in implantable cardioverter defibrillator (ICD) technology to extend battery life, improvements in patient monitoring to avoid needless shocks, the introduction of quadripolar lead devices to improve device programming and to improve therapy effectiveness, and development of magnetic resonance imaging (MRI)-safe ICDs. ICDs are implanted in patients who are at high risk for sudden cardiac arrest (SCA) due to sustained ventricular tachycardia or fibrillation.

These devices also are used to improve the heart's pumping ability in heart failure patients. ICDs are incorporated into cardiac resynchronization therapy defibrillator (CRT-D) devices, which resynchronize the contractions of both ventricles and have defibrillation capabilities. Several newer ICDs offer pacing functions, and many vendors offer wireless remote monitoring/interrogation of the device data with bedside sending units so patients do not need to come in for regular office visits.

### Quadripolar Leads Expand Therapy Options

One of the biggest innovations has been the introduction of quadripolar lead devices. The leads use four electrodes to allow more programming options for pacing and overcoming issues with lead placement. This can help optimize CRT-D therapy and decrease the number of patients who do not respond. Up to 10% of heart failure patients' left ventricular (LV) lead placements are not successful because of anatomical challenges, phrenic nerve stimulation (PNS) or poor electrical measurement.

Use of a quadripolar LV lead instead of a bipolar option during CRT can decrease complications at 6 months, according to preliminary results presented at the 2014 European Society of Cardiology (ESC) Congress. The MORE-CRT trial demonstrated the safety and efficiency of the quadripolar lead technology in providing more options to manage CRT patients. The MORE-CRT study included 1,068 heart failure patients scheduled for CRT from 63 centers in 13 countries. The study includes more than 1,000 CRT patients with either a bipolar lead or a quadripolar lead. The study showed that at 6 months, compared to controls, patients with quadripolar leads were significantly more likely to be free from a composite endpoint of both intraoperative and postoperative LV lead-related complications (85.97% vs 76.86%, P = 0.0001)—a relative risk reduction (RRR) of 40.8%. The driver of this benefit was mainly intra-operative complications, which were

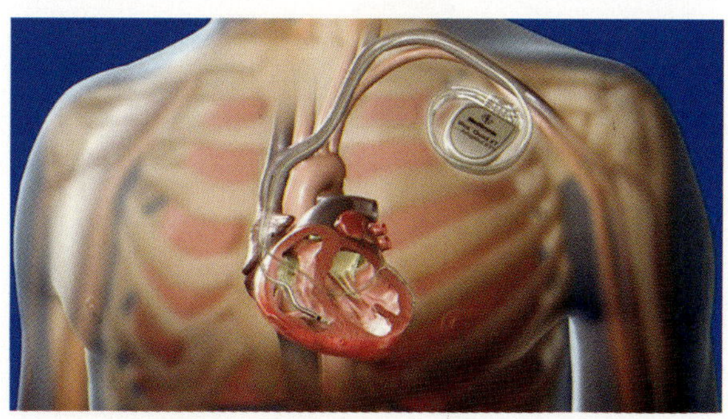

Fig. A-43: Medtronic's attain performa quadripolar lead and VivaQuad XT CRT-D system. Quadripolar leads enable more programming options to enable better patient care

reduced by more than 50% in the quadripolar group (5.98% vs. 13.73%, P<0.0001, RRR 56.4%). Additional data released in 2014 show use of quadripolar LV leads was associated with significantly reduced hospitalizations specific to heart failure and LV lead surgical revision.

Presented at Heart Rhythm 2014. The hospitalization rates and associated cost analysis of quadripolar versus bipolar CRT-D—a comparative analysis of a single-center prospective Italian registry presentation, demonstrated quadripolar leads reduced the number of hospitalizations by 53 % when compared to the nonquadripolar group. This hospitalization rate reduction translated into a statistically significant 62% reduction in overall costs for both healthcare systems and patients. St. Jude Medical was the first to gain US Food and Drug Administration (FDA) approval for a quadripolar pacing lead in January 2012, on its Unify Quadra CRT-D, which uses the Quartet left ventricular quadripolar pacing lead.

Boston Scientific received FDA approval in April 2014 for the Dynagen X4 and Inogen X4 CRT-Ds. The X4 line of quadripolar CRT-Ds offers 70% more pacing options to address high capture thresholds and PNS effectively, along with a large battery capacity and a 6-year warranty. Medtronic received FDA approval for the Attain Performa model 4298 quadripolar lead, and the Viva Quad XT and Viva Quad S CRT-D. The quadripolar lead and devices offer 16 pacing configurations and shorter spacing between the two center electrodes, and the Attain Performa model 4298 left-heart lead provides additional options for physicians to treat different patient anatomies. Medtronic launched two additional Attain Performa LV quadripolar leads in December with S-shape and straight leads to accommodate patients' varying vessel sizes and curvatures to enhance successful lead placement.

### Battery Life

Battery longevity has long been an issue with ICDs. As patients live longer, they may need to undergo surgical procedures every few years for regular battery replacements. Increased device longevity can reduce the risk of infection and other complications due to repeat replacement procedures and help minimize out-of-pocket patient expenses for avoidable replacement procedures. Boston Scientific launched a line of extended longevity (EL) battery ICDs, including the Dynagen EL and Inogen EL device models. The devices use the EnduraLife battery, developed with high-performance chemistry and advanced manufacturing capabilities to provide up to double the battery capacity of other ICDs, the vendor said. Boston Scientific said the battery life is projected to be about 12 years before a replacement is needed. The EnduraLife battery is packaged in a device up to 11% smaller and 24% thinner than other ICDs.

'Battery longevity has a direct impact on patient outcomes and the cost of care,' said Samir Saba, MD, who was the first to implant an EL ICD after FDA approval at The University of Pittsburgh Medical Center. 'The EL ICD is an important advancement that can help minimize the frequency of avoidable replacement procedures to help reduce costs and the potential for replacement-related complications.'

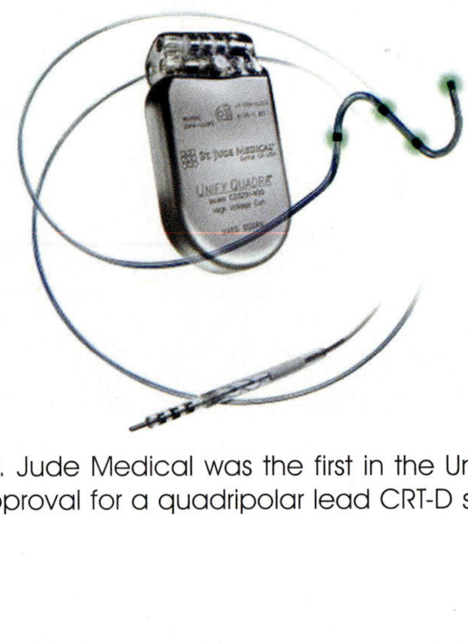

Fig. A-44: St. Jude Medical was the first in the United States to gain FDA approval for a quadripolar lead CRT-D system

## SUBCUTANEOUS ICD TECHNOLOGY

The FDA granted market clearance in October 2012 for Boston Scientifics' S-ICD system, the world's first commercially available subcutaneous ICD (S-ICD). The S-ICD sits entirely just below the skin without the need for implantable leads to be placed inside the heart. This leaves the heart and blood vessels untouched, offering patients an alternative to transvenous ICDs, which require leads to be placed in the heart itself.

'The S-ICD system establishes the first new category of cardiac rhythm management devices since the introduction of cardiac resynchronization therapy,' said Raul Weiss, MD, associate professor of clinical and cardiovascular medicine at The Ohio State University. 'Doctors now have a breakthrough treatment option that provides protection from sudden cardiac arrest without touching the heart.'

The S-ICD system is designed to provide the same protection from sudden cardiac arrest as transvenous ICDs.

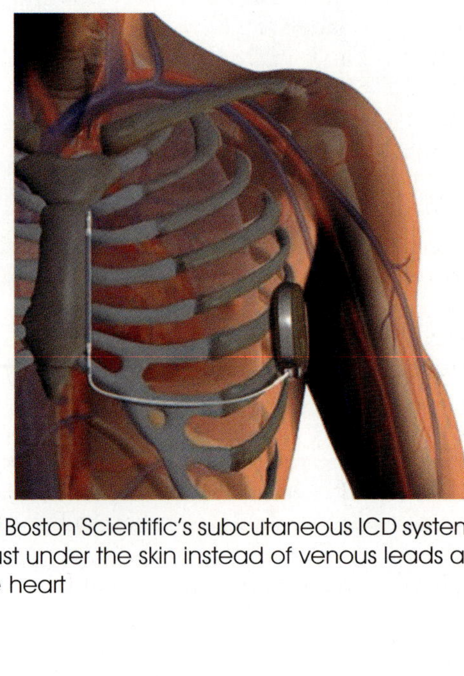

Fig. A-45: Boston Scientific's subcutaneous ICD system uses leads that run just under the skin instead of venous leads and implants inside the heart

The system has two main components—(1) the pulse generator, which powers the system, monitors heart activity and delivers a shock if needed, and (2) the electrode, which enables the device to sense the cardiac rhythm and deliver shocks when necessary. Both components are implanted just under the skin—the generator at the side of the chest and the electrode beside the breastbone. Implantation with the S-ICD system is straightforward using anatomical landmarks, without the need for fluoroscopy, eliminating patient X-ray exposure.

### External Defibrillator Offers Bridge Therapy

For patients at risk for SCA who are being evaluated for a permanent ICD, Zoll offers the LifeVest wearable external defibrillator as a temporary solution. The LifeVest allows a physician time to assess a patient's long-term arrhythmic risk and make appropriate plans. The LifeVest is lightweight and easy to wear under a patient's clothing, allowing them to return to their daily activities while having the peace of mind that they are protected from SCA. The LifeVest continuously monitors the patient's heart and, if a life-threatening heart rhythm is detected, the device delivers a treatment shock to restore normal heart rhythm. This device continuously monitors the patient's heart with dry, nonadhesive sensing electrodes to detect life-threatening abnormal heart rhythms. If a life-threatening heart rhythm is detected, the device alerts bystanders and delivers a treatment shock to restore normal heart rhythm. The entire event, from detecting a life-threatening arrhythmia to automatically delivering a treatment shock, usually occurs in less than a minute.

The LifeVest is used for a range of patient conditions or situations, including following a heart attack and before or after bypass surgery or stent placement, as well as for those with cardiomyopathy or congestive heart failure that places them at particular risk. Zoll said the LifeVest has been prescribed to more than 100,000 patients. Zoll intregrates this device with the LifeVest Network online patient data management system. It allows clinicians to monitor patient data online, downloaded from a patient's LifeVest. It gives the clinician options to customize events that generate an alert, or to be notified for a number of events, such as detected arrhythmias, treatments, patient-recorded electrocardiograms (ECGs) and patient use.

### MRI-safe ICDs

It is estimated that about 60% of ICD patients will need an MRI within 10 years of receiving a device. Until the availability of MR-conditional ICD systems, patients with devices have been contraindicated from receiving MRI scans because of potential interactions between the MRI and device function. There are several MRI-compatible ICDs now available in Europe and two undergoing FDA investigational device exemption (IDE) pivotal trials in the United States The ProMRI trial is evaluating Biotronik's DX ICD system, which gained CE mark in Europe in 2011, becoming the first MRI-compatible ICD on the market. In May 2014, Medtronic announced the first US trial implant of its Evera MRI SureScan ICD system. Medtronic gained European CE mark approval for the device in April 2014.

### Reducing Shocks

Patients' quality of life and faith in their ICDs can be significantly decreased if their ICD shocks the patient needlessly. Some vendors now include technology to help reduce inappropriate shocks. St. Jude Medical's Assura ICD and CRT portfolio features Secure Sense RV Lead Noise Discrimination, an algorithm that expands St. Jude's ShockGuard technology and offers advanced sensing options designed to reduce the incidence of inappropriate shocks. The algorithm provides advanced alerts as well as more proactively lowering the risk of lead-related complications through its ability to automatically withhold tachycardia therapy in the presence of lead noise (over-sensing of electrical signals). The technology differentiates lead noise from true ventricular tachycardia (VT) or ventricular fibrillation (VF) episodes that require life-saving therapy.

In addition, ShockGuard technology features specific programming that distinguishes between rhythms that require defibrillation therapy and those that do not, such as benign arrhythmias. DecisionTx programming offers advanced sensing technology designed to avoid sensing unwanted signals (T-waves) and more anti-tachycardia pacing options, which can convert many fast ventricular arrhythmias painlessly and avoid the need for high-voltage shocks. Medtronic's Evera MRI includes SmartShock 2.0, a shock reduction algorithm that enables the device to better differentiate between dangerous and harmless heart rhythms. Medtronic said studies estimate about 20% of patients with implantable defibrillators might experience inappropriate shocks in response to a benign arrhythmia or electrical noise sensed by the device.

Lead failure is another source of inappropriate shocks. In late 2013, Medtronic gained FDA clearance for its lead integrity alert (LIA) software for use with non-Medtronic leads. LIA can report performance issues on Durata and Riata (St. Jude Medical) and Endotak (Boston Scientific) defibrillator leads when connected to a Medtronic device.

### Reducing Implanted Hardware

Biotronik's Ilesto family of ICD/CRT-D devices includes the Ilesto DX. The platform allows for a 15% size reduction and 29% fewer components with no compromise in longevity or clinical features. It is the first defibrillator system equipped to provide full atrial diagnostic information with just one specialized defibrillator lead. The DX system offers an alternative with more monitoring capability than a single-chamber device, and without additional leads required for dual-chamber devices.

## BIO-HYBRID KIDNEY POWERED BY HEART IN THE OFFING

Washington, Feb 16 (PTI) scientists are developing a first-of its kind implantable artificial kidney with microchip filters and living cells that will be powered by the patient's own heart. 'We are creating a bio-hybrid device that can mimic a kidney to remove enough waste products, salt and water to keep a patient off dialysis,' said William H Fissell IV, from Vanderbilt University Medical Centre in US. The goal is to make it small enough, roughly the size of a soda can, to be implanted inside the body, Fissell said. The key to the device is a microchip, researchers said. 'It uses the same processes that were developed by the microelectronics industry for computers,' said Fissell. The chips are affordable, precise and make ideal filters. Researchers are designing each pore in the filter one by one based on what they want that pore to do. Each device will hold roughly fifteen microchips layered on top of each other. However, the microchips have another essential role beyond filtering, researchers said. 'They're also the scaffold in which living kidney cells will rest,' said Fissell. Researchers use live kidney cells that will grow on and around the microchip filters. The goal is for these cells to mimic the natural actions of the kidney. "We can use kidney cells that fortunately for us grow well in the lab dish, and grow them into a bioreactor of living cells that will be the only 'Santa Claus' membrane in the world—the only membrane that will know which chemicals have been naughty and which have been nice," said Fissell. 'Then they can reabsorb the nutrients your body needs and discard the wastes your body desperately wants to get rid of,' said Fissell. Since this bio-hybrid device sits out of reach from the body's immune response, it is protected from rejection. 'The issue is not one of immune compliance, of matching, like it is with an organ transplant,' said Fissell. The device operates naturally with a patient's blood flow.'We must transform that unsteady pulsating blood flow in the arteries and move it through an artificial device without clotting or damage,' he said. Researchers are using fluid dynamics to see if there are certain regions in the device that might cause clotting. They use computer models to refine the shape of the channels for the smoothest blood flow. Then they rapidly prototype the new design using 3D printing and test it to make the blood flow as smoothly as possible.

## SOON VACCINE TO LOWER CHOLESTEROL

*A vaccine that could reduce LDL cholesterol and atherosclerosis is currently being tested in human trials.*

Daily statin use to lower cholesterol may soon be a thing of the past. A new study reveals how a vaccine successfully lowered 'bad' cholesterol in mice and reduced atherosclerosis, which is a narrowing of the arteries caused by a buildup of plaque.

The vaccine is called AT04A and has already entered a human clinical trial, which is expected to deliver results by the end of this year.

If the vaccine is found to be safe and effective in humans, researchers say that it would offer a long-term therapeutic strategy for high cholesterol; rather than taking statins every day, patients could simply have an initial injection, followed by an annual booster.

According to the centers for disease control and prevention (CDC), in the United States, around *73.5 million adults* have high low-density lipoprotein (LDL) *cholesterol*. LDL cholesterol is often referred to as 'bad' cholesterol; high LDL levels can lead to *atherosclerosis*. This is the accumulation of fatty deposits, or plaque, in the arteries. Over time, plaque buildup can cause the arteries to narrow, restricting blood flow.

### Vaccine Targets PCSK9 Enzyme

High LDL cholesterol is a major risk factor for cardiovascular diseases. Statistics show that people with high LDL cholesterol are around *twice as likely* to develop *heart disease*—the leading cause of death in the United States—than those with lower LDL cholesterol.

Lifestyle changes, such as adopting a healthful diet and partaking in regular exercise, can help to lower LDL cholesterol levels, but some patients may also require medication.

Statins remain the gold standard of cholesterol-lowering therapy. This class of drugs helps to lower LDL cholesterol by inhibiting a cholesterol-producing enzyme in the liver called HMG-CoA reductase.

While statins are effective for lowering cholesterol, they are not without risk, with side effects including muscle pain and liver damage. What is more, statins need to be taken on a daily basis, a regimen that is hard for some patients to follow.

In the new *study*-recently published in the *European Heart Journal* Dr. Günther Staffler and colleagues describe the development of a vaccine that targets and blocks the activity of an enzyme called Proprotein convertase subtilisin/kexin type 9 (PCSK9).

Produced by the liver, PCSK9 is known to bind to LDL cholesterol receptors. This stops these receptors from clearing LDL cholesterol from the blood. As such, blocking PCSK9 is considered a promising strategy to lower LDL cholesterol.

### Total Cholesterol Levels Halved in Mice

Dr. Staffler and team reveal how, when injected, their AT04A vaccine produces antibodies that target PCSK9 and stop it from functioning. This increases LDL receptor activity, enabling them to clear LDL cholesterol from the blood.

The researchers tested the vaccine in mice that had high LDL cholesterol and atherosclerosis, induced by consumption of a high-fat, Western-style diet.

When injected under the skin of the rodents, the team found that the AT04A vaccine led to a 53% reduction in total cholesterol levels, compared with unvaccinated mice, as well as a 64% reduction in atherosclerosis-related blood vessel damage.

What is more, the vaccine led to a 21–28% reduction in biological markers of blood vessel *inflammation.*

Importantly, the researchers found that the antibodies produced by the vaccine remained high and functional throughout the entire 18-week study period, suggesting that it has long-term benefits.

'As antibody concentrations remained high at the end of the study, it can be assumed they would continue to reduce cholesterol levels for some time afterwards, resulting in a long-lasting effect, as has been shown in previous studies,' says Dr. Staffler.

### Human Clinical Trials Started

Based on the success of AT04A in mouse studies, a phase I clinical trial of the vaccine began in 2015, which involves 72 healthy adults. The trial is due to be complete by the end of this year.

'If these findings translate successfully into humans, this could mean that, as the induced antibodies persist for months after a vaccination, we could develop a long-lasting therapy that, after the first vaccination, just needs an annual booster,' says Dr. Staffler.

'This would result in an effective and more convenient treatment for patients, as well as higher patient compliance.'

### *Dr. Günther Staffler*

While the AT04A vaccine shows promise, researchers stress that it is very important to determine the long-term safety of this therapeutic strategy.

'In particular, reductions in total cholesterol via statins and other drugs are associated with an increase in new-onset *diabetes*,' write Prof. Ulrich Laufs, of Saarland University in Germany, and Prof. Brian Ference, of the University of Bristol in the United Kingdom, in an *editorial* linked to the study.

'Therefore, one potential safety concern for long-term lowering of LDL cholesterol with a vaccine directed against PCSK9 is the potential for an increased risk of new-onset diabetes,' they add. 'In the short-term, the LDL cholesterol-lowering effect of statins and PCSK9 inhibitors appears to far outweigh the risks of new-onset diabetes.'

## INJECTABLE ALTERNATIVES TO STATINS

According to the *US Centers for Disease Control and Prevention*, about 610,000 people die of heart disease in the United States every year. Heart disease is also the leading cause of death for both men and women. Since high cholesterol is such a widespread problem, new medications have been in the works to help control and manage it. PCSK9 inhibitors are the newest line of medications in the war against cardiovascular disease. These cholesterol-lowering injectable drugs work to increase your liver's ability to remove 'bad' LDL cholesterol from your blood and thus decrease your risk of heart attack or stroke.

### About PCSK9 Inhibitors

PCSK9 inhibitors can be used with or without the addition of a statin, however they can help reduce LDL cholesterol by as much as 75% when used in conjunction with a statin drug. This could be especially beneficial for those who can't tolerate the muscle aches and other side effects of statins or those who simply can't get their cholesterol under control by using statins alone. The recommended starting dose is 75 mg injected once every 2 weeks. This dosage may be increased to 150 mg every 2 weeks if your doctor feels your LDL levels aren't responding adequately to the smaller dose. While the research and testing results with these injection drugs are still relatively new, they show *great promise*.

### Newest Inhibitor Treatments

The *US Food and Drug Administration (FDA)* recently approved praluent (alirocumab) and repatha (evolocumab), the first cholesterol-lowering injection treatments in the new class of PCSK9 inhibitors. They're designed to be used in combination with statin therapy and dietary changes.

Praluent and repatha are for adults with heterozygous familial hypercholesterolemia (HeFH), an inherited condition that causes high levels of LDL cholesterol in the blood, and those with clinical cardiovascular disease. These drugs are antibodies that target a protein in the body called PCSK9. By inhibiting PCSK9's ability to work, these antibodies are able to get rid of LDL cholesterol from the blood and decrease overall LDL cholesterol levels.

### Newest Inhibitor Treatments

The *US Food and Drug Administration (FDA)* recently approved praluent (alirocumab) and repatha (evolocumab), the first cholesterol-lowering injection treatments in the new class of PCSK9 inhibitors. They're designed to be used in combination with statin therapy and dietary changes.

Praluent and repatha are for adults with heterozygous familial hypercholesterolemia (HeFH), an inherited condition that causes high levels of LDL cholesterol in the blood, and those with clinical cardiovascular disease.

These drugs are antibodies that target a protein in the body called PCSK9. By inhibiting PCSK9's ability to work, these antibodies are able to get rid of LDL cholesterol from the blood and decrease overall LDL cholesterol levels.

### Latest Research

Trials and research have shown positive results for both praluent and repatha. In a recent trial on repatha, participants with HeFH and others with high risk factors for heart attack or stroke lowered their LDL cholesterol by an average of 60%.

The most common reported side effects of repatha were:

- Upper respiratory tract infection
- Nasopharyngitis
- Back pain
- Flu and bruising, redness, or pain at the injection site
- Allergic reactions, including hives and rash, were also observed.

Another trial using praluent also showed favorable results. These participants, who were already using statin therapy and had HeFH or increased risk of stroke or heart attack, saw a 36–59% drop in LDL cholesterol.

*Side effects* from praluent use were similar to repatha, including:

- Pain and bruising at the injection site
- Flu-like symptoms
- Nasopharyngitis
- Allergic reactions, such as hypersensitivity vasculitis

### Cost

As is the case with most pharmaceutical advancements, these new injection drugs will come with a hefty price tag. While the cost for patients will depend on their insurance plan, wholesale costs start at $14,600 per year. In comparison, brand name statin drugs cost only $500–$700 per year, and those figures drop considerably if purchasing the generic statin form. Analysts are expecting the drugs to advance to bestseller status in record time and bring in billions of dollars in new sales.

### The Future of PCSK9 Inhibitors

Experiments are still ongoing as to the effectiveness of these injection drugs. Some health officials worry the new drugs pose the potential for neurocognitive hazards, due to some study participants reporting difficulties with confusion and the inability to pay attention.

## VACCINATION AGAINST ANGIOTENSINS FOR THE TREATMENT OF HYPERTENSION

Current vaccination approaches against hypertension target angiotensin I and angiotensin II, key components of the renin-angiotensin system. The effectiveness and long-term safety of blockade of the renin-angiotensin system with antihypertensive small-molecule drugs is well documented. Phase I/II testing of the angiotensin I vaccine PMD3117 demonstrated safety and immunogenicity in humans. While angiotensin I-specific antibodies were induced blood pressure was not lowered, presumably due to insufficient antibody levels. A second vaccine, which targets angiotensin II, has been clinically tested. Administration of CYT006-AngQb to subjects with mild-to-moderate hypertension was safe and well tolerated. After three administrations of 300 µg of the vaccine, ambulatory blood pressure was significantly reduced compared to placebo. The vaccine was particularly effective early in the morning as systolic and diastolic blood pressure were lowered by –25 mmHg and –13 mmHg, respectively. Further studies are required to show long-term safety and to assess how robust and long-lived the blood pressure reduction is. It will also be important to ascertain whether the strong reduction of blood pressure in the early morning, when most cardiovascular events occur, might result in long-term benefits over current therapies.

## CIRCADIAN RHYTHM IN CARDIOVASCULAR DISEASE

Circadian rhythms have long been recognized to occur in many biologic phenomena, including secretion of hormones as well as autonomic nervous system. There is increasing evidence that circadian rhythms have been also found in cardiovascular events, for example, myocardial infarction, sudden cardiac death as well as stroke have shown a circadian pattern of the distribution. Transient myocardial ischemia, detected by ambulatory ST-segment monitoring, is also unevenly distributed during the day. The pathophysiology and the mechanism underlying these variations are the focus of much investigation, while it is not full understood up to date. Heart rate, blood pressure, neural and humoral vasoactive factors such as plasma norepinephrine levels and renin activity, and probably also contractility are increased in the morning hours, indicating that increase in myocardial oxygen demand contribute importantly to the increased prevalence of ischemia in the morning. Our recent study found that circadian rhythm of

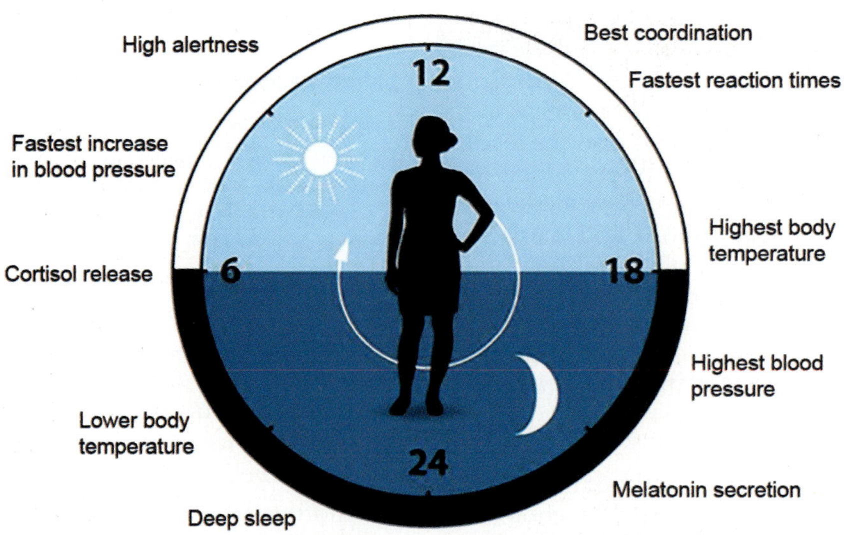


**Fig. A-46:** Physiological changes in circadian rhythm

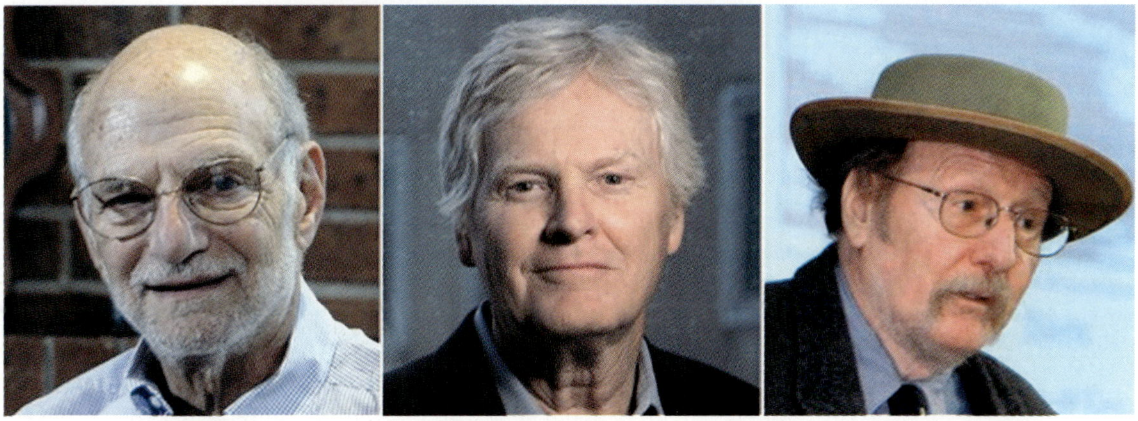

Dr. Rosbash Dr. Young Dr. Hall CreditBill

**Fig. A-47:** Nobel prize is awarded to three Americans for work on circadian rhythm

ischemic threshold detected by repetitive exercise treadmill tests in patients with chronic coronary artery disease is also apparently associated with levels of plasma ET-1. This information should enable better understanding as well as treatment on patients on circadian variation of cardiovascular events.

Some of the workers have found that cardiovascular surgeries conducted afternoon had better outcome than performed during early morning period.

## NOBEL PRIZE IN MEDICINE IS AWARDED TO THREE AMERICANS FOR WORK ON CIRCADIAN RHYTHM

Jeffrey C. Hall, Michael Rosbash and Michael W. Young are the joint winners of the 2017 Nobel Prize in physiology or medicine, winning for their discoveries about how internal clocks and biological rhythms govern human life. The three Americans won 'for their discoveries of molecular mechanisms controlling the circadian rhythm,' the Nobel Foundation says. From the Nobel Assembly at Karolinska Institutet, which *announced the prize* early Monday morning.

'Using fruit flies as a model organism, this year's Nobel laureates isolated a gene that controls the normal daily biological rhythm. They showed that this gene encodes a protein that accumulates in the cell during the night, and is then degraded during the day. Subsequently, they identified additional protein components of this machinery, exposing the mechanism governing the self-sustaining clockwork inside the cell. We now recognize that biological clocks function by the same principles in cells of other multicellular organisms, including humans. 'With exquisite precision, our inner clock adapts our physiology to the dramatically different phases of the day. The clock regulates critical functions such as behavior, hormone levels, sleep, body temperature and metabolism.'

Hall, 72, was born in New York and has worked at institutions from the University of Washington to the California Institute of Technology. For decades, he was on the faculty at Brandeis University in Waltham, west of Boston; more recently, he has been associated with the University of Maine.

Rosbash, 73, was born in Kansas City, Mo., and studied at the Massachusetts Institute of Technology and at the University of Edinburgh in Scotland. Since 1974, he has been on faculty at Brandeis University in Waltham, Mass.

Young, 68, was born in Miami, Fla., and earned his doctoral degree at the University of Texas in Austin. He then worked as a postdoctoral fellow at Stanford University in Palo Alto before joining the faculty at the Rockefeller University in 1978.

## ENDOVASCULAR REPAIR OF COMPLEX AORTIC ANEURYSMS

### Thoracic Endovascular Aortic Repair

Endovascular aortic aneurysm repair (EVAR) has been shown to reduce blood loss, operative time, length of hospital stay, mortality, and morbidity compared with open surgical repair of infrarenal abdominal aortic aneurysms (AAAs).

Anatomical constraints limit the use of EVAR in 30–40% of patients, because of short necks, excessive angulation, or frank aneurysm involvement of aortic side branches such as supra-aortic trunks (arch aneurysms), visceral arteries (thoracoabdominal and pararenal aneurysms), or the internal iliac arteries.

'Fenestrated and branched stent-grafts allow incorporation of aortic side branches and preservation of end-organ perfusion while achieving aneurysm exclusion with a total endovascular approach,' says Gustavo S. Oderich, MD, director of endovascular therapy and a vascular surgeon at Mayo Clinic's campus in Rochester, Minnesota. Single-center reports, multicenter registries, and systematic reviews indicate that the technique is reproducible with high rates of technical success and low morbidity and mortality.

Open conventional repair remains the standard treatment for patients with complex aortic aneurysms, but this necessitates extensive dissection, higher clamp site, prolonged visceral ischemia and more extensive recons-

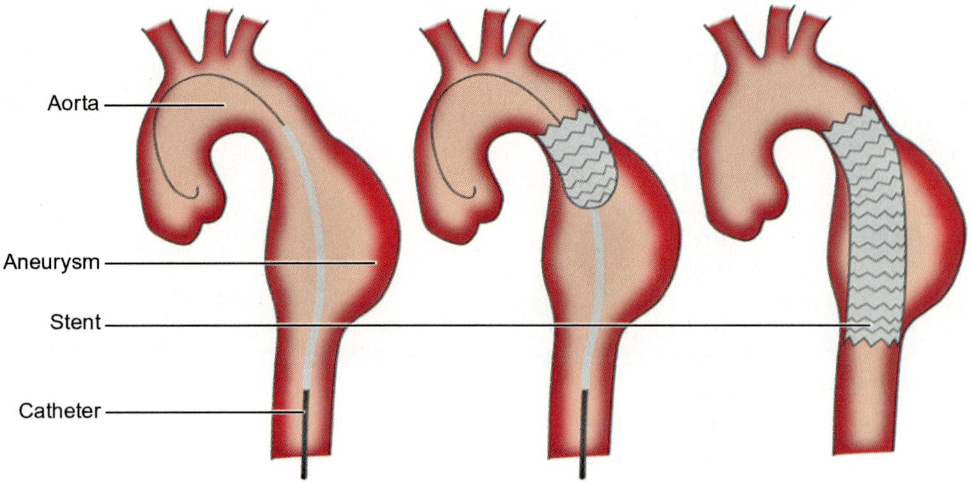


**Fig. A-48:** Thoracic endovascular aortic repair (TEVAR)

truction. While contemporary series have shown that open repair of thoracoabdominal aortic aneurysms (TAAAs) can be performed with mortality rates in the range of 5–15% in high-volume centers, analyses of national and regional data sets have demonstrated more-ominous results. In the study by Rigberg and associates on 797 medicare beneficiaries who underwent elective open TAAA repair in California, the mortality rate was 19% at 30 days and 31% at 1 year.

Dr. Oderich and colleagues at Mayo Clinic have reported the results of 5,798 medicare patients who underwent open repair in the United States. Mortality increased from 15% for patients ages 60–70 years to 30% for those older than 80 years. Overall, a third of the patients were dismissed home and the remainder required prolonged recovery in rehabilitation centers or nursing homes.

## SCIENTISTS CREATED A PIG-HUMAN HYBRID EMBRYO FOR HUMAN ORGAN TRANSPLANTATION

Scientists at the Salk Institute in California have created a part-human, part-pig embryo. Bioethicist Arthur Caplan

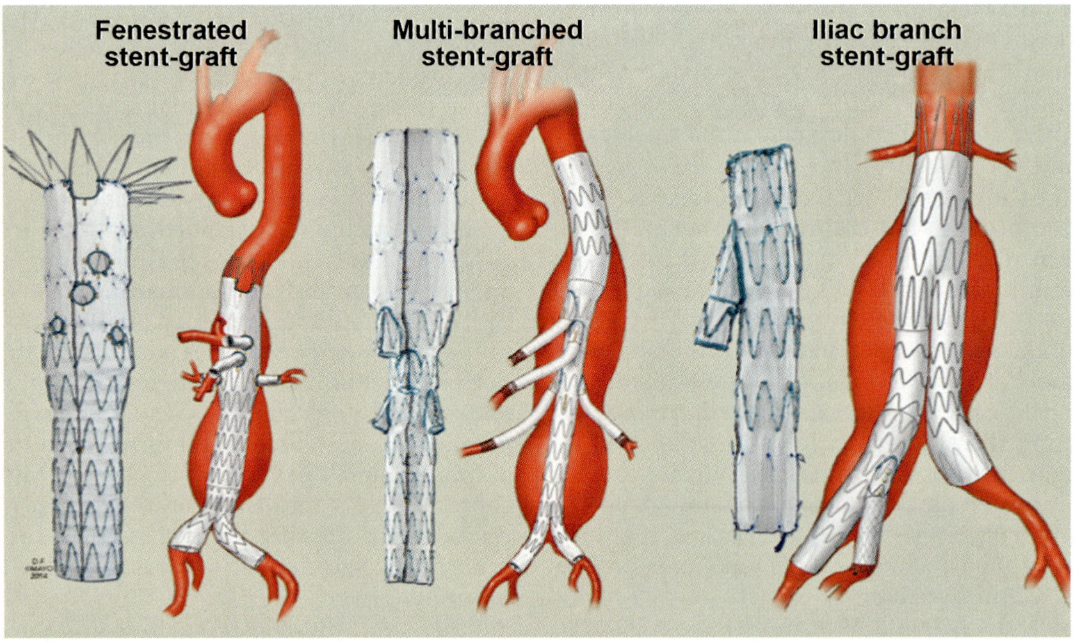


**Fig. A-49:** Thoracic endovascular aortic repair (TEVAR). Endovascular options for branch incorporation include fenestrated branched devices for pararenal aneurysms, multi-branched devices for thoracoabdominal aneurysms, and iliac branch devices for aortoiliac aneurysms

told us about the ethical concerns involved in mixing human and animal DNA.

An experiment *reported on Thursday in Cell*, a peer-reviewed scientific journal, announced a purported breakthrough in bioengineering; the successful creation of an embryo with both human and pig DNA (and to be clear, the artwork above is just a photo of a sculpture). The results, 'raise the possibility of xeno-generating transplantable human tissues and organs towards addressing the worldwide shortage of organ donors,' according to the paper. But while the embryo was only allowed to develop for a few days, the genesis of this early-stage creature revives an uncomfortable debate about whether animal-human hybrids are, well, horrifying monsters waiting to happen.

In November 2015, shortly after the National Institutes of Health (NIH) put a hold on its own experiments that combined human and animal cells, the federal government *hosted a meeting of the minds* to discuss that very question. More specifically, the NIH feared 'the specter of an intelligent mouse stuck in a laboratory somewhere screaming 'I want to get out,' NIH ethicist David Resnik, *told Technology Review magazine*.

NIH may have been acting out of an abundance of caution, but there are still potentially icky dilemmas to work out. We still don't know how these early-stage bundles of fetal cells translate into human parts on or inside a pig. Some areas for human cells, like the stomach, are less troubling than if they materialized in, say, the brain. To find out we're on the verge of a horror movie scenario, I talked to medical ethicist Arthur Caplan of New York University's Langone Medical Center. He told me more oversight for scientists like Wu might be a good idea, but not for the reason I thought he would. He also said we're kinda-sorta, already animal-human hybrids.

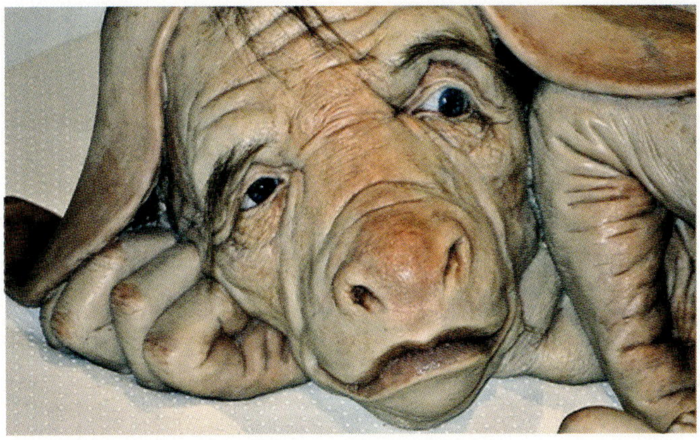

**Fig. A-50:** Scientists at the Salk Institute in California have created a part-human, part-pig embryo

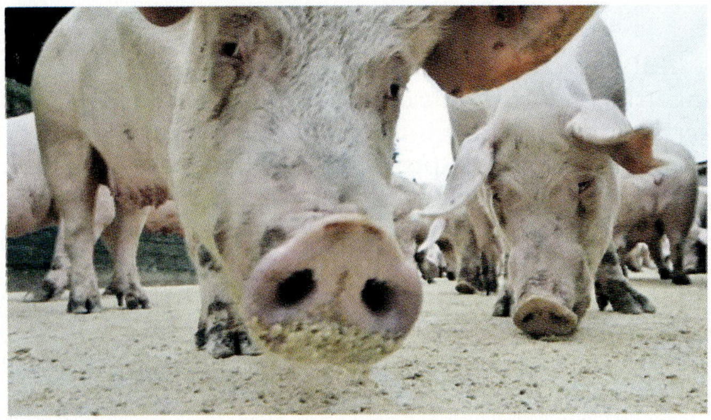

**Fig. A-51:** Scientists have successfully transplanted human stem cells into pigs that were genetically modified not to reject them in a major breakthrough for stem cells treatments

## TRANSPLANT BREAKTHROUGH AS SCIENTISTS IMPLANT HUMAN STEM CELLS INTO PIGS GENETICALLY MODIFIED TO ACCEPT THEM

- New line of pigs do not reject transplants
- Will allow for future research on stem cell therapies
- Pigs are much closer to humans than many other test animals

Scientists have successfully transplanted human stem cells into pigs that were genetically modified not to reject them. The cells were able to thrive, raising hopes of potential stem cells treatments for debilitating diseases. The breakthrough could also aid in developing treatments for patients suffering from severe immune deficiency.

### What is the Technique?

The team of researchers implanted human pluripotent stem cells in a special line of pigs developed by Randall Prather, an MU Curators Professor of reproductive physiology. Prather created the pigs with immune systems that allow the pigs to accept all transplants or grafts without rejection. Once the scientists implanted the cells, the pigs did not reject the stem cells and the cells thrived.

One of the biggest challenges for medical researchers studying the effectiveness of stem cell therapies is that transplants or grafts of cells are often rejected by the hosts.

This rejection can render experiments useless, making research into potentially life-saving treatments a long and difficult process.

'The rejection of transplants and grafts by host bodies is a huge hurdle for medical researchers,' said Michael Roberts at the University of Missouri.

By establishing that these pigs will support transplants without the fear of rejection, we can move stem cell therapy research forward at a quicker pace.

'Hopefully this means that we are one step closer to therapies and treatments for a number of debilitating human diseases.' The team of researchers implanted human pluripotent stem cells in a special line of pigs developed by Randall Prather, an MU Curators Professor of reproductive physiology.

Prather created the pigs with immune systems that allow the pigs to accept all transplants or grafts without rejection.

Researchers created the pigs with immune systems that allow the pigs to accept all transplants or grafts without rejection.

Once the scientists implanted the cells, the pigs did not reject the stem cells and the cells thrived.

Prather says achieving this success with pigs is notable because pigs are much closer to humans than many other test animals. 'Many medical researchers prefer conducting studies with pigs because they are more anatomically similar to humans than other animals, such as mice and rats,' Prather said.

Physically, pigs are much closer to the size and scale of humans than other animals, and they respond to health threats similarly. 'This means that research in pigs is more likely to have results similar to those in humans for many different tests and treatments.'

## HEART CELLS TRANSFORMED INTO 'BIOLOGICAL PACEMAKER'

### New Biological Pacemaker

In healthy people, a small region of the heart, called the sinoatrial node, fires the electrical impulses that determine *heart rate*. If this region is not working properly, people can develop heart rhythm problems, and have symptoms such as fatigue, fainting or even cardiac arrest. Such patients may have electronic pacemakers put in to monitor the heart rhythm, which sends electrical pulses to keep the heart beating normally.

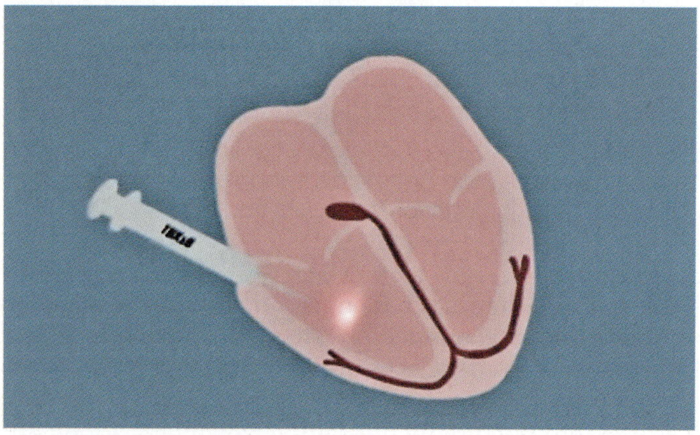

Fig. A-52: Gene therapy is a procedure where genes (or segments of DNA) are inserted into a cell and the cell then takes up the gene and incorporates it into its own genome

In the study, the researchers used pigs with a condition called complete heart block, in which the heart beats very slowly. The researchers injected a gene called TBX18 into a small area of the heart muscle. This gene converted this area of heart muscle cells into sinoatrial node cells.

'In essence, we create a new sinoatrial node in a part of the heart that ordinarily spreads the impulse, but does not originate it,' study researcher Dr. Eduardo Marbán, director of the Cedars-Sinai Heart Institute, said in news conference about the findings. 'The newly created node then takes over as a functional pacemaker, bypassing the need for implanted electronics and hardware.'

Within a few days, the pigs that received the TBX18 gene had faster *heartbeats* than pigs that did not receive the gene. In addition, the hearts of pigs with the biological pacemaker were able to speed up during exercise, and slow down during rest much better than the hearts of pigs without the biological pacemaker. The pigs with the TBX18 gene were also more physically active than the pigs without the gene, according to the study.

The treatment was designed to be temporary, and the researchers tested it for only 2 weeks. Toward the end of the study, the treatment was slightly less effective, likely because, over time, the pigs' bodies started to reject cells with the injected virus. The researchers are now testing how long the treatment lasts.

### Future Research

The new findings 'represent a critical step toward potentially filling an important clinical niche and provide an encouraging indication that a biological pacemaker might eventually be ready for human translation,' Dr. Nikhil Munshi and Eric Olson, of the University of Texas Southwestern Medical Center, wrote in an editorial accompanying the study in the journal.

However, some questions still need to be addressed. In the study, a small amount of virus ended up in the pigs' spleens and lungs after it was injected, and so future research is needed to see whether this low level of infection has long-term consequences, the editorial said.

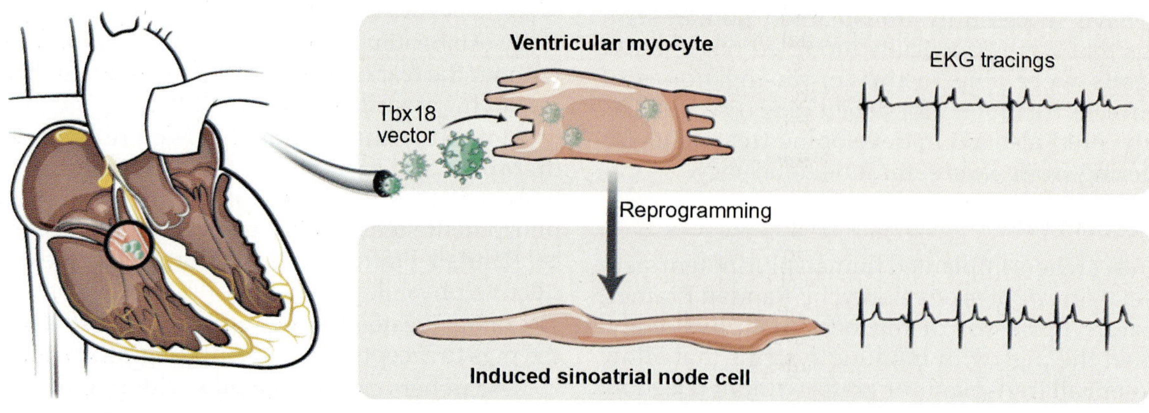


Fig. A-53: Tbx18 adenovirus reprograms heart muscle cells into sinoatrial node cells. Reprogrammed cells then generate electrical impulses to restore normal heart rate. Image from Science 345(6194):268–9

In addition, it could be problematic if the virus ends up in multiple places in the heart and forms more than one biological pacemaker. 'If multiple pacemaker foci were to form, there would be the potential for 'competition' between the foci, and the concern would be that competing pacemakers would be less efficient in setting a consistent heart rate," Munshi told Live Science.

**Table A-3:** Antiarrhythmic drugs

| Class | Mechanism of action | Effects | Clinical applications | Pharmacokinetics, toxicities, interactions |
|---|---|---|---|---|
| **Class IA** | | | | |
| Procainamide | $I_{Na}$ (primary) and $I_{Kr}$ (secondary) blockade | Slows conduction velocity and pacemaker rate • prolongs action potential duration and dissociates from $I_{Na}$ channel with intermediate kinetics • direct depressant effects on sinoatrial (SA) and atrioventricular (AV) nodes | Most atrial and ventricular arrhythmias drug of second choice for most sustained ventricular arrhythmias associated with acute myocardial infarction | Oral, IV, IM • Eliminated by hepatic metabolism to *N*-acetyl-procainamide (NAPA) and renal elimination • NAPA implicated in torsade de pointes in patients with renal failure • *Toxicity:* Hypotension • long-term therapy produces reversible lupus-related symptoms |
| *Disopyramide: Similar to procainamide but significant antimuscarinic effects; may precipitate heart failure* | | | | |
| *Quinidine: Similar to procainamide but more toxic (cinchonism, torsade); rarely used* | | | | |
| **Class 1B** | | | | |
| Lidocaine | Sodium channel ($I_{Na}$) blockade | Blocks activated and inactivated channels with fast kinetics • does not prolong and may shorten action potential | Terminate ventricular tachycardias and prevent ventricular fibrillation after cardioversion | IV • first-pass hepatic metabolism reduce dose in patients with heart failure or liver disease • *Toxicity:* Neurologic symptoms |
| *Mexiletine: Orally active congener of lidocaine; used in ventricular arrhythmias, chronic pain syndromes* | | | | |
| **Class 1C** | | | | |
| Flecainide | Sodium channel ($I_{Na}$) blockade | Dissociates from channel with slow kinetics no change in action potential duration | Supraventricular arrhythmias in patients with normal heart • do not use in ischemic conditions (postmyocardial infarction) | Oral • hepatic, and kidney metabolism • half life ~ 20 h • *Toxicity:* Proarrhythmic |
| *Propafenone: Orally active, weak-blocking activity; supraventricular arrhythmias; hepatic metabolism* | | | | |
| *Moricizine: Phenothiazine derivative, orally active; ventricular arrhythmias, proarrhythmic. Withdrawn in USA.* | | | | |
| **Class 2** | | | | |
| Propranolol | β-Adrenoceptor blockade | Direct membrane effects (sodium channel block) and prolongation of action potential duration • slows SA node automaticity and AV nodal conduction velocity | Atrial arrhythmias and prevention of recurrent infarction and sudden death | Oral, parenteral • duration 4–6 h • *Toxicity:* Asthma, AV blockade, acute heart failure • *Interactions:* With other cardiac depressants and hypotensive drugs |
| *Esmolol: Short-acting, IV only; used for intraoperative and other acute arrhythmias* | | | | |
| **Class 3** | | | | |
| Amiodarone | Blocks $I_{Kr}$, $I_{Na}$, $I_{Ca\text{-}L}$ channels, β adrenoceptors | Prolongs action potential duration and QT interval • slows heart rate and AV node conduction • low incidence of torsade de pointes | Serious ventricular arrhythmias and supraventricular arrhythmias | Oral, IV • variable absorption and tissue accumulation • hepatic metabolism, elimination complex and slow • *Toxicity:* Bradycardia and heart block in diseased heart, peripheral vasodilation, pulmonary and hepatic toxicity |

*Contd...*

*Contd...*

| Class | Mechanism of action | Effects | Clinical applications | Pharmacokinetics, toxicities, interactions |
|---|---|---|---|---|
| | | | | • hyper- or hypothyroidism. • *Interactions:* Many, based on CYP metabolism |
| Dofetilide | $I_{Kr}$ block | Prolongs action potential, effective refractory period | Maintenance or restoration of sinus rhythm in atrial fibrillation | Oral • renal excretion • *Toxicity:* Torsade de pointes (initiate in hospital) • *Interactions:* Additive with other QT-prolonging drugs |
| *Sotalol: β-Adrenergic blocker, direct action potential prolongation properties, use for ventricular arrhythmias, atrial fibrillation* | | | | |
| *Ibutilide: Potassium channel blocker, may activate inward current; IV use for conversion in atrial flutter and fibrillation* | | | | |
| *Dronedarone: Investigational amiodarone derivative; multichannel actions, reduces mortality in patients with atrial fibrillation* | | | | |
| *Vernakalant: Investigational, multichannel actions in atria, prolongs atrial refractoriness, effective in atrial fibrillation* | | | | |
| **Class 4** | | | | |
| Verapamil | Calcium channel ($I_{Ca-L}$ type) blockade | Slows SA node automaticity and AV nodal conduction velocity • decreases cardiac contractility • reduces blood pressure | Supraventricular tachycardias | Oral, IV • hepatic metabolism • caution in patients with hepatic dysfunction • *Toxicity and interactions:* See Chapter 12 |
| *Diltiazem: Equivalent to verapamil* | | | | |
| **Miscellaneous** | | | | |
| Adenosine | Activates inward rectifier $I_K$ • blocks $I_{Ca}$ | Very brief, usually complete AV blockade | Paroxysmal supraventricular tachycardias | IV only • duration 10–15 • *Toxicity:* Flushing, chest tightness, and dizziness • *Interactions:* Minimal |
| Magnesium | Poorly understood • interacts with $Na^+$, $K^+$ ATPase, $K^+$ and $Ca^{2+}$ channels | Normalizes or increases plasma $Mg^{2+}$ | Torsade de pointes • digitalis-induced arrhythmias | IV • duration dependent on dosage • *Toxicity:* Muscle weakness in overdose |
| Potassium | Increases $K^+$ permeability, $K^+$ currents | Slows ectopic pacemakers • slows conduction velocity in heart | Digitalis-induced arrhythmias • arrhythmias associated with hypokalemia | Oral, IV • *Toxicity:* Re-entrant arrhythmias, fibrillation or arrest in overdose |

**Table A-4:** Guideline identifies four statin benefit group

| | Four statin benefit group | High intensity (Atorvastatin 80/40 mg) | Moderate intensity (Atrovastatin 20/10 mg) |
|---|---|---|---|
| 1 | Secondary prevention with clinical ASCVD initiate or continue | ✓ | |
| 2 | Age >21 years, LDL-C >190 mg/dl | ✓ | |
| 3A | DM age 40–75 years with estimated 10 years ASCVD score ≥7.5% | ✓ | |
| 3B | Diabetes with LDL-C 70–189 mg/dl | | ✓ |
| | Without diabetes and LDL-C 70–189 mg/dl | | |
| 4 | Adults 40–75 years, without or with clinical ASCVD, estimated 10 years ASCVD risk score ≥7.5% | | ✓ |

**A patient centric approach to treatment**

- ♥ Identified 4 statin benefit groups based on risk factors and not LDL-C targets for high intensity or moderate intensity statin therapy
- ♥ Diabetics irrespective of LDL-C (70–189 mg/dl), guidelines recommend. Moderate intensity stain therapy and in those with ASCVD (Athero sclerotic cardio vascular disease) risk factor >7.5–High intensity statin therapy
- ♥ The guidelines do not recommended nonstatin therapy for acheiving cholesterol targets.

**Flowchart A-1:** Latest drug treatment of hypercholestrolemia according to new ACC/AHA guidelines (2013–2014)

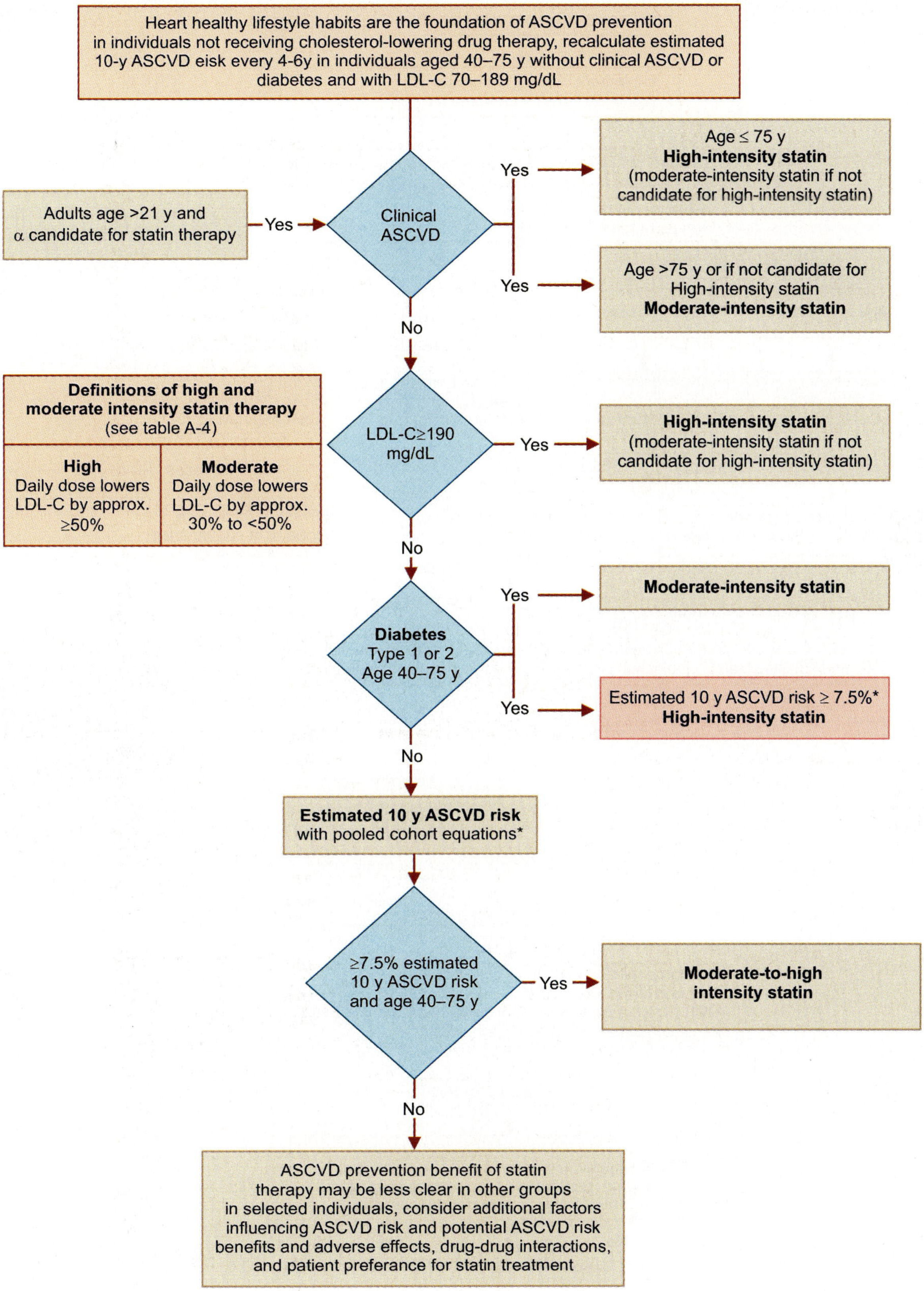

**Flowchart A-2:** 2014 Hypertension guideline management algorithm

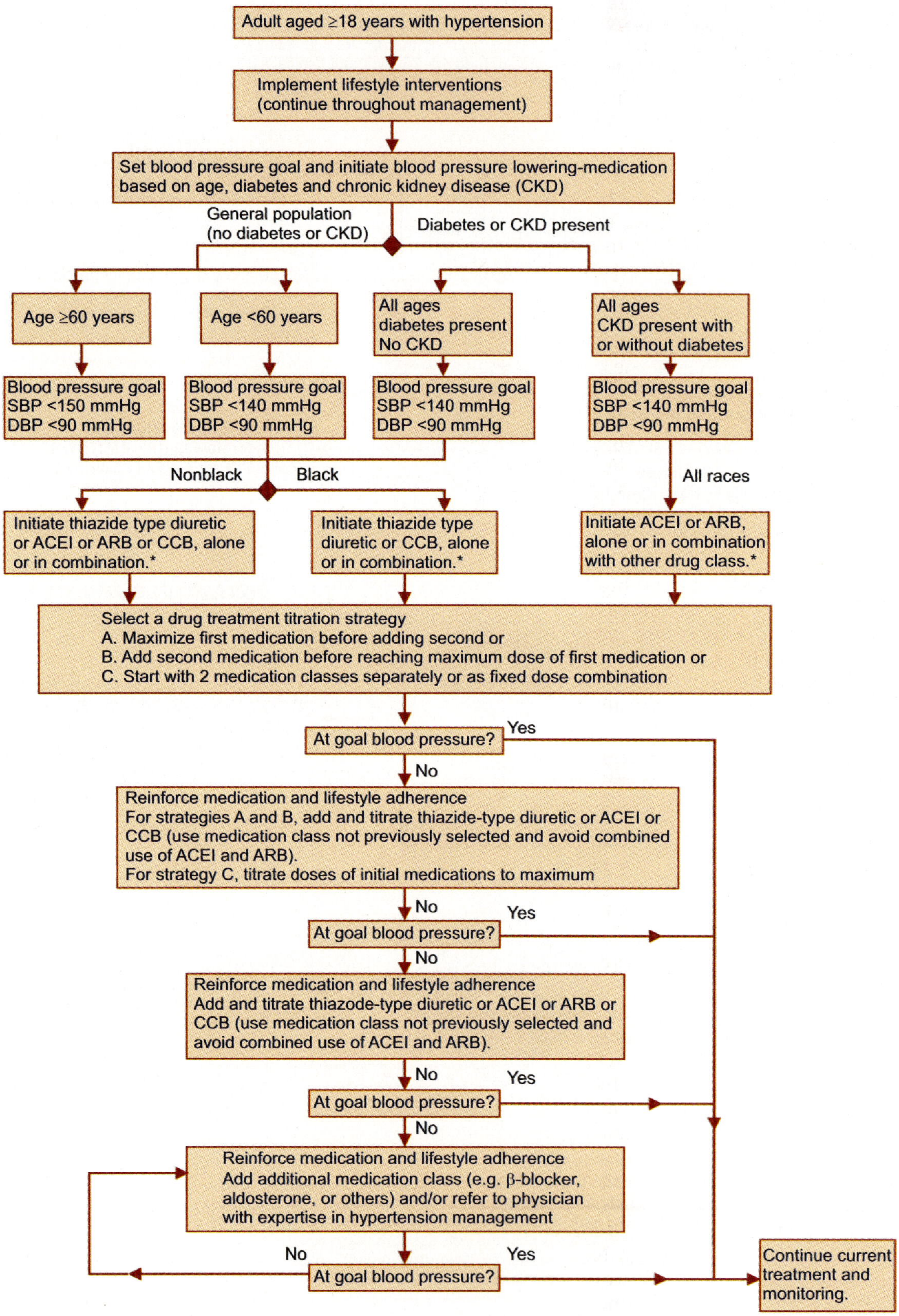


SBP=systolic blood pressure; DBP=diastolic blood pressure; ACEI=angiotensin-converting enzyme; ARB=angiotensin receptor blocker; CCB=calcium channel blocker. aACEIs and ARBs should not be used in combination

## IIT GUWAHATI TEAM DEVELOPS SILK PATCH TO REPAIR DAMAGED HEART TISSUE

### By Prasad Ravindranath Posted on August 12, 2017

'The heart cells grew and proliferated filling the membrane 7–10 days after it was seeded with cells,' say Biman Mandal and Shreya Mehrotra.

Unlike current scaffolds, the 3D patch has high cell density, a foremost requirement for heart tissue.

Scientists at the Indian Institute of Technology (IIT) Guwahati have fabricated a 3D cardiac tissue patch using silk protein membranes seeded with heart muscle cells. The patch can potentially be used for regenerating damaged heart tissue. 'The 3D patch that we fabricated can be implanted at the site of damage to help the heart regain normal function. It can also be used for sealing holes in the heart,' says Prof. Biman Mandal from the Department of Biosciences and Bioengineering, IIT Guwahati, who led the research.

Cardiac tissue gets permanently damaged when oxygen supply is reduced or cut off during heart attack. The damaged portion gets scarred and does not contract and relax leading to a change in the shape of the heart over time and reduced pumping capacity. While grafts currently available fail to mimic the structure and the function of the native heart tissue as well as maintain high cell numbers, the patch developed by the IIT Guwahati researchers scores over them on many counts. The results were published in the Journal of Materials Chemistry. The team led by Prof. Mandal tested both mulberry (*Bombyx mori*) and non-mulberry (*Antheraea assama*) silk to fabricate the membrane.

## NONINVASIVE CARDIAC RADIATION FOR ABLATION OF VENTRICULAR TACHYCARDIA

Recent advances have enabled noninvasive mapping of cardiac arrhythmias with electrocardiographic imaging and noninvasive delivery of precise ablative radiation with stereotactic body radiation therapy (SBRT). We combined these techniques to perform catheter-free, electrophysiology-guided, noninvasive cardiac radioablation for ventricular tachycardia.

Investigators targeted arrhythmogenic scar regions by combining anatomical imaging with noninvasive electrocardiographic imaging during ventricular tachycardia that was induced by means of an implantable cardioverter–defibrillator (ICD). SBRT simulation, planning, and treatments were performed with the use of standard techniques. Patients were treated with a single fraction of 25 Gy while awake. Efficacy was assessed by counting episodes of ventricular tachycardia, as recorded by ICDs. Safety was assessed by means of serial cardiac and thoracic imaging.

Results obtained from April through November 2015, five patients with high-risk, refractory ventricular tachycardia underwent treatment. The mean noninvasive ablation time was 14 minutes (range, 11 to 18). During the 3 months before treatment, the patients had a combined history of 6577 episodes of ventricular tachycardia. During a 6-week postablation 'blanking period' (when arrhythmias may occur owing to postablation inflammation), there were 680 episodes of ventricular tachycardia. After the 6-week blanking period, there were 4 episodes of ventricular tachycardia over the next 46 patient-months, for a reduction from baseline of 99.9%. A reduction in episodes of ventricular tachycardia occurred in all five patients. The mean left ventricular ejection fraction did not decrease with treatment. At 3 months, adjacent lung showed opacities consistent with mild inflammatory changes, which had resolved by 1 year.

It is therefore inferred that patients with refractory ventricular tachycardia, noninvasive treatment with electrophysiology-guided cardiac radioablation markedly reduced the burden of ventricular tachycardia (Funded by Barnes–Jewish Hospital Foundation and others).

## TELOMERES AND TELOMERASE IN CARDIOVASCULAR DISEASES

### Cardiovascular Risk Factors

The amount of telomere lost during each cell division varies among people. Previous evidence indicated that increased oxidative stress and chronic inflammation are associated with a higher telomere loss and accelerated telomere shortening. Several common risk factors for CVD such as smoking, diabetes mellitus, hypercholesterolemia, hypertension, obesity, physical inactivity, alcohol consumption and psychosocial problems have been associated with short TL. However, the mechanism underlying the association of telomere shortening with these risk factors remains hypothetical. Most studies have reported that telomere shortening is associated with these risk factors through increased tissue inflammation and oxidative stress. For example, animal studies demonstrated that hyperglycemia attenuates nitric oxide production in endothelial cells, promotes inflammation and oxidative stress, and accelerates LTL shortening and vascular atherosclerotic processes. In additional, we found disrupted circadian rhythm results in loss of rhythmic telomerase activities with shortened TL and premature aging in mice. Similar observations also showed in the emergency physicians working in rotating shifts.

## BCG VACCINE IN TYPE I DIABETES MELLITUS

BCG vaccine could restore proper immune response in type 1 diabetes Faustman's team was the first to document type 1 diabetes reversal in mice and in a subsequent phase I trial demonstrated successful human clinical results who had received the BCG vaccination. Long-term data from the study is expected to be published later this year. Now a 5-year, 150-person, phase II trial is enrolling to assess whether repeat BCG vaccination can improve or even reverse advanced type 1 diabetes in adults. Earlier this year Belgian biotech company, Imcyse, announced they will begin human trials across Europe of a separate type 1 diabetes vaccine, with results expected later.

## BIBLIOGRAPHY


1. Autier P, Boniol M, Pizot C, Mullie P. Vitamin D status and ill health: a systematic revie. Lancet Diabetes Endocrinol 2014;2:76–89.
2. Avolio A. "Central Aortic Blood Pressure and Cardiovascular Risk: A Paradigm Shift?," Hypertension 2008;51:1470–1.
3. Botha JS, Scheffer C, Lubbe WW, Doubell AF. Auto-nomous auscultation of the human heart employing a precordial electrophonocardiogram and ensemble empirical mode decomposition. Australas Phys Eng Sci Med 2010;33(2): 171–83.
4. Boutouyrie P, Achouba A, Trunet P, Laurent S, and for the EXPLOR Trialist Group, "Amlodipine-Valsartan Combination Decreases Central Systolic Blood Pressure More Effectively Than the Amlodipine-Atenolol Combination: The EXPLOR Study," Hypertension 2010;55:1314–22.
5. Christine Landlinger, Marianne G Pouwer, Claudia Juno, José WA van der Hoorn, Elsbet J Pieterman, J Wouter Jukema, Guenther Staffler, Hans MG Princen, Gergana Galabova. The AT04A vaccine against proprotein convertase subtilisin/kexin type 9 reduces total cholesterol, vascular inflammation, and atherosclerosis in APOE*3Leiden.CETP mice. European Heart Journal, 2017.
6. De Bruyne B, Pijls NH, Kalesan B, et al. Fractional flow reserve–guided PCI versus medical therapy in stable coronary disease. (FAME-2) study. N Engl J Med 2012;367: 991–1001.
7. Di Mario C, Borgia F. Assimilating the current clinical data of fully bioabsorbable stents. EuroIntervention 2009;5(Suppl F):F103–F108.
8. FDA approves first artificial aortic heart valve placed without open-heart surgery, FDA, 11/2011.
9. First TAVR with FDA nod, www.thebeatingedge.org, 11/2011.
10. Garg S, Serruys PW. Coronary stents: looking forward. J Am Coll Cardiol 2010;56:S43–S78.
11. Gaskin PR, Owens SE, Talner NS, Sanders SP, Li JS. Clinical auscultation skills in pediatric residents. Pediatrics 2000; 105(6):1184–7.
12. Gaur S, Achenbach S, Leipsic J, et al. Rationale and design of the HeartFlowNXT (HeartFlow analysis of coronary blood flow using CT angiography: NeXt sTeps) study. J Cardiovasc Comput Tomogr 2013;7:279–88.
13. Geva T, Hegesh J, Frand M. Reappraisal of the approach to the child with heart murmurs: is echocardiography mandatory? Int J Cardiol 1988;19(1):107–13.
14. Guanlan Xu, Junqin Chen, Gu Jing, Anath Shalev. Preventing cell loss and diabetes with calcium channel Blockers. Diabetes 2012 DOI: 10.2337/db11–0955.
15. Hoffman JI. Incidence of congenial heart disease: I. Postnatal incidence. Pediatr Cardiol 1995;16(3):103–13.
16. Indian guidelines on hypertension JAPI 2013;61.
17. Joner M, Nakazawa G, Finn AV, et al. Endothelial cell recovery between comparator polymer-based drug-eluting stents. J Am Coll Cardiol 2008;52:333–42.
18. Koo BK, Erglis A, Doh JH, et al. Diagnosis of ischemia-causing coronary stenoses by noninvasive fractional flow reserve computed from coronary computed tomographic angiograms. Results from the prospective multicenter DISCOVER-FLOW (Diagnosis of Ischemia-Causing Stenoses Obtained via Noninvasive Fractional Flow Reserve) study. J Am Coll Cardiol 2011;58:1989–97.
19. Leon MB, Smith CR, et al. Transcatheter Aortic-Valve Implantation for Aortic Stenosis in Patients Who Cannot Undergo Surgery, N Engl J Med 2010;363:1597–607.
20. Lowe A, Harrison W, El-Aklouk E, Ruygrok P, Al-Jumaily AM. "Non-invasive model-based estimation of aortic pulse pressure using suprasystolic brachial pressure waveforms," Journal of biomechanics 2009;42:2111–5.
21. Maier W. Exercise-induced coronary artery vasodilation is not impaired by stent placement. Circ 2002;105:2373–7.
22. Mancia G, Fagard R, Narkiewicz K, Task Force Members, et al. ESH/ESC Guidelines for the management of arterial hypertension: the Task Force for the management of arterial hypertension of the European Society of Hypertension (ESH) and of the European Society of Cardiology (ESC) J Hypertens 2013;1281–357.
23. McCrindle BW, Shaffer KM, Kan JS, Zahka KG, Rowe SA, Kidd L. Factors prompting referral for cardiology evaluation of heart murmurs in children. Arch Pediatr Adolesc Med 1995;149(11):1277–9.
24. Min JK, Leipsic J, Pencina MJ, et al. Diagnostic accuracy of fractional flow reserve from anatomic CT angiography. JAMA 2012;308:1237–45.
25. Norgaard BL, Leipsic J, Sengupta S, et al. Quantitative assess-ment of image quality for determination of FFR by coronary computed tomography angiography (abstr). J Cardiovasc Comput Tomogr 2013;3 (Suppl):233.
26. Ormiston J, Serruys PWS. Bioabsorbable coronary stents. Circ Cardiov Interv 2009;2:255–60.
27. PA James S, Oparil BL Carter, et al. Evidence-based guideline for the management of high blood pressure in adults: report from the panel members appointed to the Eighth Joint National Committee (JNC 8) JAMA 2014, 2013;284–427.
28. Payne RA, Wilkinson IB, Webb DJ. "Arterial Stiffness and Hypertension: Emerging Concepts," Hypertension 2009;55: 9–14.
29. Pelech AN. The physiology of cardiac auscultation. Pediatr Clin North Am 2004;51(6):1515–1535, vii-viii.
30. Rajakumar K, Weisse M, Rosas A, et al. Comparative study of clinical evaluation of heart murmurs by general pediatricians and pediatric cardiologists. Clin Pediatr 1999;38(9): 511–8.
31. Rajasree S, Rajpal K, Kartha CC, et al. Serum 25-hydroxy vitamin D3 levels are elevated in south indian patients with ischemic heart disease Eur J Epidemiol 2001;17:567–71.
32. Reddy VY, Holmes D, Doshi SK, Neuzil P, Kar S. Safety of percutaneous left atrial appendage closure: results from the Watchman Left Atrial Appendage System for Embolic Protection in Patients with AF (PROTECT AF) clinical trial and the Continued Access Registry. Circulation 2011;123:417–24.
33. Roman MJ, Devereux RB, Kizer JR, Lee ET, Galloway JM, Ali T, Umans JG, Howard BV. "Central Pressure More Strongly Relates to Vascular Disease and Outcome than Does Brachial Pressure. The Strong Heart Study," Hypertension HYPERTENSIONAHA 2007;107:089–078.
34. Roman MJ, Devereux RB, Kizer JR, Okin PM, Lee ET, Wang W, Umans JG, Calhoun D, Howard BV, "High Central Pulse Pressure is Independently Associated With Adverse Cardiovascular Outcome: The Strong Heart Study," J Am Coll Cardiol 2009;54:1730–4.

35. Sick PB. Initial worldwide experience with the WATCHMAN left atrial appendage system for stroke prevention in atrial fibrillation. J Am Coll. Cardiol 2007;49:1490–5.
36. Smith CR, Leon MB, et. al. Transcatheter versus Surgical Aortic-Valve Replacement in High-Risk Patients, N Engl J Med 2011;364:2187–98, (see video in article).
37. Smythe JF, Teixeira OP, Vlad P, Demers PP, Feldman W. Initial evaluation of heart murmurs: are laboratory tests necessary? Pediatrics 1990;86(4):497–500.
38. Stefanini GG, Kalesan B, Serruys PW, et al. Long-term clinical outcomes of biodegradable polymer biolimus-eluting stents versus durable polymer sirolimus-eluting stents in patients with coronary artery disease (LEADERS).
39. Stettler C, Wandel S, Allemann S, et al. Outcomes associated with drug-eluting and bare-metal stents: a collaborative network meta-analysis. Lancet 2007;370:937–48.
40. Svensson LG, Dewey T, et al. United States Feasibility Study of Transcatheter Insertion of a Stented Aortic Valve by the Left Ventricular Apex, Ann Thorac Surg 2008;86:46–55.
41. Waksman R. The disappearing stent: when plastic replaces metal. Circulation 2012;125:2291–4.
42. Wentzel JJ, Whelan DM, van der Giessen WJ, et al. Coronary stent implantation changes 3-D vessel geometry and 3-D shear stress distribution. J Biomech 2000;33:1287–95.
43. Wilkinson IB, Prasad K, Hall IR, Thomas A, MacCallum H, Webb DJ, Frenneaux MP, Cockcroft JR, "Increased central pulse pressure and augmentation index in subjects with hypercholesterolemia," J Am Coll Cardiol 2002;39,:1005–11.
44. Wilson GJ, Nakazawa G, Schwartz RS, et al. Comparison of inflammatory response after implantation of sirolimus- and paclitaxel-eluting stents in porcine coronary arteries. Circulation 2009;120:141–9.

# Index

## Symbols



## A

## B



## C

## D



## E

## L



## M



## N



## O



## P

## Q



## R

## S



## T

## U



## V



## W



## Y